ANTIMICROBIAL
THERAPY AND VACCINES

EDITORS

Victor L. Yu

Thomas C. Merigan, Jr.
Steven L. Barriere

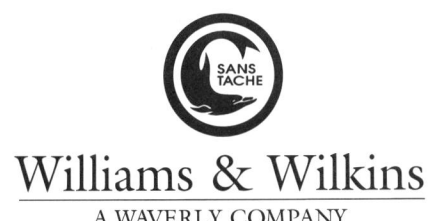

Williams & Wilkins
A WAVERLY COMPANY

BALTIMORE • PHILADELPHIA • LONDON • PARIS • BANGKOK
BUENOS AIRES • HONG KONG • MUNICH • SYDNEY • TOKYO • WROCLAW

ANTIMICROBIAL THERAPY AND VACCINES

ANTIMICROBIAL THERAPY AND VACCINES

EDITORS

Victor L. Yu, MD

Professor of Medicine
University of Pittsburgh
Chief, Infectious Disease Section
VA Medical Center
Pittsburgh, Pennsylvania

Thomas C. Merigan, Jr, MD

George and Lucy Becker Professor of Medicine
Director, Center for AIDS Research
Stanford University Medical Center
Stanford, California

Steven L. Barriere, PharmD

Director, Clinical Affairs
Gilead Sciences
Foster City, California

ASSOCIATE EDITORS

Alan M. Sugar, MD

Professor of Medicine
Boston University School of Medicine
Evans Memorial Department of Clincal Research
Department of Medicine
Boston, Massachusetts

Didier Raoult, MD

Professor and Chairman
Faculté de Médicine
Unité des Rickettsies
CNRS UPRESA 6020
Marseille, France

Charles Peloquin, MD

Director, Infectious Disease Pharmacokinetics Laboratory
National Jewish Medical and Research Center
Adjoint Associate Professor
Schools of Pharmacy and Medicine
University of Colorado
Denver, Colorado

Michael Iseman, MD

Professor of Medicine and Infectious Diseases
University of Colorado School of Medicine
Chief, Clinical Mycobacterial Service
Division of Infectious Diseases
National Jewish Medical and Research Center
Denver, Colorado

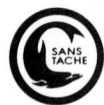

Editor: Jonathan W. Pine, Jr.
Managing Editor: Molly L. Mullen
Marketing Manager: Peter Darcy
Project Editor: Kathy Gilbert

Copyright 1999 Williams & Wilkins

351 West Camden Street
Baltimore, Maryland 21201-2436 USA

Rose Tree Corporate Center
1400 North Providence Road
Building II, Suite 5025
Media, Pennsylvania 19063-2043 USA

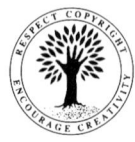

Printed in the United States of America

Antimicrobial therapy and vaccines / Victor L. Yu, Thomas C. Merigan, Steven L. Barriere,
    editors ; Alan M. Sugar, Didier Raoult, Michael Iseman, associate editors.
        p.   cm.
    Includes bibliographical references and index.
    ISBN 0-683-30061-X
    1. Anti-infective agents.   2. Communicable diseases—Chemotherapy.   I. Yu, Victor L.
II. Merigan, Thomas C., 1934–   .   III. Barriere, Steven L.
    [DNLM: 1. Anti-Infective Agents—therapeutic use.   2. Vaccines—therapeutic use.
3. Bacteria—drug effects.   4. Fungi—drug effects.   5. Viruses—drug effects.
QV 250A6311   1999]
RM267.A575   1999
616.9′0461—dc21
DNLM/DLC
for Library of Congress   98-36941
                                                             CIP

To purchase additional copies of this book, call our customer service department at **(800)
638–0672** or fax orders to **(800) 447–8438.** For other book services, including chapter
reprints and large quantity sales, ask for the Special Sales department.

Canadian customers should call **(800) 665–1148,** or fax **(800) 665–0103.** For all other calls
originating outside of the United States, please call **(410) 528–4223** or fax us at **(410)
528–8550.**

Visit Williams & Wilkins on the Internet: **http://www.wwilkins.com** or contact our customer service department at **custserv@wwilkins.com**. Williams & Wilkins customer service
representatives are available from 8:30 am to 6:00 pm, EST, Monday through Friday, for
telephone access.

                                             99 00 01 02
                             1 2 3 4 5 6 7 8 9 10

PREFACE

Changes in antimicrobial agent therapy for infectious diseases are evolving at a rate in concert with developing antimicrobial resistance as well as new and emerging human pathogens. The rate is so rapid that no textbook of infectious diseases or medicine has attempted to keep up with this dizzying pace.

Physicians and pharmacists are now relying more on the medical literature to prescribe antimicrobial agents in difficult or unusual clinical situations, but recent information useful for patient management is difficult to obtain. Thus, we have created a new textbook unparalleled in its comprehensiveness with respect to antimicrobial agent therapy and vaccines. The structure of the book is designed for easy use by the clinician and pharmacist and includes two major sections: *(a)* microorganisms, with emphasis on infectious disease syndromes and difficult clinical situations, and *(b)* antimicrobial agents.

Rapid updating will be critically important to a textbook dealing with therapy, so an electronic version of this textbook is being created that will be available on the Internet and in CD-ROM format. The Internet version will allow frequent updates and rapid searches to optimize its utility; in addition, focused Medline searches can be conducted through the Internet version.

The authors put forth an unprecedented effort in making this textbook comprehensive and clinically oriented. They are especially thanked for their forbearance in creating a textbook with a new format.

We thank Molly Mullen and Jonathan Pine from Williams & Wilkins for shepherding this book into publication.

If you wish to comment or criticize any of the recommendations made in this book, please write me at the following address: Victor L. Yu, MD, Infectious Disease Section, VA Medical Center, University Drive C, Pittsburgh, PA 15240, or e-mail me at vly+@pitt.edu. If you notice that a particular pathogen or antimicrobial agent has not been covered in this textbook, please let me know; feel free to suggest experts who could write authoritatively on the subject.

Even as you read this Preface to the First Edition, the second edition is being prepared. New parasite and antiparasite drug sections headed by Dr Geoffrey Edwards (Editor) and Drs Rainer Weber and Nicholas J. White (Associate Editors) are being added. Fifteen new chapters on other bacteria, viruses, and fungi will also be added. Finally, commentaries and reviews on topical issues have been commissioned for the second edition.

You, the reader, are the final arbiter of the value of this textbook. We wish to hear from you.

Victor L. Yu
Editor-in-Chief

CONTRIBUTORS

Jeffrey R. Aeschlimann, PharmD
Research Fellow, Infectious Diseases
Pharmacotherapy
Pharmacy Practice
Wayne State University
Detroit, Michigan

Ban Mishu Allos, MD
Assistant Professor of Medicine and Preventive Medicine
Department of Medicine
Vanderbilt University School of Medicine
Nashville, Tennessee

Neal M. Ampel, MD
Associate Professor
Department of Medicine
University of Arizona
Director, HIV Clinical Services
Tucson VAMC
Tucson, Arizona

Elias J. Anaissie, MD
Director for Clinical Affairs
Myeloma and Transplantation Research Center
University of Arkansas for Medical Sciences
Little Rock, Arkansas

Fred Y. Aoki, MD
Professor of Medicine, Medical Microbiology, and
Pharmacology and Therapeutics
University of Manitoba School of Medicine
Winnipeg, Manitoba, Canada

Donald Armstrong, MD
Professor of Medicine
Cornell University Medical College
Chief, Infectious Disease Service
Memorial Sloan-Kettering Cancer Center
New York, New York

Ann M. Arvin, MD
Professor of Pediatrics, Microbiology and Immunology
Stanford University Medical Center
Department of Pediatrics
Stanford, California

Shai Ashkenazi, MD
Director, Unit of Infectious Diseases
Schneider Children's Medical Center
Petah Tiova, Israel
Associate Professor
Sackler School of Medicine
Tel Aviv University
Tel Aviv, Israel

Johan S. Bakken, MD, FACP
Consultant in Infectious Diseases
The Duluth Clinic
Associate Professor
Department of Family Medicine
University of Minnesota, Duluth
Duluth, Minnesota

Steven L. Barriere, PharmD
Director, Clinical Affairs
Gilead Sciences
Foster City, California

Christiane Bébéar, MD
Professor of Bacteriology
Laboratoire de Bactériologie,
Centre Hospitalier Régional de Bordeaux,
Bordeaux Cedex, France

Suzanne R. Belfiglio, PharmD
Clinical Pharmacist
Department of Pharmacy
The University of Pittsburgh Medical Center
Pittsburgh, Pennsylvania

E. Bergogne-Berezin, MD
Professor of Microbiology
Paris University VII
Bichat-Claude Bernard Hospital
Paris, France

Steven L. Berk, MD
Professor and Chairman
Department of Internal Medicine
East Tennessee State University
James H. Quillen College of Medicine
Johnson City, Tennessee

Shaun E. Berning, PharmD
Clinical Pharmacist
Department of Medicine
National Jewish Medical and Research Center
Adjoint Assistant Professor
School of Pharmacy
University of Colorado
Denver, Colorado

Martin J. Blaser, MD
Addison B. Scoville Professor of Medicine
Director, Division of Infectious Diseases
Professor of Microbiology and Immunology
Vanderbilt University School of Medicine
Staff Physician
VA Medical Center
Nashville, Tennessee

Suzanne F. Bradley, MD
Associate Professor
Department of Internal Medicine
University of Michigan
Staff Physician
GRECC
VA Medical Center
Ann Arbor, Michigan

Itzhak Brook, MD, MSc
Professor of Pediatrics
Georgetown University School of Medicine
Washington, DC

June M. Brown, BS
Microbiologist
Meningitis and Special Pathogens Branch
Division of Bacterial and Mycotic Diseases
National Center for Infectious Diseases
Centers for Disease Control and Prevention
Public Health Service
U.S. Department of Health and Human Services
Atlanta, Georgia

André J. Bryskier, MD
Head of Clinical Pharmacology, Anti-infectives
Hoechst Marion Roussel
Department of Pharmacology
Romainville, France

Sandra J. Burgess, PharmD
Barnes-Jewish Hospital
St. Louis, Missouri

Thomas Butler, MD
Professor
Department of Medicine
Texas Tech University
Lubbock, Texas

Frank M. Calia, MD
Vice Dean, School of Medicine
Professor of Medicine
Department of Medicine
University of Maryland at Baltimore
Baltimore, Maryland

Kerstin E. Calia, MD
Clinical and Research Fellow
Infectious Disease Unit
Massachusetts General Hospital
Boston, Massachusetts

Donald R. Carrigan, PhD
Herpesvirus Diagnostics, Inc.
Greenfield, Wisconsin

Keith A.V. Cartwright, MA, BM, FRCPath
Professor
Public Health Laboratory
Gloucestershire Royal Hospital
Gloucester, United Kingdom

Feng-Yee Chang, MD, DSc
Associate Professor
Department of Medicine
National Defense Medical Center
Chief
Department of Infectious Diseases
Tri-Service General Hospital
Taipei, Taiwan

Shan-Chwen Chang, MD, PhD
Chief, Section of Infectious Diseases
Department of Internal Medicine
National Taiwan University Hospital
Taipei, Taiwan

Casey Chen, DDS, PhD
Assistant Professor of Periodontology
School of Dentistry
University of Southern California
Los Angeles, California

Joseph W. Chow, MD
Associate Professor of Medicine
Division of Infectious Diseases
Wayne State University School of Medicine
Staff Physician
Medical Service
Detroit VA Medical Center
Detroit, Michigan

Laurent Christin, MD
Clinical Instructor
Department of Medicine
Section of Infectious Diseases
Boston Medical Center
Boston, Massachusetts

Yin Ching Chuang, MD
Division of Infectious Disease
Department of Medicine
National Cheng Kung University Hospital
Associate Professor
Department of Internal Medicine
National Cheng Kung University Medical College
Tainan, Taiwan

Cornelius J. Clancy, MD
Instructor in Medicine
Department of Medicine
Division of Infectious Diseases
University of Florida College of Medicine
Gainesville, Florida

David L. Coleman, MD
Professor, Infectious Disease Section
Department of Medicine
Yale University School of Medicine
New Haven, Connecticut
Chief, Medical Service
VA Connecticut Healthcare System
West Haven, Connecticut

Rebecca L. Coleman, PharmD
Associate Clinical Director
Clinical Research
Gilead Sciences, Inc.
Foster City, California
Associate Clinic Professor
Department of Pharmacy
University of California, San Francisco
San Francisco, California

Jacques Couvreur, MD
Associate Professor
Department of Pediatric Immunology
Armand Trousseau Hospital
Institut de Puériculture
Laboratoire de la Toxoplasmose
Paris, France

Clyde S. Crumpacker, MD
Professor of Medicine
Harvard Medical School
Division of Infectious Diseases
Beth Israel Deaconess Medical Center
Boston, Massachussetts

Charles L. Daley, MD
Assistant Professor of Medicine
Department of Medicine
University of California, San Francisco
San Francisco, California

Ross J. Davidson, MD
Department of Microbiology
Mount Sinai Hospital
University of Toronto
Toronto, Ontario, Canada

Catherine F. Decker, MD
Staff Physician, Infectious Diseases
HIV Unit
National Naval Medical Center
Bethesda, Maryland

Cindy P. Dougherty, PharmD
Deputy Chief, Drug Services
National Center for Infectious Diseases
Centers for Disease Control and Prevention
Atlanta, Georgia

Cherie L. Drenzek, DVM, MS
Viral and Rickettsial Zoonoses Branch
Division of Viral and Rickettsial Diseases
National Center for Infectious Diseases
Centers for Disease Control and Prevention
Atlanta, Georgia

Richard H. Drew, MS, RPh
Clinical Pharmacist, Infectious Diseases
Department of Medicine
Duke University Medical Center
Durham, North Carolina

George L. Drusano, MD
Professor of Medicine and Pharmacology
Departments of Medicine and Pharmacology
Albany Medical College
Albany, New York

J. Stephen Dumler, MD
Assistant Professor of Pathology
Department of Pathology
Johns Hopkins Medical Institutions
Baltimore, Maryland

Michel Dupon, MD
Professor of Infectious Diseases
Département de Maladies Infectieuses et Médecine
Interne
Hôpital Pellegrin-Tripode
Bordeaux, France

Bertrand F. Dupont, MD
Professor of Infectious and Tropical Diseases
Institut Pasteur Hospital
National Reference Center for Antifungals and Fungal
Infections
Institut Pasteur
Paris, France

Geoffrey Edwards, BSc, PhD
Senior Lecturer
Department of Pharmacology and Therapeutics
University of Liverpool
Liverpool, Merseyside, United Kingdom

Ricardo Espinoza-Araya, MD
Internal Medicine, Infectious Diseases Section
Hospital Urgencia, Asistencia Publica
Santiago, Chile

Solly Faine, MD, PhD, FRCPA
Emeritus Professor
Department of Microbiology
Monash University
Melbourne, Victoria, Australia
Director
MediSci Consulting and Writing
Armadale, Victoria, Australia

Lori E. Fantry, MD, MPH
Assistant Professor
Department of Internal Medicine
University of Maryland
Baltimore, Maryland

Jeremy Farrar, BSc, MB BS, MRCP, DPhil
Senior Lecturer,
University of Oxford
The University of Oxford–Wellcome Trust Clinical Research Unit
The Centre for Tropical Disease
Ho Chi Minh City, Viet Nam

Daniel Fekade, MD
Associate Professor of Medicine
Department of Internal Medicine
Faculty of Medicine
Addis Ababa University
Addis Ababa, Ethiopia

Thomas Fekete, MD
Associate Professor of Medicine
Section of Infectious Diseases
Temple University School of Medicine
Philadelphia, Pennsylvania

Thomas M. File, Jr, MD, MS
Professor of Internal Medicine
Northeastern Ohio Universities
College of Medicine
Rootstown, Ohio
Chief, Infectious Disease Section
Summa Health System
Akron, Ohio

Karl P. Fischer, MSc
Scientist, GlaxoWellcome-Heritage Research Institute
Department of Microbiology and Immunology
University of Alberta, Edmonton, Alberta, Canada

Margaret A. Fischl, MD
Comprehensive AIDS Program
Director
University of Miami School of Medicine
Miami, Florida

Douglas N. Fish, PharmD, BCPS
Assistant Professor
University of Colorado School of Pharmacy
Clinical Specialist, Infectious Diseases and Critical Care
University of Colorado Health Sciences Center
University of Colorado Health Sciences Center
Department of Pharmacy Practice, School of Pharmacy
Denver, Colorado

John F. Flaherty, Jr, PharmD
Professor of Clinical Pharmacy
Department of Clinical Pharmacy
School of Pharmacy
University of California, San Francisco
San Francisco, California

Courtney V. Fletcher, PharmD
Professor
College of Pharmacy
University of Minnesota
Minneapolis, Minnesota

David N. Fredricks, MD
Division of Infectious Diseases
Stanford University
Stanford, California

Collin Freeman, MD
Assistant Professor of Medicine
Clinical Pharmacology
University of Missouri Kansas City, School of Medicine
Kansas City, Missouri

Ian R. Friedland, MD
Assistant Professor
Department of Pediatrics
University of Texas Southwestern Medical Center
Dallas, Texas

John E. Fuchs, Jr, PharmD
Assistant Professor
Department of Internal Medicine
University of Texas Medical Branch
Galveston, Texas

Dale N. Gerding, MD
Chief, Medical Service
VA Chicago, Lakeside Division
Professor and Associate Chair
Department of Medicine
Northwestern University Medical Center
Chicago, Illinois

Mae F. Go, MD
Staff Physician
Medical Service/Digestive Diseases
Veterans Affairs Medical Center
Houston, Texas

Ellie J. C. Goldstein, MD
Director
R. Malden Research Laboratory
Santa Monica–UCLA Medical Center
Santa Monica, California
Clinical Professor of Medicine
UCLA School of Medicine
Los Angeles, California

Fred W. Goldstein, MD
Laboratoire de Microbiologie Médicale
Fondation Hôpital Saint-Joseph
Paris, France

Eduardo Gotuzzo, MD, FACP
Principal Professor of Medicine
Director, Tropical Medical Institute Alexander von
Humboldt
Cayetano Heredia University
Chairman
Department of Tropical and Infectious Diseases
Cayetano Heredia National Hospital
Lima, Peru

David Y. Graham, MD
Professor of Medicine
Department of Medicine
Professor
Department of Molecular Virology
Baylor College of Medicine
Chief Gastroenterology
VA Medical Center
Houston, Texas

John R. Graybill, MD
Professor of Medicine and Chief, Infectious Disease
University of Texas Health Science Center
Division of Infectious Disease
San Antonio, Texas

J. Thomas Grayston, MD
Professor
Department of Epidemiology
School of Public Health and Community Medicine
University of Washington
Seattle, Washington

Harry Greenberg, MD
Professor of Medicine and Microbiology and Immunology
Associate Chair, Department of Medicine
Chief of Gastroenterology
Medical Investigator-PAUAHCS
Stanford University Medical School
Stanford, California

David E. Griffith, MD
Professor of Medicine
The University of Texas Health Center at Tyler
Director of Medical Affairs
Center for Pulmonary Infectious Disease Control
Tyler, Texas

Andreas H. Groll, MD
Visiting Associate
Immunocompromised Host Section
Pediatric Oncology Branch
National Cancer Institute
National Institutes of Health
Bethesda, Maryland

Richard L. Guerrant, MD
Thomas H. Hunter Professor of International Medicine
Chief, Division of Geographic and International Medicine
University of Virginia School of Medicine
Charlottesville, Virginia

Gregory W. Hammond, MD, FRCP(C)
Director, Public Health Branch
Manitoba Health,
Winnipeg, Manitoba, Canada

H. Hunter Handsfield, MD
Professor of Medicine
University of Washington
Harborview Medical Center
Director, STD Control Program
Seattle–King County Department of Public Health
Seattle, Washington

Daniel H. Havlichek, Jr, MD
Associate Professor of Medicine and Microbiology
College of Human Medicine
Department of Microbiology
Michigan State University
East Lansing, Michigan

Frederick G. Hayden, MD
Stuart S. Richardson Professor of Clinical Virology
Professor of Internal Medicine and Pathology
University of Virginia School of Medicine
Charlottesville, Virginia

Qiushui He, MD
Senior Investigator
Department of Pediatrics
Turku University Hospital
National Public Health Institute Department
Turku, Finland

David W. Hecht, MD
Associate Professor of Medicine, Microbiology, and Molecular
Biology
Loyola University Medical Center
Maywood, Illinois

Maria Hedberg, PhD
Associate Professor
Department of Immunology, Microbiology, Pathology and
Infectious Diseases
Karolinska Institute
Huddinge University Hospital
Stockholm, Sweden

Leonid Heifets, MD, PhD, ScD
Director, Mycobacteriology Laboratory
Department of Medicine
National Jewish Medical and Research Center
Professor
Department of Microbiology
University of Colorado Health Sciences Center
Denver, Colorado

Mark A. Herbert, MD
Medical Research Council Clinical Research Training Fellow
Molecular Infectious Diseases Group
Institute for Molecular Medicine
Department of Paediatrics
John Radcliffe Hospital
Oxford, United Kingdom

Monto Ho, MD
Professor of Medicine, Pathology and Microbiology
University of Pittsburgh School of Medicine
Chair, Department of Infectious Disease and
Microbiology
Graduate School of Public Health
University of Pittsburgh
Pittsburgh, Pennsylvania

Sharon Hunt Gerardo, PhD
Research Microbiologist
R. M. Alder Research Laboratory
Santa Monica–UCLA Medical Center
Santa Monica, California

Michael D. Iseman, MD
Professor of Medicine and Infectious Diseases
University of Colorado School of Medicine
Chief, Clinical Mycobacterial Service
Division of Infectious Diseases
National Jewish Medical and Research Center
Denver, Colorado

Lisa A. Jackson, MD, MPH
Research Assistant Professor
Department of Epidemiology
School of Public Health and Community Medicine
University of Washington
Seattle, Washington

Richard F. Jacobs, MD, FAAP
Horace C. Cabe Professor of Pediatrics
Chief, Pediatric Infectious Diseases
University of Arkansas for Medical Sciences
Arkansas Children's Hospital
Little Rock, Arkansas

Stuart Johnson, MD
Staff Physician, Infectious Disease Section
VA Lakeside Medical Center
Assistant Professor
Department of Medicine
Northwestern University
Chicago, Illinois

Thomas P. Kanyok, PharmD
Assistant Professor
College of Pharmacy
University of Illinois at Chicago
Chicago, Illinois
Consultant
World Bank/UNDP/WHO
Special Programs for Research and Training in Tropical
Diseases
Geneva, Switzerland

Patricia Kauffman, MD
Office of the Medical Examiner
Philadelphia, Pennsylvania

Carol A. Kauffmann, MD
Chief, Infectious Diseases
VA Medical Center
Professor of Internal Medicine
University of Michigan Medical School
Ann Arbor, Michigan

Daryl J. Kelly, PhD
Chief
Department of Rickettsial Diseases
Walter Reed Army Institute of Research
Washington, DC

Elias N. Kiwan, MD
Postdoctoral Fellow
Myeloma and Transplantation Research Center
University of Arkansas for Medical Sciences
Little Rock, Arkansas

Wen Chien Ko, MD
Physician
Division of Infectious Diseases
National Cheng Kung University Hospital
Senior Lecturer
Department of Medicine
National Cheng Kung University, Medical College
Tainan, Taiwan

Jane E. Koehler, MD
Assistant Professor of Medicine
Division of Infectious Diseases
University of California, San Francisco
San Francisco, California

Joyce A. Korvick, MD
Medical Officer
Division of Antiviral Drug Products
Food and Drug Administration
Rockville, Maryland
Infectious Disease Attending Physician
Department of Medicine
VA Medical Center
Washington, DC

Bruce Kreter, PharmD
International Clinical Project Director
Anti-Infective Clinical Research and Development
Rhône-Poulenc Rorer
Collegeville, Pennsylvania

F. Marc LaForce, MD
Professor of Medicine
University of Rochester
Physician-in-Chief
Department of Medicine
The Genesee Hospital
Rochester, New York

Selwyn D. R. Lang, MBChB, FRACP, FRCPA
Clinical Microbiologist and Infectious Diseases Physician
Department of Microbiology and Medicine
Middlemore Hospital
Auckland, New Zealand

Catherine Leport, MD
Professeur des Universités
Hôpital Bichat-Claude Bernard
Service des Maladies Infectieuses et Tropicales
Paris, France

Matthew E. Levison, MD
Allegheny University of the Health Sciences
Department of Medicine
Division of Infectious Diseases
Philadelphia, Pennsylvania

Milena L. Lewis, MD
Clinical Associate Professor of Medicine
New York University School of Medicine
Pulmonary Disease Section
New York, New York

Christian Lienhardt, MD, DTM, MSc
TB Research Unit
Medical Research Council Laboratories
Fajara, Banjul
The Gambia

Benjamin A. Lipsky, MD
Associate Professor
Department of Medicine
University of Washington
Hospital Epidemiologist
Director, General Internal Medicine Clinic
VA Puget Sound Health Care System
Seattle, Washington

Gabriel Lopez-Berestein, MD
Professor of Medicine and Internist
Chief, Section of Immunobiology and Drug Carriers
Department of Bioimmunotherapy
M. D. Anderson Cancer Center
Houston, Texas

Donald E. Low, MD, FRCPC
Microbiologist-in-Chief
Department of Microbiology
Mount Sinai and Princess Margaret Hospitals
University of Toronto
Toronto, Ontario, Canada

Mang M. Ma, MD, FRCPC
Assistant Professor
Division of Gastroenterology and Hepatology
Department of Medicine
University of Alberta
Edmonton, Alberta, Canada

Sheldon M. Markowitz, MD, MS
Chief, Medical Service
Veterans Affairs Medical Center
Professor of Internal Medicine, Microbiology, and Immunology
Department of Internal Medicine
Medical College of Virginia
Richmond, Virginia

Thomas J. Marrie, MD, FRCPC, FACP
Professor of Medicine
Departments of Medicine and Microbiology
Dalhousie University
Queen Elizabeth II Health Sciences Centre
Halifax, Nova Scotia, Canada

Henry Masur, MD
Chief, Critical Care Medicine Department
Warren Grant Magnuson Clinical Center
National Institutes of Health
Bethesda, Maryland

M. Maurin, MD, PhD
Clinical Microbiology
Unité des Ricketties
Université de la Méditerranée
Faculté de Médicine
Marseille, France

Keith P. W. J. McAdam, MA, MBBChir, FRCP
Director
Medical Research Council Laboratories
Fajara, Banjul
The Gambia

George H. McCracken, MD
Professor of Pediatrics
The Sarah M. and Charles E. Seay Chair in Pediatric Infectious Diseases
University of Texas Southwestern Medical Center
Dallas, Texas

Peggy S. McKinnon, MD
Clinical Assistant Professor of Pharmacy
Department of Pharmacy Practice, Wayne State University
Department of Pharmacy Services and the Anti-Infective Research Laboratory,
Detroit Receiving Hospital
Detroit, Michigan

Julia A. McMillan, MD
Associate Professor of Pediatrics
Johns Hopkins University School of Medicine
Baltimore, Maryland

Michael M. McNeil, MD
Medical Epidemiologist
Mycotic Diseases Branch
National Center for Infectious Diseases
Centers for Disease Control
Atlanta, Georgia

Thomas C. Merigan, Jr, MD
Director, Center for AIDS Research
Stanford University Medical Center
Stanford, California

Jussi Mertsola, MD
Associate Professor
Department of Pediatrics
Turku University Hospital
Finland

Richard A. Miller, MD
Associate Professor
Department of Medicine
University of Washington
Chief, Infectious Diseases Section
Infectious Diseases/Medicine
VA Puget Sound Health Care System
Seattle, Washington

Ayesha Mirza, MD
Instructor in Pediatrics
Division of Infectious Diseases
Louisiana State University School of Medicine
New Orleans, Louisiana

Abdolghader Molavi, MD
Professor of Medicine
Department of Medicine
Allegheny University of the Health Sciences
Philadelphia, Pennsylvania

Sara G. Monroe, MD
Associate Professor
Division of Infectious Disease
Medical College of Virginia
Richmond, Virginia

John S. Moran, MD, MPH
STD Advisor
HIV/AIDS Prevention Project
Ministry of Health
Jakarta, Indonesia
Medical Epidemiologist
National Center for HIV, STD and TB Prevention
Centers for Disease Control and Prevention
Atlanta, Georgia

Anne B. Morris, MD
Assistant Professor of Medicine and Obstetrics and Gynecology
Department of Medicine
Division of Infectious Diseases
Baystate Medical Center
Tufts University School of Medicine
Springfield, Massachusetts

Arthur J. Morris, BSc(Hons), MD
Clinical Microbiologist
Microbiology Laboratory
Green Lane Hospital
Auckland, New Zealand

Gene D. Morse, PharmD, FCCP, BCPS
Professor
Pharmacy Practice
State University of New York at Buffalo
Director
Laboratory for Antiviral Research
Amherst, New York

Richard E. Moxon, PhD
Professor of Paediatrics
Molecular Infectious Diseases Group
Institute for Molecular Medicine
Department of Paediatrics
John Radcliffe Hospital
Oxford, United Kingdom

Robert R. Muder, MD
Chief, Infection Control
VA Pittsburgh Healthcare System
Associate Professor of Medicine
University of Pittsburgh School of Medicine
Infectious Disease Section
Pittsburgh, Pennsylvania

Lütfiye Mülazimoglu, MD
Associate Professor of Infectious Diseases and Clinical
Microbiology
Marmara University School of Medicine
Istanbul, Turkey

Profesor Dr. Ricardo Negroni
Mycology Unit
Francisco Javier Muñiz Hospital
Buenos Aires City, Argentina

M. Hong Nguyen, MD
Assistant Professor of Medicine
Department of Medicine
Division of Infectious Diseases
University of Florida College of Medicine
Chief, Infectious Disease Section
VA Medical Center
Gainesville, Florida

David P. Nicolau, PharmD
Coordinator for Research
Department of Medicine
Division of Infectious Diseases
Hartford Hospital
Hartford, Connecticut

Carl Erik Nord, MD, PhD
Professor and Chairman
Department of Immunology, Microbiology, Pathology, and
Infectious Diseases
Karolinska Institute
Huddinge University Hospital
Stockholm, Sweden

Diana L. Nunley, MD
Associate Professor
Department of Internal Medicine
James H. Quillen College of Medicine
Johnson City, Tennessee

Elizabeth Olek, DO
Post-Doctoral Fellow
Section of Infectious Disease
Boston Medical Center
Boston, Massachusetts

Robert Orenstein, DO
Assistant Professor of Medicine
Virginia Commonwealth University/Medical College of
Virginia
Director HIV/AIDS Program
Hunter Holmes McGuire Veterans Affairs Medical
Center
Richmond, Virginia

Peter G. Pappas, MD
Associate Professor
Department of Medicine
University of Alabama at Birmingham
Birmingham, Alabama

Valerie Parkas, MD
Instructor of Medicine
Division of Infectious Diseases
Mount Sinai School of Medicine
New York, New York

Joseph G. Pastorek II, MD, FACOG, FACS
Coeditor, Medscape, Women's Health
Louisiana Representative for OBGYN.net
Metairie, Louisiana

David L. Paterson, MBBS, FRACP
Infectious Diseases Physician
J. J. Sullivan, N. J. Nicolaides and Partners
Brisbane, Queensland, Australia

Thomas F. Patterson, MD
Associate Professor of Medicine
The University of Texas Health Science Center at San
Antonio
San Antonio, Texas

David A. Pegues, MD
Assistant Professor
Department of Medicine
UCLA School of Medicine
Los Angeles, California

Charles A. Peloquin, PharmD
Director, Infectious Disease Pharmacokinetics Laboratory
National Jewish Medical and Research Center
Adjoint Associate Professor
Schools of Pharmacy and Medicine
University of Colorado
Denver, Colorado

Beulah E. Perdue, PharmD, BCPS
Antimicrobial Coordinator
Clinical Specialist, Infectious Diseases and HIV
Medicine
University of Maryland Medical System
Clinical Assistant Professor
University of Maryland School of Pharmacy
Department of Pharmacy Services
University of Maryland Medical System
Baltimore, Maryland

John R. Perfect, MD
Associate Professor of Medicine
Department of Medicine
Duke University Medical Center
Durham, North Carolina

Piero Periti, MD
Professor of Chemotherapy
Department of Pharmacology
University of Florence
Florence, Italy

Marion G. Peters, MD
Associate Professor of Medicine
Chief of Hepatology
Department of Medicine
Washington University School of Medicine
St. Louis, Missouri

Raymond D. Pitetti, MD
Fellow
Department of Pediatric Emergency Medicine
Children's Hospital of Pittsburgh
Pittsburgh, Pennsylvania

Pierre J. Plourde, MD, FRCPC
Director, Infection Control
Department of Infectious Diseases
St. Boniface Hospital
Assistant Professor
Department of Internal Medicine
University of Manitoba
Winnipeg, Manitoba, Canada

Ronald E. Polk, PharmD
Professor of Pharmacy and Medicine
School of Pharmacy
Virginia Commonwealth University
Medical College of Virginia Campus
Richmond, Virginia

Richard B. Pollard, MD
Professor
Department of Internal Medicine, Microbiology, Immunology, and Pathology
The University of Texas Medical Branch
Galveston, Texas

William G. Powderly, MD, FRCPI
Associate Professor of Medicine
Co-Director, Division of Infectious Diseases
Washington University
St. Louis, Missouri

Sandra L. Preston, PharmD
Assistant Professor of Medicine
Departments of Medicine and Pharmacology
Albany Medical College
Albany, New York

John P. Quinn, MD
Associate Professor of Medicine
Department of Medicine
University of Illinois at Chicago
Chicago, Illinois

Richard Quintiliani, Jr, MD
Director, Anti-Infective Research and Pharmacoeconomic Studies
Hartford Hospital
Hartford, Connecticut
Professor of Medicine
University of Connecticut School of Medicine
Farmington, Connecticut

D. Raoult, MD
Professor and Chairman
Faculté de Médicine
Unité des Rickettsies
CNRS UPRESA 6020
Marseille, France

Annette C. Reboli, MD
Associate Professor of Medicine
Department of Medicine
Division of Infectious Diseases
University of Medicine and Dentistry of New Jersey
Robert Wood Johnson Medical School at Camden
Camden, New Jersey

David A. Relman, MD
Assistant Professor
Departments of Medicine, Microbiology, and Immunology
Stanford University School of Medicine
Stanford, California
Staff Physician
Veterans Affairs Palo Alto Health Care System
Palo Alto, California

John H. Rex, MD
Associate Professor of Medicine
Division of Infectious Diseases
Department of Internal Medicine
Center for the Study of Emerging and Reemerging Pathogens
University of Texas Medical School
Houston, Texas

John Richens, MA, MSc, FRCPE
Lecturer
Sexually Transmitted Diseases
University College London
London, United Kingdom

William J. Riebel, MD
Director
Department of Infectious Diseases
Lakewood Hospital
Lakewood, Ohio
Clinical Instructor
Department of Medicine
Case Western Reserve University
Cleveland, Ohio

John D. Rihs, BS
Supervisor
Department of Microbiology
VA Pittsburgh Health Care System
Pittsburgh, Pennsylvania

Jason Rosé, PhD
Postdoctoral Fellow in Microbiology and Immunology
Stanford University School of Medicine
Stanford, California

Ted Rosen, MD
Professor of Dermatology
Baylor College of Medicine
Chief, Dermatology Service
Houston VA Medical Center
Houston, Texas

Mark E. Rupp, MD
Assistant Professor of Medicine
Department of Internal Medicine
The University of Nebraska Medical Center
Omaha, Nebraska

Charles E. Rupprecht, VMD, MS, PhD
Chief, Rabies Section
Viral and Rickettsial Zoonoses Branch
Division of Viral and Rickettsial Diseases
National Center for Infectious Diseases
Centers for Disease Control and Prevention
Atlanta, Georgia

Michael J. Rybak, PharmD, FCCP, FIDSA
Professor of Pharmacy and Medicine
Pharmacy Practice, Division of Infections Diseases
Wayne State University
Director, Anti-Infective Research Laboratory
Detroit Receiving Hospital
University Health Center
Detroit, Michigan

Stephen L. Sacks, MD, FRCPS
Professor, Department of Pharmacology and Therapeutics
Faculty of Medicine
University of British Columbia
President and CEO
Viridae Clinical Sciences, Inc.
Vancouver, British Columbia, Canada

Maurice R. Scavizzi, MD
Professor, Head of Department
Department of Bacteriology, Virology
University of Paris
Faculty of Medicine/Avicemme Hospital
Bobigny, France

Klaus P. Schaal, MD
Director, Institute for Medical Microbiology and Immunology
University of Bonn
Bonn, Germany

Julius Schachter, PhD
Professor of Laboratory Medicine
Department of Laboratory Medicine
University of California, San Francisco
San Francisco, California

Jerome J. Schentag, PharmD
SUNY at Buffalo School of Pharmacy
The Clinical Pharmacokinetics Laboratory
Millard Fillmore Health System
Buffalo, New York

David Schlossberg, MD
Professor of Medicine
Jefferson Medical College
Director, Department of Medicine
Episcopal Hospital
Philadelphia, Pennsylvania

James Scott, PharmD
Program Director, Infection Management Division
Clinical Pharmacokinetics Laboratory
Millard Fillmore Health System
Buffalo, New York

Brian Scully, MBBS
Division of Infectious Diseases
Department of Medicine
College of Physicians and Surgeons of Columbia University
Columbia Presbyterian Hospital
New York, New York

Carlos Seas, MD
Attending Physician
Department of Tropical and Infectious Diseases
Cayetano Heredia National Hospital
Lima, Peru

Teshale Seboxa, MD, MSC (CTM)
Associate Professor of Medicine
Department of Internal Medicine
Faculty of Medicine
Addis Ababa University
Addis Ababa, Ethiopia

Daniel J. Sexton, MD
Professor
Department of Medicine
Division of Infectious Diseases
Duke University Medical Center
Durham, North Carolina

Eugene D. Shapiro, MD
Professor of Pediatrics and Epidemiology
Department of Pediatrics
Yale University School of Medicine
New Haven, Connecticut

David M. Shlaes, MD, PhD
Vice President
Infectious Disease Research
Wyeth Ayerst Research
Pearl River, New York

Andrew J. H. Simpson MB,BSMSc MRCPath
Wellcome Clinical Senior Lecturer
Nuffield Department of Clinical Medicine
University of Oxford
Radcliffe Hospital
Headington
Oxford, United Kingdom

Nina Singh, MD
Chief, Transplant Infectious Diseases
Infectious Diseases Section
Veterans Affairs Medical Center
Pittsburgh, Pennsylvania

Jack D. Sobel, MD
Professor of Medicine
Chief, Division of Infectious Diseases
Department of Internal Medicine
Wayne State University School of Medicine
Chief, Section of Infectious Diseases
Harper Hospital
Detroit Medical Center
Detroit, Michigan

Wladimir Sougakoff
Assistant Professor of Microbiology
Service de Bactériologie-Hygiéne
Faculté de Médecine Pitié-Salpêtrière
Paris, France

Harold C. Standiford, MD, FACP
Deputy Director Medical Care
VA Maryland Health Care System
Professor of Medicine
University of Maryland School of Medicine
Baltimore, Maryland

Russell W. Steele, MD
Professor and Vice Chairman
Division Head, Infectious Diseases
Department of Pediatrics
Louisiana State University School of Medicine
New Orleans, Louisiana

Gary E. Stein, PharmD
Associate Professor of Medicine and Pharmacology
Department of Medicine
Michigan State University
East Lansing, Michigan

Dennis P. Stevens, MD, PhD
Infectious Disease Section
Veterans Affairs Medical Center
Boise, Idaho
Department of Medicine
University of Washington
School of Medicine
Seattle, Washington

Alan M. Sugar, MD
Professor of Medicine
Boston University School of Medicine
Evans Memorial Department of Clinical Research
Department of Medicine
Boston, Massachusetts

Susan Swindells, MD
Associate Professor of Medicine
Department of Internal Medicine–Infectious Diseases
University of Nebraska Medical Center
Omaha, Nebraska

James S. Tan, MD
Head, Infectious Disease Section
Professor and Vice-Chairman
Department of Internal Medicine
Northeastern Ohio Universities
Rootstown, Ohio
Chairman, Department of Medicine
Summa Health System
Akron, Ohio

Nathan M. Thielman, MD, MPH
Assistant Professor
Division of Infectious Diseases
Department of Medicine
Medical University of South Carolina
Charleston, South Carolina

Graham A. Tipples, PhD
Research Scientist, Viral and Zoonotic Diseases
Bureau of Microbiology
Laboratory Centre for Disease Control
Edmonton, Alberta, Canada

Michael L. Towns, MD
Associate Medical Director
Becton Dickinson
Microbiology Systems
Sparks, Maryland

Edmond C. Tramont, MD
Professor and Director
Medical Biotechnology Center
University of Maryland Biotechnology Institute
Baltimore, Maryland

John J. Treanor, MD
Associate Professor of Medicine
Department of Medicine
Infectious Diseases Unit
University of Rochester
Rochester, New York

Gordon M. Trenholme, MD
Director
Section of Infectious Disease
Rush-Presbyterian-St Luke's Medical Center
Chicago, Illinois

Carmelita U. Tuazon, MD
Professor of Medicine
Department of Medicine
George Washington University Medical Center
Washington, D.C.

John Turnidge, MBBS, FRACP, FRCPA
Director, Microbiology and Infectious Diseases
Women's and Children's Hospital
Adelaide, South Australia

David L. J. Tyrrell, MD, PhD, FRCPC
Dean, Faculty of Medicine
Director, GlaxoWellcome-Heritage Research Institute
University of Alberta
Edmonton, Alberta, Canada

Hillar Vellend, MD
Professor, Department of Medicine
Faculty of Medicine, University of Toronto
Mount Sinai Hospital
Toronto, Ontario, Canada

Emanuel N. Vergis, MD
Instructor in Medicine
University of Pittsburgh Medical Center
Pittsburgh, Pennsylvania

Jan Verhoef, MD, PhD
Professor of Clinical Microbiology
Medical Microbiology
Eykman-Winkler Institute
Utrecht, The Netherlands

David H. Walker, MD
Professor and Chairman
Department of Pathology
Director, WHO Collaborating Center for Tropical Diseases
University of Texas Medical Branch
Galveston, Texas

Thomas L. Wallace, PhD
Director, Pharmacology
Preclinical Development
Aronex Pharmaceuticals, Inc.
The Woodlands, Texas

Richard J. Wallace, Jr, MD
Professor of Medicine
Chairman, Department of Microbiology
John Chapman Professorship in Microbiology
Acting Director, Center for Pulmonary Infectious Disease Control
The University of Texas Health Center at Tyler
Tyler, Texas

Thomas J. Walsh, MD
Senior Investigator
Chief, Immunocompromised Host Section
Pediatric Oncology Branch
National Cancer Institute
Bethesda, Maryland

Frederick C. S. Wang
Assistant Professor of Medicine
Harvard Medical School
Brigham and Women's Hospital
Boston, Massachusetts

Lauri Welles, MD
Clinical Associate
HIV and AIDS Malignancies Branch
National Cancer Institute
Bethesda, Maryland

Melinda Wharton, MD, MPH
Chief, Child Vaccine Preventable Diseases Branch
Epidemiology and Surveillance Division
National Immunization Program
Centers for Disease Control and Prevention
Atlanta, Georgia

Joseph L. Wheat, MD
Department of Medicine
Wishard Memorial Hospital
Indianapolis, Indiana

Nicholas J. White, DSc, MD, FRCP
Professor
Nuffield Department of Clinical Medicine
University of Oxford
John Radcliffe Hospital
Headington, Oxford, United Kingdom
Wellcome-Mahidol University Oxford Tropical Medicine
Research Programme
Faculty of Tropical Medicine
Mahidol University
Bangkok, Thailand

Paul L. Williams, MD
Visalia Medical Clinic, Inc.
Visalia, California

Edward S. Wong, MD
Hospital Epidemiologist
McGuire Veterans Affairs Hospital
Associate Professor of Medicine
Medical College of Virginia
Richmond, Virginia

Craig A. Wood, MD
Associate Professor of Medicine
Allegheny University Hospitals, Hahnemann
Philadelphia, Pennsylvania

Martin J. Wood, MD
Senior Clinical Lecturer
University of Birmingham
Heartlands Hospital
Birmingham, United Kingdom

Robert Yarchoan, MD
Head, Retroviral Diseases Section
Department of Medicine Branch
National Cancer Institute
Bethesda, Maryland

Edward J. Young, MD
Chief of Staff
VA Medical Center
Professor of Medicine and Microbiology and Immunology
Baylor College of Medicine
Houston, Texas

Victor L. Yu, MD
Professor of Medicine
University of Pittsburgh
Chief, Infectious Disease Section
VA Medical Center
Pittsburgh, Pennsylvania

CONTENTS

PART B
Mycobacterial Species 492

SECTION I

Bacteria and Antibacterial Agents

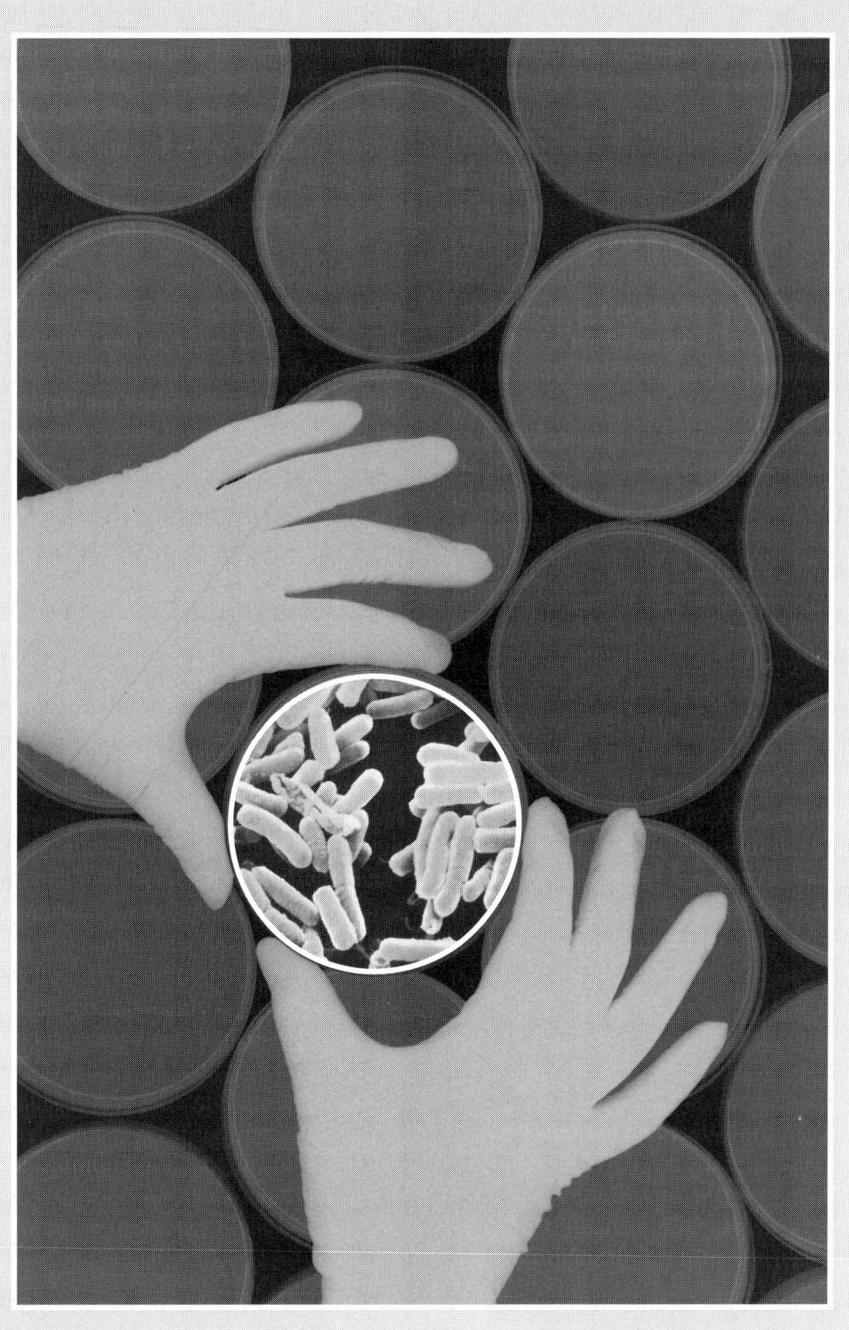

PART A

Standard Bacteria

Acinetobacter Species

E. Bergogne-Berezin

GENERAL DESCRIPTION

Acinetobacter spp. are strictly aerobic Gram-negative bacilli commonly present in soil and water as free-living saprophytes; they are also isolated as commensals from skin, throat, and various secretions of healthy people (15).

Epidemiology

Strains of *Acinetobacter* are widely distributed in nature and can be found in virtually 100% of soil and fresh-water samples when appropriate culture techniques are used (2, 15). As non-fastidious organisms, they utilize a wide variety of substrates as sole carbon source. *Acinetobacter* strains can also be isolated from food and form part of the normal flora of fresh meats; they may contribute to the spoilage of refrigerated meats. In the hospital environment, the organism has been found in moist situations such as room cold-air humidifiers, tap water, hand-washing basins, water baths, moist respirometers, and all types of ventilatory equipment that are capable of aerosolizing the organism.

Normal individuals have been shown to carry *Acinetobacter*, indicating that the source of nosocomial infections might be endogenous as well as from the external environment. Like *Pseudomonas aeruginosa*, *Acinetobacter* forms part of the bacterial flora of the skin and is found in the axillae, groin, and toe webs of normal individuals; the organism can colonize the oral cavity, the respiratory tract, and the normal intestine and is carried in hospitals by staff and patients.

Microbiology

Acinetobacter strains are nonfermentative, nonfastidious, aerobic Gram-negative coccobacilli, usually found in diploid formation or in chains of variable length. They are not motile (*akinetos,* "unable to move") but the cells display a "twitching motility." Strictly aerobic, they grow well on all common media, at temperatures between 20 and 30°C, but for most strains the optimum is 33 to 35°C. Growth at 41 and 44°C can occur for a few species and is a discriminating character between species. Identification of *Acinetobacter* spp. is based upon oxidase-negative, catalase-positive, indole-negative, nitrate-negative test results with production or no production of acid from D-glucose, D-ribose, D-xylose, and L-arabinose (used oxidatively as carbon sources).

The nomenclature of *Acinetobacter* spp. changed considerably over the years: designated *Bacterium anitratum, Herellea vaginicola, Mima polymorpha* (Debord, 1939), *Achromobacter, Alcaligenes, Neisseria, Micrococcus calcoaceticus, Diplococcus,* B5W, and *Cytophaga* (16), the genus *Acinetobacter* (Brisou and Prvt, 1954) comprised one species, *A. calcoaceticus,* and two varieties, *anitratus* (formerly *H. vaginicola*) and *lwoffi* (formerly *M. polymorpha*) until 1986 (5).

By using modern methods of taxonomy (genetic transformations, DNA hybridizations and RNA sequence comparisons), the classification proposed by Bouvet and Grimont (5) identified 19 genomic species including *A. baumannii* (formerly *A. calcoaceticus* var. *anitratus* and *A. glucidolytica non liquefaciens*), *A. haemolyticus, A. junii, A. johnsonii* and *A. radioresistens.* The new definition of *Acinetobacter* is based on phenotypic characters (biotyping) and identification of genomic species.

Most studies support the initial observation that *A. baumannii* is the main species associated with outbreaks of nosocomial infections (5); other species, *A. haemolyticus, A. junii, A. lwoffi,* can be associated with clinical infections; they can be natural inhabitants of human skin, and with repeated isolation, these non-*baumannii* species must be considered as potential pathogens (2).

SUSCEPTIBILITY IN VITRO

Since their recognition as significant human pathogens, one of the most striking features of *Acinetobacter* spp. has been their extraordinarily rapid response to challenge with new antibiotics.

Overview of Clinical Resistance

Since 1975, successive surveys have reported increasing resistance in clinical isolates of *Acinetobacter* spp. periodically (3, 24). High proportions of strains have become resistant to older antibiotics; many *Acinetobacter* strains are now resistant to most commonly used antibacterial drugs, including aminopenicillins, ureidopenicillins, cephalosporins of the first (cephalotin) and second (cefamandole) generations, cephamycins such as cefoxitin, most aminoglycosides-aminocyclitols, chloramphenicol, and tetracyclines. Contrasting data are sparsely distributed in the literature for some antibiotics: minocycline and doxycycline were cited in one study as the most active of 21 antibiotics tested, including 10 β-lactams, 3 aminoglycosides, and nalidixic acid (22). Differences in susceptibilities of *Acinetobacter* isolates could be attributable to environmental factors such as the different patterns of antibiotic usage that exist in Japan (22), the United States (27), France (3), Germany (24), or Spain (28).

Among various factors associated with the increasing resistance of *Acinetobacter* spp. to antibiotics, an increased incidence of the most resistant species (*A. baumannii*) may also have changed the reported overall antibiotic resistance of clinical isolates of *Acinetobacter*. Other *Acinetobacter* spp., i.e., *A. lwoffi, A. johsonii, A. haemolyticus,* and *A. junii,* can be isolated from the hospital environment but are involved less frequently in nosocomial infection and show variable susceptibility to antibacterial agents. Resistance patterns in different countries are reported in Table 1.

Antibiotic Resistance in *Acinetobacter:* Therapeutic Problems

Several reviews have focused on therapeutic problems caused in ICUs by *Acinetobacter* strains resistant to aminoglycosides and most β-lactams, except for imipenem (6, 20, 27). In one report (29), two series of isolates obtained over a period of 2 to 3 years had changing susceptibility patterns over time. In 1989, 144 strains isolated from nosocomial infections were susceptible to co-trimoxazole, polymyxin B, doxycycline, ceftazidime, and imipenem, and the authors mentioned that ceftazidime and imipenem had been pre-

scribed widely for treating patients with *Acinetobacter* infections. In 1991–1992, strains resistant to imipenem, ceftazidime, amikacin, and all other antibiotics tested routinely were isolated; polymyxin B and sulbactam were the only agents that retained activity. In five patients who received ampicillin plus sulbactam, resolution of infections and eradication of the resistant organisms was achieved. A high level of resistance to ampicillin and cefoperazone was observed in vitro, whereas these drugs combined with sulbactam provided favorable results in this particular study.

ANTIMICROBIAL THERAPY
Drugs of Choice

Until in vitro susceptibility results are available, empiric first-line therapy for serious *Acinetobacter* infections could include the carbapenems or third-generation cephalosporins, depending on the hospital's susceptibility profile of *Acinetobacter* spp. Once susceptibility results are available, many drugs could be found appropriate. The most useful drugs are described below.

β-Lactams

β-Lactams have been widely used in the treatment of *Acinetobacter* infections for the last two decades. A multicenter sur-

TABLE 1 • Evolution and Current Resistance Patterns in *Acinetobacter spp.*[a]

	Bichat-Claude Bernard University Hospital									France[b]	Germany[c]	Spain[d]
	1975 (%)	1980 (%)	1985 (%)	1991 (%)	1992 (%)	1993 (% ICU)	1993 (%)	1994[e] (%)	1995 (%)	1991 (%)	1993 (n = 95) (%)	1993 (n = 54) (%)
β-Lactams												
Ampicillin	83	94	98	100	—	—	—	—	—	—	91	98
Carbenicillin ticarcillin	16	70	72	77.5	40.4	46	42.9	39.4	36.4	44	—	70
Mezlocillin piperacillin	—	80	92	88	82.7	94	—	—	—	—	36	67
Aztreonam	85	93	90	90	—	—	—	—	—	—	54	98
Imipenem	—	—	0	2	2.3	5	6.9	4.6	0.7 (1.6)[f]	0.6	0	0
Cephalosporin 2nd gen.	90	95	98	98	—	—	—	—	96.7	—	99	—
Cefotaxime	—	55	84.5	95	91.5	98	95	97.4	86.1	—	32	69
Ceftazidime	—	19	45.5	92	82.4	91	88	94	—	76	32	45
Moxalactam	—	90	90	92	—	—	—	—	—	—	—	—
Aminoglycosides												
Gentamicin	12	81	84	80	74	88	78	77.6	78.8 (90.5)[e]	69.5	98	67
Tobramycin	12	22	47	76	58	61	65	66	—	62	98	50
Netilmicin	—	16	49	85	64.5	79	73	62	87.5 (76.2)[e]	44.5	—	34
Amikacin	—	2.5	39	78	68	81	69	61	62.2 (76.2)[e]	55	64	28
Kanamycin	17	67	70	89	—	—	—	—	—	—	—	—
Fluoroquinolones												
Pefloxacin			19	75	75	83	63	73	82.2 (92.1)[e]	85	—	—
Ciprofloxacin			18	70	—	—	—	—	—	80	94	30
Ofloxacin			20	67	—	—	—	—	—	—	—	28
Norfloxacin			87	95	—	—	—	—	—	—	—	82

[a]Data for *A. baumannii.*

[b]After Joly-Guillou (1992).

[c]After Seifert et al. (1993).

[d]After Vila et al. (1992).

[e]Joly-Guillou (personal communication).

[f]% Resistant in ICU.

vey in France included 6 centers in 1988 and 12 centers from 1989 to 1992; 3450 *Acinetobacter* isolates were tested for susceptibility/resistance to ticarcillin, cefotaxime, ceftazidime, and imipenem. The results of this survey are described below.

Ticarcillin. Carboxypenicillins were initially very active in *Acinetobacter* infections (3). From 1975 to 1985, the proportion of strains resistant to carboxypenicillins rose from 16 to 72% (Table 1). Over the 4-year period of surveillance (1988–92), ticarcillin resistance decreased significantly, from 53% in 1988 to 25% in 1992. This observation gives ticarcillin (with potential addition of a β-lactamase inhibitor) a rejuvenated place in the anti-*Acinetobacter* armamentarium.

Third-Generation Cephalosporins

Ceftazidime. Initially seen as the cephalosporin of reference against *Acinetobacter,* the survey showed a slow and progressive increase in resistance of *A. baumannii* to ceftazidime, from a high of 72% resistant strains in 1988, to 80% in 1992–1993, and reaching 86% in 1994–95 (Table 1).

Cefotaxime. Among third-generation cephalosporins, cefotaxime has always been less active than ceftazidime. Decreasing efficacy with a significantly higher level of resistance than that of ceftazidime was seen, reaching up to 92% resistant strains in 1992–93 and 96.7 to 98% in 1994–95.

Comments. The place of third-generation cephalosporins in the treatment of *Acinetobacter* infections is currently restricted to documented *Acinetobacter* infections with susceptibility testing indicating persistent susceptibility to third-generation cephalosporins, mainly to ceftazidime (rare non–cephalosporinase producers: 8–15% of clinical strains). Empiric therapy of *Acinetobacter* nosocomial infection can include ceftazidime with a rapid switch to another β-lactam such as carbapenem (imipenem, meropenem) in case of clinical deterioration.

Imipenem. Imipenem is often considered the drug of choice for *Acinetobacter* infection. The above-mentioned national survey showed a low level of resistance to imipenem, except in 1988, when 5% of strains were resistant or intermediate to imipenem, although only 2% of strains were "fully resistant" (MIC >8 mg/L). The latter observation corresponded with the emergence and spread in a few hospitals of *Acineto-bacter* strains with diminished susceptibility to imipenem. The frequency of imipenem-resistant strains in 1992 was 4% (including 2.5% intermediate strains), but surveys since 1993 have noted a return to full susceptibility to imipenem (MICs 0.03–1.0 mg/L), with only 0.5 to 0.7% imipenem-resistant strains (Table 1). Imipenem remains a drug of choice, widely used in the treatment of *Acinetobacter* infections.

β-Lactamase Inhibitors

Of the available β-lactamase inhibitors, clavulanic acid and sulbactam have been introduced and widely used in medical practice in combination with aminopenicillins or cephalosporins, and a newly developed compound, tazobactam, has also been investigated. β-lactamase inhibitors have poor intrinsic antibacterial activities, although sulbactam is intrinsically active against *Acinetobacter* spp. (2). Sulbactam was less active than tazobactam against ticarcillin-resistant strains (MIC range, 1–32 mg/L), but both were active by themselves against ticarcillin-susceptible strains, with geometric mean MICs of sulbactam and tazobactam of 2.1 and 6.5 mg/L, respectively (personal observation). The inhibitory activities of these β-lactamase inhibitors against the β-lactamases produced by *Acinetobacter* strains were examined. Clavulanic acid caused a significant decrease in the MICs for the ticarcillin-resistant strains (MIC_{50}, 112 mg/L) but not a true reversion to susceptibility. The MIC for ticarcillin-resistant strains (breakpoint > 64 mg/L) fell to susceptible levels in combination with tazobactam (geometric mean MIC, 33.02 mg/L); sulbactam in combination with ticarcillin reduced the MICs of ticarcillin to a lower geometric mean MIC of 15.5 mg/L. A more recent multicenter investigation has confirmed these data (Table 2).

The sulbactam-ticarcillin combination shows an interesting potential therapeutic activity, with a slight improvement of activity on addition of clavulanic acid. These results are related to the intrinsic activity of sulbactam against *Acinetobacter* and the specific inhibitory power of this β-lactamase inhibitor against the β-lactamases of *Acinetobacter* in addition to the activity of ticarcillin.

TABLE 2 • In Vitro Activities of β-Lactams and β-Lactamase Inhibitors against Clinical Isolates of *A. baumannii* (after Joly-Guillou 1996)

Antibiotics	E Test (n = 257)		Agar Dilution (n = 197)	
	%R[a] + I[b]	MIC 50%	%R[a] + I[b]	MIC 50%
Ticarcillin	67	32	—	—
Ticarcillin + clavulanate	64	24	50.2	16
Ticarcillin + sulbactam	—	—	33.5	2
Ticarcillin + clavulanate + sulbactam	—	—	18.8	2
Ampicillin + sulbactam	37.4	2	—	—
Piperacillin + tazobactam	—	—	52.3	32
Ceftazidime	77.6	12	—	—
Imipenem	11.4	0.38	0	0.125

[a] R, resistant.

[b] I, intermediate.

Newer β-Lactams

Recent studies have compared cefepime, cefpirome, and a new carbapenem, meropenem, with drugs mentioned above (personal unpublished data). One study tested 60 *A. baumannii* isolates against ceftazidime, cefpirome, and imipenem; the MICs of cefpirome were slightly lower (geometric mean MIC, 3.6 mg/L) than those of ceftazidime (4.0 mg/L) for fully susceptible *Acinetobacter* strains, while the MIC_{90}s for 25 strains (penicillinase-cephalosporinase producers) were 128 and 64 mg/L with ceftazidime and cefpirome, respectively. Strains that produced only a cephalosporinase behaved variably in the presence of these drugs but were predominantly resistant, with MICs ranging from 16 to 128 mg/L. Imipenem and meropenem inhibited most *Acinetobacter* strains, with MIC values of 0.5 mg/L. For cephalosporinase producers, the MIC_{90} of imipenem was slightly higher (1 mg/L), but for 10 strains with diminished susceptibility to imipenem, the MIC_{90} was 4 mg/L, with a geometric mean MIC of 1.8 mg/L. Twenty-five non–*A. baumannii* strains were variably susceptible, with 60% of *A. haemolyticus* and *A. lwoffi* isolates inhibited by 4 mg/L and 1 mg/L of cefpirome and imipenem, respectively.

Aminoglycosides

Resistance to streptomycin, gentamicin, tobramycin, and kanamycin arose quite suddenly in 1975 (3), and since then, after the development of newer aminoglycosides, resistance to netilmicin and amikacin has also been observed (6). All types of aminoglycoside-modifying enzymes have been found in *Acinetobacter* spp., and up to 75% of isolates in some series had mechanisms of resistance to aminoglycosides (Table 1). In France, the triple inactivating-enzyme combination of adenylase AAD(2″)-I plus phosphorylase APH(3′)-VI plus acetylase AAC(3) is particularly common, while other combinations have included AAC(6′)-I, AAC(3)-I, AAD(2″)-I, and APH(3′)-VI. The latter enzyme, found at a high incidence, causes amikacin resistance (6). An international survey of 1189 aminoglycoside-resistant strains found that 34.8% of them produced at least three enzymes, and various combinations of enzymes have been observed (G. Miller, personal communication). Amikacin and a newer aminoglycoside, isepamicin, are the least inactivated drugs; recently, 66 and 62% of strains were reported to be resistant to these two aminoglycosides, respectively, (vs. 74% for gentamicin) (Lambert 1996, personal communication).

Fluoroquinolones

Since 1985, the new fluoroquinolones have been used increasingly for the treatment of severe nosocomial infections caused by multiply resistant bacteria, especially those compounds that can be administered parenterally (pefloxacin, ciprofloxacin). Comparison of the in vitro susceptibilities of *Acinetobacter* strains collected before and after the introduction of new quinolones showed MIC values for recent strains five- to tenfold higher for pefloxacin, ciprofloxacin, and ofloxacin. The newer compounds (temafloxacin and sparfloxacin) did not show significantly better activity than previous compounds, and the most active fluorinated quinolone against clinical iso-

lates of *Acinetobacter* remains ofloxacin. The proportions of fully susceptible strains ranged from 18 to 70% for pefloxacin, ciprofloxacin, and ofloxacin in 1993, depending on the country (Table 1). In France, the proportions of resistant strains were stable in 1995. However, in killing curves for *A. baumannii* in the presence of four fluoroquinolones, sparfloxacin showed significantly better bactericidal activity than temafloxacin, while ciprofloxacin and pefloxacin were bacteriostatic only (14).

Combination Therapy

Based the high incidence of resistance of *Acinetobacter* spp. to major antibiotic classes as seen above, monotherapy is not advisable. Most recent studies have recommended either extended-spectrum penicillins, third-generation cephalosporins, or imipenem, aminoglycosides, and/or fluoroquinolones in various combinations (to be tested in the laboratory prior to clinical use).

First-Line Combination Therapy

A clinical survey showed that preferred combinations included imipenem and amikacin (56%) or ceftazidime and an aminoglycoside (17%) (13). These combinations are synergistic in vitro, particularly in a rather late phase (>6 h), by inhibiting regrowth as was shown in a study of 20 aminoglycoside-resistant *A. baumannii* strains (30). Combinations of aminoglycosides with imipenem at concentrations similar to serum levels (amikacin, 16 mg/L; imipenem, 8 mg/L) were yielded killing curves showing enhanced killing for 45 to 75% of strains. Other in vitro studies of bactericidal activities of β-lactams combined with aminoglycosides have confirmed this in vitro synergy (28). Similarly, another in vitro study detected synergy by checkerboard titrations with combinations of imipenem plus amikacin or tobramycin against 14 *Acinetobacter* isolates resistant to at least two aminoglycosides (19). The clinical relevance of these combinations has been confirmed (8, 17).

Second-Line Combination Therapy

Fluoroquinolones have been increasingly used in *Acinetobacter* infections, and ceftazidime combined with a quinolone was prescribed in 11% of cases. A previous study in our hospital showed imipenem to be used as monotherapy in 20% of 33 nosocomial infections, imipenem in combination with amikacin in 40%, and pefloxacin plus amikacin or tobramycin (depending on the antibiogram) in 20% of cases; treatment failure and death (caused by *Acinetobacter* infection and/or underlying disease) occurred in 17% of patients who received antibiotics. Many similar studies can be found in the medical literature (17, 20).

Other Combinations

Combinations of aminoglycosides and fluoroquinolones have often shown indifferent or additive effects, both in vitro and in clinical trials (21). Ciprofloxacin plus imipenem is the combination used most frequently in our own hospital. In vitro killing curves of this combination demonstrate synergy and bactericidal activity against *Acinetobacter* isolates, and this combination has yielded favorable patient outcomes in *Acinetobacter* pneumonia (8). Combining either imipenem or ciprofloxacin with an aminoglycoside, enhanced killing for 45 to 75% and 15 to 35%, respectively, of tested strains in another study (14).

Unusual Combinations

Sulbactam. The role of sulbactam as a β-lactamase inhibitor in association with its intrinsic antibacterial activity, in combinations with β-lactams and/or an aminoglycoside should be defined and may offer a new therapeutic approach to *Acinetobacter* infections. Enhanced killing of resistant *A. baumannii* isolates by combinations of ticarcillin-sulbactam-netilmicin has been confirmed (Joly-Guillou, personal communication). Combinations of piperacillin-tazobactam-sulbactam or ticarcillin-clavulanic acid-sulbactam, although rather unconventional, may potentially have clinical relevance.

Rifampicin. The surprising activity of rifampicin against *Acinetobacter* (MIC range, 2–4 mg/L) described above may give rifampicin a role, provided that it is part of a synergistic combination to avoid or reduce the risk of spontaneous mutation to rifampicin resistance (4).

Management of Special Situations

Acinetobacter has been isolated from various types of opportunistic infections including septicemia, pneumonia, endocarditis, meningitis, skin and wound sepsis, and urinary tract infections (17). The main infections are in the lower respiratory tract, bacteremia, and urinary tract infections, but among the most difficult-to-treat infections, meningitis and endocarditis require specific management.

Meningitis

Nosocomial meningitis is not an infrequent manifestation of *Acinetobacter* infection. Meningitis due to this organism has been reported after neurosurgical procedures, and rare cases of primary meningitis, especially in children, also occur. *Acinetobacter* meningitis may result from introduction of the organism directly into the central nervous system (CNS) following intracranial surgery, as well as from indwelling ventriculostomy tubes or cerebrospinal fluid fistulae in patients receiving antimicrobial therapy. Siegman-Igra et al. (25) reviewed 25 cases of nosocomial *Acinetobacter* meningitis secondary to invasive procedures. In seven patients, ureidopenicillin plus an aminoglycoside was used as empirical therapy. In 16 other patients, local amikacin injections were added to the initial regimen. Eighteen of 21 patients who received appropriate therapy recovered from infection, whereas 2 patients receiving inappropriate treatment died, as well as 2 patients who died before being treated. Segev et al. (23) used intravenous pefloxacin at a dosage of 800 mg twice daily in four patients with *Acinetobacter* meningitis; eradication resulted in all four patients, with a mean CSF pefloxacin concentration of 8.8 mg/L. In a series of eight cases of nosocomial *Acinetobacter* meningitis, all isolates were resistant to cefotaxime, ceftriaxone, ceftazidime, ureidopenicillins, ciprofloxacin, and gentamicin, and seven strains

were resistant to imipenem. For all strains, the MIC of ampicillin/sulbactam was 8/4 mg/L or less, and the MIC of sulbactam was 4 mg/L for two strains. All patients were treated with ampicillin/sulbactam (2 g/1 g every 6 h or 2 g/1 g every 8 h). Of the eight patients, six were cured and two died of meningitis (12).

Endocarditis

In the literature (17), in patients with native valve endocarditis, the underlying cardiac conditions included rheumatic heart disease (30%), congenital heart disease (20%), or bicuspid aortic valve (10%). Some 25% percent of cases were associated with dental procedures, 16% followed open heart surgery, and single cases occurred in drug users, burns, and septic abortion. *Acinetobacter* endocarditis is also seen in patients with prosthetic valves. Empiric treatment should include broad-spectrum antibiotic therapy. Gradon et al. (11) reviewed 15 cases of *Acinetobacter* endocarditis; 66% were cured with various antibiotic combinations, but the latest reported patient was treated successfully by monotherapy with imipenem.

Newer Drugs with Anti-*Acinetobacter* Activity

Beside preparing new derivatives of existing drugs, research in the pharmaceutical industry today also focuses on identification of new targets in the bacterial cell. Proteins vital to bacteria are known, and the corresponding genes have been cloned. Thus either semisynthetic modifications of known antibacterials or preparation of completely new inhibitors of vital bacterial function are "in the pipeline."

Levofloxacin

A new fluoroquinolone, levofloxacin, the L-isomer of ofloxacin has shown MICs lower than that of ofloxacin and ciprofloxacin against *A. baumannii*. Its bactericidal activity was similar to that of ofloxacin and ciprofloxacin, but in combination with amikacin, an early (5 h) and strong bactericidal activity (6 log CFU decrease) was observed in a recent study (10), and synergism was reported (1). Pharmacokinetic studies and clinical trials with levofloxacin are in progress.

RU 59863

A new parenteral cephalosporin containing a catechol moiety has shown significant in vitro activity against *Acinetobacter* spp. Compared with ceftazidime, cefpirome, and imipenem, this new compound has shown higher activity against susceptible strains and against penicillinase producers than ceftazidime and cefpirome (MICs of 0.125–0.5 vs. 1.4 and 0.5–4 mg/L, respectively). It also exhibited better activity against strains with higher MICs for ceftazidime and cefpirome (imipenem remained the most active drug) (personal data, unpublished).

New Approaches, New Targets

Protegrins. "Protegrins" are antibacterial peptides with a wide spectrum that have been isolated from pig leukocytes. They are formed of chains of 16 to 18 homologous aminoacids with a disulfide bridge between cysteines (1–4 and 2–3). Many

Gram-negative bacteria are susceptible to protegrins, but data on their potential activity against *Acinetobacter* spp. are not yet available (data from international conference on staphylococci and staphylococcal infections, Aix-les-Bains, June 1996).

Cecropins-Magainins.   Some antibiotic peptides widely distributed in nature and identified in insects and in mammalians act as membrane-active agents in bacterial cells by disrupting cell membrane permeability. Among magainins are selected antimicrobial peptides exhibiting bactericidal activity against many species, Gram-positive and Gram-negative bacteria, as well as fungi and protozoa (31). One of these compounds, MSI-78, has shown interesting in vitro activity against *Acinetobacter baumannii,* with MICs ranging between 2 and 8 mg/L. Some of these compounds are being evaluated at an early stage, and one (magainin-2) has been shown to act synergistically with standard antibiotics in Gram-negative bacterial infections (9).

CONCLUSION

Acinetobacter infections remain difficult to treat and occur in patients who are generally fragile, aged, and immunodepressed, which makes treatment even more difficult. However clinicians have at their disposal bactericidal combinations of active antibiotics. Each patient must be examined carefully, and each isolate of *Acinetobacter* should be tested with all potentially active drugs and their combinations. To overcome resistance problems, newer drugs, either derivatives of existing antibiotics or totally new compounds with new bacterial targets, are expected to complete the anti-*Acinetobacter* armamentarium.

REFERENCES

1. Bajaksouzian S, Visalli MA, Jacobs MR, Appelbaum PC. Activity of levofloxacin, ofloxacin and ciprofloxacin, alone and combined with amikacin, against *Acinetobacter* species. Antimicrob Agents Chemother 1997;41:1073–1076.
2. Bergogne-Berezin E, Towner J. *Acinetobacter* spp. as nosocomial pathogens: microbiological, clinical and epidemiological features. Clin Microbiol Rev 1996;9:148–165.
3. Bergogne-Berezin E. Resistance of *Acinetobacter* spp. to antimicrobials. Overview of clinical resistance patterns and therapeutic problems. In: Bergogne-Berezin E, Joly-Guillou L, Towner KJ, eds. *Acinetobacter—*microbiology, epidemiology, infection, management. Boca Raton, FL: CRC Press, 1996:133–183.
4. Bergogne-Berezin E, Joly-Guillou ML. An underestimated nosocomial pathogen, *Acinetobacter calcoaceticus.* J Antimicrob Chemother 1985;16:535–538.
5. Bouvet PJM, Grimont PAD. Taxonomy of the genus *Acinetobacter* with the recognition of *Acinetobacter baumannii* sp. nov., *Acinetobacter haemolyticus* sp. nov., *Acinetobacter johnsonii* sp nov., and *Acinetobacter junii* sp. nov. and emended descriptions of *Acinetobacter calcoaceticus* and *Acinetobacter lwoffi.* Int J Syst Bacteriol 1986;36:228–240.
6. Buisson Y, Tran Van Nhieu G, Ginot L, Bouvet P, Fhill H, Driot L, Meyran M. Nosocomial outbreaks due to amikacin-resistant tobramycin sensitive *Acinetobacter* species: correlation with amikacin usage. J Hosp Infect 1990;15:83–93.
7. Cefai C, Richards J, Gould FK, McPeake P. An outbreak of *Acinetobacter* respiratory tract infection resulting from incomplete disinfection of ventilatory equipment. J Hosp Infect 1990;15:117–182.
8. Chastre J, Trouillet JL, Vuagnat A, Joly-Guillou ML. Nosocomial pneumonia caused by *Acinetobacter* spp. In: Bergogne-Berezin E, Joly-Guillou L, Towner KJ, eds. *Acinetobacter—*microbiology, epidemiology, infection, management. Boca Raton, FL: CRC Press, 1996:117–132.
9. Darveau RP, Cunningham MD, Seachord CL, Cassiano-Clough L, Cosand WL, Blake J, Watkins CS. Beta-lactam antibiotics potentiate magainin-2 antimicrobial activity in vitro and in vivo. Antimicrob Agents Chemother 1991;35:1153–1159.
10. Decr D, Benoit C, Joly-Guillou ML, Bergogne-Berezin E, Bryskier A. In vitro activity and bactericidal activity of levofloxacin (LEVX) alone or in combination with amikacin against *Acineto*bacter spp. in comparison with ofloxacin (OFL) and ciprofloxacin (CIP) [Abstract E 100]. 35th ICAAC, San Francisco, 1995.
11. Gradon JD, Chapnick EK, Lutwick LI. Infective endocarditis of a native valve due to Acinetobacter: case report and review. Clin Infect Dis 1992;14:1145–1148.
12. Jimenez-Mejias ME, Pachon J, Becerril B, Palomino-Nicas J, Rodriuez-Coacho A, Revuelta M. Treatment of multidrug resistant *Acinetobacter baumannii* meningitis with ampicillin/sulbactam. Clin Infect Dis 1997;24:932–935.
13. Joly-Guillou ML, Decr D, Wolff M, Bergogne-Berezin E. *Acinetobacter* spp: clinical epidemiology in 89 intensive care units. A retrospective study in France during 1991 [Abstract Cj1]. 2nd International Conference on the Prevention of Infection (CIPI), Nice, 4–5 May 1992.
14. Joly-Guillou ML, Bergogne-Berezin E. In vitro activity of sparfloxacin, pefloxacin, ciprofloxacin and temafloxacin against clinical isolates of *Acinetobacter* spp. J Antimicrob Chemother 1992;29:466–468.
15. Joly-Guillou ML, Brun-Buisson C. Epidemiology of *Acinetobacter* spp.: surveillance and management of outbreaks. In: Bergogne-Berezin E, Joly-Guillou L, Towner KJ, eds. *Acinetobacter—*microbiology, epidemiology, infection, management. Boca Raton, FL: CRC Press, 1996:71–100.
16. Juni E. Genus III. *Acinetobacter.* Brisou and Prévot, 1954. In: Krieg NR, Hold JG, eds. Bergey's manual of systematic bacteriology, vol 1. Baltimore: Williams & Wilkins, 1984:303–307.
17. Levi I, Rubinstein E. *Acinetobacter* infections. Overview of clinical features. In: Bergogne-Berezin E, Joly-Guillou L, Towner KJ, eds. *Acinetobacter—*microbiology, epidemiology, infection, management. Boca Raton, FL: CRC Press, 1996:101–115.
18. Lye WC, Lee EJ, Ang KK. *Acinetobacter* peritonitis in patients on CAPD: characteristics and outcome. Adv Peritoneal Dialysis 1991;7:176–179.
19. Marques MB, Brookings ES, Moser SA, Sonke PB, Waites KB. Comparative in vitro antimicrobial susceptibilities of nosocomial isolates of *Acinetobacter baumannii* and synergistic activities of nine antimcrobial combinations. Antimicrob Agents Chemother 1997;41:881–885.
20. Muller-Serieys C, Lesquoy JB, Perez E, Fichelle A, Bougeois B, Joly-Guillou ML, Bergogne-Berezin E. Infections nosocomiales à *Acinetobacter:* épidémiologie et difficultés thérapeutiques. Presse Med 1989;18:107–110.
21. Neu HC. Synergy and antagonism of combinations with quinolones. Eur J Clin Microbiol Infect Dis 1991;10:255–261.
22. Obana Y, Nishino T, Tanino T. In vitro and in vivo activities of antimicrobial agents against *Acinetobacter calcoaceticus.* J Antimicrob Chemother 1985;15:441–448.

23. Segev S, Rosen N, Joseph G, Alpern-Elran H, Rubinstein E. Pefloxacin efficacy in Gram-negative bacillary meningitis. J Antimicrob Chemother 1990;26(Suppl B):187–4192.
24. Seifert H, Baginski R, Schulze A, Pulverer G. Antimicrobial susceptibility of *Acinetobacter* species. Antimicrob Agents Chemother 1993;37:750–753.
25. Siegman-Igra Y, Bar Yosef S, Gorea A, Avram J. Nosocomial *Acinetobacter* meningitis secondary to invasive procedures: report of 25 cases and review. Clin Infect Dis 1993;17:843–849.
26. Struelens MJ, Carlier E, Maes N, Serruys E, Quint WGV, Van Belkum A. Nosocomial colonization and infection with multi-resistant *Acinetobacter baumanii:* outbreak delineation using DNA macrorestriction analysis and PCR-fingerprinting. J Hosp Infect 1993;25:15–32.
27. Thornsberry C, Marler JK, Brown SD, Yee C, Bouchillon SK, Rich T. Clinical *Acinetobacters:* which species? what susceptibility [Abstract]? 33d ICAAC, New Orleans, 1993.
28. Vila J, Marcos A, Marcos F, Abdalla F, Bergara Y, Reig R, Gomez-Lus R, Jimenez de Anta T. In vitro antimicrobial production of β-lactamases, aminoglycoside-modifying enzymes and chloramphenicol acetyltranferase by and susceptibility of clinical isolates of *Acinetobacter baumannii.* Antimicrob Agents Chemother 1993;37:138–141.
29. Urban C, Go E, Mariano N, et al. Effect of sulbactam in infections caused by imipenem-resistant *Acinetobacter calcoaceticus* biotype *anitratus.* J Infect Dis 1993;67:448–451.
30. Xirouchaki E, Giamarellou H. In vitro interactions with imipenem or ciprofloxacin against aminoglycoside resistant *Acinetobacter baumannii.* J Chemother 1992;4:263–267.
31. Zasloff M. Magainins, a class of antimicrobial peptides from Xenopus skin: isolation, characterization of two active forms and partial CDNA of a precursor. Proc Natl Acad Sci USA 1987;84:5449–5453.

Actinobacillus Species

●

Selwyn D. R. Lang and Arthur J. Morris

GENERAL DESCRIPTION
Microbiology

Actinobacillus actinomycetemcomitans is the only species in this genus that is commonly pathogenic for humans. It is part of the normal oral flora, and infection is endogenously acquired. *Actinobacillus ureae* (formerly *Pasteurella ureae*) and *A. hominis* are also principally associated with humans and have occasionally caused disease (18, 21, 49).

Actinobacillus equuli, A. equuli–like bacterium, *A. lignierensis,* and *A. suis* have their reservoirs in the mouths of animals and are uncommonly causes of infection in humans, including those following bites, e.g., by horses and sheep (3, 8, 36). Little is published on the susceptibility patterns of *Actinobacillus* spp. other than *A. actinomycetemcomitans,* but what there is suggests that the uncommonly encountered species are unlikely to be more resistant. Kingsland and Guss (21) describe *A. ureae* as susceptible to most commonly used antibiotics and Benaoudia et al. (3) note that their isolate of *A. lignierensis* was susceptible to penicillin, amoxicillin/clavulanic acid, cefotaxime, chloramphenicol, tetracycline, rifampicin, cotrimoxazole, and pefloxacin but resistant to clindamycin and aminoglycosides. The rest of this chapter is restricted to *A. actinomycetemcomitans.*

A. actinomycetemcomitans is a fastidious, nonmotile, nonencapsulated, slow-growing, capnophilic, Gram-negative coccobacillus. It is a commensal of the human mouth and can be recovered on culture of oral secretions in up to 20% of healthy people and in the great majority of those with local-ized juvenile periodontitis (15, 24, 32). *A. actinomycetemcomitans* grows slowly at 37°C, aerobically or anaerobically, in standard broth media or on noninhibitory solid media provided there is an atmosphere of approximately 5% carbon dioxide. The need to incubate cultures for 2 to 3 weeks before reporting them as negative has been emphasized (47); however, the mean time for blood cultures to become positive in 13 cases of prosthetic valve endocarditis was 5.5 days (range, 2–9 days) (13). In liquid media, the organism tends to adhere to the walls of the bottle; on agar, colonies generally become visible after 24 hours, reaching approximately 3 mm diameter after several days. Initially smooth, domed, and translucent, they become corrugated, star-shaped, and notably sticky and may pit the agar.

A. actinomycetemcomitans is typically catalase positive and oxidase negative, although occasional strains produce oxidase. It reduces nitrates to nitrites and is urease and indole negative. It ferments glucose and maltose but not lactose or sucrose. King and Tatum (20) identified two biochemical groups: one fermenting mannitol but not xylose and the other xylose but not mannitol. Subsequently, several biotypes and serotypes have been described, and serotyping has been used to demonstrate that an isolate causing endocarditis was likely to have originated from the patient's oral flora (37). These classifications, however, appear to have little relevance to antimicrobial susceptibility.

The distinctive name *A. actinomycetemcomitans* originates from it having been first isolated in association with *Actino-*

myces israelii from patients with cervicofacial actinomycosis (22). It has subsequently been confirmed as present in at least 30% of actinomycotic lesions (19). For many years *A. actinomycetemcomitans* was not considered an independent pathogen; however, in 1951 it was reported as the sole pathogen in a human case of "lumpy jaw" (43). In 1962 King and Tatum reviewed 27 blood isolates (20).

Clinical Manifestations

A well-documented case of native valve endocarditis due to *A. actinomycetemcomitans* was reported by Mitchell in 1964 (27), and Page and King (33) considered that 23 of 25 patients with *A. actinomycetemcomitans* bacteremia had good evidence for the diagnosis of bacterial endocarditis. Prosthetic valve endocarditis due to *A. actinomycetemcomitans* was first described in 1972 (42). Currently, physicians associate *A. actinomycetemcomitans* and other members of the HACEK group *(Haemophilus, Cardiobacterium, Eikenella,* and *Kingella)* primarily with bacterial endocarditis. In a review of 56 cases of endocarditis due to Gram-negative bacteria, infections were caused by *Haemophilus* (18), *Cardiobacterium* (6), *A. actinomycetemcomitans* (4), *Eikenella* (2), and *Kingella* (2) (11). In dentistry, the emphasis is on its apparent involvement in the pathogenesis of localized juvenile periodontitis and acute necrotizing ulcerative gingivitis (2, 25, 28, 34, 35, 38).

Other infections in which *A. actinomycetemcomitans* has been implicated (and usually isolated in pure culture) include brain abscess (39, 52), endophthalmitis (17, 40), lymphadenitis (14), septic arthritis (7, 29), vertebral osteomyelitis (19), tenosynovitis (4), pacemaker infection (45), pericarditis (16, 52), pneumonia (30, 46, 51, 52), empyema, chest wall and subphrenic collections (5, 6), septicemia during pregnancy (41), and urinary tract infection (19).

SUSCEPTIBILITY IN VITRO
Single Agents

A. actinomycetemcomitans is usually susceptible to second- and third-generation cephalosporins, mezlocillin, aminoglycosides, fluoroquinolones, cotrimoxazole, rifampicin, chloramphenicol, tetracyclines, and azithromycin (Table 1). Susceptibility to penicillin, amoxicillin, ampicillin, ticarcillin, and piperacillin is more variable (Table 1). The addition of clavulanic acid to amoxicillin confers no advantage against this organism because it does not produce β-lactamase (33). *A. actinomycetemcomitans* is usually resistant to erythromycin and to clindamycin and is predictably resistant to methicillin and to vancomycin (Table 1).

Two studies have investigated the bactericidal activity of various antibiotics against several strains of *A. actinomycetemcomitans* (10, 28). Eng et al. examined killing kinetics for 20 isolates following a case of endocarditis that developed despite vancomycin and erythromycin prophylaxis. Penicillin (range MIC, 0.02–4 μg/mL), gentamicin (0.1–10 μg/mL), and ciprofloxacin (0.001–0.5 μg/mL) showed the greatest reduction in colony-forming units (−4 logs) after 24 hours incubation in an antibiotic concentration four times the MIC. Cefotaxime (range MIC, 0.2–0.5 μg/mL), cefoxitin (0.2–4 μg/mL), cotri-

moxazole (0.08/5–1.6/100 μg/mL), and erythromycin (0.12–4 μg/mL) showed less bactericidal activity. Only vancomycin (range MIC, 16–120 μg/mL) was associated with a total absence of bactericidal activity. Unfortunately, this paper does not report conventional MBCs (10). Miyake et al. determined both MICs and MBCs of tetracyclines, macrolides, clindamycin, fluoroquinolones, and metronidazole for 11 isolates of *A. actinomycetemcomitans* (28). The MBCs of the fluoroquinolones were the same or little higher than their MICs. In contrast, MBCs of tetracycline, minocycline, erythromycin, and clindamycin were several times their MICs. Metronidazole appeared to have bactericidal activity, but both MICs and MBCs were high (MIC$_{50}$ = MBC$_{50}$ = 64 μg/mL). Horowitz et al. determined both MIC and MBC values of penicillin G, ampicillin, cefazolin, tetracycline, and chloramphenicol for a single clinical isolate of *A. actinomycetemcomitans*. MBC values were four times the MIC in the case of the β-lactam antibiotics, twice the MIC in the case of chloramphenicol, and sixteen times the MIC in the case of tetracycline (16).

Combination Agents

Yogev et al. showed that rifampicin and ceftriaxone shared the lowest MIC$_{90}$ value (1.6 μg/mL) for 24 clinical isolates of *A. actinomycetemcomitans* (50). They therefore tested combinations of rifampicin with various β-lactam antibiotics. No combination was consistently synergistic against the 12 isolates tested. Antagonism was seen as often as synergy when rifampicin was combined with penicillin but was not seen in combination with cephalosporins (cephapirin or ceftriaxone). Indifference or addictive effects were seen with rifampicin plus penicillin against 4 of 12 isolates, with rifampicin plus ceftriaxone against 9 of 12 isolates, and with rifampicin plus cephapirin against all 12 isolates (50). These authors note the absence of previous studies to determine which combinations of antibiotics are synergistic against *A. actinomycetemcomitans* and caution against empirical use of most single agents or any combination to treat *A. actinomycetemcomitans* infection without laboratory backing (50).

Pavicic et al. studied various antimicrobials in combination with either metronidazole or its hydroxymetabolite against five *A. actinomycetemcomitans* strains (35). β-Lactam antibiotics (penicillin G, cefixime, and moxalactam) as well as ciprofloxacin acted synergistically with both metronidazole and its hydroxymetabolite, whereas erythromycin, tetracycline, and tobramycin showed indifferent or only additive effects. They concluded that ciprofloxacin or cefixime might be used in combination with metronidazole to treat periodontitis in patients allergic to penicillins (35).

Surprisingly, very few investigators have reported on the effect of combining an aminoglycoside with a β-lactam against *A. actinomycetemcomitans*. Grace et al. demonstrated synergy between ampicillin and gentamicin by the checkerboard technique for a single isolate with ampicillin MIC, MBC = 4 mg/L and gentamicin MIC, MBC = 4 mg/L, but subsequently treated the patient with ceftriaxone (MIC, MBC < 0.12 mg/L) and gentamicin (13). In their review of the literature they found only two reports of *A. actinomycetem-*

TABLE 1 • In Vitro Susceptibilities of *Actinobacillus actinomycetemcomitans*

Antibiotic	n	Range	MIC$_{50}$	MIC$_{90}$	Breakpoint[a]	% Susceptible	Reference
Amikacin	24	0.8–>25	6.25	25	≤16		50
Streptomycin	37	0.75–12.5	1.5	3			33
Amoxicillin clavulanate	<14	0.06–0.5	0.25	0.5	≤8/4	100	12
Ampicillin	<14	0.06–0.5	0.25	0.5			12
Ampicillin	24	≤0.1–>25	1.6	25			50
Ampicillin	37	0.37–>100	>100	>100			33
Penicillin	37	0.75–>100	>100	>100			33
Penicillin	<14	0.06–0.5	0.25	0.5			12
Penicillin	24	≤0.1–>25	3.1	12.5			50
Piperacillin	24	0.4–>25	12.5	>25	≤16		50
Ticarcillin	24	0.2–>25	6.2	12.5	≤16		50
Cefadroxil	<14	0.25–16	8	16			12
Ceftriaxone	24	≤0.1–3.1	0.2	1.6	≤8	100	50
Cefuroxime	<14	0.6–2	0.25	2	≤8	100	12
Cephalexin	<14	0.5–16	4	8			12
Cephapirin	24	≤0.1–6.2	0.4	3.1			50
Chloramphenicol	24	0.4–6.2	0.8	3.1	≤8	100	50
Chloramphenicol	37	≤0.3–1.5	0.75	1.5	≤8	100	33
Ciprofloxacin	<14	≤0.03–0.06	<0.03	0.06	≤1	100	12
Enoxacin	11	≤0.03–1	0.12	0.5	≤2	100	28
Ofloxacin	<14	≤0.03–0.25	0.06	0.06	≤2	100	12
Ofloxacin	11	≤0.03–0.125	0.06	0.06	≤2	100	28
Sparfloxacin	11	≤0.50–0.125	≤0.50	0.06			28
Tosufloxacin	11	≤0.50	≤0.50	≤0.50			28
Erythromycin	11	1–32	2	16	≤0.5	0	28
Erythromycin	79	0.5–8	4	8	≤0.5	6	34
Azithromycin	79	≤0.25–2	1	2	≤2	100	34
Clindamycin	11	0.25–>64	4	>64	≤0.5		28
Rifampicin	24	≤0.1–3.1	0.8	1.6	≤1		50
Minocycline	11	0.125–4	0.25	2	≤4	100	28
Tetracycline	37	0.37–3.1	3.1	3.1	≤4	100	33
Tetracycline	<14	0.5–4	2	4	≤4	100	12
Tetracycline	11	0.5–8	1	4	≤4		28
Tetracycline	24	0.2–12.5	0.8	3.1	≤4		50
Metronidazole	11	8–>64	64	>64			28

Modified from references 12, 28, 33, 34, and 50.

[a] Current NCCLS interpretive standards for susceptibility (μg/mL) (50).

comitans endocarditis that included synergy studies. One showed an additive effect between ampicillin and gentamicin by time-kill curve, and the other, absence of synergy between ampicillin and streptomycin (13).

ANTIMICROBIAL THERAPY
Bacterial Endocarditis

Despite the paucity of evidence of synergy between penicillin or ampicillin and aminoglycosides against *A. actinomycetemcomitans*, most patients with *A. actinomycetemcomitans* endocarditis, whether native or prosthetic valve disease, have been treated with this combination for 4 to 6 weeks with largely satisfactory outcomes (9, 13, 19, 26). The overall mortality rate was approximately 25% and is not increased with prosthetic valve involvement (13, 26). In the series reported by Grace et al., only 1 of 13 patients with *A. actinomycetemcomitans* prosthetic valve endocarditis died, and only 2 required surgical intervention during treatment (13). Thus recovery of *A. actinomycetemcomitans* in prosthetic valve endocarditis is not itself an indication for valve replacement (13).

The use of combination treatment once the isolate is shown to be *A. actinomycetemcomitans* is more a matter of "usual practice" than scientifically based. Cefamandole has been used successfully as monotherapy for *A. actinomycetemcomitans* prosthetic valve endocarditis (13). Ceftriaxone has excellent activity against most strains of *A. actinomycetemcomitans* (50), and its use is endorsed by an ad hoc writing group of the American Heart Association (48). Yogev et al. found synergy in vitro between rifampicin and both penicillin and ceftriaxone, but not consistently and the combination of rifampicin and penicillin was just as commonly antagonistic (50). The combination of ceftriaxone and rifampicin would seem reasonable but has not been clinically evaluated.

For the patient who is allergic to β-lactam antibiotics, the most suitable agent is likely to be a fluoroquinolone. Prosthetic valve endocarditis due to *A. actinomycetemcomitans* was successfully treated with oral ciprofloxacin 750 mg every 12 hours for 8 weeks. The MIC of ciprofloxacin for the isolate was 0.019 mg/L, and the steady-state serum concentration achieved was 4.1 mg/L (1). The inappropriateness of vancomycin or erythromycin as treatment or prophylaxis for endocarditis due to *A. actinomycetemcomitans* was emphasized by a report of endocarditis developing in a patient with penicillin allergy who was given prophylaxis with both vancomycin and erythromycin. Unfortunately, vancomycin (2 g/day) was also chosen as empirical treatment. There was no clinical response, and the patient died. *A. actinomycetemcomitans* was recovered from blood cultures incubated for more than 14 days, including those taken during vancomycin treatment and just before death (10). Since *A. actinomycetemcomitans* is also resistant to clindamycin, currently recommended prophylactic regimens for penicillin-allergic patients will not be effective against this organism.

Periodontitis

Periodontal disease is not caused by a single pathogen, but *A. actinomycetemcomitans* appears to have an important contributory role (28). Tetracycline has been widely used as treatment but lacks bactericidal activity for most strains of *A. actinomycetemcomitans,* and the clinical response has been variable (34). Sequential administration of amoxicillin/clavulanic acid and doxycycline has been advocated (25). Azithromycin has been shown to be more active in vitro than erythromycin (34), and synergy has been demonstrated with either β-lactams or ciprofloxacin in combination with metronidazole or its metabolite (35). Because of their excellent bactericidal activity against *A. actinomycetemcomitans,* fluoroquinolones are likely to find a role in the treatment of periodontitis, albeit in combination with antibiotics having activity against anaerobes.

Other Infections

A wide variety of more or less serious infections due to *A. actinomycetemcomitans* are reported in the literature, including endophthalmitis (40), cerebral abscess (39), septicemia during pregnancy (41), pulmonary and chest wall infection (5, 30, 46, 51), pericarditis (52, 16), septic arthritis (7, 29), and chronic lymphadenitis (14). *A. actinomycetemcomitans* is also encountered in its traditional role as a companion to *Actinomyces* spp. in actinomycosis (23, 30, 44, 52). A wide variety of treatments have been used, generally successfully. The repeated message is that laboratory susceptibility testing of *A. actinomycetemcomitans* is essential to enable treatment appropriate for a particular isolate and site of infection because susceptibility varies considerably, especially to β-lactam agents.

REFERENCES

1. Babinchak TJ. Oral ciprofloxacin therapy for prosthetic valve endocarditis due to *Actinobacillus actinomycetemcomitans*. Clin Infect Dis 1995;21:1517–1518.
2. Baker PJ, Wilson ME. Effect of clindamycin on neutrophil killing of gram-negative periodontal bacteria. Antimicrob Agents Chemother 1988;32:1521–1527.
3. Benaoudia F, Escande F, Simonet M. Infection due to *Actinobacillus lignieresii* after a horse bite (letter). Eur J Clin Microbiol Infect Dis 1994;13:439–440.
4. Burgess RC. Chronic tensonovitis caused by *Actinobacillus actinomycetemcomitans*. J Hand Surg 1987;12:294.
5. Chao C-L, Chang S-C, Sheu J-C, Luh K-T. Transdiaphragmatic *Actinobacillus actinomycetemcomitans* infection; case report. Clin Infect Dis 1994;19:958–960.
6. Chen A-C, Liu C-C, Yao W-J, Chen C-T, Wang J-Y. *Actinobacillus actinomycetemcomitans* pneumonia with chest wall and subphrenic abscess. Scand J Infect Dis 1995;27:289–290.
7. Cuende E, de Pablos M, Gomez M, Burgaleta S, Michaus L, Vesga JC. Coexistence of pseudogout and arthritis due to *Actinobacillus actinomycemcomitans*. Clin Infect Dis 1996; 23: 657–658.
8. Dibb WL, Dieranes A, Tonjum S. *Actinobacillus lignieresii* infection after a horse bite. Br Med J 1981;283:583–584.
9. Ellner JJ, Rosenthal MS, Lerner PI, McHenry MC. Infective endocarditis caused by slow-growing, fastidious, gram-negative bacteria. Medicine 1979;58:145–158.
10. Eng RHK, Smith SM, Goldstein EJC, Miyasaki KT, Quah S-E, Buccini F. Failure of vancomycin prophylaxis and treatment for *Actinobacillus actinomycetemcomitans* endocarditis. Antimicrob Agents Chemother 1986;29:699–700.
11. Geraci JE, Wilson WR. Endocarditis due to gram-negative bacteria: report of 56 cases. Mayo Clin Proc 1982;57:145–148.
12. Goldstein EJC, Citron DM. Comparative activities of cefuroxime, amoxicillin-clavulanic acid, ciprofloxacin, enoxacin, and ofloxacin against aerobic and anaerobic bacteria isolated from bite wounds. Antimicrob Agents Chemother 1988;32:1143–1148.
13. Grace CJ, Levitz RE, Katz-Pollack H, Brettman LR. *Actinobacillus acetinomycetemcomitans* prosthetic valve endocarditis. Rev Infect Dis 1988;10:922–929.
14. Hammerberg O, Gregson DB, Gopaul D, Lampe H. Recurrent cervical and submandibular lymphadenitis due to *Actinobacillus actinomycetemcomitans*. Clin Infect Dis 1993;17:1077–1078.
15. Holmes B, Pickett MJ, Hollis DG. Unusual Gram-negative bacteria, including *Capnocytopaga, Eikenella, Pasteurella* and *Streptobacillus*. In: Murray PR, Baron EJ, Pfaller MA, Tenover FC, Yolken RH, eds. Manual of clinical microbiology. 6th ed. Washington, DC: American Society for Microbiology, 1995: 499–508.
16. Horowitz EA, Pugsley MP, Turbes PG, Clark RB. Pericarditis caused by *Actinobacillus actinomycetemcomitans*. J Infect Dis 1987;155:152–153.
17. Ishak MA, Zablit KV, Dumas J. Endogenous endophthalmitis caused by *Actinobacillus actinomycetemcomitans*. Can J Ophthalmol 1986;21:284–286.
18. Kaka S, Lunz R, Klugman KP. *Actinobacillus (Pasteurella) ureae* meningitis in a HIV-positive patient. Diagn Microbiol Infect Dis 1994;20:105–107.
19. Kaplan AH, Weber DJ, Oddone EZ, Perfect JR. Infection due to *Actinobacillus actinomycetemcomitans:* 15 cases and review. Rev Infect Dis 1989;11:46–63.
20. King EO, Tatum HW. *Actinobacillus actinomycetemcomitans* and *Haemophilus aphrophilis*. J Infect Dis 1962;111:85–94.
21. Kingsland RC, Guss DA. *Actinobacillus ureae* meningitis: case report and review of the literature. J Emergency Med 1995;13: 623–627.
22. Klinger R. Untersuchungen uber menschliche Aktinmykose. Zentralbl Bakteriol Mikrobiol Hyg 1912;62:191–200.
23. Kuijper EJ, Wiggerts HO, Jonker GJ, Schaal KP, de Gans J. Disseminated actinomycosis due to *Actinomyces meyeri* and *Actinobacillus actinomycetemcomitans*. Scand J Infect Dis 1992;24: 667–672.

24. McGowan IE, Steinberg JP. Other Gram-negative bacilli. In: Mandell GL, Bennett JE, Dolin R, eds. Principles and practice of infectious diseases. 4th ed. New York: Churchill Livingstone, 1995:2106–2118.

25. Matisko MW, Bissada NF. Short-term sequential administration of amoxicillin/clavulanate potassium and doxycycline in the treatment of recurrent/progressive periodontitis. J Periodontol 1993;64:553–558.

26. Meyer DJ, Gerding DN. Favorable prognosis of patients with prosthetic valve endocarditis caused by gram-negative bacilli of the HACEK group. Am J Med 1988;85:104–107.

27. Mitchell RG, Gillespie WA. Bacterial endocarditis due to an *Actinobacillus*. J Clin Pathol 1964;17:511–512.

28. Miyake Y, Tsuruda K, Okuda K, Widowati, Iwamoto Y, Suginaka H. In vitro activity of tetracyclines, macrolides, quinolones, clindamycin and metronidazole against periodontopathic bacteria. J Periodont Res 1995:30:290–293.

29. Molina F, Echániz A, Durán MT, Diz-Lois F. Infectious arthritis of the knee due to *Actinobacillus actinomycetemcomitans* [Letter]. Eur J Clin Microbiol Infect Dis 1994;13:687–689.

30. Morris JF, Sewell DL. Necrotising pneumonia caused by mixed infection with *Actinobacillus actinomycetemcomitans* and *Actinomyces israelii:* case report and review. Clin Infect Dis 1994; 18:450–452.

31. National Committee for Clinical Laboratory Standards. Methods for dilution antimicrobial susceptibility tests for bacteria that grow aerobically—fourth edition; approved standard. NCCLS document M7-A4. Wayne, PA, 1997.

32. Nerad JL, Snydman DR. Miscellaneous Gram-negative bacilli: *Actinetobacter, Cardiobacterium, Actinobacillus, Chromobacterium, Capnocytopaga,* and others. In: Gorbach SL, Bartlett JG, Blacklow NR, eds. Infectious diseases. Philadelphia: WB Saunders, 1992:1543–1555.

33. Page MI, King EO. Infection due to *Actinobacillus actinomycetemcomitans* and *Haemophilus aphrophilus.* N Engl J Med 1966;275:181–188.

34. Pajukanta R, Asikainen S, Saarela M, Alaluusua S, Jousimies-Somer H. In vitro activity of azithromycin compared with that of erythromycin against *Actinobacillus actinomycetemcomitans.* Antimicrob Agents Chemother 1992;36:1241–1243.

35. Pavicic MJAMP, van Winkelhoff AJ, de Graaff J. In vitro susceptibilities of *Actinobacillus actinomycetemcomitans* to a number of antimicrobial combinations. Antimicrob Agents Chemother 1992;36:2634–2638.

36. Peel MM, Hornidge KA, Luppino M, Stacpoole AM, Weaver RE. *Actinobacillus* spp. and related bacteria in infected wounds of humans bitten by horses and sheep. J Clin Microbiol 1991; 29:2535–2538.

37. Pierce CS, Bartholomew WR, Amsterdam D, Neter E, Zambon JJ. Endocarditis due to *Actinobacillus actinomycetemcomitans* serotype c and patient immune response. J Infect Dis 1984;149: 479.

38. Preus HR, Zambon JJ, Duanford RG, Genco RJ. The distribution and transmission of *Actinobacillus actinomycetemcomitans* in families with established adult periodontitis. J Periodontol 1994; 65:2–7.

39. Renton TF, Danks J, Rosenfeld JV. Cerebral abscess complicating dental treatment. Case report and review of the literature. Aust Dent J 1996;41:12–15.

40. Schmidt ME, Smith MA, Levy CS. Endophthalmitis caused by unusual gram-negative bacilli: three case reports and review. Clin Infect Dis 1993;17:686–690.

41. Shalini S, Ganesh P, Anand AR. *Actinobacillus actinomycetemcomitans* septicemia during pregnancy [Letter]. Int J Gynaecol Obstet 1995;51:57–58.

42. Stauffer JL, Goldman MJ. Bacterial endocarditis due to *Actinobacillus actinomycetemcomitans* in a patient with a prosthetic aortic valve. Calif Med 1972;117:59–63.

43. Thjoha TL, Sydnes S. *Actinobacillus actinomycetemcomitans* as the sole infecting agent in human being. Acta Pathol Microbiol Scand 1951;28:27–35.

44. Tyrrell J, Noone P, Prichard JS. Thoracic actinomycosis complicated by *Actinobacillus actinomycetemcomitans:* case report and review of literature. Respir Med 1992;86:341–343.

45. van Winkelhoff AJ, Overbeek BP, Pavicic MJAMP, van den Bergh JPA, Ernst JPMG, de Graaff J. Long-standing bacteremia caused by oral *Actinobacillus actinomycetemcomitans* in a patient with a pacemaker. Clin Infect Dis 1993;16:216–218.

46. Venkataramani A, Santo-Domingo NE, Main DM. *Actinobacillus actinomycetemcomitans* pneumonia with possible septic embolisation [Letter]. Chest 1994;105:645–646.

47. Wilson ME. Prosthetic valve endocarditis and paravalvular abscess caused by *Actinobacillus actinomycetemcomitans* [Letter]. Rev Infect Dis 1989;11:665–667.

48. Wilson WR, Karchmer AW, Dajani AS, Taubert KA, Bayer A, Kaye D, Bisno AL, Ferrieri P, Shulman ST, Durack DT. Antibiotic treatment of adults with infective endocarditis due to streptococci, enterococci, staphylococci, and HACEK microorganisms. JAMA 1995;274:1706–1713.

49. Wüst J, Gubler J, Mannheim W, von Graevenitz A. *Actinobacillus hominis* as a causative agent of septicemia in hepatic failure [Letter]. Eur J Clin Microbiol Infect Dis 1991;10:693–694.

50. Yogev R, Shulman D, Shulman ST, Glogowski WG. In vitro activity of antibiotics alone and in combination against *Actinobacillus actinomycetemcomitans.* Antimicrob Agents Chemother 1986; 29:179–181.

51. Yuan A, Yang P-C, Lee L-N, Chang D-B, Kuo S-H, Luh K-T. *Actinobacillus actinomycetemcomitans* pneumonia with chest wall involvement and rib destruction. Chest 1992;101: 1450–1452.

52. Zijlstra EE, Swart GR, Godfroy FJM, Degener JE. Pericarditis, pneumonia and brain abscess due to a combined *Actinomyces-Actinobacillus actinomycetemcomitans* infection. J Infect 1992; 25:83–87.

Actinomycoses[1]

●

Michael M. McNeil and Klaus P. Schaal

GENERAL DESCRIPTION

Actinomycosis is a subacute to chronic bacterial disease characterized by slowly progressing suppurative fibrosing inflammation, development of draining sinus tracts that may discharge characteristic "sulfur granules," and direct dissemination via contiguous tissues. It most commonly involves the cervicofacial area, thorax, or abdomen, including the pelvis, but rarely also the central nervous system (CNS), skin, or bone (64, 66). The disease is worldwide in distribution and more common in males.

The etiology of human actinomycoses is complex in two respects: the principal etiological agents of the disease do not belong to a single species, but to a variety of different members of the genera *Actinomyces, Propionibacterium,* and *Bifidobacterium.* Furthermore, essentially all of the typical actinomycotic lesions contain between 1 and 10 bacterial species in addition to the pathogenic actinomycetes (27, 28, 35, 62). These concomitant bacteria apparently act as synergis-tic pathogens that strengthen the comparatively low invasive power of the pathogenic actinomycetes and are in particular responsible for the early symptoms of the disease and for treatment failures (52). Since the etiologic term "actinomycosis" therefore circumscribes a polyetiologic inflammatory syndrome rather than a disease attributable to a single pathogen, it appears to be more appropriate to refer to this group of closely related conditions as "actinomycoses" in the plural.

Nearly all of the microbes etiologically involved in the development of human actinomycoses belong to the indigenous microflora of the human mucous membranes, in particular in the oral cavity, but also in the gastrointestinal and female genital tracts. Thus, most members of the actinomycotic flora possess low inherent pathogenicity so that local tissue ischemia resulting from circulatory or vascular diseases, crush injuries, or foreign bodies or from the reducing and necrotizing capacity of simultaneously present additional microbes is necessary for the infection to establish itself in tissues and to invade surrounding healthy areas. In consequence, apart from "punch actinomycoses" following human bites or fistfight injuries, the disease is always endogenous in origin and therefore neither liable to cause outbreaks nor to be transmitted from person to person.

Microbiology

Of the 20 species of the genus *Actinomyces* currently recognized, 11 may cause disease in humans (25, 62). Although the most common agents in human actinomycosis are *A. israelii* and *A. gerencseriae,* at least four other *Actinomyces* species (*A. naeslundii, A. viscosus, A. odontolyticus,* and *A. meyeri*), *Propionibacterium propionicum* (formerly *Arachnia propionica*), and *Bifidobacterium dentium* (formerly *Actinomyces eriksonii*) may also be involved. *Actinomyces bovis* causes granulomatous infections in cattle; however, this species has never been proven to be a human pathogen, and earlier reports of human *A. bovis* infections most probably were due to *A. israelii* (3, 35).

Members of the genera *Actinomyces, Propionibacterium,* and *Bifidobacterium* are morphologically similar, anaerobic to less stringently anaerobic (provided by Fortner's method) (16), nonsporulating, Gram-positive bacteria that tend to form branching rods and filaments and have a fermentative type of carbohydrate metabolism. Filamentous, microscopic colonies of *Actinomyces* species can be detected within 2 to 4 days of anaerobic incubation at 36 ± 1°C. Mature colonies require 7 to 14 days to develop. Characters that differentiate these three genera from each other and from other anaerobically growing nonsporulating Gram-positive bacteria are derived from cell wall or whole-cell analysis, acid end-product analysis, and certain physiologic tests. These last tests are particularly necessary for differentiating between the various *Actinomyces* species (59), but rapid and reliable identification to the species level may also be achieved by using serologic techniques such as direct or indirect immunofluorescence.

Actinomycosis-producing actinomycetes may be distinguished from aerobic, filamentous bacteria such as *Nocardia* species, *Rothia dentocariosa,* or *Corynebacterium (Bacterionema) matruchotii* by the type of carbohydrate metabolism (nocardiae are aerobes), by differences in cell wall composition (nocardiae and *C. matruchotii* contain *meso*-diaminopimelic acid, arabinose, and galactose as well as mycolic acids in their walls), by partial acid-fastness and aerial filaments (nocardiae), and by resistance to penicillin (nocardiae). *R. dentocariosa,* which is often difficult to distinguish from aerobically growing *Actinomyces* species, is characterized by its ability to reduce nitrate as well as nitrite.

Characteristic actinomycotic lesions usually do not develop in the absence of concomitant flora that may consist of aerobic and/or anaerobic species (36, 62). Aerobic cultures chiefly yield coagulase-negative staphylococci, *Staphylococcus aureus,* α-hemolytic and β-hemolytic streptococci as well as *Enterobacteriaceae* from abdominal and pelvic actinomycoses; whereas, anaerobic cultures chiefly yield *Actinobacillus (Haemophilus) actinomycetemcomitans* (25% of cases).

[1]Use of trade names and commercial sources is for identification only and does not imply endorsement by the U.S. Public Health Service or the U.S. Department of Health and Human Services.

Clinical Manifestations

Cervicofacial Actinomycosis

Cervicofacial actinomycosis is the most common form. Characteristic risk factors are poor oral hygiene resulting in periodontal abscesses or dental decay; orofacial trauma; foreign bodies penetrating the mucosal barrier such as bone splinters, fish bones or spicules of grass or grain; and dental procedures. One to several weeks after dental extraction or mouth trauma, or spontaneously, the infection typically causes a painful, indurated cutaneous and soft tissue swelling ("woody" fibrosis) or presents as typical odontogenic abscess. The slowly enlarging inflammatory mass is most frequently located in tissue adjacent to the body of the mandible (53.6%) but may also involve cheek (16.4%), chin (13.3%), ramus and angle of the mandible (10.7%), upper jaw (5.7%), and mandibular joint (0.3%) (24). Over ensuing weeks to months, the overlying skin may develop a bluish discoloration and become adherent, and the mass may become fluctuant and develop draining extra- or intraoral sinuses that may extrude sulfur granules. Trismus may be prominent early in the patient's course; however, cervical lymphadenopathy is uncommon. Direct extension may involve the tongue, sinuses, and meninges and, rarely, contribute to periostitis or osteomyelitis of the mandible (55).

Thoracic Actinomycosis

Actinomycosis of the lung and pleura is usually secondary to aspiration but rarely may occur secondary to hematogenous dissemination. A low-grade pneumonitis develops that tends to invade the pleura, possibly resulting in empyema necessitatis and a draining chest wall fistula(e) (29). Prior to pleural invasion, the patient's symptoms may be minimal and nonspecific (malaise, weakness); however, progression of infection may be associated with fever, productive cough (rarely hemoptysis), and weight loss, which may be severe. Pleuropulmonary actinomycosis may be complicated by direct extension into the mediastinum, pericardium, thoracic vertebrae, or subphrenic spaces, occasionally leading to paravertebral or even psoas abscesses. Pulmonary actinomycosis may disseminate hematogenously, and multiple subcutaneous nodules or neurologic symptoms resulting from a brain abscess may be the presenting manifestation of the disease.

Gastrointestinal Actinomycosis

Actinomycosis of the gastrointestinal tract most commonly develops in the ileocecal region, but it may also primarily involve the esophageal, gastric, or anorectal areas (7). There is often a previous history of appendicitis. Fever, abdominal pain, a palpable mass, and development of an external sinus may be the presenting features. Alternatively, the diagnosis may be considered only after an indurated draining sinus fails to heal following surgical drainage of a presumed appendiceal abscess. Purulent drainage may contain sulfur granules. In some patients, a primary ileocecal infection may cause secondary pelvic actinomycosis.

Pelvic Actinomycosis

Pelvic actinomycosis has been recognized with increasing frequency. Predisposing factors include intrauterine devices (IUDs), contaminated pessaries, prolapse of the uterus, and septic abortion (13). Symptoms may include pelvic pain, leukorrhea, menorrhagia, and amenorrhea, associated with fever, malaise, weakness, and weight loss, in any combination. Actinomycosis should be considered in any woman with a history of IUD use who presents with abdominal pain or a pelvic mass. Recently, Fiorino reviewed 92 cases of actinomycotic abscesses associated with IUD use or intravaginal foreign bodies (15). The patients had a mean age of 37 years (range, 20–77) and had been using an IUD for an average of 8 years. Presenting symptoms included abdominal pain and weight loss, and these patients frequently demonstrated vaginal discharge, fever, anemia, and leukocytosis. Almost 90% of patients were found at surgery to have uni- or bilateral tuboovarian abscesses. Other organs were commonly involved by the inflammatory process directly, or indirectly by adhesions or compression, in particular the large and small bowel, bladder, ureters, and liver.

Actinomycosis of the Central Nervous System

Actinomycoses of the brain and the spinal cord are rare conditions. CNS involvement may follow thoracic or abdominal infections by hematogenous spread or may result from direct dissemination of a cervicofacial lesion. It usually presents as a brain abscess that depending on its localization may lead to a headache, increased intracranial pressure, focal seizures, hemiparesis, aphasia, ataxia, or abnormal reflexes.

Actinomycosis of the Bone and Skin

In contrast to animal actinomycoses, osseous involvement is very uncommon in humans. It usually results from direct extension of an adjacent soft tissue focus leading to periostitis and finally to localized areas of bone destruction surrounded by areas of increased bone density. The mandible, ribs, and spine are the bones most frequently involved.

Cutaneous actinomycotic infections are extremely rare and mostly result from wounds that were contaminated with saliva or dental plaque material, either by human bites or as a consequence of fistfight trauma. Hematogenous spread to the skin has also been observed. The clinical picture of these cutaneous or wound actinomycoses (punch actinomycoses) is very similar to that of the cervicofacial form (58).

Diagnosis

A definitive diagnosis cannot be made solely on clinical grounds. The diagnosis of actinomycosis may be difficult and often depends on a heightened level of clinical suspicion and prior notification of the clinical laboratorian and pathologist. Bronchoscopy and bronchoalveolar lavage fluid examination and culture may be useful in thoracic actinomycosis (8, 33). Detection of the causative agents on Gram stain or by biopsy and culture from an appropriately obtained specimen is needed. Exudates and biopsy material are particularly suitable for examination and should be cultured promptly under anaerobic conditions.

After a sample is obtained, it should be examined by standard histologic methods, anaerobic culture for 2 weeks, and immunofluorescence if available. Culture is the least reliable method of verifying infection (in Fiorino's series only 35% of cultures were positive for fermentative actinomycetes (15)) when standard aerobic and anaerobic culture techniques are used. However, an 86% success rate has been reported for samples cultured in the presence of metronidazole, which inhibits the growth of faster growing anaerobes (70), and as indicated by the overall number of culture-proven cases (35, 53, 60) and the percentage of culture-positive IUD specimens (11, 12), even better results may be obtained when transparent agar media, Fortner's (16) method for producing a semianaerobic atmosphere, and microscopic examination of the cultures for up to 14 days of incubation at $36 \pm 1°C$ are used (60). The last procedure also facilitates detection of actinomycete colonies among a usually large number of various colony types of concomitant microbes.

Because of the polymicrobial nature of the disease, culture and Gram staining of abscess aspirates, sinus discharge, bronchial secretions, or biopsy specimens may have important implications for the choice of adjunctive antibiotics. Microorganisms may be scarce in pathologic specimens, so detection may require diligent searching of multiple tissue sections (43). The presence of sulfur granules is highly suggestive but not diagnostic of disease. These sulfur granules are visible with the unaided eye (diameter up to 1 mm) as yellowish to reddish to brownish particles that consist of spherical segments of filamentous actinomycete microcolonies, various concomitant bacteria, and surrounding tissue reaction material, in particular polymorphonuclear granulocytes. Serodiagnosis of actinomycosis by detection of precipitating or other antibodies has not been a particularly useful diagnostic test (19, 60). Demonstration of pathogenic actinomycetes from smears of lesions by immunofluorescence is a more promising technique.

SUSCEPTIBILITY IN VITRO
Single Drug(s)

In vitro antimicrobial susceptibility testing of fermentative actinomycetes is rarely required, as these results are quite predictable (35, 37, 45, 63). In addition, in vitro activity may not correlate with clinical outcome (e.g., streptomycin; see below). One study examined 74 strains (seven species); minimum inhibitory concentrations (MICs) for penicillin G were 0.03 to 0.5 µg/mL for all strains of *A. israelii* and 0.06 to 0.5 µg/mL for all other actinomycetes, except for one strain of *A. naeslundii* and three of four *A. bovis* strains (MIC, 1.0 µg/mL) (37). Erythromycin was the most active antimicrobial agent in vitro (MIC, 0.12 µg/mL or less). Cephaloridine, minocycline, and clindamycin were also very active in vitro (MIC, 0.003 to 1.0 µg/mL); for a few strains other than *A. israelii*, the MIC for clindamycin ranged from 2.0 to 8.0 µg/mL. The MIC for cephalothin, ampicillin, lincomycin, tetracycline, doxycycline, and chloramphenicol was within the therapeutic range for all strains of *A. israelii* and most other species. Metronida-

zole displayed conspicuously unimpressive in vitro activity, as did the aminoglycosides (36, 45). Lerner found that both *Actinomyces* and *P. propionicum* are highly susceptible to penicillin G, erythromycin, clindamycin, and minocycline and that cephalothin, ampicillin, lincomycin, tetracycline, and chloramphenicol are also active at therapeutic concentrations (36). Peabody and Seabury (48) reviewed in vitro and clinical data up to 1960 for sulfadiazine, streptomycin, erythromycin, chloramphenicol, and the tetracyclines. Cures had been achieved with each alone or in combinations; in vitro data suggest that *Actinomyces* are inhibited by chloramphenicol (0.005 to 0.01 µg/mL), erythromycin (0.005 to 0.1 µg/mL), and several tetracyclines. Even streptomycin, considerably less active in vitro, produced excellent clinical results in some cases. Cures have been reported with isoniazid and even stilbamidine (48). In addition, rifampin therapy for suspected tuberculosis may mask undiagnosed pulmonary actinomycosis (30).

From the short review of the literature given above and numerous additional reports published during the past 40 years, it must be concluded that many details concerning both the in vitro susceptibility of fermentative actinomycetes to antibacterial drugs and the clinical efficacy of these drugs are still controversial. Schaal and Pape (63) demonstrated convincingly that the results of in vitro susceptibility tests of fermentative actinomycetes are highly dependent on the individual test procedures used. For instance, with the agar dilution test, the use of different commercial agar media changed the MICs of *P. propionicum* for ampicillin, tetracycline, and gentamicin by two to three dilutions. Such discrepancies may even be more pronounced when the results of agar dilution and broth dilution techniques are compared. Disk-diffusion methods are in general not suitable for testing fermentative actinomycetes, at least as far as the slow-growing anaerobic strains are concerned (63).

Different results concerning the clinical efficacy of certain antibacterial drugs may be related to differences in the definition of clinical cure, difficulties in diagnosing human actinomycoses unambiguously, and insufficient characterization of the concomitant actinomycotic flora. The last factor is of particular clinical importance (45) because several characteristic companions of the pathogenic fermentative actinomycetes differ greatly in their antibiotic susceptibility patterns from the actinomycetes themselves. This is especially true for certain black-pigmented *Bacteroidaceae*, *Bacteroides* species sensu stricto, and *A. actinomycetemcomitans*, but also for aerobically growing members of the synergistic flora such as *Staphylococcus aureus* or *Enterobacteriaceae*. Thus, at least 5% of black-pigmented *Bacteroidaceae*, 10% of *A. actinomycetemcomitans* strains, and more than 30% of members of the genus *Bacteroides* sensu stricto are highly resistant to benzylpenicillin. Therapeutically sufficient susceptibility is only exhibited by 80% of the black-pigmented *Bacteroidaceae*, 60% of *A. actinomycetemcomitans* strains, and a few percent of the *Bacteroides* species (45). A detailed description of the in vitro susceptibility of the common concomitant bacterial species to antibiotics is beyond the scope of this chapter. However, strict anaerobes are usually susceptible to nitroimidazoles (e.g., metronidazole) or clindamycin and also to aminopenicillins combined with β-lactamase inhibitors, and carbapenems (e.g., imipenem). *A. actinomycetemcomitans,* although often resistant or only moderately susceptible to penicillin G, is nearly always susceptible to aminopenicillins such as ampicillin or amoxicillin. The susceptibility patterns of staphylococci and *Enterobacteriaceae* cannot be predicted and thus individual susceptibility test results are required for optimal treatment. Moreover, all fermentative actinomycetes are resistant to metronidazole, and *A. actinomycetemcomitans* is usually resistant to lincomycins including clindamycin (45). As aminoglycosides (e.g., gentamicin, tobramycin, amikacin) are not active against anaerobes both in vitro and in vivo, these drugs may only be considered when the concomitant flora contains *Enterobacteriaceae* or other Gram-negative aerobically growing rods that are resistant to combinations of aminopenicillins with β-lactamase inhibitors.

Combination Drugs

There are no data on the efficacy of antimicrobial combinations and synergism studies for fermentative actinomycetes.

ANTIMICROBIAL THERAPY
General Drug(s) of Choice

Penicillin in high doses, given over a period of weeks to months, has long been considered the antimicrobial therapy of choice for deep-seated actinomycoses. Prolonged treatment with large doses of the drug is required to achieve drug serum concentrations high enough to ensure drug penetration into areas of fibrosis and suppuration and possibly to penetrate the granules themselves (26). The standard recommendations for penicillin therapy are to administer intravenous penicillin G, (150,000–200,000 U/kg/day or 10–20 million U/day in divided doses for adults) for 4 to 6 weeks (or for at least 3–4 weeks after the patient appears cured), followed by oral penicillin (e.g., phenoxymethylpenicillin, 2–4 g/day, to patient tolerance) for 6 to 12 additional months or even longer to prevent relapse. Complications in a given patient—such as dissemination, critical locations (e.g., CNS involvement), or inability to perform definitive surgery—may alter or extend this regimen (73). Clinical resistance to this type of penicillin G treatment may not be a major problem; however, clinical failures have been reported and apparently considerably more therapeutic problems were not published in the literature following penicillin G therapy alone (17, 58). In addition, there have been observations that appear to support the development of acquired resistance to penicillin (5). Garrod claimed that unsuccessful penicillin treatment might be accompanied by increased in vitro resistance; the MICs for two strains of *A. israelii* increased from 0.03 U/mL to 0.2 U/mL and more than 0.5 U/mL, respectively (18). Boand and Novak (5) found that strains of *A. bovis* (probably *A. israelii*) did not adapt readily to penicillin with serial passage in subinhibitory concentrations of the drug, although four of six strains developed two- to fourfold resistance. In vivo development of acquired antimicrobial resistance by *Actinomyces* species, particularly to penicillin G, has not been reported subsequently. When the response to penicillin is poor, a search should be made for an undrained abscess, although it is more likely that unsatisfactory therapeutic results are due to the presence of resistant concomitant bacterial species.

The therapeutic concept outlined above is primarily based on the view that the antimicrobial chemotherapy must be directed principally or even solely against the pathogenic fermentative actinomycetes. Considering the impressive amount of bacteriologic data indicating that human actinomycoses are essentially always synergistic mixed infections, modification of this concept is at least worthy of discussion. Pulverer and Schaal (52) as well as several other authors have reported on characteristic clinical treatment failures of penicillin G therapy. These findings could be related to the presence either of *A. actinomycetemcomitans* or of β-lactamase-producing *Bacteroides* species, *Staphylococcus aureus,* or *Enterobacteriaceae.* Since *Bacteroides* species or *Enterobacteriaceae* are commonly found as concomitant organisms in abdominal and pelvic actinomycoses, the latter usually do not respond well to penicillin G treatment. In contrast, β-lactamase producers as well as penicillin G–resistant strains of *A. actinomycetemcomitans* are uncommon in the cervicofacial form of the disease, so that many of these patients may be effectively treated with high doses of benzylpenicillin.

Compared with narrow-spectrum penicillins, the aminopenicillins are similarly active against the pathogenic fermentative actinomycetes, but clearly much more effective against *A. actinomycetemcomitans* both in vitro and in vivo. Thus, therapy with comparatively high doses of aminopenicillins such as ampicillin or amoxicillin (4–8 g/day for adults) effectively helps to avoid the characteristic treatment failures or relapses of cervicofacial infections caused by *A. actinomycetemcomitans.* However, aminopenicillins are also susceptible to β-lactamases, so the presence of bacterial β-lactamase producers may impair their therapeutic efficacy. Therefore, general treatment schemes for human actinomycoses should include drugs that are effective not only against the causative actinomycetes and *A. actinomycetemcomitans* but also against potential producers of β-lactamases such as *Staphylococcus aureus,* various Gram-negative anaerobes of the family *Bacteroidaceae,* and in the case of abdominal and pelvic actinomycoses, certain *Enterobacteriaceae.*

On the basis of the above considerations, the current recommendations for antibiotic treatment of human actinomycoses in Germany, according to which several hundred cases were treated essentially without any therapeutic failure or relapse, are as follows (58). For cervicofacial actinomycoses, a combination of amoxicillin and clavulanic acid is the treatment of choice. The standard dose is 2.2 g amoxicillin plus clavulanic acid every 8 h for 1 week and then a lower dose of 1.1 g of the same combination every 8 h for another week. Only rarely will delayed clinical improvement of long-term chronic cervicofacial infections indicate that antibiotic treatment of 3 or even 4 weeks duration is required. Parenteral administration of the drugs is recommended; prolonged oral treatment was never found to be necessary (58). For thoracic actinomycoses, the same therapeutic scheme may be sufficient. Although no reduction in the initial dose is needed, antimicrobial therapy is usually continued for 3 to 4 weeks. In addition, patients with either advanced chronic pulmonary or abdominal disease may require the addition of 2 g ampicillin every 8 h to increase the aminopenicillin tissue levels (ampicillin is used in addition to amoxicillin to avoid possible side effects associated with high doses of amoxicillin). Treatment of abdominal and pelvic actinomycoses occasionally demands the combination of amoxicillin/clavulanic acid with an aminoglycoside such as tobramycin or gentamicin to inhibit resistant concomitant *Enterobacteriaceae*.

Special Situations

Endocarditis

Cardiac infection caused by *Actinomyces* species is rare, occurring in less than 2% of reported cases (32). This usually follows local extension of adjacent intrathoracic infective foci (most commonly pulmonary lesions); thus, endocardial involvement is usually secondary to involvement of the myocardium and pericardium. In their recent review of eight cases (seven from the literature) of primary actinomycotic endocarditis, Lam et al. (32) found that the disease affects all ages and occurs predominantly in males. No specific clinical feature distinguishes primary actinomycotic endocarditis from bacterial endocarditis caused by other organisms. In 63% of cases, blood cultures were positive, but detailed information on the species of actinomycetes and possible concomitant organisms etiologically involved is not available.

The recommended initial therapy is high doses of parenteral penicillin (38). Five patients reviewed by Lam et al. received penicillin in daily doses ranging from 60,000 to 20 million units; duration of treatment ranged from 4 weeks to 10 months (32). In addition, these investigators opted to treat their patients with a 6-week course of intravenous penicillin (18 million units daily) followed by 6 months of oral medication. Both the optimal duration of therapy and the optimal choice of drug in these patients are unknown; Gutschik (20) suggested at least a 4-week course of parenteral penicillin followed by a 4- to 6-week course of oral penicillin. But, despite the use of several alternative agents to penicillin for other forms of actinomycosis, their effectiveness for treatment of endocarditis has not been shown (3). In Lam's series, surgical intervention in actinomycotic endocarditis occurred in 50% of patients (32). With penicillin therapy, the survival rate was 80% (four of five patients). Four patients died because the diagnosis was missed or because ineffective antibiotics were administered. However, the prognosis overall was considered to be good with early diagnosis and appropriate antibiotic therapy.

CNS Involvement

CNS involvement by actinomycosis has been recently reviewed in detail (67). Types of CNS lesions include, in order of frequency, brain abscess, meningitis or meningoencephalitis, subdural empyema, and epidural abscess. For nonmeningitic lesions, the clinical presentation is commonly that of a "space-occupying lesion." Optimal management in these patients comprises adequate surgical drainage and prolonged (4–6 months) antimicrobial therapy (67). In Smego's review of 70 reported cases of CNS actinomycosis (67), several classes of antimicro-

bial agents were used for therapy. In most cases (62%), penicillin G was included in the antibiotic regimen. Other agents included sulfonamides, chloramphenicol, erythromycin, tetracycline, minocycline, streptomycin, ampicillin, gentamicin, metronidazole, isoniazid, potassium iodide, and bacitracin and polymyxin (the last two agents both administered introperatively into the abscess cavity or operative site, as well as intrathecally). The median duration of antimicrobial therapy was 2.3 months (range, 2 weeks to 22 months); however, the mean duration for survivors was 4.9 months. Surgical procedures were performed in conjunction with antimicrobial therapy in most of these patients, with the exception of those with meningitis. These procedures included total excision of lesions, open surgical drainage, and closed needle aspiration of lesions. Among these patients, the overall rate of clinical improvement or cure was 72%; however, neurologic sequelae (seizures, motor or sensory deficits, aphasia, deafness, cerebellar ataxia, and visual field defects) were seen in 54% of treated survivors (67). Importantly, relapse occurred in only one patient (23). Initially this patient responded to needle aspiration drainage and combination penicillin G, chloramphenicol, sulfadiazine, and tetracycline (given for an unknown duration) but relapsed after 29 months, with evidence of multiple brain abscesses at surgery. Nevertheless, with surgical excision of these lesions and penicillin G (again for an unreported duration), the patient made a complete recovery. The severity of these infections is apparent from Smego's findings. Despite therapy, the overall mortality from these infections was 28%, and 54% of survivors had neurologic sequelae. A poor prognosis was correlated with disease onset more than 2 months before diagnosis and treatment, no antimicrobial therapy, no surgery, and needle aspiration drainage of abscess lesions (67).

Acquired Immunodeficiency Syndrome (AIDS)

Manfredi et al. (39) describe two patients with progressive oropharyngeal actinomycosis despite apparent appropriate antimicrobial and operative management and briefly review other AIDS-associated cases. Cervicofacial actinomycosis (72, 76) and esophageal, endobronchial, and pulmonary infection have been reported (6, 31, 68). Secondary infection of cytomegalovirus (CMV) esophagitis in two AIDS patients has also been reported (51). However, actinomycosis is not considered an AIDS-defining opportunistic infection.

Alternative Therapy

First-line antimicrobial agents for use as alternative oral or parenteral therapy in patients with actinomycosis include tetracyclines, erythromycin, clindamycin, and imipenem (48, 58). Tetracyclines may be used in the nonpregnant penicillin-allergic patient and have been reported to be possibly as effective as penicillin in the cervicofacial form of the disease (40). Doxycycline in combination with penicillin has been used successfully in the therapy for muscular actinomycosis in an alcoholic patient and in women with salpingitis (9, 50). Erythromycin also appears to be an acceptable alternative to penicillins (37). Clindamycin orally for a 16-day course has been used in combination with surgical incision and drainage of infected foci in patients with acute mandibular actinomycosis (2, 46) and in a penicillin-allergic patient with osteomyelitis of the thoracic spine (4). However, clindamycin resistance is common in *A. actinomycetemcomitans* (45), so treatment failures may occur when this organism is present in the concomitant flora. In addition, Morris and Sewell (42) reported a patient with mixed anaerobic necrotizing pneumonia that did not respond clinically to clindamycin. The patient subsequently developed disseminated infection, and clindamycin-resistant *A. actinomycetemcomitans* and *A. israelii* were isolated; the patient was subsequently successfully treated with a regimen consisting of penicillin, ciprofloxacin, and cefazolin. Imipenem may be the most appropriate alternative for penicillins given its high in vitro and in vivo efficacies against both the fermentative actinomycetes and many of the common concomitant species. However, to date, this drug has only rarely been used to treat actinomycotic infections, although it has been used effectively in a diabetic patient with relapsing abdominothoracic actinomycosis unresponsive to a combination of surgery and 4- to 6-week courses of intravenous penicillin G (10) and in a patient with thoracic actinomycosis (77). Additional alternative drugs that supposedly led to complete cure in selected actinomycosis patients include ciprofloxacin (a prolonged course of this therapy in a patient with a 20-year history of actinomycosis with extensive abdominal and pelvic disease unresponsive to penicillin therapy resulted in an unexpected clinical response (41)) and ceftriaxone (administered intravenously once daily on an outpatient basis to a woman with pleural disease and chest wall muscle infection (65)). Oral cephalexin and the semisynthetic penicillins oxacillin and dicloxacillin are considerably less active against fermentative actinomycetes in vitro and probably best avoided (36). There is one report of chloramphenicol therapy for actinomycosis (69).

Combination Therapy

Since concomitant bacteria resistant to penicillin or other β-lactam first-line drugs are quite common, the combination of ampicillin and metronidazole or clindamycin has been suggested (14, 63). However, metronidazole alone is not suitable for treating actinomycotic infections because fermentative actinomycetes are generally resistant to this drug (36, 45). In particular, abdominal or thoracic infections that may more frequently contain β-lactamase-producing *Bacteroides* species and/or *Enterobacteriaceae* may benefit from addition of metronidazole or clindamycin and an aminoglycoside as a fourth drug (58, 61).

ENDPOINTS FOR MONITORING THERAPY
Laboratory

Antimicrobial susceptibility testing (minimal inhibitory concentration, minimum bactericidal concentration) and monitoring pre- and postdose serum drug (penicillin, amoxicillin) levels are probably not indicated in the routine management of this infection since the fermentative actinomycetes are almost uniformly susceptible to penicillins. However, clinical nonresponse by a patient to penicillin therapy despite in vitro susceptibility usually indicates coinfection with other resistant microbes.

Imaging Studies

The use of modern radiographic and imaging studies has doubtlessly contributed significantly to improved early recognition and the overall survival of patients with all forms of actinomycosis during the last decade. In addition to providing an earlier diagnosis of actinomycotic infections, repeated imaging studies may be very useful for monitoring a patient's response to antimicrobial therapy, so that the need for possible surgical intervention can be reevaluated.

Chest Radiography

In patients with thoracic actinomycosis, the chest radiograph appearance may be extremely variable. A triad of chronic consolidation, pleural effusion, and rib periostitis may be present (74). Development of a pleural effusion without evidence of parenchymal disease in a patient with underlying chronic pulmonary disease may be a significant finding and suggests a need for diagnostic pleural fluid analysis (22). Alternatively, parenchymal lesions mimicking a tumor may be present or cavitary disease resembling tuberculosis may occur. Evidence of adjacent rib erosions may be another useful radiographic sign suggesting formation of an empyema (54).

Other Imaging Studies

A computed tomographic (CT) scan may be an extremely useful diagnostic test. Intracerebral actinomycotic lesions may show a characteristic ring-shaped contrast enhancement with a low-density center and low-density perifocal edema. The usefulness of abdominal CT examinations has recently been reviewed by Ha (10 patients with abdominal CT) (21). Radionuclide scanning (i.e., radionuclide angiography in two cases of hepatic actinomycosis, and bone and gallium scintigraphy in a patient with polyostotic actinomycosis of the upper limb) has been reported (1, 71). In addition, magnetic resonance imaging has been reported to be useful in pelvic actinomycosis in association with IUD use (47, 49), cervicofacial actinomycosis (56), primary CNS actinomycosis (57), and actinomycosis with multiple liver abscesses (44).

CONTROVERSIES, CAVEATS, OR COMMENTS
Empirical Antimicrobial Therapy

Empirical antimicrobial therapy may mask the clinical manifestations of actinomycosis, since actinomycetes are extremely susceptible to penicillin and other broad-spectrum antibiotics, and is not recommended.

Surgery

Early effective antimicrobial therapy may obviate the need for surgery or facilitate a more conservative surgical approach. The indications for surgery for patients with actinomycosis must be individualized on the basis of the nature and extent of disease, the presence of complications, and the patient's clinical response to specific antimicrobial therapy. In addition to antibiotic therapy, optimal management of actinomycosis likely may include surgical drainage of empyema and large abscesses and excision of sinus tracts and recalcitrant fibrotic lesions (75). Recently, Fiorino reported that a preoperative diagnosis was made in only 17% of patients with pelvic actinomycosis and emphasized the need for heightened clinical suspicion and aggressive diagnostic evaluation (smear, culture, and biopsy) of these patients (15). Although some infected patients require extensive surgery, the conservative management approach may avoid hysterectomy or salpingooophorectomy (i.e., sterilizing procedures) for women of childbearing age.

Detection of Actinomyces on Cervical Smear

Among users of IUDs, the incidence of Papanicolaou smears positive for actinomycetes has ranged from 0 to 31% (mean, 7%) (15). Possible explanations for such variability include differing levels of stringency applied to the evaluation of these smears and misinterpretation of smear findings. Given this variability in *Actinomyces* detection on Papanicolaou smear, other methods have been suggested to yield more consistent results, including endometrial biopsy specimens, cultures of material adherent to IUDs, and the use of immunofluorescence to evaluate cervical smears. Cultures of material adherent to an IUD and of cervical secretions collected immediately after removal of an IUD revealed fermentative actinomycetes in 8% (12) to nearly 15% (64) of the specimens examined. The following species were identified: *A. israelii*, 41.2%; *A. gerencseriae*, 17.3%; *A. naeslundii*, 4.9%; *A. odontolyticus*, 2.5%; *A. viscosus*, 18.5%; *A. meyeri*, 3.7%; *P. propionicum*, 1.2%; *B. dentium*, 1.2%; and *R. dentocariosa*, 1.2% (total number of isolates: 81) (62). Studies using current methods of actinomycetes detection have shown an increased risk of infection with increased duration of IUD use (15). Currently, the relationship between a Papanicolaou smear positive for actinomycetes and eventual development of pelvic actinomycosis is unclear, and there appears to be no indication for antibiotic treatment in the asymptomatic patient with an incidental finding of actinomycetes on routine cervical smear (12, 15). As summarized by Fiorino (15), a consensus recommendation has been to remove the IUD and repeat the smear in 6 weeks to verify clearance of the organism, in which case the IUD may be reinserted. However, there is no valid evidence that such an approach prevents development of pelvic actinomycosis.

REFERENCES

1. Adams BK, Crosner JH. Bone and gallium scintigraphy in polyostotic actinomycosis of the upper limb. Clin Nucl Med 1994;19:254–256.
2. Badgett JT, Adams G. Mandibular actinomycosis treated with oral clindamycin. Pediatr Infect Dis J 1987;6:221–223.
3. Benhoff DF. Actinomycosis: diagnosis and therapeutic considerations and a review of 32 cases. Laryngoscope 1984;94:1198–1217.
4. Birley HD, Teare EL, Utting JA. Actinomycotic osteomyelitis of the thoracic spine in a penicillin-sensitive patient [Letter]. J Infect 1989;19:193–194.
5. Boand A, Novak M. Sensitivity changes of *Actinomyces bovis* to penicillin and streptomycin. J Bacteriol 1949;57:501–508.
6. Cendan I, Klapholz A, Talavera W. Pulmonary actinomycosis. A cause of endobronchial disease in a patient with AIDS. Chest 1993;103:1886–1887.
7. Cintron JR, Del Pino A, Duarte B, Wood D. Abdominal actinomycosis. Dis Colon Rectum 1996;39:105–108.
8. Coodley EL, Yoshinaka R. Pleural effusion as the major manifestation of actinomycosis. Chest 1994;106:1615–1617.
9. Coppens L, Ibebeke B, Widelec J, Lustman F. Muscular actinomycosis in the back. Acta Clin Belg 1996;51:94–96.
10. Edelmann M, Cullman W, Novak KH, Kozuschek W. Treatment of abdominothoracic actinomycosis with imipenem. Eur J Clin Microbiol 1987;6:194–195.
11. Eibach HW, Bolte A, Pulverer G, Schaal KP, Küpper G. Klinische Relevanz und pathognomische Bedeutung der Aktinomyzetenbesiedlung von Intrauterinpessaren. Geburtshilfe Frauenheilkd 1989;49:972–976.
12. Eibach HW, Neuhaus W, Günther W, Bolte A, Pulverer G, Schaal KP. Clinical relevance and pathognomonic significance of actinomycotic colonization of intrauterine pessaries. Int J Feto-Mat Med 1992;5:40–42.
13. Evans DT. *Actinomyces israelii* in the female genital tract: a review. Genitourin Med 1993;69:54–59.
14. Ewig S, Schaal KP, Steudel A, Nikorowitsch R, von Kampis J, Staib P, Vaupel HA. 42 jähriger Patient mit Fieber und einem palpablen abdominellen Tumor. Internist 1993;34:59–62.
15. Fiorino AS. Intrauterine contraceptive device-associated actinomycotic abscess and actinomycetes detection on cervical smear. Obstet Gynecol 1996;87:142–149.
16. Fortner J. Ein einfaches Plattenverfahren zur Züchtung strenger Anaerobier. Zentralbl Bakteriol Parasitenk Hyg Abt I Orig 1928;108:155–159.
17. Garland SM, Rawling D. Pelvic actinomycosis in association with an intrauterine device. Aust NZ J Obstet Gynecol 1993;33:96–98.
18. Garrod LP. The sensitivity of *Actinomyces israelii* to antibiotics. Br Med J 1952;1:1263–1264.
19. Georg LK, Coleman RM, Brown JM. Evaluation of an agar gel precipitin test for the serodiagnosis of actinomycosis. J Immunol 1968;100:1288–1292.
20. Gutschik E. Endocarditis caused by *Actinomyces viscosus*. Scand J Infect Dis 1976;8:271–274.
21. Ha HK, Lee HJ, Kim H, Ro HJ, Park YH, Cha SJ, Shinn KS. Abdominal actinomycosis: CT findings in 10 patients. AJR 1993;161:791–794.
22. Heffner JE. Pleuropulmonary manifestations of actinomycosis and nocardiosis. Semin Respir Infect 1988;3:352–361.
23. Heineman HS, Braude AI. Anaerobic infection of the brain: observations of eighteen cases of brain abscess. Am J Med 1963;35:682–697.
24. Herzog S. Retrospektive Untersuchungen zur Klinik, Therapie und Bakteriologie der zervikofazialen Aktinomykosen an der Zahn- und Kieferklinik der Universität zu Köln von 1952–1975—Auswertung der Aufzeichnungen von 317 Patienten. Thesis, Köln 1981.
25. Hillier S, Moncla BJ. Anaerobic gram-positive nonsporeforming bacilli and cocci. In: Balows A, Hausler WJ Jr, Herrmann, KL, Isenberg HD, Shadomy HJ, eds. Manual of clinical microbiology. 5th ed. Washington, DC: American Society for Microbiology, 1991:522–537.
26. Holm P. Some investigations into the penicillin sensitivity of human-pathogenic actinomycetes and some comments on penicillin treatment of actinomycosis. Acta Pathol Microbiol Scand 1948;25:376–404.
27. Holm P. Studies on the aetiology of human actinomycosis. I. The "other microbes" of actinomycosis and their importance. Acta Pathol Microbiol Scand 1950;27:736–751.
28. Holm P. Studies on the aetiology of human actinomycosis. II. Do

the "other microbes" of actinomycosis possess virulence? Act Pathol Microbiol Scand 1951;28:391–406.

29. Hooker TP, Hammond M, Corral K. Empyema necessitatis: review of the manifestations of thoracic actinomycosis. Cleve Clin J Med 1992;59:542–548.

30. King JW, White MC. Pulmonary actinomycosis: rapid improvement with isoniazid and rifampin. Arch Intern Med 1981;141:1234–1235.

31. Klaphotz A, Talavera W, Rorat E, Salsitz E, Widrow C. Pulmonary actinomycosis in a patient with HIV infection. Mt Sinai J Med 1989;56:300–303.

32. Lam S, Samraj J, Rahman S, Hilton E. Primary actinomycotic endocarditis: case report and review. Clin Infect Dis 1993;16:481–485.

33. Lenoir P, Gilbert L, Goossens A, Tempels D, Alexander M, Dab I. Bronchoscopic diagnosis of an unusual presentation of pulmonary actinomycosis. Pediatr Pulmonol 1993;16:138–140.

34. Lentze F. Zur antibiotischen Therapie der Aktinomykose. Fortschr Kiefer Gesichtschir 1957;3:306–313.

35. Lentze F. Die Aktinomykose und die Nocardiosen. In: Grumbach A, Bonin O, eds. Die Infektionskrankheiten der Menschen und ihre Erreger, vol I. 2nd ed. Stuttgart: Georg Thieme, 1969:83–92.

36. Lerner PI. Susceptibility of pathogenic actinomycetes to antimicrobial compounds. Antimicrob Agents Chemother 1974;5:302–309.

37. Lerner PI. The lumpy jaw. Cervicofacial actinomycosis. Infect Dis Clin North Am 1988;2:203–220.

38. MacNeal WJ, Blevins A, Duryee AW. Clinical arrest of endocardial actinomycosis after forty-four million units of penicillin. Am Heart J 1946;31:668–676.

39. Manfredi R, Mazzoni A, Marinacci G, Nanetti A, Chiodo F. Progressive intractable actinomycosis in patients with AIDS. Scand J Infect Dis 1995;27:405–407.

40. Martin MV. Antibiotic treatment of cervicofacial actinomycosis for patients allergic to penicillin: a clinical and in vitro study. Br J Oral Maxillofac Surg 1985;23:428–434.

41. McFarlane DJ, Tucker LG, Kemp RJ. Treatment of recalcitrant actinomycosis with ciprofloxacin. J Infect 1993;27:177–180.

42. Morris JF, Sewell DL. Necrotizing pneumonia caused by a mixed infection with *Actinobacillus actinomycetemcomitans* and *Actinomyces israelii:* case report and review. Clin Infect Dis 1994;18:450–452.

43. Muller-Holzner E, Ruth NR, Abfalter E, Schrocksnadel H, Dapunt O, Martin-Sances L, Nogales FF. IUD-associated pelvic actinomycosis: a report of five cases. Int J Gynecol Pathol 1995;14:70–74.

44. Nazarian LN, Spencer JA, Mitchell DG. Multiple actinomycotic liver abscesses: MRI appearances with etiology suggested by abdominal radiography. Case report. Clin Imaging 1994;18:119–122.

45. Niederau W, Pape W, Schaal KP, Höffler U, Pulverer G. Zur Antibiotikabehandlung der menschlichen Aktinomykosen. Dtsch Med Wochenschr 1982;107:1279–1283.

46. Nielsen PM, Novak A. Acute cervico-facial actinomycosis. Int J Oral Maxillofac Surg 1987;16:440–444.

47. O'Connor KF, Bagg MN, Criley MR, Schabel SI. Pelvic actinomycosis associated with intrauterine devices. Radiology 1989;170:559–560.

48. Peabody JW Jr, Seabury JH. Actinomycosis and nocardiosis; a review of basic differences in therapy. Am J Med 1960;28:99–115.

49. Perkow JH, Wigton T, Yardon EL, Graham J, Wool N, Wilbanks GD. Disseminated pelvic actinomycosis presenting as metastatic carcinoma; association with the Progestasert intrauterine device. Rev Infect Dis 1991;13:1115–1119.

50. Persson E, Brihmer C. *Actinomyces israelii*-associated salpingitis. Eur J Obstet Gynecol Reprod Biol 1986;21:173–175.

51. Poles MA, McMeeking AA, Scholes JV, Dieterich DT. *Actinomyces* infection of a cytomegalovirus esophageal ulcer in two patients with acquired immunodeficiency syndrome. Am J Gastroenterol 1994;89:1569–1572.

52. Pulverer G, Schaal KP. Medical and microbiological problems in human actinomycoses. In: Ortiz-Ortiz L, Bojalil LF, Yakoleff V, eds. Biological, biochemical, and biomedical aspects of actinomycetes. Orlando, FL: Academic Press, 1984:161–170.

53. Pulverer G, Schaal KP. Human actinomycoses. Drugs Exp Clin Res 1984;X(3):187–196.

54. Ray MS, Feldman S. Mixed *Fusobacterium* and *Actinomyces* pulmonary infection. Case report. Clin Pediatr 1989;28:426–428.

55. Roth M, Montone KT. Actinomycosis of the paranasal sinuses: a case report and review. Head Neck Surg 1996;114:818–821.

56. Sa'do B, Yoshiura K, Yuasa K, Ariji Y, Kanda S, Oka M, Katsuki T. Multimodality imaging of cervicofacial actinomycosis. Oral Surg Oral Med Oral Pathol 1993;76:772–782.

57. Salvati M, Ciappetta P, Raco A, Antico M, Artizzi S. Primary intracranial actinomycosis: report of a case and review of the literature. Zentralbl Neurochir 1991;52:95–98.

58. Schaal KP. Actinomycoses. In: Weatherall DJ, Ledingham JGG, Warrell DA, eds. Oxford textbook of medicine, vol 1. 3rd ed. Oxford: Oxford University Press, 1996:680–686.

59. Schaal KP. Laboratory diagnosis of actinomycete diseases. In: Goodfellow M, Mordarski M, Williams ST, eds. The biology of the actinomycetes. London: Academic Press, 1984:425–456.

60. Schaal KP. The genera *Actinomyces, Arcanobacterium,* and *Rothia.* In: Balows A, Trüper HG, Dworkin M, Harder W, Schleifer KH, eds. The prokaryotes. A handbook on the biology of bacteria: ecophysiology, isolation, identification, applications. 2nd ed. New York: Springer, 1992:850–905.

61. Schaal KP, Beaman BL. Clinical significance of actinomycetes. In: Goodfellow M, Mordarski M, Williams ST, eds. The biology of the actinomycetes. London: Academic Press, 1983:389–424.

62. Schaal KP, Lee HJ. Actinomycete infections in humans—a review. Gene 1992;115:201–211.

63. Schaal KP, Pape W. Special methodological problems in antibiotic susceptibility testing of fermentative actinomycetes. Infection 1980;8(Suppl 2):176–182.

64. Schaal KP, Pulverer G. Epidemiologic, etiologic, diagnostic, and therapeutic aspects of endogenous actinomycetes infections. In: Ortiz-Ortiz L, Bojalil LF, Yakoleff V, eds. Biological, biochemical, and biomedical aspects of actinomycetes. New York: Academic Press, 1984:13–32.

65. Skoutelis A, Petrochilos J, Bassaris H. Successful treatment of thoracic actinomycosis with ceftriaxone. Clin Infect Dis 1994;19:161–162.

66. Slack JM, Gerencser MA. *Actinomyces*, filamentous bacteria. Minneapolis: Burgess Publishing, 1975.

67. Smego RA Jr. Actinomycosis of the central nervous system. Rev Infect Dis 1987;9:855–865.

68. Spencer GM, Roach D, Skucas J. Actinomycosis of the esophagus in a patient with AIDS: findings on barium esophagograms. AJR 1993;161:795–796.

69. Stokes JF, Gray IR, Stokes EJ. *Actinomyces muris* endocarditis treated with chloramphenicol. Br Heart J 1951;13:247–251.

70. Traynor RM, Parrat D, Duguid HLD, Duncan ID. Isolation of actinomycetes from cervical specimens. J Clin Pathol 1981;34: 914–916.
71. Ueno K, Kabuti H, Haseda Y, Yamuda T, Nakagawa M. Radionuclide angiography in two cases of hepatic actinomycosis. Clin Nucl Med 1986;11:44–48.
72. Watkins KV, Richmond AS, Langstein IM. Nonhealing extraction site due to *Actinomyces naeslundii* in patient with AIDS. Oral Surg Oral Med Oral Pathol 1991;71:675–677.
73. Weese WC, Smith IM. A study of 57 cases of actinomycosis over a 36-year period. Arch Intern Med 1975;135:1562–1568.
74. Wilson DC. Remond AO. An unusual cause of thoracic mass. Arch Dis Child 1990;65:991–992.
75. Wolgemuth SD, Gaddy MC. Surgical implications of actinomycosis. South Med J 1986;79:1574–1578.
76. Yeager BA, Hoxie J, Weismann RA, Greenberg MS, Bilaniuk LT. Actinomycosis in the acquired immunodeficiency syndrome-related complex. Arch Otolaryngol Head Neck Surg 1986;112: 1293–1295.
77. Yew WW, Wong PC, Wong CW, Chau CH. Use of imipenem in the treatment of thoracic actinomycosis [Letter]. Clin Infect Dis 1994;19:983–984.

Aeromonas Species

●

Wen Chien Ko and Yin Ching Chuang

GENERAL DESCRIPTION

The genus *Aeromonas* is a member of family *Vibrionaceae* (31). They are oxidase-producing Gram-negative rods that grow on MacConkey agar and ferment carbohydrates (67). Separation from *Vibrio* species, another member of family *Vibrionaceae,* depends on resistance to the O/129 compound, no growth in 6% NaCl, and absence of ornithine decarboxylase (except in *A. veronii* biovar *veronii*) (23).

In nature, *Aeromonas* spp. are widely distributed in fresh and salt water and are also found in food (53), treated drinking or raw water (41), and hospital water supply systems (58). Aeromonads can cause nosocomial infections (10, 44).

The taxonomy for genus *Aeromonas* is evolving. Formerly, mesophilic aeromonads were grouped as "*Aeromonas hydrophila* complex" and then separated into three major phenospecies groups: *A. hydrophila, A. caviae,* and *A. sobria* (1). This phenospecies grouping scheme is adopted here to be consistent with previous reports; however, the scheme does not reflect the genetic diversity of this genus. At least 14 DNA hybridization groups (genomospecies) are recognized within the genus *Aeromonas* (28). Only three species (*A. sobria, A. eucrenophila* and *A. encheleia*) are not recovered from clinical material (29). Unique phenotypic characters that can reliably differentiate between *A. allosaccharophila* and other phenospecies are lacking (43). Whether differences in clinical manifestations and antibiotic susceptibility exist among those genomospecies remains unresolved.

The genus *Aeromonas* also displays antigenic diversity. Several clinically important serogroups have been defined by the serotyping system of Sakazaki and Shimada (59). Three serogroups, O:11, O:16 and O:34, predominated among clinical isolates from miscellaneous sites (28). Putative virulence factors among bacteremic isolates include resistance to complement-mediated lysis, protease and hemolysin activities, and production of siderophores (32).

SUSCEPTIBILITY IN VITRO

Aeromonads are usually sensitive in vitro to third-generation cephalosporins, aminoglycosides, chloramphenicol, tetracycline, and trimethoprim-sulfamethoxazole (38, 48), aztreonam, quinolones (6, 38), imipenem, and meropenem (9). They are uniformly resistant to ampicillin (except *A. trota*). Piperacillin shows variable activity and was more active than other penicillins (46). Combination of a β-lactamase inhibitor and a β-lactam, such as sulbactam-ampicillin (36), tazobactam-piperacillin, and clavulanate-ticarcillin (14), does not enhance the antibacterial activity. Resistance to third-generation cephalosporins, aminoglycosides, tetracycline, or trimethoprim-sulfamethoxazole is increasing in clinical *Aeromonas* isolates in Taiwan (37), as shown in Table 1. Activity of the first or second-generation cephalosporins is variable (34); there are not only interspecies differences (6, 32, 46, 48) but also geographic variability. In general, *A. hydrophila* is the most resistant and *A. sobria* the most susceptible species. The most striking variability was seen for cephalothin, particularly more active against *A. sobria* than *A. hydrophila* or *A. caviae,* and use of this property for phenospecies identification has been suggested (48).

Given the unpredictable susceptibility of *Aeromonas* species, selection of antibiotic therapy must be guided by in vitro testing. However, discrepancies exist between various in vitro susceptibility tests. Detection of resistance to β-lactam drugs by the Vitek AutoMicrobic System is weak for a small number of *Aeromonas* strains, compared with the standard agar dilution test (63). Clinical physicians in hospitals using this system should avoid ineffective β-lactams. Disk-diffusion

TABLE 1 • Variation in MIC$_{50}$\MIC$_{90}$ (μg/mL) of Three *Aeromonas* Species for Antibiotics among Reports

Antibiotics	Motyl[a]			Morita[b]			Burgos[c] (Spain)			Ko[d] (Taiwan)		
	A. hydrophila (n = 20)	*A. caviae* (n = 20)	*A. sobria* (n = 20)	*A. hydrophila* (n = 101)	*A. caviae* (n = 12)	*A. sobria* (n = 69)	*A. hydrophila* (n = 87)	*A. caviae* (n = 412)	*A. sobria* (n = 23)	*A. hydrophila* (n = 142)	*A. caviae* (n = 32)	*A. sobria* (n = 59)
Amikacin	≤2\2	≤2\2	≤2\≤2							4\8	2\4	4\8
Ampicillin	≥16\≥16	≥16\16	≥16\≥16	>256\>256	>256\>256	>256	64\128	64\>128	128\>128	256\>512	128\>512	256\>512
Aztreonam				1\0.5	≤0.06\0.12	≤0.06\0.12	≤0.06\0.25	≤0.06\0.25	≤0.06\0.13	0.06\4	0.06\0.5	0.03\0.12
Cefazolin							16\>128	32\>128	8\32			
Cefoperazone	≤4\4	≤4\4	≤4\≤4	2\16	1\8	1\4						
Cefotaxime	≤2\2	≤2\2	≤2\≤2	2\8	1\4	1\4	0.13\0.5	0.25\1	≤0.06\0.25	0.5\32	0.25\32	0.06\32
Cefoxitin	≤2\32	≤2\8	≤2\≤2	8\64	4\16	1\8	2\128	8\128	1\2			
Ceftriaxone				1\8	1\4	0.5\2				1\128	0.5\32	0.006\4
Cefuroxime				2\16	2\4	1\8				2\128	8\128	0.5\32
Cephalothin	≥32\≥32	≥32\≥32	≤2\≥32							>128\>128	>128\>128	8\>128
Chloramphenicol	≤1\≤1	≤1\≤1	≤1\≤1				1\4	2\4	1\4			
Ciprofloxacin							≤0.06\≤0.06	≤0.06\≤0.06	≤0.06\≤0.06	0.008\0.5	0.004\0.06	0.008\0.25
Gentamicin	≤0.5\1	≤0.5\1	≤0.5\1							1\8	1\4	2\8
Imipenem				0.5\4	0.25\0.5	0.5\2				2\4	0.12\0.25	2\8
Mezlocillin	≤16\256	≤16\16	≤16\256				4\16	4\16	4\128			
Moxalactam	≤4\4	≤4\4	≤4\4	1\8	1\4	1\4						
Ofloxacin							≤0.06\≤0.06	≤0.06\≤0.06	≤0.06\≤0.06	0.06\4	0.06\1	0.03\0.5
Piperacillin	≤8\256	≤8\16	≤8\64	64\128	32\128	16\128	2\4	2\8	0.5\32	0.03\0.5	0.03\0.5	0.015\0.5
Tetracycline	≤1\≤1	≤1\≤1	≤1\≤1				0.25\8	0.5\2	0.5\16	4\32	2\64	8\64
Ticarcillin				128\128	128\128	64\128	16\64	16\128	128\>128	32\512	16\256	64\512
Tobramycin	2\≥8	≤0.5\1	≤0.5\4							1\32	2\16	2\32
Trimethoprim-sulfamethoxazole	≤1\≤1	≤1\≤1	≤1\≤1				8\128	4\>128	0.5\2	0.5\128	2\128	1\256

[a]Strains from New York City and Thailand (48).

[b]Strains from Japan, Southeast Asia, mainland China (46).

[c]Ref. 6.

[d]Ref. 37.

techniques show good correlation with the agar dilution method for β-lactam agents (except for amoxicillin-clavulanate) and non-β-lactam agents (38).

Most *Aeromonas* isolates in reports dealing with in vitro susceptibility fall into three major phenospecies (6, 36, 38, 46, 48). The susceptibility profiles of less frequently encountered genomospecies such as *A. salmoncida, A. media,* or *A. trota* have been poorly documented; more clinical isolates need to be investigated. Different susceptibility patterns in the three *Aeromonas* phenospecies among previous reports might reflect geographic variability in susceptibility or be related to different proportions of genomospecies among the three major phenospecies.

Most studies dealing with β-lactamases of *Aeromonas* species focus on the chromosomally encoded β-lactamases; little is known about plasmid-encoded enzymes. Although a self-transferable plasmid encoding TEM-like β-lactamase was recently found in a clinical isolate of *A. caviae* (62), its expression was deficient in the parental isolate, and thus its role in mediating clinical resistance to β-lactams was not clear. Also, *Aeromonas* strains from India with multiple antimicrobial resistance encoded by plasmids were reported (8), which challenges the initial impression that antimicrobial resistance by plasmid-mediated β-lactamases is not a problem for *Aeromonas* species (34).

Aeromonads are known to be able to produce chromosomally encoded β-lactamases, and expression of genes encoding these enzymes is induced by some β-lactams (26). Moreover, three coexistent β-lactamases were found in *A. salmonicids* (20), *A. sobria* (70), and *A. hydrophila* (21). Two of the enzymes (a penicillinase and a cephalospoinase) can hydrolyze nitrocefin, but the third (a metallo-β-lactamase with carbapenemase activity) cannot, making it undetectable by conventional methods (21, 73). The metallocarbapenemase from *Aeromonas* species has been studied extensively (21, 70, 73); clinically detectable resistance to imipenem has been rare, although a fatal infection caused by an imipenem-resistant *Aeromonas* strain has been described (18). Although the clinical relevance of these enzymes is unclear, possibly the genes encoding these enzymes may be transferred between nonmotile and motile virulent aeromonads (21), and derepressed mutants selected by the pressure of antibiotics and coinducibility of multiple β-lactamases could cause one *Aeromonas* strain to become resistant to many β-lactam agents (70).

Combination antibiotics therapy has been evaluated in vitro (40). The combination of amikacin plus carbenicillin or piperacillin was synergistic in vitro and had the highest bactericidal activity. Synergy studies have not yet been evaluated in animal models or clinical studies.

ANTIMICROBIAL THERAPY
Gastrointestinal Infection

The most common clinical manifestation of *Aeromonas*-associated infections in humans is gastrointestinal infection. The enteropathogenicity of *Aeromonas* has been questioned. There is no universal agreement on the pathogenic role of various putative enterotoxins (27), and only 2 of 57 healthy volunteers developed diarrhea after ingesting a high dose of a virulent strain (45). However, numerous reports document predominant growth of *Aeromonas* from the feces of persons with diarrhea (15, 25, 50–51, 71), and patients infected with aeromonads in the gastrointestinal tract produced intestinal secretory antibodies against the homologous strains (33). This gastrointestinal illness has several clinical presentations: acute watery diarrhea (often with vomiting), dysenteric diarrhea, chronic diarrhea, choleraic diarrhea, and traveler's diarrhea (31). Complications related to *Aeromonas* gastroenteritis, including small bowel obstruction (4) and hemolytic-uremic syndrome (5), have been reported.

Aeromonas-associated gastroenteritis in immunocompetent persons is usually acute and self-limited; therefore, antimicrobial therapy is not routinely recommended. For those with intractable diarrhea, serious illness, or high risk of systemic infection, especially patients with hematologic malignancy or hepatobiliary diseases, therapy with effective antibiotics seems reasonable, although it is not supported by well-designed clinical surveys, (24). Treatment of chronic diarrhea with trimethoprim-sulfamethoxazole (60) and acute diarrhea in a putative outbreak with ciprofloxacin (52) have been reported. Nevertheless, because of the lack of controlled clinical trials and the increasing antibiotic resistance in *Aeromonas* species, the optimal regimen for such infections is uncertain. Considering other copathogens that cause bacterial gastroenteritis (e.g., *Salmonella, Shigella, Campylobacter, Escherichia coli,* or *Vibrio* species), the fluoroquinolones might be preferred for severe gastroenteritis if *Aeromonas* infection is suspected.

Soft-Tissue Infections

Musculoskeletal and soft-tissue infections, ranging from cellulitis (61, 68), furunculosis (19), skin nodules (73), soft-tissue abscesses (16, 68), and infected lacerations (68) to necrotizing fasciitis (2), ecthyma gangrenosum (19, 35, 49, 72), osteomyelitis (68), and myonecrosis (16, 47, 66) are common presentations. The clinical manifestations and outcomes of *Aeromonas*-associated soft-tissue infections vary with the immune status of the host. Most patients with *Aeromonas*-related wounds or soft-tissue infections showed antecedent water-related trauma and polymicrobial infections, suggesting environmental contamination (16, 64, 68). Antibiotics with or without debridement were necessary. In immunocompetent individuals, infections were localized and not associated with bacteremia, so favorable outcomes were uniform.

In immunocompromised hosts, notably patients with hepatic cirrhosis, *Aeromonas*-associated soft-tissue infections can be fulminant and fatal. Necrotizing fasciitis, myonecrosis, or both (myofascial necrosis), with or without soft-tissue gas formation (66), have been the characteristic presentations. Typically, patients experienced minor injuries or had unrecognizable wounds in their extremities while handling seafood or fishing gear. Within 24 hours, rapid, centripetal progression of pain, erythema, and swelling accompanied by hemorrhagic bullae developed. Subsequent septic shock, acute renal failure, and disseminated intravascular coagulation were noted, if not treated early. Such infections, rarely seen in nonimmunocompromised persons (22), were frequently monomicrobial and accompanied by bacteremia. In addition to appropriate antibacterial agents, early treatment with aggressive surgical debridement or amputation of the affected extremity is often necessary.

Thus, for a patient with a posttraumatic wound and a history of freshwater or seafood contact, empirical therapy with a third-generation cephalosporin, trimethoprim-sulfamethoxazole, doxycycline, or ciprofloxacin (16) may be indicated. In southern Taiwan, because of similar dermatologic presentations in necrotizing fasciitis caused by *Vibrio vulnificus* or *Aeromonas* species, cefotaxime (2 g every 6 h) is used as first-line therapy, with the addition of minocycline (i.v., 100 mg every 12 h) for suspected *V. vulnificus* infections. With the concern about potential selection of stable derepression of chromosomally encoded β-lactamase by β-lactam agents in *Aeromonas* species, β-lactam therapy is not recommended as a first choice (57). In vitro emergence of β-lactam resistance due to derepression of β-lactamase has been documented in only one report (3). In our experience with *Aeromonas* bacteremias, emergence of β-lactam resistance was quite unusual (36). Amundson et al. proposed a different therapeutic approach and suggested the use or addition of antibiotics such as tetracycline that suppress protein synthesis for suspected *Aeromonas* infections (2). In animal models of toxin-mediated streptococcal myositis, treatment with clindamycin and erythromycin were more effective than penicillin (65). However, the role of putative virulence factors such as hemolysins or proteases (7) in invasive infections remains unclear. Given the absence of data favoring such an approach and the theoretical risk of antagonism between bacteriostatic and bactericidal antibiotics, we do not recommend such an approach.

We recommend broad-spectrum bactericidal antibiotics, such as third-generation cephalosporins, aztreonam, imipenem, meropenem, or fluoroquinolones, with or without an aminoglycoside, as first-line therapy for severe *Aeromonas* soft-tissue infections, particularly in compromised patients. The optimal antimicrobial agent varies by geographic region and requires consideration of the local susceptibility pattern of *Aeromonas* strains. Therapy should be modified according to the in vitro results of the microbiology laboratory for any individual case. Surgical debridement and removal of infected foci such as prostheses are usually necessary.

Bacteremia

Aeromonas bacteremia, although reported in immunocompetent persons (17), usually occurs in patients with underlying illnesses. Patients with hematologic malignancy who are neutropenic or patients with hepatobiliary diseases are at particularly high risk (13, 19, 36). Primary bacteremia is not uncommon, although the presumed portal of entry in such cases is the gastrointestinal tract. Sepsis caused by *Aeromonas* is clinically indistinguishable from that caused by other Gram-negative bacilli. Because of bacteremic spread, invasive soft-tissue infection such as necrotizing fasciitis usually involves more than one site. Occasionally, a compartment syndrome is seen. A history of exposure to fresh or marine water or consumption of raw or semicooked seafood is helpful, when present. Some

cases are hospital acquired, and water storage tanks in hospitals are potential sources (58). Most bacteremia is caused by *A. hydrophila* and *A. sobria* (12, 30). The case fatality rate ranges from 28 to 46%. Spontaneous bacterial peritonitis, hypotension on admission, association with diabetes mellitus, and high Pugh's score are predictors of poor outcomes in cirrhotic patients with *Aeromonas* bacteremias (36).

Combination therapy with an aminoglycoside and a cephalosporin has been suggested as appropriate for *Aeromonas* bacteremias (19), but clinical trials documenting this recommendation have never been performed. A recent large-scale observation study found that combination treatment showed no additional therapeutic benefit over treatment with an appropriate β-lactam drug in nonneutropenic patients with Gram-negative bacteremia (42). In our experience, selection of a derepressed mutant during β-lactam therapy for *Aeromonas* bacteremia was rarely encountered (5%, 3 of 58 episodes of monomicrobial *Aeromonas* bacteremias treated with a β-lactam alone or in combination with a aminoglycoside; unpublished data). Therefore, for *Aeromonas* bacteremia, we recommend a β-lactam agent: cefotaxime 1 to 2 g every 6 h; ceftriaxone 1 to 2 g every 12 h; moxalactam 1 to 2 g every 8 h. The duration of therapy should be no less than 10 to 14 days. Other bactericidal β-lactam agents, such as aztreonam (2 g every 8 h), imipenem (0.5 g every 6 h), meropenem (0.5–1 g every 8 h), or fluoroquinolones (i.v. ciprofloxacin 200 mg every 12 h) may be reasonable alternatives. The potential emergence of antibiotic resistance during treatment should be kept in mind.

Specific Infections

Meningitis

Meningitis caused by *Aeromonas* species is rare. In a review article by Parras, overall, eight cases were reported from 1960 to 1993 (56). Three patients died. Diarrhea may or may not be present and is usually secondary to bacteremia and sometimes associated with skin manifestations. High-dose third-generation cephalosporins (cefotaxime 2 g every 4 h or ceftriaxone 2 g every 12 h), with or without aminoglycosides, are recommended for treatment of aeromonad meningitis.

Endocarditis

Two cases of *Aeromonas* endocarditis involving the aortic valve have been reported (11, 54). Both patients were elderly with chronic underlying illness. Although endocarditis was controlled by β-lactam-aminoglycoside combination therapy (carbenicillin plus gentamicin and cefazolin plus gentamicin), both died of the underlying illness. Given the favorable bacteriologic outcome in these two reported cases, combination therapy with an aminoglycoside plus a β-lactam seems reasonable. Fluoroquinolones may be useful if the patient has an allergy to β-lactam agents or there is concern about inducible β-lactam resistance.

Eye Infections

Aeromonas eye infections are rare and usually related to traumatic exposure to water or a contact lens. Exogenous endophthalmitis, keratitis, blepharoconjunctivitis, periocular cellulitis, and dacryocystitis have been seen. The onset of endophthalmitis is rapid and often results in enucleation. Outcomes for other ophthalmic infections are usually good. Therefore, early recognition of endophthalmitis in patients having eye injuries associated with environmental contamination is critical for preventing the serious sequelae of *Aeromonas* eye infections. Lipophilic drugs (e.g., chloramphenicol, trimethoprim-sulfamethoxazole, and tetracyclines) show reasonably good vitreous penetration (55), but a bactericidal agent (e.g., trimethoprim-sulfamethoxazole) might be more reliable for severe invasive infections. Ciprofloxacin is promising in systemic treatment of Gram-negative bacterial endophthalmitis (39). In addition to vitrectomy, intravitreous administration of amikacin or ceftazidime plus systemic administration of ciprofloxacin or trimethoprim-sulfamethoxazole, if active in vitro, is the preferred regimen.

COMMENTS

As the number of immunocompromised hosts increase, infections caused by *Aeromonas* species will certainly be encountered more frequently in patients exposed to fresh or marine water. Not surprisingly, traumatic *Aeromonas* infections are often associated with other bacteria, and empirical therapy should use broad-spectrum antibiotics. Traditional biochemical markers do not reveal the complex taxonomic grouping in the genus *Aeromonas*. Identification of the various geonomospecies would help in elucidating the environmental distribution, antibiotic susceptibility, and clinical presentation for each genomospecies. The geographic and interspecies diversity of antibiotics susceptibilities in the genus *Aeromonas* heighten the importance of in vitro susceptibility testing in guiding antibiotic selection.

REFERENCES

1. Altwegg M, Geiss HK. Aeromonas as a human pathogen. Crit Rev Microbiol 1989;16:253–286.
2. Amundson DE, Weiss PJ, Anderson MD, Myers M. Severe *Aeromonas* infection in a patient with alcoholic cirrhosis of the liver. Infect Med 1994;11:769–771.
3. Bakken JS, Sanders CC, Clark RB, Hori M. β-lactam resistance in *Aeromonas* spp. caused by inducible β-lactamase active against penicillins, cephalosporins and carbapenems. Antimicrob Agents Chemother 1988;32:1314–1319.
4. Block K, Braver JM, Farraye FA. *Aeromonas* infection and intramural intestinal hemorrhage as a cause of small bowel obstruction. Am J Gastroenterol 1994;89:1902–1903.
5. Bogdanovic R, Cobeljic M, Markovic M, Nikolic V, Ognjanovic M, Sarjanovic L, Makic D. Haemolytic-uraemic syndrome assciated with *Aeromonas hydrophila* enterocolitis. Pediatr Nephrol 1991;5:293–295.
6. Burgos A, Quindos G, Martinez R, Rojo P, Cisterna R. In vitro susceptibility of *Aeromonas caviae, Aeromonas hydrophila* and *Aeromonas sobria* to fifteen antibacterial agents. Eur J Clin Microbiol Infect Dis 1990;9:413–417.
7. Cahill MM. Virulence factors in motile *Aeromonas* species. J Appl Bacteriol 1990;69:1–16.
8. Chaudhury A, Nath G, Shukla BN, Sanyal SC. Biochemical characterisation, enteropathogenicity and antimicrobial resistance plasmids of clinical and environmental *Aeromonas* isolates. J Med Microbiol 1996;44:434–437.
9. Clark RB. Antibiotic susceptibilities of the *Vibrionaceae* to meropenem and other antimicrobial agents. Diagn Microbiol Infect Dis 1992;15:453–455.
10. Cookson BD, Houang ET, Lee JV. The use of a biotyping system to investigate an unusual clustering bacteremias caused by *Aeromonas* species. J Hosp Infect 1984;5:205–209.
11. Davis WA 2d, Kane JG, Gargusi VF. Human *Aeromonas* infection: a review of the literature and a case report of endocarditis. Medicine 1978;57:267–277.
12. Dryden M, Munro R. *Aeromonas* septicemia: relationship of species and clinical features. Pathology 1989; 21:111–114.
13. Duthie R, Ling TW, Cheng AFB, French GL. *Aeromonas* septicemia in Hong Kong species distribution and associated disease. J Infect 1995;30:241–244.
14. Fass RJ, Prior RB. Comparative in vitro activities of piper-acillin-tazobactam and ticarcillin-clavulanate. Antimicrob Agents Chemother 1989;33:1268–1274.
15. George WL, Nakata MM, Thompson J, White ML. *Aeromonas*-related diarrhea in adults. Arch Intern Med 1985;145:2207–2211.
16. Gold WL, Salit IE. *Aeromonas hydrophila* infections of skin and soft tissue: report of 11 cases and review. Clin Infect Dis 1993;16:69–74.
17. Golik A, Leonov Y, Schlaeffer F, Gluskin I, Lewinsohn G. *Aeromonas* species bacteremia in nonimmunocompromised hosts: two case reports and a review of the literature. Isr J Med Sci 1990;26:87–90.
18. Gonzalez-Barca E, Ardanuy C, Carratala J, Sanchez A, Fernandez-Sevilla A, Granena A. Fatal myofascial necrosis due to imipenem-resistant *Aeromonas hydrophila*. Scand J Infect Dis 1997;29:91–92.
19. Harris RL, Fainstein V, Elting L, Hopfer RL, Bodey GP. Bacteremia caused by *Aeromonas* species in hospitalized cancer patients. Rev Infect Dis1985;7:314–320.
20. Hayes MV, Thomson CJ, Amyes SGB. Three β-lactamases isolated from *Aeromonas salmonicida,* including a carbapenemase not detectable by conventional methods. Eur J Clin Microbiol Infect Dis 1994;13:805–811.
21. Hayes MV, Thomson CJ, Amyes SGB. The 'hidden' carbapenemase of *Aeromonas hydrophila*. J Antimicrobiol Chemother 1996;37:33–44.
22. Heckerling PS, Stine TM, Pottage JC, Levin S, Harris AA. *Aeromonas hydrophila* myonecrosis and gas gangrene in a nonimmunocompromised host. Arch Intern Med 1983;143:2005–2007.
23. Hickman-Brenner FW, MacDonald KL, Steigerwalt AG, Fanning GR, Brenner DJ, Farmer JJ 3d. *Aeromonas veronii,* a new ornithine decarboxylase-positive species that may cause diarrhea. J Clin Microbiol 1987;25:900–906.
24. Holmberg SD, Farmer JJ 3d. *Aeromonas hydrophila* and *Plesiomonas shigelloides* as causes of intestinal infections. Rev Infect Dis 1984;6:633–639.
25. Holmberg SD, Schell WL, Fanning GR, Wachsmuth IK, Hickman-Brenner FW, Blake PA, Brenner DJ, Farmer JJ 3d. *Aeromonas* intestinal infections in the United States. Ann Intern Med 1986;105:683–689.
26. Iaconis JP, Sanders CC. Purification and characterization of inducible β-lactamases in *Aeromonas* spp. Antimicrob Agents Chemother 1990;34:44–51.
27. Janda JM. Recent advances in the study of the taxonomy, pathogenicity, and infectious syndromes associated with the genus *Aeromonas*. Clin Microbiol Rev 1991;4:397–410.

28. Janda JM, Abbott SL, Carnahan M. *Aeromonas* and *Plesiomonas*. In: Murrray PR, Baron EJ, Pfaller MA, Tenover FG, Yolken RH, eds. Manual of clinical microbiology. 6th ed. Washington, DC: American Society for Microbiology 1995:477–482.

29. Janda JM, Abbott SL, Khashe S, Kellogg GH, Shimada T. Further studies on biochemical characteristics and serologic properties of the genus *Aeromonas*. J Clin Microbiol 1996;34: 1930–1933.

30. Janda JM, Brenden R. Importance of *Aeromonas sobria* in *Aeromonas* bacteremia. J Infect Dis 1987;155:589–591.

31. Janda JM, Duffey PS. Mesophilic aeromonads in human disease: current taxonomy, laboratory identification, and infectious disease spectrum. Rev Infect Dis 1988;10:980–997.

32. Janda JM, Guthertz LS, Kokka RP, Shimada T. *Aeromonas* species in septicemia: laboratory characteristics and clinical observations. Clin Infect Dis 1994;19:77–83.

33. Jiang ZD, Nelson A, Mathewson JJ, Ericsson CD, DuPont HL. Intestinal secretory immune response to infection with *Aeromonas* species and *Plesiomonas shigelloides* among students from the United States in Mexico. J Infect Dis 1991; 164:979–982.

34. Jones BL, Wilcox MH. *Aeromonas* infections and their treatment. J Antimicrob Chemother 1995;35:453–461.

35. Ketover BP, Young LS, Armstrong D. Septicemia due to *Aeromonas hydrophila:* clinical and immunologic aspects. J Infect Dis 1973;127:284–290.

36. Ko WC, Chuang YC. *Aeromonas* bacteremia: review of 59 episodes. Clin Infect Dis 1995;20:1298–1304.

37. Ko WC, Yu KW, Liu CY, Huang CT, Leu HS, Chuang YC. Increasing antibiotic resistance in clinical isolates of *Aeromonas* strains in Taiwan. Antimicrob Agents Chemother 1996;40: 1260–1262.

38. Koehler JM, Ashdown LR. In vitro susceptibilities of tropical strains of *Aeromonas* species from Queensland, Australia, to 22 antimicrobial agents. Antimicrob Agents Chemother 1993;37: 905–907.

39. Kowalski RP, Karenchak LM, Eller Aw. The role of ciprofloxacin in endophthalmitis therapy. Am J Ophthalmol 1993;116:695–699.

40. Lai HC, Tsai WC. Antibiotics combination effect on the clinical isolates of *Aeromonas hydrophila*. Chin J Microbiol Immunol 1990;23:44–52.

41. LeChevallier MW, Seidler RJ, Evans TM. Enumeration and characterization of standard plate count bacteria in chlorinated and raw water supplies. Appl Environ Microbiol 1980;40:922–930.

42. Leibovici L, Paul M, Ponznanski O, Drucker M, Samra Z, Konigsberger H, Pitlik M. Monotherapy versus β-lactamaminoglycoside combination treatment for gram-negative bacteremia: a prospective, observational study. Antimicrob Agents Chemother 1997;41:1127–1133.

43. Martinez-Murcia AJ, Esteve C, Garay E, Collins MD. *Aeromonas allosaccharophila* sp. nov., a new mesophilic member of the genus *Aeromonas*. FEMS Microbiol Lett 1992;91: 199–206.

44. Mellersh AR, Norman P, Smith GH. *Aeromonas hydrophila:* an outbreak of hospital infection. J Hosp Infect 1984;5: 425–430.

45. Morgan DR, Johnson PC, Dupont HL, Satterwhite TK, Wood LV. Lack of correlation between known virulence properties of *Aeromonas hydrophila* and enteropathogenicity for humans. Infect Immun 1985;50:62–65.

46. Morita, K, Watanbe N, Kurata S, Kanamori M. β-Lactam resistance of motile *Aeromonas* isolates from clinical and environment sources. Antimicrob Agents Chemother 1994;38:353–355.

47. Moses AE, Leibergal M, Rahav G, Perouansky M, Or R, Shapiro M. *Aeromonas hydrophila* myonecrosis accompanying mucormycosis five years after bone marrow transplantation. Eur J Clin Microbiol Infect Dis 1994;14:237–240.

48. Motyl MR, McKinley G, Janda JM. In vitro susceptibilities of *Aeromonas hydrophila, Aeromonas sobria,* and *Aeromonas caviae* to 22 antimicrobial agents. Antimicrob Agents Chemother 1985;28:151–153.

49. Moyes CD, Sykes PA, Rayner JM. *Aeromonas hydrophila* septicemia producing ecthyma gangrenosum in a child with leukemia. Scand J Infect Dis 1977;9:151–153.

50. Moyer NP. Clinical significance of *Aeromonas* species isolated from patients with diarrhea. J Clin Microbiol 1987;25: 2044–2048.

51. Namdari H, Bottone EJ. Microbiologic and clinical evidence supporting the role of *Aeromonas caviae* as a pediatric enteric pathogen. J Clin Microbiol 1990;28:837–840.

52. Nathwani D, Laing RB, Harvey G, Smith CC. Treatment of symptomatic enteric *Aeromonas hydrophila* infection with ciprofloxacin. Scand J Infect Dis 1991;23:653–654.

53. Nishikawa Y, Kishi T. Isolation and characterization of motile *Aeromonas* from human, food and environmental specimens. Epidemiol Infect 1988;101:213–223.

54. Ong KR, Sordillo EA, Frankel E. Unusual case of *Aeromonas hydrophila* endocarditis. J Clin Microbiol 1991;29:1056–1057.

55. Papastamelos AG, Tunkel AR. Antibacterial agents in infections of the central nervous system and eye. Infect Dis Clin North Am 1995;9:615–637.

56. Parras F, Diaz MD, Reina J, Moreno S, Guerrero C. Meningitis due to *Aeromonas* species: case report and review. Clin Infect Dis 1993;17:1058–1060.

57. Paterson DL. Antibiotic-induced antimicrobial resistance in *Aeromonas* spp [Letter]. Med J Australia 1997;166:165.

58. Picard B, Goullet P. Seasonal prevalence of nosocomial *Aeromonas hydrophila* infection related to *Aeromonas* in hospital water. J Hosp Infect 1987;10:152–155.

59. Sakazaki R, Shimada T. O-Serogrouping scheme for mesophilic *Aeromonas* strains. Jpn J Med Sci Biol 1984;37:247–255.

60. San Joaquin VH, Pickett DA. *Aeromonas*-associated gastroenteritis in children. Pediatr Infect Dis J 1988;7:53–57.

61. Sanger JR, Yousif NJ, Matloub HS. *Aeromonas hydrophila* upper extremity infection. J Hand Surg 1989;14:719–721.

62. Sayseed S, Saunders JR, Edwards C, Corkill JE, Hart CA. Expression of *Aeromonas caviae bla* genes in *Escherichia coli*. J Antimicrob Chemother 1996;38:435–441.

63. Schadow KH, Giger DK, Sanders CC. Failure of the Vitek AutoMicrobic System to detect beta-lactam resistance in *Aeromonas* species. Am J Clin Pathol 1993;100:308–310.

64. Semel JD, Trenholme G. *Aeromonas hydrophila* water-associated traumatic wound infections: a review. J Trauma 1990; 30:324–327.

65. Stevens DL, Gibbons AE, Bergstrom R, Winn V. The Eagle effect revisited: efficacy of clindamycin, erythromycin, and penicillin in the treatment of streptococcal myositis. J Infect Dis 1988;158:23–28.

66. Vukmir RB. *Aeromonas hydrophila:* myofascial necrosis and sepsis. Intensive Care Med 1992;18:172–174.

67. von Graevenitz A, Altwegg M. *Aeromonas and Plesiomonas*. In: Balows A, Hausler WJ Jr, Herrmann KL, Isenberg HD, Shadomy HJ, eds. Manual of clinical microbiology. 15th ed. Washington, DC: American Society for Microbiology, 1991: 396–401.

68. Voss LM, Rhodes KH, Johnson KA. Musculoskeletal and soft tissue *Aeromonas* infections: an environmental disease. Mayo Clin Proc 1992; 67:422–427.
69. Walsh TR, Gamblin S, Emery DC, Mac Gowan AP, Bennett PM. Enzyme kinetics and biochemical analysis of ImiS, the metallo-β-lactamases from *Aeromonas sobria* 163a. J Antimicrob Chemother 1996;37:423–431.
70. Walsh TR, Payne DJ, MacGowan AP, Bennett PM. A clinical isolate of *Aeromonas sobria* with three chromosomally mediated inducible β-lactamases: a cephalosporinase, a penicillinase and a third enzyme, displaying carbapenemase activity. J Antimicrob Chemother 1995;35:271–279.
71. Wilcox MH, Cook AM, Eley A, Spencer RC. *Aeromonas* spp as a potential cause of diarrhoea in children. J Clin Pathol 1992; 45:959–963.
72. Wolff RL, Wiseman SL, Kitchens CS. *Aeromonas hydrophila* bacteremia in ambulatory immunocompromised hosts. Am J Med 1980;68:238–242.
73. Young DF, Barr RJ. *Aeromonas hydrophila* infection of skin. Arch Dermatol 1981;117:224.

Alcaligenes Species

●

Selwyn D. R. Lang and Arthur J. Morris

GENERAL DESCRIPTION
Microbiology

The nomenclature of *Alcaligenes* has been described as "confused as any in current clinical taxonomy" (15). That adopted here follows Bruckner and Colonna (4): *A. faecalis* subsp. *faecalis* formerly *A. odorans, Pseudomonas odorans,* CDC group VI; *A. xylosoxidans* formerly *A. xylosoxidans* spp. *xylosoxidans, A. denitrificans* subsp. *xylosoxidans,* CDC group IIIa, IIIb; *A. denitrificans* formerly *A. denitrificans* subsp. *denitrificans,* CDC group Vc; and *A. piechaudii.*

Members of the genus *Alcaligenes* are motile, nonfermentative, oxidase- and catalase-positive, Gram-negative bacilli that grow overnight on most solid media, including MacConkey, under aerobic conditions. *A. denitrificans* can also grow anaerobically in the presence of nitrate. Colonies are typically small with a thin, irregular, spreading edge. Those of *A. faecalis* subsp. *faecalis* commonly have a fruity odor (hence the previous name *A. odorans*) and cause green discoloration of blood agar. The name *Alcaligenes* denotes the production of alkaline reactions with carbohydrates. *A. xylosoxidans* is the exception, acidifying OF glucose and OF xylose. *A. faecalis* subsp. *faecalis* and *A. piechaudii* differ from *A. xylosoxidans* and *A. denitrificans* in their ability to grow in 6.5% salt. *A. piechaudii* reduces nitrate to nitrite, but no further, whereas *A. faecalis* ssp. *faecalis* cannot reduce nitrate but can covert nitrite to nitrogen.

Alcaligenes species are ubiquitous in soil and water and are sufficiently commonly encountered as colonists of the gastrointestinal tract to be regarded as endogenous flora. Colonization is facilitated by contamination of fluids in use in hospitals, including soaps and disinfectants, and devices such as nebulizers, pressure transducers, incubators, and humidifiers. Under these circumstances, it is sometimes difficult to distinguish between colonization and infection. However, with the exception of *A. piechaudii,* whose purported pathogenicity appears to be supported by a single case report (21), *Alcaligenes* species are occasionally recovered in pure culture from normally sterile sites and are recognized as significant pathogens, particularly in the immunocompromised host and the hospital environment. The great majority of clinical reports implicate *A. xylosoxidans.*

Clinical Manifestations

The literature on treatment of infections due to *Alcaligenes* species consists of case reports and reviews of case reports. Infections include bacteremia (5, 14, 16, 23), meningitis (7, 8), prosthetic joint infection (25), sternal osteomyelitis (26), corneal ulceration (24), chronic otitis media (21), lung abscess (11), and endocarditis (6). Most of these were adult patients who had underlying malignancy or were otherwise immunocompromised. There are several reports of neonatal infections, especially bacteremia and meningitis, and including maternal-fetal transfer (12). Two series have reported colonization and infection with *A. xylosoxidans* in children with cystic fibrosis (9, 18). Dunne et al. reported an epidemiologic investigation of 16 cases of *A. xylosoxidans,* of which 8 occurred in patients with cystic fibrosis (9). Recently, Moissenet et al. reported that 8 of 120 children with cystic fibrosis were persistently colonized with *A. xylosoxidans* for a mean of 3.5 years, despite various antibiotic treatments including intravenous ticarcillin, piperacillin, ceftazidime, and imipenem, oral trimethoprim-sulfamethoxazole and ciprofloxacin, and nebulized colistin (18).

SUSCEPTIBILITY IN VITRO
A. xylosoxidans (recently *A. xylosoxidans* subsp. *xylosoxidans*)

Three published studies (3, 10, 13) provide MIC_{50} and MIC_{90} data for a wide range of antibiotics for clinical isolates of *A. xylosoxidans* (Table 1). The most consistently active antibiotics

TABLE 1 • **Susceptibilities of _Alcaligenes xylosoxidans_**

Antibiotic	n	Range	MIC$_{50}$	MIC$_{90}$	Breakpoint[a]	% Susceptible	Reference
Amikacin	33	8–125	128	128	≤16		10
Gentamicin	33	4–64	64	64	≤4		10
Gentamicin	16	256	256	256	≤4	0	3
Gentamicin	15	1->64	>64	>64	≤4		13
Kanamycin	16	64–512	128	256	≤16	0	3
Netilmicin	33	8–64	64	64	≤8		10
Netilmicin	16	64–256	128	256	≤8	0	3
Tobramycin	33	16–64	32	64	≤4	0	10
Amidinocillin	33	32->256	256	>256			10
Ampicillin	33	16->128	32	>128	≤8	0	10
Amoxicillin	16	32–512	64	256	≤8	0	3
Amoxicillin clavulanate	16	16–64	32	64	≤8/4	0	3
Amoxicillin clavulanate	33	4->128	16	64	≤8/4		10
Piperacillin	33	0.5->128	0.5	64	≤16		10
Piperacillin	16	0.5–8	4	8	≤16	100	3
Piperacillin	15	≤2->256	≤2	256	≤16		13
Temocillin	33	64->256	>256	>256			10
Ticarcillin	15	≤2->256	4	>256	≤16		13
Ticarcillin	16	4–512	16	128	≤16		3
Ticarcillin clavulanate	16	2–16	4	8	≤16/2	100	3
Ticarcillin clavulanate	33	0.25–64	1	32	≤16/2		10
Ticarcillin clavulanate	15	≤2–128	≤2	128	≤16/2		13
Cefamandole	33	4–128	16	32	≤8		10
Cefazolin	33	16–128	128	128	≤8	0	10
Ceforanide	33	4–256	256	256			10
Cefotaxime	33	8–64	32	64	≤8		10
Cefotaxime	16	64–256	256	256	≤8	0	3
Cefotaxime	15	16->64	64	>64	≤8	0	13
Cefotetan	33	16–256	128	256	≤16	10	10
Cefoxitin	16	256	256	256	≤8	0	3
Ceftazidime	33	1–64	4	16	≤8		10
Ceftazidime	15	2->64	8	16	≤8		13
Ceftriaxone	33	2–128	32	64	≤8		10
Cefuroxime	33	32–128	64	64	≤8	0	10
Cephalothin	16	128–256	128	256	≤8	0	3
Aztreonam	16	32–64	64	64	≤8	0	3
Aztreonam	15	32->64	64	>64	≤8	0	13
Imipenem	33	0.25–4	0.5	2	≤4	100	10
Imipenem	15	1->16	2	8	≤4		13
Meropenem	15	0.25–4	1	4			13
Ciprofloxacin	33	1–64	4	16	≤1		10
Ciprofloxacin	16	2–8	4	8	≤1	0	3
Ciprofloxacin	15	1->8	4	>8	≤1		13
Norfloxacin	33	8–64	32	64			10
Ofloxacin	33	1–64	4	32	≤2		10
Pefloxacin	33	1–64	4	32			10
Pipemidic acid	16	512	512	512			3
Nalidixic acid	16	128	128	128			3
Trimethoprim-sulfamethoxazole[b]	33	0.12–64	0.2	16	≤2/38		10

Modified from (3, 10, 13)

[a] Current NCCLS interpretive standards for susceptibility (μg/mL) (19).

[b] Trimethoprim-sulfamethoxazole tested in a ratio of 1:19. Concentration refers to the trimethoprim component.

among those tested were imipenem, meropenem, trimethoprim-sulfamethoxazole, piperacillin, ticarcillin/clavulanate, and ceftazidime. All isolates were resistant to aminoglycosides, ampicillin, amoxicillin, amdinocillin, and aztreonam; most were resistant to first-, second-, and third-generation cephalosporins (other than ceftazidime) and to the quinolones. These are in keeping with the results of a small series of isolates tested by

Auckenthaler et al. (2). Addition of clavulanic acid to amoxicillin and to ticarcillin reduced the mean MICs of these antibiotics such that most isolates were susceptible to ticarcillin-clavulanate in vitro (Table 1).

A more detailed study of the susceptibility of 56 clinical isolates and 2 reference strains of _A. xylosoxidans_ to 12 β-lactam antibiotics, and of the effect of β-lactamase inhibitors, was conducted by Mensah et al. (17). All strains produced β-lactamase, but two phenotypic classes of activity were observed: 41 strains produced β-lactamase inhibited by cloxacillin (type S) but not by clavulanic acid, and the other 17 (type R) strains showed β-lactamase activity inhibited by clavulanic acid. Tables 2 and 3 show the susceptibilities of these two groups of isolates. All were susceptible to imipenem and to moxalactam. The 41 type S strains were highly sensitive to ticarcillin, piperacillin, and azlocillin. Susceptibility to cephalosporins was more variable. These strains were highly resistant to cefuroxime and cefoxitin, resistant to cefotaxime and cefamandole, and susceptible to cefoperazone and cef-

TABLE 2 • Susceptibilities of Cloxacillin-Sensitive β-Lactamase-Producing *Alcaligenes xylosoxidans*

Antibiotic	n	Range	MIC$_{50}$	MIC$_{90}$	Breakpoint[a]	% Susceptible
Amoxicillin	41	4–64	8	64	≤8	
Amoxicillin clavulanate[b]	41	2–32	4	8	≤8/4	
Azlocillin	41	≤0.12–2	0.25	0.5		
Piperacillin	41	≤0.12–1	0.5	0.5	≤16	100
Piperacillin tazobactam[c]	41	≤0.12–1	0.5	0.5	≤16/4	100
Ticarcillin	41	0.25–8	1	4	≤16	100
Ticarcillin clavulanate[b]	41	0.25–2	1	1	≤16/2	100
Cefamandole	41	4–64	16	32	≤8	
Cefoperazone	41	0.5–4	2	4	≤16	100
Cefoperazone clavulanate[b]	41	≤0.12–4	2	2	≤16	100
Cefotaxime	41	16–128	64	64	≤8	0
Cefotaxime clavulanate[b]	41	16–64	64	64	≤8	0
Cefoxitin	41	64–>256	256	256	≤8	0
Ceftazidime	41	1–16	4	8	≤8	
Ceftazidime clavulanate[b]	41	1–16	4	8	≤8	
Cefuroxime	41	>256	>256	>256	≤8	0
Cefuroxime clavulanate[b]	41	>256	>256	>256	≤8	0
Moxalactam	41	0.25–8	2	4	≤8	100
Imipenem	41	1–4	2	2	≤4	100

Modified from (17).

[a] Current NCCLS interpretive standards for susceptibility (μg/mL) (19).

[b] Clavulanate (2 μg/mL).

[c] Tazobactam (4 μg/mL).

TABLE 3 • Susceptibilities of Cloxacillin/Clavulanic Acid–Susceptible β-Lactamase-Producing *Alcaligenes xylosoxidans*

Antibiotic	n	Range	MIC$_{50}$	MIC$_{90}$	Breakpoint[a]	% Susceptible
Amoxicillin	17	>256	>256	>256	≤8	0
Amoxicillin clavulanate[b]	17	≤2–128	64	128	≤8/4	
Azlocillin	17	4–64	32	64		
Piperacillin	17	4–128	32	64	≤16	
Piperacillin tazobactam[c]	17	0.5–16	1	4	≤16/4	100
Ticarcillin	17	64–>256	>256	>256	≤16	0
Ticarcillin clavulanate[b]	17	0.5–64	16	64	≤16/2	
Cefamandole	17	16–256	32	128	≤8	0
Cefoperazone	17	16–128	64	128	≤16	
Cefoperazone clavulanate[b]	17	1–8	2	8	≤16	100
Cefotaxime	17	64–>256	64	>256	≤8	0
Cefotaxime clavulanate[b]	17	32–>256	64	>256	≤8	0
Cefoxitin	17	128–>256	256	>256	≤8	0
Ceftazidime	17	2–32	16	32	≤8	
Ceftazidine clavulanate[b]	17	2–16	4	8	≤8	
Cefuroxime	17	>256	>256	>256	≤8	0
Cefuroxime clavulanate[b]	17	>256	>256	>256	≤8	0
Moxalactam	17	0.5–8	2	2	≤8	100
Imipenem	17	1–2	2	2	≤4	100

Adapted from (17).

[a] Current NCCLS interpretive standards for susceptibility (μg/mL) (19).

[b] Clavulanate (2 μg/mL).

[c] Tazobactam (4 μg/mL).

tazidime. In the case of the type R strains (Table 3), clavulanic acid potentiated amoxicillin, ticarcillin, cefoperazone, and to a lesser extent ceftazidime, but not cefuroxime or cefotaxime; tazobactam potentiated piperacillin. The authors note in their discussion that isolates resistant to penicillins are also resistant to sulfonamides; however, others have found no cross-resistance with trimethoprim-sulfamethoxazole (8).

A. denitrificans, A. faecalis subsp. faecalis, and A. piechaudii

These organisms are less commonly encountered clinically and there is a relative paucity of in vitro susceptibility data. Tables 4, 5, and 6 show what has been reported (3). The antibiogram for A. denitrificans isolates (Table 4) does not differ significantly from that for A. xylosoxidans (Table 1). A. faecalis subsp. faecalis isolates (Table 5) were less resistant to cephalosporins than A. xylosoxidans, and clavulanate rendered most susceptible to amoxicillin and to ticarcillin. Piperacillin had slightly greater intrinsic activity than ticarcillin but was not investigated in combination with tazobactam. The quinolones showed variable activity. All were resistant to aztreonam, and most to the aminoglycosides. A. piechaudii isolates showed a resistance pattern similar to that of A. faecalis subsp. faecalis but were more markedly resistant to cefoxitin and cefotaxime (Table 6).

Jorgensen et al. reported that all 14 isolates of Alcaligenes species (other than A. xylosoxidans) in their series were susceptible to mero- penem (MIC$_{90}$ 0.25 µg/mL) and to imipenem

TABLE 4 • In Vitro Susceptibilities of *Alcaligenes denitrificans*

Antibiotic	n	Range	MIC$_{50}$	MIC$_{90}$	Breakpoint[a]	% Susceptible
Amoxicillin	10	0.5–512	32	128	≤8	
Amoxicillin clavulanate[b]	10	0.5–128	16	32	≤8/4	
Piperacillin	10	0.125–1024	1	4	≤16	
Ticarcillin	10	0.125–256	8	64	≤16	
Ticarcillin clavulanate[b]	10	0.125–256	2	4	≤16/2	
Cefotaxime	10	0.125–256	64	128	≤8	
Cefoxitin	10	0.125–256	128	256	≤8	
Cephalothin	10	0.125–128	32	128	≤8	
Aztreonam	10	32–64	32	64	≤8	0
Ciprofloxacin	10	0.125–8	2	8	≤1	
Pipemidic acid	10	8–512	256	512		
Nalidixic acid	10	2–128	128	256		
Gentamicin	10	0.125–256	128	256	≤4	
Kanamycin	10	0.125–512	128	256	≤16	
Netilmicin	10	0.125–256	128	256	≤8	

Modified from (3).

[a] Current NCCLS interpretive standards for susceptibility (µg/mL) (19).

[b] Clavulanate (2 µg/mL).

TABLE 5 • In Vitro Susceptibilities of *Alcaligenes faecalis* subsp. *faecalis*

Antibiotic	n	Range	MIC$_{50}$	MIC$_{90}$	Breakpoint[a]	% Susceptible
Amoxicillin	34	2–1024	16	64	≤8	
Amoxicillin clavulanate[b]	34	0.5–128	2	4	≤8/4	
Piperacillin	34	1–256	4	16	≤16	
Ticarcillin	34	1–512	16	64	≤16	
Ticarcillin clavulanate[b]	34	0.5–32	2	8	≤16/2	
Cefotaxime	34	0.5–128	2	8	≤8	
Cefoxitin	34	2–128	4	8	≤8	
Cephalothin	34	2–128	8	32	≤8	
Aztreonam	34	32	32	32	≤8	0
Ciprofloxacin	34	0.5–8	2	4	≤1	
Pipemidic acid	34	8–512	256	256		
Nalidixic acid	34	128	128	128		
Gentamicin	34	32–512	32	64	≤4	
Kanamycin	34	4–512	128	256	≤16	
Netilmicin	34	1–256	8	16	≤8	

Modified from (3).

[a] Current NCCLS interpretive standards for susceptibility (µg/mL) (19).

[b] Clavulanate (2 µg/mL).

TABLE 6 • In Vitro Susceptibilities of *Alcaligenes piechaudii*						
Antibiotic	n	Range	MIC$_{50}$	MIC$_{90}$	Breakpoint[a]	% Susceptible
Amoxicillin	5	4–64	16	32	≤8	
Amoxicillin clavulanate[b]	5	1–2	2	2	≤8/4	100
Piperacillin	5	0.5–1	0.5	1	≤16	100
Ticarcillin	5	8–32	8	16	≤16	100
Ticarcillin clavulanate[b]	5	1–4	2	2	≤16/2	100
Cefotaxime	5	64	64	64	≤8	0
Cefoxitin	5	64	64	64	≤8	0
Cephalothin	5	8–16	8	16	≤8	
Aztreonam	5	16	16	16	≤8	0
Ciprofloxacin	5	2–8	2	4	≤1	0
Pipemidic acid	5	256	256	256		
Nalidixic acid	5	2–32	4	8		
Gentamicin	5	16–128	32	64	≤4	0
Kanamycin	5	8–32	8	8	≤16	
Netilmicin	5	2–32	4	8	≤8	

Modified from (3).

[a] Current NCCLS interpretive standards for susceptibility (μg/mL) (19).

[b] Clavulanate (2 μg/mL).

(MIC$_{90}$ 1 μg/mL) (13). In contrast, the MIC$_{90}$ of meropenem and of imipenem for 15 isolates of *A. xylosoxidans* were 4 μg/mL and 8 μg/mL, respectively (13).

In summary, *Alcaligenes* species are susceptible to the carbapenems imipenem and meropenem. Most isolates are susceptible to trimethoprim-sulfamethoxazole, piperacillin (especially with tazobactam), and ticarcillin/clavulanate. Susceptibility to cephalosporins varies; moxalactam and ceftazidime are the most active. There are no data for cefpirome and other "fourth-generation" cephalosporins. Tetracyclines, chloramphenicol, macrolides, and quinolones show variable activity. *Alcaligenes* species are generally resistant to aminoglycosides, ampicillin, penicillin, and rifampicin (22).

A. xylosoxidans (and perhaps other *Alcaligenes* species also) is commonly tolerant to many antibiotics including trimethoprim-sulfamethoxazole, ticarcillin, mezlocillin, piperacillin, and cefoperazone (1, 20). Tolerance is of potential importance in patients with endocarditis, meningitis, neutropenic sepsis, or prosthetic device infection, conditions in which bactericidal activity is deemed relevant. Most case reports of treatment of infections due to *Alcaligenes* species do not describe bactericidal titers. However, a titer of 1:16 was obtained in the cerebrospinal fluid (CSF) of a patient successfully treated with a combination of ceftazidime, gentamicin, and trimethoprim-sulfamethoxazole (7). There are very few reports of the effects of combinations of antibacterial agents against *Alcaligenes* species, other than β-lactam plus β-lactamase inhibitor and trimethoprim plus sulfamethoxazole. Despite resistance to amikacin, synergy has been reported with amikacin plus ceftazidime, a combination used successfully to treat intravascular catheter-related sepsis due to *A. xylosoxidans* in a child with AIDS (5). Since in this case synergy was detected by disk-diffusion testing and bactericidal titers were not reported, it is not certain whether the combination was bactericidal.

ANTIMICROBIAL THERAPY

There are no large series and no randomized controlled trials. On the basis of in vitro data, carbapenems are likely to replace trimethoprim-sulfamethoxazole as the agents of first choice for serious infections due to *Alcaligenes* species. Piperacillin with or without tazobactam and ticarcillin with clavulanate are alternatives. A β-lactamase-hyperproducing variant of *A. xylosoxidans* has been selected in vivo in a patient treated initially with piperacillin and pefloxacin. The CSF cultures were still positive after a month of therapy. Although the therapy was changed to trimethoprim-sulfamethoxazole, the patient (who had acute lymphoblastic leukemia) died a few days later (8). Combination therapy with ceftazidime and amikacin for 14 days was used successfully in treating Broviac catheter–related sepsis when the catheter was not removed (5). If synergy (as shown in vitro in this case) can be shown with an aminoglycoside, then combination therapy could be considered.

REFERENCES

1. Arroyo JC, Jordan W, Lema MW, Brown A. Diversity of plasmids in *Actinobacter xylosoxidans* isolates responsible for a seemingly common source nosocomial outbreak. J Clin Microbiol 1987;25:1952–1955.
2. Auckenthaler R, Michea-Hamzehpour M, Pechere JC. In vitro activity of newer quinolones against aerobic bacteria. J Antimicrob Chemother 1986;17(Suppl B):29–39.
3. Bizet C, Tekaia F, Philippon A. In vitro susceptibility of *Alcaligenes faecalis* compared with those of other *Alcaligenes* spp. to antimicrobial agents including seven beta-lactams [Letter]. J Antimicrob Chemother 1993;32:907–910.
4. Bruckner DA, Colonna P. Nomenclature for aerobic and facultative bacteria. Clin Infect Dis 1997;25:1–10.
5. Cieslak TJ, Raszka WV. Catheter-associated sepsis due to *Alcaligenes xylosoxidans* in a child with AIDS [Letter]. Clin Infect Dis 1993;16:592–593.

6. Cohen PS, Maguire JH, Weinstein L. Infective endocarditis caused by gram-negative bacteria: a review of the literature, 1945–1977. Prog Cardiovasc Dis 1980;22:205–242.

7. D'Amato RF, Salemi M, Mathews A, Cleri DJ, Reddy G. *Achromobacter xylosoxidans* (*Alcaligenes xylosoxidans* subs. *xylosoxidans*) meningitis associated with gunshot wound. J Clin Microbiol 1988;26:2425–2426.

8. Decre D, Arlet G, Danglot C, Lucet J-C, Fournien G, Bergogne-Berezin E, Philippon A. A beta-lactamase-overproducing strain of *Alcaligenes denitrificans* subsp. *xylosoxidans* isolated from a case of meningitis. J Antimicrob Chemother 1992;30:769–779.

9. Dunne WM Jr, Maisch S. Epidemiological investigation of infections due to *Alcaligenes* species in children and patients with cystic fibrosis: use of repetitive element-sequence polymerase chain reaction. Clin Infect Dis 1995;20:836–841.

10. Glupcynski H, Hansen W, Freney J, Yourassowsky E. In vitro susceptibility of *Alcaligenes denitrificans* subsp. *xylosoxidans* to 24 antimicrobial agents. Antimicrob Agents Chemother 1988;32:276–278.

11. Gradon JD, Mayrer AR, Hayes J. Pulmonary abscess associated with *Alcaligines xylosoxidans* in a patient with AIDS [Letter]. Clin Infect Dis 1993;17:1071–1072.

12. Hearn YR, Gander RM. *Achromobacter xylosoxidans* an unusual neonatal pathogen. Am J Clin Pathol 1991;96:211–214.

13. Jorgensen JH, Maher LA, Howell AW. Activity of meropenem against antibiotic-resistant or infrequently encountered gram-negative bacilli. Antimicrob Agents Chemother 1991;35:2410–2414.

14. Legrand C, Anaissie E. Bacteremia due to *Achromobacter xylosoxidans* in patients with cancer. Clin Infect Dis 1992;14:479–484.

15. McGowan JE, Steinberg JP. Other gram-negative bacilli. In: Mandell GL, Bennet JE, Dolin R, eds. Principles and practice of infectious diseases. 4th ed. New York: Churchill Livingstone, 1995:2106–2116.

16. Mandell WF, Garvey GJ, Neu HC. *Achromobacter xylosoxidans* bacteremia. Rev Infect Dis 1987;9:1001–1005.

17. Mensah K, Philippon A, Richard C, Nevot P. Susceptibility of *Alcaligenes denitrificans* subspecies *xylosoxidans* to beta-lactam antibiotics. Eur J Clin Microbiol Infect Dis 1990;9:405–409.

18. Moissenet D, Baculard A, Valcin M, Marchand V, Tournier G, Garbarg-Chenon A, Vu-Thien H. Colonisation by *Alcaligenes xylosoxidans* in children with cystic fibrosis: a retrospective clinical study conducted by means of molecular epidemiological investigation. Clin Infect Dis 1997;24:274–275.

19. National Committee for Clinical Laboratory Standards. Methods for dilution antimicrobial susceptibility tests for bacteria that grow aerobically—fourth edition; approved standard. NCCLS document M7-A4. Wayne, PA: NCCLS, 1997.

20. Olson DA, Hoeprich PD. Post-operative infection of an aortic prosthesis with *Achromobacter xylosoxidans*. West J Med 1982;136:153–157.

21. Peel MM, Hibberd AJ, King BM, Williamson HG. *Alcaligenes piechaudii* from chronic ear discharge. J Clin Microbiol 1988;26:1580–1581.

22. Schoch PE, Cunha BA. Nosocomial *Achromobacter xylosoxidans* infection. Infect Control Hosp Epidemiol 1988;9:84–87.

23. Spear JB, Fuhrer J, Kirby BD. *Achromobacter xylosoxidans* (*Alcaligenes xylosoxidans* subsp. *xylosoxidans*) bacteremia associated with a well-water source: a case report and review of the literature. J Clin Microbiol 1988;26:598–599.

24. Tayeri T, Kelly LD. *Alcaligenes faecalis* corneal ulcer in a patient with cicatricial pemphigoid. Am J Ophthalmol 1993;115:255–256.

25. Taylor P, Fischbein L. Prosthetic knee infection due to *Achromobacter xylosoxidans*. J Rheumatol 1992;19:992–993.

26. Walsh RD, Klein NC, Cunha BA. *Achromobacter xylosoxidans* osteomyelitis [Letter]. Clin Infect Dis 1993;16:176–178.

Anaerobes

●

Maria Hedberg and Carl Erik Nord

GENERAL DESCRIPTION
Anaerobic Gram-Positive Nonsporeforming Rods and Anaerobic Gram-Positive Cocci Excluding *Clostridial spp*

The anaerobic Gram-positive cocci and anaerobic Gram-positive nonsporeforming rods such as *Actinomyces, Bifidobacterium, Eubacterium, Lactobacillus,* and *Propionibacterium* species are, for the most part, components of the normal flora of the mucosal surfaces and, to a lesser extent, the skin. They are generally considered to be of relatively low virulence and are especially prevalent in infections associated with predisposing or underlying conditions such as previous surgery, malignancy, immunodeficiency, diabetes, and presence of foreign bodies.

These opportunistic pathogens are seldom recovered as single isolates (2). They are often mixed with other anaerobic or aerobic bacteria. The infections in which this group of microorganisms most often have been recovered are chronic otitis media and sinusitis, aspiration pneumonia, intraabdominal infections, gynecologic infections, and skin and soft tissue infections.

Actinomycosis is an uncommon bacterial infection that has a characteristic chronic indolent course. *Actinomyces* species are relatively often recovered from female genital tract infections, especially in women using an intrauterine contraceptive device. Pelvic actinomycosis associated with an intrauterine device can mimic pelvic malignancy. If the diagnosis of actinomycosis can be obtained preoperatively, antibiotic treatment may lead to complete resolution (7, 18). *Actinomyces* species are also isolated from patients with anaerobic pleuropulmonary infections and from skin and soft-tissue abscesses in intravenous drug abusers (*A. odontolyticus*) and non–intravenous drug abusers (*Actinomyces* sp.) (4).

Bifidobacteria are seldom encountered in clinical materials. *Bifidobacterium dentium* seems to be the only *Bifidobacterium* with pathogenic potential. It has been isolated from dental caries, feces, and vagina of humans and from lower respiratory tract specimens. *B. longum* and *B. breve* are occasionally found in clinical materials (11). Meningitis caused by *B. breve* has been reported (19).

Eubacteria are not frequently isolated from clinical specimens. They have been reported from anaerobic pleuropulmonary infections and intrauterine contraceptive device–associated infections (4), in mixed cultures from abscesses and wounds, and infections at different sites such as head and neck, thorax, bone, skin, and pelvis (11).

The pathogenic potential of lactobacilli is very low, and infections caused by these bacteria are rare, in spite of their ubiquitous presence in the gastrointestinal tract and their widespread consumption in fermented milk. In a study of lactobacilli and bacteremia by Saxelin (23), lactobacilli were identified in eight patients among 3317 blood culture isolates. There was no evidence that any particular species or subspecies of *Lactobacillus* was the cause of the infection.

Lactobacillus spp. are sometimes recovered from anaerobic pleuropulmonary infections (4). They can also cause other human diseases such as dental caries, rheumatic vascular disease, septicemia, and infective endocarditis. In elderly and immunocompromised patients, they have been identified as potential emerging pathogens, particularly in patients receiving broad-spectrum antibiotic therapy. In infective endocarditis, *L. rhamnosus* and *L. paracasei* subsp. *paracasei* are frequently isolated, which suggests that they may have greater pathogenic potential than other *Lactobacillus* species or may just reflect their relatively high numbers in the oral cavity (10).

Propionibacterium species are frequently recovered from mixed infections of the skin, acne vulgaris, and infections linked to operative procedures or foreign bodies (11). They have also been reported from cases of chronic infectious endophthalmitis following extracapsular cataract extraction (9). Propionibacteria are dominating in conjunctival cultures from children and adults.

The Gram-positive anaerobic cocci are seen particularly in oral and dental infections, head and neck infections, and other infections related to the oropharyngeal flora as well as in female genital tract infections, where they are the most common anaerobic isolates. They are also one of the major groups isolated from patients with pulmonary (*P. micros, P. anaerobius,* and *P. magnus*) and intraabdominal infections (*P. micros*) and are frequently isolated from diabetic foot ulcers (*P. magnus, P. prevotii, P. anaerobius* and *P. asaccharolyticus*) (4, 6). The three species of *Peptostreptococcus* most commonly seen in clinical specimens from the intestinal and genital tracts are *P. magnus, P. anaerobius,* and *P. asaccharolyticus. P. prevotii* and *P. tetradius* are also clinically important peptostrepto-

cocci. *P. micros* has been found in periodontal and peritonsillar infections (16, 17).

Anaerobic Gram-Negative Rods Excluding *Bacteroides*

Gram-negative anaerobic bacilli are the anaerobes most commonly encountered in clinical infections. Pigmented and nonpigmented *Prevotella* species are, after the *Bacteroides fragilis* group, the most commonly encountered anaerobic bacteria in human infections.

The pigmented anaerobic Gram-negative rods consist of species of the genera *Prevotella* and *Porphyromonas*. Nine species of these genera are found in human clinical material. Eight of these species originate mostly from the oral cavity (*Prevotella corporis, Prevotella denticola, Prevotella intermedia, Prevotella loeschii, Prevotella melaninogenica, Prevotella nigrescens, Porphyromonas endodontalis* and *Porphyromonas gingivalis*), while one (*Porphyromonas asaccharolytica*) is prevalent in the urogenital and intestinal tracts.

Some of the pigmented *Porphyromonas* and *Prevotella* species are important pathogens in oral, dental, and bite infections. They are also isolated from infections of the head, neck, and lower respiratory tract and from gynecologic infections. *Prevotella corporis, P. intermedia* and *Porphyromonas asaccharolytica* have been reported in peritonsillar abscesses, suggesting that these species may have a role in the pathogenesis of this type of infection. Some 84% of the positive cultures in peritonsillar abscesses have been reported to contain anaerobic bacteria (17). Periodontal diseases are often associated with a subgingival microflora comprising specific potentially pathogenic microorganisms. The most important periodontal pathogens associated with adult periodontitis are considered to be the black-pigmented *Porphyromonas gingivalis* and *Prevotella intermedia* (15).

Prevotella bivia and *Prevotella disiens* are nonpigmented and found in female genital tract infections and less frequently in respiratory tract infections (12).

The fusobacteria are normally found in the oropharyngeal and intestinal tracts. They are often isolated from severe infections such as peritonsillar abscesses, head and neck infections, brain abscesses, meningitis, gynecologic infections, and intraabdominal abscesses. *F. nucleatum* is the *Fusobacterium* species most commonly encountered in clinical infections. *F. necrophorum, F. varium,* and *F. mortiferum* are also common clinical isolates. *F. necrophorum* is a very virulent species causing severe infections, most often in children or young adults, originating from pharyngotonsillitis. The microorganism is encountered frequently in mixed infections and, therefore, synergism between *F. necrophorum* and other pathogens may play an important role in infections (25). *F. necrophorum* has been encountered in peritonsillar abscesses in pure cultures (17). Fusobacteria are also associated with refractory and recurrent periodontitis (15).

Three chemotherapy-induced neutropenic hematologic patients with severe systemic infection by *F. nucleatum* were recently reported (14). The infection was considered to be promoted by a combination of chemotherapy-induced mucositis, which served as a portal entry for the systemic infection, and the antibiotic regimen (vancomycin) used in these patients.

ANTIMICROBIAL SUSCEPTIBILITY IN VITRO

During the past years, an increasing resistance to different antimicrobial agents in anaerobic bacteria has been observed. Anaerobic bacteria are naturally resistant to certain antibiotics, including the aminoglycosides and the quinolones, and many now exhibit resistance to several β-lactam agents as well. Resistance to β-lactam agents is most often caused by production of β-lactamases, enzymes that inactivate β-lactam compounds by hydrolysis. Changes in the penicillin-binding proteins (PBPs) or blocked penetration of drug into the active site via alteration of the bacterial outer membrane pores are also decreasing susceptibility to β-lactam agents. Resistance is more common in Gram-negative than in Gram-positive anaerobic isolates. Patterns of susceptibility vary in different geographic areas and even in different hospitals in the same city, depending on antibiotic-prescribing practices. Four groups of drugs are active against almost all anaerobic bacteria of clinical significance: nitroimidazoles, carbapenems, chloramphenicol, and combinations of β-lactam drugs with a β-lactamase inhibitor (ampicillin/sulbactam, amoxicillin/clavulanic acid, piperacillin/tazobactam) (Table 1).

The antimicrobial activity of clindamycin is directed against most anaerobic bacteria, and clindamycin is therefore often used for treatment of anaerobic infections. It is not active against enterococci and aerobic Gram-negative rods. Perorally administered clindamycin causes marked ecologic disturbances in the normal oropharyngeal and intestinal microflora, and resistant clostridia and enterococci are frequently isolated during and after treatment.

Metronidazole is an antimicrobial agent that is often used for treatment and prophylaxis of anaerobic infections. Anaerobic bacteria sensitive to metronidazole include peptostreptococci, clostridia, bacteroides, fusobacteria, prevotella, and porphyromonas. A few clinical anaerobic strains resistant to metronidazole have been reported (20).

Chloramphenicol is a bacteriostatic, highly effective, broadspectrum antimicrobial agent. The drug is very active against many Gram-positive and Gram-negative bacteria and has excellent activity against anaerobic bacteria. Chloramphenicol is specially indicated for use in seriously ill patients. It passes the blood-brain barrier well and it can be bactericidal against common meningeal pathogens such as *Streptococcus pneumoniae,* *Neisseria meningitidis,* and *Haemophilus influenzae.* The major side effect is bone marrow toxicity, which complicates the use of chloramphenicol.

Since the bacteria in anaerobic infections are often mixed with aerobic microorganisms, combinations of two antimicrobial agents may be used to treat these infections, when microbiologic analyses reveal two or more pathogenic species with different susceptibility patterns. In certain situations, the pharmacologic properties of the drugs and whether or not they are bactericidal are important considerations. Central nervous system infections require use of a drug that crosses the bloodbrain barrier well. In such infections and in endocarditis, the bactericidal activity is important (5). Most of the drugs that are active against anaerobes have good bactericidal activity, except chloramphenicol. Antimicrobial agents prescriptions must always be based on distinct clinical and microbiologic diagnoses, and the clinical benefits must always be expected to outweigh potential ecologic disadvantages and other side effects of the treatment.

Most *Peptostreptococcus* (96%) isolates are susceptible to β-lactam agents, although MICs as high as 64 mg/L have been reported for ticarcillin and cefotaxime (11). Decreased susceptibility to penicillins in *Peptostreptococcus* spp. was demonstrated by Baquero (1). In a study by Duerden (3), all except

---

TABLE 1 • In Vitro Susceptibility to Antimicrobial Agents of Anaerobic Bacteria (Not Including *Bacteroides* sp. or *Clostridium* sp.)[a]

Bacteria	PcV	Amox	Amox/Clav	Cefox	Imi	Clinda	Metro	Chloram
Gram-positive bacteria								
Peptostreptococci	S/V	S/V	S/V	S	S	V	V	S
Eubacteria	S	S	S	S	S	S	R	S
Actinomyces	S	S	S	S	S	S	R	S
Bifidobacteria	S	S	S	S	S	S	R	S
Lactobacilli	S	S	S	S	S	S	R	S
Propionebacteria	S	S	S	S	S	S	R	S
Gram-negative bacteria								
Fusobacteria	V	V	S	S	S	S	S	S
Porphyromonas	V	V	S	S	S	S	S	
Prevotella	V	V	S	S	S	S	S	S

Data adapted from Duerden (3), Finegold (6), Wexler and Doern (27), Wexler et al. (28), and Yao and Moellering (29).

[a] PcV, phenoxymethylpenicillin; Amox, amoxicillin; Amox/Clav, amoxicillin/clavulanic acid; Cefox, cefoxitin; Imi, imipenem; Clinda, clindamycin; Metro, metronidazole; Chloram, chloramphenicol.

S, generally susceptible; R, generally resistant; V, variable.

two of 25 *Peptostreptococcus* isolates were susceptible to penicillin. The two resistant strains had MIC values above 16 mg/L, and neither strain was susceptible to amoxicillin/clavulanate. β-Lactam resistance in Gram-positive cocci seems not to be due to β-lactamase production, but rather to PBP modifications that frequently involve cross-resistance to cefoxitin and β-lactamase inhibitor combinations. Compared with β-lactam agents, clindamycin and metronidazole are slightly less active against peptostreptococci (84 and 88% of isolates, respectively) (11). Macrolide-lincosamide resistance has been shown to be inducible in *Peptostreptococcus* strains, and highly resistant populations of *P. asaccharolyticus* (MIC > 8 mg/L) to erythromycin (29.6% resistant strains) and clindamycin (22.2% resistant strains) have also been documented (22). Recent multicenter studies have reported that the incidence of resistance to clindamycin in *Peptostreptococcus, Prevotella, Porphyromonas* and *Fusobacterium* strains is about 10% (8).

Information on antimicrobial susceptibility of anaerobic nonspore forming Gram-positive rods is limited compared with the information available on other anaerobic bacterial groups. In general, members of this bacterial group are susceptible to benzylpenicillin, carbenicillin, and chloramphenicol. Clindamycin, erythromycin, and tetracycline are active against 60 to 94% of isolates tested in this group of bacteria, and the rods are commonly resistant to nitroimidazoles (11).

Resistance is increasingly common among anaerobic Gram-negative rods. Approximately one-third of *Prevotella* species are β-lactamase producers (12), and β-lactamase production among oral pigmented *Prevotella* species is also frequently present in young children. β-Lactamase production has been studied among different ribotypes of *P. melaninogenica* isolated from the oral cavity of young children and their mothers. Some 76% of the strains isolated from the children and 69% of the strains isolated from their mothers turned out to be β-lactamase producers (13). Most strains are still susceptible to clindamycin and metronidazole, while resistant strains to tetracycline have been reported.

The fusobacteria have become more resistant to antimicrobial agents during the last years. Penicillin-resistant strains due to β-lactamase production have been found as well as clindamycin-resistant strains. The fusobacterial isolates are still susceptible to β-lactam agents combined with β-lactamase inhibitors. Metronidazole is also active against all strains (4).

Most anaerobic Gram-negative rods are susceptible to metronidazole, but there are exceptions. In a Colombian population, metronidazole lacked activity against *Fusobacterium* strains (45% resistant strains), *Prevotella* strains, and *Porphyromonas* strains (25% resistant strains) isolated from patients with periodontitis (16). The clinical implication of these findings is unknown.

ANTIMICROBIAL AGENTS
Drugs of Choice

The anaerobic Gram-positive nonsporeforming rods are susceptible to β-lactam agents, including penicillins, cephalosporins, carbapenems, and β-lactam/β-lactamase inhibitor combinations that are used for the treatment of infections caused by these microorganisms. Lactobacilli may be resistant to cephalosporins (27). Clindamycin can be given to patients allergic to β-lactam agents, while metronidazole is inactive against most isolates. All strains are susceptible to chloramphenicol.

Most peptostreptococci are normally susceptible to penicillins, cephalosporins, and β-lactam/β-lactamase inhibitor combinations recommended for treatment of infections involving these cocci (27). Clindamycin and metronidazole are less active against peptostreptococci but can be used in most infections. Peptostreptococci resistant to metronidazole are usually microaerophilic.

Thirty percent of *Porphyromonas* and *Prevotella* strains produce β-lactamases that inactivate penicillin. The combination of a β-lactam agent with a β-lactamase inhibitor is active against these strains and has been used for treatment of infections caused by them (4). The anti-*Pseudomonas* penicillins ticarcillin, mezlocillin, and piperacillin are active against 70% of *Prevotella* and *Porphyromonas* species (27).

Fusobacterium strains have also been reported to produce β-lactamase. Resistance to β-lactam agents is relatively frequent among fusobacteria, about 20 to 30% in Europe and 40% in the United States (8). β-Lactam-resistant strains of *F. nucleatum* are most often seen, but resistant *F. varium* and *F. mortiferum* strains have also been isolated. Some strains of these species produce β-lactamases. β-Lactamase-producing *F. nucleatum* strains have been isolated from the tonsils during penicillin treatment (26). As *Fusobacterium* species are intrinsically resistant to erythromycin, which is often the alternative antibiotic for the treatment of upper respiratory tract infections in patients allergic to penicillin, a combination of erythromycin or penicillin with metronidazole provides protection against both the aerobic and anaerobic pathogens. Alternatively, clindamycin or a β-lactam agent in combination with a β-lactamase inhibitor can be effective.

Special Situations
Anaerobic Endocarditis

Peptostreptococci and *Bacteroides fragilis* most often cause anaerobic endocarditis. In patients with prosthetic heart valves, vascular grafts, or intravascular prosthesis, endovascular infections caused by lactobacilli, propionibacteria, and bifidobacteria have been reported. Benzylpenicillin is considered the agent of choice for treatment of endocarditis caused by peptostreptococci, lactobacilli, propionibacteria, and bifidobacteria (4).

Anaerobic Pericarditis

Anaerobic bacteria have only rarely been isolated from pericardial fluid. In a review by Skiest (24), 30 cases of pericarditis were reported in which at least one specific type of anaerobic bacteria was implicated. The anaerobes were isolated from the pericardial fluid in 27 cases and from the blood in 3 cases (in these 3 cases, cultures of purulent pericardial fluid were sterile). The following anaerobic organisms were isolated: *Bacteroides* species (including *Prevotella* species), "anaerobic streptococci," *Clostridium* species, peptostreptococci, *Fusobacterium* species, and *Bifidobacterium* species. The mortality rate was 52%. No firm conclusion concerning the impact of treatment on outcome could be drawn because of the small number of cases. Cases due to actinomyces were excluded from the review. For patients with odontogenic infections, esophageal diseases, anaerobic pleuropulmonary infections, intraabdominal infections, or pelvic infections, purulent pericarditis may be caused by anaerobic bacteria. In all cases of pericarditis, the source of the organism infecting the pericardium should be sought, and initial antimicrobial therapy should include antibiotics directed against anaerobic bacteria (24).

Anaerobic Meningitis

Anaerobic bacteria are an uncommon cause of meningitis. Anaerobic bacterial meningitis occurs in older children and adults with chronic sinusitis, chronic otitis media, or bowel diseases. Benzylpenicillin is recommended for treatment of meningitis due to peptostreptococci and propionibacteria (4). Chloramphenicol has also been used. Recently, meropenem was shown to be useful for treatment of pneumococcal meningitis. It may thus also be used for peptostreptococcal meningitis (21).

Anaerobic Liver Abscess

From liver abscesses the following anaerobic bacteria are most often isolated: peptostreptococci, bacteroides, and fusobacteria. The most common sources are biliary tract and other intraabdominal infections. Successful treatment of liver abscess requires drainage of the abscess and appropriate antimicrobial therapy. If the underlying source of infection such as bowel perforation or bile duct obstruction must be controlled, surgical drainage is indicated. Empirical antimicrobial treatment is recommended, starting before surgical drainage. A combination of an aminoglycoside plus metronidazole or clindamycin gives optimal coverage for the aerobic and anaerobic bacteria involved. Carbapenems like imipenem and meropenem have also been used successfully for treatment of these infections (21).

CONCLUSION

During the last years, resistance to different antimicrobial agents by anaerobic bacteria has been reported more frequently (8). While other groups of anaerobic bacteria have remained substantially stable in their susceptibility patterns, the *Bacteroides* genus and new genera *Prevotella* and *Porphyromonas* have become increasingly resistant to many antianaerobic agents such as penicillins and cephalosporins as their use has become more widespread. Antimicrobial agents commonly used in the treatment of anaerobic infections are β-lactam antibiotics (carbapenems), metronidazole, and β-lactam compounds (ampicillin, amoxicillin, ticarcillin, and piperacillin) in combination with a β-lactamase inhibitor such as clavulanic acid, sulbactam, or tazobactam. The treatment of anaerobic infections must be individualized, taking into account the site, type, extent, and severity of the infection. The patient's condition and the nature of the infecting organism are also of great importance.

REFERENCES

1. Baquero F, Reig M. Resistance of anaerobic bacteria to antimicrobial agents in Spain. Eur J Clin Microbiol Infect Dis 1992; 11:1016–1020.
2. Brook I, Frazier EH. Significant recovery of nonsporulating anaerobic rods from clinical specimens. Clin Infect Dis 1993; 16:476–480.
3. Duerden BI. Role of the reference laboratory in susceptible testing of anaerobes and a survey of isolates referred from laboratories in England and Wales during 1993–1994. Clin Infect Dis 1995;20(Suppl 2):S180–186.
4. Finegold SM, Wexler HM. Present status of therapy for anaerobic infections. Clin Infect Dis 1996;23:S9–S14.
5. Finegold SM. Anaerobic infections in humans. Anaerobe 1995; 1:3–9.
6. Finegold SM. Overview of clinically important anaerobes. Clin Infect Dis 1995;20(Suppl 2):S205–207.
7. Fiorino AS. Intrauterine contraceptive device-associated actinomycotic abscess and Actinomyces detection on cervical smear. Obstetrics and Gynecology 1996;87:142–149.
8. García-Rodríguez JA, García-Sánches JE, Muños-Bellido JL. Antimicrobial resistance in anaerobic bacteria: current situation. Anaerobe 1995;1:69–80.
9. Hall GS, Pratt-Rippin K, Meisler DM, Washington JA, Roussel TJ, Miller D. Minimum bactericidal concentrations of *Propionibacterium acnes* isolates from cases of chronic endophthalmitis. Diagn Microbiol Infect Dis 1995;21:187–190.
10. Harty DWS, Oakey HJ, Patrikakis M, Hume EBH, Knox KW. Pathogenic potential of lactobacilli. Int J Food Microbiol 1994; 24:179–189.
11. Hillier SH, Moncla BJ. *Peptostreptococcus, Propionibacterium, Eubacterium,* and other nonsporeforming anaerobic Gram-positive bacteria. In: Murray PR, Baron EJ, Pfaller MA, Tenover FC, Yolken RH, eds. Manual of clinical microbiology. Washington, DC: American Society for Microbiology 1995:587–602.
12. Jousimies-Somer HR, Summanen PH, Finegold SM. *Bacteroides, Porphyromonas, Prevotella, Fusobacterium,* and other anaerobic Gram-negative bacteria. In: Murray PR, Baron EJ, Pfaller MA, Tenover FC, Yolken RH, eds. Manual of clinical microbiology Washington, DC: American Society for Microbiology 1995:603–620.
13. Könönen E, Saarela M, Kanervo A, Karjalainen J, Asikainen S, Jousimies-Somer H. β-Lactamase production and penicillin susceptibility among different ribotypes of *Prevotella melaninogenica* simultaneously colonizing the oral cavity. Clin Infect Dis 1995;20(Suppl 2):S364–366.
14. Landsaat PM, van der Lelie H, Bongaerts G, Kuijper EJ. *Fusobacterium nucleatum,* a new invasive pathogen in neutropenic patients? Scand J Infect Dis 1995;27:83–84.
15. Listgarten MA, Lai CH, Young V. Microbial composition and pattern of antibiotic resistance in subgingival microbial samples from patients with refractory periodontitis. J Periodontol 1993; 64:155–161.
16. Mefía GI, Botero A, Rojas W, Robledo JA. Refractory periodontitis in a Colombian population: predominant anaerobic bacterial flora and antibiotic susceptibility. Clin Infect Dis 1995; 20(Suppl 2):S311–313.
17. Mitchlemore IJ, Prior AJ, Montgomery PQ, Tabaqchali S. Microbiological features and pathogenesis of peritonsillar abscesses. Eur J Clin Microbiol Infect Dis 1995;14:870–877.
18. Muller-Holzner E, Ruth NR, Abfalter E, Schrocksnadel H, Dapunt O, Martin-Sances L, Nogales FF. IUD-associated pelvic actinomycosis: a report of five cases. Int J Gynecol Pathol 1995;14:70–74.
19. Nakazava T, Kaneko K, Takahashi H, Inoue S. Neonatal meningitis caused by *Bifidobacterium breve.* Brain Dev 1996; 18: 160–162.

20. Nord CE. In vitro activity of quinolones and other antimicrobial agents against anaerobic bacteria. Clin Infect Dis 1996;23 (Suppl 1):S15–18.
21. Norrby SR, Newell PA, Faulkner KL, Lesky W. Safety profile of meropenem: international clinical experience based on the first 3125 patients treated with meropenem. J Antimicrob Chemother 1995;36(Suppl A):S207–223.
22. Reig M, Moreno A, Baquero F. Resistance in *Peptostreptococcus* spp. to macrolides and lincosamides: inducible and constitutive phenotypes. Antimicrob Agents Chemother 1992;36:662–664.
23. Saxelin M, Chuang NH, Chassy B, Rautelin H, Mäkelä PH, Salminen S, Gorbach SL. Lactobacilli and bacteremia in southern Finland, 1989–1992. Clin Infect Dis 1996;22:564–566.
24. Skiest DJ, Steiner D, Werner M, Garner JG. Anaerobic pericarditis: case report and review. Clin Infect Dis 1994;19:435–440.
25. Tan ZL, Nagaraja TG, Chengappa MM. *Fusobacterium necrophorum* infections: virulence factors, pathogenic mechanism and control measures. Vet Res Commun 1996;20:113–1140.
26. Tunér K, Lindqvist L, Nord CE. Purification and properties of a novel β-lactamase from *Fusobacterium nucleatum*. Antimicrob Agents Chemother 1985;27:943–947.
27. Wexler HM, Doern GV. Susceptibility testing of anaerobic bacteria. In: Murray PR, Baron EJ, Pfaller MA, Tenover FC, Yolken RH eds. Manual of clinical microbiology. Washington, DC: American Society for Microbiology, 1995:1350–1355.
28. Wexler HM, Molitoris E, Molitoris D, Finegold SM. In vitro activities of trovafloxacin against 557 strains of anaerobic bacteria. Antimicrob Agents Chemother 1996;40:2232–2235.
29. Yao JDC, Moellering RC, Jr. Antibacterial agents. In: Murray PR, Baron EJ, Pfaller MA, Tenover FC, Yolken RH eds. Manual of clinical microbiology. Washington, DC: American Society for Microbiology, 1995:1281–1307.

Bacillus anthracis

●

F. Marc LaForce

GENERAL DESCRIPTION

Bacillus anthracis is a nonmotile, sporulating, Gram-positive rod that grows well on blood agar. Individual colonies are gray-white, rough, and sticky when teased with a bacteriologic loop. Susceptibility to a γ-bacteriophage confirms the identity of the organism. Serologic diagnosis is possible with use of a sensitive and specific indirect microhemagglutination test. All virulent strains are pathogenic for mice.

Systemic anthrax is largely a disease of herbivores, and humans become accidentally infected through contact with contaminated animals or their products (10). Thus, the organism has three distinct cycles: (*a*) multiplication of spores in the soil, (*b*) animal infection, and (*c*) human disease. *B. anthracis* can be part of normal soil flora and can undergo bursts of local multiplication that increase the density of organisms in the soil and facilitate infection in grazing animals. Spores may persist in the soil for long periods of time.

The clinical manifestations of human anthrax are quite striking. Cutaneous anthrax, the most common form of the disease, begins as a small, painless, pruritic papule that within 2 days enlarges, develops vesicles, and ulcerates to form an eschar. Cultures of the vesicular fluid are usually positive. Prompt antibiotic treatment, while not stopping the progression of the local infection to eschar formation, is associated with low mortality rates (1%).

Pulmonary anthrax, now a rare disease, follows inhalation of infectious doses of anthrax spores. During the first 3 days, symptoms mimic influenza, but patients become dramatically more ill when dyspnea and hypoxemia develop. Chest x-rays show a wide mediastinum secondary to hemorrhagic mediastinitis. About half of all patients develop secondary anthrax meningitis, and virtually all cases end fatally. Pharyngeal and gastrointestinal anthrax follow ingestion of grossly contaminated and undercooked meat. Pharyngeal ulcers and brawny edema of the neck result from local oropharyngeal multiplication of anthrax bacilli. Gastrointestinal anthrax follows the intestinal absorption of anthrax bacilli and transport of bacteria to mesenteric lymph nodes, with development of hemorrhagic adenitis, ascites, and septicemia. Mortality rates from pharyngeal and gastrointestinal anthrax are high ($\approx$40%).

Overwhelming infection by *B. anthracis* results in uncontrolled intravascular multiplication and a fatal toxemia characterized by hypotension and hemorrhage. For example, during the 12-hour period preceding death of guinea pigs infected with anthrax bacilli, the number of bacteria in the blood rises from 3×10^5 to 1×10^9 organisms/mL. If antibiotics are given after intravascular bacterial counts reach 10^6 organisms/mL, experimental animals die despite a massive reduction in bacterial numbers. Furthermore, sterile blood from these doomed guinea pigs reproduces a fatal toxemic syndrome when given to normal guinea pigs (12).

Human anthrax in the United States is now a rare disease, with fewer than one case per year reported to the CDC over the last 20 years. Inhalation anthrax is now a disease mainly of historic interest, but epidemics of gastrointestinal anthrax continue to be sporadically reported from developing countries.

SUSCEPTIBILITY IN VITRO
Single Drug

B. anthracis is widely susceptible to a variety of antibiotics including penicillin, chloramphenicol, tetracycline, erythromycin, streptomycin, and the fluoroquinolones. Only two contemporary papers have described the in vitro antimicrobial susceptibility of *B. anthracis* (2, 8) (Table 1). Lightfoot et al. (8) studied 70 strains isolated in England, of which 33 were epidemiologically different, while Doganay and Aydin (2) characterized 22 strains from central Turkey. MICs in both studies were determined by agar dilution technique, and results were comparable across both studies. None of the Turkish strains and two strains from the British study were resistant to penicillin. First-generation cephalosporins had excellent activity against *B. anthracis,* but there was considerable resistance to second- and third-generation cephalosporins. All isolates were sensitive to chloramphenicol, tetracycline, streptomycin, gentamicin, vancomycin, and ciprofloxacin.

Combination Drugs

There are no published studies that have evaluated in vitro susceptibility of *B. anthracis* to antibiotic combinations.

ANTIMICROBIAL THERAPY DOSES, DURATION

Penicillin remains the drug of choice for the treatment of cutaneous anthrax. In 1929, Fleming first reported that penicillin could inhibit the growth of anthrax bacilli in vitro and that animals pretreated with penicillin were resistant to anthrax infection. Organisms are rapidly cleared from skin lesions; 25 patients with cutaneous anthrax and positive initial cultures of blister fluid were given 2 million units of penicillin G intravenously and the blister fluid was cultured hourly (10); 5 h after the initiation of therapy, all of the cultures were negative. The duration of therapy with penicillin is not well established, and in the absence of controlled observations, parenteral therapy with penicillin for 5 to 7 days is generally recommended.

Erythromycin, tetracycline, and chloramphenicol are also effective therapy for cutaneous anthrax and are alternative drugs for penicillin-sensitive patients (5).

Single-dose oral therapy with doxycycline has also been evaluated clinically (11). Some 33 patients with cutaneous anthrax were treated with a single oral dose of doxycycline and observed in a hospital setting for 3 days. There was dramatic clinical improvement, and all patients were bacteriologically negative by the fourth day. The authors propose that cutaneous anthrax in adults can be safely treated with a single 500-mg oral dose of doxycycline, while children and adolescents could be treated with single doses of 100 to 300 mg orally.

Because patients with pulmonary anthrax present late in the course of their illness, virtually all cases are fatal irrespective of antibiotic therapy. However, the concept that pulmonary anthrax is uniformly fatal is worth reconsidering because there were at least 11 survivors in the Sverdlovsk outbreak (9). There are so few well-studied cases of gastrointestinal and pharyngeal anthrax that specific recommendations about antibiotic treatment other than intravenous penicillin G (2 million units intravenously every 3 h) cannot be made at this time.

No reliable recommendations can be made on the role of combination therapy, although one animal study suggested that combination therapy with penicillin and streptomycin was better than treatment with either agent alone (6).

VACCINES

Prevention of anthrax has largely depended on the use of vaccines, since widespread decontamination of infected soil is impractical. Sterne vaccine is a live, toxigenic, unencapsulated avirulent animal strain that is widely used as a veterinary vaccine. The main limitation to its use in humans is safety; its use is sometimes associated with necrosis at the inoculation site. Because of safety concerns, these spore vaccines have generally not been used as human vaccines except in Russia, where a live spore vaccine has been developed for human use and is

---

TABLE 1 • **Antibiotic Susceptibility of *Bacillus anthracis* (μg/mL)**

| | Source of Strains | | | | | |
| | England (3) | | | Turkey (4) | | |
	Range	50%[a]	90%[b]	Range	50%[a]	90%[b]
Penicillin	0.015–0.64	0.06	0.125	0.015–0.03	0.015	0.015
Amoxicillin	0.03–0.64	0.06	0.125	0.015–0.03	0.015	0.015
Cefuroxime	1–64	32	64	16–64	64	64
Gentamicin	0.06–0.5	0.125	0.25	0.03–0.25	0.06	0.125
Streptomycin	0.5–4	1.0	1.0	1–4	2	4
Erythromycin	0.25–1.0	0.5	1.0	Not done	Not done	Not done
Tetracycline	0.06–1.0	0.125	0.125	Not done	Not done	Not done
Chloramphenicol	2.0–4.0	4.0	4.0	1–2	2	2
Ciprofloxacin	0.03–0.06	0.06	0.06	0.03–0.06	0.03	0.06
Cefotaxime	Not done	Not done	Not done	8–32	32	32
Aztreonam	Not done	Not done	Not done	>128	>128	>128
Vancomycin	Not done	Not done	Not done	0.25–1.0	1.0	1.0

[a] Dose at which 50% of strains are inhibited.

[b] Dose at which 90% of strains are inhibited.

considered highly effective. A nonliving anthrax vaccine produced by the Biologics Products Program, Michigan Department of Public Health, has been field tested and is highly effective under field conditions (1). The vaccine is an aluminum hydroxide–adsorbed cell-free filtrate of cultures of a strain of anthrax bacillus that produces protective antigen (PA) in the relative absence of lethal factor (LF) and edema factor (EF).

Indications

Anthrax vaccine is recommended for persons whose occupations require frequent contact with imported animal products likely to be contaminated with anthrax spores and for laboratory workers who perform studies using *B. anthracis*.

Doses and Schedules

The current recommendation for anthrax vaccine consists of 0.5 mL administered subcutaneously at 0, 2, and 4 weeks and 6, 12 and 18 months, followed by yearly boosters.

Adverse Effects

Local reactions are common after receipt of anthrax vaccine, with about one-third of recipients reporting some type of reaction (1). Most of these reactions were minor, with less than 1% reporting systemic symptoms.

ENDPOINTS FOR MONITORING THERAPY

Case fatality rates as high as 20% have been reported for untreated cutaneous anthrax, but with appropriate antibiotic treatment, fatalities are now unusual. However, cutaneous lesions, even if promptly treated with antibiotics, continue to progress through the eschar phase. Surgical removal of these lesions is not recommended. Inhalation anthrax is virtually always diagnosed late in its course, and antibiotic therapy, even when given in heroic doses, is unsuccessful. Gastrointestinal and meningeal anthrax are also serious infections with high fatality rates.

COMMENTS

The extensive epidemic of inhalation anthrax that occurred in Sverdlosk, Russia, in 1979, following accidental release of anthrax spores from a biologic weapons laboratory, resulted in more than 60 deaths due to inhalation and has increased interest in the question of postexposure prophylaxis (9). Earlier studies in experimental animals had shown that treatment with penicillin beginning 1 day after aerosol exposure to anthrax spores was protective during the 5 to 10 days of drug therapy,

but animals died when the antibiotic was discontinued (4). In more recent studies, Friedlander et al. challenged monkeys with aerosolized anthrax spores. Beginning 1 day after exposure, groups of animals were given penicillin, ciprofloxacin, or doxycycline for 30 days. A fourth group was immunized with anthrax vaccine after exposure and treated with doxycycline. All antibiotic regimens completely protected animals while they were on therapy and provided better long-term protection than the shorter 5- and 10-day treatment protocols. All animals that were immunized and treated with doxycycline survived. When these monkeys were rechallenged with airborne anthrax spores, all succumbed except those who had been immunized (3). These data offer convincing proof that postexposure prophylaxis is effective, particularly when combined with active immunization.

REFERENCES

1. Brachman PS, Gold H, Plotkin SA, Fekety FR, Werrin M, Ingraham NR. Field evaluation of a human anthrax vaccine. Am J Public Health 1962;52:632–645.
2. Doganay M, Aydin N. Antimicrobial susceptibility of *Bacillus anthracis*. Scand J Infect Dis 1991;23:333–335.
3. Friedlander AM, Welkos SL, Pitt MLM, et al. Postexposure prophylaxis against experimental inhalation anthrax. J Infect Dis 1993;167:1239–1242.
4. Gochenour WS, Gleiser CA, Tigertt WD. Observations on penicillin prophylaxis of experimental inhalation anthrax in the monkey. J Hyg (London) 1962;60:29–33.
5. Gold H. Anthrax: a report of one hundred seventeen cases. Arch Intern Med 1955;96:387–396.
6. Jones WI, Klein F, Lincoln RE, Walker JS, Mahlandt BG, Dobbs JP. Antibiotic treatment of anthrax infection in mice. J Bacteriol 1967;94:609–614.
7. LaForce FM. Anthrax. Clin Infect Dis 1994;19:1009–1014.
8. Lightfoot NF, Scott RJD, Turnbull BCB. Antimicrobial susceptibility of *Bacillus anthracis*. Salisbury Med Bull Suppl 1990;68:95–98.
9. Meselson M, Guillemin J, Hugh-Jones M, et al. The Sverdlovsk anthrax outbreak of 1979. Science 1994;266:1202–1208.
10. Ronaghy HA, Azadeh B, Kohout E, Dutz W. Penicillin therapy of human cutaneous anthrax. Curr Ther Res 1972;14:721–725.
11. Saggar SN, Joseph MM, Bell WJ. Treatment of cutaneous anthrax with a single oral dose of doxycycline. East Afr Med J 1974;51:889–894.
12. Smith H, Keppie J, Stanley JL, Harris-Smith PW. The chemical basis of the virulence of *Bacillus anthracis*. IV. Secondary shock as the major factor of death in guinea pigs from anthrax. Br J Exp Pathol 1955;36:323–335.

Bacillus (Non-*anthracis*) Species

●

Carmelita U. Tuazon

Bacillus spp. are aerobic sporeforming rods that stain Gram positive. They are widely distributed in the environment, although their primary habitat is the soil. Except for few species, the large majority have no pathogenic potential and have never been associated with disease in man or animals.

Members of the genus have significant microbiologic uses (20). Numerous enzymes, antibiotics, and other metabolites have medical, agricultural, pharmaceutical, and other industrial applications. Examples of antibiotics formed by *Bacillus* spp. include bacitracin by *B. licheniformis* or *B. subtilis,* polymyxin by *B. polymyxa,* and gramicidin by *B. brevis.* Certain strains of *Bacillus* have been used as biologic controls in antibiotics and other assays.

Although *Bacillus* spp. have not been considered major human pathogens, with recent advances in medical technology and increased number of immunosuppressed patients, they have been increasingly recognized as opportunistic pathogens in the hospitalized patient. Most clinical laboratories do not speciate *Bacillus* spp. because they are often considered a contaminant. The clinical microbiology laboratory and/or physician should recognize the clinical setting in which further workup of the organism is important.

SUSCEPTIBILITY IN VITRO

Selection of antibiotics for the treatment of serious *Bacillus* infections is based on susceptibility in vitro. More recent studies on the in vitro susceptibilities of *Bacillus* spp. have been reported (4, 21). A microbiologic study of 89 strains of *Bacillus* spp. isolated from clinical blood cultures was performed (21). Species of the isolates were determined by the API 50 CA and API 20E systems. The most common clinically significant isolate was *B. cereus.* Other strains isolated include *B. megaterium, B. polymyxa, B. pumilus, B. subtilis, B. circulans, B. amyloliquifaciens,* and *B. licheniformis.*

All strains of *B. cereus* were susceptible to imipenem, vancomycin, chloramphenicol, gentamicin, and ciprofloxacin by the microdilution susceptibility method (Table 1). Most strains were resistant to clindamycin, cefazolin, and cefotaxime. Disk-diffusion susceptibility revealed that *B. cereus* strains were resistant to all penicillins, oxacillin, and cephalosporins with the exception of mezlocillin. Activity of clavulanic acid was not enhanced by combination with ticarcillin. Many strains were susceptible to erythromycin and tetracycline.

Over 95% of non–*B. cereus* strains were susceptible to imipenem, vancomycin, LY 146032, and ciprofloxacin (Table 1). Between 75 and 90% of strains were susceptible to penicillin, oxacillin, cefazolin, cefotaxime, and chloramphenicol. *B. circulans* and *B. polymyxa* were more likely than other non–*B. cereus* to be resistant to penicillin, oxacillin, cefazolin, and cefotaxime. Using the disk-diffusion method, many non–*B. cereus* strains were susceptible to penicillin, cephalosporins, and trimethoprim-sulfamethoxazole (21).

Another study of in vitro susceptibilities of ocular *B. cereus* isolates demonstrated that clindamycin, gentamicin, and vancomycin are all relatively effective against *B. cereus* as single agents (4). In a checkerboard in vitro synergy study, the clindamycin-gentamicin combination demonstrated a higher rate of bactericidal synergy than vancomycin-gentamicin (60% vs. 40%). Such bactericidal effect may be important clinically in disease states (e.g., endophthalmitis) in which host immune response to infection results in end-organ damage and in immunocompromised hosts who have been shown to be at risk of developing *B. cereus* infections.

ANTIMICROBIAL THERAPY

Isolation of *Bacillus* organism requires careful clinical evaluation to determine the significance of the finding. Certain risk factors have been associated with significant *Bacillus* infections, including intravenous drug abuse, sickle cell disease, foreign devices (e.g., indwelling intravascular catheters, central nervous system shunts, breast implants, pacemakers), immunosuppression from malignancy, neutropenia, and corticosteroid therapy (2, 14).

Based on in vitro data, the drug of choice for serious infections caused by *Bacillus* spp. is vancomycin, since *B. cereus* is the most common isolate. Clinically, both vancomycin and clindamycin have yielded successful outcomes. Whether monotherapy is adequate or combination therapy is better has not been addressed in in vitro models or clinical trials. Other drugs that are highly active and likely to be bactericidal include imipenem, ciprofloxacin, and gentamicin. Tetracycline, chloramphenicol, clindamycin, and erythromycin have activity against *Bacillus* species. Most *Bacillus* strains are resistant to broad-spectrum cephalosporins and ticarcillin-clavulanate. Empirical coverage with the latter agents should be avoided in immunocompromised patients whose blood cultures yield Gram-positive aerobic *Bacillus* until susceptibility testing results are available.

Serious infections caused by *Bacillus* species include ocular infections, endocarditis, bacteremia and septicemia, pneumonia, meningitis, musculoskeletal infections (19), infections associated with injuries from motor vehicle accidents and road trauma (22), and gunshot injuries (9). Systemic antibiotic therapy is usually required for most serious *Bacillus* infections.

A self-limited illness that presents as food poisoning caused by *B. cereus* requires no antimicrobial therapy. Treatment is

TABLE 1 • Antimicrobial Susceptibility of *Bacillus* spp. Isolates		
Organism	Drug	MIC (μg/mL)
Bacillus cereus	Mezlocillin	≤1–32
	Cefazolin	0.5–>64
	Cefotaxime	16–>128
	Imipenem	≤0.25–4
	Vancomycin	≤0.25–2
	LY146032	≤0.25–4
	Chloramphenicol	2–4
	Clindamycin	0.25–2
	Gentamicin	≤0.25–2
	Ciprofloxacin	≤0.25–1
Non–*B. cereus*	Penicillin	≤0.03–>8
	Mezlocillin	≤1–> 128
	Oxacillin	≤0.125–>16
	Cefazolin	≤0.5–32
	Cefotaxime	≤1–>128
	Imipenem	≤0.25–16
	Vancomycin	≤0.25–4
	Chloramphenicol	1–32
	Clindamycin	≤0.125–>16
	Ciprofloxacin	≤0.25–1

Adapted from Weber DJ et al (21).

usually symptomatic, and fluid replacement may be indicated for patients who are severely dehydrated. The main preventive measure for *B. cereus* gastroenteritis is proper food handling.

Ocular Infections

B. cereus has been recently recognized as a primary pathogen in ocular infections (3, 19). Endophthalmitis is a serious illness that can result in visual compromise within 12 to 48 hours after inoculation (5, 13). Early diagnosis is important for successful treatment. A high index of suspicion is required with a patient who presents with ocular infection after trauma or in the setting of drug abuse. Because of the serious sequelae of panophthalmitis, an aggressive approach with early vitrectomy and vitreal instillation of appropriate antibiotic is indicated (5, 19). Both local and systemic antibiotics are used. Antibiotics administered systemically, intravitreally, topically, and via periocular routes are used in conjunction with surgical intervention. An aminoglycoside (either gentamicin or tobramycin) administered locally and systemically was found inadequate to eradicate the infection (7). Clindamycin or vancomycin with or without aminoglycoside is appropriate before the results of culture are known, since *B. cereus* is the predictable isolate. Clindamycin and gentamicin seem to be favored by ophthalmologists. Clindamycin has moderate-to-good activity against *B. cereus* and, when administered subconjunctivally or parenterally, reaches therapeutic levels in the iris, choroid, and vitreous. Intravitreal administration is favored, and a combination of 200 to 400 μg of gentamicin and 450 μg of clindamycin is recommended (5). In addition, 8 μg/mL of gentamicin and 9 μg/mL of clindamycin can be added to the vitrectomy infusion fluid (10). Intravitreal dexamethasone to control the destructive inflammation and early

vitrectomy have been recommended in the management of endophthalmitis caused by *B. cereus*.

Endocarditis

Endocarditis caused by *Bacillus* organisms is a well-recognized complication of intravenous drug abuse (14, 18, 19). Rarely, it has been isolated from patients with underlying valvular disease. Since *B. cereus* is the most common isolate, empirical use of penicillin is usually not effective. Antibiotic therapy with vancomycin or clindamycin has achieved high cure rates in *Bacillus* endocarditis. Intravenous drug abusers with endocarditis caused by *Bacillus* species have responded well to clindamycin. Other patients with underlying valvular heart disease and pacemakers have required surgery in addition to antibiotic therapy (15). In this series, most patients with *Bacillus* endocarditis were treated with clindamycin.

Bacteremia

Intravascular devices are the common source of positive blood cultures for *Bacillus* species. In patients with positive blood cultures for *Bacillus,* a decision has to be made whether the organism is causing disease. In most cases, especially if the patient is asymptomatic, the bacteremia is limited and requires no antimicrobial therapy, emphasizing that the process is relatively benign. A recent report on an AIDS patient with *B. cereus* bacteremia also emphasizes the low morbidity associated with this condition (1). Appropriate therapy can be readily instituted once a decision has been made that a clinically significant infection is present. Usually infections have an indolent course, and institution of antimicrobial therapy can await specific sensitivity results. For immunosuppressed patients with chronic indwelling catheters, recent experience suggests that catheters should be promptly removed to prevent recurrent bacteremia in addition to administering antibiotic therapy (2). Depending on how ill the patient is, antibiotics (e.g., vancomycin with or without gentamicin) may be given until susceptibility results become available.

Musculoskeletal Infections

Musculoskeletal infections caused by *Bacillus* species have been reported. Necrotizing fasciitis was described in a leukemic patient and in a patient with sickle cell disease (14, 18). Antibiotic therapy alone is not sufficient, multiple surgical debridement is usually required, and rarely amputation may be necessary. Antibiotic therapy should be tailored according to the species. Again, if the patient is critically ill, vancomycin plus gentamicin is a reasonable initial regimen.

Acute vertebral osteomyelitis caused by *B. cereus* has been reported in drug abusers and most likely introduced via the bloodstream by contaminated heroin and/or paraphernalia (17). Chronic osteomyelitis has usually been related to accidental trauma, and infection is usually difficult to eradicate and requires multiple surgical procedures. Vertebral osteomyelitis caused by *B. cereus* has responded well to prolonged intravenous antibiotic therapy (18).

Therapy for chronic osteomyelitis can be quite prolonged, as it was in a 13-year-old girl who developed osteomyelitis of the femur caused by *Staphylococcus aureus* and was subsequently superinfected with *B. cereus*. She was treated with vancomycin for 6 months (12).

Meningitis

A wide variety of *Bacillus* species have been isolated from cerebrospinal fluid (CSF) of patients who had spinal anesthesia, subdural hematoma, ventricular shunts, and parameningeal foci of infections (e.g., otitis and mastoiditis). Any foreign body such as a ventricular shunt must be removed to eradicate the infection. Initial therapy is with intravenous vancomycin with or without aminoglycoside and can be adjusted when susceptibility results become available. Supplemental intraventicular or intrathecal instillation of vancomycin may be required in patients who respond poorly. Intrathecal doses of 3 to 5 mg of vancomycin may be used in addition to parenteral antibiotics (16).

In the treatment of central nervous system (CNS) infections, the ability of the antibiotic to penetrate the CNS must be considered. Clindamycin does not reach significant levels in the CSF, even with meningitis. Vancomycin appears to be the preferred drug for serious CNS infections. In certain settings (e.g., brain abscesses), prolonged antibiotic treatment may be required. A 3-year-old patient with acute lymphocytic leukemia who developed multiple brain abscesses and meningitis was treated successfully with antibiotics alone (6). Surgical excision of the abscesses was precluded by their number and locations. The patient was treated with intravenous vancomycin and gentamicin for 3 weeks, and then rifampin was substituted for gentamicin for a total treatment of more than 8 weeks. The abscesses were completely resolved on follow-up computed tomographic (CT) scan studies.

DOSAGE AND DURATION OF THERAPY

For deep-seated infections caused by *B. cereus,* optimal dosages of clindamycin and vancomycin are indicated. In patients with *Bacillus* endocarditis, vancomycin (1 g every 12 h) may be used, with dosage adjusted to achieve peak therapeutic levels of 30 to 40 μg/mL and trough levels of 5 to 10 μg/mL. Gentamicin (3–5 mg/kg/day in divided dosages) is adjusted to peak therapeutic levels of 4 to 10 μg/mL and trough levels of 1 to 2 μg/mL. Gentamicin may be used in combination with vancomycin, especially in left-sided endocarditis. In the setting of drug abuse, vancomycin or clindamycin can be used; both have been proven efficacious with successful outcomes. Dosage of clindamycin may vary from 600 to 900 mg every 6 to 8 hours depending on the severity of the illness.

The same antibiotics may be used for osteomyelitis, and the duration of treatment may be longer, depending on the adequacy of surgical debridement. Treatment can be as long as 6 months, depending on healing of wounds and fractures (12). Clindamycin may be preferred for osteomyelitis because higher levels of drug are achieved in bone tissues.

For ocular infections, doses of clindamycin or vancomycin in combination with gentamicin are similar to those outlined above for the treatment of deep-seated infections. In addition, intraocular administration of antibiotics as described above is equally important. Clindamycin is preferred by ophthalmologists because of good penetration in ocular tissues and on the basis of limited in vitro synergy data.

In patients with uncomplicated bacteremia, dosages for either vancomycin or clindamycin are as stated above. Duration of treatment can vary from 7 to 14 days, depending on the severity of the illness and underlying host defense impairment.

Depending on the clinical setting, one may prefer to use vancomycin rather than clindamycin; for example, in a nosocomially acquired infection when there is concern about *Clostridium difficile* colitis as a complication. Newer drugs (e.g., imipenem and quinolones) appear to be active, but more experience is needed in their use. There has been limited experience with the use of oral antibiotics in the treatment of *B. cereus* infections. A patient who developed severe wound infection with bacteremia caused by *B. cereus* was treated successfully with ciprofloxacin 750 mg every 12 hours for almost 3 months (8). Doxycycline was used to treat Hickman catheter–associated bacteremia caused by *B. cereus* in a patient with non-Hodgkins lymphoma (11).

After completion of recommended parenteral antibiotics treatment, the clinician may choose to extend treatment with oral antibiotics in such settings as chronic osteomyelitis and soft tissue infections. Oral ciprofloxacin or clindamycin are reasonable choices.

ENDPOINTS FOR MONITORING THERAPY

To monitor response to therapy, clinical parameters can be followed such as resolution of fever and feeling of well-being. Involved sites such as skin and soft tissues for decreased tenderness, swelling, or erythema can be examined. In addition, blood cultures should be repeated to ensure clearance of any bacteremia. With endocarditis, follow-up echocardiography to assess the size of vegetation and/or valve function (including prosthetic valves) may be useful. CT scans may help in detecting recurrent emboli in cases of endocarditis or in detecting loculated infections. Although a nonspecific parameter, the erythrocyte sedimentation rate may be helpful, especially with endocarditis, osteomyelitis, or other deep-seated infections. When adequate debridement has been performed, persistent isolation of *Bacillus* species is an indication for repeat susceptibility testing to ensure that the organism remains sensitive to the antibiotic being administered.

REFERENCES

1. Ball SC, Sepkowitz K. Infection due to *Bacillus cereus* in an injection drug user with AIDS: bacteremia without morbidity. Clin Infect Dis 1994;19:216–217.
2. Cotton DJ, Gill VJ, Marshall DJ, Gress J, Thaler M, Pizzo PA. Clinical features and therapeutic interventions in 17 cases of Bacillus bacteremia in an immunosuppresed patient population. J Clin Microb 1987;25:672–674.
3. Drobniewski FA. *Bacillus cereus* and related species. Clin Microb Rev 1993;6:324–338.
4. Gigantelli JW, Torres Gomez J, Osato MS. In vitro susceptibilities of ocular *Bacillus cereus* isolates to clindamycin, gentamicin and vancomycin alone or in combination. Antimicrob Agents Chemother 1991;35:201–202.
5. Hemady R, Zaltas M, Paton B, Foster CS, Baker AS. Bacillus

endophthalmitis: new series of 10 cases and review of the literature. Br J Ophthalmol 1990;74:26–29.

6. Jenson HB, Levy Sr, Duncan C, McIntosh S. Treatment of multiple brain abscesses caused by *Bacillus cereus*. Pediatr Infect Dis J 1989;8:795–798.

7. Kervick GN, Flynn HW, Alfonso E, Miller D. Antibiotic therapy for Bacillus species infections. Am J Opthalmal 1990;110: 683–687.

8. Kemmerly SA, Pankey GA. Oral ciprofloxacin therapy for *Bacillus cereus* wound infection and bacteremia. Clin Infect Dis 1993;16:189.

9. Krause A, Freeman R, Sisson PR, Murphy OM. Infection with *Bacillus cereus* after close-range gunshot injuries. J Trauma 1996;41:546–548.

10. Morgan BS, Larson B, Peyman GA, West CS. Toxicity of antibiotic combinations for vitrectomy infusion fluid. Ophthalmic Surg 1979;10:74–77.

11. Saleh RA, Schorin MA. Bacillus sepsis is associated with Hickman catheters in patients with neoplastic disease. Pediatr Infect Dis J 1987;6:851–856.

12. Schricker ME, Thompson GH, Schreiker JR. Osteomyelitis due to *Bacillus cereus* in an adolescent: case report and review. Clin Infect Dis 1994;18:863–867.

13. Shamsuddin D, Tuazon CU, Levy C, Curtin J. *Bacillus cereus* panophthalmitis: source of the organism. Rev Infect Dis 1982; 4:97–103.

14. Sliman R, Rehm S, Shlaes DM. Serious infections caused by Bacillus sp. Medicine (Baltimore) 1987;66:218–223.

15. Steen MK, Bruno-Murtha LA, Chaux G, Lazar H, Mernard S, Sulis C. *Bacillus cereus* endocarditis: report of a case and review. Clin Infect Dis 1992;14:945–946.

16. Swayne RS, Rampling A, Newsom SWB. Intraventricular vancomycin for treatment of shunt associated ventriculitis. J Antimicrob Chemother 1987;19:249–253.

17. Tuazon CU, Hill R, Sheagen SN. Microbiologic study of street heroin and injection paraphernalia. J Infect Dis 1974;129: 327–329.

18. Tuazon CU, Murray HW, Levy C, Solny M, Curtin JA, Sheagren JN. Serious infections from Bacillus sp. JAMA 1979;241: 1137–1145.

19. Tuazon CU. Other Bacillus species In: Mandell, Bennett, Dolin, eds. Principles and practice of infectious diseases. New York: Churchill Livingstone, 1994:1890–1894.

20. Turnbull P, Kramer J, Melling J. Bacillus. In: Topley and Wilson principles of bacteriology, virology and immunity. 8th ed. London: Edward Arnold, 1990:185–210.

21. Weber DJ, Saviteer SM, Rutala WA, et al. In vitro susceptibility of Bacillus spp. to selected antimicrobial agents. Antimicrob Agents Chemother 1988;32:642–645.

22. Wong MT, Dolan MJ. Significant infections due to Bacillus species following abrasions associated with motor vehicle-related trauma. Clin Infect Dis 1992;15:855–857.

Bacteroides fragilis Group

●

David W. Hecht

GENERAL DESCRIPTION
Microbiology

Bacteroides spp. are nonsporeforming Gram-negative bacilli that are part of the human resident flora. Microbiologically, they are distinguished from other genera by growth in 20% bile. At present, the *Bacteroides fragilis* group consists of 10 species: *B. fragilis* (the most frequent isolate), *B. distasonis*, *B. thetaiotaomicron*, *B. vulgatus*, *B. ovatus*, *B. eggerrthii*, *B. merdae*, *B. stercoris*, *B. uniformis*, and *B. caccae*. Since 1990, many organisms previously designated as *Bacteroides* have been reclassified (see chapter on anaerobes other than *Bacteroides*). *Bacteroides,* the predominant genus in the human intestine, are important in numerous metabolic activities and may provide some protection from invasive pathogens. All 10 species are usually isolated from the colon, although infections caused by or associated with them can include virtually any organ.

Isolation and identification of *Bacteroides* spp. pose a hurdle to many clinical laboratories; most only identify the genus. Other laboratories may identify *B. fragilis* species and lump all others into the *B. fragilis* group. Further, if more than three anaerobic organisms are isolated in a clinical specimen, many laboratories do not perform further identification. Those laboratories that do identify *Bacteroides* frequently do not perform susceptibility testing. Lack of identification and susceptibility testing of anaerobes can be attributed in part to its expense and the lack of timeliness in providing relevant information to the clinician (42). Thus, choice of therapy for infections that may involve *Bacteroides* is empirical.

Clinical Manifestations

Nearly any infection involving *Bacteroides* spp. includes abscess formation, and they are frequent isolates in polymicrobial infections. Typical sites of polymicrobial infections involving *Bacteroides* include the abdomen and pelvis, perirectal area, skin and soft tissue, and solid organs. Although isolation of *Bacteroides* spp. as the sole pathogen can occur, it is unusual. Single-organism isolation most commonly associated with *Bacteroides* involves endocarditis, meningitis, septic arthritis, and osteomyelitis (32).

SUSCEPTIBILITY IN VITRO

In general, *Bacteroides* spp. grow well on enriched media in an anaerobic environment. Aerotolerance is greater in this genus than with more fastidious anaerobes. Historically, susceptibility testing of *Bacteroides* has used a variety of media and methods. The National Committee for Clinical Laboratory Standards (NCCLS) recommends the agar dilution method as the reference standard (66). The testing medium recommended is *Brucella* agar supplemented with lysed sheep blood, vitamin K_1, and hemin, which supports the growth of virtually all anaerobes. This method is generally time consuming and expensive to perform, leading to its infrequent use. Alternative methods include a limited agar dilution or a broth microdilution technique, although the latter method has not been well standardized to agar dilution (2, 47). In addition to the NCCLS-approved methods, the Food and Drug Administration (FDA) has also approved use of the E-test gradient method, which is a more rapid but somewhat expensive method (18, 81). Currently, the NCCLS recommends testing to monitor susceptibility patterns as a guide for empirical antibiotic choice for individual patients when there is known resistance of a particular species, failure of a usual regimen, a pivotal role of the antimicrobial agent in determining outcome, and the need for long-term therapy. In particular, susceptibility testing is indicated for isolates from brain abscess, meningitis, osteomyelitis, joint infections, infection of prosthetic devices or vascular grafts, and refractory bacteremia (66).

For the purpose of this chapter, in vitro data for each of the antibiotics were chosen from published studies using NCCLS agar dilution or broth microdilution methodology. Intermediate and susceptible breakpoints for each antibiotic with activity against *Bacteroides* were set by the NCCLS (66). The intermediate range was established because of the difficulty in reading endpoints and the clustering of MICs at breakpoint concentrations. With maximum dosages of appropriate antibiotics, organisms with susceptible or intermediate endpoints are generally considered amenable to therapy. Susceptibility among the different species of the *B. fragilis* group can vary significantly. Table 1 contains susceptibility results from various recent publications for the most frequently isolated species.

Penicillins

Penicillin-hydrolyzing activity in *B. fragilis* group members was first recognized in 1968 (74). More than 90% of clinical isolates produce β-lactamases that are predominantly active against cephalosporins, have high activity, are cell associated, and are produced constituitively (3, 22, 69, 102). Thus most *Bacteroides* isolates are resistant to penicillin G and ampicillin but may remain susceptible to cephamycins and extended-spectrum penicillins. Table 1 illustrates the comparative activities of ticarcillin and piperacillin. Ticarcillin is moderately active against *B. fragilis* group members, while piperacillin demonstrates significantly greater activity. However, recent data demonstrates steadily decreasing activity of piperacillin over the period of 1990 to 1994, noted by increasing MIC_{50} and MIC_{90} values (90). Susceptibility may range from 30 to 90%, depending on the species tested (46), with *B. thetaiotaomicron* and *B. distasonis* the most resistant.

Penicillins Plus β-Lactamase Inhibitors

Most of the β-lactamases produced by *B. fragilis* group members are inhibited by sulbactam, clavulanic acid, and tazobactam. As a result, nearly all isolates of the *B. fragilis* group are susceptible to ampicillin/sulbactam, ticarcillin/clavulanate, and piperacillin/tazobactam. All three combinations demonstrate very potent activity against members of the *B. fragilis* group, although strains of *B. distasonis* that do not produce β-lactamases have somewhat higher MIC values (Table 1) (55, 108). Susceptibility of *Bacteroides* to these agents has not changed significantly from 1990 to 1994 (90).

Cephalosporins

Three cephamycins (cefoxitin, cefotetan, cefmetazole) and two extended-spectrum cephalosporins (ceftizoxime, moxalactam) have demonstrated generally good activity against *B. fragilis* group members, although marked differences among species can be noted for some agents. Cefoxitin is the most potent in this class, with 90% of strains below the susceptible or indeterminate breakpoint, although resistance has been noted to occur in clusters (21). Its activity is similar against all members of the *B. fragilis* group. The two other cephamycins, cefotetan and cefmetazole, have activity similar to that of cefoxitin against *B. fragilis*. However, their activity against the non-*fragilis* members of the *B. fragilis* group is significantly lower and species dependent (Table 1) (20). Ceftizoxime has been shown to have activity against most *Bacteroides* spp. Early studies demonstrated activity similar to that of cefoxitin, but more-recent data suggest resistance to this agent is increasing (45, 68, 90, 107). Moxalactam also has excellent in vitro activity but is little used because of serious side effects. Broad-spectrum cephalosporins, including cefaclor, cefuroxime, cefotaxime, cetazidime, cefpodoxime, and cefepime have generally poor activity against the *B. fragilis* group and are generally not considered effective against these organisms (92).

Carbapenems

The carbapenems, imipenem and meropenem, are resistant to hydrolysis by a number of β-lactamases, including those of *Bacteroides* spp. Thus, both agents demonstrate excellent activity against all species within the *B. fragilis* group. MIC_{90} values for both imipenem and meropenem are 2 μg/mL or less (46, 75, 90). Overall, the susceptibility of *B. fragilis* group members to the carbapenems is 99.5% in the United States. Most resistant strains produce a zinc metalloenzyme β-lactamase (52). The significantly higher levels of resistance reported in Japan is attributed to significantly greater use of imipenem in that country (5). Resistance to carbapenems also confers cross-resistance to all β-lactam agents, including the β-lactam/β-lactamase inhibitor combinations.

Clindamycin

Historically, *B. fragilis* group members have been highly susceptible to clindamycin and its predecessor lincomycin (20,

TABLE 1 • Comparative Activity of Antimicrobial Agents against *B. fragilis* Group Species

Antibiotic	NCCLS Breakpoints[a] (S, I)	B. fragilis			B. distasonis			B. thetaiotamicron			B. ovatus			B. vulgatus		
		MIC$_{50}$	MIC$_{90}$	Range	MIC$_{50}$	MIC$_{90}$	Range	MIC$_{50}$	MIC$_{90}$	Range	MIC$_{50}$	MIC$_{90}$	Range	MIC$_{50}$	MIC$_{90}$	Range
Ticarcillin	(32,64)	32	≥128	NA[b]	≥128	≥128	NA	64	≥128	NA	64	≥128	NA	32	≥128	NA
Piperacillin	(32,64)	16	256	NA	64	≥128	NA	32	≥128	NA	32	≥128	NA	64	≥128	NA
Cefoxitin	(16,32)	8	32	2–≥56	16	32	4–256	8	16	1–≥256	8	16	2–64	4	16	2–64
Cefotetan	(16,32)	8	64	2–≥256	128	≥256	4–≥256	64	≥256	1–≥256	64	128	2–128	4	128	2–256
Ceftizoxime	(32,64)[d]	64	≥128	4–≥256	32	≥256	1–≥256	64	256	1–≥256	32	256	4–≥256	16	128	1–≥256
Imipenem	(4,8)	0.5	0.5	0.015–4	0.06	0.25	0.015–0.25	0.5	1	0.03–4	0.125	0.25	0.015–0.5	0.25	0.5	0.015–0.5
Meropenem	(4,8)	0.5	0.5	0.015–4	0.06	0.25	0.015–0.25	0.5	1	0.03–4	0.125	0.25	0.015–0.5	0.25	0.5	0.015–0.5
Amoxicillin/clavulanate	(4,8)	1	4	0.25–4	2	32	0.125–32	1	2	0.125–4	2	8	0.25–16	2	8	0.25–8
Ampicillin/sulbactam	(8,16)	2	8	NA	8	32	NA	4	16	NA	4	16	NA	4	16	NA
Piperacillin/tazobactam	(32,64)	0.5	4	NA	8	32	NA	8	16	NA	8	16	NA	8	16	NA
Ticarcillin/clavulanate	(32,64)	1	8	NA	16	64	NA	4	16	NA	4	16	NA	2	8	NA
Clindamycin	(2,4)	0.5	128	0.06–≥128	2	≥128	0.06–≥128	4	≥128	0.06–≥128	2	≥128	0.06–≥128	0.06	≥128	0.03–≥128
Chloramphenicol[c]	(8,16)	—	≤8	NA	—	≤8	NA	—	≤8	NA	—	≤8	NA	—	≤8	NA
Metronidazole	(8,16)	0.5	0.5	0.25–1	0.5	0.5	0.25–1	0.5	1	0.25–1	0.5	1	0.25–1	0.5	0.5	0.25–1
Trovafloxacin	(2,4)	0.25	2	0.25–2	0.5	1	0.125–1	0.5	2	0.25–4	1	2	0.125–2	0.25	4	0.125–4

Data based upon various published studies.

[a] S, I; susceptible and intermediate breakpoints in µg/mL.

[b] Not available.

[c] Drug tested only at screening dilutions.

[d] Breakdowns are (16, 32) using broth microdilution.

34). Throughout the 1970s, clindamycin demonstrated the greatest activity with an MIC_{90} of 4 μg/mL or less for most clinical isolates (96). However, by the late 1970s, isolates with high-level resistance to clindamycin emerged (83). In 1979, three laboratories reported identification of a clindamycin-resistance gene on transferable plasmids (84). Further, these genes shared more than 95% homology among their coding sequences (77). Subsequently, resistance among *Bacteroides* spp. has increased in the United States and worldwide. In one report, resistance at four Chicago area medical centers exceeded 25% (45). High-level clindamycin resistance is now reported worldwide (6). Among the different species, *B. fragilis* and *B. vulgatus* are the most susceptible (MIC_{50} = 1 and 0.25 μg/mL, respectively), although the MIC_{90} for both species has exceeded 256 (46). A national survey has confirmed a rising trend in resistance among all members of the *B. fragilis* group from 1990 to 1994 (90).

Chloramphenicol

Chloramphenicol is very active against all members of the *B. fragilis* group. Resistance has been reported rarely and is due to inactivation by either a nitroreductase or chloramphenicol acetyltransferase, and resistance transfer has been reported (10, 44, 82). Use of the this drug for clinical infections involving anaerobes is generally limited, primarily because of concerns about toxicity.

Aminoglycosides

Bacteroides are uniformly resistant to aminoglycosides. This is likely due to a failure to transport the aminoglycosides into bacterial cells and their inability to reach the ribosomal target site (14).

Metronidazole

Nitroimidazoles, including metronidazole, have high activity against *Bacteroides,* with MIC_{90} values of 1 μg/mL or less (64). They are bactericidal and penetrate well into abscesses, frequently making them ideal candidates in therapy. Resistance to metronidazole is extremely rare and has been limited primarily to strains isolated in France (79). The resistance determinant has been localized to two different transferable plasmids (78), suggesting that resistance may increase over time.

Fluoroquinolones

The activity of several fluoroquinolones has been evaluated against anaerobes including the *B. fragilis* group. Ciprofloxacin, ofloxacin, levofloxacin, sparfloxacin, and grepafloxacin have generally fair-to-poor activity against members of the *B. fragilis* group, with MIC_{90} values that range from 2 to 32 μg/mL, although they demonstrate greater activity against non-*Bacteroides* anaerobes (41, 49). Trovafloxacin is a new trifluoronaphthyridone that demonstrates significantly greater activity against all members of the *B. fragilis* group (MIC_{90} = 0.39–2 μg/mL) (48, 93). Investigational agents, including DU6859a and clinafloxacin, also appear very active in vitro and await results of clinical trials (110, 111).

Tetracyclines

Once a mainstay in therapy of anaerobic infections in the 1960s, more than 80% of *Bacteroides* isolates are now resistant to tetracyclines (30). Tetracycline derivatives, the glycylcyclines, demonstrate excellent in vitro activity but are still in early investigational studies (109).

ANTIMICROBIAL THERAPY

The principles of treatment for infection involving members of the *B. fragilis* group are (*a*) making the environment inhospitable for anaerobic bacterial proliferation, (*b*) checking the spread of anaerobic bacteria into healthy tissues, (*c*) neutralizing the toxins of anaerobes, and (*d*) supportive care (31). Control of the local environment includes debriding necrotic tissue, draining pus collections, and improving oxygenation. For intraabdominal abscesses, this can be performed via surgery or percutaneously. Failure of a patient to improve within 48 hours after initial drainage is an indication for repeat radiographic scanning and drainage, or laparotomy. When a drain has been placed, criteria for removal of the catheter include clinical resolution of sepsis, minimal drainage from catheter, and radiographic evidence of abscess resolution.

Antimicrobial therapy is an important adjunct to removal of infected tissues. Most infections involving *B. fragilis* are polymicrobial, involving aerobes and anaerobes. Thus, antibiotic therapy usually requires activity against both *B. fragilis* and enteric Gram-negative and/or Gram-positive organisms, depending upon the site of isolation. In general, maximum dosages of antimicrobial agents recommended by the manufacturers are suggested for infections involving *B. fragilis* group members (66).

Intraabdominal and Pelvic Infections

B. fragilis is isolated in 70% of cases of intraabdominal infection involving abscesses (7). Early on, animal models demonstrated the importance of anaerobes, particularly *B. fragilis,* in intraabdominal infection and abscess formation (70). The first clinical trial in humans, reported in 1973, compared cephalothin/kanamycin with clindamycin/kanamycin (103). The infectious complication rate due to anaerobes noted in the cephalothin/kanamycin group was 21%, compared with 2% in the clindamycin/kanamycin group. This study established that treatment of the anaerobe was important, and clindamycin/aminoglycoside became the "gold standard" to which other regimens were compared. Treatment of facultative bacteria is also important (17, 26). Interested readers are referred to an excellent review for a summary of comparative clinical trials (43). Of particular note are the studies that do not require an aminoglycoside in combination with clindamycin, and the use of monotherapy (61, 65).

Drugs of Choice

Table 2 lists suitable agents determined to be effective in clinical trials, either as monotherapy or in combination. Monotherapy with a carbapenem (imipenem, 500 mg i.v. q. 6 h; meropenem, 1 g i.v. q. 8 h), β-lactam/β-lactamase inhibitor combinations (ampicillin/sulbactam 3 g i.v. q. 6 h; ticarcillin/

TABLE 2 • Comparative Antimicrobial Trials for Treatment of Intraabdominal and Pelvic Infections

Intraabdominal

Cefoxitin ± aminoglycoside vs. clindamycin + aminoglycoside	(25, 67, 101)
Ceftizoxime vs. cefoxitin	(7)
Piperacillin vs. cefoxitin	(62)
Ampicillin/sulbactam vs. clindamycin + aminoglycoside	(95)
Imipenem vs. clindamycin + aminoglycoside	(85, 91)
Aztreonam + clindamycin vs. clindamycin + aminoglycoside	(8, 113)
Aztreonam + clindamycin vs. imipenem	(23)
Ticarcillin/clavulanate vs. clindamycin + aminoglycoside	(35)
Piperacillin/tazobactam vs. imipenem	(9)
Piperacillin/tazobactam vs. clindamycin + aminoglycoside	(76)
Meropenem vs. clindamycin + tobramycin	(19)
Meropenem vs. cefotaxime + metronidazole	(57)

Pelvic

Piperacillin vs. cefoxitin	(99)
Piperacillin vs. clindamycin + gentamicin	(38)
Piperacillin/tazobactam vs. clindamycin + gentamicin	(100)
Ampicillin/sulbactam vs. clindamycin	(60)
Imipenem vs. clindamycin + gentamicin	(59)
Meropenem vs. clindamycin + gentamicin	(50)

clavulanate 3.1 g i.v. q. 8 h; piperacillin/tazobactam 3.375 g i.v. q. 6 h), or metronidazole (500 mg i.v. or p.o. q. 6 h) combined with either an aminoglycoside or a third-generation cephalosporin could be considered the most active. Clindamycin (900 mg i.v. q. 8 h)/aminoglycoside, piperacillin (3 g i.v. q. 6 h)/aminoglycoside, cefoxitin (2 g i.v. q. 6 h), cefotetan (2 g i.v. q. 12 h), and ceftizoxime (2 g i.v. q. 8 h) might now be considered second-line therapy because of concerns about resistance among aerobic and anaerobic organisms. Among the quinolones, trovafloxacin (300 mg i.v. q.d., 200 mg p.o. q.d.) has demonstrated activity equivalent to that of imipenem (unpublished data submitted to FDA) and has recent FDA approval for complicated intraabdominal infections. The principle behind all agents listed as monotherapy or in combination is to treat *B. fragilis,* other anaerobes, and *Enterobacteriaceae.* However, the choice of antimicrobial therapy may require modification depending upon the clinical setting. For example, a patient who develops an intraabdominal infection while in hospital may be colonized with more-resistant Gram-negative organisms, such as *Pseudomonas* or resistant *Enterobacter* spp.

Antimicrobial therapy for pelvic infections involving *Bacteroides* spp. is similar to intraabdominal therapy. Polymicrobial infections that include *B. fragilis* group organisms and involve the female genital tract and pelvis include soft-tissue infection following episiotomy, postpartum endometritis, pelvic abscess, tuboovarian abscess, and acute pelvic inflammatory disease. Most agents listed in Table 2 have demonstrated similar clinical efficacy against *B. fragilis* as part of a polymicrobial infection in this setting (60, 98, 100). Failures associated with these regimens are usually due to *Enterococcus.* A specific regimen is recommended for pelvic inflammatory disease. Current recommendations from the Centers for Disease Control and Prevention include cefoxitin (2 g i.v. q. 6 h) or cefotetan (2 g i.v. q. 12 h) plus doxycycline (100 mg p.o. b.i.d.), or clindamycin (900 mg i.v. q. 8 h) plus gentamicin followed by doxycycline (15). These regimens are recommended for treatment of *Chlamydia trachomatis* and *Neisseria gonorrhoeae* in addition to *B. fragilis* and other anaerobes.

Bacteremia

B. fragilis is the most common anaerobe isolated from blood cultures, although the frequency of positive cultures is decreasing overall (11, 24, 106). In virtually all cases, isolation of a member of the *B. fragilis* group from blood indicates underlying infection (106) and is associated with 60% mortality if untreated (16). The source of bacteremia is most commonly intraabdominal, female genital tract, or soft tissue (33, 36, 72).

Drug of Choice

Empirical antimicrobial therapy of *Bacteroides* bacteremia includes parenteral agents that are effective against *B. fragilis* and aerobic organisms, depending upon the source of bacteremia (Table 2). Specific choices of an agent against *Bacteroides* should be guided by local patterns of resistance or susceptibility results for the isolate. *Bacteroides* strains demonstrating higher MICs have been correlated with treatment failure (89). Identification and drainage of the source of bacteremia remains a mainstay of nonantibiotic therapy.

Skin and Soft Tissue

B. fragilis is not considered part of the normal skin flora. However, these organisms are an important cause of disease when soft tissues are damaged and in diabetes. The most serious infections involving *B. fragilis* include synergistic necrotizing fasciitis and Fournier's gangrene. Other infections include wound infections following abdominal or pelvic surgery, pilonidal cysts, decubitus wounds, and diabetic foot ulcers (39,94). The role of anaerobes in uncomplicated diabetic foot infection has been debated, with only 13% of these infections associated with anaerobes (mostly Gram-positive) in one study (4, 37).

Drug of Choice

Treatment of *B. fragilis* in serious soft tissue infection requires parenteral therapy resembling that used for abdominal infections (Table 2). Thus, empirical coverage for Gram-negative and Gram-positive anaerobes plus enteric Gram-negative organisms is required. Empirical coverage for *Staphylococcus aureus* and streptococci may be considered in more serious infections until culture results are available. Ampicillin/sulbactam (3 g i.v. q. 6 h) with or without an aminoglycoside, ticarcillin/clavulanate (3.1 g i.v. q. 8 h), piperacillin/tazobactam (3.375 g i.v. q. 6 h), imipenem (500 mg i.v. q. 6 h) or meropenem (1 g i.v. q. 8 h), or a combination of metronidazole (500 mg i.v. or p.o. q. 6 h)/aminoglycoside (if staphylococci or streptococci are not suspected) may be suitable for empirical therapy. Patients who have been hospitalized may have resistant Gram-negative aerobic bacteria as well and the antimicrobial choice should be modified accordingly. Changes in the empirical regimen should be guided by culture results. For less serious soft tissue infections, such as the diabetic foot, parenteral or oral agents can be used. Currently, recommendations for empirical parenteral therapy include β-lactam/β-lactamase inhibitor combinations (ampicillin/sulbactam 3 g i.v. q. 6 h); ticarcillin/clavulanate (3.1 g i.v. q. 8 h); piperacillin/tazobactam (3.375 g i.v. q. 6 h), clindamycin (900 mg i.v. q. 8 h) plus a third-generation cephalosporin or fluoroquinolone, cefoxitin (2 g i.v. q. 6 h) or ceftizoxime (2 g i.v. q. 8 h) or metronidazole (500 mg i.v. or p.o. q. 6 h) plus a fluoroquinolone (ciprofloxacin 750 mg p.o. b.i.d.; ofloxacin, 200 mg p.o. b.i.d.) (37). Therapy may also require coverage for *Pseudomonas,* depending upon culture results. Examples of effective oral therapy include clindamycin (300 mg p.o q.i.d.) or metronidazole (250–500 mg p.o. q.i.d.) in combination with a fluoroquinolone, or monotherapy with amoxicillin/clavulanate (500 mg p.o. t.i.d. or 875 mg p.o. b.i.d.), or trovafloxacin (200 mg p.o. q.d.) when *Bacteroides* spp. are involved (37, 56, 73).

Special Situations

Bacteroides spp. can be the sole cause of infection in certain rare clinical situations, requiring special consideration. Endocarditis, osteomyelitis, septic arthritis, and meningitis are four such examples. In addition, brain abscesses caused by *B. fragilis* alone or in a mixed infection require special consideration. In all circumstances, antibiotic susceptibility of *B. fragilis* should be tested to determine the most appropriate antibiotic.

Endocarditis, Pericarditis, and Vascular Graft Infections

Bacteroides fragilis is one of the most common causes of anaerobic infective endocarditis, although overall quite rare. It is usually associated with large valvular vegetations and peripheral embolization (33). Thrombophlebitis and congestive heart failure are common complications as well (64). Mortality is reported to be as high as 46% (28).

Drug of Choice

Bactericidal antimicrobials are indicated in treatment of anaerobic infective endocarditis. In experimental endocarditis due to *B. fragilis,* metronidazole alone or in combination with clindamycin was superior to clindamycin or cefoxitin alone (40). The potent activity of carbapenems and possibly β-lactam/β-lactamase inhibitors may also prove effective. In a recent report of one patient, imipenem was administered, followed by a combination of ampicillin/clavulanate and metronidazole with a successful outcome (54).

   B. fragilis is an extremely rare cause of pericarditis, mycotic aneurysm, and vascular graft infection. All three clinical situations are associated with high mortality, and no specific data on antimicrobial efficacy are available (86, 88). This author suggests choosing the most potent antimicrobial that is bactericidal (such as metronidazole) in conjunction with appropriate surgical intervention.

Meningitis

B. fragilis is a rare cause of meningitis in the absence of brain abscess and is found most commonly in neonates as a result of congenital malformations, necrotizing enterocolitis, bowel perforation, or shunts. Anaerobes are so rare a cause of meningitis that clinical laboratories do not routinely culture cerebrospinal fluid for them. Thus, the only clue may be positive blood cultures (27).

Drug of Choice

Treatment of *B. fragilis* meningitis requires bactericidal therapy with metronidazole (500 mg i.v. or p.o. q. 6 h). Because of limited or unknown penetration of β-lactam/β-lactamase inhibitors and imipenem, these agents cannot be recommended (71, 104, 105). Further, *B. fragilis* meningitis treated with chloramphenicol has resulted in death or failure that required a change to metronidazole. Chloramphenicol failure is likely due to its bacteriostatic activity against *B. fragilis.* Some authors have measured bactericidal activity during therapy as a guide (27). Meropenem has recently been approved for treatment of meningitis; its efficacy against *B. fragilis* in this setting is unknown.

Septic Arthritis

In the largest review of anaerobic septic arthritis, 20 of 180 cases were caused by *B. fragilis* (29). Of the *Bacteroides* cases, most were from hematogenous spread, with the knee as the most commonly involved joint. Prosthetic joints appear more susceptible to anaerobic infection, primarily with peptostreptococci followed by *B. fragilis* (13,63).

Drug of Choice

Therapy for joint infections is directed at the *B. fragilis* group species and its susceptibility. Given the limited clinical experience, metronidazole (500 mg i.v. or p.o q. 6 h), carbapenems (imipenem, 500 mg i.v. q. 6 h; meropenem, 1 g i.v. q. 8 h), and β-lactam/β-lactamase inhibitor combinations (ampicillin/sulbactam, 3 g i.v. q. 6 h; ticarcillin/clavulanate, 3.1 g i.v. q. 8 h; piperacillin/tazobactam, 3.375 g i.v. q. 6 h) are suitable empirical choices until susceptibility results are obtained. Duration of therapy is usually 4 to 6 weeks. Prosthetic joints usually require removal, followed by 4 to 6 weeks of antibiotic therapy. A recent case of *B. fragilis* septic arthritis in a patient with sickle cell disease was treated successfully with 4 weeks of metronidazole and chloramphenicol (58).

Brain Abscess

B. fragilis is frequently isolated as a component of a mixed infection in brain abscesses. Previous studies have reported *Bacteroides* to be isolated as frequently as 20 to 60% from culture, associated with a number of other pathogens (particularly streptococci) (12,97). This high percentage represents inclusion of organisms formerly classified as *Bacteroides*.

Drug of Choice

Historically, treatment of brain abscess has included penicillin (20–24 million units/day) and chloramphenicol (1 g i.v. q. 6 h) as empirical therapy (97). However, while penicillin remains a mainstay of therapy, chloramphenicol has been largely replaced with metronidazole. Metronidazole (500 mg i.v. or p.o q. 6 h) provides several advantages, including its bactericidal activity and excellent concentration in brain abscess pus (1, 53, 87, 97). It is not affected by steroids, and the superior outcomes may reflect degradation of chloramphenicol in pus. No randomized trials have been conducted to compare these two agents. Patients suspected of having staphylococci as a component of the abscess should be treated with nafcillin in place of penicillin, along with metronidazole. Alternatives for penicillin-allergic patients include cefotaxime (3 g i.v. q. 8 h). Duration of therapy, when surgery is performed, depends upon clinical and radiologic response. Generally, 4 to 6 weeks of therapy are required. When surgical drainage is not performed, longer duration may be attempted (6–8 weeks). Although some patients respond to medical management alone, most require surgical therapy. Aspiration and drainage by stereotaxic computed tomographic (CT) guidance may suffice in conjunction with antibiotics for stable patients without progressive neurologic signs (80).

Osteomyelitis

The site of infection is important when *B. fragilis* is suspected as part of a polymicrobial aerobic/anaerobic osteomyelitis. Trauma and direct spread from contiguous foci are the principle factors indicating development of anaerobic osteomyelitis. *B. fragilis* is most frequently associated with osteomyelitis when peripheral vascular disease secondary to diabetes is present (4). Using careful culture techniques, 70% of diabetes-associated osteomyelitis cases are polymicrobial, with *B. fragilis* as the second most common anaerobe isolated (112).

Drug of Choice

Treatment requires identification of the infecting organism from bone and susceptibility testing of *B. fragilis* group isolates, when possible (13). Empirical therapy should be based upon knowledge of resistance of the *Bacteroides* spp. and coinfecting organisms. Agents that may be suitable as monotherapy or in combination include cefoxitin (2 g i.v. q. 6 h), clindamycin (600–900 mg i.v. q. 8 h), metronidazole (500 mg q. 6–8 h), β-lactam/β-lactamase inhibitors (ampicillin/sulbactam, 3 g i.v. q. 6 h; ticarcillin/clavulanate, 3.1 g i.v. q. 8 h; piperacillin/tazobactam 3.375 g i.v. q. 6 h), and carbapenems (imipenem, 500 mg i.v. q. 6 h; meropenem, 1 g i.v. q. 8 h). Trovafloxacin may be an alternative therapeutic choice, although data are not yet available. Therapy should continue for 4 to 6 weeks, although prolonged oral therapy including amoxicillin/clavulanate (500 mg p.o. t.i.d. or 875 mg p.o. b.i.d.) may be required when vascular insufficiency is not corrected.

Alternative Therapy

Hyperbaric oxygen treatment has been advocated as an adjunct for more serious infections involving *B. fragilis* group and other anaerobes. Despite its use, data supporting its role in the treatment of *B. fragilis* infections are not conclusive (51).

COMMENTS

The role of *B. fragilis* has been well established for many types of infection. However, as a component of a polymicrobial infection, it is difficult to determine if the organism is always playing a dominant role. In the most serious infections involving *B. fragilis,* there appears to be good correlation between susceptibility test results and clinical response. However, it is more difficult to correlate specific susceptibility results with clinical outcomes in individual cases. The clinical outcome may be difficult to assess for many reasons. Some patients may respond without antimicrobial therapy or to inappropriate chemotherapy, with or without surgical intervention. The effects of surgical drainage, debridement, and other procedures are also important. Improper surgical management may result in poor clinical outcome even when antimicrobial therapy is adequate, and proper surgical management may result in a good outcome despite inappropriate antimicrobial therapy (66).

REFERENCES

1. Alderson D, Strong AJ, Ingham HR, Selkon JB. Fifteen year review of the mortality of brain abscess. Neurosurgery 1981; 8:1–6.
2. Aldridge KE, Schiro DD. Major methodology-dependent discordant susceptibility results from *Bacteroides fragilis* group isolates but not other anaerobes. Diagn Microbiol Infect Dis 1994;20:135–142.
3. Anderson JD, Sykes RB. Characterisation of a β-lactamase obtained from a strain of *Bacteroides fragilis* resistant to β-lactamase antibiotics. J Med Microbiol 1973;6:201–206.
4. Bamberger DM, Daus GP, Gerding DN. Osteomyelitis in the feet of diabetic patients. Am J Med 1987;83:653–660.
5. Bandoh K, Ueno K, Watanabe K, Kato N. Susceptibility patterns and resistance to imipenem in the *Bacteroides fragilis* group species in Japan: a 4-year study. Clin Infect Dis 1993;16: S382–S386.
6. Baquero F, Reig M. Resistance of anaerobic bacteria to antimicrobial agents in Spain. Eur J Clin Microbiol Infect Dis 1992; 11:1016–1020.
7. Bennion RS, Thompson JE, Baron EJ, Finegold SM. Gangrenous and perforated appendicitis with peritonitis: treatment and bacteriology. Clin Ther 1990;12:S31–S44.
8. Birolini D, Moraes MF, Soare de Souza O. Aztreonam plus clindamycin vs tobramycin plus clindamycin for the treatment of intra-abdominal infections. Rev Infect Dis 1985;7:S724–S728.
9. Brismar B, Malmborg AS, Tunevall G, Wretlind B, Bergman L, Mentzing LO, Nystrom PO, Kihlstrom E, Backstrand B, Skau T, Kasholm-Tengve B, Sjoberg L, Olsson-Liljequist B, Tally FP, Gatenbeck L, Eklund AE, Nord CE. Piperacillin-tazobactam versus imipenem-cilastatin for treatment of intra-abdominal infections. Antimicrob Agents Chemother 1992;36:2766–2773.
10. Britz ML, Wilkinson RG. Chloramphenicol acetyl-transferase of *Bacteroides fragilis*. Antimicrob Agents Chemother 1978;14: 105–111.

11. Brook I. Anaerobic bacterial bacteremia: 12-year experience in two military hospitals. J Infect Dis 1989;160:1071–1075.

12. Brook I. Aerobic and anaerobic bacteriology of intracranial abscesses. Pediatr Neurol 1992;8:210–214.

13. Brook I, Frazier EH. Anaerobic osteomyelitis and arthritis in a military hospital: a 10-year experience. Am J Med 1993;94:21–28.

14. Bryan LE, Kowand SK, Van Den Elzen JM. Mechanism of aminoglycoside antibiotic resistance in anaerobic bacteria, *Clostridium perfringens* and *Bacteroides fragilis.* Antimicrob Agents Chemother 1979;15:7–13.

15. Centers for Disease Control. Sexually transmitted diseases treatment guidelines. MMWR 1993;42:75–81.

16. Chow AW, Guze LB. Bacteroidaceae bacteremia: clinical experiences with 112 patients. Medicine 1974;53:93–123.

17. Chow AW, Marshall JR, Guze LB. A double-blind comparison of clindamycin with penicillin plus chloramphenicol in treatment of septic abortion. J Infect Dis 1977;135:S35–S39.

18. Citron DM, Ostavari A, Karlsson A, Goldstein EJC. Evaluation of the epsilometer (E-test) for susceptibility testing of anaerobic bacteria. J Clin Microbiol 1991;29:219–2203.

19. Condon RE, Walker AP, Sirinek KR, White PW, Fabian TC, Nichols RL, Wilson SE. Meropenem versus tobramycin plus clindamycin for treatment of intraabdominal infections: results of a prospective, randomized, double-blind clinical trial. Clin Infect Dis 1995;21:544–550.

20. Cuchural GJ, Tally FP, Jacobus NV, Aldridge KE, Cleary TJ, Finegold SM, Hills GB, Iannini PB, O'Keefe JP, Pierson CL, Crook DW, Russo TA, Hecht DW. Susceptibility of *Bacteroides fragilis* group in the United States: analysis by site of isolation. Antimicrob Agents Chemother 1988;32:717–722.

21. Cuchural GJ, Tally FP, Jacobus NV, Marsh PK, Mayhew JW. Cefoxitin inactivation by *Bacteroides fragilis.* Antimicrob Agents Chemother 1983;34:936–940.

22. Darland C, Birnbaum J. Cefoxitin resistance to beta-lactamase: a major factor for susceptibility of *Bacteroides fragilis* to the antibiotic. Antimicrob Agents Chemother 1975;9:725–734.

23. de Groot HGW, Hustinx PA, Lampe AS, Oosterwijk WM. Comparison of imipenem/cilastatin with the combination of aztreonam and clindamycin in the treatment of intra-abdominal infections. J Antimicrob Chemother 1993;32:491–500.

24. Dorsher CW, Rosenblatt JE, Wilson WR, Ilstrup DM. Anaerobic bacteremia: decreasing rate over a 15-year period. Rev Infect Dis 1991;13:633–636.

25. Drusano GL, Warren WJ, Saah AJ, Caplan ES, Tenney JH, Hansen S, Granados J, Standiford HC, Miller EH Jr. A prospective randomized controlled trial of cefoxitin versus clindamycin-aminoglycoside in mixed anaerobic-aerobic infections. Surg Gynecol Obstet 1982;154:715–720.

26. el-Sefi TA, el-Awadi JM, Shehata MI, Al-Hindi MA. The place of antibiotics in the prevention of post-appendicectomy sepsis: a prospective study of 400 cases. Int Surg 1986;71:18–21.

27. Feder HM. *Bacteroides fragilis* meningitis. Rev Infect Dis 1987;9:783–786.

28. Felner JM, Dowell VR, Jr. Anaerobic bacterial endocarditis. N Engl J Med 1970;283:1188–1192.

29. Finegold SM. Bone and joint infections. In: Finegold SM, ed. Anaerobic bacteria in human disease. New York: Academic Press, 1977:433–453.

30. Finegold SM. Therapy and prognosis in anaerobic infections. In: Finegold SM, ed. Anaerobic bacteria in human disease. New York: Academic Press, 1977:534–562.

31. Finegold SM. Therapy of anaerobic infections. In: Finegold SM, George WL, eds. Anaerobic infections in humans. Orlando, FL: Academic Press, 1989:793–818.

32. Finegold SM. General aspects of anaerobic infection. In: Finegold SM, George WL, eds. Anaerobic infections in humans. San Diego: Academic Press, 1989:137–149.

33. Finegold SM, George WL, Mulligan ME. Anaerobic infections. Part I. DM 1985;31:1–77.

34. Finegold SM, Harada NE, Miller LG. Lincomycin: activity against anaerobes and effect on normal human fecal flora. Antimicrob Agents Chemother 1966;1965:659–667.

35. Fink MP, Helsmoortel CM, Arous EJ, Doern GV, Moriarty KP, Fairchild PG, Townsend PL. Comparison of the safety and efficacy of parenteral ticarcillin/clavulanate and clindamycin/gentamicin in serious intra-abdominal infections. J Antimicrob Chemother 1989;24:147–156.

36. Galpin JE, Chow AW, Bayer AS, Guze LB. Sepsis associated with decubitus ulcers. Am J Med 1976;61:346–350.

37. Gerding DN. Foot infections in diabetic patients: the role of anaerobes. Clin Infect Dis 1995;20:S283–S288.

38. Gilstrap LC, Maier RC, Gibbs RS, Connor KD, St Clair PJ. Pipercillin versus clindamycin plus gentamicin for pelvic infections. Obstet Gynecol 1984;64:762–765.

39. Giuliano A, Lewis F Jr, Hudley K, Blaisdell FW. Bacteriology of necrotizing fasciitis. Am J Surg 1977;134:52–56.

40. Goldman PL, Durack DT, Petersdorf RG. Effect of antibiotics on the prevention of experimental *Bacteroides fragilis* endocarditis. Antimicrob Agents Chemother 1978;14:755–760.

41. Goldstein EJC. Patterns of susceptibility to fluoroquinolones among anaerobic bacterial isolates in the United States. Clin Infect Dis 1993;16:S377–381.

42. Goldstein EJC, Citron DM, Goldman RJ, Claros MC, Hunt-Gerrado S. United States national hospital survey of anaerobic culture and susceptibility methods, II. Anaerobe 1995;1:309–314.

43. Gorbach SL. Antibiotic treatment of anaerobic infections. Clin Infect Dis 1994;18:S305–S310.

44. Hecht DW, Malamy MH, Tally FP. Mechanisms of resistance and resistance transfer in anaerobic bacteria. In: Finegold SM, George WL, eds. Anaerobic infections in humans. Orlando, FL: Academic Press, 1989:

45. Hecht DW, Osmolski JR, O'Keefe JP. Variation in the susceptibility of *Bacteroides fragilis* group isolates from six Chicago hospitals. Clin Infect Dis 1993;16:S357–360.

46. Hecht DW, Lederer L. Effect of choice of medium on the results of in vitro susceptibility testing of eight antibiotics against the *Bacteroides fragilis* group. Clin Infect Dis 1995;20:S346–349.

47. Hecht DW, Lederer L, Osmolski JR. Susceptibility results for the *Bacteroides fragilis* group: comparison of the broth microdilution and agar dilution methods. Clin Infect Dis 1995;20:S342–S345.

48. Hecht DW, Osmolski JR. Comparison of activities of trovafloxacin (CP-99,219) and five other agents against 585 anaerobes with use of three media. Clin Infect Dis 1996;23:S44–S50.

49. Hecht DW, Wexler HM. In vitro susceptibility of anaerobes to quinolones in the United States. Clin Infect Dis 1996;23:52–58.

50. Hemsell DL, Martens MG, Faro S, Gall S, McGregor JA. A multicenter study comparing intravenous meropenem with clindamycin plus gentamicin for the treatment of acute gynecologic and obstetric pelvic infections in hospitalized women. Clin Infect Dis 1997;24:S222–S230.

51. Hirn M, Niinikoski J, Lehtonen O. Effect of hyperbaric oxygen

and surgery on experimental multimicrobial gas gangrene. Eur Surg Res 1993;25:265–269.

52. Hurlbut S, Cuchural GJ, Tally FP. Imipenem resistance in *Bacteroides distasonis* mediated by a novel β-lactamase. Antimicrob Agents Chemother 1990;34:117–120.

53. Ingham HR, Selkon JB, Roxby CM. Bacteriological study of otogenic cerebral abscesses: chemotherapeutic role of metronidazole. Br Med J 1977;2:991–993.

54. Jackson RT, Dopp AC. *Bacteroides fragilis* endocarditis. South Med J 1988;81:781–782.

55. Jacobs MR, Spangler SK, Appelbaum PC. β-Lactamase production, β-lactam sensitivity and resistance to synergy with clavulanate of 737 *Bacteroides fragilis* group organisms from thirty-three US centers. J Antimicrob Chemother 1990;26:361–370.

56. Karchmer AW, Gibbons GW. Foot infections in diabetes: evaluation and management. In: Remington JS, Swartz MN, eds. Current clinical topics in infectious diseases. Boston: Blackwell Scientific, 1994:7–10.

57. Kempf P, Bauernfeind A, Muller A, Blum J. Meropenem monotherapy versus cefotaxime plus metronidazole combination treatment for serious intra-abdominal infections. Infection 1996;24:473–479.

58. Konstantopoulos K, Avlami A, Demarongona K, Sideris G, Rekoumi L, Stefanou J, Voskaridou E, Loukopoulos D. Bacteroides fragilis arthritis in a sickle cell-thalassaemia patient. Scand J Infect Dis 1194;26:495–497.

59. Larsen JW, Gabel-Hughes K, Kreter B. Efficacy and tolerability of imipenem-cilastatin versus clindamycin + gentamicin for serious pelvic infections. Clin Ther 1992;14:90–96.

60. Martens mG, Faro S, Hammill HA, Smith D, Riddle G, Maccato M. Ampicillin/sulbactam versus clindamycin in the treatment of postpartum endomyometritis. South Med J 1990;83:408–413.

61. Meller JL, Reyes HM, Loeff DS, Federer L, Hall JR. One-drug versus two-drug antibiotic therapy in pediatric perforated appendicitis: a prospective randomized study. Surgery 1991;110: 764–768.

62. Najem AZ, Kaminski CR, Spillert CR, Lazaro EJ. Comparative study of parenteral piperacillin and cefoxitin in the treatment of surgical infections of the abdomen. Surgery 1983;157:423–425.

63. Nakata MM, Lewis RP. Anaerobic bacteria in bone and joint infections. Rev Infect Dis 1984;6:165–170.

64. Nastro LJ, Finegold SM. Endocarditis due to anaerobic gram-negative bacilli. Am J Med 1973;54:482–496.

65. Nathens AB, Rotstein OD. Antimicrobial therapy for intraabdominal infection. Am J Surg 1996;172:S1–S6.

66. National Committee for Clinical Laboratory Standards. Methods for antimicrobial susceptibility testing of anaerobic bacteria. 4th ed. Approved standard M11-A4. Villanova, PA: National Committee for Clinical Laboratory Standards, 1997.

67. Nichols RL, Smith JW, Klein DB, Trunkey DD, Cooper RH, Adinolfi MF, Mills J. Risk of infection after penetrating abdominal trauma. N Engl J Med 1984;311:1065–1070.

68. O'Keefe JP, Venezio FR, DiVincenzo CA, Shatzer KL. Activity of newer beta-lactam agents against clinical isolates of *Bacteroides fragilis* and other *Bacteroides* species. Antimicrob Agents Chemother 1987;31:2002–2004.

69. Olsson B, Nord CE, Wadstrom T. Formation of beta-lactamase in *Bacteroides fragilis:* Cell-bound and extracellular activity. Antimicrob Agents Chemother 1976;9:727–735.

70. Onderdonk AB, Weinstein WM, Sullivan NM, Bartlett JG, Gorbach SL. Experimental intra-abdominal abscesses in rats: quantitative bacteriology of infected animals. Infect Immun 1974;10: 1256–1259.

71. Patey O, Breuil J, Fisch A, Burnat C, Vincent-Ballareau F, Dublanchet A. *Bacteroides fragilis* meningitis: report of two cases. Rev Infect Dis 1990;12:364–365.

72. Peraino VA, Cross SA, Goldstein EJC. Incidence and clinical significance of anaerobic bacteremia in a community hospital. Clin Infect Dis 1993;16:S288–S291.

73. Peterson LR, Lissack LM, Canter K, Fasching CE, Clabots C, Gerding DN. Therapy of lower extremity infections with ciprofloxacin in patients with diabetes mellitus, peripheral vascular disease, or both. Am J Med 1989;86:801–808.

74. Pinkus G, Veto G, Braude AI. *Bacteroides* penicillinase. J Bacteriol 1968;96:1437–1438.

75. Pitkin D, Sheikh W, Wilson S, Hemsell D, Nichols R, Nadler H, Dowzicky M. Comparison of the activity of meropenem with that of other agents in the treatment of intraabdominal, obstetric/gynecologic, and skin and soft tissue infections. Clin Infect Dis 1995;20:S372–S375.

76. Polk HC, Fink MP, Laverdiere M, Wilson SE, Garber GE, Barie PS, Hebert JC, Cheadle WG. Prospective randomized study of piperacillin/tazobactam therapy of surgically treated intraabdominal infection. Am Surg 1993;59:598–605.

77. Rasmussen J, Odelson D, Macrina F. Complete nucleotide and transcription of ermF, a macrolide-lincosamide-streptogramin B resistance determinant from *Bacteroides fragilis*. J Bacteriol 1986;168:523–533.

78. Reyssett G, Haggoud A, Su W, Sebald M. Genetic and molecular analysis of pIP417 and pIP419: Bacteroides plasmids encoding 5-nitroimidazole resistance. Plasmid 1992;27:181–190.

79. Reyssett G, Su W, Sebald M. Genetics of 5-nitroimidazole resistance in *Bacteroides*. In: Sebald M, ed. Genetics and molecular biology of anaerobic bacteria. New York: Springer-Verlag, 1993:494–504.

80. Rosenblatt J. Antimicrobic susceptibility of anaerobic bacteria. In: Finegold SM, George WL, eds. San Diego: Academic Press, 1989:715–727.

81. Rosenblatt J, Gustafson DR. Evaluation of the E test for susceptibility testing of anaerobic bacteria. Diagn Microbiol Infect Dis 1995;22:279–284.

82. Rotimi V, Duerden B, Hafiz S. Transferable plasmid mediated antibiotic resistance in *Bacteroides*. J Med Microbiol 1981;14: 359–370.

83. Salaki JS, Black R, Tally FP, Kislak JW. *Bacteroides fragilis* resistant to clindamycin. Am J Med 1976;60:426–428.

84. Salyers AA, Schoemaker NB, Guthrie EP. Recent advances in Bacteroides genetics. CRC Crit Rev Microbiol 1987;14:49–71.

85. Scandinavian Study Group. Imipenem-cilastatin versus gentamicin-clindamycin for treatment of serious bacterial infections. Lancet 1983;1:868–871.

86. Sioson P, Brown RB. Successful medical treatment of an infected prosthetic aortic graft. West J Med 1993;158:301–303.

87. Sjolin J, Eriksson N, Arneborn P, Cars O. Penetration of ceftizoxime and desacetylcefotaxime into brain abscesses in humans. Antimicrob Agents Chemother 1991;35:2606–2610.

88. Skiest DJ, Steiner D, Werner M, Garner JG. Anaerobic pericarditis: case report and review. Clin Infect Dis 1994;19: 435–440.

89. Snydman DR, Cuchural GJ, McDermott L, Gill M. Correlation of various in vitro testing methods with clinical outcomes in patients with *Bacteroides fragilis* group infections treated with cefoxitin: a retrospective analysis. Antimicrob Agents Chemother 1992;36:540–544.

90. Snydman DR, McDermott L, Cuchural GJ, Hecht DW, Iannini PB, Harrell LJ, et al. Analysis of trends in antimicrobial

resistance patterns among clinical isolates of Bacteroides fragilis group species from 1990 to 1994. Clin Infect Dis 1996;23: S54–S65.

91. Solomkin JS, Dellinger EP, Christou NV, Busuttil RW. Results of a multicenter trial comparing imipenem cilastatin to tobramycin-clindamycin for intra-abdominal infections. Ann Surg 1990;212:581–591.

92. Spangler SK, Jacobs MR, Appelbaum PC. Activity of WY-49605 compared with those of amoxicillin, amoxicillin-clavulanate, imipenem, ciprofloxacin, cefaclor, cefpodoxime, cefuroxime, clindamycin, and metronidazole against 384 anaerobic bacteria. Antimicrob Agents Chemother 1994;38: 2599–2604.

93. Spangler SK, Jacobs MR, Appelbaum PC. Activity of CP 99,219 compared with those of ciprofloxacin, grepafloxacin, metronidazole, cefoxitin, piperacillin, and piperacillin-tazobactam against 489 anaerobes. Antimicrob Agents Chemother 1994;38:2471–2476.

94. Stone HH, Martin JJ Jr. Synergistic necrotizing cellulitis. Ann Surg 1972;175:702.

95. Study Group of Intra-Abdominal Infections. A randomized controlled trial of ampicillin plus sulbactam vs gentamicin plus clindamycin in the treatment of intra-abdominal infections. Rev Infect Dis 1986;8:S533–S538.

96. Sutter VL. In vitro susceptibility of anaerobes: comparison of clindamycin and other antimicrobial agents. J Infect Dis 1977; 135:S7–S12.

97. Swartz MN. Central nervous system infections. In: Finegold SM, George WL, eds. Anaerobic infections in humans. San Diego: Academic Press, 1989:155–212.

98. Sweet RL. Role of cephamycins in obstetrics and gynecology. J Reprod Med 1990;35:S1064–S1069.

99. Sweet RL, Robbie MO, Ohm-Smith M, Hadley WK. Comparative study of piperacillin versus cefoxitin in the treatment of obstetrics and gynecologic infections. Am J Obstet Gynecol 1983;145:342–349.

100. Sweet RL, Roy S, Faro S, O'Brien WF, Sanfilippo JS, Seidlin M, The Piperacillin/Tazobactam Study Group. Piperacillin and tazobactam versus clindamycin and gentamicin in the treatment of hospitalized women with pelvic inflammation. Obstet Gynecol 1994;83:280–286.

101. Tally FP, McGowan K, Kellum JM, Gorbach SL, O'Donnell TF. A randomized comparison of cefoxitin with or without

amikacin and clindamycin plus amikacin in surgical sepsis. Ann Surg 1981;193:318–323.

102. Tally FP, O'Keefe JP, Sullivan NM, Gorbach SL. Inactivation of cephalosporins by *Bacteroides*. Antimicrob Agents Chemother 1979;16:565–571.

103. Thadepalli H, Gorbach SL, Broido PW, Norsen J, Nyhus L. Abdominal trauma, anaerobes, and antibiotics. Surg Gynecol Obstet 1973;137:270–276.

104. Unhanand M, Mustafa MM, McCracken GH, Nelson JD. Gram-negative enteric bacillary meningitis: a twenty-one year experience. J Pediatr 1993;122:15–21.

105. Warner JF, Perkins RL, Cordero L. Metronidazole therapy of anaerobic bacteremia, meningitis and brain abscess. Arch Intern Med 1979;139:167–169.

106. Weinstein MP, Reller LB, Murphy JR, Lichtenstein KA. The clinical significance of positive blood cultures: a comprehensive analysis of 500 episodes of bacteremia and fungemia in adults. I. Laboratory and epidemiologic observations. Rev Infect Dis 1983;5:35–53.

107. Wexler HM, Finegold SM. Media-and method-dependent variation in MIC values of ceftizoxime for clinical isolates of the *Bacteroides fragilis* group. Clin Ther 1990;12(Suppl C):13–24.

108. Wexler HM, Molitoris E, Finegold SM. Effect of B-lactamase inhibitors on the activities of various B-lactam agents against anaerobic bacteria. Antimicrob Agents Chemother 1991;25: 1219–1224.

109. Wexler HM, Molitoris E, Finegold SM. In vitro activities of two new glycylcyclines, N,N-dimethylglycylamido derivatives of minocycline and 6-demethyl-6-deoxytetracycline, against 339 strains of anaerobic bacteria. Antimicrob Agents Chemother 1994;38:2513–2515.

110. Wexler HM, Molitoris E, Reeves D, Finegold SM. In vitro activity of DU-6859a against anaerobic bacteria. Antimicrob Agents Chemother 1994;38:2504–2509.

111. Wexler HM, Molitoris E, Reeves D, Finegold SM. In-vitro activity of clinafloxacin (CI-960) and PD 131628–2 against anaerobic bacteria. J Antimicrob Chemother 1994;34:579–584.

112. Wheat LJ, Allen SD, Henry M, Kernak CB, Siders JA, Kueber T, Fineberg N, Norton J. Diabetic foot infections: bacteriologic analysis. Arch Intern Med 1986;146:1935–1940.

113. Williams RR, Hotchkin D. Aztreonam plus clindamycin versus tobramycin plus clindamycin in the treatment of intraabdominal infections. Rev Infect Dis 1991;13:S629–S633.

Bordetella pertussis and Other Species

●

Jussi Mertsola and Qiushui He

GENERAL DESCRIPTION
Microbiology

Bordetella pertussis, a small Gram-negative coccobacillus, is the most important cause of pertussis. *B. parapertussis* causes

a similar, but often milder, type of cough with posttussive vomiting. *B. bronchiseptica* and *B. avium* are important pathogens in wild and domestic animals. *B. bronchiseptica, B. holmesii,* and *B. hinzii* have been rarely found in immunocompromised patients (53). Variants of *B. bronchiseptica* have recently been found in immunized children in Italy, suggesting that there might be some "intermediate strains" of *Bordetella* that can cause significant illness in humans (57).

B. pertussis has many virulence factors. Several are important in adhesion of the bacteria to the respiratory epithelium, whereas others have toxic properties (34). Filamentous hemagglutinin (FHA), pertactin (PRN), and fimbriae (FIM) are adhesion proteins that have been used as antigens in new acellular pertussis vaccines. Pertussis toxin (PT) is considered to play an essential role in this disease. It is a hexameric protein with an A-promoter and a pentameric B-oligomer. PT has a wide variety of biologic activities. The A-promoter induces the ADP-ribosylation of Gi proteins, which leads to chronic activation of the GTP second-messenger system. This results in intracellular activation of the cells, finally paralyzing the normal functions of the target cells. Tracheal cytotoxin is a specific peptidoglycan fragment that causes ciliostasis and damage to the ciliated epithelial cells (34). The toxicity of this cytotoxin is mediated by intracellular production of interleukin-1 and nitric oxide (33). Also PT can induce nitric oxide via interferon-γ (56). It could be speculated that selective inhibitors of inducible nitric oxide synthase may have an unique therapeutic application in pertussis.

B. pertussis has a notable capacity to alternate between virulent and avirulent forms (16). It has been speculated that in the late stage of pertussis disease, *B. pertussis* bacteria may be in a avirulent phase that represents a pathogenically dormant state in the situation when the host immune response has developed. Bacteria may use this as a strategy for immune evasion and persistence within the host. This is of a hypothetical concern if new acellular vaccines are to consist of antigens produced only during the virulent phase (16).

Classically, *B. pertussis* infection is considered not to be an invasive disease but merely a local process on the epithelial surfaces. The organisms can, however, survive in vitro in HeLa and mouse kidney cells and also in vivo in alveolar macrophages in a mouse model (9, 17). Friedman et al. showed long-term survival of *B. pertussis* organisms in vitro in human macrophages (23). The important, but yet open, clinical question is, does this intracellular survival of *B. pertussis* exist during pertussis disease? Recently, intracellular bordetellae were found in macrophages of bronchoalveolar lavage samples from three children with HIV infections (7). Knowledge of intracellular survival of *B. pertussis* in humans has clinical implications in development of vaccines and in use of other preventive and therapeutic strategies.

Epidemiology

It is estimated that there are 40 million cases of pertussis, causing 360,000 deaths annually (1). In the prevaccine era in the United States, pertussis was the leading cause of death from communicable disease among children less than 14 years of age (47). Pertussis is a highly contagious respiratory disease. Transmission of the disease is airborne and usually results from contact with an infected coughing patient. In households, the spread is 90 to 100%. In these settings, even 50% of fully immunized persons develop subclinical or symptomatic infection.

Several studies from countries with high vaccination coverage showed that pertussis has shifted to older age groups, indicating that lifelong immunity from pertussis immunization and childhood pertussis does not exist (27, 59). When adults with cough of more than 4 weeks' duration were tested in Australia, 26% had serologic findings indicating recent pertussis infection (55). Nennig et al. studied adults with prolonged cough for 2 weeks or longer and found a prevalence of 12.4% (51). The incidence was estimated to be 176 per 100,000 persons per year. Adults as a source of transmission of pertussis in households is stressed by a report of 23 infants who died in pertussis in 16 families (65). Thirteen (81%) were exposed to others in their homes who had cough before the onset of cough in those children. Adults accounted for at least 46% of those contacts. In a prospective contact study in 122 households in Germany, 15% of the sources were adults (64).

Diagnosis

In unvaccinated infants, the clinical diagnosis of pertussis is relatively easy. The knowledge of symptoms is critical because physical examination is generally uninformative. Mainly for the purpose of conducting clinical vaccine efficacy trials, a case definition for pertussis was agreed upon in a WHO consensus conference in Geneva in 1992. This definition requires that a patient have laboratory evidence of *B. pertussis* infection and a paroxysmal cough for 21 days or longer. Laboratory confirmation of a household member could also be used as an indirect evidence of pertussis in a patient fulfilling the clinical criteria. Case determination is difficult, however, because clinical pertussis is a highly variable disease and with the WHO criteria, the diagnosis of several pertussis cases will be missed (10, 32).

Because mild and atypical cases of pertussis are often encountered, laboratory diagnosis of pertussis is highly important. Culture has remained the gold standard of diagnosis. Specimens should be taken from the posterior nasopharynx, preferably by intranasal aspiration or by swab. Calcium alginate swabs are better than Dacron, rayon, or cotton wool swabs (42). The specimens should be plated immediately onto selective media, and charcoal supplemented with 10% horse blood and 40 mg/L of cephalexin is currently the medium of choice (36). Bordetellae are first identified by colony morphology and Gram staining. *B. parapertussis* grows faster than *B. pertussis* and is oxidase negative, whereas *B. pertussis* is oxidase positive. The two species are also identified by slide agglutination with antisera. In addition, *B. parapertussis* shows urease activity and pigment formation on tyrosine agar.

Culture positivity is often highest during the first 2 weeks of illness, and cultures are seldom positive if cough has lasted more than 4 weeks. Usually the sensitivity of culture is less than 50% (better in unvaccinated infants), and false-negative results are common. The direct fluorescent antibody test (DFA) from nasopharyngeal secretions is rapid but often lacks specificity.

Recently several polymerase chain reaction (PCR) assays have been developed for rapid diagnosis of *B. pertussis* infection (48). Usually two types of samples, nasopharyngeal aspirates or nasopharyngeal swabs (taken as for cultures) have been used. PCR results are available in 1 to 2 days, and this method usually detects about four times more positive samples than culture (30, 31). Also, when effective antimicrobial therapy is started several days before the specimen is collected, the patient is likely to be PCR positive but culture negative (20).

Enzyme immunoassay (EIA) for detection of immunoglobulin IgM, IgA, and IgG antibodies to *B. pertussis* is particularly useful in diagnosis during the late stage of the disease when other tests are negative (49, 62). The strict criteria for seropositivity often decrease the sensitivity to a level of 50 to 70%. Even with the use of various purified antigens (PT, FHA, PRN) and measurement of different antibody classes, no single test has proven to be sensitive enough to be used alone. Although EIA has its limitations, it is a practical aid in recognizing small local outbreaks in older children and adults (47). In immunized persons, laboratory confirmation of the diagnosis of pertussis is difficult, and combinations of culture, PCR, and EIA serology should be used. Epidemiologic data and laboratory-confirmed contact patients often help in making the diagnosis.

Complications

Pertussis is most severe in young infants. In an analysis of pertussis cases in 1989 to 1991 in the United States, 69% of infants under 6 months of age were hospitalized, 16% had pneumonia, 1.8% had seizures, 0.2% had encephalopathy, and deaths occurred in 0.4% (5). Although the disease is milder in older children, even in the age group of 5 to 9 years, 1.4% had seizures and 1 of 704 patients died. The risk of complications during pertussis is much higher than any risk attributed to the significant adverse effects of the whole-cell pertussis vaccine (12).

ANTIMICROBIAL SUSCEPTIBILITY IN VITRO

Antimicrobial susceptibility testing of the fastidious species *B. pertussis* and *B. parapertussis* is not standardized (38). The methods used have been widely divergent. Testing by broth dilution has usually resulted in higher MICs than testing by agar dilution (38). In addition to different broth media used, the inoculum has varied 100-fold, and different sources of blood with different concentrations have been used. Other variables have been the incubation atmosphere and period of time used.

Erythromycin has been a drug of choice, and until recently, there has been no need for routine susceptibility testing of *B. pertussis,* since all strains have been susceptible to erythromycin. In 1994, the first erythromycin-resistant strain was isolated from a 2-month-old infant in Arizona (46). Hoppe and Tschirner have recommended use of Mueller-Hinton broth supplemented with 5% horse blood for testing the activity of erythromycin (41). The erythromycin-containing plates should be incubated in ambient air for 48 hours for *B. parapertussis* and 72 hours for *B. pertussis*. Recently, the E-test was evaluated as an alternative to agar dilution testing (36). Standardization of test methods is especially needed if erythromycin-resistant strains become more common, and it is needed for studying new antimicrobial agents.

In vitro, the new macrolides show similar activity against *B. pertussis*. Usually *B. parapertussis* is more resistant than *B. pertussis* against all these macrolides in in vitro conditions (Table 1) (45). Tuomanen et al. proposed that the bvg locus of *B. pertussis,* which determines phase transition in these organisms, also controls the cell wall hydrolases (61). Virulent strains of *B. pertussis* grow much more slowly than avirulent strains and might thus be more difficult to kill with antibiotics. However, penem antibiotics, which rapidly kill even slowly growing organisms, killed a slowly growing virulent strain of *B. pertussis* in vitro at more than twice the rate of erythromycin (61).

Several quinolones (especially ciprofloxacin and temafloxacin) are also very active against *B. pertussis* and *B. parapertussis* in vitro (Table 1). Other agents showing good in vitro activity against *B. pertussis* are piperacillin and mezlocillin, ceftazidime, cefotaxime, and ceftriaxone (Table 1). The in vitro data on cotrimoxazole is difficult to interpret because of the large discrepancies in the test results (39).

Antimicrobial Therapy

In older children, especially those previously immunized, and adults, the diagnosis is often difficult. Usually treatment should be initiated to prevent spread of the disease, even when the patient has had cough for weeks. After 4 to 5 weeks, about 5 to 10% of patients are still culture positive, and 30 to 40% have positive PCR results (30). If treatment is started later than 2 weeks after the onset of symptoms, it often has no significant clinical effect on the patient's symptoms.

Drug of Choice

Erythromycin for 14 days is the standard treatment recommended by the American Academy of Pediatrics (14); in Canada, 10 days treatment has been recommended (29). Recently Halperin et al. showed that 7 days treatment with erythromycin estolate is as effective as 14 days treatment (29). However, the mean age of their patients was about 7 years, and 88% of them had received at least the primary series of immunizations. The 7-day treatment of infants needs further studies. Erythromycin estolate is preferred, at a dose of 40 mg/kg/day (maximum, 2 g/day). If erythromycin ethylsuccinate or stearate is used, the dose is 20 to 40 mg/kg/day (36). Erythromycin is usually given in four divided doses (47). Hoppe et al. treated 190 culture-positive children with a two-dose regimen of estolate or with three doses of ethylsuccinate per day and had relapse rates of only 2% and 1%, respectively (35). Most patients were treated during the first 2 weeks after onset of coughing. After completion of the treatment, 82% and 75% of the parents, respectively, judged the clinical condition as cured or improved. Baraff showed that erythromycin therapy eliminated *B. pertussis* from the nasopharynx in 2 to 7 days (mean, 3.6 days) and in the study by Bergqvist, none of the patients had positive cultures 5 days after initiation of erythromycin treatment (3, 4).

Cotrimoxazole is considered an alternative for those who do not tolerate erythromycin, but controlled clinical data supporting this therapy are limited (36).

New macrolides are superior to erythromycin in terms of

TABLE 1 • Antimicrobial Susceptibility (μg/mL) of *Bordetella pertussis* and *B. parapertussis*

Antimicrobial Agent	B. pertussis		B. parapertussis	
	MIC (range)	MIC$_{90}$	MIC (range)	MIC$_{90}$
Macrolides[a]				
Azithromycin	0.015–0.03	0.015	0.125–0.25	0.125
Clarithromycin	≤0.008–0.03	0.03	0.25	0.25
Dirithromycin	0.03	0.03	0.125	0.125
Erythromycin	≤0.008–0.03	0.03	0.25	0.25
Josamycin	0.06–0.5	0.06	1	1
Roxithromycin	≤0.008–0.03	0.03	0.25	0.25
Miscellaneous[b]				
Ciprofloxacin	0.03–0.25	0.06	0.06	0.06
Enoxacin	0.5	0.5	0.5	0.5
Fleroxacin	0.06–0.125	0.125	0.25	0.25
Lomefloxacin	0.125–0.25	0.25	0.25	0.25
Ofloxacin	0.125–0.5	0.125	0.125	0.125
Pefloxacin	0.25–0.5	0.5	0.25–0.5	0.5
Temafloxacin	0.06	0.06	0.06	0.06
Penicillin G	≤0.1–12.5			
Ampicillin	0.063->32	0.24		
Amoxicillin	0.5			
Piperacillin	≤0.003–0.006			
Cephalexin	12.5–125			
Cefaclor	12->64			
Cefuroxime	1.5–6	5.3		
Ceftazidime	0.16–0.5	0.29		
Ceftriaxone	0.06–0.125	0.1		
Cefotaxime	0.16–0.78	0.3		
Aztreonam	4			
Cotrimoxazole	0.006/0.125–32/640			
Clindamycin	0.25->8			
Doxycycline	≤0.06->2			
Gentamycin	0.063–16			
Imipenem	≤0.06->8	0.05		
Rifampicin	≤0.006->2	0.125		
Tetracycline	≤0.1–16	0.25		

[a] Modified from Hoppe JE, Eichhorn A. Activity of new macrolides against *Bordetella pertussis* and *Bordetella parapertussis*. Eur J Clin Microbiol Infect Dis 1989;8:653–654.

[b] Modified from Hoppe JE, Haug A. Antimicrobial susceptibility of *Bordetella pertussis* (part I). Infection 1988;16:126–130 and Hoppe JE, Simon CG. In vitro susceptibilities of *Bordetella pertussis* and *Bordetella parapertussis* to seven fluoroquinolones. Antimicrob Agents Chemother 1990;34:2287–2288.

absorption, acid stability, and tissue penetration. Their in vitro activity against *B. pertussis* is good (Table 1). Recently, one small study showed promising results with clarithromycin (10 mg/kg/day twice a day for 7 days; 9 children) or azithromycin (10 mg/kg/day, once a day for 5 days; 8 children) (2). Eradication rates at 7 days after treatment were 100% in both groups. Cultures were taken from some patients 3 to 4 days after treatment, and eradication had occurred in 5 of 8 and in 4 of 5 children, respectively. Although the results are encouraging, further studies are needed before these agents can be recommended for routine treatment of pertussis.

Based on in vitro results, quinolones could also be an alternative for adults, but clinical data on their efficacy are lacking. Piperacillin and third-generation cephalosporins could, in theory, be used as combination therapy with erythromycin for patients with severe secondary infections (usually pneumonia). In one retrospective analysis, all deaths due to severe pneumonia and septicemia in hospitalized pertussis patients were caused by Gram-negative organisms other than *B. pertussis* (24).

Adjunctive Therapy

Infants have the highest risk of complications (usually related to hypoxia during paroxysms), and they should be hospitalized with continuous electronic monitoring. Assessing the need to provide oxygen, stimulation during bradycardia, and suctioning requires skilled personnel. Large-volume feedings are avoided, but maximal nutrition is provided. Antimicrobial therapy should be initiated on the basis of clinical suspicion (47).

There is no convincing evidence of efficacy of cough suppressants, salbutamol, antihistamines, or corticosteroids in the treatment of pertussis (8, 18, 44). Hyperimmune serum was widely used and regarded as beneficial in the 1930s and 1950s, but later studies showed little or no effect of this treatment in pertussis. More recent, but limited, data indicate that treatment with specific immunoglobulin with high antitoxin concentration has a beneficial effect in treatment of this disease (26, 43).

Chemoprophylaxis and Control Measures

Drug of Choice

Several reports show a wide spread of pertussis in families, schools, nursing homes, and hospitals. Erythromycin prophylaxis (same dose and duration as in treatment) is recommended in Canada and in the United States for all household and other close contacts of pertussis patients regardless of their immunization status (14, 50). A contact is defined as a person living in the same household, attending the same day-care center, or sharing the same air space for more than 1 hour (50). Health care workers who have used appropriate protective measures, such as masks, were not considered contacts.

Assessing the real benefits of erythromycin prophylaxis is difficult because early treatment of index cases also reduces the spread of pertussis effectively. The beneficial effect of early treatment of the index case in the household was clearly shown during an acellular pertussis vaccine efficacy trial in Mainz, Germany. Early use of erythromycin, for treatment and/or for prophylaxis, reduced the spread (63). A study by Steketee et al. during an outbreak showed that with early use of erythromycin the infectivity rate was 16%, compared with 75% for late use of this antibiotic (58). A retrospective cohort study by de Serres showed that when prophylaxis was used before the onset of a secondary case, the attack rate was 4% in families, compared with 35% if the family already had a secondary case (19). Granström showed that if a mother has pertussis at the time of labor, she can safely be allowed to nurse her infant if both mother and baby are given erythromycin (25). In this instance, the father and siblings at home should also receive prophylaxis. The patient with pertussis should be placed in respiratory isolation for 5 days after initiation of erythromycin, or for 3 weeks after the onset of paroxysmal cough if antimicrobial therapy is not given (14). Asymptomatic adult contacts who are on prophylaxis can return to work (63).

Christie et al. implemented a vigorous 15-point control plan to reduce spread of pertussis in hospitals (13). This included a program of early diagnosis, treatment, and prevention for employees; immediate isolation of all patients with respiratory illnesses that might prove to be pertussis; wearing of masks by patients, visitors, and personnel in the test referral center where pertussis cultures were performed; restriction of patient travel and visitors; and restrictions in the employees' child-care service. The new epidemiologic data indicates that pertussis is also common but often unrecognized in adults in the population outside the hospital, and therefore the control plans have to be practical (11). Wide use of erythromycin has problems, and one small analysis indicated that less than 50% of health care workers in prophylaxis completed the 14-day course (11). The general value and practicality of wide use of prophylaxis in the community is questionable. It is important to increase awareness of pertussis disease in adults and school-children in the population, to start treatment early in the cat-arrhal phase of pertussis, and to give prophylaxis to those at high risk if infected (infants, other high-risk patients).

During outbreaks, the importance of proper immunizations in children must be stressed. The recommended series should be completed. Children who are less than 7 years old and have received a third dose 6 months or more before exposure or a fourth dose 3 years or more before exposure, could be given a booster dose (47). In the future, acellular vaccines may also be used in older age groups to decrease and prevent endemic circulation of *B. pertussis*.

ENDPOINTS FOR MONITORING THERAPY

Follow-up cultures after therapy are usually not needed.

PREVENTION BY IMMUNIZATION
Whole-Cell Pertussis Vaccines

Whole-cell vaccines prepared from killed whole-cell *B. pertussis* bacteria have been used for decades. Local and systemic side effects, the major disadvantage of whole-cell vaccines, resulted in declining vaccination rates in several countries such as Japan, Germany, Italy, Sweden, and the United Kingdom. Subsequently, large epidemics occurred in these countries. Therefore, extensive efforts have been made to develop less reactogenic acellular vaccines (12).

Acellular Pertussis Vaccines

Acellular vaccines are based on bacterial components, and at present, four main components including PT (pertussis toxin), FHA (filamentous hemagglutinin), PRN (pertactin), and FIM (fimbriae) are considered suitable candidates (Table 2). All acellular vaccines for clinical evaluation contain inactivated PT in different concentrations, and several vaccines have one or more of the other three components in varying amounts.

Acellular vaccines containing PT and FHA were first developed in Japan and have been extensively used there since 1981. The reported reactogenicity of these vaccines is low, and their efficacy is by the fact that pertussis has remained "well-controlled" in Japan after introduction of the new vaccines.

During the last 10 years, nine controlled efficacy trials of acellular vaccines have been carried out in Germany, Italy, Senegal, and Sweden (34, 54). The acellular vaccines used in these trials were from different manufacturers, and either a whole-cell DTP vaccine or a DT vaccine served as control. In most trials, three doses were administered before 6 months of age. The results are summarized in Table 2. The efficacy trials proved that acellular vaccines can prevent pertussis disease and give less adverse reactions than whole-cell vaccines (15). However, several important issues remain.

What are optimal antigens and their quantities in an acellular vaccine? PT is considered to be the most important protective antigen and is included in all the currently available vaccines. Without a clinical efficacy trial, the efficacy of the vaccine is difficult to predict because studies have not identified a correlation between the serum antibody levels and protection. In addition, not even the amount of antigen in some vaccines correlates with mean antibody levels elicited by these antigens. Comparisons between the studies should be done

TABLE 2 • Results from Pertussis Vaccine Efficacy Trials

Manufacturer	Components[a]	Vaccination regimen (months)	Site	Efficacy (95% CI)[b]
Amvax	PT	3, 5, 12	Göteborg	71 (63–78)
Pasteur Merieux	PT, FHA	2, 4, 6	Senegal	86 (71–93)
Pasteur Merieux	Whole cell	2, 4, 6	Senegal	96 (87–94)
Connaught (US)-Biken	PT, FHA	2, 4, 6	Munich	96 (78–99)[c]
Behringwerke	Whole cell	2, 4, 6	Munich	97 (79–100)[d]
SmithKline Beecham	PT, FHA	2, 4, 6	Stockholm	59 (51–66)
Connaught (Canada)	PT, FHA, PRN, FIM	2, 4, 6	Stockholm	85 (81–89)
Connaught (Canada)	Whole cell	2, 4, 6	Stockholm	48 (37–58)
SmithKline Beecham	PT, FHA, PRN	2, 4, 6	Rome	84 (76–90)
Chiron Biocine	PT[e]–, FHA, PRN	2, 4, 6	Rome	84 (76–90)
Connaught (Canada)	Whole cell	2, 4, 6	Rome	36 (14–52)
SmithKline Beecham	PT, FHA, PRN	3, 4, 5	Mainz	89 (77–95)
Behringwerke	Whole cell	3, 4, 5	Mainz	97 (83–100)
Lederle-Takeda	PT, FHA, PRN, FIM	3, 4, 5, 15–18	Erlangen	82 (73–87)[d]
Lederle	Whole cell	3, 4, 5, 15–18	Erlangen	91 (85–94)[d]

Modified from Hewlett EL. Pertussis: current concepts of pathogenesis and prevention. Pediatr Infect Dis J 1997;16:S78–S84.

[a] PT, pertussis toxin; FHA, filamentous hemagglutinin; PRN, pertactin; FIM, fimbriae.

[b] Using the WHO case definition unless otherwise noted.

[c] Using the WHO clinical case definition and positive culture.

[d] Using a modified WHO case definition.

[e] Genetically toxoided PT.

with caution, but the results indicate that addition of FHA, PRN, or FIM to the inactivated PT component conveyed modest additional efficacy (10, 28, 34). The peroxide-detoxified PT vaccine clearly protected against what might be considered moderately severe pertussis but was less effective against mild disease (34, 60). A significant benefit of FHA, PRN, and especially FIM has been observed with respect to long-term protection against pertussis disease (52).

How rapidly does pertussis immunity wane after immunization with different vaccines? It is not known if circulating antibodies are protective, and even less is known about the role of cell-mediated immunity in protection against pertussis. *B. pertussis* remains localized to the respiratory tract throughout the course of the disease, suggesting that a potent local immune response may be highly effective in clearing infection (6). This, however, is difficult to measure in humans. Plotkin and Cadoz suggest that there are likely to be multiple protective factors rather than a single protective correlate (54). To eradicate the organism, the best vaccine should provide long-lasting protection not only against disease but also against both colonization and infection.

What are the mechanisms of the local reaction often seen after booster immunizations? The reactions tend to be more frequent after a booster dose when the child has been immunized with an acellular vaccine, but less so if the primary immunizations were done with a whole-cell vaccine.

Is there interference with reactogenicity and immunogenicity when the vaccines are used in combination? Combined vaccines including antigens against diphtheria, tetanus, *B. pertus-*

sis, Haemophilus influenzae type b, hepatitis B, and inactivated poliovirus have been developed. At present, the effect of combining antigens in the same dose of vaccine on reactogenicity and immune responses is poorly understood. Recently, it has been discovered that antibody response against *H. influenzae* type b is reduced in some combined acellular vaccines (21, 22).

From an economical and a practical point of view, the new acellular vaccines should not be too expensive in comparison with whole-cell vaccines. This is crucial for developing countries.

General

Acellular pertussis vaccines are highly effective against pertussis disease. Several developed countries, including Germany and Italy, have recently taken acellular vaccines into their primary immunization programs. In the United States, two acellular pertussis vaccines have been licensed by the Food and Drug Administration for the initial three-dose series (15). Recent efficacy trials indicate that at least some whole-cell pertussis vaccines are as effective as the new acellular vaccines (Table 2). Therefore, some countries may continue to use the potent whole-cell vaccines. In these situations, acellular vaccines are also needed for continuous booster immunizations, which are important for elimination of pertussis in the older population.

REFERENCES

1. Anonymous. Pertussis vaccines. The International Vaccine Institute Newsletter 1996;2:3–8.

2. Aoyama T, Sunakawa K, Iwata S, Takeuchi Y, Fujii R. Efficacy of short-term treatment of pertussis with clarithromycin and azithromycin. J Pediatr 1996;129:761–764.

3. Baraff LJ, Wilkins J, Wehrle PF. The role of antibiotics, immunizations, and adenoviruses in pertussis. Pediatrics 1978;61:224–230.

4. Bergquist SO, Bernander S, Dahnsjö H, Sundelöf B. Erythromycin in the treatment of pertussis: a study of bacteriologic and clinical effects. Pediatr Infect Dis J 1987;6:458–461.

5. Black S. Epidemiology of pertussis. Pediatr Infect Dis J 1997;16:S85–S89.

6. Brennan MJ, Shahin RD. Pertussis antigens that abrogate bacterial adherence and elicit immunity. Am J Respir Crit Care Med 1996;154:S145–S149.

7. Bromberg K, Tannis G, Steiner P. Detection of Bordetella pertussis associated with the alveolar macrophages of children with human immunodeficiency virus infection. Infect Immun 1991;59:4715–4719.

8. Broomhall J, Herxheimer A. Treatment of whooping cough: the facts. Arch Dis Child 1984;59:185–187.

9. Cheers C, Gray DF. Macrophage behaviour during the complaisant phase of murine pertussis. Immunology 1969;17:875–887.

10. Cherry JD. Comparative efficacy of acellular pertussis vaccines: an analysis of recent trials. Pediatr Infect Dis J 1997;16:S90–S96.

11. Cherry JD. Nosocomial pertussis in the nineties. Infect Control Hosp Epidemiol 1995;16:553–555.

12. Cherry JD, Brunell PA, Golden GS, Karzon DT. Report of the task force on pertussis and pertussis immunization–1988. Pediatrics 1988;81:S939–S984.

13. Christie CDC, Glover AM, Willke MJ, Marx ML, Reising SF, Hutchinson NM. Containment of pertussis in the regional pediatric hospital during the greater Cincinnati epidemic of 1993. Infect Control Hosp Epidemiol 1995;16:556–563.

14. Committee on Infectious Diseases, American Academy of Pediatrics. Pertussis. Report of the Committee on Infectious Diseases. 24th ed. Elk Grove Village, IL: American Academy of Pediatrics, 1997:394–407.

15. Committee on Infectious Diseases, American Academy of Pediatrics. Acellular pertussis vaccine: recommendations for use as the initial series in infants and children. Pediatrics 1997;99:282–288.

16. Coote JG. Antigenic switching and pathogenicity: environmental effects on virulence gene expression in Bordetella pertussis. J Gen Microbiol 1991;137:2493–2503.

17. Crawford JG, Fishel GW. Growth of Bordetella pertussis in tissue culture. J Bacteriol 1959;77:465–474.

18. Danzon A, Lacroix J, Infante-Rivard C, Chicoine L. A double-blind clinical trial on diphenhydramine in pertussis. Acta Paediatr Scand 1988;77:614–615.

19. de Serres G, Boulianne N, Duval B. Field effectiveness of erythromycin prophylaxis to prevent pertussis within families. Pediatr Infect Dis J 1995;14:969–975.

20. Edelman K, Nikkari S, Ruuskanen O, He Q, Viljanen M, Mertsola J. Detection of Bordetella pertussis by polymerase chain reaction and culture in the nasopharynx of erythromycin-treated infants with pertussis. Pediatr Infect Dis J 1996;15:54–57.

21. Edwards KM, Decker MD. Combination vaccines consisting of acellular pertussis vaccines. Pediatr Infect Dis J 1997;16:S97–S102.

22. Eskola J, Olander R-M, Hovi T, Litmanen L, Peltola S, Kayhty H. Randomised trial of the effect of co-administration with acellular pertussis DTP vaccine on immunogenicity of Haemophilus influenzae type b conjugate vaccine. Lancet 1996;348:1688–1692.

23. Friedman RL, Nordensson K, Wilson L, Akporiaye ET, Yocum DE. Uptake and intracellular survival of Bordetella pertussis in human macrophages. Infect Immun 1992;60:4578–4585.

24. Gan VN, Murphy TV. Pertussis in hospitalized children. Am J Dis Child 1990;144:1130–1134.

25. Granström G, Sterner G, Nord CE, Granström M. Use of erythromycin to prevent pertussis in newborns of mothers with pertussis. J Infect Dis 1987;155:1210–1214.

26. Granström M, Olinder-Nielsen AM, Holmblad P, Mark A, Hanngren K. Specific immunoglobulin for treatment of whooping cough. Lancet 1991;338:1230–1233.

27. Grimpel E, Begue P, Anjak I, Njamkepo E, Francois P, Guiso N. Longterm human serum antibody responses after immunization with whole-cell pertussis vaccine in France. Clin Diagn Lab Immunol 1996;3:93–97.

28. Gustafsson L, Hallander HO, Olin P, Reizenstein E, Storsaeter J. A placebo-controlled trial of a two and five component acellular and a US licensed whole-cell pertussis vaccine. N Engl J Med 1996;334:349–355.

29. Halperin SA, Bortolussi R, Langley JM, Miller B, Eastwood BJ. Seven days erythromycin estolate is as effective as fourteen days for the treatment of Bordetella pertussis infections. Pediatrics 1997;100:65–71.

30. He Q, Schmidt-Schläpfer G, Just M, et al. Impact of polymerase chain reaction on clinical pertussis research: Finnish and Swiss experiences. J Infect Dis 1996;174:1288–1295.

31. He Q, Viljanen MK, Nikkari S, Lyytikäinen R, Mertsola J. Outcomes of Bordetella pertussis infection in different age-groups of an immunized population. J Infect Dis 1994;170:873–877.

32. Heininger U, Cherry JD, Eckhardt T, Lorenz C, Christenson P, Stehr K. Clinical and laboratory diagnosis of pertussis in the regions of a large vaccine efficacy trial in Germany. Pediatr Infect Dis J 1993;12:504–509.

33. Heiss LN, Lancaster JR, Corbett JA, Goldman WE. Epithelial autotoxicity of nitric oxide: role in the respiratory cytopathology of pertussis. Proc Natl Acad Sci USA 1994;91:267–270.

34. Hewlett EL. Pertussis: current concepts of pathogenesis and prevention. Pediatr Infect Dis J 1997;16:S78–S84.

35. Hoppe JE, and The Erythromycin Study Group. Comparison of erythromycin estolate and erythromycin ethylsuccinate for treatment of pertussis. Pediatr Infect Dis J 1992;11:189–193.

36. Hoppe JE. Update on epidemiology, diagnosis, and treatment of pertussis. Eur J Clin Microbiol Infect Dis 1996;15:189–193.

37. Hoppe JE, Eichhorn A. Activity of new macrolides against Bordetella pertussis and Bordetella parapertussis. Eur J Clin Microbiol Infect Dis 1989;8:653–654.

38. Hoppe JE, Haug A. Antimicrobial susceptibility of Bordetella pertussis (part I). Infection 1988;16:126–130.

39. Hoppe JE, Haug A. Treatment and prevention of pertussis by antimicrobial agents (part II). Infection 1988;16:148–152.

40. Hoppe JE, Simon CG. In vitro susceptibilities of Bordetella pertussis and Bordetella parapertussis to seven fluoroquinolones. Antimicrob Agents Chemother 1990;34:2287–2288.

41. Hoppe JE, Tschirner T. Comparison of media for agar dilution susceptibility testing of Bordetella pertussis and Bordetella parapertussis. Eur J Clin Microbiol Infect Dis 1995;14:775–779.

42. Hoppe JE, Weiss A. Recovery of Bordetella pertussis from four kinds of swabs. Eur J Clin Microbiol 1987;6:203–205.

43. Ichimaru T, Ohara Y, Hojo M, Miyazaki S, Harano K, Totoki T. Treatment of severe pertussis by administration of specific

gamma globulin with high titers anti-toxin antibody. Acta Paediatr 1993;82:1076–1078.

44. Krantz I, Norrby SR, Trollfors B. Salbutamol vs. placebo for treatment of pertussis. Pediatr Infect Dis J 1985;4:638–640.

45. Kurzynski TA, Boehm DM, Rott-Pettri JA, Schell RF, Allison PE. Antimicrobial susceptibilities of Bordetella species isolated in a multicenter pertussis surveillance project. Antimicrob Agents Chemother 1988;32:137–140.

46. Lewis K, Saubolle MA, Tenover FC, Rudinsky MF, Barbour SD, Cherry JD. Pertussis caused by an erythromycin-resistant strain of Bordetella pertussis. Pediatr Infect Dis J 1995;14:388–391.

47. Long SS. Bordetella pertussis (pertussis) and other species. In: Long SS, Pickering LK, Prober CG, eds. Principles and practice of pediatric infectious diseases. New York: Churchill Livingstone, 1997:976–986.

48. Meade BD, Bollen A. Recommendations for use of the polymerase chain reaction in the diagnosis of Bordetella pertussis infections. J Med Microbiol 1994;41:51–55.

49. Mertsola J, Ruuskanen O, Eerola E, Viljanen MK. Intrafamilial spread of pertussis. J Pediatr 1983;103:359–363.

50. National Advisory Committee on Immunization, Advisory Committee on Epidemiology and Canadian Pediatric Society. Management of people exposed to pertussis and control of pertussis outbreaks. Can Med Assoc J 1990;143:751–753.

51. Nenning ME, Shinefield HR, Edwards KM, Black SB, Fireman BH. Prevalence and incidence of adult pertussis in an urban population. JAMA 1996;275:1672–1674.

52. Olin P. Commentary: the best acellular pertussis vaccines are multicomponent. Pediatr Infect Dis J 1997;16:517–519.

53. Parton R. New perspectives on Bordetella pathogenicity. J Med Microbiol 1996;44:233–235.

54. Plotkin SA, Cadoz M. The acellular pertussis vaccine trials: an interpretation. Pediatr Infect Dis J 1997;16:508–517.

55. Robertson PW, Goldberg H, Jarvie BH, Smith DD, Whybin LR. Bordetella pertussis infection: a cause of persistent cough in adults. Med J Aust 1987;147:522–525.

56. Sakurai S, Kamachi K, Konda T, Miyajima N, Kohase M, Yamamoto S. Nitric oxide induction by pertussis toxin in mouse spleen cells via gamma interferon. Infect Immun 1996;64:1309–1313.

57. Stefanelli P, Mastrantonio P, Hausman SZ, Giuliano M, Burns DL. Molecular characterization of two Bordetella bronchiseptica strains isolated from children with coughs. J Clin Microbiol 1997;35:1550–1555.

58. Steketee RW, Wassilak SGF, Adkins WN, Burstyn DG, Manclark CR, Berg J, Hopfensperger D, Schell WL, Davis JP. Evidence for a high attack rate and efficacy of erythromycin prophylaxis in a pertussis outbreak in a facility for the developmentally disabled. J Infect Dis 1988;157:434–440.

59. Thomas MG. Epidemiology of pertussis. Rev Infect Dis 1989;11:255–262.

60. Trollfors B, Taranger J, Lagergard T, Lind L, Sundh V, Zackrisson G, Lowe CU, Blackwelder W, Robbins JB. A placebo-controlled trial of a pertussis-toxoid vaccine. N Engl J Med 1995;333:1045–1050.

61. Tuomanen E, Schwartz J, Sande S. The vir locus affects the response of Bordetella pertussis to antibiotics: phenotypic tolerance and control of autolysis. J Infect Dis 1990;162:560–563.

62. Viljanen MK, Ruuskanen O, Granberg C, Salmi TT. Serological diagnosis of pertussis: IgM, IgA and IgG antibodies against Bordetella pertussis measured by enzyme-linked immunosorbent assay (ELISA). Scand J Infect Dis 1982;14:117–122.

63. Weber DJ, Rutala WA. Management of healthcare workers exposed to pertussis. Infect Control Hosp Epidemiol 1994;15:411–415.

64. Wirsing von König CH, Postels-Multani S, Bock HL, Schmitt HJ. Pertussis in adults: frequency of transmission after household exposure. Lancet 1995;346:1326–1329.

65. Wortis N, Strebel PM, Wharton M, Bardenheier B, Hardy IRB. Pertussis deaths: report of 23 cases in the United States, 1992 and 1993. Pediatrics 1996;97:607–612.

Borrelia burgdorferi

●

Eugene D. Shapiro and David L. Coleman

GENERAL DESCRIPTION

Lyme disease is caused by the spirochete *Borrelia burgdorferi,* a fastidious, microaerophilic bacterium that replicates very slowly and requires special media to grow in the laboratory (110). *B. burgdorferi* is transmitted by *Ixodid* ticks—in the United States, primarily *Ixodes scapularis* (previously called *Ixodes dammini*), the deer tick. In the United States most cases of Lyme disease occur in southern New England, southeastern New York, New Jersey, eastern Pennsylvania, eastern Maryland, Delaware, and parts of Minnesota and Wisconsin.

Pathogenesis

The pathogenesis of Lyme disease is incompletely understood. In contrast to infections caused by bacteria that elaborate or contain classic toxins, *B. burgdorferi* does not produce a toxin (11). In addition, the number of organisms found in infected tissues is relatively small. These observations suggest a complex interaction between organism and host in the pathogenesis of Lyme disease.

B. burgdorferi can be found in the skin at the site of the bite after inoculation by the tick. The organism spreads centrifugally through the extracellular matrix and induces a mild inflammatory reaction manifest clinically as erythema migrans (51). The organism disseminates hematogenously to the heart, the central nervous system, and other sites shortly after inoculation. *B. burgdorferi* can adhere to a variety of mesenchymal cells and penetrates cell monolayers through intercellular junctions or, occasionally, through the cytoplasm of cells (118). In vitro, the organism grows within macrophages, endothelial cells, and fibroblasts (34, 64, 69). The ability of the organism to survive within these cell types in vivo is unknown.

After infection, IgM antibodies develop over a 3- to 6-week period, and IgG is detectable within 4 to 12 weeks after infection. Antibody is required to kill the spirochete via the classic complement pathway (53).

Direct invasion of the synovium by the organism is likely to be responsible for the symptomatic arthritis in Lyme disease. Without treatment, the organism may persist in the joint for months and may produce chronic arthritis (102). The role of autoimmunity in Lyme arthritis in humans has not been proved. However, it does appear that autoimmunity may be important in some patients, since *B. burgdorferi* was not detected in the synovial fluid of patients with recurrent Lyme arthritis who had received a standard course of antimicrobial treatment (77). In addition, chronic arthritis appears to be associated with certain HLA types (111).

The experimental data on the potential pathogenic role of outer surface protein A (OspA) are conflicting. In an animal model of antigen-induced arthritis, an extract of *B. burgdorferi* that contained OspA induced arthritis in the knee (38). In contrast, mice made transgenic for both OspA and OspB develop arthritis after exposure to *B. burgdorferi* that is similar to the arthritis that develops in nontransgenic control mice (32).

The pathogenesis of the neuropathy associated with Lyme disease also is unclear. *B. burgdorferi* does not appear to be present in affected nerves. Antiaxonal antibodies have been identified in patients with Lyme disease (97). Antiaxonal antibodies similar to those found in patients with Lyme disease have been shown to alter axonal transport (95). In addition to these findings in peripheral nerves, cerebrospinal fluid of patients with Lyme disease contains antibodies reactive with myelin basic protein (33, 124). The role of these antibodies in the pathogenesis of the neurologic manifestations of Lyme disease is unknown.

Clinical Aspects

The clinical manifestations of Lyme disease generally are divided into early localized disease, early disseminated disease, and late disease (110). Early localized disease is manifest by the characteristic rash, erythema migrans. The most common manifestation of early disseminated disease is multiple erythema migrans (often accompanied by fever and flulike symptoms), although patients may have cranial neuritis (especially facial nerve palsy), carditis, radiculoneuropathy, or meningitis. The classic manifestation of late Lyme disease is arthritis. Acrodermatitis atrophicans and lymphocytoma (which usually affects the breast or the earlobe) are rare manifestations of late Lyme disease, especially in the United States. Encephalopathy is another very uncommon manifestation of late Lyme disease.

A host of other abnormalities have been associated with Lyme disease. However, because the association is often based on positive antibody test results that may be inaccurate or coincidental (see below), the causal relationship to Lyme disease is uncertain.

Diagnosis

Misdiagnosis is a major problem and is the most common cause of treatment failure (31, 112). In the absence of the characteristic rash, diagnosis of Lyme disease may be difficult, since the other clinical manifestations of Lyme disease are not specific. Because the sensitivity of culture for *B. burgdorferi* is poor and patients must undergo an invasive procedure such as biopsy or lumbar puncture to obtain appropriate tissue or fluid for culture, such procedures are indicated only in rare circumstances. Consequently, confirmation of Lyme disease without erythema migrans usually depends on demonstration of antibodies to *B. burgdorferi* in the patient's serum.

Both the sensitivity and specificity of antibody tests for Lyme disease vary substantially (9, 10, 45). The accuracy of prepackaged kits, used by most commercial laboratories in the United States, is poor (8–10, 14, 45). The use of Western immunoblots improves the specificity of serologic testing for Lyme disease (26), although the accuracy of commercial kits also is substantially worse than that of tests performed by reference laboratories. Official recommendations from the Second National Conference on Serologic Diagnosis of Lyme Disease are that clinicians use a two-step procedure when ordering antibody tests for Lyme disease—first, a sensitive screening test, either an enzyme-linked immunosorbent assay (ELISA) or an immunofluorescent assay (IFA) and, if that result is positive or equivocal, a Western immunoblot to confirm the result (6). If the ELISA or the IFA is negative, an immunoblot is not necessary. Antibody tests generally are not useful for the diagnosis of early localized Lyme disease, since only a minority of patients with solitary erythema migrans have a positive test result (35, 37).

The predictive value of antibody tests (even of very accurate tests) is highly dependent on the prevalence of the infection among patients who are tested. Because many lay persons as well as many physicians erroneously believe that nonspecific symptoms alone (e.g., headache, fatigue, or arthralgia) may be manifestations of Lyme disease, patients with only nonspecific symptoms frequently are tested for Lyme disease (57). However, because the specificity of the tests is poor (the specificity of even excellent antibody tests for Lyme disease rarely exceeds 90%), some patients who do not have Lyme disease will test positive; the overwhelming majority (>95%) of patients with only nonspecific symptoms will have false-positive test results (90). Lyme disease is the cause of the nonspecific symptoms in very few (if any) such patients.

Even though a symptomatic patient has a positive serologic test result for antibodies to *B. burgdorferi,* Lyme disease may not be the cause of that patient's symptoms. In addition to the possibility that the result is falsely positive (a common occurrence), the patient may have been infected with *B. burgdorferi* previously, and the symptoms may be unrelated to that previous infection. Once serum antibodies to *B. burgdorferi* develop, they may persist for many years despite adequate treatment and clinical cure of the disease (30). In addition, because a substantial proportion of people who become infected with *B. burgdorferi* never develop symptoms (41, 109), in endemic areas a background rate of seropositivity will exist among patients who have never had clinically apparent Lyme disease. When patients with previous Lyme disease (whether asymptomatic and untreated or clinically apparent and adequately treated) develop any kind of symptoms and are tested for antibodies against *B. burgdorferi*, their symptoms may erroneously be attributed to active Lyme disease. Clinicians should not routinely order antibody tests for Lyme disease in either patients who have not been in endemic areas or patients with only nonspecific symptoms.

SUSCEPTIBILITY IN VITRO AND IN VIVO

Results of in vitro and in vivo antimicrobial susceptibility tests for *B. burgdorferi* have been conflicting. Agents that appear to be quite active in vitro have been ineffective in vivo. The discrepancy between in vitro and in vivo activity has been most notable for the macrolide antibiotics (84). Moreover, antibiotics with good activity both in vitro and in animal models have not necessarily been effective in treating humans with Lyme disease. For example, roxithromycin has good activity in vitro (MBC, 0.06–0.25 µg/mL) and has been effective for treating gerbils infected with *B. burgdorferi*. However, treatment with roxithromycin failed in 5 of 19 patients with early Lyme disease (42). Therefore, the results of in vitro and in vivo susceptibility tests should not be used to guide therapy in the same manner in which they are used for many other bacterial infections.

The in vitro susceptibility tests use macro- or microdilution methods in standard Barbour-Stoenner-Kelly medium. The spirochetes are inoculated at a concentration of 10^5 organisms/mL and are incubated for 3 to 8 days at 32 to 34° C. Absence of spirochetes by darkfield microscopy after the initial 7-day incubation period is used to determine the minimal inhibitory concentration (MIC). An aliquot of medium is subcultured for an additional 7 to 42 days and then examined microscopically to determine the minimal bactericidal concentration (MBC). The results of in vitro susceptibility tests of *B. burgdorferi* may be influenced by the following factors (22, 47, 56, 73):

1. Strain of the organism
2. Prior passage of the organism in vitro
3. Duration of incubation before determination of the MIC or the MBC

In more recent studies, investigators have evaluated the susceptibility of multiple different strains of the organism, have standardized the preparation of laboratory strains, and have incubated the organisms for 7 days prior to determination of the MIC and for 7 to 21 days prior to determination of the MBC (22, 56). The most active agents in vitro are the tetracyclines, clarithromycin, amoxicillin, cefotaxime, and ceftriaxone (22, 47, 56).

In vivo susceptibility testing has been conducted primarily in gerbils (92), hamsters (47), rats (12), rabbits (70), and mice (71). The animals are inoculated intradermally or intraperitoneally with 10^4 to 10^8 organisms and then treated with standard antibiotic regimens. Hamsters may be treated with cyclophosphamide prior to inoculation to induce immunosuppresion (5). The animals are sacrificed and tissues are subcultured and examined histologically for the presence of spirochetes. In the hamster model of hind paw inoculation (5), therapeutic efficacy is determined by measuring the reduction in swelling of the paws.

The results of antimicrobial susceptibility testing using animal models of borrelial infection may be influenced by the following factors:

1. Species of animal used
2. Strain of *B. burgdorferi*
3. Method used to detect surviving organisms

The most active agents in vivo are ceftriaxone, clarithromycin, and the tetracyclines (5, 71).

The basis for the occasional discrepancy between in vitro and in vivo results of antimicrobial susceptibility tests for *B. burgdorferi* is unknown. The organism may persist intracellularly where antibiotic agents may vary widely in their effectiveness (34, 64, 69). For example, *B. burgdorferi* persists within fibroblasts where it may avoid the antimicrobial effects of ceftriaxone (34). The organism may also interact with host factors to alter its pathogenicity. For example, addition of cytokines to the culture medium enhances the pathogenicity of *B. burgdorferi* (39, 40).

Selection of appropriate antimicrobials to treat *B. burgdorferi* should be based on results of clinical trials in addition to studies conducted in vitro or in animal models. Reliance solely on either in vitro susceptibility results or data from animal models may lead to the use of ineffective antimicrobial agents.

ANTIMICROBIAL THERAPY
General

Choice of treatment for Lyme disease depends on the manifestations of the illness. Although there is substantial evidence that treatment of Lyme disease, whatever the stage, usually is highly effective, there are few controlled clinical trials comparing different doses of medication and/or different durations of treatment. In addition, the "success rates" of treatment that have been reported in various studies are highly dependent on the definition of cure. Many studies classified patients as treatment failures if they had any symptoms, even nonspecific symptoms such as fatigue or intermittent arthralgia, after antimicrobial treatment was discontinued. Clearly, some patients have such nonspecific symptoms that persist for some time after treatment (23, 94). There is no evidence that such nonspecific symptoms indicate that the previous treatment was inadequate or that additional antimicrobial treatment is necessary. Indeed, in the vast majority of patients these symptoms resolve in a matter of weeks without additional antimicrobial treatment. Treatment with nonsteroidal antiinflammatory agents may be helpful for arthralgia or headache. Recommended treatment for Lyme disease is shown in Table 1 (2, 85, 96).

TABLE 1 • Antimicrobial Treatment of Lyme Disease

---

1. Early disease

  a. Erythema migrans and disseminated early disease (including facial nerve palsy)

    Doxycycline, 100 mg b.i.d. for 14–30 days (for children: 3–4 mg/kg/day divided b.i.d.; do not use in children <8 years of age), or amoxicillin, 500 mg t.i.d. (for children: 50 mg/kg/day divided t.i.d.) for 14–30 days

    Alternative agents for those who cannot take either amoxicillin or doxycycline are cefuroxime axetil, 500 mg bid (for children: 30 mg/kg/day divided b.i.d.) or erythromycin, 250–500 mg q.i.d. (for children: 30–50 mg/kg/day divided q.i.d.) or tetracycline, 500 mg q.i.d. (for children: 25–50 mg/kg/day divided q.i.d.)

  b. Meningitis

    Ceftriaxone, 2 g/day in a single dose (for children: 50–80 mg/kg/day in a single dose for 14–21 days administered i.v. or i.m.), or penicillin G, 14–20 million units/day administered i.v. divided q. 4 h (for children: 200,000–400,000 units/kg/day divided q. 4 h administered i.v.) for 14–21 days

    An alternative agent is cefotaxime, 10–12 g/day divided q. 8 h (for children: 150 mg/kg/day divided q. 8 h) administered i.v.

2. Late disease

  a. Arthritis

    Initial treatment is the same as for early disease except treat for 30 days; if symptoms fail to resolve after 2 months or there is a recurrence, either repeat a course of an orally administered antimicrobial or treat as for meningitis for 2–4 weeks

  b. Neurologic disease[a]

    Same as for meningitis.

---

[a] For facial nerve palsy, see 1a.

Children under 8 years of age and pregnant women should not be treated with either doxycycline or tetracycline because they may cause permanent discoloration of the teeth of children or a fetus. Patients who are treated with doxycycline should be alerted to the risk of drug-related, sun-induced dermatitis. Some patients with Lyme disease who receive antimicrobial treatment develop a Jarisch-Herxheimer reaction, marked by increased fever, myalgia, and chills, within 48 hours after treatment is begun (72). The symptoms, presumably a reaction to bacteriolysis and release of bacterial products, usually resolves within 1 to 3 days. Antimicrobial treatment should not be stopped. Nonsteroidal antiinflammatory agents may be useful in treating the symptoms of the Jarisch-Herxheimer reaction as well as the myalgia, arthralgia, headache, and other symptoms of Lyme disease.

Early Localized Disease

The goals of treatment of early localized disease are to alleviate symptoms and to prevent development of either early disseminated or late Lyme disease. Early studies found penicillin and tetracycline to be effective in the treatment of early Lyme disease (105, 106). Subsequently, it was shown that treatment of early Lyme disease with doxycycline, amoxicillin, or cefuroxime was as or more effective than treatment with penicillin or tetracycline and could be administered in fewer daily doses. Overall success rates ranged from 90 to 100% with these drugs. Although in most studies treatment was administered for 3 weeks, some patients were cured with 10 days of treatment (67). Optimal duration of treatment is unknown. In most instances, persons who developed objective neurologic manifestations of Lyme disease despite treatment had symptoms suggesting that early neurologic involvement was present at the time that treatment was initiated. Treatment appears to sterilize skin lesions rapidly (75). Limited data on treatment of patients with Lyme disease with macrolide antibiotics, including erythromycin, azithromycin, and clarithromycin, suggest that these drugs may not be as effective as the above-cited agents, and should be reserved for patients with contraindications to the preferred drugs (20, 62, 67, 106).

Early Disseminated Disease

Patients with early disseminated Lyme disease manifest as either multiple erythema migrans or cranial neuritis (including seventh nerve palsy) can be treated for 21 to 28 days with the same agents used to treat early localized disease (21, 37, 85). In the only comparative clinical trial of treatment of patients with disseminated Lyme disease (without meningitis), there were no significant differences in the outcomes of patients treated with doxycycline (100 mg b.i.d. for 21 days) or with ceftriaxone (2 g q.d. for 14 days) (21). Both regimens were extremely efficacious. Because of lower cost and fewer side effects, treatment with doxycycline (or another oral agent such as amoxicillin) is recommended.

Treatment of patients with facial palsy has been controversial (93). Some experts believe that a patient with facial palsy due to Lyme disease should undergo lumbar puncture, and if the results of the cerebrospinal fluid analyses are abnormal, the patient should be treated parenterally with antibiotics. Although there is evidence that B. burgdorferi may affect the central nervous system in patients with early Lyme disease (60)—even among patients with no apparent neurologic involvement (54)—there is little evidence that parenterally administered treatment necessarily is indicated. On the contrary, substantial evidence indicates that orally administered therapy is highly effective (15, 21, 25, 37, 48, 54, 96). Nevertheless, this remains an area of controversy. There is no evidence that use of corticosteroids improves the outcomes of patients with facial nerve palsy due to Lyme disease (15).

Patients with Bannwarth's syndrome (radiculoneuritis) have been treated successfully with ceftriaxone and cefotaxime as well as with doxycycline (18, 24, 82, 89). There is some evidence that corticosteroids are effective for treatment of patients with painful radiculitis (80). Most experts recommend that patients with meningitis be treated parenterally with ceftriaxone, cefotaxime or penicillin, although there are reports of successful treatment with orally administered tetracycline or doxycycline (3, 24, 18, 81, 82, 87).

There are no clinical trials of treatment of carditis with antimicrobials and no evidence that antimicrobial treatment hastens the resolution of carditis. There are reports of resolution of carditis after both orally and parenterally administered antimicrobial treatment as well as after no antimicrobial treatment (13, 59, 79, 86, 105, 120). Temporary cardiac pacing may be necessary in patients with high-grade heart block. Nevertheless, experts generally recommend 2 to 3 weeks of parenteral treatment for patients with symptomatic carditis with high-grade heart block, although patients with only mild manifestations or in whom low-grade heart block is an incidental finding may be treated orally (85, 96). Corticosteroids may be useful if there is any delay in the resolution of the heart block (68).

Late Disease

Lyme arthritis can be treated effectively with either orally administered or parenterally administered treatment (18, 37, 44, 96, 108, 113, 114, 119). There is evidence that treatment with an oral antimicrobial is more cost-effective than parenteral treatment (27). In most instances the arthritis resolves within 2 months. In some patients, the arthritis persists or recurs. Such patients should be treated with another course of antibiotics—some would repeat a course of an orally administered antimicrobial, while others would initiate parenteral treatment with a drug such as ceftriaxone. Rarely, patients with Lyme disease may develop chronic or recurrent arthritis; there appears to be an association with certain HLA types and this apparent autoimmune disease that is triggered by infection with *B. burgdorferi* (111). There is little evidence of persistent infection in patients with chronic or recurrent arthritis who have received adequate antimicrobial treatment (77). Patients with chronic arthritis unresponsive to antimicrobial treatment have been treated with remitting agents, such as hydroxychloroquine, or with synovectomy (19, 89, 99, 103, 113).

There is controversy about the entity of late neurologic Lyme disease (sometimes called either chronic or tertiary neuroborreliosis). Although some well-documented cases of patients with late neurologic Lyme disease (91) exist, there are also many poorly substantiated reports. There are no clinical trials of treatment. Most experts recommend a course (2–4 weeks) of a parenterally administered antimicrobial such as ceftriaxone (96).

Unusual Manifestations
Ocular Disease. A wide range of ocular manifestations of Lyme disease have been reported (49, 55). While the most commonly reported ocular manifestations are relatively minor (e.g., conjunctivitis) and respond to standard, orally administered regimens, occasionally more serious ocular disease, including retinitis, has been reported. There are no clinical trials of treatment. Successful treatment of intraocular Lyme borreliosis with ceftriaxone has been reported (117).

Borrelial Lymphocytoma and Acrodermatitis Atrophicans. Lyme disease skin manifestations of borrelial lymphocytoma and acrodermatitis atrophicans are seen primarily in Europe (7, 46) and are rare in the United States, presumably because of regional, strain-specific differences in the organism. Lymphocytoma, a dense inflammatory infiltrate of lymphocytes that occurs at the site of inoculation of the organism, is usually treated with orally administered drugs. Either doxycycline, penicillin, or amoxicillin, administered for 2 weeks, has been effective (7, 46, 114). Acrodermatitis atrophicans, a late manifestation of Lyme disease, is a chronic, sclerotic skin lesion. In a clinical trial, 3 to 4 weeks of orally administered penicillin or doxycycline was more effective than a 2-week course of ceftriaxone (1, 50). Hence, patients with acrodermatitis atrophicans should be treated for 4 weeks with either doxycycline or amoxicillin.

Special Situations

Pregnancy
Because clinical syndromes caused by congenital infection have been recognized with other spirochetal infections such as syphilis, there has been substantial concern about the possible transmission of *B. burgdorferi* from an infected pregnant woman to her unborn fetus. Although there are case reports in which *B. burgdorferi* has been identified from several abortuses and from a few live-born children with congenital anomalies, the placentas, abortuses, and tissues in which the spirochete was identified showed no histologic evidence of inflammation (69, 88, 123). In addition, no consistent pattern of congenital malformations (as would be expected in a "syndrome" due to congenital infection) has been identified. In longitudinal studies of pregnant women who developed Lyme disease that were conducted by the Centers for Disease Control, the adverse outcomes that occurred could not be attributed to infection with *B. burgdorferi* (66). Furthermore, two serosurveys and a prospective study that were conducted in endemic areas showed no significant differences in the prevalence of congenital malformations among the offspring of women with serum antibodies against *B. burgdorferi* and the offspring of those without such antibodies (74, 116, 125). Moreover, in a large-scale survey, no children with neurologic abnormalities attributable to Lyme disease could be identified by child neurologists in endemic areas (36).

There is no definite evidence that congenital disease caused by *B. burgdorferi* exists, although existence of such a syndrome also has not been ruled out (101). If it does exist, congenital Lyme disease must be extremely rare. Consequently, in theory, pregnant women who develop Lyme disease should not be treated differently than others with Lyme disease. There is no evidence that either longer courses of treatment or parenteral treatment is indicated for pregnant women with early

Lyme disease. However, because of the potential adverse effects of tetracyclines on the fetus, these antimicrobials (including doxycycline) should be avoided. Consequently, amoxicillin is the drug of choice to treat pregnant women with uncomplicated Lyme disease. Cefuroxime and erythromycin are alternative agents for women who are allergic to penicillin.

Tick Bites

Physicians in endemic areas often are asked whether a patient who is bitten by a deer tick should receive antimicrobial prophylaxis. There is substantial evidence that the risk of Lyme disease after a recognized deer tick bite, even in hyperendemic areas, does not exceed 1 to 2% (92). Presumably this is because ticks must be infected with *B. burgdorferi* (only a minority of ticks are infected) and, even then, the infected tick must feed for 48 hours or longer before the risk of transmission of *B. burgdorferi* becomes substantial (83). There is evidence that nearly 75% of persons who remove ticks do so before the tick has fed for 48 hours (29).

Investigators who conducted different randomized, double-blind clinical trials in which more than 600 subjects bitten by deer ticks were treated with either a placebo or an antibiotic (penicillin, tetracycline, or amoxicillin) concluded that routine antimicrobial prophylaxis is not warranted (4, 16, 92). A meta-analysis also found no statistically significant benefit to prophylactic treatment for tick bites (122).

Ascertaining whether the tick is infected, using tests such as the polymerase chain reaction (PCR), is not useful. While testing ticks with PCR may provide important epidemiologic information, the predictive values for infection of humans of either a positive or a negative PCR are unknown. Routine serologic testing of persons bitten by a deer tick also is not indicated. Among more than 1000 subjects who have been followed in prospective studies after recognized tick bites, none has been reported to have developed either late disease or latent infection (i.e., asymptomatic seroconversion, the clinical significance of which is unknown). Moreover, serologic tests for Lyme disease do not have a high enough specificity to be useful for screening (90).

Seropositive Persons Who Are Asymptomatic

Although antibody tests for Lyme disease are not sufficiently accurate to be used for screening and should never be ordered for asymptomatic patients (14, 90), occasionally physicians are confronted with asymptomatic patients with positive results of antibody tests for *B. burgdorferi*. In many instances these are false-positive results, but in some instances the test result may be accurate (see section above on diagnosis). There are not adequate data to know whether asymptomatic persons with antibodies to *B. burgdorferi* should be treated. Presumably, one would be concerned about the possible development of late neurologic disease in such patients. However, if the purpose of treatment is to eradicate *B. burgdorferi* from the central nervous system, orally administered antimicrobials are not likely to be effective. On the other hand, it seems unreasonable to commit such patients to an expensive and inconvenient course of treatment with a parenterally administered drug such as ceftriaxone without evidence that they risk poor outcomes without treatment.

Alternative Therapy

Alternative drugs for persons who cannot tolerate the usual medications are listed in Table 1.

ENDPOINTS FOR MONITORING THERAPY

The most appropriate endpoint for monitoring the effects of treatment is careful clinical evaluation of the patient. Laboratory tests generally are not helpful. Antibodies against *B. burgdorferi* may develop, persist, or even rise in concentration despite adequate treatment and clinical cure of the patient. Symptoms such as fatigue, arthralgia, and myalgia sometimes persist for some time after completion of a course of treatment for Lyme disease. These nonspecific symptoms (which may accompany or follow more specific symptoms and signs of Lyme disease but almost never are the sole manifestations of Lyme disease) usually resolve over a period of weeks. There is little evidence that such symptoms are related to persistence of *B. burgdorferi,* and there is no evidence that either repeated or prolonged courses of antimicrobials speed the resolution of such symptoms. A number of possible reasons exist for persistence of symptoms after a patient is treated for Lyme disease (98). It is critical to differentiate patients with nonspecific subjective complaints from those with objective evidence of an abnormality (e.g., synovitis). It is unlikely that additional or prolonged antimicrobial treatment will benefit patients in whom subjective symptoms persist or recur despite appropriate antimicrobial treatment. Indeed, clear recommendations against such practice have been given by expert panels sanctioned by both the Infectious Diseases Society of America and the American College of Rheumatology (61). Moreover, such treatment is not cost-effective (58).

CONTROVERSIES

There have been efforts to characterize Lyme disease as a difficult-to-treat infection that often leads to chronic symptoms unresponsive to anything but very prolonged antimicrobial treatment. Current evidence indicates that the vast majority of patients with Lyme disease respond well to conventional courses of antimicrobial treatment. Moreover, there is evidence that prolonged courses of treatment do more harm than good (28, 58, 61). Other diagnoses should be considered for persons who fail to respond to conventional treatment. If objective abnormalities persist for several months despite adequate courses of antimicrobial treatment, the patient should be referred to an appropriate specialist experienced in the treatment of Lyme disease.

REFERENCES

1. Aberer E, Breier F, Stanek G, Schmidt B. Success and failure in the treatment of acrodermatitis chronica atrophicans. Infection 1996;24:85–87.
2. Abramowicz M. Treatment of Lyme disease. Med Letter 1997;39:47–48.
3. Ackley A Jr, Lupovici M. Lyme disease meningitis treated with tetracycline. Ann Intern Med 1986;105:630–631.

4. Agre F, Schwartz R. The value of early treatment of deer tick bite for the prevention of Lyme disease. Am J Dis Child 1993; 147:945–947.

5. Alder J, Mitten M, Jarvis K, Gupta P, Clement J. Efficacy of clarithromycin for treatment of experimental Lyme disease in vivo. Antimicrob Agents Chemother 1993;37:1329–1335.

6. Anonymous. Recommendations for test performance and interpretation from the second national conference on serologic diagnosis of Lyme disease. MMWR 1995;44:590.

7. Asbrink E, Hovmark A. Early and late cutaneous manifestations in *Ixodes*-borne borreliosis. Ann NY Acad Sci 1988;539:4–15.

8. Bacterial Zoonoses Branch, Centers for Disease Control. Evaluation of serologic tests for Lyme disease: report of a national evaluation. Lyme Disease Surveillance Summary 1991;2:1–3.

9. Bakken LL, Case KL, Callister SM, Bourdeau NJ, Schell RF. Performance of 45 laboratories participating in a proficiency testing program for Lyme disease serology. JAMA 1992;268: 891–895.

10. Bakken LL, Callister SM, Wand PJ, Schell RF. Interlaboratory comparison of test results for detection of Lyme disease by 516 participants in the Wisconsin State Laboratory of Hygiene/College of American Pathologists proficiency testing program. J Clin Microbiol 1997;35:537–543.

11. Barbour A, Hayes SF. Biology of Borrelia species. Microbiol Rev 1986;50:381–400.

12. Barthold SE, Moody KD, Terwilliger GA, Duray PH, Jacoby RO, Steere AC. Experimental Lyme arthritis in rats infected with Borrelia burgdorferi. J Infect Dis 1988;157:842–846.

13. Bedell SE, Pastor BM, Cohen SI. Symptomatic high grade heart block in Lyme disease. Chest 1981;79:236–237.

14. Burlington DB. FDA public health advisory: assays for antibodies to *Borrelia burgdorferi:* limitations, use, and interpretation for supporting a clinical diagnosis of Lyme disease [1997–520-050]. Washington, DC: US Government Printing Office, 1997.

15. Clark JR, Carlson RD, Sasaki CT, Pachner AR, Steere AC. Facial paralysis in Lyme disease. Laryngoscope 1985;95:1341–1345.

16. Costello CM, Steere AC, Pinkerton RE, Feder HM Jr. A prospective study of tick bites in an endemic area for Lyme disease. J Infect Dis 1989;159:136–139.

17. Dattwyler RJ, Halperin JJ, Pass H, Luft BJ. Ceftriaxone as effective therapy in refractory Lyme disease. J Infect Dis 1987; 155:1322–1325.

18. Dattwyler RJ, Halperin JJ, Volkman DJ, Luft BJ. Treatment of late Lyme borreliosis—randomised comparison of ceftriaxone and penicillin. Lancet 1988;1:1191–1194.

19. Dattwyler RJ, Volkman DJ, Conaty SM. Amoxycillin plus probenecid versus doxycycline for treatment of erythema migrans borreliosis. Lancet 1990;336:1404–1406.

20. Dattwyler RJ, Grunwaldt E, Luft BJ. Clarithromycin in treatment of early Lyme disease: a pilot study. Antimicrob Agents Chemother 1996;40:468–469.

21. Dattwyler RJ, Luft BJ, Kunkel MJ, Finkel MF, Wormser GP, Rush TJ, Grunwaldt E, Agger WA, Franklin M, Oswald D, Cockey L, Maladorno D. Ceftriaxone compared with doxycycline for the treatment of acute disseminated Lyme disease. N Engl J Med 1997;337:289–294.

22. Dever LL, Jorgensen JH, Barbour AG. Comparative in vitro activities of clarithromycin, azithromycin, and erythromycin against *Borrelia burgdorferi.*. Antimicrob Agents Chemother 1993;37:1704–1706.

23. Dinerman H, Steere AC. Lyme disease associated with fibromyalgia. Ann Intern Med 1992;117:281–285.

24. Dotevall L, Alesitig K, Hanner P, Norkrans G, Hagberg L. The use of doxycycline in nervous system *Borrelia burgdorferi* infection. Scand J Infect Dis 1988;53(Suppl):74–79.

25. Dotevall L, Hagberg L. Penetration of doxycycline into cerebrospinal fluid in patients treated for suspected Lyme neuroborreliosis. Antimicrob Agents Chemother 1989;33:1078–1080.

26. Dressler F, Whalen JA, Reinhardt BN, Steere AC. Western blotting in the serodiagnosis of Lyme disease. J Infect Dis 1993;167: 392–400.

27. Eckman MH, Steere AC, Kalish RA, Pauker SG. Cost effectiveness of oral as compared with intravenous antibiotic therapy for patients with early Lyme disease or Lyme arthritis. N Engl J Med 1997;337:357–363.

28. Ettestand PJ, Campbell GL, Welbel SF, Genese CA, Spitalny KC, Marchetti CM, Dennis DT. Biliary complications in the treatment of unsubstantiated Lyme disease. J Infect Dis 1995; 171:356–361.

29. Falco RC, Fish D, Piesman J. Duration of tick bites in a Lyme disease-endemic area. Am J Epidemiol 1996;143:187–192.

30. Feder HM Jr, Gerber MA, Luger SW, Ryan RW. Persistence of serum antibodies to *Borrelia burgdorferi* in patients treated for Lyme disease. Clin Infect Dis 1992;15:788–793.

31. Feder HM Jr, Hunt MS. Pitfalls in the diagnosis and treatment of Lyme disease in children. JAMA 1995;274:66–68.

32. Fikrig E, Tao H, Chen M, Barthold SW, Flavell RA. Lyme borreliosis in transgenic mice tolerant to *Borrelia burgdorferi* OspA or B. J Clin Invest 1995;96:1706–1714.

33. Garcia-Monco JC, Coleman JL, Benach JL. Antibodies to myelin basic protein in Lyme disease. J Infect Dis 1988;158: 667–668.

34. Georgilis K, Peacocke M, Klempner MS. Fibroblasts protect the Lyme disease spirochete, *Borrelia burgdorferi,* from ceftriaxone in vitro. J Infect Dis 1992;166:440–444.

35. Gerber MA, Shapiro ED. Diagnosis of Lyme disease in children. J Pediatr 1992;121:157–162.

36. Gerber MA, Zalneraitis EL. Childhood neurologic disorders and lyme disease during pregnancy. Pediatr Neurol 1994;11:41–43.

37. Gerber MA, Shapiro ED, Burke GS, Parcells VJ, Bell GL. Lyme disease in children in southeastern Connecticut. N Engl J Med 1996;335:1270–1274.

38. Gondolf KB, Mihatsch M, Curschellas E, Dunn JJ, Batsford SR. Induction of experimental allergic arthritis with outer surface proteins of *Borrelia burgdorferi*. Arthritis Rheum 1994;37: 1070–1077.

39. Guner ES. Retention of *B. burgdorferi* pathogenicity and infectivity after multiple passages in a co-culture system. Experientia 1994;50:54–59.

40. Guner ES. Complement evasion by the Lyme disease spirochete *Borrelia burgdorferi* grown in host-derived tissue co-cultures: role of fibronectin in complement resistance. Experientia 1996;52:364–372.

41. Hanrahan JP, Benach JL, Coleman JL, Bosler EM, Morse DL, Cameron DJ, Edelman R, Kaslow RA. Incidence and cumulative frequency of endemic Lyme disease in a community. J Infect Dis 1984;150:489–496.

42. Hansen K, Hovmark A, Lebech AM, Lebech K, Olsson I, Halkier-Sorensen L, Olsson E, Asbrink E. Roxithromycin in Lyme borreliosis: discrepant results of an in vitro and in vivo animal susceptibility study and a clinical trial in patients with erythema migrans. Acta Derm Venereol (Stockh) 1992;72:297–300.

43. Hansen K, Madsen JK. Myocarditis associated with tickborne *Borrelia burgdorferi* infection. Lancet 1986;2:1323–1324.

44. Hassler D, Zöller L, Haude M, Hufnagel H-D, Heinrich F, Sonntag H-F. Cefotaxime versus penicillin in the late stage of Lyme disease—prospective, randomized therapeutic study. Infection 1990;18:24–28.

45. Heideberg CW, Osterholm MT. Serologic tests for antibody to *Borrelia burgdorferi*:. another Pandora's box for medicine [Editorial]? Arch Intern Med 1990;150:732–733.

46. Hovmark A. Role of *Borrelia burgdorferi* in lymphocytomas and sclerotic skin lesions. Clin Dermatol 1993;11:363–367.

47. Johnson RC, Kodner C, Russel M. In vitro and in vivo susceptibility of the Lyme disease spirochete *Borrelia burgdorferi*, to four antimicrobial agents. Antimicrob Agents Chemother 1987; 31:164–167.

48. Karlsson M, Hammers S, Nilsson-Ehle I, Malmborg A-S, Wretlind B. Concentrations of doxycycline and penicillin G in sera and cerebrospinal fluid of patients treated for neuroborreliosis. Antimicrob Agents Chemother 1996;40:1104–1107.

49. Kauffmann DJH, Wormser G. Ocular Lyme disease: case report and review of the literature. Br J Ophthalmol 1990;74:325–327.

50. Kaufman LD, Gruber BL, Phillips ME, Benach JL. Late cutaneous Lyme disease: acrodermatitis chronic atrophicans. Am J Med 1989;86:828–830.

51. Kimsey RB, Spielman A. Motility of Lyme disease spirochetes in fluid as viscous as the extracellular matrix. J Infect Dis 1990; 162:1205–1208.

52. Kishaaba RG, Weinhouse E, Chusid MJ, Nudel DB. Lyme disease presenting as heart block. Clin Pediatr 1988;27:291–293.

53. Kochi SK, Johnson RC. Role of immunoglobulin G in killing of *Borrelia burgdorferi* in the classical complement pathway. Infect Immun 1988;56:314–321.

54. Kuiper H, de Jongh BM, van Dam AP, Dodge DE, Ramselaar ACP, Spanjaard L, Dankert J. Evaluation of central nervous system involvement in Lyme borreliosis patients with a solitary erythema migrans lesion. Eur J Clin Microbiol Infect Dis 1994; 13:379–387.

55. Lesser RL, Kornmehal EW, Pachner AR, Kattah J, Hedges TR 3d, Newman NM, Ecker PA, Glassman MI. Neuroophthalmologic manifestations of Lyme disease. Ophthalmology 1990;97: 699–706.

56. Levin JM, Nelson JA, Segreti J, Harrison B, Benson CA, Strle F. In vitro susceptibility of *Borrelia burgdorferi* to 11 antimicrobial agents. Antimicrob Agents Chemother 1993;37:1444–1446.

57. Ley C, Le C, Olshen EM, Reingold AL. The use of serologic tests for Lyme disease in a prepaid health plan in California. JAMA 1994;271:460–463.

58. Lightfoot RW, Luft BJ, Rahn DW, Steere AC, Sigel LH, Zoschke DC, Gardner P, Britton MC, Kaufman RL. Empiric parenteral antibiotic treatment of patients with fibromyalgia and fatigue and a positive serologic result for Lyme disease: a cost-effectiveness analysis. Ann Intern Med 1993;119:503–509.

59. Lorincz I, Lakos A, Kovacs P, Varvolgyi C, Polgar P, Worum F. Temporary pacing in complete heart block due to Lyme disease: a case report. Pacing Clin Electrophysiol 1989;12:1433–1436.

60. Luft BJ, Steinman CR, Neimark HC, Muralidhar B, Rush T, Finkel MF, Kunkel M, Dattwyler RJ. Invasion of the central nervous system by *Borrelia burgdorferi* in acute disseminated infection. JAMA 1992;267:1364–1367.

61. Luft BJ, Gardner P, Lightfoot RW Jr, Joint Committee of the American College of Rheumatology and the Council of the Infectious Diseases Society of America. Appropriateness of parenteral antibiotic treatment for patients with presumed Lyme disease. Clin Infect Dis 1994;18:112.

62. Luft BJ, Dattwyler RJ, Johnson RC, Luger SW, Bosler EM, Rahn DW, Masters EJ, Grunwaldt E, Gadgil SD. Azithromycin compared with amoxicillin in the treatment of erythema migrans. A double-blind, randomized, controlled trial. Ann Intern Med 1996;124:785–791.

63. Luger SW, Paparone P, Wormser GP, Nadelman RB, Grunwaldt E, Gomez G, Wisniewski M, Collins JJ. Comparison of cefuroxime axetil and doxycycline in treatment of patients with early Lyme disease associated with erythema migrans. Antimicrob Agents Chemother 1995;39:661–667.

64. Ma Y, Sturrock A, Weis J. Intracellular localization of *Borrelia burgdorferi* within human endothelial cells. Infect Immun 1991;59:671–678.

65. MacDonald AB, Benach JL, Burgdorfer W. Stillborn following maternal Lyme disease. NY State J Med 1987;87:615–616.

66. Markowitz LE, Steere AC, Benach JL, Slade JD, Broome CV. Lyme disease during pregnancy. JAMA 1986;255:3394–3396.

67. Massarotti EM, Luger SW, Rahn DW, Messner RP, Wong JB, Johnson RC, Steere AC. Treatement of early Lyme disease. Am J Med 1992;92:396–403.

68. McAlister HF, Klementowicz PT, Andrews C, Fisher JD, Feld M, Furman S. Lyme carditis: an important cause of reversible heart block. Ann Intern Med 1989;110:339–345.

69. Montgomery RR, Nathanson MH, Malawista SE. The fate of *Borrelia burgdorferi*, the agent for Lyme disease, in mouse macrophages. Destruction, survival, recovery. J Immunol 1993; 150:909–915.

70. Moody KD, Barthold SW, Terwilliger GA. Lyme borreliosis in laboratory animals: effect of host species and in vitro passage level of *Borrelia burgdorferi*. Am J Trop Med Hyg 1990;43: 87–92.

71. Moody KD, Adams RL, Barthold SW. Effectiveness of antimicrobial treatment against *Borrelia burgdorferi* infection in mice. Antimicrob Agents Chemother 1994;38:1567–1572.

72. Moore JA. Jarisch-Herxheimer reaction in Lyme disease. Cutis 1987;39:397–398.

73. Mursic VP, Wilske B, Schierz G, Holmburger M, Suss E. In vitro and in vivo susceptibility of *Borrelia burgdorferi*. Eur J Clin Microbiol 1987;6:424–426.

74. Nadal D, Hunziker UA, Bucher HU, Hitzig WH, Duc G. Infants born to mothers with antibodies against *Borrelia burgdorferi* at delivery. Eur J Pediatr 1989;148:426–427.

75. Nadelman RB, Nowakowski J, Forseter G, Bittker S, Cooper D, Goldberg N, McKenna D, Wormser GP. Failure to isolate *Borrelia burgdorferi* after antimicrobial therapy in culture-documented Lyme borreliosis associated with erythema migrans: report of a prospective study. Am J Med 1993;94:583–588.

76. Nadelman RB, Luger SW, Frank E, Wisniewski M, Collins JJ, Wormser GP. Comparison of cefuroxime axetil and doxycycline in the treatment of early Lyme disease. Ann Intern Med 1992; 117:273–280.

77. Nocton JJ, Dressler F, Rutledge BJ, Rys PN, Persing DH, Steere AC. Detection of *Borrelia burgdorferi* DNA by polymerase chain reaction in synovial fluid from patients with Lyme arthritis. N Engl J Med 1994;330:229–234.

78. Nowakowski J, Nadelman RB, Forseter G, McKenna D, Wormser GP. Doxycycline versus tetracycline therapy for Lyme disease associated with erythema migrans. J Am Acad Dermatol 1995;32:223–227.

79. Olson LJ, Okafor EC, Clements IP. Cardiac involvement in Lyme disease: manifestations and management. Mayo Clin Proc 1986;61:745–749.

80. Pfister H-W, Einhaupl KM, Franz P, Garner C. Corticosteroids for radicular pain in Bannwarth's syndrome. Ann NY Acad Sci 1988;539:485–487.

81. Pfister H-W, Preac-Mursic V, Wilske B, Einhäupl KM. Cefotaxime vs. penicillin G for acute neurologic manifestations in Lyme borreliosis: a prospective randomized study. Arch Neurol 1989;46:1190–1194.

82. Pfister H-W, Preac-Mursic V, Wilske B, Schielke E, Sorgel F, Einhäupl KM. Randomised comparison of ceftriaxone and cefotaxime in Lyme neuroborreliosis. J Infect Dis 1991;163: 311–318.

83. Piesman J. Dynamics of Borrelia burgdorferi transmission by nymphal .Ixodes dammini ticks. J Infect Dis 1993;167: 1082–1085.

84. Preac-Mursic V, Wilske B, Schierz G, Suss E, Gross B. Comparative antimicrobial activity of the new macrolides against Borrelia burgdorferi. Eur J Clin Microbiol 1989;8:651–653.

85. Rahn DW, Malawista SE. Lyme disease: recommendations for diagnosis and treatment. Ann Intern Med 1991;114:1472–1481.

86. Reznick JW, Braunstein DB, Walsh RL, Smith CR, Wolfson PM, Gierke LW, Gorelkin L, Chandler FW. Lyme carditis: electrophysiologic and histopathologic study. Am J Med 1986; 81:923–927.

87. Rohacova H, Hancil J, Hulinska D, Mailer H, Havlik J. Ceftriaxone in the treatment of Lyme neuroborreliosis. Infection 1996;24:88–90.

88. Schlesinger PA, Duray PH, Burke BA, Steere AC, Stillman MT. Maternal-fetal transmission of the Lyme disease spirochete, Borrelia burgdorferi. Ann Intern Med 1985;103:67–68.

89. Schoen RT, Aversa JM, Rahn DW, Steere AC. Treatment of refractory chronic Lyme arthritis with arthroscopic synovectomy. Arthritis Rheum 1991;34:1056–1060.

90. Seltzer EG, Shapiro ED. Misdiagnosis of Lyme disease: when not to order serologic tests. Pediatr Infect Dis J 1996;15: 762–763.

91. Shadick NA, Phillips CA, Logigian EL, Steere AC, Kaplan RF, Berardi VP, Duray PH, Larson MG, Wright EA, Ginsburg KS. The long-term clinical outcomes of Lyme disease: a population-based retrospective cohort study. Ann Intern Med 1994;121: 560–567.

92. Shapiro ED, Gerber MA, Holabird N, Berg AT, Feder HM, Bell GL, Rys PR, Persing DH: a controlled trial of antimicrobial prophylaxis for Lyme disease after deer-tick bites. N Engl J Med 1992;327:1769–1773.

93. Shapiro ED, Gerber MA. Lyme disease and facial nerve palsy: more questions than answers [Editorial]. Arch Pediatr Adolesc Med 1997;151(2):1183–1184.

94. Sigal LH. Experience with the first one hundred patients referral to a Lyme disease referral center. Am J Med 1987;88:577–581.

95. Sigal LH, Tatum A. Lyme disease patients' serum contains IgM antibodies to Borrelia burgdorferi that cross-react with neuronal antigens. Neurology 1988;38:1439–1442.

96. Sigal LH. Current recommendations for the treatment of Lyme disease. Drugs 1992;43:683–699.

97. Sigal LH. The flagellin of Borrelia burgdorferi, the causative agent of Lyme disease, cross-reacts with a human axonal 64,000 molecular weight protein. J Infect Dis 1993;167:1372–1378.

98. Sigal LH. Persisting complaints attributed to chronic Lyme disease: possible mechanisms and implications for management. Am J Med 1994;96:365–374.

99. Sigal LH. Management of Lyme disease refractory to antibiotic therapy. Rheum Dis Clin North Am 1995;21:217–230.

100. Sigal LH. The Lyme disease controversy: social and financial costs of misdiagnosis and mismanagement. Arch Intern Med 1996;156:1493–1500.

101. Silver HM. Lyme disease during pregnancy. Infect Dis Clin North Am 1997;11:93–97.

102. Snydman DR, Schenkein DP, Berardi VP, Lastavica CC, Pariser KM. Borrelia burgdorferi in joint fluid in chronic Lyme arthritis. Ann Intern Med 1986;104:798–800.

103. Steere AC, Gibofsky A, Patarroyo ME, Winchester RJ, Hardin JA, Malawista SE. Chronic Lyme arthritis: clinical and immunogenetic differentiation from rheumatoid arthritis. Ann Intern Med 1979;90:896–901.

104. Steere AC, Batsford WP, Weinberg M, Alexander J, Berger HJ, Wolfson S, Malawista SE. Lyme carditis: cardiac abnormalities of Lyme disease. Ann Intern Med 1980;93:8–16.

105. Steere AC, Malawista SE, Newman JH, Spieler PN, Bartenhagen NH. Antibiotic therapy in Lyme disease. Ann Intern Med 1980;93:1–8.

106. Steere AC, Hutchinson GJ, Rahn DW, Sigal LH, Craft JE, DeSanna ET, Malawista SE. Treatment of the early manifestations of Lyme disease. Ann Intern Med 1983;99:22–26.

107. Steere AC, Pachner AR, Malawista SE. Neurologic abnormalities of Lyme disease: successful treatment with high-dose intravenous penicillin. Ann Intern Med 1983;99:767–772.

108. Steere AC, Green J, Schoen RT, Taylor E, Hutchinson GJ, Rahn DW, Malawista SE. Successful parenteral penicillin therapy of established Lyme arthritis. N Engl J Med 1985;312:869–874.

109. Steere AC, Taylor E, Wilson ML, Levine JF, Spielman A. Longitudinal assessment of the clinical and epidemiological features of Lyme disease in a defined population. J Infect Dis 1986;154:294–300.

110. Steere AC. Lyme disease. N Engl J Med 1989;321:586–596.

111. Steere AC, Dwyer E, Winchester R. Association of chronic Lyme arthritis with HLA-DR4 and HLA-DR2 alleles. N Engl J Med 1990;323:219–223.

112. Steere AC, Taylor E, McHugh GL, Logigian EL. The overdiagnosis of Lyme disease. JAMA 1993;269:1812–1826.

113. Steere AC, Levin RE, Molloy PJ, Kalish RA, Abraham JH III, Liu NY, Schmid CH. Treatment of Lyme arthritis. Arthritis Rheum 1994;37:878–888.

114. Steere AC. Diagnosis and treatment of Lyme arthritis. Med Clin North Am 1997;81:179–194.

115. Strle F, Maraspin V, Pleterski-Rigler D, Lotric-Furlan S, Ruzic-Sabljic E, Jurca T, Cimperman J. Treatment of borrelial lymphocytoma. Infection 1996;24:80–84.

116. Strobino BA, Williams CL, Abid S, Chalson R, Spierling P. Lyme disease and pregnancy outcome: prospective study of two thousand prenatal patients. Am J Obstet Gynecol 1993;169: 367–375.

117. Sutthorp-Schulten MSA, Kuiper H, Kijlstra A, van Dam AP, Rothova A. Long-term effects of ceftriaxone treatment on intraocular Lyme borreliosis. Am J Ophthalmol 1993;116: 571–575.

118. Szczepanski A, Furie MB, Benach JL, Lane BP, Fleit HB. Interaction between Borrelia burgdorferi and endothelium in vitro. J Clin Invest 1990;85:1637–1647.

119. Valesová M, Mailer H, Havlik J, Hulinska D, Hercogova J. Long-term results in patients with Lyme arthritis following treatment with ceftriaxone. Infection 1996;24:100–104.

120. van der Linde MR, Crijns HJGM, de Koning J, Hoogkamp-Korstanje JA, de Graaf JJ, Piers DA, van der Galien A, Lie KI. Range of atrioventricular conduction disturbances in Lyme

borreliosis: a report of four cases and review of other published reports. Br Heart J 1990;63:162–168.

121. Vlay SC. Complete heart block due to lyme disease [Letter]. N Engl J Med 1986;315:1418.

122. Warshafsky S, Nowakowski J, Nadelman RB, Kamer RS, Peterson SJ, Wormser GP. Efficacy of antibiotic prophylaxis for prevention of Lyme disease. J Gen Intern Med 1996;11: 329–333.

123. Weber K, Bratzke H, Neubert U, Wilske B, Duray PH. *Borre-*

lia burgdorferi in a newborn despite oral penicillin for Lyme borreliosis during pregnancy. Pediatr Infect Dis J 1988;7: 286–289.

124. Weder B, Wiedershiem P, Matter L, Steck A. Chronic progressive neurologic involvement in Borrelia burgdorferi infection. J Neurol 1987;234:40–43.

125. Williams CL, Benach JL, Curran AS, Spierling P, Medici F. Lyme disease during pregnancy: a cord blood serosurvey. Ann NY Acad Sci 1988;539:504–506.

Borrelia Species

Teshale Seboxa and Daniel Fekade

GENERAL DESCRIPTION

Relapsing fevers are caused by arthropod-borne spirochetes of the genus *Borrelia*. There are two epidemiologic forms: one occurs in epidemic outbreaks and the other is a zoonosis. Louse-borne (epidemic) relapsing fever is caused by *B. recurrentis* and is transmitted only between humans by the body louse, *Pediculus humanus* var. *corporis*. Tick-borne relapsing fever is caused by more than 15 *Borrelia* species. *B. duttoni* and *B. crocidurae* are the predominant strains in Africa. *B. hermsi, B. turicatae,* and *B. parkeri* cause endemic relapsing fever in parts of the United States and Central and South America. *B. presica* and *B. hispanica* cause disease in some parts of Asia and the Mediterranean, respectively.

Borrelia are slender, actively motile organisms; 10 to 20 μm long, 0.2 to 0.5 μm wide, with 4 to 10 loose coils. Several species of tick-borne *Borrelia* and recently *B. recurrentis* have been cultivated and propagated in artificial media (19). However, in vitro and in vivo culture for diagnosis is difficult and not always successful.

SUSCEPTIBILITY IN VITRO

Because of the difficulty of cultivating the organism, little information is available about in vitro antimicrobial susceptibility. *B. recurrentis* had been considered noncultivable until recently. Cutler grew the organism from an Ethiopian patient in BSK II medium, and it has now survived several passages in vitro (9).

This strain was highly susceptible to tetracycline (MIC and MBC, 0.006 μg/mL), penicillin (MIC, 0.2 mg/mL; MBC, 0.75 mg/mL), and erythromycin (MIC, 0.04 μg/mL, MBC < 0.02 μg/mL). In contrast, *B. hermsii* and *B. turicatae* strains have an MIC for tetracycline of 1 to 4 mg/mL and an MBC of 2 to 4 μg/mL.

ANTIBIOTIC THERAPY

Tetracycline, penicillin, erythromycin, and chloramphenicol are effective in vivo for the treatment of relapsing fevers (1, 3, 4, 7, 10, 12, 15, 22, 28, 31, 33). In patients with louse-borne relapsing fever, single-dose tetracycline (500 mg) or doxycycline (100 mg) by mouth is effective in clearing spirochetes from the circulation in 2 to 4 h (7, 27, 28). Although there were no blood smear–positive relapses during 1 to 2 weeks of follow-up, over one-third of patients had recurrent fever, perhaps due to low levels of spirochetemia. Single-dose doxycycline (100 mg) also effectively cleared spirochetes from the circulation in patients with tick-borne relapsing fever. This was associated with a relapse rate of less than 1% at 2 weeks of follow-up (11).

In a randomized clinical trial, single-dose minocycline was as effective as doxycycline in terminating an attack of tick-borne relapsing fever, however no definite conclusions could be made about relapses because very few patients had sufficient follow-up (12). A patient with tick-borne relapsing fever was reported to have relapsed several weeks after treatment with single-dose doxycycline (21).

Single-dose penicillin treatment of both forms of relapsing fevers (procaine penicillin, 100,000–600,000 units i.m.) resulted in slower clearance of spirochetemia, up to 24 h, with failure/relapse rates of 2 to 16% (1, 3, 15, 24, 28, 31). Tetracycline clears the spirochetes rapidly and is associated with few or no relapses, but it induces more frequent and severe Jarisch-Herxheimer reactions than penicillin (7, 12, 18, 28, 30, 31, 33).

As the reaction is associated with high mortality and relapses are clinically mild and easy to treat, the treatment of choice for relapsing fever is combination therapy with immediate procaine penicillin (400,000–600,000 units intramuscularly) followed by tetracycline (500 mg every 6 h) or doxycycline (100 mg daily) for 2 more days (3, 4, 10, 15, 16, 22, 28, 31). However, single-dose tetracycline (500 mg) or doxycycline (100 mg) is adequate treatment for most patients in areas with limited health care resources (11, 12, 27).

Alternative therapy for pregnant women, children, and patients allergic to penicillin is erythromycin (250–500 mg) as a single dose (7, 20, 25, 28).

ENDPOINTS FOR MONITORING THERAPY

Untreated, mortality ranges from 30 to 70%; with treatment, mortality is 1 to 5% (5). Spirochetes are cleared from the circulation by 24 h following administration of antibiotics.

THE JARISCH-HERXHEIMER REACTION

Although a number of antimicrobial agents are effective for the treatment of relapsing fevers; antimicrobial treatment is followed by a severe and sometimes life-threatening Jarisch-Herxheimer reaction (5, 6, 12, 18, 23, 31, 33, 34). The reaction occurs 1 to 2 h after antimicrobial treatment, is distressing to the patient, and carries a case fatality of about 5% (5, 35). Clinically, the reaction is characterized by a rise in temperature, pulse, and respiratory rate, often accompanied by rigors. This is followed by a more prolonged phase in which patients develop hypotension or frank shock.

The clinical and pathophysiologic changes of the Jarisch-Herxheimer reaction resemble a classic endotoxin reaction (17, 34). It is associated with a transient, but marked, rise in cytokine levels coinciding with the chills phase of the reaction (26). Circulating levels of tumor necrosis factor-α (TNF-α), interleukin-6 (IL-6), and interleukin-8 were found to increase by four- to sixfold from admission levels. Peak cytokine concentrations are correlated with the severity of the reaction (8).

Attempts to prevent the reaction with acetaminophen or hydrocortisone were not successful (7, 34). Meptazinol, an opiate antagonist, ameliorated some of the symptoms but did not suppress the reaction (32). In an open clinical trial, pretreatment with pentoxyfilline, which had been shown to reduce cytokine production both in vitro and in vivo, failed to prevent either the reaction or the associated cytokine response (29). In a randomized, double-blind, placebo-controlled trial, pretreatment with ovine polyclonal antibody against TNF-α reduced the incidence of the Jarisch-Herxheimer reaction in louse-borne relapsing fever patients from 90% in controls to 45% in the treatment group (14). Peak rises in temperature, pulse, respiratory rate, and systolic blood pressure were higher among the controls than in the treated group. Levels of TNF-α, IL-6, and IL-8 (but not IL-1β) were significantly lower among those treated than in controls. This form of therapy might be relevant for other septicemic illnesses (2, 13).

REFERENCES

1. Barclay AJ, Coulter JB. Tick-borne relapsing fever in central Tanzania. Trans R Soc Trop Med Hyg 1990;84:852–856.
2. Beutler B, Munford RS. Tumor necrosis factor and the Jarisch-Herxheimer reaction. N Engl J Med 1996;335:347–348.
3. Borgnolo G, Hailu B, Ciancarelli A, Almaviva M, Woldemariam T. Louse-borne relapsing fever. Trop Geogr Med 1993;45:66–69.
4. Borgnolo G, Denku B, Chiabrera F, Hailu B. Louse-borne relapsing fever in Ethiopian children: a clinical study. Ann Trop Paediatr 1993;13:165–171.
5. Bryceson ADM, Parry EHO, Perine PL, Warrell DA, Vukotich D, Leithead CS. Louse-borne relapsing fever: a clinical and laboratory study of 62 cases in Ethiopia and a reconsideration of the literature. Q J Med 1970;39:129–170.
6. Butler TC. Relapsing fever: new lessons about antibiotic action. Ann Intern Med 1985;102:397–399.
7. Butler T, Jones PK, Wallace CK. Borrelia recurrentis infection: single dose antibiotic regimens and management of the Jarisch-Herxheimer reaction. J Infect Dis 1978;137:573–577.
8. Coxon RE, Fekade D, Knox k, Melka A, Daniel A. Griffin GE, Warrell DA. The effect of polyclonal antibody fragments to tumor necrosis factor on the cytokine response during the Jarisch-Herxheimer reaction of louse borne relapsing fever. Q J Med 1997;90:213–221.
9. Cutler SJ, Fekade D, Hussein K, Knox K, Melka A, Cann K, Emilanus AR, Warrell DA, Wright DJM. Successful in vitro cultivation of Borrelia recurrentis [Letter]. Lancet 1994;343:242.
10. Daniel E, Beyene H, Tessema T. Relapsing fever in children—demographic, social and clinical features. Ethiop Med J 1992;30:207–214.
11. de-Clercq AG, Meheus AZ, de-Pierpont E, Nyirashema C. Single-dose doxycycline treatment of tick-borne relapsing fever. East Afr Med J 1975;52:428–429.
12. De Pierpont E, Goubau PF, Verhgaen J, Vandepitte J. Single dose minocycline and doxycycline treatment of tick borne relapsing fever: a double blind clinical trial in Rwanda. Ann Soc Belg Med Trop 1983;63:357–361.
13. Dinarello CA, Gelfand JA, Wolff SM. Anticytokine strategies in the treatment of the systemic inflammatory response syndrome. JAMA 1993;269:1829–1835.
14. Fekade D, Knox K, Hussein K, Melka A, Lalloo G, Coxen RE, Warrel DA. Prevention of the Jarish-Herxheimer reaction by treatment with antibodies against tumor necrosis factor α. N Engl J Med 1996;335:311–315.
15. Gebrehiwot T, Fiseha A. Tetracycline versus penicillin in the treatment of louse-borne relapsing fever. Ethiop Med J 1992;30:175–178.
16. Goubau PF Relapsing fevers. A review. Ann Soc Belg Med Trop 1984;64:335–361.
17. Griffin GE, Negussie Y, Fekade D, Morlese J, Forrester T, Remick DG. The Jarish-Herxheimer reaction: a paradigm of cytokine cascade. In: Griffin GE, ed. Cytokines and infection. Bailliere's clinical infectious diseases, 1994:65–74.
18. Horton JM, Blaser MJ. The spectrum of relapsing fever in the Rocky Mountain. Arch Intern Med 1985;145:871–875.
19. Kelly RT. Cultivation and physiology of relapsing fever borreliae. In: Johnson RC, ed. The biology of parasitic spirochetes. New York: Academic Press, 1976:87–94.
20. Le CT. Tick-borne relapsing fever in children. Paediatrics 1980;66:963–966.
21. Liles WC, Spach DH. Late relapse of tick-borne relapsing fever following treatment with doxycycline [Letter]. West J Med 1993;158:200.
22. Mekasha A. Louse borne relapsing fever in children. J Trop Med Hyg 1992;95:206–209.
23. Melkert PW. Fatal Jarish-Herxheimer reaction in a case of tick borne relapsing fever misdiagnosed as lobar pneumonia. Trop Geogr Med 1987;39:92.
24. Melkert PW. Mortality in high risk patients with tick-borne relapsing fever analysed by the Borrelia-index. East Afr Med J 1991;68:875–879.
25. Melkert PW, Stel HV. Neonatal Borrelia infections (relapsing fever): report of 5 cases and review of the literature. East Afr Med J 1991;68:999–1005.
26. Negussie Y, Remick DG, Deforge LE, Kunkel SL, Eynon A, Griffin GE. Detection of plasma tumor necrosis factor, inter-

leukins 6, and 8 during the Jarisch-Herxheimer reaction of relapsing fever. J Exp Med 1992;175:1207–1212.

27. Perine PL, Kraus DW, Awoke S, McDade JE. Single dose doxycycline treatment of louse borne relapsing fever and epidemic typhus. Lancet 1974;ii:742–744.

28. Perine PL, Teklu B. Antibiotic treatment of louse-borne relapsing fever in Ethiopia: a report of 377 cases. Am J Trop Med Hyg
1983;32:1096–1100.

29. Remick DJ, Negussie Y, Morlesse J, Forrester T, Fekade D,
Griffin GE. Pentoxyfilline fails to prevent the Jarish-Herxheimer
reaction or associated cytokine release. J Infect Dis 1996;174:
627–630.

30. Salih SY, Mustafa D. Louse-borne relapsing fever: II. Combined
penicillin and tetracycline therapy in 160 Sudanese patients.
Trans R Soc Trop Med Hyg 1971;71:49–51.

31. Seboxa T, Rahlenbeck SI. Treatment of louse-borne relapsing

fever with low dose penicillin or tetracycline: a clinical trial.
Scand J Infect Dis 1995;27:29–31.

32. Teklu B, Habte-Michael A, Warrell DA, White NJ, Wright DJM.
Meptazinol diminishes the Jarisch-Herxheimer reaction of relapsing fever. Lancet 1983;1:835–839.

33. Warrell DA, Perine P, Krause D, Bing D, MacDougal S. Pathophysiology and immunology of the Jarisch-Herxheimer like reaction of louse-borne relapsing fever: comparison of tetracycline
and slow-release penicillin. J Infect Dis 1983;147:898–909.

34. Warrell DA, Pope HM, Parry EHO, Perine PL, Bryceson ADM.
Cardiorespiratory disturbances associated with infective fever in
man: studies of Ethiopian louse-borne relapsing fever. Clin Sci
1970;39:123–145.

35. Zein AZ. Louse borne relapsing fever: mortality and frequency
of the Jarish-Herxheimer reaction. J R Soc Health 1987;4:
146–147.

Brucella Species

Edward J. Young

GENERAL DESCRIPTION

Brucellosis is a disease of domestic and wild animals (zoonosis) that is transmittable to humans. The disease exists worldwide, especially in the Mediterranean basin, the Arabian
peninsula, the Indian subcontinent, and in parts of Mexico and
Central and South America. In the United States, the incidence
of human brucellosis declined dramatically after WWII, associated with programs to control bovine brucellosis and enforcement of laws requiring pasteurization of milk (260). Once
a disease principally affecting persons engaged in the livestock industry, the epidemiology of brucellosis has changed in
recent years toward a foodborne infection, associated primarily with consumption of unpasteurized dairy products originating abroad (46, 236).

Four species of *Brucella* are pathogenic for man. They are
closely related genetically, but for reasons that are not entirely
clear, each species shows a predilection for certain natural host
animals: *B. abortus* (cattle), *B. melitensis* (goats and sheep), *B.
suis* (swine), and *B. canis* (dogs). Human brucellosis is a systemic infection with protean clinical manifestations. Characteristically, patients present with fever, sweats, fatigue, and
joint pains. Abnormal physical findings are few, with the exception of occasional hepatosplenomegaly. *Brucella* species
are facultative intracellular pathogens that can survive and
replicate within phagocytic cells of the host. Following inoculation into the body, organisms rapidly localize within
macrophages of the reticuloendothelial system where they can

give rise to localized complications (256). Humoral antibodies are raised early in infection; however, recovery from brucellosis depends on the generation of cell-mediated immunity.
A variety of antimicrobial agents have activity against *Brucella* species, but the results of in vitro susceptibility tests do
not always correlate with clinical efficacy of the drug. This is
believed to be due, in part, to the intracellular localization of
the organism, which provides it some protection against host
defenses and antimicrobial drug effects. For this reason,
prolonged therapy with more than one drug is generally required to achieve a cure (224).

SUSCEPTIBILITY IN VITRO

Working with *Brucella* species is a risk to laboratory personnel,
and level 3 biohazard precautions are required. Periodic serologic testing of personnel handling brucellae is also advised.

Brucella species have relatively simple nutritional requirements; however, they grow slowly in vitro. They can be cultured on any peptone-based media supplemented with serum,
including blood and chocolate agar. Some strains of *Brucella*
require supplemental CO_2, especially for primary isolation.
Historically, susceptibility testing of *Brucella* species has used
a variety of media, inoculum concentrations, incubation times,
and atmospheric conditions. An acceptable approach is the
National Committee for Clinical Laboratory Standards (NC-
CLS 1987) method modified to substitute trypticase soy broth
(TSB) for Mueller-Hinton broth (MHB) supplemented with

6% CO_2 (239, 240). Tilton et al. examined the effects of TSB versus MHB on susceptibility testing of various organisms and found only slight variations with the number of organisms/drug combinations (241). In our experience, with TSB, there is little variation in minimal inhibitory concentration (MIC) among *Brucella* strains (158). Alternatively, Hall recommended Albimi Brucella broth and an atmosphere of 10% CO_2 for susceptibility studies (107). By convention, a test inoculum of 5×10^5 to 1×10^6 CFU of bacteria incubated at 35°C for 48 hours is generally used. The endpoint (MIC) is defined as the lowest dilution of the antimicrobial agent that completely inhibits growth.

To test for synergy between combinations of antimicrobial agents, most authors recommend conventional checkerboard techniques using reagents, inocula, and conditions of incubation similar to those used for standard MIC tests (133). The nature of the ensuing interaction between antimicrobial agents is determined by the fractional inhibitory concentration index (FIC index) with antagonism defined as an FIC index of 2.0 or more, indifference as between 0.5 and 2.0, and synergy as 0.5 or less (169).

Another method of testing the susceptibility of *Brucella* species to antimicrobial agents, singly or in combination, uses the rate of bacterial killing in vitro (205). The rate of killing is determined by using an inoculum of 10^5 CFU/mL in tubes containing broth. The antimicrobial agents are tested at concentrations four times the respective MIC, either singly or in combinations. After incubation for 48 hours, aliquots are removed at timed intervals (0 to 96 h) and mixed with warm molten agar in 10^3 to 10^5 dilutions, and the number of CFUs is determined by the pour plate method.

Finally, a variety of laboratory animal models have been used to test the benefit of antimicrobial agents against *Brucella* species in vivo. Although animal models have been no more predictive of clinical success than in vitro methods for certain antimicrobial agents (183), they have been used to study novel delivery systems, such as liposome encapsulation (85), and to confirm the superiority of combination therapy for brucellosis (139, 216, 217).

Single Drug Susceptibility

Penicillins

As early as 1944, crude penicillin was shown to be active in vitro against *Brucella* species, but the effect was least against strains of *B. melitensis* (244). When crystalline penicillin G was tested against various *Brucella* species, the MIC_{50} value was 12.5 μg/mL, and the MIC_{90} value exceeded 100 μg/mL (107). Ampicillin was found to be more active than penicillin G by several investigators (104, 107, 158, 175). The inhibitory concentrations for ampicillin ranged from 0.5 to 8 μg/mL, with the MIC_{50} between 0.5 and 1.0 μg/mL. Since it is estimated that serum concentrations in the range of 4 to 5 μg/mL can be achieved with ampicillin, it should be therapeutic for some, but not all, *Brucella* strains. Consequently, it is not surprising that clinical results with ampicillin and amoxacillin in the treatment of human brucellosis have been disappointing (73, 163, 202). The semisynthetic penicillins (methicillin, naf-

cillin, oxacillin), and the ureidopenicillins (carbenicillin, piperacillin) are much less active than ampicillin against *Brucella* species, with MIC_{90} values of 12 and 32 μg/mL, respectively (107, 158).

Cephalosporins

There are wide variations in the activities of cephalosporin antibiotics against *Brucella* species. The first-generation cephalosporins, which have a limited Gram-negative spectrum, are similar to penicillin G, with generally high MIC values (Table 1). Although structurally related to the cephalosporins, moxalactam has a considerably broader spectrum of activity (252). In two series, moxalactam had high MIC values (Table 1); however, some *Brucella* isolates have been shown to be susceptible, and a child infected with *B. canis* was successfully treated with this agent (242). In addition, after intravenous administration, moxalactam achieves a cerebrospinal fluid (CSF) concentration of approximately 18.5% of the serum level, and it has been used successfully to treat meningitis caused by highly sensitive strains of *Haemophilus influenzae* type b (125). Before moxalactam is used to treat human brucellosis, the infecting strain of *Brucella* must be shown to be highly sensitive.

Among the third-generation cephalosporins, cefotaxime, ceftizoxime, and ceftriaxone were found to have activity against *Brucella melitensis* (Table 1). Like moxalactam, these drugs achieve reasonably good levels in the CSF in the presence of inflamed meninges (167). In addition, the novel β-lactam antibiotic *N*-formimidoyl thienamycin (imepenam) was shown to be active in vitro against 98 strains of *B. melitensis*, with an MIC_{50} value of 0.25 μg/mL (102); however, there have been no clinical studies with this drug in patients with brucellosis. Ceftriaxone, on the other hand, was shown to inhibit 95 strains of *B. melitensis*, with MIC values in the range of 0.25 to 1.0 μg/mL (173), yet when used clinically, the results were disappointing (39). Using a dose of 4 g/day of ceftriaxone intravenously, 30.8% of 14 patients in one study failed to respond (13), and using a dose of 2 g/day intramuscularly in another study, only 1 of 8 patients was cured (137). The reasons for the lack of clinical effectiveness of β-lactam antibiotics that inhibit *Brucella* species in vitro is not clear; however, penicillin and cephalosporins cannot be considered first-line drugs for the treatment of human brucellosis (36).

Macrolides

The macrolide antibiotic erythromycin has been shown to have some activity in vitro against *Brucella* species. One-half of 27 strains of various species of *Brucella* were inhibited by 0.15 μg/mL of erythromycin, and all strains were inhibited by 2.5 μg/mL in one study (107). In another study, the range of inhibitory concentrations was 0.5 to 8 μg/mL (158). In a recent report, the MIC range for erythromycin was 0.2 to 16 μg/mL against 62 strains of *Brucella* species (89). Thus it is not surprising that when erythromycin was used as monotherapy in the treatment of human brucellosis, the relapse rate was unacceptably high (44, 145, 246, 247). Even when erythromycin was used in combination with streptomycin, the results were poor, and the incidence of gastrointestinal side ef-

TABLE 1 • Minimal Inhibitory Concentrations (μg/mL) of Cephalosporins against *Brucella* Species

Drug	Hall (107)		Mortensen (158)			Palenque (173)		
	MIC$_{50}$	MIC$_{100}$	MIC$_{50}$	MIC$_{90}$	(Range)	MIC$_{50}$	MIC$_{90}$	(Range)
Cephalothin	12.5	>100	8	32	(1–64)	NT	NT	
Cephaloridine	12.5	>100	NT		NT	NT	NT	
Cephalexin	12.5	>100	NT		NT	NT	NT	
Cefoxitin	NT	NT	4	16	(2–16)	NT	NT	
Cefamandole	NT	NT	16	32	(4->64)	NT	NT	
Moxalactam	NT	NT	8	16	(1–16)	16	16	(4–16)
Cefotaxime	NT	NT	1	2	(≤0.5–4)	1	2	(0.5–2)
Cefoperazone	NT	NT	16	16	(≤1–16)	16	32	(4–64)
Ceftizoxime	NT	NT	NT		NT	0.5	1	(0.5–1)
Cefuroxime	NT	NT	NT		NT	32	32	(8–64)
Aztreonam	NT	NT	NT		NT	128	>256	(64->256)
Ceftriaxone	NT	NT	NT		NT	0.5	1	(0.25–1)
Ceftazidime	NT	NT	NT	NT		32	32	(16–32)

Brucella species and no. strains tested

	Hall (107)	Mortensen (158)	Palenque (173)
B. abortus	7	4	0
B. melitensis	2	7	83
B. suis	10	2	0
B. canis	4	2	0

fects was high (73). In an extensive review of the chemotherapy of human brucellosis, Hall reported an overall relapse rate with erythromycin treatment, alone or in combination with other drugs, of 27% (108).

Among the newer macrolides, dirithromycin and roxithromycin are similar in activity in vitro to erythromycin (MIC ranges, 0.5 to 16 μg/mL and 0.1 to 32 μg/mL, respectively) (89). In contrast, azithromycin and clarithromycin have in vitro activity against *Brucella* species many times greater than that of erythromycin (MIC ranges, 0.1 to 4 μg/mL and 0.06 to 8 μg/mL, respectively) (89, 135, 191). These drugs achieve good serum levels after oral administration, and their tissue concentrations exceed serum levels by as much as 100-fold. Furthermore, azithromycin is concentrated within phagocytic cells (neutrophils and macrophages) without interfering with the bactericidal activities of the cell (164). Such properties suggest that azithromycin and clarithromycin might be useful in treating brucellae that are known to survive and multiply within host cells. However, azithromycin was found to be less effective than doxycycline in eradicating brucellosis in a mouse model of brucellosis (69), raising serious questions about its clinical usefulness. To date, there have been no clinical trials of newer macrolides in human brucellosis.

Chloramphenicol

Chloramphenicol is mentioned only because it has some activity in vitro against *Brucella* species, and it found limited use for human brucellosis during the 1940s and 1950s (108). The in vitro activity of chloramphenicol against *Brucella* species is variable, with a range of MIC values from 1.25 to 5 μg/mL (107, 158). Among 47 patients treated with chloramphenicol from the literature, the rate of relapse was 32%. In view of this high relapse rate, the potential for serious hematologic side ef-

fects (some fatal) (94), and the availability of safer and more effective drugs, chloramphenicol cannot be considered appropriate therapy for human brucellosis (67, 201).

Tetracyclines

The tetracyclines remain the most active and clinically effective antibiotics for the treatment of brucellosis, and they are the standard against which all other drugs are measured. Although differences in the in vitro activity of tetracycline analogues against *Brucella* species were reported (78, 202, 233), since 1955 tetracycline HCl has been the most commonly used drug for treating human brucellosis (108, 140). Tetracycline achieves a serum level of about 4 μg/mL after an oral dose of 500 mg, whereas, the long-acting analogues doxycycline and minocycline achieve a prolonged serum level of 2.5 μg/mL following an oral dose of 200 mg (232). Doxycycline is almost completely absorbed and has a prolonged half-life due to its slow rate of renal excretion. In addition, doxycycline is the only tetracycline compound that can be used in patients with renal insufficiency, since it is excreted from the gastrointestinal tract under these conditions (251). The low MIC values against *Brucella* species (Table 2), the convenience of once-daily dosing, and the low rate of gastrointestinal side effects, make doxycycline now the preferred tetracycline analogue for treating human brucellosis. These factors notwithstanding, the use of tetracyclines as monotherapy for human brucellosis is complicated by a relapse rate between 8 and 39%. The high relapse rates are dramatically reduced when doxycycline is combined with other drugs, such as streptomycin (relapse rate, 4.5%) or rifampin (relapse rate, 8.4%) (108).

A major drawback to the use of tetracyclines is the permanent staining of teeth in young children. Consequently, tetracyclines are contraindicated for brucellosis in pregnant

TABLE 2 • Minimal Inhibitory Concentrations (μg/mL) of Tetracyclines against *Brucella* Species

Drug	No. Strains Tested	MIC$_{90}$ (Range)[a]	(Ref.)
Tetracycline	27	0.03 (0.001–0.07)	(107)
	98	0.39 (0.1–0.5)	(102)
	15	0.25 (≤0.13–0.25)	(158)
	95	0.25 (0.06–0.25)	(39)
	47	0.04 (0.001–0.6)	(131)
	358	0.25 (0.06–0.5)	(135)
	105	0.25 (0.06–0.25)	(189)
	62	0.2 (0.01–0.2)	(90)
Minocycline	27	0.3 (0.01–0.3)	(107)
	86	0.4 (NR)	(205)
	85	0.4 (NR)	(18)
Doxycycline	27	0.3 (0.01–0.3)	(107)
	95	0.12 (0.06–0.25)	(39)

[a] NR, not reported.

TABLE 3 • Minimal Inhibitory Concentrations (μg/mL) of Aminoglycosides against *Brucella* Species

Drug	No. Strains Tested	MIC$_{90}$ (Range)[a]	(Ref.)
Streptomycin	27	2.5 (0.02–5.0)	(107)
	8	4.0 (1.0–4.0)	(158)
	95	0.5 (0.12–1.0)	(39)
	47	2.5 (0.15–5.0)	(131)
	86	3.1 (NR)	(205)
	146	1.0 (0.5–2.0)	(190)
	62	0.2 (0.01–0.2)	(90)
Gentamicin	27	0.4 (0.02–2.5)	(107)
	15	1.0 (0.25–2.0)	(158)
	105	0.25 (0.12–0.5)	(189)
	146	0.25 (0.12–0.5)	(190)
Kanamycin	27	2.5 (0.02–5.0)	(107)
Tobramycin	15	2.0 (0.5–4.0)	(158)
Amikacin	15	2.0 (1.0–4.0)	(158)

[a] NR, not reported.

women and children under 8 years of age. In this regard, doxycycline binds less to calcium than do other tetracyclines and may cause dental complications less frequently (84, 232).

Aminoglycosides

Streptomycin, the first aminoglycoside antibiotic discovered, was shown to have activity in vitro against *Brucella* species (MIC values, 1–5 μg/mL) (92, 107, 131, 158, 189, 205). Streptomycin is rapidly absorbed after intramuscular injection and reaches a peak serum concentration of 20 to 40 μg/mL after a 1-g dose (152). However, when streptomycin was used as monotherapy for patients with brucellosis, it soon became evident that it was ineffective (82, 118, 187, 195). In addition, occasional streptomycin-resistant strains were isolated from patients treated with streptomycin alone (106, 261). Consequently, streptomycin was used in combination with other drugs, initially sulfadiazine, and later tetracycline (108). For many years the standard therapy for human brucellosis was tetracycline (500 mg four times daily by mouth) given for 4 to 6 weeks, plus streptomycin (1 g/day intramuscularly) given for the first 2 weeks (2, 108, 140). The discrepancy between in vitro methods for evaluating antibiotic efficacy is illustrated by bacterial killing rate studies showing that streptomycin exhibits the most rapid rate (complete killing of log$_{10}$ CFU at 4 times MIC in 8 h) against *B. melitensis* (205).

Studies comparing the in vitro activity of other aminoglycosides with streptomycin have shown that gentamicin is more active, kanamycin and tobramycin are equivalent, and amikacin is less active (Table 3). Netilmicin, an aminoglycoside derived from sisomycin, was reported to have an MIC value of 0.6 μg/mL against *Brucella* species (152); however, when netilmicin was used in combination with doxycycline to treat brucellosis, the rates of failure and relapse were unacceptably high (22%) (221). Spectinomycin, another aminoglycoside antibiotic, was shown to have activity against *Brucella* species (MIC values, 1–5 μg/mL), but it is only bacteriostatic, and it has not been used to treat human brucellosis (58).

Gentamicin has rarely been used as monotherapy for brucellosis (170), but it has been shown to be effective when combined with other drugs, such as doxycycline (150). Although aminoglycosides must be administered parenterally, once-daily dosing has improved efficacy and reduced the incidence of toxic side effects (95, 168, 262). Streptomycin combined with tetracycline (153) or doxycycline (25) has been the "gold standard" for comparison of other antibiotic regimens for the treatment of human brucellosis. No such trials have compared streptomycin and gentamicin. Most authorities believe that gentamicin can be used in place of streptomycin; however, no comparative trials of the two drugs have been published. A prospective study, sponsored by the World Health Organization (WHO), comparing gentamicin and streptomycin in combination with doxycycline is currently under way.

Trimethoprim/Sulfamethoxazole (Cotrimoxazole)

Trimethoprim, a 2,4-diamino-5-(3′,4′,5′-trimethoxy benzyl) pyrimidine, is a potent inhibitor of dihydrofolate reductase. The antimicrobial action of trimethoprim is potentiated by combination with sulfamethoxazole. The synergistic action of trimethoprim/sulfamethoxazole (TMP-SMX) depends somewhat on the sensitivity of the organism to each drug. Cotrimoxazole is available in a fixed combination in a ratio of 1:5 (80 mg trimethoprim, 400 mg sulfamethoxazole). Double-strength tablets, quarter-strength (pediatric dose) tablets, and an intravenous preparation (16 mg/mL trimethoprim, 80 mg/mL sulfamethoxazole) are also available. After oral administration of a single-strength tablet, the peak level of trimethoprim is 3.5 μg/mL after about 2 to 4 h. The CSF concentration of trimethoprim is approximately 40% of the serum concentration (264).

Cotrimoxazole has clinical efficacy against facultative intracellular pathogens, such as *Salmonella typhi* and *Salmonella paratyphi,* and two patients were treated successfully in 1970 (75). Lal et al. treated four patients with brucellosis and showed that the MIC values for TMP-SMX was greater than those of either drug alone (134). Additional patients with brucellosis were treated with cotrimoxazole (62, 96, 111), but the rates of relapse ranged from 4 to 37.5%.

In vitro susceptibility of *Brucella* species to TMP-SMX, individually or in combination, has been reported with variable results (Table 4). Although some patients have been treated successfully with cotrimoxazole (237), relapse rates in excess of 40% have been reported in open trials (20) and in a prospective comparative study (22). In addition, strains of *Brucella* species resistant to cotrimoxazole have been reported (15). Nevertheless, cotrimoxazole is a useful alternative in the treatment of brucellosis when the use of tetracyclines is contraindicated (e.g., in children and in pregnancy) (140). Cotrimoxazole has yielded good results when used in combination with other drugs such as doxycycline (156) and streptomycin (15).

Rifampin

Rifampin is a semisynthetic derivative of rifamycin B, a macrocyclic antibiotic produced by the mold *Streptomyces mediterranei*. The drug is remarkably lipid soluble and accumulates in eukaryotic cells. It exerts its antimicrobial effect by inhibiting DNA-dependent RNA polymerase. Rifampin is almost completely absorbed after oral ingestion and reaches a peak serum concentration of 7 to 10 μg/mL after a dose of 600 mg. Rifampin penetrates tissues well, and levels of 1.3 μg/mL are found in the CSF in the presence of inflamed meninges (77). Since plasma clearance is via the enterohepatic circulation, rifampin can be used in patients with renal insufficiency; however, drug-induced hepatitis and cholestatic jaundice have been reported, especially in alcoholics and patients treated with isoniazid (INH). Rifampin induces hepatic microsomal enzymes, which can result in accelerated metabolism of some other drugs, such as warfarin, oral contraceptives, glucocorticoids, digoxin, quinidine, and oral hypoglycemics (28). Accelerated clearance of doxycycline caused by rifampin was cited as a possible explanation for relapses of brucellosis in patients treated with this combination of drugs (55).

The in vitro susceptibility of *Brucella* species to rifampin has

been documented by numerous investigators (Table 5), and it has been shown to be effective in experimental animal models of brucellosis (183, 216). Corbel reported that rifampin was bactericidal at concentrations four times the MIC; however, rifampin-resistant variants occurred frequently irrespective of the antibiotic concentration (59). Although rifampin has been used as monotherapy for human brucellosis (34, 57, 174), relapses (147) and the emergence of rifampin-resistant strains (66) have led to its use primarily in combination with other drugs (140).

Fluoroquinolones

Quinolones are derivatives of nalidixic acid, an oral agent introduced in 1963 to treat urinary infections. Nalidixic acid was only weakly active against *Brucella* species, (MIC$_{90}$, 64 μg/mL) and serum concentrations were too low to be effective in brucellosis (108, 138, 215). In the 1980s, development of fluorine- and piperazinyl-substituted derivatives with greater antimicrobial activities and extended spectra, renewed interest in this class of drugs (115). Quinolones block bacterial DNA synthesis by inhibiting the enzyme DNA gyrase (116). Quinolones are well absorbed after oral administration, and following a 400 mg dose, serum levels range from 1.5 μg/mL for norfloxacin to 5.8 μg/mL for perfloxacin. The drug is concentrated in macrophages and neutrophils, but penetration into CSF is low except for perfloxacin (40% of serum) and ofloxacin (90% of serum) (115).

The quinolones have greater activity in vitro against *Brucella* species than nalidixic acid (Table 6), but the MIC$_{90}$ values vary for each compound and to some extent for *Brucella* isolates. Newer quinolones, such as fleroxacin, lomefloxacin, and clinafloxacin, have MIC$_{90}$ values similar to those listed in Table 6. Although minimal bactericidal concentration (MBC) values are said to be one to four dilutions above MIC values, one study found that quinolones lacked bactericidal activity at pH levels comparable to those within the cell (88). In a murine model of brucellosis, treatment with ciprofloxacin, ofloxacin, and perfloxacin failed to cure infected animals despite drug serum levels that should have been therapeutic (216). Results were also generally disappointing when monotherapy with quinolones

---

TABLE 4 • Minimal Inhibitory Concentrations (μg/mL) of Cotrimoxazole against *Brucella* Species

Drug	No. Strains Tested	MIC$_{90}$ (Range)[a]	(Ref.)
Cotrimoxazole	160	3.15 (3.15–10.5)	(42)
	98	32 (8–128)	(102)
	15	1/19[b] (≤0.25/4.5–1/19)	(158)
	95	0.25 (0.06–0.5)	(39)
	47	5.0 (5.0–25)	(131)
	86	6.3 (NR)	(205)
	105	1.0 (0.12–1.0)	(189)
	146	1.0 (0.12–1.0)	(190)
	62	4/76 (0.1/1.9–4/76)	(90)
	116	1.0 (0.25–1.0)	(188)

[a] NR, not reported.

[b] Values shown for trimethoprim/sulfamethoxazole components.

TABLE 5 • Minimal Inhibitory Concentrations (μg/mL) of *Rifampin* against *Brucella* Species

Drug	No. Strains Tested	MIC$_{90}$ (Range)[a]	(Ref.)
Rifampin	27	1.25 (0.02–12.5)	(107)
	107	≤2.5 (0.018–10)	(59)
	98	0.5 (0.06–1.0)	(102)
	8	1.0 (0.06–1.0)	(158)
	95	0.5 (0.12–4.0)	(39)
	47	1.25 (0.02–2.5)	(131)
	86	4.0 (NR)	(205)
	105	1.0 (0.12–1.0)	(189)
	62	1.0 (0.1–4.0)	(90)
	146	1.0 (0.12–1.0)	(190)
	116	1.0 (0.25–1.0)	(188)

[a] NR, not reported.

TABLE 6 • **Minimal Inhibitory Concentrations (μg/mL) of Selected Quinolones against *Brucella* Species**			
Drug	**No. Strains Tested**	**MIC$_{90}$ (Range)^a**	**(Ref.)**
Ciprofloxacin	68	1.0 (0.5–1.0)	(97)
	95	0.5 (0.12–0.5)	(39)
	62	0.5 (NR)	(91)
	22	0.78 (0.39–0.78)	(31)
	47	2.5 (1.25–2.5)	(131)
	86	0.8 (NR)	(205)
	146	0.5 (0.06–0.5)	(190)
	105	0.5 (0.06–0.5)	(189)
	116	0.5 (0.25–2.0)	(188)
	123	0.5 (0.25–0.5)	(90)
Norfloxacin	68	8.0 (2.0–8.0)	(97)
	62	4.0 (1.0–4.0)	(91)
	146	0.5 (0.12–0.5)	(190)
	105	4.0 (0.12–>4.0)	(189)
Ofloxacin	62	1.0 (NR)	(91)
	28	0.78 (0.39–0.78)	(31)
	47	0.3 (0.02–0.3)	(131)
	86	2.5 (NR)	(205)
Perfloxacin	62	4.0 (2.0–4.0)	(91)
	86	3.1 (NR)	(205)
	146	0.5 (0.06–0.5)	(190)
	105	4.0 (0.06–>4)	(189)

^{a} NR, not reported.

was used to treat human brucellosis. In a study from Turkey, 12 patients received ofloxacin (200 mg twice daily) for varying periods of time, with no failures or relapses (31). When this study was extended to 21 patients, the relapse rate was 16% (3). In contrast, a group of patients in Israel treated with ciprofloxacin (750 or 1000 mg twice daily) for 6 weeks had a relapse rate of 66% (136). Similarly, another study from Turkey reported 12 patients treated with ciprofloxacin (500 mg thrice daily) for 3 to 6 weeks, with a relapse rate of 21% (68). Although prompt clinical improvement occurred, four patients failed to respond or relapsed (25%) (18). In addition, one patient had bacteremia that persisted for 3 weeks, and the isolate showed increasing MIC values to ciprofloxacin (17). Consequently, monotherapy of brucellosis with quinolones is not recommended; however, ofloxacin combined with rifampin was reported to yield satisfactory results (4).

Combinations of Drugs

Penicillin and Sulfathiazole
Of historic interest, T'Ung reported that penicillin combined with a small amount of sulfathiazole inhibited some strains of *Brucella* species more effectively than either drug alone (244). Although these drugs are no longer used to treat brucellosis, this early study suggested that combinations of drugs might be synergistic against *Brucella* species.

Tetracycline and Streptomycin or Gentamincin
Tetracycline and streptomycin were reported to act synergistically in inhibiting intracellular replication of *B. abortus* in primary cell cultures. Tetracycline, bacteriostatic at concentrations

of 0.5 to 1.0 μg/mL, became bactericidal when combined with 10 μg/mL of streptomycin (199). In vivo synergy between tetracycline and streptomycin was also reported in a murine model of brucellosis (114); however, using BALB/c mice infected with *B. melitensis,* Domingo et al. found the combination of doxycycline and streptomycin to be no more effective than doxycycline alone in reducing CFUs in the spleen (70).

Attempts to demonstrate synergy in vitro between tetracycline and streptomycin have been less successful. Robertson et al. studied 25 strains of *B. abortus* and were unable to demonstrate synergy between tetracycline and streptomycin (202). Using conventional checkerboard microdilutions of combinations of tetracycline and streptomycin, Mortensen et al. were unable to demonstrate synergy for 5 of 8 strains of *Brucella* species. In three cases this combination of drugs was actually antagonistic as calculated by the FIC index. Combinations of tetracycline and gentamicin were indifferent for eight *Brucella* strains tested (158). Ariza et al. studied the antimicrobial sensitivity patterns of *B. melitensis* strains recovered from patients with bacteriologic relapse. No differences in antibiotic susceptibility were noted between original isolates and relapse strains. Synergism for the antibiotic combinations used could not be assessed because of the very low MIC values of tetracycline and doxycycline for these isolates (24).

Rubinstein et al. used agar plate dilutions and broth dilution methods to study combinations of antibiotics against 15 strains of *B. melitensis.* They found that no combinations of minocycline, ciprofloxacin, rifampin, or streptomycin exhibited synergy against any of the strains tested. In contrast, when bacterial killing rates were compared, streptomycin in combination with minocycline, rifampin, or ciprofloxacin exhibited the fastest killing of *B. melitensis* (205).

Tetracycline and Rifampin
Using conventional checkerboard microdilution techniques, Mortensen et al. reported that the combination of tetracycline and rifampin was synergistic for 6 of 8 strains of *Brucella* species and indifferent for 2 strains (158).

Trimethoprim and Sulfamethoxazole
TMP-SMX (cotrimoxazole) is compounded as a fixed combination containing 80 mg trimethoprim and 400 mg sulfamethoxazole; however, each component has been tested against *Brucella* species alone and together. Lal et al. reported that MIC values for two strains of *B. abortus* declined from 15 μg/mL for trimethoprim and 3 μg/mL for sulfamethoxazole individually to 0.05 μg/mL for trimethoprim and 1.0 μg/mL for sulfamethoxazole when the drugs were combined (134). Using an agar dilution method with a heavy inoculum of *B. abortus,* Robertson et al. reported that 25 strains had MIC values of 32 μg/mL for trimethoprim and 2 μg/mL for sulfamethoxazole. When the drugs were combined, the MIC values were reduced to 2 μg/mL for trimethoprim and 0.125 μg/mL for sulfamethoxazole, indicating 16-fold synergy (202). Shir and Michel also reported synergy between trimethoprim and sulfamethoxazole for 25 strains of *Brucella* species from Israel (218).

ANTIMICROBIAL THERAPY
General

In 1958 the Expert Committee on Brucellosis of the WHO concluded that treatment of human brucellosis (*a*) shortened the clinical course of the disease, (*b*) lessened complications, and (*c*) reduced fatalities (253). Spink likened brucellosis to tuberculosis, another facultative intracellular pathogen, which produces an illness characterized by persistence of organisms within the tissues of a host rendered hypersensitive to antigens of the organism (227). Spink also showed that mice infected with *B. melitensis* (5×10^5 to 1×10^6 CFUs) developed a chronic infection of the reticuloendothelial system and that treatment with tetracycline alone for less than 3 to 6 months did not entirely eradicate the disease (230). Such experimental data plus clinical reports showing rates of relapse of 15 to 30% with single drug therapy (108), led to the conclusion that prolonged treatment with combinations of drugs was required to achieve a cure in human brucellosis. Consequently, in 1965, the WHO recommended a regimen of tetracycline (500 mg four times daily by mouth) for 4 to 6 weeks plus streptomycin (1 g/day intramuscularly) given for the first 1 to 3 weeks (254). Although some reports did not find a significant difference in relapse rates between tetracycline alone and tetracycline plus streptomycin (73), combination therapy generally reduces the rate of relapse in brucellosis below 10% in both adults (67, 108, 140) and children (150).

When doxycycline became available, which can be given once or twice daily with fewer gastrointestinal side effects, it largely replaced tetracycline HCl as the preferred tetracycline for treating human brucellosis. Based on a few reports showing good activity of rifampin against *Brucella* species, in 1986 the WHO recommended the combination of doxycycline (200 mg/d) plus rifampin (600–900 mg/d) for at least 6 weeks as the preferred treatment for brucellosis (255).

In recent years, numerous clinical trials have compared various combinations of drugs in patients with brucellosis (Table 7). Most studies were prospective and used random enrollment of patients into each treatment regimen. Only the study by Ariza et al. (25) was double-blind. Patients suffering from neurobrucellosis and infective endocarditis were excluded. Therapeutic *failure* was defined as the persistence of characteristic signs and symptoms of the disease, with or without persistent bacteremia, or the discontinuation of treatment due to serious untoward side effects of one or more of the drugs. *Relapse* was defined as the recurrence of characteristic signs and symptoms of the disease with or without recurrent bacteremia at some time after the completion of therapy. Follow-up periods varied among the studies, but in most cases were for 12 months or more posttreatment.

Although these studies differed in design, drug combinations compared, doses of drugs administered, and lengths of treatment, certain observations can be made from the data. The efficacy of the combination of tetracycline in a dose of 2 g/day by mouth plus streptomycin in a dose of 1 g/day intramuscularly improved with the duration of treatment. For example, when the two drugs were given for 21 days and 14 days, respectively, the relapse/failure rate was 37% (2). In contrast, when the same combination of drugs was administered for 30

TABLE 7 • Clinical Trials Comparing Antimicrobial Combinations for the Treatment of Brucellosis

Drugs (doses) Duration (days)[a]	No. Patients Treated	No. Failed/Relapsed	Rate (%)	(Ref.)
Tetracycline (2 g/day)30 + streptomycin (1 g/day)21	28	2	(7.1)	(23)
Doxycycline (200 mg/day)30 + rifampin (15 mg/kg/day)30	18	7	(38.9)	(23)
Tetracycline (2 g/day)21 + streptomycin (1 g/day)14	27	10	(37)	(2)
Doxycycline (200 mg/day)45 + streptomycin (1 g/day)21	53	2	(3.8)	(2)
Doxycycline (200 mg/day)45 + rifampin (900 mg/day)45	65	3	(4.6)	(2)
Doxycycline (200 mg/day)30 + streptomycin (1 g/day)21	59	5	(8.5)	(53)
Doxycycline (200 mg/day)45 + rifampin (15 mg/kg/day)45	52	7	(13.5)	(53)
Doxycycline (200 mg/day)45 + streptomycin (1 g/day)15	51	3	(5.8)	(25)
Doxycycline (200 mg/day)45 + rifampin (15 mg/kg/day)45	44	6	(13.6)	(25)
Doxycycline (200 mg/day)45 + rifampin (600 mg/day)45	30	1	(3.3)	(4)
Ofloxacin (400 mg/day)45 + rifampin (600 mg/day)45	31	2	(6.5)	(4)
Doxycycline (200 mg/day)45 + streptomycin (1 g/day)14	40	3	(7.5)	(156)
Doxycycline (200 mg/day)45 + streptomycin (1 g/day)21	44	1	(2.3)	(156)
Doxycycline (200 mg/day)45 + rifampin (900 mg/day)45	46	6	(13)	(156)
Doxycycline (200 mg/day)45 + streptomycin (1 g/day)14	94	7	(7.4)	(222)
Doxycycline (200 mg/day)45 + rifampin (15 mg/kg/day)45	100	24	(24)	(222)
Doxycycline (200 mg/day)45 + streptomycin (1 g/day)14	38	3	(7.9)	(220)
Doxycycline (200 mg/day)45 + rifampin (15 mg/kg/day)21	38	12	(31.6)	(220)
Tetracycline (NR)90 + streptomycin (NR)21	102	4	(3.9)	(15)
Tetracycline (NR)90 + cotrimoxazole (NR)21	96	10	(10.4)	(15)
Cotrimoxazole (NR)90 + streptomycin (NR)21	31	3	(9.7)	(15)
Cotrimoxazole (NR)90 + rifampin (NR)21	4	1	(25)	(15)
Doxycycline (200 mg/day)45 + gentamicin (5 mg/kg/day)7	17	1	(5.9)	(223)
Doxycycline (200 mg/day)30 + gentamicin (5 mg/kg/day)7	35	8	(22.9)	(223)

[a] NR, not reported.

and 21 days, respectively, the rate of relapse/failure was reduced to 7% (23). Al Majid et al. reported a retrospective review of treatment using tetracycline and streptomycin, but they failed to include the doses used (15). Assuming that standard doses of each drug were used, it appears that continuing tetracycline and streptomycin for 90 days and 21 days, respectively, further reduced the failure/relapse rate to 3.9%. Furthermore, as might be expected, substituting doxycycline at a dose of 200 mg/day for tetracycline (2 g/day) in combination with streptomycin (1 g/day) resulted in comparable success, and the length of treatment again appeared to be more important than the tetracycline compound used. For example, when doxycycline was used for 45 days and streptomycin for 21 days, the relapse/failure rates in two studies were 3.8 and 2.3%, respectively (2, 156). However, shortening the length of streptomycin administration to 14 days (156, 222) and 15 days (25) resulted in relapse/failure rates of 7.5%, 7.4% and 5.8%, respectively. Similarly, shortening the duration of doxycycline from 45 to 30 days yielded a relapse/failure rate of 8.5% (53).

The results of studies comparing doxycycline plus streptomycin with doxycycline plus rifampin generally favored the doxycycline/streptomycin combination (Table 7). With the exception of the studies by Acocella et al. (2) and Akova et al. (4), in which both drugs were administered for 45 days with relapse/failure rates of 4.6 and 4.3%, respectively, all other studies in which doxycycline plus rifampin was given for 45 days resulted in relapse/failure rates ranging from 13 to 24% (25, 53, 156, 222). In the study by Ariza et al. in which doxycycline plus rifampin were administered for 30 days, the relapse/failure rate was 38.9% (22). Two other randomized trials comparing doxycycline/rifampin and doxycycline/streptomycin obtained similar results, with relapse rates of 13 and 7%, respectively (132, 203). Luzzi et al. analyzed the data from reports comparing doxycycline/streptomycin with doxycycline/rifampin and concluded that the chances of failure and relapse were significantly lower with doxycycline/streptomycin by about 70% (151). The differences between high and low relapse/failure rates with doxycycline/rifampin cannot be explained on the basis of dosage of the drugs, although the importance of the length of treatment appears obvious. In treating brucellosis with oral agents, patient compliance is always a concern when prolonged administration is required. Whether or not compliance had any effect on these data is unknown.

Retrospective data comparing TMP-SMX (cotrimoxazole) in combination with other drugs in the treatment of brucellosis clearly showed them to be less effective than tetracycline or doxycycline plus streptomycin (15). Although the drug doses were not specified, these data are consistent with reports showing that cotrimoxazole alone is also less effective than tetracycline plus streptomycin (21, 22).

Although quinolone monotherapy for human brucellosis is clearly associated with an unacceptably high rate of failure/relapse (138), Akova concluded that ofloxacin plus rifampin administered for 6 weeks was as effective as doxycycline plus rifampin (4). Additional studies using quinolones in combination with other drugs are required before their role in the treatment of brucellosis is fully defined.

The combination of doxycycline for 6 weeks plus streptomycin for 2 weeks remains the most commonly used and most effective treatment for human brucellosis (50, 129, 160, 223). In the United States, access to streptomycin has become limited, although it is still available for the treatment of tuberculosis. Availability notwithstanding, streptomycin appears to be less active in vitro against *Brucella* species than gentamicin (Table 3). A report from Peru indicated that 21% of clinical isolates of *B. melitensis* were resistant to streptomycin (MIC range, 0.125 to 16 μg/mL), whereas none were resistant to gentamicin (MIC range, 0.25 to 2.0 μg/mL) (43). Many clinicians now substitute gentamicin for streptomycin in treating patients with brucellosis; however, few studies have compared the two aminoglycosides and the optimal duration of gentamicin administration remains undefined. Lubani et al. reported success using a regimen of gentamicin (5 mg/kg/day) for 5 days in combination with doxycycline or oxytetracycline for 3, 5, or 8 weeks to treat children with brucellosis (150). Solera et al. treated two cohorts of patients infected with *B. melitensis;* the first received doxycycline (200 mg/day) for 45 days plus gentamicin (5 mg/kg/day) as a single intramuscular injection for 7 days. Only 1 of 17 patients in this cohort relapsed (relapse rate, 5.9%), and this patient was found to be HIV positive. The second cohort of 35 patients received the same dose of doxycycline for only 30 days plus the same dose of gentamicin. In this group, the relapse rate was 22.9% (223). These data further illustrate the importance of prolonged antibiotic administration and also support the notion that gentamicin is comparable to, if not better than, streptomycin. Subsequently, Abramson et al. reported 15 children with brucellosis: 5 received gentamicin for 5 days and cotrimoxazole for 3 weeks and 10 received gentamicin for 5 days and doxycycline for 3 weeks. The relapse rates were unacceptably high in both groups (60 and 20%, respectively); however, this report simply underscores the importance of prolonged versus short-term therapy and is not evidence against gentamicin per se (1). The study currently proposed by the WHO to compare streptomycin and gentamicin in combination with doxycycline should provide additional data on the efficacy of gentamicin and define the appropriate dosage and treatment duration.

Drug of Choice

The treatment of choice for human brucellosis is the combination of doxycycline (200 mg/day orally) for 6 weeks plus streptomycin (1 g/day intramuscularly) for 3 weeks. Most authorities consider that gentamicin (5 mg/kg/day) intravenously or intramuscularly as a single injection can be used in place of streptomycin; however, the duration of gentamicin administration is unclear. Although 5- and 7-day regimens of gentamicin have been used, we advise no fewer than 10 days. As additional data become available, this recommendation is subject to change. Many clinicians prefer to administer rifampin (600–900 mg/day orally) for the remainder of the 6 weeks after discontinuing gentamicin, but this regimen has not been studied in comparative trials. The second-choice regimen consists of doxycycline (200 mg/day orally) plus rifampin

(600–900 mg/day orally), with both drugs administered for 45 days. Cotrimoxazole and quinolones can be used in special situations (see below); however, neither drug is considered first-line treatment.

Special Situations

Neurobrucellosis

Depression and mental inattention are common complaints of patients with brucellosis; however, direct invasion of the central nervous system (CNS) occurs in less than 5% of cases (260). A variety of nervous system complications have been reported in brucellosis, including meningitis (41, 159, 165, 178), meningoencephalitis (141, 142, 250), myelitis/radiculoneuronitis (7, 29, 30, 83, 213), brain abscess (103, 209), spinal epidural abscess (155, 181, 234), demyelinating syndromes (7, 213), and meningovascular syndromes (165). Meningitis is the most frequent CNS complication, and it can be acute or chronic.

Treatment of neurobrucellosis poses special problems because of the need to achieve high concentrations of antimicrobial drugs in the CSF. Unfortunately, the drugs most commonly used to treat brucellosis do not penetrate the blood/brain barrier in sufficient concentrations to treat Gram-negative meningitis effectively. Bouza et al. reviewed cases of brucella meningitis in the literature from 1975 to 1985. Among 78 cases, only 17 reports contained sufficient data to be analyzed, and they added 7 cases to this number (41). A variety of antimicrobial drug combinations were used for varying periods of time. The authors could reach no conclusions about the ideal treatment of neurobrucellosis. Accordingly, in keeping with current practice, they suggested that the combination of tetracycline (or doxycycline) with streptomycin, rifampin, or both, appeared to offer the best results. Rifampin achieves high concentrations in CSF, and its penetration into cells appears to warrant its inclusion in the treatment of all cases of neurobrucellosis, a conclusion also reached by Mousa et al. (159).

TMP-SMX also penetrates the blood/brain barrier well, but when used alone, it is associated with high failure/relapse rates. Nevertheless, regimens containing tetracycline, rifampin, and cotrimoxazole have been reported to be effective in cases of brucella meningitis (7, 16, 30, 165, 204).

Just as there is no agreement on the combinations of drugs for brucella meningitis, there is no consensus on the optimum duration of therapy. Most authorities agree that therapy needs to be prolonged: no less than 6 to 8 weeks and often for 6 to 8 months (16, 30, 41, 213). Clinical and serologic responses and improvements in CSF parameters are used to monitor the course of treatment (259). Another point of disagreement is the value of administering corticosteroids in addition to antimicrobial drugs for brucella meningitis. Most authorities do not use steroids; others add them in "complicated cases" despite no definitive proof of their efficacy (41). Surgical intervention is rarely needed in the treatment of neurologic complications of brucellosis; however, large brain abscesses (27) and especially abscesses of the spinal epidural space can progress rapidly and should be surgically decompressed.

Brucella Endocarditis

Infective endocarditis was reportedly the most common cause of death from brucellosis in the preantibiotic era (32, 71, 179, 211, 225). Infection of the heart valves occurs in less than 2% of patients with brucellosis; however, in countries where the disease is enzootic, 4 to 8% of cases of infective endocarditis are caused by *Brucella* species (12, 81). Brucella endocarditis has been reported on native and prosthetic heart valves (14, 80, 146, 172). The aortic valve is infected more often than the mitral valve. Mycotic aneurysms of the brain (11), the aorta, and other vessels are secondary complications, especially with *B. suis* infection (65, 87, 110,144).

Infective endocarditis presents a special problem because of the need for bactericidal concentrations of drugs within vegetations. Although there are reports of the successful treatment of brucella endocarditis with antibiotics alone, most patients have required drug therapy combined with valve replacement surgery (14, 45, 51, 113, 123, 177, 186, 210). Although tetracyclines are considered only bacteriostatic, combination with an aminoglycoside results in rapid killing of *Brucella* species (205). In patients who were reportedly cured with antibiotics alone, combinations of tetracycline plus streptomycin, oxytetracycline plus gentamicin, doxycycline plus rifampin, and tetracycline, streptomycin, and rifampin were used for periods ranging from 6 weeks to 9 months (5, 35, 49, 76, 119, 184). In patients who underwent valve replacement, tetracycline and streptomycin combined with other drugs, such as TMP/SMZ or rifampin, were given postoperatively for periods as short as 2 weeks and as long as 13 months (mean, 3.5 months) (121).

Consequently, the optimal therapy for brucella endocarditis remains to be determined. Nevertheless, combination therapy with tetracycline (or doxycycline) plus an aminoglycoside (streptomycin or gentamicin) and another drug such as cotrimoxazole or rifampin, usually with valve replacement, offers a reasonable chance for cure. The optimal duration of therapy for endocarditis is also unknown, but prolonged treatment (at least 8 weeks) is generally recommended (121).

Brucella Pericarditis

Pericarditis complicating brucellosis is rare, but it has been reported distinct from endocarditis (60, 98, 245). Treatment of pericarditis does not differ from therapy of uncomplicated brucellosis except that pericardiocentesis may be required for cases of tamponade.

Brucellosis in Children

Brucellosis in children was once considered rare, and when it occurred, the symptoms were said to be mild (105). These findings were based on studies of *B. abortus* infection, which is principally occupation related, occurring mainly in working adults. In contrast, infection with *B. melitensis* is primarily foodborne (46, 109, 236), and in countries where *B. melitensis* is enzootic, childhood brucellosis is common (79). Reports of complications of brucellosis in children prove that the disease is similar in patients of all ages (6, 9, 10, 148, 149, 248).

Tetracycline compounds are contraindicated for children under 8 years of age, owing to the risk of permanent staining of teeth. Consequently, other drugs have been investigated for use in children and pregnant women with brucellosis. Lubani et al. reported a prospective multicenter study of 1100 children with brucellosis in Kuwait (150). The data (Table 8) indicate that doxycycline is more effective than oxytetracycline or rifampin when given as monotherapy, even when treatment was continued for weeks. Cotrimoxazole (in a fixed combination of trimethoprim and sulfamethoxazole) used alone was associated with an unacceptably high rate of failure/relapse. Treatment with combinations of drugs was superior to single-drug therapy, especially when the combination included an aminoglycoside (streptomycin or gentamicin), and better results were obtained when therapy exceeded 3 weeks. Although successful results were reported in this study using gentamicin (5 mg/kg/day) for only 5 days, others have questioned such short-term aminoglycoside therapy. Sanchez-Tamayo et al. reported high relapse rates in childhood brucellosis when gentamicin was given for only 5 days in combination with doxycycline for 3 weeks (relapse rate, 23.8%) or with cotrimoxazole for 3 weeks (relapse rate, 30.8%) (208). Abramson et al. also reported high relapse rates in a small number of children treated with gentamicin for 5 days in combination with doxycycline for 3 weeks (relapse rate, 20%) or cotrimoxazole for 3 weeks (relapse rate, 60%) (1). Although the optimal duration of gentamicin treatment has not yet been established, the value of prolonged combination therapy over monotherapy is well illustrated by Gottesman et al. who reported relapse rates of 43% with monotherapy and 14% with combinations of drugs (99).

On the basis of available data, children 8 years of age and older with brucellosis, like adults, benefit most from a long-term course of therapy consisting of tetracycline (30 mg/kg/day) four times daily by mouth or doxycycline (5 mg/kg/day twice daily by mouth) administered for 45 days, combined with streptomycin (30 mg/kg/day) once daily intramuscularly administered for 21 days. As with adults, it appears that gen-tamicin can be substituted for streptomycin with treatment given for at least 10 days; however, additional experience is needed to confirm this regimen.

For children under 8 years of age, for whom tetracycline therapy is contraindicated, satisfactory results have been obtained using TMP-SMX (8/40 mg/kg/day) twice daily for 45 days plus streptomycin (30 mg/kg/day) for 21 days or gentamicin (5mg/kg/day) once daily intramuscularly for 7 days (150, 214). Others have recommended the use of rifampin (15 mg/kg/day) in combination with cotrimoxazole or streptomycin (8, 33, 54).

Brucellosis during Pregnancy

Brucellosis in animals is characterized by chronic infection, and in pregnant animals, brucellae localize in the uterus where they replicate within trophoblasts, leading to abortion. Intratrophoblastic replication occurs with *B. abortus* in cows, with *B. melitensis* in goats, with *B. suis* in swine, and with *B. canis* in dogs (19). Localization of *B. abortus* in the pregnant ruminant uterus has been attributed to its content of the 4-carbon alcohol erythritol, which is a growth stimulant for *B. abortus* in vitro (127, 219). Erythritol is not found in the human uterus (243), and human amniotic fluid contains antibrucella activity (122). Nevertheless, abortion can occur in brucella-infected pregnant women, although it may not be more common than abortion caused by any bacteremic infection (229, 258).

Treatment of pregnant women with brucellosis poses special problems, since tetracyclines are contraindicated owing to the risk of tooth staining, possible inhibition of bone growth, and potential birth defects. Consequently, some authorities favor cotrimoxazole despite the fact that the manufacturer does not recommend its use in pregnant women or nursing mothers (126, 129, 130). Seoud et al. reported six patients with brucellosis during pregnancy: one terminated pregnancy in the first trimester, one suffered a spontaneous abortion at 12 weeks of gestation,

---

TABLE 8 • Comparison of Antimicrobial Drugs for the Treatment of Childhood Brucellosis

Drugs	Failure/Relapse Rates (%) by Length of Therapy (weeks)		
	3	**5**	**8**
Oxytetracycline (30 mg/kg/day) q.i.d.	(9.2)	(8.8)	(3.1)
Doxycycline (5 mg/kg/day) b.i.d.	(8.0)	(6.7)	(0.0)
Oxytetracycline (30 mg/kg/day) q.i.d. + streptomycin (1 g/day) 21 day	(2.1)	(0.0)	(0.0)
Doxycycline (5 mg/kg/day) b.i.d. + streptomycin (1 g/day) 21 day	(0.0)	(0.0)	(0.0)
Oxytetracycline (30 mg/kg/day) q.i.d. + gentamicin (5 mg/kg/day) 5 day	(0.0)	(0.0)	(0.0)
Cotrimoxazole (10/50 mg/kg/day) b.i.d.	(30)	(29.7)	(28.6)
Cotrimoxazole (10/50 mg/kg/day) b.i.d. + streptomycin (1 g/day) 21 day	(2.6)	(2.0)	(0.0)
Cotrimoxazole (10/50 mg/kg/day) b.i.d. + gentamicin (5 mg/kg/day) 5 day	(0.0)	(0.0)	(0.0)
Rifampin (20 mg/kg/day) b.i.d.	(5.4)	(5.0)	(3.3)
Rifampin (20 mg/kg/day) b.i.d. + streptomycin (1 g/day) 21 day	(6.7)	(0.0)	(0.0)
Rifampin (20 mg/kg/day) b.i.d. + gentamicin (5 mg/kg/day) 5 day	(0.0)	(0.0)	(0.0)
Rifampin (20 mg/kg/day) b.i.d. + cotrimoxazole (10/50 mg/kg/day) b.i.d.	(7.7)	(7.7)	(0.0)
Rifampin (20 mg/kg/day) b.i.d + oxytetracycline (30 mg/kg/day) q.i.d	(5.0)	(6.7)	(0.0)
Cotrimoxazole (10/50 mg/kg/day) b.i.d + oxytetracycline (30 mg/kg/day) q.i.d	(7.7)	(4.0)	(0.0)

Data modified from Lubani MM, Dudin KI, Sharda DC, Manandhar DS, Araj GF, Hafez HA, Al-Saleh QA, Helin I, Salhi MM. A multicenter therapeutic study of 1100 children with brucellosis. Pediatr Infect Dis J 1989;8:75–78, with permission.

and four carried to term, delivering healthy babies after treatment with cotrimoxazole (2 tablets/day) for 3 to 6 weeks (212).

Currently, the optimal treatment of pregnant women with confirmed brucellosis is unclear; however, most authorities recommend cotrimoxazole, rifampin, or a combination of the two for 4 to 6 weeks with close fetal monitoring (100). Addition of gentamicin for the initial 5 to 7 days of treatment has not been studied but seems warranted based on the results in childhood brucellosis.

Brucella canis Infection

Although *B. canis* has been found in canines worldwide, it remains the least frequent cause of human brucellosis. Since it was first shown to be a human pathogen in 1967, most human infections with *B. canis* have been laboratory acquired (157). The first case acquired outside the laboratory was reported in 1972 in a woman with an infected German shepherd dog (235). The clinical manifestations of human *B. canis* infection do not appear to differ from those with other *Brucella* species (37, 161, 185). A variety of antibiotics have been used to treat the infection, including moxalactam (242), ampicillin plus streptomycin (235), and tetracycline plus streptomycin (200, 206). Consequently, human infection with *B. canis* does not pose special problems, and treatment is similar to that for infection with other *Brucella* species.

Postexposure Prophylaxis

With the widespread use of live brucella vaccines for the immunization of cattle with *B. abortus* strain 19 and of sheep and goats with *B. melitensis* strain Rev-1, accidental human self-inoculation is a common problem. Although the vaccines are attenuated for animals, they can cause brucellosis in humans (228); however, the risk appears to be low, considering the millions of doses of vaccine administered annually. Most vaccine accidents involve needle-stick injuries suffered while injecting animals. Consequently, strain 19 disease is an occupational hazard for veterinarians, animal health technicians, and vaccine producers (38, 171). Individuals with preexisting antibodies to brucella usually suffer only a self-limited skin reaction at the inoculation site, which is believed to be immunologically mediated (258). Since most veterinarians lack antibodies to brucella, vaccine accidents can result in clinical brucellosis (207); however, since the amount of vaccine inoculated is usually small, the risk of infection by the intradermal route appears to be low. Of greater concern is accidental spraying of vaccine into the eyes. Conjunctival inoculation is an extremely efficient method of transmitting brucellosis, and human infection by this route has been reported (258).

Some experts have recommended a 10- to 20-day course of tetracycline as prophylaxis for vaccine accidents (162); however, there are no data to support the efficacy of such treatment. In a series of patients with accidental exposure to *Brucella* species in a laboratory, prophylaxis with sulfadiazine, streptomycin, or sulfadiazine plus penicillin did not appear to alter the course of infection (117). On the basis of available data, we recommend the following approach to management of patients with accidental self-inoculation of live brucella vaccine:

1. Needle-stick injuries: local wound care, tetanus toxoid booster (if indicated), serum sample for SAT to obtain baseline status of brucella antibodies. The use of prophylactic antibiotics is left to the discretion of the physician and the patient, based on the type of wound, the vaccine involved (*B. abortus* strain 19 *may* be less hazardous than *B. melitensis* Rev-1), the amount of vaccine injected, and the level of concern on the part of the patient. If *B. melitensis* Rev-1 vaccine is involved or if the patient desires antibiotics, we recommend a course of doxycycline (200 mg/day) by mouth for 45 days plus rifampin (600 mg/day) by mouth for 45 days.

2. Conjunctival inoculation: in addition to local eye care (copious lavage with water) and baseline serum for SAT, this route is so efficient in transmitting brucellosis that we recommend treatment with doxycycline (200 mg/day) by mouth for 6 weeks, plus streptomycin (1 g/day) intramuscularly for 21 days or gentamicin (5 mg/kg/day) intramuscularly for 10 days. A recent report on potential biologic warfare agents, including *Brucella* species, recommends a 3-week course of doxycycline plus rifampin as chemoprophylaxis for any inadvertent inoculations, regardless of the route (86).

CONTROVERSIES AND UNCERTAINTIES

Chronic Brucellosis

Perhaps no aspect of brucellosis engenders more controversy than chronic brucellosis. The problem is not whether the condition exists, but rather obtaining a consensus on a definition and making the diagnosis. Some authors have considered that patients who experience a prolonged delay before the diagnosis of brucellosis suffer from chronic infection. There is no evidence to support the concept that prolonged symptoms before diagnosis represent chronic infection; however, the longer the disease exists before therapy, the greater the opportunity for infection to become localized within an organ or tissues. Another problem of definition is whether or not complaints that persist following therapy and can be attributed to chronic infection.

In 1934, when brucellosis was widespread in the United States, the bacteriologist Alice Evans called attention to the syndrome of "neurasthenia," pointing out that its clinical manifestations could not always be distinguished from chronic brucellosis (72). Others followed Evans' lead, using patient's complaints, a positive intradermal test with brucella antigen, and a "response" to vaccine therapy to define chronic brucellosis (101). This situation is now recognized as analogous to the "chronic fatigue syndrome." Patients who feel chronically fatigued and have serum antibodies to brucella do not a priori suffer from chronic brucellosis (52).

In 1951, Spink studied more than 100 patients with brucellosis, in an attempt to define chronic brucellosis (226). The patients were classified into three groups: *acute, subacute,* and *chronic.* Among those classified acute, symptoms resolved within 3 months of treatment. Among those classified subacute, symptoms persisted from 3 to 12 months, and continued illness was associated with persistent or recurrent (relapse) bacteremia. A few patients lacked objective clinical or laboratory evidence of disease, and they appeared to suffer from delayed convalescence. Among those classified chronic, one-half had objective evidence of illness (e.g., episodes of fever) and evidence of localized infection, (e.g., spondylitis, osteomyelitis, septic arthritis, meningitis, and intraabdominal abscess). The remaining half lacked objective evidence of infection and appeared to represent delayed convalescence. Whereas patients with objective signs of chronic brucellosis benefited from antibiotics (with or without surgical intervention), those lacking objective signs of disease did not. In studying the response of patients to laboratory-acquired brucellosis, Imboden et al. showed that patients with delayed convalescence from brucellosis were more likely to have had a premorbid propensity for depression and to have suffered a major traumatic event before their illness than patients who recovered normally (120).

Relapse and chronic localized infection are well-recognized complications of acute brucellosis (26, 154, 193); however, more often than not, continued complaints following treatment represent delayed convalescence. Management of such patients is sometimes complicated by workmans' compensation claims in which the patient may have other reasons for claiming ill health. Although it has been reported that titers of agglutinating antibodies can be low or absent in chronic brucellosis (128), the presence of so-called blocking antibodies can result in false-negative serologic results (263). It is now clear that patients with relapse or chronic brucellosis have persistently elevated levels of IgG antibodies (26, 93, 180, 259), which is an important laboratory clue for making the diagnosis.

Relapse of brucellosis can be treated with the same antibiotics used initially, since the organisms generally have the same antibiotic susceptibility patterns (24). Treatment of chronic localized brucellosis may require prolonged administration of antibiotics, and when deep tissue abscesses are present, can require surgical drainage.

Immune Modulators

Some authors claim that chronic brucellosis is characterized by immune suppression (48, 182, 238), suggesting a role for immunostimulatory drugs such as levamisole. Levamisole is an adjuvant when administered with brucella vaccines in mice (196, 197) and in cattle (47, 56, 124); however, it did not improve clearance of bacteria from the tissues of brucella-infected mice (257). In a small number of patients with alleged chronic brucellosis, levamisole plus tetracycline reportedly improved symptoms and restored lymphocyte reactivity to mitogens; however, no controls treated with tetracycline alone were included (198). Another group of seven patients with alleged chronic brucellosis received antibiotics plus levamisole and were said to show improved cellular reactivity and "earlier" improvement in clinical symptoms (194). Once again, no controls were included in the study. Another uncontrolled study of levamisole alone in patients with presumed chronic brucellosis claimed similar results (40).

Levamisole is approved for adjuvant chemotherapy after surgical resection of advanced colon cancer; however, claims for its efficacy in the treatment of a variety of other diseases have not withstood vigorous scientific scrutiny (143). More important, levamisole can have serious side effects, including agranulocytosis; therefore, it should not be used for unapproved conditions until there is convincing evidence of efficacy from rigorously controlled studies.

Vaccine Therapy

In the preantibiotic era, a variety of *Brucella* antigens were used in an attempt to ameliorate or cure the disease (63). Vaccine therapy, using phenol-killed organisms and other preparations was given allegedly to increase the titer of antibodies or to "desensitize" the hypersensitive host. Despite claims of efficacy, the Expert Committee of the WHO found insufficient evidence to confirm the efficacy of vaccine therapy (253).

Although cases of human brucellosis caused by *B. abortus* strain 19 vaccine have been documented (231), Russian workers once used a less virulent variant of strain 19, termed 19-BA, for immunization of humans at high risk of contracting brucellosis (249). Although few details were reported, apparently no cases of clinical brucellosis were caused by strain 19-BA at doses of 4 to 5×10^8 CFU administered subcutaneously or by scarification (61). Strain 19-BA has also been used to potentiate the effects of cyclophosphamide in patients with various malignancies (64). Even at doses as high as $2.5 - 10^{10}$ CFU subcutaneously, strain 19-BA produced few side effects and no cases of clinical brucellosis. Studies using variants of *B. abortus* are in stark contrast to reports of *B. melitensis* Rev-1 vaccine, which, when administered to volunteers, produced clinical infection in a high proportion of cases (176). The data available provide little evidence to support the efficacy of vaccine therapy for brucellosis. Moreover, vaccination of humans with the available live *Brucella* vaccines can potentially cause the disease and should be unnecessary if appropriate measures are taken to eradicate brucellosis in animals and to eliminate foodborne infection by pasteurizing milk.

REFERENCES

1. Abramson O, Abu-Rashid M, Gordischer R, Yagupsky P. Failure of short antimicrobial treatments for human brucellosis. Antimicrob Agents Chemother 1997;41:1621–1622.
2. Acocella G, Bertrand A, Beytout J, Durrande JB, Rodriguez J-AG, Kosmidis J, Micoud M, Rey M, Roux J, Stahl J-P. Comparison of three different regimens in the treatment of acute brucellosis: a multinational study. J Antimicrob Agents Chemother 1989;23:433–439.
3. Akalin HE, Unal S, Gur D, Baykal M. Ofloxacin in the treatment of brucellosis [Abstract no. 90]. Proceedings of the Third International Symposium on Quinolones, Vancouver, Canada, 1990.
4. Akova M, Uzun D, Akalin HE, Hayran M, Unal S, Gur D. Quinolones in treatment of human brucellosis: comparative trial of ofloxacin-rifampin versus doxycycline-rifampin. Antimicrob Agents Chemother 1993;37:1831–1834.
5. Almer L-O. A case of brucellosis complicated by endocarditis and disseminated intravascular coagulation. Acta Med Scand 1985;217:139–140.
6. Alvarez de Buergo M, Gomez Reino FJ, Gomez Reino JJ. A long term study of 22 children with brucellar arthritis. Clin Exp Rheum 1990;8:609–612.

7. Al-Deeb SM, Yaqub BA, Sharif HS, Phadke JG. Neurobrucellosis: clinical characteristics, diagnosis, and outcome. Neurology 1989;39:498–501.

8. Al-Eissa Y, Kambal AM, Al-Nasser MN, Al-Habib SA, Al-Fawaz IM, Al-Zamil FA. Childhood brucellosis: a study of 102 cases. Pediatr Infect Dis J 1990;9:74–79.

9. Al-Eissa Y, Al-Nasser M. Haematologic manifestations of childhood brucellosis. Infection 1993;21:23–26.

10. Al-Eissa YA. Unusual suppurative complications of brucellosis in children. Acta Pediatr 1993;82:987–992.

11. Al-Harthi SS. Association of brucella endocarditis with intracerebral hemorrhage. Int J Cardiol 1987;16:214–216.

12. Al-Harthi SS. The morbidity and mortality pattern of *Brucella* endocarditis. Int J Cardiol 1989:25:321 324.

13. Al-Idrissi HY, Uwaydah AK, Danso KT, Qutub H, Al-Mousa MS. Ceftriaxone in the treatment of acute and subacute human brucellosis. J Intern Med Res 1989;17:363–368.

14. Al-Kasab S, Al-Fagih MR, Al-Yousef S, Ali Khan MA, Ribeiro PA, Nazzal S, Al-Zaibag M. Brucella infective endocarditis. J Thorac Cardiovasc Surg 1988;95:862–867.

15. Al-Majed SA, Al-Aska AK, Al-Mitwalli A, Al-Wazzan A, Al-Arfaj H, Al-Anazi A. Use of antibiotics in the treatment of human brucellosis. Curr Ther Res 1996;57:175–180.

16. Al-Orainey I, Laajam MA, Al-Aska AK, Rajapakse CN. Brucella meningitis. J Infect 1987;14:141–145.

17. Al-Sibai MB, Qadri SMH. Development of ciprofloxacin resistance in *Brucella melitensis*. J Antimicrob Chemother 1990;25: 302–303.

18. Al-Sibai MB, Halim MA, El-Shaker MM, Khan BA, Qadri SMH. Efficacy of ciprofloxacin in the treatment of *Brucella melitensis* infections. Antimicrob Agents Chemother 1992;36:150–152.

19. Anderson TD, Cheville NF. Ultrastructural morphometric analysis of *Brucella abortus*-infected trophoblasts in experimental placentitis. Am J Pathol 1986;124:226–237.

20. Ariza J, Gudiol F, Rufi G, Priu R. Tratamiento de la brucelosis aguda con trimethoprim-sulfamethoxazole. Med Clin (Barc) 1977;69:437–441.

21. Ariza J, Gudiol F, Dominguez C. Tratamiento de la brucelosis aguda con TMP-SMZ. In: Baquero F, ed. Proceedings of the 1st Mediterranean Congress of Chemotherapy. Madrid: Mediterranean Congress of Chemotherapy, 1978:769–775.

22. Ariza J, Gudiol F, Pallares R, Rufi G, Fernandez-Viladrich P. Comparative trial of co-trimoxazole versus tetracycline-streptomycin in treating human brucellosis. J Infect Dis 1985; 152:1358–1359.

23. Ariza J, Gudiol F, Pallares, R, Rufi G, Fernandez-Viladrich P. Comparative trial of rifampin-doxycycline versus tetracycline-streptomycin in the therapy of human brucellosis. Antimicrob Agents Chemothar 1985;28:548–551.

24. Ariza J, Bosch J, Gudiol F, Linares J, Fernandez-Viladrich P, Martin R. Relevance of in vitro antimicrobial susceptibility of *Brucella melitensis* to relapse rate in human brucellosis. Antimicrob Agents Chemother 1986;30:958–960.

25. Ariza J, Gudiol F, Pallares R, Viladrich PF, Rufi G, Corredoira J, Miravitlles MR. Treatment of human brucellosis with doxycycline plus rifampin or doxycycline plus streptomycin. Ann Intern Med 1992;117:25–30.

26. Ariza J, Corredoira J, Pallares R, Viladrich PF, Rufi G, Pujol M, Gudiol F. Characteristics of and risk factors for relapse of brucellosis in humans. Clin Infect Dis 1995;20:1241–1249.

27. Ayala-Gaytan J, Ortegon-Baqueiro H, de la Maza M. *Brucella melitensis* cerebellar abscess. J Infect Dis 1989;160:730–731.

28. Baciewicz AM, Self TH. Rifampin drug interactions. Arch Intern Med 1984;144:1667–1671.

29. Bahemuka M, Shemena AR, Panayiotopoulos CP, Al-Aska AK, Obeid T, Daif AK. Neurological syndromes of brucellosis. J Neurol Neurosurg Psych 1988;51:1017–1021.

30. Bashir R, Al-Kawi MZ, Harder EJ, Jinkins J. Nervous system brucellosis. Diagnosis and treatment. Neurology 1985;35: 1576–1581.

31. Baycal M, Akalin HE, Firat M, Serin A. In vitro activity and clinical efficacy of ofloxacin in infections due to *Brucella melitensis*. Rev Infect Dis 1989;11(Suppl 5):S993–S994.

32. Beebe RT, Meneely JK. *Brucella melitensis* endocarditis. Am Heart J 1949;38:788–791.

33. Benjamin B, Annobil SH. Childhood brucellosis in southwestern Saudi Arabia: a 5-year experience. J Trop Pediatr 1992;38: 167–172.

34. Bertrand A, Roux J, Janbon J, Jourdan J, Jonquet O. Traitement de la brucellose par la rifampicine. Nouv Presse Med 1979;8: 3635–3639.

35. Bertrand A, Lepeu G, Jonquet O, Janbon F, Jourdan J. L'endocardite brucellienne: aspects cliniques et immunologiques. Sem Hop Paris 1982;58:275–279.

36. Bertrand A. Traitement antibiotique de la brucellose. Presse Med 1994;23:1128–1131.

37. Blankenship RM, Sanford JP. *Brucella canis*. A cause of undulant fever. Am J Med 1975;59:424–426.

38. Blasco JM, Diaz R. *Brucella melitensis* Rev-1 vaccine as a cause of human brucellosis. Lancet 1993;342:805.

39. Bosch J, Linares J, Lopez de Goicoechea MJ, Ariza J, Cisnal MC, Martin R. In vitro activity of ciprofloxacin, ceftriaxone and five other antimicrobial agents against 95 strains of *Brucella melitensis*. J Antimicrob Chemother 1986;17:459–461.

40. Boura P, Raptopoulou-Gigi M, Acriviadis E, Goulis G. Reevaluation of the effect of levamisole in chronic brucellosis: in vitro and in vivo effect on monocyte phagocytosis. J Immunopharmacol 1984;6:135–146.

41. Bouza E, Garcia de la Torre M, Parras F, Guerrero A, Rodriguez-Creixems M, Gobernado J. Brucella meningitis. Rev Infect Dis 1987;9:810–822.

42. Bushby SRM. Trimethoprim-sulfamethoxazole: in vitro microbiological aspects. J Infect Dis 1973;128(Suppl):S442–S462.

43. Carrillo C, Gotuzzo E, Adachi J, Tolmos J. Sensibilidad antimicrobiana in vitro de cepas de *Brucella melitensis* aisladas en una area endemica (Lima, Peru). Rev Esp Quimioter 1993;6:309–313.

44. Cassano A, Barletta R. Erythromycin in the treatment of human brucellosis. Riforma Med 1954;68:953–956.

45. Chaptal PA, Lepeu G, Grolleau R, Jonquet O, Bertrand A. Cause rare de remplacement valvulaire: l'endocardite brucellienne. Ann Chir Thorac Cardiovasc 1982;36:678–681.

46. Chomel BB, DeBess EE, Manigiamele DM, Reilly KF, Farver TB, Sun RK, Barrett LR. Changing trends in the epidemiology of human brucellosis in California from 1973 to 1992: a shift toward foodborne transmission. J Infect Dis 1994;170:1216–1223.

47. Chukwu CC. Serological response of cattle following *Brucella abortus* strain 19 vaccination and simultaneous administration of levamisole. Int J Zoonoses 1985;12:196–202.

48. Chung SCS. Immunosuppression in chronic brucellosis. Ir J Med Sci 1978;147:103–107.

49. Cisneros JM, Pachon J, Cuello JA, Martinez A. *Brucella* endocarditis cured by medical treatment. J Infect Dis 1989;160:907.

50. Cisneros JM, Viciana P, Colmenero J, Pachon J, Martinez C, Alarcon A. Multicenter prospective study of treatment of

Brucella melitensis brucellosis with doxycyline for 6 weeks plus streptomycin for 2 weeks. Antimicrob Agents Chemother 1990; 34:881–883.

51. Cleveland JC, Suchor RJ, Dague J. Destructive aortic valve endocarditis from *Brucella abortus:* survival with emergency aortic valve replacement. Thorax 1978;33:616–618.

52. Cluff LE. Medical aspects of delayed convalescence. Rev Infect Dis 1991;13(Suppl 1):S138–S140.

53. Colmenero Castillo JD, Hernandez Marquez S, Reguera Iglesias JM, Cabrera Franquelo F, Rius Diaz F, Alonso A. Comparative trial of doxycycline plus streptomycin versus doxycyline plus rifampin for the therapy of human brucellosis. Chemotherapy 1989;35:146–152.

54. Colmenero JD, Reguera JM, Cabrera FP, Cisneros JM, Orjuela DL, Fernandez-Crehuet J. Serology, clinical manifestations and treatment of brucellosis in different age groups. Infection 1990; 18:152–156.

55. Colmenero JD, Fernandez-Gallardo LC, Agundez JAG, Sedeno J, Benitez J, Valverde E. Possible implications of doxycycline-rifampin interaction for treatment of brucellosis. Antimicrob Agents Chemother 1994;38:2798–2802.

56. Confer AW, Hall SM, Espe BH. Transient enhancement of the serum antibody response to *Brucella abortus* strain 19 in cattle treated with levamisole. Am J Vet Res 1985;46:2440–2446.

57. Conti R, Parenti F. Rifampin therapy for brucellosis, flavobacterium meningitis and cutaneous leishmaniasis. Rev Infect Dis 1983;5(Suppl):S600–S605.

58. Corbel MJ. The in vitro sensitivity of *Brucella* strains to spectinomycin. Br Vet J 1974;130:446–452.

59. Corbel MJ. Determination of the in vitro sensitivity of *Brucella* strains to rifampin. Br Vet J 1976;132:266–275.

60. Cuisinier Y, Blanc P, Doumetx JJ, Virot P, Chabanier A, Delhoume B, Bensaid J. Pericardite au cours de la brucellose. Nouv Presse Med 1982;11:3352–3353.

61. Dafni I. Control of brucellosis in the USSR. Retuah Veterinarith 1963;20:41–43.

62. Daikos GK, Papapolyzos N, Marketos N, Mochlas S, Kastanakis S, Papasteriadis E. Trimethoprim-sulfamethoxazole in brucellosis. J Infect Dis 1973;128(Suppl):S731–S733.

63. Dalrymple-Champneys W. Brucella infection and undulant fever in man. London: Oxford University Press, 1960:147–150.

64. Dazord L, Martin A, Le Rest R. Phase I study of immunotherapy by live *Brucella abortus* (strain 19-BA) in cancer patients. Cancer Treat Rep 1984;68:417–418.

65. De Gowin EL, Carter JR, Borts IH. A case of infection with *Brucella suis,* causing endocarditis and nephritis: death from rupture of mycotic aneurysm. Am Heart J 1945;30:77–87.

66. De Rautlin de la Roy YM, Grignon B, Grollier G, Coindreau MF, Becq-Giraudon B. Rifampin resistance in a strain of *Brucella melitensis* after treatment with doxycycline and rifampin. J Antimicrob Chemother 1986;18:648–649.

67. Di Nola F, Soranzo ML. Terapia della brucellosi. Minerva Med 1986;77:1647–1662.

68. Dogany M, Aygen B. Use of ciprofloxacin in the treatment of brucellosis. Eur J Clin Microbiol Infect Dis 1992;11:74–75.

69. Domingo S, Gastearena I, Vitas AI, Lopez-Goni I, Dios-Vieitez C, Diaz R, Gamazo C. Comparative activity of azithromycin and doxycycline against *Brucella* spp. infection in mice. J Antimicrob Chemother 1995;36:647–656.

70. Domingo S, Diaz R, Gamazo C. Antibiotic treatment induces an increase of specific antibody levels in *Brucella melitensis* infected mice. FEMS Immunol Med Microbiol 1995;12:91–96.

71. Dudley Hart F, Morgan A, Lacey B. *Brucella abortus* endocarditis. Br Med J 1951;1:1048–1053.

72. Evans AC. Chronic brucellosis. JAMA 1934;103:665–667.

73. Farid Z, Miale A, Omar MS, Van Peenen PFD. Antibiotic treatment of acute brucellosis caused by *Brucella melitensis*. J Trop Med Hyg 1961;64:157–163.

74. Farid Z, Bassily S, Omar MS. Ampicillin ("Penbritin") in the treatment of acute *Brucella melitensis* septicemia and *Salmonella typhi* urinary carriers. J Trop Med Hyg 1967;20:95–98.

75. Farid Z, Hassan A, Wahab MFA, Sanborn WR, Kent DC, Yassa A, Hathout SE. Trimethoprim-sulfamethoxazole in enteric fevers. Br Med J 1970;3:323–324.

76. Farid Z, Trabolsi B. Successful treatment of two cases of brucella endocarditis. Br Med J 1985;291:110.

77. Farr BM. Rifamycins. In: Mandell GL, Bennett JE, Dolin R, eds. Principles and practice of infectious diseases. 4th ed. New York: Churchill Livingstone, 1995:317–329.

78. Farrell ID, Hinchliffe PM, Robertson L. Sensitivity of *Brucella* spp. to tetracycline and its analogues. J Clin Pathol 1976;29: 1097–1100.

79. Feiz J, Sabbaghian H, Miralai M. Brucellosis due to *B. melitensis* in children. Clin Pediatr 1978;12:904–907.

80. Fernandez-Guerrero ML, Martinell J, Aguado JM, Ponte MC, Fraile J, Rabago G. Prosthetic valve endocarditis caused by *Brucella melitensis*. Arch Intern Med 1987;147:1141–1143.

81. Fernandez-Guerrero ML. Zoonotic endocarditis. Infect Dis Clinics North Am 1993;7:135–152.

82. Finch GH. Streptomycin therapy in undulant fever. Am J Med 1947;2:485–490.

83. Fincham RW, Sahs AL, Joynt RJ. Protean manifestations of nervous system brucellosis. JAMA 1963;184:269–275.

84. Forti G, Renincori C. Doxycycline and the teeth. Lancet 1969; 1:782.

85. Fountain MW, Weiss SJ, Fountain AG, Shen A, Lenk RP. Treatment of *Brucella canis* and *Brucella abortus* in vitro and in vivo by stable plurilamellar vesicle-encapsulated aminoglycosides. J Infect Dis 1985;152:529–535.

86. Franz DR, Jahrling PB, Friedlander AM, McClain DJ, Hoover DL, Bryne WR, Pavlin JA, Christopher GW, Eitzen EM. Clinical recognition and management of patients exposed to biological warfare agents. JAMA 1997;278:399–411.

87. Fudge TL, Ochsner JL, Ancalmo N, Mills NL. Surgical resection of multiple aortic aneurysms due to *Brucella suis*. Surgery 1977;81:236–238.

88. Garcia-Rodriguez JA, Garcia Sanchez JE, Trujillano I. Lack of effective bactericidal activity of new quinolones against *Brucella* spp. Antimicrob Agents Chemother 1991;35:756–759.

89. Garcia-Rodriguez JA, Munoz Bellido A, Fresnadillo JL, Trujillano I. In vitro activities of new macrolides and rifapentine against *Brucella* spp. infection in mice. J Antimicrob Chemother 1995;36:647–656.

90. Garcia-Rodriguez JA, Garcia Sanchez JE, Trujillano I, Garcia Sanchez E, Garcia Garcia MI, Fresnadillo MJ. Susceptibilities of *Brucella melitensis* isolates to clinafloxacin and four other new fluoroquinolones. Antimicrob Agents Chemother 1995;39: 1194–1195.

91. Garcia-Sanchez JE Trujillano I, Munoz Bellido JL. In vitro activities of new quinolones against *Brucella melitensis*. Rev Infect Dis 1989;11(Suppl 5):S992–S993.

92. Gargani G, Pacetti AM. Sensitivity of 115 strains of the genus *Brucella* to some antibiotics (cephalosporins, ureidopenicillins and aminoglycosides). Chemioterapia 1986;5:7–13.

93. Gazapo E, Gonzalez Lahoz JG, Subiza JL, Baquero M, Gil J, dela Concha EG. Changes in IgM and IgG antibody concentrations in brucellosis over time: importance for diagnosis and follow-up. J Infect Dis 1989;159:219–225.

94. Gigli G, Sicca GT. Sul comportamento della crasi ematica in ammalati di maltese trattai con cloramfenicolo. Rass Fisiopatol Clin 1950;22:1075–1094.

95. Gilbert DN. Once-daily aminoglycoside therapy. Antimicrob Agents Chemother 1991;35:399–405.

96. Giunchi G, deRosa F, Fabiani F. Trimethoprim-sulfamethoxazole combination in the treatment of acute human brucellosis. Chemotherapy 1971;16:332–335.

97. Gobernado M, Canton E, Santos M. In vitro activity of ciprofloxacin against *Brucella melitensis*. Eur J Clin Microbiol Infect Dis 1984;3:371.

98. Gomez-Huelgas R, deMora M, Porras JJ, Nuno E, SanRoman CM. *Brucella* and acute pericarditis: fortuitous or casual association? J Infect Dis 1986;154:544.

99. Gottesman G, Vanunu D, Maayan MC, Lanf R, Uziel Y, Sagi H, Wolach B. Childhood brucellosis in Israel. Pediatr Infect Dis J 1996;15:610–615.

100. Gotuzzo E, Carrillo C. Brucella. In: Gorbach SL, Bartlett JH, Blacklow NR, eds. Infectious diseases. Philadelphia: WB Saunders, 1992:1513–1521.

101. Griggs JF. Chronic brucellosis: diagnostic points noted in one hundred cases. Calif West Med 1943;58:118–124.

102. Gutierrez Altes A, Diez Enciso M, Pena Garcia P, Campos Bueno A. In vitro activity of N-formimidoyl thienamycin against 98 clinical isolates of *Brucella melitensis* compared with those of cefoxitin, rifampin, tetracycline, and co-trimoxazole. Antimicrob Agents Chemother 1982;21:501–503.

103. Guvenc H, Kocabay K, Okten A, Bektas S. Brucellosis in a child complicated with multiple brain abscesses. Scand J Infect Dis 1989;21:333–336.

104. Gwynn MN, Rolinson GN. Bactericidal action of amoxicillin alone and in combination with gentamicin and rifampin against *Brucella melitensis*. J Infection 1980;2:61–65.

105. Hagenbush OE, Frei CF. Undulant fever in children. Am J Clin Pathol 1947;11:497–515.

106. Hall WH, Spink WW. In vitro sensitivity of *Brucella* to streptomycin; development of resistance during streptomycin treatment. Proc Soc Exp Biol Med 1946;64:403–406.

107. Hall WH, Manion RE. In vitro susceptibility of *Brucella* to various antibiotics. Appl Microbiol 1970;20:600–604.

108. Hall WH. Modern chemotherapy for brucellosis in humans. Rev Infect Dis 1990;12:1060–1099.

109. Halling SM, Young EJ. Brucella. In: Hui YH, Gorham JR, Murrell KD, Cliver DO, eds. Foodborne disease handbook, vol I, Diseases caused by bacteria. New York: Marcel Dekker, 1994:63–69.

110. Hansmann GH, Schenken JR. Melitensis meningo-encephalitis. Mycotic aneurysm due to Brucella melitensis var. porcine. Am J Pathol 1932;8:435–439.

111. Hassan A, Erian MM, Farid Z, Hathout SD, Sorensen K. Trimethoprim-sulfamethoxazole in acute brucellosis. Br Med J 1971;3:159–160.

112. Hatala R, Dinh T, Cook DJ. Once-daily aminoglycoside dosing in immunocompetent adults: a meta-analysis. Ann Intern Med 1996;124:717–725.

113. Heibig J, Beall AC Jr, Myers R, Harder E, Feteih N. *Brucella* aortic endocarditis corrected by prosthetic valve replacement. Am Heart J 1983;106:594–596.

114. Heilman FR. The effect of combined treatment with aureomycin and dihydrostreptomycin on brucella infection in mice. Proc Staff Meeting Mayo Clinic 1949;24:133–137.

115. Hooper DC, Wolfson JS. Fluoroquinolone antimicrobial agents. N Engl J Med 1991;324:384–394.

116. Hooper DC. Quinolones. In: Mandell GL, Bennett JE, Dolin R, eds. Principles and practice of infectious diseases. 4th ed. New York: Churchill Livingstone, 1995:364–376.

117. Howe C, Miller ES, Kelly EH, Bookwalter HL, Ellingson HV. Acute brucellosis among laboratory workers. N Engl J Med 1947;236:741–747.

118. Howe C, Heyl JT. Streptomycin treatment in acute brucellosis: report of a case with review of the literature. N Engl J Med 1948;238:431–434.

119. Hudson RA. *Brucella abortus* endocarditis: a case. Circulation 1957;16:411–413.

120. Imboden JB, Canter A, Cluff LE, Trever RW. Brucellosis. III. Psychologic aspects of delayed convalescence. Arch Intern Med 1959;103:406–414.

121. Jacobs F, Abramowicz D, Vereerstraeten P, Le Clerc JL, Zech F, Thys JP. Brucella endocarditis: the role of combined medical and surgical treatment. Rev Infect Dis 1990;12:740–744.

122. Jankowski RP, Aikins HE, Vahrson H, Gupta KG. Antibacterial activity of amniotic fluid against *Staphylococcus aureus, Candida albicans* and *Brucella abortus*. Arch Gynaekol 1977;222:275–281.

123. Jeroudi MO, Halim MA, Harder EJ, Al-Sibai MB, Ziady G, Mercer EN. Brucella endocarditis. Br Heart J 1987;58:279–283.

124. Kaneene JMB, Okino FC, Anderson RK, Muscoplat CC, Johnson DW. Levamisole potentiation of antigen specific lymphocyte blastogenic response in *Brucella abortus* exposed but nonresponsive cattle. Vet Immunol Immunopathol 1981;2:75–85.

125. Kaplan SL, Mason EO Jr, Garcia H, Kvernland SJ, Loiselle EM, Anderson DC, Mintz AA, Feigin RD. Pharmacokinetics and cerebrospinal fluid penetration of moxalactam in children with bacterial meningitis. J Pediatr 1981;98:152–157.

126. Kelly RT, Bibbins B. Pregnancy and brucellosis. Texas Med 1987;83:39–41.

127. Keppie J, Williams AE, Witt K, Smith H. The role of erythritol in the tissue localization of the brucellae. Br J Exp Pathol 1965;46:104–108.

128. Kerr WR, Coghlin JD, Payne DJH, Robertson L. The laboratory diagnosis of chronic brucellosis. Lancet 1966;2:1181–1183.

129. Khan MY. Brucellosis: observations on 100 patients. Ann Saudi Med 1986;6:19–23.

130. Khan MY. Outcome of *Brucella melitensis* infection in pregnancy [Abstract no. 1370]. Interscience Conf Antimicrob Agents Chemother 1988.

131. Khan MY, Dizon M, Kiel FW. Comparative in vitro activities of ofloxacin, difloxacin, ciprofloxacin, and other selected antimicrobial agents against *Brucella melitensis*. Antimicrob Agents Chemother 1989;33:1409–1410.

132. Kosmidis J, Karagounis A, Tselentis J, et al. The combination rifampin-doxycycline in brucellosis is better than the WHO regimen. Chemoterapia 1982;1(Suppl 4):107.

133. Krogstadt DJ, Moellering RC. Combinations of antibiotics, mechanisms of interaction against bacteria. In: Lorian V, ed. Antibiotics in laboratory medicine. Baltimore: Williams & Wilkins, 1980:300–305.

134. Lal S, Modawal KK, Fowles ASE, Peach B, Popham RD. Acute brucellosis treated with trimethoprim and sulfamethoxazole. Br Med J 1970;3:256–257.

135. Landinez R, Linares J, Loza E, Martinez-Beltran J, Martin R, Baquero F. In vitro activity of azithromycin and tetracycline against 358 clinical isolates of *Brucella melitensis*. Eur J Clin Microbiol Infect Dis 1992;11:265–267.

136. Lang R, Raz R, Sacks T, Shapiro M. Failure of prolonged treatment with ciprofloxacin in acute brucellosis. J Antimicrob Chemother 1990;26:841–846.

137. Lang R, Dugan R, Potasman I, Einhorn M, Raz R. Failure of ceftriaxone in the treatment of acute brucellosis. Clin Infect Dis 1992;14:506–509.

138. Lang R, Rubinstein E. Quinolones for the treatment of brucellosis. J Antimicrob Chemother 1992;29:357–363.

139. Lang R, Shasha B, Rubinstein E. Therapy of experimental murine brucellosis with streptomycin alone and in combination with ciprofloxacin, doxycycline, and rifampin. Antimicrob Agents Chemother 1993;37:2333–2336.

140. Lang R, Banai M, Lishner M, Rubinstein E. Brucellosis. Int J Antimicrob Agents 1995;5:203–208.

141. Larbrisseau A, Maravi E, Aguilera F, Martinez-Lage JM. The neurological complications of brucellosis. Can J Neurol Sci 1978;5:369–376.

142. Lastra TDV. Epidemiology and neurological manifestations of brucellosis. In: Bogaert LV, Kafer JP, Poch GF, eds. Tropical neurology. Buenos Aires: Lopez Libreros Editions, 1961:302–325.

143. Laurie JA, Moertel CG, Fleming TR, Wieand HS, Leigh JE, Rubin J, McCormack GW, Gerstner JB, Krook JE, Malliard J, Twito DI, Morton RF, Tschetter LK, Barloe JF. Surgical adjuvant therapy of large-bowel carcinoma: an evaluation of levamisole and the combination of levamisole and fluorouracil. J Clin Oncol 1989;7:1447–1456.

144. Layman TE, January LE. Mycotic left ventricular aneurysm involving the fibrous atrioventricular body. Am J Cardiol 1967;20:423–427.

145. Leon AP, Cano C. Action of Ilotycin against *Brucella* and employed with streptomycin in the treatment of human brucellosis. Rev Inst Salubr Enferm Trop 1954;14:5–17.

146. Lezaun R, Teruel J, Maitre MJ, Artaza M. *Brucella* endocarditis on double valvular prosthesis. Postgrad Med J 1980;56:119–120.

147. Lloren-Terol J, Busquets RM. Brucellosis treated with rifampin. Arch Dis Child 1980;55:486–488.

148. Lubani M, Sharda D, Helin I. Brucella arthritis in children. Infection 1986;14:233–236.

149. Lubani MM, Dudin KI, Araj GF, Manandhar DS, Rashid FY. Neurobrucellosis in children. Pediatr Infect Dis J 1989;8:79–82.

150. Lubani MM, Dudin KI, Sharda DC, Manandhar DS, Araj GF, Hafez HA, Al-Saleh QA, Helin I, Salhi MM. A multicenter therapeutic study of 1100 children with brucellosis. Pediatr Infect Dis J 1989;8:75–78.

151. Luzzi GA, Brindle R, Sockett PN, Solera J, Klenerman P, Warrell DA. Brucellosis: imported and laboratory-acquired cases, and an overview of treatment trials. Trans R Soc Trop Med Hyg 1993;87:138–141.

152. Madkour MM. Brucellosis. Boston: Butterworths, 1989:219–243.

153. Magill GB, Kilough JM. Oxytetracycline-streptomycin therapy in brucellosis due to *Brucella melitensis*. Arch Intern Med 1953;91:204–211.

154. Martin WJ, Nichols DR, Beahrs OH. Chronic localized brucellosis. Arch Intern Med 1961;107:143–148.

155. Montejo M, Merino J, Alberola I, Martinez E, Noguerales F, Aguirre C. Absceso epidural brucelosico. Med Clin (Barc) 1983;80:187–188.

156. Montejo JM, Alberola I, Glez-Zarate P, Alvarez A, Alonso J, Canovas A, Aguirre C. Open, randomized therapeutic trial of six antimicrobial regimens in the treatment of human brucellosis. Clin Infect Dis 1993;16:671–676.

157. Morisset R, Spink WW. Epidemic canine brucellosis due to a new species, *Brucella canis*. Lancet 1969;2:1000–1002.

158. Mortensen JE, Moore DG, Clarridge JE, Young EJ. Antimicrobial susceptibility of clinical isolates of *Brucella*. Diagn Microbiol Infect Dis 1986;5:163–169.

159. Mousa ARM, Koshy TS, Araj GF, Marafie AA, Muhtaseb SA, Al-Mudallal DS, Busharetulla MS. Brucella meningitis: presentation, diagnosis and treatment. A prospective study of ten cases. Q J Med 1986;60:873–885.

160. Mousa ARM, Elhag KM, Khogali M, Marafie AA. The nature of brucellosis in Kuwait: study of 379 cases. Rev Infect Dis 1988;10:211–217.

161. Munford RS, Weaver RE, Patton C, Feeley JC, Feldman RA. Human disease caused by *Brucella canis*. A clinical and epidemiologic study of two cases. JAMA 1975;231:1267–1269.

162. McCullough NB. Medical care following accidental injection of *Brucella abortus,* strain 19, in man. J Am Vet Med Assoc 1963;143:617–618.

163. McDivitt DG. Ampicillin in the treatment of brucellosis: a controlled therapeutic trial. Br J Ind Med 1970;27:67–71.

164. McDonald PJ, Pruul H. Phagocyte uptake and transport of azithromycin. Eur J Clin Microbiol Infect Dis 1991;10:828–833.

165. McLean D, Russell N, Khan MY. Neurobrucellosis: clinical and therapeutic features. Clin Infect Dis 1992;15:582–590.

166. National Committee for Clinical Laboratory Standards. Methods for determining bactericidal activity of antimicrobial agents. Proposed guideline M26-P. Villanova, PA: NCCLS, 1987.

167. Neu HC. The new beta-lactamase stable cephalosporins. Ann Intern Med 1982;97:408–419.

168. Nicolau DP, Freeman CD, Belliveau PP, Nightingale CH, Ross JW, Quintiliani R. Experience with a once-daily aminoglycoside program administered to 2,184 adult patients. Antimicrob Agents Chemother 1995;39:650–655.

169. Norden CW, Wentzel H, Keleti E. Comparison of techniques for measurement of in vitro antibiotic synergism. J Infect Dis 1979;140:629–633.

170. Novotny Z, Moeschlin S. Klinisch Erfahrungen mit dem Breifspekimantibiotik Gentamizin (1969–1970). Schweiz Med Wochenschr 1972;102:24–27.

171. Olle-Goig J, Canela-Soler J. An outbreak of *Brucella melitensis* infection by airborne transmission among laboratory workers. Am J Public Health 1987;77:335–338.

172. O'Meara JB, Eykyn S, Jenkins BS, Braimbridge MV, Phillips I. *Brucella melitensis* endocarditis: successful treatment of an infected prosthetic mitral valve. Thorax 1974;29:377–381.

173. Palenque E, Otero JR, Noriega AR. In vitro susceptibility of *Brucella melitensis* to new cephalosporins crossing the blood-brain barrier. Antimicrob Agents Chemother 1986;29:182–183.

174. Pandolfo GP, Villegas C. Tratamiento dela brucelosis con rifampicina: estudio de 21 enfermos. Dia Med 1970;42:215–220.

175. Papapolizos N, Tsiana-Papastergiou A, Ioannou O, Katsensis I, Kritikos A. Amoxycillin in the treatment of acute brucellosis. J Infect 1988;2:161–163.

176. Pappagianis D, Elberg SS, Crouch D. Immunization against brucella infection. Effects of graded doses of viable attenuated *Brucella melitensis* in humans. Am J Epidemiol 1966;84: 21–25.

177. Pazderka E, Jones JW. *Brucella abortus* endocarditis. Successful treatment of an infected aortic valve. Arch Intern Med 1982;142:1567–1568.

178. Pedro-Pons A, Foz M, Codina A, Rey C. Neurobrucellosis (estudio de 41 casos). Rev Clin Esp Eur Med 1972;159:55–62.

179. Peery TM, Belter LF. Brucellosis and heart disease. II. Fatal brucellosis: a review of the literature and report of new cases. Am J Pathol 1960;36:673–697.

180. Pellicer T, Ariza J, Foz A, Pallares R, Gudiol F. Specific antibodies detected during relapse of human brucellosis. J Infect Dis 1988;157:918–924.

181. Perez-Calvo J, Matamala C, Sanjoaquin I, Rodriguez-Benavente A, Ruiz-Laiglesia F, Bueno-Gomez J. Epidural abscess due to acute *Brucella melitensis* infection. Arch Intern Med 1994;154:1410.

182. Person JM, Frottier J, Le Garrec Y, Barrat F, Bastin R, Pilet C. Exploration of the cellular mediated immunity by the blastogenesis test during chronic brucellosis in human. Comp Immun Microbiol Infect Dis 1987;10:1–8.

183. Phillipon AM, Plommet MG, Kazmierczak A, Marly JL, Nevot PA. Rifampin in the treatment of experimental brucellosis in mice and guinea pigs. J Infect Dis 1977;136:482–488.

184. Platt P, Gray J, Carson P. Brucella endocarditis—a successfully treated case. J Infect 1980;2:275–278.

185. Polt SS, Dismukes WE, Flint A, Schaefer J. Human brucellosis caused by *Brucella canis*. Ann Intern Med 1982;97:717–719.

186. Pratt DS, Tenny JH, Bjork CM, Reller LB. Successful treatment of *Brucella melitensis* endocarditis. Am J Med 1978;64: 897–900.

187. Pulaski EJ, Amspacher WH. Streptomycin therapy in brucellosis. Bull US Army Med Dept 1947;7:221–225.

188. Qadri HSM, Ayub A, Ueno Y, Saldin H. Susceptibility of *Salmonella typhi* and *Brucella melitensis* to the new fluoroquinolone rufloxacin (MF934). Chemotherapy 1993;39: 311–314.

189. Qadri HSM, Akhter J, Ueno Y, Saldin H. In vitro activity of eight fluoroquinolones against clinical isolates of *Brucella melitensis*. Ann Saudi Med 1993;13:37–40.

190. Qadri HSM, Ueno Y. Susceptibility of *Brucella melitensis* to the new fluoroquinolone PD131628: comparison with other drugs. Chemotherapy 1993;39:128–131.

191. Qadri HSM, Halim MA, Ueno Y, Abumustafa FM, Postle AG. Antibacterial activity of azithromycin against *Brucella melitensis*. Chemotherapy 1995;41:253–256.

192. Quinton TJ, Stalker MR. Endocarditis due to *Brucella abortus*. Can Med Assoc J 1946;55:50–52.

193. Radolf DJ. Brucellosis: don't let it get your goat! Am J Med Sci 1994;307:64–75.

194. Raptopoulou-Gigi M, Boura P, Valcanos N, Goulis G. Conventional therapy and levamisole in the management of chronic brucellosis. J Infect Dis 1983;147:1123–1124.

195. Reimann HA, Price AH, Elias WF. Streptomycin for certain systemic infections and its effect on the urinary and fecal flora. Arch Intern Med 1945;76:269–277.

196. Renaux G, Renaux M. Effect immuno-stimulant d'un imidothiazole dans l'immunisation des souris contra l'infection par *Brucella abortus*. C R Acad Sci 1971;2720:349–350.

197. Renaux G, Renaux M. Stimulation of anti-*Brucella* vaccination

198. Renaux M, Renaux G. Brucellosis, immunosuppression, and levamisole. Lancet 1977;1:372.

199. Richardson M, Holt JN. Synergistic action of streptomycin with other antibiotics on intracellular *Brucella abortus* in vitro. J Bacteriol 1962;84:638–646.

200. Rifkin GD, Supena RB, Axelson JA. *Brucella canis* bacteremia: a case with negative *B. canis* agglutinins. Am J Med Sci 1978;276:113–115.

201. Rizzo-Naudi J, Griscti-Soler N, Ganado W. Human brucellosis: an evaluation of antibiotics in the treatment of brucellosis. Postgrad Med J 1967;43:520–526.

202. Robertson I., Farrell ID, Hinchliffe PM. The sensitivity of *Brucella abortus* to chemotherapeutic agents. J Med Microbiol 1973;6:549–557.

203. Rodriguez M, Gamo A, Moreno J. Evaluacion de dos regimenes diferentes en el tratamiento de la brucelosis: rifampicina-doxyciclina vs. estreptomicina-doxyciclina. Resultados preliminares. N Arch Fac Med 1985;43:171–175.

204. Roldan A, Molina JA, Fernandez A, Zancada F, Gutierrez A. TMP/SMZ in the treatment of brucellar meningitis. Rev Infect Dis 1988;10:1233–1234.

205. Rubinstein E, Lang R, Shasha B, Hagar B, Diamanstein L, Joseph G, Anderson M, Harrison K. In vitro susceptibility of *Brucella melitensis* to antibiotics. Antimicrob Agents Chemother 1991; 35:1925–1927.

206. Rumley RL, Chapman SW. *Brucella canis:* an infectious cause of prolonged fever of undetermined origin. South Med J 1986;79:626–628.

207. Sadusk JF Jr, Browne AS, Born JL. Brucellosis in man, resulting from *Brucella abortus* (strain 19) vaccine. JAMA 1957; 164:1325–1328.

208. Sanchez-Tamayo T, Colmenero JD, Martinez-Cortes F, Moreiras A, Ramos-Diaz JC, Garcia-Martin FJ, Martinez Valverde A. Failure of short-term antimicrobial therapy in childhood brucellosis. Pediatr Infect Dis J 1997;16:323–324.

209. Santini C, Baiocchi P, Berardelli A, Venditti M, Serra P. A case of brain abscess due to *Brucella melitensis*. Clin Infect Dis 1994;19:977–978.

210. Schvarcz R, Svedenhag J, Radegran K. A case of *Brucella melitensis* endocarditis successfully treated by a combination of surgical resection and antibiotics. Scand J Infect Dis 1995; 27:641–642.

211. Scott RW, Saphir O. Brucella melitensis (abortus) bacteremia associated with endocarditis. Am J Med Sci 1928;175:66–69.

212. Seoud M, Saade G, Awar G, Uwaydah M. Brucellosis in pregnancy. J Reprod Med 1991;36:441–445.

213. Shakir RA, Al-Din ASN, Araj GF, Lulu AR, Mousa AR, Saadah MA. Clinical categories of neurobrucellosis. Brain 1987;110:213–223.

214. Sharda DC, Lubani M. A study of brucellosis in childhood. Clin Pediatr 1986;25:492–495.

215. Sharma B. Treatment of brucellosis by nalidixic acid. Lancet 1965;1:1171–1173.

216. Shasha B, Lang R, Rubinstein E. Therapy of experimental murine brucellosis with streptomycin, co-trimoxazole, ciprofloxacin, ofloxacin, perfloxacin, doxycycline, and rifampin. Antimicrob Agents Chemother 1992;36:973–976.

217. Shasha B, Lang R, Rubinstein E. Efficacy of combinations of doxycycline and rifampin in the therapy of experimental mouse brucellosis. J Antimicrob Chemother 1994;33:545–551.

in mice by tetramisole, a phenyl-imidothiazole salt. Infect Immun 1973;8:544–548.

218. Shir Y, Michel J. Susceptibility of *Brucella* strains to antibiotics. Pathol Biol 1984;32:381–383.

219. Smith H, Williams AE, Pearce JH, Keppie J, Harris-Smith PW, Fitz-George RB, Witt K. Foetal erythritol: a cause of the localization of *Brucella abortus* in bovine contagious abortion. Nature 1962;193:47–49.

220. Solera J, Medrano F, Rodriguez M, Geijo P, Paulino J. Ensayo terapeutico comparativo y multicentrico de rifampicina y doxiciclina frente a estreptomicina y doxiciclina en la brucelosis humana. Med Clin (Barc) 1991;96:649–653.

221. Solera J, Espinoza A, Geijo P, Martinez-Alfaro E, Saez L, Sepulveda MA, Ruiz-Ribo MD. Treatment of human brucellosis with netilmycin and doxycycline. Clin Infect Dis 1996; 22:441–445.

222. Solera J, Rodriguez-Zapata M, Geijo P, Largo J, Paulino J, Saez L, Martinez-Alfaro E, Sanchez L, Sepulveda MA, Ruiz-Ribo MD. Doxycycline-rifampin versus doxycycline-streptomycin in treatment of human brucellosis due to *Brucella melitensis*. Antimicrob Agents Chemother 1995;39:2061–2067.

223. Solera J, Espinoza A, Martinez-Alfaro E, Sanchez L, Geijo P, Navarro E, Escribano J, Fernandez JA. Treatment of human brucellosis with doxycycline and gentamicin. Antimicrob Agents Chemother 1997;41:80–84.

224. Solera J, Martinez-Alfaro E, Espinoza A. Recognition and optimum treatment of brucellosis. Drugs 1997;53:245–256.

225. Spink WW, Titrud LA, Kabler P. A case of brucella endocarditis with clinical, bacteriologic, and pathologic findings. Am J Med Sci 1942;203:797–801.

226. Spink WW. What is chronic brucellosis? Ann Intern Med 1951;35:358–374.

227. Spink WW. Some biologic and clinical problems related to intracellular parasitism in brucellosis. N Engl J Med 1952;247: 603–610.

228. Spink WW, Thompson H. Human brucellosis caused by *Brucella abortus,* strain 19. JAMA 1953;153:1162–1165.

229. Spink WW. The nature of brucellosis. Minneapolis: University of Minnesota Press, 1956:188.

230. Spink WW, Bradley M. Persistent parasitism in experimental brucellosis: attempts to eliminate brucellae with long-term tetracycline therapy. J Lab Clin Med 1960;55:535–547.

231. Spink WW, Hall WH, Finstad J. Immunization with viable *Brucella* organisms. Bull WHO 1962;26:409–419.

232. Standiford HC. Tetracyclines and chloramphenicol. In: Mandell GL, Bennett JE, Dolin R, eds. Principles and practice of infectious diseases. 4th ed. New York: Churchill Livingstone, 1995:306–317.

233. Steigbigel NH, Reed CW, Finland M. Susceptibility of common pathogenic bacteria to several tetracycline antibiotics in vitro. Am J Med Sci 1968;255:179–195.

234. Sumner JW. Epidural abscess secondary to brucellosis ("Brucella suis"). US Armed Forces Med J 1950;1:218–221.

235. Swenson RM, Carmichael LE, Cundy KR. Human infection with *Brucella canis*. Ann Intern Med 1972;76:435–438.

236. Taylor JP, Perdue JN. The changing epidemiology of human brucellosis in Texas, 1977–1986. Am J Epidemiol 1989;130: 160–165.

237. Thapar MK, Young EJ. Urban outbreak of goat cheese brucellosis. Pediatr Infect Dis J 1986;5:640–643.

238. Thornes RD. The anergy of chronic human brucellosis. J Ir Med Assoc 1977;70:480–483.

239. Thornberry C, Anhalt J, Barry A, Gerlach EH, Hossom H, Jones RN, Matsen JM, Moellering RC, Norton R. Methods for dilution antimicrobial susceptibility testing for bacteria that grow aerobically, tentative standards, M7-T. Villanova, PA: National Committee for Clinical Laboratory Standards, 1983.

240. Thornberry C, Swenson JM, Baker CN, et al. Susceptibility testing of fastidious and unusual pathogens. Antimicrob Newslett 1987;4:47–55.

241. Tilton RC, Liberman L, Gerlach EH. Microdilution antibiotic susceptibility test: examination of certain variables. Appl Microbiol 1973;26:658–660.

242. Tosi MF, Nelson TJ. *Brucella canis* infection in a 17-month-old child successfully treated with moxalactam. J Pediatr 1982;101: 725–727.

243. Tripathi KK, Bhatnager L, Seiftge D, Jankowski RP, Aikins HE, Gupta KG. On the growth of *Brucella* species in the presence of erythritol in defined and undefined media and amniotic fluid of human, cow and sheep. Zentralbl Bakteriol 1977;237: 324–329.

244. T'Ung T. In vitro action of penicillin alone and in combination with sulfathiazole on *Brucella* organisms. Proc Soc Exp Biol Med 1944;56:8–11.

245. Ugartemendia MC, Curos-Abadal A, Pujol-Rakosnik M, Pujadas-Capenany R, Escriva-Montserrat E, Jane-Pesquer J. *Brucella melitensis* pericarditis. Am Heart J 1985;109:1108.

246. Urteaga BO, Larrea RP, Calderon MJ. Biologic cycle of *Brucella* as a basis for treatment of human brucellosis. Experimental studies with Ilotycin. Arch Peruanos Patol Clin (Lima) 1954;8:437–460.

247. Urteaga BO, Larrea RP, Calderon MJ. Erythromycin in human brucellosis. Antibiot Med 1955;1:513–522.

248. Vallejo JG, Stevens AM, Dutton RV, Kaplan SL. Hepatosplenic abscesses due to *Brucella melitensis:* report of a case involving a child and review of the literature. Clin Infect Dis 1996;22:485–489.

249. Vershilova PA. The use of live vaccine for vaccination of human beings against brucellosis in the USSR. Bull WHO 1961;24:85–89.

250. Weissenborn K, Wiehler ST, Malin J-P. Meningoenzephalitis durch Brucella-abortus-infektion. Dtsch Med Wochenschr 1987;112:57–59.

251. Whelton A. Tetracyclines in renal insufficiency: resolution of a therapeutic dilemma. Bull NY Acad Med 1978;54:223–226.

252. Winston DJ, Busuttil RW, Kurtz TO, Young LS. Moxalactam therapy for bacterial infections. Arch Intern Med 1981;141: 1607–1612.

253. Joint FAO/WHO Expert Committee on Brucellosis. WHO Tech Rep Ser 148. 3rd report. Geneva, 1958.

254. Joint FAO/WHO Expert Committee on Brucellosis. WHO Tech Rep Ser 289. 4th report. Geneva, 1965.

255. Joint FAO/WHO Expert Committee on Brucellosis. WHO Tech Rep Ser 740. 6th report. Geneva, 1986.

256. Young EJ. Human brucellosis. Rev Infect Dis 1983;5:821–842.

257. Young EJ. Effects of levamisole in murine brucellosis. J Infect Dis 1987;156:530–531.

258. Young EJ. Clinical manifestations of human brucellosis. In: Young EJ, Corbel MJ, eds. Brucellosis: clinical and laboratory aspects. Boca Raton, FL: CRC Press, 1989:110.

259. Young EJ. Serologic diagnosis of human brucellosis: analysis of 214 cases by agglutination tests and review of the literature. Rev Infect Dis 1991;13:359–372.

260. Young EJ. An overview of human brucellosis. Clin Infect Dis 1995;21:283–289.

261. Yow EM, Spink WW. Experimental studies on the action of

streptomycin, aureomycin, and chloromycetin on *Brucella*. J Clin Invest 1949;28:871–885.

262. Zhanal GG, Hoban DJ, Harding GKM. The postantibiotic effect: a review of in-vitro and in-vivo data. Ann Pharmacother 1991;25:153–163.

263. Zineman HH, Glenchur H, Hall WH. Chronic renal brucellosis. Report of a case with studies of blocking antibodies and precipitins. N Engl J Med 1961;265:872–875.

264. Zinner SH, Mayer KH. Sulfonamides and trimethoprim. In: Mandell GL, Bennett JE, Dolin R, eds. Principles and practice of infectious diseases. 4th ed. New York: Churchill Livingstone, 1995:354–364.

Burkholderia cepacia

●

David A. Pegues

GENERAL DESCRIPTION

Burkholderia (formerly *Pseudomonas*) *cepacia* is a plant pathogen that is ubiquitous in the environment (5). The organism is an obligate aerobic Gram-negative rod that does not ferment glucose, is catalase positive, and grows well on standard laboratory media. Isolation of *B. cepacia* from specimens with mixed flora is enhanced by use of selective media, such as PC medium (12).

Historically regarded as an organism of low pathogenicity, the incidence of nosocomial *B. cepacia* infections appears to be increasing (18). Based upon data from the Centers for Disease Control and Prevention, from 1989 to 1996, 589 *B. cepacia* isolates associated with nosocomial infections were reported from hospitals participating in the National Nosocomial Infections Surveillance System (R. Gaynes, personal communication, 1997). The most frequent infections were pneumonia (57.5%), urinary tract infection (11.1%), and bloodstream infection (9.8%). *B. cepacia* infections were reported most commonly from patients on medicine (45.2%), general surgery (20.5%), and cardiac surgery (13.2%) services.

B. cepacia can survive for long periods in water or disinfectants, including povidone-iodine, and outbreaks of *B. cepacia* infection have been linked to a variety of contaminated medications, solutions, and disinfectants and to inadequate disinfection of reusable medical devices (1, 26). Outbreaks of bloodstream infection, (particularly associated with intravenous catheters), urinary tract infection, respiratory tract infection (particularly associated with nebulized medications), wound infection, peritonitis, septic arthritis, and conjunctivitis and cases of neonatal meningitis and brain abscess associated with *B. cepacia* have been reported (2, 15, 16, 26, 31, 34). *B. cepacia* also has emerged as an important cause of respiratory infections among patients with cystic fibrosis (CF) and those with chronic granulomatous disease. The clinical distinction between infection and colonization, particularly of the respiratory tract, is often difficult. When *B. cepacia* is isolated from the blood of multiple patients within a short time, pseudobacteremia due to extrinsic contamination of blood culture bottles should be considered (29).

SUSCEPTIBILITY IN VITRO AND IN VIVO
Single Drug

B. cepacia is intrinsically resistant to a wide range of antimicrobial agents, including polymyxin, first- and second-generation cephalosporins, aminoglycosides, and carboxypenicillins (e.g., carbenicillin, azlocillin, and ticarcillin). Antimicrobial agents effective against *B. cepacia* in vitro include trimethoprim-sulfamethoxazole, minocyline, chloramphenicol, ureidopenicillins, ceftazidime, ciprofloxacin, and carbapenems (Table 1). Meropenem appears to have greater activity in vitro against *B. cepacia* than does imipenem (11).

The most common mechanism of resistance in *B. cepacia* is decreased porin-mediated outer membrane permeability and production of aminoglycoside-modifying enzymes (6, 36). Resistance to β-lactam drugs is usually mediated by constitutively expressed or easily induced chromosomal β-lactamases (36). Less commonly, resistance is due to plasmid-mediated β-lactamases of the TEM class (cephalosporinases) or to alterations in the penicillin-binding proteins (e.g., piperacillin resistance). Resistance to β-lactam drugs also can be increased in vitro by incubation in 5% CO_2, a condition that may mimic the mileu of the lung in cystic fibrosis (10). A carbapenem-hydrolyzing metallo-β-lactamse has recently been isolated from a clinical strain of *B. cepacia* that is particularly effective in hydrolyzing impenem (3). *B. cepacia* represented 6% of imipenem-resistant and 9% of amikacin-resistant Gram-negative blood isolates, respectively, obtained from patients in New Jersey hospitals during the period 1992–1995 (44).

B. cepacia isolates from patients with cystic fibrosis appear to be more resistant than isolates from other patients, which may reflect the frequent exposure of patients with cystic fibrosis to antimicrobial agents (Table 2). In a study comparing 110 *B. cepacia* isolates from patients without cystic fibrosis with 20 isolates from patients with cystic fibrosis, the cystic fibrosis isolates were less susceptible to all antibiotics tested, including meropenem, ceftazidime, chloramphenicol, trimethoprim-sulfamethoxazole, and two investigational fluoroquinolones (Table 2) (23). Ceftazidime and piperacillin appear to have the

TABLE 1 • Results of Antimicrobial Susceptibility Testing of 96 _B. cepacia_ Isolates, UCLA Medical Center, 1984–1996

Agent	Number of Isolates Tested	MIC (μg/mL)			
		MIC_{50}	MIC_{90}	MIC Range	Percentage of Isolates Susceptible
Cefotaxime	24	16	>32	2–>32	45.8
Ceftazidime	70	4	16	1–>32	82.9
Ceftizoxime	43	4	32	≤0.5–>32	81.4
Ciprofloxacin	69	1	4	≤0.25–8	59.4
Imipenem	93	8	>8	≤0.25–>8	45.2
Piperacillin	96	≤8	64	≤8–512	79.2
Piperacillin-tazobactam	26	≤8/4	16/4	≤8/4–256/4	88.5
Trimethoprim-sulfamethoxazole	96	≤1/20	≤1/20	≤1/20–>4/80	94.8

greatest activity in vitro against _B. cepacia_ isolates from patients with cystic fibrosis. Of 73 isolates collected from the sputum of patients from Michigan CF Centers, 92% were susceptible to ceftazidime (MIC_{50} ≤ 4 mg/mL and MIC_{90} = 16 mg/mL), 89% to piperacillin, 85% to mezlocillin, and 40% to ciprofloxacin (4). However, ceftazidime and piperacillin have been associated with clinical failures despite in vitro susceptibility (13).

None of the currently available antimicrobial agents have been effective in eradicating _B. cepacia_ pulmonary colonization in patients with cystic fibrosis. The discrepancy between in vitro susceptibility testing results and the clinical response to antimicrobial therapy among patients with cystic fibrosis may be due to a variety of factors including altered pharmacokinetics, failure to deliver drug to the bronchiectatic lung, failure to penetrate across the bronchial mucosa in sufficient concentration into abnormally viscous bronchial secretions, high colony counts of organisms (>10^7 CFU/mL), and local factors such as decreased pH and increased concentration of divalent cations that impair phagocytic activity in the lung.

Combination Drugs

Limited information is available on in vitro synergy of combination antimicrobial therapy against _B. cepacia_ (20, 21, 38). Among 16 tobramycin- and ticarcillin-resistant isolates of _B. cepacia_ evaluated in one study, the combination of imipenem and ciprofloxacin was synergistic for 7 (44%) isolates, and the combination of imipenem, ciprofloxacin, and rifampicin was synergistic for 12 (75%) (21). In addition, a preliminary study demonstrated a significant (≥0.5 h) postantibiotic effect of ceftazidime, ciprofloxacin, imipenem, and piperacillin against sensitive _B. cepacia_ isolates when the agents were administered at their MIC breakpoints (22). The clinical significance of the synergy and postantibiotic effect in the treatment of pulmonary infection in cystic fibrosis remains to be defined.

ANTIMICROBIAL THERAPY
Drug of Choice

Clinical studies comparing various agents in the treatment of _B. cepacia_ infection are not currently available. Published expe-

TABLE 2 • In Vitro Activity of Selected Antimicrobial Agents for Isolates of _B. cepacia_ from Non–Cystic Fibrosis and Cystic Fibrosis Patients

Agent	Strains from Non–Cystic Fibrosis Patients				Strains from Cystic Fibrosis Patients				Ref
	Number Tested	MIC (μg/mL)			Number Tested	MIC (μg/mL)			
		MIC_{50}	MIC_{90}	MIC Range		MIC_{50}	MIC_{90}	MIC Range	
Ceftazidime	29	8	16	<0.03–16	26	8	>64	2–>64	39
	110	2	4	0.06–>128	20	8	32	1–>128	23
	—				34	4	16	0.5–>64	19
Chloramphenicol	110	16	32	1–128	20	16	64	2–>128	23
Ciprofloxacin	29	2	16	<0.03–64	26	2	64	0.25–64	39
	110	1	2	<0.06–128	20	8	128	0.25–128	23
	—				34	4	16	<0.06–16	19
Imipenem	29	8	32	<0.03–>64	26	16	>64	1–>64	39
	—				34	16	32	2–>64	19
Levofloxacin	29	4	16	<0.03–32	26	2	16	0.25–64	39
Meropenem	110	2	4	<0.06–16	20	2	16	1–16	23
Mezlocillin	—				34	64	>64	1–>64	19
Ofloxacin	29	4	32	<0.03–32	26	2	32	0.5–>64	39
Piperacillin	29	8	32	2–>64	26	8	>64	4–>64	39
Piperacillin-tazobactam	29	8	32	2–>64	26	8	>64	4–>64	39
Trimethoprim-sulfamethoxazole	110	4	32	4–128	20	32	128	4–>128	23
	29	4	16	0.25–>64	26	32	>64	4–>64	39

rience is especially limited with respect to treatment of *B. cepacia* infection in patients who do not have cystic fibrosis. Based upon in vitro susceptibility data, ceftazidime, imipenem, meropenem, ciprofloxacin, piperacillin, mezlocillin, chloramphenicol, and trimethoprim-sulfamethoxazole have the greatest activity against *B. cepacia*. Data from synergy studies and the potential for emergence of resistance while on monotherapy suggest that therapy for serious *B. cepacia* infection should include two parenteral antimicrobial agents administered at standard doses. The choice of agents should be guided by results of in vitro susceptibility testing, and the duration of therapy should be based upon assessment of the clinical and microbiologic response.

Special Situations

Cystic Fibrosis

Each year, approximately 3% of all U.S. patients with cystic fibrosis have *B. cepacia* isolated from respiratory secretions, almost all of whom are previously colonized with mucoid *Pseudomonas aeruginosa* (27). Pulmonary infection of cystic fibrosis patients with *B. cepacia* most often results in chronic endobronchial colonization with an large numbers of organisms (10^7 CFU/mL). Acquisition of *B. cepacia* has been associated with deterioration of pulmonary function and earlier death among some patients with cystic fibrosis and with a rapidly fatal necrotizing pneumonia, especially among those with more advanced pulmonary disease or those who have undergone lung transplantation (9, 24, 41, 42). Evidence suggests that *B. cepacia* can be transmitted, directly or indirectly, to patients with cystic fibrosis during hospitalization, while attending CF clinic, and during social gatherings, including camp (14, 25, 32, 33). When hospitalized, cystic fibrosis patients with *B. cepacia* should be isolated from those who are not colonized by means of cohorting in CF units or use of contact precautions (17, 35).

Patients with cystic fibrosis experience periodic exacerbations of pulmonary infections, typically manifested by increased pulmonary symptoms and sputum production. Recommended therapy includes 14 to 21 days of parenteral therapy with two antimicrobials, intensified chest physiotherapy to promote airway clearance, and bronchodilator administration (37). Because of reports of poor clinical response to ceftazidime and piperacillin, parenteral chloramphenicol (15–20 mg/kg every 6 h), trimethoprim-sulfamethoxazole (5 mg trimethoprim/kg and 25 mg sulfamethoxazole/kg every 6 h), or both are recommended currently for treatment of pulmonary exacerbations when *B. cepacia* is the sole respiratory pathogen. Serum chloramphenicol levels should be monitored. However, most cystic fibrosis patients with *B. cepacia* also have respiratory colonization with *P. aeruginosa*. In this situation, choice of antimicrobial therapy should be based upon results of susceptibility testing of each of the strains and may include combination therapy with ceftazidime and ciprofloxacin (or chloramphenicol or trimethoprim-sulfamethoxazole at the above doses). The role of maintenance oral therapy in reducing the incidence of exacerbations of pulmonary infections associated with *B. cepacia* has not been defined, but trimethoprim-sulfamethoxazole (children: 4 mg trimethoprim/kg and 20 mg sulfamethoxazole/kg every 12 h; adults: 160 mg trimethoprim and 800 mg sul-

famethoxazole every 12 h) has been recommended when oral therapy is used (37).

Several small studies have examined combination therapy against *B. cepacia* in patients with cystic fibrosis. Combination therapy with temocillin (mean dose, 3 g/day) and an aminoglycoside for a mean duration of 12 days resulted in objective clinical improvement following 9 of 12 treatment courses administered to five patients colonized with *both P. aeruginosa* and *B. cepacia* (43). All *B. cepacia* isolates were resistant to the aminoglycoside, while most were susceptible in vitro to temocillin; *P. aeruginosa isolates* were susceptible to both agents. Despite clinical response, sputum colony counts of *B. cepacia* were unchanged or were reduced only tenfold following 11 of 12 treatment courses. In another study, large doses of ceftazidime (200 mg/kg/day) administered alone (4 courses), with tobramycin (9 courses), or with piperacillin (4 courses) failed to reduce sputum colony counts of *B. cepacia* in 17 of 18 treatment courses administered to cystic fibrosis patients, despite in vitro susceptibility of all *B. cepacia* strains to ceftazidime (13). In 7 of the courses, *B. cepacia* was the sole respiratory isolate, while *B. cepacia* and one or more strains of *P. aeruginosa* were isolated in the remaining 11 courses. Clinical improvement was seen in only 8 treatment courses; eight patients failed, and four patients died. In a third small uncontrolled study, patients colonized with *B. cepacia* alone and those colonized with *B. cepacia* and *P. aeruginosa* had similar improvement in lung function and inflammatory markers, including white blood count and C-reactive protein, following treatment of pulmonary infection exacerbations with combination antimicrobial therapy, despite in vitro resistance of the *B. cepacia* isolates (30). In each of these studies, clinical improvement may have reflected reduction of the endobronchial load of *P. aeruginosa* or other susceptible organism(s), as no microbiologic effect on *B. cepacia* sputum counts was seen following almost all of the treatment courses.

Chronic Granulomatous Disease

B. cepacia also has emerged as an important cause of infection, including pneumonia, septicemia, and soft tissue abscesses, among patients with chronic granulomatous disease (28, 40). The pathogenicity of *B. cepacia* in chronic granulomatous disease appears to be due to the ability of the organism to resist neutrophil-mediated nonoxidative killing (40). Because *B. cepacia* may be difficult to isolate and identify early in the course of invasive infection in patients with chronic granulomatous disease, it is important to consider *B. cepacia,* especially in patients with culture-negative pneumonia. The initial empirical antimicrobial regimen for invasive infections in patients with chronic granulomatous disease should include ceftazidime and trimethoprim-sulfamethoxazole (5 mg trimethoprim/kg and 25 mg sulfamethoxazole/kg every 6 h) or a similar agent with broad-spectrum antimicrobial activity (40). Prophylactic antimicrobial therapy benefits patients with chronic granulomatous disease, and oral trimethoprim-sulfamethoxazole (children: 4 mg trimethoprim/kg and 20 mg sulfamethoxazole/kg every 12 h; adults: 160 mg trimethoprim and 800 mg sulfamethoxazole every 12 h) is the regimen of choice.

Other Special Situations

Data are limited on the treatment of central nervous system infections with *B. cepacia*. In one report, an adult with *B. cepacia* brain abscess secondary to chronic suppurative otitis media required prolonged (>6 months) antimicrobial therapy with ceftazidime (3 g intravenously every 6–8 hours) and oral ciprofloxacin (400 mg twice daily) as well as multiple surgical drainage procedures for cure (16). In a second report, an infant developed *B. cepacia* meningitis associated with a Holter ventriculoatrial shunt following perioperative skin antisepsis with a contaminated aqueous chlorhexidene solution. The infection responded to removal of the infected device and treatment with intravenous chloramphenicol and trimethoprim-sulfamethoxazole (2). This and other reports emphasize that management of *B. cepacia* infection associated with indwelling medical devices such as central nervous system shunts, central venous catheters, and peritoneal dialysis catheters may require removal of the device in addition to antimicrobial therapy (29, 31).

Alternative Therapy

B. cepacia is resistant to the commonly used inhaled antimicrobials (e.g., tobramycin, colistin, polymyxin). However, inhaled amiloride may have antimicrobial activity against *B. cepacia*, exhibiting a postantibiotic effect and potentiating the effect of tobramycin in vitro despite negligible activity against *B. cepacia* by standard MIC testing at neutral pH (7). Addition of verapamil reduced the tobramycin MIC markedly against isolates of *B. cepacia* in another study (8). Together, these findings suggest that drugs such as amiloride and verapamil that inhibit the bacterial multidrug resistance efflux protein may be worth evaluating as new treatment strategies for endobronchial *B. cepacia* infection.

ENDPOINTS OF THERAPY

Among cystic fibrosis patients, objective response to therapy for exacerbations of pulmonary infection associated with *B. cepacia* can be monitored by improved pulmonary functions, decreased inflammatory markers such as white blood count, and weight gain. Unlike treatment of exacerbations associated with *P. aeruginosa*, a decreased density of *B. cepacia* in the sputum is infrequently seen, and eradication of endobronchial *B. cepacia* colonization is rarely, if ever, achieved. Although information about the treatment of pulmonary infection associated with *B. cepacia* is limited, several preliminary conclusions can be drawn: (*a*) neither in vitro susceptibility nor resistance reliably predicts clinical response to antimicrobial therapy; (*b*) clinical response does not correlate with bacteriologic response; and (*c*) antimicrobial therapy should not be withheld from patients with cystic fibrosis because of in vitro resistance.

CONTROVERSIES, CAVEATS, AND COMMENTS

Although much has been learned about the epidemiology and pathogenicity of *B. cepacia*, particularly in cystic fibrosis patients, further investigation is needed to define the relationship between in vitro susceptibility and clinical response to therapy, the role of inhaled agents in treating endobronchial infection, and the role of synergistic combination therapy. Development of new agents with in vitro and in vivo activities against *B. cepacia* would be an important advance in the management of patients with cystic fibrosis.

REFERENCES

1. Anderson RL, Vess RW, Carr JH, Bond WW, Panlilio AL, Favero MS. Investigations of intrinsic *Pseudomonas cepacia* contamination in commercially manufactured povidone-iodine. Infect Control Hosp Epidemiol 1991;12:297–302.
2. Bassett DCJ, Dixon JAS, Hunt GH. Infection of Holter valve by *Pseudomonas*-contaminated chlorhexidine. Lancet 1973;I: 1263–1264.
3. Baxter IA, Lambert PA. Isolation on partial purification of a carbapenem-hydrolysing metallo-beta-lactamase from *Pseudomonas cepacia*. FEMS Microbiol Lett 1994;122:251–256.
4. Bhakta DR, Learder I, Jacobson R, Robinson-Dunn B, Honicky RE, Kumar A. Antibacterial properties of investigational, new, and commonly used antibiotics against isolates of *Pseudomonas cepacia* in Michigan. Chemotherapy 1992;38:319–323.
5. Burkholder WH. Sour skin, a bacterial rot of onion bulbs. Phytopathology 1959;40:115.
6. Burns JL, Clark DK. Salicylate-inducible antibiotic resistance in *Pseudomonas cepacia* with absence of pore-forming outer membrane protein. Antimicrob Agents Chemother 1992;36: 2280–2285.
7. Cohn RC, Rudzienski L. In vitro suppression of *Pseudomonas cepacia* after limited exposure to subinhibitory concentratios of amiloride and 5-(N,N-hexamethylene) amiloride. Pediatr Pulmonol 1994;17:336–339.
8. Cohn RC, Rudzienski L, Putman RW. Verapamil-tobramycin synergy in *Pseudomonas cepacia* but not *Pseudomonas aeruginosa*. Chemotherapy 1995;41:330–333.
9. Corey M, Farewell V. Determinants of mortality from cystic fibrosis in Canada 1970–1989. Am J Epidemiol 1996;143: 1007–1017.
10. Corkill JE, Deveney J, Pratt J, Shears P, Smyth A, Heaf D, Hart CA. Effect of pH and CO_2 on in vitro susceptibility of *Pseudomonas cepacia* to beta-lactams. Pediatr Res 1994;35: 299–302.
11. Edwards JR, Turner PJ. Laboratory data which differentiate meropenem and imipenem. Scand J Infect Dis 1995;96 (Suppl): 5–10.
12. Gilligan PH, Gage PA, Bradshaw LM, Schidlow DV, DeCicco BT. Isolation medium for the recovery of *Pseudomonas cepacia* from respiratory secretions of patients with cystic fibrosis. J Clin Microbiol 1995;22:5–8.
13. Gold R, Jin E, Levison H, Isles A, Fleming PC. Ceftazidime alone and in combination in patients with cystic fibrosis: lack of efficacy in treatment of severe respiratory infecitons caused by *Pseudomonas cepacia*. J Antimicrob Chemother 1983;12(Suppl A):331–336.
14. Govan JRW, Brown PH, Maddison J, Doherty CJ, Nelson JW, Dodd M, Greening AP, Webb AK. Evidence for transmission of *Pseudomonas cepacia* by social contact in cystic fibrosis. Lancet 342;1993:15–19.
15. Hamill RJ, Houston ED, Gorghiou PR, Wright CE, Koza MA, Cadle RM, Goepfert PA, Lewis DA, Zenon GJ, Clarridge JE. An outbreak of *Burkholderia* (formerly *Pseudomonas*) *cepacia* respiratory tract colonization and infection associated with nebulized albuterol therapy. Ann Intern Med 1995;122:762–766.

16. Hobson R, Gould I, Govan J. *Burkholderia (Pseudomonas) cepacia* as a cause of brain abscesses secondary to chronic suppurative otitis media. Eur J Clin Microbiol Infect Dis 1995;14: 908–911.

17. Hospital Infections Control Practices Advisory Committee. Guideline for isolation precautions in hospitals. Infect Control Hosp Epidemiol 1996;17:53–80.

18. Jarvis WR, Olson D, Tablan O, Martone WJ. The epidemiology of nosocomial *Pseudomonas cepacia* infections. Eur J Epidemiol 1987;3:233–236.

19. Klinger JD, Aronoff SC. In vitro activity of ciprofloxacin and other antibacterial agents against *Pseudomonas aeruginosa* and *Pseudomonas cepacia* from cystic fibrosis patients. J Antimicrob Chemother 1985;15:679–684.

20. Kumar A, Wofford-McQueen R, Gordon RC. In vitro activity of multiple antimicrobial combinations against *Pseudomonas cepacia* isolates. Chemotherapy 1989;35:246–253.

21. Kumar A, Wofford-McQueen R, Gordon RC. Ciprofloxacin, imipenem and rifampicin: in-vitro synergy of two and three drug combinations against *Pseudomonas cepacia*. J Antimicrob Chemother 1989;23:831–835.

22. Kumar A, Hay MB, Maier GA, Dyke JW. Post-antibiotic effect of ceftazidime, ciprofloxacin, imipenem, piperacillin and tobramycin for *Pseudomonas cepacia*. J Antimicrob Chemother 1992;30:597–602.

23. Lewin C, Doherty C, Govan J. In vitro activities of meropenem, PD 127391, PD 131628, ceftazidime, chloramphenicol, cotrimoxazole, and ciprofloxacin against *Pseudomonas cepacia*. Antimicrob Agents Chemother 1993;37:123–125.

24. Lewin LO, Byard PJ, Davis PB. Effect of *Pseudomonas cepacia* colonization on survival and pulmonary function of cystic fibrosis patients. J Clin Epidemiol 1990;43:125–131.

25. LiPuma JJ, Dasen SE, Nielson DW, Stern RC, Stull TL. Person-to-person transmission of *Pseudomonas cepacia* between patients with cystic fibrosis. Lancet 1990;336:1094–1096.

26. Martone WJ, Tablan OC, Jarvis WR. The epidemiology of nosocomial epidemic *Pseudomonas cepacia* infections. Eur J Epidemiol 1987;3:222–232.

27. Moss RB. Cystic fibrosis: pathogenesis, pulmonary infection, and treatment. Clin Infect Dis 1995;21:839–851.

28. O'Neill KM, Herman JH, Modlin JF, Moxon ER, Windelstein JA. *Pseudomonas cepacia*: an emerging pathogen in chronic granulomatous disease. J Pediatr 1986;108:940–942.

29. Panlilio AL, Beck-Sague CM, Siegel JD, Anderson RL, Yetts SY, Clark NC, Duer PN, Thomassen KA, Vess RW, Hill BC, Tablan OC, Jarvis WR. Infections and pseudoinfection due to povidone-iodine solution contaminated with *Pseudomonas cepacia*. Clin Infect Dis 1992;14:1078–1083.

30. Peckham D, Crouch S, Humphreys H, Lobo B, Tse A, Knox AJ. Effect of antibiotic treatment on inflammatory markers and lung function in cystic fibrosis patients with *Pseudomonas cepacia*. Thorax 1994:803–807.

31. Pegues DA, Carson LA, Anderson RL, Norgard MJ, Argent TA, Jarvis WR, Woernle CH. Outbreak of *Pseudomonas cepacia* bacteremia in oncology patients. Clin Infect Dis 1993:16:407–411.

32. Pegues DA, Schidlow DV, Tablan OC, Carson LA, Clark NC, Jarvis WR. Possible nosocomial transmission of *Pseudomonas cepacia* in patients with cystic fibrosis. Arch Pediatr Adolesc Med 1994;148:805–812.

33. Pegues DA, Carson LA, Tablan OC, FitzSimmons SC, Roman SB, Miller JM, Jarvis WR. Acquisition of *Pseudomonas cepacia* at summer camps for patients with cystic fibrosis. J Pediatr 1994;124:694–702.

34. Pegues CF, Pegues DA, Ford DS, Hibberd PL, Carson LA, Raine CM, Hooper DC. *Burkholderia cepacia* respiratory tract acquisition: epidemiology and molecular characterization of a large nosocomial outbreak. Epidemiol Infect 1996:116–3309–3317.

35. Pitt TL, Govan JRW. *Pseudomonas cepacia* and cystic fibrosis. PHLS Microbiol Digest 1993;10:69–72.

36. Prince A. Antibiotic resistance of *Pseudomonas* species. J Pediatr 1986;198:830–834.

37. Ramsey BW. Management of pulmonary disease in patients with cystic fibrosis. N Engl J Med 1996;335:179–188.

38. Rubio TT. Ciprofloxacin: comparative data in cystic fibrosis. Am J Med 1987;82(Suppl 4A):185–188.

39. Spangler SK, Visalli MA, Jacobs MR, Appelbaum PC. Susceptibilities of non-*Pseudomonas aeruginosa* gram-negative nonfermentative rods to ciprofloxacin, ofloxacin, levofloxacin, D-ofloxacin, sparfloxacin, ceftazidime, piperacillin, piperacillin-tazobactam, trimethoprim-sulfamethoxazole, and imipenem. Antimicrob Agents Chemotherapy 1996;40:772–775.

40. Speert DP, Bond M, Woodman RC, Curnutte JT. Infection with *Pseudomonas cepacia* in chronic granulomatous disease: role of nonoxidative killing by neutrophils in host defense. J Infect Dis 1994;170:1524–1531.

41. Steinbach S, Sun L, Jiang R-Z, Flume P, Gilligan P, Egan TM, Goldstein R. Transmissibility of *Pseudomonas cepacia* infection in clinic patients and lung-transplant recipients with cystic fibrosis. N Engl J Med 1994;331:981–987.

42. Tablan OC, Martone WJ, Doershuk CF, Stern RC, Thomassen MJ, Klinger JD, White JW, Carson LA, Jarvis WR. Colonization of the respiratory tract with *Pseudomonas cepacia* in cystic fibrosis: risk factors and outcomes. Chest 1987;91:527–532.

43. Taylor RFH, Gaya H, Hodson ME. Temocillin and cystic fibrosis: outcome of intravenous administration in patients infected with *Pseudomonas cepacia*. J Antimicrob Chemother 1992;29:341–344.

44. Tokars JI, Paul SM, Crane GL, Cetron MS, Finelli L, Jarvis WR. Secular trends in blood stream infection due to antimicrobial-resistant bacteria in New Jersey hospitals, 1991–1995. Am J Infect Control 1997;25:395–400.

Burkholderia pseudomallei and *B. mallei*

●

Andrew J. H. Simpson and Nicholas J. White

There are several members of the genus *Burkholderia* (formerly *Pseudomonas*) (33), but only three are considered significant human pathogens: *B. pseudomallei,* the cause of melioidosis; *B. mallei,* the cause of glanders; and *B. cepacia,* a cause of opportunistic lung infection in cystic fibrosis patients. This chapter discusses the treatment of infections caused by *B. pseudomallei* and *B. mallei.*

MELIOIDOSIS: GENERAL DESCRIPTION

Melioidosis is an infection caused by the motile, aerobic, Gram-negative bacterium *Burkholderia* (formerly *Pseudomonas*) *pseudomallei.* The disease was first recognized in Rangoon, Burma, among injecting morphia addicts in 1911 (30) and is now known to be endemic to a large part of Southeast Asia and northern Australia (17). Sporadic cases have been described elsewhere, mainly in the tropics. The organism is an environmental saprophyte found in wet soil in particular, for example in rice paddies. In endemic areas it may be a leading cause of community-acquired septicemia; in Ubon Ratchatani in northeast Thailand, it is responsible for approximately 20% of such cases per year (7).

Clinical aspects of the disease have been reviewed elsewhere (15, 25). Briefly, the disease may involve almost any organ system, with acute septicemic infection, disseminated disease, or lung infection the most common presentations, but chronic suppurative infections also occur. Abscess formation is common, particularly in the lungs, liver, and spleen. Children may present with a specific syndrome of localized parotid abscesses (11). Patients with underlying diabetes mellitus (particularly if poorly controlled) or renal disease (including renal calculi) are at increased risk of infection.

Antibiotic Susceptibility

B. pseudomallei is resistant in vitro to many antibiotics, including penicillins, aminopenicillins, many cephalosporins (2), macrolides, and most aminoglycosides (21), including gentamicin. Kanamycin is reported to have some activity. *B. pseudomallei* is susceptible to some third-generation cephalosporins such as ceftazidime (3, 12) and to ureidopenicillins (3), carbapenems (23), chloramphenicol, trimethoprim-sulfamethoxazole (4), and fluoroquinolones (3, 31). Cefotaxime and ceftriaxone show some activity (3). *B. pseudomallei* is unusual among pseudomonads in that it is also susceptible to tetracyclines (10, 34) and the combination of amoxicillin and clavulanic acid (co-amoxiclav, Augmentin) (14). The β-lactams and fluoroquinolones possess bactericidal activity, whereas chloramphenicol, tetracyclines, trimethoprim, and sulfamethoxazole are bacteriostatic only (12). The carbapenems and fluoro-

quinolones also exert a postantibiotic effect against *B. pseudomallei* (27); however, the MICs for the fluoroquinolones are relatively high, and doubts over their effectiveness have been raised. The carbapenems appear to be among the most active antibiotics currently available, with biapenem and imipenem showing the greatest activity (23). They also appear to be active against strains that are resistant to either ceftazidime or amoxicillin-clavulanic acid (23).

ANTIMICROBIAL THERAPY
General

B. pseudomallei is resistant to the first-line agents used in many hospitals worldwide to treat community-acquired septicemias (i.e., penicillin-aminoglycoside combinations). In endemic areas, therefore, many patients may receive ineffective empirical therapy.

Quadruple or conventional therapy with intravenous chloramphenicol (100–150 mg/kg/day), doxycycline (4–6 mg/kg/day), and trimethoprim-sulfamethoxazole (8–12 and 40–60 mg/kg/day, respectively) was the mainstay of therapy for many years (20). However this regimen was associated with a mortality of approximately 70 to 80% in septicemic melioidosis (7, 28) in addition to its considerable potential for toxicity.

Ceftazidime is a third-generation cephalosporin with activity against *Pseudomonas* species. One open, prospective, randomized trial compared high-dose intravenous ceftazidime with use of conventional therapy in severe melioidosis in patients over 10 years old (29). The trial was conducted in northeastern Thailand. Ceftazidime was associated with a 50% reduction in mortality, to less than 40% in patients who survived for a minimum of 48 h (29). There was no difference in mortality during the first 48 h of treatment. Ceftazidime was given at a dose of 120 mg/kg/day (usual dose, 2 g 8 hourly) for a minimum of 7 days. Lower doses were given in patients with renal failure. Of 161 patients entered into the study, 65 had culture-proven melioidosis, and 54 (83%) of these patients were septicemic. As a result of this trial, ceftazidime became the acute treatment of choice for severe melioidosis.

Another trial (24) in northeastern Thailand, conducted on two sites, compared conventional therapy with use of a combination of intravenous ceftazidime (100 mg/kg/day) and trimethoprim-sulfamethoxazole (8/40 mg/kg/day) for a minimum of 10 days, with similar results to those of the previous trial. Some 64 patients were subsequently shown to have culture-proven severe melioidosis; 3 patients suffered severe adverse reactions (2 in the conventional treatment group, 1 to the trimethoprim-sulfamethoxazole component in the other group). There have been no trials comparing intravenous ceftazidime with use of this ceftazidime-trimethoprim-sulfamethoxazole combination.

One large trial of high-dose intravenous ceftazidime (120 mg/kg/day) versus high-dose co-amoxiclav (160 mg/kg/day) for a minimum of 7 days has been reported (26). This open, randomized, controlled trial involved 212 culture-positive patients. Overall mortality was the same in both groups (47%); however, the treatment failure rate was significantly higher for co-amoxiclav (23% vs. 5%). Both drugs were well tolerated and appeared safe at the doses used. The authors concluded that co-amoxiclav was an effective acute treatment but that ceftazidime remained the drug of choice. Co-amoxiclav has a broader antibacterial spectrum than ceftazidime and hence may be the more appropriate of the two agents as empirical therapy for community-acquired septicemias in endemic areas.

While high-dose ceftazidime remains the treatment of choice at present, trials of ceftazidime against the carbapenem antibiotic imipenem (50 mg/kg/day; normal dose, 1 g 8 hourly) are currently under way. It is too early to assess the relative merits of the carbapenems in vivo, although in vitro studies indicate that these agents are highly promising (23). Preliminary clinical experience with imipenem in northeastern Thailand is also very encouraging; it appears to be an effective treatment, but we await trial results.

Combination parenteral therapy (e.g., ceftazidime and co-trimoxazole) has been recommended by some authors (24, 25). As with the treatment of tuberculosis, this has the theoretical advantage of reducing the emergence of resistant strains during therapy (12). This is known to occur, but it is not clear whether it is of clinical importance. Whether such combination therapy would prevent this phenomenon is unknown, but the appearance of resistant strains during conventional four-drug therapy provides evidence against this. Unlike tuberculosis, the emergence of resistant strains does not have public health implications, as human-human transmission is rare, and patients are not regarded as infectious. There are also worries about the potential for in vivo antagonism between these antibiotic combinations, which can be demonstrated in vitro (13), although clinical evidence is lacking. We do not recommend combination therapy at present.

Special Situations

Empirical Treatment

In endemic areas, patients presenting with conditions consistent with melioidosis require early treatment that will cover infection with *B. pseudomallei*. The same applies to patients from, or those with a travel history to, endemic areas. Penicillin-aminoglycoside combinations are therefore not advisable. If the diagnosis is not clear, broad-spectrum agents that have activity include co-amoxiclav, ceftriaxone, or imipenem. Ceftazidime should usually be substituted once the diagnosis has been confirmed.

Relapse

Relapses are common (8) and should be treated as for first episodes. Mortality and morbidity in relapsed cases are similar to that in first episodes (8). Frequently, the antimicrobial

susceptibility pattern of the relapse isolate is unchanged, but repeat susceptibility testing is mandatory. Development of resistance during treatment has been described for all of the commonly used agents (ceftazidime, co-amoxiclav, chloramphenicol, trimethoprim, sulfamethoxazole, and doxycycline) (12, 18).

Adjunctive Therapy

Appropriate supportive measures should be instituted in acutely ill patients. Surgical drainage of large abscesses is indicated. Frequently drainage is not possible because multiple small abscesses are present, particularly in the liver or spleen. Isolation of patients is not necessary.

Oral Treatment

Nonsevere infections with *B. pseudomallei* can be treated with oral antibiotics. There are very few reports of studies of oral treatment in nonsevere melioidosis. Much of the current knowledge and practice stems from studies of oral maintenance therapy (see next section).

Maintenance Treatment

Following successful acute treatment of melioidosis, a substantial risk of relapse remains, with similar morbidity and mortality to first episodes (8). Prolonged maintenance therapy is necessary for all patients (8). Most experience has been gained with oral conventional antibiotics (i.e., chloramphenicol, doxycycline, and trimethoprim-sulfamethoxazole). Treatment courses of 8 weeks have been associated with a relapse rate of 23% (8), but 20-week courses have reduced this to under 10%.

Conventional oral therapy was compared with oral co-amoxiclav in one randomized study (22). Relapse rates after 20 weeks of therapy were 4% and 16%, respectively. Doses were chloramphenicol (40 mg/kg/day in 4 divided doses), doxycycline (4 mg/kg/day in 2 divided doses), and trimethoprim-sulfamethoxazole (10 mg and 50 mg/kg/day, respectively, in 2 divided doses), or co-amoxiclav (amoxicillin 30 mg/kg/day, clavulanic acid 15 mg/kg/day) plus amoxicillin (30 mg/kg/day). Chloramphenicol was given for the first 8 weeks of therapy only. The authors concluded that co-amoxiclav was safer and better tolerated but possibly less effective. Either regimen may be used for maintenance therapy. Not surprisingly, there were considerable problems with compliance; the conventional regimen involves taking up to 14 tablets or capsules, and co-amoxiclav, 12 capsules per day. Cost is also an important consideration in choice of regimen; co-amoxiclav costs approximately 15 times as much as the conventional regimen. However, co-amoxiclav should be considered the treatment of choice for children or pregnant women.

Fluoroquinolone therapy (with either ciprofloxacin or ofloxacin) appears unsatisfactory, with a relapse rate approaching 30% despite prolonged treatment (9). Fluoroquinolones should thus be considered only third-line agents.

There remains an urgent need for simple, cheap, less-toxic regimens for maintenance treatment of melioidosis. Failure of compliance with complex regimens remains a major risk factor for relapse (8). Clinical experience with other regimens is limited (e.g., cotrimoxazole alone or in combination with doxycycline). Comparative trials of doxycycline alone versus conventional oral therapy are currently under way. New oral agents are required, but they are unlikely to be cheap. Whether newer oral cephalosporins or penems (32) will be clinically useful remains to be determined.

ENDPOINTS FOR THERAPY

Whichever parenteral agents are used for first-line therapy for moderate or severe melioidosis, the therapeutic response is usually slow, with a median time to defervescence of 9 to 10 days (26). A minimum of 10 to 14 days of parenteral therapy should be given and continued until there is clear evidence of a clinical response. Some patients may require several weeks of parenteral treatment. It is important not to switch to an alternative regimen too early simply because a patient maintains fever after several days of treatment—this does not necessarily imply treatment failure.

Following a satisfactory response to parenteral antibiotics, all patients should receive oral maintenance therapy. Oral treatment, including maintenance therapy, as discussed above, should be continued for 12 to 20 weeks.

Treatment Failure

Failure of parenteral treatment, defined as development of septic shock more than 72 h after starting treatment, development of new abscesses, fever that persists without signs of resolution for 14 days, or blood cultures remaining positive 7 or more days after starting appropriate therapy, is common and may require a change of treatment. Sputum cultures may remain positive for *B. pseudomallei* for several weeks despite adequate therapy, and this does not necessarily indicate failure. Suitable second-line parenteral agents include co-amoxiclav and imipenem.

PROPHYLAXIS

Human-to-human transmission of *B. pseudomallei* appears to be very rare. Occasional laboratory-acquired infections have been reported, but very little is known about the appropriateness, dose, or duration of prophylaxis. There is no documented experience with primary prophylaxis, and it is not advised for contacts of known cases (16). A case may be made for offering secondary prophylaxis in certain circumstances (e.g., following a laboratory accident involving cultures of the organism), but such instances can only be assessed on their individual merits. An oral agent such as co-amoxiclav would be most suitable in such a situation.

Vaccines

There are no available vaccines at present.

BURKHOLDERIA MALLEI INFECTIONS

Human infection with *B. mallei*, the cause of glanders and farcy in equine animals, is rare and usually confined to those in contact with infected animals (25). The organism is also a considerable hazard to laboratory workers. It is closely related to *B. pseudomallei*, and the disease has similarities to melioidosis, ranging from acute septicemic disease to localized chronic suppurative infection and carrying a high mortality rate. It is transmissible from human to human, and patients should be isolated.

Susceptibility in Vitro

Although there are few studies, the organism is reported to be susceptible in vitro to tetracyclines (6), sulfonamides, aminoglycosides, trimethoprim-sulfamethoxazole (1), some cephalosporins, imipenem (19), and ciprofloxacin (5).

Treatment

Few data exist on the treatment of human infection because of the rarity of the disease. Treatment similar to that for melioidosis is probably most appropriate; that is, high-dose ceftazidime (120 mg/kg/day). There is no information on how long treatment should be continued.

CONCLUSION

Ceftazidime remains the treatment of choice for acute severe melioidosis. High-dose parenteral treatment (120 mg/kg/day; normal dose, 2 g 8 hourly) should be given for at least 10 to 14 days and continued until there has been a clinical response to therapy. Co-amoxiclav is a suitable alternative. Imipenem also appears to be effective. Nonsevere infections can be treated with oral antibiotics.

Oral maintenance therapy is required for 12 to 20 weeks following an acute infection, with either conventional antibiotics in combination (chloramphenicol, doxycycline, and trimethoprim-sulfamethoxazole) or co-amoxiclav alone.

Human infection with *B. mallei* should be treated acutely in a manner similar to melioidosis treatment.

REFERENCES

1. Al-Izzi SA, Al-Bassam LS. In vitro susceptibility of Pseudomonas mallei to antimicrobial agents. Comp Immunol Microbiol Infect Dis 1989;12:5–8.
2. Ashdown LR, Frettingham RJ. In vitro activity of various cephalosporins against *Pseudomonas pseudomallei*. J Infect Dis 1984;150:779–780.
3. Ashdown LR. In-vitro activity of newer β-lactam and quinolone antimicrobial agents against *Pseudomonas pseudomallei*. Antimicrob Agents Chemother 1988;32:1435–1436.
4. Bassett DCJ. The sensitivity of *Pseudomonas pseudomallei* to trimethoprim and sulphamethoxazole in vitro. J Clin Pathol 1971;24:798–800.
5. Batmanov VP. Sensitivity of Pseudomonas mallei to fluoroquinolones and their efficacy in experimental glanders [Russian]. Antibiot Khimioter 1991;36:31–34.
6. Batmanov VP. Sensitivity of Pseudomonas mallei to tetracyclines and their effectiveness in experimental glanders [Russian]. Antibiot Khimioter 1994;39:33–37.
7. Chaowagul W, White NJ, Dance DA, Wattanagoon Y, Naigowit P, Davis TM, Looareesuwan S, Pitakwatchara N. Melioidosis: a major cause of community-acquired septicemia in north-eastern Thailand. J Infect Dis 1989;159:890–899.
8. Chaowagul W, Suputtamongkol Y, Dance DAB, Rajchanuvong A, Pattara-arechachai J, White NJ. Relapse in melioidosis: incidence and risk factors. J Infect Dis 1993;168:1181–1185.

9. Chaowagul W, Suputtamongkol Y, Smith MD, White NJ. Oral fluoroquinolones for maintenance treatment of melioidosis. Trans R Soc Trop Med Hyg 1997;91:599–601.

10. Chau PY, Ng WS, Leung YK, Lolekha S. In vitro susceptibility of strains of Pseudomonas pseudomallei isolated in Thailand and Hong Kong to some newer beta-lactam antibiotics and quinolone derivatives. J Infect Dis 1986;153:167–170.

11. Dance DAB, Davies TME, Wattanagoon Y, Chaowagul W, Saipan P, Looareesuwan S, Wuthiekanun V, White NJ. Acute suppurative parotitis caused by *Pseudomonas pseudomallei* in children. J Infect Dis 1989;159:654–660.

12. Dance DAB, Wuthiekanun V, Chaowagul W, White NJ. The antimicrobial susceptibility of Pseudomonas pseudomallei. Emergence of resistance in vitro and during treatment. J Antimicrob Chemother 1989;24:295–309.

13. Dance DAB, Wuthiekanun V, Chaowagul W, White NJ. Interactions in vitro between agents used to treat melioidosis. J Antimicrob Chemother 1989;24:311–316.

14. Dance DAB, Wuthiekanun V, Chaowagul W, White NJ. The activity of amoxycillin/clavulanic acid against *Pseudomonas pseudomallei*. J Antimicrob Chemother 1989;24:1012–1014.

15. Dance DAB. Melioidosis. Rev Med Microbiol 1990;1:143–150.

16. Dance DAB, Suputtamongkol Y, Chaowagul W, White NJ. Prophylaxis for contacts of melioidosis. J Infect 1990;21:222–223.

17. Dance DAB. Melioidosis: the tip of the iceberg? Clin Microbiol Rev 1991;4:52–60.

18. Dance DAB, Wuthiekanun V, Chaowagul W, Suputtamongkol Y, White NJ. Development of resistance to ceftazidime and co-amoxiclav in *Pseudomonas pseudomallei*. J Antimicrob Chemother 1991;28:321–324.

19. Iliukhin VI, Alekseev VV, Antonov IuV, Savchenko ST, Lozovaia NA. Effectiveness of treatment of experimental glanders after aerogenic infection [Russian]. Antibiot Khimioter 1994;39:45–48.

20. Leelarasamee A, Bovornkitti S. Melioidosis: review and update. Rev Infect Dis 1989;11:413–425.

21. McEniry DW, Gillespie SH, Felmingham D. Susceptibility of Pseudomonas pseudomallei to new beta-lactam and aminoglycoside antibiotics. J Antimicrob Chemother 1988;21:171–175.

22. Rajchanuvong A, Chaowagul W, Suputtamongkol Y, Smith MD, Dance DAB, White NJ. A prospective comparison of co-amoxyclav and the combination of chloramphenicol, doxycycline, and co-trimoxazole for the oral maintenance treatment of melioidosis. Trans R Soc Trop Med Hyg 1995;89:546–549.

23. Smith MD, Wuthiekanun V, Walsh AL, White NJ. In-vitro activity of carbapenem antibiotics against β-lactam susceptible and resistant strains of *Burkholderia pseudomallei*. J Antimicrob Chemother 1996;37:611–615.

24. Sookpranee M, Boonma P, Susaengrat W, Bhuripanyo K, Punyagupta S. Multicenter prospective randomized trial comparing ceftazidime plus co-trimoxazole with chloramphenicol plus doxycycline and co-trimoxazole for treatment of severe melioidosis. Antimicrob Agents Chemother 1992;36:158–162.

25. Stanford JP. Pseudomonas species (including melioidosis and glanders). In: Mandell GL, Bennett JE, Dolin R, eds. Principles and practice of infectious diseases. 4th ed. 1995. New York: Churchill Livingstone.

26. Suputtamongkol Y, Rajchanuwong A, Chaowagul W, Dance DAB, Smith MD, Wuthickanun V, Walsh AL, Pukrittayakamee S, White NJ. Ceftazidime vs. amoxicillin/clavulanate in the treatment of severe melioidosis. Clin Infect Dis 1994;19:846–853.

27. Walsh AL, Smith MD, Wuthiekanun V, White NJ. Postantibiotic effects and *Burkholderia (Pseudomonas) pseudomallei:* evaluation of current treatment. Antimicrob Agents Chemother 1995;39:2356–2358.

28. White NJ, Dance DAB. Clinical and laboratory studies of malaria and melioidosis. Trans R Soc Trop Med Hyg 1988;82:15–20.

29. White NJ, Dance DAB, Chaowagul W, Wattanagoon Y, Wuthiekanun V, Pitakwatchara N. Halving of mortality of severe melioidosis by ceftazidime. Lancet 1989;2:697–701.

30. Whitmore A. An account of a glanders-like disease occurring in Rangoon. J Hyg 1913;13:1–34.

31. Winton MD, Everett ED, Dolan SA. Activities of five new fluoroquinolones against Pseudomonas pseudomallei. Antimicrob Agents Chemother 1988;32:928–929.

32. Woodcock JM, Andrews JM, Brenwald NP, Ashby JP, Wise R. The in-vitro activity of faropenem, a novel oral penem. J Antimicrob Chemother 1997;39:35–43.

33. Yabuuchi E, Kosako Y, Oyaizu H, Yano I, Hotta H, Hashimoto Y, Ezaki T, Arakawa M. Proposal of Burkholderia gen. nov. and transfer of seven species of the genus Pseudomonas homology group II to the new genus, with the type species Burkholderia cepacia (Palleroni and Holmes 1981) comb. nov. Microbiol Immunol 1992;36:1251–1275.

34. Yamamoto T, Naigowit P, Dejsirilert S, Chiewsilp D, Kondo E, Yokota T, Kanai K. In vitro susceptibilities of Pseudomonas pseudomallei to 27 antimicrobial agents. Antimicrob Agents Chemother 1990;34:2027–2029.

Calymmatobacterium granulomatis

John Richens

MICROBIOLOGY

Calymmatobacterium granulomatis is a pleomorphic Gram-negative coccobacillus believed to be the etiologic agent of granuloma inguinale (now often known by the alternative name donovanosis), a tropical infection, characterized principally by cutaneous ulcers of the anogenital and inguinal regions. Little is known about this organism, which will not grow on conventional media. The first successful isolation was reported by Anderson in 1943 (1). Only 15 successful isolations have been described in published articles, and only one of these in the past 30 years (19). The diagnosis of the granuloma inguinale depends primarily on demonstrating the presence of intracellular organisms (termed *Donovan bodies*) within lesions with the typical clinical appearance of the disease.

C. granulomatis is found mainly within large histiocytes. The logical choice of therapy is thus an antibiotic with good activity against Gram-negative bacteria, with good lipid solubility, which is capable of achieving a high intracellular:extracellular concentration ratio. As with other intracellular infections, all attempts to identify a successful form of single-dose therapy have failed, and relapse is fairly common following therapy. Granuloma inguinale may in the future prove a suitable infection for treatment with liposome-encapsulated antibiotics.

On the basis of serologic studies (30), *C. granulomatis* appears to share antigens with *Klebsiella,* which is consistent with the observation that the infection that bears the closest histologic resemblance to granuloma inguinale is another tropical granulomatous disease, rhinoscleroma, the agent of which, *Klebsiella rhinoscleromatis,* is also found predominantly intracellularly. Recent comparison of gene sequences further supports the relationship between *C. granulomatis* and *Klebsiella* species (3).

SUSCEPTIBILITY IN VITRO AND IN VIVO

Only three papers report results of in vitro experiments with chemotherapeutic agents (4, 7, 29). Chen et al. (7) demonstrated that streptomycin, penicillin, chlortetracycline, and chloramphenicol have additive effects against *C. granulomatis* in vitro when administered in combination (Table 1).

Numerous unsuccessful attempts have been made to find an animal model for donovanosis. In 1931, DeMonbreun et al. reported successful infection of the eyelids of macaques with tissue taken from human lesions of donovanosis, but these lesions resolved spontaneously (10). It has not been possible so far to assess antibiotic activity against *C. granulomatis* in an animal model.

ANTIMICROBIAL THERAPY

Drugs of Choice

Table 2 summarizes data from the most important therapeutic trials. For a comprehensive bibliography of drug trials for

granuloma inguinale up to 1991, readers are referred to a recent review by the author (34).

Drugs of the tetracycline group have been used extensively in the treatment of granuloma inguinale for many years, generally with excellent results. Many published guidelines for the treatment of granuloma inguinale (e.g., World Health Organization, Centers for Disease Control) recommend use of tetracyclines as first-choice therapy. Individual well-documented cases of tetracycline resistance have been reported (26), and the drug appeared ineffective in infections contracted in Vietnam (37). It may be assumed that the different forms of tetracycline have equivalent efficacy. Doxycycline is now generally preferred over alternatives for ease of administration (twice daily).

Excellent results with cotrimoxazole have been reported from India (21) and Africa (23). Two treatment failures with cotrimoxazole were reported from South America (28).

Chloramphenicol is widely used for treatment of granuloma inguinale in Papua New Guinea (24), generally with excellent results. Lengthy experience with the use of chloramphenicol for a variety of infections in Papua New Guinea has shown that hematologic toxicity is rare in this population. While chloramphenicol may be considered a treatment of choice in Melanesians, concerns about potential toxicity limit its use elsewhere. Recent work from South America suggests that thiamphenicol, a congener of chloramphenicol that has the convenience of once-daily administration and reputedly does not carry the risk of hematological toxicity, is of comparable efficacy (17).

Recent studies from Australia indicate that ceftriaxone can give good results in chronic relapsing patients who have failed to respond to a variety of other antibiotics (25) and that weekly or daily azithromycin has useful activity that may make it a valuable drug for use in poorly compliant patients (5). In India, an initial study using norfloxacin showed good results (33).

Erythromycin and lincomycin both give good results in granuloma inguinale, although only a few trials have been conducted and experience is limited. Streptomycin was for many years the main drug used in the treatment of granuloma inguinale. It continued in use in India up to 1971 (22), and more recently, it has been evaluated in combination with tetracycline (23; see below). Most clinicians now prefer to select antibiotics with less toxicity and greater ease of administration. Gentamicin also shows useful activity but has not been used much (24).

Ampicillin gave good results when used in American soldiers in Vietnam (6), but results in other trials have been poor. A treatment failure with ampicillin was reported by Johnson in 1991 (18). On the strength of available evidence, ampicillin cannot be recommended as first-line treatment.

Combination Therapy

Only one trial has been reported comparing monotherapy with combination therapy in the treatment of granuloma inguinale (23). In this study, streptomycin with tetracycline was compared with cotrimoxazole, and no significant difference in outcome was noted in the two groups. Good results in the treat-

---

TABLE 1 • Bactericidal Concentrations of Antibiotics against *C. granulomatis* Reported by Chen (1951)

Antibiotic	Bactericidal Concentration (per mL of medium)
Streptomycin	0.2 μg
Penicillin G	1 unit
Chlortetracycline	5 μg
Chloramphenicol	10 μg

From Chen CH, Dienst RB, Greenblatt RB. Antibiotics versus *Donovania granulomatis.* Am J Syphilis 1951;35:383–392.

TABLE 2 • Key Trials of Antibiotics for Treatment of Granuloma Inguinale[a]

Drug	Dose	Route	Duration	M:F	Total Patients	Smear Positive	Relapse	Time to Smear Negative	Time to Heal	Ref
Ampicillin	500 mg q.i.d.	O	2–4 weeks		31	67%				6
Chloramphenicol	500 mg–1 g 6 h	O	5–20 days	0/23	23		2	2–4 days		13
	2–4 g every 3–4 days	IM	8–12 days	20/23	43	43	5	1–7 days	7–30 days	14
	500 mg q.i.d.	O	10–55 days		50		1	av. 7 days	av. 17 days	24
Thiamphenicol	2.5g stat, then 500 mg b.i.d.	O	1–3 weeks	26/8	34	34		1–3 weeks	1–3 weeks	17
Cotrimoxazole	160/800 mg, b.i.d.	O	Mean 12.5 days	84/32	116	116	2	5 days	7–22 days	21
	160/800 mg, b.i.d.	O	20–49 days	19/1	20	16			2–5 weeks	36
	160/800 mg, b.i.d.	O	14 days	12/6	18	18			7–21 days	23
Erythromycin	1–300 mg 6 h	O	16–37 days	5/4	9	9	1		9–30 days	35
Lincomycin	500 mg q.i.d.	O	14 days		5					6
Streptomycin	0.3–1 g 4 h	IM	6–46 days		23	23	3	5–9 days		12
	0.3–4 g/day	IM	5–62 days	32/16	48	48	3	2–11 days	av. 3 weeks	20
	1 g b.i.d.	IM	3–70 days	146/81	227	219	1	av. 6 days		31
	1 g b.i.d.	IM	av. 12.5 days	83/39	122					22
Gentamicin	1 mg/kg t.i.d.	IM	Mean 22 days		9			Mean 12 days	Mean 22 days	24
Tetracyclines										
Minocycline	200 mg stat, then 100 mg b.i.d.	O	15–45 days	5/1	6	6			15–90 days	38
	100–300 mg/day	O	max 58 days	1/9	10	10				8
Oxytetracycline	2–3 g/day	O	2–29 days		32	32	2	4–5 days		11
Tetracycline hydrochloride	1 g/day	O	20 days	14/6	20	20		5–7 days	25–45 days	32
Norfloxacin	400 mg b.i.d.	O	2–11 days	10/0	10	10		8 by 3 days	Mean 7.3 days	33
Ceftriaxone	1 g o.d.	IM/IV	10 days	4/8	12	8	5			25
Azithromycin	1 g per week or 500 mg daily	O	1–4 weeks	4/7	11	9	0			5
Antibiotic combinations										
Streptomycin with tetracycline	1 g/day 500 mg 6 h	IM O	14 days 14 days	7/6	13	13			7–21 days	23
Erythromycin with lincomycin	500 mg q.i.d. 500 mg q.i.d.	O O	10–14 days 10–14 days	0/4	4	4			"rapid"	2

[a]Abbreviations: av, average; b.i.d., twice daily; h, hourly; IM, intramuscular; IV, intravenous; O, oral; q.i.d., 4 times daily; t.i.d., 3 times daily; top, topical; o.d., once daily; max, maximum; M:F, male:female ratio.

ment of pregnant women with a combination of erythromycin and lincomycin were reported from Australia (2). Small numbers of patients have been treated with combinations of streptomycin plus penicillin or chloramphenicol and with chloramphenicol plus tetracycline.

The efficacy of antibiotics in the treatment of granuloma inguinale has largely been assessed in small-scale open trials. No randomized comparisons of therapy have been reported, and the trial of streptomycin and tetracycline compared with cotrimoxazole described above (23) is one of a very small number of nonrandomized comparisons published. Published treatment guidelines tend to favor antibiotics of the tetracycline group over alternatives but do not offer explicit reasons for adopting this choice. On the basis of the published data shown in Table 2 and known adverse reaction profiles, the following antibiotics should be considered first-line therapies for granuloma inguinale: cotrimoxazole, erythromycin, tetracyclines, fluorinated quinolones, ceftriaxone, or azithromycin. The dosage used in reported trials is shown in Table 2. In gen-

eral, most antibiotics are given at conventional dosage. Most clinicians continue therapy until lesions heal, and some extend the treatment period in the hope of reducing relapse. One or 2 weeks of therapy often suffices for small early lesions. Therapy may need to be continued for 2 to 3 months for female patients with extensive pelvic infection.

Special Situations

Pregnancy

During pregnancy, granuloma inguinale tends to extend rapidly and to show diminished responsiveness to antibiotic therapy. Many of the reported cases of hematogenous dissemination (a rare complication with a potentially fatal outcome) have been linked to tearing of an infected cervical lesion during delivery. Cordero described one such patient who responded well to combination treatment with streptomycin and minocycline (9). Many first-line antibiotics are contraindicated in pregnancy, but erythromycin is considered safe for use in pregnancy, and satisfactory results among pregnant women have been reported with erythromycin alone (15) or in combination with lincomycin (2).

Granuloma Inguinale in Patients with HIV

Jardim et al. described two patients with HIV infection who failed to respond to extended treatment with combinations of cotrimoxazole, tetracycline, and thiamphenicol (16). This suggests that such patients may require vigorous treatment with high-dose parenteral combination regimens. In a recent study from South Africa, 18 pregnant women with HIV and donovanosis did not differ significantly in outcome from women without HIV (15).

Alternative Therapies and Supplementary Measures

Second-line drugs that may be considered for patients failing to respond to, or intolerant of, the first-line drugs listed above include ampicillin, chloramphenicol, thiamphenicol, lincomycin, streptomycin, and gentamicin. Prior to the introduction of antibiotics, the following treatments were used with success in treatment of granuloma inguinale: intravenous potassium antimony tartrate and other trivalent antimonials, surgical excision of lesions, diathermic fulguration, local treatment with podophyllin, ultraviolet radiation, and radiotherapy (34).

Adjunctive surgical measures are required for patients with complications such as abscess formation, fistulae, strictures, and elephantiasis (27). Surgery carries the risk of disseminating active infections if carried out without antibiotic cover.

Patients with extensive malodorous ulcers benefit from addition of penicillin to treatment regimens and from bathing ulcers in solutions of dilute potassium permanganate.

ENDPOINTS FOR MONITORING THERAPY

Patients can be monitored clinically by observing the healing and reepithelialization of ulcers. Repeat smears may be made from lesions to monitor the disappearance of Donovan bodies, though this is rarely undertaken outside the context of clinical trials. Follow-up should ideally be extended up to 18 months, as late relapse may occur.

ADDITIONAL MANAGEMENT ISSUES

As granuloma inguinale is sexually transmitted, management should always address the issues of partner management, health education, and screening for other sexually transmitted infections, especially syphilis, which often accompanies granuloma inguinale. Exposed sexual partners should be offered examination and treated if lesions are found. Epidemiologic treatment can be offered to asymptomatic exposed individuals who are concerned about becoming infected.

REFERENCES

1. Anderson K. The cultivation from granuloma inguinale of a microorganism having the characteristics of Donovan bodies in the yolk sac of chick embryos. Science 1943;97:560–561.
2. Ashdown LR, Kilvert GT. Granuloma inguinale in northern Queensland. Med J Aust 1979;1:146–148.
3. Bastian I, Bowden FJ. Amplification of *Klebsiella*-like sequences from biopsy samples from patients with donovanosis. Clin Infect Dis 1996;23:1328–1330.
4. Beveridge WIB. The action of antimony and some other bacteriostatic substances on *Donovania granulomatis* isolated in the chick embryo. J Immunol 1946;53:215–223
5. Bowden FJ, Mein J, Plunkett C, Bastian I. Pilot study of azithromycin in the treatment of genital donovanosis. Genitourin Med 1996;72:17–19.
6. Breschi LC, Goldman G, Shapiro SR. Granuloma inguinale in Vietnam: successful therapy with ampicillin and lincomycin. J Am Vener Dis Assoc 1975;1:118–120.
7. Chen CH, Dienst RB, Greenblatt RB. Antibiotics versus *Donovania granulomatis*. Am J Syphilis 1951;35:383–392.
8. Cordero FA. Evaluación clínica de la minociclina en dermatología y en venéreología. Rev Col Med 1972;23:149–154.
9. Cordero FA. Granuloma venereo. Su manifestacion clinica en genitales y otras partes del organismo. Med Cutanea Ibero Latin Am 1975;3:125–132.
10. DeMonbreun WA, Goodpasture WE. Infection of monkeys with Donovan organisms by injections of tissue from human lesions of granuloma inguinale. Am J Trop Med 1931;11:311–323.
11. Greenblatt RB, Barfield WE, Dienst RB, West RM. Terramycin in the treatment of granuloma inguianle. J Vener Dis Info 1951;32:113–115.
12. Greenblatt RB, Kupperman HS, Dienst RB. Streptomycin in the therapy of granuloma inguinale. Proc Soc Exp Biol Med 1947; 56:1–6.
13. Greenblatt RB, Wammock VS, Dienst RB, West RM. Chloromycetin in the therapy of granuloma inguinale. Am J Obstet Gynecol 1950;59:1129–1133.
14. Harb FW, Simpson WG, Wood CE. Intramuscular injections of chloromycetin in the treatment of granuloma inguinale. J Vener Dis Info 1951;32:177–181.
15. Hoosen AA, Mphatsoe M, Kharsany AB, Moodley J, Bassa A, Bramdev A. Granuloma inguinale in association with pregnancy and HIV infection. Int J Gynaecol Obstet 1996;53:33–38.
16. Jardim ML, Barros ER, Silveira M. Donovanose em pacientes portadores de AIDS. Relato de dois casos. An Bras Dermatol Sifilogr 1990;65:175–177.
17 Jardim ML, Melo ZD. Tratamento da donovanose com o tianfenicol. An Bras Dermatol Sifilogr 1990;65:93–94.
18. Johnson SH, Cherubin C. Case report. Infect Dis Newslett 1991;10:14–15.
19. Kharsany AB, Hoosen AA, Kiepiela P, Naicker T, Sturm AW. Culture of Calymmatobacterium granulomatis. Clin Infect Dis 1996;22:391.
20. Kupperman HS, Greenblatt RB, Dienst RB. Streptomycin in the therapy of granuloma inguinale. JAMA 1948;136:84–89.
21. Lal S, Garg BR. Further evidence of the efficacy of co-trimoxazole in granuloma venereum. Br J Vener Dis 1980;56:412–413.
22. Lal S. Continued efficacy of streptomycin in the treatment of granuloma inguinale. Br J Vener Dis 1971;47:454–455.
23. Latif AS, Mason PR, Paraiwa E. The treatment of donovanosis (granuloma inguinale). Sex Transm Dis 1988;15:27–29.
24. Maddocks I, Anders EM, Dennis E. Donovanosis in Papua New Guinea. Br J Vener Dis 1976;52:190–196.
25. Merianos A, Gilles M, Chuah J. Ceftriaxone in the treatment of chronic donovanosis in central Australia. Genitourin Med 1994; 70(2):84–89.
26. Pariser RJ. Tetracycline-resistant granuloma inguinale. Arch Dermatol 1997;113:988.

27. Parkash S, Radhakrishna K. Problematic ulcerative lesions in sexually transmitted diseases: surgical management. Sex Transm Dis 1986;13:127–133.
28. Pradinaud R, Grosshans E, Basset A, Bertin C. Étude de 24 cas de donovanose en Guyane Francaise. Bull Soc Pathol Exot Filiales 1981;74:30–36.
29. Rake G, Dunham W. Action of disinfectant, chemotherapeutic, and antibiotic agents on the organism of granuloma inguinale. Am J Syphilis 1947;31:610–617.
30. Rake G. The antigenic relationships of *Donovania granulomatis* (Anderson) and the significance of this organism in granuloma inguinale. Am J Syphilis Gonorrhea Vener Dis 1948;32:150–158.
31. Rajam RV, Rangiah PN. Further observations on streptomycin therapy in venereal granuloma. Indian J Vener Dis Dermatol 1952;18:1–8.
32. Rajam RV, Rangiah PN, Sowmini CN, Krishnamoorthy N. Tetracyclene (Achromycin) in venereal diseases. The Antiseptic 1956;53:9–19.
33. Ramanan C, Sarma PSA, Ghorpade A, Das M. Treatment of donovanosis with norfloxacin. Int J Dermatol 1990;29:298–299.
34. Richens J. The diagnosis and treatment of donovanosis (granuloma inguinale). Genitourin Med 1991;32:441–452.
35. Robinson HM, Cohen MM. Treatment of granuloma inguinale with erythromycin. J Invest Dermatol 1953;20:407–409.
36. Rosen T, Tschen JA, Ramsdell W, Moore J, Markham B. Granuloma inguinale. J Am Acad Dermatol 1984;11:433–437.
37. Shapiro SR, Breschi LC. Venereal disease in Vietnam: clinical experience at a major military hospital. Milit Med 1974;139:374–379.
38. Velasco JE, Miller E, Zaias N. Minocycline in the treatment of venereal disease. JAMA 1972;22:1323–1325.

Campylobacter Species

●

Ban Mishu Allos and Martin J. Blaser

GENERAL DESCRIPTION

Campylobacters are spiral or comma-shaped Gram-negative bacteria that usually produce an acute gastrointestinal illness. In developed countries, campylobacters are the most frequently identified bacterial cause of diarrhea. In developing countries, *Campylobacter* infection produces substantial morbidity and mortality among young children. A large proportion of traveler's diarrhea also is caused by infection with *Campylobacter*. In the United States, more than 99% of reported *Campylobacter* isolates are *C. jejuni* (97). In other parts of the world, such as South Africa, non-*jejuni Campylobacter* species are identified more frequently and may account for almost 50% of campylobacters isolated (Table 1) (50). As isolation techniques for detection of these "atypical" *Campylobacter* species are improved, there is greater appreciation of the importance of these organisms as pathogens.

Campylobacters are motile via unipolar or bipolar flagellae. They are slowly growing organisms that require 72 to 96 h for isolation from stools. Isolation from blood takes even longer; up to 2 weeks may be required for certain species (64). Although some *Campylobacter* species and Campylobacter-like organisms, such as *C. fetus, Helicobacter cinaedi,* and *H. fennelliae,* grow best at 37°C, the optimal temperature for *C. jejuni* growth is 42°C. Because most *C. jejuni* strains are resistant to cephalothin, they may be isolated from stools using a cephalothin-containing medium. Such *Campylobacter*-selective media permit the growth of most *C. jejuni* strains while in-

hibiting growth of other stool organisms. However, many non-*jejuni Campylobacter* species and even some *C. jejuni* strains are susceptible to cephalothin and cannot be identified on media containing this antibiotic. Therefore, culturing stools on an antibiotic-free medium using a filtration technique may be a better way to isolate these organisms. The filtration technique takes advantage of the small size of *Campylobacter* species; 0.45- to 0.65-μm filters allow passage of *Campylobacter* while retaining other stool flora.

SUSCEPTIBILITY IN VITRO
Single Agents

Campylobacters are susceptible in vitro to a wide variety of antimicrobial agents (40, 117, 118, 122). Macrolides, quinolones, aminoglycosides, and nitrofurans are the most active agents against *C. jejuni* and *C. coli* (49, 92, 110, 116). In special circumstances, as when a patient is intolerant of many agents or when a strain has an unusual antibiotic resistance pattern, alternative agents such as chloramphenicol may be used; nearly all campylobacters are susceptible to chloramphenicol (81, 84). Clindamycin usually is effective against *Campylobacter* (32), although this drug is not recommended for young children. Imipenem also is active against *Campylobacter* and may be used in serious infections. Aminoglycosides are effective in the treatment of *Campylobacter* infection; in most studies, resistance to gentamicin has not been observed (4, 7, 77). In contrast, from 10 to 69% of campylobacters are resistant to tetracyclines (80, 81).

TABLE 1 • **Clinical Presentations and Antimicrobial Agents of Choice for Treatment of Infection with Pathogenic Campylobacters and Related Organisms**

Organism	Principal Clinical Presentation	Antimicrobial Agent(s) of Choice
C. jejuni	Gastroenteritis	Erythromycin
C. fetus	Bacteremia	Aminoglycoside plus ampicillin
C. upsaliensis	Gastroenteritis	Fluoroquinolones
C. hyointestinalis	Gastroenteritis	Erythromycin
H. cinaedi	Proctocolitis; enterocolitis	Fluoroquinolones
H. fennelliae	Proctocolitis; enterocolitis	Fluoroquinolones
C. lari	Gastroenteritis	Erythromycin

Ampicillin and amoxicillin have activity against *Campylobacter,* but in general, rates of resistance are too high for these drugs to be useful. Furthermore, the organism may produce β-lactamase (40), making the use of ampicillin or amoxicillin suboptimal, especially in serious infections. More than 20% of strains in India are resistant to ampicillin (9, 65, 73). In Spain, the rate of resistance to ampicillin has ranged from 18 to 69% (66). Resistance is thought to be chromosomally mediated (73). Campylobacters are almost always susceptible to ampicillin-clavulanic acid (32); however, relatively high doses are required to be effective (48). Even in areas with very high rates of resistance to β-lactam antibiotics, imipenem displayed high in vitro activity against *Campylobacter* strains (81).

Although campylobacters are microaerophilic, not anaerobes, some but not all strains may be susceptible to metronidazole (10). *C. jejuni* is not susceptible to most cephalosporins, although other non-*jejuni* campylobacters often are (32, 109). However, even *C. jejuni* may be moderately susceptible to other cephalosporins including cefotaxime, ceftazidime, and cefpirome (16, 110). Campylobacters are inherently resistant to trimethoprim, vancomycin, and rifampin. Interestingly, however, rifabutin exhibits some anti-*Campylobacter* activity (47); indeed, the incidence of *Campylobacter* infection among patients with AIDS who were treated with rifabutin prophylaxis was reported to be lower than that in untreated controls (75).

Combination Therapy

Because combination therapy is not required and rarely used to treat most *Campylobacter* infections, there are few data on in vitro susceptibilities to combinations of agents.

ANTIMICROBIAL THERAPY

The most important tenet of treatment of patients with acute gastroenteritis due to *C. jejuni* or any other microbe is not treatment with antibiotics, but maintenance of proper hydration and electrolyte balance. In nearly all cases, this can be accomplished by encouraging proper oral intake of liquids; occasionally, intravenous fluids are required, especially in the very young or elderly.

Most *Campylobacter* infections produce a self-limited illness and do not require treatment with antimicrobial agents. Young children in Thailand infected with *Campylobacter* and treated with erythromycin experienced no decrease in duration of diarrhea compared with untreated *Campylobacter*-infected controls (104). However, in another study, Peruvian children with bloody diarrhea caused by *Campylobacter* infection recovered more quickly if they were treated with erythromycin soon after the onset of symptoms (85). Nevertheless, although antimicrobial therapy begun on the day of onset of diarrhea reduces the number of days of excretion of bacteria in stools (33, 71), when initiated on the second or third day of illness (the time when most patients with uncomplicated enteritis seek medical care) antibiotics may not have a significant impact on the duration of illness. Patients in whom antibiotic therapy is indicated include those with bloody stools, high fevers, prolonged symptoms (lasting >1 week), worsening symptoms, or relapses. Antibiotics should also be administered promptly to patients with human immunodeficiency virus (HIV) infection or other states of immunocompromise. Because pregnant women may experience severe consequences of *C. jejuni* infection, including septic abortion or stillbirths, and because their neonates are in effect compromised hosts, pregnant women also should be treated with antimicrobial agents.

Drugs of Choice

After a brief flirtation in which fluoroquinolones were considered as the treatment of choice for *Campylobacter* infections, the rapidly increasing resistance of campylobacters to these agents has made erythromycin once again the optimal therapy. Years of testing for antimicrobial resistance in many parts of the world has demonstrated that the resistance rate to erythromycin among human *C. jejuni* isolates has changed very little (66, 77, 92, 119). In the Netherlands and Spain, the rate of erythromycin resistance is negligible (25, 81). In most developed countries, the rate of resistance has remained under 10% (14, 99, 121).

The rate of erythromycin resistance (range, 15 to 93%) is substantially higher among *C. coli* strains (37, 81, 104, 122). Very high rates of resistance (>50% for *C. jejuni,* >90% for *C. coli*) have been reported from institutionalized children in developing countries such as Thailand (104), but rates remain quite low in others, such as in an Indian study (73). Local patterns of antibiotic use in both humans and animals may explain these differences.

The mechanism of *Campylobacter*'s resistance to erythromycin probably is a point mutation in a ribosomal protein gene (26). The use of macrolide antibiotics analogous to erythromycin (e.g., tylosin) to increase weight gain in swine intended for human consumption may have contributed to the emergence of erythromycin resistance among *C. coli* (14). Swine are an important host for *C. coli.*

Other advantages of erythromycin include its low cost, safety, ease of administration, and narrow spectrum of activity. Unlike the fluoroquinolones and tetracyclines, erythromycin may be used safely in children and pregnant women and is less likely than many agents to exert an inhibitory effect on other fecal flora. Erythromycin stearate is acid resistant, stable, and incompletely absorbed. Therefore, in addition to its systemic effects, it may be capable of exerting a contact effect throughout the bowel (93). The recommended dose in adults is 500 mg orally two times per day for 5 days. For children, the recommended dose is 40 mg per kg per day in two divided doses for 5 days.

Alternative Therapies

Fluoroquinolones

Fluroquinolones have been considered among the agents of choice for empirical treatment of traveler's diarrhea and of bacterial gastroenteritis in general. Ciprofloxacin was superior to placebo in the treatment of community-acquired gastroenteritis, even when no organisms were isolated (20). However, after initial interest in the use of these agents, they are no longer considered appropriate for treatment of *Campylobacter* infections because of increasing primary resistance. Not surprisingly, secondary (in vivo) resistance to quinolones emerges rapidly in patients requiring prolonged treatment (1, 87). However, even in healthy hosts with limited illnesses, an initially susceptible strain may become resistant after only a brief (<2 weeks) duration of therapy (2, 33, 124).

Although primary quinolone resistance is still uncommon in some areas, resistance is increasing rapidly in most parts of the world (73). In Spain, *C. jejuni* isolates resistant to ciprofloxacin increased from 7.5% in 1989 to 57% in 1992; among *C. coli* strains, the rate of resistance increased from 14 to 43% (66). Similarly, in Sweden, *C. jejuni* resistance to quinolones increased from 2% in 1988 to 29% in 1992–1993 (91) despite a stable rate (<2%) from 1978 to 1988 (92).

The rapid increase in the proportion of *Campylobacter* strains resistant to fluoroquinolones observed since the 1990s has occurred partly because of the common and indiscriminate use of these agents (80) and agents that induce cross-resistance (e.g, enrofloxacin). Enrofloxacin (a newer quinolone marketed for veterinary use) recently has been extensively used in food animals including poultry (26) and swine (120). Of 209 *Campylobacter* strains isolated from surface water, sewage, and poultry abattoir drain water, quinolone resistance was highest in isolates from the poultry drain water (46). Indeed, increasing *C. jejuni* and *C. coli* resistance to fluoroquinolones parallels that seen in strains isolated from poultry (26, 77). Interestingly, although *Campylobacter* and *Salmonella* occupy the same niche in poultry flocks, use of these agents has not produced a similar resistance pattern among salmonellae (79).

The mechanism of resistance to fluoroquinolones among campylobacters is due to point mutations in DNA gyrase (87, 103). This may be primary (usually due to use of the drug in food animals) (2, 77) or secondary (emergence of resistance, during therapy, in a previously susceptible strain) (87). Newer fluoroquinolones (such as DU-6859a) may be active against campylobacters (108), but it is likely that these agents also will be ineffective against strains already resistant to ciprofloxacin and ofloxacin because of cross-resistance. Fluoroquinolones are not recommended for use in children less than 8 years old.

Nalidixic Acid

In theory, strains resistant to ciprofloxacin should always be resistant to nalidixic acid, the parent compound of the fluorinated 4-quinolones. In actuality, nalidixic acid resistance commonly, but not invariably, crosses with resistance to ciprofloxacin. Eleven percent of *C. jejuni* strains resistant to nalidixic acid are nevertheless, susceptible to ciprofloxacin (81). In general, however, resistance to this agent has paralleled the increasing resistance to fluoroquinolones. In Spain, currently, resistance to nalidixic acid ranges from 28 to 55% (81, 86, 120), and it is not clinically useful.

New Macrolides

The newer macrolides—azithromycin, clarithromycin, and dirithromycin—have excellent in vitro activity against *Campylobacter* (44, 45, 98, 123). In contrast, roxithromycin is not as effective (86). In Spain, the rate of resistance to macrolide antibiotics was stable (<3%) over a 5-year period, whereas the resistance rate to fluoroquinolones rose dramatically (86), which probably reflects their relative use among food animals. Although the new macrolides achieve higher concentrations in tissue and may be superior to erythromycin in vitro, they provide little clinical advantage over erythromycin and are considerably more expensive (78). Macrolide resistance has been observed in some communities. For example, among U.S. troops stationed in Thailand, 31% of *Campylobacter* isolates were resistant to both azithromycin and erythromycin (63). In these situations, macrolide resistance may be due to the importance of humans as the principal reservoir for campylobacters in certain developing countries. In such places (e.g., Thailand) macrolides are dispensed without prescriptions and are commonly given to children. Strains resistant to erythromycin will also be resistant to these newer macrolides (32).

Tetracyclines

Plasmids are responsible for the increasing level of *Campylobacter* resistance to tetracyclines. Up to 69% of campylobacters are now resistant to tetracycline (66, 84, 118). The rate of resistance is higher for *C. coli* than for *C. jejuni* (81, 84). More than 80% of tetracycline-resistant strains possess a conjugative plasmid that mediates resistance to this drug (7, 101, 102, 104, 106, 107).

Chloramphenicol

Chloramphenicol remains a useful alternative to erythromycin for treatment of *C. jejuni* infections, because of both its effectiveness and low cost. *C. jejuni* are almost always susceptible to chloramphenicol (38, 59, 118, 121), although a small proportion of *C. coli* strains are resistant (84). Occasional resistance is mediated by production of chloramphenicol acetyl transferase, which is encoded on a transferable plasmid (84, 100). This agent should never be used routinely but can be reserved for patients who have recurrent infections, who are immunocompromised, or who have extraintestinal infections.

Cephalosporins

Nearly all *C. jejuni* and *C. coli* strains are resistant to first-generation cephalosporins such as cephalothin, cefazolin, and cefuroxime (120). They are moderately susceptible to cefotaxime, ceftazidime, cefpirone, and the new fourth-generation cephalosporin, cefpirome (16).

Aminoglycosides and Imipenem

Resistance rates to aminoglycosides and imipenem among *Campylobacter* species have remained under 1%. These agents should be used only in patients with extraintestinal infections.

SPECIAL SITUATIONS
Campylobacter Infection among Travelers

C. jejuni is an important cause of diarrhea among persons traveling from highly industrialized countries to developing areas. During the fall and winter, *C. jejuni* infection may be the most common bacterial cause of traveler's diarrhea in certain locales (28, 56). Antibiotic prophylaxis for persons traveling to high-risk areas is not recommended except in very specific clinical situations. Instead, travelers should be advised to practice ordinary precautions such as drinking only treated or bottled water, avoiding raw foods of animal origin, and eating only cooked or peeled fruits and vegetables. If diarrhea accompanied by fever develops, antimotility agents such as loperamide should not be used, as a paradoxical worsening of symptoms may occur due to intestinal invasion with *Campylobacter*, *Salmonella*, or *Shigella* (21). If antibiotic treatment of traveler's diarrhea is considered necessary and if *Campylobacter* infection is suspected, erythromycin is a better choice than fluoroquinolones. However, fluoroquinolones remain active against many other bacterial causes of traveler's diarrhea (e.g., *Salmonella*, *Shigella*, enterotoxigenic *Escherichia coli*); if these organisms are suspected or if the patient did not travel to a place with a high rate of *Campylobacter*-resistance to quinolones, then these agents may be considered. Nevertheless, as *Campylobacter* and other Gram-negative bacteria worldwide become increasingly resistant to fluoroquinolones, even this recommendation will soon be outdated.

Life-Threatening *Campylobacter* Infections

Campylobacter infections usually may be treated with a single agent; combination therapy is infrequently required. One exception may be when it is necessary to treat a life-threatening, blood-borne *Campylobacter* infection with systemic complications. In such cases, it might be reasonable to treat with an aminoglycoside and imipenem while awaiting susceptibility results. This therapy can be individually tailored. Because aminoglycosides are ineffective treatment for gut infections, to eradicate an intestinal focus of infection, a luminal agent such as erythromycin may be added.

Campylobacter Infection during Pregnancy

Most *Campylobacter* infections in pregnant women are mild and self-limited, with no severe adverse consequences for the mother or baby (125, 126). However, neonatal sepsis and death can occur if a woman is infected during the third trimester, as babies can be infected during birth if the mother is excreting *Campylobacter* at the time of delivery (6, 41, 88).

Neonates may experience only benign infection, but they also may develop severe enteritis or meningitis (34, 36, 112). Even earlier in pregnancy, infection with *C. jejuni* may produce spontaneous abortion or premature labor (89). Therefore, all *Campylobacter* infections in pregnant women should be promptly treated with antibiotics. Fluoroquinolones and tetracyclines are not recommended in this setting because these agents are not safe for the developing fetus. Erythromycin is the drug of choice; for women with a history of hypersensitivity to erythromycin, amoxicillin-clavulanate should be used. However, although crythromycin, chloramphenicol, and amoxicillin-clavulanate have no known teratogenic effects, controlled trials in pregnant women establishing their safety have not been done.

Campylobacter and AIDS

Campylobacter infections as well as other common foodborne infections occur at a high rate among persons infected with HIV. The reported incidence of *Campylobacter* infections among persons infected with HIV in Los Angeles was almost 40 times higher than that observed in the general population (95). The prevalence of *Campylobacter* infections among hospitalized HIV-infected persons was 2.2% (61), substantially higher than the expected rate among HIV antibody-negative hospitalized patients. In addition to an increased incidence and prevalence, the severity and duration of *Campylobacter* infections are more likely to be increased among HIV-infected persons (70, 95). Bacteremia was detected in 17% of *C. jejuni*–infected HIV antibody–positive patients (61). Other campylobacters and *Campylobacter*-like organisms (e.g., *C. hyointestinalis*, *H. cinaedi*, *H. fennelliae*) also are far more common among homosexual men. Therefore, HIV-infected persons should almost always receive antibiotics for *Campylobacter* enteritis. Furthermore, because of differences in optimal treatments, species determination should be done whenever *Campylobacter* is isolated, especially in patients with persistent, recurrent, or severe infections.

Defects in humoral immunity may contribute to the persistence and severity of *Campylobacter* infections among patients with AIDS. Chronic campylobacter infections lasting several months despite repeated courses of antibiotics are commonly seen among patients with AIDS (11, 22, 61, 70), although brief infections occur as well. Initial resistance to antibiotics used, acquisition of resistance during therapy, and insufficient duration of therapy may play a role in some treatment failures. Close monitoring with repeated culture and susceptibility testing and prolonged treatment (e.g., many months or lifelong) may be necessary in some patients. *Campylobacter* infection should be considered in the differential diagnosis of AIDS patients with persistent diarrhea even if the organism is not identified in stools. Failure to culture *Campylobacter* from stools does not rule out their presence, as the organisms are sometimes difficult to isolate. Zidovudine, a commonly used antiretroviral agent among HIV-infected persons, has no in vitro activity against *Campylobacter*, although activity against salmonella has been documented (24).

Campylobacter Infection in Other Immunocompromised States

Although the serum-resistant organism *C. fetus* is a known opportunist in immunocompromised persons, *C. jejuni,* which usually is serum susceptible, also can produce bacteremia and severe illness in such patients. Patients with acquired or congenital hypogammaglobulinemia may develop severe recurrent *Campylobacter* enteritis (3, 54, 58, 72). Hypogammaglobulinemic patients also are particularly susceptible to extraintestinal *C. jejuni* infections (e.g., bacteremia, skin infections, osteomyelitis), suggesting that immunoglobulins are important in the defense against *Campylobacter* infections (17, 39, 96, 111). Indeed, in one study of 41 hypogammaglobulinemic patients, 5 (12%) had experienced at least one episode of documented *C. jejuni* septicemia (43).

Patients with hypogammaglobulinemia likely lack serum bactericidal activity against *Campylobacter*, as the organism usually is serum susceptible (12). Therefore, treatment with antibiotics alone may fail to eradicate the infection. Although administration of immunoglobulin IgG preparations has not restored serum bactericidal activity against *Campylobacter* in hypogammaglobulinemic patients (27, 43), this activity may be restored by infusions of plasma substitution therapy (8, 27, 43). Perhaps this is because plasma substitution therapy restores IgM, which is most efficient for complement activation leading to serum killing (12). Combination treatment with immunoglobulin (plasma) and antimicrobial therapy may be needed to achieve cure in certain patients.

For very ill patients with sepsis, immunocompromise, or both, use of an intravenous agent such as imipenem, to which *Campylobacter* is exquisitely susceptible, may be needed. An aminoglycoside plus an antibiotic effective against gut infection also may be used in seriously ill patients with normal renal function (see above).

TREATMENT OF ATYPICAL *CAMPYLOBACTER* INFECTIONS
Campylobacter fetus

C. fetus usually causes serious extraintestinal infections, most commonly in immunocompromised hosts (35). Typical clinical presentations include bacteremia, vascular infections, abscesses, and central nervous system (CNS) infections (15, 62). *C. fetus* also causes perinatal infection and fetal loss in both humans and animals (89). Because of the serious nature of these infections, treatment with a single agent is not recommended; treatment with erythromycin alone may not eradicate *C. fetus* bacteremia. Aminoglycosides, ampicillin, and third-generation cephalosporins are effective against serious *C. fetus* infections (67).

C. fetus bacteremias may be successfully treated with 2 weeks of treatment, but at least in part reflecting the population affected, relapses are not uncommon. Relapsing or persistent infections, however, require prolonged use of antimicrobial agents. When treating endocarditis or other vascular infections caused by *C. fetus,* an aminoglycoside may be added to the regimen. Four to 6 weeks of antimicrobial therapy is required. CNS infections due to *C. fetus* should be treated with a drug that penetrates the blood-brain barrier (e.g., chloramphenicol or ampicillin) for 2 to 3 weeks.

Campylobacter upsaliensis

C. upsaliensis infection usually causes a diarrheal illness (69); however, immunocompromised persons are more likely than others to develop bacteremia (18, 51, 69). As with uncomplicated gastroenteritis caused by *C. jejuni* infection, many *C. upsaliensis* infections do not require specific antimicrobial therapy. Because a large proportion of *C. upsaliensis* isolates are resistant to erythromycin (19), when drug therapy is required, fluoroquinolones are considered the agents of choice (74). Other effective agents include doxycycline, cefotaxime, and Augmentin (69).

Campylobacter hyointestinalis

Infection with *C. hyointestinalis* produces watery, nonbloody diarrhea, especially in homosexual men (23, 60). Infections also may be asymptomatic. All clinical isolates tested have been susceptible to erythromycin (23). Other antimicrobial agents with in vitro activity against *C. hyointestinalis* include metronidazole, nitrofurantoin, ampicillin, and aminoglycosides.

Helicobacter cinaedi and *Helicobacter fennelliae*

Infections with *H. cinaedi* and *H. fennelliae* (formerly called *Campylobacter*-like organisms) cause proctocolitis or enterocolitis in homosexual men or bacteremia in immunocompromised persons (52, 68, 76). These organisms are commonly resistant to erythromycin and many also are resistant to clindamycin and trimethoprim-sulfamethoxazole (31, 50). In vitro data suggest that effective antimicrobial agents include fluoroquinolones, ampicillin, gentamicin, doxycycline, tetracycline, ceftriaxone, rifampin, streptomycin, chloramphenicol, and nalidixic acid (31). Fluoroquinolones have documented in vivo efficacy (83) and are the drug of choice. Resistance may emerge following failure of treatment with fluoroquinolones, especially in immunocompromised hosts.

Campylobacter lari

Infections with *C. lari* may cause gastroenteritis in immunocompetent hosts or bacteremia in immunocompromised ones (13, 55). Uncomplicated gastrointestinal infections do not require antimicrobial therapy. If antibiotics are required, care should be taken to choose an appropriate agent. *C. lari* is resistant to all cephalosporins, penicillin, vancomycin, and trimethoprim-sulfamethoxazole. As with *C. jejuni,* increased reports of fluoroquinolone resistance have made these agents less useful (29). *C. lari* is susceptible to erythromycin, chloramphenicol, clindamycin, aminoglycosides, and imipenem (29, 90).

Other Campylobacters and Related Organisms

Campylobacter mucosalis is not an important human pathogen; however, it has substantial economic impact because it causes proliferative enteritis in pigs and lambs (53, 57). Nevertheless, isolation of C. mucosalis from the blood of a human has been reported; the organism was susceptible to cephalothin, nalidixic acid, erythromycin, doxycycline, and chloramphenicol (94). Two patients with *C. mucosalis*–induced diarrhea have been reported; both recovered completely with no antimicrobial therapy (30). *C. concisus, C. rectus,* and *Wolinella curva* are associated with periodontal disease in humans (114) but also may cause gastrointestinal illness. Most of these organisms are susceptible to both cephalothin and nalidixic acid (113). *Arcobacter butzleri, A. skirrowi,* and more rarely *A. cryaerophila* have been associated with diarrheal disease in humans, especially among children (42, 105, 115). In vitro assays have demonstrated the resistance of these organisms to cephalothin and their susceptibility to nalidixic acid (82). *C. doylei* may cause diarrhea in very young children; the organism also has been isolated from blood (5, 50). Most *C. doylei* strains are susceptible to both nalidixic acid and cephalothin.

ENDPOINTS FOR MONITORING THERAPY

Most patients with *Campylobacter* infection who require antimicrobial therapy respond promptly to treatment. Repeat cultures with drug susceptibility testing should be performed on any patient with worsening symptoms, symptoms lasting longer than 1 week, or bloody stools or high fevers despite therapy. If such testing is not immediately available, empirical change or adding to the antimicrobial regimen may be required for patients who are seriously ill and not responding to therapy. Even in severely ill patients, 1 week usually suffices to eradicate infection. However, in patients with persistent or recurrent infections, especially immunocompromised patients, prolonged use of antibiotics (perhaps months) may be required. Documentation of eradication of bacteria from stools of pregnant women is needed because there may be severe consequences to the neonate if the mother is still excreting *Campylobacter* at the time of delivery.

REFERENCES

1. Adler-Mosca H, Altwegg M. Fluoroquinolone resistance in *Campylobacter jejuni* and *Campylobacter coli* isolated from human faeces in Switzerland. J Infect 1991;23:341–342.
2. Adler-Mosca H, Lüthy-Hottenstein J, Martinetti Lucchini G, Burnens A, Altwegg M. Development of resistance to quinolones in five patients with campylobacteriosis treated with norfloxacin or ciprofloxacin. Eur J Clin Microbiol Infect Dis 1991;10:953–957.
3. Ahnen DJ, Brown WR. *Campylobacter* enteritis in immunodeficient patients. Ann Intern Med 1982;96:187–189.
4. Akhtar SQ. Antimicrobial sensitivity and plasmid-mediated tetracycline resistance in Campylobacter jejuni isolated in Bangladesh. Chemotherapy 1988;34:326–331.
5. Albert MJ, Tee W, Leach A, Asche V, Penner JL. Comparison of a blood-free medium and a filtration technique for the isolation of *Campylobacter* spp. from diarroeal stools of hospitalized patients in central Australia. J Med Microbiol 1992;37:176–179.
6. Anders BJ, Lauer BA, Paisley JW. *Campylobacter* gastroenteritis in neonates. Am J Dis Child 1981;135:900–902.
7. Ansary A, Radu S. Conjugal transfer of antibiotic resistances and plasmids from *Campylobacter jejuni* clinical isolates. FEMS Microbiol Lett 1992;91:125–128.
8. Autenrieth I, Schuster V, Ewald J, Harmsen D, Kreth HW. An unusual case of refractory *Campylobacter jejuni* infection in a patient with X-linked agammaglobulinemia: successful combined therapy with maternal plasma and ciprofloxacin. Clin Infect Dis 1996;23:526–531.
9. Ayyagari A, Ganju S, Sharma P, Pancholi UK, Panigrahi D, Agarwal KC, Walia BN. Detection of *Campylobacter coli* in diarrhoeal and non-diarrhoeal children in India. J Diarrhoeal Dis Res 1984;2:228–231.
10. Bannatyne RM, Jackowski J, Karmali MA. Susceptibility of *Campylobacter* species to metronidazole, its bioactive metabolities and tinidazole. Infection 1987;15:457–458.
11. Bernard E, Roger PM, Carles D, Bonaldi CV, Fournier JP, Dellamonica P. Diarrhea and *Campylobacter* infections in patients infected with human immunodeficiency virus. J Infect Dis 1989;159:3–4.
12. Blaser MJ, Smith PF, Kohler PA. Susceptibility of *Campylobacter* isolates to the bactericidal activity in human serum. J Infect Dis 1985;151:227–235.
13. Borczyk A, Thompson S, Smith D, Lior H. Water-borne outbreak of *Campylobacter laridis*-associated gastroenteritis. Lancet 1987;i:164–165.
14. Brunton WA, Wilson A, Macrae RM. Erythromycin-resistant campylobacters. Lancet 1978;ii:1385.
15. Carbone KM, Heinrich MC, Quinn TC. Thrombophlebitis and cellulitis due to *Campylobacter fetus* ssp. *fetus*. Medicine 1985;64:244–250.
16. Cheng AFB, Ling TKW, Lam AW, Fung KSC, Wise R. The antimicrobial activity and β-lactamase stability of cefpirome, a new fourth-generation cephalosporin in comparison with other agents. J Antimicrob Chemother 1993;31:699–709.
17. Chusid MJ, Coleman CM, Dunne MW. Chronic asymptomatic *Campylobacter* bacteraemia in a boy with X-linked hypogammaglobulinemia. Pediatr Infect Dis J 1987;6:943–944.
18. Chusid MJ, Wortmann DW, Dunne WM. "*Campylobacter upsaliensis*" sepsis in a boy with acquired hypogammaglobulinemia. Diagn Microbiol Infect Dis 1990;13:367–369.
19. da Silva-Tatley FM, Lastovica AJ, Steyn LM. Plasmid profiles of "*Campylobacter upsaliensis*" isolated from blood cultures and stools of pediatric patients. J Med Microbiol 1992;37:8–14.
20. Dryden MS, Gabb RJE, Wright SK. Empirical treatment of severe acute community-acquired gastroenteritis with ciprofloxacin. Clin Infect Dis 1996;22:1019–1025.
21. DuPont HL, Hornick RB. Adverse effect of Lomotil therapy in shigellosis. JAMA 1973;226:1525–1528.
22. Dworkin B, Wormser GP, Abdoo RA, Cabello F, Aguero ME, Sivak SL. Persistence of multiply antibiotic-resistant *Campylobacter jejuni* in a patient with the acquired immune deficiency syndrome. Am J Med 1986;80:965–970.
23. Edmonds P, Patton CM, Griffin PM, Barrett TJ, Schmid GP, Baker CN, Lambert MA. *Campylobacter hyointestinalis* associated with human gastrointestinal disease in the United States. J Clin Microbiol 1987;25:685–691.
24. Elwell LP, Ferone R, Freeman GA, Fyfe JA, Hill JA, Ray PH, Richards CA, Singer SC, Knick VB, Rideout JL. Antibacterial activity and mechanism of action of 3'-azido-3'-deoxythymidine (BW A509U). Antimicrob Agent Chemother 1987;31:274–280.
25. Endtz HP, Broeren M, Mouton RP. In vitro susceptibility of quinolone-resistant *Campylobacter jejuni* to new macrolide antibiotics. Eur J Clin Microbiol Infect Dis 1993;12:48–50.
26. Endtz HP, Ruijs GJ, van Klingeren B, Jansen WH, van der Reyden T, Mouton RP. Quinolone resistance in *Campylobacter* isolated from man and poultry following the introduction of fluoroquinolones in veterinary medicine. J Antimicrob Chemother 1991;27:199–208.

27. Endtz HP, Van der Meer JWM, Mouton RP. *Campylobacter jejuni* bacteraemia in hypogammaglobulinaemia: emergence of ciprofloxacin resistance and results of serum bactericidal assays. In: Kaijser B, Falsen E, eds. Proceedings of the Fourth International Workshop on Campylobacter Infections. Küngalve, Sweden, University of Göteburg; 1988:150–151.

28. Ericsson CD, DuPont HL. Travelers' diarrhea: approaches to prevention and treatment. Clin Infect Dis 1993;16:616–626.

29. Evans TG, Riley D. *Campylobacter laridis* colitis in a human immunodeficiency virus-positive patient treated with a quinolone. Clin Infect Dis 1992;15:172–173.

30. Figura N, Guglielmetti P, Zanchi A, Partini N, Armellini D, Bayeli PF, Bugnoli M, Verdani S. Two cases of *Campylobacter mucosalis* enteritis in children. J Clin Microbiol 1993;31: 727–728.

31. Flores BM, Fennell CL, Holmes KK, Stamm WE. In vitro susceptibility of *Campylobacter*-like organisms to twenty antimicrobial agents. Antimicrob Agents Chemother 1985;28: 188–191.

32. Gomez-Garces JL, Cogollos R, Alos JI. Susceptibilities of fluoroquinolone-resistant strains of *Campylobacter jejuni* to 11 oral antimicrobial agents. Antimicrob Agent Chemother 1995;39: 542–544.

33. Goodman LJ, Trenholme GM, Kaplan RL, Segreti J, Hines D, Petrak R, Nelson JA, Mayer KW, Landau W, Parkhurst GW. Empiric antimicrobial therapy of domestically acquired acute diarrhea in urban adults. Arch Intern Med 1990;150:541–546.

34. Goossens H, Henocque G, Kremp L, Rocque J, Boury R, Alanio G, Vlaes L, Hemelhof W, Van den Borre C, Macart M. Nosocomial outbreak of *Campylobacter jejuni* meningitis in newborn infants. Lancet 1986;2:146–149.

35. Guerrant RL, Lahita RG, Winn EC, Jr., Roberts RB. Campylobacteriosis in man: pathogenic mechanisms and review of 91 bloodstream infections. Am J Med 1978;65:584–592.

36. Hershkowici S, Barak M, Cohen A, Montag J. An outbreak of *Campylobacter jejuni* infection in a neonatal intensive care unit. J Hosp Infect 1987;9:54–59.

37. Hirschl AM, Wolf D, Berger J, Rotter ML. In vitro susceptibility of *Campylobacter jejuni* and *Campylobacter coli* isolated in Austria to erythromycin and ciprofloxacin. Int J Med Microbiol 1990;272:443–447.

38. Itoh T, Takahashi M, Kai A, Takano I, Saito K, Ohashi M. Fluoroquinolone resistance in *Campylobacter* spp. isolated from human stools and poultry products. Lancet 1990;335:787

39. Johnson RJ, Nolan C, Wang SP, Shelton WR, Blaser MJ. Persistent *Campylobacter jejuni* infection in an immunocompromised patient. Ann Intern Med 1984;100:832–834.

40. Karmali MA, De Grandis S, Fleming PC. Antimicrobial susceptibility of *Campylobacter jejuni* with special reference to resistance patterns of Canadian isolates. Antimicrob Agents Chemother 1981;19:593–597.

41. Karmali MA, Norrish B, Lior H, Heyes B, Monteath A, Montgomery H. *Campylobacter* enterocolitis in a neonatal nursery. J Infect Dis 1984;149:874–877.

42. Keihlbauch JA, Brenner DJ, Nicholson MA, et al. *Campylobacter butzleri* sp. nov. isolated from humans and animals with diarrheal illness. J Clin Microbiol 1991;29:376–385.

43. Kerstens PJSM, Endtz HP, Meis JF, Oyen WJ, Koopman RJ, Van den Broek PJ, Van der Meer JW. Erysipelas-like skin lesions associated with *Campylobacter jejuni* septicemia in patients with hypogammaglobulinemia. Eur J Clin Microbiol Infect Dis 1992;11:842–847.

44. Kirst HA, Sides GD. New directions for macrolide antibiotics: pharmacokinetics and clinical efficacy. Antimicrob Agents Chemother 1989;33:1419–1422.

45. Kitzis MD, Goldstein FW, Miégi M, Acar JF. In vitro activity of azithromycin against various gram-negative bacilli and anaerobic bacteria. Antimicrob Agents Chemother 1990;25:15–18.

46. Koenraad PM, Jacobs-Reitxma WF, Van der Laan T, Beumer RR, Rombouts FM. Antibiotic susceptibility of Campylobacter isolates from sewage and poultry abattoir drain water. Epidemiol Infect 1995;115:475–483.

47. Kunin CM. Antimicrobial activity of rifabutin. Clin Infect Dis 1996;22(Suppl 1):S3–S13.

48. Lachance N, Gaudreau C, Lamonthe F, Turgeon F. Susceptibilities of β-lactamase-positive and -negative strains of *Campylobacter coli* to β-lactam agents. Antimicrob Agent Chemother 1993;37:1174–1176.

49. Lariviere LA, Gaudreau CL, Turgeon FF. Susceptibility of clinical isolates of *Campylobacter jejuni* to twenty-five antimicrobial agents. J Antimicrob Chemother 1986;18:681–685.

50. Lastovica AJ, Le Roux E. Prevalence and distribution of *Campylobacter* spp. in the diarrhoeic stools and blood cultures of pediatric patients. Acta Gastroenterol Belg 1993;56:34

51. Lastovica AJ, Le Roux E, Penner JL. "*Campylobacter upsaliensis*" isolated from blood cultures of pediatric patients. J Clin Microbiol 1989;27:657–659.

52. Laughon BE, Vernon AA, Druckman DA, Fox R, Quinn, TC, Polk BF, Bartlett JG. Recovery of *Campylobacter* species from homosexual men. J Infect Dis 1988;158:464–467.

53. Lawson GHK, Rowland AC. *Campylobacter sputorum* subsp. *mucosalis*. In: Butzler JP, ed. *Campylobacter* infection in man and animals. Boca Raton, FL: CRC Press, 1984:207–225.

54. Lever AM, Dolby JM, Webster AD, Price AB. Chronic *Campylobacter* colitis and uveitis in patient with hypogammaglobulinaemia. Br Med J 1984;288:531.

55. Lindblom GB, Johny M, Khalil K, Mazhar K, Ruiz-Palacios GM, Kaijser B. Enterotoxigenicity and frequency of *Campylobacter jejuni, C. coli,* and *C. laridis* in human and animal stool isolates from different countries. FEMS Microbiol Lett 1990;54:163–168.

56. Mattila L, Siitonen A, Kyroseppa H, Kryonseppa H, Simula I Oksanen P, Stenvik M, Salo P, Peltola H. Seasonal variation in etiology of travelers' diarrhea. Finnish-Moroccan Study Group. J Infect Dis 1992;165:385–388.

57. Megraud F, Elharrif Z. Isolation of *Campylobacter* species by filtration. Eur J Clin Microbiol 1985;4:437–438.

58. Melamed I, Bujanover Y, Igra YS, Schwartz D, Zakuth V, Spirer Z. *Campylobacter* enteritis in normal and immunodeficient children. Am J Dis Child 1983;137:752–753.

59. Michel J, Rogol M, Dickman D. Susceptibility of clinical isolates of *Campylobacter jejuni* to sixteen antimicrobial agents. Antimicrob Agent Chemother 1983;23:796–797.

60. Minet J, Growbois B, Megraud F. *Campylobacter hyointestinalis:* an opportunistic enteropathogen? J Clin Microbiol 1988; 26:2659–2660.

61. Molina JM, Casin I, Hausfater P, Giretti E, Welker Y, Decazes J, Garrait V, Lagrange P, Modai J. Campylobacter infections in HIV-infected patients: clinical and bacteriological features. AIDS 1995;9:881–885.

62. Morrison VA, Lloyd BK, Chia JKS, Tuazon CU. Cardiovascular and bacteremic manifestations of *Campylobacter fetus* infection: case report and review. Rev Infect Dis 1990;12:387–392.

63. Murphy GS, Echeverria P, Jackson LR, Arness MK, LeBron C, Pitarangsi C. Ciprofloxacin- and azithromycin-resistant

Campylobacter causing traveler's diarrhea in U.S. troops deployed to Thailand in 1994. Clin Infect Dis 1995;22:868–869.

64. Nachamkin I. *Campylobacter* and *Arcobacter*. In: Murray PR, Baron EJ, Pfaller MA, Tenover FC, Yolen RH, eds. Manual of clinical microbiology. Washington, DC: American Society for Microbiology, 1995:483–491.

65. Nair GB, Pal SC. Biotype characterization and antibiotic sensitivity of *Campylobacter* from human and non-human sources in Calcutta. Indian J Med Res 1985;81:357–363.

66. Navarro F, Miro E, Mirelis B, Prats G. *Campylobacter* spp antibiotic susceptibility. J Antimicrob Chemother 1993;32:906–907.

67. Neuzil K, Wang E, Haas D, Blaser MJ. Persistence of *Campylobacter fetus* bacteremia associated with absence of opsonizing antibodies. J Clin Microbiol 1994;32:1718–1720.

68. Orlicek SL, Welch DF, Kuhls TL. Septicemia and meningitis caused by *Helicobacter cinaedi* in a neonate. J Clin Microbiol 1993;31:569–571.

69. Patton CM, Shaffer N, Edmonds P, Barrett TJ, Lambert MA, Baker C, Perlman DM, Brenner DJ. Human disease associated with "*Campylobacter upsaliensis*" (catalase-negative or weakly positive *Campylobacter* species) in the United States. J Clin Microbiol 1989;27:66–73.

70. Perlman DM, Ampel NM, Schifman RB, Cohn DL, Patton CM, Aguirre ML, Wang WL, Blaser MJ. Persistent *Campylobacter jejuni* infections in patients infected with the human immunodeficiency virus (HIV). Ann Intern Med 1988;108:540–546.

71. Petruccelli BP, Murphy GS, Sanchez JL, Walz S, DeFraites R, Gelnett J, Haberberger RL, Echeverria P, Taylor DN. Treatment of traveler's diarrhea with ciprofloxacin and loperamide. J Infect Dis 1992;165:557–560.

72. Pönkä A, Tilvis R, Kosunen TU. Prolonged *Campylobacter* gastroenteritis in a patient with hypogammaglobulinaemia. Acta Med Scand 1983;213:159–160.

73. Prasad KN, Mathur SK, Dhole TN, Ayyagari A. Antimicrobial susceptibility and plasmid analysis of *Campylobacter jejuni* isolated from diarrhoeal patients and healthy chickens in northern India. J Diarrhoeal Dis Res 1994;12:270–273.

74. Preston MA, Simor AE, Walmsley SL, Fuller SA, Lastovica AJ, Sandstedt K, Penner JL. In vitro susceptibility of "*Campylobacter upsaliensis*" to twenty-four antimicrobial agents. Eur J Clin Microbiol Infect Dis 1990;9:822–824.

75. Pulik M, Leturdu F, Lionnet F, Genet P, Petitdidier C, Touahri T. Rifubutin prevents Campylobacter infection in patients with AIDS. Clin Infect Dis 1996;23:1197–1198.

76. Quinn TC, Goodell SE, Fennell CL, Wang SP, Schuffler MD, Holmes KK, Stamm WE. Infections with *Campylobacter jejuni* and *Campylobacter*-like organisms in homosexual men. Ann Intern Med 1984;101:187–192.

77. Rautelin H, Renkonen OV, Kosunen TU. Emergence of fluoroquinolone resistance in *Campylobacter jejuni* and *Campylobacter coli* in subjects from Finland. Agents Chemother 1991;35:2065–2069.

78. Rautelin H, Renkonen OV, Kosunen TU. Azithromycin resistance in *Campylobacter jejuni* and *Campylobacter coli*. Eur J Clin Microbiol Infect Dis 1993;12:864–865.

79. Reina J. Resistance to fluoroquinolones in *Salmonella* non-*typhi* and Campylobacter spp. Lancet 1992;340:1035–1036.

80. Reina J, Borrell N, Serra A. Emergence of resistance to erythromycin and fluoroquinolones in thermotolerant *Campylobacter* strains isolated from feces 1987–1991. Eur J Clin Microbiol Infect Dis 1992;11:1163–1166.

81. Reina J, Ros MJ, Serra A. Susceptibilities to 10 antimicrobial agents of 1,220 *Campylobacter* strains isolated from 1987 to 1993 from feces of pediatric patients. Antimicrob Agents Chemother 1994;38:2917–2920.

82. Russell RG, Kiehlbauch JA, Gebhart CJ, DeTolla LJ. Uncommon Campylobacter species in infant Macaca nemestrina monkeys housed in a nursery. J Clin Microbiol 1992;30:3024–3027.

83. Sacks LV, Labriola AM, Gill VJ, Gordin FM. Use of ciprofloxacin for successful eradication of bacteremia due to *Campylobacter cinaedi* in a human immunodeficiency virus-infected patient. Rev Infect Dis 1993;13:1066–1068.

84. Sagara H, Mochizuki A, Okamura N, Nakaya R. Antimicrobial resistance of *Campylobacter jejuni* and *Campylobacter coli* with special reference to plasmid profiles of Japanese clinical isolates. Antimicrob Agents Chemother 1987;31:713–719.

85. Salazar-Lindo E, Sack RB, Chea-Woo E, Kay BA, Piscoya ZA, Leon-Barua R, Yi A. Early treatment with erythromycin of *Campylobacter jejuni*-associated dysentery in children. J Pediatr 1986;109:357–360.

86. Sánchez R, Fernández-Baca V, Díaz MD, Muñoz P, Rodríguez-Créixems M, Bouza E. Evolution of susceptibilities of *Campylobacter* spp. to quinolones and macrolides. Antimicrob Agents Chemother 1994;38:1879–1882.

87. Segreti J, Gootz TD, Goodman LJ, Parkhurst GW, Quinn JP, Martin BA, Trenholme GM. High-level quinolone resistance in clinical isolates of *Campylobacter jejuni*. J Infect Dis 1992;165:667–670.

88. Simor AE, Ferro S. *Campylobacter jejuni* infection occurring during pregnancy. Eur J Clin Microbiol Infect Dis 1990;9:142–144.

89. Simor AE, Karmali MA, Jadavji T, Roscoe M. Abortion and perinatal sepsis associated with *Campylobacter* infection. Rev Infect Dis 1986;8:397–402.

90. Simor AE, Wilcox L. Enteritis associated with *Campylobacter laridis*. J Clin Microbiol 1987;25:10–12.

91. Sjögren E, Lindblom GB, Kaijser B. Rapid development of resistance to quinolones in *Campylobacter* in Sweden. Acta Gastroenterol Belg 1993;56:10.

92. Sjögren E, Kaijser B, Werner M. Antimicrobial susceptibilities of *Campylobacter jejuni* and *Campylobacter coli* isolated in Sweden: a 10-year follow-up report. Antimicrob Agent Chemother 1992;36:2847–2849.

93. Skirrow MB, Blaser MJ. *Campylobacter jejuni*. In: Blaser MJ, Smith PD, Ravdin JI, Greenberg HB, Guerrant RL, eds. Infections of the gastrointestinal tract. New York: Raven Press, 1995:825–848.

94. Soderstrom C, Schalen C, Walder M. Septicaemia caused by unusual *Campylobacter* species (*C. laridis* and *C. mucosalis*). Scand J Infect Dis 1991;23:369–371.

95. Sovillo FJ, Lieb LE, Waterman SH. Incidence of campylobacteriosis among patients with AIDS in Los Angeles County. J Acquired Immune Defic Syndr 1991;4:598–602.

96. Spelman DW, Davidson N, Buckmaster ND, Spicer WI, Ryan P. *Campylobacter* bacteraemia: a report of 10 cases. Med J Aust 1986;145:503–505.

97. Tauxe RV, Hargrett-Bean N, Patton CM, Wachsmuth IK. *Campylobacter* isolates in the United States, 1982–1986. MMWR CDC Surveill Summ 1988;37:1–14.

98. Taylor DE, Chang N. In vitro susceptibilities of *Campylobacter jejuni* and *Campylobacter coli* to azithromycin and erythromycin. Antimicrob Agents Chemother 1991;35:1917–1918.

99. Taylor DE, Chang N, Garner RS, Sherburne R, Mueller L. Incidence of antibiotic resistance and characterization of plasmids in

Campylobacter jejuni strains isolated from clinical sources in Alberta, Canada. Can J Microbiol 1986;32:28–32.

100. Taylor DE, Courvalin P. Mechanisms of antibiotic resistance in *Campylobacter* species. Antimicrob Agents Chemother 1988; 32:1107–1112.

101. Taylor DE, De Grandis SA, Karmali MA, Fleming PC. Transmissible plasmids from *Campylobacter jejuni*. Antimicrob Agents Chemother 1981;19:831–835.

102. Taylor DE, Garner RS, Allan BJ. Characterization of tetracycline resistance plasmids from *Campylobacter jejuni* and *Campylobacter coli*. Antimicrob Agents Chemother 1983;24:930–935.

103. Taylor DE, Ng LK, Lior H. Susceptibility of *Campylobacter* species to nalidixic acid, enoxacin, and other DNA gyrase inhibitors. Agents Chemother 1985;28:708–710.

104. Taylor DN, Blaser MJ, Echeverria P, Pitarangsi C, Bodhidatta L, Wang WL. Erythromycin-resistant *Campylobacter* infections in Thailand. Antimicrob Agents Chemother 1987;31: 438–442.

105. Taylor DN, Diehlbauch JA, Tee W, Pitarangsi C, Echeverria P. Isolation of group 2 aerotolerant *Campylobacter* species from Thai children with diarrhea. J Infect Dis 1991;163:1062–1067.

106. Tenover FC, Bronsdon MA, Gordon KP, Plorde JJ. Isolation of plasmids encoding tetracycline resistance from *Campylobacter jejuni* strains isolated from simians. Antimicrob Agents Chemother 1983;23:320–322.

107. Tenover FC, Williams S, Gordon KP, Nolan C, Plorde JJ. Survey of plasmids and resistance factors in *Campylobacter jejuni* and Campylobacter coli. Antimicrob Agents Chemother 1985; 27:37–41.

108. Tomayko JF, Korten V, Murray BE. DU-6859a, a new fluoroquinolone agent. Comparative in vitro activity against enteric pathogens and multiresistant outpatient *Escherichia coli*. Diagn Microbiol Infect Dis 1994;20:45–47.

109. Van der Auwera P, Scorneaux B. In vitro susceptibility of *Campylobacter jejuni* to 27 antimicrobial agents and various combinations of β-lactams with clavulanic acid or sulbactam. Antimicrob Agent Chemother 1985;28:37–40.

110. Van der Auwera, Scorneaux B. In vitro susceptibility of *Campylobacter jejuni* to 27 antimicrobial agents and various combinations of β-lactams with clavulanic acid or sulbactam. Amtimicrob Agent Chemother 1985;28:37–40.

111. Van der Meer JWM, Mouton RP, Daha MR, Schuurman RKB. *Campylobacter jejuni* bacteraemia as a cause of recurrent fever in a patient with hypogammaglobulinaemia. J Infect 1986;12: 235–239.

112. van Dijk WC, van der Straaten PJC. An outbreak of *Campylobacter jejuni* infection in a neonatal intensive care unit. J Hosp Infect 1988;11:91–99.

113. Vandamme P, De Ley J. Proposal for a new family, *Campylobacteraceae*. Int J Syst Bacteriol 1991;41:451–455.

114. Vandamme P, Falsen E, Rossau R, Hoste B, Tytgat R, De Ley J. Revision of *Campylobacter, Helicobacter,* and *Wolinella* taxonomy: emendation of generic descriptions and proposal of Arcobacter gen. nov. Int J Syst Bacteriol 1991;41:88–103.

115. Vandamme P, Pugina P, Benzi G, Van Etterijek R, Vlaes L, Kersters K, Butzler JP, Lior H, Lauwers S. Outbreak of recurrent abdominal cramps associated with *Arcobacter butzleri* in an Italian school. J Clin Microbiol 1992;30:2335–2337.

116. Vanhoof R, Goossens H, Coignau H, Stas G, Butzler JP. Susceptibility pattern of *Campylobacter jejuni* from human and animal origins to different antimicrobial agents. Antimicrob Agent Chemother 1982;21:990–992.

117. Vanhoof R, Hubrechts JM, Roebben E, Nyssen HJ, Nulens E, Leger J, DeSchepper N. The comparative activity of perfloxacin, enoxacin, ciprofloxacin and 13 other antimicrobial agents against enteropathogenic microorganisms. Infection 1986;14:294–298.

118. Vanhoof R, Vanderlinden MP, Dierickx R, Lauwers S, Yourassowsky E, Butzler JP. Susceptibility of *Campylobacter fetus* subsp. jejuni to twenty-nine antimicrobial agents. Antimicrob Agents Chemother 1978;14:553–556.

119. Varoli O, Gatti M, Montella MT, La Placa M. Observations on strains of *Campylobacter* spp. isolated in 1989 in northern Italy. Microbiologica 1991;14:31–35.

120. Velázquez JB, Jiménez A, Chomón B, Villa TG. Incidence and transmission of antibiotic resistance in *Campylobacter jejuni* and *Campylobacter coli*. J Antimicrob Chemother 1995; 35:173–178.

121. Walder M, Forgren A. Erythromycin-resistant campylobacters. Lancet 1978;ii:1201

122. Wang WL, Reller LB, Blaser MJ. Comparison of antimicrobial susceptibility patterns of *Campylobacter jejuni* and *Campylobacter coli*. Antimicrob Agents Chemother 1984;26:351–353.

123. Wintermeyer SM, Abdel-Rahman SM, Nahata MC. Dirithromycin: a new macrolide [Abstract]. Ann Pharmacother 1996;30:1141–1149.

124. Wistrom J, Jertborn M, Ekwall E, Norlin K, Soderquist B, Stromberg A, Lundholm R, Hogevik H, Lagergren L, Englund G. Empiric treatment of acute diarrheal disease with norfloxacin. A randomized placebo-controlled study. Ann Intern Med 1992;117:202–208.

125. Wong SK, Tam AC, Yuen KY. *Campylobacter* infection in the neonate: case report and review of the literature. Pediatr Infect Dis 1990;9:665–669.

126. Youngs ER, Roberts C. *Campylobacter* carriage and pregnancy. Br J Obstet Gynaecol 1985;92:541–542.

Capnocytophaga Species

●

Hillar Vellend

GENERAL DESCRIPTION

Capnocytophaga species constitute part of the normal oral microflora of humans and animals. It is a long, thin Gram-negative rod that is slow growing, is facultatively anaerobic, and requires enrichment with CO_2 (5–10%) for optimum growth (capnophilic).

Clinical isolates of *Capnocytophaga* species are classified into two broad groups, dysgonic fermenter-1 (DF-1) and DF-2 (16). The species within the DF-1 group include *C. gingivalis, C. ochracea* and *C. sputigena.* The two species in the DF-2 group include *C. canimorsus* and *C. cynodegmi.*

The DF-1 group is thought to have a role in the pathogenesis of various forms of periodontal disease. Systemic infections have been reported in patients with severe chemotherapy-induced granulocytopenia and oral ulcerations (3, 11). These *Capnocytophaga* species have also been reported to cause a wide variety of infections in immunocompetent hosts, including bacteremia, endocarditis, pericardial abscess, mediastinal abscess, septic arthritis, osteomyelitis, endophthalmitis, peritonitis and suppurative lymphadenitis (20). Peripartum infections have been described, leading to chorioamnionitis and sepsis in the newborn (17).

DF-2 organisms, especially *C. canimorsus,* have been associated with severe sepsis following dog (and occasionally cat) bites, particularly in patients who have undergone splenectomy for a variety of reasons or who are chronic alcoholics (8, 9, 21).

SUSCEPTIBILITY IN VITRO

There have been relatively few recent studies of the in vitro antimicrobial susceptibilities of *Capnocytophaga* species (2, 7, 15, 22, 25, 27). Prior to 1987, β-lactamase-producing strains of *Capnocytophaga* spp. were rare (<2%). However, in the 1990s there have been increasing reports of serious infections due to β-lactamase-producing strains. Indeed, one report from Canada (22) demonstrated β-lactamase production in 6 of 19 (32%) isolates studied in their laboratory in Vancouver. These strains were almost all from the DF-1 group. A similar high incidence of β-lactamase positivity (7 of 26 strains) was observed in a recent report from France (19). β-lactamase-negative strains remain highly susceptible ($MIC_{90} \leq 1.0$ μg/mL) to penicillin, amoxicillin, amoxicillin/clavulanate, piperacillin, ticarcillin, and imipenem. First-generation cephalosporins (cephalothin, cefazolin) are relatively less active ($MIC_{90} \leq 8$–32 μg/mL). Second-generation cephalosporins (cefamandole, cefuroxime, cefoxitin) are more active ($MIC_{90} \leq 2$–8 μg/mL), but third-generation cephalosporins (cefotaxime, ceftriaxone, ceftazidime, ceftizoxime) are usually very active ($MIC_{90} \leq 0.5$–4.0 μg/mL).

Antibiotics other than β-lactams that are very active against *Capnocytophaga* spp. include clindamycin ($MIC_{90} \leq 0.03$ μg/mL) and most fluoroquinolones (ciprofloxacin, ofloxacin, pefloxacin; $MIC_{90} \leq 0.5$ μg/mL). All *Capnocytophaga* spp. are resistant to vancomycin ($MIC_{90} \geq 16$ μg/mL), metronidazole ($MIC_{90} \geq 16$ μg/mL), trimethoprim ($MIC_{90} > 64$ μg/mL), aminoglycosides (gentamicin, amikacin; $MIC_{90} > 64$ μg/mL) and aztreonam ($MIC_{90} > 64$ μg/mL).

β-Lactamase-producing strains are most susceptible to amoxicillin/clavulanic acid ($MIC_{90} = 1.0$ μg/mL), imipenem ($MIC_{90} = 0.25$ μg/mL), clindamycin ($MIC_{90} = 0.015$ μg/mL), and ciprofloxacin ($MIC_{90} = 1.0$ μg/mL). Such strains are usually more resistant to all cephalosporins (22) than β-lactamase-negative strains. Older studies (26) documented susceptibility to erythromycin ($MIC_{90} = 1.0$ μg/mL), tetracycline ($MIC_{90} = 1$ μg/mL), and chloramphenicol ($MIC_{90} = 8$ μg/mL), but in recent case reports (5, 13), erythromycin resistance appears to be common.

There are no data on in vitro susceptibility to combinations of antibiotics.

There are only three published reports of in vitro susceptibility testing of the DF-2 group of *Capnocytophaga* (7, 9, 27). The results of these studies are similar to susceptibility data for *Capnocytophaga* spp. except that there are no reports of β-lactamase-producing *C. canimorsus.*

ANTIMICROBIAL THERAPY
Drug of Choice

In view of the increasing prevalence of β-lactamase-producing strains of *Capnocytophaga* spp., it is prudent to treat patients with serious infections with ampicillin plus sulbactam (or other β-lactam + β-lactamase-inhibitor combinations) or a third-generation cephalosporin such as cefotaxime or ceftriaxone. Initial empirical treatment of the febrile neutropenic patient with such widely used combinations as cefazolin plus gentamicin or vancomycin plus amikacin may result in failure to adequately treat *Capnocytophaga* sp. bacteremia.

There are no data to support the use of combination drug therapy.

Special Situations

Endocarditis

Only seven cases of *Capnocytophaga* sp. endocarditis have been reported in the English-language literature. Successful treatment was accomplished with 4 weeks of ampicillin (2 g intravenously 4 hourly) plus metronidazole (1 g orally twice daily) (10); penicillin G (20 MU/day intravenously) (4); clindamycin (600 mg intravenously, four times daily) (1); and penicillin plus netilmicin (21).

Fulminant Postsplenectomy Sepsis

Fulminant postsplenectomy sepsis is due to *C. canimorsus,* and the treatment of choice remains penicillin or ampicillin.

Meningitis

Both purulent and lymphocytic meningitis have been reported with *C. canimorsus.* Successful treatment has been achieved with penicillin (5 MU thrice daily for 15 days) (18) and ampicillin (150 mg/kg daily for 3 weeks) (6). There are no reports of meningitis due to β-lactamase-producing strains, but empirical treatment with ceftriaxone or cefotaxime should be effective.

Endophthalmitis

A recent report of *Capnocytophaga* endophthalmitis recommended that one of the third-generation cephalosporins (e.g., ceftriaxone, 2 g/day) should be the antibiotic of choice (24).

Alternative Therapy

In the "penicillin-allergic" patient, clindamycin or ciprofloxacin are effective alternatives to β-lactam antibiotics.

ENDPOINTS FOR MONITORING THERAPY

In general, there are no unique endpoints for monitoring therapy for infections due to *Capnocytophaga* spp. Treatment duration must be guided by clinical response and host characteristics (e.g., neutropenia).

CONTROVERSIES

Several authors (12, 21) have suggested that prophylactic antibiotics should be administered to all at-risk patients who seek medical attention following a dog bite. This recommendation is particularly applicable to patients who have undergone splenectomy and are at risk of overwhelming infection due to *C. canimorsus.* However, the cost-effectiveness of routine use of such drugs as amoxicillin with or without clavulanic acid is questionable.

REFERENCES

1. Adair JC, Banks DD, Call GK. Stroke due to Capnocytophaga endocarditis. Rev Infect Dis 1991;13:341–342.
2. Arlet G, Pors M-J S-L, Casin IM, Ortenberg M, Perol Y. In vitro susceptibility of 96 Capnocytophaga strains, including a β-lactamase producer, to new β-lactam antibiotics and six quinolones. Antimicrob Agents Chemother 1987;31:1283–1284.
3. Baquero F, Fernandez J, Dronda F, Erice A, Perez de Oteiza J, Reguera JA, Reig M. Capnophilic and anaerobic bacteremia in neutropenic patients: an oral source. Rev Infect Dis 1990;12 (Suppl 2):S157–160.
4. Baranda MM, Arrieta VA, Almaraz JH, Rodriguez MP, Oraeta MA, Errasti CA. Two cases of Capnocytophaga bacteremia, one with endocarditis [Letter]. Can Med Assoc J 1984;130:1420.
5. Bilgrami S, Bergstrom SK, Peterson DE, Hill DR, Dainiak N, Quinn JJ, Ascensao JL. Capnocytophaga bacteremia in a patient with Hodgkin's disease following bone marrow transplantation: a case report and review. Clin Infect Dis 1992;14:1045–1049.
6. Blanche P, Sicard D, Meyniard O, Ratovohery D, Brun T, Paul G. Capnocytophaga canimorsus lymphocytic meningitis in an immunocompetent man who was bitten by a dog. Clin Infect Dis 1994;18:654–655.
7. Bremmelgaard A, Pers C, Kristiansen JE, Korner B, Heltberg O, Frederiksen W. Susceptibility testing of Danish isolates of Capnocytophaga and CDC group DF-2 bacteria. APMIS 1989; 97:43–48.
8. Brenner DJ, Hollis DG, Fanning GR, Weaver RE. Capnocytophaga canimorsus sp. nov. (formerly CDC group DF-2), a cause of septicemia following dog bite, and C. cynodegmi sp. nov., a cause of localised wound infection following dog bite. J Clin Microbiol 1989;27:231–235.
9. Butler T, Weaver RE, Ramani TKV, Uyeda CT, Bobo RA, Ryu JS, Kohler RB. Unidentified gram-negative rod infection: a new disease of man. Ann Int Med 1977;86:1–5.
10. Buu-Hoi AY, Joundy S, Acar JF. Endocarditis caused by Capnocytophaga ochracea. J Clin Microbiol 1988;26: 1061–1062.
11. Campbell JR, Edwards MS. Capnocytophaga species infection in children. Pediatr Infect Dis J 1991;10:944–948.
12. Cummings P. Antibiotics to prevent infection in patients with dog bite wounds: a meta analysis of randomized trials. Ann Emerg Med 1994;23:335–340.
13. Duong M, Besancenot JF, Neuwirth C, Buisson M, Chavanet P, Portier H. Vertebral osteomyelitis due to Capnocytophaga species in immunocompetent patients: report of two cases and review. Clin Infect Dis 1996;22:1099–1101.
14. Foweraker JE, Hawkey PM, Heritage J, Van Landuyt HW. Novel β-lactamase from Capnocytophaga sp. Antimicrob Agents Chemother 1990;34:1501–1504.
15. Hawkey PM, Smith SD, Haynes J, Malnick H, Forlenza SW. In vitro susceptibility of Capnocytophaga species to antimicrobial agents. Antimicrob Agents Chemother 1987;31:331–332.
16. Holmes B, Pickett MJ, Hollis DG. Unusual gram-negative bacteria, including Capnocytophaga, Eikenella, Pasteurella, and Streptobacillus. In: Murray PR, Baron EJ, Pfaller MA, Tenover FC, Yolken RH, eds. Manual of clinical microbiology. 6th ed. Washington, DC: American Society for Microbiology Press, 1995:503.
17. Iralu JV, Roberts D, Kazanjian PH. Chorioamnionitis caused by Capnocytophaga: case report and review. Clin Infect Dis 1993; 17:457–461.
18. Kristensen KS, Winthereik M, Rasmussen ML. Capnocytophaga canimorsus infection after dog-bite. Lancet 1991;337: 849.
19. Mory F, Lozniewski A, Del Galloc C, Lemozy J, Weber M. In vitro activity of β-lactamase inhibitors against clinical Capnocytophaga sp. strains [Abstract no. E90]. In: Abstracts of the 35th Interscience Conference on Antimicrobial Agents and Chemotherapy. San Francisco, 1995.
20. Parenti DM, Snydman DR. Capnocytophaga species: infections in nonimmunocompromised and immunocompromised hosts. J Infect Dis 1985;151:140–147.
21. Pers C, Gahrn-Hansen B, Frederiksen W. Capnocytophaga canimorsus septicemia in Denmark, 1982–1995: review of 39 cases. Clin Infect Dis 1996;23:71–75.
22. Roscoe DL, Zemcov SJV, Thornber D, Wise R, Clarke AM. Antimicrobial susceptibilities and β-lactamase characterization of Capnocytophaga species. Antimicrob Agents Chemother 1992; 36:2197–2200.
23. Roscoe D, Clarke A. Resistance of Capnocytophaga species to β-lactam antibiotics [Letter]. Clin Infect Dis 1993;17: 284–285.

24. Rubsamen PE, McLeish WM, Pflugfelder S, Miller D. Capnocytophaga endophthalmitis. Ophthalmology 1993;100: 456–459.

25. Rummens JL, Gordts B, Van Landuyt HW. In vitro susceptibility of Capnocytophaga species to 29 antimicrobial agents. Antimicrob Agents Chemother 1986;30:739–742.

26. Sutter VL, Pyeatt D, Kwok YY. In vitro susceptibility of Capnocytophaga strains to 18 antimicrobial agents. Antimicrob Agents Chemother 1981;20:270–271.

27. Verghese A, Hamati F, Berk S, Franzus B, Berk S, Smith JK. Susceptibility of dysgonic fermenter 2 to antimicrobial agents in vitro. Antimicrob Agents Chemother 1988;32:78–80.

Cardiobacterium hominis

Selwyn D. R. Lang and Arthur J. Morris

GENERAL DESCRIPTION
Microbiology

Cardiobacterium hominis is a slow-growing, fastidious, capnophilic, Gram-negative bacillus represented by the "C" in "HACEK", an acronym for *Haemophilus* species, *Actinobacillus actinomycetemcomitans, C. hominis, Eikenella corrodens* and *Kingella* species (4). All these organisms have the propensity to cause endocarditis, but in the case of *C. hominis,* this disease is, with rare exceptions, its only pathologic manifestation.

C. hominis was first isolated from a patient with endocarditis and described as a *Pasteurella*-like organism, designated "CDC group II-D" (17). It was given the name *C. hominis* in 1964 (15) and is the single species in the genus. *C. hominis* is a member of the normal upper respiratory flora in humans and may be found only rarely on other mucosal surfaces. It has not been isolated from animals, soil, water, or hospital equipment.

In the clinical laboratory, *C. hominis* is recovered almost exclusively from blood cultures from patients with endocarditis. Although growth in modern commercial media is usually detectable after 3 to 5 days, incubation for 2 to 3 weeks is recommended before reporting a culture as negative (19). Gram staining and subculturing is essential, since there is likely to be no visible change in blood culture medium. The Gram-stained organisms tend to retain crystal violet at one or both poles, giving a Gram-variable lollipop or dumbbell appearance. They are typically clustered in rosettes.

C. hominis grows on blood or chocolate agar at 35°C when there is adequate humidity and an atmosphere enriched by CO_2. It will seldom grow on MacConkey agar or other enteric media. Small, glistening, opaque colonies become apparent after 2 or 3 days, but occasionally up to 2 weeks, and with further incubation these may pit the agar. *C. hominis* is oxidase positive, catalase negative, nitrate negative, urease negative, and indole positive. The positive indole reaction is useful in distinguishing *C. hominis* from other "HACEK" organisms, though *Suttonella indologenes* (formerly *Kingella indologenes*) is also indole positive.

Clinical Manifestations

Although *C. hominis* was responsible for only 2 of 1989 cases of endocarditis accumulated from 13 published series before 1983, it accounted for 14 of 111 cases in case reports of endocarditis due to "unusual organisms" (1). Between 1962 and 1991 only 54 cases of *C. hominis* endocarditis were reported in the literature (5, 21), and a few have been added since. Most, perhaps all, have involved previously abnormal valves or prosthetic valves (1, 2, 4, 5, 8, 13, 14, 16, 20). Endocarditis due to *C. hominis* tends to be exceptionally low grade and insidious, but with a tendency to form large friable vegetations associated with frequent embolic complications (13, 20). Meningitis and intracranial mycotic aneurysm secondary to endocarditis (3, 7) and an abdominal abscess (12) are exceptional examples of *C. hominis* causing infection outside the cardiovascular system.

SUSCEPTIBILITY IN VITRO

Susceptibility testing of *C. hominis* can be difficult owing to the fastidious nature and slow growth rate of the organism. However, susceptibility testing should be performed because the result is never entirely predictable.

There are no published studies of antibiotic susceptibilities of large numbers of *C. hominis* tested in parallel against a range of antibiotics. Table 1 summarizes representative susceptibilities of several strains to a range of antibiotics (20). Notably, all 22 isolates tested against penicillin were susceptible; however, one isolate developed resistance to ampicillin during treatment. There are very few published data on the bactericidal activity of antibiotics for *C. hominis*. Chloramphenicol has been noted to achieve bactericidal titers in serum of 1:32 in a patient with *C. hominis* infection successfully treated with this drug (11). Vogt et al. reported MIC/MBC (μg/mL) for a single isolate: penicillin, 0.06/0.06; mezlocillin, 0.5/0.5; tobramycin, 1/2; imipenem, 0.06/0.25; and ciprofloxacin, 0.06/0.06 (18). Their patient developed renal toxicity while receiving treatment with mezlocillin and gentamicin, relapsed on mezlocillin alone, and was cured by two courses

TABLE 1 • In Vitro Susceptibilities of *Cardiobacterium hominis**

Antimicrobial Agent	n	Representative MIC (μg/mL)[a]	Breakpoint[b]	n (%) Susceptible
Penicillin	22	0.05		22 (100%)
Ampicillin	16	<0.4		15 (94%)
Oxacillin	3	NA[c]		2 (67%)
Carbenicillin	5	<1.6	≤16	5 (100%)
Cephalothin	11	<0.4	≤8	11 (100%)
Chloramphenicol	17	1.25	≤8	17 (100%)
Colistin	2	NA		2 (100%)
Trimethoprim-sulfamethoxazole	3	NA	≤2/38	3 (100%)
Sulfonamide	1	NA		0 (0%)
Tetracycline	19	0.25	≤4	19 (100%)
Erythromycin	14	NA	≤0.5	11 (79%)
Gentamicin	9	<0.8	≤4	8 (89%)
Kanamycin	6	<0.8	≤16	1 (17%)
Streptomycin	14	1.6		14 (100%)
Tobramycin	2	NA	≤4	2 (100%)
Rifampin	1	NA	≤1	1 (100%)
Vancomycin	3	25	≤4	1 (33%)
Clindamycin	2	5	≤0.5	0 (0%)

Modified from Wormser GP, Bottone EJ. *Cardiobacterium hominis:* review of microbiologic and clinical features. Rev Infect Dis 1983;5:680–691.

[a] MIC_{50}, MIC_{90} and MIC range not reported.

[b] Current NCCLS interpretive standards for susceptibility (μg/mL) (10).

[c] NA, data not available.

of ciprofloxacin. Both peak and trough sera were rapidly bactericidal while the patient received ciprofloxacin.

Le Quellec et al. reported the first case of infection with a β-lactamase-producing strain of *C. hominis* (6). β-Lactamase production was confirmed by a chromogenic cephalosporin test. Susceptibility to both amoxicillin and ticarcillin was restored in the presence of clavulanic acid. This isolate was resistant to cefotaxime, piperacillin, erythromycin, trimethoprim-sulfamethoxazole, and gentamicin, but susceptible to imipenem, tetracycline, rifampicin, and vancomycin.

ANTIMICROBIAL THERAPY
General

An ad hoc writing group for the American Heart Association (19) notes the emergence of β-lactamase-producing strains within the HACEK group of organisms and recommends cefotaxime or ceftriaxone as the drugs of choice for treatment of HACEK endocarditis. The recommended dose of ceftriaxone is 2 g once daily intravenously or intramuscularly. Their preferred alternative is combination treatment with ampicillin and gentamicin, providing the isolate does not produce β-lactamase. The recommended dose of ampicillin is 12 g/day intravenously, either continuously or in 6 equally divided doses, and that of gentamicin is 1 mg/kg intramuscularly or intravenously 8-hourly. Monotherapy with ampicillin is no longer recommended. The recommended duration of treatment is 3 to 4 weeks for native valve disease and 6 weeks when a prosthetic valve is involved. These recommendations are necessarily made on the basis of scanty published data. Until relatively recently, a penicillin alone or in combination with an aminogly-

coside was used almost routinely. Serum bactericidal titers in patients given penicillin alone have ranged from 1:256 to 1:2560, and the average duration of treatment for cured patients was 37 days, with a range of 12 to 49 days (20). Twenty-seven (87%) of 31 patients with *C. hominis* endocarditis, including all 4 patients with prosthetic heart valve involvement, were cured (20).

A successful outcome has been reported in 10 patients with *C. hominis* infection of prosthetic valves (8, 9). Of these, four underwent valve replacement for hemodynamic reasons. Treatment regimens ranged from ampicillin or ceftriaxone alone for 4 weeks to penicillin or ampicillin plus gentamicin for almost 6 weeks. In a review of 22 cases of infective endocarditis due to *C. hominis,* Robison et al. reported a bacteriologic cure in all but one patient, from whom *Enterococcus* species, not *C. hominis,* was recovered from vegetations on the valve at postmortem (13).

Alternative Regimens

There are few precedents for managing infection due to isolates resistant to penicillins or cephalosporins, or for treating patients unable to tolerate these antibiotics. In those with penicillin and cephalosporin allergies, aztreonam, fluoroquinolones, and trimethoprim-sulfamethoxazole are suggested as alternatives. Gentamicin alone for 6 weeks has been reported to be successful (2). Le Quellec et al. successfully treated endocarditis due to an unusually resistant isolate with rifampicin plus vancomycin, followed by rifampicin 600 mg twice daily together with amoxicillin-clavulanate 1 g intravenously 8-hourly (6). Vogt et al. used ciprofloxacin 200 mg twice daily for 5 weeks in two patients who relapsed while being treated with mezlocillin. The patient's serum was rapidly bactericidal for the organism during treatment with ciprofloxacin alone (18).

REFERENCES

1. Ben-Chetrit E, Nashif M, Levo Y. Infective endocarditis caused by uncommon bacteria. Scand J Infect Dis 1983;15:179–183.
2. Botha P, Venter M. *Cardiobacterium hominis* as a cause of bacterial endocarditis [Letter]. S Afr Med J 1996;86:91.
3. Francioli PB, Roussianos D, Glauser MP. *Cardiobacterium hominis* endocarditis manifesting as bacterial meningitis. Arch Intern Med 1983;143:1483–1484.
4. Geraci JE, Wilson WR. Endocarditis due to gram-negative bacteria: report of 56 cases. Mayo Clin Proc 1982;57:145–148.
5. Kiwan Y, Shubaiber H, Chungh T. *Cardiobacterium hominis* endocarditis. J Cardiovasc Surg 1989;30:281–283.
6. Le Quellec A, Bessis D, Perez C, Ciurana AJ. Endocarditis due to β-lactamase-producing *Cardiobacterium hominis* [Letter]. Clin Infect Dis 1994;19:994–995.
7. Lin BH-J, Vieco PT. Intracranial mycotic aneurysm in a patient with endocarditis caused by *Cardiobacterium hominis*. Can Assoc Radiol J 1995;46:40–42.
8. Marques MT, Barreira R, Almeida M, Gil V. *Cardiobacterium hominis* prosthetic valve endocarditis diagnosed in Portugal [Letter]. Ann Biol Clin 1995;53:299–300.
9. Meyer DJ, Gering DN. Favorable prognosis of patients with prosthetic valve endocarditis caused by gram-negative bacilli of the HACEK group. Am J Med 1988;85:104–107.
10. National Committee for Clinical Laboratory Standards. Methods for dilution antimicrobial susceptibility tests for bacteria that grow aerobically. 4th ed. Approved standard. NCCLS document M7-A4. Wayne, PA: NCCLS, 1997.
11. Rahal JJ Jr, Simberkoff MS. Bactericidal activity of chloramphenicol in endocarditis and meningitis [Abstract no. 5]. Program and abstracts of the 17th Interscience Conference on Antimicrobial Agents and Chemotherapy. Washington, DC: American Society for Microbiology, 1977.
12. Rechtman DJ, Nadler JP. Abdominal abscess due to *Cardiobacterium hominis* and *Clostridium bifermentans*. Rev Infect Dis 1991;13:418–419.
13. Robison WJ, Vitelli AS. Infectious endocarditis by *Cardiobacterium hominis*. South Med J 1985;78:1020–1021.
14. Savage DD, Kagen RL, Young NA, Horvath AE. *Cardiobacterium hominis* endocarditis: description of two patients and characterization of the organism. J Clin Microbiol 1977;5:75–80.
15. Slotnich IJ, Dougherty M. Further characterization of an unclassified group of bacteria causing endocarditis in man: *Cardiobacterium hominis* gen. et sp. nov. Antonie von Leeuwenhoek J Microbiol Serol 1964;30:261–272.
16. Taveras JM III, Campo R, Segal N, Urena PE, Lacayo L. Apparent culture-negative endocarditis of the prosthetic valve caused by *Cardiobacterium hominis*. South Med J 1993;86:1439–1440.
17. Tucker DN, Slotnick IJ, King EO. Endocarditis caused by a Pasteurella-like organism. Report of four cases. N Engl J Med 1962;267:913–916.
18. Vogt K, Klefisch F, Hahn H, Schmutzler H. Antibacterial efficacy of ciprofloxacin in a case of endocarditis due to *Cardiobacterium hominis*. Zentralbl Bakteriol 1994;281:80–84.
19. Wilson WR, Karchmer AW, Dajani AS, Taubert KA, Bayer A, Kaye D, Bisno AL, Ferrieri P, Shulman ST, Durack DT. Antibiotic treatment of adults with infective endocarditis due to streptococci, enterococci, staphylococci, and HACEK organisms. JAMA 1995;274:1706–1713.
20. Wormser GP, Bottone EJ. *Cardiobacterium hominis:* review of microbiologic and clinical features. Rev Infect Dis 1983;5:680–691.
21. Zehtner E, Seifert H, Petit M, Plum G, Peters G, Diehl V. Protrahierter verlauf einer Cardiobacterium hominis-endokarditis. Dtsch Med Wochenschr 1991;116:768–771.

Chromobacterium violaceum

Selwyn D. R. Lang and Arthur J. Morris

GENERAL DESCRIPTION
Microbiology and Epidemiology

Chromobacterium violaceum is a straight or slightly curved, facultatively anaerobic, motile, Gram-negative bacillus. It is catalase and oxidase positive and urease negative. Most strains produce a violet pigment, violacein, which is insoluble in water. This pigment confers a deep violet to black color to colonies. It is the only violet-colored pathogen of man. Not all strains are pigmented (18, 31), and some strains may produce pigmented and nonpigmented colonies on the same plate (5,

19, 37). The pigment interferes with interpretation of the oxidase test, but this may be overcome by testing a subculture grown under anaerobic conditions in which pigment production is suppressed (11). *C. violaceum* produces hydrogen cyanide, and a faint cyanide smell may be detectable.

C. violaceum was first described by Bergonzini 1881 (10). The first description of naturally occurring disease was made in 1905 by Wodey, who reported it caused fatal infection in water buffaloes in the Philippines (10). It has also been reported to cause infections in pigs and liver and lung abscesses in monkeys (10, 37, 38). The first recognized human cases occurred in Malaysia in 1927 and were reported in the 1950s (10, 13). Previous names have included *Bacillus violaceus, B. violaceus manilae,* and *C. janthinium.*

C. violaceum is a normal inhabitant of soil and water (21). It grows best at 20 to 37°C, and almost all infections have been acquired in tropical and subtropical regions between latitudes 35°N and 35°S. Most infections in the United States have occurred in the southeast, in Florida and Louisiana. Rare exceptions to acquisition in subtropical regions have been reported from the northeast (18, 31). Almost all cases in the United States have occurred in June through September; however, one case occurred in January (34). Other countries and regions where infection with *C. violaceum* has been recognized include Argentina, Brazil, India, Malaysia, Senegal, Singapore, Thailand, Vietnam, and Northern Australia.

In the past, it is likely that *C. violaceum* was isolated but not recognized as a pathogen (26, 30). In some cases, authors have specifically mentioned that the initial isolate was considered a contaminant (14, 37). All isolates of *C. violaceum* from clinical specimens should be regarded as clinically significant until proven otherwise.

Clinical Manifestations

Infection due to *C. violaceum* is uncommon; when it occurs, there is usually a clear history of exposure to water. Exposures have included wading in a pool of rain water (3); insect bites after wading through stagnant water in a drainage ditch (22); insect bites or wasp stings while in water (11, 20); scuba diving (14); trauma associated with either a fresh or salt water source (5, 9, 22), e.g., coral injury (23); skin abrasions from carrying damp carpet (8); and in four cases, near drowning (17, 18, 29, 32), which in two instances occurred 6 to 8 weeks before presentation (29, 32). Eye infections have followed inoculation of mud or muddy water (7, 28). *C. violaceum* should be included in the differential diagnosis of infections following exposure to water or soil.

Clinical disease often presents as a skin lesion or cellulitis, with or without regional or diffuse lymphadenopathy. Dissemination to multiple sites with a fulminant septicemic illness is common. The initial lesions and lymphadenopathy may be present for days or weeks before the systemic disease occurs. The illness may be clinically indistinguishable from melioidosis (17, 35). Abscesses may be present in single or multiple organs, including skin and spleen. The organs most commonly involved are lungs and liver (2, 4, 5, 7, 8, 10, 17, 19, 23, 24, 26, 28–30, 32, 34, 38), and provisional diagnoses have included amebic hepatitis (5, 30). Skin lesions may develop or progress despite appropriate antimicrobial therapy.

In addition to this typical syndrome of *C. violaceum* infection, other infections have included a breast abscess without a known environmental source (37), superinfection of a sacral decubitus ulcer in a patient with acute myelocytic leukemia (6), periorbital cellulitis (28), eye infections as the primary site of infection or as a complication of septicemia (7, 28), septic arthritis (25), osteomyelitis (36), neonatal meningitis (27), and urinary tract infection (30). Although *C. violaceum* was recovered from stool of two patients with diarrhea, its role as a cause of diarrhea is not established (30).

Several infections have been reported in patients with chronic granulomatous disease (7, 14, 15, 28, 31), which led to the suggestion that patients with *C. violaceum* infection should be evaluated for the presence of an underlying neutrophil dysfunction syndrome (14). Deficiency of polymorphonuclear leukocyte glucose-6-phosphate-dehydrogenase and neutrophil dysfunction was described in a 3-year-old who died of *C. violaceum* sepsis (16). Most of those investigated, however, will not have any detectable deficiency of host defenses.

In several patients, altered mental status led to lumbar puncture and cerebrospinal fluid (CSF) culture. In some, there was a CSF leukocytosis; *C. violaceum,* however, has only been recovered once from CSF (27). There are two reported cases of meningitis on gross examination at autopsy (28, 35), and in one of these patients, computed tomographic (CT) scanning before death showed three brain lesions (35).

Fatal relapse after discontinuing antimicrobial therapy has been reported in three patients. One was treated for more than 4 weeks with mezlocillin (MIC and MBC, 64 μg/mL) and gentamicin (MIC and MBC, 1 μg/mL), achieving a serum bactericidal titer of 1:16. Two weeks after finishing treatment, the patient developed clinical evidence of septic arthritis and died suddenly of septic shock due to *C. violaceum* (11). The second case was a child apparently cured by a 3-week course of gentamicin and imipenem, initially in combination with chloramphenicol. Two days after treatment was stopped, he relapsed, and blood cultures subsequently grew *C. violaceum* (22). He died 2 days later. In the third case, relapse occurred in a patient with multiple liver abscesses, 4 days after a 10-day course of chlortetracycline that had brought about clinical improvement and resolution of fever. A positive culture was obtained from a liver abscess the day before death (30). No specific comment is made in these three reports on the susceptibility patterns of the early and later isolates, so it is unknown if antimicrobial resistance played a part in these fatalities. In another report, one patient had two separate episodes of infection 20 months apart (20). The patient had an abnormality of leukocyte function.

SUSCEPTIBILITY IN VITRO

C. violaceum should be considered resistant to penicillin, amoxicillin, amoxicillin-clavulanate, ampicillin, cephalothin, cefamandole, and vancomycin (1, 4, 7–11, 19, 22, 23, 28, 31, 34, 35, 37). Although many authors repeat the statement that *C. violaceum* is always susceptible to chloramphenicol, tetracycline, and the aminoglycosides, this is not correct. Apart from the quinolones, imipenem, and doxycycline, susceptibility to all other agents varies and must be determined on an isolate-by-isolate basis. Disk susceptibility results can serve as a reliable preliminary guide, but for serious disease, selection of the best agent requires knowledge of MIC and possibly MBC data for the agents being considered for therapy for the particular isolate of *C. violaceum.*

Only one study has evaluated the in vitro activity of several antimicrobial agents against a collection of clinical isolates (1). In this study, 24 agents were tested against 11 strains (Table 1). The quinolones had the lowest MICs and were active against all isolates. All isolates were also susceptible to imipenem and doxycy-

TABLE 1 • **In Vitro Susceptibilities of *Chromobacterium violaceum***

Antibiotic	n	Range	MIC$_{50}$	MIC$_{90}$	Breakpoint[a]	(%) Susceptible	Ref
Mezlocillin	11	0.5–64	8	32	≤16	—	1
Piperacillin	11	4–64	16	32	≤16	—	1
Ticarcillin	11	2–128	64	64	≤16	—	1
Ticarcillin-clavulanate	11	0.5–128	32	64	≤16/2	—	1
Apalcillin	11	1–32	8	32	—	—	1
Cefamandole	11	≥128	≥128	≥128	≤8	0	1
Cefoperazone	3	≥128	NA[b]	NA	≤8	0	33
Cefotaxime	11	2–128	8	128	≤8	—	1
Cefotaxime	3	64–≥128	NA	NA	≤8	0	33
Cefotetan	11	2–64	16	32	≤16	—	1
Cefoxitin	11	2–128	16	128	≤8	—	1
Cefsulodin	3	≥128	NA	NA	—	—	33
Ceftazidime	3	≥128	NA	NA	≤8	0	33
Ceftizoxime	11	4–64	64	64	—	—	1
Ceftriaxone	11	0.5–>128	4	>128	≤8	—	1
Cephalothin	11	≥128	≥128	≥128	≤8	0	1
Moxalactam	3	≤0.06–0.5	NA	NA	≤8	100	33
Imipenem	11	0.5–4	2	4	≤4	100	1
Imipenem	3	4–64	NA	NA	≤4	—	33
Aztreonam	11	0.5–16	2	16	≤8	—	1
Aztreonam	3	32–≥128	NA	NA	≤8	0	33
Ciprofloxacin	11	≤0.008	≤0.008	≤0.008	≤1	100	1
Norfloxacin	11	≤0.008	≤0.008	≤0.008	—	—	1
Pefloxacin	11	≤0.008–0.032	0.016	0.016	—	—	1
Nalidixic acid	11	1–4	1	2	—	—	1
Amikacin	11	0.25–128	16	64	≤16	—	1
Amikacin	3	≥64	NA	NA	≤16	0	33
Gentamicin	11	≤0.016–16	2	4	≤4	—	1
Gentamicin	3	≥64	NA	NA	≤4	0	33
Tobramycin	11	0.063–32	4	16	≤4	—	1
Chloramphenicol	11	2–16	8	16	≤8	—	1
Trimethoprim-sulfamethoxazole[c]	11	≤0.016–8	0.5	4	≤2/38	—	1
Doxycycline	11	1–4	1	2	≤4	100	1
Rifampin	11	1–32	8	16	≤1	—	1
Vancomycin	11	≥128	≥128	≥128	≤4	0	1

Modified from references 1, 33.

[a] Current NCCLS interpretative standards for susceptibility (μg/mL).

[b] NA, not applicable.

[c] Trimethoprim-sulfamethoxazole tested in a ratio of 1:19. The concentration refers to the trimethoprim component.

cline. Gentamicin had the best activity, and with an MIC$_{90}$ of 4 μg/mL was 4 and 16 times more active than tobramycin and amikacin, respectively. Chloramphenicol and trimethoprim-sulfamethoxazole each inhibited at least 50% of the strains. Activity varied among the β-lactam agents tested. Addition of clavulanate did not improve the activity of ticarcillin. Moreover, time kill studies showed that addition of clavulanate decreased the killing activity of ticarcillin at subinhibitory concentrations. There was good correlation, 94%, between disk susceptibility results and broth microdilution, and only 17 of 286 determinations had discrepant results; 16 of these were minor errors in which one method produced a moderately susceptible result while the other produced a susceptible or resistant result (1).

Aldridge et al. also tested for the bactericidal activity of various agents by testing at 0.5, 1, and 4 times the MIC. Ciprofloxacin was the most bactericidal compound, followed by gentamicin, doxycycline, and ticarcillin (1). Mezlocillin and chloramphenicol were the least bactericidal.

A β-lactamase induction test was performed on one isolate and was positive (1). The same phenomenon was also observed in an isolate from a recently published case (23) (Paul S, Morris A, unpublished observation). These results suggest that strains of *C. violaceum* may have stably derepressed mutants that produce β-lactamase constitutively in large amounts. If this is so, therapy with extended-spectrum penicillins and late-generation cephalosporins may tend to select for resistant subpopulations. To date, emergence of resistance to ceftazidime and to carbenicillin has been reported in one patient each (35, 37), and resistance has emerged in vitro to mezlocillin in one isolate (1). Further studies are needed to determine if this type of β-lactamase is of clinical importance.

ANTIMICROBIAL THERAPY

C. violaceum infection has a high mortality. In a recent review of North American cases, there were 15 (65%) deaths among the 24 cases (22). Many of the patients who died, however, re-

TABLE 2 • Summary of Antimicrobial Therapy Used in Survivors of *Chromobacterium violaceum* Infection[a]

	Age	Sex	Disease	Initial Therapy	Main Therapy	Discharge Therapy	Comment	Ref
1	10	M	Skin ulcer, lymphadenopathy, orbital cellulitis	Nafcillin i.v., tobramycin i.v.	Nafcillin i.v., chloramphenicol i.v., carbenicillin i.v.	NS[b]	CGD[c]	7
2	35	M	Skin abscess, septicemia, liver abscesses	Flucloxacillin i.v., gentamicin i.v., metronidazole i.v	Chloramphenicol i.v. 12 days, gentamicin i.v. 26 days, imipenem i.v. 26 days	Ciprofloxacin 750 mg p.o. b.d. for 8 weeks	No immune defect found	8
3	15	M	Lymphadenopathy, bacteremia	Gentamicin i.v., chloramphenicol i.v., clindamycin i.v.	Gentamicin i.v. 3 weeks, chloramphenicol i.v. 3 weeks, then gentamicin i.v. 3 weeks, tetracycline p.o. 3 weeks	Sulfisoxazole p.o. daily, duration not stated	CGD	14
4	5	F	Skin pustules, cellulitis, lymphadenopathy		Tobramycin i.v. chloramphenicol	NS	CGD	15
5	56	M	Septicemia, skin pustules, liver abscesses	Amoxicillin i.v., gentamicin i.v., metronidazole i.v.	Chloramphenicol i.v., tetracycline, gentamicin i.v., cotrimoxazole[d], then gentamicin i.v., ciprofloxacin 4 weeks	Ciprofloxacin p.o. for 12 weeks	No immune deficit found	17
6	13	M	Skin ulcers	Penicillin i.v., gentamicin i.v.	Chloramphenicol 20 days cotrimoxazole 20 days	NS	Abnormal leukocyte function; second episode 20 months later, also successfully treated with 21 days of chloramphenicol and cotrimoxazole	20
7	27	M	Deep neck tissue infection	Amoxicillin-clavulanate i.v.	Chloramphenicol i.v. 6 days, amikacin i.v. 6 days, then ciprofloxacin i.v. 4 days, p.o. 3 days	Ciprofloxacin 750 mg p.o. b.d. for 10 weeks	Surgical debridement of deep neck tissue required	23
8	9 mo	F	Furuncles, septic arthritis	NS	NS	NS	Surgical debridement required	25
9	9	M	Skin abscess, orbital cellulitis	Nafcillin i.v., tobramycin i.v.	Carbenicillin i.v., chloramphenicol i.v.	NS	CGD	28
10	49	M	Skin lesions, septicemia, liver abscesses		Chloramphenicol 24 days, ticarcillin i.v. 24 days, gentamicin i.v. 24 days	Doxycycline p.o. for 2 weeks		29
11	17 mo	M	Pustule, lymphadenopathy		Chloramphenicol i.v.	Cotrimoxazole p.o. for at least 6 months	Surgical debridement performed; CGD	31
12	53	M	Pustules, liver abscesses	Cephalothin i.v., gentamicin i.v.	Chloramphenicol i.v., carbenicillin i.v., ampicillin i.v. all for ~ 3 weeks	Doxycycline p.o. duration NS		32
13	24	M	Liver abscesses	Erythromycin i.v.	Tobramycin i.v. ~ 4 weeks piperacillin i.v. ~ 4 weeks	Cotrimoxazole p.o. for 2 weeks	No immune deficit detected	34

continued

TABLE 2 • Summary of Antimicrobial Therapy Used in Survivors of *Chromobacterium violaceum* Infection[a]

	Age	Sex	Disease	Initial Therapy	Main Therapy	Discharge Therapy	Comment	Ref
14	3	F	Skin ulcer, cellulitis, popliteal mass		Gentamicin i.v., ceftazidime i.v., then gentamicin i.v., cotrimoxazole p.o.	NS	Ceftazidime susceptibility changed between initial and later isolates	35
15	3	M	Pustules, septicemia, osteomyelitis	Gentamicin i.v., ampicillin i.v.	Gentamicin i.v., ticarcillin i.v., cotrimoxazole, chloramphenicol	Cotrimoxazole p.o. duration NS		12, 36
16	17	F	Breast abscess	Methicillin i.v.	Carbenicillin i.v. ~ 11 days gentamicin i.v. 16 days	NS	Surgical drainage; carbenicillin susceptibility changed between initial and later isolates	37

[a] Where sufficient detail is given in the original report on the route and duration of therapy, this is provided. Initial therapy refers to empirical therapy given before *C. violaceum* was recovered. Main therapy refers to the agents used for all or most of the definitive course for *C. violaceum* infection.

[b] NS, not stated.

[c] CGD, the patient had chronic granulomatous disease.

[d] Cotrimoxazole, trimethoprim-sulfamethoxazole.

ceived antimicrobial therapy too late in the disease to influence outcome.

A summary of the 16 survivors of *C. violaceum* infection is given in Table 2. No details of antimicrobial therapy were provided for one survivor (25). One case has been reported twice (12, 36). Empirical therapy was initiated in 11 of the 16 patients and included an aminoglycoside in 8. Initial therapy included specific β-lactam cover for *Staphylococcus aureus* in 6 patients, reflecting the common presence of cutaneous infection. The most commonly used antimicrobial agent was chloramphenicol (12 patients), followed by various aminoglycosides (10 patients). The combination of chloramphenicol with an aminoglycoside was used in 7 survivors. Other agents used in combination with chloramphenicol were carbenicillin (3 patients) and trimethoprim-sulfamethoxazole (1 patient). Chloramphenicol was used as monotherapy in 1 patient (31). The 3 patients who did not receive chloramphenicol all received an aminoglycoside in combination with other agents: tobramycin and piperacillin; gentamicin, ceftazidime, and trimethoprim-sulfamethoxazole; and gentamicin and carbenicillin (Table 2).

Clinical experience thus favors the use of chloramphenicol and an aminoglycoside. In vitro data, however, show that neither agent has particularly good activity against *C. violaceum*. The time kill data of Aldridge et al. suggest that most of the killing activity of such a combination would be provided by the aminoglycoside (1). Many of the infections treated with the combination of chloramphenicol and an aminoglycoside occurred either before the quinolones were available or before their excellent activity against *C. violaceum* was known.

The best therapeutic regimen is unknown, and although we favor ciprofloxacin and gentamicin, the most frequently used combination in survivors has been chloramphenicol and an aminoglycoside. Ciprofloxacin and gentamicin was used as the main component of therapy in one patient (17). Given the severity of infection caused by this organism and the very low risk of side effects with this combination, we also recommend it for use in children.

Prolonged treatment may be necessary to manage disseminated infection and prevent fatal relapse. This perception may account for the high proportion of patients who received ongoing treatment after discharge from the hospital. Nine of 17 (53%) survivors were discharged on a course of oral antimicrobial therapy. The agents used have been ciprofloxacin, trimethoprim-sulfamethoxazole, doxycycline, and sulfisoxazole in three, three, two, and one patient respectively (Table 2). When the duration of therapy was explicitly stated, it ranged from 2 to 12 weeks. When ciprofloxacin was used it was continued for 8, 10, and 12 weeks (Table 2).

COMMENT

Because fatal relapse has occurred following clinical improvement or apparent cure and because lung or liver abscesses are commonly present, we recommend continuing oral therapy after discharge. The optimal duration of therapy is unknown, and although courses as short as 2 weeks have been used, we recommend the use of an oral agent to complete a total course of therapy of the order of 8 to 12 weeks. The initial therapeutic choice may be based on disk susceptibility results, but formal MIC testing is recommended to help determine a definitive treatment regimen.

REFERENCES

1. Aldridge KE, Valainis GT, Sanders CV. Comparison of the in vitro activity of ciprofloxacin and 24 other antimicrobial agents against clinical strains of *Chromobacterium violaceum*. Diagn Microbiol Infect Dis 1988;10:31–39.
2. Annapurna F, Reddy SVR, Kumari PL. Fatal infection by *Chromobacterium violaceum*: clinical and bacteriological study. Indian J Med Sci 1979;33:8–10.
3. Black ME, Shahan J. *Bacillus violaceus* infection in a human being. JAMA 1938;110:1270–1271.
4. Blereau RP. Septicemia and death caused by *Chromobacterium violaceum*. South Med J 1980;73:1093–1094.
5. Dauphinais RM, Robben GG. Fatal infection due to *Chromobacterium violaceum*. Am J Clin Pathol 1968;50:592–597.
6. Dreizen S, McCredie KB, Bodey GP, Keating MJ. Unusual mucocutaneous infections in immunosuppressed patients with leukemia—expansion of an earlier study. Postgrad Med 1986; 79:287–294.
7. Feldman RB, Stern GA, Hood CI. *Chromobacterium violaceum* infection of the eye: a report of two cases. Arch Ophthalmol 1984;102:711–713.
8. Georghiou PR, O'Kane GM, Siu S, Kemp RJ. Near-fatal septicaemia with *Chromobacterium violaceum*. Med J Aust 1989; 150:720–721.
9. Hassan H, Suntharalingam S, Dhillon KS. Fatal *Chromobacterium violaceum* septicaemia. Singapore Med J 1993;34: 456–458.
10. Johnson WM, DiSalvo AF, Steuer RR. Fatal *Chromobacterium violaceum* septicaemia. Am J Clin Pathol 1971;56:400–406.
11. Kaufman SC, Ceraso D, Schugurensky A. First case report from Argentina of fatal septicemia caused by *Chromobacterium violaceum*. J Clin Microbiol 1986;23:956–958.
12. Lee TS, Wright BD. Fulminating chromobacterium septicaemia presenting as respiratory distress syndrome. Thorax 1981; 36:557–559.
13. Lesslar JE. Cited in: Sneath PHA, Whelan JPF, Singh RB, Edwards D. Fatal infection by *Chromobacterium violaceum*. Lancet 1953;2:276–277.
14. Macher AM, Casale TB, Fauci AS. Chronic granulomatous disease of childhood and *Chromobacterium violaceum* infections in the southeastern United States. Ann Intern Med 1982;97:51–55.
15. Macher AM, Casale TB, Gallin JI, Boltansky H, Fauci AS. *Chromobacterium violaceum* infections and chronic granulomatous disease [Letter]. Ann Intern Med 1983;98:259.
16. Mamlock RJ, Mamlock V, Mills GC, Daeschner CW, Schmalstieg FC, Anderson DC. Glucose-6-phosphate dehydrogenase deficiency, neutrophil dysfunction and *Chromobacterium violaceum* sepsis. J Pediatr 1987;111:852–854.
17. Martin J, Brimacombe J. *Chromobacterium violaceum* septicaemia: the intensive care management of two cases. Anaesth Intensive Care 1992;20:88–90.
18. Myers J, Ragasa DA, Eisele C. *Chromobacterium violaceum* septicaemia in New Jersey. J Med Soc NJ 1992;79:212–213.
19. Ognibene AJ, Thomas E. Fatal infection due to *Chromobacterium violaceum* in Vietnam. Am J Clin Pathol 1970;54: 607–610.
20. Petrillo VF, Severo V, Santos MM, Edelweiss EL. Recurrent infection with *Chromobacterium violaceum*: first case report from South America. J Infect 1984;9:167–169.

21. Pitlik S, Berger SA, Huminer D. Nonenteric infections acquired through contact with water. Rev Infect Dis 1987;9:54–63.

22. Ponte R, Jenkins SG. Fatal *Chromobacterium violaceum* infections associated with exposure to stagnant waters. Pediatr Infect Dis J 1992;11:583–586.

23. Roberts SA, Morris AJ, McIvor N, Ellis-Pegler, R. Infection of the deep tissues of the neck by *Chromobacterium violaceum* in a traveller. Clin Infect Dis 1997;25:334–335.

24. Ruiz CJ. Multiple abscesses and death due to *Chromobacterium violaceum*—Florida. MMWR 1974;23:378.

25. Sagin DD, Tan PT, Dolkadir J. *Chromobacterium violaceum* septicaemia in Malaysia [Letter]. Singapore Med J 1994;35:426.

26. Schattenberg HJ, Harris WH. A definitive and unique occurrence of rapidly fatal infection caused by *Bacillus violaceus manilae*. JAMA 1941;117:2069–2070.

27. Shetty M, Venkatesh A, Shenoy S, Shivananda PG. *Chromobacterium violaceum* meningitis—a case report. Indian J Med Sci 1987;41:275.

28. Simo F, Reuman PD, Martinez FJ, Ayoub EM. *Chromobacterium violaceum* as a cause of periorbital cellulitis. Pediatr Infect Dis J 1984;3:561–563.

29. Sinnot JT, Yangco G, Feldman DH, Gunn RA. Chromobacteriosis—Florida. MMWR 1981;29:613–615.

30. Sneath PHA, Whelan JPE, Singh RB, Edwards D. Fatal infection by *Chromobacterium violaceum*. Lancet 1953;ii:276–277.

31. Sorenson RU, Jacobs MR, Shurin SB. *Chrombacterium violaceum* adenitis acquired in the northern United States as a complication of chronic granulomatous disease. Pediatr Infect Dis 1985;4:701–702.

32. Starr AJ, Cribbett LS, Poklepovic J, Friedman H, Ruffolo EH. *Chromobacterium violaceum* presenting as a surgical emergency. South Med J 1981;74:1137–1139.

33. Strandberg DA, Jorgensen JH, Drutz DJ. Activities of aztreonam and new cephalosporins against infrequently isolated gram-negative bacilli. Antimicrob Agents Chemother 1983;24:282–286.

34. Suarez AE, Wenokur B, Johnson JM, Saravolatz LD. Nonfatal chromobacterial sepsis. South Med J 1986;79:1146–1148.

35. Ti T-Y, Tan WC, Chong APY, Lee EH. Nonfatal and fatal infections caused by *Chromobacterium violaceum*. Clin Infect Dis 1993;17:505–507.

36. Tucker RE, Winter WG, Wilson HD. Osteomyelitis associated with *Chromobacterium violaceum* sepsis. J Bone Joint Surg 1979;61A:949–951.

37. Victorica B, Baer H, Ayoub EM. Successful treatment of systemic *Chromobacterium violaceum* infection. JAMA 1974;230:578–580.

38. Wilkey IS, McDonald A. A probable case of *Chromobacterium violaceum* infection in Australia. Med J Aust 1983;2:39–40.

Chryseobacterium Species

•

Selwyn D. R. Lang and Arthur J. Morris

GENERAL DESCRIPTION
Microbiology and Epidemiology

During the long and complex history of the genus *Flavobacterium,* most of its original members have been reclassified (8, 70, 79). The most recent change of clinical relevance is the transfer of two species to the new genus *Chryseobacterium* (79). *Chryseobacterium* spp. are obligatively aerobic, nonmotile, oxidase-positive, catalase-positive, glucose-oxidizing Gram-negative bacilli. They are slender slightly curved or straight rods, sometimes showing slight clubbing at the ends (41). Although the genus name *Chryseobacterium* refers to the production of yellow pigment, some strains, especially *C. meningosepticum,* are not pigmented or only weakly so (54, 58). The species of medical importance are *C. meningosepticum* (previously *F. meningosepticum* and CDC group IIa), *C. indologenes* (previously *F. indologenes* and CDC group IIb), and *C. odoratum*. The former two species are indole positive, the latter is not. In one study of biologic characteristics, all *C. meningosepticum* but not *C. indologenes* strains formed a diffusable yellow-green pigment at room temperature, whereas all *C. indologenes* but no *C. meningosepticum* strains had yellow to orange colonies at 48 h (58). Biochemical reactions separating the indole-positive species depend on the methods and reagents used (58). *Chryseobacterium odoratum* produces a fruity odor and until recently was in taxonomic limbo (8). It is now in the genus *myroides*, but the name chryseobacterium has been retained in this chapter.

Two main genomic groups, I and II (with group II having four subgroups II:1 to II:4) and 6 serotypes, A–F, have been described within *C. meningosepticum*. Serotype C is reported to account for 63% of neonatal infections (11). Otherwise, these divisions have no relevance for the type of infection, the possible source of infection, or choice of therapy. Where susceptibility results have been compared between genetic subgroups, considerable overlap in susceptibility has been found (15). Nevertheless, ribotyping is useful for showing strain relatedness within groups and between clinical isolates involved in nosocomial infection (21).

The natural habitats of *Chryseobacterium* spp. are soil,

plants, food, and environmental water (11, 59, 70). They can grow or remain viable in nonnutrient fluids and are reported resistant to common concentrations of chlorine in water (2, 61). Cutaneous infection has followed exposure to stagnant street water (13), and pneumonia has followed wading barefoot in muddy surface water (5).

Within hospitals, *Chryseobacterium* isolates, mostly *C. meningosepticum,* may colonize the respiratory tract of neonates (17, 31) and adult patients in intensive care (14). Epidemics have occurred in neonatal units (17, 26, 31). They have been recovered in a diverse array of moist, inanimate locations in hospitals, including disinfectants, peritoneal dialysis fluids, medication vials, respiratory equipment, flower vases, tap water, ice, spray heads, and scrub sinks.

Recovery of *C. meningosepticum* should raise the possibility of an environmental source. The occurrence of two or more infections should prompt a search for a common source. Several investigations have identified a source or a faulty process and thereby prevented further infections; e.g., a faulty drain (17), contaminated chlorhexidine solution (22), water sources in a cardiothoracic operating room (9), and inadequate processing of nebulizer tubing (61). The organism has been recovered from hose water used to extinguish a burning child who subsequently developed sepsis (69). On occasion, widespread possible sources of infection have been found in washbasins, sinks, suction apparatus and air-conditioning humidifiers (56). Disappointingly, many investigations have not identified a source (12, 14, 51, 72, 83). Environmental *Chryseobacterium* spp. isolates should be typed to show their relatedness to the outbreak strain to ensure that the actual source has been identified.

Clinical Manifestations of *C. meningosepticum*

C. meningosepticum accounts for 1 to 2% of Gram-negative nonfermentative bacilli isolated in microbiologic cultures (11, 34). There are only 323 reports of positive cultures in the literature, of which approximately 59% represented true infection, and over 60% of these affected infants less than 3 months of age (11).

C. meningosepticum is best known for causing severe meningitis in premature and newborn infants (17, 26, 30, 40, 45, 49, 51, 60, 77, 83). Ventriculitis is always present (45). The mortality exceeds 50% (11), and the morbidity in survivors (e.g., hydrocephalus) is also high (11, 17, 44, 49, 51, 60, 63, 83): 84% of those with reported neonatal infection due to *C. meningosepticum* have meningitis; 13%, sepsis; and 3%, pneumonia (11).

In contrast to the predominance of meningitis among neonatal infections, pneumonia (40%) is the most common type of *C. meningosepticum* infection in the postneonatal period, followed by sepsis (24%), meningitis (18%), and others (18%) (11). Among the 68 cases reported in the literature, 32 of 50 (64%) were reported to be immunocompromised, and 16 of 55 died, giving an overall case fatality rate of 29% (11). Most of these infections were hospital acquired, but community-acquired infection with *C. meningosepticum* is also reported (2, 5, 13, 74, 78).

The various infections reported due to *C. meningosepticum* include bacteremia (16, 29, 32, 61); bacteremia following operations (9, 56) or polypectomy (46); possible relapsing Hickman catheter–related sepsis (64); endophthalmitis (47, 67); community-acquired pneumonia (5); pneumonia in adults, children, infants, and neonates in intensive care units (14, 17, 61, 75, 76); intraabdominal abscess (61); peritonitis complicating continuous ambulatory peritoneal dialysis (42, 53); native and prosthetic endocarditis (38, 66, 68, 84); adult meningitis (32, 41, 43, 44, 51, 52, 63); and meningitis following head and neck surgery (7, 18, 29). Cutaneous infection is rare but may occur with bacteremia (2) or without (13) or follow human or animal bites (27).

Many adults with severe infection have been immunocompromised by a range of underlying conditions including carcinoma, tuberculosis, leukemia, aplastic anemia, or congenital immunodeficiency (43, 44, 46, 52, 63, 72). In adults without significant underlying disease, the prognosis is much better; for example, in one study in which bacteremia followed the injection of contaminated medicine during surgery, all patients improved without antimicrobial therapy with activity against *C. meningosepticum* (56). Meningitis following head and neck surgery in immunocompetent adults also has a good prognosis (7, 18, 29).

SUSCEPTIBILITY IN VITRO

Chryseobacterium species have an unusual susceptibility pattern in that they are almost always resistant to agents commonly chosen to treat aerobic Gram-negative bacilli. They are usually resistant to aminoglycosides and β-lactams, including antipseudomonal penicillins and late-generation cephalosporins. All isolates tested have produced a β-lactamase (4, 10). There is some evidence that the β-lactamase of these species is a metallo-β-lactamase (10), which is supported by the resistance of the genus to carbapenems (10, 12, 35, 39, 64, 73). Although addition of clavulanate appears to confer little advantage over ticarcillin alone (39), amoxicillin-clavulanate was significantly more active than ampicillin (27). *Chryseobacterium* spp. are exceptional among aerobic Gram-negative bacilli in that vancomycin is sometimes clinically effective.

In the study that determined MICs for the greatest number of isolates (100), combining *Chryseobacterium* spp. and *C. odoratum,* none of the antibiotics tested had MIC_{90}s greater than its susceptibility breakpoint. Only minocycline and piperacillin had MIC_{50}s exceeding the breakpoint, although ciprofloxacin and ofloxacin came close to this (35). These findings are supported by consistent MICs obtained in two smaller studies (39, 82) (Table 1).

Other investigators (1, 12, 15, 23, 48, 64, 73) have reported MICs for *C. meningosepticum,* the most frequently pathogenic *Chryseobacterium* spp. (Table 2). The most consistently active of the non–β-lactam antibiotics were rifampicin (range MIC, 0.2–3.1 μg/mL; breakpoints, ≤1, ≥4 μg/mL), trimethoprim-sulfamethoxazole (≤.0.15–>6.4; ≤2, ≥8), minocycline (0.5–4; ≤4, ≥16), doxycycline (1–32; ≤4, ≥16), ofloxacin (0.06–4; ≤2, ≥8), ciprofloxacin (0.1–6.25; ≤1, ≥4), teicoplanin (8–32; ≤8, ≥32), vancomycin (3.1–50; ≤4, ≥32). Clindamycin (range MIC 0.025–16 μg/mL, breakpoints ≤0.5, ≥4 μg/mL) was more active than erythromycin (0.1–200

TABLE 1 • In vitro susceptibilities of *Chryseobacterium* species

Antibiotic	n	Range	MIC$_{50}$	MIC$_{90}$	Breakpoint[a]	% Susceptible	Ref
Gentamicin	19	4->64	>64	>64	≤4		39[b]
Gentamicin	28	32->128	64	>128	≤4	0	1[c]
Cefazolin	28	128->128	128	>128	≤8	0	1
Cefmenoxime	22	6.25->100	100	>100	—	—	82[d]
Cefotaxime	19	4->64	64	>64	≤8	—	39
Cefoxitin	28	4–64	8	16	≤8	—	1
Cefsulodin	22	100->100	>100	>100	—	—	82
Ceftazidime	22	6.25->100	>100	>100	≤8	—	82
Ceftazidime	19	1->64	>64	>64	≤8	—	39
Cephalothin	28	128->128	>128	>128	≤8	0	1
Aztreonam	19	>64	>64	>64	≤8	—	39
Imipenem	19	2->16	>16	>16	≤4	—	39
Meropenem	19	2->16	16	>16	—	—	39
Tetracycline	28	16–64	32	64	≤4	0	1
Ampicillin	28	64->128	>128	>128	—	—	1
Piperacillin	19	≤2–256	64	128	≤16	—	39
Ticarcillin	19	32->256	256	>256	≤16	—	39
Ticarcillin-clavulanate	19	8->256	128	>256	≤16/2	—	39
E1040	22	0.78->100	50	>100	—	—	82
Ciprofloxacin	19	0.25->8	1	4	≤1	—	39
Rifampicin	28	0.25–2	1	2	≤1	—	1
Erythromycin	28	32->128	128	>128	≤0.5	0	1
Chloramphenicol	28	64–128	128	128	≤8	0	1
Clindamycin	28	0.5–8	4	8	≤0.5	—	1
Trimethoprim-sulfamethoxazole[e]	28	0.15–1.25	0.62	1.25	≤2/38	100	1
Sulfamethoxazole	28	32–128	128	128	—	—	1
Vancomycin	28	8–16	16	16	≤4	0	1

Modified from references 1, 39, 82.

[a] Current NCCLS interpretive standards for susceptibility (μg/mL) (55).

[b] The 19 isolates tested were *C. meningosepticum* (10), *C. indologenes* (8), and one unspeciated.

[c] The 28 isolates tested were *C. meningosepticum* (6) and other species (22).

[d] No information provided on the species tested.

[e] Trimethoprim-sulfamethoxazole tested in a ratio of 1:19. Concentration refers to the trimethoprim component.

μg/mL, ≤0.5, ≥8). With the exception of clarithromycin (Table 2), activity of the newer macrolides against *C. meningosepticum* has not been reported. Minocycline and doxycycline were much more active than tetracycline. Only the occasional isolate was susceptible to chloramphenicol.

Piperacillin was the most active of the penicillins. In one series of 52 isolates, all were susceptible (range MIC, 1.6–12.5 μg/mL; breakpoints, ≤16, ≥128 μg/mL) (15). However, others found isolates of intermediate susceptibility (23) or resistant (12). Of the cephalosporins, cefoperazone, cefotaxime, ceftrizoxime, and ceftriaxone showed similar activity, with some isolates highly susceptible and many of intermediate susceptibility. Ceftazidime, and the first- and second-generation cephalosporins were generally less active. Few isolates have been tested against the monobactam aztreonam (12, 73) or against carbapenems (12, 15, 64, 73), but neither of these groups of β-lactams appear particularly promising.

In a study of seven distinct isolates of *C. meningosepticum*, clavulanic acid was shown to lower the MICs of β-lactam antibiotics to a varying extent, ranging from 2- to 64-fold, with the greatest reduction with cephalosporins, particularly ceftazidime (62). Clavulanic acid itself had an MIC of 8 mg/L for all seven isolates. None of the strains appeared to harbor plasmids, but a broad-substrate, constitutive, chromosomal β-lactamase was detected, probably a class IV enzyme of the Sykes and Matthew classification. The importance of this enzyme for resistance to β-lactam antibiotics remains uncertain (62). There appear to be no studies that compare other β-lactam/β-lactamase inhibitor combinations with the β-lactam antibiotic alone. Piperacillin-tazobactam showed poor activity against nine isolates tested (64) (Table 2). Eight of 12 isolates were reported susceptible to cefoperazone-sulbactam (25).

Although some authors have reported isolates of *Chryseobacterium* species susceptible to, for example, erythromycin (4, 45, 63, 84) and amikacin, the MICs or zones of inhibition do not match quoted current NCCLS breakpoints for susceptibility; e.g., an amikacin MIC of 80 μg/mL, well above the current breakpoint of ≤16 μg/mL (29, 55). This inappropriate statement regarding susceptibility was borne out by therapeutic failure with amikacin (29). Thus statements in the older literature about the susceptibility of single isolates should be regarded with skepticism, particularly if the comment has been based on disk-testing results and is at odds with the data contained in Tables 1–4.

TABLE 2 • **In Vitro Susceptibilities of *Chryseobacterium meningosepticum***

Antibiotic	n	Range	MIC$_{50}$	MIC$_{90}$	Breakpoint[a]	% Susceptible	Ref
Amikacin	9	≤2–>64	64	>4	≤16	22	64
Amikacin	18	≥64	NS[b]	NS	≤16	0	12
Amikacin	10	≥64	>64	NS	≤16	0	23
Amikacin	8	8–64	32	32	≤16	—	73
Amikacin	41	16–>128	64	>128	≤16	—	19
Gentamicin	9	1–>16	>16	>16	≤4	11	64
Gentamicin	18	2–≥16	NS	NS	≤4	6	12
Gentamicin	10	16–>64	>64	NS	≤4	0	23
Gentamicin	8	16–32	16	16	≤4	0	73
Gentamicin	41	8–>128	64	>128	≤4	0	19
Kanamycin	10	>64	>64	NS	≤16	0	23
Netilmicin	52	6.25–>200	200	>200	≤8	—	15
Netilmicin	10	>64	>64	NS	≤8	0	23
Netilmicin	41	32–>128	>128	>128	≤8	0	19
Streptomycin	10	≥64	>64	NS	—	—	23
Tobramycin	18	8–≥16	NS	NS	≤4	0	12
Tobramycin	10	>64	>64	NS	≤4	0	23
Ampicillin	18	16–≥32	NS	NS	—	—	12
Ampicillin	52	2–>200	100	200	—	—	15
Ampicillin	10	64–>128	128	NS	—	—	23
Mecillinam	10	>128	>128	NS	—	—	23
Penicillin	52	6.25–100	50	50	—	—	15
Penicillin	10	16–>128	64	NS	—	—	23
Apalcillin[c]	9	8–128	32	32	—	—	64
Azlocillin	10	32–64	64	NS	—	—	23
Carbenicillin	10	>128	>128	NS	≤16	0	23
Mezlocillin	18	≤16–≥256	NS	NS	≤16	67	12
Mezlocillin	10	8–>128	32	NS	≤16	—	23
Piperacillin	18	≤8–≥256	NS	NS	≤16	28	12
Piperacillin	52	1.6–12.5	6.25	12.5	≤16	100	15
Piperacillin	10	8–128	16	NS	≤16	—	23
Piperacillin	41	1–32	4	8	≤16	—	19
Piperacillin-tazobactam	9	2–>128	64	64	≤16/4	22	64
Ticarcillin	18	≤16–≥256	NS	NS	≤16	22	12
Ticarcillin	10	>128	>128	NS	≤16	0	23
Cefamandole	10	32–128	64	NS	≤8	0	23
Cefazolin	18	≥32	NS	NS	≤8	0	12
Cefazolin	10	≥128	>128	NS	≤8	0	23
Cefepime	12	0.03–>256	8	>256	≤8	—	48
Cefoperazone	8	16–32	32	32	≤16	—	73
Cefoperazone	41	16–>128	32	64	≤16	—	19
Cefotaxime	12	0.015–>256	64	>256	≤8	—	48
Cefotaxime	52	1.6–50	12.5	25	≤8	—	15
Cefotaxime	10	16–64	32	NS	≤8	0	23
Cefotaxime	8	16–64	16	32	≤8	0	73
Cefotaxime	41	16–>128	32	128	≤8	0	19
Cefoxitin	18	8–≥32	NS	NS	≤8	11	12
Cefoxitin	10	4–64	8	NS	≤8	—	23
Cefsulodin	8	≥128	≥128	≥128	—	—	73
Ceftazidime	12	0.12–>256	32	>256	≤8	—	48
Ceftazidime	18	≤8–≥32	NS	NS	≤8	6	12
Ceftazidime	52	6.25–200	50	100	≤8	—	15
Ceftazidime	8	≥128	≥128	≥128	≤8	0	73
Ceftazidime	41	2–>128	>128	>128	≤8	—	19
Ceftizoxime	8	2–32	4	16	≤8	—	73
Ceftriaxone	12	0.03–>256	64	>256	≤8	—	48
Ceftriaxone	18	16–≥64	NS	NS	≤8	0	12
Ceftriaxone	41	16–>128	64	128	≤8	0	19
Cefuroxime	52	25–>200	200	>200	≤8	0	15
Cefuroxime	10	≥128	≥128	NS	≤8	0	23

continued

TABLE 2 • In Vitro Susceptibilities of *Chryseobacterium meningosepticum*

Antibiotic	n	Range	MIC$_{50}$	MIC$_{90}$	Breakpoint[a]	% Susceptible	Ref
Cephalothin	52	25–>200	200	>200	≤8	0	15
Cephalothin	10	64–>128	128	NS	≤8	0	23
Cephalothin	41	>128–>128	>128	>128	≤8	0	19
Moxalactam	10	16–>128	64	NS	≤8	0	23
Moxalactam	8	16–64	16	32	≤8	0	73
Moxalactam	41	8–>128	64	128	≤8	—	19
Aztreonam	18	≤8–≥32	NS	NS	≤8	11	12
Aztreonam	8	≥128	≥128	≥128	≤8	0	73
Aztreonam	41	128–>128	>128	>128	≤8	0	19
Biapenem	9	4–8	8	8	—	—	64
Imipenem	18	≥16	NS	NS	≤4	0	12
Imipenem	8	16–32	16	32	≤4	0	73
Imipenem	41	1–128	64	64	≤4	—	19
Meropenem	9	8–>8	8	>8	—	—	64
Thienamycin	52	1.6–50	25	50	—	—	15
Chloramphenicol	52	6.25–>200	50	100	≤8	—	15
Chloramphenicol	10	32≥64	64	NS	≤8	0	23
Clindamycin	9	0.5–8	4	8	≤0.5	11	64
Clindamycin	52	0.025–3.1	0.8	3.1	≤0.5	—	15
Clindamycin	10	0.5–16	1	NS	≤0.5	—	23
Ciprofloxacin	9	0.5–2	1	2	≤1	67	64
Ciprofloxacin	18	<0.5–2	NS	NS	≤1	94	12
Ciprofloxacin	52	0.1–6.25	0.8	3.1	≤1	—	15
Ciprofloxacin	41	0.5–16	1	8	≤1	—	19
Clinafloxacin	9	0.12–1	0.25	0.5	—	—	64
DU-6859a	9	1–>4	2	>4	—	—	64
Ofloxacin	9	0.06–0.25	0.25	0.25	≤2	100	64
Ofloxacin	18	≤1–4	NS	NS	≤2	83	12
Ofloxacin	41	1–8	2	4	≤2	—	19
Colistin	10	>64	>64	NS	—	—	23
Trimethoprim-sulfamethoxazole[d]	18	≤0.5–4	NS	NS	≤2/38	72	12
Trimethoprim-sulfamethoxazole	10	3.2–>6.4	>6.4	NS	≤2/38	0	23
Trimethoprim	41	1–>16	8	>16	—	—	19
Erythromycin	52	0.1–200	0.8	3.1	≤0.5	—	15
Erythromycin	10	4–32	8	NS	≤0.5	0	23
Erythromycin	41	8–>128	16	>128	≤0.5	0	19
Clarithromycin	9	1.5–16	6	8	≤2	11	64
Everninomicin	9	2–8	2	2	—	—	64
Fusidic acid	52	3.1–>200	100	>200	—	—	15
Rifampicin	52	0.2–3.1	0.8	3.1	≤1	—	15
Rifampicin	9	0.5–1	1	1	≤1	100	64
Doxycycline	9	1–16	2	4	≤4	89	64
Doxycycline	10	1–32	4	NS	≤4	—	23
Minocycline	10	0.5–4	1	NS	≤4	100	23
Minocycline	41	1–8	2	4	≤4	—	19
Tetracycline	52	25–200	100	100	≤4	—	15
Tetracycline	10	32–>64	64	NS	≤4	0	23
Vancomycin	9	8–32	16	16	≤4	0	64
Vancomycin	52	3.1–50	12.5	50	≤4	—	15
Vancomycin	10	8–32	16	NS	≤4	0	23
Vancomycin	41	4–32	16	16	≤4	—	19
Teicoplanin	9	8–32	8	16	≤8	56	64
Teicoplanin	41	8–64	16	32	≤8	—	19

Modified from references 12, 15, 19, 23, 48, 64, 73.

[a]Current NCCLS interpretive standards for susceptibility (μg/mL) (55).

[b]NS, not stated.

[c]Apalcillin in combinations with a β-lactamase inhibitor, Ro48–1220 (4 μg/mL).

[d]Trimethoprim-sulfamethoxazole tested in a ratio of 1:19. Concentration refers to the trimethoprim component.

Relatively few isolates of *C. indologenes* (Table 3) and *F. odoratum* (Table 4) are reported as series tested against various antibiotics. Overall, the pattern of resistance is similar to that of *C. meningosepticum*. In the case of *C. indologenes*, ceftazidime appears to be relatively active, although the reason is not certain. *C. odoratum* has been shown to produce a β-lactamase distinct from that produced by *C. meningosepticum* (65). It is exceptionally resistant to almost all antibiotics reported to have been tested, with the exceptions of minocycline (19) and doxycycline (23). We are not aware of any studies for synergy between unrelated antibiotics against *C. meningosepticum, C. indologenes,* or *C. odoratum.*

Correlation between Disk or E-Test Testing and MIC Results

An early study compared disk-diffusion testing with agar dilution (1). The data showed that for many agents, the interpretive disk zone diameters did not accurately predict the susceptibility of *Chryseobacterium* spp. as determined by the agar dilution method (1). For example, 3 strains tested susceptible to erythromycin by disk testing when the MICs were 32 to 128 μg/mL, and a further 11 tested in the intermediate range by disk when the MICs were 32 μg/mL or higher; for gentamicin, all 28 were resistant (MICs >32 μg/mL), but 2 tested susceptible and 13 were intermediate by disk testing; and although all vancomycin MICs were 8 to 16 μg/mL, all 28 tested susceptible, with zones of 12 mm or more, by disk testing. These results and those of others have led to the recommendation that the MIC should be measured directly, to avoid very major and major errors in reporting *Chryseobacterium* susceptibility results (1, 19, 80, 81, 85).

One study evaluated 100 isolates and compared the MIC results from agar dilution testing with E-test MICs (35). Compared with the agar dilution method, the E-test produced higher piperacillin, cefotaxime, and amikacin MICs for 43 to 56% of isolates and lower ofloxacin and ciprofloxacin MICs for 26% of isolates for each quinolone. For significant percentages of isolates, the E-test MICs of ceftazidime (36%), cefotaxime (46%), and amikacin (48%) exceeded the highest concentration by the agar dilution method. The poorest correlation between methods was found for piperacillin, with only 84% agreement (MICs within one $\log_2$ dilution). For piperacillin, 56% of the isolates tested had higher E-test MICs. When the NCCLS breakpoint for piperacillin susceptibility was applied, there were 17% major errors, that is, a susceptible isolate classified as resistant. The authors suggest that any E-test piperacillin MIC between 16 and 128 μg/mL should be tested by another procedure (35).

Chryseobacterium indologenes

The largest series of *C. indologenes* bacteremia was reported from Taiwan (36). Twelve episodes were reported, six patients had ventilator-associated pneumonia, two patients had primary bacteremia, and one patient each had pyonephrosis, peritonitis, biliary tract infection, and surgical wound infection. Five patients (42%) had malignancies, and three (25%) had multiple burns. Polymicrobial bacteremia was common (67%), and the two deaths (17%) were in this group. In a nonfatal case of bacteremia in a patient with advanced carcinoma of the breast, the portal of entry was assumed to be an intravenous line or an open eroded wound (71). Peritonitis due to *C. indologenes* was reported in a patient on CAPD who was receiving treatment with ciprofloxacin, to which the organism was susceptible in vitro (3).

Chryseobacterium odoratum

F. odoratum is uncommonly encountered in the clinical laboratory and still less commonly pathogenic. Of 24 isolates identified over a decade at the Central Public Health Laboratory, Colindale, London, 2 from amputation stumps and 3 from urine were possibly, but not definitely, opportunistic pathogens (33). Rare instances of serious infection caused by *C. odoratum* are cellulitis and bacteremia in a patient on prednisone (6), bacteremic necrotizing fasciitis in a patient with hepatitis B virus and related to cirrhosis (37), right-sided bacterial endocarditis in a patient on long-term hemodialysis (24), and ventriculitis in a 6-week-old infant (50).

ANTIMICROBIAL THERAPY

Because almost all strains of *C. meningosepticum, C. indologenes,* and *C. odoratum* are resistant to agents commonly used to treat Gram-negative bacillary infections, discussion can be limited to a short list of agents that have been used effectively or show promise on the basis of in vitro testing. The most challenging type of infection (and one not uncommonly due to *C. meningosepticum*) is meningitis. Vancomycin was the most effective agent used in an early outbreak, including nine cases of neonatal meningitis (26). Four of six patients given vancomycin intravenously, intrathecally, or both survived, whereas all three given other regimens died. A neonate with *C. meningosepticum* meningitis given intravenous vancomycin (MIC/MBC, 12.5 μg/mL) became afebrile within 24 h, and her cerebrospinal fluid (CSF) sterile within 3 days (30). She had previously failed to respond to treatment with several other antibiotics, including erythromycin (MIC/MBC, 1.5/>100 μg/mL). The bactericidal activity of vancomycin for this organism is likely to be relevant to a successful outcome in meningitis. However, vancomycin penetrates CSF somewhat erratically; hence, intrathecal and intraventricular administration have been advocated (34).

Rifampicin is probably the single most reliably active agent against *C. meningosepticum* (Table 2). Rifampicin was used as treatment in the only substantial series of neonatal *C. meningosepticum* meningitis, with a uniformly good outcome (45). All seven patients were treated with rifampicin (20 mg/kg 12-hourly intramuscularly plus 2–5 mg intraventricularly each day), and all survived. With intramuscular dosing alone, penetration into the ventricular fluid was poor (0.5–1.5 μg/mL), but 20 to 24 h after intraventricular dosing, levels ranged from 3.1 to 85.5 μg/mL. A note of caution: in one case, the organism became resistant to rifampicin after 3 days. This patient was subsequently treated with intraventricular

TABLE 3 • In Vitro Susceptibilities of *Chryseobacterium indologenes*

Antibiotic	n	Range	MIC$_{50}$	MIC$_{90}$	Breakpoint[a]	% Susceptible	Ref
Amikacin	12	32->128	64	>128	≤16	0	36
Amikacin	10	8–64	16	NS[b]	≤16	—	23
Amikacin	4	2–32	8	32	≤16	—	73
Amikacin	59	32–128	128	>128	≤16	0	19
Gentamicin	12	8->128	64	>128	≤4	0	36
Gentamicin	10	2–16	8	NS	≤4	—	23
Gentamicin	4	1–16	4	16	≤4	—	73
Gentamicin	59	8->128	128	>128	≤4	0	19
Kanamycin	10	≥64	≥64	NS	≤16	0	23
Netilmicin	12	64->128	>128	>128	≤8	0	36
Netilmicin	10	8–64	16	NS	≤8	—	23
Netilmicin	59	16->128	>128	>128	≤8	0	19
Streptomycin	10	2->64	8	NS	—	—	23
Tobramycin	10	≥64	≥64	NS	≤4	0	23
Penicillin	18	2->128	>128	>128	—	—	27
Penicillin	10	4–128	8	NS	—	—	23
Ampicillin	10	8->128	16	NS	—	—	23
Ampicillin	18	1->128	>128	>128	—	—	27
Amoxicillin-clavulanate	18	1–32	32	32	≤8/4	11	27
Mecillinam	10	64->128	128	NS	—	—	23
Azlocillin	10	0.5–16	2	NS	—	—	23
Carbenicillin	10	32->128	32	NS	≤16	0	23
Mezlocillin	10	1–8	4	NS	≤16	100	23
Piperacillin	12	1–8	2	4	≤16	100	36
Piperacillin	10	0.25–4	1	NS	≤16	100	23
Piperacillin	59	1->128	4	128	≤16	—	19
Ticarcillin	10	16->128	32	NS	≤16	—	23
Cefadroxyl	18	8->128	>128	>128	—	—	27
Cefamandole	10	64->128	128	NS	≤8	0	23
Cefazolin	10	32->128	64	NS	≤8	0	23
Cefoperazone	12	4->128	8	16	≤16	92	36
Cefoperazone	4	2–8	4	8	≤16	100	73
Cefoperazone	59	2->128	16	>128	≤16	—	19
Cefotaxime	12	16->128	32	64	≤8	0	36
Cefotaxime	10	2–32	8	NS	≤8	—	23
Cefotaxime	4	1–32	16	32	≤8	—	73
Cefotaxime	59	4->128	64	>128	≤8	—	19
Cefoxitin	10	4–64	8	NS	—	≤8	23
Cefsulodin	4	≥128	≥128	≥128	—	—	73
Ceftazidime	12	2->128	8	8	≤8	92	36
Ceftazidime	4	0.5–4	2	4	≤8	100	73
Ceftazidime	59	2->128	8	32	≤8	—	19
Ceftizoxime	4	4–32	16	32	≤8	—	73
Ceftriaxone	12	16->128	32	64	≤8	0	36
Ceftriaxone	59	16->128	32	>128	≤8	0	19
Cefuroxime	18	1->128	>128	>128	≤8	6	27
Cefuroxime	10	16->128	32	NS	≤8	0	23
Cephalexin	18	8->128	>128	>128	—	—	27
Cephalothin	12	32->128	>128	>128	≤8	0	36
Cephalothin	10	16->128	64	NS	≤8	0	23
Cephalothin	59	32->128	>128	>128	≤8	0	19
Moxalactam	12	32->128	64	>128	≤8	0	36
Moxalactam	10	16–64	16	NS	≤8	0	23
Moxalactam	4	8–32	8	32	≤8	—	73
Moxalactam	59	32->128	64	128	≤8	0	19
Aztreonam	12	>128	>128	>128	≤8	0	36
Aztreonam	4	≥128	≥128	≥128	≤8	0	73
Aztreonam	59	>128	>128	>128	≤8	0	19
Imipenem	12	32->128	64	64	≤4	0	36
Imipenem	4	4–32	4	32	≤4	—	73
Imipenem	59	1->128	64	>128	≤4	—	19
Chloramphenicol	10	32->64	32	NS	≤8	0	23
Clindamycin	12	4	4	4	≤0.5	0	36

continued

TABLE 3 • **In Vitro Susceptibilities of *Chryseobacterium indologenes***

Antibiotic	n	Range	MIC$_{50}$	MIC$_{90}$	Breakpoint[a]	% Susceptible	Ref
Clindamycin	10	0.13–>64	0.5	NS	≤0.5	—	23
Ciprofloxacin	12	0.5–128	1	32	≤1	67	36
Ciprofloxacin	18	0.5–1	0.5	0.5	≤1	100	27
Ciprofloxacin	59	0.25–128	2	128	≤1	—	19
Enoxacin	18	0.5–4	1	2	≤2	94	27
Ofloxacin	12	2–64	2	32	≤2	50	36
Ofloxacin	18	0.25–2	0.25	1	≤2	100	27
Ofloxacin	59	0.5–64	8	64	≤2	—	19
Trimethoprim-sulfamethoxazole[c]	12	0.5–16	2	16	≤2/38	50	36
Trimethoprim-sulfamethoxazole	10	0.2–1.6	0.4	NS	≤2/38	100	23
Trimethoprim	59	0.25–16	4	16	—	—	19
Erythromycin	12	64–>128	>128	>128	≤0.5	0	36
Erythromycin	10	1–16	2	NS	≤0.5	0	23
Erythromycin	59	8–>128	128	>128	≤0.5	0	19
Doxycycline	10	1–8	4	NS	≤4	—	23
Minocycline	12	2–16	4	4	≤4	92	36
Minocycline	10	1–4	1	NS	≤4	100	23
Minocycline	59	1–16	4	8	≤4	—	19
Tetracycline	18	4–32	16	32	≤4	29	27
Tetracycline	10	4–32	16	NS	≤4	—	23
Vancomycin	12	2–128	16	16	≤4	8	36
Vancomycin	10	16–>64	16	NS	≤4	0	23
Vancomycin	59	2–>128	16	16	≤4	—	19
Teicoplanin	12	32–64	32	64	≤8	0	36
Teicoplanin	59	16–>128	32	32	≤8	0	19
Colistin	10	>64	>64	NS	—	—	23

Modified from references 19, 23, 27, 36, 73.

[a]Current NCCLS interpretive standards for susceptibility (μg/mL) (55).

[b]NS, not stated.

[c]Trimethoprim-sulfamethoxazole tested in a combination of 1:19. Concentration refers to the trimethoprim component.

erythromycin and it took 10 days for the CSF to become sterile, versus 2 to 6 days for the other six patients.

Oral rifampicin alone (10 mg/kg 12 hourly) achieved prompt CSF sterilization in an infant whose CSF had been culture positive for 8 days while on erythromycin, gentamicin, and chloramphenicol therapy (85). A 10-day course cured the meningitis, and the child was developmentally normal at 12 months of age. In the early part of this infant's course, sequential CSF isolates, obtained before rifampicin therapy, developed decreased susceptibility not only to erythromycin, but also to clindamycin, doxycycline, and trimethoprim-sulfamethoxazole, even through the patient received none of these latter agents (85). The susceptibility to rifampicin (MIC/MBC of 0.5/1 μg/mL), however, did not change.

Resistance to erythromycin was also reported in the course of treatment; this patient was treated successfully by substituting intravenous and intraventricular rifamycin for intravenous and intraventricular erythromycin (63). Rifampicin is ordinarily regarded as having bactericidal antibacterial activity, but this is not necessarily so for *C. meningosepticum*. Its MIC was 0.39 μg/mL and MBC 25 μg/mL for an isolate causing neonatal meningitis. Despite this, the patient was successfully treated with intravenous and intraventricular rifampicin (20). The first successfully treated adult with *C. meningosep-*

ticum meningitis was given oral rifampicin together with parenteral cefoperazone and chloramphenicol (18). All four adults previously reported had died.

Because of its relatively good activity against *C. meningosepticum* and excellent penetration into the CSF, trimethoprim-sulfamethoxazole might be considered useful for treatment of meningitis due to this organism. There is, however, a surprising paucity of clinical data. Eight of nine patients with neonatal sepsis due to *C. meningosepticum* were successfully treated with trimethoprim-sulfamethoxazole, but none of these were proven to have meningitis (49). However, anecdotal evidence for its effectiveness in *C. meningosepticum* meningitis is available (44, 57).

Empirical treatment with minocycline has been recommended because of good in vitro activity against the great majority of isolates, good penetration into CSF, and the availability of a parenteral formulation (11). Unfortunately, this antibiotic cannot be used in young children or pregnant women because it may cause discoloration of the permanent teeth. Since it is primarily bacteriostatic, combination with another active agent such as rifampicin seems advisable. At present, these considerations are academic as there is very little reported use of minocycline to treat *C. meningosepticum* infections (11). Other antibiotics used to treat *C. meningosepticum* meningitis

TABLE 4 • In Vitro Susceptibilities of *Chryseobacterium odoratum*

Antibiotic	n	Range	MIC$_{50}$	MIC$_{90}$	Breakpoint[a]	% Susceptible	Ref
Amikacin	5	>64	>64	NS[b]	≤16	0	23
Amikacin	17	64->128	>128	>128	≤16	0	33
Amikacin	6	>128	>128	NS	≤16	0	19
Gentamicin	5	>64	>64	NS	≤4	0	23
Gentamicin	26	64->128	>128	>128	≤4	0	33
Gentamicin	6	>128	>128	NS	≤4	0	19
Kanamycin	5	>64	>64	NS	≤16	0	23
Kanamycin	26	>128	>128	>128	≤16	0	33
Netilmicin	5	>64	>64	NS	≤8	0	23
Netilmicin	6	>128	>128	NS	≤8	0	19
Streptomycin	5	>64	>64	NS	—	—	23
Streptomycin	26	64->128	>128	>128	—	—	33
Tobramycin	5	>64	>64	NS	≤4	0	23
Tobramycin	17	>128	>128	>128	≤4	0	33
Ampicillin	5	1->128	16	NS	—	—	23
Ampicillin	26	4->128	32	128	—	—	33
Penicillin	5	1->128	4	NS	—	—	23
Mecillinam	5	>128	>128	NS	—	—	23
Azlocillin	5	16->128	16	NS	—	—	23
Carbenicillin	5	8->128	128	NS	≤16	—	23
Carbenicillin	26	32->128	128	>128	≤16	0	33
Mezlocillin	5	8->128	16	NS	≤16	—	23
Piperacillin	5	16->128	16	NS	≤16	—	23
Piperacillin	6	4->128	>128	NS	≤16	—	19
Ticarcillin	5	1->128	64	NS	≤16	—	23
Cefamandole	5	≥128	≥128	NS	≤8	0	23
Cefuroxime	5	128	128	NS	≤8	0	23
Cefazolin	5	≥128	≥128	NS	≤8	0	23
Cefoperazone	6	16->128	>128	NS	≤16	—	19
Cefotaxime	5	64-128	64	NS	≤8	0	23
Cefotaxime	6	64->128	>128	NS	≤8	0	19
Cefoxitin	5	16-64	32	NS	≤8	0	23
Ceftazidime	6	4->128	>128	NS	≤8	—	19
Ceftriaxone	6	128->128	>128	NS	≤8	0	19
Cephaloridine	26	1-128	8	16	—	—	33
Cephalothin	5	64->128	64	NS	≤8	0	23
Cephalothin	6	128->128	>128	NS	≤8	0	19
Moxalactam	5	8-128	32	NS	≤8	—	23
Moxalactam	6	16-64	64	NS	≤8	0	19
Aztreonam	6	32->128	>128	NS	≤8	0	19
Imipenem	6	8-32	16	NS	≤4	0	19
Chloramphenicol	5	4-32	32	NS	≤8	—	23
Chloramphenicol	26	4->128	16	32	≤8	—	33
Clindamycin	5	0.13-1	0.5	NS	≤0.5	—	23
Ciprofloxacin	6	1-64	32	NS	≤1	—	19
Ofloxacin	6	2-64	32	NS	≤2	—	19
Colistin	5	>64	>64	NS	—	—	23
Trimethoprim-sulfamethoxazole[c]	5	0.4->6.4	>6.4	NS	≤2/38	—	23
Trimethoprim-sulfamethoxazole	26	0.2->6.4	3.2	6.4	≤2/38	—	33
Sulfamethoxazole	26	1->128	>128	>128	—	—	33
Trimethoprim	6	4->16	>16	NS	—	—	19
Erythromycin	5	4	4	NS	≤0.5	0	23
Erythromycin	26	<1->128	2	4	≤0.5	—	33
Erythromycin	6	64->128	>128	NS	≤0.5	0	19
Minocycline	5	0.5-2	0.5	NS	≤4	100	23
Minocycline	6	2-8	2	NS	≤4	—	19
Doxycycline	5	0.5-8	1	NS	≤4	—	23
Tetracycline	5	4->64	64	NS	≤4	—	23
Tetracycline	26	4-128	64	128	≤4	—	33
Vancomycin	5	32->64	>64	NS	≤4	0	23

continued

TABLE 4 • In Vitro Susceptibilities of *Chryseobacterium odoratum*

Antibiotic	n	Range	MIC$_{50}$	MIC$_{90}$	Breakpoint[a]	% Susceptible	Ref
Vancomycin	6	16–64	64	NS	≤4	0	19
Teicoplanin	6	16–>128	>128	NS	≤8	0	19
Polymyxin B	26	64–>128	>128	>128	—	—	33
Nalidixic acid	26	8–32	8	16	—	—	33

Modified from references 19, 23, 33.

[a]Current NCCLS interpretive standards for susceptibility (μg/mL) (55).

[b]NS, not stated.

[c]Trimethoprim-sulfamethoxazole tested in a ratio of 1:19. Concentration refers to the trimethoprim component.

successfully include ampicillin (MIC, 6–12 μg/mL) (7), ciprofloxacin (MIC, 0.19 μg/mL) (28), and a combination of vancomycin (MIC/MBC, 25/25 μg/mL) plus rifampicin (MIC/MBC, 0.2/0.4 μg/mL) (78).

Of the agents discussed, rifampicin particularly and vancomycin were well tried and relatively effective. Previous treatment regimens involving combinations of chloramphenicol, erythromycin, tetracycline, and penicillin were generally ineffective (51). It is important to determine the MIC and preferably the MBC of the agent chosen in any particular instance. Disk testing cannot be relied on (19, 85). Similar principles apply to the choice of therapy for *C. meningosepticum* infections at other sites and for infections due to *C. indologenes* (80).

C. odoratum is exceptionally resistant, and of the antibiotics tested in vitro, minocycline appears most active (11). However, there is insufficient clinical experience in treating infections due to *F. odoratum* to justify recommendations.

REFERENCES

1. Aber RC, Wennersten C, Moellering RC Jr. Antimicrobial susceptibility of flavobacteria. Antimicrob Agents Chemother 1978;14:483–487.
2. Abter EIM, Lutwick LI, Torrey MJ, Mann R. Cellulitis associated with bacteremia due to *Flavobacterium meningosepticum* [Letter]. Clin Infect Dis 1993;17:929–930.
3. Akl ZA, Stern L, Romagnoli MF, Della-Latta P. *Flavobacterium* group IIb peritonitis in a patient on chronic ambulatory peritoneal dialysis [Letter]. Perit Dial Int 1996;16:331–332.
4. Altmann G, Bogokovsky B. In vitro sensitivity of *Flavobacterium meningosepticum* to antimicrobial agents. J Med Microbiol 1971;4:296–299.
5. Ashdown LR, Previtera S. Community acquired *Flavobacterium meningosepticum* pneumonia and septicemia [Letter]. Med J Aust 1992;156:69–70.
6. Bachman KH, Sewell DL, Strausbaugh LJ. Recurrent cellulitis and bacteremia caused by *Flavobacterium odoratum*. Clin Infect Dis 1996;22:1112–1113.
7. Bagley DH, Alexander JC, Gill VJ, Dolin R, Ketcham AS. Late *Flavobacterium* species meningitis after craniofacial exenteration. Arch Intern Med 1976;136:229–231.
8. Bernardet J-F, Segers P, Vancanneyt M, Berthe F, Kersters K, Vandamme P. Cutting a gordian knot: emended classification and description of the genus *Flavobacterium*, emended description of the family *Flavobacteriaceae*, and proposal of *Flavobacterium hydatis* nom. nov. (Basonym, *Cytophaga aquatilis* Strohol and Tait 1978). Int J Syst Bacteriol 1996;46:128–148.
9. Berry WB, Morrow AG, Harrison DC, Hochstein HD, Himmelsbach CK. Flavobacterium septicemia following intracardiac operations: clinical observations and identification of the source of infection. J Thorac Cardiovasc Surg 1963;45:476–481.
10. Blahova J, Hupkova M, Krcmery V, Kubonova K. Resistance to and hydrolysis of imipenem in nosocomial strains of *Flavobacterium meningosepticum* [Letter]. Eur J Clin Microbiol Infect Dis 1994;13:833.
11. Bloch KC, Nadarajah R, Jacobs R. *Chryseobacterium meningosepticum:* an emerging pathogen among immunocompromised adults. Report of 6 cases and literature review. Medicine 1997;76:30–41.
12. Bolash NK, Liu HH. Quinolone susceptibility of multiply-resistant *Flavobacterium meningosepticum* clinical isolates in one urban hospital. Drugs 1995;49(Suppl 2):168–170.
13. Bolivar R, Abramovits W. Cutaneous infection caused by *Flavobacterium meningosepticum* [Letter]. J Infect Dis 1989;159:150–151.
14. Brown RB, Phillips D, Barker MJ, Pieczarka R, Sands M, Teres D. Outbreak of nosocomial *Flavobacterium meningosepticum* respiratory infections associated with use of aerosolized polymyxin B. Am J Infect Control 1989;17:121–125.
15. Bruun B. Antimicrobial susceptibility of *Flavobacterium meningosepticum* strains identified by DNA-DNA hybridization. Acta Pathol Microbiol Immunol Scand (B) 1987;95:95–101.
16. Burnakis TG, Mioduch J, LeBar WD, Yalamanchi RR. Sepsis from *Flavobacterium meningosepticum*, an uncommon pathogen with unusual susceptibility patterns. South Med J 1986;79:518–519.
17. Cabrera HA, Davis GH. Epidemic meningitis of the newborn caused by Flavobacteria. I. Epidemiology and bacteriology. Am J Dis Child 1961;101:289–295.
18. Chan KH, Chau PY, Wang RYC, Huang CY. Meningitis caused by *Flavobacterium meningosepticum* after transsphenoidal hypophysectomy with recovery. Surg Neurol 1983;20:294–296.
19. Chang J-C, Hsueh P-R, Wu J-J, Ho S-W, Hsieh W-C, Luh K-T. Antimicrobial susceptibility of flavobacteria as determined by agar dilution and disk diffusion methods. Antimicrob Agents Chemother 1997;41:1301–1306.
20. Chandrika T, Adler SP. A case of neonatal meningitis due to *Flavobacterium meningosepticum* successfully treated with rifampin. Pediatr Infect Dis 1982;1:40–41.
21. Colding H, Bangsborg J, Fiehn N-E, Bennekov T, Bruun B. Ribotyping for differentiating *Flavobacterium meningosepticum* isolates from clinical and environmental sources. J Clin Microbiol 1994;32:501–505.
22. Coyle-Gilchrist MM, Crewe P, Roberts G. *Flavobacterium*

meningosepticum in the hospital environment. J Clin Pathol 1976;29:824–826.

23. Fass RJ, Barnishan J. In vitro susceptibilities of nonfermentative Gram-negative bacilli other than *Pseudomonas aeruginosa* to 32 antimicrobial agents. Rev Infect Dis 1980;2:841–853.

24. Ferrer C, Jakob E, Pastorino G, Juncos LI. Right-sided bacterial endocarditis due to *Flavobacterium odoratum* in a patient on chronic hemodialysis. Am J Nephrol 1995;15:82–84.

25. Fujita J, Hata Y, Shozo I. Respiratory infection caused by *Flavobacterium meningosepticum* [Letter]. Lancet 1990;335:544.

26. George RM, Cochran CP, Wheeler WE. Epidemic meningitis of the newborn caused by flavobacteria. II. Clinical manifestations and treatment. Am J Dis Child 1961;101:296–304.

27. Goldstein EJC, Citron DM. Comparative activities of cefuroxime, amoxicillin-clavulanic acid, ciprofloxacin, enoxacin, and ofloxacin against aerobic and anaerobic bacteria isolated from bite wounds. Antimicrob Agents and Chemother 1988;32:1143–1148.

28. Green SDR, Ilunga F, Cheesbrough JS, Tillotson GS, Hichens M, Felmingham D. The treatment of neonatal meningitis due to gram-negative bacilli with ciprofloxacin: evidence of satisfactory penetration into the cerebrospinal fluid. J Infect 1993;26:253–256.

29. Harrington SP, Perlino CA. *Flavobacterium meningosepticum* sepsis: disease due to bacteria with unusual antibiotic susceptibility. South Med J 1981;74:764–766.

30. Hawley HB, Gump DW. Vancomycin therapy of bacterial meningitis. Am J Dis Child 1973;126:261–264.

31. Hazuka BT, Dajani AS, Talbot K, Keen BM. Two outbreaks of *Flavobacterium meningosepticum* type E in a neonatal intensive care unit. J Clin Microbiol 1977;6:450–455.

32. Hirsh BE, Wong B, Kiehn TE, Gee T, Armstrong D. *Flavobacterium meningosepticum* bacteremia in an adult with acute leukemia. Use of rifampin to clear persistent infection. Diagn Microbiol Infect Dis 1986;4:65–69.

33. Holmes B, Snell JJS, Lapage SP. *Flavobacterium odoratum:* a species resistant to a wide range of antimicrobial agents. J Clin Pathol 1979;32:73–77.

34. Holmes B. Identification and distribution of *Flavobacterium meningosepticum* in clinical material. J Appl Bacteriol 1987;62:29–41.

35. Hsueh P-R, Chang J-C, Teng L-J, Yang P-C, Ho S-W, Hsieh W-C, Luh K-T. Comparison of E test and agar dilution method for antimicrobial susceptibility testing of *Flavobacterium* isolates. J Clin Microbiol 1997;35:1021–1023.

36. Hsueh P-R, Hsiue T-R, Wu J-J, Teng L-J, Ho S-W, Hsieh W-C, Luh K-T. *Flavobacterium indologenes* bacteremia: clinical and microbiological characteristics. Clin Infect Dis 1996;23:550–555.

37. Hsueh P-R, Wu J-J, Hsiue T-R, Hsieh W-C. Bacteremic necrotising fasciitis due to *Flavobacterium odoratum*. Clin Infect Dis 1995;21:1337–1338.

38. Johnson DC. *Flavobacterium* infective endocarditis and prosthetic heart valve. Bol Assoc Med PR 1980;72:126–134.

39. Jorgensen JH, Maher LA, Howell AW. Activity of meropenem against antibiotic-resistant or infrequently encountered gram-negative bacilli. Antimicrob Agents Chemother 1991;35:2410–2414.

40. Kaplan M, Goldberg MD, Tauber Z, Solomon F, Sompolinsky D. Successful treatment of neonatal *Flavobacterium meningosepticum* infection. Eur J Pediatr 1983;140:337–338.

41. King EO. Studies on a group of previously unclassified bacteria associated with meningitis in infants. Am J Clin Pathol 1959;31:241–247.

42. Korzets Z, Maayan MC, Bernheim J. Flavobacterial peritonitis in patients treated by peritoneal dialysis. Nephrol Dial Transplant 1995;10:280–283.

43. Krebs S, Blanche P, Bouscary D, Gauther E, Dreyfus F, Sicard D, Blanchard H. *Flavobacterium meningosepticum* meningitis in an adult with acute leukaemia [Letter]. Postgrad Med J 1996;72:187–188.

44. Lapage SP, Owen RJ. *Flavobacterium meningosepticum* from cases of meningitis in Botswana and England. J Clin Pathol 1973;26:747–749.

45. Lee EL, Robinson MJ, Thong ML, Puthucheary SD, Ong TH, Ng KK. Intraventricular chemotherapy in neonatal meningitis. J Pediatr 1977;91:991–995.

46. Lee M, Munoz J. Septicemia occurring after colonscopic polypectomy in a splenectomized patient taking corticosteroids. Am J Gastroenterol 1994;89:2245–2246.

47. LeFrancois M, Baum JL. *Flavobacterium endophthalmitis* following keratoplasty. Use of a tissue culture medium-stored cornea. Arch Ophthalmol 1976;94:1907–1909.

48. Lim V, Halijah M. A comparative study of the in vitro activity of cefepime and other cephalosporins. Malays J Pathol 1993;15:65–68.

49. Linder N, Korman SH, Eyal F, Michel J. Trimethoprim sulphamethoxazole in neonatal *Flavobacterium meningosepticum* infection. Arch Dis Child 1984;59:582–584.

50. Macfarlane DE, Baum-Thureen P, Crandon I. *Flavobacterium odoratum* ventriculitis treated with intraventricular cefotaxime. J Infect 1985;11:233–238.

51. Madruga M, Zanon U, Pereira GMN, Galvao AC. Meningitis caused by *Flavobacterium meningosepticum*. The first epidemic outbreak of meningitis in the newborn in South America. J Infect Dis 1970;121:328–330.

52. Mani RM, Kuruvila KC, Batliwala PM, Damle PN, Shirgaonkar GV, Soni RP, Vyas PR. *Flavobacterium meningosepticum* as an opportunist. J Clin Pathol 1978;31:220–222.

53. Marnejon T, Watanakunakorn C. *Flavobacterium meningosepticum* septicemia and peritonitis complicating CAPD [Letter]. Clin Nephrol 1992;38:176–177.

54. McGowan JE, Steinberg JP. Other gram-negative bacilli. In: Mandell GL, Bennett JE, Dolin R, eds. Principles and practice of infectious diseases. 4th ed. New York: Churchill Livingstone, 1995:2106–2116.

55. National Committee for Clinical Laboratory Standards. Methods for dilution antimicrobial susceptibility tests for bacteria that grow aerobically. 4th ed. Approved standard. NCCLS document M7-A4, Wayne, PA: NCCLS, 1997.

56. Olsen H, Frederiksen WC, Siboni KE. *Flavobacterium meningosepticum* in 8 non-fatal cases of postoperative bacteraemia. Lancet 1965;1:1294–1296.

57. Overturf GD. Use of trimethoprim-sulfamethoxazole in pediatric infections: relative merits of intravenous administration. Rev Infect Dis 1987;9:168–176.

58. Pickett MJ. Methods for identification of flavobacteria. J Clin Microbiol 1989;27:2309–2315.

59. Pitlik S, Berger SA, Huminer D. Nonenteric infections acquired through contact with water. Rev Infect Dis 1987;9:54–63.

60. Plotkin SA, McKitrick JC. Nosocomial meningitis of the newborn caused by Flavobacterium. JAMA 1966;198:194–196.

61. Pokrywka M, Viazanko K, Medvick J, Knabe S, McCool S, Pasculle AW, Dowling JN. A *Flavobacterium meningosepticum*

outbreak among intensive care patients. Am J Infect Control 1993;21:139–145.

62. Raimondi A, Moosdeen F, Williams JD. Antibiotic resistance pattern of *Flavobacterium meningosepticum*. Eur J Clin Microbiol Infect Dis 1986;5:461–463.

63. Rios I, Klimek JJ, Maderazo E, Quintiliani R. *Flavobacterium meningosepticum* meningitis. Report of selected aspects. Antimicrob Agents Chemother 1978;14:444–447.

64. Sader HS, Jones RN, Pfaller MA. Relapse of catheter-related *Flavobacterium meningosepticum* bacteremia demonstrated by DNA macrorestriction analysis. Clin Infect Dis 1995;21:997–1000.

65. Sato K, Fujii T, Okamoto R, Inoue M, Mitsuhashi S. Biochemical properties of beta-lactamase produced by *Flavobacterium odoratum*. Antimicrob Agents Chemother 1985;27:612–614.

66. Schiff J, Suter LS, Gourley RD, Sutliff WD. Flavobacterium infection as a cause of bacterial endocarditis. report of a case, bacteriologic studies, and review of the literature. Ann Intern Med 1961;53:499–506.

67. Schmidt ME, Smith MA, Levy CS. Endophthalmitis caused by unusual gram-negative bacilli: three case reports and review. Clin Infect Dis 1993;17:686–690.

68. Sexton DJ, Houk PC, Grantham RN. Successful treatment of prosthetic valve endocarditis due to *Flavobacterium meningosepticum* [Letter]. South Med J 1985;78:1267–1268.

69. Sheridan RL, Ryan CM, Pasternack MS, Weber JM, Tompkins RG. Flavobacterial sepsis in massively burned pediatric patients. Clin Infect Dis 1993;17:185–187.

70. Shewan JM, McMeekin TA. Taxonomy (and ecology) of *Flavobacterium* and related genera. Ann Rev Microbiol 1983;37:233–252.

71. Siegman-Igra Y, Schwartz D, Soferman G, Konforti N. *Flavobacterium* group 11b bacteremia: report of a case and review of *Flavobacterium* infections. Med Microbiol Immunol 1987;176:103–111.

72. Skapek SX, Jones WS, Hoffman KM, Kuskie MR. Sinusitis and bacteremia caused by *Flavobacterium meningosepticum* in a sixteen-year-old with Shwachman Diamond syndrome. Pediatr Infect Dis J 1992;11:411–413.

73. Strandberg DA, Jorgensen JH, Drutz DJ. Activities of aztreonam and new cephalosporins against infrequently isolated Gram-negative bacilli. Antimicrob Agents and Chemother 1983;24:282–286.

74. Sundin D, Gold BD, Berkowitz FE, Schwartz DA, Goo D. Community-acquired *Flavobacterium meningosepticum* meningitis, pneumonia, and septicemia in a normal infant. Pediatr Infect Dis J 1991;10:73–76.

75. Tam AYC, Yung RWH, Fu K-H. Fatal pneumonia caused by *Flavobacterium meningosepticum*. Pediatr Infect Dis J 1989;8:252–254.

76. Teres D. ICU-acquired pneumonia due to *Flavobacterium meningosepticum*. JAMA 1974;228:732.

77. Thong ML, Puthucheary SD, Lee EL. *Flavobacterium meningosepticum* infection: an epidemiological study in a newborn nursery. J Clin Pathol 1981;34:429–433.

78. Tizer KB, Cervia JS, Dunn A-M, Stavola JJ, Noel GJ. Successful combination vancomycin and rifampin therapy in a newborn with community-acquired *Flavobacterium meningosepticum* neonatal meningitis. Pediatr Infect Dis J 1995;14:916–917.

79. Vandamme P, Bernardet J-F, Segers P, Kersters R, Holmes B. New perspectives in the classification of flavobacteria: description of *Chryseobacterium* gen. nov., *Bergeyella* gen. nov., and *Empedobacter* nom. rev. Int J Syst Bacteriol 1994;44:827–831.

80. von Graevenitz A, Grehn M. Susceptibility studies on *Flavobacterium* 11-b. FEMS Microbiol Lett 1977;2:289–292.

81. von Graevenitz A. *Acinetobacter, Alcaligenes, Moraxella*, and other nonfermentative gram-negative bacteria. In: Murray PR, Baron EJ, Pfaller MA, Tenover FC, Yolken RH, eds. Manual of clinical microbiology. 6th ed. Washington, DC: American Society for Microbiology, 1995:520–532.

82. Watanabe N-A, Katsu K, Moriyama M, Kitoh K. In vitro evaluation of E1040, a new cephalosporin with potent antipseudomonal activity. Antimicrob Agents Chemother 1988; 32:693–701.

83. Watson KC, Krogh JG, Jones DT. Neonatal meningitis caused by *Flavobacterium meningosepticum* type F. J Clin Pathol 1966;19:79–80.

84. Werthamer S, Weiner M. Subacute bacterial endocarditis due to *Flavobacterium meningosepticum*. Am J Clin Pathol 1972; 57:410–412.

85. Winslow DL, Pankey GA. Successful therapy with rifampicin—*Flavobacterium meningosepticum* meningitis developing while on erythromycin therapy. Del Med J 1982;54: 575–579.

Citrobacter Species

Shan-Chwen Chang

GENERAL DESCRIPTION

Citrobacter species, aerobic enteric Gram-negative bacilli, are commonly found in water, soil, food, and the intestinal tracts of animals and humans. This genus was proposed in 1932 by Werkman and Gillen (35). Before 1993, only three species, *Citrobacter freundii, Citrobacter koseri* (*Citrobacter diver-* sus), and *Citrobacter amalonaticus,* were recognized. *C. freundii* is the type species in this genus, and the later two species have been called other names. *C. koseri* was accepted to replace the name *C. diversus* by the Judicial Commission of the International Committee on Systematic Bacteriology in 1993 (22). In the same year, Brenner et al. classified *Citrobacter* into 11 genospecies by DNA hybridization: *C. freundii, C. koseri, C. amalonaticus, C.farmeri, C. youngae, C. braakii, C. werkmanii, C. sedlakii,* and unnamed genospecies 9, 10 and 11 (6). However, most studies of clinical cases or antimicrobial susceptibilities were based on the previous classification and focused on *C. freundii* and *C. koseri* (*C. diversus*), the two most commonly isolated species in this genus.

In early years, *Citrobacter* isolated from clinical specimens were considered environmental contaminants or harmless colonizers, but gradually it was recognized as a true human pathogen (1, 17). Like other *Enterobacteriaceae, Citrobacter* can cause a wide spectrum of infections in humans, such as infections in the urinary tract, respiratory tract, wounds, bone, peritoneum, endocardium, meninges, and bloodstream (24). Among the various sites of infection, the urinary tract is the most common, followed by the respiratory tract, and skin/soft tissues. *C. koseri* can cause an unusually severe form of neonatal meningitis, associated with necrotizing encephalitis and brain abscesses (13, 23). Many *Citrobacter* infections are nosocomially acquired; however, they can also be community acquired. According to data from the National Nosocomial Infection Surveillance (NNIS) Study, during 1986–1989, *Citrobacter* accounted for 2% of total nosocomial infections (32). Among 1441 nosocomial *Citrobacter* infection patients, 812 had urinary tract infection, 321 had surgical wound infection, 226 had pneumonia, and 82 had bloodstream infection.

SUSCEPTIBILITY IN VITRO AND IN VIVO
Single Drug

Different species of *Citrobacter* demonstrate different antimicrobial susceptibility profiles. *C. freundii* is generally much more resistant to antimicrobial agents than *C. koseri* (*C. diversus*), with *C. amalonaticus* having a susceptibility profile intermediate between those two species. In the 1970s, isolates of *C. koseri* (*C. diversus*) were usually resistant to ampicillin and carbenicillin but susceptible to cephalothin; in contrast, isolates of *C. freundii* were usually susceptible to ampicillin and carbenicillin but resistant to cephalothin (18, 21, 25). This characteristic was even proposed for use in species identification (34). However, *C. freundii* has become more resistant to many antimicrobial agents, including ampicillin and carbenicillin, so classification of species by antibiotic susceptibility pattern is no longer valid.

Current isolates of *C. koseri* (*C. diversus*) remain more susceptible than *C. freundii* to various anti-Gram-negative agents, except ampicillin. However, isolates of *C. freundii* in recent years have demonstrated resistance not only to traditional agents such as ampicillin, carbenicillin, and cephalothin, but also to newer agents such as piperacillin, third-generation cephalosporins, and monobactams. Table 1 shows the antimicrobial susceptibilities of *Citrobacter* isolates obtained from blood cultures from M.D. Anderson, Houston, Texas. *C. freundii* is more resistant than *C. koseri* to most antimicrobial agents (30). The minimum inhibitory concentrations (MICs) of various antimicrobial agents for *C. freundii* were higher than those of *C. koseri*. Aminoglycosides (gentamicin, netilmicin, amikacin), fluoroquinolones (enoxacin, ciprofloxacin), and car-

bapenems (imipenem) were the most active agents against both *C. freundii* and *C. koseri* (30).

Other fluoroquinolones and carbapenems, such as fleroxacin, levofloxacin, lomefloxacin, sparfloxacin, meropenem, and biapenem, also displayed good in vitro activity against *Citrobacter* (4, 9, 16, 29, 38). These new fluoroquinolones usually have MIC_{90}s of 1 μg/mL or less against *Citrobacter* and the new carbapenems have MIC_{90}s of 0.125 μg/mL or less in most studies. Some newer parenteral cephems, such as cefepime and cefpirome, also have good in vitro activity against *Citrobacter* (MIC_{50}s ≤ 0.125 μg/mL; MIC_{90}s ≤8 μg/mL) (5, 20, 27).

As for oral β-lactam agents, penicillins and first- and second-generation cephalosporins do not have activity against most *C. freundii* isolates but may have activity against some *C. koseri* isolates. Some newer or third-generation oral cephalosporins, such as cefixime, cefpodoxime proxetil, cefprozil, cefetamet pivoxil, and ceftibuten, have good activity against *C. koseri* but only moderate or poor activity against *C. freundii* (7, 11, 36, 37). The MIC_{90}s for *C. koseri* are usually 4 μg/mL or less, but for *C. freundii* they usually exceed 16 μg/mL.

β-lactamase production is a common phenomenon in both *C. freundii* and *C. koseri* isolates. The β-lactamase produced by *C. freundii* is a type I β-lactamase that is not inhibited by clavulanic acid, sulbactam, and tazobactam. Therefore, for *C. freundii,* the MICs of β-lactam antibiotics in combination with a β-lactamase inhibitor, such as ampicillin plus sulbactam, amoxicillin plus clavulanic acid, ticarcillin plus clavulanic acid, and piperacillin plus tazobactam, are similar or identical to those of the β-lactam antibiotics alone (8, 26).

Other agents, such as tetracycline, chloramphenicol, and trimethoprim/sulfamethoxazole showed good antimicrobial activities in previous studies or case reports, although few data exist about their antimicrobial activities against isolates after 1990. Disk susceptibility tests in the National Taiwan University Hospital generally showed in vitro resistance to tetracycline, chloramphenicol, and trimethoprim/sulfamethoxazole in *C. freundii* isolates (Table 2). These agents appear to have good in vitro activity against *C. koseri*; however, the number of strains of *C. koseri* in this hospital, however, is too small to allow any conclusions about the activity of tetracycline, chloramphenicol, and trimethoprim/sulfamethoxazole against *C. koseri*. One study from Belgium also demonstrated 100% susceptibility of 23 strains of *C. koseri* to trimethoprim/sulfamethoxazole (3).

In summary, aminoglycosides, fluoroquinolones, carbapenems, and some newer cephems (including cefepime and cefpirome) have the highest in vitro antimicrobial activities against *C. freundii*. There are high proportions of resistance to other agents. For *C. koseri* (*C. diversus*), in addition to aminoglycosides, fluoroquinolones, carbapenems, and newer cephems (cefepime and cefpirome), many other agents, such as the third-generation cephalosporins, aztreonam, piperacillin, piperacillin plus tazobactam, and some new oral cephems (including cefixime, cefpodoxime proxetil, cefprozil, cefetamet pivoxil, and ceftibuten) also have good in vitro activities.

combination of an aminoglycoside with a fluoroquinolone, a carbapenem or a "fourth-generation" cephalosporin could be as effective as, or better than, a third-generation cephalosporin in combination with an aminoglycoside in the treatment of *Citrobacter* infection. It is also not really known whether there is any difference between treatment of *Citrobacter* infections and treatment of other *Enterobacteriaceae* infections. Recommendations in the literature for treatment of *Citrobacter* meningitis are based largely on the authors' personal experience, published case reports, and general experience with Gram-negative bacillary meningitis. Therefore, more studies on the in vitro and in vivo efficacy of various agents, alone or in combination, would be helpful in determining the most appropriate treatment of *Citrobacter* infections.

REFERENCES

1. Altman G, Sechter I, Cahan D, Gerichter CB. *Citrobacter diversus* isolated from clinical material. J Clin Microbiol 1976;3: 390–392.
2. Aoyama H, Fujimaki K, Sato K, Fujii T, Inoue M, Hirai K, Mitsuhashi S. Clinical isolate of *Citrobacter freundii* highly resistant to new quinolones. Antimicrob Agents Chemother 1988;32: 922–924.
3. Arens S, Verhaegen J, Verbist L. Differentiation and susceptibility of *Citrobacter* isolates from patients in a university hospital. Clin Microbiol Infect 1997;3:53–57.
4. Balfour JA, Todd PA, Peter DH. Fleroxacin: a review of its pharmacology and therapeutic efficacy in various infections. Drugs 1995;49:794–850.
5. Barradell LB, Bryson HM. Cefepime: a review of its antibacterial activity, pharmacokinetic properties and therapeutic use. Drugs 1994;47:471–505.
6. Brenner DJ, Grimont PAD, Steigerwalt AG, Fanning GR, Ageron E, Riddle CF. Classification of citrobacteria by DNA hybridization: designation of *Citrobacter farmeri* sp. nov., *Citrobacter youngae* sp. nov., *Citrobacter breakii* sp. nov., *Citrobacter werkmanii* sp. nov., *Citrobacter sedlakii* sp. nov., and three unnamed *Citrobacter* genospecies. Int J Syst Bacteriol 1993;43:645–658.
7. Bryson HM, Brogden RN. Cefetamet pivoxil: a review of its antibacterial activity, pharmacokinetic properties and therapeutic use. Drugs 1993;45:589–621.
8. Bryson HM, Brogden RN. Piperacillin/tazobactam: a review of its antibacterial activity, pharmacokinetic properties and therapeutic potential. Drugs 1994;47:506–535.
9. Davis R, Bryson HM. Levofloxacin: a review of its antibacterial activity, pharmacokinetics and therapeutic efficacy. Drugs 1994; 47:677–700.
10. Drelichman VD, Band JD. Bacteremias due to *Citrobacter diversus* and *Citrobacter freundii:* incidence, risk factors and clinical outcome. Arch Intern Med 1985;145:1808–1810.
11. Frampton JE, Brogden RN, Langtry HD, Buckley MM. Cefpodoxime proxetil: a review of its antibacterial activity, pharmacokinetic properties and therapeutic potential. Drugs 1992;44: 889–917.
12. Gootz TD, Jackson DB, Sherris JC. Development of resistance to cephalosporins in clinical strains of *Citrobacter* sp. Antimicrob Agents Chemother 1984;25:591–595.
13. Graham DR, Band JD. *Citrobacter diversus* brain abscess and meningitis in neonates. JAMA 1981;245:1923–1925.
14. Greene GR, Heitlinger L, Madden JD. *Citrobacter ventriculitis*

in a neonate responsive to trimethoprim-sulfamethoxazole. Clin Pediatr 1983;22:515–517.
15. Haimi-Cohen Y, Amir J, Weinstock A, Varsano I. The use of imipenem-cilastatin in neonatal meningitis caused by *Citrobacter diversus*. Acta Paediatr 1993;82:530–532.
16. Hoban DJ, Jones RN, Yamane N, Frei R, Trilla A, Pignatari AC. In vitro activity of three carbapenem antibiotics: comparative studies with biapenem (L-627), imipenem, and meropenem against aerobic pathogens isolated worldwide. Diagn Microbiol Infect Dis 1993;17:299–305.
17. Hodges GR, Degener CE, Barnes WG. Clinical significance of *Citrobacter* isolates. Am J Clin Pathol 1978;70:37–40.
18. Holmes B, King A, Phillips I, Lapage SP. Sensitivity of *Citrobacter freundii* and *Citrobacter koseri* to cephalosporins and penicillins. J Clin Pathol 1974;27:729–733.
19. Jacobson KL, Cohen SH, Inciardi JF, King JH, Lippert WE, Iglesias T, VanCouwenberghe CJ. The relationship between antecedent antibiotic use and resistance to extended-spectrum cephalosporins in group I β-lactamase-producing organisms. Clin Infect Dis 1995;21:1107–1113.
20. Jones RN, Pfaller MA, Allen SD, Gerlach EH, Fuchs PC, Aldridge KE. Antimicrobial activity of cefpirome: an update compared to five third-generation cephalosporins against nearly 6000 recent clinical isolates from five medical centers. Diagn Microbiol Infect Dis 1991;14:361–364.
21. Jones SR, Ragsdale AR, Kutscher E, Sanford JP. Clinical and bacteriologic observations on a recently recognized species of *Enterobacteriaceae, Citrobacter diversus*. J Infect Dis 1973; 128:563–565.
22. Judicial Commission of the International Committee on Systematic Bacteriology. Opinion 67. Rejection of the name *Citrobacter diversus* Werkman and Gillen 1932. Int J Syst Bacteriol 1993;43:392.
23. Kline MW. *Citrobacter* meningitis and brain abscess in infancy: epidemiology, pathogenesis, and treatment. J Pediatr 1988;113: 430–434.
24. Lipsky BA, Hook EW III, Smith AA, Plorde JJ. *Citrobacter* infections in humans: experience at the Seattle Veterans Administration Medical Center and a review of the literature. Rev Infect Dis 1980;2:746–760.
25. Lund ME, Matsen JM, Blazevic DJ. Biochemical and antibiotic susceptibility studies of hydrogen sulfide-negative *Citrobacter*. Appl Microbiol 1974;28:22–25.
26. Marshall SA, Aldridge KE, Allen SD, Fuchs PC, Gerlach EH, Jones RN. Comparative antimicrobial activity of piperacillin-tazobactam tested against more than 5000 recent clinical isolates from five medical centers: a reevaluation after five years. Diagn Microbiol Infect Dis 1995;21:153–168.
27. Neu HC, Chin NX, Huang HB. In vitro activity and β-lactamase stability of FK-037, a parenteral cephalosporin. Antimicrob Agents Chemother 1993;37:566–573.
28. Nicolle LE. Prior antimicrobial therapy and resistance of *Enterobacter, Citrobacter* and *Serratia* to third generation cephalosporins. J Hosp Infect 1988;11:321–327.
29. Sader HS, Jones RN. Antimicrobial activities of the new carbapenem biapenem compared to imipenem, meropenem and other broad-spectrum beta-lactam drugs. Eur J Clin Microbiol Infect Dis 1993;12:384–391.
30. Samonis G, Ho DH, Gooch GF, Rolston KVI, Bodey GP. In vitro susceptibility of *Citrobacter* species to various antimicrobial agents. Antimicrob Agents Chemother 1987;31:829–830.
31. Samonis G, Anaissie E, Elting L, Bodey GP. Review of *Cit-*

robacter bacteremia in cancer patients over a sixteen-year period. Eur J Clin Microbiol Infect Dis 1991;10:479–485.

32. Schaberg DR, Culver DH, Gaynes RP. Major trends in the microbial etiology of nosocomial infection. Am J Med 1991;91 (Suppl 3B):72–75S.

33. Shih CC, Chen YC, Chang SC, Luh KT, Hsieh WC. Bacteremia due to *Citrobacter* species: significance of primary intraabdominal infection. Clin Infect Dis 1996;23:543–549.

34. Southern PM Jr, Bagby MK. Antimicrobial susceptibility patterns (antibiograms) as an aid in differentiating *Citrobacter* species. Am J Clin Pathol 1977;67:187–189.

35. Werkman CH, Gillen GF. Bacteria producing trimethylene glycol. J Bacteriol 1932;23:167–182.

36. Wiseman LR, Benfield P. Cefprozil: a review of its antibacterial activity, pharmacokinetic properties, and therapeutic potential. Drugs 1993;45:295–317.

37. Wiseman LR, Balfour JA. Ceftibuten: a review of its antibacterial activity, pharmacokinetic properties and clinical efficacy. Drugs 1994;47:784–808.

38. Wiseman LR, Wagstaff AJ, Brogden RN, Bryson HM. Meropenem: a review of its antibacterial activity, pharmacokinetic properties and clinical efficacy. Drugs 1995;50:73–101.

Clostridium botulinum

Cindy P. Dougherty

Clostridium botulinum is an anaerobic, sporeforming, Gram-positive bacillus that is widely distributed. It is present in soil, water, dust, and the gastrointestinal tracts of numerous mammalian, avian, and marine species (2, 6). Several strains of *C. botulinum* exist, but they all share a common property of producing potent neurotoxins that can potentially cause botulism, a disease that can result in paralysis and death.

Seven serologically related but immunologically distinct neurotoxins, designated A to G, have been identified. These neurotoxins, among the most potent known, are heat-labile, high-molecular-weight proteins with a human lethal dose in the range of 5 to 50 ng/kg (8). Neurotoxins A, B, E (and rarely F) have been implicated in illness among humans; types C and D primarily affect other mammals and birds. Their mechanism of action is to block presynaptic release of acetylcholine at skeletal muscle neuromuscular junctions and at autonomic nervous system neuroeffector junctions. The blockade of acetylcholine release results in muscle weakness and paralysis and variable autonomic deficits. Since *C. botulinum* neurotoxins do not cross the blood-brain barrier, botulism does not affect central nervous system cholinergic nerve endings (2).

PATHOPHYSIOLOGY OF BOTULISM

Acetylcholine is released normally from nerve endings in response to the propagation of an action potential over the presynaptic membrane. *C. botulinum* neurotoxins interfere with this process. The polypeptide neurotoxins have a high affinity for receptor sites on the presynaptic cholinergic membrane, and they bind irreversibly with those proteins. They enter the nerve ending by the process of endocytosis and, in ways that are not yet understood, block the release of acetylcholine in response to the stimulus of the action potential. Evidence suggests that the toxins inhibit vesicle-release sites on the presynaptic membrane. Once the toxin is internalized, it may act as an enzyme to convert host proteins into inhibitory proteins that interfere with acetylcholine release (2).

CLINICAL SYNDROMES OF BOTULISM

Three distinct forms of botulism are recognized clinically: foodborne, wound, and infant. The course of the disease may be affected by host factors, the amount of toxin ingested, and if and when botulinum antitoxin is given.

Foodborne Botulism

The classic form of the disease is associated with ingestion of food that is contaminated with preformed neurotoxins. More than 90% of foodborne botulism results from eating improperly preserved home-canned foods (2). Most cases follow intoxication with type A (60%), type B (30%), or type E (10%) botulinum toxin (3); type A toxin has been associated with more-severe disease and a higher fatality rate than either type B or type E (12).

The presumptive diagnosis of botulism is based on neurologic signs and symptoms of the patient rather than laboratory test results. Treatment must be initiated before confirmatory evidence is available, and evidence may be lacking in about 12% of the laboratory investigations (6). Foodborne botulism is confirmed by detecting toxin in the patient's serum, gastric contents, or feces or in suspected food.

An important clinical aspect of botulism is the patient's normal mental functioning, the absence of sensory abnormalities, and the presence of autonomic dysfunctions. This is consistent with toxin inactivation of peripheral cholinergic synapses of the somatic and visceral motor nerves only (2, 6). Treatment includes supportive intensive care, including mechanical ventilation and use of therapeutic antitoxin.

Wound Botulism

Wound botulism has become increasingly common in recent years. This form of botulism occurs when the neurotoxin, produced in wounds contaminated with *C. botulinum,* is absorbed systemically and disseminated throughout the body. Most cases of wound botulism are now associated with subcutaneous injection of street drugs that result in formation of abscesses (2). The diagnosis is best made by isolating the *C. botulinum* organism from a wound specimen, since toxin is not usually detected in serum and is never found in the patient's stool (2). Management of the patient includes respiratory support, administration of antitoxin, surgical debridement of the wound, and usually antibiotic therapy. Penicillin is frequently recommended to eradicate *C. botulinum* from the wound, although the efficacy of antibiotics is not proven. Results of wound culture may indicate the use of a different antibiotic (1, 8, 10).

Infant Botulism

Infant botulism is characterized by the presence of some of the same signs and symptoms as foodborne and wound botulism. It is considered a separate entity because the infant ingests the spores and, unlike adults, is incapable of inhibiting their growth and multiplication. More than 90% of cases occur in infants younger than 6 months (3).

The absence of bowel movements in an infant is an early symptom of botulism and can persist for as long as 3 weeks before other symptoms appear (2). Most children are afebrile with an admitting diagnosis of sepsis or failure to thrive (2, 6). Cranial nerve function deficits are the most valid indicators of infant botulism, although the patient's history and response to rapid repetitive myelography (EMG) play important diagnostic roles. Recovery of clostridial organisms and toxin from the stool confirms the diagnosis. Serum toxin levels in infants are not high enough to measure, and cerebrospinal fluid is normal (3, 6).

When sepsis and botulism are possible diagnoses in the infant, and if antibiotic therapy is initiated for presumptive sepsis, ampicillin plus cefotaxime or ceftriaxone (10) are the best choice, since aminoglycosides may contribute to neuromuscular blockade (3, 11). Once the diagnosis of botulism is made, antibiotics are not recommended for clearing toxigenic organisms from the infant's intestines, since release of toxin in the gut through bacterial cell lysis may worsen neurologic symptoms (6, 11). Treatment is usually restricted to supportive care with particular attention to nutritional supplementation and respiratory support (2, 6, 11).

A few rare cases of botulism have occurred in which adults have suffered a similar colonization of the gastrointestinal tract by clostridial organisms. Unique to most cases of adult "infant botulism" is a patient history of abdominal surgery, gastrointestinal tract abnormalities, or recent antibiotic treatment (7).

DIAGNOSIS

Botulism is probably underdiagnosed because many clinicians are unfamiliar with the illness, and symptoms are mistaken for more common clinical entities. The differential diagnosis for botulism includes myasthenia gravis, Guillain-Barré syndrome, stroke, bacterial and chemical food poisoning, tick paralysis, chemical intoxication, mushroom poisoning, medication reactions, sepsis, poliomyelitis, diphtheria, and nervous system infections (2, 3, 6).

BOTULINUM ANTITOXIN

Administration of botulinum antitoxin is used as routine therapy in suspected cases of botulism and botulinum toxin exposure in humans. However, with adequate supportive care, even severe cases of botulism can be handled successfully without administration of the antitoxin. One licensed antitoxin product, Botulinum Antitoxin, trivalent (types A, B, E) is currently available in the United States. It is manufactured by Pasteur Mérieux Connaught and is distributed by the Centers for Disease Control and Prevention (CDC). The antitoxin is a refined and concentrated preparation of horse globulins modified by enzymatic digestion and contains 0.4% phenol as a preservative.

Botulinum antitoxin is used to prevent or treat botulism by neutralizing botulinum neurotoxins circulating in the individual. The antitoxin has no effect on toxin already bound to the nerve receptors; therefore, clinical symptoms may not improve immediately. However, administration of antitoxin may stop the progression of symptoms. The amount of circulating antitoxin needed to counteract botulism toxin poisoning is not known, and the efficacy of treatment depends on the time interval between onset of symptoms and administration of the antitoxin (package insert, Connaught 1988). To be most effective, treatment should be initiated as soon as a firm clinical diagnosis is made, even in the absence of laboratory confirmation (2, 6).

Botulinum antitoxin and intensive respiratory support are the mainstays of treatment in both foodborne and wound botulism. Many reports in the literature show that antitoxin therapy has a beneficial effect on survival and shortens the course of illness, especially if antitoxin is received within 24 h of the onset of symptoms (8, 9). However, clinicians must consider other conditions that present with neurologic signs and symptoms consistent with botulism. They must also recognize that hypersensitivity reactions and serum sickness can result from administration of an equine product.

A heptavalent equine antitoxin has been produced and is currently being tested in humans under an Investigational New Drug application (IND). This antitoxin has the ability to neutralize seven serotypes of *C. botulinum* toxins (A, B, C, D, E, F, G).

Treatment of infant botulism usually requires meticulous supportive care, and administration of botulinum antitoxin is not recommended. Studies have shown that the antitoxin has little effect on the outcome of infantile botulism because antitoxin only binds circulating toxin, and infants have very low levels of serum toxin. Another reason to avoid the use of equine antitoxin, since there is favorable prognosis without it, is the risk of adverse reactions and of sensitizing the patient against equine serum at such an early age (2, 6, 11).

Since 1989, the California Department of Health Services (Berkeley) has been studying the use of a pentavalent botulism immune globulin (types A, B, C, D, and E), derived from human serum of immunized volunteer donors. If the product proves efficacious, it may become the treatment of choice for infants with botulism (4, 6).

Dosage

Each vial (10 mL) of botulinum antitoxin, trivalent, contains at least 7500 IU of type A, 5500 IU of type B, and 8500 IU of type E antitoxins. For years the CDC and published literature have recommended use of two vials of antitoxin for the treatment of patients with suspected cases of botulism. However, circulating antitoxin levels measured in patients after treatment indicate that one vial of trivalent antitoxin contains more than 100 times the amount needed to neutralize the largest amount of circulating toxin ever measured at CDC, and antitoxins persist in the circulation with a half-life of 5 to 7 days (6; CDC, unpublished data). Due to this and decreased availability of the botulinum antitoxin, CDC now recommends using one vial of trivalent (A, B, E) antitoxin intravenously. CDC does not recommend the use of intramuscular antitoxin (CDC, unpublished data).

Contraindications

There are essentially no "absolute" contraindications to the use of antitoxin. In patients with a history of a severe hypersensitivity reaction to equine serum or any component of the product, the risks and benefits must be considered carefully before administration of antitoxin.

The package insert for botulinum antitoxin, trivalent (equine), describes most aspects of administration of the product, such as tests for sensitivity to serum or antitoxin along with a schedule for desensitization in sensitive persons, description and treatment of serum reactions, and important instructions for injecting the antitoxin.

THERAPEUTIC USES OF BOTULINUM TOXIN AND TOXOID

A licensed product, *C. botulinum* toxin A, is used to treat a range of conditions in which deliberately induced paralysis of particular muscles benefits the patient. This toxin has been effective in the treatment of blepharospasm, spasmodic torticollis, hemifacial spasm, strabismus, and other focal dystonias.

Administration of minute amounts of botulinum toxin A into specific skeletal muscles causes localized muscle weakness or paralysis lasting from 4 to 12 months. The procedure may be repeated when necessary. Some investigators are concerned that multiple injections may elicit antibody production, thereby reducing the beneficial and therapeutic effects of the toxin (2, 5).

A pentavalent botulinum toxoid, approved for investigational human use, is manufactured by the Michigan State Department of Public Health. This toxoid is used to vaccinate laboratorians who work with the botulinum toxin or organisms and is available through the CDC Drug Service (6, 9).

SUMMARY

Supportive intensive care and the use of therapeutic antitoxin are the only treatments available for botulism. If botulism is suspected in a patient, the physician should contact the Centers for Disease Control and Prevention (CDC) for consultation on diagnosis and treatment (404-639-2888). An epidemiologist will authorize release of trivalent (A, B, E) botulinum antitoxin from the appropriate PHS Quarantine station for treatment (CDC, unpublished data).

REFERENCES

1. Centers for Disease Control and Prevention. Wound botulism—California, 1995. MMWR 1995;44:889–892.
2. Davis LE. Botulinum toxin: from poison to medicine. West J Med 1993;158:25–29.
3. Ferrari ND, Weisse ME. Botulism. Adv Pediatr Infect Dis 1995;10:81–91.
4. Grabenstein JD. Immunoantidotes: II. One hundred years of antitoxins. Hosp Pharm 1992;27:637–646.
5. Hambleton P. *Clostridium botulinum* toxins: a general review of involvement in disease, structure, mode of action and preparation for clinical use. J Neurol 1992;239:16–20.
6. Hatheway CL. Botulism: the present status of the disease. Curr Top Microbiol Immunol 1995;195:55–75.
7. McCroskey LM, Hatheway CL. Laboratory findings in four cases of adult botulism suggest colonization of the intestinal tract. J Clin Microbiol 1988;26:1052–1054.
8. Mechem CC, Walter FG. Wound botulism. Vet Hum Toxicol 1994;36:233–237.
9. Middlebrook JL. Protection strategies against botulinum toxin. Adv Exp Med Biol 1995;383:93–98.
10. Sanford JP, Gilbert DN, Moellering RC Jr, Sande MA, eds. The Sanford guide to antimicrobial therapy. 27th ed. Dallas: Antimicrobial Therapy, 1997.
11. Schmidt RD, Schmidt TW. Infant botulism: a case series and review of the literature. J Emerg Med 1992;10:713–718.
12. Woodruff BA, Griffin PM, McCroskey LM, Smart JF, Wainwright RB, Bryant RG, Hutwagner LC, Hatheway CL. Clinical and laboratory comparison of botulism from toxin types A, B, and E in the United States, 1975–1988. J Infect Dis 1992;166:1281–1286.

Clostridium difficile

●

Stuart Johnson and Dale N. Gerding

GENERAL DESCRIPTION

Infection with *Clostridium difficile* is associated with clinical manifestations ranging from asymptomatic colonization, non-specific watery diarrhea, and pseudomembranous colitis to toxic megacolon (29). This enteric pathogen has several unique epidemiologic associations that should be remembered when considering therapeutic options. Hospitalization and anti-microbial therapy are the best-documented risk factors for *C. difficile*–associated diarrhea and reflect important steps in the pathogenesis of this disease.

First, the association with hospitalization reflects the fact that *C. difficile* infection is acquired and that hospitals and other chronic-care institutions are major reservoirs for this infection (29). Where surveillance has been conducted, *C. difficile* diarrhea is found to be endemic in most tertiary hospitals, and large outbreaks continue to occur (55). Stool culture surveillance of hospitalized patients indicates that *C. difficile* infection is extremely common, and careful epidemiologic typing studies have demonstrated that most of these infections are acquired exogenously (37, 46, 58). In fact, the risk of *C. difficile* acquisition is directly associated with the length of hospital stay (14). After 3 weeks of hospitalization in one study, one-third of initially noncolonized patients were culture positive, most of whom were asymptomatic (14). In this setting, detection of *C. difficile* by culture is only presumptive evidence of associated disease. Detection of *C. difficile* toxins by cell culture assay or enzyme-linked immunosorbent assay (ELISA) is more specific for disease, but assessment of clinical symptoms is equally important in making therapeutic decisions. In addition, attempts at eradicating carrier state are ineffective with metronidazole and only temporarily effective with vancomycin; therefore, treatment of asymptomatic patients is not recommended (38).

Second, this infection is seen almost exclusively in patients who are currently receiving, or have recently received, antimicrobial therapy (45). Disruption of indigenous bacterial flora resident in the intestinal tract by antimicrobial therapy (or, occasionally, by chemotherapy) is a critical element in the pathogenesis of *C. difficile*–associated disease (73). Bacteria indigenous to the host's intestinal tract prevent establishment of most nonindigenous organisms and potential pathogens. This protection, or "colonization resistance," can be overcome by enteric pathogens that use specific virulence mechanisms (e.g., epithelial invasion by salmonellae). However, the identified virulence factors of *C. difficile* (toxins) are not sufficient themselves to allow *C. difficile* to overcome colonization resistance. In contrast, once *C. difficile* infection has been established, recovery of colonization resistance may be significantly delayed, as shown by the high rate of relapse following initially effective therapy (29, 36). With the understanding that this infection is a complication of antimicrobial therapy, an important therapeutic intervention to remember is discontinuation of the offending drug or switching therapy to a potentially less predisposing agent such as (intravenous) aminoglycoside, vancomycin, or metronidazole (28). Simply discontinuing the offending agent may be the only intervention necessary in 15% of patients with *C. difficile* diarrhea (64). More commonly, *C. difficile* diarrhea becomes a prolonged illness unless it is recognized and treated with specific antimicrobial therapy.

SUSCEPTIBILITY IN VITRO AND IN VIVO

Although *C. difficile* isolates are highly resistant to some agents commonly implicated in precipitating *C. difficile* diarrhea (e.g., cephalosporins), other implicated antimicrobials (e.g., penicillin G and ampicillin) show marked activity against *C. difficile* in vitro (19). For other antimicrobial agents, different *C. difficile* isolates show marked heterogeneity in susceptibility (e.g., clindamycin). Therefore, factors other than antimicrobial susceptibility in vitro are important in determining the risk of *C. difficile* diarrhea. When analyzing the in vitro susceptibility of *C. difficile* to agents used specifically for treatment of *C. difficile* diarrhea, one must also consider the achievable antimicrobial concentrations at the site of infection—the colonic mucosa.

Single Drug

Table 1 lists the relative susceptibilities of *C. difficile* to various agents used to treat or proposed to treat *C. difficile* diarrhea. With the exception of rifampin, metronidazole is one of the most active agents available and is bactericidal over a wide range of concentrations in vitro (44). Almost all isolates are susceptible to metronidazole concentrations of 1 μg/mL or less, with a typical minimal inhibitory concentration for 50% of strains tested (MIC_{50}) of 0.3 μg/mL (3, 13, 19, 21). Tinidazole, a related compound, is slightly less active (3, 39). *C. difficile* isolates are somewhat less susceptible to vancomycin (compared with metronidazole), with a typical MIC_{50} of 1 μg/mL, and occasional isolates are found with MICs of 8 or 16 μg/mL (12, 19). However, fecal vancomycin concentrations are typically in the 100 to 1000 μg/g range with oral therapy (38), and there is no evidence that isolates with the higher MIC values exhibit clinical resistance. In vitro kinetic studies demonstrated that whereas vancomycin was bactericidal for *C. difficile* at concentrations close to the MIC of the isolate, vancomycin exerted a bacteriostatic effect at higher concentrations typical of levels in the feces during therapy (44). This observation may partially explain the failure to eradicate

TABLE 1 • In Vitro Susceptibility of *Clostridium difficile* to Potential Therapeutic Antimicrobial Agents

Agent	n	MIC (μg/mL)		Range	Reference
		MIC$_{50}$	MIC$_{90}$		
Rifampin	55	<0.001	0.002	<0.001–0.002	Bacon 1991 (2)
Metronidazole	50	0.29	0.6	0.25–1.0	Bannatyne 1987 (3)
Ramoplanin[a]	70	0.25	0.5	0.12–1.0	Biavsco 1991 (8)
Tiacumicin B[a]	15	0.25	0.25	0.12–0.5	Swanson 1991 (63)
Tiacumicin C[a]	15	0.5	1.0	0.25–1.0	Swanson 1991 (63)
Teicoplanin	70	0.5	0.5	0.25–1.0	Biavsco 1991 (8)
Vancomycin	70	1.0	2.0	1.0–2.0	Biavsco 1991 (8)
Tinidazole[a]	50	0.55	3.74	0.5–4.0	Bannatyne 1987 (3)
Bacitracin	110	(MIC mode = 16 μg)		8.0–32.0	Young 1985 (75)
Fusidic acid	20	(17/20 susceptible to 10 μg, disk testing)			Burdon 1979 (7)

[a]Investigational agents.

C. difficile following initially effective therapy. In addition, relapse of *C. difficile* diarrhea has not been associated with development of vancomycin resistance (26). Teicoplanin, a related glycopeptide, is somewhat more active in vitro than vancomycin (8, 53).

The Syrian golden hamster has been used for susceptibility testing of *C. difficile* in vivo (4, 21). *C. difficile* infection in the hamster is a model of human infection, including the susceptibility to colonization at an early age that is lost with establishment of the indigenous flora (57). After 2 weeks of age, infection (colonization or disease) is totally dependent on antimicrobial exposure. The main site of disease in the antibiotic-treated hamster is the cecum, which is proportionately much larger in rodents than in humans, but which serves functions similar to that served by the human colon, the site of disease in humans. Although the results of in vivo testing depend on the strain of *C. difficile* used and the experimental design (63), several common themes have been documented by most investigators. First, the mortality of untreated *C. difficile* diarrhea in hamsters is close to 100%. Second, all antimicrobial agents that have shown treatment efficacy in vivo can also be used to precipitate the disease in hamsters. Third, while both vancomycin and metronidazole protect infected hamsters during therapy, once therapy is discontinued, the organism and cytotoxin become detectable in the stool, and the animals succumb within 2 to 9 days (4, 21). When strict animal housing/handling methods have been used in these experiments, mortality rates drop, suggesting that these animals are still susceptible following vancomycin treatment and that conventionally housed hamsters reacquire the organism from their environment (21). More recently, vancomycin was shown to protect hamsters in a dose-dependent manner, and tiacumicin B, an investigational macrolide, was more active than vancomycin in these experiments (63).

Combination Drugs

Rifampin has been tested in combination with various agents against *C. difficile* in vitro. Although this drug is the most active single agent tested in vitro, resistance develops quickly (20). When defined as a 4-fold reduction in the MIC for both agents,

one study demonstrated synergy with the rifampin/metronidazole combination in 68% of isolates tested, with rifampin/vancomycin in 38% of isolates, and with vancomycin/metronidazole in 68% of isolates (20). A more recent study demonstrated only partial synergy with rifampin/metronidazole in 38% of isolates tested and with rifampin/vancomycin in 4% of isolates, using a fractional inhibitory concentration (FIC) index of 0.51 to 0.75 as the definition of partial synergy (2). However, full synergy (FIC <0.50) was demonstrated with rifampin/bacitracin in 85% of isolates tested.

ANTIMICROBIAL THERAPY
General

As shown in Table 2, metronidazole, vancomycin, teicoplanin, and fusidic acid have all demonstrated greater than 90% efficacy in randomized comparative trials of *C. difficile* diarrhea treatment. The most clinical experience has been with vancomycin and metronidazole. Metronidazole, unlike vancomycin, is well absorbed, and fecal concentrations are low or absent in treated patients without diarrhea (1, 35, 38). However, bactericidal fecal concentrations are present in patients with *C. difficile* diarrhea and decrease as the diarrhea improves, suggesting that metronidazole may diffuse from the serum compartment directly through inflamed colonic mucosa or that reduced intestinal transit time results in increased absorption (7).

Although vancomycin was originally considered the drug of choice by several experts, metronidazole is now the preferred first-line agent for several reasons. First, the efficacy of metronidazole has been confirmed in a recent prospective randomized trial demonstrating high cure rates and similar clinical relapse rates, compared with vancomycin and teicoplanin (71). The earlier prospective comparison of metronidazole and vancomycin (64) has been criticized because patients with positive stool cultures and negative stool toxin assays were included in the study, and several reviews have cautioned reserving metronidazole for less severe cases of *C. difficile* diarrhea (23). Cure and relapse rates in the recent study (71) and in the earlier prospective study (64) were the same when patients with pseudomembranous colitis documented by en-

TABLE 2 • **Randomized, Comparative Trials of Oral Therapy for *Clostidium difficile* Diarrhea**

Agent	Regimen	Patients Studied	Cure Rate (%)	Relapse Rate[a] (%)	Time to Resolution (days)	References
Metronidazole	500 mg t.i.d. × 10 days	31	94	16	3.2	Wenisch 1996 (71)
	250 mg q.i.d. × 10 days	42	95	5	2.4	Teasley 1983 (64)
Vancomycin	500 mg t.i.d. × 10 days	31	94	16	3.1	Wenisch 1996 (71)
	500 mg q.i.d. × 10 days	87	100	15	2.6–3.6	Teasley 1983, deLalla 1992, Dudley 1986 (64, 17, 18)
	125 mg q.i.d. × 7 days	21	86	29	4.2	Young 1985 (75)
	125 mg q.i.d. × 5 days	12	75	NS	<5.0	Mogg 1980 (49)
Teicoplanin	400 mg b.i.d. × 10 days	28	96	7	2.8	Wenisch 1996 (71)
	100 mg b.i.d. × 10 days	26	96	8	3.4	deLalla 1992 (17)
Fusidic acid	500 mg t.i.d. × 10 days	29	93	28	3.8	Wenisch 1996 (71)
Bacitracin	20k–25k U qid × 7–10 days	36	78	28	2.5–4.1	Dudley 1986, Young 1985 (18, 75)
Colestipol	10 g q.i.d. × 5 days	14	36	NS	<5.0	Mogg 1980 (49)
Placebo	— × 5 days	14	21	NS	<5.0	Mogg 1980 (49)

Adapted from Gerding DN, Johnson S, Peterson LR, Mulligan ME, Silva J Jr. Society for Healthcare Epidemiology of America position paper on *Clostridium difficile*-associated diarrhea and colitis. Infect Control Hosp Epidemiol 1995;16:459–477.

[a]NS, not stated, only bacteriologic follow-up reported.

doscopy were analyzed separately, suggesting that severity of disease does not influence the response to metronidazole. Another recent report also documented similar cure and relapse rates; however, in this retrospective study, duration of symptoms was shorter in patients treated with vancomycin than for those who received metronidazole (3 vs. 4.6 days, respectively) (72). Neither of the two prospective studies showed any difference in the time to response between patients treated with these two agents (64, 71). Because the response rates to either metronidazole or vancomycin are so high, a prospective study of enormous patient size would be necessary to demonstrate any subtle differences in clinical efficacy. Clinical experience with metronidazole for *C. difficile* diarrhea was recently reviewed at one institution over a 10-year period in which metronidazole was emphasized as first-line therapy (70, 13), and 17% of patients received metronidazole, vancomycin, and no treatment, respectively (52). The drug intolerance rate, treatment failure rate, and relapse rate for 632 metronidazole-treated patients were 1, 2, and 6%, respectively.

Second, metronidazole is the least expensive treatment for *C. difficile* diarrhea, at a cost of $4.00 for a 10-day treatment course (250 mg four times daily) compared with $175.00 or $873.00 for a 10-day course of vancomycin (125 mg or 500 mg four times daily) (local Chicago, IL, pharmacy costs). Third, concern over the increase in vancomycin resistance among enterococci and (potentially) other important hospital-acquired pathogens has led to the recommendation that vancomycin use be limited. In particular, the Hospital Infection Control Practices Advisory Committee (HICPAC) has suggested that oral vancomycin be reserved for the treatment of patients who fail to respond to metronidazole or for severe, potentially life-threatening illness (34). This recommendation has, in general, received widespread acceptance, and most experts now recommend metronidazole as the initial specific agent of choice except for particular situations (24, 29). Long-term follow-up of more than 700 women who received metronidazole for vaginal trichomoniasis did not demon-

strate increased cancer-related morbidity or mortality (6), despite evidence of carcinogenic potential in some rodent studies. The safety of metronidazole in children has not been proven (24), and metronidazole is a pregnancy category B drug. Despite having no FDA approval for this indication, we believe that metronidazole should be considered the drug of choice for *C. difficile* diarrhea.

Vancomycin was the first effective therapy for *C. difficile* diarrhea and has been the drug with which all subsequent therapies have been compared (23). Cure rates close to 100% for vancomycin at a dosage of 500 mg given three to four times daily for 10 days have been documented in all prospective studies reported (Table 2). This response rate drops to 75% when the regimen is decreased to 125 mg four times daily for 5 days (Table 2). However, there were no treatment failures when the "lower-dose" vancomycin regimen (125 mg four times daily) was given for 10 days (22). Despite the predictably high fecal levels achieved and its remarkable clinical efficacy, about 15% of treated patients still relapse (Table 2). Teicoplanin has now demonstrated efficacy similar to that achieved with vancomycin and metronidazole in two prospective clinical studies, at two different doses given twice a day for 10 days (17, 71). Fusidic acid has now been studied prospectively, and although similar high cure rates were demonstrated, the clinical relapse rate was higher than for those treated with teicoplanin (71). Fusidic acid was also associated with a higher rate of side effects (gastrointestinal discomfort) than vancomycin and teicoplanin therapy. Clinical cure rates and *C. difficile* eradication rates with bacitracin are somewhat lower than with vancomycin (18, 75), and bacitracin should be considered a second-line agent in the treatment of *C. difficile* diarrhea. Treatment with the ion-exchange resin colestipol is clearly inferior to the agents described above (49) and is not recommended for initial treatment.

The optimal dosage of most effective treatments for *C. difficile* diarrhea has not been determined, but 10 days of therapy appears necessary to achieve cure rates of 90%. Based on available data, we recommend the following dosages; metronidazole 250 mg four times daily or 500 mg three times daily and vancomycin 125 mg four times daily. Further studies are necessary before teicoplanin (71, 74) and fusidic acid (16, 71) dosage recommendations can be made. All therapies should be administered orally, and antiperistaltic agents should not be administered. An early controlled trial indicated that phenoxylate-atropine (Lomotil) used alone was deleterious to patients with *C. difficile* diarrhea (51), and anecdotal reports suggest that its use may predispose to toxic megacolon (15, 27). Loperamide has also been implicated in toxic megacolon (68). A recent retrospective study did not demonstrate any different response in patients who received antimotility agents (usually loperamide or codeine phosphate) in conjunction with specific therapy (72), but carefully designed prospective studies must be conducted before any general recommendations can be made regarding the use of antimotility agents for *C. difficile* diarrhea.

Special Situations

Diarrhea Recurrence

It is apparent from Table 2 that most people respond to treatment for *C. difficile* diarrhea. Recurrence of diarrhea after initially effective therapy is extremely common, however, occurring at rates of 5 to 30% regardless of the initial treatment regimen, similar to the experience with the hamster model of *C. difficile* diarrhea. As mentioned above, the mechanism of diarrhea recurrence may differ following metronidazole or vancomycin therapy as a result of decreasing metronidazole fecal levels on resolution of diarrhea or the bacteriostatic effect of vancomycin on *C. difficile* at the high concentrations achieved during therapy (44). In addition, diarrhea recurrence may be due to relapse of the original infecting strain or due to exogenous reinfection with a new strain (36). There is no evidence that recurrence is due to acquisition of resistance to the initial therapeutic agent, and the first relapse should be treated in the same manner as the first episode.

A small group of patients suffer multiple recurrences of *C. difficile* diarrhea, frustrating the physician as well as the patient. Typically, these patients respond promptly to treatment after each recurrent episode but redevelop symptoms and positive stool assays within 1 to 2 weeks after discontinuation of treatment. As mentioned above, nearly all cases of *C. difficile* diarrhea are precipitated by antimicrobial disruption of normal intestinal flora. It is possible that the specific agent used to treat the initial episode of diarrhea is the precipitating agent for the recurrent episode. Empirical strategies that have been used to manage patients with multiple recurrences of *C. difficile* diarrhea are listed in Table 3 and discussed below under "Alternative Therapy."

Severe Ileus/Toxic Megacolon

The most serious manifestation of *C. difficile* disease is toxic megacolon, which paradoxically may present without diarrhea (50, 52). Treatment of patients with toxic megacolon or severe illness is difficult and controversial, but several attempts have been made to achieve effective antimicrobial concentrations at the site of infection when the oral route is compromised. Some authors advocate treatment with intravenous metronidazole or intravenous vancomycin at dosages of 2 g/day, or placement of a long catheter in the small intestine and instillation of vancomycin (61). Another approach is to administer vancomycin by rectal enema (30, 52, 54). A strategy used successfully at one institution in six patients with severe ileus included vancomycin administered by nasogastric tube and by retention enema plus intravenous metronidazole (Table 4) (52). Surgical intervention is indicated when patients with toxic megacolon do not respond to medical treatment or when colonic perforation is suspected (50). Colonic diversions and partial or complete colectomies have been performed, but mortality is high (50). Although efficacy has been difficult to assess, subtotal colectomy with sparing of the rectal stump appears to be the preferred surgical option (15, 50).

Alternative Therapy

When Oral Therapy Is Not Possible

Although several options exist for the treatment of *C. difficile* diarrhea (Table 2), all well-studied regimens use oral therapy. When the oral route is compromised, intravenous therapy may be considered. Colonic concentrations of vancomycin are negligible after intravenous administration, and there is little support for this option. Fecal concentrations of metronidazole, however, are similar when metronidazole is given orally or in-

TABLE 3 • Empirical Treatment Strategies for Patients with Multiple Recurrences of *C. difficile* Diarrhea

Strategy	References
Saccharomyces boulardii	McFarland 1994, Surawicz 1989 (47, 62)
Lactobacillus	GG Biller 1995, Gorbach 1987 (9, 31)
Rectal infusion of feces or a synthetic fecal bacterial flora	Tvede, 1989, Schwan 1983, Bowden 1982 (67, 59, 10)
Administration of a nontoxigenic *C. difficile* strain	Seal, 1987 (60)
Vancomycin and rifampin combination	Buggy 1987 (11)
Vancomycin in tapering doses	Tedesco 1985 (66)
Cholestyramine	Monico 1992, Pruksananonda 1989, Kunimoto 1986, Tedesco 1982 (48, 56, 41, 65)
Intravenous gamma globulin	Hassett 1995, Warny 1995, Leung 1991 (33, 70, 43)
Whole bowel irrigation	Liacouras 1996 (42)
No treatment with careful observation	Gerding 1995, Bartlett 1992 (29, 5)

travenously in the setting of acute *C. difficile* diarrhea (7). Anecdotal experience supports intravenous metronidazole therapy for *C. difficile* diarrhea (7, 40), but this therapy alone may be inadequate in patients with severe adynamic ileus (32). Therefore, in patients with severe manifestations of *C. difficile* disease, other methods to ensure effective antimicrobial concentrations at the site of infection should also be considered (Table 4).

Patients with Multiple Diarrhea Recurrences

Several strategies have been explored for managing patients with multiple recurrences (Table 3). None of these regimens has proven efficacy, and although the first four therapeutic agents listed are not commercially available, they may eventually be the preferred strategies to deal with this select group of difficult-to-manage patients. Part of the rationale behind the first four strategies listed is an attempt to avoid further antibiotic therapy and allow the normal colonic flora to reestablish itself. Of these biotherapeutic approaches, treatment with the yeast *Saccharomyces boulardii* is probably the best studied. In the initial report of 13 patients with multiple diarrhea recurrences who received vancomycin for 10 days and *S. boulardii* for 28 days, 11 patients had no further recurrences (62). More recently, a randomized, placebo-controlled study showed that *S. boulardii* in combination with standard therapy was more effective than standard therapy alone in preventing recurrences in patients who had a history of more than one *C. difficile* diarrhea episode (47). Other, nonantimicrobial, biotherapeutic approaches tested on small groups of patients in open trials include treatment with *Lactobacillus* GG (9, 31), rectal infusion of feces from normal hosts (10, 59), and infusion of a mixture of bacteria simulating a normal flora (67). An additional novel approach that was partially successful in two patients was introduction of a nontoxigenic strain of *C. difficile* (60).

Two other antimicrobial approaches that have been studied in small open trials include combination therapy with vancomycin (125 mg orally, four times a day) and rifampin (600 mg orally, twice daily) for 7 days (11) and treatment with a tapering dose of vancomycin over 21 days followed by pulse therapy for the next 21 days (66). Cholestyramine, an anion-exchange binding resin has also been anecdotally reported as useful in this setting (41, 48, 56, 65); however, efficacy of anion-exchange binding resins in the treatment of primary *C. difficile* diarrhea has been poor (Table 1). The proposed mechanism of action is the binding of *C. difficile* toxins, but vancomycin is also bound, and cholestyramine has a nonspecific constipating effect.

Intravenous administration of immune globulin (IVIG) may also benefit a subgroup of patients with multiple relapses of *C. difficile* diarrhea (33, 43, 70). In two studies, patients had low levels of serum antitoxin A IgG (43, 70), and the patient in the third study had selective IgG1 deficiency (33). A recent report suggested that whole bowel irrigation with a polyethylene glycol solution (Golytely) followed by a course of vancomycin was successful in terminating multiple relapses of *C. difficile* colitis in two young children (42). Finally, no treatment with careful observation has also been advocated in selected patients (5, 29).

ENDPOINTS FOR MONITORING THERAPY

The only endpoint useful in monitoring therapy for *C. difficile* diarrhea is clinical evaluation of patient symptoms. Treatment with specific therapy (Table 2) should be given for 10 days and discontinued. If the patient does not respond after 5 to 6 days of specific therapy, an empirical switch to an alternate drug may be considered (e.g., vancomycin for metronidazole), but the initial diagnosis should also be reconsidered. Positive stool cultures for *C. difficile* at the completion of therapy is moderately predictive of relapse (69), but it is strongly recommended that stool cultures and toxin assays not be performed if the patient's symptoms have resolved (25, 29). Positive test results alone often lead clinicians to inappropriately prolong therapy or switch therapy to a different agent. Clinical relapses occur frequently, but final resolution of symptoms in most patients likely depends on reestablishing the normal colonic flora, and further antibiotic therapy potentially delays the recovery of this flora.

COMMENTS

In summary, *C. difficile* diarrhea and colitis are complications of antimicrobial therapy, and the indigenous bacterial flora of the intestinal tract provide a critical element of host defense against this pathogen. Once *C. difficile* diarrhea is suspected on clinical grounds (patient has recently received antimicrobial therapy, particularly with recent hospitalization), the following general principles of therapy should be considered (29). First, discontinue the offending antibiotic, if possible. This may be the only intervention necessary in 17% of patients (52). In contrast, if the patient is seriously ill, empirical therapy should be administered after a stool specimen has been obtained for diagnostic assay. Second, specific therapy should be administered orally. Third, nearly all patients respond to specific therapy, but the mean time to response is 2 to 4 days (Table 2). Fourth, treat for 10 days and do not perform test of cure assays if the patient has responded. Finally, until better data become available, avoid antiperistaltic agents.

TABLE 4 • **Empirical Treatment Protocol for *Clostridium difficile*-Infected Patients with Severe Ileus**

Vancomycin	500 mg per rectum every 6 h[a], plus
Vancomycin	500 mg via NG tube every 6 h[b], plus
Metronidazole	500 mg i.v. every 6 h

From Olson MM, Shanholtzer CJ, Lee JT Jr, Gerding DN. Ten years of prospective *Clostridium difficile*-associated disease surveillance and treatment at the Minneapolis VA Medical Center, 1982–1991. Infect Control Hosp Epidemiol 1994;15:371–381.

[a]Liquid intravenous formulation diluted in 100 mL of normal saline; insert #18 Foley catheter into rectum 4 to 8 inches, fill the balloon to 30 mL, gently pull catheter down, instill vancomycin, and clamp catheter for 60 min, deflate balloon and remove catheter.

[b]Liquid intravenous formulation diluted with at least 10 mL of fluid; clamp nasogastric tube for 60 min after each instillation.

REFERENCES

1. Arabi Y, Dimock F, Burdon DW, Alexander-Williams J, Keighley MRB. Influence of neomycin and metronidazole on colonic

microflora of volunteers. J Antimicrob Chemother 1979;5: 531–537.

2. Bacon AE, McGrath S, Fekety R, Holloway WJ. In vitro synergy studies with *Clostridium difficile*. Antimicrob Agents Chemother 1991;35:582–583.

3. Bannatyne R, Jackowski J. Susceptibility of *Clostridium difficile* to metronidazole, its bioactive metabolites and tinidazole. Eur J Clin Microbiol 1987;6:505.

4. Bartlett JG. Treatment of antibiotic-associated pseudomembranous colitis. Rev Infect Dis 1984;6(Suppl 1):S235–S241.

5. Bartlett JG. The 10 most common questions about *Clostridium difficile*-associated diarrhea/colitis. Infect Dis Clin Pract 1992;1: 254–259.

6. Beard CM, Noller KL, O'Fallon WM, Kurland LT, Dahlin DC. Cancer after exposure to metronidazole. Mayo Clin Proc 1988; 63:147–153.

7. Bolton RP, Culshasw MA. Fecal metronidazole concentrations during oral and intravenous therapy for antibiotic-associated colitis due to *Clostridium difficile*. Gut 1986;27:1169–1172.

8. Biavasco F, Manso E, Varaldo PE. In vitro activities of ramoplanin and four glycopeptide antibiotics against clinical isolates of *Clostridium difficile*. Antimicrob Agents Chemother 1991;35: 195–197.

9. Biller JA, Katz AJ, Flores AF, Buie TM, Gorbach SL. Treatment of recurrent *Clostridium difficile* colitis with *Lactobacillus* GG. J Pediatr Gastroenterol Nutr 1995;21:224–226.

10. Bowden TA, Mansberger AR, Lykins LE. Pseudomembranous enterocolitis: mechanism of restoring floral homeostasis. Am Surg 1981;47:178–183.

11. Buggy BP. Fekety R, Silva J Jr, Therapy of relapsing *Clostridium difficile*-associated diarrhea and colitis with the combination of vancomycin and rifampin. J Clin Gastroenterol 1987;9: 155–159.

12. Burdon DW, Brown DJ, Youngs DJ, Arabi Y, Shinagawa N, Alexander-Williams J, Keighley MRB. Antibiotic susceptibility of *Clostridium difficile*. J Antimicrob Chemother 1979;5: 307–310.

13. Clabots CR, Shanholtzer CJ, Peterson LR, Gerding DN. In vitro activity of efrotomycin, ciprofloxacin, and six other antimicrobials against *Clostridium difficile*. Diagn Microbiol Infect Dis 1987;6:49–52.

14. Clabots CR, Johnson S, Olson MM, Peterson LR, Gerding DN. Acquisition of *Clostridium difficile* by hospitalized patients: evidence for colonized new admissions as the source of infection. J Infect Dis 1992;166:561–567.

15. Cone JB, Wetzel W. Toxic megacolon secondary to pseudomembranous colitis. Dis Colon Rectum 1982;25:478–482.

16. Cronberg S, Castor B, Thorén A. Fusidic acid for the treatment of antibiotic-associated colitis induced by *Clostridium difficile*. Infection 1984;12:276–279.

17. deLalla F, Nicolin R, Rinaldi E, Scarpellini P, Rigoli R, Manfrin V, Tramarin A. Prospective study of oral teicoplanin versus oral vancomycin for therapy of pseudomembranous colitis and *Clostridium difficile*-associated diarrhea. Antimicrob Agents Chemother 1992;36:2192–2196.

18. Dudley MN, McLaughlin JC, Carrington G, Frick J, Nightingale CH, Quintiliani R. Oral bacitracin versus vancomycin therapy for *Clostridium difficile*-induced diarrhea: a randomized, double-blind trial. Arch Intern Med 1986;146:1101–1104.

19. Dzink J, Bartlett JG. In vitro susceptibility of *Clostridium difficile* isolates from patients with antibiotic-associated diarrhea or colitis. Antimicrob Agents Chemother 1980;17:695–698.

20. Ensminger PW, Counter FT, Thomas LJ, Lubbehusen PP. Sus-

ceptibility, resistance development, and synergy of antimicrobial combinations against *Clostridium difficile*. Curr Microbiol 1982;7:59–62.

21. Fekety F, Silva J, Toshniwal R, Allo M, Armstrong J, Browne R, Ebright J, Rifkin G. Antibiotic-associated colitis: Effects of antibiotics on *Clostridium difficile* and the disease in hamsters. Rev Infect Dis 1979;1:386–397.

22. Fekety R, Silva J, Kauffman C, Buggy B, Deery G. Treatment of antibiotic-associated *Clostridium difficile* colitis with oral vancomycin: Comparison of two dosage regimens. Am J Med 1989;86:15–19.

23. Fekety R, Shah AB. Diagnosis and treatment of *Clostridium difficile* colitis. JAMA 1993;269:71–75.

24. Fekety R. Guidelines for the diagnosis and management of *Clostridium difficile*-associated diarrhea and colitis. Am J Gastroenterol 1997;92:739–750.

25. Finegold SM, George WL. Therapy directed against *Clostridium difficile* and its toxins: complications of therapy. In: Rolfe RD, George WL, eds. *Clostridium difficile:* its role in intestinal disease. New York: Academic Press, 1988:341–357.

26. George WL, Volpicelli NA, Stiner DB, Richman DD, Liechty EJ, Mok HYI, Finegold SM. Relapse of pseudomembranous colitis after vancomycin therapy. N Engl J Med 1979;301:414–415.

27. George WL, Rolfe RD, Finegold SM. Treatment and prevention of antimicrobial agent-induced colitis and diarrhea. Gastroenterol 1980;79:366–372.

28. Gerding DN, Olson MM, Johnson S, Peterson LR, Lee JT Jr. *Clostridium difficile* diarrhea and colonization following treatment with abdominal infection regimens containing clindamycin or metronidazole. Am J Surg 1990;159:212–217.

29. Gerding DN, Johnson S, Peterson LR, Mulligan ME, Silva J Jr. Society for Healthcare Epidemiology of America position paper on *Clostridium difficile*-associated diarrhea and colitis. Infect Control Hosp Epidemiol 1995;16:459–477.

30. Goodpasture HC, Dolan PJ Jr, Jacobs ER, Meridith WT. Pseudomembranous enterocolitis and antibiotics. Kans Med 1986;87:133–146.

31. Gorbach SL, Chang T-W, Goldin B. Successful treatment of relapsing *Clostridium difficile* colitis with *Lactobacillus* GG. Lancet 1987;ii:1519.

32. Guzman R, Kirkpatrick J, Forward K, Lim F. Failure of parenteral metronidazole in the treatment of pseudomembranous colitis. J Infect Dis 1988;158:1146.

33. Hassett J, Meyers S, McFarland L, Mulligan ME. Recurrent *Clostridium difficile* infection in a patient with selective IgG1 deficiency treated with intravenous immune globulin and *Saccharomyces boulardii*. Clin Infect Dis 1995;20(Suppl 2): S266–S268.

34. Hospital Infection Control Practices Advisory Committee (HICPAC). Recommendations for preventing the spread of vancomycin resistance. Infect Control Hosp Epidemiol 1995;16: 105–113.

35. Høverstad T, Carlstedt-Duke B, Lingaas E, Midtvedt T, Norin KE, Saxerholt H, Steinbakk M. Influence of ampicillin, clindamycin, and metronidazole on faecal excretion of short-chain fatty acids in healthy subjects. Scand J Gastroenterol 1986; 21:621–628.

36. Johnson S, Adelmann A, Clabots CR, Peterson LR, Gerding DN. Recurrences of *Clostridium difficile* diarrhea not caused by the original infecting organism. J Infect Dis 1989; 159:340–343.

37. Johnson S, Clabots CR, Linn FV, Olson MM, Peterson LR, Gerding DN. Nosocomial *Clostridium difficile* colonization and disease. Lancet 1990;336:97–100.

38. Johnson S, Homann SR, Bettin KM, Quick JN, Clabots CR, Peterson LR, Gerding DN. Treatment of asymptomatic *Clostridium difficile* carriers (fecal excretors) with vancomycin, metronidazole or placebo. Ann Intern Med 1992;117:297–302.

39. Jokipii AMM, Jokipii L. Comparative activity of metronidazole and tinidazole against *Clostridium difficile* and *Peptostreptococcus anaerobius*. Antimicrob Agents Chemother 1987;31: 183–186.

40. Kleinfeld DI, Sharpe RJ, Donta ST. Parenteral therapy for antibiotic-associated pseudomembranous colitis. J Infect Dis 1988; 157:389.

41. Kunimoto D, Thomson ABR. Recurrent *Clostridium difficile*-associated colitis responding to cholestyramine. Digestion 1986; 33:225–228.

42. Liacouras CA, Piccoli DA. Whole-bowel irrigation as an adjunct to the treatment of chronic, relapsing *Clostridium difficile* colitis. J Clin Gastroenterol 1996;22:186–189.

43. Leung DYM, Kelly CP, Boguniewicz M, Pothoulakis C, LaMont JT, Flores A. Treatment with intravenously administered gamma globulin of chronic relapsing colitis induced by *Clostridium difficile* toxin. J Pediatr 1991;118:633–637.

44. Levett PN. Time-dependent killing of *Clostridium difficile* by metronidazole and vancomycin. J Antimicrob Chemother 1991; 27:55–62.

45. Manabe YC, Vinetz JM, Moore RD, Merz C, Charache P, Bartlett JG. *Clostridium difficile* colitis: an efficient clinical approach to diagnosis. Ann Intern Med 1995;123:835–840.

46. McFarland LV, Mulligan M, Kwok RYY, Stamm WE. Nosocomial acquisition of *Clostridium difficile*-associated infection. N Engl J Med 1989;320:204–210.

47. McFarland LV, Surawicz CM, Greenberg RN, Fekety R, Elmer GW, Moyer KA, Melcher SA, Bowen KE, Cox JL, Noorani Z, Harrington G, Rubin M, Greenwald D. A randomized placebo-controlled trial of *Saccharomyces boulardii* in combination with standard antibiotics for *Clostridium difficile* disease. JAMA 1994;271:1913–1918.

48. Moncino MD, Falletta JM. Multiple relapses of *Clostridium difficile*-associated diarrhea in a cancer patient: successful control with long-term cholestyramine therapy. Am J Pediatr Hematol Oncol 1992;14:361–364.

49. Mogg GAG, Arabi Y, Youngs D, Johnson M, Bentley S, Burdon DW, Keighley MRB. Therapeutic trials of antibiotic associated colitis. Scand J Infect Dis 1980;(Suppl 22):41–45.

50. Morris JB, Zollinger RM, Stellato TA. Role of surgery in antibiotic-induced pseudomembranous colitis. Am J Surg 1990; 160:535–539.

51. Novak E, Lee JG, Seckman CE, Phillips JP, DiSanto AR. Unfavorable effect of atropine-diphenoxylate (Lomotil) therapy in lincomycin-caused diarrhea. JAMA 1976;235:1451–1454.

52. Olson MM, Shanholtzer CJ, Lee JT Jr, Gerding DN. Ten years of prospective *Clostridium difficile*-associated disease surveillance and treatment at the Minneapolis VA Medical Center, 1982–1991. Infect Control Hosp Epidemiol 1994;15:371–381.

53. Pantosti A, Luzzi I, Cardines R, Gianfrilli P. Comparison of the in vitro activities of teicoplanin and vancomycin against *Clostridium difficile* and their interactions with cholestyramine. Antimicrob Agents Chemother 1985;28:847–848.

54. Pasic M, Jost R, Carrel T, Von Segesser L, Turina M. Intracolonic vancomycin for pseudomembranous colitis. N Engl J Med 1993;329:583.

55. Pear SM, Williamson TH, Bettin KM, Gerding DN, Galgiani JN. Decrease in nosocomial *Clostridium difficile*-associated diarrhea by restricting clindamycin use. Ann Intern Med 1994;120: 272–277.

56. Pruksananonda P, Powell KR. Multiple relapses of *Clostridium difficile*-associated diarrhea responding to an extended course of cholestyramine. Pediatr Infect Dis J 1989;8:175–178.

57. Rolfe RD, Iaconis JP. Intestinal colonization of infant hamsters with *Clostridium difficile*. Infect Immun 1983;42:480–486.

58. Samore MH, DeGirolami PC, Tlucko A, Lichtenberg DA, Melvin ZA, Karchmer AW. *Clostridium difficile* colonization and diarrhea at a tertiary care hospital. Clin Infect Dis 1994; 18:181–187.

59. Schwan A, Sjolin S, Trottestam U, Aronsson B. Relapsing *Clostridium difficile* enterocolitis cured by rectal infusion of normal faeces. Scand J Infect Dis 1984;16:211–215.

60. Seal D, Borriello SP, Barclay F, Welch A, Piper M, Bonnycastle M. Treatment of relapsing *Clostridium difficile* diarrhea by administration of a non-toxigenic strain. Eur J Clin Microbiol 1987;6:51–53.

61. Silva J Jr. Update on pseudomembranous colitis. West J Med 1989;151:644–648.

62. Surawicz CM, McFarland LV, Elmer G, Chin J. Treatment of recurrent *Clostridium difficile* colitis with vancomycin and *Saccharomyces boulardii*. Am J Gastroenterol 1989;84: 1285–1287.

63. Swanson RN, Hardy DJ, Shipkowitz NL. In vitro and in vivo evaluation of tiacumicins B and C against *Clostridium difficile*. Antimicrob Agents Chemother 1991;35:1108–1111.

64. Teasley DG, Gerding DN, Olson MM, Peterson LR, Gebhard RL, Schwartz ML, Lee JT Jr. Prospective randomized trial of metronidazole versus vancomycin for *Clostridium difficile*-associated diarrhea and colitis. Lancet 1983;ii:1043–1046.

65. Tedesco FJ. Treatment of recurrent antibiotic-associated pseudomembranous colitis. Am J Gastroenterol 1982;77:220–221.

66. Tedesco FJ, Gordon D, Fortson WC. Approach to patients with multiple relapses of antibiotic-associated pseudomembranous colitis. Am J Gastroenterol 1985;80:867–868.

67. Tvede M, Rask-Madsen J. Bacteriotherapy for chronic relapsing *Clostridium difficile* diarrhea in six patients. Lancet 1989;i: 1156–1160.

68. Walley T, Milson D. Loperamide related toxic megacolon in *Clostridium difficile* colitis. Postgrad Med J 1990;66:582.

69. Walters BAJ, Roberts R, Stafford R, Seneviratne E. Relapse of antibiotic associated colitis: endogenous persistence of *Clostridium difficile* during vancomycin therapy. Gut 1983;24:206–212.

70. Warny M, Denie C, Delmee M, Lefebvre C. Gamma globulin administration in relapsing *Clostridium difficile*-induced pseudomembranous colitis with a defective antibody response to toxin A. Acta Clin Belg 1995;50:36–39.

71. Wenisch C, Parschalk B, Hasenhundl M, Hirschl AM, Graninger W. Comparison of vancomycin, teicoplanin, metronidazole, and fusidic acid for the treatment of *Clostridium difficile*-associated diarrhea. Clin Infect Dis 1996;22:813–818.

72. Wilcox MH, Howe R. Diarrhoea caused by *Clostridium difficile*: response time for treatment with metronidazole and vancomycin. J Antimicrob Chemother 1995;36:673–679.

73. Wilson KH. The microecology of *Clostridium difficile*. Clin Infect Dis 1993;16(Suppl 4):S214–S218.

74. Wiström J, and the Swedish CDAD Study Group. Treatment of *Clostridium difficile* associated diarrhea and colitis with an oral preparation of teicoplanin; a dose finding study. Scand J Infect Dis 1994;26:309–316.

75. Young GP, Ward PB, Bayley N, Gordon D, Higgins G, Trapani JA, McDonald, MI, Labrooy J, Hecker R. Antibiotic-associated colitis due to *Clostridium difficile*: double-blind comparison of vancomycin with bacitracin. Gastroenterol 1985;89:1038–1045.

Clostridium Species

•

Itzhak Brook

GENERAL DESCRIPTION

Organisms of the genus *Clostridium* are important members of human anaerobic gastrointestinal and cervical-vaginal flora that can be found in soil, decaying vegetation, and marine sediments and therefore have the potential of causing endogenous and exogenous infections (16). Infections caused by these organisms range from a variety of localized wound contamination to overwhelming systemic disease (3, 4).

The major disease entities caused by *Clostridium* include intestinal disorders, deep tissue suppurative infections, skin and soft tissue infections, and bacteremias. Most of the resulting diseases are mediated through production of potent extracellular toxins (13). The ability to form spores is often an important factor in the epidemiology of these infections. Many infections caused by *Clostridium* spp. are polymicrobic and include other aerobic and anaerobic bacteria. Of the 90 known *Clostridium* spp. at least 30 are associated with human disease. *C. perfringens,* the most important species, accounts for 20 to 40% of all isolates. Speciation is based mostly on cellular morphology, spore location (central, terminal, or subterminal), biochemical reactions, gas-liquid chromatography for fermentation products, and demonstration of production of lecithinase (or α-toxin by *C. perfringens*) and lipase (by *C. sporogenes, C. novyi,* and *C. botulinum* (21). Identification of the specific species of *Clostridium* from clinical infection is important, as the presence of some may indicate underlying bowel pathology (*C. septicum*) (7), require antitoxin administration (*C. perfringens*), or show increased resistance to certain antimicrobials (*C. ramosum, C. innocuum,* and *C. clostridioforme*). The susceptibility of *Clostridium* spp. needs to be monitored to verify current susceptibility. In serious infections, susceptibility tests of isolated *Clostridium* spp. should be performed, to ensure proper use of antimicrobials.

SUSCEPTIBILITY IN VITRO AND IN VIVO
Single Drugs

C. perfringens as well as most other *Clostridium* spp. is generally, but not universally, susceptible to penicillin-G, amoxicillin, ticarcillin, piperacillin, cefazolin, cefoxitin, cefotetan, third-generation cephalosporins, chloramphenicol, clindamycin, erythromycin, metronidazole, imipenem, meropenem, tetracycline, vancomycin, rifampin, and combinations of penicillins and β-lactamase inhibitors (1, 2, 5, 9, 11, 14, 22). Rifampin and chloramphenicol occasionally lack bactericidal activity against *C. perfringens* (22). Cefoxitin is less effective against *Clostridium* spp. than most other cephalosporins. Recent data indicate increasing resistance of *C. perfrigens* as

well as other species to antimicrobials (1, 2); *C. ramosum, C. innocuum,* and *C. clostridioforme* show increased resistance to penicillin (16–26%), cefoxitin (22–48%), other cephalosporins (20%), clindamycin (5–30%), and metronidazole (11–12%). *C. innocuum* is resistant to cephalosporins, and only moderately susceptible to penicillin (90%) and vancomycin (90%). *C. clostridioforme* resistance was noted to penicillin (26–90%), cephalothin (17%), cefoxitin (48%), chloramphenicol (33%), clindamycin (30%), and tetracycline (55%) (1, 20).

C. sordellii and *C. septicum* posses susceptibility similar that of *C. perfringens,* although occasional strains are resistant to extended-spectrum penicillins and clindamycin. *C. tertium* displays resistance to third-generation cephalosporins (2, 15). Decreased affinity for penicillin-binding proteins was found for strains of *C. perfringens,* and β-lactamase production has been observed with *C. ramosum, C. butyricum,* and *C. clostridioforme.* A transferable, plasmid-mediated resistance to tetracycline, chloramphenicol, and erythromycin-clindamycin was observed with *C. perfringens.*

In vivo studies demonstrated that drugs other than penicillin were more effective in treatment of clostridial infection. In mice, clindamycin, metronidazole, rifampin, and tetracycline were more efficacious than penicillin in the treatment of fulminate gas gangrene caused by *C. perfrigins* (17). Protein synthesis inhibitors (tetracycline, metronidazole, rifampin, clindamycin, and chloramphenicol) were better inhibitors of toxin synthesis than cell wall–active agents (penicillin). Compared with penicillin, a combined, superior, rapid bacterial killing and ability to suppress toxin production was noted with clindamycin, rifampin, and metronidazole (18).

Combination of Drugs

The combination of penicillin and clindamycin was found to be more efficacious than single therapy with metronidazole, clindamycin, rifampin, or penicillin. In contrast, the combination of penicillin and metronidazole was deleterious (19).

ANTIMICROBIAL THERAPY

Current recommendations for treatment are based on many retrospective studies in humans and several studies in animal models. Penicillin-G in a dose of 20 million units a day in adults and 100,000 to 250,000 units/kg/day intravenously every 4 h in children is the treatment of choice for serious infections due to *C. perfringens, C. sordellii* and *C. septicum,* such as bacteremia and intraabdominal, gall bladder, genital tract, pulmonary, central nervous system, and soft tissue infections. In cases of penicillin allergy or concern about resistance, other antibiotics should be considered. All isolates of serious infections should be tested for in vitro efficacy because of the possible recovery of resistant strains. Alternative drugs to penicillin are chloramphenicol (12.5–25 mg/kg q. 6 h for adults and children, p.o/i.v./i.m.; maximal dose, 4 g/day for adults), clindamycin (150–450 mg q. 6 h, p.o./i.v./i.m. for adults; 25–40 mg/kg/day q. 6–8 h for children), metronidazole (7.5 mg/kg q. 6 h p.o./i.v./i.m. for adults and children; maximal daily dose, 4.0 g/day in adults), tetracycline (250–500 mg q. 6 h p.o./i.v./i.m. for adults; maximal dose, 2 g; for children >9 years, 15–20 mg/kg/day i.v. q. 6 h or 25–50 mg/kg/day p.o. q. 6 h), vancomycin (15 mg/kg q. 12 h or 6–8 mg/kg q. 6 h i.v., maximal daily dose 2 g in adults; 10 mg/kg q. 6 h i.v. in children), imipenem (0.5–1 g q. 6–8 h i.v./i.m. in adults, maximal daily dose 2 g; and 15–25 mg/kg q. 6 h i.v./i.m. in children), and meropenem) 0.5–1.0 g q. 8 h i.v. for adults; 40 mg/kg/day q. 8 h i.v. for children). Cefoxitin is less active than most other cephalosporins against clostridia. Since *C. ramosum, C. butyricum* and *C. clostridioforme* can produce β-lactamase, penicillin cannot be the drug of choice for these organisms. Similarly, third-generation cephalosporins should not be used for *C. tertium*.

In clinical situations that involve polymicrobial infections, coverage against other potential pathogens, aerobic and anaerobic, should be included. This can be achieved by choosing single therapy with an antimicrobial that possesses wider coverage (e.g., imipenem) or by additional agents that cover other organisms (e.g., an aminoglycoside or quinolone for *Enterobacteriaceae,* or a penicillinase-resistant penicillin for *Staphylococcus aureus*). The impact of the animal studies that show improved efficacy of combination therapy with penicillin and clindamycin is not obvious. However, use of such a combination in serious clostridial myonecrosis (gas gangrene) should be considered (19).

Enteric diseases due to histotoxic clostridia include *C. perfringens* food poisoning and enteritis necroticans. Clostridial food poisoning generally does not require antibiotic therapy. The antibiotics preferred in enteritis necroticans and neutropenic enterocolitis are penicillin G, metronidazole, or chloramphenicol.

Clostridial bacteremia may not always require therapy, as it may be transitory or may only represent specimen contamination (6, 12). However, there are instances of clinically significant clostridial bacteremia without toxin involvement. This usually occurs in gynecologic, intraabdominal (including biliary and intestinal), and soft tissue (i.e., decubitus ulcer, myonecrosis) infections in which the organisms originate from the flora of the infected site. Treatment of central nervous system infection requires the use of antimicrobials with good penetration through the blood-brain barrier.

Antitoxin for gas gangrene is no longer commercially available in the United States, as it was not found to be effective and was associated with severe allergic reactions. However it is still recommended by some authorities. The use of hyperbaric oxygen in the treatment of gas gangrene is also controversial.

ENDPOINTS OF MONITORING THERAPY

Improvements and resolution of the infections are determined through a variety of clinical and laboratory tests. In the case of bacteremia, the lack of recovery of organisms from the blood is an important end point. The disappearance of hemolysis and reduction in the number of white blood cells are important signs of improvement. Improvement in intra-abdominal, biliary tract, genital and pulmonary infections can be judged through clinical and radiographic resolution of the infection — returns the gastrointestinal and pulmonary system to normal function, and disappearance of purulence. Central nervous system infection can be followed by repeated lumbar punctures and radiography. In the cases of subcutaneous tissue infection, return of the tissue to normal color and blood perfusion and resolution of the purulent inflammation are desired. The disappearance of the gas formation in the inflamed tissue (determined clinically or radiographically) are important clues.

CAVEATS AND COMMENTS

Surgery, debridement, and fluid management are important integral parts of any therapy of clostridial infection. Surgery is important in treatment of clostridial myonecrosis or gas gangrene. Amputation may be required in rapidly spreading infection of a limb. Repeated debridement may be required. Other modalities that are controversial are the use of polyvalent gas gangrene antitoxin and hyperbaric oxygen (8).

Even though cephalosporins and clindamycin are effective in vitro, their clinical efficacy is uncertain, and clinical failures have been noted with cephalosporins (10). Although clindamycin showed superior efficacy in animal models, clostridia other than *C. perfringens* showed increased resistance (1, 2). Penicillin is still the drug of choice for clostridial infection.

REFERENCES

1. Alexander CJ, Citron DM, Brazier JS, Goldstein EJC. Identification and antimicrobial resistance patterns of clinical isolates of *Clostridium clostridioforme, Clostridium innocuum* and *Clostridium ramosen* compared with these of clinical isolates of *Clostridium perfringens.* J Clin Microbiol 1995;33:3209–3215.
2. Brazier JS, Levitt PN, Stannard AL, Phillips KD, Willis AT. Antibiotic susceptibility of clinical isolates of *Clostridia.* J Antimicrob Chemother 1985;15:181–185.
3. Brook I. Pediatric anaerobic infections: diagnostic and management. St Louis: CV Mosby, 1989.
4. Finegold SM. Anaerobic bacteria in human disease. New York: Academic Press, 1977.
5. Gabay EL, Rolfe RD, Finegold SM. Susceptibility of *Clostridium septicum* to 23 antimicrobial agents. Antimicrob Agents Chemother 1981;20:852–853.
6. Gorbach SL, Thadepalli H. Isolation of *Clostridium* in human infections: evaluation of 114 cases. J Infect Dis 1985;131: S81–S85.
7. Kornbluth A., Danzig JB, Bernstien JH, *Clostridium septicum* infection and associated malignancy. Medicine 1989;68:30–37.
8. Lober B. Gas gangrene and other clostridium associated diseases. In: Mandell GL, Bennett JE, Dolin R, eds. Principle and practice of infectious diseases. 4th ed. New York: Churchill Livingstone, 1995:2182–2194.

9. Marrie TJ, Haldane EV, Swantee CA, Kerr EH. Susceptibility of anaerobic bacteria to nine antimicrobial agents and demonstration of decreased susceptibility of *Clostridium perfringens* to penicillin. Antimicrob Agents Chemother 1981;19:51–55.

10. Mohr JA, Griffiths W, Holm R, Garcia-Moral C, Flournoy DJ. Clostridial myonecrosis (gas gangrene) during cephalosporin prophylaxis. JAMA. 1978;239:847–849.

11. Musial CE, Rosenblatt JE. Antimicrobial susceptibilities of anaerobic bacteria isolated at the Mayo Clinic during 1982 thorough 1987: comparison with results from 1977 through 1981. Mayo Clinic Proc 1989;64:392–399.

12. Ramsay AM. The significance of *Clostridium welchii* in the cervical swab and blood-stream infection in post partum sepsis. J Obstet Gynaecol 1949;56:247–248.

13. Rood JI, Cole ST. Molecular genetics and pathogens of *Clostridium perfringens*. Microbiol Rev 1991;55:621–648.

14. Schwartzman JD, Reller LB, Wang W-L. Susceptibility of *Clostridium perfringens* isolated from human infections to twenty antibiotics. Antimicrob Agents Chemother 1977;11:695–697.

15. Spera RV Jr, Kaplan MH, Allen SL. *Clostridium sordellii* bacteremia: case report and review. Clin Infect Dis 1992;15:950–954.

16. Smith LDS. The pathogenic anaerobic bacteria. Springfield, IL: Charles C Thomas, 1975.

17. Stevens DL, Mitten JE, Laine BM. Comparison of clindamycin, rifampin, tetracycline, metronidazole, and penicillin for efficacy in prevention of experimental gas gangrene due to *Clostridium perfringens*. J Infect Dis 1987;155:220–228.

18. Stevens DL, Maier KA, Mitten JE. Effect of antibiotics on toxin production and viability of *Clostridium perfringens*. Antimicrob Agents Chemother 1987;31:213–218.

19. Stevens DL, Laine BM, Mitten JE. Comparison of single and combination antimicrobial agents for prevention of experimental gas gangrene caused by *Clostridium perfringens*. Antimicrob Agents Chemother 1987;31:312–316.

20. Sutter VL, Finegold SM. Susceptibility of anaerobic bacteria to 23 antimicrobial agents. Antimicrob Agents Chemother 1976; 10:736–752.

21. Summanen P, Baron EJ, Citron DM, Strong CA, Wexler HM, Finegold SM. Wadsworth anaerobic bacteriology manual. 5th ed. Belmont, CA: Star Publishing, 1993.

22. Traub WH, Comparative in-vitro bactericidal activity of 24 antimicrobial drugs against *Clostridium perfringens*. Chemotherapy 1990;36:127–135.

Clostridium tetani

●

Jeremy Farrar

GENERAL DESCRIPTION
Epidemiology

Tetanus was first described in Egypt over 3000 years ago and was prevalent throughout the ancient world. Despite the availability of passive immunization since 1893 and effective active vaccination since 1923, tetanus remains a major health problem in the developing world and is still encountered in the developed world. There are between 800,000 and 1 million deaths due to tetanus each year, of which approximately 400,000 are due to neonatal tetanus (17). Some 80% of these deaths occur in Africa and Southeast Asia, and it remains endemic in 90 countries worldwide (49). Incomplete vaccine deployment among the population at risk is the major factor, but quality of tetanus toxoid and how it is stored is also important. Fifteen lots in use from eight manufacturers in seven countries were found to have potency values below WHO requirements (17).

Microbiology

The *Clostridium* genus is a diverse group of anaerobic spore-forming Gram-positive bacilli. They are widely distributed in the environment and are found in the intestinal flora of domestic animals, horses, chickens, and man. Endospores are produced that are wider than the bacillus, giving rise to the characteristic drumstick shape. The most noteworthy toxin-mediated diseases associated with infection by this genus are tetanus (*C. tetani*) and botulism (*C. botulinum*).

C. tetani is an obligate anaerobic bacillus, which is Gram positive if processed immediately, but which may stain inconsistently from tissue samples (7). The bacilli are 2 μm × 0.5 μm in size and usually occur singly although occasionally in chains. They possess flagella and are motile when young. Older organisms lose their flagella after development of a spore. The spores are extremely stable, and although boiling for 15 min kills most, some survive unless autoclaved at 120°C, 15 psi, for 15 min, which ensures sterility.

Although anaerobic, the organisms can be cultured in the presence of air, providing a low redox potential is maintained within the growth medium. For routine surface culture, an agar medium with brain heart medium is adequate. Agglutination identification is possible, and ten serotypes have been defined; although of little use clinically, this may be useful in investigation of an outbreak. In routine practice, few attempts are made to culture *C. tetani*: it is difficult to culture, a positive result does not indicate if the organism contains the toxin-producing plasmid, and *C. tetani* may be present without disease in patients with protective immunity. Similarly, there have been very few attempts to quantify the toxin load and assess the prognostic significance of this. If large amounts are produced, the toxin may be transported by blood and the lymphatics as well as by direct entry into nerve fibers; hence the effects of the toxin are more rapid and have wider dissemination.

The toxin is encoded on a 75-kb plasmid and transcribed as a single polypeptide with a molecular weight of 150,000; the complete amino acid sequence of the toxin is known (18–20). The polypeptide undergoes posttranslational cleavage into two subchains, a heavy and a light chain, linked by a disulfide bond. The carboxyl-terminal part of the H chain mediates attachment to gangliosides (GD1b and GT1b) on peripheral nerves; subsequently the toxin is internalized (11). It then is then moved from the peripheral nervous system to the central nervous system (CNS) by retrograde axonal flow and transsynaptic spread. The light chain of the toxin acts as a zinc metallopeptidase, which cleaves synaptobrevin (40); a single base-pair mutation in the light chain abolishes this proteolytic activity (33). Synaptobrevin is an integral membrane component of synaptic vesicles. When cleaved, these vesicles containing the inhibitory neurotransmitter γ-aminobutyric acid (GABA) cannot fuse with the presynaptic membrane and release their contents into the synaptic cleft. The α motor neurons are thus under no inhibitory control and undergo sustained excitatory discharge, causing the characteristic motor spasms of tetanus. The toxin exerts its effects on the spinal cord, brainstem, and peripheral nerves, at neuromuscular junctions, and directly on muscles. To what extent cortical and subcortical structures are involved remains unknown; certainly the toxin is a potent convulsant when injected into the cortex of experimental animals.

The autonomic nervous system is also affected by tetanus toxin, causing cardiac arrhythmias, severe sweating, and labile blood pressure. This is extremely difficult to manage and is a common cause of sudden death. As a consequence, catecholamine levels are high, which may contribute to the high incidence of acute renal dysfunction seen in severe tetanus (13).

Clinical Manifestations

Tetanus typically follows deep penetrating wounds where anaerobic bacterial growth is facilitated. The most common portals of infection are wounds on the lower limbs, postpartum or postabortion infections of the uterus, nonsterile intramuscular injections, and compound fractures. However, even minor trauma can lead to disease, and in up to 30% of cases, no portal of entry is apparent (8). Tetanus has been reported following a myriad of injuries, including intravenous and intramuscular injections, acupuncture, and ear piercing and even from toothpicks. It can follow chronic infections such as otitis media (16, 38) and has been reported with a decubitus ulcer (34). Tetanus acquired following intramuscular injection with quinine is associated with a higher mortality than other modes of acquisition (50). Patients who have injuries more commonly associated with tetanus—deep wounds contaminated with dirt or feces—should have the wound cleaned and be given antitoxin as well as active immunization.

The incubation period (the time from inoculation to the first symptom) can be as short as 24 h or as long as many months after inoculation with *C. tetani*. This interval reflects the dis-

tance the toxin must travel within the nervous system and may be related to the quantity of toxin released. The period of onset is the time between the first symptom and the start of spasms. These periods are important prognostically: the shorter the incubation period or period of onset, the more severe the disease. Trismus (lockjaw), the inability to open the mouth fully owing to rigidity of the masseters, is often the first symptom. Generalized tetanus, the most common form of the disease, presents with pain, headache, stiffness, rigidity, opisthotonus, laryngeal obstruction, and spasms that may be induced by minor stimuli such as noise or touch or by simple medical and nursing procedures such as intravenous and intramuscular injections, suction, or catheterization. The spasms are excruciatingly painful and can be uncontrollable, leading to respiratory arrest and death. Tetanus can be localized at the site of injury, causing local rigidity and pain. This form has the lowest mortality, although cephalic tetanus is a local form with a higher mortality.

The diagnosis is a clinical one, relatively easy to make in areas where tetanus is seen frequently, but often delayed in the developed world where cases are seen infrequently (41). The differential includes tetany, strychnine poisoning, drug-induced dystonic reactions, rabies, and orofacial infection.

SUSCEPTIBILITY IN VITRO

The paucity of information on the bacteria in vitro means very little is known about antimicrobial sensitivity patterns, important if resistance were to develop in *C. tetani*.

ANTIMICROBIAL THERAPY

Penicillin remains the standard therapy for tetanus in most parts of the world. The dose is 100,000 to 200,000 IU/kg/day intramuscularly or intravenously for 7 to 10 days. Johnson and Walker were the first to report that intravenous administration of penicillin could cause convulsions and went on to show, in animal models, that penicillin caused myoclonic convulsions when applied directly to the cortex (29). Penicillin became the standard model for induction of experimental focal epilepsy. The structure of penicillin, distant to the β-lactam ring, is similar to that of GABA, the principal inhibitory neurotransmitter in the CNS. Penicillin therefore acts as a competitive antagonist to GABA. Penicillin does not readily cross the blood-brain barrier, but in high cumulative doses, it can cause CNS hyperexcitability. In tetanus, this side effect of penicillin could synergize with the action of the toxin in blocking transmitter release at GABA neurons.

Metronidazole is a safe alternative and may now be considered the drug of choice. The dose is 400 mg rectally every 6 h, or 500 mg every 6 hours intravenously, for 7 to 10 days. Following rectal administration, metronidazole is rapidly bioavailable and causes fewer spasms than repeated intravenous or intramuscular injections. Ahmadsyah and Salim were the first to compare penicillin and metronidazole and showed a reduction in mortality in the metronidazole group (7 vs. 24%) (2). In a much larger study, Yen recruited over 1000 patients and showed that there was no significant difference in mortality between the penicillin and metronidazole groups (50). However, the 533 patients randomized to metronidazole required fewer muscle relaxants and sedatives than the 572 patients randomized to penicillin. This may be explained by the action of penicillin at GABA-nergic synapses and may therefore apply to the third-generation cephalosporins. The structure of these drugs is similar to that of penicillin, and ceftazidime can induce absence seizures with spike and wave discharges (27). If metronidazole is available and applicable, it should be considered the drug of choice in the treatment of tetanus. Erythromycin, tetracycline, vancomycin, clindamycin, doxycycline, and chloramphenicol would be alternatives to penicillin and metronidazole if they were unavailable or unusable in individual patients (5, 9). Little or no indication exists for the use of other antibiotics in the management of tetanus. An up-to-date assessment of the antimicrobial sensitivity patterns of clinical isolates of *C. tetani* is needed.

VACCINES
Therapy

Passive immunization with human or equine tetanus immunoglobulin shortens the course and may reduce the severity of tetanus. The human antiserum is isolated from a pool of plasma derived from healthy human tetanus-immune donors and has a half-life of 24.5 to 31.5 days. The equine (or bovine) form, widely available throughout the developing world, has a higher incidence of anaphylactic reactions, has a half-life of only 2 days, but is much cheaper to produce. In established cases, patients should receive equine antitoxin (500–1000 IU/kg) intravenously or intramuscularly. Anaphylactic reactions occur in 20% of cases; in 1% they are severe enough to warrant adrenaline, antihistamines, steroids, and intravenous fluids. If available, 3000 to 6000 IU of human antitetanus immunoglobulin should be given intramuscularly; this has a lower incidence of side effects. Antitetanus toxin was first used in 1893, and the incidence of disease among soldiers in World War I dropped dramatically following its introduction. Although the antiserum affects only circulating and unbound toxin (demonstrated in the serum of only 10% of patients at presentation and in 4% of cerebrospinal fluid (47)), it should be administered to all patients with tetanus. Whether it should also be infiltrated locally at the portal of entry is unclear and should be examined prospectively. For prophylaxis, 1500 to 3000 IU equine or 250 to 500 IU human antitetanus immunoglobulin should be given.

Passive immunization should be administered as soon as possible after the injury; once the toxin is bound and internalized, it clearly has no effect. The blood level of passive antitoxin to protect a man against tetanus is approximately 0.1 IU/mL. When 3000 IU is administered intramuscularly, maximum levels are reached in 24 to 48 h, and adequate levels are maintained for 10 to 15 days. It is not easy to assess the optimal dose of antisera to give for prophylaxis. Extrapolation from animal work suggests that these doses are too low and that 50,000 IU would afford greater protection; however, at such doses the incidence of side effects is higher. The side effects can be either acute anaphylactic reactions or delayed serum sickness. The former has an estimated incidence of 1 per 200,000 individuals; the overall frequency of all reactions

is approximately 5%. The incidence of immediate reactions can be reduced by simultaneous (or 15 min prior to use) injection with an antihistamine (promethazine). Use of the Besredka rapid desensitization method does not necessarily prevent anaphylactic reactions. Use of human tetanus immunoglobulin is very rarely associated with anaphylactic reactions, creates protective immunity of longer duration, and permits use of lower doses (500–1000 IU). It is the passive immunization of choice; unfortunately, it remains unaffordable in many parts of the world.

Complete human immunoglobulin now can be engineered in vitro and designed for specific antigens (32). This raises the possibility of producing human antibodies specific for the tetanus toxin, free from the risks of infection, easy to store, and potentially available at a cost affordable in the developing world. Owing to its smaller size, it is possible that the antigen-binding domain of the immunoglobulin, the Fab fragment, may gain better access to the toxin and so enhance neutralization. Fab fragments can be produced from donors, but the engineered approach to antibody production would facilitate this.

Intrathecal therapy with antitetanus serum has been subjected to a number of clinical trials. A meta-analysis has concluded that there is currently no evidence of a beneficial effect in neonates or adults using equine or human tetanus immune globulin and that the safety of their use intrathecally remains unproved (1).

In addition to passive immunization, active vaccination needs to be administered to all patients not previously vaccinated, so-called active-passive immunization. This adds to the short-term immunity (passive) and to long-term humoral and cellular immunity (active). As the former is declining, the latter appears and thus avoids a window of nonprotection. Experimental work in animals shows that the toxoid starts acting a few hours after injection, before a humoral response is detectable. Presumably, the toxoid saturates the ganglioside receptors and prevents wild-type toxin binding. The toxoid and human (or equine) antitetanus immunoglobulin should be administered at different sites on the body to prevent interaction at the injection site. If both are to be administered together no more than 1000 IU human or 5000 IU equine should be administered; higher doses can neutralize the immunogenicity of the toxoid.

Prevention

Tetanus toxoid is produced by formaldehyde treatment of the toxin; its immunogenicity is improved by absorption with aluminium hydroxide. Alum-absorbed tetanus toxoid is very effective at preventing tetanus, with a failure rate of 4 per 100 million immunocompetent individuals. In the United Kingdom and United States, it is administered to children between 2 and 6 months of age (3 doses at 4-week intervals), with boosters at 15 months (U.S.) and at 4 years (U.K. and U.S.). A further dose is recommended in both the United States and United Kingdom within 5 to 10 years (Table 1). Serum antitoxin levels above 0.01 units/mL are considered protective, although a number of cases have been reported in patients with

TABLE 1 • Vaccination Schedules[a]

Vaccine	
	Children under 7 years
1-DPT	6–8 weeks
2-DPT	4–8 weeks after previous dose
3-DPT	4–8 weeks after previous dose
4-DPT	1 year after previous dose
Booster-DPT	4–6 years of age
	Adults and children not previously vaccinated
1-Td	At presentation
2-Td	4–8 weeks after previous dose
3-Td	6 months–1 year after previous dose
Booster-Td	Every 10 years after previous dose
	Pregnant women previously vaccinated
Booster-TT	During first 6 months of pregnancy
	Pregnant women not previously vaccinated
1-TT	First encounter during pregnancy
2-TT	4 weeks after previous dose

From Peter G, Halsey NA, Marcuse EK, Pickering LK, eds. American Academy of Paediatrics. 1994 Red book: report of the Committee on Infectious Diseases. Illinois: American Academy of Paediatrics.

[a]Abbreviations: DPT, diphtheria and tetanus toxoid and pertussis absorbed; Td, tetanus and reduced-dose diphtheria toxoids absorbed; TT, tetanus toxoid.

protective serum antibody levels (12, 14, 35). A protective antibody level is attained after the second dose, but a third dose ensures longer-lasting immunity. To maintain adequate levels of protection, additional booster doses should be administered every 10 years.

Reactions to the tetanus toxoid are estimated to occur in 1 in 50,000 injections, although most are not severe: local tenderness, edema, flulike illness, and low-grade fever are most frequently encountered. Severe reactions such as the Guillain-Barré syndrome and acute relapsing polyneuropathy are rare (23, 25).

In recent years, there have been a number of reports from Australia and the United States of tetanus occurring in patients over the age of 50 (26). In a survey from the United States, 59% of women and 27% of men from an urban geriatric care center did not have adequate antitetanus titers (3). For every child in the United States who dies of a vaccine-preventable disease, about 400 adults die of such a disease (22). There is a strong argument for introduction of a vaccination strategy for immunization of all adults at the age of 50.

Neonatal tetanus can be prevented by immunization of women during pregnancy. Two or three doses of absorbed toxin should be given, with the last dose at least 1 month prior to delivery. Immunity is passively transferred to the fetus, and protective antibodies will persist long enough to protect the baby. There is no evidence of congenital anomalies associated with tetanus toxin administered during pregnancy (43).

The influence of human immunodeficiency virus (HIV) infection on the transplacental transfer of tetanus-specific maternal IgG is of critical importance. Polyclonal hyperimmunoglobulinemia is common in HIV and may limit the transfer of protective maternal antibodies, as may HIV infection per se. Antitetanus antibody levels were lower in babies born to 46 HIV infected women than in an HIV-negative control group, although they were still above 0.01 IU/ml (15). Approximately 10% of babies born to mothers with a placenta heavily infected with *Plasmodium falciparum* may fail to acquire protective levels of tetanus antibody despite adequate maternal levels (6). The antibody response to tetanus vaccination is reduced in HIV-infected adult individuals with a CD4+ lymphocyte count of 300×10^6/L (31). HIV-infected individuals who completed their vaccination course prior to acquisition of HIV should maintain adequate levels of protection against tetanus.

ENDPOINTS AND PROGNOSIS

A number of groups have attempted to devise a scoring system to assess prognoses; the Dakar and Phillips scores are two examples (Tables 2 and 3). Both of these scoring systems are relatively simple schemes that take into account the incubation period and/or the period of onset as well as neurologic and cardiac manifestations. The Phillips score also factors in the state of immune protection. The more clinical grading system developed by Urwardia is also useful (Table 4).

The common complications in tetanus, such as noscomial infection, bed sores, tracheal stenosis, and gastrointestinal hemorrhage, are often attributable to prolonged periods in intensive care. Secondary infections are a frequent complication, most commonly associated with the lower respiratory tract, catheterization, and wound sepsis. Gram-negative organisms, particularly *Klebsiella* and *Pseudomonas* are common. *Proteus* and staphylococcal infections are also frequently encountered. Rigorous attention to sterile technique and infection control is essential in a tetanus intensive care unit.

TABLE 2 • Prognostic Scoring Systems in Tetanus: Dakar Score

Prognostic Factor	Score 1	Score
Incubation period	<7 days	≥7 days or unknown
Period of onset	<2 days	≥2 days
Entry site	Umbilicus, burn, uterine, open fracture, surgical wound, IM injection	All others plus unknown
Spasms	Present	Absent
Fever	>38.4°C	<38.4°C
Tachycardia	Adult >120 beats/min	Adult <120 beats/min
	Neonate >150 beats/min	Neonate <150 beats/min
Total Score		

TABLE 3 • Prognostic Scoring Systems in Tetanus: Phillips Score

Factor	Score
Incubation Time	
<48 hours	5
2–5 days	4
5–10 days	3
10–14 days	2
>14 days	1
Site of infection	
Internal and umbilical	5
Head, neck, and body wall	4
Peripheral proximal	3
Peripheral distal	2
Unknown	1
State of protection	
None	10
Possibly some or maternal immunization in neonatal patients	8
Protected >10 years ago	4
Protected <10 years ago	2
Complete protection	0
Complicating factors	
Injury or life-threatening illness	10
Severe injury or illness not immediately life threatening	8
Injury or non-life-threatening illness	4
Minor injury or illness	2
ASA grade 1	0
Total Score	

In addition, there are also problems unique to the disease. Cardiac and hemodynamic problems resulting from sympathetic overactivity are seen in a significant number of patients with severe disease. β-Blockers, magnesium, clonidine, and labetolol have been used to treat autonomic dysfunction, with mixed success (28, 30, 44, 48). The most complete work on the hemodynamic complications, by Urwadia, has shown that the mortality in severe disease can be substantially reduced by careful attention to the patient's hemodynamic and respiratory state (45). This seminal work deserves further attention, in particular elucidating the causes of sudden death that occurs despite intensive monitoring. Acute renal dysfunction and failure is a common complication and is probably secondary to markedly labile blood pressure and severe autonomic dysfunction rather than to rhabdomyolysis or myoglobinuria. The pathology is acute tubular necrosis (42). The consequent metabolic derangement inevitably worsens the cardiac function, and hence, the renal failure should be treated early with appropriate renal support, either hemofiltration or dialysis. Unfortunately, in most centers where tetanus is seen, neither of these renal support systems are available. Other complications include hematemesis, compression fractures of vertebrae, constipation, and pulmonary emboli.

Respiratory failure, hemodynamic disturbance, and septicemia are the most common causes of death. In those who survive, sequelae include contractures, chest deformities, fits, myoclonus, and the consequences of hypoxia. There is essentially very little information on follow-up of patients after tetanus, particularly with regard to cognitive function. In one of the few studies to examine this question, Anlar et al. found enuresis, mental retardation, and growth delay to be frequent after neonatal tetanus (4). This aspect of tetanus deserves further research.

ADJUNCTIVE THERAPY

The mainstay of management is supportive, with adequate ventilatory support, sedation, and muscle relaxation. The respiratory state should be assessed, the airway secured, and ventilation initiated if necessary. A tracheostomy should be performed as soon as possible in generalized tetanus; this allows maintenance of the airway during laryngeal spasms and facilitates removal of secretions. Patients may need to be sedated and paralyzed if mechanical ventilation is available. A nasogastric tube should be inserted, and the wound cleaned and debrided if necessary.

Pyridoxine (vitamin B_6) is a coenzyme with glutamate decarboxylase in the production of GABA from glutamic acid and increases GABA levels in animal models. In an unblinded open trial, 20 neonates with tetanus were treated with pyridoxine (100 mg/day) and compared with retrospective records. Mortality was reduced in the pyridoxine-treated group (21). The role of pyridoxine in the management of neonatal tetanus should be reexamined in a blind randomized trial.

Steroids have been shown to be of benefit in tetanus; however, as is often the case in studies on this disease, the trials have not recruited enough patients to be convincing or have been inadequately controlled. In two studies, betamethasone reduced the mortality, but only in small numbers of patients (10, 39). Steroids should not be administered routinely in the management of tetanus until further blinded, controlled studies are conducted with sufficient numbers to show significant differences.

TABLE 4 • Prognostic Scoring Systems in Tetanus: Grading of Severity

Grade 1 (mild):	Mild-to-moderate trismus, generally increased tone, no respiratory distress, no spasms, and no dysphagia
Grade 2 (moderate):	Moderate trismus, marked rigidity, short-lasting spasms, tachypnea ≥35/min, mild dysphagia
Grade 3 (severe):	Severe trismus, generalized increased tone, reflex spontaneous or prolonged spasms, respiratory distress with tachypnea ≥40/min, apneic spells, severe dysphagia, tachycardia ≥120/min, moderate increase in autonomic nervous system dysfunction
Grade 4 (very severe):	Features of grade 3, plus severe autonomic dysfunction, persistent labile blood pressure and pulse rate.

From Udwadia FE. Tetanus. New York: Oxford University Press, 1994.

Adequate sedation is essential in tetanus, but is a double-edged sword. Benzodiazepines are the most commonly used sedative agents. Diazepam has a wide margin of safety; can be given orally, rectally, or intravenously; and is a sedative, an anticonvulsant, and a muscle relaxant. It is also cheap and available in most parts of the world. However, it has a long cumulative half-life (72 h) and has active metabolites, in particular, oxazepam and demethyldiazepam. Invariably, in the doses required to achieve adequate control of spasms (often up to 3–8 mg/kg/day in adults), respiratory depression, coma, and medullary depression are common. Establishing the correct therapeutic window is extremely difficult, particularly in patients who require prolonged support. Midazolam and propofol are alternatives, but these are often not available or not affordable in regions where tetanus is seen frequently (24, 36). Neuromuscular blocking agents such as pancuronium and vecuronium are used in centers with adequate facilities for mechanical ventilation. Tetanus patients require sedation in addition to muscle paralysis.

COMMENTS

The World Health Assembly resolved to eliminate neonatal tetanus by 1995. Three years after the deadline, the infection still kills over 400,000 babies a year. A safe, effective vaccine has been available for most of this century. If any one disease epitomizes the health care disparity between north and south and the difficulties in overcoming that inequality, then tetanus is that disease. It is entirely preventable, worldwide. The priorities must be in prevention: universal vaccination and development of simpler immunization schedules with longer protection. However, for the foreseeable future, hospitals in many parts of the developing world will continue to see large numbers of patients with tetanus. Sadly, much of this ideal therapeutic approach is not applicable in hospitals where the vast majority of the worldwide cases of tetanus are seen. Adequate sedation and muscle relaxation is only possible if there are adequate facilities for ventilation, and equine antitoxin is much cheaper to produce than human.

Further work on pragmatic solutions applicable in these countries is needed to reduce the high mortality. A better understanding of *C. tetani,* the toxin, its effects on the central and autonomic nervous systems, and cardiac and respiratory function is needed. There is a tendency to accept a high mortality from tetanus; Udwadia and his colleagues have shown in India that it is possible to reduce the mortality substantially, even in the absence of full-fledged intensive care units (46).

REFERENCES

1. Abrutyn E, Berlin JA. Intrathecal therapy in tetanus. A meta-analysis. JAMA 1991;266:2262–2267.
2. Ahmadsyah I, Salim A. Treatment of tetanus: an open study to compare the efficacy of procaine penicillin and metronidazole. Br Med J 1985;291:648–650.
3. Alagappan K, Rennie W, Kwiatkowski T, Falck J, Silverstone F, Silverman R. Seroprevalence of tetanus antibodies among adults older than 65 years. Ann Emerg Med 1996;28:18–21.
4. Anlar B, Yalaz K, Dizmen R. Long term prognosis after neonatal tetanus. Dev Med Child Neurol 1989;31:76–80.
5. Bleck TP. Review: Pharmacology of tetanus. Clin Neuropharmcol 1986;9:103.
6. Reduced transfer of tetanus antibodies with placental malaria. Lancet 1994;343:208–209.
7. Cato EP, George WL, Finegold SM. Genus Clostridium praemozski 1880, 23AL. In: Smeath PHA, Mair NS, Sharpe ME, et al., eds. Bergey's manual of systemic bacteriology, vol II. Baltimore: Williams & Wilkins, 1986:1141–1200.
8. Centers for Disease Control. Tetanus–United States, 1985–1986. MMWR 1987;36:477–481.
9. Chambers HF, Sande MA. Antimicrobial agents. In: Hardman JG, Limbird LE, eds. The pharmacological basis of therapeutics. 9th ed. 1996;43:1029–1225.
10. Chandy ST, Peter JV, John L. Betamethasone in tctanus patients: an evaluation of its effects on the mortality and morbidity. JAPI 1992;10:373–376.
11. Collee JG, van Heyningen S. Systemic toxigenic diseases (tetanus, botulism). In: Duerden BI, Draser BS, eds. Anaerobes and human disease. London: Edward Arnold, 1990:372–394.
12. Crone NE, Reder AT. Severe tetanus in immunised patients with high anti-tetanus titres. Neurology 1992;42:761–764.
13. Daher EF, Abdulkader RCRM, Motti E, Marcondes M, Sabbage E, Burdmann EA. Prospective study of tetanus-induced acute renal dysfunction: role of adrenergic overactivity. Am J Trop Med Hyg 1997;57:610–614.
14. de Moraes-Pinto MI, Oruamabo RS, Igbagiri FP. Neonatal tetanus despite immunisation and protective antitoxin antibody. J Infect Dis 1995;171:1076–1077.
15. de Moraes-Pinto MI, Almeida ACM, Kenj G, Filgueiras TE, Tobias W, Santos AMN, Carneiro-Sampaio MMS, Farhat CK, Milligan P, Johnson P, Hart CA. Placental transfer and maternal acquired neonatal IgG immunity in human immunodeficiency virus infection. J Infect Dis 1996;173:1077–1084.
16. DeSouza CE, Karnard DR, Tilve GH. Clinical and bacteriological profile of the ear in otogenic tetanus: a case control study. J Laryngol Otol 1992;106:1051–1054.
17. Dietz V, Milstien JB, van Loon F, Cochi S, Bennett J. Performance and potency of tetanus toxoid: implications for eliminating neonatal tetanus. Bull WHO 1996;74:619–28.
18. Eisel U, Jarausch W, Goretzki K, Henschen A, Engels J, Weller U, Hudel M, Habermnn E, Niemann H. Tetanus toxin: primary structure, expression in E. coli, and homology with botulinum toxins. EMBO J 1986;5:2495–2502.
19. Fairweather NF, Lyness VA. The complete nucleotide sequence of tetanus toxin. Nucleic Acids Res 1986;14:7809–7812.
20. Finn CJ, Silver RP, Habig WH, Hardegree MC, Zon G, Garon CF. The structural gene for tetanus neurotoxin is on a plasmid. Science 1984;224:881–884.
21. Godel JC. Trial of pyridoxine therapy for tetanus neonatorum. J Infect Dis 1982;145:547–549.
22. Grabenstein JD. Status and future of vaccines for adults. Am J Health Syst Pharm 1997;54:379–387.
23. Grouleau G. Tetanus. Emerg Med Clin North Am 1992;10(2):351–360.
24. Gyasi HK, Fahr J, Kurian E, Mathew M. Midazolam for prolonged intravenous sedation in patients with tetanus. Middle East J Anesthesiol 1993;12:135–141.
25. Halliday PL, Bauer RB. Polyradiculitis secondary to immunisation with tetanus and diphtheria toxoids. Arch Neurol 1983;40:56–57.
26. Heath TC, Smith W, Capon AG, Hanlon M, Mitchell P. Tetanus in an older Australian population. Med J Aust 1996;164:593–596.

27. Jackson G, Berkovic SL. Ceftazidime encephalopathy: absence status and toxic hallucinations. J Neurol Neurosurg Psychiatry 1992;55:333–334.
28. James MFM, Manson EDM. The use of magnesium infusions in the management of very severe tetanus. Intensive Care Med 1985;11:5–12.
29. Johnson HC, Walker A. Intraventricular penicillin. JAMA 1945;127:217–219.
30. King WW, Cave DR. Use of esmolol to control autonomic instability of tetanus. Am J Med 1991;91:425–428.
31. Kroon FP, van DJ, Labadie J, van Loom A, van Furth R. Antibody response to diphtheria, tetanus, and poliomyelitis vaccines in relation to the number of CD4+ T lymphocytes in adults infected with human immunodeficiency virus. Clin Infect Dis 1995;21:1197–1203.
32. Larrick JW, Wallace EF, Coloma MJ, Bruderer U, Lang AB, Fry KE. Therapeutic human antibodies derived from PCR amplification of B-cell variable regions. Immunol Rev 1992;130:69–85.
33. Li Y, Foran P, Fairweather NF. A single mutation in the recombinant light chain of tetanus toxin abolishes its proteolytic activity and removes the toxicity seen after reconstitution with native heavy chain. Biochemistry 1994;33:7014–7020.
34. Luisto M. Unusual and iatrogenic sources of tetanus. Ann Chir Gynaecol 1993;82:25–29.
35. Maselle SY, Matre R, Mbise R, Hofstad T. Neonatal tetanus despite protective serum antitoxin concentration. FEMS Microbiol Immunol 1991;3:171–175.
36. Orko R, Rosenberg PH, Himberg JJ. Intravenous infusion of midazolam, propofol and vecuronium in a patient with severe tetanus. Acta Anaesthesiol Scand 1988;32:590–592.
37. Peter G, Halsey NA, Marcuse EK, Pickering LK, eds. American Academy of Paediatrics. 1994 Red book: report of the Committee on Infectious Diseases. Illinois: American Academy of Paediatrics.
38. Patel JC, Kale PA, Mehta BC. Octogenic tetanus: a study of 922 cases. In: Patel JC, ed. Proceedings, 1st International Conference on Tetanus, Bombay, 1965.
39. Paydas S, Akoglu TF, Akkiz H, Ozer FL, Burgut R. Mortality-lowering effect of systemic corticosteroid therapy in severe tetanus. Clin Ther 1988;10:276–280.
40. Schiavo G, Benfenati F, Poulain B, Rossetto O, Polverino P, DasGupta BR, Montecucco C. Tetanus and botulinum-B neurotoxins block neurotransmitter release by proteolytic cleavage of synaptobrevin. Nature 1992;359:832–835.
41. Schon F, O'Dowd L, White J, Begg N. Tetanus: delay in diagnosis in England and Wales. J Neurol Neurosurg Psychiatry 1994;57:1006–1007.
42. Seedat YK, Omar MAK, Seedat MA, Wessley A, Pather M. Renal failure in tetanus. Br Med J 1981;282:360–361.
43. Silveira CM, Caceres VM, Dutra MG, Lopes-Cameol J, Castilla EE. Safety of tetanus toxoid in pregnant women: a hospital-based case control study of congenital anomalies. Bull WHO 1995;73:605–608.
44. Sutton DN, Tremlett MR, Woodcock TE, Nielsen MS. Management of autonomic dysfunction in severe tetanus: the use of magnesium sulphate and clonidine [see comments]. Intensive Care Med 1990;16:75–80.
45. Udwadia FE, Sunavala JD, Jain MC, D'Costa R, Jain PK, Lall A, Sekhar M, Udwadia ZF, Kapadia F, Kapur KC. Haemodynamic studies during the management of severe tetanus. Q J Med 1992;83:449–460.
46. Udwadia FE. Tetanus. New York: Oxford University Press, 1994.
47. Veronesi R. Clinical picture. In: Veronesi R, ed. Tetanus: important new concepts. Amsterdam: Excerpta Medica, 1981:183–206.
48. Wesley AG, Hariparsad D, Pather M, Rocke DA. Labetalol in tetanus. The treatment of sympathetic nervous system overactivity. Anaesthesia 1983;38:243–249.
49. Whitman C, Belgharbi L, Gasse F, Torel C, Mattei V, Zoffmann H. Progress towards the global elimination of neonatal tetanus. World Health Stat Q 1992;45:248–256.
50. Yen LM, Dao LM, Day NPJ, Waller DJ, Bethell DB, Son LH, Hien TT, White NJ. The role of quinine in the high mortality of intramuscular injection in tetanus. Lancet 1994;344:786–787.
51. Yen LM, Dao LM, Day NPJ, Bethell DB, Son LH, Hien TT, White NJ, Farrar JJ. Management of tetanus: a comparison of penicillin and metronidazole. Symposium of antimicrobial resistance in southern Viet Nam, 1997.

Corynebacterium diphtheriae

•

Melinda Wharton

GENERAL DESCRIPTION

In temperate climates, infections due to *Corynebacterium diphtheriae* typically present as respiratory disease, characterized by pharyngeal, laryngeal, or tracheal pseudomembrane formation. Death may result from airway obstruction or from effects of a powerful exotoxin produced by toxigenic strains of *C. diphtheriae,* resulting in myocarditis, paralysis, renal failure, disseminated intravascular coagulation, or cardiovascular collapse. However, other virulence factors exist in addition to diphtheria toxin, because respiratory disease with pseudomembrane may occur following infection with nontoxigenic strains.

Prior to the introduction and widespread use of diphtheria toxoid vaccine in the United States and other developed countries, diphtheria was an epidemic disease that was a major cause of childhood death. In most developed countries, diphtheria is now recognized only rarely; in the United States, only 41 cases were reported between 1980 and 1995 (5). Following several decades of excellent control of diphtheria, a major epidemic began in the former Soviet Union in 1990 (15, 23).

In tropical climates, infection with *C. diphtheriae* more commonly results in cutaneous infection. It is believed that because toxin is poorly absorbed from skin, complications due to toxin such as myocarditis and neuropathy are relatively uncommon following cutaneous infection. In developed countries, cutaneous diphtheria is most commonly identified among substance abusers, immigrants from developing countries, and travelers; however, the diagnosis is not commonly sought, and other cases could go unrecognized.

Infection with nontoxigenic *C. diphtheriae* strains may occasionally produce other clinical syndromes. Clusters of endocarditis due to nontoxigenic *C. diphtheriae* have been reported (29, 31), and sporadic cases also occur (19).

SUSCEPTIBILITY IN VITRO AND IN VIVO

In vitro, *C. diphtheriae* isolates are generally highly susceptible to erythromycin as well as to other newer macrolides (Table 1)(3, 11a, 12, 30a). Resistance to erythromycin has been reported in Canada and the United States. In Canada, nontoxigenic *C. diphtheriae* biotype mitis from 2 patients with chronic superficial skin lesions who had previously been treated with erythromycin and lincomycin were found to be highly resistant to both antimicrobials, although both remained fully sensitive to penicillin G (18). During the diphtheria outbreak in Seattle in the 1970s, erythromycin was used extensively for treatment. Nontoxigenic *C. diphtheriae* biotype mitis isolates from patients with cutaneous diphtheria were found to have inducible resistance to both erythromycin and clindamycin when grown in the presence of subinhibitory concentrations of erythromycin (8). This resistance was plasmid mediated (26), and homology was demonstrated between this plasmid and plasmids found in skin coryneforms, suggesting that it may have originated in skin flora (27). After 1978, use of erythromycin for treatment of skin lesions among the at risk population was no longer recommended, and the frequency of erythromycin resistance of clinical isolates of *C. diphtheriae* decreased dramatically (16).

Few clinical trials of antimicrobial agents for treatment of diphtheria have been reported. Parenteral penicillin followed by oral penicillin and parenteral erythromycin followed by oral erythromycin appeared to be equally effective in eliminating the organism from the pharynx of hospitalized patients with diphtheria, although randomization was terminated early because of adverse reactions among erythromycin-treated patients (21). In a randomized study, oral erythromycin was more effective in eliminating the carrier state than a single intramuscular injection of benzathine penicillin (22).

Ciprofloxacin and other fluoroquinolones have demonstrated excellent in vitro activity against *C. diphtheriae,* but no clinical data are available on experience with these agents in treatment of diphtheria.

High level resistance to rifampin has been demonstrated in biotype gravis strains recovered from patients in Estonia, but the treatment history of the patients was unknown (20). Tetracycline resistance has been reported in Indonesia, where tetracycline was often used for empiric treatment of infections (25). Ampicillin tolerance of *C. diphtheriae* biotype mitis strains from patients with endocarditis has been reported (9).

ANTIMICROBIAL THERAPY
Respiratory Diphtheria

The mainstay of treatment of respiratory diphtheria is diphtheria antitoxin; antimicrobial therapy is of secondary importance. Treatment should begin with intramuscular procaine penicillin (25,000–50,000 units/kg/day for children and 1.2 million units/day for adults, in two divided doses) or intravenous erythromycin (40–50 mg/kg/day, with a maximum dose of 2 g/day) until the patient can swallow comfortably. At that point, oral erythromycin in four divided doses or oral penicillin V (125–250 mg four times per day) may be substituted to complete a total 14-day course of treatment (10). In mild cases, oral treatment may be used for the entire course (30).

CARRIERS

Persons infected with *C. diphtheriae* who do not have signs and symptoms of diphtheria should be treated with antimicrobials to eradicate the organism and prevent further spread. A single dose of intramuscular benzathine penicillin (600,000 units for children less than 6 years of age and 1.2 million units for persons 6 years of age or older) or a 7- to 10-day course of oral erythromycin (40 mg/kg/day for children; 1 g/day for adults) is recommended (10). Although there is some evidence that erythromycin may be more effective in eliminating carriage (22), intramuscular benzathine penicillin may be preferred if compliance is doubtful (10).

Following completion of treatment, cultures should be obtained, and if the organism persists, a second course of antimicrobial therapy (erythromycin for 10 days) should be provided, and specimens submitted for follow-up culture.

PROPHYLACTIC TREATMENT OF CONTACTS

To prevent further spread of *C. diphtheriae* infection, prophylactic antimicrobial treatment of close contacts is recommended, regardless of vaccination status, as soon as samples are obtained for culture. Surveillance for signs and symptoms of diphtheria should be maintained for 7 days, and diphtheria toxoid vaccination status reviewed; if indicated, diphtheria toxoid should be administered. A single dose of intramuscular benzathine penicillin (600,000 units for children less than 6 years of age and 1.2 million units for persons 6 years of age and older) or a 7- to 10-day course of oral erythromycin (40 mg/kg/day for children; 1 g/day for adults) is recommended. Intramuscular benzathine penicillin may be preferred if compliance is doubtful (10). Persons found to be infected with *C. diphtheriae* should have another specimen obtained for culture a minimum of 2 weeks after completion of antimicrobial therapy. Persons who continue to harbor the organism after treatment with either penicillin or erythromycin should receive an additional 10-day course of oral erythromycin and follow-up specimens should be obtained for culture to ensure that the organism has been eradicated.

TABLE 1 • **In Vitro Susceptibility of *Corynebacterium diphtheriae***

Antimicrobial	N[a]	Source	MIC range (mg/L)	Reference
Ampicillin	14	U.S.	0.1–0.4	11a
	192[b]	Iran and U.K.	0.05–0.8	30a
	83	N.I.S.	0.25–1.0	20
Azithromycin	3	—[c]	0.03–0.06	3
Cefuroxime	83	N.I.S.	0.5–2.0	20
Cephalexin	14	U.S.	0.8–1.6	11a
Cephaloridine	192[b]	Iran and U.K.	0.05–0.4	30a
Cephalothin	14	U.S.	0.2–0.4	11a
Cephapirin	14	U.S.	0.2–0.4	11a
Chloramphenicol	14	U.S.	0.4–1.6	11a
	83	N.I.S.	1	20
Ciprofloxacin	10	U.K.	0.12–0.5	12
	83	N.I.S.	0.12	20
Clarithromycin	3	—[c]	0.016–0.03	3
Clindamycin	192[b]	Iran and U.K.	0.025–0.5	30a
Dirithromycin	3	—[c]	0.03–0.06	3
Enoxacin	10	U.K.	1–2	12
Erythromycin	14	U.S.	0.0125–0.05	11a
	192[b]	Iran and U.K.	0.0125–0.5	30a
	3	—[c]	0.008–0.016	3
	83	N.I.S.	≤0.06	20
Gentamicin	14	U.S.	0.4–1.6	11a
	83	N.I.S.	≤0.12–0.5	20
Josamycin	3	—[c]	0.06–0.25	3
Kanamycin	14	U.S.	0.8–3.1	11a
Lincomycin	14	U.S.	0.4–0.8	11a
	192[b]	Iran and U.K.	0.1–0.8	30a
Naladixic acid	10	U.K.	32–64	12
Neomycin	192[b]	Iran and U.K.	0.025–0.4	30a
Norfloxacin	10	U.K.	0.5–2	12
Ofloxacin	10	U.K.	0.25–1	12
Oxacillin	14	U.S.	1.6–3.1	11a
Oxytetracycline	192[b]	Iran and U.K.	0.4–1.6	30a
Pefloxacin	10	U.K.	0.5–1	11a
Penicillin	14	U.S.	0.05–0.2	11a
	192[b]	Iran and U.K.	0.025–0.4	30a
	83	N.I.S.	0.12–0.5	20
Rifampin	14	U.S.	0.0125–0.05	11a
	83	N.I.S.	≤0.06–≥2.0	20
Roxithromycin	3	—[c]	0.03–0.06	3
Tetracycline	14	U.S.	0.4–0.8	11a
	83	N.I.S.	0.5	20
Trimethoprim	83	N.I.S.	0.12–≥2.0	20

[a]Number of isolates tested.

[b]Includes one isolate of *Corynebacterium ulcerans*.

[c]Source of isolates not stated.

Cutaneous Diphtheria

First-line antimicrobial agents for treatment of cutaneous diphtheria are penicillin or erythromycin. Topical application of bacitracin or gentian violet has been recommended, and administration of antitoxin has been recommended for patients with extended, multiple lesions and pseudomembrane formation (17). Lesions should be vigorously cleaned with soap and water.

Endocarditis

For treatment of endocarditis due to *C. diphtheriae,* penicillin and an aminoglycoside has been recommended (19). Most re-

ported cases have been associated with nontoxigenic *C. diphtheriae* without associated respiratory disease; antitoxin is not required for treatment of patients with invasive disease due to nontoxigenic strains.

ANTITOXIN FOR TREATMENT OF DIPHTHERIA

Antitoxin is the mainstay of diphtheria treatment. Because the prognosis improves with early administration of diphtheria antitoxin, a decision to treat with antitoxin usually must be made on the basis of a presumptive diagnosis in the absence of culture confirmation.

Currently available diphtheria antitoxin is of equine origin, and testing for hypersensitivity to horse serum is essential prior to administration. Any history of previous administration of horse serum or possible allergy should be sought prior to administering antitoxin.

The patient should be tested for hypersensitivity by skin or eye test prior to administration of antitoxin. During testing, a syringe loaded with a 1:1000 solution of epinephrine should be ready and available for emergency use. For skin testing, 0.1 mL of a 1:100 dilution of diphtheria antitoxin in physiologic saline is injected intracutaneously. After 20 minutes, a wheal of 1 cm or more is read as a positive test result. If there is a history of allergy to equine serum, the dose should be reduced (0.05 mL of a 1:1,000 dilution administered intracutaneously). For the eye test, one drop of a 1:10 dilution of diphtheria antitoxin in physiologic saline is instilled in the lower lid of one eye, and in the other eye, 1 drop of physiologic saline is instilled as a control. After 20 minutes, conjunctivitis and lacrimation indicate a positive result; if test results are positive, the eye should be treated with 1 drop of a 1:100 solution of epinephrine. Neither a negative skin test result nor a negative eye test result precludes subsequent reactions to diphtheria antitoxin.

The recommended dosage of diphtheria antitoxin depends on the duration and extent of disease. For anterior nasal diphtheria, 10,000 to 20,000 units is recommended; for tonsillar diphtheria, 15,000 to 25,000 units; for pharyngeal or laryngeal diphtheria of 48-h duration or less, 20,000 to 40,000 units; for nasopharyngeal diphtheria, 40,000 to 60,000 units; and for extensive disease of 3 days or greater duration or for any patient with brawny swelling of the neck, 80,000 to 120,000 units. The preferred route of administration is intravenous because toxin is more rapidly neutralized; antitoxin may also be administered by intramuscular injection, but reaching peak antitoxin levels may be delayed for several days. For intravenous administration, antitoxin should be diluted in 500 mL of saline and administered by intravenous drip with a slow rate during the first 30 min of infusion. During administration of diphtheria antitoxin the patient must be carefully monitored, and the infusion stopped if signs of shock appear. Epinephrine (0.1–0.3 mL of a 1:1,000 dilution) may be added to the solution. If administered intramuscularly, antitoxin is injected into the buttocks without dilution.

If the patient is sensitive to horse serum, the indications for diphtheria antitoxin should be reconsidered; if indicated, antitoxin can be administered following desensitization by either the intravenous or intradermal, subcutaneous, and intramuscular route. Standard desensitization protocols are published (7).

Diphtheria antitoxin is no longer available commercially in the United States, but can be obtained for treatment of suspected cases from the Centers for Disease Control and Prevention (6) (Contact the diphtheria duty officer, Child Vaccine Preventable Diseases Branch, Epidemiology and Surveillance Division, National Immunization Program, CDC, at 404/639–8255 during regular business hours or 404/639–2889 at all other times). All suspected diphtheria cases should be reported to local and state health departments.

VACCINES

Diphtheria is preventable by vaccination with diphtheria toxoid, administered in combination with tetanus toxoid and pertussis vaccine or with tetanus toxoid alone. Preparations of diphtheria toxoid for use in adults contain a lower concentration of diphtheria toxoid than those for use in children.

The routine vaccination schedule for children comprises five doses of diphtheria and tetanus toxoids and pertussis vaccine (DTaP, with acellular pertussis vaccine, or DTP, with whole cell pertussis vaccine). Three primary doses are administered during the first year of life at 2, 4, and 6 months of age. To maintain adequate immunity during preschool years, the fourth (first booster) dose is recommended for children aged 15 to 18 months. The fourth dose should be administered 6 months or more after the third. The fifth (second booster) dose is recommended for children aged 4 to 6 years to confer continued protection against disease during the early years of schooling. A fifth dose is not necessary if the fourth dose in the series is administered on or after the fourth birthday (1).

Adult-formulation diphtheria and tetanus toxoid (Td) is available for use among persons 7 years of age or older. The primary series consists of three doses of Td vaccine, with the second dose given 4 to 8 weeks after the first and the third dose given 6 to 12 months after the second. Immunity induced by both diphtheria and tetanus toxoids diminishes with time, and booster vaccination with Td is recommended at 10-year intervals throughout life, following administration of a primary series. Administration of the first Td booster vaccination at 11 to 12 years has recently been recommended.

Three preparations of acellular pertussis vaccine and diphtheria and tetanus toxoids are licensed in the United States: Tripedia (Connaught Laboratories, Inc.) and Infanrix (SmithKline Beecham) for the first four doses and ACEL-IMUNE (Wyeth-Lederle Vaccines and Pediatrics) for all five doses. TriHIBit (ActHIB reconstituted with Tripedia) is currently licensed for the fourth dose of the vaccination series. Licensure of additional acellular pertussis vaccines for use in young children is anticipated.

Diphtheria toxoid–containing vaccines are administered intramuscularly. The preferred injection sites are the anterolateral aspect of the thigh in young infants or the deltoid muscle of the upper arm if muscle mass is adequate.

Contraindications to further administration of DTaP or DTP are an immediate anaphylactic reaction and encephalopathy not attributable to another identifiable cause occurring within 7 days after vaccination. Because of the importance of tetanus vaccination, persons who experience anaphylactic reactions may be referred to an allergist for evaluation and (if specific allergy can be demonstrated) desensitized to tetanus toxoid. In cases of acute encephalopathy, further administration of pertussis vaccine is contraindicated, and DT vaccine (pediatric-formulation diphtheria and tetanus toxoids) should be administered for the remaining doses in the vaccination schedule (1).

CONTROVERSIES, CAVEATS, OR COMMENTS

During the recent diphtheria epidemic in the former Soviet Union, the World Health Organization recommended a dosage schedule for diphtheria antitoxin similar to that recommended above (4). This was in conflict with standard practice in the former Soviet Union, where dosages in excess of 1,000,000 units were recommended for treatment of patients with severe disease. Although data from clinical trials are limited, there is some evidence that doses of antitoxin much lower even than currently recommended by WHO may be just as effective as higher dosages (2, 11).

Development of a human diphtheria immune globulin has been sought but has proven difficult because even in immune persons, high titers of diphtheria antitoxin are not maintained (14). In the future, such a product may make obsolete the currently available equine antitoxin. Development of a human monoclonal antibody with diphtheria toxin–neutralizing activity has been reported (13).

The role of steroids in prevention of diphtheria toxin–mediated complications remains controversial. While standard in some centers in the former Soviet Union (24), in one clinical trial there was no evidence that steroid therapy prevented myocarditis or neuritis complicating diphtheria (28).

REFERENCES

1. Advisory Committee on Immunization Practices. Pertussis vaccination: use of acellular pertussis vaccines among infants and young children—recommendations of the Advisory Committee on Immunization Practices (ACIP). MMWR 1997;46(no. RR-7):1–25.
2. Agarwal SK, Gupta OP, Mital VN, Pandey RC, Kuman P. An evaluation of the therapeutic efficacy of low dose of antitoxin in the treatment of diphtheria. J Indian Med Assoc 1982;79:1–4.
3. Bauernfeind A. In-vitro activity of dirithromycin in comparison with other new and established macrolides. J Antimicrob Chemother 1993;31(Suppl C):39–49.
4. Begg N. Manual for the management and control of diphtheria in the European region. The Expanded Programme on Immunization in the European Region of WHO. Copenhagen: WHO, 1994.
5. Bisgard KM, Hardy IRB, Popovic T, Strebel PM, Wharton M, Chen RT, Hadler SC. Respiratory diphtheria in the United States, 1980–1995. Am J Public Health 1998;88;787–791.
6. CDC. Availability of diphtheria antitoxin through an investigational new drug protocol. MMWR 1997;47:380.
7. Committee on Infectious Diseases. 1997 Redbook: report of the Committee on Infectious Diseases. 24th ed. Elk Grove Village, IL: American Academy of Pediatrics, 1997:43–45.
8. Coyle MB, Minshew BH, Bland JA, Hsu P. Erythromycin and clindamycin resistance in Corynebacterium diphtheriae from skin lesions. Antimicrob Agents Chemother 1979;16:525–527.
9. Dupont C, Turner L, Rouveix E, Nicolas MH, Dorra M. Endocardite à Corynebacterium diphtheriae tolérante à l'amoxicilline. Presse Med 1995;24:1135.
10. Farizo KM, Strebel PM, Chen RT, Kimbler A, Cleary TJ, Cochi SL. Fatal respiratory disease due to Corynebacterium diphtheriae: case report and review of guidelines for management, investigation, and control. Clin Infect Dis 1993;16:59–68.
11. Gandhi MJ. ADS dosage in diphtheria. J Indian Med Assoc 1966;46:152–154.
11a. Gordon RC, Yow MD, Clark DJ, Stephenson WB. In vitro susceptibility of Corynebacterium diphtheriae to thirteen antibiotics. Applied Microbiology 1971;21:548–549.
12. Grüneberg RN, Felmingham D, O'Hare MD, Robbins MJ, Perry K, Wall RA, Ridgway GL. The comparative in-vitro activity of ofloxacin. J Antimicrob Chemother 1988;22(Suppl C):9–19.
13. Gupta KC, Agha R, Santos E, Brodeur BR. Isolation of human monoclonal antibodies binding to B fragment of diphtheria toxin. Hum Antibod Hybridomas 1992;3:25–31.
14. Gupta RK, Griffin P, Xu J, Rivera R, Thompson C, Siber GR. Diphtheria antitoxin levels in U.S. blood and plasma donors. J Infect Dis 1996;173:1493–1497.
15. Hardy IRB, Dittman S, Sutter RW. Current situation and control strategies for resurgence of diphtheria in the newly independent states of the former Soviet Union. Lancet 1996;347:1739–1744.
16. Harnisch JP, Tronca E, Nolan CM, Turck M, Holmes KK. Diphtheria among alcoholic urban adults: a decade of experience in Seattle. Ann Intern Med 1989;111:71–82.
17. Höfler W. Cutaneous diphtheria. Int J Dermatol 1991;30:845–847.
18. Jellard CH, Lipinski AE. Corynebacterium diphtheriae resistant to erythromycin and lincomycin. Lancet 1973;1:156.
19. Lortholary O, Buu-Hoï A, Gutmann L, Acar J. Corynebacterium diphtheriae endocarditis in France. Clin Infect Dis 1993;17:1072–1074.
20. Maple PAC, Efstratiou A, Tseneva G, Rikushin Y, Deshevoi S, Jahkola M, Vuopio-Varkila J, George RC. The in-vitro susceptibilities of toxigenic strains of C. diphtheriae isolated in northwestern Russia and surrounding areas to ten antimicrobials. J Antimicrob Chemother 1994;34:1037–1040.
21. McCloskey RV, Eller JJ, Green M, Mauney CU, Richards SEM. The 1970 epidemic of diphtheria. Ann Intern Med 1971;75:495–503.
22. McCloskey RV, Green MJ, Eller J, Smilack J. Treatment of diphtheria carriers: benzathine penicillin, erythromycin and clindamycin. Ann Intern Med 1974;81:788–791.
23. Popovic T, Kombarova SY, Reeves MW, Nakao H, Mazurova IK, Wharton M, Wachsmuth IK, Wenger JD. Molecular epidemiology of diphtheria in Russia, 1985–1994. J Infect Dis 1996;174:1064–1072.
24. Rakhmanova AG, Lumio J, Groundstroem K, Valova E, Nosikova E, Tanasijchuk T, Saikku J. Diphtheria characteristics in St. Petersburg: clinical characteristics of 1,860 adult patients. Scand J Infect Dis 1996;28:37–40.
25. Rockhill RC, Sumaro, Hadiputranto H, Siregar SP, Muslihun B. Tetracycline resistance of Corynebacterium diphtheriae isolated from diphtheria patients in Jakarta, Indonesia. Antimicrob Agents Chemother 1982;21:842–843.
26. Schiller J, Groman N, Coyle M. Plasmids in Corynebacterium diphtheriae and diphtheroids mediating erythromycin resistance. Antimicrob Agents Chemother 1980;18:814–821.
27. Serwold-Davis TM, Groman NB. Mapping and cloning of Corynebacterium diphtheriae plasmid pNG2 and characterization of its relatedness to plasmids from skin coryneforms. Antimicrob Agents Chemother 1986;30:69–72.
28. Thisyakorn U, Wongvanich J, Kumpeng V. Failure of corticosteroid therapy to prevent diphtheritic myocarditis or neuritis. Pediatr Infect Dis J 1984;3:126–128.
29. Tiley SM, Kociuba KR, Heron LG, Munro T. Infective endocarditis due to non-toxigenic Corynebacterium diphtheriae: report of seven cases and review. Clin Infect Dis 1993;16:271–275.
30. Wilson APR. Treatment of infection caused by toxigenic and non-toxigenic strains of Corynebacterium diphtheriae. J Antimicrob Chemother 1995;35:717–720.
30a. Zamiri I, McEntegart MG. The sensitivity of diptheria bacilli to eight antibiotics. J Clin Pathol 1972;25:716–717.
31. Zuber PLF, Gruner E, Altwegg M, von Graevenitz A. Invasive infection with non-toxigenic Corynebacterium diphtheriae among drug users. Lancet 1992;339:1359.

Corynebacteria other than
Corynebacterium diphtheriae

Richard A. Miller and Benjamin A. Lipsky

The genus *Corynebacterium* encompasses a heterogeneous collection of Gram-positive rod-shaped bacteria (4). They are related to mycobacteria and nocardia, with which they share many biochemical characteristics. Historically, species were often classified as corynebacteria solely on the basis of morphologic characteristics, and the group as a whole was referred to as "diphtheroids" or "coryneform bacilli." Renewed interest in taxonomy, augmented by genetic sequencing, has led to reevaluation of the classification of many species, with the result that several have been removed from this genus (e.g., *Arcanobacterium haemolyticum* and *Rhodococcus equi*). We have attempted to use the currently accepted terminology, but future revisions are inevitable. Table 1 lists some of the species that have been recently renamed and their older designations.

With the exception of *C. diphtheriae,* the corynebacteria were long regarded as nonpathogenic commensals and environmental contaminants. This view was refuted by growing recognition over the last two decades of the pathogenic role of many species of corynebacteria in human and animal illnesses. While they remain relatively uncommon causes of disease in healthy individuals, they have emerged as important pathogens in immunocompromised hosts and in association with implantable medical devices.

IDENTIFICATION AND TAXONOMY

Corynebacteria are rod-shaped, nonsporeforming, often pleomorphic bacteria that take up Gram's stain somewhat more weakly than many other Gram-positive bacteria. This often results in a "Gram-variable" or even Gram-negative appearance if decolorization is excessive. They are nonmotile and aerobic (or facultatively anaerobic); none are obligate anaerobes. Corynebacteria are catalase positive and, with one exception, contain characteristic mycolic acids in their cell walls. The corynebacterial mycolic acids are closely related to one another (>85% similarity) but more distantly related to the mycolic acids found in mycobacteria, *Rhodococcus,* and *Nocardia.*

No special specimen collection or handling procedures are required. All clinically significant species of corynebacteria grow readily in complex growth media containing serum, such as blood agar. Specialized media (e.g., tellurite agar or Loeffler's medium) are most often used to detect *C. diphtheriae* but also support the growth of many other corynebacteria. Staining organisms from a colony or broth media often show unusual geometric groupings that may resemble "Chinese characters." Assigning a clinical isolate to a specific species can be difficult and time consuming. Traditional typing based on biochemical characteristics is being supplanted by chromatographic analysis of cell wall fatty acids (8). Although several species of corynebacteria are capable of producing toxins, assays for specific toxin production are generally applied only to isolates of *C. diphtheriae.* The clinical implication of these microbiologic characteristics is that the clinician is often notified of the isolation of a "diphtheroid" several days before the exact species can be identified.

CLINICAL SIGNIFICANCE OF *CORYNEBACTERIUM* SPECIES

Little is known about the natural epidemiology of most species of corynebacteria. Some species appear to be human skin or oropharyngeal commensals. Others are zoonotic commensals or occasional pathogens. Still others may be components of the environmental microbiota, either in the natural world or in specialized niches in the hospital setting. Assessing their role as human pathogens is complicated by the frequent isolation of nondiphtheria corynebacteria in specimens from nonsterile sites. The ubiquitous presence of corynebacteria on normal skin complicates interpreting their clinical significance, even when isolated from normally sterile body fluids or from surgical specimens. This is especially true if only a single culture is positive. The most difficult decision in treating a corynebacterial infection is often determining whether or not the *Corynebacterium* isolate is a pathogen. Table 2 provides some guidelines to help in assessing the clinical significance of a *Corynebacterium* isolate, but in the end, each case must be individually analyzed.

With the exception of *C. diphtheriae,* none of the corynebacteria produces a unique illness that permits clinical diagnosis of a corynebacterial infection prior to receiving the results of cultures and Gram-stained smears. Similarly, epidemic clusters of nondiphtheria corynebacterial disease are unknown, with the possible exception of nosocomial *C. jeikeium* infections (19). Corynebacteria have been identified as causative agents in a wide range of infections, including endocarditis of native and prosthetic valves, bacteremia and sepsis (particularly in immunocompromised hosts), infections associated with implanted medical devices (including venous access catheters and cerebrospinal shunts), pharyngitis, pneumonia, otitis media, septic arthritis, osteomyelitis, neonatal sepsis and meningitis, peritonitis associated with continuous ambulatory peritoneal dialysis, wound infections, soft-tissue infections, lymphadenitis, and urinary tract infections.

TABLE 1 • Corynebacteria Nomenclature

Current Designation	Previous or Alternative Name(s)
Corynebacterium pseudotuberculosis	Corynebacterium ovis
Corynebacterium pseudodiphtheriticum	Corynebacterium hofmannii
Arcanobacterium haemolyticum	Corynebacterium haemolyticum
C. afermentans subsp. lipophilum	CDC group ANF-1
Bifidobacterium adolescentis	Corynebacterium group E
Corynebacterium urealyticum	CDC group D2
Actinomyces pyogenes	Corynebacterium pyogenes

SUSCEPTIBILITY IN VITRO

Broth microdilution assays are most commonly used with corynebacteria, although disk-diffusion testing appears to yield similar results for most antibiotics, with the possible exception of penicillin. One study (25) suggests using streptococcal susceptibility criteria rather than those for *Listeria*, but no formal guidelines have been issued. The streptococcal guidelines are more stringent, especially with respect to penicillin susceptibility, and their usage would result in more isolates being reported as resistant or intermediate to penicillin.

Antimicrobial susceptibility is highly variable within and between species. Antibiotic selection should be based on the results of sensitivity testing of each individual patient's isolate, when possible. When empirical antibiotic therapy is necessary, some generalizations can help when the microbiology laboratory reports the isolation of a "diphtheroid" with "sensitivities to follow."

Virtually all corynebacteria are susceptible to the glycopeptide antibiotics vancomycin and teichoplanin. Minimal inhibitory concentrations (MICs) to these two agents are usually similar, but there is much more clinical experience with vancomycin. Doxycycline is also highly active against most strains, except for occasional isolates of *C. jeikeium, C. ure-*

alyticum, C. striatum, and some nonspeciated strains. Until recently, penicillin (and other β-lactam agents) and erythromycin were generally active against corynebacteria other than *C. jeikeium* and *C. urealyticum.* Unfortunately, recent studies have demonstrated increasing levels of resistance to these agents in a wide range of *Corynebacterium* species, as well as variable sensitivity to clindamycin, quinolones, aminoglycosides, and the newer macrolides (azithromycin and clarithromycin) (22). Addition of the β-lactamase inhibitor clavulanic acid did not affect the MICs to β-lactam antibiotics (7).

ANTIMICROBIAL THERAPY
General Guidelines

Recommendations for antimicrobial therapy of corynebacterial infections are largely empirical. Because these infections are sporadic and infrequent, conventional controlled therapeutic trials have never been conducted. Thus, recommendations must be based on compilations of reported cases and the results of in vitro susceptibility testing (7, 22, 25). Interpreting the results of susceptibility testing is further complicated by the absence of standardized methodology and susceptibility criteria (8) and the lack of documented correlation between in vitro susceptibility and clinical response. Fortunately, clinical failure of therapy with an antibiotic to which the organism was sensitive in vitro is rare.

On the basis of in vitro observations, vancomycin should be included in the empirical treatment regimen of all life-threatening infections caused by "diphtheroids." To minimize the unnecessary use of glycopeptide antibiotics, the need for continued vancomycin therapy must be reassessed once sensitivity testing results become available. Vancomycin is also indicated in empirical therapy of serious but not life-threatening infections of the urinary tract, especially if nephrolithiasis is present (because of the likelihood of *C. urealyticum*), and in hospitalized neutropenic patients (in whom *C. jeikeium* is common). For other serious infections requiring parenteral therapy, empirical regimens should include a β-lactam antibi-

TABLE 2 • Guidelines for Assessing the Clinical Significance of a *Corynebacterium* Isolate

Almost certainly significant, treatment mandatory:
   Isolation of the same species from more than two blood cultures, regardless of the presence of other possible pathogens
   Isolation from a specimen from a normally sterile site obtained during surgery or by another aseptic procedure (e.g., aspiration of ascites, pleura, joint, or CSF) in a patient with a compatible clinical syndrome
Probably significant, treatment mandatory because of severity of illness:
   Isolation in one culture of blood or other normally sterile body fluid from a patient with sepsis or signs of impending sepsis
   Isolation in one blood culture from a febrile immunocompromised patient if no other cause for fever is identified
   Isolation as the sole organism in one blood culture from a patient with clinical or echocardiographic evidence of endocarditis
Possibly significant, treatment or further diagnostic evaluation indicated:
   Isolation as the sole organism in one blood culture from a febrile patient with a prosthetic heart valve but no other signs of endocarditis
   Isolation in conjunction with other possible pathogens from a normally sterile body fluid or site
   Repeated isolation from a potentially contaminated site (e.g., urine, tracheal aspirate)
Probably not significant, do not treat unless further evidence supports a pathogenic role:
   Isolation in conjunction with other, known pathogenic organisms from oropharyngeal swabs, sputum, genital swabs, skin lesions, urine
   Isolation from improperly obtained blood culture or from a normally sterile specimen yielding other probable contaminants

otic (e.g., a penicillin or a cephalosporin). The semisynthetic penicillins such as oxacillin are less active in vitro and should be avoided. First-generation cephalosporins such as cephalothin are generally at least as active as second- or third-generation agents. For less serious infections, especially those involving skin, soft tissue, or upper respiratory tract, oral therapy with doxycycline is the most logical choice. An oral macrolide or β-lactam are acceptable alternatives.

Dosage and duration of therapy are determined by the site and seriousness of the infection. Combinations of antibiotics (e.g., vancomycin-rifampin, vancomycin-gentamicin) have not been shown more effective than single agents and cannot be recommended for empirical therapy. Definitive cure of corynebacterial infection of prosthetic devices often requires surgical removal of the foreign body, but in most instances, this does not have to be done emergently.

GUIDELINES FOR INFECTIONS DUE TO SPECIFIC *CORYNEBACTERIUM* SPECIES
Corynebacterium aquaticum

The relatively uncommon human pathogen *C. aquaticum* has been implicated in several serious infections, including endocarditis, bacteremia, peritonitis (in association with peritoneal dialysis), and neonatal infections. Water-borne transmission was suspected in some cases. While many strains are broadly susceptible, resistance to β-lactams is reported, sometimes in up to 50% of isolates. Nonetheless, most reported patients have responded to therapy with penicillin or ampicillin, often in combination with an aminoglycoside. Ampicillin (or penicillin) alone or combined with gentamicin, appears to be the treatment of choice if the organism is known to be susceptible. Given the prevalence of penicillin resistance, vancomycin should be used initially in life-threatening infections, pending the results of sensitivity testing.

Corynebacterium bovis

C. bovis, a commensal inhabitant of the bovine udder is found as a contaminant in raw milk. The most common clinical illness attributed to *C. bovis* has been prosthetic valve endocarditis, but it has also been reported to cause otitis media, cerebrospinal fluid (CSF) shunt infections, meningitis, epidural abscess, and skin infections. A history of animal contact or raw milk consumption has not been elicited in most reported cases, so the mechanism of acquisition of infection is uncertain. All reported isolates have been susceptible to vancomycin, and most have been sensitive to rifampin and erythromycin. MICs to penicillin have been variable. Vancomycin is the drug of choice for endocarditis, meningitis, and other serious infections, although parenteral penicillin or ampicillin are preferable if the organism is susceptible. Infections of the skin or upper respiratory tract can be treated with oral erythromycin.

Corynebacterium jeikeium

C. jeikeium is an important pathogen of immunocompromised hosts (19). Primary risk factors for invasive disease include prolonged hospitalization, neutropenia, prior treatment with antibiotics, and disruption of the integument (wounds, intra-

venous catheters). Skin colonization, particularly of the axilla and groin, has been documented in 40 to 82% of hospitalized patients with malignancies. Several hospital case clusters have been associated with high carriage rates on the hands of ward staff as well as environmental contamination of room surfaces and air. The results of epidemiologic studies have both favored and disputed nosocomial transmission (11, 12).

Initial reports of *C. jeikeium* infections stressed septicemia and wound infections as the most common clinical manifestations. More recently, *C. jeikeium* has been accepted as a cause of endocarditis (upward of 30 cases, some involving native valves), bacteremia, pneumonia, skin and soft-tissue infections, intravenous catheter-related infections, and ventriculoperitoneal shunt infections (5, 9).

A distinguishing characteristic of *C. jeikeium* is its constitutive resistance to most antibiotics. The extent of broad-spectrum antimicrobial resistance may have been slightly exaggerated by the use of antibiotic-containing selective media for the isolation of *C. jeikeium* in most early studies, but this is clearly the most resistant *Corynebacterium* species. All isolates have been sensitive to vancomycin, but only 15% are susceptible to erythromycin, and 18% to penicillin (25). Many isolates are susceptible to rifampin, doxycycline, and ciprofloxacin, although quinolone resistance seems to be increasing. Virtually all successfully treated patients reported in the literature have received vancomycin, which must be regarded as the drug of choice for *C. jeikeium* infections. Doxycycline might be an acceptable alternative for minor infections in noncompromised hosts, but there is no clinical experience with this treatment. Alternative therapy would have to be determined by sensitivity testing. Cure of most *C. jeikeium* infections associated with prosthetic valves or invasive lines has required removal of the foreign body. Successful therapy of CSF shunts infected with *C. jeikeium* has been achieved with combined intravenous and intrathecal vancomycin for 10 days followed by removal of the original shunt hardware and continuation of intrathecal (with or without intravenous) vancomycin for an additional 6 to 14 days (9). The authors of this study did not report the dose of intrathecal vancomycin they used, but a dose of 3 to 5 mg (in adults) should produce adequate CSF drug levels. The optimal timing for installation of a new shunt apparatus is uncertain, but it can often be successfully accomplished at the same time the original shunt is removed.

Corynebacterium minutissimum

C. minutissimum is best known as the putative etiologic agent of erythrasma, a common and relatively mild skin condition characterized by brownish macules in intertriginous areas. Risk factors for erythrasma include male sex and diabetes mellitus. The clinical diagnosis is made by demonstrating coral-red fluorescence of characteristic lesions when illuminated with ultraviolet (Wood's) light. The etiologic role of *C. minutissimum* has not been unequivocally established, and another species of corynebacteria may be the true etiologic agent. Alternatively, erythrasma may be a common result of infection by any of several diphtheroid species.

More-serious infections with *C. minutissimum* have been

recently reported, including soft-tissue abscesses, bacteremia, and endocarditis. Erythrasma has traditionally been treated with oral erythromycin (250 mg four times a day for 5–7 days). Topical clindamycin (2% aqueous solution) is an alternative. Sensitivity testing results have been reported for relatively few isolates, but erythromycin resistance is surprisingly common (>70% in one series). It has been postulated that certain biotypes (propionic acid producing) of *C. minutissimum* are broadly resistant. Among the few reported patients with invasive disease, some were successfully treated with vancomycin or penicillin, while others failed therapy with β-lactam agents. Based on these anecdotes and in vitro data, vancomycin should be the drug of choice for invasive disease, with penicillin or ampicillin as alternative choices if the organism is demonstrated to be sensitive.

Corynebacterium pseudodiphtheriticum

C. pseudodiphtheriticum can be found in the pharyngeal flora of healthy adults. It does not produce toxins and has not been associated with pharyngitis, but its growth characteristics, colonial morphology, and appearance in Gram-stained smears resemble those of *C. diphtheriae,* occasionally resulting in an incorrect presumptive diagnosis of diphtheria (10). *C. pseudodiphtheriticum* is most often encountered as a pathogen in infections of the lower respiratory tract in both immunocompetent and compromised hosts (1, 14, 16). In one patient with AIDS, *C. pseudodiphtheriticum* was associated with a lung abscess, mimicking the clinical syndrome observed with *Rhodococcus equi* in these patients. It has also been reported causing endocarditis (of both prosthetic and native valves), suppurative lymphadenitis, and cutaneous infections.

Most strains of *C. pseudodiphtheriticum* are broadly susceptible to β-lactam antibiotics. Penicillin or ampicillin should be regarded as the agent of choice for pulmonary infections caused by *C. pseudodiphtheriticum*. Addition of an aminoglycoside is often recommended for treating *C. pseudodiphtheriticum* endocarditis but has not been proven necessary for cure (16). Alternative agents for respiratory tract disease include clindamycin, a macrolide (erythromycin, azithromycin), or a fluoroquinolone, although occasional strains are resistant in vitro to some or all of these agents. Clinical treatment failures are very rare and usually occur in the setting of rapidly fatal comorbid conditions. Endocarditis in a patient with documented hypersensitivity to penicillin is probably best managed by desensitization, although vancomycin may be an effective alternative therapy.

Corynebacterium pseudotuberculosis

C. pseudotuberculosis is a well recognized pathogen of domestic and wild animals. Infection can produce pneumonia or suppurative lymphadenitis in several species, most commonly sheep and goats but also horses, cattle, and deer. Contact with sheep (or their hides or offal) has been reported in over 80% of cases of human infection with *C. pseudotuberculosis,* and other cases have been linked to ingestion of raw milk. Almost all strains of *C. pseudotuberculosis* produce a dermonecrotic toxin. This exotoxin is a phospholipase D, similar in activity

(though immunologically distinct) to the phospholipase D present in the venom of *Loxosceles reclusa,* the brown recluse spider. Some strains are also capable of producing diphtheria toxin.

The most common manifestation of *C. pseudotuberculosis* infection in humans is suppurative granulomatous lymphadenitis. Some cases of pneumonia caused by *C. pseudotuberculosis* have been reported. One patient with cervical adenitis had mild exudative tonsillitis, but diphtheria-like pharyngitis has not been reported. Most tested isolates have shown susceptibility to a broad range of antibiotics, including penicillin, cephalosporins, tetracycline, erythromycin, and chloramphenicol. Successful therapy of suppurative lymphadenitis has required both surgery (lymph node excision and drainage of purulent material) and antibiotics, usually erythromycin or tetracycline. A notable feature of human disease with *C. pseudotuberculosis* is its tendency for local recurrence after apparent clinical resolution. Many of the published case reports stress the need for prolonged antibiotic therapy (often 6–12 weeks), repeated surgical exploration with excision and drainage of purulence or necrotic tissue, and long-term clinical follow-up to identify late relapse (18).

Corynebacterium striatum

C. striatum appears to be a component of the normal flora of the anterior nares and skin (especially above the waist). It has been reported as a causative agent in lower respiratory tract infections, bacteremia, endocarditis, intravenous catheter-related infections, chorioamnionitis, conjunctivitis, meningitis (posttraumatic), and peritonitis associated with peritoneal dialysis (15, 23, 24). Most cases are believed to arise from invasion by endogenous strains, but molecular strain typing of hospital isolates of *C. striatum* have established its role as a nosocomial pathogen in two intensive care unit outbreaks. Transmission between patients apparently occurred through transient carriage on the hands of medical personnel.

C. striatum is susceptible to vancomycin, rifampin, and aminoglycosides, and most strains are sensitive to penicillin, ciprofloxacin, and imipenem. Erythromycin resistance has been reported. Penicillin remains the drug of choice for sensitive strains, but vancomycin is a reasonable choice for empirical therapy of serious infections such as meningitis and endocarditis, pending the results of sensitivity testing.

Corynebacterium ulcerans

Like *C. pseudotuberculosis, C. ulcerans* is a zoonotic pathogen. It can produce bovine mastitis with concomitant contamination of the milk but is often simply a component of the normal intestinal flora in horses and cattle. Human cases occur most commonly during the summer and are often, but not always, associated with exposure to livestock. Many strains of *C. ulcerans* produce diphtheria toxin, and some produce a dermonecrotic toxin similar or identical to that of *C. pseudotuberculosis*. In contrast to the disease syndromes characteristic of *C . pseudotuberculosis,* however, *C. ulcerans* is predominantly a pathogen of the oropharynx and lower respiratory tract in humans. The pharyngitis is generally mild, but can on occasion mimic diphtheria, including its neurologic and cardiac abnormalities. Lower respiratory tract involvement can manifest as a nonspecific pneumonia or as pulmonary nodules comprised of necrotizing, granulomatous inflammation. Cutaneous and soft-tissue disease have also been reported.

In vitro sensitivity testing of *C. ulcerans* strains demonstrates their susceptibility to a broad range of antimicrobial agents. Published patients were usually treated successfully with either erythromycin or penicillin. Diphtheria antitoxin would probably benefit patients with severe toxigenic *C. ulcerans* pharyngitis, but there is no published experience with this treatment.

Corynebacterium urealyticum

As implied by its name, urease activity is the distinguishing characteristic of *C. urealyticum*. Its environmental reservoir is poorly defined, but it can colonize human skin, where it is found in up to one-third of hospitalized patients. When it produces human disease, *C. urealyticum* is almost exclusively associated with infections of the upper and lower urinary tract and complications arising from these infections (3, 17, 20). The overwhelming majority of reported patients were hospitalized (or had recently been hospitalized), were immunocompromised, had recently undergone instrumentation of the urologic tract, and had received antibiotics. Half had a history of a urologic disorder.

Alkaline-encrusted cystitis, an unusual clinical syndrome, is frequently associated with *C. urealyticum* infection (20). This chronic inflammatory disease of the bladder is marked by deposition of struvite (ammonium magnesium phosphate) on the bladder surface, with ulceration and localized necrosis of the bladder mucosa. The bladder wall becomes edematous and rigid. These changes, which are often irreversible, have also been associated with infection by other urea-splitting bacteria, such as *Proteus* spp. Patients with alkaline-encrusted cystitis complain of gross hematuria, cloudy urine, and passage of gritty material or small stones in the urine, in addition to the usual cystitis symptoms of dysuria and suprapubic pain. Low-grade fever may be present. Pyuria is common, and the urine invariably has an alkaline pH and contains struvite crystals. The clinical presentation and urinalysis findings are generally sufficient to make the diagnosis of alkaline-encrusted cystitis, but cystoscopy can be useful in confirming the diagnosis and for therapy (see below). Fewer than 5% of reported *C. urealyticum* infections have involved sites outside the urinary tract, including bacteremia, wound infection, endocarditis, peritonitis, and respiratory tract infection (21, 26).

Antimicrobial sensitivity testing has shown *C. urealyticum* to be among the more resistant species of corynebacteria. All strains tested have been susceptible to vancomycin. Fluoroquinolones, such as ciprofloxacin, are active against most isolates, but susceptibility to rifampin, tetracycline, erythromycin, nitrofurantoin, and gentamicin is variable. Vancomycin and the fluoroquinolones retain their antimicrobial activity at alkaline pH, unlike many other antibiotics. Based on reported clinical efficacy, vancomycin (or possibly teicoplanin (6)) is the antibiotic of choice, but when oral therapy is an option, tetra-cycline or a fluoroquinolone are acceptable alternatives. Prolonged antibiotic therapy as well as cystoscopic or surgical resection of struvite deposits is necessary for cure of alkaline-encrusted cystitis.

Corynebacterium xerosis

C. xerosis is found on the skin and mucosal surfaces of the nasopharynx and has been associated with only a few cases of human disease. Endocarditis, mediastinitis, pneumonia, and infection of CSF shunts have been reported (2, 13). Vancomycin and tetracycline are the most consistently active agents in vitro; sensitivity to penicillin and erythromycin is variable. Almost all reported cases have been treated successfully with parenteral penicillin (or ampicillin) or vancomycin. Doxycycline might be an acceptable alternative when oral therapy is appropriate.

Corynebacterium spp. Associated with Rare Cases of Human Disease

Several other *Corynebacterium* spp., including *C. accolens, C. afermentans* subsp. *lipophilum, C. pilosum, C. seminale,* and members of coryneform groups A-4, ANF-3, and G-2, have been linked to rare cases of human infection. Most of the isolates tested have shown in vitro sensitivity to a broad range of antimicrobial agents.

REFERENCES

1. Ahmed K, Kawakami K, Watanabe K, Mitsushuma H, Hagatake T, Matsumoto K. *Corynebacterium pseudodiphtheriticum:* a respiratory tract pathogen. Clin Infect Dis 1995;20:41–46.
2. Arisoy E, Turkey M, Demmler G, Dunne W Jr. *Corynebacterium xerosis* ventriculoperitoneal shunt infection in an infant; report of a case and review of the literature. Pediatr Infect Dis J 1993;12:536–538.
3. Bravo-Garcie M, Aguado J, Morales J, Noriega A. Influence of external factors in resistance of *Corynebacterium urealyticum* to antimicrobial agents. Antimicrob Agents Chemother 1996;40:497–499.
4. Coyle M, Lipsky B. Coryneform bacteria in infectious diseases: clinical and laboratory aspects. Clin Microbiol Rev 1990;3:227–246.
5. DeBriel D. Langs JC, Rougeron G, Chabot P, Le Faou A. A multiresistant corynebacteria in bacteriuria: a comparative study of the role of *Corynebacterium* group D2 and *Corynebacterium jeikeium*. J Hosp Infect 1991;17:35–43.
6. Estorc JJ, de la Coussaye JE, Viel EJ, Bouziges N, Ramuz M, Eledjam JJ. Teicoplanin treatment of alkaline encrusted cystitis due to *Corynebacterium* group D2. Eur J Med 1992;1:183–184.
7. Funke G, Punter V, Von Graevenitz A. Antimicrobial susceptibility patterns of some recently established coryneform bacteria. Antimicrob Agents Chemother 1996;40:2874–2878.
8. Funke G, Von Graevenitz A, Claridge JE III, Bernard KA. Clinical microbiology of coryneform bacteria. Clin Microbiol Rev 1997;10:125–129.
9. Greene K, Clark R, Zabramski M. Ventricular CSF shunt infections associated with *Corynebacterium jeikeium:* report of three cases and review. Clin Infect Dis 1993;16:139–141.
10. Izurieta HS, Strebel PM, Youngblood T, Hollis DG, Popovic T. Exudative pharyngitis possibly due to *Corynebacterium*

pseudodiphtheriticum, a new challenge in the differential diagnosis of diphtheria. Emerging Infect Dis 1997;3:65–68.

11. Kerry-Williams SM, Noble WC. Plasmids in group JK coryneform bacteria isolated in a single hospital. J Hyg (Cambridge) 1986;97:255–263.

12. Khabbaz RF, Kaper JB, Moody MR, Schimpff SC, Tenney JH. Molecular epidemiology of group JK *Corynebacterium* on a cancer ward: lack of evidence for patient-to-patient transmission. J Infect Dis 1986;154:95–99.

13. Lortholary O, Buu-Hoi A, Fagon JY, Pierre J, Slama M, Gutmann L, Acar JF. Mediastinitis due to multiply resistant *Corynebacterium xerosis.* Clin Infect Dis 1993;16:172.

14. Manzella J, Kellogg J, Parsey KS. *Corynebacterium pseudodiphtheriticum:* a respiratory tract pathogen in adults. Clin Infect Dis 1995;20:37–40.

15. Martinez-Martinez L, Pascual A, Bernard K, Suarez A. Antimicrobial susceptibility pattern of *Corynebacterium striatum.* Antimicrob Agents Chemother 1996:40:2671–2672.

16. Morris A, Guild I. Endocarditis due to *Corynebacterium pseudodiphtheriticum:* five case reports, review, and antibiotic susceptibilities of nine strains. Rev Infect Dis 1991;13:887–892.

17. Nebreda-Mayoral T, Munoz-Bellido JL, Garcia-Rodrigues JA. Incidence and characteristics of urinary tract infections caused by *Corynebacterium urealyticum* (*Corynebacterium* group D2). Eur J Clin Microbiol Infect Dis 1994;13:600–604.

18. Peel MM, Palmer GG, Stacpoole AM, Kerr TG. Human lymphadenitis due to *Corynebacterium pseudotuberculosis:* report of ten cases from Australia and review. Clin Infect Dis 1997;24:185–191.

19. Schoch P, Unna B. The JK diphtheroids. Infect Control 1986;7:466–469.

20. Soriano F, Aguado J, Ponte C, Fernandez-Roblas R, Rodriguez-Tudela J. Urinary tract infection caused by *Corynebacterium* group D2: report of 82 cases and review. Rev Infect Dis 1990;12:1019–1034.

21. Soriano F, Ponte C, Ruis P, Zapardiel J. Non-urinary tract infections caused by multiple antibiotic-resistant *Corynebacterium urealyticum.* Clin Infect Dis 1993;17:890–891.

22. Soriano F, Zapardiel J, Nieto E. Antimicrobial susceptibilities of *Corynebacterium* species and other non-spore forming gram-positive bacilli to 18 antimicrobial agents. Antimicrob Agents Chemother 1995;39:208–214.

23. Watkins D, Chahine A, Creger R, Jacobs M, Lazarus H. *Corynebacterium striatum:* a diphtheroid with pathogenic potential. Clin Infect Dis 1993;17:21–25.

24. Weiss K, Labbe AC, Laverderiere M. *Corynebacterium striatum* meningitis: case report and review of an increasingly important *Corynebacterium* species. Clin Infect Dis 1996;23:1246–1248.

25. Weiss K, Laverdiere M, Rivest R. Comparison of antimicrobial susceptibilities of *Corynebacterium* species by broth microdilution and disk diffusion methods. Antimicrob Agents Chemother 1996;40:930–933.

26. Wood C, Pepe R. Bacteremia in a patient with non-urinary tract infection due to *Corynebacterium urealyticum.* Clin Infect Dis 1994;19:367–368.

Edwardsiella tarda

Selwyn D. R. Lang and Arthur J. Morris

GENERAL DESCRIPTION
Microbiology and Epidemiology

The genus *Edwardsiella* comprises three species and a biogroup: *E. tarda, E. hoshinae, E. ictaluri* and *E. tarda* biogroup I. Almost all human infections are caused by *E. tarda.* This organism has previously been called "bacterium 1483-59," the "Asakusa group," and the "Bartholomew group" (8). The species name *tarda* refers to its inability to ferment most carbohydrates.

Edwardsiella spp. inhabit fresh water and animals that live there, including turtles, fish, alligators, toads, and lizards (8, 10, 17, 22). Human infections have been linked to animals and fish (7, 13, 24). *E. tarda* causes a variety of diseases in animals, including emphysematous putrefaction of catfish, enteritis in penguins, and visceral disease in eels (8). Recovery of biogroup I has been limited to environmental water and snakes.

Edwardsiella spp. are motile, oxidase-negative, catalase-positive, Gram-negative bacilli in the family Enterobacteriaceae. The biochemical profile varies very little between strains, although rare strains with single atypical reactions cause human disease, e.g., sucrose-positive strains (27). *E. tarda* is biochemically most similar to *Salmonella* spp.; it produces hydrogen sulfide. Because it is sucrose and lactose negative, it grows on most selective and differential agars as colonies that can be picked out as requiring workup as a potential enteric pathogen. Biogroup I isolates do not produce hydrogen sulfide, and ferment sugars that *E. tarda* does not, e.g., sucrose and mannitol.

Clinical Manifestations

Most (>80%) reported cases of *E. tarda* infection are gastrointestinal (2, 6, 8). Exceptionally, enterocolitis with bloody diarrhea, multiple ulcerations of the colon and rectum, and nodularity of the terminal ileum has been reported

(12). Of the remaining cases, wound infections (~10%) and bacteremia (~5%) are the most common (4, 7–9, 28). Underlying liver disease has been noted in 50% of septicemic cases (8). In several cases, wound infection or cellulitis has followed puncture injuries by catfish spines (1, 4, 7), and in one, a puncture wound from stepping on remnants of a snake (18). An injury sustained in lake water (25), association with aquariums (13, 24) and eating raw fish (16), seafood (29), or snake (15) have also been implicated in infection with *E. tarda*. Other reported infections include cholecystitis (27), peritonitis (4), osteomyelitis (18), pneumonia, genitourinary including tuboovarian abscess (16), infected vascular prosthesis (5), neonatal and adult meningitis (15, 21, 23), and liver abscesses (9, 30). An association between *E. tarda* osteomyelitis (18) and meningitis (21) and underlying sickle cell disease has been suggested. The possibility of human-to-human transmission has been raised by an outbreak of eight cases in two day-care centers where no common source of infection could be found (6) and by a cluster of three cases in one family (29).

SUSCEPTIBILITY IN VITRO

Four formal in vitro studies have been performed (Table 1). Resistance to antimicrobial agents commonly used for therapy of Gram-negative sepsis is uncommon. All 29 isolates tested by Reinhardt et al. were susceptible to quinolones, tetracycline, chloramphenicol, trimethoprim and sulfamethoxazole (either as single agents or in combination), gentamicin, and cefotaxime (20). Almost all the activity of trimethoprim-sulfamethoxazole is due to the trimethoprim component (20). Although the ampicillin MIC_{90} was low (0.5 µg/mL), all 29 isolates produced a β-lactamase detected by the cephinase test (20). This discrepancy, also reported by others (3, 19), requires explanation before β-lactams such as ampicillin or amoxicillin can be regarded as reliably active for therapeutic purposes (19). A fourfold or greater decrease in MIC was noted when tazobactam was added to piperacillin (8 of 22 isolates) and clavulanate to ticarcillin (11 of 22 isolates) but not when clavulanate was added to amoxicillin or when sulbactam was added to ampicillin or to cefoperazone (3). Another study, involving 10 isolates, showed all isolates to be susceptible to imipenem, aztreonam, cefotaxime, ciprofloxacin, norfloxacin, gentamicin, and doxycycline (19).

The bactericidal activity of antibiotics for *E. tarda* has seldom been investigated. Reger et al. reported that aztreonam, cefotaxime, ciprofloxacin, and norfloxacin had MBCs equal to MICs for 80% or more of 10 isolates; MBCs of ampicillin, imipenem, piperacillin, and gentamicin exceeded MICs for 50% or more, and MBCs of clindamycin and doxycycline exceeded MBCs for all isolates (19). MICs and MBCs (mg/L) for a single clinical isolate from a patient with endocarditis were ampicillin, 0.095/0.095; cephalothin, 0.19/0.39; chloramphenicol, 12.5/50; kanamycin, 0.95/1.9; polymyxin B, 100/100; and tetracycline, 0.95/50 (11).

Resistance to methicillin, cloxacillin, lincomycin, and clindamycin appears to be the rule, whereas resistance to penicillin G and erythromycin is variable (26). We are unaware of any

published report of the activity of vancomycin against *E. tarda*. No published studies have investigated synergy between antibiotics against *E. tarda*.

ANTIMICROBIAL THERAPY

Infections due to *E. tarda* are sufficiently uncommon that there have been no comparative trials of their treatment with any of the numerous antibiotics to which they are almost always susceptible. Gastrointestinal infections usually resolve spontaneously, and antibiotic treatment is not required (8). However, trimethoprim-sulfamethoxazole (two single-strength tablets 6 hourly) was given to a patient with severe invasive enterocolitis, relieving symptoms within 48 h and rendering subsequent stool cultures negative (12). Amoxicillin has also been used with prompt resolution of symptoms (13). On the basis of in vitro data and their excellent track record against other enteric pathogens, the fluoroquinolones would be expected to be effective.

A wide variety of antibiotic regimens have been used in the treatment of extraintestinal disease, especially septicemia, due to *E. tarda*. The choices often reflect local preferences for empirical regimens begun before *E. tarda* has been isolated. In a review of 16 cases of bacteremic *E. tarda* infection (28), 7 patients died, for a case fatality rate of 44%. However, of the 10 for whom antibiotic treatment was recorded, 7 survived, 6 of whom received combination treatment: β-lactam plus aminoglycoside plus chloramphenicol for 4 patients; β-lactam plus aminoglycoside, 1; and chloramphenicol plus aminoglycoside, 1. The other survivor was treated with ampicillin alone. Of the 3 who died despite treatment, 1 received ampicillin plus gentamicin, 1 cephalothin alone, and 1 (with meningitis), a combination of penicillin, streptomycin, chloramphenicol, and sulfadiazine, which the authors speculate may have been antagonistic (15). A comprehensive review published 4 years later was able to add only one further bacteremic case to those described by Wilson et al. (8).

More-recent regimens used successfully in serious infections have included sequential imipenem, ceftriaxone, and ciprofloxacin to treat multiple liver abscesses (30), imipenem alone for 6 weeks after a short initial course of combination treatment for an infected vascular prosthesis (5), and a 6-week course of amoxicillin, clavulanate, and ciprofloxacin for *E. tarda* septicemia in a cirrhotic patient (29).

On the basis of in vitro activity and very limited anecdotal data, second- or third-generation cephalosporins and fluoroquinolones are likely to become antibiotics of choice for treating serious infection due to *E. tarda*. This said, only occasional isolates are resistant to ampicillin, tetracycline, chloramphenicol, and trimethoprim-sulfamethoxazole, all of which have been used successfully in treatment. The fact that all strains produce a β-lactamase enzyme raises some questions about the appropriateness of monotherapy with amoxicillin, ampicillin, ticarcillin, or piperacillin, even though there is no evidence that the enzyme confers significant resistance to these antibiotics. Penicillin G and erythromycin have variable-to-poor activity and should not be used to treat *E. tarda* infections. *E. tarda* is invariably resistant to cloxacillin, lincomycin, and clindamycin (27). In the absence of published

TABLE 1 • In Vitro Susceptibilities of *Edwardsiella tarda*

Antibiotic	n	Range	MIC$_{50}$	MIC$_{90}$	Breakpoint[a]	% Susceptible	Ref
Amikacin	22	1–8	2	4	≤16	100	3
Amikacin	86	1–8	4	4	≤16	100	26
Gentamicin	29	1–2	2	2	≤4	100	20
Gentamicin	22	1–2	1	1	≤4	100	3
Gentamicin	10	NS[b]	0.625	0.625	≤4	100	19
Gentamicin	86	0.5–4	1	2	≤4	100	26
Tobramycin	22	0.25–1	1	1	≤4	100	3
Tobramycin	86	0.5–4	1	2	≤4	100	26
Amoxicillin	22	0.5–4	0.5	1	≤8	100	3
Amoxicillin-clavulanate	22	0.5/0.25–4/2	0.5/0.25	1/0.5	≤8/4	100	3
Ampicillin	29	0.125–1	0.25	0.5	≤8	100	20
Ampicillin	10	NS	0.1	0.1	≤8	100	19
Ampicillin	86	0.5–≥16	1	4	≤8	—	26
Ampicillin	22	0.12–1	0.25	0.25	≤8	100	3
Ampicillin-sulbactam	22	0.12/0.06–1/0.5	0.25/0.12	0.25/0.12	≤8/4	100	3
Carbenicillin	86	8–512	8	8	≤16	—	26
Piperacillin	10	NS	0.1	0.1	≤16	100	19
Piperacillin	22	0.12–0.5	0.25	0.5	≤16	100	3
Piperacillin-tazobactam	22	0.12/0.015–0.5/0.06	0.25–0.03	0.25/0.03	≤16/4	100	3
Ticarcillin	22	0.5–8	8	8	≤16	100	3
Ticarcillin-clavulanate	22	0.5/2–4/2	2/2	4/2	≤16/2	100	3
Cefamandole	22	≤0.06	≤0.06	≤0.06	≤8	100	3
Cefamandole	86	1–8	1	1	≤8	100	26
Cefoperazone	22	≤0.06–0.12	≤0.06	≤0.06	≤16	100	3
Cefoperazone-sulbactam	22	≤0.25/0.03–0.12/0.06	≤0.06/0.03	≤0.06/0.03	≤16	100	3
Cefotaxime	29	≤0.063	≤0.063	≤0.063	≤8	100	20
Cefotaxime	22	≤0.06–1	≤0.06	≤0.06	≤8	100	3
Cefotaxime	10	NS	0.01	0.01	≤8	100	19
Cefotaxime	86	2	2	2	≤8	100	26
Cefoxitin	22	0.25–4	0.5	0.5	≤8	100	3
Cefoxitin	86	1–2	1	1	≤8	100	26
Ceftazidime	22	≤0.06–8	≤0.06	0.25	≤8	100	3
Ceftriaxone	22	≤0.06–0.5	≤0.06	≤0.06	≤8	100	3
Cephalothin	22	1–8	2	2	≤8	100	3
Cephalothin	86	1–≥64	8	≥16	≤8	—	26
Aztreonam	22	≤0.06	≤0.06	≤0.06	≤8	100	3
Aztreonam	10	NS	0.012	0.012	≤8	100	19
Imipenem	22	0.12–0.5	0.25	0.25	≤4	100	3
Imipenem	10	NS	0.156	0.156	≤4	100	19
Chloramphenicol	29	0.5–1	1	1	≤8	100	20
Chloramphenicol	86	0.5–≥32	1	≥32	≤8	—	26
Ciprofloxacin	29	≤0.063	≤0.063	≤0.063	≤1	100	20
Ciprofloxacin	22	≤0.06	≤0.06	≤0.06	≤1	100	3
Ciprofloxacin	10	NS	0.0001	0.0001	≤1	100	19
Enoxacin	29	≤0.063–0.25	≤0.063	0.125	≤2	100	20
Norfloxacin	29	≤0.063	≤0.063	≤0.063	—	—	20
Norfloxacin	10	NS	0.01	0.01	—	—	19
Nalidixic acid	29	1–4	2	2	—	—	20
Trimethoprim-sulfamethoxazole[c]	29	≤0.063–0.13	≤0.063	0.13	≤2/38	100	20
Sulfamethoxazole	29	2.4–38	19	38	—	—	20
Trimethoprim	29	≤0.063–1	0.25	0.25	—	—	20
Tetracycline	29	0.5–1	1	1	≤4	100	20
Tetracycline	86	0.25–≥16	0.5	≥16	≤4	—	26
Doxycycline	10	NS	0.31	0.31	≤4	100	19
Clindamycin	10	NS	12.5	12.5	≤0.5	0	19
Polymyxin B[d]	29	8–>256	>256	>256	—	—	20
Colistin	29	1–>128	128	>128	—	—	20

Modified from references 3, 19, 20, 26.

[a] Current NCCLS interpretive standards for susceptibility (μg/mL) (14).

[b] NS, not stated.

[c] Trimethoprim-sulfamethoxazole tested in a ratio of 1:19. Concentration refers to the trimethoprim component.

[d] MIC in Units/mL.

data to the contrary, we assume resistance to glycopeptides and metronidazole.

REFERENCES

1. Banks AS. A puncture wound complicated by infection with *Edwardsiella tarda.* J Am Podiatr Med Assoc 1992;82:529–531.
2. Bockemühl J, Pan-Urai R, Burkhardt F. *Edwardsiella tarda* associated with human disease. Pathol Microbiol 1971;37: 393–401.
3. Clark RB, Lister PD, Janda JM. In vitro susceptibilities of *Edwardsiella tarda* to 22 antibiotics and antibiotic-β-lactamase-inhibitor agents. Diagn Microbiol Infect Dis 1991;14:173–175.
4. Clarridge JE, Musher DM, Fainstein V, Wallace RJ Jr. Extraintestinal human infection caused by *Edwardsiella tarda.* J Clin Microbiol 1980;11:511–514.
5. Coutlée F, Saint-Jean LA, Plante R. Infection with *Edwardsiella tarda* related to a vascular prosthesis [Letter]. Clin Infect Dis 1992;14:621–622.
6. Desenclos J-CA, Conti L, Junejo S, Klontz KC. A cluster of *Edwardsiella tarda* infection in a day-care center in Florida [Letter]. J Infect Dis 1990;162:782–783.
7. Hargreaves JE, Lucey DR. Life-threatening *Edwardsiella tarda* soft-tissue infection associated with catfish puncture wound [Letter]. J Infect Dis 1990;162:1416–1417.
8. Janda JM, Abbott SL. Infections associated with the genus *Edwardsiella:* the role of *Edwardsiella tarda* in human disease. Clin Infect Dis 1993;17:742–748.
9. Jordon GW, Hadley WK. Human infection with *Edwardsiella tarda.* Ann Intern Med 1969;70:283–288.
10. Kourany M, Vasquez MA, Saenz R. Edwardsiellosis in man and animals in Panamá: clinical and epidemiological characteristics. Am J Trop Med Hyg 1977;26:1183–1190.
11. Le Frock JL, Klainer AS, Zuckerman K. *Edwardsiella tarda* bacteremia. South Med J 1976;69:188–190.
12. Marsh PK, Gorbach SL. Invasive enterocolitis caused by *Edwardsiella tarda.* Gastroenterology 1982;82:336–338.
13. Nagel P, Serritella A, Layden TJ. *Edwardsiella tarda* gastroenteritis associated with a pet turtle. Gastroenterology 1982;82: 1436–1437.
14. National Committee for Clinical Laboratory Standards. Methods for dilution antimicrobial susceptibility tests for bacteria that grow aerobically. 4th ed. Approved standard. NCCLS document M7-A4, Wayne, PA: NCCLS, 1997.
15. Okubadejo OA, Alausa KO. Neonatal meningitis caused by *Edwardsiella tarda.* Br Med J 1968;3:357–358.
16. Pien FD, Jackson MT. Tuboovarian abscess caused by *Edwardsiella tarda.* Am J Obstet Gynecol 1995;173:964–965.
17. Pitlik S, Berger SA, Huminer D. Nonenteric infections acquired through contact with water. Rev Infect Dis 1987;9:54–63.
18. Rao KRP, Shah J, Rajashekaraiah KR, Patel AR, Miskew DB, Fennewald PS. *Edwardsiella tarda* osteomyelitis in a patient with SC hemoglobinopathy. South Med J 1981;74: 288–292.
19. Reger PJ, Mockler DF, Miller MA. Comparison of antimicrobial susceptibility, β-lactamase production, plasmid analysis and serum bactericidal activity in *Edwardsiella tarda, E. ictaluri* and *E. hoshinae.* J Med Microbiol 1993;39:273–281.
20. Reinhardt JF, Fowlston S, Jones J, George WL. Comparative in vitro activities of selected antimicrobial agents against *Edwardsiella tarda.* Antimicrob Agents Chemother 1985;27:966–967.
21. Sachs JM, Pacin M, Counts GW. Sickle hemoglobinopathy and *Edwardsiella tarda* meningitis. Am J Dis Child 1974;128: 387–388.
22. Sechter I, Shmilovitz M, Altmann G, Seligmann R, Kretzer B, Braunstein I, Gerichter CB. *Edwardsiella tarda* isolated in Israel between 1961 and 1980. J Clin Microbiol 1983;17:669–671.
23. Sonnenwirth AC, Kallus BA. Meningitis due to *Edwardsiella tarda:* first report of meningitis caused by *E. tarda.* Am J Clin Pathol 1968;49:92–95.
24. Vandepitte J, Lemmens P, De Smert L. Human edwardsiellosis traced to ornamental fish. J Clin Microbiol 1983;17:165–167.
25. Vartian CV, Septimus EJ. Soft-tissue infection caused by *Edwardsiella tarda* and *Aeromonas hydrophilia* [Letter]. J Infect Dis 1990;161:816.
26. Waltman WD, Shotts EB. Antimicrobial susceptibility of *Edwardsiella tarda* from the United States and Taiwan. Vet Microbiol 1986;12:277–282.
27. Walton DT, Abbott SL, Janda JM. Sucrose-positive *Edwardsiella tarda* mimicking a biogroup 1 strain isolated from a patient with cholelithiasis. J Clin Microbiol 1993;31:155–156.
28. Wilson JP, Waterer RR, Wofford JD, Chapman SW. Serious infections with *Edwardsiella tarda.* Arch Intern Med 1989;149: 208–210.
29. Wu M-S, Shyu R-S, Lai M-Y, Huang G-T, Chen D-S, Wang T-H. A predisposition toward *Edwardsiella tarda* bacteremia in individuals with preexisting liver disease [Letter]. Clin Infect Dis 1995;21:705–706.
30. Zighelboim J, Williams TW Jr, Bradshaw MW, Harris RL. Successful medical management of a patient with multiple hepatic abscesses due to *Edwardsiella tarda.* Clin Infect Dis 1992;14: 117–120.

Eikenella corrodens

●

Casey Chen, Michael L. Towns, and Ellie J. C. Goldstein

GENERAL DESCRIPTION

Eikenella corrodens is a facultative, capnophilic, Gram-negative rod that often exhibits a "corroding" colony morphology on agar surface but may yield noncorroding colonies. Due to changes in taxonomy, there may be confusion when reading the literature about *E. corrodens*. Eiken provided a detailed study of "corroding bacilli" and proposed a species name "*Bacteroides corrodens*" to accommodate these organisms (9) but unknowingly included genetically distinct facultative and obligate anaerobes. The facultative anaerobes were later transferred to a new species, *Eikenella corrodens* (25). The obligate anaerobes were renamed *Bacteroides ureolyticus* (24), which is of uncertain taxonomic status and may actually be a *Campylobacter*. Currently only one species is recognized within the genus *Eikenella*. However, an *Eikenella*-like oral strain was identified as a distinct species within the genus according to 16S rRNA sequence data analysis (8). Other organisms that can "corrode" the agar and can be confused with *E. corrodens* include *Kingella kingae, Kingella oralis,* and *Campylobacter rectus*.

E. corrodens is part of the normal oral microbiota (5, 23) and is frequently found in supra- and subgingival dental plaque, on the surface of the tongue, tonsils, buccal mucosa, and in saliva (6). Individuals commonly harbor multiple genetically distinct oral *E. corrodens,* but the significance of this clonal diversity is not known (3, 4). The organism has been increasingly recognized in recent years as a human pathogen (Table 1) (5). Predisposing factors for infections due to *E. corrodens* may include malignancy, diabetes, trauma, gastric ulcers, dental abscess, congenital heart disease, alcoholism, intravenous drug abuse, and coinfection with streptococci. The most common *E. corrodens* infections occur in the head, neck, and extremities. These infections are most likely caused by a direct inoculation of oral *E. corrodens* to the infection sites or from spreading of infections from the oral cavity through tissue spaces to other anatomic sites. For example, direct inoculation may explain the common occurrence of *E. corrodens* infections in clenched-fist injuries or in skin infections of intravenous drug abusers who practiced skin popping (injecting the drug under the skin rather than into a vein) and often put their mouth to the injection sites. *E. corrodens* infections involving gastrointestinal and genital tracts have also been reported. Oral sex was identified as a predisposing factor in a few cases of infections involving the genital tract, also suggesting direct inoculation of the organism into infection sites. Dental manipulation often causes transient bacteremia that could provide a hematogenous route for *E. corrodens* to cause infections in distant body sites. *E. corrodens* infections of the heart valves, eye, and brain are relatively rare. However, a high mortality rate is reported in brain abscess involving this organism.

E. corrodens is a slow-growing organism and may be easily overgrown by other organisms on primary cultures. It may take 7 to 10 days to become evident on agar. In the era of cost containment and automated systems, many laboratories discard their blood cultures in 5 days and may therefore fail to identify this organism. For this reason, it seems possible that *E. corrodens* may be the cause of certain cases of culture-negative bacteremia and endocarditis. The organism should be considered a potential pathogen in any orally contaminated infection or when antimicrobial therapy fails with agents to which *E. corrodens* is resistant. Effective medical management of patients who have infections with *E. corrodens* requires knowledge of the antimicrobial susceptibility profile of this organism. The following discussion represents a sound basis for medical management of infections caused by *E. corrodens* based on the antimicrobial susceptibility profile and case studies from the literature.

SUSCEPTIBILITY IN VITRO

E. corrodens has a unique antibiotic susceptibility profile. Table 2 displays the antimicrobial susceptibility profile of *E. corrodens* from various studies (2, 13, 15, 17–20, 22). It is usually susceptible to β-lactam antibiotics such as penicillin, amoxicillin, and ampicillin but is resistant to penicillinase-resistant penicillin (dicloxacillin, methicillin, nafcillin) and displays variable susceptibilities to cephalosporins.

E. corrodens is usually resistant to first-generation cephalosporins (e.g., cephalexin, cefazolin) but susceptible to second- and third-generation agents (e.g., cefoxitin, cefuroxime). The organism is susceptible to quinolones as well as tetracyclines, trimethoprim-sulfamethoxazole, chloramphenicol, and rifampin. *E. corrodens* is resistant to lincosamides (clindamycin and lincomycin) and nitroimidazole (metronidazole) and is moderately resistant to aminoglycosides (streptomycin and gentamicin). In vitro activity of macrolides against *E. corrodens* has been reported as variable; the organism is usually resistant to erythromycin, roxithromycin, and clarithromycin but susceptible to azithromycin. The new ketolides (RMH-3004 and RU-66647) show good activity against *E. corrodens*.

Penicillin-resistant strains of *E. corrodens* have been isolated from human clinical specimens (41, 42). The mechanisms of resistance were either through plasmid-mediated β-lactamase similar to those found in *Neisseria* species (37) or due to a non-plasmid-mediated 2a (Bush type) β-lactamase (29). Lacroix and Walker (30) further noted that a periodontal strain (EC-38) not only produced β-lactamase but had a partial Tn 3 transposon that encoded for streptomycin resistance.

TABLE 1 • Infections Due to *E. corrodens*

Central nervous system
  Brain abscess, meningitis, subdural empyema

Head and neck
  Eye, ear, and nose: dacryocystitis, lacrimal abscess, conjunctivitis, orbital cellulitis, keratitis, otitis, nasal abscess
  Oral cavity: alveolar abscess, submandibular gland abscess, parotitis, peritonsillar abscess
  Upper and lower jaws, sinuses: chronic diffusing sclerosing osteomyelitis of the mandible, maxillary osteitis, maxillary sinusitis,
    frontal sinusitis, cervicofacial actinomycosis
  Others: thyroiditis, thyroid abscess, branchial arch cyst infections, mastoid osteitis, facial abscess, forehead cellulitis, facial wounds

Chest
  Pneumonia, empyema, pulmonary abscess, chest wall wounds, mediastinitis

Abdominal cavity
  Subdiaphragmatic abscess, pancreatic abscess, spleen abscess, abdominal abscess, appendicitis, sacral abscess, esophagus
    empyema, pelvic abscess, peritoneal abscess, liver abscess, abdominal wounds

Cardiovascular system
  Bacteremia/septicemia, endocarditis, vascular prosthesis infections

Extremities
  Bite wounds, paronychia, skin abscess, foot amputation stump, ankle arthritis, osteomyelitis

Genitourinary and reproductive systems
  Cervicitis, Bartholin's abscess, perirectal abscess, inguinal abscess, chorioamnionitis

E. corrodens strains carrying a plasmid that confers resistance to tetracycline have been reported (28). It is difficult to be certain whether the susceptibility profile of *E. corrodens* has changed significantly over the past 10 to 15 years. Since the susceptibility testing methodology for this organism is not as straightforward as that for many other organisms, it is also difficult to compare results from individual case reports. However, the prevalence of penicillin-resistant stains has been reported to be 10.5% for penicillin and 9.2% for ampicillin among 107 recent clinical isolates (1). Resistance was presumed to be due to β-lactamase, since the resistant strains were susceptible to amoxicillin/clavulanate. This finding suggests that penicillin-resistant strains are not unusual. The possible emergence of penicillin-resistant *E. corrodens* strains will affect the choice of antimicrobial therapy against this organism, particularly in serious cases such as endocarditis.

ANTIMICROBIAL THERAPY
General

Although the clinical course of *E. corrodens* infections varies widely and depends on the site of infection, two general features are noted. First, *E. corrodens* infection is often indolent. Patients may complain of a mild discomfort lasting for several days or weeks prior to seeking medical treatment. A prompt microbial diagnosis is occasionally difficult because *E. corrodens* may not grow well in all types of blood culture media. Difficulty in culture identification of *E. corrodens* may preclude timely and effective therapy and further prolong the illness.

Second, an infection involving *E. corrodens* is commonly polymicrobial. Coinfections of *E. corrodens* with α-hemolytic streptococci and group C β-hemolytic streptococci are well recognized (2). *E. corrodens* and *Actinomyces* have been identified as common coinfecting organisms in chronic diffuse sclerosing osteomyelitis of the mandible (33). A strong association between subgingival *E. corrodens* and *Actinobacillus actinomycetemcomitans* in juvenile periodontitis has also been suggested. Experiments in animal models indicated a synergism in causing infections between streptococci and *E. corrodens* (2) and between *Actinomyces* and *E. corrodens* (26). Other reported coinfecting organisms include *Staphylococcus aureus*, *Bacteroides*, *Enterococcus*, *Fusobacterium*, *Haemophilus*, *Pseudomonas aeruginosa*, *Klebsiella*, *Enterobacter*, *Eubacterium*, *Peptostreptococcus*, *Escherichia coli*, and *Candida*. Many of these coinfecting organisms are part of the normal microbiota of the infection sites.

Drug of Choice

Single antibiotic therapy is effective against *E. corrodens* if the organism is the sole pathogen involved (11, 12, 14, 16). For oral outpatient therapy, penicillin (250–500 mg orally q.i.d.), amoxicillin (500 mg orally t.i.d. with food), and amoxicillin/clavulanic acid (375–875 orally b.i.d. with food) should be considered the first choice against infections due to *E. corrodens*. Several cephalosporins such as cefotaxime and cefoxitin are also effective. Tetracycline, quinolones (both contraindicated in children and pregnant women) and sulfa-trimethoprim should be considered for patients with an allergic reaction to penicillin.

There is no clear evidence to suggest that combination therapy with different antibiotics has enhanced clinical efficacy over monotherapy. Some patients with infective endocarditis have received combination therapy with a β-lactam antibiotic and an aminoglycoside. However, *E. corrodens* is frequently resistant to aminoglycosides, casting some doubt on whether combination therapy is necessary in the absence of studies of synergistic interaction between these antibiotics. These organisms are notoriously resistant to both clindamycin and metronidazole, two agents that frequently are given as empirical therapy for presumed mixed aerobic/anaerobic infections.

Specific Infections
Bite Wounds

Human bite wounds, especially clenched-fist injuries, are one of the more common infections due to *E. corrodens*. Bite

TABLE 2 • Comparative Activity of Antimicrobial Agents against *E. corrodens*

Antibiotics	MIC$_{50}$ (mg/mL)	MIC$_{90}$ (mg/mL)	Range (mg/mL)	Antibiotics	MIC$_{50}$ (mg/mL)	MIC$_{90}$ (mg/mL)	Range (mg/mL)
β-Lactams				Sparfloxacin	0.015	0.03	0.008–0.03
Imipenem	0.12	0.25	0.12–0.25	Ofloxacin	0.03	0.03	0.015–0.125
Moxalactam	0.03	0.25	0.3–1	Amifloxacin	0.003	0.06	0.15–1
Cefotaxime	0.06	0.5	0.016–1	Norfloxacin	0.03	0.06	0.15–0.5
Amoxicillin/	0.5	0.5	0.125–0.5	Difloxacin	0.06	0.125	0.008–0.5
clavulanic acid				Enoxacin	0.06	0.125	0.03–2
Cefoxitin	0.5	0.5	0.25–1	Trovafloxacin	0.06	0.06	0.008–0.25
Ampicillin	0.5	1	0.5–4	Nalidixic acid	1	2	0.25–16
Mezlocillin	0.12	1	0.06–32	Cinoxacin	2	2	0.5–16
Ceftriaxone	0.25	1	0.016–2	Tetracyclines			
Ticarcillin	1	2	0.25–4	Tetracycline	0.5	2.0	0.5–2.0
Penicillin G	1.25	2.5	0.6–5	Doxycycline	1	2	0.25–4
Loracarbef	4	4	0.015–8	Macrolides			
Cefoperazone	0.5	4	0.25–32	Erythromycin	2	4	0.06–4
Bacampicillin	2	4	2–8	Azithromycin	1	2	0.06–4
Piperacillin	0.25	4	0.06–32	Roxithromycin	32	32	4–>32
Cefprozil	8	8	0.06–8	Clarithromycin	2	4	0.125–4
Cephaloridine	16	16	8–32	Ketolides			
Cephapirin	8	16	8–16	HMR-3004	0.25	0.5	0.03–1.0
Cefazolin	8	16	4–32	HMR-3647	0.5	1	0.03–1.0
Cephalothin	16	32	8–32	Lincosamides			
Cefaclor	8	32	4–32	Clindamycin	32	64	16–>128
Cefamandole	16	64	8–64	Lincomycin	>100	>100	>100
Cephradine	64	64	32–128	Glycopeptides			
Cefadroxil	>64	>64	0.25–>64	Vancomycin	32	64	4–64
Methicillin	>16	>16	8–>16	Aminoglycosides			
Cephalexin	>64	>64	0.125–>64	Streptomycin	8	16	8–>16
Dicloxacillin	>128	>128	64–>128	Gentamicin	4	4	4–8
Quinolones				Nitroimidazoles			
DU-6859a	0.002	0.004	0.001–0.008	Metronidazole	>100	>100	>100
Moxifloxacin	0.016	0.06	0.008–0.125	Trimethoprim-	0.125	0.25	0.06–0.5
Ciprofloxacin	0.015	0.015	0.008–0.06	sulfamethoxazole			
Levofloxacin	0.015	0.015	0.015–0.03	Chloramphenicol	2	4	1–>16
Ofloxacin	0.015	0.03	0.008–0.125	Rifampin	2	4	1–8
				Synercid	90	16	0.06–16

Data based on various published reports.

wounds to the hand are particularly troublesome as they are often insidious and may result in loss of function and permanent limitation of the range of motion of a "knuckle," osteomyelitis, septic arthritis, and other serious complications. This is partly due to the failure of clinicians to identify *E. corrodens* from the infection sites. One study of 21 patients with hand infections due to *E. corrodens* noted that "patients given empirical therapy ineffective against *E. corrodens* had a high incidence of complications, while proper therapy was associated with good recovery" (12). Sound principles of management of bite wounds should be followed carefully (11). Aerobic and anaerobic cultures are recommended for moderate-to-severe bite wounds. Antimicrobial therapy should be given for moderate or severe bite wounds (especially when bones, a joint, or a prosthetic joint may be involved), bite wounds to the hand, cat bites, and deep puncture wounds. Antibiotic therapy is also recommended in patients with serious predisposing diseases. Infected wounds require longer courses of antibiotics consistent with the type of infection. Clinical follow-up within 24 hours after the initial visit is essential. Patients who experience increased pain, swelling, or cellulitis or possible extension into a joint or bone should be considered for hospitalization.

The clinician should empirically select antimicrobial agents against the most likely offending organisms based on the literature (11) and modify the antimicrobial regimen based on microbial culture and susceptibility data when they become available. Empirical therapy should provide broad coverage against these organisms. Amoxicillin/clavulanic (Augmentin; 875 mg orally b.i.d. with food, or 375 mg b.i.d. if the patient weighs less than 120 pounds) or ampicillin/sulbactam (Unasyn; 1.5–3.0 g intravenously q. 6 h) provide excellent coverage in these cases. In the penicillin-allergic patient, tetracycline (250–500 mg orally q.i.d.) or doxycycline (100 mg orally b.i.d.) provides adequate coverage for adult patients awaiting culture results. Also, quinolones should be considered as the sole antibiotic or as part of combination therapy for adult patients with an allergic reaction to penicillin. The duration of therapy should be 10 to 14 days in uncomplicated cases. More severe infections such as septic arthritis or osteomyelitis require longer courses of therapy. Antimicrobial therapy is not the definitive treatment in the management of these infections. Surgical evaluation and debridement are important aspects of therapy to prevent or treat possible serious deep space infections such as septic arthritis or osteomyelitis. The reader is referred to a review paper on bite wound management for further discussion on this topic (11).

Endocarditis

E. corrodens is member of the HACEK group (*Haemophilus* species, *A. actinomycetemcomitans, Cardiobacterium hominis, E. corrodens,* and *Kingella* species) of organisms that may cause infective endocarditis of either undamaged or prosthetic valves in otherwise healthy individuals, in subjects with predisposing factors such as intravenous drug abusers, or subjects with poor dentition following dental procedures (35).

Since there have been fewer than 20 cases of endocarditis caused by *E. corrodens* reported in the literature, it is difficult to make any firm recommendations on therapy, but some generalizations can be made. Based on the literature, high doses of penicillin (18–24 million units/day) or ampicillin (12 g/day) should be given in combination with an aminoglycoside at doses to achieve peak serum levels of 5 to 10 μg/mL while awaiting susceptibility results. If the organism is shown to be susceptible to both antibiotics, then combination therapy could be continued for at least 2 weeks, followed by an additional 2 to 4 weeks with the β-lactam alone. If the organism is found to be resistant to the aminoglycoside, then treatment should be continued with the β-lactam antibiotic alone for the duration of therapy. *E. corrodens* usually displays moderate resistance to aminoglycosides. Although endocarditis caused by *E. corrodens* has been successfully treated with combination therapy consisting of a β-lactam antibiotic and an aminoglycoside, additional benefit from the use of aminoglycoside has not been demonstrated clearly.

Alternatively, a third-generation cephalosporin, such as ceftriaxone, could be used with or without aminoglycoside for a similar duration. This is probably the best regimen for a patient with a history of type II penicillin allergy (not anaphylactic type) as well as for patients in whom outpatient treatment is being considered. The few patients with prosthetic valve endocarditis due to this organism were cured with medical treatment alone without valve replacement (34).

ENDPOINTS FOR MONITORING THERAPY

There are no data to suggest that any radiographic or laboratory studies are beneficial in monitoring a patient's response to therapy. Evaluation of treatment is based solely on the clinical response to the predetermined course of therapy. There have been rare reports of relapse in endocarditis requiring a second course of therapy (38). The patient must be monitored closely both on and off therapy.

CAVEATS AND COMMENTS

E. corrodens may be suspected in prolonged infections with a history that suggests the oral flora as the source of infection and with a poor response to common antibiotic regimens against anaerobic infections such as clindamycin, metronidazole, or penicillinase-resistant penicillin. However, because infections by *E. corrodens* may occur in any body site and do not exhibit pathognomonic signs or symptoms, microbial diagnosis is essential for definitive diagnosis and effective therapy.

We noted general agreement between the in vitro susceptibility profile of *E. corrodens* and the in vivo efficacy of antimicrobial agents against infections caused by this organism. Our personal experience is supported by various reports that documented the failure of first-generation cephalosporins (cephalexin, cefazolin, cephalothin), penicillinase-resistant penicillins (e.g., dicloxacillin, methicillin), erythromycin, and clindamycin in the treatment of *E. corrodens* infections (7, 10, 12, 21, 31, 40). The clinical efficacy of aminoglycosides in treating infections by *E. corrodens* is not clear, although case reports showed some success in treating endocarditis with a combination therapy involving aminoglycosides and penicillins. The use of antimicrobial agents without microbial analysis may be problematic if *E. corrodens* is the unknown organism of the infection. The occurrence of antibiotic-resistant strains of *E. corrodens* may be more common than previously recognized. Routine antibiotic susceptibility testing of *E. corrodens,* once cultivated, is recommended.

REFERENCES

1. Alcala L, Garcia-Garrote F, Gijon P, Pelaez T, Munoz P, Bouza E. *Eikenella corrodens* antimicrobial susceptibility in recent years [Abstract no. 121]. Intersci Conf Antimicrob Agents Chemother 1995.
2. Brooks GF, O'Donoghue JM, Rissing JP, Soapes K, Smith JW. *Eikenella corrodens,* a recently recognized pathogen: infections in medical-surgical patients and in association with methylphenidate abuse. Medicine 1974;53:325–342.
3. Chen C, Ashimoto A. Clonal diversity of oral *Eikenella corrodens* within individual subjects by arbitrarily primed PCR. J Clin Microbiol 1996;34:1837–1839.
4. Chen C, Sunday GJ, Zambon JJ, Wilson ME. Restriction endonuclease analysis of oral and nonoral isolates of *Eikenella corrodens.* J Clin Microbiol 1990;28:1265–1270.
5. Chen C, Wilson ME. *Eikenella corrodens* in human oral and non-oral infections: a review. J Periodontol 1992;63:941–953.
6. Chen CK, Dunford RG, Reynolds HS, Zambon JJ. *Eikenella corrodens* in the human oral cavity. J Periodontol 1989;60: 611–616.
7. Cohen JD, Maile TD. Tobramycin and cephalothin for the treatment of suspected sepsis in neutropenic patients with cancer. J Infect Dis 1977;134:S175–S176.
8. Dewhirst FE, Chen CK, Paster BJ, Zambon JJ. Phylogeny of species in the family *Neisseriaceae* isolated from human dental plaque and description of *Kingella oralis* sp. nov [corrected] [published erratum appears in Int J Syst Bacteriol 1994;44:376]. Int J Syst Bacteriol 1993;43:490–499.
9. Eiken M. Studies on an anaerobic, rod-shape Gram-negative microorganism: *Bacteroides corrodens* n. sp. Acta Pathol Microbiol Scand 1958;43:404–416.
10. Geraci JE, Herman PE, Washington Jr JA. *Eikenella corrodens* endocarditis. Mayo Clin Proc 1974;49:950–953.
11. Goldstein EJC. Bite wounds and infection [see comments]. Clin Infect Dis 1992;14(3):633–638.
12. Goldstein EJC, Barones MF, Miller TA. *Eikenella corrodens* in hand infections. J Hand Surg (Am) 1983;8(5 Pt 1):563–567.
13. Goldstein EJC, Citron DM. Comparative susceptibilities of 173 aerobic and anaerobic bite wound isolates to sparfloxacin, temafloxacin, clarithromycin, and older agents. Antimicrob Agents Chemother 1993;37:1150–1153.
14. Goldstein EJC, Citron DM, Finegold SM. Dog bite wounds and

infection: a prospective clinical study. Ann Emerg Med 1980;9: 508–512.

15. Goldstein EJC, Nesbit CA, Citron DM. Comparative in vitro activities of azithromycin, Bay y 3118, levofloxacin, sparfloxacin, and 11 other oral antimicrobial agents against 194 aerobic and anaerobic bite wound isolates. Antimicrob Agents Chemother 1995;39:1097–1100.

16. Goldstein EJC, Richwald GA. Human and animal bite wounds. Am Fam Physician 1987;36:101–109.

17. Goldstein EJC, Citron DM, Gerardo SH, Hudspeth M, Merriam CV. Comparative in vitro activity of DU-6859a, levofloxacin, ofloxacin, sparfloxacin, and ciprofloxacin against 388 aerobic and anaerobic bite wound isolates. Antimicrob Agents Chemother 1997; in press.

18. Goldstein EJC, Citron DM, Hudspeth M, Gerardo SH, Merriam CV. In vitro activity of Bay 12-8039, a new 8-methoxy quinolone, compared to 11 other oral antimicrobial agents against 390 aerobic and anaerobic human and animal bite wound isolates. Antimicrob Agents Chemother 1997; in press.

19. Goldstein EJC, Citron DM, Vagvolgyi AE, Gombert ME. Susceptibility of *Eikenella corrodens* to newer and older quinolones. Antimicrob Agents Chemother 1986;30:172–173.

20. Goldstein EJC, Gombert ME, Agyare EO. Susceptibility of *Eikenella corrodens* to newer beta-lactam antibiotics. Antimicrob Agents Chemother 1980;18:832–833.

21. Goldstein EJC, Kirby BD, Finegold SM. Isolation of *Eikenella corrodens* from pulmonary infections. Am Rev Resp Dis 1979; 119:55–58.

22. Goldstein EJC, Sutter VL, Finegold SM. Susceptibility of *Eikenella corrodens* to ten cephalosporins. Antimicrob Agents Chemother 1978;14:639–641.

23. Goldstein EJC, Tarenzi LA, Agyare EO, Berger JR. Prevalence of *Eikenella corrodens* in dental plaque. J Clin Microbiol 1983;17:636–639.

24. Jackson FL, Goodman YE. *Bacteroides ureolyticus,* a new species to accommodate strains previously identified as "*Bacteroides corrodens,* anaerobic." Int J Syst Bacteriol 1978;28:197–200.

25. Jackson FL, Goodman YE. Transfer of facultatively anaerobic organism *Bacteroides corrodens* Eiken to a new genus, *Eikenella.* Int J Syst Bacteriol 1972;22:73–77.

26. Jordan HV, Kelly DM. Persistence of associated gram-negative bacteria in experimental actinomycotic lesions in mice. Infect Immun 1983;40:847–849.

27. Joshi N, Obryan T, Appelbaum PC. Pleuropulmonary infections caused by *Eikenella corrodens* [see comments]. Rev Infect Dis 1991;13:1207–1212.

28. Knapp JS, Johnson SR, Zenilman JM, Roberts MC, Morse SA. High-level tetracycline resistance resulting from TetM in strains of *Neisseria* spp., *Kingella denitrificans,* and *Eikenella corrodens.* Antimicrob Agents Chemother 1988;32: 765–767.

29. Lacroix JM, Walker C. Characterization of a beta-lactamase found in *Eikenella corrodens.* Antimicrob Agents Chemother 1991;35:886–891.

30. Lacroix JM, Walker CB. Identification of a streptomycin resistance gene and a partial Tn3 transposon coding for a beta-lactamase in a periodontal strain of *Eikenella corrodens.* Antimicrob Agents Chemother 1992;36:740–743.

31. Lutwick LI. Pancreatic abscess with *Haemophilus influenzae* and *Eikenella corrodens.* JAMA 1976;236:2091–2092.

32. Mandell RL, Ebersole JL, Socransky SS. Clinical immunologic and microbiologic features of active disease sites in juvenile periodontitis. J Clin Periodontol 1987;14:534–540.

33. Marx RE, Carlson ER, Smith BR, Toraya N. Isolation of *Actinomyces* species and *Eikenella corrodens* from patients with chronic diffuse sclerosing osteomyelitis. J Oral Maxillofac Surg 1994;52:26–33 discussion 33–34.

34. Meyer DJ, Gerding DN. Favorable prognosis of patients with prosthetic valve endocarditis caused by gram-negative bacilli of the HACEK group. Am J Med 1988;85:104–107.

35. Patrick WD, Brown WD, Ian Bowmer AM, Sinave CP. Infective endocarditis due to *Eikenella corrodens:* case report and review of the literature. Can J Infect Dis 1990;1:139–142.

36. Perez-Pomata MT, Dominguez J, Horcajo P, Santidrian F, Bisquert J. Spleen abscess caused by *Eikenella corrodens.* Eur J Clin Microbiol Infect Dis 1992;11:162–163.

37. Rotger R, Garcia Valdes E, Trallero EP. Characterization of a beta-lactamase-specifying plasmid isolated from Eikenella corrodens and its relationship to a commensal Neisseria plasmid. Antimicrob Agents Chemother 1986;30:508–509.

38. Sobel JD, Carrizosa J, Ziobrowski TF, Gluckman SJ. Polymicrobial endocarditis involving *Eikenella corrodens.* Am J Med Sci 1981;282:41–44.

39. Stamboulian D. Outpatient treatment of endocarditis in a clinic-based program in Argentina. Eur J Clin Microbiol Infect Dis 1995;14:648–654.

40. Suwanagool S, Rothkopf MM, Smith SM, LeBlanc D, Eng R. Pathogenicity of *Eikenella corrodens* in humans. Arch Intern Med 1983;143:2265–2268.

41. Trallero EP, Arenzana JMC, Eguiluz GC, Larrucea JT. β-Lactamase-producing *Eikenella corrodens* in an intraabdominal abscess. J Infect Dis 1986;153:379.

42. Walker CB, Pappas JD, Tyler KZ, Cohen S, Gordon JM. Antibiotic susceptibilities of periodontal bacteria. In vitro susceptibilities to eight antimicrobial agents. J Periodontol 1985;56(11 Suppl):67–74.

Enterobacter Species

●

John P. Quinn

GENERAL DESCRIPTION
Microbiology and History

Enterobacter species are motile, aerobic, Gram-negative bacilli belonging to the family *Enterobacteriaceae*. The major species are *Enterobacter cloacae, E. aerogenes,* and *E. agglomerans*. They first achieved wide notoriety as pathogens in 1976 following a nationwide outbreak of septicemia in 378 patients at 25 hospitals, resulting from contaminated intravenous solutions (25). Because they can replicate in glucose-containing parenteral fluids, they continue to cause sporadic outbreaks of this type (33).

Epidemiology

Enterobacter infections are increasing in frequency, particularly in intensive care units (ICUs). Using data from the National Nosocomial Infection Surveillance (NNIS) survey from the Centers for Disease Control (CDC), collected between 1986 and 1989, Schaberg (31) reported that *Enterobacter* was the fifth leading cause of ICU infections in the United States and the third most common cause of nosocomial pneumonia overall.

In early studies of the epidemiology of *Enterobacter* infections, emphasis was placed on horizontal transmission in hospitals. A landmark study in 1987 by Flynn et al. (14) emphasized the importance of *Enterobacter* arising from a patient's endogenous gut flora causing subsequent infection. In this study of 87 patients undergoing cardiac surgery, all patients underwent surveillance cultures before and after surgery. Cefazolin prophylaxis was administered to all patients. Some 23% of patients were colonized on admission, and 49% of patients were colonized by 72 h after surgery. Of those colonized, 72% had increased numbers of organisms isolated following cefazolin prophylaxis. Of 12 nosocomial infections due to *Enterobacter* in this group of patients, 9 were due to strains detected colonizing the gut preoperatively.

In a more recent study using a consensus PCR technique for molecular typing of strains, Davin-Regli et al. (10) studied 185 clinical isolates of *E. aerogenes* collected from two ICUs over a 1-year period from a hospital in France. A ubiquitous clone was found responsible for two-thirds of epidemiologically related transmissions in these units.

SUSCEPTIBILITY IN VITRO

In a recent report of 33,869 Gram-negative isolates (16.1% *Enterobacter*) from 396 ICUs in the United States sampled between 1990 and 1993 in the Intensive Care Unit Surveillance Study, emerging resistance to extended-spectrum cephalosporins was a problem in both *Enterobacter* and *Klebsiella* (20).

Resistance in *Enterobacter* increased from 30.8% to 38.3% between 1990 and 1993. Teaching hospitals with 500 beds or more were significantly more likely to yield resistant isolates (Table 1).

A recent report from eight hospitals in the United States participating in the NNIS system under the auspices of the CDC analyzed resistance rates among *Enterobacter* isolates from outpatients and inpatients (3). A clear gradient of increasing ceftazidime resistance rates was noted. The prevalence of ceftazidime resistance was 12% among community isolates, versus 26% among nosocomial isolates. Within these hospitals, resistance rates were consistently higher among ICU isolates (36 vs. 26%).

Mechanisms of β-Lactam Resistance in *Enterobacter*

The saga of *Enterobacter* as a nosocomial pathogen is closely linked to the logarithmic increase in the use of extended-spectrum cephalosporins in the 1980s. A series of reports emphasized the proclivity of members of this genus to acquire broad β-lactam resistance during therapy with extended-spectrum cephalosporins (7, 29).

An illustrative paper is the work of Chow et al. (7) reporting 129 cases of *Enterobacter* bacteremia at six medical centers in the United States. The mean age of infected patients was 59 years. Almost all patients had concomitant illnesses predisposing to *Enterobacter* sepsis. For example, 42% of patients had undergone recent major surgery, and 40% were mechanically ventilated. When first isolated in the laboratory, 29% of the strains were resistant to all β-lactams other than carbapenems. As shown in Table 2, 36 of 37 resistant isolates came from patients exposed to prior antibiotic therapy. In two-thirds of those patients, prior therapy had included extended-spectrum cephalosporins. This difference was highly statistically significant compared with other agents.

As shown in Table 3, an additional six patients acquired broad β-lactam resistance during therapy with an extended-spectrum cephalosporin. Five of these six patients were receiving concomitant aminoglycoside therapy. This high incidence compared unfavorably with 0 of 50 patients receiving other β-lactams (e.g., imipenem or broad-spectrum penicillins). In this study, infections due to a multiresistant strain were associated with a mortality rate twice that associated with those due to susceptible strains (32 vs. 16%).

In each case of emergence of resistance during therapy, DNA typing techniques demonstrated strain identity. Posttherapy resistant isolates produced up to 5000 times more chromosomal β-lactamase activity than susceptible pretherapy isolates. This observation has been made in numerous other studies (29).

TABLE 1 • **Rates of Resistance to Ceftazidime in Selected Bacteria, As Determined by Surveillance of Intensive Care Units, 1990–1993[a]**

Variable	*Klebsiella pneumoniae*		*Enterobacter* Species		*Pseudomonas aeruginosa*	
	No. of Strains Tested	Percent Resistant	No. of Strains Tested	Percent Resistant	No. of Strains Tested	Percent Resistant
Overall resistance	4100	5.8	5381	32.0	6675	14.2
Site of recovery						
Urine	958	5.2	583	37.4[b]	996	9.3
Blood	417	6.5	394	35.7	370	12.7
Respiratory tract	1885	5.9	3102	31.0	3888	15.2[c]
Wounds	120	14.2[d]	220	35.5	262	15.6
Miscellaneous	720	4.4	1092	29.9	1159	15.3
Hospital status						
Teaching	2521	7.3[e]	3330	32.6	4235	15.5[e]
Nonteaching	1579	3.4	2051	30.9	2440	12.0
No. of beds						
<200	142	2.1	135	23.7	194	19.1
200–500	2173	3.8	2766	29.8	3398	12.3
>500	1785	8.6[f]	2480	34.9[f]	3083	16.1

From Itokazu GS, Quinn JP, Bell-Dixon C, Kahan FM, Weinstein RA. Antimicrobial resistance rates among aerobic gram-negative bacilli recovered from patients in intensive care units: evaluation of a national postmarketing surveillance program. Clin Infect Dis 1996;23:779–784. With permission.

[a]Data exclude outlier hospitals and were analyzed with use of the χ^2 test.

[b]$P < .01$ (urine vs. other sites).

[c]$P < .007$ (respiratory tract vs. other sites).

[d]$P < .001$ (wounds vs. other sites).

[e]$P < .001$ (teaching vs. nonteaching hospitals).

[f]$P < .0003$ (>500 beds vs. other hospital sizes).

Therapy with extended-spectrum cephalosporins often selects for mutants that hyperproduce type I chromosomal β-lactamase. These mutants occur spontaneously at frequencies of about 10^7. A comprehensive review of the molecular biology of this phenomenon is beyond the scope of this work; the interested reader is referred to the excellent review of Ehrhardt and Sanders (13).

Recent surveys indicate that the prevalence of resistance to extended-spectrum cephalosporins among *Enterobacter* isolates is slowly increasing over time. Jacobson et al. (21) demonstrated broad resistance to β-lactams in 31% of *Enterobacter cloacae* in their hospital and showed that prior therapy with an extended-spectrum cephalosporin was responsible for much of this resistance, not only in *Enterobacter,* but also among other type-1-β-lactamase-producing pathogens (e.g., *Pseudomonas aeruginosa, Serratia marcascens,* and *Citrobacter* species).

Plasmid-mediated extended-spectrum β-lactamases (ESBLs) are responsible for the explosive rise in the prevalence of extended-spectrum cephalosporin resistance in *Klebsiella* and *E. coli* (22). These enzymes have been detected in *Enterobacter* but are very uncommon (27).

ANTIMICROBIAL THERAPY
General Drug of Choice

β-Lactams
Extended-Spectrum Cephalosporins. All of the so-called third-generation cephalosporins and the monobactams (e.g., aztreonam) have approximately the same risk of emergence of resistance during therapy of *Enterobacter* infections. The data

on preventing this type of resistance by use of concomitant aminoglycoside therapy are mixed. Jacobson et al. (21) found a lower incidence of emergence of resistance to extended-spectrum cephalosporins among patients treated with concomitant aminoglycoside therapy, while Chow et al. did not (7).

A new group of broad cephalosporins, the so-called fourth-generation compounds, (e.g., cefepime and cefpirome) usually retain their activity against *Enterobacter* strains resistant to third-generation cephalosporins (32). The basis for this retained

TABLE 2 • **Association of Previously Administered Antibiotics with Multiresistant *Enterobacter* in the Initial Blood Culture**

Antibiotic[a]	Multiresistant *Enterobacter* Isolate *n/N* (%)	P Value
Any antibiotic		
Yes	36/103 (35)	
No	1/26 (4)	.002
Third-generation cephalosporin		
Yes	22/32 (69)	
No	14/71 (20)	.001

From Chow JW, Fine MJ, Shlaes DM, Quinn JP, Hooper DC, Johnson MP, Ramphal R. Wagener MM, Miyashiro DK, Yu VL. *Enterobacter* bacteremia: clinical features and emergence of antibiotic resistance during therapy. Ann Intern Med 1991;115:585–590. With permission.

[a]Antibiotics received in the 2 weeks before the initial positive blood culture.

TABLE 3 • Emergence of Resistance during Antibiotic Therapy for *Enterobacter* Bacteremia

Patient	Antibiotics Used	Emergence of Resistance to Drug	MIC[a] before Therapy (μg/mL)	MIC after Therapy (μg/mL)	Duration of Therapy When Resistance Was Seen (days)	Source of Second Positive Culture	*Enterobacter* spp.	Outcome
1	Cefotaxime	Cefotaxime	≤4	>32	16	Intraabdominal abscess	*E. cloacae*	Survived
2	Ceftazidime, tobramycin	Ceftazidime	≤2	>16	18	Blood	*E. cloacae*	Survived
3	Ceftazidime, gentamicin	Ceftazidime	≤2	>16	5	Blood	*E. cloacae*	Survived
4	Cefotaxime, amikacin	Cefotaxime	≤4	>32	6	Blood	*E. aerogenes*	Died
5	Ceftizoxime	Ceftizoxime	8	32	4	Blood	*E. cloacae*	Survived
6	Cefotaxime, gentamicin	Cefotaxime	8	32	7	Blood	*E. aerogenes*	Survived
7	Piperacillin, tobramycin	Tobramycin	≤0.25	8	8	Two central venous catheters	*E. cloacae*	Survived

From Chow JW, Fine MJ, Shlaes DM, Quinn JP, Hooper DC, Johnson MP, Ramphal R, Wagener MM, Miyashiro DK, Yu VL. *Enterobacter* bacteremia: clinical features and emergence of antibiotic resistance during therapy. Ann Intern Med 1991;115:585–590. With permission.

[a]MIC, minimal inhibitory concentration.

activity is (*a*) faster penetration through outer membrane porin proteins, (*b*) superior stability to chromosomal β-lactamases, and (*c*) enhanced binding to critical penicillin-binding proteins in *Enterobacter* compared with older cephalosporins (4, 5).

In a recent report, Sanders et al. (30) described successful therapy with cefepime of 17 infections due to *Enterobacter* strains resistant to third-generation cephalosporins. These patients had infections at a variety of sites. All patients responded clinically, and bacteriologic eradication was documented in 88%.

Cefpirome is structurally similar to cefepime and has roughly comparable activity against *Enterobacter* strains, including those displaying resistance to third-generation cephalosporins (23). Fewer data are available on the clinical efficacy of this agent against multiresistant Gram-negative pathogens.

Broad-Spectrum Penicillins. Piperacillin is slightly less active than extended-spectrum cephalosporins against *Enterobacter;* in the ISS study, 67% were susceptible to ceftazidime versus 63% to piperacillin. In the Chow study, no patient receiving piperacillin experienced treatment failure due to emergence of resistance. In contrast, Jacobson et al. reported a statistically significant association of prior piperacillin therapy with broad β-lactam resistance.

Carbapenems. Carbapenems display superb activity against a wide variety of enteric Gram-negative pathogens, including *Enterobacter* (28). Strains of *Enterobacter, Citrobacter,* and *Pseudomonas aeruginosa* that are resistant to extended-spectrum cephalosporins on the basis of hyperproduction of type I β-lactamase typically remain susceptible to carbapenems. Resistance to carbapenems in *Enterobacter* is rare (1% of NNIS isolates in 1992) (17), presumably because *Enterobacter* isolates require two separate mutations to acquire carbapenem resistance: loss of porin proteins plus hyperproduction of β-lactamase (24). Carbapenem resistance among

Enterobacter isolates does not appear to be increasing over time.

In the series of Chow et al., none of 17 patients receiving imipenem for *Enterobacter* bacteremia had resistant organisms emerge during therapy. The new carbapenem, meropenem, has activity comparable to that of imipenem against *Enterobacter* and ought to prove effective in the therapy of these infections (9, 12).

Aminoglycosides

In the survey of 5451 isolates of *Enterobacter* collected from 396 ICUs in the United States between 1950 and 1993, 98% were susceptible to amikacin and 93% were susceptible to gentamicin and tobramycin. These rates were stable over the time period. In the Chow study, only 1 of 89 patients receiving aminoglycoside therapy failed treatment because of emergence of resistance during therapy.

Trimethoprim-Sulfamethoxasole

A few series have examined the susceptibility of *Enterobacter* isolates to trimethoprim-sulfamethoxasole (TMP-SMX) (16, 34, 37) and reported susceptibility rates in excess of 90%. This agent is used infrequently in the treatment of *Enterobacter* infections.

A report of *Enterobacter* bacteremia among pediatric patients emphasized the importance of central venous catheters as a portal of entry (63% of cases) and the excellent activity of TMP-SMX (91% susceptible) (18). Use of TMP-SMX in the therapy of *Enterobacter* meningitis is discussed below under "Special Situations."

Quinolones

In the ISS survey of 5451 *Enterobacter* isolates from 396 American ICUs collected between 1990 and 1993, ciprofloxacin was effective against 96% of strains. The newer quinolones such as ofloxacin, levofloxacin, and sparfloxacin vary in their activity against *Enterobacter* (6, 19, 38); in one study, sparfloxacin was the most active quinolone tested against *Enterobacter* (6).

It is reasonable to anticipate that quinolone resistance rates will increase over time as these agents are increasingly used to treat serious *Enterobacter* infections. Davin-Regli et al. (11) raised a cautionary note in their report of an outbreak of *Enterobacter hormachei* infections among patients in a French hospital who had been treated with quinolones. Over a 1-year period, 21 resistant isolates were detected. All were shown to be clonally related using the random amplification of DNA technique.

Special Situations

Meningitis

Enterobacter is an uncommon cause of meningitis, with two exceptions: postneurosurgical meningitis and neonatal meningitis. A recent review of TMP-SMX therapy for *Enterobacter* meningitis yielded excellent results (37). In this retrospective study, 13 patients with *Enterobacter* meningitis complicating trauma or neurosurgical procedures were treated with TMP-SMX with or without other agents (extended-spectrum cephalosporins, aminoglycosides, chloramphenicol), and all were cured.

Enterobacter sakazakii (formerly yellow-pigmented *Enterobacter cloacae*) is a sporadic cause of neonatal meningitis (36). In a review of 15 cases published in 1988, risk factors for a fatal outcome included prematurity and low birth weight. Overall, about 50% of cases end in death, and all survivors have severe neurologic sequelae. About half of reported patients have cyst or abcess formation. The epidemiology of this organism is poorly understood. *E. sakazakii* has been isolated from infant formula, but molecular typing techniques have not confirmed that these strains are the source of disease (35).

Pneumonitis

Enterobacter species are the third most common cause of nosocomial Gram-negative bacillary respiratory infections; as with other aerobic Gram-negative rods, risk factors include severity of illness, mechanical ventilation, and prior antibiotic exposure (7). Distinguishing colonization from infection is extremely difficult unless the patient has the same strain of *Enterobacter* isolated from respiratory secretions and bloodstream or pleural fluid. No data exist to guide therapy for respiratory *Enterobacter* infections other than the general guidelines outlined above in the discussion of the bacteremia study.

Syndromes Associated with Unusual Species of *Enterobacter*

Although the vast majority of Enterobacter infections are due to *E. cloacae, E. aerogenes,* and *E. agglomerans,* occasionally other species occur in discrete syndromes. The specific association of *E. sakazakii* with neonatal meningitis is one example.

E. cancerogenus (formerly *E. taylorae*) is an uncommon species that is a sporadic cause of a variety of nosocomial infections (1). More recently, this organism has been reported to cause community-acquired infection complicating severe trauma or crush injuries (1). In this report, 5 cases were described among trauma victims. All isolates were obtained from soft tissue and/or blood samples on admission to the hospital, suggesting possible acquisition from soil. All isolates in this report were susceptible to extended-spectrum cephalosporins and quinolones.

COMMENTS

Enterobacter is an increasingly important nosocomial pathogen. The incidence of infections due to this organism is rising, and broad β-lactam resistance is an increasing problem. A number of agents offer promise for treatment of *Enterobacter* infections. Among the β-lactams, the so-called fourth-generation cephalosporins and carbapenems are attractive options. Aminoglycosides retain good activity but usually require combination with another agent. Quinolones are highly active. Trimethoprim-sulfamethoxasole is underused as therapy for *Enterobacter* infections and is especially promising in the treatment of meningitis.

REFERENCES

1. Abbott S, Janda JM. *Enterobacter cancerogenus* ("Enterobacter taylorae") infections associated with severe trauma or crush injuries. Microb Infect Dis 1997;359–361.
2. Andresen J, Asmar BI, Dajani AS. Increasing *Enterobacter* bacteremia in pediatric patients. Pediatr Infect Dis J 1994;13:787–792.
3. Archibald L, Phillips L, Monnet D, Mcgowan J, Tenover F, Gaynes R. Antimicrobial resistance in isolates from inpatients and outpatients in the United States: increasing importance of the intensive care unit. Clin Infect Dis 1997;27;211–215.
4. Bellido F, Pechere J, Hancock RE. Novel method for measurement of outer membrane permeability to new beta-lactams in intact *Enterobacter cloacae* cells. Antimicrobial Agents Chemother 1991;35:68–72.
5. Bellido F, Pechere J, Hancock RE. Reevaluation of the factors involved in the efficacy of new beta-lactams against *Enterobacter cloacae*. Antimicrob Agents Chemother 1991:35:73–78.
6. Canton E, Peman J, Jimenez MT, Ramon MS, Gobernado M. In vitro activity of sparfloxacin compared with those of five other quinolones. Antimicrob Agents Chemother 1992:558–565.
7. Chow JW, Fine MJ, Shlaes DM, Quinn JP, Hooper DC, Johnson MP, Ramphal R. Wagener MM, Miyashiro DK, Yu VL. *Enterobacter* bacteremia: clinical features and emergence of antibiotic resistance during therapy. Ann Intern Med 1991;115:585–590.
8. Chow JW, Yu VL, Shlaes DM. Epidemiologic perspectives on *Enterobacter* for the infection control professional. Am J Infect Control 1994;22:195–201.
9. Colardyn F, Faulkner K. Intravenous meropenem versus imipenem/cilastatin in the treatment of serious bacterial infections in hospitalized patients. J Antimicrob Chemother 1996;38: 523–537.
10. Davin-Regli A, Monnet D, Saux P, Bosi C, Charrel R, Barthelemy A, Bollett C. Molecular epidemiology of *Enterobacter aerogenes* acquisition: one-year prospective study in two intensive care units. J Clin Microbiol 1996;4:1474–1480.
11. Davin-Regli A, Bosi C, Charrel R, Ageron E, Papazian L, Grimont P, Cremieux A, Bollett C. A nosocomial outbreak due to *Enterobacter cloacae* strains with the *E. hormaechei* genotype in patients treated with fluoroquinolones. J Clin Microbiol 1997; 4:1008–1010.

12. Edwards JR. Meropenem: a microbiological overview. J Antimicrob Chemother 1995;36(Suppl A):1–17.
13. Ehrhardt AF, Sanders CC. Beta-lactam resistance amongst *Enterobacter* species. J Antimicrob Chemother 1993;32(Suppl B):1–11.
14. Flynn DM, Weinstein RA, Nathan C, Gaston MA, Kabins SA. Patients' endogenous flora as the source of "nosocomial" *Enterobacter* in cardiac surgery. J Infect Dis 1987;156:363–368.
15. Fung-Tomc J, Dougherty TJ, DeOrio FJ, Simich-Jacobson V, Kessler RE. Activity of cefepime against ceftazidime- and cefotaxime-resistant gram-negative bacteria and its relationship to beta-lactamase levels. Antimicrob Agents Chemother 1989;33:498–502.
16. Gallagher PG. *Enterobacter* bacteremia in pediatric patients. Rev Infect Dis 1990;12:808–812.
17. Gaynes P, Culver DH. Resistance to imipenem among selected gram-negative bacilli in the United States. Infect Control Hosp Epidemiol 1992;13:10–14.
18. Giamarellou H, Voutsinas D, Xirouchaki. Comparative in vitro activity of sparfloxacin against 275 multiresistant clinical isolates. J Chemother 1992;4:12–15.
19. Hoban DJ, Jones RN, Harrell LJ, Knudson M, Sewell D. The North American component (the United States and Canada) of an international comparative MIC trial monitoring resistance. Diagn Microbiol Infect Dis 1993;17:157–161.
20. Itokazu GS, Quinn JP, Bell-Dixon C, Kahan FM, Weinstein RA. Antimicrobial resistance rates among aerobic gram-negative bacilli recovered from patients in intensive care units: evaluation of a national postmarketing surveillance program. Clin Infect Dis 1996;23:779–784.
21. Jacobson KL, Cohen SH, Inciardi JF, King JH, Lippert WE, Iglesias T, VanCouwenberghe CJ. The relationship between antecedent antibiotic use and resistance to extended-spectrum cephalosporins in group I beta-lactamase-producing organisms. Clin Infect Dis 1995;21:1107–1113.
22. Jacoby FA, Medeiros AA. More extended-spectrum beta-lactamases. Antimicrob Agents Chemother 1991;35:1697–1704.
23. Jones RN, Pfaller MA, Allen SD, Gerlach EH, Fuchs PC, Aldridge KE. Antimicrobial activity of cefpirome: an update compared to five third-generation cephalosporins against nearly 6000 recent clinical isolates from five medical centers. Diagn Microbiol Infect Dis 1991;14:361–364.
24. Livermore DM. Mechanisms of resistance to beta-lactam antibiotics. Scand J Infect Dis 1991;78(Suppl):7.
25. Maki DG, Rhame FS, Mackel DC, Bennett JV. Nationwide epidemic of septicemia caused by contaminated intravenous products. Am J Med 1976;60:471–485.
26. Martinez-Beltran J, Canton R, Linares J, Garcia de Lomas J, Gimeno C, Tubau F, Baquero F. Multicentre comparative study on the antibacterial activity of FK-037, a new parental cephalosporin. Eur J Clin Microbiol Infect Dis 1995;14: 244–252.
27. Neuwirth C, Siebor E, Lopez J, Pechinot A, Kazmierczak A. Outbreak 0f TEM-24 producing *Enterobacter aerogenes* in an intensive care unit and dissemination of the extended-spectrum beta-lactamase to other members of the family *Enterobacteriaceae*. J Clin Microbiol 1996;1:76–79.
28. Norrby SR. Carbapenems. Med Clin North Am 1995;79(4): 745–759.
29. Sanders CC. Beta-lactamases of gram-negative bacteria: new challenges for new drugs. Clin Infect Dis 1992;14:1089–1099.
30. Sanders WE, Tenney JH, Kessler RE. Efficacy of cefepime in the treatment of infections due to multiply resistant *Enterobacter* species. Clin Infect Dis 1996;23:454–461.
31. Schaberg T, Lode H, Raffenberg M, Mauch H. Lower respiratory tract infection in the intensive care unit: consequences of antibiotic resistance for choice of antibiotic. Microb Drug Resist 1995;1:163–167
32. Segreti J, Levin S. Bacteriologic and clinical applications of a new extended-spectrum parental cephalosporin. Am J Med 1996;100(Suppl 6A):45S 1991;35:976–982.
33. Verschraegen G, Claeys G, Delanghe M, Pattyn P. Serotyping and phage typing to identify *Enterobacter cloacae* contaminating total parental nutrition. Eur J Clin Microbiol Infect Dis 1988;7:306–307.
34. Watanakunakorn C, Weber J. *Enterobacter* bacteremia: a review of 58 episodes. Scand J Infect Dis 1989;21:1–8.
35. Nazarowec-White M, Farber J. *E sakazakii:* a review. Int J Food Microbiol 1997;34:103–113.
36. Willis J, Robinson J. *Enterobacter sakazakii* meningitis in neonates. Pediatr Infect Dis J 1988;3:197–199.
37. Wolff MA, Young CL, Ramphal R. Antibiotic therapy for *Enterobacter* meningitis: a retrospective review of 13 episodes and review of the literature. Clin Infect Dis 1993;16: 772–777.
38. Yuk-Fong Liu P, Lau YJ, Hu BS, Shyr JM, Shi ZY, Tsai WS, Lin YH, Tseng CY. Comparison of susceptibility to extended-spectrum beta-lactam antibiotics ciprofloxacin among gram-negative bacilli isolated from intensive care units. Diagn Microbiol Infect Dis 1995;22:285–291.

Enterococcus Species

●

Joseph W. Chow and David M. Shlaes

GENERAL DESCRIPTION

Enterococcus species are Gram-positive, facultatively anaerobic cocci that are found in the gastrointestinal tract of most healthy adults (82). *E. faecalis* and *E. faecium* are the most common species that cause infection. All the other enterococcal species together probably constitute less than 5% of enterococcal infections (38, 100). These other species associated with human infections include *E. gallinarum*, *E. casseliflavus*, *E. avium*, *E. durans*, *E. raffinosus*, *E. hirae*, *E. pseudoavium*, *E. malodoratus*, and *E. mundtii* (28, 38, 42, 72, 91, 92, 115).

SUSCEPTIBILITY IN VITRO

Agents with varying degrees of in vitro activity against enterococci include the penicillins (especially penicillin, ampicillin, and piperacillin), glycopeptides (vancomycin and teicoplanin), carbapenems (imipenem and meropenem), aminoglycosides, tetracyclines (tetracycline and doxycycline), quinolones (including ciprofloxacin, sparfloxacin, and clinafloxacin), chloramphenicol, and rifampin. The penicillins and glycopeptides have the best activity, and ampicillin typically has greater in vitro killing ability than vancomycin (13). Enterococci have intrinsic low-level resistance to the aminoglycosides due to the decreased ability of these agents to penetrate the cell wall, but this can be overcome by the addition of cell wall–active agents (e.g., penicillins and glycopeptides) that result in synergistic killing of the organisms (77). Antimicrobial agents in various stages of development such as the streptogramin combination quinupristin/dalfopristin (17, 49, 106), the glycylcyclines (26, 36, 106), the oxazolidinones (27), the fluoroquinolone trovafloxacin (20, 105, 106), the oligosaccharide everninomicin (117), and the 2-pyridones (1, 32) also exhibit in vitro activity against enterococci.

ANTIMICROBIAL THERAPY

A number of enterococcal infections such as urinary tract, soft tissue, and intraabdominal infections and perhaps some cases of septic arthritis can be treated with a single antimicrobial agent, especially when the patient has normal host defenses (75, 82, 97). Some studies suggest that many cases of enterococcal bacteremia without endocarditis can also probably be treated with a single agent (39, 42, 68), although they did not adjust the analyses for the source of bacteremia, which may be an important factor in determining outcome (47). However, other studies suggest that combination therapy may be more effective than monotherapy for serious infections such as bacteremia (75, 82, 88). In one prospective, observational study of 110 serious enterococcal infections (which included bacteremias, endocarditis, cholangitis, abscesses, skin and soft tissue infections, bone and joint infections, and ventriculitis), 71% of patients who received appropriate combination therapy (cell wall–active agent plus aminoglycoside) achieved clinical cure, compared with 53% of patients who received an appropriate single agent ($P = .08$) (92).

For monotherapy, the drug of choice is ampicillin (MIC usually two- to fourfold lower than penicillin). β-Lactamase-producing enterococci had been a concern, since they are resistant to ampicillin but are not detected by routine ampicillin susceptibility testing (83, 84). However, it appears now that they are rare, and many hospitals that have screened for β-lactamase production in enterococci for several years have not found any (38). If isolated, they can be treated with ampicillin/sulbactam. If the organism is resistant to ampicillin, a glycopeptide such as vancomycin may be used for monother-

apy. For simple urinary tract infections, a quinolone with a low MIC for a particular isolate might be considered as an alternative, but caution must be exerted since enterococcal superinfections have occurred in patients treated with ciprofloxacin for infections caused by other bacteria (29, 122). Imipenem offers no advantage over ampicillin against β-lactamase-negative enterococci in vitro or in animal endocarditis models (6, 22, 103). We have seen a few *E. faecalis* isolates that are susceptible to ampicillin (MIC = 0.5–1.0 µg/mL) but relatively resistant to imipenem (MIC ≥ 8.0 µg/mL). However, in situations such as empirical therapy for complex intraabdominal infections in which coverage that includes enterococci may be prudent, imipenem (or piperacillin/tazobactam or ampicillin/sulbactam) might be substituted for regimens that contain ampicillin. A case control study has suggested that empirical therapy for enterococci be especially considered for hepatobiliary or pancreatic infection, in which both the prevalence of enterococci and the rate of enterococcal bacteremia are high (18).

Endocarditis

Combination therapy is necessary to achieve optimal killing of enterococci and is definitely indicated for enterococcal endocarditis, in which patients who received a synergistic combination of a cell wall–active agent plus an aminoglycoside demonstrated a better outcome than those who received monotherapy (23, 35, 51, 69, 71, 75, 82, 119). Cell wall–active antimicrobial agents such as the penicillins and glycopeptides, when combined with aminoglycosides, produce a synergistic bactericidal effect against susceptible strains of enterococci because of enhanced intracellular penetration of the aminoglycoside (78).

Penicillin plus streptomycin has been the most studied combination regimen for enterococcal endocarditis. No direct studies comparing the efficacy of penicillin (or ampicillin) plus streptomycin with that of penicillin plus gentamicin are available, although there has been some suggestion that streptomycin may be more effective than gentamicin in treatment of enterococcal endocarditis (118). This stemmed from a study of streptomycin-resistant enterococcal endocarditis, in which 16 of 20 (80%) patients treated with penicillin plus gentamicin were cured versus 33 of 36 (92%) treated with penicillin plus streptomycin for streptomycin-susceptible enterococci in the same study (118). This higher relapse rate in patients treated with penicillin plus gentamicin was also higher than the relapse rate among patients treated with penicillin plus streptomycin in previous studies (51, 69, 71). Streptomycin has traditionally been given intramuscularly, which involves greater pain for the patient, although intravenous streptomycin given to a few patients seemed to be well tolerated (80). Streptomycin is predominantly ototoxic, and gentamicin is primarily nephrotoxic; while nephrotoxicity is often reversible, ototoxicity often is not (119). Gentamicin serum levels are more readily available to aid in monitoring for potential toxicity, and gentamicin is less expensive than streptomycin. Enough patients have now been treated successfully with penicillin (or ampicillin) plus gentamicin that it is now well accepted (71,

75, 99, 119). For these reasons, gentamicin has replaced streptomycin as the more commonly used aminoglycoside.

The recommended streptomycin dosing in enterococcal endocarditis is 7.5 mg/kg intramuscularly every 12 h, with a goal of peak serum levels of 15 to 30 µg/mL (71, 119). Gentamicin is usually given at 1 mg/kg intravenously every 8 h, with a goal of peak serum levels of 3 µg/mL or above (71, 119). Treatment should continue for at least 4 weeks. Patients with symptoms of greater than 3 months duration before initiation of appropriate therapy and patients with prosthetic valve endocarditis should receive antimicrobial therapy for at least 6 weeks (99, 118). Animal data do not support the use of once-daily dosing of aminoglycosides in enterococcal endocarditis (30, 70).

The combination of vancomycin plus an aminoglycoside has not been as extensively studied, so vancomycin should be used only when the patient has a significant history of allergy to the penicillins (119). Addition of ciprofloxacin to a regimen of ampicillin plus gentamicin was associated with cure in a case of relapsing *E. faecalis* endocarditis (101).

Meningitis

Due to the severity of this infection, most experts would concur that enterococcal meningitis should be treated with combination therapy (7, 75, 82). However, in contrast to endocarditis, abundant clinical information showing unequivocally that combination therapy is superior to monotherapy is not available in meningitis. In a review of enterococcal meningitis, 30 of 32 cases had data on antibiotic therapy (109). Most patients (20 of 30) received penicillin or ampicillin plus an aminoglycoside (three patients also received intrathecal gentamicin); there was only one death in this group, compared with one death in the group of four patients who received penicillin or ampicillin alone (109). One patient failed his initial regimen of ampicillin plus chloramphenicol but recovered when the chloramphenicol was replaced by gentamicin (109). One severely ill patient received chloramphenicol plus gentamicin and subsequently died (109).

Therapy for Strains Resistant to Aminoglycosides

High-level gentamicin resistance (MICs > 500–2000 µg/mL) in enterococci is usually due to the presence of the *aac(6′)-aph(2″)* gene (3, 31). This gene encodes a bifunctional enzyme that modifies the aminoglycoside and eliminates synergism between a cell wall–active agent (e.g., ampicillin or vancomycin) and gentamicin, plus virtually all clinically available aminoglycosides except streptomycin. High-level streptomycin resistance can be caused by either a gene that encodes the streptomycin-modifying enzyme ANT(6)-I or by a change in the ribosome binding site and also eliminates synergism with the cell wall–active agents (25, 52, 89). Nosocomial isolates that possess genes for high-level resistance to both gentamicin and streptomycin are not uncommon (19, 38, 116).

Treatment of patients with endocarditis caused by enterococci with high-level resistance to aminoglycosides is associated with a high incidence of failure or relapse (74). Therapy for strains resistant to all aminoglycosides is usually limited to the use of ampicillin alone. Vancomycin alone is potentially less efficacious. In an in vitro study, both vancomycin and teicoplanin were bacteriostatic and not bactericidal against *E. faecalis* with high-level gentamicin resistance, and antagonism was often seen when either agent was combined with ciprofloxacin (112). In the same study, ampicillin alone was bactericidal against 8 of 13 *E. faecalis* strains, and ampicillin plus ciprofloxacin was bactericidal against all 13 (112). In a rabbit endocarditis model with a β-lactamase-producing, high-level gentamicin resistant *E. faecalis* strain, ampicillin/sulbactam reduced bacterial titers in vegetations more effectively than vancomycin after 7 days, although neither regimen could sterilize the heart valve (57). Duration of therapy with ampicillin alone is not known, but the observation that valve cultures at surgery are positive after as much as 1 month of ampicillin therapy suggests that longer courses than the traditional 4 to 6 weeks (e.g., 8–12 weeks) should be strongly considered (23, 50, 119). Continuous, rather than intermittent, infusion of ampicillin might prove beneficial, since there are data showing its greater efficacy in sterilizing cardiac vegetations and improving the survival rate in a rat endocarditis model (110). Cardiac valve replacement may well be required for a cure in many of these patients (23, 74, 99, 119).

Although high-level aminoglycoside resistance is synonymous with resistance to synergism, there are rare enterococci with gentamicin MICs below 500 µg/mL that are also resistant to the synergistic effect of a cell wall–active agent plus gentamicin. Moellering et al. detected several *E. faecalis* with gentamicin MICs of only 8 µg/mL that are resistant to ampicillin-gentamicin synergism but susceptible to ampicillin-tobramycin synergism (76). Hayden et al. reported five *E. faecium* with gentamicin MICs between 4 and 32 µg/mL that are resistant to ampicillin-gentamicin synergism (46). The mechanisms of these resistance phenotypes have not yet been determined. A novel gentamicin resistance gene, *aph(2″)-Ic*, has been found in *E. faecalis, E. faecium*, and *E. gallinarum* isolates (14). This gene compromises ampicillin-gentamicin synergism but confers a gentamicin MIC of only 256 µg/mL. If these three enterococcal phenotypes become more prevalent, synergy testing of a cell wall–active agent combined with gentamicin may be indicated in such selected clinical situations as enterococcal endocarditis or meningitis to confirm the efficacy of the antimicrobial combination used for therapy.

Heretofore, only gentamicin and streptomycin have been used for high-level aminoglycoside testing in enterococci, since the *aac(6′)-aph(2″)* gene confers high-level resistance to virtually all the clinically available aminoglycosides (including gentamicin, amikacin, tobramycin, netilmicin, and kanamycin) except for streptomycin. A second gene, *aph(2″)-Id,* that confers high-level gentamicin resistance has now been detected (114). This gene also confers resistance to tobramycin, netilmicin, and kanamycin, but not to amikacin. Studies performed on the *E. casseliflavus* from which the gene was isolated showed synergistic killing with the combination of ampicillin and amikacin (113). Molecular epidemiologic studies show that 17 of 108 enterococcal isolates with high-level gentamicin resistance possess the *aph(2″)-Id* gene, and not the bifunctional gene *aac(6′)-aph(2″)* (113).

Therefore, a small percentage of enterococcal isolates with high-level gentamicin resistance might be susceptible to the combination of a cell wall–active agent plus amikacin.

Therapy for Strains Resistant to Penicillins and Glycopeptides but Susceptible to Aminoglycosides

Enterococci resistant to both the penicillins and glycopeptides have provided a therapeutic challenge since these cell wall–active agents may no longer be combined with aminoglycosides in the synergistic combination proven most efficacious against enterococci. High-level penicillin resistance in enterococci is due to modification of penicillin-binding proteins, especially overproduction of a penicillin-binding protein (PBP 5) that has low affinity for the penicillins but is able to substitute for the functions of the susceptible penicillin-binding proteins when they are inhibited by the β-lactam agents (2, 33, 40, 61, 62, 108). For an *E. faecium* strain resistant to penicillin (MIC = 200 μg/mL) but susceptible to gentamicin, no in vitro synergistic bactericidal activity was observed when penicillin was combined with gentamicin, and the combination did not significantly lower bacterial counts in vegetations in a rat endocarditis model, compared with no therapy (9). However, Torres et al. have found in vitro synergism when high levels of penicillin are combined with gentamicin against some *E. faecium* isolates with high-level penicillin resistance (MIC ≥ 128 μg/mL) but low-level gentamicin resistance. Synergism was exhibited in 9 of 12 strains (penicillin MIC = 200 μg/mL) when penicillin (100 μg/mL) was combined with gentamicin (5 μg/mL) (111). In addition, synergism was seen in all three strains for which the penicillin MIC was 400 μg/mL when penicillin at 200 μg/mL was combined with gentamicin at 5 μg/mL (111). Thus, for certain enterococcal strains, synergism may be limited chiefly by the achievable penicillin serum concentration. Since a 1-h intravenous infusion of 5 million units of penicillin G can achieve a peak serum concentration of 135 μg/mL (81), the authors conclude that some *E. faecium* strains with penicillin MICs between 50 and 200 μg/mL and susceptible to gentamicin may be treated with high doses of penicillin in combination with gentamicin (111). These findings for penicillin have been assumed to be true for ampicillin, also, because the two agents have the same mechanism of action. Since peak ampicillin serum levels of 40 to 71 μg/mL can be attained after a 1-g intravenous dose, and levels of 109 to 150 μg/mL can be attained after a 2-g intravenous dose (94), some enterococci with ampicillin MICs as high as 64 μg/mL (or perhaps even 128 μg/mL) may prove to be susceptible to ampicillin-gentamicin synergism if high-dose ampicillin (1–2 g/dose) is used.

Glycopeptide resistance in enterococci is due to synthesis of modified peptidoglycan precursors that have decreased affinity for vancomycin and teicoplanin (4, 59). Most glycopeptide-resistant clinical isolates have the VanA or VanB phenotype. Strains with the VanA phenotype have high-level resistance to both vancomycin (MICs = 64–>1024 μg/mL) and teicoplanin (MICs = 16–512 μg/mL), while strains with the VanB phenotype have varying levels of resistance to vancomycin (MICs = 4–1024 μg/mL) but are susceptible to teicoplanin (4, 59). *E.*

gallinarum, E. casseliflavus, and *E. flavescens* strains are intrinsically resistant to vancomycin (MICs = 4–32 μg/mL) but remain susceptible to teicoplanin and have the VanC phenotype (59, 86, 98). In a rat endocarditis model, teicoplanin was actually more efficacious than vancomycin against a β-lactamase-producing strain with high-level gentamicin resistance (120). Teicoplanin plus gentamicin produced in vitro bactericidal synergism against an *E. faecalis* resistant to vancomycin but susceptible to teicoplanin and gentamicin (5). When the combination was used in a rabbit endocarditis model, vegetations were sterilized in 25% of the rabbits, and no mutants with increased glycopeptide resistance were isolated (5). In an open trial of teicoplanin therapy for enterococcal endocarditis, 5 of 7 patients treated with teicoplanin alone and 6 of 7 patients treated with teicoplanin plus an aminoglycoside were cured (104). In a study of teicoplanin therapy for endocarditis caused by Gram-positive bacteria, five patients with *E. faecalis* endocarditis were treated with teicoplanin alone, and all five were cured (95). Intrathecal teicoplanin has been used successfully to treat *E. faecium* meningitis (66). However, teicoplanin resistance can be selected for in vitro with both *E. faecalis* and *E. faecium* strains (45), and teicoplanin-resistant *E. faecalis* mutants have arisen during teicoplanin therapy in a rabbit endocarditis model (5). Resistance to teicoplanin has emerged in vivo during vancomycin therapy for *E. faecium* (VanB phenotype) bacteremia (45).

For strains truly resistant to ampicillin, vancomycin, and teicoplanin but still susceptible to aminoglycosides, several options have been suggested. The combination of ciprofloxacin plus rifampin plus gentamicin was used with success in two cases of enterococcal bacteremia (65). Ciprofloxacin plus gentamicin, ciprofloxacin plus rifampin, and ciprofloxacin plus rifampin plus gentamicin all showed bactericidal activity in time-kill studies (65). The newer quinolones with greater in vitro potency than ciprofloxacin against enterococci, such as clinafloxacin, sparfloxacin, and trovafloxacin (24, 93, 106), may prove in the future to be better therapeutic choices than ciprofloxacin.

Penicillin plus vancomycin plus gentamicin has produced in vitro synergistic killing against some clinical enterococcal isolates (107). In an *E. faecium* strain for which a synergistic bacteriostatic effect between penicillin and vancomycin was demonstrated in vitro, the triple combination of high-dose penicillin plus vancomycin and gentamicin proved effective in a rabbit endocarditis model, although a bacterial subpopulation resistant to penicillin/vancomycin synergism was frequently isolated from vegetations at the end of therapy (10). In a subsequent study using the same model, the triple combination of ceftriaxone/vancomycin/gentamicin was even more effective in reducing bacterial counts than the combination of either penicillin/vancomycin/gentamicin or penicillin/teicoplanin/gentamicin; still, a subpopulation resistant to ceftriaxone/vancomycin synergism emerged in 10 to 20% of the animals (11). Other investigators have not found the triple combination of ampicillin/vancomycin/gentamicin to be reliably bactericidal in vitro against highly ampicillin-resistant, vancomycin-resistant, gentamicin-susceptible *E. faecium* strains (34).

Therapy for Strains Resistant to Penicillins, Glycopeptides, and Aminoglycosides

Antimicrobial therapeutic options for strains resistant to the penicillins, glycopeptides, and aminoglycosides are extremely limited. The combinations of ampicillin (or penicillin) plus vancomycin, imipenem plus vancomycin, and ceftriaxone plus vancomycin (or teicoplanin) have shown in vitro bacteriostatic synergism against some enterococci resistant to penicillin, glycopeptides, and aminoglycosides (43, 58). However, bacteriostatic synergism may be limited to specific strains (41, 44, 46), and bactericidal synergism has not been shown with these combinations (12, 44, 46, 55, 58).

Ampicillin plus ciprofloxacin has produced in vitro synergistic killing against some of these multiresistant strains that were still susceptible to ciprofloxacin, but in a rabbit endocarditis model, this combination did not significantly reduce bacteria in vegetations (55, 56). A case of clinical failure (despite valve replacement) with ampicillin plus ciprofloxacin therapy for enterococcal endocarditis has been described (60). The combination of ampicillin plus clinafloxacin was bactericidal against 7 of 12 isolates of *E. faecium* resistant to ampicillin and vancomycin (8), and penicillin plus clinafloxacin significantly reduced vegetation bacterial counts in a rabbit endocarditis model (121). Ciprofloxacin plus novobiocin was bactericidal in a time-kill study and significantly decreased bacterial counts in vegetations in a rabbit endocarditis model (55, 96).

Various other bacteriostatic antimicrobials with less in vitro activity than the penicillins, glycopeptides, and aminoglycosides have been tried either alone or in combination against multiresistant enterococci. Chloramphenicol therapy for multiresistant enterococci in 16 severely ill patients in one study showed somewhat encouraging results (87). Eight of 14 patients in whom a clinical response could be determined showed improvement. Four patients were treated with rifampin in addition to chloramphenicol; most patients received other antibiotics that alone do not have activity against enterococci. Eleven of the 16 patients had a drainage procedure or debridement performed. In a study of *E. faecium* infections in liver transplant recipients, chloramphenicol was used as monotherapy in 16 cases, and 6 patients died (90). Single cases of successful therapy using chloramphenicol alone or in combination with vancomycin or rifampin have also been reported (54, 92).

Intravenous doxycycline used alone for 2 weeks in a patient with catheter-related sepsis and probable endocarditis resulted in clearing of the bacteremia, but the patient subsequently died of congestive heart failure (54). Oral doxycycline for 2 weeks plus removal of the Hickman catheter presumed to be the source of the bacteremia was successful in treating a patient with *E. faecium* bacteremia (79). An immunocompromised patient with vancomycin- and ampicillin-resistant *E. faecium* bacteremia who appeared to fail therapy with quinupristin/dalfopristin plus gentamicin was cured with 5 days of intravenous tetracycline followed by 2 months of oral doxycycline (with occasional periods of intravenous tetracycline when he could not tolerate oral therapy) (48).

The new streptogramin combination quinupristin/dalfopristin has been used for treatment of *E. faecium*, but not *E.*

faecalis, which are intrinsically resistant to the combination. Among 15 cases of multiresistant *E. faecium* infection treated with quinupristin/dalfopristin, 3 patients were cured of their infection, 5 had recurrence of the infection, and in 7 the outcome was indeterminate (21). Blood cultures became negative for enterococcus during treatment in all patients with bacteremia. However, catheters were removed in the patients with catheter-related bacteremia prior to therapy, so it is not known whether removal of catheters alone would have been curative (21). Vancomycin-resistant *E. faecium* (VREF)-associated mortality was significantly lower in a group of 20 patients with VREF bacteremia treated with quinupristin/dalfopristin than in a historical cohort of 42 patients with VREF bacteremia treated with other agents (64). Successful treatment with quinupristin/dalfopristin for *E. faecium* peritonitis, ventriculitis, aortic graft infection, and prosthetic valve endocarditis has also been reported (37, 53, 67, 85, 102). However, *E. faecium* strains resistant to quinupristin/dalfopristin can be selected in vitro without difficulty (73). Furthermore, superinfection with *E. faecalis* bacteremia has occurred during quinupristin/dalfopristin therapy for *E. faecium* bacteremia (15), and increased resistance to quinupristin/dalfopristin has emerged during therapy for *E. faecium* bacteremia (16, 63).

COMMENTS

In short, infections caused by enterococci resistant to the penicillins, glycopeptides, and aminoglycosides pose a difficult therapeutic dilemma at this time, since no alternative antimicrobial regimen has been proven more efficacious than another. Still, there may be clinical settings in which the patient will recover even when no appropriate antimicrobial therapy is available. For example, line-related bacteremias might sometimes be treatable with line removal alone (39, 53). Surgical site infections, skin and soft tissue infections, and intraabdominal abscesses may at times be manageable by surgical debridement and drainage alone (18, 39, 53). It remains to be seen whether the newer quinolones, glycylcyclines, oxazolidinones, everninomicin, and the 2-pyridones will prove to be significant improvements on the current agents used for treating multiresistant enterococci.

REFERENCES

1. Alder J, Clement J, Meulbroek J, Shipkowitz N, Mitten M, Jarvis K, Oleksijew A, Hutch T Sr, Paige L, Flamm B, Chu D, Tanaka K. Efficacies of ABT-719 and related 2-pyridones, members of a new class of antibacterial agents, against experimental bacterial infections. Antimicrob Agents Chemother 1995;39:971–975.
2. Al-Obeid S, Gutmann L, Williamson R. Modification of penicillin-binding proteins of penicillin-resistant mutants of different species of enterococci. J Antimicrob Chemother 1990;26:613–618.
3. Arduino RC, Murray BE. Enterococci: antimicrobial resistance. In: Mandell GL, Douglas RG, Bennett JE, eds. Update to principles and practice of infectious diseases. New York: Churchill Livingstone, 1993:3–15.
4. Arthur M, Courvalin P. Genetics and mechanisms of glycopeptide resistance in enterococci. Antimicrob Agents Chemother 1993; 37:1563–1571.

5. Aslangul E, Baptista M, Fantin B, Depardieu F, Arthur M, Courvalin P, Carbon C. Selection of glycopeptide-resistant mutants of VanB-type *Enterococcus faecalis* BM4281 in vitro and in experimental endocarditis. J Infect Dis 1997;175:598–605.

6. Auckenthaler R, Wilson WR, Wright AJ, Washington JA II, Durack DT, Geraci JE. Lack of an in vivo and in vitro bactericidal activity of N-formimidoyl thienamycin against enterococci. Antimicrob Agents Chemother 1982;22:448–452.

7. Bayer AS, Seidel JS, Yoshikawa TT, Anthony BF, Guze LB. Group D enterococcal meningitis: clinical and therapeutic considerations with report of three cases and review of the literature. Arch Intern Med 1976;136:883–886.

8. Burney S, Landman D, Quale JM. Activity of clinafloxacin against multidrug-resistant *Enterococcus faecium*. Antimicrob Agents Chemother 1994;38:1668–1670.

9. Bush LM, Calmon J, Cherney CL, Wendeler M, Pitsakis P, Poupard J, Levison ME, Johnson CC. High-level penicillin resistance among isolates of enterococci. Ann Intern Med 1989;110:515–520.

10. Caron F, Lemeland J-F, Humbert G, Klare I, Gutmann L. Triple combination penicillin-vancomycin-gentamicin for experimental endocarditis caused by a highly penicillin- and glycopeptide-resistant isolate of *Enterococcus faecium*. J Infect Dis 1993; 168:681–686.

11. Caron FM, Pestel M, Kitzis M-D, Lemeland J-F, Humbert G, Gutmann L. Comparison of different β-lactam-glycopeptide-gentamicin combinations for an experimental endocarditis caused by a highly β-lactam-resistant and highly glycopeptide-resistant isolate of *Enterococcus faecium*. J Infect Dis 1995;171: 106–112.

12. Cercenado E, Eliopoulos GM, Wennersten CB, Moellering RC Jr. Absence of synergistic activity between ampicillin and vancomycin against highly vancomycin-resistant enterococci. Antimicrob Agents Chemother 1992;36:2201–2203.

13. Cercenado E, Eliopoulos GM, Wennersten CB, Moellering RC Jr. Influence of high-level gentamicin resistance and beta-hemolysis on susceptibility of enterococci to the bactericidal activities of ampicillin and vancomycin. Antimicrob Agents Chemother 1992;36:2526–2528.

14. Chow JW, Zervos MJ, Lerner SA, Thal LA, Donabedian SM, Jaworski DD, Tsai S, Shaw KJ, Clewell DB. A novel gentamicin resistance gene in *Enterococcus*. Antimicrob Agents Chemother 1997;41:511–514.

15. Chow JW, Davidson A, Sanford E III, Zervos MJ. Superinfection with *Enterococcus faecalis* during quinupristin/dalfopristin therapy. Clin Infect Dis 1997;24:91–92.

16. Chow JW, Donabedian SM, Zervos MJ. Emergence of increased resistance to quinupristin/dalfopristin during therapy for *Enterococcus faecium* bacteremia. Clin Infect Dis 1997;24:90–91.

17. Collins LA, Malanoski GJ, Eliopoulos GM, Wennersten CB, Ferraro MJ, Moellering RC Jr. In vitro activity of RP59500, an injectable streptogramin antibiotic, against vancomycin-resistant gram-positive organisms. Antimicrob Agents Chemother 1993;37:598–601.

18. Cooper GS, Shlaes DM, Jacobs MR, Salata RA. The role of *Enterococcus* in intraabdominal infections: case control analysis. Infect Dis Clin Pract 1993;2:332–339.

19. Coque TM, Arduino RC, Murray BE. High-level resistance to aminoglycosides: comparison of community and nosocomial fecal isolates of enterococci. Clin Infect Dis 1995;20:1048–1051.

20. Coque TM, Singh KV, Murray BE. Comparative in-vitro activity of the new fluoroquinolone trovafloxacin (CP-99,219) against Gram-positive cocci. J Antimicrob Chemother 1996;37: 1011–1016.

21. Dever LL, Smith SM, DeJesus D, Masurekar M, Patel D, Kaminski ZC, Johanson WG Jr. Treatment of vancomycin-resistant *Enterococcus faecium* infections with an investigational streptogramin antibiotic (quinupristin/dalfopristin): a report of fifteen cases. Microb Drug Resist 1996;2:407–413.

22. Eliopoulos GM, Eliopoulos CT. Therapy of enterococcal infections. Eur J Clin Microbiol Infect Dis 1990;9:118–126.

23. Eliopoulos GM. Aminoglycoside resistant enterococcal endocarditis. Infect Dis Clin North Am 1993;7:117–133.

24. Eliopoulos GM, Eliopoulos CT. Activity in vitro of the quinolones. In: Hooper DC, Wolfson JS, eds. Quinolone antimicrobial agents. 2nd ed. Washington, DC: American Society for Microbiology, 1993:161–194.

25. Eliopoulos GM, Farber BF, Murray BE, Wennersten C, Moellering RC Jr. Ribosomal resistance of clinical enterococcal isolates to streptomycin. Antimicrob Agents Chemother 1984;25:398–399.

26. Eliopoulos GM, Wennersten CB, Cole G, Moellering RC. In vitro activities of two glycylcyclines against gram-positive bacteria. Antimicrob Agents Chemother 1994;38:534–541.

27. Eliopoulos GM, Wennersten CB, Gold HS, Moellering RC Jr. In vitro activities of new oxazolidinone antimicrobial agents against enterococci. Antimicrob Agents Chemother 1996;40: 1745–1747.

28. Facklam RR, Collins MD. Identification of *Enterococcus* species isolated from human infections by a conventional test scheme. J Clin Microbiol 1989;27:731–734.

29. Fang G, Brennen C, Wagener M, Swanson D, Hilf M, Zadecky L, DeVine J, Yu VL. Use of ciprofloxacin versus use of aminoglycoside for therapy of complicated urinary tract infection: prospective, randomized clinical and pharmacokinetic study. Antimicrob Agents Chemother 1991;35:1849–1855.

30. Fantin B, Carbon C. Importance of the aminoglycoside dosing regimen in the penicillin-netilmicin combination for treatment of *Enterococcus faecalis*-induced experimental endocarditis. Antimicrob Agents Chemother 1990;34:2387–2391.

31. Ferretti JJ, Gilmore KS, Courvalin P. Nucleotide sequence analysis of the gene specifying the bifunctional 6′-aminoglycoside acetyltransferase 2″-aminoglycoside phosphotransferase enzyme in *Streptococcus faecalis* and identification and cloning of gene regions specifying the two activities. J Bacteriol 1986;167:631–638.

32. Flamm RK, Vojtko C, Chu DTW, Li Q, Beyer J, Hensey D, Ramer N, Clement JJ, Tanaka SK. In vitro evaluation of ABT-719, a novel DNA gyrase inhibitor. Antimicrob Agents Chemother 1995;39:964–970.

33. Fontana R, Aldegheri M, Ligozzi M, Lopez H, Sucari A, Satta G. Overproduction of a low-affinity penicillin-binding protein and high-level ampicillin resistance in *Enterococcus faecium*. Antimicrob Agents Chemother 1994;38:1980–1983.

34. Fraimow HS, Venuti E. Inconsistent bactericidal activity of triple-combination therapy with vancomycin, ampicillin, and gentamicin against vancomycin-resistant, highly ampicillin-resistant *Enterococcus faecium*. Antimicrob Agents Chemother 1992;36:1563–1566.

35. Francioli P. Antibiotic treatment of streptococcal and enterococcal endocarditis: an overview. Eur Heart J 1995;16(Suppl B):75–79.

36. Fraise AP, Brenwald N, Andrews JM, Wise R. In vitro activity of two glycylcyclines against enterococci resistant to other agents. J Antimicrob Chemother 1995;35:877–881.

37. Furlong WB, Rakowski TA. Therapy with RP 59500 (quinupristin/dalfopristin) for prosthetic valve endocarditis due to enterococci with vanA/vanB resistance patterns. Clin Infect Dis 1997;25:163–164.

38. Gordon S, Swenson JM, Hill BC, Pigott NE, Facklam RR, Cooksey RC, Thornsberry C, Enterococcal Study Group, Jarvis WR, Tenover FC. Antimicrobial susceptibility patterns of common and unusual species of enterococci causing infections in the United States. J Clin Microbiol 1992;30:2373–2378.

39. Graninger W, Ragette R. Nosocomial bacteremia due to *Enterococcus faecalis* without endocarditis. Clin Infect Dis 1992; 15:49–57.

40. Grayson ML, Eliopoulos GM, Wennersten CB, Ruoff KL, De Girolami PC, Ferraro MJ, Moellering RC Jr. Increasing resistance to β-lactam antibiotics among clinical isolates of *Enterococcus faecium:* a 22-year review at one institution. Antimicrob Agents Chemother 1991;35:2180–2184.

41. Green M, Binczewski B, Pasculle AW, Edmund M, Barbadora K, Kusne S, Shlaes DM. Constitutively vancomycin-resistant *Enterococcus faecium* resistant to synergistic β-lactam combinations. Antimicrob Agents Chemother 1993;37:1238–1242.

42. Gullberg RM, Homann SR, Phair JP. Enterococcal bacteremia: analysis of 75 episodes. Rev Infect Dis 1989;11:74–85.

43. Gutmann L, Al-Obeid S, Billot-Klein D, Guerrier M-L, Collatz E. Synergy and resistance to synergy between β-lactam antibiotics and glycopeptides against glycopeptide-resistant strains of *Enterococcus faecium*. Antimicrob Agents Chemother 1994;38: 824–829.

44. Handwerger SD, Perlman C, Altarac D, McAuliffe V. Concomitant high-level vancomycin and penicillin resistance in clinical isolates of enterococci. Clin Infect Dis 1992;14:655–661.

45. Hayden MK, Trenholme GM, Schultz JE, Sahm DF. In vivo development of teicoplanin resistance in a VanB *Enterococcus faecium* isolate. J Infect Dis 1993;167:1224–1227.

46. Hayden M, Koenig GI, Trenholme GM. Bactericidal activities of antibiotics against vancomycin-resistant *Enterococcus faecium* blood isolates and synergistic activities of combinations. Antimicrob Agents Chemother 1994;38:1225–1229.

47. Hoge CW, Adams J, Buchanan B, Sears SD. Enterococcal bacteremia: to treat or not to treat, a reappraisal. Rev Infect Dis 1991;13:600–605.

48. Howe RA, Robson M, Oakhill A, Cornish JM, Millar MR. Successful use of tetracycline as therapy of an immunocompromised patient with septicaemia caused by a vancomycin-resistant enterococcus. J Antimicrob Chemother 1997;40:144–145.

49. Johnson CC, Slavoski L, Schwartz M, May P, Pitsakis PG, Shur AL, Levison ME. In vitro activity of RP59500 (quinupristin/dalfopristin) against antibiotic-resistant strains of *Streptococcus pneumoniae* and enterococci. Diagn Microbiol Infect Dis 1995; 21:169–173.

50. Kaye D. Treatment of infective endocarditis. Ann Intern Med 1996;124:606–608.

51. Koenig MG, Kaye D. Enterococcal endocarditis: report of nineteen cases with long-term follow-up data. N Engl J Med 1961;264:257–264.

52. Krogstad DJ, Korfhagen TR, Moellering RC Jr, Wennersten C, Swartz MN, Perzynski S, Davies J. Aminoglycoside-inactivating enzymes in clinical isolates of *Streptococcus faecalis:* an explanation for antibiotic synergism. J Clin Invest 1978;62: 480–486.

53. Lai KK. Treatment of vancomycin-resistant *Enterococcus faecium* infections. Arch Intern Med 1996;156:2579–2584.

54. Lam S, Singer C, Tucci V, Morthland VH, Pfaller MA, Isenberg HD. The challenge of vancomycin-resistant enterococci: a clinical and epidemiologic study. Am J Infect Control 1995;23: 170–180.

55. Landman D, Mobarakai NK, Quale JM. Novel antibiotic regimens against *Enterococcus faecium* resistant to ampicillin, vancomycin, and gentamicin. Antimicrob Agents Chemother 1993; 37:1904–1908.

56. Landman D, Quale JM, Mobarakai N, Zaman MM. Ampicillin plus ciprofloxacin therapy of experimental endocarditis caused by multidrug-resistant *Enterococcus faecium*. J Antimicrob Chemother 1995;36:253–258.

57. Lavoie SR, Wong ES, Coudron PE, Williams DS, Markowitz SM. Comparison of ampicillin-sulbactam with vancomycin for treatment of experimental endocarditis due to a β-lactamase-producing, highly gentamicin-resistant isolate of *Enterococcus faecalis*. Antimicrob Agents Chemother 1993;37:1447–1451.

58. Leclercq R, Bingen E, Su QH, Lambert-Zechovski N, Courvalin P, Duval J. Effects of combinations of β-lactams, daptomycin, gentamicin, and glycopeptides against glycopeptide-resistant enterococci. Antimicrob Agents Chemother 1991;35:92–98.

59. Leclercq R, Courvalin P. Resistance to glycopeptides in enterococci. Clin Infect Dis 1997;24:545–556.

60. Lee PYC, Das SS, Stevens PJ. Achieving bactericidal therapy and high-level aminoglycoside resistance. J Antimicrob Chemother 1993;31:608–609.

61. Ligozzi M, Pittaluga F, Fontana R. Identification of a genetic element (*psr*) which negatively controls expression of *Enterococcus hirae* penicillin-binding protein 5. J Bacteriol 1993;175: 2046–2051.

62. Ligozzi M, Pittaluga F, Fontana R. Modification of penicillin-binding protein 5 associated with high-level ampicillin resistance in *Enterococcus faecium*. Antimicrob Agents Chemother 1996;40:354–357.

63. Linden PK, Pasculle AW, Manez R, Kramer DJ, Fung JJ, Pinna AD, Kusne S. Differences in outcomes for patients with bacteremia due to vancomycin-resistant *Enterococcus faecium* or vancomycin-susceptible *E. faecium*. Clin Infect Dis 1996;22: 663–670.

64. Linden PK, Pasculle AW, McDevitt D, Kramer DJ. Effect of quinupristin/dalfopristin on the outcome of vancomycin-resistant *Enterococcus faecium* bacteraemia: comparison with a control cohort. J Antimicrob Chemother 1997;39(Suppl A):145–151.

65. Livornese LL Jr, Dias S, Samel C, Romanowski B, Taylor S, May P, Pitsakis P, Woods G, Kaye D, Levison ME, Johnson CC. Hospital-acquired infection with vancomycin-resistant *Enterococcus faecium* transmitted by electronic thermometers. Ann Intern Med 1992;117:112–116.

66. Losonsky GA, Wolf A, Schwalbe RS, Nataro J, Gibson CB, Lewis EW. Successful treatment of meningitis due to multiply resistant *Enterococcus faecium* with a combination of intrathecal teicoplanin and intravenous antimicrobial agents. Clin Infect Dis 1994;19:163–165.

67. Lynn WA, Clutterbuck E, Want S, Markides V, Lacey S, Rogers TR, Cohen J. Treatment of CAPD-peritonitis due to glycopeptide-resistant *Enterococcus faecium* with quinupristin/dalfopristin. Lancet 1994;344:1025–1026.

68. Maki DG, Agger WA. Enterococcal bacteremia: clinical features, the risk of endocarditis, and management. Medicine (Baltimore) 1988;67:248–269.

69. Mandell GL, Kaye D, Levison ME, Hook EW. Enterococcal endocarditis: an analysis of 38 patients observed at the New York

Hospital-Cornell Medical Center. Arch Intern Med 1970;125: 258–264.

70. Marangos MN, Nicolau DP, Quintiliani R, Nightingale CH. Influence of gentamicin dosing interval on the efficacy of penicillin-containing regimens in experimental *Enterococcus faecalis* endocarditis. J Antimicrob Chemother 1997;39:519–522.

71. Megran, DW. Enterococcal endocarditis. Clin Infect Dis 1992;15:63–71.

72. Mellman RL, Spisak GM, Burakoff R. *Enterococcus avium* bacteremia in association with ulcerative colitis. Am J Gastroenterol 1992;87:337–338.

73. Millichap J, Ristow RA, Noskin GA, Peterson LR. Selection of *Enterococcus faecium* strains with stable and unstable resistance to the streptogramin RP 59500 using stepwise in vitro exposure. Diagn Microbiol Infect Dis 1996;25:15–20.

74. Moellering RC Jr. The enterococcus: a classic example of the impact of antimicrobial resistance on therapeutic options. J Antimicrob Chemother 1991;28:1–12.

75. Moellering RC Jr. Emergence of enterococcus as a significant pathogen. Clin Infect Dis 1992;14:1173–1178.

76. Moellering RC Jr, Murray BE, Schoenbaum SC, Adler J, Wennersten CB. A novel mechanism of resistance to penicillin-gentamicin synergism in *Streptococcus faecalis*. J Infect Dis 1980;141:81–86.

77. Moellering RC Jr, Weinberg AN. Studies on antibiotic synergism against enterococci. II. Effect of various antibiotics on the uptake of ¹⁴C-labelled streptomycin by enterococci. J Clin Invest 1971;50:2580–2584.

78. Moellering RC Jr, Wennersten C, Weinberg AN. Studies on antibiotic synergism against enterococci. I. Bacteriologic studies. J Lab Clin Med 1971;77:821–828.

79. Moreno F, Jorgensen JH, Weiner MH. An old antibiotic for a new multiple-resistant *Enterococcus faecium*? Diagn Microbiol Infect Dis 1994;20:41–43.

80. Morris JT, Cooper RH. Intravenous streptomycin: a useful route of administration. Clin Infect Dis 1994;19:1150–1151.

81. Mouton Y, Deboscker Y. Les beta-lactamines. Encycl Med Chir Paris Ther 1983;25007:B10–20.

82. Murray BE. The life and times of the enterococcus. Clin Microbiol Rev 1990;3:46–65.

83. Murray BE, Singh KV, Markowitz SM, Lopardo HA, Patterson JE, Zervos MJ, Rubeglio E, Eliopoulos GM, Rice LB, Goldstein FW, Jenkins SG, Caputo GM, Nasnas R, Moore LS, Wong ES, Weinstock G. Evidence for clonal spread of a single strain of β-lactamase-producing *Enterococcus (Streptococcus) faecalis* to six hospitals in five states. J Infect Dis 1991;163:780–785.

84. Murray BE. β-Lactamase-producing enterococci. Antimicrob Agents Chemother 1992;36:2355–2359.

85. Nachtman A, Verma R, Egnor M. Vancomycin-resistant *Enterococcus faecium* shunt infection in an infant: an antibiotic cure. Microb Drug Resist 1995;1:95–96.

86. Navarro F, Courvalin P. Analysis of genes encoding D-alanine-D-alanine ligase-related enzymes in *Enterococcus casseliflavus* and *Enterococcus flavescens*. Antimicrob Agents Chemother 1994;38:1788–1793.

87. Norris AH, Reilly JP, Edelstein PH, Brennan PJ, Schuster MG. Chloramphenicol for the treatment of vancomycin-resistant enterococcal infections. Clin Infect Dis 1995;20:1137–1144.

88. Noskin GA, Peterson LR, Warren JR. *Enterococcus faecium* and *Enterococcus faecalis* bacteremia: acquisition and outcome. Clin Infect Dis 1995;20:296–301.

89. Ounissi H, Courvalin P. Appendix B. Nucleotide sequences of streptococcal genes. In: Ferretti JJ, Curtis R III, eds. Streptococcal genetics. Washington, DC: American Society for Microbiology, 1987:275.

90. Papanicolaou GA, Meyers RR, Meyers J, Mendelson MH, Lou W, Emre S, Sheiner P, Miller C. Nosocomial infections with vancomycin-resistant *Enterococcus faecium* in liver transplant recipients: risk factors for acquisition and mortality. Clin Infect Dis 1996;23:760–766.

91. Patel R, Keating MR, Cockerill FR III, Steckelberg JM. Bacteremia due to *Enterococcus avium*. Clin Infect Dis 1993;17: 1006–1011.

92. Patterson JE, Sweeney AH, Simms M, Carley N, Mangi R, Sabetta J, Lyons RW. An analysis of 110 serious enterococcal infections: epidemiology, antibiotic susceptibility, and outcome. Medicine (Baltimore) 1995;74:191–200.

93. Perri MB, Chow JW, Zervos MJ. In vitro activity of sparfloxacin and clinafloxacin against multidrug-resistant enterococci. Diagn Microbiol Infect Dis 1993;17:151–155.

94. Physicians' desk reference. 51st ed. Montvale, NJ: Medical Economics Company, 1997:2035.

95. Presterl E, Graninger W, Georgopoulos A. The efficacy of teicoplanin in the treatment of endocarditis caused by Gram-positive bacteria. J Antimicrob Chemother 1993;31:755–766.

96. Quale JM, Landman D, Mobarakai N. Treatment of experimental endocarditis due to multidrug resistant *Enterococcus faecium* with ciprofloxacin and novobiocin. J Antimicrob Chemother 1994;34:797–802.

97. Raymond NJ, Henry J, Workowski KA. Enterococcal arthritis: case report and review. Clin Infect Dis 1995;21:516–522.

98. Reynolds PE, Snaith HA, Maguire AJ, Dutka-Malen S, Courvalin P. Analysis of peptidoglycan precursors in vancomycin-resistant *Enterococcus gallinarum* BM4174. Biochem J 1994;301:5–8.

99. Rice LB, Calderwood SB, Eliopoulos GM, Farber BF, Karchmer AW. Enterococcal endocarditis: a comparison of prosthetic and native valve disease. Rev Infect Dis 1991;13:1–7.

100. Ruoff KL, de la Maza L, Murtagh MJ, Spargo JD, Ferraro MJ. Species identities of enterococci isolated from clinical specimens. J Clin Microbiol 1990;28:435–437.

101. Sacher HL, Miller WC, Landau SW, Sacher ML, Dixon WA, Dietrich KA. Relapsing native-valve enterococcal endocarditis: a unique cure with oral ciprofloxacin combination drug therapy. J Clin Pharmacol 1991;31:719–721.

102. Sahgal VS, Urban C, Mariano N, Weinbaum F, Turner J, Rahal JJ. Quinupristin/dalfopristin (RP 59500) therapy for vancomycin-resistant *Enterococcus faecium* aortic graft infection: case report. Microb Drug Resist 1995;1:245–247.

103. Scheld WE, Keeley JM. Imipenem therapy of experimental *Staphylococcus aureus* and *Streptococcus faecalis* endocarditis. J Antimicrob Chemother 1983;12(Suppl D):65–78.

104. Schmit JL. Efficacy of teicoplanin for enterococcal infections: 63 cases and review. Clin Infect Dis 1992;15:302–306.

105. Sefton AM, Maskell JP, Rafay AM, Whiley A, Williams JD. The in-vitro activity of trovafloxacin, a new fluoroquinolone, against Gram-positive bacteria. J Antimicrob Chemother 1997; 39(Suppl B):57–62.

106. Shonekan D, Handwerger S, Mildvan D. Comparative in-vitro activities of RP59500 (quinupristin/dalfopristin), CL 329,998, CL 331,002, trovafloxacin, clinafloxacin, teicoplanin and vancomycin against Gram-positive bacteria. J Antimicrob Chemother 1997;39:405–409.

107. Shlaes DM, Etter L, Gutmann L. Synergistic killing of vancomycin-resistant enterococci of classes A, B, and C by combinations of vancomycin, penicillin, and gentamicin. Antimicrob Agents Chemother 1991;35:776–779.

108. Signoretto C, Boaretti M, Canepari P. Cloning, sequencing and expression in *Escherichia coli* of the low-affinity penicillin-binding protein of *Enterococcus faecalis*. FEMS Microbiol Lett 1994;123:99–106.

109. Stevenson KB, Murray EW, Sarubbi FA. Enterococcal meningitis: report of four cases and review. Clin Infect Dis 1994;18:233–239.

110. Thauvin C, Eliopoulos GM, Willey S, Wennersten C, Moellering RC Jr. Continuous-infusion ampicillin therapy of enterococcal endocarditis in rats. Antimicrob Agents Chemother 1991;31:139–143.

111. Torres C, Tenorio C, Lantero M, Gastañares M-J, Baquero F. High-level penicillin resistance and penicillin-gentamicin synergy in *Enterococcus faecium*. Antimicrob Agents Chemother 1993;37:2427–2431.

112. Tripodi M F, Utili R, Rambaldi A, Locatelli A, Rosario P, Florio A, Ruggiero G. Unorthodox antibiotic combinations including ciprofloxacin against high-level gentamicin resistant enterococci. J Antimicrob Chemother 1996;37:727–736.

113. Tsai SF, Zervos MJ, Clewell DB, Donabedian SM, Sahm DF, Chow JW. A new high-level gentamicin resistance gene, *aph(2″)-Id*, in *Enterococcus* spp. Antimicrob Agents Chemother 1998;42:1229–1232.

114. Tsai S, Zervos MJ, Donabedian S, Clewell DB, Chow JW. Nucleotide sequence analysis of a new gentamicin resistance gene in *Enterococcus casseliflavus* [Abstract]. Abstracts of the 97th general meeting of the American Society for Microbiology, Miami Beach, FL, May 4–8, 1997. Washington, DC: American Society for Microbiology, 1997:A-128.

115. Van Goethem GF, Louwagie BM, Simoens MJ, Vandeven JM, Verhaegen JL, Boogaerts MA. *Enterococcus casseliflavus* septicaemia in a patient with acute myeloid leukaemia. Eur J Clin Microbiol Infect Dis 1994;13:519–520.

116. Watanakunakorn C. Rapid increase in the prevalence of high-level aminoglycoside resistance among enterococci isolated from blood cultures during 1989–1991. J Antimicrob Chemother 1992;30:289–293.

117. Willey BM, Sachse L, Mustachi B, McGeer A, Low DE. Comparative in vitro activities of a new oligosaccharide, everninomicin (SCH27899), against clinical enterococci [Abstract]. Abstracts of the 36th Interscience Conference on Antimicrobial Agents and Chemotherapy, New Orleans, LA, September 15–18, 1997. Washington, DC: American Society for Microbiology, 1997:F-237.

118. Wilson WR, Wilkowske CJ, Wright AJ, Sande MA, Geraci JE. Treatment of streptomycin-susceptible and streptomycin-resistant enterococcal endocarditis. Ann Intern Med 1984;100:816–823.

119. Wilson WR, Karchmer AW, Dajani AS, Taubert KA, Bayer A, Kaye D, Bisno AL, Ferrieri P, Shulman ST, Durack DT. Antibiotic treatment of adults with infective endocarditis due to streptococci, enterococci staphylococci, and HACEK microorganisms. JAMA 1995;274:1706–1713.

120. Yao JDC, Thauvin-Eliopoulos C, Eliopoulos GM, Moellering RC Jr. Efficacy of teicoplanin in two dosage regimens for experimental endocarditis caused by a β-lactamase-producing strain of *Enterococcus faecalis* with high-level resistance to gentamicin. Antimicrob Agents Chemother 1990;34:827–830.

121. Zaman MM, Landman D, Burney S, Quale JM. Treatment of experimental endocarditis due to multidrug-resistant *Enterococcus faecium* with clinafloxacin and penicillin. J Antimicrob Chemother 1996;37:127–132.

122. Zervos MJ, Bacon AE III, Patterson JE, Schaberg DR, Kauffman CA. Enterococcal superinfection in patients treated with ciprofloxacin. J Antimicrob Chemother 1988;21:113–115.

Erysipelothrix rhusiopathiae

•

Annette C. Reboli

GENERAL DESCRIPTION

Erysipelothrix rhusiopathiae is a slender, pleomorphic, nonsporulating, Gram-positive rod. It is found worldwide. It has been reported as a commensal or a pathogen in a wide variety of vertebrate and invertebrate species including swine, sheep, turkeys, ducks, and fish. The risk of human infection with *E. rhusiopathiae* is closely related to the opportunity for exposure to the organism. Most human cases are related to occupational exposure. Those at greatest risk include fishermen, butchers, slaughterhouse workers, veterinarians, and housewives. The or-

ganism is communicable from animals to humans, generally by direct cutaneous contact. There are a few reports of bacteremia that occurred after ingestion of undercooked pork.

Three well-defined clinical entities have been described in humans: (*a*) a localized cutaneous form known as erysipeloid, (*b*) a generalized cutaneous form, and (*c*) a bacteremic form that is often associated with endocarditis (8). Erysipeloid is a cellulitis. Because of its mode of acquisition (i.e., contact with infected animals, fish, or their products, with organisms gaining entrance via cuts or abrasions on the skin), lesions are usually confined to the hands and fingers. Erysipeloid is painful and may have a throbbing or burning quality. The incubation period is approximately 5 to 7 days. The lesion is violaceous and slightly elevated, with well-defined borders. As it spreads peripherally, the central area clears. Lymphadenopathy and lymphangitis occur in approximately one-third of cases. Systemic symptoms are uncommon, with low-grade fevers and arthralgias occurring in only 10% of cases. Features that help to distinguish erysipeloid from staphylococcal or streptococcal cellulitis include the absence of suppuration, the violaceous color, the lack of pitting edema, and the disproportionate pain seen with erysipeloid.

The diffuse cutaneous form is rare. In this situation, the cutaneous lesion progresses proximally from the site of inoculation or appears at remote areas. Vesicles and bullae may be present. There are often systemic manifestations such as fever and arthralgias, but blood cultures are usually negative. The clinical course is much more protracted than in erysipeloid, and recurrences are not unusual.

Systemic infection with *Erysipelothrix* is uncommon. It rarely develops from localized infection. Over 60 cases of bacteremia with *E. rhusiopathiae* have been reported, with a very high incidence of endocarditis (90%) among them (6, 13). All reported cases of endocarditis, except one, have involved native valves (7). *Erysipelothrix* endocarditis correlates highly with occupation (animal exposure), affects more males than females (which probably reflects occupational exposure), exhibits a peculiar aortic valve trophism, and is associated with significant mortality (overall rate, 38%). Approximately 40% of patients have a history of an antecedent skin lesion or a concurrent characteristic skin lesion of erysipeloid (6). In nearly 60% of patients, *Erysipelothrix* endocarditis apparently developed on previously normal heart valves. The clinical picture with respect to fever, emboli, peripheral skin stigmata of endocarditis, splenomegaly, hematuria, and mycotic aneurysm is similar for *Erysipelothrix* endocarditis and endocarditis caused by other bacteria. The most common complication of *Erysipelothrix* endocarditis, congestive heart failure, was present in approximately 80% of patients (3). Very few cases of endocarditis have occurred in immunocompromised patients, but a history of ethanol abuse was present in one-third. There has been a recent suggestion that bacteremia due to *E. rhusiopathiae* without endocarditis occurs more frequently than previously believed and that bacteremia may be occurring with increased frequency in immunocompromised patients, while endocarditis usually occurs in immunocompetent patients (5). Brain abscess, osteomyelitis, and chronic arthritis have also been reported (8).

Routine blood culture techniques are adequate for specimen collection and organism growth in suspected cases of bacteremia or endocarditis. Because organisms are located only in deeper parts of the skin in cases of erysipeloid, aspirates or biopsy specimens from the edge of the lesion are needed to recover the organism. Biopsies should include the entire thickness of the dermis (12). *E. rhusiopathiae* must be differentiated from other Gram-positive bacilli, in particular from *Actinomyces* (*Corynebacterium*) *pyogenes* and *Arcanobac-*terium (*Corynebacterium*) *haemolyticum,* and from *Listeria monocytogenes*. The first two organisms are β-hemolytic on blood agar and do not produce hydrogen sulfide in the butt of triple-sugar iron agar slants, whereas *E. rhusiopathiae* may be α-hemolytic but is never β-hemolytic, and most *Erysipelothrix* strains produce hydrogen sulfide, which causes a blackened butt on triple-sugar iron agar slants. The catalase test should be performed and motility examined to distinguish *E. rhusiopathiae* from *L. monocytogenes*. *E. rhusiopathiae* is catalase negative and nonmotile, while *L. monocytogenes* is catalase positive and motile. The neomycin susceptibility test can also be used to distinguish the two organisms. *E. rhusiopathiae* is resistant to neomycin, whereas *L. monocytogenes* is susceptible (11). *E. rhusiopathiae* has occasionally been misidentified as a viridans streptococcus, and since it decolonizes readily, as a Gram-negative rod it has also been dismissed as a contaminant.

SUSCEPTIBILITY IN VITRO

Because of the small number of reported cases of systemic human infection with *E. rhusiopathiae,* antibiotic susceptibility data are limited. Overall, *E. rhusiopathiae* is very susceptible to penicillins and to cephalosporins (6, 16, 18). Penicillin and imipenem were the most active of 16 agents tested by a macrodilution method in cation-supplemented Mueller-Hinton broth with 5% horse blood (18). Additional blood was required because some *E. rhusiopathiae* strains showed poor growth in Mueller-Hinton broth in preliminary testing. Penicillin and imipenem were inhibitory or bactericidal for all ten isolates tested at concentrations of 0.01 and 0.06 μg/ml, respectively. The next most active antibiotics were cefotaxime and piperacillin, which were bactericidal at concentrations of 0.12 and 0.25 μg/ml, respectively. Clindamycin and quinolones are also active against *E. rhusiopathiae*. Although clindamycin was inhibitory for all isolates tested with an MIC range of 0.01–1μg/ml, it was usually not bactericidal. Of the fluoroquinolones, only pefloxacin and ciprofloxacin were tested (18). Ciprofloxacin was superior to pefloxacin and showed MIC and MBC results similar to those obtained with β-lactam antibiotics. Chloramphenicol, erythromycin, and tetracycline are inhibitory for many *E. rhusiopathiae* isolates. Emergence of *E. rhusiopathiae* strains that are resistant to these three antibiotics is arising as a consequence of animals eating antibiotic-containing feed (16).

Susceptibility of *E. rhusiopathiae* to vancomycin has been determined by disk diffusion or by MIC testing in eight isolates from systemic human infection reported in the medical literature and nine isolates from swine (6, 7, 15, 17, 18). Virtually all isolates of *E. rhusiopathiae* are resistant to vancomycin (MIC 25 μg/ml). Teicoplanin and daptomycin appear to be somewhat more active than vancomycin. These agents were inhibitory for a human isolate at 4 and 2 μg/ml respectively (18). They were not bactericidal. Trimethoprim-sulfamethoxazole and aminoglycosides are inactive against *E. rhusiopathiae*. Mechanisms of resistance are unknown although *E. rhusiopathiae* is known to have plasmids.

ANTIMICROBIAL THERAPY
General

Despite being ubiquitous in nature, infection with *Erysipelothrix* is rare. In humans, *E. rhusiopathiae* manifests itself primarily as a skin disease. Except for one case of erysipeloid in a sheep farmer with coexisting orf, all other reported cases have been monomicrobial (1). Based on in vitro susceptibility data and on clinical experience reported in the literature, penicillin G is the drug of choice for infections caused by *E. rhusiopathiae* (6, 8). Alternatives to penicillin have seldom been used in therapy. Cephalosporins are an alternative for the penicillin allergic patient. Use of quinolones, in particular, ofloxacin or ciprofloxacin, may be considered in *Erysipelothrix* infections when the patient is allergic to β-lactams. Clindamycin may be used if the patient does not have endocarditis. Tetracyclines and erythromycin are another alternative if susceptibility is documented. Resistance to vancomycin and to gentamicin is important because these agents are often used empirically to treat bacteremia due to gram-positive organisms or in those who are allergic to β-lactams.

Specific Infections
Erysipeloid

Erysipeloid usually resolves without treatment within three to four weeks. Intramuscular penicillin has been shown to shorten the course of erysipeloid from an average of 17.4 to 2 days (9). The optimum dosage and duration of penicillin therapy for erysipeloid have not been defined ; oral penicillin at a dose of one gram per day for five to seven days is probably adequate for most uncomplicated cases. Although data on the quinolones and *Erysipelothrix* infections are minimal, ofloxacin at 200 mg orally twice a day was successful in curing erysipeloid (4).

Bacteremia/Endocarditis

Because of the high rate of endocarditis among cases of bacteremia, most of the cases of bacteremia reported in the literature have been treated with at least two weeks of parenteral penicillin G at doses of 12–20 million units per day often followed by one to two weeks of oral penicillin or amoxicillin (5, 10). Patients with the diffuse cutaneous form should probably be treated like the bacteremic patients with at least two weeks of intravenous penicillin G (12 million units daily). Two cases of bacteremia in penicillin allergic immunocompromised hosts were treated successfully with either clindamycin alone for two weeks or erythromycin for six weeks with rifampin for three weeks (1, 14).

The recommended antibiotic therapy for endocarditis is 12 to 20 million units of penicillin G per day in divided doses for 4 to 6 weeks. Synergy with aminoglycosides has not been demonstrated. Shorter causes consisting of 2 weeks of IV penicillin followed by 2–4 weeks of oral penicillin have been reported to be successful (12).

Other Focal Infections

There is a paucity of data in the literature on the treatment of serious focal infections such as brain abscess and bone and joint infections. Brain abscess should be treated with high dose intravenous penicillin for at least six weeks and until resolution by CT scan. Although not established as such by reports in the literature, the author recommends ofloxacin at 400 mg orally twice a day or ciprofloxacin orally twice a day for six weeks for treatment of osteomyelitis.

ENDPOINTS FOR MONITORING THERAPY

Because of the limited clinical experience with this organism, therapeutic response should be monitored clinically.

COMMENTS

Despite antibiotic therapy, mortality is about 38% in cases of endocarditis, with most deaths attributed to complications of endocarditis (6). Over one third of the patients with endocarditis reported in the literature required valve replacement (6).

REFERENCES

1. Berg RA. *Erysipelothrix rhusiopathiae*. South Med J 1984;77: 1614.
2. Connor MP, Green AD. Erysipeloid infection in a sheep farmer with coexisting orf. J Infect 1995;30:161–163.
3. Fliegelman RM, Cohen RS, Zakhireh B. *Erysipelothrix rhusiopathiae* endocarditis: report of a case and review of the literature. J Am Osteopath Assoc 1985;85:39–42.
4. Fritzen T, Marx E, Uy J. Treatment of surgical infections with a modern quinolone: Therapy of soft tissue infections and pneumonia with ofloxacin. Infection 1986;14(Suppl 4):S293.
5. García-Restoy E, Espejo E, Bella F, Llebot J. Bacteremia due to *Erysipelothrix rhusiopathiae* in immunocompromised hosts without endocarditis. Rev Infect Dis 1991;13:1252–1253.
6. Gorby GL, Peacock JE Jr. *Erysipelothrix rhusiopathiae* endocarditis: microbiologic, epidemiologic, and clinical features of an occupational disease. Rev Infect Dis 1988;10:317–325.
7. Grandsen WR, Eykyn SJ. *Erysipelothrix rhusiopathiae* endocarditis. Rev Infect Dis 1988;10:1228.
8. Grieco MH, Sheldon C. *Erysipelothrix rhusiopathiae*. Ann NY Acad Sci 1970;174:523–532.
9. King PF. Erysipeloid. Survey of 115 cases. Lancet 1946;ii: 196–198.
10. Ognibene FP, Cunnion RE, Gill V, Ambrus J, Fauci AS, Parrillo JE. *Erysipelothrix rhusiopathiae* bacteremia presenting as septic shock. Am J Med 1985;78:861–864.
11. Reboli AC, Farrar WE. The genus *Erysipelothrix*. In: Balows A, Truper HG, Dworkin M, Harder W, Schleifer KH, Editors. The prokaryotes. A handbook on the biology of bacteria: ecophysiology, isolation, identification, applications. New York: Springer-Verlag, 1992;1629–1642.
12. Reboli AC, Farrar WE. *Erysipelothrix rhusiopathiae:* An occupational pathogen. Clin Microbiol Rev 1989;2:354–359.
13. Reboli AC, Farrar WE. *Erysipelothrix rhusiopathiae*. In: Mandell GL, Bennett JE, Dolin R, eds. Principals and practice of infectious diseases. New York: Churchill Livingstone, 1995;4: 1894–1896.
14. Shumack SL, McDonald S, Baer P. Erysipelothrix septicemia in an immunocompromised host. Can Med Assoc J 1987;136:273.
15. Simberkoff MS, Rahal JJ Jr. Acute and subacute endocarditis due to *Erysipelothrix rhusiopathiae*. Am J Med Sci 1973;266: 53–57.

16. Takahashi T, Sawada T, Ohmae K. Antibiotic resistance of *Erysipelothrix rhusiopathiae* isolated from pigs with chronic swine erysipelas. Antimicrob Agents Chemother 1984;25:385–386.

17. Venditti M, Gelfusa V, Tarasi A, Brandimarte C, Serra P. An-timicrobial susceptibilities of *Erysipelothrix rhusiopathiae*. Antimicrob Agents Chemother 1990;2038–2040.

18. Venditti M, Gelfusa V, Castelli F, Brandimarte C, Serra P. *Erysipelothrix rhusiopathiae* endocarditis. Eur J Clin Microbiol Infect Dis 1990;9:50–52.

Escherichia coli

●

Nathan M. Thielman and Richard L. Guerrant

GENERAL DESCRIPTION

In 1885 Theodor Escherich described *Escherichia coli* and named the organism *Bacterium coli commune*. Nine years later he noted its role as a human pathogen and postulated that the organism was responsible for ascending urinary tract infections in young women (99). *E. coli* is nearly ubiquitous and is present in virtually all animal and human intestinal tracts (105). In humans, it is the major aerobic organism residing in the intestine, typically with about 10^6 to 10^9 colony-forming units per gram of stool (9, 18). The organism is also found in soil and water, usually as a result of fecal contamination. The clinically important strains of *E. coli* are not morphologically or biochemically distinct from those that reside as commensal gut flora, although, as indicated below, certain serogroups may predominate in given types of *E. coli* infections. In addition to its important role in causing watery, inflammatory, and hemorrhagic diarrheal illnesses, *E. coli* is a major cause of neonatal meningitis (38), nosocomial bacteremia, and surgical site infections and is the leading cause of urinary tract infections (24).

The organism is a short Gram-negative bacillus that grows readily on simple culture media or synthetic media with minimal nutrients; glucose or glycerol is often sufficient. Except for many of the enteroinvasive strains, *E. coli* is typically first identified in the microbiology laboratory as a lactose-fermenting Gram-negative rod. It is oxidase negative, produces indole, does not ferment citrate, and demonstrates a positive methyl red test and a negative Voges-Proskauer reaction.

E. coli strains can be typed according to their somatic lipopolysaccharide (O), capsular (K), and flagellar (H) antigens. At least 173 O, 80 K, and 56 H antigen types have been described (63). Certain O serogroups may predominate for the various types of enteric *E. coli* infections (Table 1). Most notable among these is *E. coli* O157, one of the major serogroups seen in enterohemorrhagic *E. coli* infections. For some *E. coli* infections elsewhere, certain K antigens have predominated. For example, K1 encapsulated strains constitute approximately 80% of *E. coli* causing neonatal meningitis (85). The association of particular serotypes with different disease patterns has proven useful for linking specific virulence factors (e.g., the various toxins, adhesins, and invasive properties) to pathogenicity.

The various classes of antibiotics that effectively inhibit *E. coli* are represented in Figure 1. Best understood among these are β-lactam antibiotics, which disrupt cell wall synthesis by binding to and inhibiting the penicillin-binding proteins essential for transpeptidation and carboxypeptidation reactions in cell wall peptidoglycan synthesis. β-Lactams cross the outer membrane into the periplasm via pores composed of porin proteins. Of several porin types expressed by *E. coli*, OmpC and OmpF are most important for the uptake of β-lactams, and decreased expression of these porins by *E. coli* elevates the MICs of many β-lactams (45). Once within the periplasmic space, β-lactams may be cleared by hydrolysis or covalent binding to β-lactamases or nonessential penicillin-binding proteins. Quinolones interfere with DNA supercoiling and promote DNA gyrase–mediated double-stranded DNA breakage (60). Resistance in *E. coli* has been observed in isolates with alterations in the A subunit of DNA gyrase at amino acid 83 (serine → tryptophan) (107) and in *E. coli* with decreased expression of porin outer-membrane protein OmpF (32, 33). In addition, an active efflux mechanism combined with decreased outer membrane permeability has been associated with decreased susceptibility of *E. coli* to norfloxacin (17). Both aminoglycosides and chloramphenicol inhibit *E. coli*, the former by binding irreversibly, and the later by binding reversibly, to the larger 50S subunit of the 70S bacterial ribosomes. Chloramphenicol resistance has been associated both with the presence of the enzyme chloramphenicol acetyltransferase, which acetylates the antibiotic to an inactive diacetyl derivative (93), and with an active efflux mechanism (48). In laboratory isolates of *E. coli*, resistance to aminoglycosides may develop because of impaired uptake and aminoglycoside phosphorylation (70), although enzymatic modification by acetylation of an amino group is considered the most common mechanism. Sulfonamides and trimethoprim interferes with bacterial folic acid synthesis by inhibiting tetrahydropteric acid synthetase and dihydrofolate reductase, respectively. Several mechanisms

TABLE 1 • Serogroup Clustering of Different Types of *E. coli* Infections	
Type of *E. coli* Infection	**Some Predominant Serogroups**
Enteric	
Enterotoxigenic (ETEC)	O groups: 1, 6,7, 8,9, 11, 12, 15, 20, 25, 27, 60, 63, 75, 78, 80, 85, 88, 89, 99, 101, 109, 114, 115, 128, 139, 148, 149, 153, 159, 166, 167
Enterohemorrhagic (EHEC)	O groups: 157, 26, 103, 111, 113, + about 50 others
Enteroinvasive (EIEC)	O groups: 11, 28, 29, 112, 115, 121, 124, 136, 143, 144, 147, 152, 164, 173
Enteropathogenic (EPEC)	O groups: 18, 26, 44, 55, 86, 111, 114, 119, 125, 126, 127, 128, 142, 157, 158
Enteroaggregative (EAggEC)	O groups: 3, 15, 44, 51, 77, 78, 86, 91, 92, 111, 113, 126, 141, 146
Diffusely adherent (DAEC)	O groups: 75, 11, 15, 126
Urinary tract infection	O:K:H groups: O1:K1:H7, O4:K12:H5, O4:K12:H1, O6:K13:H1, and others
Bacteremia	O:K:H groups: O4:K12:H5, O2:K2:H1, O2:K1:H4, O1:K1:H-, O75:K5:H5, and others
Central nervous system	O:K:H groups: O18ac:K1:H7, O7:K1:H1, O2:K1:H6, O16:K1:H6, O83:K1:H4, and others

may account for the trimethoprim-sulfamethoxazole resistance rates ranging from the teens in the United States and western Europe to up to 63% in Thailand for *E. coli* (106). These include alterations of substrate enzymes or their overproduction, loss of bacterial drug-binding capacity, and decreased cell permeability (34, 98).

SUSCEPTIBILITY IN VITRO

Table 2 lists in vitro activity data for a broad range of antimicrobial agents against *E. coli* from multiple studies published since 1987. The range of minimum inhibitory concentrations (MICs), along with MIC_{50} and MIC_{90} data,

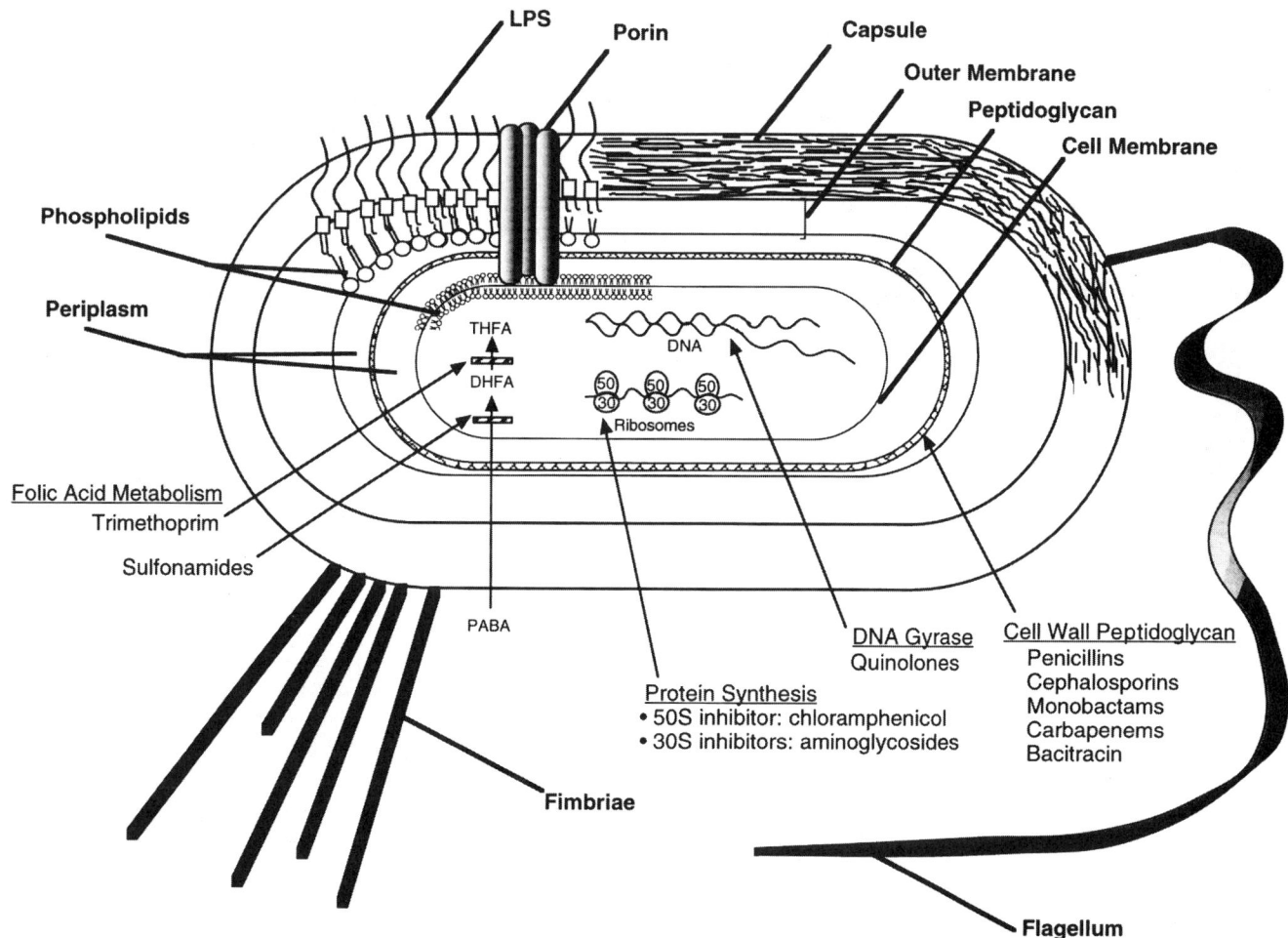

FIGURE 1. Schematic representation of *E. coli* with sites of action of various antibiotics. *LPS,* lipopolysaccharide; *mRNA,* messenger RNA; *PABA, p*-aminobenzoic acid; *DHFA,* dihydrofolic acid; *THFA,* tetrahydrofolic acid.

TABLE 2 • In Vitro Susceptibility of *Escherichia coli* to Antimicrobials[a]

Antibiotic	n	Range (µg/mL)	MIC$_{50}$(µg/mL)	MIC$_{90}$(µg/mL)	Reference
Amikacin	108	0.78–12.5	1.56	3.13	52
Amikacin	373	≤0.5–16	2	4	101
Amoxicillin	10	<2->128	>128	>128	80
Amoxicillin and clavulanic acid	100	≤2->64	16	32	87
Amoxicillin and clavulanic acid	44	—	2/1	4/2	56
Amoxicillin and clavulanic acid	10	<2–16	4	16	80
Ampicillin	512	2->128	8	16	83
Aztreonam	20	≤0.032–0.5	0.062	0.125	3
Aztreonam	373	≤1->64	≤1	≤1	101
Aztreonam	108	≤0.008–4	0.03	0.12	46
Cefaclor	44	—	1	2	56
Cefaclor	10	1–16	4	16	80
Cefaclor	98	1–256	2	16	44
Cefadroxil	44	—	4	4	56
Cefepime	108	≤0.008–2	0.01	0.12	46
Cefepime	373	≤0.5->64	≤0.5	≤0.5	101
Cefepime	105	0/008–1	0.03	0.06	49
Cefepime	98	<0.06–0.5	<0.06	0.12	44
Cefepime	43	0.025–6.25	0.05	0.20	95
Cefixime	44	—	0.12	0.5	56
Cefotaxime	108	≤0.008–8	0.06	0.12	46
Cefotaxime	98	<0.06–64	<0.06	0.12	44
Cefotaxime	15	0.015–0.25	0.06	0.12	29
Cefotaxime	528	0.03–8.0	0.006	0.25	19
Cefotaxime	512	≤0.01–4	0.06	0.13	83
Cefotaxime	373	≤0.5->64	≤0.5	≤0.5	101
Cefpirome	43	0.025–6.25	0.10	0.20	95
Cefprozil	10	1–16	2	8	80
Ceftazidime	43	0.10–100	0.20	0.78	95
Ceftazidime	20	0.062–0.25	0.125	0.25	3
Ceftazidime	27	0.05–0.39	0.1	0.2	4
Ceftazidime	108	0.03–4	0.12	0.5	46
Ceftazidime	108	0.025–0.78	0.10	0.20	62
Ceftazidime	98	<0.06–64	0.12	0.25	44
Ceftazidime	40	0.05–0.78	0.2	0.39	61
Ceftazidime	15	0.03–1	0.25	0.5	29
Ceftazidime	528	0.03–16	0.006	0.25	19
Ceftazidime	373	≤0.5->64	≤0.5	≤0.5	101
Cefpirome	108	≤0.008–2	0.03	1	46
Cefpirome	40	0.025–0.78	0.05	0.2	61
Ceftriaxone	27	0.025–0.1	0.05	0.05	4
Ceftriaxone	98	<0.006–64	<0.006	0.12	44
Ceftriaxone	32	0.008–0.25	0.03	0.06	37
Ceftriaxone	373	≤0.5->64	≤0.5	≤0.5	101
Cefuroxime	44	—	1	2	56
Cefuroxime	10	1–16	4	8	80
Cefuroxime	100	≤2–64	4	16	87
Cefuroxime	98	0.25–256	4	16	44
Cephalexin	98	2–256	8	16	44
Cephalexin	100	≤2–≥64	4	64	87
Cephalexin	10	4–8	4	8	80
Cephalexin	44	—	4	4	56
Cephalothin	512	1->128	8	16	83
Cephalothin	100	4->64	32	>64	87
Ciprofloxacin	20	≤0.008	≤0.008	≤0.008	3
Ciprofloxacin	29	≤0.03	≤0.03	≤0.03	16
Ciprofloxacin	108	≤0.006–1.56	0.012	0.025	52
Ciprofloxacin	98	<0.06–32	<0.06	0.12	44
Ciprofloxacin	528	0.008–0.5	0.015	0.03	19
Ciprofloxacin	373	≤0.12->16	≤0.12	≤0.12	101
Ciprofloxacin	100	≤0.006–0.78	0.013	0.025	16

continued

TABLE 2 • **In Vitro Susceptibility of** *Escherichia coli* **to Antimicrobials**[a]

Antibiotic	n	Range (μg/mL)	MIC$_{50}$(μg/mL)	MIC$_{90}$(μg/mL)	Reference
Ciprofloxacin	40	0.012–0.2	0.025	0.025	35
Ciprofloxacin	32	0.002–0.03	0.008	0.003	37
Clarithromycin	10	8–>64	16	32	80
Doxycycline	10	<0.5–>32	1	2	80
Enoxacin	20	≤0.008–0.06 3	0.016	0.032	3
Erythromycin	10	All >32	>32	>32	80
Fleroxacin	108	0.05–25	0.10	0.20	52
Gentamicin	20	0.25–4	0.5	1.0	3
Gentamicin	108	0.20–>100	0.78	0.78	52
Gentamicin	512	0.25–4	1	1	83
Gentamicin	373	≤1–>64	≤1	≤1	101
Imipenem	20	0.125–0.5	0.25	0.25	3
Imipenem	108	0.05–0.78	0.10	0.20	52
Imipenem	108	0.01–0.25	0.12	0.25	46
Imipenem	32	0.06–0.25	0.12	0.25	37
Imipenem	15	0.03–0.5	0.25	0.5	29
Imipenem	528	0.06–2.0	0.06	0.25	19
Imipenem	373	≤0.12–>16	≤0.12	≤0.12	101
Lomefloxacin	40	0.1–1.56	0.2	0.2	35
Lomefloxacin	29	≤0.03–0.12	0.12	0.12	16
Mecillinam	512	0.13–>128	0.5	1	83
Meropenem	32	0.02–0.06	0.03	0.06	37
Minocycline	108	0.78–>100	3.13	50	52
Nalidixic acid	512	1–>128	2	4	83
Nitrofurantoin	512	2–128	16	16	83
Norfloxacin	20	≤0.008–0.032	≤0.008	0.016	3
Norfloxacin	100	0.013–3.13	0.05	0.10	16
Norfloxacin	108	0.012–6.25	0.05	0.10	52
Norfloxacin	512	≤0.01–1	0.06	0.06	83
Ofloxacin	40	0.05–0.78	0.1	0.1	35
Ofloxacin	20	≤0.008–0.032	≤0.008	0.016	3
Ofloxacin	29	≤0.03–0.12	0.06	0.06	16
Ofloxacin	108	0.025–12.5	0.05	0.10	52
Piperacillin/tazobactam	373	≤2–>256	≤2	4	101
Piperacilin/tazobactam	528	0.25–128.0	1.0	2.0	29
Piperacillin	373	≤2–≤256	≤2	>256	101
Piperacillin	15	0.25–>128	32	>128	29
Piperacillin	20	0.5–>256	1.0	256	3
Sparfloxacin	40	0.1–1.56	0.39	0.78	35
Sparfloxacin	29	≤0.03	0.03	0.03	16
Sulfamethoxazole	512	5–512	32	512	83
Temafloxacin	100	0.025–6.25	0.10	0.20	57
Tosufloxacin	108	≤0.006–3.13	0.025	0.05	52
Ticarcillin/ clavulanic acid	528	0.25–>256	2.0	32	19
Ticarcillin/ clavulanic acid	373	≤2–>256	≤2	64	101
Tobramycin	20	0.5–16	0.5	1.0	3
Trimethoprim	512	≤0.06–>64	0.25	0.5	83
TMP-SMX	512	0.25–>128	1	2	83
TMP-SMX	20	≤0.063/1.19–0.5/9.5	0.125/2.38	0.25/4.75	3
Zidovudine	9	0.031–1	0.125	—	89
ddl	9	31–>62.5	62.5		89

[a]All studies reported reflect clinical isolates except that of ref 88, in which trimethoprim-resistant isolates from stools of children attending day-care centers were selected for study.

representing minimum concentrations that inhibit 50 and 90% of strains, respectively, are given for each.

Emerging Trends in Resistance of Differing Types of *E. coli* Infections

The factors associated with the emergence of antibiotic resistance in *E. coli* have been studied in more depth and breadth than perhaps in any other species. These factors include, of course, direct ingestion of food and water harboring resistant strains, as well as incidental fecal-oral cross-contamination (which frequently occurs among children in day-care centers, households, hospitals, and in settings where sanitation is poor), selective ecologic pressure exerted by various antimicrobials, and regional differences in susceptibility patterns.

Regional Trends

Shortly after the introduction of trimethoprim and trimethoprim-sulfamethoxazole (TMP-SMX) in the 1970s, the emergence of trimethoprim resistance in fecal *E. coli* was reported among travelers to Mexico who were taking trimethoprim or TMP-SMX for the prophylaxis of traveler's diarrhea (55). In contrast, several studies in the United States and elsewhere documented little or no emergence of trimethoprim- or TMP-SMX-resistant *E. coli* (30, 31, 66, 91), and it was hypothesized that the widespread use of TMP-SMX over the counter in Mexico may have contributed to this initial observation (55). In a subsequent study of travelers to Mexico not taking prophylactic antimicrobial agents, resistance to ampicillin, chloramphenicol, kanamycin, streptomycin, sufonamides, tetracycline, trimethoprim, and TMP-SMX, but not gentamicin, increased significantly over time (54). Whereas no trimethoprim/TMP-SMX-resistant isolates were found prior to travel, by the final week in Mexico 57% of individuals harbored trimethoprim- and TMP-SMX-resistant strains. Another study demonstrated resistance to TMP-SMX in 40% of clinical *E. coli* isolates in 1983 in Chile and Thailand, compared with 8% of concurrent *E. coli* isolates in the United States (53). More recently, Calva et al. studied 20 healthy children from a periurban community in Mexico and found that 90% of *E. coli* isolates were resistant to ampicillin, 77% were resistant to trimethoprim, and 62% were resistant to tetracycline (10). Simultaneous resistance to more than one antibiotic by an *E. coli* isolate was observed in 88% of stool samples.

In a well-designed study, Lester et al. (42) clearly identified regional differences spanning three continents in carriage of resistant *E. coli*. Using identical microbiologic techniques, the resistance profiles of *E. coli* in stool samples from untreated healthy children in Boston were compared with similar source populations in Caracas, Venezuela, and in Qin Pu, China. While 21 of 39 children in Boston had no resistant colonies, all but 1 of 41 children in Caracas and all but 2 of 53 in Qin Pu carried resistant strains of *E. coli*. In all three cities, over half the resistant isolates were resistant to more than one agent, and resistance to three or more antimicrobials was found in only 6% of colonies from Boston, but 42% and 30% of colonies from Qin Pu and Caracas, respectively.

Day-Care Centers, Households, and Communities

Like numerous other organisms, such as *Cryptosporidium*, hepatitis A, and *Giardia* (26, 96), *E. coli* is readily spread among children in day-care centers. Not surprisingly, children in day-care centers (many of whom receive frequently receive antimicrobials) have been found to harbor increased numbers of antibiotic resistant *E. coli*. Reves et al. (78) reported that 19% of children in seven day-care centers in Houston were colonized with trimethoprim-resistant *E. coli* at a time when resistance among clinical isolates, even among nosocomial strains, was comparatively low, ranging from 7 to 13% in four hospitals in Boston, St. Louis, and Houston. In a subsequent study, the prevalence of trimethoprim-resistant fecal *E. coli* isolates among children in day-care centers was 30%, compared with 6% among control children and 8% among medical students.

Significant risk factors for colonization with resistant strains were enrollment of over 40 diapered children and age less than 12 months (77). Trimethoprim-resistant *E. coli* are easily spread within day-care centers and among household members of children attending day-care centers who are colonized with such strains. A 13-fold increase in colonization rates was observed in household members of colonized center children versus those of noncolonized children, and mothers and siblings tended to be colonized more than fathers (35 and 30% vs. 12%) (25). Of note, among trimethoprim-resistant isolates, (many of which were also resistant to sufisoxazole, streptomycin, and ampicillin) from these children, cefuroxime, cephalexin, and amoxicillin-clavulanic acid remained generally active at concentrations achievable in urine; 77% of isolates, however, were resistant to cephalothin (87).

Spread of trimethoprim-resistant *E. coli* to family members of outpatients being treated with trimethoprim has also been observed (82), and multiresistant *E. coli* isolates with the same antibiograms and serogrouping have been associated with epidemic infections in the community (71).

Clinical *E. coli* Isolates

Bloodstream and Nosocomial Isolates. Paralleling the changes in resistance ecology in the communities, clinical isolates of *E. coli* have demonstrated increased resistance to several antimicrobials in recent decades. The pattern of initial susceptibility to a new antibiotic followed by gradual emergence of resistance was first demonstrated in *E. coli* in the 1960s. After introduction of the new β-lactam ampicillin early in that decade, plasmid-mediated β-lactamase resistance emerged, and by the late 1960s, 30 to 50% of hospital-acquired *E. coli* were resistant (59). More recently, there have been reports of extended-spectrum β-lactamases in clinical *E. coli* isolates, and fluoroquinolone resistance is increasing markedly with the widespread use of these drugs in the community (68).

Among nosocomial *E. coli* isolates reported in the National Nosocomial Infections Surveillance (NNIS) system, ampicillin resistance increased from 28.8% in 1987 to 38.4% in 1994, and ciprofloxacin resistance increased from 0.3% in 1989 to 1.4% in 1994 (Fig. 2) (106). In a 1991 study of antibiotic susceptibility patterns among clinical isolates from 39 French intensive care units at teaching hospitals (36), more than 95% of *E. coli* isolates were susceptible to ceftriaxone, ceftazidime, aztreonam, imipenem, gentamicin, tobramycin, and ciprofloxacin. Only 58% of strains were susceptible to piperacillin, and 90% to cefoxitin.

Durand-Gasselin et al. reported on changing susceptibility patterns from 1987 to 1992 among clinical *E. coli* isolates on a hematology unit in France. Amoxicillin susceptibility decreased from 62 to 37%; amoxicillin-clavulanic acid, 85 to 47%; piperacillin, 63 to 43%; and gentamicin, 96 to 89%, while cefotaxime, tobramycin, and amikacin susceptibility patterns changed very little. Ciprofloxacin susceptibility decreased from 100% in 1990 to 93% in 1992 (21). Among 474 episodes of *E. coli* bacteremia studied in one hospital in Spain, 95% of isolates remained susceptible to cefoxitin, cefotaxime, gentamicin, tobramycin, and amikacin (103).

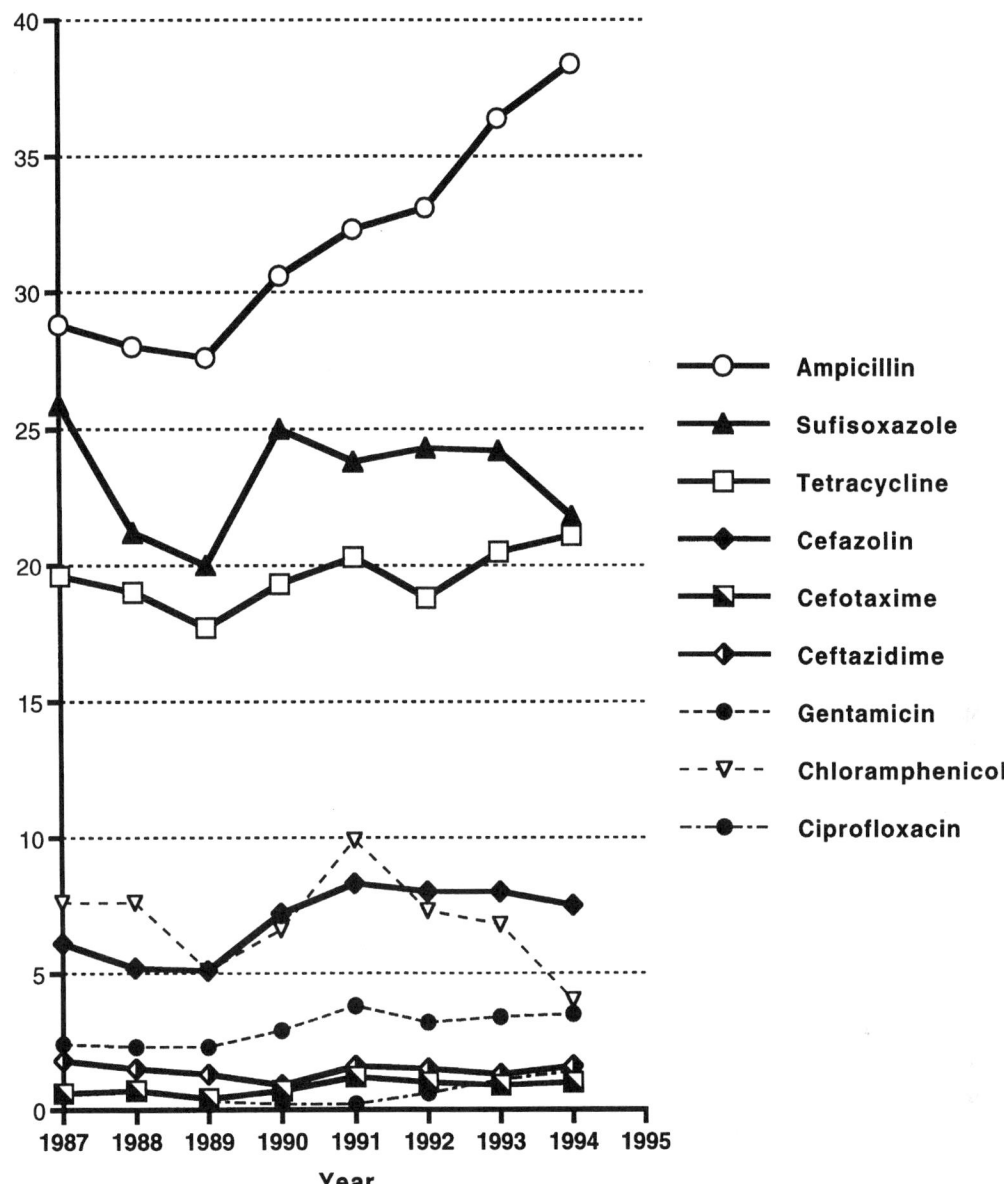

FIGURE 2. Trends in antimicrobial susceptibility of *E. coli* isolated reported to the NNIS system during 1986 to 1994. Data from Wiedemann B, Grimm H, Lorian V, eds. Susceptibility to antibiotics: species incidence and trends. Baltimore: Williams & Wilkins, 1996:900–1168. (*NNIS,* National Nosocomial Infections Surveillance.)

Although resistance of *E. coli* to fluoroquinolones was initially exceedingly rare, with MICs typically below 0.1 μg/mL, several reports have identified an even more disturbing trend in fluoroquinolone resistance than that reflected in the NNIS data and the Durand-Gasselin study. Among 23 cancer patients receiving prophylactic norfloxacin, new fluoroquinolone-resistant *E. coli* strains were subsequently isolated in 8 patients, and 1 patient developed fluoroquinolone-resistant *E. coli* bacteremia (12). In a separate analysis, 37% of *E. coli* bacteremic episodes in neutropenic patients with cancer were due to quinolone-resistant species (11). MICs for norfloxacin and ciprofloxacin ranged from 16 to 128 μg/mL and 8 to 64 μg/mL, respectively. All 13 patients with quinolone-resistant *E. coli* bacteremia had received prophylaxis with norfloxacin (compared with 1 of 22

patients with bacteremia due to susceptible *E. coli*), implicating fluoroquinolone prophylaxis in neutropenic patients as a significant risk factor for quinolone-resistant *E. coli* bacteremia. Because fecal carriage of resistant strains emerges rapidly in these patients (3 to 35 days, mean 10 for 8 of 23 patients) and occurs even in patients with no recent hospitalization or exposure to quinolones, it is likely that a significant reservoir of fluoroquinolone-resistance exists in the general population (12). Another study (68) documented an increase of *E. coli* bacteremia with ciprofloxacin-resistant strains from 0% in 1988 to 7.5% in 1992 and found a significant correlation between the incidence of ciprofloxacin-resistant *E. coli* bacteremia and the increased use of fluoroquinolones in the community; prior fluoroquinolone use was an independent risk factor. The lack of strong clonal relationships among such isolates (41, 62) provides indirect corroborative evidence of increasing background colonization in the general population, likely related to widespread use of fluoroquinolones in the community.

Although still relatively infrequent, extended-spectrum β-lactamases of both chromosomal and plasmid origin have been identified among blood culture isolates of *E. coli* with reduced susceptibility or resistance to cefotaxime, ceftazidime, and/or aztreonam (72).

Diarrhea Isolates.   Susceptibility data from the differing types of *E. coli* specifically associated with diarrhea are limited because most microbiology laboratories do not screen for diarrheagenic *E. coli* other than *E. coli* O157. It is not clear if antimicrobial susceptibility patterns of these diarrheagenic *E. coli* simply mimic those of nonpathogenic strains from the local community. Multidrug resistance to sulfonamides, tetracycline, trimethoprim, and ampicillin was identified in 53% of 49 enterotoxigenic *E. coli* (ETEC) strains isolated from British troops deployed in Saudi Arabia in 1990–1991 (108). Among 220 ETEC isolates from U.S. travelers to Guadalajara, Mexico, between 1987 and 1989, none were resistant to aztreonam, norfloxacin, ciprofloxacin, gentamicin, or furazolidone. High-level resistance to TMP-SMX was seen in 7% of *E. coli* (6). In Nigerian children with both ETEC (62 isolates) and enteropathogenic *E. coli* (EPEC) (100 isolates) associated diarrhea, high rates of resistance to many antibiotics were noted, including trimethoprim (35% and 42% of ETEC and EPEC strains, respectively), sulfamethoxazole (81%, 90%), ampicillin (58%, 41%), tetracycline (88%, 93%), and cephalothin (47%, 56%) (40). More than 93% of these isolates, however, were reported as sensitive to nalidixic acid. Notably, 41% of ETEC isolates in this study contained transmissible toxigenic

factors, raising the concern that toxigenic strains could become more populous with the increased used of antimicrobials to which the same organisms are resistant (40). *En block transfer* of both antibiotic resistance and toxigenic determinants has been demonstrated in vitro with a heat-labile toxin–producing equine strain (88).

Table 3 illustrates the differences in EPEC susceptibility reported since 1989 in various geographic regions (40, 43, 51, 86). Although there is some variability among EPEC identification methods and in vitro susceptibility testing between these studies, overall, both the African isolates and those from Singapore appear more resistant than those collected and studied in the United States (which were collected from 1950 to 1983). These differences may reflect again the influence of differing sanitation conditions as well as Darwinian selective pressure on the microbial flora from variable exposure to antimicrobials.

Enteroaggregative *E. coli* (EaggEC) isolates from Mexico, Chile, Peru, and Thailand studied by Yamamoto et al. (110) showed marked resistance in vitro to sulfamethoxazole, ampicillin, and chloramphenicol; 35% were highly resistant to trimethoprim, and all trimethoprim-resistant strains were also resistant to sulfamethoxazole. Fluoroquinolones, cefixime, and gentamicin all showed good activity against the EAggEC strains.

Most *E. coli* O157:H7 isolates are susceptible in vitro to antibiotics such as ampicillin, carbenicilllin, gentamicin, cephalothin, chloramphenicol, quinolones, trimethoprim, and TMP-SMX (27, 65, 75, 97).

Urinary Isolates.   As with the aforementioned *E. coli* pathogens and colonizers, urinary *E. coli* isolates have seen similar increased resistance to aminopenicillins and TMP-SMX over the past two decades. For example, among the thou-

---

TABLE 3 • Antimicrobial Resistance among Enteropathogenic *E. coli* strains

Antibiotic	U.S. Outbreaks[a] n = 28	Nairobi, Kenya[b] n = 78	Ibadan, Nigeria[c] n = 100	Singapore[d] n = 83
Oxytetracycline	—	100	—	—
Tetracycline	39	—	88	67
Ampicillin	39	100	58	41
Chloramphenicol	11	94	70	27
TMP-SMX	0	73	35	30
Sulfamethoxazole	—	—	81	—
Gentamicin	—	9	85	0
Streptomycin	64	—	—	67
Cefazolin	—	5	—	—
Cephalothin	32	—	47	—
Cefamandole	—	3	—	—
Cefotaxime	—	0	—	—
Ceftriaxone	—	—	—	0
Amikacin	—	3	—	—
Nalidixic acid	0	0	4	—

[a]EPEC serotype strains, resistance determined by single-disk diffusion (Moyenuddin et al., 1989).

[b]EPEC identified by EAF probe positivity, resistance determined by Neosensitab system (Ericsson HM and Sherris JC, 1971).

[c]EPEC identified serologically; resistance determined by disk diffusion (Lamikanra et al., 1990).

[d]EPEC identified serologically; resistance determined by disk diffusion (Lim et al., 1992).

sands of isolates from various general practices and hospitals in London, amoxicillin sensitivity declined from 84–91% to 57–66% from 1971 to 1989, and TMP-SMX sensitivity dropped from 97–99% to 78–83% (28). In a recent U.S. study of 183 bacteremic urinary tract infections in community hospitals, the in vitro susceptibility of cefazolin, ceftriaxone, gentamicin, aztreonam, TMP-SMX, and ciprofloxacin were all highly favorable (1). Although the quinolones remain an important drug of choice for urinary tract infections with *E. coli*, a disturbing trend in resistance patterns over time has emerged in some regions. Among 9934 isolates tested over a 10-year period in Spain, ciprofloxacin resistance (MIC $\geq$ 4 mg/L) increased from 0.8% in 1989 to 7.1% in 1992 (69).

ANTIMICROBIAL THERAPY

Despite the concerning trends in antimicrobial resistance among *E. coli* isolates worldwide, a growing armamentarium of antimicrobial agents provides multiple options for treating *E. coli* infections. Ironically, these newer agents are more readily available and affordable in developed nations where *E. coli* resistance is less of a problem than in the developing world. As with other *Enterobacteriaceae*, where and when available, antimicrobial testing of the infecting strain should direct therapy. In other situations, knowledge of recent local susceptibility patterns is useful for guiding treatment. In general, monotherapy with TMP-SMX, third-generation cephalosporins, and fluoro-

quinolones as drugs of choice is recommended for known infections with *E. coli*, although many broad-spectrum agents (such as β-lactam/β-lactamase inhibitor combinations and the carbapenems) remain highly active.

Special Situations

Urinary Tract Infections

Because *E. coli* accounts for nearly 80% of uncomplicated lower and upper urinary tract infections, practical management of *E. coli* urinary tract infections follows general empirical guidelines recently summarized (92) and presented in Table 4.

Enteric *E. coli* Infections

Placebo-controlled trials published in the early 1980s demonstrated the effectiveness of tetracycline, TMP-SMX, and trimethoprim alone in decreasing the duration of diarrhea in either naturally acquired ETEC infection or in volunteers experimentally infected with the organism (20, 50). As noted above, the high rates of TMP-SMX resistance throughout much of the developing world have prompted most authorities to now recommend fluoroquinolones for treatment (and, according to some, prophylaxis) of traveler's diarrhea, although TMP-SMX remained active for 93% of isolates in some areas of Mexico as recently as 1992 (5). Multiple studies have demonstrated the efficacy of fluoroquinolones in treatment of

TABLE 4a • Treatment Options for *E. coli* Urinary Tract Infections

Condition	Mitigating Circumstances	Treatment[a]	Duration
Acute uncomplicated cystitis in women	None	Oral TMP-SMX, trimethoprim, or fluoroquinolone	3 days
	Diabetes, symptoms for > 7 days, recent UTI, use of diaphragm, age > 65 years	Oral TMP-SMX, trimethoprim, or fluoroquinolone	Consider 7-day regimen
	Pregnancy	Oral: amoxicillin, macrocrystalline nitrofurantoin, cefpodoxime, or TMP-SMX[b]	Consider 7-day regimen
Acute uncomplicated pyelonephritis in women	Mild to moderate illness, no nausea or vomiting	Outpatient: TMP-SMX or fluoroquinolone	10 to 14 days
	Severe illnes or possible urosepsis	Hospitalization: parenteral TMP-SMX, ceftriaxone, ciprofloxacin, ofloxacin, levofloxacin—followed by oral TMP-SMX, or fluoroquinolone	Parenteral therapy until defervescence Oral therapy $\times$ 14 days
	Pregnancy	Hospitalization: parenteral ceftriaxone, aztreonam or TMP-SMX[c]—followed by oral cephalosporin or TMP-SMX[b]	Parenteral therapy until defervescence Oral therapy $\times$ 14 days
Complicated UTI[c]	Mild to moderate illness	Outpatient therapy: oral fluoroquinolone	10–14 days
	Severe illness or possible urosepsis	Hospitalization: parenteral ceftriaxone, ciprofloxacin, ofloxacin, aztreonam—followed by oral TMP-SMX or fluoroquinolone	Parenteral therapy until defervescence Oral therapy $\times$ 14–21 days

Adapted and modified from Stamm W, Hooton T. Management of urinary tract infections in adults. N Engl J Med 1993;329:1328–1334.

[a]See Table 4b for dosing information.

[b]TMP-SMX is not approved for use in pregnancy.

[c]Such as UTI associated with obstruction at any site in urinary tract, foreign body in urinary tract, evidence of voiding dysfunction (postvoid residual urine >100 mL or vesicoureteral reflux), recent invasive urologic procedure, renal transplant recipient, azotemia, surgically created ileal loop, UTI in males (24).

TABLE 4b • Oral and Parenteral Regimens for *E. coli* Urinary Tract Infections

Drug	Typical Adult Dose	Interval
Oral regimens		
TMP-SMX	160/800 mg	q. 12 h
Trimethoprim	100 mg	q. 12 h
Fluoroquinolones		
Ciprofloxacin	250 mg	q. 12 h
Norfloxacin	400 mg	q. 12 h
Ofloxacin	200 mg	q. 12 h
Lomefloxacin		400 mg q.d.
Enoxacin	400 mg	q. 12 h
Levofloxacin	250 mg	q. 12 h
Macrocrystalline nitrofurantoin	100 mg	q.i.d.
Amoxicillin	250 mg	q. 8 h
Cefpodoxime	100 mg	q. 12 h
Parenteral regimens		
TMP-SMX	160 mg/800 mg	q. 12 h
Ciprofloxacin	200–400 mg	q. 12 h
Ofloxacin	200–400 mg	q. 12 h
Ceftriaxone	1–2 g	Daily
Ampicillin	1 g	q. 6 h
Aztreonam	1 g	q. 8–12 h

TABLE 5 • Summary of Clinical Data Addressing Antimicrobial Therapy in Enterohemorrhagic *E. coli* Infections

Retrospective series

- No change in duration of symptoms in 11 of 23 Oregon patients receiving antibiotics (tetracycline or erythromycin) (79)
- No change in duration of symptoms in 37 of 80 Washington patients receiving antibiotics and no change in progression with HUS[a] (antibiotic history in 5 of 10 with HUS vs. 32 of 65 without) (64)
- No significant change in duration of symtoms in 9 of 28 patients receiving antibiotics in sporadic cases collected by CDC (7.5 vs 8.5 days) (76)
- 5 of 8 secondary cases in a nursing home outbreak received prior abx vs. 12 of 114 who remained well (RR10.3), and antibiotic use after onset of symptoms was associated with increased mortality (13)
- 5 of 8 patients with HUS received TMP-SMX vs. 0 of 7 without HUS in Utah institutional outbreak (67)
- 2 of 28 HUS patients had >24-h use of "appropriate" antibiotics vs. 29 of 73 without HUS (P = .001) (14)

Prospective series

- No significant change in clinical symptoms or HUS in 2 of 22 children receiving TMP-SMX vs. 4 of 25 not receiving TMP-SMX in a prospective randomized controlled trial (74)

[a] HUS, hemolytic-uremic syndrome.

traveler's diarrhea, including the subgroups infected with ETEC (22, 47, 84, 102). Short-course quinolone therapy for 3 days has documented efficacy in patients with traveler's diarrhea (47, 109), and Salam et al. recently demonstrated that single-dose (500 mg) ciprofloxacin therapy decreases the duration of diarrhea in travelers from 50 to 21 h (84). Ciprofloxacin resistance has emerged in multidrug-resistant *E. coli* isolates from travelers treated with ciprofloxacin (109).

The role of antimicrobial therapy for other enteric *E. coli* infections is less clear. Several reports suggest the efficacy of antibiotics in managing EPEC infections, but the only controlled trial specifically addressing EPEC infections was with 49 Ethiopian children in whom a single serotype predominated (100). Complete resolution of diarrhea was reported within 3 days in 73% of patients receiving TMP-SMX (and 76% in those receiving mecillinam) versus 7% in controls. Bacteriologic cure was confirmed in 53% of those receiving antibiotics versus none in the control group. Orally administered neomycin has been reported effective in some patients (58, 81) but not others (6, 7). In addition to rehydration therapy and antibiotics, parenteral nutritional supplementation may be helpful in the severely malnourished patient with EPEC infection (81). The efficacy of antimicrobials in the treatment of EAggEC has not been evaluated.

The role of antimicrobial therapy in EHEC disease is unclear. In vitro exposure of EHEC to sublethal concentrations of TMP-SMX, ciprofloxacin, and tetracycline has been reported to increase Shiga-like toxin production (104), but whether this phenomenon occurs in vivo is unknown. Summarized in Table 5 are the results of several clinical studies addressing the efficacy and safety of antibiotics. The association of antibiotics with increased risk of death in nursing home pa-

tients (13) and progression to hemolytic-uremic syndrome (HUS) in the institutional outbreak (67) in the retrospective studies may reflect allocation bias (i.e., those more ill to begin with were the ones to receive antibiotics) or true adverse events. Unfortunately, the prospective study, which found no difference in clinical symptoms or progression to HUS had limited statistical power owing to its small numbers and thus may have missed a true difference in the two groups. Further studies are needed to definitively address antimicrobial therapy in EHEC disease.

Bacillary dysentery associated with EIEC typically responds to appropriate antimicrobials targeting shigellosis. As with *Shigella* species and other *E. coli,* antibiotic susceptibility patterns vary geographically, and ampicillin and TMP-SMX may not be effective. Resistance to third-generation cephalosporins and quinolones, including nalidixic acid, is less common (73).

Prostatitis

As with urinary tract infections, *E. coli* are a leading cause of acute and chronic prostatitis, and the same antimicrobial regimens apply (Table 4). Because drugs that do not normally enter prostate tissue are effective in the acutely inflamed prostate, agents and regimens used for bacteremia (see below) are appropriate for acute prostatitis (39, 90). Chronic or recurring prostatitis can be treated with agents used for complicated urinary tract infections (Table 4), but relapses because of poor diffusion of many drugs into the prostatic parenchyma, altered prostatic pH with infection, or persistently infected calculi

(39) warrant chronic suppression with low doses of TMP-SMX, quinolones, nitrofurantoin, or naladixic acid (90).

Bacteremia

E. coli is often the most frequent species isolated in blood cultures of patients with septicemia and is the leading Gram-negative cause of bacteremia (behind staphylococci and streptococci). *E. coli* bacteremia in children may present without fever, especially in neonates, and is often community acquired, ampicillin resistant (especially in neonates), and associated with underlying immune deficiency, urinary infection, or lesions in the gastrointestinal tract (8); it carries approximately 18% mortality. Because of the frequency of resistance to ampicillin and other agents, a third-generation cephalosporin is the treatment of choice, pending susceptibility results.

Meningitis

Neonatal meningitis may be due to *E. coli* and is treated with a third-generation cephalosporin.

Mixed Intraabdominal Infections

In humans, the pharmacodynamic activity of cefotaxime plus metronidazole against *E. coli* is superior to that of ampicillin-sulbactam or cefoxitin (and less expensive), making this an excellent choice of drugs for empirical coverage of uncomplicated intraabdominal infections.

REFERENCES

1. Ackermann R, Monroe P. Bacteremic urinary tract infection in older people. J Am Geriatr Soc 1996;44:927–933.
2. Anonymous. National Nosocomial Infections Surveillance (NNIS) report: data summary from October 1986–April 1996.
3. Arguedas A, Akaniro J, Stutman H, Marks M. In vitro activity of tosufloxacin, a new quinolone, against respiratory pathogens derived from cystic fibrosis sputum. Antimicrob Agents Chemother 1990;34:2223–2227.
4. Arisawa M, Sekine Y, Shimizu S, Takano H, Angehrn P, Then R. In vitro and in vivo evaluation of Ro 09-1428, a new parenteral cephalosporin with high antipseudomonal activity. Antimicrob Agents Chemother 1991;35:653–659.
5. Bandres J, Mathewson J, Ericsson C, DuPont H. Trimethoprim/sulfamethoxazole remains active against enterotoxigenic Escherichia coli and Shigella species in Guadalajara, Mexico. Am J Med Sci 1992;303:289–291.
6. Bartlett A, Torun B, Morales C, Cano F, Cruz J. Oral gentamicin is not effective treatment for persistent diarrhea. Acta Paediatr Suppl 1992;381:149–154.
7. Bhatnagar S, Bhan M, Sazawal S, Gupta U, George C, Arora N, Kashyap D. Efficacy of massive dose oral gentamicin therapy in nonbloody persistent diarrhea with associated malnutrition. J Pediatr Gastroenterol Nutr 1992;15:117–124.
8. Bonadio W, Smith D, Madagame E, Machi J, Kini N. Escherichia coli bacteremia in children. A review of 91 cases in 10 years. Am J Dis Child 1991;145:671–674.
9. Bonten M, Stobberingh E, Philips J, Houben A. High prevalence of antibiotic resistant Escherichia coli in faecal samples of students in the south-east of the Netherlands. J Antimicrob Chemother 1990;26:585–592.
10. Calva J, Sifuentes-Osornio J, Ceron C. Antimicrobial resistance in fecal flora: longitudinal community-based surveillance of children from urban Mexico. Antimicrob Agents Chemother 1996;40:1699–1702.
11. Carratala J, Fernandez-Sevilla A, Tubau F, Callis M, Gudiol F. Emergence of quinolone-resistant Escherichia coli bacteremia in neutropenic patients with cancer who have received prophylactic norfloxacin. Clin Infect Dis 1995;20:557–560; discussion 5.
12. Carratala J, Fernandez-Sevilla A, Tubau F, Dominguez M, Gudiol F. Emergence of fluoroquinolone-resistant Escherichia coli in fecal flora of cancer patients receiving norfloxacin prophylaxis. Antimicrob Agents Chemother 1996;40:503–505.
13. Carter A, Borczyk A, Carlson J, Harvey B, Hockin J, Karmali M, Krishnan C, Korn D, Lior H. A severe outbreak of Escherichia coli O157:H7–associated hemorrhagic colitis in a nursing home. N Engl J Med 1987;317:1496–1500.
14. Cimolai N, Carter J, Morrison B, Anderson J. Risk factors for the progression of Escherichia coli O157:H7 enteritis to hemolytic-uremic syndrome [published erratum appears in J Pediatr 1990;116:1008] [see comments]. J Pediatr 1990;116:589–592.
15. Clausen C, Christie D. Chronic diarrhea in infants caused by adherent enteropathogenic Escherichia coli. J Pediatr 1982;100:358–361.
16. Clement J, Tanaka S, Alder J, Vojtko C, Beyer J, Hensey D, Ramer N, McDaniel D, Chu D. In vitro and in vivo evaluations of A-80556, a new fluoroquinolone. Antimicrob Agents Chemother 1994;38:1071–1078.
17. Cohen S, Hooper D, Wolfson J, Souza K, McMurry L, Levy S. Endogenous active efflux of norfloxacin in susceptible Escherichia coli. Antimicrob Agents Chemother 1988;32:1187–1191.
18. Conway P, Macfarlane G. Microbial ecology of the human large intestine. In: Gibson G, ed. London: CRC Press, 1995:1–24.
19. Daley D, Mulgrave L, Munro R, Neville S, Smith H, Dimech W. An evaluation of the in vitro activity of piperacillin/tazobactam. Pathology 1996;28:167–172.
20. DuPont H, Reves R, Galindo E, Sullivan P, Wood L, Mendiola J. Treatment of travelers' diarrhea with trimethoprim/sulfamethoxazole and with trimethoprim alone. N Engl J Med 1982;307: 841–844.
21. Durand-Gasselin B, Leclercq R, Girard-Pipau F, Deharvengt M, Rochant H, Astier A, Duval J, Cordonnier C. Evolution of bacterial susceptibility to antibiotics during a six-year period in a haematology unit [see comments]. J Hosp Infect 1995;29:19–33.
22. Ericsson C, Johnson P, DuPont H, Morgan D, Bitsura J, dela-Cabada F. Ciprofloxacin or trimethoprim-sulfamethoxazole as initial therapy for travelers' diarrhea. A placebo-controlled, randomized trial. Ann Intern Med 1987;106:216–220.
23. Ericsson C, Sherris J. Antibiotic sensitivity testing. Report of an international collaborative study. Acta Pathol Microbiol Scand 1971;Sect B, Suppl 2.
24. Falagas M, Gorbach S. Practice guidelines: urinary tract infections. Infect Dis Clin Pract 1995;4:241–257.
25. Fornasini M, Reves R, Murray B, Morrow A, Pickering L. Trimethoprim-resistant Escherichia coli in households of children attending day care centers. J Infect Dis 1992;166:326–330.
26. Goodman R, Osterholm M, Granoff D, Pickering L. Infectious diseases and child day care. Pediatrics 1984;74:134–139.
27. Griffin P, Ostroff S, Tauxe R, Greene K, Wells J, Lewis J, Blake P. Illnesses associated with Escherichia coli O157:H7 infections. A broad clinical spectrum [Review; 41 refs]. Ann Intern Med 1988;109:705–712.

28. Gruneberg R. Changes in the antibiotic sensitivities of urinary pathogens, 1971–1989. J Antimicrob Chemother 1990;26(Suppl F):3–11.

29. Gu J, Chin N, Neu H. In vitro activity of an oxycephem OCP 9–176 compared with its sulfur analog and other beta-lactams. Diagn Microbiol Infect Dis 1991;14:135–140.

30. Guerrant R, Wood S, Krongaard L, Reid R, Hodge R. Resistance among fecal flora of patients taking sulfamethoxazole-trimethoprim or trimethoprim alone. Antimicrob Agents Chemother 1981;19:33–38.

31. Gurwith M, Brunton J, Lank B, Harding G, Ronald A. A prospective controlled investigation of prophylactic trimethoprim/sulfamethoxazole in hospitalized granulocytopenic patients. Am J Med 1979;66:248–256.

32. Hooper D, Wolfson J, Bozza M, Ng E. Genetics and regulation of outer membrane protein expression by quinolone resistance loci nfxB, nfxC, and cfxB. Antimicrob Agents Chemother 1992;36:1151–1154.

33. Hooper D, Wolfson J, Souza K, Ng E, McHugh G, Swartz M. Mechanisms of quinolone resistance in Escherichia coli: characterization of nfxB and cfxB, two mutant resistance loci decreasing norfloxacin accumulation. Antimicrob Agents Chemother 1989;33:283–290.

34. Huovinen P. Trimethoprim resistance [Review; 94 refs]. Antimicrob Agents Chemother 1987;31:1451–1456.

35. Ito T, Otsuki M, Nishino T. In vitro antibacterial activity of Q-35, a new fluoroquinolone. Antimicrob Agents Chemother 1992;36:1708–1714.

36. Jarlier V, Fosse T, Philippon A. Antibiotic susceptibility in aerobic gram-negative bacilli isolated in intensive care units in 39 French teaching hospitals (ICU study). Intensive Care Med 1996;22:1057–1065.

37. Kessler R, Fung-Tomc J, Kolek B, Minassian B, Huczko E, Gradelski E, Bonner D. In vitro activity of BMS-181139, a new carbapenem with potent antipseudomonal activity. Antimicrob Agents Chemother 1995;39:380–385.

38. Klein J, Feigin R, McCracken G. Report of the task force on diagnosis and management of meningitis. Pediatrics 1986;78:959–982.

39. Krieger JN. Mandell GL, Prostatitis, epididymitis and orchitis. In: Bennett JE, Dolin R, eds. Principles and practice of infectious diseases. 4th ed. New York: Churchill Livingstone, 1995:1098–1103.

40. Lamikanra A, Ako-Nai A, Ola J. Transmissible trimethoprim resistance in strains of Escherichia coli isolated from cases of infantile diarrhoea. J Med Microbiol 1990;32:159–162.

41. Lehn N, Stowerhoffmann J, Kott T, Strassner C, Wagner H, Kronke M, Schneiderbrachert W. Characterization of clinical isolates of Escherichia coli showing high levels of fluoroquinolone resistance. J Clin Microbiol 1996;34:597–602.42.

42. Lester S, del Pilar Pla M, Wang F, Perez Schael I, Jiang H, O'Brien T. The carriage of Escherichia coli resistant to antimicrobial agents by healthy children in Boston, in Caracas, Venezuela, and in Qin Pu, China [see comments]. N Engl J Med 1990;323:285–289.

43. Lim Y, Ngan C, Tay L. Enteropathogenic Escherichia coli as a cause of diarrhoea among children in Singapore. J Trop Med Hyg 1992;95:339–342.

44. Liu Y, Huang W, Cheng D. Antibacterial activity of cefepime in vitro. Chemotherapy 1994;40:384–390.

45. Livermore D. Permeation of beta-lactam antibiotics into Escherichia coli, Pseudomonas aeruginosa, and other gram-negative bacteria [Review; 59 refs]. Rev Infect Dis 1988;10:691–698.

46. Martinez-Beltran J, Canton R, Linares J, Garcia de Lomas J, Gimeno C, Tubau F, Baquero F. Multicentre comparative study on the antibacterial activity of FK-037, a new parenteral cephalosporin. Eur J Clin Microbiol Infect Dis 1995;14:244–252.

47. Mattila L, Peltola H, Siitonen A, Kyronseppa H, Simula I, Kataja M. Short-term treatment of traveler's diarrhea with norfloxacin: a double-blind, placebo-controlled study during two seasons. Clin Infect Dis 1993;17:779–782.

48. McMurry L, George A, Levy S. Active efflux of chloramphenicol in susceptible Escherichia coli strains and in multiple-antibiotic-resistant (Mar) mutants. Antimicrob Agents Chemother 1994;38:542–546.

49. Menard R, Molinas C, Arthur M, Duval J, Courvalin P, Leclercq R. Overproduction of 3′-aminoglycoside phosphotransferase type I confers resistance to tobramycin in Escherichia coli. Antimicrob Agents Chemother 1993;37:78–83.

50. Merson M, Sack R, Islam S, Saklayen G, Huda N, Huq I, Zulich A, Yolken R, Kapikian A. Disease due to enterotoxigenic Escherichia coli in Bangladeshi adults: clinical aspects and a controlled trial of tetracycline. J Infect Dis 1980;141:702–711.

51. Moyenuddin M, Wachsmuth I, Moseley S, Bopp C, Blake P. Serotype, antimicrobial resistance, and adherence properties of Escherichia coli strains associated with outbreaks of diarrheal illness in children in the United States. J Clin Microbiol 1989;27:2234–2239.

52. Muratani T, Inoue M, Mitsuhashi S. In vitro activity of T-3761, a new fluoroquinolone. Antimicrob Agents Chemother 1992;36:2293–2303.

53. Murray B, Alvarado T, Kim K, Vorachit M, Jayanetra P, Levine M, Prenzel I, Fling M, Elwell L, McCracken G, et al. Increasing resistance to trimethoprim-sulfamethoxazole among isolates of Escherichia coli in developing countries. J Infect Dis 1985;152:1107–1113.

54. Murray B, Mathewson J, DuPont H, Ericsson C, Reves R. Emergence of resistant fecal Escherichia coli in travelers not taking prophylactic antimicrobial agents. Antimicrob Agents Chemother 1990;34:515–518.

55. Murray B, Rensimer E, DuPont H. Emergence of high-level trimethoprim resistance in fecal Escherichia coli during oral administration of trimethoprim or trimethoprim-sulfamethoxazole. N Engl J Med 1982;306:130–135.

56. Murray P. Antimicrobial activity of seven oral antibiotics against selected community- and hospital-acquired pathogens. Clin Ther 1991;13:224–231.

57. Nakanishi N, Inoue M, Inoue K, Yamaguchi T, Mitsuhashi S. In vitro activity of temafloxacin hydrochloride (TA-167 or A-62254), a new fluorinated 4-quinolone. Chemotherapy 1990;36:345–355.

58. Nelson J. Duration of neomycin for enteropathogenic Escherichia coli diarrheal disease: a comparative study of 113 cases. Pediatrics 1971;48:248–258.

59. Neu H. The emergence of bacterial resistance and its influence on empiric therapy [Review; 95 refs]. Rev Infect Dis 1983;5 (Suppl 1):S9–20

60. Neu H. Quinolone antimicrobial agents. [Review] [99 refs]. Annu Rev Med 1992;43:465–486.

61. Nishino T, Otsuki M, Hatano K, Nishihara Y. In vitro and in vivo antibacterial activities of FK037, a new parenteral cephalosporin. Chemotherapy 1994;40:167–182.

62. Oethinger M, Conrad S, Kaifel K, Cometta A, Bille J, Klotz G, Glauser M, Marre R, Kern W. Molecular epidemiology of fluoro-quinolone-resistant Escherichia coli bloodstream isolates from patients admitted to European cancer centers. Antimicrob Agents Chemother 1996;40:387–392.

63. Orskov F, Orskov I. Escherichia coli serotyping and disease in man and animals [Review]. Can J Microbiol 1992;38:699–704.

64. Ostroff S, Kobayashi J, Lewis J. Infections with Escherichia coli O157:H7 in Washington State. The first year of statewide disease surveillance [see comments]. Jama 1989;262:355–359.

65. Pai C, Gordon R, Sims H, Bryan L. Sporadic cases of hemorrhagic colitis associated with Escherichia coli O157:H7. Clinical, epidemiologic, and bacteriologic features. Ann Intern Med 1984;101:738 742.

66. Pancoast S, Hyams D, Neu H. Effect of trimethoprim and trimethoprim-sulfamethoxazole on development of drug-resistant vaginal and fecal floras. Antimicrob Agents Chemother 1980;17:263–268.

67. Pavia A, Nichols C, Green D, Tauxe R, Mottice S, Greene K, Wells J, Siegler R, Brewer E, Hannon D, et al. Hemolytic-uremic syndrome during an outbreak of Escherichia coli O157:H7 infections in institutions for mentally retarded persons: clinical and epidemiologic observations. J Pediatr 1990; 116:544–551.

68. Pena C, Albareda J, Pallares R, Pujol M, Tubau F, Ariza J. Relationship between quinolone use and emergence of ciprofloxacin-resistant Escherichia coli in bloodstream infections. Antimicrob Agents Chemother 1995;39:520–524.

69. Perez-Trallero E, Urbieta M, Jimenez D, Garcia-Arenzana J, Cilla G. Ten-year survey of quinolone resistance in Escherichia coli causing urinary tract infections. Eur J Clin Microbiol Infect Dis 1993;12:349–351.

70. Perlin M, Lerner S. High-level amikacin resistance in Escherichia coli due to phosphorylation and impaired aminoglycoside uptake. Antimicrob Agents Chemother 1986;29:216–224.

71. Phillips I, Eykyn S, King A, Gransden W, Rowe B, Frost J, Gross R. Epidemic multiresistant Escherichia coli infection in West Lambeth Health District. Lancet 1988;1:1038–1041.

72. Pornull K, Goransson E, Rytting A, Dornbusch K. Extended-spectrum beta-lactamases in Escherichia coli and Klebsiella spp. in European septicaemia isolates. J Antimicrob Chemother 1993;32:559–570.

73. Prado D, Lopez E, Liu H, Devoto S, Woloj M, Contrini M, Murray B, Gomez H, Cleary T. Ceftibuten and trimethoprim-sulfamethoxazole for treatment of Shigella and enteroinvasive Escherichia coli disease. Pediatr Infect Dis J 1992;11:644–647.

74. Proulx F, Turgeon J, Delage G, Lafleur L, Chicoine L. Randomized, controlled trial of antibiotic therapy for Escherichia coli O157:H7 enteritis. J Pediatr 1992;121:299–303.

75. Ratnam S, March S, Ahmed R, Bezanson G, Kasatiya S. Characterization of Escherichia coli serotype O157:H7. J Clin Microbiol 1988;26:2006–2012.

76. Remis R, MacDonald K, Riley L, Puhr N, Wells J, Davis B, Blake P, Cohen M. Sporadic cases of hemorrhagic colitis associated with Escherichia coli O157:H7. Ann Intern Med 1984; 101:624–626.

77. Reves R, Fong M, Pickering L, Bartlett Ad, Alvarez M, Murray B. Risk factors for fecal colonization with trimethoprim-resistant and multiresistant Escherichia coli among children in day-care centers in Houston, Texas. Antimicrob Agents Chemother 1990;34:1429–1434.

78. Reves R, Murray B, Pickering L, Prado D, Maddock M, Bartlett Ad. Children with trimethoprim- and ampicillin-resistant fecal Escherichia coli in day care centers. J Infect Dis 1987;156: 758–762.

79. Riley L, Remis R, Helgerson S, McGee H, Wells J, Davis B, Hebert R, Olcott E, Johnson L, Hargrett N, et al. Hemorrhagic colitis associated with a rare Escherichia coli serotype. N Engl J Med 1983;308:681–685.

80. Ritchie D, Hopefl A, Milligan T, Byrne J, Maddux M. In vitro activity of clarithromycin, cefprozil, and other common oral antimicrobial agents against gram-positive and gram-negative pathogens. Clin Ther 1993;15:107–113.

81. Rothbaum R, McAdams A, Giannella R, Partin J. A clinico-pathologic study of enterocyte-adherent Escherichia coli: a cause of protracted diarrhea in infants. Gastroenterology 1982; 83:441–454.

82. Rydberg J, Cederberg A. Intrafamilial spreading of Escherichia coli resistant to trimethoprim. Scand J Infect Dis 1986;18: 457–460.

83. Rylander M, Norrby S, Svard R. Norfloxacin versus co-trimoxazole for treatment of urinary tract infections in adults: microbiological results of a coordinated multicentre study. Scand J Infect Dis 1987;19:551–557.

84. Salam I, Katelaris P, Leigh-Smith S, Farthing M. Randomised trial of single-dose ciprofloxacin for travellers' diarrhoea [see comments]. Lancet 1994;344:1537–1539.

85. Schiffer M, Oliveira E, Glode M, McCracken GJ, Sarff L, Robbins J. A review: relation between invasiveness and the K1 capsular polysaccharide of Escherichia coli [Review; 61 refs]. Pediatr Res 1976;10:82–87.

86. Senerwa D, Mutanda L, Gathuma J, Olsvik O. Antimicrobial resistance of enteropathogenic Escherichia coli strains from a nosocomial outbreak in Kenya. Acta Pathol Microbiol Immunol Scand 1991;99:728–734.

87. Singh K, Reves R, Pickering L, Murray B. Comparative in vitro activities of amoxicillin-clavulanic acid, cefuroxime, ceph-alexin, and cephalothin against trimethoprim-resistant Escherichia coli isolated from stools of children attending day-care centers. Antimicrob Agents Chemother 1990;34: 2047–2049.

88. Singh M, Sanyal S, Yadav J. Enterotoxigenic drug resistant plasmids in animal isolates of Escherichia coli and their zoonotic importance. J Trop Med Hyg 1992;95:316–321.

89. Sperber S, Feibusch E, Damiani A, Weinstein M. In vitro activities of nucleoside analog antiviral agents against salmonellae. Antimicrob Agents Chemother 1993;37:106–110.

90. Stamey TA. Pathogenesis and treatment of urinary tract infections. 1st ed. Baltimore: Williams & Wilkins, 1980.

91. Stamm W, Counts G, Wagner K, Martin D, Gregory D, McKevitt M, Turck M, Holmes K. Antimicrobial prophylaxis of recurrent urinary tract infections: a double-blind, placebo-controlled trial. Ann Intern Med 1980;92:770–775.

92. Stamm W, Hooton T. Management of urinary tract infections in adults. N Engl J Med 1993; 329:1328–1334.

93. Standiford H. Tetracyclines and chloramphenicol. In: Mandell GL, Bennett JE, Dolin R, eds. Principles and practice of infectious diseases. 4th ed. New York: Churchill Livingstone, 1995: 306–317.

94. Sullivan M, Nightingale C, Quintiliani R, Sweeney K. Comparison of the pharmacodynamic activity of cefotaxime plus metronidazole with cefoxitin and ampicillin plus sulbactam. Pharmacotherapy 1995;15:479–486.

95. Tanaka M, Otsuki M, Nishino T. In vitro and in vivo activities of

DQ-2556 and its mode of action. Antimicrob Agents Chemother 1992;36:2595–2601.

96. Tangermann R, Gordon S, Wiesner P, Kreckman L. An outbreak of cryptosporidiosis in a day-care center in Georgia. Am J Epidemiol 1991;133:471–476.

97. Tarr P, Neill M, Christie D, Anderson D. Escherichia coli O157:H7 hemorrhagic colitis [Letter]. N Engl J Med 1988; 318:1697.

98. Then R. Mechanisms of resistance to trimethoprim, the sulfonamides, and trimethoprim-sulfamethoxazole [Review; 60 refs]. Rev Infect Dis 1982;4:261–269.

99. Thielman N, Guerrant R. Escherichia coli. Princ Pract Clin Bacteriol 1997:373–388.

100. Thoren A, Wolde-Mariam T, Stintzing G, Wadstrom T, Habte D. Antibiotics in the treatment of gastroenteritis caused by enteropathogenic Escherichia coli. J Infect Dis 1980;141: 27–31.

101. Thornsberry C, Brown S, Yee Y, Bouchillon S, Marler J, Rich T. In-vitro activity of cefepime and other antimicrobials: survey of European isolates. J Antimicrob Chemother 1993;32(Suppl B):31–53.

102. Thornton S, Wignall S, Kilpatrick M, Bourgeois A, Gardiner C, Batchelor R, Burr D, Oprandy J, Garst P, Hyams K. Norfloxacin compared to trimethoprim/sulfamethoxazole for the treatment of travelers' diarrhea among U.S. military personnel deployed to South America and West Africa. Mil Med 1992;157:55–58.

103. Vazquez F, Mendoza M, Viejo G, Mendez F. Survey of Escherichia coli septicemia over a six-year period. Eur J Clin Microbiol Infect Dis 1992;11:110–117.

104. Walterspiel J, Ashkenazi S, Morrow A, Cleary T. Effect of subinhibitory concentrations of antibiotics on extracellular Shiga-like toxin I. Infection 1992;20:25–29.

105. Wanke C, Swartz M. Remington J, eds. Enteropathogenic and enteroaggregative strains of Escherichia coli: clinical features of infection, epidemiology, and pathogenesis. Cambridge, MA: Blackwell Science; 1995:230–252.

106. Wiedemann B, Grimm H. Lorian V, eds. Susceptibility to antibiotics: species incidence and trends. Baltimore: Williams & Wilkins, 1996:900–1168.

107. Willmott C, Maxwell A. A single point mutation in the DNA gyrase A protein greatly reduces binding of fluoroquinolones to the gyrase-DNA complex. Antimicrob Agents Chemother 1993;37:126–127.

108. Willshaw G, Cheasty T, Rowe B, Smith H, Faithfull-Davies D, Brooks T. Isolation of enterotoxigenic Escherichia coli from British troops in Saudi Arabia. Epidemiol Infect 1995;115: 455–463.

109. Wistrom J, Gentry L, Palmgren A, Price M, Nord C, Ljungh A, Norrby S. Ecological effects of short-term ciprofloxacin treatment of travellers' diarrhoea. J Antimicrob Chemother 1992;30: 693–706.

110. Yamamoto T, Echeverria P, Yokota T. Drug resistance and adherence to human intestines of enteroaggregative Escherichia coli. J Infect Dis 1992;165:744–749.

Francisella tularensis

●

Richard F. Jacobs

GENERAL DESCRIPTION

Tularemia is an epizootic infection caused by *Francisella tularensis* (19). Any age, sex, or race is universally susceptible to infection (12, 28, 52). Tularemia is primarily a disease of wild animals that is transmitted to humans by a contaminated environment or ectoparasites. Infection is incidental and usually the result of interaction with biting or bloodsucking insects, wild animals, or their environment (7, 9, 12). Tularemia is a common illness in certain geographic regions of the southeastern to midwestern United States with highly endemic areas, including Arkansas, Oklahoma, and Missouri (17, 26, 59). The illness is characterized by six clinical syndromes: ulceroglandular, glandular, oropharyngeal, oculoglandular, gastrointestinal (typhoidal), and pneumonic (5, 6, 16). The most common syndrome presents with an ulcerative lesion at the site of inoculation and regional lymphadenopathy/lymphadenitis (ulceroglandular tularemia). Systemic manifestations with pneumonia, typhoidal tularemia, or fever without localizing findings present a more challenging differential diagnosis (4, 8, 15, 21).

F. tularensis is the etiologic agent of tularemia and, with rare exception, the only disease produced by this genus. The organism is a small, Gram-negative, pleomorphic, nonmotile, nonsporeforming coccobacillus measuring 0.2×0.2 to 0.7 μm. It is a nonpiliated strict aerobe that infects the host as a facultatively intracellular bacterium. The two main biovars, *F. tularensis* biovar *tularensis* (type A) and *F. tularensis* biovar *palearctica* (type B) are found in the United States (29). Type A produces the more serious disease in humans, with an untreated fatality rate of approximately 5%, and is found in the North American continent. Type B produces a milder, often subclinical, disease and has usually been associated with water or aquatic mammals. Recent evidence of more serious disease and an increased incidence have been found in Scandinavian countries, eastern Europe, and Siberia (24, 61). In nature, it is a rather hardy organism persisting for weeks to months in mud, water, and decaying animal carcasses (29). Animal reservoirs include wild rabbits, sheep, beavers, and muskrats. Animal bites, including those from cats and squirrels, have transmitted infection (14, 20, 37, 48). Numerous biting and blood-sucking insects can serve as vectors. Ticks and wild rabbits are the source of most human cases in endemic areas (26, 27).

Ticks pass the organism to their offspring via a transovarian route. The organism is found in tick feces but not in salivary glands. In the United States, the disease can be carried by *Dermacentor andersoni* (Rocky Mountain wood tick), *Dermacentor variabilis* (American dog tick), *Dermacentor occidentalis* (Pacific Coast dog tick), and *Amblyomma americanum* (Lone Star tick). Most cases of tularemia result from blood meals taken by embedded ticks (27, 39). Tularemia is most likely to occur in adult males, and person-to-person transmission rarely, if ever, occurs. The organism is transmitted mainly in the spring and summer; however, continued transmission in winter months has been documented. The organism is extremely infectious. The most common portal of entry for human infection is through skin or mucous membranes, either directly through the bite of a tick or other arthropods or via inapparent abrasions. Inhalation or ingestion of *F. tularensis* can also result in infection (51). Although more than 10^8 organisms are usually required to produce infection via the oral route (oropharyngeal or gastrointestinal tularemia), fewer than 50 organisms result in infection when injected into the skin (ulceroglandular/glandular tularemia) or inhaled (pneumonia) (42, 27). Following inoculation into the skin, the organism multiplies locally and, after 2 to 5 days (range, 1–10 days), produces an erythematous, tender, or pruritic papule. The papule rapidly enlarges and forms an ulcer with a black base. The bacteria spread to regional lymph nodes, producing lymphadenopathy, and may spread further with bacteremia. With bacteremia, organisms are cleared from the blood by the phagocytic cells of the reticuloendothelial system and may survive intracellularly for long periods of time. Biosafety level 2 is recommended for clinical laboratory work with suspected material, and biosafety level 3 is required for culturing the organism in large quantities.

MICROBIOLOGY

Culture and isolation of *F. tularensis* are difficult (46, 62). In a study of over 1000 human cases, 84% of which were serologically confirmed, the organism was isolated in only 10%. The medium of choice is cysteine-glucose-blood agar. Good growth has also been achieved on modified Mueller-Hinton broth, chocolate agar supplemented with IsoVitale X, and modified charcoal–yeast extract agar. The requirement of cysteine and enriched medium for stimulated growth has traditionally served as a useful characteristic for presumptive identification of *F. tularensis*. Recently, strains of *F. tularensis* have been described that on primary isolation failed to demonstrate a requirement for cysteine-enriched media but grew well on conventional laboratory medium (3). Therefore, isolation of a strictly aerobic, tiny, weakly staining, Gram-negative coccobacillus that lacks the aforementioned growth requirements may represent strains of *F. tularensis*. A heavy inoculum on appropriate medium will yield a growth mass in 18 h, while individual colonies may require 2 to 4 days. Overgrowth by contaminating microorganisms can be reduced by incorporating penicillin (100 to 500 U/mL) into the medium.

Direct isolation can be achieved from infected ulcer scrapings, lymph node biopsy specimens, gastric washings, sputum, and blood cultures. Colonies are blue-gray, round, smooth, and slightly mucoid. On media containing blood, a small zone of O-hemolysis usually surrounds the colony. Direct application of slide agglutination tests or direct fluorescent antibody using commercially available antisera can be performed on culture suspensions for identification. Although biochemical reactions are of no particular value, fermentation of glycerol or evidence of citrulline ureadase production may serve to differentiate biovar type A from type B. Polymerase chain reaction testing for *F. tularensis* DNA has been used to demonstrate the infection, with blood used as the primary source for detection (34). However, this test has not been shown to be more sensitive than direct culturing and remains, at this time, a research tool.

Tularemia is most frequently confirmed by serology (27, 28). In a standard tube agglutination test, a titer of less than 1:20 is not considered diagnostic because nonspecific cross-reactions are common at this level. A single titer of 1:160 should be interpreted as a presumptive positive result. A fourfold increase in titer is considered diagnostic. Late in infection, titers into the thousands are common, and titers of 1:20 to 1:80 may persist for years. A microagglutination test that may be up to 100 times more sensitive than the standard tube agglutination test is currently used in clinical microbiology laboratories. Enzyme-linked immunosorbent assays have proven useful in detecting both antibodies and antigens (55). Analysis of urine for *F. tularensis* antigen has shown promising results in clinical trials but is not widely available. Although extremely rare, *F. philomiragia* and *F. tularensis* biovar *novicida* have been associated with human disease and can cause serologic cross-reactions.

ANTIMICROBIAL SUSCEPTIBILITY IN VITRO

In vitro studies have shown *F. tularensis* to be susceptible to a wide range of antimicrobial agents, many of which have not been studied for the treatment of patients with tularemia. Several articles have reported the details of antimicrobial susceptibility testing; the methods used differed by investigator (2, 39, 40, 57, 61). Such testing showed no difference between type A and type B strains of *F. tularensis* (39). The results of tests with isolates from ticks and from humans are summarized in Tables 1 and 2, respectively.

In light of the in vitro susceptibility data reported by Baker, Hossis, and Thornsberry in 1985 and by Markowitz et al. in 1985, it appears that the third-generation cephalosporins or amikacin would be effective against tularemia. However, Cross and Jacobs have compiled data showing that ceftriaxone is ineffective for the treatment of tularemia (11) (Table 3). In eight documented cases of tularemia, patients were initially treated empirically with ceftriaxone for adenitis and pneumonia, but the condition of all patients worsened. With institution of standard therapy for tularemia, symptoms resolved quickly. These results indicate that in vitro data on *F. tularensis* do not always correlate with clinical response. Of interest are the markedly lower MICs of ceftazidime compared with those of

TABLE 1 • Antimicrobial Susceptibility of *Francisella tularensis* Isolates from Ticks.

Drug	Result (mg/mL)		
	MIC_{50}	MIC_{50}	MIC_{90}
Cefotaxime	0.5	2	4
Moxalactam	≤0.12	≤0.12	0.25
Cefoperazone	8	16	>32
Ceftazidime	0.25	≤0.5	≤0.5
Ceftriaxone	0.5	2	8
Streptomycin	4	2	4
Gentamicin	1	1	2
Amikacin	2	1	2
Tobramycin	—	1	2
Netilmicin	—	1	2
Tetracycline	1	2	2
Doxycycline	2	—	—
Chloramphenicol	0.5	1	1
Rifampin	0.5	—	—
Erythromycin	2	1	2
Clindamycin	—	>2	>2
Rifampin	—	0.5	1
Vancomycin	—	>16	16

Table modified and adapted from references 2 and 39.

TABLE 2 • Antimicrobial Susceptibility of *Francisella tularensis* Isolates from Patients

Drug	Result (μg/mL)[a]	
	MIC	MBC
Erythromycin	0.5, 1	0.5, 1
Tetracycline	0.5, 0.5	0.5, 0.5
Chloramphenicol	1, 1	1, 1
Trimethoprim-sulfamethoxazole	6	6
Gentamicin	0.2, 1	0.2, 1
Clindamycin	8, 8	8, 16

Adapted from Westerman EL, McDonald J. Tularemia pneumonia mimicking Legionnaires' disease: isolation of organism on CYE agar and successful treatment with erythromycin. South Med J 1983;76:1169–1170.

[a] Listing two values indicates two isolates.

ceftriaxone. However, no patients treated with ceftazidime have yet been reported, and given the disappointing results obtained with ceftriaxone, cephalosporins should not be used until their clinical efficacy has been demonstrated. Similarly, no case reports have documented the efficacy of amikacin.

Syrjala et al. determined the in vitro susceptibility of 10 strains of *F. tularensis* to ciprofloxacin, norfloxacin, ofloxacin, and pefloxacin (Table 4) (57). They noted a narrower range among the MBCs of ciprofloxacin and norfloxacin for the various strains, suggesting that these agents may be preferable to others in this class.

ANTIMICROBIAL THERAPY
Streptomycin

Streptomycin (7.5 to 10 mg/kg every 12 h intramuscularly) is considered the drug of choice in adults (13, 18) and (in a dose of 30–40 mg/kg/day divided into two daily doses intramuscularly) children. Following a clinical response in 3 to 5 days, the

dose can be reduced in children to 10 to 15 mg/kg/day in two divided doses. Therapy is typically continued for 7 to 10 days; however, in mild-to-moderate cases of tularemia with 48 to 72 h of afebrile course, 5 to 7 days of therapy have been used successfully. A reference review identified 224 patients who received streptomycin as the primary therapeutic agent (8, 14, 21, 22, 27, 31, 41) (Table 3). Of these 224 patients, 217 were treated successfully, 1 became more ill, and 6 died. No instances of relapse were noted. Some patients received other antibiotics either before or concurrently with streptomycin, but in no case were these other agents considered effective against tularemia.

Evans et al. described one patient whose infection worsened despite treatment with streptomycin and one patient who died after experiencing a Jarisch-Herxheimer-like reaction to streptomycin (15). The latter reaction is attributed to excess antigen resulting from the drug's "bactericidal efficiency" and leading to exacerbation of signs and symptoms. Continuation of therapy usually results in the patient's recovery (12). No instances of this reaction to other drugs were reported.

Giddens et al. in 1957 reported the use of streptomycin in 141 cases of tularemia. Most patients received 1 to 3 g of streptomycin or dihydrostreptomycin daily. The duration of fever was the best indicator of response; the patient's temperature usually fell within 3 days, but duration ranged from 1 to 40 days. The

TABLE 3 • Summary of the Results of Antimicrobial Treatment of Tularemia

Drug (no. of articles reviewed)	Total	Cure	(%)	Relapse	Deterioration	Death	Not Stated
Streptomycin (8)	224	217	(97)	0	1	6	0
Gentamicin (21)	36	31	(86)	2	2	1	0
Chloramphenicol (7)	43	33	(77)	9	1	0	0
Tobramycin (4)	6	3	(50)	0	0	2	1
Tetracycline (13)	50	44	(88)	6	0	0	0
Ceftriaxone (1)	8	0		0	8	0	0
Imipenem/cilastatin (1)	1	0	(100)	0	0	0	0
Ciprofloxacin (2)	5	5	(100)	0	0	0	0
Norfloxacin (1)	1	1	(100)	0	0	0	0

Modified from Enderlin G, Morales L, Jacobs RF, Cross JT. Streptomycin and alternative agents for the treatment of tularemia: review of the literature. Clin Infect Dis 1994;19:42–47.

TABLE 4 • Susceptibility of 10 Isolates of *Francisella tularensis* to Quinolones

Drug	Mean MBC ± SE (μg/mL)
Ciprofloxacin	0.13 ± 0.04
Norfloxacin	0.24 ± 0.07
Ofloxacin	2.16 ± 0.78
Pefloxacin	0.51 ± 0.50

Modified from Syrjala H, Schildt R, Raisainene S. In vitro susceptibility of *Francisella tularensis* to fluoroquinolones and treatment of tularemia with norfloxacin and ciprofloxacin. Eur J Clin Microbiol Infect Dis 1991;10:68–70.

authors concluded that doses of streptomycin above 2 g in adults provided no additional benefit. In this series, five patients treated with streptomycin died (mortality, 3%), as did six patients treated with other antibiotics. Renal dysfunction was the most serious complication, occurring in 6 of these 11 patients. Typhoidal tularemia was the most frequent fatal form of infection. The authors reported a mortality of 33% among 169 patients treated before streptomycin became available (21).

Gentamicin

Gentamicin at a dose of 1.7 mg/kg intramuscularly or intravenously every 8 hours is also effective (13). The published experience in adults is based on two reports of nine patients and an additional eight patients receiving effective treatment with gentamicin (13, 25, 40). In the second report, fever was present in all patients treated with gentamicin and all eight became afebrile within 24 to 72 h (40). Other symptoms, such as tender lymphadenitis and pharyngitis, also responded within 24 to 72 h of starting gentamicin therapy in a recent pediatric study (11). With the recent advent of home intravenous therapy for hospitalized patients, intravenous gentamicin is an option. Recently, the use of once-daily gentamicin for other infections has been reported, but no data on using once-daily gentamicin for tularemia currently exist. Virtually all strains of *F. tularensis* are susceptible to streptomycin and gentamicin.

In successfully treated patients, temperature response usually occurs within 2 days, but skin lesions and lymph nodes may take 1 to 2 weeks to heal. When therapy is not initiated within several days to weeks of illness, the temperature response may be delayed. Relapses are very uncommon with streptomycin or gentamicin therapy (47). Relapses did not occur in any of the patients recently described with gentamicin therapy. Twenty-one articles described 36 patients who received gentamicin (1, 5, 6, 14–16, 20, 23, 25, 26, 30, 36, 38, 40, 44–46, 48, 49, 56, 58) (Table 3). Of these patients, 31 had their infections cured, 2 experienced a relapse, 2 became more ill, and 1 died. Of the 31 successfully treated patients, 13 received gentamicin only, 10 received gentamicin along with other antibiotics not effective against tularemia, 4 received gentamicin after the failure of therapy with a tetracycline or chloramphenicol, and 1 received gentamicin but also received tetracycline on discharge, despite the resolution of disease. Of the articles reviewed, that by Mason et al. in 1980 reported the largest-scale experience with gentamicin treatment—9 patients.

Gallivan et al. in 1980 reported a case of ulceroglandular tularemia that resulted in the death of a 65-year-old man. The patient presented with a 5-day history of spiking fever, shaking chills, and a nonhealing ulcer on his left hand. After 10 days of hospitalization, he reported abdominal pain and underwent exploratory laparotomy; he developed progressive bilateral pneumonitis postoperatively. Treatment with cephalothin and gentamicin was started 15 days after the onset of symptoms. Therapy with doxycycline and streptomycin was begun after antibody to *F. tularensis* was detected. Pneumonitis worsened; disseminated intravascular coagulation and renal failure developed. The patient died 28 days into the disease.

Evans et al. in 1985 described two patients, one of whom had chronic lymphocytic leukemia and was admitted with a rectal temperature of 105°F, diffuse pneumonia, and septic shock. Blood cultures were positive for *F. tularensis,* and treatment with gentamicin was initiated. Because of a dramatic response, gentamicin therapy was stopped after 6 days, but relapse occurred 17 days later. The second patient had been gravely ill, with fever, confusion, pneumonia, and hepatitis. This patient did not respond to 4 days of treatment with gentamicin and responded only slowly after the regimen was changed to streptomycin.

Lovell et al. in 1986 reported a case of glandular tularemia in a 13-month-old child; diagnosis and initiation of appropriate therapy were delayed for 43 days. The patient responded to 9 days of treatment with gentamicin and ampicillin. However, 5 days after discharge, he experienced a relapse, with tularemic meningitis. The infecting organism was not identified until the patient's second admission, when cerebrospinal cultures yielded *F. tularensis.* He was successfully treated with a 2-week course of chloramphenicol.

Roy et al. in 1989 reported on a 42-year-old man admitted to the hospital with a 7-day history of fever, anorexia, malaise, nonproductive cough, and diarrhea. The patient was treated with erythromycin and gentamicin for coverage of tularemic pneumonia and legionella infection. His respiratory status deteriorated, and administration of gentamicin was discontinued after 24 hours. Therapy with rifampin was initiated for increased coverage of legionella pneumonia. Tularemia was later diagnosed on the basis of positive cultures, and the patient made slow but steady progress. He was discharged during a course of treatment with doxycycline.

Chloramphenicol

A total of 7 articles reported on 43 patients who received chloramphenicol (5, 12, 15, 21, 23) (Table 3). Of these patients, 33 had their infections cured, 1 became more ill, and 9 experienced a relapse. Of the 33 patients whose therapy was successful, 31 received chloramphenicol only, and 2 received both chloramphenicol and gentamicin. The 1 patient whose condition worsened and the 9 patients who had relapses received chloramphenicol only.

Dienst in 1963 reported cures of tularemia in 16 patients treated with chloramphenicol, although the condition of 1 patient later worsened and 1 patient's infection relapsed. The latter patient responded to a continuation of chloramphenicol therapy. Evans et al. in 1985 described three patients whose infections relapsed after discontinuation of treatment with chloramphenicol; these infections were cured by streptomycin therapy. Jacobs and Narain in 1983 described four children treated with chloramphenicol. One infection was cured, but three relapsed within 72 hours of the completion of a 7- to 10-day course of therapy.

Parker et al. in 1950 described a 27-year-old man with pneumonic tularemia who was treated with chloramphenicol beginning on day 6 of disease. An initial oral dose of 3 g was followed by doses of 1 g every 8 h. The patient was afebrile and asymptomatic after 36 h, and therapy was discontinued after 5 days. On the 17th day, a relapse resulted in initiation of a second course of treatment with chloramphenicol (total, 10 g); the patient became asymptomatic after 12 h. Two days after discontinuation of this second course, recrudescence was again documented. A third course of chloramphenicol (18 g over 7 days) was curative. In another case, a 35-year-old patient with uleroglandular tularemia presented with fever, chills, and headache. An initial dose of 3.5 g of chloramphenicol was followed by doses of 0.5 g every 4 hours for 5 days; the patient defervesced. Three days later, fever and symptoms returned. Therapy with chloramphenicol was reinstituted for 4 more days, and the patient's condition improved.

Tobramycin

Four articles described six cases of tularemia in which tobramycin was used (6, 30, 46, 60) (Table 3). Three patients recovered and two patients died; the outcome of the remaining patient was not stated. All six patients were severely ill, with complications including sepsis, diabetes, rhabdomyolysis, and renal failure. The total duration of tobramycin therapy was not stated in four cases.

Kaiser et al. in 1985 described the death of a 63-year-old woman with a 7-day history of fever, chills, cough, malaise, myalgias, lethargy, and confusion. The patient had symptoms suggesting typhoidal tularemia and developed renal failure secondary to rhabdomyolysis. She was initially treated with cefazolin and tobramycin and became afebrile within 24 h. The therapeutic regimen was changed to chloramphenicol and cefotaxime because of the need for dialysis on day 6. The patient subsequently developed disseminated intravascular coagulation and died.

Provenza et al. in 1986 described the death of a 75-year-old woman who was septic upon presentation to the hospital after several weeks of symptoms. The patient had renal insufficiency and hypertension. She was initially treated with vancomycin, tobramycin, and corticosteroids and died 2 days after admission.

Tetracycline

A total of 13 articles described 50 patients treated with tetracycline (7, 8, 15, 26, 33, 35, 38, 40, 45, 50, 54, 61, 62) (Table 3). Forty-four patients had their infections cured, while six patients had a relapse. Of the 44 successfully treated patients, 31 received tetracycline alone, 3 received tetracycline and gentamicin, and 10 received tetracycline and other antibiotics not effective against tularemia. Of the 6 patients with relapses, 2 were treated with tetracycline and other antibiotics not effective against tularemia, 3 with tetracycline alone, and 1 with tetracycline and streptomycin.

Caruso et al. in 1983 reported on a 38-year-old woman who presented with a 9-day history of oropharyngeal tularemia that was treated initially with ampicillin and then with erythromycin. Approximately 22 days after the onset of symptoms, therapy with tetracycline (250 mg orally every 6 h) and streptomycin (500 mg intramuscularly every 12 h) was initiated. The duration of therapy was not stated. This patient was readmitted 2 months later with enlarged cervical nodes and was treated with chloramphenicol and gentamicin. The wounds stopped draining after 2 weeks and healed after 2 months; cultures were negative. Adenitis with late suppuration of regional lymph nodes has been reported in successfully treated cases, although drainage of these nodes reveals necrotic tissue that is sterile (28).

Evans et al. in 1985 reported three relapses of infections treated with tetracycline and described two of these instances. One case involved a 13-year-old girl whose oropharyngeal tularemia was treated first with cefaclor and then with tetracycline. She continued to have low-grade fever and tender lymph nodes, and her regimen was changed to streptomycin. Her fever responded to this therapy, but her lymphadenopathy persisted. The other case involved a 72-year-old man with uleroglandular tularemia who defervesced 24 h after the start of tetracycline therapy. Administration of the drug was inadvertently discontinued, and fever returned. After tetracycline therapy was reinitiated, the patient defervesced and his pneumonia cleared. He later received a course of streptomycin, but further details were not given.

Penn and Kinassewitz in 1987 described two patients whose infections relapsed despite tetracycline therapy. Both patients received fewer than 7 days of therapy and had underlying medical conditions (e.g., diabetes) that may have contributed to the relapse.

Quinolones

Syrjala, Schildt, and Raisainene in 1991 reported on three patients with pneumonic tularemia and one with uleroglandular tularemia who were successfully treated with ciprofloxacin (750 mg twice daily). These authors also described one patient with uleroglandular tularemia who responded to therapy with norfloxacin (400 mg twice daily for 10 days). Neither the severity of illness nor the presence of underlying complications was discussed. All five patients responded to treatment within 48 h, and no relapses occurred within 6 months.

Scheel et al. in 1992 reported the case of a veterinarian with uleroglandular tularemia. He treated himself intermittently with doxycycline and then with amoxicillin for 10 days, but his adenitis persisted. He switched back to doxycycline for 3 weeks, and his condition improved. However, 3 days after the completion of doxycycline therapy, the infection relapsed. After presenting for treatment, the patient received ciprofloxacin (75 mg twice daily) for 2 weeks. The axillary adenitis resolved; no signs of relapse were detected at a follow-up examination 2 months later.

Imipenem/Cilastatin

Lee et al. in 1991 described a patient who had pneumonic tularemia with renal failure and chronic obstructive airway disease, as well as alcohol-related cardiomyopathy. Although seriously ill, the patient responded to therapy with imipenem/cilastatin (500 mg intravenously every 8 h for 14 days). No relapse was evident at a 1-year follow-up examination.

OUTCOME

Late lymph node suppuration may occur in up to 40% of children regardless of the treatment received (29). These nodes have typically been found to contain sterile necrotic lymph node tissue without evidence of active infection. If untreated, symptoms of tularemia usually last 1 to 4 weeks but may continue for months. The mortality of severe untreated infection, which includes all untreated tularemia pneumonia and typhoidal tularemia cases, can be as high as 30%. However, the overall mortality rate for untreated tularemia is less than 8%. Mortality is less than 1% with appropriate treatment and is often associated with long delays in diagnosis and treatment. Following tularemia, there is usually lifelong immunity (29).

PREVENTION

Prevention of tularemia is based on avoidance of exposure to biting and bloodsucking insects (28). Vaccination of high-risk populations who primarily work with, and are exposed to, large quantities of cultured organisms can be effective. Avoidance of skinning wild animals, especially rabbits, and wearing gloves while handling animal carcasses decreases the risk of transmission. Use of insect repellents and tick-attachment preparations and prompt removal of ticks can be helpful. Prophylactic treatment of patients exposed to embedded tick bite exposures has not been proven effective in preventing tularemia. However, in patients known to be exposed to large quantities of organisms (laboratory exposure) who are incubating *F. tularensis,* early treatment has prevented development of significant clinical disease (51).

REFERENCES

1. Alford RH, John JT, Bryant RE. Tularemia treated successfully with gentamicin. Am Rev Respir Dis 1972;106:265–268.
2. Baker CN, Hossis DG, Thornsberry C. Antimicrobial susceptibility testing of *Francisella tularensis* with a modified Mueller-Hinton broth. J Clin Microbiol 1985;22:212–215.
3. Bernard K, Tessier S, Winstanley J, Chang D, Borczyk A. Early recognition of atypical *Francisella tularensis* strains lacking a cysteine requirement. J Clin Microbiol 1994;32:551.
4. Butler T. Plague and tularemia. Pediatr Clin North Am 1979;26:355–366.
5. Caruso VG, Caruso AP, Panebianco RJ. Oropharyngeal tularemia. NY State J Med 1983;83:226–227.
6. Centers for Disease Control. Tularemic pneumonia—Tennessee. MMWR 1983;32:262–269.
7. Centers for Disease Control. Outbreak of tick-borne tularemia—South Dakota. MMWR 1984;33:601–602.
8. Cox SK, Everett ED. Tularemia: an analysis of 25 cases. Mo Med 1981;78:70–74.
9. Craven RB, Barnes AM. Plague and tularemia. Infect Dis Clin North Am 1991;5:165–175.
10. Cross JT, Jacobs RF. Tularemia: treatment failures with outpatient use of ceftriaxone. Clin Infect Dis 1993;17:976–980.
11. Cross JT, Schutze GE, Jacobs RF. Treatment of tularemia with gentamicin in pediatric patients. Pediatr Infect Dis J 1995;14:151–152.
12. Dienst FT Jr. Tularemia: a perusal of three hundred thirty-nine cases. J La State Med Soc 1963;115:114–127.
13. Enderlin G, Morales L, Jacobs RF, Cross JT. Streptomycin and alternative agents for the treatment of tularemia: review of the literature. Clin Infect Dis 1994;19:42–47.
14. Evans ME, McGee ZA, Hunter PT, Schaffner W. Tularemia and the tomcat. JAMA 1981;246:1343.
15. Evans ME, Gregory DW, Schaffner W, McGee ZA. Tularemia: a 30-year experience with 88 cases. Medicine (Baltimore) 1985;64:251–269.
16. Everett ED, Templer JW. Oropharyngeal tularemia. Arch Otolaryngol 1980;106:237–238.
17. Finley CR, Hamilton BW, Hamilton TR. Tularemia: a review. Mo Med 1986;83:741–743.
18. Foshay L, Pasternack AB. Streptomycin treatment of tularemia. JAMA 1946;130:393–398.
19. Francis E. Tularemia, Francis 1921: a new disease of man. JAMA 1922;78:1015–1018.
20. Gallivan MVE, Davis WA II, Garagusi VF, Paris AL, Lack EE. Fatal cat-transmitted tularemia: demonstration of the organism in tissue. South Med J 1980;73:240–242.
21. Giddens WR, Wilson JW Jr, Dienst FT Jr, Hargrove MD. Tularemia: an analysis of one hundred forty-seven cases. J La State Med Soc 1957;109:93–98.
22. Gourdeau M, Lamothe F, Ishak M, Cote J, Breton, G, Villeneuve JP, D'Amico P. Hepatic abscess complicating ulceroglandular tularemia. Can Med Assoc J 1983;129:1286–1288.
23. Halperin SA, Gast T, Ferrieri P. Oculoglandular syndrome caused by *Francisella tularensis.* Clin Pediatr (Phila) 1985;24:520–522.
24. Hoel T, Scheel O, Nordahl SHG, Sandvik T. Water and airborne *Francisella tularensis* biovar palaearctica isolated from human blood. Infection 1991;19:348–350.
25. Jackson RT, Lester JP. Case report. Tularemia presenting as unresponsive pneumonia: Diagnosis and therapy with gentamicin. J Tenn Med Assoc 1978;71:189–191.
26. Jacobs RF, Narain JP. Tularemia in children. Pediatr Infect Dis J 1983;2:487–491.
27. Jacobs RF, Condrey YM, Yamauchi T. Tularemia in adults and children: A changing presentation. Pediatrics 1985;76:818.
28. Jacobs RF. Tularemia. Clinical Reviews in Pediatric Infectious Disease 1985:165–170.
29. Jacobs RF. Tularemia. In: Kasper D, ed. Harrison's principles of internal medicine. In press.
30. Kaiser AB, Rieves D, Price AH, Gelfand MR, Parrish RE, Decker MD, Evans ME. Tularemia and rhabdomyolysis. JAMA 1985;253:241–243.
31. Larson BW, Jacobson HJ. Tularemia with unusual laboratory characteristics in South Dakota children. SD J Med 1984;37:5–10.
32. Lee HC, Horowitz E, Linder W. Treatment of tularemia with imipenem/cilastatin sodium. South Med J 1991;84:1277–1278.
33. Leggiadro RJ, Kenigsberg K, Annunziato D. Tick-borne ulceroglandular tularemia. NY State J Med 1983;83:1053–1054.
34. Long GW, Oprandy JJ, Narayanan RB, Fortier AH, Porter KR,

Nacy CA. Detection of *Francisella tularensis* in blood by polymerase chain reaction. J Clin Microbiol 1993;31:152–154.

35. Lopez CE, Kornblatt AN, Sikes RK, Hanes OE. Tularemia: review of eight cases of tick-borne infection and the epidemiology of the disease in Georgia. South Med J 1982;75:404–407.

36. Lovell VM, Cho CT, Lindsey NJ, Nelson PL. *Francisella tularensis* meningitis: a rare clinical entity. J Infect Dis 1986;154:916–918.

37. Magee JS, Steele RW, Kelly NR, Jacobs RF. Tularemia transmitted by a squirrel bite. Pediatr Infect Dis J 1989;8:123–125.

38. Marcus DM, Frederick AR Jr, Hodges T, Allan JD, Albert DM. Typhoidal tularemia. Arch Ophthalmol 1990;108:118–119.

39. Markowitz LE, Hynes NA, de la Cruz P, Campos E, Barbaree JM, Plikaytis BD, Mosier D, Kaufmann AF. Tick-borne tularemia: an outbreak of lymphadenopathy in children. JAMA 1985;254:2922–2925.

40. Mason WL, Eigelsbach HT, Little SF, Bates JH. Treatment of tularemia, including pulmonary tularemia, with gentamicin. Am Rev Respir Dis 1980;121:39–45.

41. Miller RP, Bates JH. Pleuropulmonary tularemia: a review of 29 patients. Am Rev Respir Dis 1969;99:31–41.

42. Overholt EL, Tigertt WD, Kadull PJ, Ward MK, Charkes MD, Rene RM, Salzman TE, Mallory S. An analysis of forty-two cases of laboratory-acquired tularemia: treatment with broad-spectrum antibiotics. Am J Med 1961;30:785–806.

43. Parker R, Lister L, Bauer R, Hall HE, Woodward TE. Use of chloramphenicol (chloromycetin) in experimental and human tularemia. JAMA 1950;143:7–11.

44. Parkhurst JB, San Joaquin VH. Tonsillopharyngeal tularemia: a reminder [Letter]. Am J Dis Child 1990;144:1070–1071.

45. Penn RL, Kinasewitz GT. Factors associated with a poor outcome in tularemia. Arch Intern Med 1987;147:265–268.

46. Provenza JM, Klotz SA, Penn RL. Isolation of *Francisella tularensis* from blood. J Clin Microbiol 1986;24:453–455.

47. Risi GF, Pombo DJ. Relapse of tularemia after aminoglycoside therapy: case report and discussion of therapeutic options. Clin Infect Dis 1995;20:174–175.

48. Rowland MD, Griffiths DW. The spider as a possible source of tularemia [Letter]. JAMA 1988;260:33.

49. Roy TM, Fleming D, Anderson WH. Tularemic pneumonia mimicking Legionnaires' disease with false-positive direct fluorescent antibody stains for *Legionella*. South Med J 1989;82:1429–1431.

50. Ryan-Poirier K, Whitehead PY, Leggiadro RJ. An unlucky rabbit's foot? Pediatrics 1990;85:598–600.

51. Sawyer WD, Dangerfield HG, Hogge AL, Crozier D. Antibiotic prophylaxis and therapy of airborne tularemia. Bacteriol Rev 1966;30:542–548.

52. Scheel O, Sandivik T, Hoel T, Aasen S. Tularemia in Norway. A clinical and epidemiological review. Tidsskr Nor Laegeforen 1992;112:635–637.

53. Scheel O, Reiersen R, Hoel T. Treatment of tularemia with ciprofloxacin. Eur J Clin Microbiol Infect Dis 1992;11:447–448.

54. Scully RE, Mark EJ, McNeely BU. Case records of the Massachusetts General Hospital. Weekly clinicopathological exercises. Case 27–1985. N Engl J Med 1985;313:36–42.

55. Syrjala, Koskela HP, Ripatti T, Salminen A, Herva E. Agglutination and ELISA methods in the diagnosis of tularemia in different clinical forms and severities of the disease. J Infect Dis 1986;153:142–145.

56. Syrjala H, Koskela P, Kujala P, Mylyla V. Guillain-Barre syndrome and tularemia pleuritis with high adenosine deaminase activity in pleural fluid. Infection 1989;171:152–153.

57. Syrjala H, Schildt R, Raisainene S. In vitro susceptibility of *Francisella tularensis* to fluoroquinolones and treatment of tularemia with norfloxacin and ciprofloxacin. Eur J Clin Microbiol Infect Dis 1991;10:68–70.

58. Tarpay M. Tularemic pharyngitis [Letter]. Pediatr Infect Dis 1983;2:266.

59. Taylor JP, Istre GR, McChesney TC, Satalowich FT, Parker RL, McFarland LM. Epidemiologic characteristics of human tularemia in the southwest-central states. 1981–1987. Am J Epidemiol 1991;133:1032.

60. Tilley WAS, Garman RW, Stone WJ. Tularemia complicated by acute renal failure. South Med J 1983;7i6:273–274.

61. Uhari M, Syrjala H, Salminen A. Tularemia in children caused by *Francisella tularensis* biovar *palaearctica*. Pediatr Infect Dis J 1990;9:80–83.

62. Westerman EL, McDonald J. Tularemia pneumonia mimicking Legionnaires' disease: isolation of organism on CYE agar and successful treatment with erythromycin. South Med J 1983;76:1169–1170.

Gemella Species

●

William J. Riebel

GENERAL DESCRIPTION

Gemellae ("little twin") are catalase-negative, Gram-positive cocci that appear to cause diseases similar to those caused by the oral or viridans streptococci, with which they are commonly confused (8). Currently, two species are assigned to the genus, based on DNA-DNA homology (43), 16S RNA sequencing (46, 68), and phenotypic analysis (7). Information concerning gemellae comes mainly from individual case reports and survey studies of streptococcal-type organisms; most isolates are still probably misidentified in clinical microbiology laboratories. In clinical practice, the reported identity of isolates should generally be questioned because of the lack of verification of accuracy of commercial identification systems and the variability in biochemical test results when different media and methodologies are used (60). In addition to confusion with oral streptococci and neisseriae, gemellae usually possess pyrrolidonylarylamidase (PYR), which could lead to confusion with enterococci (29). Furthermore, gemellae and nutritionally variant streptococci overlap in physiologic characteristics (29), which could also have therapeutic implications, since some infections due to nutritionally variant streptococci and enterococci may be best treated by combination therapies. Gemellae can be found in polymicrobial infections that are often related to their sites of colonization, but this review focuses on single-isolate reports.

Gemella haemolysans, so named because of its hemolytic colony pattern on rabbit-blood agar, was originally considered a *Neisseria* species (7, 63). Microscopically it appears in tetrads, clusters, and short chains, with adjacent sides of its coccal shape flattened. It is considered Gram positive, but due to very easy decolorization it frequently appears Gram negative or Gram variable. It is a part of the oropharyngeal flora, found in 30% of pharyngeal cultures when sought (6, 8). Endocarditis (2, 10, 11, 13, 16, 17, 32, 39, 42, 44, 48, 53, 61), meningitis (3, 36, 50, 51), bacteremia of unclear source (9, 15, 29), bacteremic pneumonia (29), and prosthetic joint infection (25) have been reported.

G. morbillorum (of the disease *morbilli* or measles) was transferred from the *Streptococcus* genus in the late 1980s, although it previously had been classified as an anaerobe because of its growth preferences (6, 43, 46). Similar to *G. haemolysans,* strains can show adjacent-side flattening and easy decolorization on Gram staining, but it can also be variably sized and elongated to rodlike morphology (7, 8). *G. morbillorum* was initially isolated from the foot, nose, and eyes of measles patients (65), hence its name, but it has also been isolated from the upper respiratory tract, intestinal tract, and genitourinary tract (8, 33, 37, 57, 69). *G. morbillorum* has been reported to cause numerous infections: endocarditis (1, 5, 14, 19, 20, 24, 28, 30, 31, 40, 41, 45, 47, 49, 52, 62, 64), infected left atrial myxoma (67), a possible subacute pericarditis (18), intravascular dialysis shunt infections (4, 54), bacteremia of uncertain source (12, 26, 29, 33), meningitis (12, 34), sinusitis (12, 66), brain abscess (22, 28), neck space abscesses (12, 55, 56), pneumonia and/or empyema (12, 21, 28, 35, 38, 56), breast abscess (12), septic arthritis and or bone and joint infections (27, 28, 33, 54), and urinary or genital infections (12, 28, 56, 57, 59).

SUSCEPTIBILITY
In Vitro and in Vivo

No large-scale studies of in vitro susceptibility of *G. haemolysans* have been reported. Susceptibilities seem to be similar those of oral streptococci; MICs for five strains are listed in Table 1 (13). In this and most other reports, penicillin has been active, with MICs and MBCs below 0.01 μg/mL (10, 13, 32); however, relative penicillin resistance (MIC = 1 μg/mL) has also been reported (42). Resistance to trimethoprim and sulfamethoxazole is often found, as is resistance to aminoglyco-

TABLE 1 • MICs (μg/mL) of *Gemella haemolysans* to 21 Antimicrobial Agents

Drug	Geometric Mean	Range
Penicillin	0.007	0.003–0.015
Ampicillin	0.007	0
Oxacillin	0.5	0.25–1
Cephalothin	0.125	0.062–0.5
Cefamandole	0.125	0
Cefotaxime	0.007	0.007–0.015
Tetracycline	0.25	0.12–4
Minocycline	0.25	0.06–1
Chloramphenicol	1	0.5–1
Erythromycin	0.15	0.015–64
Clindamycin	0.06	0.015–0.25
Pristinamycin	0.12	0.06–0.12
Rifampin	0.003	0.0005–0.003
Vancomycin	0.5	0
Streptomycin	8	2–16
Kanamycin	4	1–16
Gentamicin	2	0.5–4
Tobramycin	2	1–4
Amikacin	8	2–32
Sulfonamides	>128	—
Trimethoprim	>128	—

From Buu-Hoi A, Sapoetra A, Branger C, Acar JF. Antimicrobial susceptibility of *Gemella haemolysans* isolated from patients with subacute endocarditis. Eur J Microbiol 1982;1:102–106.

sides and polymyxin B; most strains are susceptible to the cephalosporins, chloramphenicol, erythromycin, clindamycin, and rifampin (3, 8, 10, 13, 25, 42, 50, 53). All strains have been susceptible to vancomycin with the exception of one reported by a reputable laboratory. This isolate was fully glycopeptide resistant as well as resistant to erythromycin and tetracycline and relatively resistant to penicillin (58).

There is no summary data on in vitro susceptibility of *G. morbillorum.* Case report information generally notes penicillin susceptibility, with MICs less than or equal to 0.06 μg/mL (5, 20, 49, 54, 64). When reported, all strains have been vancomycin susceptible; isolates generally have been susceptible to cephalosporins, chloramphenicol, erythromycin, clindamycin, and tetracyclines (5, 8, 45, 54, 66). Cefotaxime resistance was reported in a single isolate of *G. morbillorum* in one series (23). One strain was reported to be penicillin tolerant (49), and one strain, ceftriaxone tolerant (31). More recently, one strain was reported to be fully penicillin resistant, with an MIC of 4 μg/mL or higher (66).

Combination Therapy

Synergy was found between penicillin or vancomycin and gentamicin or streptomycin for all five strains of *G. haemolysans* in one study using killing curve and checkerboard titration methodologies (13). Checkerboard synergy for penicillin and gentamicin was also demonstrated for a strain of penicillin-tolerant *G. morbillorum* (49), but ceftriaxone and netilmicin showed no synergy against a ceftriaxone-tolerant strain (31). There have been no synergy reports of penicillin plus rifampin or fusidic acid.

ANTIMICROBIAL THERAPY
Drug of Choice

Penicillin is the general drug of choice for monotherapy, although the synergistic activity of penicillin with gentamicin and streptomycin makes combination therapy attractive in endocarditis. However, due to reports of variability on all drugs tested for both *Gemella* species, the drug of choice would best be directed by in vitro susceptibility data. In addition to bacteriostatic information, bactericidal data are useful in directing therapy for endocarditis and meningitis. Recommendations that apply to treatment of oral streptococcal infections probably apply to infections due to gemellae.

Special Situations

Endocarditis and Endovascular Infection

At least 17 cases of infective endocarditis due to *G. haemolysans* have been reported (2, 10, 11, 13, 16, 17, 32, 39, 42, 44, 48, 53, 61). One case was interestingly associated with elevated ASO and anti-DNase-B serum antibodies, which was eliminated by preabsorption with a gemella antigen (11). Cases have been attributed to both dental origin (13, 17, 32) and colonic origin (39). Most clinicians chose the combination of penicillin and an aminoglycoside to treat this condition (10, 32, 42). Courses of antibiotics generally equaled or exceeded 28 days; 2-week combination therapy was not reported. Erythromycin-rifampin combination therapy was reported to sterilize the blood within 8 days, but progressive prosthetic valvular insufficiency necessitated valve replacement (53). Vancomycin and fusidic acid were used prior to penicillin and an aminoglycoside with initial success (32). Cefuroxime and gentamicin combination therapy for 14 days followed by 5 days of cefuroxime and ciprofloxacin and subsequent oral erythromycin for an unspecified time was successful in one patient with neutropenia due to β-lactams (61). β-Lactam therapy was somewhat abbreviated in this patient with success (61).

Surveys of streptococcal infections and case reports have reported at least 29 cases of infective endocarditis due to *G. morbillorum*, all of which have been subacute when specified (1, 5, 14, 20, 24, 28, 30, 31, 40, 41, 45, 47, 49, 52, 62, 64, 67). Many have been thought to arise from dental or saliva-related bacteremias (5, 20, 24, 31, 49, 62), and one from a colonic source (45). Treatment has generally been successful with penicillin plus an aminoglycoside for 4 weeks (5, 49) or with penicillin for 4 weeks and an aminoglycoside for 2 weeks (14, 45). A case of either endocarditis or an infected aortic graft that recurred after penicillin monotherapy was cured with penicillin and rifampin combination therapy (20). Two week combination therapy with ceftriaxone (2 g) plus netilmicin (4 mg/kg) daily was successful in only one of two cases in which it was tried (31); in the patient that failed clinically and microbiologically, cure was achieved with ceftriaxone for 2 weeks followed by an unspecified dose of oral amoxicillin for 2 weeks plus netilmicin for 20 days. This isolate was ceftriaxone tolerant, and in vitro synergy was not found with the ceftriaxone and netilmicin combination. Penicillin for 1 week followed by 3 weeks of vancomycin was successful for a

hemodialysis arteriovenous shunt infection without graft excision (4), and vancomycin monotherapy for 6 weeks plus graft excision cured a dialysis shunt infection versus a mitral valve endocarditis (54).

It is not clear whether penicillin alone would suffice in endocarditis or endovascular infection due to either *G. haemolysans* or *G. morbillorum* or whether penicillin plus an aminoglycoside would be required. Since this combination is usually synergistic in vitro for both species and has been generally successful, its use would appear optimal for at least the initial 2 weeks, perhaps aiming for peak serum gentamicin levels of only about 3 μg/mL. Vancomycin and gentamicin or streptomycin were also synergistic when tested against *G. haemolysans*, making these combinations potentially useful as well, although the enhanced risk of renal toxicity and ototoxicity may limit use of these combinations to treatment failures or prosthetic valve infections. Long-acting cephalosporins such as ceftriaxone with or without aminoglycosides also deserve therapeutic consideration in endocarditis. Due to failures of therapy in cases due to β-lactam-tolerant strains, either an MBC or a serum bactericidal titer should probably be obtained in endocarditis.

Central Nervous System Infections

G. haemolysans has been reported in at least four cases of meningitis (3, 36, 50, 51), all involving cerebrospinal fluid (CSF) leaks, usually following procedures that violated the blood-brain barrier. Therapy was successful in all cases: cefotaxime followed by penicillin for 14 days (3), piperacillin for 3 weeks (50), and cefotaxime for 2 weeks (36). Spontaneously occurring meningitis due to *G. morbillorum* was successfully treated with ampicillin and chloramphenicol combination therapy (34). However, a case of sinusitis and brain abscess was rapidly fatal (22). Penicillin or a CSF-penetrating third-generation cephalosporin would seem the drugs of choice for meningitis due to gemellae, although chloramphenicol also seems reasonable.

Alternative Therapy

A case of bacteremia with a penicillin-resistant *G. morbillorum*, due to either an infected subcutaneous intravenous infusion device or a sinusitis, resolved after an ampicillin–clavulanic acid regimen was changed to 14 days of vancomycin (66). Because of this and since vancomycin has proven useful in endovascular infections due to *G. morbillorum* (4, 54), vancomycin would be a good alternative antimicrobial for treating serious gemellae infections in persons who cannot take penicillin. For less-severe infections, single-drug β-lactam therapy is generally recommended, although macrolide or clindamycin treatment has been effective (12) and would probably suffice. Combination therapy should be reserved for endocarditis. Chloramphenicol or a CNS-penetrating cephalosporin may be useful in CNS infections.

ENDPOINTS FOR MONITORING THERAPY

There are no recommendations for monitoring therapeutic endpoints specific to infections due to *Gemella* species; guidelines that apply to infections due to streptococci should generally be followed.

CAVEATS AND COMMENTS

Despite the statement that penicillin is the drug of choice for gemella infections, like *Streptococcus pneumoniae* and the oral streptococci, gemellae have been reported resistant to penicillin. Multiresistance to clindamycin, erythromycin, and even vancomycin has also been reported, as has β-lactam tolerance. Therapy should be directed by accurate in vitro susceptibility testing for all significant gemella isolates.

The preference for penicillin and aminoglycoside combination therapy in endocarditis due to *Gemellae* species must be viewed as only that. Although penicillin and aminoglycoside combination therapy is synergistic in most isolates thus far tested and these combinations have usually been given in reported cases of endocarditis, monotherapy still may be adequate as long as bactericidal activity can be ensured.

REFERENCES

1. Abboud R, Friart A. 2 cases of isolated tricuspid endocarditis following colonic intervention. Acta Clin Belg 1995;50:242–245.
2. Aoki Y, Tazawa S, Nakamura Y, Matsumoto H, Ohta A, Harumi K. Isolation and identification of *Gemella haemolysans* from a septic patient with heart failure. Kansenshogaku Zasshi 1982;56:715–723.
3. Aspevall O, Hillebrant E, Linderoth B, Rylander M. Meningitis due to *Gemella haemolysans* after neurosurgical treatment of trigeminal neuralgia. J Infect Dis 1991;23:503–505.
4. Bannatyne RM, Fong I. *Gemella morbillorum* infection in an arteriovenous shunt. Clin Microbiol Newslett 1992;14:7–8.
5. Bell E, McCartney AC. *Gemella morbillorum* endocarditis in an intravenous drug abuser. J Infect 1992;25:110–112.
6. Berger U. Prevalence of *Gemella haemolysans* on the pharyngeal mucosa of man. Med Microbiol Immunol 1985;174:267–274.
7. Berger U, Pervanidis A. Differentiation of *Gemella haemolysans* from *Streptococcus morbillorum*. Zentralbl Bakteriol Hyg A 1986;261:311–321.
8. Berger U. The genus *Gemella*. In: Balows A, Truper HG, Dworkin M, Harder W, Schleifer KH, editors. The prokaryotes: a handbook on the biology of bacteria: ecophysiology, isolation, identification, applications. 2nd ed. New York: Springer-Verlag, 1992:1643–1653.
9. Blin C, Vialette V, Tenaillon A, Fischer D, Cosson G. Septicémie à *Gemella haemolysans*. Med Mal Infect 1984;14:163–165.
10. Brack MJ, Avery PG, Hubner PJB, Swann RA. *Gemella haemolysans:* a rare and unusual cause of endocarditis. Postgrad Med J 1991;67:210–212.
11. Breathnach AS, Gould FK, Bain HH, Aucken HM. *Gemella haemolysans* endocarditis associated with a raised anti-streptolysin-o titre. J Infect 1997;37:87–88.
12. Brook I, Frazier EH. Microaerophilic streptococci as a significant pathogen: a twelve year review. J Med 1994;25:129–144.
13. Buu-Hoi A, Sapoetra A, Branger C, Acar JF. Antimicrobial susceptibility of *Gemella haemolysans* isolated from patients with subacute endocarditis. Eur J Microbiol 1982;1:102–106.
14. Calopa M, Rubio F, Aguilar M, Peres J. Giant basilar aneurysm in the course of subacute bacterial endocarditis. Stroke 1990;21:1625–1627.
15. Carles-Giraud D, Dellamonica P, Monnier B, Duplay H. Septicemié à *Gemella haemolysans*. A propos d'une observation. Med Mal Infect 1982;12:255–256.
16. Casado JL, Calderon C, Quereda C, Fortun J, Loza E. Endocarditis caused by *Gemella haemolysans* with a formation of a perivalvular abscess. Enferm Infecc Microbiol Clin 1995;13:127–128.
17. Chatelain R, Croize J, Rouge P, Massot C, Dabernat H, Auvergnat JC, Buu-Hoi A, Stahl JP, Bimet F. Isolement de *Gemella haemolysans* dans trois cas d'endocardites bactériennes. Med Mal Infect 1982;12:25–30.
18. Condoluci D, Chessa M, Butera G, Cipriani A, Pelargonio S. Pericarditis caused by *Gemella morbillorum*. Description of a case. Minerva Pediatr 1995;47:545–547.
19. Cooksey RC, Thompson FS, Facklam RR. Physiological characterization of nutritionally variant streptococci. J Clin Microbiol 1979;10:326–330.
20. Coto H, Berk SL. Endocarditis caused by *Streptococcus morbillorum*. Am J Med Sci 1984;287:54–58.
21. da Costa CTKA, Porter C, Parry K, Morris A, Quoraishi AH. Empyema thoracis and lung abscess due to *Gemella morbillorum*. Eur J Clin Microbiol Infect Dis 1996;15:75–77.
22. Debast SB, Koot R, Meis JFGM. Infections caused by *Gemella morbillorum*. Lancet 1993;342:177.
23. Devlin HR, Boskovski L. The synergistic effect of cefotaxime and desacetylcefotaxime against clinical isolates of anaerobic bacteria. Drugs 1988;35(Suppl 2):45–50.
24. Durack DT, Kaplan EL, Bisno AL. Apparent failures of endocarditis prophylaxis. Analysis of 52 cases submitted to a national registry. JAMA 1983;250:2318–2322.
25. Eggelmeijer F, Petit P, Dijkmans BAC. Total knee arthroplasty infection due to *Gemella haemolysans*. Br J Rheumatol 1992;31:67–69.
26. Elting ES, Bodey GP, Keefe BH. Septicemia and shock syndrome due to viridans streptococci: a case control study of predisposing risk factors. Clin Infect Dis 1992;14:1201–1207.
27. von Essen R, Ikavalko M, Forsblum B. Isolation of *Gemella morbillorum* from joint fluid. Lancet 1993;342:177–179.
28. Facklam RR. Physiological differentiation of viridans streptococci. J Clin Microbiol 1977;5:184–201.
29. Facklam R, Elliott JA. Identification, classification, and clinical relevance of catalase-negative, gram-positive cocci, excluding the streptococci and enterococci. Clin Microbiol Rev 1995;8:479–495.
30. Francioli P, Etienne V, Hoigné R, Thys JP, Gerber A. Treatment of streptococcal endocarditis with a single daily dose of ceftriaxone for 4 weeks: efficacy and out-patient feasibility. JAMA 1992;267:264–267.
31. Francioli P, Ruch W, Stamboulian D. Treatment of streptococcal endocarditis with a single daily dose of ceftriaxone and netilmicin for 14 days: a prospective multicenter study. Clin Infect Dis 1995;21:1406–1410.
32. Frésard A, Michel VP, Rueda X, Aubert G, Dorche G, Lucht F. *Gemella haemolysans* endocarditis. Clin Infect Dis 1993;16:586–587.
33. Gallis HA. Viridans and beta-hemolytic (non-group a, b and d) streptococci. In: Mandell GL, Douglas RG, Bennett JE, editors. Principles and practice of infectious diseases. 3rd ed. New York: Churchill Livingstone, 1990:1563–1572.
34. Garavelli PL. Meningitis caused by *Streptococcus morbillorum*. Minerva Med 1990;81(Suppl 7–8):69.
35. Garcia del Busto A, Moreno R, Ferrandiz A. Empyema caused by *Gemella morbillorum*. Med Clin (Barc) 1995;104:196–197.
36. Garcia-Markos JA, Meseguer M, Baquero F, Hellin T, Martinez-Luengas F, Gimeno C. Meningitis due to *Gemella haemolysans*. Clin Microbiol Newslett 1992;14:142–143.

37. Haffajee AD, Dzink JL, Socransky SS. Effect of modified Widman flap surgery and systemic tetracycline on the subgingival microbiota of periodontal lesions. J Clin Periodontol 1988;15:255–257.

38. Hayashi Y, Ito G. A case of bacterial empyema caused by *Gemella morbillorum*. Kansenshogaku Zasshi 1996;70:259–263.

39. Helft G, Tabone X, Metzger JP, Vacheron A. *Gemella haemolysans* endocarditis with colonic carcinoma. Eur J Med 1993; 2:369–370.

40. Holland J, Wilson R, Cumpston N. *Gemella morbillorum* prosthetic valve endocarditis. NZ Med J 1996;109:367.

41. Kerr JR, Webb CH, McGimpsey JG, Campbell NP. Infective endocarditis due to *Gemella morbillorum* complicating hypertrophic obstructive cardiomyopathy. Ulster Med J 1994;63:108–110.

42. Kaufhold A, Franzen D, Lutticken R. Endocarditis caused by *Gemella haemolysans*. Infection 1989;6:385–387.

43. Kilpper-Bälz R, Schleifer KH. Transfer of *Streptococcus morbillorum* to the genus *Gemella* as *Gemella morbillorum* comb. nov. Int J Syst Bacteriol 1988;38:442–443.

44. Laudat P, Cosnay P, Icole B, Raoult A, Raynaud P, Brochier M. Endocardite á *Gemella haemolysans:* une nouvelle observation. Med Mal Infect;14:159–161.

45. Lopez-Dupla M, Creus C, Navarro O Raga X. Association of *Gemella morbillorum* endocarditis with adenomatous polyps and carcinoma of the colon: case report and review. Clin Infect Dis 1996;22:379–380.

46. Ludwig W, Weizenegger R, Kilpper-Bälz R, Schleifer KH. Phylogenetic relationships of anaerobic streptococci. Int J Syst Bacteriol 1988;38:15–18.

47. Martin MJ, Wright DA, Jones AR. A case of *Gemella morbillorum* endocarditis. Postgrad Med 1995;71:188.

48. Matsis PP, Easthope RN. *Gemella haemolysans* endocarditis. Aust NZ J Med 1994;24:417–418.

49. Maxwell S. Endocarditis due to *Streptococcus morbillorum*. J Infect 1989;18:67–72.

50. May T, Amiel C, Lion C, Weber M, Gerard A, Canton P. Meningitis due to *Gemella haemolysans*. Eur J Clin Microbiol Infect Dis 1993;12:644–645.

51. Mitchell RG, Teddy PJ. Meningitis due to *Gemella haemolysans* after radiofrequency trigeminal rhizotomy. J Clin Pathol 1985; 38:558–560.

52. Molina M, Ortega G, Bermudo J, Ruiz J. Endocarditis and renal abscess caused by *Gemella morbillorum*. Enferm Infecc Microbiol Clin 1995;13:263–264.

53. Morea P, Toni M, Bressan M, Stritoni P. Prosthetic valve endocarditis by *Gemella haemolysans*. Infection 1991;19:446.

54. Omran Y, Wood CA. Endovascular infection and septic arthritis caused by *Gemella morbillorum*. Diagn Microbiol Infect Dis 1993;16:131–134.

55. Pradeep R, Ali M, Encarnacion CF. Retropharyngeal abscess due to *Gemella morbillorum*. Clin Infect Dis 1997;24:284–285.

56. Prévot AR, Turpin A, Kaiser P. Les bactéries anaérobies. Paris: Dunod; 1967.

57. Rabe LK, Winterscheid KK, Hillier SL. Association of viridans streptococci from pregnant women with bacterial vaginosis and upper genital tract infection. J Clin Microbiol 1988;26: 1156–1160.

58. Reed C, Efstratious A, Morrison D, Woodford N. Glycopeptide-resistant *Gemella haemolysans* from blood. Lancet 1993;342: 927–928.

59. Ruoff K, Fishman JA, Calderwood SB, Kunz LJ. Distribution and incidence of viridans streptococcal species in routine clinical specimens. Am J Clin Pathol 1983;80:854–858.

60. Ruoff K. Gemella: a tale of two species (and five genera). Clin Microbiol Newslett 1990;12:1–4.

61. Samuel L, Bloomfield P, Ross P. *Gemella haemolysans* prosthetic valve endocarditis. Postgrad Med J 1995;71:188.

62. Terada H, Miyahara K, Sohara H, Sonoda M, Uenomachi H, Sanada J, Arima T. Infective endocarditis caused by an indigenous bacterium (*Gemella morbillorum*). Intern Med 1994;33: 628–631.

63. Thjøtta T, Bøe J. *Neisseria haemolysans:* a haemolytic species of *Neisseria trevisian*. Acta Pathol Microbiol Scand 1938;37 (Suppl):527–541.

64. Tuazon CU, Gill V, Gill F. Streptococcal endocarditis: single vs. combination antibiotic therapy and role of various species. Rev Infect Dis 1986;8:54–60.

65. Tunnicliff R. The cultivation of a micrococcus from blood in pre-eruptive and eruptive stages of measles. JAMA 1917;68: 1028–1030.

66. Vasishtha S, Isenberg HD, Sood SK. *Gemella morbillorum* as a cause of septic shock. Clin Infect Dis 1996;22:1084–1086.

67. Wang TD, Chang SC, Chiang IP, Luh KT, Lee YT. Infected left atrial myxoma caused by *Gemella morbillorum*. Scand J Infect Dis 1996;28:633–634.

68. Whitney AM, O'Connor SP. Phylogenetic relationship of *Gemella morbillorum* to gemella haemolysans. Int J Syst Bacteriol 1993;43:832–838.

69. Willcox MD, Irwin AM, Jacques NA, Knox KW. Enumeration of oral streptococci on media containing different concentrations of sodium and potassium ions. J Dent Res 1991;70:1375–1379.

Haemophilus ducreyi

●

Pierre J. Plourde

GENERAL DESCRIPTION

Haemophilus ducreyi, a fastidious Gram-negative bacillus causing chancroid, is a sexually transmitted pathogen associated with the sexual transmission of human immunodeficiency virus (HIV). Chancroid is commonly seen in sexually transmitted disease (STD) clinics in Africa, Asia, and Latin America, where its incidence exceeds that of syphilis. In North America, chancroid was considered a relatively rare STD until a large increase in prevalence occurred in the late 1980s (5). Most cases of chancroid in the United States have been reported from California, Florida, Georgia, Louisiana, New York, and Texas, occurring primarily in heterosexual men and women from lower socioeconomic groups who consistently report recent exchange of sex for drugs or money.

Chancroid typically presents with painful, nonindurated, usually purulent genital ulcers, without initial vesicular lesions characteristic of genital herpes. Inguinal adenopathy, often unilateral and tender, occurs in approximately 50% of patients, with about half of these progressing to suppurative adenopathy known as buboes. Untreated, the infection eventually resolves spontaneously in 1 to 3 months. A successful therapeutic response is usually manifested by decreased ulcer tenderness and pain within 48 to 72 h. Complete epithelialization of successfully treated ulcers is usually achieved in 7 to 14 days but may take up to 28 days in 5 to 10% of patients. Buboes may continue to suppurate with eventual formation of inguinal ulcers. Persistent buboes do not usually necessitate further antimicrobial therapy and rupture may be prevented by timely needle aspiration through adjacent normal skin. HIV seropositivity and, in a few instances, an intact foreskin have been associated with increased likelihood of treatment failure.

Diagnosis of chancroid is complicated by difficulties encountered in isolating the organism in culture as well as its clinical presentation, which can be very similar to genital herpes viral infection, with which it is most commonly confused. Specific selective enriched culture media that are generally available only in specialized reference laboratories have sensitivities ranging from less than 50% to over 80%. Nonculture diagnostic antigen-detection tests including DNA probes and PCR currently under investigation may be more sensitive, but for the moment are research tools only. Hence, in most clinical settings, the diagnosis of chancroid remains a clinical diagnosis of exclusion.

SUSCEPTIBILITY IN VITRO

In general, minimal inhibitory concentrations (MICs) to cephalosporins, macrolides, and quinolones for *H. ducreyi* are favorable, of the order of 0.125 μg/mL or less (Table 1). Repeated observations have revealed that a successful therapeutic response requires antibiotic regimens that produce blood or tissue levels of the drug above its MIC for *H. ducreyi* for at least 36 to 48 h. This can be achieved by administering an antibiotic of short half-life for 5 to 7 days or by giving a single dose of an agent with a long half-life. Single-dose regimens are preferred over multidose regimens because compliance is a major contributor to successful STD control. However, there is a higher failure rate with single-dose regimens in HIV-seropositive patients (7).

Virtually all strains of *H. ducreyi* carry a plasmid-mediated tetracycline-resistance determinant and β-lactamase. Therefore *H. ducreyi* is inherently resistant to both tetracyclines and penicillins. Although trimethoprim in combination with sulfonamides used to be a highly efficacious treatment recommended as either a single dose or a short-course (3 to 5 days) therapy worldwide (11), it can no longer be recommended as resistance to both trimethoprim and sulfonamides exceeds 50% in many parts of Asia and sub-Saharan Africa (3, 10, 12). This resistance may be chromosomally mediated, as a trimethoprim/sulfonamide-associated plasmid has not been identified.

ANTIMICROBIAL THERAPY

The recommended first-line therapy for chancroid according to the Centers for Disease Control and Prevention (CDC) STD treatment guidelines is one of three regimens: azithromycin 1 g orally in a single dose, ceftriaxone 250 mg intramuscularly in a single dose, or erythromycin base 500 mg orally four times a day for 7 days. Amoxicillin 500 mg plus clavulanic acid 125 mg orally three times a day for 7 days or ciprofloxacin 500 mg orally twice a day for 3 days are recommended as alternative regimens (4). Amoxicillin clavulanate has not been studied as extensively as the other regimens. Recent in vitro data suggesting an increasing level of resistance to amoxicillin clavulanate in strains from both the United States and Thailand has led to some caution regarding use of this antibiotic for the treatment of chancroid (8).

Of the cephalosporins, ceftriaxone has received the most study, and for the most part has consistently demonstrated high clinical and microbiologic efficacy (near 100%) for over one decade, at a single dose of 250 mg intramuscularly (9, 12). However, a recent publication from Nairobi revealed dismal efficacy with ceftriaxone, with documented clinical and microbiologic

TABLE 1 • In Vitro Sensitivities of *Haemophilus ducreyi* (8, 10)			
Antimicrobial Agent	MIC$_{50}$ (μg/mL)	MIC$_{90}$ (μg/mL)	MIC Range (μg/mL)
Penicillin G	64.0	64.0	0.25–64.0
Amoxicillin clavulanate	2.0	8.0	0.03–16.0
Trimethoprim-sulfamethoxazole	1.0	32.0	0.015–64.0
Tetracycline	16.0	32.0	2.0–64.0
Ceftriaxone	0.004	0.004	0.002–0.25
Cefixime	0.06	0.25	0.015–0.5
Erythromycin	0.008	0.125	0.002–4.0
Azithromycin	0.004	0.03	0.002–0.06
Ciprofloxacin	0.004	0.004	0.002–2.0
Ofloxacin	0.008	0.008	0.004–0.125
Fleroxacin	0.008	0.125	0.004–0.125

failure rates of 35 and 28%, respectively (13). The authors observed that HIV seropositivity and the presence of a foreskin may have contributed to this high failure rate. Nevertheless, clinical failure in HIV-negative, circumcised men was still unacceptably high at 25%. Ceftriaxone MICs in this study were universally below 0.008 µg/ml. Further studies will be necessary to assess the efficacy of single-dose ceftriaxone for the treatment of chancroid, especially in HIV-infected populations.

Macrolide antibiotics have also enjoyed success in treating chancroid for several years without any significant evidence of the emergence of resistance. The World Health Organization (WHO) recommends erythromycin 500 mg orally three times a day for 7 days as first-line therapy for chancroid, with some countries in sub-Saharan Africa recommending doses as low as 250 mg three times a day for 7 days to lower the cost of therapy (7). Although lower-dose regimens of erythromycin may be more economically feasible in the developing world, they should be recommended with caution because clinical efficacy of lower-dose regimens has ranged from 80 to 90% (1, 2, 6, 7). Azithromycin, with lower MICs to *H. ducreyi* than erythromycin and a very favorable pharmacokinetic profile resulting in clinical and microbiologic cures rates exceeding 90% when administered in a single oral dose make this an ideal choice for treatment of chancroid (9). However, caution must be advised once again with HIV-positive uncircumcised men who demonstrated a clinical failure rate of 24% in another study from Nairobi (15).

Since quinolones have consistently demonstrated very low MICs against *H. ducreyi* in vitro, they have also received considerable attention with respect to the treatment of chancroid. The WHO recommends ciprofloxacin 500 mg orally, administered as a single dose, as the second-line therapy after erythromycin. Studies using ciprofloxacin performed prior to 1990 consistently revealed clinical and microbiologic cure rates of 95 to 100% with regimens ranging from 500 mg twice a day for 3 days (recommended by CDC) to 500 mg in a single oral dose (1). More-recent attempts at administering a long-acting quinolone in a single dose have produced mixed results. Oral fleroxacin 400 mg in a single dose resulted in a clinical success rate of 94% in culture-positive HIV-negative men from Nairobi (10). However, cure rates in HIV-infected men have been disappointingly low at 68%, even when a multidose regimen of 400 mg once daily for 5 days was used (14).

ENDPOINTS FOR MONITORING THERAPY

Successful therapy should reveal markedly reduced tenderness, absence of purulence, and partial reepithelialization of ulcers at a follow-up evaluation 7 days after initiation of therapy. Although female sex workers have been identified as an important reservoir of chancroid, efficacy of currently recommended regimens have not been evaluated in women. Such evaluation is needed.

IMMUNOSUPPRESSION, PRECAUTIONS, COSTS, AND SYNDROMIC MANAGEMENT

Although several studies have suggested that immunosuppression secondary to HIV infection may worsen the clinical efficacy of antimicrobials used for treatment of chancroid,

none have actually systematically measured immunologic function in study participants. A recent publication from Rwanda also disputed the adverse impact of HIV on the therapy of chancroid, demonstrating equivalent clinical cure rates of 75 to 80% in HIV-negative and HIV-positive men, respectively, treated with a single 500-mg dose of ciprofloxacin (3). These investigators also did not find any correlation between CD4+ lymphocyte counts and clinical efficacy. Nevertheless, the CDC still recommends that if no clinical improvement is noted 7 days after initiation of a first-line agent, consideration should be given to the possibility of coinfection with HIV. Other causes of clinical failure include another diagnosis (especially herpes genitalis), noncompliance (which should not be the case with single-dose regimens), and resistance to the prescribed antimicrobial.

There are no major contraindications to the administration of ceftriaxone for chancroid, although intramuscular administration may not always be optimal. Although minimal cross-reactivity exists between the penicillins and third-generation cephalosporins, caution should be exercised in patients with a history of severe allergic reactions to penicillin. Erythromycin is contraindicated in individuals taking terfenadine, and theophylline levels may be increased when coadministered with erythromycin. Azithromycin should not be taken with food or antacids containing magnesium or aluminum, which may interfere with absorption. Quinolones are contraindicated in pregnancy and in persons less than 18 years of age. When cost is a factor, erythromycin and ciprofloxacin have the most favorable profiles, averaging under U.S.$5.00 per treatment, while ceftriaxone costs approximately U.S.$10.00 per treatment, with azithromycin being the most expensive choice at over U.S.$30.00.

A syndromic approach to the management of genital ulcers has been adopted by many developing countries. This essentially consists of treating all chancroidlike genital ulcers at first contact with the health care system with antibiotics that are effective against both syphilis and chancroid, the two most common treatable causes of genital ulcers in most developing countries. First-line treatment recommended for chancroid is usually erythromycin. In the absence of adequate laboratory facilities, it is hoped that this approach will lead to better control of genital ulcer diseases worldwide. Chancroid is largely controlled in most developed countries and has been eradicated in several outbreak situations. The strong epidemiologic association between chancroid and HIV infection in several developing countries emphasizes the urgency of focusing resources on control of chancroid. Availability of cost-effective, inexpensive, easily administered regimens for the treatment of chancroid is crucial to worldwide control of HIV transmission. Successful control of outbreaks require prompt identification and treatment of patients with simple antibiotic regimens followed by aggressively pursuing treatment of all recent sexual contacts within the previous 7 to 10 days, combined with sensitive and appropriate prevention educational messages. Dramatic reductions in the number of cases in the United States in the past 5 years and several successful eradications of *H. ducreyi* from local outbreaks in various North American cities in the past 10 years have demonstrated that at least theoretically, it may be possible to completely eradicate *H. ducreyi* as a cause of genital ulcer disease.

REFERENCES

1. Ballard RC, Duncan MO, Fehler HG, Dangor Y, Exposto FL, Latif AS. Treating chancroid: summary of studies in southern Africa. Genitourin Med 1989;65:54–57.
2. Behets FM, Liomba G, Lule G, Dallabetta G, Hoffman IF, Hamilton HA, Moeng S, Cohen MS. Sexually transmitted diseases and human immunodeficiency virus control in Malawi: a field study of genital ulcer disease. J Infect Dis 1995;171: 451–455.
3. Bogaerts J, Kestens L, Martinez Tello W, Akingeneyc J, Mukantabana V, Verhaegen J, Van Dyck E, Piot P. Failure of treatment for chancroid in Rwanda is not related to human immunodeficiency virus infection: in vitro resistance to *Haemophilus ducreyi* to trimethoprim-sulphamethoxazole. Clin Infect Dis 1995;20: 924–930.
4. Centers for Disease Control and Prevention. Sexually transmitted diseases treatment guidelines. MMWR 1993;42(RR-14): 20–22.
5. Centers for Disease Control and Prevention. Sexually transmitted disease surveillance, 1993. U.S. Department of Health and Human Services, Atlanta, Georgia, 1994.
6. Choudhri SH, Nasio J, Nagelkerke NJ, Plummer FA, Ronald AR. Treatment of chancroid with low dose erythromycin in a population with high HIV seroprevalence. Canadian J Infect Dis 1995;6(Suppl B):40B.
7. Kimani J, Bwayo JJ, Anzala AO, MacLean I, Mwatha A, Choudhri SH, Plummer FA, Ronald AR. Low dose erythromycin regimen for the treatment of chancroid. East Afr Med J 1995; 72:645–648.
8. Knapp JS, Back AF, Babst AF, Taylor D, Rice RJ. In vitro susceptibilities of isolates of *Haemophilus ducreyi* from Thailand and the United States to currently recommended and newer agents for treatment of chancroid. Antimicrob Agents Chemother 1993; 37:1552–1555.
9. Martin DH, Sargent SJ, Wendel GD Jr, McCormack WM, Spier NA, Johnson RB. Comparison of azithromycin and ceftriaxone for the treatment of chancroid. Clin Infect Dis 1995;21:409–414.
10. Plourde PJ, D'Costa LJ, Agoki E, Ombette J, Ndinya-Achola JO, Slaney LA, Ronald AR, Plummer FA. A randomized, double-blind study of the efficacy of fleroxacin versus trimethoprim-sulphamethoxazole in men with culture-proven chancroid. J Infect Dis 1992;165:949–952.
11. Plummer FA, Nsanze H, D'Costa LJ, Karasira P, Maclean IW, Ellison RH, Ronald AR. Single-dose therapy of chancroid with trimethoprim-sulfametrole. N Engl J Med 1983;309:67–71.
12. Taylor DN, Pitarangsi C, Echeverria P, Panikabutra K, SuvongseC. Comparative study of ceftriaxone and trimethoprim-sulphamethoxazole for the treatment of chancroid in Thailand. J Infect Dis 1985;152:1002–1006.
13. Tyndall M, Malisa M, Plummer FA, Ombetti J, Ndinya-Achola JO, Ronald AR. Ceftriaxone no longer predictably cures chancroid in Kenya. J Infect Dis 1993;167:469–471.
14. Tyndall MW, Plourde PJ, Agoki E, Malisa W, Ndinya-Achola JO, Plummer FA, Ronald AR. Fleroxacin in the treatment of chancroid: an open study in men seropositive or seronegative for the human immunodeficiency virus type 1. Am J Med 1993; 94(3A):85S–88S.
15. Tyndall MW, Agoki E, Plummer FA, Malisa W, Ndinya-Achola JO, Ronald AR. Single dose azithromycin for the treatment of chancroid: a randomized comparison with erythromycin. Sex Transm Dis 1994;21:231–234.

Haemophilus influenzae

●

Mark A. Herbert and Richard E. Moxon

GENERAL DESCRIPTION

Haemophilus influenzae is a small, nonmotile, nonsporeforming, Gram-negative pleomorphic rod that can be either encapsulated (serotypes a–f) or unencapsulated. *H. influenzae* normally exists as a commensal in the human upper respiratory tract but can cause disease, either by invasion of the bloodstream or by contiguous spread. Invasive disease has the most serious consequences, including meningitis, epiglottitis, and bacteremia, and is principally caused by *H. influenzae* type b (104, 178). Lower respiratory tract infections, otitis media, and sinusitis are predominantly caused by contiguous spread of unencapsulated *H. influenzae* (139). The two disease patterns overlap so that unencapsulated *H. influenzae* occasionally invades, especially in immunocompromised persons, the elderly, and neonates; conversely, *H. influenzae* type b accounts for a minor percentage of localized infection. *H. influenzae* also causes cellulitis, osteomyelitis, septic arthritis, cholecystitis, endocarditis, pericarditis, acute exacerbations of chronic bronchitis or cystic fibrosis, genitourinary infections, and neonatal-maternal sepsis (17, 94, 132, 139, 203).

Before introduction of *H. influenzae* type b vaccination, 20 to 50 per 100,000 children in Europe and North America developed invasive disease (104), and even 500 per 100,000 in some susceptible populations (187). The impact of disease can be gauged from a meningitis mortality of 6 to 12% in the tropics (46, 208) and less then 5% in developed countries (135). Neurologic sequelae occur in up to 20% of survivors in the tropics and up to 14% in industrialized nations (189). Immunization has almost eradicated invasive type b disease in countries that have implemented national vaccination programs (1); but the vaccine does not protect against unencapsulated *H. influenzae* or other capsular types. Children under 5 years old are principally affected; infection in adults is unusual. The incidence of *H. influenzae* invasive disease in adults is 0.2 to 1.7 per 100,000. In Barcelona, 30% were *H. influenzae* type b, 3% type f, and 67% unencapsulated. Seventy percent or more adults have an underlying predisposing illness (52, 64, 179, 188). Neonatal-maternal infections in one study occurred in 0.64 per 1000 births in 1979–84 but increased to 2.38 per 1000 in 1985–87 (160).

SUSCEPTIBILITY IN VITRO
Single-Drug Therapy

Ampicillin

Prior to the 1970s, all isolates of *H. influenzae* were uniformly susceptible to ampicillin or amoxicillin (142, 143, 180), but in 1972, *H. influenzae* containing the TEM-1 β-lactamase was first recognized in Europe. By 1973, TEM-1 was reported as a cause of treatment failure in *H. influenzae* meningitis. A second β-lactamase, ROB-1, emerged later (167) and now accounts overall for 8% of ampicillin resistance, 13% in North America compared with 0.3% in France (115). β-Lactamases have now been documented in *H. influenzae* in virtually all parts of the world and are present in over 95% of ampicillin-resistant isolates (105), and respiratory outbreaks of ampicillin-resistant unencapsulated *H. influenzae* have been reported (2, 89). Resistance has increased to a level that curtails ampicillin's usefulness (Table 1) (37). In studies spanning 1986 to 1993, the prevalence of ampicillin resistance in *H. influenzae* type b has been twice that in unencapsulated *H. influenzae,* 14 to 64% in type b versus 8 to 34% in unencapsulated isolates (Table 1) (52, 83, 105, 120, 157–159). The prevalence of resistance in unencapsulated *H. influenzae* from urogenital and neonatal sources is low, an indication that ampicillin is still useful for maternal and neonatal infections (160). The β-lactamase inhibitors clavulanate, sulbactam, and tazobactam are active against *H. influenzae* harboring TEM-1 and reduce the minimal inhibitory concentration (MIC) by 8- to 64-fold. Between 0.1 and 2.6% of all *H. influenzae* isolates have developed resistance through alterations in penicillin-binding proteins (PBPs) 3, 4, and 5 (36,

73, 115, 178). Most are unencapsulated strains isolated from sputum of patients with chronic lung disease (50, 157), but they have also been implicated in meningitis and endocarditis treatment failure (123). They are insensitive to β-lactamase inhibitors and have decreased susceptibility to some oral cephalosporins. Further mutations in PBPs may lead to third-generation cephalosporin resistance, but it has not yet been reported. Extended-spectrum β-lactamases that are found in *Enterobacteriaceae* and confer third-generation cephalosporin and carbapenem resistance have not spread to *H. influenzae* (71).

Chloramphenicol

Chloramphenicol resistance, mediated by chloramphenicol acetyltransferase in more than 90% of resistant *H. influenzae,* emerged in 1976 (50). In North America, the prevalence is less than 1% (Table 1) (58, 193) and in much of Europe it is less than 5%; however, in pockets of Europe and Asia, resistance has become a major problem, reaching 24.9% in Spain, 10.9% in Belgium, and 8 to 36% in Thailand (105, 120, 158), and outbreaks of chloramphenicol-resistant *H. influenzae* type b have occurred (26). Chloramphenicol-resistant isolates are often multidrug resistant. Chloramphenicol is still considered a valuable drug for susceptible *H. influenzae* (135). Bone marrow suppression is almost always dose related and reversible, and permanent hematologic toxicity is extremely rare.

Cephalosporins

During the 1980s, as a result of excellent in vitro activity and cerebrospinal fluid penetration, third-generation cephalosporins became the preferred treatment for invasive *H. influenzae* disease (30). First-generation cephalosporins (e.g., cefaclor and cephalexin) have limited activity against *H. influenzae* (Table 2) (50, 157). Cefaclor resistance has a prevalence of 1.4 to 5.5% in North America and 2% in Europe. Second- and third-generation oral cephalosporins, cefuroxime axetil, cefamandole, cefixime, ceftibuten, and cefpodoxime proxetil have MICs below 0.5 μg/mL. Resistance is generally less than 2% for cefuroxime and cefamandole, and resistance to newer cephalosporins has not been documented (163). Cefotaxime, ceftazidime, ceftriaxone, and moxalactam all have excellent cerebrospinal fluid penetra-

TABLE 1 • **World Prevalence of Antibiotic Resistance, Combined Percentages for Unencapsulated and Type b *H. influenzae***

	Canada 1985–87	U.S. 1986	U.S. 1988	U.S. 1995	U.K. 1986	Europe 1983–92	Asia 1991–92	Taiwan
Ampicillin	19.3	20	16.5	38.9	6.2	<2–30[a]	1–35	51
Amox/clav	1.7		0.2	4.5		0–2		
Chloramphenicol	0.04	0.5	0	0.2	1.7	0.6–25	8–36	28
TMP-SMX	3.8	0.9	0.7	9	4.6	4–30	9–11	49
Tetracycline	1.3	2.3	2.1	1.3	2.7	<2–25		37
Rifampicin	1	0.7		0.3		1		
Cefaclor	1.4	5.5	1.1	18.3		≤5		
Cefuroxime	0.7	3	0.2	6.4		0–2		3
Cefamandole	0.1	10	1.3					10

Data from references 35, 50, 55, 56, 58, 76, 83, 105, 105, 107, 115, 120, 157, 159, 178, 199.

[a] Highly variable percentage depending on European country examined.

TABLE 2 • MIC$_{90}$ (μg/mL) for *H. influenzae*

Amoxicillin or ampicillin	0.5
Amoxicillin-clavulanate	0.5/0.25
Chloramphenicol	0.5
Gentamicin	1
Kanamycin	0.5–1
Trimethoprim-sulfisoxazole	0.5/4
Tetracycline	0.5
Azithromycin	0.06–4
Clarithromycin	2–16
Roxithromycin	8–32
Erythromycin	4–32
Cefaclor	2–8
Cephalexin	8–32
Cephradine	8–32
Cefamandole	0.03–2
Cefuroxime	0.2–3
Cefpodoxime	0.06–2
Cefixime/ceftibuten	<0.5
Cefotaxime	0.004–0.06
Ceftriaxone	0.004–0.03
Ceftazidime	0.03–0.25
Ceftizoxime	0.001–3
Ciprofloxacin	0.012
Sparfloxacin	0.06
Ofloxacin	0.06
Meropenem	0.015–1
Imipenem	0.06–2
Aztreonam	0.1–0.5
Rifampicin	1

Data from references 6, 30, 34, 50, 65, 69, 99, 109, 113, 119, 122, 133, 155, 178, 180, 190, 201, 206.

tion and are extraordinarily active against *H. influenzae* (MICs usually <0.1 μg/mL) (69, 99).

Macrolides and Azalides

In vitro susceptibility testing of many antibiotics is confounded by the fastidious growth of *H. influenzae*. The composition of media, the concentration of CO_2 during incubation (11), and the bacterial inoculation density all affect results of disk-diffusion tests; breakpoints vary between laboratories, and discrepancies in reported prevalence of resistance are common (50, 151, 193). Breakpoints for erythromycin range from 0.5 to 4 μg/mL, whereas 8 μg/mL for *H. influenzae* cultured on Haemophilus Test Media has been proposed by the National Committee for Clinical Laboratory Standards (NCCLS) (59). Consequently, 90% erythromycin resistance is reported in Barcelona (105), but only 1.1% in Austria (50). Even where *H. influenzae* is deemed susceptible to erythromycin, the MICs of isolates are usually high, between 2 and 8 μg/mL (average, 6.4 μg/mL; Table 2). *H. influenzae* appears to have an inherent resistance to erythromycin, which should thus theoretically have a limited role in treatment. Azithromycin and clarithromycin are considerably more active (84, 96, 151, 152), whereas roxithromycin has activity similar to that of erythromycin (74, 122).

Clarithromycin is metabolized to 14-OH-clarithromycin, which is two to four times more active than clarithromycin itself (18); thus in vitro susceptibility testing with only the par-

ent drug inaccurately reflects in vivo sensitivity (12). Clarithromycin and 14-OH-clarithromycin have additive effects against 82% of *H. influenzae* isolates and are synergistic against 8%. Guidelines for disk-diffusion interpretation suggested by the NCCLS (103) do not include addition of 14-OH-clarithromycin to clarithromycin-containing disks, partly because the most appropriate concentration of metabolite and the ratio to parent drug are unknown. An alternative proposal is to increase the clarithromycin breakpoint to take account of the greater in vivo activity (96).

Tetracycline and Aminoglycosides

Both tetracycline and aminoglycosides are active against *H. influenzae*, and resistance has low prevalence, but the availability of more efficient and safer drugs has limited their use. Tetracycline resistance is a plasmid-encoded, energy-dependent process similar to the class B efflux system of resistance in *Enterobacteriaceae*. It is frequently associated with ampicillin and chloramphenicol resistance. Areas of high tetracycline resistance in the world are Spain (25.4%), Belgium (17.8%), and Thailand (36%) (50). Aminoglycoside resistance in *H. influenzae* involves drug modification and inactivation or alteration of the ribosomal target. Aminoglycosides used in broad-spectrum therapy of acute exacerbations of cystic fibrosis are initially effective, but *H. influenzae* becomes resistant swiftly.

Newer Broad-Spectrum Antimicrobials

Fluoroquinolones, aztreonam, moxalactam, and carbapenems are used to treat neutropenic and other highly susceptible patients with infections of unknown etiology. These agents are all extremely active against *H. influenzae*, but *H. influenzae* is an infrequent cause of sepsis in such patients (24). Quinolones are likely to be used with increasing frequency where multidrug resistance exists. Resistance to quinolones has been reported but is rare and does not at present restrict empirical use of this class of drug (10, 40, 79).

Combination Therapy

Trimethoprim-sulfamethoxazole

H. influenzae develops resistance through overproduction or altered structure of dihydrofolate reductase (49). Trimethoprim-sulfamethoxazole resistance has low prevalence in North America and the United Kingdom, but has become significant in Spain and Asia (Table 1) (105). A polysaccharide capsule confers tolerance to trimethoprim-sulfamethoxazole in some *H. influenzae* type b; that is, they have an MBC of 4 to 76 μg/mL or more but a low MIC of 0.03 to 0.6 μg/mL or less. One consequence is that a proportion of *H. influenzae* type b with virulence potential may persist in the nasopharynx of carriers after trimethoprim-sulfamethoxazole therapy, whereas relatively benign unencapsulated strains may be eradicated (207).

Rifampicin (Plus or Minus Cephalosporin)

Resistance emerges rapidly in *H. influenzae* after a 4-day course of prophylactic rifampicin; nevertheless, the community prevalence of resistance is low (≤1%), perhaps reflecting the infrequent use of this drug for treatment. No rifampicin-resistant invasive disease has yet been documented (180). When rifampicin is used in treatment, it is often coadministered with a cephalosporin, and these two drugs exhibit synergy against *H. influenzae* (78).

Erythromycin-Sulfisoxazole

This combination appears to have little advantage over erythromycin, which alone is of unproven efficacy.

Multiple Drug Resistance

In the late 1970s, chloramphenicol combined with ampicillin was the treatment of choice for life-threatening *H. influenzae* infections. *H. influenzae* resistant to both ampicillin and chloramphenicol were first recovered in Thailand in 1980. In most areas of Europe and North America, multidrug resistance has a prevalence of only 0.6%, but the prevalence of multidrug resistance in Barcelona is 45% in type b isolates and 57% in type b causing meningitis; in Taiwan it is 51% in *H. influenzae* type b (24, 30, 64). Multidrug resistance is encoded by at least three distinct but similar plasmids (30) and can potentially spread with ease (53, 116).

Summary of in Vitro Sensitivities

Over the course of two decades, the prevalence of ampicillin-resistant *H. influenzae* has increased markedly, and it is twice as frequent in type b as in unencapsulated *H. influenzae*. Fortunately, resistance to other antimicrobials has not escalated at a comparable rate. Amoxicillin-clavulanate, cefuroxime axetil, and cefpodoxime proxetil remain active, and rates of resistance to trimethoprim-sulfamethoxazole, chloramphenicol, cefaclor, tetracycline, azithromycin, and clarithromycin are generally low (prevalence, 1–5%) with geographic exceptions. Third-generation cephalosporins are uniformly active, and a variety of broad-spectrum drugs that are usually reserved for compromised patients are highly effective (30). Interpretive criteria for cefaclor, loracarbef, cefprozil, and cefixime resistance have recently been revised for testing on Haemophilus Test Medium (57).

SUSCEPTIBILITY IN VIVO

Determinants of in vivo susceptibility are drug pharmacokinetics (see below), the activity of metabolites, and postantibiotic effects. Bactericidal assays using volunteers' or patients' serum or cerebrospinal fluid previously used to confirm that the pathogen deemed susceptible in vitro is indeed killed in vivo are little used as a clinical tool for *H. influenzae* infections.

In developing antimicrobials for *H. influenzae* infections, animals have been vital in determining drug kinetics and efficacy, for example, the rabbit meningitis model (126, 163). Clarithromycin has greater efficacy than azithromycin in murine *H. influenzae* pulmonary infections and otitis media in gerbils (152). In the rabbit meningitis model, imipenem treatment of ampicillin/chloramphenicol-resistant *H. influenzae* reduced the bacterial load by only 49% in 24 h, compared with 92% for cefotaxime and ceftriaxone (168). Although interpretation should be cautious, animal models may guide therapeutic choice for newer drugs, but such information contributes little to data derived from drug trials in man.

Postantibiotic effects have been most elegantly demonstrated for azithromycin and clarithromycin by analysis of *H. influenzae* growth curves after incubation in broth containing antibiotics at concentrations 10 times the MIC, removing the antibiotics by washing, and then allowing growth to restart in broth containing antibiotics at concentrations equivalent to 0.1 to 0.3 times the MIC (145). Reduced growth rates were observed for up to 19.6 h after a 2-h incubation at 10 times the MIC followed by 0.3 times the MIC. Clarithromycin had a shorter postantibiotic effect than azithromycin. 14-OH-Clarithromycin and desacetyl cefotaxime are active metabolites and consequently the parent compounds have greater in vivo efficacies than expected from bacterial killing studies conducted in vitro.

ANTIMICROBIAL THERAPY
General

The antibiotics used for known or presumptive *H. influenzae* infections can be categorized into several groups:

1. Those with minimal activity against *H. influenzae* (erythromycin)
2. Those active against *H. influenzae* but with unfavorable pharmacokinetics or side effects that limit their usefulness (aminoglycosides and tetracycline)
3. Those active against susceptible *H. influenzae* that cannot be used where antibiotic resistance prevalence is high (ampicillin, chloramphenicol, tetracycline and trimethoprim-sulfamethoxazole)
4. Highly active agents with good tissue penetration appropriate for therapy of noninvasive infections (second- and third-generation oral cephalosporins, azithromycin, and clarithromycin)
5. Extremely active agents with reliable cerebrospinal fluid penetration, used in the treatment of invasive disease (third-generation parenteral cephalosporins)
6. Oral cephalosporins still being assessed for their full potential in *H. influenzae* infections (cefpodoxime proxetil, ceftibuten, cefetamet)
7. Newer agents to which *H. influenzae* is highly susceptible (fluoroquinolones, aztreonam, and carbapenems); the reliability of cerebrospinal fluid penetration has often not been fully established

Special Situations

Meningitis

H. influenzae meningitis is predominantly caused by *H. influenzae* type b in children under 5 years old. Unencapsulated *H. influenzae* is an infrequent meningitis pathogen in neonates and immunocompromised persons and where there is a basilar skull fracture or cerebrospinal fluid fistula. Cerebrospinal fluid penetration, a major determinant of drug choice, can be estimated from antibiotic concentrations in volunteers (without meningeal inflammation) and in patients (with inflammation) following parenteral antibiotic administration (Table 3). Meningeal inflammation markedly affects penetration, so that at the start of treatment, hydrophilic antibiotics such as β-lactams achieve bactericidal levels in cerebrospinal fluid, but as recovery ensues, penetration declines, and concentrations fall

TABLE 3 • Some Reported Drug Concentrations in Body Compartments following Therapeutic Doses of Antibiotics (µg/mL)

Drug	Cerebrospinal Fluid	Respiratory Tract	Middle Ear Fluid
Penicillin V			6
Ampicillin	0.3	0.25–0.6	0.2–2.2
Amoxicillin	2	0.9–7.2	1.8–2.3
Clavulanate		1–1.6	
Sulbactam	4.2	0.3	
Erythromycin			0.6
Sulfisoxazole			3.7
Trimethoprim			1.9
Sulfamethoxazole			17
Chloramphenicol	5.7		
Ciprofloxacin	0.35–0.56		
Rifampicin	0.27		
Cephradine	<1.5	1.3	
Cephalexin		0.3	
Cefuroxime	0.3–21.7	2.4	
Cefotaxime	1–15	0.6	
Ceftriaxone	1–13.5[a]	1.9–27	
Ceftazidime	1–30	5.6–7	
Cefpodoxime		1.1	
Cefpriome		7.2	
Cefamandole	0.94		
Cefixime	0.2–11.7	<0.2–2.4	
Azithromycin		9	
Clarithromycin		9–17	
Aztreonam	3		
Imipenem	2.1[b]		
Meropenem	2.8		

Data from references 32, 34, 80, 110, 119, 122, 124, 133, 141, 156.

[a]Up to 58.

[b]Up to 8.6 in early phase of acute bacterial meningitis.

to about 0.5 to 2% of peaks in serum (163). Lipophilic drugs such as chloramphenicol and rifampicin enter the cerebrospinal fluid adequately even in the absence of inflammation. Serum protein binding inversely correlates with meningeal penetration, and although cefotaxime is highly protein bound, cerebrospinal fluid levels are high enough for therapeutic success (15, 163). As the cerebrospinal fluid is physiologically "hidden" from the immune system and bacterial killing is impaired, a bactericidal antimicrobial is prefered to a bacteriostatic one. The speed of cerebrospinal fluid sterilization is proportionate to the neurologic sequelae rate (44), and microbial killing is maximal when antibiotic concentrations are 10 to 20 times higher than the MBC (Tables 2 and 3).

Clavulanate and other β-lactamase inhibitors reach therapeutic levels in cerebrospinal fluid and are active against most ampicillin-resistant *H. influenzae* type b. Chloramphenicol has outstanding cerebrospinal fluid penetration; however, geographic variations in resistance, largely unjustified apprehension about side effects of chloramphenicol, and the perceived comparative safety of cephalosporins have led to declining use of chloramphenicol. Third-generation cephalosporins are extremely active against *H. influenzae* causing meningitis, with achievable cerebrospinal fluid concentrations 100 to several 1000 times greater than the MIC (25, 33) and are the preferred

antibiotics for meningitis treatment (14, 15, 28, 99, 125). Cefotaxime or ceftriaxone treatment of meningitis may result in fewer neurologic sequelae than chloramphenicol therapy (148) or are at least as effective as the combination of chloramphenicol and ampicillin (3, 87, 100, 146, 164). Ampicillin and chloramphenicol may be preferred in countries were the per capita expenditure on health care is low (191). In many such countries, even when the individual prevalence of ampicillin resistance or chloramphenicol resistance is high, the prevalence of combined ampicillin/chloramphenicol resistance is often low (148).

Initial studies of cefuroxime in meningitis indicated equivalent efficacy to cefotaxime or ceftriaxone, but delayed cerebrospinal fluid sterilization is more frequent with cefuroxime (9 vs. 0% at 24 h, or 12 vs. 2% at 18–36 h), with reports of cerebrospinal fluid cultures remaining positive until the 5th day of treatment, and breakthrough or secondary bacteremia, mastoiditis, and epiglottitis occurring between 10 and 17 days after the start of therapy (114, 127, 173). Hearing impairment is more common after cefuroxime therapy (18 vs. 11%, or 17 vs. 4%), and third-generation cephalosporins have been found consistently better (13, 200, 205). Oral cephalosporins are considered inadequate therapy for meningitis because breakthrough meningitis has been reported in children receiving cephalexin, cefaclor, and cephamandole for otitis media (50, 162). However, the role of oral cefixime in meningitis needs further evaluation (141).

Carbapenems and aztreonam penetrate into the cerebrospinal fluid, but levels may be unreliable (128). Imipenem-cilastatin, but not meropenem, result in more convulsions during meningitis therapy than third-generation cephalosporins (109, 110, 204). Fluoroquinolones have a potential future role in *H. influenzae* meningitis: they penetrate cerebrospinal fluid well, and limited reports indicate that they are efficacious in meningitis. Perfloxacin and ciprofloxacin have been most studied (130). Aztreonam or fluoroquinolones are being considered as alternative therapies for *H. influenzae* meningitis (163).

Current dosage recommendations, based on measured serum and cerebrospinal fluid concentrations, rate of bacterial killing in cerebrospinal fluid, and drug side effects, are given in Table 4.

TABLE 4 • Recommended Drug Dosages for Meningitis

Drug	Total Daily Dose (mg/kg/day)	
	Adults (dosing interval, h)	Children (dosing interval, h)
Ampicillin	12 (4)	200–400 (3–6)
Chloramphenicol	4–6 (6)	75–100 (6–8)
Cefotaxime	8–12 (6–8)	200 (6)
Ceftazidime	6 (8)	75–150 (6–8)
Ceftriaxone	4 (12–24)	100 (12–24)
Meropenem	3 (8)	120 (8)
Rifampicin	0.6 (24)	10–20 (12–24)
Dexamethasone		0.6 (6)

Data from references 91 and 163.
Adult doses are listed as g/day and children doses are listed as mg/kg/day.

Cerebrospinal Fluid Shunt Infections

H. influenzae rarely causes meningitis in patients with cerebrospinal fluid shunts. In one analysis of 27 cases, 22 were caused by *H. influenzae* type b and 5 by unencapsulated *H. influenzae* (202). In one review, most pathogens infecting cerebrospinal fluid shunts did so within 30 weeks of the last neurosurgical operation, whereas *H. influenzae* infections occurred later, 33 weeks to 4 years after surgery (166), indicating that shunt infection by *H. influenzae* is usually blood borne as is meningitis in children without shunts. Meningitis in patients with cerebrospinal fluid shunts who have not had recent surgery should be treated with antimicrobials that cover *H. influenzae*. Treatment of any shunt infection often necessitates removal of the shunt with a period of externalization before replacement. However, apparent successful treatment of some *H. influenzae* infections with antibiotics alone has been reported, including treatment with a combination of rifampicin and ceftriaxone (90, 91, 166) and with cefotaxime followed by ampicillin (202). A large multicenter study would be necessary to determine whether *H. influenzae* shunt infections are particularly amenable to therapy without surgical intervention.

Lower Respiratory Tract Infections

Pneumonia has been estimated to cause over 3 million deaths in children under 5 years of age in developing countries (194). In industrialized countries, the incidence of pneumonia is about 40 per 1000 preschool children and 9 per 1000 in those 9 to 15 years old. Worldwide, *H. influenzae* is the second most common bacterial pathogen in community-acquired pneumonia (176). Unencapsulated strains cause most *H. influenzae* pneumonia, especially in the elderly and in those with chronic respiratory diseases such as acute exacerbations of chronic bronchitis, cystic fibrosis, and bronchiectasis. *H. influenzae* type b accounts for less than 2% of bacterial pneumonia in hospitalized patients and mainly occurs in young children. *H. influenzae* is one of five bacteria that most frequently cause acute bronchitis, although the most common etiology is viral. Seventy percent of parapneumonic effusions occur in children under 2 years old, and in children between 7 and 24 months old, *H. influenzae* is the most common pathogen; 90% are *H. influenzae* type b and 10% are unencapsulated strains (68). Effusions caused by *H. influenzae* type b are particularly likely to progress to empyema.

Empirical therapeutic regimens for community-treated pneumonia are directed at *H. influenzae* and *Streptococcus pneumoniae* (± atypical bacteria) and include either a second-generation cephalosporin (± erythromycin), amoxicillin plus a β-lactamase inhibitor, or one of the newer macrolides, azithromycin or clarithromycin. Second-generation are often replaced by third-generation cephalosporins for hospitalized patients.

Antibiotic concentrations considered to represent those in the lower respiratory tract during infection are measured in mucosal biopsies obtained during bronchoscopy (80), in bronchial secretions obtained during intubation (32), and in lung tissues and tonsillar tissue procured during thoracic surgery and tonsillectomy (67, 124) (Table 3).

The increased prevalence of β-lactam resistance (56, 58) and reports of ampicillin-resistant outbreaks (89) have curtailed the usefulness of ampicillin or amoxicillin. Amoxicillin/clavulanate or amoxicillin/sulbactam (42), show good distribution into the lung and remain useful in the treatment of lower respiratory tract infections, with more than 80% satisfactory outcomes for treatment of a range of pathogens (86, 98). Ampicillin-resistant unencapsulated *H. influenzae* with altered PBPs are almost all obtained from lower respiratory tract infections, but at present, the prevalence of *H. influenzae* with this type of resistance is not high enough to alter therapeutic choice. Reports of significant resistance to trimethoprim-sulfamethoxazole and tetracycline in *S. pneumoniae* limit the use of these drugs for empirical treatment of lower respiratory tract infection, even when *H. influenzae* is the suspected pathogen. The prevalence of resistance to these drugs among respiratory unencapsulated *H. influenzae* isolates remains low (54).

Oral first-generation cephalosporins, cephalexin, cephradine, and cefadroxil, were all previously considered useful for lower respiratory tract infection therapy but have been replaced by cephalosporins with increased activity against *H. influenzae* and improved pharmacokinetics.

The second-generation cephalosporins, cefuroxime, cefuroxime axetil, and cephamandole are insensitive to the TEM-1 β-lactamase. Cefaclor has limited use because of protracted skin reactions, especially in children; its clinical efficacy is indistinguishable from that of many other antibiotics (66, 192), but the bacteriologic cure rate was only 61% versus 93.5% with azithromycin (47). Cefaclor and cefuroxime have produced clinical cure/improvement in 93 to 95% of adults with pneumonia or acute exacerbations of chronic bronchitis and are as efficient as amoxicillin (39), though 1 in 10 patients with proven *H. influenzae* lower respiratory tract infection treated with cefuroxime and 2 of 5 receiving cefaclor are not bacteriologically cured.

Oral third-generation cephalosporins, cefixime, ceftibuten, and cefpodoxime proxetil are licensed for treatment of lower respiratory tract infections, but such broad-spectrum antimicrobials should be reserved when narrower-spectrum agents are available. Cefixime has a long half-life, 3 h compared with 0.5 h for cefaclor (122), and can be given once daily for lower respiratory tract infections. Cefixime does not penetrate well into sputum but reaches useful levels in bronchial mucosa (Table 5). In comparative trials, cefixime had an efficacy similar to that of amoxicillin/clavulanate, cefaclor, cephalexin, cefuroxime axetil, and clarithromycin; in noncomparative studies it had a high clinical cure/improvement rate for lower respiratory tract infections, up to 96% in a large multicenter study of acute bronchitis or acute exacerbations of chronic bronchitis in adults, especially when the pathogen was *H. influenzae* (122, 144). Cefixime may have a specific role in the future when the antibiotic is switched from intravenous to oral administration when broad-spectrum antibiotic cover has been initiated empirically with a third-generation cephalosporin. Ceftibuten has less activity against *S. pneumoniae,* limiting its role as an empirical agent, whereas cefpodoxime proxetil is the most active of this group against all respiratory tract

TABLE 5 • **Dosages of Antibiotics Used in *H. influenzae* Pneumonia and Otitis Media**

Drug	Total Daily Dose (mg/kg/day)[a]	
	Adults (dosing interval, h)	Children (dosing interval, h)
Ampicillin	4 g (6)	50–100 (6)
Amoxicillin	1.5 g (8)	30–60 (8)
Trimethoprim-sulfamethoxazole	320 mg (12)	8 (12)
Cefaclor	1.5 g (8)	40 (8)
Cefuroxime	500 (12)	30 (12)
Third-generation cephalosporins	As for meningitis	As for meningitis
Cefixime	200–400 (12–24) mg	8 (12–24)
Ceftibuten	400 (24) mg	9 (24)
Cefpodoxime	200–400 (12) mg	8 (12)
Azithromycin	500 (24) mg	200–400 mg/day (24)
Clarithromycin	500 (12) mg	15 (12)
Ciprofloxacin	0.5–1.5 (12)	10–20 (12)

Compiled from references 72, 95, 122, 140, 154.

[a] Or as indicated on table.

pathogens. Cure/improvement rates of cephalosporins for lower respiratory tract infections and acute exacerbations of chronic bronchitis are similar to rates achieved with conventional antibiotics, except for first-generation cephalosporins. Cefpodoxime has an efficacy similar to that of conventional antibiotics and to parenteral cephalosporins, with 90 to 100% satisfactory clinical response rates in lower respiratory tract infections, 80% cure in acute exacerbations of chronic bronchitis, and 91 to 100% in community-acquired pneumonia where *H. influenzae* is the second commonest pathogen (72).

Third-generation parenteral cephalosporins, cefotaxime, ceftriaxone, ceftazidime, ceftizoxime, and others, are used for severe and life-threatening pneumonia. *H. influenzae* is extremely sensitive to these agents, as are most community-acquired respiratory pathogens, and achievable lung concentrations are high, well above the MIC$_{90}$ of *H. influenzae,* and remain so for the duration of the dosing interval. Ceftriaxone has the advantage of once-daily administration. Cefpirome is reserved for severe sepsis and the treatment of complicated lower respiratory tract infection.

Azithromycin and clarithromycin have proven efficacy in upper and lower respiratory tract infections and can be considered as alternatives to amoxicillin/clavulanate, erythromycin plus a sulfonamide, or a cephalosporin (82, 151, 152). They attain particularly high tissue and intracellular concentrations. Azithromycin tissue concentrations can be up to 100 times serum levels. The half-life in tissue is 4 days, and levels remain above the MIC$_{90}$ for up to 10 days after a 3-day course (67, 118). Clinical cure/improvement rates for lower respiratory tract infection range from 90 to 100% for azithromycin and clarithromycin (47, 66, 97, 129, 140, 144, 151, 152). Bacteriologic cure rates in the same studies were 72 to 100% (84). The efficacy of both was at least comparable to that of amoxicillin/clavulanate, cefaclor, cefixime, and cefuroxime (45, 66, 93, 129, 144, 151, 152, 174). Development of azithromycin resistance was shown to contribute to disease recurrence 1 month after treatment of chronic bronchitis (152).

Fluoroquinolones are characterized by their broad antibacterial spectrum, with excellent activity against *H. influenzae,* and rapid bactericidal action. Particularly ciprofloxacin, but also sparfloxacin (93), and norfloxacin (102), have been extensively prescribed in lower respiratory tract infection. For *H. influenzae,* cure rates exceed 90% (65). In cystic fibrosis, fluoroquinolones are used to treat acute exacerbations (95) or in maintenance treatment (92) but are primarily directed at *Pseudomonas* superinfection. *H. influenzae,* particularly unencapsulated strains, is a common pathogen in young cystic fibrosis patients (131). Unencapsulated *H. influenzae* is rarely cultured consecutively from the same cystic fibrosis patient for more than a few months and in most is rapidly cleared from sputum with conventional therapy such as amoxicillin/clavulanate (134). In the unusual circumstance of persistent *H. influenzae* infection, use of fluoroquinolones would be appropriate. General guidelines for the treatment of infective exacerbations in cystic fibrosis are to make a microbiologic diagnosis when possible before initiating treatment, use high-dose bactericidal antibiotics for 14 days, avoid prophylactic regimens (except for maintenance therapy in chronic *Pseudomonas* infections) (92), be aware of altered pharmacokinetics in cystic fibrosis patients (especially, increased total body clearance of β-lactams and hence shorter half-life and lower sputum concentrations), and aim to eradicate *H. influenzae* in the lower respiratory tract whenever present (94, 95).

Parapneumonic Effusion and Empyema

The presence of an effusion demands a diagnostic thoracentesis and an empyema requires drainage; in one large retrospective study of 227 patients, 21 of 40 empyemas caused by *H. influenzae* were deemed too small for closed drainage and were treated by needle aspiration. Antibiotics were given for a median duration of 13 days (68). Antibiotic choice should be the same as for invasive *H. influenzae* type b disease, usually a parenteral cephalosporin. Therapeutic doses of cefuroxime, cefotaxime, and ceftriaxone all result in pleural fluid concentrations of up to 7 μg/mL (119), well above the MIC for *H. influenzae.*

Acute Exacerbations of Chronic Bronchitis

More than 50% of bacterial isolates from the sputum of patients with chronic bronchitis are unencapsulated *H. influenzae*. Antibiotics are given to treat acute exacerbations of chronic bronchitis when they occur or given as long-term prophylaxis or as suppressive therapy in advanced disease. The benefit of antibiotics has been extremely difficult to demonstrate conclusively, partly because many acute exacerbations of chronic bronchitis are of viral origin, because patients enrolled in trials are at very different stages of disease, and because improvement often occurs without antibiotics (139). Consequently, comparative studies demonstrate only marginal differences between antibiotics. There is little solid evidence on which to make a choice between amoxicillin, amoxicillin/clavulanate, trimethoprim-sulfamethoxazole, tetracycline, erythromycin, chloramphenicol, and cefaclor or other oral cephalosporin. Suboptimal pharmacokinetics in the lungs of patients with chronic bronchitis and higher antibiotic resistance rates may also contribute to the poor responses. Newer antibiotics with excellent in vitro activity against *H. influenzae* should be more effective, but this is seldom demonstrated (4). Because of the difficulty in interpreting comparative trials, amoxicillin alone is still recommended by some for acute exacerbations of chronic bronchitis. A more logical choice would be amoxicillin/clavulanate or a cephalosporin.

Recommended dosages of antibiotics for *H. influenzae* pneumonia are given in Table 5.

Otitis Media and Sinusitis

H. influenzae causes 10 to 30% of acute otitis media; *S. pneumoniae*, 20 to 40% (9). In chronic otitis media, *H. influenzae* predominates (15 vs. 7% with *S. pneumoniae*), and the rate of β-lactamase-producing *H. influenzae* is up to three times higher than in acute otitis media. More than 90% of *H. influenzae* are unencapsulated (139), and 15 to 30% of them produce β-lactamases (147); only a minor percentage are *H. influenzae* type b. *H. influenzae* is a primary pathogen in the now rare but serious intracranial complications of chronic otitis media, mastoiditis and subdural empyema. Sinusitis has a comparable pathogenesis and microbiology (139) and is treated similarly.

Ampicillin-resistant *H. influenzae* strains are widely prevalent. Although it would seem logical to abandon amoxicillin in preference to other antimicrobials, for many physicians, amoxicillin remains the first choice for treatment of acute otitis media (108). One recommendation is to use alternatives to amoxicillin only if two treatment failures occur in any one winter season. It is difficult to establish that amoxicillin has reduced efficacy, because so many bouts of acute otitis media are caused by viruses, and even when *H. influenzae* or other bacteria are recovered by tympanocentesis, spontaneous resolution of acute otitis media is common. Comparison of drugs is impeded by lack of a universal definition of otitis media, difficulty in making bacteriologic diagnoses, and often no clear outcome measures within studies. The penetration of amoxicillin and alternative antibiotics into middle ear effusions is given in Table 3 (119).

Clinical comparative studies in the treatment of otitis media have identified little difference between amoxicillin, amoxicillin/clavulanate (61, 121, 147), trimethoprim-sulfamethoxazole (112, 175, 177), erythromycin-sulfisoxazole (112, 165), cefaclor (27, 121, 147), cefixime (27), cefprozil, cefuroxime, cefpodoxime, clarithromycin, and azithromycin (27, 38, 149, 151). In general, the numbers of patients in trials of otitis media therapy are too small to assess equivalence of two agents, which often requires several times the number of patients needed to demonstrate a difference between drugs. Thus, most studies conclude that no difference between two antibiotics can be shown but do not predict with confidence that two antibiotics are equally efficacious (108). The situation is exemplified by the continued use of erythromycin. *H. influenzae* has inherent resistance to erythromycin in vitro, and erythromycin penetrates less well than most other antibiotics into middle ear effusions; yet trials do not show it to be less effective (112, 165). Comparative trials of maxillary sinusitis treatment similarly show little difference between antibiotics (31, 106, 185). The clinician's choice of antibiotic in otitis media therefore rests on knowledge of each drug's pharmacokinetics and the sensitivity of *H. influenzae* (and other pathogens) to the various antibiotics (Tables 2 and 3) as well as palatability and administration frequency.

In general, cefaclor appears to have lower efficacy than cefuroxime axetil, cefixime, or amoxicillin/clavulanate. Cefixime has exceptional stability against *H. influenzae* β-lactamases. Drugs with questionable efficacy—erythromycin, cefaclor, and possibly amoxicillin (alone)—should perhaps be avoided in preference to those with predicted better in vivo efficacy—amoxicillin/clavulanate, cefuroxime axetil, cefixime, cefprozil, ceftibuten, and cefpodoxime proxetil.

Table 5 gives some recommended dosages of antibiotics for otitis media.

OTHER INFECTIONS

H. influenzae type b is one of the principal causes of bacteremic infection in young children; in addition to meningitis, *H. influenzae* type b may cause orbital cellulitis and epiglottitis (77), vertebral osteomyelitis (16), septic arthritis, psoas abscess (48), rarely septicemia, and very rarely endocarditis. If *H. influenzae* type b is the pathogen in apparently localized disease, likelihood of systemic spread and another concurring focus is high. For example, in *H. influenzae* type b infections, 75% of patients with pneumonia have bacteremia, and 15% have meningitis; 30% with empyema have meningitis; and 50% with infective endocarditis have pneumonia or meningitis (68).

Unencapsulated *H. influenzae* causes mainly localized disease, otitis media, sinusitis, acute tracheobronchitis, and conjunctivitis (139). Occasionally, unencapsulated *H. influenzae* strains are implicated in invasive disease; one of the most serious manifestations of which is Brazilian purpuric fever, a rare fulminant septicemic illness with a case-fatality rate of more than 60% (85, 184). Unencapsulated *H. influenzae*, especially biotype IV, causes invasive neonatal-maternal infections (29, 203) with endometritis (160) leading to bacteremia in the mother and fulminant septicemia and meningitis in the premature neonate (117, 139). Localized disease has been reported in the genitourinary tract, presenting as urinary tract infection (60, 132, 160, 197), urethritis (183), orchidoepididymitis, Bartholin abscess (196), cervicovaginitis, salpingitis (75), and spontaneous abortion (160). Meningitis can be caused by unencapsulated *H. influenzae,* especially when there is a breach of the meninges, either after trauma (182) or due to congenital sinuses (161).

Whether it is an unencapsulated or type b *H. influenzae* that causes infection, the treatment for invasive disease is as for meningitis, usually with a third-generation cephalosporin. Cefotaxime penetrates well into bone (62) and joints, with joint fluid concentrations 2 h after administration greater than that in serum (e.g., 29 μg/mL), and penetrates into skin (2–6.3 μg/mL), and the genitourinary tract. Bone and joint infections require 3 to 6 weeks of therapy (181). Ceftriaxone penetrates into bone efficiently and has been given once daily in the community after resolution of the acute stages of disease (25, 43).

VACCINES

One of the most successful chapters in the history of vaccinology was development of the *H. influenzae* type b vaccine and its introduction into North America, Finland, and the United Kingdom from 1989 to 1992 and subsequently into many other European countries and Australia (23, 88). The *H. influenzae* type b vaccine is being considered for incorporation into the Extended Programme for Immunisation to provide protection against childhood pneumonia (81), and meningitis in developing countries (70, 81, 136–138).

Conjugate vaccines consist of the polyribosyl phosphate (PRP) capsule derived from *H. influenzae* type b covalently attached to a protein carrier. Four commercial conjugate vaccines are available: Act-Hib (Pasteur Merieux) is formulated from native PRP linked to tetanus toxoid (PRP-T); HibTITER (Lederle) is a PRP oligosaccharide connected to CRM197, a mutant diphtheria toxoid; PedvaxHIB (Merck, Sharp and Dohme) is a native PRP attached to the outer membrane protein complex of serogroup b *Neisseria meningitidis* (PRP-OMP); and ProHIBit is composed of sized PRP linked to the diphtheria toxoid (PRP-D) (111). All have been extensively evaluated in trials in man (51, 63, 169, 170, 195), and the reduction in invasive *H. influenzae* type b disease as well as carriage has been impressive (7, 8). PRP-T in the U.K. has a protective efficacy in infants of over 98% and is protective after just two doses (22). PRP-D appears to be the least immunogenic, and though efficacious in Finland, it was not protective in Alaskan Eskimos, perhaps as a result of a younger age of presentation. PRP-OMP is the most immunogenic after just one dose of vaccine and may be the best choice for immunization in the developing world. Within countries that have national vaccination coverage, it is still too early to determine whether vaccination will diminish carriage and transmission enough to eliminate *H. influenzae* type b.

Indications

H. influenzae type b vaccine should be considered for prevention of invasive disease in all infants. Invasive disease occurs at a younger age in many children in developing countries; 44% of *H. influenzae* type b meningitis occurs before 6 months of age, compared with 5 to 12% in Europe (19). Consequently, in such countries, the efficacy of the vaccine may be reduced because more disease is occurring prior to the age at which immunization is protective; although this does not seem to be borne out by recent studies in the Gambia (138).

Doses and Schedules

Single doses of PRP-T, PRP-OMP, and PRP-D contain 10, 15, and 20 μg of PRP, respectively. HbOC consists of 10 μg of oligosaccharide. Each dose is administered in a volume of 0.5 mL, given intramuscularly. Primary courses of 3 doses are given in the first few months of life: e.g., in months 2, 3, 4; 2, 4, 6; or 3, 4, 5. In North America, a booster dose is recommended at 12 to 15 months of age, whereas the experience in the U.K. is that vaccination may afford long-term protection without the need for a booster (21).

Adverse Effects

No association with major adverse events has been reported in the first 5 to 8 years of use. *H. influenzae* type b disease may still occur in partially vaccinated infants and in children with immune deficiencies. Vaccine failures should be considered for immunologic investigations.

ENDPOINTS FOR MONITORING THERAPY

A 7-day course of parenteral antibiotics is satisfactory for most cases of uncomplicated *H. influenzae* meningitis (125, 127), but conventionally, 10 days has been recommended. There are no long-term comparisons of sequelae rates for 10-day, 7-day, or shorter regimens (127). It is prudent to continue antibiotics for 7 to 10 days, depending on severity, or for 3 to 5 days after effervescence of fever and signs of meningitis. A repeat lumbar puncture is considered unnecessary, except when pyrexia and clinical state have not improved after 48 hours or more of therapy.

Duration of therapy for lower respiratory tract infection is dictated by disease severity. As a guide, 7 or more days, or 3 to 5 days after pyrexia recedes is appropriate for hospital-acquired pneumonia. Intravenous therapy can be switched to the oral route after there has been no fever for 24 to 48 h. For oral therapy of community-acquired pneumonia, 5 to 7 days is usually satisfactory, though a 3-day course of a newer macrolide/azalide may also be adequate.

A 10-day course of antibiotics for acute otitis media has become standard, based on the necessity to treat group A streptococcal pharyngitis for this duration. However, a single intramuscular dose of ceftriaxone, which produces therapeutic levels for 3 days, or 3 days of azithromycin or 5 days of cefaclor are as effective as 10 days of amoxicillin or amoxicillin/clavulanate (149). The 10-day rationale has not been adopted in Europe, where 5 to 7 days of therapy is considered sufficient for uncomplicated acute otitis media. Adenoidectomy, antihistamines, and decongestants are of unproven benefit in chronic otitis media, and the appropriate time for myringotomy with ventilation tube insertion is an area of contention. The effectiveness of treatment is assessed by the presence of otoscopic findings, pyrexia, and symptoms at 48 h and by repeat otoscopy at the end of therapy.

Resolution of symptoms and pyrexia at about 48 h is a useful guide to the effectiveness of therapy for most *H. influenzae* infections.

CONTROVERSIES

Dexamethasone

For *H. influenzae* meningitis, it is generally agreed that dexamethasone therapy significantly reduces the incidence of sensorineural deafness (171). Although a 1989 meta-analysis of all studies concluded that there was no benefit, scrutiny of selected studies from Dallas and Switzerland did show an advantage (172). In a large prospective study, the incidence of hearing loss was 3.3% in dexamethasone recipients and 15.5% in controls, whereas the recent meta-analysis determined the incidence of neurologic or audiologic sequelae in steroid and nonsteroid groups to be 7 and 16%, respectively. Routine use of empirical dexamethasone for pediatric meningitis remains controversial because a clear benefit in *S. pneumoniae* and *N. meningitidis* meningitis has not been established. In many countries, *H. influenzae* type b has been virtually eradicated by implementation of national vaccination, so administration of steroids to meningitis patients before microbial diagnosis is likely to be less beneficial than in the nonvaccinating countries where *H. influenzae* still predominates (198). Steroids must be given before the first dose of antibiotic (20). Cerebrospinal fluid parameters return to normal faster with dexamethasone treatment, yet dexamethasone does not affect cerebrospinal fluid sterilization or cephalosporin concentrations (172). Dexamethasone therapy has been associated with rebound fever and carries a 0.5% risk of significant bleeding in the absence of coagulopathy (204). Dexamethasone 0.15 mg/kg 6 hourly for 4 days is the standard regimen; some consider a 2-day course effective (186), and 2 days may be associated with less secondary fever (153).

Rifampicin Prophylaxis

The risk of *H. influenzae* type b invasive disease in an unvaccinated household contact is 500 to 800 times higher than that in the general population and is greatest in infants under 2 years old (41). Rifampicin prophylaxis is recommended for all household contacts of a patient with *H. influenzae* type b meningitis if there is an infant under 2 years old or an immunocompromised person in the house (150). Where necessary, all children should have their vaccinations brought up to date (101). Rifampicin eradicates *H. influenzae* from the nasopharynx in 95% of carriers and is given on the presumption that clearing carriage prevents infection. Only one prospective study, however, has clearly shown a benefit (5, 41). In countries with *H. influenzae* vaccination programs, the benefits may be marginal. Ceftriaxone clears nasopharyngeal carriage and when used for treatment, eliminates the need for rifampicin prophylaxis in the index case. When a single child has meningitis in a day-care center, the role of prophylaxis is controversial; one proposal is to give rifampicin to all unvaccinated children under 2 years old

if contact has been for 25 h or more per week or if a second case arises within 60 days (150).

REFERENCES

1. Adams WG, Deaver KA, Cochi SL. Decline of childhood Haemophilus influenzae type b (Hib) disease in the Hib vaccine era. JAMA 1993;269:221–226.
2. Anderson JR, Smith MD, Kibbler CC. A nosocomial outbreak due to non-encapsulated Haemophilus influenzae: analysis of plasmids coding for antibiotic resistance. J Hosp Infect 1994;27: 17–27.
3. Aronoff SC, Reed MD, O'Brien CA, Blumer JL. Comparison of the efficacy and safety of ceftriaxone to ampicillin/chloramphenicol in the treatment of childhood meningitis. J Antimicrob Chemother 1984;13:143–151.
4. Ball P, Tillotson G, Wilson R. Chemotherapy for chronic bronchitis. Controversies. Presse Med 1995;24:189–194.
5. Band JD, Fraser DW, Ajello G. Prevention of Hemophilus influenzae type b disease. JAMA 1984;251:2381–2386.
6. Baquero F. Trends in antibiotic resistance of respiratory pathogens: an analysis and commentary on a collaborative surveillance study. J Antimicrob Chemother 1996;38:117–132.
7. Barbour ML, Booy R, Crook DW. Haemophilus influenzae type b carriage and immunity four years after receiving the Haemophilus influenzae oligosaccharide-CRM197 (HbOC) conjugate vaccine. Pediatr Infect Dis J 1993;12:478–484.
8. Barbour ML, Mayon WR, Coles C. The impact of conjugate vaccine on carriage of Haemophilus influenzae type b. J Infect Dis 1995;171:93–98.
9. Barnett ED, Klein JO. The problem of resistant bacteria for the management of acute otitis media. Pediatr Clin North Am 1995; 42:509–517.
10. Barriere SL, Hindler JA. Ciprofloxacin-resistant Haemophilus influenzae infection in a patient with chronic lung disease. Ann Pharmacother 1993;27:309–310.
11. Barry AL, Fuchs PC. Influence of the test medium on azithromycin and erythromycin regression statistics. Eur J Clin Microbiol Infect Dis 1991;10:846–849.
12. Barry AL, Schultheiss TS, Brown SD, Fuchs PC. Reassessment of methods for testing the susceptibility of Haemophilus influenzae to clarithromycin. J Antimicrob Chemother 1996;37:845–847.
13. Bass JW, Person DA, Fonseca RJ. Cefuroxime versus ceftriaxone for bacterial meningitis. J Pediatr 1990;116:488–490.
14. Baumgartner JD, Glauser MP. Single daily dose treatment of severe refractory infections with ceftriaxone. Cost savings and possible parenteral outpatient treatment. Arch Intern Med 1983;143:1868–1873.
15. Begue P, Floret D, Mallet E, et al. Pharmacokinetics and clinical evaluation of cefotaxime in children suffering with purulent meningitis. J Antimicrob Chemother 1984;14(Suppl B):161–165.
16. Beltrani VP, Echols RM, Vedder DK. Vertebral osteomyelitis caused by Haemophilus influenzae. J Infect Dis 1987;156: 391–394.
17. Bendig JW, Barker KF, O'Driscoll JC. Purulent salpingitis and intra-uterine contraceptive device-related infection due to Haemophilus influenzae. J Infect 1991;22:111–112.
18. Bergeron MG, Bernier M, L'Ecuyer J. In vitro activity of clarithromycin and its 14-hydroxy-metabolite against 203 strains of Haemophilus influenzae. Infection 1992;20:164–167.
19. Bijlmer HA. World-wide epidemiology of Haemophilus influenzae meningitis; industrialized versus non-industrialized countries. Vaccine 1991;9 suppl:s5–9.

20. Bonadio WA. Dexamethasone therapy for bacterial meningitis. Pediatrics 1996;97:286–287.

21. Booy R, Heath PT, Slack MP, Begg N, Moxon ER. Vaccine failures after primary immunisation with Haemophilus influenzae type-b conjugate vaccine without booster [see comments]. Lancet 1997;349:1197–1202.

22. Booy R, Hodgson S, Carpenter L. Efficacy of Haemophilus influenzae type b conjugate vaccine PRP-T. Lancet 1994b;344:362–366.

23. Booy R, Kroll S. Bacterial meningitis in children. Curr Opin Pediatr 1994a;6:29–35.

24. Bouffet E, Fuhrmann C, Frappaz D, et al. Once daily antibiotic regimen in paediatric oncology. Arch Dis Child 1994;70:484–487.

25. Bradley JS. Ceftriaxone in Haemophilus influenzae type b meningitis. JAMA 1988;259:2851–2852.

26. Brightman CA, Crook DW, Kraak WA, et al. Family outbreak of chloramphenicol-ampicillin resistant Haemophilus influenzae type b disease. Lancet 1990;335:351–352.

27. Brogden RN, Campoli RD. Cefixime. A review of its antibacterial activity. Pharmacokinetic properties and therapeutic potential. Drugs 1989;38:524–550.

28. Cabellos C, Viladrich PF, Verdaguer R, et al. A single daily dose of ceftriaxone for bacterial meningitis in adults: experience with 84 patients and review of the literature. Clin Infect Dis 1995;20:1164–1168.

29. Campognone P, Singer DB. Neonatal sepsis due to nontypable Haemophilus influenzae. Am J Dis Child 1986;140:117–121.

30. Campos J, Garcia TS. Comparative susceptibilities of ampicillin and chloramphenicol resistant Haemophilus influenzae to fifteen antibiotics. J Antimicrob Chemother 1987;19:297–301.

31. Casiano RR. Azithromycin and amoxicillin in the treatment of acute maxillary sinusitis. Am J Med 1991;91:27s–30s.

32. Cazzola M, Gabriella MM, Polverino M. Pulmonary penetration of ceftazidime. J Chemother 1995;7:50–54.

33. Chadwick EG, Yogev R, Shulman ST, et al. Single-dose ceftriaxone pharmacokinetics in pediatric patients with central nervous system infections. J Pediatr 1983;102:134–137.

34. Cherubin CE, Eng RH, Norrby R. Penetration of newer cephalosporins into cerebrospinal fluid. Rev Infect Dis 1989;11:526–548.

35. Chiu CH, Ou JT, Su HC. Serotypes, biotypes and antibiotic susceptibility of 126 clinical isolates of Haemophilus influenzae. J Formosan Med Assoc 1995;94:351–354.

36. Clairoux N, Picard M, Brochu A. Molecular basis of the non-beta-lactamase-mediated resistance to beta-lactam antibiotics in strains of Haemophilus influenzae isolated in Canada. Antimicrob Agents Chemother 1992;36:1504–1513.

37. Cohen ML. Epidemiology of drug resistance: implications for a post-antimicrobial era. Science 1992;257:1050–1055.

38. Coles SJ, Addlestone MB, Kamdar MK, Macklin JL. A comparative study of clarithromycin and amoxycillin suspensions in the treatment of pediatric patients with acute otitis media. Infection 1993;21:272–278.

39. Cooper TJ, Ladusans E, Williams PE. A comparison of oral cefuroxime axetil and oral amoxicillin in lower respiratory tract infections. J Antimicrob Chemother 1985;16:373–378.

40. Corkill JE, Percival A, McDonald P, Bamber AI. Detection of quinolone resistance in Haemophilus spp. J Antimicrob Chemother 1994;34:841–844.

41. Cuevas LE, Hart CA. Chemoprophylaxis of bacterial meningitis. J Antimicrob Chemother 1993;31(Suppl B):79–91.

42. Cunha BA. Ampicillin/sulbactam in lower respiratory tract infections: a review. Clin Ther 1991;13:714–726.

43. Dagan R, Phillip M, Watemberg NM, Kassis I. Outpatient treatment of serious community-acquired pediatric infections using once daily intramuscular ceftriaxone. Pediatr Infect Dis J 1987;6:1080–1084.

44. Dajani AS, Pokowski LH. Delayed cerebrospinal fluid sterilization, in vitro bactericidal activities, and side effects of selected beta-lactams. Scand J Infect Dis Suppl 1990;73:31–42.

45. Daniel R. Simplified treatment of acute lower respiratory tract infection with azithromycin: a comparison with erythromycin and amoxycillin. European Azithromycin Study Group. J Int Med Res 1991;19:373–383.

46. Daoud AS, Al-Sheyyab M, Batchoun RG. Bacterial meningitis: still a cause of high mortality and severe neurological morbidity in childhood. J Trop Pediatr 1995;41:308–310.

47. Dark D. Multicenter evaluation of azithromycin and cefaclor in acute lower respiratory tract infections. Am J Med 1991;91:31s–35s.

48. Davies D, King SM, Parekh RS, D'Angelo G. Psoas abscess caused by Haemophilus influenzae type B. Pediatr Infect Dis J 1991;10:411–412.

49. de Groot R, Chaffin DO, Kuehn M, Smith AL. Trimethoprim resistance in Haemophilus influenzae is due to altered dihydrofolate reductase(s). Biochem J 1991a;274:657–662.

50. de Groot R, Dzoljic DG, van KB. Antibiotic resistance in Haemophilus influenzae: mechanisms, clinical importance and consequences for therapy. Eur J Pediatr 1991b;150:534–546.

51. Decker MD, Edwards KM, Bradley R, Palmer P. Comparative trial in infants of four conjugate Haemophilus influenzae type b vaccines. J Pediatr 1992;.

52. Deulofeu F, Nava JM, Bella F. Prospective epidemiological study of invasive Haemophilus influenzae disease in adults. Eur J Clin Microbiol Infect Dis 1994;13:633–638.

53. Dimopoulou ID, Kraak WA, Anderson EC. Molecular epidemiology of unrelated clusters of multiresistant strains of Haemophilus influenzae. J Infect Dis 1992;165:1069–1075.

54. Doern GV. Trends in antimicrobial susceptibility of bacterial pathogens of the respiratory tract. Am J Med 1995b;99:3s–7s.

55. Doern GV, Brueggemann AB, Pierce G, Holley HJ, Rauch A. Antibiotic resistance among clinical isolates of Haemophilus influenzae in the United States in 1994 and 1995 and detection of beta-lactamase-positive strains resistant to amoxicillin-clavulanate: results of a national multicenter surveillance study. Antimicrob Agents Chemother 1997;41:292–297.

56. Doern GV, Jones RN. Antimicrobial susceptibility testing of Haemophilus influenzae, Branhamella catarrhalis, and Neisseria gonorrhoeae. Antimicrob Agents Chemother 1988b;32:1747–1753.

57. Doern GV, Jones RN, Gerlach EH. Revised disk diffusion interpretive criteria for cefaclor, loracarbef, cefprozil and cefixime when testing Haemophilus influenzae on haemophilus test medium. Eur J Clin Microbiol Infect Dis 1994;13:481–489.

58. Doern GV, Jorgensen JH, Thornsberry C. National collaborative study of the prevalence of antimicrobial resistance among clinical isolates of Haemophilus influenzae. Antimicrob Agents Chemother 1988a;32:180–185.

59. Doern GV, Jorgensen JH, Thornsberry C, Snapper H. Disk diffusion susceptibility testing of Haemophilus influenzae using haemophilus test medium. Eur J Clin Microbiol Infect Dis 1990;9:329–336.

60. Elcuaz R, Castillo M, Pena MJ. Urinary tract infection caused by

Haemophilus influenzae and Haemophilus parainfluenzae. Enferm Infecc Microbiol Clin 1992;10:315–316.

61. Engelhard D, Cohen D, Strauss N, Sacks TG, Jorczak SL, Shapiro M. Randomised study of myringotomy, amoxycillin/clavulanate, or both for acute otitis media in infants. Lancet 1989;2:141–143.

62. Eron LJ, Park CH, Hixon DL. Ceftriaxone therapy of bone and soft tissue infections in hospital and outpatient settings. Antimicrob Agents Chemother 1983;23:731–737.

63. Eskola J, Peltola H, Takala AK. Efficacy of Haemophilus influenzae type b polysaccharide-diphtheria toxoid conjugate vaccine in infancy. N Engl J Med 1987;317:717–722.

64. Farley MM, Stephens DS, Brachman PJ. Invasive Haemophilus influenzae disease in adults. A prospective, population-based surveillance. CDC Meningitis Surveillance Group. Ann Intern Med 1992;116:806–812.

65. Finch RG. The role of new quinolones in the treatment of respiratory tract infections. Drugs 1995;2:144–151.

66. Fong IW, Laforge J, Dubois J, Small D, Grossman R, Zakhari R. Clarithromycin versus cefaclor in lower respiratory tract infections. The Canadian Bronchitis Study Group. Clin Invest Med 1995;18:131–138.

67. Foulds G, Johnson RB. Selection of dose regimens of azithromycin. J Antimicrob Chemother 1993;31(Suppl E):39–50.

68. Freij BJ, Kusmiesz H, Nelson JD, McCracken GJ. Parapneumonic effusions and empyema in hospitalized children: a retrospective review of 227 cases. Pediatr Infect Dis 1984;3:578–591.

69. Frenkel LD. Once-daily administration of ceftriaxone for the treatment of selected serious bacterial infections in children. Pediatrics 1988;82:486–491.

70. Funkhouser A, Steinhoff MC, Ward J. Haemophilus influenzae disease and immunization in developing countries. Rev Infect Dis 1991;13(Suppl 6):s542–554.

71. Garau J. Beta-lactamases: current situation and clinical importance. Intensive Care Med 1994;20(Suppl 3):s5–9.

72. Geddes AM. Cefpodoxime proxetil in the treatment of lower respiratory tract infections. Drugs 1991;3:34–40.

73. Georgopapadakou NH. Penicillin-binding proteins and bacterial resistance to beta-lactams. Antimicrob Agents Chemother 1993;37:2045–2053.

74. Goldstein FW, Emirian MF, Coutrot A, Acar JF. Bacteriostatic and bactericidal activity of azithromycin against Haemophilus influenzae. J Antimicrob Chemother 1990;25(Suppl A):25–28.

75. Golledge CL. Urinary tract infection caused by Haemophilus parainfluenzae. J Infect 1991;22:98.

76. Gomez J, Ruiz GJ, Hernandez CJ, Nunez ML, Canteras M, Valdes M. Antibiotic resistance patterns of Streptococcus pneumoniae, Haemophilus influenzae and Moraxella catarrhalis: a prospective study in Murcia, Spain, 1983–1992. Chemotherapy 1994;40:299–303.

77. Gonzalez-Valdepena H, Wald ER, Rose E, Ungkanont K, Casselbrant ML. Epiglottitis and Haemophilus influenzae immunization: the Pittsburgh experience—a five-year review. Pediatrics 1995;96:424–427.

78. Gordon RC, Wofford MR, Shu K. In vitro synergism of rifampin-cephalosporin combinations against Haemophilus influenzae type b. Eur J Clin Microbiol Infect Dis 1990;9:201–205.

79. Gould IM, Forbes KJ, Gordon GS. Quinolone resistant Haemophilus influenzae. J Antimicrob Chemother 1994a;33:187–188.

80. Gould IM, Harvey G, Golder D. Penetration of amoxicillin/clavu-lanic acid into bronchial mucosa with different dosing regimens. Thorax 1994b;49:999–1001.

81. Greenwood B. Epidemiology of acute lower respiratory tract infections, especially those due to Haemophilus influenzae type b, in The Gambia, west Africa. J Infect Dis 1992;165(Suppl 1):s26–8.

82. Guay DR. Macrolide antibiotics in paediatric infectious diseases. Drugs 1996;51:515–536.

83. Hammond ML, Norriss MS. Antibiotic resistance among respiratory pathogens in preschool children. Med J Aust 1995; 163:239–242.

84. Hardy DJ, Guay DR, Jones RN. Clarithromycin, a unique macrolide. A pharmacokinetic, microbiological, and clinical overview. Diagn Microbiol Infect Dis 1992;15:39–53.

85. Harrison LH, da SG, Pittman M, Fleming DW, Vranjac A, Broome CV. Epidemiology and clinical spectrum of Brazilian purpuric fever. Brazilian Purpuric Fever Study Group. J Clin Microbiol 1989;27:599–604.

86. Haruta T, Kuroki S, Okura K. Bacteriological, pharmacokinetic and clinical studies of sulbactam/ampicillin in the pediatric field. Jpn J Antibiot 1989;42:719–724.

87. Hatch D, Overturf GD, Kovacs A, Forthal D, Leong C. Treatment of bacterial meningitis with ceftazidime. Pediatr Infect Dis 1986;5:416–420.

88. Heath PT, Moxon ER. Haemophilus influenzae type b vaccination. Postgrad Doctor Middle East 1995;18:396–402.

89. Hekker TA, van dSA, Kempers J, Namavar F, van Alphen L. A nosocomial outbreak of amoxycillin-resistant non-typable Haemophilus influenzae in a respiratory ward. J Hosp Infect 1991;19:25–31.

90. Hellbusch LC, Penn RG. Cerebrospinal fluid shunt infections by unencapsulated Haemophilus influenzae. Childs Nerv Syst 1989;5:315–317.

91. Hellbusch LC, Penn RG. Treatment of haemophilus influenzae type B cerebrospinal fluid shunt infection with ceftriaxone and rifampin: case report. Nebr Med J 1995;80:27–29.

92. Hodson ME. Maintenance treatment with antibiotics in cystic fibrosis patients. Sense or nonsense? Neth J Med 1995;46:288–292.

93. Hoepelman AI, Sips AP, van-Helmond Jl. A single-blind comparison of three-day azithromycin and ten-day co-amoxiclav treatment of acute lower respiratory tract infections. J Antimicrob Chemother 1993;31(Suppl E):147–152.

94. Hoiby N. Cystic fibrosis: infection. Schweiz Med Wochenschr 1991;121:105–109.

95. Hoiby N, Pedersen SS, Jensen T, Valerius NH, Koch C. Fluoroquinolones in the treatment of cystic fibrosis. Drugs 1993;3:98–101.

96. Hoover WW, Barrett MS, Jones RN. Clarithromycin in vitro activity enhanced by its major metabolite, 14-hydroxyclarithromycin. Diagn Microbiol Infect Dis 1992;15:259–266.

97. Hosie J, Quinn P, Smits P, Sides G. A comparison of 5 days of dirithromycin and 7 days of clarithromycin in acute bacterial exacerbation of chronic bronchitis. J Antimicrob Chemother 1995;36:173–183.

98. Iwata S, Yamada K, Sato Y. Clinical studies on sulbactam/ampicillin in the field of pediatrics. Jpn J Antibiot 1989;42:598–611.

99. Jacobs RF, Kearns GL. Cefotaxime and desacetylcefotaxime in neonates and children: a review of microbiologic, pharmacokinetic, and clinical experience. Diagn Microbiol Infect Dis 1989;12:93–9.

100. Jacobs RF, Wells TG, Steele RW, Yamauchi T. A prospective randomized comparison of cefotaxime vs ampicillin and chloramphenicol for bacterial meningitis in children. J Pediatr 1985;107:129–33.

101. Jones DM. Chemoprophylaxis of meningitis. Trans R Soc Trop Med Hyg 1991;1:44–45.

102. Jones RN, Barrett MS, Erwin ME. In vitro antimicrobial activity of sparfloxacin compared with numerous other quinolone compounds. Diagn Microbiol Infect Dis 1991;14:319–330.

103. Jones RN, Doern GV, Gerlach EH, Hindler J, Erwin ME. Validation of NCCLS macrolide (azithromycin, clarithromycin, and erythromycin) interpretive criteria for Haemophilus influenzae tested with the Haemophilus test medium. National Committee for Clinical Laboratory Standards. Diagn Microbiol Infect Dis 1994;18:243–249.

104. Jordens JZ, Slack MP. Haemophilus influenzae: then and now. Eur J Clin Microbiol Infect Dis 1995;14:935–948.

105. Jorgensen JH. Update on mechanisms and prevalence of antimicrobial resistance in Haemophilus influenzae. Clin Infect Dis 1992;14:1119–1123.

106. Karma P, Pukander J, Penttila M. The comparative efficacy and safety of clarithromycin and amoxycillin in the treatment of outpatients with acute maxillary sinusitis. J Antimicrob Chemother 1991;27(Suppl A):83–90.

107. Kayser FH, Morenzoni G, Santanam P. The Second European Collaborative Study on the frequency of antimicrobial resistance in Haemophilus influenzae. Eur J Clin Microbiol Infect Dis 1990;9:810–817.

108. Klein JO. Current issues in upper respiratory tract infections in infants and children: rationale for antibacterial therapy. Pediatr Infect Dis J 1994;13(Suppl 1):s5–9.

109. Klugman KP, Dagan R. Carbapenem treatment of meningitis. Scand J Infect Dis Suppl 1995a;96:45–48.

110. Klugman KP, Dagan R. Randomized comparison of meropenem with cefotaxime for treatment of bacterial meningitis. Meropenem Meningitis Study Group. Antimicrob Agents Chemother 1995b;39:1140–1146.

111. Kniskern PJ, Marburg S, Ellis RW. Haemophilus influenzae type b conjugate vaccines. Pharm Biotechnol 1995;6:673–694.

112. Krause PJ, Owens NJ, Nightingale CH. Penetration of amoxicillin, cefaclor, erythromycin-sulfisoxazole, and trimethoprim-sulfamethoxazole into the middle ear fluid of patients with chronic serous otitis media. J Infect Dis 1982;145: 815–821.

113. Lambert ZN, Mariani KP, Doit C. In-vitro bactericidal activity of four oral antibiotics against pathogens responsible for acute otitis media in children. J Hosp Infect 1992;.

114. Lebel MH, Hoyt MJ, McCracken GJ. Comparative efficacy of ceftriaxone and cefuroxime for treatment of bacterial meningitis. J Pediatr 1989;114:1049–1054.

115. Levy J. Antibiotic resistance in Europe and the current use of antibiotics in severe pediatric infections. Scand J Infect Dis Suppl 1990;73:23–29.

116. Levy J, Verhaegen G, De MP, Couturier M, Dekegel D, Butzler JP. Molecular characterization of resistance plasmids in epidemiologically unrelated strains of multiresistant Haemophilus influenzae. J Infect Dis 1993;168:177–187.

117. Lim CT, Parasakthi N, Puthucheary SD. Neonatal meningitis due to non-encapsulated Haemophilus influenzae in a set of twins—a case report. Singapore Med J 1994;35:104–105.

118. Lode H, Schaberg T. Azithromycin in lower respiratory tract infections. Scand J Infect Dis Suppl 1992;83:26–33.

119. Lorian V. Antibiotics in laboratory medicine. 4th ed. Baltimore: Williams & Wilkins, 1996.

120. Machka K, Braveny I, Dabernat H. Distribution and resistance patterns of Haemophilus influenzae: a European cooperative study. Eur J Clin Microbiol Infect Dis 1988;7:14–24.

121. Marchant CD, Shurin PA, Johnson CE, Murdell PD, Feinstein JC, Fulton D, Flexon P, Carlin SA, Van HG. A randomized controlled trial of amoxicillin plus clavulanate compared with cefaclor for treatment of acute otitis media. J Pediatr 1986;109: 891–896.

122. Markham A, Brogden RN. Cefixime. A review of its therapeutic efficacy in lower respiratory tract infections. Drugs 1995; 49:1007–1022.

123. Markowitz SM. Isolation of an ampicillin-resistant, non-beta-lactamase-producing strain of Haemophilus influenzae. Antimicrob Agents Chemother 1980;17:80–83.

124. Martin C, Ragni J, Lokiec F. Pharmacokinetics and tissue penetration of a single dose of ceftriaxone (1,000 milligrams intravenously) for antibiotic prophylaxis in thoracic surgery. Antimicrob Agents Chemother 1992;36:2804–2807.

125. Martin E, Hohl P, Guggi T. Short course single daily ceftriaxone monotherapy for acute bacterial meningitis in children: results of a Swiss multicenter study. Part I: Clinical results. Infection 1990;18:70–77.

126. McColm AA, Ryan DM. Therapeutic activity of ceftazidime and eleven other beta-lactam antibiotics against experimental Haemophilus influenzae, type b meningitis. J Antimicrob Chemother 1984;13:517–520.

127. McCracken GJ, Nelson JD, Kaplan SL, Overturf GD, Rodriguez WJ, Steele RW. Consensus report: antimicrobial therapy for bacterial meningitis in infants and children. Pediatr Infect Dis J 1987;6:501–505.

128. McCracken GJ, Sakata Y, Olsen KD. Aztreonam therapy in experimental meningitis due to Haemophilus influenzae type b and Escherichia coli K1. Antimicrob Agents Chemother 1985;27:655–656.

129. Mertens JC, van BP, Asin HR. Double-blind randomized study comparing the efficacies and safeties of a short (3-day) course of azithromycin and a 5-day course of amoxicillin in patients with acute exacerbations of chronic bronchitis. Antimicrob Agents Chemother 1992;36:1456–1459.

130. Modai J. Potential role of fluoroquinolones in the treatment of bacterial meningitis. Eur J Clin Microbiol Infect Dis 1991; 10:291–295.

131. Moller LV, Regelink AG, Grasselier H. Multiple Haemophilus influenzae strains and strain variants coexist in the respiratory tract of patients with cystic fibrosis. J Infect Dis 1995;172: 1388–1392.

132. Morgan MG, Hamilton MJ. Haemophilus influenzae and H. parainfluenzae as urinary pathogens. J Infect 1990;20:143–145.

133. Motohiro T, Oki S, Tsumura N. Basic and clinical study of meropenem in pediatric field. Jpn J Antibiot 1992;45: 1356–1384.

134. Mouton JW, Kerrebijn KF. Antibacterial therapy in cystic fibrosis. Med Clin North Am 1990;74:837–850.

135. Moxon ER. Haemophilus influenzae. In: Principles and practice of infectious diseases, vol 2. 4th ed. New York: Churchill Livingstone, 1995:2039–2045.

136. Mulholland EK, Byass P, Campbell H. The immunogenicity and safety of Haemophilus influenzae type b-tetanus toxoid conjugate vaccine in Gambian infants. Ann Trop Paediatr 1994;14:183–188.

137. Mulholland EK, Hoestermann A, Ward JI, Maine N, Ethevenaux C, Greenwood BM. The use of Haemophilus influenzae type b-tetanus toxoid conjugate vaccine mixed with diphtheria-tetanus-pertussis vaccine in Gambian infants. Vaccine 1996;14: 905–909.

138. Mulholland K, Hilton S, Adegbola R, Usen S, Oparaugo A, Omosigho C, Weber M, Palmer A, Schneider G, Jobe K, Lahai G, Jaffar S, Secka O, Lin K, Ethevenaux C, Greenwood B. Randomised trial of Haemophilus influenzae type-b tetanus protein conjugate for prevention of pneumonia and meningitis in Gambian infants. Lancet 1997;349:1191–1197.

139. Murphy TF, Apicella MA. Nontypable Haemophilus influenzae: a review of clinical aspects, surface antigens, and the human immune response to infection. Rev Infect Dis 1987; 9:1–15.

140. Myburgh J, Nagel GJ, Petschel E. The efficacy and tolerance of a three-day course of azithromycin in the treatment of community-acquired pneumonia. J Antimicrob Chemother 1993;31 (Suppl E):163–169.

141. Nahata MC, Kohlbrenner VM, Barson WJ. Pharmacokinetics and cerebrospinal fluid concentrations of cefixime in infants and young children. Chemotherapy 1993;39:1–5.

142. Nathwani D, Wood MJ. Penicillins. A current review of their clinical pharmacology and therapeutic use. Drugs 1993;45: 866–894.

143. Neu HC. The crisis in antibiotic resistance. Science 1992;257: 1064–1073.

144. Neu HC, Chick TW. Efficacy and safety of clarithromycin compared to cefixime as outpatient treatment of lower respiratory tract infections. Chest 1993;104:1393–1399.

145. Odenholt-Tornqvist I, Lowdin E, Cars O. Postantibiotic effects and postantibiotic sub-MIC effects of roxithromycin, clarithromycin, and azithromycin on respiratory tract pathogens. Antimicrob Agents Chemother 1995;39:221–226.

146. Odio CM, Faingezicht I, Salas JL, Guevara J, Mohs E, McCracken GJ. Cefotaxime vs. conventional therapy for the treatment of bacterial meningitis of infants and children. Pediatr Infect Dis 1986;5:402–407.

147. Odio CM, Kusmiesz H, Shelton S, Nelson JD. Comparative treatment trial of Augmentin versus cefaclor for acute otitis media with effusion. Pediatrics 1985;75:819–826.

148. Peltola H, Anttila M, Renkonen OV. Randomised comparison of chloramphenicol, ampicillin, cefotaxime, and ceftriaxone for childhood bacterial meningitis. Finnish Study Group. Lancet 1989;1:1281–1287.

149. Pestalozza G, Cioce C, Facchini M. Azithromycin in upper respiratory tract infections: a clinical trial in children with otitis media. Scand J Infect Dis Suppl 1992;83:22–25.

150. Peter G. 1994 Red book: report of the Committee on Infectious Diseases. 23rd ed. Elk Grove Village, IL: American Academy of Pediatrics, 1994.

151. Peters DH, Clissold SP. Clarithromycin. A review of its antimicrobial activity, pharmacokinetic properties and therapeutic potential. Drugs 1992a;44:117–164.

152. Peters DH, Friedel HA, McTavish D. Azithromycin. A review of its antimicrobial activity, pharmacokinetic properties and clinical efficacy. Drugs 1992b;44:750–799.

153. Pichard E, Gillis D, Aker M, Engelhard D. Rebound fever in bacterial meningitis: role of dexamethasone dosage. Isr J Med Sci 1994;30:408–411.

154. Pichichero ME. Resistant respiratory pathogens and extended-spectrum antibiotics. Am Fam Physician 1995;52:1739–1746.

155. Piscitelli SC, Danziger LH, Rodvold KA. Clarithromycin and azithromycin: new macrolide antibiotics [published erratum appears in Clin Pharm 1992;11:308]. Clin Pharm 1992;11: 137–152.

156. Poirier R. Comparative study of clarithromycin and roxithromycin in the treatment of community-acquired pneumonia. J Antimicrob Chemother 1991;27:109–116.

157. Powell M, McVey D, Kassim MH, Chen HY, Williams JD. Antimicrobial susceptibility of Streptococcus pneumoniae, Haemophilus influenzae and Moraxella (Branhamella) catarrhalis isolated in the UK from sputa. J Antimicrob Chemother 1991;28:249–259.

158. Powell M, Williams JD. In-vitro activity of cefaclor, cephalexin and ampicillin against 2458 clinical isolates of Haemophilus influenzae. J Antimicrob Chemother 1988;21:27–31.

159. Powell M, Yeo SF, Seymour A. Antimicrobial resistance in Haemophilus influenzae from England and Scotland in 1991. J Antimicrob Chemother 1992;29:547–554.

160. Quentin R, Musser JM, Mellouet M. Typing of urogenital, maternal, and neonatal isolates of Haemophilus influenzae and Haemophilus parainfluenzae in correlation with clinical source of isolation and evidence for a genital specificity of H. influenzae biotype IV. J Clin Microbiol 1989;27:2286–2294.

161. Rajeshwari K, Sharma A. Remediable recurrent meningitis. Indian Pediatr 1995;32:491–496.

162. Raucher HS, Murphy RJ, Barzilai A. Meningitis occurring during therapy for otitis media with cephalexin and cefaclor. Am J Dis Child 1982;136:745–746.

163. Rockowitz J, Tunkel AR. Bacterial meningitis. Practical guidelines for management. Drugs 1995;50:838–853.

164. Rodriguez WJ, Puig JR, Khan WN, Feris J, Gold BG, Sturla C. Ceftazidime vs. standard therapy for pediatric meningitis: therapeutic, pharmacologic and epidemiologic observations. Pediatr Infect Dis 1986;5:408–415.

165. Rodriguez WJ, Schwartz RH, Khan WN, Gold AJ. Erythromycin-sulfisoxazole for persistent acute otitis media due to ampicillin-resistant Haemophilus influenzae. Pediatr Infect Dis 1983;2:27–29.

166. Ronan A, Hogg GG, Klug GL. Cerebrospinal fluid shunt infections in children. Pediatr Infect Dis J 1995;14:782–786.

167. Rubin LG, Medeiros AA, Yolken RH, Moxon ER. Ampicillin treatment failure of apparently beta-lactamase-negative Haemophilus influenzae type b meningitis due to novel beta-lactamase. Lancet 1981;2:1008–1010.

168. Sakata Y, McCracken GJ, Thomas ML, Olsen KD. Pharmacokinetics and therapeutic efficacy of imipenem, ceftazidime, and ceftriaxone in experimental meningitis due to an ampicillin- and chloramphenicol-resistant strain of Haemophilus influenzae type b. Antimicrob Agents Chemother 1984;25:29–32.

169. Santosham M, Hill J, Wolff M. Safety and immunogenicity of a Haemophilus influenzae type b conjugate vaccine in a high risk American Indian population. Pediatr Infect Dis J 1991;10: 113–117.

170. Santosham M, Wolff M, Reid R. The efficacy in Navajo infants of a conjugate vaccine consisting of Haemophilus influenzae type b polysaccharide and Neisseria meningitidis outer-membrane protein complex. N Engl J Med 1991;324:1767–1772.

171. Schaad UB, Kaplan SL, McCracken GJ. Steroid therapy for bacterial meningitis. Clin Infect Dis 1995;20:685–690.

172. Schaad UB, Lips U, Gnehm HE. Dexamethasone therapy for bacterial meningitis in children. Swiss Meningitis Study Group. Lancet 1993;342:457–461.

173. Schaad UB, Suter S, Gianella BA. A comparison of ceftriaxone

and cefuroxime for the treatment of bacterial meningitis in children. N Engl J Med 1990;322:141–147.

174. Schleupner CJ, Anthony WC, Tan J, File TM, Lifland P, Craig W, Vogelman B. Blinded comparison of cefuroxime to cefaclor for lower respiratory tract infections. Arch Intern Med 1988; 148:343–348.

175. Schwartz RH, Rodriguez WJ, Khan WN, Mann R, Barsanti RG, Ross S. Trimethoprim-sulfamethoxazole in the treatment of otitis media caused by ampicillin-resistant strains of Haemophilus influenzae. Rev Infect Dis 1982;4:514–516.

176. Selwyn BJ. The epidemiology of acute respiratory tract infection in young children: comparison of findings from several developing countries. Coordinated Data Group of BOSTID Researchers. Rev Infect Dis 1990;12(Suppl 8):s870–888.

177. Shurin PA, Pelton SI, Donner A. Trimethoprim-sulfamethoxazole compared with ampicillin in the treatment of acute otitis media. J Pediatr 1980;96:1081–1087.

178. Slack M. Haemophilus. In: Topley and Wilson's principles of bacteriology, virology and immunology, vol 2. 8th ed. London: Edward Arnold, 1990:355–381.

179. Slater LN, Guarnaccia J, Makintubee S, Istre GR. Bacteremic disease due to Haemophilus influenzae capsular type f in adults: report of five cases and review. Rev Infect Dis 1990;12: 628–635.

180. Smith AL. Antibiotic resistance in pediatric pathogens. Infect Dis Clin North Am 1992;6:177–195.

181. Sonnen GM, Henry NK. Pediatric bone and joint infections. Diagnosis and antimicrobial management. Pediatr Clin North Am 1996;43:933–947.

182. Stewart BT, Kaye AH. Delayed cerebrospinal fluid rhinorrhoea: a case report. Aust NZ J Surg 1992;62:818–20.

183. Sturm AW. Haemophilus influenzae and Haemophilus parainfluenzae in nongonococcal urethritis. J Infect Dis 1986;153: 165–167.

184. Swaminathan B, Mayer LW, Bibb WF. Microbiology of Brazilian purpuric fever and diagnostic tests. Brazilian Purpuric Fever Study Group. J Clin Microbiol 1989;27:605–608.

185. Sydnor AJ, Gwaltney JJ, Cocchetto DM, Scheld WM. Comparative evaluation of cefuroxime axetil and cefaclor for treatment of acute bacterial maxillary sinusitis. Arch Otolaryngol Head Neck Surg 1989;115:1430–1433.

186. Syrogiannopoulos GA, Lourida AN, Theodoridou MC. Dexamethasone therapy for bacterial meningitis in children: 2- versus 4-day regimen. J Infect Dis 1994;169:853–858.

187. Takala AK. Epidemiologic characteristics and risk factors for invasive Haemophilus influenzae type b disease in a population with high vaccine efficacy. Pediatr Infect Dis J 1989;8: 343–346.

188. Takala AK, Eskola J, van Alphen L. Spectrum of invasive Haemophilus influenzae type b disease in adults. Arch Intern Med 1990;150:2573–2576.

189. Taylor HG, Mills EL, Ciampi A, du BR, Watters GV, Gold R, MacDonald N, Michaels RH. The sequelae of Haemophilus influenzae meningitis in school-age children. N Engl J Med 1990;323:1657–1663.

190. Teigen K, Lingaas E. In vitro activity of 9 antimicrobial agents against 177 strains of Haemophilus influenzae isolated from hospitalized patients. APMIS 1990;98:753–757.

191. Tetanye E, Yondo D, Bernard BA. Initial treatment of bacterial meningitis in Yaounde, Cameroon: theoretical benefits of the ampicillin-chloramphenicol combination versus chloramphenicol alone. Ann Trop Paediatr 1990;10:285–291.

192. Tilyard MW, Dovey SM. A randomized double-blind controlled trial of roxithromycin and cefaclor in the treatment of acute lower respiratory tract infections in general practice. Diagn Microbiol Infect Dis 1992;15(Suppl):97s–101s.

193. Tremblay LD, L'Ecuyer J, Provencher P, Bergeron MG. Susceptibility of Haemophilus influenzae to antimicrobial agents used in Canada. Canadian Study Group. Can Med Assoc J 1990;143:895–901.

194. UNICEF. The state of the world's children 1994. Oxford: Oxford University Press, 1994.

195. Vadheim CM, Greenberg DP, Partridge S, Jing J, Ward JI. Effectiveness and safety of an Haemophilus influenzae type b conjugate vaccine (PRP-T) in young infants. Kaiser-UCLA Vaccine Study Group. Pediatrics 1993;92: 272–279.

196. van Bosterhaut B, Buts R, Veys A, Piot P. Haemophilus influenzae bartholinitis. Eur J Clin Microbiol Infect Dis 1990;9: 442.

197. Vazquez F, Andres MT, Palacio V. Isolation of Haemophilus influenzae and Haemophilus parainfluenzae in genitourinary infections: a 4-year review. Enferm Infecc Microbiol Clin 1996; 14:181–185.

198. Wald ER, Kaplan SL, Mason EJ. Dexamethasone therapy for children with bacterial meningitis. Meningitis Study Group. Pediatrics 1995;95:21–28.

199. Weinberg GA, Spitzer ED, Murray PR, Ghafoor A, Montgomery J, Tupasi TE, Granoff DM. Antimicrobial susceptibility patterns of Haemophilus isolates from children in eleven developing nations. BOSTID Haemophilus Susceptibility Study Group. Bull WHO 1990;68:179–184.

200. Weiss D, Glaser JH. Ceftriaxone versus cefuroxime for treatment of bacterial meningitis. J Pediatr 1990;116: 488–490.

201. Williams JD. Spectrum of activity of azithromycin. Eur J Clin Microbiol Infect Dis 1991;10:813–820.

202. Wong GW, Oppenheimer SJ, Vaudry W. CSF shunt infection by unencapsulated Haemophilus influenzae. Clin Infect Dis 1993;17:519–520.

203. Wong SN, Ng TL. Haemophilus influenzae septicaemia in the neonate: report of two cases and review of the English literature. J Paediatr Child Health 1991;27:113–115.

204. Wong VK, Wright HJ, Ross LA, Mason WH, Inderlied CB, Kim KS. Imipenem/cilastatin treatment of bacterial meningitis in children. Pediatr Infect Dis J 1991;10:122–125.

205. Wrenn K. Ceftriaxone versus cefuroxime for meningitis in children. N Engl J Med 1990;322:1821.

206. Yeo SF, Chiew YF, Fung CP. Susceptibility of Haemophilus influenzae isolates with known resistance mechanisms to five cephalosporins. Chemotherapy 1996;42:85–89.

207. Yogev R, Moxon ER. Elaboration of type b capsule by Haemophilus influenzae as a determinant of pathogenicity and impaired killing by trimethoprim-sulfamethoxazole. J Clin Invest 1982;69:658–665.

208. Zaki M, Daoud AS, ElSaleh Q, West PW. Childhood bacterial meningitis in Kuwait. J Trop Med Hyg 1990;93:7–11.

Helicobacter pylori

●

Mae F. Go and David Y. Graham

GENERAL DESCRIPTION

For the past 80 years, peptic ulcer disease has been attributed to the dictum "no acid, no ulcer." The discovery of *Helicobacter pylori* and its pivotal role in the pathogenesis of peptic ulcer has led to a revolution in concepts regarding the pathogenesis and management of peptic ulcer disease. It is now evident that while acid plays a role in ulcerogenesis, successful treatment of *H. pylori* infection results in the cure of most peptic ulcers.

H. pylori infection is a ubiquitous infection afflicting more than half the world's population. The prevalence of the infection is highest in those born in less developed countries and in those of low socioeconomic class in developed countries. Factors associated with increased prevalence of the infection include untreated water source, crowded living conditions, and poor sanitation. *H. pylori* infection causes chronic gastritis; infection without histologic disease has not been reported. Against the background of gastritis, a proportion of those infected will develop symptomatic disease, such as peptic ulcer or gastric malignancy (gastric adenocarcinoma or gastric MALT lymphoma). Most of the United States population with *H. pylori* infection remains asymptomatic, but one in six will develop peptic ulcer disease; the risk of gastric cancer is much lower. In the developing world, both ulcer disease and gastric cancer remain common. Gastric adenocarcinoma is the second most common cause of cancer-related death worldwide.

H. pylori infection has been reported to be essentially universal in antral-predominant gastritis. When nonsteroidal antiinflammatory drug use is excluded, it is associated with at least 95% of duodenal or gastric ulcers, 95% of MALT lymphoma, and 85% of those with gastric cancer. In February 1994, the NIH Consensus Development Conference concluded that the data were sufficient to show that *H. pylori* was the cause of most cases of peptic ulcer disease and declared that all ulcer patients with *H. pylori* infection should receive antimicrobial therapy (47). In June 1994, the International Agency for Research on Cancer Working Group of the World Health Organization classified *H. pylori* as a group I, or definite, human carcinogen (32). Successful treatment of *H. pylori* infection is now a medical goal because cure of the infection leads to healing of gastritis, cure of duodenal and gastric ulcer, and remission of most cases of gastric B-cell lymphoma (gastric MALT lymphoma). There is also speculation that if the infection is cured early enough in individuals with intestinal metaplasia, the malignant potential may be reversed.

MICROBIOLOGY

H. pylori is a Gram-negative spiral bacterium with multiple (~6) monopolar flagella, occupying a unique niche, the human stomach. *H. pylori* has great affinity for gastric and gastriclike epithelium. A number of virulence factors have been identified. For example, flagella are important for the microorganism to remain in the mucous layer overlying the gastric epithelium. *H. pylori* also express large quantities of a high-specific-activity urease that is essential in the initial colonization of gastric mucosa (9). Urease may produce acid tolerance by generation of ammonia produced by cleavage of urea, allowing adaptation and survival in the human stomach. Long-term survival in the acid environment of the gastric milieu may be regulated by ionic pumps in the membrane of the microorganism and the gastric H-K ATPase pump allowing selective adaptation to different pH environments (40, 42). *H. pylori* can be cultured on various types of media (26), but growth is better on solid substrates than in liquid medium. The bacterium requires a microaerophilic environment with high humidity for optimal growth.

DIAGNOSIS

While the infection is very common in many gastroduodenal diseases, its presence should be confirmed before treatment is initiated (6). A systemic immune response occurs with *H. pylori* infection, resulting in production of specific IgG antibodies that can be measured in serum or whole blood. Testing for IgG antibodies to the microorganism is the least expensive method for initial diagnosis of the infection in the patient who has not been previously treated. These tests have 85 to 95% sensitivity and about 90% specificity. The most sensitive antibody tests are based on the multiwell enzyme-linked immunosorbent assay (ELISA) tests that are generally sent to a laboratory. Rapid immunoassays using serum or whole blood are also available in which *H. pylori* status can be determined within 5 to 20 min. Examples of these tests are the FlexSure HP from SmithKline Diagnostics (San Jose, CA) and the QuickVue from Quidel (San Diego, CA). Both appear to be highly sensitive and specific (19). Serologic tests are rapid, accurate, inexpensive, and widely available. Use of antibody tests is limited by the slow decline in antibody titers after cure of the infection (6–12 months or even years after treatment) and thus these tests can not be used to follow up the patient in the early posttreatment period. Whole blood tests detecting IgG antibodies have recently become available, but their sensitivity and specificity appear slightly lower than the serum tests.

One caveat regarding serologic testing is that "in-house" ELISA of unknown specificity and sensitivity that have not been approved by the Food and Drug Administration (FDA) are widely available. If serum samples are sent out for *H. pylori* serology, one should confirm that the test used is FDA approved and, ideally, has been evaluated in a similar population. Current tests that examine for the presence of anti–*H. pylori* IgG as well as IgA and IgM titers are unapproved, correlate poorly with the presence or absence of *H. pylori* infection, and are not recommended. Receipt of results of IgA or IgM testing for *H. pylori* is one way to alert the clinician that they are dealing with a laboratory that uses tests of unknown accuracy.

Urea breath tests (UBTs) are based on the large quantities of urease produced by *H. pylori*. The patient ingests a small quantity of carbon-labeled urea (either the stable isotope ^{13}C-urea or the radioactive ^{14}C-urea). If *H. pylori* is present, the microorganism will hydrolyze the labeled urea, which can be measured in the breath by excess labeled $^{13}CO_2$ or $^{14}CO_2$. Both the ^{13}C-urea breath test (MERETEK UBT Breath Test, Houston, TX) and the ^{14}C-urea breath test (PYtest, Tri-Med, Lexexa, KS) are sensitive and specific for *H. pylori* detection and have been approved by the FDA. The ^{13}C-urea breath test has an accuracy of 95% both before and after treatment of *H. pylori* infection (33).

Endoscopic tests include culture, histology, and the rapid urease test and require gastric tissue. While culture is the "gold standard" for many infectious diseases, it is not recommended for the routine diagnosis of *H. pylori* infection because the microorganism is fastidious and culture is labor intensive. If antimicrobial resistance becomes a significant problem, culture becomes important to select the appropriate therapy.

Advantages of histology for detection of *H. pylori* infection include the permanent record of the degree, type, and location of inflammation as well as assessment of *H. pylori* infection. Many stains are useful for detecting the organism, including hematoxylin and eosin, Giemsa, Warthin-Starry, and the recently described Genta stain (12). Most studies have established that the experience and interest of the histopathologist are crucial for proper interpretation of the histologic specimens. Hematoxylin and eosin staining alone may be unsatisfactory because low-density microorganisms are often undetected (11, 46); many histopathologists feel that the Giemsa stain is highly reliable. The Warthin-Starry and Genta stains are silver stains that enhance the visibility of *H. pylori* and are recommended particularly to confirm cure of infection.

Rapid urease tests are based on production of urease by the microorganism. Gastric biopsy specimens are placed in a urea-containing substrate with a color indicator. Urea hydrolysis increases the pH, causing a color change that signifies the presence of the organism. Results can be read within 1 to 24 h, depending on the test used. Rapid urease testing has a 90 to 95% sensitivity and specificity and is comparable to histology for detection of the infection (60). Gastric biopsy specimens should be obtained from areas of abundant *H. pylori;* these include the antrum and corpus of the stomach (11, 58).

ANTIMICROBIAL THERAPY

H. pylori is susceptible to numerous antimicrobial agents when tested in vitro (41). However, susceptibility in vitro does not predict clinical efficacy. Single-drug therapy has proven poor for curing *H. pylori* infections, but a number of multidrug combination therapies have been effective. The best therapy is unknown, as large multicenter clinical trials comparing competing therapies are virtually nonexistent. Recommendations have often been based upon summary data using information obtained from small clinical trials often published in abstract form. Nevertheless, a number of regimens that reliably cure most *H. pylori* infections have now been demonstrated.

The goals of antiulcer therapy include relieving the pain, healing the ulcer (antisecretory therapy), and curing the infection (antimicrobial therapy) (17, 21). The names of various therapies have become confusing as multiple drugs are used for different purposes (ulcer healing vs. antimicrobial effect). The tendency has been to name therapies according to the number of drugs used, irrespective of whether each was integral to the antimicrobial effect. This has been further complicated by the fact that there are a number of different "triple therapies." We will use terminology with letters to describe therapies. For example, the historic treatment proposed by Borody in 1989 (5, 13) consisting of the combination of bismuth, metronidazole, and tetracycline is denoted as BMT triple therapy in this chapter. Clarithromycin can be successfully substituted for metronidazole in BMT triple therapy, producing BCT triple therapy. Addition of a proton pump inhibitor (either omeprazole or lansoprazole) to BMT triple therapy yields BMT quadruple therapy or bismuth-metronidazole-tetracycline–proton pump inhibitor quadruple therapy. Hundreds of studies evaluating various anti–*H. pylori* therapies have been published, but this chapter focuses on therapies that have been or are under evaluation in the United States. Cure rates in European studies have not been consistently reproducible in the United States or in large multicenter trials (49, 52, 53).

GENERAL

The optimum therapy for *H. pylori* infection would be effective, inexpensive, simple, of short duration, and without side effects. Failure to treat the infection successfully should also be associated with a low frequency of acquired resistance to the antimicrobials used. The antimicrobial should be as specific as possible to prevent development of antibiotic resistance among other microflora. No therapy meets all these objectives. The drugs that have been used in successful therapies approved by the FDA are listed in Table 1. Ampicillin cannot be substituted for amoxicillin. Amoxicillin can be substituted for tetracycline in BMT triple therapy (bismuth-metronidazole-amoxicillin, or BMA triple therapy) but with some loss of effectiveness (7). Oxytetracycline can be substituted for tetracycline hydrochloride (3), but doxycycline and chlortetracycline cannot. Erythromycin, azithromycin, or dirithromycin cannot substitute for clarithromycin (5). Preliminary data suggest that spiramycin may be an acceptable substitute for clarithromycin (bismuth-metronidazole-spiramycin, or BMS triple therapy) (2). Bismuth nitrate, subsalicylate, and citrate appear similarly effective. The new compound, ranitidine bismuth citrate (Tritec,

TABLE 1 • Regimens Approved by the U.S. FDA for Treatment of *H. pylori* Infection

Antimicrobial Agent	Dosage	Efficacy	Duration	Name
1. Omeprazole[a] clarithromycin with antisecretory drug	40 mg q. a.m. 500 mg t.i.d. (4–8 weeks)	70–80%	14 days	Dual OC
2. RBC[b], clarithromycin plus RBC	400 mg b.i.d. 500 mg t.i.d. 400 mg b.i.d. for additional 2 weeks	70—85%	14 days	Dual RBC/C
3. Bismuth subsalicylate[c, d] metronidazole tetracycline HCl with antisecretory drug	2 tablets q.i.d. 250 mg t.i.d. 500 mg q.i.d. (4–8 weeks)	>90%	14 days	BMT triple
4. Lansoprazole[a] amoxicillin clarithromycin	30 mg b.i.d. 1000 mg b.i.d. 500 mg b.i.d.	80–95%	14 days	LAC triple

[a]Omeprazole 20 mg b.i.d. and lansoprazole 30 mg b.i.d. are equivalent.

[b]RBC, ranitidine bismuth subcitrate (Tritec).

[c]Pepto-Bismol or bismuth subcitrate can be substituted.

[d]A modification is the packaged combination Helidac.

GlaxoWellcome), provides a bismuth that is soluble in acid and may have an advantage over other bismuth preparations. This theoretical advantage has not been evaluated in head-to-head comparisons. Azithromycin is being evaluated in clinical trials in the United States to examine its usefulness in combination therapies to cure *H. pylori* infection. Azithromycin studies published to date have been conducted outside the United States and have shown mixed results: some studies suggest good cure rates while others demonstrate poor results.

A number of antimicrobial combinations achieve cure rates between 80 and 100% (Tables 1 and 2). Current multidrug regimens must be considered "recipes" because changes in dose, dosing interval, or formulation may result in significantly poorer results. *H. pylori* is an infection of a mucosal surface and as such is outside the body. The stomach, because of its acidity, rapid emptying, and frequent shedding of its mucous lining, is a very hostile place for antibiotics to function effectively. *H. pylori* organisms are not only outside the body but they are encased in

TABLE 2 • Emerging Regimens for Treatment of *H. pylori* Infection

Antimicrobial Agent	Dosage	Efficacy	Duration	Name
1. Bismuth subsalicylate[a] clarithromycin tetracycline HCl with antisecretory drug	2 tablets q.i.d. 500 mg t.i.d. 500 mg q.i.d. (4–8 weeks)	>90%	14 days	BCT triple
2. Bismuth subsalicylate[b, c] metronidazole tetracycline HCl with PPI[d]	2 tabs q.i.d. 250 mg t.i.d. 500 mg q.i.d. (4 weeks)	>90%	14 days	BMT quadruple
3. Metronidazole omeprazole[d] clarithromycin continue omeprazole	500 mg b.i.d 20 mg b.i.d. 250 mg b.i.d. (20 mg daily, additional 2 weeks)	>90%	14 days	MOC triple
4. Omeprazole[d] amoxicillin clarithromycin continue omeprazole	20 mg b.i.d. 1000 mg b.i.d. 500 mg b.i.d. (20 mg daily, additional 2 weeks)	80–95%	14 days	OAC triple
5. Bismuth subsalicylate[b] metronidazole amoxicillin with antisecretory drug	2 tablets q.i.d. 250 mg t.i.d. 500 mg q.i.d. (4–8 weeks)	>80%	14 days	BMA triple

[a]This regimen can be used in patients with suspected metronidazole resistance.

[b]Pepto-Bismol, or bismuth subcitrate can be substituted

[c]A modification is the packaged combination Helidac.

[d]Omeprazole 20 mg b.i.d. and lansoprazole 30 mg b.i.d. are equivalent.

thick mucus. The low pH environment may also adversely affect antimicrobial effectiveness. Tetracycline, bismuth, and metronidazole appear to be largely pH independent antimicrobials, whereas the effectiveness of amoxicillin and the macrolides (clarithromycin and possibly azithromycin) is enhanced by increasing the pH (25, 36). Inhibition of acid secretion has the advantage of increasing intragastric pH, but it is difficult or impossible to increase the pH reliably above the 3 to 5 range for any length of time. Antisecretory agents inhibit acid secretion and thus may limit the ability of the antimicrobial to be carried along as acid is secreted into the stomach.

Combinations of a proton pump inhibitor (omeprazole, lansoprazole, or pantoprazole) and a single antimicrobial are less effective than combinations in which it is included with two antimicrobials. The combination of a proton pump inhibitor and amoxicillin proved very sensitive to external factors, and success rates have varied widely, with a worldwide average of about 50% (24). Increasing the dose of amoxicillin or proton pump inhibitor did not increase the reliability of this combination, and it has largely been abandoned. The results of the omeprazole/amoxicillin therapy for *H. pylori* infection are largely unprecedented for a bacterial infection susceptible to the antibiotics used. For example, the same combination of antibiotics used to treat infections with susceptible organisms in different countries, or even different gastroenterology units within the same country, gave markedly different results. These results demonstrated how little is known about the pharmacology of antimicrobials in the stomach and how much more information is needed for rational development of therapies for this important infection.

While cigarette smoking does not have a direct effect on the development of ulcers, it may influence the efficacy of certain anti–*H. pylori* therapies. Dual therapy with various doses of omeprazole and amoxicillin have shown lower cure rates in smokers than in nonsmokers (65 and 83%, respectively; *P* = .003) (35). It has been suggested that BMT triple therapy may be less effective in smokers (8), but that has not been our experience (23). However, no difference in cure rates was detected in *H. pylori*–infected smokers and nonsmokers who were treated with clarithromycin and omeprazole (71 vs. 77%); furthermore, no difference in ulcer recurrence (12%) was seen in smokers and nonsmokers treated with this dual therapy (1).

The reader must be aware that data regarding individual therapies for *H. pylori* have generally been reported from small trials; direct multicenter comparisons of sufficient size between different regimens are still unavailable. Two triple therapies and one quadruple therapy have the best results worldwide (BMT triple therapy; metronidazole-clarithromycin–proton pump inhibitor triple therapy; and BMT–proton pump inhibitor quadruple therapy) (Tables 1 and 2). BMT triple therapy, with or without an antisecretory drug, has been used in a number of studies with 90 or more patients and has consistently yielded cure rates in the range of 85 to 95% (4, 8, 16, 18, 22, 31). Metronidazole-resistant *H. pylori* responds less well, with cure rates between 60 and 80%, but will not greatly affect the outcome unless metronidazole-resistant strains are prevalent in the population (18, 23).

Caveats relating to BMT therapy are that the pharmacist must be alerted, the patient educated, and that both tetracycline and bismuth are given with meals. While both meals and bismuth theoretically reduce the effectiveness of tetracycline, in practice, the convenience and prolonged residence in the stomach at high concentration makes it desirable to give them in this manner. The patient must also be alerted to the fact that any bismuth preparation may cause darkening of the stool and this should not be confused with bleeding. For all therapies, patients must understand the importance of taking all of the medication, not stopping when they feel better. All the drugs should be begun at the same time (i.e., to follow the recipe) because sequential addition of agents may lead to an increase in the frequency of metronidazole-resistant *H. pylori*.

The four regimens approved for use by the FDA (Table 1) include two dual therapies, omeprazole-clarithromycin and ranitidine bismuth citrate–clarithromycin, and while both appear effective (70–80%), they are less so than the proton pump inhibitor triple therapies, BMT triple therapy, or BMT–proton pump inhibitor quadruple therapy. Both dual therapies can be improved by addition of a third drug (e.g., metronidazole or tinidazole). The third approved therapy is a version of BMT triple therapy. The fourth approved therapy is a triple therapy that includes amoxicillin, clarithromycin, and lansoprazole. This regimen differs from the first three in being a twice-a-day therapy for only 14 days.

While there is no single "right choice," a regimen with a high cure rate should be chosen. The choice depends on cost, availability, and whether metronidazole or clarithromycin resistance is suspected. If the patient has received clarithromycin-based therapy in the past, one should assume that the microorganism is clarithromycin-resistant until proven otherwise by culture, and macrolides should be avoided. In the United States, the results of therapy for peptic ulcer, even prior to *H. pylori,* have generally been inferior to results in Europe, and it is unclear whether results from Europe are directly transferable to the United States. In Europe, the tendency has been to give therapy for 7 days, while in the United States therapy has been administered for 2 weeks. Randomized controlled trials with sufficient sample sizes have not been done to compare durations of therapy or whether proton pump inhibitors offer a significant advantage over H_2-receptor antagonists for therapies that require pH control. We recommend that if an active ulcer is being treated, anti–*H. pylori* therapy should be given for 2 weeks and antisecretory therapy continued for a total of 6 weeks (16, 18) (Table 3). If omeprazole-containing anti–*H. pylori* therapy is prescribed, one can switch to a less expensive H_2-receptor antagonist during the last 4 weeks of therapy. Patients are seen at the end of antimicrobial therapy to ascertain whether problems have occurred and to evaluate compliance. They are seen again after 4 to 6 weeks to evaluate the effectiveness of therapy by endoscopy or preferably the urea breath test. This standard protocol eliminates the need to remember whether the regimen is 1 or 2 weeks in duration, adequate antisecretory therapy is given to reliably heal the ulcer, and patients continue to take medication and are more likely to return for follow up.

Multiple reasons can explain failure of *H. pylori* treatment,

TABLE 3 • Evaluation of the Patient with *H. pylori* Disease

1. Before checking *H. pylori* status of the individual, the decision should have been made to treat for cure if the infection is present.
2. Confirm presence of infection: serology, urea breath test, histology, or rapid urease test.
3. Treat with combination therapy with cure rate of 90% or better.
4. If active ulcer disease is present, treat with antisecretory agent for a total of 4 to 6 weeks to ensure healing of ulcer in addition to the 2 weeks of antimicrobial agents.
5. For confirmation of cure and if malignancy is not suspected, the urea breath test can be performed 4 or more weeks after completion of therapy. Proton pump inhibitors should be discontinued for at least 1 week prior to testing.

such as use of an inappropriate therapy (e.g., use of doxycycline instead of tetracycline or erythromycin instead of clarithromycin). Compliance can be a problem if the patient does not appreciate the need for continuing the regimen for the prescribed duration even though symptoms have disappeared. While the large number of pills in some combination therapies poses a potential problem in compliance, if the patient realizes the importance of taking all prescribed pills and is aware of potential side effects, excellent compliance is the rule.

Side Effects

Because of the multiple drugs included in anti–*H. pylori* treatment, a number of different side effects may be experienced by the patient. The most common one is nausea, which can result from almost any drug. Clarithromycin given in doses greater than 1 g/day may cause a taste disturbance. Patients treated with bismuth salts have dark stools; they should be warned that this is not blood in the stool but the bismuth. Diarrhea may occur in some patients. Penicillin allergy should be excluded if an amoxicillin regimen is being prescribed. Some women develop vaginitis after treatment with tetracycline. The patient with renal disease may need decreased doses of clarithromycin. In general, these side effects occur in about 20 to 30% of patients and are mild and transient; they do not lead to decreased compliance if the patient has been made aware of them. Severe side effects such as pseudomembranous colitis are rare.

Antimicrobial Resistance

Antimicrobial resistance has become an important problem in most infectious diseases. To date, acquired resistance by *H. pylori* has usually concerned only mutational resistance at the chromosomal level. However, there is no assurance that plasmid-mediated resistance will not occur, since many *H. pylori* strains contain plasmids. Acquired resistance has been demonstrated in four groups of antimicrobial agents: nitroimidazoles, macrolides, fluoroquinolones, and rifampicins. Resistance to tetracycline (44) and amoxicillin (unpublished observations) has also been demonstrated in naturally occurring *H. pylori* isolates.

Metronidazole has been one of the cornerstone drugs in combination therapies, but increasing resistance is being ob-

served worldwide because of its widespread use. Resistance to metronidazole in the United States is probably about 30%, but it will be much more common if the subpopulation includes immigrants from developing countries where this drug is empirically dispensed. Metronidazole resistance has escalated from 60 to 75% in some developing countries (39); it continues to increase even in developed countries (14). Although the cellular events resulting in metronidazole resistance in *H. pylori* are still being unraveled, some potential genes in the metabolic pathway for the metronidazole mechanism are being characterized (15, 28). Metronidazole resistance develops less often when metronidazole is given with bismuth or a second antimicrobial drug. While the levels of metronidazole resistance vary, with MIC values from 16 mg/L to more than 512 mg/L, cutoff values that predict treatment failure for any of the combination therapies remain undetermined.

Metronidazole resistance may be considered as occurring in two forms in relation to outcome: laboratory evidence of metronidazole resistance (laboratory resistance) and metronidazole resistance acquired following an attempt to treat the infection (acquired resistance). It is our impression that infection with strains with acquired resistance are much more difficult to cure with a metronidazole-containing regimen than those with only laboratory resistance. We suggest that authors report success rates of therapy with respect to sensitive and resistant strains and in relation to laboratory and acquired resistance (18).

Clarithromycin is another antimicrobial agent with a significant role in *H. pylori* combination therapies. The antibacterial spectrum of clarithromycin is similar to that of erythromycin, but it is more effective against *H. pylori*, is more acid stable, and is better absorbed. *H. pylori* resistance remains low, but increased resistance is also being observed in some locations (59). Three single-point mutations in the 23S rRNA have been identified that reduce clarithromycin binding to a ribosomal target and confirm clarithromycin resistance (50, 57). Specific single-base mutations can be correlated with a lower or higher MIC (50). In the presence of clarithromycin resistance, cure rates with clarithromycin-containing therapies fall remarkably (0–25%) (18). Because of the potential for development of resistance, neither metronidazole nor clarithromycin should be administered as monotherapies.

Reinfection after Apparently Successful Therapy

Reinfection in adults is rare in studies in developed countries (e.g., 10, 20, 43, 51). There are few data on children or reinfection rates in developing countries. Most early reinfection (within the first year) is actually misidentified failure of the therapy to cure the original infection (54). It has been reported that reinfection in 0.1 to 1.0% of patients occurred at endoscopy (37), but endoscopic transmission of *H. pylori* has not been shown in the United States where stringent high-level disinfection of endoscopes and accessories is the rule. Endoscopic transmission is a particularly important potential problem in countries or endoscopy units where routine high-level disinfection of endoscopes and accessories is not performed. Endoscopy should not be performed to follow up therapy if endoscopically transmitted reinfection cannot be prevented.

Treatment of Patients Who Have Failed Therapy

There are now many combination therapies that effectively cure *H. pylori* infection, but no therapy thus far has 100% efficacy. The success rates listed in Tables 1 and 2 apply to the general population unless there are many who have been exposed multiple times to a particular antimicrobial agent. If a patient is from a developing country, there is high likelihood that metronidazole-resistant *H. pylori* may be present, and a nonmetronidazole regimen should be selected. The most common reasons for treatment failure in the patient who has been treated with an effective regimen include antimicrobial resistance and noncompliance. If the patient has been previously exposed to metronidazole or clarithromycin, *H. pylori* resistance to these drugs may have developed. Clarithromycin can substitute for metronidazole, but clarithromycin resistance is generally not overcome by other drugs such as tetracycline or amoxicillin, so a nonclarithromycin regimen should be selected.

The compliant patient who has failed an initial anti–*H. pylori* regimen should be treated with a different regimen. At this time one must assume antimicrobial resistance exists. If the standard BMT was used, clarithromycin can be substituted for metronidazole in this same regimen or a different nonmetronidazole regimen can be prescribed. If clarithromycin resistance is suspected, a metronidazole or amoxicillin regimen should be used for the second treatment. The patient who has failed appropriate treatment twice should undergo endoscopic evaluation to assess for organic disease and have gastric biopsy for antimicrobial susceptibility testing. Although most microbiology laboratories do not perform *H. pylori* testing routinely, they may do this on special occasions or the biopsy specimens can be sent to specialized laboratories in research centers. Antimicrobial susceptibility testing should evaluate susceptibility to metronidazole, clarithromycin, amoxicillin, and tetracycline. Both microdilution and the epsilometer agar-diffusion gradient test (E-Test, AB Biodisk) can be used (27, 55). Thus far, *H. pylori* resistance to bismuth has not been demonstrated. The patient can then be treated with a regimen with antimicrobials to which the *H. pylori* isolate is susceptible. The rare patient resistant to all regimens should be treated with a maintenance antisecretory drug.

Other classes of drugs are being evaluated in combination therapies for *H. pylori* treatment. Furazolidone is an inexpensive antimicrobial under review for use in developing countries because of its potential efficacy and low cost. Ketolides, a new class of drugs distantly related to the macrolides, may be useful in future anti–*H. pylori* therapies.

ENDPOINTS FOR MONITORING THERAPY

Cure of *H. pylori* infection is defined as the inability to detect *H. pylori* 4 or more weeks after treatment. As a result of clinical experience, successful treatment (cure or eradication) is now defined as absence of detectable organisms 4 weeks or more after therapy (16, 30) (Table 4). Sampling earlier than 4 weeks after the end of antimicrobial therapy is associated with an unacceptably high rate of false-negative results, since failure to detect the organism during this period may reflect suppression of the infection rather than cure. The combination of several different tests increases the confidence that the infection has been cured (30). Cure is also associated with a very low rate of reinfection.

Serologic testing in the early posttreatment period is problematic because the IgG titers decline very slowly over months to years even after successful treatment. The urea breath test is the most useful follow-up test if malignancy is not suspected, as it is noninvasive, highly accurate before and after treatment, and inexpensive compared with endoscopy. Proton pump inhibitors should be stopped for at least 1 week before testing, as these drugs can suppress *H. pylori* growth and yield a false-negative result.

POTENTIAL ROLE OF VACCINATION

The ubiquity of *H. pylori* infection and its association with multiple gastroduodenal diseases makes it a public health hazard. Because of the high prevalence of the infection worldwide, it is not economically feasible or practical to attempt to cure each infected individual with antimicrobial therapy. Furthermore, widespread use of antimicrobial combination therapy would likely result in increased antimicrobial resistance. Therefore, vaccines have been under development for not only cure but also prevention of the infection. Several animal models have been developed with *Helicobacter* species that produce gastritis similar to that in the human host (38). Antigens from whole cells and recombinant proteins have conferred protection in the mouse–*H. felis* model. Immunization to cure established infection has also been successful in the mouse–*H. felis* model (29, 38, 45). Specific antigens and adjuvants are being evaluated. Phase I trials have been completed showing safety of urease recombinant antigens in human volunteers (34). Improvement and safety of mucosal adjuvants such as the cholera toxin subunit and *E. coli* toxin also continue.

TABLE 4 • **Criteria for Cure of *Helicobacter pylori* Infection**

Clinical
1. Absence of duodenal or gastric ulcer recurrence
2. Risk of developing a duodenal or gastric ulcer less than that of a control population (for those who have not had duodenal or gastric ulcer)

Laboratory
Noninvasive
1. Continued fall of anti–*H. pylori* antibody titer in serologic tests
2. Continued negative urea breath tests

Invasive
1. *H. pylori* not cultured from at least two gastric mucosal biopsy specimens, one from the antrum
2. *H. pylori* not detected on gastric mucosal biopsy specimens (at least one antral) using sensitive special stains
3. Continued improvement in the histology of the gastric mucosa toward normal; clearance of polymorphonuclear infiltration

CONTROVERSIES OR CAVEATS

As public awareness about the links between *H. pylori* infection, peptic ulcer, and gastric cancer increases, physicians will be under increasing pressure from patients to test for infection. However, we believe that it is inappropriate to test patients for infection unless one is prepared to inform the patient about the potential consequences of infection and offer therapy. The physician must inform the patient that the infection damages the structure and function of the stomach, can lead to peptic ulcer and gastric cancer, can potentially be transmitted to others in the community, and in fact has no known beneficial effects for the host or for society. Thus, our guiding principle is "Do not test, if you are not willing to treat." Whom then, should we be willing to treat? Based on the available evidence, we should treat all patients with active or previous peptic ulcer disease, because ulcer patients with *H. pylori* infection are those most likely to benefit from anti–*H. pylori* therapy, as ulcer disease can be cured. It has also been confirmed that the rule "no ulcer no complications" is also true. Because of the high frequency of dyspepsia in the population and frequent difficulty in distinguishing between an ulcer and nonulcer dyspepsia by symptoms alone, the issue of curing *H. pylori* infection in nonulcer dyspeptics remains controversial. *H. pylori* infection is as common in the nonulcer dyspepsia population as it is in the general population. The risks and benefits of routine testing of patients with dyspepsia for *H. pylori* infection are unclear, as the few prospective studies evaluating long-term symptom improvement after *H. pylori* cure have not demonstrated lasting benefit (long-term symptom improvement) in most patients (56).

We recommend that all first-degree relatives of gastric cancer patients should be tested and, if infected, treated. A recent decision analysis study suggests that cure of the infection in a high-risk population such as Japanese-Americans may be cost-effective (48). Otherwise, unless children are present in the family, transmission of *H. pylori* infection is probably uncommon among adults.

REFERENCES

1. Bardhan KD, Graham DY, Hunt RH, O'Morain CA. Effects of smoking on cure of *H. pylori* infection and duodenal ulcer recurrence in patients treated with clarithromycin and omeprazole. Helicobacter 1997;2:27–31.
2. Berstad A, Berstad K, Wilhelmsen I, Hatlebakk JG, Nesje LB, Hausken T. Spiramycin in triple therapy of *Helicobacter pylori*-associated peptic ulcer disease. An open pilot study with 12-month follow-up. Aliment Pharmacol Ther 1995;9: 197–200.
3. Berstad A, Hatlebakk JG Wilhelmsen I, Berstad K, Bang Ch J, Nysaeter G, Hausken T, Weberg R, Nesje LB, Hjartholm AS. Follow-up on 242 patients with peptic ulcer disease one year after eradication of *Helicobacter pylori* infection. Hepatogastroenterology 1995;42:655–659.
4. Borody TJ, Andrews P, Mancuso N, McCauley D, Jankiewicz E, Ferch N, Shortis NP, Brandl S. *Helicobacter pylori* reinfection rate, in patients with cured duodenal ulcer. Am J Gastroenterol 1994;89:529–532.
5. Borody TJ, Cole P, Noonan S, Morgan A, Lenne J, Hyland L, Brandl S, Borody EG, George LL. Recurrence of duodenal ulcer and *Campylobacter pylori* infection after eradication. Med J Aust 1989;151:431–435.
6. Brown KE, Peura DA. Diagnosis of *Helicobacter pylori* infection. Gastroenterol Clin North Am 1993;22:105–117.
7. Chiba N, Rao RV, Rademaker JW, Hunt RH. Meta-analysis of the efficacy of antibiotic therapy in eradicating *Helicobacter pylori*. Am J Gastroenterol 1992;87:1716–1727.
8. Cutler AF, Schubert TT. Patient factors affecting *Helicobacter pylori* eradication with triple therapy. Am J Gastroenterol 1993; 88:505–509.
9. Eaton KA, Brooks CL, Morgan DR, Krakowka S. Essential role of urease in pathogenesis of gastritis induced by *Helicobacter pylori* in gnotobiotic piglets. Infect Immun 1991;59:2470–2475.
10. Forbes GM, Glaser ME, Cullen DJE, Warren JR, Christiansen KJ, Marshall BJ, Collins BJ. Duodenal ulcer treted with *Helicobacter pylori* eradication: seven year follow-up. Lancet 1994; 343:258–260.
11. Genta RM, Graham DY. Comparison of biopsy sites for the histopathologic diagnosis of *Helicobacter pylori*: a topographic study of *H. pylori* density and distribution. Gastrointest Endosc 1994a;40:342–345.
12. Genta RM, Robason GO, Graham DY. Simultaneous visualization of *Helicobacter pylori* and gastric morphology. Hum Pathol 1994b;25:221–226.
13. George LL, Borody TJ, Andrews P, Devine M, Moore-Jones D, Walton M, et al. Cure of duodenal ulcer after eradication of *Helicobacter pylori*. Med J Aust 1990;153:145–149.
14. Goddard AF, Logan RPH. Antimicrobial resistance and *Helicobacter pylori*. J Antimicrob Chemother 1996;37:639–643.
15. Goodwin A, Veldhuyzen van Zanten S, Hoffman PS. Cloning of a metronidazole-resistance locus from *Helicobacter pylori*. Gut 1996;39(Suppl 2):A8.
16. Graham DY. A reliable cure for *Helicobacter pylori* infection? Gut 1995;37:154–156.
17. Graham DY. Evolution of concepts regarding *Helicobacter pylori*: from a cause of gastritis to a public health problem [Editorial]. Am J Gastroenterol 1994a;89:469–472.
18. Graham DY, de Boer WA, Tytgat GN. Choosing the best anti-*Helicobacter pylori* therapy: effect of antimicrobial resistance. Am J Gastroenterol 1996;91:1072–1076.
19. Graham DY, Evans DJ Jr, Peacock J, Baker JT, Schrier WH. Comparison of rapid serological tests (FlexSure HP and QuickVue) with conventional ELISA for detection of *Helicobacter pylori* infection. Am J Gastroenterol 1996;91:942–948.
20. Graham DY, Genta RM. Reinfection with *H. pylori*. In: Hunt RH, Tytgat GNJ, eds. *Helicobacter pylori*: basic mechanisms to clinical cure. Boston: Kluwer Academic Publishers, 1993: 113–120.
21. Graham DY, Karttunen TJ, Genta RM. The evaluation of treatment of *H. pylori* infections: strategies for the design of clinical trials. Endosc Digest 1994;6:991–1006.
22. Graham DY, Lew GM, Klein PD, Evans DG, Evans DJ, Saeed ZA, Malaty HM. Effect of treatment of *Helicobacter pylori* on the long-term recurrence of gastric or duodenal ulcers: a randomized controlled study. Ann Intern Med 1992;116:705–708.
23. Graham DY, Lew GM, Malaty HM, Evans DG, Evans DJ Jr, Klein PD, Alpert LC, Genta RM. Factors influencing the eradication of *Helicobacter pylori* with triple therapy. Gastroenterology 1992;102:493–496.
24. Graham KS, Malaty HM, El-Zimaity HMT, Genta RM, Cole RA, Al-Assi M, Yousfi MM, Neil GA, Graham DY. Variability with omeprazole-amoxicillin combinations for treatment of infection. Am J Gastroenterol 1995;90:1415–1418.

25. Gustavson LE, Kaiser JF, Edmonds AL, Locke CS, DeBartolo ML, Schneck DW. Effect of omeprazole on concentrations of clarithromycin in plasma and gastric tissue at steady state. Antimicrob Agents Chemother 1995;39:2078–2083.

26. Hachem CY, Clarridge JE, Evans DG, Graham DY. Comparison of agar based media for primary isolation of *Helicobacter pylori*. J Clin Pathol 1995;48:714–716.

27. Hachem CY, Clarridge JE, Reddy R, Flamm R, Evans DG, Tanaka SK, Graham DY. Antimicrobial susceptibility testing of *Helicobacter pylori*: comparison of E-Test, broth microdilution, and disk diffusion for ampicillin, clarithromycin, and metronidazole. Diagn Microbiol Infect Dis 1996;24:37–41.

28. Hoffman PS, Goodwin A, Johnsen J, Magee K, Veldhuyzen van Zanten SJ. Metabolic activities of metronidazole-sensitive and resistant strains of *Helicobacter pylori*: repression of pyruvate oxidoreductase and expression of isocitrate lyase activity correlate with resistance. J Bacteriol 1996;178:4822–4829.

29. Hook-Nikanne J, Aho P, Karkkainen P, Kosunen TU, Salaspuro M. The *Helicobacter felis* mouse model in assessing anti-Helicobacter therapies and gastric mucosal prostaglandin E_2 levels. Scand J Gastroenterol 1996;31:334–338.

30. Hopkins RJ, Girardi LS, Turney EA. Relationship between *Helicobacter pylori* eradication and reduced duodenal and gastric ulcer recurrence: a review. Gastroenterology 1996;110: 1244–1252.

31. Hosking SW, Ling TK, Yung MY, Cheng A, Chung SC, Leung JW, Li AK. Randomised controlled trial of short term treatment to eradicate *Helicobacter pylori* in patients with duodenal ulcer. Br Med J 1992;305:502–504.

32. IARC Working Group on the Evaluation of Carcinogenic Risks to Humans. *Helicobacter pylori*. In: Schistosomes, liver flukes and *Helicobacter pylori*: views and expert opinions of an IARC Working Group on the Evaluation of Carcinogenic Risks to Humans. Lyon: IARC, 1994:177–240.

33. Klein PD, Malaty HM, Martin RF, Graham KS, Genta RM, Graham DY. Noninvasive detection of *Helicobacter pylori* infection in clinical practice: the ^{13}C urea breath test. Am J Gastroenterol 1996;91:690–694.

34. Kreiss C, Buclin T, Cosma M, Corthesy-Theulaz I, Michetti P. Safety of oral immunisation with recombinant urease in patients with *Helicobacter pylori* infection [Letter]. Lancet 1996;347: 1630–1631.

35. Labenz J, Leverkus F, Borsch G. Omeprazole plus amoxicillin for cure of *Helicobacter pylori* infection. Scand J Gastroenterol 1994;29:1070–1075.

36. Lambert JR. Pharmacology of the gastric mucosa: a rational approach to *Helicobacter* polytherapy [Editorial]. Gastroenterology 1996;111:521–523.

37. Langenberg W, Rauws EA, Oudbier JH, Tytgat GN. Patient-to-patient transmission of *Campylobacter pylori* infection by fiberoptic gastroduodenoscopy and biopsy. J Infect Dis 1990; 161:507–511.

38. Lee A, Buck F. Vaccination and mucosal responses to *Helicobacter pylori* infection. Aliment Pharmacol Ther 1996;10 (Suppl 1):129–138.

39. Ling TKW, Cheng AFB, Sung JJY, Yiu PYL, Chung SSC. An increase in *Helicobacter pylori* strains resistant to metronidazole: a five-year study. Helicobacter 1996;1:57–61.

40. Matin A, Zychlinsky E, Keyhan M, Sachs G. Capacity of *Helicobacter pylori* to generate ionic gradients at low pH is similar to that of bacteria which grow under strongly acidic conditions. Infect Immun 1996;64:1434–1436.

41. McNulty CAM, Dent JC, Ford GA, Wilkinson SP. Inhibitory concentrations against *Campylobacter pylori* in gastric mucosa. J Antimicrob Chemother 1988;22:729–738.

42. Meyer-Rosberg K, Scott DR, Rex D, Melchers K, Sachs G. The effect of environmental pH on the proton motive force of *Helicobacter pylori*. Gastroenterology 1996;111:887–900.

43. Miehlke S, Bayerfoerffer E, Lehn N, Mannes GA, Hoechter W, Weingart J, Sommer A, Heldwein W, Mueller-Lissner S, Baestlein E, Ruckdeschel G, Koepcke W, Stolte M. Recurrence of duodenal ulcers during five years of follow-up after cure of *Helicobacter pylori* infection. Eur J Gastroenterol Hepatol 1995;7:975–978.

44. Midolo P, Korman MG, Turnidge JD, Lambert JR. *Helicobacter pylori* resistance to tetracycline. Lancet 1996;347:1194–1195.

45. Mohammadi M, Redline R, Nedrud J, Czinn S. Role of the host in pathogenesis of *Helicobacter*-associated gastritis: *H. felis* infection of inbred and congenic mouse strains. Infect Immun 1996;64:238–245.

46. Molyneux AJ, Harris MD. *Helicobacter pylori* in gastric biopsies—should you trust the pathology report? J R Coll Physicians Lond 1993;27:119–120.

47. NIH consensus development panel on *Helicobacter pylori* in peptic ulcer disease. *Helicobacter pylori* in peptic ulcer disease. JAMA 1994;272:65–69.

48. Parsonnet J, Harris RA, Hack HM, Owens DK. Modelling of cost-effectiveness of *Helicobacter pylori* screening to prevent gastric cancer: a mandate for clinical trials. Lancet 1996; 348:150–154.

49. Penston JG. Review article: clinical aspects of *Helicobacter pylori* eradication therapy in peptic ulcer disease. Aliment Pharmacol Ther 1996;10:469–486.

50. Stone G, Shortridge D, Flamm RK, Versalovic J, Beyer J, Idler K, Zulawinski L, Tanaka SK. Identification of a 23S rRNA gene mutation in clarithromycin-resistant *Helicobacter pylori*. Helicobacter 1996;1:227–228.

51. Tatsuta M, Iishi H, Yokota Y. Effects of *Helicobacter pylori* infection healing and recurrence of gastric ulcers. Am J Gastroenterol 1995;90:406–410.

52. Unge P. Review of *Helicobacter pylori* eradication regimens. Scand J Gastroenterol 1996;31(Suppl 215):74–81.

53. van der Hulst RWM, Keller JJ, Rauws EAJ, Tytgat GNJ. Treatment of *Helicobacter pylori* infection: a review of the world literature. Helicobacter 1996;1:6–19.

54. van der Hulst RWM, Koycu B, Keller JJ, Feller M, Rauws EAJ, Dankert J, Tytgat GNJ. *H. pylori* reinfection after successful eradication analyzed by RAPD or RFLP. Gastroenterology 1996;110:A284.

55. Vasquez A, Valdez Y, Gilman RH, McDonald JJ, Westblom TU, Berg D, Mayta H, Gutierrez V, and the Gastrointestinal Physiology Working Group of Universidad Peruana Cayetano Heredia and the Johns Hopkins University. Metronidazole and clarithromycin resistance in *Helicobacter pylori* determined by measuring MICs of antimicrobial agents in color indicator egg yolk in a miniwell format. J Clin Microbiol 1996;34:1232–1234.

56. Veldhuyzen van Zanten SJO, Cleary C, Talley NJ, Peterson TC, Nyren O, Bradley LA, Verlinden M, Tytgat GNJ. Drug treatment of functional dyspepsia: a systematic analysis of trial methodology with recommendations for design of future trials. Am J Gastroenterol 1996;91:660–673.

57. Versalovic J, J, Shortridge D, Kibler K, Griffey MV, Beyer J, Flamm RK, Tanaka SK, Graham DY, Go MF. Mutations in 23S ribosomal RNA are associated with clarithromycin resistance in

Helicobacter pylori. Antimicrob Agents Chemother 1996;40: 477–480.

58. Woo JS, El-Zimaity HMT, Genta RM, Yousfi MM, Graham DY. The best gastric site for obtaining a positive rapid urease test. Helicobacter 1996;1:256–259.

59. Xia HX, Keane CT, O'Morain CA. A 5-year survey of metron-

idazole and clarithromycin resistance in clinical isolates of *Helicobacter pylori.* Gut 1996;39(Suppl 2):A6.

60. Yousfi MM, El-Zimaity HM, Cole RA, Genta RM, Graham DY. Detection of *Helicobacter pylori* by rapid urease tests: is biopsy size a critical variable? Gastrointest Endosc 1996;96: 222–224.

Kingella Species

Michael L. Towns

GENERAL DESCRIPTION

Kingella spp. are small, fastidious, capnophilic, facultatively anaerobic, Gram-negative coccobacilli that normally colonize the mucosal surfaces of the upper respiratory tract in man (16). *Kingella* are members of the *Neisseriaceae* family and currently consist of two species: *K. kingae* and *K. denitrificans. Kingella indologenes* has been reclassified as *Suttonella indologenes.* Although *K. kingae* has been reported to cause most *Kingella* infections in man, the other species have also been reported to cause disease. It has been suggested that most infectious disease syndromes associated with these organisms result from a transient bacteremia originating from the oropharynx with subsequent metastatic seeding of endocardium, bones, and joints most commonly, with less likely involvement elsewhere (12).

Effective medical management of patients who have or may have infections with these organisms requires knowledge of the typical antimicrobial susceptibility profile as well as clinical data based on effective antimicrobial regimens for treating the various infectious disease syndromes associated with these organisms. The following discussion represents a sound basis for medical management of patients with infections due to *Kingella* spp.

SUSCEPTIBILITY IN VITRO AND IN VIVO

Table 1 depicts susceptibility data for a number of antimicrobial agents that might be used empirically or definitively to treat a patient with an infection caused by *Kingella* spp. The data were taken from two publications in which standard agar-dilution testing was performed. Most data in the literature, however, have been obtained from disk-diffusion susceptibility testing, which not only is not standardized for these organisms but also is likely to produce false-susceptible results for these slow-growing, fastidious organisms. With this caveat, a few other antibiotic profiles and comments are as follows:

1. Although these results show uniform susceptibility to ampicillin and penicillin, there are rare reports of β-lactamase activity (14), and therefore it would be prudent to test

a clinically significant strain for β-lactamase activity. If the strain was shown to be β-lactamase positive, then a β-lactam/ β-lactamase inhibitor combination could be used, although there has been a rare report of a methicillin-resistant strain (4).

2. *K. kingae* isolates are susceptible to tetracyclines; however, high-level tetracycline resistance has been detected in 16% of *K. denitrificans* isolates (8).

3. Most isolates are resistant to clindamycin (similar to *Eikenella corrodens*) (1).

4. Most strains are susceptible (90%+) to trimethoprim/sulfamethoxazole (1).

ANTIMICROBIAL THERAPY
General

Penicillin (or ampicillin) in conjunction with an aminoglycoside is currently considered the drug of choice for treatment of documented *Kingella* infections (2, 3). Monotherapy with ampicillin or penicillin, however, has been used with clinical success and there is no clear evidence to suggest that combination therapy affords any enhanced clinical efficacy. Since there have been rare reports of β-lactamase activity in both *K. kingae* and *K. denitrificans* (11), combination therapy with a β-lactam and β-lactamase inhibitor would be expected to be clinically useful in this situation. β-Lactamase activity has not been reported in any *S. indologenes* isolates thus far.

Specific Infections
Infective Endocarditis

Kingella spp. are considered members of the HACEK group of organisms (*Haemophilus* spp., *Actinobacillus actinomycetemcomitans, Cardiobacterium hominis, E. corrodens,* and *Kingella* spp.), which may cause infective endocarditis of either native or prosthetic valves in intravenous drug abusers or those with poor dentition or following dental procedures (13). Antimicrobial therapy for this infection has usually involved using a β-lactam such as ampicillin or penicillin, with or without an aminoglycoside, for 4 weeks in the case of native valvular disease or 6 weeks with prosthetic valve endocarditis. Since

TABLE 1 • In Vitro Activity of 11 Antimicrobial Agents against *K. kingae*

Antibiotic	MIC$_{50}$ (μg/mL)	MIC$_{90}$ (μg/mL)	MIC Range (μg/mL)
Ampicillin	0.004	0.008	0.004–0.06
Penicillin G	0.008	0.015	0.004
Cephalothin	0.25	0.25	0.125–0.25
Cefuroxime	0.008	0.03	0.008–0.06
Ceftriaxone[a]	≤0.008	0.06	≤0.008–0.06
Ceftriaxone[b]	0.015	0.015	0.008–0.015
Chloramphenicol	0.5	1.0	0.25–2.0
Ciprofloxacin[a]	0.06	1.0	0.03–4.0
Ciprofloxacin[b]	0.004	0.004	≤0.002–0.008
Gentamicin[a]	2.0	4.0	0.5–8.0
Gentamicin[b]	0.06	0.5	0.03–0.5
Erythromycin	0.125	0.5	0.06–1.0
Imipenem	0.03	0.03	≤0.008–0.03
Meropenem	≤0.008	0.015	≤0.008–0.12

[a]Data from Clark RB, Joyce SE. Activity of meropenem and other antimicrobial agents against uncommon Gram-negative organisms. J Antimicrob Chemother 1993;32:233–237.

[b]Data from Jensen KT, Schonheyder H, Thomsen VF. In-vitro activity of β-lactam and other antimicrobial agents against *Kingella kingae*. J Antimicrob Chemother 1994;33:635–640.

fewer than 30 cases have been reported in the literature, it is difficult to make any firm recommendations on therapy, but some generalizations can be made.

Since infective endocarditis with *Kingella* spp. progresses rapidly despite its susceptibility to antimicrobial agents and since there have been rare reports of β-lactamase-producing strains, it is prudent to treat a patient with known *Kingella* endocarditis with a β-lactamase-resistant antibiotic and an aminoglycoside until results of antimicrobial susceptiblity testing are known. If the strain is shown to be susceptible to penicillin and is β-lactamase negative, then penicillin in high doses (18–24 million units/day) or ampicillin (12 g/day) can be given, with or without an aminoglycoside, for 4 to 6 weeks. In practice, this regimen has been used more than any other. Alternately, since these organisms have been shown to be exquisitely susceptible to the third-generation cephalosporins, ceftriaxone, with or without an aminoglycoside, can also be used for a similar duration. Indeed, the Committee on Rheumatic Fever, Endocarditis, and Kawasaki Disease has recommended ceftriaxone (2 g daily i.v. or i.m) for 4 weeks in cases of native valve endocarditis and

for 6 weeks in cases of prosthetic valve endocarditis due to this organism and other HACEK organisms, although only limited clinical data support this recommendation (6, 15). This regimen, however, does have the advantage of being appropriate for patients with a history of mild penicillin allergy, as well as for patients for whom outpatient treatment is being considered. The few reported patients with prosthetic valve endocarditis due to these organisms were cured with medical treatment alone, without requiring valve replacement (10).

Osteoarticular Infections

Osteoarticular infections are the most common infectious disease syndromes associated with *Kingella* (7). These infections, which more commonly affect infants and young children, include septic arthritis, osteomyelitis, and discitis. Of the three, septic arthritis is the most common. These infections are thought to arise from a transient bacteremia during an upper respiratory infection, as trauma or other predisposing factors for these infectious diseases have not been identified. These infections are discussed together because medical management is similar, although the length of therapy differs.

Successful medical management of these infections requires isolation of the causative organism from the site of infection and accurate antimicrobial susceptibility testing. The principal pathogen causing these infectious diseases in children and adults is *Staphylococcus aureus*, which most likely would be treated with a β-lactamase-stable β-lactam or with vancomycin if methicillin resistant. There have been reports of *Kingella* isolates that are oxacillin and vancomycin resistant, and these would not be treated effectively with either of these antimicrobial regimens if empirical therapy were used for *S. aureus*.

Septic arthritis has been treated with standard doses of an intravenous β-lactam such as ampicillin, penicillin, cefuroxime, or cefotaxime until there is clinical improvement, typically in 5 days to 2 weeks, and only occasionally more, followed by an additional 2 to 4 weeks of an oral antibiotic such as amoxicillin, penicillin VK, or dicloxicillin at maximum doses (Table 2).

Osteomyelitis or discitis, however, usually requires longer treatment courses with similar antibiotics at standard dosages for 2 to 4 weeks of intravenous therapy, followed by an additional 1 to 6 months of oral β-lactam antimicrobial therapy (Table 2). The optimum drug(s) and duration of therapy for these infections currently remain unknown.

TABLE 2 • Antimicrobial Dosages for Adults and Children in Osteoarticular Infections

Antibiotic	Adult	Children
Ampicillin	1.0 g i.v. q. 6 h	25 mg/kg i.v. q. 6 h
Penicillin G	12–18 M units/day i.v. divided q. 4–6 h	200,000 units/kg/day i.v. divided q. 6 h
Cefuroxime	1.5 g i.v. q. 8 h	150 mg/kg/day i.v. divided q. 8 h
Cefotaxime	2.0 g i.v. q. 6 h	150 mg/kg/day i.v. divided q. 8 h
Amoxicillin	500 mg p.o. q. 8 h	40 mg/kg/day p.o. divided q. 6 h
Penicillin VK	500 mg p.o. q. 6 h	50 mg/kg/day p.o. divided q. 6 h
Dicloxacillin	500 mg p.o. q. 6 h	50 mg/kg/day

Alternative Therapy

Although ampicillin and penicillin are the drugs of choice for susceptible *Kingella* isolates, the cephalosporins are acceptable alternatives, especially in patients with a history of type II penicillin allergy. There are no clinical data (even anecdotal) on which alternative antibiotics might be useful clinically in children with a history of a potentially severe type I penicillin or other β-lactam allergy. Based on susceptibility data, aztreonam or trimethoprim/sulfamethoxazole might be effective if the isolate is susceptible. In adults, ciprofloxacin and probably the other quinolones as well as aztreonam or trimethoprim/sulfamethoxazole would likely be effective if the organism was shown to be susceptible, although again, there are no clinical data on which to base a recommendation.

ENDPOINTS FOR MONITORING THERAPY

In most instances, clinical response to therapy is used to judge when therapy has been successfully completed in patients with infections due to *Kingella*. In one case, a serum bactericidal titer (Schlicter test) was used in a child to determine whether the oral antibiotic regimen prescribed had resulted in a high enough bactericidal titer to be effective (7). There simply have not been enough cases to determine whether this test should be routinely recommended in these instances. Finally, in a few cases, the fall in the erythrocyte sedimentation rate (ESR), or C-reactive protein, was used to determine the response to the initial intravenous therapy, prior to switching the patient to an oral antibiotic regimen. Again, there are not adequate data to make this a universal recommendation, and indeed, many cases of osteoarticular infections with these organisms are not associated with a high ESR or CRP at the beginning of therapy.

CAVEATS

Infectious disease syndromes caused by *Kingella* spp. are relatively uncommon and thus there are limited clinical data to make firm therapeutic recommendations for all possible circumstances in which these organisms may be involved. In addition, there are no recent papers describing treatment of these infections with newer antimicrobial agents. Once-daily third-generation cephalosporins, such as ceftriaxone, might be the best choice of parenteral therapy for not only infective endocarditis but also osteoarticular infections, especially for outpatient therapy. Unfortunately, the clinical data are inadequate to support a recommendation at this time. Fortunately, these infections, with the exception of infective endocarditis, are usually indolent and appear to respond favorably to a variety of antimicrobial agents.

REFERENCES

1. Amir J, Shockelford PG. *Kingella kingae* intervertebral disk infection. J Clin Microbiol 1991;29:1083–1086.
2. Bartlett JG. Tables of antimicrobial agents. In: Gorbach SL, Bartlett JG, Blacklow N, eds. Infectious diseases. Philadelphia: WB Saunders, 1992.
3. Bartlett JG. Pocket book of infectious disease therapy. Baltimore: Williams & Wilkins, 1996.
4. Clark RB, Joyce SE. Activity of meropenem and other antimicrobial agents against uncommon Gram-negative organisms. J Antimicrob Chemother 1993;32:233–237.
5. Clement JL, Berard J, Cahuzac JP, Gaubert J. *Kingella kingae* osteoarthritis and osteomyelitis in children. J Pediatr Orthop 1988;8:59–61.
6. Francioli P, Etienne J, Hoigne R, Thys JP, Gerber A. Treatment of streptococcal endocarditis with a single daily dose of ceftriaxone sodium for four weeks. JAMA 1992;267:264–267.
7. de Groot RD, Glover D, Clausen C, Smith AL, Wilson CB. Bone and joint infections caused by *Kingella kingae:* six cases and review of the literature. Rev Infect Dis 1988;10:998–1004.
8. Jensen KT, Schonheyder H, Thomsen VF. In-vitro activity of β-lactam and other antimicrobial agents against *Kingella kingae.* J Antimicrob Chemother 1994;33:635–640.
9. Knapp JS, Johnson SR, Zenilman JM, Roberts MC, Morse SA. High-level tetracycline resistance resulting from TetM in strains of *Neisseria* spp., *Kingella denitrificans,* and *Eikenella corrodens.* Antimicrob Agents Chemother 1988;32:765–767.
10. Meyer DJ, Gerding DN. Favorable prognosis of patients with prosthetic valve endocarditis caused by gram-negative bacilli of the HACEK group. Am J Med 1988;85:104–107.
11. Minamoto GY, Sordillo EM. *Kingella denitrificans* as a cause of granulomatous disease in a patient with AIDS [Letter]. Clin Infect Dis 1992;15:1052–1053.
12. Morrison VA, Wagner KF. Clinical manifestations of *Kingella kingae* infections: case report and review. Rev Infect Dis 1989;11:776–782.
13. Scheld WM, Sande MA. Endocarditis and intravascular infections. In: Mandell GL, Bennett, JE, Dolin R, eds. Principles and practice of infectious diseases. 4th ed. New York: Churchill Livingstone, 1995.
14. Sordillo EM, Rendel M, Sood R, Belinfanti J, Murray O, Brook D. Septicemia due to β-lactamase-positive *Kingella kingae.* Clin Infect Dis 1993;17:818–819.
15. Wilson WR, Karchmer AW, Dajani AS, Taubert KA, Bayer A, Dyae D, Bisno AL, Ferrieri P, Shulman ST, Durack DT. Antibiotic treatment of adults with infective endocarditis due to streptococci, enterococci, staphylococci, and HACEK microorganisms. JAMA 1995;274:1706–1713.
16. Yagupsky P, Dagan R, Prajgrod F, Merires M. Respiratory carriage of *Kingella kingae* among healthy children. Pediatr Infect Dis J 1995;14:673–678.

Klebsiella Species

David L. Paterson and Gordon M. Trenholme

GENERAL DESCRIPTION

The genus *Klebsiella* consists of nonmotile, aerobic and facultatively anaerobic, Gram-negative rods. Six species have been associated with human disease (91). *K. pneumoniae* and *K. oxytoca* are the two most commonly isolated from clinical specimens. *K. ornithinolytica, K. planticola, K. ozaenae,* and *K. rhinoscleromatis* are rarely isolated. *K. pneumoniae* is similar to *K. oxytoca* biochemically, although *K. oxytoca* is indole positive. Both produce capsules that appear macroscopically as mucoid colonies when grown on media rich in carbohydrates.

Community-acquired infections due to *K. pneumoniae* include urinary tract infections (cystitis, pyelonephritis, prostatitis), hepatobiliary infections (cholangitis, liver abscess), and pneumonia. Community-acquired pneumonia due to *K. pneumoniae* classically occurs as a fulminant lobar disease in alcoholic men (119), although this syndrome is now very rare in Western countries (150). Meningitis, endophthalmitis, and endocarditis are less common infections produced by this organism.

K. oxytoca can produce community-acquired infections similar to those produced by *K. pneumoniae* but is substantially less common. *K. rhinoscleromatis* produces rhinoscleroma, a rare granulomatous infiltration of the mucosa of the nose and upper respiratory system (6). Recent cases have been reported in patients with human immunodeficiency virus (HIV) infection and in immigrants from parts of the world where the disease is endemic (197, 251). *K. ozaenae* may be related to a form of chronic atrophic rhinitis called ozena. *K. ozaenae* is also considered to be an opportunistic pathogen in immunocompromised hosts (67, 149, 244). *K. ornithinolytica* and *K. planticola* are rare causes of disease (175).

K. pneumoniae and *K. oxytoca* are also regarded as important causes of nosocomial infections. Between 40 and 60% of episodes of *Klebsiella* bacteremia are nosocomial (149, 110, 196, 269), and *Klebsiella* bacteremia accounts for at least 4% of all nosocomial bacteremias (220). Nosocomial bloodstream infections due to *Klebsiella* species may be secondary to infection of the urinary tract, intravascular catheters, surgical wounds, or respiratory tract (196). Nosocomial urinary tract infections appear to be increasing in frequency (37). One recent study showed that *Klebsiella* species were the most commonly isolated organism in nosocomial urinary tract infections, accounting for 25% of all infections (55). *K. pneumoniae* is also a common cause of nosocomial pneumonia occurring more than 3 days after admission (271). Mechanical ventilation and immunosuppression are major risk factors (150, 271).

Acquisition of plasmid-mediated extended-spectrum β-lactamase (ESBL) producing *K. pneumoniae* has become a major problem in many hospitals. Numerous molecular epidemiologic studies have shown a single clone or a single gene to be responsible for outbreaks (29, 84, 105, 192, 222). The bowel is the major site of colonization, with infection of the urinary tract, respiratory tract, and wounds being widely reported. Bacteremia has occurred, with substantial mortality (173, 196). Risk factors for the presence of ESBL-producing *K. pneumoniae* include prior use of oxyimino β-lactams; presence of an indwelling urinary catheter, feeding tube, or central venous catheter; poor health status; intensive care unit admission; and nursing home residence. Infection with ESBL-producing *K. pneumoniae* has important implications, because of resistance to multiple antibiotics and potential transfer of plasmids to other organisms, such as *Escherichia coli* and *Citrobacter freundii* (42).

SUSCEPTIBILITY IN VITRO AND IN VIVO
In Vitro Studies

K. pneumoniae

An overview of the susceptibility of *K. pneumoniae* to antimicrobial agents is given in Table 1. *K. pneumoniae* is intrinsically resistant to penicillin, ampicillin, amoxicillin, oxacillin, carbenicillin, and ticarcillin, with mean minimum inhibitory levels ranging from 200 to more than 1000 mg/L (54). Mechanisms of resistance include intrinsic chromosomal production of β-lactamase and acquisition of plasmids containing the genetic material to produce SHV and TEM β-lactamases (219, 242). β-lactamase inhibitors such as clavulanic acid (186), sulbactam (90), and tazobactam (10, 92, 152) are active against the SHV-1 and TEM-1 β-lactamases of *K. pneumoniae*. Recently two clinical isolates were described that were resistant to amoxicillin-clavulanate because of a change in the amino acid sequences of a TEM enzyme (156, 187).

Although almost all isolates of *K. pneumoniae* were initially considered susceptible to cephalosporins, recent studies have shown variable susceptibility to this antibiotic class. Several large surveys published in the 1990s detail susceptibility of *K. pneumoniae* to third-generation cephalosporins. In Europe, susceptibility to third-generation cephalosporins has ranged from 100% in Finland (12) to 84.3% in London (163) and 86.7% in France (234). In North America, susceptibility to third-generation cephalosporins has ranged from 99.8% in Canada (249) to 97.4% in the United States (43). In Australia, 96% of 5514 isolates were susceptible to ceftazidime (24). In some areas, resistance to third-generation cephalosporins has risen dramatically in recent years. One hospital in the United States had an increase in ceftazidime resistance from 1% in 1987–1989 to 40% in 1990–1991 (43). The marked increase

TABLE 1 • **Susceptibility of *K. pneumoniae* to Antimicrobial Agents**

Antibiotic	MIC$_{50}$ (mg/L)	MIC$_{90}$ (mg/L)	Range (mg/L)
Penicillins			
Ticarcillin	256	>512	NS[a]
Piperacillin	4	>256	0.5->512
Penicillins plus β-lactamase inhibitors			
Amoxicillin-clavulanate	1	2	0.25–8
Ticarcillin-clavulanate	2	32	1–256
Ampicillin-sulbactam	4	16	2->16
Piperacillin-tazobactam	4	16	1–512
First-generation cephalosporins			
Cefazolin	2	4	1–128
Cephalexin	16	32	8–64
Cefadroxil	8	16	4–32
Cephradine	8	64	4–128
Second-generation cephalosporins			
Cefamandole	2	2	2->32
Cefprozil	1	8	0.5–128
Cefaclor	1	4	0.5–64
Loracarbef	0.5	1	0.12–32
Cefuroxime	2	16	1–32
Cefoxitin	2	8	1–16
Cefotetan	0.25	0.5	0.12->32
Cefmetazole	1	2	0.5–16
Third-generation cephalosporins			
Cefotaxime	0.12	0.25	0.016->128
Ceftriaxone	0.12	0.25	0.016->128
Cefixime	0.03	0.25	0.016–0.5
Cefpodoxime	0.12	0.5	0.12–32
Ceftazidime	0.12	0.25	0.03->128
Cefepime	0.12	0.25	0.03->128
Cefpirome	0.06	1	0.06–1
Other β-lactams			
Imipenem	0.06	0.5	0.06–8
Meropenem	0.06	0.06	0.06–8
Aztreonam	0.5	0.5	0.5->32
Aminoglycosides			
Gentamicin	0.25	2	0.06->128
Tobramycin	0.25	2	0.06->128
Amikacin	0.25	2	0.06–32
Netilmicin	0.12	0.12	0.12–2
Streptomycin	0.5	15.6	0.12–0.500
Quinolones			
Ciprofloxacin	0.06	0.25	0.016–16
Clinafloxacin	0.015	0.03	0.008–0.03
Enoxacin	0.12	0.25	0.06–2
Levofloxacin	0.03	0.06	0.016–0.06
Norfloxacin	0.12	0.25	0.06–0.5
Ofloxacin	0.12	0.12	0.03->32
Sparfloxacin	0.12	0.12	0.016–1
Other antibiotics			
Azithromycin	8	16	NS
Erythromycin	64	>64	NS
Rifampin	32	NS	NS
Chloramphenicol	4	8	0.12–500
Trimethoprim (TMP)	0.5	8	0.005->25
Sulfamethoxazole (SMX)	16	NS	NS
TMP/SMX	0.01/0.25	1.56/3.12	<0.01/0.25–25/500
Nalidixic acid	8	16	4–64
Fusidic acid	32	NS	NS
Mupirocin	64	128	NS
Tetracycline	0.12	2	0.12–500
Quinupristin-dalfopristin	>32	>32	NS

Collated from references 21, 28, 30, 45, 56, 64, 68, 118, 125, 132, 139, 171, 174, 182, 185, 207, 208, 223, 228, 255, 264, 272, 273, 274, 277.

[a]NS, not specified.

in resistance of *K. pneumoniae* to cephalosporins is attributed to the spread of plasmid-mediated ESBLs.

Plasmid-mediated ESBLs were first described in Germany in 1983 (148). They were subsequently described in France (42, 233), and by the late 1980s, numerous outbreaks had occurred in the United States (173, 184, 205, 211), Great Britain (131, 229), Australia (84, 179), and many other parts of the world (71, 127, 202, 216).

ESBLs are plasmid-mediated enzymes that confer resistance to third-generation cephalosporins such as cefotaxime, ceftriaxone, and ceftazidime, as well as the monobactam aztreonam (202). The cephamycins (cefoxitin, cefotetan, and cefmetazole) and the carbapenems (imipenem and meropenem) are not hydrolyzed by most ESBLs (202).

The molecular basis of ESBLs is mutation within the common plasmid-mediated SHV-1, TEM-1, and TEM-2 β-lactamases (128). The amino acid configuration around the active site of these enzymes is altered, thus expanding their spectrum of activity. A change in only one amino acid in the structure of a TEM β-lactamase may dramatically alter susceptibility to cephalosporins. At least 40 such modifications of the TEM and SHV β-lactamases have been described in *K. pneumoniae* (44). An up-to-date listing of TEM and SHV β-lactamases is maintained on the Internet by George Jacoby and Karen Bush and is linked to http://www.asmusa.org.

Some plasmid-mediated ESBLs produced by *K. pneumoniae* have been described that are unrelated to TEM or SHV. Three such β-lactamases are responsible for resistance to cephamycins (20, 22, 195). (Cephamycin resistance can also occur because of the loss of outer-membrane porins mediating permeability to cefoxitin (193).) There are two reports of plasmid-mediated β-lactamases with hydrolytic activity closely resembling that of class I chromosomal cephalosporinases (121, 257). The first of these enzymes (designated LAT-1) was resistant to third-generation cephalosporins, aztreonam, and cephamycins, as well as to β-lactam/clavulanate and sulbactam combinations (257). The second β-lactamase (designated MOX-1) conferred resistance to broad-spectrum β-lactams such as moxalactam, flomoxef, ceftizoxime, cefotaxime, and ceftazidime. Clavulanate was able to competitively inhibit the enzyme's activity (121).

An ESBL produced by *K. pneumoniae* has been recently described that is resistant to the actions of the β-lactamase inhibitor tazobactam (209). Hyperproduction of SHV-5 β-lactamase, leading to resistance to β-lactam/β-lactamase inhibitor combinations (amoxicillin–clavulanic acid, ampicillin-sulbactam, piperacillin-tazobactam, ceftazidime–clavulanic acid) has been reported (99). A β-lactamase inhibitor–resistant *K. pneumoniae* isolate that retained susceptibility in vitro to cephalosporins has also recently been isolated (26).

The plasmids containing ESBLs frequently carry aminoglycoside-modifying enzymes (95). One study of 120 ESBL-producing *K. pneumoniae* showed the percentages of strains resistant to various aminoglycosides to be as follows: 100% dibekacin, 89% sisomicin, 84% gentamicin, 84% tobramycin, 78% netilmicin, 65% streptomycin, 65% kanamycin, 57% spectinomycin, 48% neomycin, and 19% amikacin (95). The aminoglycoside-modifying enzymes most frequently associated with TEM and SHV type ESBLs were AAC(3)V, APH(3″), and APH(3′)I (95).

Susceptibility of ESBL-producing *K. pneumoniae* to antimicrobial agents is given in Table 2. The carbapenems (meropenem and imipenem) are the most active agents in vitro. Virtually all tested strains have been susceptible to these agents. Quinolones, cephamycins, "fourth-generation" cephalosporins (e.g., cefepime), piperacillin-tazobactam, and some aminoglycosides also have useful in vitro activity against ESBL-producing *K. pneumoniae*. However, in recently described outbreaks, approximately 40% of isolates were resistant to ciprofloxacin, cefepime, and piperacillin-tazobactam (51, 210, 222). Unlike resistance to other antibiotics, quinolone resistance is not plasmid mediated (35).

K. oxytoca

K. oxytoca has antibiotic resistance profiles similar to those of *K. pneumoniae*. Like *K. pneumoniae*, *K. oxytoca* can contain plasmid-mediated ESBLs (127). In addition, *K. oxytoca* can contain ESBLs encoded by a chromosomal gene (7, 98, 126). One such enzyme confers low-level resistance to third-generation cephalosporins such as cefotaxime but higher-level resistance to aztreonam. The enzyme has 40% amino acid homology with TEM-type β-lactamases and is inhibited by clavulanate (7).

K. rhinoscleromatis

In vitro studies have been performed on 23 clinical isolates of *K. rhinoscleromatis* submitted to the Centers for Disease Control and Prevention between 1956 and 1987 (201). All isolates were inhibited by and killed by amoxicillin-clavulanate, ciprofloxacin, cefuroxime, and cefpodoxime in clinically achievable concentrations (201). Ciprofloxacin had the greatest in vitro activity of any of the above. Forty-five percent of isolates were susceptible to ampicillin. β-Lactamase production is suggested by the disparity between the ampicillin and amoxicillin-clavulanate results. All 23 isolates were susceptible to trimethoprim-sulfamethoxazole, but the combination was bactericidal for only 65% of isolates. Tetracycline at 4 mg/L or less inhibited 87% of isolates and was bactericidal at this concentration for 52%. Streptomycin at 1 mg/L or less inhibited and killed 21 of 23 isolates; 2 isolates were resistant to streptomycin at 32 mg/L. Only 27% of isolates were inhibited and killed by rifampin at concentrations of 1 mg/L or less, although all isolates were killed by 4 mg/L or less. Cephalexin at 4 mg/L or less inhibited all isolates and killed all but one. Chloramphenicol inhibited all isolates but was not bactericidal.

K. ozaenae

Limited in vitro data exist on antibiotic susceptibility of *K. ozaenae*. Goldstein (104) performed antibiotic susceptibility testing by the agar dilution method on 21 isolates. Some 95% of the 21 isolates were susceptible to cephalothin; 90% of 20 isolates were susceptible to gentamicin; 90% of 9 isolates were susceptible to amikacin; and 88% of 8 isolates were susceptible to kanamycin. Only 26% of 19 isolates were susceptible to

TABLE 2 • Susceptibility of ESBL-Producing *K. pneumoniae* to Antimicrobial Agents

Antibiotic	MIC$_{50}$ (mg/L)	MIC$_{90}$ (mg/L)	Range (mg/L)
Penicillins			
Ticarcillin	16384	32768	NS[a]
Piperacillin	256	512	16–256
Penicillins plus β-lactamase inhibitors			
Amoxicillin-clavulanate	8	16	0.25–16
Ticarcillin-clavulanate	64	64	16–>64
Ampicillin-sulbactam	16	128	8–>128
Piperacillin-tazobactam	4	32	0.5–>128
Cefotaxime-clavulanate	0.5	2	0.25–2
Ceftazidime-clavulanate	0.5	1	0.06–2
Cefotaxime-sulbactam	8	32	0.25–32
First-generation cephalosporins			
Cefazolin	128	512	16–512
Second-generation cephalosporins			
Cefamandole	256	512	16–512
Cefoxitin	8	32	4–64
Cefotetan	0.5	2	0.03–64
Third-generation cephalosporins			
Cefotaxime	32	64	0.03–256
Ceftriaxone	32	64	4–64
Ceftazidime	256	512	0.25–512
Cefepime	8	256	0.25–256
Cefpirome	16	64	0.25–128
Other β-lactams			
Imipenem	0.12	0.5	0.03–2
Meropenem	0.06	0.5	0.03–1
Aztreonam	32	128	0.25–512
Aminoglycosides			
Gentamicin	8	>16	0.5–>16
Amikacin	4	16	NS
Quinolones			
Ciprofloxacin	0.25	16	0.03–>8
Ofloxacin	1	16	0.06–16
Others			
Trimethoprim (TMP)	>4	>4	1–>4
Sulfamethoxazole (SMX)	76	76	38–76

Collated from references 25, 52, 56, 130, 200.

[a]NS, not specified.

ampicillin, and 21% of 14 isolates susceptible to tetracycline. All of three isolates were susceptible to chloramphenicol, and one of two isolates was susceptible to tobramycin. Murray et al. (180) examined 16 strains of *K. ozaenae*. All were susceptible to cephalothin, chloramphenicol, tetracycline, gentamicin, streptomycin, kanamycin, and amikacin. Less than 20% were susceptible to ampicillin and carbenicillin. The one isolate of *K. ozaenae* tested by Strampfer et al. (239) was susceptible to cefotaxime, and the isolate tested by Chowdhury and Stein (67), to ciprofloxacin.

Interestingly, the first report of plasmid-mediated resistance to broad-spectrum cephalosporins was an isolate of *K. ozaenae* in Germany, analyzed in 1983 (145, 203). No subsequent isolates of ESBL-producing *K. ozaenae* have been reported.

Combination Drugs

Addition of β-lactamase inhibitors to β-lactams is well known to result in enhanced activity of the β-lactams against β-lactamase-producing strains of *K. pneumoniae*. Several groups have found that the combination of piperacillin with tazobactam has greater activity than ticarcillin and clavulanate against piperacillin-resistant *K. pneumoniae* (152, 248, 261).

Synergy has been frequently found in vitro between β-lactams and aminoglycosides against *K. pneumoniae* (Table 3). There are three studies in which no synergy was demonstrated between β-lactams and aminoglycosides—ceftazidime and netilmicin (153), ceftazidime and amikacin (263), and cefepime and gentamicin (122).

Synergy has been less frequently observed in vitro between combinations of β-lactams. It has rarely, if ever, been observed between combinations of the commonly used third-generation cephalosporins, extended-spectrum penicillins, or the carbapenems, imipenem and meropenem. Conversely, only one study described antagonism between β-lactams (278); it occurred in a single strain only.

Four studies investigated interactions between β-lactams

TABLE 3 • Studies in Which Synergy Was Shown by β-Lactams and Aminoglycosides against *K. pneumoniae*

Reference	Number of Isolates Examined	Antibiotic Combination Used	% Isolates in Which Synergistic Effect Achieved
Penicillins			
11	18	Piperacillin + netilmicin	89%
278	39	Azlocillin + amikacin	51%
141	4[a]	Carbenicillin + gentamicin	100%
141	4[a]	Carbenicillin + tobramycin	100%
142	86	Carbenicillin + gentamicin	21%
81	53	Mezlocillin + tobramycin	51%
81	53	Piperacillin + tobramycin	53%
Cephalosporins			
278	39	Cefotaxime + amikacin	77%
141	4[a]	Cephalothin + gentamicin	100%
141	4[a]	Cephalothin + tobramycin	75%
100	16	Cefamandole + amikacin	46%
100	16	Cefamandole + gentamicin	46%
142	20	Cefazolin + amikacin	65%[b], 80%[c]
170	27	Cephalothin + gentamicin	70%
142	20	Cefazolin + amikacin	55%[b], 80%[c]
Other β-lactams			
96	6	Imipenem + gentamicin	17%
96	6	Imipenem + amikacin	17%
96	6	Meropenem + gentamicin	33%
96	6	Meropenem + amikacin	33%

[a]Carbenicillin- or cephalothin-resistant strains only examined.

[b]Synergy assessed by checkerboard.

[c]Synergy assessed by kill curves.

and quinolones against *K. pneumoniae* (63, 96, 109, 124). No synergy was demonstrated between ciprofloxacin and ceftibuten, ciprofloxacin and meropenem, or ciprofloxacin and piperacillin (96, 109, 124). One of six strains tested displayed synergy between ciprofloxacin and imipenem, whereas five of the six displayed additive effects only (96). Antagonism was seen in one isolate tested at low ciprofloxacin:piperacillin concentration ratios only (124).

Interaction between quinolones and aminoglycosides against *K. pneumoniae* has been seldom studied. The combination of ciprofloxacin and gentamicin resulted in more rapid killing of some strains of *K. pneumoniae* in one study (270). Neither synergy nor antagonism was observed with the combination of pefloxacin and amikacin (262).

Chloramphenicol has been found antagonistic to gentamicin for most *K. pneumoniae* strains tested (194). One study showed an increase in the MIC of aminoglycosides when clindamycin was used in combination against *K. pneumoniae* isolates (15). Erythromycin shows neither synergy nor antagonism when combined with gentamicin, cefamandole, or ampicillin against the vast majority of strains of *K. pneumoniae* (70).

A novel combination is the addition of salicylate to cultures of *K. pneumoniae* (79, 80). The synergistic activity of imipenem and amikacin was significantly increased by salicylate (79). The MICs of aminoglycosides for *K. pneumoniae* were lowered 2- to 4-fold in the presence of salicylate, possibly by facilitation of aminoglycoside transport through the cytoplasmic membrane (80); addition of salicylate increased the MIC for most other antibiotics (79).

Studies on the in vitro use of combination drugs against ESBL-producing strains of *K. pneumoniae* are limited. Guerillot et al. (109) found no synergy between ceftibuten and netilmicin. Roussel-Delvallez et al. (215) found that while cefotaxime and sulbactam had no bactericidal effect in combination against ESBL-producing strains of *K. pneumoniae*, the addition of amikacin to this regimen resulted in a bactericidal effect. When used alone, cefepime resulted in a 2-log decrease at 6 h, but at 24 h, regrowth had occurred (87). Combination of cefepime with amikacin (4 mg/L) resulted in a 4-log decrease at 6 h; furthermore, there were no surviving bacteria at 6 h when cefepime was combined with amikacin at higher concentration (8 mg/L).

Two studies have suggested that synergy may occur when ciprofloxacin is added to β-lactam antibiotics in vitro against ESBL-producing strains of *K. pneumoniae*. Addition of ciprofloxacin to imipenem and to the combination of cefotaxime and sulbactam has been found synergistic (8). The antimicrobial combinations of ciprofloxacin plus either cefpirome or cefipime resulted in a 4-log decrease in ESBL-producing *K. pneumoniae* (87).

In Vivo Studies (Animal Studies)

Single Drug

Most studies of animal models have involved a single isolate of *K. pneumoniae*, and applicability to humans is limited. In vivo studies have revealed that β-lactam antibiotics to which *K. pneumoniae* is susceptible in vitro are effective in animal models of infection. More-recent cephalosporins (e.g., cefpirome and cefepime) appear to be more effective than earlier cephalosporins (144, 253). Of the β-lactams tested, cefazolin and the extended-spectrum penicillins (e.g., piperacillin) appear less effective (17, 250, 255). The dosing interval of β-lactams has a major impact on efficacy in animal models. When ceftazidime was used in leukopenic rats with experimental *K. pneumoniae* sepsis, continuous infusion of the antibiotic was more effective than dosing at 6 hourly intervals (213).

Addition of β-lactamase inhibitors to β-lactams may provide additional clinical activity against *K. pneumoniae*. In vivo studies have shown that tazobactam and clavulanic acid are superior to sulbactam (152). The efficacies of piperacillin-tazobactam and ticarcillin-clavulanate were nearly the same in a mouse model of infection (97).

Imipenem has consistently shown very strong killing activity against *K. pneumoniae* in vivo (212, 255). Meropenem is as effective as imipenem in systemic infection with *K. pneumoniae* in mice (113). No postantibiotic effect has been seen with imipenem in *K. pneumoniae* infections (108).

Aminoglycosides have been shown to be highly effective against *K. pneumoniae* in experimental septicemia in neutropenic mice (250). Postantibiotic effect was well demonstrated (108, 204).

Animal models have shown that quinolones may be superior to aminoglycosides or cephalosporins against experimental *K. pneumoniae* infections (155, 214, 250). Oral ciprofloxacin was shown to be very effective (38), although a recent study showed that intravenous ciprofloxacin has greater therapeutic efficacy in experimental murine respiratory tract infection (189).

Novel therapies that have met with some success in animal studies include use of gentamicin or ceftazidime entrapped in polymer-coated liposomes (16), combination of antibiotic treatment with the thrombin inhibitor recombinant hirudin (77), use of antithrombin III (78), monoclonal antibody against *Klebsiella* capsular polysaccharide (114, 167), and human hyperimmune intravenous immunoglobulin (74).

A small number of studies have explored which antibiotics are most effective against infection with ESBL-producing isolates of *K. pneumoniae*. Rice et al. (212) showed that cefoperazone, cefotaxime, cefpirome, and ceftazidime were ineffective in a rat intraabdominal abscess model. Addition of a β-lactamase inhibitor resulted in significant improvement. In contrast, in a rabbit endocarditis model, addition of sulbactam at high dose was not sufficient to restore activity of ceftriaxone against an ESBL-producing strain (47). Piperacillin in combination with tazobactam, and ticarcillin in combination with clavulanate, had equal efficacy in a rat model of intraabdominal abscess (246). Overall, treatment outcome against experimental infections with ESBL-producing isolates of *K. pneumoniae* has been best with imipenem (209, 212, 246).

Combination Drugs

A number of studies have shown the combination of β-lactam and aminoglycoside to be more effective in vivo than either drug alone against single isolates. The combination of ceftriaxone and gentamicin was shown to be superior to either drug alone in an animal model of endocarditis (166). The combination of piperacillin/tazobactam/gentamicin was also found more effective in animal models than piperacillin/tazobactam alone (172). Similarly, the combination of amikacin and imipenem resulted in significantly better survival in neutropenic rats with *Klebsiella* sepsis than either drug alone (53).

Fewer data exist on other antibiotic combinations in animal studies. Trautmann et al. (250) showed that ciprofloxacin and ceftazidime in combination were more effective than ciprofloxacin alone. The same did not hold true for ciprofloxacin and gentamicin (250).

ANTIMICROBIAL THERAPY
General Drug of Choice

Klebsiella pneumoniae Bacteremia

The in vitro data presented above shows that a wide range of β-lactams, aminoglycosides, quinolones, and other antibiotics may be potentially useful in the treatment of serious infections with *K. pneumoniae*. No randomized trials of treatment of bacteremia with *K. pneumoniae* have been performed. Eleven studies of large numbers of patients with *K. pneumoniae* that have included details on outcome of antimicrobial therapy have been reported (31, 33, 94, 101, 110, 149, 176, 245, 258, 267, 269). Several found that no antibiotic therapy or inappropriate therapy was associated with very high mortality (31, 110, 245, 258, 267, 269). The data from the observational studies performed are insufficient to determine which aminoglycosides, quinolones, cephalosporins, extended-spectrum penicillins, or carbapenems might be clinically superior.

A number of studies assessed whether combination antibiotic therapy is superior to single-drug therapy (31, 94, 101, 149, 176). Of these studies, two determined that the combination of an aminoglycoside and a cephalosporin or extended-spectrum penicillin resulted in greater clinical benefit than either agent alone (31, 94). The only prospective study found a benefit of combination therapy only in the subgroup of patients who were most severely ill, particularly those who experienced hypotension within 72 h prior to, or on the day of, the first positive blood culture (149).

As initial therapy of patients with suspected bacteremia due to *K. pneumoniae* is empirical, antimicrobial therapy should be selected on the basis of local susceptibility patterns of isolates causing bacteremia. Once *Klebsiella* bacteremia is confirmed, therapy may be modified. In critically ill patients, antimicrobials with high intrinsic activity against *K. pneumoniae* should be chosen. Third-generation cephalosporins, aztreonam, carbapenems, aminoglycosides, or quinolones satisfy this requirement. In addition, some authorities would use combination therapy with a β-lactam agent and an aminoglycoside for all patients with bacteremia. However, aminoglycosides should not be used for combination therapy if the isolate is resistant to the aminoglycoside. If an aminoglycoside is used, consideration should be given to once-daily dosing of the aminoglycoside. The exact duration of therapy of *K. pneumoniae* bacteremia has not been determined, but at least 10 days of therapy is reasonable. As with other Gram-negative organisms producing bacteremia, low mortality is seen in patients with *K. pneumoniae* bacteremia secondary to a urinary tract infection. Although published experience is very limited, monotherapy with trimethoprim-sulfamethoxazole or piperacillin has been associated with higher mortality than other agents (149). Earlier experience with trimethoprim-sulfamethoxazole in the treatment of serious *K. pneumoniae* infections was also less favorable than that with aminoglycosides, for example (107).

Klebsiella pneumoniae Pneumonia

Community-acquired *K. pneumoniae* pneumonia in alcoholics has a mortality exceeding 50%, regardless of treatment (133). Fortunately this disease is quite rare in the United States—nosocomial infection now predominates (48, 149). Effective therapy for severe community-acquired *K. pneumoniae* pneumonia consists of empirical treatment with coverage against Gram-negative organisms, aggressive ventilation, and clinical and radiologic surveillance for surgically treatable entities such as pulmonary gangrene, lung abscess, and empyema (111, 147, 177). Third-generation cephalosporins or quinolones provide coverage against most community-acquired *K. pneumoniae*. Macrolides (including azithromycin) have no useful activity against *K. pneumoniae*. The superiority of combinations of third-generation cephalosporins and aminoglycosides was demonstrated in one study (111) but not in others (133, 135). Clinical outcome when chloramphenicol and aminoglycosides are used in combination has been poor (119).

Antimicrobial therapy for nosocomial pneumonia due to *K. pneumoniae* depends on local susceptibility patterns. As opposed to patients with bacteremia, the susceptibility of pulmonary isolates may be available at initiation of therapy for nosocomial pneumonia. However, patients with nosocomial pneumonia are frequently elderly, debilitated, and hospitalized in intensive care units and may have received prior antibiotics. In these circumstances, antibiotics with high intrinsic activity against *K. pneumoniae* should be chosen. In addition, multiple organisms are frequently isolated from respiratory tract specimens of patients with nosocomial pneumonias. Thus, a regimen that includes imipenem, third-generation cephalosporins, aminoglycosides, or quinolones is favored. Although the superiority of combination therapy is debatable, if combination therapy is used, a combination of a β-lactam and an aminoglycoside to which the isolate is susceptible should be chosen rather than a combination of two β-lactam agents. In treatment of Gram-negative pneumonia with an aminoglycoside, it is very important to avoid subtherapeutic serum levels (178). Thus, maximal doses of the aminoglycoside should be initiated. Endotracheal aminoglycosides have been used in addition to systemic therapy in the treatment of Gram-negative pneumonia (39). Although, pathogens were eradicated from sputum more frequently using this mode of therapy, no significant difference in clinical outcome was seen.

K. pneumoniae pneumonia should be treated for at least 14 days. Computed tomography of the chest may be useful if a patient is slow to respond to exclude entities treated by drainage or debridement (e.g., empyema or abscess) (177). If a patient improves rapidly on intravenous therapy, sequential therapy with an oral quinolone to which the isolate is susceptible was shown to be safe in most circumstances (102, 252).

Klebsiella pneumoniae Urinary Tract Infections

Uncomplicated urinary tract infections (UTIs) with *K. pneumoniae* can be treated with any oral antibiotic commonly used to treat UTIs, except ampicillin. Published series including patients with *K. pneumoniae* describe use of trimethoprim-sulfamethoxazole, trimethoprim alone, ofloxacin, nitrofurantoin, norfloxacin, enoxacin, ciprofloxacin, cephalexin, cefadroxil, and amoxicillin/clavulanic acid in uncomplicated UTI (1, 36, 73, 86, 120, 134). Monotherapy with any of the drugs mentioned is likely to be effective against susceptible urinary tract isolates. One study found trimethoprim-sulfamethoxazole to be more effective and less expensive than nitrofurantoin, cefadroxil, or amoxicillin (120). Therapy for 3 days is sufficient (120, 206).

Complicated UTIs due to *K. pneumoniae* have been successfully treated with an oral quinolone or intravenous aminoglycosides, third-generation cephalosporins, imipenem, aztreonam, or ticarcillin-clavulanate (9, 221, 236). In general, intravenous agents should be used until fever has resolved; oral therapy with a quinolone can then follow for a total duration of 14 to 21 days (236). Correction of an underlying anatomic abnormality or removal of a urinary catheter is also frequently necessary.

Klebsiella pneumoniae Cholangitis/Liver Abscess

After the urinary tract, the biliary tree is the most common portal of entry of *K. pneumoniae* bacteremia. The combination of a β-lactam and an aminoglycoside has been the gold standard of empirical treatment of cholangitis for many years, although few comparative studies are available to determine that this is indeed the optimal treatment (162). Most studies of therapeutic efficacy in this group of patients include multiple different organisms and are not specific for *K. pneumoniae*. Ciprofloxacin as monotherapy has been found as effective as combination therapy with ampicillin, ceftazidime, and metronidazole in the treatment of acute suppurative cholangitis (241). In this study, *E. coli*, *Klebsiella* spp., and *Enterococcus* spp. predominated. This group also found that ciprofloxacin produced higher biliary concentrations than ceftazidime, cefoperazone, imipenem, or netilmicin (158). Biliary decompression is often required as adjunctive treatment of the underlying cause of the cholangitis. Antibiotics should be administered for a minimum of 10 days.

In Asian countries particularly, *K. pneumoniae* bacteremia is frequently associated with hepatic abscess (60, 154, 164, 267). Successful treatment usually consists of appropriate antibiotics plus drainage. The combination of clindamycin or ampicillin/sulbactam with either an aminoglycoside, a third-generation cephalosporin, aztreonam, or a quinolone may be used. Imipenem as monotherapy is another alternative. Taiwanese authors, who have the most experience with this disease, recommend that therapy be given for 2 to 4 weeks for a solitary abscess or as long as 6 weeks for multiple abscesses (58). The precise duration of therapy can be determined by ultrasonographic progress and resolution of fever and leukocytosis.

Klebsiella oxytoca

Antibiotic susceptibilities and treatment guidelines for *K. oxytoca* are virtually identical to those for *K. pneumoniae*. Outcomes are very similar to those with *K. pneumoniae*. The mortality rate at 14 days of *K. oxytoca* bacteremia was 21% (149).

Klebsiella rhinoscleromatis

Treatment of rhinoscleroma consists of a combination of prolonged antimicrobial therapy (at least 6–8 weeks, but sometimes months or years) and surgical debridement to relieve obstruction of the respiratory tract or cosmetic deformity (6). No randomized controlled trials have determined optimal antimicrobial therapy. Nonantibiotic treatments that have been used include mercurials, caustics (e.g., zinc chloride, silver nitrate, and salicylic acid), arsenicals, and methylene blue (6). Streptomycin, the first antibiotic used successfully, suffers from the need for intravenous or intramuscular use, nephrotoxicity, and ototoxicity (6). Combination with tetracycline has allowed lower doses of streptomycin to be used, thus lowering toxicity (2). Failure with this regimen has been reported (251). Use of aminoglycosides other than streptomycin has rarely been mentioned.

Despite reported clinical failure of sulfonamides in the 1940s (201), TMP-SMX has been used successfully (5, 157, 197). Three case reports of quinolone use in the treatment of rhinoscleroma have been published (14, 197, 251). Avery (14) reported a patient who had partially responded to 6 weeks of tetracycline and TMP-SMX but achieved pathologic and bacteriologic resolution during treatment with oral ciprofloxacin (500 mg twice daily for 3 months). Trautmann (251) described a patient who was unsuccessfully treated with streptomycin and tetracycline but responded to a 3-month course of oral ciprofloxacin (750 mg every 12 h). The granuloma was then surgically removed. Paul et al. (197) described a patient with HIV infection who responded well to TMP/SMX given for 25 days but was then changed to ofloxacin (400 mg daily). The ofloxacin was continued for 60 days with clinical cure.

Despite high cost, the quinolone class and ciprofloxacin in particular appear to have a number of advantages over other antibiotics for the treatment of *K. rhinoscleromatis* infections. Ciprofloxacin is the most effective antibiotic in vitro (201), achieves high concentrations in nasal secretions (75), can be orally administered, and can concentrate and kill microorganisms within macrophages (260). From the limited data available, response should be expected after 1 month of therapy, although a total of 2 to 3 months of therapy is reasonable because of the tendency of the condition to relapse (14).

Klebsiella ozaenae

There have been no randomized trials in the treatment of *K. ozaenae* infections. Ozena has been successfully treated with ciprofloxacin (for 1–3 months) and with intravenous aminoglycosides (82, 188). The clinical outcome and treatment of patients with serious infections with *K. ozaenae* are detailed in Table 4. As the data are limited, treatment should be based on antibiotic susceptibility results and consideration of the site of infection.

TABLE 4 • Treatment and Clinical Outcome of Patients with Serious Infections Due to *K. ozaenae*

Reference	Site[a]	Antibiotic[a]	Outcome
180	Blood, CSF	GENT, CARB, AMP	Died
180	Blood	AMP, GENT, DOXY	Survived
67	Blood, Liver	AMP-SUL	Survived
239	Brain	CHLOR, CEFTAZ, AMP	Died
129	Cornea	CARB, TOBRA (top)	Abscess healed
244	CSF	CEFOTAX	Survived
244	CSF	CEFOTAX	Survived

[a]CSF, cerebrospinal fluid; AMP, ampicillin; AMP-SUL, ampicillin-sulbactam; CARB, carbenicillin; CEFOTAX, cefotaxime; CEFTAZ, ceftazidime; CHLOR, chloramphenicol; DOXY, doxycycline; GENT, gentamicin; TOBRA, tobramycin; top, administered topically and by subconjunctival injection.

Special Situations

Klebsiella pneumoniae Meningitis

K. pneumoniae meningitis in adults occurs extremely rarely as a community-acquired infection but more commonly as a nosocomial disease complicating shunts and other devices (243). No randomized controlled treatment trials have been carried out, but it seems probable that in the absence of ESBL production, third-generation cephalosporins are the drugs of choice for *K. pneumoniae* meningitis, because of their superior penetration into the cerebrospinal fluid (CSF) (62) and their excellent activity against the organism. One animal study (27) suggested that ceftriaxone is superior to cefotaxime, but this has not been confirmed in humans. However, there is more published clinical experience with cefotaxime than with ceftriaxone for *K. pneumoniae* meningitis. Cherubin et al. (61) described successful use of cefotaxime in 14 cases of *K. pneumoniae* meningitis. Large doses are traditionally used (cefotaxime, up to 2 g every 4 h; ceftriaxone, 2 g twice daily). No studies have been conducted on duration of treatment, although 3 weeks has been recommended because of significant relapse rates in those treated with shorter courses of therapy (256). Although dexamethasone may be used as an adjunct to antibiotics in treatment of bacterial meningitis, no data exist on its use in *K. pneumoniae* meningitis.

K. pneumoniae is a relatively common cause of neonatal meningitis in developing countries (accounting for 28% of cases in one series) but is less common in developed areas (4, 231). Cefotaxime is the preferred therapy because there is more clinical experience with it than with ceftriaxone (93, 183). Cefotaxime should not be used alone as empirical treatment of neonatal meningitis because it does not cover *Listeria monocytogenes*. However, because of its superior CSF penetration, it is preferred over aminoglycosides in the treatment of neonatal meningitis when bacteriologic diagnosis of *K. pneumoniae* has been confirmed.

If ceftriaxone or cefotaxime cannot be used, meropenem is a reasonable alternative. Meropenem is very active against *K. pneumoniae* (228) and also has excellent CSF penetration (123, 181). In addition, it has a low incidence of neurologic side effects such as seizures when used in the treatment of bacterial meningitis (146, 191, 225). However, only one published instance of its use against *K. pneumoniae* meningitis exists (106).

Ventriculoperitoneal shunt infections due to *K. pneumoniae* and other Gram-negative bacilli have traditionally had high mortality (227). However, a recent study that combined antibiotics and shunt removal described a 100% cure rate in 23 such infections (237). In this study, ceftriaxone sterilized CSF more rapidly than intravenous aminoglycosides.

Trimethoprim-sulfamethoxazole penetrates effectively into the CSF (159) and is generally microbiologically active against *K. pneumoniae*. Recent published experience with this drug is limited, but papers from the early 1980s documented both clinical success (115, 159) and failure (160, 224). There is a small amount of published experience with imipenem in the treatment of *K. pneumoniae* meningitis. In the presence of meningeal inflammation, CSF concentrations of imipenem of 0.8 to 2.6 mg/L have been recorded (13). This is three to ten times higher than the MIC_{90} (0.25 mg/L) (228). However, seizures, the most serious toxic effect seen with imipenem, are more likely in patients with central nervous system disorders (46). There are two case reports of successful use in *K. pneumoniae* meningitis without development of seizure activity (13, 76); in one of these studies, imipenem was given for only 3 days, with cefotaxime and pefloxacin used for a further 18 days (13).

There are numerous instances of relapse of meningitis when chloramphenicol has been used for *K. pneumoniae* meningitis (18, 165, 259). Some have attributed chloramphenicol failure to antibiotic antagonism (40, 41). In vitro, chloramphenicol interfered with the activity of cefotaxime and several other β-lactams (40). One case report of clinical failure in meningitis described use of chloramphenicol plus cefotaxime (41).

There are single case reports of successful treatment of *K. pneumoniae* meningitis with aztreonam (138), cefoperazone (88), ciprofloxacin (217), and pefloxacin (226). However, for a variety of pharmacokinetic reasons, these drugs would only be used in *K. pneumoniae* meningitis if treatment with the superior agents described above was impossible or had failed.

Klebsiella pneumoniae Endophthalmitis

There have been numerous reports of *K. pneumoniae* endophthalmitis, many occurring in patients with diabetes mellitus (168). There is also a strong association between *K. pneumoniae* endophthalmitis and concurrent hepatic abscess (59, 66, 112); more than 50% of patients with *K. pneumoniae* endophthalmitis have hepatic abscess. The prognosis for a good visual recovery after treatment for *K. pneumoniae* endophthalmitis is extremely poor; more than 85% of reported patients had a visual outcome worse than ability to count fingers (49, 59, 60, 65, 66, 83, 103, 116, 117, 161, 168, 169, 232, 238). The few successfully treated patients had a correct diagnosis within 24 h of ocular disease presentation and received aggressive antimicrobial therapy (59, 66). *K. pneumoniae* endophthalmitis may present days after appropriate treatment for *K. pneumoniae* bacteremia and hepatic abscess has been started (59).

Each of the previously reported patients who had successful treatment for *K. pneumoniae* endophthalmitis received

both intravenous and local ocular antimicrobial therapy (59, 66, 164, 232). Local ocular therapy involved intravitreal antibiotics in all but two of the patients treated successfully. Some authors successfully used combination intravitreal therapy with cefazolin (2 mg) and gentamicin (4 mg); others used monotherapy with intravitreal amikacin (0.4–0.5 mg) (66). Ceftazidime (2.25 mg) could also be used (23).

Comparative trials of treatment for endophthalmitis suggesting that intravitreal therapy alone is as effective as combined intravitreal/intravenous therapy have not included patients with *K. pneumoniae* endophthalmitis (89, 198). In view of the generally poor results with this infection, both intravitreal and intravenous antibiotics should be used to treat *K. pneumoniae* endophthalmitis. The penetration of systemically given antibiotics into the eye is variable, however. Third-generation cephalosporins can achieve peak vitreous levels of at least 2 mg/L (32, 230, 266). Aminoglycosides penetrate the vitreous reasonably well after repetitive systemic dosing (19). Oral ciprofloxacin can achieve vitreous concentrations of 0.2 to 0.5 mg/L (85, 137). A single dose of 0.5 g of imipenem resulted in a mean vitreous level of 0.2 mg/L 2 to 4 h after infusion. This increased to approximately 2 mg/L after a 1-g dose (3).

Of the above choices, clinical experience in treating endophthalmitis with intravenous antibiotics has been greatest with ceftazidime or aminoglycosides, particularly amikacin (89).

Klebsiella pneumoniae Endocarditis

K. pneumoniae endocarditis is extremely rare. One study associated *Klebsiella* endocarditis with high mortality (275). Nine cases of *Klebsiella* endocarditis in which antibiotic treatment was detailed are in the medical literature (34, 50, 69, 136, 190, 218, 247, 265, 268). Of these nine patients, four survived and five died. All of those who survived this infection received combination antibiotic therapy with an aminoglycoside and another antibiotic (69, 190, 247, 268). Three of the four who survived also underwent valve replacement surgery. Only one of the five patients who died received valve replacement surgery (34).

Klebsiella endocarditis should be treated with a combination of intravenous aminoglycoside and β-lactam antibiotic, most likely a third-generation cephalosporin. Early consideration of cardiac surgery is essential. There are few data to guide duration of therapy, but 6 weeks seems reasonable (247).

Alternative Therapy

Treatment guidelines for patients who cannot take the first-choice agents because of allergy or renal insufficiency are given in Table 5. Guidelines for treatment of infections with ESBL-producing organisms are given below.

Few formal studies on the treatment of serious infections with ESBL-producing *K. pneumoniae* have been performed. Therapy with third-generation cephalosporins or aminoglycosides to which the organism is resistant is likely to be unsuccessful. In a recent study of bacteremia with organisms producing ESBLs, only 1 of 19 patients who received appropriate therapy died, versus 5 of 12 who received inappropriate therapy (222). In the treatment of bacteremia with ESBL-producing

TABLE 5 • Recommended Treatment for Clinical Diseases Caused by Non-ESBL-Producing _K. pneumoniae._

	First-Line Therapy	Alternative if Previous Anaphylactic Reaction to Cephalosporins or Penicillin
Bacteremia	Cefotaxime	Ciprofloxacin
Pneumonia	Cefotaxime	Ciprofloxacin
Urinary tract infection	Ciprofloxacin	Ciprofloxacin
Meningitis	Ceftriaxone	Trimethoprim-sulfamethoxazole
Endocarditis	Ceftriaxone + gentamicin	Ciprofloxacin + gentamicin
Endophthalmitis	Ceftazidime + intravitreal amikacin	Ciprofloxacin + amikacin
Liver abscess	Ceftriaxone	Ciprofloxacin

K. pneumoniae, carbapenem use (meropenem or imipenem) is associated with lower mortality than use of other antibiotics that are active in vitro against the organism (196). Quinolones or amikacin, while associated with less favorable results than carbapenems, have also been used successfully, particularly in combination with other agents. Concomitant resistance to ciprofloxacin restricts empirical use of this agent when an ESBL-producing organism is suspected. The lack of data in patients treated with a fourth-generation cephalosporin (cefepime or cefpirome) or the combination of a β-lactam plus a β-lactamase inhibitor limits their usage. Failure to treat ESBL-producing _K. pneumoniae_ bacteremia successfully appears higher with such agents than with imipenem (51, 196).

Complicated UTIs may be due to ESBL-producing strains of _K. pneumoniae._ Treatment regimens for such UTIs vary, depending on antibiotic susceptibilities, but third-generation cephalosporins have been surprisingly successful. This is probably related to the high urinary concentration of the antibiotics.

Three cases of nosocomial meningitis due to ESBL-producing _K. pneumoniae_ have been described (76, 106, 235). One patient was successfully treated with a combination of intrathecal catheter removal, high-dose intravenous imipenem (8 g/day), and two intrathecal infusions of amikacin (50 mg) (76). Previous treatment with intravenous ceftazidime, amikacin, and then lower-dose imipenem (2, then 4 g/day) had failed. A patient with postneurosurgery meningitis was unsuccessfully treated with imipenem and ceftazidime. Substitution of these antibiotics with meropenem was successful (106). One unsuccessfully treated patient with meningitis due to ESBL-producing _K. pneumoniae_ failed on intravenous ceftazidime and amikacin (235). Based on in vitro activity and pharmacokinetics, meropenem should be considered the agent of choice until further data are available.

Treatment in children should follow the same guidelines as in adults. Imipenem has been shown to be well tolerated by preterm and severely ill neonates with ESBL-producing _K. pneumoniae_ infection (240). Of the 70 neonates in one study, only 2 (2.5%) had seizures (240), and both infants had underlying cranial abnormalities.

ENDPOINTS FOR MONITORING THERAPY

Generally, the standard clinical endpoints are used to determine the adequacy of therapy for _K. pneumoniae_ infections. After initiation of therapy, a favorable response is signified by res-

olution of systemic and local symptoms and signs of infection. In patients with primary or secondary bacteremia, blood cultures should become negative. For UTIs, urine cultures should become negative. Repeat sputum culture to show clearance of the pathogen is rarely necessary for patients with pneumonia. Chest x-rays frequently take weeks to resolve completely.

In patients with Gram-negative meningitis, a repeat spinal tap after 48 to 72 h may help to document microbiologic clearance. The duration of therapy after an initial favorable clinical response is generally empirical. Pneumonia, bacteremia, and UTIs require at least 10 days of therapy. Meningitis should be treated for 21 days.

If fever recurs during therapy, a superinfection or a drug allergy should be considered. Many patients infected with _K. pneumoniae_ have serious underlying illnesses that predispose them to superinfection.

CONTROVERSIES, CAVEATS, AND COMMENTS

Attempts to control the spread of ESBL-producing _K. pneumoniae_ have concentrated on antibiotic restriction. Restriction of ceftazidime use coupled with increased use of imipenem or piperacillin/tazobactam has been proposed as a means of controlling the spread of ESBL-producing organisms. This strategy was successful at one institution but resulted in an increase in isolates of imipenem-resistant _Acinetobacter._ Others have suggested vigorous isolation procedures.

A recent study of patients bacteremic with ESBL-producing _K. pneumoniae_ and _E. coli_ showed that almost all community-acquired infections were among nursing home residents with very low functional levels (222). This study also indicated that horizontal transmission occurred in intensive care units. A previous study of nursing home residents colonized with ESBL-producing organisms correlated colonization with use of trimethoprim/sulfamethoxazole. Vigorous enforcement of hand washing and glove use by those caring for any febrile, debilitated patient receiving tube feedings or who has a central line is reasonable. In addition, attempts to restrict the use of aztreonam, ceftazidime, and other broad-spectrum cephalosporins seems warranted (72, 199).

REFERENCES

1. Abbas AM, Chandra V, Dongaonkar PP, Goel PK, Kacker P, Patel NA, Shrivastava OP, Thakkar B, Tillotson GS. Ciprofloxacin versus amoxycillin/clavulanic acid in the treatment of urinary

tract infections in general practice. J Antimicrob Chemother 1989;24:235–239.

2. Acuna RT. Endoscopy of the air passages with special reference to scleroma. Ann Otol Rhinol Laryngol 1973;82:765–769.

3. Adenis JP, Mounier M, Salomon JL, Denis F. Human vitreous penetration of imipenem. Eur J Ophthalmol 1994;4:115–117.

4. Adhikari M, Coovadia YM, Singh D. A 4-year study of neonatal meningitis: clinical and microbiological findings. J Trop Pediatr 1995;41:81–85.

5. Altman G, Ostfeld E, Zohar S, et al. Rhinoscleroma. Isr J Med Sci 1977;13:62.

6. Andraca R, Edson RS, Kern EB. Rhinoscleroma: a growing concern in the United States? Mayo Clinic experience. Mayo Clin Proc 1993;68:1151–1157.

7. Arakawa Y, Ohta M, Kido N, Mori M, Ito H, Komatsu T, Fujii Y, Kato N. Chromosomal beta-lactamase of *Klebsiella oxytoca*, a new class A enzyme that hydrolyses broad-spectrum beta-lactam antibiotics. Antimicrob Agents Chemother 1989;33:63–70.

8. Archambaud M, Labau E, Clave D, Suc C. Bactericidal effect of cefotaxime-sulbactam and imipenem combined with gentamicin and/or ciprofloxacin against CTX-1 producing *Klebsiella pneumoniae*. Pathol Biol 1989;37:534–539.

9. Arcieri G, August R, Becker N, Doyle C, Griffith E, Gruenwaldt G, Heyd A, O'Brien B. Clinical experience with ciprofloxacin in the USA. Eur J Clin Microbiol 1986;5:220–225.

10. Aronoff SC, Jacobs MR, Johenning S, Yamabe S. Comparative activities of the beta-lactamase inhibitors YTR 830, sodium clavulanate, and sulbactam combined with amoxicillin or ampicillin. Antimicrob Agents Chemother 1984;26:580–582.

11. Arpi M, Jorgensen PE, Pedersen HF. In vitro studies of the synergism of piperacillin and netilmicin against blood culture isolates. Chemotherapy 1986;32:68–74.

12. Arstila T, Auvinen H, Houvinen P. Beta-lactam resistance among *Escherichia coli* and *Klebsiella* species blood culture isolates in Finnish hospitals. Finnish Study Group for Antimicrobial Resistance. Eur J Clin Microbiol Infect Dis 1994;13: 468–474.

13. Aubert G, Jacquemond G, Pozzetto B, Duthel R, Boylot D, Brunon J, Dorche G. Pharmacokinetic evidence of imipenem efficacy in the treatment of *Klebsiella pneumoniae* nosocomial meningitis. J Antimicrob Chemother 1991;28:316–317.

14. Avery RK, Salman SD, Baker AS. Rhinoscleroma treated with ciprofloxacin: a case report. Laryngoscope 1995;105:854–856.

15. Baltch AL, Smith RP, Hammer MC, Conroy JV, Michelson PB. Antimicrobial effect of clindamycin in combination with aztreonam or aminoglycosides against *Klebsiella* spp. J Antimicrob Chemother 1991;27:303–310.

16. Bakker-Woudenberg IA, Ten Kate MT, Stearne-Cullen LE, Woodle MC. Efficacy of gentamicin or ceftazidime entrapped in liposomes with prolonged blood circulation and enhanced localization in *Klebsiella pneumoniae* infected lung tissue. J Infect Dis 1995;171:938–947.

17. Bakker-Woudenberg IA, van den Berg JC, Michel MF. Therapeutic activities of cefazolin, cefotaxime, and ceftazidime against experimentally induced *Klebsiella pneumoniae* pneumonia in rats. Antimicrob Agents Chemother 1982;22:1042–1050.

18. Barriere SL, Conte JE. Emergence of multiple antibiotic resistance during the therapy of *Klebsiella pneumoniae* meningitis. Am J Med Sci 1980;279:61–65.

19. Barza M, Kane A, Baum J. Comparison of the effects of continuous and intermittent systemic administration on the penetration of gentamicin into infected rabbit eyes. J Infect Dis 1983; 147:144–148.

20. Bauernfeind A, Chong Y, Schweighart S. Extended spectrum beta-lactamase in *Klebsiella pneumoniae* including resistance to cephamycins. Infection 1989;17:316–321.

21. Bauernfeind A, Jungwirth R, Schweighart S. In vitro activity of meropenem, imipenem, the penem HRE 664 and ceftazidime against clinical isolates from West Germany. J Antimicrob Chemother 1989;24(Suppl A):73–84.

22. Bauernfeind A, Stemplinger I, Jungwirth R, Giamarellou H. Characterization of the plasmidic beta-lactamase CMY-2, which is responsible for cephamycin resistance. Antimicrob Agents Chemother 1996;40:221–224.

23. Baum J. Infections of the eye. Clin Infect Dis 1995;21:479–488.

24. Bell J, Turnidge J. National Antimicrobial Resistance Surveillance Program, 1995 report. Canberra: National Health and Medical Research Council, 1995.

25. Bercion R, Meyran M, Labia R, Thabaut A. Comparative activities of 15 beta-lactam antibiotics against 590 strains of *Klebsiella pneumoniae* according to the production of beta-lactamase. Pathol Biol 1991;39:353–360.

26. Bermudes H, Jude F, Arpin C, Quentin C, Morand A, Labia R. Characterization of an inhibitor-resistant TEM (IRT) beta-lactamase in a novel strain of *Klebsiella pneumoniae*. Antimicrob Agents Chemother 1997;41:222.

27. Beskid G, Christenson JG, Cleeland R, DeLorenzo W, Trown PW. In vivo activity of ceftriaxone (Ro 13–9904), a new broad-spectrum semisynthetic cephalosporin. Antimicrob Agents Chemother 1981; 20:159–167.

28. Biedenbach DJ, Sutton LD, Jones RD. Antimicrobial activity of CS-940, a new trifluorinated quinolone. Antimicrob Agents Chemother 1995;39:2325–2330.

29. Bingen EH, Desjardins P, Arlet G, Bourgeois F, Mariani-Kurkdjian P, Lambert-Zechovsky NY, Denamur E, Philippon A, Elion J. Molecular epidemiology of plasmid spread among extended broad spectrum beta-lactamase producing *Klebsiella pneumoniae* isolates in a pediatric hospital. J Clin Microbiol 1993;31: 179–184.

30. Blondeau JM, Yaschuk Y, and the Canadian Ciprofloxacin Study Group. Canadian Ciprofloxacin Susceptibility Study: comparative study from 15 medical centers. Antimicrob Agents Chemother 1996;40:1729–1732.

31. Bodey GP, Elting LS, Rodriquez S, Hernandez M. *Klebsiella* bacteremia. A 10-year review in a cancer institution. Cancer 1989;64:2368–2376.

32. Boisjoly HM, Jotterand VH, Bazin R, et al. Metastatic *Pseudomonas* endophthalmitis following bronchoscopy. Can J Ophthalmol 1987;22:378–380.

33. Bonadio WA. *Klebsiella pneumoniae* bacteremia in children. Fifty-seven cases in ten years. Am J Dis Child 1989;143: 1061–1063.

34. Bortolotti U, Thiene G, Milano A, Pannizon G, Valente M, Galluci V. Pathological study of infective endocarditis on Hancock porcine bioprostheses. J Thorac Cardiovasc Surg 1981;81: 934–942.

35. Bradford PA, Cherubin CE, Idemyor V, Rasmussen BA, Bush K. Multiply resistant *Klebsiella pneumoniae* strains from two Chicago hospitals: identification of the extended-spectrum TEM-12 and TEM-10 ceftazidime hydrolyzing beta-lactamases in a single isolate. Antimicrob Agents Chemother 1994;38: 761–766.

36. Brogden RN, Carmine AA, Heel RC, et al. Trimethoprim: a review of its antibacterial activity, pharmacokinetics and therapeutic use in urinary tract infections. Drugs 1982;23:405–430.

37. Bronsema DA, Adams JR, Pallares R, Wenzel RP. Secular trends in rates and etiology of nosocomial urinary tract infections at a university hospital. J Urol 1993;150:414–416.

38. Brook I, Elliott TB, Ledney GD. Quinolone therapy of *Klebsiella pneumoniae* sepsis following irradiation: comparison of pefloxacin, ciprofloxacin and ofloxacin. Radiat Res 1990;122: 215–217.

39. Brown RB, Kruse JA, Counts GW, Russell JA, Christou NV, Sands ML. Double-blind study of endotracheal tobramycin in the treatment of gram-negative bacterial pneumonia. The endotracheal tobramycin study group. Antimicrob Agents Chemother 1990;34:269–272.

40. Brown TH, Alford RH. Antagonism by chloramphenicol of broad-spectrum beta-lactam antibiotics against *Klebsiella pneumoniae*. Antimicrob Agents Chemother 1984;25:405–407.

41. Brown TH, Alford RH. Failure of chloramphenicol and cefotaxime therapy in *Klebsiella* meningitis: possible role of antibiotic antagonism. South Med J 1985;78:869–871.

42. Brun-Buisson C, Legrand P, Philippon A, Montravers F, Ansquer M, Duval J. Transferable enzymatic resistance to third-generation cephalosporins during nosocomial outbreak of multiresistant *K. pneumoniae*. Lancet 1987;302–306.

43. Burwen DR, Banerjee SN, Gaynes RP, et al. Ceftazidime resistance among selected nosocomial Gram-negative bacilli in the United States. J Infect Dis 1994;170:1622–1625.

44. Bush K, Jacoby G. Nomenclature of TEM beta-lactamases. J Antimicrob Chemother 1997;39:1–3.

45. Bushby SRM. Trimethoprim-sulfamethoxazole: in vitro microbiologic aspects. J Infect Dis 1973;128(Suppl):442–467.

46. Calandra GB, Ricci FM, Wang C et al. Safety and tolerance comparison of imipenem-cilastatin to cephalothin and cefazolin. J Antimicrob Chemother 1983;12(Suppl D):79–87.

47. Caron F, Gutmann L, Bure A, Pangon B, Vallois JM, Pechinot A, Carbon C. Ceftriaxone-sulbactam combination in rabbit endocarditis caused by a strain of *Klebsiella pneumoniae* producing extended-broad-spectrum TEM-3 beta-lactamase. Antimicrob Agents Chemother 1990;34:2070–2074.

48. Carpenter JL. *Klebsiella* pulmonary infections: occurrence at one medical center and review. Rev Infect Dis 1990;12:672–682.

49. Casanova C, Lorente JA, Carrillo F, Perez-Rodriguez E, Nunez N. *Klebsiella pneumoniae* liver abscess associated with septic endophthalmitis. Arch Intern Med 1989;149:1467.

50. Case records of the Massachusetts General Hospital. Case 36–1980. N Engl J Med 1980;303:628–636.

51. Casellas JM, Goldberg M, Tome G, Merino S, Gilardoni M, San Juan J, Rolon M, Bauernfeind A. Is cefipime a reliable alternative for the treatment of infections due to extended spectrum beta-lactamase producer strains isolated in Argentina [Abstract E89]? Program and Abstracts of the 36th Interscience Conference of Antimicrob Agents Chemother, New Orleans, 1996.

52. Cavallo JD, Fabre R, Crenn Y, Meyran M. In vitro activity of meropenem and seven other beta-lactam antibiotics against *K. pneumoniae* and enterobacteriaceae producing beta-lactamases with extended spectrum. Pathol Biol 1994;42:365–368.

53. Chadwick EG, Shulman ST, Yogev R. Correlation of antibiotic synergy in vitro and in vivo: use of an animal model of neutropenic gram-negative sepsis. J Infect Dis 1986;154: 670–675.

54. Chambers HF, Neu HC. Penicillins. In: Mandell GL, Bennett JE, Dolin R, eds. Principles and practice of infectious diseases. 4th ed. New York: Churchill Livingstone, 1995.

55. Chan RK, Lye WC, Lee EJ, Kumarasinghe G. Nosocomial urinary tract infection: a microbiological study. Ann Acad Med Singapore 1993;22:873–877.

56. Chanal C, Sirot D, Chanal M, Cluzel M, Sirot J, Cluzel R. Comparative in-vitro activity of meropenem against clinical isolates including *Enterobacteriaceae* with expanded-spectrum beta-lactamase. J Antimicrob Chemother 1989;24(Suppl A):133–141.

57. Chanal CM, Sirot DL, Petit A, Labia R, Morand A, Sirot JL, Cluzel RA. Multiplicity of TEM-derived beta-lactamases from *Klebsiella pneumoniae* strains isolated at the same hospital and relationships between the responsible plasmids. Antimicrob Agents Chemother 1989;33:1915–1920.

58. Chang FY, Chou MY, Fan RL, Shaio MF. A clinical study of *Klebsiella* liver abscess. Taiwan I Hsueh Hui Tsa Chih 1988;87: 282–287.

59. Chee SP, Ang CL. Endogenous *Klebsiella* endophthalmitis—a case series. Ann Acad Med Singapore 1995;24:473–478.

60. Cheng DL, Liu YC, Yen MY, Liu CY, Wang RS. Septic metastatic lesions of pyogenic liver abscess. Their association with *Klebsiella pneumoniae* bacteremia in diabetic patients. Arch Intern Med 1991;151:1557–1559.

61. Cherubin CE, Corrado ML, Nair SR, Gombert ME, Landesman S, Humbert G. Treatment of Gram-negative bacillary meningitis: role of the new cephalosporin antibiotics. Rev Infect Dis 1982;4(Suppl):S453–S464.

62. Cherubin CE, Eng RH, Norrby R, Modai J, Humbert G, Overturf G. Penetration of newer cephalosporins into cerebrospinal fluid. Rev Infect Dis 1989;11:526–548.

63. Chin NX, Neu HC. In-vitro activity of FCE 22101 and synergy studies with other antimicrobial agents. J Antimicrob Chemother 1989;23(Suppl C):95–101.

64. Chin N, Novelli A, Neu HC. In vitro activity of lomefloxacin (SC-47111; NY-198), a difluoroquinolone 3-carboxylic acid, compared with those of other quinolones. Antimicrob Agents Chemother 1988;32:656–662.

65. Chiu CT, Lin DY, Liaw YF. Metastatic septic endophthalmitis in pyogenic liver abscess. J Clin Gastroenterol 1988;10: 524–527.

66. Chou FF, Kou HK. Endogenous endophthalmitis associated with pyogenic hepatic abscess. J Am Coll Surg 1996;182:33–36.

67. Chowdhury P, Stein DS. Pyogenic hepatic abscess and septic pulmonary emboli associated with *Klebsiella ozanae* bacteremia. South Med J 1992;85:638–641.

68. Clarke AM, Zemcov SJ. Clavulanic acid in combination with ticarcillin: an in-vitro comparison with other beta-lactams. J Antimicrob Chemother 1984;13:121–128.

69. Cohen PS, Maguire JH, Weinstein L. Infective endocarditis caused by Gram negative bacteria: a review of the literature, 1945–1977. Prog Cardiovasc Dis 1980;22:205–242.

70. Cohn JR, Jungkind DL, Baker JS. In vitro antagonism by erythromycin of the bactericidal action of antimicrobial agents against common respiratory pathogens. Antimicrob Agents Chemother 1980;18:872–876.

71. Cookson B, Johnson AP, Azadin B, Paul J, Hutchinson G, Kaufmann M, Woodford N, Malde M, Walsh B, Yousif A. International inter- and intrahospital patient spread of a multiple antibiotic resistant strain of *Klebsiella pneumoniae*. J Infect Dis 1995;171:511–513.

72. Coulter C, Faoagali JC, Doige S, Bodman J, George N. Hand culture surveillance to investigate transmission of epidemic extended spectrum beta-lactamase producing *Klebsiella pneumoniae* in a major intensive care unit [Abstract]. Aust NZ J Med 1995;25:572.

73. Cox CE. A comparison of the safety and efficacy of lomefloxacin

and ciprofloxacin in the treatment of complicated or recurrent urinary tract infections. Am J Med 1992;92:82S–86S.

74. Cryz SJ, Furer E, Sadoff JC, Fredeking T, Que JU, Cross AS. Production and characterization of a human hyperimmune intravenous immunoglobulin against *Pseudomonas aeruginosa* and *Klebsiella* species. J Infect Dis 1991;163:1055–1061.

75. Darouiche R, Perkins B, Musher D, Hamill R, Tsai S. Levels of rifampin and ciprofloxacin in nasal secretions: correlations with MIC_{90} and eradication of nasopharyngeal carriage of bacteria. J Infect Dis 1990;162:1124–1127.

76. De Champs C, Guelon D, Joyon D, Sirot D, Chanal M, Sirot J. Treatment of a meningitis due to an *Enterobacter aerogenes* producing a derepressed cephalosporinase and a *Klebsiella pneumoniae* producing an extended-spectrum beta-lactamase. Infection 1991;19:181–183.

77. Dickneite G, Czech J. Combination of antibiotic treatment with the thrombin inhibitor recombinant hirudin for the therapy of experimental *Klebsiella pneumoniae* sepsis. Thromb Haemost 1994;71:768–772.

78. Dickneite G, Paques EP. Reduction of mortality with antithrombin III in septicemic rats: a study of *Klebsiella pneumoniae* induced sepsis. Thromb Haemost 1993;69:98–102.

79. Domenico P, Hopkins T, Cunha BA. The effect of sodium salicylate on antibiotic susceptibility and synergy in *Klebsiella pneumoniae*. J Antimicrob Chemother 1990;26:343–351.

80. Domenico P, Hopkins T, Schoh PE, Cunha BA. Potentiation of aminoglycoside inhibition and reduction of capsular polysaccharide production in *Klebsiella pneumoniae* by sodium salicylate. J Antimicrob Chemother 1990;25:903–914.

81. Downs JT, Andriole VT, Ryan JL. Synergism of azlocillin, mezlocillin, piperacillin in combination with tobramycin against *Klebsiella* and *Pseudomonas*. Yale J Biol Med 1986; 59:11–16.

82. Dudley JP. Atrophic rhinitis: antibiotic treatment. Am J Otolaryngol 1987;8:387–390.

83. Ebisuno S, Miyai M. A case of *Klebsiella pneumoniae* endophthalmitis metastasized from prostatitis. Hinyokika Kiyo 1994; 40:625–627.

84. Eisen D, Russell EG, Tymms M, Roper EJ, Grayson ML, Turnidge J. Random amplified polymorphic DNA and plasmid analyses used in the investigation of an outbreak of multiresistant *Klebsiella pneumoniae*. J Clin Microbiol 1995; 33:713–717.

85. El Baba FZ, Trousdale MD, Garderman J, et al. Intravitreal penetration of oral ciprofloxacin in humans. Ophthalmology 1992; 99:483–486.

86. Elhanan G, Tabenkin H, Yahalom R, Raz R. Single dose fosfomycin trometamol versus 5-day cephalexin regimen for treatment of uncomplicated lower urinary tract infections in women. Antimicrob Agents Chemother 1994;38:2612–2614.

87. Elkhaili H, Kamili N, Linger L, Leveque D, Pompei D, Monteil H, Jehl F. In vitro time-kill curves of cefepime and cefpriome combined with amikacin, gentamicin or ciprofloxacin against *Klebsiella pneumoniae* producing extended-spectrum betalactamase. Chemotherapy 1997;43:245–253.

88. Ellis-Pegler RB, Lang SD. Cefoperazone in Klebsiella meningitis: a case report. Drugs 1981;22(Suppl 1):69–71.

89. Endophthalmitis vitrectomy study group. Results of the endophthalmitis vitrectomy study. Arch Ophthalmol 1995;113: 1479–1496.

90. English AR, Retsema JA, Girard AE, et al. CP-45 899, a betalactamase inhibitor that extends the antibacterial spectrum of

beta-lactams: initial bacteriological characterization. Antimicrob Agents Chemother 1978;14:414.

91. Farmer JJ III. *Enterobacteriaceae:* introduction and identification. In: Murray PR, ed. Manual of clinical microbiology. 6th ed. Washington, DC: American Society for Microbiology Press, 1995.

92. Fass RJ, Prior RB. Comparative in vitro activity of piperacillin-tazobactam and ticarcillin-clavulanate. Antimicrob Agents Chemother 1989;33:1268–1274.

93. Feigin RD, McCracken GH, Klein JO. Diagnosis and management of meningitis. Pediatr Infect Dis J 1992:11;785–814.

94. Feldman C, Smith C, Levy H, Ginsburg P, Miller SD, Koornhof HJ. *Klebsiella pneumoniae* bacteraemia at an urban general hospital. J Infect 1990;20:21–31.

95. Fernandez-Rodriguez A, Canton R, Perez-Diaz JC, Martinez-Beltran J, Picazo JJ, Baquero F. Aminoglycoside-modifying enzymes in clinical isolates harboring extended spectrum betalactamases. Antimicrob Agents Chemother 1992;36:2536–2538.

96. Ferrara A, Grassi G, Grassi FA, Piccioni PD, Gialdroni Grassi G. Bactericidal activity of meropenem and interactions with other antibiotics. J Antimicrob Chemother 1989;24(Suppl A):239–250.

97. Fournier J-L, Ramisse F, Jacolot AC, Szatanik M, Petitjean OJ, Alonso J-M, Scavizzi MR. Assessment of two penicillins plus beta-lactamase inhibitors versus cefotaxime in treatment of murine *Klebsiella pneumoniae* infections. Antimicrob Agents Chemother 1996;40:325–330.

98. Fournier B, Roy PH, Lagrange PH, Philippon A. Chromosomal beta-lactamase genes of *Klebsiella oxytoca* are divided into two main groups, (BLA)OXY-1 and (BLA)OXY-2. Antimicrob Agents Chemother 1996;40:454–459.

99. French GL, Shannon KP, Simmons N. Hospital outbreak of *Klebsiella pneumoniae* resistant to broad-spectrum cephalosporins and beta-lactam-beta-lactamase inhibitor combinations by hyperproduction of SHV-5 beta-lactamase. J Clin Microbiol 1996;34:358–363.

100. Fu KP, Neu HC. A comparative study of the activity of cefamandole and other cephalosporins and analysis of the beta-lactamase stability and synergy of cefamandole with aminoglycosides. J Infect Dis 1978;137(Suppl):S38–S50.

101. Garcia de la Torre M, Romero-Vivas J, Martinez-Beltran J, Guerrero A, Meseguer M, Bouza E. *Klebsiella* bacteremia: an analysis of 100 episodes. Rev Infect Dis 1985;7:143–150.

102. Gentry LO, Rodriguez-Gomez G, Kohler RB, Khan FA, Rytel MW. Parenteral followed by oral ofloxacin for nosocomial pneumonia and community-acquired pneumonia requiring hospitalization. Am Rev Respir Dis 1992;145:31–35.

103. Glassman RM, Lieberman TT, Friedman AH, Fuchs W, Meltzer MA, Gabrilove L. Endogenous *Klebsiella* endophthalmitis: case report. Mt Sinai J Med 1989;56:326–329.

104. Goldstein EJC, Lewis RP, Martin WJ, Edelstein PH. Infections caused by *Klebsiella ozaenae:* a changing disease spectrum. J Clin Microbiol 1978;8:413–418.

105. Gouby A, Neuwirth C, Bourg G, Bouziges N, Carles-Nurit MJ, Despaux E, Ramuz M. Epidemiological study by pulsed field gel electrophoresis of outbreak of extended spectrum beta-lactamase producing *Klebsiella pneumoniae* in a geriatric hospital. J Clin Microbiol 1994;32:301–305.

106. Gould IM, MacKenzie FM, Thomson C. Multi-resistant *Klebsiella* in Grampian. Lancet 1995;345:122.

107. Grose WE, Bodey GP, Rodriguez V. Sulfamethoxazole-trimethoprim for infections in cancer patients. JAMA 1977; 237:352.

108. Gudmundsson S, Erlendsdottir H, Gottfredsson M, Gudmundsson A. The post-antibiotic effect induced by antimicrobial combinations. Scand J Infect Dis Suppl 1990;74:80–93.

109. Guerillot F, Carret G, Flandrois JP. A statistical evaluation of the bactericidal effects of ceftibuten in combination with aminoglycosides and ciprofloxacin. J Antimicrob Chemother 1993;32:685–694.

110. Haddy RI, Lee M, Sangal SP, Walbroehl GS, Hambrick CS, Sarti GM. *Klebsiella pneumoniae* bacteremia in the community hospital. J Fam Pract 1989;28:686–690.

111. Hammond JM, Potgieter PD, Linton DM, Forder AA. Intensive care management of community-acquired *Klebsiella pneumoniae.* Respir Med 1991;85:11–16.

112. Han SH. Review of hepatic abscess from *Klebsiella pneumoniae.* An association with diabetes mellitus and septic endophthalmitis. West J Med 1995;162:220–224.

113. Harabe E, Kawai Y, Kanazawa K, Otsuki M, Nishino T. In vitro and in vivo antibacterial activities of meropenem, a new carbapenem antibiotic. Drugs Exp Clin Res 1992;18:37–46.

114. Held TK, Trautmann M, Mielke ME, Neudeck H, Cryz SJ, Cross AS. Monoclonal antibody against *Klebsiella* capsular polysaccharide reduces severity and hematogenic spread of experimental *Klebsiella pneumoniae* pneumonia. Infect Immun 1992;60:1771–1778.

115. Hickstein DD, Dillon JT. *Klebsiella pneumoniae* meningitis. Intravenous trimethoprim-sulfamethoxazole treatment. JAMA 1982;248:1212–1213.

116. Hidaka T, Yokata T, Tamura K. A case of liver abscess associated with endophthalmitis caused by *Klebsiella pneumoniae.* Kansenshogaku Zasshi 1993;67:76–80.

117. Higashi T, Makino Y, Katsurada K. A case of gas-containing liver abscess with multiple metastatic lesions. Kansenshogaku Zasshi 1995;69:1017–1020.

118. Hoban DJ, Jones RN, Yamane N, Frei R, Trilla A, Pignatari AC. In vitro activity of three carbapenem antibiotics. Comparative studies with biapenem (L-627), imipenem and meropenem against aerobic pathogens isolated worldwide. Diag Microbiol Infect Dis 1993;17:299–305.

119. Hoffman NR, Preston FS. Friedlander's pneumonia. A report of 11 cases and appraisal of antibiotic therapy. Dis Chest 1968; 53:481–486.

120. Hooton TM, Winter C, Tiu F, Stamm WE. Randomized comparative trial and cost analysis of 3-day antimicrobial regimens for treatment of acute cystitis in women. JAMA 1995;273: 41–45.

121. Horii T, Arakawa Y, Ohta M, Ichiyama S, Wacharotayankun R, Kato N. Plasmid-mediated AmpC-type beta-lactamase isolated from *Klebsiella pneumoniae* confers resistance to broad-spectrum beta-lactams, including moxalactam. Antimicrob Agents Chemother 1993;37:984–990.

122. Hubner J, Hartung D, Kropec A, Daschner FD. Combination effect of SCE-2787 and cefepime with aminoglycosides on nosocomial gram-negative bacteria. Infection 1991;19:186–189.

123. Hutchison M, Faulkner KL, Turner PJ, Haworth SJ, Sheikh W, Nadler H, Pitkin DH. A compilation of meropenem tissue distribution data. J Antimicrob Chemother 1995;36(Suppl A): 43–56.

124. Hyatt JM, Nix DE, Stratton CW, Schentag JJ. In vitro pharmacodynamics of piperacillin, piperacillin-tazobactam, and ciprofloxacin alone and in combination against *Staphylococcus aureus, Klebsiella pneumoniae, Enterobacter cloacae,* and *Pseudomonas aeruginosa.* Antimicrob Agents Chemother 1995; 39:1711–1716.

125. Inderlied CB, Lancero MG, Young LS. Bacteriostatic and bactericidal in-vitro activity against clinical isolates, including *Mycobacterium avium* complex. J Antimicrob Chemother 1989; 24(Suppl A):85–99.

126. Inoue M, Maejima T, Sanai S, Okamoto R, Hashimoto H. Purification and properties of a chromosomal beta-lactamase from *Klebsiella oxytoca.* J Antibiot 1991;44:435–440.

127. Jacoby GA, Medeiros AA. More extended-spectrum beta-lactamases. Antimicrob Agents Chemother 1991;35:1697–1704.

128. Jacoby GA, Sutton L. Properties of plasmids responsible for production of extended-spectrum beta-lactamases. Antimicrob Agents Chemother 1991;35:164–169.

129. Janda WM, Hellerman DV, Zeiger B, Brody BB. Isolation of *Klebsiella ozaenae* from a corneal abscess. Am J Clin Pathol 1985;83:655–657.

130. Jett BD, Ritchie DJ, Reichley R, Bailey TC, Sahm DF. In vitro activities of various beta-lactam antimicrobial agents against clinical isolates of *Escherichia coli* and *Klebsiella* species resistant to oxyimino cephalosporins. Antimicrob Agents Chemother 1995;39:1187–1190.

131. Johnson AP, Weinbren MJ, Ayling-Smith B, Du Bois SK, Amyes SGB, George RC. Outbreak of infection in two UK hospitals caused by a strain of *Klebsiella pneumoniae* resistant to cefotaxime and ceftazidime. J Hosp Infect 1992;20:97–103.

132. Jones RN, Barry AL, Thornsberry C. In vitro studies of meropenem. J Antimicrob Chemother 1989;24(Suppl A):9–29.

133. Jong GM, Hsiue TR, Chen CR, Chang HY, Chen CW. Rapidly fatal outcome of bacteremic *Klebsiella pneumoniae* pneumonia in alcoholics. Chest 1995;107:214–217.

134. Karachalios GN. Randomized comparative study of amoxicillin-clavulanic acid and co-trimoxazole in the treatment of acute urinary tract infections in adults. Antimicrob Agents Chemother 1985;28:693–694.

135. Karnad A, Alvarez S, Berk SL. Pneumonia caused by Gram negative bacilli. Am J Med 1985;79:61–67.

136. Kenevan RJ, Zinneman HH. Bacterial endocarditis 1963 to 1973. Observations on incidence, course and treatment at Minneapolis Veterans Administration Hospital. Minn Med 1975; 58:663–667.

137. Keren G, Ahalel A, Bartou E, et al. The intravitreal penetration of orally administered ciprofloxacin in humans. Invest Ophthalmol Vis Sci 1991;32:2388–2392.

138. Kilpatrick M, Girgis N, Farid Z, Bishay E. Aztreonam for treating meningitis caused by gram-negative rods. Scand J Infect Dis 1991;23:125–126.

139. King A, Boothman C, Phillips I. Comparative in-vitro activity of meropenem on clinical isolates from the United Kingdom J Antimicrob Chemother 1989;24(Suppl A):31–45.

140. Klastersky J. Concept of empiric therapy with antibiotic combinations. Indications and limits. Am J Med 1986;80:2–12.

141. Klastersky J, Henri A, Vandenborre L. Antimicrobial activity of tobramycin and gentamicin used in combination with cephalothin and carbenicillin. Am J Med Sci 1973;266:13–21.

142. Klastersky J, Meunier-Carpentier F, Prevost JM, Staquet M. Synergism between amikacin and cefazolin against *Klebsiella:* in vitro studies and effect on the bactericidal activity of serum. J Infect Dis 1976;134:271–276.

143. Klastersky J, Swings G, Vandenborre L, Weerts D, De Maertelaer V. Effectiveness of the carbenicillin-cephalothin combination against gram-negative bacilli. Am J Med Sci 1973;265: 45–53.

144. Klesel N, Isert D, Limbert M, Seibert G, Winkler I, Schrinner

E. Comparative effects of cefpirome (HR 810) and other cephalosporins on experimentally induced pneumonia in mice. J Antibiot 1986;39:971–977.

145. Kliebe C, Nies BA, Meyer JF, Tolxdorff-Neutzling RM, Wiedemann B. Evolution of plasmid-coded resistance to broad-spectrum cephalosporins. Antimicrob Agents Chemother 1985; 28:302–307.

146. Klugman KP, Dagan R. Randomized comparison of meropenem with cefotaxime for treatment of bacterial meningitis. Meropenem Meningitis Study Group. Antimicrob Agents Chemother 1995;39:1140–1146.

147. Knight L, Fraser RG, Robson HG. Massive pulmonary gangrene: a severe complication of Klebsiella pneumonia. Can Med Assoc J 1975;112:196–198.

148. Knothe H, Shah P, Krcmery V, Antal M, Mitsuhashi S. Transferable resistance to cefotaxime, cefoxitin, cefamandole and cefuroxime in clinical isolates of Klebsiella pneumoniae and Serratia marcescens. Infection 1983;11:315–317.

149. Korvick JA, Bryan CS, Farber B, Beam TR Jr, Shenfeld L, Muder RR, Weinbaum D, Lumish R, Gerding DN, Wagener MM. Prospective observational study of Klebsiella bacteremia in 230 patients: outcome for antibiotic combinations versus monotherapy. Antimicrob Agents Chemother 1992;36:2639–2644.

150. Korvick JA, Hackett AK, Yu VL, Muder RR. Klebsiella pneumonia in the modern era: clinicoradiographic correlations. South Med J 1991;84:200–204.

151. Kremer I, Gaton DD, Baniel J, Servadio C. Klebsiella metastatic endophthalmitis—a complication of shock wave lithotripsy. Ophthalmic Surg 1990;21:206–208.

152. Kuck NA, Jacobus NV, Petersen N, Weiss WJ, Testa RT. Comparative in vitro and in vivo activities of piperacillin combined with the beta-lactamase inhibitors tazobactam, clavulanic acid and sulbactam. Antimicrob Agents Chemother 1989;33: 1964–1969.

153. LeBel M, Pellerin M, Bergeron MG. Serum bactericidal activity of ceftazidime increased by netilmicin. Drug Intell Clin Pharm 1985;19:932–936.

154. Lee KH, Hui KP, Tan WC, Lim TK. Klebsiella bacteraemia: a report of 101 cases from National University Hospital, Singapore. J Hosp Infect 1994;27:299–305.

155. Leggett JE, Ebert S, Fantin B, Craig WA. Comparative dose-effect relations at several dosing intervals for beta-lactam, aminoglycoside and quinolone antibiotics against gram-negative bacilli in murine thigh-infection and pneumonitis models. Scand J Infect Dis 1990;74(Suppl):179–184.

156. Lemozy J, Sirot D, Chanal C, Huc C, Labia R, Dabernat H, Sirot J. First characterization of inhibitor-resistant TEM (IRT) beta-lactamases in Klebsiella pneumoniae strains. Antimicrob Agents Chemother 1995;39:2580–2582.

157. Lenis A, Ruff T, Diaz JA, Chandour EG. Rhinoscleroma. South Med J 1988;81:1580–1582.

158. Leung JW, Ling TK, Chan RC, Cheung SW, Lai CW, Sung JJ, Chung SC, Cheng AF. Antibiotics, biliary sepsis and bile duct stones. Gastrointest Endosc 1994;40:716–721.

159. Levitz RE, Dudley MN, Quintiliani R, Mullany LD, Nightingale CH. Cerebrospinal fluid penetration of trimethoprim-sulfamethoxazole in two patients with gram-negative bacillary meningitis. J Antimicrob Chemother 1984a;13:400–401.

160. Levitz RE, Quintiliani R. Trimethoprim-sulfamethoxazole for bacterial meningitis. Ann Intern Med 1984b;100:881–890.

161. Liao HR, Lee HW, Leu HS, Lin BJ, Juang CJ. Endogenous Klebsiella pneumoniae endophthalmitis in diabetic patients. Can J Ophthalmol 1992;27:143–147.

162. Lipsett PA, Pitt HA. Acute cholangitis. Surg Clin North Am 1990;70:1297–1312.

163. Liu PY, Gur D, Hall LM, Livermore DM. Survey of the prevalence of beta-lactamases amongst 1000 gram-negative bacilli isolated consecutively at the Royal London Hospital. J Antimicrob Chemother 1992;30:429–447.

164. Liu YC, Cheng DL, Lin CL. Klebsiella pneumoniae liver abscess associated with septic endophthalmitis. Arch Intern Med 1986;146:1913–1916.

165. Madhavan T, Kiani D, Saravolatz L, Burch K, Mellinger RC. Recurrent Klebsiella meningitis following trans-sphenoidal hypophysectomy for Nelson's syndrome. Chloramphenicol resistance during relapse. Henry Ford Hosp Med J 1980;28: 142–144.

166. Mainardi JL, Zhou XY, Goldstein F, Mohler J, Farinotti R, Gutmann L, Carbon C. Activity of isepamicin and selection of permeability mutants to beta-lactams during aminoglycoside therapy of experimental endocarditis due to Klebsiella pneumoniae CF 104 producing an aminoglycoside acetyltransferase 6′ modifying enzyme and a TEM-3 beta-lactamase. J Infect Dis 1994; 169:1318–1324.

167. Mandine E, Salles MF, Zalisz R, Guenounou M, Smets P. Murine monoclonal antibodies to Klebsiella pneumoniae protect against lethal endotoxemia and experimental infection with capsulated K. pneumoniae. Infect Immun 1990;58:2828–2833.

168. Margo CE, Mames RN, Guy JR. Endogenous Klebsiella endophthalmitis. Report of two cases and review of the literature. Ophthalmology 1994;101:1298–1301.

169. Martinez M, Castro F, Ocasio R, Vazquez G, Ramirez Ronda CH. Septic endophthalmitis associated with bacteremia and liver abscess caused by Klebsiella pneumoniae. Bol Asoc Med PR 1991;83:485–486.

170. Masuda G, Nakamura K, Yajima T, Saku K. Bacteriostatic and bactericidal activities of beta-lactam antibiotics enhanced by the addition of low concentrations of gentamicin. Antimicrob Agents Chemother 1980;17:334–336.

171. Matsumoto T, Tateda K, Ishii Y, Ohno A, Miyazaki S, Yamaguchi K. In vitro and in vivo antibacterial activities of broad spectrum quinolones against clinical bacterial isolates. Drugs 1995;49(Suppl 2):219–221.

172. Mentec H, Vallois JM, Bure A, Saleh-Mghir A, Jehl F, Carbon C. Piperacillin, tazobactam and gentamicin alone or combined in an endocarditis model of infection by a TEM-3 producing strain of Klebsiella pneumoniae or its susceptible variant. Antimicrob Agents Chemother 1992;36:1883–1889.

173. Meyer KS, Urban C, Eagan JA, Berger BJ, Rahal JJ. Nosocomial outbreak of Klebsiella infection resistant to late-generation cephalosporins. Ann Intern Med 1993;119:353–358.

174. Molinari G, Schito GC. Comparative in vitro activity of BAY Y 3118 with other fluoroquinolones. Drugs 1995;49(Suppl 2):222–225.

175. Monnet D, Freney J, Brun Y, Boeufgras JM, Fleurette J. Difficulties in identifying Klebsiella strains of clinical origin. Int J Med Microbiol 1991;274:456–464.

176. Montgomerie JZ, Ota JK. Klebsiella bacteremia. Arch Intern Med 1980;140:525–527.

177. Moon WK, Im JG, Yeon KM, Han MC. Complications of Klebsiella pneumonia: CT evaluation. J Comput Assist Tomogr 1995;19:176–181.

178. Moore RD, Smith CR, Lietman PS. Association of aminoglycoside plasma levels with therapeutic outcome in Gram-negative pneumonia. Am J Med 1984;77:657–662.

179. Mulgrave L, Attwood PV. Characterization of an SHV-5 related extended broad spectrum beta-lactamase in Enterobacteriaceae from Western Australia. Pathology 1993;25:71–75.

180. Murray KA, Clements BH, Keas SE. *Klebsiella ozaenae* septicemia associated with Hansen's disease. J Clin Microbiol 1981;14:703–705.

181. Nairn K, Shepherd GL, Edwards JR. Efficacy of meropenem in experimental meningitis. J Antimicrob Chemother 1995;36 (Suppl A):73–84.

182. Nakane T, Iyobe S, Sato K, Mitsuhashi S. In vitro antibacterial activity of DU-6859a, a new fluoroquinolone. Antimicrob Agents Chemother 1995;39:2822–2826.

183. Naqvi SH, Maxwell MA, Dunkle LM. Cefotaxime therapy of neonatal gram-negative bacillary meningitis. Pediatr Infect Dis 1985;4:499–502.

184. Naumovski L, Quinn JP, Miyashiro D, Patel M, Bush K, Singer SB, Graves D, Palzkill T, Arvin AM. Outbreak of ceftazidime resistance due to a novel extended spectrum beta-lactamase in isolates from cancer patients. Antimicrob Agents Chemother 1992;36:1991–1996.

185. Neu HC, Chin N, Gu JW. The in-vitro activity of new streptogramins, RP 59500, RP 57669 and RP 54476, alone and in combination. J Antimicrob Chemother 1992;30(Suppl A):83–94.

186. Neu HC, Fu KP. Clavulanic acid: a beta-lactamase inhibiting beta-lactamase. Antimicrob Agents Chemother 1978;14:650–655.

187. Nicolas-Chanoine MH. Inhibitor-resistant beta-lactamases. J Antimicrob Chemother 1997;40:1–3.

188. Nielsen BC, Olinder-Nielsen AM, Malmborg AS. Successful treatment of ozena with ciprofloxacin. Rhinology 1995;33:57–60.

189. Nishino T, Obana Y. Therapeutic efficacy of intravenous and oral ciprofloxacin in experimental murine infections. Chemotherapy 1996;42:140–145.

190. Noble RC, Cooper RM, Jarvis AL, Caples PL, Todd EP. Trimethoprim-sulfamethoxazole therapy for infective endocarditis. South Med J 1981;74:1299–1303.

191. Norrby SR, Newell PA, Faulkner KL, Lesky W. Safety profile of meropenem: international clinical experience based on the first 3125 patients treated with meropenem. J Antimicrob Chemother 1995;36(Suppl A):207–223.

192. Nouvellon M, Pons JL, Sirot D, Combe ML, Lemeland JF. Clonal outbreaks of extended spectrum beta-lactamase producing strains of *Klebsiella pneumoniae* demonstrated by antibiotic susceptibility testing, beta-lactamase typing, and multilocus enzyme electrophoresis. J Clin Microbiol 1994;32:2625–2627.

193. Pangon B, Bizet C, Bure A, Pichon F, Philippon A, Regnier B, Gutmann L. In vivo selection of acephamycin-resistant, porin-deficient mutant of *Klebsiella pneumoniae* producing a TEM-3 beta-lactamase. J Infect Dis 1989;159:1005–1006.

194. Panwalker AP, Trager GM, Porembski PE. *Klebsiella* species: antimicrobial susceptibilities, bactericidal kinetics, and in vitro inactivation of beta-lactam antibiotics. Antimicrob Agents Chemother 1980;18:877–881.

195. Papanicolaou GA, Medeiros AA, Jacoby GA. Novel plasmid-mediated beta-lactamase (MIR-1) conferring resistance to oxyimino- and alpha-methoxy beta-lactams in clinical isolates of *Klebsiella pneumoniae*. Antimicrob Agents Chemother 1990;34:2200–2209.

196. Paterson DL, Ko WC, Mohapatra S, Von Gottberg A, Mulazimoglu L, Casellas JM, Klugman KP, Trenholme GM, Wagener MM, Yu VL. *Klebsiella pneumoniae* bacteremia: impact of extended spectrum beta-lactamase (ESBL) production in a global study of 216 patients. Abstracts of the 37th Interscience Conference on Antimicrob Agents Chemother, Toronto, Canada, 1997.

197. Paul C, Pialoux G, Dupont B et al. Infection due to *Klebsiella rhinoscleromatis* in two patients infected with human immunodeficiency virus. Clin Infect Dis 1993;16:441–442.

198. Pavan PR, Otaiza EE, Hughes BA, Avni A. Exogenous endophthalmitis initially treated without systemic antibiotics. Ophthalmology 1994;101:1289–1296.

199. Pena C, Pujol M, Ardanuy C, et al. Impact of third generation cephalosporin restriction on the control of an extended-spectrum beta-lactamase producing *Klebsiella pneumoniae* outbreak in intensive care unit [Abstract]. Proceedings of the 36th ICAAC, New Orleans, 1996.

200. Pena C, Pujol M, Ricart A, Ardanuy C, Ayats J, Linares J, Garrigosa F, Ariza J, Gudiol F. Risk factors for faecal carriage of *Klebsiella pneumoniae* producing extended spectrum beta-lactamase (ESBL-KP) in the intensive care unit. J Hosp Infect 1997;35:9–16.

201. Perkins BA, Hamill RJ, Musher DM, O'Hara C. In vitro activities of streptomycin and 11 oral antimicrobial agents against clinical isolates of *Klebsiella rhinoscleromatis*. Antimicrob Agents Chemother 1992;36:1785–1787.

202. Philippon A, Labia R, Jacoby G. Extended-spectrum beta-lactamases. Antimicrob Agents Chemother 1989;33:1131–1136.

203. Podbielski A, Melzer B. Nucleotide sequence of the gene encoding the SHV-2 beta-lactamase (blaSHV-2) of *Klebsiella ozaenae*. Nucleic Acids Res 1990;18:4916.

204. Queiroz ML, Bathirunathan N, Mawer GE. Influence of dosage interval on the therapeutic response to gentamicin in mice infected with *Klebsiella pneumoniae*. Chemotherapy 1987;33:68–76.

205. Quinn JP, Miyashiro D, Sahm D, Flamm R, Bush K. Novel plasmid-mediated beta-lactamase (TEM-10) conferring selective resistance to ceftazidime and aztreonam in clinical isolates of *Klebsiella pneumoniae*. Antimicrob Agents Chemother 1989;33:1451–1456.

206. Raz R, Rottensterich E, Boger S, Potasman I. Comparison of single-dose administration and three-day course of amoxicillin with those of clavulanic acid for treatment of uncomplicated urinary tract infection in women. Antimicrob Agents Chemother 1991;35:1688–1690.

207. Reeves DS, Bywater MJ, Holt HA, White LO. In-vitro studies with ciprofloxacin, a new 4-quinolone compound. J Antimicrob Chemother 1984;13:333–346.

208. Retsema J, Girard A, Schelkly W, Manousos M, Anderson M, Bright G, Borovoy R, Brennan L, Mason R. Spectrum and mode of action of azithromycin (CP-62,993), a new 15-membered ring macrolide with improved potency against gram-negative organisms. Antimicrob Agents Chemother 1987;31:1939–1947.

209. Rice LB, Carias LL, Bonomo RA, Shlaes DM. Molecular genetics of resistance to both ceftazidime and beta-lactam-beta-lacatamase inhibitor combinations in *Klebsiella pneumoniae* and in vivo response to beta-lactam therapy. J Infect Dis 1996;173:151–158.

210. Rice LB, Eckstein EC, De Vente J, Shlaes DM. Ceftazidime-resistant *Klebsiella pneumoniae* isolates recovered at the Cleveland Department of Veterans Affairs Medical Center. Clin Infect Dis 1996;23:118–124.

211. Rice LB, Willey SH, Papanicolaou GA, Medeiros AA, Eliopoulos GM, Moellering RC, Jacoby GA. Outbreak of ceftazidime

resistance caused by extended spectrum beta-lactamases at a Massachusetts chronic-care facility. Antimicrob Agents Chemother 1990;34:2193–2199.

212. Rice LB, Yao JD, Klimm K, Eliopoulos GM, Moellering RC. Efficacy of different beta-lactams against an extended spectrum beta-lactamase producing *Klebsiella pneumoniae* strain in the rat intra-abdominal abscess model. Antimicrob Agents Chemother 1991;35:1243–1244.

213. Roosendaal R, Bakker-Woudenberg IA, van den Berghe-van Raffe M, Michel MF. Continuous versus intermittent administration of ceftazidime in experimental *Klebsiella pneumoniae* pneumonia in normal and leukopenic rats. Antimicrob Agents Chemother 1986;30:403–408.

214. Roosendaal R, Bakker-Woudenberg IA, van den Berghe-van Raffe M, Vink-van den Berg JC, Michel MF. Comparative activities of ciprofloxacin and ceftazidime against *Klebsiella pneumoniae* in vitro and in experimental pneumonia in leukopenic rats. Antimicrob Agents Chemother 1987;31:1809–1815.

215. Roussel-Delvallez M, Sirot D, Berrouane Y, Goffart M, Gourde B, Wallet F, Courcol RJ. Bactericidal effect of beta-lactams and amikacin alone or in association against *Klebsiella pneumoniae* producing extended spectrum beta-lactamase. J Antimicrob Chemother 1995;36:241–246.

216. Sanders CC, Sanders WE. Beta-lactam resistance in Gram-negative bacteria: global trends and clinical impact. Clin Infect Dis 1992;15:824–839.

217. Sarkar S, Singh M, Narang A. Successful treatment of hospital acquired *Klebsiella pneumoniae* meningitis in a neonate with ciprofloxacin. Indian Pediatr 1993;30:913–914.

218. Satterwhite TK, McGee ZA, Schnaffer W, Friesinger GC, Mishu M, Collins RD. Infection of an avulsed papillary muscle tip simulating bacterial endocarditis. Am Heart J 1973;86:107–111.

219. Sawai T, Yamagishi S, Mitsuhashi S. Penicillinases of *Klebsiella pneumoniae* and their phylogenetic relationship to penicillinases mediated by R factors. J Bacteriol 1973;115:1045–1054.

220. Schaberg DR, Culver DH, Gaynes RP. Major trends in the microbial etiology of nosocomial infection. Am J Med 1991;91:725–755.

221. Schentag JJ, Vari AJ, Winslade NE, Swanson DJ, Smith IL, Simons GW, Vigano A. Treatment with aztreonam or tobramycin in critical care patients with nosocomial Gram negative pneumonia. Am J Med 1985;78:34–41.

222. Schiappa DA, Hayden MK, Matushek MG, Hashemi FN, Sullivan J, Smith KY, Miyashiro D, Quinn JP, Weinstein RA, Trenholme GM. Ceftazidime-resistant *Klebsiella pneumoniae* and *Escherichia coli* bloodstream infection: A case-control and molecular epidemiologic investigation. J Infect Dis 1996;174:529–536.

223. Schito GC, Sanna A, Chazzi C, Ravizzola G, Leone F, Molinari G, Menozzi MG, Pirali F. In vitro activity of meropenem against clinical isolates in a multicentre study in Italy. J Antimicrob Chemother 1989;24(Suppl A):57–72.

224. Schmidt U, Sen P, Kapila R, Louria DB. Clinical evaluation of intravenous trimethoprim/sulfamethoxazole for serious infections. Rev Infect Dis 1982;4:332–337.

225. Schmutzhard E, Williams KJ, Vukmirovits G, Chmelik V, Pfausler B, Featherstone A. A randomised comparison of meropenem with cefotaxime or ceftriaxone for the treatment of bacterial meningitis in adults. Meropenem Meningitis Study Group. J Antimicrob Chemother 1995;36(Suppl A):85–97.

226. Segev S, Rosen N, Joseph G, Elran HA, Rubinstein E. Pefloxacin efficacy in gram-negative bacillary meningitis. J Antimicrob Chemother 1990;26(Suppl B):187–192.

227. Sells CJ, Shurtleff DB, Loeser JD. Gram-negative cerebrospinal fluid shunt-associated infections. Pediatrics 1977;59:614–618.

228. Sentochnik DE, Eliopoulos GM, Ferraro MJ, Moellering RC. Comparative in vitro activity of SM7338, a new carbapenem antimicrobial agent. Antimicrob Agents Chemother 1989;33:1232–1236.

229. Shannon KP, King A, Phillips I, Nicolas MH, Philippon A. Importance of organisms producing broad-spectrum SHV-group beta-lactamases in the United Kingdom. J Antimicrob Chemother 1990;25:343–351.

230. Sharir M, Triester G, Kneer J, Rubinstein E. The intravitreal penetration of ceftriaxone in man following systemic administration. Invest Ophthalmol Vis Sci 1989;30:2179–2183.

231. Shattuck KE, Chonmaitree T. The changing spectrum of neonatal meningitis over a fifteen-year period. Clin Pediatr 1992;31:130–136.

232. Sipperley JO, Shore JW. Septic retinal cyst in endogenous *Klebsiella* endophthalmitis. Am J Ophthalmol 1982;94:124–125.

233. Sirot D, Sirot J, Labia R, Morand A, Courvalin P, Darfeuille-Michaud A, Perroux R, Cluzel R. Transferable resistance to third-generation cephalosporins in clinical isolates of *Klebsiella pneumoniae*: identification of CTX-1, a novel beta-lactamase. J Antimicrob Chemother 1987;20:323–334.

234. Sirot DL, Goldstein FW, Soussy CJ, Courtieu AL, Husson MD, Lemozy J, et al. Resistance to cefotaxime and seven other beta-lactams in members of the family *Enterobacteriaceae*: a 3-year survey in France. Antimicrob Agents Chemother 1992;36:1677–1681.

235. Smith CE, Tillman BS, Howell AW, Longfield RN, Jorgensen JH. Failure of ceftazidime-amikacin therapy for bacteremia and meningitis due to *Klebsiella pneumoniae* producing an extended spectrum beta-lactamase. Antimicrob Agents Chemother 1990;34:1290–1293.

236. Stamm WE, Hooton TM. Management of urinary tract infections in adults. N Engl J Med 1993;329:1328–1334.

237. Stamos JK, Kaufman BA, Yogev R. Ventriculoperitoneal shunt infections with Gram-negative bacteria. Neurosurgery 1993;33:858–862.

238. Stotka JL, Rupp ME. *Klebsiella pneumoniae* urinary tract infection complicated by endophthalmitis, perinephric abscess, and ecthyma gangrenosum. South Med J 1991;84:790–793.

239. Strampfer MJ, Schoch PE, Cunha BA. Cerebral abscess caused by *Klebsiella ozaenae*. J Clin Microbiol 1987;25:1553–1554.

240. Stuart RL, Turnidge J, Grayson ML. Safety of imipenem in neonates. Pediatr Infect Dis J 1995;14:804–805.

241. Sung JJ, Lyon DJ, Suen R, Chung SC, Co AL, Cheng AF, Leung JW, Li AK. Intravenous ciprofloxacin as treatment for patients with acute suppurative cholangitis: a randomized, controlled clinical trial. J Antimicrob Chemother 1995;35:855–864.

242. Sykes RB, Matthew M. The beta-lactamases of gram-negative bacteria and their role in resistance to beta-lactam antibiotics. J Antimicrob Chemother 1976;2:115–157.

243. Tang LM, Chen ST. *Klebsiella pneumoniae* meningitis: prognostic factors. Scand J Infect Dis 1994:26:95–102.

244. Tang LM, Chen ST. *Klebsiella ozaenae* meningitis: report of two cases and review of the literature. Infection 1994;22:58–61.

245. Terman JW, Alford RH, Bryant RE. Hospital-acquired *Klebsiella* bacteremia. Am J Med Sci 1972;264:191–196.

246. Thauvin-Eliopoulos C, Tripodi F, Cole G, Moellering RC, Eliopoulos GM. Efficacies of piperacillin-tazobactam and cefepime in rats with experimental intra-abdominal abscesses due to an extended-spectrum beta-lactamase-producing strain of *Klebsiella pneumoniae.* Antimicrob Agents Chemother 1997; 41:1053–1057.

247. Thomas MG, Rowland-Jones S, Smyth E. *Klebsiella pneumoniae* endocarditis. J R Soc Med 1989;82:114–115.

248. Thomson KS, Weber DA, Sanders CC, Sanders WE. Beta-lactamase production in members of the family *Enterobacteriaceae* and resistance to beta-lactam-enzyme inhibitor combinations. Antimicrob Agents Chemother 1990;34:622–627.

249. Toye BW, Scriver SR, Low DE. Canadian survey of antimicrobial resistance in *Klebsiella* spp. And *Enterobacter* spp. The Canadian Antimicrobial Resistance Study Group. J Antimicrob Chemother 1993;32(Suppl B):81–86.

250. Trautmann M, Bruckner O, Marre R, Hahn H. Comparative efficacy of ciprofloxacin, ceftazidime and gentamicin, given alone or in combination, in a model of experimental septicemia due to *Klebsiella pneumoniae* in neutropenic mice. Infection 1988;16:49–53.

251. Trautmann M, Held T, Ruhnke M, Schnoy N. A case of rhinoscleroma cured by ciprofloxacin. Infection 1993;21: 403–406.

252. Trenholme GM, Schmitt BA, Spear J, Gvazdinskas LC, Levin S. Randomized study of intravenous/oral ciprofloxacin versus ceftazidime in the treatment of hospital and nursing home patients with lower respiratory tract infections. Am J Med 1989; 87:116S–118S.

253. Tsai YH, Bies M, Leitner F, Kessler RE. Therapeutic studies of cefepime (BMY 28142) in murine meningitis and pharmacokinetics in neonatal rats. Antimicrob Agents Chemother 1990; 34:733–738.

254. Tsuji M, Ishii Y, Ohno A, Miyazaki S, Yamaguchi K. In vitro and in vivo antibacterial activities of S-1090, a new oral cephalosporin. Antimicrob Agents Chemother 1995;39:2544–2551.

255. Tsuji A, Kaneko Y, Yamaguchi K, Goto S. Correlation between the in vitro and in vivo effects of fourteen beta-lactam compounds in mice with systemic infection. Chemotherapy 1994; 40:324–332.

256. Tunkel AR, Scheld WM. Acute meningitis. In: Mandell GL, Bennett JE, Dolin R, eds. Principles and practice of infectious diseases. 4th ed. New York: Churchill Livingstone, 1995.

257. Tzouvelekis LS, Tzelepi E, Mentis AF, Tsakris A. Identification of a novel plasmid-mediated beta-lactamase with chromosomal cephalosporinase characteristics from *K. pneumoniae.* J Antimicrob Chemother 1993;31:645–654.

258. Umsawasdi T, Middleman EA, Luna M, Bodey GP. *Klebsiella* bacteremia in cancer patients. Am J Med Sci 1973;265: 473–482.

259. Unhanand M, Mustafa MM, McCracken GH, Nelson JD. Gram-negative enteric bacillary meningitis: a twenty-one year experience. J Pediatr 1993;122:15–21.

260. van den Broek PJ. Antimicrobial drugs, microorganisms, and phagocytes. Rev Infect Dis 1989;11:213–245.

261. Van der Auwera P, Duchateau V, Lambert C, Husson M, Kinzig M, Sorgel F. Ex vivo pharmacodynamic study of piperacillin alone and in combination with tazobactam, compared with ticarcillin plus clavulanic acid. Antimicrob Agents Chemother 1993;37:1860–1868.

262. Van der Auwera P, Klastersky J, Lieppe S, Husson M, Lauzon D, Lopez AP. Bactericidal activity and killing rate of serum from volunteers receiving pefloxacin alone or in combination with amikacin. Antimicrob Agents Chemother 1986;29:230–234.

263. Van Laethem Y, Lagast H, Klastersky J. Serum bactericidal activity of ceftazidime and cefoperazone alone or in combination with amikacin against *Pseudomonas aeruginosa* and *Klebsiella pneumoniae.* Antimicrob Agents Chemother 1983;23:435–439.

264. Verbist L. In vitro activity of piperacillin, a new semisynthetic penicillin with an unusually broad spectrum of activity. Antimicrob Agents Chemother 1978;13:349–357.

265. Wallace AG, Young G, Osterhout S. Treatment of acute bacterial endocarditis by valve excision and replacement. Circulation 1965;31:450–453.

266. Walstad R, Blika S, Nielsen E, Halvorsen T. The penetration of ceftazidime into the inflamed rabbit eye. Scand J Infect Dis 1987;19:131–135.

267. Wang LS, Lee FY, Cheng DL, Liu CY, Hinthorn DR, Jost PM. *Klebsiella pneumoniae* bacteremia: analysis of 100 episodes. J Formosan Med Assoc 1990;89:756–763.

268. Watanakunakorn C. *Klebsiella oxytoca* endocarditis after transurethral resection of the prostate gland. South Med J 1985;78:356–357.

269. Watanakunakorn C, Jura J. *Klebsiella* bacteremia: a review of 196 episodes during a decade (1980–1989). Scand J Infect Dis 1991;23:399–405.

270. Weiss D, Trautmann M, Wagner J, Borner K, Hahn H. Ciprofloxacin: a comparative evaluation of its bactericidal activity in human serum against four enterobacterial species. Drugs Exp Clin Res 1986;12:889–894.

271. Wiblin RT. Nosocomial pneumonia. In: Wenzel RP, ed. Prevention and control of nosocomial infections. 3rd ed. Baltimore: Williams & Wilkins, 1997.

272. Wiedemann B, Zuhlsdorf M. Antibacterial properties of meropenem towards clinical isolates, beta-lactamase producers and laboratory mutants. J Antimicrob Chemother 1989;24(Suppl A):197–205.

273. Wise R, Andrews JM, Bedford KA. Clavulanic acid and CP-45,889: a comparison of their in vitro activity in combination with penicillins. J Antimicrob Chemother 1980;6:197–206.

274. Wise R, Pagella PG, Cacchetti V, Fravolini A, Tabarrini O. In vitro activity of MF 5137, a new potent 6-aminoquinolone. Drugs 1995;49(Suppl 2):272–273.

275. Woo KS, Lam YM, Kwok HT, Tse LK, Vallance-Owen J. Prognostic index in prediction of mortality from infective endocarditis. Int J Cardiol 1989;24:47–54.

276. Woodcock JM, Andrews JM, Boswell FJ, Brenwald NP, Wise R. In vitro activity of BAY 12–8039, a new fluoroquinolone. Antimicrob Agents Chemother 1997;41:101–106.

277. Zhang Y-Y, Wang F, Zhang J, Zhu D, Zhou L. In vitro antibacterial activity of levofloxacin. Drugs 1995;49(Suppl 2): 274–275.

278. Zinner SH, Klastersky J, Gaya H, Bernard C, Ryff JC. In vitro and in vivo studies of three antibiotic combinations against gram-negative bacteria and *Staphylococcus aureus.* Antimicrob Agents Chemother 1981;20:463–469.

Legionella Species

●

Emanuel N. Vergis and Victor L. Yu

GENERAL DESCRIPTION
Microbiology

Legionella are Gram-negative, aerobic, unencapsulated bacilli that are nutritionally fastidious, requiring special media for growth. *L. pneumophila* is responsible for up to 85% of cases of pneumonia, with the non-*pneumophila* species responsible for the remaining 15%. These include, in order of decreasing incidence, *L. micdadei, L. bozemanii, L. dumoffii,* and *L. longbeachae* (105).

Clinical Manifestations

Pneumonia is the predominant clinical manifestation due to *Legionella* infection. The symptomatic presentation is that of pneumonia and is nonspecific. However, prominent hallmarks of Legionnaires' disease are high fever (>40°C) and gastrointestinal symptoms including diarrhea. Hyponatremia (serum Na < 130 meq/L) occurs significantly more often in Legionnaires' disease than in pneumonia of other etiology. The heart is the most common extrapulmonary site of infection, with numerous reported cases of myocarditis, pericarditis, postcardiotomy syndrome, and prosthetic valve endocarditis (67). Other extrapulmonary manifestations occur rarely and include sinusitis, wound and soft tissue infection, pancreatitis, peritonitis, and pyelonephritis.

Pontiac fever is a nonpneumonic infection caused principally by *L. pneumophila* serogroup 1, but *L. pneumophila* serogroups 6 and 7, *L. feeleii,* and *L. micdadei* have also been implicated (114). Malaise, fatigue, and myalgias are the most common symptoms, and fever is the most common physical finding. The illness is self-limited and does not require antimicrobial treatment.

Laboratory

When reviewing antibiotic efficacy studies in humans, the method of diagnosis is critical in evaluating the credibility of the study. Isolation of the organism from culture on selective media is the gold standard. Diagnosis by direct fluorescent antibody stain of sputa or by urinary antigen is also acceptable. Diagnosis by a single elevated serologic result is weak, since this test may be nonspecific.

SUSCEPTIBILITY IN VITRO AND IN VIVO

Susceptibility results in vitro for *Legionella* spp. are not readily interpretable since no standardized method exists, and correlation between in vitro results and clinical outcome is tenuous and often contradictory. An interesting facet of *Legionella* susceptibility testing is that circumstantial evidence in early outbreaks of Legionnaires' disease suggested that erythromycin or tetracyclines were more effective than other antimicrobial agents; testing methodologies of in vitro susceptibility favored those methods that showed that erythromycin/tetracycline were more effective than β-lactam or aminoglycoside agents.

It is now accepted that the intracellular location of this pathogen is relevant to the efficacy of the antimicrobial agent. Antibiotics capable of achieving intracellular concentrations higher than the MIC were more likely to be clinically efficacious than antibiotics with inferior intracellular penetration (51). Susceptibility of *Legionella* species to antimicrobial drugs has been based on three laboratory methods: standard dilution testing in agar or broth, intracellular models in vitro, and animal models of *Legionella* infection.

Dilution Testing in Vitro

Dilutional methods for extracellular susceptibility testing are considered less relevant than other methods (intracellular in vitro, animal models), since many antibiotics that are active extracellularly perform poorly in intracellular models. However, extracellular susceptibility testing does provide a screening test to determine which antimicrobial agents are likely to have clinical potential. *Legionella* are grown either in supplemented buffered yeast extract (BYE) broth or in supplemented buffered charcoal–yeast extract agar (BCYE). Antimicrobial agents are added in increasing concentrations. MICs and MBCs are assessed after 1 to 5 days of incubation.

MIC determinations of antibiotics on BCYE agar may be up to tenfold those when BYE broth is used. This difference in MICs is due to the inhibitory effect of BCYE on antibiotic activity. Reasons postulated for this inhibitory effect include: (*a*) acid pH of the media, (*b*) iron content of the media, (*c*) absorption of the antibiotics by charcoal, or (*d*) the autoclaving process (25). Although buffered starch–yeast extract (BSYE) agar is less inhibitory than BCYE, growth is better, endpoints are easier to interpret, and results are more consistent for BCYE (86).

Intracellular Models in Vitro

Several in vitro intracellular models have been developed: guinea pig peritoneal or alveolar macrophages (26, 36, 59, 112), human peripheral blood monocytes and monocyte-derived macrophages (88, 110), human neutrophils (2), and tissue culture models using HeLa cells (44), MRC-5 human fetal lung fibroblast cells (101), and the macrophage-like cell lines U937 (89) and HL-60 (102). Antimicrobial agents are added to the *Legionella*-infected cells and the degree of inhibition of intracellular bacterial growth is determined by quantifying bacterial concentration (25). Subsequent removal of the antimicrobial agent and recording the time required for re-growth of the bacteria in the tissue or cell culture gives a measure of the intracellular activity of the antimicrobial agent. Edelstein classified antimicrobial agents as not inhibitory (growth of intracellular *L. pneumophila* occurs despite presence of antimicrobial agent), reversibly inhibitory (slow regrowth of *L. pneumophila* occurs after antimicrobial agent removal from the culture), or cidal or causing prolonged inhibition of growth after the antimicrobial agent is removed (29).

Animal Models of *Legionella*

Models of respiratory tract infections (15, 38, 111) and peritonitis (22, 32) have been developed. Pneumonia produced in animals is pathophysiologically more appealing than experimental *Legionella* infection induced by intraperitoneal inoculation. *Legionella* peritonitis results in localized infection without histopathologic evidence of disseminated (pulmonary, splenic, hepatic) disease (40). Antimicrobial agents presumed clinically effective (erythromycin, tetracycline) have been effective in the animal models, while those considered clinically ineffective (gentamicin, cefoxitin) are also inactive in animal models. Disadvantages of animal models include the differing pharmacokinetics in animals and humans and the expense and logistics involved.

Macrolides

Erythromycin

Erythromycin's apparent clinical success was bolstered by studies in experimental animals showing its superiority over other antibiotics including penicillin, tetracycline, chloramphenicol, and gentamicin. The fact that *Legionella* is an intracellular pathogen provided the biologic basis for the success of erythromycin given its relatively high intracellular penetration (50).

Legionella pneumophila was susceptible to erythromycin when tested by in vitro dilution methods (Tables 1 and 2). Growth of *L. pneumophila* was inhibited by erythromycin within guinea pig alveolar macrophages (26–31), guinea pig peritoneal macrophages (59), peripheral blood monocytes (18), human promyelocytic leukemic cells (HL-60) (102, 103), and macrophage-like cells (89). Erythromycin was also active in animal models of pneumonia (32, 96, 100) and guinea pig models of peritonitis (22, 40) (Table 3).

The non-*pneumophila* species were also susceptible to erythromycin when tested by in vitro dilution methods (Tables 1 and 2). Growth of *L. micdadei* and *L. bozemanii* within peripheral blood monocytes (18) and HL-60 cells (102, 103) was inhibited by erythromycin.

Azithromycin

Azithromycin appeared to be the most active macrolide in vitro against *Legionella* (Tables 1 and 2). By in vitro dilution methods, azithromycin was more active against *L. pneumophila* than erythromycin (54, 79, 102), clarithromycin (11), roxithromycin (11), and dirithromycin (54, 79, 102).

Azithromycin was more active than erythromycin, clarithromycin, roxithromycin, and dirithromycin in inhibiting the growth of *L. pneumophila* within HL-60 cells (102) and erythromycin in inhibiting growth within guinea pig alveolar macrophages (26). In two studies in a guinea pig model of *Legionella* pneumonia, azithromycin resulted in 100% survival, whereas erythromycin resulted in 33% survival, and no therapy resulted in 0% survival (37, 38). In a mouse model of pneumonia, azithromycin was superior to erythromycin in clearing *Legionella* (33).

For the non-*pneumophila* species, by in vitro dilution methods, azithromycin was more active than erythromycin (102), roxithromycin (54), and dirithromycin (54, 79, 102) (Tables 1 and 2). Azithromycin was more active than erythromycin in inhibiting the growth of *L. micdadei* within peripheral blood monocytes (18) and clarithromycin, roxithromycin, and dirithromycin within HL-60 cells (102).

Clarithromycin

In only a few in vitro dilution studies, clarithromycin was more active than azithromycin (54, 79, 102). Clarithromycin was more active in vitro dilution studies against *L. pneumophila* than roxithromycin and dirithromycin (54, 79, 102) (Tables 1 and 2).

In a guinea pig model of *Legionella* pneumonia, clarithromycin resulted in 100% survival, whereas no treatment resulted in 0% survival (38) (Table 3).

For the non-*pneumophila Legionella* species, by in vitro dilution methods, clarithromycin was more active than erythromycin, azithromycin, roxithromycin, and dirithromycin (54, 79, 102) (Tables 1 and 2). Clarithromycin was more active than azithromycin and roxithromycin in inhibiting the growth of *L. micdadei* and *L. bozemanii* within HL-60 cells (102).

Roxithromycin

In only a few in vitro dilution studies, roxithromycin was more active than azithromycin (54, 79, 102). Roxithromycin was more active in vitro against *L. pneumophila* than erythromycin, dirithromycin (54, 59, 79, 102), and josamycin (60) (Tables 1 and 2).

Roxithromycin was more active than erythromycin, clarithromycin, and dirithromycin in inhibiting the growth of *L. pneumophila* within guinea pig peritoneal macrophages (59) and HL-60 cells (102). In a guinea pig model of *Legionella* pneumonia, roxithromycin was more active than either erythromycin or josamycin, resulting in 80% survival compared with 40 and 20% survival for erythromycin and josamycin, respectively (60) (Table 3).

For the non-*pneumophila Legionella* species, by in vitro dilution methods, roxithromycin was more active than erythromycin, azithromycin, dirithromycin (54, 79, 102), and josamycin (60) (Tables 1 and 2). Roxithromycin was active in inhibiting the growth of *L. micdadei* and *L. bozemanii* within HL-60 cells (102).

Dirithromycin

In in vitro dilution methods, dirithromycin was less active against *L. pneumophila* than erythromycin, clarithromycin, azithromycin, and roxithromycin (54, 79, 102) (Tables 1 and 2).

TABLE 1 • Susceptibility of *Legionella* spp. to Antimicrobial Agents by in Vitro Agar Dilution Method

Species	MIC$_{50}$ (μg/mL)	MIC$_{90}$ (μg/mL)	MIC Range (μg/mL)	References
Erythromycin				
L. pneumophila (serogroups 1–8)	0.015–1.0	0.03–2.0	0.008–1.0	(11, 22, 23, 26, 41, 79)
Legionella spp.	0.10–0.50	0.25–1.0	<0.0015–2.0	(11, 23, 26, 28, 32, 45, 55)
L. micdadei	0.06–1.0	0.25	0.06–0.25	(11, 18, 23, 45, 54)
L. bozemanii	0.12–2.0	—	—	(11, 45, 54)
L. dumoffii	0.25	0.50	0.25–0.50	(23, 45, 54)
L. longbeachae	0.25–1.0	0.50	0.008–0.50	(11, 23, 79)
L. gormanii	0.12	—	—	(45, 54)
Azithromycin				
Legionella spp.	0.03–0.50	0.06–2.0	0.016–4.0	(11, 26, 54)
L. pneumophila (serogroups 1, 2, 5, 6)	0.06–1.5	0.50–1.0	0.03–2.0	(11, 26, 38, 79)
L. longbeachae	0.50–1.0	0.50	0.06–0.50	(11, 79)
L. micdadei	0.12–1.0	—	—	(11, 18, 54)
L. bozemanii	0.50–1.0	—	—	(11, 54)
L. dumoffii	0.25	—	—	(54)
L. gormanii	0.25	—	—	(54)
Clarithromycin				
Legionella spp.	0.016–0.25	0.06–2.0	≤0.016–2.0	(11, 54)
L. pneumophila (serogroups 1, 2, 5, 6)	0.03–0.5	00.06–2.0	0.03–2.0	(11, 38, 79)
L. longbeachae	0.12–0.25	0.12	0.03–0.25	(11, 79)
L. micdadei	0.12–0.50	—	—	(11, 54)
L. bozemanii	0.12–0.50	—	—	(11, 54)
L. dumoffii	0.12	—	—	(54)
L. gormanii	0.12	—	—	(54)
14-OH Clarithromycin				
Legionella spp.	0.06	0.12	0.03–0.50	(54)
L. micdadei	0.12	—	—	(54)
L. bozemanii	0.06	—	—	(54)
L. dumoffii	0.12	—	—	(54)
Dirithromycin				
Legionella spp.	1.0	4.0	0.25–4.0	(54)
L. pneumophila (serogroups 1, 2, 5)	0.50	8.0	0.25–8.0	(79)
L. longbeachae	8.0	8.0	0.25–16	(79)
L. bozemanii	2.0	—	—	(54)
L. dumoffii	4.0	—	—	(54)
L. gormanii	1.0	—	—	(54)
Josamycin				
Legionella spp.	0.25–0.50	0.25–1.0	0.0625–1.0	(96)
L. pneumophila	—	—	0.25–0.50	(96)
L. micdadei	—	—	≤0.0313–0.50	(96)
L. bozemanii	—	—	0.125–0.50	(96)
L. dumoffii	—	—	0.125–0.50	(96)
L. longbeachae (*serogroups 1, 2*)	—	—	≤0.0313–0.25	(96)
L. gormanii	—	—	≤0.0313–0.0625	(96)
L. jordanis	—	—	≤0.0313–0.5	(96)
L. wadsworthii	—	—	*0.125–0.50*	(96)
Roxithromycin				
Legionella spp.	0.06–0.25	0.125–1.0	0.016–2.0	(11)
L. pneumophila (serogroups 1, 2, 5, 6)	0.12–0.50	0.25–2.0	0.06–2.0	(11, 59, 79)
L. longbeachae	0.06–0.50	0.50	0.12–0.50	(11, 79)
L. micdadei	0.125–1.0	—	—	(11)
L. bozemanii	0.12–0.25	—	—	(11, 54)
L. dumoffii	0.12	—	—	(54)
L. gormanii	0.25	—	—	(54)
Ciprofloxacin				
L. longbeachae	≤0.004–1.0	0.01–0.06	≤0.004–0.06	(11, 23, 79)
L. pneumophila (serogroups 1–8)	≤0.03–2.0	0.01–2.0	≤0.004–4.0	(11, 23, 26, 41, 79)
Legionella spp.	0.01–1.0	0.03–2.0	≤0.004–4.0	(11, 23, 26, 32, 45, 54, 55)
L. micdadei	0.01–1.0	0.03	0.01–0.03	(11, 23, 45, 54)
L. dumoffii	0.01–0.06	0.03	0.01–0.03	(23, 45, 54)
L. bozemanii	0.015–1.0	—	—	(11, 45, 54)
L. gormanii	0.03	—	—	(45, 54)

continued

TABLE 1 • Susceptibility of *Legionella* spp. to Antimicrobial Agents by in Vitro Agar Dilution Method

Species	MIC$_{50}$ (μg/mL)	MIC$_{90}$ (μg/mL)	MIC Range (μg/mL)	References
Enoxacin				
L. pneumophila	0.125	—	—	(12)
Fleroxacin				
Legionella spp.	0.06	0.06	0.005–0.06	(45)
L. micdadei	0.03	—	—	(45)
L. bozemanii	0.03	—	—	(45)
L. dumoffii	0.03	—	—	(45)
L. gormanii	0.03	—	—	(45)
Grepafloxacin				
Legionella spp.	0.015	0.015	0.008–0.03	(91)
Levofloxacin				
L. pneumophila	0.03	—	—	(12)
Lomefloxacin				
Legionella spp.	0.06	0.12	0.03–0.12	(45)
L. micdadei	0.03–0.06	—	—	(45)
L. bozemanii	0.06	—	—	(45)
L. dumoffii	0.12	—	—	(45)
L. gormaii	0.03	—	—	(45)
Ofloxacin				
L. pneumophila	0.015–0.03	0.015	0.015	(12, 41, 59)
L. micdadei	0.03–0.06	—	—	(45)
L. bozemanii	0.03	—	—	(45)
L. dumoffii	0.06	—	—	(45)
L. gormanii	0.03	—	—	(45)
Pefloxacin				
L. pneumophila (serogroup 1)	0.50	—	—	(22)
Rufloxacin				
L. pneumophila	0.12	0.25	0.06–0.25	(41)
Sparfloxacin				
L. pneumophila (serogroups 1–8)	≤0.004	≤0.004	≤0.004–0.01	(23, 32, 55)
L. micdadei	≤0.004	≤0.004	≤0.004	(23)
Legionella spp.	≤0.004–0.50	0.008–1.0	≤0.004–2.0	(23, 55)
L. dumoffii	0.01	0.01	0.008–0.01	(23)
L. longbeachae	0.008	0.01	≤0.004–0.01	(23)
Trovafloxacin				
L. pneumophila (serogroups 1–8)	≤0.004	<0.004	≤0.004–0.008	(23)
L. micdadei	≤0.004	<0.004	≤0.004	(23)
L. dumoffii	≤0.004	<0.004	≤0.004–0.008	(23)
L. longbeachae	≤0.004	<0.004	≤0.004	(23)
Legionella spp.	≤0.004	<0.004	≤0.004	(23)
Amoxicillin				
L. pneumophila (serogroups 1, 2, 5)	0.25–0.50	2.0	0.12–2.0	(79)
L. longbeachae	0.50–1.0	>2.0	0.25–2.0	(79)
Amoxicillin/clavulanate				
L. pneumophila (serogroups 1, 2, 5)	0.06–0.25	0.25	0.06–0.50	(79)
L. longbeachae	0.25–0.50	1.0	0.25–1.0	(79)
Piperacillin/tazobactam				
L. longbeachae	0.06	0.12	0.015–0.12	(79)
L. pneumophila (serogroups 1, 2, 5)	0.25	0.50	0.06–0.50	(79)
Imipenem				
L. longbeachae	≤0.03	0.03	0.015–0.06	(11, 79)
L. pneumophila (serogroups 1, 2, 5, 6)	0.03–0.125	0.06	≤0.015–0.25	(11, 79)
Legionella spp.	0.03–0.50	0.06–1.0	≤0.03–2.0	(11, 45)
L. micdadei	0.125–0.25	—	—	(11, 45)
L. bozemanii	0.25–1.0	—	—	(11, 45)
L. dumoffii	4.0	—	—	(45)
Imipenem				
L. gormanii	1.0	—	—	(45)
Meropenem				
Legionella spp.	≤0.06	0.12	≤0.06–0.125	(54)
L. micdadei	≤0.06	—	—	(54)
L. bozemanii	≤0.06	—	—	(54)
L. dumoffii	0.12	—	—	(54)
L. gormanii	0.12	—	—	(54)

continued

TABLE 1 • Susceptibility of *Legionella* spp. to Antimicrobial Agents by in Vitro Agar Dilution Method

Species	MIC$_{50}$ (μg/mL)	MIC$_{90}$ (μg/mL)	MIC Range (μg/mL)	References
Rifampicin				
Legionella spp.	≤0.002–0.03	≤0.002–0.03	≤0.002–0.03	(11, 23, 45, 54, 55)
L. pneumophila (serogroups 1–8)	≤0.002–0.004	≤0.004–0.008	≤0.0004–0.008	(11, 23, 59, 79)
L. micdadei	0.008	0.008	0.008	(11, 23, 45, 54)
L. dumoffii	0.008–0.015	0.01	≤0.004–0.03	(11, 23, 45, 54)
L. longbeachae	≤0.002–0.004	0.01	≤0.004–0.01	(11, 23, 79)
L. bozemanii	≤0.002–0.004	—	—	(11, 23, 45, 54)
L. gormanii	0.015	—	—	(45, 54)
Clindamycin				
Legionella spp.	4.0	8.0	2.0->8.0	(54)
L. micdadei	4.0–8.0	—	—	(54)
L. bozemanii	4.0	—	—	(54)
L. dumoffii	4.0	—	—	(54)
L. gormanii	4.0	—	—	(54)
Trimethoprim/sulfamethoxazole				
Legionella spp.	0.50	0.50	≤0.03–1.0	(54)
L. micdadei	0.50	—	—	(54)
L. bozemanii	≤0.03	—	—	(54)
L. dumoffii	≤0.03	—	—	(54)
L. gormanii	≤0.03	—	—	(54)
Doxycycline				
Legionella spp.	1.0	2.0	0.12–2.0	(54)
L. micdadei	0.12–0.25	—	—	(54)
L. bozemanii	1.0	—	—	(54)
L. dumoffii	1.0	—	—	(54)
L. gormanii	2.0	—	—	(54)
Tetracycline				
Legionella spp.	8.0	8.0	1.0->8.0	(54)
L. micdadei	0.25–1.0	—	—	(54)
L. bozemanii	4.0	—	—	(54)
L. dumoffii	4.0	—	—	(54)
L. gormanii	4.0	—	—	(54)

Dirithromycin was less active than erythromycin, azithromycin, and roxithromycin in inhibiting growth of *L. pneumophila* within HL-60 cells (102).

For the non-*pneumophila Legionella* species, by in vitro dilution methods, dirithromycin was less active than erythromycin, clarithromycin, azithromycin, and roxithromycin (54, 79, 102) (Tables 1 and 2). Dirithromycin was more active than clarithromycin, roxithromycin, and azithromycin in inhibiting growth of *L. micdadei* and *L. bozemanii* within HL-60 cells (102).

Josamycin

In in vitro dilution studies, josamycin was less active than erythromycin and roxithromycin (60, 96) against *L. pneumophila* (Tables 1 and 2).

In a guinea pig model of pneumonia, josamycin (20% survival) was more active than no treatment (0% survival) but less active than erythromycin (40% survival) and roxithromycin (80% survival) (60) (Table 3). In another guinea pig model of pneumonia, josamycin was the least active agent studied, resulting in 0% survival; erythromycin, rifampin, and ofloxacin resulted in 60, 90, and 100% survival, respectively (96) (Table 3).

For the non-*pneumophila Legionella* species, by in vitro dilution methods, josamycin was less active than erythromycin and roxithromycin (60, 96) (Tables 1 and 2).

Quinolones

Quinolone agents were more active than all macrolides by all in vitro and in vivo methods. Ciprofloxacin, enfloxacin, grepafloxacin, levofloxacin, ofloxacin, pefloxacin, rufloxacin, sparfloxacin, and trovafloxacin were all active by in vitro dilution methods (Tables 1 and 2).

The quinolones were more active than erythromycin in irreversibly inhibiting the growth of *L. pneumophila* within guinea pig alveolar macrophages (30–32), peripheral blood monocytes (96), guinea pig peritoneal macrophages (59), and HL-60 cells (103).

Ciprofloxacin, levofloxacin, pefloxacin, sparfloxacin, and trovafloxacin were more active than erythromycin or no therapy in guinea pig models of pneumonia (30–32, 94–96) and of peritonitis (22) (Table 3).

For the non-*pneumophila Legionella* species, by in vitro dilution methods, ciprofloxacin, fleroxacin, grepafloxacin, lomefloxacin, sparfloxacin, temafloxacin, and trovafloxacin were more active than erythromycin (23, 54, 79, 95, 96, 103), clarithromycin (54, 79, 91), azithromycin (54, 79), roxithromycin (54), dirithromycin (54), and josamycin (96) (Tables 1 and 2). Ciprofloxacin, levofloxacin, and ofloxacin were more active than erythromycin in inhibiting intracellular growth of *L. micdadei* and *L. bozemanii* within HL-60 cells (103).

TABLE 2 • **Susceptibility of** *Legionella* **spp. to Antimicrobial Agents by in Vitro Broth Dilution Method**

Species	MIC$_{50}$ (μg/mL)	MIC$_{90}$ (μg/mL)	MIC Range (μg/mL)	References
Erythromycin				
L. pneumophila	0.125–0.25	0.37–0.408	<0.062–1.0	(26, 28, 32, 41, 59, 90, 102)
Legionella spp.	0.06	0.10	≤0.06–0.50	(26, 28)
L. micdadei	—	—	1.0	(18, 102)
L. bozemanii	—	—	0.25	(18, 102)
Azithromycin				
L. pneumophila	0.06–1.39	1.65–2.77	0.12–7.80	(26, 90, 102)
L. micdadei	—	—	0.50	(102)
L. bozemanii	—	—	0.25q	(102)
Clarithromycin				
L. pneumophila	0.007	0.008–0.013	<0.001–0.125	(90, 102)
L. micdadei	—	—	0.125	(102)
L. bozemanii	—	—	0.03	(102)
Dirithromycin				
L. pneumophila	—	—	0.50–8.0	(102)
L. micdadei	—	—	4.0	(102)
L. bozemanii	—	—	8.0	(102)
Roxithromycin				
L. pneumophila	0.0625	—	0.06–0.25	(59, 102)
L. micdadei	—	—	1.0	(102)
L. bozemanii	—	—	0.125	(102)
Ciprofloxacin				
Legionella spp.	0.016	0.032	0.008–0.032	(26, 30)
L. pneumophila serogroup 1	0.0079–0.06	—	—	(26, 32, 59, 90)
Levofloxacin				
Legionella spp	0.016	0.032	0.008–0.032	(30)
Ofloxacin				
Legionella spp	0.032	0.064	0.016–0.064	(30, 59)
L. pneumophila (serogroup 1)	0.157	—	—	(30, 59)
Sparfloxacin				
L. pneumophila (serogroup 1)	≤0.003	—	—	(32)
Piperacillin				
L. pneumophila (serogroup 1)	0.25	—	—	(59)
Imipenem				
L. pneumophila (serogroup 1)	0.0157	—	—	(59)
Rifampicin				
L. pneumophila	0.0000043–0.001	0.000012–0.0028	<0.001–0.062	(59, 90)
Doxycycline				
L. pneumophila	1.76–2.48	3.65–4.95	0.24–31.25	(90)
Minocycline				
L. pneumophila (serogroup 1)	0.0313	—	—	(59)

Rifampicin (Rifampin)

Rifampicin is highly active in vitro against *Legionella* when tested by in vitro dilution methods (Tables 1 and 2). Using in vitro dilution methods, rifampicin was more active than macrolides (11, 23, 45, 54, 59, 79, 90, 91, 95, 96, 110), quinolones (11, 23, 45, 54, 59, 79, 90, 91, 95, 96, 110), β-lactam agents with or without β-lactamase inhibitors (59, 79), carbapenems (11, 45, 54, 59, 79), tetracyclines (45, 54, 59, 90), aminoglycosides (59), clindamycin (54), and trimethoprim-sulfamethoxazole against *L. pneumophila* (54) (Tables 1 and 2).

Rifampicin was more active than erythromycin, quinolones, β-lactams, carbapenems, and gentamicin in inhibiting growth of *L. pneumophila* within guinea pig peritoneal macrophages (59) and erythromycin, pefloxacin, cefoxitin, doxycycline, and trimethoprim-sulfamethoxazole within monocytes (110). In a guinea pig model of pneumonia, rifampicin was more active than ofloxacin, erythromycin, josamycin, and no treatment, resulting in 100% survival, compared with 0 to 90% for the other agents (96) (Table 3). In another guinea pig model of pneumonia, rifampicin was less active, resulting in 62.5% survival,

TABLE 3 • **Activity of Antimicrobial Agents in in Vivo Animal Model**

Species	Antimicrobials	Animal Model	Effect	References
L. pneumophila serogroup 1	Erythromycin	Guinea pig pneumonia	10–90% survival	(32, 60, 81, 94, 96)
		Guinea pig peritonitis	33–100% survival	(20, 40)
		Rat pneumonia	Significant decrease in bacterial load in lung	(100)
	Azithromycin	Guinea pig pneumonia	100% survival	(38)
	Clarithromycin	Guinea pig pneumonia	100% survival	(38)
	Josamycin	Guinea pig pneumonia	0–20% survival	(60, 96)
	Ciprofloxacin	Guinea pig pneumonia	50–80% survival	(94, 95)
	Levofloxacin	Guinea pig pneumonia	100% survival	(30)
	Ofloxacin	Guinea pig pneumonia	70–100% survival	(30, 31, 94, 96)
	Pefloxacin	Guinea pig peritonitis	100% survival	(22)
		Guinea pig pneumonia	87.5% survival	(81)
	Sparfloxacin	Guinea pig pneumonia	100% survival	(32, 94)
	Trovafloxacin	Guinea pig pneumonia	100% survival	(31)
L. pneumophila serogroup 1	Rifampicin	Guinea pig pneumonia	62.5–90% survival	(81, 96)
		Guinea pig peritonitis	67–100% survival	(100)
	Amoxicillin/ clavulanate	Rat pneumonia	Significant decrease in bacterial load in lung	(100)
	Ticarcillin/ clavulanate	Rat pneumonia	Significant decrease in bacterial load in lung	(100)
	Amoxicillin	Rat pneumonia	No decrease in bacterial load in lung	(100)
	Ticarcillin	Rat pneumonia	No decrease in bacterial load in lung	(100)
	Minocycline	Guinea pig pneumonia	75–87.5% survival	(81)
		Guinea pig peritonitis	33–67% survival	(77)
	Doxycycline	Guinea pig pneumonia	75% survival	(81)
	Tetracycline	Guinea pig peritonitis	17% survival	(40)
	Chloramphenicol	Guinea pig peritonitis	33% survival	(40)
	Penicillin	Guinea pig peritonitis	0% survival	(40)
	Aminoglycosides	Guinea pig peritonitis	0–33% survival	(40, 77)
L. micdadei	Erythromycin	Guinea pig pneumonia	70% survival	(84)
	Rifampicin	Guinea pig pneumonia	60% survival	(84)
	Trimethoprim- sulfamethoxazole	Guinea pig pneumonia	60% survival	(84)
	Doxycycline	Guinea pig pneumonia	40% survival	(84)
	Penicillin	Guinea pig pneumonia	30% survival	(84)
	Cefazolin	Guinea pig pneumonia	30% survival	(84)
	Chloramphenicol	Guinea pig pneumonia	20% survival	(84)
	Gentamicin	Guinea pig pneumonia	20% survival	(84)
	Cefoxitin	Guinea pig pneumonia	0% survival	(84)

compared with 75 to 87.5% for pefloxacin, erythromycin, and the tetracyclines (81) (Table 3).

By in vitro dilution methods, rifampicin was more active than the macrolides and quinolones (23, 54, 79, 95, 96), β-lactam agents with or without β-lactamase inhibitors, carbapenems (54, 79), clindamycin, and trimethoprim-sulfamethoxazole (54) against the non-*pneumophila Legionella* species (Tables 1 and 2).

Combination therapy in vitro with rifampicin and other antimicrobial agents is discussed below.

Trimethoprim-Sulfamethoxazole

By in vitro dilution methods, trimethoprim-sulfamethoxazole was more active than azithromycin, dirithromycin, doxycycline, and clindamycin but less active than rifampicin, ciprofloxacin,

clarithromycin, roxithromycin, and meropenem against *L. pneumophila* (54) (Tables 1 and 2).

Trimethoprim-sulfamethoxazole was more active than doxycycline and cefoxitin in inhibiting growth of *L. pneumophila* within human monocyte-derived macrophages (110); however, it was less active than rifampicin, pefloxacin, and erythromycin in the same study.

For the non-*pneumophila Legionella* species, by in vitro dilution methods, trimethoprim-sulfamethoxazole was more active than the macrolides, ciprofloxacin, meropenem, doxycycline, and clindamycin (54) (Table 1). In a guinea pig model of *L. micdadei* pneumonia, trimethoprim-sulfamethoxazole was more active than erythromycin, rifampin, doxycycline, penicillin, chloramphenicol, gentamicin, cefazolin, cefoxitin, and no treatment, resulting in 60 to 100% survival, compared with to 0 to 90% survival for the other agents (84) (Table 3).

Tetracycline/ Doxycycline/Minocycline

The tetracyclines are the least active of the agents used for Legionnaires' disease when assessed by in vitro dilution methods (Tables 1 and 2). The tetracyclines were less active than the macrolides (54, 90, 110), quinolones (45, 54, 59, 90), rifampicin (45, 54, 59, 90, 110), carbapenems (45, 54, 59), and trimethoprim-sulfamethoxazole (54) (Tables 1 and 2).

Doxycycline was less active than rifampicin, erythromycin, pefloxacin, trimethoprim-sulfamethoxazole, and cefoxitin in inhibiting growth of *L. pneumophila* within monocytes (110). In a guinea pig model of *Legionella* pneumonia, doxycycline was more active than rifampicin, resulting in 75% survival, compared with 62.5% survival for rifampicin (81) (Table 3). In the same study, doxycycline was less active than pefloxacin and erythromycin (75 to 87.5% survival). In a guinea pig model of *Legionella* peritonitis, tetracycline was less active than erythromycin, rifampicin, chloramphenicol, and gentamicin, resulting in 17% survival compared with 33 to 100% survival for the other agents (40) (Table 3). In another guinea pig model of *Legionella* peritonitis, minocycline was more active than rifampicin, amikacin, tobramycin, gentamicin, and no treatment, resulting in 50% survival compared with 0 to 33% for the other agents (77) (Table 3).

For the non-*pneumophila Legionella* species (except *L. micdadei*), by in vitro dilution methods, doxycycline was less active than rifampicin, ciprofloxacin, macrolides, meropenem, and trimethoprim-sulfamethoxazole (54) (Tables 1 and 2). In a guinea pig model of *L. micdadei* pneumonia, doxycycline was more active than erythromycin, rifampicin, penicillin, gentamicin, chloramphenicol, cefazolin, cefoxitin or no treatment, resulting in 40 to 90% survival compared with to 0 to 70% survival for the other agents (84) (Table 3).

β-Lactam Agents

By in vitro dilution methods, amoxicillin (79), amoxicillin/ clavulanic acid (12, 79), piperacillin (59), piperacillin/ tazobactam (79), ceftazidime (59), and ceftizoxime (59) were more active than erythromycin, azithromycin, dirithromycin, and enoxacin against *L. pneumophila* (Tables 1 and 2).

However, ceftizoxime, ceftazidime, and piperacillin did not inhibit growth of *L. pneumophila* within guinea pig peritoneal macrophages (59), nor did ampicillin inhibit growth of *L. pneumophila* within a macrophage-like cell line (89). Ampicillin/ sulbactam inhibited growth of *L. pneumophila* within a macrophage-like cell line (89). In a rat model of pneumonia, amoxicillin/clavulanic acid and ticarcillin/ clavulanic acid (100) were more active than amoxicillin, ticarcillin, or no treatment in reducing the counts of *L. pneumophila* in the lungs of the animals (Table 3).

For the non-*pneumophila Legionella* species, by in vitro dilution methods, piperacillin/tazobactam (79) was more active than erythromycin, azithromycin, roxithromycin, and dirithromycin (Tables 1 and 2). However, amoxicillin/clavulanic acid, and amoxicillin (79) were less active than the macrolides against the non-*pneumophila Legionella* species (Tables 1 and 2).

Carbapenems

The carbapenems were active in vitro against *Legionella* when tested by the in vitro dilution method (Table 1) but less active than the quinolones and rifampin. Imipenem (45, 54, 59) and meropenem (54) were more active than the macrolides, β-lactam/β-lactamase inhibitors, doxycycline, gentamicin, and clindamycin against *Legionella* (Tables 1 and 2). Although imipenem was active by in vitro dilution methods, it was ineffective in a guinea pig model of pneumonia (24).

Clindamycin

Clindamycin is less active than the macrolides, quinolones, meropenem, and trimethoprim-sulfamethoxazole against the *Legionella* species (54) (Table 1).

Combination of Antimicrobial Agents in Vitro or in Vivo

Macrolide-Rifampicin

The combination of erythromycin and rifampicin was synergistic for two isolates of *L. pneumophila* in time-kill curve studies (6, 7). In a checkerboard method, the combination of erythromycin and rifampicin proved synergistic against 20% (4 of 20) *L. pneumophila* strains and was indifferent against the remainder (73). The combination of erythromycin and rifampicin was effective in reducing the number of rifampicin-resistant *Legionella* strains by both the checkerboard (73) and the time-kill curve method (7).

Quinolone-Rifampicin

The combination of ciprofloxacin and rifampicin was synergistic (time-kill curve) against one isolate of *L. pneumophila* (7). The combination of ciprofloxacin and rifampicin was indifferent against 80% (16 of 20) *L. pneumophila* strains in a checkerboard method (73). The combination of ciprofloxacin and rifampicin did not eradicate the rifampicin-resistant subpopulation of *L. pneumophila* (73). The combinations of levofloxacin and rifampicin and ofloxacin and rifampicin were synergistic (time-kill curve) (6).

Macrolide-Quinolone

Rapid bactericidal activity of the combination of erythromycin and ciprofloxacin was seen by time-kill curve analysis. The subpopulation of ciprofloxacin-resistant *L. pneumophila* was reduced (7). These results were similar to those obtained with the combination of erythromycin and rifampicin, raising the possibility of using ciprofloxacin with erythromycin if rifampicin was poorly tolerated (7). The combination of erythromycin and ciprofloxacin was indifferent (checkerboard) but was effective in reducing the subpopulations of ciprofloxacin- and erythromycin-resistant *L. pneumophila* (73).

The combinations of erythromycin and ciprofloxacin, erythromycin and levofloxacin, and clarithromycin and ciprofloxacin were additive or indifferent (checkerboard) against 12 to 79% of *L. pneumophila* isolates (68). The combinations of azithromycin and ciprofloxacin, azithromycin and levofloxacin, and clarithromycin (and its metabolite) and levofloxacin were synergistic or partially synergistic (checkerboard) against 6 to 47% of *L. pneumophila* isolates (68, 69).

The combinations of erythromycin and levofloxacin, erythromycin and ciprofloxacin, clarithromycin and levofloxa-cin, azithromycin and ciprofloxacin, azithromycin and levofloxacin, and clarithromycin and ciprofloxacin were synergistic or partially synergistic (checkerboard) against 14 to 28% of non-*pneumophila Legionella* isolates (68). These same combinations were additive or indifferent (checkerboard) against 4 to 42% of non-*pneumophila Legionella* isolates (68). No antagonism (checkerboard) was observed.

Macrolide–β-Lactam
By the time-kill curve method (7), the combination of erythromycin and amoxicillin reduced the colony count of *L. pneumophila* after 75 h of incubation to below the level of detection.

Quinolone-Cephalosporin
The combination of fleroxacin with desacetyl cefotaxime inhibited growth of *L. pneumophila* within guinea pig alveolar macrophages (27). A prolonged postantibiotic effect was observed with the combination.

ANTIMICROBIAL THERAPY
Macrolides

Erythromycin
Erythromycin was historically the drug of choice on the basis of retrospective review of *Legionella* outbreaks (4, 39, 58, 64). In the 1976 Philadelphia outbreak, the mortality rate was 11% (2 of 18) in patients treated with erythromycin compared with 28% (51 of 85) in patients treated with cephalothin, penicillins, aminoglycosides, or chloramphenicol (39). Mortality rates in those treated with erythromycin or tetracycline were on average half of those seen in untreated patients (24). Striking clinical improvement was apparent in 83% (5 of 6) of patients failing therapy with β-lactam antibiotics with or without aminoglycosides when therapy with erythromycin was initiated during an outbreak of Legionnaires' disease in Columbus, OH (4). A lower mortality rate has been observed in nosocomial Legionnaires' disease in patients treated with erythromycin than in those given other antibiotics (9, 57, 58). However, clinical and microbiologic failures of erythromycin therapy have been reported (19, 47, 83, 92, 108). Despite widespread use, emergence of resistance in vitro has not been seen for macrolides.

Erythromycin is generally a safe antibiotic. The principal toxicities of erythromycin are irritative such as dose-related gastrointestinal discomfort (abdominal cramps, nausea, vomiting, diarrhea) and thrombophlebitis at the infusion site (104). The large volume of normal saline infusate required for the 4-g dose can be problematic in patients with compromised left ventricular function or impaired renal ability. Symptomatic ototoxicity (tinnitus or hearing loss confirmed by audiograms) was documented in 21% (5 of 24) of patients with pneumonia receiving erythromycin at the 4-g dose, in 0% (0 of 6) receiving erythromycin at the 2-g dose and in 0% (0/15) receiving other antibiotics. Ototoxicity was significantly related to high peak concentration and high serum concentration time curve

(AUC) as a function of decreased total systemic clearance. Ototoxicity resolved in all patients within 6 to 14 days after discontinuation of therapy.

Azithromycin
In a series of noncomparative studies, 46 nonimmunosuppressed patients with community-acquired Legionnaires' disease diagnosed by serology (37 patients) or urinary antigen (9 patients) were treated with oral azithromycin (total dose, 1.5 g over 1–5 days). The authors reported a surprising 100% cure rate (62, 63, 76). Intravenous azithromycin (500 mg on day 1 and 250 mg daily for 13 days) initiated after clinical failure with trimethoprim-sulfamethoxazole, erythromycin, cefotaxime, and rifampicin resulted in clinical cure in a case report (19).

In a prospective, randomized trial, intravenous azithromycin (500 mg daily for 2–5 days) followed by oral drug (500 mg daily to complete a total of 10 days of therapy) resulted in 92% cure (11 of 12). The comparative regimen of cefuroxime plus erythromycin resulted in 88% cure (7 of 8). Diagnosis was confirmed by sputum culture, polymerase chain reaction, and fourfold seroconversion (109).

Clarithromycin
In one noncomparative study, oral clarithromycin (500–1000 mg twice daily for up to 27 days) was reportedly efficacious in patients with presumed Legionnaires' disease. However, interpretation was clouded by the uncertain criteria for diagnosis and the fact that most patients received prior or concurrent antibiotics with activity against *Legionella* (46).

In a prospective, randomized trial, intravenous clarithromycin (500 mg twice daily for 3–5 days) followed by oral drug (500 mg twice daily to complete a total of 10 days of therapy) resulted in 100% cure (6 of 6) of patients with serologically confirmed Legionnaires' disease. There were no cases of Legionnaires' disease in the comparative regimen of amoxicillin/clavulanic acid (42).

Dirithromycin
In a prospective, randomized trial, oral dirithromycin (500 mg daily for up to 18 days) and oral erythromycin resulted in 100% clinical improvement in three patients with serologic evidence of Legionnaires' disease (65). In a prospective, randomized multicenter trial, oral dirithromycin (500 mg daily for 10 to 14 days) resulted in 86% (12 of 14) cure in patients with serologic evidence of Legionnaires' disease. Oral erythromycin resulted in 70% (7 of 10) cure rate in patients with serologically confirmed Legionnaires' disease (53).

Josamycin
In one noncomparative trial of nonsevere community-acquired pneumonia, oral josamycin (1000 mg twice daily for 5 days) resulted in 100% (4 of 4) cure in patients with serologically confirmed Legionnaires' disease (70).

Roxithromycin
In a prospective, randomized trial, oral roxithromycin (150 mg twice daily for 10 to 14 days) resulted in 100% (2 of 2) cure in

patients with Legionnaires' disease (both patients had mixed infections with either *S. pneumonia* or *M. catarrhalis*). In the comparative regimen, oral sparfloxacin resulted in treatment failure in one patient with serologically confirmed Legionnaires' disease (82).

The macrolides have the potential of interacting with other drugs by interfering with their hepatic route of metabolism through the cytochrome P-450 enzyme system (85). An important drug interaction exists with tacrolimus (formerly FK-506) and cyclosporine, immunosuppressive agents used in solid organ transplants, whose metabolism is mediated by the cytochrome P-450 system. The 14-membered lactone ring of the macrolides complexes with the cytochrome P-450 3A isoenzymes thereby inactivating the metabolism of tacrolimus and cyclosporine. Azithromycin differs somewhat since it has a 15-membered ring structure and is known to not form complexes with the cytochrome P-450 3A isoenzymes. Azithromycin is therefore less likely to interfere with the metabolism of drugs that are hepatically metabolized through the cytochrome P-450 system; clinical studies have not yet been conducted to confirm this hypothesis (85).

Quinolones

Ciprofloxacin

Monotherapy with ciprofloxacin was described as clinically effective in 80% (8 of 10) of critically ill or immunocompromised patients with community- and nosocomially acquired Legionnaires' disease (108). In this same study, 40% (4 of 10) of the patients were initially unresponsive to treatment with erythromycin and rifampin, but treatment with ciprofloxacin resulted in clinical cure in 75% (3 of 4) of these nonresponders. Diagnosis of Legionnaires' disease was confirmed by direct immunofluorescence stain (DFA) and serology (108).

Anecdotal clinical reports have shown that therapy with ciprofloxacin is effective for Legionnaires' disease in solid organ transplant recipients receiving cyclosporine (49, 98, 99). Clinical failures of ciprofloxacin treatment have been reported in three cases in which a low dosage of 400 mg daily was given (61, 108).

Ofloxacin

Intravenous and oral ofloxacin have been used successfully in the treatment of Legionnaires' disease. In one noncomparative trial, intravenous ofloxacin (200 mg every 12 h for a minimum of 5 days) followed by oral drug (200 mg every 12 h for up to 29 days) cured a patient with Legionnaires' disease (diagnostic details not provided) (75). In another noncomparative study, oral ofloxacin (400 mg twice daily for 10 days) resulted in cure in a patient with serologically confirmed Legionnaires' disease (43). Clinical failure of ofloxacin treatment was reported in a human immunodeficiency virus (HIV)-infected patient receiving a low dosage of 200 mg twice daily (97).

Sparfloxacin

In four prospective, randomized trials, oral sparfloxacin (400 mg on day 1 followed by 200 mg daily for 10–14 days) resulted in 75% (3 of 4) cure in patients with serologically confirmed Legionnaires' disease. The comparative regimens (amoxicillin/clavulanic acid, amoxicillin, amoxicillin plus ofloxacin, erythromycin) resulted in 59% (10 of 17) cure in patients with serologically confirmed Legionnaires' disease (3, 66, 82, 87).

In a prospective, randomized trial, oral sparfloxacin (400 mg on day 1 followed by 200 mg daily for up to 10 days) yielded a bacteriologic response in two patients with Legionnaires' disease, diagnosed by a positive sputum culture in one patient and by a positive urinary antigen in the other (17).

Trovafloxacin

In two prospective, randomized trials of intravenous alatrofloxacin (prodrug of trovafloxacin; 200 mg daily for 2–7 days) followed by oral trovafloxacin (200 mg daily to complete a total of 7 to 14 days of therapy), resulted in 77% (10 of 13) cure of patients with serologically confirmed Legionnaires' disease. The comparative regimens (intravenous ciprofloxacin plus ampicillin followed by oral ciprofloxacin plus amoxicillin, ceftriaxone followed by oral cefpodoxime) resulted in 86% (12 of 14) cure of the patients with serologically confirmed Legionnaires' disease. The cure rates were not significantly different.

Levofloxacin

In a prospective, randomized trial, intravenous and/or oral levofloxacin (500 mg daily for 7–14 days) resulted in 80% cure (4 of 5) in patients with serologically confirmed Legionnaires' disease (35). The control regimen of ceftriaxone and/or cefuroxime axetil with or without erythromycin or doxycycline resulted in 67% (2 of 3) cure in patients with serologically confirmed Legionnaires' disease.

Grepafloxacin

In one open-label, noncomparative trial, oral grepafloxacin (600 mg daily for 10 days) resulted in 100% (13 of 13) cure in patients with serologically confirmed *Legionella* pneumonia (107).

Fleroxacin

In a prospective, randomized trial, oral fleroxacin (400 mg daily for 10 days) resulted in 100% (3/3) cure in patients with serologically confirmed Legionnaires' disease. The comparative regimen, oral doxycycline, resulted in 100% (1 of 1) cure in a patient with serologically confirmed Legionnaires' disease (80).

Rifampicin (Rifampin)

Rifampicin monotherapy has been discouraged because of theoretical concerns about emergence of resistance to the drug during therapy. In a retrospective review of cases of severe Legionnaires' disease, addition of rifampicin (1200–2400 mg daily) to erythromycin resulted in a mortality rate of 25% (5 of 20), compared with a mortality rate of 35% (7 of 20) in patients treated with erythromycin alone (21). In the same study, combination therapy with erythromycin, rifampicin, and/or pefloxacin resulted in a mortality rate of 15% (3 of 20), suggesting that addition of rifampicin to anti-*Legionella* antibiotics may improve clinical outcome. On the other hand, in a retrospective study, 15 patients with Legionnaires' disease were treated with a combination of erythromycin and rifampicin (300–600 mg twice daily) resulting in a cure rate of 67% (10 of 15), whereas erythromycin alone yielded a comparable cure rate of 80% (12 of 15) (52); however, patients who are more severely ill are likely to receive combination therapy.

Anecdotal reports show that addition of rifampicin to erythromycin may improve the clinical outcome of *L. bozemanii* infection in immunosuppressed patients (34).

Trimethoprim-Sulfamethoxazole

There are anecdotal reports of treatment success with trimethoprim-sulfamethoxazole in two patients with nosocomial Legionnaires' disease (58) and in one patient failing therapy with erythromycin and rifampin (92). High-dose trimethoprim-sulfamethoxazole (400 mg trimethoprim and 200 g sulfamethoxazole by mouth every 8 h) appeared effective in two nosocomial cases of Legionnaires' disease (58). One patient who failed erythromycin plus rifampin was successfully treated with two double-strength tablets (a total of 320 mg trimethoprim and 1600 mg sulfamethoxazole) (92).

Tetracyclines

In the 1976 Philadelphia outbreak, the mortality rate was 10% (3 of 30) in patients who were treated with tetracycline (500 mg four times a day), compared with 11% (2 of 18) for erythromycin, 23% (16 of 71) for penicillins, 30% (3 of 10) for chloramphenicol, 41% (20 of 49) for cephalothin, and 36% (9 of 25) for aminoglycosides (39). Oral tetracycline (500 mg four times a day) resulted in rapid resolution of fever within 3 days of commencing therapy in a patient with Legionnaires' disease—a response comparable to that observed with erythromycin (72).

Therapy with tetracycline (2 g/day) was effective in curing one patient with relapsing Legionnaires' disease after three separate episodes had failed to respond to treatment with β-lactam antibiotics and aminoglycosides (1).

In a prospective, randomized trial, oral doxycycline (100 mg twice daily for 10 days) resulted in 100% (1 of 1) cure in a patient with serologically confirmed Legionnaires' disease (80). The comparative regimen of oral fleroxacin resulted in 100% (3 of 3) cure in patients with serologically confirmed Legionnaires' disease.

Two case reports document the effectiveness of doxycycline therapy (200–400 mg/day) for Legionnaires' disease that was initially unresponsive to β-lactam antibiotics and cephalosporins (14, 56).

Addition of intravenous tetracycline (dose and duration not known) was effective therapy for pneumonia due to *L. bozemanii* initially unresponsive to erythromycin (93).

Clindamycin

Intravenous clindamycin (900 mg every 6 h) was successful in treating cavitary disease in an immunosuppressed patient with Legionnaires' disease (10).

β-Lactam Agents

Based on retrospective review of outbreaks of Legionnaires' disease in Philadelphia in 1976, Columbus, OH, in 1977, and Los Angeles in 1977–78, antibiotics such as ampicillin, penicillin, and cephalothin as well as other cephalosporins were relatively ineffective (4, 39, 58). Numerous anecdotal case reports have also demonstrated the relative lack of clinical efficacy of penicillins (penicillin, piperacillin) and cephalosporins (cephaloridine, cephalothin) in treating Legionnaires' disease (1, 10, 14, 56).

Failures of ticarcillin and ampicillin therapy for infection with *L. micdadei* (92) and of cefamandole for *L. bozemanii* pneumonia (93) have been reported. Progressive disease due to *L. maceachernii* was reported, despite treatment with ampicillin, flucloxacillin, and imipenem (71).

Several case reports describe failure of β-lactam/β-lactamase inhibitor combinations including amoxicillin-clavulanic acid (19, 48, 61), ticarcillin-clavulanic acid, and ampicillin-sulbactam (29).

Carbapenems

Imipenem was reported to be effective in treatment of Legionnaires' disease in several anecdotal reports (8, 13). Successful treatment of four patients with serologically confirmed Legionnaires' disease with imipenem in a pilot study was reported (8). However, clinical failures of imipenem have occurred (5, 71, 113).

Drug of Choice

The new macrolides, especially azithromycin, have displaced erythromycin as the macrolide of choice. The new macrolides have more potent intracellular activity and superior penetration into lung tissue, alveolar macrophages, and white blood cells. Furthermore, their improved pharmacokinetic properties permit once- or twice-daily dosing. Gastrointestinal toxicity is significantly lower for the new macrolides than for erythromycin.

Although oral therapy has proven effective in treating Legionnaires' disease (62), given the gastrointestinal manifestations so prominent in some patients, parenteral therapy is preferred to remove the possibility of incomplete gastrointestinal absorption. Parenteral therapy should be given until there is an objective clinical response—often as short as 3 days. Then therapy can be concluded with oral agents for a total 10- to 14-day course. Azithromycin need be given only for 7 to 10 days (109). A 21-day course has been recommended for immunosuppressed patients. Dosages of commonly used antibiotics are given in Table 4.

For empirical therapy of the hospitalized patient with community-acquired pneumonia, azithromycin as monotherapy has been tentatively recommended by the American Thoracic Society/Infectious Diseases Society of America Consensus Committee (78). Note that azithromycin and the other new macrolides provide coverage against the other common pathogens of community-acquired pneumonia, including the other "atypical" pathogens (*Mycoplasma pneumoniae, Chlamydia pneumoniae*) and typical pathogens (*Streptococcus pneumoniae, Haemophilus influenzae, Moraxella catarrhalis,* and *Staphylococcus aureus*).

For nosocomial pneumonias and nursing home pneumonias in which *Legionella* is considered a potential pathogen, the

TABLE 4 • Antibiotic Doses for *Legionella* Infection

Antimicrobial Agent	Dosage[a]
Azithromycin	500 mg[b] orally or intravenously every 24 h
Clarithromycin	500 mg orally or intravenously[c] every 12 h
Roxithromycin	500 mg orally every 12 h
Erythromycin	1000 mg intravenously every 6 h 500 mg orally every 6 h
Dirithromycin	500 mg orally every 24 h
Levofloxacin	500 mg[b] orally or intravenously every 24 h
Ciprofloxacin	400 mg intravenously every 12 h 750 mg orally every 12 h
Ofloxacin	400 mg orally or intravenously every 12 h
Doxycycline	100 mg[b] orally or intravenously every 12 h
Minocycline	100 mg[b] orally or intravenously every 12 h
Tetracycline	500 mg orally or intravenously every 6 h
Trimethoprim/ sulfamethoxazole	160/800 mg intravenously every 8 h 160/800 mg orally every 12 h
Rifampin	300–600 mg orally or intravenously every 12 h

[a] Dosages are based on clinical experience, not on controlled trials.

[b] We recommend doubling the first dose.

[c] Intravenous form not available in the United States.

quinolones (especially ciprofloxacin, levofloxacin, and trovafloxacin) may be the empirical drugs of choice. The quinolones also provide coverage against the Gram-negative bacilli, common pathogens in the hospital or nursing home setting.

For transplant recipients in whom *Legionella* is a potential pathogen, we recommend a quinolone, especially ciprofloxacin, levofloxacin, or trovafloxacin as the drug of choice. The macrolides (but not azithromycin) interact with the immunosuppressive agents, cyclosporine and tacrolimus, used in transplantation.

SPECIAL SITUATIONS

Nosocomial *Legionella* prosthetic valve endocarditis has been described in seven patients (106). The infecting organisms isolated from blood, sternal wound, and valve cultures included *L. pneumophila* in three patients, *L. dumoffii* in three patients, and both *L. pneumophila* and *L. dumoffii* in one patient. The combination of erythromycin and rifampicin was given successfully for 6 to 14 months to five patients who also had replacement of the prosthetic valve; two of these patients were cured (no evidence of continued infection), and three patients had a clinical response (defervescence and improvement in signs and symptoms). Treatment with erythromycin and rifampicin alone for 5 to 6 months effected cure in one patient and clinical improvement in the other (106). For patients with prosthetic valve endocarditis, we recommend combination therapy: quinolone

combined with rifampicin or a new macrolide (e.g., azithromycin) combined with rifampicin. The optimal duration of therapy is unknown, but we would administer at least 3 months of therapy if the infected valve was resected and at least 6 months if it was not.

For patients with other forms of extrapulmonary disease, we recommend a new macrolide or quinolone for 14 to 21 days; combination therapy with the addition of rifampicin might be considered in invasive disease.

Legionella infection is uncommon in patients with AIDS. However, cavitating pneumonia and bacteremia due to *L. pneumophila* was reported (74). In this particular patient with cavitary Legionnaires' disease and positive sputum cultures, bacteremia recurred 4 months after concluding an 8-week course of combination therapy with macrolides and rifampin. Retreatment with erythromycin led to prompt defervescence. In patients with AIDS, we recommend continuing several weeks of oral maintenance antimicrobial agent therapy until the infiltrates on chest radiographs resolve. Close follow-up for detection of possible recurrence is necessary after discontinuation of therapy.

ENDPOINTS OF MONITORING THERAPY

A clinical response (e.g., defervescence) is generally seen within 3 days of initiation of appropriate antibiotic therapy. Improvement on chest radiograph lags behind clinical improvement by several days. In one study of nosocomial pneumonia, 29% of patients showed progression of infiltrate despite erythromycin administration. At 12 weeks, 50% of patients still showed abnormalities on chest radiographs (16).

Mortality rates for Legionnaires' disease vary, depending on the underlying disease and its severity, presence of immunosuppression, severity of pneumonia, and timing of administration of appropriate antimicrobial therapy. Immunosuppressed patients who have not received appropriate antimicrobial therapy have the highest mortality rates (>80%) (58). Mortality among this group is 24 to 37% even when appropriately treated. Mortality rates in community-acquired Legionnaires' disease in immunocompetent patients range from 0 to 11% with appropriate therapy, and as high as 31% if untreated. If a patient with Legionnaires' disease experiences clinical failure confirmed by positive sputum cultures, we recommend combination therapy that includes rifampicin for a prolonged duration of 3 weeks or more.

REFERENCES

1. Aderka D, Garfinkel D, Bagrad H, Torton M, Goldwasser R, Pinkhas J. Relapsing legionella pneumonia. Respiration 1982; 43:317–320.
2. Anderson R, Joone G, vanRensburg CE. An in vitro evaluation of the cellular uptake and intraphagocytic bioactivity of clarithromycin (A-56268, TE-031), a new macrolide antimicrobial agent. J Antimicrob Chemother 1988;22:923–933.
3. Aubier M, Lode H, Gialdroni-Grassi G, Huchon G, Hosie J, Legakis N, Regamey C, Segev S, Vester R, Wijnands WJ, Tolstuchow N. Sparfloxacin for the treatment of community-acquired pneumonia: a pooled data analysis of two studies. J Antimicrob Chemother 1996;37:73–82.

4. Baird IM, Fay D, Thompson RL, Gordon NE, Murcko LG. Case report: Clinical manifestations and treatment of Legionnaires' disease. Am J Med Sci 1979;227:223–232.
5. Bally F, Burdet L, Zanetti G. Personal Communication, 1997.
6. Baltch AL, Smith RP, Ritz W. Inhibitory and bactericidal activities of levofloxacin, ofloxacin, erythromycin, and rifampin used singly and in combination against Legionella pneumophila. Antimicrob Agents Chemother 1995;39:1661–1666.
7. Barker JE, Farrell ID. The effects of single and combined antibiotics on the growth of Legionella pneumophila using time-kill studies. J Antimicrob Chemother 1990;26:45–53.
8. Beasley CRW, Humble MW, O'Donnell TV. Imipenem in the treatment of Legionella pneumonia. Aust NZ J Med 1985;15: 456.
9. Brown A, Yu VL, Elder EM. Nosocomial outbreak of Legionnaires' disease at the Pittsburgh Veterans Administration Medical Center. Trans Assoc Am Physicians 1980;93:52–59.
10. Buggy BP, Saravolatz LD. Treatment of Legionella pneumophila lung abscess with clindamycin. Clin Infect Dis 1995;20:1158–1162.
11. Chen SCA, Paul ML, Gilbert GL. Susceptibility of Legionella species to antimicrobial agents. Pathology 1993;25:180–183.
12. Cherubin CE, Eng RHK, Smith SM, Tan EN. A comparison of antimicrobial activity of ofloxacin, L-ofloxacin, and other oral agents for respiratory pathogens. Diagn Microbiol Infect Dis 1992;15:141–144.
13. Chiodini PL, Barker J. Successful treatment of Legionella pneumonia with imipenem. Lancet 1984;i:401.
14. Cunha BA, Jonas M. Legionnaires' disease treated with doxycycline. Lancet 1981;ii:1107.
15. Davis GS, Winn WC Jr, Gump DW, Craighead JE, Beaty HN. Legionnaires' pneumonia after aerosol exposure in guinea pigs and rats. Am Rev Respir Dis 1982;126:1050–1057.
16. Domingo C, Roig J, Planas F, Bechini TM, Morera J. Radiographic appearance of nosocomial Legionnaires' disease after erythromycin treatment. Thorax 1991;46:633–666.
17. Donowitz GR, Brandon ML, Salisburgy JP, Harman CP, Tipping DM, Urick AE, Talbot GH. Sparfloxacin versus cefaclor in the treatment of patients with community-acquired pneumonia: a randomized, double-masked, comparative, multicenter study. Clin Ther 1997;19:936–953.
18. Donowitz GR, Earnhardt KI. Azithromycin inhibition of intracellular Legionella micdadei. Antimicrob Ag Chemother 1993;37:2261–2264.
19. Dorrell L, Fulton B, Ong ELC. Intravenous azithromycin as salvage therapy in a patient with Legionnaires' disease. Thorax 1994;49:620–621.
20. Dournon E, Mayaud C, Wolff M, et al. Comparison of the activity of three antibiotic regimens in severe Legionnaires' disease. J Antimicrob Chemother 1990;26:129–139.
21. Dournon E, Mayaud C, Wolff M, Schlemmer B, Samuel D, Sollet J, Levasseur-Rajagopalan P. Comparison of the activity of three antibiotic regimens in severe Legionnaires' disease. J Antimicrob Chemother 1990;26(Suppl B):129–139.
22. Dournon EP, Rajagopalan JL, Vilde JL, Pocidalo JJ. Efficacy of pefloxacin in comparison with erythromycin in the treatment of experimental guinea pig legionellosis. J Antimicrob Chemother 1986;17(Suppl B):41–48.
23. DuBois J, St.Pierre C. An in vitro susceptibility study of trovafloxacin against Legionella species [Abstract E075]. Intersci Conf Antimicrob Agents Chemother, New Orleans, 1996.
24. Edelstein PH. Legionnaires' disease [Letter]. N Engl J Med 1998;338:200–201.
25. Edelstein PH. Antimicrobial chemotherapy for Legionnaires' disease: a review. Clin Infect Dis 1995;21(Suppl 3):S265–276.
26. Edelstein PH, Edelstein MAC. In vitro activity of azithromycin against clinical isolates of Legionella species. Antimicrob Agents Chemother 1991;35:180–181.
27. Edelstein PH, Edelstein MAC. In vitro activity of RO 23-9424 against clinical isolates of Legionella species. J Antimicrob Chemother 1992;36:2559–2561.
28. Edelstein PH, Edelstein MAC. In vitro activity of RP 74501-RP74502, a novel streptogramin antimicrobial mixture against clinical isolates of Legionella species. Antimicrob Agents Chemother 1993;37:908–910.
29. Edelstein PH, Edelstein MAC. In vitro extracellular and intracellular activities of clavulanic acid and those of piperacillin and ceftriaxone alone and in combination with tazobactam against clinical isolates of Legionella species. Antimicrob Agents Chemother 1994;38:200–204.
30. Edelstein PH, Edelstein MAC, Lehr KH, Ren J. In-vitro activity of levofloxacin against clinical isolates of Legionella spp., its pharmacokinetics in guinea pigs, and use in experimental Legionella pneumophila pneumonia. J Antimicrobial Chemother 1996;37:117–126.
31. Edelstein PH, Edelstein MAC, Ren J, Polzer R, Gladue RP. Activity of trovafloxacin (CP-99, 219) against Legionella isolates: in vitro activity, intracellular accumulation, and killing in macrophages, and pharmacokinetics and treatment of guinea pigs with L. pneumophila pneumonia. Antimicrob Agents Chemother 1996;40:314–331.
32. Edelstein PH, Edelstein MAC, Weidenfeld J, Dorr MB. In vitro activity of sparfloxacin (CI-978; AT-4140) for clinical Legionella isolates, pharmacokinetics in guinea pigs, and use to treat guinea pigs with L. pneumophila pneumonia. Antimicrob Agents Chemother 1990;34:2122–2127.
33. Engleberg NC, McClain MS, Legendre M, Brieland JK. Macrolide-azalide efficacy against chronic pulmonary legionellosis in BALB/c gamma-interferon knock-out mice [Abstract A39]. 97th annual meeting of the American Society for Microbiology, Miami Beach, 1997.
34. Fang GD, Yu VL, Vickers RM. Disease due to Legionellaceae (other than Legionella pneumophila): historical, microbiological, clinical and epidemiological review. Medicine 1989;68: 116–139.
35. File TM, Segreti J, Dunbar L, Player R, Kohler R, Williams RR, Kojak C, Rubin A. A multicenter, randomized study comparing the efficacy and safety of intravenous and/or oral levofloxacin versus ceftriaxone and/or cefuroxime axetil in the treatment of adults with community-acquired pneumonia. Antimicrob Agents Chemother 1997;41:1965–1972.
36. Fitzgeorge RB, Featherstone ASR, Baskerville A. The effect of ofloxacin on the intracellular growth of Legionella pneumophila in guinea pig alveolar phagocytes. J Antimcrob Chemother 1988;22:53–57.
37. Fitzgeorge RB, Featherstone ASR, Baskerville A. Efficacy of azithromycin in the treatment of guinea pigs infected with Legionella pneumophila by aerosol. J Antimicrob Chemother 1990; 25(Suppl A):101–108.
38. Fitzgeorge RB, Lever S, Baskerville A. A comparison of the efficacy of azithromycin and clarithromycin in oral therapy of experimental airborne Legionnaires' disease. J Antimicrob Chemother 1993;31:171–176.
39. Fraser DW, Tsai T, Ornstein W, et al. Legionnaires' disease: description of an epidemic of pneumonia. N Engl J Med 1977; 297:1189–1197.

40. Fraser DW, Wachsmuth IK, Bopp C, Feeley JC, Tsai TF. Antibiotic treatment of guinea-pigs infected with agent of Legionnaires' disease. Lancet 1978;1:175–178.

41. Furneri PM, Bazzano M, Campo L, Cesana M, Tempera G. In vitro activity of rufloxacin against Listeria monocytogenes, Legionella pneumophila, and Chlamydia trachomatis. Chemotherapy (Basel) 1994;40:104–108.

42. Genne D, Siegrist HH, Humair L, Janin-Jaquat B, de Torrente A. Clarithromycin versus amoxicillin-clavulanate in the treatment of community-acquired pneumonia. Eur J Clin Microbiol Infect Dis 1997;16:783–788.

43. Gentry LO, Lipsky B, Farber MO, Tucker B, Rodriguez-Gomez C. Oral ofloxacin therapy for lower respiratory tract infection. South Med J 1992;85:14–18.

44. Goldini P, Castellani-Pastoris M, Cattani L, Peluso C, Sinibald L, Orsi N. Effect of monesin on the invasiveness and multiplication of Legionella pneumophila. J Med Microbiol 1995; 42:269–275.

45. Gooding BB, Erwin ME, Barasett MS, Johnson MS, Johnson DM, Jones RN. Antimicrobial activities of two investigational fluoroquinolones (CI-960 and E4695) against over 100 Legionella sp. isolates. Antimicrob Agents Chemother 1992;36: 2049–2050.

46. Hamedani P, Ali J, Hafeez S, et al. The safety and efficacy of clarithromycin in patients with Legionella pneumonia. Chest 1991;100:1503–1506.

47. Hays JH, Hinthorn DR, Chanko A, Liu C. Failure of oral erythromycin therapy for Legionnaires' disease in a renal transplant recipient. South Med J 1981;74:1422–1433.

48. Hohl P, Buser U, Frei R. Fatal legionella pneumophila pneumonia: treatment failure despite early sequential oral-parenteral amoxicillin-clavulanic acid therapy. Infection 1992;20:51–52.

49. Hooper TL, Gould FK, Swinburn CR, et al. Ciprofloxacin: a preferred treatment for Legionella infections in patients receiving cyclosporine A [Letter]. J Antimicrob Chemother 1988;22: 952–953.

50. Horwitz MA. Toward an understanding of host and bacterial molecules mediating L. pneumophila pathogenesis. In: Barbaree JM, Breiman RF, Dufour AP, eds. Legionella—current status and emerging perspectives. Washington, DC: American Society for Microbiology, 1993:55–62.

51. Horwitz MA, Silverstein SC. Intracellular multiplication of Legionnaires' disease bacteria (Legionella pneumophila) in human monocytes is reversibly inhibited by erythromycin and rifampin. J Clin Invest 1983;71:15–26.

52. Hubbard RB, Mathur RM, MacFarlane JT. Severe community-acquired Legionella pneumonia: treatment, complications and outcome. Q J Med 1993;86:327–332.

53. Jacobson K. Clinical efficacy of dirithromycin in pneumonia. J Antimicrob Chemother 1993;31:121–129.

54. Johnson DM, Erwin ME, Barrett MS, Gooding BB, Jones RN. Antimicrobial activity of ten macrolide, lincosamine and streptogramin drugs tested against Legionella species. Eur J Clin Microbiol Infect Dis 1992;11:751–755.

55. Jones RN. Activity of sparfloxacin (AT-4140), PD 127391 and PD 131628 against Legionella spp. J Antimicrob Chemother 1991;389–390.

56. Keys TF. A sporadic case of pneumonia due to Legionnaires' disease. Mayo Clin Proc 1977;52:657–660.

57. Keys TF. Therapeutic considerations in the treatment of Legionella infection. Semin Respir Infect 1987;2:270–273.

58. Kirby BD, Snyder K, Meyer R, Finegold SM. Legionnaires' disease: report of 65 nosocomially acquired cases and a review of the literature. Medicine 1980;59:188–205.

59. Kitsukawa K, Hara J, Saito A. Inhibition of Legionella pneumophila in guinea pig peritoneal macrophages by new quinolone, macrolide, and other antimicrobial agents. J Antimicrob Chemother 1991;27:343–353.

60. Kohno S, Koga H, Yamaguchi K, Masaki M, Inoue Y, Dotsu Y, et al. A new macrolide, TE-031 (A-56268), in treatment of experimental Legionnaires' disease. J Antimicrob Chemother 1989;24:397–405.

61. Kurz RW, Graninger W, Egger TP, Pichler H, Tragl KH. Failure of treatment of Legionella pneumophila with ciprofloxacin. J Antimicrob Chemother 1988;22:389–391.

62. Kuzman I, Oreskovicic K, Schowald S, Culig S. Azithromycin in the treatment of community acquired LD [Abstract 10.29]. Fourth International Conference on the Macrolides, Azalides, Streptogramins, and Ketolides, Barcelona, Jan 21–23, 1998.

63. Kuzman I, Soldo I, Schonwald S, Culig J. Azithromycin for treatment of community-acquired pneumonia caused by Legionella pneumophila: a retrospective study. Scand J Infect Dis 1995;27:503–505.

64. Lattimer GL, Rhodes LV. Legionnaires' disease: clinical findings and one-year follow-up. JAMA 1978;240:1169–1171.

65. Liippo K, Tala E, Puolijoki H, Bruckner OJ, Rodrig J, Smits JPH. A comparative study of dirithromycin and erythromycin in bacterial pneumonia. J Infection 1994;28:131–139.

66. Lode H, Garau J, Grassi C, Hosie J, Huchon G, Legakis N, Segev S, Wijnands G. Treatment of community-acquired pneumonia: a randomized comparison of sparfloxacin, amoxycillin-clavulanic acid and erythromycin. Eur Respir J 1995;8:1999–2007.

67. Lowry PW, Tompkins LS. Nosocomial legionellosis: a review of pulmonary and extrapulmonary syndromes. Am J Infect Control 1993;21:21–27.

68. Martin SJ, Pendland SL, Chen C, Schreckenberger P, Danziger LH. In vitro synergy testing of macrolide-quinolone combinations against 41 clinical isolates of Legionella. Antimicrob Agents Chemother 1996;40:1419–1421.

69. Martin SJ, Pendlard SL, Chen C, Schreckenberger PC, Danziger LH. In vitro synergy of clarithromycin and its 14-hydoxy metabolite in combination with levofloxacin or ciprofloxacin against 42 clinical isolates of Legionella [Abstract W.04]. Fourth International Conference on the Macrolides, Azalides, Streptogramins, and Ketolides, Barcelona, Jan 21–23, 1998.

70. Mensa J, Trilla A, Moreno A, Vidal J, Espaulella J, Soriano E, Garcia San Miguel J. Five-day treatment of non-severe, community-acquired pneumonia with josamycin. J Antimicrob Chemother 1993;31:749–754.

71. Merrell WH, Moritz A, Butt HL, Barnett G, Eather EW, Bishop JM. Isolation of Legionella maceachernii from an immunocompromised patient with severe underlying disease. Med J Aust 1991;155:415–417.

72. Miller AC. Erythromycin in Legionnaires' disease: a reappraisal. J Antimicrob Chemother 1981;7:217–222.

73. Moffie BG, Mouton RP. Sensitivity and resistance of L. pneumophila to some antibiotics and combination of antibiotics. J Antimicrob Chemother 1988;22:457–462.

74. Morley JN, Crocker Smith L, Baltch AL, Smith RP. Recurrent infection due to Legionella pneumophila in a patient with AIDS. Clin Infect Dis 1994;19:1130–1132.

75. Moutan Y, Leroy O, Beuscart C, Sivery B, Senneville E, Chidiac C, et.al. Efficacy of intravenous ofloxacin: a French multicentre

trial in 185 patients. J Antimicrobial Chemother 1990;26(Suppl D):115–121.

76. Myburgh J, Nagel GJ, Petschel E. The efficacy and tolerance of a three-day course of azithromycin in the treatment of community-acquired pneumonia. J Antimicrob Chemother 1993;31:163–169.

77. Nash P, Sideman L, Pidcoe V, Kleger B. Minocycline in Legionnaires' disease. Lancet 1978;i:45.

78. Neiderman MS, Yu VL. ATS/IDSA consensus on management of community-acquired pneumonia. Unknown 1998;

79. Nimmo GR, Bull JZ. Comparative susceptibility of Legionella pneumophila and Legionella longbeachae to 12 antimicrobial agents. J Antimicrob Chemother 1995;36:219–223.

80. Norrby R. Atypical pneumonia in the Nordic countries: aetiology and clinical results of a trial comparing fleroxacin and doxycycline. J Antimicrob Chemother 1997;39:499–508.

81. Nowicki M, Paucod JC, Bornstein N, Meuginier H, Isoard P, Fleurette J. Comparative efficacy of five antibiotics on experimental airborne legionellosis in guinea pigs. J Antimicrob Chemother 1988;22:513–9.

82. Ortgvist A, Valtonen M, Cars O, Wahl M, Saikku P, Jean C. Oral empiric treatment of community-acquired pneumonia: a multicenter, double-blind, randomized study comparing sparfloxacin with roxithromycin. Chest 1996;110:1499–1506.

83. Parker MM, Macher AM, Shelhamer JH, Balow JE. Unresponsiveness of Legionella bozemanii pneumonia to erythromycin administration despite in vitro susceptibility. Am Rev Respir Dis 1983;128:955–956.

84. Pasculle AW, Dowling JN, Frola FN, McDevit DA, Levi MA. Antimicrobial therapy of experimental Legionella micdadei pneumonia in guinea pigs. Antimicrob Agents Chemother 1985; 28:730–734.

85. Paterson DL, Singh N. Interactions between tacrolimus and antimicrobial agents. Clin Infect Dis 1997;25:1430–1440.

86. Pendland SL, Martin SJ, Chen C, Schreckenberger PC, Danziger LH. Comparison of charcoal and starch based media and inoculum sizes for growth and susceptibility of 42 clinical isolates of *Legionella* to erythromycin, clarithromycin, 14-hydroxy clarithromycin, levofloxaciin, and ciprofloxacin [Abstract 1027]. Fourth International Conference on the Macrolides, Azalides, Streptogramins, and Ketolides, Barcelona, Jan 21–23, 1998.

87. Portier H, May TH, Proust A, French Study Group. Comparative efficacy of sparfloxacin in comparison with amoxycillin plus ofloxacin in the treatment of community-acquired pneumonia. J Antimicrob Chemother 1996;37:83–91.

88. Rajagopalan-Levasseur P, Dournon E, Dameron G, Vilde J-L, Pocidalo J. Comparative postantibacterial activities of pefloxacin, ciprofloxacin, and ofloxacin against intracellular multiplication of Legionella pneumophila serogroup 1. Antimicrob Agents Chemother 1990;34:1733–1738.

89. Ramirez JA, Summersgill JT, Miller RD, Myers TL, Ruff MJ. Comparative study of the bactericidal activity of ampicillin/sulbactam and erythromycin against intracellular Legionella pneumophila. J Antimicrob Chemother 1993;32:93–99.

90. Reda C, Quaresima T, Castellani Pastoris M. In-vitro activity of six intracellular antibiotics against Legionella pneumophila strains of human and environmental origin. J Antimicrob Chemother 1994;33:757–764.

91. Ridgway GL, Salman H, Robbins MJ, Dencer C, Felmingham D. The in-vitro activity of grepafloxacin against chlamydia spp., mycoplasma spp., ureaplasma urealyticum and legionella spp. J Antimicrob Chemother 1997;40:31–34.

92. Rudin JE, Evans TL, Wing EJ. Failure of erythromycin in treatment of Legionella micdadei pneumonia. Am J Med 1984;76: 318–320.

93. Ruiz-Santana S, Aguado-Bourrey JM, Narvaez-Bermejo JM, Gonzalez-Mediero G. Legionella bozemanii pneumonia and tetracycline. Ann Intern Med 1986;105:969–970.

94. Saito A, Gaja M. In vitro and in vivo activities of sparfloxacin in legionella infections. Drugs 1995;49:250–252.

95. Saito A, Koga H, Shigeno H, Watanabe K, Mori K, Kohno S, Shigeno Y, Suzuyama Y, Yamaguchi K, Hirota M, Hara K. The antimicrobial activity of ciprofloxacin against Legionella species and the treatment of experimental legionella pneumonia in guinea pigs. J Antimicrob Chemother 1986;18: 251–260.

96. Saito A, Sawatari K, Fukuda Y, Nagasawa M, Koga H, Tomonaga A, Nakazato H, Fujita K, Shigeno Y, Suzuyama Y, Yamaguchi K, Izumik K, Hara K. Susceptibility of *Legionella pneumophila* to ofloxacin in vitro and in experimental Legionella pneumonia in ginea pigs. Antimicrob Agents Chemother 1985; 28:15–20.

97. Salord JM, Matsiota-Bernard P, Staikowsky F, Kirstetter M, Frottier J, Nauciel C. Unsuccessful treatment of Legionella pneumophila infection with a fluoroquinolone. Clin Infect Dis 1993;17:518–519.

98. Shah A, Check F, Baskin S. Legionnaires' disease and acute renal failure: case report and review. Clin Infect Dis 1992;14: 204–207.

99. Singh N, Muder RR, Yu VL, Gayowski T. Legionella infection in liver transplant recipients: implications for management. Transplantation 1993;56:1549–1551.

100. Smith GM, Abbott KH, Wilkinson MJ, Sutherland R. A rat model of Legionella pneumophila pneumonia for efficacy studies with beta-lactam antibiotics. In: Barbaree JM, Breiman RF, Dufour AP, eds. Legionella: current status and emerging perspectives. Washington, DC: American Society for Microbiology, 1993:19–22.

101. Stokes DH, Wilkinson MJ, Tyler J, Slocomb B, Sutherland R. Bactericidal effects of amoxycillin/clavulanic acid against intracellular Legionella pneumophila in tissue culture studies. J Antimicrob Chemother 1989;23:547–556.

102. Stout JE, Arnold B, Yu VL. Comparative activity of azithromycin, clarithromycin, roxithromycin, dirithromycin, quinopristin/dalfopristin, and erythromycin against Legionella species by broth microdilution and intracellular susceptibility testing in HL-60 cells. J Antimicrob Chemother 1997;41:289–291.

103. Stout JE, Arnold B, Yu VL. Comparative activity of ciprofloxacin, ofloxacin, levofloxacin, and erythromycin against legionella species by broth microdilution and intracellular susceptibility testing in HL-60 cells. Diagn Microbiol Infect Dis 1998;30:37–43.

104. Stout JE, Yu VL. Current concepts: legionellosis. N Engl J Med 1997;337:682–687.

105. Swanson DJ, Sung RJ, Fine MJ, Orloff J, Chu SY, Yu VL. Erythromycin ototoxicity: prospective assessment with serum concentrations and audiograms in a study of patients with pneumonia. Am J Med 1992;92:61–68.

106. Tompkins LS, Roessler BJ, Redd SC, et al. Legionella prosthetic-valve endocarditis. N Engl J Med 1988;318:530–535.

107. Topkis S, Swarz H, Breisch SA, Maroli AN. Efficacy and safety of grepafloxacin 600 mg daily for 10 days in patients with community-acquired pneumonia. Clin Ther 1997:975–988.

108. Unertl KE, Lenhart FP, Forst H, Vogler G, Wilm V, Ehret W, Ruckdeschel G. Brief report: ciprofloxacin in the treatment of legionellosis in critically ill patients including those cases

unresponsive to erythromycin. Am J Med 1989;87(Suppl 5A):128S–131S.

109. Vergis EN, Phillips J, Bates JH, File TM, Tan JS, Sarosi GA, Grayston JT, Yu VL. A prospective, randomized, multicenter trial of azithromycin versus cefuroxime plus erythromycin for community-acquired pneumonia in hospitalized patients. Proceedings of the 35th annual meeting of the Infectious Diseases Society of America, San Francisco, Sept 13–16, 1997.

110. Vilde VL, Dournon E, Rajagopalan P. Inhibition of Legionella pneumophila multiplication within human macrophages by antimicrobial agents. Antimicrob Agents Chemother 1986;30: 743–748.

111. Winn WC Jr, Davis GS, Gump DW, Craighead JE, Beaty HN. Legionnaires' pneumonia after intratracheal inoculation of guinea pigs and rats. Lab Invest 1982;47:568–578.

112. Yoshida SI, Mizuguchi Y. Antibiotic susceptibility of Legionella pneumophila Philadelphia-1 in cultured guinea-pig peritoneal macrophages. J Gen Microbiol 1984;130: 901–906.

113. Yu VL, Stout JE. Legionnaires' disease—reply [Letter]. N Engl J Med 1998;338:201.

114. Yu VL, Vergis EN. Legionellosis. In: Fishman AP, Elias JA, Fishman JA, Grippi MA, Kaiser LR, Senior RN, eds. Fishman's pulmonary diseases and disorders. 3rd ed. New York: McGraw-Hill, 1998:2235–2246.

Leptospira Species

●

Solly Faine

MICROBIOLOGY

Leptospirosis is a ubiquitous zoonosis. The causal bacteria are leptospires, spirochetes that are members of the genus *Leptospira*, comprising at least 8 pathogenic species, with others yet to be formally published. The current main species names are *borpetersenii, inadai, interrogans, kirschneri, noguchii, santarosai,* and *weilii*. Within these species are about 200 serovars, forming groups whose characteristic antigens are related to immunity and used in serodiagnosis. Several of the serovars appear in two or more species (7, 9–11). Leptospires are slow-growing bacteria (doubling time, about 6 h) that can be readily cultivated in laboratories using special liquid media and strict aseptic technique. The conventional media contain long-chain fatty acids essential for growth and a detoxicant of fatty acids, usually serum albumin.

Most tests of susceptibility of leptospires to antibiotics were conducted many years ago in media containing serum. More-recent tests of both newer and older antibiotics in oleate-albumin media suggest that the composition of the test medium is not important. The earlier tests were often carried out on only one isolate, designated by serovar, without authentication and of unspecified provenance, before species were recognized. Nevertheless, repeated testing in many laboratories gives confidence in the reliability of the results. Patients treated as suggested by the susceptibility tests in the literature recover well, better than without antibiotic therapy.

Epidemiology

All leptospires can live freely in the environment as well as in the renal tubules and sometimes the genital tracts of carrier animals, themselves survivors of infection. The most important carrier animals for infections in humans are rodents (especially rats of various types), dogs, pigs, and cows. Leptospires excreted in urine from carrier animals survive in moist conditions such as surface water, soil, or mud. They enter the body through skin abrasions, by inhalation of aerosols, or through the conjunctiva. Humans are at risk in their work or leisure activities through direct contact with animals or indirectly via contaminated water or urine. The highest risks occur in agricultural workers in moist conditions throughout the world; rice-planters and harvesters, miners, travelers, soldiers, canoeists, swimmers, animal attendants, milkers, and meat workers are most at risk. In Western temperate countries, most people with leptospirosis are infected through milking cows (serovar *hardjo*), slaughtering or maintaining pigs (serovars *pomona, tarassovi*), or exposure to domestic or agricultural conditions in which there is heavy rodent infestation, sometimes after civil or military emergencies that destroy effective rat control. In Asia, serovar *lai* is currently predominant.

Clinical Manifestations

The main clinical features in humans are grouped into two ill-defined and overlapping forms, depending on the serovar (7–9, 11, 12). Both forms start suddenly with severe headache, fever of 39°C or higher, excruciating muscle tenderness (especially in the back and calves), red eyes (vascular dilatation, not inflammation), and sometimes photophobia or meningism. The so-called mild or influenzal type progresses in the following 3 to 7 days with transient nitrogen retention, rarely jaundice, occasionally a rash, and meningitis or abdominal pains mimicking an acute abdominal surgical emergency. Recovery is almost invariable in 2 to 3 weeks, and fatalities are so rare that there are no recorded autopsy observations. In the severe (also known as the icteric, renal, or hemorrhagic) form, the patient's condition deteriorates rapidly, so that the initial phase of 3 to 7 days is followed by increasing interstitial nephritis, liver failure and jaundice, myocarditis, or severe respiratory distress syndrome denoting pulmonary hemorrhages ranging from small to massive and fatal. Antibiotic treatment in itself cannot reverse the pathologic changes once established. Clinical supportive and symptomatic treatments are essential adjuncts to chemotherapy (7, 8, 11, 12).

SUSCEPTIBILITY IN VITRO AND IN VIVO

Leptospires are not usually tested for susceptibility in individual cases, for several reasons. Leptospires are not usually isolated from patients because they grow slowly, and the culture is not available until it is too late to influence management. Antibiotic resistance has been reported in the laboratory in experimental conditions, but there are no well-authenticated reports of isolation from a patient or the environment of a leptospire resistant to an antibiotic expected to have therapeutic value. Because of their slow growth, many fewer generations and mutational events can be expected during an infection with leptospires than during conventional bacterial infections. Plasmids and phages have not been reported in pathogenic leptospires, and the mechanisms governing genetic variability are obscure.

Leptospires are sensitive to most antibiotics (β-lactams, cephalosporins, aminoglycosides, macrolides) but not to chloramphenicol, vancomycin, rifampicin, and metronidazole (7) (Table 1). Combined therapy to overcome development of resistance is not indicated, and there are no tests of combinations of antibiotics useful in human medicine.

ANTIMICROBIAL THERAPY

Although there is still some dispute about the value of penicillin therapy, it is valuable and the drug of choice where it is not contraindicated, given early in infection. To be effective, antibiotic treatment should be instituted as early as possible, even before the diagnosis is certain, and within the first 7 to 10 days after infection (not 7–10 days after diagnosis, onset of symptoms, or hospitalization), since leptospires are removed from the tissues by natural immune mechanisms after that time. In most studies of hospitalized jaundiced patients, the illness on admission was near or past its 10th day after infection. High doses (6–8 megaunits of benzyl [crystalline] penicillin daily, in divided doses, intramuscularly or intravenously) are recommended. Alternatively, 4 to 5 megaunits of equal parts of procaine penicillin and crystalline penicillin are given daily intramuscularly, reducing the dose by half after the fever subsides, for a total of 5 to 7 days, continuing 1.5 megaunits of procaine penicillin daily until 2 days after albuminuria ceases (6). Gendron et al. (14) reported successfully using 10 to 20 megaunits/day routinely. A well-controlled study in severe leptospirosis patients, using 6 megaunits/day (1.5 megaunits 6-hourly) intravenously, showed that the treatment, even if begun late, was effective in improving all measurable parameters in the patients (22). A contrary result was obtained in another careful analysis (5), and a short prophylactic course of an unspecified dose of an undefined penicillin preparation failed to protect against a laboratory infection

with a leptospire of the Icterohaemorrhagiae serogroup (15). Despite these negative findings, penicillin as described remains the recommended treatment. Defervescence can be expected within 24 h (2–4, 6–8, 11, 17).

There are no special situations; the general recommendations apply.

Alternative antibiotics for those allergic to penicillin include erythromycin (250 mg 6-hourly for 5 days). A controlled trial of doxycycline given in 100-mg oral doses twice daily showed that it reduced the severity and duration of illness (16). Tetracyclines have been recommended (in doses of 500 mg tetracycline immediately, followed by 250 mg 8-hourly orally, intramuscularly, or intravenously if the patient is vomiting or unable to absorb orally, for 24 h, then 250–500 mg 6-hourly for 6 days), but they cannot be recommended nowadays when alternatives are available. The use of tetracyclines is contraindicated in the presence of renal failure because it is nephrotoxic; likewise, they should not be used in pregnant women or children because of their effects on developing teeth and bone. There is no apparent advantage currently in using newer, more expensive, and more toxic antibiotics. A recent experimental animal trial confirmed these observations (1).

MONITORING THERAPY, AND PROGNOSIS

Most patients with leptospirosis recover in 2 to 6 weeks if not jaundiced, but they may not be fit to return to a normal life for a further 4 weeks. The death rate in jaundiced patients may be very low if penicillin treatment is begun early and if renal and liver failure, myocarditis, and pulmonary hemorrhages can be treated successfully. Death rates in recent well-treated and well-documented studies were 0, 2.5, or 5.7% (5, 14, 22). Patients who recover from the severe forms, including renal failure and jaundice, can expect complete recovery. A certain proportion of patients may need support for psychologic and mental problems for 1 to 2 years or more after their illness, and 10% of patients or more complain of recurring, persistent headaches and uveitis for some years (18).

Jarisch-Herxheimer (JH) reactions may follow institution of penicillin therapy. In typical examples, fever rose to 37.8 to 38.4°C with severe rigors and hypotension, 4 to 5 h after institution of intravenous penicillin therapy (20, 21). The mechanism of the JH reaction in leptospirosis is not established. Toxins released by lysis of the leptospires by antibiotic may induce cytokines. Treatment with penicillin released limulus lysate–active material in some patients, independent of (and in the absence of) a JH reaction. Management of the JH reaction is supportive and symptomatic; its effects are temporary and should not contraindicate antibiotic therapy (13, 21).

Chemoprophylaxis

Doxycycline hyclate, given orally in a 200-mg single dose weekly, protected military personnel exposed to risks of leptospirosis (19).

Reinfection

Patients cannot be reinfected and do not develop a second infection with the same serovar so long as they maintain even a

TABLE 1 • Susceptibilities of Leptospires[a] to Antibiotics in Vitro

Antibiotic[b]	Sensitivity[c]	Concentration[b] (μg/mL)
Amikacin	S	1.56–12.5
Amoxicillin	S	0.5
Ampicillin	S	0.025
Carbomycin	S	10–100
Cefmetazole	S	1–0.78
Cefotaxime	S	0.05–0.1
Ceftizoxime	S	0.05–0.2
Cephalothin	S	6.25
Cephalothin	S	3.13
Cephalothin	S	0.78–6.25
Chloramphenicol	R	>4000
Chloramphenicol	S	20
Chloramphenicol	I	100
Chloramphenicol	R	2000
Chlortetracycline	S	1.0–20
Chlortetracycline	I	50
Ciprofloxacin	S	0.6
Dihydrostreptomycin	S	0.3
Erythromycin	S	0.001–0.01
Erythromycin	S	0.00002
Erythromycin	S	0.63
Erythromycin	S	0.025
Erythromycin	S	15
Erythromycin	S	0.11
Kanamycin	S	0.25–0.5
Kanamycin	S	3.13–12.5
Lincomycin	S	2.5
Methicillin	S	6.6
Metronidazole	S	100
Minocycline	S	0.08–0.625
Moxalactam	S	0.2–0.78
Novobiocin	S	20
Oxytetracycline	S	1.0
Oxytetracycline	S	110
Oxytetracycline	S	0.25
Penicillin, benzyl	S	0.005–0.2
Penicillin V	S	0.2
Penicillin G	S	10.0
Pipericillin	S	0.39–0.78
Polymyxin	S	10
Sulfamethoxy-pyridazine	R	>2000
Streptomycin	S	3.5–20
Streptomycin	S	0.2–0.4
Streptomycin	S	0.39 >100
Tetracycline	S	0.04–4
Tetracycline	S	10

Antibiotic[b]	Sensitivity[c]	Concentration[b] (μg/mL)
Tobramycin	S	1.56–6.25
Tobramycin	S	6.25
Tobramycin	S	1.56
Tropolon compounds	S	0.52
Vancomycin	R	50–200
Vancomycin	R	10
Viomycin	R	>500

Serovar: *hardjo;* species: *interrogans*, in oleate-albumin medium at 29°C

Antibiotic[b]	Sensitivity[c]	Concentration[b]
Ampicillin	S	≥1.0
Chloramphenicol	R	>10.0 <100
Colimycin	S	>1.0 <10.0
Doxycycline	S	>1.0 <10.0
Erythromycin	S	≥1.0
Ethambutol	R	>100.0
Furadantin	R	>10.0 <100
Gentamicin	S	>1.0 <10.0
INH	R	>100.0
Keflex	R	>10.0 <100
Keflin	R	>10.0 <100
Lincomycin	S	≥1.0
Neomycin	R	>10.0 <100
PAS	R	>100.0
Polymyxin	R	>10.0 <100
Rifampicin	R	>100.0
Streptomycin	S	≥1.0
Terramycin	S	>1.0 <10.0
Tetracycline	S	≥1.0
Tetracycline	S	≥1.0
Vancomycin	R	>100.0

Summarized and modified with permission from Faine S. Leptospira and leptospirosis. Boca Raton, FL: CRC Press, 1994. (The extended table [Chapter 4, Table 4, pp. 56–67] includes details of strains and species, susceptibilities, test conditions, and references to the original tests.)

[a]Serovars: *australis, autumnalis, ballum, bataviae, budapest, canicola, copenhageni, grippotyphosa, hebdomadis, icterohaemorrhagiae, kremastos, pomona, pyrogenes, robinsoni, saxkoebing, sejroe, tarassovi, zanoni,* and various unspecified serovars, mostly tested in serum media at 28 or 30°C.

[b]Interpretations, names of antibiotics, concentrations, and names of leptospires are generally those used by the authors.

[c]Sensitivity: S, sensitive; R, resistant; I, intermediate.

low level of agglutinating antibodies in their serum. There is a dearth of information about reinfection once antibody has fallen below detectable levels. Second infections are usually with a different serovar. Exacerbation of leptospirosis due to development of resistance to antibiotic in an individual patient has never been reported. Leptospirosis in patients infected with the human immunodeficiency virus (HIV) proceeds as in normal individuals.

REFERENCES

1. Alt DP, Bolin CA. Preliminary evaluation of antimicrobial agents for treatment of Leptospira interrogans serovar pomona infection in hamsters and swine. Am J Vet Res 1996;57:59–62.
2. Benzi Cipelli R, Gorini O, Caligaris S, Lanzarini P, Milano F, Orsolini P, Filice G. In vitro sensitivity of 3 strains of Leptospira interrogans to 3 different antibiotics, Boll Ist Sieroter Milan 1989;68:17–23.
3. Biegel E, Mortensen H, Gaub J. [Leptospirosis in the Ribe County 1980–1991]; Leptospirose i Ribe Amt 1980–1991. Ugeskr Laeger 1995;157:157–161.
4. Brouqui P, Barnton G, Raoult D. Les leptospiroses. Encycl Méd Chir 9:1990;1–10.
5. Edwards CN, Nicholson GD, Hassell TA, Everard CO, Callender J. Leptospirosis in Barbados. A clinical study. West Indian Med J 1990;39:27–34.
6. Faine S. Guidelines for the control of leptospirosis [Offset publication]. Geneva: World Health Organization, 1982.

7. Faine S. Leptospira and leptospirosis. Boca Raton, FL: CRC Press, 1994.
8. Faine S. Leptospirosis. In: Hoeprich PD, Jordan MC, Roland AR, eds. Infectious diseases. 5th ed. Philadelphia: JB Lippincott, 1994:619–625.
9. Faine S. Leptospira. In: Balows A, Duerden BI, eds. Topley and Wilson's microbiology and microbial infections. 9th ed. Collier LH, ed., vol 2, Systematic bacteriology. London: Arnold, 1997: 1287–1303.
10. Faine S. Leptospirosis. In: Evans AS, Brachman PS, eds. Bacterial infections of humans. Epidemiology and control. 3rd ed. New York: Plenum Medical, 1997, in press.
11. Faine S. Leptospirosis. In: Hausler WJ, Sussman M, eds. Topley and Wilson's microbiology and microbial infections. 9th ed. Collier LH, ed., vol 3, Bacterial infections. London: Arnold, 1997:849–869.
12. Farr RW. Leptospirosis. Clin Infect Dis 1995;21:1–6.
13. Friedland JS, Warrell DA. The Jarisch-Herxheimer reaction in leptospirosis: possible pathogenesis and review [see comments]. Rev Infect Dis 1991;13:207–210.
14. Gendron Y, Prieur J, Gaufroy X, Gras C. Les leptospiroses en Polynesie Francaise: étude de 120 observations. (Leptospirosis in French Polynesia; 120 case reports.) Med Trop (Mars) 1992; 52:21–27.
15. Gilks CF, Lambert HP, Broughton ES, Baker CC. Failure of penicillin prophylaxis in laboratory acquired leptospirosis. Postgrad Med J 1988;64:236–238.
16. McClain JBL, Ballou WR, Harrison SM, Steinweg DL. Doxycycline therapy for leptospirosis. Ann Intern Med 1984;100: 696–698.
17. Roura Carrasco J, Pila Perez R, Caveda Estela O, Pila Pelaez R. 1. Estudio clinico de la leptospirosis humana. A proposito de 215 casos. (A clinical study of human leptospitosis. Apropos 215 cases). Rev Clin Esp 1992;190:389–392.
18. Shpilberg O, Shaked Y, Maier MK, Samra D, Samra Y. Long-term follow-up after leptospirosis. South Med J 1990;83:405–407.
19. Takafuji ET, Kirkpatrick JW, Miller RN, Karwacki JJ, Kelley PW, Gray MR, McNeill KM, Timboe HL, Kane RE, Sanchez JL. An efficacy trial of doxycycline chemoprophylaxis against leptospirosis. N Engl J Med 1984;310:497–500.
20. Vaughan C, Cronin CC, Walsh EK, Whelton M. The Jarisch-Herxheimer rection in leptospirosis. Postgrad Med J 1994;70: 118–121.
21. Watt G, Padre LP, Tuazon M, Calubaquib C. Limulus lysate positivity and Herxheimer-like reactions in leptospirosis: a placebo-controlled study. J Infect Dis 1990;162:564–567.
22. Watt G, Padre LP, Tuazon ML, Calubaquib C, Santiago E, Ranoa CP, Laughlin LW. Placebo-controlled trial of intravenous penicillin for severe and late leptospirosis. Lancet 1988; 1:433–435.

Leuconostoc Species

●

Ricardo Espinoza-Araya

GENERAL

Leuconostoc spp. are Gram-positive cocci normally found in vegetables, milk, and dairy products. Although the organism has been isolated from the human gastrointestinal tract, it is not part of the normal human flora (25). It was considered a nonpathogen until 1985, when the first cases of infection in humans were reported (2). *Leuconostoc* spp. grow in pairs and produce α-hemolysis in sheep-blood agar. They are catalase-negative, facultative anaerobes. At least five biochemically distinct species of *Leuconostoc* have been isolated from human sources, including: *L. mesenteroides, L. lacti, L. citreum, paramesenteroides, L. pseudomesenteroides,* and *L. cremoris* (9). The first two of the above species are the most commonly isolated *Leuconostoc* species in clinical samples. *Leuconostoc* spp. can be confused with streptococci, especially with *Streptococcus* viridans and enterococci. Gas production during glucose fermentation and failure of *Leuconostoc* to hydrolyze arginine distinguishes them from *Streptococcus* species (8, 9, 19). Their Gram stain appearance and resistance to vancomycin should raise the possibility of their presence.

SUSCEPTIBILITY IN VITRO

In vitro, the most striking feature of *Leuconostoc* spp. is their intrinsic resistance to vancomycin ($MIC_{90} > 256$ μg/mL). Although *Leuconostoc* and vancomycin-resistant enterococcus are not related organisms, both share the same mechanism of resistance to vancomycin; their cell walls are deficient in the terminal D-alanine-D-alanine that is the receptor for glycopeptide antibiotics. Instead a terminal D-alanine-D-lactate is found within the cell wall (7, 17).

Leuconostoc spp. are susceptible to many antibiotics, despite being resistant to vancomycin. Almost 100% of *Leuconostoc* spp. are susceptible to erythromycin and clindamycin ($MIC_{90} < 0.06$ μg/mL). Aminoglycosides are also very active, and gentamicin is the most active agent of this group ($MIC_{90} < 0.05$ μg/mL) (Table 1).

Although only 6% of strains are susceptible at the streptococcal break point of 0.1 μg/mL (27), penicillin has been recommended by some as the antibiotic of choice since concentrations exceeding the MIC are usually obtainable (1, 21). Cephalothin is somewhat more active than the second- and

TABLE 1 • Susceptibility of 43 Strains of *Leuconostoc* spp.					
Antibiotics	MIC Range (µg/mL)	MIC$_{50}$ (µg/mL)	MIC$_{90}$ (µg/mL)	Breakpoint conc. (µg/mL)	% Susceptible
Vancomycin	256->256	>256	>256	≤4	0
Teicoplanin	128->256	>256	>256	≤4	0
Penicillin	0.03-2	0.5	1	≤0.12	6
Ampicillin	0.03-2	1	2	≤0.12	2
Cephalothin	0.12-32	4	16	≤8	87
Cefuroxime	≤0.25-32	8	16	≤8	66
Cefotaxime	≤0.25-64	8	16	≤8	66
Ceftazidime	4->128	64	128	≤8	17
Imipenem	0.06-8	2	8	≤4	81
Erythromycin	≤0.015-0.06	0.03	0.06	≤0.5	100
Clindamycin	≤0.008-2	0.015	0.06	≤0.5	98
Gentamicin	≤0.25-0.5	<0.25	0.5	≤4	100
Tobramycin	≤0.25-2	0.5	1	≤4	100
Doxycycline	0.25-16	4	8	≤4	91
Chloramphenicol	2-16	4	8	≤8	98
Rifampin	0.06-64	1	8	≤1	55
Ciprofloxacin	0.5-4	2	4	≤1	24
Trimethoprim	<0.5-16	4	8	≤8	98
Trimethroprim-sulfamethoxazole	0.03-16	1	4	≤2	70

Modified from Swenson JM, Facklam RR, Thornsberry C. Antimicrobial susceptibility of vancomycin-resistant *Leuconostoc, Pediococcus,* and *Lactobacillus* species. Antimicrob Agent Chemother 1990;34:543–549.

third-generation cephalosporins. Interestingly, trimethoprim alone is more active than trimethoprim-sulfamethoxazole (27).

The in vitro data are very limited for combination therapy. The activity of penicillin G combined with streptomycin or gentamicin was evaluated for killing curves; both combinations were synergistic for 6 of 8 strains studied (2).

ANTIMICROBIAL THERAPY
General Drug of Choice

The most commonly used antibiotics reported in the literature are penicillins, with 31% (10 of 32) of reported patients receiving only penicillins: 7, penicillin G (1, 2, 5, 15, 16, 24); 1, amoxicillin (3); 1, nafcillin (16); and 1, amoxicillin/clavulanate (10). Therapy with penicillin was successful in 9 (3 patients with catheter infection, 3 with bacteremia, 3 with pneumonia); 1 patient with bacteremia died secondary to staphylococcal meningitis (15). An additional 7 patients received penicillins in combination with another antibiotic: 2 with meningitis (1 treated with chloramphenicol and penicillin (4), and another treated with cefotaxime, chloramphenicol, and penicillin (11)) and 1 patient with endocarditis treated with gentamicin and penicillin (14). The other 4 patients with catheter-related infection were treated successfully with combinations of aminoglycosides and penicillins (6, 16, 23, 24, 25). The only death clearly attributable to *Leuconostoc* was the patient with *Leuconostoc* meningitis (11).

In mild or moderately severe cases, penicillin could be the first choice, if the identity of the organism is confirmed. However, we recommend susceptibility testing in vitro, at least to penicillin, clindamycin, erythromycin, and aminoglycosides. If the clinical response is unsatisfactory, one can switch to the agent most active in vitro. Since the MICs of penicillin are relatively high, doses of 12 to 16 million units/day are advisable to obtain higher serum concentrations.

Alternative Therapy

Clindamycin is an excellent alternative antibiotic (Table 1). Two patients were successfully treated with this antibiotic: one with dental abscess (28) and another with catheter-related infection (18).

Special Situations

Catheter-Related Infections

The most common infection (47%, 15 of 32) associated with *Leuconostoc* spp. is catheter-related infection (1, 3, 6, 16, 18, 20, 22, 23, 25). Among 15 patients reported in the literature, 3 were treated successfully without specific antibiotics (1, 16), and 3 were treated successfully with antibiotics with the catheter left in place (2, 23, 25). However, most were treated with both antibiotics and removal of the catheter. In fact, one patient with persistent bacteremia despite antibiotic treatment ultimately required removal of the catheter for cure (3). Amoxicillin (3), ampicillin (20), penicillin (1, 16, 25), and clindamycin (18) have been used successfully to treat catheter-related bacteremia. The outcome of this infection has been uniformly good. No deaths have been associated directly to *Leuconostoc* catheter-related infection.

Primary Bacteremia

Bacteremia without an obvious source has been the second most frequent clinical presentation of *Leuconostoc* infection (2, 5, 15, 16). Two of six patients with primary bacteremia died from their infections (15). Ampicillin and gentamicin, penicillin, and nafcillin were used successfully. One patient receiving gentamicin and one receiving penicillin with gentamicin died, but the causes of death were probably multifactorial; blood cultures in both became negative on therapy.

Pneumonia

Pneumonia occurred usually in immunosuppressed patients including AIDS or transplant recipients. Three of six patients with pneumonia due to *Leuconostoc* infection died of their infection (5, 10, 12, 13, 24). Two patients were successfully treated with penicillin (5, 23), and one was successfully treated with amoxicillin/clavulanate intravenously (10). Unsuccessful therapies included teicoplanin and gentamicin (12), trimethropim-sulfamethoxazole (5), and a combination of ceftazidime and ciprofloxacin (13).

Combination Therapy

Eight patients have been treated with combination therapy. The most commonly used combination therapy was penicillin combined with an aminoglycoside. Combination therapy in 5 patients, one with endocarditis and four with catheter-related infection, yielded uniformly good outcomes (6, 14, 16, 23, 25).

Two patients with meningitis received combination therapy: one received penicillin and chloramphenicol (4) and the other received penicillin, cefotaxime, and chloramphenicol (11). The latter patient died from the *Leuconostoc* meningitis; the bacterium was isolated once in cerebrospinal fluid (CSF) during therapy and then cleared from the CSF, but the CSF neutrophil count and protein concentration increased progressively despite therapy. A patient with a pneumonia died after receiving only 2 days of ciprofloxacin and ceftazidime (13). Combination therapy with penicillin and aminoglycoside has some support in vitro and in anecdotal case reports. Therefore, addition of an aminoglycoside (gentamicin) to penicillin therapy might be considered if the patient has a poor clinical response to monotherapy.

REFERENCES

1. Bernaldo de Quirùs JCL, Muûoz P, Cercenado E, Hernandez Sampelayo T, Moreno S, Bouza E. *Leuconostoc* species as a cause of bacteremia: two case reports and a literature review. Eur J Clin Microbiol Infect Dis 1991;10:505–509.
2. Buu-Hoi A, Branger C, Acar JF. Vancomycin-resistant streptococci or *Leuconostoc* sp. Antimicrob Agents Chemother 1985; 28:458–460.
3. Carapetis J, Bishop S, Davis J, Bell B, Hogg G. *Leuconostoc* sepsis in association with continuous enteral feeding: two case reports and a review. Pediatr Infect Dis J 1994;13:816–823.
4. Coovadia YM, Solwa Z, Van Den Ende J. Meningitis caused by vancomycin-resistant *Leuconostoc* sp. J Clin Microbiol 1987; 25:1784–1785.
5. Coovadia YM, Solwa Z, Van Den Ende J. Potential pathogenicity of *Leuconostoc*. Lancet 1988;1:306.
6. Dhodapkar KM, Henry NK. *Leuconostoc* bacteremia in an infant with short-gut syndrome: case report and literature review. Mayo Clin Proc 1996;71:1171–1174.
7. Elisha BG, Courvalin P. Analysis of genes encoding D-alanine: D-alanine ligase-related enzymes in *Leuconostoc* mesenteroides and Lactobacillus spp. Gene 1995;152:79–83.
8. Facklam R, Hollis D, Collins MD. Identification of gram-positive coccal and coccobacillary vancomycin-resistant bacteria. J Clin Microbiol 1989;27:724–730.
9. Facklam R, Elliott JA. Identification, classification, and clinical

relevance of catalase-negative, gram-positive cocci, excluding the streptococci and enterococci. Clin Microbiol Rev 1995;8: 479–495.
10. Ferrer S, de Miguel G, Domingo P, Pericas R, Prats G. Pulmonary infection due to *Leuconostoc* species in a patient with AIDS. Clin Infect Dis 1995;21:225–226.
11. Friedland IR, Snipelisky M, Khoosal M. Meningitis in a neonate caused by *Leuconostoc* sp. J Clin Microbiol 1990;28:2125–2126.
12. Giacometti A, Ranaldi R, Siquini FM, Scalise G. *Leuconostoc* citreum isolated from lung in AIDS patient. Lancet 1993;342: 622.
13. Giraud P, Attal M, Lemouzy J, Huguet F, Schlaifer D, Pris J. *Leuconostoc,* a potential pathogen in bone marrow transplantation. Lancet 1993;341:1481–1482.
14. Gollcdge CL. Bacteremia due to *Leuconostoc* species. Clin Microbiol Newslett 1989;11:29–30.
15. Golledge CL. Infection due to *Leuconostoc* species. Rev Infect Dis 1991;13:184–185.
16. Handwerger S, Horowitz H, Coburn K, Kolokathis A, Wormser G. Infection due to *Leuconostoc* species: six cases and review. Rev Infect Dis 1990;12:602–610.
17. Handwerger S, Pucci MJ, Volk KJ, Liu J, Lee MS. Vancomycin-resistant *Leuconostoc* mesenteroides and Lactobacillus casei synthesize cytoplasmic peptidoglycan precursors that terminate in lactate. J Bacteriol 1994;176:260–264.
18. Hardy S, Ruoff KL, Catlin EA, Santos JI. Catheter-associated infection with a vancomycin-resistant gram positive coccus of the *Leuconostoc* sp. Pediatr Infect Dis J 1988;7:519–520.
19. Isenberg HD, Vellozzi EM, Shapiro J, Rubin LG. Clinical laboratory challenges in the recognition of *Leuconostoc* spp. J Clin Microbiol 1988;26:479–483.
20. Jimenez-Mejias ME, Becerril B, Gomez-Cia T, Del Nozal M, Palomino-Nicas J. Bacteremia caused by *Leuconostoc cremoris* in a patient with severe burn injuries. Eur J Clin Microbiol Infect Dis 1997;16:533–535.
21. Moellering RC. Enterococcus species, Streptococcus bovis and *Leuconostoc* species. In: Mandell GL, Bennett JE, Dolin R, eds. Principles and practices of infectious disease. 4th ed. New York: Churchill Livingstone, 1995:1832–1835.
22. Martinez-Martinez L, Saavedra JM, Conejo MC. Bacteremia caused by *Leuconostoc* spp. Clin Microbiol Newslett 1992;14: 102–104.
23. Noriega FR, Kotloff KL, Martin MA, Schwalbe RS. Nosocomial bacteremia caused by Enterobacter sakazakii and *Leuconostoc* mesenteroides resulting from extrinsic contamination of infant formula. Pediatr Infect Dis J 1990;9:447–449.
24. Peters VB, Bottone EJ, Barzilai A, Hyatt A, Blank S, Hodes DS. Leuconostoc species bacteremia in a child with acquired immunodeficiency syndrome. Clin Pediatr 1992;31:699–701.
25. Rubin LG, Vellozzi E, Shapiro J, Isenberg HD. Infection with vancomycin resistant "streptococci" due to Leuconostoc species. J Infect Dis 1988;157:216.
26. Ruoff KL, Kuritzkes DR, Wolfson JS, Ferraro MJ. Vancomycin-resistant gram-positive bacteria isolated from human sources. J Clin Microbiol 1988;26:2064–2068.
27. Swenson JM, Facklam RR, Thornsberry C. Antimicrobial susceptibility of vancomycin-resistant *Leuconostoc*, Pediococcus, and Lactobacillus species. Antimicrob Agent Chemother 1990; 34:543–549.
28. Wenocur HS, Smith MA, Vellozi EM, Shapiro J, Isenberg HD. Odontogenic infection secondary to *Leuconostoc* species. J Clin Microbiol 1988;26:893–894.

Listeria monocytogenes

●

Valerie Parkas and Donald Armstrong

GENERAL DESCRIPTION

Listeria monocytogenes is a Gram-positive, nonsporeforming aerobic bacillus. The organism is widespread throughout nature, found in soil, water, and many food products. Clinical infection with *L. monocytogenes* can occur in the general population but is more common in neonates, pregnant women, the elderly, and immunosuppressed patients such as transplant recipients, patients on corticosteroids, and patients with the acquired immunodeficiency syndrome. Clinically, infection with *L. monocytogenes* can be divided into five syndromes: infections in pregnancy, granulomatosis infantiseptica, sepsis of unknown origin, meningoencephalitis, and focal infections (Table 1).

SUSCEPTIBILITY IN VITRO AND IN VIVO

Until recently, this organism was thought to be universally susceptible to antibiotics active against Gram-positive bacteria. However, the first resistant *L. monocytogenes* was isolated in 1988 in France; this isolate was resistant to chloramphenicol, erythromycin, tetracycline, and streptomycin (23). Since then, there have been several reports of resistant strains of *L. monocytogenes* (22, 24). The in vitro susceptibilities of 49 clinical strains of *L. monocytogenes* were evaluated against 22 antimicrobial agents (5): all of the strains were susceptible to penicillin, ampicillin, vancomycin, gentamicin, tetracycline, ciprofloxacin, imipenem, and trimethoprim-sulfamethoxazole, and they were all resistant to the cephalosporins. Susceptibility testing was also done on 621 strains of *L. monocytogenes* from cases of human infection between 1987 and 1990 in England, and all strains were uniformly susceptible to ampicillin, imipenem, chloramphenicol, and gentamicin (18); 13 strains were resistant to tetracycline, and 1 was resistant to erythromycin. Eleven hundred isolates, 60 from human infections and the remaining majority from food or the environment, were collected from a worldwide distribution and susceptibility testing was performed (8). All strains were susceptible to ampicillin, gentamicin, chloramphenicol, vancomycin, and erythromycin. Thirty-seven clinical strains were resistant to tetracycline, and one strain from the environment was resistant to trimethoprim. The authors believe that the increasing resistance to the tetracyclines may be secondary to the widespread use of this antibiotic class in animal feed. In vitro testing of isolates of *L. monocytogenes* against single antibiotics shows that resistance remains low. Nevertheless, resistance is increasing, with tetracycline resistance becoming more common, multidrug resistance increasing, and, in this series, the first report of trimethoprim resistance. For all of these reasons, susceptibility testing for all cases of human listeriosis is now necessary.

As mentioned above, strains of *L. monocytogenes* are susceptible to a wide variety of antibiotics by disk sensitivity testing; however, many of these antibiotics are bacteriostatic against this organism (27), including erythromycin, tetracycline, chloramphenicol, and rifampin. The β-lactam antibiotics are often described as bacteriostatic against *Listeria,* when indeed they show delayed in vitro bactericidal activity. The aminoglycosides and the combination drug trimethoprim-sulfamethoxazole are bactericidal against *Listeria.*

Combinations of drugs have also been widely tested in vitro against *Listeria.* Ampicillin or penicillin in combination with an aminoglycoside has been found both synergistic and bactericidal. In addition, trimethoprim-sulfamethoxazole is also a synergistic and bactericidal combination in vitro. Macgowan et al. compared the activities of nine combinations of antibiotics and found gentamicin in combination with either ampicillin, trimethoprim, or vancomycin to be the most synergistic in bactericidal tests. Combinations containing rifampin were the least effective (19).

Animal models have been used widely to study the treatment of listerial infections. A model of *Listeria* meningitis in rabbits revealed that ampicillin has greater bactericidal activity than penicillin. The same model also shows that addition of the aminoglycoside gentamicin to either penicillin or ampicillin improves the results. Not surprisingly, ampicillin and gentamicin is the most effective combination in this rabbit model of *Listeria* meningitis (26). Twenty-four antibiotics have been evaluated in a murine model of *Listeria* meningitis (29). Parenteral amoxicillin shows high therapeutic efficacy with low acute toxicity to the central nervous system. Ampicillin and penicillin G are also quite effective, while the cephalosporins are ineffective in this model. Erythromycin, clindamycin, and chloramphenicol were all active in vitro but inactive or only weakly active in the murine model. The tetracyclines were the most active but displayed severe toxicity to the murine central nervous system.

Two other models of *Listeria* infection in mice with compromised defense mechanisms have also been developed. The first model uses dextran sulfate to destroy the function of the macrophage system, and the second uses a mouse congenitally lacking virtually all functional T lymphocytes (13). In both of these models, bacteriologic cure was not obtained with ampicillin. Thus, the benefit obtained from an antibiotic in an immunologically normal mouse infected with *Listeria* is not the same in an immunocompromised mouse. The implication for the treatment of *Listeria* in the immunosuppressed patient is that prolonged treatment and bactericidal antibiotic regimens may be required. Trimethoprim-sulfamethoxazole was highly

TABLE 1 • Clinical Syndromes Caused by *Listeria monocytogenes*

Syndrome	Presentation
1. Infection in pregnancy	Fever, chills, ± back pain in a pregnant woman (usually in the third trimester)
2. Granulomatosis infantiseptica	Fever, weakness, cardiopulmonary failure in a neonate who has been infected transplacentally
3. Sepsis	Neonates (after 7 days of age) or adults with fever and chills
4. Meningoencephalitis	Variable presentation in neonates (after 7 days of age) and adults, but generally fever, mental status changes
5. Focal infections	Ulcerating skin lesions, purulent conjunctivitis, endocarditis, osteomyelitis, peritonitis, hepatitis, lymphadenitis, prosthetic joint infection, spinal/brain abscess, cholecystitis

active in another murine model of listerial infection in which normal mice were infected with *Listeria*, but in T cell–deficient mice, only transient reduction of bacterial counts was achieved (16). In yet another mouse model of listerial infection in which the animals were given steroids to induce immunosuppression, animals treated for 3 days with ampicillin were bacteriologically cured, whereas those treated for 3 days with ciprofloxacin remained infected (30). More recently, both liposome-entrapped ampicillin and ampicillin linked to nanoparticles were used as drug delivery systems in a murine model of *Listeria* infection. Both delivery systems were more effective than free ampicillin in the treatment of *Listeria* in this model (11). Further investigation of these improved drug delivery systems is necessary as listerial infections in immunosuppressed patients can be quite difficult to eradicate.

ANTIMICROBIAL THERAPY

There have been no controlled trials to establish a drug of choice or an optimal duration of therapy for specific *Listeria* infections. Thus, optimal antibiotic therapy for listeriosis in humans remains controversial. Recommendations are compiled from in vitro testing, animal models, and clinical experience (Table 2). Ampicillin is regarded as the first-line antibiotic for the treatment of *Listeria* infections; however, some experts advocate the use of penicillin rather than ampicillin (2).

Bacteremia

In a series of 46 patients with primary *Listeria* bacteremia (21), 33% had an underlying malignancy, 24% had undergone a renal transplant, 13% were pregnant, 11% had liver disease, and 11% had no underlying disease. Antibiotic treatment primarily included ampicillin or penicillin. Eighty-nine percent

survived the infection. Death occurred only in those with an underlying malignancy, and in this group the mortality was 33%. The authors believe that many in this group had undocumented central nervous system involvement. Ampicillin alone is considered appropriate treatment for uncomplicated bacteremia, but for bacteremia in a patient with severe immunosuppression, most experts prefer a combination of ampicillin with an aminoglycoside. Because of the bactericidal synergism of ampicillin and gentamicin against *Listeria* and because of the animal model data, this combination is first line in the treatment of serious listerial infections. However, there have been no controlled trials in humans comparing use of ampicillin alone with use of a combination of ampicillin and gentamicin. Patients with bacteremia and no evidence of meningitis (normal cerebrospinal fluid [CSF]) can be treated for 2 weeks. Recurrence has been noted after 2 weeks of therapy in immunosuppressed patients, however, so an additional 1 or 2 weeks of treatment may be prudent. High doses of ampicillin (200 mg/kg/day divided every 4 h) and gentamicin (5 mg/kg/day divided every 8 h) are recommended for proper treatment of complicated bacteremia (17).

Meningitis

L. monocytogenes has a predilection for infecting the central nervous system, especially the meninges. In 1990, the Centers for Disease Control reported *L. monocytogenes* to be the fifth most common cause of bacterial meningitis. In neonates, it is among the three most common causes of bacterial meningitis, and it is the most common pathogen causing bacterial meningitis in patients on corticosteroids and recipients of organ transplants (17). In a series of patients with *Listeria* meningitis (21), the mortality was 30% overall. Upon further review,

TABLE 2 • Recommended Treatment for Infections Caused by *Listeria monocytogenes*

Clinical Syndrome	Antibiotic	Dose (i.v.)	Alternative Therapy	Duration (weeks)
Bacteremia	Ampicillin	200 mg/kg div q. 4 h	TMP-SMX	2
Meningitis	Ampicillin + gentamicin	200 mg/kg div q. 4 h 5 mg/kg div q. 8 h	TMP-SMX	3
Rhomboencephalitis	Ampicillin + gentamicin	200 mg/kg div q. 4 h 5 mg/kg div q. 8 h	TMP-SMX	6
Endocarditis	Ampicillin + gentamicin	200 mg/kg div q. 4 h 5 mg/kg div q. 8 h	TMP-SMX	4
Infection in pregnancy	Ampicillin	200 mg/kg div q. 4 h	Ampicillin desensitization	2
Neonatal infection	Ampicillin + gentamicin	50–100 mg/kg q. 8 h 5 mg/kg div q. 12 h	Ampicillin desensitization	2

however, the mortality was 60% in patients with an underlying malignancy and only 13% in patients with no underlying disease. The combination of ampicillin and an aminoglycoside is recommended for treatment of meningitis. Patients with meningitis should be treated with high doses of these agents (doses as outlined for bacteremia) and should receive at least 3 weeks of treatment. Repeat lumbar puncture to document improved CSF parameters is usually recommended. Although parenteral gentamicin can obtain adequate levels in the CSF, some experts advocate intraventricular gentamicin for refractory cases (2). No controlled trials have evaluated addition of intraventricular gentamicin to combination intravenous ampicillin and gentamicin therapy, but intraventricular therapy should be considered when intravenous therapy is failing.

Rhomboencephalitis

In a review of listerial infections (21), of the 186 cases of adult listeriosis, 6.5% were nonmeningitic central nervous system infections. Five of the 12 patients died, and the survivors often had marked neurologic deficits. Since patients were treated with a variety of antibiotic regimens and the number of cases was small, conclusions about treatment remain difficult. Most experts agree that rhomboencephalitis or brain abscess requires at least 6 weeks of treatment with close radiographic follow-up (17, 21). Again, high-dose ampicillin with an aminoglycoside is advocated.

Endocarditis

In the aforementioned review of *Listeria* infections in adults (21), endocarditis accounted for 7% of listerial infections. Most patients had known underlying cardiac abnormalities that predisposed them to endocarditis. Most were treated with long courses of penicillin or ampicillin, and the mortality was 36%. Treatment of *Listeria* native valve endocarditis should include high-dose ampicillin and gentamicin for at least 4 weeks. Prosthetic valve endocarditis may require surgical intervention in addition to antimicrobial therapy (25).

Infection in Pregnancy

During pregnancy, especially in the third trimester, cell-mediated immunity declines, and the pregnant female is at risk for listeriosis. In a review of listeria bacteremia, 13% of the 46 patients were pregnant (21). The infection quite commonly results in premature labor or septic spontaneous abortion. After this occurrence, the infection is usually self-limited in the female. A recent case report shows that early diagnosis and initiation of antibiotic therapy in a pregnant woman with listeriosis may increase the chances of delivering a healthy baby (15). In this report, high-dose ampicillin was given to the infected pregnant patient for 3 days prior to premature labor and continued for a total duration of 2 weeks.

Neonatal Infection

Listerial infections in children are usually divided into two categories: early onset and late onset. Early-onset infections occurring in the neonate have been termed *granulomatosis infantiseptica,* in which the neonate has septicemia, pneumonia, and often widespread microabscesses. The recommended treatment is ampicillin (50–100 mg/kg q. 8 h) and gentamicin (5 mg/kg/day divided q. 12 h) for at least 2 weeks. Late-onset infection appears in full-term children at least 1 week after delivery and is more typical of an adult infection, with bacteremia or meningitis being the most common manifestation. Again, treatment consists of ampicillin and gentamicin.

ALTERNATE THERAPY

When ampicillin or penicillin is not an option because the patient cannot tolerate either of these drugs, treatment decisions become more difficult. Trimethoprim-sulfamethoxazole is thought to be a good alternative in penicillin-allergic patients (12, 17). The data both from the laboratory and from clinical experience support use of this combination drug. In vitro bactericidal effects of trimethoprim-sulfamethoxazole have been shown to be equivalent to those of ampicillin combined with gentamicin (28). A recent review reported eight patients with *Listeria* infection treated with trimethoprim-sulfamethoxazole. Although most of these patients with listerial bacteremia or meningitis were immunosuppressed, treatment was successful. In these patients, trimethoprim-sulfamethoxazole was administered either parenterally or orally from 14 to 49 days. (When using trimethoprim-sulfamethoxazole to treat listeriosis, a dose of 15 mg/kg/day divided every 6 h should be used.) Because clinical data for treatment of listerial infections with trimethoprim-sulfamethoxazole are limited, definite conclusions are difficult. The results are, however, encouraging; this combination drug is bactericidal in vitro, has performed well in animal models, and has good central nervous system penetration. Clinical results are thus far comparable to those achieved with ampicillin and gentamicin. For patients unable to tolerate the penicillins, trimethoprim-sulfamethoxazole is thought to be the best alternative for treating listerial infections.

In serious listerial infections in immunocompromised patients who are penicillin allergic, many experts advocate ampicillin desensitization. Certainly if the patient is failing treatment with trimethoprim-sulfamethoxazole, desensitization is the best option. In certain populations such as pregnant woman and neonates, trimethoprim-sulfamethoxazole is contraindicated. Thus, treatment options are limited in a patient with listeriosis who is penicillin allergic and who also cannot receive trimethoprim-sulfamethoxazole. For these patients, ampicillin desensitization is the best option.

Vancomycin has also been used successfully to treat listerial infections in penicillin-allergic patients (6, 9). A recent review identified eight cases of listerial infection treated with vancomycin. Courses of treatment ranged from 2 to 12 weeks, and six of the patients were clinically and bacteriologically cured. The remaining two required surgical removal of infected vascular access devices for cure (4). In vitro testing consistently shows *L. monocytogenes* to be quite sensitive to vancomycin, which is bacteriostatic against this organism but has been shown to be bactericidal and synergistic when combined with an aminoglycoside (6,19). However, clinical experience with vancomycin is variable. A recent report of development of *Listeria* meningitis in a patient on therapeutic doses of vancomycin as well as reports of treatment failures argue against the use of vancomycin for the treatment of these infections (3, 10).

In the past, chloramphenicol was considered the first-line antibiotic in penicillin-allergic patients with listeriosis. It should no longer be used to treat these infections, as its use is associated with a high relapse rate and a high mortality rate (17, 20). Cephalosporins also should not be used to treat *Listeria* infections; they are inactive in vitro and there have been many documented treatment failures (1, 9). The newer cephalosporins, including the fourth-generation agents, are also inactive in vitro (5). Of the macrolides, clarithromycin is the most active in vitro against *L. monocytogenes* (5), but given the bacteriostatic nature of these agents, the poor central nervous system penetration, and documented clinical failures with erythromycin, it is prudent to avoid these agents when treating listeriosis (9). The tetracyclines are also not recommended because they are bacteriostatic, penetrate the central nervous system poorly, and have been ineffective clinically (9, 17). Ciprofloxacin is the most active quinolone against *L. monocytogenes*. It however has variable central nervous system penetration, poor results when tested in animal models (30), and extremely limited clinical experience and thus cannot be recommended. *L. monocytogenes* is highly sensitive to rifampin, and although bacteriostatic, it has performed well in animal studies (14) and has the theoretical advantage of enhanced intracellular killing. Unfortunately there are few data on the use of rifampin in human listeriosis.

REFERENCES

1. Allerberger FJ, Dierich MP. Listeriosis and cephalosporins [Letter]. Clin Infect Dis 1992;15:177.
2. Armstrong D. *Listeria monocytogenes*. In: Mandell GL, Bennett JE, Dolin R, eds. Principles and practice of infectious diseases. New York: Churchill Livingstone, 1995:1880–1885.
3. Baldassarre JS, Ingerman MJ, Nansteel J, Santoro J. Development of *Listeria* meningitis during vancomycin therapy [Letter]. J Infect Dis 1991;164:221–222.
4. Blatt SP, Zajac RA. Treatment of *Listeria* bacteremia with vancomycin [Letter]. Rev Infect Dis 1991;13:181–182.
5. Blazquez R, Pelaez T, Munoz P, Sanchez R, Rodriguez-Creixems M, Bouza E. Activity in vitro of 22 antimicrobial agents against clinical isolates of *Listeria monocytogenes*. Clin Microb Infect 1996;2:63–64.
6. Bonacorsi S, Doit C, Aujard Y, Blot P, Bingen E. Successful antepartum treatment of listeriosis with vancomycin plus netilmicin. Clin Infect Dis 1993;17:139–140.
7. Bortolussi R, Evans J. Listeriosis. In: Feigin RD, Cherry JD, eds. Pediatric infectious diseases. Philadelphia: WB Saunders, 1992: 1180–1185.
8. Charpentier E, Gerbaud G, Jacquet C, Rocourt J, Courvalin P. Incidence of antibiotic resistance in *Listeria* species. J Infect Dis 1995;172:277–281.
9. Cherubin CE, Appleman MD, Heseltine PNR, Khayr W, Stratton CW. Epidemiological spectrum and current treatment of Listeriosis. Rev Infect Dis 1991;13:1108–1114.
10. Dryden MS, Jones NF, Phillips I. Vancomycin therapy failure in
11. Fattal E, Rojas J, Youssef M, Couvreur P, Andremont A. Liposome-entrapped ampicillin in the treatment of experimental murine listeriosis and salmonellosis. Antimicrob Agents Chemother 1991;35:770–772.
12. Gellin BG, Broome CV. Listeriosis. JAMA 1989;261(9): 1313–1320.
13. Hof H, Emmerling P, Seeliger HPR. Murine model for therapy of listeriosis in the compromised host. Effect of ampicillin. Chemotherapy 1981;27:214–219.
14. Hof H, Emmerling P. Murine model for therapy of listeriosis in the compromised host. Effect of rifampicin. Chemotherapy 1984;30:125–130.
15. Kalstone C. Successful antepartum treatment of listeriosis. Am J Obstet Gynecol 1991;164:57–58.
16. Kawaler B, Hof H. Murine model for therapy of listeriosis in the compromised host. Cotrimoxazole. Chemotherapy 1985;31: 366–371.
17. Lorber B. Listeriosis. Clin Infect Dis 1997;24:1–9.
18. MacGowan AP, Reeves DS, McLauchlin J. Antibiotic resistance of *Listeria monocytogenes*. Lancet 1990;336:513–514.
19. MacGowan AP, Holt HA, Reeves DS. In-vitro synergy testing of nine antimicrobial combinations against *Listeria monocytogenes*. J Antimicrob Chemother 1990;25:561–566.
20. MacGowan AP. Listeriosis—the therapeutic options [Letter]. J Antimicrob Chemother 1990;26:721–722.
21. Nieman RE, Lorber B. Listeriosis in adults: a changing pattern. Report of eight cases and review of the literature, 1968–1978. Rev Infect Dis 1980;2:207–227.
22. Papa A, Alexiou-Daniel S, Danielidis BD, Antoniadis A. Multiresistant strain of *Listeria monocytogenes* in Greece. Clin Microb Infect 1996;2:64–65.
23. Poyart-Salmeron C, Carlier C, Trieu-Cuot P, Courtieu AL, Courvalin P. Transferable plasma-mediated antibiotic resistance in *Listeria monocytogenes*. Lancet 1990;335:1422–1426.
24. Quentin C, Thibaut MC, Horovitz J, Bebear C. Multiresistant strain of *Listeria monocytogenes* in septic abortion [Letter]. Lancet 1990;336:375.
25. Rao N. *Listeria* prosthetic valve endocarditis [Letter]. J Thorac Cardiovasc Surg 1989;98:303–306.
26. Scheld WM, Fletcher DD, Fink FN, Sande MA. Response to therapy in an experimental rabbit model of meningitis due to listeria monocytogenes. J Infect Dis 1979;140(3):287–294.
27. Scheld WM. Evaluation of rifampin and other antibiotics against *Listeria monocytogenes* in vitro and in vivo. Rev Infect Dis 1983;5(Suppl 3):S593–S599.
28. Spitzer PG, Hammer SM, Karchmer AW. Treatment of *Listeria monocytogenes* infection with trimethoprim-sulfamethoxazole: case report and review of the literature. Rev Infect Dis 1986;8: 427–430.
29. Tsai YH, Hirth RS, Leitner F. A murine model for listerial meningitis and meningoencephalomyelitis: therapeutic evaluation of drugs in mice. Chemotherapy 1980;26:196–206.
30. Van Ogtrop ML, Mattie H, Sekh BR, Van Strijen E, Van Furth R. Comparison of the antibacterial efficacies of ampicillin and ciprofloxacin against experimental infections with *Listeria monocytogenes* in hydrocortisone treated mice. Antimicrob Agents Chemother 1992;36(11):2375–2380.

Moraxella catarrhalis

●

Diana L. Nunley and Steven L. Berk

During the 1960s and early 1970s *Moraxella catarrhalis* was classified as *Neisseria catarrhalis*—a nonpathogenic inhabitant of the upper respiratory tract. In 1970, *Neisseria catarrhalis* was reclassified as a member of the genus *Branhamella*. A heightened appreciation for *Branhamella catarrhalis* as a true pathogen occurred during the 1970s. Presently, *Branhamella catarrhalis* has been delegated to the genus *Moraxella* and has been renamed *Moraxella catarrhalis*.

GENERAL DESCRIPTION

M. catarrhalis has been implicated in a diverse array of pediatric and adult infections. *M. catarrhalis* is the third most common bacterial agent in pediatric acute otitis media and maxillary sinusitis—surpassed only by *Streptococcus pneumoniae* and *Haemophilus influenzae* (23). In adult patients, *M. catarrhalis* is responsible for acute exacerbations of chronic bronchitis and bronchopneumonia in the elderly and immunocompromised (37). Bacteremia with and without endocarditis (42), septic arthritis (17, 56), meningitis (62, 30), conjunctivitis (13,45), and acute urethritis (24, 55) have been less commonly associated with *M. catarrhalis* infection.

As appreciation of the pathogenicity of *M. catarrhalis* increased, investigations revealed production of a chromosomally mediated β-lactamase. In 1977, β-lactamase-producing strains of *M. catarrhalis* were recovered in Sweden, France, and England (54, 60, 63). Review of earlier strains from the Centers of Disease Control, Atlanta, Georgia revealed initial β-lactamase-producing strains only as far back as 1976 (77). Further investigations revealed that β-lactamase producing strains have spread rapidly throughout the world.

The β-lactamases associated with *M. catarrhalis* are unique among β-lactamase classes defined by Richmond and Sykes (66). *M. catarrhalis* produces two enzymes, BRO-1 and BRO-2, which hydrolyze penicillin, ampicillin, methicillin, and cefaclor. These enzymes have much more activity against penicillinase-susceptible penicillins than against cephalosporins (60). Since these β-lactamases are strongly membrane-associated and are present in small amounts, their activity is limited and easily neutralized by β-lactamase inhibitors (25, 29). BRO-1 is present in approximately 90% of β-lactamase-producing isolates, with BRO-2 present in the remaining 10% (14, 28, 58). BRO-1-producing isolates are more resistant to ampicillin than BRO-2 producers (34, 52). BRO-1 production levels are also generally double or triple those of BRO-2.

Resistance to non-β-lactam antimicrobials has also been reported, but specific mechanisms have not been well characterized. Inherent resistance to vancomycin (2, 74), trimethoprim (1), and clindamycin (25, 79) has been documented. Resistance to tetracycline and erythromycin was reported initially in 1983

by Kallings (44). Since then, trends in the spread of resistance to erythromycin and tetracycline have been slow. Relatively high minimal inhibitory concentrations (MICs) of amoxicillin and cephalosporins for β-lactamase-negative strains of *M. catarrhalis* also reflect further mechanisms of resistance that have not been elucidated. Adaptations in cellular targets or permeability may operate in these situations (34). Recently, resistance to complement-mediated killing was identified as a virulence factor of *M. catarrhalis* (39, 43). *M. catarrhalis* isolates from patients manifesting clinical disease were more likely to be serum resistant than were colonizing strains.

SUSCEPTIBILITY IN VITRO AND IN VIVO

The heightened appreciation of *M. catarrhalis* as a pathogen coupled with the organism's recent and progressive β-lactamase production has made vigilant monitoring of antibiotic susceptibility essential. Due to the high incidence of β-lactamase production, testing for β-lactamase activity should be routine in all *M. catarrhalis* isolates of clinical importance.

Susceptibility testing for *M. catarrhalis* is medium and inoculum dependent. Carefully standardized media and methodologies must be used when comparing susceptibility data to ensure accurate results. Broth microdilution is considered a "gold standard" in susceptibility testing. The in vitro activity of various antimicrobial agents against *M. catarrhalis* is expressed in MICs. Table 1 summarizes MIC data from a recent international study. MICs are a single piece of information that must be interpreted in conjunction with other factors such as the achievable concentration of an antimicrobial at the site of infection, host factors, necessity for bactericidal activity, and breakpoint criteria to arrive at a sound therapeutic decision. It is tempting to equate in vitro potency of an antimicrobial agent with the clinical response rate. In truth, susceptibility in vitro does not predict a clinically favorable outcome, although resistance in vitro generally does predict clinical failure. In vitro studies aid in identifying specific areas that require close scrutiny in judging clinical efficacy.

Although many excellent studies have compared MICs of antimicrobial agents, fewer studies have addressed the bactericidal activity of these drugs against *M. catarrhalis*. Determination of an antimicrobial agent's bactericidal activity against a particular organism is problematic. Issues such as antibiotic tolerance, growth phase, antibiotic carryover, and degradation rates can all affect results (81).

Single Drug

Penicillin

Studies by Barbar and Waterforter in 1962 revealed *M. catarrhalis* to be highly sensitive to penicillin V. By 1983, a widening range of MICs for penicillin V was reported for both

TABLE 1 • MIC Distribution of European and U.S. *M. catarrhalis* Isolates for 1992 and 1993 (*n* = 818)

Antibiotic	0.03	0.06	0.12	0.25	0.5	1	MIC 2	4	8	16	32	64
Penicillin	119[a]	18[a]	2[a]	17[b]	36[b]	160[b]	95[b]	60[b]	85[b]	224[b]	nt	nt
Amoxicillin	nt	152[a]	56[a]	153[a]	78[b]	111[b]	126[b]	104[b]	26[b]	4[b]	8[b]	nt
Amoxicillin/clavulanate	nt	471[a]	177[a]	154[a]	14[a]	2[a]	0[a]	0[a]	0[b]	0[b]	0[b]	nt
Cefaclor[b]	nt	nt	nt	179[a]	267[a]	296[a]	51[a]	16[a]	7[a]	2[c]	0[b]	0[b]
Cefuroxime	nt	nt	nt	96[a]	283[a]	226[a]	197[a]	15[a]	1[c]	0[b]	0[b]	0[b]
Cefixime	nt	nt	471[a]	210[a]	136[a]	1[a]	0[a]	0[b]	0[b]	0[b]	0[b]	nt
Ceftriaxone	nt	nt	458[a]	70[a]	158[a]	122[a]	9[a]	1[a]	0[a]	0[c]	0[c]	0[b]
Erythromycin	nt	129[a]	622[a]	48[a]	11[a]	3[c]	2[c]	3[c]	0[b]	0[b]	0[b]	nt
Clarithromycin	nt	728[a]	72[a]	8[a]	3[a]	3[a]	3[a]	1[c]	0[b]	0[b]	0[b]	nt
Azithromycin	nt	795[a]	13[a]	2[a]	6[a]	1[a]	1[a]	0[c]	0[b]	0[b]	0[b]	nt
Doxycycline	nt	nt	nt	810[a]	4[a]	3[a]	1[a]	0[d]	0[c]	0[b]	0[b]	nt
Chloramphenicol	nt	nt	nt	157[a]	615[a]	45[a]	1[a]	0[a]	0[a]	0[c]	0[b]	0[b]
Ciprofloxacin	628[a]	171[a]	15[a]	3[a]	0[a]	1[a]	0[a]	0[b]	0[b]	0[b]	nt	nt
Ofloxacin	49[a]	305[a]	445[a]	15[a]	3[a]	0[a]	0[a]	1[c]	0[b]	0[b]	nt	nt
Cotrimoxazole	nt	nt	nt	nt	796[a]	176[a]	4[a]	1[c]	0[b]	0[b]	0[b]	0[b]

[a]Sensitive.

[b]Resistant.

[c]Intermediate.

β-lactamase producers and non-β-lactamase producers (9, 44). MICs varied from less than 0.125 to 8 mg/L for non-β-lactamase producers. MICs for β-lactamase-producing strains ranged from 1 to more than 16 mg/L. Most recently, a study of community-acquired respiratory isolates from 15 centers in Europe and the United States (6) revealed 83% penicillin resistance, with an MIC breakpoint of 0.25 mg/L; 92% of U.S. isolates were resistant, compared with 79.4% of European isolates. All β-lactamase-producing strains had MICs above 0.25 mg/L, consistent with resistance. Of interest, 8.3% of β-lactamase-negative isolates from Europe were resistant, while all U.S. isolates had MICs below 0.06 mg/L and were uniformly sensitive.

Ampicillin/Amoxicillin

In general, ampicillin has greater in vitro activity against β-lactamase-producing *M. catarrhalis* than penicillin. Kallings (44) and Bronson et al. (9) reported an MIC range of 0.005 to 0.5 mg/L for β-lactamase (−) strains and an MIC range of 1 to 4 mg/L for β-lactamase (+) strains. A wide range of MICs for ampicillin has been reported, with both β-lactamase (−) and β-lactamase (+) strains. Careful scrutiny is necessary when evaluating ampicillin MICs in β-lactamase (+) strains with regard to achievable serum levels of ampicillin. Kovatch et al. (47) noted that ampicillin MICs in β-lactamase (+) strains were inoculum dependent. Interpretation of antimicrobial susceptibility may also depend upon changing MIC breakpoints. Kibsey et al. (46) found 56% resistance to ampicillin in 100 strains of *M. catarrhalis* by disk-diffusion testing. These same isolates showed 95% resistance with the broth microdilution technique. These discrepancies were reconciled with changes in breakpoint criteria from the 1990 NCCLS tables to 1992 NCCLS tables.

Fung et al. (34) found the ampicillin MIC_GM for BRO-1 producers to be 25 times that for nonproducers of β-lactamase.

BRO-2 producers were only 4 times higher than nonproducers. Spencer and Wheat (71) found an ampicillin MIC range of 0.06 to more than 8 mg/L for *M. catarrhalis* and an MIC$_{90}$ above 8 mg/L. Berk and Kalbfleisch (6) observed 55.9% amoxicillin resistance in 818 study isolates. Amoxicillin resistance was higher in U.S. isolates (73%) than in European isolates (49%). The European MIC$_{GM}$ was 0.44 mg/L in comparison to the U.S. MIC$_{GM}$ of 0.98 mg/L. Nonproducers of β-lactamase from Europe had MICs of amoxicillin ranging from 0.06 to 1.0 mg/L. Five strains were resistant to amoxicillin with MICs of 0.5 mg/L. U.S. nonproducing strains were uniformly sensitive with MICs of 0.06 mg/L.

Cephalosporins

Most studies have shown that β-lactamase production by *M. catarrhalis* confers only a modest effect on in vitro antibiotic susceptibilities to cephalosporins. Isolates with BRO-1 enzyme production are less susceptible to cephems than are BRO-2 and nonproducing isolates. Previous studies by Barry (5) and Fung et al. (33) revealed twofold increases in MICs for β-lactamase producers versus nonproducers. A similar relationship between enzyme production and waning cephalosporin susceptibility was noted by Berk and Kalbfleisch (6). MICs for cefaclor, cefuroxime, and ceftriaxone for β-lactamase producers were twice those for nonproducers.

Doern et al. (27) reported no substantial difference in antibiotic susceptibility to loracarbef between BRO-1 and BRO-2 producers. Nash et al. (57) found *M. catarrhalis* BRO-1 producers had two- to fourfold increased MICs for cefixime, cefuroxime, cephalexin, and cefaclor; BRO-2 production had a minimal effect on MIC interpretations. An antibiotic susceptibility study by Fung et al. (34) also noted two- to fourfold higher MICs for cefaclor, cefixime, loracarbef, and cefetamet for BRO-1 producers, compared with BRO-2 producers and nonproducers. This study also suggested that cefetamet and cefaclor were least affected by BRO-1 enzyme production. Berk and Kalbfleisch (6) reported cefixime to have a smaller difference in MICs for β-lactamase producers and nonproducers. In vitro studies of BRO-1 and BRO-2 producers by Ikeda et al. (41) revealed that cefaclor was hydrolyzed as rapidly as penicillin and amoxicillin, while cefixime was a poor substrate. Fung et al. (34) also reported cefixime to be 3 to 10 times more active against *M. catarrhalis* than loracarbef, cefaclor, and cefetamet. Stefani et al. (72) found that cefixime inhibited 90% of β-lactamase-producing and non-β-lactamase-producing strains of *M. catarrhalis* at less than 1 mg/L. Cefixime exhibited greater in vitro activity against *M. catarrhalis* than cefaclor; 4% of isolates were resistant to cefaclor, and 10% showed intermediate susceptibility (72).

Lambert-Zechowsky et al. assessed the bactericidal activity of cefaclor against 10 β-lactamase-producing strains of *M. catarrhalis* (49). An MIC range of 8 to 64 mg/L with an MIC_{90} of 16 mg/L was reported for cefaclor. No bactericidal activity was noted with cefaclor at 5 h, and no appreciable killing occurred at 24 h. A time killing study using 30 β-lactamase (+) isolates of *M. catarrhalis* found early bactericidal activity with cefixime (7). Bacterial regrowth occurred overnight with cefaclor at its Cmax. Prompt hydrolysis of cefaclor by the β-lactamase of *M. catarrhalis* probably accounts for this observation (7). Serum bactericidal activity of cefuroxime axetil, cefetamet pivoxil, and ceftibuten against 10 strains of *M. catarrhalis* was studied by Lemmen et al. (51). Cefuroxime axetil possessed the greatest serum bactericidal activity against *M. catarrhalis*, with 80% killing at a titer of 1:8 or above after 2 hours. Cefetamet pivoxil and ceftibufen provided 60% killing at a titer of 1:8 or above after 2 h. A similar study with clarithromycin and cefaclor revealed 10% killing of *M. catarrhalis* at a titer of 1:8 after 2 h with cefaclor; no activity was detected with cefaclor at 6 h (50).

Macrolides

Erythromycin resistance was initially reported from Sweden in 1983 (44). Slevin et al. (70) from New Zealand and Davies and Maesen (22) from the Netherlands also reported reduced susceptibility to erythromycin. Brown et al. (11) confirmed a similar trend in U.S. isolates. A 3.6% incidence of erythromycin resistance was found in 305 U.K. isolates in 1991 (64). Fung et al. (33) reported comparable results in a study of 413 *M. catarrhalis* isolates from England and Scotland. Subsequent reports from Struelens et al. (73), Nash et al. (57), Spencer and Wheat (71), Stefani et al. (72), and Forsgren and Walder (31) identified no resistant strains in more than 450 isolates studied. Of the 818 isolates tested by Berk and Kalbfleish (6), none exhibited erythromycin resistance. Eight strains from Europe had intermediate susceptibility to erythromycin and MICs above 0.5 mg/L. No in vitro bactericidal activity for erythromycin or erythromycin combined with sulfisoxazole was found by Lambert-Zechowsky (49). A bacteriostatic effect was observed.

The in vitro activity of roxithromycin was studied in 188 clinical isolates of *M. catarrhalis* (71). An MIC range of 0.06 to 0.25 mg/L and an MIC_{90} of 0.25 mg/L was determined for roxithromycin. An MIC_{90} of 1 mg/L was reported by Hardy et al. (38) on 17 isolates of *M. catarrhalis*.

A study by Humphreys et al. (40) assessed the sensitivity of 223 strains of *M.catarrhalis* in the United Kingdom to clarithromycin (by Stokes method); 94.9% of β-lactamase (−) strains were judged sensitive to clarithromycin while 97.9% of β-lactamase (+) strains were sensitive. Similar percentages were found for erythromycin. Barry (5) found the macrolide and azalide agents to have considerable activity again 55 β-lactamase (+) and (−) strains of *M. catarrhalis*. European and U.S. isolates of *M. catarrhalis* (6) had an MIC_{90} of 0.12 mg/L for clarithromycin, with only one isolate of intermediate susceptibility (MIC = 4 mg/L). Azithromycin MIC_{90} was 0.06 mg/L, with no resistant isolates noted.

The serum bactericidal activity of clarithromycin against 10 isolates of *M. catarrhalis* was evaluated by Lemmen et al. (50). Clarithromycin exhibited some activity, with approximately 30% of *M. catarrhalis* isolates dying at a titer of 1:8 at 2 h; only 20% killing was noted at 6 h.

Tetracyclines

Tetracycline resistance was initially reported in Swedish isolates by Kallings et al. (44). By 1988, tetracycline resistance has increased to 15% in the Netherlands (22), and Zheng and Cao reported 43% resistance in China (82). Tetracycline-resistant isolates were also recovered in the United States by 1988 (11). Wallace et al. (76) identified the Tet B resistance determinant in two resistant strains of *M. catarrhalis* but found in vitro transfer of this determinant problematic. The slow spread of tetracycline resistance may best be explained by this finding.

An antimicrobial sensitivity study of 305 *M. catarrhalis* isolates by Powell et al. (64) found less than 4% resistance to tetracycline. Spencer and Wheat (71) reported an MIC range of 0.25 to more than 8 mg/L of tetracycline and an MIC_{90} of 1 mg/L. Wallace et al. (76) reported an MIC_{90} of 0.25 mg/L. Berk and Kalbfleisch (6) found all 818 isolates of *M. catarrhalis* to be highly susceptible to doxycycline. Only four European isolates had MICs above 0.5 mg/L.

Fluoroquinolones

Quinolones have considerable respiratory tissue penetration and are known to exhibit a postantibiotic effect, which make them efficacious in the treatment of respiratory tract infections. Ball and Tillotson (3) reviewed 37 published clinical trials of ciprofloxacin treatment in patients with lower respiratory tract infections; 74 patients with *M. catarrhalis* lower respiratory tract infections were treated with ciprofloxacin, with an eradication percentage of 96%. The 22 published cases of bronchitis revealed an eradication percentage of 95.4% for ciprofloxacin.

Struelens et al. (73) found ciprofloxacin and ofloxacin to have lower MICs against all 46 *M. catarrhalis* isolates (71.7% β-lactamase producers) than nine other commonly used agents. Bourgeois and Bingen (8) reported an MIC_{90} of 0.12 mg/L for ofloxacin and an MIC_{90} of 0.06 mg/L for ciprofloxacin. Wallace et al. (76) reported an MIC_{90} of 0.015 mg/L for ciprofloxacin. Most published MIC_{90}s for ciprofloxacin have been 0.06 mg/L or less. Berk and Kalbfleisch (6) found all *M. catarrhalis* isolates in their centers sensitive to ciprofloxacin (MIC_{90} = 0.06 mg/L). One U.S. isolate had intermediate sensitivity to ofloxacin (MIC = 4 mg/L). Ofloxacin had an MIC_{90} of 0.06 mg/L as well.

A highly ciprofloxacin-resistant strain of *M. catarrhalis* was isolated from the sputum of a patient who received six courses of oral ciprofloxacin over a 6-month period (18). Ciprofloxacin MIC by E-Test (AB Biodisk, Sweden) was 8 mg/L. MICs by agar dilution were 4 mg/L for ciprofloxacin, 8 mg/L for norfloxacin, and 4 mg/L for ofloxacin. The mechanism of resistance is yet unknown. Possible explanations include decreased permeability to quinolones, decreased affinity of DNA gyrase for quinolones, or active efflux of the antimicrobial agent (18).

Fluoroquinolones have favorable in vitro bactericidal activity against *M. catarrhalis* (8). Concentration-dependent killing was observed, with 24-h bactericidal activity noted for both ciprofloxacin and ofloxacin. Krasemann et al. (48) also found bactericidal activity with ciprofloxacin at 0.25 mg/L (Cmax/8) against β-lactamase (+) strains of *M. catarrhalis*.

Combination Drugs

Amoxicillin/Clavulanate

The β-lactamase activity of *M. catarrhalis* is counteracted by β-lactamase inhibitors such as sulbactam and clavulanic acid (1, 25, 59). Alvarez et al. (2) found that testing β-lactamase producers for ampicillin susceptibility in the presence of clavulanic acid resulted in significantly lower MICs. Cooper et al. (16) found both BRO-1 and BRO-2 producers of β-lactamase to be inhibited by low concentrations of clavulanic acid. A study of 375 *M. catarrhalis* isolates from England and Scotland in 1991 found MICs of amoxicillin/clavulanate ranging from 0.008 to 0.25 mg/L for β-lactamase producers and from 0.008 to 0.06 mg/L for nonproducers, while others found similar results (MIC ranges, ≤0.03–0.06 for nonproducers and ≤0.03–0.25 mg/L for β-lactamase producers) (5, 33).

Studies by Struelens et al. (73) and Powell et al. (64) found no *M. catarrhalis* strains resistant to amoxicillin/clavulanate in a total of 351 isolates tested. Berk and Kalbfleisch (6) tested 818 *M. catarrhalis* strains from Western Europe and the United States and found all susceptible to amoxicillin/clavulanate as well. The MIC_{90} of amoxicillin/clavulanate was quite low (0.12 mg/L). A time killing study performed on five β-lactamase producers by Yourassowsky et al. (81) reported MICs of amoxicillin/clavulanate of 0.03 to 0.12 mg/L.

In vitro bactericidal activity of amoxicillin/clavulanate for 30 β-lactamase (+) strains of *M. catarrhalis* was studied by Bingen et al. (7), who found an MIC_{90} of 0.5 mg/L for amoxicillin/clavulanate (range, 0.06–0.5 mg/L). Rapid bactericidal activity (<24 h) was found for amoxicillin/clavulanate against *M. catarrhalis*. Bactericidal activity takes on particular relevance when treating immunocompromised patients or patients with deep-seated infectious processes such as endocarditis, osteomyelitis, meningitis, and bacteremia.

Trimethoprim/Sulfamethoxazole or Cotrimazole

Despite the inherent resistance of *M. catarrhalis* to trimethoprim, most isolates are sensitive to trimethoprim in combination with sulfamethoxazole (2, 26, 74). Resistance to the combination of trimethoprim and sulfamethoxazole (TMP/SMX) was reported by Slevin et al. (70) in New Zealand and by Robledano et al. (68) in Spain.

Wallace et al. (76) reported an MIC_{90} of 0.25 mg/L for TMP/SMX and a MIC_{90} 4.0 mg/L for sulfisoxazole. Spencer and Wheat (71) found an MIC range of 0.5:0.025 to >8:0.4 mg/L for sulfamethoxazole-trimethoprim (19:1). An MIC_{90} above 8:0.4 mg/L was found for the combination. Fung et al. (33) evaluated 413 clinical isolates of *M. catarrhalis* and found uniform resistance to trimethoprim (MICs, 2–128 mg/L). Sulfamethoxazole MICs were 0.06 to 128 mg/L with a breakpoint of 32 mg/L or above. Some 6.5% of *M. catarrhalis* isolates were resistant to 32 mg/L or less of sulfamethoxazole in combination with trimethoprim. In contrast, Riley et al. (67) detected no *M. catarrhalis* isolates requiring more than 32 mg/L of sulfamethoxazole for inhibition.

Humphreys et al. (40) found 62% of 223 *M. catarrhalis* strains sensitive to cotrimazole. Berk and Kalbfleisch (6) found all isolates susceptible to cotrimazole (MIC_{90} = 0.5 mg/L). A trend toward rising MICs of cotrimazole has been noted as well as sporadic resistance.

ANTIMICROBIAL THERAPY

Upper Respiratory Tract Infection

M. catarrhalis is a recognized pathogen in pediatric upper respiratory infections such as otitis media, sinusitis, and pharyngitis. Treatment is generally empirical and usually includes oral medications (which may be available in liquid formulation) for 10 days. Second- and third-generation cephalosporins, trimethoprim-sulfamethoxazole, and amoxicillin/clavulanate are considered first-line agents. Erythromycin and the newer macrolides and azalides have considerable activity against *M. catarrhalis* but questionable performance against *H. influenzae*. Selection of the optimal antimicrobial agent must take into account other possible pathogens, since infections may be polymicrobial and acceptable material for culture may not be readily available. Tetracyclines and fluoroquinolones are not recommended for treatment in children because of their potential for adverse reactions. Recent studies comparing the clinical efficacy of a single intramuscular dose of ceftriaxone with 7- to 10-day courses of oral antimicrobial therapy for acute otitis media have shown comparable outcomes (4, 12, 36, 75). Single-dose parenteral therapy may be advantageous when vomiting may cause suboptimal absorption of oral formulations or poor compliance is anticipated.

Lower Respiratory Tract Infection

Lower respiratory tract infections may involve acute exacerbations of tracheobronchitis or pneumonia in patients with chronic respiratory disease and various immunologic derangements such as long-term steroid usage, alcoholism, hypogammaglobulinemia, and neutropenia. Mixed infection with other respiratory pathogens such as *S. pneumoniae* and *H. influenzae* are common. The diagnosis of lower respiratory infection due to *M. catarrhalis* may be made on the basis of Gram stain and culture of expectorated sputum. These evaluations may be problematic in patients with chronic bronchitis and in the very young or old. A documented *M. catarrhalis* lower respiratory infection may be treated with second-generation cephalosporins, trimethoprim-sulfamethoxazole, erythromycin, β-lactamase inhibitor combinations (ampicillin/sulbactam or amoxicillin/clavulanate), or tetracyclines as first-line agents. Empirical treatment prior to culture confirmation of *M. catarrhalis* must cover other possible pathogens and generally includes broad-spectrum agents such as second- and third-generation cephalosporins. The duration of therapy is generally 10 to 14 days, depending on the patient's clinical response.

Bacteremia

The clinical features of *M. catarrhalis* bacteremia vary somewhat from the pediatric to adult population and from the immunocompetent to the immunodeficient host. Most patients have underlying disease and associated respiratory tract infections. Bacteremia may be present in normal hosts (particularly children) with otitis media and sinusitis. Selection of antimicrobial therapy depends upon the patient's clinical presentation and immune status. Neutropenic patients should receive broad-spectrum agents as empirical parenteral therapy to cover Gram-positive and Gram-negative pathogens. Immunocompetent patients may receive parenteral second- or third-generation cephalosporins or ampicillin/sulbactam. Fluoroquinolones could be used as second-line options for patients allergic to penicillin or β-lactam antibiotics and in streamlining therapy from parenteral to oral formulations. Prompt antibiotic therapy should be initiated whenever *M. catarrhalis* is isolated from blood. *M. catarrhalis* may have significant pathogenicity even in an immunocompetent host. The recommended duration of therapy for bacteremia without associated endocarditis is 14 days.

Bacteremia with endocarditis usually produces a continuous bacteremia with numerous positive blood cultures. Endocarditis due to *M. catarrhalis* is a rare entity and there is limited clinical experience in treating this serious and life-threatening infection. Therapeutic decisions are best guided by in vitro susceptibility testing and determination of β-lactamase activity. Empirical therapy may be necessary while awaiting in vitro susceptibility testing results and should consist of β-lactamase-stable antimicrobial agents with bacteriocidal activity. Second- and third-generation cephalosporins are attractive options since more experience has been gained recently in using these agents in the treatment of endocarditis (32). The most recently reported *M. catarrhalis* endocarditis (61) was treated with a parenteral broad-spectrum cephalosporin with defervescence within 48 h and had a favorable clinical outcome. Treatment options for patients sensitive to penicillin and other β-lactam antibiotics are best guided by in vitro susceptibility testing. Possible options include aminoglycosides, fluoroquinolones, erythromycin, and chloramphenicol. Fluoroquinolones and aminoglycosides are reasonable options for combination therapy since these agents exert a postantibiotic effect and are bacteriocidal. Experience with the use of fluoroquinolones and erythromycin in endocarditis is limited. Fluoroquinolones should only be used when established treatments are not possible or have failed.

Meningitis

M. catarrhalis meningitis has been reported only sporadically since 1908. Questions have been raised regarding the possible misidentification of *M. catarrhalis* in the cerebrospinal fluid in the early cases. *Neisseria meningitidis* shares many microbiologic similarities with *M. catarrhalis*. It is possible, however, that the paucity of cases since that time may reflect a natural change in the spectrum of this disease. Due to the small number of clinically documented cases of *M. catarrhalis* meningitis, recommendations regarding therapy should be drawn primarily from in vitro susceptibility data. This is best illustrated in the recent report of a case of neonatal meningitis in which the isolate was sensitive only to ceftazidime, amikacin, netilmicin, and erythromycin (21). Previous patients have been treated with combinations of various agents such as penicillin, chloramphenicol, and sulfa. The fact that most *M. catarrhalis* isolates are presently β-lactamase producers suggests use of β-lactamase-stable antimicrobial agents. The recent recommendations for empirical use of a third-generation cephalosporin in combination with vancomycin for bacterial meningitis in which penicillin-resistant *S. pneumoniae* is suspected should provide reasonable coverage for *M. catarrhalis*. Third-generation cephalosporins have excellent central nervous system (CNS) penetration and favorable efficacy against *M. catarrhalis,* while vancomycin has no activity against this organism. Treatment options for patients allergic to β-lactam antimicrobials are chloramphenicol and trimethoprim-sulfamethoxazole. Tetracyclines and fluoroquinolones have contraindications in pediatric patients, where most *M. catarrhalis* meningitis has been documented. Fluoroquinolones also have variable CNS penetration and should only be considered when more-accepted therapy has been futile.

Bone and Joint Infection

M. catarrhalis has been implicated in vertebral osteomyelitis (65) and septic arthritis (17, 56) on rare occasion. Empirical coverage with a second- or third-generation cephalosporin is reasonable unless Gram stains of the infected material suggest staphylococcus. Fluoroquinolones are also reasonable therapeutic options in adults, particularly when streamlining from intravenous to oral therapy or when intravenous access is problematic.

Eye Infection

M. catarrhalis has been reported as an etiologic agent in ophthalmia neonatorum (35), adult conjunctivitis (13, 45), and keratitis (78). Treatment of ocular infections such as conjunctivitis and keratitis is usually initiated while awaiting culture confirmation. Gram stains of conjunctival secretions or corneal scrapings direct empirical therapy. Ideally, antimicrobial agents are applied topically in concentrated formulations for enhanced penetration. Subconjunctival injection, continuous lavage, or parenteral therapy may be used when keratitis

TABLE 2 • Adult Doses

Agents	Route	Dose	Infection	Frequency	Duration (days)	Pregnancy Category
Cefprozil	p.o.	500 mg	Bronchitis/sinusitis	q. 12 h	10–14[b]	B
Cefuroxime axetil	p.o.	250–500 mg[3]	Bronchitis/sinusitis/pneumonia[3]	q. 12 h	10–14[b]	B
Cefuroxime	i.v.	750 mg–1.5 g[3/4/5]	Pneumonia[3]/bacteremia[4]/ Bone & joint[5]	q. 8 h	10–14[b]	B
Cefixime	p.o.	400 mg	Bronchitis/sinusitis/pneumonia	q. 24 h	10–14[b]	B
Cefpodoxime	p.o.	200 mg	Bronchitis/sinusitis/pneumonia	q. 12 h	10–14[b]	B
Ceftriaxone	i.v. or i.m.	1–2 g max; 2 g q. 12 h[6]	Pneumonia/meningitis[6]/ Bone & joint	q. 12–24 h	10–14[b]	B
Amoxicillin/ clavulanate	p.o.	250–500 mg[3]	Bronchitis/sinusitis/pneumonia[3]	q. 8 h	10–14	B
Ampicillin/sulbactam	i.v./i.m.	1.5–3.0 g	Pneumonia	q. 6 h	10–14	B
Trimethoprim/ sulfamethoxazole TMP/SMX	p.o. i.v.[3]	1 DS tab 5 mg/kg i.v. (TMP)	Bronchitis/sinusitis Pneumonia[3]	q. 12 h q. 6 h	10–14	Caution Contraindicated at term
Erythromycin	p.o.	250 mg/333[a] mg/500 mg	Bronchitis/sinusitis/pneumonia	q. 6/8/12 h[a]	10–14	B estolate contraindicated
Erythromycin	i.v.[3]	500 mg–1 gm	Pneumonia[3]	q. 6 h	10–14	B
Clarithromycin	p.o.	250 mg–500 mg	Bronchitis/sinusitis/pneumonia	q. 12 h	10–14	C/contraindicated
Azithromycin	p.o.	500 mg day 1/250 mg day 2–5	Bronchitis/sinusitis	q. 24 h	5	B
Azithromycin	i.v.[3]	500 mg	Pneumonia[3]	q. 24 h (2–5)	7–10 total i.v./p.o.	B
Ciprofloxacin	p.o./i.v.	500–750 mg p.o./400 mg i.v.	Bronchitis/sinusitis/pneumonia/ bacteremia/bone & joint	q. 12 h	10–14[b]	C/contraindicated
Ofloxacin	p.o./i.v.	400 mg p.o./ 400 mg i.v.	Bronchitis/sinusitis/pneumonia/ bacteremia/bone & joint	q. 12 h	10–14[b]	C/contraindicated
Levofloxacin	p.o./i.v.	500 mg p.o./ 500 mg i.v.	Bronchitis/sinusitis/pneumonia/ bacteremia/bone & joint	q. 24 h	10–14[b]	C/contraindicated
Tetracycline	p.o.	250–500 mg	Bronchitis/sinusitis	q. 6 h	10–14	Contraindicated
Doxycycline	p.o.	200 mg 1st day/ 100 mg q. day	Bronchitis/sinusitis/pneumonia	q. 12–24 h	10–14	Contraindicated
Doxycycline	i.v.	100 mg	Pneumonia	q. 12 h	10–14	Contraindicated
Chloramphenicol	i.v.	100 mg/kg/d[7]	Meningitis[7]	q. 6 h	10–14[b]	Caution— especially at term
Chloramphenicol	i.v. 50 mg–75 mg/kg/day		Bacteremia/pneumonia	q. 6 h	10–14[b]	Caution— especially at term

[a]Preparation dependent.

[b]Bone infections and bacteremia with associated endocarditis require longer therapy.

is present. Parenteral therapy is usually necessary when deep corneal ulcers pose a threat of perforation. Parenteral second- and third-generation cephalosporins and aminoglycosides are effective options. Topical therapies are not judged on the basis of MIC determinations, which apply to the achievable serum levels of antimicrobial agents. Therapeutic options should, however, have bactericidal activity for *M. catarrhalis,* limited toxicity to ocular tissues, and a low risk of emergence of resistance. Topical aminoglycosides, erythromycin, and tetracycline can be used. Topical fluoroquinolones are generally reserved for severe conjunctivitis. Topical therapy is usually applied every 2 to 4 h for 7 to 10 days.

Periocular infection with *M. catarrhalis* has been reported in a patient with pediatric bacteremia with preseptal cellulitis (69). Parenteral therapy with a second- or third-generation

cephalosporin, trimethoprim-sulfamethoxazole, or chloramphenicol should be initiated in the pediatric population. Tetracycline or fluoroquinolones could be used as well in adults. Antimicrobial therapy may be further refined when the results of susceptibility and β-lactamase testing are available.

Peritonitis Associated with Continuous Ambulatory Peritoneal Dialysis

M. catarrhalis has been associated with bacterial peritonitis in patients receiving continuous ambulatory peritoneal dialysis (CAPD) (15, 19, 20, 53). Therapeutic decisions for *M. catarrhalis* peritonitis are best directed by antimicrobial susceptibility testing results and determination of β-lactamase production. The intraperitoneal route is preferred for CAPD patients, and second- and third-generation cephalosporins

TABLE 3 • Pediatric Doses

Agents	Route	Dose	Infection	Frequency	Duration
Cefprozil	p.o.	30 mg/kg q. d[1], 15 mg/kg q. d.[2]	Acute otitis media[1]/pharyngitis/ sinusitis/bronchitis	q. 12 h	10–14 days[a]
Cefuroxime axetil	p.o.	30–40 mg/kg/day[1]/ 20 mg/kg/day[2]	Acute otitis media[1]/pharyngitis[2] sinusitis/bronchitis/pneumonia	q. 12 h	10–14 days[a]
Cefuroxime	i.v.	100–150 mg/kg/day[5/6]	Pneumonia[4]/bacteremia[5]/ bone & joint[6]	q. 8 h	10–14 days[a]
Cefixime	p.o.	8 mg/kg/day[1]	Acute otitis media[1]/pharyngitis sinusitis/bronchitis/pneumonia	q. 24 h	10–14 days[a]
Cefpodoxime	p.o.	10 mg/kg/day[1] (NTE 400 mg/day[1])	Acute otitis media[1]/pharyngitis Sinusitis/bronchitis/pneumonia	q. 12 h	10–14 days[a]
Ceftriaxone	i.v. or IM	50mg/kg to 75–100 mg/kg/day[7b]	Acute otitis media[1]/bronchitis/ pneumonia/meningitis[7] bacteremia/bone & joint	Single dose[1] to 12 h[7]	10–14 days[a]
Amoxicillin/clavulanate	p.o.	40/6.4–20/6. 4 mg/kg/day	Acute otitis media[1]/bronchitis/ pneumonia/pharyngitis/sinusitis	q. 8 h	10–14 days[a]
Ampicillin/sulbactam	i.v. or i.m. Not recommended if < 12 years of age	25–50 mg/kg q6° 50–100 mg/kg[7] q6	Pneumonia[4]/meningitis[7]/ bacteremia[5]/bone & joint[6]	q. 6 h	10–14 days[a]
Trimethoprim/ sulfamethoxazole TMP/SMX	p.o. i.v.[4/6/7]	8 mg/kg/day (TMP)[1] 5 mg/kg q. 6 h (TMP)	Acute otitis media[1]/bronchitis/ pneumonia[4] Meningitis[7]/bacteremia[6]/sinusitis	q. 12 h q. 6 h	10–14 days 10–14 days
Erythro-sulfisoxazole	p.o.	40 mg/kg/day[1]	Acute otitis media[1]/bronchitis/ pneumonia/pharyngitis/sinusitis	q. 6–8 h	10–14 days
Erythromycin	p.o.	30–40 mg/kg/day	Acute otitis media[1]/bronchitis/ pneumonia/pharyngitis/sinusitis	q. 6/8/12 h	10–14 days
Erythromycin	i.v.	15–40 mg/kg/day	Pneumonia[4]	q. 6 h	10–14 days
Clarithromycin	p.o.	7.5 mg/kg/day	Acute otitis media[1]/bronchitis/ pneumonia/pharyngitis/sinusitis	q. 12 h (NTE 500 mg dose)	10–14 days
Azithromycin	p.o.	10 mg/kg/day, then 5 mg/kg/day 2–5 days	Acute otitis media[1]/bronchitis/ pneumonia/sinusitis/pharyngitis	q. 24 h	5 days dosing
Chloramphenicol	i.v.	50–75 mg/kg/day	Bacteremia	q. 6 h	10–14 days[a]
Chloramphenicol	i.v.	100 mg/kg/day[7]	Meningitis[7]	q. 6 h	10–14 days[a]

[a]Bone infections and bacteremia with associated endocarditis require longer therapy.

[b]100 mg/kg primary dose for meningitis not to exceed 4 g then 100/kg/day not to exceed (4 g/day).

are well tolerated. Aminoglycosides and trimethoprim-sulfamethoxazole are also acceptable options, especially for patients with β-lactam allergy. Initial and maintenance doses should be adjusted to maintain an antimicrobial concentration above the MIC for *M. catarrhalis* for the duration of the dosing interval. The duration of intraperitoneal therapy usually ranges from 10 to 21 days and depends upon a functioning catheter. Systemic therapy should be initiated if the intraperitoneal route is not available.

CAVEATS AND COMMENTS

Clinicians presently face a challenging era with rapid emergence of antibiotic-resistant bacteria. Prudent use of antibiotics in the managed-care environment with formulary restrictions must be balanced with the delivery of safe and effective therapy without risk to the patient. Optimal therapy involves prompt identification of the pathogen whenever possible, targeted therapy based on antibiotic susceptibility studies, and adequate doses and duration of treatment.

In clinical situations in which *M. catarrhalis* is a pathogen, bacterial cultures may be difficult to obtain (i.e., tympanocentesis, transtracheal aspirate, or sinus aspirates). Therapeutic intervention may be empirical, particularly in the ambulatory setting. Treatment decisions will be based upon the severity of the infection, likelihood of resistance in the suspected pathogens, and clinician awareness and understanding of antibiotic resistance.

The prevalence of β-lactamase-producing strains of *M. catarrhalis* approaching 100% in some U.S. centers, should draw attention to the clinical evidence regarding treatment failures with penicillin and ampicillin therapy. Empirical use of penicillin, ampicillin, or amoxicillin is not advised in treating presumed *M. catarrhalis* infections. The progressive spread of resistance among other respiratory pathogens such as *S. pneumoniae* and *H. influenzae* also makes empirical use of these agents obsolete. In summary, β-lactamase-producing strains of *M. catarrhalis* should not be treated with penicillin, ampicillin, or amoxicillin regardless of MICs suggesting susceptibility.

Other concerns regarding the indirect pathogenic potential of *M. catarrhalis* warrant mention as well. Brook (10) and others have postulated that β-lactamase production by *M. catarrhalis* may prevent eradication of other bacteria such as *H. influenzae* and group A streptococci because of inactivation of penicillinase-susceptible penicillins. Yamada et al. (80) developed a simple agar double-layer method to evaluate the influence of β-lactamase-producing organisms such as *M. catarrhalis* on the disk susceptibility of other pathogens to various antibiotics. While evaluating *S. pneumoniae, Streptococcus pyogenes,* and *H. influenzae,* Yamada et al. found reduced inhibition zones for various drugs in the presence of β-lactamase-producing *M. catarrhalis.*

The relatively high MICs of amoxicillin for β-lactamase (−) isolates of *M. catarrhalis* noted by Berk and Kalbfleisch (6) suggest additional modes of resistance necessitating further study.

Data from various studies suggest that β-lactamase production by *M. catarrhalis* has a limited effect on the in vitro susceptibility to oral or parenteral cephalosporins. In general, second- and third-generation cephalosporin resistance is unusual in *M. catarrhalis.* A trend toward cefaclor resistance may be in progress, with intermediate susceptibility of *M. catarrhalis* strains being reported in different areas. Studies assessing serum bactericidal activity by Lambert-Zechowsky (49), Bingen et al. (7), and Lemmen et al. (50) failed to reveal any bactericidal activity of cefaclor as well. Resistance to erythromycin and tetracycline have been reported, but to date, spread has been slow. With increasing use of newer macrolides in the United States, further progression of *M. catarrhalis* resistance to these agents may be forthcoming.

The effect of selective antibiotic pressure on development of resistance is best shown in the recent report by Cunliffe et al. (18) of a highly ciprofloxacin resistant strain of *M. catarrhalis.* To date fluoroquinolones have very low MICs against *M. catarrhalis* isolates, but this could change with further fluoroquinolone use.

Various oral and parenteral therapeutic agents are available for treatment of *M. catarrhalis* infection. Table 2 lists adult doses for common infections caused by *M. catarrhalis;* Table 3 lists pediatric doses. Selecting an antibiotic for empirical use involves consideration of *M. catarrhalis* sensitivity data as well as data for *S. pneumoniae* and *H. influenzae.* Constraints on therapy imposed by drug-resistant *S. pneumoniae* and coverage for *H. influenzae* are more likely. Once microbiologic confirmation and sensitivity profiles are available, use of a narrower-spectrum agent may be possible.

The choice of oral or parenteral therapy depends on the severity of illness and the patient's immune status and ability to retain oral medications. Special consideration should be given to the bactericidal activity of different therapeutic options when immunosuppression, deep-seated infection, or the potential for bacteremia or meningitis exists.

REFERENCES

1. Ahmad F, McLeod DT, Croughan MJ, Calder MA. Antimicrobial susceptibility of Branhamella isolates from bronchopulmonary infections. Antimicrob Agents Chemother 1984;26: 424–425.

2. Alvarez S, Jones M, Holtsclaw-Berk S, Guarderas J, Berk SL. In vitro susceptibilities and β-lactamase production of 53 clinical isolates of Branhamella catarrhalis. Antimicrob Agents Chemother 1985;27:646–647.

3. Ball AP, Tillotson GS. Lower respiratory tract infection therapy—the role of ciprofloxacin. J Int Med Res 1995;23:315–327.

4. Barnett ED, Tule DW, Klein JO, Cabral HJ, Kharasch SJ, and the Greater Boston Otitis Media Study Group. Comparison of ceftriaxone and trimethoprim-sulfamethoxazole for acute otitis media. Pediatrics 1997;99:23–28.

5. Barry AL. In vitro potency of nine orally administered antimicrobial agents against three respiratory tract pathogens. Eur J Clin Microbiol Infect Dis 1992;11:867–869.

6. Berk SL, Kalbfleisch JH. Antibiotic susceptibility patterns of community acquired respiratory isolates of Moraxella catarrhalis in western Europe and in the USA. J Antimicrob Chemother 1996;38(Suppl A):85–96.

7. Bingen E, Bourgeois F, Chardon H, Doit C, Lambert-Zechovsky, N. Killing kinetics of five orally administered antibiotics at clinically achievable concentrations against Moraxella catarrhalis. Eur J Clin Microbiol Infect Dis 1992;11:923–926.

8. Bourgeois F, Bingen E. Killing kinetics of five fluroquinolones against Moraxella catarrhalis at clinically achievable concentrations. J Antimicrob Chemother 1994;33:364–365.

9. Bronson JE, Larsson P, Zachrisson G. Antibiotic susceptibility of bacteria commonly isolated from the upper respiratory tract. Infection 1983;11:287–288.

10. Brook I. Pathogenicity of Branhamella catarrhalis in respiratory tract infections. Immunol Allergy Pract 1988;10:342–348.

11. Brown BA, Wallace RJ Jr, Flanagan CW, Wilson RW, Luman JI, Redditt SD. Tetracycline and erythromycin resistance among clinical isolates of Branhamella catarrhalis. Antimicrob Agents and Chemother 1989;33:1631–1633.

12. Chamberlain JM, Boenning DA, Ochsenschlager DW, Klein BL. Single dose ceftriaxone versus 10 days of ceclor for otitis media. Clin Pediatr 1994;33:642–646.

13. Chin AT. Branhamella catarrhalis conjunctivitis. Can Med Assoc J 1983;129:922–926.

14. Christensen JJ, Keiding J, Bruun B. Antimicrobial susceptibility and β-lactamase characterization of Branhamella catarrhalis isolates from 1983/1984 and 1988. APMIS 1990;98:1039–1044.

15. Contreras MR, Ash SR, Swick SD, Grutzner J. Peritonitis due to Moraxella (Branhamella) catarrhalis in a diabetic patient receiving peritoneal dialysis. South Med J 1993;86:589–590.

16. Cooper CE, Slocombe B, White AR. Effect of low concentration of clavulanic acid on the in-vitro activity of amoxicillin against β-lactamase producing Branhamella catarrhalis and Hemophilus influenzae. J Antimicrob Chemother 1990;26:371–380.

17. Craig DB, Wehrle PA. Branhamella catarrhalis septic arthritis. J Rheumatol 1983;10:985–986.

18. Cunliffe NA, Emmanuel FX, Thomson CJ. Lower respiratory tract infection due to ciprofloxacin resistant Moraxella catarrhalis J Antimicrob Chemother 1995;36:273–274.

19. Dadone C, Redaelli B. Branhamella catarrhalis peritonitis in CAPD: an avoidable complication? Peritoneal Dial Int 1991;11: 185.

20. Damari NN, Chin ATL. Branhamella catarrhalis peritonitis in a continuous ambulatory peritoneal dialysis patient. Nephron 1987;45:160–161.

21. Daoud A, Abuekteish F, Masaadeh H. Neonatal meningitis due

to Moraxella catarrhalis and review of the literature. Ann Trop Paediatr 1996;16:199–201.

22. Davies BI, Maesen FP. The epidemiology of respiratory tract pathogens in southern Netherlands. Eur Respir J 1988;1: 415–420.

23. Doern GV. Branhamella catarrhalis—an emerging human pathogen. Diagn Microbiol Infect Dis 1986;4:191–201.

24. Doern GV, Gantz NM. Isolation of Branhamella (Neisseria) catarrhalis from men with urethritis. Sex Transm Dis 1982;9: 202–204.

25. Doern GV, Siebers KG, Hallick LM, Morse SA. Antibiotic susceptibility of beta-lactamase-producing strains of Branhamella (Neisseria) catarrhalis. Antimicrob Agents and Chemother 1980;17:24–29.

26. Doern GV, Tubert TA. In vitro activities of 39 antimicrobial agents for Branhamella catarrhalis and comparison of results of different quantitative susceptibility test methods. Antimicrob Agents and Chemother 1988;32:259–261.

27. Doern GV, Vantour R, Parker D, Tubert T, Torres B. In vitro activity of loracarbef (LY163892) a new oral carbacephem antimicrobial agent, against respiratory isolates of Haemophilus influenzae and Moraxella catarrhalis. Antimicro Agents Chemother 1991;35:1504–1507.

28. Eliasson I, Kamme C, Vang M, Waley SG. Characterization of cell-bound papain-soluble beta-lactamases in Bro-1 and Bro-2 producing strains of Moraxella (Branhamella) catarrhalis and Moraxella nonliquifaciens. Eur J Clin Microbiol Infect Dis 1992;11:313–321.

29. Farmer T, Reading C. Beta-lactamases of Branhamella catarrhalis and their inhibition by clavulanic acid. Antimicrob Agents and Chemother 1982;21:506–508.

30. Feigin RD, San Joaquin V, Middelkamp JN. Purpura fulminans associated with Neisseria catarrhalis septicemia and meningitis. Pediatrics 1969;44:120–123.

31. Forsgren A, Walder M. Antimicrobial susceptibility of bacterial isolates in south Sweden including a 13 year follow-up study of some respiratory tract pathogens. APMIS 1994;102(3):227–235.

32. Francioli PB. Ceftriaxone and outpatient treatment of infective endocarditis. In: Wilson WR, Steckelberg JM, eds. Infectious disease clinics of North America. Philadelphia: WB Saunders 1993;7:97–115.

33. Fung CP, Powell M, Seymour M, Yuan T, Williams JD. The antimicrobial susceptibility of Moraxella catarrhalis isolated in England and Scotland in 1991. J Antimicrob Chemother 1992;30:47–55.

34. Fung CP, Yeo SF, Livermore DM. Susceptibility of Moraxella catarrhalis isolates to β-lactamase antibiotics in relation to β-lactamase pattern. J Antimicrob Chemother 1994;33:215–222.

35. Garvey RJP, Reed TAG. Ophthalmia neonatorum due to Branhamella (Neisseria) catarrhalis. Case reports. Br J Vener Dis 1981;57:346.

36. Gehanno P, Tailleve M, Deims P, Jacquet P, Hoareau J, Gojon D, Pascarel J, Kosowski A. Short-course cefotaxime compared with five-day co-amoxyclav in acute otitis media in children. J Antimicrob Chemother 1990;26(Suppl A):29–36.

37. Hager H, Verghese A, Alvarez S, Berk SL. Branhamella catarrhalis respiratory infections. Rev Infec Dis 1987;9:1140–1149.

38. Hardy DJ, Hensey DM, Beyer JM, Vojtko C, McDonald EJ, Fernandes PB. Comparative in vitro activities of new 14-, 15-, and 16- membered macrolides. Antimicrob Agents Chemother 1988;32:1710–1719.

39. Hol C, Verduin CM, Van Dijke EE, Verhoef J, Fleer A, Van Dijk

H. Complement resistance is a virulence factor of Branhamella (Moraxella) catarrhalis. FEMS Immunol Med Microbiol 1995; 11:207–211.

40. Humphreys JE. Smith EG, Coles SJ. A clarithromycin sensitivity survey in the United Kingdom using Stokes' method. J Antimicrob Chemother 1993;32:341–342.

41. Ikeda F, Yokota Y, Mine Y, Yamada T. Characterization of BRO enzymes and beta-lactamase transfer of Moraxella (Branhamella) catarrhalis isolated in Japan. Chemotherapy 1993;39: 88–95.

42. Ioannidis John PA, Worthington M, Griffiths JK, Snydman DR. Spectrum and significance of bacteremia due to Moraxella catarrhalis. Clin Infect Dis 1995;21:390–397.

43. Jordan K L, Berk, SH, Berk SL. A comparison of serum bactericidal activity and phenotypic characteristics of bacteremia pneumonia-causing strains, and colonizing strains of Branhamella catarrhalis. Am J Med 1990;88(Suppl 5A):28S–32S.

44. Kallings I. Sensitivity of Branhamella catarrhalis to oral antibiotics. Drugs 1986:31(Suppl 3):17–22.

45. Kawakami Y, Segawa K, Kanai M. A case of acute catarrhal conjunctivitis due to Branhamella catarrhalis. Microbiol Immunol 1983;27:641–643.

46. Kibsey PC, Rennie RP, Rushton JE. Disk diffusion versus broth micro dilution susceptibility testing of Haemophilus species and Moraxella catarrhalis using seven oral antimicrobial agents: application of updated susceptibility guidelines of the National Committee for Clinical Laboratory Standards. J Clin Microbiol 1994;32:2786–2790.

47. Kovatch AL, Wald ER, Michaels RH. β-lactamase producing Branhamella catarrhalis causing otitis media in children. J Pediatr 1983;102:261–264.

48. Krasemann C, Rohrig M, Cullman B. Bactericidal kinetics of ciprofloxacin and β-lactams against strains of Branhamella catarrhalis and Haemophilus influenzae. Eur J Clin Microbiol Infect Dis 1990;10(Suppl S):356–357.

49. Lambert-Zechovsky N, Mariani-Kurkdjian P, Doit C, Bourgeois F, Bingen E. In vitro bactericidal activity of four oral antibiotics against pathogens responsible for acute otitis media in children. J Hosp Infect 1992;22(Suppl A):89–97.

50. Lemmen SW, Anding K, Engels I, Daschner FD. Bactericidal activity of clarithromycin and ceclor against Streptococcus pneumoniae and Moraxella catarrhalis in healthy volunteers. J Antimicrob Chemother 1994;33:673–674.

51. Lemmen SW, Hauer T, Anding K, Engels I, Daschner FD. Serum bactericidal activity against Moraxella catarrhalis and Streptococcus pneumoniae after administration of four oral cephalosporins in health volunteers. J Antimicrob Chemother 1995;35:233–235.

52. Luman I, Wilson RW, Wallace RJ Jr, Nash DR. Disk diffusion susceptibility of Branhamella catarrhalis and relationship of β-lactam zone size to β-lactamase production. Antimicrob Agents Chemother 1986;30:774–776.

53. MacArthur RD. Branhamella catarrhalis peritonitis in two continuous ambulatory dialysis patients. Peritoneal Dial Int 1990; 10:169–171.

54. Malmvall BE, Brorsson JE, Johnsson J. In vitro sensitivity to penicillin V and beta-lactamase production of Branhamella catarrhalis. J Antimicrob Chemother 1977;3:374–375.

55. McCague JJ, McCague NJ, Altman CC. Neisseria catarrhalis urethritis: a case report. J Urol 1976;115:471.

56. Melendez PR, Johnson RH. Bacteremia and septic arthritis caused by Moraxella catarrhalis. Rev Infect Dis 13(3):428–429.

57. Nash DR, Flanagan C, Steele LC, Wallace RJ Jr. Comparison of the activity of cefixime and activities of other oral antibiotics against adult clinical isolates of Moraxella (Branhamella) catarrhalis containing BRO-1 and BRO-2 and Haemophilus influenza. Antimicrob Agents Chemother 1991;35:192–4.

58. Nash DR, Wallace RJ Jr, Steingrube VA, Shurin PA. Isoelectric focusing of beta-lactamases from sputum and middle ear isolates of Branhamella catarrhalis recovered in the United States. Drugs 1986;31(Suppl 3):48–54.

59. Ninane G, Joly J, Kraytman M, Piot P. Bronchopulmonary infection due to β-lactamase producing Branhamella catarrhalis treated with amoxycillin/clavulanic-acid. Lancet 1978;(8083):257.

60. Percival A, Corkill JE, Rowlands J, Sykes RB. Pathogenicity of and beta-lactamase production of Branhamella (Neisseria) catarrhalis. Lancet 1977;(8049)1175.

61. Periyakoil V, Krasner C. Moraxella catarrhalis bacteremia as a cause of erythema nodosum. Clin Infect Dis 1996;23:650–651.

62. Pfister LE, Gallagher MV, Potterfield TG, Brown DW. Neisseria catarrhalis bacteremia with meningitis. JAMA 1965;193:399–401.

63. Philippon A, Riou JY, Guibourdenche M, Sotolongo F. Detection, distribution and inhibition of Branhamella catarrhalis β-lactamases. Drugs 1986;31(Suppl 3):64–69.

64. Powell M, McVey D, Kassim MH, Chen HY, Williams JD. Antimicrobial susceptibility of Streptococcus pneumoniae, Haemophilus influenza, and Moraxella (Branhamella) catarrhalis isolated in the UK from sputa. J Antimicrob Chemother 1991;28:249–259.

65. Prallet B, Lucht F, Alexandre C. Vertebral osteomyelitis due to Branhamella catarrhalis. Rev Infect Dis 1991;13:769.

66. Richmond MH, Sykes RB. The beta-lactamases of gram negative bacteria and their physiologic role. Adv Microbiol Physiol 1973;9:31–88.

67. Riley TV, Digiovanni C, Hoyne GF. Susceptibility of Branhamella catarrhalis to sulphamethoxazole and trimethoprim. J Antimicrob Chemother 1987;19:39–43.

68. Robledano L, Rivera MJ, Otal I, Gomez-Lus R. Enzymatic modification of amino glycoside antibiotics by Branhamella catarrhalis carrying an R-factor. Drugs Exp Clin Res 1989;13(3):137–143.

69. Rotta AT, Asmar BI. Moraxella catarrhalis bacteremia and preseptal cellulitis. South Med J 1994;87:541–542.

70. Slevin NJ, Aitken J, Thornley PE. Clinical and microbiological features of Branhamella catarrhalis bronchopulmonary infections. Lancet 1984;(8380):782–783.

71. Spencer RC, Wheat PF. In vitro activity of roxithromycin against Moraxella catarrhalis. Diagn Microbiol Infect Dis 1991;15:63S–65S.

72. Stefani S, Pellegrino MB, D'Amico G, Privitera A, Privitera O, Maccarrone G, Russo G, Nicoletti G. In vitro activity of a new broad spectrum beta-lactamase-stable oral cephalosporin, cefixime, in comparison with other drugs, against Haemophilus influenza, Haemophilus parainfluenza, Moraxella catarrhalis and Streptococcus pneumoniae. Chemotherapy 1992;38:36–45.

73. Struelens MJ, Nonhoff C, Llontie M, Delannoy P, Lanis G, Van Pelt H, Serruys E. In vitro activity of commonly used oral antimicrobial agents against community isolates of respiratory pathogens. Acta Clin Belg 1991;46:283–289.

74. Sweeney KG, Verghese A, Needham CA. In vitro susceptibilities of isolates from patients with Branhamella catarrhalis pneumonia compared with those of colonizing strains. Antimicrob Agents Chemother 27:499–502.

75. Varsano I, Frydman M, Amir J, Alpert G. Single dose intramuscular dose of ceftriaxone as compared to 7-day amoxicillin therapy for acute otitis media in children: a double-blind clinical trial. Chemotherapy 1988;34(Suppl 1):39–46.

76. Wallace RJ Jr, Nash DR, Steingrube VA. Antibiotic susceptibilities and drug resistance in Moraxella (Branhamella) catarrhalis. Am J Med 1990;88(Suppl 5A):46S–50S.

77. Wallace RJ Jr, Steingrube VA, Nash DR, Hollis DG, Flanagan CW, Brown BA, et al. BRO β-lactamases of Branhamella catarrhalis and subgenus Moraxella, including evidence for chromosomal β-lactamase transfer by conjugation in B. catarrhalis, M. nonliquefaciens, and M. lacunata. Antimicrob Agents Chemother 1989;33:1845–1854.

78. Wilhelmus KR, Peacock J, Coster DJ. Branhamella keratitis. Br J Ophthalmol 1980;64:892.

79. Winstanley TG, Spencer RC. Moraxella catarrhalis: antibiotic susceptibility with special reference to trimethoprim. J Antimicrob Chemother 1986;18:425–426.

80. Yamada T, Yokota Y, Ikeda F, Mine Y, Kitada T. Antibacterial activity of cefixime against Streptococcus pneumoniae, Streptococcus pyogenes, and Haemophilus influenza in the presence of Moraxella (Branhamella) catarrhalis. Chemotherapy 1992;38:28–35.

81. Yourassowsky E, Van der Linden MP, Crokaert F. Killing rate and growth rate comparison for newer beta-lactamase stable oral beta-lactams against Streptococcus pneumoniae, Haemophilus influenza and Moraxella catarrhalis. Chemotherapy 1992;38:7–13.

82. Zheng XT, Cao Y. β-lactamase producing Branhamella in Beijing, China. Pediatr Infect Dis J 1988;7:744.

Morganella Species

●

Robert Orenstein and Edward S. Wong

GENERAL DESCRIPTION

The third genus within the tribe Proteeae is *Morganella*. These microorganisms share many of the clinical and therapeutic attributes of their fellow Proteeae, *Providencia* and *Proteus*. Originally described in 1906 in children with diarrhea by the British microbiologist H. de R. Morgan, today *Morganella* are most often nosocomial pathogens recovered from the urinary tract of patients with long-term catheters (4, 29, 30).

Morganella are motile, non–lactose fermenters previously classified as *Proteus morganii* due to their urease activity and presence of phenyalanine deaminase. They grow as flat, colorless, 2- to 3-mm nonswarming colonies on MacConkey's and sheep-blood agar. In addition to their inability to swarm, *Morganella* are differentiated from the genus *Proteus* by their lack of H_2S production or gelatin hydrolysis, their ability to ferment mannose, and presence of the enzyme ornithine decarboxylase (10). On the basis of genetic studies, *Proteus morganii* was reclassified as *Morganella morganii* (5). Varying biochemical features separate the three current Proteeae. Currently, two subspecies, *M. morganii* subsp. *morganii* and *M. morganii* subsp. *siboni* are recognized on the basis of both biochemical and genetic features (15).

Morganella infections are rarely seen in healthy hosts. Infections due to *Morganella* have been reported to cause diabetic foot infections (31), decubitus ulcer infections (27), septic arthritis (16), meningitis (14), middle ear infections (13), gastroenteritis and traveler's diarrhea (2), urinary tract infections (UTIs) (38), conjunctivitis, pneumonia, peritonitis and bacteremia (15), and chorioamnionitis (7).

Clinical infections due to *Morganella* are uncommon and most often involve the urinary tract in patients with recurrent UTIs or those who have received multiple antimicrobial agents. Often these are elderly patients in nursing homes with asymptomatic bacteriuria. *Morganella* is the fifth leading cause of UTI in nursing home patients (28). In a study of 20 patients with chronic indwelling urinary catheters, Warren et al. found *Morganella* bacteriuria in 19% of weekly specimens and a mean duration of bacteriuria of 3.3 weeks (37). Like *Providencia,* some strains of *Morganella* possess the MR/K hemagglutinin that enhances adherence to urinary catheters (25). Once having gained access to the urinary tract, *Morganella* appears to persist for less time than *Providencia* in catheterized patients—only one-fourth of bacteriuric episodes were of 1-week duration, whereas the median duration for *Providencia* bacteriuria was 9 weeks (37). Additionally, *Morganella* produces urease that predisposes to encrustation of urinary catheters (36).

Morganella may rarely cause bacteremia. In a multicenter study of 2084 cases of bacteremia in Britain, *Morganella* ac-

counted for 1% of cases and 4 deaths (20). Muder reported *Morganella* as the cause of up to 3% of bacteremias in a nursing home, arising primarily from either urinary tract or soft tissue infections (27).

SUSCEPTIBILITY IN VITRO

Morganella, like its fellow Proteeae possesses several mechanisms of antibiotic resistance. Resistance may be mediated by constitutive (derepressed) or inducible, class C β-lactamases. Most *Morganella* possess AmpC β-lactamases that are inducible in the presence of β-lactam antibiotics (6). These enzymes may lead to expression of high-level resistance in the presence of enzyme-inducing antibiotics. As a result, agents such as ampicillin, amoxicillin, and first-generation cephalosporins are ineffective. Second-generation cephalosporins such as cefuroxime are also ineffective against *Morganella,* with MIC_{90}s ranging from 16 to 64 μg/mL (21, 39). Cefoxitin, though a potent β-lactamase inducer appears more stable against *Morganella* than *Enterobacter* (19).

A second mechanism of β-lactam resistance in *Morganella* is the chromosomally mediated hyperproduction of β-lactamases. Mutations at the ampD locus lead to derepression of the β-lactamase and permanent production of excessive enzyme levels. These derepressed strains continuously produce β-lactamase without a need for an inducing antibiotic. The extended-spectrum penicillins and third-generation cephalosporins are generally active against *Morganella* that have inducible enzymes but not the constitutive hyperproducers. Addition of clavulanic acid or sulbactam to these agents fails to enhance their activity against derepressed organisms. Thus the MICs of ticarcillin and ticarcillin-clavulanate against *Morganella* are the same (11). Tazobactam, on the other hand, enhances the activity of piperacillin against derepressed strains. Hence, the combination of piperacillin plus tazobactam is five times more active than piperacillin alone (19).

The third-generation cephalosporins ceftriaxone, cefotaxime, and ceftazidime are more active against *Morganella,* with MIC_{90}s ranging from 0.03 to 32 μg/mL (3). The MICs for cefotaxime and ceftazidime are 0.015 and 0.06 μg/mL for inducible strains but 4 and 8 μg/mL for constitutive hyperproducers, respectively (19).

The most active β-lactam antibiotics against the derepressed and inducible isolates are cefipime and cefpirome. These agents are the most β-lactamase stable and have MICs against the derepressed isolates of 1 to 4 μg/mL versus more than 64 μg/mL for cefotaxime (3). Cefipime appears to be the most active cephalosporin (MIC_{90}s, 0.03–0.25 μg/mL). Washington found MIC_{90}s to cefipime below 1 μg/mL for all isolates (39); Kessler found that 100% of isolates had MICs below 8 μg/mL and that cefipime was more active than ceftazidime, ceftriaxone, or imipenem (17). This increase in cefipime activity is due to the limited effect of constitutive β-lactamase production compared with the other cephalosporins. MICs for aztreonam range between 0.06 and 0.12 μg/mL (29). Meropenem appears to be the most active of the carbapenems, even against imipenem-resistant isolates (33).

A third mechanism of resistance has recently begun to appear in *Morganella* strains due to extended-spectrum β-lactamase production (personal communication, Coudron 1997). Since 1990, *Morganella* isolates possessing the extended spectrum TEM 13 enzyme have been reported (22). In a 1992 survey of 1000 isolates of *Enterobacteriaceae,* Liu found several *Morganella* isolates possessing either SHV, TEM, or OXA plasmid-mediated β-lactamases (18).

Aminoglycosides are usually active against *Morganella*. In 1997, at the Richmond VA Medical Center, 89 and 100% of 55 *Morganella* isolates were susceptible to gentamicin and amikacin, respectively (Coudron, personal communication). Between 71 and 100% of *Morganella* isolates from the Medical College of Virginia remained susceptible to aminoglycosides (20). At the Mayo Clinic, 91 and 98% of 163 isolates of *M. morganii* were reported susceptible to less than 2 μg/mL of gentamicin and less than 8 μg/mL of amikacin, respectively (9). Aminoglycoside resistance among *Morganella* is rare and mediated by a variety of complex combinations of enzymes, the most frequent of which is the modifying enzyme ANT(2″)-I, which confers resistance to gentamicin, tobramycin, and kanamycin (24).

The fluoroquinolones are highly active against *Morganella*, with the MIC$_{90}$s for most isolates below 0.25 μg/mL (21). Ciprofloxacin is twice as active as ofloxacin in vitro (21). In a study of 390 clinical isolates, 97% were ciprofloxacin susceptible (1).

Trimethoprim-sulfamethoxazole is also active against some *Morganella* (MIC$_{50}$, 0.06 μg/mL; MIC$_{90}$, 16 μg/mL) (21).

ANTIMICROBIAL THERAPY

Therapeutic choices for infections due to *Morganella* are primarily based upon in vitro susceptibility data, since little information is available from clinical trials. The antibiotic of choice depends upon the milieu in which the infection occurs, the site of infection, and the prevalence of resistant isolates. The *Medical Letter* has suggested a third-generation cephalosporin as the drug of choice for *Morganella* infections (23). For nursing home residents with catheter-related UTIs, a third-generation cephalosporin such as ceftriaxone that can be given once daily, an oral fluoroquinolone, or trimethoprim-sulfamethoxazole may be used in an effort to reduce hospitalization and costs.

Nosocomially acquired infections due to *Morganella* may be associated with multiple mechanisms of resistance. In this case, an agent such as cefipime or a carbapenem may be the antibiotic of choice. In highly resistant infections, addition of an aminoglycoside may be helpful. Polymicrobial soft tissue infections of the diabetic foot or decubitus ulcers involving *Morganella* should be treated with a broad-spectrum combi-

nation such as piperacillin-tazobactam, a third-generation cephalosporin or aztreonam plus clindamycin or a fourth-generation cephalosporin or fluoroquinolone plus an antianaerobic agent.

TABLE 1 • Comparative Activity of Antibiotic against *Morganella morganii*				
Antibiotic	No. Isolates	MIC$_{50}$	MIC$_{90}$	Reference
Amoxicillin	9	128	128	32
Amoxicillin-clavulanate	39	64	>64	21
	16	>64	>64	21
Ticarcillin	165	<1	16	11
Ticarcillin-clavulanate	165	<1	16	11
Cefaclor	16	>64	>64	5
	39	>64	>64	21
Cefuroxime	39	>64	>64	21
	62	>16	>16	39
	19	1	4	34
Cefoxitin	9	16	512	32
	39	8	>64	21
Cefixime	19	0.008	0.008	34
	16	2	32	35
Cefpodoxime	19	0.06	0.5	34
Ceftriaxone	39	0.5	8	21
	33	<0.03	2	17
Cefotaxime	9	8	16	32
	33	0.06	2	17
Ceftazidime	9	8	32	32
	62	<0.25	<0.25	39
	33	0.25	2	17
Cefipime	62	<0.25	<0.25	39
	33	0.03	0.12	17
Cefoperazone	33	1	16	17
Imipenem	33	2	4	17
TMP-SMX[a]	39	0.06	16	21
Fleroxacin	39	0.06	0.12	21
Ciprofloxacin	39	0.06	0.06	21
Ofloxacin	39	0.12	0.25	21
Lomefloxacin	39	0.12	0.25	21

[a]TMP-SMX, trimethoprim-sulfamethoxazole.

REFERENCES

1. Acar JF, Goldstein FW. Trends in bacterial resistance to fluoroquinolones. Clin Infect Dis 1997;24(Suppl 1):S67–73.
2. Ahren CM, Jertborn M, Herclik L, Kaijser B, Svennerholm AM. Infection with bacterial enteropathogens in Swedish travellers to Southeast Asia—a prospective study. Epidemiol Infect 1990; 105:325–333.
3. Binfiglio G, Stefani S, Nicoletti G. In vitro activity of cefpirome against beta-lactamase-inducible and stably derepressed Enterobacteriaceae. Chemotherapy 1994;40:311–316.
4. Braunstein H, Tomasulo M. Identification of Proteus morgani and distinction from other Proteus species. Am J Clin Pathol 1975;69:905–908.
5. Brenner DJ, Farmer JJ III, Fanning GR, Steigerwalt AG, Klykken P, Wathen HG, Hickman FW, Ewing WH. Deoxyribonucleic acid relatedness of Proteus and Providencia. Int J Syst Bacteriol 1978;28:269–282.
6. Bush K, Jacoby GA, Medeiros AA. A functional classification scheme for beta-lactamases and its correlation with molecular structure. Antimicrob Agents Chemother 1995;39:1211–1233.

7. Carmona F, Fabregues F, Alvarez R, Vila J, Cararach V. A rare case of chorioamnionitis by Morganella morganii complicated by sepsis and ARDS. Eur J Obstet Gynecol Reprod Biol 1992;45:67–70.

8. DiPersio JR, Krafczyk TL. In vitro activity of netilmicin, gentamicin, tobramycin and amikacin against glucose fermenting and nonfermenting bacteria. Chemotherapy 1980;26:323.

9. Edson RS, Terrell CL. The aminoglycosides. Mayo Clin Proc 1991;66:1158.

10. Farmer JJ III. Enterobacteriaceae: introduction and identification. In: Murray PR, Baron EJ, Pfaller MA, Tenover FC, Yolken RH, eds. Manual of clinical microbiology. 6th ed. Washington, DC: American Society for Microbiology, 1995:438–449.

11. Fuchs PC, Barry AL, Jones RN. In vitro activity and disk susceptibility of Timentin: Current status. Am J Med 1985;(Suppl 5B):25–32.

12. Fuchs PC, Barry AL, Sewell DL. Antibacterial activity of WY-49605 compared with those of the other oral agents and selection of disk content for disk diffusion and susceptibility testing. Antimicrob Agents Chemother 1995;39:1472–1479.

13. Haddad J Jr, Inglesby TV Jr, Addonizio L. Head and neck infections in pediatric cardiac transplant patients. Ear Nose Throat J 1995;74:422–425.

14. Isaacs RD, Ellis-Pegler RB. Successful treatment of Morganella morganii meningitis with pefloxacin mesylate. J Antimicrob Chemother 1987;20:769–770.

15. Jensen KT, Fredericksen W, Hickman-Brenner FW, Steigerwalt AG, Riddle CF, Brenner DJ. Recognition of Morganella subspecies with proposal of M. morganii subsp. morganii and M. morganii subsp. sibonii. Int J Syst Bacteriol 19:613–620.

16. Katz LM, Lewis RJ, Borenstein DG. Successful joint arthroplasty following Proteus morganii (Morganella morganii) septic arthritis: a four-year study. Arthritis Rheum 1987;30:583–585.

17. Kessler RE, Fung-Tomc J. Susceptibility of bacterial isolates to beta-lactam antibiotics from US clinical trials over a 5-year period. Am J Med 1996;100(Suppl 6A):13S–19S.

18. Liu PY, Gur D, Hall LM, Livermore DM. Survey of the prevalence of beta-lactamases amongst 1000 gram-negative bacilli isolated consecutively at the Royal London Hospital. J Antimicrob Chemother 1992;30:429–447.

19. Livermore DM. Beta-lactamases in laboratory and clinical resistance. Clin Microbiol Rev 1995;8:557–584.

20. Markowitz SM. Urinary tract specimens. In: Dalton HP, Nottebart HC, eds. Interpretive medical microbiology. New York: Churchill Livingstone, 1986:564–570.

21. Markowitz SM, Williams DS, Hanna CB, Parker JL, Pierce MA, Steele JC Jr. A multicenter comparative study of the in vitro activity of fleroxacin and other antimicrobial agents. Chemotherapy 1995;41:477–486.

22. Medeiros AA. Evolution and dissemination of beta-lactamases accelerated by generations of beta-lactam antibiotics. Clin Infect Dis 1997;24(S1)S19–45.

23. Medical Letter. The choice of antibacterial drugs. Med Lett 1996;38:25–30.

24. Miller GH, Sabatelli FJ, Hare RS, Glupczynski Y, Mackey P, Shlaes D, et al. The most frequent aminoglycoside resistance mechanisms—changes with time and geographic area: a reflection of aminoglycoside usage patterns? Clin Infect Dis 1997;24(Suppl 1):S46–62.

25. Mobley HLT, Chippendale GR, Tenney JH, Mayrer A, Crisp LJ, Penner JL, Warren JW. MR/K hemagglutination of Providencia stuartii correlates with adherence to catheters and with persistence in catheter-associated bacteriuria. J Infect Dis 1988;157:264–271.

26. Morgan HR. Upon the bacteriology of the summer diarrhea of infants. Br Med J 1906;1:908–912.

27. Muder RR, Brennen C, Wagener MM, Goetz AM. Bacteremia in a long term care facility: a five year prospective study of 163 consecutive episodes. Clin Infect Dis 1992;14:647–654.

28. Nicolle LE, Strausbaugh LJ, Garibaldi RA. Infections and antibiotic resistance in nursing homes. Rev Clin Microbiol 1996;9:1–17.

29. Parry MF. Aztreonam susceptibility testing. A retrospective analysis. Am J Med 1990;88(3C);7S–11S.

30. Penner JL, Hennessy JN. O-antigen grouping of Morganella morganii (Proteus morganii) by slide agglutination. J Clin Microbiol 1979;10:8–13.

31. Pereira A, Monteagudo J, Mazzara R, Reverter JC, Castillo R. Anti-K1 of the IgA class associated with Morganella morganii infection. Transfusion 1989;29:549–551.

32. Piddock LJV, Walters RN, Jin YF, Turner HL, Gascoyne-Binzi DM, Hawkey PM. Prevalence and mechanism of resistance to 'third-generation' cephalosporins in clinically relevant isolates of Enterobacteriaceae from 43 hospitals in the U.K., 1990–1991. J Antimicrobial Chemother 1997;39:177–187.

33. Pitkin DH, Sheikh W, Nadler H. Comparative in vitro activity of meropenem versus other extended-spectrum antimicrobials against randomly chosen and selected resistant clinical isolates tested in 26 North American centers. Clin Infect Dis 1997;24(Suppl 2):S238–248.

34. Riess G, Andres J, Thornber D, Wise R. In vitro activity of RU 29246, the active compound of the cephalosporin prodrug ester HR 916. Antimicrob Agents Chemother 1992;36:2360–2364.

35. Sewell D, Barry A, Allen S, Fuchs P, McLaughlin J, Pfaller M. Comparative antimicrobial activities of the penem WY-49605 (SUN5555) against recent clinical isolates from five US medical centers. Antimicrob Agents Chemother 1995;39:1591–1595.

36. Stamm W. Catheter-associated urinary tract infections: epidemiology, pathogenesis, and prevention. Am J Med 1991;91(3B):65S–71S.

37. Warren JW, Tenney JH, Hoopes JM, Muncie HL, Anthony WC. A prospective microbiologic study of bacteriuria in patients with chronic indwelling urethral catheters. J Infect Dis 1982;146:719–723.

38. Warren JW. Catheter-associated bacteriuria in long term care facilities. Infect Control Hosp Epidemiol 1994;15:557–562.

39. Washington JA, Jones RA, Gerlach EH, Murray PR, Allen SD, Knapp CC. Multicenter comparison of in vitro activities of FK-037, cefepime, ceftriaxone, ceftazidime, and cefuroxime. Antimicrob Agents Chemother 1993;37:1696–1700.

40. Wiseman LR, Wagstaff AJ, Brogden RN, Bryson HM. Meropenem. A review of its antibacterial activity, pharmacokinetic properties and clinical efficacy. Drugs 1995;1:73–101.

Neisseria gonorrhoeae

●

John S. Moran and H. Hunter Handsfield

GENERAL DESCRIPTION
Transmission

The gonococcus is a fragile bacterium adapted to growth on mucous membranes. Its fragility limits its transmissibility to direct, or nearly direct, contact between mucous membranes. The requirement for such intimate contact to permit transmission makes gonorrhea a classic sexually transmitted disease (STD). Sexual transmission via penile-vaginal, penile-rectal, or penile-pharyngeal contact accounts for the vast majority of cases.

It is remarkable that the gonococcus, which is too fragile to be transmitted by food, water, air, or (with very rare exceptions) fomites remained a very common infection in most of the world in the preantibiotic era despite sometimes strenuous efforts to control its transmission. Only since the introduction of antimicrobials has gonorrhea been controlled in some populations. It is, perhaps, even more remarkable, given the natural susceptibility of gonococci to small concentrations of a wide variety of antimicrobials, that 50 years after the discovery of penicillin, gonorrhea remains a common infection in much of the world.

Natural History

Most gonococcal infections produce symptoms that lead the infected person to seek treatment or, if asymptomatic, resolve without treatment. However, infection can ascend the reproductive tract, threatening fertility in both sexes. Rarely, infection spreads beyond the initial site of infection to the joints, skin, endocardium, or meninges. Antimicrobial therapy very rapidly eradicates infection from the urethra (14) and, presumably, from other sites as well.

SUSCEPTIBILITY IN VITRO AND IN VIVO
In Vitro Data

The gonococcus is a model of adaptability, having developed resistance to sulfonamides, penicillins, tetracyclines, and (very recently) fluoroquinolones. Nevertheless, any individual gonococcal strain has a high probability of being susceptible to a single dose of any of a large number of antimicrobials, and all gonococci remain susceptible to single doses of several of the newer cephalosporins. Table 1 shows some recent MIC values from around the world for the antimicrobials most useful against the gonococcus.

Relationship between in Vitro Susceptibility and Clinical Outcome

Studies of subjects experimentally infected with gonorrhea strains of known penicillin susceptibility and treated with various doses of penicillin showed that eradication of urethral in-fections in men treated with penicillin was associated with the presence of plasma antimicrobial levels 3 to 4 times the MIC of the infecting strain for 7 to 10 h (15).

More recently, it has been shown that high cure rates (>97.5%) in clinical trials of fluoroquinolones and cephalosporins for the treatment of urogenital and rectal infections are associated with serum or plasma antimicrobial concentrations at least four times the MIC_{90} of the infecting strains, persisting for at least 10 h (20). For pharyngeal infection, high cure rates (80%) are associated with high serum or plasma antimicrobial levels that persist for at least 20 h.

CRITERIA FOR SELECTION OF ANTIMICROBIAL THERAPY

Efficacy and safety are, of course, the most important criteria for selecting a regimen for the treatment of uncomplicated gonorrhea. Other considerations are acceptability to the patient, contraindications, and cost.

Efficacy

Only the most effective regimens should be used. Using any regimen with a significant failure rate obligates the prescriber to reexamine patients after treatment to ensure that they are no longer infectious. Such follow-up would be expensive and, in many cases, impossible. Fortunately, many safe regimens exist that cure essentially 100% of infections. With several safe and effective antigonococcal regimens to choose from, it has been proposed that the minimal standard of efficacy for uncomplicated urogenital or rectal infections should be a proven efficacy of at least 95% in summed clinical trials with a 95% confidence interval that excludes values below 95% (20).

Note that the last three regimens listed in Table 2 do not meet this criterion. Note also that many regimens that meet this criterion are not recommended.

Safety

In the single doses used for the treatment of gonorrhea, the recommended antimicrobials are all safe; hypersensitivity reactions are the greatest concern.

Acceptability to the Patient

The recommended regimens are all well tolerated. The main consideration is route of administration: oral versus intramuscular.

Contraindications

The cephalosporins and spectinomycin have few contraindications. Fluoroquinolones, on the other hand, are contraindicated for children under 17 years of age and for pregnant

TABLE 1 • In Vitro Activities of Some Antimicrobials against *N. gonorrhoeae*

Antimicrobial	MIC$_{50}$ (µg/mL)	MIC$_{90}$ (µg/mL)	Number of Strains	Source of Isolates (country and year)[a]	Reference
Cephalosporins					
Cefixime	0.015	0.064	164	Kenya 1989–90	24
	<0.001	0.03	328	Thailand 1990	4
	0.016	0.031	79	Japan 1992–93	30
	0.015	0.06	>30,000	USA 1988–94	9
	<0.002	0.008	150	Germany 1988–92	27
	≤0.015	≤0.015	104	United Kingdom n.r.	18
Cefotaxime	0.03	1	134	Philippines 1989	5
	0.03	0.06	333	Thailand 1990	4
	0.031	0.125	79	Japan 1992–93	30
	0.008	0.015	130	Tanzania 1992	33
	≤0.015	0.03	104	United Kingdom n.r.	18
Cefotetan	—	0.5	150	USA 1989	34
Cefoxitin	0.5	1	129	USA 1987	7
	1	2	402	Spain 1988–89	23
	1	4	134	Philippines 1989	5
	1	2	332	Thailand 1990	4
Cefpodoxime	0.008	0.03	54	USA nonPPNG (n.r.)	8
	0.008	0.06	23	USA PPNG (n.r.)	8
	0.03	2	134	Philippines 1989	5
	0.03	0.125	331	Thailand 1990	4
Ceftizoxime	0.004	0.016	89	Germany (n.r.)	17
	0.008	0.25	137	Philippines 1989	5
	0.015	0.03	333	Thailand 1990	4
Ceftriaxone	0.004	0.016	89	Germany (n.r.)	17
	≤0.004	0.008	213	Congo-Kinshasa 1988	31
	0.0018	0.0037	402	Spain 1988–89	23
	0.008	0.06	134	Philippines 1989	5
	0.015	0.06	164	Kenya 1989–90	24
	0.008	0.03	333	Thailand 1990	4
	0.016	0.063	79	Japan 1992–93	30
	0.002	0.19	57	South Africa 1990–93	3
	0.004	0.015	>30,000	USA 1988–1994	9
Cefuroxime	0.03	0.06	402	Spain 1988–89	23
	0.125	2	135	Philippines 1989	5
	0.5	1	333	Thailand 1990	4
	0.03	0.125	150	Germany 1988–92	27
	0.06	0.25	130	Tanzania 1992	33
Quinolones					
Ciprofloxacin	0.0009	0.0018	402	Spain 1988–89	23
	0.004	0.25	135	Philippines 1989	5
	0.015	0.015	40	Kenya 1989–90	24
	0.004	0.008	329	Thailand 1990	4
	0.004	0.008	>30,000	USA 1988–94	9
	≤0.002	0.008	388	Sweden 1988–89	1
	0.004	0.008	251	Côte d'Ivoire 1992–93	32
	0.004	0.015	952	Congo-Kinshasa 1988–1993	32
	0.004	0.015	1085	Rwanda 1989–90	32
	0.002	0.047	57	South Africa 1990–93	3
	0.008	0.015	130	Tanzania 1992	33
	0.031	0.5	79	Japan 1992–93	30
	<0.002	0.004	150	Germany 1988–92	27
	≤0.004	0.06	104	United Kingdom n.r.	18
Enoxacin	0.03	0.06	126	USA non-PPNG, non-TRNG 1986–87	22
	0.25	2	79	Japan 1992–93	30
Lomefloxacin	0.016	0.032	196	Canada PCN-sensitive 1988	28
	0.125	1.0	79	Japan 1992–93	30
Norfloxacin	0.03	0.12	213	Congo-Kinshasa 1988	31
	0.06	0.125	332	Thailand 1990	4
	0.5	2	69	Japan 1992	29
	0.016	0.06	388	Sweden 1988–89	1
	0.06	0.125	130	Tanzania 1992	33

continued

TABLE 1 • In Vitro Activities of Some Antimicrobials against *N. gonorrhoeae*

Antimicrobial	MIC$_{50}$ (μg/mL)	MIC$_{90}$ (μg/mL)	Number of Strains	Source of Isolates (country and year)[a]	Reference
Ofloxacin	0.0039	0.0078	100	USA (n.r.)	10
	0.03	0.06	402	Spain 1988–89	23
	0.038	0.625	139	Philippines 1989	5
	0.038	0.075	333	Thailand 1990	4
	0.125	1	79	Japan 1992–93	30
	0.008	0.03	150	Germany 1988–92	27
Miscellaneous					
Azithromycin	0.125	0.25	69	Japan 1992	29
	0.125	0.25	>7,000	USA 1992–94	9
	0.5	1	130	Tanzania 1992	33
	0.125	0.25	150	Germany 1988–92	27
	0.12	0.25	104	United Kingdom n.r.	18
Spectinomycin	32	32	213	Congo-Kinshasa 1988	31
	16	16	402	Spain 1988–89	23
	16	16	187	USA 1989–90	25
	32	32	105	Kenya 1989–90	24
	32	32	117	Philippines 1989	5
	64	64	305	Thailand 1990	4
	16	32	130	Tanzania 1992	33
	4	8	150	Germany 1988–92	27
	16	16	79	Japan 1992–1993	30
	32	64	104	United Kingdom n.r.	18

[a] n.r. indicates that dates of specimen isolation were not reported.
PPNG = penicillinase-producing Neisseriae gonnorrhoeae.

women. These contraindications are based on extrapolation from animal studies, not on any human studies or clinical experience. Studies of children with cystic fibrosis treated with multiple doses of fluoroquinolones have shown no evidence of toxicity (11, 12, 26).

Cost

Cost is an important consideration for public STD clinics. In general, the fluoroquinolones can be purchased for a lower per treatment cost ($2–$4) than can the cephalosporins ($3–$12) or spectinomycin.

Efficacy against incubating syphilis should not be an important consideration in the United States for two reasons: (*a*) there is no evidence that incubating syphilis is common among gonorrhea patients in the United States and (*b*) patients treated for gonorrhea should, in general, be treated presumptively for

Chlamydia trachomatis infection as well and recommended antichlamydia regimens are likely to eradicate incubating syphilis.

Efficacy against concurrent *C. trachomatis* infection is not an important consideration because none of the recommended antigonococcal regimens is effective against chlamydia.

ANTIMICROBIAL THERAPY

Almost all clinical data are from clinical trials of therapy for uncomplicated infections. Most subjects are men with urethral gonorrhea. Fewer subjects are women with cervical or urethral infections, and even fewer have rectal or pharyngeal gonorrhea. The site of infection is related to clinical outcome. A systematic review of published trials of various antimicrobial regimens for the biological cure of uncomplicated *N. gonorrhoeae* infection found that modern antigonococcal agents eradicate infections of the urethra, cervix, and rectum more reliably than infection of

TABLE 2 • Aggregated Results of Clinical Trials

Drug Regimen	Pharyngeal Infections		Urogenital and Rectal Infections	
	% Cured	95% CI	% Cured	95% CI
Ciprofloxacin 500 mg	97.2	85.5–100	99.8	98.7–100
Ceftriaxone 250 mg	98.8	94.2–100	99.2	98.8–99.5
Ciprofloxacin 250 mg	89.0	82.3–95.8	99.2	98.6–99.8
Azithromycin 2 g	100	82.3–100	99.2	97.3–99.9
Ceftriaxone 125 mg	93.7	84.5–98.2	99.1	98.7–99.8
Ofloxacin 400 mg	88.0	68.8–97.5	98.4	97.2–99.8
Cefixime 800 mg	80.0	51.9–95.7	98.4	95.9–99.6
Spectinomycin 2 g	51.8	38.7–64.9	98.2	97.6–99.0
Cefixime 400 mg	100	63.1–100	97.1	96.1–99.3
Cefpodoxime proxetil 200 mg	78.9	54.4–94.0	96.5	94.3–98.6
Cefuroxime axetil 1g	56.9	42.3–70.6	96.2	94.7–97.5
Azithromycin 1 g	100	29.2–100	95.2	91.4–98.9

the pharynx (19). Cure rates were 96.4% for the male urethra, 98.4% for the female urethra, 98.0% for the cervix, 97.9% for the female rectum, and 95.3% for the male rectum. Cure rates were significantly lower for infections of the pharynx: 83.7% in females and 79.2% in males.

There is a close relationship between efficacy at the pharynx and efficacy at other sites, so that one can be confident that the regimens most effective against urogenital and rectal infections will be efficacious against pharyngeal infections as well. An exception to this relationship is spectinomycin (2 g i.m.), which is highly effective against urogenital and rectal infections but relatively ineffective against pharyngeal infection.

Table 2 summarizes the results of clinical trials of the most promising antigonococcal regimens. For a more comprehensive summary (87 regimens) see reference 20. These same data are shown graphically in Figure 1. Note that only agents 99% or more effective for urogenital and rectal infections can be relied upon to cure pharyngeal infections (i.e., have been shown to cure 90% or more).

Regimens Recommended for the Treatment of Uncomplicated Gonococcal Infections of the Cervix, Urethra, and Rectum in Adults and Adolescents.

First-Line Therapy
The following single-dose regimens have been shown to be safe and highly effective for treatment of cervical, urethral, and rectal infections among adult men and women: ceftriaxone 125 mg intramuscularly, cefixime 400 mg orally, ciprofloxacin 500 mg orally, or ofloxacin 400 mg orally.

Ceftriaxone in a single injection of 125 mg provides sustained, high bactericidal levels in the blood. Extensive clinical experience indicates that it is safe and effective for the treatment of uncomplicated gonorrhea at all sites, curing 99.1% of uncomplicated urogenital and anorectal infections in published clinical trials. (A 250-mg dose is also acceptable, but so large a dose is unnecessary.)

Cefixime has an antimicrobial spectrum similar to that of ceftriaxone, but the 400-mg oral dose does not provide as high nor as sustained a bactericidal level as does 125 mg of ceftriaxone. In published clinical trials, the 400-mg dose cured 97.1% of uncomplicated urogenital and anorectal infections. The advantage of cefixime is that it can be administered orally. An 800-mg dose may be slightly more effective but is less well tolerated.

Ciprofloxacin is very active against most strains of *N. gonorrhoeae* and, at a dose of 500 mg, provides sustained bactericidal levels in the blood that have cured 99.8% of uncomplicated urogenital and anorectal infections in published clinical trials. It is safe, is relatively inexpensive, and can be administered orally. Although numerous studies have shown that a 250-mg dose is also highly effective (curing 99.2% of uncomplicated urogenital and anorectal infections in published trials), these studies were done in populations free of fluoro-

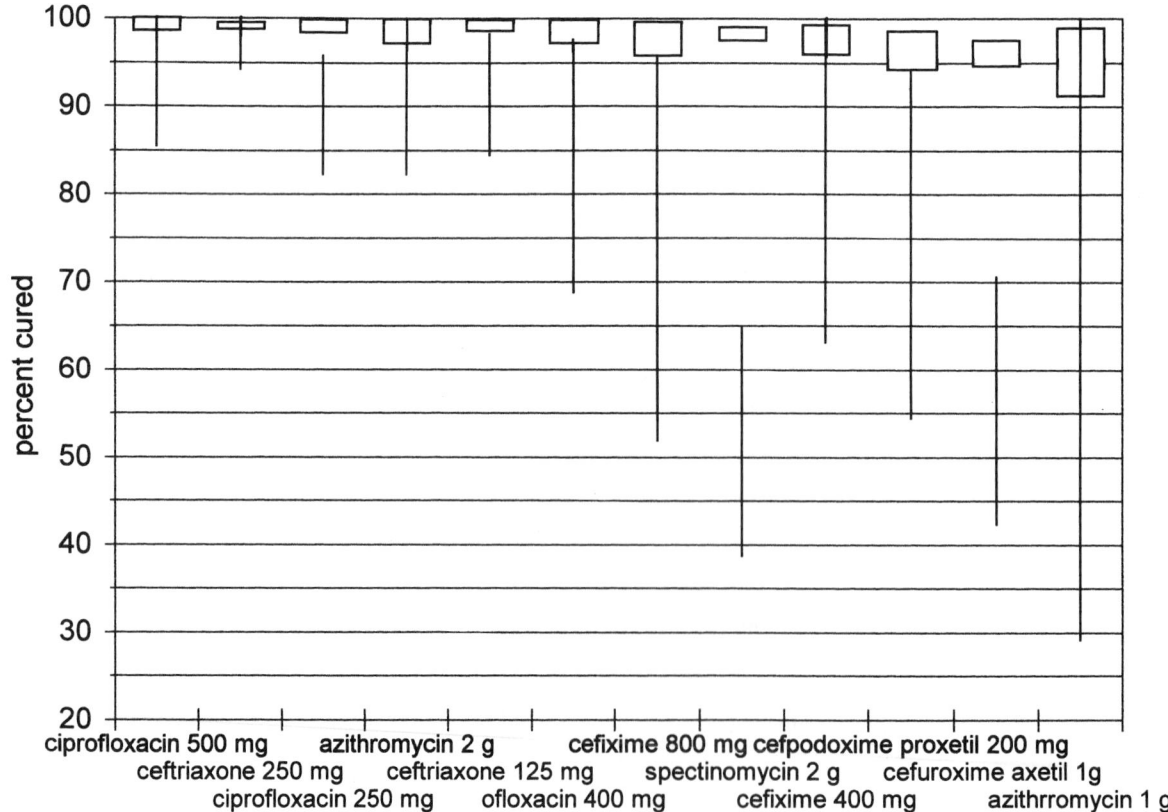

FIGURE 1. Efficacy of various antigonococcal regimens in clinical trials. *Boxes:* 95% confidence intervals for urogenital and rectal infections. *Lines:* 95% confidence interval for pharyngeal infections.

quinolone-resistant strains. In view of the recent emergence of quinolone-resistant *N. gonorrhoeae* and the fact that the 250-mg dose is not significantly safer, cheaper, or better tolerated than the 500-mg dose, the 500-mg dose is recommended (21). Because quinolone-resistant *N. gonorrheae* is becoming common in some Asian countries, fluoroquinolones should not be used to treat infections acquired from someone who may have been infected in Asia.

Ofloxacin is also very active against most strains of *N. gonorrhoeae* and has favorable pharmacokinetics. The 400-mg oral dose has been very effective for the treatment of uncomplicated urogenital and anorectal infections, curing 98.4% in published clinical trials. As is the case with other fluoroquinolones, ofloxacin should not be used if the infection was acquired from someone who may have been infected in Asia.

For patients who can tolerate neither cephalosporins nor fluoroquinolones, spectinomycin (2 g i.m. in a single dose) is an acceptable alternative. Spectinomycin is expensive in the United States and must be given by injection, but it has been effective in published clinical trials, curing 98.2% of uncomplicated urogenital and anorectal infections, and resistance remains rare in the United States (9) and elsewhere.

Alternative Therapy

There are several acceptable alternatives to the five regimens listed above. These include single-dose injectable cephalosporin regimens other than ceftriaxone (125 mg i.m.) that have been shown to be safe and highly effective against uncomplicated urogenital and anorectal infections. These are ceftizoxime (500 mg i.m.), cefotaxime (500 mg i.m.), cefotetan (1 g i.m.), and cefoxitin (2 g i.m.) with probenecid (1 g p.o.). None of these injectable cephalosporins offers any advantage over ceftriaxone, and there is less clinical experience with them for the treatment of uncomplicated gonorrhea. There are no acceptable cephalosporin alternatives to cefixime 400 mg for the oral treatment of gonorrhea. Neither cefuroxime axetil 1 g nor cefpodoxime proxetil 200 mg have been shown to cure more than 95% of uncomplicated urogenital and anorectal infections with a 95% confidence interval that excludes 95%. The overall cure rate for cefuroxime axetil 1 g has been only 96.2% with a lower 95% confidence limit of 94.7%, and the overall cure rate for cefpodoxime proxetil 200 mg has been 96.5% with a lower 95% confidence limit of 94.3% (Table 2). Single-dose, quinolone alternatives to ciprofloxacin (500 mg p.o.) and ofloxacin (400 mg p.o.) include enoxacin (400 mg p.o.); lomefloxacin (400 mg p.o.); and norfloxacin (800 mg p.o.). They are safe and effective for the treatment of uncomplicated gonorrhea, but they are less active in vitro and less well studied in vivo, and none offers any advantage over ciprofloxacin (500 mg p.o.) or ofloxacin (400 mg p.o.). Azithromycin (2 g p.o.) is highly effective against uncomplicated gonococcal infection but is expensive and causes gastrointestinal distress too often to be recommended for the treatment of gonorrhea. At an oral dose of 1 g, azithromycin is insufficiently effective, curing only 95.2% of subjects in published studies.

The list above is not a comprehensive list of all effective treatment regimens. Many other antimicrobials are active against *N. gonorrhoeae*. However, some agents have not been well studied (e.g., sparfloxacin, levofloxacin), and others are not very effective (e.g., kanamycin, cotrimoxazole, thiamphenicol).

Regimens Recommended for the Treatment of Uncomplicated Gonococcal Infections of the Pharynx in Adults and Adolescents

Gonococcal infections of the pharynx are more difficult to eradicate than are infections at urogenital and anorectal sites. Few antigonococcal regimens can be relied upon to cure them more than 90% of the time. The most effective are single doses of ceftriaxone 125 (or 250) mg intramuscularly and ciprofloxacin 500 mg orally.

Pelvic Inflammatory Disease

The syndrome of pelvic inflammatory disease (PID) results when infection ascends the reproductive tract from the cervix to the fallopian tubes and ovaries. Although PID is the most common complication of genital gonococcal infection, it can be caused by other microbes as well; therapy of PID should cover not only *N. gonorrhoeae*, but also *C. trachomatis*, anaerobes, Gram-negative facultative bacteria, and streptococci.

The Division of STD Prevention of the Centers for Disease Control and Prevention (CDC) recommends the following parenteral regimens for the treatment of PID: (*a*) cefotetan (2 g i.v. every 12 h) or cefoxitin (2 g i.v. every 6 h), either accompanied by doxycycline (100 mg p.o. or i.v. every 12 h), (*b*) clindamycin (900 mg i.v. every 8 h) plus gentamicin (2 mg/kg i.v. or i.m. as a loading dose, followed by 1.5 mg/kg every 8 h) (2). Alternative parenteral regimens are (*a*) ofloxacin (400 mg p.o. or i.v. every 12 h) plus metronidazole (500 mg i.v. every 8h), (*b*) ampicillin/sulbactam (3 g i.v. every 6 h) plus doxycycline (100 mg p.o. or i.v. every 12 h), or (*c*) ciprofloxacin (200 mg i.v. every 12 h) plus doxycycline (100 mg i.v. every 12 h) plus metronidazole (500 mg i.v. every 8 h). Parenteral therapy may be discontinued 24 h after the patient shows clinical improvement and replaced with an oral regimen of 100 mg doxycycline 2 times a day for 14 days unless a tuboovarian abscess is present, in which case doxycycline may be supplemented with clindamycin or metronidazole.

The CDC also recommends the following oral regimens: (*a*) ofloxacin 400 mg orally 2 times a day for 14 days plus metronidazole 500 mg orally 2 times a day for 14 days, (*b*) a single dose of a parenteral cephalosporin (either ceftriaxone 250 mg i.m., cefoxitin 2 g i.m. with 1 g of probenecid p.o. given concurrently, or another third-generation cephalosporin) plus doxycycline 100 mg orally 2 times a day for 14 days.

Of the antimicrobials recommended for the treatment of PID, the third-generation cephalosporins (especially ceftriaxone) and the fluoroquinolones are the most active against *N. gonorrhoeae* (except where fluoroquinolone-resistant *N. gonorrhoeae* are common). However, all regimens are likely to eradicate *N. gonorrhoeae*, since they include multiple doses and combinations of antimicrobials with activity against gonococci.

Gonococcal Conjunctivitis in Adults and Adolescents

Only one study of the treatment of gonococcal conjunctivitis among adults has been published in recent years (13). In that study, all 12 patients responded well to a single 1-g injection of ceftriaxone. The CDC recommends that a single 1-g dose of ceftriaxone be administered intramuscularly and the infected eye lavaged with saline solution once (2).

Disseminated Gonococcal Infections in Adults and Adolescents

Disseminated gonococcal infection results from gonococcal bacteremia, often resulting in petechial or pustular, acral skin lesions, asymmetric arthralgias, tenosynovitis, or septic arthritis—and is occasionally complicated by perihepatitis and, very rarely, by endocarditis or meningitis. No studies of the treatment of disseminated gonococcal infection have been published in the past 10 years. The CDC's recommendations for treatment of disseminated gonococcal infection are based on the opinions of experts. Despite the lack of experimental or even observational studies of the efficacy of the recommended regimens, it is reassuring to note that no reports of treatment failures have been published since these recommendations were first made by the CDC in 1989.

The CDC recommends hospitalization for initial therapy, especially for patients who cannot be relied on to comply with treatment, for those for whom the diagnosis is uncertain, and for those who have purulent synovial effusions or other complications. Patients should be examined for clinical evidence of endocarditis and meningitis. If endocarditis and meningitis are ruled out, patients should initially be treated with ceftriaxone (1 g i.m. or i.v. every 24 h). Acceptable alternatives are cefotaxime (1 g i.v. every 8 h) or ceftizoxime (1 g i.v. every 8 h). Patients allergic to β-lactam drugs may be treated initially with spectinomycin (2 g i.m. every 12 h). Parenteral treatment should be continued for 24 to 48 h after improvement begins; then therapy may be switched to cefixime (400 mg p.o. 2 times a day) or ciprofloxacin (500 mg p.o. 2 times a day) to complete a full week of antimicrobial therapy. For gonococcal endocarditis or meningitis, initial therapy should be with 1 to 2 g of ceftriaxone intravenously every 12 h, and therapy should be continued for 10 to 14 days for meningitis and for at least 4 weeks for endocarditis.

Gonococcal Infections among Infants

Ophthalmia Neonatorum

Gonococcal ophthalmia is likely when typical Gram-negative diplococci are found in conjunctival exudate. Presumptive treatment for *N. gonorrhoeae* is appropriate in infants with conjunctivitis without gonococci in a Gram-stained smear if their mothers are at high risk of gonorrhea. In all cases, conjunctival exudate should be cultured for *N. gonorrhoeae* so that a definitive diagnosis can be made and for antibiotic susceptibility testing. A definitive diagnosis is important because of the public health and social consequences of a diagnosis of gonorrhea. Infants diagnosed with gonococcal ophthalmia should be admitted to the hospital and evaluated for signs of disseminated infection (e.g., sepsis, arthritis, and meningitis). The CDC

recommends that gonococcal neonatal ophthalmia be treated with 25 to 50 mg/kg ceftriaxone intravenously or intramuscularly in a single dose, not to exceed 125 mg. Ceftriaxone should be administered cautiously to hyperbilirubinemic infants, especially those born prematurely. Topical antibiotic therapy alone is inadequate and is unnecessary if systemic treatment is administered. Simultaneous infection with *C. trachomatis* should be considered when a patient does not respond satisfactorily.

Disseminated Gonococcal Infection and Gonococcal Scalp Abscesses among Newborns

Sepsis, arthritis, and meningitis are rare complications of neonatal gonococcal infection. Infection of the scalp may result from fetal monitoring. Recommended treatment is with ceftriaxone (25–50 mg/kg/day i.v. or i.m.) in a single daily dose for 7 days or for 10 to 14 days if meningitis is documented. An alternative is cefotaxime (25 mg/kg i.v. or i.m.) every 12 h for the same length of time.

Prophylactic Treatment for Infants Whose Mothers Have Gonococcal Infection

Infants born to mothers who have untreated gonorrhea but who have no evidence of infection themselves should be treated with a single dose of ceftriaxone (25–50 mg/kg i.v. or i.m., not to exceed 125 mg).

CDC Recommendations for the Treatment of Gonococcal Infections among Children

Children who weigh more than 45 kg should be treated with one of the regimens recommended for adults.

Children who weigh less than 45 kg who have uncomplicated vulvovaginitis, cervicitis, urethritis, pharyngitis, or proctitis should be treated with a single dose of ceftriaxone (125 mg i.m.). If ceftriaxone cannot be given, an acceptable alternative is spectinomycin (40 mg/kg; maximum, 2 g; i.m.) in a single dose. Spectinomycin is unreliable against pharyngeal infections. Some experts use cefixime to treat gonococcal infections in children because it can be administered orally as a tablet or liquid; however, there are no published reports of its safety or effectiveness for this purpose.

Children who weigh less than 45 kg who have bacteremia or arthritis should be treated with ceftriaxone (50 mg/kg; maximum, 1 g) intramuscularly or intravenously in a single dose daily for 7 days. Children who weigh less than 45 kg who have meningitis should be treated with ceftriaxone (50 mg/kg; maximum, 1 g) intramuscularly or intravenously in a single dose daily for 10 to 14 days.

SPECIAL CONSIDERATIONS
Multidose Regimens for Uncomplicated Infections

There are so many safe and effective single-dose regimens that multidose regimens, with which some patients may have trouble complying, have no role.

Combination Therapies

There are so many safe and effective single-agent regimens that combination regimens, with their increased risk of adverse drug reactions, are unnecessary. For complicated infections, treatment with a higher dose of a single agent (e.g., 1 g instead of 125 mg of ceftriaxone for ophthalmia) or with multiple doses of a single agent (e.g., 4 weeks of therapy with ceftriaxone for endocarditis) is recommended rather than adding a second antigonococcal agent.

Penicillins and Tetracyclines

High-level, plasmid-mediated resistance to penicillin (PPNG) and tetracycline have been reported from all the populated continents. In the United States, 6.8% of a sample of over 5000 isolates collected in 1995 were PPNG, and 8.6% were tetracycline resistant (6). In some parts of the world, most strains carry resistance plasmids. For example, 85 of 86 gonococcal strains isolated in the Indonesian port of Surabaya in 1993 carried plasmids for tetracycline or penicillin resistance or both (16). Although there may be communities where penicillin and tetracycline remain useful for the treatment of locally acquired gonorrhea, such communities are rare, and we have therefore excluded penicillin and tetracycline regimens from our discussion.

Pregnancy

Quinolones are contraindicated in pregnant women. Those infected with *N. gonorrhoeae* should be treated with a cephalosporin or, if they cannot tolerate a cephalosporin, should be treated with spectinomycin intramuscularly.

HIV Infection

Persons with HIV infection and gonococcal infection should receive the same treatment as persons not infected with HIV.

Allergy, Intolerance, or Adverse Reactions

Persons who cannot tolerate cephalosporins or quinolones should, in general, be treated with spectinomycin. However, since spectinomycin is unreliable against pharyngeal infections (curing only 52% of infections in published studies), patients who are treated with spectinomycin and suspected or known to have pharyngeal infection should undergo a pharyngeal culture 3 to 5 days after treatment to verify eradication of their infection.

ENDPOINTS FOR MONITORING

The goals of therapy are to prevent complications and to render the individual noncontagious. For uncomplicated urogenital or rectal infections, the recommended regimens are so close to 100% effective that no follow-up is needed if symptoms resolve. For pharyngeal infections, only the most effective regimens (e.g., ciprofloxacin 500 mg and ceftriaxone 125 mg) are more than 90% effective (Table 2). However, most experts believe that pharyngeal infections are self-limited and not highly contagious, so follow-up cultures are not routinely recommended. For infections at other sites (e.g., the eye) and for disseminated infection, clinical resolution of signs and symptoms is used as an endpoint, since there is little concern about persistent asymptomatic infection that would, in any case, not be readily transmissible.

CONTROVERSIES, CAVEATS, COMMENTS
Dual Therapy for Gonorrhea and Chlamydial Infection

Because persons with gonorrhea are generally at high risk of being infected with *C. trachomatis* as well, persons treated for gonorrhea should, in general, also be treated with a regimen effective against genital *C. trachomatis* infection (e.g., doxycycline 100 mg p.o. 2 times a day for 7 days or azithromycin 1 g p.o. once). Routine dual therapy without testing can clearly be cost-effective where chlamydial infection accompanies 20 to 40% of gonococcal infections because chlamydia therapy is safe and costs so little (e.g., $0.50 to $1.50 for doxycycline) compared with the cost of testing. Some experts believe that routine use of dual therapy has significantly decreased the prevalence of chlamydial infection. In addition to its value as a strategy for the control of chlamydial infection, dual therapy may have secondary benefits. Because most gonococci in the United States are susceptible to the antimicrobial regimens recommended for the treatment of uncomplicated *C. trachomatis* infection, routine cotreatment may hinder development of antimicrobial-resistant *N. gonorrhoeae*.

Since the introduction of dual therapy, chlamydial infection prevalence has dropped in some populations, and testing for chlamydial infection has become quicker, more sensitive, and more widely available. Where rates of coinfection are low, some clinicians may prefer to test for chlamydia rather than treat presumptively. However, presumptive treatment is indicated for patients who may not return for test results.

Quinolone-Resistant *N. gonorrhoeae*

Cases of gonorrhea caused by *N. gonorrhoeae* resistant to fluoroquinolones have been reported sporadically from many parts of the world, including North America, and are becoming widespread in parts of Asia. However, as of February 1997, quinolone-resistant *N. gonorrhoeae* remained very rare in the United States: less than 0.03% of 3449 isolates collected by the Gonococcal Isolate Surveillance Project in the first three quarters of 1996 had ciprofloxacin MICs of 1.0 μg/mL or above (2). This study sample is drawn from 26 cities and includes approximately 1.3% of all gonococcal infections reported among men in the United States. As long as quinolone-resistant *N. gonorrhoeae* comprise less than 1% of all *N. gonorrhoeae* strains isolated at each of the 26 study cities, the fluoroquinolone regimens recommended here can be used with confidence. However, importation of quinolone-resistant *N. gonorrhoeae* is likely to continue, and the prevalence of quinolone-resistant *N. gonorrhoeae* in the United States may well increase in the future to a point at which fluoroquinolones can no longer be relied upon to eradicate gonococcal infections.

OTHER MANAGEMENT CONSIDERATIONS
Screening for Syphilis

Persons treated for gonorrhea should be screened for syphilis by serology when first seen. Treatment regimens including ceftriaxone or a 7-day course of doxycycline or erythromycin may cure incubating syphilis, but few data are available on either the efficacy of these regimens against incubating syphilis or the prevalence of incubating syphilis among patients diagnosed with gonorrhea.

Disease Reporting

Gonorrhea is a reportable disease in the United States.

Importance of a Definitive Diagnosis in Children

N. gonorrhoeae infection in children is often due to sexual abuse. Therefore, only standard culture procedures for the isolation of *N. gonorrhoeae* should be used for children beyond the neonatal period.

Management of Sex Partners

Recent sexual contacts of persons treated for gonorrhea should generally be tested for gonorrhea and treated presumptively. If found to be infected, they should be advised to refer their recent sex partners.

Follow-Up

Persons with uncomplicated gonorrhea who are treated with any of the recommended regimens need not return for a test of cure. Those whose symptoms persist after treatment should be evaluated by culture for *N. gonorrhoeae,* and any gonococci isolated should be tested for antimicrobial susceptibility. Infections detected after treatment with one of the recommended regimens are more likely to be reinfections than treatment failures.

REFERENCES

1. Bygdeman SM, Rudén A-K, Jonsson A, Lidbrink P, Olofsson M-B, Bäckman, Gästrin B, Kallings I, Ramberg M, Rylander M, Wretlind B. Antibiotic susceptibility, serovars and auxotypes of gonococcal isolates in Stockholm. Relation to geographical origin of the infection. Int J STD AIDS 1993;4:33–40.
2. Centers for Disease Control and Prevention (CDC). 1998 Guidelines for Treatment of Sexually Transmitted Diseases. MMWR 1998; 47 (no. RR-1).
3. Chenia HY, Pillay B, Hoosen AA, Pillay D. Antibiotic susceptibility patterns and plasmid profiles of penicillinase-producing *Neisseria gonorrhoeae* strains in Durban, South Africa, 1990–1993. Sex Transm Dis 1997;24:18–22.
4. Clendennen TE, Echeverria E, Saengeur S, Kees ES, Boslego JW, Wignall FS. Antibiotic susceptibility survey of *Neisseria gonorrhoeae* in Thailand. Antimicrob Agents Chemother 1992; 36:1682–1687.
5. Clendennen TE 3d, Hames CS, Kees ES, Price FC, Rueppel WJ, Andrada AB, Espinosa GE, Kabierra G, Wignal FS. In vitro antibiotic susceptibilities of *Neisseria gonorrhoeae* isolates in the Philippines. Antimicrob Agents Chemother 1992;36:277–282.
6. Division of STD/HIV Prevention. Sexually transmitted disease surveillance, 1995. Atlanta: Centers for Disease Control and Prevention (CDC), 1996.
7. Fekete T, Serfass DA, Lafredo SC, Cundy KR. Susceptibility to cephalosporins of penicillin-susceptible and penicillin-resistant strains of *Neisseria gonorrhoeae* from Philadelphia. Antimicrob Agents Chemother 1989;33:164–166.
8. Fekete T, Woodwell J, Cundy KR. Susceptibility of *Neisseria gonorrhoeae* to cefpodoxime: determination of MICs and disk diffusion zone diameters. Antimicrob Agents Chemother 1991;35: 497–499.
9. Fox KK, Knapp JS, Holmes KK, Hook EW III, Judson FN, Thompson SE, Washington JA, Whittington WL. Antimicrobial resistance in *Neisseria gonorrhoeae* in the United States 1988–1994: the emergence of decreased susceptibility to fluoroquinolones. J Infect Dis 1997; 175:1396–1403.
10. Glatt AE, Cummings M, McCormack W. In vitro activity of temafloxacin compared with those of other agents against 100 clinical isolates of *Neisseria gonorrhoeae*. Antimicrob Agents Chemother 1992;36:1131–1132.
11. Green SD. Indications and restrictions of fluoroquinolone use in children. Br J Hosp Med 1996;56:420–423.
12. Grenier B. Use of fluoroquinolones in children. An overview. Adv Antimicrob Antineopl Chemother 1992;11–2:135–140.
13. Haimovici R, Roussel TJ. Treatment of gonococcal conjunctivitis with single-dose intramuscular ceftriaxone. Am J Ophthalmol 1989;107:511–514.
14. Haizlip J, Isbey SF, Hamilton HA, Jerse AE, Leone PA, Davis RH, Cohen MS. Time required for elimination of *Neisseria gonorrhoeae* from the urogenital tract in men with symptomatic urethritis: comparison of oral and intramuscular single-dose therapy. Sex Transm Dis 1995;22:145–148.
15. Jaffee HW, SchroeterAL, Reynolds GH, Zaidi AA, Martin JE, Thayer JD. Pharmacokinetic determinants in penicillin cure of gonococcal urethritis. Antimicrob Agents Chemother 1979;15: 587–591.
16. Joesoef MR, Knapp JS, Idajadi A, Linnan M, Barakbah Y, Kambodji A, O'Hanley PJ, Moran JS Antimicrobial susceptibility of *Neisseria gonorrhoeae* strains isolated in Surabaya, Indonesia. Antimicrob Agents Chemother 1994;38:2530–2533.
17. Korting HC, Abeck D. One-shot treatment of uncomplicated gonorrhoea with third-generation cephalosporins with differing serum half-life. Results of a controlled trial with ceftriaxone and cefotaxime. Chemotherapy 1989;35:441–448.
18. Lewis DA, Ison CA, Livermore DM, Chen HY, Hooi AY, Wisdon AR. A one-year survey of *Neisseria gonorrhoeae* isolated from patients attending an east London genitourinary medicine clinic: antibiotic susceptibility patterns and patients' characteristics. Genitourin Med 1995:71:13–17.
19. Moran JS. Treating uncomplicated *Neisseria gonorrhoeae* infections: is the anatomic site of infection important? Sex Transm Dis 1995;22:39–47.
20. Moran JS, Levine WC. Drugs of choice for the treatment of uncomplicated gonococcal infections. Clin Infect Dis 1995;20 (Suppl 1):S47–65.
21. Moran JS. Ciprofloxacin for gonorrhea—250 mg or 500 mg? Sex Transm Dis 1996;23:165–167.
22. Pabst KM, Siegel NA, Smith S, Black JR, Handsfield HH, Hook EW. Multicenter, comparative study of enoxacin and ceftriaxone for treatment of uncomplicated gonorrhea. Sex Transm Dis 1989;16:148–151.
23. Perea EJ, García-López JL, Martín R, Calmet M, Cisterna R. Estébanez V, Vázquez JA, Martín Luengo F, Altuna A, Merino C, Rodríquez Torres A. Sensibilidad a antimicrobianos de 402 cepas de *Neisseria gonorrhoeae* aisladas en 7 ciudades de España. Enferm Infecc Microbiol Clin 1991;9:619–623.
24. Plourde PJ, Tyndall M, Agoki E, Ombette J, Slaney LA, D'Costa LJ, Ndinya-Achola JO, Plummer FA. Single-dose cefixime versus single-dose ceftriaxone in the treatment of antimicrobial-resistant *Neisseria gonorrhoeae* infection. J Infect Dis 1992; 166:919–922.
25. Portilla I, Lutz B, Montalvo M, Mogabgab WJ. Oral cefixime versus intramuscular ceftriaxone in patients with uncomplicated gonococcal infections. Sex Transm Dis 1992;19:94–98.

26. Schaad UB. Use of quinolones in children and articular risk. Arch Pediatr 1996;3:183–184.

27. Schäfer V, Enzensberger R, Schneider C, Rickmann J, Nitschke-Özbay H, Brade V. Epidemiology of penicillin-resistant *Neisseria gonorrhoeae* in Frankfurt, Germany. Eur J Clin Microbiol Infect Dis 1995;14:914–918.

28. Talbot H, Romanowski B. In vitro activities of lomefloxacin, tetracycline, penicillin, spectinomycin, and ceftriaxone against *Neisseria gonorrhoeae* and *Chlamydia trachomatis*. Antimicrob Agents Chemother 1989;33:2049–2051.

29. Tanaka M, Kumazawa J, Matsumoto T, Kobayashi I. High prevalence of *Neisseria gonorrhoeae* strains with reduced susceptibility to fluoroquinolones in Japan. Genitourin Med 1994:70:90–93.

30. Tananka M, Matsumoto T, Kobayashi I, Uchino U, Kumazawa J. Emergence of in vitro resistance to fluoroquinolones in *Neisseria gonorrhoeae* isolated in Japan. Antimicrob Agents Chemother 1995;39:2367–2370.

31. Van Dyck E, Rossau R, Duhamel M, Behets F, Laga M, Nzila M, Bygdeman S, Van Heuverswijn H, Piot P. Antimicrobial susceptibility of *Neisseria gonorrhoeae* in Zaire: high level plasmid-mediated tetracycline resistance in Central Africa. Genitourin Med 1992;68:111–116.

32. Van Dyck E, Crabbé F, Nzila N, Bogaerts J, Munyabikali J-P, Ghys P, Diallo M, Laga M. Increasing resistance of *Neisseria gonorrhoeae* in West and Central Africa: consequences on therapy of gonococcal infection. Sex Transm Dis 1997;24:32–37.

33. West B, Changalucha J, Grosskurth H, Mayaud P, Gabone RM, Ka-Gina G, Mabey R. Antimicrobial susceptibility, auxotype and plasmid content of *Neisseria gonorrhoeae* in Northern Tanzania: emergence of high level plasmid mediated tetracycline resistance. Genitourin Med 1995;71:9–12.

34. Youssef RZ, Murray M, Holmes B, Mogabgab WJ. Cefotetan therapy for gonococcal urethritis and cervicitis. Sex Transm Dis 1990;17:99–101.

Neisseria meningitidis

●

Keith A. V. Cartwright

GENERAL DESCRIPTION

Neisseria meningitidis is a fastidious Gram-negative diplococcus that colonizes and invades only man. Its normal habitat is the posterior nasopharynx. Carriage is rare in infants and young children, rises to a peak of about 25 to 30% in the late teens, and then declines slowly in older age groups; overall carriage rates are about 10% (13). Carriage may be of long duration—often more than a year. Perhaps surprisingly, most meningococci are not very infectious; transmission from person to person is by the respiratory route and generally only results from prolonged close contact. In a very small proportion of individuals, the organisms breach the nasopharyngeal mucosal barrier shortly after colonization and cause invasive disease. Meningococcal pathogenicity varies enormously from strain to strain. Most strains are incapable of causing disease in immunocompetent individuals, and most older children and adults are immune to systemic infection.

Epidemiology

Meningococci can be divided into *serogroups* on the basis of structural differences in the capsular polysaccharide, a major virulence factor; only well-capsulated strains have the potential to invade. Strains can be further classified into *types* and *subtypes* based on variations in the class 2/3 and class 1 outer membrane proteins, respectively.

Almost all meningococcal disease in immunocompetent individuals is caused by strains of three serogroups: A, B, and C. Serogroup A disease dominates in sub-Saharan Africa and some other tropical countries. In higher-latitude countries in-

cluding the North American continent and most of Europe, disease due to serogroups B and C predominates. Attack rates vary widely by region, by country, and over time.

Overall disease rates in higher-latitude countries are often about 1 to 2 per 10^5 population, but higher rates are not uncommon from time to time (37). Meningococci can cause clusters of cases, or outbreaks, which are usually due to strains of a single clonal type. Disease attack rates are highest in the very young, peaking at about age 7 months, then falling steadily to age 10 years, followed by a second and smaller peak in those in their late teens (29). The disease incidence in adults is low. The sex ratio of cases usually shows a small male preponderance.

Infants, among whom the prevalence of protective antibodies is low, only rarely acquire meningococci; when they do, the chances of invasive disease are high. The second disease peak in teenagers and young adults may be due to the peak of carriage and, more importantly, the peak of acquisition that occurs around this age.

Massive pancontinental epidemics due to serogroup A strains occur in sub-Saharan Africa (the so-called meningitis belt) at intervals of about 5 to 10 years, with attack rates of 100 per 10^5 population or more. These are due to introduction and dissemination of new meningococcal clones within susceptible populations (2).

Pathogenesis

Natural Immunity

Natural protection against invasive meningococcal infection is associated with acquisition of protective bactericidal antibodies.

Most infants are protected transiently by passively transferred maternal antibodies. As protection wanes, susceptibility to infection rises rapidly. Bactericidal antibodies are acquired progressively by exposure to various bacteria that express noncapsular antigens in common with meningococci. Later in life, immunity is sustained by exposure to many immunizing organisms including nonpathogenic meningococci.

Invasive Disease

Meningococci breaching the nasopharyngeal mucosa may reach the bloodstream, where they may shed large amounts of endotoxin, the main effector of tissue damage. Although the blood-brain barrier is normally highly effective in excluding bacteria, most (75–80%) patients with invasive meningococcal disease have meningitis. Liberation of endotoxin into the subarachnoid space provokes a marked cytokine-mediated inflammatory response that causes the blood-brain barrier to become "leaky" and facilitates penetration of antibiotics. As meningeal inflammation subsides, the penetration of antibiotics into the subarachnoid space declines progressively (36, 45). Therefore, when treating bacterial meningitis of any etiology, antibiotic doses must be kept high throughout the period of parenteral treatment.

Meningococcal Septicemia and Other Clinical Syndromes

In 10 to 20% of cases of invasive disease, meningococci remain restricted to the bloodstream and cause septicemia, a more serious illness. The mortality in vigorously treated meningococcal meningitis is about 2 to 4%, whereas mortality in septicemia without meningitis is 20 to 40%. Most deaths occur within the first 24 to 48 h. Occasionally, meningococci cause other clinical syndromes including pneumonia, pericarditis, conjunctivitis, endophthalmitis, septic arthritis, pelvic infection, or a chronic low-grade septicemia.

SUSCEPTIBILITY IN VITRO

Meningococci continue to demonstrate exquisite sensitivity in vitro to the antibiotics commonly used in empirical treatment of bacterial meningitis. Typical inhibitory concentrations for relevant antibiotics are given in Table 1. Many newer β-lactam antibiotics also exhibit high activity against meningococci but either offer no particular advantages over currently used agents or have yet to be evaluated adequately in clinical trials.

Antibiotics for the Treatment of Meningitis

In addition to being safe and showing a high level of activity against meningococci in vitro, antibiotics for the treatment of meningitis must be able to penetrate the inflamed meninges and reach the subarachnoid space (7). Some of the factors determining such penetration are listed in Table 2 (55). All antibiotics given for the treatment of bacterial meningitis must be administered, at least initially, by the parenteral route, normally intravenously. In uncomplicated bacterial meningitis, consideration of intrathecal treatment is rarely if ever needed. Misinterpretation of intrathecal penicillin G doses by junior medical

TABLE 1 • Meningococcal Inhibitory Concentrations of Antibiotics Commonly Used in the Treatment of Bacterial Meningitis

Antibiotic	MIC_{50} (mg/L)	MIC_{90} (mg/L)	Range (mg/L)	% Strains Resistant
Penicillin G[a]	0.032	0.05	0.016–1.28	0
Ampicillin/ amoxycillin[a]	0.075	0.2	0.016–2.0	0
Cefotaxime	<0.008	<0.008	<0.008	0
Ceftriaxone	<0.002	<0.002	<0.008	0
Chloramphenicol	0.75	1.0	—	0

Data adapted from Emmerson 1985 (18), Enting 1996 (19), and Kaczmarksi 1997 (32).

[a]Three β-lactamase producing clinical isolates have been described (see text).

staff continues to result in occasional avoidable deaths due to massive overdosing and penicillin encephalopathy.

Penicillin G (Benzylpenicillin)

With its high intrinsic activity and outstanding safety record, penicillin G remains the drug of choice for treatment of all types of invasive meningococcal disease. The England and Wales Meningococcal Reference Unit first drew attention to a small but increasing proportion (3.1% in 1989) of clinical isolates of meningococci showing reduced sensitivity to penicillin G (minimum inhibitory concentrations (MICs) between 0.16 and 1.28 mg/L) (28, 61). Reports of similar prevalences followed from the North and South American continents and from the Netherlands, but Spanish workers reported a far higher prevalence of 20 to 40%, and in the U.K., the proportion of clinical isolates showing reduced sensitivity has continued to increase (11% in 1995) (32).

Spratt et al. showed that the reduced sensitivity was due to a decreased affinity of meningococcal penicillin-binding protein 2 for penicillin G, caused by transformation of the meningococcal *pen A* gene by nucleotide sequences most probably originating in the commensal *Neisseria flavescens* (57). Clinical concerns eased when it became clear that such strains continued to respond to standard treatment (26, 65), though treatment failure was documented in a patient with meningitis due to a

TABLE 2 • Factors Increasing the Penetration of Antibiotics into the Subarachnoid Space

Antibiotic Related	Host Related
Low protein binding	Meningeal inflammation
Hydrophobicity	Blockage of CSF efflux pump (e.g., by probenecid)
Low molecular weight	
Neutral surface isoelectric charge	

Modified from Schmidt T, Täuber MG. Pharmacodynamics of antibiotics in the therapy of meningitis: infection model observations. J Antimicrob Chemother 1993;31(Suppl D):61–70.

meningococcus of reduced sensitivity to penicillin who received a relatively low dose of penicillin G (64).

There have been very occasional anecdotal reports of isolation of β-lactamase-producing strains of meningococci from clinical sources (9, 17, 23), and a plasmid-borne gonococcal β-lactamase has been transferred to a meningococcus in the laboratory (11). As yet, no adverse clinical outcomes have been caused by such strains.

ANTIMICROBIAL THERAPY
Prehospital Treatment
Effect of Oral Antibiotic Therapy
In its early clinical stages, meningococcal meningitis is very hard to differentiate from more trivial respiratory infections. Thus, up to 50% of patients with what is later confirmed to be meningococcal disease, receive oral antibiotic treatment prior to admission to the hospital, often with agents to which the invading meningococcus is sensitive in vitro (24). It is not known how many cases of invasive meningococcal disease are aborted by such treatment. Oral antibiotic treatment may fail to prevent further progression of meningococcal disease because of intrinsic lack of activity of the antibiotic against the invading strain, failure of absorption from the bowel, or failure in distribution.

Prehospital Parenteral Antibiotic Treatment
Most (8, 14, 41) but not all (47) authorities are persuaded that early parenteral antibiotic treatment improves outcome substantially in meningococcal disease. Some uncertainty remains because no prospective, randomized, placebo-controlled studies stratified by disease severity (a key determinant of outcome) have been reported. Preadmission parenteral antibiotic therapy is recommended in many countries. Primary care doctors in the U.K. are advised by the Chief Medical Officer to carry penicillin G (which has a half-life of about 3 years in the doctor's bag) at all times and to use it as soon as the possibility of meningococcal disease is recognized. The same advice applies if the patient is admitted to the hospital via the Accident & Emergency Department (Emergency Room). Penicillin G should be given swiftly, ideally by the intravenous route. The doses are probably not critical, but those recommended in the U.K. are

Adults and children aged 10 years and over: 1200 mg
Children aged 1 to 9 years: 600 mg
Children under 1 year of age: 300 mg

Penicillin Anaphylaxis and Allergy
The only contraindication is a history of penicillin anaphylaxis, which is very rare, with an estimated incidence of around 0.01% (25), and **not** penicillin allergy, which is commoner, though greatly overdiagnosed (51, 60). Intravenous chloramphenicol, if available, can be used in patients with a history of penicillin anaphylaxis. The dose is 1.2 g for adults and 25 mg/kg in children under 12 years of age. A parenteral cephalosporin is another alternative; the true rate of cross-sensitivity with penicillin G is not known accurately but is probably low (33).

Routes of Antibiotic Administration.   Gaining access to a vein may be difficult in profoundly shocked patients, in infants and small children, or in patients being treated in poorly lit surroundings. In such circumstances, the intramuscular route can be used but may not be so effective, particularly in shocked patients. Regardless of whether a dose of parenteral antibiotic has been given, the patient should be transferred to the hospital as quickly as possible.

Inpatient Treatment
Diagnostic Considerations
The question facing the admitting hospital doctor is often not How do I treat this case of invasive meningococcal disease? but, How do I treat this case of possible meningitis or septicemia that may be meningococcal? If the patient has fever and a hemorrhagic rash, meningococcal disease is the most likely diagnosis. Other causes of fever with purpura (6) may need to be excluded. Unless meningococcal disease has been confirmed by visualization of Gram-negative diplococci in a sample of cerebrospinal fluid (CSF) or, better, by culture from a deep site such as blood or CSF, it is wise to commence a broad-spectrum antibiotic regime.

Empirical Antibiotic Treatment of Bacterial Meningitis
Many antibiotics and combinations have been advocated for the empirical treatment of suspected bacterial meningitis. Selection of particular combinations will be influenced by the age, clinical history, and overall condition of the patient; by pharmacokinetic factors; and by a range of local factors including the incidence of invasive *Haemophilus influenzae* type b (Hib) disease (depending on whether Hib vaccines have been introduced) and the prevalence of penicillin-resistant pneumococci and of other types of bacterial meningitis and septicemia in the community.

Penicillin G or ampicillin, initially accompanied by chloramphenicol, or monotherapy with cefotaxime or ceftriaxone are all suitable empirical treatments for bacterial meningitis in children (excluding neonates) (21, 46), though chloramphenicol and cefuroxime (46, 53) appear to be inferior single agents. In practice, use of chloramphenicol with or without a β-lactam for the treatment of bacterial meningitis has declined rapidly, at least in the United States (34), while the simplicity of single daily dosing with ceftriaxone has undoubtedly contributed to its increasing use both in empirical treatment of bacterial meningitis and in confirmed meningococcal disease. The relative expense of both cefotaxime and ceftriaxone may continue to restrain their use in developing countries. Dosages for all these agents are given in Table 3.

Empirical antibiotic treatment of community-acquired pyogenic meningitis in immunocompetent adults should take into account the possibility of a wider range of potential pathogens including *Listeria monocytogenes*.

Effect of Prehospital Parenteral Antibiotic Treatment on Inpatient Investigations
Administration of penicillin G prior to hospital admission reduces considerably the chances of isolating a meningococcus

TABLE 3 • **Dosages of Antibiotics Commonly Used in the Treatment of Bacterial Meningitis**

Antibiotic	Total Daily Dose	No. of Daily Doses
Penicillin G	Adults and children > 12 years: 9.6–14.4 g	4–6
	Children 1 month– 12 years: 180–300 mg/kg	4–6
Ampicillin	250 mg/kg	4
Cefotaxime	200 mg/kg	4–6
Ceftriaxone	80–100 mg/kg	1–2
Chloramphenicol	75–100 mg/kg	4

from a deep site (usually blood or CSF), though isolation of meningococci from nasopharyngeal swabs is unaffected (15) and offers a good chance of obtaining a meningococcus for sensitivity testing and for epidemiologic purposes (66). Establishing as swiftly as possible whether a meningococcal infection is presenting primarily as septicemia or meningitis will help guide inpatient management. Development of improved nonculture methods of diagnosis, including polymerase chain reaction (PCR) of CSF (43) and peripheral blood (42) and better serologic tests (30), means that antibiotic treatment should never be withheld while diagnostic specimens are collected. Optimizing treatment must always have priority over diagnostic niceties.

Inpatient Management of Suspected Meningococcal Disease

General aspects of the prehospital and inpatient management of meningococcal disease have been reviewed recently in two complementary U.K. articles (31, 48) that deal with isolation nursing, microbiologic investigations, collection of appropriate clinical information for audit, and management in the community.

Once meningococcal disease has been confirmed in either child or adult, penicillin G monotherapy is effective, cheap, and exerts minimum selective pressure on the patient's (and the hospital's) indigenous bacterial flora. It remains the drug of choice.

Alternative Antibiotic Therapy

A number of different antibiotics and regimens are suitable alternatives for the treatment of invasive meningococcal disease, and choice depends on local circumstances. The likelihood of encountering truly resistant (β-lactamase-producing) meningococci is so low throughout the world that penicillin G (given in adequate dosage, see above) can be recommended strongly for the antibiotic monotherapy of confirmed meningococcal meningitis or septicemia. Alternative single agents in allergic patients are ceftriaxone, cefotaxime, or (if the patient is allergic to all β-lactams) chloramphenicol. Doses are the same as those used for empirical treatment of bacterial meningitis of unknown etiology (Table 3).

Duration of Parenteral Antibiotic Treatment

There are few hard data on which to base a recommendation for the duration of antibiotic treatment. If the CSF is resampled during treatment, it is usually sterile within 24 to 36 h. Despite this, 7 days of treatment are still normally recommended for meningococcal meningitis (21, 39, 44) though shorter courses of 4 days may suffice in uncomplicated cases (38), and single-dose treatment with long-acting penicillin or chloramphenicol has been used in Nigeria with some success. Antibiotic treatment of meningococcal septicemia is often prolonged because the patients are sicker, even though the bloodstream is likely to be sterilized more rapidly than the CSF.

Elimination of Meningococcal Nasopharyngeal Carriage

Chloramphenicol and most β-lactam antibiotics are not completely effective in eliminating meningococci from the nasopharynx (1, 5). In the U.K., patients recuperating from meningococcal disease are given a course of a chemoprophylactic antibiotic (see below) just prior to discharge from the hospital. Others do not consider the small risk of persistent carriage to be worth specific treatment (5, 66).

Prophylaxis of Close Contacts

Close contacts of patients with meningococcal disease are at increased risk of developing infection themselves. Though the relative risk for household contacts is very high (500–1000×), albeit transiently, the absolute risk is very low—only 1 to 2% of all cases of meningococcal disease are secondary (16). Part of the management of an acute case is the identification and antibiotic treatment of the close contact group, normally the immediate family and any additional mouth-kissing contacts such as boyfriends and girlfriends.

Close contacts should be identified as swiftly as possible, given accurate information on the symptoms and signs of meningococcal disease, and offered chemoprophylaxis. The antibiotics used to eliminate meningococci from the nasopharynx and the recommended dosage regimens are listed in Table 4. Detailed advice on the practicalities of using the different chemoprophylactic antibiotics was set out recently (48).

If the index case strain is of serogroup A or C, vaccine should be offered in addition to chemoprophylaxis. When prevention of secondary cases rests solely on antibiotic chemoprophylaxis, contacts must be reminded that prophylaxis can fail; secondary cases may then occur weeks or months after the index case (58). Familiarity with the symptoms and signs of meningococcal disease may then be lifesaving.

Guidance on management of clusters of cases has been updated recently in both the United States and the United Kingdom in the light of recent experience (3, 59). Expert advice should be sought when clusters of cases occur within families, day-care centers, schools and universities, military training establishments, or wider communities. Principles of management underpinning intervention are the definition of logical at-risk groups and the calculation of disease attack rates relative to the surrounding community.

TABLE 4 • **Dosage Regimens of Antibiotics Commonly Used for Meningococcal Chemoprophylaxis**

Antibiotic	Treatment Group	Dose	Route and Frequency	% Strains Resistant
Rifampicin	Adults and children over 12 years	600 mg		
	Children 6–12 years	300 mg		
	Children 1–5 years	150 mg	Oral, twice daily for 2 days	<1
	Infants 3–11 months	40 mg		
	Infants 0–2 months	20 mg		
Ciprofloxacin	Adults (not licensed in children)	500 mg	Oral, single dose	<1
Ceftriaxone	Adults	250 mg		
	Children under 12 years	125 mg	Intramuscular, single dose	<1

Data adapted from PHLS Meningococcal Infections Working Group and Public Health Medicine Environmental Group. Control of meningococcal disease: guidance for consultants in communicable disease control. Commun Dis Rep 1995;5:R189–195.

VACCINES
Indications

Purified polysaccharide vaccines for the prevention of meningococcal disease due to serogroups A, C, Y, and W-135 are available commercially. In the U.S. and the U.K., bivalent vaccines containing the A and C polysaccharides are the most widely used. A quadrivalent product containing A, C, Y, and W-135 polysaccharides is also available but is used less frequently. These nonconjugated vaccines have two principal drawbacks: they do not stimulate memory lymphocytes and therefore give only short-term protection, and they are not immunogenic in infants, the age group with the highest disease attack rate. For these two reasons they are not suitable for programs of universal childhood immunization.

Despite these deficiencies, bivalent A+C nonconjugated vaccines have a number of indications, including

- Protection of close contacts of sporadic cases of meningococcal disease caused by the homologous serogroup; close contacts are normally defined as household contacts, mouth-kissing contacts, and medical or paramedical staff carrying out mouth-to-mouth resuscitation
- Mass vaccination of members of closed or semiclosed communities (schools, universities, military recruit training establishments, etc.) following clusters of cases caused by the homologous serogroup
- Mass vaccination of members of wider communities during prolonged clusters or outbreaks of disease caused by strains of serogroup A or C
- Protection of travelers to endemic or epidemic meningococcal disease areas (e.g., sub-Saharan Africa) or to countries requiring evidence of vaccination as a condition of entry (Saudi Arabia requires vaccination of all incoming travelers during the Haj religious festival, and visitors to Mecca at any time)

Younger persons (who are less likely to have acquired natural protection), those making prolonged visits, those traveling "rough" or to "skid road" areas, and those who are functionally or surgically asplenic are at higher than average risk and should be targeted specifically. Other groups for whom vaccination may be indicated include medical and paramedical staff providing clinical care to patients during an epidemic caused by serogroup A or C meningococci and laboratory staff exposed regularly to live cultures of serogroup A or C meningococci.

Quadrivalent A, C, Y, W-135 vaccine can be used for any of the indications listed above for the bivalent vaccine but is specifically indicated for protection of contacts of patients with disease due to strains of serogroup Y or W-135 (both very rare causes of invasive meningococcal disease). When invasive meningococcal disease is caused by strains of serogroups other than A, B, or C, patients (and their first-degree relatives) should undergo careful investigation, as there is a high prevalence of immunologic abnormality, most frequently a deficiency of a terminal complement component (C5 through C9) (22).

Patients with the extremely rare condition of properdin deficiency and a consequent very high lifetime risk of fatal meningococcal disease can (in theory) be protected from meningococcal disease caused by vaccine serogroups and should be offered the quadrivalent vaccine.

Doses and Schedules

The dose of each of these vaccines is 0.5 mL; administration is by the intramuscular route, and a single dose only is needed. Protection wanes after about 3 years. Revaccination, if necessary, is acceptable, but there is little published experience of repeated revaccination. Because of their lack of efficacy in infants and younger children, vaccination with any of the nonconjugated meningococcal polysaccharide vaccines is not recommended for children under the age of 18 months.

Adverse Effects

Both the bivalent and quadrivalent nonconjugated polysaccharide vaccines are extremely safe. They cause slight redness and swelling at the site of injection in about 1% of recipients. In a study of 1.2 million children vaccinated in Canada with a nonconjugated A+C vaccine, the incidence of allergic reactions was 9.2 per 100,000 doses, and for anaphylaxis, 0.1 per 100,000 doses (68).

Vaccine Developments

Protein-polysaccharide-conjugated serogroup A and C vaccines that are expected be immunogenic in infants and young children and to confer long-term immunity are currently undergoing clinical trial in a number of countries. Initial results are highly encouraging (20).

The immune response to serogroup B meningococcal infection is not directed toward the capsular polysaccharide, and vaccines using this antigen are ineffective. Several candidate vaccines for prevention of serogroup B meningococcal disease, which are based on a number of alternative surface-expressed meningococcal components, are at various stages of development and clinical evaluation (4). Though long-term prospects for effective serogroup B vaccines are good, successful vaccines still appear to be some years away.

ENDPOINTS FOR MONITORING THERAPY

Monitoring of peripheral blood to check for sterility and to ensure that antibiotic levels are satisfactory is not normally undertaken in meningococcal disease. The margin between the therapeutic and toxic concentrations of the antibiotics most frequently used in treatment is very wide. There is a greater risk that antibiotic concentrations in the subarachnoid space may not be adequate and therefore at least a theoretical case for resampling CSF during the course of treatment to check for sterility (52). However, lumbar puncture is not without risk (56, 67), and resampling CSF is not part of routine management in the U.K. unless the patient's clinical condition is giving cause for concern.

CONTROVERSIES, CAVEATS, OR COMMENTS
"Frapper Fort ou Frapper Doucement?"

Concerns have been expressed for years that release of endotoxin from Gram-negative bacteria following first administration of antibiotics may cause clinical deterioration (12, 50). Endotoxin release from meningococci may be slower when the bacteria are exposed to lethal doses of chloramphenicol, a bacteriostatic antibiotic, than to penicillin G, a bactericidal agent (40, 49), but this laboratory observation is of uncertain clinical relevance. Brandtzaeg et al. treated a small series of Norwegian patients with meningococcal disease with an initial combination of penicillin G and chloramphenicol; in all, plasma levels of endotoxin fell, despite presumed rapid death of circulating meningococci (10).

Dexamethasone

Dexamethasone given prior to, or concurrently with, the first dose of parenteral antibiotic is associated with improved outcome in bacterial meningitis due to Hib (35) and to other organisms (54, 63); its use is also supported by animal models of bacterial meningitis. It is postulated to act by blocking the inflammatory cytokine cascade normally initiated by release of endotoxin from dead and dying meningococci (27). Dexamethasone can be advocated in meningococcal meningitis if treatment starts at the same time as, or very soon after, the first parenteral dose of antibiotic, but not in meningococcal

septicemia (41). Its lack of efficacy in septicemia, combined with its potential toxicity, mandate clearly against its widespread use as part of prehospital treatment given at a time when the diagnosis is not certain. When used in the inpatient setting, a 2-day course (0.15 mg/kg i.v. 6 hourly) is probably sufficient (62).

A number of experimental immunomodulators are currently undergoing clinical evaluation.

REFERENCES

1. Abramson JS, Spika JS. Persistence of *Neisseria meningitidis* in the upper respiratory tract after intravenous therapy for systemic meningococcal disease. J Infect Dis 1985;151:370–371.
2. Achtman M. Global epidemiology of meningococcal disease. In: Cartwright K, ed. Meningococcal disease. Chichester: John Wiley & Sons, 1995:159–175.
3. Advisory Committee on Immunization Practices. Control and prevention of serogroup C meningococcal disease: evaluation and management of outbreaks. MMWR, in press.
4. Ala'Aldeen DAA, Cartwright KAV. *Neisseria meningitidis*: vaccines and vaccine candidates. J Infect 1996;33:153–157.
5. Alvez F, Aguilera A, Garcia-Zabarte A, Castro-Gago M. Effect of chemoprophylaxis on the meningococcal carrier state after systemic infection. Pediatr Infect Dis J 1991;10:700.
6. Anonymous. Fever with purpura. Lancet 1990;335:889–890.
7. Barling RWA, Selkon JB. The penetration of antibiotics into cerebrospinal fluid and brain tissue. J Antimicrob Chemother 1978;4:203–227.
8. Begg N. Reducing mortality from meningococcal disease. Br Med J 1992;305:133–134.
9. Botha P. Penicillin-resistant *Neisseria meningitidis* in Southern Africa. Lancet 1988;i:54.
10. Brandtzaeg P, Kierulf P, Gaustad P, Skulberg A, Bruun JN, Halvorsen S, Sorensen E. Plasma endotoxin as a predictor of multiple organ failure and death in systemic meningococcal disease. J Infect Dis 1989;159:195–204.
11. Brett MSY. Conjugal transfer of gonococcal β-lactamase and conjugative plasmids to *Neisseria meningitidis*. J Antimicrob Chemother 1989;24:875–879.
12. Buxton Hopkin DA. Frapper fort ou frapper doucement: a Gram-negative dilemma. Lancet 1978;ii:1193–1194.
13. Cartwright KAV, Stuart JM, Jones DM, Noah ND. The Stonehouse survey: nasopharyngeal carriage of meningococci and *Neisseria lactamica*. Epidemiol Infect 1987;99:591–601.
14. Cartwright K, Strang J, Gossain S, Begg N. Early treatment of meningococcal disease. Br Med J 1992;305:774.
15. Cartwright K, Reilly S, White D, Stuart J. Early treatment with parenteral penicillin in meningococcal disease. Br Med J 1992; 305:143–147.
16. Cooke RPD, Riordan T, Jones DM, Painter MJ. Secondary cases of meningococcal infection among close family and household contacts in England and Wales, 1984–7. Br Med J 1989;298: 555–558.
17. Dillon JR, Pauzé M, Yeung K-H. Spread of penicillinase-producing and transfer plasmids from the gonococcus to *Neisseria meningitidis*. Lancet 1983;i:779–781.
18. Emmerson AM, Lamport PA, Reeves DS, Bywater MJ, Holt HA, Wise R, Andrews J, Hall MJ. The in vitro antibacterial activity of ceftriaxone in comparison with nine other antibiotics. Curr Med Res Opin 1985;9:480–493.
19. Enting RH, Spanjaard L, van de Beek D, Hensen EF, de Gans J,

Dankert J. Antimicrobial susceptibility of *Haemophilus influenzae, Neisseria meningitidis* and *Streptococcus pneumoniae* isolates causing meningitis in The Netherlands, 1993–4. J Antimicrob Chemother 1996;38:777–786.

20. Fairley CK, Begg N, Borrow R, Fox AJ, Jones DM, Cartwright K. Conjugate meningococcal serogroup A and C vaccine: reactogenicity and immunogenicity in UK infants. J Infect Dis 1996;174:1360–1363.

21. Feigin RD, McCracken GH, Klein JO. Diagnosis and management of meningitis. Pediatr Infect Dis J 1992;11:785–814.

22. Fijen CA, Kuijper EJ, Hannema AJ, Sjøholm AG, van Putten JP. Complement deficiencies in patients over ten years old with meningococcal disease due to uncommon serogroups. Lancet 1989;ii:585–588.

23. Fontanals D, Pineda V, Pons I, Rojo JC. Penicillin-resistant betalactamase producing *Neisseria meningitidis* in Spain. Eur J Clin Microbiol Infect Dis 1989;8:90–91.

24. Goldacre MJ. Acute bacterial meningitis in childhood: aspects of prehospital care in 687 cases. Arch Dis Child 1977;52:501–503.

25. Idsøe O, Guthe T, Willcox RR, De Weck AL. Nature and extent of penicillin side-reactions, with particular reference to fatalities from anaphylactic shock. Bull WHO 1968;38:159–188.

26. Jackson LA, Tenover FC, Baker C, Plikaytis BD, Reeves MW, Stocker SA, Weaver RE, Wenger JD and the Meningococcal Disease Study Group. Prevalence of *Neisseria meningitidis* relatively resistant to penicillin in the United States, 1991. J Infect Dis 1994;169:438–441.

27. Jafari HS, McCracken GH. Dexamethasone therapy in bacterial meningitis. Pediatr Ann 1994;23:83–88.

28. Jones DM, Sutcliffe EM. Meningococci with reduced susceptibility to penicillin. Lancet 1990;i:863–864.

29. Jones DM, Mallard RH. Age incidence of meningococcal infection, England and Wales 1984–1991. J Infect 1993;27:83–88.

30. Jones DM, Kaczmarski EB. Meningococcal infections in England and Wales: 1994. Commun Dis Rep 1995;5:R125–130.

31. Kaczmarski EB, Cartwright KAV. Control of meningococcal disease: guidance for microbiologists. Commun Dis Rep 1995;5:R196–198.

32. Kaczmarski EB. Meningococcal disease in England and Wales: 1995. Commun Dis Rep 1997;7:R55–59.

33. Kishiyama JL, Adelman DC. The cross-reactivity and immunology of β-lactam antibiotics. Drug Safety 1994;10:318–327.

34. Klass PE, Klein JO. Therapy of bacterial sepsis, meningitis and otitis media in infants and children: 1992 poll of directors of programs in pediatric infectious diseases. Pediatr Infect Dis J 1992;11:702–705.

35. Lebel MH, Freij BJ, Syrogiannopoulos GA, Chrane DF, Hoyt MJ, Stewart SM, Kennard BD, Olsen KD, McCracken GH. Dexamethasone therapy for bacterial meningitis: results of two double-blind, placebo-controlled trials. N Engl J Med 1988;319:964–971.

36. Love WC, McKenzie P, Lawson JH, Pinkerton IW, Jamieson WM, Stevenson J, Roberts W, Christie AB. Treatment of pneumococcal meningitis with cephaloridine. Postgrad Med J 1970;46(Suppl):155–159.

37. Lystad A, Asen S. Epidemiology of meningococcal disease in Norway 1975–91. NIPH Ann 1991;14:57–64.

38. Martin E, Hohl P, Guggi T, Kayser FH, Fernex M, and Members of the Swiss Multicenter Meningitis Study Group. Short course single daily ceftriaxone monotherapy for acute bacterial meningitis in children: results of a Swiss multicenter study. Part I: clinical results. Infection 1990;18:70–77.

39. McCracken GH, Nelson JD, Kaplan SL, Overturf GD, Rodriguez WJ, Steele RW. Consensus report: antimicrobial therapy for bacterial meningitis in infants and children. Pediatr Infect Dis J 1987;6:501–505.

40. Mellado MC, Rodriguez-Contreras R, Mariscal A, Luna JD, Delgado Rodriguez M, Galvez-Vargas R. Effect of penicillin and chloramphenicol on the growth and endotoxin release by *N. meningitidis*. Epidemiol Infect 1991;106:283–288.

41. Nadel S, Levin M, Habibi P. Treatment of meningococcal disease in childhood. In: Cartwright K, ed. Meningococcal disease. Chichester: John Wiley & Sons, 1995:207–243.

42. Newcombe J, Cartwright K, Palmer WH, McFadden J. PCR of peripheral blood for diagnosis of meningococcal disease. J Clin Microbiol 1996;34:1637–1640.

43. Ni H, Knight AI, Cartwright K, Palmer WH, McFadden J. Polymerase chain reaction for diagnosis of meningococcal meningitis. Lancet 1992;340:1432–1434.

44. O'Neill P. Meningitis. How long to treat bacterial meningitis. Lancet 1993;341:530.

45. Oppenheimer S, Beaty HN, Petersdorf RG. Pathogenesis of meningitis. VIII. Cerebrospinal fluid and blood concentrations of methicillin, cephalothin and cephaloridine in experimental pneumococcal meningitis. J Lab Clin Med 1969;73:535–543.

46. Peltola H, Anttila M, Renkonen O-V. Randomised comparison of chloramphenicol, ampicillin, cefotaxime, and ceftriaxone for childhood bacterial meningitis. Lancet 1989;i:1281–1287.

47. Peltola H. Early meningococcal disease: advising the public and the profession. Lancet 1993;342:509–510.

48. PHLS Meningococcal Infections Working Group & Public Health Medicine Environmental Group. Control of meningococcal disease: guidance for consultants in communicable disease control. Commun Dis Rep 1995;5:R189–195.

49. Prins JM, Speelman P, Kuijper EJ, Dankert J, van Deventer SJH. No increase in endotoxin release during antibiotic killing of meningococci. J Antimicrob Chemother 1997;39:13–18.

50. Reilly J, Rivalier E, Compagnon A, Laplane R, Du Buit H. Sur la pathogénie de la dothiénentéric. La fièvre typhoide expérimentale. Ann Med 1935;37:182, 241.

51. Saxon A, Beall GN, Rohr AS, Adelman DC. Immediate hypersensitivity reactions to beta-lactam antibiotics. Ann Intern Med 1987;107:204–215.

52. Schaad UB. Treatment of bacterial meningitis. Eur J Clin Microbiol 1986;5:492–497.

53. Schaad UB, Suter S, Gianella-Borradori A, Pfenninger J, Auckenthaler R, Bernath O, Cheseaux J-J, Wedgwood J. A comparison of ceftriaxone and cefuroxime for the treatment of bacterial meningitis in children. N Engl J Med 1990;322:141–147.

54. Schaad UB, Lips U, Gnehm HE, Blumberg A, Heinzer I, Wedgwood J. Dexamethasone therapy for bacterial meningitis in children. Lancet 1993;342:457–461.

55. Schmidt T, Täuber MG. Pharmacodynamics of antibiotics in the therapy of meningitis: infection model observations. J Antimicrob Chemother 1993;31(Suppl D):61–70.

56. Slack J. Coning and lumbar puncture. Lancet 1980;ii:474–475.

57. Spratt BG, Zhang Q-Y, Jones DM, Hutchison A, Brannigan JA, Dowson CG. Recruitment of a penicillin-binding protein gene from *Neisseria flavescens* during the emergence of penicillin resistance in *Neisseria meningitidis*. Proc Natl Acad Sci USA 1989;86:8988–8992.

58. Stuart JM, Cartwright KAV, Robinson PM, Noah ND. Does eradication of meningococcal carriage in household contacts

prevent secondary cases of meningococcal disease? Br Med J 1989;298:569–570.

59. Stuart JM, Monk PN, Lewis DA, Constantine C, Kaczmarski EB, Cartwright KAV. Management of clusters of meningococcal disease. Commun Dis Rep 1997;7:R3–R4.

60. Surtees SJ, Stockton MG, Gietzen TW. Allergy to penicillin: fable or fact? Br Med J 1991;302:1051–1052.

61. Sutcliffe EM, Jones DM, El-Sheikh S, Percival A. Penicillin-insensitive meningococci in the UK. Lancet 1988;i:657–658.

62. Syrogiannopoulos GA, Lourida AN, Theodoridou MC, Pappas IG, Babilis GC, Economidis JJ, Zoumboulakis DJ, Beratis NG, Matsaniotis NS. Dexamethasone therapy for bacterial meningitis in children: 2- versus 4-day regimen. J Infect Dis 1994;169: 853–858.

63. Townsend GC, Scheld WM. The use of corticosteroids in the management of bacterial meningitis in adults. J Antimicrob Chemother 1996;37:1051–1061.

64. Turner PC, Southern KW, Spencer NJB, Pullen H. Treatment failure in meningococcal meningitis. Lancet 1990;335:732–733.

65. Uriz S, Pineda V, Grau M, Nava JM, Bella F, Morera MA, Fontanals D, Font B, Marti C, Deulofeu F, Calderon A, Duran P, Matas E, Garau J. *Neisseria meningitidis* with reduced sensitivity to penicillin: observations in 10 children. Scand J Infect Dis 1991;23:171–174.

66. Weis N, Lind I. Pharyngeal carriage of *Neisseria meningitidis* before and after treatment of meningococcal disease. J Med Microbiol 1994;41:339–342.

67. Wylie P, Stevens DS, Drake W III, Stuart JM, Cartwright K. The epidemiology and clinical management of meningococcal disease in Gloucestershire. Br Med J 1997;315:774–779.

68. Yergeau A, Alain L, Pless R, Robert Y. Adverse events temporally associated with meningococcal vaccines. Can Med Assoc J 1996;154:503–507.

Nocardia Species[1]

●

Michael M. McNeil and June M. Brown

MICROBIOLOGY

Nocardia species are widely geographically distributed soil bacteria that usually cause chronic progressive infections. These infections may be localized or disseminated and are more common and generally more serious in severely immunocompromised and debilitated patients. Invasive *Nocardia* infections may be an important cause of death and infectious disease in immunocompromised solid organ transplant recipients. Severe infections with *Nocardia* species have also been reported in patients with human immunodeficiency virus (HIV) infection (50, 51). Recent in vitro and in vivo studies, clinical observations, and taxonomic developments indicate that antimicrobial therapy must be adjusted to the particular species of *Nocardia* present, to individual strain antimicrobial susceptibility patterns, and to the site and type of infection (4, 49).

Nocardiosis is difficult to diagnose clinically, radiologically, and histopathologically. A definitive diagnosis depends on the isolation and identification of *Nocardia* species. Making the diagnosis often involves invasive techniques and may take up to 2 or 3 weeks. Recent data derived from modern taxonomic methods have changed the taxonomy of the actinomycetes, leaving the genus *Nocardia* a relatively homogeneous taxon (13, 52). Three major pathogenic *Nocardia* species, *N. farcinica, N. nova,* and *N. pseudobrasiliensis,* were recently

characterized. *N. farcinica* and *N. nova* were separated from the *N. asteroides* complex, and *N. pseudobrasiliensis* from *N. brasiliensis,* primarily on the basis of DNA-DNA hybridization, 16S rRNA sequence analysis, antimicrobial susceptibility and biochemical profiles, and (to a lesser degree) high-performance liquid chromatography (13, 34, 42, 68, 77, 81, 82, 85, 86, 88).

Use of molecular technology for species identification and epidemiologic subtyping of the *Nocardia* species has been limited by the lack of simple and rapid assays. Rapid molecular identification and typing methods that may be useful include random amplified polymorphic DNA and a combination polymerase chain reaction–restriction fragment length polymorphism analysis (22, 74).

Nocardia microorganisms are filamentous rods that show right-angled branching both in culture and in tissues. For culture, they require aerobic conditions, but growth on blood agar may be slow, and incubation for periods longer than 48 h is usually necessary. As cultures enter the stationary phase, the filaments tend to fragment into coccobacillary forms. Although the organisms are Gram positive, many strains have a low affinity for this stain and give a faint beaded appearance with alternating positive and negative areas. Since the *Nocardia* are weakly acid fast, the most useful acid-fast stain is the modified Kinyoun method (5). The Brown-Brenn modification of Gram stain and the Gomori methenamine stain are useful in demonstrating the organisms in histopathologic preparations from tissue (11).

[1]Use of trade names and commercial sources is for identification purposes only and does not imply endorsement by the U.S. Public Health Service or the U.S. Department of Health and Human Services.

TABLE 1 • Characteristics Used to Differentiate the Medically Important *Nocardia* species[a]

Characteristic	*N. asteroides complex[b]*	*N. brasiliensis*	*N. pseudobrasiliensis*	*N. otitidiscaviarum*	*N. transvalensis*
Decomposition of					
Adenine	−	−	+	−	v
Casein	−	+	+	−	−
Hypoxanthine	−	+	+	+	+
Tyrosine	−	+	+	−	−
Xanthine	−	−	−	+	v
Acid produced from:					
Adonitol (ribitol)	−	−	−	−	+
L-Arabinose	−	−	−	v	−
i-Erythritol	−	−	−	−	+
D-Galactose	v	+	+	−	+
D-Glucose	+	+	+	+	+
i-*myo*-Inositol	−	+	+	+	v
D-Mannitol	−	+	+	v	v
L-Rhamnose	v	−	−	−	−
D-Sorbitol (D-glucitol)	−	−	−	−	v
D-Trehalose	v	+	+	v	v
Production of:					
Nitrate reductase	+	+	−	+	+
Urease	+	+	+	+	+

Data from Steingrube et al. (74) and Ruimy et al. (68).

[a] +, 90% or more of the strains are positive; v, 11 to 89% of the strains are positive; −, 10% or less of the strains are positive.

[b] The *N. asteroides* complex includes *N. nova, N. farcinica,* and *N. asteroides* sensu stricto, four unnamed taxa.

Characteristics used to separate the clinically important *Nocardia* species are listed in Table 1. Gram stain, the presence of aerial filaments, decomposition of substrates, and acid production from carbohydrates, as previously described, are used to differentiate the members of the genus *Nocardia* (5, 68, 74).

Of importance, the *N. asteroides* complex responsible for most invasive human infections has been separated into four new taxa (*N. farcinica, N. nova* and two unnamed taxa, previously included in *N. asteroides* sensu stricto) (Table 2). *N. farcinica* is particularly important to distinguish since it has increased virulence and differs in its antimicrobial susceptibility test results and its epidemiology (80). Additional tests used to separate *N. asteroides* complex isolates further as *N. farcinica, N. nova,* and *N. asteroides* sensu stricto include comparison of growth on tryptone-glucose-yeast agar at 35 and 45°C for 1 day, hydrolysis of acetamide, production of acid from L-rhamnose, arylsulfatase production, and disk-diffusion susceptibility tests using Mueller-Hinton agar and commercial disks of cefamandole (30 μg) and tobramycin (10 g) (82, 86). Additional tests used to separate *N. pseudobrasiliensis* from *N. brasiliensis* include mycolic acid patterns, decomposition of adenine, nitrate reduction, susceptibility to ciprofloxacin and/or clarithromycin, and resistance to minocycline (68, 81).

Since *Nocardia* species infections are very often sporadic, information from randomized clinical trials comparing the clinical efficacy of specific antimicrobial agents is lacking. Reports have been limited to antimicrobial susceptibility test results of clinical isolates, usually from reference laboratories, animal studies, and case summaries. Interpretation of these data may be complicated by several factors. When data are from a reference laboratory that is likely to receive referral isolates from patients who are intolerant of therapy or for whom therapy has failed, there is a potential for bias in their interpretation. Also, often it is difficult to compare in vitro susceptibility results with data reported by other investigators because of differences in methodology, e.g., lack of interlaboratory standardization of inocula (10^4 vs. 10^2 CFU/mL), use of a broth microdilution method versus agar-dilution or disk-diffusion methods, or use of different breakpoints of resistance (7, 70, 82, 85, 86). In addition, the results of some of these reported studies may vary because no distinction was made between *N. nova* and *N. asteroides* sensu stricto strains (7, 70) or between *N. brasiliensis* and *N. pseudobrasiliensis* (55, 81, 68).

Nocardia species act as facultative intracellular organisms within macrophages (2, 16), where they inhibit the fusion of phagosomes with the lysosomes. In addition, human neutrophils and monocytes have been shown not to kill these organisms (23). Therefore, for optimal therapy for these intracellular microorganisms, it may be important to choose antimicrobial agents that can penetrate the cell. However, demonstrated ability of a drug to enter cells does not guarantee activity. The microenvironment and intracellular distribution of the organisms and antimicrobial agent, and interactions between antimicrobial agent, pathogenic organism, and host cell all contribute to the therapeutic result (18).

SUSCEPTIBILITY IN VITRO AND IN VIVO

Six major classes of antimicrobial compounds are currently in clinical use: the sulfonamides, the aminoglycosides, the β-lactams (penicillins, carbapenems, and cephalosporins)

TABLE 2 • **Characteristics Used to Differentiate the Groups within the *Nocardia asteroides* Complex**[a]

Characteristic	*N. asteroides* sensu stricto				*N. farcinica*	*N. nova*
	I	II	IV	VI		
Resistance[b] to						
Amikacin (MIC,≥8 μg/mL)	−	−	+	−	−	−
Gentamicin (MIC,≥4 μg/mL)	−	+	+	−	+	±
Kanamycin (MIC,≥16 μg/mL)	−	−	+	±	+	±
Tobramycin (zone,<20 mm)	−	−	+	−	+	±
Ciprofloxacin (MIC,≥4 μg/mL)	+	−	−	+	−	+
Ampicillin (MIC,≥4 μg/mL)	±	±	NT	+	+	−
Amoxicillin–clavulanic acid (MIC,≥64/32 μg/mL)	NT	NT	NT	NT	−	+
Cefamandole (zone, <20mm)	−	−	−	−	+	−
Cefotaxime (MIC,≥64 μg/mL)	−	−	−	−	+	−
Ceftriaxone (MIC,≥64 μg/mL)	−	−	−	−	+	−
Imipenem (MIC,≥16 μg/mL)	±	NT	NT	−	±	−
Erythromycin (zone,<30 mm)	+	+	+	+	+	−
Growth at 45°C (2 days)	±	−	−	±	+	−
Hydrolysis of acetamide	−	−	−	±	+	−
Arylsulfatase production	−	−	−	−	−	±
Acid production from:						
D-Galactose	−	−	+	±	±	±
L-Rhamnose	−	±	−	±	+	−
D-Sorbitol	±	−	±	−	−	−
D-Trehalose	±	±	+	±	−	±
Specific PCR-RFLP pattern	+	+	+	+	+	+
Specific HPLC pattern	−	−	−	−	−	+

Data were previously reported by Wallace et al. (82, 85, 86) and Steingrube et al. (74).

[a] +, 90% or more of the strains are positive; −, 10% or less of the strains are positive; ±, 11 to 89% of the strains are positive; NT, not tested; PCR-RFLP, polymerase chain reaction–restriction fragment length polymorphism; HPLC, high-performance liquid chromatography.

[b] Strains were considered resistant when the MIC was equal to or greater than the breakpoint (61); strains were considered resistant when the disk-zone size was less than 20 mm (86) and less than 30 mm for erythromycin (74).

and the β-lactam/β-lactamase inhibitors, the quinolones, the macrolides, and the tetracyclines (Table 3).

Single Drug(s)

General Drug of Choice

Sulfamethoxazole inhibits bacterial synthesis of dihydrofolic acid by competing with *p*-aminobenzoic acid. Trimethoprim blocks the production of tetrahydrofolic acid from dihydrofolic acid by binding to, and reversibly inhibiting, the essential enzyme dihydrofolate reductase. Thus, trimethoprim-sulfamethoxazole (TMP-SMX) blocks two consecutive steps in the biosynthesis of nucleic acids and proteins (Table 3). Sulfamethoxazole and trimethoprim have intermediate and high intracellular penetration of human polymorphonuclear leukocytes (PMNs), respectively (25, 38) (Table 3). For trimethoprim, in particular, this may be connected to its efficacy in combination with sufamethoxazole in treating intracellular pathogens (38). Sulfonamides (or the combination TMP-SMX) are the therapy of choice for nocardiosis (28, 50, 72, 85). Certain *N. asteroides* complex isolates may be susceptible to sulfonamides or TMP-SMX, and response to treatment may be attained in 90% or more of cases if the infection is confined to pleuropneumonia (72). However, in patients with disseminated disease to the central nervous system (CNS) or with depressed cell-mediated immunity such as occurs in renal transplant recipients and HIV-in-

fected patients, several factors may complicate therapy (1, 4, 26, 32, 35, 40, 43, 44, 50, 59, 69, 73, 75, 93).

One factor is the frequent occurrence of patient intolerance or side effects with the most commonly used drug combination, TMP-SMX; this occurs in HIV-infected patients with either *Pneumocystis carinii* (35, 43) or *Nocardia* species infections (75) and in renal transplant recipients with nocardiosis (1, 93). In these patient populations, adverse reactions such as rash, fever, and neutropenia have been reported in 44 to 80% of cases (35, 43). Hepatic toxicity, reported rarely with TMP-SMX, has occurred in 20% of patients with acquired immunodeficiency syndrome (AIDS), and the probability of toxicity is further increased by its prolonged use as prophylactic therapy (35).

Another factor is resistance of the infecting microorganism to drug therapy (TMP-SMX and alternative agents or drug therapy combinations) (14, 26, 32, 44, 69, 73). In a recent review of nocardiosis in AIDS, TMP-SMX was used as therapy for 50% of patients; however, 90% of these patients were nonresponsive and died (50). The need for prolonged antimicrobial therapy (6–12 months routinely) to prevent recurrences of the infection and lifetime prophylactic therapy in AIDS patients further increases the possibility of development of drug resistance (40). In a review of 19 patients on TMP-SMX for *P. carinii* prophylaxis, 2 patients developed *Nocardia* infections (40). Also, an infection caused by a TMP-SMZ-resistant *N.*

TABLE 3 • Characteristics of Some Antimicrobial Agents Used Clinically[a]

Class and Microbial Agent (s)	Route of Administration	Drug Concentration Intracellular/ Extracellular Ratio	Mechanism of Action	Drug Interactions	Side Effects
Aminoglycosides Amikacin	Parenteral	<1 (79) and 2 to 4 after 72 h of incubation (78) in macrophages and fibroblasts	Bactericidal activity results from action on 30S ribosomal subunit to produce faulty protein synthesis	Calcium, sodium bicarbonates, β-lactams, and heparin	Nephro- and ototoxicity
β-Lactams		<1 in PMNs and macrophages after prolonged incubation (79)	Bactericidal activity results from interference with construction of bacterial cell wall by inhibition of transpeptidases responsible for catalysis of peptido-glycan cross-linking	Allopurinol, bacteriostatic antibiotics (chloramphenicol, sulfonamides, or tetracyclines) may interfere with bactericidal effect of ampicillin, and probenecid Aminoglycosides	Gastrointestinal and hypersensitivity reactions
Penicillins Ampicillin	Oral/parenteral				
Carbapenem Imipenem	Parenteral				

Cephalosporins
    Cefotaxime
    Ceftriaxone
    Cefixime
    Cefuroxime
	Parenteral
	Parenteral
	Oral
	Oral/parenteral				

β-Lactam-β-lactamase inhibitor Amoxicillin–clavulanic acid	Oral		Bactericidal activity results from the ability of clavulanic acid to inactivate a wide variety of β-lactamases by blocking the active sites of these enzymes and thus protects amoxicillin from degradation	Probenecid, allopurinol, antabuse, and ampicillin	Gastrointestinal and hypersensitivity reactions
Macrolides Erythromycin	Oral/parenteral	16 to 32 in alveolar macrophages (41) and 2 to 10 in PMNs (10)	Bactericidal activity results from inhibition of protein synthesis by binding 50S ribosomal subunit	Theophylline, digoxin, oral anticoagulants, ergotamine	Gastrointestinal irritation, transient CNS reactions, and cardiac arrhythmias
Quinolones Ciprofloxacin	Oral/parenteral	2 to 8 in macrophages and fibroblasts (10)	Bactericidal activity results from gyrase inhibition required to fold DNA strands	Theophylline, magnesium-aluminum antacids, and other cations (calcium, zinc, and iron)	Gastrointestinal, CNS, and skin/allergic reactions
Sulfonamides Sulfamethoxazole	Oral	1.7 in PMN (25)	Bacteriostatic activity results from the inhibition of the folate pathway	Thiazides, warfarin, phenytoin, and cyclosporine	Hepatoxicity, myelosuppression, and gastrointestinal, allergic skin, hematologic, neurologic, and psychiatric reactions
Trimethoprim	Oral	4.1 in PMN (25) and 9 at 37° C and 13 at 25° C (38) in PMNs			
TMP-SMX					
Tetracyclines	Oral/parenteral	7.1 in PMNs (25)	Bacteriostatic activity results from inhibition of protein synthesis		
Doxycycline	Oral/parenteral			Antacids and anticoagulant therapy	Gastrointestinal reactions and renal toxicity
Minocycline	Oral/parenteral			Bacteriostatic drugs may interfere with with bactericidal action of penicillin	Hypersensitivity reactions and i.v. minocycline may cause thrombophlebitis

Adapted from Physicians' Desk Reference (65) except where referenced.

[a] PMN, polymorphonuclear leukocytes; CNS, central nervous system; and i.v., intravenous.

nova strain was reported in a leukemic child placed on TMP-SMX prophylaxis for *P. carinii* infection (59).

A third factor is the lack of information on newer oral alternative antimicrobial agents or combinations that might improve the outcome of patients with *Nocardia* species infection. The results of our susceptibility study using a microdilutional technique in 98 patient isolates of *N. asteroides* complex, including 10 reference strains, are given in Table 4. All *N. asteroides* sensu stricto isolates were susceptible to sulfamethoxazole and to TMP-SMX. These isolates were usually susceptible to dapsone (8% resistant). *N. farcinica* isolates were usually susceptible to TMP-SMX (7% resistant), sulfamethoxazole (11%), and dapsone (14%). *N. nova* isolates were usually susceptible to TMP-SMX (11% resistant), sulfamethoxazole (11%), and dapsone (6%). In addition, the results of minimum inhibitory concentration (MIC) ranges—the MIC_{50}, and the MIC_{90} of four experimental folate pathway antagonists that were provided by Jacobus Pharmaceutical, Princeton, NJ—were consistent for each of these experimental drugs with most strains of *N. farcinica, N. nova,* and *N. asteroides* sensu stricto. WR99210 was the most active, with an MIC_{90} for *N. farcinica* strains of 0.5 µg/mL, an MIC_{90} for *N. nova* strains of 0.125 µg/mL, and an MIC_{90} for *N. asteroides* sensu stricto strains of 2 µg/mL. The prodrug of WR99210, PS-15, was slightly less active: the MIC_{90} for all three *Nocardia* species strains was 4 µg/mL. Cycloguanil and its prodrug, proguanil, showed much less activity for the three *Nocardia* species. The MIC_{90} for both *N. farcinica* and *N. asteroides* sensu stricto strains was 512 µg/mL or greater. Cycloguanil and proguanil were more active, with MIC_{90}s for *N. nova* strains of 128 µg/mL and 64 µg/mL, respectively.

Studies by Boiron and Provost (7) and Schaal et al. (70) found a high degree of resistance to TMP-SMX in *N. farcinica* strains and a lesser degree of resistance in *N. asteroides* sensu stricto strains. These discrepancies with our data may reflect differences in methodology or differences in the geographic origin of strains. Nevertheless, in general, our study results agreed with those of Wallace and colleagues in their recent evaluations of antimicrobial susceptibilities of *N. farcinica, N. nova,* and *N. asteroides* sensu stricto (82, 85, 86). However, an important exception was the increase in resistance detected in our study of *N. farcinica* and *N. nova* to sulfamethoxazole and TMP-SMX (Table 4). In a previous study, we found all isolates of *N. brasiliensis* to be susceptible to sulfamethoxazole and TMP-SMX (55). These results are in good agreement with the data of other investigators (4, 70). In contrast to *N. brasiliensis,* all *N. otitidiscaviarum* isolates in the latter studies and in a further study by Boiron and Provost were resistant to sulfamethoxazole and TMP-SMX (4, 7, 70).

Alternative Antimicrobial Agents
Aminoglycosides.   Amikacin and the most recent aminoglycosides are semisynthetic compounds designed to have potent antibacterial activity and minimal potential aminoglycoside-associated nephro- and ototoxicity (Table 3). They are bactericidal agents that inhibit bacterial protein synthesis by binding irreversibly to the bacterial 30S ribosomal subunit (Table 3). With the exception of *N. transvalensis* (53) and *N.*

asteroides sensu stricto group IV (Tables 2 and 5), all *Nocardia* species have low MICs to amikacin in vitro (1, 15, 27, 85) (Tables 4 and 5). Two new aminoglycosides, SCH 21420 and SCH 22591 (Schering Corp., Kenilworth, NJ), had low MICs to all *Nocardia* species (MIC_{90} for *N. asteroides* complex was 2–4 µg/mL and MIC_{50} for both *N. brasiliensis* and *N. otitidiscaviarum* was 1–2 µg/mL), but their minimal bactericidal concentration (MBC) values were high (44). Despite low MICs, this class of antimicrobial agents has been reported to penetrate poorly into macrophages and neutrophils (79) (Table 3). However, most of these reports were short-term (1–6 h) experiments; the incubation time may have been too short to obtain detectable intracellular levels (78). Furthermore, the intracellular:extracellular (I:E) ratio increased from less than 1 to 2 to 4 after 72-h incubation (78) (Table 3). In a mouse model study using a biochemically typical *N. asteroides* sensu stricto strain and *N. farcinica* strain, amikacin, amoxicillin-clavulanic acid, and minocycline proved therapeutically more effective than sulfadiazine (70).

β-Lactams.   The vast majority of *Nocardia* strains in our study had intermediate to high resistance to the β-lactam antimicrobial agents currently in use (Tables 4 and 5). This may be predominantly due to production of the potent β-lactamases identified in pathogenic nocardiae (47). These enzymes appear to be especially active in members of the species *N. farcinica, N. asteroides* (group VI, unnamed taxon), *N. brasiliensis,* and *N. otitidiscaviarum* (70, 83). Only 44% of *N. nova* isolates were susceptible to ampicillin (Tables 4 and 5).

All *N. farcinica* isolates were resistant to cefixime. Most isolates were resistant to cefamandole (70%), cefuroxime (64%), cefotaxime (82%), and ceftriaxone (86%) (Table 4). Although all isolates of *N. nova* were resistant to cefixime, they were usually susceptible to cefamandole (17% resistant), cefotaxime (6%), and ceftriaxone (11%). All isolates of *N. nova* were susceptible to the oral cephalosporin cefuroxime. Most *N. asteroides* sensu stricto isolates were resistant to cefixime (87%); isolates were less frequently resistant to cefamandole (29%). These isolates were usually susceptible to cefuroxime (6% resistant), cefotaxime (2%), and ceftriaxone (2%).

In another study of 12 clinical isolates of *N. asteroides,* Gutmann et al. (36) found the oral cephalosporin cefuroxime to have the best activity of the cephalosporins tested, followed by cefotaxime.

Carbapenems are a unique class of β-lactam agents with the widest spectrum of antimicrobial activity of the currently available antimicrobial agents. Structurally, they differ from other β-lactams in the unique stereochemistry of the hydroxyethyl side chain that confers stability against β-lactamases. Imipenem (*N*-formimidoyl thienamycin), a semisynthetic derivative of thienamycin, was the first carbapenem antimicrobial agent developed for clinical use. The drug is metabolized and inactivated in the kidneys by a dehydropeptidase-I (DHP-I) enzyme found in the brush borders of proximal renal tubular cells. To achieve adequate concentrations in serum and urine, a DPH-I inhibitor, cilastatin, was developed and is combined with imipenem in a 1:1 dosage ratio for clinical use (Table 3). Other members of this class currently undergoing

TABLE 4 • Antimicrobial Susceptibility of *Nocardia farcinica*, *N. nova*, and *N. asteroides* Sensu Stricto Isolates[a]

MIC (μg/mL) in Broth

Antimicrobial Agent	50%			90%			Geometric Mean[b]			Range			Breakpoint (μg/mL)[c]			% Resistant Isolates		
	Nf	Nn	Na	Nf	Nn	Na	Nf	Nn	Na	Nf	Nn	Na	Nf	Nn	Na	Nf	Nn	Na
Ampicillin	>32	4	8	>32	8	>32	49	2	6	32->32	≤0.25-16	≤0.25-16	≥4	≥4	≥4	100	56	73
Amoxicillin/ clavulanic acid	16/8	64/32	8/4	32/16	64/32	64/32	12/6	48/24	8/4	2/1-64/32	2/1-64/32	≤0.5/0.25->64/32	≥32/16	≥32/16	≥32/16	29	94	33
Cefuroxime	32	1	<1	64	4	8	30	1	2	4->64	≤1-32	≤1-32	≥32	≥32	≥32	64	0	6
Cefotaxime	64	4	2	>64	16	16	66	4	2	32->64	≤0.5-64	<0.5-64	≥64	≥64	≥64	82	6	2
Ceftriaxone	>64	4	2	>64	16	8	45	5	2	8->64	≤1-64	≤1-64	≥64	≥64	≥64	86	11	0
Cefixime	>64	64	16	>64	>64	>64	111	49	26	64->64	8->64	≤1->64	≥4	≥4	≥4	100	100	87
Imipenem	8	<0.25	2	>32	0.5	32	7	0.3	2	0.5-32	≤0.25->32	≤0.25->32	≥16	≥16	≥16	36	0	23
Amikacin	1	<0.25	<0.25	1	>0.25	1	1	0.25	0.4	≤0.25-2	≤0.25	≤0.25-4	≥64	≥64	≥64	0	0	0
Erythromycin	16	0.25	4	>16	0.5	>16	14	0.3	3	1->16	1->16	×0.13->16	≥8	≥8	≥8	86	0	40
Minocycline	2	1	1	8	4	8	2	1.6	1	0.5-16	0.25-8	0.13->16	≥16	≥16	≥16	4	0	6
Doxycycline	4	4	2	8	8	16	4	4	2	1-16	1->16	0.13->16	≥16	≥16	≥16	14	6	12
Ciprofloxacin	1	8	8	8	>8	>8	1	8	3	0.25-≥8	4->8	0.06->8	≥4	≥4	≥4	32	100	62
Rifampin	>32	2	32	>32	>32	>32	42	8	3	≤0.25->32	≤0.5->32	≤0.5->32	≥4	≥4	≥4	93	50	73
Sulfamethoxazole	8	32	4	32	8	16	7	2.3	4	≤1-128	≤1->128	≤1-32	>32	>32	>32	11	11	0
Dapsone	8	4	2	>32	8	32	8	3.5	5	1->32	≤0.5->32	≤0.5->32	>32	>32	>32	14	6	8
PS-15	4	2	2	4	4	4	2	1.8	2	≤0.063->4	0.5-4	0.5->4						
WR99210	≤0.063	≤0.063	≤0.063	0.5	0.08	2	0.2	0.08	0.2	≤0.063-2	≤0.063-4	0.063-4						
Cycloguanil	512	64	256	>512	128	>512	512	60	194	128->512	16-256	≤8->512						
Proguanil	128	32	64	512	64	>512	132	37	60	32->512	16-128	≤8->512						
Trimethoprim	4	8	4	>32	32	>32	5	7	5	1->32	1->32	≤0.5->32	≥16	≥16	≥16	82	39	2
TMP-SMX	0.5/9.55	0.06/1.19	0.25/4.8	2/38	0.5/9.5	1/19	0.5/9.5	0.17/3.2	0.22/4.18	1.19-4/76	≤0.06/1.19->8/152	1.19-1/19	>2/38	>2/38	>2/38	7	11	0

Zone of Inhibition (mm) on Disk

	Arithmetic Mean			Range			Breakpoint (mm)			% Resistant Isolates		
	Nf	Nn	Na	Nf	Nn	Na	Nf	Nn	Na	Nf	Nn	Na
Cefamandole (30 μg)	12	53	38	6-46	6-90	6-50	≤14	≤14	≤14	70	17	29
Tobramycin (10 μg)	7	24	37	6-22	6-46	6-40	≤14	≤14	≤14	96	33	25

[a] Modified from McNeil MM, Brown JM, Hutwagner LC, Schiff TA. Evaluation of therapy for *Nocardia asteroides* complex infections. Infect Dis Clin Pract 1995;4:287–292. Nf, *N. farcinica* (23 clinical isolates, five reference strains); Nn, *N. nova* (16 clinical isolates, two reference strains); Na, *N. asteroides* sensu stricto (49 clinical isolates, three reference strains).

[b] Estimated value (next highest twofold value was used when calculating geometric mean of values that were greater than the highest concentration tested).

[c] Breakpoint for resistance from National Committee for Clinical Laboratory Standards (61).

TABLE 5 • Antimicrobial Susceptibility of Two Unnamed Taxa of *Nocardia asteroides* Sensu Stricto[a]

Antimicrobial agent	MIC (μg/mL) in broth										% Resistant Isolates	
	50%		90%		Geometric Mean[b]		Range		Breakpoint (μg/mL)[c]			
	Na (I)	Na (VI)	Na (I)	Na (VI)	Na (I)	Na (VI)	Na (I)	Na (VI)	Na (I)	Na (VI)	Na (I)	Na (VI)
Ampicillin	4	32	8	>32	4	30	1–8	16–>32	≥4	≥4	86	100
Amoxicillin/clavulanic acid	4/2	32/16	16/8	64/32	3.2/1.6	20/10	≤0.5/0.25–16/8	1/0.5–>64/32	≥32/16	≥32/16	0	61
Cefuroxime	2	1	4	16	2	2	≤1–4	≤1–32	≥32	≥32	0	11
Cefotaxime	2	2	4	8	2	3	0.5–16	1–64	≥64	≥64	0	6
Ceftriaxone	≤1	2	4	8	3	3	≤1–16	≤1–64	≥64	≥64	0	6
Cefixime	64	>64	>64	>64	32	45	0.5–>64	0.5–>64	≥64	≥64	71	61
Imipenem	1	4	4	16	1	5	≤0.25–>32	≤0.25–>32	≥16	≥16	14	11
Amikacin	0.5	0.5	2	1	1	0.5	≤0.25–4	≤0.25–1	≥16	≥16	0	0
Erythromycin	>16	16	>16	>16	24	12	8–>16	2–>16	≥8	≥8	100	72
Minocycline	1	2	8	8	3	2	1–16	≤0.13–>16	≥16	≥16	14	6
Doxycycline	8	2	16	8	7	2	0.25–>8	0.13–>16	≥16	≥16	43	6
Ciprofloxacin	8	8	8	>8	4	2	0.25–>8	0.13–>8	≥4	≥4	71	83
Rifampin	>32	32	>32	>32	24	24	4–>32	0.5–>32	≥4	≥4	100	94
Sulfamethoxazole	8	4	32	16	32	5	2–>32	1–16	>32	>32	0	0
Dapsone	4	4	8	32	4	4	2–16	1–>32	≥32	≥32	0	17
PS-15	2	2	2	4	2	2	1–4	1–>4				
WR99210	0.125	0.125	2	2	0.26	0.35	≤0.063–2	≤0.063–4				
Cycloguanil	128	512	>512	>512	388	338	128–>512	8–>512				
Proguanil	64	64	128	>512	97	97	32–>512	8–>512				
Trimethoprim	8	4	16	32	9.7	6.5	2–>32	2–>32	≥16	≥16	43	33
TMP-SMX	0.5/9.5	0.25/4.80	0.5/9.5	0.5/9.5	0.15/2.80	0.2/4.4	≤0.06/1.19–1/19	≤0.06/1.19–1/19	>2/38	>2/32	0	0

	Zone of Inhibition (mm) on Disk							
	Arithmetic Mean		Range		Breakpoint (mm)			
	Na (I)	Na (VI)	Na (I)	Na (VI)	Na (I)	Na (VI)	Na (I)	Na (VI)
Cefamandole (30 μg)	35	47	0–50	0–50	≤14	≤14	57	89
Tobramycin (10 μg)	40	45	0–34	0–40	≤14	≤14	86	89

[a] Na (I) (7 clinical isolates); Na (VI) (18 clinical isolates).

[b] Estimated value (next highest twofold value was used when calculating geometric mean of values that were greater than the highest concentration tested).

[c] Breakpoint for resistance from National Committee for Clinical Laboratory Standards (61).

preclinical evaluation or clinical trials include meropenem and biapenem. These agents are thought to be resistant to the action of DPH-I without the need for a DHP-I inhibitor. Most isolates in our study were susceptible to the carbapenem imipenem, particularly, *N. nova* (100%) (Table 4). The resistance of *N. farcinica* isolates was high (36%), followed by *N. asteroides* sensu stricto resistance (23%) (Table 4). Our MIC results for *N. nova* correlated with those of a study of 22 isolates of this species, but that study found less resistance for *N. asteroides* and *N. farcinica* than in our study (90). Most isolates of *N. brasiliensis* and *N. otitidiscaviarum* have been reported resistant to imipenem (66, 90). However, *N. brasiliensis* isolates were less frequently resistant to one of the new carbapenems, meropenem, which has also been shown to have intermediate activity against *N. otitidiscaviarum* isolates (90). As with other β-lactams, the in vivo activity of imipenem may be affected by poor penetration into macrophages (Table 3).

Macrolides. The macrolides are a class of antimicrobial agents with bactericidal activity due to inhibiting bacterial protein synthesis by binding to the 50S ribosomal subunit (Table 3). However, in general, poor results were seen with these agents in our study (Table 4), despite their good penetration into phagocytes (Table 3). The isolates of *N. nova* are an exception: these isolates are always susceptible to erythromycin (82) (Table 4).

The inconsistency in results (40% resistance) between our study given in Table 4 and the results (>90% resistance) given in Table 2 for *N. asteroides* sensu stricto isolates reported in the literature may reflect different methodology (broth microdilutions vs. disk diffusion) or a different species distribution.

Quinolones. Quinolones, also called fluoroquinolones, are a group of synthetic agents related to an older synthetic agent, nalidixic acid. Norfloxacin, the first of the fluorinated compounds to be introduced, was (in contrast to nalidixic acid) bactericidal and had less ocular toxicity. Currently, in addition to norfloxacin, there are four new quinolones approved by the Food and Drug Administration for use in the United States: ciprofloxacin, ofloxacin, lomefloxacin, and enoxacin. Fleroxacin is expected to be approved in the near future. These agents have proved effective against most *N. asteroides* complex; however, the MICs of each quinolone varied greatly depending on the species (44). This variability may reflect the different permeabilities of each species to the antimicrobial agent. Most isolates of *N. nova*, *N. otitidiscaviarum*, and *N. brasiliensis* were resistant to ciprofloxacin and to experimental quinolones (6, 68, 81). However, the recently described taxon *N. pseudobrasiliensis* is susceptible to ciprofloxacin (68, 81). One experimental carboxyquinolone, PD 117558 (Warner Lambert Pharmaceutical Research, Ann Arbor, MI), was exceptional: all isolates tested (including the *N. asteroides* complex, *N. otitidiscaviarum,* and *N. brasiliensis*) were susceptible (6).

These agents can be taken orally and reach high concentrations in the bloodstream. They also have little or no associated toxicity, even when prolonged therapy is required. More and more quinolone derivatives are becoming available and each derivative has a different serum half-life. Quinolones inhibit bacterial DNA gyrase and are not subject to alteration or

degradation by plasmid-mediated mechanisms (Table 3). Quinolones can be given orally, and ciprofloxacin and the newer experimental fluoroquinolones—tosufloxacin (T-3262) (91), grepafloxacin (89), PD 117596 and PD 127391 (44), and PD 117558 (6)—may be administered parenterally. The marked intracellular penetration of ciprofloxacin, ofloxacin, and pefloxacin (I:E ratios, >8, >7, and 6.9, respectively) into the alveolar macrophages should allow effective therapy for pathogens in respiratory infections (10, 63) (Table 3).

Tetracyclines. Tetracyclines are bacteriostatic agents that inhibit bacterial protein synthesis (Table 3). These antibiotics have high PMN penetration (I:E = 7.1) (25). All isolates of *N. nova* in our study were susceptible to minocycline, and most *N. asteroides* sensu stricto and *N. farcinica* were susceptible (6 and 4% resistance, respectively) (Table 4). Our results for minocycline correlated well with data of other investigators (1, 36, 70). Minocycline resistance of the recently separated *N. pseudobrasiliensis* may have contributed to the reports in the literature of *N. brasiliensis's* resistance to this agent (81). In one study, 25% of *N. brasiliensis* isolates were resistant (55). In the 1995 Wallace study, 60% of the invasive disease isolates of *N. brasiliensis* that were resistant to minocycline were identified as *N. pseudobrasiliensis,* the new taxon (81). All isolates of *N. otitidiscaviarum* were susceptible to minocycline in studies by Schaal et al. (70) and Boiron and Provost (7).

Combination Drugs

The β-lactam/β-lactamase inhibitor combination amoxicillin–clavulanic acid presents an approach to the problem of β-lactamase-induced resistance to antibiotics. Clavulanic acid is a β-lactam that is structurally related to the penicillins and possesses the ability to inactivate a wide variety of β-lactamases by blocking the active site of the enzyme (Table 3). In our study, *N. nova* was usually resistant to amoxicillin–clavulanic acid (94%); *N. asteroides* sensu stricto and *N. farcinica* isolates were less frequently resistant (33 and 29%, respectively) (Table 4). Another species of *Nocardia, N. otitidiscaviarum,* was reported to be resistant to amoxicillin–clavulanic acid (4, 7, 70). In vitro studies assessing potential synergy with β-lactam/β-lactamase inhibitor combinations showed that 11 ampicillin-resistant strains of *N. asteroides* became susceptible to these drugs in the presence of clavulanic acid (47). Furthermore, Wallace et al. (83) showed that amoxicillin resistance in *N. brasiliensis* could be reduced in the presence of clavulanic acid. The triple combination of amoxicillin plus clavulanic acid plus amikacin was reported to be superior to each agent alone in reducing the infective burden of microorganisms in tissue in vivo in a murine model (70). However, the organisms studied were other members of the *N. asteroides* complex and did not include *N. nova* or *N. otitidiscaviarum.*

ANTIMICROBIAL THERAPY
General Drug of Choice

Sulfonamides (with or without trimethoprim) have been the mainstay of antimicrobial therapy for human nocardiosis. TMP-SMX is frequently used for this infection; however, this usage may not be as much related to properties of synergism or better efficacy than sulfonamide treatment alone as to favorable pharmacokinetics (effective penetration of cerebrospinal fluid (CSF)) and general familiarity among clinicians. For most patients with nocardiosis, clinical improvement is expected within 7 to 10 days after initiation of empirical therapy with sulfonamides (with or without trimethoprim). The route of drug administration for infected patients may be influenced by their overall clinical status. In addition, a serum level estimation at least once following institution of antimicrobial therapy may be useful to confirm adequate drug absorption and to provide a basis for any necessary dosage adjustment to achieve the recommended levels in blood of 100 to 150 μg/mL approximately 2 h after an oral dose. It is recommended that therapy with sulfonamides be given at a high dose (3–6 g/day) for extended periods (6–12 months). While primary cutaneous nocardiosis may be cured by a 1- to 3-month course of antimicrobial therapy and uncomplicated pulmonary nocardiosis may respond to therapy for 6 months or less, therapy for 12 months or more is usually required for disseminated infection or when the patient is immunocompromised. In addition, HIV-infected patients should receive long-term maintenance suppressive therapy. Also, in organ transplant patients treated with the commonly used antirejection medication cyclosporine, TMP-SMX may cause reversible cyclosporine-induced nephrotoxicity (Table 3).

Special Situations

Endocarditis

Ertl et al. (21) described three patients with aortic valve prostheses who developed nocardial endocarditis. Two of these patients died before specific antimicrobial therapy could be instituted. In the third patient, the successful outcome was attributed to the combination of the following: the causative agent *N. farcinica* was identified early; abscesses did not occur in vital organs; an effective bactericidal antibiotic regimen was instituted; and the infected aortic valve prosthesis was surgically replaced (21). After receipt of a prosthetic heart valve, this patient was slow to recover and developed intermittent fever that did not respond to treatment with cefadroxil, amoxicillin, mezlocillin, or tobramycin. After the isolate was identified as *N. farcinica,* the treatment was changed to oral sulfadiazine (12 g/day), which produced unacceptable gastrointestinal side effects. Intravenous treatment was started with amikacin (250 mg, 2–4 times/day) and a combination of 5 g of amoxicillin plus 5 g of clavulanic acid every 8 h. This combination only temporarily reduced the patient's fever and leukocyte counts. Therapy was then changed to intravenous imipenem (1.5 g) and amikacin (500 mg) every 6 h to maintain serum bactericidal concentrations, which were monitored during therapy. With this treatment, the patient recovered quickly and was discharged without further antibiotic therapy. Three months later, the patient was readmitted, and blood cultures were again positive for *N. farcinica* that was still susceptible to imipenem and amikacin. These antimicrobial agents were reinstituted, and the patient's aortic valve was surgically replaced. Postoperatively, the patient recovered quickly without fever or an elevated erythrocyte sedimentation rate (21). Results from in vitro and in vivo experiments as well as the results in this case suggest that treatment of human nocardial endocarditis can be improved by the combination of a β-lactam compound (e.g., imipenem) and amikacin (70).

Meningitis

Nocardiae have a specific predilection for invading the CNS (4). Dissemination to the CNS is noted in 25% of reported cases of nocardial infections (3). Brain abscess is the most common clinical manifestation of CNS infection, and although CSF culture has been positive in up to 20% of these cases, meningitis itself is considered uncommon (8). In 1991, Bross and Gordon (8) reviewed 28 cases that fulfilled at least one the following criteria for meningitis: isolation of *Nocardia* species from CSF or meningeal cultures; concurrent culture-positive extrameningeal nocardial infection with histopathologic evidence of meningitis at autopsy and no evidence of another infectious etiology; and concurrent culture-positive extrameningeal nocardial infection with two of the following signs suggesting meningitis: head/neck pain, lethargy/confusion, and stiff neck.

The typical findings in CSF studies were increased leukocytes (83% of cases, >500 leukocytes/mm^3) with a predominance of neutrophils; hypoglycorrhachia (64%, <40 mg glucose/dL); and elevated protein level (61%, >100 mg/dL). In this review the authors cited the following difficulties in establishing the etiologic agent as a *Nocardia* species: Gram stains of CSF are often negative and cultures are discarded prematurely or may demonstrate growth too late to be clinically useful (8). Eighteen of 21 (86%) culture-positive nocardial meningitis cases in this series were caused by *N. asteroides* complex, 2 were due to *N. brasiliensis,* and 1 was due to *N. otitidiscaviarum.* All survivors were treated with some form of sulfonamide except one patient who received minocycline, and there was no difference noted with respect to the infecting species. Further, as noted by these authors, the utility of using large volumes of CSF or concentration techniques to enhance the yield of *Nocardia* species from CNS has not been well studied.

Most in vitro susceptibility studies have suggested that sulfonamides, minocycline, amikacin, imipenem, and the quinolones are the most active agents. Combination testing has revealed synergy of TMP and SMX, and this combination appears to penetrate the blood-CSF barrier and achieve high CSF concentrations (76). Another study suggested that antimicrobial combinations should include at least one of the cephalosporins or ciprofloxacin (64). Several cephalosporins reach the CSF in concentrations adequate to inhibit *Nocardia* in vitro, but cefuroxime appears to be the most active (76). Although amikacin may be active in vitro against most *Nocardia* species, it penetrates the blood-CSF barrier poorly; therefore, it is sometimes necessary to administer this agent directly into CSF (76). Other authors have suggested that use of a combination of a cell wall–active agent plus amikacin might yield a bactericidal synergism that would enhance intracellular uptake of amikacin (20).

Alternative Therapy

There is scant information concerning the effectiveness of newer oral alternative antimicrobial agents or combinations of antimicrobial agents that might improve the outcome of *Nocardia*-infected patients. Alternative oral drug therapy for *Nocardia* infections may include the cephalosporins cefixime and cefuroxime or dapsone; these may potentially avoid some of the problems incurred by TMP-SMX. Dapsone, a long-acting oral sulfone, is known to be therapeutic for human *Mycobacterium leprae* infections, and recently, its effectiveness in the treatment and prophylaxis of *P. carinii* pneumonia has been reported (56). In addition, efficacy of dapsone in treating chronic nocardial mycetoma infections has been reported (39). Thus, dapsone may be potentially useful in the therapy of other *Nocardia* species infections. Its mechanism of action is identical to that of the sulfonamides. Although there is considerable clinical trial experience with this drug in the treatment of human leprosy with respect to the occurrence and severity of clinical side effects, to our knowledge, ours are the only in vitro antimicrobial susceptibility data that may assist in predicting its potential effectiveness for the therapy of *Nocardia* species infections (Tables 4 and 5).

Four promising folate pathway antagonists have been evaluated for the therapy of other infections: cycloguanil chloride, WR99210 (a triazine inhibitor of dihydrofolate reductase) and their respective prodrugs, proguanil, and PS-15 (9, 33). PS-15, the biguanide precursor of WR99210, was designed and synthesized to circumvent the adverse gastrointestinal symptoms and poor absorption found in clinical pharmacologic trials of WR99210 in humans. Analysis of plasma drug concentrations by high-performance liquid chromatography showed that monkeys converted PS-15 into its active metabolite WR99210 (19). If these drugs with suggested in vitro activity demonstrate in vivo activity against *Nocardia* species isolates, they could represent new alternative therapy for patients with these infections.

Clinical experience shows that aminoglycosides are both efficacious and safe when used and monitored conventionally. The conventional amikacin dosage regimen (7.5 mg/kg every 12 h) should be adjusted so that the peak serum levels (determined on samples drawn 60 min after the start of a 30- to 60-min infusion) are high enough to be bactericidal, and trough levels (on samples drawn within 30 min of the next dose) are low enough to avoid toxicity. The safety and efficacy of conventional aminoglycoside dosing regimens have been proven in clinical trials. The newer approach of a single daily dosage has many theoretical benefits including improved efficacy, decreased toxicity, and pharmacoeconomic advantages. However, there is limited experience with once-daily dosage of aminoglycosides in patients with normal renal function and even less experience in those with impaired function. Issues regarding dosing, combination therapy, and proper monitoring for efficacy and toxicity need to be evaluated in clinical trials (17). Serum aminoglycoside levels in patients with impaired renal function must be monitored to provide adequate therapy and reduce toxicity. Specifically, the status of the patient's renal function should be estimated by measuring the serum creatinine concentration or calculating the endogenous creatinine clearance rate (24).

The first successful use of surgical debridement followed by amikacin in the treatment of nocardiosis was in 1980 in a renal transplant recipient (93). Other favorable treatment outcomes were reported with amikacin and surgical drainage or debridement in a patient with a pancreatic *N. asteroides* abscess and in a patient with primary cutaneous *N. farcinica* infection (57, 71).

Only rarely have nocardial infections been treated with macrolides, possibly because of the lack of availability of antimicrobial susceptibility studies and species identification in the past. The value of antimicrobial susceptibility studies and species identification was recently illustrated in a cardiac transplant recipient with pneumonia caused by *N. nova*. When TMP-SMX was not tolerated, the patient was treated successfully with the macrolide clarithromycin (60).

Rarely have the quinolones been used for therapy for nocardiosis. Only two patients with *N. asteroides* sternotomy infection have reportedly been treated successfully with ofloxacin (92). In addition, ciprofloxacin (to which the patient's isolate showed only intermediate susceptibility in vitro) was administered late and unsuccessfully to a renal transplant patient with disseminated *N. farcinica* infection to the brain; amikacin had been avoided for this patient because of the risk of associated nephrotoxicity (58).

In our study, minocycline showed in vitro activity comparable to that of folate pathway antagonists. Also, minocycline was as effective as sulfonamides in eliminating a large inoculum of *N. asteroides* from mice after intraperitoneal injection of a suspension in mucin (1). On the other hand, in a mouse model of cerebral nocardiosis, minocycline did not eradicate intracerebral microorganisms, and its effects were no different from those of the saline control (32). Despite these in vivo results, there is adequate support in the literature for using minocycline to treat cerebral infection effectively on the basis of the drug's excellent in vitro activity (45, 46, 87). For example, although the diagnosis in a case of cerebral *Nocardia asteroides* infection in an AIDS patient was presumptive, a computed tomographic (CT) scan of the brain showed a right frontal lobe abscess that progressed to involve the right parietal lobe. With this progression, the previous treatment (sulfadiazine 1.5 g every 6 h and intravenous imipenem 500 mg every 6 h) was discontinued, and oral minocycline (200 mg every 12 h) was increased to 300 mg in combination with intravenous ceftriaxone (2 g every 12 h), an antimicrobial agent that is likely to achieve adequate CSF concentrations (45, 46). After 5 weeks of therapy with minocycline and ceftriaxone, the patient's brain lesions almost completely resolved, as evidenced by CT scan (46). This case suggests that in a patient with AIDS and a presumptive nocardial cerebral infection, antibiotic treatment alone was successful without surgical intervention.

Since all reported isolates of *N. otitidiscaviarum* have been susceptible to minocycline, some authors recommend that optimal therapy for these infections should include the combination of minocycline with an aminoglycoside demonstrated to have a low MIC, such as amikacin and kanamycin (4). However, like the folate pathway antagonists, minocycline is bacteriostatic, and prolonged therapy may be associated with toxicity.

Combination Therapy

Generally, a combination of two or more antimicrobial agents is selected to achieve one or more of the following goals: to attain the broadest possible spectrum of activity for empirical therapy of potentially infected persons; to minimize drug toxicity by using relatively low doses of two or more agents with additive efficacies but independent toxicities; to minimize emergence of strains resistant to a single agent; and to exploit the possibility of synergistic inhibitory or bactericidal activities (20).

Different combinations of amikacin with ceftriaxone, erythromycin, sulfisoxazole, imipenem, cefotaxime, and clarithromycin were clinically efficacious in three bone marrow recipients. Isolates from two of these patients were identified as *N. nova;* the third, as *N. asteroides* sensu stricto (12). Favorable clinical outcomes with the combination of imipenem and amikacin were reported for a patient with nocardial endocarditis of an aortic valve prosthesis, caused by *N. farcinica* (21), and for a patient with primary cutaneous *N. farcinica* infection following heart transplantation (67). In addition, combining amikacin with imipenem and surgical excision resulted in a successful clinical outcome in a patient with cerebral nocardiosis (48). In another study, seven of eight patients with disseminated nocardiosis were treated with amikacin in combination with other effective antimicrobial agents for 2 to 12 months (26). These patients received drug combinations that included cefuroxime (2 patients), cefuroxime and TMP-SMX (2 patients), cefuroxime plus the amoxicillin–clavulanic acid combination (2 patients), and TMP-SMX plus minocycline (1 patient). All patients were considered cured at follow-up after 2 years. Because of good in vitro and in vivo responses and confirmation of the clinical usefulness of imipenem, amoxicillin–clavulanic acid, and amikacin in patients, the combination of either imipenem or amoxicillin–clavulanic acid together with amikacin may become the antibiotic choice for management of human nocardiosis (30, 31, 70).

In other experimental studies that used antimicrobial combinations that demonstrated synergy in vitro, the combinations of amikacin and either imipenem or amoxicillin–clavulanic acid, or cefotaxime and either amikacin or imipenem, were found to be efficacious (4, 29, 32, 70). In a study of CNS nocardiosis in a murine model, these combinations were shown to be statistically superior to single-agent therapy (30). However, despite their efficacy in vitro and in vivo, the above combinations of antimicrobial agents require parenteral administration and are limited by the effects of long-term toxicity with amikacin (84). However, amikacin and imipenem have bactericidal activity, in contrast to the bacteriostatic activity of the sulfonamides. In addition, the weak in vivo activity of sulfonamides may help explain treatment failures with these drugs and the recommendation for long-term, high-dosage therapy.

ENDPOINTS FOR MONITORING THERAPY
General

Clinical improvement is the best and most comprehensive guide to the adequacy of therapy; however, it is often difficult to monitor objectively. For infections requiring long-term therapy, such as endocarditis, clinical improvements may also be prolonged. Close monitoring of serum antibiotic levels may be extremely useful clinically. In addition, maintaining the antibiotic level at the site of infection above the in vitro MIC of the organism is vitally important, particularly when host defenses are reduced or absent. The primary reason for serum drug level monitoring is to attain therapeutic levels quickly but not exceed them. Nephrotoxicity may be associated with prolonged treatment with amikacin, and ototoxicity is associated with both total cumulative dose and prolonged treatment (62).

Pulmonary Disease

In pulmonary nocardiosis, the chest radiograph typically shows some consolidation, multiple nodular lesions, and cavitation or abscesses over both lung fields. A CT scan of the lungs may show abscess formation and other important features earlier than the plain chest radiograph. Philpott-Howard (64) found that patients who received appropriate antimicrobial agents and improved clinically may yield *Nocardia* in their sputum for the first 2 to 3 weeks of therapy, which suggests that sputum cultures may not be useful for monitoring early response to therapy in these patients.

Central Nervous System Disease

In most cases of cerebral nocardiosis, the antimicrobial agents given initially intravenously for 5 to 7 days were then continued orally for a total of 8 to 10 weeks or longer until abscesses were resolved on CT scan (64). In a series of three patients with brain abscesses who were receiving immunosuppressive therapy at the time of diagnosis of nocardial infection, the abscess was accurately located by CT scans, but CT-guided sterotactic aspiration was required for diagnosis and treatment (37). In two of these patients, the authors attributed their clinical success to early abscess evacuation and prolonged antibiotic therapy. Patient response to therapy was satisfactorily monitored by CT scan.

Studies for routine monitoring of CSF infections should include CSF leukocyte count, glucose and protein levels, and results of smears and culture (8).

CONTROVERSIES, CAVEATS, OR COMMENTS

Although the results of animal studies are usually thought to be more relevant clinically than in vitro data, it is difficult to compare data between animal studies because of differences in dosage and route of inoculation (4, 32, 70). Beaman et al. (4) recently reported an experimental murine nocardiosis model that has provided data for evaluating various antimicrobial agents as treatments for this infection (see above). Colony counts of *N. asteroides* in various target organs, assessed over time, provide quantitative endpoints for assessing both the comparative bactericidal efficacy of these agents and the timing of bactericidal activity. Results from this animal model show that imipenem and amikacin are superior to other antimicrobial agents, including TMP-SMX (29, 30, 31, 70); this finding has also been supported by clinical observations of infected persons (70).

Our study found that despite interspecies differences in antimicrobial susceptibility, the folate pathway antagonists, sulfamethoxazole, TMP-SMX, dapsone, amikacin, minocycline, and amoxicillin–clavulanic acid may all be effective in patients with *Nocardia* species infections. The experimental folate pathway antagonist WR99210 has excellent in vitro activity against all strains of *N. farcinica, N. nova,* and *N. asteroides* sensu stricto. Thus, this agent, via its prodrug PS-15, may offer a desirable alternative therapy for multidrug-resistant *N. farcinica* infections. Moreover, in vitro studies with the experimental carboxyquinolone PD 117558 suggest that this drug may be effective against *N. asteroides* complex, *N. brasiliensis,* and *N. otitidiscaviarum* (6). Furthermore, meropenem, because of its in vitro activity against *N. brasiliensis* and *N. otitidiscaviarum,* may also be an effective carbapenem for treatment of these infections (90).

Although in vitro activity does not always correlate with clinical response, these data may aid in formulating new recommendations for the treatment of clinical infections. Because of good in vitro and in vivo responses and the confirmation of clinical usefulness in patients, a combination of either imipenem or amoxicillin–clavulanic acid together with amikacin has great potential for becoming the antibiotic choice for management of human nocardiosis (30, 31, 70). However, before alternative drugs—such as dapsone and WR99210 via PS-15, and the carboxyquinolone PD 117558—and combination of either imipenem or amoxicillin–clavulanic acid with amikacin can be recommended as therapy for *Nocardia* spp. infections (e.g., in HIV-infected patients who do not tolerate sulfonamides), their efficacy and potential toxicity should ideally be evaluated in controlled clinical trials.

If a patient remains febrile during antimicrobial therapy, it is important to consider various factors, such as treatment failure, drug fever, a sequestered abscess (which may require surgical drainage), and a coexistent or secondary opportunistic infection with another pathogen.

REFERENCES

1. Bach MC, Gold O, Finland M. Activity of minocycline against *Nocardia asteroides:* comparison with tetracycline in agar-dilution and standard disc-diffusion tests and with sulfadiazine in an experimental infection of mice. J Lab Clin Med 1973;81:787–793.
2. Beaman BL. Interaction of *Nocardia asteroides* at different phases of growth with in vitro-maintained macrophages obtained from lungs of normal and immunized rabbits. Infect Immun 1979;26:355–361.
3. Beaman BL, Beaman L. *Nocardia* species: host-parasite relationships. Clin Microbiol Rev 1994;7:213–264.
4. Beaman BL, Boiron P, Beaman L, Brownell GH, Schaal K, Gombert ME. *Nocardia* and nocardiosis. J Med Vet Mycol 1992;30:317–331.
5. Berd D. Laboratory identification of clinically important aerobic actinomycetes. Appl Microbiol 1973;25:665–681.
6. Berkey P, Moore D, Rolston K. In vitro susceptibilities of *Nocardia* species to newer antimicrobial agents. Antimicrob Agents Chemother 1988;32:1078–1079.
7. Boiron P, Provost F. In-vitro susceptibility testing of *Nocardia* spp. and its taxonomic implication. J Antimicrob Chemother 1988;22:623–629.
8. Bross JE, Gordon G. Nocardial meningitis: case report and review. Rev Infect Dis 1991;13:160–165.
9. Canfield CJ, Milhous WK, Ager AL, Rossan RN, Sweeney TR, Lewis NJ, Jacobus DP. PS-15: a potent, orally active antimalarial from a new class of folic acid antagonists. Am J Trop Med Hyg 1993;49:121–126.
10. Carlier MB, Scorneaux B, Jenebergh A, Tulkens PM. Uptake and subcellular distribution of 4-quinolones in phagocytes [Abstract 622]. Proceedings of the 27th Interscience Conference on Antimicrobial Agents Chemotherapy, Washington, 1987.
11. Chandler FW, Kaplan W, Ajello L. A color atlas and textbook of histopathology of mycotic diseases. London: Wolfe Medical Publications, 1980:333.
12. Choucino C, Goodman SA, Greer JP, Stein RS, Wolff SN, Dummer JS. Nocardial infection in bone marrow transplant recipients. Clin Infect Dis 1996;23:1012–1019.
13. Chun J, Goodfellow M. A phylogenetic analysis of the genus *Nocardia* with 16S rRNA gene sequences. Int J Syst Bacteriol 1995;45:240–245.
14. Cockerill FR, Edson RS, Roberts GD, Waldorf JC. Trimethoprim/sulfamethoxazole-resistant *Nocardia asteroides* causing hepatic abscesses. Am J Med 1984;77:558–560.
15. Dalovisio JR, Pankey GA. In vitro susceptibility of *Nocardia asteroides* to amikacin. Antimicrob Agents Chemother 1978;3:1–8.
16. Davis-Scibiensky C, Beaman BL. Interaction of *Nocardia asteroides* with rabbit alveolar macrophages: association of virulence, viability, ultrastructural damage and phagosome-lysosome fusion. Infect Immun 1980;28:610–619.
17. Dew RB III, Susla GM. Once-daily aminoglycoside treatment. Infect Dis Clin Pract 1996;5:12–24.
18. Donowitz GR. Tissue directed antibiotics and intracellular parasites: complex interaction of phagocytes, pathogens, and drugs. Clin Infect Dis 1994;19:926–930.
19. Edstein MD, Corcoran KD, Shanks GD, Ngampochjana M, Hansukjariya P, Sattabongkot J, Webster HK, Rieckmann KH. Evaluation of WR250417 (a proguanil analog) for causal prophylactic activity in the *Plasmodium cynomolgi-Macaca mulatta* model. Am J Trop Med Hyg 1994;50:181–186.
20. Eliopoulos GM, Eliopoulos CT. Antibiotic combinations: should they be tested? Clin Microbiol Rev 1988;1:139–156.
21. Ertl G, Schaal KP, Kochsiek K. Nocardial endocarditis of an aortic prosthesis. Br Heart J 1987;57:384–386.
22. Exmelin L, Malbruny B, Vergnaud M, Provost F, Boiron P, Morel C. Molecular study of nosocomial nocardiosis outbreak involving heart transplant recipients. J Clin Microbiol 1996;34:1014–1016.
23. Filice GA, Beaman BL, Krick JA, Remington JS. Effect of human neutrophils and monocytes on *Nocardia asteroides:* failure of killing despite occurrence of the oxidative metabolic burst. J Infect Dis 1980;142:432–438.
24. Gilbert DN, Bennett WM. Use of antimicrobial agents in renal failure. In: Moellering RC, Kaye D, eds. Antibacterial agents: pharmacodynamics, pharmacology, new agents. Infect Dis Clin North Am 1989;3:517–531
25. Gmunder FK, Seger RA. Chronic granulomatous disease: mode of action of sulfamethoxazole/trimethoprim. Pediatr Res 1981;15:1533–1537.
26. Goldstein FW, Hautefort B, Acar JF. Amikacin-containing regimens for treatment of nocardiosis in immunocompromised patients. Eur J Clin Microbiol 1987;6:198–200.
27. Gombert ME. Susceptibility of *Nocardia asteroides* to various antibiotics, including newer beta lactams, trimethoprim-sulfamethoxazole, amikacin, and N-formimidoyl thienamycin. Antimicrob Agents Chemother 1982;21:1011–1012.

28. Gombert ME. Antimicrobial management of *Nocardia asteroides* infection. Infect Med 1994;11:448–452.
29. Gombert ME, Aulicino TM. Synergism of imipenem and amikacin in combination with other antibiotics against *Nocardia asteroides*. Antimicrob Agents Chemother 1983;24:810–811.
30. Gombert ME, Aulicino TM, duBouchet L, Silverman GE, Sheinbaum WM. Therapy of experimental cerebral nocardiosis with imipenem, amikacin, trimethoprim-sulfamethoxazole, and minocycline. Antimicrob Agents Chemother 1986;30:270–273.
31. Gombert ME, Berkowitz LB, Aulicino TM, duBouchet L. Therapy of pulmonary nocardiosis immunocompromised mice. Antimicrob Agents Chemother 1990;34:1766–1768.
32. Gombert ME, duBouchet L, Aulicino TM, Berkowitz LB. Antimicrobial synergism in the therapy of experimental cerebral nocardiosis. J Antimicrob Chemother 1989;24:39–43.
33. Gonzalez AH, Berlin OGW, Bruckner DA. In-vitro activity of dapsone and two potentiators against *Mycobacterium avium* complex. J Antimicrob Chemother 1989;24:19–22.
34. Goodfellow M, Orchard VA. Antibiotic sensitivity of some nocardioform bacteria and its value as a criterion for taxonomy. J Gen Microbiol 1974;83:375–387.
35. Gordin FM, Simon GL, Wofsy CB, Mills J. Adverse reactions to trimethoprim-sulfamethoxazole in patients with the acquired immune deficiency syndrome. Ann Intern Med 1984;100:495–499.
36. Gutmann L, Goldstein FW, Kitzis MD, Hautefort B, Darmon C, Acar JF. Susceptibility of *Nocardia asteroides* to 46 antibiotics, including 22 β-lactams. Antimicrob Agents Chemother 1983; 23:248–251.
37. Hall WA, Martinez J, Dummer S, Lunsford LD. Nocardial brain abscess: diagnostic and therapeutic use of stereotactic aspiration. Surg Neurol 1987;28:114–118.
38. Hand WL, King-Thompson NL, Holman JW. Entry of roxithromycin (RU 965), imipenem, cefotaxime, trimethoprim, and metronidazole into human polymorphonuclear leukocytes. Antimicrob Agents Chemother 1987;31:1553–1557.
39. Hay RJ, Mahgoub ES, Leon G, Al-Sogair S, Welsh O. Mycetoma. J Med Vet Mycol 1992;30:41–49.
40. Javaly K, Horowitz HW, Wormser GP. Nocardiosis in patients with human immunodeficiency virus infection. Medicine 1992; 71:128–138.
41. Johnson JD, Hand WL, Francis JB, King-Thompson N, Corwin RW. Antibiotic uptake by alveolar macrophages. J Lab Clin Med 1980;95:429–439.
42. Kampfer P, Dott W, Kroppenstedt RM. Numerical classification and identification of some nocardioform bacteria. J Gen Appl Microbiol 1990;36:309–331.
43. Kelly JW, Dooley DP, Lattuada CP, Smith CE. A severe, unusual reaction to trimethoprim-sulfamethoxazole in patients with immunodeficiency virus. Clin Infect Dis 1992;14:1034–1039.
44. Khardori N, Shawar R, Gupta R, Rosenbaum B, Rolston K. In vitro antimicrobial susceptibilities of *Nocardia* species. Antimicrob Agents Chemother 1993;37:882–884.
45. Kim J, Minamoto GY, Grieco MH. Nocardial infection as a complication of AIDS: report of six cases and review. Rev Infect Dis 1991;13:624–629.
46. Kim J, Minamoto GY, Hoy CD, Grieco MH. Presumptive cerebral *Nocardia asteroides* infection in AIDS: treatment with ceftriaxone and minocycline. Am J Med 1991;90:656–658.
47. Kitzis MD, Gutmann L, Acar JF. In vitro susceptibility of *Nocardia asteroides* to 21 β-lactam antibiotics, in combination with three β-lactamase inhibitors, and its relationship to the β-lactamase content. J Antimicrob Chemother 1985;15:23–30.
48. Krone A, Schaal KP, Brawanski A, Schuknecht B. Nocardial cerebral abscess cured with imipenem/amikacin and enucleation. Neurosurg Rev 1989;12:333–340.
49. Lerner PL. Nocardiosis. Clin Infect Dis 1996;22:891–905.
50. Long PF. A retrospective study of *Nocardia* infections associated with the acquired immune deficiency syndrome (AIDS). Infection 1994;22:362–364.
51. Lucas SB, Hounnou A, Peacock C, Beaumel A, Kadio A, De Cock KM. Nocardiosis in HIV-positive patients: an autopsy study in West Africa. Tuber Lung Dis 1994;75:301–307.
52. McNeil MM, Brown JM. The medically important aerobic actinomycetes: epidemiology and microbiology. Clin Microbiol Rev 1994;7:357–417.
53. McNeil MM, Brown JM, Georghiou PR, Allworth AM, Blacklock ZM. Infections due to *Nocardia transvalensis:* clinical spectrum and antimicrobial therapy. Clin Infect Dis 1992;15: 453–463.
54. McNeil MM, Brown JM, Hutwagner LC, Schiff TA. Evaluation of therapy for *Nocardia asteroides* complex infections. Infect Dis Clin Pract 1995;4:287–292.
55. McNeil MM, Brown JM, Jarvis WR, Ajello L. Comparison of species distribution and antimicrobial susceptibility of aerobic actinomycetes from clinical specimens. Rev Infect Dis 1990;12: 778–783.
56. Medina I, Mills J, Leoung G, Hopewell PC, Lee B, Modin G, Benowitz N, Wofsy CB. Oral therapy for *Pneumocystis carinii* pneumonia in the acquired immunodeficiency syndrome. N Engl J Med 1990;323:776–882.
57. Meier B, Metzer U, Muller F, Sigenthaler W, Luthy R. Successful treatment of pancreatic *Nocardia asteroides* abscess with amikacin and surgical drainage. Antimicrob Agents Chemother 1986;29:150–151.
58. Miksits K, Stoltenberg G, Neumayer HH, Spiegel H, Schaal KP, Cervos-Navarro J, Distler A, Stein H, Hahn H. Disseminated infection of the central nervous system caused by *Nocardia farcinica*. Nephrol Dial Transplant 1991;6:209–214.
59. Miron D, Dennehy PH, Josephson SL, Forman EN. Catheter-associated bacteremia with *Nocardia nova* with secondary pulmonary involvement. Pediatr Infect Dis J 1994;13:416–417.
60. Monteforte JS, Wood CA. Pneumonia caused by *Nocardia nova* and *Aspergillus fumigatus* after cardiac transplantation. Eur J Clin Microbiol Infect Dis 1993;12:112–114.
61. National Committee for Clinical Laboratory Standards. Methods for dilution antimicrobial susceptibility tests for bacteria that grow aerobically (M7-A2) 1990. Villanova, PA: National Committee for Clinical Laboratory Standards, 1990.
62. Parker S, Davey PG. Practicalities of once-daily aminoglycoside dosing. J Antimicrob Chemother 1993;31:4–8.
63. Perea EJ. Ofloxacin concentrations in tissues involved in respiratory tract infections. J Antimicrob Chemother 1990;26:55–60.
64. Philpott-Howard J. Update on human nocardiosis. Rev Med Microbiol 1993;4:207–214.
65. Physicians' desk reference. 51st ed. Montvale, NJ: Medical Economics Company, 1997.
66. Poonwan N, Kusum M, Mikami Y, Yazawa K, Tanaka Y, Genoi T. Pathogenic *Nocardia* isolated from clinical specimens including those of AIDS patients in Thailand. Eur J Epidemiol 1995;11:507–512.
67. Rees W, Schuler S, Hummel M, Hempel S, Moller J, Hetzer R. Primary cutaneous *Nocardia farcinica* infection after heart transplantation: a case report. J Thorac Cardiovasc Surg 1995; 109: 181–183.

68. Ruimy R, Riegel P, Carlotti A, Boiron P, Bernardin G, Monteil H, Wallace RJ Jr, Christen R. *Nocardia pseudobrasiliensis* sp. nov., a new species of *Nocardia* which groups bacterial strains previously identified as *Nocardia brasiliensis* and associated with invasive diseases. Int J Syst Bacteriol 1996;46:259–264.

69. Schaal KP, Lee HJ. Actinomycete infection in humans—a review. Gene 1992;115;201–211.

70. Schaal KP, Schutt-Gerowitt H, Goldmann A. In vitro and in vivo studies on the efficacy of various antimicrobial agents in the treatment of human nocardiosis. In: Szabo G, Biro S, Goodfellow M. eds. Biological, biochemical, and biomedical aspects of actinomycetes, part B. Budapest: Akademiai Kiado, 1986:619–633.

71. Schiff TA, McNeil MM, Brown JM. Cutaneous *Nocardia farcinica* infection in a nonimmunocompromised patient: case report and review. Clin Infect Dis 1993;16:756–760.

72. Smego RD, Moeller MB, Gallis HA. Trimethoprim-sulfamethoxazole therapy for *Nocardia* infections. Arch Intern Med 1983;143:711–717.

73. Stamm AM, McFall DW, Dismukes WE. Failure of sulfonamides and trimethoprim in the treatment of nocardiosis. Arch Intern Med 1983;143;383–385.

74. Steingrube VA, Brown BA, Gibson JL, Wilson RW, Brown J, Blacklock Z, Jost K, Locke S, Ulrich RF, Wallace RJ Jr. DNA amplification and restriction endonuclease analysis for differentiation of 12 species and taxa within the *Nocardia asteroides* complex and taxa of *Nocardia,* including recognition of four new taxa within the *Nocardia asteroides* complex. J Clin Microbiol 1995;33:3096–3101.

75. Telzak EE, Hii J, Polsky B, Kiehn TE, Armstrong D. *Nocardia* infection in the acquired immunodeficiency syndrome. Diagn Microbiol Infect Dis 1989;12:517–519.

76. Thea D, Barza M. Use of antibacterial agents in infections of the central nervous system. Infect Dis Clin North Am 1989;3: 553–570.

77. Tsukamura M. Numerical taxonomy of the genus *Nocardia*. J Gen Microbiol 1969;56:265–287.

78. Tulkens PM. Intracellular distribution and activity of antibiotics. Eur J Clin Microbiol Infect Dis 1991;10:100–106.

79. van den Broek PJ. Antimicrobial drugs, microorganisms and phagocytes. Rev Infect Dis 1989;11:213–245.

80. Wallace RJ Jr, Brown BA, Brown JM, McNeil MM. Taxonomy of *Nocardia* Species [Letter]. Clin Infect Dis 1994;18:476.

81. Wallace RJ Jr, Brown BA, Blacklock Z, Ulrich R, Jost K, Brown JM, McNeil MM, Onyi G, Steingrube VA, Gibson J. New *Nocardia* taxon among isolates of *Nocardia brasiliensis* associated with invasive disease. J Clin Microbiol 1995;33:1528–1533.

82. Wallace RJ Jr, Brown BA, Tsukamura M, Brown JM, Onyi GO. Clinical and laboratory features of *Nocardia nova*. J Clin Microbiol 1991;29:2407–2411.

83. Wallace RJ Jr, Nash DR, Johnson WK, Steele LC, Steingrube VA. B-Lactam resistance in *Nocardia brasiliensis* is mediated by B-lactamase and reversed in the presence of clavulanic acid. J Infect Dis 1987;156:959–966.

84. Wallace RJ Jr, Septimus EJ, Musher DM, Berger MB, Martin RR. Treatment of experimental nocardiosis in mice: comparison of amikacin and sulfonamide. J Infect Dis 1979;140:244–248.

85. Wallace RJ Jr, Steele LC, Sumter G, Smith JM. Antimicrobial susceptibility patterns of *Nocardia asteroides*. Antimicrobiol Agents Chemother 1988;32:1776–1779.

86. Wallace RJ Jr, Tsukamura M, Brown BA, Brown J, Steingrube VA, Zhang Y, Nash DR. Cefotaxime-resistant *Nocardia asteroides* strains are isolates of the controversial species *Nocardia farcinica*. J Clin Microbiol 1990;28:2726–2732.

87. Wren MV, Savage AM, Alford RH. Apparent cure of intracranial *Nocardia asteroides* infection by minocycline. Arch Intern Med 1979;139:249–250.

88. Yano I, Imaeda T, Tsukamura M. Characterization of *Nocardia nova*. Int J Syst Bacteriol 1990;40:170–174.

89. Yazawa K, Mikami Y. In-vitro antimicrobial activity of the new fluoroquinolones, grepafloxacin, against pathogenic *Nocardia* spp. J Antimicrob Chemother 1995;35:541–544.

90. Yazawa K, Mikami Y, Ohashi S, Miyaji M, Ichihara Y, Nishimura C. In-vitro activity of new carbapenem antibiotics: comparative studies with meropenem, L-627 and imipenem against pathogenic *Nocardia* spp. J Antimicrob Chemother 1992; 29: 169–172.

91. Yazawa K, Mikami Y, Uno J. In vitro susceptibility of *Nocardia* spp. to a new fluoroquinolone, tosufloxacin (T-3262). Antimicrob Agents Chemother 1989;33:2140–2141.

92. Yew WW, Wong PC, Kwan SYL, Chan CY, Li MSK. Two cases of *Nocardia asteroides* sternotomy infection treated with ofloxacin and a review of other active antimicrobial agents. J Infect 1991;23:297–230.

93. Yogev R, Greenslade T, Firlit CF, Lewy P. Successful treatment of *Nocardia asteroides* infection with amikacin. J Pediatr 1980; 96:771–3.

Oerskovia Species

●

John D. Rihs

GENERAL DESCRIPTION

The genus *Oerskovia* belongs to the class *Actinomycetales* and includes two species *Oerskovia turbata* and *Oerskovia xanthineolytica*. These organisms were first isolated from the soil by Orskov in 1938. *Oerskovia* species are nocardia-like bacteria that are branched, Gram-positive bacilli, oxidase negative, catalase positive, and non–acid fast. Unlike *Nocardia* species, these organisms fragment into small motile rods, do not produce aerial mycelia, and possess a cell wall with large amounts of galactose. Colonies are glistening, bright yellow and produce branched vegetative hyphae on nutrient agar.

There have been 14 documented reports of infections due to *Oerskovia* species: 8 involving *O. xanthineolytica*, 4 caused by *O. turbata*, and 2 in which the species was not identified. Thirteen of the 14 cases have involved compromised patients with chronic underlying conditions. The one exception was a farmer who developed endophthalmitis related to a penetrating injury with a metallic object (5). Association of *Oerskovia* infection with a foreign body is well documented. Eleven of the 14 infections have involved foreign bodies. In addition to the above-mentioned case of endophthalmitis, there has been one case of homograft valve endocarditis (12), one meningitis due to an infected ventriculoperitoneal shunt (6), one prosthetic joint infection (4), two cases of peritonitis from infected peritoneal catheters (1, 13), and five bacteremias from central venous catheters (3, 7–10). Only three reports did not confirm the presence of a foreign body with infection (2, 11, 14).

These reports demonstrated the use of a wide range of antibiotics, different routes of administration and duration, monotherapy and combination therapy, and removal and nonremoval of foreign objects. These organisms have low virulence, and despite patients with persistent symptoms and a lingering course, no deaths occurred, and all patients were eventually cured of their infections.

IN VITRO SUSCEPTIBILITY

In vitro data on the clinical isolates has shown them all to be susceptible to vancomycin. Six of seven isolates were susceptible to trimethoprim-sulfamethoxazole. Eight of nine isolates were either susceptible or moderately susceptible to ampicillin. Five of six were susceptible to amikacin, and five of five tested sensitive to imipenem. The few isolates tested to rifampin have all been susceptible. Susceptibility to the following antibiotics has been variable: penicillin, erythromycin, cephalothin, tetracycline, clindamycin, ciprofloxacin, and gentamicin. The organism is resistant to the semisynthetic penicillins. A summary of the antimicrobial susceptibilities of 12 clinical isolates is shown in Table 1.

ANTIMICROBIAL THERAPY
Drug of Choice

Vancomycin appears to be the drug of choice on the basis of in vitro testing and clinical experience thus far. The usual adult daily intravenous dose is 2 g divided either as 500 mg every 6 h or 1 g every 12 h. Patient factors such as age, obesity, and impaired renal function call for a modification of the usual adult daily dose. In children, the usual intravenous dose is 10 mg/kg given every 6 h. In neonates and young infants, an initial dose of 15 mg/kg is recommended, followed by 10 mg/kg every 12 h for neonates in the first week of life and every 8 h thereafter up to the age of 1 month. Monitoring vancomycin serum concentrations is recommended in the very young, the elderly, the seriously ill, and patients with impaired renal function.

TABLE 1 • Antimicrobial Susceptibilities of Twelve Clinical Isolates

Drug	Isolates												A[a]
Penicillin	R	S	S	MS	S	—	S	R	R	R	R	—	5/10
Ampicillin	S	S	S	MS	—	MS	S	R	—	—	MS	S	8/9
Oxacillin	—	—	—	—	—	R	—	R	—	R	—	—	0/4
Cephalothin	S	—	—	S	R	—	S	—	S	—	R	S	6/8
Erythromycin	R	S	—	MS	S	R	R	MS	—	R	R	S	5/10
Clindamycin	—	R	—	—	S	—	R	MS	—	R	R	—	2/6
Tetracycline	R	S	—	S	—	R	S	S	S	R	S	—	6/9
Gentamicin	S	R	—	S	—	R	R	S	—	R	—	S	4/8
Amikacin	S	—	—	S	—	S	—	—	—	R	S	S	5/6
Ciprofloxacin	—	—	—	R	—	R	—	S	S	R	R	—	2/6
Rifampin	—	—	S	—	—	—	—	S	—	—	—	S	3/3
Imipenem	—	—	—	S	—	MS	—	S	—	—	S	S	5/5
TMP/SMX[b]	—	—	S	S	—	S	S	S	—	S	R	—	6/7
Vancomycin	—	S	S	S	S	S	S	S	S	S	S	S	11/11
References	2	5	6	8	3	13	14	10	1	9	4	7	

[a]Number of strains susceptible/total strains tested.

[b]TMP/SMX, trimethoprim-sulfamethoxazole.

Special Situations
Endocarditis

One report of endocarditis involving *Oerskovia* species has appeared in the literature (12), a case of homograft valve endocarditis in a patient whose aortic valve was replaced because of severe aortic insufficiency associated with ankylosing spondylitis. Three different antibiotic regimens over a 6-month period (penicillin; ampicillin and erythromycin; and ampicillin and trimethoprim-sulfamethoxazole) failed to eradicate the infection. Cure was only achieved after the infected homograft was replaced with a prosthetic valve and the patient was treated with oral trimethoprim-sulfamethoxazole for 12 weeks along with 6 weeks of parenteral ampicillin and 6 weeks of oral amoxicillin.

Meningitis

A case of meningitis resulted from an infected ventriculoperitoneal shunt in a patient with hydrocephalus (6). The patient was initially treated with 12 million units of penicillin per day and clinically improved. However, the ventricular fluid remained positive. The penicillin dose was increased to 24 million units daily, and rifampin was added. After 5 days and persistent infection, the shunt was replaced with a shunt on the opposite side. Antibiotic therapy was continued for 10 days after the surgery and resulted in a bacteriologic cure. Failure to cure this infection prior to removal may have resulted from poor antibiotic penetration into the cerebrospinal fluid and a relatively short duration.

Catheter-Associated Infections

Seven patients have been associated with catheter infections. Two of these patients initially failed antibiotic therapy despite in vitro susceptibility to the agents. A 3-year-old patient with acute myelogenous leukemia developed bacteremia from an infected Broviac catheter (8). Despite antimicrobial therapy with amikacin, blood cultures remained positive, and the catheter was removed. A patient with peritonitis caused by an infected peritoneal dialysis catheter was treated with vancomycin and gentamicin (13). After repeated positive cultures of the peritoneal effluent, the peritoneal catheter was removed. These accounts suggest that foreign body removal is often necessary for cure and should be a part of the initial therapy. On the other hand, some success with antibiotic cures in catheter-associated infections has been achieved. In three cases, central venous catheters were sterilized using vancomycin alone. Two of these patients had catheter-related sepsis due to infected Groshong catheters (9, 10), and one patient had an infected Hickman catheter that was being used for home total parenteral nutrition (3). Antibiotics alone were used to cure a forth patient with peritonitis. Vancomycin intraperitoneally, tobramycin intramuscularly, and oral doxycycline were used to clear the infected peritoneal dialysis catheter infection (1).

Alternative Therapy

Alternative therapy includes trimethoprim-sulfamethoxazole or ampicillin. The daily intravenous dose for trimethoprim-sulfamethoxazole is 8 to 10 mg/kg (based on the trimethoprim component), given in two to four equally divided doses every 6, 8, or 12 h. Trimethoprim-sulfamethoxazole is contraindicated in infants less than 2 months of age, and a reduced dosage should be used for patients with impaired renal function. Intravenous ampicillin can be given at 150 to 200 mg/kg per day in equally divided doses every 3 to 4 h.

COMMENTS

Patient management can be particularly problematic when a foreign body is present. For best results, the recommended course of action is removal of the foreign body, debridement if necessary, and antibiotic therapy. Patients with a removable focus can be treated with a 10- to 14-day course. However, because of the nonaggressive nature of these infections, an antibiotic trial seems appropriate when removal of the foreign material is undesirable. The duration of therapy may have to be extended if the foreign body is not removed.

There is no evidence to support any combination regimen over monotherapy.

REFERENCES

1. Borra S, Kleinfeld M. Peritonitis caused by *Oerskovia xanthineolytica* in a patient on chronic ambulatory peritoneal dialysis (CAPD). Am J Kidney Dis 1996;27:458.
2. Cruickshank JG, Gawler AH, Shaldon C. *Oerskovia* species: rare opportunistic pathogens. J Med Microbiol 1979;12:513–515.
3. Guss WJ, Ament ME. *Oerskovia* infection caused by contaminated home parenteral nutrition solution. Arch Intern Med 1989; 149:1457–1458.
4. Harrington RD, Lewis CG, Aslanzadeh J, Stelmach P, Woolfrey AE. *Oerskovia xanthineolytica* infection of a prosthetic joint: case report and review. J Clin Microbiol 1996;34:1821–1824.
5. Hussain Z, Gonder JR, Lannigan R, Stoakes L. Endophthalmitis due to *Oerskovia xanthineolytica*. Can J Ophthalmol 1987;22: 234–236.
6. Kailath EJ, Goldstein E, Wagner FH. Case report: meningitis caused by *Oerskovia xanthineolytica*. Am J Med Sci 1988; 295:216–217.
7. Lair MI, Bentolila S, Grenet D, Cahen P, Honderlick P. *Oerskovia turbata* and *Comamonas acidovorans* bacteremia in a patient with AIDS. Eur J Clin Microbiol Infect Dis 1996:15:424–425.
8. LeProwse CR, McNeil MM, McCarty JM. Catheter-related bacteremia caused by *Oerskovia turbata*. J Clin Microbiol 1989:27: 571–572.
9. Maguire JD, McCarthy MC, Decker CF. *Oerskovia xanthineolytica* bacteremia in an immunocompromised host: case report and review. Clin Infect Dis 1996;22:554–556.
10. McDonald CL, Chapin-Robertson K, Dill SR, Martino RL. *Oerskovia xanthineolytica* bacteremia in an immunocompromised patient with pneumonia. Diagn Microbiol Infect Dis 1994;18: 259–261.
11. Reina J, Liompart I, Altes J. An axillary abscess produced by *Oerskovia turbata* in an AIDS patient. Rev Clin Esp 1991;188: 485–486.
12. Reller LB, Maddoux GL, Eckman MR, Pappas G. Bacterial endocarditis caused by *Oerskovia turbata*. Ann Intern Med 1975; 83:664–666.
13. Rihs JD, McNeil MM, Brown JM, Yu VL. *Oerskovia xanthineolytica* implicated in peritonitis associated with peritoneal dialysis: case report and review of *Oerskovia* infections in humans. J Clin Microbiol 1990;28:1934–1937.
14. Truant AL, Satishchandrn V, Eisenstaedt R, Richman P, McNeil MM. *Oerskovia xanthineolytica* and methicillin resistant *Staphylococcus aureus* in a patient with cirrhosis and variceal hemorrhage. Eur J Clin Microbiol Infect Dis 1992;11:950–951.

Pasteurella multocida and Other Species

●

Sharon Hunt Gerardo and Ellie J. C. Goldstein

MICROBIOLOGY

Pasteurella are pleomorphic, coccoid to bacillary, (0.2–0.4 × 0.4–2.0 μm), nonmotile, facultatively anaerobic, Gram-negative bacteria. On Gram stain, they may occur singly or in pairs or short chains. They may be mistaken for *Haemophilus* species or with the closely related *Actinobacillus* species. *Pasteurella* species grow on blood and chocolate agar but do not grow on MacConkey agar.

Pasteurella species have been isolated from a variety of animals either as saprophytes in the nasopharynx or gastrointestinal tract, or as primary pathogens (Table 1). Human diseases associated with *Pasteurella,* first reported in 1913, are listed in Table 2. Although most human disease is associated with some form of animal contact, most commonly a dog bite or cat bite or scratch (32, 50, 93), cases have been reported unassociated with known animal contact (50, 52–53, 94).

Pasteurella multocida (multocida, L. adj., *multus,* "many"; L. adj. *cidus,* "kill"; M.L. fem. adj. "many killing," referring to potential fatal pathogenicity in many species of animals) has been the predominant species isolated from human infections. Recent advances in molecular biologic methods have led to suggested taxonomic changes for this genus (Table 3), e.g., limiting the genus to 11 genetically closely related taxa, including establishment of several new species that have been isolated from human and animal sources, and acceptance of three subspecies of *P. multocida* (68–69). These subspecies and new species, which can be differentiated by routine biochemical testing, may have different ecologic niches and different propensities for tissue invasion and pathogenic potentials.

IN VITRO SUSCEPTIBILITY

Pasteurella susceptibility data from various studies are reported in Table 4. *Pasteurella* are generally susceptible to penicillin G, its derivatives (penicillin V, ampicillin, amoxicillin, carbenicillin, ticarcillin, piperacillin, and mezlocillin), and second- and third-generation cephalosporins. Isolated instances of penicillin resistance have been noted (4), including some that produce an ROB-1 β-lactamase that is mediated by a nonconjugative plasmid (77). The β-lactamase inhibitor combinations (e.g., amoxicillin/clavulanate and ampicillin/sulbactam) are also quite efficacious in vitro. Dicloxacillin, oxacillin, and nafcillin may not achieve adequate blood levels compared to the MIC in order to be active against pasteurella.

Confusion about cephalosporin activity (particularly the first-generation oral agents) against *Pasteurella* may arise because of the disparity in susceptibility to intravenous and oral preparations. Most laboratories report susceptibility to either cephalothin or cefazolin, which achieve much higher serum levels

than their oral counterparts, cephalexin, cefadroxil, and cefaclor, and the unsuspecting physician may extrapolate this data inappropriately (34). Of the cephalosporins (Table 4), isolates are uniformly susceptible to concentrations achieved by both oral and intravenous cefuroxime. Cefoxitin and cefamandole are uniformly active as well. Cefotaxime, ceftriaxone, cefixime, and cefpodoxime are generally more active than cefuroxime, with as much as a fourfold dilution difference. All isolates reported are susceptible to cefprozil and loracarbef; however, some isolates have cefprozil MICs close to the National Committee for Clinical Laboratory Standards (NCCLS) breakpoint (≤8 μg/mL).

While some isolates may be susceptible to erythromycin, a significant percentage are resistant to it or have MICs near the breakpoint. Roxithromycin shows poor activity against *Pasteurella*. Azithromycin appears to be active against most *Pasteurella* species at achievable concentrations and is more active than clarithromycin. Both of these macrolides have better activity than erythromycin (40). Some strains of *P. canis* and *P. dagmatis* are more resistant to clarithromycin than to azithromycin (40). The new ketolides, RU 64004 and RU 66647, appear to have better activity than azithromycin and clarithromycin, with MIC_{90}s of 0.5 and 1.0 μg/mL, respectively (41a).

All isolates are uniformly susceptible to the tetracyclines, with minocycline and doxycycline slightly more active than tetracycline. Likewise, all isolates are susceptible to the quinolones (ofloxacin, ciprofloxacin, enoxacin, sparfloxacin, temafloxacin, trovafloxacin, levofloxacin, DU-6859a, Bay 12-8039, and Bay y3118), with enoxacin somewhat less active than the other quinolones tested. In contrast, the aminoglycosides demonstrated borderline or variable results; most isolates are resistant to amikacin and streptomycin or have MICs near the NCCLS breakpoint (gentamicin and tobramycin).

Of the other antimicrobial agents tested, chloramphenicol was the most active and showed good activity against *Pasteurella* isolates. Sulfamethoxazole-trimethoprim and sulfadiazine demonstrated moderate activity, with MICs at or near the breakpoint established for urinary tract isolates. Rifampin, likewise, showed moderate activity against *Pasteurella* isolates, with MICs at or near the breakpoint. Clindamycin was usually inactive.

No data exist regarding the occurrence of synergy or antagonism of antimicrobial agents against *P. multocida*.

ANTIMICROBIAL THERAPY
General: Drug of Choice

There have been few clinical studies to determine the efficacy of antimicrobial agents against *P. multocida*. Most studies

TABLE 1 • Animal Sources of *Pasteurella* Species			
Animals from Which *Pasteurella* Species Have Been Isolated		**Animal Sources of *Pasteurella* Implicated in Human Disease**	
Dog	Horse	Dog	Guinea pig
Cat	Pig	Wolf	Opossum
Tiger	Mouse	Cat	Tasmanian devil
Lion	Rat	Tiger	Bird
Panther	Mink	Lion	Fish
Lynx	Rabbit	Panther	
Cattle	Guinea pig	Cattle	
Buffalo	Syrian hamster	Horse	
Bison	Wild birds & raptors	Pig	
Sheep	Fowl	Rat	
Reindeer	Monkey	Rabbit	
Tortoise			

Data from references 5, 9 13, 15, 18, 21, 31, 32, 50, 52, 60, 68, 69, 82, 86, 93–96.

have been of limited numbers of dog and cat bite wounds or anecdotal reports of success or failure with a particular agent. Most authors have noted the efficacy of penicillin or amoxicillin clavulanate in animal bite wounds (36, 93). The latter appears to offer an advantage over penicillin, since many of these infections are multibacterial and include other elements of the biting animal's flora, many of which may produce β-lactamase (8, 32). Older reports noted the efficacy of chloramphenicol, an agent that is currently infrequently used because of potential toxicity. The efficacy of tetracyclines and sulfamethoxazole-trimethoprim has also been noted (41a, 81). Many infections are multibacterial, so the antibacterial agent(s) selected must cover all components.

Human infections with *Pasteurella* may be divided into three categories: (*a*) skin and soft-tissue, and bone and joint infections, commonly following animal bites or scratches; (*b*) oral and respiratory infection, usually in patients with chronic pulmonary disease; and (*c*) serious invasive infection, such as meningitis, intraabdominal infection, or ocular infections, which may or may not be related to animal bites.

Skin and Soft-Tissue Infections

Most skin and soft-tissue infections with *Pasteurella* result from a bite or scratch inflicted by a dog or cat (1, 21, 24, 30, 32, 36, 50, 93–94). Infection generally becomes symptomatic (warmth, tenderness, erythema, pain, and purulent discharge) within 12 to 72 h (19). Most infections manifest as cellulitis localized to the area of the injury. An abscess may form at the site of penetration. There have also been reports of localized wound infection in patients with open wounds or lesions not resulting from an animal bite or scratch, e.g., decubitis or stasis ulcers (48, 94), postoperative surgical wounds (14, 83), and nontuberculous mycobacterial suppurating lymphadenitis (45). In most cases, licking of the wound by pet animals was the likely source of entry. Thus, *Pasteurella* can probably infect areas of broken skin regardless of the cause of injury. Penicillin and its derivatives are effective in treating these infections. Cephalothin and ciprofloxacin have been used with therapeutic success in the penicillin-allergic patient (14, 75).

TABLE 2 • Human Diseases Associated with Various *Pasteurella* Species

Skin and soft tissue infection
  Bites
  Cellulitis
  Abscess
  Open wound infection

Bone and joint infection
  Osteomyelitis
  Septic arthritis
  Bursitis
  Tenosynovitis

Oral and respiratory infection
  Tonsillitis
  Sinusitis
  Pharyngitis
  Bronchitis
  Tracheobronchitis
  Epiglottitis
  Mastoiditis
  Pneumonia
  Empyema
  Submandibular abscess
  Otitis media
  Ludwig's angina
  Pulmonary fibrosis

Serious invasive disease
  Cardiovascular system
    Bacteremia
    Septic shock
    Endocarditis
    Pericarditis
  Central nervous system
    Meningitis
    Subdural empyema
    Brain abscess
  Gastrointestinal tract
    Peritonitis
    Omental and peritoneal abscess
    Liver abscess
    Spleen abscess
  Genitourinary tract
    Renal abscess
    Vaginitis
    Cervicitis
    Bartholin gland abscess
    Urinary tract infection
    Cystitis
    Pyelonephritis
    Infected ileal loop
    Epididymitis
    Salpingitis
    Tuboovarian abscess
    Chorioamnionitis
    Opuerperal infection
    In utero infection

Ocular
  Endophthalmitis
  Conjunctivitis
  Keratitis
  Corneal ulcer

Data from references 2–3, 6, 10, 12, 14, 17, 21, 23, 28–29, 46–48, 50, 54, 56–57, 62, 71, 73, 78–79, 83, 88, 89, 92, 94, 97.

TABLE 3 • New Taxonomic Classification of *Pasteurella* Species

Proposed species of *Pasteurella* sensu stricto	Comment
Pasteurella multocida subsp. *multocida*	Most common isolate, especially from cat bites; may produce a toxin
Pasteurella multocida subsp. *septica*	Associated with more serious infections including meningitis
Pasteurella multocida subsp. *gallicida*	Animal pathogen
Pasteurella dagmatis	Prior *Pasteurella* "gas," *Pasteurella* new species 1, *Pasteurella pneumotropica* type Henriksen group; isolated from dogs and cats, as well as human bite wound infections
Pasteurella gallinarum	
Pasteurella canis	Prior *P. multocida* biotype 6 ("dog type" strains); biotype 1 isolated from dogs and dog bite wounds (indole positive); biotype 2 isolated from calves (indole negative); may produce a toxin
Pasteurella stomatis	Isolated from the respiratory tracts of dogs and cats
Pasteurella avium	Prior *Haemophilus avium;* V-factor requirement varies; isolated from chickens and calves
Pasteurella volantium	Prior *Haemophilus avium;* V-factor required; isolated from domestic fowl and humans
Pasteurella anatis	Bisgaard taxon 1; isolated from the intestinal tracts of ducks
Pasteurella langaa	Bisgaard taxon 4; isolated from the respiratory tracts of chickens
Pasteurella species A (provisional)	Prior *Haemophilus avium;* V-factor required
Pasteurella species B (provisional)	Unknown clinical significance; includes dulcitol positive strains of *P. multocida* biotype 6

Species with Low Homology to *Pasteurella* sensu stricto	Comment
Pasteurella testudinis	More closely related to *Actinobacillus* group
Pasteurella pneumotropica	More closely related to *Actinobacillus* group
Pasteurella ureae	More closely related to *Actinobacillus* group
Pasteurella haemolytica	More closely related to *Actinobacillus* group
Pasteurella aerogenes	Taxonomic position unknown
Pasteurella bettyae	Prior *P. bettii, Pasteurella* biotype 1, CDC Group HB-5; isolated from human Bartholin gland abscesses and human finger infections; taxonomic position unknown
Pasteurella caballi	First isolated from horses
Pasteurella "SP" Group	Isolated from guinea pigs
Pasteurella lymphangitidis	Bovine lymphangitis group, isolated from lymphangitis in cattle; taxonomic position unknown
Pasteurella mairi	Associated with swine abortion
Pasteurella trehalosi	Associated with septicemia in lambs; low DNA homology with accepted *Pasteurella* species, but 16S rRNA sequence homology clusters with *Pasteurella* species

Data from references 5, 18, 20, 68, 69, 82, 85–86.

Joint and Bone Infections

Serious joint and bone infections, generally following an animal bite or scratch, may be caused by *Pasteurella*. Although septic arthritis generally involves a joint in proximity to the site of injury, it may also involve a joint directly inoculated by the bite or (via bacteremia) even one away from the wound. Osteomyelitis is most commonly preceded by significant wound infection and cellulitis. Combined septic arthritis and osteomyelitis infection is almost always preceded by cat bites of the hand, resulting in osteomyelitis of the phalanx and interphalangeal arthritis. Most patients with this type of infection generally have a poor functional outcome (93). Penicillin and its derivatives are used most often to treat these infections. In the penicillin-allergic patient, cefotaxime has been used after surgery to remove an infected knee arthroplasty (44). Intravenous ceftriaxone followed by oral amoxicillin/clavulanate has been successfully used to treat subacute osteomyelitis (19). Pefloxacin has also shown good activity in these types of infections (12).

Oral and Respiratory Tract Infections

Colonization or infection of the human respiratory tract by *Pasteurella* is generally associated with traumatic animal exposure.

In man, a variety of oral and respiratory infections with *Pasteurella* have been reported, including sinusitis, pharyngitis, and epiglottitis (80, 94); tonsillitis or peritonsillar abscess (73, 94, 100); Ludwig's angina (23); submandibular abscess (94); bronchitis and tracheobronchitis (48, 94); pneumonia (22, 46, 94, 98); congenital pneumonia (3); pneumonia with lung abscess and empyema (48); lung abscess (62); empyema (94); pulmonary fibrosis (48); septicemia with peritonitis and empyema (29); otitis media and mastoiditis (94); and an unusual case of otitis media with Bell's palsy (74). Penicillin and its derivatives are effective in treating these types of infections (74, 80). Alternate therapeutic choices have included cefotaxime (23), cefazolin (98), and amoxicillin/clavulanate (62). In an unusual case of a patient with probable IgA nephropathy, recurring tonsillitis (thought due to reinfection from her pet cat) was effectively treated with cefaclor and ceftriaxone (first infection), ceftriaxone and penicillin (second infection), and cefaclor, ciprofloxacin, ceftriaxone, doxycycline and rifampin (third infection) (73).

Bacteremia and Cardiovascular System Infections

Pasteurella bacteremia is uncommon but has been reported (7, 11, 26, 27, 30, 49, 63, 66, 94). Septic shock may result, even

TABLE 4 • Summary of the Activity of Various Antimicrobial Agents against *Pasteurella* Species

β-Lactams (Penicillins) and β-Lactam plus β-Lactam Inhibitors

Antimicrobial Agent	Reference	No.	Species	MIC$_{50}$	MIC$_{90}$	Range	S	I	R
Penicillin G	4	82		0.25	0.25	0.125–0.5	≤2	—	≥4
	34	20	*P. multocida*		0.1				
	35	20	*P. multocida*	0.125	0.125	≤0.03–0.125			
	37	16	*P. multocida*	0.125	0.25	≤0.03–0.25			
	38	29	*Pasteurella* sp.	0.125	0.5	≤0.03–32			
	40	55	*Pasteurella* sp.	0.06	0.06	0.03–0.5			
	42	22	*P. multocida*	≤0.06	0.25	<0.06–32			
	84	13–15	*P. multocida*	0.8					
	87	14	*P. multocida*	1.6					
	94	19	*P. multocida*	0.125	0.125				
Penicillin VK	94	15	*P. multocida*	0.25	0.5		NA	NA	NA
Amoxicillin[a]	4	82	*P. multocida*	0.125	0.25	0.06–0.25	≤2	—	≥4
Amoxicillin/clavulanate	34	20	*P. multocida*		0.2		≤8/4	16/8	≥32/16
	35	20	*P. multocida*	0.125	0.25	≤0.03–0.5	8/4		
	37	16	*P. multocida*	0.25	0.25	0.125–0.25			
Ampicillin[a]	34	20	*P. multocida*		0.2		≤2	—	≥4
	35	20	*P. multocida*	0.125	0.25	≤0.03–0.25			
	85	13–15	*P. multocida*	0.2					
	87	14	*P. multocida*	0.8					
	94	19	*P. multocida*	0.25	0.25				
	41a	31	*Pasteurella* sp.	0.06	0.125	≤0.016–0.125			
Dicloxacillin	84	13–15	*P. multocida*	6.2			NA	NA	NA
	87	14	*P. multocida*	12.5					
	94	19	*P. multocida*	8	16				
Oxacillin	42	22	*P. multocida*	1	8	<0.06–>64	NA	NA	NA
Nafcillin	94	19	*P. multocida*	4	4		≤2	—	≥4
Ticarcillin	94	19	*P. multocida*	0.5	0.5		≤16	32–64	≥128
Mezlocillin	94	19	*P. multocida*	0.06	0.125		≤16	32–64	≥128

Cephalosporins and Other Cephems

Antimicrobial Agent	Reference	No.	Species	MIC$_{50}$	MIC$_{90}$	Range	S	I	R
Cefalexin[b]	34	20	*P. multocida*		4		≤8	16	≥32
	35	20	*P. multocida*	4	4	0.25–4			
	38	29	*Pasteurella* sp.	2	2	0.5–16			
	42	22	*P. multocida*	0.25	1	≤0.06–2			
	49	35	*P. multocida*	2.56	5.12	1.28–10.24			
	84	13–15	*P. multocida*	3.1					
	87	14	*P. multocida*	6.3					
	94	19	*P. multocida*	4	16				
Cephalothin[b]	37	16	*P. multocida*	0.25	0.25	0.125–25	≤8	16	≥32
	94	19	*P. multocida*	2	4				
Cefadroxil[b]	34	20	*P. multocida*		8		≤8	16	≥32
	35	20	*P. multocida*	4	8	0.5–16			
	38	29	*Pasteurella* sp.	4	4	0.06–8			
	49	35	*P. multocida*	5.12	10.24	5.12–20.48			
Cefaclor[b]	4	82	*P. multocida*	2	8	1–8	≤8	16	≥32
	49	35	*P. multocida*	0.64	2.56	0.32–2.56			
	94	19	*P. multocida*	4	32				
Cephapirin[b]	94	19	*P. multocida*	0.5	2		≤8	16	≥32
Cefazolin	94	19	*P. multocida*	1	2		≤8	16	≥32
Cefoxitin	94	15	*P. multocida*	1	2		≤8	16	≥32
Cefamandole	94	19	*P. multocida*	0.125	1		≤8	16	≥32
Cefuroxime[c]	4	82	*P. multocida*	0.125	0.25	0.125–1	≤8	16	≥32
	34	20	*P. multocida*		0.25				
	35	20	*P. multocida*	0.125	0.25	≤0.03–0.25			
	40	55	*Pasteurella* sp.	0.06	0.06	0.016–0.125			
	49	35	*P. multocida*	0.16	1.28	0.08–2.56			
Cefotaxime	4	82	*P. multocida*	0.06	0.125	<0.03–0.125	≤8	16–32	≥64
	94	19	*P. multocida*	0.06	0.06				
	41a	31	*Pasteurella* sp.	≤0.016	≤0.016	≤0.016–0.016			

continued

TABLE 4 • Summary of the Activity of Various Antimicrobial Agents against *Pasteurella* Species

Cephalosporins and Other Cephems

Antimicrobial Agent	Reference	No.	Species	MIC_{50}	MIC_{90}	Range	S	I	R
Ceftriaxone	4	82	*P. multocida*	0.06	0.125	≤0.03–0.125	≤8	16–32	≥64
Cefixime	4	82	*P. multocida*	0.03	0.06	≤0.03–0.5	≤1	2	≥4
Cefpodoxime	4	82	*P. multocida*	0.03	0.06	<0.03–0.125	≤2	4	≥8
	40	55	*Pasteurella* sp.	0.03	0.03	0.016–0.06			
	41a	31	*Pasteurella* sp.	0.03	0.03	≤0.016–0.06			
Cefprozil	38	29	*Pasteurella* sp.	0.25	0.5	0.125–8	≤8	16	≥32
Loracarbef	38	29	*Pasteurella* sp.	0.25	0.25	0.06–1	≤8	16	≥32
Cefcanel	49	35	*P. multocida*	0.08	0.32	0.08–0.64	NA	NA	NA
Moxalactam	94	19	*P. multocida*	0.25	0.25		≥8	16–32	≥64

Macrolides

Antimicrobial Agent	Reference	No.	Species	MIC_{50}	MIC_{90}	Range	S	I	R
Erythromycin	37	16	*P. multocida*	2	4	1–4	≤0.5	1–4	≥8
	38	29	*Pasteurella* sp.	2	4	0.5–4			
	42	22	*P. multocida*	1	4	≤0.06–>32			
	84	13–15	*P. multocida*	3.1					
	87	14	*P. multocida*	3.1					
	94	19	*P. multocida*	4	8				
	41	31	*Pasteurella* sp.	4	4	1–4			
Clarithromycin	37	16	*P. multocida*	2	2	1–2	≤2	4	≥8
	40	55	*Pasteurella* sp.	1	2	0.125–8			
	41a	31	*Pasteurella* sp.	2	2	0.25–4			
Azithromycin	38	29	*Pasteurella* sp.	1	2	0.25–2	≤2	4	≥8
	40	55	*Pasteurella* sp.	0.125	0.25	0.03–0.5			
	41a	31	*Pasteurella* sp.	1	1	0.06–1			
RU-64004	41a	31	*P. multocida*	0.5	0.5	0.06–0.5	NA	NA	NA
RU-66647	41a	31	*P. multocida*	1	1	0.125–1	NA	NA	NA

Tetracyclines

Antimicrobial Agent	Reference	No.	Species	MIC_{50}	MIC_{90}	Range	S	I	R
Doxycycline[d]	38	29	*Pasteurella* sp.	0.125	0.125	≤0.125–0.5	≤4	8	≥16
	40	55	*Pasteurella* sp.	0.06	0.125	0.03–0.5			
Tetracycline[d]	34	20	*P. multocida*		0.5		≤4	8	≥16
	35	20	*P. multocida*	0.5	0.5	0.25–1			
	37	16	*P. multocida*	0.5	0.5	0.25–1			
	84	13–15	*P. multocida*	0.8					
	87	14	*P. multocida*	0.09					
	94	19	*P. multocida*	0.25	0.5				
	41a	31	*Pasteurella* sp.	0.25	0.5	0.125–1			
Minocycline[d]	38	22	*P. multocida*	0.25	0.25	≤0.06–4	≤4	8	≥16
	94	19	*P. multocida*	0.25	0.25				

Quinolones

Antimicrobial Agent	Reference	No.	Species	MIC_{50}	MIC_{90}	Range	S	I	R
Ciprofloxacin	35	20	*P. multocida*	≤0.03	<0.03	≤0.03–≤0.03	≤1	2	≥4
	37	16	*P. multocida*	≤0.03	≤0.03	≤0.03–≤0.03			
	38	29	*Pasteurella* sp.	0.008	0.015	≤0.005–0.125			
	39	54	*Pasteurella* sp.	0.004	0.004	0.002–0.008			
	40	55	*Pasteurella* sp.	0.008	0.008	0.002–0.016			
Ofloxacin	35	20	*P. multocida*	≤0.03	0.06	≤0.03–0.25	≤2	4	≥8
	37	16	*P. multocida*	≤0.03	0.06	≤0.03–0.06			
	38	29	*Pasteurella* sp.	0.03	0.06	≤0.015–0.125			
	39	54	*Pasteurella* sp.	0.016	0.03	0.008–0.06			
	40	55	*Pasteurella* sp.	0.016	0.03	0.008–0.06			
Enoxacin	35	20	*P. multocida*	0.12	0.5	<0.03–0.5	≤2	4	≥8
Sparfloxacin	37	16	*P. multocida*	≤0.03	≤0.03	≤0.03–≤0.03	NA	NA	NA
	38	29	*Pasteurella* sp.	0.004	0.008	≤0.004–0.015			
	39	54	*Pasteurella* sp.	0.002	0.004	0.001–0.016			
	40	55	*Pasteurella* sp.	0.002	0.004	0.001–0.016			
Temafloxacin	37	16	*P. multocida*	≤0.03	≤0.03	≤0.03–≤0.03	NA	NA	NA
Levofloxacin	38	29	*Pasteurella* sp.	0.015	0.015	≤0.008–0.06	NA	NA	NA
	39	54	*Pasteurella* sp.	0.008	0.016	0.004–0.016			
	40	55	*Pasteurella* sp.	0.008	0.016	0.004–0.016			
	41b	31	*Pasteurella* sp.	0.016	0.03	0.008–0.03			

continued

TABLE 4 • **Summary of the Activity of Various Antimicrobial Agents against *Pasteurella* Species**

Quinolones

Antimicrobial Agent	Reference	No.	Species	MIC$_{50}$	MIC$_{90}$	Range	S	I	R
Trovafloxacin	41b	55	*Pasteurella* sp.	0.008	0.03	0.002–0.125	NA	NA	NA
DU-6859a	39	54	*Pasteurella* sp.	0.001	0.004	0.001–0.016	NA	NA	NA
Bay 12-8039	40	55	*Pasteurella* sp.	0.008	0.016	0.004–0.06	NA	NA	NA
Bay y3118	38	29	*Pasteurella* sp.	0.004	0.008	≤0.004–0.008	NA	NA	NA

Aminocyclitols

Antimicrobial Agent	Reference	No.	Species	MIC$_{50}$	MIC$_{90}$	Range	S	I	R
Amikacin	94	19	*P. multocida*	32	32		≤16	32	≥64
Streptomycin	94	19	*P. multocida*	32	32		NA	NA	NA
Gentamicin	94	19	*P. multocida*	2	2		≤4	8	≥16
Tobramycin	94	19	*P. multocida*	4	4		≤4	8	≥16

Others

Antimicrobial Agent	Reference	No.	Species	MIC$_{50}$	MIC$_{90}$	Range	S	I	R
Chloramphenicol	84	13–15	*P. multocida*	0.4			≤8	16	≥32
	87	14	*Pasteurella* sp.	1.6					
	94	19	*P. multocida*	0.25	0.5				
Trimethoprim/ sulfamethoxazole	38	29	*Pasteurella* sp.	0.06	0.25	≤0.03–0.25	≤2/38	—	≥4/76
	42	22	*P. multocida*	0.5	2	≤0.06–8			
	94	19	*P. multocida*	0.5	1				
Rifampin	94	19	*P. multocida*	0.5	1		≤1	2	≥4
Sulfadiazine	94	19	*P. multocida*	4	128		NA	NA	NA
Clindamycin	84	13–15	*P. multocida*	25			≤0.5	1–2	≥4
	87	14	*P. multocida*	25					
	94	19	*P. multocida*	16	32				

[a] Ampicillin MIC breakpoints representative of ampicillin and amoxicillin.

[b] Cephalothin MIC breakpoints representative of cephalothin, cephapirin, cefalexin, cefaclor, and cefadroxil.

[c] MIC breakpoints for cefuroxime for oral drug.

[d] Tetracycline MIC breakpoints representative of tetracycline, doxycycline and minocycline.

in previously healthy individuals (67, 79). Bacteremia with *Pasteurella,* which frequently accompanies serious infections, has been associated with disseminated intravascular coagulation (10), biliary sepsis with Waterhouse-Friderichsen syndrome (54), and peritonitis and empyema (29). Although rare, endocarditis and purulent pericarditis have been noted as complications of *Pasteurella* sepsis (51, 93–94). Penicillin and its derivatives are commonly used to treat these infections. Alternate and combination therapies have included cefuroxime (26), ceftazidime and penicillin (66), ampicillin/clavulanate and ofloxacin followed by ampicillin (7), and penicillin and amoxicillin (67).

Central Nervous System Infections

Multiple cases of *Pasteurella* meningitis have been described (50, 57, 64, 71, 94). *Pasteurella* meningitis tends to occur at the extremes of life: 50% of cases involve infants under the age of 1 year, and 30% involve adults over the age of 60 years (94). In addition to age, alcohol abuse may be a predisposing factor (65). Meningitis can also occur in healthy individuals following mastoidectomy (17). Brain abscesses (59, 94) and subdural empyema (94) due to *Pasteurella* have also been noted. Effective therapy is based on early recognition of the possibility of in-

fection with *Pasteurella* and prompt initiation of treatment with penicillin, ampicillin, or a third-generation cephalosporin (57).

Intraabdominal Infections

Serious intraabdominal infections involving *Pasteurella* have been reported, the most common being peritonitis (50, 56, 61). Omental or appendiceal abscesses, liver abscess, and splenic abscess have also been noted (88, 94). Cirrhosis and thalassemia can be underlying conditions that predispose one to serious intraabdominal infection. Effective therapeutic choices include penicillin, its derivatives, and third-generation cephalosporins. Prophylactic therapy with one of the β-lactam agents is recommended for cirrhotic patients prior to endoscopy or in those who have sustained an animal bite or scratch (56). Secondary prevention for recurrent disease should be considered and may consist of norfloxacin or trimethoprim-sulfamethoxazole, to which *Pasteurella* is usually sensitive (56).

Genitourinary Tract Infections

A variety of *Pasteurella* genitourinary tract infections have been reported. Weber (94) cites cases of cystitis, pyelonephritis, infected ileal loop, renal abscess, vaginitis, cervicitis, Bartholin gland abscess, and epididymitis. Chorioamnionitis

(94, 97), tuboovarian abscess (89), salpingitis (78), colonization of the cervical canal and opuerperal infection (3), and in utero infection (92) have been noted. *Pasteurella* is also thought to be responsible for a human stillbirth (90). Successful therapeutic combinations have included ampicillin, gentamicin, and metronidazole followed by amoxicillin/clavulanate (78); ampicillin, gentamicin, and clindamycin (89); and cefuroxime and metronidazole followed by cephadroxil and metronidazole (3).

Ocular Infection

Ocular infection with *Pasteurella* can be a serious sequela to direct inoculation with *Pasteurella* following injury to the eye. Conjunctivitis (47, 94), keratitis and corneal ulcer (47, 76, 94), and endophthalmitis (91, 94) have been described. There is an insufficient number of cases to establish optimal therapy. Despite aggressive therapeutic and surgical intervention, the outcome is often poor for these types of *Pasteurella* infections.

Infection with Other Pasteurella Species

Although *P. multocida* is the most common *Pasteurella* species isolated from human infections, *P. canis, P. dagmatis, P. stomatis,* and *P. pneumotropica* have been isolated from wound infections and abscesses following dog and cat bites (21, 50, 72, 99). *P. dagmatis* was also reported in cases of severe cellulitis, groin abscess, throat abscess, and septicemia (27, 50). *P. pneumotropica* has been isolated from patients with severe infections, including meningitis (65), pneumonia (16) and endocarditis (2). Similarly, *P. haemolytica, P. ureae,* and *P. gallinarum* have been associated with cases of endocarditis (2). *P. ureae* was reported as the responsible infectious agent in an HIV-positive patient with meningitis (55). The first report of human infection with *P. caballi* involved an infected wound on a veterinary surgeon (5). Local wound infection and severe arthritis with tendon necrosis following a guinea pig bite was attributed to *Pasteurella* "SP" group (60). *P. aerogenes* was isolated from the ears and throat of a stillbirth and from the vaginal vault of the mother (90). These case reports indicate that most *Pasteurella* species are capable of causing human infection given exposure and the proper conditions. Infection with these other *Pasteurella* species can be effectively treated with penicillin, its derivatives, and third-generation cephalosporins.

Special Situations

Problems arise in the highly penicillin allergic patient, especially if the patient is pregnant or a juvenile, when fluoroquinolones and tetracyclines are contraindicated. In such cases, determining the degree and severity of allergy may be important. Several β-lactam agents have efficacy in vitro but have not been studied clinically. We have used cefoxitin in more than 20 pateints over the years, with good success, and expect that therapy might also be successful with other, newer, oral and parenteral cephalosporin agents. First-generation oral cephalosporins (e.g., cephalexin) and β-lactamase-stable penicillins such as dicloxacillin have been associated with therapeutic failure (25, 42–43, 94, Goldstein, personal experience) and should be avoided.

Alternative Therapy

Azithromycin looks promising for therapy on the basis of in vitro data; however, clinical trials are lacking. Clarithromycin has also never been studied. There are numerous anecdotal reports of erythromycin failure in bite wounds and against *P. multocida.* Nevertheless, there may be instances that require erythromycin use, and these patients should be warned about the risk of failure and be clinically monitored more closely.

Obviously, the choice of any agent depends on its pharmacokinetics and its ability to penetrate in good concentrations to the infected site. Thus, in non–bite wound infections due to *P. multocida,* there are other considerations besides those noted above, including the multibacterial nature of many of these infections.

ENDPOINTS FOR MONITORING THERAPY

Standard clinical endpoints are used to monitor the efficacy of therapy. In early therapy of animal bite wounds, some believe that a 3- to 5-day course of oral antimicrobial agents, along with good wound care (irrigation and elevation), diminishes the risk of infection, especially in high-risk wounds (36). Such high-risk wounds include those to the hand, multiple punctures, those associated with preexisting edema of the traumatized area, those in compromised hosts, and those with pain out of proportion to the injury. Infected wounds that result in cellulitis are treated for 10 to 14 days, depending upon response. Abscesses, of course, need to be drained. Those that involve the bone (osteomyelitis) or joint (septic arthritis) require longer therapy, often from 4 to 6 weeks, plus ancillary therapeutic measures. Endpoints include the resolution of erythema for cellulitis and return of normal mobility for those involving the joints. Noninfectious complications can include compartment syndrome, posttraumatic synovitis, and permanent loss of range of motion of a joint.

CONTROVERSIES

The most controversial area involves the efficacy of "prophylaxis" in patients who present less than 8 h after injury, without established infection. This has never been studied on a large scale. The authors favor its use in moderate-to-severe wounds or those with special characteristics noted above (36), whereas others eschew its use. There is also no agreement about the "best" antimicrobial agent, the efficacy (or lack thereof) of erythromycin, or the agent to use in the penicillin-allergic patient, especially if pregnant or a juvenile. It is unlikely to be studied in the future because of funding restrictions. In addition, there is marked variability in wound severity and the wound care applied to patients, which also limits the design of many studies.

REFERENCES

1. Acay MC, Oral ET, Yenigün M, Sahin A. *Pasteurella multocida* ulceration on the penis. Int J Dermatol 1993;32:519–520.
2. Al Fadel Saleh M, Al-Madan MS, Erwa HH, Sohel SZ, Sanyal SK. First case of human infection caused by *Pasteurella gallinarum* causing infective endocarditis in an adolescent 10 years after surgical correction for truncus arteriosus. Pediatrics 1995;5:944–948.
3. Andersson S, Larinkari U, Vartia T, Forsblom B, Saarela M, Rautio M, Seppälä I, Schildt R, Kivijärvi A, Haavistok H,

Jousimies-Somer H. Fatal congenital pneumonia caused by cat-derived *Pasteurella multocida*. Pediatr Infect Dis J 1994;3:74–75.

4. Avril JL, Mesnard R, Donnio P-Y. In-vitro activities of penicillin, amoxycillin and certain cephalosporins, including cefpodoxime, against human isolates of *Pasteurella multocida*. J Antimicrobiol Chemother 1991;28:473–474.

5. Bisgaard M, Heltberg O, Frederiksen W. Isolation of *Pasteurella caballi* from an infected wound on a veterinary surgeon. APMIS 1991; 99:291–294.

6. Braithwaite BD, Giddins G. *Pasteurella multocida* infection of a total hip arthroplasty: A case report. J Arthroplasty 1992;7: 309–310.

7. Brivet FM, Guibert, Barthélémy P, Lepicard A, Naveau S, Dormont J. *Pasteurella multocida* sepsis after hemorrhagic shock in a cirrhotic patient: possible role of endoscopic procedures and gastrointestinal translocation. Clin Infect Dis 1994;18:842–843.

8. Brook I. Microbiology of human and animal bite wounds in children. Pediatr Infect Dis J 1987;6:29–32.

9. Burdge DR, Scheifele D, Speert DP. Serious *Pasteurella multocida* infections from lion and tiger bites. JAMA 1985;253: 3296–3297.

10. Caldeira L, Dutschmann L, Carmo G, Abreu J, Sousa G. Fatal *Pasteurella multocida* infection in a systemic lupus erythematosus patient. Infection 1993;4:254–255.

11. Carr RJ, Gonzalez G, Lin T. Fatal *Pasteurella* septicemia associated with herpes zoster lesions. J Am Board Fam Pract 1994; 7:245–247.

12. Chevalier X, Martigny J, Avouac B, Larget-Piet B. Report of 4 cases of *Pasteurella multocida* septic arthritis. J Rheumatol 1991;18:1890–1892.

13. Chua J, Spelman D. Animal bites and infections. Aust Fam Physician 1989;18:1010–1012.

14. Cook PP. Persistent postoperative wound infection with *Pasteurella multocida:* case report and literature review. Infect 1995;23:252.

15. Corredoira JC, Viladrich PF, Verdaguer R, Gudiol F. Soft-tissue *Pasteurella multocida* infection caused by a fish bone puncture. Eur J Clin Microbiol Infect Dis 1990;1:155–156.

16. Cuadrado-Gómez LM, Arranz-Caso JA, Cuadros-Gonzalez J, Albarran-Hernandez R. *Pasteurella pneumotropica* pneumonia in a patient with AIDS. Clin Infect Dis 1995;21:445–446.

17. Dammeijer PF, McCombe AW. Meningitis from canine *Pasteurella multocida* following mastoidectomy. J Laryngol Otol 1991;105:571–572.

18. De Ley J, Mannheim W, Mutters R, Piechulla K, Tytgat R, Segers P, Bisgaard M, Frederiksen W, Hinz K-H, Vanhoucke N. Inter- and intrafamilial similarities of rRNA cistrons of the *Pasteurellaceae*. Int J Syst Bacteriol 1990;40:126–137.

19. Desai SS, Groves RJ, Glew R. Subacute *Pasteurella* osteomyelitis of the hand following dog bite. Orthopedics 1990;13:653–656.

20. Dewhirst FE, Paster BJ, Olsen I, Fraser GJ. Phylogeny of 54 representative strains of species in the family *Pasteurellaceae* as determined by comparison of 16S rRNA sequences. J Bacteriol 1992;174:2002–2013.

21. Dibb WL, Digranes A. Characteristics of 20 human *Pasteurella* isolates from animal bite wounds. Acta Path Microbiol Scand (B) 1981;89:127–141.

22. Drabick JJ, Gassner RA Jr, Saunders NB, Hadfield TL, Rogers LC, Berg BW, Drabick CJ. *Pasteurella multocida* pneumonia in a man with AIDS and nontraumatic feline exposure. Chest 1993;103:7–11.

23. Dryden MS, Dalgiesh D. *Pasteurella multocida* from a dog causing Ludwig's angina. Lancet 1996;347:123.

24. El-Gadi SMA, Estreich S, Davidson EAF. Syphilitic aortic aneurysm and squamous cell carcinoma of the penis: a case report. Int J STD AIDS 1995;6:356–360.

25. Ellenbaas RM, McNabney WK, Robinson WA. Prophylactic oxacillin in dog bite wounds. Ann Emerg Med 1982;11: 248–251.

26. Ernst AA, Sanders WM. A case of unexpected *Pasteurella multocida* bacteremia. J Emerg Med 1990;8:437–440.

27. Fajfar-Whetstone CJT, Coleman L, Biggs DR, Fox BC. *Pasteurella multocida* septicemia and subsequent *Pasteurella dagmatis* septicemia in a diabetic patient. J Clin Microbiol 1995; 33:202–204.

28. Fahmy FS, Morgan MS, Saxby PJ. *Pasteurella* tenosynovitis following a dog bite. Injury 1994;25:262–263.

29. Fernández-Esparrach G, Mascaro J, Rota R, Valerio L. Septicemia, peritonitis, and empyema due to *Pasteurella multocida* in a cirrhotic patient. Clin Infect Dis 1994;18:486.

30. Francis DP, Holmes MA, Brandon G. *Pasteurella multocida* infections after domestic animal bites and scratches. JAMA 1975; 233:42–45.

31. Georghiou PR, Mollee TF, Tilse MH. *Pasteurella multocida* infection after a Tasmanian devil bite. Clin Infect Dis 1992;14: 1266–1267.

32. Goldstein EJC, Citron DM, Wield B, Blachman U, Sutter VL, Miller TA, Finegold SM. Bacteriology of human and animal bite wounds. J Clin Microbiol 1978;8:667–672.

33. Goldstein EJC, Citron DM, Vagvolgyi AE, Finegold SM. Susceptibility of bite wound bacteria to seven oral antimicrobial agents, including RU-985, a new erythromycin: considerations in choosing empiric therapy. Antimicrob Agents Chemother 1986;29:556–559.

34. Goldstein EJC, Citron DM, Richwald GA. Lack of in vitro efficacy of oral forms of certain cephalosporins, erythromycin, and oxacillin against *Pasteurella multocida*. Antimicrob Agents Chemother 1988;32:213–215.

35. Goldstein EJC, Citron DM. Comparative activities of cefuroxime, amoxicillin-clavulanic acid, ciprofloxacin, enoxacin, and ofloxacin against aerobic and anaerobic bacteria isolated from bite wounds. Antimicrob Agents Chemother 1988;32:1143–1148.

36. Goldstein EJC. Bite wounds and infections. Clin Infect Dis 1992;14:633–640.

37. Goldstein EJC, Citron DM. Comparative susceptibilities of 173 aerobic and anaerobic bite wound isolates to sparfloxacin, temafloxacin, clarithromycin, and older agents. Antimicrob Agents Chemother 1993;37:1150–1153.

38. Goldstein EJC, Nesbitt CA, Citron DM. Comparative in vitro activities of azithromycin, Bay y3118, levofloxacin, sparfloxacin, and 11 other oral antimicrobial agents against 194 aerobic and anaerobic bite wound isolates. Antimicrob Agents Chemother 1995;39:1097–100.

39. Goldstein EJC, Citron DM, Hunt Gerardo S, Hudspeth M, Merriam CV. Comparative in vitro activity of DU-6859a, levofloxacin, ofloxacin, sparfloxacin, and ciprofloxacin against 387 aerobic and anaerobic bite wound isolates. Antimicrob Agents Chemother 1997;41:1193–1195.

40. Goldstein EJC, Citron DM, Hudspeth MK, Hunt Gerardo S, Merriam CV. In vitro activity of Bay 12–8039, a new 8-methoxy quinolone, compared to 11 other oral antimicrobial agents against 390 aerobic and anaerobic human and animal bite wound isolates. Antimicrob Agents Chemother 1997;41(7):1552–1557.

41a. Goldstein EJC, Citron Om, Hunt Gerardo S, Hindspeth M, Merriam CV. Activities of HMR (RU 64004) and HMR 3647 (RU 66647) compared to those of erythromycin, azithromycin, clarithromycin, roxithromycin, and eight other antimicrobial agents unusual aerobic and anaerobic human and animal bite pathogens isolated from skin and soft tissue infections in humans. Antimicrob Agents Chemother 1988;42 (b);1127–1132.

41b. Goldstein EJC, Citron DM, Hudspeth MK, Hunt Gerardo S, Merriam CV. Trovafloxacin compared to levofloxacin, ofloxacin, ciprofloxacin, azithromycin, and clarithromycin against unusual aerobic and anaerobic human and animal bite wound pathogens. J Antimicrob Chemother. 1998;41:391–396.

42. Goldstein RW, Goodhart G. *Pasteurella multocida* infection after animal bite. N Engl J Med 1986;315:460.

43. Gómez-Reino JJ, Shah M, Gorevic P, Lusskin R. *Pasteurella multocida* arthritis. J Bone Joint Surg 1980;62A:1212–1213.

44. Guion TL, Sculco TR. *Pasteurella multocida* infection in total knee arthroplasty. J Arthroplasty 1992;7:157–160.

45. Heaton PAJ. *Pasteurella multocida* infection complicating nontuberculous mycobacterial lymphadenitis. Pediatr Infect Dis J 1995;14:157.

46. Henderson JAM, Rowsell HC. Fatal *Pasteurella multocida* pneumonia in an IgA-deficient cat fancier. West J Med 1989;150: 208–210.

47. Ho AC, Rapauno CJ. *Pasteurella multocida* keratitis and cor-neal laceration from a cat scratch. Ophthalmic Surg 1993;24: 346–348.

48. Holloway WJ, Scott EG, Adams YB. *Pasteurella multocida* infection in man. Am J Clin Pathol 1969;51:705–708.

49. Holst E, Rollof J, Miörner H. In vitro activities of cefcanel and some other cephalosporins against *Pasteurella multocida*. Antimicrob Agents Chemother 1989;33:2142–2143.

50. Holst E, Rollof J, Larsson L, Nielsen JP. Characterization and distribution of *Pasteurella* species recovered from infected humans. J Clin Microbiol 1992;30:2984–2987.

51. Hombal SM, Dincsoy HP. *Pasteurella multocida* endocarditis. Am J Clin Pathol 1992;98:565–568.

52. Hubbert WT, Rosen MN. I. *Pasteurella multocida* infection due to animal bite. Am J Public Health 1970;60:1103–1108.

53. Hubbert WT, Rosen MN. *Pasteurella multocida* infection in man unrelated to animal bite. Am J Public Health 1970;60: 1109–1117.

54. Ip M, Teo JGC, Cheng AFB. Waterhouse-Friderichsen syndrome complicating primary biliary sepsis due to *Pasteurella multocida* in a patient with cirrhosis. J Clin Pathol 1995;48: 775–777.

55. Kaka S, Lung R, Klugman KP. *Actinobacillus* (*Pasteurella*) *ureae* meningitis in an HIV-positive patient. Diagn Microbiol Infect Dis 1994;20:105–107.

56. Koch CA, Mabee CL, Robyn JA, Koletar S, Metz EN. Exposure to domestic cats: risk factor for *Pasteurella multocida* peritonitis in liver cirrhosis? Am J Gastroenterol 1996;91:1447–1449.

57. Kumar A, Kannampuzha P. Septic arthritis due to *Pasteurella multocida*. South Med J 1992;85:329–330.

58. Levin JM, Talan DA. Erythromycin failure with subsequent *Pasteurella multocida* meningitis and septic arthritis in a cat-bite victim. Ann Emerg Med 1990;19:1458–1461.

59. Li Z, Ahao B, Feng Z. Brain abscess due to *Pasteurella multocida*. Kansenshogaku Zasshi 1994;68:403–406.

60. Lion C, Conroy MC, Dupuy ML, Escande F. *Pasteurella* "SP" group infection after a guinea pig bite. Lancet 1995;346: 901–902.

61. London RD, Bottone EJ. *Pasteurella multocida*: zoonotic cause of peritonitis in a patient undergoing peritoneal dialysis. Am J Med 1991;91:202–204.

62. Machiels P, Haxhe J-P, Triguax J-P, Delos M, Shoevaerdts J-C, Vandenplas O. Chronic lung abscess due to *Pasteurella multocida*. Thorax 1995;50:1017–1018.

63. Majeed H, Verghese A, Rivera RR. The cat and the catheter. N Engl J Med 1995;332:338.

64. Miller JJ, Gray BM. *Pasteurella multocida* meningitis presenting as fever without a source in a young infant. Pediatr Infect Dis J 1995;14:331–332.

65. Minton EJ. *Pasteurella pneumotropica*: meningitis following a dog bite. Postgrad Med J 1990;66:125–126.

66. Morris JT, McAllister CK. Bacteremia due to *Pasteurella multocida*. South Med J 1992;85:442–443.

67. Murray AE, Mills SF. Rapid development of shock following cat scratch injury in a previously fit middle aged woman. J Infect 1991;22:307–308.

68. Mutters R, Piechulla K, Hinz K-H, Mannheim W. *Pasteurella avium* (Hinz and Kunjara 1977) comb. nov. and *Pasteurella volantium* sp. nov. Int J Syst Bacteriol 1985;35:5–9.

69. Mutters R, Ihm P, Pohl S, Frederiksen W, Mannheim W. Reclassification of the genus *Pasteurella* Trevisan 1887 on the basis of deoxyribonucleic acid homology, with proposals for the new species *Pasteurella dagmatis, Pasteurella canis, Pasteurella stomatis, Pasteurella anatis*, and *Pasteurella langaa*. Int J Syst Bacteriol 1985;35:309–322.

70. Orton DW. *Pasteurella multocida*: bilateral septic knee joint prosthesis from a distant cat bite. Ann Emerg Med 1984;13: 1065–1067.

71. Parry CM, Cheesbrough JS, O'Sullivan G. Meningitis due to *Pasteurella multocida*. Rev Infect Dis 1991;13:187.

72. Pouëdras P, Donnio PY, Tulzo YL, Avril JL. *Pasteurella stomatis* infection following a dog bite. Eur J Clin Microbiol Infect Dis 1993;12:65.

73. Ramdeen GD, Smith RJ, Smith EA, Baddour LM. *Pasteurella multocida* tonsillitis: case report and review. Clin Infect Dis 1995;20:1055–1057.

74. Rapp MF, Potter CR, Graham DR. *Pasteurella multocida* otitis media complicated by facial palsy. Otolaryngol Head Neck Surg 1990;102:290–292.

75. Richards CAL, Emmanuel FXS. Treatment of *Pasteurella multocida* cellulitis with ciprofloxacin. J Infect 1992;24: 216–217.

76. Robinson JD, Kosoko O, Mason RP, Cowan CL. *Pasteurella multocida* corneal ulcer following a baseball injury. J Natl Med Assoc 1989;5:609–610.

77. Rosenau A, Labigne A, Escande F, Courcoux P, Philippon A. Plasmid-mediated ROB-1 β-lactamase in *Pasteurella multocida* from a human specimen. Antimicrob Agents Chemother 1991; 35:2419–2422.

78. Rowe J, Mikuta J. Cat-scratch salpingitis. N Engl J Med 1992; 327:1395–1396.

79. Ruiz-Irastorza G, Garea C, Alonso JJ, Hernandez JL, Aguirrebengoa K, Alonso J, Aguirre C. Septic shock due to *Pasteurella multocida* subspecies *multocida* in a previously healthy woman. Clin Infect Dis 1995;21:232–234.

80. Rydberg J, White P. *Pasteurella multocida* as a cause of acute epiglottitis. Lancet 1993;341:381.

81. Sands M, Ashley R, Brown R. Trimethoprim/sulfamethoxazole therapy of *Pasteurella multocida* infection. J Infect Dis 1989; 160:353–354.

82. Schlater LK, Brenner DJ, Steigerwalt AG, Moss CW, Lambert MA, Packer RA. *Pasteurella caballi,* a new species from equine clinical specimens. J Clin Microbiol 1989;27:2169–2174.

83. Shewring DJ, Rushforth GF. A bizarre postoperative wound infection. Br Med J 1990;300:1557.

84. Shikuma CC, Overturf GD. Antibiotic susceptibility of *Pasteurella multocida*. Eur J Clin Microbiol 1985;4:518–519.

85. Sneath PHA, Stevens M. *Actinobacillus rossii* sp. nov., *Actinobacillus seminis* sp. nov., nom. rev., *Pasteurella bettii* sp. nov., *Pasteurella lymphangitidis* sp. nov., *Pasteurella mairi* sp. nov., and *Pasteurella trehalosi* sp. nov. Int J Syst Bacteriol 1990; 40(2):148–153.

86. Snipes KP, Biberstein EL. *Pasteurella testudinis* sp. nov.: a parasite of desert tortoises (*Gopherus agassizi*). Int J Syst Bacteriol 1982;32:201–210.

87. Stevens DK, Higbee JW, Oberhoffer TR, Everett ED. Antibiotic susceptibilities of human isolates of *Pasteurella multocida*. Antimicrob Agents Chemother 1979;16:322–324.

88. Talbodec N, Bottelin E, Boruchowicz A, Merlier O, Paris J-C, Colombel J-F. Splenic abscess associated with *Pasteurella multocida* in an immunocompetent patient. J Clin Gastroenterol 1995;21:76–78.

89. Teng FY, Cardone JT, Au AH. *Pasteurella multocida* tuboovarian abscess in a virgin. Obstet Gynecol 1996;87(5 Pt 2):883.

90. Thorsen P, Møller BR, Arpi M, Bremmelgaard A, Frederiksen W. *Pasteurella aerogenes* isolated from stillbirth and mother. Lancet 1994;343:485–486.

91. Vartian CV, Septimus EJ. Endophthalmitis due to *Pasteurella multocida* and CDC EF-4. J Infect Dis 1989;160:733.

92. Waldor M, Roberts D, Kazajian. In utero infection due to *Pasteurella multocida* in the first trimester of pregnancy: case report and review. Clin Infect Dis 1992;14:497–500.

93. Weber DJ, Hansen AR. Infections resulting from animal bites. Infect Dis Clin North Am 1991;5:663–680.

94. Weber DJ, Wolfson JS, Swartz MN, Hooper DC. *Pasteurella multocida* infections. Report of 34 cases and review of the literature. Medicine 1984;63:133–154.

95. Wilson MA, Duncan RM, Nordholm GE, Berlowski BM. Serotypes and DNA fingerprint profiles of *Pasteurella multocida* isolated from raptors. Avian Dis 1995;39:94–99.

96. Wilson MA, Duncan RM, Nordholm GE, Berlowski BM. *Pasteurella multocida* isolated from wild birds of North America: a serotype and DNA fingerprint study of isolates from 1978 to 1993. Avian Dis 1995;587–593.

97. Wong GP, Cinolai N, Dimmick JE, Martin TR. *Pasteurella multocida* chorioamnionitis from vaginal transmission. Acta Obstet Gynecol Scand 1992;71:384–387.

98. Yedwab B, Carmichael JK, Grenet E. Pneumonia caused by *Pasteurella multocida*. J Fam Pract 1990;31:313–314.

99. Zbinden R, Sommerhalder P, von Wartburg U. Co-isolation of *Pasteurella dagmatis* and *Pasteurella multocida* from cat-bite wounds. Eur J Clin Microbiol Infect Dis 1988;7:203–204.

100. Zhao G, Galina L, Hanyanun W, Pijoan C. Human tonsillitis associated with porcine *Pasteurella multocida* infection. Lancet 1993;342:491.

Plesiomonas shigelloides

●

Selwyn D. R. Lang and Arthur J. Morris

GENERAL DESCRIPTION
Microbiology and Epidemiology

Plesiomonas shigelloides was previously known as *Aeromonas shigelloides*. The genus name *Plesiomonas* is derived from the Greek for "neighbor," reflecting that it was considered to be related to the genus *Aeromonas* where it once resided. More-recent studies have shown it to be more closely related to *Proteus* spp. (28). Other names have included C27, *Pseudomonas shigelloides, Vibrio shigelloides,* and *Fergusonia shigelloides* (13). *Plesiomonas shigelloides* is the only species in the genus.

Plesiomonas shigelloides is a motile, facultatively anaerobic, Gram-negative, oxidase-positive, nitrate-reducing bacillus (23). It possesses two to five polar flagella. It grows readily on enteric agars such as MacConkey, deoxycholate, and Hektoen as a lactose nonfermenter. Its positive oxidase reaction distinguishes it from the *Enterobacteriaceae*. A positive ornithine decarboxylase differentiates it from most *Aeromonas* spp. and fermentation of inositol differentiates it from both *Aeromonas* spp. and *Vibrio* spp. (23). Many different enrichment methods have been used in attempts to increase the recovery of *P. shigelloides* from stool (37). In one study the best yield was obtained following 24-h enrichment in bile-peptone broth (37). Using this method, 4% of patients with diarrhea in Bangladesh have *P. shigelloides* recovered as the sole bacterial pathogen (47). Such a high rate, however, is clearly location dependent.

Asymptomatic stool carriage in adults is rare, and *P. shigelloides* is not considered part of the normal human gastrointestinal flora. It has been recovered from both fresh and salt water. Infection has been associated with ingestion of seafood (18, 22, 24, 29); untreated water (24); travel, especially to Mexico, Central America and Southeast Asia (18, 24); and trauma involving either water exposure (8, 9) or fish handling (13, 15). Neonatal infection is thought to follow perinatal exposure. Some mothers of infected neonates have been shown to have infection or genital colonization with *P. shigelloides*. Other mothers with infected infants had recently consumed uncooked seafood (2, 27, 46). Dual infection with *Aeromonas* sp. also indicates water and soil are the environmental niche for *P. shigelloides* (9).

Clinical Manifestations

Most infections are either gastrointestinal or a septicemic illness that in neonates is often accompanied by meningitis. Most

TABLE 1 • In Vitro Susceptibilities of *Plesiomonas shigelloides*

Antibiotic	n	Range	MIC$_{50}$	MIC$_{90}$	Breakpoint[a]	% Susceptible	Ref.
Amdinocillin	4	≤0.5–32	≤0.5	1			5
Amoxicillin	29	0.06–≥64	64	≥128	≤8	7	7
Amoxicillin	14	1–>32	>32	>32	≤8		1
Amoxicillin-clavulanate	29	≤0.06/0.03–8/4	2/1	4/2	≤8/4	100	7
Ampicillin	17	2–32	8	16	≤8		38
Ampicillin	72	32–≥256	128	256	≤8	0	25
Ampicillin	29	0.25–≥128	≥128	≥128	≤8	3	7
Ampicillin	4	8–32	8	8	≤8		5
Ampicillin-sulbactam	29	0.25/0.12–4/2	1/0.5	2/1	≤8/4	100	7
Piperacillin	72	8–≥256	≥256	≥256	≤16	3	25
Piperacillin	29	≤0.06–≥64	64	≥128	≤16	7	7
Piperacillin-tazobactam	29	≤0.06/0.0075–1/0.125	0.25/0.03	1/0.125	≤16/4	100	7
Ticarcillin	72	64–≥128	≥128	≥128	≤16	0	25
Ticarcillin	29	0.5–≥128	≥128	≥128	≤16	4	7
Ticarcillin-clavulanate	29	0.5/2–4/2	1/2	2/2	≤16/2	100	7
Mezlocillin	29	0.125–≥128	≥128	≥128	≤16	14	7
Carbenicillin	72	128–≥512	256	512	≤16	0	25
Cefaclor	14	0.5–4	1	1	≤8	100	1
Cefamandole	72	≤1–4	≤1	≤1	≤8	100	25
Cefamandole	29	≤0.06–0.5	≤0.06	0.25	≤8	100	7
Cefazolin	72	≤1–8	≤1	≤1	≤8	100	25
Cefetamet	14	≤0.06–0.12	≤0.06	0.12			1
Cefoperazone	72	≤1–8	≤1	≤1	≤16	100	25
Cefoperazone	29	≤0.06–8	1	4	≤16	100	7
Cefoperazone-sulbactam	29	≤0.06/0.03–0.5/0.25	0.125/0.06	0.25/0.125	≤16/8	100	7
Cefotaxime	17	≤0.063–0.125	≤0.063	≤0.063	≤8	100	38
Cefotaxime	72	≤8	≤8	≤8	≤8	100	25
Cefotaxime	29	≤0.06–4	≤0.06	≤0.06	≤8	100	7
Cefoxitin	72	≤4	≤4	≤4	≤8	100	25
Cefoxitin	29	1–4	2	4	≤8	100	7
Ceftazidime	72	≤1	≤1	≤1	≤8	100	25
Ceftazidime	29	≤0.06–1	≤0.06	≤0.06	≤8	100	7
Ceftriaxone	72	≤1	≤1	≤1	≤8	100	25
Ceftriaxone	29	≤0.06	≤0.06	≤0.06	≤8	100	7
Cefuroxime	29	≤0.06–0.125	≤0.06	≤0.06	≤8	100	7
Cephalexin	14	2–16	4	8			1
Cephalothin	72	≤8	≤8	≤8	≤8	100	25
Cephalothin	29	0.5–2	1	2	≤8	100	7
Aztreonam	29	≤0.06	≤0.06	≤0.06	≤8	100	7
Imipenem	29	≤0.06–0.25	≤0.06	0.125	≤4	100	7
Chloramphenicol	17	0.25–8	0.5	1	≤8	100	38
Chloramphenicol	72	≤4	≤4	≤4	≤8	100	25
Ciprofloxacin	17	≤0.063	≤0.063	≤0.063	≤1	100	38
Ciprofloxacin	72	≤1	≤1	≤1	≤1	100	25
Ciprofloxacin	29	≤0.06	≤0.06	≤0.06	≤1	100	7
Ciprofloxacin	<19	<0.001–0.015	0.004	0.008	≤1	100	3
Ciprofloxacin	13	≤0.06	≤0.06	≤0.06	≤1	100	20
Enoxacin	17	≤0.063–0.25	≤0.063	0.125	≤2	100	38
Enoxacin	4	≤0.5	≤0.5	≤0.5	≤2	100	5
Enoxacin	<19	0.03–0.125	0.06	0.125	≤2	100	3
Norfloxacin	17	≤0.063–0.125	≤0.063	≤0.063			38
Norfloxacin	72	≤0.1–1	≤0.1	≤0.1			25
Norfloxacin	4	≤0.5	≤0.5	≤0.5			5
Norfloxacin	<19	<0.015–0.06	0.03	0.06			3
Ofloxacin	<19	0.008–0.03	0.015	0.015	≤2	100	3
Pefloxacin	<19	<0.015–0.06	0.015	0.06			3
Pipemidic acid	<19	0.125–0.5	0.125	0.25			3
Erythromycin	72	4–32	16	16	≤0.5	0	25
Erythromycin	4	16–32	32	32	≤0.5	0	5
Erythromycin	13	0.5–14	1	4	≤0.5		20
Furazolidone	4	≤0.5	≤0.5	≤0.5			5
Amikacin	72	8–64	16	32	≤16	54	25
Amikacin	29	≤0.06–16	0.25	8	≤16	100	7
Gentamicin	17	2–8	4	8	≤4		38

continued

TABLE 1 • **In Vitro Susceptibilities of *Plesiomonas shigelloides***

Antibiotic	n	Range	MIC$_{50}$	MIC$_{90}$	Breakpoint[a]	% Susceptible	Ref.
Gentamicin	72	4–16	4	6	≤8	57	25
Gentamicin	29	1–8	4	8	≤4	86	7
Gentamicin	13	2–12	3	10	≤4		20
Tobramycin	72	4–8	4	6	≤4	36	25
Tobramycin	29	≤0.06–8	≤0.06	1	≤4	97	7
Kanamycin	13	0.4–10	0.6	8	≤16	100	20
Netilmicin	72	2–4	4	4	≤8	100	25
Nalidixic acid	17	0.25–2	0.5	0.5			38
Nalidixic acid	<19	0.5–2	1	2			3
Doxycycline	4	≤0.5	≤0.5	≤0.5	≤4	100	5
Tetracycline	17	0.25–2	0.5	0.5	≤4	100	38
Tetracycline	72	≤1–64	≥1	32	≤4	68	25
Tetracycline	13	0.25–2.4	0.5	1	≤4	100	20
Trimethoprim-sulfamethoxazole[b]	17	≤0.063–0.125	0.125	0.125	≤2/38	100	38
Trimethoprim-sulfamethoxazole[b]	72	≤0.1–0.5	≤0.1	0.5	≤2/38	100	25
Trimethoprim-sulfamethoxazole[b]	4	0.05	0.05	0.05	≤2/38	100	5
Trimethoprim	17	0.25–4	1	4			38
Trimethoprim	72	≤1	≤1	≤1	≤8	100	25
Trimethoprim	4	≤0.5–2	≤0.5	≤0.5			5
Sulfisoxazole	72	≤32–≥512	32	256			25
Sulfamethoxazole	17	4.75–19	9.5	19			38
Bicozamycin	4	16	16	16			5

Modified from references 1, 3, 5, 7, 20, 25, 38

[a]Current NCCLS interpretive standards for susceptibility (μg/ml) (32).

[b]Trimethoprim-sulfamethoxazole tested in a ratio of 1:19. The concentration refers to the trimethoprim component.

reports have concerned gastrointestinal infections (4, 18, 22, 24, 29, 33). Diarrheal disease ranges from a secretory-type to one compatible with invasive infection, although the pathogenic mechanisms are not known (17, 18, 24). Disease occurs within 2 days of ingesting uncooked seafood (18), and most develop the disease within 5 days of consuming untreated water or infected seafood (24). Disease resolves slowly, with a mean duration of 11 days in one study (18). In another study 76 and 36% of patients were symptomatic for more than 2 and 4 weeks, respectively (24). Symptoms vary but include abdominal pain or cramps (84–100%), nausea and/or vomiting (32–40%), headache and dehydration (32%), and fever (18–30%) (18, 24). Although bacteremia has been reported in association with intestinal infection, this is uncommon (10, 22, 31, 33, 35, 40).

Approximately 80% of patients with *P. shigelloides* bacteremia have been immunocompromised either by age (i.e., neonates), hyposplenism due to either splenectomy or sickle cell disease, or alcoholic liver disease (8, 10, 13, 16, 21, 27, 31, 40). Survival of bacteremia is more common in those considered immunocompetent (~75%) than in the immunocompromised (~30%) (27).

Meningitis is virtually restricted to infants (2, 11, 12, 34, 41); however, at least one case of meningitis has been reported in an adult (19). Meningoencephalitis is also reported (42). Other types of infection (many of which have accompanied bacteremia) are not common but include biliary tract infection and cholecystitis (6, 26), small bowel overgrowth syndrome (36), endophthalmitis (9), septic arthritis (16, 22), cellulitis with or without compartment syndrome (13, 15, 30), infected pleural effusion (21), pyometria (45), and osteomyelitis (22).

SUSCEPTIBILITY IN VITRO

The results of seven in vitro studies are summarized in Table 1. *P. shigelloides* is usually susceptible to chloramphenicol, trimethoprim-sulfamethoxazole, the quinolones, cephalosporins, aztreonam, and imipenem (3, 4, 7, 18, 20, 25, 38, 43, 44, 47). Tetracycline and aminoglycoside susceptibility is variable. In six studies, the proportion of strains susceptible to tetracycline ranged from 39 to 100%, median 89% (18, 20, 25, 38, 43, 47). For gentamicin, 50 to 100% of strains are susceptible (7, 18, 20, 25, 38, 43, 47); for tobramycin, 36 to 97% (7, 25); for amikacin, between 54 and 100% (7, 25, 43); and for netilmicin, 94 to 100% (25, 43). Activity in the combination agent trimethoprim-sulfamethoxazole is essentially due to the trimethoprim component alone (18, 25, 39). Production of a β-lactamase that confers resistance to penicillin, ampicillin, amoxicillin, carbenicillin, ticarcillin, and piperacillin is essentially invariable (4, 7, 18, 25, 39). Addition of a β-lactamase inhibitor—clavulanate, sulbactam, or tazobactam—restores susceptibility to amoxicillin, ampicillin, and piperacillin, respectively (7).

ANTIMICROBIAL THERAPY

Gastroenteritis has developed in patients taking ampicillin for reasons other than diarrhea (18). This observation and the organism's β-lactamase production means this class of agent should not be used for therapy for any type of infection caused by *P. shigelloides*. Patients with *P. shigelloides* diarrhea have improvement or resolution of their symptoms after taking an antimicrobial agent to which the strain is susceptible (4, 18, 24, 31, 39). Norfloxacin or trimethoprim are recommended for gastrointestinal infection; however, there are no prospective trial data to indicate how therapy may improve symptoms.

Antimicrobial therapy with local debridement if necessary is required for a successful outcome in extraintestinal disease. If treatment with a cephalosporin (with or without an aminoglycoside) is ineffective, consider using ciprofloxacin. Ciprofloxacin brought about prompt lysis of fever in an infected bone marrow transplant patient who had failed to respond to combination therapy with amikacin and ceftazidime (27).

Although neonatal infection with *P. shigelloides* has a 50% mortality, most infants who survive do so without sequelae (14); in this review of 10 cases of neonatal septicemia and meningitis, only 1 of 5 survivors suffered sequelae. This infant developed extensive multilocular brain cysts and lack of sensory evoked potentials and died when respiratory support was withdrawn (42). Cefotaxime appears to be the treatment of choice for neonatal septicemia and meningitis due to *P. shigelloides*. Four of 10 patients who received cefotaxime alone or as a component of the initial treatment regimen survived, whereas 5 of the remaining 6 who initially received regimens not including cefotaxime (commonly ampicillin plus aminoglycoside) died (14). Addition of aminoglycoside, to which the isolate has been shown to be susceptible, or therapy with ciprofloxacin could be considered if response to cefotaxime alone is poor.

REFERENCES

1. Angehrn P, Hohl P, Then RL. In vitro antibacterial properties of cefetamet and in vivo activity of its orally absorbable ester derivative, cefetamet pivoxil. Eur J Clin Microbiol Infect Dis 1989;8: 536–543.
2. Appelbaum PC, Bowen AJ, Adhikari M, Robins-Browne RM, Koornhof HF. Neonatal septicemia and meningitis due to *Aeromonas shigelloides*. J Pediatr 1978;92:676–677.
3. Auckenthaler R, Michea-Hamzehpour M, Pechere JC. In-vitro activity of newer quinolones against aerobic bacteria. J Antimicrob Chemother 1986;17(Suppl B):29–39.
4. Brenden RA, Miller MA, Janda JM. Clinical disease spectrum and pathogenic factors associated with *Plesiomonas shigelloides* infections in humans. Rev Infect Dis 1988;10:303–316.
5. Carlson JR, Thornton SA, DuPont HL, West AH, Mathewson JJ. Comparative in vitro activities of ten antimicrobial agents against bacterial enteropathogens. Antimicrob Agents Chemother 1983; 24:509–513.
6. Claesson BEB, Holmlund DEW, Lindhagen CA, Matzsch TW. *Plesiomonas shigelloides* in acute cholecystitis: a case report. J Clin Microbiol 1984;20:985–987.
7. Clark RB, Lister PD, Arneson-Rotert L, Janda JM. In vitro susceptibilities of *Plesiomonas shigelloides* to 24 antibiotics and antibiotic-β-lactamase-inhibitor combinations. Antimicrob Agents Chemother 1990;34:159–160.
8. Clark RB, Westby GR, Spector H, Soricelli RR, Young CL. Fatal *Plesiomonas shigelloides* septicaemia in a splenectomised patient. J Infect 1991;23:89–92.
9. Cohen KL, Holyk PR, McCarthy LR, Peiffer RL. *Aeromonas hydrophila* and *Plesiomonas shigelloides* endophthalmitis [Letter]. Am J Ophthalmol 1983;96:403–404.
10. Curti AJ, Lin JH, Szabo K. Overwhelming post-splenectomy infection with *Plesiomonas shigelloides* in a patient cured of Hodgkins disease. Am J Clin Pathol 1985;83:522–524.
11. Dahm LJ, Weinberg AG. *Plesiomonas (Aeromonas) shigelloides* septicemia and meningitis in the neonate. South Med J 1980;73:393–394.
12. Dudley AG, Mays W, Sale L. *Plesiomonas (Aeromonas) shigelloides* meningitis in a neonate—a case report. J Med Assoc Ga 1982;71:775–776.
13. Ellner PD, McCarthy LR. *Aeromonas shigelloides* bacteremia: a case report. Am J Clin Pathol 1973;59:216–218.
14. Fujita K, Shirai M, Ishioka T, Kakuya F. Neonatal *Plesiomonas shigelloides* septicemia and meningitis: a case and review. Acta Paediatr Jpn 1994;36:450–452.
15. Gopal V, Burns FE. Cellulitis and compartment syndrome due to *Plesiomonas shigelloides:* a case report. Milit Med 1991; 156:43.
16. Gordon DL, Philpot CR, McGuire C. *Plesiomonas shigelloides* septic arthritis complicating rheumatoid arthritis. Aust NZ J Med 1983;13:275–276.
17. Herrington DA, Tzipori S, Robins-Browne RM, Tall BD, Levine MM. In vitro and in vivo pathogenicity of *Plesiomonas shigelloides*. Infect Immun 1987;55:979–985.
18. Holmberg SD, Wachsmuth IK, Hickman-Brenner FW, Blake PA, Farmer JJ III. *Plesiomonas* enteric infections in the United States. Ann Intern Med 1986;105:690–694.
19. Horst H, Kohlhase B, Konopatzki I. Eitrige meningitis durch *Plesiomonas shigelloides*. Dtsch Med Wochenschr 1982;107: 1238–1239.
20. Hossain MS, Hossain A. Effect of antibiotics on serum bactericidal action on *Plesiomonas shigelloides* by normal human serum. Bangladesh Med Res Counc Bull 1994;20:117–122.
21. Humphreys, H, Keogh B, Keane CT. Septicemia and pleural effusion due to *Plesiomonas shigelloides*. Postgrad Med J 1986; 62:663–664.
22. Ingram CW, Morrison AJ, Levitz RE. Gastroenteritis, sepsis, and osteomyelitis caused by *Plesiomonas shigelloides* in an immunocompetent host: case report and review of the literature. J Clin Microbiol 1987;25:1791–1793.
23. Janda JM, Abbott SL, Carnahan AM. *Aeromonas* and *Plesiomonas*. In: Murray PR, Barron EJ, Pfaller MA, Tenover FC, Yolken RH, eds. Manual of clinical microbiology. 6th ed. Washington, DC: American Society for Microbiology, 1995:477–482.
24. Kain KC, Kelly MT. Clinical features, epidemiology, and treatment of *Plesiomonas shigelloides* diarrhea. J Clin Microbiol 1989;27:998–1001.
25. Kain KC, Kelly MT. Antimicrobial susceptibility of *Plesiomonas shigelloides* from patients with diarrhea. Antimicrob Agents Chemother 1989;33:1609–1610.
26. Korner RJ, MacGowan AP, Warner B. The isolation of *Plesiomonas shigelloides* in polymicrobial septicaemia originating from the biliary tree. Zentralbl Bakt 1992;277:334–339.
27. Lee ACW, Yuen KY, Ha SY, Chiu DCK, Lau YL. *Plesiomonas shigelloides* septicemia: case report and literature review. Paed Hem Onc 1996;13:265–269.
28. MacDonell MT, Colwell RR. Phylogeny of the Vibrionaceae,

and recommendation for two new genera, *Listonella* and *Shewanella*. Syst Appl Microbiol 1985;6:171–182.

29. Martin DL, Gustafson TL. *Plesiomonas* gastroenteritis in Texas [Letter]. JAMA 1985;254:2063.

30. McCracken AW, Barkley R. Isolation of *Aeromonas* species from clinical sources. J Clin Pathol 1972;25:970–975.

31. McNeeley D, Ivy P, Craft JC, Cohen I. *Plesiomonas:* biology of the organism and diseases in children. Pediatr Infect Dis 1984;3: 176–181.

32. National Committee for Clinical Laboratory Standards. Methods for dilution antimicrobial susceptibility tests for bacteria that grow aerobically. 4th ed. Approved standard. NCCLS document M7-A4. Wayne, PA: NCCLS, 1997.

33. Nolte FS, Poole RM, Murphy GW, Clark C, Panner BJ. Proctitis and fatal septicemia caused by *Plesiomonas shigelloides* in a bisexual man. J Clin Microbiol 1988;26:388–391.

34. Pathak A, Custer JR, Levy J. Neonatal septicemia and meningitis due to *Plesiomonas shigelloides*. Pediatrics 1983;71:389–391.

35. Paul R, Siitonen A, Karkkainen P. *Plesiomonas shigelloides* bacteremia in a healthy girl with mild gastroenteritis. J Clin Microbiol 1990;28:1445–1446.

36. Penn RG, Giger DK, Knoop FC, Preheim LC. *Plesiomonas shigelloides* overgrowth in the small intestine. J Clin Microbiol 1982;15:869–872.

37. Rahim Z, Kay BA. Enrichment for *Plesiomonas shigelloides* from stools. J Clin Microbiol 1988;26:789–790.

38. Reinhardt JF, George WL. Comparative in vitro activities of selected antimicrobial agents against *Aeromonas* species and *Plesiomonas shigelloides*. Antimicrob Agents Chemother 1985;27: 643–645.

39. Reinhardt JF, George WL. *Plesiomonas shigelloides*-associated diarrhea. JAMA 1985;253:3294–3295.

40. Riley PA, Parasakthi N, Abdullah WA. *Plesiomonas shigelloides* bacteremia in a child with leukemia [Letter]. Clin Infect Dis 1996;23:206–207.

41. Su S, Ee CK. *Plesiomonas shigelloides* meningitis in newborn. Singapore Paediatr 1981;23:156–158.

42. Terpeluk C, Goldmann A, Bartmann P, Pohlandt F. *Plesiomonas shigelloides* sepsis and meningoencephalitis in a neonate. Eur J Pediatr 1992;151:499–501.

43. Visitsunthorn N, Komolpis P. Antimicrobial therapy in *Plesiomonas shigelloides*-associated diarrhea in Thai children. Southeast Asian J Trop Med Public Health 1995;26:86–90.

44. von Graevenitz A, Bucher C. The effect of *N*-formimidoyl thienamycin, ceftazidime, cefotiam, ceftriaxone and cefotaxime on non-fermentative gram-negative rods, *Aeromonas, Plesiomonas* and *Enterobacter agglomerans*. Infection 1982;10:293–298.

45. von Graevenitz A, Mensch AH. The genus *Aeromonas* in human bacteriology: report of 30 cases and review of the literature. N Engl J Med 1968;278:245–249.

46. Waecker NJ, Davis CE, Bernstein G, Spector SA. *Plesiomonas shigelloides* septicemia and meningitis in a newborn. Paediatr Infect Dis J 1988;7:877–879.

47. Zeaur R, Akbar A, Bradford AK. Prevalence of *Plesiomonas shigelloides* among diarrhoeal patients in Bangladesh. Eur J Epidemiol 1992;5:753–756.

Proteus Species

●

Edward S. Wong and Sheldon M. Markowitz

GENERAL DESCRIPTION
Microbiology

Proteus is a member of the tribe *Proteeae*, which includes *Morganella* and *Providentia*. The genus *Proteus* includes several species: *P. mirabilis, P. vulgaris, P. penneri,* and *P. myxofaciens*. *Proteus* are easily identified by biochemical characteristics that they share with other members of the tribe: positive methyl red reaction, negative Voges-Proskauer reaction, phenylalanine deaminase production, growth on KCN, and urease production (8). On culture plates, *Proteus* species are distinguished by their ability to swarm. Virtually all *P. mirabilis* strains are indole-negative. In contrast, other *Proteus* species and other members of the tribe are indole positive.

Ninety percent of the strains of *Proteus* isolated in the clinical laboratory are *P. mirabilis*. The remaining 10% are identified as either *P. vulgaris* or *P. penneri*. The latter, formerly known as indole-negative *P. vulgaris* is being identified more frequently from clinical specimens, usually as a nosocomial

pathogen (14). *P. myxofaciens* has not been associated with infections in man.

Proteus is a member of the *Enterobacteriaceae* family and a resident of the gastrointestinal tract. *P. mirabilis* can be found as normal flora in approximately 50% of randomly selected individuals. It can be found to colonize the vaginal introitus prior to onset of bacteriuria and thus, like *Escherichia coli, Proteus* causes urinary tract infections by ascending from the rectum to the periurethra and bladder (39). Not surprisingly, most common infections caused by *P. mirabilis* are urinary tract infections, both among outpatients and inpatients.

Pathogenesis

Proteus possesses several virulence factors that explain its uropathogenic potential (19). It has pili or fimbriae for adherence to uroepithelium and elaborates cytotoxic hemolysins that lyse red cells and release iron, a bacterial growth factor. Proteus possesses flagella for motility and produces urease, which spits urea and raises urinary pH. The alkaline pH promotes precipitation of magnesium-ammonium phosphate salts and formation of struvite stones. Silverman (38) observed that 40 of 46 patients with struvite stones were in fact infected with *P. mirabilis*. Once formed, stones can obstruct the urinary tract, leading to renal involvement, parenchymal damage, and possibly septicemia. Infected stones can act as a nidus for chronic persistent or recurrent infections.

Epidemiology

Most *Proteus* infections are nosocomial (1, 2, 46). The two most common risk factors associated with nosocomial urinary tract infections are indwelling Foley catheterization and genitourinary tract manipulation (2, 46). *P. mirabilis* is the causative organism for community-acquired urinary tract infections 2 to 14% of the time (11, 44). Among urinary tract infections acquired during hospitalization, *P. mirabilis* ranks seventh, accounting for 5% of nosocomial infections (35). *Proteus* is also found in postoperative wound infections, infected decubiti, and skin and skin structure infections (2). At Boston City Hospital, respiratory tract infections with *Proteus* were infrequently encountered (6%): most had underlying tracheostomy (2). One-quarter of the 116 cases of infection were associated with *Proteus* bacteremia (1). Bacteremic patients were characterized by older age (median, 64–75 years), serious underlying diseases, and recent interventions, most commonly indwelling Foley catheterization or central venous access (2, 46).

In a review of 176 cases of *Proteus* bacteremia from a large community teaching hospital, most (56.8%) patients came from a nursing home with an indwelling Foley catheter and had infected urine as the source of their bacteremia (46). In this study, overall mortality was 29%, with an attributable mortality rate of 25%.

SUSCEPTIBILITY IN VITRO
Proteus mirabilis

Chromosomal β-lactamase production in *P. mirabilis* either does not exist or is negligible; thus *P. mirabilis* is one of the most susceptible members of the *Enterobacteriaceae* family to β-lactam antibiotics (4). Ampicillin, amoxicillin, and other extended-spectrum penicillins are all active against *P. mirabilis* (Table 1). In 1971, the minimal inhibitory concentration (MIC) required to inhibit *P. mirabilis* encountered at Boston City Hospital was 3.1 and 6.3 µg/mL for 50 and 66% of the isolates, respectively (1). *P. mirabilis* can acquire resistance to ampicillin through acquisition of plasmid-mediated β-lactamases (TEM type) (21), and in some parts of the world, this is quite common (32). For example, in Jordan, only 38% of 200 clinical isolates of *P. mirabilis* tested were susceptible to ampicillin (28). In the United States, however, resistance has remained low at approximately 10% (32). In Watanakunakorn and Perni's (46) review of 176 cases of *P. mirabilis* bacteremia, 83% of the isolates were susceptible to ampicillin. In the United Kingdom, a survey of antimicrobial susceptibility patterns over an 8-year period revealed no change in the susceptibility of 638 isolates of *Proteus* to ampicillin (23). The authors did note a decline in the susceptibility to trimethoprim between 1984 and 1988, but this reversed itself by 1990.

TABLE 1 • **Comparative Activity of Antibiotics against *Proteus mirabilis***

Antibiotic	No. Isolates[a]	MIC$_{50}$	MIC$_{90}$	Reference
Ampicillin	209	3.1	—	1
	30	—	>128	15
Ticarcillin	NA	<1	<1	31
	NA	—	2	7
	617	<1	<1	10
Piperacillin	NA	—	2	7
	134	0.5	8	43
Ticarcillin/clavulanate	617	<1	<1	10
Piperacillin/tazobactam	NA	—	2	7
Amoxicillin/clavulanate	102	1	4	24
	52	1	—	36
Cephalothin	30	>128	>128	15
Cefazolin	NA	—	16	30
Cefsulodin	NA	—	>128	30
Cefaclor	102	1	8	24
Cefoxitin	10	8	16	16
Cefuroxime	102	0.5	2	24
	236	0.5	1	45
	30	—	8	15
Cefotaxime	135	0.03	0.03	43
	30	0.12	2	15
	NA	—	0.1	31
	538	0.2	—	34
Ceftriaxone	236	≤.03	≤.03	45
	NA	—	0.05	31
	102	0.5	0.5	24
Ceftazidime	236	≤.25	≤.25	45
	538	0.6	—	34
	NA	—	0.2	31
Cefoperazone	NA	—	1	31
Aztreonam	25	<0.1	<0.1	42
	10	0.125	0.125	16
Imipenem	139	2	4	43
	1398	—	4	6
Meropenem	1398	—	0.13	6
Cefepime	236	≤0.25	≤0.25	45
	538	0.04	—	34
Cepirone	538	0.06	—	34
Gentamicin	139	1	4	43
Trimethoprim/ sulfamethoxaxole	102	0.06	16	24
Ciprofloxacin	102	0.06	0.12	24
	NA	0.06	0.13	48
Ofloxacin	102	0.06	0.5	24
	NA	0.1	0.2	48
Fleroxacin	102	0.06	0.5	24
Lomefloxacin	102	0.12	0.5	24
Nalidixic acid	NA	2	8	48
Norfloxacin	NA	0.01	0.5	48
Enoxacin	NA	0.4	0.8	48

[a]NA, not available.

Resistance to ampicillin by acquisition of plasmid-mediated β-lactamases generally confers resistance to the narrow-spectrum first-generation cephalosporins and extended-spectrum penicillins, such as carbenicillin and ticarcillin, but generally does not affect the organism's susceptibility to second- or third-generation cephalosporin antibiotics. In the studies by Washington et al. (45) and Markowitz et al. (24), the MIC_{90} of cefuroxime of a combined 338 isolates of *P. mirabilis* was 2 μg/mL or less.

The third-generation cephalosporins and the recently available new cephalosporin, cefepime, are the even more active. The MIC_{50}s and MIC_{90}s of cefotaxime, ceftizoxime, cefmenoxime, cefoperazone, ceftriaxone, ceftazidime, and aztreonam against *P. mirabilis* are all less than 1 μg/mL (45). Similarly, the new "fourth-generation" cephalosporins, cefepime and cepirone, show high activity against *P. mirabilis,* with MIC_{50}s and MIC_{90}s below 1 μg/mL (45).

Imipenem is also active against *P. mirabilis*. MIC_{90}s range from 2 to 4 μg/mL (20). This is relatively high compared with the activity of other third-generation cephalosporins but still well below the breakpoint for resistance ($\geq$16 μg/mL). *P. vulgaris* as well as *Morganella morganii* and other members of Proteae tribe apparently exhibit the same phenomenon (30). The explanation for the lower activity of imipenem against *Proteus* is not known. The main target of imipenem is the penicillin-binding protein 2 (PBP-2) of bacteria. Neu (31) postulated that the lower activity of imipenem might be due to the lower number of PBP-2 sites in *Proteae*.

Since its initial recognition in 1983, resistance to third-generation antibiotics on the basis of production of extended-spectrum β-lactamases (ESBLs) has become increasingly prevalent among *Klebsiella, Enterobacter,* and other members of the *Enterobacteraciae* family (34). It is rare among *P. mirabilis* and in fact, had not been reported until Mariotte in 1994 described five isolates that were resistant to extended-spectrum cephalosporins, including the monobactam aztreonam. These isolates were susceptible to cephamycins and carbapenems, a susceptibility profile typical of ESBLs. The authors isolated a β-lactamase closely related to TEM-3/CTX-1 type from all five isolates and transferred the plasmid by conjugation experiments to *Escherichia coli*.

P. mirabilis are generally susceptible to aminoglycosides. The MIC_{50} of *P. mirabilis* to gentamicin in Adler's study from the 1970s was 0.8 μg/mL, making it the most active antibiotic against *P. mirabilis* available at that time (1). Apparently, resistance through acquisition of aminoglocoside-modifying enzymes has not occurred to any great extent among *P. mirabilis* over the years since the 1970s. Gerding (13) compared the susceptibility patterns of *P. mirabilis* to aminoglycosides over a 6-year observation period and noticed minimal change in the MICs. Overall susceptibility in this study averaged 97%.

The fluoroquinolone antibiotics are gaining increasing use. As a class, these antibiotics are very active against *P. mirabilis* with MIC_{90}s ranging from 0.1 to 0.5 μg/mL (9, 24).

Proteus vulgaris

Proteus vulgaris is much more resistant to antibiotics than *P. mirabilis*. *P. vulgaris* is usually resistant to ampicillin and first-generation cephalosporins (Table 1). It is generally susceptible to extended-spectrum carboxypenicillins and ureidopenicillins, and addition of β-lactamase inhibitors to these broad-spectrum penicillins enhances their activity. For example, addition of clavulanic acid to ticarcillin lowers the MIC_{50} and MIC_{90} from 4 and 8 μg/mL to less than 0.5 and 1 μg/mL, respectively (10).

The cephamycins, cefoxitin and cefotetan, are active against *P. vulgaris,* but cefuroxime and other second-generation cephalosporins are not (22). The activity of third- and later-generation cephalosporins is variable against *P. vulgaris*. Ceftazidime, aztreonam, and cefepime are highly active, with MIC_{50}s below 1 μg/mL, and consequently, more than 90% of isolates of *P vulgaris* tested are susceptible to these antibiotics (42, 45). The MICs of cefoperaxone, ceftriaxone, and imipenem against *P. vulgaris* are higher and consequently, a greater percentage of isolates are resistant (42, 6). In recent surveys, 30 to 35% of *P. vulgaris* tested by Markowitz (24) and Washington (45) were resistant to ceftriaxone.

P. vulgaris possesses an inducible class A chromosomal β-lactamase, which explains its variable susceptibility to β-lactam antibiotics (22). Ampicillin, amoxicillin, and first-generation cephalosporins strongly induce production of this β-lactamase, resulting in high MICs and resistance (Table 2). Extended-spectrum carboxypenicillins, ureidopencillins, cefotaxime, and ceftriaxone are weak inducers, and thus they retain activity against *P. vulgaris*. Strains of *P. vulgaris* that have a mutation in regulatory genes produce high-levels of this enzyme and are resistant to β-lactam antibiotics, even those that weakly induce β-lactamase, such as extended-spectrum penicillins and ceftriaxone.

The enzyme is not active against ceftazidime, cephamycins, or aztreonam, and these antibiotics retain their activity even against derepressed mutants that produce high levels (22). The enzyme is also susceptible to the activity of β-lactamase inhibitors, hence its classification in group 2e by Bush (3).

Aminoglycosides and fluoroquinolones are very active against *P. vulgaris* (26, 47). Ninety-seven and 99% of more than 1200 isolates of *P. vulgaris* tested in 1991 by the Institutes for Microbiology Research proved susceptible to gentamicin and ciprofloxacin, respectively (personal communication). Trimethoprim-sulfamethoxazole is also highly active, with an MIC below 0.25 μg/mL (24).

ANTIMICROBIAL THERAPY

In most clinical laboratories, isolation of *P. mirabilis* outnumbers isolation of *P. vulgaris* by a ratio of 10:1. This is fortuitous, since *P. mirabilis* is the more antibiotic susceptible of the two. *P. mirabilis* can be treated with any number of antibiotics, but the antibiotic of choice on the basis of efficacy and low cost is ampicillin (27). In most centers in the United States, 80 to 90% of *P. mirabilis* isolates are susceptible to ampicillin. Alternative antibiotics, including use in the treatment of ampicillin resistant *P. mirabilis,* include aminoglycosides, trimethoprim-sulfamethoxazole, extended-spectrum penicillins, second- or third-generation cephalosporins, and the fluoroquinolones. Third- and fourth-generation cephalosporins and quinolones are extremely active against *P. mirabilis* but are expensive compared with aminoglycosides or trimethoprim-sulfamethoxazole, and they offer no clear therapeutic advantages in treating mild to moderately severe infections, especially urinary tract infections.

Because of an inducible cephalosporinase, *P. vulgaris* are usually resistant to ampicillin, amoxicillin, and first-generation cephalosporins (22). The enzyme is also active against cefuroxime, cefotaxime, and ceftriaxone, and thus, isolates that produce

TABLE 2 • Comparative Activity of Antibiotics against *Proteus vulgaris*

Antibiotic	No. Isolates[a]	MIC$_{50}$	MIC$_{90}$	Reference
Ampicillin	22	—	>128	15
Ticarcillin	49	8	32	10
Ticarcillin/ clavulanic acid	49	≤1	≤1	10
Amoxicillin/ clavulanic acid	9	16	—	36
Cefaclor	9	0.12	—	36
	11	>64	>64	24
Cefuroxime	21	>16	>16	36
	11	>64	>64	24
Cefoxitin	11	16	32	16
Cefotaxime	226	0.05	—	34
	11	<.1	5.5	42
Ceftriaxone	21	0.25	>64	45
	11	64	>64	24
Ceftazidime	226	0.08	—	34
	21	<.25	<.25	45
	11	<.1	<.1	42
Cefoperazone	11	1.4	5.8	42
Aztreonam	11	0.125	0.25	16
	11	<.1	<.1	42
Imipenem	377	—	4	6
Meropenem	377	—	0.25	6
Cefepime	21	<.25	<.25	45
	226	0.05	—	34
Cefpirone	226	0.09	—	34
	11	8	8	24
Gentamicin	6	0.4	—	26
Tobramycin	11	1	4	16
	6	0.4	—	26
Amikacin	11	2	8	16
	6	1.0	—	26
Trimethoprim/ sulfamethoxazole	11	0.12	0.25	24
Ciprofloxacin	11	0.06	0.06	24
	NA	0.02	0.06	48
Ofloxacin	11	0.12	0.25	24
	NA	0.1	0.16	
Floroxacin	11	0.12	0.25	24
Lomefoxacin	11	0.25	0.5	24
Nalidixic acid	NA	4	8	48
Norfloxacin	NA	0.1	0.4	48
Enoxacin	NA	0.4	1.6	48

[a]NA, not available.

high levels of this enzyme on the basis of induction or mutation are resistant to these antibiotics. Disturbing recent surveys report 30% prevalence of resistance of *P. vulgaris* to ceftriaxone (24, 45). The enzyme has little activity against cephamycins and thus, cefoxitin and cefetetan can be used to treat *P. vulgaris*. Carboxy- and ureidopenicillins are also active, and addition of β-lactamase inhibitors such as sulbactam, clavulanic acid, or tazobactam to extended-spectrum antibiotics enhances the usefulness of this class of antibiotics against *P. vulgaris* (10).

Third-generation cephalosporins are recommended for the treatment of *P. vulgaris* infections (27). Within this class, ceftazidime and aztreonam must be considered the drugs of choice because they are highly active, with MIC$_{50}$s that are usually less than 1μg/mL, and they are resistant to the hydrolytic activity of class A β-lactamase (22).

Imipenem is active against both *P. mirabilis* and *P. vulgaris*, with MIC$_{50}$s ranging from 2 to 4 μg/mL. These MICs are relatively high compared with the activity of imipenem against other Gram-negative bacteria. However they fall within the susceptible range, and the overwhelming majority of infections caused by *Proteus* respond to imipemem, although clinical failures have been reported (37, 5). Meropenem, a recently introduced carbapenem, is more potent then imipenem against *Enterobacteriaceae*, including *P. mirabilis* and *P. vulgaris* (6). However, it has only recently been marketed, and there is little clinical experience with this new antibiotic.

Aminoglycosides are extremely active against *P. vulgaris* as well as *P. mirabilis* (26). Despite its efficacy and low cost, the use of aminoglycosides in the treatment of Gram-negative bacillary infections has been largely supplanted by the use of third-generation cephalosporins. In seriously ill patients, however, experts do recommend adding an aminoglycoside to a third-generation cephalosporin or a quinolone for its additive or synergistic activity (27).

Trimethoprim-sulfamethoxazole is active against both species of *Proteus*. It may be an especially good choice for treatment of urinary tract infections caused by *Proteus* (40). In treatment trials that compared β-lactam antibiotics (ampicillin) and trimethoprim-sulfamethoxazole in uncomplicated and complicated urinary tract infections, trimethoprim-sulfamethoxazole has generally been more efficacious, even though causative organisms isolated in these studies proved to be susceptible to both antibiotics (19, 40).

Urinary tract infections in nursing home patients or hospitalized patients are often associated with indwelling Foley catheters and are more likely to be caused by the more antibiotic-resistant indole-positive *P. vulgaris* or *P. penneri* rather than indole-negative *P. mirabilis* (12). *P. vulgaris* and *P penneri* are likely to be susceptible to trimethoprim-sulfamethoxazole. Because of older age and concomitant underlying disease, persons in this population often have some impairment in renal clearance. The last concern often leads clinicians away from a sulfur-containing antibiotic or aminoglycosides in considering treatment of *Proteus* infections.

Norfloxacin, ciprofloxacin, ofloxacin, and the recently released levofloxacin have excellent activity against indole-negative and -positive *Proteus*. They have been used successfully in short-course (3-day) treatment of uncomplicated urinary tract infections and longer courses for complicated urinary tract infections caused by *Proteus* (47). Because of their expense, however, they are generally not used as first-line drugs but are reserved for treatment of β-lactam-resistant infections or treatment in a β-lactam-allergic patient.

REFERENCES

1. Adler JL, Burke JP, Martin DF, Finland M. Proteus infections in a general hospital. I. Biochemical characteristics and antibiotic susceptibility of the organisms. With special reference to proticine typing and the Dienes phenomenon. Ann Intern Med 1971; 75:517–530.

2. Adler JL, Burke JP, Martin DF, Finland M. Proteus infections in a general hospital. II. Some clinical and epidemiologic characteristics. With an analysis of 71 cases of Proteus bacteremia. Ann Intern Med 1971;75:531–536.

3. Bush K, Jacoby GA, Mederios AA. A functional classification scheme for beta-lactamases and its correlation with molecular structure. Antimicrob Agents Chemother 1995;39:1211–1233.

4. Chen HY, Bonfiglio G, Allen M, Piper D, Edwardson T, McVey D, Livermore DM. Multicentre survey of the in-vitro activity of piperacillin/tazobactam against bacteria from hospitalized patients in the British Isles. J Antimicrob Chemother 1993;32: 247–266.

5. Chiodini PL, Geddes AM, Smith EG, Conlon CP, Farrel ID. Imipenem/cilastatin in the treatment of serious bacterial infections. Rev Infect Dis 1985;7(Suppl 3):S490–S495.

6. Edwards JR, Turner PJ. Laboratory data which differentiate meropenem from imipenem. Scand J Infect Dis Suppl 1995;96: 5–10.

7. Eliopoulos GM, Klimm K, Ferraro MJ, Jacoby GA, Moellering RC. Comparative in vitro activity of piperacillin combined with the beta-lactamase inhibitor tazobactam (YTR 830). Diagn Microbiol Infect Dis 1989;12:481–488.

8. Farmer JJ. Enterobacteriaceae: introduction and identification. In: Murray PR, Baron EJ, Pfaller MA, Tenover FC, Yolken RH, eds. Manual of clinical microbiology. Washington, DC: American Society for Microbiology Press, 1995:438–449.

9. Fu KP, Lafredo SC, Folendo B, Isaacson DM, Barett JF, Tobia AJ, Rosenthale ME. In vitro and in vivo antibacterial activities of levofloxacin (L-ofloxacin), an optically active ofloxacin. Antimicrob Agents Chemother 1992;36:860–866.

10. Fuchs PC, Barry AL, Jones, RN. In vitro and disk susceptibility of Timentin: current status. Am J Med 1985;79(Suppl 5B): 25–32.

11. Gallager DJ, Montgomerie JZ, North JD, Acute infections of the urinary tract and the urethral syndrome in general practice. Br Med J 1965;1:622–624.

12. Gaynes RP, Weinstein RA, Chamberlin W, Kabbins SW. Antibiotic-resistant flora in nursing home patients admitted to the hospital. Arch Intern Med 1985;145:1804–1807.

13. Gerding DN, Larson TA. Resistance surveillance programs and the incidence of gram-negative bacillary resistance to amikacin form 1967 to 1985. Am J Med 1986;80(Suppl 6B):22–28.

14. Hickman FW, Steigerwalt AG, Harmer JJ III, Brenner DJ. Identification of *Proteus penneri* sp. nov., formerly known as *Proteus vulgaris* indole negative or as *Proteus vulgaris* biogroup 1. J Clin Microbiol 1982;15:1097–1102.

15. Hopefl AW. Aztreonam—an overview. Drug Intell Clin Pharm 1985;19:171–175.

16. Jacobus NV, Ferreira MC, Barza M. In vitro activity of aztreonam, a monobactam antibiotic. Antimicrob Agents Chemother 1982;22:832–838

17. Jacoby GA, Archer GL. New mechanisms of bacterial resistance to antimicrobial agents. N Engl J Med 1991;324:601–612.

18. Johnson HR, Lyons MF II, Pearce W, Gorman P, Roberts PL, White N, Brust P, Olsen R, Gnann JW, Stamm WE. Therapy for women hospitalized with acute pyelonephritis: a randomized trial of ampicillin versus trimethoprim-sulfamethoxazole for 14 days. J Infect Dis 1991;163:325–330.

19. Johnson JR. Virulence factors in *Escherichia coli* urinary tract infection. Clin Microbiol Rev 1991;4:80–128.

20. Jones RN. Review of the in vitro spectrum of activity of imipenem. Am J Med 1985;78(Suppl 6A):22–32.

21. Liu PY, Gur D, Hall MC, Livermore DM. Survey of the prevalence of β-lactamases amongst 1000 gram-negative bacilli isolated consecutively at the Royal London Hospital. J Antimicrob Chemother 1992;30:429–447.

22. Livermore DM. β-lactamases in laboratory and clinical resistance. Clin Microbiol Rev 1995;8:557–584.

23. MacGowan AP, Brown NM, Holt HA, McCulloch SY, Reeves DS. An eight year survey of the antimicrobial susceptibility patterns of 85,971 bacteria isolated from patients in a district general hospital and the local community. J Antimicrob Chemother 1993;31:543–547.

24. Markowitz SM, Williams DS, Hanna CB, Parker JL, Pierce MA, Steele JCH Jr. A multicenter comparative study of the in vitro activity of fleroxacin and other antimicrobial agents. Chemother 1995;41:477–486.

25. Mariotte S, Nordmann P, Nicolas MH. Extended-spectrum β-lactamase in *Proteus mirabilis*. J Antimicrob Chemother 1994; 33:925–935.

26. Moellering RC Jr. In vitro antibacterial activity of the aminoglycosides antibiotics. Rev Infect Dis 1983;(Suppl 3): S212–S230.

27. Medical Letter. The choice of antibacterial drugs. Med Lett 1996;38(Issue 971):25–30.

28. Na'was TE, Mawajdeh S, Dababneh A, al-Omari A. In vitro activities of antimicrobial agents against Proteus species from clinical specimens. Br J Biomed Sci 1994;51:95–99.

29. Neu HC. The new beta-lactamase-stable cephalosporins. Ann Intern Med 1982;97:408–419

30. Neu HC. Carbapenems: special properties contributing to their activity. Am J Med 1985;78(Suppl 6A);33–40.

31. Neu HC. β-Lactam antibiotics: structural relationships affecting in vitro activity and pharmacologic properties. Rev Infect Dis 1986;8(Suppl 3):S237–S259.

32. O'Brien TF and members of Task Force 2. Resistance of bacteria to antibacterial agents: report of task force 2. Rev Infect Dis 1987; 9(Suppl 3):S244–S260.

33. Sanders CC, Sanders WE Jr. Beta-lactam resistance in gram-negative bacteria: global trends and clinical impact. Clin Infect Dis 1992;15:824–839.

34. Sanders CC. Cefepime: the next generation? Clin Infect Dis 1993;17:369–379.

35. Schaberg DR, Culver DH, Gaynes RP. Major trends in the microbial etiology of nosocomial infection. Am J Med 1991;91(Suppl 3B):72S–75S.

36. Sewell D, Barry A, Allen S, Fuchs P, McLaughlin J, Pfaller M. Comparative antimicrobial activities of the penem WY-49605 (SUN5555) against recent clinical isolates from five U.S. medical centers. Antimicrob Agents Chemother 1995;39:1591–1595.

37. Shah PM. Clinical experience with imipenem/cilastatin: analysis of a multicenter study. Rev Infect Dis 1985;7(Suppl 3): S471–S475.

38. Silverman DE, Stamey TA. Management of infectious stones: the Stanford experience. Medicine 1983;62:44.

39. Stamey TA. Pathogenesis and treatment of urinary tract infections. Baltimore: Williams & Wilkins, 1980.

40. Stamm WE, McKevitt M, Counts GW. Acute renal infection in women: treatment with trimethoprim-sulfamethoxazole or ampicillin for two or six weeks: a randomized trial. Ann Intern Med 1987;106:341–345.

41. Stamm WE, Hooton TM. Management of urinary tract infections in adults. N Engl J Med 1993;329:1328–1334.

42. Sykes RB, Bonner DP, Bush K, Georgopapadakou BH. Aztreonam (SQ26,776), a synthetic monobactam specifically

active against aerobic gram-negative bacteria. Antimicrob Agents Chemother 1982;21:85–92.

43. Thornsberry C, Yee YC. Comparative activity of eight antimicrobial agents against clinical bacterial isolates from the United States, measured by two methods. Am J Med 1996;100(Suppl 6A):26S–38S.

44. Wallmark G, Arremark I, Telander B. *Staphylococcus saprophyticus:* a frequent cause of acute urinary tract infections among female outpatients. J Infect Dis 1978;138:791.

45. Washington JA, Jones RN, Gerlach EH, Murray PR, Allen SD, Knapp CC. Multicenter comparison of in vitro activities of FK-037, cefepime, ceftriaxone, ceftazidime, and cefuroxime. Antimicrob Agents Chemother 1993;37:1696–1700.

46. Watanakunakorn C, Perni SC. *Proteus mirabilis* bacteremia: a review of 176 cases during 1980–1992. Scand J Infect Dis 1994; 24:361–367.

47. Wolfson JS, Hooper DC. Treatment of genitourinary tract infections with fluoroquinolones: activity in vitro, pharmacokinetics, and clinical efficacy in urinary tract infections and prostatitis. Antimicrob Agents Chemother 1989;33:1655–1661.

48. Wolfson JS, Hooper DC. Fluoroquinolone antimicrobial agents. Clin Microbiol Rev 1989;2:378–424.

Providencia Species

●

Robert Orenstein and Edward S. Wong

GENERAL DESCRIPTION

The *Providencia* are a genus of *Enterobacteriaceae* within the tribe *Proteeae* that are closely related clinically and microbiologically to the genus *Proteus*. Though not as common a community pathogen as *Proteus*, *Providencia* are highly resistant urinary tract pathogens frequently found in chronically catheterized patients.

The tribe *Proteeae* is distinguished from other *Enterobacteriaceae* by the presence of the enzyme phenylalanine deaminase, which enables them to deaminate phenylalanine to produce phenylpyruvic acid (6, 35). *Providencia* spp. grow as colorless, flat, 2- to 3-mm, nonswarming colonies on MacConkey's and sheep-blood agar. Originally, *Providencia* was distinguished from the genus *Proteus* by the lack of urease activity. However, because of considerable overlap among the various species of *Providencia* and *Proteus*, differential biochemical tests are required for accurate speciation. Biochemical characteristics and DNA relatedness studies have led to the five currently recognized species of *Providencia*: *P. alcalifaciens*, *P. rettgeri*, *P. rustigianii*, *P. stuartii*, and *P. heimbachae*. The most frequently isolated species in the clinical laboratory and the principal human pathogen in the genus is *P. stuartii*.

Infections due to *Providencia* are uncommon in healthy hosts. *P. stuartii* and *P. rettgeri* are most often associated with urinary tract infections (UTIs) in individuals with long-term urinary catheters. *P. alcalifaciens* is an uncommon agent of invasive diarrhea in children. *P. rustigianii*, previously considered *P. alcalifaciens* biogroup 3, is rarely isolated from stool specimens (15); its role in human infections is unclear. No human infections have been reported with the animal pathogen *P. heimbachae*.

Of the *Providencia*, *P. stuartii* is reported most commonly from patients with nosocomially acquired UTIs (14, 16, 18, 19, 30, 33, 37, 41). *P. stuartii* was isolated from 61% of 619 bacteriuric episodes at two nursing homes (37). *P. stuartii* is a frequent cause of UTIs in long-term catheterized patients but rarely found in noncatheterized or short-term catheterized patients (9). *P. stuartii* appears to have an enhanced ability to adhere to, and persist on, biofilms of the inner lumen of urinary catheters. Unlike strains of adherent *Escherichia coli* commonly found in community-acquired UTIs, these isolates adhere to the catheter rather than to the urinary epithelium (8). Strains of *Providencia* that possess the MR/K (mannose-resistant *Klebsiella*-like fimbriae) hemagglutinin have increased adherence to catheters but not to uroepithelial cells (23). Outbreaks of UTIs due to *Providencia* have been associated with contaminated leg bags. In one outbreak of *Providencia* UTIs in 14 patients, the reservoir of infection was traced to reused urinals used to empty condom catheter drainage bags (7).

Risk factors and the reservoirs for transmission of *Providencia* are largely unknown. The urinary tract appears to be the primary reservoir for this infection in nosocomial outbreaks. Wenzel et al. identified these organisms as an important airborne cause of burn wound infections and bacteremia (39). In two burn unit outbreaks, *Providencia* was resistant to amikacin and silver sulfadiazine agents frequently used to inhibit growth of *P. aeruginosa* (27, 39). In a review from Belgium of 48 infections due to *Providencia* in neurosurgical and cancer patients, preceding gentamicin use, gastrointestinal tract decontamination with oral antibiotics and indwelling urinary or endotracheal tubes were identified as predisposing factors (18); 80% of these patients had received antibiotics prior to the isolation of *Providencia*. Selective pressure from the use of antibiotics is believed responsible for the emergence of aminoglycoside resistance worldwide (22).

Respiratory tract infections due to *Providencia* are rare and are generally seen in those with instrumentation of the respiratory tree. Though it might be anticipated that *Providencia* pneumonia would arise hematogenously from a urinary tract source, Wenzel et al. demonstrated that high airborne concentrations of *Providencia* could be found in the rooms of patients colonized with these organisms in their sputa. All patients with *Providencia* pneumonia had experienced endotracheal instrumentation (39).

Bacteremia due to *Providencia* is also uncommon. Most bacteremias have occurred in the setting of prior UTI or burn wound infection (27, 39). Despite their frequency as urinary tract pathogens in the chronically catheterized elderly, *Providencia* account for only 0.8 to 3% of hospital acquired bacteremias (18, 33, 41). A review of bacteremias in 49 patients at a community hospital reported an incidence of 0.17 *P. stuartii* bacteremias per 1000 admissions. Two-thirds of patients were men, with a mean age of 75 years. Ninety-six percent of these patients came from a nursing home, 92% had chronic indwelling Foley catheters, and 82% had concurrent bacteriuria with this organism. Despite the frailty of these patients, their in-hospital mortality was only 24% (41).

Infections due to *P. rettgeri* parallel those of *P. stuartii*. Though rarely the causative agent of wound infections, abscesses, or bloodstream or respiratory tract infections, *P. rettgeri* is frequently associated with antibiotic-resistant UTIs in debilitated elderly patients (2). Urease production by *P. rettgeri* may predispose patients to development of urinary struvite stones and was the reason it was previously misclassified as *Proteus rettgeri*.

Providencia are not commonly found as lower intestinal tract flora. However, both *P. stuartii* and *P. alcalifaciens* have been isolated from feces of neonates and British travelers, with diarrhea in the absence of other enteropathogens (13). Recent studies from children with diarrhea in Brazil demonstrated the ability of *P. alcalifaciens* to invade both HeLa and Hep 2 cells (13).

SUSCEPTIBILITY IN VITRO

Considerable variation in antibiotic susceptibility patterns exists among the species of *Providencia*. *P. alcalifaciens* and *P. rustigianii* are most susceptible, whereas *P. stuartii* and *P. rettgeri* are most resistant to antimicrobial agents. Though clinical data are limited on infections due to *P. rustigianii* and *P. alcalifaciens*, most isolates remain susceptible to ampicillin, carbenicillin, cephalosporins, and aminoglycosides (15, 28). This contrasts with the uropathogens *P. rettgeri* and *P. stuartii*, which have acquired numerous mechanisms of antibiotic resistance. These latter two organisms can persist in the catheterized urinary tract and, under selective pressure of numerous antimicrobials, develop resistance to virtually all classes of antibiotics.

P. stuartii, the most common clinical isolate, possesses the broadest spectrum of resistance, spanning several classes of antibiotics including the β-lactam agents, aminoglycosides, sulfonamides, tetracyclines, chloramphenicol, and most recently the fluoroquinolones. Resistance may be either chromosomal or plasmid mediated and may be transferable among other *Enterobacteriaceae*. In the 1960s, many isolates were ampicillin susceptible. However by the 1970s, over 70% of *Providencia* isolates had acquired ampicillin resistance. Addition of the β-lactamase inhibitor clavulanic acid to amoxicillin did not improve amoxicillin's activity against *P. stuartii*. Most isolates have an MIC_{90} above 64 μg/mL (5, 20). The introduction of carbenicillin was considered a major advance in the treatment of these resistant infections, but by the mid 1980s, most *P. stuartii* had acquired plasmid-mediated resistance to the extended-spectrum penicillins. The β-lactamase inhibitors sulbactam and clavulanic acid appear to add little protection against the β-lactamases of *P. stuartii;* however, tazobactam is active against the type 1 β-lactamases of *Providencia*.

Resistance is widespread among first-generation cephalosporins and emerging to second-generation agents such as cefuroxime and cefoxitin (3, 21). Recent studies show an MIC_{50} for cefuroxime of 32 μg/mL and an MIC_{90} above 128 μg/mL, with only 50 to 80% of *P. stuartii* isolates still susceptible (5, 20, 41). At present, resistance to third-generation cephalosporins is rare, and they are considered the drugs of choice for infections due to *Providencia*. Some recent isolates have been reported to possess inducible Bush type 1 chromosomally mediated β-lactamases that may increase resistance to these agents (4, 31). Introduction of the expanded-spectrum cephalosporin cefipime, which appears resistant to extended-spectrum β-lactamases, may prove useful in isolates that have acquired this trait (31). In a study of over 400 isolates of *Providencia*, the mean MIC_{50} for cefipime was 0.03 μg/mL (31). An alternative to the cephalosporins for multiply resistant *Providencia* are the carbapenems. Imipenem-cilastatin and meropenem are both very active against all *Providencia*, inhibiting almost 100% of isolates (29, 40, 41). In a study of bacteremias due to *P. stuartii*, the most effective agents in vitro were imipenem, ceftizoxime, aztreonam, ceftazidime, and amikacin (41).

The aminoglycosides gentamicin and tobramycin are no longer reliable for treatment of serious UTIs due to *P. stuartii*. Resistance to gentamicin and tobramycin is now widespread among *P. stuartii* and *P. rettgeri* because of chromosomal and plasmid-borne aminoglycoside-modifying enzymes. In *P. stuartii*, the aminoglycoside acetyltransferase enzymes are encoded by chromosomal genes that are not usually well expressed. Mutants that express high levels of this enzyme account for the significant spread of resistant strains. The most common aminoglycoside-modifying enzyme found in U.S. isolates is AAC(2')-I (22). Studies in the 1960s and early 1970s found isolates of *Providencia* to be gentamicin susceptible, but with increased aminoglycoside use in the 1970s, resistance became widespread. Over 40% of isolates from bacteremic patients in a community hospital in Ohio were gentamicin resistant (41). In hospitals with limited amikacin use, this agent remains useful. However, Wenzel et al. reported a significant number of amikacin-resistant *P. stuartii* isolates from a burn unit in which this agent was widely used for *Pseudomonas* infections (39).

Since most infections due to *Providencia* originate in the catheterized urinary tracts of elderly nursing home patients,

TABLE 1 • Comparative Activity of Antibiotics against *Providencia stuartii*

Antibiotic	No. Isolates	MIC$_{50}$	MIC$_{90}$	Reference
Amoxicillin	10	>16	>16	12
Amoxicillin-clavulanate	202	>128	>128	5
	34	32	64	20
	10	>16	>16	12
Ticarcillin	24	—	>512	36
	59	<1	>64	11
Ticarcillin-clavulanate	24	—	16	36
	59	<1	32	11
Cephalothin	363	>128	>128	28
Cefaclor	202	>128	>128	5
	9	>64	—	32
	34	>64	>64	20
	10	>16	>16	12
	34	4	>64	20
	10	4	>16	12
Cefoxitin	363	4	64	28
Cefixime	9	0.5	—	32
	34	0.5	8	20
	10	0.06	0.12	12
Cefpodoxime	202	2	32	5
Cefetamet	202	1	32	5
Cefamandole	363	4	32	28
Cefotaxime	10	0.12	4	17
	20	—	0.63	40
	—	0.07	—	31
Ceftriaxone	10	0.03	2	17
	34	0.5	8	20
Cefoperazone	10	2	32	17
Ceftazidime	10	0.25	0.5	10
	20	—	0.97	40
	—	0.17	—	31
Cefipime	10	0.03	1	17
	435	0.04	—	31
Imipenem	10	1	2	17
	20	—	2.24	40
Meropenem	20	—	0.11	40
Gentamicin	363	8	32	28
	20	—	>32	40
Tobramycin	363	8	32	28
TMP-SMX[a]	34	16	16	20
Ciprofloxacin	20	—	1.11	40
	202	4	64	5
	17	0.06	0.12	10
	34	0.12	8	20
	10	0.06	4	12
Ofloxacin	17	0.25	0.5	10
	34	0.5	8	20
Levofloxacin	17	0.12	0.25	10
Norfloxacin	17	0.25	0.25	10
Lomefloxacin	34	0.5	8	20
Fleroxacin	34	0.25	4	20

[a]TMP-SMX, trimethoprim-sulfamethoxazole.

TABLE 2 • Comparative Activity of Antibiotics against *Providencia rettgeri*

Antibiotic	No. Isolates	MIC$_{50}$	MIC$_{90}$	Reference
Amoxicillin	10	>16	>16	12
Amoxicillin-clavulanate	19	>64	>64	20
	10	>16	>16	12
Piperacillin	60	0.5	64	29
Cephalothin	104	>128	>128	28
Cefaclor	19	>64	>64	20
	10	>16	>16	12
Cefuroxime	19	2	>64	20
	10	1	8	12
Cefoxitin	104	4	16	28
Cefixime	19	0.5	32	20
	10	<0.03	0.25	12
Cefamandole	104	0.25	4	28
Cefotaxime	67	0.125	2	29
	20	—	0.24	40
Ceftriaxone	19	0.5	8	20
Ceftazidime	15	0.06	0.5	10
	67	0.06	4	29
	15	<0.25	1	38
	20	—	0.34	40
Cefipime	15	<0.25	1	38
Imipenem	88	1	2	29
	20	—	1.47	40
Meropenem	20	—	0.10	40
	88	0.06	0.125	29
Gentamicin	104	<0.5	4	28
	30	1	32	29
Tobramycin	104	<0.5	4	28
	29	0.5	16	29
TMP-SMX[a]	19	16	16	20
Ciprofloxacin	20	—	0.09	40
	15	0.03	0.12	10
	19	0.06	0.25	20
	10	0.03	1	12
Ofloxacin	15	0.25	0.5	10
	19	0.25	2	20
Levofloxacin	15	0.12	0.5	10
Norfloxacin	15	0.12	0.5	10
Lomefloxacin	19	0.25	1	20
Fleroxacin	19	0.12	0.5	20

[a]TMP-SMX, trimethoprim-sulfamethoxazole

oral antibiotics active against these organisms would be expected to help limit hospitalizations, morbidity, and costs. In a study of 255 isolates of *Providencia* (202 *P. stuartii*, 40 *P. rettgeri*, 13 *P. alcalifaciens*) from nursing home patients, the

extended-spectrum oral cephalosporins cefetamet and cefpodoxime were more active than the quinolone ciprofloxacin (3, 5). For the more resistant and prominent *P. stuartii*, the most effective oral agents studied were cefetamet (72% susceptible) and cefpodoxime (53% susceptible). Other agents frequently used for UTIs such as ciprofloxacin, cefuroxime, cefaclor, and amoxicillin-clavulanate were much less active (5).

Providencia spp. are susceptible to most quinolones. Ciprofloxacin is the most active (MIC$_{90}$, 0.12 µg/mL) and is twice as active against *P.stuartii* than levofloxacin in vitro (10, 20). *Providencia rettgeri* and *P. stuartii* have however developed fluoroquinolone resistance. In a multicenter study of 169 isolates of *P. stuartii*, only 64% of isolates were ciprofloxacin susceptible (1). An international study revealed even more disturbing results with only 41, 39, 38, and 69% of isolates susceptible to lomefloxacin in France, Italy, Spain, and Argentina, respectively (1).

ANTIMICROBIAL THERAPY

The initial management step in patients with indwelling urinary catheters should be removal of the catheter if possible. Therapy of infections with *Providencia* depends upon the species isolated. Since *P. rustigianii* and *P. alcalifaciens* remain susceptible to ampicillin, trimethoprim-sulfamethoxazole, first- and second-generation cephalosporins, and aminoglycosides, there are many therapeutic options for these uncommon pathogens.

P. stuartii and *P. rettgeri,* on the other hand, are urinary pathogens that are becoming more multiply antibiotic resistant. Since they are the most frequent clinical isolates and since some laboratories may not speciate these, initial empirical therapy should be directed at these highly resistant organisms. Although some references suggest use of an extended-spectrum penicillin, aminoglycoside, trimethoprim-sulfamethoxazole, or a fluoroquinolone as initial therapy, caution should be used because of emerging resistance to all of these. Woods and Watanakunakorn found amikacin, ceftizoxime, imipenem, aztreonam, and ceftazidime to be most active against bloodstream isolates of *P. stuartii* in the 1980s and early 1990s. Less than 50% of these isolates were susceptible to gentamicin, piperacillin, mezlocillin, ticarcillin, or trimethoprim-sulfamethoxazole (41). The initial empirical choice in serious infections should be a third-generation cephalosporin such as ceftriaxone, ceftazidime, cefotaxime, ceftizoxime, cefipime, or aztreonam, with consideration given to adding an aminoglycoside such as amikacin. In health care settings in which extended-spectrum β-lactamases prevail, a carbapenem may be preferred. Isolates resistant to third-generation cephalosporins can be treated with imipenem, meropenem, or amikacin. In an uncomplicated UTI, initial therapy with a single daily parenteral dose of ceftriaxone or one of the extended-spectrum oral cephalosporins—cefpodoxime, cefetamet, or oral ciprofloxacin—could be considered in an effort to decrease the need for hospitalization.

REFERENCES

1. Acar JF, Goldstein FW. Trends in bacterial resistance to fluoroquinolones. Clin Infect Dis 1997;24(Suppl 1):S67–73.
2. Arroyo JV, Sonnenwirth AC, Liebhaber H. *Proteus rettgeri* infections: a review. J Urol 1977;117:115–117.
3. Biedenbach DJ, Jones R. Predictive accuracy of disk diffusion test for *Proteus vulgaris* and *Providencia* species against five newer orally administered cephalosporins, cefdinir, cefetamet, cefprozil, cefuroxime and loracarbef. J Clin Microbiol 1994;32:559–562.
4. Bush K, Jacoby GA, Medeiros AA. A functional classification scheme for beta-lactamases and its correlation with molecular structure. Antimicrob Agents Chemother 1995;39:1211–1233.
5. Cornaglia G, Frugoni S, Mazzariol A, Piacentini E, Berlusconi A, Fontana R. Activities of oral antibiotics on Providencia strains isolated from institutionalized elderly patients with urinary tract infections. Antimicrob Agents Chemother 1995;39: 2819–2821.
6. Ewing WH, Tanner KE, Dennard DA. The Providence group: an intermediate group of enteric bacteria. J Infect Dis 1954;94: 134–140.
7. Fierer J, Ekstrom M. An outbreak of *Providencia stuartii* urinary tract infections. Patients with condom catheters are a reservoir of the bacteria. JAMA 1981;245:1553–1555.
8. Fletcher M, Oppenheimer S, Warren JW. Colonization of urinary catheters by *Escherichia coli* and *Providencia* stuartii in a laboratory model system. J Urol 1994;152:232–236.
9. Flournoy DJ. Incidence of bacteria from clean catch and catheterized urine of nursing home residents. J Okla State Med Assoc 1993;86:550–552.
10. Fu KP, Lafredo SC, Foleno B, Isaacson DM, Barrettt JF, Tobia AJ, Rosenthale ME. In vitro and in vivo antibacterial activities of levofloxacin (l-ofloxacin), an optically active ofloxacin. Antimicrob Agents Chemother 1992;36:860–868.
11. Fuchs PC, Barry AL, Jones RN. In vitro activity and disk susceptibility of Timentin: current status. Am J Med 1985;(Suppl 5B):25–32.
12. Fuchs PC, Barry AL, Sewell DL. Antibacterial activity of WY-49605 compared with those of the other oral agents and selection of disk content for disk diffusion and susceptibility testing. Antimicrob Agents Chemother 1995;39:1472–1479.
13. Guth BEC, Perrella E. Prevalence of invasive ability and other virulence associated characteristics in *Providencia alcalifaciens* strains isolated in Sao Paulo, Brazil. J Med Microbiol 1996; 45:459–462.
14. Hawkey PM. Providencia stuartii: a review of a multiply antibiotic-resistant bacterium. J Antimicrob Chemother 1984;13: 209–226.
15. Hickman-Brenner FW, Farmer JJ, Steigerwalt AG, Brenner DJ. *Providencia rustigianii*: a new species in the family Enterobacteriaceae formerly known as Providencia alcalifaciens biogroup 3. J Clin Microbiol 1983;17:1057–1060.
16. Janis B, Evans RG, Hoeprich PD. *Providence bacillus* bacteremia and septicopyemia. Am J Med 1968;45:943–947.
17. Kessler RE, Fung-Tomc J. Susceptibility of bacterial isolates to Beta-lactam antibiotics from US clinical trials over a 5-year period. Am J Med 1996;100(Suppl 6A):13S–19S.
18. Klastersky J, Bogaerts AM, Noterman J, VanLaer E, Daneau D, Mouawad E. Infections caused by *Providence bacilli*. Scand J Infect Dis 1974;6:153–160.
19. Kocka FE, Srinivasan S, Mowjood M, Kantor HS. Nosocomial multiply resistant *Providencia stuartii*: a long-term outbreak with multiple biotypes and serotypes at one hospital. J Clin Microbiol 1980;11:167–169.
20. Markowitz SM, Williams DS, Hanna CB, Parker JL, et al. A multicenter comparative study of the in vitro activity of fleroxacin and other antimicrobial agents. Chemotherapy 1995;41:477–486.
21. McHale PJ, Keane CT, Dougan G. Antibiotic resistance in *Providencia stuartii* isolated in hospitals. J Clin Microbiol 1981;13: 1099–1104.
22. Miller GH, Sabatelli FJ, Hare RS, Glupczynski Y, Mackey P, Shlaes D, et al. The most frequent aminoglycoside resistance mechanisms—changes with time and geographic area: a reflection of aminoglycoside usage patterns? Clin Infect Dis 1997; 24(Suppl 1):S46–62.
23. Mobley HLT, Chippendale GR, Tenney JH, Mayrer A, Crisp LJ, Penner JL, Warren JW. MR/K hemagglutination of *Providencia stuartii* correlates with adherence to catheters and with persistence in catheter-associated bacteriuria. J Infect Dis 1988;157: 264–271.

24. Mobley HLT, Chippendale GR, Tenney JH, Warren JW. Adherence to uroepithelial cells of *Providencia stuartii* isolated from the catheterized urinary tract. J Gen Microbiol 1986;132:2863–2872.

25. Muller HE, O'Hara M, Fanning GR, Hickman-Brenner FW, Swenson JM, Brenner DL. *Providencia heimbachae*, a new species of *Enterobacteriaceae* isolated from animals. Int J Syst Bacteriol 1986;36:252–256.

26. Overturf GD, Wilkins J, Ressler R. Emergence of resistance of *Providencia stuartii* to multiple antibiotics: speciation and biochemical characterization of *Providencia*. J Infect Dis 1974; 129:353–357.

27. Overturf GD, Zawacki BE, Wilkins J. Emergence of resistance to amikacin during treatment of burn wounds: the role of antimicrobial susceptibility testing. Surgery 1976;79:224–228.

28. Penner JL, Preston MA. Differences among *Providencia* species in their in vitro susceptibilities to five antibiotics. Antimicrob Agents Chemother 1980;18:868–871.

29. Pitkin DH, Sheikh W, Nadler H. Comparative in vitro activity of meropenem versus other extended-spectrum antimicrobials against randomly chosen and selected resistant clinical isolates tested in 26 North American centers. Clin Infect Dis 1997;24 (Suppl 2):S238–248.

30. Rahav G, Pinco E, Silbaq F, Bercovier H. Molecular epidemiology of catheter-associated bacteriuria in nursing home patients. J Clin Microbiol 1994;32:1031–1034.

31. Sanders CC. Cefepime: the next generation. Clin Infect Dis 1993;17:369–379.

32. Sewell D, Barry A, Allen S, Fuchs P, McLaughlin J, Pfaller M. Comparative antimicrobial activities of the penem WY-49605 (SUN5555) against recent clinical isolates from five US medical centers. Antimicrob Agents Chemother 1995;39: 1591–1595.

33. Solberg CO, Matsen JM. Infections with Providence bacilli. A clinical and bacteriologic study. Am J Med 1971;50:241–246.

34. Stuart CA, Wheeler KM, Rustigian R, Zimmerman A. Biochemical and antigenic relationships of the paracolon bacteria. J Bacteriol 1943;45:101–119.

35. Stuart CA, Wheeler KM, McGann V. Further studies on one anaerogenic paracolon organism, type 29911. J Bacteriol 1946; 52:431–438.

36. Sutherland R, Beale AS, Boon RJ, Griffin KE, Slocombe B, et al. Antibacterial activity of ticarcillin in the presence of clavulanate potassium. Am J Med 1985;79(Suppl 5B):13–24.

37. Warren JW. *Providencia stuartii*: a common cause of antibiotic-resistant bacteriuria in patients with long-term indwelling catheters. Rev Infect Dis 1986;8:61–67.

38. Washington JA, Jones RA, Gerlach EH, Murray PR, Allen SD, Knapp CC. Multicenter comparison of in vitro activities of FK-037, cefepime, ceftriaxone, ceftazidime, and cefuroxime. Antimicrob Agents Chemother 1993;37:1696–1700.

39. Wenzel RP, Hunting KJ, Osterman CA, Sande MA. *Providencia stuartii*, a hospital pathogen: potential factors for its emergence and transmission. Am J Epidemiol 1976;104:170–180.

40. Wiseman LR, Wagstaff AJ, Brogden RN, Bryson HM. Meropenem. A review of its antibacterial activity, pharmacokinetic properties and clinical efficacy. Drugs 1995;1:73–101.

41. Woods TD, Watanakunakorn C. Bacteremia due to *Providencia stuartii*: review of 49 episodes. South Med J 1996;89:221–224.

Pseudomonas aeruginosa

●

Victor L. Yu and David L. Paterson

GENERAL DESCRIPTION
Microbiology

Pseudomonas aeruginosa is an aerobic Gram-negative bacterium. Like many environmental bacteria, *P. aeruginosa* lives in slime-enclosed biofilms that allow survival and replication within human tissues and medical devices. The biofilm protects *P. aeruginosa* from host-produced antibodies and phagocytes and contributes to antibiotic resistance of this organism.

Epidemiology

The organism thrives in moist environments such as soil and water. It can be found in large numbers in fresh fruits and vegetables. Human colonization begins within the gastrointestinal tract, with subsequent spread to moist cutaneous sites such as the perineum and axilla. *P. aeruginosa* is an opportunistic pathogen that rarely causes disease in healthy persons. While animal models suggest that both humoral and cell-mediated immunity are involved in host defense against *P. aeruginosa,* the most important host defense is the neutrophil. Numerous underlying diseases (cystic fibrosis), hematologic malignancy, or predisposing factors (burns, mechanical ventilation) are linked to *P. aeruginosa* infection; however, the clinical risk factor most frequently associated with severe infections is neutropenia.

SUSCEPTIBILITY IN VITRO

Over the past two decades, numerous antibacterial agents with potent in vitro activity against *P. aeruginosa* have been developed. They include the third-generation cephalosporins (cefoperazone, cefsulodin, ceftazidime), fourth-generation cephalosporins (cefepime, cefpirome, cefclidin), extended-spectrum penicillins (ticarcillin, piperacillin, azlocillin), monobactams (aztreonam), carbapenems (imipenem, meropenem), and quinolones (ciprofloxacin, enoxacin) (Table 1). Addition

TABLE 1 • **Minimum Inhibitory Concentrations of _Pseudomonas aeruginosa_ for Selected Antibiotics**

Antibiotic	MIC (mg/L)		
	MIC$_{50}$	MIC$_{90}$	Range
Extended-spectrum penicillins			
Piperacillin	4	64	1->128
Ticarcillin	32	128	1->128
Carbenicillin	64	256	8–512
Mezlocillin	64	256	1->128
Extended-spectrum penicillins plus β-lactamase inhibitors			
Piperacillin-tazobactam[a]	4	64	1->128
Ticarcillin-clavulanate[a]	32	128	1->128
Cephalosporins			
Third-generation			
Ceftazidime	2	8	0.5–128
Cefsulodin[b]	4	16	2->128
Cefoperazone	8	32	0.25->128
Cefotaxime	16	64	0.25->64
Ceftriaxone	16	64	0.25->64
Moxalactam	16	128	1->128
Fourth-generation			
Cefclidin[b]	0.78	6	0.25–50
Cefepime	4	16	1–32
Cefpirome	16	32	4->128
Other β-lactams			
Meropenem	1	2	0.06–16
Imipenem	2	8	0.5–256
Aztreonam	8	16	0.5–256
Quinolones			
Clinafloxacin[b]	0.06	0.25	0.03–1
Tosufloxacin[b]	0.25	1	0.06–4
Ciprofloxacin	0.5	2	0.06–4
Fleroxacin[b]	0.5	2	0.25–16
Ofloxacin	1	2	0.25–32
Norfloxacin	2	8	0.2–32
Lomefloxacin	2	4	0.5–8
Enoxacin[b]	2	8	0.05–8
Sparfloxacin	1	4	0.5–8
Aminoglycosides			
Tobramycin	2	4	0.25->512
Gentamycin	4	16	2->512
Amikacin	8	16	1–128
Isepamicin	8	16	1–128
Netilmicin	8	32	1–64

[a]Footnotes: Adapted from 8,20,51,78,83

[b]Investigational in the United States.

of β-lactamase inhibitors to extended-spectrum penicillins and cephalosporins has expanded the antibacterial spectra of these agents against Gram-positive and Gram-negative organisms; however, the antipseudomonal activity of ticarcillin/clavulanate and piperacillin/tazobactam has not been significantly enhanced. The β-lactamases of _P. aeruginosa_ are not generally inhibited by tazobactam or clavulanate. A small number of strains producing the β-lactamases PSE-1, PSE-3, PSE-4, CARB-4, and OXA-6 may be susceptible to these β-lactamase inhibitors (52).

β-Lactam Antibiotics

Piperacillin and ceftazidime are the most active penicillin and cephalosporin in vitro, respectively (Table 1). The major mechanism of resistance to β-lactam antibiotics is β-lactamase production. Both plasmid-mediated and chromosomally mediated β-lactamases occur. Plasmid-mediated β-lactamases are responsible for resistance to the penicillins but not to the cephalosporins or the carbapenems (20). Monotherapy with either aztreonam or the antipseudomonal cephalosporins or penicillins can result in selection of stably depressed mutants (induction) that produce massive amounts of chromosomally mediated β-lactamase (68). Although there are rare exceptions, the vast majority of β-lactamases produced by _P. aeruginosa_ are not affected by the β-lactamase inhibitors sulbactam, clavulanate, or tazobactam.

Other mechanisms of resistance to β-lactams are rare. Alteration in penicillin-binding proteins is a very rare cause of resistance that has emerged with therapy for _P. aeruginosa_ in patients with cystic fibrosis (33). Apart from the loss of a protein described above, decreased permeability of the bacterial outer membrane to β-lactams accounts for some of the relative resistance of _P. aeruginosa_ to β-lactams (3).

Carbapenems

The carbapenems are highly active in vitro against _P. aeruginosa_ and often remain active against strains resistant to other β-lactam agents and aminoglycosides. Imipenem and meropenem are not inactivated by any of the plasmid-mediated or chromosomally mediated β-lactamases described above. Plasmid-mediated metallo-β-lactamases have been described, however, that confer resistance to imipenem (57, 71, 81). Although rare at present, increased selective pressure from carbapenem use will likely result in a much larger problem of plasmid-mediated metallo-β-lactamases in the future (64). Strains of _P. aeruginosa_ resistant to the carbapenems can also be associated with lowered permeability of the bacterial outer membrane by loss of a porin protein (63). Cross-resistance to other β-lactams does not occur because the channel associated with this porin protein facilitates passage of carbapenems at low concentrations but not other β-lactams (76).

Aminoglycosides

The most active aminoglycoside in vitro against _P. aeruginosa_ is tobramycin, but the aminoglycoside with lowest frequency of resistant strains is amikacin. Aminoglycoside resistance in _P. aeruginosa_ is most commonly due to aminoglycoside-modifying enzymes (aminoglycoside-inactivating enzymes) that are coded by genes on plasmids or the chromosome. Modification of the aminoglycoside by these enzymes results in poor binding to the ribosome, the site of action of aminoglycosides. At least 14 different aminoglycoside-modifying enzymes can be produced by _P. aeruginosa_ (67). Reduced uptake of the aminoglycoside into bacteria has also been described as a mode of resistance in _P. aeruginosa_. In some cases this has been the mechanism of emergence of resistance during therapy. Cross-resistance for all aminoglycosides generally results, but the level of resistance is lower than that resulting from enzymatic modification.

Quinolones

Ciprofloxacin is the most active quinolone against *P. aeruginosa*. Resistance of *P. aeruginosa* to quinolones is chromosomally mediated. No clinical isolates exhibiting plasmid-mediated resistance have been found. Quinolones act by inhibiting the activity of DNA gyrase enzymes. Resistance to quinolones can result from mutations in the chromosomal genes that code for these gyrases (38). Another mechanism of resistance is decreased penetration of the outer membrane of the organism (38).

Multidrug Resistance

In vitro resistance to multiple classes of antibiotics, particularly that arising after treatment with a single antimicrobial agent, has been seen with *P. aeruginosa* (61). In some circumstances, this may be due to synergy between enhanced production of β-lactamases and decreased outer membrane permeability. More prominence is now given, however, to energy-dependent efflux of antibiotics by *P. aeruginosa*. A single operon facilitates resistance to quinolones, β-lactams, tetracycline, and chloramphenicol via drug efflux (61). Outer membrane proteins may be involved in this energy-dependent process.

ANTIMICROBIAL THERAPY

Antibiotic selection for treatment of *P. aeruginosa* is often problematic for the clinician. Clinical efficacy does not necessarily correlate with in vitro antibiotic susceptibility or in vivo studies in animals. Prospective, randomized, clinical trials of therapeutic agents for *Pseudomonas* infections are few, most involving empirical therapy in febrile neutropenic patients. Strain differences, presence of a protective mucoid capsule, and the ability of the organism to develop resistance while on therapy also complicate antibiotic selection.

Combination Therapy of β-Lactam plus Aminoglycoside Agents

Demonstration of in vitro synergy with antipseudomonal penicillin and aminoglycoside agents and the development of resistance with monotherapy prompted use of combination antibiotic therapy for serious *Pseudomonas* infections. A number of studies of Gram-negative bacteremia have suggested (but not proved) that combination therapy that is synergistic in vitro is therapeutically superior to combination therapy that is not. However, few studies focus only on *P. aeruginosa* infection (2, 16, 17, 37). In one retrospective study of 18 patients with *P. aeruginosa* bacteremia, synergistic combination of carbenicillin plus aminoglycoside (as determined by the checkerboard method) was successful in 83%, while nonsynergistic (additive) combination therapy was successful in none (2). But, in two later studies, no improvement in outcome was seen for combinations that were synergistic versus those that were not (as determined by the checkerboard method) (17, 37). The study by Hilf et al. found a trend toward improved out-

come for patients receiving antipseudomonal drug combinations synergistic in vitro by time-kill curve methods ($P < .10$) (37).

In a prospective observational study by Hilf et al. of 200 consecutive patients with *P. aeruginosa* bacteremia, combination therapy was significantly better than monotherapy in improving outcome (37). Mortality was significantly higher in patients given monotherapy (47%) than in those given combination therapy (27%). The most common combination used was piperacillin or ticarcillin combined with tobramycin or gentamicin. The monotherapy group was dominated by patients given an aminoglycoside alone. A randomized study of 550 patients with febrile neutropenia comparing ceftazidime alone with combination antibiotics showed equivalent outcomes in the two groups (60); however, this sample of 550 patients included only 12 *P. aeruginosa* bacteremias. In an EORTC study of neutropenic patients including 34 patients with *P. aeruginosa* bacteremia, ceftazidime plus 9 days of amikacin was superior to ceftazidime plus only 3 days of amikacin ($P = .06$) (28). In a large-scale observational study of Gram-negative bacteremia, empirical therapy (defined as antibiotics given within 48 h of obtaining the positive blood culture) resulted in significantly lower mortality for *P. aeruginosa* bacteremia if it was a combination of β-lactam plus aminoglycoside rather than a β-lactam alone (54).

Rifampin is synergistic in vitro with an antipseudomonal penicillin and aminoglycoside against *P. aeruginosa* (75, 80, 89). A prospective randomized trial of 121 patients was conducted to determine if addition of rifampin to the combination of antipseudomonal β-lactam and aminoglycoside would improve outcome in patients with *P. aeruginosa* bacteremia (49). Rifampin significantly increased the bacteriologic cure rate (2% failure for the three drugs vs. 14% failure for the two drugs) but did not improve mortality.

Double β-Lactam Agent Therapy

Combination of two antipseudomonal β-lactam agents has also been evaluated as empirical therapy in the febrile neutropenic host (25). Advantages include lower frequency of side effects related to aminoglycoside use, especially nephrotoxicity. Theoretical disadvantages to double β-lactam agent therapy include the absence of in vitro synergy that might be found with a β-lactam/aminoglycoside combination, and potential induction of β-lactamases that would inactivate one of the β-lactam agents.

Double β-lactam therapy has proved inferior to the β-lactam/aminoglycoside combination in animal models (43). One study in humans showed emergence of resistance in 40% (2 of 5) of cases in one series of *P. aeruginosa* infection treated with double β-lactams (85). In two studies comparing a moxalactam/piperacillin combination with moxalactam/amikacin, the response rate was superior for the aminoglycoside-containing regimen, although sample sizes were small (25, 85). Thus, the bulk of data suggests that double β-lactam agent therapy offers no advantage. Indeed, this combination should possibly be avoided if there is a high likelihood of *P. aeruginosa* infection.

Dosing

Standard doses are listed in Table 2. For ciprofloxacin, an intravenous dose of 400 mg every 8 h is recommended instead of the standard dose of 400 mg every 12 h.

Minimum bactericidal concentrations (MBCs) for the β-lactam agents are generally twofold higher than minimum inhibitory concentrations (MICs). The rate of bactericidal activity of β-lactams does not increase substantially once concentrations exceed four times the MIC (20). β-Lactams do not exhibit a postantibiotic effect against *P. aeruginosa,* with the notable exception of the carbapenems. Thus, high drug concentrations do not kill *P. aeruginosa* any faster than low concentrations, and bacterial regrowth begins very soon after serum and tissue levels fall below the MIC. Theoretically, the duration of time that serum levels exceed the MIC is the pharmacokinetic parameter that best correlates with in vivo efficacy of the β-lactams. Thus, many investigators have advocated continuous infusion of antipseudomonal β-lactams to ensure that serum levels exceed the MIC virtually all of the time; this approach awaits clinical validation (20).

Aminoglycosides exhibit concentration-dependent bactericidal activity and also produce prolonged postantibiotic effects (PAEs). This supports the practice of once-daily aminoglycoside dosing. For typical daily doses, tobramycin achieves the highest AUC (area under the serum concentration–time curve) to MIC_{50} ratio, followed by isepamicin, gentamicin, and amikacin. Once-daily dosing should increase the peak serum level:MIC ratio (C_{max}:MIC_{50}) for a given total daily dose of drug. The magnitude of the peak serum level also affects the emergence of resistant transport-deficient mutants of *P. aeruginosa*. While a few studies in animal models support the advantage of once-daily dosing (20), it awaits confirmation in clinical studies.

As with the aminoglycosides, the AUC:MIC and peak serum level:MIC ratios can be used to estimate the relative in vivo activity of the quinolones. For typical daily dosages, ciprofloxacin has the highest values, followed by fleroxacin and ofloxacin.

For *P. aeruginosa* bacteremia and deep-seated infections, we recommend use of any of the antipseudomonal penicillins or cephalosporins in combination with an aminoglycoside. For the aminoglycoside component of combination therapy, we prefer tobramycin, although its in vitro superiority has not been demonstrable in clinical trials. Carbapenems often continue to be active against organisms resistant to the other β-lactam agents. Ciprofloxacin, the only oral agent with proven efficacy, is a useful alternative in patients who are allergic to β-lactam agents.

SPECIFIC SITUATIONS
Skin and Soft-Tissue Infection

Folliculitis

Folliculitis due to *P. aeruginosa* results from exposure to contaminated water, particularly hot tubs, whirlpools, or swim-

---

TABLE 2 • Dosing of Antipseudomonal Drugs for Adults and Children with Normal Renal and Hepatic Function

Drug	Adult	Child	Infant
β-Lactams			
Penicillins			
Piperacillin	4 g q. 4–6 h	50 mg/kg q. 4–6 h[a]	50 mg/kg q. 4–12 h[a]
Piperacillin-tazobactam	3.375 g q. 6 h	80 mg/kg q. 8 h[a]	80 mg/kg q. 8–12 h[a]
Ticarcillin	3 g q. 4 h	40 mg/kg q. 4–6 h	75 mg/kg q. 12 h[a]
			75–100 mg/kg q. 8 h[c]
Ticarcillin-clavulanate	3.1 g q. 4–6 h	50 mg/kg q. 4–6 h[a]	50 mg/kg q. 4–12 h[a]
Cephalosporins			
Ceftazidime	1–2 g q. 8 h	30–50 mg/kg q. 8 h[d]	30 mg/kg q. 12 h
Other β-lactams			
Aztreonam	2 g q. 6–8 h	30 mg/kg q. 6–8 h	30 mg/kg q. 6–12 h[a]
Imipenem	0.5–1 g q. 6–8 h	10–15 mg/kg q. 6 h[a]	20 mg/kg q. 8–24 h[a]
Meropenem	1 g q. 8 h	20–40 mg/kg q. 8 h	20–40 mg/kg q. 8–24 h
Aminoglycosides			
Gentamicin	4–7 mg/kg q. 24 h	1–2.5 mg/kg q. 8 h[e]	2.5 mg/kg q. 8–24 h
Tobramycin	4–7 mg/kg q. 24 h	1–2.5 mg/kg q. 8 h[e]	2.5 mg/kg q. 8–24 h
Amikacin	5 mg/kg q. 8 h or 7.5 mg/kg q. 12 h	5 mg/kg q. 8 h	7.5–10 mg/kg q. 8–24 h
Quinolones			
Ciprofloxacin IV	400 mg q. 8–12 h	200–400 mg q. 12 h[a, f]	No data

[a]Dosages in infants and children under 12 years of age have not been clearly established.

[b]Use 75 mg/kg q. 12 h for infants under 2000 g body weight aged 0–7 days.

[c]Use 75 mg/kg q. 8 h for infants under 2000 g body weight but over 7 days old or in infants over 2 grams body weight aged 0–7 days; for infants over 2000 g body weight over 7 days old use 100 mg/kg q. 8 h.

[d]A maximum of 6 g/day should be used.

[e]In children with cystic fibrosis 2.5–3.5 mg/kg q. 8 h of gentamicin or tobramycin may be required.

[f]Many authorities do not recommend ciprofloxacin use in children.

ming pools. Normal hosts with intact skin are affected, predominantly in body sites covered by bathing suits. The disease is mild and self-limiting. Exposure of the head and external auditory canal may result in facial folliculitis or otitis externa. In healthy persons, lesions resolve spontaneously and scarring is rare, so no treatment may be necessary. Topical 0.1% polymyxin B has been useful.

Cellulitis and Pyoderma

Cellulitis due to *P. aeruginosa* occurs at sites of damage to the dermal barrier, such as puncture sites or surgical wounds. Pyoderma occurs when a preexisting skin lesion becomes colonized and subsequently invaded by *P. aeruginosa*. *Pseudomonas* infection can also occur in patients with underlying exfoliative skin diseases, venous stasis ulcers, and eczema. Severity of infection may range from localized cellulitis to a necrotizing gangrenous process with associated bacteremia in immunocompromised hosts. *P. aeruginosa* can be cultured from the purulent discharge, but clinical manifestations of erythema, tenderness, or heat should be present to differentiate infection from colonization. Infection may be acute and invasive or may follow a chronic indolent course. Long-term antipseudomonal therapy (e.g., oral ciprofloxacin) may be necessary for cure.

Toenail and Web

The moist interdigital areas of the feet are ideal sites for colonization with *P. aeruginosa*. When these areas become infected with dermatophytes or suffer other trauma to the dermal barrier, secondary bacterial invasion can readily occur. Treatment involves cleaning and debriding the infected skin and avoiding wetness. Therapy with dilute acetic acid can successfully suppress *P. aeruginosa*.

The green nail syndrome has been described when digits suffer prolonged immersion in water. Paronychial infection with *P. aeruginosa* leads to pyocyanin pigment staining of the adjacent nail. This benign condition can be treated by local measures such as removal of the onycholytic portion of the nail and avoiding wetness. In addition, therapy with dilute acetic acid (0.25–1%) or 0.1% polymyxin B can be used (1). Pigmentation may persist for many months following therapy.

Burns

Pseudomonas colonization of severe burn wounds is hospital acquired and usually accompanies colonization at other body sites (55). Colonization is abetted by broad-spectrum antibiotics, both topical and systemic. Cultures of the burn wound may not differentiate wound colonization from true invasive disease. Results from biopsy and quantitative cultures may be useful in differentiating infection from colonization (84). *Pseudomonas* infections typically occur several weeks after the initial burn, when normal skin flora is replaced by hospital flora. "Burn sepsis" is occasionally associated with positive blood cultures.

Topical agents are frequently used to prevent infection of burn wounds. Several topical antibiotic agents are available—silver sulfadiazine and mafenide (Sulfanylon). Outbreaks of sulfadiazine-resistant organisms have occurred in burn units in which silver sulfadiazine was used. Used prophylactically, it may delay *P. aeruginosa* colonization for more than 7 days. Mafemide has better eschar penetration than silver sulfadiazine. Early and frequent debridement of necrotic tissue and excision of infected burn wounds is probably more important than topical therapy in preventing infection.

Patients with overt infection should be treated aggressively with parenteral antibiotics. An aminoglycoside/β-lactam combination is recommended. Antibiotic susceptibility testing is critical for antibiotic choice, since nosocomial strains may be multiply resistant. Patients with significant burns have dramatic alterations in pharmacokinetics of most drugs. The risk in most patients may be undertreatment rather than antibiotic toxicity (87). The applicability of once-daily dosing of aminoglycosides in burn patients is unknown but is possibly advantageous. Individualized pharmacokinetic dosing with monitoring of aminoglycoside serum concentrations is recommended.

Soft-Tissue Infection in Immunocompromised Hosts

Ecthyma gangrenosum is a cutaneous manifestation of invasive infection due to *P. aeruginosa,* often associated with bacteremia and sepsis. Skin lesions may be multiple, with rapid evolution through stages of macules, nodules, vesicles, and ulcerative eschars.

Necrotizing fasciitis has been well described in neutropenic and diabetic hosts (53). In patients with facial cellulitis, the mucous membrane of the mouth is often the initial site of infection with subsequent spread to subcutaneous tissue and blood. Rapid progression to gangrene mandates vigorous surgery including extensive debridement and resection (53, 82). Combination antipseudomonal antibiotic therapy is necessary. Leukocyte transfusions or colony-stimulating factors are often used. Mortality is high, even with aggressive antibiotic therapy and surgical resection.

Pneumonia

Based on isolation of the organism from sputum culture, *P. aeruginosa* ranks as a leading cause of nosocomial pneumonia in the United States (15). Risk factors for development of *P. aeruginosa* pneumonia are (*a*) mechanical ventilation in an intensive care setting; (*b*) cancer, especially with concomitant neutropenia; (*c*) hypogammaglobulinemia; and (*d*) cystic fibrosis.

In intubated hospitalized patients, the diagnosis of *Pseudomonas* pneumonia is complicated by the inability of sputum cultures to differentiate between mucosal colonization and invasive disease. An observed increase in the quantity and purulence of respiratory secretions, combined with isolation and culture of the organism and appearance of systemic symptoms (fever) can justify therapy directed at *P. aeruginosa*.

No randomized controlled studies of therapy of *Pseudomonas* pneumonia have been performed. A prospective observational study of 28 cases of bacteremically confirmed *Pseudomonas* pneumonia demonstrated that survival rates were significantly better in patients receiving combination β-lactam/aminoglycoside therapy than in patients receiving monotherapy (mainly with aminoglycosides) (37).

The role of aminoglycosides for *Pseudomonas* pneumonia has been debated. Penetration of aminoglycosides into respiratory secretions is poor (7). Furthermore, reduced pH and presence of inflammatory cells in infected patients can limit the activity of aminoglycosides (10). Thus, local therapy via endotracheal administration has been applied. Small open studies of endotracheally administered aminoglycosides showed that this mode of administration improves bacteriologic and clinical outcome in nosocomial pneumonia (47, 70, 72). However, in a randomized study, endotracheally administered tobramycin led to significantly better bacteriologic eradication than placebo but no benefit in clinical outcome (13).

Quinolones have not been found to be synergistic with β-lactam agents or aminoglycosides in animal models of pneumonia (45). Ciprofloxacin is comparable to ceftazidime for monotherapy of nosocomial *Pseudomonas* pneumonia (36, 44). In a prospective, randomized, double-blind trial of ciprofloxacin versus imipenem in patients with nosocomial pneumonia, ciprofloxacin proved bacteriologically and clinically superior (29). However, when *P. aeruginosa* was the causative agent, bacteriologic failure (about 60%) and emergence of in vitro resistance (about 40%) was common in both groups (29).

Thus, for the bacteremic, immunosuppressed, or critically ill patient with *Pseudomonas* pneumonia, combination therapy is recommended. The current standard would be an antipseudomonal β-lactam agent combined with an aminoglycoside. A β-lactam agent combined with ciprofloxacin would presumably be less toxic, and controlled evaluation of this regimen seems warranted.

Endocarditis

Factors predisposing to *Pseudomonas* endocarditis include the presence of a prosthetic valve or other intravascular foreign body, underlying malignancy, chemotherapy, prolonged neutropenia, and intravenous drug use. Of these, intravenous drug use accounts for most cases, with regional epidemics in Midwestern U.S. cities (40, 41).

The specific heart valve involved is important with respect to clinical manifestations, therapy, and prognoses (41). Infection of the tricuspid valve represents the mildest form of endocarditis. The presentation is usually subacute, owing in large part to lower bacterial densities resulting from lower oxygen tension on the right side of the heart. Cure with antibiotic therapy alone is the rule, and valvulectomy is seldom indicated. Infection of the mitral valve presents more acutely, with more severe systemic manifestations. Valvular dysfunction may lead to congestive heart failure. Optimal treatment involves combined antibiotic and surgical therapy. Infection of the aortic valve is the most severe, with an acute, often fulminant, onset. Sepsis with multiple septic emboli, congestive heart failure, renal failure, and early death is common. Successful outcome requires rapid institution of aggressive antibiotic therapy combined with early replacement of the aortic valve. Even with combined medical and surgical therapy, survival in one series was only 38% (41).

Infection of prosthetic valves by *Pseudomonas* differs both clinically and pathologically from native valve infection. Surgical removal of infected prosthetic material and necrotic tissue is considered essential for cure.

An aminoglycoside combined with an antipseudomonal β-lactam remains the regimen of choice for most cases of endocarditis. Because of the high morbidity, Detroit investigators have recommended an aggressive dosing regimen for aminoglycosides (74). Their loading regimen consisted of gentamicin or tobramycin (8 mg/kg/day) given in three divided doses, regardless of underlying renal function. Thereafter, doses are adjusted to maintain peak serum aminoglycoside concentrations of 12 to 15 µg/mL and trough levels of 0 to 2 µg/mL. Patients treated in this manner were less than 45 years of age and without significant comorbidities. Even so, ototoxicity and nephrotoxicity were common, although the latter was usually reversed with discontinuation of the aminoglycoside. In patients with preexisting renal compromise, total aminoglycoside dosage and dosing intervals must be adjusted on the basis of serum concentrations. Once-daily aminoglycoside dosing has theoretical advantages over a multiple dosing regimen, but this remains to be confirmed.

The use of quinolones to treat *Pseudomonas* endocarditis has not been well studied, but anecdotal reports suggest that ciprofloxacin can be effective in patients intolerant of aminoglycosides (21, 79).

Ear Infection

Simple External Otitis

Simple external otitis is associated with warm, humid atmospheric conditions, aural water exposure, and ear canal trauma. *P. aeruginosa* is the most frequent organism isolated from the drainage associated with acute external otitis and is reported in up to 50% of cases (14). Local therapy is usually adequate. Crusts, scales, and debris must be evacuated from the ear canal. Wicks are commonly used. Topical antibiotics active in vitro against *P. aeruginosa* such as colistin sulfate, neomycin sulfate, aminoglycosides, and ciprofloxacin are preferred. A double-blind study found that antiseptic drops (aluminum acetate) that were inactive in vitro against *P. aeruginosa* were as effective as topical gentamicin (19).

Malignant External Otitis

Malignant (necrotizing) external otitis is a subset of osteomyelitis caused by *P. aeruginosa* in which the temporal bone and skull base are involved (34). The most important predisposing factor is the combination of advanced age (above 60 years) and diabetes mellitus. Classic signs of infection including fever, leukocytosis, and systemic toxicity are notably absent, thus making diagnosis difficult. Otalgia followed by severe and often excruciating headache is the most common presenting symptom. Cranial nerve dysfunction, especially facial nerve palsy, is a late complication. Diagnosis rests on abnormal findings of the temporal bone and skull on computed tomographic scan, an elevated erythrocyte sedimentation rate (often exceeding 100 mm/h), and isolation of *P. aeruginosa* from the external auditory canal or mastoid in a patient with a recalcitrant headache. Recurrence is the major complication, since mortality has decreased substantially with the advent of effective antipseudomonal therapy (32).

Interestingly, oral ciprofloxacin therapy (750 mg twice daily) appears to be as effective as parenteral combination antipseudomonal therapy (32, 65, 66). Duration should be 4 to 10 weeks, depending on the severity of infection at initiation of therapy. The erythrocyte sedimentation rate is useful in monitoring responsiveness to therapy. Hyperbaric oxygen has been used in anecdotal reports, but efficacy is uncertain (23). Surgery is rarely necessary except for local debridement or excision of accessible foci of infection such as polypectomy or removal of sequestrum.

Bone and Joint Infection

Community-acquired cases of *Pseudomonas* osteomyelitis are uncommon but can occur in intravenous drug users in the context of *P. aeruginosa* bacteremia. Superinfection of diabetic foot ulcers and direct inoculation via puncture wounds of the foot may result in *P. aeruginosa* alone or in combination with other bacteria. Antibiotic therapy with adjunctive surgical debridement is the current standard. Most cases of *P. aeruginosa* osteomyelitis can be treated with single-antibiotic therapy consisting of an antipseudomonal β-lactam or quinolone (22, 26). Immunosuppressed patients with associated *P. aeruginosa* bacteremia should receive a combination of β-lactam agent and aminoglycoside. Duration of therapy is prolonged (4–6 weeks), dating from initiation of therapy or from the last major surgical debridement. In the absence of vascular compromise or diabetes mellitus, a 4-week course of antibiotics may be adequate (42). In chronic osteomyelitis, in which prolonged therapy is needed (e.g., 6–10 weeks), oral ciprofloxacin can play a major role as single-agent therapy. This should follow adequate debridement, hardware removal, and an initial course of 4 to 6 weeks of parenteral therapy. The use of oral monotherapy will be limited by the extent of emergence of resistant organisms (4, 5).

Urinary Tract Infection

Urinary tract infection due to *Pseudomonas aeruginosa* is related to urinary tract catheterization or instrumentation, chronic prostatitis, renal stones, or prior antibiotic therapy. Uncomplicated urinary tract infection in females is relatively rare. Infections are often persistent and difficult to treat. Treatment regimens depend upon a number of variables including presence or absence of systemic sepsis, site of involvement, presence of structural abnormalities including indwelling urinary catheters, and previous antibiotic use. In general, the organism can be difficult to eradicate, unless the predisposing factors that led to infection are eliminated.

Uncomplicated symptomatic urinary tract infection in the patient with no structural abnormality can be treated with carbenicillin or ciprofloxacin for 3 to 5 days. The asymptomatic patient with an indwelling urinary catheter should not be treated with antibiotics. Treatment will lead to either replacement of the *P. aeruginosa* with another organism resistant to the drug or emergence of a *P. aeruginosa* strain resistant to the antibiotic in question. Systemic antibiotics should be reserved for patients with fever or evidence of sepsis. The catheter should be removed or replaced if at all possible. Intermittent catheterization may be considered in the patient with urinary obstruction or a neurogenic bladder. Combination of an antipseudomonal β-lactam plus an aminoglycoside is recommended for urosepsis for 10 days. Two to 3 weeks of therapy should be given for pyelonephritis and longer for intrarenal or perinephric abscess.

The patient with recurrent symptomatic infections and whose focus of infection can not be removed is a difficult problem. One approach is to use acute parenteral therapy for 7 to 10 days, followed by chronic suppression with ciprofloxacin for 4 to 6 weeks. Subsequent emergence of resistant organisms has been common with prolonged oral quinolone therapy, however (5, 30). Prostatitis due to *P. aeruginosa* is also difficult to treat; therapy with an oral quinolone for 6 to 12 weeks is often necessary.

Eye Infections

P. aeruginosa infections of the eye are rare but, when they occur, can be serious.

Corneal Ulceration and Keratitis

P. aeruginosa is a common cause of corneal ulceration, usually in contact lens wearers. Topical ticarcillin and piperacillin are often used. Topical tobramycin is often preferred over gentamicin and amikacin because of superiority in vitro (which should be confirmed in the laboratory). Amikacin can be used for strains resistant in vitro to tobramycin. Both tobramycin and gentamicin are commercially available as a 0.3% solution (3 mg/mL). Fortification with the intravenous preparation (40 mg/mL) to 13.6 mg/mL may be advantageous because of increased diffusion into the tissues and anterior chamber. Multiple and frequent instillation topically is recommended for severe infections, especially for initial therapy (e.g., every 15–30 min). As an alternative, a collagen shield reconstituted with 0.3% tobramycin and placed onto the eye releases antibiotic over several hours (88).

The quinolones have also proven useful (48, 77). Although ciprofloxacin is more active in vitro, ofloxacin has greater ocular tissue penetration. Fortification of the commercial preparation (0.3%, 3.0 mg/mL) of ofloxacin is possible by using the intravenous preparation (ciprofloxacin is near its saturation limit with the commercial preparation) (12, 88).

Granulocyte colony-stimulating factor given parenterally was useful in an anecdotal report of a human immunodeficiency virus (HIV) patient with leukopenia (88).

Endophthalmitis

Endophthalmitis caused by *P. aeruginosa* is a medical emergency. The most common predisposing factor is postoperative infection after cataract surgery. If treatment is delayed, return of retinal function is poor, despite antibiotics. Systemic therapy is required in addition to ocular administration. Direct injection of antipseudomonal antibiotics into the anterior chamber and vitreous cavity is usually necessary. Retinal necrosis may occur if antibiotic concentrations are excessive. Cipro-

TABLE 3 • Antipseudomonal Antibiotic Formulations for Keratitis and Corneal Ulceration

Drug	Suggested Concentrations (mg/mL)	Comments
Amikacin[a]	14–50	Use 50 mg/mL
Ciprofloxacin	3	Commercial preparation
Gentamicin	3	Commercial preparation
Gentamicin[b]	13.6	
Piceracillin[a, c]	7–100	Use 50 mg/mL
Ticarcillin[a, c]	7–100	Use 50 mg/mL
Tobramycin[b]	3	Commercial preparation
Vancomycin[a, c]	33–50	Use 33 mg/mL

From Zloty P, Belin MW. Ocular infections caused by *Pseudomonas aeruginosa*. In: Baltch AL, Smith RD, eds. *Pseudomonas aeruginosa* infections and treatment. New York: Marcel Dekker, 1994, with permission.

[a]Preservative-free normal saline should be used to formulate topical solutions for ocular use from intravenous preparations.

[b]Formulations using intravenous concentrates and commercial preparation together. Fortification of a commercial ocular aminoglycoside with the intravenous preparation usually results in a concentration of 13.6 mg/mL.

[c]pH buffering will decrease discomfort and local irritation.

floxacin, ceftazidime, and imipenem have better intraocular penetration than aminoglycosides.

Meningitis

P. aeruginosa is a rare cause of meningitis. Mortality is high, especially if infection results from bacteremia in an immunosuppressed host, underlying endocarditis, or malignant otitis externa. Cure is more likely if the meningitis results from neurosurgical procedures involving ventricular shunts, drains, or reservoirs.

Ceftazidime has been widely used because of its in vitro activity and ability to penetrate the cerebrospinal fluid (30). Carbapenems, with excellent in vitro activity against *P. aeruginosa* and ability to penetrate into the cerebrospinal fluid, are a useful alternative, especially when resistant organisms are present. However, the high doses of imipenem required may be associated with central nervous system toxicity, most notably seizures. Meropenem also reaches high concentrations in the cerebrospinal fluid and has been successful in treating *P. aeruginosa* meningitis (18, 59). Central nervous system toxicity due to meropenem was not seen in an animal model of meningitis (59).

Addition of an aminoglycoside can be justified on the basis of synergistic interaction or prevention of ceftazidime resistance. Anecdotal reports, however, have not clearly shown enhanced efficacy with addition of an aminoglycoside. This may be due to poor penetration of the aminoglycosides into cerebrospinal fluid. Thus, intrathecal or intraventricular, as well as intravenous administration of aminoglycosides may be required for maximal effect.

Ciprofloxacin has been successfully used in anecdotal reports (39, 56, 69, 86). However, given its relatively poor pen-

etration into the cerebrospinal fluid, ciprofloxacin usage should be confined to situations involving life-threatening β-lactam drug allergies or the presence of documented β-lactam-resistant organisms (58). In one case of recurrent meningitis, a ciprofloxacin dose of 800 mg every 8 h (49 mg/kg/day) was used successfully (86). Ciprofloxacin concentration in the CSF was 2.6 μg/mL, while the MIC for this multidrug-resistant organism was 0.5 to 1.0 μg/mL.

APPROACHES TO CLINICAL SYNDROMES

Febrile Neutropenic Host

Conventional empirical therapy of the febrile neutropenic host has generally involved use of an antipseudomonal β-lactam agent in combination with an aminoglycoside. The superior in vitro activity of the new β-lactam and fluoroquinolone agents has renewed interest in monotherapy. A number of prospective randomized studies have compared monotherapy with newer β-lactam agents or ciprofloxacin with combination regimens. In most studies, monotherapy has proven equally efficacious, but the number of documented *P. aeruginosa* infections, especially *P. aeruginosa* bacteremia, has been small. When the presence of *P. aeruginosa* has been documented, outcome has been predictably poor regardless of the regimen used (27). Most investigators, including ourselves, have preferred combination antibiotic therapy when *P. aeruginosa* bacteremia has been documented.

Maximal survival for disseminated *P. aeruginosa* infections with bacteremia requires early administration of antibiotic therapy (6, 9, 11, 37, 50). Thus, the strategy of adding an aminoglycoside when *P. aeruginosa* is isolated following prior empirical administration of a single antipseudomonal agent may be inadequate given any delay. This issue requires further clarification. On the other hand, for a number of reasons, the frequency of *P. aeruginosa* infection has been steadily declining in this patient population, and the issue of combination antibiotic therapy for *P. aeruginosa* has been supplanted by increasing concern about Gram-positive bacterial and fungal infections.

AIDS

Pseudomonas aeruginosa infections involving virtually any body site have been described in HIV-infected patients (31, 46) and may be the first indication of underlying immune dysfunction. *P. aeruginosa* is the most frequently isolated Gram-negative bacillus in bacteremias in HIV-infected patients, even more common than *Salmonella*.

Hospitalized HIV-infected patients are at higher risk of acquiring nosocomial *P. aeruginosa* infections than other hospitalized immunocompromised patients (31). Community-acquired *P. aeruginosa* pneumonia in an apparently healthy individual should prompt testing for HIV. Pneumonia due to *P. aeruginosa* tends to be less fulminant in AIDS patients than in other immunocompromised patients. Unusual radiographic patterns such as lobar consolidation and interstitial infiltrates are commonly seen and may be indistinguishable from more common pulmonary pathogens in HIV patients such as *Pneumocystis carinii* (31).

TABLE 4 • Ocular Penetration of Antipseudomonal Antibiotics after a Single Intravenous Dose

Antibiotic	Dosage (i.v.)	Aqueous (μg/mL)	Vitreous (μg/mL)
Amikacin	7.5 mg/kg	—[a]	—[a]
Gentamicin	1 mg/kg	<.08	—[a]
Tobramycin	1 mg/kg	3.4	
Imipenem	1 g	2.99	2.53
Ceftazidime	2 g	3.4–11.0	No data
Ciprofloxacin	400 mg	0.8	0.1–0.04
	750 mg oral	0.18	0.06–0.28

From Zloty P, Belin MW. Ocular infections caused by *Pseudomonas aeruginosa*. In: Baltch AL, Smith RD, eds. *Pseudomonas aeruginosa* infections and treatment. New York: Marcel Dekker, 1994: . With permission.

[a]Not detected.

An antipseudomonal β-lactam in combination with an aminoglycoside should be considered first-line therapy. Development of resistance during treatment is well documented, even with combination therapy. Relapses are common, even after an apparently successful treatment course. A prolonged course of oral ciprofloxacin may prevent relapse. An anecdotal case of relapsing pseudomonal pneumonia was successfully controlled with nebulized colistin used as prophylaxis (35). In cases of relapse, an unrecognized focus of infection should be sought (e.g., sinus, bone, abscess) (46).

Cystic Fibrosis

P. aeruginosa is the predominant respiratory tract pathogen in patients with cystic fibrosis (73). A large proportion of the isolates are mucoid with a slime coating, which makes them relatively resistant to opsonization, phagocytosis, and antibacterial agents and increases their adherence to respiratory tract cells. Once colonization occurs, eradication is unlikely, and chronic colonization predicts a poorer prognosis (73).

Patients, usually children, typically have hacking cough with copious sputum production. Respiratory insufficiency can lead to decreased quality of life and ultimately death. Antibiotic therapy is generally used for patients with pulmonary exacerbation, although a few investigators have questioned its necessity (73). Parenteral antipseudomonal therapy consisting of a β-lactam agent (e.g., piperacillin or ceftazidime) combined with an aminoglycoside (e.g., tobramycin) is standard. Monotherapy is often used, but rapid emergence of resistance is common. Home-based parenteral therapy has obvious advantages for these chronically infected patients with intermittent exacerbations. Oral ciprofloxacin has proven as effective as parenteral antipseudomonal agents, but emergence of resistant isolates has limited its widespread use. Aerosolized therapy with β-lactam agents, aminoglycosides, and colistin, has been used alone or in combination with parenteral agents (73), although emergence of antibiotic-resistant strains is a concern with monotherapy.

Cystic fibrosis patients metabolize aminoglycosides, β-lactam agents, and trimethoprim-sulfamethoxazole more rapidly than normal individuals, necessitating higher doses of antibi-

otics (62). Ciprofloxacin pharmacokinetics are not affected, however, and dosing adjustments are not necessary (24).

ADJUNCTIVE

Alternative therapeutic modalities to antimicrobial agents such as immunotherapy and cytokine modulation are currently under investigation but are not expected to be commercially available for some years.

REFERENCES

1. Agger WA, Mardan A. *Pseudomonas aeruginosa* infections of intact skin. Clin Infect Dis 1995;20:302–308.
2. Anderson ET, Young LS, Hewitt W. Antimicrobial synergism in the therapy of gram-negative rod bacteremia. Chemotherapy 1978;24:45–54.
3. Angus BL, Carey AM, Caron DA, Kropinski AMB, Hancock REW. Outer membrane permeability in *Pseudomonas aeruginosa;* comparison of wild-type with an antibiotic supersucceptible mutant. Antimicrob Agents Chemother 1982;21:299–309.
4. Aquado JH, Arjona R, Valle R, Moreno J. Prolonged oral ciprofloxacin treatment of recalcitrant and severe osteomyelitis [Abstract 980]. 30th Interscience Conference on Antimicrobial Agents and Chemotherapy, Atlanta, 1990.
5. Ball P. Emergent resistance to ciprofloxacin amongst *Pseudomonas aeruginosa* and *Staphylococcus aureus:* clinical significance and therapeutic approaches. J Antimicrob Chemother 1990;16(Suppl F):165–169.
6. Baltch AL, Griffin PE. *Pseudomonas aeruginosa* bacteremia: a clinical study of 75 patients. Am J Med Sci 1977;274:119–129.
7. Bergogne-Berezin E. Pharmacokinetics of antibiotics in respiratory secretions. In: Pennington JE, ed. Respiratory infections: diagnosis and management. 2nd ed. New York: Raven Press, 1984.
8. Biederbach DJ, Sutton RD, Jones RD. Antimicrobial activity of CS-940, a new trifluorinated quinolone. J Infect Dis 1984;149:257–263.
9. Bisbe J, Gatell JM, Puig J, Martinez JA, de Anta Jemines M, Soriano E. *Pseudomonas aeruginosa* bacteremia: univariate and multivariate analyses of factors influencing the prognosis in 122 patients. Rev Infect Dis 1988;10:629–635.
10. Bodem C, Lampton D, Miller E, Everett E. Endobronchial pH. Relevance to aminoglycoside activity in gram-negative bacillary pneumonia. Am J Respir Dis 1983;127:39–41.
11. Bodey GP, Jadeja L, Elting L. Pseudomonas bacteremia. Retrospective alalysis of 410 episodes. Arch Intern Med 1985;145:1621–1629.
12. Bowe BE, Snyder JW, Eiiferman RA. An in vitro study of the potency and stability of fortified opthalmic antibiotic preparations. Am J Ophthalmol 1991;111:686–689.
13. Brown RB, Kruse JA, Counts GWJA, Christou NV, Sands M. Double-blind study of endotracheal tobramycin in the treatment of gram-negative bacterial pneumonia. Antimicrob Agents Chemother 1990;34:269–272.
14. Cassisi N, Cohn A, Davidson T, Witten BR. Diffuse otitis externa: clinical and microbiological findings in the course of a multicenter study on a new otic solution. Ann Otol Rhinol Laryngol Suppl 1977;86:1–16.
15. Centers for Disease Control. Guidelines for prevention of nosocomial pneumonia. MMWR 1997;46:4RR–7RR.
16. Chan EL, Zabrinsky RJ. Determination of synergy by two methods with eight antimicrobial combinations against tobramycin-

susceptible and tobramycin-resistant strains of *Pseudomonas aeruginosa*. Diagn Microbiol Infect Dis 1987;6:157–164.

17. Chandrasekar PH, Crane LR, Bailey EJ. Comparison of the activity of antibiotic combinations in vitro with clinical outcome and resistance emergence in serious infections by *Pseudomonas aeruginosa* in nonneutropenic patients. Antimicrob Chemother 1987;9:321–329.

18. Chmelik V, Gutvirth J. Meropenem treatment of post-traumatic meningitis due to *Pseudomonas aeruginosa*. J Antimicrob Chemother 1993;32:922–929.

19. Clayton MI, Osborne JE, Rutherford P, Rivron RP. A double-blind, randomized, prospective trial of a topical antiseptic versus a topical antibiotic in the treatment of otorrhea. Clin Otolaryngol 1990;15:7–10.

20. Craig WA, Ebert SC. Antimicrobial therapy in *Pseudomonas aeruginosa* infections. In: Baltch AL, Smith RP, eds. *Pseudomonas aeruginosa* infections and treatment. New York: Marcel Dekker, 1994:441–518.

21. Daikos GL, Kathpalia S, Lolans V, Jackson GG, Fossilien E. Long-term oral ciprofloxacin: experience in the treatment of incurable infective endocarditis. Am J Med 1988;84:786–790.

22. Dan M, Sigeman-Igra Y, Pitlik S, Raz R. Oral ciprofloxacin treatment of *Pseudomonas aeruginosa* osteomyelitis. Antimicrob Agents Chemother 1990;34:849–852.

23. Davis JC, Gates GA, Lerner C, Davis MG, Mader JT, Dinesman A. Adjuvant hyperbaric oxygen in malignant external otitis. Arch Otolaryngol Head Neck Surg 1992;118:89–93.

24. Davis RL, Koup JR, Williams-Warren J, Weber A, Heggen L, Stempel D, Smith AL. Pharmacokinetics of ciprofloxacin in cystic fibrosis. Antimicrob Agents Chemother 1987;32:915–919.

25. Dejace P, Klatersky J. Comparative review of combination therapy: two beta-lactams versus beta-lactam plus aminoglycoside. J Med 1986;80(Suppl 6B):29–38.

26. Dellamonica P, Bernard E, Etesse H, Garaffo R, Drugeon HB. Evaluation of pefloxacin, ofloxacin, and ciprofloxacin in the treatment of 39 cases of chronic osteomyelitis. Eur J Clin Microbiol Infect Dis 1989;8:1024–1030.

27. DePauw BE. New empiric regimens for febrile neutropenic patients. Curr Opin Infect Dis 1993;6:725–730.

28. EORTC International Antimicrobial Therapy Group. Ceftazidime combined with short or long course of amikacin for empirical therapy of gram-negative bacteremia in cancer patients with granulocytopenia. N Engl J Med 1987;317:1692–1698.

29. Fink MP, Snydman DR, Niederman MS, Leeper KV, Johnson RH, Heard SO, Wunderink RG, Caldwell JW, Schentag JJ, Siami GA, Zameck RL, Haverstock DL, Reinhart HH, Echols RM. Treatment of severe pneumonia in hospitalized patients: results of a multicenter, randomized, double-blind trial comparing intravenous ciprofloxacin with imipenem-cilastatin. Antimicrob Agents Chemother 1994;38:547–557.

30. Fong IW, Tomkins KB. Penetration of ceftazidime into the CSF of patients with and without evidence of meningitis. Antimicrob Agents Chemother 1984;26:115–119.

31. Franzetti F, Cernuschi M, Esposito R, Moroni M. *Pseudomonas* infections in patients with AIDS and AIDS-related complex. J Int Med 1992;231:437–443.

32. Giamarellou H. Malignant otitis externa: the therapeutic evolution of a lethal infection. J Antimicrob Chemother 1992;30:745–51.

33. Godrey AJ, Byran LE, Rabin HR. Beta-lactam-resistant *Pseudomonas aeruginosa* with modified penicillin-binding proteins emerging during cystic fibrosis treatment. Antimicrob Agents Chemother 1981;19:705–711.

34. Grandis JR, Yu VL. *Pseudomonas aeruginosa* infection of the ear. In: Baltch AL, Smith RP, eds. *Pseudomonas* infections and treatment. New York: Marcel Dekker, 1994:

35. Green ST, Nathwani D, Gourley Y, McMenamin J, Goldberg DJ, Kennedy DH. Nebulized colistin (polymyxin E) for AIDS-associated *Pseudomonas aeruginosa* pneumonia. Int J STD AIDS 1992;3:130–131.

36. Haddow A, Greene S, Heinz G, Wantuck D. Ciprofloxacin (intravenous/oral) versus ceftazidime in lower respiratory tract infections. Am J Med 1989;87(Suppl 5A):113S–115S.

37. Hilf M, Yu VL, Sharp J, Zuravleff JJ, Korvick JA, Muder RR. Antibiotic therapy for *Pseudomonas aeruginosa* bacteremia: outcome correlations in a prospective study of 200 patients. Am J Med 1989;87:540–546.

38. Hooper DC, Wolfson JS. Mechanisms of bacterial resistance to quinolones. In: Hooper DC, Wolfson JS, eds. Quinolone antimicrobial agents. 2nd ed. Washington, DC: American Society for Microbiology, 1993:

39. Isaacs D, Stack MPE, Wilkinson AR, Westwood AW. Successful treatment of *Pseudomonas* ventriculitis with ciprofloxacin. J Antimicrob Chemother 1986;17:535–538.

40. Jackson GG, Riff LJ. *Pseudomonas* bacteremia: pharmacologic and other bases for failure of treatment with gentamicin. J Infect Dis 1971;124:S185–198.

41. Jackson GG. Infective endocarditis caused by *Pseudomonas aeruginosa*. In: Baltch AL, Smith RP, eds. *Pseudomonas aeruginosa* infection and treatment. New York: Marcel Dekker, 1994:129–158.

42. Jacobs RF, McCarthy R, Elser J. *Pseudomonas* osteochondritis complicating puncture wounds of the foot in children—a 10 year evaluation. J Infect Dis 1989;4:657–661.

43. Johnson DE, Thompson B. Efficacy of single-agent therapy with azlocillin, ticarcillin, and amikacin and beta-lactam/amikacin combinations for the treatment of *Pseudomonas aeruginosa* bacteremia in granulocytopenic rats. Am J Med 1986;89(Suppl 5C):53–58.

44. Kahn FA, Basin R. Sequential intravenous-oral administration of ciprofloxacin vs. ceftazidime in serious bacterial respiratory tract infection. Chest 1989;96:528–537.

45. Kemmerich B, Small G, Pennington JE. Comparative evaluation of ciprofloxacin, enoxacin, and ofloxacin in experimental *Pseudomonas aeruginosa* infections. Antimicrob Chemother 1986;29:395–399.

46. Kielholner M, Atmar RL, Hamill RJ, Musher DM. Life-threatening *Pseudomonas aeruginosa* infections in patients with human immunodeficiency virus infection. Clin Infect Dis 1992;14:403–411.

47. Klatersky J, Huysmans D, Weerts C, Hensgens C, Daneou D. Endotracheally administered gentamicin for the prevention of infections of the respiratory tract in patients with tracheostomy: a double blind study. Chest 1974;65:650–654.

48. Knauf HP, Silvany R, Southern PM, Risser RC, Wilson SE. Susceptibility of corneal and conjunctival pathogens to ciprofloxacin. Cornea 1996;15:66–71.

49. Korvick JA, Peacock JE, Muder RR, Wheeler RR, Yu VL. Addition of rifampin to combination antibiotic therapy for *Pseudomonas aeruginosa* bacteremia: prospective trial using the Zelen protocol. Antimicrob Agents Chemother 1992;36:620–625.

50. Korvick J, Yu VL, Hilf M. Susceptibility of 100 blood isolates of *Pseudomonas aeruginosa* to 19 antipseudomonal antibiotics: old and new. Diagn Microbiol Infect Dis 1987;7:107–111.

51. Kovacs K, Yu VL. Antipseudomonal antimicrobial agent therapy. Drugs Today 1994;30:155–170.

52. Kuck NA, Jacobus NV, Petersen N, Weiss WJ, Testa RT. Comparative in vitro and in vivo activities of piperacillin combined with the beta-lactamase inhibitors tazobactam, clavulanic acid and sulbactam. Antimicrob Agents Chemother 1989;33:1964–1969.

53. Kusne S, Eibling DE, Yu VL, et al. Gangrenous cellulitis associated with gram-negative bacilli in pancytopenic patients: dilemma with respect to effective therapy. Am J Med 1988;85:490–494.

54. Leibovici L, Paul M, Poznanski O, Drucker M, Samm Z, Koningsberger H, Pitlick SD. Monotherapy versus beta-lactam aminoglycoside combination treatment for gram-negative bacteremia: a prospective observational study. Antimicrob Agents Chemother 1997;41:1127–1133.

55. McManus AT, Mason AD, McManus WF. Twenty-five year review of Pseudomonas aeruginosa bacteremia in a burn center. Eur J Clin Microbiol 1985;4:219–226.

56. Millar M, Bransby-Zachary M, Tompkins D, Hawkey P, Gibson R. Ciprofloxacin for Pseudomonas aeruginosa meningitis. Lancet 1986;I:1325.

57. Minami S, Akama M, Araki H, Watanabe Y, Narita H, Iyobe S, Mitsuhashi S. Imipenem and cephem resistant Pseudomonas aeruginosa carrying plasmids coding for class B beta-lactamase. J Antimicrob Chemother 1996;37:433–444.

58. Nau R, Prange H, Martell J, Sharifi S, Kolenda H, Birchner J. Penetration of ciprofloxacin into the cerebrospinal fluid of patients with uninflamed meninges. J Antimicrob Chemother 1990;15:965–973.

59. Patel JB, Giles RB. Meropenem: evidence of lack of proconvulsive tendency in mice. J Antimicrob Chemother 1989;24(Suppl A):125–1332.

60. Pizzo PA, Hathorn JW, Hiemenz J. A randomized trial comparing ceftazidime alone with combination antibiotic therapy in cancer patients with fever and neutropenia. N Engl J Med 1986;315:552–558.

61. Poole K. Bacterial multidrug resistance—emphasis on efflux mechanisms and Pseudomonas aeruginosa. J Antimicrob Chemother 1994;34:453–456.

62. Prandota J. Drug disposition in cystic fibrosis: progress in understanding pathophysiology and pharmacokinetics. Pediatr Infect Dis J 1987;6:1111–1126.

63. Quinn JP, DiVincenzo CA, Lerner SA. Resistance to imipenem in Pseudomonas aeruginosa: clinical experience and biochemical mechanisms. Rev Infect Dis 1988;10:892–898.

64. Rasmussen BA, Bush K. Carbapenem-hydrolyzing beta-lactamases. Antimicrob Agents Chemother 1997;41:223–232.

65. Rubin J, Yu VL. Malignant external otitis: insights into pathogenesis, clinical manifestations, diagnosis and therapy. Am J Med 1988;85:391–398.

66. Rubin JG, Stoehr G, Yu VL, Muder RR, Matador A, Kamerer DB. Efficacy of oral ciprofloxacin plus rifampin for treatment of malignant external otitis. Arch Otolaryngol Head Neck Surg 1889;115:1063–1069.

67. Sabath LD. Biochemical and physiologic basis for susceptibility and resistance of Pseudomonas aeruginosa to antimicrobial agents. Rev Infect Dis 1984;6(Suppl 3):S643–656.

68. Sanders CC. Chromosomal cephalosporinases responsible for multiple resistance to newer beta-lactam antibiotics. Annu Rev Microbiol 1987;41:573–593.

69. Schonwald S, Beus I, Lisic M, Car V, Gmajricki B. Brief report: ciprofloxacin in the treatment of gram-negative bacillary meningitis. Am J Med 1989;87(Suppl 5A):248S–249S.

70. Schuller JP, Coppens I, Klatersky J. Effectiveness of mezlocillin and endotracheally administered sisomicin with or without parenteral sisomicin in the treatment of gram-negative bronchopneumonia. J Antimicrob Chemother 1982;9:63–68.

71. Senda CC, Arakawa Y, Nakashima K, Ito H, Ichiyama S, Shimikata K, Kato N, Ohta M. Multifocal outbreaks of metallo-beta-lactamase-producing Pseudomonas aeruginosa resistant to broad-spectrum beta-lactams, including carbapenem. Antimicrob Agents Chemother 1996;40:349–353.

72. Sorensen VJ, Horst H, Obeid F, Bivens B. Endotracheal aminoglycoside in gram negative pneumonia. Am Surg 1986;52:391–394.

73. Speert DP. Pseudomonas aeruginosa infection in patients with cystic fibrosis. In: Baltch AL, Smith RD, eds. Pseudomonas aeruginosa infection and treatment. New York: Marcel Dekker, 1994.

74. Tablan OC, Reyes MP, Rintelmann WF, Lerner AM. Renal and auditory toxicity of high-dose, prolonged therapy with gentamicin and tobramycin in P. aeruginosa endocarditis. J Infect Dis 1984;149:257–263.

75. Traub WH, Spohr M, Bauer D. Pseudomonas aeruginosa: in vitro susceptibility to antimicrobial drugs, single and combined, with and without defibrinated human blood. Chemotherapy 1988;34:284–297.

76. Trias J, Dufresne J, Levesque RC, Nikaido H. Decreased outer membrane permeability in imipenem-resistant mutants of Pseudomonas aeruginosa. Antimicrob Agents Chemother 1989;33:1202–1206.

77. Tsai AC, Tseng MC, Cheng SW, Hu FR. Clinical evaluation of ciprofloxacin ophthalmic solution in the treatment of refractory bacterial keratitis. J Formosan Med Assoc 1995;94:760–764.

78. Tsuji M, Isahii Y, Ohno A, Yamaguchi K. In vitro and in vivo antibacterial activities of S-1090, a new oral cephalosporin. Antimicrob Agents Chemother 1995;39:2544–2551.

79. Uzun O, Erdal Akalin H, Unal S, Demirin M, Yorgancioglu AC, Ugurlu B. Long-term oral ciprofloxacin in the treatment of prosthetic valve endocarditis due to Pseudomonas aeruginosa. Scand J Infect Dis 1992;24:707–800.

80. Valdes JM, Baltch A, Smith RP, et al. The effect of rifampicin or the in vitro activity of cefopirime or ceftazidime in combination with aminoglycosides against Pseudomonas aeruginosa. J Antimicrob Chemother 1990;25:575–584.

81. Watanabe M, Iyobe S, Inoue M, Mitsuhashi S. Transferable imipenem resistance in Pseudomonas aeruginosa. Antimicrob Agents Chemother 1991;35:147–151.

82. Weinbren MJ, Forgeson G, Helenglass G, Jameson B, Powles R. Unusual presentation of Pseudomonas infection. Br Med J 1988;297:1034–1035.

83. Wiedemann B, Grimm H. Susceptibility to antibiotics. Species incidence and trends. In: Lorian V, ed. Antibiotics in laboratory medicine. 4th ed. Baltimore: Williams & Wilkins, 19xx:900–1168.

84. Williams HB, Breidenbach WC, Callaghan WB. Are burn wound biopsies obsolete? A comparative study of bacterial quantitation in burn patients using the absorbent disc and biopsy techniques. Ann Plast Surg 1984;13:388–395.

85. Winston DJ, Barnes RC, Ho WG, Young LS, Champlin RE, Gate RP. Moxalactam plus piperacillin versus moxalactam plus amikacin in febrile granulocytopenia patients. Am J Med 1984;77:442–450.

86. Wong-Beringer A, Beringer P, Lovett MA. Successful treatment of multidrug-resistant *Pseudomonas aeruginosa* meningitis with high-dose ciprofloxacin. Clin Infect Dis 1997;25:936–937.

87. Zaske D, Chin T, Kohls PR, Solem LD, Strate RG. Initial dosage regimens of gentamicin in patients with burns. J Burn Care Rehabil 1991;12:46–50.

88. Zloty P, Belin MW. Ocular infections caused by *Pseudomonas aeruginosa*. In: Baltch AL, Smith RD, eds. *Pseudomonas aeruginosa* infections and treatment. New York: Marcel Dekker, 1994:

89. Zuravleff JJ, Yu VL, Yee RB. Ticarcillin-tobramycin-rifampin: in vitro synergy of the triplet combination against *Pseudomonas aeruginosa*. J Lab Clin Med 1983;101:896–902.

Roseomonas Species

●

John D. Rihs

GENERAL DESCRIPTION

Roseomonas is a newly described genus of pink-pigmented, Gram-negative, oxidative bacteria, which includes three named species, *R. gilardii, R. cervicalis,* and *R. fauriae* and three unnamed genomospecies (3). These bacteria can be differentiated from *Methylobacterium* species (which appear to be their closest phenotypic and genotypic relatives) by their inability to oxidize methanol, assimilate acetamide, and absorb long-wavelength light.

Roseomonas species have been isolated from human sources such as blood, genitourinary sites, wounds, respiratory tract, body fluids, eye, and bone (3, 4). Nearly half of the isolates have been from blood. For most of the isolates, very little clinical information is available, and their pathogenic role remains unclear. In those cases in which information is available, most patients were severely debilitated or immunocompromised hosts with a clinical presentation of sepsis. This group of organisms appears to be of low virulence, and no deaths have been directly attributed to *Roseomonas* infections.

IN VITRO SUSCEPTIBILITIES

All species have been susceptible to the aminoglycosides and imipenem. All but one strain of genomospecies 5 tested susceptible to tetracycline. Most isolates are resistant to the broad-spectrum penicillins. The penicillins containing β-lactamase inhibitors are more active in vitro. Fifteen of 23 isolates of genomospecies 1 tested sensitive to amoxicillin-clavulanate, and 20 of 23 were sensitive to ticarcillin-clavulanate. All isolates from genomospecies 2 through 6 tested sensitive to both. Most isolates are also resistant to the cephalosporin agents. Only a few isolates of genomospecies 1 were sensitive to any of the cephalosporins. The seven isolates of genomospecies 2 were all sensitive to cefoxitin but resistant to all other cephalosporins. The five isolates of genomospecies 3 were sensitive to cefoxitin, cefotetan, and ceftazidime. The three isolates of genomospecies 4 were sensitive to cefoxitin, cefotetan, and cefotaxime. The three isolates of genomospecies 5 were sensitive to cefotetan, cefotaxime, ceftriaxone, and ceftazidime. The isolates were generally not susceptible to the sulfonamides or aztreonam but generally were susceptible to the quinolones. A summary of 42 clinical isolates is shown in Table 1.

ANTIMICROBIAL THERAPY
Drug of Choice

The empirical drug of choice is gentamicin. All clinical isolates tested have been susceptible. Organisms within the genus *Methylobacterium* are also susceptible in vitro to gentamicin. Standard doses of aminoglycosides used for Gram-negative sepsis can be used. Once-daily dosing is probably acceptable given the relative lack of virulence of *Roseomonas,* although postantibiotic effect (PAE) has not been studied.

Special Situations
Bacteremia

Bacteremia is the most common presentation. Patients generally appear septic and typically are severely immunocompromised. In most cases the source of the bacteremia is not demonstrated. Since these organisms are of low virulence, when the source of the bacteremia is uncertain, a short course of 7 to 10 days is recommended.

Catheter-Associated Infection

Sepsis due to an infected Hickman catheter was reported in a patient with chronic intestinal pseudoobstruction requiring home total parenteral nutrition (2). A regimen of gentamicin and cefuroxime initially failed despite in vitro susceptibility to these agents. Blood cultures remained negative only after the Hickman line was removed.

Osteomyelitis

One case of vertebral osteomyelitis has been reported (1). A 55-year-old man with chronic steroid-dependent lung disease presented with back pain of 5 months' duration. Magnetic resonance imaging showed enhancement of the T4-T5 disk space with an inflammatory paravertebral mass. Two computed tomography (CT)-guided percutaneous needle aspirations

TABLE 1 • Antimicrobial Susceptibilities of the Six Genomospecies

Drug[a]	No. of Strains Sensitive in Genomospecies					
	1 (n = 23)	2 (n = 7)	3 (n = 5)	4 (n = 3)	5 (n = 3)	6 (n = 1)
Ampicillin	4	0	0	0	1	1
Carbenicillin	7	0	0	0	2	1
Mezlocillin	0	0	0	0	1	0
Ticarcillin	7	0	0	0	2	0
Piperacillin	0	0	0	0	1	0
Amox/clavulanate	15	7	5	3	3	1
Ticar/clavulanate	20	7	5	3	3	1
Cephalothin	0	0	0	2	2	0
Cefazolin	5	0	0	0	2	0
Cefoxitin	1	7	5	3	1	1
Cefotetan	2	0	5	3	3	1
Cefuroxime	0	0	1	1	0	1
Cefotaxime	1	0	3	3	3	1
Ceftriaxone	1	0	0	1	3	0
Ceftazidime	0	0	5	1	3	1
Gentamicin	23	7	5	3	3	1
Tobramycin	23	7	4	3	3	1
Amikacin	23	7	5	3	3	1
Sulfamethoxazole	0	4	4	1	3	1
Trimeth/sulfa	2	5	4	1	2	1
Tetracycline	23	7	5	3	2	1
Aztreonam	0	0	2	1	3	1
Ciprofloxacin	15	7	5	3	3	1
Norfloxacin	19	7	5	3	3	1
Imipenem	23	7	5	3	3	1
Nitrofurantoin	1	0	2	0	0	0

[a]Amox, amoxicillin; Ticar, ticarcillin; Trimeth/sulfa, trimethoprim-sulfamethoxazole.

showed evidence of osteomyelitis but did not reveal any pathogens on culture. An open biopsy was performed 4 weeks after the initial procedure. Cultures of this material grew *Roseomonas*. Ceftriaxone was started empirically. Susceptibility results showed the isolate to be resistant to ceftriaxone, ceftazidime, mezlocillin, and piperacillin and susceptible to ofloxacin, ciprofloxacin, imipenem, and gentamicin. The patient was switched to oral ofloxacin and completed a 6-week course of therapy. Follow-up examinations revealed stable neurologic findings but little pain relief. Further studies could not be performed because of progressive respiratory deterioration, ventilatory failure, and death.

Alternative Therapy

Alternative therapy includes doxycycline or ticarcillin/clavulanate. The usual adult dosage of doxycycline is 200 mg on the first day, given as one or two infusions, followed by 100 or 200 mg daily, with the 200-mg doses given in one or two infusions. The recommended dosage for children above 8 years of age and below 100 pounds is 2 mg/lb on the first day, given in one or two infusions, and then daily doses of 1 to 2 mg/lb given as

one or two infusions. The normal adult dose should be used for children over 100 pounds. Doxycycline is not recommended for children under 8 years of age.

The usual recommended dose of ticarcillin/clavulanate for an average (60-kg) adult is 3.1 g given every 4 to 6 h. For patients with renal insufficiency, an initial loading dose of 3.1 g should be followed by doses based on creatinine clearance and type of dialysis.

REFERENCES

1. Nahass RG, Wisneski R, Herman DJ, Hirsh E, Goldblatt K. Vertebral osteomyelitis due to *Roseomonas:* case report and review of the evaluation of vertebral osteomyelitis. Clin Infect Dis 1995;21:1474–1476.

2. Richardson JD. Failure to clear a *Roseomonas* line infection with antibiotic therapy. Clin Infect Dis 1997;25:155.

3. Rihs JD, Brenner DJ, Weaver RE, Steigerwalt AG, Hollis DG, Yu VL. *Roseomonas,* a new genus associated with bacteremia and other human infections. J Clin Microbiol 1993;31:3275–3283.

4. Struthers M, Wong J, Janda JM. An initial appraisal of the clinical significance of *Roseomonas* species associated with human infections. Clin Infect Dis 1996;23:729–733.

Salmonella typhi and *paratyphi*

Nicholas J. White

GENERAL DESCRIPTION

Typhoid and paratyphoid fevers are commonly grouped together under the collective term *enteric fever*. Typhoid is caused by *Salmonella typhi* (strictly termed *S. enterica* subspecies *enterica* serotype typhi) and paratyphoid is caused by either *Salmonella paratyphi* A, B, or C. *S. paratyphi* B is also known as *S. schottmuelleri,* and *S. paratyphi* C as *S. hirschfeldii*. These salmonelloses are highly adapted infections of man, with no animal or environmental reservoir. Occasionally other salmonellae may cause an enteric feverlike syndrome. Typhoid fever was once a major cause of morbidity and mortality throughout the world, with a case fatality rate of approximately 15% (45, 83). Over the past century, the infection has been largely eradicated from more affluent temperate countries, although it remains a major infection in tropical areas of the world. Precise estimates of the mortality and morbidity of infectious diseases in poor countries are notoriously unreliable, but a recent estimate suggested that there are approximately 33,000,000 cases of typhoid each year, with 600,000 deaths (91).

Epidemiology

Typhoid and paratyphoid are transmitted mainly by the fecal-oral route. In most cases, an asymptomatic carrier of *S. typhi* or an individual who has recently recovered from the infection continues to excrete large numbers of organisms in the stool and contaminates food or drink, either through direct food handling, through transfer of bacteria by flies and other insects, or by contamination of potable water. Approximately 10% of patients recovering from typhoid fever excrete *S. typhi* in the stool for 3 months, and in the past, 2 to 3% became permanent carriers. These infections thus have great potential for epidemic spread (145, 150).

In the tropics, enteric fever tends to be more common during the hot dry seasons, sometimes continuing on to the early part of the rainy season. In some areas, the incidence of typhoid may be as high as 1,000 cases per 100,000 population per year. In such areas, typhoid is predominantly a disease of children, and stool excretion of *S. typhi* during and after infection is the main source of the infection. In temperate countries, persistent carriers are a more important reservoir of infection (83). For travelers the highest attack rates are associated with visits to Peru (17 per 10^5 visits), India ($11/10^5$ visits), and Pakistan ($10/10^5$ visits). Although Indonesia has a reported annual incidence up to 1%, the attack rate for travelers is low. In general, the mortality of enteric fever is low (<1%) where antibiotics are available, but in poorer areas or in the context of natural disasters, war, migrations, large concentrated refugee populations, and other privations, the mortality may rise to 10 to 30%, despite antibiotic therapy.

A number of factors increase the risk of salmonella infections. Disease-related (achlorhydria) or iatrogenic (antacids, H_2 blockers, proton pump inhibitors) reduction in stomach acidity or gut pathology (surgery, inflammatory bowel disease, malignancy, antibiotics) increases susceptibility to infection. Disease-related or iatrogenic immunosuppression and several other infections, notably schistosomiasis, malaria (103), histoplasmosis, and bartonellosis, are associated with an increased risk of salmonella infections. Typhoid is more common and more severe at the extremes of age. Neonatal typhoid (usually acquired from the mother) may follow a fulminant course, often with meningitis (16, 34). Patients with hemoglobinopathies, particularly sickle cell disease, are also at increased risk.

Clinical Features

The clinical features of enteric fever vary considerably between different geographic regions. In many areas, typhoid becomes the leading differential diagnosis of a patient with a fever that has lasted for more than 1 week. The clinical features of typhoid and paratyphoid fever are generally similar, although paratyphoid tends to be a milder infection (45). Most patients with enteric fever present with a nonspecific gradual onset of an influenza-like illness, although *S. typhi* infection can present with fever and a bewildering array of signs and symptoms ranging from nonmetastatic central nervous system syndromes including psychosis and cerebellar ataxia (152), to focal involvement of bone (51), liver (57, 92, 135), spleen (8), testes (170), meninges (100, 141), vascular prostheses, atheromatous plaques, etc. (157).

In general, the enteric fevers are subacute infections with an incubation period of approximately 7 to 14 days (range, 3–60 days) following exposure. The illness begins insidiously, with nonspecific signs and symptoms of fever (122), headache, muscle and joint aches, malaise, lassitude, anorexia, and often a dry cough (sometimes associated with a sore throat) (139). The spleen enlarges, but lymphadenopathy is not usually prominent. There may be a few rose spots (sparse, pink, maculopapular lesions that blanch with pressure and fade after 2 or 3 days) on the thorax or abdomen (usually less than 10), but these are often unnoticed (particularly in dark-skinned patients). In paratyphoid fever rose spots may be more prominent. The classic "stepladder fever" of typhoid is unusual, although the fever does become higher as the disease progresses, until it levels, fluctuating between 39 and 40°C. Mild chills and sweating are common, but true rigors are rare. Relative bradycardia is considered common in typhoid, although in many series this has not been a feature of the disease. Abdominal complaints are common, and either diarrhea or constipation may occur. There is usually some abdominal discomfort, and even in the first week of the disease, the patient may notice passage per rectum of a small amount of blood or melena. Normal bowel habit is unusual in typhoid. Diarrhea (129) is more common in infants (21) and in patients with AIDS. Constipation occurs in approximately 40% of patients. A fulminant onset with a septic shock presentation may occur, but is unusual.

The clinical evolution of typhoid is divided classically into weeks (45). During the first week, the fever rises gradually and, in the second week, reaches a high plateau. By the second week the patient has become progressively weaker, has lost weight, and has often developed the characteristic affect from which typhoid derives its name (typhoid means "like typhus," from the Greek *typhos* meaning "smoke," referring to the clouding of the sensorium in these infections). The patient remains apathetic or depressed, anergic, often confused and withdrawn while lying in bed, yet sleep does not come easily. By the third week of infection, if untreated, a dangerous stage is reached in which either intestinal perforation or hemorrhage becomes more likely as the necrotic Peyer's patches either erode through the wall of the terminal ileum (24) or penetrate a large blood vessel. In large series reported before the chloramphenicol era, intestinal hemorrhage occurred in 7 to 21% of cases and intestinal perforation in 0.7 to 4.7% (45). In the antibiotic era, the incidence of perforation has fallen slightly to approximately 3% of cases, and intestinal bleeding now occurs in less than 2%, although figures still vary considerably from series to series. The risk of both hemorrhage and perforation increases from the middle of the second week. In the third week of the illness, the patient is often withdrawn, obtunded, or intermittently delirious. The abdomen becomes distended, and there may be vomiting and abdominal pain. Right upper quadrant pain may indicate cholecystitis or cholangitis (3% of cases); lower quadrant pain with signs of peritoneal irritation may indicate perforation. Complications in the third and fourth week also include pneumonia (139), adult respiratory distress syndrome (31), development of acute psychosis, coma (23, 120), myocarditis (118), pericarditis, orchitis (170), venous thrombosis (64), splenic rupture (7), and occasional renal failure (140). If the patient survives this phase of illness, a gradual recovery follows.

As the duration of infection is an important determinant of the risk of severe complications, a delay in receiving appropriate antibiotic treatment may have serious consequences. In some endemic areas, multidrug resistance (and thus delayed treatment with effective antimicrobials) has led to increased mortality, particularly in infants (16).

Diagnosis

The clinical diagnosis of typhoid or paratyphoid is confirmed by culture of the organism from blood, bone marrow, or another nongastrointestinal site. Isolation of the organism from duodenal secretions or stool of a febrile patient also suggests enteric fever (although fever from a different infection may occur in someone who has recently recovered from typhoid or is a chronic carrier). Stool cultures are positive in approxi-

mately 60% of children and 25% of adults (66). Excretion of *S. typhi* in the stool is more likely with higher blood bacterial counts, and children tend to have higher bacteremias than adults. Blood cultures are positive in 60 to 80% of patients, with yields maximized by taking a large volume of blood. The median bacterial count is 1 CFU/mL (161). Approximately two-thirds of these organisms are within phagocytic cells and thus located in the buffy coat (130, 161). Blood bacterial counts decline as the disease progresses. Bone marrow culture increases the diagnostic yield from blood cultures by approximately 30% (49, 66, 84, 86). Biopsy specimens taken from the rose spots are also usually culture positive. *S. typhi* is usually present in the duodenum and can be recovered by the string test (86). This is also useful for identifying chronic gallbladder carriers (65). *S. typhi* is sometimes excreted in the urine and occasionally causes urinary tract infections, particularly if there are structural abnormalities of the urinary tract (105). In areas where *S. haematobium* is endemic, such as Egypt, urinary tract carriers outnumber enteric carriers of *S. typhi*. Urine antigen tests have been described recently (40) but have not been evaluated sufficiently. Several polymerase chain reaction methods have been described but are not used widely (144, 171). Serologic diagnosis is widely relied upon. The Widal test, which measures antibody titers to the somatic O and flagellar H antigens is used widely, although there are very divergent views on its utility. In several well-documented epidemics Widal results were usually negative.

SUSCEPTIBILITY IN VITRO

S. typhi and *S. paratyphi* A, B, and C are susceptible in vitro to a variety of antibiotics. However, in vivo response is not always predicted accurately from in vitro susceptibility, largely because the bacteria are predominantly found intracellularly, within phagocytic cells (41). For example, the aminoglycosides are highly effective in vitro but ineffective in vivo because of their poor penetration into cells and susceptibility to the acid pH inside the phagolysosomes containing ingested bacteria. The in vitro susceptibility profile to antimicrobial drugs is shown in Table 1. In general, in vitro susceptibility testing to the agents commonly used for treatment of typhoid does predict the clinical response, although in endemic areas patients with mild typhoid may improve following administration of an antibiotic to which the organism is shown subsequently to be resistant in vitro. This represents self-cure and natural resolution of the infection and explains why therapeutic responses in semiimmune persons are always superior to those in nonimmune subjects. As *S. typhi* and *S. paratyphi* are obligate infections of man, no appropriate animal models exist in which to test treatment regimens. In general, *S. typhimurium* in a murine model has been used to assess pathophysiology and host defense mechanisms but not treatment responses.

Chloramphenicol

Chloramphenicol has been the treatment of choice for typhoid and paratyphoid fevers since 1948, when Woodward and Smadel first demonstrated its effectiveness in Malaya while evaluating the new antibiotic in the treatment of scrub typhus (168). A patient in their trials proved to have typhoid, and instead

TABLE 1 • Minimum Inhibitory Concentrations (μg/mL) for Selected Antibiotics against _Salmonella typhi_

Antibiotic	"Sensitive Isolates"		"MDR Isolates"	
	MIC$_{50}$	MIC$_{90}$	MIC$_{50}$	MIC$_{90}$
Penicillin G	4	8		
Ampicillin	0.5	1.0	>256	>256
Amoxicillin–clavulanic acid	0.5	1.0	8	8
Piperacillin	0.5	1		
Piperacillin-tazobactam	0.5	1		
Ticarcillin	2	4		
Azlocillin	8	8		
Mezlocillin	2	2		
Mecillinam	0.125	0.125	1*	2*
Cefuroxime	2	4		
Cefoperazone	1	4		
Cefoxitin	1	4		
Ceftriaxone	0.06	0.125	0.06	0.125
Ceftazidime	0.25	0.25		
Cefepime	0.06	0.125		
Cefpirome	0.06	0.06		
Cefixime	0.06	0.06		
Ceftizoxime	0.06	0.125		
Aztreonam	0.125	0.25		
Imipenem	0.25	0.5		
Meropenem	0.06	0.06		
Azithromycin	8	8	8	8
Rifampicin	8	16		
Trimethoprim	0.125	0.25	128	>256
Sulfamethoxazole	4	16	>256	>256
Chloramphenicol	4	8	>256	>256
Tetracycline	1	1	>256	>256
Gentamicin	0.25	2.0		
Nalidixic acid	4	8	4	8
Norfloxacin	0.06	0.25	0.06	0.25
Ciprofloxacin	0.015	0.03	0.015	0.03
Ofloxacin	0.06	0.125	0.06	0.125
Pefloxacin	0.125	0.125	0.125	0.125
Fleroxacin	0.06	0.125	0.06	0.125

of the normally protracted debilitating fever, he responded well to the treatment. Chloramphenicol has reduced the mortality of typhoid from 20% to less than 1%, and the duration of fever from 2 to 4 weeks to 4 to 5 days. It is the gold standard with which other antibiotics should be compared. Chloramphenicol has excellent cellular penetration and is extensively distributed in the body. Chloramphenicol-sensitive stains of _S. typhi_ typically have MICs between 0.75 and 5 μg/mL (Table 1). Thiamphenicol (in which the _p_-nitro group of the benzene ring of chloramphenicol is substituted by a methylsulfonyl group) has been used less frequently but has given similar clinical results.

Ampicillin, Amoxicillin, and Trimethoprim-Sulfamethoxazole

There have been many open evaluations and several comparisons of these drugs in typhoid fever (94, 123). In general, results with ampicillin, amoxicillin, or trimethoprim-sulfamethoxazole have been similar to or slightly inferior to those with chloramphenicol. They have emerged as effective

and acceptable alternatives, with trimethoprim-sulfamethoxazole holding a slight advantage over ampicillin, although most authorities still prefer chloramphenicol, particularly for severe infections (36). Ampicillin and amoxicillin have been the treatment of choice in pregnancy and in neonates. MICs for ampicillin are typically 0.25 to 5 μg/mL (MIC$_{90}$, 1), either similar or one dilution lower for amoxicillin, and 0.125 to 0.5 μg/mL for trimethoprim (Table 1). Although synergy can be demonstrated with sulfonamides in vitro, and most clinical experience is with trimethoprim-sulfamethoxazole, the importance of synergy in determining treatment response in enteric fever is unclear. Some authorities consider trimethoprim alone to be equally effective and less toxic. Unfortunately, strains that are simultaneously resistant to all of these first-line drugs have become widespread in recent years (112, 121). The third-generation cephalosporins and the fluoroquinolones have been used increasingly as multidrug resistance has spread (9, 30, 75, 143).

Resistance to Chloramphenicol, Ampicillin, and Trimethoprim

Resistance to chloramphenicol, ampicillin, and trimethoprim-sulfamethoxazole is usually plasmid mediated. Resistance to chloramphenicol was reported within 2 years of its original introduction but was not a major problem until the early 1970s (27, 36, 80). The extensively documented epidemic in Mexico (71, 113, 159) involved chloramphenicol-resistant _S. typhi_ that in a few cases were also resistant to the other first-line antimicrobials. Over the following 20 years, similar chloramphenicol-resistant organisms were reported in many other countries (3, 11, 27, 28, 37, 38, 63, 70). With increasing use of ampicillin (or amoxicillin) and trimethoprim-sulfamethoxazole as alternatives (136), resistance to these antibiotics developed also (10, 50, 59, 125, 134). Resistance was shown to be transmitted by a single "R" factor (plasmid) (37, 69, 70, 114), which also often encoded resistance to tetracyclines, sulfonamides, and the aminoglycosides. In some countries, particularly those such as Thailand and Vietnam where trimethoprim-sulfamethoxazole was used widely but chloramphenicol was not, the prevalence of chloramphenicol resistance fell before the arrival of multidrug resistance in the early 1990s. In recent years, multidrug resistance has been reported from the Americas, North and South Africa, and the Middle East, although the biggest problems are in the Indian subcontinent, Southeast Asia, and China (6, 9, 46, 78, 108, 109, 121, 125, 151, 166). In many countries where typhoid fever is endemic, the proportion of MDR isolates has increased steadily and they now comprise the majority of strains isolated. In a few areas (e.g., parts of India) the proportion appears to have decreased again (148). Resistance is usually associated with a single large plasmid varying in M_r between approximately 90×10^6 and 120×10^6, which is of the incompatibility group H complex (usually H1) (125, 149). DNA probes identifying these plasmid-encoded resistance genes have been used for molecular typing in epidemiologic investigations (79).

The mechanism of resistance to chloramphenicol is usually production of chloramphenicol acetyltransferase. For ampicillin, it is production of β-lactamase (usually TEM1, and therefore inhibited by clavulanic acid). Other mechanisms may contribute in addition, as MDR strains are more resistant to amoxicillin-clavulanic acid than sensitive isolates (Table 1). Trimethoprim and sulfamethoxazole resistance is mediated by alteration in the enzyme targets dihydrofolate reductase and dihydropteroate synthase, respectively, usually related to point mutations in the respective genes. MICs for resistant isolates are typically above 125 to 256 µg/mL for all three first-line antibiotics. *S. typhi* carrying MDR plasmids appears to be at least as virulent, and possibly more virulent, than fully drug-sensitive strains (161).

Third-Generation Cephalosporins

MDR strains of *S. typhi* remain sensitive to third-generation cephalosporins, fluoroquinolone antibiotics, aztreonam, and the carbapenems (5, 39, 60, 104, 108, 112, 126, 143, 147, 156, 165). Ceftriaxone has been the most widely used of the third-generation cephalosporins, although several studies used oral cefixime, which is also very active. MICs for both drugs are typically 0.06 µg/mL.

Fluoroquinolones

S. typhi, and *S. paratyphi* A, B, and C are usually extremely sensitive to the fluoroquinolone antibiotics. In time-kill studies, the fluoroquinolones are significantly more rapidly bactericidal than the third-generation cephalosporins. In general, MICs for the individual fluoroquinolones against *S. typhi* and *S. paratyphi* parallel those against other *Enterobacteriaceae*. In vivo, these are the most active drugs, with the most rapid response rates and the highest cure rates. Although the earlier compounds enoxacin, cinoxacin, and norfloxacin have proved effective in the treatment of typhoid, they have usually given inferior results, presumably because of poor oral bioavailability (111, 132). Norfloxacin occupies an intermediate position; it is more active in vivo than enoxacin and cinoxacin but less effective than the newer fluoroquinolones.

Unfortunately quinolone resistance has now been reported in *S. paratyphi* A (29) and, more importantly, in *S. typhi,* in both southern India and Vietnam (48, 127). As in *S. typhimurium* and other bacteria, fluoroquinolone resistance is usually associated with single point mutations in the "quinolone resistance–determining region" of the *gyrA* gene (26, 74). This is not plasmid mediated and does not appear to be transferable. The most commonly identified mutation has been a serine to phenylalanine substitution at position 83 (26, 162). Less common have been aspartate to tyrosine or glycine at position 87. Reduced susceptibility to quinolones without these mutations has also been reported, suggesting an alternative mechanism of resistance. *S. typhi* containing these *gyrA* mutations shows reduced susceptibility to fluoroquinolones, although the MICs are often still below the breakpoint for resistance, and on disk susceptibility testing, zone sizes may still indicate full susceptibility. Compared with fluoroquinolone-sensitive strains, MICs are commonly two or three dilutions higher (ofloxacin MIC$_{90}$ = 0.5 µg/mL compared with 0.06–0.125 µg/mL for quinolone-sensitive strains), but greater discrimination is found in tests with nalidixic acid. With a nalidixic acid disk, these fluoroquinolone-resistant strains are resistant, with MICs of 32

µg/mL or higher, compared with 4 to 8 µg/mL for sensitive isolates. In a recent series from Vietnam, the mean (SD) zone diameter around an ofloxacin 5-µg disk was 30 (3) mm with nalidixic acid–sensitive organisms (N = 381), and 22.5 (2) mm around the 14 nalidixic acid–resistant organisms (*P* < .001) (162). As these nalidixic acid–resistant isolates are effectively fluoroquinolone resistant in vivo, nalidixic acid–disk testing with a 30-µg disk should be routine when evaluating *S. typhi* or *S. paratyphi* susceptibility. To date, only single point mutations have been encountered, but double mutations conferring high-level fluoroquinolone resistance (as in other *Enterobacteriaceae*) can be expected. Resistance to third-generation cephalosporins is extremely rare.

Other Drugs

Mecillinam (Amdinocillin)

Mecillinam is available as either the parenteral formulation or a prodrug, pivmecillinam, for oral use. 6-β-Amidinopenicillin is very active against ampicillin-sensitive strains of *S. typhi* with MICs typically 0.2 µg/mL. Although it is more stable than ampicillin against the β-lactamases produced by MDR strains, MICs are higher (typically, 0.8–2 µg/mL). Mecillinam used alone for the treatment of typhoid, has yielded relatively low cure rates and high rates of stool carriage (93). Mecillinam binds to PBP2, and in vitro synergy can be shown with other β-lactam antibiotics. Combinations of mecillinam with ampicillin or pivmecillinam with pivampicillin given for 10 to 14 days have given good clinical results, although in the former study, stool carriage rates were also very high. These double β-lactam combinations have been little used in recent years.

Furazolidone

Furazolidone, an inexpensive nitrofuran derivative, has been available for many years in tropical countries and has been used extensively for enteric infections (137). Although inferior to chloramphenicol in sensitive infections, it retains sensitivity against MDR strains of *S. typhi*. Furazolidone was recently shown effective in an uncontrolled study of 56 children with MDR typhoid, although fever clearance was slow: mean (SD), 5.9 (1.6) days; range, 3 to 10 days (98, 137). However, oral bioavailability is very poor, and in the absence of further information, furazolidone cannot be recommended for enteric fever unless other more effective drugs are not available.

Aztreonam

The monobactam aztreonam is highly active against *S. typhi* in vitro, with MIC$_{90}$s of 0.25 µg/mL (44, 72). Despite good results in earlier uncontrolled trials, aztreonam (6 g/day for 10 days) proved inferior to chloramphenicol (50 mg/kg/day for 14 days) in 44 adults in Peru with uncomplicated chloramphenicol-sensitive enteric fever. Mean (SD) fever clearance was slower, 6.6 (3.6) days versus 4.5 (2.3) days, and seven patients failed, versus none in the chloramphenicol group (72).

Azithromycin

Although the macrolides and lincosamides generally have little or no activity against salmonellae, the new macrolide, azithromycin, does have in vivo activity against *S. typhi* despite MICs that are typically between 4 and 8 μg/mL. *S. typhi* exhibits tolerance to this antimicrobial, with an MBC:MIC ratio that commonly exceeds 8. In vivo activity may result from its over 100-fold concentration in leukocytes. Clinical results with azithromycin have been mixed (153, 164). Initial enthusiasm was dampened by a recent report from Egypt in which three of the first four patients treated failed.

Antimicrobial Pharmacokinetics in Enteric Fever

Chloramphenicol. Oral chloramphenicol, either as crystalline base or as the palmitate ester, is well absorbed in uncomplicated enteric fever (14). Intravenous or intramuscular chloramphenicol succinate is a biologically inactive prodrug for the active base. Systemic bioavailability of chloramphenicol base following intravenous administration of the succinate is between 50 and 80%. Plasma concentration profiles vary considerably between individuals.

In Pakistan, Bhutta et al. studied children receiving either 75 or 100 mg/kg/day of intravenous chloramphenicol succinate (19, 20) and, 48 h after starting treatment, found mean (SD) peak levels of 15.4 (6.1) and 19.9 (12.2) μg/mL, respectively, and trough levels of 8.8 (7.7) and 5.4 (2.6) μg/mL, respectively. In an unrandomized study, Ti et al. in Singapore compared plasma concentrations following equivalent doses of oral and intravenous chloramphenicol in 11 and 15 patients, respectively; plasma concentrations were approximately 50% lower in the parenteral group. Using a regimen of 60 mg/kg daily orally or intravenously until defervescence followed by 40 mg/kg/day to complete 14 days treatment in 31 Bangladeshi adults and children, Islam et al. (89) found trough serum chloramphenicol concentrations on day 3 of 5 to 57 μg/mL (median, 18 μg/mL) and on day 7 of 5 to 40 μg/mL (median, 20 μg/mL). Concentrations above 20 μg/mL are known to suppress erythropoiesis (107). Thus even intravenous administration shows considerable interindividual variability.

The greatest controversy has surrounded intramuscular administration of chloramphenicol. Since 1970, following the study of du Pont et al. in patients with Rocky Mountain spotted fever or volunteers with induced typhoid, it has been generally recommended that chloramphenicol not be given by intramuscular injection because of poor bioavailability. In this relatively small study (only 4 in the oral group and 13 in the intramuscular group), plasma chloramphenicol levels after oral administration were approximately twice those following intramuscular administration of chloramphenicol sodium succinate (52). Later authors have pointed out that this difference can be explained fully by the incomplete systemic bioavailability of chloramphenicol base following administration of the succinate prodrug. Subsequently, Shann et al. studied 57 children in Papua New Guinea with a variety of infections and showed that both peak serum concentrations and chloramphenicol AUC values were similar following intramuscular and intravenous chloramphenicol sodium succinate (138). In a recent randomized comparison in 29 Nepalese adults with suspected uncomplicated typhoid or paratyphoid fever given 30 mg/kg of succinate ester, mean (SD) peak plasma chloram-

phenicol concentrations following intramuscular administration were 7.8 (3.6) μg/mL, compared with 16.2 (9.1) μg/mL following intravenous administration, but AUC values did not differ significantly with the two routes of administration, indicating similar bioavailability (2). In the 16 culture-positive patients, chloramphenicol plasma clearance correlated weakly with measures of liver blood flow (indocyanine green clearance) and metabolic function (antipyrine clearance) but was unrelated to glomerular filtration rate (iothalamate clearance).

Ceftriaxone. Trough plasma ceftriaxone concentrations following an intravenous dose of 3 g/day usually exceed 11 μg/mL (which corresponds approximately to an unbound concentration of 0.5 μg/mL); concentrations at least eight times the usual MIC are achieved (1).

Ofloxacin. The pharmacokinetic properties of intravenous and oral ofloxacin have been studied recently in children with MDR typhoid fever (14). The median (95% CI) peak serum concentrations following an intravenous infusion of 7.5 mg/kg were 8.7 (7.6–9.7) μg/mL and 5.5 (4.7–6.3) μg/mL, respectively. These were 10 to 100 times higher than the maximum MICs for nalidixic acid sensitive *S. typhi*. The mean (95%) estimated oral bioavailability was 91% (74–109%). Although systemic clearance values were slightly higher than reported previously in adults with other infections, these data suggest that dose regimens should be the same in adults and children.

Combination Drugs

The only combination of drugs used widely for the treatment of typhoid and paratyphoid fevers is trimethoprim-sulfamethoxazole. Combination of ampicillin with chloramphenicol proved no more effective than chloramphenicol alone (123). The use of combinations to prevent the emergence of resistance (e.g., fluoroquinolones) has not been evaluated.

ANTIMICROBIAL THERAPY
General Points

Most patients with typhoid or paratyphoid fevers have uncomplicated infections and present with a febrile illness. Most can take oral treatment. The proportion of patients who present with complicated infections varies considerably; for example in Nepal and Vietnam, most patients with typhoid have uncomplicated infections and many can still walk despite having positive blood cultures. In contrast, in Jakarta, Indonesia, severe infections are relatively common, particularly in children, and often present with encephalopathy or shock (85). These patients obviously require parenteral treatment.

With the extensive spread of MDR *S. typhi*, chloramphenicol can no longer be considered the drug of choice for suspected enteric fever, unless the background prevalence of resistant strains in the area where the infection was acquired is known to be very low (75, 124). In uncomplicated infections, the median time to fever clearance in fully sensitive infections is usually 4 to 5 days. It is not uncommon for blood cultures to remain positive up to the third day of treatment with chloramphenicol in a fully sensitive infection. The fluoroquinolones sterilize the blood more rapidly, and in general, fever clearance times range between 3 and 5 days with this group of drugs (166) (Table 2).

TABLE 2 • Fluoroquinolone Efficacy in Enteric Fever

Drug	Reference	Dosage	Patients	Clinical Cure (%)	Micro Cure (%)	Mean (SD) FCT (days)	Relapse Rate (%)
Ofloxacin	Morelli et al. 1992 (111)	300 mg t.i.d., 15 days	30	100	100	2.6	0
Pefloxacin	Morelli et al. 1992 (111)	400 mg t.i.d., 15 days	36	100	100	3.7	0
Ciprofloxacin	Morelli et al. 1992 (111)	500 mg t.i.d., 15 days	20	100	100	3.3	0
Enoxacin	Morelli et al. 1992 (111)	300 mg t.i.d., 15 days	20	80	80	4.6	0
Norfloxacin	Morelli et al. 1992 (111)	400 mg t.i.d.	20	60	60	4.6	0
Norfloxacin	Sarma & Durairaj 1991 (132)	400 mg b.d., 7 days	20	100	100	3.7 (0.5)	0
Ciprofloxacin	Uwayda et al. 1992 (155)	500 mg b.d., 7–10 days	34	100	100	4.9 (1.7)	0
Ciprofloxacin	Uwayda et al. 1992 (155)	750 mg b.d., 7–10 days	28	100	100	5.2 (2.2)	4
Fleroxacin	Arnold et al. 1993 (12)	400 mg o.d., 7 days	28	83	96	4	17
Fleroxacin	Arnold et al. 1993 (12)	400 mg o.d., 14 days	35	100	97	4	0
Ciprofloxacin	Wallace et al. 1993 (163)	500 mg b.d., 7 days	20	100	100	4	0
Fleroxacin	Hien et al. 1994 (82)	400 mg o.d., 7 days	15	100	100	3.4 (1.7)	0
Ofloxacin	Smith et al. 1994 (142)	200 mg b.d., 5 days	22	100	100	3.4 (1.0)	0
Ciprofloxacin	Alam et al. 1995 (5)	500 mg b.d., 10 days	35	100	100	4.2 (1.9)	0
Ciprofloxacin	Alam et al. 1995 (5)	500 mg b.d., 14 days	34	100	100	4.9 (2.6)	0
Ofloxacin	Hien et al. 1995 (81)	15 mg/kg/day, 3 days	118	100	100	2.5 (0.9)	0
Ofloxacin	Hien et al. 1995 (81)	10 mg/kg/day, 5 days	110	100	100	3.0 (0.9)	1
Fleroxacin	Duong et al. 1995 (53)	400 mg o.d., 5 days	41	97.5	100	3.4 (1.5)	4
Fleroxacin	Duong et al. 1995 (53)	400 mg o.d., 3 days	22	100	100	3.7 (1.2)	0
Ofloxacin	Vinh et al. 1996 (160)	15 mg/kg/d, 3 days	47	96	100	4.5 (2.5)	0
Ofloxacin	Vinh et al. 1996 (160)	15 mg/kg/d, 2 days	53	89	98	4.5 (2.7)	2
Pefloxacin	Unal et al. 1996 (154)	400 mg b.d., 7 days	24	100	100	3.4 (1.0)	4
Pefloxacin	Unal et al. 1996 (154)	400 mg b.d., 5 days	22	100	96	3.1 (1.0)	0
Ofloxacin	Chinh et al. 1997 (43)	15 mg/kg/day, 3 days	53	89	100	4.0 (1.4)	2
Ofloxacin	Chinh et al. 1997 (43)	15 mg/kg/day, 2 days	47	98	98	4.0 (1.8)	0

Fever lasting 1 week following fluoroquinolone treatment is rare, and usually indicates nalidixic acid resistance. With third-generation cephalosporins, fever clearance times have been longer, generally ranging between 5 and 8 days (68, 82, 142, 163) (Table 3). Recent studies with short-course fluoroquinolone treatment suggest that the duration of fever does not reliably reflect the duration of infection. Two-day treatments with fluoroquinolones, which have over 85% treatment efficacy (160), are associated with a fever clearance time of 4 to 5 days; that is, the patient is febrile for a longer period than the treatment is given. Patients with background immunity respond better to treatment than do nonimmunes. Oligosymptomatic patients with mild fever usually respond rapidly and have a low incidence of relapse. In a recent study from Nepal, high plasma concentrations of proinflammatory cytokines, reflecting a more severe infection, were associated with delayed response to antimicrobial treatment and increased risk of relapse (33).

Drug of Choice

In the past, chloramphenicol and trimethoprim-sulfamethoxazole have given equivalent results in randomized trials and were considered equivalent first-line treatments (47, 136). Ampicillin has given either equal or slightly inferior therapeutic results and is considered acceptable empirical therapy (116) of particular value in eradication of chronic gallbladder carriage. Amoxicillin is certainly as good as ampicillin and, with better oral bioavailability and less iatrogenic diarrhea, may be considered preferable when cost is not a limiting factor.

There are insufficient studies with trimethoprim alone to conclude that it can be substituted for trimethoprim-sulfamethoxazole; small studies do suggest equivalence (62, 106). The risk of serious drug toxicity (hepatitis, erythema multiforme) is 30 to 50% lower with trimethoprim alone. However, in many endemic areas, formulations of trimethoprim alone are unavailable.

The newer fluoroquinolones have proved the most effective drugs for treatment of enteric fever (81, 82, 142). They have given the highest cure rates and the lowest carrier rates, without significant adverse effects, in treatment courses as short as 2 days (160). This compares with the general recommendation of 2- to 3-week courses of either chloramphenicol, trimethoprim-sulfamethoxazole, or ampicillin (amoxicillin). Short-course fluoroquinolone therapy is particularly effective in epidemic containment (81).

The clinical trials are reviewed in Table 2. There have been a total of 19 randomized trials involving the newer fluoroquinolones (i.e., excluding cinoxacin, enoxacin, and norfloxacin), which together have enrolled and treated 788 patients with culture-confirmed enteric fever (>95% *S. typhi*, and mostly MDR). Mean fever clearance times have ranged between 2.5 and 5.2 days, and 767 of the patients had clinical and microbiologic cures, giving an overall pooled cure rate of 97.3% (95% CI, 96–98%). Over half the studies reported no relapses (i.e., median relapse rate, 0%). Of the 591 patients for whom follow-up stool cultures were reported, only 1 (0.2%) was identified as a carrier in these series. This compares with

TABLE 3 • Third-Generation Cephalosporin Efficacy in Enteric Fever

Drug	Reference	Dosage	Patients	Clinical Cure (%)	Micro Cure (%)	Mean (SD) FCT (days)	Relapse Rate (%)
Cefotaxime	Soe et al. 1987 (143)	200 mg/kg/day	6–14 days	61	82	—	6
Ceftriaxone	Islam et al. 1988 (90)	3–4 g/day, 7 days	32	91	100	4–>14	6
Ceftriaxone	Lasserre et al. 1991 (99)	3 g/day,3 days	19	95	100	3–13	11
Ceftriaxone	Lasserre et al. 1991 (99)	4 g/day, 3 days	20	100	100	4–11	0
Ceftriaxone	Wallace et al. 1993 (163)	3 g/day, 7 days	22	73	100	5.2	5
Ceftriaxone	Islam et al. 1993 (89)	4 g/day, 5 days	28	79	100	—	4
Ceftriaxone	Hien et al. 1994 (82)	2 g/day, 5 days	15	87	93	6.7 (3.1)	0
Ceftriaxone	Smith et al. 1994 (142)	3 g/day, 3 days	25	72	92	8.2 (3.6)	4
Ceftriaxone	Bhutta et al. 1994 (18)	65 mg/kg/day, 14 days	25	88	88	8.0 (4.1)	14
Cefixime	Bhutta et al. 1994 (18)	20 mg/kg/day, 12+ days	50	100	100	5.3 (1.5)	4
Cefixime	Girgis et al. 1994 (68)	10 mg/kg/day, 14 days	25	88	96	8.3 (3.7)	4
Cefixime	Girgis et al. 1995 (67)	7.5 mg/kg b.d., 14 days	50	100	100	5.3	6
Cefixime	Girgis et al. 1995 (67)	50–70 mg/kg daily, 5 days	43	100	100	3.9	5

a rate of approximately 3% with other drugs and strongly suggests that fluoroquinolones prevent the carrier state. Ofloxacin has been the most extensively evaluated fluoroquinolone, although ciprofloxacin, fleroxacin, and pefloxacin have all given similar results. There is no reason a priori to suspect that other drugs in the same class with good oral bioavailability would give inferior responses. All have excellent activity in vitro. Norfloxacin, cinoxacin, and enoxacin have insufficient systemic bioavailability and should not be used to treat enteric fever if the newer agents are available.

Nine randomized trials have involved third-generation cephalosporins. These have enrolled and treated 322 patients (Table 3). Mean fever clearance times have ranged from 5.2 to 8.3 days. Overall, 280 patients responded well, giving a pooled clinical and microbiologic cure rate of 79% (95% CI, 83–90%). The median relapse rate in these series following cephalosporin treatment was 4%. Thus the fluoroquinolones are clearly superior to oral or parenteral third-generation cephalosporins in MDR typhoid (166). There are insufficient comparative studies with chloramphenicol, trimethoprim-sulfamethoxazole, or ampicillin (amoxicillin) in fully sensitive *S. typhi* and *S. paratyphi* infections for firm conclusions, but the available data suggest that the fluoroquinolones are superior. Even in areas where resistance is unusual, the fluoroquinolones offer the advantages of a very well tolerated short-course treatment with very low relapse and carrier rates, and efficacy should the infection prove subsequently to be resistant to the other antibiotics.

Dose and Duration of Treatment

Chloramphenicol treatment of typhoid fever with a total adult dose below 15 g or a treatment duration less than 10 days has been associated with an increased incidence of complications (56, 58, 128). The importance of dose and duration of treatment in preventing relapse is less clear. In early studies, relapse was generally more common following chloramphenicol than with no antibiotic treatment at all, but this reflected the eventual acquisition of immunity following self-cure and did not take into account the morbidity associated with a pro-

tracted illness nor the hazards of intestinal hemorrhage or perforation (56, 58). In general, chloramphenicol, trimethoprim-sulfamethoxazole, and ampicillin have all been prescribed for between 14 and 21 days. It is often recommended that the dose of oral or parenteral chloramphenicol should be reduced by 30% at the time of, or shortly after, defervescence (from 50 to 35 mg/kg/day; usual adult dose, from 3 to 2 g/day). Since the introduction of third-generation cephalosporins and fluoroquinolones, the duration of treatment in clinical trials has progressively shortened. With the fluoroquinolones, treatment courses of 2 days in Vietnam have given cure rates that are similar to those following longer courses, and regimens of ofloxacin at 10 mg/kg/day have given results equivalent to those with 15 mg/kg/day. Although further studies are required in other areas, these data suggest a considerable margin of safety for longer courses of fluoroquinolone treatment. (Treatment regimens are summarized in Table 4.)

Treatment of Children

In areas where resistance is unusual, chloramphenicol, trimethoprim-sulfamethoxazole, or ampicillin (amoxicillin) may all be used. MDR typhoid fever in children has been treated successfully with third-generation cephalosporins, although parenteral ceftriaxone is impractical and oral cefixime has given slow responses with mean times to fever clearance over 5 days (67). In a recent comparative study in 138 Vietnamese children with uncomplicated typhoid fever, oral ofloxacin proved significantly better than oral cefixime, with median (95% CI) fever clearance times of 102 h (78–108) and 177 h (150–204), respectively, and failure rates of 3% and 21%, respectively (Phuong CXT, personal communication).

In many countries, typhoid and paratyphoid fevers are predominantly infections of children (76). Fluoroquinolones are generally considered to be contraindicated in children because of their potential for arthropathogenicity. In immature experimental animals, principally beagle dogs, the fluoroquinolones cause damage to the cartilaginous endplates of long bones. There is no evidence that a similar process of joint damage occurs in humans, but until recently, caution has dictated that

TABLE 4 • Antibiotics of Choice and Alternative Treatments

	Endemic Area	Nonimmune
Uncomplicated enteric fever	Ofloxacin or ciprofloxacin orally 7.5 mg/kg b.i.d for 3 days or 5 mg/kg b.i.d for 5 days[a]	Ofloxacin or ciprofloxacin orally 5 mg/kg b.i.d for 5–7 days[a]
Severe typhoid[b]	Ofloxacin or ciprofloxacin 5 mg/kg infused over 30–60 min every 12 h until oral treatment can be substituted; continue same dose for 10–14 days	Ofloxacin or ciprofloxacin 5 mg/kg infused over 30–60 min every 12 h until oral treatment can be substituted; continue same dose for 10–14 days; immunocompromised patients should receive at least 3 weeks of treatment
Carriers	Adults: Ofloxacin or ciprofloxacin 7.5 mg/kg b.i.d. for 4 weeks Children: Amoxicillin 60 mg/kg/day for 6–8 weeks plus probenecid	

Alternative Treatments	Uncomplicated Enteric Fever	Severe Typhoid
Chloramphenicol	50 mg/kg/day in 4 divided oral doses for 14 days	Chloramphenicol succinate 75 mg/kg/day i.v. or i.m. in 4 divided doses until oral treatment can be substituted; then 50 mg/kg/day orally for 14–21 days
Ampicillin/amoxicillin	Amoxicillin 60 mg/kg or ampicillin 100 mg/kg/day in 4 divided oral doses for 14 days	Ampicillin 100 mg/kg/day in 4 divided doses for 14–21 days
Trimethoprim/sulfamethoxazole	8/40 mg/kg/day in 2 divided oral doses (corresponding in adults to 3 tablets b.i.d.); after defervescence reduce by one-third, to complete 14 days	Intravenous dose regimen similar to the oral regimen
Cefixime/ceftriaxone	Cefixime 20 mg/kg/day in 4 divided oral doses for 7–10 days	Ceftriaxone 60 mg/kg/day i.v. or i.m. for at least 5 days, then if possible switch to oral therapy to complete 14–21 days of treatment

[a]Pefloxacin or fleroxacin have both proved very effective as well (Table 2). The best treatment for quinolone-resistant typhoid remains uncertain.

[b]Dexamethasone 3 mg/kg i.v. stat followed by 1 mg/kg 6-hourly for 48 h should be given to patients with encephalopathy or shock unrelated to perforation or hemorrhage.

alternative drugs be used in children. However, in areas with MDR typhoid, there are no satisfactory orally administered alternatives for children (13, 17, 54, 110, 119). Fluoroquinolones have been evaluated in children with infections caused by other non-*typhi* MDR salmonellae without complications (42, 73, 97). Recent large studies in Vietnam have evaluated fluoroquinolones given for 1 week or less in the treatment of uncomplicated typhoid fever in adults and children (81, 160). In total, over 500 Vietnamese children under 14 years of age have been enrolled in prospective randomized comparisons, and both short- and long-term follow-up that has concentrated on joint or skeletal toxicity revealed no evidence of adverse effects (15, 146). In a recent controlled comparison, 326 children received either short-course ofloxacin (total dose, 45 mg/kg over 3 days) or a longer duration of ciprofloxacin (total dose, 140 mg/kg over 7–10 days). These children were compared with control children from the same location and of the same age who had not received any fluoroquinolones. Over a 2-year period of follow-up, there were no short- or long-term adverse effects and no evidence of impaired growth; indeed, children who received the higher dose (ciprofloxacin) showed significantly increased growth (height velocity) during the first year of the study, compared with untreated healthy controls (15). Taken together, these data suggest that short courses of

fluoroquinolones are safe and effective in children with MDR typhoid and should now be the treatment of choice. Given their other advantages in this potentially life-threatening disease and their safety profile not only in typhoid but also in children treated for other infections (notably protracted high dosages in cystic fibrosis) (42, 73, 133), there seems no reason to withhold fluoroquinolones from children with drug-sensitive enteric fever (167).

Treatment of Pregnant Women

Ampicillin or amoxicillin is considered the treatment of choice for enteric fever in pregnancy. Ciprofloxacin or ofloxacin should be given for MDR infections or, before sensitivities are available, to women coming from areas where these strains are prevalent. Treatment can then be changed to ampicillin if the infecting organism is sensitive (101).

Severe Typhoid

Severe typhoid carries a high mortality. There are two different syndromes. The first represents severe infection with a heavy bacterial load. The patient may present with septic shock or complications including acute renal failure, hepatic dysfunction (57, 135), myocardial failure (118), disseminated intravascular coagulation (32, 95), or encephalopathy (120).

The encephalopathic presentation is particularly common in Java, where it was associated with a mortality of 56% (85). The second presentation is the culmination of a steady downhill progression and results from a focal necrotic process in the terminal ileum. The debilitated patient displays either signs of acute blood loss or peritonitis, indicating intestinal hemorrhage or perforation, respectively (4, 24, 157), usually in the third or fourth week of disease. The clinical diagnosis of perforation can be difficult, as localized abdominal discomfort with guarding and rebound may occur without evident perforation in typhoid.

In severe typhoid, the objective of treatment is to save life and manage complications as early as possible. Although there was a period when conservative management of intestinal perforation was considered acceptable, opinion now strongly favors immediate surgery (24, 35). Patients with severe typhoid need intensive care. Cardiovascular monitoring should be started, and blood should be cross-matched. Plasma electrolytes and renal function should be monitored, and the patient examined frequently for signs of intestinal blood loss or peritonitis. The mortality of intestinal perforation has been reduced significantly by prompt resuscitation, with vigorous fluid administration to restore the intravascular volume and use of parenteral broad-spectrum antibiotics to treat the fecal peritonitis (22, 77, 158). These should cover aerobic and anerobic bacteria. The choice of antibiotic depends on which drug is being used for typhoid treatment. If fluoroquinolones or third-generation cephalosporins are being used, then metronidazole or clindamycin should be added. The combination of metronidazole and third-generation cephalosporin gives inadequate enterococcal coverage, and ampicillin may be required in addition. With the other drugs (ampicillin, trimethoprim-sulfamethoxazole, or chloramphenicol), both an aminoglycoside and metronidazole should be added.

Intestinal Perforation

If perforation is suspected, nasogastric suction should be started, and the patient resuscitated. Plain abdominal films should be obtained to look for subdiaphragmatic air. Once the hemodynamic status is stabilized, a laparotomy should be performed. Both small and large bowel should be examined. The choice of surgical procedure depends on the extent of ulceration and the state of the bowel wall. Either resection or wedge excision of the ulcer with single- or double-layer closure of the perforation can be performed. Areas where the bowel wall looks friable or an ulcer is about to penetrate may also need preemptive surgery.

Intestinal hemorrhage

In most cases, intestinal bleeding can be managed with fluid replacement and transfusion, preferably of fresh blood. Uncontrolled hemorrhage may necessitate surgery. Intraarterial vasopressin has also been used to control bleeding.

Drug Treatment of Severe Typhoid

There have been no recent randomized controlled trials of the specific antibiotic treatment of severe typhoid. The agents used for oral treatment of uncomplicated typhoid may all be given parenterally, and all are effective (54). Our current preference is for intravenous fluoroquinolones; we currently use ofloxacin at a dose of 5 mg/kg 12-hourly by intravenous infusion. The optimum duration of treatment has also not been determined. Our recommendation is to give 7 to 14 days of antibiotic treatment in severe typhoid. In a double-blind randomized placebo-controlled trial of severe typhoid (defined as shock or coma) conducted in Jakarta, high-dose corticosteroids (dexamethasone 3 mg/kg to start, followed by 1 mg/kg 6-hourly for 48 h) reduced mortality from 56% (10 of 18) to 10% (2 of 20).

The Immunocompromised Patient

Immunocompromised patients with typhoid or paratyphoid fever have a high rate of relapse and should not receive short-course treatment, although the optimum duration of treatment has not been established. Empirically, the duration of treatment should be proportional to the degree of immunosuppression. A 3- to 6-week course of fluoroquinolones should suffice in mildly compromised patients. In patients with AIDS, between 6 weeks and 8 months of fluoroquinolone treatment have been given. The fluoroquinolones and zidovudine show synergistic antibiotic activity against *S. typhi* in vitro. In patients infected with sensitive organisms, trimethoprim-sulfamethoxazole prophylaxis in AIDS also helps to prevent relapse and allows a shorter course of fluoroquinolones (3 weeks) to be given. There are insufficient data in this important area to provide confident treatment recommendations.

Focal Infections

The management of focal infections with *S. typhi* or *S. paratyphi* is similar to that of infections with the other salmonellae. The basic principles of drainage of pus, if possible, and long-course antibiotic treatment are unchanged. Again, the fluoroquinolones have emerged as the drugs of choice in these infections

The Carrier State

Treatment in uncomplicated typhoid is directed toward preventing progression to severe disease and complications, reducing the incidence of relapse, and preventing the carrier state. As asymptomatic carriers are a major source of infection, elimination of carriers has major epidemiologic importance. The carrier state occurs in up to 10% of patients (usually 3%) receiving conventional treatments and in less than 1% of patients receiving fluoroquinolones. Carriers are people who excrete organisms in the stool or urine for more than 3 months following an acute infection. Following chloramphenicol treatment, the proportion of carriers at the end of 3 months is approximately 4%, falling to 3% at 1 year (45). The carrier state is more likely in adults and more likely in females than males. Carriers are usually asymptomatic, although they have an increased risk of gallbladder cancer. High serum levels of antibody to the Vi antigen are useful diagnostically. Carriers may continue to excrete *S. typhi* throughout their lives. Stool excretion is intermittent and varies in intensity, with stool bacterial counts of up to 10^{10} *S. typhi* per gram of feces.

The fecal carrier state results from chronic infection of the gallbladder and is strongly linked to cholelithiasis. Management may therefore require a combination of medical and surgical treatment.

Compared with the large amount of information on the treatment of enteric fever, there is relatively little information on the treatment of *S. typhi* carriers. Chloramphenicol does not seem to be effective. High-dose ampicillin or amoxicillin (14 days of intravenous treatment or 3 months of oral treatment in combination with probenecid) have given the best results. Phillips reviewed three studies (115) and concluded that eradication of the carrier state was obtained in 34 (71%) of 48 patients who had received 4 g of ampicillin/day for 28 days. Others have reported lower cure rates. Carriage in patients with gallstones is often not eradicated with this regimen and may require cholecystectomy (55). Recent experience with the fluoroquinolones suggests that these drugs may become the treatment of choice for chronic carriers. Ferreccio et al. reported cure in 10 of 12 Chilean adult patients (61) given ciprofloxacin (750 mg twice daily for 28 days). Equally good results have been obtained elsewhere (131).

VACCINES

For over 100 years, heat-killed, phenol-treated whole organisms (either *S. typhi* alone or combined with *S. paratyphi* A and B) have been used as vaccines. These vaccines are usually administered by subcutaneous injection. Monovalent whole-cell typhoid vaccine contains not less than 10^9 heat-killed, phenol-preserved *S. typhi* bacteria/mL. These whole-cell vaccines have given 50 to 77% protection, but unpleasant local and systemic side effects are common, with fever in up to 30% and local pain and swelling in up to 60% of those vaccinated. Approximately 25% of vaccine recipients are sufficiently unwell to miss school or work. An acetone-inactivated vaccine that may be given either by subcutaneous or intramuscular injection has been shown to be both more effective and more toxic. In a recent study, 5 of 25,000 military personnel who received the acetone-inactivated vaccine by intramuscular injection required hospitalization.

Most of the protective efficacy of the phenol- and acetone-inactivated vaccines derives from their Vi antigen content, which has led to development of a parenteral purified Vi antigen vaccine. Two vaccines have now largely superseded the older crude vaccines: the purified parenteral Vi capsular polysaccharide antigen (117) and an oral live attenuated bacterium (Ty21a) (102). Both have a protective efficacy between 65 and 70%, with immunity lasting between 3 and 7 years (96), and they are generally well tolerated (8). These vaccines are generally not deployed in endemic areas. Several vaccines are under development including live attenuated *S. typhi* containing autotrophic mutations, which may be more immunogenic than Ty21a and could therefore be given in a single immunizing dose (87).

In general, typhoid vaccines have not been deployed widely in endemic areas; most usage is in travelers. The currently available parenteral Vi antigen and oral live attenuated Ty21a vaccines give similar levels of protective efficacy, and there is little to choose between the two. Neither give 100% protection, and neither vaccine is considered to have adequate protective efficacy in children under 18 months of age. The Ty21a is not generally recommended under the age of 6. Thus the Vi vaccine should be used for younger children. Local and systemic reactions to parenteral typhoid vaccine begin within hours and lasts for up to 3 days. Subjects receiving typhoid vaccines should be warned about potential side effects (Table 5).

Typhoid immunization is advised for laboratory workers handling the organisms and travelers to countries in Africa, some parts of Eastern Europe, Asia, Oceania, Central and South America, and the Caribbean where sanitation and hygiene is poor. Typhoid immunization may not be necessary for

---

TABLE 5 • Typhoid Vaccines

Vaccine	Dose	Adverse Effects	Comments
Vi capsular polysaccharide vaccine	Single dose 0.5 mL of 50 μg/mL vaccine by i.m. or deep s.c. injection	Local pain, erythema and fever may occur 1–3 days after administration	Children < 18 months may show suboptimal response; repeat every 3 years
Ty 21a oral live attenuated vaccine	1 capsule to be swallowed with cold or lukewarm drink on days 1, 3, and 5	Usually none; nausea, vomiting, abdominal cramps, headache, fever, allergic reactions; rarely: anaphylaxis	Contraindicated in patients who are immunosuppressed either by disease or drugs; inactivated by antibiotics; capsules must be refrigerated; not recommended for children <6 years; provides protection 7–10 days after last dose, and in endemic areas this lasts for 3 years in most cases, but for travelers who are not repeatedly exposed, protection may last for only 1 year; do not give mefloquine until 3 days after last dose, and administration of oral polio vaccine should be separated by at least 3 weeks

individuals making short trips and staying in good accommodation. Typhoid immunization is *not* recommended for contacts of known carriers or for epidemic containment.

Contraindications

Typhoid vaccines should not be given during an acute febrile illness if there has been a previous reaction to the same vaccine or to pregnant women (unless there is clear indication). The oral Ty21a vaccine should not be given to patients who have a disease or drug treatment causing immunosuppression (including those who are HIV positive). The oral Ty21a vaccine also should not be given to patients receiving antibiotics, and efficacy is reduced if coadministered with mefloquine prophylaxis. A gap of 3 days between mefloquine and the vaccine is recommended (25, 88). There is a theoretical risk of interference in local immune responses if oral polio vaccine is coadministered with Ty21a; a gap of 3 weeks between the two is recommended.

Prevention

A high prevalence of typhoid reflects poor sanitation and hygiene. The most efficient preventive methods involve providing clean potable water and effective sewage disposal. Typhoid carriers should be identified, treated, and prevented from preparing food until their carrier state has been eradicated. For the individual, prevention entails avoiding potentially contaminated food or water. Dairy products, meat, and shellfish are all potential sources of infection. Nonbottled drinks, ice, uncooked food (apart from fruit and vegetables that can be shelled or peeled), and some desserts (particularly ice cream from an unreliable source) are all potentially contaminated.

MONITORING RESPONSE TO TREATMENT
Clinical Follow-Up

Patients should be observed in the hospital until their temperature has been normal for at least 1 day and they are able to sit and eat. Fever in typhoid is slow to resolve, even with appropriate antibiotic treatment, although the patient often begins to feel better within 1 or 2 days. Recent recommendations that treatment should be deemed to have failed if the fever persists for more than 5 days are too strict (47), as many patients are cured despite fever clearance longer than this. As can be seen from Table 3, most patients treated effectively with third-generation cephalosporins have fever clearance beyond 5 days. Fever clearance is usually defined as the time until the oral temperature has fallen below 37.5°C and remained below this level for at least 24 h. The most important parameter to observe is the patient's general well-being. If patients are brighter, able to sit and take some food or even walk, then the physician can afford to wait; but if their general condition is deteriorating, they are becoming more withdrawn, pulse and fever are rising, and the abdomen is becoming more distended or painful, then intravenous treatment should be substituted and continued beyond 5 days. In practice, the therapeutic options are limited, particularly with MDR typhoid. Parenteral treatment should always be given if there is any doubt about the oral route of administration.

Patients with severe typhoid should be admitted to an intensive care unit and monitored closely. Development of a perforation or hemorrhage does not indicate treatment failure within 1 week of starting treatment, although perforation requires surgical intervention and broadening of antimicrobial coverage.

Microbiologic Follow-Up

Following treatment with chloramphenicol, trimethoprim-sulfamethoxazole, or ampicillin (amoxicillin), it is not unusual for blood cultures to remain positive for several days despite clinical improvement. Occasionally, blood cultures have been positive in the second and third weeks of disease despite full in vitro sensitivity to the antibiotic being given. With fluoroquinolone treatment, it is unusual for blood cultures to be positive after the first 24 h of treatment, and a positive day 3 culture indicates significant risk of subsequent treatment failure.

In routine clinical practice, it is not necessary to repeat blood cultures in patients who are clearly responding to treatment. If the patient does not respond or deteriorates, then cultures should be taken again, and if fever persists for 7 days, even with a clinical response, cultures should be repeated. Sites other than blood or stool should be recultured on the 3rd and 7th day following the start of treatment. To identify *S. typhi* carriers, convalescent stool samples should be obtained in all patients. Three separate samples should taken at 3- to 7-day intervals beginning 1 month after completion of treatment. Patients with repeated positive cultures should be educated about the public health risk they pose, placed on antibiotic treatment, and reviewed at monthly intervals.

RECOMMENDATIONS, CAVEATS, AND CONTROVERSIES

The newer fluoroquinolone antibiotics should be the treatment of choice for MDR typhoid fever at all ages. Most available data concern ofloxacin studied in Vietnam. There is ample evidence in that country to support a treatment course of 3 days (15 mg/kg/day usually given as two doses per day) in previously healthy individuals. Although 2-day regimens have not proved significantly inferior, cure rates have been slightly lower than with the 3- to 5-day regimens. These short-course regimens have not been evaluated outside the endemic areas, and it remains possible that background immunity or other unidentified host factors contribute significantly to these excellent clinical responses. Until further trials are conducted in other countries, it would be prudent to give ofloxacin for 5 or 7 days in a dose of 10 mg/kg/day. Recent pharmacokinetic studies support a twice-daily dose regimen. Further studies are needed to define the importance of concentration-dependent killing and postantibiotic effect with this class of compounds to determine whether a once-daily regimen would be equally or more effective. However, in the absence of such information, a twice-daily regimen is recommended currently. Although the clinical trial data are very encouraging and indicate therapeutic superiority of the fluoroquinolones in the treatment of enteric fever and prevention of the carrier state, it is not certain how effective they are at preventing complications of typhoid. More information is also needed on the optimum treatment duration for immunocompromised patients.

Whether fluoroquinolones should become the treatment of choice for all typhoid and paratyphoid fever and also for eradication of the carrier state remains unresolved. My opinion is that they should. However, in countries where the quinolones are still considered contraindicated in children, then either trimethoprim-sulfamethoxazole or chloramphenicol remain satisfactory treatments for drug-sensitive infections. Given for 2 weeks, chloramphenicol has been associated with relapse rates between 10 and 25%, compared with failure rates below 5% with the fluoroquinolones. However, there are insufficient randomized comparative trials between the fluoroquinolones and the conventional first-line drugs in the treatment of drug-sensitive infections to define the extent of the advantage. Depending on the source of antibiotics, a 3-day course of fluoroquinolones is only slightly more expensive than a 2-week course of chloramphenicol or trimethoprim-sulfamethoxazole.

For MDR typhoid or paratyphoid fever, the oral third-generation cephalosporins are effective, although in randomized comparative trials both parenteral ceftriaxone and oral cefixime have proved clinically inferior to ofloxacin. Nevertheless, these remain an alternative and may be of particular value for the treatment of nalidixic acid (quinolone)-resistant *S. typhi*. Fortunately these infections have been confined to India and Vietnam, but with increasing use of fluoroquinolones, they can be expected to spread. The cure rate with short-course fluoroquinolone treatments in nalidixic acid–sensitive typhoid consistently exceeds 95%. However, if the organisms are nalidixic acid resistant, then whether or not they are reported as sensitive to the fluoroquinolones, failure rates are approximately 50%. In some of these patients, extending the fluoroquinolone treatment course to 7 or 10 days results in a clinical response. Third-generation cephalosporins are the only available alternatives, and they are associated with slow resolution of fever and symptoms and a relapse rate of approximately 20%. Nearly all nalidixic acid–resistant isolates of *S. typhi* have also been fully resistant to chloramphenicol, trimethoprim-sulfamethoxazole, and ampicillin. Preliminary trials with azithromycin suggest that this is a weakly active compound that could be considered an alternative. Although in theory amoxicillin–clavulanic acid might be considered an alternative to the fluoroquinolones, as ampicillin resistance is usually mediated by a TEM1 plasmid–encoded β-lactamase, preliminary clinical trials with this drug in MDR typhoid have proved disappointing. There are no randomized comparative trials on which to make categorical recommendations for the treatment of quinolone-resistant typhoid.

REFERENCES

1. Acharya G, Crevoisier C, Butler T, Ho M, Tiwari M, Stoeckel K, Bradley CA. Pharmacokinetics of ceftriaxone in patients with typhoid fever. Antimicrob Agents Chemother 1994;38:2415–2418.
2. Acharya GP, Davis TME, Ho M, Harris S, Chataut C, Acharya S, Tuladhar NR, Kafle KE, Pokhrel B, Nosten F, Dance DAB, Smith A, Weber A, White NJ. Factors affecting the pharmacokinetics of parenteral chloramphenicol in enteric fever. J Antimicrob Chemother 1997;40:91–98.
3. Agarwals C. Chloramphenicol resistance of *Salmonella species* in India 1959–61. Bull WHO 1962;27:331–335.
4. Akgun Y, Bac B, Boylu S, Aban N, Tacyildiz I. Typhoid enteric perforation. Br J Surg 1995;82:1512–1515.
5. Alam MN, Haq SA, Das KK, Baral PK, Mazid MN, Siddique RU, Rahman KM, Hasan Z, Khan MA, Dutta P. Efficacy of ciprofloxacin in enteric fever: comparison of treatment duration in sensitive and multidrug-resistant *Salmonella*. Am J Trop Med Hyg 1995;53:306–311.
6. Albert MJ, Haider K, Nahar S, Kibriya AKNG, Hossain MA. Multiresistant *Salmonella typhi* in Bangaladesh. J Antimicrob Chemother 1991:154–155.
7. Ali G, Kamili MA, Rashid S, Mansoor A, Lone BA, Allaqaband GQ. Spontaneous splenic rupture in typhoid fever. Postgrad Med J 1994;70:513–514.
8. Allal R, Kastler B, Gangi A, Bensaid AH, Bouali O, Cherrak C, Brun F, Dietemann JL. Splenic abscesses in typhoid fever: US and CT studies. J Comput Assist Tomogr 1993;17:90–93.
9. Anand AC, Kataria VK, Singh W, Chatterjee SK. Epidemic multiresistant enteric fever in eastern India. Lancet 1990;352.
10. Anderson ES. The problem and implications of chloramphenicol resistance in the typhoid bacillus. J Hyg (Cambridge) 1975;24:289–299.
11. Anderson ES, Smith HR. Chloramphenicol resistance in the typhoid bacillus. Br Med J 1972;3:329–331.
12. Arnold K, Hong CS, Nelwan R, Trujillo IZ, Kadio A, Barros MA, de Garis S. Randomised comparative study of fleroxacin and chloramphenicol in typhoid fever. Am J Med 1993; 1994 (Suppl):195–200.
13. Bavdekar A, Chaudhari M, Bhave S, Pandit A. Ciprofloxacin in typhoid fever. Indian J Pediatr 1991;58:335–339.
14. Bethell DB, Day NP, Dung NM, McMullin C, Loan HT, Tam DTH, Minh LTH, Linh NTM, Dung NQ, Vinh H, MacGowan AP, White LO, White NJ. Pharmacokinetics of oral and intravenous ofloxacin in children with multi-drug resistant typhoid fever. Antimicrobial Agents Chemother 1996;40:2167–2172.
15. Bethell DB, Hien TT, Phi LT, Day NP, Vinh H, Duong NM, Len NV, Chuong LV, and White NJ. The effects on growth of single short courses of fluoroquinolone. Arch Dis Child 1996:7444–7446.
16. Bhutta ZA. Impact of age and drug resistance on mortality in typhoid fever. Arch Dis Child 1996;75:214–217.
17. Bhutta ZA. Therapeutic aspects of typhoidal salmonellosis in childhood: the Karachi experience. Ann Trop Paediatr 1996;16:299–306.
18. Bhutta ZA, Khan IA, Molla AM. Therapy of multidrug-resistant typhoid fever with oral cefixime vs. intravenous ceftriaxone. Pediatr Infect Dis J 1994;13:990–994.
19. Bhutta ZA, Naqvi SH, Durrani S, Suria A. Chloramphenicol therapy of typhoid fever. JPMA J Pak Med Assoc 1991;41:26–30.
20. Bhutta ZA, Naqvi SH, Durrani S, Suria A. Chloramphenicol therapy of typhoid fever and its relationship to hepatic dysfunction. J Trop Paediatr 1991;37:320–322.
21. Bhutta ZA, Naqvi SH, Razzaq RA, Farooqui BJ. Multidrug-resistant typhoid in children: presentation and clinical features. Rev Infect Dis 1991;13:832–836.
22. Bissett IP. Typhoid enteric perforation [Letter]. Br J Surg 1996;83:1478–1479.
23. Biswal N. Neurological manifestations of typhoid fever in children [Letter]. J Trop Pediatr 1994;40:190.

24. Bitar R, Tarpley J. Intestinal perforation in typhoid fever: a historical and state-of-the-art review. Rev Infect Dis 1985;7: 257–271.

25. Brachman PS Jr, Metchock B, Kozarsky PE. Effects of antimalarial chemoprophylactic agents on the viability of the Ty21a typhoid vaccine strain [Letter]. Clin Infect Dis 1992;15: 1057–1058.

26. Brown JC, Shanahan PMA, Jesudason MV, Thomson CJ, Amyes SGB. Mutations responsible for reduced susceptibility to 4-quinolones in clinical isolates of multi-resistant salmonella typhi in India. J Antimicrobial Chemother 1996;37:891–900.

27. Brown JD, Mo DH, Rhoades ER. Chloramphenicol-resistant *Salmonella typhi* in Saigon. JAMA 1975;231:161–166.

28. Brown JD, Mo DH, Rhoades ER. Chloramphenicol-resistant *Salmonella typhi* in Saigon. JAMA 1975;231:162–166.

29. Brown NM, Millar MR, Frost JA, Rowe B. Ciprofloxacin resistance in *Salmonella paratyphi* A. J Antimicrob Chemother 1994;33:1258–1259.

30. Bryan JP, Rocha H, Scheld WM. Problems in salmonellosis: rationale for clinical trials with newer β-lactam agents and quinolones. Rev Infect Dis 1986;8:189–207.

31. Buczko GB, McLean J. Typhoid fever associated with adult respiratory distress syndrome. Chest 1994;105:1873–1874.

32. Butler T, Bell WR, Levin J, Linh NN, Arnold K. Typhoid fever; studies of blood coagulation, bacteremia, and endotoxemia. Arch Intern Med 1978;138:407–410.

33. Butler T, Ho M, Acharya G, Tiwari M, Gallati H. Interleukin-6, gamma interferon, and tumor necrosis factor receptors in typhoid fever related to outcome of antimicrobial therapy. Antimicrob Agents Chemother 1993;37:2418–2421.

34. Butler T, Islam S, Kabir I, Jones PK. Patterns of morbidity and mortality in typhoid fever dependent on age and gender: review of 552 hospitalized patients with diarrhea. Rev Infect Dis 1991; 13:85–90.

35. Butler T, Knight J, Nath SK, Speelman P, Roy SK, Azad MA. Typhoid fever complicated by intestinal perforation: a persisting fatal disease requiring surgical management. Rev Infect Dis 1985;7:244–256.

36. Butler T, Linh NN, Arnold K, Adickman MD, Chau DM, Muoi MM. Therapy of antimicrobial-resistant typhoid fever. Antimicrob Agents Chemother 1977;11:645–650.

37. Butler T, Linh NN, Arnold K, Pollack M. Chloramphenicol resistant typhoid fever in Vietnam associated with R factor. Lancet 1973;2:983–985.

38. Calder JF. Chloramphenicol resistance in typhoid. Br Med J 1972;3:645.

39. Carbon C, Weber P, Levy M, Boussougant Y, Cerf N. Short-term ciprofloxacin therapy for typhoid fever. J Infect Dis 1987; 155:833.

40. Chaicumpa W, Ruangkunaporn Y, Burr D, Chongsanguan M, Echeverria P. Diagnosis of typhoid fever by detection of *Salmonella typhi* antigen in urine. J Clin Microbiol 1992;30: 2513–2515.

41. Chang HR, Vladoianu I, Pechere J. Effects of ampicillin, ceftriaxone, chloramphenicol, pefloxacin and trimethoprim-sulphamethoxazole on *Salmonella typhi* within human monocyte-derived macrophages. Antimicrob Chemother 1990;26: 689–694.

42. Cheesbrough JS, Ilunga Mwema F, Green SD, Tillotson GS. Quinolones in children with invasive *Samonellosis*. Lancet 1991;338:127.

43. Chinh NT, Solomon T, Thong MX, Ly NT, Hoa NTT, Wain J, Diep TS, Day NPJ, Phi LT, Parry CM, White NJ. Short courses of ofloxacin for the treatment of enteric fever. Trans R Soc Trop Med Hyg 1997;91:347–349.

44. Choo KE, Ariffin WA, Ong KH, Sivakumaran S. Aztreonam failure in typhoid fever. Lancet 1991;337:498.

45. Christie AB. Typhoid and paratyphoid fevers. In: Christie AB. Infectious diseases: epidemiology and clinical practice. 3rd ed. Edinburgh: Churchill Livingstone, 1984:47–102.

46. Coovadia YM, Gathiram V, Bhamjee A, Garret RM, Mlisana K, Pillay N, Madlalose T, Short M. An outbreak of multiresistant *Salmonella typhi* in South Africa. Q J Med 1992;82:91–100.

47. Corrado ML, DuPont HL, Cooperstock M, Fekety R, Murray DM. Evaluation of new anti-infective drugs for the treatment of typhoid fever. Clin Infect Dis 1992;15(Suppl 1):S236–240.

48. Daga MK, Sarin K, Sarkar R. A study of culture positive multidrug resistant enteric fever-changing pattern and emerging resistance to ciprofloxacin. J Assoc Physicians India 1994;42: 599–600.

49. Dance DA, Richens J, Ho M, Acharya G, Pokhrel B, Tuladhar NR. Blood and bone marrow cultures in enteric fever. J Clin Pathol 1991;44.

50. Datta N, Richards H, Datta C. *Salmonella typhi* in vivo acquire resistant to both chloramphenicol and co-trimoxazole. Lancet 1981;1:1181–1183.

51. Declercq J, Verhaegen J, Verbist L, Lammens J, Stuyck J, Fabry G. *Salmonella typhi* osteomyelitis. Arch Orthop Trauma Surg 1994;113:232–234.

52. Du Pont H, Hornick RB, Weiss CF, Snyder MJ, Woodward TE. Evaluation of chloramphenicol acid succinate therapy of induced typhoid fever and Rocky Mountain spotted fever. N Engl J Med 1970;282:53–57.

53. Duong NM, Chau NVV, Anh DCV, Hoa NTT, Tam DTH, Ho VA, Hai DT, Hien TT, Arnold K. Short course fleroxacin in the treatment of typhoid fever. JAMA South East Asia 1995;11 (Suppl):21–25.

54. Dutta P, Rasaily R, Saha MR, Mitra U, Bhattacharya SK, Bhattacharya MK, Lahiri M. Ciprofloxacin for treatment of severe typhoid fever in children. Antimicrob Agents Chemother 1993; 37:1197–1199.

55. Edelman R, Levine MM. Summary of an international workshop on typhoid fever. Rev Infect Dis 1986;8:329–349.

56. El Ramli. Chloramphenicol in treatment of enteric group of fevers. J Egypt Med Assoc 1950;33:40–46.

57. El Newihi HM, Alamy ME, Reynolds TB. Salmonella hepatitis: analysis of 27 cases and comparison with acute viral hepatitis. Hepatology 1996;24:516–519.

58. El Ramli AH. Chloramphenicol in treatment of enteric fever. Lancet 1950;1:618–620.

59. El-Sherbini A. An outbreak of typhoid fever resistant to chloramphenicol and other drugs in Gharbeya Governorate in Egypt. J Trop Pediatr 1992;38:331–334.

60. Eykyn SJ, Williams H. Treatment of multi-resistant *Salmonella typhi* with oral ciprofloxacin. Lancet 1987;2:1407–1408.

61. Ferreccio C, Morris JG, Valdivieso C, Prenzel I, Sotomayor V, Drusano GL, Levine MM. The efficacy of ciprofloxacin in the treatment of chronic typhoid carriers. J Infect Dis 1988;157: 1235–1239.

62. Gargalianos P, Jackson PT, Herzog C, Geddes AM. Trimethoprim in enteric fever. J Antibicrob Chemother 1986;18:277–283.

63. Geddes AM, Goodall JAD. Chloramphenicol resistance in the typhoid bacillus. Br Med J 1972;3:525.

64. Ghosh JB, Samanta S. Venous thrombosis in enteric fever [Letter]. Indian Pediatr 1994;31:230–231.

65. Gilman RH, Islam S, Rabbani H, Ghosh H. Identification of gallbladder typhoid carriers by a string device. Lancet 1979: 795–796.

66. Gilman RH, Terminel M, Levine MM, Hernandez-Mendoza P, Hornick RB. Relative efficacy of blood, urine, rectal swab, bone-marrow, and rose-spot cultures for recovery of *Salmonella typhi* in typhoid fever. Lancet 1975;i:1211–1213.

67. Girgis NI, Sultan Y, Hammad O, Farid Z. Comparison of the efficacy, safety and cost of cefixime, ceftriaxone and aztreonam in the treatment of multidrug-resistant *Salmonella typhi* septicemia in children. Pediatr Infect Dis J 1995;14:603–605.

68. Girgis NI, Tribble DR, Sultan Y, Farid Z. Short course chemotherapy with cefixime in children with multidrug-resistant *Salmonella typhi* septicaemia. J Trop Paediatr 1995;41:364–365.

69. Goldstein FW, Chumpitaz JC, Guevara JM, Papadopoulou B, Acar JF, Vieu JF. Plasmid-mediated resistant to multiple antibiotics in *Salmonella typhi*. J Infect Dis 1986;153:261–266.

70. Goldstein W, Chumpitaz JC, Guevara JM, Papadopoulou B, Acar JF, Vieu JF. Plasmid mediated resistance to multiple antibiotics in *Salmonella typhi*. J Infect Dis 1986;153:261–266.

71. Gonzalez-Cortes A, Bessudo D, Sanchez-leyva R, Fragoso R, Hinojosa M, Becerril P. Water-borne transmission of chloramphenicol-resistant *Salmonella typhi* in Mexico. Lancet 1973;2: 605–607.

72. Gotuzzo E, Echevarria J, Carrillo C, Sanchez J, Grados P, Maguina C, DuPont HL. Randomized comparison of aztreonam and chloramphenicol in treatment of typhoid fever. Antimicrob Agents Chemother 1994;38:558–562.

73. Green SD, Ilunga FM, Numbi A, Cheesbrough JS, Tillotson GS. An open study of ciprofloxacin for the treatment of proven or suspected extra intestinal salmonellosis in African children: a preliminary report. Adv Antimicrob Antineoplast Chemother 1992;11:181–187.

74. Griggs DJ, Hall MC, Jin YF, Piddock LJ. Quinolone resistance in veterinary isolates of *Salmonella*. J Antimicrob Chemother 1994;33:1173–1189.

75. Gulati S, Marwaha RK, Prakash D, Ayyagari A, Singhi S, Kumar L, Singhi P, Walia BN. Multi-drug-resistant *Salmonella typhi*—a need for therapeutic reappraisal. Ann Trop Paediatr 1992;12: 137–141.

76. Gupta A. Multidrug-resistant typhoid fever in children: epidemiology and therapeutic approach. Pediatr Infect Dis J 1994; 13:134–140.

77. Haefeli WE, Ott R, Bircher AJ, Burnens AP. Hair loss following typhoid fever: a forgotten phenomenon [Letter]. Clin Infect Dis 1995;20:723–724.

78. Harnet PN, Mcleod S, Auyong Y, Brown S, Krishnan C. Emergence in Ontario, Canada, of multiresistant *Salmonella typhi* from South Asia. Lancet 1992;340:177.

79. Hermans PW, Saha SK, van Leeuwen WJ, Verbrugh HA, van Belkum A, Goessens WH. Molecular typing of *Salmonella typhi* strains from Dhaka (Bangladesh) and development of DNA probes identifying plasmid-encoded multidrug-resistant isolates. J Clin Microbiol 1996;34:1373–1379.

80. Herzog C, Wood MJ. Chloramphenicol resistance in *Salmonella typhi*. Lancet 1982;658–659.

81. Hien TT, Bethell DB, Hoa NT, Wain J, Diep TS, Phi LT, Cuong BM, Duong NM, Thanh PT, Walsh AL, Day NP, White NJ. Short course of ofloxacin for treatment of multidrug-resistant typhoid. Clin Infect Dis 1995;20:917–923.

82. Hien TT, Duong NM, Ha HD, Hoa NT, Diep TS, Phi LT, Arnold K. A randomized comparative study of fleroxacin and ceftriax-

one in enteric fever. Trans R Soc Trop Med Hyg 1994;88: 464–465.

83. Hoffman SL. Typhoid fever. In: Strickland GT, ed. Hunter's tropical medicine. 6th ed. Philadelphia: WB Saunders, 1984: 282–296.

84. Hoffman SL, Edman DC, Punjabi NH, Lesmana M, Cholid A, Sundah S, Harahap J. Bone marrow aspirate culture superior to streptokinase clot culture and 8 ml 1:10 blood-to-broth ratio blood culture for diagnosis of typhoid fever. Am J Trop Med Hyg 1986;35:836–839.

85. Hoffman SL, Punjabi NH, Kumala S, Moechtar MA, Pulungsih SP, Rivai AR, Rockhill RC, Woodward TE, Loedin AA. Reduction of mortality in chloramphenicol-treated severe typhoid fever by high-dose dexamethasone. N Engl J Med 1984;310:82–88.

86. Hoffman SL, Punjabi NH, Rockhill RC, Sutomo A, Rivai AR, Pulungsih SP. Duodenal string-capsule culture compared with bone-marrow, blood, and rectal-swab cultures for diagnosing typhoid and paratyphoid fever. J Infect Dis 1984;149:157–161.

87. Hohmann EL, Oletta CA, Killeen KP, Miller SI. phoP/phoQ-deleted *Salmonella typhi* (Ty800) is a safe and immunogenic single dose typhoid fever vaccine in volunteers. J Infect Dis 1996;173:1408–1414.

88. Horowitz H, Carbonaro CA. Inhibition of the *Salmonella typhi* oral vaccine strain, Ty21a, by mefloquine and chloroquine [Letter]. J Infect Dis 1992;166:1462–1464.

89. Islam A, Butler T, Kabir I, Alam NH. Treatment of typhoid fever with ceftriaxone for 5 days or chloramphenicol for 14 days: a randomized clinical trial. Antimicrob Agents Chemother 1993; 37:1572–1575.

90. Islam S, Butler T, Kabir I, Alam NH. Treatment of typhoid fever with ceftriaxone for 5 days or chloramphenicol for 14 days: a randomized clinical trial. Antimicrob Agents Chemother 1993;37:1572–1575.

91. Ivanoff B. Typhoid fever: global situation and WHO recommendations. Southeast Asian J Trop Med Public Health 1995; 26(Suppl 2):1–6.

92. Jagadish K, Patwari AK, Sarin SK, Prakash C, Srivastava DK, Anand VK. Hepatic manifestations in typhoid fever. Indian Pediatr 1994;31:807–811.

93. Jones DA, Kudlac H, Edwards IR. Pivmecillinam and relapse of typhoid fever. J Infect Dis 1982;145:773–777.

94. Kamat SA. Evaluation of trimethoprim-sulphamethoxazole and chloramphenicol in enteric fever. Br Med J 1970;3:240–243.

95. Khosla SN, Anand A, Singh U, Khosla A. Haematological profile in typhoid fever. Trop Doct 1995;25:156–158.

96. Klugman KP, Koornhof HJ, Robbins JB, Le Cam NN. Immunogenicity, efficacy and serological correlate of protection of *Salmonella typhi* Vi capsular polysaccharide vaccine three years after immunization. Vaccine 1996;14:435–438.

97. Kubin R. Safety and efficacy of ciprofloxacin in paediatric patients—review. Infection 1993;21:413–421.

98. Kumar AS, Legori M, Sathy N, Mathew R. Furazolidone in typhoid fever—correlation of clinical efficacy with serum bactericidal activity. Indian Pediatr 1995;32:533–538.

99. Lasserre R, Sangalang RP, Santiago L. Three-day treatment of typhoid fever with two different doses of ceftrione, compared to 14-day therapy with chloramphenicol: a randomized trial. J Antimicrob Chemother 1991;28:765–772.

100. Lecour H, Santos L, Oliveira M, Pereira A, Simoes J. *Salmonella typhi* meningitis. Scand J Infect Dis 1994;26:103–104.

101. Leung D, Venkatesan P, Boswell T, Innes JA, Wood MJ. Treatment of typhoid in pregnancy [Letter]. Lancet 1995;346:648.

102. Levine MM, Ferreccio C, Black RE, Germanier R. Large-scale field trial of TY21A live oral typhoid vaccine in enteric-coated capsule formulation. Lancet 1987:1049–1052.

103. Mabey DC, Brown A, Greenwood BM. *Plasmodium falciparum* malaria and salmonella infections in Gambian children. J Infect Dis 1987;155:1319–1321.

104. Mandal B. Treatment of multiresistant typhoid fever. Lancet 1990;336:1383.

105. Mathai E, John TJ, Rani M, Mathai D, Chacko N, Nath V, Cherian AM. Significance of *Salmonella typhi* bacteriuria. J Clin Microbiol 1995;33:1791–1792.

106. McCendrick MW, Geddes AM, Farrell ID. Trimethoprim in enteric fever. Br Med J 1981;282:364–368.

107. McCurdy PR. Plasma concentration of chloramphenicol and bone marrow suppression. Blood 1963;21:323–325.

108. Mikhail IA, Haberger RL, Farid Z, Girgis NI, Woody JL. Antibiotic-multiresistant *Salmonella typhi* in Egypt. Trans R Soc Trop Med Hyg 1989;83:921.

109. Mirza SH, Beeching NJ, Hart CA. The prevalence and clinical features of multi-drug resistant *Salmonella typhi* infections in Baluchistan, Pakistan. Ann Trop Med Parasitol 1995;89:515–519.

110. Mishra S, Patwari AK, Anand BK, Pillai PK, Aneja S, Chandra J, Sharma D. Multidrug resistant typhoid fever: therapeutic considerations. Indian J Pediatr 1992;29:443–448.

111. Morelli G, Mazzoli S, Tortoli E, Simonetti MT, Perruna S, Postiglione A. Fluoroquinolones versus chloramphenicol in the therapy of typhoid fever: a clinical and microbiological study. Ther Res 1992;52:532–542.

112. Mourad AS, Metwally M, Nour Ei Deen A, Threlfall EJ, Rowe B, Mapes T, Hedstrom R, Bourgeois AL, Murphy JR. Multiple-drug-resistant *Salmonella typhi*. Clin Infect Dis 1993;17:135–136.

113. Ollarte J, Galindo E. *Salmonella typhi* resistant to chloramphenicol, ampicillin, and other antimicrobial agents: strains isolated during an extensive typhoid fever epidemic in Mexico. Antimicrob Agents Chemother 1973;4:597–607.

114. Paniker CKJ, Vimala KN. Transferable chloramphenicol resistance in *Salmonella typhi*. Nature 1972;239:109–110.

115. Phillips WE. Treatment of chronic typhoid carriers with ampicillin. JAMA 1970;1971:913–915.

116. Pillay N, Adams EB, North-Coombes D. Comparative trial of amoxycillin and chloramphenicol in treatment of typhoid fever in adults. Lancet 1979;2:333–334.

117. Plotkin SA, Bouveret Le Cam N. A new typhoid vaccine composed of the Vi capsular polysaccharide. Arch Intern Med 1995;155:2293–2299.

118. Prabha A, Mohanan, Pereira P, Raghuveer CV. Myocarditis in enteric fever. Indian J Med Sci 1995;49:28–31.

119. Pradhan KM, Arora NK, Jena A, Susheela AK, Bhan MK. Safety of ciprofloxacin therapy in children: magnetic resonance images, body fluid levels of fluoride and linear growth. Acta Paediatr 1995;84:555–560.

120. Rajeshwari K, Yadav S, Puri RK, Khanijo CM, Sethi Y. Cerebritis in typhoid fever. Indian Pediatr 1995;32:1305–1307.

121. Rao PS, Rajashekar V, Varghese GK, Shivananda PG. Emergence of multidrug-resistant *Salmonella typhi* in rural southern India. Am J Trop Med Hyg 1993;48:108–111.

122. Richens J, Smith T, Mylius T, Spooner V. An algorithm for the clinical differentiation of malaria and typhoid: a preliminary communication. Papua New Guinea Med J 1992;35:298–302.

123. Robertson RP, Wahab MFA, Raasch FO. Evaluation of chlor-

amphenicol and ampicillin in *Salmonella* enteric fever. N Engl J Med 1968;278:171–175.

124. Rowe B, Threlfall EJ, Ward LR. Does chloramphenicol remain the drug of choice for typhoid? Epidemiol Infect 1987;98:379–383.

125. Rowe B, Ward LR, Threlfall EJ. Spread of multiresistant *Samonella typhi*. Lancet 1990;336:1065.

126. Rowe B, Ward LR, Threlfall EJ. Treatment of multiresistant typhoid fever. Lancet 1991;337:1422.

127. Rowe B, Ward LR, Threlfall EJ. Ciprofloxacin-resistant *Salmonella typhi* in the UK [Letter]. Lancet 1995;346:1302.

128. Rowland HAK. The complications of typhoid fever. J Trop Med Hyg 1961;64:143.

129. Roy SK, Speelman P, Butler T, Nath SK, Rahman H, Stoll BJ. Diarrhea associated with typhoid fever. J Infect Dis 1985;151:1138–1143.

130. Rubin FA, McWhirter PD, Burr D, Punjabi NH, Lane E, Kumala S, Sudarmono P, Pulungsih SP, Lesmana M, Tjaniadi P, Sukri N, Hoffman SL. Rapid diagnosis of typhoid fever through identification of *Salmonella typhi* within 18 hours of specimen acquisition by culture of the mononuclear cell-platelet fraction of blood. J Clin Microbiol 1990;28:825–827.

131. Samnalkorpi K, Lahdevirta J, Makela T, Rostila T. Treatment of chronic salmonella carrier with ciprofloxacin. Lancet 1987;2:164–165.

132. Sarma PS, Durairaj P. Randomized treatment of patients with typhoid and paratyphoid fevers using norfloxacin or chloramphenicol. Trans R Soc Trop Med Hyg 1991;85:670–671.

133. Schaad UB. Toxicity of quinolones in paediatric patients. Adv Antimicrob Antineoplast Chemother 1992;11(Suppl):259–265.

134. Schwalbe RS, Hage CW, Morris JG, O-hanlon PN, Crawford RA, Gilligan PH. In vivo selection for transmissible drug resistance in *Salmonella typhi* during antimicrobial therapy. Antimicrob Agents Chemother 1990;34:161–163.

135. Schwartz E, Jenks NP, Shlim DR. 'Typhoid hepatitis' or typhoid fever and acute viral hepatitis. Trans R Soc Trop Med Hyg 1994;88:437–438.

136. Scregt JN, Rubidge CJ. Trimethoprim and sulphamethoxazole in typhoid fever in children. Br Med J 1971;3:738–741.

137. Sethuraman S, Mahamood M, Kareem S. Furazolidone in multi-resistant childhood typhoid fever. Ann Trop Paediatr 1994;14:321–324.

138. Shann F, Linnemann V, MacKenzie A, Barker J, Gratten M, Crinis N. Absorption of chloramphenicol sodium succinate after intramuscular administration in children. N Engl J Med 1985;313:410–414.

139. Sharma AM, Sharma OP. Pulmonary manifestations of typhoid fever. Chest 1992;101:1144–1146.

140. Sitprija V, Pipatanagul V, Boonpucknavig V, Boonpucknavig S. Glomerulitis in typhoid fever. Ann Intern Med 1974;81:210–213.

141. Smith CE, Marsden AT. Fatal meningitis in typhoid fever treated with chloramphenicol. Lancet 1951;iii:430–435.

142. Smith MD, Duong NM, Hoa NT, Wain J, Ha HD, Diep TS, Day NP, Hien TT, White NJ. Comparison of ofloxacin and ceftriaxone for short-course treatment of enteric fever. Antimicrob Agents Chemother 1994;38:1716–1720.

143. Soe GB, Overturf GD. Treatment of typhoid fever and other systemic salmonelloses with cefotaxime, ceftriaxone, cefoperazone, and other newer cephalosporins. Rev Infect Dis 1987;9:719–736.

144. Song J, Cho H, Park MY, Na DS, Moon HB, Pai CH. Detection of *Salmonella typhi* in the blood of patients with typhoid

fever by polymerase chain reaction. J Clin Microbiol 1993;31: 1439–1443.

145. Spika JS, Waterman SH, Soo Hoo GW, St Louis ME, Pacer RE, James SM, Bissett ML, Mayer LW, Chiu JY, Hall B, Greene K, Potter ME, Cohen ML, Blake PA. Chloramphenicol-resistant *Salmonella newport* traced through hamburger to dairy farms. N Engl J Med 1987;316:566–570.

146. Sridhar CB, Kulkarni RD. Reassessment of frequency of occurrence of typhoid fever and cost efficacy analysis of antibiotic therapy. J Assoc Physicians India 1995;43:679–684.

147. Stanley PJ, Flegg PJ, Mandoul BK, Geddes AM. Open study of ciprofloxacin in enteric fever. J Antimicrob Chemother 1989; 23:789–791.

148. Takkar VP, Kumar R, Takkar R, Khurana S. Resurgence of chloramphenicol sensitive *Salmonella typhi*. Indian Pediatr 1995;32:586–587.

149. Taylor DE, Chumpitaz JC, Goldstein F. Variability of *IncHI1* plasmids from *Salmonella typhi* with special reference to Peruvian plasmids encoding resistance to trimethoprim and other antibiotics. Antimicrobial Agents Chemother 1985;28:452–455.

150. Thong K, Cheong Y, Puthucheary S, Koh C, Pang T. Epidemiologic analysis of sporadic *Salmonella typhi* isolates and those from outbreaks by pulsed-field gel electrophoresis. J Clin Microbiol 1994;32:1135–1141.

151. Threlfall EJ, Ward LR, Frost JA, Rowe B. Typhoid fever and other salmonellosis: a changing pattern of drug susceptibilities. Southeast Asian J Trop Med Publ Hlth 1995;26:13–15.

152. Trevett AJ, Nwokolo N, Lightfoot D, Naraqi S, Kevau IH, Temu PI, Igo JD. Ataxia in patients infected with *Salmonella typhi* phage type D2: clinical, biochemical and immunohistochemical studies. Trans R Soc Trop Med Hyg 1994;88:565–568.

153. Tribble D, Girgis N, Habib N, Butler T. Efficacy of azithromycin for typhoid fever. Clin Infect Dis 1995;21:1045–1046.

154. Unal S, Hayran M, Tuncer S, Gur D, Uzun O, Adova M, Akalin HE. Treatment of enteric fever with pefloxacin for 7 days versus 5 days: a randomized clinical trial. Antimicrobial Agents Chemother 1996;40:2898–2900.

155. Uwaydah AK, Al Soub H, Matar I. Randomized prospective study comparing two dosage regimens of ciprofloxacin for the treatment of typhoid fever. J Antimicrob Chemother 1992;30: 707–711.

156. Uwaydah AK, Matar I, Chacko KC, Davidson JC. The emergence of antimicrobial resistant *Salmonella typhi* in Qatar: epi-

demiology and therapeutic implications. Trans R Soc Trop Med Hyg 1991;85:790–782.

157. van Basten JP, Stockenbrugger R. Typhoid perforation. Trop Geogr Med 1994;46:336–339.

158. van Basten JP, Stockenbrugger R. Typhoid perforation. A review of the literature since 1960. Trop Geogr Med 1994;46: 336–339.

159. Vazquez C, Calderon E, Rodriguez RS. Chloramphenicol-resistant strain of *Salmonella typhosa*. N Engl J Med 1972;286: 12–20.

160. Vinh H, Wain J, Hanh VTG, Nga CG, Chinh MT, Bethell DB, Hoa NTT, Diep TS, Dung NM, White NJ. Two or three days of ofloxacin treatment for uncomplicated multidrug-resistant typhoid fever in children. Antimicrobial Agents Chemother 1996;40:958–961.

161. Wain J, Diep ST, Ho VA, Walsh AL, Hoa NTT, Parry CM, White NJ. Quantitation of bacteria in blood of typhoid fever patients and relationship between counts and clinical features, transmissibility, and antibiotic resistance. J Clin Microbiol 1988;36:1683–1687.

162. Wain J, Hoa NTT, Chinh NT, Vinh H, Everett MJ, Diep TS, Dung NM, Day NP, White NJ, Piddock LJ, Parry CM. Quinolone resistant *Salmonella typhi* from Vietnam; molecular basis of resistance and clinical response to treatment. Clin Infect Dis 1997;25(6):1404–1410.

163. Wallace MR, Yousif AA, Mahroos GA, Mapes T, Threlfall EJ, Rowe B, Hyams KC. Ciprofloxacin versus ceftriaxone in the treatment of multiresistant typhoid fever. Eur J Clin Microbiol Infect Dis 1993;12:907–910.

164. Wallace MR, Yousif AA, Habib NF, Tribble DR. Azithromycin and typhoid [Letter]. Lancet 1994;343:1497–1498.

165. Wang F, Gu XJ, Zhang MF, Tai TY. Treatment of typhoid fever with ofloxacin. J Antibicrob Chemother 1989;23:785–788.

166. White NJ, Parry CM. The treatment of typhoid fever. Curr Opin Infect Dis 1996;9:298–302.

167. White NJ, Dung NM, Vinh H, Bethell D, Hien TT. Fluoroquinolone antibiotics in children with multidrug resistant typhoid [Letter]. Lancet 1996;348:547.

168. Woodward TE, Smadel JE. The management of typhoid fever and its complications. Ann Intern Med 1964;60:144–149.

170. Zafar J, Abbas S, Qayyum A, Ahmed N, Hussain S, Qazi RA. Typhoid orchitis. JPMA J Pak Med Assoc 1995;45:106–107.

171. Zhu Q, Lim CK, Chan YN. Detection of *Salmonella typhi* by polymerase chain reaction. J Appl Bacteriol 1996;80:244–251.

Serratia marcescens

Edward S. Wong and Sheldon M. Markowitz

GENERAL DESCRIPTION

Serratia marcescens is an opportunistic pathogen whose clinical importance has only been appreciated in the last three decades. While *Serratia* is a rare cause of community-acquired infections, it has become an important nosocomial pathogen. According to the National Nosocomial Infections Surveillance Study (NNIS), *Serratia* is responsible for 2% of infections occurring in hospitals (2).

Serratia is a member of *Enterobacteriaceae* family. *Serratia* spp. are motile and do not ferment lactose (or only very slowly) or produce H_2S on a triple-sugar-iron slant. They are Voges-Proskauer positive and can use citrate as a sole carbon source (17). The genus *Serratia* contains multiple species but only one, *S. marcescens,* has been consistently associated with human disease. There are currently nine other members of the genus, including *S. odifera, S. liquifasciens,* and *S. rubidaea,* but these have rarely caused infections in man. *S. marcescens* does not ferment L-arabinose, which can differentiate it from these other species with the exception of *S. entomophila,* which is not found in human clinical specimens.

Prior to the 1960s, *Serratia* were presumed to be nonpathogenic, and because of their distinctive red pigmentation on culture, *Serratia* were used as indicator organisms to study wind and water currents and released in bus terminals and subways to study population susceptibility to germ warfare (62). *Serratia*'s potential to cause infections in man only became recognized after reports of this organism causing postoperative wound infections (43), nosocomial pneumonias (41), endocarditis among drug addicts (35), bacteremias (60), and cellulitis (3) were published. It is now recognized as an important pathogen of nosocomial urinary tract infections, particularly among patients with indwelling Foley catheters or who have had recent genitourinary instrumentation. Numerous nosocomial outbreaks of urinary tract infections have been reported, with problems traced to improper catheter care and contaminated urinary drainage devices or specific-gravity-measuring devices (1, 28, 44, 52).

Outpatient infections involving *Serratia* are rare. *Serratia* is an infrequent cause of otitis and sinusitis. Septic arthritis in the outpatient setting has been reported following diagnostic and therapeutic intraarticular injections (11, 36). In one such outbreak, use of an antiseptic solution contaminated with *Serratia* prior to injection was implicated (36). *Serratia* is also a rare cause of endocarditis. In the 1970s, *S. marcescens* was the most frequent cause of Gram-negative endocarditis among intravenous drug addicts in San Francisco (35). In retrospect, the sheer number of cases is unusual, and the geographic clustering to San Francisco remains unexplained. The frequency has since subsided, although sporadic cases of *Serratia* endocarditis still occasionally occur (20).

Unlike other members of the *Enterobacteriaceae* family, the predominant site of colonization for *Serratia* is not the gastrointestinal tract but the urinary or respiratory tract (1, 28). When infection control techniques are poor, these sites often serve as reservoirs for transmission to other patients, as suggested by outbreak investigations in which close proximity to patients infected or colonized with *Serratia* was identified as a risk factor for acquisition (28, 51).

SUSCEPTIBILITY IN VITRO
Single Drugs

Isolates of *S. marcescens* from the 1960s were uniformly susceptible to aminoglycosides. Some 98% of the strains tested by Cabrera (5) were susceptible to kanamycin. Thornton and Andriole (56) and Wilkowske et al. (59) reported that more than 97% of strains were susceptible to gentamicin at 1 µg/mL or less. Beginning in the 1970s, however, gentamicin resistance began to be noted in *Serratia*. Meyer et al. (33) reported that the prevalence of gentamicin resistance among clinical isolates recovered in their general hospital was 50%. Yu (64) reported that 24% of 140 nosocomial *S. marcescens* identified from 1968 through 1977 were gentamicin resistant. None of the *Serratia* isolates from 1968 to 1974 exhibited resistance; gentamicin resistance was observed only after 1974. Emergence of resistance to gentamicin paralleled the overall increased use of gentamicin in their hospital. Specifically, antecedent exposure to gentamicin for 2 days or more predisposed patients to acquiring gentamicin-resistant *Serratia*. Markowitz and Sibilla, in 1980, similarly reported that 37% of clinically significant isolates of *Serratia* from a urban teaching hospital were resistant to gentamicin.

The gentamicin-resistant *Serratia* were generally resistant to other aminoglycosides, including streptomycin, kanamycin, and tobramycin. They were, however, susceptible to amikacin. Bodey (2) noted that 48 of 50 isolates of *S. marcescens* were sensitive to concentrations of amikacin of 6.25 µg/mL or less. Meyer et al. (33) found 100% of *S. marcescens* isolates to be sensitive to amikacin. Similarly, 100% of the isolates tested by Markowitz and Sibilla (29) were susceptible to concentrations of amikacin safely achievable in serum ($\leq$25 µg/mL).

Gentamicin-resistant *Serratia* were often resistant to multiple other antibiotics as well. Schaberg et al. (52) noted that the *Serratia* responsible for outbreaks in four hospitals was resistant to what was then all currently available parenteral antibiotics (chloramphenicol, tetracycline, sulfonamide, ampicillin, cephalothin, carbenicillin, kanamycin, streptomycin, and gentamicin). Craven et al. (10) reported an outbreak involving 222 patients caused by *Serratia* that was resistant to ampicillin, cephalothin, chloramphenicol, colistin, gentamicin, and kanamycin. Similarly, Olexy et al. (40) reported a small cluster of infections caused by *S. marcescens* resistant to ampicillin, cephalothin, carbenicillin, sulfonamide, trimethoprim, streptomycin, kanamycin, gentamicin, tobramycin, neomycin, polymyxin B, and tetracycline.

In mating experiments, Schaberg et al. (51) were able to transfer resistance to kanamycin, tetracycline, chloramphenicol, streptomycin, ampicillin, and carbenicillin from a multiply-resistant *Serratia* donor to recipient *Escherichia coli* with a transfer frequency of 10^{-5}, confirming that the resistance was plasmid mediated. John and McNeill (23) identified a 41-megadalton plasmid from 92% of multiply-drug resistant *S. marcescens* isolated from an outbreak in a neurosurgical unit. This plasmid was found by conjugation experiments to encode resistance to ampicillin, carbenicillin, tetracycline, kanamycin, gentamicin, and tobramycin. Analysis of DNA fragment profiles of this plasmid after endonuclease digestion revealed the pattern from multiple isolates to be identical, suggesting that the outbreak was due to intrahospital spread of a single strain.

Serratia is uniformly resistant to ampicillin, cephalothin, and carboxypenicillins (Table 1). The mechanism of resistance is likely a plasmid-mediated β-lactamase that is common among *Enterobacteriaceae*. The acylampicillins, azlocillin, mezocillin,

TABLE 1 • Comparative Activity of Antibiotics against *Serratia marcescens*

Antibiotic	No. Isolates[a]	MIC_{50}	MIC_{90}	Reference
Gentamicin	71	1.0	16.0	55
Amoxicillin/ clavulanic acid	78	64	>64	30
Trimethoprim- sulfamethoxazole	78	0.25	1.0	30
Cefazolin	NA	>128	>128	38
Cefaclor	78	>64	>64	30
Cefoxitin	70	≥25	≥100	30
Cefuroxime	88	>16	>16	57
	78	>64	>64	30
Cefoperazone	44	2	16	24
	NA	—	16	38
Moxalactam	NA	—	4	38
Cefotaxime	71	0.5	32	55
	400	0.5	—	48
	44	0.5	4	24
	NA	—	4	38
Ceftazidime	24	1.0	2.0	
	400	0.29	—	48
	44	0.25	0.5	24
	71	0.25	8	55
	NA	—	2	38
	88	<.25	1	56
Ceftriaxone	69	0.25	16	56
	88	<0.5	8	57
	44	0.5	4	24
	78	0.5	8	30
	NA	—	4	38
Aztreonam	113	—	1.6	53
	18	1	2	21
Cefepime	70	0.12	8	55
	88	<.25	0.5	57
	400	0.15	—	48
	44	0.12	0.5	24
Cefpirone	400	0.11	—	48
Imipenem	71	1	2	55
	44	0.5	1	24
Meropenem	764	—	0.25	13
	46	0.3	0.06	27
Norfloxacin	24	0.5	1	14
Ofloxacin	24	0.5	1	14
	78	0.5	4.0	30
	NA	0.04	1.6	61
Levofloxacin	24	0.25	0.5	14
Ciprofloxacin	24	0.25	0.5	14
	78	0.25	4.0	30
	NA	<0.1	1.0	61
Lomefloxacin	78	0.5	8.0	30
Fleroxacin	78	0.25	2.0	30
Enoxacin	NA	0.8	6.3	61

[a] NA, not available.

and piperacillin, are more resistant to hydrolysis of β-lactamase and thus show more activity against this *Serratia*. However, the activity is variable, depending on the amount of β-lactamase being produced, and even piperacillin, the most active of the extended-spectrum penicillins against *Serratia*, is effective against only 50% of *Serratia* isolates (12).

Like *Enterobacter* and *Pseudomonas*, *Serratia* are capable of producing a chromosomal β-lactamase (4, 47 or 49). Induction of this chromosomal enzyme by exposure to β-lactam antibiotics leads to resistance to first- and second-generation cephalosporins.

Third-generation cephalosporins and the recently introduced "fourth-generation" cephalosporins, cefepime and cefpirone, are stable to the hydrolytic activity of both plasmid-mediated and low levels of chromosomal β-lactamase (47). Not surprisingly, they are highly active against *S. marcescens* (Table 1). Cefotaxime and ceftriaxone have low minimal inhibitory concentrations ($MIC_{50} < 1$ μg/mL) and achieve high serum levels. The monobactam aztreonam is also very active, with an MIC_{90} below 1.6 μg/mL (53).

The carbapenams, imipenem and meropenem, resist inactivation by most of the known plasmid-mediated and chromosomal β-lactamases, including ezymes produced by *Serratia* (13, 47, or 49). Both carbapenems have MIC_{50}s against *Serratia* of 1 μg/mL or less and would be expected to be very effective against *Serratia* (13, 27).

Fluoroquinolones inhibit bacteria via their effect on DNA gyrase, an essential enzyme for replication (19). All the quinolones are active against Gram-negative bacteria, including *Serratia*. Ciprofloxacin and levofloxacin, however, appear to be the two most active of the class against *S. marcescens*, with MIC_{90}s of 0.5 μg/mL (14, 19).

Antibiotic Combinations

When multiantibiotic-resistant *Serratia* was prevalent in the 1970s, investigators examined various combinations of antibiotics, looking for synergistic activity. Weinstein et al. (58) looked at carbenicillin in combination with either gentamicin or amikacin. Fu and Neu (15) combined an aminoglycoside (netilmicin, gentamicin, or amikacin) with an extended-spectrum penicillin (carbenicillin, ticarcillin, axlocillin, or mezlocillin). Miller et al. (34) looked at addition of carbenicillin, cefamandole, cefoxitin, or cefuroxime to aminoglycosides against *Serratia*. These combinations showed in vitro synergistic activity against *S. marcescens*, defined by a fourfold drop in the MIC of two drugs together compared with each drug alone.

Other combinations have also been tested. Thomas (54) showed in vitro synergism between sulfamethoxazole, trimethoprim, and polymyxin against an epidemic strain of *S. marcescens* resistant to each drug alone. In vivo, this drug combination effected clinical improvement or microbiologic cure in 4 of 6 patients infected with *Serratia*. Polymyxin B and rifampin also appear to have synergistic activity (42).

β-Lactamase inhibitors, clavulanate, sulbactam, and tazobactam, covalently bind β-lactamases before they can degrade β-lactam antibiotics (39). Addition of a β-lactam inhibitor to a β-lactam antibiotic should thus improve overall activity against organisms producing β-lactamase, including *Serratia*. Testing 73 isolates of *S. marcescens* recovered from our clinical microbiology laboratory, we found that addition of sulbactam and clavulanate to ampicillin and ticarcillin increased the coverage from 16 and 59% to 38 and 68% of the isolates, respectively (unpublished data). β-Lactamase inhibitors however do not affect chromosomal β-lactamases

(39). These combination antibiotics offer no additional advantage over the antibiotic alone in the treatment of *Serratia* secreting chromosomal β-lactamases.

ANTIMICROBIAL THERAPY
General

Until gentamicin resistance began to emerge in the mid-1970s, aminoglycosides, particularly gentamicin, were considered the drugs of choice for treatment of infections caused by *S. marcescens*. Gentamicin-resistant *Serratia* were often cross-resistant to other aminoglycosides, including kanamycin and tobramycin, but they often remained susceptible to amikacin. Yu (62) and Craven et al. (10) reported good clinical responses when amikacin was used to treat gentamicin-resistant *Serratia*. Unfortunately, amikacin resistance among *Serratia* has also been noted. In the report by Craven et al. (10), amikacin resistance even emerged during therapy.

In the past decade, overall use of aminoglycosides has declined. Coincident with this decline, and perhaps related to it, is the reemergence of activity of aminoglycosides against *Serratia*. In 1980, Markowitz noted that 63% and 100% of *Serratia* isolates were susceptible to gentamicin and amikacin, respectively. More recently, Thornsberry and Yee (55) reported that 89% of 71 isolates of *S. marcescens* tested were susceptible to gentamicin. These isolates were gathered from multiple hospitals across the United States, and thus the results are broadly representative.

Despite improved activity, however, aminoglycosides are unlikely to regain their previous role as the drugs of choice against *Serratia*, given the availability of new antibiotics with equal, if not better, activity against *Serratia* and concerns among clinicians about the aminoglycosides' potential for nephrotoxicity and ototoxicity. As a result, aminoglycosides have largely been relegated to a secondary role, to be used in combination with another antibiotic in the treatment of moderate-to-severe infections in critically ill patients.

Currently, the new cephalosporins must be considered drugs of choice for treating infections caused by *S. marcescens* (16). With MIC_{50}s generally below 1 μg/mL and high peak serum levels and safety profiles, any of the third generation cephalosporins such as ceftazidime, ceftriaxone, cefotaxime, ceftizoxime, or cefoperazone should be highly effective in the treatment of *S. marcescens* infections (63). The monobactam aztreonam also has good activity against *Serratia*. Cox (9) used aztreonam to treat 17 patients with complicated urinary tract infections with *S. marcescens*. At a dose of 0.5 g twice daily, 16 of the 17 patients were cured.

Carbapenems and fluoroquinolone antibiotics are also highly active against *Serratia* (13, 14). However, in most institutions the purchasing cost of these drugs exceeds the cost of equally effective third-generation cephalosporins. For this reason, carbapenems and quinolones are often restricted for use only when *S. marcescens* is resistant to third-generation cephalosporins.

TABLE 2 • Antimicrobial Therapy for *Serratia marcescens*

Antibiotic	Usual Dose	Comments
Cephalosporins		
Third generation: Considered the treatment of choice for *Serratia,* often combined with gentamicin or amikacin		
Cefotaxime	1–2 g q. 4–8 h	
Ceftriaxone	1–2 g q. 24 h	
Ceftazidime	1–2 g q. 8 h	
Aztreonam	1–2 g q. 6–8 h	
Imipenem	0.5–1 g q. 6 h	Active against ESBL- and chromosomal β-lactamase-producing *Serratia*
Meropenem	1 g q. 8 h	
Fourth generation		
Cefipeme	1 g q. 12 h	Active against ESBL- and chromosomal β-lactamase-producing *Serratia*
Fluoroquinolones: Also very active against *Serratia,* can be used as first- or second-line therapy		
Ciprofloxacin	400 mg q. 12 h	Oral formulations can be used in UTIs
Ofloxacin	200–400 mg q. 12 h	
Levofloxacin	500 mg q. 24 h	
Norfloxacin	400 mg p.o. b.i.d.	No i.v. formulation, only for UTIs
Aminoglycosides: Usually active, but no longer treatment of choice; usually combined with third-generation cephalosporins in serious infections; not to be used alone except in UTIs		
Gentamicin	3–5 mg/kg/day × SD/day or q. 8 h	Most experience of aminoglycosides
Tobramycin	3–5 mg/kg/day × SD/day or q. 8 h	
Amikacin	15 mg/kg/day × SD/day or q. 12 h	Usually active against gentamicin-resistant *Serratia*
Miscellaneous		
Trimethoprim-sulfamethoxazole	1 DS p.o. b.i.d. 5–10 mg/kg (trimethoprim) i.v. q. 8 h	Usually active; ok for UTI but little experience with use as sole agent for more serious infections
Rifampin	600 mg q. 24 h	Limited experience but used in combination with another agent

Special Situations

Emergence of Resistance to Third-Generation Cephalosporins

With the widespread reliance on use of β-lactam antibiotics, the frequency of resistance to third-generation cephalosporins has risen steadily among Gram-negative bacteria, including *Serratia* (18). One mechanism for this resistance is a mutation in the genes encoding the common TEM, SHV, and OXA β-lactamases (32, 47). The resultant enzymes differ from their parent compounds often by only one or two amino acids but greatly expand the spectrum of hydrolyzing activity to include third-generation cephalosporins, including the monobactams, hence the name "extended-spectrum β-lactamases" (ESBLs). ESBLs first appeared in England, Germany, and France in the early 1980s (26). They did not appear in the United States until 1986. *Klebsiella* and *Enterobacter* are the two most common organisms to harbor ESBLs, but these enzymes have also been detected in clinical isolates of *E. coli, Serratia, Citrobacter, Salmonella,* and *Morganella* (32).

Despite numerous published outbreaks, the prevalence of ESBL production among *Enterobacteriaceae* is unknown, in part because routine susceptibility testing may fail to detect it (47). Isolates harboring ESBL may have a higher MIC than usually encountered at an institution, for example, an MIC of ceftazidime above 1 μg/mL, but the MIC remains below the resistant range. Thus, the organism appears less susceptible but not frankly resistant, thereby going unnoticed.

The prevalence of ESBL in published reports from around the world varies greatly, ranging from 1 to 74% (47). In the United States, the prevalence is believed to be much lower, although a recent report suggests it may be higher than previously thought. Using isoelectric focusing and double-disk potentiation, Coudron et al. (8) detected a 16% incidence of ESBL production among *Enterobacteriaceae* from clinical specimens submitted from the intensive care unit of a large Veterans Affairs hospital. The most frequent producer of ESBL was *Enterobacter aerogenes* (27%), but *S. marcescens* strains with ESBL were also detected.

Serratia strains producing ESBL are resistant to ceftazidime, cefotaxime, ceftriaxone, and aztreonam. They remain susceptible to cephamycins cefoxitin and cefotetan and carbapenems imipenem and meropenem (47). Since β-lactamase inhibitors continue to bind these variant β-lactamases, combination antibiotics that include a β-lactamase inhibitor such as Augmentin, Timentin, and Zosyn continue to be effective against ESBL-producing *Serratia* (18). Fluoroquinolones inhibit bacterial growth through a different mechanism (DNA gyrase) and remain active against ESBL-producing *Serratia*.

Not all resistance to third-generation cephalosporins is due to ESBL production. *S. marcescens* possesses a chromosomally encoded cephalosporinase that is inducible by cephalosporins (4, 47). As a Bush group 1 enzyme, this cephalosporinase is not inhibited by clavulanic acid or other β-lactamase inhibitors (4). It will bind and hydrolyze cephamycins, making cefoxitin and cefotetan ineffective for treatment. Production of high levels of this enzyme by either induction, gene amplification, or mutation in the regulatory gene would also lead to resistance to many third-generation cephalosporins including the monobactams (47).

Currently, the carbapenems must be considered the drugs of choice against *Serratia* that is resistant to third-generation cephalosporins. The carbapenems are resistant to the hydrolyzing activity of both chromosomal β-lactamases and ESBLs (22). However, imipenem resistance among *S. marcescens,* although infrequent, has been reported (37, 41). The mechanism of resistance is either production of a metallo-β-lactamase (Bush group 3) or change in porin size that drastically lowers penetration of the antibiotic into the periplasmic space (44).

An alternative to imipenem in the treatment of *S. marcescens* resistant to third-generation cephalosporins is cefepime, one of the new "fourth-generation cephalosporins recently approved for marketing. This new cephalosporin is active against Gram-negative bacteria producing either ESBL or chromosomal group 1 β-lactamase (48).

Treatment of *S. marcescens* Endocarditis

In San Francisco during the 1970s, up to 14% of addict-associated endocarditis in the city was associated with *S. marcescens* (35). This clustering has since resolved, but endocarditis caused by *Serratia* occasionally still occurs, with two of the highest risk groups being intravenous drug users and patients who recently underwent prosthetic valve surgery. Because overall mortality with *Serratia* endocarditis is high, approaching 50%, most experts recommend using more than one antibiotic in treating this serious infection (7). This recommendation is based on experimental and clinical evidence. In the rabbit model of endocarditis, combination antibiotics are generally more effective in reducing bacteremia, sterilizing vegetations, and preventing relapse. Clinically, in the reports from San Francisco, patients with *S. marcescens* endocarditis who were treated with aminoglycosides in combination with carbenicillin or chloramphenicol fared better than patients treated with aminoglycosides alone (35).

Treatment of *S. marcescens* Infections in Neutropenic Patients

Infected compromised patients who are neutropenic generally have poorer outcomes than their immunocompetent counterparts with the same infections (25). The choice of antibiotics is especially critical in neutropenia, because these patients lack the cellular immune mechanisms that are key to defending the host (2). In neutropenic patients, aminoglycosides alone are considered suboptimal therapy for Gram-negative infections. Saito et al. (46) reviewed their experience with the treatment of 118 cases of *Serratia* bacteremia at the M. D. Anderson Cancer Center. They observed that despite in vitro susceptibility of *S. marcescens* to aminoglycosides, monotherapy with an aminoglycoside was substantially less effective than regimens that included other antibiotics, generally β-lactam antibiotics (60 vs. 86%, $P = .08$).

REFERENCES

1. Allen SD, Conger KB. *Serratia marcescens* infection of the urinary tract: a nosocomial problem. J Urol 1969;101:621–623.

2. Bodey GP. Antibiotics in patients with neutropenia. Arch Intern Med 1984;144:1845–1851.

3. Brenner DE, Lookingbill DP. *Serratia marcescens* cellulitis. Arch Dermatol 1977;113:1599–1600.

4. Bush K, Jacoby GA, Mederios AA. A functional classification scheme for beta-lactamases and its correlation with molecular structure. Antimicrob Agents Chemother 1995;39:1211–1233.

5. Cabrera HA. An outbreak of *Serratia marcescens* and its control. Arch Intern Med 1969;123:650–655.

6. Centers for Disease Control. National nosocomial infection study report. Annual summary 1979; issued March 1982.

7. Chambers HF, Mills J. Endocarditis associated with intravenous drug abuse. In: Sande MA, Kaye D, Root RK, eds. Endocarditis. New York: Churchill Livingstone, 1984:183–200.

8. Coudron PE, Williams D, Markowitz SM. Prevalence of extended spectrum beta-lactamases (ESBL) in *Enterobacter aerogenes* from Richmond, VA [Abstract C-202]. 96th American Society for Microbiology general meeting, Washington, DC, 1996.

9. Cox CE. Aztreonam therapy for complicated urinary tract infections caused by multidrug-resistant bacteria. 1985;7(Suppl 4): S767–S771.

10. Craven PC, Jorgensen JH, Kasper RL, Drutz DJ. Amikacin therapy of patients with multiply antibiotic-resistant *Serratia marcescens* infections. Development of increasing resistance during therapy. Am J Med 1977;62:66–74.

11. Dorwar BB, Abrutyn E, Schumacher HR. Serratia arthritis. JAMA 1973;225:1642–1643.

12. Drusano GL, Schimpff SC, Hewitt WL. The acylampicillins: mexlocillin, piperacillin, and azlocillin. Rev Infect Dis 1984;6: 13–32.

13. Edwards JR, Turner PJ. Laboratory data which differentiate meropenem from imipenem. Scand J Infect Dis Suppl 1995;96: 5–10.

14. Fu KP, Lafredo SC, Folendo B, Isaacson DM, Barrett JF, Tobia AJ, Rosenthale ME. In vitro and in vivo antibacterial activities of levofloxacin (L-ofloxacin), an optically active ofloxacin. Antimicrob Agents Chemother 1992;36:860–866.

15. Fu KP, Neu HC. The comparative synergistic activity of amikacin, gentamicin, netilmicin and azlocillin, mezlocillin, carbenicillin, and ticarcillin against *Serratia marcescens*. J Antibiot 1978;31:135–140.

16. Garzone P, Lyon J, Yu VL. Third-generation and investigational cephalosporins; II Microbiologic review and clinical summaries. Drug Intell Clin Pharm 1983;17:615–622.

17. Gilchrist MJR. Enterobacteriaceae: opportunistic pathogens and other genera. In: Murray PR, Baron EJ, Pfaller MA, Tenover FC, Yolken RH, eds. Manual of clinical microbiology. Washington, DC: American Society for Microbiology Press, 1995:457–467.

18. Gold HS, Moellering RC. Antimicrobial-drug resistance. N Engl J Med 1996;335:1445–1453.

19. Hooper DC, Wolfson JS. Fluoroquinolones antimicrobial agents. N Engl J Med 1991;324:384–394.

20. Hyams KC, Mader JT, Pollard RB, Parks DH, Thomson PD, Reinarz JA. Serratia endocarditis in a pediatric burn patient. Cure with cefotaxime. JAMA 1981;246:983–984.

21. Jacobus NV, Ferreira MC, Barza M. In vitro activity of aztreonam, a monobactam antibiotic. Antimicrob Agents Chemother 1982;22:832–838.

22. Jacoby GA, Carreras I. Activities of β-lactam antibiotics against *Escherichia coli* strains producing extended-spectrum β-lactamases. Antimicrob Agents Chemother 1990;34:858–862.

23. John JF Jr, McNeill WF. Characteristics of *Serratia marcescens* containing a plasmid coding for gentamicin resistance in nosocomial infections. J Infect Dis 1981;143:810–817.

24. Kessler RE, Fung-Tomc J. Susceptibility of bacterial isolates to β-lactam antibiotics from U.S. clinical trials over a 5-year period. Am J Med 1996;100(Suppl 6A):3S–12S.

25. Klatersky J, Glauser MP, Schmpff SC, Zinner SH, Gaya H, and European Organization for Research on Treatment of Cancer Antimicrobial Therapy Project Group. Prospective randomized comparison of three antibiotic regimens for empirical therapy of suspected bacteremic infections in febrile granulocytopenic patients. Antimicrob Agents Chemother 1986;29:263–270.

26. Knothe H, Shah P, Krcmery V, Antal M, Mitsuhashi S. Transferable resistance to cefotaxime, cefoxitin, cefamandole and cefuroxime in clinical isolates of *Klebsiella pneumoniae* and *Serratia marcescens*. Infection 1983;11:315–317.

27. MacGowan AP, Bowker KE, Bedford KA, Holt HA, Reeves DS, Hedges A. The comparative inhibitory and bactericidal activities of meropenem and imipenem against *Acinetobacter* spp. and Enterobacteriaceae resistant to second generation cephalosporins. J Antimicrob Chemother 1995;35:333–337.

28. Maki DG, Hennekens CG, Phillips CW, et al. Nosocomial urinary tract infections with *Serratia marcescens:* an epidemiologic study. J Infect Dis 1973;128:579–562.

29. Markowitz SM, Sibilla DJ. Comparative susceptibilities of clinical isolates of *Serratia marcescens* to newer cephalosporins, alone and in combination with various aminoglycosides. Antimicrob Agents Chemother 1980;18:651–655.

30. Markowitz SM, Williams DS, Hanna CB, Parker JL, Pierce MA, Steele JCH Jr. A multicenter comparative study of the in vitro activity of fleroxacin and other antimicrobial agents. Chemotherapy 1995;41:477–486.

31. Meyer RD, Lewis RP, Carmalt ED, Finegold SM. Amikacin therapy for serious gram-negative bacillary infections. Ann Intern Med 1975;83:790–800.

32. Medeiros AA. Evolution and dissemination of β-lactamases accelerated by generations of β-lactam antibiotics. Clin Infect Dis 1997;24(Suppl 1):S19–45.

33. Meyer RD, Lewis RP, Halter J, White M. Gentamicin-resistant *Pseudomonas aeruginosa* and *Serratia marcescens* in a general hospital. Lancet 1976;1:580–583.

34. Miller MA, Yousuf M, Griffin PS, Barlett M, Crane JK. In vitro activity of cefamandole, cefoxitin, cefuroxime, and carbenicillin, alone and in combination with aminoglycosides against *Serratia marcescens*. Microbiol Immunol 1979;23:955–964.

35. Mills J, Drew E. *Serratia marcescens* endocarditis: a regional illness associated with intravenous drug abuse. Ann Intern Med 1976;84:29–35.

36. Nakashima AK, McCarthy A, Martone WJ, Anderson RL. Epidemic septic arthritis caused by *Serratia marcescens* and associated with a benzalkonium chloride antiseptic. J Clin Microbiol 1987;25:1014–1018.

37. Nass T, Livermore DM, Nordmann P. Characterization of an LysR family protein, SmeR from *Serratia marcescens* S6, its effect on expression of the carbapenem-hydrolyzing β-lactamase Sme-1, and comparison of this regulator with other β-lactamases regulators. Antimicrob Agents Chemother 1995;39:629–637.

38. Neu HC. The new beta-lactamase-stable cephalosporins. Ann Intern Med 1982;97:408–419.

39. Neu HC. Contribution of beta-lactamases to bacterial resistance and mechanisms to inhibit beta-lactamases. Am J Med 1985;79 (Suppl 5B).

40. Olexy VM, Bird TJ, Grieble HG, Farrand SK. Hospital isolates

of *Serratia marcescens* transferring ampicillin, carbenicillin, and gentamicin resistance to other gram-negative bacteria including *Pseudomonas aeruginosa.* Antimicrob Agents Chemother 1979;15:93–100.

41. Osano E, Arakawa Y, Wacharotayankun R, Ohta M, Horii T, Ito H, Yoshimura F, Kato N. Molecular characterization of an enterobacterial metallo β-lactamase found in a clinical isolate of *Serratia marcescens* that shows imipenem resistance. Antimicrob Agents Chemother 1994;38:71–78.

42. Ostenson RC, Fields BT, Nolan CM. Polymyxin B and rifampin: new regimen for multiresistant *Serratia marcescens* infections. Antimicrob Agents Chemother 1977;12:655–659.

43. Richards NM, Levitsky S. Outbreak of *Serratia marcescens* infections in a cardiothoracic surgical intensive care unit. Ann Thorac Surg 1975;19:503–513.

44. Rasmussen BA, Bush K. Carbapenem-hydrolyzing β-lactamases. Antimicrob Agents Chemother 1997;41:223–232.

45. Rutala WA, Kennedy VA, Loflin HB, Sarubbi FA Jr. *Serratia marcescens* nosocomial infections of the urinary tract associated with urine measuring containers and urinometers. Am J Med 1981;70:659–663.

46. Saito H, Elting L, Bodey GP, Berkey P. Serratia bacteremia: review of 118 cases. Rev Infect Dis 1989;11:912–920.

47. Sanders CC. Beta-lactamases of gram-negative bacteria: new challenges for new drugs. Clin Infect Dis 1992;14:1089–1099.

48. Sanders CC. Cefepime: the next generation? Clin Infect Dis 1993;17:369–379.

49. Sanders CC, Sanders WE Jr. Beta-lactam resistance in gram-negative bacteria: global trends and clinical impact. Clin Infect Dis 1992;15:824–839.

50. Sanders CV Jr, Luby JP, Johanson WG Jr, Barnett JA, Sanford JP. *Serratia marcescens* infections from inhalation therapy medications: nosocomial outbreak. Ann Intern Med 1970;73:15–21.

51. Schaberg DR, Highsmith AK, Wachsmuth IK. Resistance plasmid transfer by *Serratia marcescens.* Antimicrob Agents Chemother 1977;11:449–450.

52. Schaberg DR, Weinstein RA, Stamm WE. Epidemics of nosocomial urinary tract infections caused by multiply resistant gram-negative bacilli: epidemiology and control. J Infect Dis 1976;133:363–366.

53. Sykes RB, Bonner DP, Bush K, Georgopapadakou BH. Aztreonam (SQ26,776), a synthetic monobactam specifically active against aerobic gram-negative bacteria. Antimicrob Agents Chemother 1982;21:85–92.

54. Thomas FE, Leonard JM, Alford RH. Sulfamethoxazole-trimethoprim-polymyxin therapy of serious multiple drug-resistant Serratia infections. Antimicrob Agents Chemother 1976;9:201–207.

55. Thornsberry C, Yee Y C. Comparative activity of eight antimicrobial agents against clinical bacterial isolates from the United States, measured by two methods. Am J Med 1996;100(Suppl 6A):26S–38S.

56. Thornton GF, Andriole VT. Antibiotic sensitivities of nonpigmented *Serratia marcescens* to gentamicin and carbenicillin. J Infect Dis 1969;119:393–394.

57. Washington JA, Jones RN, Gerlach EH, Murray PR, Allen SD, Knapp CC. Multicenter comparison of in vitro activities of FK-037, cefepime, ceftriaxone, ceftazidime, and cefuroxime. Antimicrob Agents Chemother 1993;37:1696–1700.

58. Weinstein RJ, Yound LS, Hewitt WL. Comparison of methods for assessing in vitro antibiotic synergism against Pseudomonas and Serratia. J Lab Clin Med 1975;86:853–862.

59. Wilkowske CJ, Washington JA II, Martin WJ, Ritts RE Jr. *Serratia marcescens:* biochemical characteristics, antibiotic susceptibility patterns, and clinical significance. JAMA 1970:214:2157–2162.

60. Wilfert JN, Barrett FF, Kass EH. Bacteremia due to *Serratia marcescens.* N Engl J Med 1968;279:286–289.

61. Wolfson JS, Hooper DC. Fluoroquinolone antimicrobial agents. Clin Microbiol Rev 1989;2:378–424.

62. Yu VL. *Serratia marcescens:* historical perspective and clinical review. N Engl J Med 1979;300:887–893.

63. Yu VL. Serratia infection in a surgical patient. Infect Surg 1984:127–132.

64. Yu VL, Oakes CA, Axnick KJ, Merigan TC. Patient factors contributing to the emergence of gentamicin-resistant *Serratia marcescens.* Am J Med 1979;66:468–472.

Shigella Species

●

Shai Ashkenazi

GENERAL DESCRIPTION

Shigellosis, the clinical illness caused by bacteria of the genus *Shigella,* is usually characterized by acute diarrhea (with or without blood or mucus), high fever, and general toxicity (19). Shigellae spread through the fecal-oral route, and because of the low infectious dose (10–100 organisms), person-to-person transmission is common. Transmission by contaminated food, drinking water, swimming pools, and flies has also been documented.

Shigellae are small, nonmotile, Gram-negative rods that belong to the family *Enterobacteriaceae.* They do not ferment lactose or do so slowly. The genus *Shigella* includes four species or serogroups: *S. dysenteriae,* group A; *S. flexneri,* group B; *S. boydii,* group C; and *S. sonnei,* group D. Species classification is important regarding treatment of shigellosis because the species differ in geographic distribution and antimicrobial susceptibility. In developed countries,

S. sonnei is the most common species, and its relative prevalence is increasing (6, 23). In developing countries, *S. flexneri* is most frequent, with outbreaks often caused by *S. dysenteriae,* which are often resistant to multiple antimicrobial agents (35, 36, 45).

SUSCEPTIBILITY IN VITRO AND IN VIVO

The major problem in treating shigellosis is the increasing antimicrobial resistance of *Shigella* species (5, 12). Although initially susceptible to most antimicrobial agents including sulfonamides, nowadays most isolates are resistant to the usually recommended antibiotics (Table 1), and even multiple resistance is frequent (7, 11, 17, 30, 31). High resistance rates were first reported in developing countries but have rapidly spread to developed countries, initially among travelers, day-care centers, and Native American reservations (2, 21, 44, 49). Seasonality in antimicrobial resistance of shigellae has been reported, with winter isolates significantly more resistant than summer isolates to ampicillin, trimethoprim-sulfamethoxazole (TMP-SMX), or both (7). The frequent use of antibiotics during winter months may play a role.

Another problem is that not all antimicrobial agents that are active against *Shigella* species in vitro are also efficacious in vivo, clinically or bacteriologically (24, 41). Though the reasons for this disparity are not always clear, it mandates that recommendations for antimicrobial therapy be based not only on in vitro susceptibility but also on clinical studies, preferably randomized and double blinded.

Sulfonamides and Trimethoprim-Sulfamethoxazole (TMP-SMX)

Sulfonamides were the first antimicrobial agents used in the 1940s to treat shigellosis effectively. Today, however, most shigellae isolates are resistant to sulfonamides.

Several controlled studies have documented the efficacy of TMP-SMX (5, 41). Compared with ineffective therapy in patients with culture-proven shigellosis, TMP-SMX yielded a clinical response (absence of fever and appearance of formed stool without blood or mucus after 48 h of therapy) in about 97%, and a bacteriologic response (eradication of shigellae from the stool by day 3 of therapy) was noted in about 94%. For several decades, TMP-SMX was the drug of choice for shigellosis in adults and children. It is still recommended as such in several textbooks, though most isolates of *Shigella* species have shown increasing resistance to this agent in more and more locations, particularly in Asia, Africa, and South America. Reports have come from Bangladesh (30), India (15, 45), Thailand (36, 47), Saudi Arabia (28), Israel (7), Kenya (32), Somalia (16), and Brazil (34). Studies in the United States (44), Germany (2), and Spain (49) have emphasized high TMP-SMX resistance among travelers with shigellosis, and in 1985, in the United States, a high resistance rate of 21% was noted in Native American populations (21). Resistance is now spreading to developed countries, as well (23, 30, 50). In Canada, TMP-SMX resistance of *Shigella* increased from 3% in 1978 to about 30% in 1990 (23). A random sampling of *Shigella* isolates in 1995, performed by the Centers for Disease Control and Prevention (CDC) in the United States, showed 37% resistance to TMP-SMX (17), compared with only 7% in 1985–86 (44). In 1990, Wharton reported an outbreak of shigellosis in the United States that was multiply resistant to ampicillin, tetracycline, and TMP-SMX. TMP-SMX resistance is now high for all *Shigella* species, with a particularly alarming increase for *S. sonnei,* the most common species in developed countries (7).

Aminopenicillins

Studies in the 1960s and 1970s showed good results with ampicillin against shigellosis, both in vitro and in vivo. Controlled studies comparing ampicillin with either placebo or ineffective therapy such as unabsorbed neomycin confirmed its therapeutic benefit, with clinical efficacy ranging between 87 and 100% and bacteriologic efficacy between 83 and 94% (41).

TABLE 1 • **In Vitro Antimicrobial Resistance of *Shigella* Isolates in Various Geographic Locations According to Selected Recent Publications**

Reference	Country	Year Isolates Obtained	Percentage Resistance to[a]		
			AMP	TMP-SMX	NAL
Cook 1996	U.S.A.	1995	67	37	0
Khan 1996	Bangladesh	1995–96	73	80	51
Ashkenazi 1995	Israel	1991–92	81	90	0.3
Thapa 1995	India	—	83	66	—
Lima 1995	Brazil	1988–93	90	84	8
Lin 1992	Taiwan	1982–87	52	10	25
Harnett 1990	Canada	1990	52	34	0
Kruse 1992[b]	Kenya	1990–91	54	95	2
Kagalwalla 1992	Saudi Arabia	1985–90	54	72	—
Thisyakorn 1992	Thailand	1990	90	81	—
Lolekha 1991	Thailand	1988	87	89	0
Tauxe 1990	U.S.A.	1985–6	32	7	0.4

[a] AMP, ampicillin; TMP-SMX, trimethoprim-sulfamethoxazole; N, nalidixic acid.

[b] Patients with AIDS.

As with TMP-SMX, however, most *Shigella* isolates are currently resistant to ampicillin (Table 1). High resistance rates have been noted in both developing and developed countries. In the United States, the report of ampicillin resistance of *Shigella* isolates increased from 32% in 1985–86 to 73% in 1995 (30, 44). Therefore, ampicillin can no longer be recommended as appropriate empirical antibiotic treatment against shigellosis. Although the resistance of *Shigella* species to ampicillin is usually mediated by β-lactamase, the efficacy of combining aminopenicillins with β-lactamase inhibitors remains to be proven.

Amoxicillin is similar to ampicillin in its in vitro activity against *Shigella* strains. A single open study compared the efficacy of amoxicillin (25 or 50 mg/kg/day) and ampicillin (50 mg/kg/day) for shigellosis; amoxicillin was inferior in terms of longer diarrhea and persistence of shigellae in stool cultures. It was concluded that amoxicillin is ineffective against shigellosis.

Cephalosporins

Controlled studies have shown that first- and second-generation cephalosporins, including cephalexin, cefamandole, and cefaclor, are ineffective against shigellosis, often despite in vitro susceptibility of the pathogen (41). Their main limitation is delayed eradication of shigellae from stool specimens.

The third-generation cephalosporins hold promise. Most *Shigella* isolates have shown susceptibility in vitro (7, 48). Among this group, ceftriaxone has been the most extensively investigated. A comparative study in children showed that parenteral ceftriaxone (50 mg/kg/day) yielded a good clinical response and 100% eradication of the pathogen after 5 days (48). A single dose of ceftriaxone, though clinically efficacious, showed a high rate of bacteriologic failure; two doses were comparable to five doses, both clinically and bacteriologically (20). Ceftriaxone has been suggested as the treatment of choice for children with severe shigellosis, especially those who are hospitalized (37). Its high efficacy may be related to excretion of the active agent in bile, with enterohepatic circulation, leading to high levels of the drug within the gastrointestinal tract.

Less definitive conclusions have been drawn for other third-generation cephalosporins. Clinical and bacteriologic failure of cefotaxime therapy was reported in a child with *S. flexneri*, despite in vitro susceptibility (MIC 0.0098 (μg/mL) (24). Of the two oral agents studied, ceftibuten showed promising results, despite the small number of patients investigated (12 study patients vs. 8 treated with TMP-SMX) (39), and cefixime was proven effective for relatively mild shigellosis, caused mostly by *S. sonnei* (4). Indeed, 82% of the control group who received TMP-SMX, had TMP-SMX-resistant *Shigella* isolates. Cefixime was ineffective in patients with severe shigellosis, caused mostly by *S. dysenteriae* and *S. flexneri* (43).

Quinolones

Until the end of the 1980s, nearly all *Shigella* isolates were susceptible to quinolones. In a double-blind trial in Bangladesh, 5 days of therapy with nalidixic acid yielded rapid clinical improvement, although bacteriologic eradication was somewhat slower (42). Because of its low cost and availability in suspension for children, and the high ampicillin and TMP-SMX resistance of *Shigella* species, nalidixic acid was introduced for treatment of shigellosis in developing countries.

Unfortunately, resistance to nalidixic acid appeared relatively quickly (Table 1). In 1990, 20% of *Shigella* isolates in Bangladesh were already resistant to nalidixic acid, compared with only 0.8% in 1986, before it came into widespread use (10). Resistance was particularly high (58%) for *S. dysenteriae* type 1. Nalidixic acid resistance has since been reported in other developing countries, including India (15, 46), Pakistan (3), and Taiwan (35), but it is relatively rare in developed countries.

Most *Shigella* isolates, including those resistant to nalidixic acid, are susceptible to the newer fluoroquinolones. Clinical studies have shown ciprofloxacin, norfloxacin, enoxacin, and pefloxacin to be clinically and bacteriologically effective against shigellosis (9, 13, 14, 22). Because of the relatively long half-lives of the fluoroquinolones and their high activity against shigellae in vitro, they were evaluated for short courses of therapy. Single doses of ciprofloxacin or norfloxacin were effective in the treatment of infections caused by species other than *S. dysenteriae* type 1 (8, 11). The relative resistance of this serotype to a single-dose regimen may be related to its tendency to cause more severe symptoms or to its lower in vitro susceptibility.

Recently, however, reports have appeared of reduced susceptibility and even resistance of *Shigella* isolates to the newer fluoroquinolones. In India, six *Shigella* strains resistant to nalidixic acid, ciprofloxacin, pefloxacin, and enoxacin were noted (46). Japanese investigators studied seven clinical isolates of *S. sonnei* with reduced susceptibility (MICs 16 to 32 times higher than susceptible strains) to ciprofloxacin, ofloxacin, and sparfloxacin; resistance was likely due to a mutation in the DNA gyrase subunit A gene of these strains (25), as shown also by Rahman et al. (40). Five nalidixic acid–resistant *Shigella* strains isolated in the Netherlands showed reduced susceptibility to norfloxacin (50). John et al. (27) studied the activities of six fluoroquinolones against 117 *S. sonnei* isolates. Excluding enoxacin, which had a relatively high MIC (0.25 μg/mL), all the other agents had good in vitro activity (MIC, 0.008–0.032 μg/mL).

Other Antimicrobial Agents

Despite good in vitro activity against shigellae and high fecal concentrations, nonabsorbable oral antimicrobial agents are usually ineffective against shigellosis, both clinically and bacteriologically. These include streptomycin, neomycin, kanamycin, gentamicin, and furazolidone (26, 41). Oral, poorly absorbed aztreonam (100 mg three times a day for 5 days) was found effective in travelers to Mexico suffering from bacterial diarrhea (18). Compared with placebo, aztreonam reduced the duration of both diarrhea and fecal excretion of the bacteria. However, only seven patients with *Shigella* gastroenteritis were included in the study.

Pivmecillinam is a penicillin that binds selectively to penicillin-binding protein-2 and therefore has high activity against Gram-negative bacteria, including *Enterobacteriaceae*. It was proven effective clinically against infections with *Shigella,* compared with TMP-SMX (38) or nalidixic acid (1). This antimicrobial agent is not available in the United States and in other locations. Resistance of *Shigella* strains to pivmecillinam has been reported in Bangladesh and Guatemala (38).

Azithromycin, a new azalide with broad-spectrum antimicrobial activity, was compared with ciprofloxacin for the treatment of shigellosis (30). Five-day treatment gave clinical efficacy of 82% and bacteriologic efficacy of 100% after 2 days. These results were comparable to those with ciprofloxacin (31).

ANTIMICROBIAL THERAPY
Benefits of Antimicrobial Therapy

The clinical and bacteriologic benefits of effective antimicrobial therapy against shigellosis have been proven in controlled studies by comparison with placebo or ineffective therapy (5, 41). Clinically, effective therapy shortens the duration of diarrhea and fever, resulting in a higher proportion of patients who are free of symptoms by the end of the treatment period. Concomitantly, shigellae are excreted in stools for a significantly shorter time, and excretion usually stops after 1 or 2 days. This is important epidemiologically, because infected patients are the major reservoir of shigellae, and person-to-person spread is the major mode of transmission of this infection.

The impact of antibiotic therapy on the complications of *Shigella* infections, including hemolysis, hemolytic-uremic syndrome, bacteremia, and toxic megacolon, is less clear. Complication rates are low, making them nearly impossible to study in prospective treatment trials. In developing countries, appropriate antibiotic treatment may have a significant benefit on the nutritional status and growth of children with shigellosis, because it shortens the duration of diarrhea, thereby enabling early feeding with adequate intestinal absorption.

Drugs of Choice

Most textbooks still recommend TMP-SMX as the empirical treatment of choice for shigellosis. However, most *Shigella* isolates in certain areas of Southeast Asia, the Middle East, Africa, and South America are currently resistant to TMP-SMX, as were 37% of representative *Shigella* isolates in the United States as of 1995. The treatment of choice depends, therefore, on the specific geographic location and on epidemiologic data.

Fluoroquinolones, such as ciprofloxacin, norfloxacin, ofloxacin, and pefloxacin, are now the usual treatment of choice for suspected shigellosis in adults, especially in developing countries and in travelers. Fluoroquinolones are also effective against most other causes of bacterial gastroenteritis that may be indistinguishable from shigellosis clinically, when empirical therapy is started.

Alternative Therapy

Quinolones are not approved for use in children under 17 years of age because of possible damage to the growing cartilage, as seen in animal studies. In children with severe shigellosis, parenteral ceftriaxone (i.v. or i.m.) 50 mg/kg/day in a single dose, is the treatment of choice. For milder cases and when parenteral therapy is impossible, nalidixic acid 55 mg/kg/day in four divided doses is recommended. Although nalidixic acid is a quinolone, it is approved for children older than 2 months. This is a consequence of a historical rather than a scientific precedent, as nalidixic acid was introduced and approved for use in children before the possible skeletal damage of the quinolones was known.

Shigella strains susceptible to TMP-SMX or to ampicillin should be so treated. Susceptibility can be predicted according to up-to-date microbiologic data on isolates in the community or according to results from contacts of the patient.

More data are needed for azithromycin, oral third-generation cephalosporins, and oral aztreonam before routine use can be recommended.

Duration of Treatment

The usual duration of antimicrobial treatment of shigellosis is 5 days. This is the only recommendation when TMP-SMX, ampicillin, nalidixic acid, or azithromycin is used. Shorter durations have been studied with parenteral third-generation cephalosporins and the fluoroquinolones. Two days of treatment with ceftriaxone (50 mg/kg/day in a single daily dose) in children showed very good clinical and bacteriologic efficacy (20). Since a single dose of ceftriaxone did not effectively eradicate shigellae from stools, it was concluded that 2-day treatment with ceftriaxone was safe in children. Ceftriaxone is indicated mainly in those with severe disease who require parenteral therapy.

As mentioned, a single dose of ciprofloxacin (1 g) or norfloxacin (800 mg) was effective in controlled studies in adults. During an outbreak of multiresistant *Shigella* infection in Madagascar, nalidixic acid was not available, so pefloxacin was used to treat the affected children (22). A single dose (20 mg/kg) given to 13 children resulted in rapid resolution of the diarrhea; stool cultures performed after 5 to 8 days were negative. A single fluoroquinolone dose should not be used for infections with *S. dysenteriae* type 1.

Special Situations

Patients with underlying immune deficiency disorder or neutropenia, especially those with the acquired immunodeficiency syndrome (AIDS), may have a more complicated course of shigellosis (29). These patients may have prolonged or recurrent diarrhea and systemic complications, such as septicemia; a high mortality rate has been reported. In addition, as reported in African AIDS patients, they may have infections with multiresistant *Shigella* strains. In these patients, we recommend a full course (at least 5 days, pending resolution of fever and other symptoms) of parenteral antibiotic therapy, preferably with ceftriaxone in children or adults or with fluoroquinolones (ciprofloxacin or norfloxacin) in adults only.

ENDPOINTS FOR MONITORING THERAPY

With effective antimicrobial therapy, clinical improvement (i.e. resolution of fever, diarrhea, and dysentery) is usually seen within 2 days. After 5 days, the patient is usually afebrile, with less than three nonwatery stools a day. Bacteriologically, eradication of shigellae from the stool culture is usually seen after 2 days of effective treatment. Clinical failure is defined as the presence of fever or watery diarrhea after 5 days of therapy, and bacterial failure, as a positive stool culture after 2 days.

ADJUNCTIVE THERAPY

Replacement of fluid and electrolyte losses is essential in treating patients with shigellosis. Dehydration may be caused by the high-volume watery diarrhea during the early course of the disease, or later, by the low-volume bloody diarrhea, when generalized toxicity and vomiting preclude sufficient fluid intake. Oral rehydration solutions containing glucose and electrolytes are usually efficacious, though intravenous fluids may be necessary. In certain patients, especially young children, nutritional support is also important.

Antimotility agents, such as diphenoxylate (Lomotil), prolong the duration of fever, diarrhea, and excretion of the organism in patients with *Shigella* infections and should therefore not be used when shigellosis is suspected. Intestinal motility and the constant fluid flow may actually be an important host defense mechanism for rapid clearance of the infection.

CONTROVERSIES AND CAVEATS
Treatment of Mild Cases

Shigella infections may cause only mild symptoms, such as mild watery diarrhea and low-grade fever, which resolve spontaneously within a few days. Asymptomatic infections have also been reported. The treatment of mild cases is controversial. Early treatment may enhance recovery, but its main benefit is early eradication of shigellae from stools and, thereby, prevention of secondary cases and spread of infection. Treatment of mild cases is of particular importance in patients in hospitals, day-care centers, and institutions, where spread of the infection is likely. The main disadvantage of treating mild cases is the spread of resistant strains. Cost may also be a factor in some locations. Practically, shigellosis is usually not suspected in mild cases of diarrhea unless relevant epidemiologic data are available.

Quinolones in Children

The new fluoroquinolones are not approved for use in children because of their potential cartilaginous toxicity. This finding, however, was noted in young animals when relatively high doses were used. Because of the frequent resistance to other antimicrobial agents and the relatively short treatment course, quinolone treatment in children may be required. After limited uncontrolled experience with pefloxacin for shigellosis in children (22), controlled blinded studies are currently being done. Further information is needed before quinolones can be widely recommended for shigellosis in children.

New Antimicrobial Agents

More experience and additional data are needed regarding the role of oral third-generation cephalosporins, oral aztreonam, and the newer macrolides, especially azithromycin, in the treatment of *Shigella* infections.

REFERENCES

1. Alam AN, Islam MR, Hossain MS, Mahalanabis D, Hye HK. Comparison of pivmecillinam and nalidixic acid in the treatment of acute shigellosis in children. Scand J Gastroenterol 1994; 29:313–317.
2. Aleksic S, Katz A, Aleksic V, Bockemuhl J. Antibiotic resistance of Shigella strains isolated in the Federal Republic of Germany 1989–1990. Int J Med Microbiol Virol Parasitol Infect Dis 1993;279:484–493.
3. Ambler JE, Drabu YJ, Blakemore PH, Pinney RJ. Mutator plasmid in a nalidixic acid-resistant strain of Shigella dysenteriae type 1. J Antimicrob Chemother 1993;31:831–839.
4. Ashkenazi S, Amir J, Waisman Y, Rachmel A, Garty BZ, Samra Z, Varsano I, Nitzan M. A randomized, double-blind study comparing cefixime and trimethoprim-sulfamethoxazole in the treatment of childhood shigellosis. J Pediatr 1993;123:817–821.
5. Ashkenazi S, Cleary TG. Antibiotic treatment of bacterial gastroenteritis. Pediatr Infect Dis J 1991;10:140–148.
6. Ashkenazi S, May-Zahav M, Dinari G, Gabbay U, Zilberberg R, Samra Z. Recent trends in the epidemiology of Shigella species in Israel. Clin Infect Dis 1993;17:897–899.
7. Ashkenazi S, May-Zahav M, Sulkes J, Zilberberg R, Samra Z. Increasing antimicrobial resistance of Shigella isolates in Israel during the period 1984 to 1992. Antimicrob Agents Chemother 1995;39:819–823.
8. Bassily S, Hyams KC, el Masry NA. Short-course norfloxacin and trimethoprim-sulfamethoxazole treatment of shigellosis and salmonellosis in Egypt. Am J Trop Med Hyg 1994;51:219–223.
9. Bennish ML, Salam MA, Haider R, Barza M. Therapy for shigellosis. II. Randomized, double-blind comparison of ciprofloxacin and ampicillin. J Infect Dis 1990;102:711–716.
10. Bennish ML, Salam MA, Hossain MA, Myaux J, Khan EH, Chakraborty J, Henry F, Ronsman C. Antimicrobial resistance of Shigella isolates in Bangladesh, 1983–1990: increasing frequency of strains multiply resistant to ampicillin, trimethoprim-sulfamethoxazole, and nalidixic acid. Clin Infect Dis 1992; 14:1055–1060.
11. Bennish ML, Salam MA, Khan WA, Khan AM. Treatment of shigellosis: III. Comparison of one- or two-dose ciprofloxacin with standard 5-day therapy. A randomized, blinded trial. Ann Intern Med 1992;117:727–734.
12. Bennish ML, Salam MA. Rethinking options for the treatment of shigellosis. J Antimicrob Chemother 1992;30:243–247.
13. Bhattacharya MK, Nair GB, Sen D. Efficacy of norfloxacin for shigellosis: a double-blind randomized clinical trial. J Diarrhoeal Dis Res 1992;10:146–150.
14. Bhattacharya SK, Bhattacharya MK, Dutta P, Sen D, Rasaily R, Moitra A, Pal SC. Randomized clinical trial of norfloxacin for shigellosis. Am J Trop Med Hyg 1991;45:683–687.
15. Bhattacharya MK, Bhattacharya SK, Paul M. Shigella in Calcutta during 1990–1992: antibiotic susceptibility pattern and clinical features. J Diarrhoeal Res 1994;12:121–124.
16. Casalino M, Nicoletti M, Salvia A, Colonna B, Pazzani C, Calconi A, Mohamud KA, Maimone F. Characterization of endemic Shigella flexneri strains in Somalia: antimicrobial resistance, plasmid profiles, and serotype correlation. J Clin Microbiol 1994;32:1179–1183.
17. Cook K, Boyce T, Puhr N, Tauxe R, Mintz E. Increasing antimicrobial-resistant Shigella infection in the United States [Abstract E20]. 36th Interscience Conference of Antimicrobial Agents and Chemotherapy, New Orleans, LA, Sept 1996.
18. DuPont HL, Ericson CD, Mathewson JJ, de la Cabada FJ, Con-

rad DA. Oral aztreonam: a poorly absorbed yet effective therapy for bacterial diarrhea in US travelers to Mexico. JAMA 1992; 267:1932–1935.

19. DuPont HL. Shigella. Infect Dis Clin North Am 1988;2: 599–606.

20. Eidlitz-Marcus T, Cohen YH, Nussinovitch M, Elian I, Varsano I. Comparative efficacy of two- and five-day courses of ceftriaxone for treatment of severe shigellosis in children. J Pediatr 1993;123:822–824.

21. Griffin PM, Tauxe RV, Redd SC, Puhr ND, Hargrett-Bean N, Blake PA. Emergence of highly trimethoprim-sulfamethoxazole-resistant Shigella in a Native American population: an epidemiologic study. Am J Epidemiol 1989;129:1042–1051.

22. Guyon P, Cassel-Beraud AM, Rakotonirina G, Gendrel D. Short-term pefloxacin therapy in Madagascan children with shigellosis due to multiresistant organisms [Letter]. Clin Infect Dis 1994;19:1172–1173.

23. Harnett N. High level resistance to trimethoprim, cotrimoxazole and other antimicrobial agents among clinical isolates of Shigella species in Ontario, Canada—an update. Epidemiol Infect 1992; 109:463–472.

24. Hoffman J, Kim KS. Failure of cefotaxime therapy in a child with shigellosis. Pediatr Infect Dis J 1996;15:174–175.

25. Horiuchi S, Inagaki Y, Yamamoto N, Okamura N, Imagawa Y, Nakaya R. Reduced susceptibilities of Shigella sonnei strains isolated from patients with dysentery to fluoroquinolones. Antimicrob Agents Chemother 1993;37:2486–2489.

26. Islam MR, Alam AN, Hossain MS, Mahalanabis D, Hye HK. Double-blind comparison of oral gentamicin and nalidixic acid in the treatment of acute shigellosis in children. J Trop Pediatr 1994;40:320–325.

27. John JF Jr, Atkins LT, Maple PA, Bratoeva M. Activities of newer fluoroquinolones against Shigella sonnei. Antimicrob Agents Chemother 1992;36:2346–2348.

28. Kagalwalla AF, Khan SN, Kagalwalla YA. Childhood shigellosis in Saudi Arabia. Pediatr Infect Dis J 1992;11:215–219.

29. Kenet G, Salomon F, Samra Z, Pinkhas J, Sidi Y, Arber N. Fatal Shigella sepsis in a neutropenic patient. Mt Sinai J Med 1994; 61:367–368.

30. Khan WA, Seas C, Dhar U, Salam MA, Bennish ML. Azithromycin is equivalent to ciprofloxacin in the treatment of shigellosis: results of a randomized, blinded clinical trial [Abstract LM 29]. 36th Interscience Conference of Antimicrobial Agents and Chemotherapy, New Orleans, LA, Sept 1996.

31. Khan WA, Seas C, Dhar U, Salam MA, Bennish ML. Treatment of shigellosis: v. comparison of azithromycin and ciprofloxacin. A double-blind, randomized, controlled trial. Ann Intern Med 1997;126:697–703.

32. Kruse H, Kariuki S, Soli N, Olsvik O. Multiresistant Shigella species from African AIDS patients: antibacterial resistance patterns and application of the E-test for determination of minimum inhibitory concentration. Scand J Infect Dis 1992;24:733–739.

33. Lew JF, Swerdlow DL, Dance ME. An outbreak of shigellosis aboard a cruise ship caused by a multiple-antibiotic-resistant strain of Shigella flexneri. Am J Epidemiol 1991;134:413–420.

34. Lima AA, Lima NL, Pinho MC, Barros EA, Teixeira MJ, Martins MCV, Guerrant RL. High frequency of strains multiply resistant to ampicillin, trimethoprim-sulfamethoxazole, streptomycin, chloramphenicol, and tetracycline isolated from patients with shigellosis in northeastern Brazil during the period 1988 to 1993. Antimicrob Agents Chemother 1995;39:256–259.

35. Lin SR, Chang SF. Drug resistance and plasmid profile of shigellae in Taiwan. Epidemiol Infect 1992;108:87–97.

36. Lolekha S, Vibulbandhitkit S, Poonyarit P. Response to antimicrobial therapy for shigellosis in Thailand. Rev Infect Dis 1991;13(Suppl 4):S342–346.

37. Park JW, Rogers PL. Treatment of shigellosis. J Pediatr 1991; 119:841.

38. Prado D, Liu H, Velasquez T, Cleary TG. Comparative efficacy of pivmecillinam and cotrimoxazole in acute shigellosis in children. Scand J Infect Dis 1993;25:713–719.

39. Prado D, Lopez E, Liu H, DeVoto S, Woloj M, Contrini M, Murray BE, Gomez H, Cleary TG. Ceftibuten and trimethoprim-sulfamethoxazole for treatment of Shigella and enteroinvasive Escherichia coli disease. Pediatr Infect Dis J 1992;11:644–647.

40. Rahman M, Mauff G, Levy J, Couturier M, Pulvierer G, Glasdorff N, Butzler JP. Detection of 4-quinolone resistance mutation in gyrA gene of Shigella dysenteriae type 1 by PCR. Antimicrob Agents Chemother 1994;38:2488–2491.

41. Salam MA, Bennish ML. Antimicrobial therapy for shigellosis. Rev Infect Dis 1991;13(Suppl 4):S332–341.

42. Salam MA, Bennish ML. Therapy of shigellosis. I. Randomized double blind trial of nalidixic acid in childhood shigellosis. J Pediatr 1988;113:901–907.

43. Salam MA, Seas C, Khan WA, Bennish ML. Treatment of shigellosis: IV. Cefixime is ineffective in shigellosis in adults. Ann Intern Med 1995;123:505–508.

44. Tauxe RV, Puhr ND, Wells JG, Hargrett-Bean N, Blake PA. Antimicrobial resistance of Shigella isolates in the USA: the importance of international travelers. J Infect Dis 1990;162:1107–1111.

45. Thapa BR, Ventkateswarlu K, Malik AK, Panigrahi D. Shigellosis in children from north India: a clinicopathological study. J Trop Pediatr 1995;41:303–307.

46. Thirunarayanan MA, Jesudason MV, John TJ. Resistance of shigella to nalidixic acid and fluorinated quinolones. Indian J Med Res 1993;97:239–241.

47. Thisyakorn U, Rienprayoon S. Shigellosis in Thai children: epidemiologic, clinical and laboratory features. Pediatr Infect Dis J 1992;11:213–215.

48. Varsano I, Eidlitz-Marcus T, Nussinovitch M, Elian I. Comparative efficacy of ceftriaxone and ampicillin for treatment of severe shigellosis in children. J Pediatr 1991;118:627–632.

49. Vila J, Gascon J, Abdalla S, Gomez J, Marco F, Moreno A, Corachan M, De Anta TJ. Antimicrobial resistance of Shigella isolates causing traveler's diarrhea. Antimicrob Agents Chemother 1994;38:2668–2670.

50. Voogd CE, Schot CS, van Leeuwen WJ, van Klingeren B. Monitoring of antibiotic resistance in shigellosis isoated in the Netherlands 1984–1989. Eur J Clin Microbiol Infect Dis 1992: 11:164–167.

51. Wharton M, Spiegel RA, Horan JM, Tauxe RV, Wells JG, Barg N, Herndon J, Meriwether RA, MacCormack JN, Levine RH. A large outbreak of antibiotic-resistant shigellosis at a mass gathering. J Infect Dis 1990;162:1324–1328.

Spirillum minus

●

Mark E. Rupp

HISTORY, GENERAL DESCRIPTION, AND MICROBIOLOGY

Spirillum minus is the principal cause of rat bite fever in the Eastern hemisphere but only rarely causes disease in the United States. The organism, first described by Dr. Henry Van Dyke Carter in 1887, was previously known as *Spirocheta morus muris* or *Sporozoa muris* (2). The first case description of rat bite fever due to *S. minus* in the United States was by Shattuck and Theiller in 1924 (9). In Japan, infection caused by *S. minus* is known as Sodoku from *So*, "rat" and *Doku*, "poison."

S. minus is a Gram-negative, tightly coiled spirochete measuring 0.2 to 0.5 μm by 3 to 5 μm, which possesses 2 to 6 regular spirals (4). The organism is motile by means of bipolar flagella. *S. minus* has not been cultivated on laboratory media.

EPIDEMIOLOGY AND CLINICAL PRESENTATION

The epidemiology of *S. minus* infection is similar to that of *Streptobacillus moniliformis*. Rats are frequently colonized by *S. minus* (1, 4), and infection in humans is usually acquired through a rat bite. In contrast to *S. moniliformis, S. minus* has not been described as causing disease via oral ingestion.

Generally, the bite wound heals during the 1- to 3-week incubation period. However, as the systemic phase of the illness begins (characterized by fever, chills, malaise, and headache), the bite wound becomes swollen and indurated and is often associated with regional adenopathy. A macular violaceous rash may occur involving the extremities, face, and trunk. Laboratory studies reveal leukocytosis, and up to 50% of patients have a false-positive serologic test result for syphilis (4). Diagnosis of *S. minus* infection can be proven by recovery of organisms from mice or guinea pigs, 1 to 3 weeks after intraperitoneal inoculation of infectious material from the index patient.

Without antimicrobial therapy, the fever abates over 3 to 5 days, only to recur at regular intervals of 3 to 10 days. Although relapses have been described to occur for years (10), spontaneous resolution usually occurs in 1 to 2 months. Without treatment, mortality is approximately 10% (3).

Complications of *S. minus* infection are rare. The most serious complication is endocarditis, which usually occurs in the setting of preexisting valvular abnormality (12). However, spirillar endocarditis in previously normal valves has been described (7). Other complications include myocarditis, meningitis, hepatitis, pleural effusions, conjunctivitis, epididymitis, and anemia (12).

SUSCEPTIBILITY IN VITRO AND IN VIVO
In Vitro Studies

Because *S. minus* has not been cultivated on synthetic media, no in vitro data exist regarding the susceptibility of *S. minus* to antimicrobial agents.

In Vivo Studies

Although *S. minus* can be propagated in mice or guinea pigs, there are few data from this system regarding treatment of *S. minus*. However, Heilman and Hermel clearly demonstrated the efficacy of penicillin by treating one-half of 50 infected mice with penicillin (5). Blood smears from the treated mice were negative within 2 days of starting treatment. Blood smears from all but one of the untreated mice remained positive for *S. minus* for the 30-day observation period. Tani and Takano reported treating experimentally infected mice with a variety of antimicrobial agents to determine the dosage required to prevent transmission of disease through transfusion (11). The 100% preventive dose (PD_{100}) for penicillin was 1000 units, while the PD_{100} for tetracycline, oxytetracycline, chloramphenicol, and streptomycin were 100 μg, 100 μg, more than 200 μg, and more than 100 μg, respectively.

ANTIMICROBIAL THERAPY

There are no prospective trials concerning the treatment of *S. minus*. Data are derived from anecdotal reports of treatment of single patients or small groups of patients. Prior to the availability of penicillin, arsenicals were frequently used to treat patients infected with *S. minus,* apparently, with some degree of success (13). Streptomycin and tetracycline derivatives have also reportedly been used successfully to treat *S. minus* infection (1, 6, 8).

Wheeler is credited with reporting the first use of penicillin against *S. minus* (14). Currently, penicillin is the drug of choice for treatment of spirillar rat bite fever. The organism appears to be exquisitely susceptible to penicillin, and it has been stated that only 2 doses of procaine penicillin or 1 dose of repository penicillin is adequate for cure (3). However, most authorities recommend treatment for 10 to 14 days. Initially, patients should be treated with 2.4 to 4.8 million units of penicillin G daily, delivered intravenously in 4 evenly timed doses. Following defervescence, patients can be switched to oral ampicillin or penicillin V (500 mg orally every 6 h) to finish a 10- to 14-day course. Although there are no studies for guidance, patients with relatively mild disease and no evidence of complications such as endocarditis or meningitis, can probably be treated with an oral regimen for the entire treatment course. Jarisch-Herxheimer reactions may occur during the initial stages of therapy (8).

SPECIAL SITUATIONS
Serious β-Lactam Allergy

In the event of serious penicillin allergy, a tetracycline derivative should be used in treatment of *S. minus* infection. The recommended dosage is 500 mg either orally or intravenously every 6 h or doxycycline 100 mg orally or intravenously every 12 h.

Pediatric Patients

Penicillin remains the drug of choice for pediatric patients. The dosage is 25,000 units/kg/day, divided into 4 doses. Tetracyclines should be avoided because of their association with tooth enamel agenesis and tooth staining.

Endocarditis and Central Nervous System Infection

Complications of spirillar rat bite fever are rare. Although optimal therapy for endocarditis or meningitis is unknown, high-dose penicillin is indicated at a dosage of approximately 20 million units/day divided evenly every 4 h. Although the optimum duration of therapy is unknown, on the basis of limited data, treatment of meningitis for 10 to 14 days and endocarditis for 28 days should suffice.

PREVENTION AND ANTIBIOTIC PROPHYLAXIS

In the event of a rat bite, the wound should be thoroughly cleaned, and tetanus prophylaxis administered if appropriate. Although the efficacy of prophylaxis is not proven, a prudent course of action dictates administration of amoxicillin/clavulanate at a dosage of 500 mg orally every 8 h for 3 days. In addition to *S. minus,* this regimen would cover *S. moniliformis* and other commonly encountered pathogens in bite wounds.

REFERENCES

1. Biberstein EL. Rat bite fever. In: Hubbert WT, McCulloch WF, Schnurrenberger PR, eds. Diseases transmitted from animals to man. 6th ed. Springfield, IL: Charles C Thomas, 1975;9: 186–190.
2. Carter HV. Note on the occurrence of a minute blood spirillum in an Indian rat. Sci Mem Med Off Army India. 1888;3:45–48.
3. Cook GC. Other spirochaetal diseases. In: Cook GC, ed. Manson's tropical diseases. 20th ed. London: WB Saunders, 1996; 55:958–962.
4. Gunning JJ. Rat-bite fevers. In: Hunter GW III, Swartzwelder JC, Clyde DF, eds. Tropical medicine. 5th ed. Philadelphia: WB Saunders, 1976:245–247.
5. Heilman FR, Herrell WC. Mayo Clinic Proc 1994;19:257.
6. Jellison WL, Eneboe PI, Parker RR, Hughes LE. Rat-bite fever in Montana. Public Health Rep 1949;64:1661–1665.
7. McIntosh CS, Vickers PJ, Isaacs AJ. Sprillum endocarditis. Postgrad Med J 1975;51:645–648.
8. Roughgarden JW. Antimicrobial therapy of ratbite fever. Arch Intern Med 1965;116:39–54.
9. Shattuck GC, Theiler M. Rat-bite disease in the United States with report of a case. Am J Trop Med 1924;4:453–460.
10. Taber LH, Feigin RD. Spirochetal infections. Pediatr Clin North Am 1979;26:377–413.
11. Tani T, Takano S. Prevention of *Borrelia duttonii, Trypanosoma gambionse, Spirillum minus,* and *Treponema pallidum* infections conveyable through transfusion. Jpn J Med Sci Biol 1958; 11:407.
12. Washburn RG. *Spirillum minus* (rat-bite fever). In: Mandell GL, Bennett JE, Dolin R, eds. Principles and practice of infectious diseases. New York: Churchill Livingstone, 1995;220:2155–2156.
13. Watkins CG. Ratbite fever. J Pediatr 1946;28:429–448.
14. Wheeler WE. Treatment of the rat bite fevers with penicillin. Am J Dis Child 1945;69:215–220.

Staphylococcus aureus

Feng-Yee Chang and John Turnidge

GENERAL DESCRIPTION

Staphylococcus aureus is a Gram-positive coccal bacterium; 25 to 33% of normal individuals carry its organism in the anterior nares and skin. It can colonize and infect both healthy, immunologically competent people in the community and hospitalized patients with decreased host defenses. *S. aureus* is the commonest and most important Gram-positive hospital-acquired organism. It has a high propensity to colonize abnormal skin surfaces and open wounds, where it may merely reside rather than cause active infection. Although minor skin infections such as furuncles may resolve naturally without antibiotic intervention, once *S. aureus* invades deeper structures, it often spreads hematogenously to other organ systems, leading to metastatic infection. Endocarditis and septicemia often have significant mortality despite aggressive antimicrobial therapy.

SUSCEPTIBILITY IN VITRO AND IN VIVO

Following its introduction into clinical practice in the 1940s, penicillin became the treatment of choice for infections caused by *S. aureus;* however, *S. aureus* resistant to penicillin through production of a β-lactamase (penicillinase) rapidly emerged. Since the 1970s, *S. aureus* strains resistant to the penicillinase-resistant penicillins (including nafcillin, methicillin, and oxacillin) have gradually emerged. These strains are generally multiresistant, exhibiting resistance to macrolides and lincosamines, and usually to tetracyclines and gentamicin. Methicillin-resistant *S. aureus* (MRSA) is now a common cause of nosocomial infection. The rapidity with which MRSA developed in Europe after introduction of methicillin in 1959 and its subsequent spread throughout the world have created therapeutic problems for physicians, in part because of its high propensity to acquire new resistances.

Methicillin resistance in MRSA isolates is chromosomally mediated and results, at least in part, from the presence of a modified penicillin-binding protein (PBP-2a), which has reduced affinity for methicillin and other β-lactams and hence retains critical functions necessary for cell survival (15, 20). PBP-2a is coded for by the *mec*A gene located on the staphylococcal chromosome. Resistance to all cephalosporins, antistaphylococcal penicillins, and probably all other β-lactams including β-lactamase inhibitor combinations should be assumed once methicillin resistance has been demonstrated.

Recently, a different type of MRSA was described in Australia and nearby countries. This strain is characterized by resistance to penicillin and methicillin but susceptibility to other drug classes. It appears to be principally a community-acquired organism (102, 139). Methicillin resistance is also coded for by *mec*A in these strains. Antimicrobial activity of the different antibiotics for both methicillin-susceptible *S. aureus* (MSSA) and MRSA is listed in Table 1.

Single Drugs

Penicillin G
Most staphylococci are resistant to penicillin and other β-lactamase-labile penicillins such as the aminopenicillins, carbenicillin, and the ureidopenicillins through production of β-lactamase. Only a small proportion (5–30%) of community-acquired strains of *S. aureus* do not produce a β-lactamase and remain susceptible to penicillin G. β-Lactamase-mediated resistance results from production of an extracellular enzyme by *S. aureus* that inactivates the antibiotic by opening the β-lactam ring.

Penicillinase-Resistant Penicillins
Currently, the vast majority of community-acquired *S. aureus* strains remain susceptible to the antistaphylococcal semisynthetic penicillins and first-generation cephalosporins (Table 1). The greatest stability to β-lactamase is observed with methicillin and nafcillin, followed by oxacillin, cloxacillin, dicloxacillin, and flucloxacillin. Differences in in vitro potency of the penicillin-resistant penicillins are small, with modal minimum inhibitory concentrations (MICs) in the range of 0.125 to 0.5 μg/mL (91).

Cephalosporins
Cephalosporins show variable stability to β-lactamase, depending on their chemical structure. Cephalothin is relatively resistant, while cefazolin is more sensitive to staphylococcal β-lactamase degradation (56, 136). Although this in vitro phenomenon has not been clearly demonstrated to be clinically significant, some prefer cephalothin for the treatment of life-threatening *S. aureus* infections (130). Data from animal studies suggest that cephalosporins are probably less effective than the penicillinase-resistant penicillins for treatment of serious staphylococcal infections. Cefazolin and cephalothin were less effective than nafcillin in the rabbit model of endocarditis (19, 157).

Compared with first-generation cephalosporins, the second- and third-generation cephalosporins have inferior in vitro

activity against *S. aureus*. With the exception of cefamandole, cefuroxime, and possibly cefaclor, cephalosporins of later generations generally have lower activity against staphylococci and offer no advantages in the management of staphylococcal infection. However, almost all cephalosporins have sufficient activity to provide initial coverage pending the results of laboratory investigations.

Cephalosporins are not active against MRSA strains in vivo, despite the fact that some strains may appear susceptible in routine laboratory tests.

Penicillin/β-Lactamase-Inhibitor Combinations
Staphylococcal β-lactamase is readily inhibited by the currently available β-lactamase inhibitors clavulanic acid, sulbactam, and tazobactam. Thus, combination of these inhibitors with β-lactamase-labile penicillins restores activity against penicillin-resistant, methicillin-susceptible staphylococci (Table 1). Like cephalosporins, they are not active against MRSA strains.

Carbapenems
Imipenem and meropenem have a very broad spectrum of activity that includes *S. aureus*. However, MRSA is also resistant to imipenem and meropenem (Table 1). Although some strains of MRSA appear susceptible to imipenem in vitro, they are not susceptible in vivo (11, 25).

Macrolides
In general, the macrolides show a fairly uniform activity against staphylococci (5, 7, 184). MRSA (apart from many of the Australian community-acquired type) is resistant to the macrolides (68). Resistance to erythromycin is also prevalent worldwide in community-acquired strains. The newer macrolides—dirithromycin, roxithromycin, clarithromycin, and azithromycin—have activity similar to that of erythromycin against staphylococci (Table 1). Strains resistant to erythromycin are also resistant to these newer macrolides.

Lincosamines (Clindamycin and Lincomycin)
S. aureus resistant to erythromycin often demonstrates inducible resistance to both clindamycin and lincomycin (95). MSSA is susceptible to clindamycin (MIC range, <0.06 μg/mL–0.125 μg/mL (Table 1)). Classical MRSA is resistant to clindamycin with a consistent MIC above 256 μg/mL (Table 1). In a rabbit model of endocarditis, clindamycin was associated with a relatively slow rate of eradication of organisms from the infected vegetation, and relapse was more likely in rabbits given clindamycin than in those treated with penicillin or vancomycin (144).

Fluoroquinolones
Fluoroquinolones are DNA gyrase inhibitors that are active in vitro and in vivo against *S. aureus,* including some MRSA strains (18, 60, 158). The MICs of fluoroquinolones are typically between 0.5 and 1 μg/mL for MSSA strains (Table 1). Most strains of MRSA are now resistant to fluoroquinolones (36, 152, 168). Resistance to fluoroquinolones has been found in MSSA and MRSA strains (81, 117). Both altered gyrase and

TABLE 1 • In Vitro Activity of Antimicrobial Agents against *Staphylococcus aureus*

Antibiotic	MIC (μg/mL) against MSSA[a]			MIC (μg/mL) against MRSA		
	Range	50%	90%	Range	50%	90%
Penicillins						
Penicillin	<0.06–128	16	128	32–128	64	128
Ampicillin	2.0–>32	>32	>32	4.0–>32	>32	>32
Oxacillin	0.25–2.0	0.5	1	16.0–>128	>64	>128
Nafcillin	0.25–1	0.5	1	—	—	—
Methicillin	0.5–4	1	4	8–>128	64	>64
Dicloxacillin	0.06–0.5	0.25	0.5	—	—	—
Cephalosporins						
Cephalothin	0.125–0.5	0.5	0.5	4.0–>32	>32	>32
Cefazolin	0.5–4	1	2	—	—	—
Cephalexin	4–16	8	16	128–256	>128	256
Cefaclor	1–32	4	16	>64–>128	128	>128
Cefuroxime	0.5–2	1	2	64–>128	>128	>128
Cefotaxime	0.5–>16.0	>16	>16	2.0–>32	>32	>32
Cefepime	1–8	4	4	8–>64	64	>64
Ceftazidime	4–16	8	16	16–>64	64	>64
Ceftriaxone	2–4	4	4	16–>64	>64	>64
Cefoperazone	2–4	2	4	32–>256	>256	>256
Cefixime	8–64	16	32	>32–>64	>32	>64
Cefdinir	0.125–1	0.25	1	0.5–>64	64	>64
Cefpodoxime	2–8	4	8	>64–>128	>64	>128
Flomoxef	0.12–4	0.5	4	8–>32	>32	>32
Moxalactam	2–16	8	16	>32	>32	>32
Cefpirome	0.5–2	1	2	32–128	128	128
Carbapenems						
Meropenem	0.06–1	0.12	0.12	0.5–16	8	>8
Imipenem	0.12–0.5	0.12	0.25	0.05–>16.0	4	16
Glycopeptides						
Vancomycin	0.25–2	1	2.0	0.25–4.0	2	2.0
Teicoplanin	0.25–4.0	0.5	0.5	0.5–4.0	0.5	1.0
LY264826	0.12–0.5	0.25	0.25	0.12–1.0	0.25	0.5
Macrolides						
Erythromycin	0.13–4	0.25	4	0.06–>32	>32	>32
Azithromycin	0.25–8	1	4	>128	>128	>128
Clarithromycin	0.13–4	0.25	1	0.125–>64	>64	>64
Dirithromycin	0.25–8	0.5	4	>64	>64	>64
Roxithromycin	0.13–0.16	0.5	4	>64	>64	>64
Aminoglycosides						
Gentamicin	0.06–16	0.12	0.5	0.06–64	1	32
Tobramycin	0.06–32	0.125	0.25	—	—	—
Amikacin	0.5–4	1	2	2–64	16	32
Quinolones						
Ofloxacin	0.12–1	0.5	1	0.25–32	8.0	16
Pefloxacin	0.12–2	0.5	1	0.25–128	32	128
Rufloxacin	1.0–16	1.0	4.0	1.0–>32	1.0	4.0
Sparfloxacin	<0.015–0.12	0.03	0.12	<0.015–16	4	16
Ciprofloxacin	0.03–4.0	0.5	1.0	0.25–>128	32	64
Norfloxacin	0.25–1.0	0.5	1.0	0.25–>32	0.5	1.0
β-Lactam/β-lactam inhibitors						
Amoxicillin/clavulanate	0.12–2	1	2	16–64	32	64
Ampicillin/sulbactam	0.06–2	1	2	8–32	32	32
Piperacillin-tazobactam	0.06–32	1	1	—	—	—
Miscellaneous						
Clindamycin	<0.06–0.125	0.125	0.125	>256	>256	>256
Tetracycline	0.006–124	0.25	64	—	—	—
TMP/	0.06–0.25	0.125	0.25	0.25–1	0.5	1
SMX	1.19–4.75	2.38	4.75	4.75–19	9.5	19
Fusidic acid	0.06–0.12	0.06	0.06	0.03–8	0.06	0.06
Rifampin	<0.03–>16	<0.03	1.0	<0.03–>16	>16	>16
Mupirocin	0.06–2	0.25	0.25	0.125–>256	0.25	0.5

Adapted from references 6, 7, 28, 32, 45, 54, 60, 120, 121, 128, 141, 142, 159, 170, 172, 183.

[a] MSSA, methicillin-susceptible *S. aureus;* MRSA, methicillin-resistant *S. aureus.*

energy-dependent efflux mechanisms account for the development of resistance to fluoroquinolones (81).

Glycopeptides

Until recently, MRSA strains were invariably sensitive to vancomycin and teicoplanin (Table 1). Strains with increased MICs to vancomycin were recently described in Japan (73). MICs range between 0.25 and 4 μg/mL (Table 1). However, vancomycin is slowly and incompletely bactericidal against MSSA in vitro compared with nafcillin (17, 124, 154).

Teicoplanin (not available in the United States) is another glycopeptide with a spectrum of activity similar to that of vancomycin but may be less active against some coagulase-negative staphylococci. In animal models, teicoplanin has activity equivalent to that of vancomycin for treatment of experimental endocarditis caused by both MSSA and MRSA (3, 24).

Tetracyclines

Resistance to tetracyclines is common in community-acquired strains of *S. aureus*. Some tetracycline-resistant stains appear susceptible to minocycline and doxycycline. The incidence of tetracycline resistance is 92% in classical MRSA (45). In vitro susceptibility of *S. aureus* to minocycline has been documented for a number of years (110). Minocycline and vancomycin proved equally effective in reducing bacterial density in infected vegetations in a rabbit model of MRSA endocarditis (122).

Trimethoprim-Sulfamethoxazole (TMP-SMX)

In vitro susceptibility of MRSA to TMP-SMZ varies around the world. In one study, up to 95% of classical MRSA strains were susceptible to TMP-SMX (47), while in other areas almost all strains were resistant (168). TMP-SMX was strikingly inferior to vancomycin for infection caused by either an MSSA or an MRSA strain in the rabbit model of aortic valve endocarditis (38). The numbers of bacteria in the vegetations of rabbits treated for 3 days with TMP-SMX were minimally reduced, compared with untreated controls, and no infection was sterilized, versus a rate of 70 to 80% for vancomycin.

Mupirocin

Some 414 nasal and 586 nonnasal *S. aureus* isolates, both methicillin resistant and methicillin susceptible, showed similar $MIC_{90}s$ and a susceptibility of 99.1% to the topical antimicrobial agent mupirocin (Table 1) (170).

Fusidic Acid

Fusidic acid (available in Europe and some Western Pacific countries) has a distinct Gram-positive spectrum (excluding streptococci) and is active against both MSSA and MRSA strains (172). *S. aureus* is inhibited by fusidic acid at very low concentrations, usually between 0.03 and 0.25 μg/mL, regardless of their susceptibility to methicillin or oxacillin (105, 172). Fusidic acid–resistant mutants are harbored at relatively high frequencies.

Fosfomycin

Fosfomycin is an epoxide antibiotic that has a different structure and mode of action from other antimicrobials. The MIC_{90}

for MRSA is 4 μg/mL. Fosfomycin, alone or in combination with β-lactam antibiotics, has been said to be active against MRSA in vitro (2).

Rifampin

Rifampin is highly active against staphylococci, with $MIC_{50}s$ for about 0.03 μg/mL. Resistant mutants can be easily selected in vitro and are thought to be naturally present in susceptible populations at frequencies of 10^{-6} to 10^{-7} (86, 92). Resistance to rifampin is more prevalent in classical MRSA than MSSA in some regions of the world (168).

Combination Drugs

In Vitro

Addition of gentamicin to nafcillin produces an enhanced bactericidal effect in vitro (146). The combinations of vancomycin-gentamicin and vancomycin-tobramycin were synergistic against most MSSA and MRSA strains (178). If synergism was defined as a decrease in colony counts of at least 100-fold at 24 h with the combination compared with that of the most active single drug, vancomycin-gentamicin synergism was not predictable for strains of MRSA with gentamicin MICs of 0.5 to more than 128 μg/mL (114). Moreover, a gentamicin MIC above 500 μg/mL predicted a lack of vancomycin-gentamicin synergism for strains of MRSA (114). The in vitro effect of rifampin in combination with semisynthetic penicillins, vancomycin, and aminoglycosides is highly variable (66, 165, 178, 189). For both MSSA and MRSA, minocycline-rifampin synergism has been demonstrated by checkerboard evaluation (30, 150)

Resistance in vitro does not appear to emerge if MRSA are exposed to a combination of fusidic acid and rifampin (108), and sub-MIC concentrations of trimethoprim also appear to be able to prevent selection of rifampin-resistant mutants.

In Vivo (Animal Studies)

Killing of MSSA within experimentally induced cardiac vegetations in animal models is accelerated by adding gentamicin to nafcillin (143). Some animal models favor the use of rifampin (71, 79). In animal studies, rifampin was shown to play a unique role in the complete sterilization of foreign bodies infected by *S. aureus* (31). Addition of rifampin to combination antibiotic regimens proved highly effective in an animal model of MRSA osteomyelitis (71). In experimental MRSA endocarditis in rabbits, an ampicillin/sulbactam/rifampin regimen (with a high ampicillin dosage at 625–800 mg/kg/day) was as effective as vancomycin (21). In animal models, use of quinolone combinations with rifampin may prevent resistance to both drugs (79, 147).

ANTIMICROBIAL THERAPY
Drug of Choice

Treatment of staphylococcal infections depends on the site and severity of infection and the antibiotic susceptibility pattern of the organism.

Penicillin-Susceptible *S. aureus*

Penicillin G is the drug of choice for penicillinase-negative strains because on a weight-for-weight basis, it is more active than penicillinase-resistant penicillins. Penicillin-sensitive *S. aureus* strains have not been reported to become resistant to penicillin during treatment. penicillin V and amoxicillin can both be used as oral agents for penicillin-sensitive *S. aureus*, with amoxicillin preferred when higher levels are required.

Methicillin-Susceptible *S. aureus* (MSSA)

Penicillinase-resistant penicillins are the preferred drugs for all *S. aureus* infections caused by penicillin-resistant MSSA strains. These agents have gained wide acceptance because they are bactericidal and, like other penicillins, have a low incidence of adverse reactions. A variety of penicillinase-resistant penicillins are available, including the isoxazolyl penicillins (cloxacillin, dicloxacillin, flucloxacillin, and oxacillin) for both oral and parenteral use and methicillin, oxacillin, nafcillin for parenteral use. There are no apparent differences in efficacy between these agents, and they have similar pharmacokinetic profiles.

In most countries, methicillin has been superseded by the other agents in this group because of its association with a higher incidence of adverse reactions, especially hypersensitivity and interstitial nephritis. A serious reaction to flucloxacillin, characterized by prolonged hepatic cholestasis, has been described with some frequency and has been associated with both parenteral and oral therapy (50, 166).

Cephalosporins, particularly those of the first generation, have proven useful alternatives to penicillinase-resistant penicillins, since they are relatively stable to staphylococcal β-lactamase. They are most commonly used in patients with a history of allergy or intolerance to penicillins. However, it is considered imprudent to administer them to patients with a history of accelerated reactions (e.g., angioedema or anaphylaxis). Patients with this type of history should not be given β-lactams of any class, and other antistaphylococcal agents such as clindamycin or vancomycin should be used. Cephaloridine, the cephalosporin with the greatest potency in vitro against staphylococci, has been abandoned because of the risk of nephrotoxicity and relative instability to staphylococcal β-lactamases. Suitable first-generation cephalosporins for staphylococcal infections include cephalothin, cefazolin, cefapirin, and cephradine for parenteral use and cephalexin, cefapirin, and cephradine for oral use.

Currently available combinations of penicillin/β-lactamase inhibitor include amoxicillin/clavulanic acid, ticarcillin/clavulanic acid, ampicillin/sulbactam, and piperacillin/tazobactam. These combinations have no in vitro or in vivo superiority over penicillinase-resistant penicillins, but they do have the advantage of possessing a broad spectrum of activity against Gram-negative bacteria, including anaerobes. Therefore, they should not be used as substitutes for penicillinase-resistant penicillins when staphylococci are the sole pathogens. However, their broader spectrum gives them a significant advantage when staphylococci are involved in mixed infections with enteric Gram-negative organisms and anaerobes.

Imipenem and meropenem provide adequate staphylococcal coverage in mixed infections but, again, have no role in the specific treatment of pure staphylococcal infection.

Erythromycin has been used extensively for treatment of both minor and serious staphylococcal infections. It is bacteriostatic against staphylococci and, for this reason, has generally lost favor for the management of serious and life-threatening infection, being largely supplanted by penicillinase-resistant penicillins. Moreover, the role of erythromycin in empirical treatment is further limited because of drug resistance. Nevertheless, oral erythromycin is still suitable for minor skin infections caused by *S. aureus,* especially in penicillin-allergic patients, provided the strain has demonstrated susceptibility on laboratory testing.

The newer macrolides, roxithromycin, clarithromycin, dirithromycin, and azithromycin, have activity similar to that of erythromycin against staphylococci. In general, strains resistant to erythromycin are also resistant to these newer macrolides. The latter two agents have very high tissue penetration, which may be of advantage in some sequestrated staphylococcal infections. Although there is good experience with the newer macrolides for staphylococcal skin infections, there is little experience with these drugs in the treatment of osteomyelitis. These drugs are not currently recommended for treatment of bacteremia or endocarditis. However, new intravenous formulations are under development, and future studies might alter this opinion.

Like erythromycin, lincosamines (clindamycin and lincomycin) have been available for many years and have been used frequently for treatment of staphylococcal infections. They are also bacteriostatic and have been mostly relegated to reserve agents. However, the lincosamines are perhaps more useful second-line agents than macrolides.

Clindamycin is better absorbed than lincomycin when administered orally and is the preferred agent for oral use. It demonstrates good penetration into tissues, notably bone, and oral clindamycin in particular is less likely than erythromycin to cause gastrointestinal upset at high doses. This makes clindamycin potentially useful in patients with a history of accelerated reactions to penicillins, when cephalosporins are contraindicated.

Vancomycin and teicoplanin may occasionally be considered for treatment of life-threatening staphylococcal infection in patients with a history of accelerated allergic reactions to β-lactams. It is not clear whether they are superior to macrolides or lincosamines in this setting, but they are preferred because of greater experience gained in the management of life-threatening MRSA infections. Caveats for their use are given below.

Methicillin-Resistant *S. aureus*

Vancomycin is the drug of choice for infections caused by *S. aureus* strains that are resistant to β-lactam antibiotics and for patients who are allergic to the latter drugs. However, several anecdotal reports have questioned the efficacy of vancomycin for both MSSA and MRSA (84, 98, 154). Vancomycin treatment of deep-seated staphylococcal infections such as endocarditis was reported to clear bacteremia more slowly than β-lactam treatment (98). Bacteremia was often prolonged more than 6 days in patients receiving vancomycin therapy (97, 98, 137, 154). In contrast, almost all blood cultures of patients receiving nafcillin or other β-lactams became sterile within 6 days (22, 48, 90). Relapse and treatment failure of *S. aureus* bacteremia and endocarditis were associated with vancomycin therapy (23, 27, 59, 61, 69, 154). The slower bactericidal rate has been suggested as a possible reason for the higher failure rate seen with vancomycin therapy in patients with MSSA endocarditis (154). Moreover, the recent emergence of vancomycin resistance by enterococci, observed first in the Europe and now globally (77), has been met with great apprehension.

For teicoplanin to be efficacious in the treatment of *S. aureus* endocarditis, the trough serum concentration should be maintained at 20 μg/mL during the first week of therapy (99, 101, 185). Long-term teicoplanin therapy can result in emergence of strains resistant to teicoplanin; however, these strains remain susceptible to vancomycin (80).

There are a number of alternatives for oral therapy of classical MRSA. Most experience has been gained with rifampin, fluoroquinolones, and (in countries where it is available) fusidic acid.

Vancomycin Intermediate-Resistant *S. aureus*

Sporadic cases of infection due to organisms with intermediate resistance to vancomycin have been reported in Japan and the United States. An MRSA with intermediate susceptibility to vancomycin (MIC = 8 μg/mL) was reported from Japan (73). An infant developed MRSA postoperative wound infection after heart surgery. The patient recovered and was treated with ampicillin-sulbactam in combination with arbekacin (an aminoglycoside approved for MRSA infection in Japan).

Special Situations

Suggested antibiotics, doses, and duration for treatment of *S. aureus* infections are shown in Table 2. Some special situations are discussed below.

Catheter-Related Bacteremia

Several prospective studies using semiquantitative catheter cultures have identified *S. aureus* as one of the leading causes of catheter-related bacteremia (13, 33, 35, 103, 153). More than 30% of *S. aureus* bacteremia was attributable to an infected intravascular device (44, 63, 93, 100, 119).

The optimal duration of antibiotic treatment remains unknown, although many authors advocate shorter courses of antibiotic therapy for uncomplicated catheter-related *S. aureus* bacteremia, claiming that this infection has a low rate of complications after a 2-week course of intravenous antistaphylococcal antibiotics. On the other hand, a few studies have suggested that short-course therapy is inadequate, citing experience with patients who had complications and relapse (76, 111, 129, 133, 179, 186). In a well-reasoned meta-analysis, an average late complication rate of 6.1% was found for 11 studies totaling 132 patients treated with short-course therapy for uncomplicated catheter-related *S. aureus* bacteremia (76). These investigators also estimated the rate that might be observed after 4 to 6 weeks of therapy to be in the range of 0.07 to 0.99%. In another study (not included in the meta-analysis) of 12 patients with *S. aureus* bacteremia associated with intra-venous catheter infection, three of eight patients who received 2-week treatment were considered failures: one each developed endocarditis 3 days and 7 weeks later, respectively, and one developed epidural abscess and meningitis after the first week of therapy and underwent 6 weeks of antibiotic therapy (132).

A study of *S. aureus* bacteremia in patients on chronic hemodialysis showed that less than 4 weeks of treatment was associated with a higher occurrence of primary treatment failure (definition not given) than treatment for more than 4 weeks (129). Ideally, catheters should be removed regardless of type (i.e., peripheral vs. central venous catheters, nontunneled vs. tunneled catheters). Delayed removal of the infected catheter was associated with persistence of bacteremia (104). Only 18% of those with Hickman catheter–related *S. aureus* bacteremia and only 10% of patients with exit site infections were cured without catheter removal (42). If the focus of infection has been promptly removed with rapid documented resolution of the bacteremia (<3 days), 2 weeks of antibiotic therapy with nafcillin, cefazolin, or vancomycin is likely to be enough. Serious infectious complications such as septic thrombosis, deep-seated infections, and sepsis-related death have often resulted from vascular catheter–related *S. aureus* bacteremia (131). If signs of endocarditis, metastatic infection, or prolonged bacteremia are present, longer therapy is needed. Large doses of oral dicloxacillin sodium (for MSSA) that can be taken at home for 2 weeks to supplement an initial 2-week intravenous regimen have been recommended (134). Under no circumstances should patients simply have the catheter removed without antibiotic treatment.

Endocarditis

Endocarditis caused by *S. aureus* is a very serious disease with a high rate of morbidity and mortality. Endocarditis due to *S. aureus* in nonaddicts primarily involves valves in the left side of the heart and is associated with mortality rates of 25 to 40%. By contrast, staphylococcal endocarditis occurring in addicts usually involves the tricuspid valve (right-sided endocarditis) and has a low mortality. The incidence of infective endocarditis in patients with community-acquired *S. aureus* bacteremia has ranged from 6 to 64% (8, 55, 78, 88, 93, 111, 113, 118, 151, 186).

The drugs of choice for endocarditis (Table 3) caused by MSSA are the semisynthetic penicillinase-resistant penicillins. Benzylpenicillin is preferred in the uncommon circumstance that the strain is shown to be penicillin susceptible. First-generation cephalosporins are effective alternatives, usually reserved for patients with a history of minor penicillin allergy. Vancomycin is the drug of choice for patients with life-threatening penicillin allergy and those with endocarditis due to MRSA.

Clindamycin has been used successfully for *S. aureus* endocarditis, but clinical data are limited. Relapse and treatment failure are documented (16, 29, 164, 180).

Although vancomycin is still recommended therapy for *S. aureus* endocarditis in patients with life-threatening penicillin allergy, recent experience suggests caution, as suboptimal outcomes have been associated with the use of this agent. Failure

TABLE 2 • Suggested Antibiotics, Doses, and Duration for Treatment of *Staphylococcus aureus* Infections

Infection	First-Line Antibiotics (duration)	Alternatives (duration)
Catheter-Related Bacteremia		
MSSA	1. Nafcillin/oxacillin 2 g q. 4 h i.v. ($\geq$2 weeks) 2. Cephalothin 2 g q. 4 h i.v. ($\geq$2 weeks) 3. Cefazolin 2 g q. 8 h i.v. ($\geq$2 weeks)	Vancomycin 15 mg/kg q. 12 h i.v. ($\geq$2 weeks)
MRSA	Vancomycin 15 mg/kg q. 12 h i.v. ($\geq$2 weeks)	
Infective endocarditis (Table 3)		
Meningitis		
MSSA	Nafcillin/oxacillin 2 g q. 4 h i.v. (>4 weeks)	Vancomycin 15 mg/kg q. 12 h i.v. (>4 weeks)
MRSA	Vancomycin 15 mg/kg q. 8–12 h i.v. (>4 weeks) plus rifampin 600 mg q.d. p.o. (>4 weeks)	
Osteomyelitis		
Acute osteomyelitis		
MSSA	Nafcillin/oxacillin 2 g q. 4–6 h i.v. (2–4 weeks), then 1 g q. 6 h of an oral antistaphylococcal penicillin (2–4 weeks) Cefazolin 2 g q. 8 h i.v. (2–4 weeks), then 1 g q. 6 h of an oral first generation cephalosporin (2–4 weeks)	Vancomycin 15 mg/kg q. 12 h i.v. (2–4 weeks)
MRSA	Vancomycin 15 mg/kg q. 12 h i.v. (2–4 weeks)	
Chronic osteomyelitis/ associated with orthopaedic devices		
MSSA	Nafcillin 2 g q. 4–6 h i.v. (2–6 weeks), then 1 g q. 6 h of an oral antistaphylococcal penicillin (for the remaining time $\geq$3 months) Cefazolin 2 g q. 8 h i.v. (2–6 weeks), then 1 g q. 8 h p.o. as above (for the remaining time $\geq$3 months)	Vancomycin 15 mg/kg q. 12 h i.v. (2–6 weeks)
MRSA	Vancomycin 15 mg/kg q. 12 h i.v. (2–6 weeks)	
Septic arthritis		
MSSA	Nafcillin 2 g q. 4–6 h i.v. (2 weeks), then 0.5–1 g q. 6 h p.o. as above (4 weeks) Cefazolin 2 g q. 8 h i.v. (2 weeks), then 0.5–1 g q. 6 h p.o. as above (4 weeks)	Vancomycin 1 g q. 12 h i.v. (3 weeks)
MRSA	Vancomycin 1 g q. 12 h i.v. (3 weeks)	
Pneumonia/lung abscess		
MSSA	Nafcillin 2 g q. 4–6 h i.v. (2 weeks), then 1 g q. 6 h p.o. as above (4 weeks) Cefazolin 2 g q. 8 h i.v. (2 weeks), then 1 g q. 6 h p.o. as above (4 weeks)	Vancomycin 1 g q. 12 h i.v. (2–4 weeks)
MRSA	Vancomycin 1 g q. 12 h i.v. (2–4 weeks)	
Cellulitis		
MSSA	Nafcillin 1 g q. 4–6 h i.v. (10–14 days) Cefazolin 1 g q. 8 h i.v. (10–14 days)	Vancomycin 1 g q. 12 h i.v. (10–14 days)
MRSA	Vancomycin 1 g q. 12 h i.v. (10–14 days)	

rates of approximately 40% have been documented in patients with *S. aureus* endocarditis treated with vancomycin despite right-sided involvement (154). β-Lactam desensitization should be carefully considered for MSSA endocarditis in patients with β-lactam allergy and suboptimal response to vancomycin (9).

Left-Sided Endocarditis. A minimum of 4 weeks of intravenous treatment is recommended for left-sided endocarditis (173). This duration is also recommended for *S. aureus* septicemia complicated by metastatic infection, on the presumption that endocarditis may well be present. Of 20 patients with *S. aureus* endocarditis receiving at least 4 weeks of treatment, all were cured at 1 month follow-up (132). For endocarditis

occurring on prosthetic devices, a 6-week course of a penicillin with an aminoglycoside has been recommended (173).

The combination of nafcillin and gentamicin was associated with a more rapid clearance of bacteremia in MSSA endocarditis. Addition of gentamicin for the first 2 weeks of a 6-week course of intravenous nafcillin therapy led to more rapid defervescence but did not improve the cure rate (90). However, an increased risk of renal dysfunction was observed (90). Addition of gentamicin for the first 3 to 5 days of therapy may avoid nephrotoxicity and should be considered (12). Although aminoglycosides have been added to the vancomycin regimen for MRSA endocarditis, this addition should be restricted to

TABLE 3 • Most Commonly Recommended Treatment Regimens for *Staphylococcus aureus* Endocarditis

Infection Type	Penicillin Allergy Status	Regimen
Left-sided infection with penicillin-susceptible *S. aureus* (PSSA)		
Native valve	Penicillin nonallergic	Penicillin G 1.2–1.8 g q. 4 h for 4–6 weeks ± gentamicin for 3–5 days
	Minor penicillin allergy	First-generation cephalosporin, e.g., cephalothin 2 g q. 4 h or cefazolin 2 g q. 8 h for 4 weeks ± gentamicin for 3–5 days
	Life-threatening penicillin-allergy	Vancomycin 15 mg/kg q. 12 h for 4–6 weeks ± gentamicin for 3–5 days
Prosthetic valve	Any of the above	Add rifampin and give gentamicin for 2 weeks
Left-sided infection with methicillin-susceptible *S. aureus* (MSSA)		
Native valve	Penicillin nonallergic	Penicillinase-resistant penicillin, e.g., nafcillin/oxacillin 2 g q. 4 h for 4 weeks ± gentamicin 1 mg/kg q. 8 h for 3–5 days
	Minor penicillin allergy	First-generation cephalosporin, e.g., cephalothin 2 g q. 4 h or cefazolin 2 g q. 8 h for 4–6 weeks ± gentamicin for 3–5 days
	Life-threatening penicillin-allergy	Vancomycin 15 mg/kg q. 12 h for 4–6 weeks ± gentamicin for 3–5 days
Poor response	Any of the above	Add rifampin
Prosthetic valve	Any of the above	Add rifampin and give gentamicin for 2 weeks
Left-sided infection with methicillin-resistant *S. aureus* (MRSA)		
Native valve	All	Vancomycin 15 mg/kg q. 12 h for 4 weeks ± gentamicin for 3–5 days
Poor response	All	Add rifampin
Prosthetic valve	All	Add rifampin and give gentamicin for 2 weeks
Right-sided infection (nonprosthetic)		Above regimens for 2 weeks or ciprofloxacin + rifampin for 4 weeks if no other infection focus

endocarditis caused by aminoglycoside-susceptible strains, and aminoglycoside use should be limited to 3 to 5 days (12).

For patients with MRSA endocarditis unresponsive to vancomycin, addition of rifampin and/or gentamicin (if susceptible) or the use of minocycline, trimethoprim-sulfamethoxazole, or ciprofloxacin-rifampin might be considered if the strain is susceptible, although experience with these regimens is limited (43, 53, 106).

The in vivo effect of rifampin in combination with nafcillin, oxacillin, vancomycin, or aminoglycosides is highly variable. Routine use of rifampin is not recommended for treatment of native valve *S. aureus* endocarditis. Although the addition of rifampin to vancomycin for patients with MRSA endocarditis failed to show either enhanced survival or reduced duration of bacteremia in comparison with vancomycin alone (98), it could be used as a supplemental therapy in patients who do not respond adequately to conventional antimicrobial therapy.

Breakthrough bacteremia was shown in patients with *S. aureus* endocarditis receiving teicoplanin in a graduated dosing regimen of 20 mg/kg/day for 3 days, 12 mg/kg/day for 4 days, and 7 mg/kg/day thereafter (57, 96). Teicoplanin is not currently recommended for severe *S. aureus* infection (i.e., septicemia and endocarditis).

Right-Sided Endocarditis.   Right-sided endocarditis has a high cure rate, and carefully selected regimens as short as 2 weeks have been efficacious, provided there are no other foci of infection (23, 39, 138, 163). Effective regimens have included intravenous nafcillin and tobramycin (23), intravenous cloxacillin and amikacin (163), and intravenous cloxacillin with and without gentamicin (138). Four weeks of oral ciprofloxacin plus rifampin was also shown to be effective (70).

Prosthetic Valve Endocarditis.   Because prosthetic valve staphylococcal endocarditis has a high mortality, combination therapy seems prudent. Addition of rifampin and gentamicin to the β-lactam or vancomycin is most commonly recommended, although controlled studies have not been done. Gentamicin should be given for 2 weeks rather than for 3 to 5 days. A favorable response of MRSA prosthetic valve endocarditis to minocycline therapy after unsuccessful treatment with vancomycin has been reported (94). Because of the very limited clinical data, minocycline should probably be regarded as an alternative agent for MRSA endocarditis.

Meningitis

Meningitis caused by *S. aureus* is often found in early post-neurosurgery or posttrauma in those with cerebrospinal fluid shunts (87). Other underlying conditions include diabetes mellitus, alcoholism, chronic renal failure requiring hemodialysis, intravenous drug abuse, and malignancy (62, 87, 148). Mortality rates have ranged from 14 to 77%. Like all penicillins, penicillinase-resistant penicillins show minimal penetration into the cerebrospinal fluid in the absence of inflammation, but acceptable concentrations are seen in the presence of inflammation, despite the high level of protein binding (91). Hence, recommended treatment of meningitis caused by MSSA is nafcillin or oxacillin, in a dose of 9 to 12 g/day in adults or 200 to 300 mg/kg daily in 6 divided doses in children (49, 87, 148). For MRSA and for patients allergic to penicillin, vancomycin 2 g/day for adults and 40 mg/kg daily for children in 2 divided doses is recommended. In MRSA infection, the cerebrospinal fluid should be monitored during therapy, and if the spinal fluid continues to yield viable organisms after 48 h of intravenous antibiotic therapy, then either intrathecal or intraventricular vancomycin (20 mg once daily in adults) can be added (49, 65).

Therapy for cerebrospinal fluid shunt infections caused by MRSA should include a combination of intravenous vancomycin and either oral rifampin (1200 mg/day in adults; 20 mg/kg daily in children) or intrashunt or intraventricular vancomycin at a dose of 20 mg once daily (49, 58). Many shunt infections require shunt removal to achieve a cure.

Bone and Joint Infections

Osteomyelitis and Septic Arthritis.   *S. aureus* is the most common cause of osteomyelitis in all settings, including acute hematogenous infection, chronic osteomyelitis, and prosthesis infection. Septic arthritis, an acute infection of joints, is also most commonly caused by *S. aureus*. As in other staphylococcal infections, penicillinase-resistant penicillins are considered the drugs of choice for MSSA infections, and vancomycin is recommended for acute MRSA infections. Chronic MRSA infections are probably best managed with a combination of two oral agents (e.g., rifampin plus ciprofloxacin or fusidic acid).

Acute Hematogenous Osteomyelitis.   Acute hematogenous osteomyelitis usually involves long bones in children and vertebrae in adults. Antibiotic treatment alone is usually sufficient treatment. The cure rates of adequately treated *S. aureus* hematogenous osteomyelitis are close to 90%. In general, antibiotic treatment should be continued for 4 weeks (173). Surgery is indicated only with medullary or periosteal abscess formation, persistence of fever, presence of a sequestrum, or doubt about the offending organism. Short-term parenteral antibiotic therapy (i.e., 5–9 days of intravenous therapy) followed by 14 to 26 days of oral therapy has given a cure rate of more than 90% in both adults and children (14, 162).

Chronic Osteomyelitis.   Chronic osteomyelitis with *S. aureus* usually occurs when acute osteomyelitis is not recognized early or is inadequately treated. Infection can be low grade or remain dormant for years and flair up to clinically resemble acute osteomyelitis. Surgery is usually required to remove necrotic bone and occasionally for diagnosis. Prolonged antibiotic therapy is recommended. Although the optimum duration of antibiotic therapy has never been established, most authors recommend therapy for 6 weeks to 6 months. Combination therapy with nafcillin and rifampin was studied in chronic osteomyelitis and appears to offer no additional benefit to nafcillin alone (123).

Joint Prosthetic and Fixation Device Infections.   Surgical intervention is essential in prosthetic and fixation device infections. In the acute postsurgical setting, the prosthesis or fixation device may be left in place if the joint or bone union is stable, and treated expectantly with antibiotics. In chronic or late infections, the prosthesis or fixation device must be removed to effect a cure (74, 149). When removal of the prosthesis or device is impractical, long-term suppressive therapy has been effective with agents such as cloxacillin (10) or rifampin plus a fluoroquinolone (41).

Septic Arthritis.   Medical management of septic arthritis involves the same antibiotic regimens as acute hematogenous osteomyelitis. Repeat joint aspiration will alleviate pain, allow bacteriologic monitoring, and probably reduce joint damage. Open joint drainage is generally unnecessary except for hip infections in children, where it seems to prevent necrosis of the femoral head (174).

Eradication of *S. aureus* Carriage

Use of mupirocin to eliminate nasal carriage has been associated with concomitant eradication of carriage on hands (135) and on other body sites (72). In addition, the MRSA colonization rate decreased significantly when both nares and wounds were treated with mupirocin (85).

The combination of oral trimethoprim-sulfamethoxazole, oral rifampin, and topical bacitracin has been evaluated in uncontrolled studies (140, 176, 187). Success rates of 100% were seen for MRSA nasal carriage, but lower rates of 66 to 81% were seen for extranasal sites (176, 187). Failures in patients receiving bacitracin/rifampin resulted from development of rifampin resistance (176).

Trimethoprim-sulfamethoxazole, novobiocin, ciprofloxacin, and minocycline used singly or in combination with rifampin have been tried. Rifampin-resistant staphylococci have emerged during therapy when rifampin was used as a single agent (145, 188). Combinations of trimethoprim-sulfamethoxazole plus rifampin and novobiocin plus rifampin have been used with modest success (50–75%) in eradicating MRSA nasal carriage (46, 175). Clearance of extranasal sites, especially wounds, was less successful. Resistance has emerged even for the combination regimens. Ciprofloxacin, even when combined with rifampin, has proven disappointing for eradicating MRSA nasal carriage; emergence of resistance to ciprofloxacin has been commonplace following therapy (89, 116, 126, 155, 156). Finally, minocycline plus rifampin was no more effective than rifampin alone in either eradicating nasal carriage or preventing emergence of rifampin resistance (113a).

Alternative Therapy

Alternative antibiotics with good activity against MRSA include the parenteral antibiotics, teicoplanin and fosfomycin, and the orally absorbed antibiotics, rifampin, the fluoroquinolones, and fusidic acid. Teicoplanin has a longer elimination half-life, permitting once-daily dosing, and studies suggest a lower propensity for toxicity, including that seen on coadministration with aminoglycosides. Suboptimal outcomes have been shown with *S. aureus* endocarditis in patients receiving teicoplanin (57).

The oral formulation of fusidic acid is similar to rifampin in having good oral bioavailability and good tissue penetration, and resistance can emerge during treatment. Originally promoted as a primary antistaphylococcal agent, including a topical formulation for superficial skin infections, it is now most often used for MRSA infections. It is occasionally used in combination with rifampin for continuing oral and outpatient treatment of MRSA infections. Emergence of fusidic acid resistance has been observed when the antibiotic is administered alone (127), and significant gastrointestinal intolerance limits use in some patients. The intravenous formulation, in the form of the diethanolamine salt, is usually reserved for serious infections. Its use is associated with hyperbilirubinemia in up to 50% of patients. Rifampin, which is remarkably active against *S. aureus,* cannot be used as a single agent because of the high one-step mutation rate of 10^{-7} to 10^{-8} to resistance (112).

Trimethoprim-sulfamethoxazole (TMP-SMX) has been used successfully for skin and soft tissue infections, osteomyelitis, meningitis, endocarditis, and bacteremia caused by *S. aureus* (106). It has been largely supplanted by other drugs but is effective even in life-threatening infections such as endocarditis. TMP-SMX can be a valuable alternative treatment for staphylococcal disease, particularly that caused by MRSA (106), if strains are susceptible.

Fosfomycin is used in a number of countries for treatment of staphylococcal infections, particularly parenterally for serious infection caused by MRSA strains.

Combination Therapy

Korzeniowski et al. (90) showed that eradication of bacteremia in nonaddicts with endocarditis was significantly faster with nafcillin plus gentamicin group (2.8 days (n = 19) vs. 4.1 days (n = 11)]; $P < .05$); 8 of 16 (50%) patients treated with nafcillin plus gentamicin had sterile blood cultures on day 2 compared with only 1 of 9 (11%) patients treated with nafcillin. However, the more rapid clearance of bacteremia in the nafcillin plus gentamicin group did not correlate with a more rapid clinical response (90). An increased incidence of renal dysfunction was associated with addition of gentamicin for the first 2 weeks (90).

Chambers (23) showed a cure rate of right-sided endocarditis in intravenous drug abusers of 33% (1 of 3) with vancomycin plus tobramycin versus 100% (47 of 47) with nafcillin plus tobramycin for 2 weeks.

Because of slow clearance of bacteremia and clinical failure, adding an additional antimicrobial agent to vancomycin to achieve synergistic bacterial killing for treating deep-seated staphylococcal infections has been attempted. Although combination therapy is recommended by some experts for treatment of deep-seated infections such as prosthetic valve endocarditis (115), there are no controlled trials demonstrating the superiority of the combination over vancomycin alone. Combination of vancomycin and gentamicin was reported to be more nephrotoxic than gentamicin alone (51, 52). Three studies failed to show better cure rates with combination therapy than with single-drug therapy for *S. aureus* endocarditis when the total duration of therapy was 4 to 6 weeks (1, 90, 177). Definitive guidelines for the use of vancomycin-gentamicin combination therapy for MRSA infections await results of clinical trials correlating outcome with in vitro synergy studies (114).

Aminoglycosides are considered by some authorities to have a major supportive role in endocarditis and other forms of high-grade or persistent bacteremia. Used in combination with first-line agents during the initial stabilization phase of therapy, they are suggested to shorten the duration of bacteremia (37, 90).

Rifampin has been used in combination with a semisynthetic penicillin or vancomycin for severe staphylococcal infections (82). Although rifampin has been used as supplemental therapy in patients who do not respond adequately to conventional antimicrobial therapy (53, 107), reported clinical experience is still limited. Prospective studies of these combinations, however, have demonstrated modest or no benefit (171) for most patients or no benefit at all (167). On the contrary, some clinical experience (53, 107, 160) favors addition of rifampin. Rifampin appeared to be a safe and effective addition to therapy when staphylococcal bacteremia persisted despite vancomycin treatment in neonates (160).

A combination of rifampin and ciprofloxacin cured 100% (10 of 10) intravenous drug users with right-sided *S. aureus* endocarditis (43). Clinical experience with fusidic acid and a rifampin indicates that fusidic acid resistance does not emerge readily, although strains resistant to rifampin are possible (75). As stated above, rifampin cannot be used as a single agent because of its high one-step mutation rate to resistance (112).

At present the fluoroquinolones should probably be reserved for oral treatment of infections caused by MRSA, and only used in combination with other drugs such as rifampin or fusidic acid.

When ciprofloxacin has been used as a single agent to treat staphylococcal carriage or infection, it has failed to eradicate the organism or resistance has developed in a portion of patients (64, 116).

ENDPOINTS FOR MONITORING THERAPY

Fever and breakthrough bacteremia are useful for monitoring antistaphylococcal therapy. Erythrocyte sedimentation rate (ESR) is only useful for osteomyelitis follow-up. Serum inhibitory and bactericidal titers to assess the adequacy of antibiotic therapy are often recommended for osteomyelitis and endocarditis (4, 182). Peak and trough bactericidal titers of at least 1:64 and 1:32, respectively, were suggested as good predictors of a successful therapeutic outcome in patients with infective endocarditis (181). However, the serum bactericidal titer (SBT) is subject to variation and lack of reproducibility with staphylococci (125, 161). The serum test does not predict efficacy in animal models of endocarditis (40, 67). Clinically, the test lacks precision in predicting outcome or bacteriologic failure (34, 83, 109, 181). Clinical response and results of follow-up blood cultures remain the best indicators of clinical outcome. Reanalysis of data from two large multicenter studies (181, 182) showed that outcome was strongly correlated with trough titers of SBTs. This supports the concept that the efficacy of β-lactams depends on the time above the MIC, as most patients in these studies received β-lactams as their principal therapy (169). Currently, it is not possible to define the optimal trough titer for a successful outcome.

REFERENCES

1. Abrams B, Sklaver A, Hoffman T, Greenman R. Single or combination therapy of staphylococcal endocarditis in intravenous drug abusers. Ann Intern Med 1979;90:789–791.

2. Alvarez S, Jones M, Berk SL. In vitro activity of fosfomycin, alone and in combination, against methicillin-resistant *Staphylococcus aureus*. Antimicrob Agents Chemother 1985;28:689–690.

3. Arioli V, Berti M, Candiani G. Activity of teicoplanin in localized experimental infections in rats. J Hosp Infect 1986;7(Suppl A):91–99.

4. Aspinall SL, Friedland DM, Yu VL, Rihs JD, Muder RR. Recurrent methicillin-resistant *Staphylococcus aureus* osteomyelitis: combination antibiotic therapy with evaluation by serum bactericidal titers. Ann Pharmacother 1995;29:694–697.

5. Barry AL, Fuchs PC. In vitro activities of a streptogramin (RP59500), three macrolides, and an azalide against four respiratory tract pathogens. Antimicrob Agents Chemother 1995;39:238–240.

6. Bartoloni A, Colao MG, Orsi A, Dei R, Giganti E, Parenti F. In-vitro activity of vancomycin, teicoplanin, daptomycin, ramoplanin, MDL 62873 and other agents against staphylococci, enterococci and *Clostridium difficile*. J Antimicrob Chemother 1990;26:627–633.

7. Bauernfeind A. In vitro activity of dirithromycin in comparison with other new and established macrolides. J Antimicrob Chemother 1993;31:39–49.

8. Bayer AS, Lam K, Ginzton L, Norman DC, Chiu CY, Ward JI. *Staphylococcus aureus* bacteremia: clinical, serologic, and echocardiographic findings in patients with and without endocarditis. Arch Intern Med 1987;147:457–462.

9. Bayer AS. Infective endocarditis. Clin Infect Dis 1993;17:313–320.

10. Bell SM. Further observations on the value of oral penicillins in chronic staphylococcal osteomyelitis. Med J Aust 1976;2:591–593.

11. Berry AJ, Johnson JL, Archer GL. Imipenem therapy of experimental *Staphylococcus epidermidis* endocarditis. Antimicrob Agents Chemother 1986;29:748–752.

12. Bisno AL, Dismukes WE, Durack DT, Kaplan EL, Karchmer AW, Kaye D, Rahimtoola SH, Sande MA, Sanford JP, Watanakunakorn C, Wilson WR. Antimicrobial treatment of infective endocarditis due to viridans streptococci, enterococci and staphylococci. JAMA 1989;261:1471–1477.

13. Bjornson HS, Colley R, Bower RH, Duty VP, Schwartz-Fulton JT, Fisher JE. Association between microorganism growth at the catheter insertion site and colonization of the catheter in patients receiving total parenteral nutrition. Surgery 1982;92:720–726.

14. Black J, Hunt TL, Godley PJ, Matthew E. Oral antimicrobial therapy for adults with osteomyelitis or septic arthritis. J Infect Dis 1987;155:968–972.

15. Boyce JM. Methicillin-resistant *Staphylococcus aureus*. Infect Dis Clin North Am 1989;3:901–913.

16. Burch KH, Quinn EL, Cox T, Madhavan T, Fisher E, Romig D. Intramuscular clindamycin for therapy of infective endocarditis. Am J Cardiol 1976;38:929–933.

17. Cantoni L, Glauser MP, Bille J. Comparative efficacy of daptomycin, vancomycin and cloxacillin for the treatment of *Staphylococcus aureus* endocarditis in rats and role of the test conditions in this determination. Antimicrob Agents Chemother 1990;34:2348–2353.

18. Carpenter TC, Hackbarth CJ, Chambers HF, Sande MA. Efficacy of ciprofloxacin for experimental endocarditis caused by methicillin-susceptible or -resistant strains of *Staphylococcus aureus*. Antimicrob Agents Chemother 1986;30:382–384.

19. Carrizosa J, Kobasa WD, Kaye D. Effectiveness of nafcillin, methicillin, cephalothin in experimental *Staphylococcus aureus* endocarditis. Antimicrob Agents Chemother 1979;15:735–737.

20. Chambers HF, Hartmann BJ, Tomasz A. Increased amounts of novel penicillin-binding protein in a strain of methicillin-resistant *Staphylococcus aureus* exposed to nafcillin. J Clin Invest 1985;76:325–331.

21. Chambers HF, Kartalija M, Sande M. Ampicillin, sulbactam, and rifampin combination treatment of experimental methicillin-resistant *Staphylococcus aureus* endocarditis in rabbits. J Infect Dis 1995;171:897–902.

22. Chambers HF, Korzeniowski OM, Sande MA. *Staphylococcus aureus* endocarditis: clinical manifestations in addicts and non-addicts. Medicine 1983;62:170–177.

23. Chambers HF, Miller RT, Newman MD. Right-sided *Staphylococcus aureus* endocarditis in intravenous drug abusers: two week combination therapy. Ann Intern Med 1988;109:619–624.

24. Chambers HF, Sande MA. Teicoplanin versus nafcillin and vancomycin in the treatment of experimental endocarditis caused by methicillin-susceptible or -resistant *Staphylococcus aureus*. Antimicrob Agents Chemother 1984;26:61–64.

25. Chambers HF. In vitro and in vivo antistaphylococcal activities of L-695,256, a carbapenem with high affinity for penicillin-binding protein 2a. Antimicrob Agents Chemother 1995;39:462–466.

26. Chambers HF. Methicillin-resistant staphylococci. Clin Microbiol Rev 1988;1:173–186.

27. Chang FY, Triplett P, Peacock J, Mylotte JM, Musher D, McDonald B, Wagener M, Yu VL. Prospective, multicenter study of *Staphylococcus aureus* bacteremia [Abstract 439]. Infect Dis Soc Am 35th annual meeting, San Francisco, 1997.

28. Cheng AFB, Ling TKW, Lam AW, Fung KSC, Wise R. The antimicrobial activity and beta-lactamase stability of cefpirome, a new fourth-generation cephalosporin in comparison with other agents. J Antimicrob Chemother 1993;31:699–709.

29. Cherubin CE, Nair SR. Clindamycin in infective endocarditis. JAMA 1978;239:626–627.

30. Chow JW, Hilf M, Yu VL. Synergistic interaction of antibiotics with nasal penetration to methicillin-sensitive and methicillin-resistant *Staphylococcus aureus*. J Antimicrob Chemother 1991;27:558–560.

31. Chuard C, Herrmann M, Vaudaux P, Waldvogel FA, Lew DP. Successful therapy of experimental chronic foreign-body infection due to methicillin-resistant *Staphylococcus aureus* by antimicrobial combinations. Antimicrob Agents Chemother 1991;35:2611–2616.

32. Clarke AM, Zemcov SJV. Comparative in vitro activity of biapenem, a new carbapenem antibiotic. Eur J Clin Microbiol Infect Dis 1993;12:377–384.

33. Cleri DJ, Corrado ML, Seligman SJ. Quantitative culture of intravenous catheters and other intravascular inserts. J Infect Dis 1980;141:781–786.

34. Coleman DL, Horwitz RI, Andriole VT. Association between serum inhibitory and bactericidal concentrations and therapeutic outcome in the bacterial endocarditis. Am J Med 1982;73:260–267.

35. Collignon PG, Soni N, Pearson IY, Woods WP, Munro R, Sorrell TC. Is semiquantitative culture of central vein catheter tips useful in the diagnosis of catheter-associated bacteremia? J Clin Microbiol 1986;24:532–535.

36. Cruciana M, Bassetti D. The fluoroquinolones as treatment for infections caused by gram-positive bacteria. J Antimicrob Chemother 1994;33;403–417.

37. Degener JE, Vogel M, Michel MF, Mutsaers MMA, Hop WCJ. The efficacy of the combination of teicoplanin or flucloxacillin with netilmicin in the treatment of Staphylococcus aureus bacteremia. J Antimicrob Chemother 1989;899–904.

38. deGorgolas M, Aviles P, Verdejo C, Guerrero MLF. Treatment of experimental endocarditis due to methicillin-susceptible or methicillin-resistant Staphylococcus aureus with trimethoprim-sulfamethoxazole and antibiotics that inhibit cell wall synthesis. Antimicrob Agents Chemother 1995;39:953–957.

39. DiNubile MJ. Short course antibiotic therapy for right-sided endocarditis caused by Staphylococcus aureus in injection drug users. Ann Intern Med 1994;121:873–876.

40. Drake TA, Hackbarth CJ, Sande MA. Value of serum tests in combined drug therapy of endocarditis. Antimicrob Agents Chemother 1983;24:653–657.

41. Drancourt M, Stein A, Argenson JN, Zannier A, Curvale G, Raoult D. Oral rifampin plus ofloxacin for treatment of Staphylococcus-infected orthopedic implants. Antimicrob Agents Chemother 1993;37:1214–1218.

42. Dugdale DC, Ramsey PG. Staphylococcus aureus bacteremia in patients with Hickman catheters. Am J Med 1990;89:137–141.

43. Dworkin RJ, Lee BL, Sande MA, Chambers HF. Treatment of right-sided Staphylococcus aureus endocarditis in intravenous drug users with ciprofloxacin and rifampin. Lancet 1989;ii:1071–1073.

44. Ehni WF, Reller LB. Short course therapy for catheter-associated Staphylococcus aureus bacteremia. Arch Intern Med 1989;149:533–536.

45. Eliopoulos GM, Reiszner E, Moellering RC Jr. In vitro activity of Sch 34343 against enterococci and other gram-positive bacteria. Antimicrob Agents Chemother 1985;27:28–32.

46. Ellison RT, Judson FN, Peterson LC, Cohn DL, Ehret JM. Oral rifampin and trimethoprim/sulfamethoxazole therapy in asymptomatic carriers of methicillin-resistant Staphylococcus aureus infections. West J Med 1984;140:735–740.

47. Elwell LP, Wilson HR, Knick VB, Keith BR. In vitro and in vivo efficacy of the combination trimethoprim-sulfamethoxazole against clinical isolates of methicillin-resistant Staphylococcus aureus. Antimicrob Agents Chemother 1986;29:1092–1094.

48. Eng RHK, Bishburg E, Smith SM, Scadutto P. Staphylococcus aureus bacteremia during therapy. J Infect Dis 1987;155:1331–1335.

49. Everett ED, Strausbaugh LJ. Antimicrobial agents and the central nervous system. Neurosurgery 1980;6:691–714.

50. Fairley CK, McNeil JJ, Desmond P, Smallwood R, Young H, Forbes A, Purcell P, Boyd I. Risk factors for development of flucloxacillin-associated jaundice. Br Med J 1993;306:233–235.

51. Farber BF, Moellering RC Jr. Retrospective study of the toxicity of preparations of vancomycin from 1974 to 1981. Antimicrob Agents Chemother 1983;23:138–141.

52. Fauconneau B, De Lemos E, Pariat C, Bouquet S, Courtois P, Piriou A. Chrononephrotoxicity in rat of a vancomycin and gentamicin combination. Pharmacol Toxicol 1992;71:31–36.

53. Faville RJ, Zaske DE, Kaplan EL, Crossley K, Sabath LD, Quie PG. Staphylococcus aureus endocarditis: combined therapy with vancomycin and rifampin. JAMA 1978;240:1963–1965.

54. Fernandes CJ, Benn RAV, Nimmo GR, and the Australian Group on Antimicrobial Resistance. Multi-centre collaborative study for the in vitro evaluation of new macrolides dirithromycin and erythromycyclamine. Pathology 1995;27:74–78.

55. Finkelstein R, Sobel JD, Nagler A, Merzbach D. Staphylococcus aureus bacteremia and endocarditis: comparison of nosocomial and community-acquired infection. J Med 1984;15:193–211.

56. Fong IW, Engelking ER, Kirby WMM. Relative inactivation by Staphylococcus aureus of eight cephalosporin antibiotics. Antimicrob Agents Chemother 1976;9:939–944.

57. Fortun J, Perez-Molina JA, Anon MT, Martinez-Beltran J, Loza E, Guerrero A. Right-sided endocarditis caused by Staphylococcus aureus in drug abusers. Antimicrob Agents Chemother 1995;39:525–528.

58. Gardner P, Leipzig T, Phillips P. Infections of central nervous system shunts. Med Clin North Am 1985;69:297–314.

59. Geraci JE, Wilson WR. Vancomycin therapy for infective endocarditis. Rev Infect Dis 1981;3:S250–S258.

60. Giamarellou H, Voutsinas D, Xirouchaki. Comparative in vitro activity of sparfloxacin (AT 4140, RP 64206-SPFX) against 275 multiresistant clinical isolates. J Chemother 1992;4:12–15.

61. Gopal V, Bisno AL, Silverblatt FJ. Failure of vancomycin treatment in Staphylococcus aureus endocarditis: in vivo and in vitro observations. JAMA 1976;236:1604–1606.

62. Gordon JJ, Harter DH, Phair JP. Meningitis due to Staphylococcus aureus. Am J Med 1985;78:965–970.

63. Gransden WR, Eykyn SJ, Philips I. Staphylococcus aureus bacteremia: 400 episodes in St. Thomas's Hospital. Br Med J 1984;288:300–303.

64. Greenberg RN, Kennedy DJ, Reilly PM, Luppen KL, Weinandt WT, Bollinger MR, Aguirre F, Kodesch F, Saeed AM. Treatment of bone, joint, and soft-tissue infections with oral ciprofloxacin. Antimicrob Agents Chemother 1987;31:151–155.

65. Gump DW. Vancomycin for treatment of bacterial meningitis. Rev Infect Dis 1981;3:S289–S292.

66. Hackbarth CJ, Chambers HF, Sande MA. Serum bactericidal activity of rifampin in combination with other antimicrobial agents against Staphylococcus aureus. Antimicrob Agents Chemother 1986;29:611–613.

67. Hackbarth CJ, Chambers HF, Sande MA. Serum bactericidal titer as a predictor of outcome in endocarditis. Eur J Clin Microbiol 1986;5:93–97.

68. Hardy DJ, Hensey DM, Beyer JM, Vojtko C, McDonald EJ, Fernandes PB. Comparative in vitro activities of new 14-, 15-, and 16-membered macrolides. Antimicrob Agents Chemother 1988;32:1710–1719.

69. Hartstein AI, Mulligan ME, Morthland VH, Kwok RYY. Recurrent Staphylococcus aureus bacteremia. J Clin Microbiol 1992;30:670–674.

70. Heldman AW, Hartert TV, Ray SC, Daoud EG, Kowalski TE, Pompili VJ, Sisson SD, Tidmore WC, vom Eigen KA, Goodman SN, Lietman PS, Petty BG, Flexner C. Oral antibiotic treatment of right-sided staphylococcal endocarditis in injection drug users: prospective randomized comparison with parenteral therapy. Am J Med 1996;101:68–76.

71. Henry NK, Rouse MS, Whitesell AL, McConnell ME, Wilson

WR. Treatment of methicillin-resistant *Staphylococcus aureus* experimental osteomyelitis with ciprofloxacin or vancomycin alone or in combination with rifampin. Am J Med 1987;82 (Suppl 4A):73–75.

72. Hill RLR, Duckworth GJ, Casewell MW. Elimination of nasal carriage of methicillin-resistant *Staphylococcus aureus* with mupirocin during a hospital outbreak. J Antimicrob Chemother 1988;22:377–384.

73. Hiramatsu K, Hanaki H, Ino T, Yabatu K, Oguri T, Tenover FC. Methicillin-resistant *Staphylococcus aureus* clinical strain with reduced vancomycin susceptibility. J Antimicrob Chemother 1997;40:135–136.

74. Ivey FM, Hicks CA, Calhoun JH, Mader JT. Treatment options for infected knee arthroplasties. Rev Infect Dis 1990;12: 468 478.

75. Jensen K, Lassen HCA. Combined treatment with antibacterial chemotherapeutical agents in staphylococcal infections. Q J Med 1969;38:91–106.

76. Jernigan JA, Farr BM. Short-course therapy of catheter-related *Staphylococcus aureus* bacteremia: a meta-analysis. Ann Intern Med 1993;119:304–311.

77. Johnson AP, Uttley AC, Woodford N, George RC. Resistance to vancomycin and teicoplanin: an emerging clinical problem. Clin Microbiol Rev 1990;3:280–291.

78. Julander I. Unfavourable prognostic factors in *Staphylococcus aureus* septicemia and endocarditis. Scand J Infect Dis 1985; 17:179–187.

79. Kaatz GW, Seo SM, Barriere SL, Albrecht LM, Rybak MJ. Ciprofloxacin and rifampin, alone and in combination, for therapy of experimental *Staphylococcus aureus* endocarditis. Antimicrob Agents Chemother 1989;33:1184–1187.

80. Kaatz GW, Seo SM, Dorman NJ, Lerner SA. Emergence of teicoplanin resistance during therapy of *Staphylococcus aureus* endocarditis. J Infect Dis 1990;162:103–108.

81. Kaatz GW, Seo SM, Ruble CA. Mechanisms of fluoroquinolone resistance in *Staphylococcus aureus*. J Infect Dis 1991;163: 1080–1086.

82. Kapusnik JE, Parenti F, Sande MA. The use of rifampin in staphylococcal infections: a review. J Antimicrob Chemother 1984;13:61–66.

83. Karchmer AW. Staphylococcal endocarditis: laboratory and clinical basis for antibiotic therapy. Am J Med 1985;78(Suppl 6B):116–127.

84. Karchmer AW. *Staphylococcus aureus* and vancomycin: the sequel. Ann Intern Med 1991;115:739–740.

85. Kauffman CA, Terpenning MS, He X, Zarins LT, Ramsey MA, Jorgensen KA, Sottile WS, Bradley SF. Attempts to eradicate methicillin-resistant *Staphylococcus aureus* from a long-term-care facility with the use of mupirocin ointment. Am J Med 1993;94:371–378.

86. Kerry DW, Hamilton-Miller JMT, Brumfitt W. Trimethoprim and rifampicin: in vitro activities separately and in combination. J Antimicrob Chemother 1975;1:417–427.

87. Kim JH, van der Horst C, Mulrow CD, Corey GR. *Staphylococcus aureus* meningitis: review of 28 cases. Rev Infect Dis 1989;11:698–706.

88. Knudsen AM, Rosdahl VT, Espersen F, Frimodt-Moller N, Skinhoj P, Bentzon MW. Catheter-related *Staphylococcus aureus* infections. J Hosp Infect 1993;23:123–131.

89. Korvick JA, Meek J, Mulligan M. A prospective, randomized trial of ciprofloxacin vs. ciprofloxacin/rifampin for eradication of methicillin-resistant *Staphylococcus aureus* colonization in a nursing home [Abstract 646]. 29th Interscience Conference on Antimicrobial Agents and Chemotherapy. Houston, 1989.

90. Korzeniowski O, Sande MA, the National Collaborative Endocarditis Study Group. Combination antimicrobial therapy for *Staphylococcus aureus* endocarditis in patients addicted to parenteral drugs and in nonaddicts: a prospective study. Ann Intern Med 1982;97:496–503.

91. Kucers A, Bennett NMcK. The use of antibiotics, 4th ed. London: William Heinemann, 1987.

92. Kunin CM, Brandt D, Wood H. Bacteriologic studies of rifampin, a new semisynthetic antibiotic. J Infect Dis 1969;119: 132–137.

93. Lautenschlager S, Herzog C, Zimmerli W. Course and outcome of bacteremia due to *Staphylococcus aureus*. Clin Infect Dis 1993;16:567–573.

94. Lawlor MT, Sullivan MC, Levitz RE, Quintiliani R, Nightingale CH. Treatment of prosthetic valve endocarditis due to methicillin-resistant *Staphylococcus aureus* with minocycline. J Infect Dis 1990;161:812–814.

95. Leclercq R, Courvalin P. Bacterial resistance to macrolide, lincosamide and streptogramin antibiotics by target modification. Antimicrob Agents Chemother 1991;35:1267–1272.

96. Leport C, Perronne C, Massip P, Canton P, Leclercq P, Bernard E, Lutun P, Garaud JJ, Vilde JL. Evaluation of teicoplanin for treatment of endocarditis caused by gram-positive cocci in 20 patients. Antimicrob Agents Chemother 1989;33:871–876.

97. Levine DP, Cushing RD, Jui J, Brown WJ. Community-acquired methicillin-resistant *Staphylococcus aureus* endocarditis in Detroit Medical Center. Ann Intern Med 1982;97: 330–338.

98. Levine DP, Fromm BS, Reddy BR. Slow response to vancomycin or vancomycin plus rifampin in methicillin-resistant *Staphylococcus aureus* endocarditis. Ann Intern Med 1991; 115:674–680.

99. Lewis PJ, Martino P, Mosconi G, Harding I. Teicoplanin in endocarditis: a multicentre, open European study. Chemotherapy 1995;41:399–411.

100. Libman H, Arbeit RD. Complications associated with *Staphylococcus aureus* bacteremia. Arch Intern Med 1984;144: 541–545.

101. MacGowan A, White L, Reeves D, Harding I. Retrospective review of serum teicoplanin concentrations in clinical trials and their relationship to clinical outcome. J Infect Chemother 1996; 197–208.

102. Maguire GP, Arthur AD, Boustead PJ, Dwyer B, Currie BJ. Emerging epidemic of community-acquired methicillin-resistant *Staphylococcus aureus* infection in the Northern Territory. Med J Aust 1996;164:721–723.

103. Maki DG, Weise CE, Sarafin HW. A semiquantitative culture method for identifying intravenous catheter-related infection. N Engl J Med 1977;296:1305–1309.

104. Malanoski GJ, Samore MH, Pefanis A, Karchmer AW. *Staphylococcus aureus* catheter-associated bacteremia: minimal effective therapy and unusual infectious complications associated with arterial sheath catheters. Arch Intern Med 1995;155: 1161–1166.

105. Maple PAC, Hamilton-Miller JMT, Brumfitt W. World-wide antibiotic resistance in methicillin-resistant *Staphylococcus aureus*. Lancet 1989;i:537–540.

106. Markowitz N, Quinn EL, Saravolatz LD. Trimethoprim-sulfamethoxazole compared with vancomycin for the treatment

of *Staphylococcus aureus* infection. Ann Intern Med 1992;117: 390–398.

107. Massanari RM, Donta ST. The efficacy of rifampin as adjunctive therapy in selected cases of staphylococcal endocarditis. Chest 1978;73:371–375.

108. Melchior NH. Combined in vitro activity of fusidic acid and rifampicin against methicillin-resistant *Staphylococcus aureus* strains. In: Ishigami J, ed. Recent advances in chemotherapy, antimicrobial section I. Proceedings of the 14th International Congress of Chemotherapy, Kyoto. Tokyo: University of Tokyo Press, 1985:582–583.

109. Mellors JW, Coleman DL, Andriole VT. Value of the serum bactericidal test in management of patients with bacterial endocarditis. Eur J Clin Microbiol 1986;5:67–70.

110. Minmuth JN, Holmes TM, Musher DM. Activity of tetracycline, doxycycline, and minocycline against methicillin-susceptible and -resistant staphylococci. Antimicrob Agents Chemother 1974;6:411–414.

111. Mirimanoff RO, Glauser MP. Endocarditis during *Staphylococcus aureus* septicemia in a population of non-drug addicts. Arch Intern Med 1982;142:1311–1313.

112. Moorman DR, Mandell GL. Characteristics of rifampin-resistant variants obtained from clinical isolates of *Staphylococcus aureus*. Antimicrob Agents Chemother 1981;20:709–713.

113. Mortara LA, Bayer AS. *Staphylococcus aureus* bacteremia and endocarditis. Infect Dis Clin North Am 1993;7:53–68.

113a. Muder RR, Boldin C, Brennen C, Hsieh M, Vickers RM, Mitchum K, Yee YC. A controlled trial of rifampicin plus minocycline, and rifampicin for eradication of methicillin resistant Staphylococcus aureus in long term care patients. J Antimicrob Chemother 1994;34:188–190.

114. Mulazimoglu L, Drenning SD, Muder RR. Vancomycin-gentamicin synergism revisited: effect of gentamicin susceptibility of methicillin-resistant *Staphylococcus aureus*. Antimicrob Agents Chemother 1996;40:1534–1535.

115. Mulligan ME, Murray-Leisure KA, Ribner BS, Standiford HC, John JF, Korvick JA, Kauffman CA, Yu VL. Methicillin-resistant *Staphylococcus aureus:* a consensus review of the microbiology, pathogenesis, and epidemiology with implications for prevention and management. Am J Med 1993;94:313–328.

116. Mulligan ME, Ruane PJ, Johnston L, Wong P, Wheelock JP, MacDonald K, Reinhardt JF, Johnson CC, Statner B, Blomquist I, McCarthy J, O'Brien W, Gardner S, Hammer L, Citron DM. Ciprofloxacin for eradication of methicillin-resistant *Staphylococcus aureus* colonization. Am J Med 1987;82(Suppl 4A): 215–219.

117. Murakami K, Tomasz A. Involvement of multiple genetic determinants in high-level methicillin resistance in Staphylococcus aureus. J Bacteriol 1989;171:874–879.

118. Musher DM, Lamm N, Darouiche RO, Young EJ, Hamill RJ, Landon GC. The current spectrum of *Staphylococcus aureus* infection in a tertiary care hospital. Medicine 1994;73:186–208.

119. Mylotte JM, McDermott C, Spooner JA. Prospective study of 114 consecutive episodes of *Staphylococcus aureus* bacteremia. Rev Infect Dis 1987;8:891–907.

120. Neu HC, Chin NX, Huang HB. In vitro activity and beta-lactamase stability of FK-037, a parenteral cephalosporin. Antimicrob Agents Chemother 1993;37:566–573.

121. Neu HC, Chin NX. In vitro activity and beta-lactamase stability of a new difluoro oxacephem, 6315-S. Antimicrob Agents Chemother 1986;30:638–644.

122. Nicolau DP, Freeman CD, Nightingale CH, Coe CJ, Quintiliani R. Minocycline versus vancomycin for treatment of experimen-

tal endocarditis caused by oxacillin-resistant *Staphylococcus aureus*. Antimicrob Agents Chemother 1994;38:1515–1522.

123. Norden CW, Bryant R, Palmer D, Montgomerie JZ, Wheat J, and the Chronic Staphylococcal Osteomyelitis Study Group. Chronic osteomyelitis caused by *Staphylococcus aureus:* controlled clinical trial of nafcillin therapy and nafcillin-rifampin therapy. South Med J 1986;79:947–951.

124. Pelletier LL, Baker CB. Oxacillin, cephalothin, and vancomycin tube macrodilution MBC result reproducibility and equivalence to MIC results for methicillin-susceptible and reputedly tolerant *Staphylococcus aureus* isolates. Antimicrob Agents Chemother 1988;32:374–377.

125. Pelletier LL. Lack of reproducibility of macrodilution MBCs for *Staphylococcus aureus*. Antimicrob Agents Chemother 1984; 26:815–818.

126. Peterson LR, Quick JN, Jensen B, Homann S, Johnson S, Tenquist J, Shanholtzer C, Petzel RA, Sinn L, Gerding DN. Emergence of ciprofloxacin resistance in nosocomial methicillin-resistant *Staphylococcus aureus* isolates: resistance during ciprofloxacin plus rifampin therapy for methicillin-resistant *S. aureus* colonization. Arch Intern Med 1990;150:2151–2155.

127. Price EH, Brain A, Dickinson JAS. An outbreak of infection with a gentamicin and methicillin-resistant *Staphylococcus aureus* in a neonatal unit. J Hosp Infect 1980;1:221–228.

128. Qadri SMH, Ueno Y, Postle G, Tullo D, Pedro JS. Comparative activity of the new fluoroquinolone rufloxacin (MF 934) against clinical isolates of gram-negative and gram-positive bacteria. Eur J Clin Microbiol Infect Dis 1993;12:372–377.

129. Quarles LD, Rutsky EA, Rostand SG. *Staphylococcus aureus* bacteremia in patients on chronic hemodialysis. Am J Kidney Dis 1985;6:412–419.

130. Quinn EL, Pohlod D, Madhavan T, Burch K, Fisher E, Cox F. Clinical experiences with cefazolin and other cephalosporins in bacterial endocarditis. J Infect Dis 1973;128(Suppl):S386–391.

131. Raad I, Narro J, Khan A, Tarrand J, Vartivarian S, Bodey GP. Serious complications of vascular catheter-related Staphylococcus aureus bacteremia in cancer patients. Eur J Clin Microbiol Infect Dis 1992;11:675–682.

132. Rahal JJ Jr. Preventing second-generation complications due to *Staphylococcus aureus*. Arch Intern Med 1989;149:503–504.

133. Rahal JJ Jr, Chan YK, Johnson G. Relationship of staphylococcal tolerance, teichoic acid antibody, and serum bactericidal activity to therapeutic outcome in *Staphylococcus aureus* bacteremia. Am J Med 1986;81:43–52.

134. Rahal JJ. *Staphylococcus aureus* [Letter]. N Engl J Med 1984; 311:796.

135. Reagan DR, Doebbeling BN, Pfaller MA, Sheetz CT, Houston AK, Hollis RJ, Wenzel RP. Elimination of coincident *Staphylococcus aureus* nasal and hand carriage with intranasal application of mupirocin calcium ointment. Ann Intern Med 1991; 114:101–106.

136. Regamey C, Libke RD, Engelking ER, Clarke JT, Kirby WMM. Inactivation of cefazolin, cephaloridine, and cephalothin by methicillin-sensitive and methicillin-resistant strains of *Staphylococcus aureus*. J Infect Dis 1975;131:291–294.

137. Reymann MT, Holley HP Jr, Cobbs CG. Persistent bacteremia in staphylococcal endocarditis. Am J Med 1978;65:729–737.

138. Ribera E, Gomez-Jimenez J, Cortes E, del Valle O, Planes A, Gonzalez-Alujas T, Almirante B, Ocana I, Pahissa A. Effectiveness of cloxacillin with and without gentamicin in short-term therapy for right-sided *Staphylococcus aureus* endocarditis. A randomized, controlled trial. Ann Intern Med 1996;125: 969–974.

139. Riley TV, Pearman JW, Rouse IL. Changing epidemiology of methicillin-resistant *Staphylococcus aureus* in Western Australia. Med J Aust 1995;163:412–414.

140. Roccaforte JS, Bittner MJ, Stumpf CA, Preheim LC. Attempts to eradicate methicillin-resistant *Staphylococcus aureus* colonization with the use of trimethoprim-sulfamethoxazole, rifampin and bacitracin. Am J Infect Control 1988;16:141–146.

141. Rolston KVI, Nguyen H, Messer M. In vitro activity of LY264826, a new glycopeptide antibiotic, against grampositive bacteria isolated from patients with cancer. Antimicrob Agents Chemother 1990;34:2137–2141.

142. Sader HS, Jones RN. Antimicrobial activity of the new carbapenem biapenem compared to imipenem, meropenem and other broad-spectrum beta-lactam drugs. Eur J Clin Microbiol Infect Dis 1993;12:384–391.

143. Sande MA, Courtney KB. Nafcillin-gentamicin synergism in experimental staphylococcal endocarditis. J Lab Clin Med 1976;88:118–124.

144. Sande MA, Johnson ML. Antimicrobial therapy of experimental endocarditis caused by *Staphylococcus aureus*. J Infect Dis 1975;131:367–375.

145. Sande MA, Mandell GL. Effect of rifampin on nasal carriage of *Staphylococcus aureus*. Antimicrob Agents Chemother 1975;7:294–297.

146. Sande MA, Scheld WM. Combination antibiotic therapy of bacterial endocarditis. Ann Intern Med 1980;92:390–395.

147. Schaefler S. Methicillin-resistant strains of *Staphylococcus aureus* resistant to quinolones. J Clin Microbiol 1989;27:335–336.

148. Schlesinger LS, Ross SC, Schaberg DR. *Staphylococcus aureus* meningitis: a broad-based epidemiologic study. Medicine 1987;66:148–156.

149. Schmalzried TP, Amstutz HC, Au MK, Dorey FJ. Etiology of deep sepsis in total hip arthroplasty. Clin Orthop 1992;280:200–207.

150. Segreti J, Gvazdinskas LC, Trenholme GM. In vitro activity of minocycline and rifampin against staphylococci. Diagn Microbiol Infect Dis 1989;12:253–255.

151. Shah M, Watanakunakorn C. Changing patterns of *Staphylococcus aureus* bacteremia. Am J Med Sci 1979;278:115–121.

152. Shalit I, Berger SA, Gorea A, Frimerman H. Widespread quinolone resistance among methicillin-resistant *Staphylococcus aureus* isolates in a general hospital. Antimicrob Agents Chemother 1989;33:593–594.

153. Sherertz RJ, Raad I, Belani A, Koo LC, Rand KH, Pickett DL, Straub SA, Fauerbach LL. Three-year experience with sonicated vascular catheter cultures in a clinical microbiology laboratory. J Clin Microbiol 1990;28:76–82.

154. Small PM, Chambers HF. Vancomycin for *Staphylococcus aureus* endocarditis in intravenous drug users. Antimicrob Agents Chemother 1990;34:1227–1231.

155. Smith SM, Eng RH, Tecson-Tumang F. Ciprofloxacin therapy for methicillin-resistant *Staphylococcus aureus* infections or colonizations. Antimicrob Agents Chemother 1989;33:181–184.

156. Smith SM, Eng RHK, Bais P, Fan-Harvad P, Tecson-Tumang F. Epidemiology of ciprofloxacin resistance among patients with methicillin-resistant *Staphylococcus aureus*. J Antimicrob Chemother 1990;26:567–572.

157. Steckelberg JM, Rouse MS, Tallan BM, Osmon DR, Henry NK, Wilson WR. Relative efficacies of broad-spectrum cephalosporins for treatment of methicillin-susceptible *Staphylococcus aureus* experimental infective endocarditis. Antimicrob Agents Chemother 1993;37:554–558.

158. Sullam PM, Tauber MG, Hackbarth CJ, Chambers HF, Scott KG, Sande MA. Pefloxacin therapy for experimental endocarditis caused by methicillin-susceptible or methicillin-resistant strains of *Staphylococcus aureus*. Antimicrob Agents Chemother 1985;27:685–687.

159. Sultan T, Baltch AL, Smith RP, Ritz W. In vitro activity of cefdinir (FK482) and ten other antibiotics against gram-positive and gram-negative bacteria isolated from adult and pediatric patients. Chemotherapy 1994;40:80–91.

160. Tan TQ, Mason EO Jr, Ou CN, Kaplan SL. Use of intravenous rifampin in neonates with persistent staphylococcal bacteremia. Antimicrob Agents Chemother 1993;37:2401–2406.

161. Taylor PC, Schoenknecht FD, Sherris JC, Linner EC. Determination of minimum bactericidal concentrations of oxacillin for *Staphylococcus aureus:* influence and significance of technical factors. Antimicrob Agents Chemother 1983;23:142–150.

162. Tetzlaff TR, McCracken GH Jr, Nelson JD. Oral antibiotic therapy for skeletal infections of children. J Pediatr 1978;92:485–490.

163. Torres-Tortosa M, de Cuerto M, Vergara A, Sanchez-Porto A, Perez-Guzman E, Gonzalez-Serrano M, Canneto J, Grupo de Estudio de Enfermedades Infecciosas de la Provincia de Cadiz. Prospective evaluation of a two-week course of intravenous antibiotics in intravenous drug addicts with infective endocarditis. Eur J Clin Microbiol Infect Dis 1994;13:559–564.

164. Tuazon CU, Sheagren JN. Relapse of staphylococcal endocarditis after clindamycin therapy. Am J Med Sci 1975;269: 145–148.

165. Tuazon CU, Lin MYC, Sheagren JN. In vitro activity of rifampin alone and in combination with nafcillin and vancomycin against pathogenic strains of *Staphylococcus aureus*. Antimicrob Agents Chemother 1978;13:759–761.

166. Turner IB, Eckstein RP, Riley JW, Lunzer MR. Prolonged cholestasis after flucloxacillin therapy. Med J Aust 1989;151:701–705.

167. Turnidge JD, McDonald PJ and the Staphylococcal Study Group. Multi-centre controlled trial of flucloxacillin plus rif-ampicin in serious staphylococcal infection. Interscience Conference on Antimicrobial Agents and Chemotherapy, 1986, New Orleans.

168. Turnidge JD, Nimmo GR, Francis G. Evolution of resistance in *Staphylococcus aureus* in Australian teaching hospitals. Med J Aust 1996;164:68–71.

169. Turnidge JD. Pharmacodynamics of beta-lactams. Clin Infect Dis 1997, in press.

170. Utrup LJ, Finlay JE, Rittenhouse SF, Poupard JA. Comparison of mupirocin susceptibility of nasal and nonnasal *Staphylococcus aureus* isolates. Diagn Microbiol Infect Dis 1994;20: 171–174.

171. Van Der Auwera P, Klastersky J, Thys JP, Meunier-Carpentier F, Legrand JC. Double-blind, placebo-controlled study of oxacillin combined with rifampin in the treatment of staphylococcal infections. Antimicrob Agents Chemother 1985;467–472.

172. Verbist L. The antimicrobial activity of fusidic acid. J Antimicrob Chemother 1990;25(Suppl B):1–5.

173. Waldvogel FA. *Staphylococcus aureus*. In: Mandell GL, ed. Principles and practice of infectious diseases. 4th ed. New York: Churchill Livingstone, 1995:1754–1777.

174. Waldvogel FA. Treatment of osteomyelitis and septic arthritis. Bull NY Acad Med 1982;58:733–749.

175. Walsh TJ, Standiford HC, Reboli AC, John JF, Mulligan ME, Ribner BS, Montgomerie JZ, Goetz MB, Mayhall CG, Rimland D, Stevens DA, Hansen SL, Gerard GC, Ragual RJ. Randomized double-blinded trail of rifampin with either novobiocin or trimethoprim-sulfamethoxazole against methicillin-resistant

Staphylococcus aureus colonization: prevention of antimicrobial resistance and effect of host factors on outcome. Antimicrob Agents Chemother 1993;37:1334–1342.

176. Ward TT, Winn RE, Hartstein AI, Sewell DL. Observations relating to an inter-hospital outbreak of methicillin-resistant *Staphylococcus aureus:* role of antimicrobial therapy in infection control. Infect Control 1981;2:453–459.

177. Watanakunakorn C, Baird IM. Prognostic factors in *Staphylococcus aureus* endocarditis and results of therapy with a penicillin and gentamicin. Am J Med Sci 1977;273:133–139.

178. Watanakunakorn C, Guerriero JC. Interaction between vancomycin and rifampin against *Staphylococcus aureus*. Antimicrob Agents Chemother 1981;19:1089–1091.

179. Watanakunakorn C, Tan JS, Phair JP. Some salient features of *Staphylococcus aureus* endocarditis. Am J Med 1973;54:473–478.

180. Watanakunakorn C. Clindamycin therapy of *Staphylococcus aureus* endocarditis: clinical relapse and development of resistance to clindamycin, lincomycin, and erythromycin. Am J Med 1976;60:419–425.

181. Weinstein MP, Stratton CW, Ackley A, Hawley HB, Robinson PA, Fisher BD, Alcid DV, Stephens DS, Reller LB. Multicenter collaborative evaluation of a standardized serum bactericidal test as a prognostic indicator in infective endocarditis. Am J Med 1985;78:262–269.

182. Weinstein MP, Stratton CW, Hawley HB, Ackley A, Reller LB. Multicenter collaborative evaluation of a standardized serum

183. Wiedemann B, Grimm H. Susceptibility to antibiotics: species incidence and trends. In: Lorian V, ed. Antibiotics in laboratory medicine. 4th ed. Baltimore: Williams & Wilkins, 1996:900–1168.

184. Williams JD. Spectrum of activity of azithromycin. Eur J Clin Microbiol Infect Dis 1991;10:813–820.

185. Wilson APR, Gruneberg RN, Neu H. A critical review of the dosage of teicoplanin in Europe and the USA. Int J Antimicrob Agents 1994;4(Suppl 1):1–30.

186. Wilson R, Hamburger M. Fifteen years' experience with staphylococcus septicemia in a large city hospital: analysis of fifty-five cases in the Cincinnati General Hospital 1940 to 1954. Am J Med 1957;22:437–457.

187. Winn RE. Epidemiological, bacteriological, and clinical observations on an interhospital outbreak of nafcillin-resistant *Staphylococcus aureus*. In: Nelson JD, Grassi C, eds. Current chemotherapy and infectious disease. Washington, DC: American Society for Microbiology, 1980:1096.

188. Yu VL, Goetz A, Wagener M, Smith PB, Rihs JD, Hanchett J, Zuravleff JJ. *Staphylococcus aureus* nasal carriage and infection in patients on hemodialysis: efficacy of antibiotic prophylaxis. N Engl J Med 1986;315:91–96.

189. Zinner SH, Lagast H, Klastersky J. Antistaphylococcal activity of rifampin with other antibiotics. J Infect Dis 1981;144: 365–371.

bactericidal test as a predictor of therapeutic efficacy in acute and chronic osteomyelitis. Am J Med 1987;83:218–222.

Staphylococcus epidermidis and Other Coagulase-Negative Staphylococci

Ross J. Davidson and Donald E. Low

There are many challenges in the management of patients who have cultures positive for coagulase-negative staphylococci. Foremost is determining whether or not the isolate represents the etiologic agent of an infectious process or is a contaminant. Although coagulase-negative staphylococci comprise at least 32 species, relatively few are associated with clinical disease. Even those that have been recognized as important pathogens, with the exception of *S. saprophyticus,* usually cause infection only in the presence of a foreign body and/or in a patient who is severely immunocompromised. Having decided that an infection is due to a coagulase-negative staphylococcus, the clinician is faced with finding a suitable antimicrobial regimen. Coagulase-negative staphylococci isolated from nosocomial infections are usually resistant to multiple antibiotics, thus limiting treatment options. Finally, for infections associated with a foreign body, a decision must be made regarding its removal and if not, the length of treatment. This chapter aims at aiding the physician in making these decisions.

GENERAL DESCRIPTION

Staphylococci are members of the family *Micrococcaceae.* They are Gram positive and catalase positive and occur singly and in irregular grapelike clusters (a description from which their name originates). Host factors that predispose to coagulase-negative staphylococci infections include immunosuppression and presence of a foreign body. Under any of these circumstances, no one species appears to predisposes to such infections (97). However, some species of coagulase-negative staphylococci have been associated with particular infections other than those involving immunosuppression or a foreign body. *S. saprophyticus* accounts for up to 10% of uncomplicated urinary tract infections in young women (107, 185). *S. schleiferi, S. lugdunensis,* and *S. haemolyticus* may cause native valve endocarditis (56, 106, 117). Speciation of coagulase-negative staphylococci is based on the original work of Kloos and Schleifer (98). Commercially available identification systems based on these conventional tests can provide an easy and rapid means of speciation.

With multiple isolates, it is useful to determine relatedness to aid in deciding if they are contaminants. This can be accomplished by using a combination of antibiograms and biotyping (45, 49, 69, 71, 117). Khatib et al. (96) determined the MICs of isolates to 10 antibiotics. They found that identical antibiograms were highly predictive of strain relatedness, whereas a 4-fold difference in a single MIC was not.

SUSCEPTIBILITY IN VITRO AND IN VIVO

The unpredictability of antimicrobial susceptibility and the need to identify methicillin resistance require routine susceptibility testing on all clinical isolates of coagulase-negative staphylococci. The list of antimicrobials to be tested is derived from recommendations in the National Committee for Clinical Laboratory Standards (NCCLS) (131–133). Clinical laboratories may choose from among several manual or commercial instrument-based susceptibility methods. These include disk diffusion, agar or broth microdilution, antibiotic gradient, and manual or automated commercial methods. The NCCLS Subcommittee on Antibiotic Susceptibility Testing has published documents that describe methods, contain guidelines for interpreting results, and outline quality control test criteria. These are published every 3 years with annual updates. Fortunately, with the currently available systems, susceptibility testing of staphylococci is accurate, reproducible, and predictive of clinical outcome, with the exception of methicillin resistance.

The detection of methicillin resistance is essential to determine the most effective antimicrobial. In addition to special testing methodology recommended by the NCCLS, several commercial systems are now available, including nonautomated, semiautomated, and automated ones (79, 80, 99, 100, 136).

In Vitro

Single Drugs

The coagulase-negative staphylococci most frequently associated with clinical infections share similar antimicrobial susceptibility profiles, with the exception of *S. saprophyticus* and *S. haemolyticus*. *S. saprophyticus* is typically susceptible to most antimicrobials, including the aminopenicillins. *S. haemolyticus* is not only often multidrug resistant, but may also be resistant to teicoplanin and vancomycin (162, 182). The in vitro activity of antimicrobials that have been used to treat staphylococcal infections is presented in Table 1.

Combination Drugs

Lowy et al. (119) studied the synergistic effect of antimicrobial combinations in vitro using a time-kill method. Gentamicin was the single most effective agent. Addition of vancomycin to gentamicin did not significantly improve the bactericidal activity. The combination of rifampin and vancomycin was as effective as gentamicin alone. Antagonism was observed with the combinations of gentamicin and cephalothin

or nafcillin and cephalothin and vancomycin. A further study by Lowy et al. (118) reexamined the combinations of rifampin with vancomycin or gentamicin. The combination of rifampin and gentamicin demonstrated enhanced killing in 13 of 17 strains, while the combination of rifampin and vancomycin showed enhanced killing in 13 of 25 strains. However, rifampin resistance emerged in 12 of 25 strains with the latter combination.

Clindamycin has been shown to enhance the bactericidal effect of rifampin in vitro (7). Synergy between clindamycin and rifampin was observed in 6 of 12 strains of methicillin-susceptible *S. epidermidis* examined by time-kill methodology. Svensson et al. (170) studied the effect of antimicrobial combinations on both growing and nongrowing cells of methicillin-resistant *S. epidermidis*. They demonstrated that imipenem combined with either amikacin or vancomycin displayed synergy against actively growing cells. In nongrowing cells, synergy was not observed with any combination of drugs.

In Vivo

Single and Combination Drugs

There are very few in vivo studies evaluating the efficacy of single-drug therapy, since most coagulase-negative staphylococci infections are treated with a combination of drugs. Typically, antimicrobial combinations are used to provide broad-spectrum empirical coverage or because an identified pathogen is resistant to inhibition and/or killing by conventional doses of single antimicrobials. However, the two most frequent reasons for using combination antimicrobial therapy for coagulase-negative staphylococci infections are to improve the outcome of foreign body–related infections and to prevent the emergence of resistance. Addition of gentamicin, rifampin, or both to vancomycin has improved cure rates and reduced the emergence of resistance in both animal and human studies (91, 101, 181, 187). Although rifampin combination with other agents has sometimes resulted in antagonism in vitro, the clinical relevance of such findings are unknown (67, 120).

Brandt et al. (23) compared the efficacy of cefazolin and cefpirome, alone or in combination with rifampin, with that of vancomycin, alone or in combination with rifampin, in an experimental model of methicillin-resistant coagulase-negative staphylococcal endocarditis. They found that vancomycin and cefpirome had similar activities and both were more effective than cefazolin alone. Cefpirome in combination with rifampin was more effective than cefazolin in combination with rifampin. Both cephalosporin-rifampin regimens were significantly more effective than cephalosporin or vancomycin monotherapy and were as effective as vancomycin combined with rifampin. The in vitro results were not predictive of the in vivo results. Addition of a second agent to rifampin prevented the emergence of rifampin resistance in vivo.

Blaser et al. (19) compared an in vitro pharmacodynamic model with an in vivo tissue cage infection model using several antimicrobial combinations. Both models demonstrated that rifampin combined with either vancomycin, teicoplanin, fleroxacin, or ciprofloxacin was significantly more bactericidal against adherent bacteria than netilmicin combined with van-

TABLE 1 • In Vitro Susceptibilities of the Coagulase-Negative Staphylococci

Antimicrobial Class	Drug	No. of Isolates	Susceptibility (μg/mL)		
			MIC$_{50}$	MIC$_{90}$	Range
Fluoroquinolones					
	Ciprofloxacin	163	0.25	0.5	0.06–32
	Norfloxacin	145	0.25	2	0.12–64
	Ofloxacin	139	0.25	1	0.12–64
	Sparfloxacin	69	0.12	0.25	0.12–8
	Trovafloxacin	43	0.003	1.0	0.001–8
Aminoglycosides					
	Gentamicin	18	0.03	16	0.015–32
	Tobramycin	158	<0.25	>16	<0.25->16
	Netilmicin	58	0.03	0.125	0.03–4
MLS antibiotics					
	Erythromycin	150	0.25	≥64	0.125–≥64
	Clindamycin	14	0.06	0.12	<0.06–≥64
	RP59500	43	0.25	0.5	0.25–1
β-Lactams					
	Penicillin	126	0.25	64	<0.06–64
	Amoxicillin/clavulanate	102	0.12	0.5	≤0.015–2
	Cephalexin	60	1	4	0.12–8
	Cefuroxime	95	0.5	2	0.25–128
	Ceftriaxone	160	4	16	0.06–32
	Cefixime	81	16	>64	0.06->64
	Imipenem	277	0.03	.25	0.016–2
	Meropenem	319	0.25	8	0.0075–8
Others					
	Doxycycline	58	0.5	2	0.06–16
	Vancomycin	325	1	2	0.25–4
	Teicoplanin	231	1	4	0.25–32
	Trimethoprim	20	0.25	4	0.12–4
	TMP/SMX[a]	117	0.125	0.5	0.03–4
	Rifampin	45	0.008	0.016	<0.002–0.03
	Fusidic acid	NS[b]	0.125	0.125	0.064–32

Collated from references 7, 9, 38, 75, 85, 86, 103, 115, 124, 129, 135, 153, 184, 192.

[a] Trimethoprim-sulfamethoxazole.

[b] Not stated.

comycin or daptomycin. A similar in vivo model was used by Widmer et al. (188) to study both monotherapy and combination therapy in the treatment of implant-associated infections. Rifampin monotherapy demonstrated significantly better efficacy than either ciprofloxacin or teicoplanin monotherapy or combination therapy with daptomycin and teicoplanin.

The antimicrobial regimens of amoxicillin-clavulanate, vancomycin, or teicoplanin, combined with netilmicin or amikacin were examined using an experimental subcutaneous fibrin clot model in rabbits (37). The combination of amoxicillin-clavulanate and netilmicin was highly synergistic and was more active in vivo than vancomycin alone or in combination.

ANTIMICROBIAL THERAPY
Drugs of Choice

β-Lactam Antibiotics

Coagulase-negative staphylococci may be penicillin sensitive, but most strains are resistant (>80–90%) because of production of an inducible β-lactamase (5). Staphylococcal penicillinases confer resistance to penicillins, ampicillin, amoxicillin,

azlocillin, mezlocillin, piperacillin, and ticarcillin. Staphylococci may only produce detectable amounts of enzyme after exposure to an inducing agent, generally a β-lactam, and enzyme is best detected with the chromogenic cephalosporin, acidometric, and iodometric tests (171).

If an isolate of staphylococci is β-lactamase negative, then penicillin is the drug of choice. The semisynthetic antistaphylococcal penicillins, which include methicillin, the isoxazolyl penicillins (oxacillin, cloxacillin, dicloxacillin, and flucloxacillin) and nafcillin, are derivatives of penicillin that are poorly hydrolyzed by staphylococcal β-lactamase. They are rapidly bactericidal against growing cells, with MICs below 2 mg/L for nafcillin and oxacillin, and below 8 mg/L for methicillin. There does not appear to be any significant differences in efficacy between these agents, and they have similar pharmacokinetic profiles (46, 105). These agents are the drugs of choice for treatment of staphylococcal infections unless the patient is hypersensitive to β-lactams or the infection is due to a methicillin-resistant strain (35). Their intrinsic potency is less than that of penicillin against β-lactamase-negative staphylococci. Oxacillin, cloxacillin, and flucloxacillin can be administered intravenously, 1 to 2 g every 4 to 6 h, depending on the severity of the illness. In the presence of severe renal impairment, the dose of cloxacillin or flucloxacillin should be reduced. Oxacillin dosage adjustment may not be necessary (105).

Glycopeptides

The MICs of vancomycin to staphylococci are typically less than 4 µg/mL; however, the MICs of the coagulase-negative staphylococci may be one- to twofold higher (116). Reduced susceptibility and resistance to vancomycin has been described in strains of *S. haemolyticus* (162, 182). Resistance has not been described in other staphylococcal species; however, a strain of *Staphylococcus aureus* with reduced susceptibility to vancomycin (MIC = 8 mg/L) has been described in Japan (74). These findings may warrant routine susceptibility testing of strains that fail vancomycin therapy. Vancomycin is less rapidly bactericidal than nafcillin, which may explain in part why it appears less efficacious than the β-lactams (113, 165). The dose of vancomycin in adults is 1 g every 12 h intravenously over 1 to 2 h to decrease infusion-related events such as the "red man syndrome."

Alternative Drugs

β-Lactam Antibiotics

Cephalosporins, particularly those of the first generation, are poor substrates for staphylococcal β-lactamase. However, the slow hydrolysis of cefazolin may account for failures in treatment of endocarditis and prophylaxis for cardiac surgery (95, 157). Doses of cefazolin are 1 g every 8 h. It is cleared renally, and the dose must be adjusted according to renal function.

Penicillin/β-Lactamase Inhibitor Combinations and Other β-Lactams

Although staphylococcal β-lactamases are inhibited by the currently available β-lactamase inhibitor combinations, these agents may induce β-lactamases as well as inhibit them (21). Currently available combinations include ampicillin/sulbactam, amoxicillin/clavulanic acid, ticarcillin/clavulanic acid, and piperacillin/tazobactam. These agents have no advantages over other narrower-spectrum antistaphylococcal antibiotics. The carbapenems, imipenem and meropenem, may appear in vitro to have activity against methicillin-resistant coagulase-negative staphylococci, but they are not effective in vivo (16, 34). They display good activity against methicillin-sensitive coagulase-negative staphylococci in vitro and in animal models but provide no advantage over the antistaphylococcal penicillins (16). The monobactams (e.g., aztreonam) have no activity against staphylococci.

Glycopeptides

Teicoplanin is a glycopeptide available in many countries other than those in North America. It is similar to vancomycin in mechanism of action and spectrum of activity, but its long half-life (>48 h) allows it to be given as a once-daily dose. Teicoplanin is highly protein bound (>95%), which may explain in part why it appears less efficacious than vancomycin. Early studies with teicoplanin showed a significant clinical failure rate that was thought to be due to the low doses (a loading dose of 400 mg followed by 200 mg/day) selected for initial studies (28). However, even with doses twice those used in the original study, breakthrough bacteremia occurred (58). Of greater concern is resistance and the emergence of resistance while on therapy, particularly in *S. haemolyticus* and *S. aureus* (33, 87, 116).

Macrolides, Lincosamides, and Streptogramins

Macrolides, lincosamides, and streptogramins are referred to as the MLS group of antimicrobials. Although they are chemically distinct, they are related by their mechanism of action: binding to the 50S ribosomal subunit and blocking protein synthesis. The macrolides include erythromycin, clarithromycin, and azithromycin. The lincosamides include clindamycin, and the streptogramin group consists of a combination of two chemically unrelated molecules, groups A and B. Group A compounds include streptogramin A, and group B compounds include streptogramin B.

In staphylococci, resistance to MLS antibiotics is acquired and is usually due to target modification or active efflux of the antibiotic. Methylation of the ribosome, causing target modification, confers broad cross-resistance to all macrolides, lincosamides, and streptogramin B antibiotics (the MLS_B phenotype) (110). Streptogramin A–type antibiotics are unaffected and remain active against MLS_B-resistant phenotypes.

Expression of MLS_B resistance may be constitutive or inducible. Clindamycin and streptogramin B are poor inducers of resistance and therefore in the laboratory strains will appear susceptible. However, mutations are common and may occur during treatment, resulting in a change from inducible to constitutive resistance. The second type of resistance, active efflux, involves erythromycin-inducible cross-resistance to other macrolides and streptogramin B, but not to clindamycin. This is referred to as the MS phenotype.

Macrolide antibiotics may be either bacteriostatic or bactericidal, depending on drug concentration and bacterial susceptibility (142). Clarithromycin is more active, and azithromycin less active, than erythromycin (1). Although erythromycin has been used extensively for treatment of *S. aureus* infections, there are few clinical examples in which it would be used to treat infections due to coagulase-negative staphylococci.

Clindamycin is bacteriostatic. Most strains of susceptible staphylococci are inhibited by 0.1 mg/L of clindamycin. Strains that are resistant to erythromycin but sensitive to clindamycin should be assumed to have an inducible methylase mechanism. In such circumstances, it has been recommended that clindamycin not be used (111).

RP59500 is a combination (30:70 w/w) of quinupristin (streptogramin B) and dalfopristin (streptogramin A). MICs are 0.25 to 1 mg/L for both methicillin-susceptible and methicillin-resistant staphylococci. Unlike macrolides, RP59500 is bactericidal for staphylococci. Inducible MLS_B-resistance strains remain sensitive to quinupristin because it does not induce methylase. However, if methylase is constitutively produced, quinupristin activity and its synergy with dalfopristin are lost, and failure may occur (48, 52). Therefore, as with clindamycin, caution is needed when treating a patient with coagulase-negative staphylococcus infection due to a strain resistant to erythromycin because of target modification, whether inducible or constitutive.

Trimethoprim-Sulfamethoxazole

The combination trimethoprim-sulfamethoxazole, which blocks folate synthesis, is bacteriostatic against staphylococci. Many multiresistant coagulase-negative staphylococci remain susceptible to trimethoprim-sulfamethoxazole, but susceptibility to these drugs is highly variable (176). Most of the experience in treating staphylococcal infections has been with S. aureus (6, 114, 122). Although it has been used successfully to treat staphylococcal endocarditis and meningitis, it has been as effective as vancomycin (40, 173).

Fluoroquinolones

The original fluoroquinolones had their greatest activity against Gram-negative bacteria. Shortly after their introduction, fluoroquinolone resistance became frequent in methicillin-resistant S. aureus (MRSA) and coagulase-negative staphylococci (177). This has limited the usefulness of these agents for treatment of staphylococcal infections with the exception of those due to S. saprophyticus (134).

Tetracyclines

Many strains of staphylococci are now resistant to tetracycline (168). Minocycline and doxycycline are highly lipophilic analogues that have greater staphylococcal activity and have been used in the treatment of S. saprophyticus urinary tract infections (107). Minocycline maintains its potency against many tetracycline-resistant staphylococci and is the primary agent for treatment of MRSA infections in some countries (109, 194). Strains resistant to tetracycline on the basis of ribosomal protection (TetM) are resistant to tetracycline and minocycline, whereas strains resistant on the basis of active efflux (TetK) are resistant to tetracycline and susceptible to minocycline (149, 163).

Aminoglycosides

The aminoglycosides are bactericidal inhibitors of protein synthesis. Aminoglycosides have been widely used to treat staphylococcal infections, often in combination with other antistaphylococcal agents. The major mechanism of aminoglycoside resistance in the staphylococci is drug inactivation by enzymes. Amikacin and netilmicin are the most active aminoglycosides in vitro (39, 63). They are usually used in combination with another antistaphylococcal agent.

Fusidic Acid

Fusidic acid, a steroidlike antibiotic, has been in clinical use since 1962 as a topical and oral preparation but has not been available in the United States. It is often used in combination with another antistaphylococcal agent to reduce the occurrence of resistance (3, 53, 57, 73, 83). It has retained excellent activity against S. aureus and coagulase-negative staphylococci, including methicillin-resistant strains, although there

are exceptions (51, 126, 175, 183). One of the characteristics of fusidic acid is its ability to penetrate, and be effective in, collections of pus, including cerebral abscesses. It is usually administered either orally or parenterally in a dose of 0.5 g every 8 h. The dosage for children is 20 mg/kg body weight daily. It is also available in a topical preparation.

Rifampin

Rifampin is the most active antistaphylococcal antibiotic (89). It blocks protein synthesis by inhibiting DNA-dependent RNA polymerase. High-level resistance can occur frequently as the result of a single amino acid change in the β-subunit of the RNA polymerase; thus it is always used in combination with another antistaphylococcal antibiotic. It can be given orally or parenterally in doses of 300 to 600 mg twice daily.

Specific Infectious Diseases

Catheter-Related Bacteremia

Coagulase-negative staphylococci are the most frequently isolated organisms in blood cultures, accounting for more than 40% of all nosocomial bloodstream infections. This is primarily due to the increasing use of intravascular and implanted prosthetic devices (12, 36, 155). Other populations at risk for coagulase-negative staphylococci bacteremia are the immunocompromised and low-birth-weight premature infants (64, 143).

Management of catheter-related infections has traditionally included the removal of the infected line. However, there is increasing evidence favoring conservative medical management when these infections are due to coagulase-negative staphylococci, especially in children (14, 164, 172, 191). Since these infections are typically nosocomial, vancomycin is often recommended as the antimicrobial of choice until results of susceptibility testing are available. However, Engelhard et al. (47) found that central vein catheter-related coagulase-negative staphylococcal bacteremias in febrile neutropenic bone marrow transplant patients had a benign clinical course even when vancomycin was not included in the initial empirical antimicrobial regimen and that these infections could be treated successfully without removing the catheter. Generally it is recommended that if the infection responds to therapy, treatment should be continued for 2 to 3 weeks. If the infection has not responded in 48 h, then the catheter should be removed and an abbreviated course of 5- to 14-days of antimicrobials given (68, 72, 151). In patients with central lines, catheter removal is almost always required when a tunnel infection or thrombophlebitis is present; however, most exit site infections can be managed medically.

Marr et al. (123) determined the incidence and outcome of catheter-related bacteremia in dual-lumen cuffed catheters used for vascular access in patients undergoing hemodialysis. They found that salvage attempts with antibiotics were less likely to succeed in patients with Gram-positive bacteremias than in those with Gram-negative bacteremia. They also found that antibiotic salvage attempts were sometimes successful, but more importantly, they were not associated with increased risk of complications.

Endocarditis

Prosthetic valve endocarditis (PVE) can be characterized as "early onset" if infection develops within 60 days of surgery and "late onset" if infection develops more than 60 days after surgery (22, 29, 178). However, there are several reports that nosocomial PVE due to coagulase-negative staphylococci may not become evident until many months after surgery (29, 178, 187). Coagulase-negative staphylococci account for approximately 25 to 48% of all cases of PVE, including 30 to 67% of early-onset PVE and 20 to 28% of late-onset PVE. When speciated, coagulase-negative staphylococci associated with PVE are found to be almost exclusively *S. epidermidis* (90, 91).

Coagulase-negative staphylococci associated with early-onset PVE are characteristically methicillin resistant (>80%), whereas most strains associated with late PVE are susceptible (9, 32, 90). Treatment regimens with the greatest clinical success have included vancomycin alone or in combination with rifampin, an aminoglycoside, or both, compared with a β-lactam alone or in combination with rifampin, an aminoglycoside, or both (91). A study compared the outcomes of patients with methicillin-resistant coagulase-negative staphylococcal PVE treated with 6 weeks of vancomycin and rifampin with outcomes of those receiving this regimen plus gentamicin during the first 2 weeks (92). Outcomes of the two regimens were similar (77 vs. 85% cure); however, rifampin-resistant organisms emerged with the first regimen but not with the three-drug regimen.

Current recommendations are for vancomycin and rifampin for 6 weeks with gentamicin added for the first 2 weeks of therapy (17, 18, 189). For optimal therapeutic efficacy, the peak and trough levels of vancomycin should be maintained at 25 to 35 mg/L and 10 to 15 mg/L, respectively (9, 187). Fluoroquinolones are an acceptable substitute if the organism is resistant to all of the aminoglycosides (189).

Indications for surgical intervention include increasing or refractory congestive heart failure due to prosthetic valve dysfunction, persistent fever due to invasion of annular or myocardial tissue, valve dehiscence or paravalvular regurgitation seen on echocardiography, persistent bacteremia on appropriate antimicrobial therapy, recurrent systemic embolization, and/or relapse after appropriate therapy.

Coagulase-negative staphylococci account for only 5% of cases of native valve endocarditis, which are being more frequently associated within the hospital setting (93, 159, 187). For methicillin-resistant coagulase-negative staphylococci, vancomycin for 4 to 6 weeks is advocated (18). Routine use of rifampin is not recommended for native valve endocarditis, unless patients do not respond to conventional antimicrobial therapy (189). Methicillin-sensitive coagulase-negative staphylococci strains can be treated with a β-lactam (17, 187, 189). β-Lactam-allergic individuals may be treated with a first-generation cephalosporin or vancomycin.

Central Nervous System Shunt Infections

Ventriculoperitoneal and ventriculoatrial shunt infections are the most common central nervous system (CNS) infections attributable to coagulase-negative staphylococci. Most shunt infections (70%) develop within 2 months of insertion, and almost 80% occur within 4 months (59, 147). Infants less than 6 months of age have a significantly higher incidence of shunt infections than do older infants (147). Approximately 60% of all shunt infections are due to coagulase-negative staphylococci (59, 147).

The treatment of choice for management of infected shunts is prompt and early removal of the shunt (127). Immediate replacement should not be attempted if organisms have been demonstrated in the cerebrospinal fluid or if the patient has an infected wound near the insertion site (161).

As methicillin-resistant coagulase-negative staphylococci are the predominate cause of shunt infections, vancomycin is the initial empirical drug of choice. However, parenteral vancomycin does not penetrate well into the cerebrospinal fluid. Thus treatment should consist of both intravenous vancomycin (2 g/day or 40 mg/kg/day in divided doses every 12 h) and either intrashunt or intraventricular vancomycin (10 mg once daily in children, 20 mg once daily in adults) (50). Vancomycin administration should be combined with oral rifampin (900–1200 mg/day or 20 mg/kg/day in divided doses every 8 h) (140, 152). For a proven methicillin-susceptible coagulase-negative staphylococcal shunt infection, intravenous nafcillin (9 –12 g/day or 300 mg/kg/day in divided doses every 4 h) is recommended (61). Vancomycin is still preferred for intraventricular therapy.

Endophthalmitis

Coagulase-negative staphylococci are the most common cause of endophthalmitis (70, 77, 146). The source of the infection is characteristically the endogenous flora of the ocular surface, introduced during cataract surgery, trauma, or phacoemulsification of the lens. Endophthalmitis caused by coagulase-negative staphylococci is often slow to develop, painless, and usually less virulent with better outcome than infections caused by other bacteria (139). Management of postoperative endophthalmitis due to coagulase-negative staphylococci remains controversial. Treatment options include parenteral antibiotics, intravitreal antibiotics, or vitrectomy and intraocular antibiotic (20, 55, 137). More recently, the use of steroids has been advocated, either topically, subconjunctivally, or by intravitreal injection (125, 166). The intraocular lens usually can be left in place (138). Since the source of the coagulase-negative staphylococci is often the patient's periocular skin flora, strains may be methicillin-sensitive (13). Adequate duration of intravitreal and/or subconjunctival antibiotic therapy has not been determined. Systemic antibiotics are usually administered concomitantly to reduce the concentration gradient and increase the half-life of vitreal drugs. The intravitreal and subconjunctival dose of vancomycin are 1 and 25 mg, respectively. The intravitreal and subconjunctival dose of gentamicin are 0.1 and 20 mg, respectively. The subconjunctival route of drug administration is being used less frequently.

Sternotomy and Prosthetic Joint Infections

The two most common forms of osteomyelitis due to coagulase-negative staphylococcal infection are sternal osteomyelitis following cardiothoracic surgery and infection of bone surrounding a prosthetic joint (41, 81).

Sternal osteomyelitis is due to coagulase-negative staphylococci in 30 to 45% of cases (41, 128, 130). In addition to antibiotics, treatment of superficial and deep infections includes the use of diagnostic techniques to determine the location and extent of infection so that infected bone and soft tissue can be debrided. Additional measures for management of deep infections remain controversial. Treatment options include delayed primary closure versus a muscle flap (24, 78, 195). The most appropriate antimicrobial or combination of antimicrobials and length of therapy have not been established, but usually up to 3 weeks of intravenous therapy is recommended (154).

Staphylococci are the most frequently isolated pathogens from prosthetic joint infections, with coagulase-negative staphylococci implicated in 20 to 50% of these infections (81). Conventional treatment includes long-term intravenous antibiotic therapy with one- or two-stage replacement of the infected implant (190). Use of antimicrobial-impregnated cement has been effective in reducing reinfection (62, 94). In an open-label study, Drancourt et al. (43) treated susceptible staphylococcus–infected orthopaedic implants orally with rifampin (900 mg/day) plus ofloxacin (600 mg/day). Patients with hip prosthesis infection were treated for 6 months, with removal of only unstable prostheses after 5 months of treatment; and patients with knee prosthesis infection were treated for 9 months, with removal of all prostheses after 6 months. The overall cure rate was 74%. In a subsequent nonblinded randomized study by Drancourt et al. (42), using identical treatment schedules, the previous regimen of rifampin plus ofloxacin was compared with rifampin (900 mg/day) and fusidic acid (1.5 g/day) for the first 5 days, followed by 1 g/day thereafter. Cure rates were similar in both groups, 50 and 55%, respectively.

Urinary Tract Infections

S. saprophyticus is associated with approximately 10 to 30% of all urinary tract infections in women 16 to 30 years of age (160, 185). The organism has been associated with recent menses and sexual intercourse (156). Seasonal variation in colonization has also been observed, with rates higher during the summer and fall (156, 185). In contrast to women, *S. saprophyticus* urinary tract infections in men are associated with indwelling urinary catheters or obstruction (76).

S. saprophyticus is generally susceptible to most antibiotics, including penicillins (10, 76). Although β-lactamase production in *S. saprophyticus* has been reported, the MICs of those strains are easily clinically attainable (108). Only rare resistance to methicillin has been reported (54). Treatment with trimethoprim-sulfamethoxazole, ampicillin, and nitrofurantoin is effective (169). Several studies have demonstrated that failure rates for single-dose therapy are significantly higher than those for 3- or 7-day regimens (10, 76, 158).

Continuous Ambulatory Peritoneal Dialysis Peritonitis

Infection remains the major complication of continuous ambulatory peritoneal dialysis. Coagulase-negative staphylococci account for approximately 40 to 50% of all infections (26, 66, 145). In view of the high incidence of methicillin-resistant coagulase-negative staphylococci, vancomycin should be included in empirical treatment of staphylococcal peritonitis. Therapy can be administered intraperitoneally at 20 mg/L. For methicillin-sensitive coagulase-negative staphylococci, cephalexin can be given orally (a 1-g loading dose and a maintenance dose of 500 mg every 6 h) (44). The combination of vancomycin and gentamicin intraperitoneally has been shown effective and significantly more efficacious than oral fluoroquinolone monotherapy for the treatment of coagulase-negative staphylococci peritonitis (15, 174). Intraperitoneal ciprofloxacin (20 mg/L) was as effective as intraperitoneal vancomycin plus gentamicin (60). Oral therapy with rifampin (600 mg/day) in conjunction with vancomycin may benefit refractory or recurrent peritonitis due to staphylococci (27). Both systemic and intraperitoneal routes of antimicrobial administration achieve drug levels sufficient to treat the infection; however, the intraperitoneal route is preferred (15, 144). In the absence of a tunnel infection or intraperitoneal abscess, antimicrobial treatment is usually successful without catheter removal.

Vascular Graft Infections

The incidence of vascular graft infections is about 1.5%, with coagulase-negative staphylococci accounting now for 15 to 40% of cases overall. The surgical approach to therapy for vascular graft infections has been complete excision of the graft and revascularization through a clean tissue bed with an extraanatomic bypass. For infected aortic grafts, one approach is extraanatomic bypass performed prior to graft excision, with graft resection and oversewing of the aorta performed several days later. Appropriate antibiotics are given for 6 to 8 weeks. Others have promoted a more conservative approach. Gordon et al. (65) used parenteral and oral antibiotics with minimal surgery, only when needed, and were able to preserve the aortic graft in 9 of 11 patients.

For extracavitary grafts, Calligaro et al. (30) attempted either subtotal graft excisions (for infected thrombosed grafts) or complete graft preservation (for infected nondisrupted grafts in nonseptic patients). Early aggressive wound debridement with excision of all surrounding infected tissue, wound healing by secondary intention, and appropriate antibiotics for 6 weeks parenterally resulted in partial or complete graft preservation in 85 and 71% of patients, respectively.

ALTERNATIVE THERAPY

There have been several novel approaches to preventing and treating catheter-related infections. Spafford et al. (167) were able to prevent central venous catheter–related coagulase-negative staphylococcal sepsis in neonates by adding 25 mg/L of vancomycin to the total parenteral nutrition solution. However, catheter colonization was reduced, not eliminated. Kacica et al. (88), using low-dose vancomycin prophylaxis in low-birth-weight infants, eliminated Gram-positive bacteremia. Despite the apparent short-term benefit, one must weigh the risk of possible emergence of vancomycin-resistant strains, especially with coagulase-negative staphylococci (162, 182).

The antibiotic lock technique has been used in an attempt to sterilize an infected catheter in vivo. It consists of filling and closing the catheter lumen with an antibiotic solution that acts locally, in hopes of sterilizing the device (31). Although randomized controlled trials have not been carried out, anecdotal reports have found this a promising means of preserving catheters and treating catheter-related sepsis, especially that due to coagulase-negative staphylococci (84, 104). For coagulase-negative staphylococcal infections, vancomycin (1 mg/mL dissolved in isotonic solution) is instilled for 12 h daily for 5 days (31). Modifications of this technique have included addition of heparin to prevent thrombosis and the use of fibrinolytic agents to lyse blood clots that could be foci of infection (8, 25, 82)

ENDPOINTS FOR MONITORING THERAPY

There are several reasons why defining endpoints for therapy of coagulase-negative staphylococci infections is difficult. Isolation of coagulase-negative staphylococci from a clinical specimen, including a sterile site, does not necessarily imply infection. Patients often present with minimal nonspecific signs and symptoms. Laboratory tests usually do not support a diagnosis of an infectious process or help resolve whether an isolate is a pathogen or contaminant. A single isolate from a blood culture is often thought to be of indeterminate significance or to represent contamination. Even two or three positive culture sets do not always represent true infection in the view of physicians (186). Often the initial presentation of a foreign body–associated infection is so benign that the diagnosis of infection is only entertained after a positive culture of the infected material (11, 59). Coagulase-negative staphylococci isolated from an otherwise sterile surgical site are sometimes even regarded only as a contaminant (141). Having made the diagnosis of infection, choosing appropriate therapy for an appropriate duration is plagued by the same problems. In addition, therapy assumed to have been effective may result in relapse months later, especially if the foreign body has not been removed (148, 193).

CONTROVERSIES, CAVEATS, AND COMMENTS

S. lugdunensis is suggested to differ from other coagulase-negative staphylococci in its predilection and aggressive clinical course in native valve endocarditis. A significantly higher mortality rate has been reported with *S. lugdunensis* than with other coagulase-negative staphylococci (102, 112). Surgical intervention is recommended by some authors. In one series, eight of nine patients not receiving a valve replacement died (179). If these observations prove true, it will be a compelling reason for the microbiology laboratory to perform accurate and timely speciation of blood culture isolates from patients suspected of having endocarditis.

Third-generation cephalosporins have been considered second-line agents for treatment of staphylococcal infections, despite good in vitro activity. Aldridge (2) reviewed both in vitro and in vivo studies over the last 15 years on the activity and efficacy of cefotaxime. He found that cefotaxime was highly active against methicillin-sensitive strains and that therapy of staphylococcal infections was associated with clinical cures/improvement rates ranging from 78 to 100%. This suggests that monotherapy with cefotaxime may be adequate for a mixed infection that includes staphylococci.

In an attempt to reduce sternal wound infections, Vander Salm et al. (180) carried out a nonblinded randomized study to determine the efficacy of topical application of vancomycin to the cut edges of the sternum. Sternal infection occurred in 1 of 223 patients who received vancomycin and 7 of 193 controls (*P* = .02). Possibly an agent could be evaluated that is not used systemically, such as bacitracin or ramoplanin.

Evidence is accumulating favoring use of catheters impregnated with antiseptics or antimicrobials to reduce catheter-related infections (121, 150). Maki et al. (121) found that chlorhexidine–silver sulfadiazine catheters were well tolerated and reduced the incidence of catheter-related infections. Although there were only two infections in the antiseptic catheter group, both were due to coagulase-negative staphylococci. Raad et al. (150) studied the value of central venous catheters coated with minocycline and rifampin in preventing catheter-related colonization and bloodstream infections. Colonization with coagulase-negative staphylococci was significantly reduced. There were no bloodstream infections per 1000 catheter-days with the antibiotic-coated catheters, compared with 7.34 bloodstream infections per 1000 catheter-days in the control group. Although authors of both studies argued that development of resistance to these regimens was unlikely, it is too early to make such predictions. If resistance did develop in Gram-positives, coagulase-negative staphylococci would be the most likely candidates (4).

REFERENCES

1. Clarithromycin and azithromycin. Med Lett 1992;34:45.
2. Aldridge KE. Cefotaxime in the treatment of staphylococcal infections. Comparison of in vitro and in vivo studies. Diagn Microbiol Infect Dis 1995;22:195–201.
3. Amirak ID, Li AK, Williams RJ, Noone P. A fatal infection caused by methicillin-resistant *Staphylococcus aureus* acquiring resistance to gentamicin and fusidic acid during therapy. J Infect 1981;3:50–58.
4. Archer GL, Climo MW. Antimicrobial susceptibility of coagulase-negative staphylococci. Antimicrob Agents Chemother 1994;38:2231–2237.
5. Archer GL, Scott J. Conjugative transfer genes in staphylococcal isolates from the United States. Antimicrob Agents Chemother 1991;35:2504–2504.
6. Ardati KO, Thirumoorthi MC, Dajani AS. Intravenous trimethoprim-sulfamethoxazole in the treatment of serious infection in children. J Pediatr 1979;95:801–806.
7. Arditi M, Yogev R. In vitro interaction between rifampin and clindamycin against pathogenic coagulase-negative staphylococci. Antimicrob Agents Chemother 1989;33:245–247.
8. Ascher DP, Shoupe BA, Maybee D, Fischer GW. Persistent catheter-related bacteremia: clearance with antibiotics and urokinase. J Pediatr Surg 1993;28:627–629.
9. Bailey EM, Constance TD, Albrecht LM, Rybak MJ. Coagulase-negative staphylococci: incidence, pathogenicity, and treatment in the 1990's. Ann Pharmacol 1990;24:714–719.
10. Bailey RR, Gorrie SI, Peddie BA, Davies PR. Double blind,

randomized trial comparing single dose enoxacin and trimethoprim for treatment of bacterial cystitis. NZ Med J 1987;100:
618–619.

11. Bandyk DF, Berni GA, Thiele BL, Towne JB. Aortofemoral
graft infection due to Staphylococcus epidermidis. Arch Surg
1984;119:102–108.

12. Banerjee SN, Emori TG, Culver DH. Secular trends in nosocomial primary bloodstream infections in the United States. Am J
Med 1991;91:86S–89S.

13. Bannerman TL, Rhoden DL, McAllister SK, Miller JM, Wilson
LA. The source of coagulase-negative staphylococci in the Endophthalmitis Vitrectomy Study. A comparison of eyelid and intraocular isolates using pulsed-field gel electrophoresis. Arch
Ophthalmol 1997;115:357–361.

14. Benezra D, Kiehn TE, Gold JW, Brown AE, Turnbull AD, Armstrong D. Prospective study of infections in indwelling central
venous catheters using quantitative blood cultures. Am J Med
1988;85:495–498.

15. Bennett-Jones DN, Russell GI, Barrett A. A comparison between oral ciprofloxacin and intra-peritoneal vancomycin and
gentamicin in the treatment of CAPD peritonitis. J Antimicrob
Chemother 1990;26(Suppl F):73–76.

16. Berry AJ, Johnson JL, Archer GL. Imipenem therapy of experimental *Staphylococcus epidermidis* endocarditis. Antimicrob
Agents Chemother 1986;29:748–752.

17. Bille J. Medical treatment of staphylococcal infective endocarditis. Eur Heart J 1995;16(Suppl b):8–83.

18. Bisno AL, Dismukes WE, Durack DT, Kaplan EL, Karchmer
AW, Kaye D, Rahimtoola SH, Sande MA, Sanford JP,
Watanakuuakorn C. Antimicrobial treatment of infective endocarditis due to viridans streptococci, enterococci, and staphylococci. JAMA 1989;261:1471–1477.

19. Blaser J, Vergeres P, Widmer AF, Zimmerli W. In vivo verification of in vitro model of antibiotic treatment of device-related
infection. Antimicrob Agents Chemother 1995;39:1134–1139.

20. Bohigian GM, Olk RJ. Factors associated with a poor visual result in endophthalmitis. Am J Ophthalmol 1986;101:332–341.

21. Bonfiglio G, Livermore DM. Behaviour of β-lactamase-positive
and -negative *Staphylococcus aureus* isolates in susceptibility tests
with piperacillin/tazobactam and other β-lactam/β-lactamase inhibitor combinations. J Antimicrob Chemother 1993;32: 431–444.

22. Boyce JM, Potter-Bynoe G, Steven M. A common source outbreak of *Staphylococcus epidermidis* infections among patients
undergoing cardiac surgery. J Infect Dis 1990;161:493–499.

23. Brandt CM, Rouse MS, Tallan BM, Laue NW, Wilson WR,
Steckelberg JM. Effective treatment of cephalosporin rifampin
combinations against cryptic methicillin resistant β-lactamase
producing coagulase negative staphylococcal experimental endocarditis. Antimicrob Agents Chemother 1995;39:1815–1819.

24. Bray PW, Mahoney JL, Anastakis D, Yao JK. Sternotomy infections: sternal salvage and the importance of sternal stability.
Can J Surg 1996;39:297–301.

25. Bregenzer T, Widmer AF. Bloodstream infection from a Port-A-
Cath: successful treatment with the antibiotic lock technique
[Letter]. Infect Control Hosp Epidemiol 1996;17:772.

26. Brown AL, Stephenson JR, Baker LR, Tabaqchali S. Recurrent
CAPD peritonitis caused by coagulase negative staphylococci:
re-infection or relapse determined by clinical criteria and typing
methods. Circulation 1991;18:109–122.

27. Buggy BP, Schaberg DR, Swartz RD. Intraleukocytic sequestration as a cause of persistent *Staphylococcus aureus* peritonitis.
Am J Med 1984;76:1035–1040.

28. Calain P, Krause KH, Vaudaux P, Auckenthaler R, Lew D,
Waldvogel F, Hirschel B. Early termination of a prospective,
randomized trial comparing teicoplanin and flucloxacillin for
treating severe staphylococcal infections. J Infect Dis 1987;155:
187–191.

29. Calderwood SB, Swinski FC, Karchmer AW, Buckley MJ. Risk
factors for the development of prosthetic valve endocarditis. Circulation 1985;72:31–37.

30. Calligaro KD, Veith FJ, Schwartz ML, Goldsmith J, Savarese
RP, Dougherty MJ, DeLaurentis DA. Selective preservation of
infected prosthetic arterial grafts. Analysis of a 20-year experience with 120 extracavitary-infected grafts. Ann Surg 1994;220:
461–469; discussion 469–471.

31. Caparon MG, Scott JR. Identification of a gene that regulates expression of M protein, the major virulence determinant of group
A streptococci. Proc Natl Acad Sci USA 1987;84:8677–8681.

32. Caputo GM, Singer M, White S, Weitekamp MR. Infections due
to antibiotic resistant gram positive cocci. J Gen Intern Med
1993;8:626–634.

33. Cercenado E, Garcia-Leoni ME, Diaz MD, Sanchez-Carrillo C,
Catalan P, De Quiros JC, Bouza E. Emergence of teicoplanin-
resistant coagulase-negative staphylococci. J Clin Microbiol
1996;34:1765–1768.

34. Chambers HF. In vitro and in vivo antistaphylococcal activities of
L-695,256, a carbapenem with high affinity for penicillin-binding
protein 2a. Antimicrob Agents Chemother 1995;39:462–466.

35. Chambers HF. Parenteral antibiotics for the treatment of bac-
teremia and other serious staphylococcal infections. In: Crossley
KB, Archer GL, eds. The staphylococci in human disease. New
York: Churchill Livingstone, 1997:583–601.

36. Chandrasekar PH, Brown WJ. Clinical issues of blood cultures.
Arch Intern Med 1994;154:841–849.

37. Chavanet P, Collin F, Muggeo E, Gagelin B, Chassin P, Kosmidis V, Bernard A, Kistermann JP, Portier H. The in-vivo
activity of co-amoxiclav with netilmicin against experimental
methicillin and gentamicin resistant Staphylococcus epidermidis
infection in rabbits. J Antimicrob Chemother 1993;31:129–138.

38. Cunha BA, Hussain Quadri SM, Ueno Y, Walters EA, Domenico
P. Antibacterial activity of trovafloxacin against nosocomial
gram-positive and gram-negative isolates. J Antimicrob Chemother 1997;39(Suppl B):29–34.

39. Davies AJ, Clewett J, Jones A, Marshall A. Sensitivity patterns
of coagulase-negative staphylococci from neonates. J Antimicrob Chemother 1986;17:155–160.

40. deGorgolas M, Aviles P, Verdejo C, Guerrero MLF. Treatment
of experimental endocarditis due to methicillin-susceptible or
methicillin-resisant *Staphylococcus aureus* with trimethoprim-
sulfamethoxazole and antibiotics that inhibit cell wall synthesis.
Antimicrob Agents Chemother 1995;39:953–957.

41. Dirschl DR, Almekinders LC. Osteomyelitis: common causes
and treatment recommendations. Drugs 1993;45:29–43.

42. Drancourt M, Stein A, Argenson JN, Roiron R, Groulier P,
Raoult D. Oral treatment of Staphylococcus spp. infected orthopaedic implants with fusidic acid or ofloxacin in combination
with rifampicin. J Antimicrob Chemother 1997;39:235–240.

43. Drancourt M, Stein A, Argenson JN, Zannier A, Curvale G,
Raoult D. Oral rifampin plus ofloxacin for treatment of staphy-
lococcus infected orthopedic implants. Antimicrob Agents
Chemother 1993;37:1214–1218.

44. Drew PJT, Casewell MW, Desai N. Cephalexin for the oral treatment of CAPD peritonitis. J Antimicrob Chemother 1984; 13:
153–159.

45. Dryden MS, Talsania HG, Martin S, Cunningham M, Richardson JF, Cookson B, Marples RR, Phillips I. Evaluation of methods for typing coagulase-negative staphylococci. J Med Microbiol 1992;37:109–117.

46. Egert J, Carrizosa J, Kaye D. Comparison of methicillin, nafcillin, and oxacillin in therapy of *Staphylococcus aureus* endocarditis in rabbits. J Lab Clin Med 1977;89:1262.

47. Engelhard D, Elishoov H, Strauss N, Naparstek E, Nagler A, Simhon A, Raveh D, Slavin S, Or R. Nosocomial coagulase-negative staphylococcal infections in bone marrow transplantation recipients with central vein catheter. A 5-year prospective study. Transplantation 1996;61:430–434.

48. Entenza JM, Drugeon H, Glauser MP, Moreillon P. Treatment of experimental endocarditis due to erythromycin-resistant *Staphylococcus aureus*. Antimicrob Agents Chemother 1995;39:1419.

49. Etienne J, Renaud F, Bes M, Brun Y, Greenland TB, Freney J, Fleurette J. Instability of characteristics amongst coagulase-negative staphylococci causing endocarditis. J Med Microbiol 1990; 32:115–122.

50. Everett ED, Strausbaugh LJ. Antimicrobial agents and the central nervous system. Neurosurgery 1980;6:691–714.

51. Faber M, Rosdahl VT. Susceptibility to fusidic acid among Danish *Staphylococcus aureus* strains and fusidic acid consumption. J Antimicrob Chemother 1990;25:7–14.

52. Fanti B, Leclercq R, Merle Y. Critical influence of resistance to streptogramin B-type antibiotics on activity of RP59500 (quinupristin-dalfopristin) in experimental endocarditis due to *Staphylococcus aureus*. Antimicrob Agents Chemother 1995; 39:400–405.

53. Farber BF, Yee YC, Karchmer AW. Interaction between rifampin and fusidic acid against methicillin-resistant coagulase-positive and -negative staphylococci. Antimicrob Agents Chemother 1986; 30:174–175.

54. Fass RJ, Helsel VL, Barnishan J, Ayers LW. In-vitro susceptibilities of four species of coagulase negative staphylococci. Antimicrob Agents Chemother 1986;30:545–552.

55. Ficker LA, Vickers S, Capon MR, Mellerio J, Cooling RJ. Retinal detachment following Nd:YAG posterior capsulotomy. Eye 1987;1(Pt 1):86–89.

56. Fleurette J, Bes M, Brun Y, Freney J, Forey F, Coulet M, Reverdy ME, Etienne J. Clinical isolates of *Staphylococcus lugdunensis* and *S. scheiferi*: bacteriological characteristics and susceptibility to antimicrobial agents. Res Microbiol 1989;140: 107–108.

57. Foldes M, Munro R, Sorrell TC. In-vitro effects of vancomycin, rifampicin, and fusidic acid, alone and in combination, against methicillin-resistant *Staphylococcus aureus*. J Antimicrob Chemother 1983;11:21–26.

58. Fortun J, Perez-Molina JA, Anon MT, Martinez-Beltran J, Loza E, Guerrero A. Right-sided endocarditis caused by *Staphylococcus aureus* in drug abusers. Antimicrob Agents Chemother 1995;39:525–528.

59. Forward KR, Fewer HD, Stiver HG. Cerebrospinal fluid shunt infections. A review of 35 infections in 32 patients. J Neurosurg 1983;59:389–394.

60. Friedland JS, Iveson TJ, Fraise AP. A comparison between intraperitoneal ciprofloxacin and intraperitoneal vancomycin and gentamicin in the treatment of peritonitis associated with continuous ambulatory peritoneal dialysis (CAPD). J Antimicrob Chemother 1990;26(Suppl F):77–81.

61. Gardner P, Leipzig T, Phillips P. Infections of central nervous system shunts. Med Clin North Am 1985;69:297–314.

62. Garvin KL, Evans BG, Salvati EA, Brause BD. Palacos gentamicin for the treatment of deep periprosthetic hip infections. Clin Orthop 1994;298:97–105.

63. Gill VJ, Selepak ST, Williams EC. Species identification and antibiotic susceptibilities of coagulase-negative staphylococci isolated from clinical specimens. J Clin Microbiol 1983;18: 1314–1319.

64. Gonzalez-Barca E, Fernandez-Sevilla A, Carratala J, Granena A, Gudiol F. Prospective study of 288 episodes of bacteremia in neutropenic cancer patients in a single institution. Eur J Clin Microbiol Infect Dis 1996;15:291–296.

65. Gordon A, Conlon C, Collin J, Peto T, Gray D, Hands L, Morris P. An eight year experience of conservative management for aortic graft sepsis. Eur J Vasc Surg 1994;8:611–616.

66. Gruer LD, Barlett R, Ayliffe GAJ. Species identification and antibiotic sensitivity of coagulase negative staphylococci from CAPD peritonitis. J Antimicrob Chemother 1984;13:577–583.

67. Hackbarth CJ, Chambers HF, Sande MA. Serum bactericidal activity of rifampin in combination with other antimicrobial agents against Staphylococcus aureus. Antimicrob Agents Chemother 1986;29:611–613.

68. Hampton AA, Sherertz RJ. Vascular-access infections in hospitalized patients. Surg Clin North Am 1988;68:57–71.

69. Hartstein AI, Valvano MA, Morthland VH, Fuchs PC, Potter SA, Crosa JH. Antimicrobic susceptibility and plasmid profile analysis as identity tests for multiple blood isolates of coagulase-negative staphylococci. J Clin Microbiol 1987;25:589–593.

70. Heaven CJ, Mann PJ, Boase DL. Endophthalmitis following extracapsular cataract surgery: a review of 32 cases. Br J Ophthalmol 1992;76:419–423.

71. Hébert GA, Cooksey RC, Clark NC, Hill BC, Jarvis WR, Thornsberry C. Biotyping coagulase-negative staphylococci. J Clin Microbiol 1988;26:1950.

72. Hiemenz J, Skelton J, Pizzo PA. Perspective on the management of catheter-related infections in cancer patients. Pediatr Infect Dis 1986;5:6–11.

73. Hilson GR. In vitro studies of a new antibiotic (Fucidin). Lancet 1962;1:932–933.

74. Hiramatsu K, Hanaki H, Ino T, Yabuta K, Oguri T, Tenover FC. Methicillin-resistant *Staphylococcus aureus* clinical strain with reduced vancomycin susceptibility. J Antimicrob Chemother 1997;40:135–136.

75. Hoban DJ. In-vitro activity of a new penem FCE 22101. J Antimicrob Chemother 1989;23(Suppl C):53–57.

76. Hovelius B, Mardh PA. *Staphylococcus saprophyticus* as a common cause of urinary tract infections. Rev Infect Dis 1984;6: 328–337.

77. Hughes DS, Hill RJ. Infectious endophthalmitis after cataract surgery [see comments]. Br J Ophthalmol 1994;78:227–232.

78. Hugo NE, Sultan MR, Ascherman JA, Patsis MC, Smith CR, Rose EA. Single-stage management of 74 consecutive sternal wound complications with pectoralis major myocutaneous advancement flaps. Plast Reconstr Surg 1994;93:1433–1441.

79. Hussain Quadri SM, Ueno Y, Imambaccus H, Almodovar E. Rapid detection of methicillin-resistant *Staphylococcus aureus* by crystal MRSA ID system. J Clin Microbiol 1994;32: 1830–1832.

80. Ieven M, Jansens H, Ursi D, Verhoeven J, Goosens H. Rapid detection of methicillin resistance in coagulase-negative staphylococci by commercially available fluorescence test. J Clin Microbiol 1995;33:2183–2185.

81. Inman RD, Gallegeo KV, Brause BD. Clinical and microbial features of prosthetic joint infection. Am J Med 1984;77:47–53.

82. Innes A, Burden RP, Finch RG, Morgan AG. Treatment of resistant peritonitis in continuous ambulatory peritoneal dialysis with intraperitoneal urokinase: a double-blind clinical trial. Nephrol Dial Transplant 1994;9:797–799.

83. Jensen K, Lassen HCA. Combined treatment with antibacterial chemotherapeutical agents in staphylococcal infections. Q J Med 1969;38:91–106.

84. Johnson DC, Johnson FL, Goldman S. Preliminary results treating persistent central venous catheter infections with the antibiotic lock technique in pediatric patients. Pediatr Infect Dis J 1994;13:930–931.

85. Jones RN, Barrett MS, Erwin ME. In vitro activity and spectrum of LY333328, a novel glycopeptide derivative. Antimicrob Agents Chemother 1996;41:488–493.

86. Jorgensen JH, Redding JS, Maher LA. Antibacterial activity of the new glycopeptide antibiotic SKF104662. Antimicrob Agents Chemother 1989;33:560–561.

87. Kaatz GW, Seo SM, Dorman NJ, Lerner SA. Emergence of teicoplanin resistance during therapy of *Staphylococcus aureus* endocarditis. J Infect Dis 1990;162:103–108.

88. Kacica MA, Horgan MJ, Ochoa L, Sandler R, Lepow ML, Venezia RA. Prevention of gram-positive sepsis in neonates weighing less than 1500 grams. J Pediatr 1994;125:253–258.

89. Kapusnik JE, Parenti F, Sande MA. The use of rifampicin in staphylococcal infections—a review. J Antimicrob Chemother 1984;13(Suppl C):61–66.

90. Karchmer AW. Antibiotic therapy of nonenterococcal streptococcal and staphylococcal endocarditis: current regimens and some future considerations. J Antimicrob Chemother 1988;21 (Suppl C):91–103.

91. Karchmer AW, Archer GL, Dismukes WE. *Staphylococcus epidermidis* causing prosthetic valve endocarditis: microbiologic and clinical observations as guides to therapy. Ann Intern Med 1983;98:447–455.

92. Karchmer AW, Archer GL, the Endocarditis Study Group. Methicillin resistant *Staphylococcus epidermidis* prosthetic valve endocarditis: a therapeutic trial [Abstract 476]. Abstracts of 24th Interscience Conference of Antimicrobial Agents and Chemotherapy, American Society for Microbiology, Washington, DC, 1984.

93. Kaye D. Infecting microorganism. In: Kaye D, ed. Infective endocarditis. Baltimore: University Park Press, 1976;43–54.

94. Kendall RW, Duncan CP, Beauchamp CP. Bacterial growth on antibiotic-loaded acrylic cement. J Arthrop 1995;10:817–822.

95. Kernodle DS, Classen DC, Burke JP, Kaiser AB. Failure of cephalosporins to prevent *Staphylococcus aureus* surgical wound infections. JAMA 1990;263:961–966.

96. Khatib R, Riederer KM, Clark JA, Khatib S, Briski LE, Wilson FM. Coagulase-negative staphylococci in multiple blood cultures: strain relatedness and determinants of same-strain bacteremia. J Clin Microbiol 1995;33:816–820.

97. Kloos WE, Bannerman TL. Update on clinical significance of coagulase-negative staphylococci. Clin Microbiol Rev 1994;7:117.

98. Kloos WE, Schleifer KH. Simplified scheme for routine identification of Staphylococcus species. J Clin Microbiol 1975;1:82.

99. Knapp CC, Ludwig MD, Washington JA. Evaluation of differential inoculum disk diffusion method and Vitek GPS-SA card for detection of oxacillin-resistant staphylococci. J Clin Microbiol 1994;32:433–436.

100. Knapp CC, Ludwig MD, Washington JA. Evaluation of BBL Crystal MRSA ID system. J Clin Microbiol 1994;32: 2588–2589.

101. Kobasa WD, Kaye KL, Shapiro T, Kaye D. Therapy for experimental endocarditis due to *Staphylococcus epidermidis*. Rev Infect Dis 1983;5(Suppl 3):S533–537.

102. Koh TW, Brecker SJD, Layton CA. Successful treatment of *Staphylococcus lugdunensis* endocarditis complicated by multiple emboli: a case report and review of the literature. Int J Cardiol 1996;55:193–197.

103. Kotilainen P, Nikoskelainen J, Huovinen P. Antibiotic susceptibility of coagulase-negative staphylococcal blood isolates with special reference to adherent, slime-producing Staphylococcus epidermidis strains. Scand J Infect Dis 1991;23: 325–332.

104. Krzywda EA, Andris DA, Edmiston CE Jr, Quebbeman EJ. Treatment of Hickman catheter sepsis using antibiotic lock technique. Infect Control Hosp Epidemiol 1995;16:596–598.

105. Kucers A, Bennett NM, Kemp RJ. Isoxazolyl penicillins: Oxacillin, cloxacillin, dicloxacillin and flucloxacillin. In: Anonymous. The use of antibiotics: a comprehensive review with clinical emphasis. 4th ed. Philadelphia: JB Lippincott, 1987:109–124.

106. Lambe DW Jr, Ferguson KP, Keplinger JL, Gemmell CG, Kalbfleisch JH. Pathogenicity of *Staphylococcus lugdunensis, Staphylococcus scheiferi,* and three other coagulase-negative staphylococci in a mouse model and possible virulence factors. Can J Microbiol 1990;36:455–463.

107. Latham RH, Running K, Stamm WE. Urinary tract infections in young adult women caused by *Staphylococcus saprophyticus.* JAMA 1983;250:3063.

108. Latham RH, Zeleznik D, Minshew BH, Schoenknecht FD, Stamm WE. *Staphylococcus saprophyticus* β-lactamase production and disk diffusion susceptibility testing for three β-lactam antimicrobial agents. Antimicrob Agents Chemother 1984; 26:670–672.

109. Lawlor MT, Sullivan MC, Levitz RE, Quintilliani R, Nightingale C. Treatment of prosthetic valve endocarditis due to methicillin-resistant *Staphylococcus aureus* with minocycline. J Infect Dis 1990;161:812–814.

110. Leclercq R, Courvalin P. Bacterial resistance to macrolide, lincosamide, and streptogramin antibiotics by target modification. Antimicrob Agents Chemother 1991;35:1267–1272.

111. Leclercq R, Courvalin P. Resistance to macrolides, azalides, and streptogramins. In: Neu HC, Young LS, Zinner SH, eds. The new macrolides, azalides, and streptogramins: pharmacology and clinical applications. New York: Marcel Dekker, 1993: 33–40.

112. Lessing MPA, Crook DWM, Bowler ICJ, Gribbin B. Native valve endocarditis caused by *Staphylococcus lugdunensis*. Q J Med 1996;89:855–858.

113. Levine DP, Cushing RD, Jui J, Brown WJ. Community-acquired methicillin-resistant *Staphylococcus aureus* endocarditis in the Detroit Medical Centre. Ann Intern Med 1982;97:330–338.

114. Levitz RE, Quintilliani R. Trimethoprim-sulfamethoxazole for bacterial meningitis. Ann Intern Med 1984;100:881–890.

115. Locher HH, Schlunegger H, Hartman PG, Angehrn P, Then RL. Antibacterial activities of epiprim, a new dihydrofolate reductase inhibitor, alone and in combination with dapsone. Antimicrob Agents Chemother 1996;40:1376–1381.

116. Low DE, McGeer A, Poon R. Activity of daptomycin and teicoplanin against *Staphylococcus haemolyticus and Staphylococcus epidermidis,* including evaluation of susceptibility testing recommendations. Antimicrob Agents Chemother 1989;33: 585–588.

117. Low DE, Schmidt BK, Kirpalani HM, Moodie R, Kreiswirth B, Matlow A, Ford- Jones EL. An endemic strain of *Staphylococcus haemolyticus* colonizing and causing bacteremia in neonatal intensive care unit patients. Paediatrics 1992;89: 696–700.

118. Lowy FD, Chang DS, Lash PR. Synergy of combinations of vancomycin, gentamicin, and rifampin against methicillin-resistant, coagulase-negative staphylococci. Antimicrob Agents Chemother 1983;23:932–934.

119. Lowy FD, Walsh JA, Mayers MM, Klein RS, Steigbigel NH. Antibiotic activity in vitro against methicillin-resistant *Staphylococcus epidermidis* and therapy of an experimental infection. Antimicrob Agents Chemother 1979;16:314–321.

120. Maduri-Traczcwski M, Szymczak EG, Goldmann DA. In vitro activity of penicillin and rifampin against group B streptococci. Rev Infect Dis 1983;5(Suppl 3):S586–592.

121. Maki DG, Stolz SM, Wheeler S, Mermel LA. Prevention of central venous catheter-related bloodstream infection by use of an antiseptic-impregnated catheter. A randomized, controlled trial [see comments]. Ann Intern Med 1997;127:257–266.

122. Markowitz N, Quinn EL, Saravolatz LD. Trimethoprim-sulfamethoxazole compared with vancomycin for the treatment of *Staphylococcus aureus* infection. Ann Intern Med 1992;117: 390–398.

123. Marr KA, Sexton DJ, Conlon PJ, Corey GR, Schwab SJ, Kirkland KB. Catheter-related bacteremia and outcome of attempted catheter salvage in patients undergoing hemodialysis. Ann Intern Med 1997;127:275–280.

124. Maskell JP, Tang T, Asad S, Williams JD. Comparative inhibitory and bactericidal activities of FCE 22101 against gram-positive cocci and anaerobes in vitro. J Antimicrob Chemother 1989;23(Suppl C):65–74.

125. Meredith TA, Aguilar HE, Miller MJ, Gardner SK, Trabelsi A, Wilson LA. Comparative treatment of experimental Staphylococcus epidermidis endophthalmitis. Arch Ophthalmol 1990; 108:857–860.

126. Moorhouse EC, Mulvihill TE, Jones L, Mooney D, Falkiner FR, Keane CT. The in-vitro activity of some antimicrobial agents against methicillin-resistant *Staphylococcus aureus*. J Antimicrob Chemother 1985;15:291–295.

127. Morissette I, Gourdeau M, Francoeur J. CSF shunt infections: a fifteen-year experience with emphasis on management and outcome. Can J Neurol Sci 1993;20:118–122.

128. Mossad SB, Serkey JM, Longworth DL, Cosgrove DM 3rd, Gordon SM. Coagulase-negative staphylococcal sternal wound infections after open heart operations. Ann Thorac Surg 1997; 63:395–401.

129. Mouton JW, Endtz HP, den Hollander JG, van den Braak N, Verbrugh HA. In-vitro activity of quinupristin/dalfopristin compared with other widely used antibiotics against strains isolated from patients with endocarditis. J Antimicrob Chemother 1997; 39(Suppl A):75–80.

130. Nahai F, Rand RP, Hester TR, Bostwick J3, Jurkiewicz MJ. Primary treatment of the infected sternotomy wound with muscle flaps. A review of 211 consecutive cases. Plast Reconstr Surg 1989;84:434–441.

131. National Committee for Clinical Laboratory Standards. Dilution antimicrobial susceptibility tests for bacteria that grow aerobically. Approved standard M7-A3. Villanova, PA: National Committee for Clinical Laboratory Standards, 1993.

132. National Committee for Clinical Laboratory Standards. Performance standards for antimicrobial disk susceptibility tests. Villanova, PA: National Committee for Clinical Laboratory Standards, 1993.

133. National Committee for Clinical Laboratory Standards. Performance standards for antimicrobial susceptibility testing. NCCLS document M100-S6. Villanova, PA: National Committee for Clinical Laboratory Standards, 1995.

134. Nicolle LE, Harding GKM. Susceptibility of clinical isolates of *Staphylococcus saprophyticus* to fifteen commonly used antimicrobial agents. Antimicrob Agents Chemother 1982;22: 895.

135. Norrby SR, Jonsson M. Comparative in vitro activity of PD 127,391, a new fluorinated 4-quinolone derivative. Antimicrob Agents Chemother 1988;32:1278–1281.

136. Novak SM, Hindler J, Bruckner DA. Reliability of two novel methods, Alamar and E test, for detection of methicillin-resistant *Staphylococcus aureus*. J Clin Microbiol 1993;31: 3056–3057.

137. O'Day DM, Jones DB, Patrinely J, Elliott JH. Staphylococcus epidermidis endophthalmitis. Visual outcome following noninvasive therapy. Ophthalmology 1982;89:354–360.

138. Olk RJ, Bohigian GM. The management of endophthalmitis: diagnostic and therapeutic guidelines including the use of vitrectomy. Ophthalmic Surg 1987;18:262–267.

139. Ormerod LD, Ho DD, Becker LE, Cruise RJ, Grohar HI, Paton BG, Frederick AR Jr, Topping TM, Weiter JJ, Buzney SM. Endophthalmitis caused by the coagulase-negative staphylococci. 1. Disease spectrum and outcome. Ophthalmology 1993;100: 715–723.

140. Osborn JS, Sharp S, Hanson EJ, MacGee E, Brewer JH. Staphylococcus epidermidis ventriculitis treated with vancomycin and rifampin. Neurosurgery 1986;19:824–827.

141. Perdreau-Remington F, Stefanik D, Peters G, Ludwig C, Rutt J, Wenzel R, Pulverer G. A four-year prospective study on microbial ecology of explanted prosthetic hips in 52 patients with "aseptic" prosthetic joint loosening. Eur J Clin Microbiol Infect Dis 1996;15:160–165.

142. Peters DH, Clissold SP. Clarithromycin: a review of its antimicrobial activity, pharmacokinetic properties and therapeutic potential. Drugs 1992;44:117–164.

143. Peters G, von Eiff G, Herrmann M. The changing pattern of coagulase negative staphylococci as infectious pathogens. Curr Opin Infect Dis 1995;8:S12–S19.

144. Peterson PK, Keane WF. Infections in chronic peritoneal dialysis patients. In: Remington JS, Swartz MN, eds. Current clinical topics in infectious diseases. New York: McGraw-Hill, 1985:239–260.

145. Peterson PK, Matzke GR, Keane WF. Current concepts in the management of peritonitis in continuous ambulatory peritoneal dialysis patients. Rev Infect Dis 1987;9:604–612.

146. Phillips WB 2nd, Tasman WS. Postoperative endophthalmitis in association with diabetes mellitus. Ophthalmology 1994; 101:508–518.

147. Pople IK, Bayston R, Hayward RD. Infection of cerebrospinal fluid shunts in infants: a study of etiological factors. J Neurosurg 1992;77:29–36.

148. Powers KA, Terpenning MS, Voice RA, Kauffman CA. Prosthetic joint infections in the elderly. Am J Med 1990;88: 9N–13N.

149. Poyart-Salmeron C, Trieu-Cuot P, Carlier C, Courvalin P. Nucleotide sequences specific for Tn1545-like conjugative transposons in pneumococci and staphylococci resistant to tetracycline. Antimicrob Agents Chemother 1991;35:1657–1660.

150. Raad I, Darouiche R, Dupuis J, Abi-Said D, Gabrielli A, Hachem R, Wall M, Harris R, Jones J, Buzaid A, et al. Central venous catheters coated with minocycline and rifampin for the prevention of catheter-related colonization and bloodstream infections. A randomized, double-blind trial [see comments]. The Texas Medical Center Catheter Study Group. Ann Intern Med 1997;127:267–274.

151. Raad II, Bodey GP. Infectious complications of indwelling vascular catheters. Clin Infect Dis 1992;15:197–208.

152. Ring JC, Cates KL, Belani KK, Gaston TL, Sveum RJ, Marker SC. Rifampin for CSF shunt infections caused by coagulase-negative staphylococci. J Pediatr 1979;95:317–319.

153. Rolston KVI, Ho DH, LeBlanc B, Streeter H, Dvorak T. In-vitro activity of trovafloxacin against clinical bacterial isolates from patients with cancer. J Antimicrob Chemother 1997;39 (Suppl B):15–22.

154. Rupp ME. Infections of intravascular catheters and vascular devices. In: Crossley KB, Archer GL, eds. The staphylococci in human disease. New York: Churchill Livingstone, 1997: 379–399.

155. Rupp ME, Archer GL. Coagulase-negative staphylococci: pathogens associated with medical progress [Review] [12 refs]. Clin Infect Dis 1994;19:231–243.

156. Rupp ME, Soper DE, Archer GL. Colonization of the female genital tract with *Staphylococcus saprophyticus*. J Clin Microbiol 1992;11:2975–2979.

157. Sabath LD. Reappraisal of the antistaphylococcal activities of first-generation (narrow-spectrum) and second generation (expanded-spectrum) cephalosporins. Antimicrob Agents Chemother 1989;33:407–411.

158. Saginur R, Nicolle LE. Single-dose compared with 3-day norfloxacin treatment of uncomplicated urinary tract infection in women. Canadian Infectious Diseases Society Clinical Trials Study Group. Arch Intern Med 1992;152:1233–1237.

159. Sanabria TJ, Alpert JS, Goldberg R. Increasing frequency of staphylococcal infective endocarditis: experience at a university hospital, 1981 through 1988. Arch Intern Med 1990;150: 1305–1309.

160. Schneider PF, Riley TV. *Staphylococcus saprophyticus* urinary tract infections: epidemiological data from western Australia. Eur J Epidemiol 1996;12:51–54.

161. Schoenbaum SC, Gardner P, Shillito J. Infections of cerebrospinal fluid shunts: epidemiology, clinical manifestations, and therapy. J Infect Dis 1975;131:543–552.

162. Schwalbe RS, Stapleton JT, Gilligan PH. Emergence of vancomycin resistance in coagulase-negative staphylococci. N Eng J Med 1987;316:927–931.

163. Schwarz S, Noble WC. Tetracycline resistance genes in staphylococci from the skin of pigs. J Appl Bacteriol 1994;76: 320–326.

164. Shapiro ED, Wald ER, Nelson KA, Spiegelman KN. Broviac catheter-related bacteremia in oncology patients. Am J Dis Child 1982;136:679–681.

165. Small PM, Chambers HF. Vancomycin for *Staphylococcus aureus* endocarditis in intravenous drug users. Antimicrob Agents Chemother 1990;34:122—131.

166. Smith MA, Sorenson JA, D'Aversa G, Mandelbaum S, Udell I, Harrison W. Treatment of experimental methicillin-resistant Staphylococcus epidermidis 1997;175:462–466.

167. Spafford PS, Sinkin RA, Cox C, Reubens L, Powell KR. Prevention of central venous catheter-related coagulase-negative staphylococcal sepsis in neonates. J Pediatr 1994;125:259–263.

168. Speer BS, Shoemaker NB, Salyers AA. Bacterial resistance to tetracycline: mechanisms, transfer, and clinical significance. Clin Microbiol Rev 1992;5:387–399.

169. Stamm WE, Hooton TM. Management of urinary tract infections in adults [see comments]. N Engl J Med 1993;329: 1328–1334.

170. Svensson E, Hanberger H, Nilsson LE. Pharmacodynamic effects of antibiotics and antibiotic combinations on growing and nongrowing Staphylococcus epidermidis cells. Antimicrob Agents Chemother 1997;41:107–111.

171. Swenson JM, Hindler JA, Peterson LR. Special tests for detecting antibacterial resistance. In: Murray PR, Baron EJ, Pfaller MA, Tenover FC, Yolken RH, eds. Manual of clinical microbiology. 6th ed. Washington, DC: American Society for Microbiology, 1995:1356.

172. Takasugi JK, O'Connell TX. Prevention of complications in permanent central venous catheters. Surg Gynecol Obstet 1988; 167:6–11.

173. Tamer MA, Bray JD. Trimethoprim-sulfamethoxazole treatment of multiantibiotic-resistant staphylococcal endocarditis and meningitis. Clin Pediatr (Phila) 1982;21:125–126.

174. Tapson JS, Orr KE, George JC. A comparison between oral ciprofloxacin and intraperitoneal vancomycin and netilmicin in CAPD peritonitis. J Antimicrob Chemother 1990;26(Suppl F):63–71.

175. Toma E, Barriault D. Antimicrobial activity of fusidic acid and disk diffusion susceptibility testing criteria for gram-positive cocci. J Clin Microbiol 1995;33:1712–1715.

176. Tripodi MF, Attanasio V, Adinolfi LE, Florio A, Clone P, Cuccurullo S, Utili R, Ruggiero G. Prevalence of antibiotic resistance among clinical isolates of methicillin-resistant staphylococci. Eur J Clin Microbiol Infect Dis 1994;13:148–152.

177. Trucksis M, Wolfson JS, Hooper DC. A novel locus conferring fluoroquinolone resistance in *Staphylococcus aureus*. J Bacteriol 1991;173:5854–5860.

178. Van den Broek PJ, Lampe AS, Berbee GAM. Epidemic of PVE caused by *Staphylococcus epidermidis*. Br Med J 1985;291: 949–950.

179. Vandenesch F, Etienne J, Reverdy ME, Eyken SJ. Endocarditis due to *Staphylococcus lugdunensis*: report of 11 cases and review. Clin Infect Dis 1993;17:871–876.

180. Vander Salm TJ, Okike ON, Pasque MK, Pezzella AT, Lew R, Traina V, Mathieu R. Reduction of sternal infection by application of topical vancomycin. J Thorac Cardiovasc Surg 1989; 98:618–622.

181. Vazquez GJ, Archer GL. Antibiotic therapy of experimental *Staphylococcus epidermidis* endocarditis. Antimicrob Agents Chemother 1980;17:280–285.

182. Veach LA, Pfaller MA, Barrett M, Koontz FP, Wenzel RP. Vancomycin resistance in *Staphylococcus haemolyticus* causing colonization and bloodstream infection. J Clin Microbiol 1990;28:2064–2068.

183. Verbist L. The antimicrobial activity of fusidic acid. J Antimicrob Chemother 1990;25:1–5.

184. Waites K, Rand K, Jenkins S, Yangco B, Brookings E, Gaskins D, Lewis J, Halkias K. Multicenter in vitro comparative study of fluoroquinolones after four years of widespread clinical use. Diagn Microbiol Infect Dis 1994;18:181–189.

185. Wallmark G, Arremark I, Telander B. *Staphylococcus saprophyticus*: a frequent cause of acute urinary tract infection among female outpatients. J Infect Dis 1978;138:791–797.

186. Weinstein MP, Towns ML, Quartey SM, Mirrett S, Reimer LG,

Parmigiani G, Reller LB. The clinical significance of positive blood cultures in the 1990s: a prospective comprehensive evaluation of the microbiology, epidemiology, and outcome of bacteremia and fungemia in adults. Clin Infect Dis 1997;24: 584–602.

187. Whitener C, Caputo GM, Weitekamp MR, Karchmer AW. Endocarditis due to coagulase negative staphylococci: microbiologic, epidemiologic, and clinical considerations. Infect Dis Clin 1993;7:81–96.

188. Widmer AF, Frei R, Rajacic Z, Zimmerli W. Correlation between in vivo and in vitro efficacy of antimicrobial agents against foreign body infections. J Infect Dis 1990;162: 96–102.

189. Wilson WR, Karchmer AW, Dajani AS, Taubert KA, Bayer A, Kaye D, Bisno AL, Ferrieri P, Shulman ST, Durack DT. Antibiotic treatment of adults with infective endocarditis due to streptococci, enterococci, staphylococci, and HACEK microorganisms. JAMA 1995;274:1706–1713.

190. Windsor RE, Insall JN, Urs WK, Miller DV, Brause BD. Two-stage reimplantation for the salvage of total knee arthroplasty complicated by infection. J Bone Joint Surg 1990;72:272–278.

191. Winston DJ, Dudnick DV, Chapin M, Ho WG, Gale RP, Martin WJ. Coagulase-negative staphylococcal bacteremia in patients receiving immunosuppressive therapy. Arch Intern Med 1983;143:32–36.

192. Wise R, Ashby JP, Andrews JM. In vitro activity of PD 127,391, an enhanced-spectrum quinolone. Antimicrob Agents Chemother 1988;32:1251–1256.

193. Younger JJ, Christensen GD, Bartley DL, Simmons JC, Barrett FF. Coagulase-negative staphylococci isolated from cerebrospinal fluid shunts: importance of slime production, species identification, and shunt removal to clinical outcome. J Infect Dis 1987;156:548–554.

194. Yuk JH, Dignani MC, Harris RL. Minocycline as an alternative antistaphylococcal agent. Rev Infect Dis 1991;13:1023–1024.

195. Zacharias A, Habib RH. Delayed primary closure of deep sternal wound infections. Tex Heart Inst J 1996;23:211–216.

Stenotrophomonas (*Xanthomonas*) *maltophilia*

Robert R. Muder

Stenotrophomonas (*Xanthomonas*) *maltophilia* is an nonfermentative, Gram-negative bacillus that is readily isolated from environmental sources such as soil and water. Most human isolates represent colonization rather than infection; it is, however, an opportunistic pathogen in highly debilitated patients (8, 12, 30, 33). Patients at highest risk include those with underlying malignancy, neutropenia, chemotherapy, an indwelling central catheter, and prior antimicrobial therapy. The major clinical syndrome is bacteremia; the portal of entry is typically a vascular catheter or is unknown (3, 10, 14). Other reported clinical syndromes include pneumonia (17, 33), urinary tract infection (29), soft-tissue infection (27), ocular infection (21), endocarditis (6, 13), and meningitis (15, 19).

SUSCEPTIBILITY

Methodology for in vitro determination of antimicrobial susceptibility for *S. maltophilia* is not well standardized. Results of disk diffusion, microbroth dilution, and agar dilution assays correlate poorly for a number of agents (18). There is good correlation between time-kill studies and agar dilution assays; the latter should be considered the most reliable means of determining susceptibility.

In most reports, over 90% of strains are susceptible to trimethoprim-sulfamethoxazole (4, 14). Disk diffusion and agar dilution susceptibilities correlate reasonably well for this particular combination of agents. A recent report from a major oncology center found that only 75% of strains were susceptible (28). Thus, susceptibility to trimethoprim-sulfamethoxazole should not be assumed. Most isolates are susceptible in vitro to minocycline.

Most clinical isolates of *S. maltophilia* infections are resistant to multiple agents used to treat Gram-negative infections. Resistance to β-lactam antibiotics is mediated by two unique inducible β-lactamases, a zinc-containing penicillinase (24) and a cephalosporinase (25). Some isolates appear to produce additional β-lactamases as well (20). As a consequence, many strains are resistant to extended-spectrum penicillins and third-generation cephalosporins; nearly all strains are resistant to imipenem (9, 16, 18). Most strains are susceptible to the combination of ticarcillin and the β-lactamase inhibitor clavulanic acid in vitro; however, the degree of growth inhibition depends on testing conditions (16, 18). In a murine model of *S. maltophilia* pneumonia, the efficacy of ticarcillin/clavulanic acid was similar to that of trimethoprim-sulfamethoxazole (23). Piperacillin/tazobactam is less active in vitro; only 20% of strains are susceptible by agar dilution testing (18). Ampicillin/sulbactam is generally inactive.

Most strains are resistant to aminoglycosides. The mechanism of aminoglycoside resistance is incompletely understood, but resistance may be due to a lack of permeability of the outer membrane of *S. maltophilia* (26, 31). *S. maltophilia* strains are variably susceptible to fluoroquinolones such as ciprofloxacin and ofloxacin. Emergence of resistance during quinolone therapy by an initially susceptible strain has been reported (1).

Spontaneous mutants that are resistant to multiple quinolones occur at a frequency of 10^{-5} to 10^{-7} (11); exposure to a quinolone may result in selection of the resistant clone.

Combinations of Antimicrobials

There are a limited number of in vitro studies of combinations of antimicrobial agents. The combination of carbenicillin, trimethoprim/sulfamethoxazole, and rifampin has a synergistic interaction by checkerboard broth dilution (32). The combination of carbenicillin, trimethoprim/sulfamethoxazole, and gentamicin also shows a synergistic interaction despite resistance to gentamicin by standard criteria (32). Synergistic bacterial killing occurs in vitro with ticarcillin/clavulanate plus trimethoprim/sulfamethoxazole, whether or not the isolates are susceptible to either of the two combination agents (22). Synergy may also occur with either ticarcillin/clavulanate or ceftazidime plus ciprofloxacin for strains with a ciprofloxacin MIC below 32 μg/mL (22). These reports of synergy are based on a limited number of strains.

ANTIMICROBIAL THERAPY
Drug of Choice

There are no controlled trials of therapy for *S. maltophilia* infection in humans. Therapy should be guided by the results of in vitro susceptibility testing with the caveat that the results of different testing methods may not correlate with one another; agar dilution appears to be the most reliable. Trimethoprim-sulfamethoxazole should be considered the primary therapeutic agent for susceptible strains; the daily dose should be 10 mg/kg/day based on the trimethoprim component (14). Combination therapy is warranted in life-threatening infections including bacteremia and pneumonia (see below). In a large case series (14), bacteremic patients who received at least two agents including trimethoprim-sulfamethoxazole, an extended-spectrum penicillin or a third-generation cephalosporin had a significantly lower mortality (11%) than patients who received only one of these agents (31%) or other therapies (55%).

Special Situations
Bacteremia

Most bacteremic patients have serious underlying conditions, including malignancy, immunosuppression, or neutropenia. Bacteremic patients should be treated with combination antimicrobial therapy (see below). Most bacteremias are associated with indwelling central venous catheters; removal of an infected catheter is a key component of successful treatment (3).

Pneumonia

Pulmonary infection occurs primarily in patients with malignancy or in those receiving mechanical ventilation. Patients rendered profoundly neutropenic after intensive chemotherapy for leukemia may develop fulminant pneumonia culminating in fatal pulmonary hemorrhage (2). Combination antimicrobial therapy is warranted.

Meningitis

S. maltophilia meningitis may occur in infants or as a complication of neurosurgical procedures (15, 19). Trimethoprim-sulfamethoxazole penetrates well into the cerebrospinal fluid; a limited number of patients have been treated with bacteriologic cure (13, 15, 19). One patient with postoperative meningitis was cured following a 3-week course of ciprofloxacin (5). Intraventricular drains associated with infection should be removed if possible.

Endocarditis

S. maltophilia endocarditis occurs in the setting of intravenous drug abuse or following valve replacement surgery (6, 7, 13). Complications such as valve ring abscesses and emboli are frequent; therefore, in addition to multiagent antimicrobial therapy such as trimethoprim-sulfamethoxazole and ticarcillin-clavulanate, early valve replacement is often indicated.

Ocular Infections

External infections such as keratitis and conjunctivitis predominate, although orbital cellulitis and endophthalmitis may occur (21). Most infections are preceded by surgery, corneal inflammation, or prosthetic devices including soft contact lenses. Treatment is limited by the organism's resistance to available ophthalmic antimicrobial preparations including aminoglycosides and quinolones. One should consider giving systemic therapy such as trimethoprim/sulfamethoxazole and/or ticarcillin/clavulanate in conjunction with a topical agent to which the isolate is susceptible, if available.

Combination Therapy

Neutropenic patients, and those with bacteremia or pneumonia should be treated with combination antimicrobial therapy that includes trimethoprim/sulfamethoxazole and ticarcillin/clavulanate; this combination may have synergistic bactericidal activity even if the isolate is resistant to one or both agents. Some authors recommend addition of rifampin (32) or minocycline (28) as well.

Alternative Agents

Alternative agents include ticarcillin/clavulanate (3.1 g every 6 h), a third-generation cephalosporin such as ceftazidime (2 g every 8 h), and minocycline. Selection of the agent should be based on the results of in vitro testing, with the caveat that results obtained with different testing methods may not correlate with agar dilution for agents other than trimethoprim-sulfamethoxazole. Fluoroquinolones such as ciprofloxacin or ofloxacin should not be used as single-agent therapy. Although the frequency of this phenomenon is uncertain, emergence of quinolone resistance during therapy has been reported (1). Quinolones could be considered for use as one component of multiagent chemotherapy (e.g., in place of trimethoprim/sulfamethoxazole in a sulfa-allergic patient). Synergy between ciprofloxacin and β-lactam agents appears to be unlikely if the isolate has a ciprofloxacin MIC of 32 μg/mL or higher.

ENDPOINTS FOR MONITORING THERAPY

In bacteremic patients, failure to clear the bacteremia should prompt consideration of an intravascular focus of infection, including an infected vascular catheter, septic thrombophlebitis, or endocarditis. Neutropenic patients may not clear bacteremia until the neutrophil count recovers.

REFERENCES

1. Cheng AF, Li MKW, Ling TKW, French GL. Emergence of ofloxacin-resistant *Citrobacter freundii* and *Pseudomonas maltophilia* after ofloxacin therapy. J Antimicrob Chemother 1987;20:283–285.
2. Elsner HA, Duhrsen U, Hollwitz B, Kaulfers PM, Hossfeld DK. Fatal pulmonary hemorrhage in patients with acute leukemia and fulminant pneumonia caused by *Stenotrophomonas maltophilia*. Ann Hematol 1997;155–161.
3. Elting LS, Bodey GP. Septicemia due to *Xanthomonas* species and non-*aeruginosa Pseudomonas* species: increasing incidence of catheter related infections. Medicine 1990;69:296–306.
4. Felegie TP, Yu VL, Rumans LW, Yee RB. Susceptibility of *Pseudomonas maltophilia* to antimicrobial agents, singly and in combination. Antimicrob Agents Chemother 1979;16: 833–837.
5. Girijaratnakumari T, Raja A, Ramani R, Antony B, Shivananda PG. Meningitis due to *Xanthomonas maltophilia*. J Postgrad Med 1993;39:153–155.
6. Gutierrez Rodero F, del Mar Masia M, Cortes J, Ortiz de la Tabla V, Mainar V, Vilar A. Endocarditis caused by *Stenotrophomonas maltophilia:* case report and review. Clin Infect Dis 1996;23: 1261–1265.
7. Jang TN, Wang FD, Wang LS, Liu CY, Liu IM. *Xanthomonas maltophilia* bacteremia: an analysis of 32 cases. J Formosan Med Assoc 1992;91:1170–1176.
8. Khardori N, Elting L, Wong E, Schable B, Bodey GP. Nosocomial infections due to *Xanthomonas maltophilia* (*Pseudomonas maltophilia*) in patients with cancer. Rev Infect Dis 1990;12: 997–1003.
9. Khardori N, Reuben A, Rosenbaum B, Rolston K, Bodey GP. In vitro susceptibility of *Xanthomonas* (*Pseudomonas*) *maltophilia* to newer antimicrobial agents. Antimicrob Agents Chemother 1990;34:1609–1610.
10. Krcmery V, Pichna P, Oracova E, Lacka J, Kukuckova E, Studenda M, Grausova S, Stopkova K, Krupova I. *Stenotrophomonas maltophilia* bacteremia in cancer patients; report on 31 cases. J Hosp Infect 1996;34:75–55.
11. Lecso-Bornet M, Pierre J, Sarkis-Karam D, Lubera S, Bergogne-Berezin E. Susceptibility of *Xanthomonas maltophilia* to six quinolones and study of outer membrane proteins in resistant mutants selected in vitro. Antimicrob Agents Chemother 1992; 36:669–671.
12. Marshall WF, Keating MR, Anhalt JP, Steckelberg JM. *Xanthomonas maltophilia:* an emerging nosocomial pathogen. Mayo Clin Proc 1989;64:1097–1104.
13. Muder RR, Yu VL, Dummer JS, Vinson C, Lumish RM. Infections caused by *Pseudomonas maltophilia:* expanding clinical spectrum. Arch Intern Med 1987;147:1672–1674.
14. Muder RR, Harris AP, Muller S, Edmund M, Chow JW, Papadakis K, Wagener MW, Bodey GP, Steckelberg JM. Bacteremia due to *Stenotrophomonas maltophilia:* a prospective, multicenter study of 91 episodes. Clin Infect Dis 1996;22: 508–512.
15. Nguyen MH, Muder RR. *Xanthomonas maltophilia* meningitis: case report and review of the literature. Clin Infect Dis 1994;19:325–326.
16. Neu HC, Saha G, Chin N-X. Resistance of *Xanthomonas maltophilia* to antibiotics and the effect of beta-lactamase inhibitors. Diagn Microbiol Infect Dis 1989;12:283–285.
17. Noskin GA, Grohmann SM. *Xanthomonas maltophilia* bacteremia: an analysis of factors influencing outcome. Infect Dis Clin Pract 1992;1:230–236.
18. Papdakis KA, Varivarian SE, Vassilaki ME, Anaissie EJ. *Stenotrophomonas maltophilia* meningitis: report of two cases and review of the literature. J Neurosurg 1997;87:106–108.
19. Pankuch GA, Jacobs MR, Rittenhouse SF, Appelbaum PC. Susceptibilities of 123 strains of *Xanthomonas maltophilia* to eight B-lactams (including B-lactam-B-lactamase inhibitor combinations) and ciprofloxacin tested by five methods. Antimicrob Agents Chemother 1994;38:2317–2322.
20. Paton R, Miles RS, Amyes SG. Biochemical profiles of inducible beta-lactamases produced from *Xanthomonas maltophilia*. Antimicrob Ag Chemother 1994;38:2143–2149.
21. Penland RL, Wilhelmus KR. *Stenotrophomonas maltophilia* ocular infections. Arch Opthalmol 1996;114:433–436.
22. Poulos CD, Matsumara SO, Willey BM, Low DE, McGeer A. In vitro activities of antimicrobial combinations against *Stenotrophomonas* (*Xanthomonas*) *maltophilia*. Antimicrob Agents Chemother 1995;39:2220–2223.
23. Rouse MS, Tallan BM, Henry NK, Steckelberg JM, Wilson WR. Treatment of *Xanthomonas maltophilia* experimental pneumonia in mice. Chest 1991;100(2 Suppl);147S.
24. Saino Y, Kobayashi M, Inoue M, Mitsuhashi S. Purification and properties of inducible penicillin B-lactamase isolated from *Pseudomonas maltophilia*. Antimicrob Agents Chemother 1982;22:564–570.
25. Saino Y, Inoue M, Mitsuhashi S. Purification of an inducible cephalosporinase from *Pseudomonas maltophilia* GN12873. Antimicrob Agents Chemother 1984;25:362–365.
26. Vanhoof R, Sonck P, Hannecart-Pokorni E. The role of lipopolysaccharide anionic binding sites in aminoglycoside uptake in *Stenotrophomonas* (*Xanthomonas*) *maltophilia*. J Antimicrob Chemother 1995;35:167–171.
27. Vartivarian SE, Papadakis KA, Palacios JA, Manning JT, Anaissie EJ. Mucocutaneous and soft tissue infections caused by Xanthomonas maltophilia: a new spectrum. Ann Intern Med 1994;121:969–973.
28. Vartivarian S, Anaissie E, Bodey G, Sprigg H, Rolston K. A changing pattern of susceptibility of *Xanthomonas maltophilia* to antimicrobial agents: implications for therapy. Antimicrob Agents Chemother 1994;38:624–627.
29. Vartivarian SE, Papadakis KA, Anaissie EJ. *Stenotrophomonas* (*Xanthomonas*) *maltophilia* urinary tract infection: a disease that is unusually severe and complicated. Arch Intern Med 1996;156: 433–435.
30. Victor MA, Arpi M, Bruun B, Jonsson V, Hansen MM. *Xanthomonas maltophilia* bacteremia in immunocompromised hematological patients. Scand J Infect Dis 1994;26:163–170.
31. Wilcox MH, Winstanley TG, Spencer RC. Outer membrane protein profiles of *Xanthomonas maltophilia* isolates displaying temperature-dependent susceptibility to gentamicin. J Antimicrob Chemother 1994;33:663–666.
32. Yu VL, Felegie TP, Yee RB, Paculle AW, Taylor RH. Synergistic interactions in vitro with use of three antibiotics simultaneously against *Pseudomonas maltophilia*. J Infect Dis 1980; 38:624–627.
33. Zuravleff JJ, Yu VL. Infections caused by *Pseudomonas maltophilia:* case reports and review of the literature. Rev Infect Dis 1982;4:1236–1246.

Streptobacillus moniliformis

●

Mark E. Rupp

"Rats are the most despised and contemptible parts of God's earth"

Charles Lamb, 1799

"Rats!
They fought the dogs and killed the cats,
And bit the babies in the cradles
And ate the cheeses out of vats
And licked the soup from the cooks' own ladles"

Robert Browning
The Pied Piper of Hamelin, 1888

GENERAL DESCRIPTION AND MICROBIOLOGY

It has been known for thousands of years that a febrile illness can follow the bite of a rat. In the Western hemisphere, most cases of rat-bite fever are due to *Streptobacillus moniliformis*. *S. moniliformis* is a pleomorphic Gram-negative, nonmotile, nonsporeforming, nonencapsulated microaerophilic bacillus. Although the morphology of the organism depends on the age of the culture and growth conditions, it characteristically appears as long filamentous organisms with fusiform swellings. Optimal recovery is achieved using an enriched liquid media such as trypticase-soy broth supplemented with rabbit or horse serum, incubated at 37°C in a 10% CO_2 atmosphere (5). Many commercial blood culture systems do not support the growth of *S. moniliformis* because they contain sodium-polyanethol sulfonate, which inhibits its growth at concentrations as low as 0.0125% (18, 42). When grown in thioglycolate broth, *S. moniliformis* produces characteristic "puff ball" or "bread crumb" colonies. Cell wall–deficient colonies, which have a characteristic "fried-egg" appearance on solid media, arise spontaneously and were first described by Klienberger and named L-forms in honor of the Lister Institute (16).

At the biochemical level, *S. moniliformis* is an inactive species with negative reactions for oxidase, catalase, nitrate reduction, urea, phenylalanine deamination, and gelatin liquefaction. Acid with gas formation is produced from glucose, maltose, fructose, galactose, glycogen, mannose, and starch (27). There is a high degree of conformity when testing strains of *S. moniliformis* derived from a variety of animal sources (50).

EPIDEMIOLOGY

The natural habitat of *S. moniliformis* is the respiratory passage of rodents—especially rats. The organism is carried by healthy rats, both wild and laboratory, with reported colonization rates as high as 50 to 100% (25, 24). *S. moniliformis* occasionally causes disease in rats, resulting in otitis media, conjunctivitis, and pneumonia (50).

Infection with *S. moniliformis* in humans occurs most commonly in persons living in crowded, rat-infested urban dwellings. Children appear to be at greater risk, with about 50% of cases occurring in persons under age 12 (32). Laboratory personnel working with rodents are also at increased risk of contracting rat-bite fever (1, 4, 14). Infection generally results from rat bite but has also resulted from bites or scratches due to animals that feed on, or have close contact with, rats, such as cats, dogs, pigs, and ferrets (12). Infection may also result from handling dead rats, without an apparent breach of the skin (23). In addition, a case was described in which it was hypothesized that *S. moniliformis* was inoculated across nonintact skin from an inanimate object that was colonized with the organism (9). As many as 10% of persons bitten by a rat who do not receive antibiotic prophylaxis develop rat-bite fever (33).

Oral ingestion of *S. moniliformis* can cause epidemics of an illness resembling rat-bite fever that is known as Haverhill fever or erythema arthriticum epidemicum. Such outbreaks have been linked to contaminated milk and water (22, 28).

CLINICAL MANIFESTATION

Typically, the incubation period lasts less than 10 days and is followed by abrupt onset of fever, chills, headaches, vomiting, myalgias, and arthralgias (39). At the time of presentation, the bite wound is often completely healed, and unless the history of rat bite is elicited, the diagnosis may remain obscure. Rash often develops within several days of the onset of fever and is usually macular, maculopapular, or petechial. It is most prominent on the extremities and may involve the palms and soles. Desquamation has been described (44). About 50% of patients develop septic polyarticular arthritis. The joints involved, in decreasing order of frequency, are the knees, ankles, elbows, wrists, shoulders, hips, and sternoclavicular (19, 38). Laboratory tests often reveal an elevated white blood cell count with an increased number of band-form neutrophils on the differential count. Approximately 25% of patients develop a false-positive serologic test result for syphilis (48). Complications of rat-bite fever include endocarditis (38), myocarditis (45), pericarditis (36, 2), meningitis (41, 11), pneumonia (23, 41), amnionitis (8), brain abscess (6), splenic abscess (3), liver abscess and kidney abscess (48), and prostatitis and pancreatitis (50). Mortality in untreated cases of infection due to *S. moniliformis* is approximately 10% (12), but with appropriate antimicrobial treatment, mortality is rare.

SUSCEPTIBILITY IN VITRO
In Vitro Studies

A large number of studies have reported the susceptibility of single strains of *S. moniliformis* using a variety of techniques.

There is a paucity of studies examining multiple strains. Edwards and Finch examined the susceptibility of 7 strains of *S. moniliformis* to 9 antimicrobial agents using an agar dilution method (7). The mean MICs in μg/mL were as follows: penicillin ≤ 0.015, ampicillin ≤ 0.06, cefuroxime ≤ 0.125, cefotaxime ≤ 0.05, tetra-cycline ≤ 0.5, ciprofloxacin ≤ 2.0, gentamicin ≤ 4.0, erythromycin ≤ 4.0, chloramphenicol = 8.0. Wullenweber tested the susceptibility of 13 strains of *S. moniliformis* of human, murine, and avian origin using a breakpoint microtiter assay (Radiometer, Copenhagen) (50). The organisms were susceptible to a wide variety of antibiotics including β-lactams, monobactams, carbapenems, macrolides, lincosamides, glycopeptides, rifam-pin, and tetracyclines. Indeterminate sensitivity or resistance was observed with aminoglycosides, fluoroquinolones, chlor-amphenicol, trimethoprim/sulfamethoxazole, and fusidic acid. The specific agents tested and a summary of results are shown in Table 1. Results of other studies testing single strains are generally in agreement with the two studies discussed above (1, 9, 11, 13, 14, 15, 18, 20, 21, 26, 29, 31, 36, 38, 40, 42, 43). Antibiotics examined in one or more of the studies using single strains of *S. moniliformis* that were not examined in the two larger studies are summarized in Table 2.

Two cases of infection due to *S. moniliformis* resistant to penicillin have been reported (43, 46). Both reports are somewhat suspect by current standards. In the report by Stokes et al., the organism was identified by morphology, but no biochemical tests were reported. The organism was freeze-dried, but when the investigators attempted to further characterize it, it was no longer viable. Susceptibility testing was performed by disk diffusion using disks manufactured by the authors by impregnating filter paper with the antibiotics. In the paper by Toren et al., the isolate was again identified by morphology without supporting biochemical data. The method of determining antibiotic susceptibility is not clear, and MICs were not reported. Penicillin susceptibility was simply reported as negative. Therefore, until penicillin resistance is better documented, isolates of *S. moniliformis* can be regarded as uniformly susceptible to penicillin.

In Vivo Studies

There have been no in vivo studies of the efficacy of antibiotic treatment, singly or in combination, against *S. moniliformis*.

ANTIMICROBIAL THERAPY

There are no prospective trials concerning treatment of infection due to *S. moniliformis*. All data on this subject are derived from anecdotal reports of treatment of single or small numbers of patients.

Robbins is credited with reporting the first use of penicillin against *S. moniliformis* (34). The patient was a 70-year-old man with a leg abscess and positive blood cultures for *S. moniliformis* who failed treatment with sulfathiazole but responded favorably to penicillin at a total dose of approximately 2 million units. Watkins reported 16 cases of rat-bite fever observed in St. Louis over a 8-year period and reviewed the literature with regard to antibiotic therapy (49). He concluded that "Penicillin is indicated early in the treatment of rat-bite fever after correct diagnostic procedures have been employed." Despite over 50 years of experience since this advice was printed, it should not be significantly altered in caring for patients today. In 1965, Roughgarden reviewed 62 cases of streptobacillary rat-bite fever occurring between 1918 and 1958, including 27 cases in which penicillin therapy was used, and concluded that "a consistently effective regimen for streptobacillary disease consists of a daily dosage of not less than 400,000 to 600,000 units continued for not less than seven days. If no response is obtained in two days with this program, the dosage should be raised to 1,200,000 units daily." This recommendation was for procaine penicillin G given intramuscularly.

Currently, intravenous penicillin G is thought to be more appropriate. For uncomplicated disease, low-to-moderate doses should be effective (2.4–4.8 million units/day, split evenly every 6 h). Most patients improve rapidly, and for individuals who appear well after 5 to 7 days, treatment can be switched to oral ampicillin or penicillin V (500 mg orally every 6 h) to finish 10 to 14 days of therapy. Although there are no studies to guide treatment, based on the in vitro susceptibility of *S. moniliformis* to penicillin, patients with mild disease can probably be treated with an oral regimen for the entire treatment course.

A number of antibiotics other than penicillin have been successful in treating patients with infection due to *S. moniliformis*: cefazolin, cephalothin, cephradine, flucloxacillin, oxacillin, nafcillin, ampicillin, amoxicillin/clavulanate, ticarcillin, ceftriaxone, tetracycline, clindamycin, erythromycin, and chloramphenicol. Often these agents have

---

TABLE 1 • Antibiotic Susceptibility of 13 Strains of *Streptobacillus moniliformis*

Antibiotics to which all strains were *sensitive*
  Ampicillin, azlocillin, aztreonam, cefazolin, cefixime, cefotaxime, cefoxitin, cefpirome, ceftazidime, clindamycin, erythromycin[a], fosfomycin, imipenem, meropenem, mezlocillin, mezlocillin/sulbactam, nitrofurantoin, novobiocin[a], ofloxacin, oxacillin, penicillin, piperacillin, rifampin, teicoplanin, tetracycline, vancomycin
Antibiotics to which all strains were *intermediately susceptible*
  Amikacin, chloramphenicol, ciprofloxacin, gentamicin[b], tobramycin
Antibiotics to which all strains were *resistant*
  Nalidixic acid, norfloxacin, polymyxin B, trimethoprim/sulfamethoxazole

---

Modified from Wullenweber M. *Streptobacillus moniliformis* a zoonotic pathogen. Taxonomic considerations, host species, diagnosis, therapy, geographical distribution. Lab Anim 1995;29:1–15.

[a] No clear reaction with two strains.

[b] One strain sensitive; fusidic acid yielded results varying from sensitive to intermediately susceptible.

been combined with one another, or one of these agents has been combined with an aminoglycoside. However, there are no in vivo or in vitro data to indicate synergistic activity associated with combination therapy. These cases are summarized in Table 3.

Therefore, based on the data available, the drug of choice for treatment of infections due to *S. moniliformis* is penicillin. Alternative agents for patients who are allergic to penicillin include cephalosporins (first-, second-, or third-generation agents

appear to be effective), tetracyclines, erythromycin, clindamycin, or chloramphenicol. Several in vitro studies have shown that *S. moniliformis* is resistant to sulfonamides (1, 11, 40, 50), and therapy with sulfonamides has been associated with clinical failure (11, 42). Therefore, sulfonamides are not recommended as alternatives to penicillin.

L-forms, cell wall–deficient variants, arise spontaneously in culture and have been isolated from human blood (12). Because L-form cells lack a cell wall, they are resistant to antibi-

TABLE 2 • Susceptibility of *Streptobacillus moniliformis* to Antimicrobial Agents in Studies Testing Only Single Strains

Antibiotic	Method	Result	Reference
Aureomycin	Not stated	MIC = 1 μg/mL	Petersen, 1950 (26)
	Broth dilution	MIC = 0.12 μg/mL	Hamburger, 1953 (13)
Bacitracin	Disk diffusion	Sensitive	Rygg, 1992 (40)
Carbomycin	Broth dilution	MIC = 0.12 μg/mL	Hamburger, 1953 (13)
Ceftriaxone	Broth dilution	MIC < 0.03 μg/ml	Rupp, 1992 (38)
Cephaloridine	Disk diffusion	Sensitive	Gilbert, 1971 (11)
Cephalothin	Broth diffusion	MIC < 0.03 μg/ml	Rupp, 1992 (38)
	Disk diffusion	Sensitive	Rygg, 1992 (40)
	Disk diffusion	Sensitive	Holroyd, 1988 (15)
	Not stated	Sensitive	Anderson, 1983 (1)
Flucloxacillin	Disk diffusion	Sensitive	Fordham, 1992 (9)
Kanamycin	Disk diffusion	Sensitive	Gilbert, 1971 (11)
Lincomycin	Disk diffusion	Sensitive	Gilbert, 1971 (11)
Methicillin	Disk diffusion	Sensitive	Gilbert, 1971 (11)
Neomycin	Disk diffusion	Sensitive	Rygg, 1992 (40)
Sulfonamides	Disk diffusion	Resistant	Rygg, 1992 (40)
	Disk diffusion	Resistant	Gilbert, 1971 (11)
Streptomycin	Broth dilution	MIC = 8 μg/ml	Rupp, 1992 (38)
	Disk diffusion	Sensitive	Rygg, 1992 (40)
	Disk diffusion	Sensitive	Holden, 1964 (14)

TABLE 3 • Antibiotics Other than Penicillin Used Alone or in Combination to Treat Infections Due to *Streptobacillus moniliformis*

Antibiotic Regimen	Reference
Erythromycin (relapse) followed by cephradine then clindamycin	Anderson, 1983 (1)
Cefazolin	Faro, 1980 (8)
Flucloxacillin followed by vancomycin	Fordham, 1992 (9)
Sulfonamide (failure) followed by tetracycline/penicillin	Gilbert, 1971 (11)
Chloramphenicol (failure) followed by penicillin/streptomycin	Hamburger, 1953 (13)
Tetracycline followed by penicillin	Holden, 1964 (14)
Ticarcillin/gentamicin followed by penicillin	Holroyd , 1988 (15)
Erythromycin	Konstantopoulos, 1992 (17)
Cephalothin/tetracycline	Lambe, 1973 (18)
Oxacillin/ampicillin followed by penicillin	Mandel, 1985 (19)
Penicillin/streptomycin	McCormack, 1967 (20)
Chloramphenicol	Portnoy, 1979 (29)
Nafcillin	Prager, 1994 (30)
Tetracycline (relapse) followed by penicillin	Raffin, 1979 (32)
Nafcillin/gentamicin	Rumley, 1987 (37)
Ceftriaxone/vancomycin followed by penicillin	Rupp, 1992 (38)
Penicillin/chloramphenicol	Rygg, 1992 (40)
Cotrimoxazole (failure) followed by tetracycline	Shanson, 1983 (42)
Tetracycline	Shanson, 1983 (42)
Penicillin (failure) followed by chloramphenicol	Stokes, 1951 (43)
Erythromycin (failure) followed by clindamycin then tetracycline	Taylor, 1984 (45)
Amoxicillin/clavulanate	Vasseur, 1993 (47)

otics that act upon the cell wall (i.e., β-lactams) (35). Although there is little supporting evidence, it has been postulated that persisting penicillin-resistant L-form cells may cause relapse of infection after therapy has ceased. Some authors have recommended addition of streptomycin to enhance activity against L-forms (12). Others have followed intravenous penicillin therapy with a short course of oral tetracycline (38).

SPECIAL SITUATIONS
Pediatric Patients

As mentioned above, children appear to be at increased risk for infection due to *S. moniliformis* because of their increased propensity to suffer a rat bite. Penicillin G remains the drug of choice for these infections, at a dose of 25,000 units/kg/day divided evenly every 6 h. Tetracyclines should be avoided as a secondary choice because of their association with tooth discoloration and tooth enamel agenesis. Reasonable secondary choices include cephalosporins, erythromycin, and clindamycin.

Pregnant Patients

S. moniliformis has rarely been reported to cause infection in pregnant women and has not been reported to cause transplacental infection of the fetus (8). Penicillins have been used extensively in pregnant women and neonates and are generally safe (10). Therefore, penicillin remains the drug of choice for treating *S. moniliformis* infections in pregnant patients. Cephalosporins, which have demonstrated activity against *S. moniliformis* in vitro, could be used in women allergic to penicillin. However, these agents should be used with extreme caution, if at all, in women with a history of anaphylactic reaction to penicillins. For the reasons discussed above, tetracyclines should be avoided in the treatment of pregnant women. Erythromycin is generally safe for use in pregnancy, although the estolate form should be avoided because of the risk of cholestatic hepatitis (10). Clindamycin has also been used safely in pregnant women (10). There is little change associated with pregnancy in the pharmacokinetics of this agent and the drug crosses the placenta, reaching levels approximately one-half of those in maternal serum (10). Chloramphenicol use should generally be avoided in pregnant women and children because of hematologic toxicity and the "gray baby syndrome," a syndrome of neonates, characterized by vomiting, abdominal distension, flaccidity, and circulatory collapse.

Endocarditis and Central Nervous System Infections

Endocarditis as a complication of rat-bite fever due to *S. moniliformis* occurs very rarely. A recent review found only 16 cases described in the medical literature (38). Although optimal therapy is not known, high-dose penicillin treatment is recommended (≥20 million units/day divided evenly every 4 h), particularly if the isolate is resistant to penicillin at a level of 0.1 μg/mL or above (20).

Like endocarditis, meningitis or brain abscess has been described exceedingly rarely. There are no data regarding optimal therapy, but high-dose penicillin therapy is the treatment of choice. An attractive alternative, based on limited in vitro data and their excellent penetration into the cerebrospinal fluid, are the third-generation cephalosporins, cefotaxime and ceftriaxone.

S. moniliformis Infections in Veterinary Practice

S. moniliformis causes infection in a wide variety of animals including rats, mice, spinifex hopping mice, guinea pigs, dogs, turkeys, and koalas (50). There is little information regarding therapy in animals, and the topic is beyond the scope of this chapter. The interested reader is referred to the review by Wullenweber (50).

PREVENTION AND ANTIBIOTIC PROPHYLAXIS

In the event of a rodent bite, the wound should be thoroughly cleansed, and tetanus prophylaxis administered, if warranted. Although the efficacy of antibiotic prophylaxis for rat bite is unknown, a prudent course of action would dictate administration of amoxicillin/clavulanate at a dosage of 500 mg orally every 8 h for 3 days. Other common sense precautions one should take to avoid infection with *S. moniliformis* include using caution and wearing gloves while handling laboratory rodents, eradicating rats from human dwellings, and avoiding potentially contaminated water and unpasteurized milk.

REFERENCES

1. Anderson LC, Leary SL, Manning PJ. Rat-bite fever in animal research laboratory personnel. Lab Anim Sci 1983;33:292–294.
2. Carbeck RB, Murphy TF, Britt EM. Streptobacillary rat-bite fever with massive pericardial effusion. JAMA 1967;201:703–705.
3. Chulay JD, Lankerani MR. Splenic abscess. Am J Med 1976;61:513–522.
4. Cole JS, Stoll RW, Bulger RJ. Rat-bite fever. Ann Intern Med 1969;71:979–981.
5. Dalton HP, Rupp ME. *Streptobacillus moniliformis*. Microbiology 1992;35:1–5.
6. Dijkmans BAC. Thomeer RTWM, Vielvoye GJ, Lampe AS, Mattie H. Brain abscess due to *Streptobacillus moniliformis* and *Actinobacterium meyerii*. Infection 1984;12:262–264.
7. Edwards R, Finch RG: Characterization and antibiotic susceptibilities of *Streptobacillus moniliformis*. J Med Microbiol 1986;21:39–42.
8. Faro, S, Walker C, Pierson, RL. Amnionitis with intact amniotic membranes involving *Streptobacillus moniliformis*. Obstet Gynecol 1980;55(Suppl 3):95–115.
9. Fordham JN, McKay-Ferguson E, Davis A, Blyth T. Rat bite fever without the bite. Ann Rheum Dis 1992;51:411–412.
10. Gilbert GL. Antimicrobial therapy in pregnant women and neonates. In: Infectious disease in pregnancy and the newborn infant. Chur, Switzerland: Harwood Academic Publishers, 1991:549–575.
11. Gilbert GL, Cassidy JF, Bennett N. Rat-bite fever. Med J Aust 1971;2:1131–1134.
12. Gunning JJ. Rat-bite fevers. In: Hunter GW III, Swartzwelder JC, Clyde DF, eds. Tropical medicine. 5th ed. Philadelphia: WB Saunders, 1976:246–247.
13. Hamburger M, Knowles HC. *Streptobacillus monoliformis* infection complicated by acute bacterial endocarditis. Arch Intern Med 1953;92:216–220.
14. Holden FA, MacKay JC. Rat-bite fever—an occupational hazard. Can Med J 1964;91:1–4.

15. Holroyd KJ, Reiner AP, Dick JD. *Streptobacillus moniliformis* polyarthritis mimicking rheumatoid arthritis: an urban case of rate bite fever. Am J Med 1988;85:711–714.

16. Klienberger E. The natural occurrence of pleuropneumonia-like organisms in apparent symbiosis with *Streptobacillus moniliformis* and other bacteria. J Pathol Bacteriol 1935;1:93–105.

17. Konstantopoulos K, Skarpas P, Hitjazis F, Georgakopolous D, Matrangas Y, Andreopoulou M, Koutras E. Rat bite fever in a Greek child. Scand J Infect Dis 1992;24:531–533.

18. Lambe DW Jr., McPhedran AM, Mertz JA, Stewart P. *Streptobacillus moniliformis* isolated from a case of Haverhill fever: biochemical characterization and inhibitory effect of sodium polyanethanol sulfonate. Am J Clin Pathol 1973;60:854–860.

19. Mandel DR. Streptobacillary fever: an unusual cause of infectious arthritis. Cleve Clin Q 1985;2:203–205.

20. McCormack RC, Kaye D, Hook EW. Endocarditis due to *Streptobacillus moniliformis:* a report of two cases and review of the literature. JAMA 1967;200:77–79.

21. McDermott W, Leask MM, Benoit M. *Streptobacillus moniliformis* as a cause of subacute bacterial endocarditis: report of a case treated with penicillin. Ann Intern Med 1945;23:414–423.

22. McEvoy MB, Noah ND, Pilsworth R. Outbreak of fever caused by *Streptobacillus moniliformis*. Lancet 1987:1361–1363.

23. McHugh TP, Bartlett RL, Raymond JI. Rat bite fever: report of a fatal case. Ann Emerg Med 1985;14:1116–1118.

24. Paegle RD,Tewari RP, Bernhard WN, Peters E. Microbial flora of the larynx, trachea, and large intestine of the rat after long-term inhalation of 100 per cent oxygen. Anesthesiology 1976; 44:287–290.

25. Parker F Jr, Hudson NP. The etiology of Haverhill fever (erythema arthriticum epidemicum). Am J Pathol 1926;2:357–379.

26. Petersen ES, McCullough NB, Eisele CW, Goldinger JM. Subacute bacterial endocarditis due to *Streptobacillus moniliformis*. JAMA 1950;144:144–621.

27. Piot P. *Gardnerella, Streptobacillus, Spirillum and Calymmatobacterium*. In: Balows A, Hausler WJ Jr, Herrmann KL, Isenberg HD, Shadomy HJ, eds. Manual of clinical microbiology. 5th ed. Washington, DC: American Society for Microbiology, 1991;483–487.

28. Place EH, Sutton LE. Erythema arthriticum epidemicum (Haverhill fever). Arch Intern Med 1934;54:559–684.

29. Portnoy BL, Satterwhite TK, Dyckman JD. Rat bite fever misdiagnosed as Rocky Mountain spotted fever. South Med J 1979;72:607–609.

30. Prager L, Frenck RW Jr. *Streptobacillus moniliformis* infection in a child with chicken pox. Pediatr Infect Dis J 1994;13:417–418.

31. Priest WS, Smith JM, McGee CJ. Penicillin therapy of subacute bacterial endocarditis. Arch Intern Med 1947;79:333–359.

32. Raffin BJ, Freemark M. Streptobacillary rat-bite fever: a pediatric problem. Pediatrics 1979;64:214–217.

33. Richter CP. Incidence of ratbites and rat-bite fever in Baltimore. JAMA 1945;128:324–329.

34. Robbins G. Haverhill fever following rat bite treated with penicillin. Clinics 1944;3:425.

35. Rogosa M. *Streptobacillus moniliformis* and *Spirillum minus*. In: Lennette EH, Balows A, Hausler WJ Jr, Shadomy HJ, eds. Manual of clinical microbiology. 4th ed. Washington, DC: American Society for Microbiology. 1985:400–406.

36. Roughgarden JW. Antimicrobial therapy of rat-bite fever. Arch Intern Med 1965;116:39–54.

37. Rumley RL, Patrone NA, White L. Rat-bite fever as a cause of septic arthritis: a diagnostic dilemma. Ann Rheum Dis 1987;46: 793–795.

38. Rupp ME. *Streptobacillus moniliformis* endocarditis: case report and review. Clin Infect Dis 1992;14:769–772.

39. Rupp ME. Rat-bite fever. In: Hoeprich PD, Colin MC, Ronald AR, eds. Infectious diseases. 5th ed. Philadelphia: JB Lippincott, 1994:1317–1320.

40. Rygg M, Brun CF. Rat bite fever (*Streptobacillus moniliformis*) with septicemia in a child. Scand J Infect Dis 1992;24:535–540.

41. Sens MA, Brown EW, Wilson LR, Crocker TP. Fatal *Streptobacillus moniliformis* infection in a two-month-old infant. Am J Clin Pathol 1989;91:612–616.

42. Shanson DC, Gazzard BG, Midgley J, Dixey J. *Streptobacillus moniliformis* isolated from blood in four cases of Haverhill fever. Lancet 1983;92–94.

43. Stokes JF, Gray IR,, Stokes EJ. *Actinomyces muris* endocarditis treated with chloramphenicol. Br Heart J 1951;13:247–251.

44. Taber LH, Feigin RD. Spirochetal infections. Pediatr Clin North Am 1979;26:410–411.

45. Taylor AF, Stephenson TG, Giese HA, Pettersen GR, Murray RA. Rat-bite fever in a college student—California. MMWR 1984;33:318–320.

46. Toren, DA. Mycotic rat-bite fever. Del State Med J 1953;25: 334–335.

47. Vasseur E, Joly P, Nouvellion M, Laplagne A, Lauret PH. Cutaneous abscess: a rare complication of *Streptobacillus moniliformis* infection.

48. Washburn RG. *Streptobacillus moniliformis* (rat-bite fever). In: Mandell GL, Bennett JE, Dolin R, eds. Principles and practice of infectious diseases. 4th ed. New York: Churchill Livingstone, 1995:2084–2086.

49. Watkins CG. Ratbite fever. J Pediatr 1946;28:429–448.

50. Wullenweber M. *Streptobacillus moniliformis* a zoonotic pathogen. Taxonomic considerations, host species, diagnosis, therapy, geographical distribution. Lab Anim 1995;29:1–15.

Streptococcus Group B

Ayesha Mirza and Russell W. Steele

GENERAL DESCRIPTION

Group B streptococcus was first reported as a veterinary pathogen causing bovine mastitis long before its human clinical importance was recognized. The first description of group B streptococcal human disease was three cases of fatal puerperal sepsis over 60 years ago (21). Thereafter, it was increasingly recognized as a pathogen during the neonatal period and in peripartum and febrile postpartum women. It is currently the most common cause of neonatal sepsis and many other bacterial infections during the first 6 weeks of life. In recent years, it has also been recognized as a significant pathogen in individuals with certain predisposing conditions, particularly advanced age, malignancy, diabetes, human immunodeficiency virus, and liver failure, with the risk of disease increasing as much as 30-fold in these groups (14).

ECOLOGY

Group B streptococcus can be found as part of the normal flora in the gastrointestinal and female genital tracts, periurethral area, perineal and perianal skin, and even the upper respiratory tract (38). Colonization of the lower digestive tract is most common, seen in 15 to 35% of males and females of all ages. From the lower digestive tract, bacteria intermittently colonize the genital tract and less frequently the urinary tract. It is only found on the cervix in 6% of pregnant women, although this is the site from which the neonate likely acquires the organism (8, 28).

Pregnant women probably vary in extent and duration of group B streptococcal carriage. Only a small number appear to be heavily and continually colonized during pregnancy. Intermittent carriage is more common, which well accounts for limitations in accurate prediction of carriage during labor based on cultures obtained much earlier in pregnancy. This observation is important in developing guidelines for prevention of early-onset group B streptococcal disease in neonates on the basis of maternal cultures as discussed below.

Neonatal acquisition of the organism from the mother's genital tract takes place predominantly during delivery, and 70% of babies born to culture-positive mothers become colonized. Therefore, 8 to 15% of all newborns have the potential for acquiring group B streptococcal disease (13). When maternal cultures are negative, approximately 5% (range, 1–27%) of infants may still acquire group B streptococcus as colonizing flora (3). Among neonates, the external ear is the site most frequently colonized at birth. The nose, upper respiratory tract, umbilical stump, and rectum are also colonized early. Shortly thereafter, the adult pattern of rectal carriage is established. Considerable evidence supports hospital-based acquisition by newborn infants, and subsequent nursery spread is common. However, this appears to originate predominantly from mother-infant contact rather than transmission from hospital personnel.

CLINICAL MANIFESTATIONS

Two distinct clinical syndromes in neonates have been recognized: early-onset infection occurring within the first 8 days of life, usually presenting clinically with severe pneumonia, and late-onset infection typically occurring at 3 to 4 weeks of life (range, 7 days to 3 months), manifesting as occult bacteremia, meningitis, or focal disease such as osteomyelitis, septic arthritis, and cellulitis. Virtually all cases of early-onset disease are associated with maternal group B streptococcal colonization, while only half of the cases of late-onset infection are caused by strains identified in maternal flora.

In young, healthy, nonpregnant adults, it is only an occasional pathogen associated with genitourinary infection, pneumonia, bacteremia, and soft-tissue infection, whereas in pregnant women, it is the second most common cause of urinary tract infection and a frequently isolated bacterium in cases of amnionitis, endometritis, and postpartum wound infections. Almost all of these patients have a good outcome with early recognition and adequate therapy. In nonpregnant adults however, most of whom are immunocompromised, fatal outcome is not unusual in spite of appropriate management.

Diabetes is the single most common underlying condition for severe group B streptococcal disease in adults. Other predisposing factors include advanced age, liver failure or a history of alcohol abuse, neurologic impairment, malignancy, renal failure, cardiopulmonary disease or heart failure, and pulmonary disease. Adults are more likely to die from group B streptococcal infection than are children. The presence of chronic respiratory, genitourinary, or gastrointestinal infections in patients with group B streptococcal infection suggests that the hospital is the source for acquisition of bacteremia.

SUSCEPTIBILITY IN VITRO

Group B streptococcus is highly susceptible to most classes of antibiotics including penicillins, many first- and second-generation cephalosporins (excluding cefoxitin), third-generation cephalosporins, vancomycin and imipenem (Table 1). Of the third-generation cephalosporins, ceftriaxone has the greatest activity. Most strains are also sensitive to erythromycin, chloramphenicol, and clindamycin, but they are generally resistant to tetracycline. Ciprofloxacin has moderate in vitro activity but has not yet been evaluated for clinical efficacy. Resistance to erythromycin, clindamycin, and clarithromycin occurs in 1 to

TABLE 1 • MIC$_{50}$ and MIC$_{90}$ Antimicrobial Susceptibility Concentrations for Group B Streptococci

Antimicrobial Agent	MIC (µg/mL) Range	MIC$_{50}$	MIC$_{90}$
Ampicillin	0.12–0.25	0.25	0.25
Cefamandole	≤ 0.03–0.5	0.06	0.12
Cefoxitin	0.5–8.0	4.0	4.0
Cefuroxime	≤0.03–1.0	0.06	0.06
Cephradine	0.25–4.0	2.0	2.0
Cephalexin	0.5–8.0	4.0	4.0
Cephalothin	0.06–0.5	0.25	0.25
Ceftriaxone	0.06–0.12	0.12	0.12
Cefotaxime	0.02–0.12	0.12	0.12
Cefoperazone	0.12–0.5	0.25	0.5
Ceftazidime	0.12–0.5	0.25	0.5
Clindamycin	≤0.03–0.25	0.06	0.06
Carbenicillin	0.5–1	1	1
Chloramphenicol	1.0–4.0	2.0	4.0
Colistin	8.0–>32.0	>32.0	>32.0
Doxycycline	0.12–32.0	16.0	16.0
Erythromycin	≤0.01–0.25	0.06	0.06
Gentamicin	1.0>32.0	16.0	16.0
Kanamycin	8.0–>32.0	>32.0	>32.0
Lincomycin	0.03–0.25	0.12	0.12
Methicillin	0.5–16.0	2.0	2.0
Minocycline	0.25–32.0	16.0	32.0
Mezlocillin	0.12–0.25	0.12	0.25
Moxalactam	2–8	8	8
Neomycin	4.0>32.0	32.0	>32.0
Nalidixic acid	>32.0	>32.0	>32.0
Nitrofurantoin	8.0–32.0	16.0	32
Penicillin	≤0.01–0.12	0.06	0.06
Piperacillin	0.25–0.5	0.5	0.5
Sulfa-trimethoprim	1.2/0.06–9.5/0.5	4.8/0.25	4.8/0.25
Ticarcillin	1–2	2	2
Tetracycline	0.12–>32.0	32.0	32.0
Vancomycin	0.5–2.0	0.5	0.5

3% of isolates and uniformly to nalidixic acid, trimethoprim-sulfamethoxazole, metronidazole, and aminoglycosides.

Compared with group A streptoccocci, group B streptococcus grows more rapidly and requires a longer time for killing by β-lactam antibiotics. In the presence of 1 µg/mL of ampicillin, elimination of group A strains is complete at 4 h, while sterilization of group B strains does not occur until 20 to 24 h, even at concentrations of 10 µg/mL (37). In studies using 50 times the minimal bactericidal concentration (MBC) of ampicillin, group A strains were killed within 4 hours. In contrast, virtually no killing of group B strains was observed over this time. The relatively slow bactericidal action of ampicillin on this organism may explain the difficulty in treating immunosuppressed hosts.

In Vitro and in Vivo Synergy

Synergy between ampicillin and aminoglycosides in group B streptococcal inhibition assays is well documented. Killing is much more rapid when 2 or 10 µg/mL of gentamicin is added to a cidal concentration of ampicillin. This effect is more marked when the combination contains concentrations of 10 µg/mL of gentamicin. Monitoring peak serum concentrations of

gentamicin to achieve this high level is therefore indicated. The mechanism of enhanced killing of group B streptococcus by the ampicillin-aminoglycoside combination has not been defined; it is postulated that gentamicin enters and acts on cells partially damaged by ampicillin (37). Murine animal models experimentally infected with group B streptococcus also demonstrate faster clearing of bacteremia with ampicillin and gentamicin used in combination than with ampicillin alone (12).

ANTIMICROBIAL AGENT THERAPY
General Recommendations

Since group B streptococci remain universally susceptible to penicillins, penicillin G as single therapy is considered the treatment of choice for established group B streptococcal infections (27, 31). Primary advantages over an ampicillin-gentamicin combination are its narrower spectrum of antimicrobial activity and lower cost. However, high doses of penicillin G must be used for treatment of group B streptococcal disease for two reasons. First, the MIC of penicillin G for group B streptococcus is relatively high, 4 to 10-fold greater (range, 0.01–0.4 µg/mL) than that for group A streptococcal strains. Secondly, patients are generally immunocompromised (including neonates), a factor associated with high-grade bacteremia and higher concentrations of organisms in tissue, including the cerebrospinal fluid (CSF) where 10^7 to 10^8 organisms/mL have been consistently reported. Since inoculum size greatly influences in vitro susceptibility to penicillin G, higher doses are likely required to provide bactericidal activity in vivo. This inoculum effect has also been noted with cefotaxime and imipenem.

Neonates

Low dosages of penicillin used in the 1970s may in part explain the high rate of relapse initially reported in infants (15, 24, 44, 45). Penicillin was generally given at 100,000 units/kg/day, and ampicillin with gentamicin recommended at 200 mg/kg/day and 7.5 mg/kg/day, respectively, for a period of 10 to 14 days. Following these reports, the recommended dosage of penicillin for treatment of meningitis in neonates was increased from 100,000 to 250,000 units/kg/day. Dosages in neonates of penicillin G as high as 500,000 units/kg/day or ampicillin at 300 to 400 mg/kg/day are recommended by some experts (3). While other treatment resources concur with higher dosages in neonates, they also suggest adjusting the dosage on the basis of age (Table 2).

At the present time, the accepted antimicrobial regimen for neonatal sepsis/meningitis of uncertain etiology consists of ampicillin and an aminoglycoside until the organism is identified (7). Once group B streptococcus is confirmed, treatment can be adjusted to penicillin (or ampicillin) alone.

For the infant with late-onset disease whose CSF contains Gram-positive cocci in pairs and short chains or who has a positive rapid antigen assay for group B streptococcus, it would appear prudent to begin therapy with ampicillin and gentamicin or ampicillin and a third-generation cephalosporin (ceftriaxone or cefotaxime), since it is essential to eradicate the organisms rapidly from the CSF and the synergistic or additive

TABLE 2 • **Antimicrobial Regimens Recommended for Treatment of Group B Streptococcal Infections in Neonates and Young Infants**

Site of Infection	Age	Drug	Dose/Day (Intravenous)	Duration
Bacteremia without meningitis	All	Ampicillin plus gentamicin	150–200 mg/kg 7.5 mg/kg	Initial treatment before culture results (48–72 h)
		Penicillin G	200,000 units/kg	Complete a total treatment course of 10 days
Meningitis	<7 days	Ampicillin	200–300 mg/kg/day in 3 divided doses	Initial treatment until CSF is sterile
		Gentamicin	5 mg/kg in 2 divided doses	
	<7 days	Penicillin G	250,000–400,000 u/kg/day in 3 divided doses	Complete a minimum total treatment course of 21 days
	≥7 days	Ampicillin	300–400 mg/kg/day in 4–6 divided doses	Initial treatment until CSF is sterile
		Gentamicin	7.5 mg/kg in 3 divided doses	
	≥7 days	Penicillin G in 4 divided doses	400,000 units/kg/day	Complete a minimum total treatment course of 21 days
Septic arthritis	All	Penicillin G	200,000 units/kg	2–3 weeks
Osteomyelitis	All	Penicillin G	200,000 units/kg	3–4 weeks
Endocarditis	All	Penicillin G	400,000 units/kg	4–6 weeks

TABLE 3 • **Treatment of Group B Streptococcal Infections in Adults**

Diagnosis	Antibiotic (Dose)	Alternative Dose for Penicillin-Allergic Patients	Duration
Bacteremia, soft-tissue infections	Penicillin G (10–12 million units/day)	Vancomycin	10 days
Meningitis	Penicillin G (20–30 million units/day)	Vancomycin	14–21 days
Osteomyelitis	Penicillin G (10–20 million units/day)	Vancomycin	4 weeks
Endocarditis	Penicillin G (20–30 million units/day) with an aminoglycoside for 2 weeks	Vancomycin with an aminoglycoside	6 weeks

killing effect of gentamicin combined with ampicillin may prove beneficial in the early course of the infection. In addition, *Streptococcus pneumoniae, Listeria monocytogenes,* and enterococci may resemble group B streptococcus in Gram stains of CSF, and ampicillin is the drug of choice for the latter two pathogens. A third-generation cephalosporin plus vancomycin is recommended for pneumococcus.

Older Patients

Although there has been broad experience with the successful treatment of neonatal group B streptococcal infections, much less information is available to guide clinicians in managing adults with serious invasive group B streptococcal infections (11, 18) (Table 3). Whereas ampicillin and gentamicin are acceptable as an initial empirical regimen in neonates, even broader coverage may be needed in adults to cover the range of organisms that cause serious infections, particularly in immunocompromised individuals. Initial empirical therapy, however, usually includes antimicrobials that have excellent activity against group B streptococcus, such as cefotaxime (MIC_{99} < 0.06 µg/mL) or ceftazidime (MIC_{90} < 0.5 µg/mL) often in combination with vancomycin (MIC_{90} < 0.5 µg/mL). These regimens are quite adequate, as studies have found no

evidence of improved outcome among patients who received ampicillin- or penicillin G–containing regimens compared with patients who did not receive these agents.

Endocarditis

Both acute and subacute cases of endocarditis have been described. Most occur in younger patients (mean age, ~18 years). The mitral valve is the most commonly affected (48%), followed by aortic (29%), mitral and aortic (10%), and tricuspid valves (5%). Tricuspid valve involvement is frequently seen in intravenous drug abusers. Underlying heart disease is present in more than half of the cases reported, with rheumatic heart disease being most common. Rapid valve destruction necessitating early valve replacement is a characteristic feature of this disease in adults.

The current recommendation for treatment of group B streptococcal endocarditis is penicillin (20 million units/day intravenously for 28 days). In the penicillin allergic patient, cephalothin (12 g/day intravenously) or vancomycin (2 g/day intravenously) for 28 days may be substituted. Of note is the failure of clindamycin in two presumed penicillin-allergic patients. Some have suggested that penicillin should be combined with an aminoglycoside for their synergy, but current data are not adequate to make such a recommendation. This combination should be used for cases caused by penicillin-tolerant or relatively penicillin-resistant strains. Prosthetic valve endocarditis requires early surgical intervention; medical therapy alone is usually inadequate (36).

Pneumonia

Pneumonia in patients with altered immune function is often accompanied by pleural empyema. Fatality rates from 30 to 85% are seen even with early and adequate penicillin therapy.

Bone and Joint

Arthritis and osteomyelitis seem to also occur commonly in diabetics and are generally monoarticular, affecting the knee, hip, or shoulder. High-dose penicillin (8–19.2 million units/day for 3–8 weeks) in addition to surgical drainage has been optimal. Cefazolin and cephradine for 4 to 6 weeks have also been effective. It is essential to establish an early diagnosis by needle aspiration and culture of joint fluid (3).

Skin and Soft Tissue

Most recently, skin and soft-tissue infections have accounted for one-third of infections with group B streptococcus (3). Cellulitis, foot ulcers, abscess, and infections of decubitus ulcers are the most common. Pyomyositis, blistering dactylitis, and necrotizing fasciitis have also been reported. Antimicrobial therapy along with drainage effects complete recovery in approximately 90% of these patients.

Urinary tract infections are seen in middle-aged women with underlying intrinsic alteration of urinary flow or stones. One prospective evaluation attributed 2% of all urinary tract infections to group B streptococcus (32). The isolates were susceptible to virtually all antimicrobials tested except gentamicin. Outcome in most of these cases has been poor, likely related to the well-known inability of conventional antimicrobial therapy to eradicate vaginal or enteric colonization. Penicillin remains the drug of choice in the treatment of group B streptococcus–related urinary tract infections (14).

Treatment of chorioamnionitis and intraamnionitic infection in pregnant and postpartum women requires a regimen that will cross the placenta sufficiently to begin fetal therapy. Ampicillin (2 g every 6 h) and gentamicin (1.5 mg/kg every 8 h) or ampicillin (2 g) plus sulbactam (1 g) every 6 h have been recommended (1). Gentamicin is used in higher concentrations in pregnant women because of the high renal clearance associated with pregnancy. Other treatment regimens include combinations of ticarcillin/clavulanic acid or a cephalosporin (e.g., cefuroxime or cefazolin) plus gentamicin. For penicillin-allergic patients, vancomycin plus gentamicin or a cephalosporin plus gentamicin are recommended.

Other uncommon manifestations of group B streptococcal infections in adults include meningitis, keratitis, endophthalmitis.

Duration

Parenteral therapy of 10 days duration is recommended for treatment of bacteremia, pneumonia, pyelonephritis, and soft-tissue infections. A 14-day minimum duration is recommended for treatment of meningitis, and a 4-week minimum for treatment of endocarditis or ventriculitis.

ENDPOINTS FOR THERAPY

Duration of therapy is generally based on published experience, guided by individual clinical response and follow-up cultures. Optimal results have been seen with treatment of bacteremia without a focus or with soft-tissue infection parenterally for 10 days, 2 to 3 weeks for meningitis or pyarthrosis, 3 weeks for osteomyelitis, and 4 weeks for endocarditis (3). For osteomyelitis and septic arthritis, drainage of the infected site is often an important adjunct to antimicrobial therapy. Based on previous reports of neonatal group B streptococcal meningitis relapse when treatment was given for only 10 to 14 days, some experts suggest at least 3 weeks of antimicrobial therapy for neonatal meningitis.

Acute-phase reactants are useful for monitoring response to therapy in bone and joint infection and as a guide for hospital discharge and discontinuation of antibiotics. C-reactive protein is the first to return to normal, occurring after 3 to 5 days of appropriate therapy, while the erythrocyte sedimentation rate (ESR) takes longer, generally 7 to 21 days (42). Discharge from the hospital to home parenteral antibiotic therapy can be planned when the patient is afebrile, the white blood cell count is returning to baseline, and the C-reactive protein is in the normal range. The ESR can be measured after 21 days of therapy and antibiotics discontinued if it is below 30 mm/h.

Repeat lumbar puncture 24 to 48 h into therapy is recommended in the management of infants with meningitis, to confirm response to therapy and sterilization of the CSF. Another lumbar puncture later in the course of therapy is indicated if follow-up CSF cultures were not sterile or if there is no clinical improvement.

ADJUNCTIVE THERAPY

Supportive care of the critically ill patient with group B streptococcal disease is identical to that for serious infections caused by other pathogens. This includes early recognition and treatment of shock, management of metabolic acidosis, and fluid administration. Extracorporeal membrane oxygenation has been used as rescue therapy for neonates with overwhelming group B streptococcal sepsis and pneumonia (26), and granulocyte transfusions have been used in neutrophil-depleted patients (10, 46). The potential adverse effects of granulocyte transfusions, which include graft-versus-host disease, transmission of hepatitis and cytomegalovirus, and pulmonary leukocyte sequestration, make this therapy still experimental, to be considered only in those who fail to respond to conventional treatment.

Other proposed therapies include granulocyte/macrophage-colony-stimulating factor (GM-CSF), GCSF, and intravenous immunoglobulin. Hyperimmune group B streptococcal immunoglobulin and human monoclonal antibodies to group B streptococcus are currently under development. Clearly, opsonic antibody deficiency and low total serum immunoglobulin contribute to the susceptibility of neonates and immunocompromised patients to group B streptococcus. It follows that treatment with intravenous immunoglobulin (IVIG) might be a useful adjunct to therapy. Studies using immune rabbit serum in an opsonophagocytic bactericidal assay for group B streptococcus supported this hypothesis by showing increased killing of group B streptococcus when IVIG and complement were combined (19). Similar results were seen in the type III group B streptococcal animal challenge model (23). Well designed human clinical trials are needed before any of these therapies can be endorsed.

CONTROVERSIES
Penicillin Tolerance

Defined as an MBC 16 to 32 times the MIC, the phenomenon of in vitro tolerance in group B streptococcal isolates corresponds with delayed bacterial killing. Additive rather than synergistic bactericidal activity between ampicillin and gentamicin, and possible autolytic enzyme defects in such strains. Penicillin tolerance in vitro has been noted in 4 to 6% of isolates (29). The clinical importance of this in vitro phenomenon remains ill defined, although some experts recommend that all strains of group B streptococcus be tested for tolerance before discontinuing the aminoglycoside and that combination therapy be continued for the entire course when tolerance is detected (40). Detection of tolerance depends highly on the growth medium used and the growth phase of the bacterial inoculum (29). Identification of this property is somewhat impractical, since in vitro testing is neither standardized nor available in most hospital laboratories. For patients demonstrating a good clinical response to initial therapy, demonstration of in vitro tolerance is not an indication for a change either to another class of antibiotics or to combination regimens.

Prophylactic Intravenous Immunoglobulin for Premature Neonates

A number of clinical trials have examined the protective efficacy of IVIG for early-onset group B streptococcal disease and other infections in neonates. Most important were two controlled multicenter trials (2, 5, 17). The first study randomized premature newborns weighing 500 to 1750 g to receive either placebo or 500 mg/kg of IVIG. Infusions were given between the 3rd and 7th days of life, 7 days later, and then every 14 days until a total of 5 infusions was received or the patient was discharged. There were no differences in fatality rates, but the total incidence of infections was reduced from 47 to 32% with IVIG. The largest reductions in infections were in those caused by either coagulase-negative staphylococci or *Candida* species. No significant differences for group B streptococcus were noted, but infection rates were too low to allow meaningful interpretation. A later collaborative trial (17) randomized almost 2500 infants weighing less than 1500 g to receive 500 mg/kg of IVIG or placebo within 72 h of birth and at 14-day intervals until they weighed 1800 g. In this trial, there was no difference in infection nor mortality. In summary, these two large clinical trials did not support the efficacy of high-dose IVIG in prevention of bacterial infection of premature neonates.

PREVENTION OF EARLY-ONSET GBS DISEASE IN NEONATES

Once group B streptococcal invasive disease became a major concern in the early 1970s, a number of strategies for controlling neonatal infection were examined (1, 30, 33, 34, 49). These can be divided into the following approaches: (*a*) active immunization of young or pregnant women, (*b*) passive immunization with IVIG, (*c*) treatment of group B streptococcal carriers, (*d*) early antibiotic treatment of all neonates, and (*e*) chemoprophylaxis during labor.

Immunization of Women

One fairly consistent finding with group B streptococcal invasive disease is absence of type-specific IgG antibody in the neonate (4). Maternally acquired IgG antibody in the neonate persists for 2 months. Since the presence of such antibody simply reflects passive transfer from the mother, its absence in the mother represents a focus for correction. Two strategies are presently being investigated: active immunization of antibody-negative pregnant women (6, 47) and passive immunization with specific antibody. The latter strategy has only been investigated in animal models and appears to have limited clinical applicability.

Most promising are studies examining maternal active immunization with group B streptococcal vaccines as a method of preventing neonatal invasive disease. Vaccination of non-immune women during their third trimester of pregnancy with a vaccine containing the type III polysaccharide of group B streptococcus was initially reported in 1988 (6). Low or unprotective antibody concentrations were defined as below 2 μg/mL. Some 57% of recipients responded with a rise in titer from 1.3 to 7.1 mg/mL 4 weeks after vaccination, and 80% of the infants of successfully immunized mothers retained protective levels of antibody until 1 month of age. Therefore, this vaccine would be expected to protect a maximum of only 50% of babies potentially at risk. These early studies were encouraging but indicated that a more immunogenic vaccine was needed before considering large trials to evaluate the safety and efficacy of this strategy. A conjugate antigen that covalently links group B streptococcus type III polysaccharide to a protein carrier is the likely solution and candidate vaccines are currently being developed (48). However, maternal antibody does not cross the placenta in adequate concentrations until 32 weeks' gestation. At this age, antibody concentrations are only 50% those of full-term neonates, suggesting that successful maternal immunization may still be inadequate to prevent disease in those born very prematurely.

Treatment of Group B Streptococcus Carriers

Eradication of maternal group B streptococcal colonization was a strategy first investigated two decades ago (20, 22, 25). Well-designed clinical studies used oral antibiotics to treat colonized mothers during the second or third trimester of pregnancy. In these initial trials, relapse occurred commonly and was thought to result from colonization of sexual contacts. Subsequent studies therefore included treatment of partners, but results were essentially unchanged; recolonization was still observed in two-thirds of study cases prior to rupture of membranes and onset of labor (22). These experiences suggested that prevention of neonatal disease might best be accomplished by eradicating group B streptococcus during the immediate antepartum period.

Prophylaxis of Neonates at Birth

Early administration of penicillin to prevent group B streptococcal disease in neonates has been investigated in a number of clinical studies, but results were variable. Two encouraging reports demonstrated efficacy of penicillin prophylaxis, although neither focused on high-risk populations of neonates

(16, 39, 41). In the latter study, the incidence of severe infection caused by non–group B streptococci increased, thereby negating clinical benefits of intervention.

A more recent study included an appropriate concurrent control group among neonates weighing 2000 g or less (35). Some 1187 high-risk premature neonates had blood and surface cultures obtained and were randomized to receive no treatment or 100,000 U/kg of crystalline penicillin G intramuscularly immediately after birth and every 12 h for 72 h. Treatment in this series neither prevented early-onset streptococcal disease nor reduced excess mortality associated with infection.

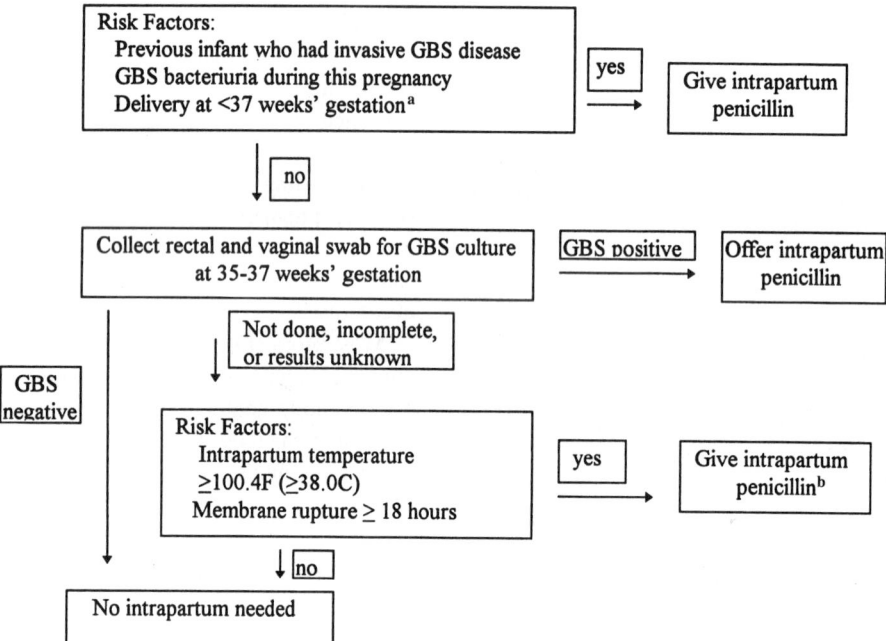

FIGURE 1. Algorithm for prevention of early-onset group B streptococcal (GBS) disease in neonates, using prenatal screening at 35–37 weeks' gestation. [a]If membranes ruptured before 37 weeks' gestation, and the mother has not begun labor, collect group B streptococcal culture and either (a) administer antibiotics until cultures are completed and the results are negative or (b) begin antibiotics only when positive cultures are available. No prophylaxis is needed if culture obtained at 35–37 weeks' gestation was negative. [b]Broader-spectrum antibiotics may be considered at the physician's discretion, based on clinical indications.

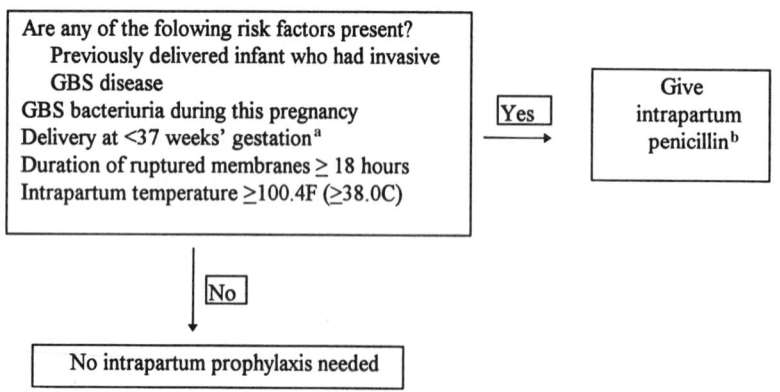

FIGURE 2. Algorithm for prevention of early-onset group B streptococcal (GBS) disease in neonates, using risk factors. [a]If membranes ruptured before 37 weeks' gestation and the mother has not begun labor, collect group B streptococcal culture and either (a) administer antibiotics until cultures are completed and the results are negative or (b) begin antibiotics only when positive cultures are available. [b]Broader-spectrum antibiotics may be considered at the physician's discretion, based on clinical indications.

TABLE 4 • **Recommended Regimens for Intrapartum Antimicrobial Prophylaxis for Perinatal Group B Streptococcal Disease**

Recommended	Penicillin G, 5 mU i.v. bolus, then 2.5 mU i.v. every 4 h until delivery
Alternative	Ampicillin, 2 g i.v. bolus, then 1 g i.v. every 4 h until delivery
If penicillin allergic	
Recommended	Clindamycin, 900 mg i.v. every 8 h until delivery
Alternative	Erythromycin, 500 mg i.v. every 6 h until delivery

Note: If patient is receiving treatment for amnionitis with an antimicrobial agent active against group B streptococci (e.g., ampicillin, penicillin, clindamycin, or erythromycin), additional prophylactic antibiotics are not needed.

Intrapartum Chemoprophylaxis

Intrapartum administration of intravenous penicillin or ampicillin to group B streptococcus–colonized mothers has been shown to decrease vertical transmission of the bacterium and to prevent neonatal disease (43). This occurs whether the mother is lightly or heavily colonized and has been documented in both low-risk and high-risk neonates. These factors only vary the incidence of disease in untreated pregnancies and therefore the relative benefits of intervention.

The best-designed and most convincing prospective, randomized, controlled clinical trial focused on pregnant women colonized with group B streptococcus and showed that intrapartum prophylaxis with intravenous ampicillin prevented at least 50% of the early-onset group B streptococcal infections in their patient population (9). A meta-analysis of seven additional trials, which included studies of carriers with and without risk factors, estimated a 30-fold reduction in early-onset group B streptococcal disease with similar chemoprophylaxis (42).

Collectively these data strongly support maternal intrapartum chemoprophylaxis, and this approach for preventing group B streptococcus has been endorsed by the American Academy of Pediatrics and by the American College of Obstetricians and Gynecologists. Two strategies are equally acceptable, one directed by culture results obtained at 35 to 37 weeks' gestation (Fig. 1) and the other based on maternal risk factors (Fig. 2).

For chemoprophylaxis based on cultures, all pregnant women should be screened at 35 to 37 weeks' gestation for group B streptococcus, using a single swab specimen from the lower vagina and anorectum and appropriate selective broth medium for transport and solid media for final recovery. Results of this culture should be recorded and be readily available when the mother begins labor.

There are two exceptions to the requirement of colonization as a prerequisite for treatment: maternal group B streptococcal bacteriuria during pregnancy or a previous neonate with invasive group B streptococcal disease. The former circumstance is appropriate since bacteriuria is strongly predictive of heavy genital colonization and early-onset disease, and the latter history is an independent variable highly associated with neonatal group B streptococcal sepsis.

Until an effective group B streptococcal vaccine is developed, selective intrapartum chemoprophylaxis should be encouraged. The preferred intrapartum chemoprophylactic regimen is intravenous penicillin G, 5 million units initially and 2.5 million units every 4 h until delivery (Table 4). Clindamycin or erythromycin may be used for women allergic to penicillin.

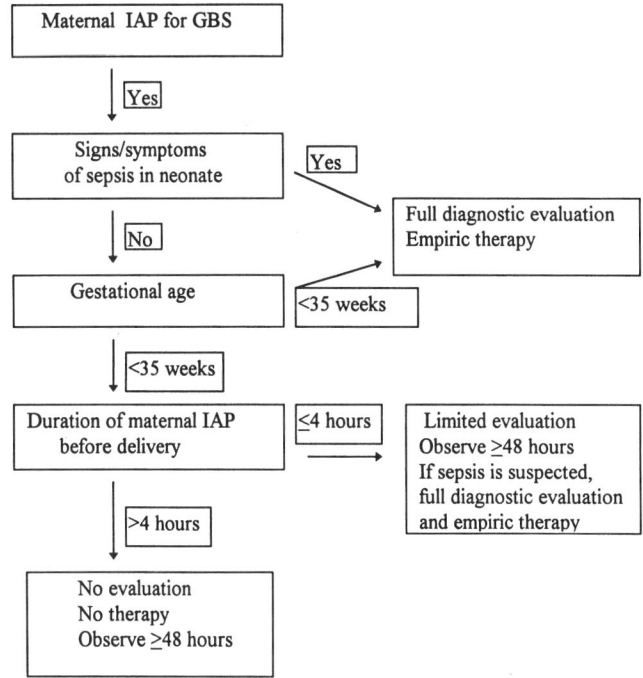

FIGURE 3. Algorithm for management of a neonate born to a mother who received intrapartum antimicrobial prophylaxis (IAP) for prevention of early-onset group B streptococcal (GBS) disease.

Management of infants whose mothers received at least two doses of intrapartum antibiotics is based on gestation and clinical assessment (Fig. 3). This algorithm is not an exclusive course of management but should be modified to include variations that incorporate individual circumstances or institutional preferences. A full diagnostic evaluation implies a complete blood count (CBC) and differential, blood culture, and chest radiograph if the neonate has respiratory symptoms. Lumbar puncture need only be performed at the discretion of the physician. Duration of therapy varies depending on blood culture and CSF results and the clinical course of the infant. If laboratory results and clinical course are unremarkable, duration of therapy may be as short as 48 to 72 h. The term *limited evaluation* for the neonate whose mother received less than 4 h of intrapartum chemoprophylaxis implies that only a CBC with a differential and a blood culture are needed. Neonates less than 35 weeks' gestation should have a complete sepsis evaluation and empirical antibiotics pending results of cultures and clinical status during this observation period. Cultures require 48 h incubation prior to being reported as negative. Asymptomatic newborns over 35 weeks' gestation can be followed without antibiotic therapy if clinically normal. Some experts recommend obtaining surface and gastric cultures for group B streptococcus in these infants. Symptomatic neonates at any gestation should undergo a sepsis work-up followed by broad-spectrum antimicrobial therapy, usually ampicillin plus gentamicin or ampicillin plus a third-generation cephalosporin.

Pediatricians are encouraged to develop their own management protocols if they disagree with any aspects of the present algorithm.

REFERENCES

1. Anonymous. Prevention of perinatal group B streptococcal disease: a public health perspective. MMWR 1996;45:RR-7.
2. Baker CJ. New uses of intravenous immune globulin in newborn infants. J Clin Immun 1990;10(Nov Suppl):47S–52S.
3. Baker CJ, Edwards MS. Group B streptococcal infections. In: Remington JS, Klein JO, eds. Infectious disease of the fetus and newborn infants. 4th ed. Philadelphia: WB Saunders, 1990: 742–811.
4. Baker CJ, Edwards MS, Kasper DL. Role of antibody to native type III polysaccharide of group B streptococcus in infant infection. Pediatrics 1981;68:544–549.
5. Baker CJ, Melish ME, Hall RT, Casto DT, Vasan U, Givner LB, and the Multicenter Group for the Study of Immune Globulin in Neonates. Intravenous immune globulin for the prevention of nosocomial infection in low-birth-weight neonates. N Engl J Med 1992;327:213–218.
6. Baker CJ, Rench MA, Edwards MS, Carpenter RJ, Hays BM, Kasper DL. Immunization of pregnant women with a polysaccharide vaccine of group B streptococcus. N Engl J Med 1988; 319:1180–1185.
7. Barton LL, Feigen RD, Lins R. Group B beta hemolytic streptococcal meningitis in infants. J Pediatr 1973;82:719–723.
8. Blumberg HM, Stephens DS, Modansky M, Erwin M, Elliot J, Facklam RR, Schuchat A, Baughman W, Farley MM. Invasive group B streptococcal disease: the emergence of serotype V. J Infect Dis 1996;173:365–373.
9. Boyer KM, Gotoff SP. Prevention of early-onset neonatal group B streptococcal disease with selective intrapartum chemoprophylaxis. N Engl J Med 1986;314:1665–1669.
10. Christensen RD, Rothstein G, Anstall HB, Bybee B. Granulocyte transfusions in neonates with bacterial infection, neutropenia and depletion of mature marrow neutrophils. Pediatrics 1982;70:1–6.
11. Colford JM, Mohle-Boetani J, Vosti KL. Group B streptococcal bacteremia in adults—five years experience and a review of the literature. Medicine 1995;74:176–190.
12. Deveikis A, Schauf V, Mizen M, Riff L. Antimicrobial therapy of experimental group B streptococcal infection in mice. Antimicrob Agents Chemother 1977;11:817–820.
13. Easmon CSF. The carrier state: group B streptococcus. J Antimicrob Chemother 1986;18(Suppl A):59–65.
14. Edwards MS, Baker CJ. Streptococcus agalactiae (group B streptococcus). In: Mandel GL, Bennett JE, Dolin R, eds. Principles and practice of infectious diseases. 4th ed. New York: Churchill Livingstone, 1995:1835–1845.
15. Eickhoff TC, Klein JO, Daly AK, Ingall D, Finland M. Neonatal sepsis and other infections due to group B beta-hemolytic streptococci. N Engl J Med 1964;271:1221–1228.
16. Ernest JM, Givner LB. A prospective, randomized, placebo-controlled trial of penicillin in preterm premature rupture of membranes. Am J Obstet Gynecol 1994;170:516–521.
17. Fanaroff AA, Korones SB, Wright LL, Wright EC, Poland RL, Bauer CB, Tyson JE, Philips III JB, Edwards W, Lucey JF, Catz CS, Shankaran S, Oh W. A controlled trial of intravenous immune globulin to reduce nosocomial infections in very-low-birth-weight infants. N Engl J Med 1994;330:1107–1113.
18. Farley MM, Harvey RC, Stull T, Smith JD, Schuchat A, Wenger JD, Stephens DS. A population based assessment of invasive disease due to group B streptococcus in nonpregnant adults. N Engl J Med 1993;328:1807–1844.
19. Fischer GW. Immunoglobulin therapy for neonatal sepsis: an overview of animal and clinical studies. J Clin Immunol 1990; 10(Nov Suppl):40S–46S.
20. Franciosi RA, Knostman JD, Zimmerman RA. Group B streptococcal neonatal and infant infections. J Pediatr 1973;82:707–718.
21. Fry RM. Fatal infections by haemolytic streptococcus group B. Lancet 1938;1:199–201.
22. Gardner SE, Yow MD, Leeds LJ, Thompson PK, Mason EO Jr, Clark DJ. Failure of penicillin to eradicate group B streptococcal colonization in the pregnant woman: a couple study. Am J Obstet Gynecol 1979;135:1062–1065.
23. Givner LB, Baker CJ. Pooled human IgG hyperimmune for type III group B streptococci: evaluation against multiple strains in vitro and in experimental disease. J Infect Dis 1991;163: 1141–1145.
24. Green PA, Singh KV, Murray BE, Baker CJ. Recurrent group B streptococcal infections in infants: clinical and microbiologic aspects. J Pediatr 1994;125:931–938.
25. Hall RT, Barnes W, Krishman L, Harris DJ, Rhodes PG, Fayez J. Antibiotic treatment of parturient women colonized with group B streptococci. Am J Obstet Gynecol 1976;124:630–634.
26. Hocker JR, Simpson PM, Rabalais GP, Stewart DL, Cook LN. Extracorporeal membrane oxygenation and early onset group B streptococcal sepsis. Pediatrics 1992;89:1–4.
27. Jacobs MR, Kelly F, Speck WT. Susceptibility of group B streptococci to 16 β-lactam antibiotics, including new penicillin and cephalosporin derivatives. Antimicrob Agents Chemother 1982; 22:897–900.
28. Katz VL. Management of group B streptococcal disease in pregnancy. Clin Obstet Gynecol 1993;36:832–842.
29. Kim KS, Yoshimori RN, Imagawa DT, Anthony BF. Importance of medium in demonstrating penicillin tolerance by group B streptococci. Antimicrob Agents Chemother 1979;16:214–216.
30. Larsen JW, Dooley SL. Group B streptococcal infections: an obstetrical viewpoint. Pediatrics 1993;91:148–149.
31. McCracken GH Jr, Ginsberg C, Chrane DF, Thomas ML, Horton LJ. Clinical pharmacology of penicillin in newborn infants. J Pediatr 1973;82:692–698.
32. Muñoz P, Coque T, Rodriquez Creixems M, Bernaldo de Quirós JCL, Moreno S, Bonza E. Group B streptococcus: a cause of urinary tract infection in nonpregnant adults. Clin Infect Dis 1992;14:492–496.
33. Ohlsson A, Myhr TL. Intrapartum chemoprophylaxis of perinatal group B streptococcal infections: a critical review of randomized controlled trials. Am J Obstet Gynecol 1994;170:910–917.
34. Paredes A, Wong P, Yow MD. Failure of penicillin to eradicate the carrier state of group B streptococcus in infants. J Pediatr 1976;89:191–193.
35. Pyati SP, Plides RS, Jacobs NM, Ramamurthy RS, Yeh TF, Raval DS, Lilien LD, Amma P, Metzger WI. Penicillin in infants weighing two kilograms or less with early-onset group B streptococcal disease. N Engl J Med 1983;308:1383–1388.
36. Roberts RB, Knieger AG, Gross KC. The species of viridans streptococci associated with microbial endocarditis: incidence

and antimicrobial susceptibilities of species of viridans strepto-coccus. J Infect Dis 1990;140:316–321.

37. Schauf V, Deveikis A, Riff L, Serota A. Antibiotic killing kinet-ics of group B streptococci. J Pediatr 1976;89:194–198.

38. Schuchat A, Wenger JD. Epidemiology of group B streptococ-cal disease: risk factors, prevention strategies and vaccine de-velopment. Epidemiol Rev 1994;16:374–402.

39. Siegel JD, McCracken GH, Threlkeld N, DePasse BM, Rosenfeld CR. Single-dose penicillin prophylaxis against neonatal group B streptococcal infection. N Engl J Med 1980;303: 769–775.

40. Siegel JD, Shannon KM, DePasse BM. Recurrent infection as-sociated with penicillin-tolerant group B streptococci: a report of two cases. J Pediatr 1981;99:920–924.

41. Steigman AJ, Bottone EJ, Hanna BA. Intramuscular penicillin administration at birth. Prevention of early-onset group B strep-tococcal disease. Pediatrics 1978;62:842–844.

42. Steele RW. Control of neonatal group B streptococcal infection. J R Soc Med 1993;86:712–715.

43. Steele RW. Prevention of group B streptococcal infection in pregnant women and neonates. Infect Med 1996;13:392–396.

44. Troug WE, Davis RF, Ray CG. Recurrence of group B strepto-coccal infection. J Pediatr 1976;89:185–186.

45. Walker ST, Santos AQ, Quintero BA. Recurrence of group B streptococcal meningitis. J Pediatr 1976;89:187–188.

46. Wheeler JG, Chauvenet AR, Johnson CA, Dillard R, Block SM, Boyle R, et al. Neutrophil storage pool depletion in septic neu-tropenic neonates. Pediatr Infect Dis J 1984;3:407–409.

47. Wessels MR, Paoletti LC, Kasper DL, DiFabio JL, Michon F, Holme K, Jennings HJ. Immunogenicity in animals of a poly-saccharide-protein conjugate vaccine against type III group B streptococcus. J Clin Invest 1990;86:1428–1433.

48. Wessels MR, Kasper DL. The changing spectrum of group B streptococcal disease. N Engl J Med 1993;328:1843–1844.

49. Yow MD, Mason EO, Leeds LJ, Thompson PK, Clark DJ, Gard-ner SE. Ampicillin prevents intrapartum transmission of group B streptococcus. JAMA 1979;241:1245–1247.

Streptococcus pneumoniae

●

Ian R. Friedland and George H. McCracken

MICROBIOLOGY

Streptococcus pneumoniae is a Gram-positive coccus that pro-duces green (α) hemolysis on blood agar. Like all streptococci, it tends to grow in chains. All pathogenic pneumococcal strains are surrounded by a polysaccharide capsule that allows the pneumococcus to evade phagocytosis, thus delaying clear-ance from the bloodstream and other body sites. More than 80 different pneumococcal capsular types have been described, and the relative frequency of each capsular type varies with age and geographic location.

EPIDEMIOLOGY

S. pneumoniae is a common cause of community-acquired lower respiratory tract infection and sepsis (bacteremia), es-pecially in the very young and the elderly. It is the most com-mon cause of otitis media and sinusitis. It is now also the most common cause of meningitis in most developed coun-tries where the *Haemophilus* conjugate vaccine has virtually eliminated that disease. Annually in the United States, pneu-mococcal infection accounts for approximately 7 million cases of otitis media, 500,000 cases of pneumonia, 50,000 cases of bacteremia, and 3000 cases of meningitis (55). Less common pneumococcal infections include peritonitis (espe-cially in patients with nephrotic syndrome), endocarditis (28), osteomyelitis, septic arthritis (1, 52), and soft-tissue in-fections.

Pneumococci are frequently carried for many months in the nasopharynx and can be found in over 40% of children (94) and in approximately 20% of adults. Highest carriage rates are observed in young children, especially those in day care. An-

tibiotic resistance rates in nasopharyngeal isolates usually ex-ceed those in isolates obtained from blood or cerebrospinal fluid (CSF) in a particular geographic location.

S. pneumoniae induces inflammation (and subsequent tis-sue damage) as a result of the release of cell wall fragments, such as peptidoglycan and teichoic acid, and intracellular pro-teins such as pneumolysin (90). Cell wall fragments are more potent inducers of inflammation than is the intact cell wall. Thus, the host reaction to the pneumococcus may be enhanced by exposure to antimicrobial agents, such as β-lactam antibi-otics, which disrupt the cell wall.

SUSCEPTIBILITY IN VITRO

Mechanisms of Antibiotic Resistance

Until the mid-1970s, pneumococci were generally highly sus-ceptible to penicillin. However in the last two decades, strains with diminished susceptibility to penicillin have been increas-ingly isolated (58). Penicillin-resistant *S. pneumoniae* (PRSP) strains are now prevalent (20–30% or above) in many parts of the United States (Table 1), Europe (e.g., Spain, France, Hun-gary), and parts of Asia and Africa. An overall penicillin re-sistance rate of 23% (range, 6–54%) was reported among 1865 strains collected in 1992–93 in a multicenter study in Europe and the United States (44). The identical rate of penicillin re-sistance was found among 1527 outpatient isolates collected in 30 U.S. centers in 1994 to 1995 (22).

Penicillin resistance results from alterations in cell wall proteins, called penicillin-binding proteins (PBPs). PBPs are responsible for elongation of peptidoglycan fragments that make up the cell wall. Generally, the number of changes in these PBPs determines the level of penicillin resistance. In particular, changes in PBP 2X are associated with high-level cephalosporin resistance (but low-level penicillin resistance), and additional alterations in PBP 2B result in high-level penicillin resistance (17, 46). Mutations in PBP genes result from acquisition of gene fragments from other streptococci, especially viridans streptococci, which co-reside with pneumococci in the oropharynx (84). The most important factors associated with PRP infections are prior antibiotic exposure (16, 18, 88), day-care attendance, and alcoholism (16). Hospitalized patients and individuals infected with the human immun-odeficiency virus are also at greater risk for PRSP infections (65, 72, 78).

Resistance to other antimicrobial agents has also become a problem in the United States and other parts of the world. Resistance to the cephalosporins has been observed in parallel to the increase in penicillin resistance in the United States and Europe (43). In a European and American multicenter study in 1992–93, the prevalence of intermediate ceftriaxone resistance was 11.2%, but less than 2% of strains were highly ceftriaxone resistant (44). Definitions of intermediate and high level ceftriaxone resistance are shown in Table 2.

Erythromycin resistance rates as high as 26% have been reported in France (40). In the United States, macrolide resistance averages approximately 10%, but rates as high as 23% occur in some locales (4), and higher rates have been reported in isolates from children with otitis media (66). A single dose of azithromycin in children has been associated with an increase in nasopharyngeal carriage of azithromycin-resistant *S. pneumoniae* (61). Resistance to trimethoprim/sulfamethoxazole exceeds 20% in parts of the United States and Europe (50). Resistance to erythromycin (and clarithromycin and azithromycin), tetracycline, and/or trimethoprim/sulfamethoxazole is often associated with penicillin resistance, or such resistance can occur independently. Recently in the United States, more than 40 and 60% of PRSP strains were reported to be resistant to erythromycin and trimethoprim/sulfamethoxazole, respectively (22, 50). Ciprofloxacin has only modest activity against *S. pneumoniae*, and resistance is close to 20% in the United States (4). Resistance rates are lower with other quinolones (e.g., sparfloxacin) that have greater intrinsic activity against pneumococci.

TABLE 1 • Pneumococcal Resistance (%) to Antibiotics in 30 Centers in the United States (1994–1995)

Antibiotic	Intermediate[a]	Resistant[a]	Any Resistance
Penicillin	14	10	24
Age < 10 years	15	12	27
Age > 20 years	13	8	21
Cefotaxime			3
Ceftriaxone			5
Cefuroxime			12
Erythromycin[b]			10
TMP-SMX			18
Rifampin			0.5
Vancomycin			0

Data adapted from Doern GV, Brueggemann A, Preston Holley H, Rauch AM. Antimicrobial resistance of *Streptococcus pneumoniae* recovered from outpatients in the United States during winter months of 1994 to 1995: results of a 30-center national surveillance study. Antimicrob Agent Chemother 1996;40:1208–1213.

[a] See Table 2 for definitions.

[b] Similar resistance rates observed with clarithromycin and azithromycin.

TABLE 2 • Definitions of Pneumococcal Resistance to β-Lactam Antibiotics and Representative Peak Serum Concentrations in Adults

Antibiotic	Definition by MIC (μg/mL)[a]			Mean Peak Serum Conc. (μg/mL)[b] (Antibiotic dosage in g)	Activity Relative to Penicillin[c]
	Susceptible	Intermediate	Resistant		
Penicillin	≤0.06	0.1–1	≥2		
Amoxicillin	≤0.5	1	≥2	7.5 (0.5)	±
Cefotaxime	≤0.5	1	≥2	130 (2)	+
Ceftriaxone	≤0.5	1	≥2	250 (2)	+
Ceftazidime	≤0.5	1	≥2	160 (2)	− −
Cefepime	≤0.5	1	≥2	130 (2)	+
Cefaclor	≤8	16	≥32	16.5 (0.5)	− −
Cefprozil	≤8	16	≥32	9.6–10.5 (0.5)	− −
Cefpodoxime	N/A[d]	N/A	N/A	4.2 (0.4)	−
Ceftibuten	N/A	N/A	N/A	15.0 (0.4)	− −
Cefixime	N/A	N/A	N/A	1.9 (0.2)	− −
Cefuroxime sodium (parenteral)	≤0.5	1	≥2	100 (1.5)	−
Cefuroxime axetil (oral)	≤4	8	≥16	4.4–9.0 (0.5)	−
Imipenem	≤0.12	0.25–0.5	≥1	52 (1)	+ +

[a] Susceptibility definitions are from references 63 and 69.

[b] Serum concentration data were obtained from references 5, 24, 26, 57, 60.

[c] ± indicates similar MICs; + indicates two- to fourfold lower MICs; ++ indicates fourfold or lower MICs; − indicates two- to fourfold greater MICs; and— indicates fourfold or greater MICs.

[d] N/A indicates that interpretive criteria are not available.

Penicillins

Pneumococcal resistance to antibiotics is categorized according to the minimum inhibitory concentration (MIC) of the antibiotic for a particular strain (Table 2). The term *penicillin-resistant Streptococcus pneumoniae* (PRSP) used herein includes both intermediately resistant *S. pneumoniae* and highly resistant *S. pneumoniae,* both defined in Table 2. The prevalence of PRSP in a recent U.S. multicenter analysis is shown in Table 1. The in vitro activity of ampicillin and amoxicillin against pneumococci is very similar to that of penicillin (74), although amoxicillin may be slightly more active than penicillin against intermediately resistant strains (44). Despite similar in vitro activities, the definitions for penicillin and amoxicillin resistance differ (Table 2). Antistaphylococcal penicillins and broad-spectrum penicillins, such as ticarcillin and piperacillin, are generally less active in vitro than penicillin G. Combinations containing β-lactamase inhibitors such as amoxicillin/clavulanate offer no advantage over the active β-lactam antibiotic alone because penicillin resistance in pneumococci is not caused by β-lactamase production.

Cephalosporins and Other β-Lactam Antimicrobials

Since all β-lactam antibiotics bind to PBPs, alterations in their number or structure are reflected by reduced susceptibility not only to penicillin but also to the cephalosporins. The activity of individual cephalosporins against resistant pneumococci can be classified relative to the activity of penicillin (Table 2). The extended-spectrum cephalosporins, with the exception of ceftazidime, are generally more active than penicillin against PRSP. However, this generalization does not apply for all strains, and susceptibility testing of individual agents being considered for therapy is essential. High-level resistance to cefotaxime or ceftriaxone (MIC ≥ 2 µg/mL) is presently uncommon in most areas but is a problem in some locations in the United States. Pneumococcal strains with ceftriaxone or cefotaxime MICs of 4 µg/mL or above are rare (0.1% in the study of Goldstein et al. (44)).

Susceptibility cutoffs for the extended-spectrum cephalosporins are low because of the difficulty in treating central nervous system (CNS) infections, in which antibiotic concentrations in CSF are diminished because of poor penetration across the blood-brain barrier. These cutoffs are unlikely to be appropriate for infections outside the CNS, and isolation of "cephalosporin-resistant" strains in patients with pneumonia or sepsis does not preclude the use of cefotaxime or ceftriaxone therapy.

The inherent activity of the oral cephalosporins against pneumococci varies and all are significantly less active against PRSP than amoxicillin. In addition, the MIC cutoffs used to define resistance vary among the cephalosporins (Table 2). Achievable serum concentrations differ markedly for individual cephalosporins given in recommended dosages. The clinical efficacy of a particular antibiotic depends on the concentration at the site of infection and the MIC for the organism. More specifically, the duration of antibiotic concentrations above the MIC for the pathogen at the site of infection (e.g., middle ear fluid in acute otitis media) is important for β-lactam antibiotics. Data presented in Table 2 illustrate that therapy based on in vitro definitions of resistance without regard to achievable serum and tissue concentration can be inappropriate. For example, a strain with a ceftriaxone MIC of 2 µg/mL would be defined as resistant but is likely to be cleared easily from the bloodstream (achievable ceftriaxone serum concentrations exceed 100 µg/mL), whereas a strain with a cefaclor MIC of 8 µg/mL would be called susceptible but is unlikely to be cleared from the middle ear, where antibiotic concentrations seldom exceed 8 µg/mL.

Imipenem is the most active β-lactam antibiotic against pneumococci (23), and even though highly penicillin-resistant strains have greater MICs to imipenem, they still fall within the susceptible range (86). Meropenem, although less active than imipenem, usually retains good activity against penicillin-resistant strains (85).

Non-β-Lactam Antimicrobials

Other antimicrobial agents, such as erythromycin, trimethoprim/sulfamethoxazole, tetracycline, and chloramphenicol may be used to treat pneumococcal infections, but resistance to these agents usually increases in parallel with penicillin resistance rates, and multiresistant strains have been problematic in some communities (see above). There is cross resistance among the macrolides, and erythromycin-resistant strains are also resistant to clarithromycin and azithromycin (67).

Vancomycin resistance has not been described among pneumococci. In the United States, most pneumococcal strains also remain susceptible to clindamycin, but in other countries such as France and South Africa, clindamycin resistance frequently accompanies macrolide resistance (macrolide-lincomycin-streptogramin resistance). Rifampin resistance is also rare in the United States, but in countries where rifampin is used frequently for treatment of tuberculosis, rifampin-resistant strains are encountered (83). Rifampin resistance can also develop during therapy (8); as a result, rifampin should not be used as a single agent for pneumococcal infections. It is not clear whether emergence of rifampin resistance can be prevented by combining rifampin with other antibiotics.

Early-generation fluoroquinolones are not particularly active against pneumococci, but newer quinolones such as levofloxacin, trovafloxacin, and to a lesser extent sparfloxacin are highly active against both penicillin-susceptible and -resistant pneumococci (4, 39, 41, 93). In contrast to many other antimicrobial agents, there is usually no association between penicillin resistance and susceptibility to vancomycin, rifampin, or the quinolones.

ANTIMICROBIAL THERAPY

Appropriate antimicrobial therapy depends on the site of infection and the antibiotic susceptibility of the causative organism. Recommendations for antimicrobial therapy are summarized in Table 3 and usual dosages for adults and children are given in Tables 4 and 5.

Pneumonia and Sepsis

Penicillin and ampicillin remain the drugs of choice for treatment of penicillin-susceptible and intermediate PRSP infec-

TABLE 3 • Recommended Therapy for Penicillin-Susceptible and -Resistant Pneumococcal Infections

Infection	Empirical Therapy[a]	Penicillin Susceptibility Known		
		Susceptible	Intermediate Resistance	High Resistance
Pneumonia or bacteremia	Ampicillin, cefuroxime, amoxicillin	Penicillin, ampicillin, amoxicillin, cefuroxime	Pencillin, ampicillin, amoxicillin, cefuroxime	Cefotaxime, ceftriaxone, high-dose ampicillin, vancomycin
Meningitis	Cefotaxime or ceftriaxone + vancomycin[b]	Cefotaxime, ceftriaxone, ampicillin or penicillin	Cefotaxime[c] or ceftriaxone + vancomycin[b]	Cefotaxime[c] or ceftriaxone + vancomycin[b]
Otitis media	Amoxicillin	Amoxicillin	Amoxicillin[d] (Avoid oral cephalosporins)	Clindamycin, high dosage amoxicillin, macrolide[e], TMP/SMX[e], or ceftriaxone[f]

[a] For suspected pneumococcal infection or confirmed pneumococcal infection pending susceptibility data.

[b] Vancomycin (15 mg/kg/dose 6-hourly in children) should be combined with a cephalosporin in areas where cephalosporin resistance occurs. Vancomycin therapy can be discontinued once the strain is confirmed to be cephalosporin susceptible.

[c] High dosage (300 mg/kg/day) recommended.

[d] Although supportive data are lacking, larger dosages (e.g., 75 mg/kg/day) should be considered.

[e] Resistance to these agents is common among highly penicillin-resistant strains.

[f] If oral therapy fails, intramuscular ceftriaxone can be given daily for 3–5 days.

TABLE 4 • Recommended Daily Dosages for Agents Commonly Used in Pneumococcal Meningitis[a]

Agent	Adult Dosage (g/day)	Pediatric Dosage (mg/kg/day)	Dosing Interval (h)
Penicillin G[b]	24 million U	200,000–300,000 U/kg	4
Ampicillin[b]	12	200–300	4–6
Cefotaxime[c]	8–12	225–300	6–8
Ceftriaxone	4	100	12–24
Vancomycin	2–3	60	6–8
Rifampin	0.6	15–20	24

[a] See Table 3 for selection of antibacterial agent.

[b] Do not use for penicillin-resistant infections.

[c] Upper range recommended in areas where cephalosporin resistance occurs.

tions. No randomized comparative therapeutic trials for PRSP pneumococcal pneumonia or bacteremia have been published, and recommendations for treating suspected pneumococcal infections (Table 3) are based on comparative in vitro susceptibility data and published clinical results. The recommendation for using penicillin or ampicillin in intermediate PRSP pneumonia is based on clinical success in children and adults and the lack of microbiologically documented treatment failures with these agents. In 208 South African children with blood culture–proved pneumococcal pneumonia or sepsis, Friedland and Klugman (30) reported similar mortality rates in children with infections caused by PRSP (mostly of intermediate resistance) strains and those infected with penicillin-susceptible strains. In a more detailed study in 108 children (34), similar clinical response rates were noted by day 3 of standard dosage therapy (usually ampicillin). In Spain, adults with PRSP pneumonia were treated successfully with high-dose ($\geq$12 million units daily) penicillin therapy (82). In a recent 10-year prospective study, mortality in 154 adults with PRSP pneumonia (including some patients with high-level PRSP) treated with penicillin or an extended-spectrum cephalosporin was not increased (73).

Of the β-lactams, only the extended-spectrum cephalosporins (excluding ceftazidime) and the carbapenems are usually equally or more active than penicillin against PRSP, and the use of other β-lactam agents for these infections could be problematic. Indeed, the only bacteriologically documented treatment failures in PRSP pneumonia involved initial treatment with ticarcillin (MIC, 64 μg/mL, (72)) and cefazolin (81). The poor activity of ceftazidime against PRSP is noteworthy, and fatalities have occurred in immunocompromised patients with PRSP pneumonia treated with ceftazidime (13). Intravenous cefuroxime, which usually retains useful activity against intermediate PRSP, has been used successfully in pediatric pneumonia and bacteremia caused by intermediate PRSP (87). In addition, intravenous cefuroxime (1500 mg every 8 h) was curative in two adult patients with pneumonia caused by strains defined as cefuroxime resistant (MICs, 2 and 4 μg/mL, (10)), emphasizing that current definitions of cephalosporin resistance are not always clinically relevant.

There is sparse information to guide the choice of antibiotic therapy for high-level PRSP. Presumably, strains in the lower range defining high-level PRSP (MICs, 2–4 μg/mL) respond adequately to high-dose intravenous penicillin or ampicillin,

TABLE 5 • **Recommended Daily Dosages of Agents Commonly Used for Treatment of Nonmeningeal Pneumococcal Infections**[a]

Agent	Route	Adult Dosage (g/day)	Pediatric Dosage (mg/kg/day)	Dosing Interval (h)
Penicillin	i.v.	4–12 million U	100,000–200,000 U/kg	4–6
Ampicillin	i.v.	4–12	100–200	6
Cefazolin	i.v.	2–6	50–100	8
Cefuroxime	i.v.	2–4.5	100–150	6–8
Cefotaxime	i.v.	2–6	100–200	8
Ceftriaxone	i.v.	1–2	75–100	24
Vancomycin	i.v.	2	30–40	6–12
Amoxicillin	p.o.	0.75–1.5	40–80	8
Cefuroxime	p.o.	0.5–1	100	12
Erythromycin	p.o.	1–2	40	6–8
Clarithromycin	p.o.	1–2	15	12
Azithromycin	p.o.	0.5 day 1, then 0.25	10	24
TMP/SMX	p.o.	0.16	8–12 (TMP)	12
Clindamycin	p.o.	0.6–1.2	20–30	6–8

[a] See Table 3 for selection of antibacterial agent. Use upper-range dosages of β-lactam antibiotics to cover penicillin-resistant strains. i.v., intravenous; p.o., per os; TMP/SMX, trimethoprim/sulfamethoxazole.

but it is unknown at what level of resistance therapy would be compromised. The extended-spectrum cephalosporins cefotaxime and ceftriaxone are usually at least as active as penicillin for high-level PRSP and are likely to be effective in most cases. The current definition for extended-spectrum cephalosporin resistance is meant to guide therapy for meningitis, and a definition appropriate for therapy for pneumonia or bacteremia has not yet been determined. Bacteriologic failure with the extended-spectrum cephalosporins in PRSP pneumonia has not been documented.

Although all pneumococcal strains are susceptible to vancomycin, there is little justification for the use of this agent in pneumococcal pneumonia (35), especially in light of the recent spread of vancomycin-resistant enterococci. Vancomycin may, however, be indicated in rare cases caused by high-level PRSP not responding satisfactorily to adequate dosages of more active β-lactam antibiotics or in patients with adverse reactions to β-lactams.

Clindamycin is also suitable for patients unable to tolerate β-lactam therapy. In North America, resistance to clindamycin is rare, but in other areas, resistance is more common. The macrolides (erythromycin, clarithromycin) and azithromycin may also be used for pneumococcal pneumonia, but resistance is a problem in certain areas. Also, high-level PRSP are more likely to be multiresistant, and caution should be exercised when using a macrolide for suspected PRSP infections.

Most of the quinolones, including ciprofloxacin, ofloxacin, lomefloxacin, and fleroxacin, have limited in vitro activity against pneumococci. Clinical failures in pneumococcal pneumonia and superinfection with resistant strains have been described with ciprofloxacin therapy (45, 80). Newer quinolones such as levofloxacin, sparfloxacin, and trovafloxacin exhibit greater intrinsic activity against pneumococci and may prove useful for therapy of pneumococcal pneumonia in adults.

Meningitis

Penicillin, chloramphenicol, and the extended-spectrum cephalosporins have proven efficacy for meningitis caused by penicillin-susceptible pneumococci. Chloramphenicol therapy may, however, be inferior to β-lactam therapy (79), especially against PRSP strains (29), and may antagonize the bactericidal activity of β-lactams against pneumococci (32). In North America, cefotaxime or ceftriaxone are used most frequently for empirical therapy of meningitis, especially in children. These agents are not only highly effective for susceptible strains but are also effective in most cases of PRSP meningitis. However, since the early 1990s, cephalosporin resistance has emerged in countries such as the United States, Spain, and France, and treatment failures with these agents in children with meningitis have been documented (48, 56, 77). The current National Committee for Clinical Laboratory Standards (NCCLS) definition for cephalosporin resistance (69) is conservative, and raising the cutpoints for resistance is being considered. Adequate responses to standard-dose cefotaxime (200–225 mg/kg/day) therapy have been described in children with cephalosporin-resistant *s. pneumoniae* (CRSP) meningitis (53, 89). High-dose cefotaxime therapy (300 mg/kg/day) has been used successfully in small numbers of adult patients with meningitis caused by CRSP (92). Thus, both treatment failure and success have been reported in patients with meningitis caused by pneumococci defined as cephalosporin resistant, but it is unclear how frequently success or failure occurs. In a recent study of children with meningitis treated with high-dose cefotaxime (300 mg/ kg/day), in vitro bactericidal activity against CRSP was tested in CSF specimens taken at various time intervals. Some CSF specimens were bactericidal for CRSP even 8 h after a dose of cefotaxime, whereas others demonstrated no bactericidal activity, emphasizing the marked interpatient variability in CSF antibiotic concentrations and consequent unreliability of cefotaxime as a single agent for CRSP meningitis (36).

The combination of a cephalosporin and vancomycin has been shown to be synergistic against β-lactam-resistant pneumococci both in vitro (33) and in the animal meningitis model (31). To overcome the possibility of treatment failure in areas where CRSP occur with some frequency (as in much of the

United States), combination therapy with a cephalosporin and vancomycin is recommended for initial empirical therapy of suspected pneumococcal meningitis (Table 3). If CRSP is isolated, this antimicrobial combination should be continued. In all other cases (including when no organism is isolated), vancomycin can be discontinued. This combination has been successful in the small number of cases reported to date. Vancomycin has not been recommended as single-agent therapy for CRSP meningitis because of reported treatment failures in adults (91). However, in children given vancomycin (60 mg/kg/day), CSF penetration appears to be reliable (59), but since clinical experience with vancomcyin as a single agent in pneumococcal meningitis is lacking, it is not recommended. Intrathecal vancomycin administration for CRSP meningitis has been reported in adults (64), but the clinical benefit of such therapy has not been documented.

Other combinations (e.g., a cephalosporin and rifampin) have been recommended for CRSP meningitis on the basis of animal studies (76), but there are no clinical data on their effectiveness in pneumococcal meningitis. Cefpirome and cefepime are new extended-spectrum cephalosporins that are usually twice as potent as ceftriaxone and cefotaxime against PRSP (6, 85) and may prove useful for treatment of meningitis. The carbapenems, especially meropenem, are also potentially useful in PRSP meningitis, but clinical experience is limited (2, 48).

The usual duration of antibiotic therapy in pneumococcal meningitis is 10 to 14 days. Ten days of therapy is probably sufficient in uncomplicated cases, but longer courses are recommended in patients with severe complications or when there is delay in eradicating the organism from the CSF. Shorter antibiotic courses (7 days) have been used in small numbers of patients with pneumococcal meningitis (54, 63), but sufficient comparative data are lacking to recommend less than 10 days of therapy.

Otitis Media and Sinusitis

The discussion of acute otitis media that follows is applicable to therapy for acute sinusitis because the pathophysiologic mechanisms of disease and the causative organisms are very similar. Therapeutic considerations in otitis media differ from those in more serious infections because the causative organism is seldom identified and otitis has a high spontaneous resolution rate. Penetration of antibiotics into middle ear fluid varies depending on the agent used, the degree of inflammation, and patient characteristics. Generally, middle ear fluid concentrations are only 20 to 50% of serum concentrations, although some agents (e.g., trimethoprim, clarithromycin, and azithromycin) achieve greater penetration (Table 6). Modest decreases in pneumococcal susceptibility can compromise the effectiveness of many oral antibacterial agents, especially when given in standard dosages. It should also be clear that current definitions of β-lactam antibiotic susceptibility (Table 2) do not correlate with achievable middle ear fluid concentrations (Table 6) or with clinical outcome.

Amoxicillin remains the antibiotic standard for initial empirical treatment of acute otitis media, even in areas with a high prevalence of antibiotic-resistant strains, because it is inexpensive, has a low rate of adverse effects, and appears to be effective for treatment of both intermediate- and high-level PRSP otitis media (7). In a recent noncomparative study, 917 children enrolled in centers in Europe, Israel, and the United States received standard-formulation amoxicillin/clavulanate therapy (40/10 mg/kg/day) for 10 days (49). The clinical response rate was independent of penicillin susceptibility; clinical cure or improvement by day 14 was observed in 20 of 22 (91%) children with highly PRSP middle ear isolates. However, a lower success rate (50%) was found at day 38 in the 8 evaluable U.S. patients with PRSP infections (not statistically significant).

In areas where PRSP infections are common, empirical use of higher dosages of amoxicillin (e.g., 75 mg/kg/day) appears reasonable despite the lack of clinical data supporting a better outcome than with standard dosage (40 mg/kg/day). Combination of amoxicillin with clavulanate offers no advantage over amoxicillin alone for treatment of resistant pneumococci, and the only potential advantage of amoxicillin/clavulanate over amoxicillin alone in otitis media is added coverage for β-lactamase-producing organisms. The possible benefit of increased dosages of amoxicillin in areas where PRSP are prevalent has led to introduction of a new formulation of amoxicillin/clavulanate (Augment BID, Smith Kline Beecham) in which the ratio of the two drugs has been increased from 7:1 in the original formulation to 14:1. Larger dosages (up to 90 mg/kg/day) of amoxicillin can be administered without increasing the dosage of clavulanate and potential adverse effects, especially diarrhea.

The oral cephalosporins are all less active than amoxicillin (Tables 2 and 6) and are likely to be less effective than amoxicillin for PRSP otitis media. Table 6 shows that many oral cephalosporins fail to achieve middle ear fluid concentrations above the MIC_{50} of intermediate PRSP strains, and agents such as ceftibuten lack reliable activity, even against penicillin-susceptible infections. Of the oral cephalosporins, only cefuroxime and cefprozil achieve middle ear fluid concentrations above the MIC_{90} for intemediate PRSP, and no oral cephalosporin appears effective for high-level PRSP (7, 12).

Non β-lactam agents that are useful for treatment of otitis media include trimethoprim/sulfamethoxazole, erythromycin/sulfamethoxazole, clarithromycin, and azithromycin. However, resistance to these agents is strongly associated with penicillin resistance, although independent resistance occurs with varying frequency. In some areas of the United States, more than 50% of PRSP isolates are resistant to either erythromycin or trimethoprim/sulfamethoxazole (7, 70). In the United States, clindamycin resistance is rare, and oral clindamycin therapy has been used successfully for multiresistant pneumococcal otitis media (7). Once-daily intramuscular ceftriaxone (for 3–5 days) has also been recommended for multiresistant infections that fail to respond to oral therapy.

Other Infections

There are few data on therapy of pneumococcal infections in other sites. Penicillin or ampicillin are the agents of choice for penicillin-susceptible infections irrespective of the site of infection. Pneumococcal endocarditis is a rare but serious con-

TABLE 6 • Serum and Middle Ear Fluid Concentrations of Antimicrobial Agents That Have Been Used for Therapy of Childhood Otitis Media and Comparative in Vitro Activity According to Pneumococcal Susceptibility to Penicillin[a]

Antibiotic	Dose (mg/kg)	Peak Concentrations (μg/mL)[b]		MIC$_{50}$, MIC$_{90}$ (μg/mL) According to Penicillin Susceptibility[c]		
		Serum	MEF	Susceptible	Intermediate	Resistant
Amoxicillin	15	13.6	5.6	0.01, 0.03	0.5, 1	4, 8
Cefaclor	15	8.5	0.5	0.5, 1	4, 16	64, 64
	15	16.8	3.8			
Cefixime	8	2.5	1.3	0.25, 0.5	2, 32	32, 32
	8	4.2	1.5			
Cefpodoxime	5	2.0	0.2	0.03, 0.06	0.5, 2	4, 32
Cefprozil	15	5.5	2.0	0.25, 0.25	1, 4	16, 32
	15	12.1	2.0			
Ceftibuten	9	6.7	4.0	4, 8	>32, >32	>32, >32
	9	12.2	9.3			
Cefuroxime	15	5.1	1.2[d]	0.03, 0.12	1, 16	8, 16
Loracarbef	15	9.3	3.9	1, 2	8, 32	32, 32
TMP/SMX	4	2.0	1.4	0.25, 1	0.25, 4	2, 4
Erythromycin	15	3.6	1.7	0.06, 0.06	0.25, 4	2, 16
Clarithromycin	7.5	1.7	2.5	≤0.03, 0.06	0.25, 8	1, 8
Azithromycin	10→5	0.2		0.12, 0.12	2, 16	2, 32
	10→5		9.4			
Clindamycin				0.06, 0.06	0.06, 0.06	0.06, 0.06
Ceftriaxone	50[e]	175		0.03, 0.06	0.012, 1	1.0, 2.0

[a] MEF, middle ear fluid; MIC$_{50}$, median MIC; MIC90, concentration inhibiting 90% of strains; TMP/SMX, trimethoprim/sulfamethoxazole.

[b] Data from references 20, 62, 70.

[c] MIC data are from middle ear isolates obtained from children in Kentucky (7) or Texas (70). Additional data are from isolates recovered from outpatients (22).

[d] After a single 250-mg dose in children aged 6 to 12 years.

[e] Single intramuscular dose (9).

dition (21, 58). In experimental animals, cefotaxime, teicoplanin, and high-dosage penicillin G effectively sterilized cardiac vegetations (27), and individual cases of PRSP endocarditis have been treated successfully with various agents (71). There are no comparative data on combination therapy for pneumococcal endocarditis. Three children with septic arthritis caused by penicillin-and-cephalosporin-resistant pneumococcal strains were recently reported (1). They received various antimicrobial agents including penicillin G, vancomycin, and clindamycin, but no conclusions can be drawn on antimicrobial efficacy from this few patients.

Combination Therapy

With the exception of meningitis (see above), there has not previously been the need to recommend combination therapy for pneumococcal infections. In vitro time-kill studies demonstrate that combinations of β-lactam agents (including penicillin, amoxicillin, cefotaxime, and cefpirome) with vancomyin or an aminoglycoside are additive or synergistic against many pneumococcal strains, including PRSP (3, 23, 33, 47). In animal models, β-lactam antibiotic and gentamicin combinations are synergistic against penicillin-susceptible (37) and -resistant pneumococcal infections (21). Synergistic interaction between cephalosporins and vancomycin has been demonstrated in different animal models (14, 31). The combination of a β-lactam antibiotic and vancomycin or an aminoglycoside could

be considered in difficult infections such as endocarditis, especially for strains with diminished susceptibility to β-lactam agents. There are, however, no clinical data to support such a recommendation, and it is unknown how combination therapy compares with an active single agent such as vancomycin or imipenem. Enhanced interactions have also been reported with combinations of cefotaxime and teicoplanin (3) or amoxicillin and fosfomycin (15). Combinations of β-lactams and rifampin have been proposed for serious infections, but rifampin has been shown to diminish the bactericidal activity of β-lactam antibiotics (19, 23, 33, 42), and there is little clinical experience with combinations incorporating rifampin.

ADJUNCTIVE THERAPY

Dexamethasone is a frequently prescribed adjunctive therapy in pediatric meningitis. In experimental meningitis, dexamethasone treatment significantly decreased activity of antibiotic therapy, especially against resistant strains (11, 77). Without steroid therapy, CSF cephalosporin concentrations may be inadequate to clear CRSP strains, but available data suggest that concomitant steroid therapy does not further reduce CSF antibiotic concentrations in children with meningitis (36, 38, 59). However, in a number of patients with CRSP meningitis, including some with strains having an MIC between 0.5 and 1.0 μg/mL, initial clinical improvement was observed, followed later by deterioration and documented failure to sterilize the CSF (64). The initial improvement may have been related to adjunctive steroid therapy, and it is important to document CSF sterilization in the first 48 to 72 h of therapy in patients with CRSP infections (or where susceptibility data are not available), especially in steroid-treated patients and in those not receiving combination antibiotic therapy.

NEW DIRECTIONS

The increasing prevalence of drug-resistant pneumococci necessitates a search for antimicrobial agents to which the organism is reliably susceptible. The only agents in common usage fitting this description are vancomycin and imipenem or meropenem, but because of increased resistance among other organisms, their overuse should be discouraged. Classes of drugs that may yield agents effective for pneumococcal infections include the fluoroquinolones (e.g., sparfloxacin, levofloxacin, trovafloxacin), streptogramins (e.g., quinupristin-dalfopristin and pyostacine (75)), ketolides (25), and oxazolidinones (86). Many such agents are under investigation, but no clinical data are yet available. It is hoped that conjugate pneumococcal vaccines administered in early infancy will reduce colonization and disease caused by susceptible and resistant organisms.

REFERENCES

1. Abbasi S, Orlicek SL, Almohsen I, Luedtke G, English BK. Septic arthritis and osteomyelitis caused by penicillin and cephalosporin-resistant *Streptococcus pneumoniae* in a children's hospital. Pediatr Infect Dis J 1996;15:78–83.
2. Asensi F, Perez-Tamarit D, Otero MC, Gallego M, Llanes S, Abadia C, Canto E. Imipenem-cilastatin therapy in a child with meningitis caused by a multiply resistant pneumococcus. Pediatr Infect Dis J 1989;12:895.
3. Bajaksouzian S, Visalli MA, Jacobs MR, Appelbaum PC. Antipneumococcal activities of cefpirome and cefotaxime, alone and in combination with vancomycin and teicoplanin, determined by checkerboard and time-kill methods. Antimicrob Agent Chemother 1996;40:1973–1976.
4. Baquero F, Loza E. Antibiotic resistance of microorganisms involved in ear, nose and throat infections. Pediatr Infect Dis J 1994;13:S9–14.
5. Barriere SL. Review of in vitro activity, pharmacokinetic characteristics, safety, and clinical efficacy of cefprozil, a new oral cephalosporin. Ann Pharmacother 1993;26:1082–1089.
6. Barry AL, Brown SD, Novick WJ. In vitro activities of cefotaxime, ceftriaxone, ceftazidime, cefpirome, and penicillin against *Streptococcus pneumoniae* isolates. Antimicrob Agent Chemother 1995;39:2193–2196.
7. Block SL, Harrison CJ, Hedrick JA, Tyler RD, Smith RA, Keegen E, Chartrand SA. Penicillin-resistant *Streptococcus pneumoniae* in acute otitis media: risk factors, susceptibility patterns and antimicrobial management. Pediatr Infect Dis J 1995;14:751–759.
8. Boswell TC, Smith EG, Ayres JG. Problems in the management of penicillin-resistant pneumococci. J Hosp Infect 1995;30:233–240.
9. Bradley JS, Compogiannis LS, Murray WE, Acosta MA, Tsu GL. Pharmacokinetics and safety of intramuscular injection of concentrated ceftriaxone in children. Clin Pharm 1992;11:961–964.
10. Caballero-Granado FJ, Palomino-Nicàs J, Pachón J, Garcia-Curiel A. Cefuroxime efficacy in treatment of bacteremic pneumonia due to penicillin-resistant and cefuroxime-resistant *Streptococcus pneumoniae*. Antimicrob Agent Chemother 1996;40:1325–1326.
11. Cabellos C, Martinez-Lacasa J, Martos A, Tubau F, Fernández A, Viladrich P, Gudiol F. Influence of dexamethasone on efficacy of ceftriaxone and vancomycin therapy in experimental pneumococcal meningitis. Antimicrob Agent Chemother 1995;39:2158–2160.
12. Cappelletty DM, Rybak MJ. Bactericidal activities of cefprozil, penicillin, cefaclor, cefixime, and loracarbef against penicillin-susceptible and -resistant *Streptococcus pneumoniae* in an in vitro pharmacodynamic infection model. Antimicrob Agent Chemother 1996;40:1148–1152.
13. Carratalià J, Marron A, Fernández-Sevilla, Liñares J, Gudiol F. Treatment of penicillin-resistant pneumococcal bacteremia in neutropenic patients with cancer. Clin Infect Dis 1997;24:148–152.
14. Chavanet P, Champliaud D, Pechinot A, Buisson M, Duong M, Neuwirth C, Kazmierczak A, Portier H. In-vivo activity and pharmacodynamics of cefotaxime in combination with vancomycin in fibrin clots infected with highly penicillin-resistant *Streptococcus pneumoniae*. J Antimicrob Agent 1996;38:655–670.
15. Chavanet P, Peyrard N, Pechinot A, Buisson M, Duong M, Neuwirth C, Kazmierczak A, Portier H. In vivo activity and pharmacokinetics of amoxicillin in combination with fosfomycin in fibrin clots infected with highly penicillin-resistant *Streptococcus pneumoniae*. Antimicrob Agent Chemother 1996;40:2062–2066.
16. Clavo-Sánchez AJ, Girón-Ganzález JA, López-Prieto, Canueto-Quintero J, Sánchez-Porto A, Vergara-Campos A, Marín-Casanova, Córdoba-Doña JA. Multivariate analysis of risk factors for infection due to penicillin-resistant and multidrug-resistant *Streptococcus pneumoniae*: a multicenter study. Clin Infect Dis 1997;24:1052–1059.
17. Coffey TJ, Dowson CG, Daniels M, Spratt BG. Genetics and molecular biology of β-lactam-resistant pneumococci. Microb Drug Resistance 1995;1:29–34.
18. Cohen R, Bingen E, Varon E, Rocque F, Brahimi N, Levy C, Boucherat M, Langue J, Geslin P. Change in nasopharyngeal carriage of *Streptococcus pneumoniae* resulting from antibiotic therapy for acute otitis media in children. Pediatr Infect Dis J 1997;16:555–560.
19. Cormican MG, Erwin ME, Jones RN. Bactericidal activity of cefotaxime, desacetylcefotaxime, rifampin, and various combinations tested at cerebrospinal fluid levels against penicillin-resistant *Streptococcus pneumoniae*. Diagn Microbiol Infect Dis 1995;22:119–123.
20. Craig WA, Andes D. Pharmacokinetics ond pharmacodynamics of antibiotics in otitis media. Pediatr Infect Dis J 1996;15:255–259.
21. Darras-Joly C, Bédos J-P, Sauve C, Moine P, Vallée E, Carbon C, Azoulay-Dupuis. Synergy between amoxicillin and gentamicin in combination against a highly penicillin-resistant and -tolerant strain of *Streptococcus pneumoniae* in a mouse pneumonia model. Antimicrob Agent Chemother 1996;40:2147–2151.
22. Doern GV, Brueggemann A, Preston Holley H, Rauch AM. Antimicrobial resistance of *Streptococcus pneumoniae* recovered from outpatients in the United States during winter months of 1994 to 1995: results of a 30-center national surveillance study. Antimicrob Agent Chemother 1996;40:1208–1213.
23. Doit CP, Bonacorsi SP, Fremaux AJ. In vitro killing activities of antibiotics at clinically achievable concentrations in cerebrospinal fluid against penicillin-resistant *Streptococcus pneu-*

moniae isolated from children with meningitis. Antimicrob Agent Chemother 1994;38:2655–2269.

24. Drusano GL, Standiford HC. Pharmacokinetic profile of imipenem/cilastatin in normal volunteers. Am J Med 1985;78: 47–53.

25. Ednie LM, Spangler SK, Jacobs MR, Appelbaum PC. Susceptibilities of 228 penicillin-and erythromycin-susceptible and -resistant pneumococci to RU 64004, a new ketolide, compared with susceptibilities to 16 other agents.

26. Fassbender M, Lode H, Schaberg T, Borner K, Koeppe P. Pharmacokinetics of new oral cephalosporins, including a new carbacephem. Clin Infect Dis 1993;16:646–653.

27. Fernandez Guerro ML, Arbol F, Verdejo C, Fernandez Roblas R, Soriano F. Treatment of experimental endocarditis due to penicillin-resistant *Streptococcus pneumoniae*. Antimicrob Agent Chemother 1994;38:1103–1106.

28. Finley J C, Davidson M, Parkinson AJ, Sullivan RW. Pneumococcal endocarditis in Alaska natives. A population-based experience, 1978 through 1990. Arch Intern Med 1992;152:1641–1645.

29. Friedland IR, Klugman KP. Failure of chloramphenicol therapy in penicillin-resistant pneumococcal meningitis. Lancet 1992; 339:405–408.

30. Friedland IR, Klugman KP. Antibiotic-resistant pneumococcal disease in South African children. Am J Dis Child 1992;146: 920–923.

31. Friedland IR, Paris M, Ehrett S, Hickey S, Olsen KD, McCracken GH. Evaluation of antimicrobial regimens for treatment of experimental penicillin-and cephalosporin-resistant pneumococcal meningitis. Antimicrob Agent Chemother 1993;10:1320–1324

32. Friedland IR, Shelton S, McCracken GH. Chloramphenicol in penicillin-resistant pneumococcal meningitis. Lancet 1993;342: 240–241.

33. Friedland IR, Paris M, Shelton S, McCracken GH, Jr. Time-kill studies of antibiotic combinations against penicillin-resistant and -susceptible *Streptococcus pneumoniae*. J Antimicrob Chemother 1994 34:231–237.

34. Friedland IR. Comparison of the response to antimicrobial therapy of penicillin-resistant and penicillin-susceptible pneumococcal disease. Pediatr Infect Dis J 1995;14:885–890.

35. Friedland IR. Antibiotic-resistant pneumococci. J Pediatr 1996; 128:862.

36. Friedland IR, Klugman KP. Cerebrospinal fluid activity against cephalosporin-resistant *Streptococcus pneumoniae* in children with meningitis treated with high-dosage cefotaxime. Antimicrob Agent Chemother 1997, in press.

37. Frimodt-Moller N, Frolund TV. Interaction between beta-lactam antibiotics and gentamicin against *Streptococcus pneumoniae* in vitro and in vivo. Acta Pathol Microbiol Immunol Scand 1987; 95:269–275.

38. Gaillard JL, Abadie V, Cheron G, Lacaille F, Mahut B, Silly C, Matha V, Coustere C, Lokiec F. Concentrations of ceftriaxone in cerebrospinal fluid of children with meningitis receiving dexamethasone therapy. Antimicrob Agent Chemother 1994:38: 1209–1210.

39. George J, Morrissey I. The bactericidal activity of levofloxacin compared with ofloxacin, D-ofloxacin, ciprofloxacin, sparfloxacin and cefotaxime against *Streptococcus pneumoniae*. J Antimicrob Chemother 1997;39:719–723.

40. Geslin P, Buu-Hoi A, Frémaux A, Acar JF. Antimicrobial resistance in *Streptococcus pneumoniae* and epidemiological survey in France, 1970–1990. Clin Infect Dis 1992;15:95–98.

41. Girard AE, Girard D, Gootz TD, Faiella JA, Cimochowski CR.

In vivo efficacy of trovafloxacin (CP-99,219), a new quinolone with extended activities against Gram-positive pathogens, *Streptococcus pneumoniae* and *Bacteroides fragilis*. Antimicrob Agent Chemother 1996;40:2210–2216.

42. Giron KP, Gross ME, Musher DM, Williams TW, Tharappel RA. In vitro antimicrobial effect against *Streptococcus pneumoniae* of adding rifampin to penicillin, ceftriaxone, or l-ofloxacin. Antimicrob Agent Chemother 1995;39:2798–2800.

43. Goldstein FW, Péan Y, Gertner J, and the Vigil'Roc Study Group. Resistance to ceftriaxone and other β-lactams in bacteria isolated in the community. Antimicrob Agent Chemother 1995; 39:2516–2519.

44. Goldstein FW, Acar JF, and the Alexander Project Collaborative Group. Antimicrobial resistance among lower respiratory tract isolates of *Streptococcus pneumoniae:* results of a 1992–93 Western Europe and USA collaborative surveillance study. J Antimicrob Chemother 1996;38(Suppl A):71–84.

45. Gordon JJ, Kauffman CA. Superinfection with *Streptococcus pneumoniae* during therapy with ciprofloxacin. Am J Med 1990; 37:89:383–384.

46. Grebe T, Hakenbeck. Penicillin-binding proteins 2b and 2× of *Streptococcus pneumoniae* are primary resistance determinants for different classes of β-lactam antibiotics. Antimicrob Agent Chemother 1996;40:829–834.

47. Gross ME, Giron KP, Septimus JD, Mason EO Jr, Musher DM. Antimicrobial activities of beta-lactam antibiotics and gentamicin against penicillin-susceptible and penicillin pneumococci. Antimicrob Agent Chemother 1995;39:1166–1168.

48. Guibert M, Chahime H, Petit J, Odièvre M, Labrune P. Failure of cefotaxime treatment in two children with meningitis caused by highly penicillin-resistant *Streptococcus pneumoniae*. Ann Paediatr 1995;84:831–833.

49. Hoberman A, Paradise JL, Block S, Burch DJ, Jacobs MR, Balanescu MI. Efficacy of amoxicillin/clavulanate potassium for acute otitis media: relation to *Streptococcus pneumoniae* susceptibility. Pediatr Infect Dis J 1996;15:955–962.

50. Hofmann J, Cetron MS, Farley MM, Baughman WS, Facklam RR, Elliott JA, Deaver KA, Breiman RF. The prevalence of drug-resistant *Streptococcus pneumoniae* in Atlanta. N Engl J Med 1995;333:481–486.

51. Jackson MJ, Rutledge J. Pneumococcal endocarditis in children. Pediatr Infect Dis J 1982;1:120–122.

52. Jacobs NM. Pneumococcal osteomyelitis and arthritis in children. Am J Dis Child 1991;145:70–74.

53. Jacobs RF, Kaplan SL, Schutze GE, Dajani AS, Leggiadro RJ, Rim C, Puri SK. Relationship of MICs to efficacy of cefotaxime in treatment of *Streptococcus pneumoniae* infections. Antimicrob Agent Chemother 1996;40:895–898.

54. Jadavji T, Biggar WD, Gold R, Prober CG. Sequelae of acute bacterial meningitis in children treated for seven days. Pediatrics 1986;78:21–25.

55. Jernigan DB, Cetron MS, Breiman RF. Minimizing the impact of drug-resistant *Streptococcus pneumoniae* (DRSP). JAMA 1996;275:206–209.

56. John CC. Treatment failure with use of a third-generation cephalosporin for penicillin-resistant pneumococcal meningitis: case report and review. Clin Infect Dis 1994;18:188–193.

57. Karchmer AW. Cephalosporins. In: Mandell GL, Bennett JE, Dolin R, eds. Principles and practice of infectious diseases. 4th ed. New York: Churchill Livingstone, 1995:247–263.

58. Klugman KP. Pneumococcal resistance to antibiotics. Clin Microbiol Rev 1990;3:171–196.

59. Klugman KP, Friedland IR, Bradley JS. Bactericidal activity against cephalosporin-resistant *Streptococcus pneumoniae* in cerebrospinal fluid of children with acute bacterial meningitis. Antimicrob Agent Chemother 1995;39:1988–1992.

60. Konishi K, Suzuki H, Hayashi M, Saruta T. Pharmacokinetics of cefuroxime axetil in patients with normal and impaired renal function. J Antimicrob Chemother 1993;31:413–420.

61. Leach AJ, Shelby-James TM, Mayo M, Gratten M, Laming AC, Currie BJ, Mathews JD. A prospective study of the impact of community-based azithromycin treatment of trachoma on carriage and resistance of *Streptococcus pneumoniae*. Clin Infect Dis 1997;24:356–362.

62. Lin C, Radwanski E, Affrime M, Cayen MN. Multiple-dose pharmacokinetics of ceftibuten in healthy volunteer. Antimicrob Agent Chemother 1995;39:356–8.

63. Lin T-Y. Chrane DF, Nelson JD, McCracken GH. Seven days of ceftriaxone therapy is as effective as ten days' treatment for bacterial meningitis. JAMA 1985;253:3559–3563.

64. Lonks JR, Durkin MR, Meyerhoff AN, Medeiros AA. Meningitis due to ceftriaxone-resistant *Streptococcus pneumoniae*. N Engl J Med 1995;332:893–894.

65. Meynard JL, Barbut F, Blum L, Guiget M, Chouaid C, Meyohas MC, Picard O, Petit JC, Frottier J. Risk factors for isolation of *Streptococcus pneumoniae* with decreased susceptibility to penicillin G from patients infected with human immunodeficiency virus. Clin Infect Dis 1996;22:437–440.

66. Morbidity and Mortality Weekly Review. Drug-resistant *Streptococcus pneumoniae*—Kentucky and Tennessee, 1993. MMWR 1994;43:23–25.

67. Moreno S, Garcia-Leoni ME, Cercenado E, Diaz MD, Bernaldo de Quirós JCL, Bouza E. Infections caused by erythromycin-resistant *Streptococcus pneumoniae:* incidence, risk factors, and response to therapy in a prospective study. Clin Infect Dis 1995;20:1195–1200.

68. National Committee for Clinical Laboratory Standards. Minimum inhibitory concentration (MIC) interpretive standards for streptococci, including *Streptococcus pneumoniae*. NCCLS document M7-A3. 1993;13(25).

69. National Committee for Clinical Laboratory Standards. Minimum inhibitory concentration (MIC) interpretive standards for streptococci, including *Streptococcus pneumoniae*. NCCLS document M7-A3. 1995;15(14).

70. Nelson CT, Mason EO, Kaplan SL. Activity of oral antibiotics in middle ear and sinus infections caused by penicillin-resistant *Streptococcus pneumoniae:* implications for treatment. Pediatr Infect Dis J 1994;12:S106–111.

71. Okumura A, Ito K, Kondo M, Takahashi H, Hayakawa F, Ogawa A, Kuno K. Infective endocarditis caused by highly penicillin-resistant *Streptococcus pneumoniae:* successful treatment with cefuzonam, ampicillin and imipenem. Pediatr Infect Dis J 1995; 14:327–329.

72. Pallares R, Gudiol F, Liñares J, Ariza J, rufi G, Murgui L, Dorca J, Viladrich PF. Risk factors and response to antibiotic therapy in adults with bacteremic pneumonia caused by penicillin-resistant pneumococci. N Engl J Med 1987;317:18–22.

73. Pallares R, Liñares J, Vadillo M, Cabellos C, Manresa F, Viladrich PF, Martin R, Gudiol F. Resistance to penicillin and cephalosporin and mortality from severe pneumococcal pneumonia in Barcelona, Spain. N Engl J Med 1995;333:474–480.

74. Pankuch GA, Jacobs MR, Appelbaum PC. Study of comparative antipneumococcal activities of ampicillin, amoxycillin, amoxycillin/clavulanate and cefotaxime against 189 penicillin-susceptible and -resistant pneumococci. J Antimicrob Chemother 1995;35:883–888.

75. Pankuch GA, Jacobs MR, Appelbaum PC. MIC and time-kill study of antpneumococcal activities of RPR 106972 (a new oral streptogramin), RP 59500 (quinupristin-dalfopristin), pyostacine (RP 7293), penicillin G, cefotaxime, erythromycin, and clarithromycin against 10 penicillin-susceptible and -resistant pneumococci. Antimicrob Agent Chemother 1996;40:2071–2074.

76. París MM, Hickey SM, Uscher MI, Shelton S, Olsen KD, McCracken GH Jr. Effect of dexamethasone on therapy of experimental penicillin- and cephalosporin-resistant pneumococcal meningitis. Antimicrob Agent Chemother 1994;38:1320–1324.

77. París MM, Ramilo O, McCracken GH, Jr. Management of meningitis caused by penicillin-resistant *Streptococcus pneumoniae*. Antimicrob Agent Chemother 1995;39:2171–2177.

78. Paul J, Kimari J, Gilks CF. *Streptococcus pneumoniae* resistant to penicillin and tetracycline associated with HIV seropositivity. Lancet 1995;346:1034.

79. Peltola H, Anttila M, Renkonen OB. Randomised comparison of chloramphenicol, ampicillin, cefotaxime, and ceftriaxone for childhood bacterial meningitis. Lancet 1989;1:1281–1287.

80. Perez-Trallero E, Garcia Arezana JM, Ayestaran I, Jiménez JM, Peris A. Therapeutic failure and selection of resistance to quinolones in a case of pneumococcal pneumonia treated with ciprofloxacin . Eur J Clin Microbiol Infect Dis 1990;9:905–906.

81. Sacho H, Klugman KP, Koornhof, Ruff P. Community-acquired pneumonia in an adult due to a multiply resistant pneumococcus. J Infect 1987;14:188–189.

82. Sanchez C, Armengol R, Lite J, Mir I, Garau J. Penicillin-resistant pneumococci and community-acquired pneumonia. Lancet 1992;339:988.

83. Schreiber JR, Jacobs MR. Antibiotic-resistant pneumococci. Pediatr Clin North Am 1995;42:519–537.

84. Sibold C, Henrichsen J, König A, Martin C, Chalkley L, Hakenbeck R. Mosaic pbpX genes of major clones of penicillin-resistant *Streptococcus pneumoniae* have evolved from pbpX genes of penicillin-sensitive *Streptococcus oralis*. Mol Microbiol 1994;12: 1013–1023.

85. Spangler SK, Jacobs MR, Appelbaum PC. Susceptibilities of 177 penicillin-susceptible and -resistant pneumococci to FK 037, cefpirome, cefepime, ceftriaxone, cefotaxime, ceftazidime, imipenem, biapenem, meropenem, and vancomycin. Antimicrob Agent Chemother 1994;38:898–900.

86. Spangler SK, Jacobs MR, Appelbaum PC. Activities of RPR 106972 (a new oral streptogramin), ceftidoren (a new oral cephalosporin), two new oxazolidinones (U-100592 and U-100766), and other oral and parenteral agents against 203 penicillin-susceptible and -resistant pneumococci. Antimicrob Agent Chemother 1996;40:481–484.

87. Tan TQ, Mason EO, Kaplan SL. Systemic infections due to *Streptococcus pneumoniae* relatively resistant to penicillin in a children's hospital: clinical management and outcome. Pediatrics 1992;90:928–933.

88. Tan TQ, Mason EO, Kaplan SL. Penicillin-resistant pneumococcal infections in children: a retrospective case-control study. Pediatrics 1993;92:761–767.

89. Tan TQ, Schutze GE, Mason EO, Kaplan SL. Antibiotic therapy and acute outcome of meningitis due to *Streptococcus pneumoniae* considered intermediately susceptible to broad-spectrum cephalosporins. Antimicrob Agent Chemother 1994;38:918–923.

90. Tuomanen EI, Austrian R, Masure HR. Pathogenesis of pneumococcal infection. N Engl J Med 1995;332:1280–1284.

91. Viladrich PF, Gudiol F, Liñares J, Pallarés R, Sabaté I, Rufí G, Ariza J. Evaluation of vancomycin for therapy of adult pneumococcal meningitis. Antimicrob Agent Chemother 1991;35:2467–2472.

92. Viladrich PF, Cabellos C, Pallarés R, Tabau F, Martinez-Lacasa J, Liñares J, Gudiol F. High doses of cefotaxime in treatment of adult meningitis due to *Streptococcus pneumoniae* with decreased susceptibilities to broad-spectrum cephalosporins. Antimicrob Agent Chemother 1996;40:218–220.

93. Visalli MA, Jacobs MR, Appelbaum PC. MIC and time-kill study of activites of DU-6859a, ciprofloxacin, levofloxacin, sparfloxacin, cefotaxime, imipenem, and vancomycin against nine penicillin-susceptible and -resistant pneumococci. Antimicrob Agent Chemother 1996;40:362–366.

94. Zenni MK, Cheatham SH, Thompson JM, Reed GW, Batson AB, Palmer PS, Holland KL, Edwards KM. *Streptococcus pneumoniae* colonization in the young child: association with otitis media and resistance to penicillin. J Pediatr 1995;127:533–537.

Streptococcus pyogenes (GABHS)

Raymond D. Pitetti and Dennis P. Stevens

Group A β-hemolytic streptococcus (*Streptococcus pyogenes*) is a major cause of significant infections in infants, children, and adults. Group A streptococcal infections have long been associated with serious morbidity and mortality, but toward the end of the 1960s, a marked decline in the incidence and severity of such infections occurred. However, over the past 10 years, there has been a resurgence in the incidence of severe, invasive group A streptococcal infections (13, 26). These include necrotizing fasciitis, myositis, scarlet fever, toxic shock syndrome, and streptococcal bacteremia. Outbreaks have even occurred in patient populations not previously thought to be at risk (13).

In addition, since the early 1980s, an increase in reports of individual cases and outbreaks of acute rheumatic fever (ARF) have been described in widely separated geographic locales. Surveys have shown that reported increases in cases of ARF have been restricted to distinct geographic locales and have not occurred nationwide (15). As a result, the treatment of GABHS infections has taken on greater importance, and investigators have searched for alternative therapies, while still relying on the first antibiotic shown effective in eradicating GABHS and preventing ARF, penicillin.

Reductions in incidence and mortality rates of ARF in the United States had begun prior to the discovery of penicillin, primarily because of improved housing, sanitation, and delivery of health care (15). However, the use of penicillin in the treatment of GABHS pharyngitis hastened the decrease in the incidence of ARF. While ARF became less of a problem in the United States, it remained a major concern in developing countries. The recent increase in incidence of ARF in the United States has occurred primarily in children of middle-class families (15). This suggests that socioeconomic factors have assumed less importance in the pathogenesis of ARF and that increased virulence of the organism may be primarily responsible for the current outbreak (31). Of particular epidemiologic interest is the resurgence of rheumatic fever in North America but not in other industrialized countries. Mucoid colonies of group A streptococci have been associated with cases of rheumatic fever in North America but not in other, developing countries. This further supports the idea that the virulence of group A streptococci has changed, resulting in the increase in ARF. Five serotypes have predominated: M-3, M-1, M-18, M-5, and M-6. Types M-1 and M-18 have been reported as most consistently mucoid (12, 15, 20).

In contrast to rheumatic fever, the increase in severe, invasive group A streptococcal infections has not been limited to North America. However, this increase has also included an association with mucoid colonies of group A streptococci.

Because group A streptococcal infections have not been reportable diseases for several decades, the true incidence is unknown. However, there has been a recognized increase in the number and severity of both suppurative and nonsuppurative complications of group A streptococcal infection. The resurgence has been partly attributed to a change in the epidemiology of group A streptococcus as well as a change in the virulence of the organism (13, 53). Some have suggested that changes in the susceptibility of group A streptococci to commonly used antibiotics may have contributed as well (13). Regardless, the increased number and severity of group A streptococcal infections present a challenge to both the general practitioner and the infectious disease specialist.

SUSCEPTIBILITY IN VITRO AND IN VIVO

Susceptibilities for commonly used antibiotics in the treatment of GABHS are presented in Table 1. Susceptibilities from Coonan and Kaplan's study were obtained from 282 pharyngeal isolates along with 43 isolates from severe or invasive group A streptococcal disease (13).

ANTIMICROBIAL THERAPY
General

Despite possible changes in virulence, group A streptococci have universally remained susceptible to penicillin since its

TABLE 1 • In Vitro Susceptibilities of *Streptococcus Pyogenes* to Common Antibiotics

Antibiotic	MIC$_{50}$ (μg/mL)	MIC$_{90}$ (μg/mL)	Range (μg/mL)	Reference
Penicillin	0.006	0.012	0.003–0.024	13
Oxacillin	0.06	0.06	≤0.03–0.25	64
Erythromycin	0.016	0.031	0.0078–8.0	13
Azithromycin	0.016	0.031	0.0078–4.0	13
Clarithromycin	0.0078	0.016	0.0039–4.0	13
Cephalothin	0.1	0.1	0.0125–0.2	13
Cefoxitin	1	1	1–4	64
Cefixime	0.25	0.5	0.078–0.5	13
Cefuroxime	≤0.03	≤0.03	≤0.03	64
Cefotaxime	≤0.03	≤0.03	≤0.03	64
Ceftriaxone	≤0.03	≤0.03	≤0.03–0.125	64
Vancomycin	0.25	0.5	0.25–0.5	5, 64
Clindamycin	0.125	0.125	0.06–0.125	64
Rifampin	0.5	0.5	≤0.03–0.5	64
Ciprofloxacin	0.256	0.5	0.016–2.0	13
Tetracycline	0.25	2	0.0039–8.0	13
Cotrimoxazole	≥64	≥64	≥64	64
Chloramphenicol	4	4	2–8	64

introduction. This is of considerable interest, since other streptococci have developed multiple antibiotic resistance, and higher concentrations of penicillin are currently required to inhibit pneumococcus. Penicillin is still considered first-line therapy in the treatment of most GABHS infections despite a recognized increase in microbiologic failure rates. Erythromycin remains the antibiotic of choice in the penicillin-allergic child for most GABHS infections. The chosen route of administration clearly depends upon the type of infection. Duration of therapy is generally 10 days. What follows is a description of GABHS infections and recommended therapy.

GABHS Pharyngitis

GABHS infections of the pharynx are the most common bacterial infections of childhood. Treatment of GABHS pharyngitis is primarily aimed at preventing nonsuppurative (in particular, rheumatic fever) and suppurative complications. Standard treatment remains penicillin VK, 25 to 50 mg/kg/day in 4 divided doses for children, or 250 to 500 mg per dose, 4 times/day for adults. However, a study conducted by Gerber et al. demonstrated that twice-a-day dosing of penicillin was as effective as four-times-a-day dosing (27). Treatment with penicillin should be continued for 10 days. Studies assessing shorter courses of penicillin have shown decreased efficacy. A clinical response is generally obtained within 24 h of beginning therapy, and most children have a negative throat culture by 48 h and can return to school at that time (3). Persistence of symptoms beyond this period may suggest development of a suppurative complication of GABHS, a lack of compliance, or the presence of another underlying disease (3).

A single injection of 1.2 million units of penicillin G benzathine given intramuscularly is as effective as enteral penicillin (6) and was for a long time the gold standard in treatment of GABHS pharyngitis. It can provide bactericidal levels against GABHS for as long as 28 days. Children who weigh less than 140 pounds (64 kg) should receive an intramuscular injection composed of 900,000 units of benzathine penicillin G and 300,000 units of procaine penicillin G.

Penicillin's efficacy in preventing rheumatic fever is well established. Prevention of rheumatic fever is thought to be achieved by eradicating the organism from the pharynx and is dependent upon prolonged, rather than high-dose, therapy. Penicillin has been shown effective when therapy is started within 9 days of onset of symptoms of GABHS pharyngitis (6, 66). Other desirable features of penicillin include lower cost, lower side effects, and a reasonably narrow antimicrobial spectrum. Recent evidence has suggested decreased susceptibility of GABHS to penicillin VK, but studies have failed to support this (19, 30). There has been no documentation of resistance in GABHS to penicillin (51). In fact, the minimal bactericidal concentration of penicillin G for GABHS has remained 0.005 μg/mL (28).

Erythromycin remains the drug of choice in patients who are allergic to penicillin. Erythromycin estolate (20–40 mg/kg/day) or erythromycin ethylsuccinate (40 mg/kg/day) given enterally in 2 to 4 divided doses has been shown as effective as penicillin in treatment of pharyngitis. However, documented cases of erythromycin-resistant GABHS have occurred in Finland, Sweden, Germany, and Japan (37, 39, 49, 68). The mechanism of resistance to erythromycin is unclear, though resistance may be plasmid mediated and may be transmitted via transduction or conjugation (26). Of interest is the recent rise and fall of resistance in Japan and Finland (33). Resistance to erythromycin in Japan had increased to 70% of all isolates, corresponding to a marked increase in macrolide use during the 1970s (21). Use of macrolides since then has declined, and a marked decrease in rates of erythromycin resistance has followed (21). Resistance rates fell to 46% in 1981 and are currently at 3% (1989) (21). In Finland, erythromycin resistance was highest among strains isolated from soft-tissue infections, was lower in pharyngeal isolates, and approached an overall rate of 25% (49).

All macrolides (erythromycin, azithromycin, clarithromycin, roxithromycin, dirithromycin) appear to be efficacious in the treatment of GABHS pharyngitis. However, a study comparing roxithromycin with erythromycin ethylsuccinate in the treatment of GABHS pharyngitis showed comparable clinical responses for both antibiotics, but a bacteriologic cure rate of only 33% for roxithromycin (38). Roxithromycin is known to achieve lower concentrations in affected tissues than other macrolides (22).

The newest macrolides, azithromycin and clarithromycin, have been shown highly effective in the treatment of GABHS pharyngitis. They provide easier dosing schedules and thus improve patient compliance. In addition, resistance among the newer macrolides has been relatively uncommon (33). However, as with other drugs used in the treatment of GABHS pharyngitis (except for penicillin), their ability to prevent episodes of rheumatic fever has not been studied (52).

Azithromycin has been shown to be efficacious in treatment

of GABHS pharyngitis when given for only 5 days (29). One recent study comparing azithromycin (20 mg/kg, once daily for 3 days) with penicillin V (125–250 mg four times daily for 10 days) showed significantly higher bacteriologic eradication rates and lower pathogen recurrence in the azithromycin group (41): 100% of the azithromycin group had a satisfactory clinical response, defined as cure or improvement, compared with 97% in the penicillin group; 5% of the azithromycin group relapsed, compared with 2% in the penicillin group (41). Azithromycin (once daily for 3 days) was also compared with clarithromcin (given twice daily for 10 days) (46). Azithromycin was again shown to be as effective, with fewer adverse effects (46).

Amoxicillin has been shown to be effective in eradicating GABHS, is more palatable, and provides easier dosing than penicillin. Though ampicillin and penicillinase-resistant penicillins are also effective in the treatment of GABHS pharyngitis, they offer no greater benefit than penicillin. Amoxicillin and ampicillin are useful in patients who have GABHS pharyngitis and a concurrent acute otitis media (3).

Oral cephalosporins have been extensively studied in the treatment of GABHS pharyngitis and have been shown highly effective. In fact, some studies have suggested greater efficacy with cephalosporins than with penicillin, possibly because of their resistance to β-lactamase-producing organisms in the pharynx (43, 45); other studies have not supported this (51). Cephalexin can be given at 30 mg/day, in four divided doses for 10 days; cefadroxil, 30 mg/kg/day, in two divided doses for 10 days; cefaclor, 30 mg/kg/day in three divided doses for 10 days; cefuroxime axetil, 15 mg/kg/day in two divided doses for 10 days; cefoxitin, 80 to 160 mg/kg/day or 4 to 12 g/day in four divided doses for 10 days; and cefixime, 8 mg/kg/day, once a day for 10 days (26). Cefaclor has been associated with a higher incidence of serum sickness than most other antibiotics. In addition, cephalosporins as a class are more expensive than penicillin, are associated with greater side effects in general, and have a broader spectrum of activity.

In many areas, tetracycline resistance occurs in a high percentage of strains; thus, this drug is not recommended for treatment of GABHS pharyngitis. Sulfonamides, including trimethoprim-sulfamethoxazole, are ineffective in the treatment of GABHS pharyngitis, though sulfadiazine has proven useful for prophylaxis in acute rheumatic fever (6, 33).

Corticosteroids have been used to treat adults with GABHS pharyngitis. A study by O'Brien et al. comparing the use of dexamethasone (10 mg intramuscularly in a single dose) with placebo, documented a significant decrease in duration and severity of pain in adults with GABHS pharyngitis (40). No documented side effects were attributed to dexamethasone (40). The use of steroids has not been studied in children. However, their use might contribute to the treatment of GABHS pharyngitis in children with severe pain and inability to swallow liquids.

Treatment failures in GABHS pharyngitis are of major concern in the prevention of rheumatic fever. Studies have reported failure rates as high as 30%, including studies of penicillin G given one time intramuscularly (30, 60). Noncompliance is thought to play a major role with oral treatments but does not account for all failures. The presence of β-lactamase-producing organisms in the pharynx has also been proposed to contribute to treatment failures with penicillin. Such organisms include *Staphylococcus aureus, Haemophilus influenzae, Haemophilus parainfluenzae, Moraxella catarrhalis,* and *Bacteroides* spp. (9). Current evidence has failed to support this (26). A study by Tanz et al. compared an antibiotic effective against both β-lactamase-producing organisms and GABHS (amoxicillin-clavulanic acid) with penicillin in patients with GABHS pharyngitis. It was hypothesized that if β-lactamase-producing organisms contributed to bacteriologic failure rates, amoxicillin-clavulanic acid should be more effective than penicillin. In fact, bacteriologic failure rates were not statistically different for either treatment group (62); 65% of patients had β-lactamase-producing flora in their pharynx. The study concluded that bacteriologic failures in the treatment of GABHS were not due solely to β-lactamase-flora colonizing a patient's pharynx (62).

Some investigators have postulated that early treatment of GABHS, within 48 h of symptoms, may alter the patient's immune system and the course of the illness. This was first proposed in the 1950s. Studies have shown that delaying therapy for 3 to 5 days results in an increase in anti–streptolysin O antibodies but have not shown that type-specific antibodies increase (23). Antibodies such as anti–streptolysin O, unlike type-specific antibodies, do not confer immunity on the host. Studies investigating development of type-specific antibodies during an acute episode of GABHS pharyngitis have shown that the antibody response may not develop until 90 days after the onset of illness (23). Complicating the issue is new evidence that suggests that type-specific antibodies may not be solely responsible for development of host immunity. Non-type-specific antibodies induced by antigenic epitopes of the M protein may play a role as well (23). At present it is unclear if delaying therapy for 2 to 3 days in patients with GABHS pharyngitis results in a significantly greater antibody rise, nor is it clear that early antibiotic therapy is a primary reason for treatment failures (24, 28). Since adequate antimicrobial therapy prevents development of suppurative and nonsuppurative complications of GABHS, most authors do not recommend delaying therapy (24).

Penicillin tolerance has been thought to play a role in some treatment failures (12), though no significant change has been reported in in vitro susceptibilities of penicillin to GABHS (25, 26, 51). Remember that tolerance is defined by in vitro studies but may not be readily applicable to in vivo effects. Exactly what role penicillin tolerance plays in bacteriologic failures is not known and deserves further study.

Some bacteriologic and clinical failures may actually represent acquisition of a new strain of GABHS. In addition, GABHS carriers with an intercurrent viral pharyngitis may be mistakenly diagnosed as patients with acute GABHS pharyngitis and thus considered treatment failures, since penicillin is ineffective in eradication of the GABHS carrier state (51).

The problem of bacteriologic and clinical failures in the treatment of GABHS pharyngitis has led some investigators to suggest that all patients should receive a test of cure at the end of their illness. However, the cost:benefit ratio of this proposal remains debatable. In addition, it raises the question of what to do with the patient who is asymptomatic but culture positive for GABHS at the end of treatment. These patients are considered GABHS carriers and do not require therapy. These patients are not at increased risk of ensuing acute pharyngitis, nor are they at increased risk of acquiring rheumatic fever (25, 63). The patient who is symptomatic and culture positive at the end of treatment for acute pharyngitis may represent either failed treatment or acquisition of a new strain of GABHS and should receive further treatment. Therapeutic alternatives to the treatment of GABHS pharyngitis that address some of the potential causes of bacteriologic failure (patient noncompliance, antimicrobial tolerance, and bacterial copathogenicity) include the use of cephalosporins, β-lactamase blockade, macrolides, and clindamycin.

Cephalosporins, as mentioned above, have activity against GABHS, are more palatable and more easily dosed, have fewer side effects, and offer greater resistance to β-lactamase-producing oropharyngeal flora. Some researchers have suggested that cephalosporins are superior to penicillin for treatment of GABHS pharyngitis (26, 28, 45). Pichichero and Margolis conducted a meta-analysis of several published studies comparing oral cephalosporins with penicillin and showed that cephalosporins had superior efficacy (44). Clinical failure rates were 5% for cephalosporins and 11% for penicillins (44). However, some investigators have questioned the methods and results of this meta-analysis and discount the findings (51). In a follow-up review to his meta-analysis, Pichichero looked at new studies comparing cephalosporins and penicillin use. Using stricter inclusion criteria, he again showed that cephalosporins had consistently lower bacteriologic (8%) and clinical failure rates (5%) than penicillin (18 and 14%, respectively) (43). Cephalosporin choices include cefadroxil, cefuroxime axetil, cefixime, and cefprozil. Cefpodoxime has been shown to be as efficacious when given for 5 days as penicillin given for 10 (28).

Amoxicillin–clavulanic acid combines β-lactamase blockade and an antimicrobial. This combination was shown superior to penicillin in its ability to eradicate streptococci from the oropharynx (28) but, as stated above, did not effectively reduced the incidence of treatment failures (62).

As mentioned above, macrolides offer an effective alternative to penicillin for management of GABHS pharyngitis. Equivalent efficacy has been shown in multiple studies. In addition, macrolides are unaffected by β-lactamases and β-lactam tolerance. Though erythromycin resistance has become a significant problem in Asia, resistance has remained at 4 to 5% for several decades in the United States. The newer macrolides offer the advantages of broader antibacterial coverage, less-frequent dosing, and higher active concentration of drug in affected tissues (28).

Clindamycin was shown to be extremely effective in the treatment of GABHS. It is unaffected by the activity of β-lactamases (26, 63) but is more expensive than penicillin and has been associated with development of pseudomembranous colitis in some patients (28).

Other alternative therapies that have been suggested to reduce the incidence of treatment failures in GABHS pharyngi-

tis include using α-streptococci to replace normal pharyngeal flora, delaying treatment of GABHS pharyngitis 48 h to promote the host's immune system (discussed above), and using topical antibiotics. The last has not been well studied.

Elimination of α-streptococci from the pharynx after therapy for acute GABHS pharyngitis has been proposed as a possible explanation for treatment failures, development of the carrier phenomenon, and frequent recurrences (63). α-Streptococci interfere strongly against GABHS (48). α-Streptococci share pharyngeal epithelial receptor sites in the posterior pharynx with GABHS, and elimination of α-streptococci may provide more attachment sites for GABHS (26). Roos et al. looked at 31 patients with recurrent GABHS pharyngitis who were given antibiotics for 10 days and then had the oropharynx sprayed with α-streptococci. None of the patients treated with α-streptococci had a recurrence of GABHS pharyngitis over a period of 3 months, while the control group had an 8% recurrence rate (48).

In patients with recurring episodes of GABHS pharyngitis or persistent, culture-positive, clinical GABHS pharyngitis, it is often necessary to change antibiotic therapy. Usually, a 10-day course of amoxicillin/clavulanate, clindamycin, or an oral cephalosporin eradicates the GABHS. Penicillin prophylaxis (penicillin V, 250 mg twice daily) during the winter and early spring was proposed for patients with recurrent GABHS pharyngitis but has not been shown to be efficacious (25).

Tonsillectomy may help reduce the number of acute infections in children with recurrent GABHS pharyngitis (42). Tonsillectomy is generally recommended for children who have 6 to 7 documented GABHS infections in a given year or 3 to 4 infections in each of 2 years (6). However, benefits of tonsillectomy have been shown to be short-lived, often providing relief from frequent episodes of pharyngitis for as little as 2 years (25, 61). Tonsils are not necessary for development of an acute episode of GABHS pharyngitis. In addition, tonsillectomy has an associated complication rate of 14% (61).

It may be desirable to eliminate the carrier state in a select group of patients. These include patients with a family history of rheumatic fever, those who have spread GABHS from family member to family member, those in outbreaks of GABHS pharyngitis in closed or semiclosed communities, those for whom tonsillectomy is being considered because of chronic streptococcal carriage or when there exists inordinate family anxiety about GABHS (24, 25, 63). In addition, recurrent episodes of GABHS pharyngitis are easier to manage when the carrier state is eliminated (63). Therapies shown to be effective in eliminating the carrier state include clindamycin (20 mg/kg/day in 3 divided doses over 10 days), amoxicillin/clavulanate given for 10 days, oral rifampin (20 mg/kg every 24 h for 4 doses) started during the last 4 days of a 10-day course of oral penicillin (24), and a combination of penicillin plus rifampin (oral rifampin 10 mg/kg every 12 h for 8 doses, with one dose of intramuscular benzathine penicillin G) (6, 24, 63). In addition, topical application of α-streptococci may eliminate the carrier state (48).

Family contacts of patients with GABHS pharyngitis should not be treated empirically, unless symptomatic, even though acquisition rates can be as high as 25% (6).

Recently, a change was reported in the specific M serotypes associated with patients with GABHS pharyngitis, which has direct implications for treatment of GABHS pharyngitis. Prior to 1979, M serotypes 4 and 12 predominated. However, during the 1980s, M serotypes 1, 3, and 18 were most frequently isolated (36). This change is significant because these particular serotypes are associated with upper respiratory infections with mild or no symptoms. As a result, during the recent outbreaks of rheumatic fever, 75% of patients had either a mild, or no, preceding upper respiratory infection (36).

Treatment of the suppurative and nonsuppurative complications of GABHS pharyngitis are described below.

Scarlet Fever

The treatment of scarlet fever is the same as that for GABHS pharyngitis, as the disease usually results from infection of the pharynx with a streptococcal strain that elaborates streptococcal pyrogenic exotoxin (6). However, scarlet fever can also result from GABHS infections at other sites, such as the skin (6).

Suppurative Complications

Peritonsillar Abscess ("Quinsy").   Peritonsillar abscess results from direct extension of group A streptococcus from an acute pharyngitis. However, a peritonsillar abscess can yield mixed flora as well. Needle aspiration or surgical drainage of the abscess as well as antimicrobials are usually required. Indications for needle aspiration include severe pain and trismus, difficulty swallowing, and poor response to antimicrobials alone. Patients can be treated orally for 10 days with either a first-generation cephalosporin such as cephalexin, clindamycin, or amoxicillin-clavulanic acid, if they appear nontoxic and can maintain adequate hydration. Some patients may require initial treatment with a parenteral antibiotic and be discharged home on oral antibiotics to complete a 10-day course. Tonsillectomy at the time of surgical incision and drainage can provide improved drainage, prevent recurrences, and permit earlier discharge. Patients with a known allergy to cephalosporins can be treated with clindamycin.

Peritonsillar Cellulitis.   Occasionally, peritonsillar cellulitis occurs without development of an abscess. Like peritonsillar abscesses, peritonsillar cellulitis results from direct extension of an acute tonsillopharyngitis and may result solely from group A streptococcus but can include mixed oral flora as well. Patients with mild symptoms who can maintain adequate hydration can be treated orally with a first- or second-generation cephalosporin such as cephalexin or cefazolin. Patients with a known allergy to cephalosporins can be treated with clindamycin. Patients with severe trismus or inadequate hydration can be treated parenterally with clindamycin or a first-generation cephalosporin such as cefazolin. Duration of therapy is generally 10 days. Tonsillectomy can ensure complete recovery and prevent recurrences.

Retropharyngeal Abscess.   Retropharyngeal abscess also occurs from direct extension of an acute pharyngitis. Causative organisms include both aerobes and anaerobes. Therapy consists of parenterally administered antimicrobials such as a first-generation cephalosporin or clindaymycin. Patients who do not respond to antimicrobial therapy or who have impaired respiratory function may require surgical incision and drainage under general anesthesia. Duration of therapy should be 10 days.

Otitis Media and Sinusitis.   Otitis media and sinusitis due to group A streptococcus normally are secondary to direct extension from a streptococcal infection occurring in the upper respiratory tract. Appropriate therapy for both is amoxicillin. With persistent infection, an appropriate alternative would be amoxicillin/clavulanate. In patients allergic to amoxicillin, erythromycin is an acceptable alternative. Oral cephalosporins can be effective as well in patients who have not had immediate hypersensitivity reactions to penicillin.

Uvulitis.   Uvulitis can occur alone or in association with acute pharyngitis or epiglottitis (34). Long known to be primarily a complication of *H. influenzae* type b infection, recent immunization strategies have greatly decreased its incidence. However, uvulitis can occur secondary to group A streptococcus, usually as a complication of an acute pharyngitis (34). Parenteral therapy should be used, directed against both group A streptococcus and *H. influenzae,* i.e., cefuroxime. Patients can be discharged on an oral antibiotic to complete a 10-day course of therapy.

Cervical Lymphadenitis.   Cervical lymphadenitis secondary to group A streptococcus infection can result from direct extension from an acute pharyngitis or direct inoculation. Since the etiologic agent is not always known, therapy is initially directed against the most common organisms, which include *S. aureus*. Therefore, a first-generation cephalosporin, such as cephalexin, or a β-lactamase-resistant penicillin should be given enterally for 10 days. If the infection persists or the patient develops signs of systemic toxicity, parenteral antibiotics should generally be used. A first-generation cephalosporin such as cefazolin, nafcillin, or clindamycin is an appropriate choice.

Meningitis and Brain Abscess.   Meningitis and brain abscesses are rare complications of group A streptococcus that can occur either from direct extension of acute pharyngitis or sinusitis or from bacteremic spread. Penicillin is still the drug of choice for treatment of known group A streptococcal meningitis or brain abscess (10). Antimicrobial therapy should be given parenterally for 10 to 14 days (10). Patients allergic to penicillin can be treated with a third-generation cephalosporin such as ceftriaxone or cefotaxime (10).

Arthritis.   Poststreptococcal reactive arthritis (PSRA) is a recognized complication of group A streptococcal infections. Antibiotic therapy aimed at the underlying focus of infection is generally all that is required. However, antiinflammatory drugs may aid patient comfort. Of concern, is the risk that a subset of patients with PSRA may develop rheumatic heart disease. Some have postulated that PSRA is part of the disease spectrum of ARF. A study by De Cunto et al. looked specifically at children with group A streptococcal pharyngitis and PSRA. Of 12 children, 1 developed rheumatic heart disease (16). Others have shown that as many as 10% of patients with PSRA who do not fulfill the criteria for ARF have gone on to develop ARF. This has led some to suggest that patients with PSRA, like patients who have had ARF, may require antimicrobial prophylaxis to prevent the occurrence of rheumatic heart disease (14). It has been recommended that these patients receive prophylaxis for 1 year, and then if no evidence of rheumatic heart disease develops, prophylaxis could be discontinued (14).

Septic arthritis secondary to group A streptococcal infection can result from direct inoculation or bacteremic spread. Therapy consists of parenteral antibiotics given for 10 to 14 days. Choices include a third-generation cephalosporin, such as ceftriaxone and cefotaxime, or nafcillin. In addition, surgical drainage of purulent material from the joint space is required.

Endocarditis. Endocarditis due to group A streptococcus was relatively common during the preantibiotic era. However, it is now rarely seen. Therapy aimed at the most common organisms in endocarditis also provides coverage for group A streptococcus and should be continued for 4 to 6 weeks. Patients with known GABHS endocarditis have been treated successfully with 6 weeks of parenterally administered penicillin (35). Of some concern, is the increasing association of severe, invasive group A streptococcal infections with intravenous drug abusers (54), which may place this segment of the population at increased risk of acquiring group A streptococcal endocarditis.

Osteomyelitis. Like septic arthritis, osteomyelitis secondary to group A streptococcal infection is known, but rare. Therapy consists of appropriate antimicrobials given parenterally to control the infection. If group A streptococcus has been identified as the etiologic agent, penicillin can be used. Patients allergic to penicillin can be treated with clindamycin, vancomycin, or cefazolin.

Liver Abscess. Liver abscesses secondary to group A streptococcal infection generally result from hematogenous spread. Therapy consists of long-term parenterally administered penicillin and surgical drainage. Initially, until an etiologic agent has been determined, a combination of a penicillinase-resistant penicillin, such as nafcillin, and an aminoglycoside should be used. Treatment should consist of 2 to 4 weeks of parenterally administered antibiotics followed by oral antibiotics to complete a 4-week course. Patients allergic to penicillin can be treated with clindamycin, vancomycin, or an appropriate first-generation cephalosporin.

Nonsuppurative Complications
Acute Rheumatic Fever. Treatment of patients with acute rheumatic fever is generally directed toward decreasing acute inflammation, decreasing fever and toxicity, controlling cardiac failure, preventing episodes of recurrent ARF after significant streptococcal upper respiratory tract infections, and preventing rheumatic heart disease. The mainstays of treatment are salicylates and corticosteroids. Neither of these agents prevents or modifies the development of rheumatic heart disease. Patients clinically diagnosed with ARF who have not received antimicrobial therapy for a recent episode of GABHS pharyngitis should receive a 10-day course of penicillin.

Primary prevention of ARF depends on accurate diagnosis of an antecedent streptococcal infection as well as adequate therapy. Penicillin given orally for 10 days or intramuscularly

one time has been shown effective in prevention of rheumatic fever. Erythromycin is considered the drug of choice for the treatment of GABHS pharyngitis in penicillin-allergic patients, but it has not been shown to prevent ARF (12). Approximately one-third of patients who develop ARF have streptococcal infections that are either subclinical or too mild to be brought to medical attention; as a result, they receive no antibiotic therapy for the infection. Recent reports have suggested that up to 75% of patients with ARF either had no history of a preceding streptococcal infection or had an infection that was so mild they did not seek medical care, unlike historically, where preceding streptococcal infections were noted to be severe (24). Of even more concern are reports of patients who develop ARF despite receiving adequate therapy for GABHS pharyngitis (15). Possible explanations for this include poor patient compliance with antibiotic therapy, a shorter latency period, documented streptococcal infections were not the cause of the resultant episodes of ARF, or currently recommended therapies for GABHS pharyngitis have become inadequate for prevention of ARF (15). The last is of greatest concern.

Only one series of studies has ever documented prevention of ARF following antimicrobial therapy for GABHS pharyngitis. These studies were conducted during the 1940s on army recruits at Fort Warren, Wyoming. Penicillin G suspended in oil, administered parenterally in a placebo-controlled study, decreased the incidence of ARF (17). Following these studies, researchers compared orally administered penicillin with parenterally administered penicillin and found equivalent bacteriologic effects. It was then assumed that bacterial eradication from the pharynx was the necessary step in prevention of ARF. As a result, penicillins as a class were assumed to be efficacious in preventing ARF (14, 33, 52). This has never been studied. No study has investigated the efficacy of other antibiotics in prevention of ARF.

Patients who develop ARF require continuous prophylaxis to prevent intercurrent and recurrent streptococcal infections and recurrent episodes of ARF. The preferred regimen consists of penicillin G benzathine, 1.2 million units given intramuscularly every 4 weeks (12). The recurrence rate of ARF with this regimen was reported to be 0.4 cases per 100 patient years of observation (6). Alternative therapies include oral sulfadiazine (1 g/day for persons over 60 lb and 0.5 g/day for those weighing less than 60 lb) or penicillin V (250 mg, twice a day). Both of these regimens are considered less effective than penicillin G benzathine. This is thought to be due to lack of patient compliance with an oral regimen. Patients who are allergic to penicillin can be treated with erythromycin stearate (250 mg, twice a day) (6).

Considerable debate has arisen over the optimal duration of prophylaxis. Some investigators previously recommended lifelong prophylaxis (12). However, the risk of recurrence of ARF decreases with patient age and the number of years since the last attack and increases with the presence of rheumatic heart disease or previous recurrences. The physician must take into account all factors when deciding when to discontinue prophylaxis. In general, it is recommended that prophylaxis continue until patients are in their early twenties and at least 5 years have passed since the most recent episode of ARF. In 1995, the Committee on Rheumatic Fever, Endocarditis, and Kawasaki Disease of the Council on Cardiovascular Disease in the Young, the American Heart Association, released a special statement on the treatment of GABHS pharyngitis and prevention of rheumatic fever. The committee recommended that patients who had rheumatic fever without rheumatic carditis should receive prophylaxis until the age of 21 or until at least 5 years had passed since their last attack. Patients who had rheumatic fever with carditis but no valvular disease should receive prophylaxis until adulthood and until at least 10 years had passed since their last attack of ARF. Patients with valvular disease should receive prophylaxis until age 40 and until at least 10 years had passed since their last attack (14).

Patients with residual rheumatic valvular disease must receive antibiotic prophylaxis whenever they undergo a surgical or dental procedure that may potentially evoke bacteremia. This is done to prevent the occurrence of bacterial endocarditis. Antimicrobial regimens recommended for the prevention of bacterial endocarditis are entirely distinct from regimens used in the prevention of ARF (14).

Currently, investigators are attempting to develop a polyvalent M-protein vaccine for the prevention of streptococcal infection and ARF.

Acute Glomerulonephritis.   Unlike rheumatic fever, acute poststreptococcal glomerulonephritis has shown no increase in incidence. Indeed, nephritogenic strains (particularly serotype M type 12) have decreased in prevalence (36). Treatment strategies in the approach to poststreptococcal acute glomerulonephritis (AGN) are directed toward management of acute problems. All patients should be treated with penicillin to eradicate the nephritogenic strain regardless of culture results of group A streptococci or immunologic tests. Paralleling the recent changes in the pathogenesis of ARF, a substantial number of patients who develop poststreptococcal AGN do not have a history of a preceding pharyngitis or soft-tissue infection (1). Penicillin-allergic patients can be treated with erythromycin in doses adequate for treatment of streptococcal pharyngitis. It is generally recommended that family members be cultured for group A streptococcus. Family members with positive cultures should be treated appropriately. Treatment of patients with poststreptococcal AGN or of family contacts is for epidemiologic purposes only. Therapy will not alter preexistent poststreptococcal AGN or prevent the disease in patients who are in the latent period. Some data suggest that antibiotic therapy may have a small effect on prevention of poststreptococcal AGN, but this has not been substantiated. However, antibiotic therapy is effective in epidemiologic efforts at eradicating nephritogenic strains of group A streptococcus. In high-risk settings during an acute epidemic of AGN, universal penicillin prophylaxis can be considered. Recurrent episodes of AGN are rare, and continuous antistreptococcal prophylaxis is generally not recommended. Long-term prognosis is generally thought to be excellent, but some studies found that up to 20% of patients develop urinary abnormalities (11).

Soft-Tissue Infections Due to GABHS

The second most common clinical manifestation of GABHS is a localized, relatively benign, infection of the skin. Recent reports have documented increased frequency and severity of invasive group A streptococcal infections of the skin and soft tissues, associated with group A streptococcal serotypes M-1 and M-3 (6). This is of considerable interest because these serotypes are more often associated with episodes of pharyngitis. Strains of group A streptococci that cause skin infections normally differ from those that cause pharyngitis and can be identified by their M serotypes. The most common streptococcal M serotypes that cause pharyngitis (types 1, 3, 5, 6, 12, 18, 19, 24 and others), including M-1 and M-3, have rarely been identified in skin lesions (6). In contrast, "skin strains" have been found to colonize the pharynx but are rarely associated with acute episodes of pharyngitis (6).

GABHS Pyoderma (Streptococcal Impetigo, Impetigo Contagiosum, Ecthyma)

Pyoderma is a term for a localized purulent infection of the skin and is used synonymously with streptococcal impetigo and impetigo contagiosa. Pyoderma is most common in children aged 2 to 5 years and occurs most commonly among economically disadvantaged children in tropical or subtropical climates but can occur in northern climates during the summer months. It normally results from direct inoculation of the skin surface with GABHS following minor trauma, abrasions, or insect bites. Often *S. aureus* can be isolated in addition to *S. pyogenes* from skin lesions of patients with pyoderma. Penicillin was effective treatment in the past but is now often associated with treatment failures. First-line therapy includes cloxacillin, cephalexin, or cefadroxil. Erythromycin is an alternative for penicillin-allergic patients but must be used with caution in regions where erythromycin-resistant strains of *S. pyogenes* and *S. aureus* are known. Therapy is continued for 10 days. Mupirocin ointment (applied to skin lesions 3 times daily for 10 days) has achieved cure rates comparable to those with enteral therapy but is more expensive (6). While rheumatic fever is not an associated complication of pyoderma, skin infections caused by nephritogenic strains of group A streptococci are the major antecedent of poststreptococcal glomerulonephritis.

Erysipelas

Erysipelas is an acute inflammation of the skin with involvement of cutaneous lymphatic vessels. It is most commonly found in infants and adults over 30 years of age. Historically, erysipelas most commonly involved the face. However, recent reports document up to 85% of infections involving the legs and feet (7). It is often preceded by a sore throat and commonly occurs at the site of a wound or surgical incision, especially when involving the trunk or extremities. The lesions are associated with fever and toxicity and are noted to spread outward. The rash itself is a scarlet-red or salmon color with well-defined borders. Blood cultures are positive in 5% of patients (7). Facial erysipelas may spontaneously resolve in 4 to 10 days (6). The mainstay of treatment remains penicillin (6). Superficial infections may be treated orally for 10 days, while more aggressive infections require parenteral therapy. Typical antimicrobial regimens include clindamycin, nafcillin, or a third-generation cephalosporin.

Cellulitis

Streptococcal cellulitis is an acute inflammation of the skin and subcutaneous tissues resulting from infection of burns, wounds, or surgical sites or following minor trauma. Symptoms include fever and toxicity and may be associated with lymphangitis or bacteremia. Cellulitis can be differentiated from erysipelas by noting that the skin lesion of cellulitis is not raised and the demarcation between involved and uninvolved skin is indistinct. Therapy should consist of a semisynthetic, penicillinase-resistant penicillin, since it is often difficult to differentiate streptococcal from staphylococcal cellulitis. In patients who are penicillin allergic, a first-generation cephalosporin may be used. Therapy can be given orally, unless there is evidence of lymphangitic spread. If lymphangitis is noted, parenterally administered antimicrobials should be used until there is marked clinical improvement. Oral antimicrobials can then be used to complete 10 days of therapy.

Necrotizing Fasciitis (Streptococcal Gangrene)

Necrotizing fasciitis is a rapidly progressing infection of the deep subcutaneous tissues and fascia with extensive and rapidly spreading necrosis. Infections often spare the skin, but 50% of patients may have associated myonecrosis. Necrotizing fasciitis is often associated with severe systemic involvement and an associated high mortality rate (57). As in other invasive streptococcal and staphylococcal skin infections, the site of inoculation is usually an area of minor trauma or the skin lesions of varicella. Like streptococcal bacteremia, there is a clear association between varicella and necrotizing fasciitis. Varicella is characterized by full-thickness dermal lesions that may induce selective immunosuppression to GABHS, though this has not been substantiated (8). Necrotizing fasciitis caused by mixed infections, involving both aerobic and anaerobic Gram-negative bacteria, is more likely to occur in the abdominal wall, following abdominal surgery or in diabetic patients.

Early and aggressive surgical debridement of the site of infection as well as appropriate antimicrobial therapy is required. Due to the "inoculum effect," penicillin may be less effective in the treatment of necrotizing fasciitis (55). Appropriate antibiotics include nafcillin and clindamycin (8). Some investigators have suggested use of hyperbaric oxygen therapy (HBO) in treatment of necrotizing fasciitis (2, 8, 58). HBO therapy may act by improving leukocyte response through oxygenation of devitalized tissue. In addition, it may aid in collagen deposition, angiogenesis, and reepithelialization (8, 58). However, HBO therapy is not without risks, and its use has not been well studied.

It was recently suggested that the use of nonsteroidal anti-inflammatory drugs (NSAIDs) in the treatment of fever in patients with GABHS infections may predispose the patient to a more severe invasive infection. NSAIDs may inhibit neutrophil function and enhance cytokine production (59). In addition, their use may mask some of the early signs and symptoms of invasive GABHS infections and has been associated with episodes of necrotizing fasciitis and toxic shock syndrome in patients with varicella (8)

Myositis/Myonecrosis

Myositis is a purulent infection of the muscles, normally occurring in the tropics and caused by *S. aureus*. Infections of the muscles are rarely caused by group A streptococcus but can occur. Infections occur following mild trauma, in toxic shock, and spontaneously. It is often difficult to differentiate streptococcal myonecrosis from necrotizing fasciitis, as the clinical features overlap, and the two entities often occur together. Fatality rates have been reported to be as high as 80 and 100% (54). Therapy includes extensive debridement of the infected muscle and parenterally administered antimicrobials. Penicillin has poor efficacy in the treatment of GABHS myonecrosis, and aggressive surgical debridement remains the most important factor in treatment (54). The failure of penicillin is attributed to decreased expression of penicillin-binding proteins during the stationary growth phase and the slow growth of group A streptococcus. This is known as the EAGLE effect and has been described elsewhere (54, 55). Clindamycin, erythromycin, and ceftriaxone have been more effective than penicillin in experimental models (54).

Lymphangitis

Lymphangitis may occur in association with cellulitis or after a clinically minor skin infection. When group A streptococcus is implicated as the etiologic agent, therapy consists of parenterally administered penicillin. When the cause of the infection is in doubt, nafcillin can be used to provide coverage for *S. aureus*. Patients allergic to penicillin can be treated with a first-generation cephalosporin, clindamycin, or vancomycin.

Puerperal Sepsis

Puerperal sepsis occurs during pregnancy or during an abortion, when group A streptococcus colonizing the patient invades the endometrium and surrounding structures as well as the lymphatics and bloodstream. Endometritis and septicemia result and can be complicated by pelvic cellulitis, thrombophlebitis, peritonitis, or pelvic abscess. Therapy consists of aggressive surgical exploration and parenterally administered penicillin or clindamycin (see section on myositis/myonecrosis). Patients allergic to penicillin can be treated with a first-generation cephalosporin, clindamycin, or vancomycin.

Vulvovaginitis

Group A streptococcus is a common cause of vulvovaginitis in the prepubertal female. Symptoms include a serous vaginal discharge, erythema of the vulvar area, and intense pruritus. Therapy consists of orally administered penicillin for 10 days. Patients allergic to penicillin can be treated with erythromycin.

Proctitis

Perianal cellulitis (proctitis or asymptomatic anal infection) has been associated with several reported outbreaks of hospital-acquired streptococcal infection. Because it is difficult to differentiate streptococcal cellulitis from staphylococcal cellulitis, it is advisable to use a first-generation cephalosporin, such as cephalexin, for therapy. Therapy should be given enterally for 10 days.

Funisitis and Omphalitis

Omphalitis is an infection of the umbilical cord and surrounding tissues. Etiologic agents include group A streptococcus, *S. aureus,* group B streptococcus, and Gram-negative enteric organisms. Combination therapy is normally provided consisting of a semisynthetic penicillin, such as oxacillin and gentamicin. Patients allergic to penicillin can be treated with a first-generation cephalosporin and gentamicin.

GABHS Toxic Shock

GABHS toxic shock usually occurs secondary to soft-tissue infections, particularly as a secondary infection of varicella lesions or as a complication of necrotizing fasciitis or myositis. However, while the upper respiratory tract is not the portal of entry in most cases, streptococcal toxic shock can follow a pharyngeal infection. Streptococcal toxic shock syndrome (TSS) must be differentiated from invasive group A streptococcal infections, which are more often a complication of a specific focus of infection and are more commonly associated with bacteremia. These two clinical entities may represent two ends of a clinical continuum.

M1 has been the predominant serotype associated with GABHS TSS, but types 3, 12, and 28 have been implicated as well (26, 32, 50). Recent interest in the pathophysiology of this disorder has focused on the role of streptococcal pyrogenic exotoxins (SPEs), extracellular products of group A streptococci that mediate not only scarlatiniform-like rashes but also multiorgan damage and shock. These toxins were rarely associated with GABHS strains in the United States until the recent increase in the number of cases of streptococcal TSS (50, 53).

SPE-A is the most common exotoxin found in the United States and has been shown to be both a superantigen and a potent inducer of tumor necrosis factor (6, 56, 67). SPE-A has been linked with the recent resurgence of severe, invasive group A streptococcal infections (4, 53). SPE-B has also been implicated but more commonly occurs in episodes of TSS in European countries (32, 50).

The patient with streptococcal TSS requires intensive management of hemodynamic abnormalities and vital functions. Patients with a soft-tissue focus of infection may require surgical intervention. Broad-spectrum antibiotic coverage should be instituted until the presence of group A streptococcus has been confirmed. Therapy may then consist of parenterally administered penicillin, with high doses recommended. Patients allergic to penicillin can be treated with a first-generation cephalosporin or vancomycin. Recently there has been some interest in using clindamycin in the treatment of GABHS TSS. In GABHS TSS, tissue destruction continues despite high concentrations of penicillin. Penicillin is known to be relatively ineffective in the treatment of soft-tissue infections with a high concentration of organisms (the EAGLE effect). This is thought to be due to the slow rate of replication of group A streptococci, decreased expression of penicillin-binding proteins, and the fact that penicillin acts by interfering with cell wall synthesis. Clindamycin inhibits protein synthesis, decreases the production of M proteins and toxins, and is unaffected by slow-growing toxin-producing streptococci. In addition, clindamycin may prevent group A streptococcus from expressing a capsule, an important virulence factor (9). A study by Brook et al. showed that by the 4th day of therapy, the frequency of capsular expression by GABHS was significantly lower in patients treated with clindamycin than in patients treated with penicillin (30). A mouse model of a soft-tissue infection with GABHS showed clindamycin to be more effective than penicillin (55). Erythromycin and ceftriaxone may also be more effective than penicillin in such cases (32).

Other proposed therapeutic interventions include the use of intravenous immunoglobulin (IVIG) and monoclonal antibodies. It is thought that IVIG may act by binding and inactivating toxins (54); however, use of IVIG in the treatment of streptococcal TSS has not been thoroughly evaluated. Investigators are studying the use of monoclonal antibodies against specific group A streptococcal toxins and the neutralization of circulating cytokines in managing invasive streptococcal disease caused by toxin-producing strains (32, 56).

Bacteremia

Accompanying the increase in number and severity of invasive group A streptococcal infections is an increase in the incidence of group A streptococcal bacteremia. There have been a number of cases associated with intravenous drug abuse as well as nosocomial outbreaks in nursing homes. Intravenous drug use has become the leading cause of GABHS bacteremia in individuals between the ages of 14 and 40 years (54). Bacteremia usually follows a cutaneous focus of infection but may follow an upper respiratory infection.

There has been increasing recognition of the association between group A streptococcal bacteremia and varicella. Up to 10% of patients with GABHS bacteremia have varicella (18). In addition, the number of children with varicella who develop GABHS bacteremia has increased (18). Doctor et al. reported an increased incidence of GABHS bacteremia in patients with varicella from 7% to 50% at their institution (18). GABHS bacteremia in varicella is thought to occur secondary to a superinfected lesion. Malignancy and immunosuppression are contributing risk factors to GABHS bacteremia.

Serotypes M-1 and M-3 have been most commonly isolated in patients with GABHS bacteremia. In addition, a relative increase in the isolation of serotypes M-1, M-3, and M-18 of GABHS in patients with GABHS bacteremia and a relative decrease in serotypes M-4 and M-12 have been reported (50). Serotypes M-1, M-3, and M-18 are more invasive and are associated with higher morbidity and mortality rates than M-4 and M-12, which are generally considered less virulent. M type 1 strains produce pyrogenic exotoxins A and B, and the latter toxin also has associated proteinase activity (36).

Therapy for GABHS bacteremia consists of parenterally administered penicillin. Patients allergic to penicillin can be treated with clindamycin, vancomycin, or a first-generation cephalosporin.

Pneumonia

Pneumonia secondary to group A streptococcus is frequently associated with preceding or concurrent viral infections such as measles, varicella, or influenza. Since the mid-1980s, the number of reports describing this association has increased. Up to 30% of patients with GABHS pneumonia have a history of group A streptococcal upper respiratory tract infection (6). Empyema develops in 40% of patients, and bacteremia in 15%. Other complications include mediastinitis, pericarditis, pneumothorax, and bronchiectasis. Therapy consists of surgical drainage of an empyema and parenteral penicillin.

COMBINATION THERAPY

In general, combination antimicrobial therapy offers no added benefit in the treatment of known GABHS infections. Antimicrobial agents possess sufficient activity in vitro to GABHS and, when initiated promptly, are effective in the treatment of such infections. However, in clinical situations in which GABHS is suspected but has not been identified (e.g., necrotizing fasciitis and TSS) antimicrobial therapy should be initiated with combinations effective against all possible pathogens.

GABHS VACCINE

Development of an effective group A streptococcal vaccine continues to be of interest; currently, none are commercially available. Proposed vaccines have focused on type-specific antibodies to M proteins, but cross-reactivity between GABHS M proteins and human myocardial tissue has raised serious safety concerns. Recent efforts have been directed at developing a vaccine against certain epitopes of the M protein that do not cross-react with myocardial tissue, providing a safer vaccine for immunizations (31, 47). In particular, researchers have looked at the conserved carboxy terminus of the M protein. Most adults develop immunity to group A streptococci, which is thought to evolve because of accumulation of antibodies to multiple serotypes. However, results of a study by Pruksakorn et al. suggest that immunity may result from long-term exposure to group A streptococci and development of antibodies to the conserved region of the M protein (47), a region that may be shared by all rheumatogenic strains of GABHS (65). A vaccine incorporating the conserved region of the M protein of group A streptococcus may stimulate a rapid rise in protective antibodies and provide safe and effective immunization.

CONCLUSION

Group A streptococcus has the unique ability to cause both acute purulent infections and nonpurulent complications that develop days after an initial infection. With a recognized increase in incidence and severity of invasive group A streptococcal infections and changes in the epidemiology of ARF, treatment of group A streptococcus has taken on even greater importance. While penicillin remains the mainstay of treatment, its use has recently been brought into question. New antibiotics and new strategies for treatment are being looked at,

and a vaccine effective against group A streptococcus is being developed. Once thought to have been relegated to simple sore throats, group A streptococcus has returned to the forefront of infectious diseases.

REFERENCES

1. Ayoub EM. Immune response to group A streptococcal infections. Pediatr Infect Dis J 1991;10:S15–19.
2. Barton LL, Jeck DT. Necrotizing fasciitis in children: report of two cases and review of the literature. Arch Pediatr Adolesc Med 1996;150:105–108.
3. Bass JW. Antibiotic management of group A streptococcal pharyngotonsillitis. Pediatr Infect Dis J 1991;10:S43–49.
4. Belani K, Schlievert PM, Kaplan EL, Ferrieri P. Association of exotoxin-producing group A streptococci and severe disease in children. Pediatr Infect Dis J 1991;10:351–354.
5. Betriu C, Sanchez A, Gomez M, Cruceyra A, Picazo JJ. Antibiotic susceptibility of group A streptococci: a 6-year follow-up study. Antimicrob Agents Chemother 1993;37(8):1717–1719.
6. Bisno AL. *Streptococcus pyogenes*. In: Mandell GL, Bennett JE, Dolin R, eds. Principles and practice of infectious diseases. 4th ed. New York: Churchill Livingstone, 1995:1786–1810.
7. Bisno AL, Stevens DL. Streptococcal infections of skin and soft tissues. N Engl J Med 1996;334:240–245.
8. Brogan TV, Nizet V, Waldhausen JHT, Rubens CE, Clarke WR. Group A streptococcal necrotizing fasciitis complicating primary varicella: a series of fourteen patients. Pediatr Infect Dis J 1995;14:588–594.
9. Brook I, Gober AE, Leyva F. In vitro and in vivo effects of penicillin and clindamycin on expression of group A beta-hemolytic streptococcal capsule. Antimicrob Agents Chemother 1995;39:1565–1568.
10. Chow JW, Muder RR. Group A streptococcal meningitis. Clin Infect Dis 1992;14:418–421.
11. Clark G, White RHR, Glasgow EF, Chantler C, Cameron JS, Gill D, Comley LA. Poststreptococcal glomerulonephritis in children: clinicopathological correlations and long-term prognosis. Pediatr Nephrol 1988;2:381–388.
12. Congeni BL. The resurgence of acute rheumatic fever in the United States. Pediatr Ann 1992;21:816–820.
13. Coonan KM, Kaplan EL. In vitro susceptibility of recent North American group A streptococcal isolates to eleven oral antibiotics. Pediatr Infect Dis J 1994;13:630–635.
14. Dajani A, Taubert K, Ferrieri P, Peter G, Shulman S, other committee members, and the Committee on Rheumatic Fever, Endocarditis and Kawasaki Disease of the Council on Cardiovascular Disease in the Young, the American Heart Association. Treatment of acute streptococcal pharyngitis and prevention of rheumatic fever: a statement for health professionals. Pediatrics 1995;96:758–764.
15. Dajani AS. Current status of nonsuppurative complications of group A streptococci. Pediatr Infect Dis J 1991;10:S25–27.
16. De Cunto CL, Giannini ED, Fink CW, Brewer EJ, Person DA. Prognosis of children with poststreptococcal reactive arthritis. Pediatr Infect Dis J 1988;7:683–686.
17. Denny FW, Wannamaker LW, Brink WR, Rammelkamp CH Jr, Custer EA. Prevention of rheumatic fever. Treatment of preceding streptococcal infection. JAMA 1950;143:151–153.
18. Doctor A, Harper MB, Fleisher GR. Group A beta-hemolytic streptococcal bacteremia: historical overview, changing incidence, and recent association with varicella. Pediatrics 1995;96:428–433.

19. Feldman S, Bisno AL, Lott L, Dodge R, Jackson RE. Efficacy of benzathine penicillin G in group A streptococcal pharyngitis: reevaluation. J Pediatr 1987;110:783–787.

20. Ferrieri P. Microbiological features of current virulent strains of group A streptococci. Pediatr Infect Dis J 1991;10:S20–24.

21. Fujita K, Murono K, Yoshikawa M, Murai T. Decline of erythromycin resistance of group A streptococci in Japan. Pediatr Infect Dis J 1994;13:1075–1078.

22. Galioto GB, Ortisi G, Mevio E, Sassella D, Bartucci F, Privitera G. Roxithromycin disposition in tonsils after single and repeated administration. Antimicrob Agents Chemother 1988; 32:1461–1463.

23. Gerber MA. Effect of early antibiotic therapy on recurrence rates of streptococcal pharyngitis. Pediatr Infect Dis J 1991;10: S56–60.

24. Gerber MA, Markowitz M. Streptococcal pharyngitis: clearing up the controversies. Contemp Pediatr 1992;Oct:118–131.

25. Gerber MA. Treatment failures and carriers: perception or problems? Pediatr Infect Dis J 1994;13:576–579.

26. Gerber MA. Antibiotic resistance in group A streptococci. Pediatr Clin North Am 1995;42:539–551.

27. Gerber MA, et al. Twice-daily penicillin in the treatment of streptococcal pharyngitis. Am J Med 1991;91:S23–30.

28. Gooch WM. Alternatives to penicillin in the management of group A streptococcal pharyngitis. Pediatr Ann 1992;21: 811–815.

29. Hooton TM. A comparison of azithromycin and penicillin V for the treatment of streptococcal pharyngitis. Am J Med 1991; 91:23S–30S.

30. Kaplan EL, Johnson DR. Eradication of group A streptococci from the upper respiratory tract by amoxicillin with clavulanate after oral penicillin V treatment failure. J Pediatr 1988;113: 400–403.

31. Klein JO. Reemergence of virulent group A streptococcal infections. Pediatr Infect Dis J 1991;10:S3–6.

32. Klein JO. Antimicrobial therapy issues facing pediatricians. Pediatr Infect Dis J 1995;14:415–418.

33. Klein JO. Management of streptococcal pharyngitis. Pediatr Infect Dis J 1994;13:572–575.

34. Kotloff KL, Wald ER. Uvulitis in children. Pediatr Infect Dis J 1983;2:392–393.

35. Liu VL, Stevenson JG, Smith AL. Group A streptococcus mural endocarditis. Pediatr Infect Dis J 1992;11:1060–1062.

36. Markowitz M. Changing epidemiology of group A streptococcal infections. Pediatr Infect Dis J 1994;13:557–560.

37. Maruyama S, Yoshioka H, Fujita K, Takimoto M Satake Y. Sensitivity of group A streptococci to antibiotics: prevalence of resistance to erythromycin in Japan. Am J Dis Child 1979;133: 1143–1145.

38. Melcher GP, et al. Comparative efficacy and toxicity of roxithromycin and erythromycin ethylsuccinate in the treatment of streptococcal pharyngitis in adults. J Antimicrob Chemother 1988;22:549–556.

39. Milatovic D. Evaluation of cefadroxil, penicillin and erythromycin in the treatment of streptococcal tonsillopharyngitis. Pediatr Infect Dis J 1991;10:S61–63.

40. O'Brien JF, Meade JL, Flak JL. Dexamethasone as adjuvant therapy for severe acute pharyngitis. Ann Emerg Med 1993; 22:212–215.

41. O'Doherty B. Azithromycin versus penicillin V in the treatment of paediatric patients with acute streptococcal pharyngitis/tonsillitis. Eur J Clin Microbiol Infect Dis 1996;15:718–724.

42. Paradise JL, Bluestone CD, Bachman RZ, Colborn DK, Bernard BS, Taylor FH, Rogers KD, Schwarzbach RH, Stool SE, Friday GA, et al. Efficacy of tonsillectomy for recurrent throat infection in severely affected children: results of parallel randomized and nonrandomized clinical trials. N Engl J Med 1984;310:674–683.

43. Pichichero ME. Cephalosporins are superior to penicillin for treatment of streptococcal tonsillopharyngitis: is the difference worth it? Pediatr Infect Dis J 1993;12:268–274.

44. Pichichero ME, Margolis PA. A comparison of cephalosporins and penicillins in the treatment of group A beta-hemolytic streptococcal pharyngitis: a meta-analysis supporting the concept of microbial copathogenicity. Pediatr Infect Dis J 1991;10:275–281.

45. Pichichero ME. The rising incidence of penicillin treatment failures in group A streptococcal tonsillopharyngitis: an emerging role for the cephalosporins? Pediatr Infect Dis J 1991;10: S50–55.

46. Pontani D. Efficacy and safety of azithromycin in the treatment of pediatric patients with acute pharyngitis due to group A beta-hemolytic streptococci [Abstract 5246]. 20th International Congress of Chemotherapy, June 29–July 3, 1997.

47. Pruksakorn S, Currie B, Brandt E, Martin D, Golbraith A, Phornphutkul C, Hunsakunachai S, Manmontri A Good MF. Towards a vaccine for rheumatic fever: identification of a conserved target epitope on M protein of group A streptococci. Lancet 1994; 344:639–642.

48. Roos K, Grahn E, Holm SE, Johansson H, Lind L. Interfering alpha-streptococci as a protection against recurrent streptococcal tonsillitis in children. Int J Pediatr Otorhinolaryngol 1993;25: 141–148.

49. Seppala H, Nissinen A, Jarvinen H, Huovinen S, Henriksson T, Herva E, Holm S, Jahkola M, Katila M, Klaukka T, Kontiairen S, Liimatainen O, Oinanen S, Passi-Metsomaa L, Huovinen P. Resistance to erythromycin in group A streptococci. N Engl J Med 1992;326:292–297.

50. Shulman ST. Invasive and toxin-related diseases caused by group A streptococci. Pediatr Infect Dis J 1991;10:S28–31.

51. Shulman ST, Gerber MA, Tanz RR, Markowitz M. Streptococcal pharyngitis: the case for penicillin therapy. Pediatr Infect Dis J 1994;13:1–7.

52. Shulman ST. Evaluation of penicillins, cephalosporins, and macrolides for therapy of streptococcal pharyngitis. Pediatrics 1996;97:S955–959.

53. Stevens DL, Tanner MH, Winship J, Swarts R, Ries K, Schlievert PM, Kaplan E. Severe group A streptococcal infections associated with a toxic shock-like syndrome and scarlet fever toxin A. N Engl J Med 1989;321:1–7.

54. Stevens DL. Invasive group A streptococcal infections: the past, present, and future. Pediatr Infect Dis J 1994;13:561–566.

55. Stevens DL, Gibbons AE, Bergstrom R, Winn V. The Eagle effect revisited: efficacy of clindamycin, erythromycin, and penicillin in the treatment of streptococcal myositis. J Infect Dis 1988;158:23–28.

56. Stevens DL, Bryant AE, Hackett SP, Chang A, Peer G, Kosanke S, Emerson T, Hinshaw L. Group A streptococcal bacteremia: the role of tumor necrosis factor in shock and organ failure. J Infect Dis 1996;173:619–626.

57. Stevens DL. Streptococcal toxic-shock syndrome: spectrum of disease, pathogenesis, and new concepts in treatment. Emerging Infect Dis 1995;1:69–78.

58. Stevens DL, Bryant AE, Yan S. Invasive group A streptococcal infection: new concepts in antibiotic treatment. Int J Antimicrob Agents 1994;4:297–301.

59. Stevens DL. Could nonsteroidal antiinflammatory drugs (NSAIDs)

enhance the progression of bacterial infections to toxic shock syndrome? Clin Infect Dis 1995;21:977–980.

60. Stillerman M. Comparison of oral cephalosporins with penicillin therapy for group A streptococcal pharyngitis. Pediatr Infect Dis J 1986;5:649–654.

61. Tanz RR, Shulman ST. Diagnosis and treatment of group A streptococcal pharyngitis. Semin Pediatr Infect Dis 1995;6: 69–78.

62. Tanz RR, Shulman ST, Sroka PA, Marubio S, Brook I, Yogev R. Lack of influence of beta-lactamase producing flora on recovery of group A streptococci after treatment of acute pharyngitis. J Pediatr 1990;117:859–863.

63. Tanz RR, Poncher JR, Corydon KE, Kabat K, Yogev R, Shulman ST. Clindamycin treatment of chronic pharyngeal carriage of group A streptococci. J Pediatr 1991;119:123–128.

64. Traub WH, Leonhard B. Comparative susceptibility of clinical groups A, B, C, F and G beta-hemolytic streptococcal isolates to 24 antimicrobial drugs. Chemotherapy 1997;43:10–20.

65. Wald ER. Acute rheumatic fever. Curr Probl Pediatr 1993;23: 264–270.

66. Wannamaker LW. The epidemiology of streptococcal infection. In: McCarty M, ed. Streptococcal infections. New York: Columbia University Press, 1953:157–175.

67. Ware JC, Eich WF, Ruben EB, Malone JA, Schlievert PM, Gray BM. Streptococcal toxic shock in three Alabama children. Pediatr Infect Dis J 1993;12:765–769.

68. Zackrisson G, Lind L, Roos K, Larsson P. Erythromycin-resistant beta-hemolytic streptococci group A in Goteborg, Sweden. Scand J Infect Dis 1988;20:419–420.

Streptococcus Species

●

James S. Tan and Thomas M. File, Jr.

"Strep" infections have been commonly associated with skin and throat infections due to group A streptococcus (*S. pyogenes*). Non–group A streptococci have also been implicated in mild-to-serious infections. Group B (*S. agalactiae*), group C and G streptococci, and viridans streptococci are known to colonize human respiratory, gastrointestinal, and genitourinary tracts. These bacteria are pathogenic under the right conditions.

Traditionally, streptococci are classified by their Lancefield group antigens and by hemolysis on blood agar. Lancefield group antigen does not correlate with the species, and classification by hemolysis is imprecise. Molecular taxonomic studies have improved classification. β-Hemolytic isolates in Lancefield groups A, C, F, and G are subdivided into large- and small-colony-forming groups. The large-colony groups possess numerous virulence mechanisms and are labeled "pyogenic." Large-colony group C streptococci are usually resistant to bacitracin, which has been used to differentiate them from group A streptococci (GABHS) in many clinical laboratories. However, some group C streptococci are susceptible to bacitracin, which may result in misidentification. Among the group G streptococci, bacitracin susceptibility has been reported to be as high as 67% (61). Trimethoprim/sulfamethoxazole disk testing has been added to improve identification. Both groups C and G streptococci are susceptible, and GABHS is resistant. For specific identification, a serogrouping reagent is used. Large-colony Lancefield group C streptococci are variably classified into one of several possible species: *S. dysgalactiae, S. equisimilis, S. zooepidemicus,* and *S. equi* (28). These species can be differentiated by microbiologic and biochemical characteristics. All but *S. dysgalactiae* commonly cause β-hemolysis in blood agar. Most clinical laboratories do not speciate group C streptococcal isolates.

The small-colony-forming groups are classified as "*S. milleri*" group or *S. intermedius* group. Although these "small-colony" organisms may possess the Lancefield group A, C, F, G, and ungroupable antigen, they are commensals and are seldom pathogenic by themselves. For example, "*S. milleri*" organisms with group A antigen can be differentiated from *S. pyogenes* by their small-colony formers and are resistant to bacitracin. "*S. milleri*" group have been considered a viridans group of streptococci. Other viridans groups include *S. mutans* group, *S. salivarius* group, *S. bovis* group, *S. sanguis* group, and *S. mitis* group (53). Formerly, "*Streptococcus* viridans" was a wastebasket term referring to streptococci that produce partial or no hemolysis on blood agar and were not groupable. The viridans group is established by exclusion of *S. pyogenes,* enterococci, pneumococci, *S. agalactiae,* and large-colony groups C and G (12) and has the following characteristics: vancomycin susceptibility, produces leucine aminopeptidase (LAP) enzyme, and does not produce pyrrolidonyl arylamidase (PYR) enzyme (53).

Group B streptococci has only one species, *S. agalactiae,* but is subclassified into 7 capsular serotypes: Ia, Ib, II, III, IV, V, and VI. Type III is most commonly associated with neonatal disease, types Ia and Ib with adult diseases (18, 65). Group B streptococcus is discussed elsewhere in this volume.

This chapter discusses the antimicrobial treatment of streptococcal infections other than those of *S. pyogenes* and *S. pneumoniae*. It discusses treatment of infections with pyogenic groups C and G and the so-called viridans group streptococci.

GROUP C AND G STREPTOCOCCI

Large-colony-forming group C streptococci and group G streptococci are part of the normal human skin and oral flora (Table 1). Human infection with groups C and G streptococci is much

TABLE 1 • Sites of Colonization and Infections in Humans; Non-Group A and Non-Group B Streptococcal Pathogens

Streptococcus	Normal Residence	Infection
Group C and G (*pyogenes*-like or large-colony-forming organisms)	Oropharyngeal flora, vagina, rectum, skin	Pharyngitis, skin infection, bacteremia, endocarditis, meningitis, osteomyelitis, septic arthritis, respiratory tract infection, puerperal infection, neonatal sepsis
Viridans groups of streptococci	Oropharynx, gastrointestinal tract, and genital tract	Endocarditis, infections in neutropenic patients
S. mutans group	Dental plaques and tooth surfaces	Dental caries, endocarditis
S. sanguis group	Dental plaques, oropharynx	Endocarditis
S. mitis	Oropharynx and gastrointestinal tract	Bacteremia and endocarditis, ARDS
S. bovis	Oropharynx, gastrointestinal, genital tract	Bacteremia and endocarditis in patients with malignancies of gastrointestinal tract especially with biotype I meningitis
S. salivarius group	Tongue and gastrointestinal tract	A frequent contaminant, rarely causes infection, bacteremia meningitis
"*S. milleri*" group *S. anginosus* *S. constellatus* *S. intermedius*	Oropharynx, gastrointestinal tract, vaginal flora, skin	Pyogenic infections, brain, liver, and appendiceal abscesses; associated with polymicrobial infection endocarditis
Nutritionally variant streptococci *S. adjacens* *S. defectivus*	Oropharynx	Endocarditis, sepsis, pancreatic abscess, otitis media eye infections (conjunctivitis, and crystalline keratopathy)

less common than with groups A and B streptococci. Groups C and G streptococci-associated pharyngitis does not differ clinically from that with GABHS. They are not associated with rheumatic fever but do cause glomerulonephritis (28). Skin infection is second most common. Other infections include puerperal and neonatal infections, bacteremia, endocarditis, meningitis, arthritis, osteomyelitis, and pneumonia (6, 8, 30, 55, 61, 63, 64). Infections with these organisms are frequently found in patients with such underlying conditions as chronic lung or heart disease, diabetes, malignancy (particularly group G streptococci), alcoholism, and immunosuppressive therapy. Group C streptococci are common pathogens in animals, and many patients with this infection have a history of animal exposure.

In Vitro Susceptibility

Penicillins, cephalosporins, carbapenems, and vancomycin are the most active antimicrobial agents against group C and G streptococci (Tables 2–4). Most strains are highly sensitive to penicillin G (MIC < 0.05 μg/mL). Strains with MICs above 0.1 μg/mL are rarely encountered (39). Broad-spectrum penicillins are also active. Rolston et al. reported MIC_{90}s of 0.03 and 0.06 μg/mL for piperacillin and azlocillin, respectively, in 44 isolates of groups C and G streptococci (48).

Cephalothin and cefotaxime are very active, with MIC_{90}s of 0.06 and 0.12 μg/mL, respectively (48). Kansenshoyaku et al. observed that all group G streptococci and 99% of group C streptococci were susceptible to 0.2 μg/mL of cephalothin (29). Other cephalosporins were less active, e.g., MIC_{90} for cephalexin was 3.13 μg/mL, and MIC_{90} for both groups C and G streptococci and MIC_{90} for cefaclor were 1.56 and 3.13

TABLE 2 • Susceptibility of Group C Streptococci from Various Reports

Antibiotic	Reference	No. of Strains	MIC_{90} μg/mL	MIC Range
Penicillin G	39	17	0.15	0.04–0.15
	29	125	0.05	≤0.006–0.05
Ampicillin	29	125	0.1	≤0.006–0.2
Amoxicillin	29	125	0.05	≤0.006–0.1
Cephalothin	29	125	0.2	0.05–0.39
Cephalexin	29	125	3.13	0.39–6.25
Cefaclor	29	125	1.56	0.39–6.25
Erythromycin	29	125	0.1	0.0125–0.39

μg/mL, respectively (29). Vancomycin is active with most isolates (MIC_{90} ≤ 0.5 mg/mL). Rolston et al. have recently reported isolates from cancer patients with MICs of 4.0 μg/mL (45). Imipenem is active against both groups C and G streptococci, all isolates evaluated by Muro et al. were susceptible (34).

Susceptibility of groups C and G streptococci to clindamycin and the macrolides is variable, with recent studies demonstrating some resistance (29, 30, 34, 46, 48). Kansenshoyaku et al. found an MIC_{90} for erythromycin of 0.1 μg/mL for both groups C and G streptococci, but 16 of 463 strains of group G streptococci had an MIC above 1.0 μg/mL (29).

Using National Committee for Clinical Laboratory Standards (NCCLS) guidelines, Muro et al. reported the in vitro susceptibilities of 113 isolates of group C streptococci and 35 isolates of group G streptococci obtained from 1992 to 1995. All were susceptible to penicillin G, ampicillin, amoxicillin/clavulanate, cefotaxime, imipenem, rifampin, and vancomycin (34). For group

TABLE 3 • Susceptibility of Group G Streptococci from Various Reports

Antibiotic	Reference	No. of Strains	MIC$_{90}$ (μg/mL)	MIC Range
Penicillin	31	20	0.017	0.0025–0.04
	29	463	0.05	≤0.0063–0.1
Amoxicillin	29	463	0.05	≤0.0063–0.2
Ampicillin	29	463	0.1	≤0.0063–0.2
	31	9	0.022	0.01–0.04
Oxacillin	50	17	0.12	0.06–0.12
Piperacillin	13	15	0.06	0.03–1.0
Cephalothin	29	463	0.2	0.025–0.2
	31	9	0.09	0.04–0.156
Cefotaxime	31	20	0.027	0.005–0.04
	31	9	0.022	0.01–0.04
Ceftazidime	13	15	0.5	0.03–32.0
Cefoxitin	31	9	0.27	0.156–0.312
Cephalexin	29	463	3.13	0.1–6.25
Cefaclor	29	463	3.13	0.1–6.25
Cefpodoxime	49	15	0.12	not reported
Vancomycin	30	20	1.13	0.312–2.5
	31	9	0.64	0.312–1.25
	50	17	0.25	0.25–0.5
	45	16	2.0	0.25–4.0
Teicoplanin	47	17	0.06	≤0.03–0.5
	45	16	0.25	0.25–0.5
LY264826	50		0.12	≤0.03–0.12
Erythromycin	46	16	0.06	≤0.03–0.12
	31	9	1.94	0.037–2.5
Clarithromycin	46	16	0.06	≤0.03–0.12
Clindamycin	46	16	0.5	≤0.03–0.5
	31	9	1.1	0.06–2
Trimethoprim/ sulfamethoxazole	47	15	0.12	0.25
Chloramphenicol	31	9	5.5	0.3–10
Ciprofloxacin	47	18[a]	1.0	0.5–2.0
	51	15[a]	2.0	0.25–2.0
	14	15	0.5	0.25–0.50
Ofloxacin	14	15	1.0	0.5–2.0
Levofloxacin	14	15	0.5	0.25–1.0
Sparfloxacin	51	15[a]	1.0	0.25–1.0
Clinafloxacin	47	15[a]	0.06	≤0.03–0.12

[a] Isolates from cancer patients.

alone. Rolston et al. found that penicillin-tolerant group C isolates were killed following addition of gentamicin to penicillin or cefotaxime (44). Lam and Bayer compared the in vitro bactericidal interaction of penicillin, cefotaxime, or vancomycin in combination with gentamicin for 20 isolates of group G streptococci. Synergism was demonstrated in each combination in 80 to 90% of isolates (31).

Antimicrobial Therapy

The response of group C or group G streptococcal infections to specific antimicrobial agents as reported in the literature is difficult to assess. Many patients in individual reports or population-based studies received multiple antibiotics with varying doses, routes of administration, and duration of therapy. There are no controlled antimicrobial efficacy trials. Most patients reported with group C or group G streptococcal infections have received a penicillin or cephalosporin (often with an aminoglycoside). Small numbers of patients have been treated with other antimicrobial agents (vancomycin, erythromycin, clindamycin, or chloramphenicol. On the basis of in vitro data as well as reported clinical experience, penicillin G is the preferred antibiotic (6, 8, 30, 55, 61, 63). Alternative agents with relatively uniform activity include ampicillin, cefotaxime, imipenem, and vancomycin. In vitro testing should be performed if clindamycin or the macrolides are considered for therapy, because of recent reports of resistance to these agents.

Because of the theoretical concern of tolerance and the probability of synergy, many authorities have recommended combination therapy using penicillin plus gentamicin for serious infectious such as sepsis and endocarditis (39, 55, 61). Such a recommendation, however, has not been substantiated by controlled studies. Watanakunakorn and Burket reported a relatively high mortality (40%) for patients with endocarditis despite penicillin susceptibility (64). This may in part be due to high association with comorbid conditions in these patients. For serious infections such as endocarditis, bacteremia, and any septic condition, penicillin (20 million units/day intravenously) is recommended. Alternatives include cefotaxime (8 g intravenously in divided doses). Vancomycin (2 g/day

C streptococci, the percentages of strains resistant to other antimicrobial agents were erythromycin and azithromycin, 9%; clindamycin, 8%; chloramphenicol, 2%; tetracycline, 17%; and trimethoprim/sulfamethoxazole, 20% (34). For group G streptococci, the percentages of strains resistant to other antimicrobial agents were erythromycin, 32%; azithromycin, 16%; clindamycin, 19%; chloramphenicol, 0%; tetracycline, 39%; and trimethoprim/sulfamethoxazole, 23% (34).

Tolerance, a condition in which bactericidal activity is more than 32 times the bacteriostatic activity, has been reported by numerous investigators. The frequency and clinical importance of tolerance is unclear (30, 61).

Synergism has been demonstrated when an aminoglycoside is added to penicillin, cefotaxime, and vancomycin. Portnoy et al. found all isolates tested to have greater killing when penicillin was combined with gentamicin than with penicillin

TABLE 4 • Susceptibility of Group C and Group G Streptococci from Two Reports

Antibiotic	Reference	No. of Strains	MIC$_{90}$ μg/mL	MIC Range
Penicillin G	48	44	0.03	0.03–0.06
Cephalothin	48	44	0.06	0.03–0.5
Cefotaxime	48	44	0.12	0.03–0.25
Piperacillin	48	44	0.03	0.03–0.5
Azlocillin	48	44	0.06	0.03–0.25
Vancomycin	48	44	0.12	0.03–0.5
Erythromycin	48	44	1.0	0.03–1.0
	35	20	0.5	0.12–1.0
Clarithromycin	35	20	0.25	0.06–1.0
Azithromycin	35	20	0.5	0.12–1.0
RP59500 Synercid-R	35	20	0.5	0.06–1.0

intravenously) may be used for patients unable to receive β-lactam agents. The duration of therapy for endocarditis is 28 days; for bacteremia or sepsis, 14 days of therapy should be adequate. There is currently no consensus on the value of adding gentamicin. We recommend gentamicin while awaiting the results of in vitro susceptibility testing. If the MIC is above 0.1 μg/mL, combination therapy should be used for the full course of therapy.

VIRIDANS STREPTOCOCCI

Viridans streptococci have been considered to have low virulence. Transient bacteremias may occur following dental manipulation and frequently are of no consequence in patients without predisposing conditions. It has been estimated that only 21% of the positive blood cultures are clinically significant (58). Viridans streptococci are the most common cause of native valve endocarditis and late-onset prosthetic valve endocarditis (56, 60, 64). They have also been associated with serious pyogenic infections, bacteremias in neutropenic patients, and septicemia/shock syndrome (also known as "α-strep shock syndrome") (3, 7, 17, 28).

S. mutans, S. sanguis, dextran-positive S. mitis (also known as S. mitior; S. mitis is used in this chapter), and S. bovis are mouth organisms associated with dental disease. They produce dextran that is associated with plaque formation and is highly associated with infective endocarditis when cultured from the blood (56). Dextran production results in glycocalyx formation that promotes adherence and serves as an adherence factor.

S. bovis is a common gastrointestinal commensal reported to cause bacteremia, endocarditis, and meningitis (41, 53). S. bovis biotype I bacteremia has been shown to be highly associated with gastrointestinal malignancies, biotype II and S. salivarius are less likely (54).

"S. milleri" group (also known as S. intermedius group) isolates have been associated with purulent infections in oral, thoracic, abdominal, and central nervous system sites (24). S. anginosus was most often found in the genitourinary and gastrointestinal tracts, S. constellatus in the chest, and S. intermedius in the central nervous system, head and neck, and abdomen, (26, 66). Singh et al. reviewed 186 S. anginosus infections and found 110 patients had at least one abscess identified. Because of this high association of abscess formation, a routine workup in "S. milleri" group bacteremia should include a search for abscess.

Antimicrobial Susceptibility

The 1995 American Heart Association guidelines for treatment of endocarditis designated viridans streptococci as penicillin susceptible, with intermediate resistance, and with high resistance. Penicillin was recommended for penicillin-susceptible viridans streptococci (68). An increasing percentage of penicillin resistance has been reported, even in serious infections, believed to be due to alteration of the penicillin-binding protein (2, 22, 24, 40, 42, 67). Alcaide et al., from Barcelona, Spain, found that 33.6% of 410 isolates were resistant to penicillin (41.5% of S. mitis, 41.7% of S. sanguis, 28.1% of S. salivarius, and 14% of S. anginosus) (2). They divided the β-lactam agents tested against the penicillin-resistant strains into three groups. In the first group, imipenem, ceftriaxone, and cefotaxime had equal or higher activity than penicillin. The second group had lower activity than penicillin: ampicillin, amoxicillin/clavulanate, piperacillin, cefuroxime, and cefpodoxime. The third group had poor in vitro activity; it includes the first-generation cephalosporins, ceftazidime, cefixime, cefaclor, ceftibuten, and oxacillin. Potgieter et al. from South Africa studied 211 isolates from blood cultures and found all to be consistently susceptible to cefotaxime, ceftriaxone, and imipenem (40). It appears that imipenem, cefotaxime, and ceftriaxone are acceptable alternatives in serious infections caused by penicillin-resistant strains, but further clinical studies are needed. When intermediate resistance (MIC = 0.25 to 2 μg of penicillin per mL) or high-level resistance (MIC ≥ 4 μg/mL) is encountered, synergism with aminoglycoside can still be achieved (11). Synergistic combination should be considered after in vitro synergism has been confirmed. A high percentage of trimethoprim/sulfamethoxazole, erythromycin, and tetracycline resistance has been reported (16, 40). In contrast, S. bovis, unlike its group D counterpart the enterococcus, is highly susceptible to penicillin.

Doern et al., reported their experience with 352 viridans group streptococci from 43 U.S. medical centers (Fig. 1) (16). They found that 13.4% had high-level resistance (MIC ≥ 4 μg/mL), and 42.9% had intermediate resistance (MIC = 0.25–2.0 μg/mL). Among the cephalosporins tested, strains appear most sensitive to ceftriaxone. Using the breakpoint of 8 μg/mL for ofloxacin, less than 1% resistance was encountered, and using a breakpoint of 2 μg/mL, less than 5% resistance. In another U.S. study, blood cultures from 47 neutropenic patients that yielded streptococci (mostly S. mitis and S. sanguis) on ciprofloxacin prophylaxis showed 38% with penicillin resistance, 54% with ceftazidime resistance, and 95% with resistance to ciprofloxacin and ofloxacin (33). Because of development of quinolone resistance, prophylactic use of quinolone in neutropenic cancer patients should be carefully evaluated. Poor susceptibility to macrolide antibiotics was demonstrated in 66 blood culture isolates from neutropenic cancer patients (1). This group of antimicrobial agents is not a good candidate for prophylaxis.

Jacobs et al. found that penicillin resistance in the "S. milleri" group is rare (27). However, Potgieter et al. reported an overall 29% penicillin resistance in the viridans group, including the "S. milleri" group (40). This group of organisms is susceptible to vancomycin, cephalosporins, clindamycin, and erythromycin but resistant to tetracyclines, sulfamethoxazole, and aminoglycosides. Synergy can usually be demonstrated with aminoglycosides (23–25, 38).

Antimicrobial Therapy

Endocarditis. Since the introduction of penicillin, the cure rate of viridans streptococcal infection has exceeded 95%. Reasons for failure include bacterial tolerance (MBC 32 times higher than MIC), inadequate antimicrobial level in the vegetation (most likely due to inadequate dosing or poor drug penetration), and heart failure. In addition to maintaining pump

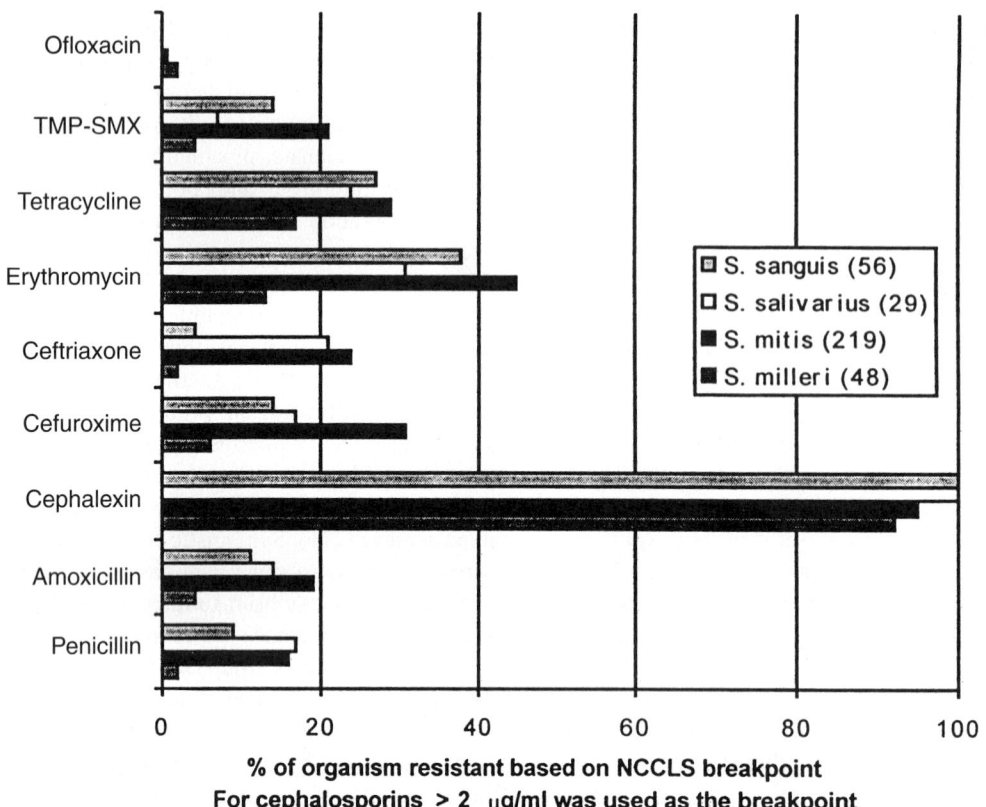

FIGURE 1. In vitro activities of selected antimicrobial agents versus 4 streptococcal species isolates from 43 U.S. medical centers from 1993–94. (Modified from Doern GV, Ferraro MJ, Brueggemann AB, Ruoff KL. Emergence of high rates of antimicrobial resistance among viridans group streptococci in the United States. Antimicrob Agents Chemother 1996;40:891–894.)

function, the major objective is eradication of the infecting viridans streptococcus. The AHA guidelines (Table 2) for treatment of native valve infection by penicillin-susceptible viridans streptococcus (MIC ≤ 0.1 μg/mL) including *S. bovis* consists of 4-week therapy with a single β-lactam agent or 2-week therapy with a combination of a β-lactam agent plus aminoglycoside. Francioli et al. recently reported successful treatment of viridans streptococci endocarditis using a 2-week course of ceftriaxone (2 g) plus netilmicin (4 mg/kg) (20). Although the guidelines recommended 4 weeks of a single β-lactam agent for the elderly, we prefer to treat with combination therapy except in the setting of either impaired renal function or high-level aminoglycoside resistance (MIC > 500 μg/mL). Gavalda et al. reported that in experimental endocarditis, once-a-day intramuscular dosing of gentamicin was as effective as multiple dosing as long as the total daily dose was 3 mg/kg (21). The overall bacteriologic failure rate is extremely low (56). Patients who were ill for more than 3 months before therapy have a higher relapse rate and a longer duration of therapy is recommended (37).

Successful oral penicillin plus intramuscular aminoglycoside therapy for penicillin-susceptible viridans streptococci has been reported (59). This form of therapy should only be tried when blood levels can be monitored and patient compliance can be ensured. For patients allergic to β-lactam

agents, vancomycin may be used. In younger patients, vancomycin clearance may be faster, thus it may be prudent to know the vancomycin half-life and adjust the dosing interval.

For patients with native valve endocarditis due to strains with MICs between 0.1 and 0.5 μg/mL, AHA (Table 5) recommends 4 weeks of treatment with penicillin plus 2 weeks of aminoglycoside therapy. If high-level resistance to aminoglycoside is present or synergism cannot be demonstrated, vancomycin should be used. Based on the study by Alcaide et al., another option is checking for susceptibility to cefotaxime, ceftriaxone, and imipenem. If the MIC is low, any of these agents may be considered. The above scenario can also apply to the highly resistant viridans streptococci, although no official recommendation is available for these organisms. Experimental studies using vancomycin plus gentamicin have shown that this combination is effective against strains that are penicillin resistant (32). Patients infected with "*S. milleri*" are at a higher risk for complications, and thus a higher dose of penicillin is recommended.

Noncardiac Sites of Infection

Clinically, "*S. milleri*" group noncardiac infections have responded well to penicillin and cephalosporins. With penicillin resistance on the rise, it is prudent to treat serious infection

---

TABLE 5 • Recommended Therapy for Viridans Streptococcal Infections

---

Endocarditis due to penicillin-susceptible viridans streptococci and *Streptococcus bovis* (MIC < 0.1 mg/mL)
  Native valve infection: use any of the following:
    1. Penicillin G 12–18 million units/day in continuous drip or 6 divided doses plus gentamicin 3 mg/kg i.v. as single dose or 3
       divided doses for 2 weeks
    2. Penicillin G 12–18 million units/day in continuous drip or 6 divided doses for 4 weeks
    3. Ceftriaxone 2 g i.v. or i.m. daily for 4 weeks
    4. Vancomycin 30 mg/kg not to exceed 2 g i.v. in 2 divided doses for 4 weeks
  Prosthetic valve infection
    Penicillin or vancomycin as 2 and 3 for 6 weeks plus gentamicin at the same dose as above for at least 2 weeks

Endocarditis due to viridans streptococci and *Streptococcus bovis* relatively resistant to penicillin G (MICs >0.1 mg/mL and <0.5
  mg/mL)[a]
    1. Penicillin 18 million U/24 h i.v. either continuously or in six equally divided doses for 4 weeks plus gentamicin 3 mg/kg i.v. as
       single dose or 3 divided doses for 2 weeks
    2. Vancomycin 30 mg/kg not to exceed 2 g i.v. in 2 divided doses for 4 weeks

Endocarditis due to viridans streptococci (MIC > 0.5 μg/mL) or NVS
    1. Aqueous crystalline penicillin G sodium, 18–30 million U/24 h i.v. either continuously or in six equally divided doses or
       ampicillin sodium 12 g/24 h i.v. either continuously or in six divided doses plus gentamicin sulfate 1 mg/kg i.m. or i.v. every 8 h
       for 4–6 weeks[a]
    2. Vancomycin[b] hydrochloride 30 mg/kg per 24 h i.v. in two equally divided doses, not to exceed 2 g/24 h unless serum levels are
       monitored, plus gentamicin sulfate (similar dose as above) for 4–6 weeks[a]

For patients with prosthetic valve endocarditis due to streptococcus
  Treat as resistant streptococcus for 6–8 weeks

For patients with bacteremia without endocarditis due to viridans group of streptococcus and NVS
    1. Penicillin G 12–18 million units i.v. continuously or in 6 divided doses for 2 weeks
    2. Ceftriaxone 2 g i.v. or i.m. daily for 2 weeks
    3. Clindamycin 300 mg i.v. or p.o. q. 8 h for 2 weeks[c]
    4. Vancomycin 30 mg/kg not to exceed 2 g i.v. in 2 divided doses for 2 weeks

For patients with meningitis due to viridans group of streptococcus or NVS
    1. Ceftriaxone 2 g i.v. or i.m. daily or cefotaxime 2 g i.v. q. 6 h for 2 weeks
    2. Penicillin 18–30 million units i.v. in 6 divided doses for 2 weeks
    3. Vancomycin 30 mg/kg not to exceed 2 g i.v. in 2 divided doses for 2 weeks

For patients with mixed infection including viridans streptococci or NVS
    1 β-lactam/β-lactamase inhibitor combinations at the recommended dose
    2. Imipenem 500–750 mg every 6–8 h i.v.
    3. Above agents or clindamycin plus gentamicin

---

[a] 4-week therapy recommended for patients with symptoms <3 months in duration; 6-week therapy recommended for patients with symptoms >3 months in duration.

[b] Vancomycin therapy is recommended for patients allergic to β-lactams; cephalosporins are not acceptable unless shown effective by susceptibility testing.

[c] Clindamycin susceptibility should not be checked.

---

with a combination of penicillin and aminoglycoside. Vancomycin or clindamycin may be used for penicillin-allergic patients. Since this group of organisms is frequently associated with abscess, an effort should be made to rule out this possibility. When abscess is present, drainage should be strongly considered. Treatment failures have been observed in patients with polymicrobial abscess who were treated with metronidazole and anti–Gram-negative rod antimicrobial agents. Because of the lack of antistreptococcal activity, "*S. milleri*" group may be isolated as the sole microbe in liver abscess (38).

Special attention should be given to neutropenic patients with viridans streptococcal bacteremia. Although it is not as common as Gram-negative and staphylococcal bacteremia, this problem is increasing because of antibiotic prophylaxis with fluoroquinolones, damage to the oral mucosa caused by chemotherapy, and neutropenia (4, 10, 43). The oral cavity is believed to be the portal of entry, especially in those with oral mucosa damage. Complications from this bacteremia include pulmonary infiltrates, adult respiratory distress syndrome, hypotension, and endocarditis. A related problem is septicemia and shock syndrome due to viridans streptococcus, which has an associated mortality rate of 11% (17). Alternatives to high-dose penicillin include vancomycin. If another β-lactam drug is used, imipenem, ceftriaxone, and cefotaxime have better activity than most other cephalosporins including ceftazidime (2, 40, 62).

Meningitis.   Streptococci rarely infect the meninges. Experience with treatment of meningitis due to these organisms is limited. The antibiotic of choice should be one with good penetration to the cerebrospinal fluid. Ceftriaxone, high-dose penicillin, or vancomycin should be effective.

Mixed Infections.   When streptococcal infection is suspected as part of a mixed infection, therapy should be directed against the mixed infection. The physician should ensure that an agent effective against viridans streptococci is part of the therapy.

NUTRITIONALLY VARIANT STREPTOCOCCI (*S. DEFECTIVUS* AND *S. ADJACENS*)

Nutritionally variant streptococci (NVS) are no longer classified under viridans streptococci. They were grouped with viridans streptococci because of some similarities to *S. mitis,* but their taxonomic status is unsettled. Unlike other streptococci NVS require pyridoxal or thiol supplementation for growth. Two species, *S. defectivus* and *S. adjacens,* are included in this group. They are found normally in the oropharynx and have been associated with bacteremia, endocarditis, and eye infections including conjunctivitis, keratitis, endophthalmitis, and infectious crystalline keratopathy (52).

In Vitro Susceptibility

In vitro susceptibility testing for this group is difficult to perform and results do not correlate well with clinical outcome. Moreover, infections due to these organisms are known to respond poorly to antibiotics (57). NVS as a rule are less susceptible to penicillin than most other streptococci, but many strains exhibit tolerance. Most strains have been reported susceptible to rifampin, clindamycin, erythromycin, chloramphenicol, and vancomycin (52). Susceptibility to tetracyclines, aminoglycosides, and cephalosporins is variable (28). Time-kill studies have shown that vancomycin and rifampin are synergistic (52).

Antimicrobial Therapy

There are two groups of streptococci that are more difficult to treat, "tolerant" organisms and NVS, which are also tolerant. As stated above, tolerant bacterial growth can be inhibited, but bacteria are not killed until the antibiotic concentration is increased by 32-fold or more.

Stein et al. reviewed 30 cases of NVS endocarditis and found that the relapse rate, bacteriologic failure, and mortality rate are higher than those of the viridans group. They believed that the slow rate of growth and the production of glycocalyx might have contributed to the lack of success (57). In addition, tolerance has been observed with penicillin and vancomycin (52). The current AHA recommendation is to treat NVS endocarditis similarly to enterococcal infection (Table 5). However, even with 6 weeks of combination therapy with penicillin and gentamicin, the failure rate is high (15).

Experimental models of endocarditis demonstrated that vancomycin or vancomycin-gentamicin combination may be used as an alternative drug in patients when penicillin-aminoglycoside combination is ineffective or contraindicated (5). Clinical experience is lacking.

SUMMARY

Recent changes in the susceptibility of streptococci have changed the attitude of clinicians toward this group of bacteria. Penicillin and many cephalosporins previously considered exquisitely active are no longer consistently effective. β-Lactam antibiotics either alone or in combination are suitable for most endocarditis patients infected with viridans streptococcus, *S. bovis,* but alternative regimens are necessary for special situations. Groups C and G streptococci respond best to the combination of a penicillin and an aminoglycoside (19). The clinician should be aware of these new developments and use MIC and synergism tests in serious infections caused by streptococci.

REFERENCES

1. Alcaide F, Carratala J, Guidol F, Martin R. In vitro activities of eight macrolide antibiotics and RP-59500 (quinupristin-dalfopristin) against viridans group streptococci isolated from blood of neutropenic cancer patients. Antimcrob Agents Chemother 1996;40:2117–2120.
2. Alcaide F, Linares J, Pallares R, et al. In vitro activities of 22 beta-lactam antibiotics against penicillin resistance and penicillin-susceptible viridans group streptococci isolated from blood. Antimicrob Agents Chemother 1995;39:2243–2247.
3. Awada A, van der Auwera P, Meunier F, Daneau D, Klastersky J. Streptococcal and enterococcal bacteremia in patients with cancer. Clin Infect Dis 1992;15:33–48.
4. Bochud P-Y, Eggiman P, Calandra T, Van Melle G, Saghafi L, Francioli P. Bacteremia due to viridans streptococcus in neutropenic patients with cancer: clinical spectrum and risk factors. Clin Infect Dis 1994;18:25–31.
5. Bouvet A. Human endocarditis due to nutritionally variant streptococci: *Streptococcus adjacens* and *Streptococcus defectivus.* Eur Heart J 1995;16(Suppl B):24–27.
6. Bradley SF, Gordon JJ, Baumgartner DD, Marasco WA, Kauffman CA. Group C streptococcal bacteremia: analysis of 88 cases. Rev Infect Dis 199a;13:270–280.
7. Broughton RA, Krafka R, Baker CJ. Non-group D alpha-hemolytic streptococci: new neonatal pathogens. J Pediatr 1981; 99:450–454.
8. Burket T, Watanakunakorn c. Group G streptococcus septic arthritis and osteomyelitis: report and literature review. J Rheumatol 1991:18:904–907.
9. Carmeli Y, Schapiro JM, Neeman D, Yinnon AM, Alkan M. Streptococcal group C bacteremia, survey in Israel and analytical review. Arch Intern Med 1995;155:1170–1176.
10. Carratala J, Alcaide F. Fernandez-Sevilla A, Corbella X, Linares J, Gudiol F. Bacteremia due to viridans streptococci that are highly resistant to penicillin: increase among neutropenic patients with cancer. Clin Infect Dis 1995;20:1169–1173.
11. Cercenado E, Diaz MD, Sanchez-Carrillo C, Vicente T, Bernado de Quiros JCL. Enhanced activity of the combination of penicillin G and gentamicin against penicillin-resistant viridans group streptococci. Antimicrob Agents Chemother 1995;39:2816–2818.
12. Coykendall AL. Classification and identification of the viridans streptococci. Clin Microbiol Rev 1989;2:315–328.
13. Dholakia N, Rolston KVI, Ho DH, et al. In vitro activity of FK-037, a novel parenteral cephalosporin against bacterial isolates from neutropenic cancer patients. Eur J Clin Microbiol Infect Dis 1994;13:679–685.

14. Dholakia N, Rolston KVI, Ho DH, et al. Susceptibility of bacterial isolates from patients with cancer to levofloxacin and other quinolones. Antimicrob Agents Chemother 1994;38:848–852.

15. Dinubile MJ. Treatment of endocarditis caused by relatively resistant nonenterococcal streptococci: is penicillin enough? Rev Infect Dis 1990;12:112–117.

16. Doern GV, Ferraro MJ, Brueggemann AB, Ruoff KL. Emergence of high rates of antimicrobial resistance among viridans group streptococci in the United States. Antimicrob Agents Chemother 1996;40:891–894.

17. Etling LS, Bodey GP, Keefe BH. Septicemia and shock syndrome due to viridans streptococci: a case control study of predisposing factors. Clin Infect Dis 1992;14:1201–1207.

18. Farley MM, Harvey C, Stull T, et al. A population-based assessment of invasive disease due to group B streptococcus in nonpregnant adults. N Engl J Med 1993;328:1807–1811.

19. Francioli P. Antibiotic treatment of streptococcal endocarditis: an overview. Eur Heart J 1995;16(Suppl B):75–79.

20. Francioli P, Ruch W, Stamboulian D, and the International Infective Endocarditis Study Group. Treatment of streptococcal endocarditis with a single daily dose of ceftriaxone and netilmicin for 14 days: a prospective multicenter study. Clin Infect Dis 1995;21:1406–1410.

21. Gavalda J, Pahissa A, Almirante B, et al. Effect of gentamicin dosing interval on therapy of viridans streptococcal experimental endocarditis with gentamicin plus penicillin. Antimicrob Agents Chemother 1995;39:2098–2103.

22. Goldfarb JG, Wormser GP, Glaser JH. Meningitis caused by multiple antibiotic resistant viridans streptococci. J Pediatr 1984;105:891–895.

23. Gomez-Garces J-L, Alos J-I, Cogolos R. Bacteriologic characteristics and antimicrobial susceptibility of 70 clinically significant isolates of Streptococcus milleri group. Diagn Microbiol Infect Dis 1994;19:69–73.

24. Gossling J. Occurrence and pathogenicity of Streptococcus milleri group. Rev Infect Dis 1988;10:257–265.

25. Horton WA, Drucker DB, Jacob AE, Hillier VF. Susceptibility of sixty-five non-oral clinical isolates of the *Streptococcus milleri* group to seven antimicrobial agents. Microbios 1992;71:12–134.

26. Jacobs JA, Pietersen HG, Stobberingh Ee, Soeters PB. Streptococcus anginosus, *Streptococcus constellatus*, and *Streptococcus intermedius*. Clinical relevance, hemolytic and serologic characteristics. Am J Clin Pathol 1995;104(5):547–553..

27. Jacobs JA, Stobberingh EE. In-vitro antimicrobial susceptibility of the *"Streptococcus milleri"* group (*Streptococcus anginosus, Streptococcus constellatus* and *Streptococcus intermedius*). J Antimicrob Chemother 1996;37:371–375.

28. Johnson CC, Tunkel AR. Viridans streptococci and groups C and G streptococci. In: Mandell GL, Bennett JE, Dolin R, eds. Principles and practice of infectious diseases. New York: Churchill Livingstone, 1995:1845–1867.

29. Kansenshogaku Z, Omuyana M, Sagayama Y, Nakajima K. An epidemiological study of group A, B, C, G hemolytic streptococci. J Jpn Assoc Infect Dis 1994;68:665–679.

30. Lam K, Bayer AS. Serious infections due to group G streptococci. Report of 15 cases with in-vitro-in-vivo correlations. Am J Med 1983;75:561–570.

31. Lam K, Bayer AS. In vitro bactericidal synergy of gentamicin combined with penicillin G, vancomycin, or cefotaxime against group G streptococci. Antimicrob Agents Chemother 1984;26:260–262.

32. Martinez F, Martin-Luengo F, Garcia A, Valdes M. Treatment with various antibiotics of experimental endocarditis caused by penicillin-resistant *Streptococcus sanguis*. Eur Heart J 1995;16:687–691.

33. McWhiney PHM, Patel S, Whiley RA, Hardies JM, Gillespie SH, Kibbler CC. Activities of potential therapeutic and prophylactic antibiotics against blood culture isolates of viridans group streptococci from neutropenic patients receiving ciprofloxacin. Antimicrob Agents Chemother 1993;37:2493–2495.

34. Muro P, Alcala L, Pelaez R, Garcia-Garrote F, Muno P, Bouza E. Erythromycin resistance in group C and group G streptococci: an analysis based on site of isolation. 36th Interscience Conference on Antimicrobial Agents and Chemotherapy, New Orleans. American Society for Microbiology, 1996:E42.

35. Neu HC, Chin N, Gu J. The in vitro activity of new streptogramins, RP57669 and RP54476, alone and in combination. J Antimicrob Chemother 1992;30(Suppl A):83–94.

36. Noble JT, Tyburske MB, Berman M, Greenspan J, Tenebaum MJ. Antimicrobial tolerance in group G streptococci. Lancet 1980;ii:982.

37. Phair JP, Tan JS. Therapy for streptococcus viridans endocarditis. In: Kaplan EL, Taranta AV, eds. Infective endocarditis. Dallas: American Heart Association, 1977:55–57.

38. Piscitelli SC, Shwed J, Schreckenberger O, Danziger LH. Streptococcus milleri group: renewed interest in an elusive pathogen. Eur J Clin Microbiol infect Dis 1992;11:491–498.

39. Portnoy D, Prentis J, Richards GK. Penicillin tolerance of human isolates of group C streptococci. Antimicrob Agents Chemother 1981;20:235–238.

40. Potgieter E, Carmichael M, Kornhof HJ, Chalkley LJ. In vitro antimicrobial susceptibility of viridans streptococci isolated from blood cultures. Eur J Clin Microbiol Infect Dis 1992;11:543–546.

41. Purdy RA, Cassidy B, Marrie TJ. Streptococcus bovis meningitis: report of 2 cases. Neurology 1990;40:1782–1784.

42. Quinn JP, DiVincenzo CA, Lucks DA, Luskin RL, Shatzer KL, Lerner SA. Serious infections due to penicillin-resistant viridans streptococci with altered penicillin-binding proteins. J Infect Dis 1988;157;764–769.

43. Richard P, Amador Del Valle G, Moreau P, et al. Viridans streptococcal bacteremia in patients with neutropenia. Lancet 1995;345:1607–1609.

44. Rolston KVI, Dholakia N, Ho DH, LeBlanc B, Dvorak T, Streeter H. In vitro activity of ramopanin, vancomycin, and teicoplanin against gram-positive clinical isolates from cancer. J Antimicrob Chemother 1984:13:389–392.

45. Rolston KVI, Dholakia N, Ho DH, LeBlanc B, Dvorak T, Streeter H. In vitro activity of ramopanin, vancomycin, and teicoplanin against gram-positive clinical isolates from cancer. J Antimicrob Chemother 1996;38:265–269.

46. Rolston KVI, Ho DH, LeBlanc B, Bodey GP. Comparative in vitro activity of new erythromycin derivative dirithromycin against gram-positive bacteria isolated from cancer patients. Eur J Clin Microbiol Infect Dis 1990;1:30–33.

47. Rolston KVI, Ho DH, LeBlanc B, Bodey GP. In vitro activity of PD127,391, a new quinolone against bacterial isolates from cancer patients. Chemotherapy 1990;36:365–372.

48. Rolston KVI, LeFrock JL, Schell RF. Activity of nine antimicrobial agents against Lancefield group C and group G streptococci. Antimicrob Agents Chemother 1982;22:930–932.

49. Rolston KVI, Messer M, Nguyen H, Ho DH, LeBlanc B, Bodey GP. In vitro activity of cefpodoxime against bacterial isolates obtained from patients with cancer. Eur J Clin Microbiol Infect Dis 1991;10:581–585.

50. Rolston KVI, Nguyen H, Messer M. In vitro activity of LY 264826, a new glycopeptide antibiotic, against gram-positive bacteria isolated from patients with cancer. Antimicrob Agents Chemother 1990;34:2137–2141.

51. Rolston KVI, Nguyen H, Messer M. LeBlanc B, Ho DH, Bodey GP. In vitro activity of sparfloxacin against clinical isolates from cancer patients. Antimicrob Agents Chemother 1990;34: 2263–2266.

52. Ruoff KL. Nutritionally variant streptococci. Clin Microbiol Rev 1991;4:184–190.

53. Ruoff KL. Dealing with viridans streptococci in the clinical laboratory: the continuing challenge. Clin Microbiol Newslett 1993;15:73–76.

54. Ruoff KL, Miller SI, Garner CV, Ferraro MJ, Calderwood SB. Bacteremia with *Streptococcus* bovis and *Streptococcus salivarius*: clinical correlates of more accurate identification of isolates. J Clin Microbiol 1989;27:305–308.

55. Salata RA, Lerner PI, Shlaes DM, Gopalakrishna KV, Wolinsky E. Infections due to Lancefield group C streptococci. Medicine 1989;68:225–239.

56. Scheld WM, Sande MA. Endocarditis and intravascular infections. In: Mandell GL, Bennett JE, Dolin R, eds. Principles and practice of infectious Diseases. New York: Churchill Livingstone, 1995:740–783.

57. Stein DS, Nelson KE. Endocarditis due to nutritionally deficient streptococci: therapeutic dilemma. Rev Infect Dis 1987; 908–916.

58. Swenson FJ, Rubin SJ. Clinical significance of viridans streptococci isolated from blood cultures. J Clin Microbiol 1982;15: 725–727.

59. Tan JS, Terhune CAJ, Kaplan S, Hamburger M. Successful two-week treatment schedule for penicillin susceptible streptococcus viridans endocarditis. Lancet 1971;2:1340–1343.

60. Threlkeld MG, Cobbs CG. Infectious disorders of prosthetic valves and intravascular devices. In: Mandell GL, Bennett JE, Dolin R, eds. Principles and practice of infectious diseases. New York: Churchill Livingstone, 1995:783–793.

61. Vartian C, Lerner PI, Shlaes DM, Gopalakrishna KV. Infections due to Lancefield group G streptococci. Medicine 1985;64:75–88.

62. Venditti M, Baiocchi P, Santini C, et al. Antimicrobial susceptibilities of Streptococcus species that cause septicemia in neutropenic patients. Antimicrob Agents Chemother 1989;33: 580–582.

63. Venezio FR, Gullber RM, Westenfelder GO, Phair JP, Cook FV. Group G streptococcal endocarditis and bacteremia. Am J Med 1986;81:29–34.

64. Watanakunakorn C, Burket T. Infective endocarditis at a large community teaching hospital 1980–1990, Medicine 1993; 72:90–102.

65. Wessels MR, Kasper DL. The changing spectrum of group B streptococcal disease. N Engl J Med 1993;328:1843–1844.

66. Whiley RA, Beighton D, Winstanley TG. *Streptococcus intermedius, Streptococcus constellatus,* and *Streptococcus anginosus* (*the Streptococcus milleri group*): associate with different body sites and clinical infections. J Clin Microbiol 1992;30:243–244.

67. Wilcox MH, Winstanley TG, Douglas CWI, Spencer RC. Susceptibility of alpha-haemolytic streptococci causing endocarditis to benzylpenicillin and ten cephalosporins. J Antimicrob Chemother 1993;32:63–69.

68. Wilson WR, Karchmer AW, Dajani AS, et al. Antibiotic treatment of adults with infective endocarditis due to streptococci, enterococci, staphylococci, and HACEK microorganisms. JAMA 1995;274:1706–1713.

Treponema pallidum

●

Lori E. Fantry and Edmund C. Tramont

GENERAL DESCRIPTION

Syphilis has afflicted mankind at least since the discovery of the New World and was one of the first infections to be treated successfully with antibiotics (63), but much remains to be learned about treatment of this devastating disease. The fundamental reason for this lack of knowledge is the need to culture *Treponema pallidum* in laboratory animals instead of routine culture media, which has made it extremely difficult to correlate clinical symptoms with presence or absence of active spirochetes and perform drug susceptibility testing, forcing us to rely on nonspecific serologic tests to gauge the effect of therapy.

However, many characteristics of the organism are well known. Syphilis is caused by a thin, tightly coiled spirochete, *T. pallidum* subspecies *pallidum* (64). It is a member of the family *Spirochaetaceae* and is related to other spirochetes including *Borrelia* and *Leptospira*. Other treponemes that cause disease in man include *T. pallidum* subspecies *pertenue,* the agent associated with yaws; *T. carateum,* the agent associated with pinta; and *T. pallidum* subspecies *endemicum,* the agent associated with nonvenereal or endemic syphilis.

Early studies in rabbits demonstrated that *T. pallidum* in early-stage disease divides every 30 to 33 h and, in later disease, takes even longer to divide (30). It has an outer membrane composed of a phospholipid bilayer with few antigenic proteins. The slow dividing time and the paucity of antigenic proteins allow the organism to evade the host immune response successfully and hence produce not only acute disease but chronic infection that may produce symptoms many years after the initial infection.

The clinical disease itself has been relatively well characterized and is divided into four stages: primary, secondary, latent, and tertiary syphilis (64). Primary syphilis typically is characterized by a painless chancre or ulcer at the site of inoculation. The lesion disappears regardless of treatment, but wide dissemination of the spirochete soon occurs, and signs and symptoms of secondary syphilis are evident. Secondary syphilis is also characterized by cutaneous diseases, but instead of a localized lesion, there is usually a widely disseminated maculopapular rash, which may also be associated with other systemic signs of disease. At this stage the antigen burden is high, and almost all patients test positive in serologic tests for syphilis. Latent syphilis is marked by a period of years in which there are no outward manifestations of disease, but the spirochete remains in the body and serologic tests for syphilis remain positive. Finally, tertiary syphilis occurs in up to 35% of untreated patients, 10 to 25 years after initial infection, with such manifestations as neurologic and cardiovascular signs and symptoms as well as benign granulomatous lesions called gummas.

SUSCEPTIBILITY IN VITRO AND IN VIVO
Single Drug

Early susceptibility testing of various antibiotics against *T. pallidum* was significant not only for the knowledge gained about specific antibiotics but also for generalities of how antibiotics work most effectively. In the rabbit model, Eagle et al. found that higher spirochete loads, associated with later-stage disease, required a longer course of therapy (15). In addition, they demonstrated that lower concentrations of antibiotics could achieve the same cure rates as higher doses if given for longer periods of time (15). Both the higher dose necessary for later-stage disease and lower-dose therapy for prolonged periods have served as basic tenants in our approach to syphilis therapy.

The first antibiotic that *T. pallidum* was shown to be susceptible to was penicillin, in the early 1940s (63). In the rabbit model, penicillin has been shown to be effective in all stages of syphilis (16). Maximal treponemicidal activity occurs with a serum concentration of penicillin of 0.36 µg/mL (15), but a dose as low as 0.002 µg/mL can clear *T. pallidum* from early lesions if given for a long enough time (34). However, viable treponemes may persist in the lymph nodes of rabbits even after early lesions are cleared (30). *T. pallidum* will regenerate if the serum penicillin concentration falls to subinhibitory levels for 18 to 24 h (30). Resistance to penicillin has not yet been found among clinical isolates (64), but there is potential for the acquisition of extrachromosomally mediated antibiotic resistance since at least one strain has been shown to contain plasmid DNA (45).

T. pallidum is also susceptible to other β-lactam antibiotics. Amoxicillin, a semisynthetic oral penicillin, inhibits *T. pallidum* at a concentration of 0.42 µg/mL, comparable to 0.018 µg/mL of penicillin (22). It is also effective in healing syphilis lesions in subcutaneously infected rabbits (46). Ceftriaxone cured early syphilis in animals (35). Ceftizoxime, another third-generation cephalosporin, also cures incubating syphilis

when given to rabbits at doses equivalent to a 1-g dose in humans (34). *T. pallidum* was inhibited by 0.004 µg/mL of ceftizoxime, compared with 0.002 µg/mL of penicillin. Likewise, cefmetazole, a second-generation cephalosporin, is treponemicidal in the rabbit model and eradicates primary syphilis as effectively as penicillin (3). The active form of a new expanded-spectrum oral cephalosporin, cefetamet, killed and lysed *T. pallidum* at a concentration of 0.05 µg/mL in another study (16). Rabbit serum did not diminish its effectiveness. It was more effective in the treatment of experimental syphilis in rabbits prior to the appearance of clinical lesions and after lesions were enlarged than immediately after the lesions became apparent.

Macrolide antibiotics are also able to inhibit *T. pallidum*. Erythromycin, the macrolide most commonly used in clinical practice, was directly compared with penicillin G and clindamycin for the treatment of rabbit skin syphilomas (6). A single injection of penicillin decreased the motile *T. pallidum* count more than 250-fold, whereas single doses of both erythromycin and clindamycin did not decrease the count significantly. Only after multiple injections of erythromycin was the motile treponeme count decrease similar to that with penicillin. Azithromycin, a newer macrolide with the advantage of daily dosing, has activity against *T. pallidum* in vitro (57) and in rabbits (36). Unlike with penicillin, resistance to macrolides has been described. A strain of *T. pallidum* resistant to erythromycin has been isolated (30).

Chloramphenicol also has some activity against *T. pallidum* but has failed to eradicate infection in rabbits (30). Other antibiotics including spectinomycin (48), quinolones (61), and clindamycin (6) have no, or very little, activity against *T. pallidum* in the animal model.

Combination Drugs

To our knowledge, there are no susceptibility data for combination therapy for syphilis.

ANTIMICROBIAL THERAPY

As in many infections, natural immunity can clear *T. pallidum* from the body without any antibiotics (26). On the other hand, in states of severe immunodeficiency, especially with cell-mediated deficits as seen in the acquired immunodeficiency syndrome (AIDS), even the most effective antibiotics will not clear *T. pallidum* (38). Antibiotics augment the immune response and do not replace it. In addition, for antibiotics to have any impact on clearing *T. pallidum,* they need to reach the sites where *T. pallidum* is viable and replicating. In 40% of patients, this occurs in the central nervous system (CNS) as well as the blood (37), and many of the current therapies recommended for syphilis do not penetrate the CNS to any significant degree (13, 14, 40, 49).

Penicillin is the best studied and still the recommended therapy for syphilis (30, 64). However, much debate remains about what dosing schedules and preparations are appropriate for the various stages and types of persons infected with *T. pallidum* (50). The original studies on penicillin treatment were performed before the modern standard of blinded-placebo or comparison controlled, randomized, clinical trials to evaluate the efficacy of therapy. In short, there have been no rigorous studies of penicillin or any other antibiotics to evaluate dose, duration, and preparation of antibiotic to achieve cure with minimal toxicity and cost. Hence, all recommendations for syphilis treatment should be regarded with skepticism. Therapy should be tailored by balancing the benefit a person would receive from a particular therapy with the inconvenience and cost of more elaborate forms of therapy. For this reason our discussion focuses on therapeutic preferences rather than rigorous recommendations.

1993 Centers for Disease Control and Prevention (CDC) Recommendations

The most recent CDC treatment recommendations were published in 1993 (Table 1). These guidelines are based on the notion that different forms of the disease should be treated with different preparations and doses of penicillin. The goal of these recommendations is to provide therapy to large numbers of patients among whom most will be cured with minimal expense, easy administration, and high compliance (30).

The CDC recommends that early syphilis, which includes primary syphilis (the stage immediately after infection, characterized by an ulcer or chancre), secondary syphilis (the later stage corresponding to spirochete dissemination and characterized by rash), and early latent syphilis (the stage up to 1 year after initial infection, when positive results in serologic tests are the only sign of infection), should be treated with one intramuscular injection of 2.4 million units of benzathine penicillin G (8). This is based on animal data showing that the minimal inhibitory concentration that cures primary lesions is easily achieved with this dose of benzathine penicillin (30). However, it does not take into consideration the fact that 40% of patients with early syphilis have CNS infection (37), and

this dose of benzathine penicillin does not penetrate the CNS to any significant degree (13, 14, 40, 49).

The CDC also recommends that patients with late syphilis (which includes latent syphilis of more than 1-year duration and tertiary syphilis, the tissue-destructive phase that appears 10 to 25 years after initial infection in 35% of untreated patients (64)) receive benzathine penicillin if they have no evidence of neurologic disease (Table 1) (8). Therapy is increased to a total dose of 7.2 million units given as 2.4 million units weekly for 3 weeks to account for the possible longer dividing time of the spirochete at this stage of disease (30).

Acknowledging the well-recognized fact the neurosyphilis is the most difficult manifestation to treat, the CDC recommends that persons with neurosyphilis be treated with 2 to 4 million units of aqueous crystalline penicillin G given intravenously every 4 h (12–24 million units daily) for 10 to 14 days. However, the designation "neurosyphilis" is vague and ill defined. Patients with typical neurologic symptoms associated with syphilis and a reactive cerebrospinal fluid (CSF) in Venereal Disease Research Laboratory (VDRL) tests are easiest to classify as having neurosyphilis, but most patients have either no symptoms or ill-defined symptoms, and many have nonspecific CSF abnormalities. Some 40% of patients with early syphilis have *T. pallidum* infection in the CNS (37), but lumbar puncture is rarely performed in asymptomatic patients with early syphilis. In fact, the CDC discourages lumbar puncture at this stage unless a patient has optic, auditory, cranial nerve, or meningeal symptoms (8). The rationale is that early invasion of the CNS by *T. pallidum* is usually insignificant and does not predict failure with benzathine penicillin.

The CDC's failure to recommend lumbar puncture in early disease may have some validity—not because CNS infection is insignificant and not worth considering in treatment decisions, but because lumbar puncture may yield little meaning-

---

TABLE 1 • CDC Guidelines for Syphilis Treatment

Stage	Patients Not Allergic to Penicillin	Allergic to Penicillin
Primary, secondary, and early latent; for early syphilis, serum concentrations must exceed 0.018 µg/mL (0.03 unit/mL) for 7–10 days	Adults: benzathine penicillin G 2.4 million units i.m. once Children: benzathine penicillin G 50,00 units/kg i.m. up to adult dose of 2.4 million units once	Nonpregnant: doxycycline 100 mg p.o. b.i.d. or tetracycline 500 mg p.o. b.i.d. × 14 days; if intolerant to doxycyline or tetracycline, then erythromycin 500 mg p.o. q.i.d. Pregnant: desensitize and then treat with penicillin
Late latent, tertiary, or syphilis of unknown duration (except neurosyphilis)	Adults: benzathine penicillin 2.4 million units × 3 administered 1 week apart for a total of 7.2 million units Children: benzathine penicillin G 50,000 units/kg administered as for adults for a total of 150,000 units/kg, not to exceed 7.2 million units	Nonpregnant; doxycycline 100 mg b.i.d. or tetracycline 500 mg q.i.d. × 28 days Pregnant: desensitize and then treat with penicillin
Neurosyphilis	Adults: penicillin G 2–4 million units i.v. every 4 h for a total of 12–24 million units/day or penicillin G procaine 2–4 million units i.m. per day plus probenicid 500 mg p.o. q.i.d. for 10–14 days	Desensitize and then treat with penicillin

ful information. A CSF white blood cell count of 6 cells or more, a protein concentration of 46 mg/dL or above, and a glucose level of 45 mg/dL or less all suggest syphilis, and a positive CSF-VDRL allegedly establishes the diagnosis (12, 37). The true "gold standard" is *T. pallidum* culture of CSF fluid in animals, but this is too expensive and labor intensive to be done in routine clinical care.

The problems with the laboratory tests currently used to diagnose and follow neurosyphilis were dramatically illustrated in the 1988 study by Lukehart et al. In this study, 4 of 12 patients (33%) with *T. pallidum* isolated from the CSF had normal cellular and protein studies, as well as a nonreactive CSF-VDRL, suggesting low sensitivity for all of these tests, even in combination (37). In addition, there was a significant number of patients in whom *T. pallidum* was not isolated from the CSF despite the fact that there were CSF abnormalities, including four patients with reactive VDRLs (37). This suggests another weakness in routine CSF studies, namely, they are not particularly specific. VDRL titers above 1:32 appeared to be the most specific of these tests and was most common in secondary syphilis.

CDC recommendations for congenital syphilis are discussed below as they are similar to our therapeutic preferences.

Therapeutic Preferences

Although benzathine penicillin is effective therapy for most persons with syphilis, we are concerned about the multiple reports of failure, especially in patients infected with the human immunodeficiency virus (HIV). It has long been known that benzathine or low-dose aqueous or procaine penicillin is not 100% successful in preventing long-term sequelae associated with syphilis. Retreatment is necessary in 5 to 10% of patients with primary or secondary syphilis treated with benzathine or low-dose aqueous, procaine penicillin (7, 50, 54, 55). Although some researchers have attributed all patients requiring retreatment to reinfection (17, 18), most experts are convinced that about half of those requiring retreatment are due to failure of initial therapy (54).

The most likely reason for treatment failures is that at least 40% of patients with early syphilis are infected with *T. pallidum* in the CNS (37), a site poorly penetrated by benzathine penicillin (13, 14, 40, 49). In most cases of syphilis, CNS infection and poor penetration of penicillin is inconsequential, since a host with an intact cell-mediated immune response can clear the infection before any neurologic damage occurs. The T cell arm of the immune system effectively clears infection in conjunction with penicillin therapy, even with inadequate penetration into the CNS. However, clearance of *T. pallidum* before neurologic damage occurs is not universal. This was first clearly demonstrated in 1976 when *T. pallidum* was isolated from the CSF despite retreatment with what was considered adequate doses of penicillin (19). Older reports also support this finding but lack some credibility since *T. cuniculi*, a treponema species found in rabbits, could not be ruled out (19). Later reports also suggest that neurologic disease can occur despite treatment with benzathine penicillin in early-stage disease in both presumably non-HIV-infected patients (30) and HIV-infected patients (5, 33, 37, 43).

Our preferred therapy for any form of syphilis in any type of patient is 2–4 million units of aqueous crystalline penicillin G given intravenously every 4 h (12–24 million units daily) for 10 to 14 days (Table 2). If outpatient treatment is desired, then 2.4 million units of aqueous procaine penicillin G can be given intramuscularly daily with probenecid (500 mg orally four times per day for 10 to 14 days).

Between 5 and 24 million units of intravenous penicillin G consistently achieved treponemicidal levels in the CSF (40, 49). Hence it would seem logical that treatment failures would be less common than with regimens that failed to penetrate the CSF to any appreciable degree. Indeed, clinical failures appear to be less common with this regimen than with benzathine penicillin, the therapy previously recommended for all stages of disease, including neurosyphilis (42). Treponemicidal levels of penicillin have not been achieved as reliably with procaine penicillin (14, 68), but supplementation with probenecid, a drug that inhibits renal excretion of natural and semisynthetic penicillins,

---

TABLE 2 • Therapeutic Preferences			
Drug and Route	**Dose**	**CSF Levels**	**Order of Preference**[a]
Aqueous penicillin G i.v.	2–4 million units q. 4–6 h for 7–10 days	Adequate	First choice
Procaine penicillin G i.m. (and probenecid)	2.4 million units q.d. for 7–10 days	Adequate	First choice
Amoxicillin p.o. (and probenecid)	3 g b.i.d. for 7–10 days	Probably adequate	Second choice
Ceftriaxone i.v.	1 g q.d. for 7–10 days	Adequate	Second choice
Doxycycline p.o.	100 mg b.i.d. for 21 days	Probably adequate	Third choice[b]
Benzathine penicillin i.m.	2.4 million units weekly for 1–3 weeks	Inadequate	Fourth choice[c]
Chloramphenicol i.v. or p.o.	500–750 mg p.o. or i.v. q.i.d. for 30 days	Excellent	Only possible indication is refractory eye disease

[a] Treatment of exposed persons is not included in this table since in many cases it is prevention rather than treatment of active disease (see text for further discussion).

[b] Not acceptable in pregnancy, congenital syphilis, or symptomatic neurosyphilis.

[c] Not acceptable in any form of neurosyphilis.

achieves treponemicidal levels (14). Since this therapy avoids the need for frequent dosing and thus hospitalization, we recommend it as an alternative in compliant patients when hospitalization is not desired by the health care provider or patient.

Both of these regimens can be used in adults with any type of syphilis. However, in neurosyphilis, even these regimens may fail (67), especially in HIV-infected patients (43), and neurologic deficits other than those associated with syphilitic meningitis and meningovascular syphilis are rarely reversed (30).

Therapeutic Alternatives

Our first alternative to penicillin is the semisynthetic penicillin amoxicillin (3.0 g orally twice a day) with probenecid (1.0 g) for 10 to 14 days (Table 2). This regimen has been used less commonly in clinical trials, and hence there is less data regarding its efficacy or lack of efficacy than for penicillin regimens. We consider it one of the better alternatives to intravenous or intramuscular penicillin since it probably achieves sufficient CSF penetration and has the convenience of oral dosing. As mentioned above, amoxicillin is treponemicidal in vitro and in the rabbit model (22). When 2 g of amoxicillin is administered to fasting adults with probenecid, a mean serum concentration of 4 μg/mL (22) can be achieved after 8 h (22). Trough serum levels in patients treated with 6 g/day given either every 4 or 8 h were 0.5 and 0.32 μg/mL, respectively. In one study, 30 patients with primary and secondary syphilis were treated with amoxicillin (1 g/day) with no failures in the 2-year follow-up period (22). In a more recent study, treatment with amoxicillin and probenecid achieved results similar to those with penicillin G benzathine (51).

Some data indicate that first- and third-generation cephalosporins, particularly ceftriaxone, are effective in treating syphilis. Ceftriaxone is recommended for treatment of early disease and neurosyphilis by some authorities (1, 8). We recommend it as second-choice therapy for any patient with syphilis (Table 2). This drug is particularly attractive since serum and CSF levels exceeding those needed to kill *T. pallidum* are easily obtained with standard dosing (34). In small numbers of patients, it has been used successfully to treat incubating (31), primary (31, 41, 53), secondary (31, 53), and latent syphilis (12). However, some data show that ceftriaxone is not as effective in HIV-infected patients with latent syphilis or neurosyphilis (12). Dowell et al. found a 20% failure rate, similar to that with benzathine penicillin, and one patient even developed symptomatic neurosyphilis when 1 to 2 g of ceftriaxone was given for 10 to 14 days.

We consider doxycycline (100 mg twice daily for 21 days) to be another effective alternative for treatment of the non-HIV-infected adult with syphilis. We are less likely to recommend this therapy to an HIV-infected adult because it is only bacteriostatic and not bacteriocidal (64). Furthermore, tetracycline and doxycycline should not be given to pregnant women and children under 8 because of potential damage to developing bones and teeth (58). Since tetracycline and doxycycline have similar spectrums of antibacterial activity, most data supporting doxycycline have been extrapolated from previous trials with tetracycline, a drug we are less inclined to recommend because

of its poor CSF penetration. Patients treated with 24 to 32 g of tetracycline for 10 to 12 days have had serologic and symptomatic responses similar to those with penicillin (17, 18, 54). One series reported a failure rate at 12 months below 4%, similar to that obtained with penicillin therapy (54). However, one small prospective observational study showed that doxycycline (100 mg twice daily for 28 days) resulted in 100, 90, 68, and 90% success rates in treating primary, early, late, and congenital syphilis, respectively, in adults (47).

Other regimens that are less desirable because of poor CSF penetration include benzathine penicillin, as discussed above, and macrolides. Despite a failure rate of only 4% at 6 months when erythromycin was used to treat early syphilis, we do not recommend this therapy because follow-up at 18 months revealed a failure rate of 14%, and this was using doses higher than that currently recommended by the CDC (54). Another macrolide, azithromycin, was shown to be effective in at least two series of patients with syphilis. In one nonrandomized study, non-HIV-infected patients with primary or secondary syphilis were treated with azithromycin (500 mg/day), with cure in 11 of 13 patients for at least 3 months (65). In another study, 100 patients with syphilis were treated with azithromycin (500 mg/day), erythromycin, or penicillin for 10 days (39). Those treated with azithromycin showed more rapid resolution both clinically and serologically, with no evidence of chronic sequelae. However, like erythromycin, azithromycin does not achieve therapeutic levels in the CSF (59), and we do not routinely recommend this therapy unless there are no other alternatives.

Chloramphenicol (2 g/day for 30 days) is another "last-resort" alternative that can be used for treatment of neurosyphilis but should not be used routinely because some animal data suggest it is less effective than other choices (64).

Special Situations

Congenital Syphilis

All infants of mothers with positive syphilis serologic test results, regardless of treatment history, should be fully evaluated for evidence of syphilis (8). These infants should be treated for congenital syphilis if they have any evidence of active disease by physical examination or x-ray, a reactive CSF-VDRL, more than 5 white blood cells/m³ or 50 mg/dL of protein in the CSF, quantitative nontreponemal serologic titers that are four times the mother's or more, or test positive for fluorescent treponemal antibody–absorbed (FTA-ABS)-19S-IgM antibody. Careful follow-up is mandatory. Since newborns often have elevated white blood cell counts, it is often impossible to rule out neurosyphilis, and these infants should be treated presumptively.

For newborns, treatment is 50,000 units/kg of aqueous crystalline penicillin G intravenously every 8 to 12 h for a total of 100,000 to 150,000 units/kg/day for 10 to 14 days. For older infants, it is usually administered every 4 to 6 h. The alternative regimen is 50,000 units/kg of procaine penicillin intramuscularly daily for 10 to 14 days. If treatment is interrupted for more than 24 h, then the full course of therapy is restarted. Children diagnosed beyond the newborn period should be treated for CNS involvement regardless of lumbar puncture results.

Otic Syphilis

Syphilitic involvement of the eye should be treated with penicillin G (12 to 24 million units/day for 10–14 days) regardless of CSF findings (10). However, regardless of dose or preparation, penicillin does not easily achieve adequate levels in the anterior chamber of the eye (64). A newborn with congenital syphilis receiving penicillin G potassium (50,000 units/kg body weight intramuscularly at 12-h intervals for 17 days after birth) had *T. pallidum* in both the aqueous humor and ground eye tissue at autopsy (26). Hence it may be prudent to consider chloramphenicol and cephalothin, antibiotics that do achieve adequate levels in the anterior chamber of the eye, as possible first-line agents (64).

Otosyphilis

Penicillin does not easily penetrate the labyrinth of the inner ear (64). Hence we recommend a more intensive course of therapy for disease involving this site. Patients are usually treated with a prolonged course of penicillin for 6 weeks to 3 months with addition of steroids (9, 11, 69). Steroids have been used both intravenously and orally, but we recommend oral prednisone 30 to 60 mg daily or every other day for 14 days, followed by a taper as tolerated by the patient (69).

HIV-Infected Patients

More-florid clinical manifestations, including symptomatic neurosyphilis early in the course of syphilis, have been well documented in persons coinfected with HIV (5, 33). In addition, multiple case reports suggest that HIV-infected patients are more likely to fail syphilis therapy than non-HIV-infected patients. HIV-infected patients with early syphilis have been reported who failed treatment with benzathine penicillin G (5, 33, 37, 44). Lukehart et al. found that *T. pallidum* could be cultured from three of three HIV-infected patients evaluated after single-dose benzathine penicillin therapy for early syphilis but could not be cultured in the only patient without HIV infection (37). In addition, retrospective chart reviews have documented treatment failures of 20% in HIV-infected patients (12, 38), significantly higher than the 5 to 10% retreatment rate reported prior to the AIDS era. Furthermore, unlike many treatment failures in immunocompetent hosts, these failures are more likely to be associated with clinical disease, especially neurosyphilis (12, 38).

The more-florid clinical manifestations and higher frequency of treatment failures are most likely due to immune dysfunction coincident with HIV that results in a significantly higher spirochete load. There is a greater likelihood that spirochetes will remain active in sequestered sites. Hence, in HIV-infected patients, we recommend only therapy that penetrates the CNS, such as high-dose penicillin or amoxicillin with probenecid, for at least 10 days.

Jarisch-Herxheimer Reaction

Treatment for syphilis is not totally benign. Along with the discomfort of intramuscular or intravenous therapy and the possibility of a drug reaction, an acute febrile response to therapy is seen in 10 to 25% of all patients and 70 to 90% of patients with secondary syphilis (64). It is rarely seen in latent syphilis and occurs to varying extents in the various forms of tertiary syphilis (52). This response, the Jarisch-Herxheimer reaction, is most commonly associated with penicillin therapy but has also been associated with other antibiotics used to treat syphilis (2). It has been correlated with the release of heat-stable pyrogens from *T. pallidum* and is seen with treatment of other spirochete infections as well (64). The clinical course is marked by abrupt onset of symptoms usually within 2 h, occasionally 24 h, after initiation of therapy (8, 64). Besides fever, clinical signs and symptoms may include chills, headache, nausea, vomiting, myalgias, tachycardia, hyperventilation, mild hypotension, vasodilation with flushing, and exacerbation and new onset of skin lesions (52). It lasts 12 to 24 h and is generally safe and self-limited (64). The exceptions are during the second half of pregnancy, when there is risk of premature labor and fetal distress (8), and during cardiovascular syphilis and neurosyphilis, when reactions are more severe and can be life threatening (64). Acetaminophen or aspirin can be used for symptomatic relief. In severe cases or those associated with cardiovascular syphilis or neurosyphilis, prednisone 60 mg often leads to prompt and dramatic decrease in fever (64).

Penicillin Desensitization

Since penicillin is the optimal therapy for syphilis, penicillin is recommended even in patients with penicillin allergies, except in those with a history of Stevens-Johnson syndrome, when the delay associated with retreatment may be harmful, and alternatives are limited. These situations include syphilis in pregnant women, infants with congenital syphilis, and adults with symptomatic neurosyphilis, since treatment must be effective as soon as possible to prevent irreversible neurologic disease. In addition, in syphilis in pregnancy and congenital syphilis, toxicity associated with the tetracyclines make this option undesirable not only in terms of possible treatment failures but also in terms of damage to bone and teeth development (58).

Anaphylactic reactions to penicillin are the principle toxicity associated with this antibiotic; they occur uncommonly, in at most 40 of 1000 treatment courses (66). In addition, the vast majority of patients who report a history of penicillin allergy do not have an allergic reaction upon rechallenge. The most reliable method of distinguishing those who will have a future reaction from those who will not is skin testing. Patients should be instructed not to take antihistamines, tricyclic antidepressants, and adrenergic drugs within a time interval appropriate for the corresponding half-life of the medication (66). For example, chlorpheniramine maleate or terfenadine should not be taken within 24 h, diphenhydramine HCL or hydroxyzine within 4 days, and astemizole within 3 weeks (8). Testing is begun by injecting skin test reagents, including negative diluent and positive histamine controls, in the epidermis on the volar surface of the forearm with a 26-gauge needle without drawing blood (66). If there is no reaction, then the same reagents are injected intradermally; if the diameter of induration exceeds 5 mm after 15 min, the result is positive.

Optimally, skin testing should include diluents with both the major and minor determinants of penicillin (66). If the skin test is negative, then there is no risk of anaphylaxis, but 1 to 3% of patients develop a mild cutaneous reaction. If the skin test is positive, then desensitization should be carried out prior to treatment, since there is a 50 to 70% risk of an acute reaction. Because minor determinants of penicillin are not commercially available in the United States, skin testing is often done with the major determinants only. In this case, if the result is negative, patients should still receive gradually increased doses of penicillin in a monitored setting, since there is still at least a 3% risk of a reaction (4).

Although desensitization can be done both orally and intravenously, oral desensitization is probably safer and certainly less expensive and easier (66). It should be performed in an intensive care setting with continuous electrocardiogram monitoring. Doses of penicillin should be gradually increased until the dose required for therapy is achieved. One-third of patients develop a transient allergic reaction during desensitization, but it is usually mild and self-limited. If mild symptoms occur, then the dose of penicillin should be stabilized until there are no signs or symptoms. If it is more severe, such as hypotension, laryngeal edema, or asthma, then the dose should be reduced at least tenfold. There should be no interruption between desensitization and treatment since the risk of an allergic reaction increases as the time from desensitization increases.

ENDPOINTS FOR MONITORING THERAPY
Non-HIV-Infected Patients

As in any disease, the primary endpoint of therapy is clinical, and a careful medical history and physical examination will determine if therapy has been successful. In primary syphilis, the patient should be examined for resolution of the chancre; in secondary syphilis, for resolution of the rash and any of the other protean disease manifestations that the patient may experience; and in early neurosyphilis, for resolution of signs and symptoms of neurologic disease. In late neurosyphilis, there is usually no reversal of signs and symptoms that are present prior to therapy, but patients should be monitored carefully for further progression of disease. During any stage of syphilis and at any time, if clinical disease persists or recurs, the patient should be retreated. He or she should also be questioned about the possibility of reinfection to ease the concern about antibiotic resistance.

However, since the disease process is clinically silent at many stages and we are unable to grow *T. pallidum* in routine culture, it is necessary to follow disease activity with surrogate markers of infection. Treponemal antibody tests, such as the FTA-ABS, the microhemagglutination assay for antibody to *T. pallidum* (MHA-TP), the *T. pallidum* hemagglutinin assay (TPH), and the treponemal immobilization test (TPI) are essential for diagnosis but are not helpful for measuring response to therapy since they are not quantified, usually remain positive for life, and do not correlate with disease activity (56). In contrast, nontreponemal or reaginic antibody tests, the rapid-plasma-reagin (RPR) and VDRL, are quantified, revert to negative in the vast majority of patients given effective therapy,

and do correlate with disease activity. The antibodies measured by these tests are IgG and IgM immunoglobulins directed against an antigen which is from *T. pallidum* itself and/or the result of an interaction between host tissues and *T. pallidum* (64). The VDRL slide test involves heating serum to 56°C and testing for its ability to flocculate a suspension of cardiolipin-cholesterol-lecithin antigen. The RPR is just a modification of this procedure.

Both the VDRL and RPR become positive shortly after initial infection, peak during the secondary or early latent stage, and then begin to decline with time (27). Without therapy, 25% of patients eventually are nonreactive in VDRL tests (27). With therapy, the vast majority of patients change from reactive to nonreactive. Fiumara found that all 196 patients with primary syphilis had nonreactive RPR titers at 1 year (17) and all 204 patients with secondary syphilis by 2 years (18). However, later studies showed that low but positive-titer VDRL or RPR results of 1:16 or less may persist despite no other evidence of treatment failure (54). In addition, Fiumara found that only 44% of 275 patients treated for late latent syphilis became seronegative (19). In another series, all patients had primary syphilis resolve both clinically and serologically, but only 55% of patients with secondary syphilis did (42).

The rate of decline in nontreponemal titers appears to be related to stage of disease, height of initial titers, and prior history of syphilis. Brown et al. found a fourfold decrease in RPR titers at 6 months and an eightfold decrease at 12 months in successfully treated patients with primary and secondary syphilis, but there was a slower decline in patients with early latent disease (7). Researchers have also found that longer duration of symptoms within a given stage is associated with slower declines in titers (7, 17, 18, 19). This is reflected in the finding that these patients have higher initial titers and that higher titers are also associated with a slower decline. In addition, patients with no prior history of syphilis have a more rapid decline in titers (7, 17, 18, 21).

Since VDRL titers are often slightly lower than RPR titers and there is significant variation in values between laboratories, results from either an RPR or VDRL test, not both, should be obtained from the same laboratory each time to monitor therapy (8). A fourfold change in titers, equivalent to a two-dilution change, is considered significant and implies a change in disease activity. For example, a change from 1:64 to 1:8 is significant, while a change from 1:64 to 1:32 is not. The frequency of serologic testing after treatment depends on the stage of disease and characteristics of the patients. Non-HIV-infected adults with syphilis should be tested at 3, 6, and 12 months (64). If syphilis lasts longer than 1 year or is of unknown duration, then serologic tests should also be run at 24 months. Infants with congenital syphilis should be checked serologically every 2 to 3 months, and those without congenital syphilis but born to infected mothers should be checked even more frequently, at 1, 2, 3, 6, and 12 months (8). In addition, pregnant women should have monthly serologic checks (8).

In most patients with syphilis, titers should decline fourfold by 3 months. When titers do not decline fourfold by 3 months in primary or secondary syphilis or by 6 months in early latent syphilis or there is a fourfold increase in titers at any evaluation, then patients should have a CSF examination and be retreated. In congenital syphilis and in infants who are seropositive only because of passive transfer of maternal antibodies and not infection, titers should decline by 3 months of age and should be nonreactive by 6 months of age. Titer, however, may decline more slowly if treatment is not initiated in the neonatal period. Occasionally, titers are still positive up to 1 year after birth. If these titers are found to be stable or increasing or are still present after 1 year of age, the child should be reevaluated fully, including a CSF examination, and retreated.

Besides a serum nontreponemal test, a lumbar puncture is recommended every 6 months after treatment for neurosyphilis, including infants with abnormal CSF analyses, until the pleocytosis has resolved or CNS nontreponemal antibodies disappear (64). Pleocytosis usually resolves before CSF protein declines, and CSF-VDRL tests may remain reactive for more than 1 year (30). If the white blood cell count is not decreased by 6 months or remains abnormal 2 years after therapy, retreatment is indicated (8). In addition, an infant who still has a positive CSF-VDRL result at 6 months of age should be retreated.

The polymerase chain reaction (PCR) test could potentially become the principle endpoint marker of disease if and when markers of active replication or viable spirochetes are validated (24).

HIV-Infected Patients

Most data indicate that HIV-infected patients do not have the same nontreponemal serologic response (VDRL and RPR) to treatment as non-HIV-infected patients. Although one small study found that HIV-infected drug users and non-HIV-infected injecting drug users (23) had similar responses to therapy, most other data suggest that nontreponemal serologic tests (VDRL and RPR) in HIV-infected patients tend to show higher nontreponemal antibody titers in secondary syphilis (32), increased rates of false-positive nontreponemal antibody titers (30), and a slower response and greater likelihood of having persistently reactive nontreponemal titers after treatment (67). A retrospective review of serologic response to therapy in patients with primary and secondary syphilis showed that HIV-infected patients with primary syphilis, but not secondary syphilis, were less likely to have a fourfold decrease in titers within 6 months than matched non-HIV-infected patients (60). Yinnon et al. found that 49 of 104 patients with all stages of disease did not have the expected fourfold decrease in titers at 6 months (67).

Other studies have shown that specific treponemal tests (FTA-ABS and MHA-TP) more often become nonreactive in HIV-infected patients than in non-HIV-infected patients, and this loss of reactivity is associated with lower T-helper lymphocyte counts (25). Of the 52 that were HIV-infected, the percentage was even higher (56%).

Whether this abnormal response to therapy is related to a true change in disease activity or represents an abnormality in immunoglobulin production remains to be determined. One would expect that HIV infection and the resultant loss of effective T-cell function would result in less ability to clear the spirochete. However, it is also possible that some of the so-called treatment failures are only a manifestation of the increased polyclonal B-cell activation found in HIV infection resulting in heighten titers of nontreponemal antibodies that fail to revert to a nonreactive pattern similar to that found in non-HIV-infected persons (60).

PROPHYLAXIS

The most effective prophylaxis against syphilis is avoiding sexual contact with persons who harbor the spirochete. Condom use during sexual intercourse can also be inferred to be protective from studies of HIV infection. Currently, prophylactic drugs are not recommended for any group of patients with syphilis except those who have been exposed to a person with syphilis, and in this population, it is unclear whether medicines prevent infection or treat very early disease—"incubating" syphilis.

We recommend that persons sexually exposed to primary, secondary, or latent syphilis of less than 1-year's duration within the previous 90 days be treated for syphilis even if they are serologically negative for syphilis. Since data suggest that therapy is most successful when initiated early and the treponemal burden is relatively low (30), this is the one instance in which treatment with 2.4 million units of benzathine penicillin is acceptable. Transmission occurs only when mucocutaneous lesions are present, usually within 1 year after initial infection (64), so contact with persons with syphilis of more than 1-year's duration is not an immediate indication for treatment (8). Instead, it is recommended that these persons be followed clinically and serologically for syphilis. Persons exposed more than 90 days prior to evaluation need not have immediate treatment, unless they are serologically positive or results will be delayed and follow-up is uncertain, because serologic tests are positive 3 months after exposure.

CONTROVERSIES, CAVEATS, AND COMMENTS

Many challenges remain in our understanding, treatment, and prevention of syphilis. Much of the challenge involves new technologies for determining the viability of *T. pallidum* and the correlate of protective immunity. Then it will be only a matter of time before we have tools to monitor treatment, better therapies, and a vaccine for prevention.

REFERENCES

1. Abramowicz M. The medical letter on drugs and therapeutics. Handbook of antimicrobial therapy. New York: The Medical Letter, 1996.
2. Anderson J, Mindel A, Tovey SJ, Williams P. Primary and secondary syphilis, 20 years experience. 3: Diagnosis, treatment, and follow up. Genitourin Med 1989;65:239–243.
3. Baker-Zander SA, Lukehart SA. Efficacy of cefmetazole in the treatment of active syphilis in the rabbit model. Antimicrob Agents Chemother 1989;33:1465–1469.
4. Beall GN. Penicillins. In: Saxon A, moderator. Immediate hypersensitivity reactions to beta-latam antibiotics. Ann Intern Med 1987;107:204–215.
5. Berry CD, Hooton TM, Collier AC, Lukehart SA. Neurological

relapse after benzathine penicillin therapy for secondary syphilis in a patient with HIV infection. N Engl J Med 1987;316:1587–1589.

6. Brause BD, Borges JS, Roberts RB. Relative efficacy of clindamycin, erythromycin, and penicillin in treatment of *Treponema pallidum* in skin syphilomas of rabbits. J Infect Dis 1976; 134:93–96.

7. Brown ST, Zaidi A, Larsen SA, Reynolds GH. Serological response to syphilis treatment: a new analysis of old data. JAMA 1985;253:1296–1299.

8. Centers for Disease Control and Prevention. 1993 Sexually transmitted diseases guidelines. MMWR 1993;42(no. rr-14):1–102.

9. Chan YM, Adams A, Ker AG. Syphilitic labyrinthitis—an update. J Laryngol Otol 1995;109:719–725.

10. Deschenes J, Seamone CD, Baines MG. Acquired ocular syphilis: diagnosis and treatment. Ann Ophthalmol 1992;24: 134–138.

11. Dobbin JM, Perkins. Otosyphilis and hearing loss: response to penicillin and steroid therapy. Laryngoscope 1983;93:1540–1542.

12. Dowell ME, Ross PG, Musher DM, Cate TR, Baughn RE. Response of latent syphilis or neurosyphilis to ceftriaxone therapy in persons infected with human immunodeficiency virus. Am J Med 1992;93:481–488.

13. Ducas J, Robson HG. Cerebrospinal fluid levels during therapy for latent syphilis. JAMA 1981;246:2583–4.

14. Dunlop EMC, Al-Egaily SS, Houang MB. Penicillin levels in blood and CSF achieved by treatment of syphilis. JAMA 1979;241:2538–2540.

15. Eagle H, Fleischman R, Magnusson AJ. The effective concentrations of penicillin in vitro and in vivo for streptococci, pneumococci, and *Treponema pallidum*. J Bacteriol 1950;59:625–643.

16. Fitzgerald TJ. Effects of cefetamet (Ro 15–8074) on *Treponema pallidum* and experimental syphilis. Antimicrob Agents Chemother 1992;36:598–602.

17. Fiumara NJ. Treatment of seropositive primary syphilis: an evaluation of 196 patients. Sex Transm Dis 1977;4:92–95.

18. Fiumara NJ. Treatment of secondary syphilis: an evaluation of 204 patients. Sex Transm Dis 1977;4:96–99.

19. Fiumara NJ. Serological responses to treatment of 128 patients with late latent syphilis. Sex Transm Dis 1979;6:243–246.

20. Fiumara NJ. Reinfection primary, secondary, and latent syphilis: the serological response after treatment. Sex Transm Dis 1980;7:111–115.

21. Fiumara NJ. Treatment of primary and secondary syphilis. Serological response. JAMA 1980;243:2500–2502.

22. Goldmeier D, Hay P. A review and update on adult syphilis, with particular reference to its treatment. Int J STD AIDS 1993;4:70–82.

23. Gourevitch MN, Selwyn PA, Davenny K, Buono D, Schoenbaum EE, Klein RS, Friedland, GH. Effects of HIV infection on the serological manifestations and response to treatment of syphilis in intravenous drug users. Ann Intern Med 1993;118: 350–355.

24. Grimprel E, Sanchez PJ, Wendel GD, Burstain JM, McCracken GH, Radolf JD, Norgard MV. Use of polymerase chain reaction and rabbit infectivity testing to detect *Treponema pallidum* in amniotic fluid, fetal and neonatal sera, and cerebrospinal fluid. J Clin Microbiol 1991;29:1711–1718.

25. Haas JS, Bolan G, Larsen SA, Clement MJ, Bacchetti P, Moss AR. Sensitivity of treponemal tests for detecting prior treated syphilis during human immunodeficiency virus infection. J Infect Dis 1990;162:862–866.

26. Hardy JB, Hardy PH, Oppenheimer EH, Ryan SJ, Sheff RN. Failure of penicillin in a newborn with congenital syphilis. JAMA 1970;212:1345–1349.

27. Hart G. Syphilis tests in diagnostic and therapeutic decision making. Ann Intern Med 1986;104:368–376.

28. Hashisaki P, Wertzberger GG, Conrad GL, Nichols CR. Erythromycin failure in the treatment of syphilis in a pregnant woman. Sex Transm Dis 1983;10:36–38.

29. Hook EW III, Baker-Zander SA, Moskovitz BL, Lukehart SA, Handsfield HH. Ceftriaxone therapy for asymptomatic neurosyphilis—case report and western blot analysis of serum and cerebrospinal fluid IgG response to therapy. Sex Transm Dis 1986;13:185–188.

30. Hook EW, Marra CM. Acquired syphilis in adults. N Engl J Med 1992;326:1060–1069.

31. Hook EW III, Roddy RE, Handsfield HH. Ceftriaxone for incubating and early syphilis. J Infect Dis 1988;158:881–884.

32. Hutchinson CM, Hook EW, Shepard M, Verley J, Rompalo AM. Altered clinical presentation of early syphilis in patients with human immunodeficiency virus infection. Ann Intern Med 1994;121:94–99.

33. Johns DR, Tierney M, Felsenstein D. Alteration in the natural history of neurosyphilis by concurrent infection with the human immunodeficiency virus. N Engl J Med 1987;316:1569–1572.

34. Korting HC, Haag R, Walter D, Riethmuller U, Meurer M. Efficacy of ceftizoxime in the treatment of incubating syphilis in rabbits. Chemotherapy 1993;39:331–335.

35. Korting HC, Walther D, Riethmuller U, Meurer M. Comparative in vitro susceptibility of *Treponema pallidum* to ceftizoxime, ceftriaxone, and penicillin G. Chemotherapy 1986;32:352–355.

36. Lukehart SA, Fohn MJ, Baker-Zander SA. Efficacy of azithromycin for therapy of active syphilis in the rabbit model. J Antimicrob Chemother 1990;25(Suppl A):91–99.

37. Lukehart SA, Hook EW III, Baker-Zander SA, Collier AC, Critchlow CW, Handsfield HH. Invasion of the central nervous system by *Treponema pallidum*: implications for diagnosis and treatment. Ann Intern Med 1988;109:855–862.

38. Malone JL, Wallace MR, Hendrick BB, LaRocco A Jr, Tonon E, Brodine SK, Bowler WA, Lavin BS, Hawkins RE, Oldfield EC 3rd. Syphilis and neurosyphilis in a human immunodeficiency virus type-1 seropositive population: evidence for frequent serologic relapse after therapy. Am J Med 1995;99:55–63.

39. Mashkilleyson AL, Gomberg MA, Mashkilleyson N, Kutin SA. Treatment of syphilis with azithromycin. Int J Sex Transm Dis AIDS 1996;7(Suppl 1):13–15.

40. Mohr JA, Griffiths W, Jackson R, Saadah H, Bird P, Riddle J. Neurosyphilis and penicillin levels in cerebrospinal fluid. N Engl J Med 1976;316:1569–1572.

41. Moorthy TT, Lee C-T, Lim K-B, Tan T. Ceftriaxone for treatment of primary syphilis in men: a preliminary study. Sex Transm Dis 1987;14:116–118.

42. Musher DM. How much penicillin cures early syphilis. Ann Intern Med 1988;109:849–851.

43. Musher DM, Baughan RE. Neurosyphilis in HIV-infected persons. N Engl J Med 1994;1516–1517.

44. Musher DM, Hamill RJ, Baughn RE. Effect of human immunodeficiency virus (HIV) infection on the course of syphilis and on the response to treatment. Ann Intern Med 1990;113: 872–881.

45. Norgard MV, Miller JN. Plasmid DNA in *Treponema pallidum* (Nichols): potential for antibiotic resistance by syphilis bacteria. Science 1981;213:553–555.

46. Onoda Y. Clinical evaluation of amoxycillin in the treatment of syphilis. J Int Med Res 1979a;7:539–545.

47. Onoda Y. Therapeutic effect of oral doxycycline on syphilis. Br J Vener Dis 1979;55:110–115.

48. Peterman TA, Zaidi AA, Lieb S, Wroten JE. Incubating syphilis in patients treated for gonorrhea: a comparison of treatment regimens. J Infect Dis 1994;170:689–692.

49. Polnikorn N, Witoonpanih W, Vorachit M, Vejjajiva S, Vejjajiva A. Penicillin concentrations in cerebrospinal fluid after different treatment regimens for syphilis. Br J Vener Dis 1980;56:363–367.

50. Rolfs RT. Treatment of syphilis, 1995. Clin Infect Dis 1995;20(Suppl 1):S23–38.

51. Rolfs RT, Joesoef MR, Hendershot EF, Rompalo AM, Augenbraun MH, Chiu M, Bolan G, Johnson SC, French P, Steen E, Radolf JD, Larsen S. A randomized trial of enhanced therapy for early syphilis in patients with and without human immunodeficiency virus infection. N Engl J Med 1997;337:307–314.

52. Rosen T, Rubin H, Ellner K, Tshen J, Cochran R. Vesicular Jarisch-Herxheimer reaction. Arch Dermatol 1989;125:77–81.

53. Schofer H, Vogt HJ, Milbradt R. Ceftriaxone for the treatment of primary and secondary syphilis. Chemotherapy 1989;35:140–145.

54. Schroeter AL, Lucas JB, Price EV, Falcone VH. Treatment for early syphilis and reactivity of serological tests. JAMA 1972;221:471–476.

55. Short DH, Knox JM, Glicksman J. Neurosyphilis, the search for adequate treatment. Arch Dermatol 1966;93:87–91.

56. Sparling PF. Diagnosis and treatment of syphilis. N Engl J Med 1971;284:642–653.

57. Stamm LV, Parish EA. In-vitro activity of azithromycin and CP-63,956 against Treponema pallidum. J Antimicrob Chemother 1990;25(Suppl A):11–14.

58. Standiford HC. Tetracyclines and chloramphenicol. In: Mandell GL, Bennett JE, Dolin R. Principles and practice of infectious diseases. 4th ed. New York: Churchill Livingstone 1995:306–317.

59. Steigbidel NH. Macrolides and clindamycin. In: Mandell GL, Bennett JE, Dolin R. Principles and practice of infectious diseases. 4th ed. New York: Churchill Livingstone 1995:334–346.

60. Telzak EE, Greenberg MSZ, Harrison J, Stoneburner RL, Schultz S. Syphilis treatment response in HIV-infected individuals. AIDS 1991;5:591–595.

61. Tartaglione TA, Hooton TM. The role of fluoroquinolones in sexually transmitted disease. Pharmacotherapy 1993;13:189–201.

62. Tramont EC. Persistence of Treponema pallidum following penicillin G therapy. Report of two cases. JAMA 1976;236:2206–2207.

63. Tramont EC. Syphilis in adults: from Christopher Columbus to Sir Alexander Fleming to AIDS. Clin Infect Dis 1995;21:1361–1371.

64. Tramont EC. Treponema pallidum (syphilis). In: Mandell GL, Bennett JE, Dolin R. Principles and practice of infectious diseases. 4th ed. New York: Churchill Livingstone 1995:2117–2133.

65. Verdon MS, Handsfield HH, Johnson RB. Pilot study of azithromycin for treatment of primary and secondary syphilis. Clin Infect Dis 1994;19:486–488.

66. Weiss ME, Adkinson NF. β-Lactam allergy. In: Mandell GL, Bennett JE, Dolin R. Principles and practice of infectious diseases. 4th ed. New York: Churchill Livingstone 1995:272–278.

67. Whiteside CM. Persistence of neurosyphilis despite multiple treatment regimens. Am J Med 1989;87:225–227.

68. Yinnon AM, Coury-Doniger P, Polito R, Reichman RC. Serological response to treatment of syphilis in patients with HIV infection. Arch Intern Med 1996;156:321–325.

69. Yoder FW. Penicillin treatment of neurosyphilis. Are recommended dosages sufficient? JAMA 1975;232:270–271.

70. Zoller M, Wilson WR, Nadol JB. Treatment of syphilitic hearing loss. Ann Otol Rhinol Laryngol 1979;88:160–165.

Treponemal Species (Nonvenereal)

Theodore Rosen

GENERAL DESCRIPTION

Microbiology

The nonvenereal treponematoses—yaws, pinta, and endemic syphilis—are caused by spirochetes that are morphologically and immunologically identical to the organism that causes venereal syphilis *(Treponema pallidum)*. Nonetheless, each disease is associated with a named microbe: yaws with *T. pallidum* subspecies *pertenue,* endemic syphilis with *T. pallidum* subspecies *endemicum,* and pinta with *T. carateum.* Indigenous cases are vanishingly rare in the industrialized countries of North America, Europe, and Asia. From a global perspective, however, the nonvenereal treponematoses constitute a significant health hazard in many developing countries. In the 1950s and 1960s, mass screening and treatment campaigns designed to eradicate these disorders were conducted under the auspices of the World Health Organization (WHO) and the United Nations Children's Fund (UNICEF). In many areas of high prevalence, such efforts were highly successful (3, 4). Nonetheless, poverty, overcrowding, poor hygiene, lack of local public health surveillance, and absence of funding for ongoing prophylactic control measures have all contributed to a resurgence of these contagious disorders, particularly yaws (9, 23, 28). The frequency and ease of international air travel may facilitate migration of infected persons into nonendemic geographic areas (7).

Epidemiology

Nonvenereal treponematoses have distinct and somewhat overlapping geographic areas of prevalence. Yaws occurs primarily in rural settings in hot and humid environments. At present, the main reservoir of yaws is in West and Central Africa (8, 17). Residual foci of infection persist in Southeast Asia and in a few countries in the Americas (Suriname, Guyana, Colombia, Venezuela, Haiti, and especially Brazil) (21). Yaws goes under many colorful local names, including *frambesia tropica* (German), *pian* (French), *buba* (Spanish), *bouba* (African dialects), and *parangi* and *paru* (Malay) (20).

Like yaws, pinta occurs in relatively remote rural settings that are warm and humid, especially in Central and South America and Mexico. Countries with historically high prevalence include Columbia, Peru, Ecuador, Venezuela, and Brazil (17). Occurrence of pinta outside the Americas is controversial. The word *pinta* means "spot" or "mark" in Spanish; synonyms for this disease include *carate, cute, enfermedad azul* (17). In the Central American countries of Nicaragua and Guatemala, afflicted individuals are called *morados,* which means "the blue ones" (17).

In contrast to pinta and yaws, endemic syphilis occurs primarily in dry, arid locales. It is seen today mostly among nomadic and seminomadic peoples in Saudia Arabia and in the immediate sub-Saharan region of Africa (Sahel) (6, 10). Endemic syphilis was once common in Eastern Europe, but it is now extremely rare in this area (24). Endemic syphilis is known most commonly as *bejel,* but is also called *njovera* or *dichuchwa* in Africa and *belesh, bishel, firjal* and *loath* in the Middle East (10, 17).

Although residual effects may persist lifelong, active nonvenereal treponematoses tend to reach peak incidence among children under 15 years of age. Yaws and pinta are thought to be passed by direct person-to-person contact with either infected skin or mucous membranes; bejel may be acquired by kissing or by contact with contaminated drinking vessels and pipes.

Clinical Manifestations

Like syphilis, these disorders undergo sequential clinical stages following inoculation. After 9 to 90 days, the "mother yaw" manifests as one or more nontender, scaly papules that later become crusted and eroded. After or during spontaneous involution of the earliest lesion(s), disseminated scaly macules, papules, and nodules appear. Constitutional symptoms may accompany skin lesions, including headache, low-grade fever, arthralgias, and generalized lymphadenopathy. Following resolution of the latter, latency begins. In about 10% of patients, late destructive lesions of skin, bone, and cartilage develop (9, 23). Neurologic and ophthalmologic complications may occur but appear to be rare (17).

The primary lesion of endemic syphilis often goes undetected as a small papule or erosion on the oropharyngeal mucosa. Widespread oropharyngeal erosions (analogous to "mucous patches" of secondary syphilis) then develop and may be accompanied by a disseminated papulosquamous skin eruption. Generalized lymphadenopathy and periostitis (especially of the long bones of the leg) may occur. Late bejel is characterized by painful osseous lesions; ulcerations of the soft palate, larynx, and nasopharynx; and destructive lesions of the nose and nasal septum. Ocular complications, especially uveitis, are possible in late endemic syphilis (27).

Pinta is unique among the nonvenereal treponematoses in having *only* skin lesions. Both primary and secondary lesions manifest as scaly papules and plaques that coalesce. Initially erythematous, these lesions develop variable dyschromia: slate-blue, violaceous, brown, gray, or black. Ultimately, pinta may manifest as complete achromia, resembling vitiligo. Cutaneous atrophy, characterized by wrinkling of the skin, may also be seen.

Diagnosis

The diagnosis of nonvenereal treponematoses depends upon detection of clinically compatible skin (bone, mucosal) lesions in a patient from an endemic region of the world who also has a positive serologic test for syphilis. All three diseases elicit the same positive serologic tests (e.g., RPR, VDRL, FTA-abs, MHA-TP) as syphilis. Exudate from early lesions can also be subjected to darkfield examination, and treponemata can be found in biopsy specimens processed with silver stains.

IN VITRO ANTIMICROBIAL SUSCEPTIBILITY PROFILE

It has been largely assumed, based on a remarkable paucity of in vitro laboratory data, that the organisms responsible for nonvenereal treponematoses remain exquisitely sensitive to penicillin. The most reliable method of assessing in vitro sensitivity consists of measuring active protein synthesis via quantitative incorporation of radiolabeled ^{35}S-methionine while freshly isolated treponemata are incubated with and without test antibiotics (25). Using this methodology, *T. pallidum* subspecies *pertenue* was found to be sensitive to penicillin, tetracycline, and erythromycin at concentrations achievable in the serum of patients receiving the drug according to recommended regimens (26). The same in vitro system demonstrated insensitivity to streptomycin (up to 500 μg/mL) and to rifampin (up to 100 μg/mL) (26).

ANTIMICROBIAL THERAPY

Penicillin is clearly the treatment drug of choice for this set of disorders. This choice is based upon clinical trials done many decades ago and often using formulations no longer in use or no longer recommended (penicillin in oil and beeswax; procaine penicillin in oil with aluminum monostearate) (5). For example, procaine penicillin achieved an 83 to 100% clinical cure for pinta treated in Mexico (16) and over 97% clinical cure rate for yaws treated in Haiti (15). Benzathine penicillin, the current recommended form of therapy, achieved cure rates of 86 to 100% when used to treat yaws in Thailand (11).

Higher cure rates were seen with dosages of 1.2 million units than with 600,000 units intramuscularly (11). For children over 10 years of age and for all adolescents and adults, the *current recommended therapy* is a single intramuscular dose of 1.2 million units of benzathine penicillin. For children under 10 years of age, the dose is reduced to 0.6 million units (5, 17).

Very little work has been done with alternative agents. For penicillin-allergic patients over the age of 12, 5 days of oral tetracycline (2.0 g/day in four divided doses) is considered the best substitute. This is based upon small series of yaws patients treated with tetracycline derivatives (aureomycin, terramycin, or oxytetracycline) in Africa (1, 2), Haiti (18, 19), and Jamaica (12–14). These studies, done some 40 years ago and not replicated recently, demonstrated cure rates from 83 to 100%. However, failures in these series may be attributed to somewhat lower dosages than would be used today as well as reliance on tetracycline derivatives that may not be as effective as either the parent drug or newer analogues. For penicillin-allergic children under 12 years of age, the recommended alternative is oral erythromycin (8–10 mg/kg, four times daily, for 15 days) (22). This is based upon the known clinical efficacy of erythromycin for most patients with venereal syphilis, not upon the results of any clinical trials. There are no studies that directly compare the efficacy of penicillin with any of the alternative agents in treatment of the nonvenereal treponematoses.

ENDPOINTS FOR MONITORING THERAPY

Efficacy of therapy is determined by disappearance of active skin lesions, healing of mucocutaneous erosions, and relief of bone/joint pain. The depigmented skin seen in late pinta usually does not revert to normal skin color (10). As with venereal syphilis, the titers of quantitative nontreponemal serological tests (RPR, VDRL) gradually decline following treatment. However, if the disease has been present for many years prior to therapy, the patient may remain serofast. Treponemal tests (MHA-TP and FTA-abs) remain positive for life.

REFERENCES

1. Ampofo O, Findlay GM. Aureomycin in the treatment of yaws and tropical ulcer in Africa. Nature 1950;165:398–399.
2. Ampofo O, Findlay GM. Terramycin in the treatment of yaws and tropical ulcer. Trans R Soc Trop Med Hyg 1951;45:261–263.
3. Anonymous. Programme for the control of the endemic treponematoses. Geneva: World Health Organization, (VDT/EXBUD/87.1) 1987.
4. Arslanagic N, Bokonjic M, Macanovic K. Eradication of endemic syphilis in Bosnia. Genitourin Med 1989;65:4–7.
5. Brown ST. Therapy for nonvenereal treponematoses: review of the efficacy of penicillin and consideration of alternatives. Rev Infect Dis 1985;7(Suppl 2):318–326.
6. Csonka G, Pace J. Endemic nonvenereal treponematosis (bejel) in Saudia Arabia. Rev Infect Dis 1985;7(Suppl 2):260–265.
7. Engelkens HJH, Oranje AP, Stolz E. Early yaws imported in the Netherlands. Genitourin Med 1989;65:316–318.
8. Englekens HJH, Judanarso J, Oranje AP, Vuzevski VD, Niemel PLA, van der Sluis JJ, Stolz E. Endemic treponematoses. Part I: Yaws. Int J Dermatol 1991;30:77–83.
9. Engelkens HJH, Niemel PLA, van der Sluis JJ, Stolz E. The resurgence of yaws. World-wide consequences. Int J Dermatol 1991;30:99–101.
10. Engelkens HJH, Niemel PLA, van der Sluis JJ, Meheus A, Stolz E. Endemic treponematoses. Part II: Pinta and endemic syphilis. Int J Dermatol 1991;30:231–238.
11. Grin EI, Guthe T, Payanandha LO, D'Mello JMF, Swaroop AS. The treponematosis control program of the WHO. The treatment of yaws with benzathine penicillin G. Am J Syphilis 1954: 38: 397–404.
12. Hill KR. The modern treatment of frambesia (yaws). West Indian Med J 1951;1:81–92.
13. Hill KR, Rhodes K, Escoffery GS, Murray CC. Frambesia (yaws) treatment with aureomycin. West Indian Med J 1951; 1:93–96.
14. Hill KR. Antibiotics other than penicillin in the treatment of yaws. Bull WHO 1953;8:107–122.
15. Hume JC, Facio G. An analysis of the results of the treatment of yaws with a single injection of procaine penicillin with 2% aluminum monostearate. Bull WHO 1956;15:1057–1085.
16. Kitchen DK. Treatment of pinta with antibiotics. Ann NY Acad Sci 1952;55:1186–1194.
17. Koff AB, Rosen T. Nonvenereal treponematoses: yaws, endemic syphilis and pinta. J Am Acad Dermatol 1993;29:519–535.
18. Loughlin EH, Joseph AA, Schaeffer K. Aureomycin in the treatment of yaws. Am J Trop Med Hyg 1951;31:20–23.
19. Loughlin EH, Joseph AA. Duvalier F. Oxytetracycline intramuscular in the treatment of yaws (pian). Antibiot Chemother 1954;4:155–164.
20. Nagreh DS. Yaws. Cutis 1986;38:303–305.
21. St John RK. Yaws in the Americas. Rev Infect Dis 1985;7(Suppl 2):266–272.
22. Sehgal VN. Leg ulcers caused by yaws and endemic syphilis. Clin Dermatol 1990;8:166–174.
23. Sehgal VN, Jain S, Bhattacharya SN, Thappa DM. Yaws control/eradication. Int J Dermatol 1994;33:16–20.
24. Spirov G. Endemic syphilis in Bulgaria. Genitourin Med 1991; 67:428.
25. Stamm LV, Bassford PJ. Cellular and extracellular protein antigens of *Treponema pallidum* synthesized during in vitro incubation of freshly extracted organisms. Infect Immunol 1985;47: 799–807.
26. Stapleton JT, Stamm LV, Bassford PJ. Potential for development of antibiotic resistance in pathogenic treponemes. Rev Infect Dis 1985;7(Suppl 2):314–317.
27. Tabbara KF, al Kaff AS, Fadel T. Ocular manifestations of endemic syphilis (bejel). Ophthalmology 1989;96:1087–1091.
28. Widy-Wirski R. Surveillance and control of resurgent yaws in the African region. Rev Infect Dis 1985;7(Suppl 2):227–232.

Vibrio cholerae and Other Species

•

Carlos Seas and Eduardo Gotuzzo

GENERAL DESCRIPTION

The scientific community has witnessed a resurgence of cholera in recent years. Epidemics of clinical cholera in endemic areas such as the Indian subcontinent and Africa occur every year. The largest epidemic during this century was reported from Latin America at the beginning of 1991 (10). A novel pathogen, *Vibrio cholerae* O139 caused an epidemic of clinical cholera in Asia in 1992, the first non-O1 vibrio to cause such a phenomenon (13). The disease caused by this novel pathogen could not be distinguished from cholera caused by O1 vibrio (18). Undoubtedly, the worst epidemic of cholera during the last decade in terms of attack and case fatality rates was reported from Zaire after a political crisis in Rwanda in 1994 (24). Additionally, multiply-resistant strains of *V. cholerae* O1 to common antimicrobials used for its treatment are becoming prevalent in endemic and epidemic areas, complicating the selection of proper antimicrobial therapy (9, 23, 43). The mainstay in the treatment of cholera is replenishment of fluids and electrolytes lost in diarrhea and vomitus. Antimicrobials play an important role as adjunctive therapy to fluid and electrolyte repletion.

SUSCEPTIBILITY IN VITRO

V. cholerae O1 is susceptible in vitro to a number of antimicrobials, including tetracycline, doxycycline, ampicillin, cephalosporins, erythromycin, chloramphenicol, cotrimoxazole, and furazolidone. O139 *V. cholerae* is susceptible to all these antimicrobials with the exception of cotrimoxazole and furazolidone. Table 1 presents data on in vitro susceptibility of O1 and O139 *V. cholerae* strains isolated from patients enrolled in clinical trials. Both O1 and O139 strains were highly susceptible to quinolones and tetracyclines including doxycycline, but 63% of O1 strains from Bangladesh were resistant to tetracycline.

An international survey to evaluate global sensitivity patterns to common antimicrobials from endemic areas of cholera including India, Bangladesh, and Peru found several subtypes of O1 and O139 strains (56). Multiple–antimicrobial agent resistance (MAR) phenotypes designated 1 and 2 were identified. MAR phenotype 1 was shared by the major susceptibility pattern of O139 and O1 El Tor Indian strains, and major susceptibility pattern A of O1 El Tor strains from Bangladesh. This pattern showed multiple resistance to chloramphenicol, furazolidone, streptomycin, and cotrimoxazole. MAR phenotype 2 was associated with major susceptibility pattern B of O1 El Tor strains from Bangladesh and was characterized by resistance to tetracycline in addition to the pattern exhibited by MAR phenotype 1. The incidence of resistance to tetracycline,

measured by disk diffusion, among O1 *V. cholerae* strains isolated from Bangladesh shows a sharp increase in recent years: 1.9% in 1990 to 85.4% in 1993, while Indian and Peruvian strains showed a high sensitivity to tetracyclines from 1991 on.

Clearly a regional susceptibility pattern to common antimicrobials is observed in endemic areas. Misuse of antimicrobials to treat diarrhea and respiratory infections by physicians and practitioners is partly responsible for the emergence of resistance. Lack of control of prescription of antimicrobials by nonphysicians plays an important role in the genesis of resistance in common bacteria as well.

ANTIMICROBIAL THERAPY

Use of antimicrobials in cholera is recommended as adjunctive therapy to fluid and electrolyte repletion (4). Several clinical trials have confirmed the utility of antimicrobials in the treatment of severe cholera. Elegant studies conducted in the sixties in India defined the role of tetracycline in the treatment of cholera (7, 31, 40, 54). Overall, these studies indicate that tetracycline reduces the duration of diarrhea by approximately 50% compared with placebo (~2 days vs. 4–5 days), reduces the volume of diarrhea by 50%, and shortens the duration of vibrio excretion to approximately 48 h (vs. 7–9 days in some studies). These achievements are especially important when treatment centers are overloaded with severely dehydrated patients, as occurs during epidemics. The rational prescription of antimicrobials not only reduces the hospital stay of patients to approximately 24 h as it did during the Peruvian cholera epidemic in 1991 (26), but also reduces the expense for fluids to rehydrate patients and all other hospital-related expenses.

From these observations, the World Health Organization recommended tetracycline 500 mg four times a day for 3 days as the treatment of choice for cholera (54). Alternative antimicrobial therapy is listed in Table 2. Tetracycline has been evaluated more recently under epidemic situations in Peru (3, 28, 30) and Dhaka (35). Battilana and Grados reported both clinical and bacteriologic cure rates of 100% in 100 cholera patients who received the standard tetracycline regimen for 3 days in an open randomized study (3). Gotuzzo et al. found that tetracycline and another quinolone, ciprofloxacin, had similar clinical and bacteriologic results in patients with moderate-to-severe dehydration in a randomized double-blind clinical trial conducted in Lima (28). In another study, Grados found that tetracycline was equivalent to trimethoprim and sulfamethoxazole in both clinical and bacteriologic parameters in patients with moderate-to-severe dehydration in Lima, Peru (30). Resistance to trimethoprim and sulfamethoxazole was observed during the study. Results from these two studies

TABLE 1 • **In Vitro Susceptibility of O1 and O139 *V. cholerae* Strains Isolated from Patients Enrolled in Clinical Trials**

Antimicrobial Agent	No. of Strains	MIC$_{50}$ (μg/mL)	MIC$_{90}$ (μg/mL)	Range	Reference
Tetracycline	12	1.56	ND[a]	1.25–2.5	Cash R, 1973
	102	ND	0.250	0.06–0.5	Gotuzzo E, 1995
Doxycycline	260[b]	ND	0.125	ND	Khan WA, 1996
Cotrimoxazole	32	1.47	ND	0.2–3.2	Cash R, 1973
Lomefloxacin	68	ND	0.06	ND	Gotuzzo E, 1994b
Ciprofloxacin	100	ND	0.007	0.0007–0.25	Gotuzzo E, 1995
	260[b]	ND	0.003	ND	Khan WA, 1996

[a]ND, not done.

[b]Includes 130 O139 strains.

TABLE 2 • **Antimicrobial Regimens for the Treatment of Cholera**

Drug	Dose Adults	Children
Tetracycline	500 mg four times daily for 3 days	50 mg/kg body weight four times daily for 3 days
Doxycycline	300 mg in single dose	Not evaluated
Furazolidone	100 mg four times daily for 3 days	5 mg/kg of body weight per day four times daily for 3 days,or 7 mg/kg as a single dose
Cotrimoxazole	160 mg of trimethoprim/800 mg of sulfamethoxazole twice daily for 3 days	8 mg of trimethoprim–40 mg of sulfamethoxazole/kg divided in two doses for 3 days
Norfloxacin	400 mg twice daily for 3 days	Not recommended
Ciprofloxacin	250 mg once daily for 3 days 1 g single dose	Not recommended

conducted under epidemic conditions were similar to those cited above from endemic countries and confirmed the previous experience with tetracycline.

Khan et al. evaluated alternatives for tetracycline-resistant vibrio endemic in the region recently (35). Ciprofloxacin (1 g, single dose) and erythromycin (500 mg four times daily) were the best alternatives; nalidixic acid and pivmecillinam were clearly ineffective. Results with tetracycline were comparable to those reported for placebo in earlier studies. Studies with tetracycline in children have also confirmed its utility in this age group (39); however, its use is not as popular as other antimicrobials because staining of permanent teeth is a major concern, although 3 days of therapy may not present a problem in this age group (40).

Several other multiple-dose regimens have been evaluated in the treatment of severe cholera, including furazolidone (11, 12, 38, 45, 46), chloramphenicol (21), trimethoprim and sulfamethoxazole (8, 21, 30, 44), doxycycline (16, 48), erythromycin (6, 35, 36), nalidixic acid (35), and pivmecillinam (35). All these drugs showed clinical and microbiologic outcomes comparable to that of tetracycline with the exception of nalidixic acid and pivmecillinam, which are more important in the treatment of shigellosis than in cholera. Erythromycin at a dose of 800 mg twice daily in adults and 40 mg/kg in two doses in children yielded better results than sulfatrimethoprim and placebo against *V. cholerae* O1 resistant to tetracyline in Somalia (6).

Single-dose regimens are preferred over multiple-dose regimens when compliance is the main concern. Furazolidone

(46), tetracycline (16, 32, 46), and doxycycline (1, 16, 37, 49) have been extensively studied in endemic areas. In general, clinical outcomes with these regimens were similar to those with multiple-dose regimens, with the exception of furazolidone, which did not differ from placebo in reducing the volume of stools and shortening the duration of diarrhea. Although it was not statistically significant, more relapses and clinical failures were reported with these regimens than with multiple-dose regimens. More-prolonged excretion of the organism was also documented with these single-dose regimens. These drawbacks should be weighed against the potential of ensuring good compliance in patients from developing countries where the acceptance of multiple-dose regimens is low.

The preferred and recommended single-dose regimen is doxycycline 300 mg. Nausea and vomiting have been reported as common side effects during therapy with single-dose doxycycline regimens. To avoid these complaints, concomitant administration of food is recommended. A more recent evaluation of this regimen against both *V. cholerae* O1 and *V. cholerae* O139 in Dhaka and Matlab, Bangladesh, confirmed its utility as an alternative to tetracycline (37). Two single-dose regimens: ciprofloxacin 1 g and doxycycline 300 mg were evaluated in a double-blind randomized trial in adult patients with severe cholera infected by both O1 and O139 *V. cholerae*. Single-dose doxycycline was clinically equivalent to ciprofloxacin in patients infected by *V. cholerae* O139 but clinically inferior in patients infected by O1 *V. cholerae*. The discrepancy in results in patients infected by different serotypes was attributed to different susceptibility patterns to tetracycline among these serotypes rather than to clinical differences. The O1 vibrio strains were more resistant to tetracycline than O139 strains. Neither significant vomiting nor nausea was observed when doxycycline was administered with light food in this trial, which included the largest number of patients so far in a single trial with doxycycline.

The appearance of strains resistant to common antimicrobials used for the treatment of cholera such as tetracyclines and cotrimoxazole in endemic areas has prompted the search for new alternatives (9, 23, 43). The fluoroquinolones have emerged as the most promising group of antimicrobials for treating enteric infections. Excellent clinical experience with quinolones in typhoid fever, shigellosis, and traveler's diarrhea has been reported around the world. Among their advantages are a broad spectrum of activity against most pathogens associated with diarrheal diseases including *Escherichia coli*, *Shigella* spp., *Salmonella* spp., *V. cholerae* O1 and O139, and *Campylobacter* spp.; very high intestinal concentrations of the active drug, several times in excess of the minimal inhibitory concentrations (MIC) for the pathogens mentioned above; easy administration including once-a-day oral regimens; and a good safety profile. A summary of relevant data from studies conducted with quinolones in patients with cholera is presented in Table 3

The first fluoroquinolone evaluated against cholera was norfloxacin. The pioneer study was conducted in Calcutta, India, and included adult patients with severe dehydration and confirmed infection by *V. cholerae* O1 (2). Patients were randomly assigned to three treatment groups; norfloxacin 400 mg twice daily, trimethoprim (160 mg)/sulfamethoxazole (800 mg) twice daily, and placebo for 5 days. Norfloxacin reduced the volume of stools, duration of diarrhea, and fluid requirements for rehydration, compared with the other two groups. Additionally, excretion of *V. cholerae* was shortened by half with norfloxacin (1–2 days) compared with the other study groups (4–5 days). The study was limited by the small number of patients included and the appearance of resistance to trimethoprim-sulfamethoxazole during the study period, which precluded adequate comparison with the standard antimicrobial regimen.

Another study with norfloxacin, conducted during the cholera epidemic in Lima, Peru, in 1991 confirmed the utility of this quinolone in the treatment of severe cholera when given in a multiple dosing regimen (26). This study included adult patients in a University Hospital in Lima who had proven infection by *V. cholerae* O1 with acute watery diarrhea and moderate-to-severe dehydration. Three study groups were tested in an open, controlled and randomized design: norfloxacin 800 mg single-dose, norfloxacin 400 mg twice daily for 3 days, and tetracycline 500 mg four times a day for 3 days. The single-dose norfloxacin arm of the study had to be stopped after an interim analysis showed more clinical and bacteriologic failures in this study group. The two multiple-dose regimens of norfloxacin and tetracycline were similar in all clinical parameters including duration of diarrhea, volume of stools, and fluid requirements for rehydration, but norfloxacin attained faster clearance of vibrio from the stools than tetracycline (18% of patients in the norfloxacin group were positive after 24 h of therapy vs. 47% in the tetracycline group). The

MIC for norfloxacin was 0.007 μg/mL. The reason for such a negative result with a single-dose regimen of an antimicrobial that reaches high luminal levels was not apparent from the trial. All strains were sensitive to norfloxacin, ruling out the possibility of resistance to explain these results. Intestinal levels were not measured in the patients included in the study. It may be speculated that in high stool purgers, norfloxacin does not reach sufficient stool concentrations when given in single-dose regimens. This hypothesis remains to be proven. Three other quinolones have been evaluated following open study designs, lomefloxacin, fleroxacin, and ofloxacin, showing excellent clinical and microbiologic results (3, 19, 27).

Ciprofloxacin is the most extensively studied quinolone to date. Studies conducted in open and double-blind and controlled designs have confirmed the excellent results with this fluoroquinolone, even when used in single-dose regimens. Two open studies conducted in Peru at the beginning of the cholera epidemic in 1991 with ciprofloxacin at 250 mg and 500 mg twice-a-day for 3 days showed clinical efficacy of 90% and microbiologic efficacy of 100% (29). Another two open studies evaluated the efficacy of ciprofloxacin in cholera caused by multiply resistant *V. cholerae* O1 in endemic areas. Khan evaluated the efficacy of ciprofloxacin 500 mg twice daily against four other regimens including erythromycin, nalidixic acid, pivmecillinam, and tetracycline in patients infected by O1 *V. cholerae* resistant to tetracycline in Bangladesh (35). Ciprofloxacin was the most effective antimicrobial in that study, considering both clinical and bacteriologic outcomes. All strains had in vitro susceptibility to ciprofloxacin as determined by disk-diffusion methods. Doganci evaluated a regimen of ciprofloxacin (1 g/day for 2 days) in 7 patients with nonsevere cholera in Ankara, Turkey, observing good clinical and bacteriologic results (19).

Ciprofloxacin was also tested against O139 *V. cholerae* in Bangladesh during the large epidemic caused by this novel pathogen in 1992 (36). An open study evaluated a single-dose regimen of ciprofloxacin (1 g) and doxycycline (300 mg) against two multiple-dose regimens of tetracycline and erythromycin (500 mg four times a day for 3 days). The single-dose ciprofloxacin group had the best overall outcome, with similar clinical efficacy to the other regimens but significantly better bacteriologic results.

Two large randomized, double-blinded, controlled studies conducted in Peru and Bangladesh have confirmed the excellent efficacy observed in the open studies with ciprofloxacin presented above. The study conducted in Peru under epidemic conditions evaluated a single daily dose of ciprofloxacin (250 mg) compared with tetracycline (500 mg four times daily) both for 3 days in patients with moderate-to-severe dehydration due to *V. cholerae* O1 infection (28). Study groups were well balanced in all baseline characteristics, almost 90% in both groups had severe dehydration on arrival. Ciprofloxacin yielded clinical and bacteriologic outcomes similar to those with tetracycline. Although not statistically different, failure rates were higher than previously reported for tetracycline and ciprofloxacin (11 and 16%, respectively). Bacteriologic cure rates were, however, very high in both study groups.

TABLE 3 • Results from Studies with Fluoroquinolones in Cholera

Quinolone	Study Design	Dosing Regimens	No. of Patients	Duration of Diarrhea (h)[a]	Clinical Cure, N(%)	Bacteriological Cure, N(%)	Ref.
Norfloxacin	1. Randomized double-blind controlled	a. Norfloxacin, 400 mg b.i.d., 3 days	13	19.2 (4.4)	NS[b]	NS	2
		b. TMP/SMX, 160/800 mg, b.i.d., 3 days	12	27.5 (4.0)	NS	NS	
		c. Placebo	12	29.3 (4.5)	NS	NS	
	2. Open randomized controlled	a. Norfloxacin, 400 mg b.i.d., 3 days	25	60.8 (18.4)	25 (74)	34 (100)	26
		b. Norfloxacin, 800 mg single dose	34	91.04 (50.1)	13 (52)	19 (76)	
		c. Tetracycline, 500 mg q.i.d., 3 days	34	61.66 (23.2)	27 (77)	31 (91)	
Lomefloxacin	Open, noncontrolled	400 mg, once per day, 3 days	68	49.6 (16.9)	61 (90)	48 (100)	27
Ofloxacin	Open, noncontrolled	400 mg/day, 2 days	42	NS	NS[c]	NS	19
Fleroxacin	Open, randomized controlled	400 mg/day, single dose	100	NS	100 (100)	100 (100)	3
Ciprofloxacin	1. Open, noncontrolled	500 mg b.i.d. 3 days	20	53.6 (14)	18 (90)	20 (100)	29
	2. Open, noncontrolled	250 mg b.i.d. 3 days	21	48.3 (14.4)	19 (90)	21 (100)	29
	3. Open, noncontrolled	1 g/day, 2 days	7	NS	NS	NS	19
	4. Open, randomized controlled	a. Ciprofloxacin 500 mg b.i.d., 3 days	15	NS[d]	14 (93)	15 (100)	35
		b. Tetracycline 500 mg q.i.d., 3 days	12	NS	5 (42)	6 (50)	
	5. Randomized double-blind controlled	a. Ciprofloxacin 250 mg once daily, 3 days	100	51.2 (17.4)	84 (84)	99 (99)	28
		b. Tetracycline 500 mg q.i.d., 3 days	102	48.0 (20.6)	91 (89)	97 (95)	
	6. Randomized double-blind controlled	a. Ciprofloxacin 1 g single dose	66	NS[e]	62 (94)	63 (95)	37
		b. Doxycycline 300 mg single dose	64	NS	47 (73)	44 (69)	
	7. Open, nonrandomized	Ciprofloxacin 1 g single dose[f]	16	41 (19)	NS[g]	NS[g]	36
	8. Randomized double-blind controlled	a. Ciprofloxacin 1 g single dose[f]	59	NS[e]	54 (92)	58 (98)	37
		b. Doxycycline 300 mg single dose	71	NS	65 (92)	56 (79)	

[a] Values are mean (SD).

[b] NS, not specified.

[c] Volume of diarrhea and excretion of vibrio were significantly reduced at the end of therapy.

[d] Patients in the ciprofloxacin group had shorter duration of diarrhea than patients in the tetracycline group (Kaplan-Meier survival curve, $P = .004$ by log rank test).

[e] Ciprofloxacin group had shorter duration of diarrhea than single-dose doxycycline group in *V. cholerae* O1–infected patients, but not in *V. cholerae* O139–infected patients (Kaplan-Meier survival curve, $P = .0451$ and $P = .435$ by log rank test, respectively).

[f] Studies conducted in O139 *V. cholerae.*

[g] Diarrhea stopped in all patients within 72 h of therapy. Stool cultures were negative for *V. cholerae* O139 during the third day of therapy.

The largest clinical trial conducted to date evaluating the efficacy of ciprofloxacin in the treatment of cholera caused by either O1 or O139 *V. cholerae* was conducted in Bangladesh (37). In this study, 260 adult male patients (130 infected by O1 and 130 infected by O139 *V. cholerae*) were randomized to receive either ciprofloxacin (1 g) or doxycycline (300 mg). Ciprofloxacin was more effective in bacteriologic outcomes than doxycycline, irrespective of the infecting serotype of *V. cholerae*, but was only superior to doxycycline in clinical outcomes against O1 *V. cholerae*–infected patients. Differences in the susceptibility to tetracycline and doxycycline of O1 vibrios explained these results; 99% of O1 isolates were susceptible to doxycycline in vitro, but only 63% were susceptible to tetracycline. The latter group had higher rates of clinical failure; 52% (14 of 27) in patients infected with tetracycline-resistant strains vs. 8% (3 of 37) of patients infected with tetracycline-sensitive strains ($P < .001$). The study also revealed new information about the efficacy of antimicrobials in patients with diarrhea. Serum and especially stool concentrations of the study drugs were determined during the study and correlated with the MICs of the infecting pathogen. Interestingly, the ratio between the peak stool concentration and the MIC of *V. cholerae* was almost 10 times higher with ciprofloxacin than with doxycycline (8690 with ciprofloxacin vs. 882 with doxycycline). Stool concentrations several times in excess of the MIC can explain the excellent bacteriologic results obtained in this study irrespective of the infecting serotype of *V. cholerae*.

What is the role of quinolones in the treatment of cholera? We believe they should be recommended for treatment of severe cholera in areas of the globe where strains resistant to other alternatives are prevalent (51). Single-dose ciprofloxacin (1 g) or single-daily dose (250 mg) for 3 days are the regimens we recommend. The use of quinolones has a number of restrictions that should be taken into account before routine use is recommended, even in areas where strains resistant to other antimicrobials are commonly found. The two most important issues are the cost of therapy and their restriction for use in children because of articular involvement reported from young animals. Although there is no conclusive evidence of toxicity in humans (50), the fluoroquinolones should be used in this age group only when no other alternative is available. Even in places where resistance is common, alternative antimicrobials such as erythromycin can be recommended for children before the quinolones. Quinolones are expensive and people from developing countries who are most affected by cholera cannot afford them. A challenge for these countries is to make quinolones available for those of low socioeconomic status.

The role of antimicrobials in the treatment of severe cholera is clearly defined. This is not the case, however, for use of antimicrobials as a prophylactic measure to curtail cholera transmission. The rationale behind its implementation is to reduce the acquisition of *V. cholerae* by household contacts of an index case by reaching high intestinal levels of antimicrobials during the period of maximum risk (52). A recent evaluation of published data on this issue concluded that implementation of prophylaxis is not feasible nor cost-effective (22). The main reason for the concern regarding its use under epidemic or endemic situations is the fact that the target population for this prophylactic measure, household contacts of index cases with clinical cholera, represents only a minority of the people exposed. El Tor *V. cholerae*, the agent of the most recent epidemics in the world, tends to produce more asymptomatic infections than the classic biotype. The ratio of asymptomatic to symptomatic people was about 20 during the Peruvian cholera epidemic in 1991. These asymptomatic people are extremely important in dissemination of the disease and definitely outnumber symptomatic persons. However, under special situations when high transmission of the disease occurs, the use of prophylaxis may be considered as an adjunctive measure along with other specific measures. Tetracyclines have been the preferred agents in these situations (33, 42), with sulfadoxine (17) and chloramphenicol (42) as alternatives.

The pharmacologic properties of the fluoroquinolones mentioned above make them an attractive group of antimicrobials for evaluation as prophylactic agents against cholera. The high concentration of ciprofloxacin in the intestinal lumen, several times in excess of the MIC of *V. cholerae*, for a prolonged time prompted its evaluation in preventing watery diarrhea and vibrio infection in household contacts of confirmed cholera infection in index cases during the Peruvian epidemic in 1991 (20). Following a randomized, double-blinded, controlled design, adult household contacts received either ciprofloxacin (250 mg, single dose) or placebo as soon as infection was confirmed in the index cases. Ciprofloxacin did not prevent development of diarrhea nor acquisition of vibrio infection among household contacts in that study. The trial lacked the statistical power to detect a difference in protective efficacy of ciprofloxacin and placebo because of a dramatic reduction in the rate of secondary transmission during the study period. However, a secondary analysis showed a trend toward faster eradication of vibrio from the stools and lower incidence of watery diarrhea in 30 patients already infected by *V. cholerae* at the time of enrollment who had received ciprofloxacin. Studies of larger sample size are needed to define the role, if any, of fluoroquinolones in the prophylaxis of cholera.

Finally, the problems associated with use of prophylactic antimicrobials should be emphasized. They include the false sense of security of recipients, the potential for inducing resistant strains, and the possibility of drug-related adverse reactions. We do not recommend routine use of antibiotic prophylaxis for prevention of cholera in either epidemic or endemic areas (53). Prophylactic use of antimicrobials may be considered under special situations when high transmission of the disease takes place. The recent epidemic of O1 cholera in Zaire might have been an opportunity to consider its implementation or to study its benefit.

ANTIMICROBIAL THERAPY FOR OTHER VIBRIO SPECIES

Treatment of other vibrio species associated with diarrheal diseases is less clearly beneficial than the treatment of O1 and O139 *V. cholerae*. The reduction in the duration of diarrhea, requirement for fluids, and excretion of vibrio O1 and O139 have not been consistently observed with other vibrio species. The diarrheal disease associated with these pathogens is usually self-limited, and replenishment of fluids is sufficient.

Infections caused by other noncholera vibrio agents, including *V. parahaemolyticus, V. vulnificus,* and *V. alginolyticus,* are localized infections with the potential of producing bacteremia. Skin and soft-tissue infections are most common, but gastroenteritis, wound infections, infections of the central nervous system, and urinary tract infections have been reported. Successful treatment using tetracyclines, a quinolone plus an aminoglycoside, or a third-generation cephalosporin has been reported (5, 41). Limited information is available on clinical trials specifically devised to treat infections caused by this kind of vibrio.

VACCINES

Controlling the spread of cholera by use of vaccines was originated soon after the etiologic agent of cholera was discovered. For a vaccine to be effective, an immune response similar to that elicited by the natural infection should be produced. Protection against vibrio is mediated by secretory immunoglobulins generated in the intestine, with antibacterial immunity being more important than the antitoxic component (34). Parenteral vaccines are no longer recommended as they induce only transient protection and are associated with side effects. Although the parenteral vaccines induce a secretory response in the intestine, a more prolonged and effective immune response is stimulated by vaccines given orally.

The ideal vaccine against cholera should be given orally (preferably in a single-dose regimen), should induce a rapid and long-lasting immune response irrespective of the age and the previous exposure to vibrio, and should be affordable by developing countries or preferably should be manufactured in endemic areas of cholera. Such a vaccine is not yet available. However, significant advances have been made in recent years with two particular kinds of oral cholera vaccines.

The most extensively studied oral cholera vaccine to date contains whole inactivated vibrio plus the B subunit. A field study conducted in Matlab, Bangladesh, showed that the overall protection after 3 years of follow-up is only 50%, with higher protection after 6 months (85%). Additionally, the protection in children below 5 years of age was only about 25% after 3 years of follow-up. Persons carrying the O blood group had lower protection against severe infection, and protection against the classic biotype was significantly better than that attained against the El Tor biotype (14). All these drawbacks along with the fact that at least two doses are needed to confer protection make this vaccine less suitable than was thought, especially for developing countries.

Live attenuated cholera vaccines are the other group of vaccines that have shown promising results in clinical trials (34). The third generation of these vaccines, CVD 103 HgR, is the most promising of this group. Studies conducted in endemic and epidemic countries showed that this vaccine elicits a significant immune response, with minimal excretion of the strain to the environment and with rates of diarrhea not different from that observed in placebo groups (15, 25). Field studies with this vaccine still in progress should answer several questions raised in trials with the oral-inactivated vaccine, such as whether the efficacy depends on age, blood group, and the biotype of *V. cholerae* and whether

protection can be attained within a few days and be long lasting.

The appearance of a new non-O1 *V. cholerae,* the O139 strain, capable of producing epidemic cholera complicates the problem further. The absence of cross-protection between O1 and O139 infections means that the whole population is at risk of acquiring cholera caused by O139 *V. cholerae.* Clearly, new vaccines including this novel strain should be evaluated for efficacy in epidemic areas.

REFERENCES

1. Alam AN, Alam NH, Ahmed T, Sack DA. Randomized double blind trial of single dose doxycycline for treating cholera in adults. Br Med J 1990;300:1619–1621.
2. Battacharya SK, Battacharya MK, Dutta P, Dutta D, De SP, Sikdar SN, Maitra A, Dutta A, Pal SC. Double-blind, randomized, controlled clinical trial of norfloxacin for cholera. Antimicrob Agents Chemother 1990;34:939–940.
3. Battilana C, Grados P. A comparative study of oral fleroxacin and tetracycline in the treatment of cholera [Abstract Is23]. 4th Western Pacific Congress on Chemotherapy and Infectious Diseases. Manila, Philippines, December 4–7, 1994:38.
4. Bennish ML. Cholera: pathophysiology, clinical features, and treatment. In: Wachsmuth IK, Blake PA, Olsvik O, eds. *Vibrio cholerae* and cholera. Molecular to global perspectives. Washington, DC: American Society for Microbiology Press, 1994:229–256.
5. Blake PA. Disease of humans (other than cholera) caused by vibrio. Annu Rev Microbiol 1980;34:341.
6. Burans JP, Podgore J, Mansour MM, Farah AH, Abbas S, Abu-Elyazeed R, Woody JN. Comparative trial of erythromycin and sulphatrimethoprim in the treatment of tetracycline resistant *Vibrio cholerae* O1. Trans R Soc Trop Med Hyg 1989;83:836–838.
7. Carpenter CCJ, Barua D, Wallace CK, Mitra PP, Sack RB, Khanra SR, Wella SA, Dans PE, Chaudhuri RN. Clinical studies in Asiatic cholera. IV. Antibiotic therapy in cholera. Bull Johns Hopkins Hosp 1966;216–229.
8. Cash RA, Northrup RS, Rahman ASMM. Trimethoprim and sulphamethoxazole in clinical cholera: comparison with tetracycline. J Infect Dis 1973;128:S749–753.
9. Cavallo JD, Niel L, Talarmin A, Dubrous P. Antibiotic sensitivity to epidemic strains of *Vibrio cholerae* and *Shigella dysenteriae* 1 isolated in Rwandan refugee camps in Zaire. Med Trop 1995;55:351–353.
10. Centers for Disease Control. Cholera—Peru, 1991. MMWR 1991; 40:108–109.
11. Chaudhury RN, Neogy KN, Sanyal SN, Gupta RK, Manji P. Furazolidone in the treatment of cholera. Lancet 1968;1:332–333.
12. Chaudhury RN, Sanyal SN, Neogy KN, Barua D, Manji P. Furazolidone in cholera. Lancet 1965;2:909.
13. Cholera Working Group. Large epidemic of cholera-like disease in Bangladesh caused by *Vibrio cholerae* O139 synonym Bengal. Lancet 1993;342:387–390.
14. Clemens JD, Sack DA, Harris JR, Van Loon F, Chakraborty J, Ahmed F, Rao MR, Khan MR, Yunus MD, Huda N, Stanton BF, Kay BA, Walter S, Eeckels R, Svennerholm AM, Holgrem J. Field trial of oral cholera vaccines in Bangladesh: results from three-year follow-up. Lancet 1990; 335:270–273.
15. Davis R, Spencer CM. Live oral cholera vaccine: a preliminary review of its pharamacology and clinical potential in providing protective immunity against cholera. Clin Immunother 1995; 4:235–247.

16. De S, Chaudhuri A, Dutta P, De SP, Pal SC. Doxycycline in the treatment of cholera. Bull WHO 1976;54:177–179.

17. Deb BC, Sengupta PG, De SP, Sil J, Sikdar SN, Pal SC. Effect of sulfadoxine on transmission of *Vibrio cholerae* infection among family contacts of cholera patients in Calcutta. Bull WHO 1976;54:171–175.

18. Dhar U, Bennish ML, Khan WA, Seas C, Khan EH, Albert MJ, Salam MA. Clinical features, antimicrobial susceptibility and toxin production in *Vibrio cholerae* O139 infection: comparison with *Vibrio cholerae* O1 infection. Trans R Soc Trop Med Hyg 1996;90:402–405.

19. Doganci L, Gün H, Baysallar M, Albay A, Cinar E, Haznedaroglu T. Short-term quinolones for successful eradication of multiply resistant *Vibrio cholerae* in adult patients. Scand J Infect Dis 1995;27:425–426.

20. Echevarria J, Seas C, Carrillo C, Mostorino R, Ruiz R, Gotuzzo E. Efficacy and tolerability of ciprofloxacin prophylaxis in adult household contacts of patients with cholera. Clin Infect Dis 1995;20:1480–1484.

21. Gharagozloo RA, Naficy AK, Mouin M, Nassirzadeh MH, Yalda R. Comparative trial of tetracycline, chloramphenicol, and trimethoprim/sulphamethoxazole in eradication of *Vibrio cholerae* El tor. Br Med J 1970;4:282.

22. Ghosh S, Sengupta PG, Gupta DN, Sirkar BK. Chemoprophylaxis studies in cholera: a review of selective works. J Commun Dis 1992;24:55–57.

23. Glass RI, Huq I, Alim ARMA, Yunus M. Emergence of multiply antibiotic-resistant *Vibrio cholerae* in Bangladesh. J Infect Dis 1980;142:939–942.

24. Goma Epidemiology Group. Public health impact of Rwandan refugee crisis: what happened in Goma, Zaire, in July 1994? Lancet 1995;345:339–344.

25. Gotuzzo E, Butron B, Seas C, Penny M, Ruiz R, Losonsky G, Lanata C, Wasserman S, Salazar E, Kaper J, Cryz S, Levine M. Safety, immunogenicity, and excretion pattern of single-dose live oral cholera vaccine CVD 103 HgR in Peruvian adults of high and low socioeconomic levels. Infect Immun 1993;61:3994–3997.

26. Gotuzzo E, Cieza J, Estremadoyro L, Seas C. Cholera. Lessons from the epidemic in Peru. Infect Dis Clin North Am 1994;8: 183–205.

27. Gotuzzo E, Carrillo C, Seas C, Cabezas C, Ruiz R. Tratamiento del cólera grave: eficacia de lomefloxacino una vez al día. Rev Esp Quimioterap 1994;7:292–295.

28. Gotuzzo E, Seas C, Echevarria J, Carrillo C, Mostorino R, Ruiz R. Ciprofloxacin for the treatment of cholera: a randomized, double-blind, controlled clinical trial of a single daily dose in Peruvian adults. Clin Infect Dis 1995;20:1485–1490.

29. Gotuzzo E, Seas C, Echevarria J, Ruiz R, Carrillo C. Oral ciprofloxacin in the treatment of cholera. Drugs 1995;49(Suppl 2): 451–453.

30. Grados P, Bravo N, Battilana C. Comparative efficacy of cotrimoxazole and tetracycline in the treatment of cholera. Bull Pan Am Health Org 1996;30:36–42.

31. Greenough WB, Gordon RS, Isenberg IS, Davies BI. Tetracycline in the treatment of cholera. Lancet 1964;1:355–357.

32. Islam MR. Single dose tetracycline in cholera. Gut 1987;28: 1029–1032.

33. Joint ICMR-GWB-WHO cholera study group. Effect of tetracycline on cholera carriers in households of cholera patients. Bull WHO 1971;45:451–455.

34. Kaper JB, Morris JG, Levine MM. Cholera. Clin Microbiol Rev 1995;8:48–86.

35. Khan WA, Begum M, Salam MA, Bardhan PK, Islam MR, Mahalanabis D. Comparative trial of five antimicrobials in the treatment of cholera in adults. Trans R Soc Trop Med Hyg 1995; 89:103–106.

36. Khan WA, Dhar U, Begum M, Salam MA, Bardhan PK, Mahalanabis D. Antimicrobial treatment of adults with cholera due to *Vibrio cholerae* O139 (synonym Bengal). Drugs 1995;49(Suppl 2):460–462.

37. Khan WA, Bennish ML, Seas C, Khan EH, Ronan A, Dhar U, Busch W, Salam MA. Randomized controlled comparison of single-dose ciprofloxacin and doxycycline for cholera caused by *Vibrio cholerae* O1 or O139. Lancet 1996;348:296–300.

38. Kobari K, Takahura I, Nakatomi M, Sogame S, Uylangeo C. Antibiotic resistant strains of El Tor Vibrio in the Philippines and the use of furalazine for chemotherapy. Bull WHO 1970;43: 365–371.

39. Lindenbaum J, Gordon RS, Hirschorn N, Akbar R, Greenough WB, Islam MR. Cholera in children. Lancet 1966;1:1066–1068.

40. Lindenbaum J, Greenough WB, Islam MR. Antibiotic therapy of cholera in children. Bull WHO 1967;37:529–538.

41. Meadors MC, Pankey GA. *Vibrio vulnificus* wound infection treated successfully with oral ciprofloxacin. J Infect Dis 1989; 20:88–89.

42. McCormack WM, Chowdhury AM, Jahangir N, Ahmed AB, Mosley WH. Tetracycline prophylaxis in families of cholera patients. Bull WHO 1968;38:787–792.

43. Mhalu FS, Mmari PW, Ijumba J. Rapid emergence of El Tor *Vibrio cholerae* resistant to antimicrobial agents during first six months of fourth cholera epidemic in Tanzania. Lancet 1979;1: 345–347.

44. Pastore G, Rizzo G, Fera G. Trimethoprim and sulphamethoxazole in the treatment of cholera. Comparison with tetracycline and chloramphenicol. Chemotherapy 1977;23:121–128.

45. Pierce NF, Banwell JG, Mitra RC, Caranasos GJ, Keimowitz JRI, Thomas J, Mondal A. Controlled comparison of tetracycline and furazolidone in cholera. Br Med J 1968;3:277–280.

46. Rabbani GH, Butler T, Shahrier M, Mazundar R, Islam MR. Efficacy of a single dose of furazolidone for treatment of cholera in children. Antimicrob Agents Chemother 1991;35:1864–1867.

47. Rabbani GH, Islam MR, Butler T, Sharier M, Alam K. Single-dose treatment of cholera with furazolidone or tetracycline in a double-blind randomized trial. Antimicrob Agents Chemother 1989,33:1447–1450.

48. Rahaman MM, Majid MA, Alam AKM, Islam MR. Effects of doxycycline in actively purging cholera patients: a double-blind clinical trial. Antimicrob Agents Chemother 1976;10:610–612.

49. Sack DA, Islam S, Rabbani GH, Islam A. Single-dose doxycycline for cholera. Antimicrob Agents Chemother 1978;14: 462–464.

50. Schaad UB, Salam MA, Aujard Y. Use of fluoroquinolones in pediatrics: consensus report of an International Society of Chemotherapy commission. Pediatr Infect Dis 1995;14:1–9.

51. Seas C, DuPont HL, Valdez LM, Gotuzzo E. Practical guidelines for the treatment of cholera. Drugs 1996;51:966–973.

52. Seas C. Gotuzzo E. Recent advances in the treatment and prophylaxis of cholera. Curr Opin Infect Dis 1996;9:380–384.

53. Seas C, Gotuzzo E. Cholera: overview of epidemiologic, therapeutic, and preventive issues learned from recent epidemics. Int J Infect Dis 1996;1:37–46.

54. Wallace CK, Anderson PN, Brown TC, Khanra SR, Lewis GH, Pierce NF, Sanyal SN, Serge SV, Waldman RH. Optimal antibiotic therapy in cholera. Bull WHO 1968;39:239–245.

55. WHO. Guidelines for cholera control. Geneva: WHO, 1993.

56. Yamamoto T, Nair GB, Albert MJ, Carrillo C, Takeda Y. Survey of in-vitro susceptibilities of *V. cholerae* O1 and O139 to antimicrobial agents. Antimicrob Agents Chemother 1995;39:241–244.

Yersinia enterocolitica

●

Maurice R. Scavizzi

GENERAL DESCRIPTION

Yersinia enterocolitica was first described in 1934 (40) as a Gram-negative coccobacillus and considered an atypical form of some well-known species or perhaps a new species. In 1939 this first isolate and four others were described as resembling *Pasteurella* (*Yersinia* now) *pseudotuberculosis* but sufficiently different to be a new species (62). *Y. enterocolitica* infection in humans has received increasing attention over the last 30 years because of its common occurrence in several countries, especially in northern and western Europe and North America (10, 17, 23, 43–45, 47, 55, 61, 70).

Microbiology

Y. enterocolitica is one of 11 species of *Yersinia*. Yersiniae are Gram-negative bacteria, members of the family *Enterobacteriaceae*. *Y. enterocolitica* has been isolated from nonclinical and clinical specimens. Stools, mesenteric lymph nodes, pharyngeal exudates, peritoneal fluid, or blood cultures may yield *Yersinia*, depending on the clinical syndrome. Many laboratories isolate *Y. enterocolitica* from contaminated material only on request because routine use of special selective media for *Y. enterocolitica* is a low-yield procedure. Most isolates can be serotyped as one of more than 50 serotypes according to somatic O antigens. Only certain biotypes and serotypes of *Y. enterocolitica* are considered invasive pathogens (i.e., serotypes 03; 05, 27; 08; 09).

A rapid polymerase chain reaction method has been developed to detect and differentiate both *Y. enterocolitica* and *Y. pseudotuberculosis* and detect their virulence-associated genes directly from cultures (19, 46, 76).

Epidemiology

Y. enterocolitica is relatively common in northern and western Europe (mainly serotypes 03 and 09), in Canada, and to a lesser extent in the United States (mainly serotypes 08 and 05, 27 (30)); however, serotype 03 is increasing as an enteric pathogen, especially in New York City and California (5, 35, 41). *Y. enterocolitica* has been isolated from nearly all parts of the world, including Asia, Africa, South America, and Australia.

Children are more often infected than adults. Transmission occurs by ingestion of contaminated food or water and, less commonly, by direct contact with infected animals or patients.

Y. enterocolitica is widely distributed in aquatic and animal reservoirs, with swine serving as a major reservoir for human pathogenic strains. In Europe, *Y. enterocolitica* is frequently isolated from pigs' tonsils and tongues at slaughterhouses; thus ingestion of undercooked pork is important in disease transmission (34). The ability of yersiniae to grow at 4°C means that refrigerated foods are sources of infection. Knowl-

edge of epidemiologic yersiniae features makes it possible to apply relevant preventive schemes against infection.

Pathogenesis

The usual means of acquisition of *Y. enterocolitica* is contaminated foods. Virulent *Y. enterocolitica* organisms initially use chromosomally mediated outer membrane proteins expressed at low temperature to promote invasion of epithelial cells; at this point, the principal gene involved in the process is *inv*, expressed maximally at 28°C. Other chromosomal gene loci, especially the *ail* gene (attachment invasion locus) are expressed mainly at 37°C (42).

Plasmid genes (plasmid pYV) (54) code for several temperature- and calcium-regulated outer membrane proteins (Yops, mainly Yad A) expressed at 37°C but not at 25°C (67, 68). In this way, bacterial invasion and their establishment within the susceptible host is facilitated. Only plasmid-positive strains are resistant to phagocytosis by polymorphonuclear leukocytes and to intracellular killing by macrophages (20). For example, the Yop B protein suppresses expression of a macrophage-derived cytokine (TNF-α)(4). Yop H acts on dephosphorylate eucaryotic proteins, especially in phagocytic cells (6). Yad A acts as an adhesin and independently enhances resistance to serum bactericidal activity (3, 38) in the same way as the ail protein (7, 52, 74). Thus virulent yersiniae attach to, and penetrate, the mucous layer overlying mucosal epithelial cells and adhere to intestinal cell brush border membranes (37). They penetrate M cells overlying Peyer's patches to gain access to and multiply (as salmonellae and shigellae do) in lamina propria, the subjacent tissue (11, 25, 26). Continued proliferation of bacteria in the lamina propria enables bacterial survival and spreads to other organs (e.g., liver, spleen, and mesenteric lymph nodes). Nonpathogenic yersiniae also cross the intestinal tract via M cells but are eliminated without disturbing the histologic structure of Peyer's patches. This pathogenic scheme indicates that yersiniae are mostly intracellular parasites, which means that the pharmacologic parameters of antibiotics, especially their intracellular diffusion, affect their in vivo efficacy.

Clinical Manifestations

Enterocolitis is the most frequent manifestation. In serious cases, perforation of the ileum may occur. Fecal excretion of *Y. enterocolitica* may continue for weeks after symptoms have subsided. Most patients with this syndrome are children. Mesenteric adenitis and/or terminal ileitis that may be clinically indistinguishable from acute appendicitis is most common in older children and adolescents.

Septicemia is less common. It is normally reported in patients with diabetes mellitus, hemoglobinopathy, hemochromatosis, cirrhosis, malignancy, renal failure, or other chronic underlying disease, or in elderly patients. To grow and establish an infection, pathogenic bacteria must obtain iron from mammalian tissues. Thus in iron-overloaded patients, systemic infection may occur. Furthermore, treatment of these patients with an iron chelator (desferrioxamine) has been particularly associated with yersiniae sepsis (13). Moreover, the serogroup 08 *Y. enterocolitica* produces and secretes its own iron chelator (siderophore) and thus requires only a low iron load in patients to ensure a systemic infection (12). All *Y. enterocolitica* pathogenic serogroups—09, 03, 05, 27 as 08—produce an iron-repressible outer membrane polypeptide that functions as a receptor for transporting chelated iron to the interior of the bacterial cell (28).

Bacterial contamination of blood for transfusion is uncommon, but in this event, morbidity and mortality are significant (septic shock and fatal bacteremia) (53). Septicemic patients may develop hepatic or splenic abscesses, osteomyelitis, wound infections, or meningitis. Endocarditis and aneurysms due to *Y. enterocolitica* have been reported. Exudative *pharyngitis, pneumonia, emphysema, and lung abscess* have also been reported (24).

Sequelae

Secondary immunologically mediated sequelae of acute *Y. enterocolitica* infection such as arthritis and erythema nodosum (the most common), Reiter's syndrome, glomerulonephritis, and myocarditis have been reported predominantly among Scandinavians (up to 30%) and in *Y. enterocolitica* serogroup 03 phage type 8 infections. The few patients who have persisting postyersinial reactive arthritis (>12 months) and patients with Reiter's syndrome are HLA-B27 positive (9); there is no clear reason for this.

Nosocomial Infections

Nosocomial *Y. enterocolitica* outbreaks of diarrheal disease have been reported (69); however, this is more likely common-source contamination than person-to-person spread.

SUSCEPTIBILITY IN VITRO AND IN VIVO

Strains exhibiting plasmid-mediated resistance to multiple antibiotics are very rare; only 15 such strains were isolated worldwide in 1982 (31) and very few since then. Thus, antibiotics known to be active against aerobic Gram-negative rods are active in vitro against *Y. enterocolitica,* with one important exception—the older β-lactam agents.

Aminoglycosides, Tetracyclines, and Fluoroquinolones

Aminoglycosides, tetracyclines, and fluoroquinolones are all regularly active in vitro (Table 1). The four main aminoglycosides, gentamicin, tobramycin, netilmicin, and amikacin, have been used for a long time; amikacin is unnecessary because of the regular absence of strains producing aminoglycoside-modifying enzymes. Doxycycline is the tetracycline that has been most used for at least two decades. Pefloxacin, ofloxacin,

TABLE 1 • In Vitro Comparative Activities of Antibiotics against *Y. enterocolitica* Clinical Isolates[a]

Antibiotic	MIC$_{50}$[b]	MIC$_{90}$[b]	Range
Ampicillin	32	64	4–128
Amoxicillin plus clavulanic acid	4	16	1–≥16
Ticarcillin	128	128	0.5–128
Piperacillin	2	4	0.25–8
Cephalothin	256	256	8–512
Cefoxitin	16	64	1–64
Cefamandole	4	8	0.5–16
Ceftazidime	0.125	0.5	0.06–1
Cefmenoxime	0.125	0.25	≤0.016–0.5
Ceftizoxime	0.06	0.25	≤0.016–1
Cefotaxime	0.06	0.25	0.03–0.5
Ceftriaxone	0.06	0.125	0.03–0.25
Aztreonam	0.5	2	0.06–2
Imipenem	0.25	0.5	0.06–0.5
Gentamicin	1	2	0.5–4
Tobramycin	1	1	0.25–4
Netilmicin	1	1	0.50–4
Amikacin	2	2	1–4
Pefloxacin	0.125	0.25	0.06–0.5
Ofloxacin	0.06	0.125	0.06–0.125
Ciprofloxacin	0.015	0.03	0.015–0.03
Tetracycline	2	4	1–4
Doxycycline	0.5	1	≤0.25–1
Cotrimoxazole	0.5	4	0.25–16

[a] Data from references 22, 30, 56, 58, 66.

[b] MIC for 50 and 90% of strains, expressed in mg/L.

and ciprofloxacin have begun to be tested against *Y. enterocolitica* and more recently used against infections due to this species (2, 29).

Cotrimoxazole

Y. enterocolitica strains are occasionally resistant to trimethoprim and/or sulfamides (e.g., 7 of 63 strains (31)).

Rifampicin and Chloramphenicol

Both rifampicin and chloramphenicol are active in vitro, but rifampicin must be restricted to mycobacterial infections as much as possible, and chloramphenicol can lead to rare but severe toxic effects.

Aminopenicillins and First-Generation Cephalosporins

For 25 years, the entire species has been shown by MIC population analysis to be resistant to these older β-lactams (58) because of production of broad-spectrum penicillinase and/or inducible cephalosporinase (15, 16). The synthesis of these two enzymes depends upon the serotype and biotype of the bacteria, which explains the different patterns of susceptibility to β-lactams among strains (14, 30, 31, 39, 51, 59). The two sorts of β-lactamase were biochemically characterized (14, 15, 59); their pIs are 5.6 for cephalosporinase, 8.5 for penicillinase in serogroup 08, 8.7 for penicillinase in serogroups 03 and 09, etc. These enzymes were shown to be chromosomally mediated.

The two genes encoding for β-lactamases were cloned individually into a plasmid vector and expressed in *Escherichia coli* (64). The gene for broad-spectrum penicillinase was cloned from a serotype 03 strain and the gene for inducible cephalosporinase was cloned from a serotype 05, 27 strain. The nucleotide sequence of a fragment from the chromosome of *Y. enterocolitica* containing the gene for penicillinase was determined (65). An open-reading-frame was identified and the amino acid sequence deduced: the broad-spectrum penicillinase of *Y. enterocolitica* is an Ambler molecular class A β-lactamase (1, 65). The nucleotide sequence of a fragment of chromosomal DNA containing both the structural gene for the cephalosporinase *(ampC)* and an adjacent gene was determined; the latter is homologous to the regulatory *ampR* gene; the *ampC* gene is homologous to other enterobacterial chromosomal cephalosporinase genes (63). Thus, the inducible cephalosporinase of *Y. enterocolitica* is an Ambler molecular class C β-lactamase (1).

Carboxypenicillins, Ureidopenicillins, Second-Generation Cephalosporins, and Amoxicillin/Clavulanic Acid

The bacteriostatic and (even more) the bactericidal activity of carboxy- and ureidopenicillins depends on whether or not the *Y. enterocolitica* strains produce penicillinase. These two groups of penicillins cannot be used habitually because most strains produce this enzyme, especially serogroups 03, 08, 09, frequent in North America and northern and western Europe (30, 59). In fact, the apparent susceptibility to piperacillin on the basis of MICs (Table 1) has to be corrected by the MBC:MIC ratio, which expressed in dilution factors ($\log_2$) was calculated to be 5 to 7 ($MBC_{50} = 64$ mg/L) (30); this agrees with the slight hydrolysis of ureidopenicillins by β-lactamases.

Similarly, cefoxitin and cefamandole with a wide range of MICs (Table 1) cannot be recommended.

Susceptibility to the combination amoxicillin/clavulanic acid varies with biotype and serotype but is most often in the intermediate range (Table 1). This may be explained by the inactivity of clavulanic acid against cephalosporinase, which partially hydrolyzes aminopenicillins. However, some isolates from Australia, New Zealand, and Canada that belong to serotype 03 phage type IXb express only penicillinase and thus are susceptible to amoxicillin/clavulanic acid (50).

Third-Generation Cephalosporins, Aztreonam, and Imipenem

Some newer β-lactams that are not actually hydrolyzed by β-lactamases have been suggested as alternatives for treatment of *Y. enterocolitica* infection on the basis of their very low MICs (Table 1) (30, 31, 73). However, an MBC:MIC ratio of 7 was calculated for aztreonam ($MBC_{50} = 32$ mg/L), and 4 to 5 for third-generation cephalosporins ($MBC_{50} = 1$ to 4 mg/L). Imipenem is the only β-lactam with a ratio of 1 ($MBC_{50} = 0.25$ mg/L) (30).

Even when in vitro susceptibility is clear (no bacterial resistance mechanism), in vivo efficacy is not guaranteed and depends more particularly on pharmacologic properties; this is the case for pathogenic yersiniae, which replicate intracellularly for the most part. In any case, the efficacy of an antibiotic is difficult to evaluate on the basis of clinical studies because it is influenced by several factors, including the severity and localization of the focus of infection, underlying diseases, the immune status of the host, interactions with other drugs, and the criteria chosen for assessing success or failure. Therefore, experimental therapeutic effects in a stringent animal model can help in interpretation of the efficacy of a drug.

ANIMAL MODELS

In experimental animal infection due to yersiniae (as with other organisms), stringent requirements have been gradually fixed and followed (8, 21, 36, 57, 60): *(a)* a strain with defined molecular characteristics of virulence, *(b)* an inoculum that ensures constant and exponential kinetics of bacteria in animal organs and a fixed interval of time for the death of the animals, *(c)* initiation of therapy when the infection is irreversibly established and histologically confirmed, *(d)* dosage regimens that achieve early concentrations in animal serum and tissues similar to those found in humans, *(e)* a treatment time that is the shortest for a change from the death of all control animals to survival of all animals treated by the effective reference drug, *(f)* periods of time between two injections of a drug that equal the time required to reach the nadir of the bacterial killing curve in animal organs from a single dose, before bacterial regrowth. In this way the efficacies of antibiotics are compared independently of the specific lengths of their in vivo activities. Drugs that fail in this animal model could perhaps succeed under less stringent conditions, but the drugs that succeed with such stringent requirements will probably succeed in humans.

This kind of animal model was used (57, 60) for murine systemic infection due to *Y. enterocolitica,* and it

- Confirmed the ineffectiveness of aminopenicillins (older β-lactams)
- Demonstrated that the efficacy of a third-generation cephalosporin, ceftriaxone, was very moderate since high doses were needed (200 mg/kg body weight); ceftriaxone appears to be the most effective of the third-generation cephalosporins, perhaps because of its specific pharmacologic properties—long half-life and good intracellular penetration (33)
- Confirmed the effectiveness of gentamicin (aminoglycoside) at moderate doses (20 mg/kg), despite the fact that these antibiotics in their active form accumulate only slowly in cells (71)
- Confirmed the effectiveness of doxycycline (tetracycline) at high doses (125 mg/kg); this can be related to two characteristics: the essentially bacteriostatic activity and the cellular penetration of these drugs
- Demonstrated that fluoroquinolones are the most effective antibiotics even at low doses (5 mg/kg of ofloxacin), perhaps because of their good penetration into the cells (71, 72)

The experimental results observed in this animal model make it clear that the pharmacologic properties of antibiotics affect their in vivo efficacy, particularly on pathogenic yersiniae, which are mostly intracellular parasites. Of course other parameters are involved in the discrepancies between the in vitro and in vivo effects of antibiotics; therapy experiments in animal models help us establish and analyze clinical studies.

ANTIMICROBIAL THERAPY

Specific antimicrobial chemotherapy is variable, depending on whether the clinical disease is self-limited or systemic and whether the host is compromised or not. The 1982 recommendations of the World Health Organization (WHO) for antibiotic treatments of infections with *Y. enterocolitica* included chloramphenicol, cotrimoxazole, gentamicin, and tetracycline (75).

Historical Perspectives

Analysis of clinical successes and failures is difficult because numerous elements linked to the patient's condition affect the effectiveness of treatment. For the last 30 years, several studies on infections and their treatment have been carried out (10, 17, 43, 44, 47, 55, 70), especially three studies at 10-year intervals using the same methods on Western European and North American patients with septicemia.

The first of these studies (45) reported cases between 1966 and 1970. Mortality was close to 50%, a high rate that can be explained by *(a)* delay in identifying *Y. enterocolitica, (b)* quasi-systematic use of an aminopenicillin in the first instance, and *(c)* interpretation of the antibiotic susceptibility tests that too frequently favored aminopenicillin activity.

The second study (61) reported 53 cases since 1970. The mortality rate was 25%, which did not vary between the early years (1970–1976) and the end of the period (1977–1982).

The third study, published in 1993, reported 53 cases since 1985 (23). The mortality rate was 7.5%. The earlier improvement followed by such spectacular progress was due to *(a)* better knowledge of *Y. enterocolitica* and its susceptibility to antibiotics (in particular, the ineffectiveness of aminopenicillins and first-generation cephalosporins), *(b)* rapid replacement aminopenicillin still often prescribed empirically by an active drug, and *(c)* measured use of active molecules.

The results of therapy in septicemias due to *Y. enterocolitica* were as follows (Table 2):

- Older β-lactams (i.e., aminopenicillins and first-generation cephalosporins) are systematically ineffective (61). Carboxy- and ureidopenicillins are active in vitro against serotype 05, 27 strains that express only cephalosporinase. But these penicillins and second-generation cephalosporins are ineffective against the vast majority of pathogenic strains that express both β-lactamases.
- Amoxicillin/clavulanic acid is ineffective in vivo on strains from the United States and northern and western Europe (23). Some strains (biotype 4, serotype 03, phage type IXb) from Australia, New Zealand, and Canada that lack the cephalosporinase are susceptible in vitro to this combination (50). Ticarcillin/clavulanic acid and piperacillin/tazobactam have not been studied; they could be active, considering what we know about resistance mechanisms.

TABLE 2 • Outcome of Antibiotic Treatment of *Y. enterocolitica* Septicemia in 43 Patients

Regimen[a]	No. of Patients with Indicated Outcome	
	Failure	Success
Benzylpenicillin	5	0
Amoxicillin	11	0
Amoxicillin plus aminoglycoside	2	0
Amoxicillin/clavulanic acid	6	0
Amoxicillin/clavulanic acid plus cotrimoxazole	1	0
Amoxicillin/clavulanic acid plus aminoglycoside	0	1
Piperacillin plus aminoglycoside	0	1
Imipenem plus aminoglycoside	1	0
Third-generation cephalosporin only	1	3
Third-generation cephalosporin plus aminoglycoside	3	14
Fluoroquinolone plus third-generation cephalosporin	0	6
Fluoroquinolone plus aminoglycoside	0	5
Fluoroquinolone only	0	4
Doxycycline	0	6[b]
Doxycycline plus aminoglycoside	2	0
Cotrimoxazole plus aminoglycoside	0	1
Rifampicin plus aminoglycoside	0	1
Total	32[c]	42

Data from Gayraud M, Scavizzi MR, Mollaret HH, Guillevin L, Hornstein MJ. Antibiotic treatment of *Yersinia enterocolitica* septicemia: a retrospective review of 43 cases. Clin Infect Dis 1993;17:405–410.

[a] According to the results of in vitro tests, all strains were categorized as intermediately susceptible or resistant to amoxicillin (MICs, 4–128 mg/l) and as susceptible, intermediately susceptible, or resistant to amoxicillin/clavulanic acid (MICs, 2–64 mg/L). All strains were resistant to benzylpenicillin. All other drugs tested were active in vitro.

[b] Apparently moderate severity of infections.

[c] Two regimens failed in four patients and four in one patient.

- The newer β-lactams, particularly third-generation cephalosporins, have been 75 to 80% successful, even when prescribed as monotherapy; the most consistently effective is ceftriaxone. Carbapenems and monobactams have been very rarely prescribed, but imipenem has an excellent bactericidal effect unlike aztreonam (30, 31).
- Aminoglycosides used in combination with an active in vitro antibiotic are 75% effective, but only two times out of five when used with an inactive in vitro antibiotic (23).
- There is a 75% success rate with tetracylines (doxycycline), but the infections treated with these drugs were only moderately serious (23).
- The rare patients treated with cotrimoxazole have shown both success and failure (23, 61). In any event, strains are not regularly susceptible (31).

Thus, failures have been reported with all the antibiotics recommended by WHO. On the other hand, 15 patients treated with fluoroquinolones alone or in association with another antibiotic were all cured (23). Moreover, apyrexia was obtained in an average of 2 days (vs. 6 days with third-generation cephalosporins). These results are similar to those obtained in the animal experiments: the bactericidal effect was much more rapid with ofloxacin at a dose of 5 mg/kg than with ceftriaxone at a dose of 200 mg/kg (60).

General

For the treatment of *Y. enterocolitica* infections the following rules could be applied. Penicillins, first- and second-generation cephalosporins, and amoxicillin/clavulanic acid must not be used against the vast majority of pathogenic yersiniae. Third-generation cephalosporins, aminoglycosides, and tetracyclines are possible agents for use on their own or in association, depending on the clinical diagnosis, the severity of the infection, and the individual case.

Drugs of Choice

Fluoroquinolones constitute the best treatment because of their *(a)* in vitro activity (2), *(b)* pharmacologic properties (18, 71, 72), *(c)* proven efficacy in animal experiments (60), and *(d)* clinical results (23, 29). Because similar results were obtained in vitro and in animal experiments for *Y. pseudotuberculosis* and *Y. pestis* (8, 36), further clinical investigations should be carried out into fluoroquinolones and these yersiniae.

The dosages in usual practice are summarized in Table 3. Choice of monotherapy or combination therapy depends on the clinical form of the infection and the state of the patient. All combinations have been tested in vitro and administered in vivo without any adverse effect (Table 2). Duration of treatment depends on the clinical form of infection and follows closely the rules used for infections due to Gram-negative bacteria.

Specific Infections

Enterocolitis and Mesenteric Adenitis

The value of antimicrobial therapy in enterocolitis and mesenteric adenitis in unclear because these infections are usually self-limited. Treatment of enterocolitis with antibiotics short-

TABLE 3 • Antibiotics and Dosages Proposed for the Treatment of *Y. enterocolitica* Infections

Antibiotic	Dosage/Day
Fluoroquinolones[a,b]	
Pefloxacin	800 mg
Ofloxacin	400 mg
Ciprofloxacin	1 g
Third-generation cephalosporins	
Cefotaxime, ceftriaxone, ceftazidime, ceftizoxime[a]	2–6 g
Cefixime[b]	800 mg
Aminoglycosides[a,c]	
Gentamicin, tobramycin	3 mg/kg
Netilmicin	4–6 mg/kg
Amikacin	15 mg/kg
Doxycycline[a,b]	200 mg

[a] Drugs are administered i.v. and/or i.m.

[b] Drugs are administered per os.

[c] Dosages are adapted to the renal function if necessary.

ened the persistence of IgG anti-*Yersinia* antibodies to about 3 months (32). Laparotomy for suspected appendicitis should be avoided when *Yersinia* infection is a likely diagnosis. Treating enterocolitis was recommended in compromised hosts (17). It is advisable to withhold desferrioxamine (when indicated) and use doxycyline (Table 2) rather than cotrimoxazole for complicated *Y. enterocolitica* gastrointestinal infection. If cotrimoxazole shows in vitro activity, in most cases it has little effect on the clinical course (duration) of *Y. enterocolitica* gastroenteritis (49).

Septicemia

Of course, antibiotic therapy is needed in systemic infections, and combination therapy is necessary in the compromised host. The drug of choice is a fluoroquinolone (pefloxacin, ofloxacin, or ciprofloxacin) in combination with a third-generation cephalosporin or an aminoglycoside. Up to now, such a treatment has been the most successful. Dosages are indicated in Table 3. Alternative therapy consisting of the conventional association between a third-generation cephalosporin (especially ceftriaxone) and an aminoglycoside has generally resulted in success but with several failures (Table 2).

ADJUNCTIVE MEASURES

Public health measures to control infection due to *Y. enterocolitica*, as with other pathogenic *Enterobacteriaceae*, should focus on the animal reservoirs. Methods of raising and slaughtering pigs can be modified to reduce contamination of meat with the contents of the oral cavity and the intestinal tract during slaughter. Because *Y. enterocolitica* can grow at 4°C, meat should not be refrigerated for prolonged periods before consumption. Consumption of uncooked meats (e.g., chitterlings) should be avoided. In dairies, care must be taken to prevent contamination of milk after pasteurization. In blood banks, suggestions have been made to reduce the incidence of contaminated transfusions (27, 48, 53).

COMMENTS AND CONTROVERSIES

The question of antimicrobial therapy in infections due to *Y. enterocolitica* has been examined from every point of view: molecular, biochemical, bacteriologic, pharmacologic, in animal experiments, and finally in clinics. Some rules are available at the present time: fluoroquinolones, third-generation cephalosporins (especially ceftriaxone), aminoglycosides, and cyclines (doxycycline) are effective drugs. They can be chosen in accordance with the clinical form, but fluoroquinolones appear now to be the most effective, particularly in systemic infections. Some authors maintain that piperacillin or cotrimoxazole can be used, but I believe that the former leads to quasi-systematic failures and that the latter is unreliably effective.

Rifampicin and phenicols are active in vitro and effective in vivo, but their use is not generally recommended because the former must be restricted to mycobacterial infections and the latter can lead to rare but severe toxic effects. Strains exhibiting plasmid-mediated resistance to multiple antibiotics are very rare, but emergence of resistant organisms is theoretically possible.

REFERENCES

1. Ambler RP. The structure of β-lactamases. Phil Trans R Soc Lond B 1980;289:321–331.
2. Auckenthaler R, Michea-Hamzempour M, Pechere JC. In vitro activity of newer quinolones against aerobic bacteria. J Antimicrob Chemother 1986;17(Suppl B):29–39.
3. Balligand G, Laroche Y, Cornelis G. Genetic analysis of virulence plasmid from a serogroup 9 *Yersinia enterocolitica* strain: role of outer membrane protein P1 in resistance to human serum and autoagglutination. Infect Immun 1985;48:782–786.
4. Beuscher HR, Rodel F, Forsberg A, Rollinghoff M. Bacterial evasion of host immune response: *Yersinia enterocolitica* encodes a suppressor for tumor necrosis factor alpha expression. Infect Immun 1995;63:1270–1277.
5. Bisset J, Powers LC, Abbott SL, Janda JM. Epidemiologic investigations of *Yersinia enterocolitica* and related species: sources, frequency, and serogroup distribution. J Clin Microbiol 1990;28:910–912.
6. Bliska JB, Clemens JC, Dixon JE, Falkow S. The *Yersinia* tyrosine phosphatase: specificity of a bacterial virulence determinant for phosphoproteins in the J774 A.1 macrophage. J Exp Med 1992;176:1625–1630.
7. Bliska JB, Falkow S. Bacterial resistance to complement killing mediated by the ail protein of *Yersinia enterocolitica*. Proc Natl Acad Sci USA 1992;89:3561–3565.
8. Bonacorsi SP, Scavizzi MR, Guiyoule A, Amouroux JH, Carniel E. Assessment of a fluoroquinolone, three β-lactams, two aminoglycosides, and a cycline in treatment of murine *Yersinia pestis* infection. Antimicrob Agents Chemother 1994;38:481–486.
9. Borg AA, Gray J, Dawes PT. Yersinia-related arthritis in the United Kingdom. A report of 12 cases and review of the literature. Q J Med (New Ser 84) 1992;304:575–582.
10. Bottone EJ. *Yersinia enterocolitica:* a panoramic view of a charismatic microorganism. CRC Crit Rev Microbiol 1977;5: 211–241.
11. Carter PB. Pathogenicity of *Yersinia enterocolitica* for mice. Infect Immun 1981;11:164–178.
12. Chambers CE, Sokol PE. Comparison of siderophore production and utilization in pathogenic and environmental isolates of *Yersinia enterocolitica*. J Clin Microbiol 1994;32:32–39.
13. Chiu HY, Flynn DM, Hoffbrand AV. Infection with *Yersinia enterocolitica* in patients with iron overload. Br Med J 1986; 292:97.
14. Cornelis G. Distribution of β-lactamases A and B in some groups of *Y. enterocolitica* and their role in resistance. J Gen Microbiol 1975;91:391–402.
15. Cornelis G, Abraham EP. β-Lactamases from *Yersinia enterocolitica*. J Gen Microbiol 1975;87:273–284.
16. Cornelis G, Wauters G, Vanderhaeghe H. Présence de β-lactamase chez *Yersinia enterocolitica*. Ann Microbiol (Paris) 1973;124B:139–152.
17. Cover TL, Aber RC. *Yersinia enterocolitica*. N Engl J Med 1989;321:16–24.
18. Easmon CFS, Crane JP, Blowers A. Effect of ciprofloxain on intracellular organisms: in vitro and in vivo studies. J Antimicrob Chemother 1986;18(Suppl D):43–48.
19. Fenwick SG, Murray A. Detection of pathogenic *Yersinia enterocolitica* by polymerase chain reaction. Lancet 1991;337: 496–497.
20. Forsberg A, Rosqvist R, Wolf-Watz H. Regulation and polarized transfer of the *Yersinia* outer proteins (Yops) involved in antiphagocytosis. Trends Microbiol 1994;2:14–19.
21. Fournier JL, Ramisse F, Jacolot AC, Szatanik M, Petitjean OJ, Alonso JM, Scavizzi MR. Assessment of two penicillines plus β-lactamase inhibitors versus cefotaxime in treatment of murine *Klebsiella pneumoniae* infections. Antimicrob Agents Chemother 1996;40:325–330.
22. Gaspar MC, Soriano F. Susceptibility of *Yersinia enterocolitica* to eight β-lactam antibiotics and clavulanic acid. J Antimicrob Chemother 1981;8:161–164.
23. Gayraud M, Scavizzi MR, Mollaret HH, Guillevin L, Hornstein MJ. Antibiotic treatment of *Yersinia enterocolitica* septicemia: a retrospective review of 43 cases. Clin Infect Dis 1993;17: 405–410.
24. Greene JN, Herndon P, Nadler JP. Case report: *Yersinia enterocolitica* necrotizing pneumonia in an immunocompromised patient. Am J Med Sci 1993;305:171–173.
25. Grützkau A, Hanski C, Naumann M. Comparative study of histopathological alterations during intestinal infection of mice with pathogenic and non-pathogenic strains of *Yersinia enterocolitica* serotype 0:8. Virchows Arch A Pathol Anat Histopathol 1993;423:97–103.
26. Hanski C, Kutschka V, Schmoranzer HP, Nauman M, Stallmach A, Hahn H, Menge H, Riechen EO. Immunohistochemical and electron microscopic study of interaction of *Yersinia enterocolitica* serotype 0:8 with intestinal during experimental enteritis. Infect Immun 1989;57:673–678.
27. Hastings JGM, Batta K, Gourevitch D, Williams MD, Rees E, Palmer M, Smilie J. Fatal transfusion reaction due to *Yersinia enterocolitica*. J Hosp Infect 1994;27:75–79.
28. Heesemann J, Hantke K, Vocke T, Saken E, Stoljiljkovic I, Berner R. Virulence of *Yersinia enterocolitica* is closely associated with siderophore production, expression of an iron-repressible outer membrane polypeptide of 65,000 Da and pesticin sensitivity. Mol Microbiol 1993;8:397–408.
29. Hoogkamp-Korstanje JAA. The possible role of quinolones in Yersiniosis. Drugs 1987;34(Suppl 1):134–138.
30. Hornstein MJ, Jupeau AM, Scavizzi MR, Philippon AM, Grimont PAD. In vitro susceptibilities of 126 clinical isolates of *Yersinia enterocolitica* to 21 β-lactam antibiotics. Antimicrob Agents Chemother 1985;27:806–811.

31. Jupeau A, Hornstein M, Philippon A, Scavizzi M. Sensibilité in vitro de *Yersinia* aux antibiotiques. Activité des β-lactamines sur *Yersinia enterocolitica*. Med Mal Infect 1982; 12:675–681.

32. Kihlstrom E, Foberg U, Bengtsson A. Intestinal symptoms and serological response in patients with complicated and uncomplicated *Yersinia enterocolitica* infections. Scand J Infect Dis 1992;24:57–63.

33. Kuhn H, Angerhn P, Havas L. Autoradiographic evidence for penetration of ^{3}H-ceftriaxone (Rocephin) into cells of spleen, liver and kidney of mice. Chemother 1986;32:102–112.

34. Lee LA, Gerber AR, Lonsway DR, Smith JD, Carter GP, Pohr ND, Parrish CM, Sikes RK, Finton RJ, Tauxe RW. *Yersinia enterocolitica* 0:3 infection in infants and children associated with the household preparation of chitterlings. N Engl J Med 1990; 322:984–987.

35. Lee LA, Taylor J, Carter GP, Quinn B, Farmer JJ III, Tauxe RV, and the *Yersinia enterocolitica* Collaboration Study Group. *Yersinia enterocolitica* 0:3: an emergence cause of pediatric gastroenteritis in the United States. J Infect Dis 1990;163:660–663.

36. Lemaitre BC, Mazigh DA, Scavizzi MR. Failure of beta-lactam antibiotics and marked efficacy of fluoroquinolones in treatment of murine *Yersinia pseudotuberculosis* infection. Antimicrob Agents Chemother 1991;35:1785–1790.

37. Mantle M, Husar SD. Adhesion of *Yersinia enterocolitica* to purified rabbit and intestinal mucin. Infect Immun 1993;61: 2340–2346.

38. Martinez R. Thermoregulation-dependent expression of *Yersinia enterocolitica* protein 1 imparts serum resistance to *Escherichia coli* K-12. J Bacteriol 1989;171:3732–3739.

39. Matthew M, Cornelis G, Wauters G. Correlation of serological and biochemical groupings of *Y. enterocolitica* with the beta-lactamases of the strains. J Gen Microbiol 1977;102:55–59.

40. McIver MA, Pike RM. Chronic glanders-like infection of face caused by an organism resembling *Flavobacterium pseudomallei* Whitmore. In: Clinical miscellany, vol 1. Cooperstone, NY: Mary Imogene Basset Hospital, 1934:16–21.

41. Metchock B, Lonsway DL, Carter GP, Lee LA, Mc Gowan JE Jr. *Yersinia enterocolitica:* a frequent seasonal stool isolate from children at an urban hospital in the southeast United States. J Clin Microb 1991;29:2868–2869.

42. Miller VL, Falkow S. Evidence for two genetic loci in *Yersinia enterocolitica* that can promote invasion of epithelial cells. Immun 1988;56:1242–1248.

43. Mollaret HH. L'infection humaine à *Y. enterocolitica*. Pathol Biol 1966;14:981–990.

44. Mollaret HH. L'infection humaine à *Y. enterocolitica* en 1970, à la lumière de 642 cas récents. Pathol Biol 1971;19:189–205.

45. Mollaret HH, Omland T, Henriksen SD, Baeroe PR, Rykner G, Scavizzi M. Les septicémies humaines à *Yersinia enterocolitica*. A propos de 17 cas récents. Presse Med 1971;79:345–348.

46. Nakajima H, Inoue M, Mori T, Itoh KI, Arakawa E, Watanabe H. Detection and identification of *Yersinia pseudotuberculosis* and pathogenic *Yersinia enterocolitica* by an improved polymerase chain reaction method. J Clin Microb 1992;30: 2484–2486.

47. Nilhen B. Studies on *Y. enterocolitica* with special reference to bacterial diagnosis and occurrence in human acute enteric disease. Acta Pathol Microbiol Scand 1969;206(Suppl):1–48.

48. Nusbacher J. *Yersinia enterocolitica* and white cell filtration. Transfusion 1992;32:597–600.

49. Pai CH, Gillis F, Tuomanen, Marks MI. Placebo-controlled double-blind evaluation of trimethoprim-sulfamethoxazole treatment of *Yersinia enterocolitica* gastroenteritis. J Pediatr 1994; 104:308–311.

50. Pham JN, Bell SM, Hardy MJ, Martin L, Guiyoule A, Carniel E. Susceptibility to β-lactam agents of *Yersinia enterocolitica* biotype 4, serotype 03 isolated in various parts of the world. J Med Microb 1995;43:9–13.

51. Pham JN, Bell SM, Lanzarone JYM. Biotype and antibiotic sensitivity of 100 clinical isolates of *Yersinia enterocolitica*. J Antimicrob Chemother 1991;28:13–18.

52. Pierson DE, Falkow S. The *ail* gene of *Yersinia enterocolitica* has a role in the ability of the organism to survive serum killing. Infect Immun 1993;61:1846–1852.

53. Pietersz RNI, Reesink HW, Pauw W. Prevention of *Yersinia enterocolitica* growth in red-blood-cells concentrates. Lancet 1992; 340:755–7556.

54. Portnoy DA, Falkow S. Virulence-associated plasmids from *Yersinia enterocolitica* and *Yersinia pestis*. J Bacteriol 1981; 148:877–883.

55. Rabson AR, Hallett AF, Koornhoff HJ. Generalized *Yersinia enterocolitica* infection. J Infect Dis 1975;131:447–451.

56. Raevuori M, Harvey SM, Pichett MJ, Martin WJ. *Yersinia enterocolitica:* in vitro antimicrobial susceptibility. Antimicrob Agents Chemother 1978;13:888–890.

57. Scavizzi MR, Alonso JM, Philippon AM, Jupeau-Vessieres AM, Guiyoule A. Failure of newer beta-lactam antibiotics for murine *Yersinia enterocolitica* infection. Antimicrob. Agents Chemother 1987;31:523–526.

58. Scavizzi M, Borgel M. Sensibilité aux antibiotiques de *Y. enterocolitica*. Med Mal Infect 1971;1,4:191–196.

59. Scavizzi MR, Bronner FD. A statistical model for the interpretation of antibiotic susceptibility tests. Int J Exp Clin Chemother 1988;11:23–42.

60. Scavizzi MR, Philippon AM, Jupeau-Vessières AM. Marked efficacy of fluoroquinolone and moderate activity of ceftriaxone in murine *Yersinia enterocolitica* infection. Int J Exp Clin Chemother 1992;5:57–60.

61. Scavizzi M, Robineau M, Hornstein M, Jupeau A. L'antibiothérapie dans les septicémies à *Yersinia enterocolitica*. Med Mal Infect 1983;13:25–30.

62. Schleigstein J, Coleman MB. An unidentified microorganism resembling *B. lignieri* and *Past. pseudotuberculosis* and pathogenic for man. NY State J Med 1939;39:1749–1753.

63. Seoane A, Francia MV, Garcia Lobo JM. Nucleotide sequence of the ampC-ampR region from the chromosome of *Yersinia enterocolitica*. Antimicrob Agents Chemother 1992; 36: 1049–1052.

64. Seoane A, Garcia Lobo JM. Cloning of chromosomal β-lactamase genes from *Yersinia enterocolitica*. J Gen Microbiol 1991; 137:141–146.

65. Seoane A, Garcia Lobo JM. Nucleotide sequence of a new class A β-lactamase gene from the chromosome of *Yersinia enterocolitica:* implications for the evolution of class A β-lactamase. Mol Gen Genet 1991;228:215–220.

66. Soriano F, Vega J. The susceptibility of Yersinia to eleven antimicrobials. J Antimicrob Chemother 1982;10:543–547.

67. Straley SC, Plano GV, Skrzypek E, Haddix PL, Fileds KA. Regulation by Ca^{2+} in the *Yersinia* low Ca^{2+} response. Mol Microbiol 1993;8:1005–1010.

68. Straley SC, Skrzypek E, Plano GV, Bliska JB. Yops of *Yersinia* spp. pathogenic for humans. Infect Immun 1993;61:3103–3110.

69. Toivanen P, Toivanen A. Does *Yersinia* produce autoimmunity? Int Arch Allergy Immunol 1994;104:107–111.

70. Toma A, Lafleur L. Survey on the incidence of *Yersinia enterocolitica* infection in Canada. Appl Microbiol 1974; 28:469–473.

71. Tulkens PM. Intracellular pharmacokinetics and activity of antibiotics. In: Neu HC, ed. Frontiers of infectious diseases: new antibacterial strategies. Edinburgh: Churchill Livingstone/Longman Group, 1990:243–259.

72. Une T, Osada Y. Penetrability of ofloxacin into cultured epithelial cells and macrophages. Drug Res 1988;38:1265–1267.

73. Verbist L. Comparison of in vitro activities of eight β-lactamase-stable cephalosporins against β-lactamase-producing Gram-negative bacilli. Antimicrob Agents Chemother 1981;19:407–413.

74. Wachtel MR, Miller VL. In vitro and in vivo characterization of an *ail* mutant of *Yersinia enterocolitica*. Infect Immun 1995; 63:2541–2548.

75. World Health Organization. Yersiniosis. Euroreports and studies, no. 60. Reports of a workshop 1982. Regional Board of Europe, Copenhagen. Geneva: World Health Organization, 1983.

76. Wren BW, Tabaqchali S. Detection of pathogenic *Yersinia enterocolitica* by the polymerase chain reaction. Lancet 1990; 336:693.

Yersinia Species

Thomas Butler

GENERAL DESCRIPTION

The genus *Yersinia* consists of three principal pathogenic species: *Y. pestis, Y. enterocolitica,* and *Y. pseudotuberculosis. Y. enterocolitica* and *Y. pseudotuberculosis* are the two principal pathogens of human nonplague yersiniosis (6). *Y. pestis* is the sole pathogen of human plague (4). *Y. enterocolitica* is covered in another chapter. This chapter is devoted to *Y. pestis* and *Y. pseudotuberculosis.* Other species that are rarely identified and have less pathogenic potential are *Y. intermedia, Y. frederickseni,* and *Y. kristensenii. Y. ruckeri* is a pathogen in fish. DNA hybridization studies indicated such close relatedness between *Y. pestis* and *Y. pseudotuberculosis* that the plague bacillus was renamed *Y. pseudotuberculosis* subspecies *pestis.* However, the older name *Y. pestis* remains in use and is used in this chapter.

The clinical presentations of nonplague yersiniosis include fever, diarrhea, abdominal pain that may mimic appendicitis, and chronic arthritis. Most patients with nonplague yersiniosis who do not have underlying illnesses or compromised immune systems recover from their illnesses in 1 to 2 weeks without the need for antimicrobial therapy. *Y. pseudotuberculosis* has its reservoirs in a variety of mammals and birds. Transmission of this infection is presumed to occur by ingestion of organisms from contact with an infected animal or common source contamination within a family, such as food or water. Most patients have been boys 5 to 15 years old. Most patients develop their illness in the winter.

The most common clinical form of plague in humans is acute febrile lymphadenitis, called bubonic plague (13). Less common forms include septicemic, pneumonic, and meningeal plague. In 1994, there was an explosive outbreak of suspected pneumonic plague in India, with more than 50 deaths, but attempts to culture *Y. pestis* from patients failed to confirm that illness was caused by the plague bacillus (5). Mortality is high in untreated plague, but early antibiotic treatment reduces mortality significantly. The major animal reservoirs are rodents, principally urban and domestic rats as well as squirrels, prairie dogs, and field mice, and less commonly rabbits, cats, and other carnivores. Transmission among animals and from animals to man occurs mainly by flea bites and less commonly by ingestion, by inhalation of infected respiratory tract secretions, and by handling infected animal tissues.

MICROBIOLOGY

Y. pseudotuberculosis is a Gram-negative, non-lactose-fermenting, urease-positive bacillus that is motile when grown at 25°C but not at 37°C (10, 11, 16). The organisms grow on blood, heart infusion, MacConkey, and SS agars at room temperature and at 37°C and in buffered saline at 4°C. Colonies are often very small after incubation for 24 h but are readily apparent at 48 h. Six serotypes (I–VI) and four subtypes of *Y. pseudotuberculosis* have been identified, with O-group I accounting for approximately 80% of human cases.

Y. pestis is a Gram-negative bipolar-staining bacillus that grows aerobically on most culture media, including blood agar and MacConkey agar (2, 7). It does not ferment lactose and forms small colonies on MacConkey agar after 24-h incubation at 35°C. On triple-sugar-iron agar, *Y. pestis* produces an alkaline slant and acid butt. It is nonmotile and negative for citrate utilization, urease, and indole.

SUSCEPTIBILITY IN VITRO

Y. pseudotuberculosis is usually sensitive in vitro to ampicillin, tetracycline, chloramphenicol, cephalosporins, and aminoglycosides. The MICs are less than 1 mg/L for all antimicrobial drugs indicated in Table 1. The susceptibility of *Y. pseudotuberculosis* to ampicillin contrasts with the resistance of *Y. enterocolitica* to ampicillin attributable to β-lactamase production by *Y. enterocolitica. Y. pestis* is susceptible in vitro to streptomycin and other aminoglycosides, tetracycline, chloramphenicol, ampicillin, cephalosporins, and fluoroquinolones. In vitro susceptibilities of *Y. pestis* indicate that virtually all antimicrobial drugs are effective (Table 1).

ANTIMICROBIAL THERAPY

Antibiotic therapy is probably not warranted in most patients with diarrhea or mesenteric adenitis due to *Y. pseudotuberculosis;* there is no evidence that antibiotics hasten clinical recovery from illness in this self-limited infection. However, patients with septicemia or immune dysfunction should receive ampicillin (100–200 mg/kg/day intravenously) or gentamicin

(3–5 mg/kg/day intravenously or intramuscularly) or tetracycline (20–30 mg/kg/day orally or intravenously in divided doses) (Table 2). Monotherapy with any of these drugs should give optimal results in this septicemic infection, even though many clinical reports describe results with combination therapies that were initiated empirically before results of blood cultures were available. The mortality in *Y. pseudotuberculosis* septicemia is 75% despite antibiotic therapy.

Early treatment of patients with plague lymphadenitis, septicemia, or pneumonia with antibiotics is life saving. Untreated plague has an estimated mortality rate of more than 50%. The β-lactam antibiotics have not yet been proven effective in clinical trials, and physicians have been reluctant to use β-lactam antibiotics for patients with plague. Streptomycin is the drug of choice for the treatment of plague lymphadenitis, septicemia, or pneumonia because it reduces the case fatality rate to less than 5%. No other drug has been shown to be more efficacious or less toxic. Streptomycin should be administered intramuscularly in two divided doses daily, totaling 30 mg per kg of body weight per day for 10 days. Most patients improve rapidly and become afebrile in about 3 days. The 10-day course of streptomycin is recommended to prevent relapses, because viable bacteria have been isolated from buboes of patients with plague during convalescence (Table 2).

For patients allergic to streptomycin or for whom an oral drug is strongly preferred, tetracycline is a satisfactory alternative. It is administered orally in a dose of 2 to 4 g/day in four divided doses for 10 days. For patients with meningitis who require a drug with good penetration into the cerebrospinal fluid and for patients with profound hypotension in whom an intramuscular infection may be poorly absorbed, chloramphenicol should be administered intravenously. This is given as a loading dose of 25 mg/kg of body weight, followed by 60 mg/kg/day in four divided doses. After clinical improvement, chloramphenicol should be continued orally to complete a total course of 10 days.

Alternative antimicrobial drugs have been used in plague with varying success. These include sulfonamides, trimethoprim-sulfamethoxazole, kanamycin, and ampicillin.

TABLE 1 • **Susceptibilities of *Y. pseudotuberculosis* and *Y. pestis* in mg/L**

Y. pseudotuberculosis[a]		Y. pestis[b]		
		MIC$_{50}$	MIC$_{90}$	Range
Amoxicillin	0.06	<0.03	0.12	<0.03–0.5
Ampicillin	—	—	—	0.1–4.9
Cefotaxime	0.015	<0.03	<0.03	≤0.03
Ceftriaxone	0.015	<0.03	<0.03	≤0.03
Chloramphenicol	—	0.5	1.0	0.06–2.0
Doxycycline	0.12	0.25	1.0	<0.03–4.0
Gentamicin	0.12	0.5	0.5	0.25–1.0
Imipenem	0.06	—	—	—
Ofloxacin	0.03	<0.03	<0.03	<0.03–0.12
Streptomycin	—	0.5	0.5	<0.03–8.0
Tetracycline	—	1.0	2.0	<0.03–2.0
TMP-SMX	—	0.03/0.59	0.06/1.18	<0.03/0.59–0.06/1.18

[a]Single human isolate (12).

[b]Combined data from 121 strains (1, 3, 8).

TABLE 2 • **Antibiotics of Choice for Infections with *Y. pseudotuberculosis* and *Y. pestis***

	Drugs of Choice	Alternatives
Y. pseudotuberculosis		
Diarrhea or mesenteric lymphadenitis without septicemia	None needed	
Septicemia	Ampicillin 100 mg/kg/day in divided doses every 6 h for 7–14 days	Cefotaxime 100–200 mg/kg/day in divided doses every 12 h for 7–14 days or gentamicin 3–5 mg/kg/day in divided doses every 8 h for 7–14 days or tetracycline 20–30 mg/kg/day in divided doses every 6 h for 7–14 days
Y. pestis		
Bubonic or septicemic or pneumonic plague	Streptomycin 30 mg/kg/day in divided doses every 12 h for 10 days or gentamicin 5 mg/kg/day in divided doses every 8 h for 10 days	Tetracycline 2–4 g/day in divided doses every 6 h for 10 days or chloramphenicol 60 mg/kg/day in divided doses every 6 h for 10 days
Plague meningitis	Chloramphenicol 25 mg/kg loading dose followed by 60 mg/kg/day in divided doses every 6 h for 10 days	

These drugs all appear to be either less effective or more toxic than streptomycin and thus should not be chosen.

An isolate from a 16-year-old boy with bubonic plague in Madagascar in 1995 was reported to be resistant to streptomycin, tetracycline, chloramphenicol, and sulfonamide but susceptible to trimethoprim (9). This patient recovered after receiving trimethoprim-sulfamethoxazole. Other than this case, antibiotic resistance in human isolates of *Y. pestis* has never been reported, nor has resistance emerged during antibiotic therapy. The antibiotics streptomycin, tetracycline, and chloramphenicol given as monotherapy are clinically very effective, and relapses are exceedingly rare. Therefore, there is no rationale for using combination therapy to treat plague (17). Other aminoglycoside antibiotics, including gentamicin, tobramycin, and amikacin, have not been used as monotherapy for plague, but the similarity of their actions and in vitro results to those of streptomycin suggests that they would be effective against plague.

Other criteria sometimes used to select antimicrobial drugs of choice are penetration into cells and bactericidal versus bacteriostatic effects. Yersiniae are intracellular organisms, and they multiply within mononuclear phagocytes. In plague, organisms are predominantly intracellular during the incubation period but break out into the extracellular space and plasma during clinical disease. The drug of choice for plague, streptomycin, as well as other aminoglycosides, penetrate poorly into cells. The aminoglycosides are bactericidal, but the bacteriostatic agents tetracycline and chloramphenicol are also clinically effective against plague. Thus, cellular penetration and bactericidal properties are not required for antimicrobials to be clinically effective.

β-lactams hold a controversial position in the treatment of *Yersinia* infections. Clinical reports going back 50 years to the early antibiotic era warned against using penicillins for plague. Clinical failures occurred, and no one has dared use any β-lactam as monotherapy for plague since that time. On the other hand, *Y. pestis* strains are uniformly susceptible to ampicillin, amoxicillin, and cephalosporins. In the animal model of murine plague, good therapeutic effects on reduction of mortality and tissue bacterial burdens were obtained with ampicillin (3) and with ceftriaxone (1). This suggests that human *Y. pestis* infection might be effectively treated with certain β-lactam antibiotics.

For *Y. pseudotuberculosis* infection, the proscription of β-lactams has not been so complete as with plague, but most clinicians are influenced by the warning against β-lactams and gravitate toward aminoglycosides or tetracyclines. In a child with lymphadenitis and serologic evidence of *Y. pseudotuberculosis* infection, cefotaxime treatment gave a rapid response, with defervescence occurring in 36 h; however, erythema nodosum on the legs persisted for 2 weeks (14). In the mouse model of *Y. pseudotuberculosis* infection, gentamicin, doxycycline, or ceftriaxone gave better results than amoxicillin (12).

The fluoroquinolones have not been evaluated yet in patients with *Yersinia* infections. In vitro susceptibilities suggest that the fluoroquinolone ofloxacin is very active, with an MIC below 0.2 mg/L. In the mouse models of infection, ofloxacin was effective against *Y. pseudotuberculosis* (12). Against *Y. pestis,* both ciprofloxacin (15) and ofloxacin (1) gave good results. Future case reports and clinical trials of fluoroquinolones as well as newer cephalosporins in the monotherapy of patients with plague and *Y. pseudotuberculosis* will be welcome.

ENDPOINTS FOR MONITORING THERAPY

For patients with *Y. pseudotuberculosis* infections, those with diarrhea or mesenteric lymphadenitis usually have self-limited infections and do not require antimicrobial therapy. Their illnesses should resolve within 7 to 14 days. Reactive arthritis has been reported to occur several weeks after the initial infection and may have a prolonged course. Synovial fluid is typically sterile. Therapy should be symptomatic treatment, such as with nonsteroidal antiinflammatory drugs. For patients with *Y. pseudotuberculosis* septicemia, the high mortality rate and likelihood of serious underlying diseases requires intensive intravenous therapy until the patient shows resolution of the sepsis by becoming afebrile and ambulatory. Although there is no evidence that combinations of antibiotics are advantageous, many patients with *Y. pseudotuberculosis* septicemia will have been started on combinations of antibiotics empirically before results of blood cultures were available. If these patients show clinical improvement on combinations, it may be desirable to continue the β-lactam (e.g., ampicillin or cefotaxime) as well as the aminoglycoside (e.g., gentamicin) until further improvement occurs. A suggested endpoint of antimicrobial therapy is at least 14 days of therapy or until the patient has been afebrile for about 3 days. Repeating blood cultures during therapy to monitor effectiveness of antimicrobial therapy is not recommended.

For patients with bubonic plague, the endpoint of antimicrobial therapy is guided by the clinical improvement of the patients. Patients effectively treated typically become afebrile within 5 days, and the continuation of therapy for a total of 10 days is advised to ensure against relapse in this much feared and potentially lethal infection. The buboes usually recede without need for local therapy. Occasionally, however, they may enlarge or become fluctuant during the first week of treatment, requiring incision and drainage. The aspirated fluid should be cultured for evidence of superinfection with other bacteria, but this material is usually sterile. The bubo resolves more slowly than the fever but should become progressively less tender during therapy. Persistence of a bubo of unchanged size should not require prolongation of therapy when the patient is afebrile and ambulatory. Repeated aspirations of the bubo for culture and repeated blood cultures during therapy to monitor effectiveness of treatment are not recommended.

VACCINES

A formalin-killed vaccine, Plague Vaccine U. S. P. is available for travelers to epidemic or hyperendemic areas, for individuals who must live and work in close contact with rodents in these areas, and for laboratory workers who must handle live *Y. pestis*. A primary series of two injections is recommended with a 1- to 3-month interval between them. Booster injections are given every 6 months for as long as ex-

whom these nominally low virulence microbes might be substantially pathogenic.

Suggested drugs for scotochromogenic mycobacterial disease are noted in Table 1.

VACCINES

No vaccines have been shown to be efficacious in the prevention of any nontuberculous mycobacterial diseases. Limited data from Scandinavia suggest that following termination of university BCG vaccination, cervical lymphadenitis due to nontuberculosis mycobacteria (NTM) occurred with increasing frequency among the unvaccinated children. From this, some people have inferred protection. While this is a plausible notion, neither the absolute increase in NTM adenitis nor a causal relationship for withdrawal of the vaccine has been proven.

ENDPOINTS FOR MONITORING

Patients receiving antimicrobial therapy should be monitored with a matrix of laboratory, clinical, and (when appropriate) radiographic criteria. Pulmonary disease is most easily assessed because of the relatively precise, quantitative, and reproducible findings on radiographic and sputum microbiologic studies. Chest x-rays or computed tomographic (CT) scans provide ready information about the locale, extent, and character of various pulmonary processes. Mycobacterial diseases inevitably cause irreversible lung damage with scarring, so the purpose of surveillance is not to await normalization but to establish trends and/or the optimal improved state. Bacteriology is a traditional endpoint for tuberculosis therapy. Therefore, it is often adopted for NTM treatment, as well. However, unlike tuberculosis (in which negative sputum cultures are vital to ensure safety from human-to-human transmission), an acceptable response for therapy of NTM disease may include clinical and radiographic improvement without conversion to culture negativity. Certainly negative cultures are a favorable sign, but some patients on treatment never achieve this status. The decision whether to reinforce the drug regimen or consider resectional surgery in this setting is complex and should be undertaken only with experienced consultants.

CONTROVERSIES, CAVEATS, AND COMMENTS

Because of the lack of structured studies, treatment of patients with infections due to these uncommon pathogens is problematic. Fundamental issues such as colonization versus infection? Treatment or not? Surgery or not? may be equivocal. Therefore, for all but straightforward cases in which patients enjoy a prompt and uncomplicated response to therapy, I believe that these patients should—at some point early in the illness—be seen by experienced consultants in referral centers. While this may sound like a conflict of interest, early errors in management may result in unrectifiable problems including acquired drug resistance and/or spread of infection.

REFERENCES

1. Berning S, Iseman M. Rifamycin-induced lupus syndrome. Lancet 1997;349:1521–1522.
2. Brown BA, Wallace RJ Jr, Onyi GO. Activities of clarithromycin against eight slowly growing species of nontuberculous mycobacteria, determined by using a broth microdilution MIC system. Antimicrob Agents Chemother 1992;36:1987–1990.
3. Davidson PT. *Mycobacterium szulgai*—a new pathogen causing infection of the lung. Chest 1976;69:799–801.
4. de Gracia J, Vidal R, Martin N, Bravo C, Gonzalez T, Riba A. Pulmonary disease caused by *Mycobacterium gordonae*. Tubercle 1989;70:135–137.
5. Douglas JG, Calder MA, Choo-Kang YFJ, Leith AG. *Mycobacterium gordonae*: a new pathogen? Thorax 1986;41:152–153.
6. Good RC, Silcox VA, Kilburn JD, Plikaytis BD. Identification and drug susceptibility test results for *Mycobacterium* spp. Clin Microbiol Newslett 1985;7:133–136.
7. Hass H, Michel J, Sacks TG. In vitro susceptibility of a mycobacteria species other that *Mycobacterium tuberculosis* to amikacin., cepholosporins, and cefoxitin, Chemotherapy 1982;28:1–5
8. Horsburgh CJ, Selik R. The epidemiology of disseminated nontuberculous mycobacterial infection in the acquired immunodeficiency syndrome (AIDS). Am Rev Respir Dis 1989; 139:4-7.
9. Joos HA, Hilty LB, Courington D, Schaefer WB, Block M. Fatal disseminated scotochromogenic mycobacteriosis in a child. AM Rev Respir Dis 1967;96:795–801
10. Lessnau K-D, Milanese S, Talavera W. *Mycobacterium gordonae*: a treatable disease in HIV-positive patients. Chest 1993; 104:1779–1785.
11. Maloney JM, Gregg CR, Stephens DS, et al. Infections caused by *Mycobacterium szulgai* in humans. Rev Infect Dis 1987; 9:1120–1126.
12. Marks J, Jenkins PA, Tsukamura M. *Mycobacterium szulgai*—a new pathogen. Tubercle 1972;53:210–214.
13. McNutt DR, Fudenberg HH. Disseminated scotochromogen infection and unusual myeloproliferative disorder. Report of a case and review of the literature. Ann Intern Med 1971;75:737–744.
14. Schaefer WB, Wolinsky E, Jenkins PA, Marks J. *Mycobacterium szulgai*—a new pathogen. Am Rev Respir Dis 1973;108: 1320–1326.
15. Wallace RJ Jr, Brown BA, Griffith DE, Girard W, Tanaka K. Reduced serum levels of clarithromycin in patients treated with multidrug regimens including rifampin or rifabutin for My-

---

TABLE 1 • Suggested Drugs for Scotochromogenic Mycobacterial Diseases

Primary Agents	Alternatives
Clarithromycin[a]	Amikacin
Rifampin (rifabutin)[a]	Streptomycin
Ethambutol	Ciprofloxacin
	Clofaximine

[a]Note predictable drug interaction between clarithromycin and the rifamycins; rifampin (>rifabutin) induced catabolism of clarithromycin, resulting in substantially reduced bioavailability (15). The clinical significance of this has not been established, but given the preeminent activity of clarithromycin against many NTMs, I would recommend checking drug levels and/or dosing clarithromycin in the high range. Conversely, clarithromycin inhibits catabolism of the rifamycins, resulting in a variety of clinical complications including uveitis, pseudojaundice, arthralgias/myalgias, and a drug-induced lupus syndrome (1).

cobacterium avium-Mycobacterium intracellulare infection. J Infect Dis 1995;171:747–750.

16. Weinberger M, Berg S, Feurstein I, Pizzo P, Witebsky F. Mycobacterium gordonae: report of a case and critical review of the literature. Clin Infect Dis 1992;14:1229–1239.

17. Weinberger M, Berg SL, Feuerstein IM, Pizzo PA, Witebsky FG. Disseminated infection with Mycobacterium gordonae: report of a case and critical review of the literature. Clin Infect Dis 1992;14:1229–1239.

18. Wolinsky E. Mycobacterial lympadenitis in childrean: a prospective study of 105 nontuberculous cases with long-term follow-up. Clin Infect Dis 1995;20:954–963.

Group IV: Rapid-Growing Mycobacteria

Michael D. Iseman

MICROBIOLOGY

The rapid-growing mycobacteria (RGMs) are genetically relatively remote from the various slow-growing mycobacteria (31). The biologic separation is reflected in several important clinical distinctions. First, dosing schedules for RGM antimicrobial agents are more frequent, commensurate with the shorter replication times. Secondly, therapy for the RGM typically involves agents without activity against the other mycobacterial pathogens (e.g., cefoxitin, erythromycin, imipenem, sulfonamides, trimethoprim, or tetracyclines). Other agents have overlapping activity against RGMs and other nontuberculosis mycobacteria (NTMs) (e.g., amikacin, clarithromycin, and ciprofloxacin), while several of the standard antituberculosis agents predictably have no activity against the RGMs, including isoniazid, pyrazinamide, and ethambutol. Finally, the RGMs may elicit a weakly granulomatous tissue response or a frankly dimorphic reaction (a combination of granulomatous and/or pyogenic features).

The RGMs predictably grow rapidly on culture medium when subcultured in the laboratory. However, on initial isolation from respiratory secretions, abscesses, or other body tissues, recovery may take several weeks.

M. abscessus, M. chelonae, M. fortuitum and M. smegmatis are the RGM species most commonly associated with human disease. M. abscessus and M. chelonae were formerly regarded as subspecies of M. chelonae, but recently have been designated distinct species (31). These mycobacteria are widely distributed in water and soil and presumably are commonly acquired from these environmental sources (8). The great majority of RGM cases, both pulmonary and extrapulmonary, have been reported from the southeast United States, notably Texas and Florida (7, 11, 32, 34–36); however, recent experience documents disease due to RGMs in all of the United States, including Alaska and Hawaii. There is no evidence of human-to-human transmission. Most data suggest that nosocomial infections with RGMs are acquired from the environment rather than devices or products that are contaminated during manufacture or packaging (34, 35).

The capacity of RGM to survive, even proliferate in water may partially explain their association with iatrogenic infections. M. chelonae in particular has been associated with water or other liquid-borne infections in a variety of medical settings including bronchoscopy (12), xenographic heart valves (20), otologic (21, 25) and ophthalmologic (18) surgery, gentian violet used to mark skin lines for plastic surgery (26), cardiac surgery (14, 19), augmentation mammaplasty prostheses (34), liposuction instruments (K Litwack, personal communication; 23), and DPTP vaccine (2). M. abscessus has also been reported in iatrogenic disease associated with renal dialysis or sternotomy for cardiac surgery (1, 17) and unlicensed preparation of adrenal extract (6). Recent reports have also documented increased numbers of soft tissue and bone infections due to M. fortuitum and M. smegmatis, including some associated with cardiac surgery (14, 17, 19), mammaplasty (34), and peritoneal dialysis (13). Shower-born colonization of the respiratory tracts of 16 patients by M. fortuitum was seen in an East Coast Veterans Administration Hospital (5).

Risk factors associated with pulmonary disease due to RGM include the unusual body habitus among females previously described in association with M. avium complex (MAC) disease—slender, mild thoracic scoliosis, pectus excavatum and/or narrowed anterior-posterior thoracic dimensions, with or without mitral valve prolapse (16). Another apparent, but not well documented, risk factor for RGM pulmonary disease is esophageal achalasia or other disorders of motility associated with vomiting (4, 11). Additional predisposing host conditions include previously damaged or scarred lungs from disorders such as prior tuberculosis, MAC disease, sarcoidosis, cystic fibrosis, rheumatoid arthritis/ankylosing spondylitis, lipoid pneumonia, and previous or coexistent disease due to MAC.

Extrapulmonary disease due to the RGMs largely takes two forms: localized–direct inoculation, typically in normal hosts, and disseminated multifocal disease, usually associated with an immunosuppressed state. Notable in the latter group is the relative paucity of disseminated RGM infection in persons with AIDS. Given the frequency with which the RGMs can be isolated from the environment, their infrequency in this group suggests to this author that an alternative immune mechanism is primarily responsible for defense against the RGMs, possibly a predominantly humoral response. Direct inoculation disease with RGM occurs both with environmental puncture wounds (10, 22–24) and with such iatrogenic procedures as injection of inflamed joints or bursae with steroids (MD Iseman, unreported data, 1997). Endocarditis may evolve in the presence of chronic infection with RGMs elsewhere (9). One case of meningitis due to *M. fortuitum* was reported in association with a puncture wound and foreign body; another patient was reported with AIDS (27).

Common host conditions associated with multifocal or disseminated RGM disease include renal failure, dialysis, organ transplantation, connective tissue disorders and other conditions treated with steroids and/or cytotoxic agents, leukemia, and lymphoma (1, 15, 30, 32).

SUSCEPTIBILITY

Like most NTM species, the RGMs show in vitro resistance to several or most of the standard antituberculosis agents. In addition, RGM species show variable patterns of susceptibility to the drugs most likely to be active against that species; for example, even wild strains (not previously exposed to antimicrobial therapy) do not have predictable in vitro susceptibility patterns.

The probabilities of in vitro susceptibility to the four major pathogenic species of RGMs are delineated in Table 1. Although these data may be assumed to be generally helpful in selecting drug regimens, the validity of in vitro susceptibility testing for RGM therapy—like that in all NTM disease—has not been proven in rigorous trials. Important variables include the methodology of the in vitro susceptibility testing technique and the choice of "critical concentrations." No evidence documents in vitro synergistic or antagonistic drug interactions. Multidrug therapy is typically used to prevent evolution of acquired drug resistance; however, the validity and utility of this practice have not been clearly demonstrated. No distinctions regarding optimal regimens in the setting of pulmonary, extrapulmonary, or disseminated disease have been made, although the understandable inference is commonly drawn that disseminated disease and/or immunocompromised hosts merit more aggressive treatment (more drugs, higher doses, and/or longer therapy).

ENDPOINTS FOR MONITORING

As noted above, patients with RGM disease should be monitored with a matrix of clinical, microbiologic, radiographic and/or other laboratory techniques. The obvious desired endpoints are clinical and microbiologic "cures," but these are difficult to achieve with most RGM disease. In particular, pulmonary disease due to *M. abscessus* and *M. chelonae* is extremely difficult to eliminate, with relapses occurring in the great majority of treated patients (11) (MD Iseman, unreported data). *M. fortuitum* pulmonary disease, due in part to the availability of long-term suppressive therapy with oral agents, may be more amenable to medical cures (11).

Reduction of cough and phlegm are the most immediate markers of clinical response. Semiquantitative enumeration of sputum smears and cultures also reflects the impact of drug therapy. Routine and computed tomographic radiography studies are useful adjuncts to stage and assess response to treatment.

Treatment for pulmonary RGM disease varies in duration. For *M. fortuitum* that is susceptible to both oral and parenteral agents, treatment may consist of an initial intensive phase of "mixed" (oral and parenteral) treatment for 6 to 12 weeks followed by 4 to 9 months of oral suppressive drugs. For *M. abscessus* disease, we typically treat for 8 to 16 weeks with a two-drug parenteral regimen directed at suppression of symptoms. Such treatment is initiated when patients find their cough, congestion, or malaise too severe to tolerate, but it is done with the explicit understanding that it is palliative, not curative. Patients are also informed that repeated use of these antibiotics entails the risk of acquired resistance to, or toxicity from, the agents employed. Also, most patients do not have good insurance coverage for home intravenous therapy, and arrangements are likely to be both expensive and awkward. Hence, such treatment is not entered into lightly.

Treatment of extrapulmonary or disseminated disease due to RGM varies according to the site and extent of infection. In some patients, simple drainage may be adequate to promote a cure of a local abscess. In others, protracted therapy with multiple antibiotics may be required to eradicate the infection. In most localized collections of RGM infection, surgical drainage is indicated. In some, radical debridement is necessary to effect cure. Identifying the extent of the abscesses associated with RGM disease is important to facilitate adequate surgical drainage or debridement. We have found magnetic

TABLE 1 • Probability of in Vitro Susceptibility of the Major RGM Pathogens to Various Antimicrobial Agents			
	Species		
Agents	M. fortuitum	M. abscessus	M. chelonae
Amikacin (kanamycin)	100%	90%	80%
Cefoxitin	80%	70%	(0–90%)[a]
Imipenem	100%	50%	60%
Clarithromycin	80%	100%	100%
Ciprofloxacin	100%	—	20%
Sulfamethoxasole	100%	—	—
Trimethoprim/Sulfa	100%	—	—
Doxycycline	50%	—	25%
Tobramycin	—	—	100%

Data from references 3, 28, 29, 33.

[a]Wallace's laboratory in Texas does not describe cefoxitin susceptibility among strains of *M. chelonae*; in fact, they regard resistance to cefoxitin as a discriminating criterion for *M. chelonae* (David Griffith, personal communication, 9/97). By contrast, in the laboratory at National Jewish, most isolates designated *M. chelonae* have cefoxitin susceptibility (Pamela Lindholm-Levy, personal communications, 9/97). The issue here probably involves both differences in speciation criteria as well as a variable in in vitro susceptibility techniques; the real "lesson" is that this remains an area with considerable uncertainty.

resonance imaging (MRI) to be useful in locating the collections in the extent of inflammatory matter. MRI is generally superior to computed tomography in characterizing soft tissue or periosteal abscesses.

Toxicity monitoring must include periodic audiometric and vestibular testing as well as blood tests for renal dysfunction for persons receiving aminoglycosides. Pharmacokinetic assessment with aminoglycosides helps reduce the likelihood of 8th nerve or renal injury. Symptomatic surveillance for diarrhea, a potential indicator of pseudomembranous colitis—especially for those receiving cefoxitin—and interval tests of hematologic and liver function are required with all RGM agents.

The role of surgery in the management of RGM disease varies according to the form and location of the infection. For cases of pulmonary disease in which there is anatomically localized disease, chemotherapy followed by resection may be useful in minimizing symptoms, slowing the progression, or (in a few cases) actually curing the disease (11; MD Iseman, unpublished data). For extrapulmonary disease, drainage or debridement of necrotic debris may promote healing of localized abscesses. Aggressive debridement has proven particularly helpful in our care of RGM infections of the hand where tendinous damage may seriously threaten function. Also, we have observed the complementary role of surgical debridement of lower extremity multinodular abscesses as described above.

Immune modulation may be appropriate in some cases. Certainly for patients whose RGM disease appears related to immunosuppressive drug therapy (steroids, cytotoxic agents, antirejection medications), reducing these agents to their minimal required dosages is desirable. We are currently evaluating the role of IFN-γ as an immunity-enhancing adjuvant for "normal hosts" with refractory pulmonary RGM disease; the data are presently insufficient to assess the utility of this treatment.

Bronchial hygiene is an essential and often overlooked element of management of patients with bronchiectatic pulmonary RGM disease. Inhaled β-agonists may be useful both for bronchodilating (a substantial portion of patients with bronchiectasis develop reversible obstructive airway dysfunction) and for accelerating ciliary activity (to help clear secretions). Purulent secretions may be cleared more effectively with the use of the Flutter-Valve or a combination of postural drainage, clapping, or vibration techniques. In addition, attention should be directed toward the potential for nonmycobacterial bronchitis with organisms such as *Pseudomonas aeruginosa,* which may require periodic intensive antibiotic therapy.

REFERENCES

1. Bolan G, Reingold AL, Carson LA, et al. Infections with *Mycobacterium chelonei* in patients receiving dialysis and using processed hemodialyzers. J Infect Dis 1985;152:1013–1019.
2. Borghans JGA, Stanford JL. *Mycobacterium chelonei* in abscesses after injection of diphtheria-pertussis-tetanus-polio vaccine. Am Rev Respir Dis 1973;107:1–8.
3. Brown BA, Wallace RJ Jr, Onyi GO, DeRosa V, Wallace RJ III. Activities of four macrolides, including clarithromycin, against *Mycobacterium fortuitum, Mycobacterium chelonae,* and *M. chelonae*-like organisms. Antimicrob Agents Chemother 1992; 36:180–184.
4. Burke DS, Ullian RB. Megaesophagus and pneumonia associated with *Mycobacterium chelonei.* A case report and a literature review. Am Rev Respir Dis 1977;116:1101–1107.
5. Burns DN, Wallace RJ Jr, Schultz ME, et al. Nosocomial outbreak of respiratory tract colonization with *Mycobacterium fortuitum:* demonstration of the usefulness of pulsed-field gel electrophoresis in an epidemiologic investigation. Am Rev Respir Dis 1991;144:1153–1159.
6. Centers for Disease Control. Infection with *Mycobacterium abscessus* associated with intramuscular injection of adrenal cortex extract—Colorado and Wyoming, 1995–1996. MMWR 1996;45:713–715.
7. Cooper JF, Lichtenstein MJ, Graham BS, Schaffner W. *Mycobacterium chelonae:* a cause of nodular skin lesions with a proclivity for renal transplant recipients. Am J Med 1989;86:173–177.
8. Falkinham JO. Epidemiology of infection by nontuberculous mycobacteria. Clin Microbiol Rev 1996;9:177–215.
9. Galil K, Thurer R, Glatter K, Barlam T. Disseminated Mycobacterium chelonae infection resulting in endocarditis. Clin Infect Dis 1996;23:1322–1323.
10. Gangadharam PR, Hsu KHK. *Mycobacterium abscessus* infection in a puncture wound. Am Rev Respir Dis 1972;106:275–277.
11. Griffith D, Girard W, Wallace RJ Jr. Clinical features of pulmonary disease caused by rapidly growing mycobacteria. An analysis of 154 patients. Am Rev Respir Dis 1993;147: 1271–1278.
12. Gubler JGH, Salfinger M, von Graevenitz A. Pseudoepidemic of nontuberculous mycobacteria due to a contaminated bronchoscope cleaning machine. Chest 1992;101:245–249.
13. Hakim A, Hisam N, Reuman PD. Environmental mycobacterial peritonitis complicating peritoneal dialysis: three cases and review. Clin Infect Dis 1993;16:426–431.
14. Hoffman PC, Fraser DW, Robicsek F, O'Bar PR, Mauney CU. Two outbreaks of sternal wound infections due to organisms of the *Mycobacterium fortuitum* complex. J Infect Dis 1981;143: 533–542.
15. Ingram CW, Tanner DC, Durack DT, Kernodle GW J, Corey GR. Disseminated infection with rapidly growing mycobacteria. Clin Infect Dis 1993;16:463–471.
16. Iseman MD, Buschman DL, Ackerson LM. Pectus excavatum and scoliosis: thoracic anomalies associated with pulmonary disease due to *M. avium* complex. Am Rev Respir Dis 1991;144: 914–916.
17. Jauregui L, Arbulu A, Wilson F. Osteomyelitis, pericarditis, mediastinitis, and vasculitis due to *Mycobacterium chelonei.* Am Rev Respir Dis 1977;115:699–703.
18. Khooshabeh R, Grange JM, Yates MD, McCartney ACE, Casey TA. A case report of *Mycobacterium chelonae* keratitis and a review of mycobacterial infections of the eye and orbit. Tuberc Lung Dis 1994;75:377–382.
19. Kuritsky JN, Bullen MG, Broome CV, Silcox VA, Good RC, Wallace RJ Jr. Sternal wound infections and endocarditis due to organisms of the *Mycobacterium fortuitum* complex. Ann Intern Med 1983;98:938–939.
20. Laskowski LF, Marr JJ, Spernoga JF, et al. Fastidious mycobacteria grown from porcine prosthetic-heart-valve cultures. N Engl J Med 1977;297:101–102.
21. Lowry PW, Jarvis WR, Oberle AD, et al. *Mycobacterium che-*

lonae causing otitis media in an ear-nose-and-throat practice. N Engl J Med 1988;319:978.

22. Meredith FT, Sexton DJ. *Mycobacterium abscessus* osteomyelitis following a plantar puncture wound. Clin Infect Dis 1996;23:651–653.
23. Newton JA Jr, Weiss PJ, Bowler WA, Oldfield EC III. Soft-tissue infection due to *Mycobacterium smegmatis*: report of two cases. Clin Infect Dis 1993;16:531–533.
24. Periyakoil V, Krasner C. *Mycobacterium abscessus* osteomyelitis following a plantar puncture wound. Clin Infect Dis 1996;23: 651–653.
25. Plemmons RM, McAllister CK, Liening DA, Garces MC. Otitis media and mastoiditis due to *Mycobacterium fortuitum:* case report, review of four cases, and a cautionary note. Clin Infect Dis 1996;22:1105–1106.
26. Safranek TJ, Jarvis WR, Carson LA, et al. *Mycobacterium chelonae* wound infections after plastic surgery employing contaminated gentian violet skin-marking solution. N Engl J Med 1987;317:197–201.
27. Santamaría-Jaúregui J, Sanz-Hospital J, Berenguer J, Muñoz D, Gómez-Mampaso E, Bouza E. Meningitis caused by *Mycobacterium fortuitum*. Am Rev Respir Dis 1984;130:136–137.
28. Stone MS, Wallace RJ, Swenson JM, Thornsberry C, Christiensen LA. An agar disk elution method for clinical susceptibility testing of *Mycobacterium marinum* and the *Mycobacterium fortuitum*-complex to sulfonamides and antibiotics. Antimicrob Agents Chemother 1983;34:486–493.
29. Swenson JM, Wallace RJ, Silcox VA, Thornsberry C. Antimicrobial susceptibility testing of 5 subgroups of *Mycobacterium*

fortuitum and *Mycobacterium chelonae*. Antimicrob Agents Chemother 1985;28:8907–811.
30. Trulock EP, Bolman RM, Genton R. Pulmonary disease caused by *Mycobacterium chelonae* in a heart-lung transplant recipient with obliterative bronchiolitis. Am Rev Respir Dis 1989;140: 802–805.
31. Wallace RJ Jr. Treatment of infections caused by rapidly growing mycobacteria in the era of newer macrolides. Res Microbiol 1996;147:30–35.
32. Wallace RJ Jr, Brown BA, Onyi GO. Skin, soft tissue, and bone infections due to *Mycobacterium chelonae chelonae:* importance of prior corticosteroid therapy, frequency of disseminated infections, and resistance to oral antimicrobials other than clarithromycin. J Infect Dis 1992;166:405–412.
33. Wallace RJ Jr, Brown BA, Onyi GO. Susceptibilities of *Mycobacterium fortuitum* biovar. *fortuitum* and the two subgroups of *Mycobacterium chelonae* to imipenem, cefmetazole, cefoxitin, and amoxicillin-clavulanic acid. Antimicrob Agents Chemother 1991;35:773–775.
34. Wallace RJ Jr, Musser JM, Hull SI, et al. Diversity and sources of rapidly growing mycobacteria associated with infections following cardiac surgery. J Infect Dis 1989;159:708–716.
35. Wallace RJ Jr, Steele LC, Labidi A, Silcox VA. Heterogeneity among isolates of rapidly growing mycobacteria responsible for infections following augmentation mammaplasty despite case clustering in Texas and other southern coastal states. J Infect Dis 1989;160:281–288.
36. Wallace RJ Jr, Swenson JM, Silcox VA, Good RC, Tschen JA, Stone MS. Spectrum of disease due to rapidly growing mycobacteria. Rev Infect Dis 1983;5:657–679.

Mycobacterium avium Complex (MAC)[1]

Joyce A. Korvick

GENERAL DESCRIPTION

Mycobacterium avium complex (MAC) infections have been noted with increasing frequency during the later half of the 20th century (37). As techniques for isolation of mycobacterial organisms improved and the rate of pulmonary tuberculosis declined, MAC was readily distinguished from *M. tuberculosis*. Clinicians have recognized MAC as a cause of pulmonary disease, often associated with predisposing chronic lung diseases: emphysema, pneumoconioses, bronchiectasis, or fibrotic lung disorders. In the 1980s, with the advent of acquired immunodeficiency syndrome (AIDS), disseminated MAC disease was documented in the most immunocompromised patients. By the early 1990s, 18 to 40% of patients with

AIDS had disseminated MAC disease (6, 37). Therapeutic interventions for MAC previously required numerous agents with considerable toxicity and limited proven efficacy. The newer macrolides have contributed substantially to the treatment of MAC infections.

Microbiology

MAC organisms are acid-fast, slow-growing, nonpigmented bacilli. Some may produce yellow pigment, which often intensifies with age. The term *Mycobacterium avium complex* refers to a serologic complex composed of 28 serovars of two species, *M. avium* and *M. intracellulare* (101). Serovars of MAC strains most frequently isolated in disseminated MAC with AIDS are 1, 4 and 8 (82). Ninety percent of disseminated MAC disease is caused primarily by *M. avium* (87). MAC pulmonary disease is frequently caused by serovars 10 and higher (*M. intracellulare*) (32).

---

[1]The comments contained herein are those of the author and do not reflect current policy of the FDA.

The colony morphology of MAC isolates varies between three types: smooth, opaque, and domed (SmD); smooth, transparent, and flat (SmT); and rough. The primary isolate of MAC from the blood is often exclusively the transparent SmT type. These variants are intrinsically more resistant to antimicrobial agents and are more virulent in animal models of MAC disease than other types (18, 63, 80, 84, 86, 88, 104).

Growth of MAC takes approximately 2 to 3 weeks with standard cell culture techniques. However, the Bactec System, a liquid medium with radiolabeled ^{14}C, can detect growth more rapidly—within 7 days (1, 33, 34). A single positive blood culture detects up to 91% of disseminated MAC (92). Negative cultures may be seen in patients with low colony counts in the early stages of dissemination. Finally, polymerase chain reaction methods are being developed for detection of MAC; however, the role of this methodology in the diagnosis and management of the disease is unclear (46). Once MAC clinical isolates are recovered, they are identified by either species-specific DNA probes from Gen-Probe or conventional biochemical or high performance liquid chromatography.

Epidemiology

The environmental reservoir for *M. avium* includes water, soil, food, and a variety of animal species (55, 97, 103). Humans may have transient or prolonged carriage of MAC in oral or bronchial secretions. Ingestion of MAC and passage through the gastrointestinal tract are common occurrences in the absence of disease (13). MAC is not spread by person-to-person contact. Specific environmental interventions that might reduce the risk of infection with MAC, have not been suggested by epidemiologic studies (38, 41, 43, 97).

The geographic distribution of MAC has been studied using skin test reactivity to the purified protein derivative Battey (PPD-B). There is cross-reactivity with the tuberculin purified protein derivative (PPD), thus resulting in some imprecision in test results. Distribution of positive skin reactivity appeared to be more frequent among military recruits coming from areas in the South and south Atlantic states (24, 85).

Current reports regarding the distribution of disseminated MAC in the United States suggest regional and seasonal variations (34, 43). Rates of disseminated MAC in European, North American, and Australian AIDS patients are between 10 and 25% (39). Disseminated MAC is less common in developing areas such as Africa. These differences may be due to several factors: smaller proportions of extremely advanced AIDS patients, protection from MAC by prior exposure to tu-

berculosis, and decreased exposure to MAC in reservoirs as recirculation water systems (43).

SUSCEPTIBILITY IN VITRO AND IN VIVO

MAC is resistant to most of the standard agents used for treatment of tuberculosis. Susceptibility testing for MAC is not standardized to date and is only available in research institutions. The precise MIC (minimum inhibitory concentration) breakpoint for resistance has not been standardized and is being evaluated by the National Committee for Clinical Laboratory Standards (NCCLS). In addition, clinical correlation with in vitro sensitivity testing has not been clearly established. Susceptibility testing is not universally recommended for initial selection of therapeutic agents. However, when the patient worsens clinically or fails prophylactic therapy, susceptibility testing may help direct selection of alternative agents (38, 93).

In vitro testing is dramatically influenced by the pH at which the test is performed and the medium used (Table 1) (28). Tween-containing broth enhances antimicrobial activity. While in vitro testing has not been standardized, there is consensus among researchers regarding certain features. A broth medium may be more reliable than agar. When using radiometric broth dilution methods, inoculum preparation is critical. An inoculum size of 10^4 to 10^5 colony-forming units (CFU)/mL has been recommended. In the absence of well-established correlations with clinical efficacy and outcome, especially in infections in AIDS patients, use of the MIC to determine resistance or susceptibility is problematic (46).

Molecular mechanisms of antimicrobial resistance are not well described for MAC. There is no evidence that MAC produces aminoglycoside- and peptide-inactivating enzymes; however, there is evidence for low-level, β-lactamase production (64, 65). Macrolide resistance has been linked to base pair substitution within the V domain of the 23S ribosomal RNA (62). This mutation appears to confer cross-resistance among the currently available macrolides

M. avium is an intracellular pathogen, therefore, the intracellular concentration of a therapeutic agent is an important consideration when evaluating the MIC. For example, azithromycin, which has a lower Cmax in the serum than clarithromycin, has a longer half-life and reaches much higher concentrations in the macrophage than clarithromycin (26, 49). Intracellular activity is often studied in the human macrophage model. With the aid of the beige mouse animal model, agents with in vitro activity are selected for human study. However, the final proof of the agent's efficacy must be demonstrated in clinical trials because of the specific pathophysiology of this disease.

ANTIMICROBIAL THERAPY

There are three common clinical syndromes caused by MAC: (*a*) lymphadenitis, (*b*) disseminated MAC in HIV (human immunodeficiency virus)-positive individuals, and (*c*) pulmonary MAC disease. Therapeutics for HIV-positive individuals include either prophylaxis or treatment, depending on the stage of the underlying disease. In general, prophylaxis with

---

TABLE 1 • Effect of pH and Inspissation of Egg Medium on the MICs of Drugs Active against MAC

Medium (pH)	MIC range (MIC$_{90}$) Clarithromycin	Rifabutin
7H11 agar (6.6)	2–32 (16)	0.5–2 (2)
Egg medium (6.6)	4–8 (8)	4–16 (16)
OADC*a*-supplemented Mueller-Hinton agar (7.3)	0.5–8 (2)	2 (2)

*a*Oleate-albumin-dextrose-catalase (28).

monotherapy is the standard, while treatment of infection requires combination therapy including a newer macrolide.

Lymphadenitis

Clinical lymphadenitis is an uncommon disease in the United States, occurring in children (72). From 1950 to 1970, *M. scrofulaceum* was the predominant cause of lymphadenitis in the United States; however, MAC became the predominant cause in the 1980s (72). There are no randomized clinical trials regarding therapy for this disease; it frequently resolves spontaneously.

HIV-Positive Individuals: Disseminated MAC Treatment

(Recommendations are summarized in Table 2.)

Disseminated MAC disease presents as a subacute process with fever, abdominal pain, diarrhea, and weight loss. Characteristic findings such as unexplained anemia and/or increased alkaline phosphatase are suggestive (53). Radiographic findings include hepatomegaly, splenomegaly, and intraabdominal or intrathoracic adenopathy. Diagnosis is made by blood culture. Median CD4+ cell counts of patients with disseminated MAC range from 10 to 20 cells/mm^3 (37, 40, 68, 90). This disease must be distinguished from those of both tuberculous and other atypical mycobacteria.

Early in the HIV epidemic, as disseminated MAC disease was being recognized, there was much debate about whether disseminated MAC was a preterminal event or a treatable disease (36, 38, 105). Early attempts at treatment with rifabutin, clofazimine, and ethionamide or ethambutol combinations were unsuccessful (31, 61). Symptomatic improvement did not correlate with microbiologic improvement, which was meager at best.

TABLE 2 • Disseminated MAC Treatment Recommendations

Duration of treatment: life-long

First-line treatment: clarithromycin 500 mg b.i.d. plus at least one other agent active against MAC (e.g., ethambutol 15 mg/kg/day, rifabutin 300 mg/day, ciprofloxacin 500–750 mg/day, amikacin); ethambutol is the preferred agent (96)

Alternatives: azithromycin is undergoing study for this indication; suggested daily doses include 600 mg plus at least one other active agent against MAC

Considerations: clofazimine is not recommended for treatment of MAC, as it has not demonstrated efficacy and may be harmful to patients

Monitoring: symptomatic assessment of the patient should demonstrate improvement within 4–6 weeks, with negative blood cultures at 12–16 weeks. If failure is suspected, blood cultures should be performed. If cultures are positive, sensitivity testing to the macrolides is recommended to direct future drug selections. Positive clinical response with negative blood cultures is the desired therapeutic outcome; however, therapy must be continued due to the presence of MAC in other extravascular sites. (See Table 7 regarding protease drug interactions)

Combination therapy was used in several case series (2, 7, 44). These reports contained similar four-drug regimens: isoniazid 300 mg, ethambutol 15 mg/kg, rifabutin 150 or 300 mg, and clofazimine 100 mg per day (one study substituted ciprofloxacin for clofazimine (97)). Six of seven and four of four patients cleared their blood of MAC, and most importantly, each of these patients had resolution of fever, night sweats, and weight loss (2, 7). The largest series was a prospective nonrandomized study of rifabutin (300–600 mg/day), clofazimine, isoniazid, and ethambutol (44). Twenty-two patients had consecutive negative blood cultures for MAC for 4 weeks or more. In 16 of these, cultures remained negative for 72 weeks.

Since MAC is so difficult to treat, four-drug combination regimens became the norm for treatment. However, the contribution of each agent to the regimen's activity was highly debated. Studies that reported the change in CFUs are summarized in Table 3. Chiu ct al. demonstrated a mean decrease of 1.5 log$_{10}$ CFU/mL MAC at 4 weeks of treatment, with 18% of the 15 patients becoming negative at 12 weeks (14). The regimen included rifampin, ciprofloxacin, ethambutol, and intravenous amikacin. Despite this success, the search for an all oral regimen continued. The California Collaborative Treatment Group (CCTG) studied such a combination: rifampin (600 mg/day), ethambutol (15 mg/kg), clofazimine (100 mg once daily), and ciprofloxacin (750 mg twice daily) (51). This regimen yielded a similar reduction in MAC CFUs (-1.4 log$_{10}$ CFU/mL) but had a better culture negativity rate at 12 weeks (42%). The oral four-drug standard was accepted among practitioners treating HIV-associated diseases, but the contribution of amikacin to the regimen was still in dispute. A randomized prospective study of the same four-drug regimen with or without intravenous amikacin demonstrated no significant contribution of amikacin to clinical or microbiologic responses above that of the four-drug regimen and, in addition, demonstrated unacceptable toxicity (73).

Desire to understand the contribution of single agents to overall activity of multidrug regimens prompted short-duration pilot studies of the microbiologic activity of single drugs. In a 4-week microbiologic study, ethambutol monotherapy was more active than clofazimine and rifampin (52). In fact, on average, CFUs increased in the rifampin group. A study of sparfloxacin alone or with ethambutol demonstrated activity, with a modest improvement for the combination (107). These studies set the stage for the macrolides. The macrolides produced between 1.5 and 3 log$_{10}$ decreases in CFUs by week 4, with rates of blood culture negativity of 41 to 56% (10, 11, 106). Investigators were stunned to find a very powerful agent.

Three studies comparing clarithromycin with placebo demonstrated the activity of clarithromycin against MAC (11, 20, 29). The largest study compared three different doses of clarithromycin (500, 1000, and 2000 mg twice daily) (11). There was a substantial microbiologic dose response. The most rapid microbiologic clearing of the blood occurred in the patients taking 2000 mg twice daily (29 days); however, this dose was poorly tolerated owing mostly to gastrointestinal toxicity, and paradoxically, survival in this group was shorter than in the two lower-dose arms of the study.

TABLE 3 • Clinical Studies of Single and Combination Agents for MAC Treatment in HIV Patients

Agent and Dose	Ref.	N	Change in $\log_{10}$ CFU/mL at Week 4	% Culture Negative by Week 12	% Reduction in Symptoms by Week 12
Azithromycin 500 mg/day	106	21	−1.2	28	—
Azithromycin 600 mg/day	10	65	−2.00	56	—
1200 mg/day			−0.60	42	
Clarithromycin 500 mg b.i.d.	11	154			
1000 mg b.i.d.		(33)[a]	−1.5	41	60
2000 mg b.i.d.		(31)[a]	−2.8	53	69
		(25)[a]	−2.7	41	75
Clofazimine 200 mg/day	52	15	−0.2	—	—
Ethambutol 15 mg/kg/day		15	−0.60	—	—
Rifampin 600 mg/day		18	+0.2	—	—
Liposomal-Gentamicin (variable 1.7–5.1 mg/kg/day)	69	21	−0.98[a]		
Sparfloxacin 200 mg/day	107	10	(4/10) −0.53		
300 mg/day		12	(3/12) −0.96		
(+ethambutol)		22	(18/22) −0.95		
Ciprofloxacin 750 mg b.i.d.	14	15	−1.5	18	60–70
Ethambutol 15 mg/kg/day					
Rifampin 600 mg/day					
Amikacin 7.5 mg/kg/day					
Ciprofloxacin 750 mg b.i.d.	51	31	−1.4	42	65–67
Ethambutol 15 mg/kg/day					
Rifampin 600 mg/day					
Clofazimine 100 mg/day					
Rifampin 600 mg/day	50	12	−0.2	—	—
Ethambutol 25 mg/kg/day					
Ciprofloxacin 750 mg b.i.d.					
or					
Placebo		12	+0.7	—	—

From Korvick JA, Benson CA. Advances in the treatment and prophylaxis of *mycobacterium avium* complex in individuals infected with human immunodeficiency virus. In: Korvick JA, Benson CA, eds. *Mycobacterium avium*-complex infection: progress in research and treatment. New York: Marcel Dekker, 1996:241–262, with permission.

[a]Available cultures.

The choice for the recommended dose of clarithromycin was then between 500 mg or 1000 mg twice daily. The 500-mg dose twice daily was recommended by the FDA for three reasons: the proportion of patients who cleared the blood of MAC was similar to that with the 1000 mg twice-daily dose, it was better tolerated, and there were fewer deaths in the 500-mg twice-daily group (60). Survival was an important consideration in selecting the dose, even though few thought it was related to clarithromycin, given the advanced stage of many of these patients. At 12 weeks of treatment, the death rates were 6% (3 of 53) for the 500-mg group compared with 25% (13 of 51) for the 1000-mg twice-daily group. Was the survival advantage dose related? A second study, comparing 500 mg twice daily with 1000 mg twice daily, in combination with other agents, showed the same results (15). In fact, the study was discontinued early because of the high rate of mortality in the 1000-mg twice-daily dose: 43% (17 of 40) versus 22% (10 of 45) deaths for the 1000-mg and 500-mg twice-daily groups, respectively. Thus, it has been clearly established that a 1000-mg twice-daily dose cannot be recommended for treatment of MAC in HIV-positive patients. Subanalysis of various parameters within these studies did not reveal a reason for the survival difference.

Resistance associated with monotherapy for disseminated MAC disease was well demonstrated in the Chaisson study (11). Bacteriologic relapses occurred in 21% of patients by week 12 and in another 26% thereafter. The bacteriologic relapses were associated with a recrudescence of symptoms and the isolation of MAC with MICs above 32 µg/mL.

Two small azithromycin dose-ranging studies demonstrated its activity against MAC (Table 3) (10, 106). MAC cleared from the blood in 28 to 56% of patients. CFU decreases were of a similar magnitude to those of clarithromycin. Currently, a large azithromycin treatment study being conducted by Pfizer is expected to define the clinical efficacy of azithromycin clearly. However, the results of a smaller VA comparative study of azithromycin (600 mg daily) and ethambutol versus clarithromycin (500 mg twice daily) and ethambutol are available (100). There were only 29 of 61 evaluable patients in the analysis at the time of presentation: 18 patients on clarithromycin and 11 patients on azithromycin. At week 16, 45% (5 of 11) of the azithromycin patients were culture negative, compared with 92% (16 of 18) patients in the clarithromycin arm. Time to clearance of MAC bacteremia was longer for the azithromycin group than for the clarithromycin group (16 vs. 4.38 weeks; $P = .0018$) (100). Although these data are provocative, follow-up data from these patients and results of the large company-sponsored studies are needed before the final comment on the efficacy of azithromycin can be made.

The Public Health Service recommends that first-line therapy for the treatment of disseminated MAC should include clarithromycin 500 mg twice daily in combination with other agents active against MAC (Table 4). Ethambutol was suggested as a useful second drug, and other drugs mentioned included clofazimine, ciprofloxacin, rifampin or rifabutin, and amikacin (94–96).

The exact number of companion agents needed to treat disseminated MAC is still debated. A Canadian study compared a four-drug regimen with a three-drug clarithromycin-containing regimen and showed superiority for the three-drug combination (90). Clarithromycin/ethambutol/rifabutin yielded a longer survival time (8.6 vs. 5.2 months) and a higher rate of clearance of bacteremia (69 vs. 29%) and was better tolerated than ciprofloxacin/clofazimine/ethambutol/rifampin. An important lesson was learned from this study. Uveitis occurred in 24 of the first 63 patients receiving rifabutin (600 mg/day). When the dose was reduced to 300 mg/day, only 3 of the 53 patients developed uveitis.

Addition of clofazimine to combination therapy of disseminated MAC in HIV-infected patients does not add to the efficacy of the regimen and may be harmful to patients. Several clinical studies have included clofazimine; most did not show much advantage, and recently, evidence regarding potential harm has come to light (12, 23, 59). A study by Chaisson et al. comparing clarithromycin plus ethambutol with and without clofazimine showed no difference in efficacy rates; however, a survival difference was detected (12). Mortality rates were higher for the three-drug group than the two-drug group (61 vs. 38%; $P = .01$). Patients in this study were not evenly balanced at baseline regarding CFUs of MAC in the blood; those in the clofazimine group had the higher counts.

Treatment of Pulmonary MAC in HIV-Negative Individuals

(Recommendations are summarized in Table 5.)

Most reported pulmonary MAC infections have been in persons with predisposing lung conditions. In the past, the most frequent clinical picture was a male smoker with chronic bronchitis or emphysema. Pulmonary tuberculosis or other infections resulting in bronchiectasis, pneumoconioses, or fibrotic lung disorders associated with rheumatoid arthritis or ankylosing spondylitis have also been associated with pulmonary MAC (16, 22, 83). Iseman et al. reported another group that appears to be at risk for pulmonary MAC, with the following features: pectus excavatum, or abnormal narrowing of the chest in the anteroposterior axis, thoracic scoliosis, and mitral valve prolapse in female patients (47).

The clinicoradiologic presentation of pulmonary MAC includes several distinctive patterns: cavitary/destructive form; multinodular bronchiectatic form; and transition/combination forms, bulitis, solitary pulmonary nodules (58, 93). The nodular bronchiectatic form tends to stay within that pattern for extended periods. This form is being recognized more frequently (78). In this series, approximately one-quarter (21 of 88 patients) had no apparent underlying disease, and 81% of these patients were women. Several other series have described a similar group of women with no underlying pulmonary disease (47, 54, 81). Radiographic abnormalities are most frequently located in the right middle lobe, lingula, and anterior segment of the right upper lobe. Clinical symptoms include cough and expectoration, with few reporting fever, chills, or weight loss. Sputum samples may grow MAC as well as other rapidly growing mycobacteria or *Pseudomonas* species.

The American Thoracic Society (ATS) criteria for pulmonary MAC diagnosis generally require two or more sputum samples demonstrating acid-fast bacilli and/or moderate to heavy growth on sputum culture (4). Other causes must have been ruled out. There is debate about the need to treat the "non-

---

TABLE 4 • Antimycrobacterial Agents Commonly Used in the Treatment of MAC Infections (51)

Agent	Adult Dose	Adverse Effects
Amikacin	7.5–15 mg/kg q.d. i.v.	Ototoxicity, nephrotoxicity
Azithromycin	500 mg/day	Nausea, diarrhea, vomiting, abdominal pain, headache, dizziness, elevations in hepatic enzymes
Ciprofloxacin	750 mg b.i.d.	Anorexia, nausea, vomiting, abdominal pain, diarrhea, rash, (rarely) mental status changes
Clarithromycin	500 mg b.i.d.[a]	Diarrhea, nausea, vomiting, elevations in hepatic enzymes, abdominal pain, renal insufficiency
Ethambutol	15 mg/kg/day	Anorexia, nausea, vomiting, diarrhea, rash, elevations in hepatic enzymes, (rarely) ocular changes–retrobulbar neuritis
Rifabutin	300 mg/day[a]	Anorexia, nausea, vomiting, diarrhea, rash, uveitis, myalgias, arthralgias, headache
Rifampin	10 mg/kg/day	Anorexia, nausea, vomiting, diarrhea, rash, elevations in hepatic enzymes

From Korvick JA, Benson CA. Advances in the treatment and prophylaxis of *mycobacterium avium* complex in individuals infected with human immunodeficiency virus. In: Korvick JA, Benson CA, eds. *Mycobacterium avium*-complex infection: progress in research and treatment. New York: Marcel Dekker, 1996:241–262, with permission. (Adapted from 45.)

[a]FDA-approved dose.

TABLE 5 • **Pulmonary MAC Treatment Recommendations**

Duration of treatment: variable; at least 1 year with clearance of sputum

First-line treatment: clarithromycin 500 mg b.i.d. with companion agents active against MAC; treatment should always include combination therapy

Second-line treatment: isoniazid, ethambutol, rifampin, and streptomycin[a] (4)

Alternative therapies: azithromycin 300–600 mg/day (not currently approved for this use, under study); combination therapies should be tailored to the sensitivity profile if the patient has failed the above regimens

Surgical resection: highly variable results, best when used in conjunction with intensive (3–4 months) chemotherapy preoperatively

Selection: drug-drug interactions, especially uveitis with rifabutin and clarithromycin

---

[a]Streptomycin is recommended for initial use in patients with extensive and/or cavitary disease; however, its exact role is unknown. In a mouse study, streptomycin was useful in preventing resistance to clarithromycin.

cavitary, stable infiltrate." The ATS recommendations suggest that these do not need to be treated. However, Iseman et al. have reported patients followed for several years who showed clear progression to cavitary disease, and thus they recommend therapy for this stage of disease (48).

Most of the data on treatment of pulmonary MAC was reported in case series. The therapies used two to five drugs (non-clarithromycin-containing regimens), with initial response rates of 55 to 100% and relapse rates of 10 to 38% (48). The only controlled trials for treatment of pulmonary MAC include one of four drugs (isoniazid, rifampin, ethambutol, and initial streptomycin), an initial 4-month monotherapy trial of clarithromycin (3), a noncomparative trial of clarithromycin-containing regimens on 50 patients with pulmonary MAC (99), and a prospective trial of azithromycin induction therapy (27). A series using clarithromycin was also reported from France (21).

Monotherapy with macrolides for pulmonary MAC demonstrated activity. While the overall results were disappointing, combination therapy results were encouraging. Dautzenberg et al. reported a series of 45 patients with pulmonary MAC without AIDS treated with clarithromycin as monotherapy (14 patients) or combination therapy (21). The companion drugs included clofazimine (18 patients), a quinolone (10 patients), ethambutol (9 patients), and/or rifampin (8 patients). The average dose of clarithromycin was higher in this study, 2000 or 1500 mg/day. At 12 months, 32 of 38 (81%) patients were culture negative, and no pulmonary relapses were seen while patients were not receiving therapy posttreatment (mean, 7 months). The incidence of acquired resistance to clarithromycin among patients treated long term was 15%. Clarithromycin (500

mg twice daily) was also evaluated as 4-month monotherapy in the induction period (98). At the end of the 4 months, 58% of 19 patients became sputum negative, and another 21% showed bacteriologic improvement.

Clarithromycin-containing combination regimens used for disseminated MAC in HIV-positive patients have shown promise for treatment of pulmonary MAC. In a controlled study of 50 patients with pulmonary MAC (99), 30 patients were given initial clarithromycin monotherapy, and the remaining 20 were given initial combination therapy (clarithromycin, ethambutol, rifampin, streptomycin; Table 6). They were treated until culture negative for 1 year; 92% (36 of 39) became sputum negative. Success rates were somewhat lower in patients who had received previous therapy than in those who had not (69 vs. 41%, respectively). Only 15% (6 of 39) of patients developed an isolate that was resistant to clarithromycin. All patients who were alive and culture negative at 12 months were culture negative at 19.1 months.

In 41% of patients treated with companion drugs, one or more were discontinued because of adverse drug events. The most common reasons for discontinuation of one of the companion study drugs included visual acuity (ethambutol), gastrointestinal symptoms (rifampin and rifabutin), leukopenia (rifabutin), and uveitis (rifabutin). Four patients who developed anterior uveitis were receiving clarithromycin and high-dose rifabutin (300–600 mg/day). The authors state that reintroduction of rifabutin at a lower dose (150–300 mg/day) allowed continuation of rifabutin in all cases.

Pharmacokinetics of clarithromycin were studied in the patients receiving rifampin (99). Clarithromycin levels were reduced significantly; however, 10 of 13 patients (77%) receiving rifampin-containing regimens were successfully treated. The drug-drug interactions between the rifamycins and clarithromycin have raised questions about the potential reduced efficacy of clarithromycin.

The usefulness of azithromycin for the treatment of pulmonary MAC is unknown. However, recently 4-month induction monotherapy was reported (27). Sputum conversion rates were lower than those for clarithromycin monotherapy at 4

TABLE 6 • **Clinical Trial Treatment Regimen for Pulmonary MAC (99)**

Drug	Dosage
Clarithromycin	500 mg/kg b.i.d.
Ethambutol	25 mg/kg daily first 2 months, then 15 mg/kg daily
Rifampin (rifabutin)	600 mg daily (if no microbiologic response occurred in the first 6 months, they were switched to rifabutin 600 mg daily)[a]
Streptomycin (ciprofloxacin)	15 mg/kg i.m. or i.v. 2–3 times per week for the first 2–4 months

Data from Wallace RJ Jr, Brown BA, Griffith DE, Girard WM, Murphy DT. Clarithromycin regimens for pulmonary *Mycobacterium avium* complex: the first 50 patients. Am J Respir Crit Care Med 1996;153:1766–1772.

[a]Consideration should be given to the 300 mg/day dose of rifabutin to avoid potential adverse events and drug interaction problems.

months (35 vs. 58%, NS). After addition of companion agents, the 6-month rate improved to 67%. The 300 mg/day dose was better tolerated than the 600 mg/day dose.

Combination therapy with clarithromycin is essential in the treatment of pulmonary MAC. The rapidity with which resistance to clarithromycin monotherapy evolves is well known (11). Additionally, combination therapy should promote increased clinical activity. Ethambutol is strongly recommended as a companion to clarithromycin.

The optimal daily dose of clarithromycin is not fully established. The Wallace study used doses of 1000 mg daily, compared with the Dautzenberg study dose of 1600 mg daily. In the former study the 4-month sputum conversion rate was 58%, compared with 100% in the latter. Higher doses are associated with more-frequent dose-limiting side effects, thus decreasing compliance.

Resectional surgery is still used occasionally to control the infection. Two series have been reported (67, 77) with varying results. While surgery can control hemoptysis and potentially protect the uninvolved lung from being infected, there are substantial risks. Serious postoperative complications can arise, including bronchopleural fistulae (67, 77). This therapy must be accompanied by intensive therapy to prevent seeding of infection.

ENDPOINTS FOR MONITORING THERAPY

Response to therapy for disseminated MAC is monitored by clinical symptoms and qualitative blood cultures. Patients should respond with resolution of fevers and chills, decreases in abnormal alkaline phosphatase levels, and a feeling of well-being within approximately 4 to 8 weeks (11). Quantitative blood cultures are a research tool used to describe the types of response to certain therapies and are not used in routine clinical practice. Response to therapy should result in a negative blood culture for MAC by 12 to 16 weeks (11). However, while the blood may be free of MAC, tissues (including the bone marrow) may still harbor the infection (19, 57, 102). Failure to clear the blood of MAC should lead the clinician to perform sensitivity testing on the clinical isolate to direct future therapeutic choices.

Responses for pulmonary MAC should be measured by negative sputum cultures. Since this is such a difficult disease to treat, as evidenced by Wallace et al. (51% sputum negative at 4 months), the approach to monitoring is similar to that for pulmonary tuberculosis. Symptomatic and radiologic improvement should be seen within 4 months. If it is not, individualized therapy decisions should be made on the basis of results of sputum culture and isolate susceptibility testing.

Prophylaxis against disseminated MAC should be monitored with blood cultures every 3 to 4 months. The interval between cultures should be modified according to the clinical status of the individual patient.

HIV-POSITIVE INDIVIDUALS: DISSEMINATED MAC PROPHYLAXIS

(Recommendations are summarized in Table 7.)

Prophylactic therapy is recommended in an effort to reduce the significant morbidity and mortality associated with dissem-

---

TABLE 7 • Disseminated MAC Prophylaxis Recommendations

Duration: prophylaxis should be initiated in individuals with CD4 cell counts < 50 cells/mm³ and continued for life

First-line prophylaxis: clarithromycin 500 mg b.i.d. or azithromycin 1200 mg once weekly (96)

Second-line prophylaxis: rifabutin 300 mg daily

Alternative: azithromycin 1200 mg weekly in combination with rifabutin 300 mg/daily

Selection: the choice should be made on the individual patient's circumstances, especially regarding concomitant drugs being taken; numerous drug-drug interactions have been reported

Drug-drug interactions: drug interactions should be considered when patients receive protease inhibitors and rifabutin therapy should be modified: rifabutin 150 mg daily with Crixivan (indinavir) (17); rifabutin is currently contraindicated with Norvir (ritonavir) (71); however, if the situation warrants, based upon the pharmacokinetic profiles, rifabutin 150 mg every other day may be used with close monitoring of the patient (9)

---

inated MAC in HIV-positive individuals. Currently, the CD4 cell count is used as an indicator for initiation of prophylactic therapy. Originally, it was recommended that HIV-positive individuals with CD4+ cell counts of 100 cells/mm³ or less should be placed on prophylaxis (94). Joint recommendations from the Centers for Disease Control and Prevention and the Infectious Diseases Society of America recommend initiation when the CD4 cell count drops to 50 cells/mm³ or below, when the risk of acquiring disease is significantly increased (96).

Clinical trials regarding prophylaxis of disseminated MAC have been completed using the following antimycobacterial agents: rifabutin (Mycobutin), clarithromycin (Biaxin), azithromycin (Zithromax), and the combination of rifabutin with either azithromycin or clarithromycin (Table 8).

In general, review of the large clinical studies reveals an advantage for rifabutin, clarithromycin, and azithromycin over the control therapy for the prevention of MAC bacteremia (Table 8). Interpretation of these advantages may be confounded by a number of factors that must be considered when making companions across studies: patient populations, duration of patient follow-up, and use of an active control arm for comparison.

Study populations that were enrolled may have changed over time. The first study of prophylaxis (initiated in 1990) compared rifabutin with placebo (70). The mean CD4+ cell count at entry in this study was 60 cells/m, while those of the other studies (clarithromycin and azithromycin) were approximately 20 cells/mm³ (9, 30, 75). Thus, a selection for patients at higher risk of infection and/or death was seen in the later studies.

To date, only one study has demonstrated a survival advantage; the study by Pierce et al. showed a survival advantage

TABLE 8 • **Clinical Studies of Disseminated MAC Prophylactic Regimens in HIV-Positive Individuals**

Agent (Reference)	Regimen Studied	MAC Events % (N)	Survival Benefit
Rifabutin (69)	Rifabutin 300 mg daily	8.5 (48/566)	No
	vs. placebo (2 studies)	17.6 (102/580)	
Clarithromycin (75)	Clarithromycin 500 mg b.i.d.	4.5 (15/343)	Yes
	vs. placebo	12.0 (41/341)	
Clarithromycin, rifabutin, combination (9)	Clarithromycin 500 mg b.i.d.	9.0 (36/398)	No
	vs. rifabutin 300 mg/day	15.0 (59/391)	
	vs. combination	7.0 (26/389)	
Azithromycin, rifabutin, combination (30)	Azithromycin 1200 mg weekly	13.9 (31/223)	No
	vs. rifabutin 300 mg/day	23.3 (52/223)	
	vs. combination	8.3 (18/218)	

for clarithromycin versus placebo (75). When comparing the studies, remember that the later two had active control arms (rifabutin) (9, 30). While rifabutin itself did not demonstrate a statistically significant difference in the Nightingale study, there were numerically fewer deaths in the rifabutin arm than with placebo; 33 and 47 deaths respectively ($P = .86$). Analysis of additional follow-up data in the rifabutin study (70) supports a survival trend for rifabutin (66). Thus, it is not completely surprising that no survival advantage was seen in the studies in which rifabutin served as the active control (9, 30). Additionally, it is of interest that combination regimens did not add to the survival advantage in either study.

Macrolide cross-resistance is an important disadvantage when monotherapy is used. To date, no rifabutin-resistant MAC breakthrough isolates have been seen (9, 30, 70). However, MAC breakthroughs in the studies of clarithromycin and azithromycin were documented. Of the 19 *M. avium* isolates recovered from treatment breakthroughs in the Pierce study, 11 were resistant to clarithromycin, an overall incidence of less than 2% for clarithromycin-resistant disease (75).

In these studies, combinations of macrolides with rifabutin did not prevent emergence of macrolide resistance. Rifabutin resistance was not found; however, breakthroughs with clarithromycin-resistant isolates were seen. Benson et al. reported clarithromycin resistance in 7 of 24 (29%) in the clarithromycin arm, compared with 4 of 15 (27%) in the combination arm and none in the rifabutin arm (9). (The breakpoint used in this study was 32 μg/mL; the Pierce study used 512 μg/mL.) There was also a trend toward higher MICs in the clarithromycin arm and the combination arm than in the rifabutin arm but no difference between clarithromycin monotherapy and the combination arm (9). Finally, Havlir et al. reported recovering resistant isolates from 2 of 11 isolates tested, both were from the azithromycin arm and were cross-resistant to clarithromycin (30).

The adverse-event profile of combination prophylactic MAC therapy leads to decreased compliance with these regimens. While there appear to be fewer MAC events with combination prophylactic regimens, especially for the combina-

tion of azithromycin and rifabutin, there were more discontinuations in that treatment group. The most frequent adverse event was gastrointestinal complaints, leading to decreased compliance with these regimens (9, 30). Therefore, the current MAC prophylaxis recommendations are for monotherapy (96).

Drug-drug interactions are very common among HIV-infected individuals because of the number of concurrent medications they receive (9). The most important interaction is between rifabutin and the protease inhibitors or rifabutin and clarithromycin, both metabolized through the CYP 3A4 enzyme of the P-450 pathway (76). Rifabutin is an enzyme inducer, and ritonavir and indinavir are enzyme inhibitors (25). Thus, rifabutin could substantially lower blood levels of the protease inhibitors, leading to a subtherapeutic dose and potential development of protease resistance by HIV. (For dosage adjustment recommendations see Table 7.)

Higher doses of rifabutin cause uveitis in HIV-positive patients (91). An attempt to optimize rifabutin therapy at higher doses was abandoned because of the increase incidence of uveitis, especially when rifabutin was used in combination with clarithromycin (89).

What is the duration for MAC prophylaxis? With the advent of the protease inhibitors and the substantial increases in CD4 cells that result from such intervention, the practice of lifelong prophylaxis is being questioned. There is concern that clonal expansion of the T-cell repertoire may not be sufficient, initially, to protect the individual against MAC (5). However, reports have described the potential unmasking of subclinical lymphadenitis in HIV-infected individuals receiving protease therapy (74, 79). This may suggest enhanced immune response as the CD4+ cells expand. This is the subject of ongoing debate.

CAVEATS AND COMMENTS

Although the macrolides have demonstrated impressive activity against MAC, compared with earlier therapies, concerns exist regarding the development of resistance. Combination therapy is the rule for treatment of pulmonary or disseminated MAC.

Monotherapy appears appropriate for the prophylaxis of MAC in persons with AIDS. Currently, few additional new drugs are on the horizon (oxazolidinones). Therapies that include immunomodulators are being studied: granulocyte/macrophage colony-stimulating factory (GM-CSF), interleukin-12, and interferon-γ. The use of new antiviral regimens including the protease inhibitors may also contribute to the management of these diseases.

REFERENCES

1. Abe C, Husojima S, Fukasawa Y, Kazumi Y, Takahashi M, Hirano K, Mori T. Comparison of MB-check, BACTEC, and egg-based media for recovery of mycobacteria. J Clin Microbiol 1992;30:878–881.

2. Agins BD, Berman DS, Spicehandler D, El-Sadr W, Simberkoff MS, Rahal JJ. Effect of combined therapy with ansamycin, clofazimine, ethambutol and isoniazid for *Mycobacterium avium* infection in patients with AIDS. J Infect Dis 1989;159:784–787.

3. Ahn C, Ann S, Anderson R, Murphy DT, Mammo A. A four-drug regimen for initial treatment of cavitary disease caused by *Mycobacterium avium* complex. Am Rev Respir Dis 1986;134:438–441.

4. American Thoracic Society. Diagnosis and treatment of disease caused by non-tuberculous mycobacteria. Am Rev Respir Dis 1990;142:940–953.

5. Autran B, Cracelain G, Li TS, Blanc C, Mathez D, Tubiana R, Katlama C, Debre P, Libowitch J. Positive effects of combined antiretroviral therapy on CD41 T cell homeostasis and function in advanced HIV disease. Science 1997;277:112–116.

6. Bacellar H, Munoz A, Hoover DR, Phair JP, Besley DR, Kingsley LA, Vermund SH, for the Multicenter AIDS Cohort Study. Incidence of clinical AIDS conditions in a cohort of homosexual men with CD41 cell counts, 100/mm³. J Infect Dis 1994:170:1284–1287.

7. Bach MC. Treating disseminated *Mycobacterium avium* intracellulare infection [Letter]. Ann Intern Med 1989;110:169–170.

8. Benson CA. Critical drug interactions with agents used for prophylaxis and treatment of *Mycobacterium avium* complex infection. Am J Med 1997;102(5C):32–36.

9. Benson CA, Williams PL, Cohn DL, Becker S, Korvick JA, Nevin T, Heifets L, Notario GF, Wynne B, Hafner R, and the ACTG 196/CPCRA 009 Protocol Team. Clarithromycin, rifabutin or the combination of clarithromycin and rifabutin for primary prophylaxis of *Mycobacterium avium* complex disease in patients with AIDS. 1997, in press.

10. Berry A, Koletar S, Williams D. Azithromycin for disseminated *Mycobacterium avium-intracellulare* in AIDS patients [Abstract 292]. The First National Conference on Human Retroviruses and Related Infections. Washington, DC: Centers for Disease Control and Prevention/National Institutes of Health, 1993.

11. Chaisson RE, Benson CA, Dube MP, Korvick JA, Elkin S, Dellerson M, Smith T, Craft CC, Sattler F, and the AIDS Clinical Trials Group Protocol 157 Study Team. Clarithromycin therapy for bacteremic *Mycobacterium avium* complex disease in patients with AIDS. Ann Intern Med 1994;121:905–911.

12. Chaisson RE, Keiser P, Pierce M, Fessel WJ, Ruskin J, Lahart C, Benson CA, Meek K, Siepman N, Craft JC. Clarithromycin and ethambutol with or without clofazimine for the treatment of bacteremic *Mycobacterium avium* complex disease in patients with HIV infection. AIDS 1997;11:311–317.

13. Chin DP, Hopewell PC, Yajko DM, Vittinghoff E, Horsburgh

CR Jr, Hadley WK, Stone EN, Nassos PS, Ostroff SM, Jacobson MA, Matkin CC, Reingold AL. *Mycobacterium avium* complex in the respiratory or gastrointestinal tract and the risk of M. avium bacteremia in patients with the human immunodeficiency virus. J Infect Dis 1994;169:289–295.

14. Chiu J, Nussbaum J, Bozzette S, Tilles JG, Young LS, Leedom J, Heseltine PNR, McCutchen JA, and the California Collaborative Treatment Group. Treatment of disseminated *Mycobacterium avium* complex infection in AIDS with amikacin, ethambutol, rifampin and ciprofloxacin. Ann Intern Med 1990;113:358–361.

15. Cohen DL, Fisher E, Franchio B, Peng G, Hodges J, Chestnut J, Child C, Gibert C, El-Sadr W, Hafner R, Ropka M, Heifets L, Clotfelter J, Munroe D, Caldwell R, Horsburgh R, CPCRA 027 protocol team. Prospective, randomized trial of four 3-drug regimens for treatment (RX) of disseminated MAC disease in AIDS (DM): excess mortality associated with high-dose clarithromycin [Abstract 659]. Abstracts of the fourth Conference on Retroviruses and Opportunistic Infections. Washington, DC, 1997.

16. Contreras M, Cheung O, Sanders D, Goldstein R. Pulmonary infection with nontuberculous mycobacteria. Am Rev Respir Dis 1988;137:149–152.

17. Crixivan (Indivir) package insert/product monograph. West Point, Pa: Merck and Co, 1996.

18. Crowle AJ, Tsang AY, Vatter AE, May MH. Comparison of 15 laboratory and patient derived strains of *Mycobacterium avium* for ability to infect and multiply in cultured human macrophages. J Clin Microbiol 1986;24:812–821.

19. DATRI 007 Study Group. *Mycobacterium avium* complex (MAC) disease in HIV-infected patients is a uniform infection of bone marrow that does not correlate with the level of infection in blood [Abstract 7]. 2nd National Conference on Human Retroviruses and Related Infections, Washington, DC, 1995.

20. Dautzenberg B, Trufflot C, Legris S, Meyohas MC, Berlie HC, Mercat A, Chevret S, Grosset J. Activity of clarithromycin against *Mycobacterium avium* infection in patients with the acquired immune deficiency syndrome: a controlled clinical trial. Am Rev Respir Dis 1991;144:564–569.

21. Dautzenberg B, Piperson D, Diot P, Truffot-Pernot C, Chauvin JP. Clarithromycin in the treatment of *Mycobacterium avium* lung infections in patients without AIDS. Chest 1995;107:1035–1040.

22. Davidson P, Khanijo V, Goble M, Moulding T. Treatment of disease due to *Mycobacterium intracellulare*. Rev Infect Dis 1981;3:1052–1059.

23. Dube M, Sattler F, Torriani F, See D, Havlir D, Kemper C, Dezfuli M, Bozzette S, Bartok A, Leedom J, Tilles J, McCutchan for the California Collaborative Treatment Group. Prevention of relapse of MAC bacteremia in AIDS: a randomized study of clarithromycin, plus clofazimine, with or without ethambutol [Abstract]. 3rd Conference on Human Retroviruses and Opportunistic Infections, Washington, DC, 1996.

24. Edwards LB, Palmer CE. Epidemiologic studies of tuberculin sensitivity. I. Preliminary results with purified protein derivatives prepared from atypical acid-fast organisms. Am J Hyg 1958;68:213–231.

25. Gerber JG. Drug interaction issues in treatment of HIV infection. HIV/AIDS Clin Insights 1996;6:1–6.

26. Gladue RP, Bright GM, Isaacson RE, Newborg MR. In vitro and in vivo uptake of azithromycin (CP-62,9331) by phagocytic cells: possible mechanism of delivery and release at sites of infection. Antimicrob Agents Chemother 1989;33:277–282.

27. Griffith DE, Brown BA, Girard W, Murphy DT, Wallace RJ Jr.

Azithromycin activity against *Mycobacterium avium* complex lung disease in HIV negative patients. Clin Infect Dis 1996; 23:983–989.

28. Grosset JH. Assessment of new therapies for infection due to the *Mycobacterium avium* complex: appropriate use of in vitro and in vivo testing. Clin Infect Dis 1994;18(Suppl 3):S233–236.

29. Gupta S, Blahunka K, Dellerson M, Craft JC, Smith T. Interim results of safety and efficacy of clarithromycin in the treatment of disseminated *Mycobacterium avium* complex (MAC) infection in patients with AIDS [Abstract]. 32rd Interscience Conference on Antimicrobial Agents and Chemotherapy, Washington, DC, 1992.

30. Havlir DV, Dube MP, Sattler FR, Forthal DN, Kemper CA, Dunne MW, Parenti DM, Lavelle JP, White AC Jr, Witt MD, Bozzette SA, McCutchan JA. Prophylaxis against disseminated *Mycobacterium avium* complex with weekly azithromycin, daily rifabutin or both. N Engl J Med 1996;335:392–398.

31. Hawkins CC, Gold JWM, Whimbey E, Kiehn TE, Brannon P, Cammarata R, Brown AE, Armstrong D. *Mycobacterium avium* complex infections in patients with acquired immunodeficiency syndrome. Ann Intern Med 1986;105:184–188.

32. Hellyer TJ, Brown IN, Dale JW, Easmon CS. Plasmid analysis of *Mycobacterium avium-intracellulare* (MAI) isolated in the United Kingdom from patients with and without AIDS. J Med Microbiol 1991;34:225–231.

33. Hoffer SE. Improved detection of *Mycobacterium avium* complex with the Bactec radiometric system. Diagn Microbiol Infect Dis 1988;10:1–6.

34. Hoffer SE, Haile M, Källenius G. A biphasic system for primary isolation of *mycobacterium* compared to solid medium and broth culture. J Med Microbiol 1992;37:332–334.

35. Hoover DR, Graham NM, Bacellar H, Murphy R, Visscher B, Anderson R, McArthur J. An epidemiologic analysis of *Mycobacterium avium* complex disease in homosexual men infected with human immunodeficiency virus type 1. Clin Infect Dis 1995;20:1250–1258.

36. Horsburgh CR, Havlik JA, Ellis DA, Kennedy E, Fann SA, Dubois RE, Thompson SE. Survival in patients with acquired immune deficiency syndrome and disseminated *Mycobacterium avium* complex infection with and without antimycobacterial chemotherapy. Am Rev Respir Dis 1991;144:557–559.

37. Horsburgh CR. *Mycobacterium avium* complex infection in the acquired immune deficiency syndrome. N Engl J Med 1991; 324:1332–138.

38. Horsburgh CR, Metchock B, Gordon SM, Havlik JA Jr, McGowan JE Jr, Thompson SE III. Predictors of survival in patients with AIDS and disseminated *Mycobacterium avium* complex disease. J Infect Dis 1994;170:573–577.

39. Horsburgh CR Jr. Epidemiology of human disease caused by *Mycobacterium avium* complex. Can J Infect Dis 1994;5(Suppl B):5B–9B.

40. Horsburgh CR, Gordin F, Schoenfelder F, Sullam P, Cohn D, Wynne B. Clinical presentation of disseminated *M. avium* complex (MAC) disease: a case controlled analysis [Abstract 147]. 35th Interscience Conference on Antimicrobial Agents and Chemotherapy, San Francisco, CA, 1995.

41. Horsburgh CR Jr, Hanson DL Jones JL, Thompson SE. Protection form *Mycobacterium avium* complex disease in human immunodeficiency virus-infected persons with a history of tuberculosis. J Infect Dis 1996;174:1212–1217.

42. Horsburgh CR Jr. Epidemiology of *Mycobacterium avium* complex disease. Am J Med 1997;102(5C):11–15.

43. Horsburgh CR Jr, Schonfelder JR, Bordin FM, Cohn DL, Sullam PM, Wynne BA. Geographic and seasonal variation in *M. avium* bacteremia among North American patients with AIDS. Am J Med Sci 1997, in press.

44. Hoy J, Mijch A, Sandland M, Grayson L, Lucas R, Dwyer B. Quadruple-drug therapy for *Mycobacterium avium-intracellulare* bacteremia in AIDS patients. J Infect Dis 1990;161: 801–805.

45. Inderleid CB, Kemper CA, Bermudez LEM. The *Mycobacterium avium* complex. Clin Microbiol Rev 1993;6:266–310.

46. Inderlied CB. Microbiology and minimum inhibitory concentration testing for *Mycobacterium avium* complex prophylaxis. Am J Med 1997;102(5C):2–10.

47. Iseman M, Buschman D, Ackerson L. Pectus excavatum and scoliosis: thoracic anomalies associated with pulmonary disease due to *M. avium* complex. Am Rev Respir Dis 1991;144: 914–916.

48. Iseman MD. Pulmonary disease due to *Mycobacterium avium* complex. In: Korvick JA, Benson CA, eds. *Mycobacterium avium*-complex infection: progress in research and treatment. New York: Marcel Dekker, 1996:45–79.

49. Ishiguro M, Koga H, Kohno S, Hayashi T, Yamaguchi K, Hirota M. Penetration of macrolides into human polymorphic nuclear leukocytes. J Antimicrob Chemother 1989;24:719–729.

50. Jacobson MA, Yajko D, Northfelt D, Charlebois E, Gary D, Brosgart C, Sanders CA, Hadley WK. Randomized, placebo controlled trial of rifampin, ethambutol and ciprofloxacin for AIDS patients with disseminated *Mycobacterium avium* complex infection. J Infect Dis 1993;168:112–119.

51. Kemper CA, Meng RC, Nussbaum J, Chiu J, Feigal D, Bartok AE, Leedom JM, Tilles JG, Deresinski SC, McCutchan JA, and the California Collaborative Treatment Group. Treatment of *Mycobacterium avium* complex bacteremia in AIDS with a four-drug oral regimen. Ann Intern Med 1992;116:466–472.

52. Kemper CA, Havlir D, Haghighat D, Dube M, Bartok AE, Sison JP, Yao Y, Yangco B, Leedom JM, Tilles JG, McCutchan A, Deresinski S. The individual microbiologic effect of three antimycobacterial agents, clofazimine, ethambutol and rifampin on *Mycobacterium avium* complex bacteremia in patients with AIDS. J Infect Dis 1994;170:157–164.

53. Kemper CA, Deresinski SC. *Mycobacterium avium* complex infection in AIDS. In: Volberding PA, Jacobson MA, eds. AIDS clinical review 1995/1996. New York: Marcel Dekker, 19xx: 153–228.

54. Kennedy T, Weber D. Nontuberculous mycobacteria: an under-appreciated cause of geriatric lung disease. Am J Respir Crit Care Med 1994;149:1654–1658.

55. Kirschner RA Jr, Parker BC, Falkinham JO III. Epidemiology of infection by nontuberculous mycobacteria. *Mycobacterium avium, Mycobacterium intracellulare,* and *Mycobacterium scrofulaceum* in acid, brown-water swamps of the southeastern United States and their association with environmental variables. Am Rev Respir Dis 1992;145:271–275.

56. Korvick JA, Benson CA. Advances in the treatment and prophylaxis of *Mycobacterium avium* complex in individuals infected with human immunodeficiency virus. In: Korvick JA, Benson CA, eds. *Mycobacterium avium*-complex infection: progress in research and treatment. New York: Marcel Dekker, 1996:241–262.

57. Lasseur C, Maugein J, Dupon M, et al. Usefulness of bone marrow aspiration culture for diagnosis of disseminated *Mycobacterium avium* complex infection (D-MAC) in patients with AIDS [Abstract D57]. Proceedings and Abstracts of the 34th

Interscience Conference on Antimicrobial Agents and Chemotherapy, Washington, DC, 1994.

58. Lynch D, Simone P, Fox M, Bucher BL, Heinig MJ. CT features of pulmonary *Mycobacterium avium* complex infection: comparison with *Mycobacterium tuberculosis*, and correlation with sputum positivity. J Computer Assist Tomogr 1995;19 (3): 353–360.

59. May T, Brel F, Beuscart C, Vincent V, Perronne C, Saint-Marc T, Dautzenberg B, Grosset J, and Curvarium Group. A French randomized open trial of 2 clarithromycin combination therapies for MAC bacteremia: first results [Abstract]. 35th Interscience Conference on Antimicrobial Agents and Chemotherapy, San Francisco, CA, 1995.

60. Food and Drug Administration Advisory Committee Meeting, Rockville, MD, May 10, 1993.

61. Masur H, Tuazon C, Gill V, Grimes G, Baird B, Fauci AS, Lane HC. Effect of combined clofazimine and ansamycin therapy on *Mycobacterium avium-Mycobacterium intracellulare* bacteremia in patients with AIDS. J Infect Dis 1987;155:127–129.

62. Meier A, Kirschner P, Springer B, Steingrub VA, Brown BA, Wallace RJ Jr, Böttger EC. Identification of mutations in 23s rRNA gene of clarithromycin-resistant *Mycobacterium intracellulare*. Antimicrob Agents Chemother 1994;38:381–384.

63. Meylan PR, Richmond DD, Kornbluth KS. Characterization and growth in human macrophages of *Mycobacterium avium* complex strains isolated from the blood of patients with acquired immunodeficiency syndrome. Infect Immun 1990;58:2564–2568.

64. Mizuguchi Y, Udou T, Yamada T. Mechanism of antibiotic resistance in *Mycobacterium intracellulare*. Microbiol Immunol 1983;27:425–431.

65. Mizuguchi Y, Ogawa M, Udou T. Morphological changes induced by beta-lactam antibiotics in *Mycobacterium avium-*intracellulare complex. Antimicrob Agents Chemother 1985; 27:541–547.

66. Moore RD, Chaisson RE. Survival analysis of two controlled trials of rifabutin prophylaxis against *Mycobacterium avium* complex in AIDS. AIDS 1995;9:1337–1342.

67. Moran J, Alexander L, Staub E, Young WG Jr, Sealy WC. Long-term results of pulmonary resection for atypical mycobacterial disease. Ann Thorac Surg 1983;35:597–604.

68. Nightingale SD, Byrd LT, Southern PM, Jockusch JD, Cal SX, Wynne BA. Incidence of *Mycobacterium avium-intracellulare* complex bacteremia in human immunodeficiency virus-positive patients. J Infect Dis 1992;165:1082–1085.

69. Nightingale SD, Saletan SL, Swenson CE, Lawrence AJ, Watson DA, Pilkiewiez FG, Silverman EG, Cal SX. Liposome-encapsulated gentamicin treatment of *Mycobacterium avium-Mycobacterium intracellulare* complex bacteremia in AIDS patients. Antimicrob Agents Chemother 1993;37:1869–1872.

70. Nightingale SD, Cameron DW, Gordin FM, Sullam PM, Cohn DL, Chaisson RE, Eron LJ, Sparti PD, Bihari B, Kaufman DL, Stern JJ, Pearce DD, Weinberg WG, LaMarca A, Siegal FP. Two controlled trials of rifabutin prophylaxis against *Mycobacterium avium* complex infection in AIDS. N Engl J Med 1993;329: 828–833.

71. Norvir (Ritonavir) package insert/product monograph. North Chicago, IL: Abbott Laboratories, 1996.

72. O'Brien RJ, Geiter LJ, Snider DE. The epidemiology of nontuberculous mycobacterial disease in the US. Results from a national survey. Am Rev Respir Dis 1987;35:1007–1014.

73. Parenti D, Ellner J, Hafner R, Williams P, Jacobs M, Hojczyk P. A phase II/III trial of rifampin (rif), ciprofloxacin (dipro), clo-fazimine (clof), ethambutol (eth), 6 amikacin (AK) in the treatment of disseminated *Mycobacterium avium* (ma) infection in HIV-infected individuals [Abstract 6]. Second National Conference on Human Retroviruses and Related Infections. Washington, DC, 1995.

74. Phillips P, Zala C, Rouleau D, Montaner JSG. Mycobacterial lymphadenitis: can highly active antiretroviral therapy (HAART) unmask subclinical infection [Abstract 351]? Abstracts of the 4th Conference on Retroviruses and Opportunistic Infections, Washington, DC, 1997.

75. Pierce M, Crampton S, Henry D, Heifets L, LaMarch A, Montecalvo M, Wormser GP, Jablonowski H, Jemsek J, Cynamon M, Yanbco BG, Notario G, Craft JC. A randomized trial of clarithromycin as prophylaxis against disseminated *Mycobacterium avium* complex infecting in patients with advanced acquired immunodeficiency syndrome. N Engl J Med 1996;335:384–391.

76. Piscilelli SC, Flexner C, Minor JR, Polis MA, Mazur H. Drug interactions in patients infected with human immunodeficiency virus. Clin Infect Dis 1996;23:685–693.

77. Pomerantz M, Madsen L, Goble M, Iseman M. Surgical management of resistant mycobacterial tuberculosis and other mycobacterial pulmonary infections. Ann Thorac Surg 1991;52: 1108–1112.

78. Prince D, Peterson D, Steiner R, Gottlieb JE, Scott R, Israel HL, Figueroa WG, Fish JE. Infection with *Mycobacterium avium* complex in patients without predisposing conditions. N Engl J Med 1989;321:863–868.

79. Race E, Adelson-Mitty J, Barlam T, Japour A. Focal inflammatory lymphadenitis (FIL) and fever following initiation of protease inhibitor (PRI) in patients with advanced HIV-1 disease [Abstract 352]. Abstracts of the 4th Conference on Retroviruses and Opportunistic Infections, Washington, DC, 1997.

80. Rastogi N, Frehel C, Ryler A, Ohayon H, Lesourd M, David HL. Multiple drug resistance in *Mycobacterium avium*: is the wall architecture responsible for the exclusion of antimicrobial agents? Antimicrob Agents Chemother 1981;20:666–677.

81. Reich J, Johnson R. *Mycobacterium avium* complex pulmonary disease. Incidence, presentation, and response to therapy in a community setting. Am Rev Respir Dis 1991;143: 1381–1385.

82. Rivoire B, Ranchoff BJ, Chatterjee D, Gaylord H, Tsang AY, Kolk AH, Aspinall GO, Brennan PJ. Generation of monoclonal antibodies to specific sugar epitopes of *Mycobacterium avium* complex serovars. Infect Immun 1989;57:3147–3158.

83. Rosensweig D, Schlueter D. Spectrum of clinical disease in pulmonary infection with *Mycobacterium avium-intracellulare*. Rev Infect Dis 1981;3:1046–1051.

84. Rulong S, Aquas AP, da Silva PP, Silva MT. Intramacrophagic mycobacterium bacilli are coated by a multiple lamellar structure: freeze fracture analysis of infected mouse liver. Infect Immun 1991;59:3895–3902.

85. Smith DT. Diagnostic and prognostic significance of the quantitative tuberculin tests. Ann Intern Med 1967;67:919–946.

86. Saito H, Tomioka H. Susceptibilies of transparent, opaque and rough colonial variants of *Mycobacterium avium* complex to fatty acids. Antimicrob Agents Chemother 1988;32: 400–402.

87. Saito H, Tomioka H, Sato K, Tasaka H, Dawson DJ. Identification of various serovar strains of *M avium* complex by using DNA probes specific for *M. avium* and *M. intracellulare*. J Clin Microbiol 1990;28:1694–1697.

88. Schaefer WB, Davis CL, Cohn ML. Pathogenicity of transpar-

ent opaque and rough variants of *Mycobacterium avium* in chickens and mice. Am Rev Respir Dis 1970;102:499–506.

89. Shafran SD, Deschenes I, Miller M, Phillips P, Toma E. Uveitis and pseudojaundice during a regimen of clarithromycin, rifabutin, and ethambutol. N Engl J Med 1994;330:438–439.

90. Shafran SD, Singer J, Zarowny DR, Phillips P, Salit I, Walmsley SL, Fong IW, Gill J, Rachlis AR, Lalonde RG, Fanning MM, Tsoukas CM. Comparison of two regimens for *Mycobacterium avium* complex bacteremia in AIDS. N Engl J Med 1996;335:377–383.

91. Siegal F, Eilbott D, Burger H, Gehan K, Davidson B, Daell AT, Weiser R. Dose-limiting toxicity of rifabutin in AIDS-related complex: syndrome of arthralgia/arthritis. AIDS 1990;4:433–441.

92. Stone BL, Cohn DL, Kane MS, et al. Utility of paired blood cultures and smears in diagnosis of disseminated *Mycobacterium avium* complex infections in AIDS patients. J Clin Microbiol 1994;32:841–842.

93. Tsukamura M. Diagnosis of disease caused by *Mycobacterium avium* complex. Chest 1991;99:667–669.

94. US Public Health Service Task Force on Prophylaxis and Treatment for *Mycobacterium avium* complex. Recommendations on prophylaxis and treatment of disseminated *Mycobacterium avium* complex for adults and adolescents infected with human immunodeficiency virus. MMWR 1993;42(RR-9):14–20.

95. USPHS/IDSA guidelines for the prevention of opportunistic infections in persons infected with HIV: an overview. Clin MMWR 1995;44(RR-8):11–34.

96. USPHS/IDSA guidelines for the prevention of opportunistic infections in persons infected with HIV: an overview. Clin MMWR Morb 1997;46(RR-12).

97. von Reyn CF, Maslow JN, Barber TW, Falkinham JO III, Arbeit RD. Persistent colonization of potable water as a source of *Mycobacterium avium* infection in AIDS. Lancet 1994;343:1137–1141.

98. Wallace RJ Jr, Brown BA, Griffith DE, Girard WM, Murphy DT, Onyi GO, Steingrube VA, Mazurek GH. Initial clarithromycin monotherapy for *Mycobacterium avium-intracellulare* complex lung disease. Am J Respir Crit Care Med 1994;149:1335–1334.

99. Wallace RJ Jr, Brown BA, Griffith DE, Girard WM, Murphy DT. Clarithromycin regimens for pulmonary *Mycobacterium avium* complex: the first 50 patients. Am J Respir Crit Care Med 1996;153:1766–1772.

100. Ward T, Rimland D, Huycke M, Kaufman C, and the VA HIV Consortium Study Group. Randomized open-label trial of azithromycin plus ethambutol vs clarithromycin plus ethambutol treatment of MAC bacteremia in AIDS [Abstract 241]. Abstracts of the 34th IDSA Conference, New Orleans, 1996.

101. Wiley EL, Parry A, Nightingale SD, Lawerence J. Detection of *Mycobacterium avium* complex in bone marrow specimens of patients with acquired immunodeficiency syndrome. Am J Clin Pathol 1994;101:446–451.

102. Wolinsky E. Nontuberculous mycobacteria and associated diseases. Am Rev Respir Dis 1979;119:107–159.

103. Woodley CL, David HL. Effect of temperature on the rate of the transparent to opaque colony type transition in *Mycobacterium avium*. Antimicrob Agents Chemother 1976;9:113–119.

104. Wayne LG, Good RC, Kirchevsky MI, Blacklock Z, David HL, Dawson D, Gross W, Hawkins J, Levy-Frebault VV, McManus. Fourth report of the cooperative open-ended study of slowly growing mycobacteria by the International Working Group on Mycobacterial Taxonomy. Int J Syst Bacteriol 1991;41:463–473.

105. Young LS. *Mycobacterium avium* complex infection. J Infect Dis 1988;157:863–867.

106. Young LS, Wiviott L, Wu M, Kolonoski P, Bolan R, Inderlied C. Azithromycin for treatment of *Mycobacterium avium-intracellulare* complex infection in patients with AIDS. Lancet 1991;388:1107–1109.

107. Young LS, WU M, Bender J, for the Sparfloxacin Study Group. Pilot study of sparfloxacin for *Mycobacterium avium* complex (MAC) bacteremia complication AIDS [Abstract 897]. Program and Abstracts of the 32nd Interscience Conference on Antimicrobial Agents and Chemotherapy, Anaheim, CA, 1992.

Mycobacterium kansasii

•

David E. Griffith and Richard J. Wallace, Jr.

GENERAL DESCRIPTION

Mycobacterium kansasii is a slowly growing species producing rough buff-colored colonies that, after exposure to light, develop yellowish pigmentation due to deposition of β-carotene crystals. Isolates produce both catalase and nitrate reductase, and they hydrolyze Tween 80. Disease-producing strains are usually highly catalase positive (17). Currently, a highly sensitive and specific commercial DNA probe (Accuprobe; GenProbe, Inc.) is available for identification of *M.* *kansasii* isolates. This method, along with high-performance liquid chromatography (HPLC) analysis of mycolic acid esters, has increasingly replaced use of colony morphology and pigmentation for early presumptive identification of the species in larger reference and state health laboratories.

M. kansasii has long been considered morphologically homogeneous. Recent genetic studies have shown major genetic diversity among *M. kansasii* isolates recovered throughout the world (14, 15). One recent DNA-based study showed the presence of five taxonomic groups among both environmental and human isolates (14). The clinical significance of these genetic subgroups remains to be defined.

M. kansasii and *M. marinum* have traditionally been grouped together because they share in vitro growth and biochemical characteristics. Unfortunately, they have little in common clinically. Current rapid diagnostic methods including the use of liquid media such as Bactec 12B broth, mycolic acid analysis, and nucleic acid probes obviate the need for traditional methods of identification that depended on type of pigment production and growth rates (Runyon classification system). Because of the clinical differences and these changes in laboratory identification techniques, *M. kansasii* and *M. marinum* are considered separately in this discussion.

SUSCEPTIBILITY IN VITRO AND IN VIVO

Previously untreated strains of *M. kansasii* are inhibited by rifampin, rifabutin, isoniazid (INH), ethambutol, ethionamide, amikacin, streptomycin, clarithromycin, and probably ciprofloxacin at concentrations readily achievable in the serum (and hence in tissues) with usual therapeutic doses (3, 8, 9, 13, 19). As with most nontuberculous mycobacteria, the MICs for most antituberculous drugs for *M. kansasii* are 10 to 100 times higher than those for *M. tuberculosis,* with the exception of rifampin, ethambutol, amikacin, and ciprofloxacin. All isolates are highly resistant to pyrazinamide. Untreated strains are highly susceptible to the rifamycins with rifampin MICs of 1.0 μg/mL or below and rifabutin MICs 0.5 μg/mL or below. Isolates of *M. kansasii* that have developed high-level (>8.0 μg/mL) resistance to rifampin usually have MICs comparable to those of rifabutin, while isolates with low-level rifampin resistance (MICs, 2.0–8.0 μg/mL) exhibit MICs for rifabutin that are similar to those of untreated wild type strains (≤0.5 μg/mL) (19). The genetic mechanism of rifampin resistance in *M. kansasii* has not been studied but presumably involves multiple mutations in the RNA polymerase gene (rpo β) as it does with *M. tuberculosis.* MICs for untreated strains of *M. kansasii* to INH generally range from 1.0 to 4.0 μg/mL (19). These MICs are 10 to 50 times higher than INH MICs for tuberculosis (≤0.1 μg/mL). MICs of *M. kansasii* for ethambutol are comparable to those of *M. tuberculosis,* and all susceptible MICs are 5.0 μg/mL or less. As with ethambutol resistance in tuberculosis, resistant MICs (>5.0 μg/mL) are associated with previous ethambutol therapy, resistance to other drugs, including rifampin, and treatment failure. The MICs of wild type strains of *M. kansasii* for streptomycin are 2.0 to 8.0 μg/mL. Acquired resistance to rifampin, ethambutol, and INH (defined as significant changes in MICs associated with treatment failure or relapse) has been demonstrated in isolates from treatment failure cases, and resistance to the first two agents is reliably demonstrated by current *M. tuberculosis* susceptibility test methods (proportion method in agar) (3, 13, 19).

The concentrations of antituberculous drugs used for routine mycobacterial susceptibility testing, including *M. kansasii,* were chosen for their usefulness with *M. tuberculosis.* Because *M. kansasii* is less susceptible to these drugs in vitro (but still susceptible to achievable blood/tissue levels of these drugs), some isolates may be reported resistant to INH at 0.2 or 1.0 μg/mL and to streptomycin at 2.0 μg/mL. These isolates are susceptible to slightly higher drug concentrations, so laboratory reports of resistance to low concentrations of these two drugs have no clinical or therapeutic significance as long as a rifampin-containing regimen is being used. Thus, when clinically indicated, INH and/or streptomycin should be used against *M. kansasii* regardless of the in vitro susceptibility results. The 1997 American Thoracic Society (ATS) statement on the nontuberculous mycobacteria recommends routine susceptibility testing of rifampin only on routine isolates to avoid this potential confusion (21).

The only drug for which resistance in vitro to a defined concentration has been regularly associated with treatment failure for *M. kansasii* is rifampin. For this reason, susceptibility testing of *M. kansasii* strains should initially include only rifampin (21). Since acquired rifampin resistance may develop during therapy and since the history of prior therapy may not be known, all initial isolates of *M. kansasii* as well as those from patients with known prior therapy should be tested with rifampin by the agar proportion method. Also, testing should be performed when the patient's sputum fails to convert from smear and/or culture positive or when a relapse occurs during therapy. For patients whose isolate is rifampin resistant, testing to all potentially useful agents, including rifabutin, ethambutol, and clarithromycin, should then be performed.

M. kansasii is also susceptible in vitro to sulfamethoxazole, amikacin, the newer quinolones, and clarithromycin, although there is limited information on the clinical usefulness of these drugs (3, 8, 19). The usual MICs for these agents include sulfamethoxazole, 4.0 μg/mL or less; amikacin, 8.0 μg/mL or less; ciprofloxacin, 0.5 to 2.0 μg/mL; and clarithromycin, 0.25 μg/mL or below. Isolates are usually resistant to high concentrations in vitro and therefore achievable levels of pyrazinamide, capreomycin, and *p*-aminosalicylic acid (PAS).

ANTIMICROBIAL THERAPY

Treatment of any *M. kansasii* infection except localized lymphadenitis (see below) requires multidrug therapy over a long period of time. There are currently no accepted intermittent or short-course treatment regimens for *M. kansasii* disease in the United States as there are for tuberculosis. The cornerstone of successful therapy for *M. kansasii* infections is inclusion of rifampin in a multidrug regimen that includes ethambutol, and (in the United States) INH. Monotherapy with rifampin (due either to patient noncompliance or inappropriate treatment recommendations) invariably leads to development of rifampin resistance, which in turn is invariably associated with treatment failure.

Special Situations

Pulmonary Disease

There have been no randomized comparative trials of treatment, comparing one drug regimen with another or with placebo, for pulmonary disease caused by *M. kansasii*. There have been, however, several retrospective and prospective studies of various treatment regimens that form a reasonable basis for drug therapy recommendations (1, 2, 4, 13) (Table 1).

TABLE 1   •   Recommended Regimens for Treatment of *M. kansasii* Infection

1. Pulmonary or disseminated disease in the immunocompetent host
   Rifampin 600 mg/day
   INH 300 mg/day
   Ethambutol 25 mg/kg/day for 2 months, then 15 mg/kg/day
   Oral medicines for 18 months with a minimum of 12 months of sputum culture negativity
   For severe disease consider adding streptomycin 0.5–1.0 g i.m. t.i.w. for the first 2–4 months of therapy or clarithromycin 500 mg
       b.i.d.
2. Pulmonary or disseminated disease in the immunocompetent host with a rifampin-resistant strain or in patients who are rifampin
   intolerant
   Clarithromycin 500 mg b.i.d.
   INH 900 mg/day (plus pyridoxine 50 mg/day)
   Ethambutol 25 mg/kg/day
   Sulfamethoxazole 1.0 g t.i.d.
   For severe disease consider streptomycin 0.5–1.0 g i.m. t.i.w. for the first 2–4 months of therapy
   Duration of therapy as above
3. Pulmonary or disseminated infection in HIV-positive patients not on protease inhibitors
   Rifampin 600 mg/day
   Ethambutol 25 mg/kg/day for 2 months, then 15 mg/kg/day
   INH 300 mg/day
   For severe disease consider streptomycin 0.5–1.0 g i.m. t.i.w. or clarithromycin 500 mg b.i.d. for the first 2–4 months of therapy
   Duration of therapy as above
4. Pulmonary or disseminated infection in HIV-positive patients on the protease inhibitor indinavir
   Clarithromycin 500 mg b.i.d.
   Rifabutin 150 mg/day
   Ethambutol 25 mg/kg/day for 2 months then 15 mg/kg/day
   INH 300 mg/day
   For severe disease consider streptomycin 0.5–1.0 g i.m. t.i.w. for the first 2–4 months of therapy.
   Duration of therapy as above
5. Pulmonary or disseminated infection in HIV-positive patients on the protease inhibitors saquinavir or ritonavir
   See 2 above
6. Lymph node disease
   Complete surgical excision of the involved nodes

The key to successful therapy of *M. kansasii* lung disease is inclusion of rifampin in a multidrug regimen. For antimycobacterial drug regimens without rifampin (and predating newer agents, such as clarithromycin), the sputum conversion rates at 6 months have ranged from 52 to 81% (10, 13). Relapse rates were approximately 10%, even in patients with an initial response.

With the inclusion of rifampin in treatment regimens, response to therapy improved dramatically. Sputum conversion rates with rifampin-containing regimens at 4 months were 100% in 180 patients from three studies (1, 2, 13). The incidence of treatment failure in these studies was 1.1%, and failure was invariably associated with development of rifampin resistance. Long-term relapse rates from these three studies of rifampin-containing regimens were also very low (0.8%).

The past and current (1997) ATS recommendation for treatment of lung disease caused by *M. kansasii* is the regimen of INH (300 mg/day), rifampin (600 mg/day), and ethambutol (25 mg/kg/day for the first 2 months, then 15 mg/kg) given daily for 18 months (18, 21). We feel that documentation of at least 12 months of negative sputum cultures is important for determining if therapy is successful.

In patients who are unable to tolerate one of these three drugs, clarithromycin appears to be a reasonable alternative based on its low MICs to *M. kansasii* and excellent activity in

vivo against other nontuberculous mycobacteria, but its role has not been established by clinical trials. An additional concern is enhanced metabolism of clarithromycin in the presence of rifampin (20). The therapeutic consequences of this interaction are not known. Azithromycin and the newer quinolones appear to be reasonable agents in this setting; however, there are no published reports of the efficacy of these drugs on which to base firm recommendations.

Three short-course treatment trials for *M. kansasii* lung disease have provided some provocative results but have not yet clearly demonstrated equivalence to the 18- to 24-month daily treatment regimens. Ahn et al. studied 40 patients and found that adding streptomycin (1 g twice weekly) for the first 3 months to INH, rifampin, and ethambutol for 12 months resulted in cure of all but 1 patient (2). A second trial sponsored by the British Medical Research Council featured ethambutol (15 mg/kg) and rifampin (450–600 mg) given daily for 9 months; 154 patients from this trial were available for analysis (11). Most patients received multiple drugs for presumed tuberculosis initially; some however, received only INH and rifampin at the start of therapy. INH was discontinued in all patients when *M. kansasii* was identified. All isolates were susceptible in vitro to rifampin and ethambutol; all were judged to be resistant in vitro to INH. Sputum conversion was achieved in 99% of patients; a 12% relapse rate was noted through 5 years follow-up. For most of these patients, relapse was attributed to medication noncompliance or severe underlying disease. This study suggests that INH does not contribute greatly to the treatment of *M. kansasii* and that 9 months may not be a long enough treatment period for this two-drug regimen.

The third study described 28 patients from France with *M. kansasii* lung disease (16). The patients were randomized to 12- or 18-month regimens. Fourteen patients received rifampin 600 mg/day, INH 300 mg/day, and ethambutol 25 mg/kg daily for the first 6 months, then rifampin and INH to complete a total of 12 months. The second group was treated with the same regimen (including 6 months of ethambutol) for 18 months. All patients converted their sputum cultures to negative. After 12 to 30 months of follow-up, only one patient (7%) in the 12-month and none in the 18-month treatment group had relapsed. The results of this study are encouraging, but it was not large enough and did not have sufficient long-term follow-up to establish 12 months of chemotherapy as the standard for treatment. Use of high-dose (25 mg/kg/day) ethambutol for 6 months is not without risk and may not be readily accepted in the United States. This study also appears to contradict the findings of the study by Jenkins et al. with respect to the importance of INH in the treatment regimen. Almost certainly, rifampin is the critical agent for efficacy, and while companion drugs may not enhance efficacy, they are essential to prevent emergence of resistance to rifampin. Both ethambutol and INH appear to be effective for this latter role. None of these studies included a macrolide, which may prove to be as active as rifampin and may provide the basis for effective short-course regimens.

For patients whose organisms have become resistant to rifampin as a result of previous therapy, a regimen of oral and injectable agents has been shown effective (3, 19). This regimen consists of high-dose daily INH (900 mg), high-dose ethambutol (25 mg/kg/day), and sulfamethoxazole (1.0 g three times per day) combined with daily or five times per week streptomycin or amikacin for the initial 2 to 3 months, followed by intermittent streptomycin or amikacin for a total of 6 months. The oral drugs are given for 12 to 15 months after sputum cultures become negative. Results with this regimen include sputum conversion in 18 of 20 patients (90%) after a mean of 11 weeks, with only one relapse (8%) among patients who are culture negative for at least 12 months while on therapy.

The above trial antedated the introduction of clarithromycin, which has been highly effective in the treatment of a number of nontuberculous mycobacteria diseases and has excellent in vitro activity against *M. kansasii*. It is reasonable that clarithromycin will be useful in the treatment of all types of *M. kansasii* disease. Clarithromycin may be especially useful in retreatment regimens for rifampin-resistant strains, perhaps allowing omission of the aminoglycoside, as a substitute for patients intolerant to one of the first-line drugs, and in the treatment regimen for all patients with *M. kansasii* infection (pulmonary and/or disseminated) (Wallace and Griffith, unpublished data). Given the success of medical regimens with rifampin-resistant *M. kansasii,* few patients require surgical resection.

Lymphadenitis

In the treatment of lymph node disease in children, all accessible nodes should be excised at the time of the initial biopsy, since the probabilities are that the etiologic agent is a nontuberculous mycobacteria, other than *M. kansasii,* for which excision is the indicated treatment (21). In some patients, complete surgical excision of involved lymph nodes may be impossible. There is, unfortunately, little published information addressing this scenario. Experience with lymphadenitis due to *Mycobacterium avium* complex (MAC) suggests that chemotherapy following incomplete surgical excision of involved nodes is associated with a high rate of success. Additionally, antibiotic therapy is likely to be required for only 6 months (5).

Disseminated Infection in Non-AIDS Patients

For treatment of disseminated disease due to *M. kansasii* in non-AIDS patients, the regimen of antimycobacterial drugs should be the same as for lung disease. It is unknown at present if drugs should be prescribed differently or for a longer period of time than for patients with lung disease. Since these patients are invariably immunocompromised, the duration of therapy depends on the reversibility of the immune deficiency.

AIDS

For patients with AIDS and pulmonary and/or disseminated *M. kansasii* infection, the treatment regimen is the same as for immunocompetent patients with *M. kansasii* pulmonary disease (Table 1). Untreated *M. kansasii* infection in these patients is essentially always fatal (7). The duration of therapy in AIDS patients remains problematic. For patients with relatively intact and stable immune function (or who recover immune function), the duration of therapy could be comparable to that for immunocompetent patients. These patients require very close clinical follow-up and monitoring. For patients with AIDS and poor immune function, the duration of treatment probably should be longer than standard therapy and perhaps lifelong in some patients.

The new class of antiretroviral drugs, the protease inhibitors, has complicated the treatment of pulmonary and disseminated *M. kansasii* disease in patients with AIDS. Rifamycins (rifampin more than rifabutin) accelerate the metabolism of all currently available protease inhibitors through induction of the hepatic P-450 cytochrome enzymes, resulting in subtherapeutic levels of the protease inhibitors. Low levels of these drugs facilitate or enhance rapid mutational resistance in HIV strains to the protease inhibitors. To complicate the situation even more, protease inhibitors retard the metabolism of rifamycins, resulting in increased serum levels of rifamycins and the potential for drug toxicity (rifabutin more than rifampin).

The issue of adverse drug interactions between protease inhibitors and rifamycins has been addressed for disease caused by *M. tuberculosis* (22). Three options were provided: (*a*) treating tuberculosis with non-rifampin-containing regimens, (*b*) substituting rifabutin for rifampin in the antituberculosis regimen, or (*c*) withholding protease inhibitors and using multiple reverse transcriptase inhibitors until patients complete a course of therapy for tuberculosis with a rifampin-containing regimen. None of these options is ideal or without risk in the setting of tuberculosis. The options are even more difficult for patients with disseminated *M. kansasii* disease, because rifampin has been the cornerstone of successful *M. kansasii* therapy (even more so than tuberculosis) and because there is less experience with rifabutin in *M. kansasii* disease than in tuberculosis.

Improvement in the underlying AIDS-induced immunosuppression would seem to be a logical priority for clearance of disseminated mycobacterial disease. Therefore, discontinuing the protease inhibitor might be the least attractive of the options. The drug regimen cited above for treatment of rifampin-resistant *M. kansasii* isolates is difficult to tolerate and of unknown efficacy in the setting of disseminated *M. kansasii* disease. An alternative approach would be substitution of rifabutin (150 mg/day) for rifampin in addition to INH and ethambutol; this strategy relies upon a minimal effect on the serum concentration of the protease inhibitor with this low dose of rifabutin, which has unproven efficacy. Addition of clarithromycin to these three drugs would also likely improve the efficacy of the regimen, although the risk of rifabutin-related toxicity would be augmented further. As with rifampin monotherapy, rifabutin monotherapy, usually as prophylaxis against *Mycobacterium avium* complex (MAC), has been associated with emergence of rifamycin (rifampin)-resistant *M. kansasii* (12). The role of other potentially useful agents such as the newer quinolones is unknown in this setting.

ENDPOINTS FOR MONITORING THERAPY

Serial sputum surveillance is the most important element of monitoring treatment of *M. kansasii* pulmonary disease. Sputum bacteriology is an indicator of medication efficacy; rendering the patient sputum-culture negative is the primary marker of success, and the time to sputum conversion may help determine the length of therapy in some patients. Sputum cultures identify relapse of disease in patients who had previously converted and provides material for in vitro susceptibility testing for patients who have relapsed. Some patients cease sputum production during therapy, making sputum analysis impossible; however, diligent effort should be made to collect sputum throughout the course of treatment. Patients failing therapy may not be recognized until therapy is discontinued unless there is careful sputum surveillance during therapy.

Periodic chest radiographs are also helpful in this setting. The chest radiograph is likely to improve slowly; thus, frequent radiographs are not necessary if the patient appears to be responding well to therapy (i.e., weight gain, improvement in cough and sputum production). Because of the potential for drug-related adverse events, patients initially require at least monthly contact with health care workers. Specific drug toxicities and monitoring recommendations have been outlined in detail (21). The inclusion of ethambutol at a dose of 25 mg/kg/day in the routine treatment regimen dictates that visual symptoms and simple visual acuity and color vision testing should be checked at least monthly. With decrease in the ethambutol dose to 15 mg/kg/day, visual acuity and red-green color discrimination need to be assessed at baseline and then

only with symptomatic changes in the patient's vision (21). The necessity for frequent patient contact to evaluate possible drug toxicity also facilitates frequent evaluation of disease symptom status.

CONTROVERSIES, CAVEATS, OR COMMENTS

The recommendation that all patients with suspected tuberculosis with a significant risk for drug resistance receive four drugs, including INH, rifampin, pyrazinamide, and ethambutol, has an additional benefit in that patients who prove to have *M. kansasii* lung disease will receive adequate (i.e., three active drugs) therapy from the outset, since pyrazinamide has little or no activity against *M. kansasii*. This treatment approach may be most important in areas with a high incidence of *M. kansasii*, such as reported by Bittner et al. (6).

M. kansasii lung disease patients would benefit from the same treatment approach as that currently used for pulmonary tuberculosis, namely, directly observed therapy to avoid emergence of acquired rifampin resistance through noncompliance. Unfortunately, in the face of competing monetary demands, it is not likely that state health departments will treat *M. kansasii* in this manner. Certainly, this process would be facilitated if there were a short course and/or intermittent regimen that was effective for treatment of *M. kansasii*. It is reasonable to hope that clinical trials, perhaps with drug combinations that include a rifamycin and a macrolide, will address this problem in the future.

REFERENCES

1. Ahn CH, Lowell JR, Ahn SA, Ahn S, Hurst GA. Chemotherapy for pulmonary disease due to *Mycobacterium kansasii:* efficacies of some individual drugs. Rev Infect Dis 1981;3: 1028–1034.
2. Ahn CH, Lowell JR, Ahn SA, Ahn SI, Hurst GA. Short-course chemotherapy for pulmonary disease caused by *Mycobacterium kansasii.* Am Rev Respir Dis 1983;128:1048–1050.
3. Ahn CH, Wallace RJ Jr, Steele LC, Murphy DT. Sulfonamide-containing regimens for disease caused by rifampin-resistant *Mycobacterium kansasii.* Am Rev Respir Dis 1987;135:10–16.
4. Banks J, Hunter AM, Campbell IA, Jenkins PA, Smith AP. Pulmonary infection with *Mycobacterium kansasii* in Wales, 1970–9: review of treatment and response. Thorax 1983;38:271–274.
5. Bergor C, Pfyffer GE, Nadal D. Treatment of nontuberculous mycobacterial lymphadenitis with clarithromycin plus rifabutin. J Pediatr 1996;128:383–386.
6. Bittner MJ, Horowitz EA, Safranek TJ, Preheim LC. Emergence of *Mycobacterium kansasii* as the leading mycobacterial pathogen isolated over a 20-year period at a midwestern Veterans Affairs hospital. Clin Infect Dis 1996;22:1109–1110.
7. Campo RE, Campo CE. *Mycobacterium kansasii* disease in patients infected with human immunodeficiency virus. Clin Infect Dis 1997;24:1233–1238.
8. Gay JD, DeYoung DR, Roberts GD. In vitro activities of norfloxacin and ciprofloxacin against *Mycobacterium tuberculosis, M. avium* complex, *M. chelonei, M. fortuitum,* and *M. kansasii.* Antimicrob Agents Chemother 1984;26:94–96.
9. Hobby GL, Redmond WB, Runyon EH, Schaefer WB, Wayne LG, Wichelhausen RH. A study of pulmonary disease associated with mycobacteria other than *M. tuberculosis:* identification and characterization of the mycobacteria. Am Rev Respir Dis 1967; 95:954–971.

10. Jenkins DE, Bahar D, Chofuas I. Pulmonary disease due to atypical mycobacteria: current concepts. Trans 19th Conf on Chemotherapy of Tuberculosis 1960:224.

11. Jenkins PA, Banks J, Campbell IA, Smith PA, Research Committee, British Thoracic Society. *Mycobacterium kansasii* pulmonary infection: a prospective study of the results of nine months of treatment with rifampicin and ethambutol. Thorax 1994;49:442–445.

12. Meynard JL, Lalande V, Meyohas MC, Petit JC, Frottier J. Rifampin-resistant *M. kansasii* infection in a patient with AIDS who was receiving rifabutin. Clin Infect Dis 1997;24:1262–1263.

13. Pezzia W, Raleigh JW, Bailey MC, Toth EA, Silverblatt J. Treatment of pulmonary disease due to *Mycobacterium kansasii:* recent experience with rifampin. Rev Infect Dis 1981;3: 1035–1039.

14. Picardeau M, Prod'holm G, Raskine L, LePennec MP, Vincent V. Genotypic characterization of five subspecies of *Mycobacterium kansasii*. J Clin Microbiol 1997;35:25–32.

15. Ross BC, Jackson K, Yang M, Sievers A, Dwyer B. Identification of a genetically distinct subspecies of *Mycobacterium kansasii*. J Clin Microbiol 1992;30:2930–2933.

16. Sauret J, Hernandez-Flix S, Castro E, Hernandez L, Ausina V, Coll P. Treatment of pulmonary disease caused by *Mycobacterium kansasii:* results of 18 vs 12 months' chemotherapy. Tuberc Lung Dis 1995;76:104–108.

17. Steadman JE. High-catalase strains of *Mycobacterium kansasii* isolated from water in Texas. J Clin Microbiol 1980;11: 496–498.

18. Wallace RJ Jr, O'Brien R, Glassroth J, Raleigh J, Dutt A. Diagnosis and treatment of disease caused by nontuberculous mycobacteria. Am Rev Respir Dis 1990;142:940–953.

19. Wallace RJ Jr, Dunbar D, Brown BA, Onyi G, Dunlap R, Ahn CH, Murphy D. Rifampin-resistant *Mycobacterium kansasii*. Clin Infect Dis 1994;18:736–743.

20. Wallace RJ Jr, Brown BA, Griffith DE, Girard W, Tanaka K. Reduced serum levels of clarithromycin in patients treated with multidrug regimens including rifampin or rifabutin for *Mycobacterium avium–M. intracellulare* infection. J Infect Dis 1995;171:747–50.

21. Wallace RJ Jr, Glassroth J, Griffith DE, Olivier KN, Cook JL, Gordin F. Diagnosis and treatment of disease caused by nontuberculous mycobacteria. Am J Respir Crit Care Med (Suppl) 1997;156:S1–S25.

22. Impact of HIV protease inhibitors on the treatment of HIV-infected tuberculosis patients with rifampin. MMWR 1996;45: 921–925.

Mycobacterium leprae

●

Christian Lienhardt and Keith P. W. J. McAdam

GENERAL DESCRIPTION

Leprosy is a chronic infectious disease of man caused by *Mycobacterium leprae*. It is a bacterial disease, mainly affecting nerves and skin but causing more widespread problems in other tissues such as eyes, mucosa of the upper respiratory tract, muscle, bones, and testes.

In 1983, the World Health Organization (WHO) estimated that there were about 11.5 million cases of leprosy in the world, but this number has dropped to 2.5 million cases today (44). The main endemic areas are the Indian subcontinent, Southeast Asia, tropical Africa, and Latin America. Man is the only commonly accepted reservoir, although natural infection has been documented in armadillos in the United States and in monkeys in Africa (40). The source of infection is the untreated lepromatous leprosy patient who can expel by aerosol 10^7 to 10^8 bacilli by coughing or sneezing. The bacilli are thought to enter the new host through the upper respiratory tract mucosa. The vast majority of people who are exposed to *M. leprae* have subclinical infection, but a few people develop the disease, depending on their ability to mount effective cellular immunity against the organism. There is no marker of infection in man, but it is estimated that 1 in 100 infected persons will eventually develop a clinical form of the disease. The incubation period ranges from 9 months to 20 years, usually 3 to 5 years for tuberculoid leprosy and 9 to 12 years for lepromatous leprosy.

M. leprae was discovered in 1873 by Armauer Hansen. It is a straight rod-shaped bacillus, 1 to 8 μm long and 0.3 μm in diameter. Its capsule is composed of two lipids, phthiocerol dimycoserosate and a phenolic glycolipid, chemically unique and antigenically specific to *M. leprae* (6). The cell wall is composed of two layers: the outer layer contains lipopolysaccharide and the inner layer peptidoglycan. Under the cell wall is a membrane composed of lipids and proteins. The cytoplasm contains storage granules, DNA, and ribosomes. *M. leprae* is an obligate intracellular parasite in man, multiplying mainly in histiocytes and Schwann cells. Its microscopic identification relies on the fact that *M. leprae* is acid and alcohol fast when stained with carbol-fuchsin.

Variability of the cell-mediated immune (CMI) response mounted by the host in response to infection with *M. leprae* determines a spectrum of bacteriologic, pathologic, immunologic, and clinical features between two polar forms, tuberculoid and lepromatous leprosy (32):

1. *Tuberculoid leprosy* is localized to one or few sites in the skin and large peripheral nerves. Skin lesions are asymmetric and hypopigmented, with well-defined margins. They are anesthetic and dry. One or few peripheral nerves are commonly enlarged. In this form, CMI is at its highest, and there are no bacilli in the lesions.

2. *Lepromatous leprosy* is the form of disease associated with an absent or low CMI response and massive bacillary multiplication. There is systemic disease, with bacillemia and multiple organ involvement. Skin lesions are of various types (nodules, papules, macules, or diffuse infiltration) and are widely disseminated, bilaterally symmetric, and usually numerous and extensive. Nerve lesions are slow to appear but can lead to deformities and handicap.

3. *Borderline leprosy* is characterized by a mixture of the signs and symptoms of the polar forms, reflecting the instability of CMI and the balance between bacillary multiplication and cellular immunity. This is the form of the disease associated with severe nerve involvement.

The clinical diagnosis is based on careful examination of the skin for depigmented anesthetic patches and search for peripheral nerve involvement. The microbiologic diagnosis relies on slit-skin smears, made from the edge of suspect lesions and from sites commonly affected (ear lobes) and stained by Ziehl-Neelson's method. The density of bacilli is recorded as the bacterial index (BI). For operational purposes, the results of skin smear are used to differentiate between paucibacillary (skin smears negative at *all* sites) and multibacillary (at least one positive skin smear at *any* site) leprosy. The biopsy specimen of the skin in an affected area will display the histologic appearance associated with the immunologic spectrum and will confirm the diagnosis.

SUSCEPTIBILITY IN VIVO

In the absence of techniques for culturing *M. leprae* in artificial media, it has been necessary to screen drugs in vivo for antimicrobial activity against *M. leprae*. In 1960, Shepard discovered that inoculation of *M. leprae* into the mouse footpad was followed by a limited multiplication of bacilli without any visible macroscopic lesion (34). This has been a milestone in the evaluation of antimicrobial activity against *M. leprae,* in particular to assess the minimal inhibitory concentration (MIC) and to distinguish bacteriostatic and bactericidal activities.

Single Drugs

Sulfones

Dapsone has been the most widely used antileprosy drug because of its low price, safety, and effectiveness. Dapsone is the parent sulfone. Its structure is very similar to the structure of the sulfonamides. As an analogue of *p*-aminobenzoic acid (PABA), dapsone prevents its use for synthesis of folic acid by competitive inhibition for dihydropteroate synthetase. The MIC, determined after inoculation in the mouse footpad system, is 0.003 μg/mL (35). In man, a single dose of 100 mg gives a blood level of about 1.5 μg/mL, 500 times the MIC. At this dose, dapsone is weakly bactericidal against *M. leprae*. At lower doses (10 mg/day), the serum concentration still exceeds the MIC, but dapsone is only bacteriostatic. Dapsone is rapidly and nearly completely absorbed when taken orally. It is then acetylated in the liver and slowly excreted through the kidneys. As acetylation is genetically determined, the half-life of the drug differs in individuals from 12 to 50 h (average, 24 h). The monoacetyl derivative (MADDS) has little or no activity against *M. leprae*. Once in the body, dapsone distributes in skin, muscles, liver, kidneys, and nerves.

Resistance to sulfones was first described in 1964 (30) and has since become an increasing problem around the world (19). Resistance probably develops as a stepwise process of mutation (14) whereby mutant bacilli resistant to increasing levels of dapsone are successively selected. Most resistance is secondary, appearing in multibacillary patients after 10 to 20 years of dapsone monotherapy. Primary resistance due to infection with dapsone-resistant *M. leprae* is less frequent and is usually present in areas of the world where dapsone has been used extensively (29).

Rifampicin

Discovered in 1967, rifampicin is a semisynthetic derivative of rifamycin SV, a broad-spectrum antibiotic of complex macrocyclic structure produced by *Streptomyces mediterranei*. Rifampicin has powerful activity against both *M. tuberculosis* and *M. leprae*.

All derivative products of rifamycin SV have a similar central macrocyclic structure, probably responsible for antibacterial activity. Rifampicin inhibits the DNA-dependent RNA polymerase by fixation on the β subunit of this enzyme, thus blocking mycobacterial RNA synthesis. The MIC is 0.3 μg/mL. After administration of one dose of 600 mg (10 mg/kg), a peak plasma concentration of 7 μg/mL is reached in 2 to 4 h, which is highly bactericidal against *M. leprae*. The biologic half-life is approximately 3 h. In man, a single dose of 600 mg renders bacilli nonviable after inoculation to mice, which corresponds to a bactericidal activity of 99 to 99.99% (31, 37).

Rifampicin resistance is rare but has been observed in patients who relapse after dapsone therapy and then are treated for long periods with rifampicin alone (11, 16). Up to now, no case of primary resistance has been reported. Persisting viable bacilli have been isolated from patients receiving rifampicin alone or in combination regimens (39).

Clofazimine

Clofazimine is a substitute iminophenazine dye that was synthesized in 1956 (Lamprene, B-663) and first used in the treatment of leprosy in 1960 (4). It is a red crystalline substance, soluble in oil and ethanol but not soluble in water. The mode of action is not totally known, but it is suggested that clofazimine inhibits DNA replication through fixation on mycobacterial DNA (7). The MIC in the mouse footpad system could not be determined because it persists in tissues for a prolonged period of time. Clofazimine has weak bactericidal activity. After 6 months of daily treatment with 100 mg, viable bacilli (after inoculation into mice footpads) are found in one-third of patients (17). In addition, clofazimine has an antiinflammatory effect that is useful in prevention and treatment of erythema nodosum leprosum (ENL) reactions.

A case of resistance to clofazimine has been reported, but this has not been confirmed up to now (41).

Thioamides

Thioamides are derivatives of isonicotinic acid, synthesized in 1956, and active against *M. tuberculosis* and *M. leprae*. There are two main molecules, ethionamide (α-ethyl-thioisonicotinamide) and prothionamide (α-propyl-thioisonicotinamide), which are very similar in terms of activity and toxicity. The mode of action is not known, but it is supposed that thioamides inhibit peptide synthesis (15). Ethionamide and prothionamide have a bactericidal effect, similar to that of dapsone. The MIC is about 0.05 µg/mL. After an oral dose of 500 mg, a peak concentration of 3 µg/mL is reached in serum in 3 h, and the half-life is 2 h (7). Thioamides have excellent tissue distribution and are metabolized in the liver. Excretion is mainly via the kidneys, with 94% of the drug in inactive form.

ANTIMICROBIAL THERAPY
General

Treatment of leprosy has evolved considerably over the past 40 years, and several effective drugs are now available, allowing an excellent prognosis if given at an early stage of the disease. The principles of combined drug therapy have been well established and multidrug therapy (MDT) is recommended by the WHO and widely used (42). Dapsone, rifampicin, clofazimine, and thioamides represent the main drugs active against *M. leprae*. Long-acting sulfamides, thiacetazone and thiambutosine, which have weak bactericidal activity, are not used anymore. Fluoroquinolones, macrolides, and cyclines have recently been demonstrated to have antileprosy activity but are not yet used routinely in antileprosy treatment regimens.

Specific Drugs

Dapsone

Dapsone is usually formulated in 100-mg tablets. It is given daily at a single dose of 100 mg for adults and 2 mg/kg body weight for children. A depot preparation of diacetyldiphenylsulfone (DADDS) is available, given at a dose of 225 mg/75 days. However, because of to the low plasma level of dapsone obtained, its use should not be recommended.

A multitude of side effects has been reported. Although rare when dapsone is used at appropriate dosages (100 mg/day), they occur much more frequently if higher doses are given (200–300 mg/day). They include headache, rash, fever, psychosis, gastrointestinal disorders, nephrotic syndrome, hemolytic anemia, agranulocytosis, hepatitis, peripheral neuropathy, methemoglobinemia, and hypoalbuminemia. The idiosyncratic DDS (or sulfone) syndrome has been described since the early days of sulfone therapy and has been reported in leprosy patients (26). It usually develops within 6 weeks of the start of treatment and manifests as rash and/or exfoliative dermatitis, generalized lymphadenopathy, hepatosplenomegaly,

fever, and hepatitis. When this syndrome occurs, dapsone should be immediately discontinued. Corticosteroids may be of benefit.

A mild hemolysis has been regularly observed in leprosy patients receiving dapsone therapy, but severe anemia is rare and is dose related. However, patients with glucose 6-phosphate dehydrogenase (G6PD) deficiency may develop severe hemolytic anemia. Methemoglobinemia can occur in patients with a congenital deficiency in NADH-dependent methemoglobin reductase. It is usually not a problem with routine doses of dapsone but may become severe with overdose. Peripheral neuropathies have been reported in patients taking high doses of the drug and are usually reversed when dapsone is discontinued. Agranulocytosis is a very rare but serious idiosyncratic effect of dapsone that has been reported in individuals taking dapsone in combination with pyrimethamine for malaria prophylaxis (28).

Rifampicin

Rifampicin is usually administered in a single daily dose of 10 mg/kg, 600 mg in adults and 450 mg in persons weighing less than 35 kg. Due to its marked bactericidal activity, rifampicin can be used intermittently, with doses ranging from 600 to 1200 mg and at intervals ranging from 1 week to 1 month (46).

After ingestion, rifampicin is rapidly absorbed on an empty stomach. It diffuses rapidly into tissues, and the concentrations obtained are at least equal to the serum concentration. It is distributed throughout the body, crosses the placental barrier, and appears in breast milk. As the drug is lipid soluble, it has excellent intracellular penetration. Rifampicin is partially eliminated in urine, but most of it enters the enterohepatic circulation where its reabsorption is interrupted by deacetylation in the liver. The drug usually produces a reddish orange discoloration of urine, feces, and lachrymal secretions, and patients should be warned of this aspect, which has no serious consequences except staining of contact lenses.

Rifampicin is usually well tolerated. Toxicity depends both on the dosage and on the interval between doses. With daily treatment, a transient elevation of hepatic transaminases (up to 2 or 3 times the normal upper limit) is often observed. Sometimes, however, especially in cases of preexisting hepatic disease or simultaneous administration of another hepatotoxic drug, transaminases may be grossly elevated. A flulike syndrome can be observed when rifampicin is used intermittently and if doses exceed 10 mg/kg. This occurs most frequently when rifampicin is given at 1- to 2-week intervals but is not common when given either daily or once a month. Current WHO multidrug therapy recommends monthly doses (600 mg). Other immunohematologic disorders may occur (e.g., hypereosinophilia, interstitial nephritis, acute tubular necrosis, thrombocytopenia, and hemolytic anemia), which demand immediate discontinuation of the drug. Other side effects include fatigue, headache, drowsiness, and rash. Teratogenicity has not been demonstrated in humans. Due to its effect on hepatic microsomal enzymes, rifampicin increases hepatic metabolism of other drugs such as corticosteroids, digoxin, quinidine, oral contraceptives, and oral hypoglycemics (1).

Clofazimine

The current preparation of clofazimine is a microcrystalline suspension in an oil-wax base, which is absorbed at about 70%. The serum concentration is variable, 0.5 to 0.7 μg/mL after a daily dose of 100 mg (2). The drug is unevenly distributed in the body; as it is lipophilic, high concentrations have been reached in fatty tissues and in cells of the reticuloendothelial system. The serum half-life is about 10 days, but the tissue half-life can be as long as 70 days. The exact mechanism of elimination is unknown, but very little is excreted in urine.

Clofazimine is available in gelatin capsules of 50 and 100 mg. The adult dose is 50 mg daily or 100 mg twice weekly, and for children, 1 mg/kg. Due to its long tissue half-life, administration of the drug can be adapted, such as the WHO-recommended scheme of 50 mg/day supplemented by 300 mg once a month.

The major side effect of clofazimine is red pigmentation of skin and conjunctiva, which varies with the initial skin color but is more troublesome in lighter-skinned people. Pigmentation usually disappears in 1 to 2 years after stopping treatment. Itching, dryness, and cracking of skin occur frequently. The more serious toxicity is with the gastrointestinal tract, giving rise to crampy abdominal pain, nausea, and diarrhea. These are less frequent, however, if capsules are given with food. High doses of clofazimine can cause severe abdominal pain. The drug appears to be safe in pregnancy, but experience so far is limited.

Thioamides

The recommended dose of thioamides is 5 to 10 mg/kg/day. The lower dose is less bactericidal but less toxic. Gastrointestinal symptoms (anorexia, nausea, vomiting, abdominal pain, diarrhea) are frequently observed, but they clear if the drug is discontinued or reduced to less than 500 mg/day. The most severe side effect is hepatotoxicity, which has been observed in 5% of patients treated with thioamides alone and in 10 to 15% of individuals treated with the combination of thioamide and rifampicin (18).

COMBINATION DRUG THERAPY

Although a minority in number, patients with multibacillary (lepromatous) leprosy are the main source of infection with *M. leprae* and those in whom drug-resistant mutants are the most easily selected. In these patients, it has been estimated that there could be as many as 10^{11} to 10^{12} acid-fast bacilli, of which only 1% (10^9–10^{10}) are viable (37). As *M. leprae* cannot be cultured in vitro, it is difficult to establish the proportion of *M. leprae* mutants that are resistant to dapsone, clofazimine, or rifampicin. By analogy with tuberculosis, the mean proportion of drug-resistant mutants within a wild strain of *M. leprae* was estimated to be 1 in 10 million organisms (13). It has thus been estimated that a multibacillary leprosy patient harbors at most 10^9 drug-susceptible organisms, 10^3 rifampicin-resistant mutants, and 10^4 dapsone-, clofazimine-, or thioamides-resistant mutants (13) (Fig. 1).

To cure a leprosy patient bacteriologically, chemotherapy must be capable of killing all viable organisms, the susceptible and the resistant mutants, and preventing selection of resistant mutants (13). Assuming that a mutant resistant to a given drug remains fully susceptible to another drug if the latter has a different mechanism of action, a combination of at least two drugs is required to kill the resistant mutants. In practice, to overcome primary and secondary resistance to dapsone, the recommendation is to use a combination of rifampicin, dapsone, and clofazimine (42). Dapsone, being poorly bactericidal, must be given daily at a dose of 100 mg in

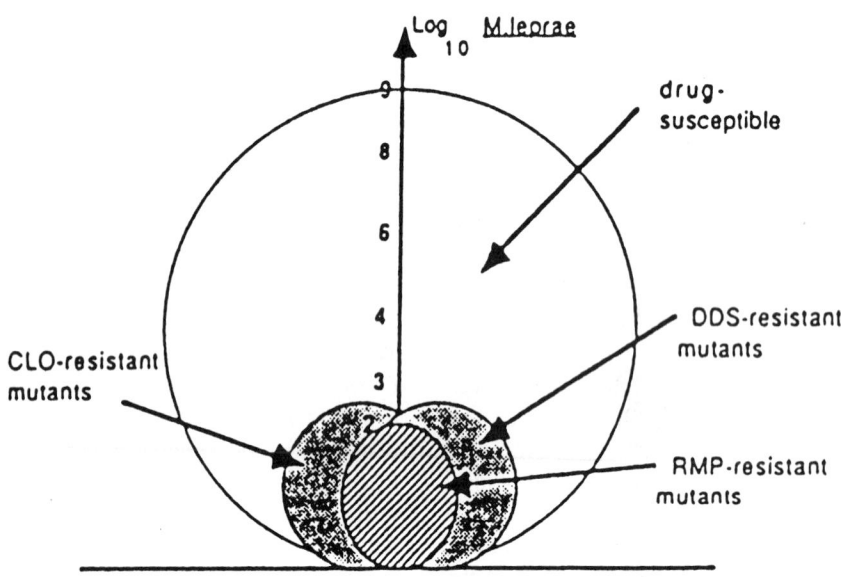

FIGURE 1. Bacillary populations in multibacillary leprosy. (From Grosset JH, Progress in the chemotherapy of leprosy. Int J Lepr 1994;62: 268–276.)

adults. Clofazimine must be given at a daily dose of 50 mg, with a monthly supplementation of 300 mg. For rifampicin, a single dose of 600 mg has been shown to kill more than 99% of susceptible organisms present at the start of treatment (36), which is equivalent to 3 to 6 months of daily treatment with dapsone and clofazimine. It was further shown that daily treatment with rifampicin was not more bactericidal than monthly treatment (38). As mutants resistant to dapsone and clofazimine are supposed to be fully susceptible to rifampicin, they are killed by the first dose of rifampicin, which has been shown to reduce the proportion of viable bacilli in multibacillary leprosy patients from 10^9 to 10^4. Thus most susceptible organisms as well as the mutants resistant to dapsone and clofazimine have been eliminated after the first dose of rifampicin. The remaining rifampicin-resistant mutants will be killed by daily doses of dapsone plus clofazimine. The combination of dapsone plus clofazimine will kill the rifampicin-resistant mutants and should be administered throughout the course of therapy.

In patients with multibacillary leprosy, the initial phase of chemotherapy considerably reduces the number of viable bacilli. The objective of the second phase of chemotherapy is then to eliminate the remaining 10^4 viable drug-susceptible bacilli, avoid selection of bacilli secondarily resistant to rifampicin, and prevent relapse after stopping treatment. It takes about 7 years to clear 10^4 bacilli in a multibacillary leprosy patient with maximum bacterial load (13, 38). Data from Mali suggest that the shorter the duration of treatment, the earlier the occurrence of relapses (27). In addition, relapses were more frequent in subjects highly bacilliferous at the start of treatment. In leprosy control programs, it is difficult to adapt the length of treatment to the bacterial load of each patient. In addition, for operational purposes, the length of treatment must be standardized for each of the main categories of leprosy patients (pauci- or multibacillary). The treatment regimens recommended for MDT are thus a compromise between theory and operational constraints.

According to the recommendations of the sixth report of the Expert Committee on Leprosy, the treatment of leprosy should be as follows (43):

Paucibacillary leprosy: rifampicin 600 mg monthly, supervised
dapsone 100 mg once daily, unsupervised given for 6 months

Multibacillary leprosy: rifampicin 600 mg monthly, supervised
dapsone 100 mg once daily, unsupervised
clofazimine 50 mg daily, unsupervised
clofazimine 300 mg monthly, supervised

This treatment is usually given for 24 months in a 36-month period or until smear negativity is obtained.

Since 1982, MDT has been extensively implemented in all leprosy endemic areas. By mid-1996, 91% of leprosy patients in the world were being treated with WHO-recommended MDT (45). The relapse rate after MDT so far is reported to be of the order of 0.1% per annum (44).

Special Situations

A major problem in leprosy is the development of reactions that, if not diagnosed and treated in time, will result in disabilities (33). There are two types of reactions: type 1, or reversal, reaction and type 2, or erythema nodosum leproticum (ENL), reaction (5, 15).

Type 1 reaction is characterized by episodes of increased inflammatory activity at sites where bacilli exist, in skin and/or nerves of patients with borderline leprosy whose immunologic status is unstable. Skin lesions flare up and become swollen. New lesions may develop, together with edema of the face, hands, and feet. Inflammation in the nerves causes pain, tenderness, and functional impairment that can lead to disability.

Type 2 reaction, ENL, occurs in multibacillary leprosy and is thought to be immune-complex mediated. ENL is characterized by the appearance in the skin of painful erythematous nodules, dome shaped, shiny, and tender, which can secondarily ulcerate. Systemic involvement is frequent, with fever, iritis, orchitis, nephritis, dactylitis, arthritis, and enlargement of nerves.

These reactions need to be recognized and treated promptly to avoid irreversible loss of nerve function (5, 25). Mild reactions, in which pain or tenderness are absent and skin lesions are minor, can be distinguished from severe reactions, characterized by the presence of severe neuritis with anesthesia and/or paralysis (type 1) or ulceration of skin accompanied by fever, iritis, and arthritis (type 2).

Mild reactions are usually treated with aspirin (600–1200 mg/day in four to six doses). Chloroquine has also been widely used for controlling mild inflammation (150 mg, three times/ day). The combination of aspirin and chloroquine is often better than either alone.

Severe reactions constitute a medical emergency and antiinflammatory treatment must be started immediately if disability is to be avoided:

Corticosteroids

In type 1 reaction, prednisolone is usually given at a starting dose of 40 to 80 mg/day, according to severity. The dose is thereafter reduced by 5 to 10 mg every 2 to 4 weeks according to the patient's response, which is best assessed clinically and through careful testing of nerve function. Immobilization of the affected limb is helpful to relieve pain and protect against nerve function loss.

Thalidomide

Thalidomide is the drug of choice for the treatment of ENL. Thalidomide and its active analogues are thought to work by partial inhibition of synthesis of tumor necrosis factor–α (TNFα). This drug is given at a daily dose of 400 mg until the reaction is controlled and then reduced gradually to 50 mg daily. This drug must *never* be given to women of childbearing age due to its disastrous teratogenic effects, causing phocomelia in the fetus if taken during the first trimester of pregnancy. If contraindicated, prednisolone should be given at a dose of 20 to 40 mg/day, and the dose adjusted according to response.

As corticosteroids suppress the immune response, it is necessary to continue antileprosy treatment while they are given or restart dapsone or clofazimine monotherapy if MDT has been completed.

Alternative Therapies

In view of the proven efficacy of WHO-MDT, the priority is to implement it as rapidly and as extensively as possible in endemic areas. Research is still necessary, however, to shorten the duration of the treatment and to improve patients' adherence to long courses of treatment. With the present drugs, there is little hope of shortening the overall duration of treatment, but compliance could be improved by developing a regimen that could be given on a monthly basis. New drugs with strong bactericidal activity are needed to develop fully supervised intermittent regimens. Three agents are now available: fluoroquinolones, minocycline, and clarithromycin.

The fluoroquinolones are nalidixic acid derivatives that inhibit DNA gyrase, an enzyme involved in DNA replication. Ofloxacin and pefloxacin have been shown to have an extremely powerful bactericidal activity on *M. leprae;* in multibacillary leprosy patients, 22 daily doses of 400 mg ofloxacin or 800 mg pefloxacin killed 99.99% of viable bacilli present at the start of treatment (12). A multicenter field trial is currently in progress under the auspices of the WHO to explore the efficacy of combined rifampicin and ofloxacin regimens.

Minocycline is the only tetracycline active against *M. leprae*. It acts on the ribosomal synthesis of proteins of *M. leprae*. In mice, its bactericidal activity is similar to that of ofloxacin (8). In man, a daily dose of 100 mg is well tolerated and kills more than 99% of viable bacilli in 1 month (21).

Clarithromycin is a new macrolide that inhibits synthesis of mycobacterial proteins. In mice, its bactericidal activity is similar to that of ofloxacin and minocycline (20). In man, given at a daily dose of 500 mg, the drug is well tolerated and kills more than 99% of viable bacilli in 1 month (21).

These 3 drugs, alone or in combination, are more active than dapsone and clofazimine and are good candidates to replace them to improve supervision and shorten duration of treatment. Recently, a single dose of clarithromycin plus minocycline with or without ofloxacin displayed bactericidal activity similar to that of 1 month of dapsone plus clofazimine (22). In addition, there is some evidence that intermittent rifampicin plus clarithromycin plus minocycline, with or without ofloxacin, administered for 12 or 24 weeks was as active as the standard multidrug regimen (23). It could thus be possible to replace the dapsone plus clofazimine component of MDT with a combination of minocycline and clarithromycin, with or without ofloxacin, which would simplify the delivery of antileprosy drugs and improve compliance. Some authors advocate daily administration of these agents as profoundly more potent than a monthly regimen (9, 10), but this has to be weighed against the problem of difficult access to health care, especially in developing countries. Further studies are currently under way to test the effect of these drug combinations.

CONTROVERSIES, CAVEATS AND COMMENTS

The introduction of multidrug therapy has had far reaching effects on the structure and strategy of leprosy control programs. The shortened course and the requirements for supervising monthly doses of rifampicin have greatly reduced the problem of compliance. However, patients with leprosy may still develop disabilities due to nerve damage, usually related to development of reactions (24, 25). Early detection of nerve damage by regular testing of nerve function is therefore a mandatory complement to MDT (3). Systematic surveillance during or after treatment is recommended to detect early signs of reactions so as to prevent disability. Optimum management of leprosy thus involves a multidisciplinary approach, including antimicrobial chemotherapy, physiotherapy, prevention of disability, and reconstructive surgery when deformity and handicap are present.

REFERENCES

1. Baciewitz AM, Self TH. Rifampicin drug interactions. Arch Intern Med 1984;144:1667–1671.
2. Banerjee DK, Ellard GA, Gammon PT, Waters MFR. Some observations on the pharmacology of clofazimine. Am J Trop Med Hyg 1974;23:1110–1115.
3. Becx-Bleuminck M, Berhe D. Occurrence of reactions, their diagnosis and management in leprosy patients treated with multidrug therapy. Experience in the leprosy control programme of the All Africa Leprosy and Rehabilitation Centre (ALERT) in Ethiopia. Int J Lepr 1992;60:173–184.
4. Browne SG, Hogerzeil LM. B663 in the treatment of leprosy: preliminary report of a clinical trial. Lepr Rev 1962;33:6–10.
5. Bryceson A, Pfaltzgraff RE. Leprosy. 3d ed. Edinburgh: Churchill Livingstone, 1990.
6. Draper. The structure of *Mycobacterium leprae*. Lepr Rev 1986; 52(Suppl 2):15–20.
7. Ellard GA. The chemotherapy of leprosy; part one. Int J Lepr 1990;58:704–716.
8. Gelber RH. Activity of minocycline in Mycobacterium leprae infected mice. J Infect Dis 1987;186:236–239.
9. Gelber RH, Murray LP, Siu P, Tsang M, Rea TH. Clarythromycine at very low levels and on intermittent administration inhibits the growth of M. leprae in lepromatous leprosy. Int J Lepr 1992;60:485–487.
10. Gelber RH, Kukuda SK, Byrd S, Murray LP, Siu P, Tsang M, Rea TH. A clinical trial of mynocycline in lepromatous leprosy. Br Med J 1992;304:91–92.
11. Grosset JH, Guelpa-Lauras CC, Bobin P, Brucker G, Cartel JL, Constant-Desportes M, Flageul B, Frederic M, Guillaume JC, Millan J. Study of 39 documented relapses of multibacillary leprosy after treatment with rifampin. Int J Lepr 1989;57:607–614.
12. Grosset JH, Ji B, Guelpa-Lauras CC, Perani EG, Ndeli L. Clinical trial of pefloxacin and ofloxacin in the treatment of lepromatous leprosy. Int J Lepr 1990;58:281–295.
13. Grosset JH. Progress in the chemotherapy of leprosy. Int J Lepr 1994;62:268–276.
14. Hastings RC. Growth of sulfone resistant Mycobacterium leprae in the food pad of mice fed with dapsone. Proc Soc Exp Biol Med 1977;156:544–545.
15. Hastings RC. Leprosy. Edinburgh: Churchill Livingstone, 1985.
16. Jacobson RR, Hastings RC. Rifampicin resistant leprosy. Lancet 1976;2:1304–1305.
17. Jamet P, Traore I, Husser JA, Ji B. Short term trial of clofazimine

in previously untreated lepromatous leprosy. Int J Lepr 1992; 60:542–548.

18. Ji B, Chen J, Wang C, Xia C. Hepatotoxicity of combined therapy with rifampicin and daily prothionamide for leprosy. Lepr Rev 1984;55:283–289.

19. Ji B. Drug resistance in leprosy—a review. Lepr Rev 1985;56: 265–278.

20. Ji B, Perani EG, Grosset JH, Effectiveness of clarithromycin or minocycline alone or in combination against Mycobacterium leprae infection in mice. Antimicrob Agents Chemother 1991; 35:575–581.

21. Ji B, Jamet P, Perani EG, Bobin P, Grosset JH. Powerful bactericidal activities of clarithromycin and minocycline against Mycobacterium leprae in lepromatous leprosy. J Infect Dis 1993, 168:188–190.

22. Ji B, Jamet P, Perani EG, Sow S, Lienhardt C, Petinon C, Grosset JH. Bactericidal activity of a single dose of clarithromycin plus minocycline with or without ofloxacin against M leprae in patients. Antimicrob Agents Chemother 1996;40:2137–2141.

23. Ji B, Perani EG, Petinon C, Grosset JH. Bactericidal activity of combinations of new drugs against *Mycobacterium leprae* in patients. Antimicrob Agents Chemother 1996;40:393–399.

24. Job CK. Nerve damage in leprosy. Int J Lepr 1989;57:532–539.

25. Lienhardt C, Fine PEM. Type 1 reaction, neuritis and disability in leprosy. What is their current epidemiological situation ? Lepr Rev 1994;65:9–33.

26. Lowe J, Smith M. The chemotherapy of leprosy in Nigeria. Int J Lepr 1949;17:181–195.

27. Marchoux Chemotherapy Study Group. Relapses in multibacillary leprosy patients after stopping treatment with rifampin-containing combined regimens. Int J Lepr 1992;60:525–535.

28. Ognibene A. Agranulocytosis due to dapsone. Ann Intern Med 1970;72:521–524.

29. Pearson JMH, Haile GS, Rees RJW. Primary dapsone-resistant leprosy. Lepr Rev 1977;48:129–132.

30. Petitt JHS, Rees RJW. Sulfone resistance in leprosy: an experimental and clinical study. Lancet 1964;2:673–674.

31. Rees RJW, Pearson JMH, Waters MFR, Experimental and clinical studies on rifampicin in the treatment of leprosy. Br Med J 1970;189–192.

32. Ridley DS, Jopling WH. Classification of leprosy according to immunity, a five-group system. Int J Lepr 1966;34:255–273.

33. Ridley DS. Reactions in leprosy. Lepr Rev 1969;40:77–81.

34. Shephard CC. The experimental disease that follows the injection of human leprosy bacilli into footpads of mice. J Exp Med 1960;112:445–454.

35. Shepard CC, Chang YT. Effect of several antileprosy drugs on multiplication of human leprosy bacilli in footpads of mice. Proc Soc Exp Biol Med 1962;109:636–638.

36. Shepard CC, Levy L, Fasal P. Rapid bactericidal effect of rifampicin on Mycobacterium leprae. Am J Trop Med Hyg 1972; 21:445–449.

37. Shepard CC, Levy L, Fasal P. Further experience with the rapid bactericidal effect of rifampicin on Mycobacterium leprae. Am J Trop Med Hyg 1974;23:1120–1124.

38. Thelep Subcommittee on Clinical Trials of the Chemotherapy of Leprosy Scientific Working Group of the UNDP/World Bank/ WHO Special Programme for Research and Training in Tropical Diseases. Persisting mycobacterium leprae among Thelep trial patients in Bamako and Chingleput. Lepr Rev 1987; 58: 325–337.

39. Waters MFR, Rees RJW, Pearson JMH, Laing ABG, Helmy HS, Gelber RH. Rifampicin for lepromatous leprosy: nine years' experience. Br Med J 1978;1:133–136.

40. Walsh GP, Meyers WM, Binford CH, et al. Leprosy—a zoonosis. Lepr Rev 1981;52(Suppl 1):77–83.

41. Warndorff van Diepen T. Clofazimine resistant leprosy: a case-report. Int J Lepr 1982;50:139–142.

42. WHO Study Group. Chemotherapy of leprosy for control programmes. Geneva: World Health Organisation, Tech Rep Ser 675, 1982.

43. WHO Expert Committee on Leprosy. Sixth report. Geneva: World Health Organisation, Tech Rep Ser 768, 1988.

44. WHO Study Group. Chemotherapy of leprosy . Geneva: World Health Organisation, Tech Rep Ser 847, 1994.

45. WHO. Progress towards the elimination of leprosy as a public health problem. WHO Weekly Epidemiol Rec 1996;20:149–156.

46. Yawalkar SJ, McDougall AC, Languillon, J et al. Once-monthly rifampicin plus daily dapsone in initial treatment of lepromatous leprosy. Lancet 1982;1:1199–1202

Mycobacterium marinum

●

David E. Griffith and Richard J. Wallace, Jr.

GENERAL DESCRIPTION

Mycobacterium marinum is a photochromogen with a growth rate intermediate between rapidly and slowly growing mycobacteria. *M. marinum* grows optimally at 28 to 30°C and fails to grow on primary isolation at 37°C, a feature that distinguishes this species from *M. kansasii*. This temperature growth restriction may explain the restriction of infection to the extremities and peripheral lymph nodes. *M. marinum* lacks catalase and nitrate reductase activities, and some, but not all, isolates hydrolyze Tween 80.

The two major risk factors for *M. marinum* infection in immunocompetent patients are exposure to *M. marinum*–infested waters and the presence of superficial cuts or abrasions. The organisms may be introduced into the skin while cleaning fresh water fish tanks ("fish tank granuloma"), by scratches or puncture wounds from saltwater fish, shrimp, fins, etc., or through abrasions in nonchlorinated swimming pools ("swimming pool granuloma") (4, 6, 9). By extension, risk factors for HIV-infected persons would be similar exposures. Although there has been no change in the prevalence and frequency of *M. marinum* infections in the developed world since the advent of the AIDS epidemic, there have been several reports of disseminated infection by *M. marinum* in patients with AIDS (12, 16).

SUSCEPTIBILITY IN VITRO AND IN VIVO

The usual MICs for active agents include rifampin, 1.0 μg/mL or less; ethambutol, 5.0 μg/mL or less; clarithromycin, 1.0 to 4.0 μg/mL or less; sulfamethoxazole, 10.0 μg/mL or less; and doxycycline and minocycline, 2.0 to 8.0 μg/mL (3, 17). Because MICs or fixed concentration susceptibilities are always the same, susceptibilities are rarely indicated for treatment of *M. marinum*. Acquired resistance with definite changes in drug susceptibility for *M. marinum* has not been reported. *M. marinum* isolates have moderately high MICs to isoniazid (4.0–16.0 μg/mL) and streptomycin and are resistant to pyrazinamide (3, 17).

ANTIMICROBIAL THERAPY

A number of treatment modalities have been used for cutaneous disease caused by *M. marinum*. These include simple observation for minor lesions, surgical excision, the use of antituberculous therapy, and the use of single antibiotic agents. Acceptable treatment regimens include monotherapy with clarithromycin 500 mg twice a day, minocycline or doxycycline at 100 mg twice a day, or trimethoprim-sulfamethoxazole (TMP-SMX) at 160/800 mg twice a day (1, 11, 13) (Table 1). Combination therapy with rifampin (600 mg) plus ethambutol (15 mg/kg) daily is also effective (5). There is limited published experience with clarithromycin (2, 7, 15); however, its in vitro activity against *M. marinum* suggests that it would be quite effective. Each regimen should be given for a minimum of 3 months. Rifampin alone has also been recommended, but there is little experience with this regimen (8).

Clinical response is generally slow with any regimen;

therefore, a minimum of 4 to 6 weeks of therapy should be given before considering that the patient may not be responding. Surgical debridement may also be important, especially for disease involving the closed spaces of the hand or disease that responds poorly to drug therapy. If a lesion is excised surgically, drug coverage during the perioperative period is generally recommended. It is not clear if chemotherapy after surgery improves treatment success.

The published experience with disseminated *M. marinum* disease in AIDS patients (or other immunocompromised patients) is limited to case reports. Hanau et al. described a patient with AIDS and sporotrichoid *M. marinum* infection who responded well to 6 months of antimycobacterial therapy, primarily rifampin and ethambutol, although the *M. marinum* infection returned soon after cessation of therapy (10). Bonnet described an AIDS patient with fluctuant nodules due to *M. marinum* who failed 5 months of ofloxacin and minocycline. The patient was subsequently changed to rifampin, ciprofloxacin, and amikacin, but she did not show a favorable clinical response until clarithromycin was added to the regimen (2). It seems prudent to treat *M. marinum* infection in immuno-compromised hosts with at least two agents, including clarithromycin (2, 10, 14). Duration of therapy in this setting is difficult to know with certainty but should be at least 6 months and, without remission of severe immunosuppression, possibly lifetime.

ENDPOINTS FOR MONITORING THERAPY

The natural history of infection with *M. marinum* is variable. Spontaneous remission, particularly when trauma is minor, is fairly common in an immunocompetent person. However, when ulceration is severe, sporotrichoid lesions appear, there is joint or tendon involvement, or cutaneous lesions occur in an immunocompromised host, chemotherapy is indicated.

REFERENCES

1. Black MM, Eykyn S. The successful treatment of tropical fish tank granuloma (*Mycobacterium marinum* infections). Arch Intern Med 1986;146:902–904.
2. Bonnet E. Clarithromycin: a potent agent against infections due to *Mycobacterium marinum*. Clin Infect Dis 1994;18:664–666.
3. Brown BA, Wallace RJ Jr, Onyi GO. Activities of clarithromycin against eight slowly growing species of nontuberculous mycobacteria, determined by using a broth microdilution MIC system. Antimicrob Agents Chemother 1992;36: 1987–1990.
4. Brown JW III, Sanders CV. *Mycobacterium marinum* infections. Arch Intern Med 1987;147:817–818.
5. Chow SP, Ip FK, Lau JH, Collins RJ, Luk KD, So YC, Pun WK. *Mycobacterium marinum* infection of the hand and wrist. J Bone Surg (Am) 1987;60-A:1161–1168.
6. Collins CH, Grange JM, Noble WC, Yates MD. *Mycobacterium marinum* infections in man. J Hyg 1985;94:135–149.
7. Dautzenberg B, Breux JP, Febvre M, Dimercurio JP, Diot P, Chauvin JP. Clarithromycin containing regimens for mycobacterial infections in 55 non AIDS patients. Am Rev Respir Dis 1992;145:A809.
8. Donta ST, Smith PW, Levitz RE, Quintiliani LR. Therapy of *Mycobacterium marinum* infections. Arch Intern Med 1986;146: 902–904.

TABLE 1 • Recommended Regimens for *M. marinum* Infection

1. Cutaneous disease in the immunocompetent host
   Clarithromycin 500 mg b.i.d.
      or
   minocycline or doxycycline 100 mg b.i.d.
      or
   TMP/SMX*[a]* at 160/800 mg b.i.d.
      or
   rifampin 600 mg plus ethambutol 15 mg/kg/day
   Administered for at least 3 months
   Consider surgical debridement for disease in the hand or
      disease responding slowly to medications
2. Disseminated disease in AIDS patients
   Combination therapy with two or more agents listed above;
      inclusion of clarithromycin recommended
   Optimal duration of therapy unknown

*[a]*TMP-SMX, trimethoprim-sulfamethoxazole.

9. Edelstein H. *Mycobacterium marinum* skin infections [Review]. Arch Intern Med 1994;154:1359–1364.

10. Hanau HH, Leaf A, Soeiro R, Weiss LM, Pollack SS. *Mycobacterium marinum* infection in a patient with the acquired immunodeficiency syndrome. Cutis 1994;54:103–105.

11. Kin R. Tetracycline therapy for atypical granuloma. Arch Dermatol 1974;110–299.

12. Lambertus MW, Mathisen GE. *Mycobacterium marinum* infection in a patient with cryptosporidiosis and the acquired immunodeficiency syndrome. Cutis 1988;41:38–40.

13. Loria PR. Minocycline hydrochloride treatment for atypical acid-fast infection. Arch Dermatol 1976;112:517–519.

14. Parent LJ, Salam MM. Disseminated *Mycobacterium marinum* infection and bacteremia in a child with severe combined immunodeficiency. Clin Infect Dis 1995;21:1325–1327.

15. Sands M, Rosenthal E, Chavan A, Snyder B. *Mycobacterium marinum* tenosynovitis treated with clarithromycin and ethambutol. Infect Dis Clin Pract 1996;5:509–510.

16. Tchornobay AM, Claudy A, Perrot JL, Levigne M, Denis M. Fatal disseminated *Mycobacterium marinum* infection. Int J Dermatol 1992;31:286–287.

17. Wallace RJ Jr, Nash DR, Steele LC, Steingrube V. Susceptibility testing of slowly growing mycobacteria by a microdilution MIC method with 7H9 broth. J Clin Microbiol 1986;24:976–981.

Mycobacterium tuberculosis Complex

●

Charles L. Daley

GENERAL DESCRIPTION

Tuberculosis is caused by any one of several mycobacterial species that belong to the *Mycobacterium tuberculosis* complex. The human pathogens are *M. tuberculosis, M. africanum,* and *M. bovis* (168). The other member of the complex, *M. microti,* is a rodent pathogen. *M. tuberculosis* is, by far, the most important of the human pathogens. Approximately one-third of the world's population, or 1.7 billion people, are thought to be infected with *M. tuberculosis* (131). Tuberculosis is the most common cause of death from an infectious or parasitic agent among individuals over 5 years of age, accounting for 3 million deaths annually. In addition, one in three AIDS patients in the world will die of tuberculosis (147). Thus, *M. tuberculosis* is one of the most important causes of morbidity and mortality worldwide. The other human pathogens, *M. bovis* and *M. africanum,* are uncommon causes of tuberculosis in most regions of the world. *M. bovis* is reported to cause approximately 3% of tuberculosis cases in San Diego (37), and *M. africanum* was recently reported to cause nearly half of the HIV-1-related tuberculosis among participants in a clinical trial in Uganda (134). Except for some variation in in vitro drug susceptibilities among the members of the *M. tuberculosis* complex, the general principles of therapy remain the same.

There are two populations for whom management of tuberculosis is often more complicated: persons coinfected with HIV-1 and patients with drug-resistant disease. HIV-1-infected patients with tuberculosis represent up to one-half of the tuberculosis cases in some areas of the United States (112). Coinfected patients are more likely to present atypically, delaying diagnosis and initiation of effective therapy. In addition, coinfected patients are often taking numerous medications, which may result in drug toxicities or interactions.

Unfortunately, the prevalence of drug-resistant tuberculosis, including multidrug-resistant disease (MDR-TB), has increased in the last few years (6, 42, 59, 60). Many of these cases of MDR-TB have occurred in HIV-1-infected populations and have been associated with high mortality rates. Treatment of MDR-TB is complicated, expensive, and associated with frequent drug toxicities and high failure and relapse rates.

Tuberculosis can develop through progression of recently acquired infection (primary disease), reactivation of latent infection, or exogenous reinfection (83). In immunocompetent individuals, approximately 3 to 10% of those with tuberculous infection develop tuberculosis in the first 1 to 2 years after infection (156), and another 5% develop tuberculosis within their lifetime. Exogenous reinfection is thought to be uncommon in immunocompetent persons residing in areas with a low prevalence of tuberculosis. In the setting of HIV-1 infection, the risk of progressing rapidly to infection once infected with *M. tuberculosis* (36), the risk of reactivation (135, 136), and the risk of exogenous reinfection (146) are all higher than in HIV-1-seronegative persons. Coinfection with HIV-1 also alters the clinical presentation of tuberculosis. Most tuberculosis occurs as pulmonary disease, with 17% occurring at an extrapulmonary site only. However, among HIV-1-infected patients, as many as 70% have evidence of extrapulmonary disease or mycobacteremia once the CD4 count is below 100 cells/mL (90).

SUSCEPTIBILITY IN VITRO

Mycobacteria of the *M. tuberculosis* complex grow slowly, dividing every 15 to 20 h (168). Because of this slow growth, it can take over 3 weeks to see visible growth on standard culture media; in radiometric culture systems, growth can be detected in as little as 10 to 14 days (138). The slow rate of growth has significant clinical implications because therapy must be begun in many patients before the diagnosis is confirmed. In addition, drug susceptibility results are seldom available at the initiation of treatment.

Drug resistance occurs in *M. tuberculosis* through chromosomal mutations that confer resistance to individual antituberculosis drugs. In vitro work suggests that these mutations occur spontaneously and at predictable rates and that mutations resulting in resistance to a particular drug are not linked to mutations resulting in resistance to other drugs (38). For example, mutations conferring resistance to isoniazid and rifampin occur with an estimated frequency of approximately 3×10^8 and 2×10^{10} mutations per bacterium per generation, respectively (38). All populations of *M. tuberculosis* therefore have a certain number of naturally occurring drug-resistant mutants, and this probability is influenced by the size of the bacterial population and the rate of replication. The probability that resistance will develop to isoniazid and rifampin in nature is the product of each of the separate probabilities, or 6×10^{18}. Even in a patient who has cavitary tuberculosis, in which the bacillary population may exceed 10^9 organisms, the probability that simultaneous mutations will occur leading to multiple resistance is exceedingly small (38). This phenomenon is the central reason for multidrug treatment of tuberculosis and the critical factor underlying acquired drug resistance.

Drug resistance is often divided into two types, primary (initial), and acquired (secondary) resistance. Primary drug resistance is defined as resistance that occurs in an individual with tuberculosis who has never been treated with antituberculosis drugs. Acquired drug resistance refers to development of resistance in an initially drug-susceptible isolate during the course of therapy. Thus, acquired drug resistance requires a mutation that leads to resistance, followed by selective pressure favoring proliferation of the mutant population. This selective pressure occurs when an inadequate regimen is prescribed, the patient does not take medications as prescribed, or there is selective malabsorption of medications. Under these circumstances, resistant mutants may flourish and become the dominant mycobacterial population.

The increasing prevalence of drug-resistant *M. tuberculosis* in recent years has increased the need for laboratories to perform drug susceptibility tests. Drug resistance can be detected by a variety of in vitro methods that are usually contingent on demonstrating growth of the organism in the presence of a critical concentration of antituberculosis drug. The two most commonly used qualitative methods are the proportion method and the BACTEC method. In the proportion method, plates of drug-free agar and agar containing critical concentrations of antituberculosis drugs are inoculated with the isolate (165). For most drugs, resistance is determined by comparing the number of colony-forming units (CFU) on drug-containing versus drug-free media, with clinically significant resistance being defined as more than 1% growth on drug-containing media relative to drug-free media.

In the BACTEC method, critical concentrations of the drugs are added to the BACTEC broth vials containing a radiolabeled substrate, allowing automated detection of growth (139). If the rate of growth of the inoculum in a drug-free vial exceeds the rate of growth of a 1:100 inoculum dilution in a drug-free vial, then the isolate is considered resistant. The BACTEC method also allows determination of minimal inhibitory concentrations (MICs), which provide the opportunity to compare the level of resistance with the concentration of a drug actually attainable in human serum (72). The clinical use of MICs in the treatment of tuberculosis is of unclear significance.

Antituberculosis drugs are traditionally divided into first- and second-line agents. The first-line agents are typically more effective and less toxic than second-line drugs. The currently available antituberculosis drugs are discussed briefly below.

First-Line Agents

At the commonly used dosages, all of the first-line agents, except ethambutol, are bactericidal for *M. tuberculosis*. However, each drug demonstrates different degrees of effectiveness because they work in different environments, under different conditions, and during different rates of growth.

Isoniazid. Isoniazid (INH), introduced in 1952, is one of the most active drugs for the treatment of tuberculosis (132). In vitro, INH inhibits most strains of *M. tuberculosis* at concentrations of 0.05 to 0.2 μg/mL, and it is bactericidal for actively growing bacilli. Resistance to INH has been associated with overproduction of the product of the *inh*A gene (5) and with mutation or deletion of *kat*G, which encodes mycobacterial catalase (174). InhA overproduction is associated with low-level resistance and cross-resistance with ethionamide, whereas *kat*G mutants express high-level resistance and are not cross-resistant to ethionamide. When given alone as monotherapy for active disease, 70% of isolates develop resistance to INH within 3 months (101).

INH is well absorbed orally, but the drug may also be given intramuscularly or intravenously, if necessary. INH penetrates readily into all body tissues and fluid. Concentrations in the central nervous system (CNS) and cerebrospinal fluid (CSF) can reach levels equal to that in the serum (74).

Rifampin (Rifampicin). Rifampin is a semisynthetic derivative of rif-amycin B, and it is a potent antimycobacterial agent, acting through inhibition of mycobacterial DNA-dependent RNA polymerase. Mutations at certain amino acid positions in the *rpo*B region may confer high-level resistance to rifampin but display MIC values of 0.25 to 0.5 μg/mL to rifabutin (9). Rifampin is widely distributed in body tissues and fluids. Because the drug is highly protein bound, adequate CSF concentrations are achieved only in the presence of meningeal inflammation (40, 74). In the setting of normal meninges, rifampin levels in the CSF may be undetectable.

Pyrazinamide. Pyrazinamide is chemically related to nicotinamide and bactericidal for *M. tuberculosis*. Susceptible strains of *M. tuberculosis* produce the enzyme pyrazinamidase, which converts pyrazinamide to pyrazinoic acid, the putatively active moiety. In most resistant strains, the level of pyrazinamidase is markedly reduced (18). *M. bovis* is intrinsically resistant to pyrazinamide. The drug is completely absorbed after an oral dose and is widely distributed throughout the body, including the CSF (55, 56, 74).

Ethambutol. Ethambutol is usually bacteriostatic against *M. tuberculosis,* with MICs of 1 to 5 μg/mL. However, at a dose of 50 μg/mL, ethambutol may become bactericidal. Although its precise mechanism of action is not known, ethambutol is known to inhibit synthesis of arabinogalactam, an essential component of the mycobacterial cell wall. Recently, investigators have documented a gene cluster involved in resistance to ethambutol (158). The drug is widely distributed throughout the body, but the CSF concentration is generally low, reaching 1 to 2 μg/mL after a dose of 25 mg/kg (7, 74).

Streptomycin. Streptomycin, an aminoglycoside, was the first effective antituberculosis agent. The drug is bactericidal to extracellular replicating tubercle bacilli and inhibits growth of tubercle bacilli at concentrations of 0.4 to 10.0 μg/mL. Mutations associated with streptomycin resistance in *M. tuberculosis* have been identified in the 16S rRNA gene (*rrs*) and the gene (*rpsL*) encoding ribosomal protein S12 (30). In the setting of meningeal inflammation, approximately 10% of the drug crosses the blood-brain barrier (74).

Second-Line Agents

Rifamycins. Two newly available rifamycins, rifabutin and rifapentine, have excellent MICs against *M. tuberculosis.* In fact, the MIC for rifabutin is 2 to 20 times lower and the MIC for rifapentine is 1.7 times lower than that of rifampin (39). Although, rifabutin has a slightly longer half-life, maximum serum concentrations are much lower than those achieved with rifampin. The extremely long half-life of rifapentine may allow once-weekly dosing. Unfortunately, there is usually cross-resistance among the rifamycins; however, *M. tuberculosis* may remain susceptible to rifabutin in a minority of rifampin-resistant strains (9, 173).

Studies have demonstrated the efficacy of rifabutin versus rifampin in a regimen containing INH, pyrazinamide, and ethambutol in both HIV-1-seropositive and -seronegative populations (100, 134). In a multinational, randomized comparative trial of rifabutin versus rifampicin, rifabutin at a dose of 150 or 300 mg/day was as effective as rifampicin (66). In addition, rifabutin has been used successfully in the treatment of multidrug-resistant tuberculosis (128).

Ethionamide. Ethionamide is chemically related to INH and also blocks the synthesis of mycolic acids. The drug is a bacteriostatic agent that inhibits most tubercle bacilli in vitro at a concentration of 2.5 mg/mL. There may be low-level cross-resistance with INH as noted above. Ethionamide is widely distributed and penetrates both normal and inflamed meninges (74).

Cycloserine. Cycloserine, an inhibitor of cell wall synthesis, is bacteriostatic for *M. tuberculosis* at concentrations of 5 to 20 μg/mL. The mechanism of drug resistance is not known. Cycloserine penetrates the blood-brain barrier extremely well (74).

p-Aminosalicylic Acid (PAS). PAS impairs folate synthesis in the tubercle bacillus and inhibits most strains in vitro at concentrations of 1 to 5 μg/mL. The mechanism of drug re-

sistance is not known. The drug is widely distributed in tissues and body fluids, except the CSF (74).

Capreomycin, Amikacin, Kanamycin. Capreomycin is a polypeptide antibiotic obtained from *Streptomyces capreolus.* There is usually no cross-resistance to streptomycin or amikacin/kanamycin. Amikacin is one of the most active aminoglycosides against *M. tuberculosis.* There is no cross-resistance between streptomycin and amikacin. Kanamycin is similar to amikacin, and cross-resistance can occur.

Quinolones. Ofloxacin and ciprofloxacin have bactericidal activity and inhibit *M. tuberculosis* at concentrations of 0.5 to 2.0 and 0.25 to 2.0 μg/mL, respectively (27, 130). Ofloxacin tends to be slightly more active in vitro than ciprofloxacin. Levofloxacin, the L-isomer of ofloxacin, has even lower MICs (0.5–0.75 μg/mL) (130). Resistance may occur from any one of several point mutations in the gyrase A subunit and typically involves all fluoroquinolones.

In a randomized controlled trial of 200 patients with sputum smear–positive tuberculosis in Tanzania, ciprofloxacin had less sterilizing activity than the combination of pyrazinamide and ethambutol (92). Most of the difference was seen in HIV-1-infected subjects. However, when ofloxacin was substituted for ethambutol, the two agents appeared to be of equal efficacy (94). Ofloxacin has been used successfully in the treatment of multidrug-resistant disease (79).

β-Lactams. All mycobacteria produce at least one β-lactamase; thus, β-lactam antibiotics are usually not effective against *M. tuberculosis.* However, β-lactam antimicrobials in combination with β-lactamase inhibitors are bactericidal in vitro against *M. tuberculosis* (34). The MIC_{90} for amoxicillin is above 32 mg/L, but with addition of clavulanic acid, the MIC_{90} decreases to 4 mg/L (171). One report suggested a possible role for this class of drugs in the treatment of highly drug resistant isolates (104).

Clofazimine. Clofazimine is a phenazine dye that has some activity against *M. tuberculosis* in vitro. It is used as a last resort in the treatment of MDR-tuberculosis.

ANTIMICROBIAL THERAPY

Soon after streptomycin became available for treatment of tuberculosis, it was recognized that monotherapy frequently resulted in treatment failure due to development of in vitro resistance to the drug (102). Addition of PAS to a regimen of streptomycin prevented development of acquired resistance to either agent and was more effective than either agent alone; however, cure rates were only in the range of 70% (14, 159). Addition of INH to streptomycin and PAS increased cure rates to 95% but required 18 to 24 months of therapy (15). Therefore, investigators began to evaluate other multidrug regimens to try to find regimens of shorter duration.

In a series of studies conducted by the British Medical Research Council (BMRC) in East Africa (49–53) and the United States Public Health Service (USPHS) (105, 106), investigators demonstrated the importance of rifampin and pyrazinamide in shortening the duration of therapy for tuberculosis. A 6-month regimen of daily INH, streptomycin, and rifampin compared favorably with the 18-month regimen of streptomycin, thiacetazone, and INH for 2 months followed by thiacetazone and INH for 16 months (53). Short-course therapy was demonstrated to be efficient in converting sputum cultures to negative, and relapse rates were low (53). Patients who relapsed after treatment with INH and rifampin, did so with organisms still sensitive to the original drugs. Addition of streptomycin to a regimen containing INH, rifampin, and pyrazinamide added little efficacy. (52, 143).

Regimens of less than 6-months' duration showed unacceptably high relapse rates among smear-positive pulmonary tuberculosis patients (54, 141, 142). However, among patients with smear-negative culture-positive disease, the relapse rate was only 2% with a 4-month regimen of streptomycin, INH, rifampin, and pyrazinamide (76). A 3-month regimen was inadequate, with a relapse rate of 13% (25).

A USPHS trial demonstrated that INH and rifampin were as effective as the standard regimen of streptomycin, INH, and ethambutol, and the rifampin-containing regimen converted the sputum cultures to negative 2 weeks faster than the standard regimen (105, 106). Addition of pyrazinamide beyond the initial 2 months was demonstrated to be unnecessary in several BMRC studies (54, 78, 142). Importantly, intermittent regimens were eventually shown to be as effective as daily regimens (77, 80, 140, 143).

Other studies from the United States and the British Thoracic Society (BTS) helped to develop our current approach to short-course therapy. INH and rifampin for 9 months was successful in 95% of smear-negative or smear-positive patients in Arkansas when given daily for 1 month followed by twice-weekly dosing (44, 47). The BTS demonstrated that INH and rifampin for 6 months, supplemented during the first 2 months with streptomycin and pyrazinamide or streptomycin and ethambutol, were as effective as a 9-month regimen of INH and rifampin with ethambutol in the first 2 months (16). USPHS Trial 21 studied daily, self-administered INH and rifampin for 6 months with pyrazinamide given during the initial 2 months (33). Ethambutol was added if INH resistance was suspected. The relapse rate was only 3.5%, despite the fact nearly 17% of the patients were felt to be nonadherent. Finally, investigators in Denver reported a very low relapse rate using a 6-month regimen that consisted of 2 weeks of daily INH, rifampin, pyrazinamide, and streptomycin followed by 6 weeks of these four drugs twice weekly, followed by 18 weeks of twice-weekly INH and rifampin (31).

In summary, several principles of therapy have emerged from the many clinical trials and the accumulated experience of experts treating tuberculosis. First and most important, at least two agents must be used in the treatment of active tuberculosis to prevent emergence of drug resistance during therapy. Second, the duration and effectiveness of a treatment regimen depend on the drugs used. The combination of INH and rifampin is the key to modern short-course therapy; addition of pyrazinamide allows us to treat predictably for 6 months. Third, intermittent therapy is as efficacious as daily therapy, which allows directly observed therapy. Fourth, although some patients relapse with short-course therapy, the great majority do so with drug-susceptible isolates. Fifth, a single drug should never be added to a failing regimen; adding a single drug to a regimen that is failing because of underlying drug resistance may result in development of resistance to the new drug. Finally, nonadherence to the treatment regimen is the most important cause of treatment failure, relapse, and acquired drug resistance.

Despite the seemingly straightforward nature of these principles, clinicians continue to make errors in the treatment of tuberculosis. Mahmoudi and Iseman (99) reported that an average of 3.9 errors were made by clinicians in the drug-resistant cases referred to National Jewish Medical and Research Center. These errors resulted in the development of significant drug resistance, which decreased the effectiveness, and increased the costs, of therapy.

Drugs of Choice

Tuberculosis must be treated with at least two drugs to which the isolate is susceptible. Duration of treatment, expected drug toxicities, and overall effectiveness depend on the drugs used. The currently available first- and second-line drugs, recommended doses, and common side effects are listed in Tables 1 and 2. The most common side effects and drug interactions are described below.

First-Line Agents

Isoniazid. INH, one of the most effective antituberculosis drugs, is generally well tolerated, with few major side effects, the most notable of which is hepatitis. Approximately 15 to 20% of individuals taking INH develop a transient mild elevation in serum aminotransferase levels (4). Such increases do not necessitate cessation of the drug. The risk of INH-related hepatitis increases with age; in persons under 20 years of age, the risk is negligible, whereas for persons over the age of 50, the frequency of hepatitis is 2.3% (95). The risk of hepatitis is increased in persons who are alcoholics, and possibly in those with chronic liver disease, and in persons taking the hepatotoxic medications. Most cases of INH-related hepatitis occur within the first 1 to 2 months of therapy, although cases have been reported at any time during the course of therapy.

Peripheral neuropathy is observed in 10 to 20% of patients given more than 5 mg/kg/day but is infrequently seen with the standard 300-mg adult dose. The risk of peripheral neuropathy is increased in persons with other underlying medical conditions that predispose to neuropathy, such as diabetes mellitus, alcoholism, HIV-1 infection, malnutrition, and end-stage renal disease. INH can also lower the seizure threshold. Coadministration of pyridoxine (B_6) can prevent development of peripheral neuropathy and may be effective with other CNS toxicities.

Rifampin. The major toxicity of rifampin is hepatitis. Elevated alkaline phosphatase and total bilirubin in someone receiving rifampin suggest a cholestatic jaundice that is typical of this drug. With higher doses given intermittently, patients may develop a flulike syndrome characterized by fever, chills, myalgias, anemia, thrombocytopenia, and occasionally acute tubular necrosis (63, 81). Although not clinically significant, patients must be warned that rifampin causes an orange discoloration of the urine, tears (which may stain soft contact lenses), semen, and other bodily fluids.

TABLE 1 • First-Line Agents

Drug	Dose[a] in mg/kg (Maximum Dose)						Adverse Reactions	Comments
	Daily		2/Week		3/Week			
	Children	Adults	Children	Adults	Children	Adults		
Isoniazid	10–20 (300 mg)	5 (300 mg)	20–40 (900 mg)	15 (900 mg)	20–40 (900 mg)	15 (900 mg)	Hepatic enzyme elevation; hepatitis; peripheral neuropathy; central nervous system (mild); drug interactions	Hepatitis risk increases with age and alcohol consumption; pyridoxine can prevent peripheral neuropathy
Rifampin	10–20 (600 mg)	10 (600 mg)	10–20 (600 mg)	10 (600 mg)	10–20 (600 mg)	10 (600 mg)	GI upset; drug interactions; hepatitis; bleeding problems; flulike symptoms; rash	Significant interactions with methadone, birth control pills, many other drugs; colors body fluids orange; may permanently discolor soft contact lenses
Pyrazinamide	15–30 (2 g)	15–30 (2 g)	50–70 (4 g)	50–70 (4 g)	50–70 (3 g)	50–70 (3 g)	Hepatitis; rash; GI upset; joint aches; hyperuricemia; gout (rare)	Treat hyperuricemia only if patient has symptoms
Ethambutol	15–25 (2.5 g)	15–25 (2.5 g)	50 (2.5 g)	50 (2.5 g)	25–30 (2.5 g)	25–30 (2.5 g)	Optic neuritis	Not recommended for children too young to be monitored for changes in vision unless tuberculosis is drug resistant
Streptomycin	20–30 (1 g)	15 (1 g)	25–30 (1 g)	25–30 (1 g)	25–30 (1.5 g)	25–30 (1.5 g)	Ototoxicity; renal toxicity	Avoid or reduce dose in adults >60 years old

Adopted from Centers for Disease Control and Prevention. Core Curriculum on Tuberculosis, 3rd ed., 1994.

[a]Children ≦12 years old: adjust weight-based dosages as weight changes.

All regimens administered 2 or 3 times a week should be used with directly observed therapy (DOT).

TABLE 2 • Second-Line Agents

Drug (Maximum Dose)	Daily Dose[a]	Adverse Reactions	Monitoring	Comments
Capreomycin	15–30 mg/kg (1 g)	Toxicity: auditory, vestibular, renal	Assess vestibular and hearing function; measure blood urea nitrogen and creatinine	After bacteriologic conversion, dosage may be reduced to 2–3 times per week
Kanamycin	15–30 mg/kg (1 g)	Toxicity: auditory, vestibular, renal	Assess vestibular and hearing function; measure blood urea nitrogen and creatinine	After bacteriologic conversion, dosage may be reduced to 2–3 times per week
Ethionamide	15–20 mg/kg (1 g)	GI upset, metallic taste, hepatotoxicity, bloating, hypersensitivity	Measure hepatic enzymes	Start with low dosage and increase as tolerated; may cause hypothyroid condition, especially if used with PAS
Para-aminosalicylic acid (PAS)	150 mg/kg (12 g)	GI upset, hypersensitivity, hepatotoxicity, sodium load	Measure hepatic enzymes; assess volume status	Start with low dosage and increase as tolerated; monitor cardiac patients for sodium load
Cycloserine	15–20 mg/kg (1 g)	Psychosis, headaches, convulsions, rash, depression, drug interactions	Assess mental status; measure serum drug levels	Start with low dosage and increase as tolerated; pyridoxine may decrease CNS effects
Ciprofloxacin	500–1000 mg/day	GI upset, drug interactions dizziness, headaches, hypersensitivity, restlessness	Drug interactions	Not approved by FDA for TB treatment; should not be used in children; avoid antacids, zinc, iron, sucralfate
Ofloxacin	400–800 mg/day	GI upset, drug interactions, dizziness, headaches, hypersensitivity, restlessness	Drug interactions	Not approved by FDA for TB treatment; should not be used in children; avoid antacids, iron, zinc, sucralfate
Amikacin	15 mg/kg	Renal toxicity, chemical imbalance, hearing loss, dizziness, vestibular dysfunction	Assess hearing function; measure renal function and serum drug levels	Not approved by FDA for TB treatment
Clofazimine	100–300 mg/day	GI upset, discoloration of skin, severe abdominal pain and organ damage due to crystal deposition	Drug interactions	Not approved by FDA for TB treatment, efficacy unproven; avoid sunlight; consider dosing at mealtime

Adopted from Centers for Disease Control and Prevention. Core Curriculum on Tuberculosis, 3rd ed., 1994.

[a]Doses for children same as for adults. Use these drugs only in consultation with a clinician experienced in the management of drug-resistant TB. Adjust weight-based dosages as weight changes.

Of all the antituberculosis drugs, the rifamycins are the most problematic because of the many drug interactions that may occur. Rifampin is a potent inducer of the hepatic cytochrome P-450 enzyme system, thus administration of rifampin may increase the metabolism of several drugs, resulting in subtherapeutic serum levels. Some examples of these medications include methadone, ketoconazole, protease inhibitors (PIs), warfarin, and steroids (10). Ketoconazole reduces rifampin serum concentrations (57).

Pyrazinamide. The most common side effects associated with pyrazinamide are nausea and vomiting. Hepatitis, which is rare at current dosages, is dose related. Pyrazinamide interferes with urate excretion, resulting in elevated uric acid levels in most patients. This elevation seldom leads to frank gout, although arthralgias are common.

Ethambutol. The major side effect of ethambutol is optic neuritis, clinically manifested as decreased visual acuity or red-green color blindness. The risk of optic neuritis is dose related, and at the usual dose of 15 mg/kg, optic neuritis is uncommon (1%) (4, 43). Because of the difficulty in measuring visual acuity in young children, ethambutol is often not used in this setting. However, when the likelihood of drug resistance is high, ethambutol should be used (160).

Streptomycin. Streptomycin has renal, acoustic, and vestibular toxicity, with vestibular toxicity being more common than with more-commonly used aminoglycosides. Vertigo and hearing loss are the most common side effects. Toxicity is dose related, and the risk increases in the elderly. As with all aminoglycosides, dosages must be adjusted in the setting of renal failure. The total cumulative dose should not exceed 120 g.

Second-Line Agents

Rifamycins. Rifabutin has been associated with development of uveitis (122). Like rifampin, rifabutin has liver enzyme–inducing properties; however, it is a less-potent inducer.

Ethionamide. The most common side effects of ethionamide involve gastrointestinal distress. Peripheral neuropathy has been occasionally reported. Reversible hepatitis occurs in approximately 5% of persons receiving this drug.

Cycloserine. Cycloserine can cause a number of neuropsychiatric disturbances, from irritability to frank psychosis, severe depression with suicidal ideation, and seizures. The drug is contraindicated in those with seizures or significant depression. The drug can also cause peripheral neuropathy. To minimize side effects, the serum level of cycloserine should be monitored closely. The dose should start low and increase every week until the target dose is reached as determined by the serum level (20 and 30 µg/mL).

***p*-Aminosalicylic Acid.** The main side effect of PAS is gastrointestinal intolerance. However, newer formulations of PAS may be better tolerated (117). When PAS is given as the sodium salt, it can result in a large salt load that may not be tolerated by patients with heart failure. PAS is associated with frequent hypersensitivity reactions characterized by fever, joint pains, and rash.

Capreomycin, Amikacin, Kanamycin. Capreomycin is a polypeptide antibiotic. Like the aminoglycosides, capreomycin can cause renal and acoustic toxicity. In general, capreomycin is better tolerated than the other injectable agents. Toxicity is reduced in intermittent regimens.

Initial Treatment Regimen in the Era of Drug Resistance

Beginning in 1986, the American Thoracic Society (ATS) and the Centers for Disease Control (CDC) recommended a three-drug regimen including INH, rifampin, and pyrazinamide (3). However, as drug-resistant strains of *M. tuberculosis* became more prevalent in the United States, this recommendation was modified. The current treatment guidelines recommend that all adult patients with tuberculosis be treated similarly, regardless of HIV serostatus (4, 23) (Table 3). A 6-month regimen consisting of INH, rifampin, pyrazinamide given for 2 months followed by INH and rifampin for 4 months is the preferred treatment for drug-susceptible organisms. Ethambutol or streptomycin should be added to the above regimen until drug susceptibility results are available unless the possibility of primary resistance to INH is less than 4%. Ethambutol (or streptomycin) can be discontinued as soon as the drug susceptibility results are known. Patients may be treated with a daily, twice-weekly, or thrice-weekly regimen.

The basic principles of treatment of tuberculosis in children and adolescents are the same as those for adults (4). Recent studies of the 6-month regimens containing pyrazinamide have produced excellent results with little toxicity. Therefore, children and adolescents should be treated with the same 6-month regimen used in adults. Because it is difficult to assess visual acuity in children less than 5 years of age, ethambutol is seldom used in this setting. However, ethambutol has been used safely in children (160).

TABLE 3 • Standard Treatment Regimens for Tuberculosis in Adults

Option	Drug[a]	Initial Phase (2 months) Dose (Max)	Frequency	Drug	Continuation Phase (4 months) Dose (Max)	Frequency
I	INH	5 mg/kg/day (300 mg)	Daily	INH	5 mg/kg/day	Daily
	RIF	10 mg/kg/day (600 mg)	Daily	RIF	10 mg/kg/day	Daily
	PZA	15–30 mg/kg/day (2 g)	Daily		or	
	EMB[b]	15 mg/kg/day	Daily	INH	15 mg/kg/day (900 mg)	2×/week
	STM[b]	15 mg/kg/day (1 g)	Daily	RIF	10 mg/kg/day (600 mg)	2×/week
II[c]	INH	5 mg/kg/day (300 mg)	Daily			
	RIF	10 mg/kg/day (600 mg)	Daily			
	PZA	15–30 mg/kg/day (2 g)	Daily			
	EMB[b]	15 mg/kg/day	Daily			
	STM[b]	15 mg/kg/day (1 g) for 2 weeks then switch to		INH	15 mg/kg/day (900 mg)	2×/week
				RIF	10 mg/kg/day (600 mg)	2×/week
	INH	15 mg/kg/day (300 mg)	2×/week			
	RIF	10 mg/kg/day (600 mg)	2×/week			
	PZA	50–70 mg/kg/day (4 g)	2×/week			
	EMB[b]	50 mg/kg/day	2×/week			
	STM[b]	25–30 mg/kg/day (1.5 g)	2×/week			
III[c]	INH	15 mg/kg/day (900 mg)	3×/week	INH	15 mg/kg/day	3×/week
	RIF	10 mg/kg/day (600 mg)	3×/week	RIF	10 mg/kg/day	3×/week
	PZA	50–70 mg/kg/day (2 g)	3×/week	PZA	50–70 mg/kg/day	3×/week
	EMB[b]	25–30 mg/kg/day	3×/week			
	STM[b]	25–30 mg/kg/day (1.5 g)	3×/week			

[a]INH, isoniazid; RIF, rifampin; PZA, pyrazinamide; EMB, ethambutol; STM, streptomycin.

[b]In areas where the INH resistance rate is not documented to be less than 4%, ethambutol or streptomycin should be added to the initial regimen until drug susceptibility to INH and RIF is demonstrated.

[c]Options II and III should be monitored by directly observed therapy (DOT).

Nonadherence to the treatment regimen is the major cause of treatment failure, relapse, and development of acquired drug resistance (169). To prevent emergence of acquired drug resistance and ensure completion of therapy, directly observed therapy (DOT) should be considered for all patients, particularly those with drug-resistant disease. DOT has been used successfully by a number of tuberculosis control programs and has been shown to be cost-effective (17, 86, 103, 169). Use of DOT was associated with a decrease in primary drug resistance, acquired drug resistance, and relapse in Tarrant County, Texas, between 1980 and 1986 (169). Nonadherence is often difficult to predict, and waiting until it has been detected may be too late.

An alternative approach to prevent acquired drug resistance (through selective ingestion of some but not all medications) is the use of combined formulations. Two combined formulations are now available in the United States: a combination of INH and rifampin (Rifamate) and a formulation of INH, rifampin, and pyrazinamide (Rifater). In two studies (78, 144), the combined formulation of INH, rifampin, and pyrazinamide was slightly less effective than a regimen in which the medications were given separately. Subsequent analyses suggested that this was due to suboptimal concentrations of rifampin in this formulation; the current form of Rifater available in the United States has increased the amount of rifampin to compensate. Combined formulations are not a substitute for DOT. If patients are to self-administer medications, combined formulations are a suitable method to lower the likelihood of ADR. However, for persons at high risk for nonadherence, the combined formulations cannot ensure adequate treatment.

Treatment in Special Circumstances
Extrapulmonary Disease

The basic principles that underlie the treatment of pulmonary disease also apply to extrapulmonary tuberculosis. Although there are few clinical therapy trials with extrapulmonary tuberculosis, current recommendations are to treat extrapulmonary disease in adults the same as pulmonary disease (4). Using a predominantly twice-weekly regimen of INH and rifampin given for 9 months, Dutt et al. reported a 95% success rate in treating 350 patients with extrapulmonary disease (45). In children, current guidelines advocate extending the duration of therapy to 12 months in patients with CNS, miliary, or bone and joint involvement (4). These guidelines are based on the clinical judgment of experts in the field; no studies document the advantage of this practice.

Tuberculosis of the Brain and Meninges.   Treatment of tuberculosis involving the brain and/or meninges can be particularly challenging because of the high frequency of neurologic sequelae and high mortality rate associated with this form of extrapulmonary disease (2, 84). Because not all of the antituberculosis medications penetrate the blood-brain barrier well, the appropriate drugs should be selected carefully (Table 4). INH (55) and pyrazinamide (41, 56, 123, 172) penetrate well into the CSF, reaching concentrations equal to those in serum. In contrast, rifampin (55, 172), ethambutol (7, 113, 124), and the aminoglycosides (55) penetrate the meninges only in the setting of inflammation. Of the second-line agents, ethionamide and cycloserine penetrate the blood-brain barrier with or without inflammation (74). Ofloxacin was shown to penetrate the CSF well in the setting of purulent meningitis (125). Because several of these drugs penetrate into the CSF only in the setting of in-

TABLE 4 • Special Situations

Drug	Pregnancy[a]	CNS TB Disease	Renal Insufficiency
INH	Safe	Good penetration	Normal clearance
Rifampin	Safe	Fair penetration; penetrates inflamed meninges (10–20%)	Normal clearance
Pyrazinamide	Avoid	Good penetration	Clearance reduced; decrease dose or prolong interval
Ethambutol	Safe	Penetrates inflamed meninges only (4–64%)	Clearance reduced; decrease dose or prolong interval
Streptomycin	Avoid	Penetrates inflamed meninges only	Clearance reduced; decrease dose or prolong interval
Capreomycin	Avoid	Penetrates inflamed meninges only	Clearance reduced; decrease dose or prolong interval
Kanamycin	Avoid	Penetrates inflamed meninges only	Clearance reduced; decrease dose or prolong interval
Ethionamide	Do not use	Good penetration	Normal clearance
p-Aminosalicylic acid	Safe	Penetrates inflamed meninges only (10–50%)	Incomplete data on clearance
Cycloserine	Avoid	Good penetration	Clearance reduced; decrease dose or prolong interval
Ciprofloxacin	Do not use	Fair penetration (5–10%); penetrates inflamed meninges (50–90%)	Clearance reduced; decrease dose or prolong interval
Ofloxacin	Do not use	Fair penetration (5–10%); penetrates inflamed meninges (50–90%)	Clearance reduced; decrease dose or prolong interval
Amikacin	Avoid	Penetrates inflamed meninges only	Clearance reduced; decrease dose or prolong interval
Clofazimine	Avoid	Penetration unknown	Clearance probably normal

[a]Safe, the drug has not been demonstrated to have teratogenic effects; Avoid, data on the drug's safety are limited or the drug is associated with mild malformations (as with the aminoglycosides); Do not use, studies show an association between the drug and premature labor, congenital malformations, or teratogenicity.

Data adapted from CUG Core Curriculum on Tuberculosis, 3rd ed., 1994.

flammation, a theoretical concern would be that coadministration of corticosteroids would result in lower CSF drug concentration. However, Kaojarern et al. reported no significant difference in CSF concentrations between patients who had received corticosteroids and those who had not (91).

There are few randomized studies to guide the treatment of tuberculous meningitis; thus, the optimum duration of treatment is not known. Prospective studies have demonstrated that short-course regimens of 6- to 12-months' duration are effective in the treatment of tuberculous meningitis (1, 2, 129, 155). Extremes of age and the level of CNS dysfunction at presentation have been associated with a poor prognosis.

INH, rifampin, and pyrazinamide should be included in the treatment regimen if possible. If INH resistance is suspected, ethambutol or streptomycin should be given during the initial treatment phase. Patients with proven INH-resistant disease should receive rifampin, ethambutol (25 mg/kg/day), pyrazinamide, and an aminoglycoside or a quinolone.

The use of corticosteroids as adjunctive treatment in tuberculous meningitis has not been studied rigorously. Corticosteroids have been shown to reduce mortality in the acute phase of disease (62, 137). In a study from China, steroid use was associated with a 50% reduction in mortality from tuberculous meningitis in patients who presented with stage 2 (neurological deficit, no coma) or 3 (both neurological deficit and coma) CNS dysfunction (137). Therefore, most authorities recommend corticosteroids in patients who present focal neurologic deficits and/or with stage 2 or 3 CNS dysfunction. Dexamethasone (or its equivalent) is given in a dose of 0.2 mg/kg for 1 to 3 weeks initially and tapered to 0.1 mg/kg and continued for a total of 2 to 3 months.

Pleural Tuberculosis. Studies have demonstrated the efficacy of short-course regimens in the treatment of pleural disease (48). A 6-month regimen consisting of INH and rifampin was shown by Dutt et al. (48) to be as effective as regimens of longer duration. Although corticosteroids hasten resolution of pleural fluid, they do not prevent pleural thickening (97).

Lymphadenitis. Prospective studies of 6- to 9-months' duration in adults (20) and 6 months of intermittent therapy in children (88) have been shown to be very effective. During the course of therapy, lymph nodes may enlarge, new nodes may appear, and nodes may spontaneously drain and create fistulas (20, 73, 98). These changes seldom denote failure, simply a vigorous immunologic reaction. Surgical resection is not usually necessary given the excellent results with chemotherapy (98). However, repeated aspirations or surgical drainage are sometimes needed for large fluctuant nodes.

Pericardial. Patients with tuberculous pericarditis should be treated with standard short-course antituberculosis therapy. Additionally, corticosteroids should be given when the diagnosis is clear. Large randomized studies have demonstrated that corticosteroids significantly reduce the risk of death from 14 to 3% and the need for repeated pericardiocentesis from 23 to 4% (154). However, corticosteroids did not decrease the need for open drainage or pericardiectomy (153). Open surgical drainage on admission has little effect on the proportion of patients dying from pericarditis or requiring subsequent pericardiectomy for constriction (153).

Bone and Joint. Treatment of tuberculosis of the bone and joints is more controversial than that of some other extrapulmonary sites. Disease affecting the spine (Pott's disease) is common and usually affects the thoracolumbar region. Most patients respond to standard short-course antituberculosis treatment, although surgery is sometimes neccessary (161, 162). Patients with evidence of cord compression, proven or suspected spinal instability due to destruction of contiguous vertebrae, or gross abscess formation should undergo surgical debridement and fixation in addition to standard chemotherapy. When tuberculosis affects another joint, chemotherapy is usually sufficient unless extensive joint destruction has occurred.

Miliary. Disseminated tuberculosis is associated with a high mortality rate, and thus, therapy should be initiated as soon as miliary disease is suspected. The standard treatment regimen should be begun. Parenteral therapy may be necessary in patients who are too ill to take oral medications. The ATS/CDC currently recommends extending therapy to 12 months in children with disseminated disease (4).

Underlying Medical Conditions
Pregnancy. INH, rifampin, and ethambutol can be used safely in the setting of pregnancy. Of the first-line agents, the one clear contraindication during pregnancy is the use of aminoglycosides; in 40 pregnancies, 17% of the babies had 8th nerve palsies, with deficits ranging from mild hearing loss to deafness (163). Given the lack of data regarding the teratogenicity of pyrazin-amide, it is not recommended in pregnant women (4). However, pyrazinamide is used throughout the world and in the treatment of drug-resistant cases in the United States. All of the antituberculosis medications are found in breast milk (150), but the dosages are small, and toxicity in the infant is not expected.

Silicosis. Silicotuberculosis requires a longer duration of therapy (82). Treatment with the standard regimen should be extended to a total of 9 to 12 months.

Renal Failure. In cases of mild renal dysfunction, INH, rifampin, and pyrazinamide may be given in the usual doses. However, in moderate-to-severe renal failure, pyrazinamide should be given in reduced dosages, or the duration between doses lengthened. Ethambutol and the aminoglycosides should have the dosages reduced, or the duration between doses lengthened and levels monitored carefully (164). The second-line agents PAS and cycloserine should also have the dosages reduced in renal failure, and cycloserine serum levels monitored closely.

Hepatic Failure. INH, rifampin, and pyrazinamide are all hepatotoxic. Although the likelihood of drug-induced hepatitis is not greater in persons with underlying liver disease, the clinical implications of further liver injury are potentially profound. Therefore, caution should be used in choosing therapy in this setting. In mild cases of tuberculosis, ethambutol and an aminoglycoside can be used. In more extensive tuberculosis, INH and rifampin should be considered, provided very close monitoring is available. Pyrazinamide is often not used in patients with significant liver disease. When serum transaminase levels are more than 5 times the upper limit of normal, a regimen of nonhepatotoxic medications should be used. Ethambutol, an aminoglycoside, a quinolone, and cycloserine could be used in this setting.

Treatment of HIV-Related Tuberculosis. Despite being immunocompromised, HIV-1-seropositive patients with tuberculosis respond well to antituberculosis therapy, as long as the regimen contains INH and rifampin. With a few notable exceptions (107), HIV-1-seropositive patients convert their sputum to negative as rapidly as seronegative cases (13), and relapses are not significantly different (26, 121). However, treatment of HIV-related tuberculosis does require close monitoring because of frequent drug toxicities and possible drug-drug interactions. In some cases, prolonging the duration of treatment is necessary. Because the margin of error is probably less in HIV-1-infected patients, 6 months should be considered the minimum duration of treatment.

It is critically important to assess the clinical and bacteriologic responses in the setting of HIV-1 infection. If there is evidence of a slow or suboptimal response, therapy should be prolonged as judged on a case-by-case basis. In addition, consideration should be given to obtaining serum levels of the antituberculosis medications, particularly rifampin (116). Recent studies have demonstrated that the serum drug levels are frequently suboptimal in AIDS patients with tuberculosis (115, 118, 119, 133). HIV-1-seropositive patients who have had breaks in therapy due to drug intolerance or nonadherence should have therapy prolonged. Antituberculosis therapy should be supplemented with pyridoxine (B_6) at 25 to 50 mg/day.

Rifampin-containing regimens are very effective in the treatment of tuberculosis regardless of the HIV-1 serostatus of the patient. In one of the first reports describing the outcome of antituberculosis therapy in 125 AIDS patients with tuberculosis, Small et al. (145), in San Francisco, demonstrated that the number of failures ($N = 1$) and relapses ($N = 3$) were low and that a poor outcome appeared to be related more to nonadherence than to which regimen was used.

More recently, Chaisson et al. (26), in Haiti, reported that an intermittent treatment regimen was as effective in HIV-1-seropositive patients as in seronegative patients with tuberculosis. Patients received supervised therapy with INH, rifampin, pyrazinamide, and ethambutol thrice weekly for 8 weeks followed by INH and rifampin, thrice weekly for 18 weeks. Relapses occurred in 5.4% of the HIV-1-seropositive and 2.8% of the seronegative patients ($P = .36$). In Kinshasa, Zaire, investigators treated tuberculosis patients with INH, rifampin, pyrazinamide, and ethambutol daily for 2 months followed by INH and rifampin twice weekly for 4 months (121). The HIV-1-seropositive patients were then randomized to receive an additional 6 months of placebo or twice-weekly INH and rifampin. After 6 months of therapy, 260 of 335 HIV-1-seropositive patients and 186 of 188 HIV-1-seronegative patients could be evaluated, and 3.8 and 2.7%, respectively, failed therapy. At 24 months, the HIV-1-seropositive patients who received the extended therapy had a recurrence rate of 1.9%, compared with 9% in the placebo group ($P < .01$). However, there was no statistically significant difference in the recurrence rates between the HIV-1-seropositive patients who took placebo (9%) and seronegative patients (5.3%). In addition, despite a lower recurrence rate in the HIV-1-seropositive subjects who received extended therapy, survival was the same as for those who did not receive the extended treatment.

A consistent finding in all the treatment studies is a high mortality rate among HIV-1-seropositive patients (26, 109, 120, 121, 145). Investigators in Nairobi, Kenya (109), reported that most deaths occurred after 1 month of treatment and were not due to tuberculosis but to other AIDS-related conditions; drug toxicities and routine bacterial pathogens were the most important causes of death. Similarly, in Zaire, of the 90 (27%) deaths in seropositive patients, only 27.8% were felt to be related to tuberculosis (120). Several investigators in sub-Saharan Africa have reported higher mortality among HIV-1-infected patients who took non-rifampin-containing regimens (109, 111, 120), highlighting the importance of rifampin-containing short-course regimens in the treatment of HIV-related tuberculosis.

In addition to the higher mortality associated with non-rifampicin-based regimens, studies have also demonstrated unacceptably high recurrence rates in the setting of HIV-1 infection (71, 120). Hawkens et al. (71), in Nairobi, Kenya, reported that the overall recurrence rate of tuberculosis was 34 times that seen in HIV-1-seronegative patients when taking a thiacetazone-based regimen. Recurrence was strongly associated with cutaneous hypersensitivity reactions due to thiacetazone.

Adverse drug reactions. Whether or not HIV-1-seropositive patients with tuberculosis have more adverse drug reactions is not clear. In studies from San Francisco, 18 to 26% of seropositive patients with tuberculosis had to have a change in therapy because of adverse drug reactions (145). Rifampin, the drug most commonly implicated, produced an adverse reaction in 12% of patients. In the previously described study from Zaire (121), 11% of the seropositive patients had a rash, but in none was treatment interrupted. Paresthesia was common (21% of patients), pointing out the need for pyridoxine when treating tuberculosis in HIV-1-seropositive individuals. On the other hand, some investigators have reported relatively low rates of drug reactions (26, 89). It is unclear why there is such a difference in the reported frequency of adverse drug reactions, although different patient populations, different degrees of immunosuppression among the patients, and different thresholds of providers to change therapy probably account for the differences. In any event, patients should be followed closely for adverse reactions and the treatment regimen changed when appropriate.

Thiacetazone has been reported to cause frequent and significant skin reactions in HIV-1-seropositive patients being treated for tuberculosis (110, 111). In one study (110), up to 20% of the HIV-1-seropositive patients on thiacetazone developed rashes, compared with 1% of the seronegative patients; the case-fatality rate was 14% in the HIV-1-seropositive persons suffering these reactions. The risk of cutaneous reactions in a randomized trial of thiacetazone and rifampin-containing regimens was nearly 10 times higher in the seropositive patients than in the seronegative patients (111). These reports prompted the WHO to abandon thiacetazone in the treatment of HIV-1-related tuberculosis (131).

Drug-drug interactions. Many different medications are prescribed for HIV-1-infected patients, particularly those with AIDS. Successful therapy for tuberculosis requires that they take an additional three to four drugs for a minimum of 6 months. Some of these antituberculosis drugs can interact adversely with medications that are commonly used by HIV-1-infected individuals, and understanding these drug-drug interactions can prevent unwanted drug toxicity and possible treatment failures.

The rifamycin derivatives (i.e., rifampin, rifabutin, rifapentine) can induce the hepatic cytochrome P-450 enzyme system, resulting in increased metabolism and decreased serum level of certain drugs (10). Medications known to be affected include fluconazole, ketoconazole, methadone, oral contraceptives, dilantin, and the protease inhibitors (see "Controversies and Uncertainties," below) (10, 24). Coadministration of rifampin with ketoconazole or fluconazole decreases the area under the curve (AUC) by approximately 80 and 20%, respectively. In a single case report, ketoconazole was felt to have impaired absorption of rifampin, resulting in low serum levels of rifampin (57). Therefore, ketoconazole and rifampin should not be given together. Rifampin and fluconazole can be used together, but the fluconazole dose may need to be increased. Peloquin et al. (119) recently reported several other possible drug-drug interactions in a small study of AIDS patients with CD4 lymphocyte counts below 200 cells/μL. These investigators demonstrated that zidovidine lowered the concentration of pyrazinamide, and pyrazinamide lowered the serum concentration of rifampin. Fluconazole increased the rifampin concentration fourfold, a finding that other investigators have not reported. Because this was a small study, these observations should be interpreted with caution.

Treatment of Drug-Resistant Tuberculosis

The treatment regimen in proved drug-resistant disease depends on the results of drug susceptibility tests (both current and prior) and the patient's previous history of treatment. Data from the National Jewish Medical Center have demonstrated that patients who have taken a drug for more than 1 month in the past have less effect from that drug, even if in vitro drug susceptibility tests show the isolate to be susceptible (64). If drug susceptibility test results are not yet available, as is true in the initiation of therapy, the drug susceptibility patterns in the community may be useful in designing a treatment regimen.

At least three drugs to which the isolate is susceptible and which the patient has never taken before should be used to initiate treatment. As more information becomes available, the regimen may need to be altered. The goal of selecting a treatment regimen is to maximize efficacy, minimize toxicity, and ensure completion of therapy. In highly resistant infections, this may be difficult to do. Table 5 lists several possible options for the treatment of drug-resistant tuberculosis depending on the drug-resistance pattern. Most clinical trials have examined the efficacy of various treatment protocols in primarily drug-susceptible cases; few studies have examined the treatment of drug-resistant patients.

Isolated Resistance to Isoniazid. Effective treatment regimens for patients with isolated INH resistance are readily available. Patients may be treated with a combination of rifampin, ethambutol (or streptomycin), and pyrazinamide for a total of 6 months (77, 141). If the patient was begun on the standard four-drug regimen, INH can be stopped when drug resistance is noted. Instead of stopping the pyrazinamide at 2 months, the drug is continued for the full 6 months along with rifampin and ethambutol (or streptomycin). The patient can also be treated with rifampin and ethambutol for 12 months (81, 175), preferably with pyrazinamide included in the regimen for at least the first 2 months or longer. Finally, one study reported low relapse rates with a regimen consisting of 6 to 9 months of rifampin and ethambutol supplemented for the first 2 months with streptomycin and pyrazinamide (157).

Some clinicians favor continuing INH despite known resistance to this agent, particularly if there is low-level resistance, in hope of killing any subpopulations that might retain some susceptibility to INH. The benefit of this practice is unclear; one study demonstrated similar rates of bacteriologic failures in patients with low-level INH resistance and patients with high-level resistance (152). Given the uncertain benefit and the well-documented risk of hepatotoxicity with INH, many experts favor stopping the drug when any level of resistance is noted. Others continue INH when the isolate shows low-level resistance.

Isolated Resistance to Rifampin. Isolated resistance to rifampin has been relatively unusual in the past. However, recent reports have described an increase in the frequency of mono-rifampin-resistant isolates among person with HIV-1 infection (11, 108). Unfortunately, the loss of rifampin from the standard treatment regimen prolongs the duration of therapy. Isolated rifampin resistance can be treated with INH and ethambutol for 18 months (8). As with isolated INH resistance, pyrazinamide should be added for at least the first 2 months of the regimen. Additionally, 9 months of INH, pyrazinamide, and streptomycin given either two or three times per week was associated with an 6% relapse rate (80).

Isolated Resistance to Ethambutol, Pyrazinamide, or Streptomycin. Isolated resistance to ethambutol, pyrazinamide, or streptomycin has little impact on the efficacy of the regimen. Loss of ethambutol or streptomycin from the regimen does not decrease the efficacy or change the total duration of therapy. Loss of pyrazinamide, however, requires prolonging the duration of therapy from 6 to 9 months.

Resistance to Two First-Line Agents (MDR-TB). Patients with MDR-TB should always be treated with at least three to four medications. The duration of therapy will depend on the agents used and the extent of disease. Some authorities recommend initial hospitalization to permit observation of toxicity and intolerance (86). At the National Jewish Center for Immunology and Respiratory Medicine, treatment is initiated with small doses that are gradually increased to the target dose over 3 to 10 days. Peak and trough serum levels are determined to optimize therapy,

TABLE 5 • **Selected Treatment Regimens for Drug-Resistant Tuberculosis**

Resistance to	Treatment Regimen	Duration of Therapy	Comments
Isoniazid[a]	Rifampin Ethambutol Pyrazinamide	6–9 months	Pyrazinamide for entire duration
Isoniazid[a]	Rifampin Ethambutol	12 months	Consider addition of pyrazinamide
Rifampin[a]	Isoniazid Ethambutol	18 months	Consider addition of pyrazinamide
Isoniazid and ethambutol[a]	Rifampin Pyrazinamide Quinolone Injectable[b]	9–12 months	
Isoniazid and rifampin[a]	Ethambutol Pyrazinamide Quinolone Injectable[b]	18 months after culture conversion	Consider surgery
Isoniazid, rifampin, ethambutol[a]	Pyrazinamide Quinolone Injectable[b] plus 2 others[c]	24 months after culture conversion	Consider surgery
Isoniazide, rifampin, pyrazinamide[a]	Ethambutol Quinolone Injectable[b] plus 2 others[c]	24 months after culture conversion	Consider surgery
Isoniazid, rifampin, ethambutol, pyrazinamide[a]	Quinolone Injectable[b] plus 3 others[c]	24 months after culture conversion	Surgery, if possible

Adapted from Iseman MD. Treatment of multidrug resistant tuberculosis. N Engl J Med 1993;329:784–791, with permission.

[a]± streptomycin resistance.

[b]Streptomycin, amikacin, kanamycin, or capreomycin. Injectable should be continued for 4–6 months, if possible.

[c]Ethionamide, cycloserine, or p-aminosalicylic acid. In some cases, rifabutin, amoxicillin/cavulanic acid, imipenem, clofazamine, thiacetazone.

since bioavailability and clearance of most antituberculosis medications is not predictable (Table 6). This is particularly important in the setting of AIDS, because of the findings noted above.

With the loss of INH and rifampin, the two most important drugs, efficacy is decreased, and therapy must be significantly prolonged. Most authorities recommend a four-drug regimen, including an injectable. The oral medications should consist of any first-line agents that are available, plus a quinolone and other second-line agents. When used as a primary agent in the treatment of tuberculosis, ethambutol should be given at a daily dose of 25 mg/kg instead of 15 mg/kg. The patient should be treated for at least 18 to 24 months. The injectable agent should be continued for 4 to 6 months or until the maximal dose has been reached. Surgical resection should be considered if culture conversion has not occurred by 6 months, particularly in patients with resistance to all first-line agents.

Alternative Therapy

Treatment of Smear and Culture Negative Pulmonary Tuberculosis. Patients with pulmonary tuberculosis who are smear and culture negative may be treated with shorter treatment regimens. Dutt and Stead (46) demonstrated that such patients may be treated with INH and rifampin for 4 months. However, the level of drug resistance in this population was extremely low, and in many circumstances, drug susceptibility test results are not available at the initiation of therapy. Therefore, in areas with over 4% resistance to INH, ethambutol (or streptomycin) should be added to the initial regimen. Furthermore, addition of pyrazinamide at initiation of therapy would likely improve the efficacy of the 4-month regimen. A 4-month regimen of isoniazid, rifampin, streptomycin, and pyrazinamide has been used successfully to treat smear and culture negative disease in Hong Kong (76).

Surgery. Resectional surgery or drainage of a tuberculous empyema (Eloesser flap) may be necessary in some patients with high-level drug resistance (87, 127). The prior probability of treatment failure, based on the extent of disease and level of drug resistance, should be used to decide whether resectional surgery is indicated. Patients with MDR-TB who have localized disease, who have failed treatment, and who have adequate pulmonary reserves, should also be considered for surgery. Iseman et al. reported that resectional surgery offered some benefit to such patients, compared with historical controls (87).

ENDPOINTS FOR MONITORING THERAPY

Patients who are being treated for tuberculosis must be monitored closely to detect possible drug toxicities and document response to therapy. Additionally, for those not receiving

TABLE 6 • Dosages and Pharmakinetics of Antituberculosis Medications

Drug	Usual Adult Daily Dosage[a]	Peak Serum Concentration (μg/mL)	Usual MIC[b] (range) (μg/mL)
First-line oral drugs			
Isoniazid	300 mg	3–5	0.01–0.025
Rifampin	600 mg	8–29	0.06–0.25
Pyrazinamide	30 mg/kg	20–60	6.2–50
Ethambutol	15–25 mg/kg	3–5	0.5–2.0
Injectable drugs			
Streptomycin	15 mg/kg	35–45	0.25–2.0
Amikacin	15 mg/kg	35–45	0.5–1.0
Kanamycin	15 mg/kg	35–45	1.5–3.0
Capreomycin	15 mg/kg	35–45	1.25–2.5
Second-line oral drugs			
Ofloxacin	400 mg b.i.d.	8–10	0.25–2.0
Ciprofloxacin	750 mg b.i.d.	3–5	0.25–2.0
Ethionamide	250 mg b.i.d. or t.i.d.	1–5	0.3–1.2
Aminosalicylic acid	3 g q.i.d.	40–70	Not known
Cycloserine	250 mg b.i.d. or t.i.d.	20–35	Not known

Adapted from Iseman MD. Treatment of multidrug resistant tuberculosis. N Engl J Med 1993;329:784–791, with permission.

[a]B.i.d., twice a day; t.i.d., three times a day; q.i.d., four times a day.

[b]MIC, minimal inhibitory concentration.

DOT, close monitoring allows assessment of adherence. Adults treated for tuberculosis should have baseline measurements of hepatic enzymes, bilirubin, serum creatinine, a complete blood count, and a platelet count (4). Given the increased frequency of tuberculosis in patients with diabetes mellitus, routine assessment of serum glucose is also justified. Serum uric acid should be measured if the patient will be receiving pyrazinamide. A baseline measurement of both visual acuity and red-green color discrimination should be obtained in all patients treated with ethambutol. Most children do not need baseline laboratory measurements except for the assessment of visual acuity for those being treated with ethambutol (4).

All patients should be monitored clinically for adverse reactions during the treatment period. Patients should be seen at least monthly, and all baseline laboratory values that were abnormal should be repeated. Some providers repeat hepatic enzymes at least once during therapy, usually after 1 month of therapy. Patients receiving ethambutol should have monthly assessments of visual acuity and red-green color perception.

For pulmonary tuberculosis, the most important parameter to monitor to assess response to therapy is the conversion of sputum smears and cultures to negative. Over 90% of patients who are treated with standard short-course therapy are culture negative after 2 months of therapy (4). Patients who remain culture positive at this juncture should have repeat drug susceptibility tests, and the patient should be placed on DOT. If the patient is already on DOT, consideration should be given to checking serum levels of the antituberculosis agents (116). Patients with pulmonary tuberculosis who have negative pretreatment sputum smears should be followed clinically and radiographically for evidence of improvement. In patients with extrapulmonary disease, the nature of the repeat evaluations depends on the site of involvement.

Monitoring for signs of nonadherence is very important. Pill counts and patient interviews may give some indication of missed doses. In addition, repeat uric acid levels, if low, may be a sign of nonadherence, since the levels are usually above baseline while taking pyrazinamide. A spot urine check to look for the orange discoloration caused by rifampin is useful and inexpensive. Finally, there are commercially available urine dipstick tests that detect INH metabolites.

PREVENTIVE THERAPY
Indications for Preventive Therapy

Preventive therapy with INH significantly reduces the risk of tuberculous infection progressing to active disease (58). When considering the use of preventive therapy, the risk of developing tuberculosis must be weighed against the development of INH-related toxicity. For some individuals infected with *M. tuberculosis,* the risk of developing disease is so high, they should be provided preventive therapy regardless of their age (4) (Table 7). For other persons, the risk of developing INH-related hepatitis outweighs the benefit of the drug in those 35 years of age or older. Close contacts of infectious patients should be given INH regardless of the result of the skin test, because it may take 2 to 10 weeks for the skin test to become positive after infection has occurred. These individuals should be retested after 10 to 12 weeks to determine if they have or have not become infected with *M. tuberculosis.*

Drug of Choice

INH is the only drug that is widely used for preventive therapy. Clinical trials have demonstrated that daily administration of INH preventive therapy for 12 months reduces the risk of developing tuberculosis by more than 90% in subjects who complete a full course of therapy (58). Six months of preven-

TABLE 7 • **Candidates for INH Preventive Therapy**[a]

Regardless of Age	Age ≤35 years
HIV positive, known or suspected	Foreign born
Close contact with infectious case	Medically underserved,
Abnormal chest radiograph[b]	low income
Medical conditions[c]	Long-term care facilities
Injection-drug users	Other high-risk populations[d]
Recent converters	

[a]Those in all categories should have a positive tuberculin skin test except for close contacts, whose skin test may be negative on initial evaluation.

[b]Abnormal chest radiograph consistent with inactive tuberculosis. Active disease has been ruled out with three negative sputum smears and cultures.

[c]Including diabetes mellitus, end-stage renal disease, chronic immunosuppressive therapy, silicosis, cancer of the head and neck, hematologic and reticuloendothelial diseases, intestinal bypass or gastrectomy, chronic malabsorption syndromes, and ≥10% below ideal body weight.

[d]Locally identified high-risk groups such as the homeless, migrant workers, and health care workers.

tive therapy also confers a high degree of protection and it is more cost-effective (149).

The benefit conferred by INH must be balanced against its known toxicities. The most important drug-related toxicity is INH-induced hepatitis. As noted above, serum aminotransferase activity is elevated in 10 to 20% of persons taking INH. In most persons, the enzyme level returns to normal despite continuing the medication. The risk of INH-induced hepatitis increases with age. In a USPHS surveillance study conducted among over 13,000 participants, the frequency of probable INH-induced hepatitis was as follows: under 20 years of age, 0 cases per 1000 persons; 20 to 34 years, 3 cases per 1000 persons; 35 to 49 years, 12 cases per 1000 persons; 50 to 64 years, 23 cases per 1000 persons; and over 64 years, 8 cases per 1000 persons (95). Daily alcohol ingestion also increased the risk of hepatitis. Some data suggest that African American and Hispanic women (and possibly postpartum women) may be at increased risk of dying from INH-induced hepatitis (148).

The other common toxicity associated with INH administration is peripheral neuropathy, which is related to pyridoxine deficiency; INH promotes urinary excretion of pyridoxine. Most patients do not need to take pyridoxine, however. Patients who have another predisposition to development of neuropathy such as diabetes mellitus, end-stage renal disease, HIV-1 infection, or alcoholism should be given pyridoxine supplementation. Additionally, pregnant women and persons with a seizure disorder should receive pyridoxine. This side effect can usually be prevented by coadministration of 10 to 50 mg of pyridoxine (B$_6$) daily.

Alternatives to INH Preventive Therapy

INH was the first form of preventive therapy proved efficacious in placebo-controlled trials (58, 85). However, animal studies (96) have demonstrated that 2 months of rifampin plus pyrazi-

namide, or 3 months of rifampin alone were more effective than 6 months of INH alone. Recent clinical data (70, 126) have also demonstrated that rifampin alone or in combination with pyrazinamide may be effective for the prevention of tuberculosis. Therefore, for contacts of patients with INH-resistant disease, rifampin (600 mg/day) should be provided for 6 months (4, 22).

Unfortunately, for contacts of patients with MDR-TB, there are no good choices for preventive therapy. The CDC has published recommendations for the management of persons exposed to MDR-TB patients (22). Decisions on preventive therapy must be based on the likelihood that the contact is newly infected with a drug-resistant strain and the likelihood that the contact, if infected, will develop tuberculosis. If, after evaluating these considerations, the contact is felt to have an intermediate-to-high likelihood of having been recently infected with a multidrug-resistant strain of *M. tuberculosis*, particularly if the individual has an increased risk for development of tuberculosis, a preventive regimen should be administered. For contacts of MDR-TB patients, two oral drugs to which the isolate is susceptible should be given for 6 to 12 months.

Patients with a positive tuberculin skin test and an abnormal chest radiograph consistent with inactive tuberculosis should be given either 12 months of INH or 4 months of INH and rifampin. Although there have been no comparative trials of these two regimens, the failure rate among such patients given the 4-month regimen is very low (46).

Dosages

Adults should receive 5 mg/kg/day of INH (maximum, 300 mg/day) given orally. Children and adolescents should receive 10 mg/kg/day. For patients receiving intermittent preventive therapy, a dose of 15 mg/kg/day (maximum, 900 mg/day) may be given twice a week. Standard dosages of INH and rifampin should be used for the 4-month regimen. For patients who will receive pyridoxine, 10 to 50 mg/day should be provided.

Duration

The current recommendations are to treat adults with 6 months of INH unless they are HIV-1 infected or have an abnormal chest radiograph consistent with old disease. In the latter circumstance, the assumption is that active disease has been ruled out (i.e., three smears and cultures for mycobacteria are negative, and active tuberculosis is no longer suspected). For patients with known or suspected HIV-1 infection and also patients with an abnormal chest radiograph, 12 months of INH are recommended. Children should be treated with 6 to 9 months of INH.

Special Circumstances

Preventive Therapy in the HIV-1 Infected

INH preventive therapy is very effective in preventing persons infected with *M. tuberculosis* from developing tuberculosis, regardless of HIV-1 serostatus. Pape et al. (114), in Haiti, conducted a randomized placebo-controlled trial of INH preventive therapy in HIV-1-infected patients. The investigators reported that patients who took placebo (pyridoxine) were approximately 6 times more likely to develop tuberculosis than those who took 1 year of INH and pyridoxine. Taking INH decreased the incidence of tuberculosis from 10.0 to 1.7 per 100 person-years (114). In addition, individuals with a positive tuberculin skin test who took INH were also less likely to progress to AIDS or die during the study period. Investigators in Zambia (166) reported that 6 months of INH preventive therapy significantly decreased the risk of tuberculosis in HIV-1-seropositive persons, but during the follow-up period, the incidence of tuberculosis increased and approached that of the placebo group. Whether these cases represented failure of the preventive regimen or exogenous reinfection is not known.

The current ATS/CDC recommendations are to provide INH (300 mg/day) for 12 months to any HIV-1-infected person with a positive tuberculin skin test (≥5 mm) who has no evidence of active tuberculosis (4, 21, 25). Therapy should be supplemented with pyridoxine (25–50 mg/day) to help prevent peripheral neuropathy.

The CDC previously recommended routine anergy testing in HIV-1-infected individuals and consideration of preventive therapy for anergic HIV-1-infected individuals who come from a population with a prevalence of tuberculous infection of 10% or above. These recommendations were based on finding high rates of tuberculosis in anergic injection-drug users, in whom tuberculosis was felt to represent reactivation disease (136). However, subsequent data have questioned the accuracy of anergy skin testing (19, 28), and data have demonstrated widely varying rates of tuberculosis among anergic individuals (35, 136). Moreover, providing INH preventive therapy to injection-drug users with a positive tuberculin skin test (and not anergic subjects) was associated with a significant decline in tuberculosis in a cohort of injection-drug users in Baltimore (68). Thus, in a low-prevalence area, it appeared that providing preventive therapy to anergic subjects was not necessary. More recently, in a placebo-controlled study, Gordin et al. (67) reported that INH preventive therapy did not alter the rates of tuberculosis. Similar data have been reported from Uganda (170). Although some experts recommend preventive therapy for anergic individuals, the efficacy of preventive therapy in this group has not been demonstrated, and decisions concerning the use of preventive therapy in these situations must be individualized (21, 25).

Twice-weekly INH for 6 months was compared with rifampicin/pyrazinamide twice-weekly for 2 months in Haiti among HIV-1-infected patients (70). There was no significant difference in the rates of tuberculosis between the three treatment groups. Investigators in Uganda (170) reported preliminary data from a randomized placebo-controlled trial of 6 months of INH, 3 months of INH/rifampin, or 3 months of INH/rifampin/pyrazinamide. The rate of tuberculosis in those taking placebo was 3.41 per 100 person-years, compared with 1.08, 1.32, and 1.73 respectively. Of note, the risk of adverse side effects was nearly two times higher in those taking the three-drug regimen than with INH alone. Thus, it is apparent that short-course preventive regimens are an effective alternative to INH preventive therapy.

HIV-1-infected individuals who are close contacts of persons with infectious tuberculosis should receive INH preventive therapy regardless of the results of the tuberculin skin test, as long as active tuberculosis has been ruled out (4, 21, 25). In addition, since exogenous reinfection has been demonstrated in AIDS patients (65, 146), preventive therapy should be given even if the person has had a prior course of preventive therapy (25).

Pregnant Women

Although pregnancy is not a contraindication to administration of INH, the drug should be withheld until after delivery in most patients. Women who are HIV-1 seropositive or who are believed to have been infected during pregnancy should receive INH during pregnancy. Although INH is secreted in breast milk, the concentration is low, and no toxicity occurs in the infant (150). Thus, INH preventive therapy should not be withheld from nursing mothers.

Monitoring Patients on Preventive Therapy

Most patients receiving INH preventive therapy require minimal monitoring, which consists of monthly symptom review (4). Patients should be questioned about the presence or absence of symptoms such as nausea, vomiting, dark urine, abdominal pain, anorexia, rash, and tingling in the hands and feet. For certain populations at increased risk of developing INH-induced hepatitis, more careful monitoring is indicated. The following patients should have baseline serum transaminases measured: patients who are over 35 years of age, have underlying chronic or acute liver disease, have had a previous reaction to INH, are HIV infected, are pregnant or postpartum, or are black or Hispanic. For these persons and those with abnormal liver function tests on the baseline measurement, periodic determinations are indicated.

CONTROVERSIES AND UNCERTAINTIES
Treatment of Tuberculosis in Patients Taking Protease Inhibitors (PIs)

Rifamycin derivatives accelerate the metabolism of the PIs, resulting in subtherapeutic levels and potential development of resistance to these important agents (24). In addition, PIs retard the metabolism of rifamycins, resulting in increased serum levels of rifamycins and the possibility of drug toxicity. These drug interactions have made many HIV care providers reticent to use rifampin when treating HIV-related tuberculosis in persons receiving PIs. However, the potential benefit of PIs must be weighed against the importance of rifampin in treating HIV-related tuberculosis. Rifampin is one of the most potent antituberculosis drugs. The loss of rifampin from the treatment regimen is likely to delay sputum conversion, delay the decrease in viral load associated with treatment, and prolong the treatment duration.

The CDC has outlined several options for the treatment of tuberculosis in patients on PIs or persons being considered for PIs (Table 8). Patients who are not currently taking PIs can be treated with the standard rifampin-containing regimen and started on PIs after completing 6 months of therapy. For patients already receiving PIs, there are at least four options: option 1 is to discontinue the PI and complete a standard short-course regimen. Option 2 is to use the standard four-drug regimen for 2 to 3 months (until drug susceptibility testing re-

TABLE 8 • Options for Treatment of Tuberculosis in HIV-1 Seropositive Patients Receiving Protease Inhibitors*

Option	Antituberculosis Therapy	Protease Inhibitor
I	Standard regimen[a]	None
II	Standard regimen for 2–3 mos then isoniazid and ethambutol for 16 mos[b]	None for 2–3 mos then start protease inhibitor
III	Standard regimen but substitute rifabutin (150 mg qd) for rifampin[c]	Indinavir or nelfinavir
IV	INH, streptomycin and pyrazimamide[c]	Any protease inhibitor

Data adapted from reference (24).

[a]Isoniazid, rifampin, pyrazinamide, ± ethambutol or streptomycin (see Table 3)

[b]Total duration of regimen is 18 months.

[c]Daily for 8 weeks then 3 × /week for 28 weeks.

sults are known and a bacteriologic response has been documented). Then the regimen can be modified to give INH and ethambutol twice weekly for 16 months (total therapy of 18 months). This regimen allows reintroduction of the PIs sooner but significantly prolongs the regimen. An additional drug (i.e., streptomycin) is recommended by some authorities because the efficacy of this regimen in HIV-seropositive patients is not known. Option 3 is to continue the PI if it is indinavir, nelfinavir or saquinavir and administer a standard 4-drug regimen containing rifabutin (150 mg/day) instead of rifampin. Rifabutin produces less induction of the P-450 system, and early study results suggest that rifabutin is just as effective as rifampin in the treatment of tuberculosis (66, 100, 134). Unfortunately, ritonavir cannot be used with this option. Another option is to use streptomycin, INH, and pyrazinamide given three times a week for 9 months (80).

Immunomodulators in the Treatment of Tuberculosis

Tuberculosis has been associated with the production of a number of cytokines, including tumor necrosis factor (TNF-α). Given the high levels of TNF-α and other cytokines that have been documented in HIV-related tuberculosis, drugs that inhibit production of TNF-α may have a role in the treatment of tuberculosis (93, 167). Pentoxifylline inhibits the synthesis of TNF-α by mononuclear phagocytes and the effect of the cytokine on target cells. In a double-blind, placebo-controlled trial, pentoxifylline was reported to be associated with a decrease in plasma HIV RNA and serum B2-microglobulin in HIV-1-infected patients with tuberculosis (167). Thalidomide also inhibits production of TNF-α. Klausner et al. (93) conducted a small randomized study in which HIV-1-infected patients with tuberculosis were treated with standard antituberculosis therapy and thalidomide or placebo. HIV-1-infected patients with tuberculosis who took thalidomide had a decrease in serum TNF-α levels and HIV-1 RNA levels. In addition, the patients who took thalidomide had significant weight gain compared with those who took placebo. Although

6 of 20 patients developed a rash, preliminary data suggest that a lower dose may decrease the risk of hypersensitivity and still provide clinical benefit (93).

Interferon-γ, a cytokine produced mainly by CD4 T-lymphocytes, can activate alveolar macrophages, which are important effector cells in host immunity against *M. tuberculosis*. Condos and colleagues (32) recently reported their experience with the use of aerosolized interferon-γ in the treatment of MDR-TB. Five patients were treated with 500 μg of interferon-γ three times a week for 1 month along with their regular antituberculosis medications. Sputum acid-fast smears became negative in all patients, and the time to positive culture increased, suggesting that the mycobacterial burden had decreased. Further studies are necessary to evaluate fully these new and exciting approaches to treatment.

Bacille Calmette-Guérin (BCG) Vaccine

BCG is derived from a strain of *M. bovis* attenuated through years of serial passage in culture. Many different BCG vaccines are available, and the efficacy of these vaccines has ranged from zero to 80%. A recent meta-analysis suggested an overall efficacy of approximately 50% (29). BCG vaccination does not prevent infection from *M. tuberculosis,* although it appears to prevent dissemination of disease in infants and young children. Recent decision analyses have suggested that BCG vaccination in health care workers would be the most effective preventive intervention in the setting of exposure to MDR-TB (12, 69, 151). However, most health care workers are not exposed to drug-resistant strains and as drug-resistant strains decline in the United States (61), the vaccine is unlikely to be used. Research continues in the search for a new and better vaccine for tuberculosis.

REFERENCES

1. Acharya VN, Kudva BT, Retnam VJ, Mehta PJ. Adult tuberculous meningitis: comparative study of different chemotherapeutic regimens. J Assoc Physicians India 1985;33:583–585.
2. Alarcon F, Escalante L, Perez Y, Banda H, Chacon G, Duenas G. Tuberculous meningitis. Short course therapy. Arch Neurol 1990;47:1313–1317.
3. American Thoracic Society. Treatment of tuberculosis and tuberculosis infection in adults and children. Am Rev Respir Dis 1986;134:355–356.
4. American Thoracic Society. Treatment of tuberculosis and tuberculosis infection in adults and children. Am Rev Respir Dis 1994;149:1359–1374.
5. Banerjee A, Dubnau E, Quemard A, Balasubramanian V, Um US, Wilson T, Callins D, de Lisle G, Jacobs WR Jr. inhA, a gene encoding a target for isonizid and ethionamide in *Mycobacterium tuberculosis*. Science 1994;263:227–230.
6. Bloch AB, Cauthen GM, Onorato IM, Dansbury KG, Kelly GD, Driver CR, Snider DE. Nationwide survey of drug-resistant tuberculosis in the United States. JAMA 1994;271:665–671.
7. Bobrowitz ID. Ethambutol in tuberculous meningitis. Chest 1972;61:629–632.
8. Bobrowitz ID. Ethambutol-isoniazid vs. streptomycin-ethambutol-isoniazid in original treatment of cavitary tuberculosis. Am Rev Respir Dis 1974;109548–553.
9. Bodmer T, Zurcher G, Imboden P, Telenti A. Mutation position and type of substitution in the beta-subunit of the RNA poly-

merase influence in-vitro activity of rifamycins in rifampicin-resistant *Mycobacterium tuberculosis*. J Antimicrob Chemother 1995;35:345–348.

10. Strayhorn VA, Baciewicz AM, Self TH. Update on rifampin drug interactions II. Arch Intern Med 1997;157:2453–2458.

11. Bradford WZ, Martin JN, Reingold AL, Schecter GF, Hopewell PC, Small PM. The changing epidemiology of acquired drug-resistant tuberculosis in San Francisco, USA. Lancet 1996;348: 928–931.

12. Brewer TF, Colditz GA. Bacille Calmette-Guerin vaccination for the prevention of tuberculosis in health care workers. Clin Infect Dis 1995;20:136–142.

13. Brindle RJ, Nunn PP, Githui W, Allen BW, Gathua S, Waiyaki P. Quantitative bacillary response to treatment in HIV-associated pulmonary tuberculosis. Am Rev Respir Dis 1993;147: 958–961.

14. British Medical Research Council. Treatment of pulmonary tuberculosis with streptomycin and para-aminosalicylic acid: a Medical Research Council investigation. Br Med J 1950;2: 1073–1085.

15. British Medical Research Council. Various combinations of isoniazid with streptomycin or with PAS in the treatment of pulmonary tuberculosis: seventh report to the Medical Research Council by their Tuberculosis Chemotherapy Trials Committee. Br Med J 1955;1:435–445.

16. British Thoracic Society. A controlled trial of six months chemotherapy in pulmonary tuberculosis. Final report: results during the 36 months after the end of chemotherapy and beyond. Br J Dis Chest 1984;78:330–336.

17. Burman WJ, Dalton CB, Cohn DL, Butler JRG, Reves RR. A cost-effectiveness analysis of directly observed therapy vs self-administered therapy for treatment of tuberculosis. Chest 1997; 112:63–70.

18. Butler WR, Kilburn JO. Susceptibility of *Mycobacterium tuberculosis* to pyrazinamide and its relationship to pyrazinamidase activity. Antimcrob Agents Chemother 1983;24:600–601.

19. Caiaffa WE, Graham NMH, Galai N, Rizzo RT, Nelson KE, Vlahov D. Instability of delayed-type hypersensitivity skin test anergy in human immunodeficiency virus infection. Arch Intern Med 1995;2111–2117.

20. Campbell IA, Ormerod LP, Friend JAR, Jenkins PA, Prescott RJ. Six months versus nine months chemotherapy for tuberculosis of lymph nodes: final results. Respir Med 1993;87:621–623.

21. Centers for Disease Control and Prevention. Anergy skin testing and preventive therapy for HIV-infected persons: revised recommendations. MMWR 1997;46(RR-15):1–10.

22. Centers for Disease Control and Prevention. Recommendations for the management of persons exposed to multidrug resistant tuberculosis. MMWR 1992;41(RR-11):59–71.

23. Centers for Disease Control and Prevention. Initial therapy for tuberculosis in the era of multidrug resistance: recommendations of the Advisory Council for the Elimination of Tuberculosis. MMWR 1993;42(RR-7):1–8.

24. Centers for Disease Control and Prevention. Clinical update: impact of HIV protease inhibitors on the treatment of HIV-infected tuberculosis patients with rifampin. MMWR 1996;45: 921–925.

25. Centers for Disease Control and Prevention. 1997 USPHS/IDSA guidelines for the prevention of opportunistic infections in persons with human immunodeficiency virus. MMWR 1997;46 (RR-12):10–12.

26. Chaisson RE, Clermont HC, Holt EA, Cantave M, Johnson MP, Atkinson J, Davis H, Boulos R, Quinn TC, Halsey NA, and the JHU-CDS Research Team. Six-month supervised intermittent tuberculosis therapy in Haitian patients with and without HIV infection. Am J Respir Crit Care Med 1996;154:1034–1038.

27. Chen CH, Shih JF, Lindholm-Levy, PJ, Heifets LB. Minimal inhibitory concentrations of rifabutin, ciprofloxacin, and ofloxacin against *Mycobacterium tuberculosis* isolated before treatment of patients in Taiwan. Am Rev Respir Dis 1989;140:987–989.

28. Chin DP, Osmond D, Page-Shafer K, Glassroth J, Rosen MJ, Reichman LB, Kvale PA, Wallace JM, Poole WK, Hopewell PC. Reliability of anergy skin testing in persons with HIV infection. Am J Respir Crit Care Med 1996;153:1982–1984.

29. Colditz GA, Brewer TG, Berkey CS, Wilson ME, Burdick E, Fineberg HV, Mosteller F. Efficacy of BCG vaccine in the prevention of tuberculosis. JAMA 1994;271:698–702.

30. Cole ST, Telenti A. Drug resistance in *Mycobacterium tuberculosis*. Eur Respir J 1995;8:701S–713S.

31. Cohn DL, Catlin BJ, Peterson KL, Judson FN, Sbarbaro. A 62-dose, 6 month therapy for pulmonary and extrapulmonary tuberculosis. A twice-weekly, directly observed, and cost-effective regimen. Ann Intern Med 1990;112:407–415.

32. Condos R, Rom WN, Schluger NW. Treatment of multidrug-resistant pulmonary tuberculosis with interferon-gamma via aerosol. Lancet 1997;349:1513–1515.

33. Combs DL, O'Brien RJ, Geiter LJ. USPHS tuberculosis short course chemotherapy trial: effectiveness, toxicity, and acceptability. The report of final results. Ann Intern Med 1990;112: 397–406.

34. Cynamon MN, Palmer GS. In vitro activity of amoxicillin in combination with clavulanic acid against *Mycobacterium tuberculosis*. Antimicrob Agents Chemother 1983;24:429–431.

35. Daley CL, Hahn JA, Hopewell PC, Moss AR, Schecter GF. Incidence of tuberculosis in injection drug users in San Francisco: impact of anergy. Am J Respir Crit Care Med 1998;157:19–22.

36. Daley CL, Small PM, Schecter GF, Schoolnik GK, McAdam RA, Jacobs WR, Hopewell PC. An outbreak of tuberculosis with accelerated progression among persons infected with the human immunodeficiency virus. An analysis using restriction-fragment-length polymorphisms. N Engl J Med 1992;326:231–235.

37. Dankner WM, Waecker NJ, Essey MA, Moser K, Thompson M, Davis CE. *Mycobacterium bovis* infections in San Diego: a clinicoepidemiologic study of 73 patients and a historical review of a forgotten pathogen. Medicine 1993;72:11–37.

38. David HL. Probability distribution of drug-resistant mutants in unselected populations of Mycobacterium tuberculosis. Appl Microbiol 1970;20:810–814.

39. Dhillon J, Mitchison. Activity in vitro of rifabutin, FCE 22807, rifapentine, and rifampin against *Mycobacterium microti* and *M. tuberculosis* and their penetration into mouse peritoneal macrophages. Am Rev Respir Dis 1992;145:212–214.

40. D'Oliveira JG. Cerebrospinal fluid concentrations of rifampin in meningeal tuberculosis. Am Rev Respir Dis 1972;106:432–437.

41. Donald PR, Seifart H. Cerebrospinal fluid pyrazinamide concentrations in children with tuberculous meningitis. Pediatr Infect Dis J 1988;7:469–471.

42. Doster B, Caras GJ, Snider DE. A continuing survey of primary drug resistance in tuberculosis, 1961 to 1968. A U.S. Public Health Service cooperative study. Am Rev Respir Dis 1976;113: 419–425.

43. Doster B, Murray FJ, Newman R, Woolpert SF. Ethambutol in the initial treatment of pulmonary tuberculosis. Am Rev Respir Dis 1973;107;177–190.

44. Dutt AK, Moers D, Stead WM. Short-course chemotherapy for tuberculosis with mainly twice-weekly isoniazid and rifampin. Am J Med 1984;77:233–242.

45. Dutt AK, Moers D, Stead WM. Short-course chemotherapy for extrapulmonary tuberculosis. Ann Intern Med 1986;104:7–12.

46. Dutt AK, Moers D, Stead WM. Smear- and culture-negative pulmonary tuberculosis: four-month short-course chemotherapy. Am Rev Respir Dis 1989;139:867–870.

47. Dutt AK, Moers D, Stead WM. Smear-negative, culture positive pulmonary tuberculosis. Am Rev Respir Dis 1990;141:1232–1235.

48. Dutt AK, Moers D, Stead WM. Tuberculous pleural effusion: 6-month therapy with isoniazid and rifampin. Am Rev Respir Dis 1992;145:1429–1432.

49. East African/British Medical Research Councils. Controlled clinical trial of short-course (6-month) regimens of chemotherapy for treatment of pulmonary tuberculosis. Lancet 1972;i:1079–1085.

50. East African/British Medical Research Councils. Controlled clinical trial of four short-course (6-month) regimens of chemotherapy for treatment of pulmonary tuberculosis. Second report. Lancet 1973;i:1331–1338.

51. East African/British Medical Research Councils. Controlled clinical trial of four short-course (6-month) regimens of chemotherapy for treatment of pulmonary tuberculosis. Third report. Lancet 1974;2:237–240.

52. East African/British Medical Research Councils Study. Controlled clinical trial of four short-course (6-month) regimens of chemotherapy for treatment of pulmonary tuberculosis. Lancet 1974;2:1100–1106.

53. East African/British Medical Research Councils Study. Results at 5 years of a controlled comparison of a 6-month and a standard 18-month regimen of chemotherapy for pulmonary tuberculosis. Am Rev Respir Dis 1977;ii:116:3–8.

54. East African/British Medical Research Councils Study. Controlled clinical trial of five short-course (4-month) chemotherapy regimens in pulmonary tuberculosis. Am Rev Respir Dis 1981;123:165–170.

55. Ellard GA, Humphries MJ, Allen BW. Cerebrospinal fluid drug concentrations and the treatment of tuberculous meningitis. Am Rev Respir Dis 1993;148:650–655.

56. Ellard GA, Humpries MJ, Gabriel M, Teoh R. Penetration of pyrazinamide into the cerebrospinal fluid in tuberculous meningitis. Br Med J 1987;294:284–285.

57. Engelhard D, Stutman HR, Marks MI. Interaction of ketoconazole with rifampin and isoniazid. N Engl J Med 1984;311:1681–1683.

58. Ferebee SH. Controlled chemoprophylaxis trials in tuberculosis. A general review. Adv Tuberc Res 1969;17:29–106.

59. Frieden TR, Fujiwara PI, Washko RM, Hamburg MA. Tuberculosis in New York City—turning the tide. N Engl J Med 1995;333:229–233.

60. Frieden TR, Sterling T, Pablos-Mendez A, Kilburn JO, Cauthen GM, Dooley SW. The emergence of drug-resistant tuberculosis in New York City. N Engl J Med 1993;328:521–526.

61. Fujiwara PI, Cook SV, Rutherford CM, Crawford JT, Glickman SE, Kreiswirth BN, Sachnev PS, Osahan SS, Ebrahimzadeh A, Frieden TR. A continuing survey of drug-resistant tuberculosis, New York City, April 1994. Arch Intern Med 1997;157:531–536.

62. Girgis NI, Zoheir F, Kilpatrick E, Sultan Y, Mikhail IA. Dexamethasone adjunctive treatment for tuberculous meningitis. Pediatr Infect Dis J 1991;10:179–183.

63. Girling DJ. Adverse reactions to rifampicin in antituberculosis regimens. J Antimicrob Chemother 1977;3:115–132.

64. Goble M, Iseman MD, Madsen LA, Waite D, Ackerson L, Horsburgh CR Jr. Treatment of 171 patients with pulmonary tuberculosis resistant to isoniazid and rifampin. N Engl J Med 1993;328:527–532.

65. Godfrey-Faussett P, Stoker NG. Aspects of tuberculosis in Africa. 3. Genetic fingerprinting for clues to the pathogenesis of tuberculosis. Trans R Soc Trop Med Hyg 1992;86:472–475.

66. Gonzalez-Montaner LJ, Natal S, Yongchaiyud P, Olliaro P, the Rifabutin Study Group. Rifabutin for the treatment of newly-diagnosed pulmonary tuberculosis: a multinational, randomized, comparative study versus rifampicin. Tuberc Lung Dis 1994;75:341–347.

67. Gordin FM, Matts JP, Miller C, Brown LS, Hafner R, John SL, Klein M, Vaughn A, Besch CL, Perez G, Szabo S, El-Sadr W. A controlled trial of isoniazid in persons with anergy and human immunodeficiency virus infection who are at high risk for tuberculosis. N Engl J Med 1997;337:315–320.

68. Graham NHM, Galai N, Nelson KE, Astemborski J, Bonds M, Rizzo RT, Sheeley L, Vlahov D. Effect of isoniazid chemoprophylaxis on HIV-related mycobacterial disease. Arch Intern Med 1996;156:889–894.

69. Greenberg PD, Lax KG, Schecter CB. Tuberculosis in house staff. A decision analysis comparing the tuberculin screening strategy with BCG vaccination. Am Rev Respir Dis 1991;143:490–495.

70. Halsey NA, Coberly JS, Desormeaux J, Lorikoff P, Atkinson J, Moulton LH, Contave M, Johnson M, Davis H, Geiter L, Johnson E, Huebner R, Boulos R, Chaisson RE. Randomized trial of isoniazid versus rifampicin and pyrazinonide for prevention of tuberculosis in HIV-1 infection. Lancet 1998;351:786–792.

71. Hawken M, Nunn P, Gathua S, Brindle R, Godfrey-Faussett P, Githui W, Odhiambo J, Batchelor B, Gilks C, Morris J. Increased recurrence of tuberculosis in HIV-1 infected patients in Kenya. Lancet 1993;342:332–337.

72. Heifets L. Qualitative and quantitative drug-susceptibility tests in mycobacteriology. Am Rev Respir Dis 1988;137:1217–1222.

73. Hill AR, Mateo F, Hudak A. Transient exacerbation of tuberculous lymphadenitis during chemotherapy in patients with AIDS. Clin Infect Dis 1994;19:774–776.

74. Holdiness MR. Cerebrospinal fluid pharmacokinetics of the antituberculosis drugs. Clin Pharmacokinet 1985;10:532–534.

75. Hong Kong Chest Service/Tuberculosis Research Centre, Madras/British Medical Research Council. A controlled trial of 2-month, 3-month, and 12-month regimens of chemotherapy for sputum-smear-negative pulmonary tuberculosis. Am Rev Respir Dis 1984;130:23–28.

76. Hong Kong Chest Service/Tuberculosis Research Centre, Madras/British Medical Research Council. A controlled trial of 3-month, 4-month, and 6-month regimens of chemotherapy for sputum-smear-negative pulmonary tuberculosis. Am Rev Respir Dis 1989;139:871–876.

77. Hong Kong Chest Service/British Medical Research Council. Five-year follow-up of a controlled trial of five 6-month regimens of chemotherapy for pulmonary tuberculosis. Am Rev Respir Dis 1987;136:1339–1342.

78. Hong Kong Chest Service/British Medical Research Council. Controlled trial of 2, 4, and 6 months of pyrazinamide in 6-month, three-times-weekly regimens for smear-positive pulmonary tuberculosis, including an assessment of a combined preparation of isoniazid, rifampin, and pyrazinamide. Am Rev Respir Dis 1991;143:700–706.

79. Hong Kong Chest Service/British Medical Research Council. A controlled study of rifabutin and an uncontrolled study of ofloxacin in the retreatment of patients with pulmonary tuberculosis resistant to isoniazid, streptomycin and rifampin. Tubercle and Lung Dis 1992;73:59–67.

80. Hong Kong Tuberculosis Chest Service/British Medical Research Council. Controlled trial of 6-month and 9-month regimens of daily and intermittent streptomycin plus isoniazid plus pyrazinamide for pulmonary tuberculosis in Hong Kong. Am Rev Respir Dis 1977;115:727–785.

81. Hong Kong Tuberculosis Treatment Services/Brompton Hospital/British Medical Research Council. A controlled trial of daily and intermittent rifampicin plus ethambutol in the retreatment of patients with pulmonary tuberculosis: results up to 30 months. Tubercle 1975;56:179–189.

82. Hong Kong Tuberculosis Treatment Services/Brompton Hospital/British Medical Research Council. A controlled clinical comparison of 6 and 8 months of antituberculosis chemotherapy in the treatment of patients with silicotuberculosis in Hong Kong. Am Rev Respir Dis 1991;143:262–267.

83. Hopewell PC, Bloom BR. Tuberculosis and other mycobacterial diseases. In: Murray JF, Nadel JA, eds. Respiratory medicine, 2nd ed. Philadelphia: WB Saunders, 1994:1094–1160.

84. Humphries MJ, Teoh R, Lau J, Gabriel M. Factors of prognostic significance in Chinese children with tuberculous meningitis. Tubercle 1990:71:161–168.

85. International Union against Tuberculosis Committee on Prophylaxis. Efficacy of various durations of isoniazid preventive therapy for tuberculosis: five years of follow-up in the IUAT trial. Bull WHO 1982;60:555–564.

86. Iseman MD. Treatment of multidrug resistant tuberculosis. N Engl J Med 1993;329:784–791.

87. Iseman MD, Madsen L, Goble M, Pomerantz M. Surgical intervention in the treatment of pulmonary disease caused by drug-resistant *Mycobacterium tuberculosis*. Am Rev Respir Dis 1990; 141:623–625.

88. Jawahar MS, Sivasubramanian S, Vijayan VK, Rmakrishnan CV, Paramasivan CN, Selvakumar V, Paul S, Tripathy SP, Prabhakar. Short course chemotherapy for tuberculous lymphadenitis in children. BMJ 1990;301:359–362.

89. Jones BE, Otaya M, Antoniskis D, et al. Prospective evaluation of antituberculosis therapy in patients with human immunodeficiency virus infection. Am J Respir Crit Care Med 1994;150: 1499–1502.

90. Jones BE, Young SMM, Antoniskis D, Davidson PT, Kramer F, Barnes PF. Relationship of the manifestations of tuberculosis to CD4 cell counts in patients with human immunodeficiency virus infection. Am Rev Respir Dis 1993;148:1292–1297.

91. Kaojarern S, Supmonchai K, Phuapradit P, Mokkhavesa C, Krittiyanunt S. Effects of steroids on cerebrospinal fluid penetration of antituberculosis drugs in tuberculous meningitis. Clin Pharmacol Ther 1991;49:6–12.

92. Kennedy N, Berger L, Curran J, Fox R, Gutman J, Kisyombe GM, Ngowi FI, Ramsay AR, Saruni AO, Sam N, Tillotson G, Uiso LO, Yates M, Gillespie SH. Randomized controlled trial of a drug regimen that includes ciprofloxacin for the treatment of pulmonary tuberculosis. Clin Infect Dis 1996;22:827–833.

93. Klausner JD, Makonkawkeyoon S, Akarasewi P, Nakata K, Kasinrerk W, Corral L, Dewar RL, Lane HC, Freedman VH, Kaplan G. The effect of thalidomide on the pathogenesis of human immunodeficiency virus type 1 and *M. tuberculosis* infection. J Acquired Immune Defic Syndr 1996;11:247–257.

94. Kohno S, Koga H, Kaku M, Maesaki S, Hara K. Prospective comparative study of ofloxacin or ethambutol for the treatment of pulmonary tuberculosis. Chest 1992;102:1815–1818.

95. Kopanoff DE, Snider DE, Caras GJ. Isoniazid-related hepatitis. Am Rev Respir Dis 1978;117:991–1001.

96. Lecoeur HF, Truffot-Pernot C, Grosset JH. Experimental short-course preventive therapy of tuberculosis with rifampin and pyrazinamide. Am Rev Respir Dis 1989;140:1189–1193.

97. Lee CH, Wang WJ, Lan RS, Tsai YH, Chiang YC. Corticosteroids in the treatment of tuberculous pleurisy. Chest 1988; 94:1256–1259.

98. Lee KC, Tami TA, Lalwani AK, Schecter G. Contemporary management of cervical tuberculosis. Laryngoscope 1992l102: 60–64.

99. Mahmoudi A, Iseman MD. Pitfalls in the care of patients with tuberculosis. Common errors and their association with the acquisition of drug resistance. JAMA 1993;270;65–68.

100. McGregor MM, Olliaro P, Wolmarans L, Mabuza B, Bredell M, Felten MK, Fourie PB. Efficacy and safety of rifabutin in the treatment of patients with newly diagnosed pulmonary tuberculosis. Am J Respir Crit Care Med 1996;154:1462–1467.

101. Medical Research Council. The treatment of pulmonary tuberculosis with isoniazid. Br Med J 1952;2:735–746.

102. Mitchison DA. Development of streptomycin resistant strains of tubercle bacilli in pulmonary tuberculosis: results of simultaneous sensitivity tests in liquid and on solid media. Thorax 1950;5:144–161.

103. Moore RD, Chaulk CP, Griffiths R, Cavalante S, Chaisson RE. Cost-effectiveness of directly observed versus self-administered therapy for tuberculosis. Am J Respir Crit Care Med 1996;154:1013–1019.

104. Nadler JP, Berger J, Nord JA, Cofsky R, Saxena M. Amoxicillin-clavulanic acid for treating drug-resistant *Mycobacterium tuberculosis*. Chest 1991;99:1025–1026.

105. Newman R, Doster B, Murray FJ, Ferebee S. Rifampin in initial treatment of pulmonary tuberculosis. Am Rev Respir Dis 1971;103:461–476.

106. Newman R, Doster B, Murray FJ, Ferebee Woolpert S. Rifampin in initial treatment of pulmonary tuberculosis. Am Rev Respir Dis 1974;216–232.

107. Nolan CM. Failure of therapy for tuberculosis in human immunodeficiency virus infection. Am J Med Sci 1992;304: 168–173.

108. Nolan CM, Williams DL, Cave MD, Eisenach KD, el-Hajj H, Hooton TM, Thompson RL, Goldberg SV. Evolution of rifampin resistance in human immunodeficiency virus-associated tuberculosis. Am J Respir Crit Care Med 1995;152:1067–1071.

109. Nunn P, Brindle R, Carpenter L, Odhiambo J, Wasunna K, Newnham R, Githui W, Gathua S, Omwega M, McAdam K. Cohort study of human immunodeficiency virus infection in patients with tuberculosis in Nairobi, Kenya. Am Rev Respir Dis 1992;146:849–854.

110. Nunn P, Kibuga D, Gathua S, Brindle R, Imalingat A, Wasunna K, Lucas S, Gilks C, Omwega M, Were J. Cutaneous hypersensitivity reactions due to thiacetazone in HIV-1 seropositive patients treated for tuberculosis. Lancet 1991;337:627–630.

111. Okwera A, Whalen C, Byekwaso F, Vjecha M, Johnson J, Huebner R, Mugerwa R, Ellner J, and the Makerere University-Case Western University of Research Collaboration. Randomized trial of thiacetazone and rifampicin-containing regimens for pulmonary tuberculosis in HIV infected Ugandans. Lancet 1994;344:1323–1328.

112. Onorato IM, McCray E, and the Field Services Branch. Prevalence of human immunodeficiency virus infection among patients attending tuberculosis clinics in the United States. J Infect Dis 1992;165:87–92.

113. Place VA, Pyle MM, de la Huerga J. Ethambutol in tuberculous meningitis. Am Rev Respir Dis 1969;99:783–785.

114. Pape JW, Jean SS, Ho JL, Hafner A, Johnson DW. Effect of isoniazid prophylaxis on incidence of active tuberculosis and progression of HIV infection. Lancet 1993;342:268.

115. Patel KB, Blemonte R, Crowe HM. Drug malabsorption and resistant tuberculosis in HIV-infected patients. N Engl J Med 1995;332:336–337.

116. Peloquin CA. Using therapeutic drug monitoring to dose the antimycobacterial drugs. Clin Chest Med 1997;18:79–87.

117. Peloquin CA, Henshaw TL, Huitt GA, Berning SE, Nitta AT, James GT. Pharmacokinetic evaluation of para-aminosalicylic acid granules. Pharmacotherapy 1994;14:40–46.

118. Peloquin CA, MacPhee AA, Berning SE. Malabsorption of antimycobacterial medications [Letter]. N Engl J Med 1993;329: 1122–1123.

119. Peloquin CA, Nitta AT, Burman WJ, Brudney KF, Miranda-Massari JR, McGuinness ME, Berning SE, Gerena GT. Low antituberculosis drug concentrations in patients with AIDS. Ann Pharmacother 1996;30:919–925.

120. Perriens JH, Colebunders RL, Karahunga C, Willame JC, Jeugmans J, Kaboto M, Mukadi Y, Pauwels P, Ryder RW, Prignot J, Piot P. Increased mortality and tuberculosis treatment failure rate among human immunodeficiency virus (HIV) seropositive compared with HIV seronegative patients with pulmonary tuberculosis treated with "standard" chemotherapy in Kinshasa, Zaire. Am Rev Respir Dis 1991;144:750–755.

121. Perriens JH, St Louis ME, Mukadi YB, Brown C, Prignot J, Pouthier F, Portaels F, Willame JC, Mandala JK, Kaboto M, Ryder RW, Roscigno G, Piot P. Pulmonary tuberculosis in HIV infected patients in Zaire: a controlled trial of treatment for either 6 or 12 months. N Engl J Med 1995;332:779–784.

122. Petrowski JT. Uveitis associated with rifabutin therapy: a clinical alert. J Am Optom Assoc 1996;67:693–696.

123. Phuapradit P, Supmonchai K Kaojarern S, Mokkhavesa C. The blood/cerebrospinal fluid partitioning of pyrazinamide: a study during the course of treatment of tuberculous meningitis. J Neurol Neurosurg Psychiatry 1990;53:81–82.

124. Pilheu JA, Maglio F, Cetrangolo R, Pleus AD. Concentration of ethambutol in the cerebrospinal fluid after oral administration. Tubercle 1971;52:117–122.

125. Pioget JC, Wolff M. Singlas E, Laisne MJ, Clair B, Regnier B, Vachon F. Diffusion of ofloxacin into cerebrospinal fluid of patients with purulent meningitis or ventriculitis. Antimicrob Agents Chemother 1989;33:933–936.

126. Polesky A, Farber HW, Gottlieb DJ, Park H, Levinson S, O'Connell JJ, McInnis B, Nieves RL, Bernardo J. Rifampin preventive therapy for tuberculosis in Boston's homeless. Am J Respir Crit Care Med 1996:154:1473–1477.

127. Pomerantz M, Madsen L, Goble M, Iseman M. Surgical management of resistant mycobacterial tuberculosis and other mycobacterial pulmonary infections. Ann Thorac Surg 1991;52: 1108–1112.

128. Pretet S, Lebeaut A, Parrot R, Truffot C, Grosset J, Dinh-Xuan AT. Combined chemotherapy including rifabutin for rifampicin and isoniazid resistant pulmonary tuberculosis. Eur Respir J 1992;5:680–684.

129. Ramachandran P, Duraipandian M, Nagarajan M, Prabhakar R, Ramakrishnan CV, Tripathy SP. Three chemotherapy studies of tuberculous meningitis in children. Tubercle 1986;67:17–29.

130. Rastogi N, Goh KS, Bryskier A, Devallois A. In vitro activities of levofloxacin used alone and in combination with first- and second-line antituberculosis drugs against *Mycobacterium tuberculosis*. Antimicrob Agents Chemother 1996;40:1610–1616.

131. Raviglione MC, Snider DE Jr, Kochi A. Global epidemiology of tuberculosis. Morbidity and mortality of a worldwide epidemic. JAMA 1995;273:220–226.

132. Robitzek EH, Selikoff IJ. Hydrazine derivatives of isonicotinic acid (Rimifon, Marsilid) in the treatment of active progressive caseous-pneumonic tuberculosis. A preliminary report. Am Rev Tuberc 1952;65:402–428.

133. Sahai J, Gallicano K, Swick L, Tailor S, Garber G, Seguin I, Oliveras L, Walker S, Rachlis A, Cameron W. Reduced plasma concentrations of antituberculosis drugs in patients with HIV infection. Ann Intern Med 1997;127:289–293.

134. Schwander S, Rusch-Gerdes S, Mateega A, Lutalo T, Tugume S, Kityo C, Rubaramira R, Mugyenyi P, Okwera A, Mugerwa R, Aisu T, Moser R, Ochen K, M'Bonye M, Dietrich M. A pilot study of antituberculosis combinations of comparing rifabutin with rifampicin in the treatment of HIV-1 associated tuberculosis. Tuberc Lung Dis 1995;76:210–218.

135. Selwyn P, Hartel D, Lewis V, Schoenbaum EE, Vermund SH, Klein RS, Walker AT, Friedland GH. A prospective study of the risk of tuberculosis among intravenous drug users with HIV infection. N Engl J Med 1989;320:545–550.

136. Selwyn P, Sckell B, Alcabes P, Friedland G, Kein R, Shoenber E. High risk of active tuberculosis in HIV-infected drug users with cutaneous anergy. JAMA 1992;268:504–509.

137. Shaw PP, Wang SM, Tung SG, Niu QW, Lu TS, Yu XC. Clinical analysis of 445 adult cases of tuberculous meningitis. Chin J Tuberc Respir Dis 1984;3:131–132.

138. Siddiqi SH, Hwangobo CC, Silcox V, Good RC, Snider DE, Middlebrook G. Rapid radiometric methods to detect and differentiate *Mycobacterium tuberculosis/M. bovis* from other mycobacterial species. Am Rev Respir Dis 1984;130:634–640.

139. Siddiqi S, Lebonate J, Middlebrook G. Evaluation of a rapid radiometric method for drug susceptibility testing of *Mycobacterium tuberculosis*. J Clin Microbiol 1981;13:908–912.

140. Singapore Tuberculosis Service/British Medical Research Council. Controlled trial of intermittent regimens of rifampin plus isoniazid for pulmonary tuberculosis in Singapore. Am Rev Respir Dis 1977;116:807–820.

141. Singapore Tuberculosis Service/British Medical Research Council. Clinical trial of six-month and four-month regimens of chemotherapy in the treatment of pulmonary tuberculosis. Am Rev Respir Dis 1979;119:579–585.

142. Singapore Tuberculosis Service/British Medical Research Council. Long term follow-up of a clinical trial of six-month and four-month regimens of chemotherapy in the treatment of pulmonary tuberculosis. Am Rev Respir Dis 1986;133:779–783.

143. Singapore Tuberculosis Service/British Medical Research Council. Five year follow-up of a clinical trial of three 6-month regimens of chemotherapy given intermittently in the continuation phase in the treatment of pulmonary tuberculosis. Am Rev Respir Dis 1988;137:1147–1150.

144. Singapore Tuberculosis Service/British Medical Research Council. Assessment of a daily combined preparation isoniazid, rifampin, and pyrazinamide in a controlled trial of three 6-month regimens for smear-positive pulmonary tuberculosis. Am Rev Respir Dis 1991;43:707–712.

145. Small PM, Schecter GF, Goodman PC, Sande MA, Chaisson RE, Hopewell PC. Treatment of tuberculosis in patients with advanced human immunodeficiency virus infection. N Engl J Med 1991;324:289–294.

146. Small PM, Shafer RW, Hopewell PC, Singh SP, Murphy MJ, Desmond E, Sierra MF, Schoolnik GK. Exogenous reinfection with multidrug-resistant *Mycobacterium tuberculosis* in patients with advanced HIV infection. N Engl J Med 1993;328:1137–1144.

147. Small PM. Tuberculosis research. Balancing the portfolio. JAMA 1996;276:1512–1513.

148. Snider DE, Caras GJ. Isoniazid-associated hepatitis deaths: a review of available information. Am Rev Respir Dis 1992;145:494–497.

149. Snider DE, Caras GJ, Koplan JP. Preventive therapy with isoniazid: cost effectiveness of different durations of therapy. JAMA 1986;255:1579–1583.

150. Snider DE, Powell KE. Should women taking antituberculosis drugs breast-feed? Arch Intern Med 1984;144:589–590.

151. Stevens JP, Danile TM. Bacille Calmette Guerin immunization of health care workers exposed to multidrug resistant tuberculosis: a decision analysis. Tuberc Lung Dis 1996;77:315–321.

152. Stewart SM, Crofton JW. The clinical significance of low degrees of drug resistance in pulmonary tuberculosis. Am Rev Respir Dis 1964:811–829.

153. Strang JIG, Kakaza HHS, Gibson DG, Allen BW, Mitchison DA, Evans DJ, Girling DJ, Nunn AJ, Fox W. Controlled clinical trial of complete open surgical drainage and of prednisolone in treatment of tuberculous pericardial effusion in Transkei. Lancet 1988;759–763.

154. Strang JIG, Kakaza HHS, Gibson DG, Girling DJ, Nunn AJ, Fox W. Controlled trial of prednisolone as adjuvant in treatment of tuberculous constrictive pericarditis in Transkei. Lancet 1987;1418–1422.

155. Sunakorn P, Pongparit S, Wongrun S. Short course chemotherapy in tuberculous meningitis: a pilot trial. J Med Assoc Thai 1980;63:340–345.

156. Sutherland I. Recent studies in the epidemiology of tuberculosis based on the risk of being infected with tubercle bacilli. Adv Tuberc Res 1976;19:1–63.

157. Swai BO, Aluoch JA, Githui WA, Thiong'o R, Edwards EA. Controlled clinical trial of a regimen of two durations for the treatment of isoniazid resistant pulmonary tuberculosis. Tubercle 1988;69:5–14.

158. Talenti A, Phillip WJ, Sreevatson S, Bernasconi C, Stockbauer KE, Wieles B, Musser JM, Jacobs WR. The emb operon, a gene cluster of *Mycobacterium tuberculosis* involved in resistance to ethambutol. Nature Med 1997;3:567–570.

159. Tempel CW, Hughes FJ, Mardis RE, Towbin MN, Dye WE. Combined intermittent regimens employing streptomycin and para-aminosalicylic acid in the treatment of pulmonary tuberculosis. Am Rev Tuberc 1951;63:295–311.

160. Trebucq A. Should ethambutol be recommended for routine treatment of tuberculosis in children? A review of the literature. Int J Tuberc Lung Dis 1997;1:12–15.

161. Twelth report of the Medical Research Council Working Party on Tuberculosis of the Spine. Controlled trial of short course regimens of chemotherapy in the ambulatory treatment of spinal tuberculosis. J Bone Joint Surg 1993;75-B:240–248.

162. Upadhyay SS, Saji MJ, Yau ACMC. Duration of antituberculosis chemotherapy in conjunction with radical surgery in the management of spinal tuberculosis. Spine 1996;21:1898–1903.

163. Varpela E, Hietalalahti J, Aro M. Streptomycin and dihydrostreptomycin during pregnancy and their effect on the child's inner ear. Scand J Respir Dis 1969;50:101–109.

164. Varughese A, Brater DC, Benet LZ, Lee C. Ethambutol kinetics in patients with impaired renal function. Am Rev Respir Dis 1986;134:34–38.

165. Vestal AL. Procedures for the isolation and identification of mycobacteria. Department of Health, Education, and Welfare, Publ no. (CDC) 76–8230, 1976;97–115.

166. Wadhawan D, Hira S, Mwansa N, Sunkutu R, Adera P, Perine P. Preventive tuberculosis chemotherapy with isoniazid (INH) among patients infected with HIV-1 [Abstract PO-B07–1114]. Ninth International Conference on AIDS in affiliation with the Fourth STD World Congress, Berlin, June 6–11, 1993.

167. Wallis RS, Nsubuga P, Whalen C, Mugerwa RD, Okwera A, Oette D, Jackson JB, Johnson JL. Ellner JJ. Pentoxifylline therapy in human immunodeficiency virus-seropositive persons with tuberculosis: a randomized, controlled trial. J Infect Dis 1996;174:727–733.

168. Wayne LG. Microbiology of the tubercle bacilli. Am Rev Respir Dis 1982;125:31–41.

169. Weis SE, Slocum PC, Blais FX, King B, Nunn M, Matney GB, Gomez E, Foresman BH. The effect of directly observed therapy on the rates of drug resistance and relapse in tuberculosis. N Engl J Med 1994;330:1179–1184.

170. Whalen CC, Johnson JL, Okwera A, Hom DL, Huebner R, Mugeny P, Mugerwa RD, Ellner JJ. A trial of three regimens to prevent tuberculosis in Ugondan adults infected with the human immunodeficiency virus. N Engl J Med 1997;337:801–808.

171. Wong CS, Palmer GS, Cynamon MH. In-vitro susceptibility of *Mycobacterium tuberculosis, Mycobacterium bovis* and *Mycobacterium kansasii* to amoxycillin and ticarcillin in combination with clavulanic acid. J Antimicrob Chemother 1988;22:863–866.

172. Woo J, Humphries M, Chan K, O'Mahony G, Teoh R. Cerebrospinal fluid and serum levels of pyrazinamide and rifampicin in patients with tuberculous meningitis. Curr Ther Res 1987:42:235–242.

173. Woodley CL, Kilburn JO. In vitro susceptibility of *Mycobacterium avium* complex and *Mycobacterium tuberculosis* strains to a spiro-piperidyl rifamycin. Am Rev Respir Dis 1982;126:586–587.

174. Zhang Y., Heym B, Allen B, Young D, Cole S. The catalase-peroxidase gene and isoniazid resistance of Mycobacterium tuberculosis. Nature 1992;358:591–593.

175. Zierski M. Prospects of retreatment of chronic resistant pulmonary tuberculosis: a critical review. Lung 1977:154:91.

PART C

Rickettsia

Coxiella burnetii

Thomas J. Marrie

MICROBIOLOGY

Coxiella burnetii is the etiologic agent of Q fever. It is a small Gram-negative bacterium that grows only in eukaryotic cells (18). Within these cells it multiplies in an acidic vacuole, pH 4.8. It can form a spore, which explains its ability to survive for extended periods in hostile environments and its marked resistance to physiochemical agents. *C. burnetii* exists in two antigenic phases, phases I and II. In animals, it exists in phase I and is extremely infectious; passage in cell culture or in embryonated eggs results in a change in surface lipopolysaccharides—phase II. This phase is much less virulent than phase I.

CLINICAL MANIFESTATIONS

Q fever has two major manifestations in man, acute and chronic infection. Acute Q fever has a variety of clinical presentations including self-limited febrile illness, pneumonia, hepatitis, meningoencephalitis, and pericarditis. Chronic Q fever is a much more serious illness and almost always means endocarditis, although infection of aortic prosthesis or aneurysm are other manifestations of chronic Q fever (18). While still not adequately described in man, it is likely that Q fever during pregnancy results in chronic uterine infection with relapse during subsequent pregnancies as it does in other female mammals (12, 21).

SUSCEPTIBILITY IN VITRO AND IN VIVO

In many of the in vitro susceptibility studies cited below, three type strains of *C. burnetii* were commonly used. Strain Nine Mile was isolated from a tick, *Dermacentor* sp., collected near Nine Mile creek, Montana, in 1935. It is a prototypic acute Q fever strain. Priscilla was isolated from a goat placenta; it is a chronic Q fever isolate. Q 212 was isolated from the brachial artery clot of a Nova Scotia, Canada, patient with Q fever endocarditis.

Determination of antimicrobial susceptibility of *C. burnetii* has been problematic, since it is an intracellular pathogen. Nevertheless, there is a long history of efforts to provide antimicrobial susceptibility data about *C. burnetii*. Three model systems have been used: chick embryos, guinea pigs, and cell cultures (29). Table 1 summarizes the results of susceptibility testing in chick embryos or guinea pigs.

In a series of studies, workers in Baca's laboratory described a cell culture model, persistently infected L929 cells, for determining susceptibility of *C. burnetii* to antibiotics (1, 2, 23, 31). The apparent advantages of the cell culture model

are convenience, more-rapid test results (24–48 h vs. 1 week), and precise control of antimicrobial concentrations, which are only approximate in in vivo systems (29). What is not certain is how closely this system mimics chronic infection in man. The cell lines, L929 (mouse fibroblasts) and J774 and P388D1 (macrophage cell lines), do develop persistent infection for periods of 250 to 1400 days (29). Furthermore, these infected cells do not require addition of normal infected cells to maintain viable populations, yet the cell cycle is similar to that of normal uninfected cells (2).

The availability of this cell model system allowed Maurin et al. (13) to make an observation that may have major implications for treatment of chronic Q fever. They found that phagolysosomal alkalinization with agents such as amantadine, chloroquine, or ammonium chloride increased the bactericidal effect of some antibiotics. These effects differed for different alkalinizing agents; for example, doxycycline plus amantadine resulted in weak bactericidal action, whereas combination with chloroquine or ammonium chloride resulted in strong antimicrobial activity (13). In contrast, the combination of pefloxacin and chloroquine was weakly bactericidal, whereas pefloxacin and ammonium chloride was much more effective (13). There was no correlation between phagolysosomal pH and the activity of rifampin (13).

Over the past few years there has been a suggestion that certain strains (whether defined by plasmid content or genomic profile following endonuclease digestion and pulse-field gel electrophoresis) of *C. burnetii* are associated with acute or chronic Q fever (5, 6, 24). There is little doubt, now that more isolates from diverse geographic areas have been studied, that there is no such association (26, 27). Yeaman and Baca (30) have shown that the plasmid content of *C. burnetii* isolates does not affect antimicrobial susceptibility.

Table 2 summarizes *C. burnetii* antimicrobial susceptibility studies in a cell culture model system. Jabrit-Aldighieri et al. (8) added another variable to the cell culture model. They used cycloheximide to block multiplication of L929 cells persistently infected with *C. burnetii*. This reduced the effectiveness of the two quinolones tested, compared with their effectiveness in untreated cells.

One of the important observations from *C. burnetii* susceptibility testing in the cell culture model is that (as might be expected) there is heterogenicity in the response of *C. burnetii* strains to antibiotics (20). Thus, of 13 strains tested, 6 were re-

TABLE 1 • Summary of Results of Antimicrobial Susceptibility Testing: *Coxiella burnetii* Using Chick Embryo or Guinea Pig Models

Ref	Author	Model System	Strain(s) Tested	Antibiotic(s) Tested	Results
7	Huebner 1948	Chick embryos Guinea pigs	Strains from patients with acute Q fever	Streptomycin	Reduced mortality
16	Ormsbee 1951	Embryonated eggs	Nine Mile	Aureomycin Terramycin Chloramphenicol Streptomycin Penicillin G	Most effective ↓ Least effective
16	Ormsbee 1951	Chick embryos	Nine Mile	Terramycin Aureomycin Erythromycin Thiocymetin	Effective Effective Ineffective Effective
9	Keren 1994	Chick embryos	Ohio 314 phase I	Minocycline Ciprofloxacin Pefloxacin Fleroxacin	Effective at 8 μg/g egg 1 μg/g egg 6 μg/g egg 1 μg/g egg

TABLE 2 • Summary of Results of Antimicrobial Susceptibility Testing: *Coxiella burnetii* Using Cell Culture Model

Ref	Author	Cell Line	Strain(s) Tested	Antibiotic(s) Tested	Results
9	Keren 1994	Vero cells	Ohio 314	Minocycline} Fleroxacin} Pefloxacin} Ciprofloxacin	95% growth inhibition at 2.5 mg/L 95% growth inhibition at 10 mg/L
28	Torres 1993	HEL cells	Nine Mile Q 212 Priscilla and 10 isolates from patients with chronic Q fever (Marseille)	Ceftriaxone Fusidic acid	Inconclusive results Authors conclude these compounds could be effective
8	Jabarit-Aldighieri 1992	L929 cells with addition of cycloheximide	Q 212 Nine Mile 13 chronic Q fever isolates	PD 127, 391} flouro-PD 131, 628} quinolones	Both quinolones more active against Nine Mile strain than against Q212 (chronic Q fever strain), but neither drug could eliminate infection
20	Raoult 1991	HEL cells	Nine Mile Q 212 Priscilla 10 chronic Q fever isolates	Amoxicillin Amikacin Erythromycin Cotrimoxazole Pefloxacin Ciprofloxacin Chloramphenicol Tetracycline Doxycycline Minocycline Rifampin	Nine Mile more susceptible than Q212 or Priscilla; all isolates were resistant to amoxicillin and amikacin; all were susceptible to rifampin, cotrimoxazole, and tetracyclines; heterogeneity of susceptibility to fluoroquinolones, chloramphenicol, and erythromycin
29, 31	Yeaman 1987	L929	Nine Mile	Penicillin G Polymyxin B Sulfamethoxazole Trimethoprim Streptomycin Gentamicin Chloramphenicol Rifampin, novobiocin Nalidixic acid Oxolinic acid Ciprofloxacin Norfloxacin Ofloxacin	Penicillin G, polymyxin B, sulfamethoxazole, trimethoprim, erythromycin, streptomycin, gentamicin—inactive; chloramphenicol, some activity; all others very active

sistant to erythromycin, and 7 were of intermediate susceptibility. Corresponding data for pefloxacin, ofloxacin, ciprofloxacin for these 13 strains were 3/0; 1/0; 8/0; 3/0. It is also apparent from Table 2 that the Nine Mile strain of *C. burnetii* is more susceptible to antibiotics than strains isolated from patients with chronic Q fever.

ANTIMICROBIAL THERAPY

Table 3 summarizes recommendations for the various types of *C. burnetii* infection.

Acute Q fever (*C. burnetii*) Pneumonia

Sobradillo et al. (25), Basque Country, Spain, carried out a prospective, randomized, double-blind study of doxycycline and erythromycin in the treatment of pneumonia presumed to be due to Q fever. Forty-eight patients were proven by serologic studies to have Q fever; 23 received 100 mg doxycycline twice daily, and 25 received erythromycin (500 mg every 6 h) for 10 days. Fever resolution was more rapid in the doxycycline-treated group (3 ± 1.6 days vs. 4.3 ± 2 days for erythromycin-treated patients; $P = .05$). The erythromycin-treated group had more gastrointestinal adverse effects (11 vs. 2 for the doxycycline-treated patients; $P < .01$). By day 40, the chest radiograph was normal in 47 of the 48 patients. The authors concluded that doxycycline was more effective than erythromycin, but they recognized the self-limiting and benign nature of most cases of pneumonia due to Q fever.

A retrospective review of 19 patients with Q fever pneumonia showed that 11 were treated with erythromycin and 8 with β-lactam antibiotics. The erythromycin-treated group became afebrile by day 3, while only 2 of the β-lactam-treated group were afebrile by this time ($P < .005$) (17).

In general, treatment of acute Q fever is not a problem clinically, since most cases are unrecognized, and recovery is uneventful. However, *C. burnetii* may occasionally cause rapidly progressive pneumonia necessitating ventilatory support. If the recommendations of the Canadian Community-Acquired Pneumonia Consensus Conference Group for treating such patients are followed, and erythromycin, rifampin, and a third-generation cephalosporin are prescribed (11), the rifampin will adequately treat severe Q fever pneumonia.

Chronic Q Fever

Chronic Q fever generally means endocarditis, although osteomyelitis and Q fever during pregnancy are other manifestations of chronic Q fever. Endocarditis is the most serious manifestation of Q fever. There is usually a considerable delay in diagnosis, and this form of Q fever carries a 37% mortality rate. Treatment of Q fever endocarditis is difficult. There are no randomized trials to provide guidance; however by trial and error and now as a result of in vitro susceptibility studies, we have arrived at regimens that provide (in conjunction with valve replacement) good cure rates.

At least two or more drugs active against *C. burnetii* should be used to treat Q fever endocarditis. Our first choice has been ciprofloxacin (750 mg twice daily, orally) plus rifampin (300 mg daily, orally). We have now treated 12 patients with this regimen, with only one failure. Therapy must be prolonged. We recommend at least 2 years—others recommend 3 years (10). The best approach is to monitor response to treatment by determining antibody titers to phase I and phase II antigens with a microimmunofluorescence test. These antibody titers should be determined for both IgG and IgA every 3 months during treatment. Declining antibody titers reflect adequate response to treatment. When the antiphase I IgA is 1:200 or less, therapy can be stopped.

There are several reports of isolation of *C. burnetii* from heart valves following months to years of treatment, especially with single antimicrobial agents (10, 14). Other antibiotic combinations that have been used successfully to treat Q fever

---

TABLE 3 • **Antimicrobial Treatment of Various Manifestations of *C. burnetii* Infection**

	Treatment[a]	Reference
Acute Q fever Pneumonia	1. Doxycycline 100 mg b.i.d. p.o. for 10 days 2. Ciprofloxacin 500 mg b.i.d. p.o. for 10 days	25
Chronic Q fever Endocaritis	1. Ciprofloxacin 750 mg b.i.d. p.o. plus rifampin 300 mg o.d. p.o.[b]	Marrie, unpublished observations
	2. Doxycycline 100 mg b.i.d. p.o. plus rifampin 300 mg o.d. p.o.[b]	Author's recommendations
	3. Doxycycline 100 mg b.i.d. p.o. plus a quinolone[b]	10
	4. Doxycycline 100 mg b.i.d. p.o. plus hydroxychloroquine 400 to 600 mg/day to achieve a chloroquine level of 1 mg/L[b]	Raoult, personal communication
Q fever in pregnancy	1. Erythromycin 500 mg q. 6 h p.o. plus rifampin 300 mg o.d. p.o. for the duration of the pregnancy After delivery, ciprofloxacin 500 mg b.i.d. p.o. plus rifampin 300 mg o.d. p.o. for 6 months	Author's recommendation
Q fever hepatitis	Can occur as an acute or chronic form; treatment is as outlined for acute Q fever; chronic Q fever hepatitis–insufficient data to make any firm recommendations about duration of treatment; would use combination therapy as listed for endocarditis	

[a] 1, first choice; 2, second choice, etc.

[b] All regimens to treat chronic Q fever must be given until IgA antiphase I antibody titer is ≤1:200; this usually requires at least 2 years.

endocarditis are doxycycline and cotrimoxazole (4) and doxycycline and quinolones (10). Addition of hydroxychloroquine (to alkalinize the phagolysosome) to doxycycline is said to be effective in the treatment of chronic Q fever (Raoult D, personal communication).

Q Fever in Pregnancy

There are very few reports of Q fever complicating pregnancy (3, 12, 21, 22). *C. burnetii* has been isolated from the placenta despite treatment of the mother for Q fever during pregnancy (3, 12). Indeed, in 24 published cases of Q fever during pregnancy (3, 12), *C. burnetii* was isolated from 12 of the 14 placentas examined. Thus in women, as in other female mammals, chronic infection of the placenta and endometrium occurs during pregnancy. This suggests that antibiotic therapy should be prolonged. In two cases (3, 22), *C. burnetii* was isolated from the placenta despite therapy with rifampin/doxycycline and erythromycin/rifampin respectively. Until further data are available, we suggest that erythromycin/rifampin be used to suppress (treat) *C. burnetii* during pregnancy and, after delivery, ciprofloxacin/rifampin or doxycycline/ciprofloxacin be given for 6 months. The infant must be monitored clinically and serologically for signs of Q fever, and a decision regarding treatment must be made on an individual basis. Clearly more data are needed before firm recommendations can be made regarding the treatment of Q fever in pregnancy. In all likelihood, however, Q fever during pregnancy is more common than is currently appreciated.

REFERENCES

1. Akporiaye ET, Rowatt JD, Aragon AS, Baca OG. Lysosomal response of a murine macrophage cell line persistently infected with *Coxiella burnetii*. Infect Immun 1983;40:1155–1162.
2. Baca OG, Scott TO, Akporiaye ET, DeBlassie R, Cussman HA. Cell cycle distribution patterns and generation times of L929 fibroblast cells persistently infected with *Coxiella burnetii*. Infect Immun 1985;47:366–369.
3. Bental T, Fejgin M, Keysary A, Rzotkiewicz S, Oron C, Nachum R, Beyth Y, Lang R. Chronic Q fever of pregnancy presenting as *Coxiella burnetii* placentitis: successful outcome following therapy with erythromycin and rifampin. Clin Infect Dis 1995;21:1318–1321.
4. Fernández-Guerrero JM, Aguado JM, Renedo G, Fraile J, Soriano F, de Villalobos E. Q fever endocarditis on porcine bioprosthetic valves. Ann Intern Med 1988;108:299–213.
5. Heinzen R, Stiegler GL, Whiting LL, Schmitt SA, Mallavia LP, Frazier ME. Use of pulse field gel electrophoresis to differentiate *Coxiella burnetii* strains. In: Hechemy KE, Paretsky D, Walker DH, Mallavia LP, eds. Rickettsiology: current issues and perspectives. Ann NY Acad Sci 1990;590:504–513.
6. Hendrix LR, Samuel JE, Mallavia LP. Differentiation of *Coxiella burnetii* isolates by analysis of restriction-endonuclease-digested DNA separated by SDS-PAGE. J Gen Microbiol 1991;137:269–276.
7. Huebner RJ, Robinson EB. Action of streptomycin in experimental infection with Q fever. Public Health Rep 1948;63:357–362.
8. Jabarit-Aldighieri N, Torres H, Raoult D. Susceptibility of *Rickettsia conorii*, *R. rickettsiae*, and *Coxiella burnetii* to PD 127, 391, PD 131, 628 pefloxacin, ofloxacin, and ciprofloxacin. Antimicrob Agents Chemother 1992;36:2529–2532.
9. Keren G, Keysary A, Goldwasser R, Rubinstein E. The inhibitory effect of fluoroquinolones on *Coxiella burnetii* growth in in vitro systems. J Antimicrob Chemother 1994;33:1254–1255.
10. Levy PY, Drancourt M, Etienne J, Auvergnat JC, Beytout J, Sainty JM, Goldstein F, Raoult D. Comparison of different antibiotic regimens for therapy of 32 cases of Q fever endocarditis. Antimicrob Agents Chemother 1991;35:533–537.
11. Mandell LA, Neiderman M, The Canadian Community-Acquired Pneumonia Consensus Conference Group. Antimicrobial treatment of community-acquired pneumonia in adults: a conference report. Can J Infect Dis 1993;4:25–28.
12. Marrie TJ. Q fever in pregnancy: report of two cases. Infect Dis Clin Pract 1993;2:207–209.
13. Maurin M, Benoliel AM, Bongrand P, Raoult D. Phagolysosomal alkalinization and the bactericidal effect of antibiotics: the *Coxiella burnetii* paradigm. J Infect Dis 1992;166:1097–1102.
14. Muhlemannn K, Matter L, Meyer B, Schopfer K. Isolation of *Coxiella burnetii* from heart values of patients treated for Q fever endocarditis. J Clin Microbiol 1995;33:428–431.
15. Ormsbee RA, Parker H, Pickens EG. The comparative effectiveness of aureomycin, terramycin, chloramphenicol, erythromycin and thiocymetin in suppressing experimental rickettsial infections in chick embryos. J Infect Dis 1955;96:162–167.
16. Ormsbee RA, Pickens EG. A comparison by means of the complement-fixation test of the relative potencies of chloramphenicol, aureomycin, and terramycin in experimental Q fever in embryonated eggs. J Immunol 1951;67:437–448.
17. Pérez-del-Molino A, Aguado JM, Riancho JA, Sampedro I, Matorras P, Gonzalez-Macias J. Erythromycin and the treatment of *Coxiella burnetii* pneumonia. J Antimicrob Chemother 1991;28:455–459.
18. Raoult D, Marrie TJ. Q fever. Clin Infect Dis 1995;20:489–496.
19. Raoult D, Raza A, Marrie TJ. Q fever endocarditis and other forms of chronic Q fever. In: Marrie TJ, ed. Q fever—the disease. Boca Raton, FL: CRC Press, 1990:180–199.
20. Raoult D, Torres H, Drancourt M. Shell-vial assay: evaluation of a new technique for determining antibiotic susceptibility, tested in 13 isolates of *Coxiella burnetii*. Antimicrob Agents Chemother 1991;35:2070–2077.
21. Raoult D, Stein A. Q fever during pregnancy—a risk for women, fetuses and obstetricians. N Engl J Med 1994;330:371.
22. Reichmann N, Raz R, Keysary A, Goldwasser R, Flatau E. Chronic Q fever and severe thrombocytopenia in a pregnant women. Am J Med 1988;85:253–254.
23. Roman MJ, Coriz PD, Baca OG. A proposed model to explain persistent infection of host cells with *C. burnetii*. J Gen Microbiol 1986;132:1415–1422.
24. Samuel JE, Frazier ME, Mallavia LP. Correlation of plasmid type and disease caused by *Coxiella burnetii*. Infect Immun 1985;49:775–777.
25. Sobradillo V, Zalacain R, Capebastegui A, Uresandi F, Corral J. Antibiotic treatment in pneumonia due to Q fever. Thorax 1992;47:276–278.
26. Stein A, Raoult D. Lack of pathotype specific gene in human *Coxiella burnetii*. Microbiol Pathog 1993;15:177–185.
27. Thiele D, Willems H, Kopf G, Krauss H. Polymorphism in DNA restriction patterns of *Coxiella burnetii* isolates investigated by pulsed field gel electrophoresis and image analysis. Eur J Epidemiol 1993;9:419–425.
28. Torres H, Raoult D. In vitro activities of ceftriaxone and fusidic

acid against 13 isolates of *Coxiella burnetii,* determined using the shell vial assay. Antimicrob Agents Chemother 1993;37:491–494.

29. Yeaman MR, Baca OG. Antibiotic susceptibility of *Coxiella burnetii.* In: Marrie TJ, ed. Q fever—the disease. Boca Raton, FL: CRC Press, 1990:213–223.

30. Yeaman MR, Boca OG. Mechanisms that may account for dif-

ferential antibiotic susceptibilities among *Coxiella burnetii* isolates. Antimicrobial Agents Chemother 1991;35:948–954.

31. Yeaman MR, Mitscher LA, Baca OG. In vitro susceptibility of *Coxiella burnetii* to antibiotics, including several quinolones. Antimicrobial Agents Chemother 1987;31:1097–1084.

Ehrlichia Species

●

Johan S. Bakken and J. Stephen Dumler

MICROBIOLOGY

Ehrlichia species are members of the family *Rickettsiaceae,* and the genus *Ehrlichia* currently counts at least 10 species (67). Ehrlichiae are obligate, Gram-negative coccobacilli that exert tropism for predominantly mammalian mononuclear and polymorphonuclear leukocytes (23, 54). Most species also require an arthropod host for parts of their life cycles. Three species are currently known to cause human disease. *E. chaffeensis* is the cause of human monocytic ehrlichiosis, whereas a granulocytic ehrlichia that has yet to be fully characterized is the cause of human granulocytic ehrlichiosis (23). Both illnesses have been primarily described in the United States, but each may also have worldwide distribution (8, 25, 57, 67). The third species, *E. sennetsu,* causes Sennetsu fever, a mononucleosis-like illness that occurs in the Far East and Malaysia (15, 32). All three agents can be cultured in vitro using mammalian continuous cell culture lines.

DIAGNOSIS

A provisional diagnosis of human ehrlichiosis may be made by recognition of characteristic clinical signs and symptoms that follow 1 to 2 weeks after tick exposure or a tick bite (6, 23, 27, 32, 66, 67). Significant laboratory changes include leukopenia, thrombocytopenia, mild elevation of serum hepatic transaminase activities, and elevated C-reactive protein (CRP) values (7, 27, 28, 34). The diagnosis is suggested by detection of characteristic intracytoplasmic leukocyte inclusions (morulae) and confirmed by a fourfold or greater IFA seroconversion or reversion in convalescent blood samples, PCR amplification of species-specific ehrlichial DNA in acute-phase blood samples, in vitro growth of the specific ehrlichial agent in cell culture, or a combination of the above tests (7, 23, 28, 34, 36, 54, 67).

Acute human ehrlichioses may present as nonspecific influenza-like illnesses without diagnostic laboratory clues such as morulae (23, 24). The clinical severity of human ehrlichioses ranges from mild to severe infection with occasional fatal outcome (7, 23, 27, 32, 34, 66), and the fatality rates of human ehrlichioses range from 1.3 to 5.0% (7, 23, 27, 32). Treatment with

an appropriate antibiotic should therefore be instituted empirically as soon as possible in patients with suspected human monocytic ehrlichiosis, since prognosis is inversely related to duration of symptoms before antibiotic therapy is instituted (15, 23, 28, 34, 40, 66). The same recommendation can be made for patients with acute human granulocytic ehrlichiosis, but published experience is limited and not as clear-cut as with human monocytic ehrlichiosis (7).

SUSCEPTIBILITY IN VITRO AND IN VIVO

All ehrlichial species recognized to date appear to be susceptible to tetracyclines and their derivatives (15, 61). Even though the three ehrlichial species that cause human disease all have been cultured in vitro, both *E. chaffeensis* and the agent of human granulocytic ehrlichiosis grow relatively slowly in vitro and at variable success rates (19, 36, 54). In vitro susceptibility tests have rarely been performed, since the testing procedures are laborious and have only recently been described. Furthermore, methods for susceptibility testing have not been standardized, and results may not be directly comparable. Most treatment recommendations have therefore been based on in vivo susceptibility testing in animal models as well as empirical antibiotic therapy and clinical treatment outcomes in humans.

In Vitro Testing

Only a handful of studies have been published on the in vitro susceptibility of ehrlichiae to antibiotic drugs. Rikihisa and Jiang (60) tested the antibiotic susceptibility of a single strain of the equine pathogen *E. risticii* cultured in murine macrophage P388D$_1$ cells and found demeclocycline and doxycycline to be very active (MIC$_{50}$s $\leq$ 0.01 µg/mL). Rifampin and tetracycline were somewhat less active (MIC$_{50}$s were 0.45–0.9 µg/ml and 1–10 µg/mL, respectively). Erythromycin and nalidixic acid were ineffective in eliminating the bacteria in macrophages; chloramphenicol was not tested (60).

Using the P388D$_1$ cell culture line and a single isolate of *E. sennetsu* (Miyayama strain) Brouqui and Raoult noted MICs of 0.125 µg/mL for doxycycline and ciprofloxacin, and 0.5

μg/mL for rifampin (13). In a separate experiment, a single strain of *E. chaffeensis* was grown in a DH 82 canine malignant histiocytic cell culture line, and doxycycline and rifampin both exerted rapid bacteriocidal effects, with MBCs in the extracellular culture medium below 0.5 and 0.125 μg/mL, respectively. Penicillin, chloramphenicol, ciprofloxacin, erythromycin, cotrimoxazole, and gentamicin were all found inactive against *E. chaffeensis;* MICs ranged from 4 to 40 μg/mL (14). Brouqui and Raoult also tested the canine pathogen *E. canis* propagated in the DH82 cell culture line and found that tetracycline and doxycycline effectively eliminated ehrlichiae from the cytoplasm of infected cells (15). Penicillin, erythromycin, chloramphenicol, gentamicin, and cotrimoxazole were all ineffective.

Granulocytic ehrlichiae were considered noncultivable in vitro until Goodman et al. published their recent landmark paper describing a culture method for the agent of human granulocytic ehrlichiosis, using a human promyelocytic continuous cell line HL60 (36). Klein et al. recently found doxycycline and rifampin to be very active against the agent of human granulocytic ehrlichiosis (MICs, 0.25 and 0.5 μg/mL, respectively) (45, 46). Trovafloxacin was also very active (MIC 0.125 μg/mL). Ciprofloxacin and chloramphenicol exerted bacteriostatic effects at 2 and 8 μg/mL, respectively, but were not bactericidal at achievable serum levels. The human granulocytic ehrlichiosis agent was resistant to cotrimoxazole, clindamycin, erythromycin, and

β-lactam drugs. No antibiotic susceptibility studies involving *E. equi* or *E. phagocytophila* have been published to date.

In Vivo Testing

Using a mouse model, Kobayashi et al. (47) tested the efficacy of various antibiotics against *E. sennetsu* and found chlortetracycline and tetracycline to be effective. Erythromycin, penicillin, and chloramphenicol were not effective, even at very high concentrations (47). Tetracycline and various derivatives have been used successfully to treat canine ehrlichiosis, but penicillin, sulfonamides, and chloramphenicol have all been ineffective (17). Delayed therapy may allow development of chronic infections in both mice and dogs.

In summary, doxycycline, tetracycline derivatives, and rifampin appear to be active against *E. risticii, E. canis, E. sennetsu, E. chaffeensis,* and the agent of human granulocytic ehrlichiosis, judged by test outcomes of in vitro susceptibility studies (Table 1). Chloramphenicol, somewhat surprisingly, appears to have no demonstrable in vitro activity against these ehrlichial species despite excellent in vivo activity against closely related rickettsial agents (66, 67). Ciprofloxacin has failed to demonstrate in vitro activity against *E. chaffeensis* but was somewhat active in vitro against the agent of human granulocytic ehrlichiosis, albeit at concentrations that may be difficult to achieve in serum or infected leukocytes.

TABLE 1 • **In Vitro Susceptibility and Clinical Efficacy of Selected Antibiotic Drugs Used for the Treatment of Acute Ehrlichial Infections**[a]

Ehrlichial Species	Mammal Host	Antibiotic Drug	MIC (μg/mL)	In Vitro Susceptibility	Clinical Efficacy	Clinical Failure	Key References[b]
E. canis	Canids	DOXY	≤2	Yes	Yes	Yes[a]	Buhles 1974
		CHLOR	>4	No	No	Yes	Brouqui 1993[b]
							Iqbal 1994
E. risticii	Equines	DOXY	≤0.03	Yes	No[d]	Unknown[d]	Rikihisa 1989[b]
		TCN	0.03	Yes	Yes	No	
		CHLOR	ND	No	Unknown	Unknown	
		RIF	0.45[b]	Yes	Unknown	Unknown	
E. sennetsu	Humans	DOXY	0.25	Yes	Yes	No	Brouqui 1990[b]
		CHLOR	>4	No	No	Unknown	McDade 1990
		RIF	0.5	Yes	Unknown	Unknown	Fine 1994
E. chaffeensis	Humans	DOXY	<0.5	Yes	Yes	No[c]	Maeda 1987
		CHLOR	>16	No	Possible	Yes	Eng 1990
		RIF	0.125	Yes	Unknown	Unknown	Brouqui 1992[b]
							Fishbein 1994
							Dumler 1995
HGE agent	Humans	DOXY	0.25	Yes	Yes	No	Dumler 1995
	Canids	CHLOR	8	No	Possible	Unknown	Wormser 1995
		RIF	0.5	Yes	Unknown	Unknown	Bakken 1996
							Goodman 1996
							Greig 1996
							Klein 1996[b]

[a] Susceptible breakpoint values have not been established for *Ehrlichiae;* ND, not done; DOXY, doxycycline; CHLOR, chloramphenicol; RIF, rifampin; TCN, tetracycline or oxytetracycline; MIC, minimum inhibitory concentration.

[b] Published in vitro antibiotic susceptibility test results.

[c] Late therapy has resulted in chronic infections.

[d] Doxycycline is toxic to horses in therapeutic concentrations.

ANTIMICROBIAL THERAPY
Sennetsu Fever

Sennetsu fever is a self-limited illness that is not known to occur in the United States. The illness often resolves without antibiotic therapy, and the prognosis is excellent. Fatal outcomes have never been described (15, 32, 51, 61, 67). Orally administered tetracycline hydrochloride or doxycycline hyclate is highly effective and should be administered for at least 7 days (32).

Human Monocytic Ehrlichiosis

Most published literature to date recommends tetracyclines and their derivatives as preferred agents for treatment (23, 27, 28, 33, 34, 49, 61, 67). Human monocytic ehrlichiosis is often a relatively mild illness that resolves even without antibiotic therapy after a variable time-course that may last from a few days to several months. Some patients have experienced a severe course, however, and the fatality rate may range from 1.3 to 5% (23, 27, 30, 34). It is generally accepted that all acutely infected patients should be treated, since it may be very difficult to predict who will have mild, self-limited illness. Furthermore, delayed treatment has been associated with more severe illness (34).

Tetracycline hydrochloride or doxycycline hyclate should be administered orally or intravenously and continued for at least 3 days after fever has abated (26, 29, 32, 43, 54, 66, 67, 70) (Table 2). Other authors have recommended minimum lengths of tetracycline therapy that have varied from 7 to 14 days (23, 28). Doxycycline rather than tetracycline has been used in most cases because of its superior body fluid penetra-

---

> **TABLE 2** • **Antibiotic Recommendations for Treatment of Human Monocytic Ehrlichiosis (HME) and Human Granulocytic Ehrlichiosis (HGE)**

1. Doxycycline hyclate: effective
   Adults: 100 mg orally or intravenously at 12-h intervals
   Children: 4.4 mg/kg/day orally or intravenously in two divided doses.
   Duration of therapy
   HME: 7–10 days, or at least 3 days after fever has abated
   HGE: 14 days
   Sennetsu fever: 7–10 days
2. Tetracycline hydrochloride: effective
   Adults: 500 mg orally in four divided doses
   Children: 25–50 mg/kg/day orally in two to four divided doses, or 0.6–1.2 g/m^2/day in two to four divided doses
   Duration of therapy: as for doxycycline hyclate
3. Chloramphenicol: possibly effective
   Adults: 500 mg orally or intravenously at 6-h intervals
   Children: 50 mg/kg/day orally or intravenously at 6-h intervals; maximum individual dose 500 mg each
   Duration of therapy
   HME: 3–10 days
   HGE: 10 days?
4. Rifampin: possibly effective
   Adults: 300 mg orally twice daily
   Children: 10 mg/kg/day orally twice daily
   Maximum individual dose 300 mg each
   Duration of therapy: Unknown

---

tion and lower frequency of gastrointestinal adverse effects (5). Both doxycycline and other tetracycline derivatives exert their effect rapidly, and most patients resolve their fever and feel markedly improved 24 to 48 h after beginning treatment (12, 23, 26, 27, 34, 40). In fact, failure to improve within 48 h after initiation of tetracycline or doxycycline therapy for presumed human monocytic ehrlichiosis should raise questions about whether the diagnosis is correct.

Published reports document that at least 170 patients with acute human monocytic ehrlichiosis have been successfully treated with doxycycline or tetracycline therapy since 1987 (27, 28, 30, 33–35, 41, 49, 59, 62, 64). In a case-controlled study, patients with human monocytic ehrlichiosis who were treated with either a tetracycline or chloramphenicol had significantly shorter intervals of fever and days to complete recovery than patients treated with other antibiotics (34). Relatively few individuals, many whom were children, were treated with only chloramphenicol. In the latter group, chloramphenicol was associated with a significantly longer interval to defervescence than tetracycline alone (34). Abramson and Givner have advocated use of tetracycline for treatment of presumed Rocky Mountain spotted fever regardless of age (1), and similar arguments have been voiced by Edwards for situations in which human monocytic ehrlichiosis is the likely diagnosis (26).

It has long been recognized that dogs treated with tetracycline late in the course of tropical canine pancytopenia (*E. canis*) frequently have relapse of infection after completion of therapy (18, 61). Although posttreatment relapse has not been described in human patients to date, four patients with documented human monocytic ehrlichiosis died either while receiving doxycycline therapy or sometime after completion of therapy (22, 27, 34). Tetracycline therapy was started late in the course of illness in each fatal case (day 9 or later), and two of the patients died more than 50 days after doxycycline or tetracycline therapy had ended. One of these patients had autopsy evidence of *E. chaffeensis* in tissue at the time of death (23). There is not sufficient information reported about the other two patients to determine whether they died while receiving tetracycline therapy (27, 34). Thus, although a tetracycline derivative or doxycycline should be considered the treatment of choice for acute human monocytic ehrlichiosis, the prognosis may worsen proportionally with delayed initiation of therapy.

Chloramphenicol is active against rickettsiae, including *Rickettsia rickettsii*, the cause of Rocky Mountain spotted fever. Because of the close phylogenetic relationship between rickettsial agents and ehrlichiae, chloramphenicol has been advocated as an alternative agent of choice for treatment of human monocytic ehrlichiosis in patients who are either intolerant or have contraindications to tetracycline therapy (9, 10, 20, 21, 27, 30, 34, 36, 40) (Table 2). Forty-one of 47 reported patients (87.2%) have been treated successfully with chloramphenicol for acute human monocytic ehrlichiosis since 1987 (9, 10, 20, 21, 27, 28, 30, 34, 36, 40, 58). Resolution of fever and clinical symptoms occurred within 2 days in most of the responders, but some patients had fever for more than 7 days after therapy had begun. Six of the 47 patients (12.8%) failed to improve with chloramphenicol therapy, and 3 of these patients died (23, 27, 30, 49). Symptoms of human monocytic ehrlichiosis often resolve after 1 to several weeks, even without specific antibiotic treatment. Furthermore, both *E. chaffeensis* and *E. canis* have been found to be resistant to chloramphenicol in vitro (14, 15). Thus, the efficacy of chloramphenicol and the role this drug should play in the treatment of human monocytic ehrlichiosis remains undefined. Patients who fail to respond promptly to chloramphenicol should receive doxycycline hyclate or tetracycline hydrochloride for definitive treatment. Children and pregnant women should receive doxycycline hyclate for as short a time as possible, perhaps no longer than 3 days after fever has resolved, to minimize the risk of adverse effects (7, 26, 67).

There are no reports describing the outcome of rifampin treatment for acute human monocytic ehrlichiosis, but *E. chaffeensis* appears to be highly susceptible to this drug in vitro (14). Thus, rifampin may be a suitable alternative drug for treatment of children under the age of 8 years, pregnant women, and patients who are allergic to tetracycline or doxycycline.

Human Granulocytic Ehrlichiosis

All published therapy recommendations for human granulocytic ehrlichiosis have been based on the response to empirical administration of doxycycline hyclate. Thirty-four of the first 41 patients diagnosed with human granulocytic ehrlichiosis at the Duluth Clinic, Duluth, MN, received doxycycline hyclate for an average of 13 days (7). One of the treated patients who was severely immunocompromised (previous splenectomy and prednisone therapy for chronic lymphocytic leukemia) started doxycycline hyclate treatment on day 14 of the acute illness. He died of fungal pneumonia 5 days after doxycycline therapy had begun, at which time there was no clinical or autopsy evidence of persistent granulocytic ehrlichiosis. In addition, Hardalo et al. described a patient who died a week after completing doxycycline hyclate therapy (38). Autopsy failed to reveal any evidence of persistent granulocytic ehrlichiosis (38). Bakken et al. reported several patients with acute human granulocytic ehrlichiosis who failed to respond to cefazolin, cefotaxime, or erythromycin; all patients rapidly resolved the infections after doxycycline hyclate therapy was initiated (6). Other reported patients have also responded well to doxycycline hyclate therapy (52, 65, 71). Goodman described an acutely infected 64-year-old man who promptly resolved fever and laboratory abnormalities following chloramphenicol administration (36). He had previously developed laryngeal edema after tetracycline therapy. Chloramphenicol is ineffective treatment for *E. equi* infections in horses (48), and since *E. equi* is closely related, or biologically identical, to the agent of human granulocytic ehrlichiosis, chloramphenicol treatment for granulocytic ehrlichiosis must be questioned. There is no published experience with the use of rifampin, clarithromycin, azithromycin, or ciprofloxacin for treatment of acute human granulocytic ehrlichiosis.

In summary, the antibiotic treatment of choice for patients with acute human granulocytic ehrlichiosis infection is doxy-cycline hyclate. Tetracycline hydrochloride should also work well, but clinical data in humans to substantiate this recommendation are limited. Patients with acute human granulocytic ehrlichiosis may have been simultaneously infected with *Borrelia burgdorferi* through the bite of *Ixodes scapularis* ticks (23, 52, 53). Thus, the recommended duration of therapy for human granulocytic ehrlichiosis has been 2 weeks, for adequate treatment of potential human granulocytic ehrlichiosis and Lyme borreliosis coinfection (6, 7, 23).

In the absence of clinical experience with active alternative drugs, it is difficult at this time to give treatment recommendations for children younger than 8 years of age, pregnant women, and individuals known to be hypersensitive to tetracyclines (7, 26). Rifampin exerts in vitro activity against *E. chaffeensis* and the agent of human granulocytic ehrlichiosis and might represent a reasonable alternative treatment choice, but clinical experience is lacking. Trovafloxacin may hold promise as an alternative agent for treating human granulocytic ehrlichiosis, but fluoroquinolones are currently not recommended for use in children and pregnant women. The questionable in vitro activity and relative lack of experience do not permit recommendation of chloramphenicol in the treatment of human ehrlichioses, especially considering the in vitro resistance observed with many veterinary ehrlichial species and the many reports of treatment failure with this drug.

REFERENCES

1. Abramson JS, Givner LB. Should tetracycline therapy be contraindicated for therapy of presumed Rocky Mountain spotted fever in children less than 9 years of age? Pediatrics 1990;86:123–124.
2. Aguero-Rosenfeld ME, Horowitz HW, Wormser GP, McKenna DF, Nowakowski J, Munoz J, Dumler JS. Human granulocytic ehrlichiosis: a case series from a medical center in New York State. Ann Intern Med 1996;125:904–908.
3. Anonymous. Chloramphenicol. In: Lambert HP, O'Grady FW. Antibiotic and chemotherapy. New York: Churchill Livingstone, 1992:136–139.
4. Anonymous. Getting a head start against ehrlichiosis. Emerg Med 1995;May:16–23.
5. Anonymous. Tetracyclines. In: American Hospital Formulary Service 94: drug information. Section 8:12.24. Bethesda, MD: American Society of Hospital Pharmacists, 1994:324–340.
6. Bakken JS, Dumler JS, Chen S-M, Eckman MR, VanEtta LL, Dumler JS. Human granulocytic ehrlichiosis in the upper midwest United States: a new species emerging? JAMA 1994;272:212–218.
7. Bakken JS, Krueth J, Wilson-Nordskog C, Tilden RL, Asanovich K, Dumler JS. Clinical and laboratory characteristics of human granulocytic ehrlichiosis. JAMA 1996;275:199–205.
8. Bakken JS, Krueth J, Tilden RL, Dumler JS, Kristiansen BE. Serological evidence of human granulocytic ehrlichiosis in Norway. Eur J Clin Microbiol Infect Dis 1996;15:829–832.
9. Barton LL, Foy TM. *Ehrlichia canis* infection in a child. Pediatrics 1989;4:580–582.
10. Barton LL, Dawson JE, Letson W, Luisiri A, Scalzo AJ. Simultaneous ehrlichiosis and Lyme disease. Pediatr Infect Dis J 1990;9:127–129.
11. Barton LL. Therapy of human ehrlichiosis reconsidered. Antimicrob Agents Chemother 1991;35:398.

12. Barton LL, Rathore MB, Dawson JE. Infection with Ehrlichia in childhood. J Pediatr 1992;6:998–1001.

13. Brouqui P, Raoult D. In vitro susceptibility of *Ehrlichia sennetsu* to antibiotics. Antimicrob Agents Chemother 1990;34:1593–1596.

14. Brouqui P, Raoult D. In vitro susceptibility of the newly recognized agent of ehrlichiosis in humans, *Ehrlichia chaffeensis*. Antimicrob Agents Chemother 1992;36:2799–2803.

15. Brouqui P, Raoult D. Susceptibility of *Ehrlichiae* to antibiotics. In: Raoult D, ed. Antimicrobial agents and intracellular pathogens. Boca Raton, FL: CRC Press, 1993:182–199.

16. Brouqui P, Raoult D. Human ehrlichiosis with features of toxic shock syndrome. Am J Med 1995;99:107.

17. Buckner RG, Ewing SA. Experimental treatment of canine ehrlichiosis and haemo-bartonellosis. J Am Vet Med Assoc 1967;150:1524–1530.

18. Buhles WC, Huxsoll DL, Ristic M. Tropical canine pancytopenia: clinical, hematologic, and serologic response of dogs to *Ehrlichia canis* infection, tetracycline therapy, and challenge inoculation. J Infect Dis 1974;130:357–367.

19. Dawson JE, Anderson BE, Fishbein DB, Sanchez JL, Goldsmith CS, Wilson KH, Duntley CW. Isolation and characterization of an *Ehrlichia* sp. from a patient diagnosed with human ehrlichiosis. J Clin Microbiol 1991;29:2741–2746.

20. Dimmitt JC, Fishbein DB, Dawson JE. Human ehrlichiosis associated with cerebrospinal fluid pleocytosis: a case report. Am J Med 1989;87:677–678.

21. Doran TI, Parmley RT, Logas PC, Chamblin S. Infection with *Ehrlichia canis* in a child. J Pediatr 1989;114:809–812.

22. Dumler JS, Sutker WL, Walker DH. Persistent infection with *Ehrlichia chaffeensis*. Clin Infect Dis 1993;17:903–905.

23. Dumler JS, Bakken JS. Ehrlichial diseases of humans: emerging tick-borne infections. Clin Infect Dis 1995;20:1102–1110.

24. Dumler JS, Bakken JS. Human granulocytic ehrlichiosis in Wisconsin and Minnesota: a frequent infection with potential for persistence. J Infect Dis 1996;173:1027–1030.

25. Dumler JS, Dotevall L, Gustafson R, Granström M. A population-based seroepidemiologic study of human granulocytic ehrlichiosis and Lyme borreliosis on the west coast of Sweden. J Infect Dis 1997;175:720–722.

26. Edwards M. Ehrlichiosis in children. Semin Pediatr Infect Dis 1994;5:143–147.

27. Eng TR, Harkess JR, Fishbein DB, Dawson JE, Greene CN, Redus MA, Satalowich FT. Epidemiologic, clinical, and laboratory findings of human ehrlichiosis in the United States, 1988. JAMA 1990;264:2251–2258.

28. Everett ED, Evans KA, Henry B, McDonald G. Human ehrlichiosis in adults after tick exposure. Diagnosis using polymerase chain reaction. Ann Intern Med 1994;120:730–735.

29. Feigin R, Snider R, Edwards M. Ehrlichiosis. In: Feigin, Cherry, eds. Textbook of pediatric infectious diseases. 3rd ed. Philadelphia: WB Saunders, 1992:1861–1865.

30. Fichtenbaum CJ, Peterson LR, Weil GJ. Ehrlichiosis presenting as a life-threatening illness with features of the toxic shock syndrome. Am J Med 1993;95:351–357.

31. Finch RG, Mandragos K. Tetracyclines. In: Lambert HP, O'Grady FW. Antibiotic and chemotherapy. New York: Churchill Livingstone, 1992:277–285.

32. Fine DP. Ehrlichiosis. In: Hoeprich, Jordan, Ronald, eds. Infectious diseases. 5th ed. Philadelphia: JB Lippincott, 1994:1281–1284.

33. Fishbein DB, Sawyer LA, Holland CJ, Hayes EB, Okoroanyanwu W, Williams D, Sikes K, Ristic M, McDade JE. Unexplained febrile illness after exposure to ticks. Infection with an *Ehrlichia?* JAMA 1987;257:3100–3104.

34. Fishbein DB, Dawson JE, Robinson LE. Human ehrlichiosis in the United States, 1985 to 1990. Ann Intern Med 1994;120:736–743.

35. Goldman DP, Artenstein AW, Bolan CD. Human ehrlichiosis: a newly recognized tick-borne disease. Am Fam Physician 1992;46:199–208.

36. Goodman JL, Nelson C, Vitale B, Madigan JE, Dumler JS, Kurtti TJ, Munderloh UG. Direct cultivation of the causative agent of human granulocytic ehrlichiosis. N Engl J Med 1996;334:209–215.

37. Greig B, Asanovich KM, Armstrong PJ, Dumler JS. Geographic, clinical, serologic, and molecular evidence of granulocytic ehrlichiosis, a likely zoonotic disease, in Minnesota and Wisconsin dogs. J Clin Microbiol 1996;34:44–48.

38. Hardalo CJ, Quagliarello V, Dumler JS. Human granulocytic ehrlichiosis in Connecticut: report of a fatal case. Clin Infect Dis 1995;21:910–914.

39. Harkess JR, Ewing SA, Brumit T, Mettry CR. Ehrlichiosis in children. Pediatrics 1991;87:199–203.

40. Harkess JR. Ehrlichiosis. Infect Dis Clin North Am 1991;5:37–51.

41. Hawkins MM. Human ehrlichiosis: a case report from the South Carolina low country. J SC Med Assoc 1995;91:228–229.

42. Heyman WR. Human ehrlichiosis. Int J Dermatol 1995;34:618–619.

43. Hornick RB. Human ehrlichiosis (spotless Rocky Mountain spotted fever). In: Bennett, Plum, eds. Cecil textbook of medicine. 20th ed. Philadelphia: WB Saunders, 1996:1733.

44. Iqbal Z, Rikihisa Y. Reisolation of *Ehrlichia canis* from blood and tissue of dogs after doxycycline treatment. J Clin Microbiol 1994;32:1644–1649.

45. Klein MB, Nelson CM, Goodman JL. Antibiotic susceptibility of the newly cultivated agent of human granulocytic ehrlichiosis (HGE) [Abstract E72]. Program and Abstracts of the 36th International Congress of Antibiotics and Chemotherapy; New Orleans, LA, September 15–18, 1996.

46. Klein MB, Nelson CM, Goodman JL. Antibiotic susceptibility of the newly cultivated agent of human granulocytic ehrlichiosis: promising activity of quinolones and rifamycins. Antimicrob Agents Chemother 1997;41:76–79.

47. Kobayashi Y, Ikeda O, Misao T. Chemotherapy of Sennetsu disease. In: Kobayashi Y, Katoura S, Misao T, eds. Progress in virology. Tokyo: Baifukan Publications, 1962:131.

48. Madigan JE, Gribble D. Equine ehrlichiosis in northern California: 49 cases (1968–1981). J Am Vet Med Assoc 1987;190:445–448.

49. Maeda K, Markowitz N, Hawley RC, Ristic M, Cox D, McDade JE. Human infection with *Ehrlichia canis,* a leukocytic ehrlichia. N Engl J Med 1987;316:853–856.

50. Magnarelli LA. Ehrlichiosis: a veterinary problem with growing epidemiologic importance. Clin Microbiol Newslett 1990;12:145–147.

51. McDade JE. Ehrlichiosis—a disease of animals and humans. J Infect Dis 1990;161:609–617.

52. Mitchell PD, Reed KD, Hoefkes JM. Immunoserologic evidence of coinfection with *Borrelia burgdorferi, Babesia microti,* and human granulocytic *Ehrlichia* species in residents of Wisconsin and Minnesota. J Clin Microbiol 1996;34:724–727.

53. Nadelman RB, Horowitz HW, Hsieh T-C, Aguero-Rosenfeld

ME, Schwartz I, Nowakowski J, Wormser GP. Simultaneous human granulocytic ehrlichiosis and Lyme borreliosis. N Engl J Med 1997;337:27–30.

54. Olson JG, Dawson JE. Ehrlichia. In: Murray, Barron, Pfaller, Tenover, Yolken. Manual of clinical microbiology. 6th ed. Washington, DC: American Society for Microbiology, 1995: 686–689.

55. Palmer JE, Benson CE, Whitlock RH. Effect of treatment with oxytetracycline during the acute stages of experimentally induced equine ehrlichial colitis in ponies. Am J Vet Res 1992;53: 2300–2304.

56. Paparone PW, Glenn WB. Lyme disease with concurrent ehrlichiosis. J Am Osteopath Assoc 1994;94:568–577.

57. Petrovec M, Furlan SL, Zupanc TA, Strle F, Brouqui P, Roux V, Dumler JS. Human disease in Europe caused by a granulocytic *Ehrlichia* species. J Clin Microbiol 1997;35:1556–1559.

58. Rathore MH. Infection due to *Ehrlichia canis* in children. South Med J 1992;85:703–705.

59. Rathore MH, Meyer K. Human ehrlichiosis in Florida. J Fla Med Assoc 1993;80:327–329.

60. Rikihisa Y, Jiang BM. In vitro susceptibility of *Ehrlichia risticii* to eight antibiotics. Antimicrob Agents Chemother 1988;32: 986–991.

61. Rikihisa Y. The tribe ehrlichiae and ehrlichial diseases. Clin Microbiol Rev 1991;4:286–308.

62. Salgado JH, Evans ME, Hoven AD, Noble RC. Ehrlichiosis in Kentucky. K Med Assoc J 1995;93:132–135.

63. Sanford JP. Human ehrlichiosis: A therapeutic and diagnostic dilemma in children. Infect Med 1993;10:18–20.

64. Simmons BP, Hughey JR. *Ehrlichia* in Tennessee. South Med J 1989;82:669.

65. Telford SR, Lepore TJ, Snow P, Warner CK, Dawson JE. Human granulocytic ehrlichiosis in Massachusetts. Ann Intern Med 1995;123:277–279.

66. Walker DH, Dumler JS. Ehrlichia chaffeensis (human ehrlichiosis) and other ehrlichiae. In: Mandell, Douglas, Bennett, eds. Infectious diseases in clinical practice. New York: Churchill Livingstone, 1994:1747–1752.

67. Walker DH, Dumler JS. Emergence of ehrlichiosis as human health problems. Emerg Infect Dis 1996;2:18–29.

68. Walker DH. Human ehrlichiosis: more trouble from ticks. Hosp Pract 1996;April 15:47–57.

69. Walker DH. Rickettsial diseases, nearly impossible to diagnose early: clues to pragmatic clinical success. Mediguide Infect Dis 1996;16:1–6.

70. Woodward TE. Ehrlichiosis. In: Harrison's principles of internal medicine. 13th ed. New York: McGraw-Hill, 1994:756.

71. Wormser G, McKenna D, Aguero-Rosenfeld M, Horowitz HE, Munoz J, Nowakowski J, Gerina G. Human granulocytic ehrlichiosis—New York, 1995. MMWR 1995;44:593–595.

Orientia tsutsugamushi[1]

●

Daryl J. Kelly

GENERAL DESCRIPTION

The scrub typhus rickettsiae are Gram-negative obligate intracellular bacteria, coccobacillary in shape, which multiply by binary fission in the cytoplasm of infected cells. Typical in vivo target cells include vascular endothelial cells and macrophages. The rickettsiae fail to grow on axenic media but grow well in cell culture, the yolk sac of embryonated eggs, and laboratory animals including the mouse. Due to major differences from other members of the genus *Rickettsia,* the genus *"Orientia" tsutsugamushi* has been proposed (26).

Scrub typhus, (synonyms: chigger-borne rickettsiosis, tsutsugamushi disease, rural typhus) is an acute zoonotic febrile illness in which humans are incidental dead-end hosts. The symptoms and signs are based upon a disseminated vasculitis involving focal infection of the endothelial vascular cells lining the small blood vessels. The agent is transmitted by the bite of infected larval trombiculid mites or "chiggers," which serve as both reservoir and vector. Infection does not occur until 6 to 8 h of infected chigger attachment, and fever begins 7 to 10 days later (18). Often a local lesion or eschar appears at the site of the chigger bite. Absence of the eschar or a rash can make the diagnosis difficult. Severity of disease depends upon the virulence of the infecting strain and age and immune status of the patient. Left untreated, the clinical disease may last for up to 2 weeks and have a mortality rate of up to 35 % (14). The disease is endemic within an area generally bordered by Papua New Guinea and Queensland, Australia, north to Kamchatka peninsula, Russia, and from Afghanistan east to the Philippines. The endemic region includes Burma, Thailand, Vietnam, Cambodia, Malaysia, India, Pakistan, Japan, Taiwan, Indonesia, China, Korea, and Pacific islands of that region.

The tetracyclines and chloramphenicol have been extremely effective agents for treatment of scrub typhus. However a recent report from Thailand of drug-resistant strains is alarming (29). Alternative agents, including rifampin, clarithromycin, and azithromycin appear promising but require further clinical evaluation.

[1]Disclaimer: The opinions and assertions contained in this paper are the private views of the authors and are not to be construed as official nor as reflecting the views of the Department of the Army, the U.S. Navy Department, the U.S. Naval Service at large, or the Department of Defense.

Specific immunity following recovery can last up to 3.5 years following reinfection with the homologous strain, but immunity is short-lived with heterologous strains (19). Isolates exhibit a high degree of antigenic diversity, complicating the development of vaccines.

SUSCEPTIBILITY IN VITRO AND IN VIVO

Since rickettsiae are obligate intracellular parasites, susceptibility testing cannot be accomplished with traditional culture methods. Experimental systems used for testing susceptibility include cell culture, the murine animal model, and embryonated eggs. In vitro cell culture tests of rickettsial susceptibility are usually performed by plaque reduction assays, dye uptake, or direct counts of infected cells. All of these assays require multiple preparation of tests at each of several concentrations of antibiotics and are not generally available.

The rickettsiostatic antibiotics chloramphenicol and the tetracyclines are traditionally used to treat scrub typhus. Cephalosporins, penicillin, and aminoglycoside antibiotics are not effective. Clinical efficacy is supported by experimental in vitro cell culture models and in vivo animal models (8, 9, 12, 15, 28). Correlation between in vitro and in vivo models is not always consistent, however, and testing methods have not yet been standardized. For example, ciprofloxacin was found to have very good activity in vivo (3, 6) but diminished in vitro susceptibility by the direct cell culture method (8; Strickman, unpublished data).

Until recently, clinically relevant antibiotic-resistant scrub typhus was unreported. Claims of antibiotic-resistant *O. tsutsugamushi* isolates recovered from patients in northern Thailand are supported by both in vitro and in vivo susceptibility testing (29). It remains possible that enhanced virulence, rather than decreased antibiotic susceptibility is contributing to the poorer clinical response to traditional antibiotics among these patients (Kelly, unpublished data). If antibiotic resistance is indeed an emerging problem, new antibiotic agents are needed for successful treatment of patients infected with these strains. Rifampin is known to be active in vitro (9) and is currently undergoing clinical evaluation in Thailand (Watt, unpublished data). The new azilide antibiotic azithromycin has been shown to be active against the doxycycline-resistant strain of *O. tsutsugamushi* (24).

ANTIMICROBIAL THERAPY
Drug of Choice

The tetracyclines and chloramphenicol are standard effective treatments for scrub typhus. As is true with all antibiotics known to be active against scrub typhus, these antibiotics are rickettsiostatic, not rickettsicidal. Patients receiving tetracycline have been reported to respond more rapidly than those receiving chloramphenicol (17) and, unless contraindicated, tetracycline is the preferred agent. Tetracycline and its longer-acting analogue doxycycline can be used interchangeably, although compliance may be better with doxycycline. The usual dose of tetracycline for adults is 500 mg every 6 h, and the usual adult oral dose of doxycycline is 200 mg once followed by 100 mg every 12 h (5). Single-dose (200 mg) doxycycline therapy has been reported to be effective (1). Although not frequently used in the United States, minocycline has been used successfully in Japan to treat scrub typhus (10, 11). Antibiotics are usually continued 7 to 15 days. Response is rapid, usually with improvement in 24 to 36 h. In general, treatment with tetracyclines is associated with favorable outcomes. Failure to defervesce within 48 h suggests an alternate diagnosis or antibiotic resistance as described by Watt (29). In earlier studies, shorter courses of tetracycline or doxycycline or initiation of therapy before day 5 of illness were sometimes associated with relapses 5 to 10 days after therapy (1, 17, 27). However, more recently, a 3-day doxycycline course was found to be as effective as a standard 7-day tetracycline course, with no relapses occurring with either regimen (22).

The tetracyclines are associated with adverse effects that limit their utility. Due to toxic effects on developing teeth and bones, tetracyclines are contraindicated in pregnancy and in

TABLE 1 • **Antibiotic Treatment Recommendations for Scrub Typhus**		
Clinical Situation	**Recommended Treatment Adults**	**Children**
Routine treatment:		
Primary	Doxycycline, 200 mg, day 1 (100 mg every 12 h), followed by 100 mg/day, 3 days[a] (single 200-mg dose may be adequate)	<100 lb: doxycycline 5 mg/kg/day, 7 days; ≥100 lb: adult dosage[b]
Alternative	Chloramphenicol, 500 mg every 6 h, 7–15 days[a, c]	Chloramphenicol, 50 mg/kg/day (divided dose every 6 h), 5 d[a, c] <1 week old, 25 mg/kg/day; 1–4 weeks old, 25 mg/kg/12 h
Alternative	Tetracycline, 25 mg/kg/day (4 divided doses) 3–7 days[b]	
Pregnancy	Chloramphenicol, 500 mg every 6 h, 7–15 days[a, c] Azithromycin 500 mg/day, 3 days[d]	
Doxycycline failure[e]	Azithromycin 500 mg/day, 3 days[d]	

[a]Relapses reported when therapy initiated before 5th febrile day. A repeated dose has been effective.

[b]Permanent tooth discoloration reported with prolonged use in children up to 8 years old (less common with doxycycline).

[c]Blood dyscrasis rarely reported.

[d]Not FDA approved for this indication.

[e]Failure to defervesce within 48 h suggests resistance; defervescence normally occurs within 24 to 36 h.

children under 12 years old. Photosensitivity and gastrointestinal symptoms are also not uncommon.

Chloramphenicol is a broad-spectrum rickettsiostatic antibiotic useful for treatment of scrub typhus (23). Usual adult dosage is 500 mg every 6 hours for 7 to 15 days, and in children, 50–75 mg/kg/day orally for 5 days. It is associated with prolonged fever following initiation of treatment (compared with tetracycline) and in rare cases causes aplastic anemia. It is therefore used as an alternative in situations in which a tetracycline is contraindicated. Patients in whom chloramphenicol therapy is initiated fewer than 5 days after onset of fever often exhibit recrudescent symptoms upon cessation of therapy (17).

Special Situations

There is currently no effective vaccine for scrub typhus. Single-dose chemoprophylaxis with either chloramphenicol (4 g weekly (20)) or doxycycline (200 mg weekly (13, 27)) has been found effective. Both can effectively suppress disease, provided treatment is continued 4 to 6 weeks after exposure, but neither drug is effective when prophylaxis is discontinued shortly after the end of exposure.

Alternative Therapy

Macrolide antibiotics such as azithromycin, clarithromycin, and erythromycin are active in vitro and in vivo against scrub typhus, but there is little clinical experience to support their routine clinical use (7, 24). Azithromycin has been used successfully to treat a few patients in Thailand, including in areas where antibiotic resistance is known to occur (Silpapojakul, Pacharee, unpublished data). Clarithromycin was used successfully at a dose of 400 mg/day for 12 to 19 days to treat three patients in Japan (7). Ciprofloxacin, 500 mg every 12 h, was also used to treat a patient in Nepal (3). The patient defervesced within 24 h. Studies are ongoing in Thailand to evaluate the clinical efficacy of rifampin (Watt, unpublished data).

ENDPOINTS FOR MONITORING THERAPY

Successful therapy is associated with rapid defervescence following initiation of treatment. Most patients become afebrile within 48 h. Failure to respond promptly should raise the suspicion of an alternate diagnosis or the possibility of antibiotic resistance. There are no useful laboratory parameters of successful treatment. Serology cannot be used, since antibody titers can continue to rise during otherwise effective therapy (10). While potentially useful in establishing diagnosis, the polymerase chain reaction (PCR) is of limited value as a treatment monitor, since circulating rickettsiae can be detected by PCR up to 8 days after initiation of antibiotic (10). Viable scrub typhus rickettsiae have been recovered from the lymph nodes of patients from 5 to 15 months after effective treatment, but spontaneous recurrence of clinical disease has not been observed (21). Specific IgM and IgG antibodies rise late in the first week of illness, and serodiagnosis can be done by the standard indirect fluorescent antibody (IFA) test, indirect immunoperoxidase (IIP) test (4), or dot-ELISA (30) (Dip-S-Ticks, Integrated Diagnostics, Balti-more, MD). The latter test was shown to be positive as early as the fifth febrile day (30).

CAVEATS AND COMMENTS

The origin of reported chloramphenicol and tetracycline resistance in Thailand is not obvious because the nature of the host-vector relationship suggests an absence of selective pressure toward drug resistance. An alternative explanation may be that these strains are more virulent, a phenomenon that has been observed in preliminary in vitro studies with strains from other regions of Thailand (Kelly, unpublished data). This issue is clinically relevant because several scrub typhus patients in the region of northern Thailand where resistance is found died while receiving appropriate antibiotic therapy (Watt, unpublished data). Use of chemoprophylaxis in such areas might present cause for concern. Currently there is no evidence of resistance occurring anywhere outside Thailand.

Disease incidence appears to be on the rise as well (16, 25). The apparent increase in Japan may be partially explained by increased use of β-antibiotics in the 1970s for treatment of febrile illnesses in place of chloramphenicol and the tetracyclines.

Scrub typhus may be difficult to diagnose as the clinical presentation can be similar to several other febrile illnesses such as dengue fever, hantavirus, leptospirosis, and typhoid. Often the pathognomic eschar is not present, or the typical rash may not be apparent if the patient has dark skin. The Weil-Felix test, while relatively specific, is somewhat insensitive, often as low as 50% early in the course of disease and should be supplanted by the more sensitive and specific IIP, IFA, or other commercial tests (2, 4, 30). However, these tests are not yet widely available. Often prompt defervescence following empirical treatment with chloramphenicol, tetracycline, or doxycycline is used to confirm the clinical impression. Thus, patients who fail to respond in typical fashion might be missed.

In view of evidence for emerging strains that respond poorly to standard treatment and possible antibiotic resistance as well as the need to identify drugs acceptable for the safe, effective treatment of children and pregnant women, continued development of new antibiotics and vaccines is needed. The possible spread of untreatable scrub typhus threatens to return us to the preantibiotic era such as occurred during World War II when tens of thousands of cases occurred in Asian and European soldiers in the Asia-Pacific region (14). While a disease described over 2000 years ago by Chinese physicians may not be classed as "emerging," an appreciation of its ubiquity and potential severity is reemerging.

REFERENCES

1. Brown GW, Saunders JP, Singh S, Huxsoll DL, Shirai A. Single dose doxycycline therapy for scrub typhus. Trans R Soc Trop Med Hyg 1978;72:412–416.
2. Chouriyagune C, Watt G, Strickman D, Jinasen R. The Weil-Felix test for the diagnosis of scrub typhus in Thailand. Intern Med 1992;8:29–33.
3. Eaton M, Cohen MT, Shlim DR, Innes B. Ciprofloxacin treatment of typhus. JAMA 1989;262:772–773.

4. Kelly DJ, Wong PW, Gan E, Chan C-T, Cowan D, Lewis GE Jr. Multi-laboratory evaluation of a scrub typhus diagnostic kit. Am J Trop Med Hyg 1990;43:301–307.

5. Maurin M, Raoult D. Optimum treatment of intracellular infection. Drugs 1996;52:45–59.

6. McClain JB, Joshi B, Rice R. Chloramphenicol, gentamycin, and ciprofloxacin against murine scrub typhus. Antimicrob Agents Chemother 1988;32:285–286.

7. Miura N, Kudoh Y, Osabe M, Shimoda T, Kohno S, Hara K. Three cases of tsutsugamushi disease successfully treated with clarithromycin. Acta Med Nagasaki 1995;40:44–47.

8. Miyamura S, Ohta T, Tamura A. Comparison of in vitro susceptibilities of *Rickettsia prowazekii*, *R. rickettsii*, *R. sibirica* and *R. tsutsugamushi* to antimicrobial agents. Nippon Saikingaku Zasshi 1989;44:717–721.

9. Miyamura S, Sato N, Tamura A. In vitro susceptibility of recent clinical isolates of *Rickettsia tsutsugamushi* to chemotherapeutic agents. Kansenshogaku Zasshi 1985;59:486–488.

10. Murai K, Okayama A, Horinouchi H, Oshikawa T, Tachibana N, Tsubouchi H. Eradication of *Rickettsia tsutsugamushi* from patients' blood by chemotherapy, as assessed by the polymerase chain reaction. Am J Trop Med Hyg 1995;52:325–327.

11. Nakagawa Y, Huruie H, Satou H, Matsumoto Y. A case of severe tsutsugamushi disease without eruption. J Jpn Assoc Infect Dis 1994;68:1433–1436.

12. Ohashi N. Susceptibility to chemotherapeutic agents. In: Kawamura A Jr, Tanaka H, Tamura A, eds. Tsutsugamushi disease. Tokyo: University of Tokyo Press, 1995:90–94.

13. Olson JG, Bourgeois AL, Fang RC, Coolbaugh JC, Dennis DT. Prevention of scrub typhus: prophylactic administration of doxycycline in a randomized double blind trial. Am J Trop Med Hyg 1980;29:989–997.

14. Philip CB. Tsutsugamushi disease (scrub typhus) in World War II. J Parasitol 1948;34:169–191.

15. Raoult D, Drancourt M. Antimicrobial therapy of rickettsial diseases. Antimicrob Agents Chemother 1991;35:2457–2462.

16. Rapmund G. Rickettsial diseases of the Far East: new perspectives. J Infect Dis 1984;149:330–338.

17. Sheehy TW, Hazlett D, Turk RE. Scrub typhus: a comparison of chloramphenicol and tetracycline in its treatment. Arch Intern Med 1973;132:77–80.

18. Shirai A, Saunders JP, Dohany AL, Huxsoll DL, Groves MG. Transmission of scrub typhus to human volunteers by laboratory-reared chiggers. Jpn J Med Sci Biol 1982;35:9–16.

19. Smadel JE. Influence of antibiotics on immunologic responses in scrub typhus. Am J Med 1954;17:246–258.

20. Smadel JE, Traub R, Frick LP, Diercks FH, Bailey CA. Chloramphenicol (chloromycetin) in the chemoprophylaxis of scrub typhus (tsutsugamushi disease) III. Suppression of overt disease by prophylactic regimens of four-week duration. Am J Hyg 1950;51:216–223.

21. Smadel JE, Ley HL, Jr, Diercks FH, Cameron JAP. Persistence of *Rickettsia tsutsugamushi* in tissues of patients recovered from scrub typhus. Am J Hyg 1952;56:294–302.

22. Song JH, Lee C, Chang WH, Choi SW, Choi JE, Kim YS, Cho SR, Ryu J, Pai CH. Short-course doxycycline treatment versus conventional tetracycline therapy for scrub typhus: a multicenter randomized trial. Clin Infect Dis 1995;21:506–510.

23. Standiford HC. Tetracyclines and chloramphenicol. In: Mandell GL, Douglas RG, Bennett JE, eds. Principles and practice of infectious diseases. 3rd ed. New York: Churchill Livingstone, 1990:284–295.

24. Strickman D, Sheer T, Salata K, Hershey J, Dasch G, Kelly D, Kuschner R. In vitro effectiveness of azithromycin against doxycycline-resistant and -susceptible strains of *Rickettsia tsutsugamushi*, etiologic agent of scrub typhus. Antimicrob Agents Chemother 1995;39:2406–2410.

25. Suto T. Rapid and accurate serologic diagnosis of tsutsugamushi disease in Japan employing the immunoperoxidase reaction In: Kazar, ed. Rickettsiae and rickettsial diseases. Bratislava: Czechoslovakia Publishing House of the Slovak Academy of Sciences, 1985:444–452.

26. Tamura A, Ohashi N, Urakami H, Miyamura S. Classification of *Rickettsia tsutsugamushi* in a new genus, *Orientia* gen. nov., as *Orientia tsutsugamushi* comb. nov. Int J Syst Bacteriol 1995;45:589–591.

27. Twartz JC, Shirai A, Selvaraju G, Saunders JP, Huxsoll DL, Groves DL. Doxycycline prophylaxis for human scrub typhus. J Infect Dis 1982;146:811–818.

28. Urakami H, Tamura A, Miyamura S. Susceptibilities of recent clinical isolates of *Rickettsia tsutsugamushi* to chemotherapeutic agents. Kansenshogaku Zasshi 1988;62:931–937.

29. Watt G, Chouriyagune C, Ruangweerayud R, Watcharapichat P, Phulsuksombati D, Jongsakul K, Teja-Isavadharm P, Bhodidatta D, Corcoran KD, Dasch GA, Strickman D. Scrub typhus infections poorly responsive to antibiotics in northern Thailand. Lancet 1996;348:86–89.

30. Weddle JR, Chan T-C, Thompson K, Paxton H, Kelly DJ, Dasch G, Strickman D. Effectiveness of a dot-blot immunoassay of anti-*Rickettsia tsutsugamushi* antibodies for serologic analysis of scrub typhus. Am J Trop Med Hyg 1995;53:43–46.

Rickettsia akari

D. Raoult and M. Maurin

GENERAL DESCRIPTION
Epidemiology

Rickettsia akari was classified in the spotted fever group rickettsiae both because it cross-reacts with other spotted fever group rickettsiae and because it is found both in the cytoplasm and the nucleus of infected eukaryotic cells. However, unlike other spotted fever group rickettsiae, it does not cross-react with *Proteus* OX-19 strain. It is the etiologic agent of rickettsialpox, a disease first described in the United States, especially in New York, in the 1940s. The disease was later characterized in the former USSR, and more recently in Slovenia.

Clinical Manifestations

Rickettsialpox is a zoonotic disease that is transmitted to humans by the painless bite of mouse mites (*Allodermanyssus sanguineus*). The organism is transmitted among mice (*Mus musculus*) by their ectoparasites. Outbreaks may occur in humans when adequate control of mouse populations and their ectoparasites is lacking.

Rickettsialpox is characterized by an incubation period of 7 to 10 days and an acute onset, typically with fever, chills, headache, myalgia, and photophobia. A red papule evolving into a vesicle with regional lymphadenopathy often develops at the site of the mite bite. A papulovesicular cutaneous rash typically supervenes 2 to 3 days after onset and becomes generalized. The formation of vesicles differentiate rickettsialpox from other spotted fever group rickettsiosis. Vesicles may then dry out to be replaced by a crust that usually does not produce a scar. The disease is considered benign, with spontaneous resolution in 2 to 3 weeks. Complications and death are very rare.

Microbiology

Rickettsiae are strict intracellular bacteria that multiply within the cytoplasm of eukaryotic cells. They escape the phagosomal compartment at the very beginning of phagosomal vacuole formation. In infected humans, the main target cells are endothelial cells. To be active, antibiotics should reach the intracellular cytoplasmic compartment of eukaryotic cells and mainly that of infected endothelial cells.

SUSCEPTIBILITY IN VITRO AND IN VIVO

Because of their obligate intracellular lifestyle, susceptibility of rickettsiae to antibiotics cannot be assessed in conventional microbiologic tests. Three types of experimental models have been developed to test the antibiotic susceptibility of rickettsiae: animal models, the embryonated egg model, and cell culture models. Animal models and the embryonated egg model were the first described; however, antibiotic doses used in these models were much higher than those usually used in humans, and therefore it is difficult to extrapolate data to the clinical situation. In vitro infected cell models have been more recently elaborated. These allow more convenient investigation of the antibiotic susceptibility of rickettsiae, and extracellular antibiotic concentrations used in these models may be compared with antibiotic concentrations obtained in human sera.

Single Drug
Animal Models

Animal models for rickettsial infections use mainly mice and guinea pigs. However, the clinical manifestations of infected animals do not usually reproduce those of human disease and may vary with the animal species investigated as well as with the rickettsial strain investigated. The reliability of animal models for rickettsial infections remains to be established.

In vivo antibiotic activity has been evaluated in mice infected with *R. akari* either intraperitoneally or intranasally and treated subcutaneously with chlortetracycline (Aureomycin) for 12 days, starting 24 h postinfection (14). Chlortetracycline (1 mg daily) allowed survival of all infected animals, whereas death occurred in two-thirds of the untreated controls, whether infected by the intraperitoneal or the intranasal route (14).

Embryonated Egg Model

In the embryonated egg model, rickettsiae were injected into the yolk sac of the eggs. This resulted in death of the embryo usually within the first week following infection. Antibiotics were administered by the same route, usually within the first hour following rickettsial inoculation. Antibiotic activity was deduced from the difference in mean survival time (DMST) of infected embryos receiving antibiotics and untreated infected controls. A rickettsiostatic effect of antibiotics allowed the embryos to survive up to the last day of experiments, usually 14 days. The rickettsiacidal activity of antibiotics was assessed from subculture of yolk sacs from surviving eggs at 14 days postinfection. Direct examination of smears prepared from infected tissues and stained with the Gimenez technique was also informative regarding the action of antibiotics. However, this model did not allow direct evaluation of the growth rate of rickettsiae.

R. akari MK strain has been used in most antibiotic susceptibility experiments. In early experiments, streptomycin was shown to display only moderate activity at high concentrations (10,000–20,000 µg/egg) (8). The activity of gentamicin was more recently evaluated against *R. akari* Hartford strain (11). Embryo death was delayed by 48 h at a concentration of 500 µg/egg (11), which confirmed the poor in

TABLE 1 • **In Vitro Antibiotic Susceptibility of *R. akari* (MK strain, and Davis # 7 strain). Minimum concentrations (μg/egg) to obtain DMST ≥ 2.5 days and MICs (μg/mL) are presented for the embryonated egg and cell culture models, respectively.**

Antibiotics	Embryonated Eggs (μg/egg)	Cell Cultures (μg/mL)	Strain	References
Amoxicillin		128	MK	Raoult, unpublished data
Streptomycin	10,000		MK	8
Dihydrostreptomycin	40,000		MK	8
Gentamicin	>500		MK	11
		8	MK	Raoult, unpublished data
Chloramphenicol	250		MK	2
	162		Davis #7	6
		30	MK	3
Thiamphenicol		1	MK	Raoult, unpublished data
Chlortetracycline	125		MK	2
		130	Davis #7	6
Oxytetracycline		15	Davis #7	6
	30		MK	9
Tetracycline		30	MK	3
Doxycycline		0.06	MK	Raoult, unpublished data
Erythromycin	290		Davis #7	6
		15	MK	3
		8	MK	Raoult, unpublished data
		16	ATCC VR-612	1
Dirithromycin		16	ATCC VR-612	1
Roxithromycin		8	ATCC VR-612	1
Azithromycin		0.25	ATCC VR-612	1
Clarithromycin		2	ATCC VR-612	1
		2	MK	Raoult, unpublished data
Josamycin		1	MK	Raoult, unpublished data
Pristinamycin		4	MK	Raoult, unpublished data
Pefloxacin		1	MK	Raoult, unpublished data
Ofloxacin		0.5	MK	Raoult, unpublished data
Ciprofloxacin		0.5	MK	Raoult, unpublished data
Rifampicin		0.25–0.5	MK	Raoult, unpublished data
Sulfamethoxazole		>8	MK	Raoult, unpublished data

vitro rickettsiostatic activity of aminoglycosides. PABA (*p*-aminobenzoic acid) was not effective at a concentration of 1000 μg/egg (8). A DMST of 2.3 days was obtained with 125 μg/egg of chloromycetin (7). Oxytetracycline (Terramycin) was more effective, with a DMST of 2.3 days at only 10 μg/egg (9). Chlortetracycline allowed embryo death delay of more than 2.5 days at concentrations of 125 μg/egg or higher (2, 6). In the same study, chloramphenicol induced a DMST of 2 days at 125 μg/egg, and 4.9 days at 250 μg per egg, showing moderate rickettsiostatic activity (2). Ormsbee et al. (6) tested the activity of chlortetracycline, oxytetracycline, erythromycin, chloramphenicol, and thiomycetin against *R. akari* (Davis #7 strain) in embryonated eggs. A DMST of 2.5 or more days was obtained with 130 μg/egg of chlortetracycline, 180 μg/egg for erythromycin, 162 μg/egg for chloramphenicol, and only 14 μg/egg with thiomycetin, and 15 μg/egg with oxytetracycline, which confirmed the high activity of tetracycline molecules.

Cell Culture Models

The primary target cells for rickettsiae are endothelial cells. However a number of eukaryotic cell lines can be infected with rickettsiae in vitro, including fibroblasts, macrophages, primary chick embryo cells, and human endothelial cells. Plaque formation in infected cell cultures was first used for numeration of viable rickettsiae (3, 4, 10, 12) and then adapted to determine their in vitro antibiotic susceptibility (3, 5, 13). The plaque assay system is currently the recommended technique, allowing evaluation of both the bacteriostatic and the bactericidal activity of antibiotics. Cell monolayers (usually Vero cells) grown in tissue culture Petri dishes are acutely infected by rocking incubation with a rickettsial inoculum. Infected cells are then overlaid with Eagle MEM with 2% fetal calf serum and 0.5% agar. Antibiotics are added at different concentrations at the same time, with no antibiotics added to drug-free controls. Petri dishes are incubated 7 to 10 days at 37°C in a 5% CO_2 atmosphere. Cell monolayers are then stained with neutral red dye, allowing visualization of the plaques. The MICs are defined as the lowest antibiotic concentration allowing complete inhibition of plaque formation, compared with a drug-free control. More recently, a new cell culture system was described by Ives et al. (1) who determined the inhibition of *Rickettsia* proliferation by comparing rickettsial growth in infected Vero cell cultures incubated in the presence of an antibiotic with that in drug-free controls. Infected cells were revealed by an indirect immunofluorescent antibody method.

Early reports, using the plaque assay system, have demonstrated that β-lactams and aminoglycosides are poorly effective against rickettsiae, including *R. akari* (3). Tetracyclines are the most effective antibiotic compounds, with MICs to doxycycline of 0.06 μg/mL. Chloramphenicol and thiamphenicol display in vitro rickettsiostatic activity (3; Raoult, unpublished data). Whereas erythromycin was shown to be poorly effective (3), the newly available macrolide compounds azithromycin and clarithromycin display lower MICs (1; Raoult, unpublished data). However, josamycin remains the most effective macrolide compound tested (Raoult, unpublished data). Nalidixic acid is poorly effective against *R. akari* (3). A more recent investigation indicates that *R. akari* (ATCC VR-612) is susceptible to the newer fluoroquinolones compounds pefloxacin, ofloxacin, and ciprofloxacin (Raoult, unpublished data).

ANTIMICROBIAL THERAPY
Drug of Choice

The conventional antibiotic regimen for spotted fever group rickettsiosis is a 7- to 10-day oral course of doxycycline 200 mg daily. There are no clinical data indicating that a single-day regimen may be sufficient to treat rickettsialpox.

Combination therapy is not indicated in common clinical presentations of rickettsialpox, which is primarily a disease with favorable spontaneous prognosis.

Alternative Therapy

The real limitation of antibiotic therapy using tetracycline compounds is the possibility of side effects, including gastric intolerance, and the possibility of dental coloration in the neonate and young child. Thus, tetracyclines are contraindicated in pregnant women and in children. Chloramphenicol for at least 1 week is classically considered an effective alternative. However it presents the potential risk of aplastic anemia and is also contraindicated in pregnant women. Although the in vitro activity of fluoroquinolones, josamycin, and the newer macrolides (azithromycin and clarithromycin) seems promising, no clinical trials are available.

REFERENCES

1. Ives TJ, Manzewitsch P, Regnery RL, Butts JD, and Kebede M. In vitro susceptibilities of *Bartonella henselae, B. quintana, B. elizabethae, Rickettsia rickettsii, R. conorii, R. akari,* and *R. prowazekii* to macrolide antibiotics as determined by immunofluorescent-antibody analysis of infected Vero cell monolayers. Antimicrob Agents Chemother 1997;41:578–582.
2. Jackson EB. Comparative efficacy of several antibiotics on experimental rickettsial infections in embryonated eggs. Antibiotics Chemother 1951;1:231–241.
3. McDade JE. Determination of antibiotic susceptibility of *Rickettsia* by the plaque assay technique. Appl Microbiol 1969; 18:133–135.
4. McDade JE, Gerone PJ. Plaque assay for Q fever and scrub typhus rickettsiae. Appl Microbiol 1970;19:963–965.
5. McDade JE, Stakebake JR, Jerone PJ. Plaque assay system for several species of *Rickettsia.* J Bacteriol 1969;99:910–912.
6. Ormsbee RA, Parker H, Pickens EG. The comparative effectiveness of chlortetracycline, terramycin, chloramphenicol, erythromycin, and thiomycetin in suppressing experimental rickettsial infections in chick embryos. J Infect Dis 1955;96: 162–167.
7. Smadel JE, Jackson EB, Cruise AB. Chloromycetin in experimental rickettsial infections. J Immunol 1949;62:49–65.
8. Smadel JE, Jackson EB, Gauld RL. Factors influencing the growth of rickettsiae. I. Rickettsiostatic effect of streotomycin in experimental infections. J Immunol 1947;57:273–284.
9. Snyder JC, Fagan R, Wells EB, Wicks HC, Miller JC. Experimental studies on the antirickettsial properties of terramycin. Ann NY Acad Sci 1950;53:362–374.
10. Weinberg EH, Stakebake JR, Gerone PJ. Plaque assay for *Rickettsia rickettsii.* J Bacteriol 1969;98:398–402.
11. White LA, Hall HE, Tzianabos T, Chappell WA. Effect of gentamicin on growth of viral, chlamydial, and rickettsial agents in mice and embryonated eggs. Antimicrob Agents Chemother 1976;10:344–346.
12. Wike DA, Tallent G, Peacock MG, Williams JC. Studies of the rickettsial plaque assay technique. Infect Immun 1972;5: 715–722.
13. Wisseman CL, Waddell AD, Walsh WT. In vitro studies of the action of antibiotics on *Rickettsia prowazekii* by two basic methods of cell culture. J Infect Dis 1974;130:564–574.
14. Wong SC, Cox HR. Action of aureomycin against experimental rickettsial and viral infections. Ann NY Acad Sci 1948;51: 290–305.

Rickettsia prowazekii

M. Maurin and D. Raoult

GENERAL DESCRIPTION
Epidemiology

Rickettsia prowazekii, a typhus group rickettsia, is the etiologic agent of epidemic or louse-borne typhus. Human-to-human transmission of the disease in most cases occurs via the human body louse (*Pediculus humanis corporis*). Both the body louse and humans may suffer and even die from *R. prowazekii* infection. Epidemic typhus was first considered a disease restricted to the human being. The observation of recurrent infection in humans, referred to as Brill-Zinsser disease, suggests man may act as a reservoir for the bacteria and explains the maintenance of the disease between epidemics. More recent data indicate that flying squirrels (*Glaucomys volans*) in North America may also represent a reservoir for *R. prowazekii* (3). The disease, referred as indigenous epidemic typhus, may be acquired from flying squirrel–parasitizing arthropods.

Epidemic typhus is considered primarily a disease of war. However, the disease is still prevalent in areas where poor socioeconomic conditions and a high prevalence of louse infestation allow human-to-human transmission of *R. prowazekii*. The present distribution of epidemic typhus corresponds to Africa, especially in the central eastern African countries (Burundi, Zaire, Rwanda), mountainous regions of South America (including Peru), the Himalayan regions, and mountainous or highland regions of North America. Most cases occur during the cold months, when heavy clothing and poor sanitary conditions allow infestation by body lice.

Clinical Manifestations

Incubation period of the disease is usually 1 to 2 weeks but can be shorter in severe forms of the disease. Prodromal symptoms include headache, arthralgia (especially in the large joints), and malaise. Onset is typically abrupt, with persistent headache, chills, and high-grade fever. Nausea and vomiting are often present. Prostration is frequent, although of variable degree. Characteristically, a cutaneous rash appears after 4 to 5 days of illness, first visible in axillae and the inner surfaces of the arms. The rash then extends to the trunk but usually does not affect the face or extremities. Early lesions are maculae, which become papulae in a few days. In more severe cases, the rash may become petechial and even hemorrhagic and necrotic. In approximately 20% of patients, the rash is absent, which hampers clinical diagnosis. Complications may occur and lead to death in about 20% of patients, a figure that may be higher in uncontrolled situations. The diversity of the rickettsial microvascular injuries in the infected patient explains the wide spectrum of clinical manifestations and life-threatening complications that may be encountered. Complications include neurologic disorders (meningitis, encephalitis, muttering delirium, coma), cardiac failure, vascular complications (mainly gangrene), intestinal complications, and renal failure.

Brill-Zinsser disease is characterized by recurrence of fever, and headaches. The clinical manifestations are similar to those of epidemic typhus, but Brill-Zinsser disease is usually milder, and the cutaneous rash is most often absent. Clinical diagnosis of Brill-Zinsser disease may be difficult when the patient's clinical history is not available. Weil-Felix reaction is negative, and compared with epidemic or murine typhus, IgG but not IgM is detected by specific serologic reactions.

Indigenous epidemic typhus has been described in the eastern United States. In this region, 15 clinical cases have been extensively described by McDade et al. (12), and Duma et al. (4). These cases occurred during the colder months, from November to March. Most patients had an abrupt onset with high fever, headache, and myalgia. A cutaneous rash was noticed in about half the patients (8 of 15). Clinical manifestations suggesting central nervous system involvement, including meningismus, confusion, delirium, and coma, were observed in 40% (6 of 15). The disease was considered milder than classical epidemic typhus, although it remains potentially life threatening.

Microbiology

Rickettsiae are strict intracellular bacteria that multiply within the cytoplasm of eukaryotic cells. They escape the phagosomal compartment at the very beginning of the phagosomal vacuole formation. In vivo, the main target cells are endothelial cells in infected humans and animals. The close association of rickettsiae with their eukaryotic cell hosts explains the possibility of chronic infection and the late resurgence of Brill-Zinsser disease. To be active, antibiotics should reach the intracellular cytoplasmic compartment where rickettsiae multiply. Probably, antibiotics do not have the ability to cure *R. prowazekii*–infected endothelial cells.

SUSCEPTIBILITY IN VITRO AND IN VIVO

Because of their obligate intracellular lifestyle, susceptibility of rickettsiae to antibiotics cannot be assessed in conventional microbiologic tests. As epidemic typhus is primarily a human disease, no animal model is available. Fever was observed in guinea pigs injected intraperitoneally with *R. prowazekii* (27); however, this model does not reproduce the clinical manifestations or the route of infection of epidemic typhus in humans. Its reliability for epidemic typhus infections has not been established. *R. prowazekii*–infected lice have been used to test the

TABLE 1 • **In Vitro Antibiotic Susceptibility of *R. prowazekii*. Minimum concentrations (mg/egg) to obtain DMST >2.5 days and MICs (µg/mL) are presented for the embryonated egg and cell culture models, respectively.**

Antibiotics	Embryonated Eggs (µg/egg)	Cell Cultures MICs (µg/mL)	Strain	References
Penicillin G	162		Breinl	15
Amoxicillin		128	Breinl	Raoult, unpublished data
Streptomycin	10,000		Breinl	19
Gentamicin		16	Breinl	Raoult, unpublished data
Chloramphenicol		1	Breinl	25
Thiamphenicol		1	Breinl	Raoult, unpublished data
Chlortetracycline	129		Breinl	15
Oxytetracycline	30		Breinl	20
	10		Breinl	15
Tetracycline		0.01–0.1	Breinl	25
Doxycycline		0.1	Breinl	25
Minocycline		0.01–0.1	Breinl	25
Erythromycin	15		Breinl	15
		0.06	Breinl	25
		2	Madrid E	7
Dirithromycin		16	Madrid E	7
Roxithromycin		1	Madrid E	7
Azithromycin		0.25	Madrid E	7
Clarithromycin		0.125	Madrid E	7
		1	Breinl	Raoult, unpublished data
Josamycin		1	Breinl	Raoult, unpublished data
Ciprofloxacin		0.5	Breinl	Raoult, unpublished data
Ofloxacin		1	Breinl	Raoult, unpublished data
Pefloxacin		1	Breinl	Raoult, unpublished data
Rifampin		0.008	Breinl	25
Sulfamethoxazole		>4	Breinl	Raoult, unpublished data

activity of antibiotics against this rickettsia. The antibiotic susceptibility of *R. prowazekii* has also been determined in the embryonated egg model and, more recently, in cell culture systems.

Single Drug

Arthropod Model
Infected body lice were used as an in vivo model to test the antibiotic susceptibility of *R. prowazekii* to antibiotics (1, 2, 9). Lice usually die from infection with *R. prowazekii*. Infected lice received either doxycycline or rifampin. Both antibiotics inhibited rickettsial growth and delayed death of infected body lice but only during antibiotic administration, which suggests that antibiotics were bacteriostatic, not bactericidal.

Embryonated Egg Model

In the embryonated egg model, rickettsiae were injected into the yolk sac of the eggs. This resulted in death of the embryo, usually within a few days following infection. Antibiotics were administered by the same route, usually within the first hour following rickettsial inoculation. Antibiotic activity was deduced from the difference in mean survival time (DMST) of infected embryos receiving antibiotics and infected untreated controls. A rickettsiostatic effect of antibiotics allowed the embryos to survive up to the last day of experiments, usually day 14. The rickettsiacidal activity of antibiotics was assessed by subculture of yolk sacs from surviving eggs at 14 days postinfection. Direct examination of smears prepared from infected tissues and

stained with the Gimenez technique has also been used to evaluate the action of antibiotics; however this does not allow direct evaluation of the growth rate of rickettsiae.

In the embryonated egg model, penicillin G and the aminoglycoside compounds streptomycin and gentamicin were not effective (19, 23). *p*-Aminobenzoic acid (PABA) was poorly effective at concentrations of 10,000 µg/egg and above (19). Chloromycetin allowed a DMST of 2.5 days or longer at concentrations of 250 µg/egg and above (18). Oxytetracycline (Terramycin) and to a lesser extent chlortetracycline (Aureomycin) and chloramphenicol were considered rickettsiostatic (15, 20). Erythromycin was found to be effective against *R. prowazekii*. However, Weiss et al. (22) demonstrated that in vitro, *R. prowazekii* could readily become resistant to this antibiotic after only 3 passages in embryonated eggs in the presence of progressively increasing erythromycin concentrations. Such results suggested the possibility of in vivo emergence of resistant strains.

Cell Culture Models
The primary target cells for rickettsiae are endothelial cells. However a number of eukaryotic cell lines can be infected with rickettsiae in vitro, including fibroblasts, macrophages, primary chick embryo cells, and human endothelial cells. Plaque formation in infected cell cultures was first used for numeration of viable rickettsiae (10, 11, 13, 21, 24) and then adapted to determine their in vitro antibiotic susceptibility (10,

13, 25). The plaque assay system is currently the recommended technique, allowing evaluation of both the bacteriostatic and the bactericidal activity of antibiotics. Cell monolayers (usually Vero cells) grown in tissue culture Petri dishes are acutely infected by rocking incubation with a rickettsial inoculum. Infected cells are then overlaid with Eagle MEM with 2% fetal calf serum and 0.5% agar. Antibiotics are added at different concentrations at the same time, with no antibiotics added to drug-free controls. Petri dishes are incubated 4 days at 37°C in a 5% CO_2 atmosphere. Cell monolayers are then stained with neutral red dye for visualization of the plaques. The MICs are defined as the lowest antibiotic concentration that completely inhibits plaque formation, compared with a drug-free growth control.

A disk assay was proposed as a convenient modification of the plaque assay. In this model, antibiotic disks are placed on the surface of the agar overlay. The diameter of the plaque formation inhibition zone around the antibiotic disk represents a measure of the antirickettsial activity of the antibiotic. Ives et al. (7) recently described a new cell culture system in which inhibition of *Rickettsia* proliferation by antibiotics was determined by comparing rickettsial growth in infected Vero cell cultures incubated in the presence of the antibiotic tested with that in drug-free controls. Infected cells were revealed by an indirect immunofluorescent antibody method.

Using the in vitro infected cell model, authors have shown that chloramphenicol, doxycycline, tetracycline, minocycline, and rifampin are effective against *R. prowazekii*, with MICs ranging from 0.005 to 1 µg/mL (14). Penicillins and cephems were considered poorly effective (14), although in earlier experiments, Wisseman et al. (26) demonstrated partial inhibition of rickettsial growth by high doses of penicillin G and spheroplast-like rickettsiae in cultures exposed to this antibiotic. Erythromycin was found effective against the Breinl strain of *R. prowazekii*, whereas the Madrid E strain was resistant (22). The newer macrolide compounds roxithromycin, azithromycin, and clarithromycin were recently tested in the immunofluorescent antibody assay (7) against the same *R. prowazekii*. Clarithromycin was the most effective compound, with MICs ten times less than that of erythromycin (0.25 and 2 µg/mL, respectively). Nalidixic acid produce only partial inhibition of plaque formation by *R. prowazekii* (10); the fluoroquinolone compounds were more effective (14; Raoult, unpublished data).

ANTIMICROBIAL THERAPY
Drug of Choice

The conventional antibiotic regimen for typhus group rickettsiosis is a 7- to 10-day oral course of doxycycline 200 mg daily. However, a single dose of 100 or 200 mg doxycycline has been reported to be as effective as conventional therapy for epidemic typhus (5, 6, 8, 16). Single-dose doxycycline therapy was more recently administered successfully, without any relapse, in patients suffering epidemic typhus in Burundi (17). Compared with the conventional antibiotic regimen, the single-dose regimen presents the advantages of being well tolerated by almost all patients and cost-effective. It is more adapted to the epidemic situation when medications and treatment facilities are limited, especially in developing countries and refugee camps. In these situations, administration of doxycycline to all suspected of having epidemic typhus should be safe and effective in preventing an epidemic of the disease. The single-dose doxycycline regimen represents the current recommendation, especially in developing countries where drugs are scarce.

Antibiotic combinations have not been tested in vitro against *R. prowazeki*. Combination therapy is not indicated, since most patients are treated easily by the single-dose doxycycline regimen. Early administration of doxycycline is critical, allowing prevention of both severe illnesses and epidemic extension of the disease.

Special Situations

In severely diseased patients, doxycycline should be administered first by the intravenous route at 200 mg daily, and 14-day duration should be considered. There is no clinical indication that other drugs should be more effective than tetracyclines, even in patients with neurologic complications.

Alternative Therapy

The real limitation of antibiotic therapy using tetracycline compounds is the possibility of side effects, including gastric intolerance, but mainly the possibility of dental coloration in the neonate and the young child. Thus, tetracyclines are contraindicated in pregnant women and children. Administration of a single dose of doxycycline usually prevents the occurrence of side effects. Although it is still contraindicated in pregnant women, it may represent a safe alternative in children.

Chloramphenicol has long been considered the main alternative for rickettsial infections. In developing countries, such as Ethiopia, chloramphenicol rather than tetracycline was administered as first-line antibiotic therapy because of its activity against both epidemic typhus and enteric fever, the difficulty of clinically differentiating these diseases, and the lack of specific diagnosis in such countries (8, 16). However, chloramphenicol presents the potential risk of aplastic anemia. Moreover, recent in vitro and in vivo data indicate that chloramphenicol has only moderate rickettsiostatic activity. Patients should be treated for at least 8 days. Death has been reported in patients with severe disease receiving chloramphenicol therapy (5).

Erythromycin is effective in vitro against *R. prowazekii*. However, as suggested by in vitro data (22), rapid in vivo selection of erythromycin-resistant mutants is possible. Failures have been reported in patients receiving erythromycin therapy (C. L. Wisseman, personal communication). No clinical data are available for the newer macrolide compounds and fluoroquinolones. Selection of resistant mutants to newer macrolides may be expected as well as for erythromycin. Cotrimoxazole has been reported to be less active than chloramphenicol or doxycycline for treatment of epidemic typhus (5) and should not be considered a safe alternative. Although fluoroquinolones display in vitro bacteriostatic activity, failure was reported using ciprofloxacin in a patient with epidemic typhus (J. P. Glauser, personal communication).

ADJUNCTIVE MEASURES

Prevention of epidemic typhus by delousing procedures is dramatically efficient and should be implemented as soon as an outbreak is suspected. Louse infestation is dramatically reduced by regularly changing and washing clothing. The World Health Organization also recommended the use of insecticides such as permethrin (1%) dusting powder. The powder should be applied in a dose of 30 to 50 g per adult (125–250 mg/m² of clothing). All clothing should be dusted inside and outside. Bedding should also be treated. Lice usually succumb to the insecticide within a few hours. When louse infestation is endemic, the treatment should be repeated every 6 weeks.

REFERENCES

1. Becla E, Krynski S. The effect of some antibiotics on *Rickettsia prowazeki* and Yersinia pseudotuberculosis in body louse *Pediculus humanus humanus*. L Wiad Parazytol 1972:599–603.
2. Boese JL, Wisseman CL, Walsh WT, Fiset P. Antibody and antibiotic action on *Rickettsia prowazeki* in body lice across the host-vector interface, with observations on strain virulence and retrieval mechanisms. Am J Epidemiol 1973;98:262–282.
3. Bozeman FM, Masiello SA, Williams MS, Elisberg BL. Epidemic typhus rickettsiae isolated from flying squirrels. Nature 1975;255:545–547.
4. Duma RT, Sonenshine DE, Bozeman FM, Veazey JM, Elisberg BL, Chadwick DP, Stoks NI, McGill TM, Miller GB, Mac Chormack JN. Epidemic typhus in the United States associated with flying squirrels. JAMA 1981;245:2318–2323.
5. Huys J, Freyens P, Kayihigi J, Van den Berghe G. Treatment of epidemic typhus. A comparative study of chloramphenicol, trimethoprim-sulphamethoxazole and doxycycline. Trans R Soc Trop Med Hyg 1973;67:718–721.
6. Huys J, Kayihigi J, Freyens P, Berghe GV. Single-dose treatment of epidemic typhus with doxycyline. Chemotherapy 1973;18:314–317.
7. Ives TJ, Manzewitsch P, Regnery RL, Butts JD, and Kebede M. In vitro susceptibilities of *Bartonella henselae*, *B. quintana*, *B. elizabethae*, *Rickettsia rickettsii*, *R. conorii*, *R. akari*, and *R. prowazekii* to macrolide antibiotics as determined by immunofluorescent-antibody analysis of infected Vero cell monolayers. Antimicrob Agents Chemother 1997;41:578–582.
8. Krause DW, Perine PL, McDade JE, Awoke S. Treatment of louse-borne typhus fever with chloramphenicol, tetracycline or doxycycline. East Afr Med J 1975;52:421–427.
9. Krynski S, Becla E. Intrahemocoelic infection of ticks *Ornothodoros moubata* (Murray) due to *Rickettsia prowazeki* and the influence of some antibiotics on growth curve of this bacteria. L Wiad Parazytol 1972;18:557–559.
10. McDade JE. Determination of antibiotic susceptibility of *Rickettsia* by the plaque assay technique. Appl Microbiol 1969;18:133–135.
11. McDade JE, Gerone PJ. Plaque assay for Q fever and scrub typhus rickettsiae. Appl Microbiol 1970;19:963–965.
12. McDade JE, Shepard CC, Redus MA, Newhouse VF, Smith JD. Evidence of *Rickettsia prowazekii* infections in the United States. Am J Trop Med Hyg 1980;29:277–284.
13. McDade JE, Stakebake JR, Jerone PJ. Plaque assay system for several species of *Rickettsia*. J Bacteriol 1969;99:910–912.
14. Miyamura S, Ohta T, Tamura A. Comparison of in vitro susceptibilities of *Rickettsia prowazekii*, *R. rickettsii*, *R. sibirica*, and *R. tsutsugamushi* to antimicrobial agents. Nippon Seirigaku Zasshi 1989;44:717–721.
15. Ormsbee RA, Parker H, Pickens EG. The comparative effectiveness of chlortetracycline, terramycin, chloramphenicol, erythromycin, and thiomycetin in suppressing experimental rickettsial infections in chick embryos. J Infect Dis 1955;96:162–167.
16. Perine PL, Krause DW, Awoke S, McDade JE. Single-dose doxycycline treatment of louse-borne relapsing fever and epidemic typhus. Lancet 1974;2:742–744.
17. Raoult D, Roux V, Ndihokubwayo JB, Bise G, Baudon D, Martet G, and Birtles R. Jail fever (epidemic typhus) outbreak in Burundi. Emerg Infect Dis 1997;3:357–360.
18. Smadel JE, Jackson EB, Cruise AB. Chloromycetin in experimental rickettsial infections. J Immunol 1949;62:49–65.
19. Smadel JE, Jackson EB, Gauld RL. Factors influencing the growth of rickettsiae. I. Rickettsiostatic effect of streptomycin in experimental infections. J Immunol 1947;57:273–284.
20. Snyder JC, Fagan R, Wells EB, Wicks HC, Miller JC. Experimental studies on the antirickettsial properties of terramycin. Ann NY Acad Sci 1950;53:362–374.
21. Weinberg EH, Stakebake JR, Gerone PJ. Plaque assay for *Rickettsia rickettsii*. J Bacteriol 1969;98:398–402.
22. Weiss E, Dressler HR. Selection of an erythromycin-resistant strain of *Rickettsia prowazekii*. Am J Hyg 1960;71:292–298.
23. White LA, Hall HE, Tzianabos T, Chappell WA. Effect of gentamicin on growth of viral, chlamydial, and rickettsial agents in mice and embryonated eggs. Antimicrob Agents Chemother 1976;10:344–346.
24. Wike DA, Tallent G, Peacock MG, Williams JC. Studies of the rickettsial plaque assay technique. Infect Immun 1972;5:715–722.
25. Wisseman CL, Waddell AD, Walsh WT. In vitro studies of the action of antibiotics on *Rickettsia prowazekii* by two basic methods of cell culture. J Infect Dis 1974;130:564–574.
26. Wisseman CL Jr, Silverman DJ, Waddell A, Brown DT. Penicillin-induced unstable intracellular formation of spheroplasts by rickettsiae. J Infect Dis 1982;146:147–158.
27. Wong SC, Cox HR. Action of aureomycin against experimental rickettsial and viral infections. Ann NY Acad Sci 1948;51:290–305.

Rickettsia rickettsii

●

David H. Walker and Daniel J. Sexton

GENERAL DESCRIPTION

Rickettsia rickettsii, the etiologic agent of Rocky Mountain spotted fever (RMSF), causes a life-threatening disease that has been reported in 48 of the United States, Canada, Mexico, Costa Rica, Panama, Colombia, and Brazil (12, 19–21, 28, 34, 36, 43, 44, 56, 67). Because of its transmission by tick bite, the disease is generally highly seasonal, reflecting the feeding activity of the tick. The natural hosts and vectors of *R. rickettsii* are ticks: *Dermacentor variabilis* (the American dog tick) in the eastern two-thirds and areas in the far west of the United States, *Dermacentor andersoni* (the Rocky Mountain wood tick) in most of the western third of the United States and Canada, *Rhipicephalus sanguineus* (the brown dog tick) in northern Mexico, and *Amblyomma cayenennse* (the cayenne cattle tick) in Brazil and Colombia (19, 20, 28). *R. rickettsii* has evolved for maintenance in the tick by transovarian transmission (16, 51). Apparent low-level pathogenicity for ticks is balanced by moderate horizontal transmission to rodents, some of which become rickettsemic at levels sufficient to infect feeding ticks (18). The microbial factors that enable the shift from relative avirulence in the tick at ambient temperature to virulence in the mammalian host at 34 to 37°C are incompletely characterized.

Microbiology

R. rickettsii is an obligately intracellular, small (0.3 $\times$ 1.0 μm), Gram-negative bacterium that resides free in the cytosol and occasionally the nucleus of endothelial and, less frequently, vascular smooth muscle cells and macrophages. The rickettsia has two major outer membrane proteins, rickettsial outer membrane protein (rOmp) A and rOmp B (7, 37). The adhesin by which *R. rickettsii* attaches to the host cell is rOmp A; rOmp B is quantitatively the major surface-exposed rickettsial protein, apparently forming a geometrical array or S-layer. The outer rickettsial membrane also contains abundant lipopolysaccharide and a 17-kDa protein with sequence similarity to lipoprotein (6, 74). Conformational epitopes on rOmp A and rOmp B are the basis for antigenic differences between *R. rickettsii* and other spotted fever group (SFG) rickettsiae (4). Although rOmp A is relatively highly conserved among all SFG rickettsiae, it is the protein with the greatest diversity identified thus far (24, 37). A domain of tandem repeat units (with 13 of them in *R. rickettsii*) appears to be the source of the greatest diversity among SFG rickettsiae. Typhus group as well as SFG rickettsiae contain the relatively highly conserved rOmp B (27).

Different isolates of *R. rickettsii* are so similar that only two strains can be designated: R strain and HLP strain (3–5). All human isolates from patients with RMSF have been antigenically indistinguishable except for limited epitope differences between strains from the eastern and western United States (4). No differences in DNA sequences have been reported among human isolates of *R. rickettsii.*

More than 40 years ago, a series of SFG isolates from ticks and humans were designated as R, S, T, or U type according to their virulence for guinea pigs (61). The primary basis for classifying rickettsial species isolated from ticks in the United States, such as *R. parkeri, R. rhipicephali, R. montana, R. bellii,* and *R. amblyommii,* has been the antigenic differences. These species also differ in virulence for guinea pigs. Such a system as proposed by Price would not be valid if current microbiologic methods are utilized (15, 17, 18, 53, 57, 58). Indeed, studies comparing human isolates from the eastern and western United States revealed that R and S strains (as determined by the method of Price) are actually present in both areas. A widely accepted explanation for the disproportionately high case-fatality rates observed during the preantibiotic era among patients in the Bitterroot Valley of western Montana, compared with much lower case-fatality rates among patients from the eastern United States, is the assumption that rickett-sial strains from the two locations were of different virulence (42, 60, 76). However, it is quite possible that the high mortality rate in patients from Montana can be explained largely by the more frequent occurrence of infection in adult males (75). Furthermore, the erroneous belief that strains of *R. rickettsii* from the eastern United States are less pathogenic is strongly refuted by the frequent occurrence of fatal cases in the East, even among children.

The HLP strain of *R. rickettsii* was originally isolated from the rabbit tick *Haemaphysalis leporispalustris* (54). It is less virulent for guinea pigs than R strain, from which it can be distinguished by monoclonal antibodies (3). As yet, no DNA sequence differences have been reported between the HLP strain and other strains of *R. rickettsii,* and the observed antigenic differences do not explain the differences in virulence. The HLP strain has never been isolated from humans, and the rabbit tick rarely bites humans. However, the possibility of human infection with HLP strain cannot be excluded. Indeed, the low mortality (3%) of RMSF in the original classical description of RMSF in Idaho by Maxey in 1899 has never been explained (49). The ability to treat this infection by inhibiting the growth of the infectious agent did not occur until nearly a half-century later in the 1940s.

SUSCEPTIBILITY IN VITRO AND IN VIVO

In vitro susceptibility testing for obligately intracellular organisms such as *R. rickettsii* has yet to be standardized and validated by studies in experimentally infected animals and in adequately controlled clinical studies. Cell cultures using fibroblasts and Vero cells, embryonated eggs, and animal models have all been used to test susceptibility of SFG rickettsiae. However, all of these methods have technical limitations. Furthermore, clinical trials of the efficacy of treatment of human rickettsial infection are arduous because of difficulties in case acquisition and recognition. Studies that have been undertaken have usually been limited because of difficulties in matching clinical cases in terms of prognostic factors such as age, length of illness prior to treatment, and severity of disease before starting treatment.

Numerous antimicrobial agents such as erythromycin, nitrofurantoin, and penicillin have been shown to exhibit antirickettsial activity in cell culture systems; yet these agents have been found clinically ineffective (77). *R. rickettsii* is susceptible to fluoroquinolones in a cell culture system. For example, the minimal inhibitory concentration (MIC) of ciprofloxacin against *R. rickettsii* is 1 μg/mL (46). Although fluoroquinolones are effective against experimental RMSF in dogs and against *R. rickettsii* in cell culture, fluoroquinolone treatment of humans with RMSF has not been reported (13, 46).

Although rifampin has not been adequately tested for in vitro activity against *R. rickettsii,* it has been shown to have in vitro activity against *R. conorii* (62).

Both tetracycline and chloramphenicol have been shown to be effective antirickettsial agents in guinea pigs and embryonated chicken eggs as well as in cultured cells. Both of these antibiotics are rickettsiostatic. It is difficult to quantitate the relative activity of the two agents against *R. rickettsii,* but in the in vitro systems used thus far, tetracycline appears to be slightly superior to chloramphenicol (50, 68, 69).

Prior to the development and introduction of tetracycline and chloramphenicol, penicillin had proven to provide no benefit in guinea pigs experimentally infected with *R. rickettsii.* Sulfonamides are not only ineffective but actually exacerbate experimental RMSF (32, 71, 73). However, an analogue of sulfonamide, *p*-aminobenzoic acid (PABA), has rickettsiostatic activity (8, 40, 41). PABA has clear therapeutic benefit in experimentally infected guinea pigs.

ANTIMICROBIAL THERAPY

In the 1940s, prior to the availability of tetracycline and chloramphenicol, PABA was used successfully to treat RMSF

(70). Because PABA is absorbed and excreted very rapidly, doses of 1 to 3 g were administered every 2 h, day and night, to maintain a blood concentration of 30 to 60 mg/dL. Bicarbonate was given to maintain a neutral or slightly alkaline urine pH to avoid precipitation of PABA in the urinary system. PABA was discontinued 48 h after defervescence or when the leukocyte count fell below 3000/μL, when the neutrophil differential was less than 25%, or when PABA crystals appeared in the urine. Although these observations were made over 50 years ago, neither the mechanism by which PABA inhibits rickettsial growth nor the mechanism by which sulfonamides exacerbate rickettsial disease has been elucidated.

For most situations, doxycycline is the drug of choice for treatment of RMSF. Chloramphenicol is the accepted alternative treatment in pregnancy, tetracycline hypersensitivity, or rare situations in which there is another contraindication to tetracycline use (35, 45). The best evaluation of antimicrobial agents in RMSF is a retrospective epidemiologic and clinical analysis of 9223 cases of RMSF reported to the Centers for Disease Control and Prevention between 1981 and 1992 (26). A tetracycline was used in 58.2% of these cases; chloramphenicol, in 19.6%; and both drugs in 9.4%. Patients treated with chloramphenicol alone had a higher case-fatality rate (8.2%) than those treated with tetracycline alone (1.6%). However, a number of obvious confounding factors make interpretation of the difference in outcome between tetracycline- and chloramphenicol-treated patients difficult. For example, chloramphenicol was used more often in children and in hospitalized patients, and chloramphenicol treatment was begun later in the course (median, 5 days) than was tetracycline therapy (median, 3 days). It is well known that RMSF is less severe in children than adults, hospitalized patients are logically more severely ill than outpatients, and late treatment is associated with a worse outcome (48). Nevertheless, statistical methods were used to compensate for these confounding factors, and after use of a logistic regression model and a subgroup analysis, the authors concluded that tetracyclines were superior to chloramphenicol in this large cohort of patients. For example, 7 (1.8%) of 390 children less than 8 years old who were treated with chloramphenicol died, compared with none of 241 children in this age group treated with tetracycline only. Furthermore, outpatients treated with tetracycline were

---

TABLE 1 • Antimicrobial Regimens for Patients with Rocky Mountain Spotted Fever

Patient Characteristics	Drug of Choice	Dose Regimen[a]
Nonpregnant adult	Doxycycline	100 mg b.i.d. i.v. or orally
Pregnant	Chloramphenicol	500 mg q.i.d. i.v. or orally maintaining monitored serum levels of 10–30 μg/mL
Child		
$\geq$45 kg	Doxycycline	100 mg b.i.d. i.v. or orally
<45 kg	Doxycycline	4.4 mg/kg/day i.v. or orally in 2 divided doses
Patient allergic to tetracyclines	Chloramphenicol	500 mg q.i.d. i.v. or orally maintaining monitored serum levels at 10–30 μg/mL in newborns, children <2 years old, and patients with hepatic disease and interacting drugs

[a]In all drug regimens, treatment should be continued until at least 48 h after defervescence and unequivocal evidence of clinical improvement.

significantly less likely to be hospitalized subsequently (11%) than those treated with chloramphenicol (30%). Despite the limitations of this retrospective study and despite the difficulties of validation of clinical details of cases that were reported passively using a standardized form, it is unlikely that better data will be forthcoming, given the relative infrequency of RMSF and the impossibility of undertaking a randomized clinical trial comparing the two agents.

For adult patients and infected children weighing more than 40 kg who are not vomiting or in a coma and are able to take oral medication, the preferred treatment for RMSF is doxycycline given in two oral doses of 100 mg daily. For smaller children, doxycycline should be given in two equally divided doses totaling 4.4 mg/kg body weight/day. An equivalent pediatric dose of tetracycline is 25 to 50 mg/kg body weight/day in four divided doses, but doxycycline is the preferred form of tetracycline therapy in children, since doxycycline binds less strongly to calcium than tetracycline and thus is less likely to stain the permanent teeth (33). Long a controversial topic, staining of teeth is unlikely to occur after one or even as many as five therapeutic courses of tetracycline. For this reason, doxycycline remains the treatment of choice for RMSF in children (39, 59). Although chloramphenicol can also be used to treat children with RMSF, routine use of chloramphenicol for empirical treatment of RMSF in children carries a small but measurable risk of fatal aplastic anemia, a complication that occurs in an estimated 1 in 25,000 to 40,000 courses of chloramphenicol treatment.

Although adults with RMSF can also be treated with oral tetracycline (2 g/day in four divided doses), doxycycline is also the preferred agent against *R. rickettsii* infection in patients above 15 years of age. Oral tetracyclines must be taken in the absence of food. Patient compliance with oral tetracycline therapy, a regimen requiring 4 doses a day, is unlikely to be as good as with doxycycline, which requires only two doses per day and can be taken with or without food. Furthermore, the cost of oral doxycycline does not differ appreciably from that of an equivalent dose of tetracycline. Photosensitization is an occasional problem when ambulatory patients are given oral doxycycline therapy. Patients should be informed of this potential side effect and advised to use sunscreen creams and to avoid prolonged skin exposure to sunlight when possible. Patients with RMSF who are seriously ill and require hospitalization and patients who are unable to take oral medications because of vomiting or altered mental status should receive parenteral therapy; the preferred agent is also doxycycline, given intravenously at the same dose (100 mg every 12 h) used for oral therapy.

Chloramphenicol (2 g/day in four divided doses for adults), either orally or intravenously, provides effective treatment when given early enough in the course of RMSF. Intramuscular administration of chloramphenicol has produced low serum levels in some, but not all, studies. In one study, intramuscular administration of chloramphenicol resulted in peak serum levels one-half to two-thirds of those seen with intravenous administration of chloramphenicol (29). The pediatric dose of chloramphenicol is 50 to 75 mg/kg body weight/day in four divided doses.

Although there are few therapeutic situations in which tetracyclines or chloramphenicol could not be used, should such an unlikely event occur, oral ciprofloxacin (1.5 g/day in two divided doses) or oral ofloxacin (400 mg/day in two divided doses) might be tried in adult patients, as these regimens have been used successfully to treat Mediterranean spotted fever (65). Except in unusual situations (e.g., cystic fibrosis), quinolones are contraindicated in children.

One study of rifampin treatment reported delayed response to treatment as well as therapeutic failures in 4 of 15 patients with Mediterranean spotted fever who were treated with rifampin. Thus it is quite possible that it would have equally disappointing activity against *R. rickettsii* (12).

SPECIAL SITUATIONS

Maternal administration of tetracycline may result in tetracycline deposition in the human fetal skeleton as early as the 11th week of gestation and temporarily inhibit bone growth (23). Tetracycline can also cause staining of the deciduous teeth of infants born to mothers who receive it after their 16th week of gestation (22). In addition, all drugs in the tetracycline class have been associated with severe hepatotoxicity and pancreatitis when given to pregnant women (45).

When chloramphenicol is given to neonates, they may develop "gray baby syndrome" consisting of abdominal distention, pallor, cyanosis, and vasomotor collapse. Although gray baby syndrome has not been reported in neonates after maternal administration of chloramphenicol, it is theoretically possible, since fetal levels of chloramphenicol reach 30 to 80% of the maternal serum level (64). Because of the potential for gray baby syndrome, many authorities advise against using chloramphenicol in women at or near term. However, if pregnant women develop RMSF, it is probably safer to treat with chloramphenicol than with doxycycline or a tetracycline (35). There is no proven teratogenicity for either chloramphenicol or tetracycline, although limb hypoplasia secondary to the use of tetracycline in the first trimester of pregnancy has been reported (23).

Because of the uncertainty of serum chloramphenicol levels owing to individual differences in absorption and metabolism, serum chloramphenicol levels should be monitored in selected situations. Serum chloramphenicol levels can be monitored by bioassay, radioenzymatic assay, competitive enzyme-linked immunoassay, or high performance chromatography. Whatever assay is used, serum levels should be maintained between 10 and 30 μg/mL. Toxic chloramphenicol levels may produce severe cardiac dysfunction (72). We do not advise monitoring serum levels in patients who receive chloramphenicol for 3 to 5 days (as is often the case in treating mild cases of RMSF or when empirical therapy is started before results of bacterial cultures and skin biopsy are available). However, monitoring chloramphenicol serum levels is advisable when treating newborns and young children (<2 years old), all patients with hepatic disease, and patients taking interacting drugs (including agents such as phenytoin, Coumadin, rifampin, and phenobarbital). Doses of chloramphenicol do not need to be modified in renal failure. Even though chloramphenicol metabolites actually accumulate in renal insufficiency, the active drug level does not depend on renal function. However, dosages of chloramphenicol should be adjusted in hepatic insufficiency (as evidenced by the presence of jaundice or ascites). In such cases, the adult dose should not exceed 2 g/day, and therapy should not exceed 10 to 14 days' duration. Chloramphenicol may produce a hemolytic anemia in patients with the Mediterranean form of glucose-6-phosphate dehydrogenase (G6PD) deficiency. However, chloramphenicol-induced hemolysis does not occur in type A G6PD deficiency (which commonly occurs in African Americans).

Patients whose differential diagnosis includes infection with *Neisseria meningitidis* may be treated with chloramphenicol to provide therapeutic coverage for these organisms and *R. rickettsii*. Alternatively, it is reasonable to combine doxycycline with an agent such as a third-generation cephalosporin (e.g., ceftriaxone) when empirical therapy is begun in a patient with illness compatible with both RMSF and meningococcemia. It is often difficult to distinguish between RMSF and another important group of tick-borne diseases: human monocytic and granulocytic ehrlichioses. In such cases, doxycycline provides therapeutic coverage for both diseases and is preferable to chloramphenicol, an agent whose antiehrlichial activity is less certain (11, 31).

Patients who develop severe illness due to RMSF often have multiorgan dysfunction. This dysfunction may manifest as renal failure, seizures, diffuse pulmonary infiltrates, or a variety of neurologic problems, ranging from altered mental status, to seizures, to coma. Such patients often require hemodynamic monitoring and careful administration of intravenous fluids and pressors. In addition, some patients develop signs and symptoms of adult respiratory distress syndrome and ultimately require ventilatory support. Patients with hypoxia, hypotension, cardiac conduction abnormalities, renal failure, and seizures usually require specialized and intensive care. Disorders of coagulation including thrombocytopenia and prolonged prothrombin and partial thromboplastin times may result in bleeding that requires transfusion. Rarely, abdominal pain may be a prominent feature of RMSF, and a small number of patients may develop signs and symptoms of peritonitis. Most of these patients can be managed medically with antirickettsial therapy and supportive care without surgical intervention.

ENDPOINTS FOR MONITORING THERAPY

Generally, patients with uncomplicated RMSF and those who are treated with an antirickettsial drug within 96 h of onset of symptoms defervesce within 48 to 72 h and rapidly exhibit evidence of clinical improvement. In general, antirickettsial therapy should be continued for at least 48 h after defervescence has occurred and until there is unequivocal evidence of clinical improvement (such as a return of appetite and general sense of well-being). Severely ill patients and especially patients with multiorgan dysfunction typically require longer to defervesce; some patients with severe illness may remain in coma, be ventilator dependent, or require amputations for gan-

grene even after rickettsiae have been cleared from the perfused parts of the body. Some patients with extensive tissue damage may die as a result of widespread tissue and organ injury even if rickettsial sterilization has occurred as a combined result of the antimicrobial therapy and the patient's immune defenses. For these patients, there is no clear endpoint for treatment. It is not possible to predict the extent of recovery after treatment of severe infection. In some patients, neurologic or organ damage may remain permanent; in other patients, even severe neurologic and renal impairment may disappear with time and supportive care (9, 24).

CONTROVERSIES AND COMMENTS

The controversy regarding the previous recommendations of the American Academy of Pediatrics and the Centers for Disease Control and Prevention that chloramphenicol should be used instead of tetracycline for the treatment of RMSF in children less than 9 years of age has been reconsidered (1). The 1995 edition of the Red Book of the American Academy of Pediatrics states, "Therefore, when comparing the benefits and risks of doxycycline and chloramphenicol in children younger than 9 years, doxycycline should be considered the drug of choice for empiric therapy of children of any age with presumed or proven RMSF" (2).

Although it is generally thought that relapse does not occur in patients who have recovered from RMSF, relapse of other SFG infections has been reported (10, 63) and there are anecdotal reports of relapse in a few patients with RMSF (30). In one instance a patient with severe RMSF was found to have viable *R. rickettsii* in a lymph node 1 year after he had recovered from his rickettsial infection (55). Another controversy surrounds the practice of prescribing a prophylactic antirickettsial drug to healthy persons giving a history of tick bite. Such prophylaxis is *not* recommended because of the very low prevalence of *R. rickettsii* in ticks and experimental evidence that the rickettsiostatic drug merely prolongs the incubation period and does not prevent the disease in prophylactically treated guinea pigs (47).

A critically important problem in treating RMSF effectively is determining which febrile patients are likely to have RMSF. Unfortunately, many patients with RMSF are erroneously treated with penicillins, cephalosporins, aminoglycosides, erythromycin, or sulfonamides because the correct diagnosis is initially not suspected or because epidemiologic and clinical clues to the correct diagnosis were either not sought or not evident. In some cases, patients initially treated with β-lactam antibiotics or sulfonamides are erroneously thought to have drug eruptions when they later manifest a rash. Such patients are not recognized as having a key clinical clue to diagnosis: rash due to rickettsia-induced vasculitis. The diagnosis of RMSF may be delayed in other patients because a rash is absent. A small percentage of patients with RMSF have delayed onset of rash. Other patients with RMSF may have atypical rashes that are either asymmetric or localized to a small area of the body surface. Still other patients never manifest a rash. Such "spotless" or "almost spotless" patients often have severe illness; some "spotless" patients succumb to their infection before the correct diagnosis is realized and before appropriate treatment can be administered (66).

There are no published criteria for hospitalization in patients with known or suspected infection with *R. rickettsii*. Certainly not all patients with RMSF require hospitalization. Many patients who are treated within 5 days of onset of illness can be safely managed as outpatients (48). However, careful clinical follow-up is mandatory for all such patients, and hospitalization is warranted if nausea or vomiting develop or if a prompt clinical response is not observed. Patients with severe thrombocytopenia, renal insufficiency, increased levels of bilirubin or aspartate aminotransferase, focal or severe neurologic signs or symptoms, and those more than 40 years of age have been shown by univariate analysis to have a worse prognosis. Of these factors, only neurologic involvement and an elevated serum creatinine level at admission were independently associated with increased mortality by multivariate analysis (24). On the basis of these data, we advise hospitalization for all patients with suspected RMSF who have renal insufficiency or any of the laboratory or clinical findings mentioned above. In addition, we advise hospitalization for patients with suspected RMSF in whom oral therapy is not suitable because of concurrent gastrointestinal symptoms such as severe nausea or vomiting.

The role of steroid therapy in the treatment of severe RMSF is unresolved. Although early uncontrolled human studies suggested benefit when steroids were used along with chloramphenicol (78), convincing evidence demonstrating benefit of steroid therapy in RMSF has never been published, and we do not advise the use of steroids even in severe cases of *R. rickettsii* infection.

REFERENCES

1. Abramson JS, Givner LB. Should tetracycline be contraindicated for therapy of presumed Rocky Mountain spotted fever in children less than 9 years of age? Pediatrics 1990;86:123.
2. American Academy of Pediatrics. 1997 Red book: report of the Committee on Infectious Diseases. 24th ed. 1997.
3. Anacker RL, List RH, Mann RE, Wiedbrauk DL. Antigenic heterogeneity in high- and low-virulence strains of *Rickettsia rickettsii* by monoclonal antibodies. Infect Immun 1986;51:653.
4. Anacker RL, Mann RE, Gonzales C. Reactivity of monoclonal antibodies to *Rickettsia rickettsii* with spotted fever and typhus group rickettsiae. J Clin Microbiol 1987;25:167.
5. Anacker RL, Philip RN, Williams JC, List RH, Mann RE. Biochemical and immunochemical analysis of *Rickettsia rickettsii* strains of various degrees of virulence. Infect Immun 1984;44:559.
6. Anderson BE, Regnery RL, Carlone GM, Tzianabos T, McDade JE, Zhang YF, Bellini WJ. Sequence analysis of the 17-kilodalton-antigen gene from *Rickettsia rickettsii*. J Bacteriol 1987;169:2385.
7. Anderson BE, McDonald GA, Jones DC, et al. A protective protein antigen of *Rickettsia rickettsii* has tandemly repeated, near-identical sequences. Infect Immun 1990;58:2760.
8. Anigstein L, Bader MN. Para-aminobenzoic acid: its effectiveness in spotted fever in guinea pigs. Science 1945;101:59.
9. Archibald L, Sexton DJ. Long-term sequelae of Rocky Mountain spotted fever. Clin Infect Dis 1995;20:1122.
10. Ash M, Smithurst BA. A case of Queensland tick typhus. Med J Aust 1995;163:167.
11. Bakken JS, Krueth J, Wilson-Nordskog C, Tilden RL, Asanovich K, Dumler JS. Clinical and laboratory characteristics of human granulocytic ehrlichiosis. JAMA 1996;275:199.
12. Bella F, Espejo E, Uriz S, Serrano JA, Alegre MD, Tort J. Randomized trial of 5-day rifampin versus 1-day doxycycline therapy for Mediterranean spotted fever. J Infect Dis 1991;164:433.
13. Breitschwerdt EB, Davidson MG, Aucoin DP, et al. Efficacy of chloramphenicol, enrofloxacin, and tetracycline for treatment of experimental Rocky Mountain spotted fever in dogs. Antimicrob Agents Chemother 1991;35:2375.
14. Burgdorfer W. Tick-borne diseases in the United States: Rocky Mountain spotted fever and Colorado tick fever. A review. Acta Trop 1977;34:103.
15. Burgdorfer W, Sexton DJ, Gerloff RK, Anacker RL, Philip RN, Thomas LA. *Rhipicephalus sanguineus:* vector of a new spotted fever group rickettsiae in the United States. Infect Immun 1975;12:205.
16. Burgdorfer W, Brinton LP. Mechanisms of transovarial infection of spotted fever rickettsiae in ticks. Ann NY Acad Sci 1975;266:61.
17. Burgdorfer W, Hayes SF, Thomas LA, Lancaster JL Jr. A new spotted fever group rickettsia from the lone star tick, *Amblyomma americanum*. In: Burgdorfer W, Anacker RL, eds. Rickettsiae and rickettsial diseases. New York: Academic Press, 1981:595.
18. Burgdorfer W. Ecological and epidemiological considerations of Rocky Mountain spotted fever and scrub typhus. In: Walker DH, ed. Biology of rickettsial diseases, vol 1. Boca Raton, FL: CRC Press, 1988:33.
19. Bustamante ME. Una neuva rickettsiosis en Mexico. Existencia de la fiebre manchada Americana en los estados de Sinaloa y Sonora. Rev Inst Salub Enferm Trop 1943;4:189.
20. Bustamante ME, Varela G, Ortiz Mariote C. II-Estudios de fiebra manchada en Mexico. Fiebre manchada en La Laguna. Rev Inst Salub Enferm Trop 1946;7:39.
21. Calero MC, Nunez JM, Silva Gotyia R. Rocky Mountain spotted fever in Panama. Report of two cases. Am J Trop Med Hyg 1952;1:631.
22. Cohlan SQ. Tetracycline staining of teeth. Teratology 1977;15:127.
23. Cohlan SQ, Beverlander G, Tiamsic T. Growth inhibition of prematures receiving tetracycline. Am J Dis Child 1963;105:454.
24. Conlon PJ, Procop GW, Fowler V, Eloubeidi MA, Smith SR, Sexton DJ. Predictors of prognosis and risk of acute renal failure in patients with Rocky Mountain spotted fever. Am J Med 1996;101:621.
25. Crocquet-Valdes PA, Weiss K, Walker DH. Sequence analysis of the 190-kDa antigen-encoding gene of *Rickettsia conorii* (Malish 7 strain). Gene 1994;140:115.
26. Dalton MJ, Clarke MJ, Holman RC, Krebs JW, Fishbein DB, Olson JG, Childs JE. National surveillance for Rocky Mountain spotted fever, 1981–1992: epidemiologic summary and evaluation of risk factors for fatal outcome. Am J Trop Med Hyg 1995;52:405.
27. Dasch GA. Isolation of species-specific protein antigens of *Rickettsia typhi* and *Rickettsia prowazekii* for immunodiagnosis and immunoprophylaxis. J Clin Microbiol 1981;14:333.
28. Dias E, Martins AV. Spotted fever in Brazil. Am J Trop Med 1939;19:103.
29. Dupont HL, Hornick CRM, Wiess CF, et al. Evaluation of chloramphenicol acid succinate therapy of induced typhoid fever and Rocky Mountain spotted fever. N Engl J Med 1970;282:53.

30. Eloubeidi MAS, Burton CS, Sexton DJ. The great imitator: Rocky Mountain spotted fever occurring after hospitalization for unrelated illnesses. South Med J 1997;90:943.

31. Fishbein DB, Dawson JE, Robinson LE. Human ehrlichiosis in the United States, 1985 to 1990. Ann Intern Med 1994;120:736.

32. Fitzpatrick FK. Penicillin in experimental spotted fever. Science 1945;102:96.

33. Fort G, Benincovi C. Doxycycline and the teeth. Lancet 1969;1: 782.

34. Fuentes LG. Primer case de fiebre de las Montanas Rocosas en Costa Rica, America Central. Rev Latinoam Microbiol 1979;21: 167.

35. Gallis HA, Agner RC, Painter CJ. Rocky Mountain spotted fever in pregnancy. NC Med J 1984;45:187.

36. Galvao MAM, Chamone CB, Olson JG, et al. Report of cases of spotted fever disease in Minas Gerais-State-Brazil-1981–1994. In: Kazar J, Toman R, eds. Rickettsiae and rickettsial diseases. Bratislava, Slovak Republic: Slovak Academy of Sciences, 1996:211.

37. Gilmore RD Jr. Comparison of the *rompA* gene repeat regions of *Rickettsiae* reveals species-specific arrangements of individual repeating units. Gene 1993;125:97.

38. Gilmore RD Jr, Cleplak W, Policastro PF, et al. The 120 kilo-dalton outer membrane protein (rOmp B) of *Rickettsia rickettsii* is encoded by an unusually long open reading frame: evidence for protein processing from a large precursor. Mol Microbiol 1991;5:2361.

39. Grossman ER, Walchek A, Freedman H. Tetracyclines and permanent teeth: the relation between dose and tooth color. Pediatrics 1971;47:567.

40. Hamilton HL. Effect of p-aminobenzoic acid on growth of rickettsiae and elementary bodies, with observations on mode of action. Soc Exp Biol Med Proc 1945;59:220.

41. Hamilton HL, Plotz H, Smadel JE. Effect of p-aminobenzoic acid on the growth of typhus rickettsiae in the yolk sac of the infected chick embryo. Report of the director of the U.S.A. Typhus Comm., Dec. 16, 1943.

42. Harden VA. Rocky Mountain spotted fever. History of a twentieth-century disease. Baltimore: Johns Hopkins University Press, 1990.

43. Hattwick MAW, O'Brien RJ, Hanson BF. Rocky Mountain spotted fever: epidemiology of an increasing problem. Ann Intern Med 1976;84:732.

44. Helmick CG, Bernard KW, D'Angelo LJ. Rocky Mountain spotted fever: clinical, laboratory, and epidemiological features of 262 cases. J Infect Dis 1984;150:480.

45. Herbert WNP, Seeds JW, Koontz WL, Cefalo RC. Rocky Mountain spotted fever in pregnancy: differential diagnosis and treatment. South Med J 1982;75:1063.

46. Jabarit-Aldighieri N, Torres H, Raoult D. Susceptibility of *Rickettsia conorii, R. rickettsii,* and *Coxiella burnetii* to PD 127,391, PD 131,638, ofloxacin, and ciprofloxacin. Antimicrob Agents Chemother 1992;36:2529.

47. Kenyon RH, Williams RG, Oster CN, Pedersen CE. Prophylactic treatment of Rocky Mountain spotted fever. J Clin Microbiol 1978;8:102.

48. Kirkland KB, Wilkinson WE, Sexton DJ. Therapeutic delay and mortality in cases of Rocky Mountain spotted fever. Clin Infect Dis 1995;20:1118.

49. Maxey EE. Some observations on the so-called spotted fever of Idaho. Med Sentinel 1899;7:433.

50. McDade JE. Determination of antibiotic susceptibility of *Rickettsia* by the plaque assay technique. Appl Microbiol 1969; 18:133.

51. McDade JE, Newhouse VF. Natural history of *Rickettsia rickettsii.* Annu Rev Microbiol 1986;40:287.

52. Ormsbee RA, Parker H, Pickens EG. The comparative effectiveness of aureomycin, terramycin, chloramphenicol, erythromycin in suppressing experimental rickettsial infections in chick embryos. J Infect Dis 1955;96:162.

53. Parker RR, Kohls GM, Cox GW, Davis GE. Observations on an infectious agent from *Amblyomma maculatum.* Public Health Rep 1939;54:1482.

54. Parker RR, Pickens EG, Lackman DB, Bell EJ, Thrailkill FB. Isolation and characterization of Rocky Mountain spotted fever rickettsiae from the rabbit tick *Haemaphysalis leporispalustris* Packard. Public Health Rep 1951;66:455.

55. Parker RT, Menon PG, Merideth AM, et al. Persistence of *Rickettsia rickettsii* in a patient recovering from Rocky Mountain spotted fever. J Immunol 1954;73:383.

56. Patino L, Afanador A, Paul JH. A spotted fever in Tobia, Colombia: preliminary report. Am J Trop Med Hyg 1937;17:639.

57. Philip RN, Casper EA, Anacker RL, Cory J, Hayes SF, Burgdorfer W, Yunker CE. *Rickettsia bellii* sp nov: a tick-borne rickettsia widely distributed in the United States that is distinct from the spotted fever and typhus biogroups. Int J Syst Bacteriol 1983;33:94.

58. Philip RN, Casper EA, Burgdorfer W, Gerloff RR, Hughes LE, Bell EJ. Serologic typing of rickettsiae of the spotted fever group by microimmunofluorescence. J Immunol 1978;121: 1961.

59. Poliak SC, Digiovanna JJ, Gross EG, Gantt G, Peck GL. Minocycline-associated tooth discoloration in young adults. JAMA 1985;254:2930.

60. Price EG. Fighting spotted fever in the Rockies. Helena, MT: Naegele Printing Co, 1948.

61. Price WH. The epidemiology of Rocky Mountain spotted fever. I. The characterization of strain virulence of *Rickettsia rickettsii.* Am J Hyg 1953;58:248.

62. Raoult D , Roussellier P, Vestris G, Tamalet J. In vitro antibiotic susceptibility of *Rickettsia rickettsii* and *Rickettsia conorii:* plaque assay and microplaque colorimetric assay. J Infect Dis 1987;155:1059.

63. Raoult D, Drancourt M. Antimicrobial therapy of rickettsial diseases. Antimicrob Agents Chemother 1991;35:2457.

64. Ross S, Burke FG, Sites J, et al. Placental transmission of chloramphenicol. JAMA 1950;142:1361.

65. Ruiz-Beltran R, Herrero-Herrero JI. Evaluation of ciprofloxacin and doxycycline in the treatment of Mediterranean spotted fever. Eur J Clin Microbiol Infect Dis 1992;11:427.

66. Sexton DJ, Corey GR. Rocky Mountain "spotless" and "almost spotless" fever: a wolf in sheep's clothing. Clin Infect Dis 1992; 15:439.

67. Sexton DJ, Corey GR, Dietze R, et al. Brazilian spotted fever in Espirito Santo, Brazil: description of a focus of infection in a new endemic region. Am J Trop Med Hyg 1993;49:222.

68. Smadel JE, Jackson EB. Chloromycetin, an antibiotic with chemotherapeutic activity in experimental rickettsial and viral infections. Science 1947;106:418.

69. Smadel JE, Jackson EB, Cruise AB. Chloromycetin in experimental rickettsial infections. J Immunol 1949;62:49.

70. Snyder JC. The treatment of the rickettsial diseases of man. In: Moulton FR, ed. Rickettsial diseases of man. Boston: Washington, Thomas, Adams & Davis, 1946:169.

71. Steinhaus EA, Parker RR. Experimental Rocky Mountain spotted fever: results of treatment with certain drugs. Public Health Rep 1943;58:351.

72. Suarez CR. Chloramphenicol toxicity associated with severe cardiac dysfunction. Pediatr Cardiol 1992;13:48.

73. Topping NH. Experimental Rocky Mountain spotted fever and endemic typhus treated with prontosil or sulfapyridine. Public Health Rep 1939;54:1143.

74. Vishwanath S. Antigenic relationships among the rickettsiae of the spotted fever and typhus group. FEMS Microbiol Lett 1991;81:341.

75. Walker DH. The role of host factors in the severity of spotted fever and typhus rickettsioses. Ann NY Acad Sci 1990;590:10.

76. Wilson LB, Chowning WM. Studies in *Pyroplasmosis hominis* ("spotted fever" or "tick fever" of the Rocky Mountains). J Infect Dis 1904;1:31.

77. Wisseman CL Jr, Silverman DJ, Waddell A, Brown DT. Penicillin-induced unstable intracellular formation of spheroplasts by rickettsiae. J Infect Dis 1982;146:147.

78. Workman JB, Hightower JA, Borges FJ, Furman JE, Parker RT. Cortisone as an adjunct to chloramphenicol in the treatment of Rocky Mountain spotted fever. N Engl J Med 1952;246:962.

Rickettsia Species

●

D. Raoult and M. Maurin

GENERAL DESCRIPTION

The number of spotted fever group rickettsioses has recently risen as new rickettsial species have been isolated using newly available cell culture methods and characterized using genomic studies, especially 16S rRNA sequencing. Spotted fever group rickettsioses now include 13 recognized human diseases: Rocky Mountain spotted fever, caused by *Rickettsia rickettsii* (see specific chapter); rickettsialpox, caused by *R. akari* (see specific chapter), and 11 other spotted fever group rickettsiosis that are summarized in Table 1. The remaining rickettsiae have only been isolated from arthropods and are presently considered nonpathogenic for humans. However, recent isolation of *R. africae* and *R. slovaca* from infected humans, subsequent to their initial isolation from ticks, demonstrates that the term *nonpathogenic* is probably misleading, and all rickettsiae may indeed be opportunistic pathogens. The spotted fever group rickettsiae presently isolated only from arthropods include *R. rhipicephali, R. montana, R. parkeri, R. belli,* and *R. amblyommi* isolated in the United States; *R. massiliae* and Mtu5 strain isolated in the Mediterranean area; *R. helvetica* isolated in Switzerland; and other strains isolated in China, the former USSR (strain S), or Asia (Indian Tick Typhus rickettsia, Pakistan strain JC880, Thai Tick Typhus rickettsia).

All of the spotted fever group rickettsiae, except *R. akari* and *R. felis,* are transmitted by ticks and have been isolated from ticks. The tick transmits rickettsiae to humans during feeding, by direct inoculation via the bite. Humans may also be infected via the tick hemolymph after crushing the tick. Ticks are both the vector and the main reservoir of tick-borne rickettsiosis, although our knowledge of the epidemiology of spotted fever group rickettsial diseases remains fragmentary. The insect vectors and geographic distributions of spotted fever group rickettsial diseases, other than Rocky Mountain

spotted fever and rickettsialpox, are summarized in Table 1. Spotted fever group rickettsioses are clinically characterized by the combination of fever, headache, myalgia, and a cutaneous maculopapular rash involving the entire body, including palms and soles. An eschar may develop at the site of the tick bite but remains most often unnoticed, with local lymphadenopathy. Incubation period is usually 4 to 7 days. Truncated clinical presentations are frequent, and a delayed seroconversion in infected patients may lead to delayed diagnosis and antibiotic therapy and thus more-profound illness.

Mediterranean spotted fever has been recognized in many parts of the world, mainly in Mediterranean areas. It is prevalent in southern Europe (France, Spain, Portugal, Italy), North Africa (Morocco, Egypt), western Africa (Ethiopia, Kenya), India, Pakistan, Israel, Russia, Georgia, and the Ukraine. Although Mediterranean spotted fever was first considered a generally benign disease, severe forms are reported in 6% of patients, and mortality may be as high as 2.5%. Malignant forms may present with petechial rash and may lead to neurologic, renal, or cardiac complications as observed in cases of Rocky Mountain spotted fever. Israeli spotted fever is typified by a lack of a characteristic cutaneous eschar at the site of the tick bite; severe, and even fatal cases have been reported. Astrakhan fever presents similarly to Israeli spotted fever, with an eschar visible in only 23% of cases (32); severe or lethal forms have not been reported.

Siberian tick typhus is distributed from Europe, across the southern regions of the former USSR, and beyond the Chinese border. The disease is characterized by frequent central nervous system involvement. Japanese spotted fever caused by *R. japonica* is confined to that country (33). An eschar is often present at the site of the vector bite, which is, in contrast to other spotted fever group rickettsiosis, often noticeable.

TABLE 1 • Spotted Fever Group Rickettsiosis Other Than Rocky Mountain Spotted Fever (due to *R. rickettsii*), and Rickettsialpox (due to *R. akari*)

Syndrome	*Rickettsia* sp.	Insect Vector	Geographic Distribution
Mediterranean spotted fever	*R. conorii*	*Rhipicephalus sanguineus* ticks	Mediterranean areas
Siberian tick typhus	*R. sibirica*	*Dermacentor* ticks	Europe, USSR, China
Israeli spotted fever	Unnamed	*R. sanguineus* ticks	Israel
Queensland tick typhus	*R. australis*	*Ixodes holocytus* ticks	Queensland (Australia)
Japanese spotted fever	*R. japonica*	Unknown	Japan
Flinders Island spotted fever	*R. honei*	Unknown	Flinder Islands (Australia)
Astrakhan fever	Unnamed	*R. sanguineus* ticks, *R. pumilio* ticks	Astrakhan region (Russia)
African tick bite fever	*R. africae*	*Amblyomma variegatum* ticks	Ethiopia, Zimbabwe
Pseudotyphus of California	R. felis	Cat fleas	Texas (US)
Spotted fever	"*Rickettsia mongolotimonae*"	*Hyalomma* ticks	France, Inner Mongolia
Spotted fever	*R. slovaca*	*Dermacentor marginatus*	France, Slovakia,

In Australia, both Queensland tick typhus and Flinders Island spotted fever are usually mild diseases. Queensland tick typhus most often corresponds to the classical clinical presentation; in patients with Flinders Island spotted fever, an eschar is rarely observed, and regional lymph node enlargement is common (1, 31).

R. africae, the agent of African tick bite fever, was first isolated from the *Amblyomma variegatum* tick in Ethiopia. The disease has been recently described in patients in Zimbabwe and in European travelers returning from this country (11). In African tick bite fever, a cutaneous rash is lacking or very transient in most cases. In some patients, eruption was vesicular.

Pseudotyphus of California, caused by *R. felis,* has been described in only one patient who presented with fever and headaches but no rash (28). This agent was previously named the ELB agent and has been isolated from cat fleas parasitizing opossums in California. A new spotted fever due to "*Rickettsia* mongolotimonae" was reported in France in 1996 (22, 38). This rickettsia was originally isolated from *Hyalomma* sp. ticks collected in Inner Mongolia, but an indistinguishable isolate was later cultured from the blood and the skin of a patient in Marseilles in March 1996, a time of year when Mediterranean spotted fever is unlikely. This patient presented with a mild disease, with only a few spots on the body and an inoculation eschar. Very recently, *R. slovaca* was isolated in our laboratory from a French patient presenting with fever, cervical lymphadenopathies, and an eschar of the scalp but without cutaneous eruption (20).

The present chapter focuses on species recognized as human pathogens and mainly *R. conorii* for which most of the experimental data on antibiotic susceptibility and/or clinical data on antibiotic therapy efficacy is available.

Microbiology

Rickettsiae are strict intracellular bacteria that multiply within the cytoplasm of eukaryotic cells. They escape the phagosomal compartment at the very beginning of phagosomal vacuole formation. The spotted fever group rickettsiae move in the cytoplasm by association with the host cell's actin filaments (perhaps explaining why spotted fever group rickettsiae are often found in the nucleus of infected cells) and readily propagate from cell to cell (manifested in vitro by formation of larger plaques in infected cells than those of the nonmotile typhus group rickettsiae). In infected humans and animals, the main target cells are endothelial cells, in which rickettsiae may induce a chronic infection. To be active, antibiotics should reach the intracellular cytoplasmic compartment of eukaryotic cells. Most antibiotics active against rickettsiae are only rickettsiostatic and may not cure endothelial cells infected with rickettsiae.

SUSCEPTIBILITY IN VITRO AND IN VIVO

Because of their obligate intracellular lifestyle, susceptibility of rickettsiae to antibiotics cannot be assessed in conventional microbiologic tests. Three experimental models have been developed to test the antibiotic susceptibility of rickettsiae: animal models, the embryonated egg model, and cell culture models. Animal models and the embryonated egg model were the first described; however, antibiotic doses used in these models were much higher than those usually used in humans, and thus it is difficult to extrapolate data to the clinical situation. In vitro infected cell models have been more recently elaborated. These allow more convenient investigation of the antibiotic susceptibility of rickettsiae, and extracellular antibiotic concentrations used in these models may be compared with antibiotic concentrations obtained in human sera.

Single Drug

Animal Models

Guinea pigs and mice were most commonly used as experimental models for testing antibiotic activity against spotted fever group rickettsiae in vivo. Rickettsiae were most often injected by the intraperitoneal or intranasal routes, which do not correspond to the natural route of human infection. Antibiotics were administered either orally or subcutaneously. Infection in animals has been assessed by the presence of fever, specific serologic response, and death ratio, compared with untreated infected controls. However, clinical manifestations in infected animals do not reproduce those of human disease, and the reliability of animal models for rickettsial infections remains to be established. *R. rickettsii,* the agent of Rocky Mountain spotted fever, was the only spotted fever group rickettsia for which antibiotic susceptibility was evaluated in an animal model, in experiments showing complete protection against fever in infected guinea pigs treated with chlortetracycline (Aureomycin) (37).

Embryonated Egg Model

In the embryonated egg model, rickettsiae were injected into the yolk sac of the eggs. This resulted in death of the embryo, usually within a few days following infection. Antibiotics were administered by the same route, usually within the first hour following rickettsial inoculation. Antibiotic activity was deduced from the difference in mean survival time (DMST) of infected embryos receiving antibiotics and infected untreated controls. A rickettsiostatic effect of antibiotics allowed the embryos to survive up to the last day of experiments, usually day 14. The rickettsiacidal activity of antibiotics was assessed by subculture of yolk sacs from surviving eggs at 14 days postinfection. Direct examination of smears prepared from infected tissues and stained with the Gimenez technique has also been used to evaluated the action of antibiotics. However, this model did not allow direct evaluation of the growth rate of rickettsiae.

In an early report, Jackson (9) showed that *R. conorii* was susceptible to chlortetracycline (DMST of 2.6 days at 125 μg/egg) and, to a lesser extent, chloramphenicol (3.8 days DMST at 500 μg/egg). More recently, pefloxacin was reported to be rickettsiostatic against *R. conorii,* with a DMST of 2.5 days when using 50 μg/egg (25).

Very few data on the antibiotic susceptibility of spotted fever group rickettsiae other than *R. rickettsii* and *R. conorii* are available. Streptomycin was not effective against *R. orientalis* at concentrations up to 20,000 μg/egg (30). Chlortetracycline and chloramphenicol displayed rickettsiostatic activity against the South African tick bite fever rickettsia and the North Queensland tick typhus rickettsia, with DMSTs of 2.5 days or more for both species at concentrations of 125 μg/egg or above for chlortetracycline and 250 μg/egg or above for chloramphenicol (9).

Cell Culture Models

The primary target cells for rickettsiae are endothelial cells. However, a number of eukaryotic cell lines can be infected with rickettsiae in vitro, including fibroblasts, macrophages, primary chick embryo cells, and human endothelial cells. Plaque formation in infected cell cultures was first used for numeration of viable rickettsiae (15, 16, 34, 35) and was then adapted to determine their in vitro antibiotic susceptibility (15, 17, 36). The plaque assay system is currently the recommended technique and allows evaluation of both the bacteriostatic and the bactericidal activity of antibiotics. Cell monolayers (usually Vero cells) grown in tissue culture Petri dishes are acutely infected by rocking incubation with a rickettsial inoculum. Infected cells are then overlaid with Eagle Minimal Essential Medium with 2% fetal calf serum and 0.5% agar. Antibiotics are added at different concentrations at the same time, with no antibiotics added to drug-free controls. Petri dishes are incubated 4 days at 37°C in a 5% CO_2 atmosphere. Cell monolayers are then stained with neutral red dye, allowing visualization of the plaques. The MICs are defined as the lowest antibiotic concentration allowing complete inhibition of plaque formation, compared with a drug-free growth control.

A disk assay was proposed as a convenient modification of the plaque assay. In this model, antibiotic disks are placed on the surface of the agar overlay. The diameter of the plaque formation inhibition zone around the antibiotic disk represents a measure of the antirickettsial activity of the antibiotic.

More recently, a microplaque colorimetric assay or dye uptake assay was described as a more convenient technique allowing accurate and more rapid determination of MICs of several strains of spotted fever group rickettsiae (26). Vero cells cultured in 96-well microtiter plates are infected with 2000 PFU of rickettsiae. Antibiotics are added at different concentrations in different rows. Drug-free rows infected with either 2000 PFU, 200 PFU, 20 PFU, or 0 PFU serve as controls. After 4-day incubation of the plates at 37°C in 5% CO_2 atmosphere, cell monolayers are washed, and neutral red dye is introduced in the wells. The optical density at 492 nm of each well is determined with a spectrophotometer. The MIC corresponds to the lowest antibiotic concentration for which the mean OD at 492 nm is lower than that of the 20-PFU controls. Comparisons between the dye uptake assay and the plaque assay for determination of MICs have given consistent results.

A new cell culture system was recently described by Ives et al. (7) who determined the inhibition of *Rickettsia* proliferation, by comparison of rickettsial growth in infected Vero cell cultures incubated in the presence of an antibiotic to that in drug-free controls. Infected cells were revealed by an indirect immunofluorescent antibody method.

A few strains of *Rickettsia conorii* have been used in in vitro antibiotic susceptibility studies, inluding Moroccan strain and strain 7 (Table 2). Tetracycline, doxycycline, chloramphenicol, and rifampin all showed bacteriostatic activity (26). Erythromycin and spiramycin were poorly effective, with MICs of 4 μg/mL and 16 to 32 μg/mL, respectively (24, 26). More recently, clarithromycin was found to be rickettsiostatic, with MICs of 2 and 4 μg/mL against *R. conorii* Moroccan strain (13) and *R. conorii* strain 7 (7), respectively. Azithromycin, roxithromycin, and dirithromycin were rather less effective, with MICs of 16 μg/mL (7). Josamycin remains the most effective macrolide compound tested (MIC, 1 μg/mL) (24). The fluoroquinolone compounds pefloxacin, ofloxacin, and ciprofloxacin were rickettsiacidal in both the plaque assay and the dye uptake assay (8, 25, 27). Sparfloxacin was more effective, with MICs of 0.25 to 0.5 μg/mL (21). More recently, levofloxacin, the *l*-isomer of ofloxacin, was

TABLE 2 • In Vitro Antibiotic Susceptibility of *R. conorii*[a]

Antibiotics	MICs in cell cultures (μg/mL)				
	Plaque Assay	Dye Uptake	IF Assay	Strain	References
Amoxicillin	128	128		Moroccan	Raoult, unpublished data
	128	128		7	Raoult, unpublished data
Gentamicin	8	8		Moroccan	Raoult, unpublished data
	8	8		7	Raoult, unpublished data
Chloramphenicol	0.5	0.25		Moroccan	26
Thiamphenicol	1	2		Moroccan	Raoult, unpublished data
	1	2		7	Raoult, unpublished data
Tetracycline	0.25	0.25		Moroccan	26
Doxycycline	0.06	0.12		Moroccan	26
	0.06	0.125		7	Raoult, unpublished data
Erythromycin	4	4		Moroccan	26, 1988
	8	8		7	Raoult, unpublished data
			8	7	7
Spiramycin	16	32		Moroccan	24
Josamycin	1	1		Moroccan	24
	0.5	0.5		7	Raoult, unpublished data
Pristinamycin	2	2		Moroccan	Raoult, unpublished data
	2	1		7	Raoult, unpublished data
Clarithromycin	2	2		Moroccan	13
	1	1		7	Raoult, unpublished data
			4	7	7
Azithromycin			16	7	7
Dirithromycin			16	7	7
Roxithromycin			16	7	7
Rifampin	0.25	0.25		Moroccan	26
	0.125	0.125		7	Raoult, unpublished data
Ciprofloxacin	0.25	0.25		Moroccan	26
	0.5	0.5		7	Raoult, unpublished data
Ofloxacin	1			Moroccan	8
	1	1		7	Raoult, unpublished data
Pefloxacin	1	0.5		Moroccan	25
	0.5	1		7	Raoult, unpublished data
Sparfloxacin	0.25	0.5		Moroccan	21
Sulfamethoxazole	>8	>8		Moroccan	Raoult, unpublished data
	>8	>8		7	Raoult, unpublished data

[a]MICs (μg/mL) are presented for *R. conorii* Moroccan and Seven strains as determined by using the plaque assay and the dye uptake assay, and for *R. conorii* ATCC VR-613 as determined by using the immunofluorescent antibody assay (IF assay).

demonstrated to be twice as active as the racemic compound ofloxacin (14).

Only a few studies on in vitro antibiotic susceptibilities of spotted fever group rickettsiae other than *R. conorii, R. rickettsii,* and *R. akari* are available. The susceptibility of ELB agent (renamed *R. felis*) was evaluated in 1995 using both the plaque assay and the dye uptake assay (19). MICs were 2 and 1 μg/mL for chloramphenicol, 0.12 and 0.06 μg/mL for doxycycline, 0.25 and 0.5 μg/mL for rifampin, and 0.5 and 1 μg/mL for erythromycin, respectively, with the plaque assay and the dye uptake assay (19). The activity of clarithromycin was evaluated against an Israelian spotted fever group rickettsia (13). MICs were 2 μg/mL using the plaque assay, and 1 μg/mL using the dye uptake assay (13). A new strain of spotted fever group rickettsiae (named Bar 29) was obtained from *Rhipicephalus sanguineus* ticks collected in Catalonia (Spain) (2). Surprisingly, multiplication of the Bar 29 strain was not inhibited by rifampin used at concentrations up to 2.0 μg/mL.

Very recently, we tested the antibiotic susceptibilities of nine rickettsial species of the spotted fever group (Raoult, unpublished data) including *R. sibirica,* Israeli spotted fever rickettsia, *R. australis, R. japonica, R. honei,* Astrakhan fever rickettsia, *R. africae, Rickettsia* "mongolotimonae," and *R. slovaca.* Antibiotic susceptibilities were highly homogeneous among the rickettsial strains tested (Table 3). Amoxicillin and gentamicin were poorly effective, with MICs ranging from 128 to 256 μg/mL and 4 to 16 μg/mL, respectively. Cotrimoxazole was not effective with MICs above 8 and 1.6 μg/mL, respectively, for sulfamethoxazole and trimethoprim, for all strains tested. Doxycycline was the most effective compound, with MICs ranging from 0.06 to 0.125 μg/mL. MICs to thiamphenicol were 0.5 to 2 μg/mL. Erythromycin and pristinamycin were poorly effective, with MICs of 2 to 8 μg/mL and 1 to 8 μg/mL, respectively. MICs to josamycin and clarithromycin ranged from 0.5 to 1 μg/mL and 0.5 to 4 μg/mL, respectively. Fluoroquinolones compounds (pefloxacin, ofloxacin, and ciprofloxacin) were rickettsiostatic, with MICs of 0.5 to 2 μg/mL. MICs to rifampin were 0.03 to 1 μg/mL.

TABLE 3 • In Vitro Antibiotic Susceptibility of Spotted Fever Group Rickettsiae Other Than *R. rickettsii*, *R. conorii*, and *R. akari*[a]

Strain	doxy	thiam	rifam	ery	clar	josa	prist	cip	ofl	pef
R. sibirica (246)	0.06	0.5	0.06	2	2	1	2	1	1	1
Israeli spotted fever rickettsia	0.06	1	0.5	4	1	0.5	1	0.5	1	1
R. australis (Phillips)	0.06	2	0.125	8	4	0.5	2	0.5	1	1
R. japonica (YM)	0.125	1	0.25	8	1	1	8	1	1	1
R. honei (RB)	0.06	2	0.5	4	1	0.5	2	1	1	1
Astrakhan fever rickettsia (A-167)	0.06	0.5	0.03	8	0.5	0.5	2	0.5	0.5	0.5
R. africae (ESF-5)	0.125	1	0.125	8	2	0.5	2	0.5	1	1
R. "mongolotimonae"	0.125	1	0.125	8	4	1	2	1	1	1
R. slovaca (13-B)	0.06	1	0.5	2	0.5	1	1	1	1	1

[a]Minimum inhibitory concentrations (μg/mL) as determined in the plaque assay are summarized; doxy, doxycycline; thiam, thiamphenicol; rifam, rifampin; ery, erythromycin; clar, clarithromycin; josa, josamycin; prist, pristinamycin; cip, ciprofloxacin; ofl, ofloxacin; pef, pefloxacin.

TABLE 4 • In Vitro Antibiotic Susceptibility of Rickettsiae Isolated Only from Ticks[a]

Strain	doxy	thiam	rifam	ery	clar	josa	prist	cip	ofl	pef
R. bellii (369L42-1)	0.125	0.5	0.06	4	4	1	2	0.5	0.5	1
R. canada (2678)	0.06	1	0.125	4	1	1	2	0.5	0.5	1
R. helvetica (C9P9)	0.125	1	0.06	2	1	0.5	2	0.25	0.5	1
R. parkeri (Maculatum)	0.25	4	0.25	4	1	0.5	2	0.25	0.25	0.5
Thai tick typhus rickettsia typhus	0.06	2	0.125	8	1	1	4	0.5	2	1
Strain Bar 29	0.06	1	2	4	2	0.5	4	0.25	0.5	0.5
R. massiliae	0.06	1	2	2	1	1	1	0.25	0.5	0.5
R. aeschlimanii	0.06	1	2	8	1	0.5	2	0.5	0.5	1
R. montana (ATCC VR-611)	0.125	2	2	8	1	2	4	1	1	1
R. rhipicephali	0.25	1	2	4	1	1	2	1	1	1

[a]Minimum inhibitory concentrations (μg/mL) as determined in the plaque assay are summarized; doxy, doxycycline; thiam, thiamphenicol; rifam, rifampin; ery, erythromycin; clar, clarithromycin; josa, josamycin; prist, pristinamycin; cip, ciprofloxacin; ofl, ofloxacin; pef, pefloxacin.

In the same study, antibiotic susceptibilities of rickettsial species isolated only from arthropods were also tested, including *R. bellii*, *R. canada*, *R. helvetica*, *R. conorii* M1 strain, *R. parkeri*, Thai tick typhus rickettsia, strain Bar 29, *R. massiliae*, *R. aeschlimanii*, *R. montana*, and *R. rhipicephali* (Table 4). Although these strains showed antibiotic susceptibility patterns comparable to the rickettsial species previously described, a heterogeneity of susceptibility to rifampin among the different species was shown. Strain Bar 29 (as previously reported), *R. massiliae*, *R. eschlimanii*, *R. montana*, and *R. rhipicephali* were more resistant to rifampin (MICs ≥ 2 μg/mL); all five rickettsial strains belong to a same phylogenetic cluster. Such results led us to speculate that heterogeneity in rifampin susceptibility among various rickettsial species and in different geographic areas may explain clinical failures using this antibiotic to treat patients suffering from rickettsial diseases.

ANTIMICROBIAL THERAPY
Drug of Choice

The conventional antibiotic regimen for spotted fever group rickettsiosis is a 7- to 10-day oral course of doxycycline 200 mg daily. However, single-day therapy with 200 mg of doxycycline twice a day has been reported to be as effective as the conventional therapy for Mediterranean spotted fever (4, 5). Compared with the conventional antibiotic regimen, the single-day regimen presents the advantages of being well tolerated in almost all patients and cost-effective. It may represent a safe alternative in children, for whom the conventional regimen is contraindicated.

Monotherapy or Combination Therapy?

Antibiotic combinations have not been tested against rickettsiae in vitro. To date, no antibiotic combination has been shown to be superior in vivo to doxycycline alone. Combination therapy is not indicated in common clinical presentations of spotted fever group rickettsiosis. In severely ill patients, early administration of doxycycline before definite diagnosis is made is critical.

Special Situations

In severely diseased patients, doxycycline should be administered first by the intravenous route at 200 mg daily, and a prolonged duration, up to 3 days following apyrexia, should be considered. There is no clinical indication that other drugs should be more effective than tetracyclines, even in patients with neurologic complications.

Alternative Therapy

The real limitation of antibiotic therapy using tetracycline compounds is the possibility of side effects including gastric intolerance, but mainly the possibility of dental coloration in the neonate and young child. Thus, tetracyclines are contraindicated in pregnant women and in children. Chloramphenicol has long been considered the main alternative for rickettsial infections. Patients should be treated at least 8 days. However, chloramphenicol presents the potential risk of aplastic anemia. Recent in vitro and in vivo data indicate that chloramphenicol has only moderate rickettsiostatic activity. Relapse was reported in an Israeli patient suffering Mediterranean spotted fever who died despite completion of the chloramphenicol therapy (29). Erythromycin is not a safe alternative for Mediterranean spotted fever (18).

Following in vitro studies, josamycin was proposed as a possible alternative to tetracyclines. The usefulness of josamycin has been assessed in a randomized trial for antibiotic therapy of Mediterranean spotted fever, both in adults and children (4). Josamycin 1 g thrice daily orally (50 mg/kg of body weight twice daily in children) was as active as single-day therapy with doxycycline (200 mg twice daily for adults, 5 mg/kg of body weight in children). In pregnant women, josamycin may also represent a safe alternative to tetracyclines.

In vitro, spotted fever group rickettsiae was isolated from ticks in cell culture systems despite adding cotrimoxazole to the culture medium (12). Moreover, plaques were larger than those of drug-free controls (D. Raoult, personal communication). Cotrimoxazole is not useful for treating rickettsiosis and potentially may worsen the outcome of the disease.

A regimen of rifampin (10 mg/kg twice daily for 5 days) was also compared with the one-day doxycycline therapy schedule, in the region of Catalonia, in Spain (3). Outcome was favorable in both groups. However, delayed apyrexia was noticed in patients receiving rifampin. Moreover four patients become apyretic only after 5 days of therapy, which is comparable to usual time of spontaneous fever resolution. In one patient, rifampin was changed for doxycycline since rifampin therapy was considered a failure. Failures have been reported in Mediterranean spotted fever patients treated with rifampin in Catalonia (3), and a strain resistant to this antibiotic (Bar 29) was recently isolated from *Rhipicephalus* ticks in this region (2). It may be hypothesized that the existence of rifampin-resistant rickettsiae in some areas may explain therapy failures when using this antibiotic as well as contradictory reports from different areas on the effectiveness of rifampin to treat rickettsial diseases. More isolates are needed to resolve this hypothesis.

More recently, fluoroquinolones, including pefloxacin, ofloxacin, and ciprofloxacin have been shown to be effective in treatment of Mediterranean spotted fever (6, 10, 23, 27). A 10- to 15-day oral regimen of ofloxacin (200 mg twice daily), pefloxacin (400 mg twice daily), or ciprofloxacin (500 mg

twice daily) has been recommended. Shorter duration of antibiotic therapy was used with ciprofloxacin (27). A 2-day regimen of 500 mg of ciprofloxacin twice daily was compared with a 2-day course of doxycycline 200 mg daily. All patients treated with ciprofloxacin resolved. However, apyrexia was delayed in the short-term ciprofloxacin therapy group, compared with the doxycycline group. Fluoroquinolones administered for 7 to 10 days may be considered a safe alternative to tetracyclines to treat spotted fevers. However, as for tetracyclines, fluoroquinolones are contraindicated in children and pregnant women.

REFERENCES

1. Baird RW, Lloyd M, Stenos J, Ross BC, Stewart RS, Dwyer B. Characterization and comparison of Australian human spotted fever group rickettsiae. J Clin Microbiol 1992;30:2896–2902.
2. Beati L, Roux V, Ortuno A, Castella J, Segura Porta F, Raoult D. Phenotypic and genotypic characterization of spotted fever group rickettsiae isolated from Catalan *Rhipicephalus sanguineus* ticks. J Clin Microbiol 1996;34:2688–2694.
3. Bella F, Espejo E, Uriz S, Serrano JA, Alegre MD, Tort J. Randomized trial of five-day rifampin versus one-day doxycycline therapy for Mediterranean spotted fever. J Infect Dis 1991; 164:433.
4. Bella F, Font B, Uriz S, Munoz T, Espejo E, Traveria J, Serrano JA, Segura F. Randomized trial of doxycycline versus josamycin for Mediterranean spotted fever. Antimicrob Agents Chemother 1990;34:937–938.
5. Bella-Cueto F, Font-Creus B, Segura-Porta F, Espejo-Arenas E, Lopez-Parez P, Munoz-Espin T. Comparative, randomized trial of one-day doxycycline versus 10-day tetracycline therapy for Mediterranean spotted fever. J Infect Dis 1987;155:1056–1058.
6. Bernard E, Carles M, Politano S, Laffont C, Dellamonica P. Rickettsiosis caused by *Rickettsia conorii*: treatment by ofloxacin. Rev Infect Dis 1989;11(Suppl 5):S989.
7. Ives TJ, Manzewitsch P, Regnery RL, Butts JD, Kebede M. In vitro susceptibilities of *Bartonella henselae, B. quintana, B. elizabethae, Rickettsia rickettsii, R. conorii, R. akari,* and *R. prowazekii* to macrolide antibiotics as determined by immunofluorescent-antibody analysis of infected Vero cell monolayers. Antimicrob Agents Chemother 1997;41:578–582.
8. Jabarit-Aldighieri N, Torres H, Raoult D. Susceptibility of *R.conorii, R.rickettsii* and *C.burnetii* to CI-960 (PD 127,391), PD 131,628, pefloxacin, ofloxacin and ciprofloxacin. Antimicrob Agents Chemother 1992;36:2529–2532.
9. Jackson EB. Comparative efficacy of several antibiotics on experimental rickettsial infections in embryonated eggs. Antibiotics Chemother 1951;1:231–241.
10. Janbon F, Jonquet O, Reynes J, Bertrand A. Use of pefloxacin in the treatment of rickettsiosis and coxiellosis. Rev Infect Dis 1989;11(Suppl 5):990–991.
11. Kelly PJ, Beati L, Mason PR, Matthewman LA, Roux V, Raoult D. *Rickettsia africae* sp nov, the etiological agent of African tick bite fever. Int J Syst Bact 1996;46:611–614.
12. Kelly PJ, Raoult D, Mason PR. Isolation of spotted fever group rickettsias from triturated ticks using a modification of the centrifugation-shell vial technique. Trans R Soc Trop Med Hyg 1991;85:397–398.
13. Maurin M, Raoult D. In vitro susceptibilities of spotted fever group rickettsiae and *Coxiella burnetii* to clarithromycin. Antimicrob Agents Chemother 1993;37:2633–2637.

14. Maurin M, Raoult D. Bacteriostatic and bactericidal activity of levofloxacin against *Rickettsia rickettsii, R. conorii,* "Israeli spotted fever group rickettsia," and *Coxiella burnetii.* Submitted for publication.

15. McDade JE. Determination of antibiotic susceptibility of *Rickettsia* by the plaque assay technique. Appl Microbiol 1969;18: 133–135.

16. McDade JE, Gerone PJ. Plaque assay for Q fever and scrub typhus rickettsiae. Appl Microbiol 1970;19:963–965.

17. McDade JE, Stakebake JR, Jerone PJ. Plaque assay system for several species of *Rickettsia.* J Bacteriol 1969;99:910–912.

18. Munoz Espin T, Lopez Pares P, Espejo Arenas E, Font Creus B, Martinez Vila I, Traveria Casanova J, Segura Porta F, Bella Cueto F. Erythromycin versus tetracycline for treatment of Mediterranean spotted fever. Arch Dis Child 1986;61:1027–1029.

19. Radulovic S, Higgins JA, Jaworski DC, Azad AF. In vitro and in vivo antibiotic susceptibilities of ELB rickettsiae. Antimicrob Agents Chemother 1995;39:2564–2566.

20. Raoult D, Berbis Ph, Roux V, Xu W, and Maurin M. A new tick-transmitted disease due to *Rickettsia slovaca.* Lancet 1997;350: 112–113

21. Raoult D, Bres P, Drancourt M, Vestris G. In vitro susceptibilities of *Coxiella burnetii, Rickettsia rickettsii,* and *Rickettsia conorii* to the fluoroquinolone sparfloxacin. Antimicrob Agents Chemother 1991;35:88–91.

22. Raoult D, Brouqui P, Roux V. A new spotted-fever-group rickettsiosis. Lancet 1996;348:412

23. Raoult D, Gallais H, de Micco P, Casanova P. Ciprofloxacin therapy for Mediterranean spotted fever. Antimicrob Agents Chemother 1986;30:606–607.

24. Raoult D, Roussellier P, Tamalet J. In vitro evaluation of josamycin, spiramycin, and erythromycin against *Rickettsia rickettsii* and *R. conorii.* Antimicrob Agents Chemother 1988; 32:255–256.

25. Raoult D, Roussellier P, Vestris G, Galicher V, Perez R, Tamalet J. Susceptibility of *Rickettsia conorii* and *R. rickettsii* to pefloxacin, in vitro and in ovo. J Antimicrob Chemother 1987;19: 303–305.

26. Raoult D, Roussellier P, Vestris G, Tamalet J. In vitro antibiotic susceptibility of *Rickettsia rickettsii* and *Rickettsia conorii:* plaque assay and microplaque colorimetric assay. J Infect Dis 1987;155:1059–1062.

27. Raoult D, Zuchelli P, Weiller PJ, Charrell C, San Marco JL, Gallais H, Casanova P. Incidence, clinical observations and risk factors in the severe form of Mediterranean spotted fever among patients admitted to hospital in Marseilles 1983–1984. J Infect 1986;12:111–116.

28. Schriefer ME, Sacci JBJ, Dumler JS, Bullen MG, Azad AF. Identification of a novel rickettsial infection in a patient diagnosed with murine typhus. J Clin Microbiol 1994;32:949–954.

29. Shaked Y, Samra Y, Maier MK, Rubinstein E. Relapse of rickettsial Mediterranean spotted fever and murine typhus after treatment with chloramphenicol. J Infect 1989;18:35–37.

30. Smadel JE, Jackson EB, Gauld RL. Factors influencing the growth of rickettsiae. I. Rickettsiostatic effect of streotomycin in experimental infections. J Immunol 1947;57:273–284.

31. Stewart RS. Flinders Island spotted fever: a newly recognised endemic focus of tick typhus in Bass Strait. Part 1. Clinical and epidemiological features. Med J Aust 1991;154:94–99.

32. Tarasevich IV, Makarova V, Fetisova NF, Stepanov A, Mistkarova E, Balayeva N, Raoult D. Astrakhan fever: new spotted fever group rickettsiosis. Lancet 1991;337:172–173.

33. Uchida T. *Rickettsia japonica,* the etiologic agent of oriental spotted fever. Microbiol Immunol 1993;37:91–102.

34. Weinberg EH, Stakebake JR, Gerone PJ. Plaque assay for *Rickettsia rickettsii.* J Bacteriol 1969;98:398–402.

35. Wike DA, Tallent G, Peacock MG, Williams JC. Studies of the rickettsial plaque assay technique. Infect Immun 1972;5:715–722.

36. Wisseman CL, Waddell AD, Walsh WT. In vitro studies of the action of antibiotics on *Rickettsia prowazekii* by two basic methods of cell culture. J Infect Dis 1974;130:564–574.

37. Wong SC, Cox HR. Action of aureomycin against experimental rickettsial and viral infections. Ann NY Acad Sci 1948;51: 290–305.

38. Yu X, Fan M, Xu G, Liu Q, Raoult D. Genotypic and antigenic identification of two new strains of spotted fever group rickettsiae isolated from China. J Clin Microbiol 1993;31:83–88.

Rickettsia typhii

●

M. Maurin and D. Raoult

GENERAL DESCRIPTION
Epidemiology

Rickettsia typhi (R. mooseri), a typhus group rickettsia, is the etiologic agent of endemic or murine typhus. Murine typhus is a flea-borne zoonosis. *R. typhi* is transmitted primarily by the rat flea, *Xenopsylla cheopis,* although lice and mites are also potential vectors. Commensal rodents (mainly *Rattus norvegicus,* and *Rattus rattus*) are considered the main reservoir of bacteria. However, other vertebrate hosts may serve as reservoirs, including house mice, shrews, opossums, skunks, and cats. Rat and rat fleas do not suffer from *R. typhi* infection, and the latter remain infected lifelong. Transovarial transmission of *R. typhi* has been demonstrated in the Oriental rat flea. Murine typhus is of worldwide distribution. It occurs primarily in ports and coastal towns where commensal rodents are prevalent.

Clinical Manifestations

The clinical manifestations of murine typhus are similar to those of epidemic typhus, although the former is usually less severe. The incubation period is usually more prolonged than that of epidemic typhus. Prodromal symptoms include headache, arthralgia, and ill feeling, with or without low-grade fever. Onset is characterized by persistent headache, high-grade fever, and a cutaneous rash predominating on the trunk. The rash is usually less apparent than in epidemic typhus and occasionally absent. Complications remain rare in murine typhus, which is considered a benign disease since complete recovery occurs spontaneously in almost all cases. *R. felis,* first considered a typhus group rickettsia, is described among the spotted fever group rickettsiae to which it has now been demonstrated to belong.

Microbiology

Rickettsiae are strict intracellular bacteria that multiply within the cytoplasm of eukaryotic cells. Endothelial cells are the primary site of their multiplication, which explains the large dissemination of bacteria within the infected host. Only antibiotics that penetrate the eukaryotic cell membrane are potentially active against rickettsiae.

SUSCEPTIBILITY IN VITRO AND IN VIVO

Because of their obligately intracellular lifestyle, susceptibility of rickettsiae to antibiotics cannot be assessed in conventional microbiologic tests. Three types of experimental models have been developed to test the antibiotic susceptibility of rickettsiae, including animal models, the embryonated egg model, and cell culture models. Animal models and the embryonated egg model were the first described; however, antibiotic doses used in these models were much higher than those usually used in humans, and therefore it is difficult to extrapolate data to the clinical situation. In vitro infected cell models have been more recently elaborated. They allow more convenient investigation of the antibiotic susceptibility of rickettsiae, and extracellular antibiotic concentrations used in these models may be compared with antibiotic concentrations obtained in human sera.

Single Drug

Animal Models

In mice infected with murine typhus rickettsiae (1), chlortetracycline and, to a lesser extent, chloramphenicol were effective and increased survival, compared with untreated infected mice. Penicillin G was not effective (22).

Embryonated Egg Model

In the embryonated egg model, rickettsiae were injected into the yolk sac of the eggs. This resulted in death of the embryo, usually within a few days following infection. Antibiotics were administered by the same route, usually at the time of rickettsial inoculation. Antibiotic activity was deduced from the difference in mean survival time (DMST) of infected embryos receiving antibiotics, compared with infected untreated controls. A rickettsiostatic effect of antibiotics allowed the embryos to survive up to the last day of experiments, usually 14 days. The rickettsiacidal activity of antibiotics was assessed by subculturing yolk sacs from surviving eggs at 14 days postinfection. Direct examination of smears prepared from in-

fected tissues and stained with the Gimenez technique were also informative regarding the action of antibiotics. This model, however, did not allow direct evaluation of the growth rate of rickettsiae.

Using the embryonated egg model, penicillin G, streptomycin, and gentamicin were not effective (5, 14, 19). PABA (*p*-aminobenzoic acid) displayed only moderate activity (4, 11, 14). Chloramphenicol allowed a DMST of 2.5 days or more at concentrations of 250 µg/egg or above (13). Oxytetracycline (Terramycin), chlortetracycline (Aureomycin), doxycycline, erythromycin, and rifampin were found to be effective against *R. typhi* (10, 16) (Table 1).

Cell Culture Models

The primary target cells for rickettsiae are endothelial cells. However, a number of eukaryotic cell lines can be infected with rickettsiae in vitro, including fibroblasts, macrophages, primary chick embryo cells, and human endothelial cells. Plaque formation in infected cell cultures was first used for numeration of viable rickettsiae (7, 8, 18, 20) and was then adapted to determine their in vitro antibiotic susceptibility (7, 9, 21). The plaque assay system is currently the recommended technique, allowing evaluation of both the bacteriostatic and the bactericidal activity of antibiotics. Cell monolayers (usually Vero cells) grown in tissue culture Petri dishes are acutely infected by rocking incubation with a rickettsial inoculum. Infected cells are then overlaid with Eagle MEM with 2% fetal calf serum and 0.5% agar. Antibiotics are added at different concentrations at the same time, with no antibiotics added in drug-free controls. Petri dishes are incubated 4 days at 37°C in a 5% CO_2 atmosphere. Cell monolayers are then stained with neutral red dye, allowing visualization of the plaques. The MICs are defined as the lowest antibiotic concentration allowing complete inhibition of plaque formation, compared with a drug-free growth control.

A disk assay was proposed as a convenient modification of the plaque assay. In this model, antibiotic disks are placed on the surface of the agar overlay. The diameter of the plaque formation inhibition zone around the antibiotic disk represents a measure of the antirickettsial activity of the antibiotic.

R. typhi strain Wilmington (ATCC VR-144) was used in most in vitro antibiotic susceptibility experiments. In early experiments using the plaque assay technique, authors showed that chloramphenicol (MIC = 1.0 µg/mL), tetracycline (MIC = 0.1 µg/mL), chlortetracycline (MIC = 1.0 µg/mL), and erythromycin (MIC = 1.0 µg/mL) were bacteriostatic against *R. typhi* (1). In contrast, penicillin G, methicillin, ampicillin, oxacillin, and cephalothin were not, which concurred with the poor activity β-lactam compounds show against rickettsial infections in vivo. The other antibiotics tested in this study were not bacteriostatic, including aminoglycosides (kanamycin, streptomycin, neomycin), novobiocin, lincomycin, viomycin, cycloserine, bacitracin, polymyxin B, sulfisoxazole, and sulfadiazine (1). Chloramphenicol was active against *R. typhi* grown in human macrophages (3). Nalidixic acid produced only partial inhibition of plaque formation by *R. typhi* (7),

TABLE 1 • **In Vitro Antibiotic Susceptibility of *R. typhi* Strain Wilmington (ATCC VR-144)**[a]

Antibiotics	Embryonated Eggs (μg/egg)	Cell Cultures MICs (μg/mL)	References
Penicillin G		100	1
Methicillin		500	1
Oxacillin		>500	1
Ampicillin		500	1
Amoxicillin		128	Raoult, unpublished data
Cephalothin		>100	1
Streptomycin	10,000		14
		>500	1
Gentamicin	500		19
		16	Raoult, unpublished data
Kanamycin		500	1
Neomycin		>250	1
Chloramphenicol		1	1
Chlortetracycline	125		10
		1	1
Oxytetracycline	50		16
	30		15
Tetracycline		0.1	1
Doxycycline	50		16
		0.125	Raoult, unpublished data
Erythromycin	50		16
	40		10
		1	1
		0.5	Raoult, unpublished data
Lincomycin		100	1
Pristinamycin		2	Raoult, unpublished data
Josamycin		1	Raoult, unpublished data
Clarithromycin		1	Raoult, unpublished data
Ciprofloxacin		1	Raoult, unpublished data
Ofloxacin		1	Raoult, unpublished data
Pefloxacin		1	Raoult, unpublished data
Sulfisoxazole		>200	1
Sulfadiazine		>500	1
Rifampin	50		16
		0.25	Raoult, unpublished data

[a] Minimum concentrations (μg/egg) to obtain DMST ≥ 2.5 days and MICs (μg/mL) are presented for the embryonated egg and cell culture models, respectively.

whereas the fluoroquinolone compounds were moderately active.

In a more recent investigation (Raoult, unpublished data), *R. typhi* was shown to be highly susceptible to doxycycline and rifampin (MICs of 0.125 and 0.25 μg/mL, respectively). Thiamphenicol and erythromycin were rickettsiostatic at concentrations of 2 and 0.5 μg/mL, respectively. Activity of josamycin and clarithromycin was comparable to that of erythromycin. The fluoroquinolones pefloxacin, ofloxacin and ciprofloxacin inhibited rickettsial growth at 1 μg/mL of extracellular concentration.

ANTIMICROBIAL THERAPY
Drug of Choice

The conventional antibiotic regimen for typhus group rickettsiosis is a 7- to 14-day oral course of doxycycline 200 mg daily. However, a single dose (100 to 200 mg) of doxycycline has been reported to be as effective as the conventional therapy for murine typhus (6), although this has been rather less documented than for epidemic typhus. This may represent the current recommendation, especially in developing countries where drugs are scarce.

Antibiotic combinations have not been tested in vitro against *R. typhi*. No antibiotic combination has been shown to be superior in vivo to doxycycline alone. Combination therapy is not indicated in common clinical presentations of epidemic typhus. Early administration of doxycycline before definite diagnosis is made is critical.

Special Situations

In severely diseased patients, doxycycline should be administered first by the intravenous route (200 mg daily), and a 14-day duration should be considered. There is no clinical indication that other drugs should be more effective than tetracyclines, even in patients with neurologic complications.

Alternative Therapy

The real limitation of the antibiotic therapy using tetracycline compounds is the possibility of side effects including gastric intolerance and dental coloration in the neonate and the young child. Thus, tetracyclines are contraindicated in pregnant women and children. As for epidemic typhus, the single-dose regimen of doxycycline may represent a safe alternative in children. Relapses of murine typhus have been reported in Israel after treatment with chloramphenicol (12). Among 72 patients suffering murine typhus, 9 (12.5 %) relapsed 3 to 8 days after completion of chloramphenicol therapy (2–3 g daily, 6–14 days). Five of the patients who relapsed became afebrile spontaneously; the remaining 4 were successfully treated with tetracycline. Chloramphenicol displays only poor rickettsiostatic activity and should not be considered a useful alternative, especially when antibiotic administration has been delayed and/or in severely ill patients. There are two reports of successful therapy for murine typhus with ciprofloxacin (2, 17). Fluoroquinolones are highly active against rickettsiae in vitro and are also active in the treatment of enteric fever, but more clinical data are needed. Fluoroquinolones are also contraindicated in the child and the pregnant woman.

REFERENCES

1. Barker LF. Determination of antibiotic susceptibility of rickettsiae and chlamydiae in BS-C-1 cell cultures. Antimicrob Agents Chemother 1968;8:425–428.
2. Eaton M, Cohen MT, Shlim DR, Innes B. Ciprofloxacin treatment of typus [Letter]. JAMA 1989;262:772–773.
3. Gambrill MR, Wisseman CL Jr. Mechanisms of immunity in typhus infections. I. Multiplication of typhus rickettsiae in human macrophage cell cultures in the nonimmune system: influence of virulence of rickettsial strains and of chloramphenicol. Infect Immun 1973;8:519–527.
4. Hamilton HL, Plotz H, Smadel JE. Effect of p-aminobenzoic acid on the growth of typhus rickettsiae in the yolk sac of infected chick embryo. Proc Soc Exp Biol Med 1945;58:255–262.
5. Jackson EB. Comparative efficacy of several antibiotics on experimental rickettsial infections in embryonated eggs. Antibiot Chemother 1951;1:231–241.
6. Krause DW, Perine PL, McDade JE, Awoke S. Treatment of louse-borne typhus fever with chloramphenicol, tetracycline or doxycycline. East Afr Med J 1975;52:421–427.
7. McDade JE. Determination of antibiotic susceptibility of *Rickettsia* by the plaque assay technique. Appl Microbiol 1969; 18:133–135.
8. McDade JE, Gerone PJ. Plaque assay for Q fever and scrub typhus rickettsiae. Appl Microbiol 1970;19:963–965.
9. McDade JE, Stakebake JR, Jerone PJ. Plaque assay system for several species of *Rickettsia*. J Bacteriol 1969;99:910–912.
10. Ormsbee RA, Parker H, Pickens EG. The comparative effectiveness of chlortetracycline, oxytetracycline, chloramphenicol, erythromycin, and thiomycetin in suppressing experimental rickettsial infections in chick embryos. J Infect Dis 1955;96:162–167.
11. Robbins ML, Bourke AR, Smith PK. The effect of certain chemicals on *Rickettsia typhi* in chick embryos. J Immunol 1950;64: 431–446.
12. Shaked Y, Samra Y, Maier MK, Rubinstein E. Relapse of rickettsial Mediterranean spotted fever and murine typhus after treatment with chloramphenicol. J Infect 1989;18:35–37.
13. Smadel JE, Jackson EB, Cruise AB. Chloromycetin in experimental rickettsial infections. J Immunol 1949;62:49–65.
14. Smadel JE, Jackson EB, Gauld RL. Factors influencing the growth of rickettsiae. I. Rickettsiostatic effect of streptomycin in experimental infections. J Immunol 1947;57:273–284.
15. Snyder JC, Fagan R, Wells EB, Wicks HC, Miller JC. Experimental studies on the antirickettsial properties of terramycin. Ann NY Acad Sci 1950;53:362–374.
16. Spicer AJ, Peacock MG, Williams JC. Effectiveness of several antibiotics in suppressing chick embryo lethality during experimental infections by *Coxiella burnetii*, *Rickettsia typhi,* and *R. rickettsii*. In: Burgdorfer W, Anacker RL, eds. Rickettsiae and rickettsial diseases. New York: Academic Press, 1981: 375–383.
17. Strand O, Stromberg A. Ciprofloxacin treatment of murine typhus. Scand J Infect Dis 1990;22:503–504.
18. Weinberg EH, Stakebake JR, Gerone PJ. Plaque assay for *Rickettsia rickettsii*. J Bacteriol 1969;98:398–402.
19. White LA, Hall HE, Tzianabos T, Chappell WA. Effect of gentamicin on growth of viral, chlamydial, and rickettsial agents in mice and embryonated eggs. Antimicrob Agents Chemother 1976;10:344–346.
20. Wike DA, Tallent G, Peacock MG, Williams JC. Studies of the rickettsial plaque assay technique. Infect Immun 1972;5:715–722.
21. Wisseman CL, Waddell AD, Walsh WT. In vitro studies of the action of antibiotics on *Rickettsia prowazekii* by two basic methods of cell culture. J Infect Dis 1974;130:564–574.
22. Wong SC, Cox HR. Action of aureomycin against experimental rickettsial and viral infections. Ann NY Acad Sci 1948;51: 290–305.

PART D

Miscellaneous

Bartonella Species

Jane E. Koehler and David A. Relman

GENERAL DESCRIPTION

There are currently nine known species of *Bartonella*, four of which have been associated with human infection: *B. henselae*, *B. quintana, B. elizabethae* and *B. bacilliformis. Bartonella henselae, B. quintana*, and *B. elizabethae* were previously classified in the genus *Rochalimaea* and considered rickettsiae but were moved to the genus *Bartonella* in 1993 and are no longer classified as rickettsial agents (2). The spectrum of disease caused by *Bartonella* species includes cat scratch disease *(B. henselae)*, bacillary angiomatosis *(B. henselae* and *B. quintana)*, bacillary peliosis *(B. henselae)*, endocarditis *(B. henselae, B. quintana,* and *B. elizabethae)*, relapsing bacteremia *(B. henselae* and *B. quintana)*, trench fever *(B. quintana)*, Oroya fever *(B. bacilliformis)*, and verruga peruana *(B. bacilliformis)* (13).

Infections occur in both immunocompromised and immunocompetent individuals, but the manifestations and response to treatment are dramatically different, depending on the immune status of the patient. Cat scratch disease, a benign, self-limited granulomatous lymphadenitis caused by *B. henselae,* occurs in immunocompetent individuals. The primary cat scratch disease lesion occurs at the site of a cat scratch, 3 to 10 days after the inoculation. Lymphadenopathy develops 2 weeks after the scratch and regresses spontaneously over the ensuing 2 to 4 months (21).

Bacillary angiomatosis and bacillary peliosis are vascular proliferative manifestations of *Bartonella* infection that occur in immunocompromised patients (30), especially those coinfected with human immunodeficiency virus (HIV). Bacillary angiomatosis infections occur most commonly late in HIV infection; in one series, the median CD_4 cell count of patients at the time of bacillary angiomatosis diagnosis was 22/mm³ (24). *B. quintana* and *B. henselae* cause bacillary angiomatosis; these lesions are most commonly noted in the skin, but also can occur in the brain, bones, subcutaneous tissues, lymph nodes, and gastrointestinal and respiratory tracts. Peliosis is a closely related vascular proliferative lesion caused by *B. henselae* infection in the liver and spleen of immunocompromised patients (26). More than half of patients with focal bacillary angiomatosis are bacteremic with the corresponding *Bartonella* species, emphasizing the systemic nature of this disease (16a).

B. bacilliformis infections occur exclusively in South America, most commonly in the Peruvian Andes at an altitude between 2500 and 8000 feet (37). The acute infection, Oroya fever, can cause a severe, potentially fatal hemolytic anemia

that is often followed by a chronic phase, verruga peruana, or Peruvian warts (7). These cutaneous lesions may be clinically indistinguishable from bacillary angiomatosis and persist for months to years, causing few symptoms.

The *Bartonella* infections most frequently encountered by physicians are bacillary angiomatosis and cat scratch disease (the latter is by far the most common, with more than 22,000 cases annually in the United States (10)). Treatment of neither bacillary angiomatosis nor cat scratch disease has been studied prospectively or systematically. The aggregate of anecdotal cases of cat scratch disease treatment does not demonstrate clearly that treatment affects outcome in immunocompetent individuals, and virtually all patients recover fully regardless of whether they receive antibiotic treatment or not. In contrast, bacillary angiomatosis and bacillary peliosis can cause death if not treated (5), and the response to antibiotic treatment is often dramatic. This difference in treatment response may be due to the number of *Bartonella* bacilli present in lesions (fewer in cat scratch disease, more numerous in bacillary angiomatosis) or the immune status of the infected individual, or both.

SUSCEPTIBILITY IN VITRO AND IN VIVO
In Vitro Susceptibilities

Bartonella species are small, Gram-negative rods that are extremely fastidious. As for many other fastidious organisms, in vitro susceptibility testing is not standardized. Additionally, there is a striking discrepancy between some of the in vitro and in vivo antibiotic susceptibility patterns obtained for *Bartonella* species. This discrepancy is especially notable for antibiotics that affect cell wall synthesis (e.g., penicillins). Most in vitro susceptibility testing reveals MIC_{90}s approximately less than 0.05 µg/mL for penicillin (22), yet we and many others have noted failures and even dramatic disease progression during treatment with this drug (15, 17). The clinical utility of MICs derived from in vitro susceptibility testing has therefore not been established, and we do not recommend routine susceptibility testing of *Bartonella* isolates to guide patient therapy.

The earliest in vitro susceptibility testing for *Bartonella* species was reported by Myers et al. in 1984 (25). They tested two *B. quintana* strains, the Fuller strain (type strain ATCC VR358) and Heliodoro strain, using the agar dilution method (antibiotics diluted with agar composed of GC agar base with IsoVitaleX supplementation). They found MIC_{50}/MIC_{90}s for penicillin of 0.024/0.035 µg/mL and 0.024/0.044 µg/mL for the two strains, respectively. The Fuller and Heliodoro strains were susceptible to erythromycin (MIC_{50}/MIC_{90}, 0.026/0.036 µg/mL and 0.033/0.040 µg/mL, respectively), doxycycline (MIC_{50}/MIC_{90}, 0.021/0.036 µg/mL and 0.095/0.115 µg/mL) and tetracycline (MIC_{50}/MIC_{90}, 0.040/0.068 µg/mL and 0.35/0.82 µg/mL).

More recently, Maurin et al. (22) reported MICs for 28 antibiotics with 14 *Bartonella* isolates, also using an agar dilution method, but using Columbia agar supplemented with 5% horse blood. They also observed susceptibility to penicillin G (MIC_{90} range, 0.015–0.06 µg/mL) for all *Bartonella* species: *B. quintana* (9 strains), *B. vinsonii* (1 strain), *B. elizabethae* (1 strain) and *B. henselae* (3 strains). All 14 *Bartonella* species and strains tested were susceptible to erythromycin, doxycycline, and rifampin. Additionally, they noted susceptibility of all *Bartonella* isolates to azithromycin and clarithromycin.

In another study, the susceptibility of *B. henselae* and *B. quintana* to five macrolides was tested using in vitro cultivation with Vero cell monolayers: all five macrolide antibiotics demonstrated activity against both these *Bartonella* species (9). Most recently, the E-Test (AB Biodisk, Solna, Sweden) was used to test the erythromycin, azithromycin, doxycycline, ciprofloxacin, rifampin, and vancomycin susceptibilities of 10 *B. henselae* isolates grown on chocolate agar (38). The susceptibilities for doxycycline, erythromycin, azithromycin, and rifampin correlated with those from agar dilution methods. Use of E-Test strips with *Bartonella* isolates streaked on fresh chocolate agar is the susceptibility testing method most accessible to a general microbiology laboratory and may be useful for comparing initial and relapse isolates for changes in susceptibility. Susceptibility testing with drug combinations has not been performed.

Recently reported animal data substantiate the role of macrolides or a tetracycline in the treatment of *Bartonella* infection. Regnery et al. experimentally infected 25 cats with *B. henselae* and then treated groups of 5 cats for 2 weeks with one of four different antibiotics: tetracycline, amoxicillin, erythromycin, or enrofloxacin, a fluoroquinolone (29). They cultured the blood of each animal at intervals after experimental infection and determined that only tetracycline or erythromycin treatment significantly decreased the titer of *B. henselae* bacilli in the blood at any time during the period after infection. There were no significant differences among the four antibiotics with regard to apparent resolution of bacteremia; however, bacteremia resolved at day 71 for tetracycline- and erythromycin-treated cats, at day 83 for control cats, and at days 98 and 127 for those treated with enrofloxacin and amoxicillin, respectively.

ANTIMICROBIAL THERAPY
Bartonella Infection in the Immunocompromised Patient

Bacillary Angiomatosis and Bacillary Peliosis

Stoler et al. described the first patient with bacillary angiomatosis in 1983, and although the disease had not been named nor the infecting bacillus identified, they treated the patient successfully with erythromycin (33). In 1987, we treated the cutaneous and osseous bacillary angiomatosis lesions of the first prospectively identified patient at San Francisco General Hospital with erythromycin; the lesions resolved completely (15). We have now treated more than 65 patients with biopsy-proven bacillary angiomatosis, and from our experience and review of the published literature on treatment of anecdotal bacillary angiomatosis (summarized in refs. 17 and 23), either one of two drugs can be confidently recommended for first-line therapy: erythromycin or doxycycline. The response to treatment appears to be equivalent whether erythromycin or doxycycline is prescribed and whether the bacillary angiomatosis is caused by *B. henselae* or *B. quintana*.

For treatment of *Bartonella* infection in the immunocompromised patient, the drug of first choice is either erythromycin (500 mg every 6 h orally or intravenously) or doxycycline (100 mg every 12 h orally or intravenously). We usually initiate therapy for bacillary angiomatosis with oral erythromycin but favor oral doxycycline over erythromycin in several situations: when poor patient compliance dictates twice-daily dosing, to achieve potentially superior central nervous system (CNS) antibiotic delivery for focal CNS *Bartonella* infection, or when severe gastrointestinal symptoms are present that could be exacerbated by oral erythromycin therapy. Rifampin also appears to have in vivo activity in patients with bacillary angiomatosis lesions, but because bacteria spontaneously develop rifampin resistance at a high rate, we do not recommend use of this antibiotic alone.

Combination therapy with addition of rifampin to either erythromycin or doxycycline is recommended for immunocompromised patients with acute, life-threatening *Bartonella* infection, including bacillary peliosis, endocarditis, or CNS disease. Failure to respond to antibiotic treatment after 7 to 10 days should prompt change of drug therapy to the other first-line drug, addition of rifampin, change to intravenous antibiotic administration, or all of these. The intravenous route is especially important in patients with severe *Bartonella* infection of the gastrointestinal tract who may have inadequate absorption of the antibiotic and symptom exacerbation by oral erythromycin therapy.

Although some anecdotal reports describe a response of *Bartonella* infection to ciprofloxacin, we have observed progression of bacillary angiomatosis lesions in patients treated with ciprofloxacin (35). In addition, we have isolated *Bartonella* species from immunocompromised patients treated with gentamicin or trimethoprim/sulfamethoxazole (16a) and would therefore not recommend treating patients with bacillary angiomatosis infection with either of these antibiotics.

It has become evident that most patients with cutaneous bacillary angiomatosis have systemic disease, and a short duration of treatment is frequently associated with relapse. At least 3 months of antibiotic treatment is recommended for patients with cutaneous bacillary angiomatosis, and 4 months for patients with bacillary peliosis (17). For patients with bacillary angiomatosis of the bone or CNS, treatment should continue for at least 4 months. After discontinuation of antibiotic therapy, patients should be monitored carefully for relapse of *Bartonella* infection in the same organ or at a new site. If relapse occurs, the patient should receive treatment and lifelong secondary prophylaxis with either doxycycline or a macrolide (11).

Alternative Therapy

For patients unable to tolerate erythromycin or doxycycline, alternative antibiotics include minocycline (100 mg orally every 12 h), used to treat bacillary angiomatosis successfully in an immunocompetent adult (36), or tetracycline (500 mg orally every 6 h), used to treat an HIV-infected patient with bacillary angiomatosis successfully (16). Experience with azithromycin is very limited; this antibiotic could be considered if a patient cannot comply with twice-daily doxycycline. Azithromycin (500 mg orally every 24 h) for 28 to 90 days was used to treat 5 of the 10 immunocompetent patients with *B. quintana* bacteremia reported by Spach et al. (32), and 1 immunocompromised patient with bacillary angiomatosis was successfully treated with 1 g orally every 24 h (8).

Bartonella Infection in the Immunocompetent Patient

Uncomplicated Cat Scratch Disease

There is no convincing evidence that antibiotic treatment affects the course of either complicated or uncomplicated cat scratch disease in the immunocompetent patient. One study (20) assessed treatment of 268 cat scratch disease patients retrospectively. Four antibiotics, rifampin, ciprofloxacin, gentamicin, and trimethoprim-sulfamethoxazole, were judged efficacious, based on 3 or more days of therapy and clinical improvement of the patient, but many of the patients had received multiple antibiotics for periods of different duration. Additional anecdotal case reports describe the response of cat scratch disease to gentamicin (1, 18) and other antibiotics, as well as failures with virtually all antibiotics. For uncomplicated cat scratch disease, treatment is not recommended.

No prospective study has been performed to demonstrate antibiotic efficacy in treatment of immunocompetent patients with uncomplicated cat scratch disease. Because the natural course of cat scratch disease is relatively benign, self-limited, and extremely variable, the practical clinical application of retrospective studies evaluating antibiotic therapy for cat scratch disease is limited. More important, as antibiotic resistance of many bacteria is increasing dramatically, treatment of uncomplicated cat scratch disease does not appear to be justified from either the standpoint of the individual patient who is likely to experience little benefit (yet would be exposed to potential antibiotic side effects) or from a public health standpoint.

Complicated Cat Scratch Disease: Retinitis, CNS Infection, and Granulomatous Hepatitis

Treatment of complicated cat scratch disease, including retinitis, granulomatous hepatitis, and encephalitis, with many different antibiotics has been reported by a number of authors. As with cat scratch disease, however, it is not clear that antibiotics have any efficacy in the treatment of these manifestations in immunocompetent patients. Wong et al. (39) report one patient with stellate neuroretinitis from whose blood *B. henselae* was isolated. However, despite receiving doxycycline and rifampin for 1 month and experiencing resolution of ophthalmologic symptoms, *B. henselae* could still be cultured from the blood of this patient.

Despite the apparent lack of demonstrated efficacy, many clinicians elect to administer intravenous antibiotics to patients ill enough to require hospitalization; in vivo experience with doxycycline and rifampin in immunocompromised patients makes this combination a reasonable choice if treatment of these patients is elected.

Relapsing Bacteremia

Clinical experience with treatment of isolated *Bartonella* bacteremia also is limited. Historically, soldiers with *B. quintana* relapsing bacteremia (trench fever) during World War I cleared the infection in the absence of antibiotic treatment. In contemporary times, one immunocompetent patient with *B. henselae* bacteremia and meningitis treated with amoxicillin for 5 days, then doxycycline for 2 weeks, and finally ceftriaxone for 10 days had positive blood cultures for the subsequent 6 weeks, despite resolution of symptoms (19). As with other *Bartonella* infections in the immunocompetent host, *Bartonella* bacteremia may be a self-limited infection. However, treatment of *Bartonella* bacteremia should be attempted, probably with doxycycline for 2 to 4 weeks. An important caveat: the patient must first be evaluated carefully for endocarditis, because this will change the duration and follow-up of antibiotic treatment.

Endocarditis

Spach et al. (31) summarized four patients with *Bartonella* endocarditis; all received antibiotic therapy with multiple drugs, three had valve replacement, and all were cured. The patient who did not require valve replacement received treatment with ceftriaxone, doxycycline, and erythromycin. The other three patients who required valve replacement did not receive treatment with a first-line antibiotic against *Bartonella* species prior to valve replacement, and whether surgery was required due to ineffective antibiotic treatment or the natural course of *Bartonella* endocarditis in these three patients is not known. In these three patients, valve replacement may have been curative.

In a series of 33 *Bartonella* endocarditis patients (27), only one surviving patient did not require valve replacement, and this patient was treated with ceftriaxone and doxycycline. The remainder of the patients received numerous other antibiotics before and after valvular surgery. *B. henselae* was isolated from one patient after completion of a course of amoxicillin and gentamicin, and we have isolated *Bartonella* species from a patient receiving similar treatment. Thus, the standard culture-negative endocarditis regimen using gentamicin plus penicillin or amoxicillin is unlikely to treat *Bartonella* endocarditis adequately.

Patients with *Bartonella* endocarditis should receive 6 weeks of antibiotic therapy, probably with two drugs (doxycycline plus rifampin or erythromycin plus rifampin), because neither first-line drug is bactericidal.

Oroya Fever and Verruga Peruana

Antibiotic treatment of patients infected with *B. bacilliformis* decreases the morbidity and mortality associated with both acute and chronic stages of infection with this pathogen. Mortality due to Oroya fever was estimated to be 40% prior to the era of antibiotics and is now estimated to be approximately 8% (7). Some patients who survive the acute infection succumb to intercurrent infection with intracellular pathogens such as *Salmonella, Toxoplasma,* and *Mycobacterium,* because of an immunodeficient state that may develop after resolution of Oroya fever (7). Thus, although penicillin treatment can attenuate the lysis of erythrocytes during the acute phase, patients in endemic regions of South America often are treated with chloramphenicol to reduce the mortality from intercurrent *Salmonella* infection. Antibiotic treatment of Oroya fever may not prevent subsequent development of verrugae (37).

Bartonella elizabethae

Only one human infection with *B. elizabethae* has been reported, in a patient with endocarditis (6). This patient defervesced during treatment with nafcillin and gentamicin but developed progressive congestive heart failure and required valve replacement.

ENDPOINTS FOR MONITORING THERAPY

Patients with cutaneous bacillary angiomatosis lesions should be evaluated for presence of *Bartonella* infection at other sites that would alter therapy duration (e.g., osseous lesions or endocarditis). Cutaneous lesions usually improve in the first several weeks of antibiotic therapy and resolve completely in 1 to 2 months, depending on the size and number of lesions. Patients with peliosis hepatis can be monitored by abdominal computed tomography (CT) scanning, and those with osseous lesions, by technetium-99m bone scans. Patients in whom antibiotic therapy has been stopped should be followed closely for recurrence of *Bartonella* infection at the original site as well as at new sites (e.g., a patient treated for osteomyelitis may develop bacteremia) (16).

An additional concern is the propensity for doxycycline to cause pill-associated ulcerative esophagitis (12). This complication, most frequently reported when a dose is taken with only a small amount of liquid or at night just before retiring, can be prevented by taking doxycycline several hours before bedtime with copious amounts of water.

A Jarisch-Herxheimer-like reaction has been described in immunocompromised patients after receiving the first several doses of antibiotics (16). Physicians should advise patients of this possible treatment complication, and patients with severe respiratory and/or cardiovascular compromise should be monitored carefully following institution of antimicrobial therapy. This reaction has occasionally been mistaken for an adverse drug reaction.

PREVENTION AND PROPHYLAXIS
Prevention of Bartonella Infection

Bartonella species often are vector borne, and control of the associated vector may help decrease incidence of these infections. The cat flea efficiently transmits *B. henselae* from cat to cat (4), which is hypothesized to facilitate creation of the large reservoir of infected cats (as many as 41% of cats are infected

in the San Francisco Bay area (14)). Fleas could potentially transmit *B. henselae* directly to humans, but this has not been documented to date, and the vast majority of human *B. henselae* infections occur following a cat scratch or bite (21). Control of cat flea infestation is recommended, especially for pets of immunocompromised patients (28). This strategy may reduce the transmission of *B. henselae* by decreasing feline infection, reducing contamination of cat claws due to scratching, and reducing the potential of direct transmission to humans via fleas. Additional recommendations for decreasing the risk of *B. henselae* infection include acquiring a mature cat, which is less likely to scratch and less likely to be bacteremic (3, 14), washing cat wounds immediately with soap and water, and avoiding rough play with the cat (11, 28).

Antibiotic treatment of cats belonging to immunocompromised individuals has been proposed, but it is not evident that *Bartonella* infection can be permanently eradicated from the feline reservoir (29). In addition, treatment usually involves orally force-feeding antibiotics to the cat, which incurs substantial risk of cat scratches and bites and is likely to increase risk of transmission of *B. henselae* to the humans involved.

B. quintana is transmitted from human to human by the body louse (34); homeless individuals are at increased risk for infestation with the body louse and thus for infection with *B. quintana*. Avoiding infestation with, and exposure to, the body louse is the only current recommendation for prevention of *B. quintana* infection. For *B. bacilliformis,* the substantial decrease of infection in endemic regions of the Peruvian Andes has been attributed not only to antibiotic treatment but also to reduction of the sandfly vector for this *Bartonella* species (37). The reservoir and vector for *B. elizabethae* remain unknown, thus there are no recommendations about prevention of infection with this species.

Prophylaxis

It is likely that *Mycobacterium avium* complex prophylaxis or treatment regimens that include a macrolide or rifabutin, or both, will provide adequate prophylaxis against *Bartonella* infection, because both of these classes of antibiotics have shown good in vivo activity against *Bartonella* species. Treatment with macrolide antibiotics was protective against B. henselae and B. quintana infection in HIV-infected patients in one study (16a).

REFERENCES

1. Bogue CW, Wise JD, Gray GF, Edwards KM. Brief report: antibiotic therapy for cat-scratch disease? JAMA 1989;262: 813–816.
2. Brenner DJ, O'Connor SP, Winkler HH, Steigerwalt AG. Proposals to unify the genera *Bartonella* and *Rochalimaea,* with descriptions of *Bartonella quintana* comb. nov., *Bartonella vinsonii* comb. nov., *Bartonella henselae* comb. nov., and *Bartonella elizabethae* comb. nov., and to remove the family *Bartonellaceae* from the order *Rickettsiales*. Int J Syst Bacteriol 1993;43: 777–786.
3. Chomel BB, Abbott RC, Kasten RW, Floyd-Hawkins KA, Kass PH, Glaser CA, Pedersen NC, Koehler JE. *Bartonella henselae* prevalence in domestic cats in California: risk factors and association between bacteremia and antibody titers. J Clin Microbiol 1995;33:2445–2450.

4. Chomel BB, Kasten RW, Floyd-Hawkins K, Chi B, Yamamoto K, Roberts-Wilson J, Gurfield AN, Abbott RC, Pedersen NC, Koehler JE. Experimental transmission of *Bartonella henselae* by the cat flea. J Clin Microbiol 1996;34:1952–1956.

5. Cockerell CJ, Whitlow MA, Webster GF, Friedman-Kien AE. Epithelioid angiomatosis: a distinct vascular disorder in patients with the acquired immunodeficiency syndrome or AIDS-related complex. Lancet 1987;2:654–656.

6. Daly JS, Worthington MG, Brenner DJ, Moss CW, Hollis DG, Weyant RS, Steigerwalt AG, Weaver RE, Daneshvar MI, O'Connor SP. *Rochalimaea elizabethae* sp. nov. isolated from a patient with endocarditis. J Clin Microbiol 1993;31: 872–881.

7. Garcia-Caceres U, Garcia FU. Bartonellosis: an immunodepressive disease and the life of Daniel Alcides Carrion. Am J Clin Pathol 1991;95(Suppl 1):S58–66.

8. Guerra LG, Neira CJ, Boman D, Ho H, Casner PR, Zuckerman M, Verghese A. Rapid response of AIDS-related bacillary angiomatosis to azithromycin. Clin Infect Dis 1993;17: 264–266.

9. Ives TJ, Manzewitsch P, Regnery RL, Butts JD, Kebede M. In vitro susceptibilities of *Bartonella henselae, B. quintana, B. elizabethae, Rickettsia rickettsii, R. conorii, R. akari,* and *R. prowazekii* to macrolide antibiotics as determined by immunofluorescent-antibody analysis of infected Vero cell monolayers. Antimicrob Agents Chemother 1997;41:578–582.

10. Jackson LA, Perkins BA, Wenger JD. Cat scratch disease in the United States: an analysis of three national databases. Am J Public Health 1993;83:1707–1711.

11. Kaplan JE. 1997 USPHS/IDSA guidelines for the prevention of opportunistic infections in persons infected with human immunodeficiency virus. MMWR 1997;46(RR-12):18.

12. Kikendall JW, Friedman AC, Oyewole MA, Fleischer D, Johnson LF. Pill-induced esophageal injury. Case reports and review of the medical literature. Dig Dis Sci 1983;28:174–182.

13. Koehler JE. *Bartonella:* an emerging human pathogen. In: Scheld WM, Armstrong D, Hughes J, eds. Emerging infections I. Washington, DC: American Society for Microbiology Press 1998:147–163.

14. Koehler JE, Glaser CA, Tappero JW. *Rochalimaea henselae* infection. A new zoonosis with the domestic cat as reservoir. JAMA 1994;271:531–535.

15. Koehler JE, LeBoit PE, Egbert BM, Berger TG. Cutaneous vascular lesions and disseminated cat-scratch disease in patients with the acquired immunodeficiency syndrome (AIDS) and AIDS-related complex. Ann Intern Med 1988;109:449–455.

16. Koehler JE, Quinn FD, Berger TG, LeBoit PE, Tappero JW. Isolation of *Rochalimaea* species from cutaneous and osseous lesions of bacillary angiomatosis. N Engl J Med 1992;327:1625–1631.

16a. Koehler JE, Sanchez MA, Garrido CS, Whitfeld MJ, Chen FM, Berger TG, Rodriguez-Barradas MC, LeBoit PE, Tappero JW. Molecular epidemiology of *Bartonella* infections in patients with bacillary angiomatosis-peliosis. N Engl J Med 1997;337:1876–1883.

17. Koehler JE, Tappero JW. Bacillary angiomatosis and bacillary peliosis in patients infected with human immunodeficiency virus. Clin Infect Dis 1993;17:612–624.

18. Lewis DE, Wallace MR. Treatment of adult systemic cat scratch disease with gentamicin sulfate. West J Med 1991;154:330–331.

19. Lucey D, Dolan MJ, Moss CW, Garcia M, Hollis DG, Wegner S, Morgan G, Almeida R, Leong D, Greisen KS, Welch DF, Slater, LN. Relapsing illness due to *Rochalimaea henselae* in immunocompetent hosts: implication for therapy and new epidemiological associations. Clin Infect Dis 1992;14: 683–688.

20. Margileth AM. Antibiotic therapy for cat-scratch disease: clinical study of therapeutic outcome in 268 patients and a review of the literature. Pediatr Infect Dis J 1992;11:474–478.

21. Margileth AM. Cat scratch disease: a therapeutic dilemma. Vet Clin North Am 1987;17:91–103.

22. Maurin M, Gasquet S, Ducco C, Raoult D. MICs of 28 antibiotic compounds for 14 *Bartonella* (formerly *Rochalimaea*) isolates. Antimicrob Agents Chemotherapy 1995;39:2387–2391.

23. Maurin M, Raoult D. Antimicrobial susceptibility of *Rochalimaea quintana, Rochalimaea vinsonii,* and the newly recognized *Rochalimaea henselae.* J Antimicrob Chemother 1993;32: 587–594.

24. Mohle-Boetani JC, Koehler JE, Berger TG, LeBoit PE, Kemper CA, Reingold AL, Plikaytis BD, Wenger JD, Tappero JW. Bacillary angiomatosis and bacillary peliosis in patients infected with human immunodeficiency virus: Clinical characteristics in a case-control study. Clin Infect Dis 1996;22: 794–800.

25. Myers WF, Grossman DM, Wisseman CLJ. Antibiotic susceptibility patterns in *Rochalimaea quintana,* the agent of trench fever. Antimicrob Agents Chemother 1984;25:690–693.

26. Perkocha LA, Geaghan SM, Yen TSB, Nishimura SL, Chan SP, Garcia-Kennedy R, Honda G, Stoloff AC, Klein HZ, Goldman RL, Van Meter S, Ferrell LD, LeBoit PE. Clinical and pathological features of bacillary peliosis hepatis in association with human immunodeficiency virus infection. N Engl J Med:1990;323: 1581–1586.

27. Raoult D, Fournier PE, Drancourt M, Marrie TJ, Etienne J, Cosserat J, Cacoub P, Poinsignon Y, Leclercq P, Sefton AM. Diagnosis of 22 new cases of *Bartonella* endocarditis. Ann Intern Med 1996;125:646–652.

28. Regnery RL, Childs JE, Koehler JE. Infections associated with *Bartonella* species in persons infected with human immunodeficiency virus. Clin Infect Dis 1995;21 Suppl 1:S94–S98.

29. Regnery RL, Rooney JA, Johnson AM, Nesby SL, Manzewitsch P, Beaver K, Olson JG. Experimentally induced *Bartonella henselae* infections followed by challenge exposure and antimicrobial therapy in cats. AJVR 1996;57:1714–1719.

30. Relman DA, Falkow S, LeBoit PE. The organism causing bacillary angiomatosis, peliosis hepatis, and fever and bacteremia in immunocompromised patients. N Engl J Med [letter] 1991;324: 1514.

31. Spach DH, Kanter AS, Daniels NA, Nowowiejski DJ, Larson AM, Schmidt RA, Swaminathan B, Brenner DJ. *Bartonella (Rochalimaea)* species as a cause of apparent "culture-negative" endocarditis. Clin Infect Dis 1995;20:1044–1047.

32. Spach DH, Kanter AS, Dougherty MJ, Larson AM, Coyle MB, Brenner DJ, Swaminathan B, Matar GM, Welch DF, Root RK, Stamm WE. *Bartonella (Rochalimaea) quintana* bacteremia in inner-city patients with chronic alcoholism. N Engl J Med 1995;332:424–428.

33. Stoler MH, Bonfiglio TA, Steigbigel RT, Pereira M. An atypical subcutaneous infection associated with acquired immune deficiency syndrome. Am J Clin Pathol 1983;80:714–718.

34. Strong RP. Trench fever: report of Commission, Medical Research Committee, American Red Cross. Oxford: Oxford University Press, 1918.

35. Tappero JW, Koehler JE. Cat scratch disease and bacillary angiomatosis [letter]. JAMA 1991;266:1938–1939.
36. Tappero JW, Koehler JE, Berger TG, Cockerell CJ, Lee T-H, Busch MP, Stites DP, Mohle-Boetani J, Reingold AL, LeBoit PE. Bacillary angiomatosis and bacillary splenitis in immunocompetent adults. Ann Intern Med 1993;118:363–365.
37. Weinman D, Kreier JP. *Bartonella* and *Grahamella*. In: Kreier JP, ed. Parasitic Protozoa. New York: Academic Press, Inc., 1977:197–233.
38. Wolfson C, Branley J, Gottlieb T. The Etest for antimicrobial susceptibility testing of *Bartonella henselae*. J Antimicrob Chemother 1996;38:963–968.
39. Wong MT, Dolan MJ, Lattuada CP Jr, Regnery RL, Garcia ML, Mokulis EC, LaBarre RA, Ascher DP, Delmar JA, Kelly JW, Leigh DR, McRae AC, Reed JB, Smith RE, Melcher GP. Neuroretinitis, aseptic meningitis, and lymphadenitis associated with *Bartonella (Rochalimaea) henselae* infection in immunocompetent patients and patients infected with human immunodeficiency virus type 1. Clin Infect Dis 1995;21: 352–360.

Chlamydia pneumoniae

●

Lisa A. Jackson and J. Thomas Grayston

GENERAL DESCRIPTION

Chlamydia are obligate intracellular bacteria that have a unique biphasic developmental cycle. The genus contains three species that are human pathogens; *C. psittaci, C. trachomatis,* and *C. pneumoniae* (TWAR). *Chlamydia* have cell walls with inner and outer membranes; replicate by binary fission; contain DNA, RNA, and ribosomes; and synthesize some proteins. They cannot, however, synthesize ATP or GTP and must rely on the host cell for ATP. The small, dense elementary body is the metabolically inactive infectious form of the organism. Elementary bodies have a rigid cell wall, resulting from disulfide cross-linking of envelope proteins, allowing survival outside the host cell. After infection of the host cell by receptor-mediated endocytosis, the elementary bodies differentiate into reticulate bodies. The reticulate body is the larger, metabolically active form of the organism. Inside the host cell, the reticulate body divides by binary fission, forming a microcolony referred to as a chlamydial inclusion. After a period of growth and division, the reticulate bodies reorganize and condense to form new elementary bodies. After host cell lysis, the elementary bodies are released to initiate new infectious cycles.

The first *C. pneumoniae* isolates were serendipitously obtained from conjunctival cultures of children during trachoma vaccine studies in the 1960s. The organism is not, however, associated with eye infection, and its role as a human pathogen was not fully defined until 1983, when the first respiratory isolate was obtained (7). Since that time, *C. pneumoniae* has been identified as an important cause of community-acquired respiratory infections, causing an estimated 10% of cases of community-acquired pneumonia and 5% of cases of bronchitis.

The first *C. pneumoniae* isolates were obtained in yolk-sac cultures, the only method then available for isolation of *Chlamydia,* and were thought to represent strains of *C. psittaci* based on inclusion morphology. After development of cell culture methods that allowed further characterization, the organism was observed to have a characteristic pear-shaped elementary body surrounded by a periplasmic space that is morphologically distinct from the round elementary bodies of *C. trachomatis* and *C. psittaci.* DNA homology studies have revealed that *C. pneumoniae* isolates have less than 5% DNA homology with *C. trachomatis* and less than 10% with *C. psittaci. C. pneumoniae* isolates are highly (>95%) related to each other, however. Since only one strain or serovar of *C. pneumoniae* has been identified, at this time the strain name, TWAR (after the designation of two of the initial isolates, TW-183 and AR-39), is synonymous with *C. pneumoniae.*

IN VITRO SUSCEPTIBILITY

The in vitro methods used for susceptibility testing of *C. pneumoniae* were adapted from those used for *C. trachomatis* and involve inoculating cell monolayers with the organism and incubating in the presence of serial dilutions of antibiotic. Most published studies of in vitro susceptibility have used cycloheximide-treated HeLa or McCoy cells, although some studies have used HL or Hep-2 cells. After the cell monolayers have been inoculated, an overlay medium containing twofold dilutions of the test antimicrobial agent is added. The infected cell monolayers are then incubated for several days and stained, usually with a genus-specific fluorescent monoclonal antibody. The minimum inhibitory concentration (MIC) for this first pass is defined as the lowest antibiotic concentration resulting in the absence of inclusions. Most investigators also determine the MIC for second passage by harvesting the cells from duplicate plates run in parallel and disrupting and passing the cells onto new monolayers. These cells are cultured in antimicrobial agent–free media and stained with fluorescent antibody for inclusion counts. The MIC for second passage is defined as the lowest antibiotic concentration that results in no inclusions after passage.

Some investigators term the MIC for second passage as the MCC (minimum chlamydicidal concentration) or the MLC (minimal lethal concentration). Methods for in vitro susceptibility testing of *C. pneumoniae* are not yet standardized, and testing methods, including the type of tissue culture system, treatment of cells prior to testing, inoculum size, and method for detection of inclusions, may vary between investigators.

A summary of the results of antimicrobial susceptibility testing from previous published reports is presented in Table 1. The results of in vitro testing indicate that, unlike *C. trachomatis, C. pneumoniae* is resistant to sulfonamides. These results also indicate that tetracyclines, macrolides, and azalides are active against *C. pneumoniae* (4, 9, 11, 15, 28). Some quinolones, particularly sparfloxacin, also appear active in vitro (4, 17).

Available data on the susceptibility of *C. pneumoniae* to β-lactams indicate that ampicillin and penicillin have high MICs on first passage but relatively low MICs on second passage. This suggests that β-lactams inhibit production of infectious particles by inhibiting the maturation of reticulate bodies to elementary bodies but do not completely inhibit replication of reticulate bodies. Accordingly, although high concentrations of antibiotic are required to produce complete absence of inclusions for the MIC on first passage, the inclusions seen in the presence of antibiotics were not viable on passage, and so much lower concentrations of antibiotic are required on second passage into antibiotic-free medium. Although resistance of *C. trachomatis* to tetracycline and erythromycin in vitro has been reported (14, 21), resistance of *C. pneumoniae* to these agents has not been described.

ANTIMICROBIAL THERAPY
General

As previously described, erythromycin, tetracycline, and doxycycline demonstrate in vitro activity against the organism, and these agents are recommended as first-line therapy of acute respiratory infections due to *C. pneumoniae*. The organism is not susceptible in vitro to penicillin, ampicillin, or sulfa drugs; therefore, these agents are not recommended for treatment of suspected *C. pneumoniae* infection. Clinical experience shows that symptoms of *C. pneumoniae* infection frequently recur after short or conventional courses of appropriate antibiotics, and persistent infection has been documented by culture after treatment. Consequently, a relatively intensive long-term course of treatment is recommended.

The drugs of choice for treatment of adults include tetracycline (500 mg four times daily for 14 days), doxycycline (100 mg twice daily for 14 days), or erythromycin (500 mg four times daily for 14 days). Erythromycin (250 mg four times daily for 21 days) may be used if the higher dose is not tolerated. Tetracyclines should not be given routinely to children under 8 years of age; therefore, erythromycin (30–50 mg/kg/day divided every 6 h) is the drug of choice in younger children.

If symptoms such as cough or malaise persist after one course of antibiotics, a second course may be useful. Unless the drug is contraindicated, tetracycline or doxycycline is recommended for the second course. Although *C. pneumoniae* infections may be prolonged, serious sequelae are rare, and most patients are expected to completely recover from their infections.

Chlamydia are slow-growing, obligately intracellular bacteria that are difficult to isolate from clinical specimens. As a result, many of the studies of respiratory infections due to *C. pneumoniae* have identified infected persons using acute and convalescent serology. This method is accurate in retrospectively identifying infected persons; however, it limits the ability of investigators to document eradication of the bacteria as a consequence of antimicrobial therapy. In the original report documenting *C. pneumoniae* as a cause of respiratory infection, infected patients were identified by both nasopharyngeal culture and serology; however, in general, cultures were not repeated posttreatment to document eradication. In that study, many patients treated with erythromycin (1 g/day orally for 5–10 days) did not have resolution of symptoms, suggesting that this therapy was inadequate. Grayston et al. then recommended either 2 g of tetracycline per day for 7 to 10 days or 1 g/day for 21 days (7).

Subsequently, Lipsky et al. reported the clinical response of patients with pneumonia and bronchitis caused by *C. pneumoniae* to ofloxacin treatment (18). Infection was defined by acute and convalescent sera. The four patients with *C. pneumoniae* infection treated with ofloxacin (400 mg twice a day for 10 days) appeared to respond clinically.

More recently, results of several clinical trials that included nasopharyngeal culture positivity as an endpoint have been reported. These types of studies allow determination of the microbiologic efficacy of antimicrobial therapy against *C. pneumoniae* infections. The first trial was a randomized controlled trial of treatment with clarithromycin (15 mg/kg body weight per day for 10 days) versus erythromycin suspension (40 mg/kg/day for 10 days) among children 3 to 12 years of age

Antibiotic	MIC on First Passage (μg/mL)	MIC on Second Passage (μg/mL)
Tetracycline	0.05–1.0	0.05–4
Doxycycline	0.05–0.5	0.125–0.5
Minocycline	0.015	NA[a]
Erythromycin	0.01–0.25	0.01–4.0
Azithromycin	0.06–1.0	0.125–2.0
Clarithromycin	0.004–0.25	0.004–2.0
Roxithromycin	0.125–0.25	0.125
Ciprofloxacin	0.25–4.0	0.25–8.0
Ofloxacin	0.5–2.0	0.5–2.0
Levofloxacin	0.125–0.5	0.125–0.25
Fleroxacin	2.0–8.0	2.0–8.0
Lomefloxacin	4	NA
Temafloxacin	0.125–4.0	0.125–4.0
Sparfloxacin	0.06–0.5	0.06–2.0
Ampicillin	>100	0.8–1.6
Penicillin	>100	0.1–0.2
Sulfisoxazole	>400	≥400
Sulfamethoxazole	>500	NA

TABLE 1 • Summary of the Results of in Vitro Susceptibility Testing of *C. pneumoniae*

[a]NA, not available.

with radiographically demonstrated community-acquired pneumonia (1). Of the 260 children enrolled in the study, 74 (28%) had evidence of infection with *C. pneumoniae* by isolation from, or PCR of, throat swab samples. Of the 33 evaluable patients with *C. pneumoniae* isolated from pretreatment nasopharyngeal cultures, bacteriologic eradication was documented in 79% (15 of 19) of those treated with clarithromycin, versus 86% (12 of 14) of those treated with erythromycin. The MICs to erythromycin and clarithromycin of isolates obtained from children positive both before and after therapy did not change during treatment (23). This suggests that persistence was not due to development of antibiotic resistance. All children with persistent infection improved clinically, with complete resolution of the chest x-rays.

In an open study of azithromycin for treatment of community-acquired respiratory infections in adults (3), *C. pneumoniae* infection was identified by culture in 16 of 62 (26%) patients with lower respiratory tract infection. All 16 culture-positive patients were treated with azithromycin at a 1.5-g total oral dose over 5 days. *C. pneumoniae* was successfully eradicated from 12 (75%) of the patients when they were seen 4 to 6 weeks after treatment. All four patients with persistent infections improved clinically.

The ability of *C. pneumoniae* to persist despite antimicrobial therapy with agents to which it is susceptible in vitro is well documented. The studies cited above demonstrate persistence of the organism after azithromycin, clarithromycin, and erythromycin treatment. In these studies, patients showed improvement of clinical symptoms despite persistent culture positivity. Hammerschlag et al. also reported several patients with acute respiratory illness and positive *C. pneumoniae* nasopharyngeal cultures who remained culture positive and symptomatic after 2 weeks of erythromycin or 30 days of tetracycline or doxycycline treatment (10). Thus, the correlations between in vitro susceptibility and nasopharyngeal eradication, and between eradication and clinical response, are not completely defined.

These more recent studies do suggest, however, that azithromycin and clarithromycin are likely to be at least as effective as doxycycline or erythromycin therapy for *C. pneumoniae* respiratory infections. These agents achieve high tissue and intracellular levels, have been demonstrated effective against *C. pneumoniae* in vitro, and are better tolerated than erythromycin, with fewer gastrointestinal side effects. They may be preferable in certain situations for treatment of *C. pneumoniae* infections. If these agents are used, the recommended dose for respiratory infections for adults is 500 mg on day 1, then 250 mg/day on days 2 through 5 for azithromycin and 500 mg twice daily for 10 to 14 days for clarithromycin. The recommended pediatric dosage of azithromycin is 5 to 12 mg/kg once daily and of clarithromycin is 15 mg/kg/day divided twice a day.

Special Circumstances

Pneumonia and bronchitis are the most common manifestations of acute infection with *C. pneumoniae;* however, the organism is also associated with other acute respiratory illnesses. It has been associated with nonpurulent sinusitis (27), and the organism has been isolated from patients with purulent sinusitis (12) as well as from children with otitis media (22). Primary pharyngitis due to *C. pneumoniae* has also been reported (13). Other reported clinical syndromes include endocarditis (19) and lumbosacral meningoradiculitis (20). Prospective assessments of treatment of upper respiratory and nonrespiratory syndromes due to *C. pneumoniae* have not been performed; therefore, recommendations for treatment are derived from those developed for the more common lower respiratory syndromes.

ENDPOINTS FOR MONITORING THERAPY

C. pneumoniae infections are, in general, diagnosed retrospectively after testing of acute and convalescent sera specimens. In addition, as described above, the organism may persist (detected by isolation or PCR of pharyngeal swab specimens) after treatment despite clinical improvement. Therefore, the clinical condition should be the primary endpoint for monitoring therapy directed against acute *C. pneumoniae* infections.

COMMENT—*C. PNEUMONIAE* AND CHRONIC INFECTIONS

Chlamydia have a predilection for causing chronic infections, which has been well described for *C. trachomatis* and has also been demonstrated for *C. pneumoniae*. Chronic *C. trachomatis* infection of fallopian tubes is associated with tubal infertility, and *C. trachomatis* DNA or antigens have been detected in a high percentage of fallopian tubal biopsy tissue from women with tubal infertility. Importantly, *C. trachomatis* antigen or DNA has been detected after antibiotic therapy. *C. trachomatis* DNA has also been identified in conjunctival scrapings from patients with chronic complications of ocular trachoma. In both of these syndromes, *C. trachomatis*–specific DNA may be detected in tissue from which the organism could not be recovered, suggesting that the organism persists in a latent state from which culture is difficult.

C. pneumoniae has recently been associated with asthma (5, 8), suggesting that chronicity may also play a role in respiratory infections. *C. pneumoniae* has also recently been associated with atherosclerotic cardiovascular disease by seroepidemiologic studies (24–26) and by direct demonstration of the organism in atheromatous plaque (2, 6, 16), suggesting that persistent *C. pneumoniae* infection may play a role in atherogenesis. Further studies are needed to determine whether antimicrobial treatment directed against *C. pneumoniae* can affect the outcomes of these chronic syndromes.

REFERENCES

1. Block S, Hedrick J, Hammerschlag MR, Cassell GH, Craft JC. *Mycoplasma pneumoniae* and *Chlamydia pneumoniae* in pediatric community-acquired pneumonia: comparative efficacy and safety of clarithromycin vs. erythromycin ethylsuccinate. Pediatr Infect Dis J 1995;14:471–477.
2. Campbell LA, O'Brien ER, Cappuccio AL, Kuo C-C, Wang S-P, Stewart D, Patton DL, Cummings P, Grayston JT. Detection of *Chlamydia pneumoniae* (TWAR) in human coronary atherectomy tissues. J Infect Dis 1995;172:585–588.

3. Cassell GL, Grayston JT, and Azithromycin Respiratory Infection Study (ARIS) Investigators. In vitro and clinical activity of azithromycin against *Mycoplasma pneumoniae* and *Chlamydia pneumoniae*. Second International Conference on the Macrolides, Azalides, and Streptogramins, Venice, Italy, 1994.

4. Cooper MA, Baldwin D, Matthews RS, Andrews JM, Wise R. In-vitro susceptibility of *Chlamydia pneumoniae* (TWAR) to seven antibiotics. J Antimicrob Chemother 1991;28:407–413.

5. Emre U, Roblin PM, Gelling M, Dumornay W, Rao M, Hammerschlag MR, Schachter J. The association of *Chlamydia pneumoniae* infection and reactive airway disease in children. Arch Pediatr Adolesc Med 1994;148:727–731.

6. Grayston JT, Kuo C-C, Coulson AS, Campbell LA, Lawrence RD, Lee MJ, Wang S-P. *Chlamydia pneumoniae* (TWAR) in atherosclerosis of the carotid artery. Circulation 1995;92:3397–3400.

7. Grayston JT, Kuo C-C, Wang S-P, Altman J. A new *Chlamydia psittaci* strain, TWAR, isolated in acute respiratory tract infection. N Engl J Med 1986;315:161–168.

8. Hahn DL, Dodge RW, Golubjatnikov R. Association of *C. pneumoniae* (strain TWAR) infection with wheezing, asthmatic bronchitis, and adult-onset asthma. JAMA 1991;266:225–230.

9. Hammerschlag MR. Antimicrobial susceptibility and therapy of infections caused by *Chlamydia pneumoniae*. Antimicrob Agents Chemother 1994;38:1873–1878.

10. Hammerschlag MR, Chirgwin K, Roblin PM, Gelling M, Dumornay W, Mandel L, Smith P, Schachter J. Persistent infection with *Chlamydia pneumoniae* following acute respiratory illness. Clin Infect Dis 1992;14:178–182.

11. Hammerschlag MR, Qumei KK, Roblin PM. In vitro activities of azithromycin, clarithromycin, l-ofloxacin, and other antibiotics against *Chlamydia pneumoniae*. Antimicrob Agents Chemother 1992;36:1573–1574.

12. Hashigucci K, Ogawa H, Suzuki T, Kazuyama Y. Isolation of *Chlamydia pneumoniae* from the maxillary sinus of a patient with purulent sinusitis. Clin Infect Dis 1992;15:570–571.

13. Huovinen P, Lahtonen R, Ziegler T, Meurman O, Hakkarainen K, Miettinen A, Arstila P, Eskola J, Saikku P. Pharyngitis in adults: the presence and coexistence of viruses and bacterial organisms. Ann Intern Med 1989;110:612–616.

14. Jones RB, Van Der Pol B, Martin DH, Shepard MK. Partial characterization of *Chlamydia trachomatis* isolates resistant to multiple antibiotics. J Infect Dis 1990;162:1309–1315.

15. Kuo C-C, Grayston JT. In vitro drug susceptibility of *Chlamydia* sp. strain TWAR. Antimicrob Agents Chemother 1988:32:257–258.

16. Kuo C-C, Grayston JT, Campbell LA, Goo YA, Wissler RW, Benditt EP. *Chlamydia pneumoniae* (TWAR) in coronary arteries of young adults (15–35 years old). Proc Natl Acad Sci USA 1995;92:6911–6914.

17. Kuo C-C, Jackson LA, Lee A, Grayston JT. In vitro activities of azithromycin, clarithromycin, and other antibiotics against *C. pneumoniae*. Antimicrobial Agents Chemother 1996;40: 2669–2670.

18. Lipsky BA, Tack KJ, Wang S-P, Kuo C-C, Grayston JT. Ofloxacin treatment of *Chlamydia pneumoniae* (strain TWAR) lower respiratory tract infections. Am J Med 1990;89:722–724.

19. Marrie TJ, Marczy M, Mann OE, Landymore RW, Raza A, Wang S-P, Grayston JT. Culture-negative endocarditis probably due to *Chlamydia pneumoniae*. J Infect Dis 1990;161:127–129.

20. Michel D, Antoine JC, Pozzetto B, Gaudin OG, Lucht F. Lumbosacral meningoradiculitis associated with *Chlamydia pneumoniae* infection. J Neurol Neurosurg Psychiatry 1992;55:511.

21. Mourad A, Sweet RL, Sugg N, Schachter J. Relative resistance to erythromycin in *Chlamydia trachomatis*. Antimicrob Agents Chemother 1980;18:696–698.

22. Ogawa H, Hashiguchi K, Kazuyama Y. Recovery of *Chlamydia pneumoniae* in six patients with otitis media and effusion. J Laryngol Otol 1992;106:490–492.

23. Roblin PM, Montalban G, Hammerschlag MR. Susceptibilities to clarithromycin and erythromycin of isolates of *Chlamydia pneumoniae* from children with pneumonia. Antimicrob Agents Chemother 1994;38:1588–1589.

24. Saikku P, Leinonen M, Tenkanen L, Linnanmake E, Ekman MR, Manninen V, Manttari M, Frick MH, Huttunnen JK. Chronic *Chlamydia pneumoniae* infection as a risk factor for coronary heart disease in the Helsinki heart study. Ann Intern Med 1992;116:273–278.

25. Saikku P, Mattila K, Nieminen MS, Makela PH, Huttunen JK, Valtonen V. Serological evidence of an association of a novel chlamydia, TWAR, with chronic coronary heart disease and acute myocardial infarction. Lancet 1988;2:983–986.

26. Thom DH, Grayston JT, Siscovick DS, Wang S-P, Weiss NS, Daling JR. Association of prior infection with *Chlamydia pneumoniae* and angiographically demonstrated coronary artery disease. JAMA 1992;268:68–72.

27. Thom DH, Grayston JT, Wang S-P, Kuo C-C, Altman J. *Chlamydia pneumoniae* strain TWAR, *Mycoplasma pneumoniae* and viral infections in acute respiratory disease in a university student health clinic population. Am J Epidemiol 1990;132:248–256.

28. Welsh L, Gaydos C, Quinn TC. In vitro activities of azithromycin, clarithromycin, erythromycin, and tetracycline against 13 strains of *Chlamydia pneumoniae*. Antimicrob Agents Chemother 1996;40:212–214.

Chlamydia psittaci

•

David Schlossberg

GENERAL DESCRIPTION

Psittacosis is a systemic infection caused by inhalation of *Chlamydia psittaci*. The source is usually an infected bird, which may be asymptomatic. Discharge from beaks, eyes, feces, and urine are all infectious and contaminate the bird's feathers and the surrounding dust. Patients may develop one of several syndromes: a mononucleosis-like illness, a typhoidal form, a nonspecific febrile illness, or atypical pneumonia. The most common signs and symptoms are fever, cough, headache, pharyngeal erythema, and rales. Particularly helpful clinical clues are hepatosplenomegaly, hemoptysis, epistaxis, rash, and relative bradycardia.

Microbiology

Like other chlamydiae, *C. psittaci* is an obligate intracellular parasite, has a cell wall resembling that of Gram-negative bacteria, and is susceptible to some antibiotics. Its developmental cycle is complex and includes two forms. An (infective) elementary body attaches to host cells and enters the cell by phagocytosis or receptor-mediated endocytosis. Phagolysosomal fusion is inhibited early, and the elementary body reorganizes into the reticulate body, which uses the host cell as an energy source. Contained in a phagosome, this dividing reticulate body enlarges and divides repeatedly by binary fusion, forming an enlarging cytoplasmic inclusion that can be stained with Giemsa or by immunofluoroscent antibodies. The enlarging and dividing reticulate body ultimately condenses back into elementary bodies, which are then released from the ruptured cell and begin the cycle anew (7, 13, 21).

SUSCEPTIBILITY IN VITRO

In vitro testing is not routinely performed; it has not been standardized, although it may be carried out in cell culture. The general process is cell culture with antibiotic-free monolayers. Endpoints are the dilution of antibiotic that prevents inclusion formation (MIC) and then identification of the highest dilution that prevents viable chlamydia from being detected in passage (MBC). Agents most active in vitro are tetracycline, doxycycline, macrolides, rifampin, quinolones, and clindamycin (2, 9, 15, 16).

ANTIMICROBIAL THERAPY
Drug of Choice

The therapy of psittacosis is primarily based on anecdotal experience in humans and animals. Controlled trials in humans are not available, and in vitro testing is not standardized to use as a basis for therapy selection. Thus, the treatment recommendations given below represent a consensus based on clinical practice, anecdotal reports, and limited in vitro data.

The tetracyclines are widely considered the drugs of choice for treatment of psittacosis, either tetracycline hydrochloride or doxycycline (5, 7, 11, 22, 24). They suppress growth and replication but do not eradicate the agent from the host (7). Although the clinical response may be dramatic, with objective and subjective improvement in 24 to 48 h, some patients respond slowly or not at all (22). Sensitivity to tetracycline appears to be universal. Resistant mutants have been seen but are extremely rare (7).

Doses administered are tetracycline hydrochloride 500 mg orally four times daily or doxycycline 100 mg twice daily orally or intravenously. Duration of therapy is usually 10 to 14 days, although some observers suggest extending the therapy to 21 days to prevent relapse. The need for therapy beyond 2 weeks is controversial (11, 26).

Special Situations

Children under the age of 8 years should be treated with erythromycin unless they are severely ill or do not respond to erythromycin, in which case tetracycline or doxycycline should be used.

Pregnant patients present a problem. Although tetracyclines are generally avoided in pregnancy, Chermon found erythromycin ineffective in a pregnant patient who improved only after delivery of the placenta. Also, the erythromycin did not appear to protect the fetus. It may be advisable to use tetracycline in these patients, although the optimal approach is unknown (3).

Endocarditis

Endocarditis presents a special difficulty because of the desirability of bactericidal therapy to eradicate valvular infection. Although there are reports of medical cures, these are infrequent and difficult to evaluate. Thus, Walker and Adgey reported a cure with doxycycline, but the patient described had also received penicillin for 3 weeks with a definite clinical response (25). Regan et al. treated a patient with erythromycin for 4 months and then doxycycline for 1 year. When the patient subsequently underwent valve replacement, there was no evidence of valvular infection. However, the patient had received penicillin and ampicillin therapy prior to the erythromycin, making it difficult to evaluate the effect of erythromycin and doxycycline therapy (19). Jariwalla et al. reported a patient treated with 16 weeks of rifampin 600 mg daily (6), but there is general concern about emergence of resistance when this drug is used alone

(21). Most authors stress the need for valve replacement or permanent antibiotic therapy for ultimate disease-free survival (8, 10, 18, 23).

Alternative Therapy

Erythromycin is the alternative therapy of choice. Controversy surrounds comparison of erythromycin with the tetracyclines. Some feel it is at least as good as tetracycline (4), while others feel it is less effective, especially for severe disease (7, 11, 24). The newer macrolides (e.g., azithromycin) may eventually prove useful, especially in view of the accumulation of azithromycin in host cells and the intracellular location of *C. psittaci* (16).

Additional potential alternatives include chloramphenicol, which has a reputation ranging from "ineffective" to a "viable alternative to tetracycline" (1, 11, 22). It probably would be acceptable with mild disease, since it is less active by weight than tetracycline, and patients have tended to respond slowly and to relapse (7).

Penicillin represents another theoretical alternative. Since chlamydia have a cell wall, a penicillin effect is not surprising. Morphologically defective forms are produced when chlamydia are exposed to penicillin, but its in vivo effectiveness does not compare with that of tetracycline. However, occasional patients treated with penicillin appear to have improved, and penicillin might be helpful in large doses, in a manner reminiscent of its effect on certain Gram-negative bacteria (7,12).

Rifampin is the most active antibiotic on a weight basis, but there are theoretical concerns about development of resistance, as noted above. Clinical data are sparse and anecdotal (6, 20).

Sulfonamides have not helped most patients in whom they have been used, unlike the situation with *C. trachomatis,* which synthesizes folate and thus is susceptible to sulfonamides. Aminoglycosides and vancomycin should *not* be used as therapy, since they permit chlamydial growth in vitro (7).

The quinolones, particularly some of the newer compounds, show promise in vitro and in animal models of psittacosis (14, 17). Their role in therapy of human infection awaits further laboratory and clinical evaluation.

Combination Therapy

There are no clinical data on combination therapy on which to base recommendations.

CONTROVERSIES OR UNCERTAINTIES

There are several uncertainties regarding the treatment of psittacosis. It is still not clear what the best approach to endocarditis is and, if the decision to replace the valve has been made, when in the course of therapy this action should be undertaken. Another area of uncertainty is the best alternative if neither tetracycline nor erythromycin can be used. Finally, as described above, the best approach for the pregnant patient and for the severely ill young patient is uncertain, regarding the advisability of assuming the risks of tetracycline therapy for efficacy that may be superior to that of erythromycin.

CAVEATS OR COMMENTS

The most important caveat regarding the treatment of psittacosis is to be sure of the diagnosis. The differential diagnosis for psittacosis is extensive, and early diagnosis is difficult. Also, if treatment is failing, the diagnosis should be secured, since patients with bird exposures may acquire other illnesses; on the other hand, not all patients with psittacosis report contact with birds.

REFERENCES

1. Covelli HD, Husky DL, Dolphin RE. Psittacosis. West J Med 1980;132:242–244.
2. Dailoux M, Ottimer C, Albert H, Weber M. In vitro sensitivity of chlamydiae to antibiotics, pathologies. Biologie 1990;38:426–430.
3. Gherman RB, Leventis LL, Miller RC. Chlamydial psittacosis during pregnancy: a case report. Obstet Gynecol 1995;86:648–650.
4. Hammers-Berggren S, Granath F, Julander I, Kalin M. Erythromycin for treatment of ornithosis. Scand J Infect Dis 1991;23:159–162.
5. Harding HB. The epidemiology of sporadic urban ornithosis. Am J Clin Pathol 1962;38:230–243.
6. Jariwalla AG, Davies BH, White J. Infective endocarditis complicating psittacosis: response to rifampin. Br Med J 1980;1:155.
7. Jawetz E. Chemotherapy of chlamydial infections. Adv Pharmacol Chemother 1979;7:253–2822.
8. Jones RB, Priest JB, Kuo C. Subacute chlamydial endocarditis. JAMA 1982;247:655–658.
9. Kimura M, Kishimoto T, Niki Y, Soejima R. In vitro and in vivo antichlamydial activities of newly developed quilone antimicrobial agents. Antimicrob Agents Chemother 1993;37:801–803.
10. Lamaury I, Sotto A, LeQuellec A, Perez C, Boussagol B, Ciurana AJ. Chlamydial psittaci as a cause of lethal bacterial endocarditis. Clin Infect Dis 1993;17:821–822.
11. MacFarlane JT, Macrae AD. Psittacosis. Med Bull 1983;39:163–167.
12. Maclachlan WWG, Crum GE, Kleinschmidt RF, Wehrle PF. Psittacosis. Am J Med Sci 1953;226:157–163.
13. McPhee SJ, Erb B, Harrington W. Psittacosis. West J Med 1987;146:91–95.
14. Miyashita N, Niki Y, Kishimoto T, Nakajimo M, Matsushima T. In vitro and in vivo activities of AM-1155, a new fluoroquinolone against *Chlamydia* spp. Antimicrob Agents Chemother 1997;41:1331–1334.
15. Murray PR, Baron EJ, Pfaller MA, Tenover FC, Yooken RH. Manual of clinical microbiology. Washington DC: American Society for Microbiology Press, 1995.
16. Niki Y, Kimura M, Miyashita N, Soejima R. In vitro and in vivo activities of azithromycin, a new azalide antibiotic against chlamydia. Antimicrob Agents Chemother 1994;38:2296–2299.
17. Niki Y, Miyashita N, Kubota Y, Nakajima M, Matsushima T. In vitro and in vivo antichlamydial activities of HSR-903, a new fluoroquinolone antibiotic. Antimicrob Agents Chemother 1997;41:857–859.
18. Oakley CM. Infective endocarditis. Br J Hosp Med 1980;24:232–234.
19. Regan RJ, Dathan JRE, Treharne JD. Infective endocarditis with glomerulonephritis associated with cat chlamydia (C. psittaci) infection. Br Heart J 1979;42:349–352.

20. Schachter J. Rifampin and chlamydial infections. Rev Infect Dis 1983;5:5562.
21. Schacter J. Chlamydial infections. N Engl J Med 1978;298: 428–434, 490–496, 540–548.
22. Schaffner W, Drutz DJ, Duncan GW, Loenig MG. The clinical spectrum of endemic psittacosis. Arch Intern Med 1967;119: 433–443.
23. Shapiro DS, Kenney SC, Johnson M, Davis CH, Knight ST, Wynick PB. Brief report: Chlamydia psittaci endocarditis diagnosed by blood culture. N Engl J Med 1992;326: 1192–1195.
24. Verweig PE, Meis JFGM, Eijk R, Melchers WJG, Galama JMD. Severe human psittacosis requiring artifical ventilation: case report and review. Clin Infect Dis 1995;20:440–442.
25. Walker LJE, Adgey AAJ. Successful treatment by doxycycline of endocarditis caused by ornithosis. Br Heart J 1987;57:58–60.
26. Young AP, Grayson ML. Psittacosis—a review of 135 cases. Med J Aust 1988;148:228–233.

Chlamydia trachomatis

●

Julius Schachter

GENERAL DESCRIPTION
Microbiology

Chlamydia trachomatis is one of four species within the genus Chlamydia (7, 8, 11). The other species include C. psittaci, the cause of psittacosis. This organism is a common pathogen of mammals and is ubiquitous in avian species, but infects humans only as a zoonosis. C. pecorum is a pathogen of sheep and cattle. C. pneumoniae is exclusively a human pathogen. It has no known animal reservoir. The same is true of those C. trachomatis strains that infect humans. A murine biovar of C. trachomatis is recognized, but it is not known to infect man.

Chlamydiae are distinguishable from all other organisms by a unique life cycle that involves transition between 2 major morphologic forms (12). The infectious particle, called the elementary body, attaches to susceptible host cells and is ingested by a process akin to receptor-mediated endocytosis. It enters the cell within an endosome and remains there throughout its life cycle. Chlamydiae inhibit phagolysosomal fusion. Once in the cell the elementary body changes, approximately 6 to 8 h after entering the cell, to the reticulate body (sometimes called an initial body). This represents the metabolically active and reproductive form of the organism. Reticulate bodies are not infectious. They divide by binary fission up to approximately 48 h into the infectious cycle. At some time between 24 and 48 h, some of the reticulate bodies reorganize again into elementary bodies and thus become infectious. Ultimately, the cell will burst, and the elementary bodies exit the host cell to infect new cells. The full cycle takes approximately 48 h for the more virulent lymphogranuloma venereum (LGV) biovar; and 72 to 96 h for the trachoma biovar.

C. trachomatis strains can be divided into three biovars. The murine biovar, as noted, does not infect humans and is not discussed further. The trachoma biovar is a pathogen of columnar and squamocolumnar cells and thus causes disease at the mucous membrane level, where such cells are found. These sites include conjunctivae, urethra, the endocervical canal, fallopian tubes, and gastrointestinal and respiratory tracts. The trachoma biovar is capable of infecting all these sites and can cause disease at each. The LGV biovar is more virulent. These strains are more invasive and can cause disease in many tissues. They obviously infect epithelial cells because the primary lesion for this infection is often in the skin. The organism subsequently invades draining lymph nodes and causes formation of buboes. These strains are readily differentiated in the laboratory because the LGV strains are capable of cell-to-cell transmission in cell culture and lethal infection following intracranial inoculation in mice. The trachoma biovar is not lethal for mice by this route and does not grow well in cell culture systems. It requires mechanical assistance (centrifugation) for efficient infection.

Several aspects of C. trachomatis microbiology are relevant to treatment. The organism is an obligate intracellular parasite and is metabolically active only after it enters the host cell. The infectious elementary body is metabolically inert and thus not affected by antibiotics. Therefore, only antibiotics that penetrate cells will be effective against C. trachomatis. Because the life cycle is so long (typically, 2–4 days), long courses of therapy are required. In addition, although C. trachomatis is a bacterium, it does not contain a peptidoglycan layer (structural rigidity appears to depend on disulfide binding among at least three outer membrane proteins). A lack of peptidoglycan predicts that β-lactam antibiotics will not be effective in treating chlamydial infections. Experience has shown that these drugs are not efficient in treating C. trachomatis infections, although high doses and long courses of therapy may be active. C. trachomatis does contain penicillin-binding sites, and in vitro, penicillin induces large, irregularly shaped, reticulate particles, as the antibiotics appear to interfere with the division process (3).

Laboratory Diagnosis

Many chlamydial infections are managed on a syndromic basis. For example, urethritis in men is often managed by ruling out gonorrhea (by Gram staining of urethral discharge or swab) and then treating for chlamydia if the smear is negative. Where specific diagnosis is required (it is always advisable), the most commonly used tests include isolation of organism in cell cultures or detection of chlamydial antigens either by enzyme immunoassays or direct fluorescent antibody staining of smears (19). Serology does not play a role in routine diagnosis of genital infection. Recently, DNA amplification tests such as polymerase chain reaction and ligase chain reaction have been introduced. These tests are far more sensitive than cell culture or antigen detection (18).

SUSCEPTIBILITY IN VITRO AND IN VIVO
Single Drug

There is no generally accepted way of determining antimicrobial susceptibility patterns for *C. trachomatis*. The general approach is to use relatively low infectious inocula in susceptible cells and to titrate the quantity of antibiotic that reduces inclusion counts by 50, 90, or 100% in that initial growth cycle (14). This is the method used to determine inhibitory levels. Cidal levels are determined by subculturing from the antibiotic-treated cells into antibiotic-free cells to determine the lowest concentration of antibiotic that prevents subsequent recovery of the organism.

The most active antibiotics against *C. trachomatis* are in the rifampin group. However, these drugs are not used clinically, because resistance develops rapidly in vitro (15).

In general, the MICs of antibiotics in cell culture systems predict the clinical responses seen in humans. Thus tetracyclines are highly active in vitro and are highly useful clinically. Macrolides show lesser activity in vitro yet are considered clinically active. Quinolones have borderline levels of activity, and some are considered clinically active, while others are not useful in treating human infections. Table 1 lists typical antimicrobial susceptibility levels for a variety of common antibiotics for *C. trachomatis*.

Combination Drugs

In general, combinations of drugs are not used for *C. trachomatis* infection. Where commonly used drugs often show synergy with other infections, activity with *C. trachomatis* appears to be additive rather than synergistic.

TABLE 1 • Minimum Inhibitory Concentration (MIC) of Antimicrobial Agents for *C. trachomatis*	
Drug	**MIC (µg or U/mL)**
Rifampin	0.005–0.25
Tetracyclines	0.03–1
Azithromycin	0.03–1
Erythromycin	0.1–1
Ofloxacin	0.5–1
Ampicillin	0.5–10
Penicillin	1–10
Sulfamethoxazole	0.5–4
Clindamycin	2–16
Spectinomycin	32–100
Gentamicin	500
Vancomycin	1000

ANTIMICROBIAL THERAPY
Drug of Choice

For many years, tetracyclines have been considered the drugs of choice for treating *C. trachomatis* infections. Doxycycline has been preferred because of the presumption of improved compliance. Courses of therapy have ranged from 7 to 21 days, depending on the disease being treated. Recommended protocols are listed in Table 2.

More recently, a single 1-g dose of oral azithromycin was shown to be as effective as week-long courses of doxycycline in treatment of uncomplicated chlamydial genital tract infection (10). This drug has also been used in treating chlamydial infections in pregnant women. In addition, a single 1-g dose of oral azithromycin was also shown to be as effective as long (30 days–6 weeks) courses of topical tetracycline ointment in the treatment of hyperendemic trachoma (2). It is likely that ultimately azithromycin will become the drug of choice in treating all chlamydial infections. Week-long courses of doxycycline and a single 1-g dose of azithromycin have been 96 to 98% effective in curing chlamydial infection as determined by isolation in cell culture (see alternative therapy).

Ofloxacin (but not all other quinolones) is effective in treating chlamydial infections. In general, erythromycin is considered the backup drug for those who cannot take tetracycline. This of course applies to settings in which azithromycin may not be used because of cost concerns.

There are special instances in which erythromycin is considered the drug of choice. For example, in treating chlamydial infections in pregnant women or in infected infants (dosages are shown in Table 2), it is considered the first-line treatment.

Azithromycin has now been shown to be highly effective in treating chlamydial infection in pregnancy. It is not a drug that is likely to be explicitly approved for use in pregnancy, but with a lack of reported complications, it will probably become accepted as the drug of choice in this setting. Until that becomes standard care, amoxicillin is considered the alternative drug for pregnant women who are erythromycin intolerant. A substantial proportion of pregnant women suffer gastrointestinal upset to the extent that it causes them to cease their courses of erythromycin. In this setting, amoxicillin is the appropriate alternative regimen and has been shown to be highly effective.

The regimens listed below are modified from the Centers for Disease Control (CDC) STD treatment guidelines (5).

Special Situations
Lymphogranuloma Venereum

The LGV biovar of *C. trachomatis* is highly invasive and can cause many different clinical manifestations, although the typical presentation in males is of inguinal buboes with or without systemic manifestations of infection (16). There is a paucity of controlled treatment trials for this disease. In general, long courses of therapy (at least 21 days) are called for. Treatment failures are not uncommon, and the usual approach is to retreat using an alternate regimen. The recommended regimen is doxycycline 100 mg twice daily for 21 days. The alternate regimens are either erythromycin, 500 mg twice daily, or sulfisoxazole, 500 mg twice daily, both for 21 days.

TABLE 2 • Treatment of Chlamydial Infections

Organism and Condition	First Choice		Second Choice	
	Drug	Dose	Drug	Dose
C. trachomatis				
Genital tract infections (e.g., urethritis, cervicitis)	Doxycycline	100 mg, b.i.d. × 1 week	Azithromycin	1 g, orally, single dose
Pregnant women	Erythromycin	250 mg, q.i.d. × 2 weeks	Amoxicillin	500 mg, t.i.d. × 1 week
Infant pneumonia	Erythromycin	10 mg/kg, q.i.d. × 2 weeks	Sulfisoxazole	37.5 mg/kg, q.i.d. × 2 weeks
Inclusion conjunctivitis (Infants)	Erythromycin	10 mg/kg, q.i.d. × 2 weeks	Sulfisoxazole	37.5 mg/kg, q.i.d. × 2 weeks
Inclusion conjunctivitis (Adults)	Tetracycline	250 mg, q.i.d. × 3 weeks	Erythromycin	250 mg, q.i.d. × 3 weeks

Genital Tract Infection

The trachoma biovar has a more limited spectrum of susceptible cells; causes diseases at mucous membranes; and is an important cause of urethritis and epididymitis in men (20). In women, it causes lower genital tract infection, and more importantly, it will infect fallopian tubes, where the resultant damage may cause such sequelae as tubal factor infertility and ectopic pregnancy (21). *C. trachomatis* is considered the most common sexually transmitted bacterial infection. It is estimated that in the United States, more than 4 million infections occur each year (4).

The recommended regimens are doxycycline, 100 mg twice daily for 7 days; or a single 1-g oral dose of azithromycin. Alternate regimens include ofloxacin, 300 mg, twice daily for 7 days; erythromycin, 500 mg, four times a day for 7 days; or erythromycin ethylsuccinate, 800 mg, four times a day for 7 days.

All cases of pelvic inflammatory disease should be treated with a regimen of multiple antibiotics that includes a drug active against *C. trachomatis*.

Pregnant Women

Treatment of chlamydial infection in pregnancy is recommended to prevent postpartum complications and perinatal infections (17). In general, the drug of choice is erythromycin (500 mg, four times a day for 7 days). Because a 2 g/day dose of erythromycin may not be well tolerated by pregnant women, an alternate regimen involves a smaller daily dose of 250 mg four times a day with treatment extended to 14 days. Similarly, erythromycin and ethylsuccinate can be used at 800 mg, orally, four times a day for 7 days; or 400 mg, orally, four times a day for 14 days. Amoxicillin at 500 mg thrice daily for 7 to 10 days is another alternate regimen.

Where relatively large numbers of patients have been tested following amoxicillin regimens, tests of cure have shown failure rates equivalent to, or less than, those seen with erythromycin (1, 6). This drug is not considered a drug of choice for treatment of chlamydial infection in pregnancy only because of the theoretical concerns that most researchers have that β-lactam drugs can often suppress, but not eradicate, chlamydial infection. That caveat has not translated into actual demonstration of persistent or inapparent infections, even though many of the tests of cure were performed late enough that such infections should have been detected.

Chlamydial Infections in Infants

Infants exposed during the birth process by passing through an infected birth canal may develop conjunctivitis and/or pneumonia (17). Conjunctivitis is typically seen in the first 3 weeks of life; pneumonia generally occurs in the first 3 to 4 months after birth. The drug of choice for treatment of these infections is erythromycin, 12.5 mg/kg, 4 times daily, for 10 to 14 days.

ENDPOINTS OF MODERN THERAPY

It is generally considered that tests of cure are not required for evaluating treatments for chlamydial infection. With adequate compliance, cure rates in the upper 90 percentile range are expected. Using single doses of oral azithromycin may remove the compliance concern. Where there may be an indication that tests of cure are important, certain caveats must be considered. With some antibiotic regimens it is possible to suppress chlamydiae and render early tests of cure inaccurate. Thus, it may be misleading to perform a test of cure 1 week after treatment has been completed. It is more prudent to wait at least 3 weeks after treatment to assess potential failures. This, of course, introduces a problem of potential reinfection. That potential is most marked in sexually transmitted infections where reexposure to untreated partners or infected others within the same group may result in a positive test result because of new infection rather than treatment failure.

Selecting the appropriate microbiologic test to assess treatment efficacy may also present a problem. Antigen detection methods have inadequate sensitivity. For a long time, culture was the only test that could be recommended. However, the use of DNA amplification procedures, particularly the revelation that urine can be an appropriate specimen for diagnosing chlamydial infection in women, suggests that urine specimens tested by LCR or PCR may be an appropriate test of cure. The caveat here is that chlamydial DNA has been detected for at least 2 to 3 weeks after treatment has begun (in the absence of recoverable viable organism by culture), thus it is necessary to wait at least that long before performing tests of cure (22).

Clinical response may be a useful endpoint but may also be misleading. For example, somewhere between 10 and 15% of men with nongonococcal urethritis do not respond to tetracycline, erythromycin, or azithromycin therapy. These men do not have persistent chlamydial infection or recurrent chlamydial infection. Typically, if they had chlamydial infection at the beginning of therapy, that infection is cured, but they have other causes (i.e., nongonococcal-nonchlamydial urethritis) of inflammation.

CONTROVERSIES

There are several areas of controversy regarding treatment to *C. trachomatis* infection. First, there is the concern about antimicrobial resistance. Some laboratory workers have generated some evidence of antibiotic resistance in clinic settings (9). These results were developed using high titer inocula in in vitro tests for susceptibility, and other workers have failed to provide evidence of tetracycline resistance. Even when there are treatment failures, the isolated strains tend to be susceptible, and infections tend to respond to second courses of therapy. Thus, at the moment, antimicrobial resistance obviously remains a possibility but is not of major concern. For example, earlier reports of relative resistance to erythromycin in vitro have not been clinically relevant (13).

Another area of controversy relates to the belief by some that chlamydia persists in nonreplicating forms in infected patients and that these forms are not affected by antibiotics. Thus, persistent chlamydial infection exists as a state, and total cure is not possible. Suffice it to say that the author does not subscribe to these beliefs.

REFERENCES

1. Alary M, Joly JR, Moutquin JM, Mondor M, Boucher M, Fortier A, Pinault JJ, Paris G, Carrier S, Chamberland H, et al. Randomised comparison of amoxycillin and erythromycin in treatment of genital chlamydial infection in pregnancy. Lancet 1994; 344:1461–1465.
2. Bailey RL, Arullendran P, Whittle HC, Mabey DC. Randomised controlled trial of single-dose azithromycin in treatment of trachoma. Lancet 1993;342:453–456.
3. Barbour AG, Amano K, Hackstadt T, Perry L, Caldwell HD. *Chlamydia trachomatis* has penicillin-binding proteins but not detectable muramic acid. J Bacteriol 1982;151:420–428.
4. Centers for Disease Control. Recommendations for the prevention and management of *Chlamydia trachomatis* infections, 1993. MMWR 1993;42:1–39.
5. Centers for Disease Control. 1993 Sexually transmitted disease guidelines. MMWR 1993;42:1–102.
6. Crombleholme WR, Schachter J, Grossman M, Landers DV, Sweet RL. Amoxicillin therapy for *Chlamydia trachomatis* in pregnancy. Obstet Gynecol 1990;75:752–756.
7. Fukushi H, Hirai K. *Chlamydia pecorum*—the fourth species of genus Chlamydia. Microbiol Immunol 1993;37:516–522.
8. Grayston JT, Kuo C-C, Campbell LA, Wang S-P. *Chlamydia pneumoniae* sp. nov. for *Chlamydia* sp. strain TWAR. Int J Syst Bacteriol 1989;39:88–90.
9. Jones RB, Van der Pol B, Martin DH, Shepard MK. Partial characterization of *Chlamydia trachomatis* isolates resistant to multiple antibiotics. J Infect Dis 1990;162:1309–1315.
10. Martin DH, Mroczkowski TF, Dalu ZA, McCarty J, Jones RB, Hopkins SJ, Johnson RB. A controlled trial of a single dose of azithromycin for the treatment of chlamydial urethritis and cervicitis. The Azithromycin for Chlamydial Infections Study Group. N Engl J Med 1992;327:921–925.
11. Moulder JW. Order Chlamydiales and family Chlamydiaceae. In: Krieg NR, ed. Manual of systematic bacteriology, vol 1. Baltimore: Williams & Wilkins, 1984:729.
12. Moulder JW. Interaction of chlamydiae and host cells in vitro. Microbiol Rev 1991;55:143–190.
13. Mourad A, Sweet RL, Sugg N, Schachter J. Relative resistance to erythromycin in *Chlamydia trachomatis*. Antimicrob Agents Chemother 1980;18:696–698.
14. Ridgway GL. Advances in the antimicrobial therapy of chlamydial genital infections. J Infect 1992;25(Suppl 1):51–59.
15. Schachter J. Rifampin in chlamydial infections. Rev Infect Dis 1983;5(Suppl 3):S562–564.
16. Schachter J, Osoba AO. Lymphogranuloma venereum. Br Med Bull 1983;39:151–154.
17. Schachter J, Sweet RL, Grossman M, Landers D, Robbie M, Bishop E. Experience with the routine use of erythromycin for chlamydial infections in pregnancy. N Engl J Med 1986;314:276–279.
18. Schachter J. Evolution of diagnostic tests for *Chlamydia trachomatis* infections [Abstract]. In: Stary A, ed. Proceedings, 3rd Meeting of the European Society for Chlamydia Research. Bologna, Italy: Societa Editrice Esculapio, 1996:243–246.
19. Stamm WE. Diagnosis of *Chlamydia trachomatis* genitourinary infections. Ann Intern Med 1988;108:710–717.
20. Stamm WE, Holmes KK. *Chlamydia trachomatis* infections of the adult. In: Holmes KK, Mardh P-A, Sparling PF, Wiesner PJ, eds. Sexually transmitted diseases. 2nd ed. New York: McGraw-Hill, 1990:258.
21. Westrom L, Joesoef R, Reynolds G, Hagdu A, Thompson SE. Pelvic inflammatory disease and fertility. A cohort study of 1,844 women with laparoscopically verified disease and 657 control women with normal laparoscopic results. Sex Transm Dis 1992;19:185–192.
22. Workowski KA, Lampe MF, Wong KG, Watts MB, Stamm WE. Long-term eradication of *Chlamydia trachomatis* genital infection after antimicrobial therapy. Evidence against persistent infection. JAMA 1993;270:2071–2075.

Mycoplasma pneumoniae

●

Julia A. McMillan

GENERAL DESCRIPTION

Mycoplasma pneumoniae is a mollicute, a class of bacteria that lack a cell wall. The class includes organisms that are both commensals and pathogens for animals and plants, but the human is the only known host for *M. pneumoniae*. Lack of a cell wall makes it possible to grow *M. pneumoniae* in the laboratory on cell-free media only if it is supplemented with sterols and other nutrients provided by yeast extract and animal serum. Laboratory isolation is tedious, and identification by culture usually cannot be accomplished until the illness has run its course. The organism does not stain reliably with vital dyes, and it is inherently resistant to cell wall–active antibiotics, the penicillins and cephalosporins. Timely diagnosis rests primarily upon clinical suspicion, though IgM antibody assays and polymerase chain reaction are increasingly used for laboratory confirmation.

   M. pneumoniae was first recognized as a human pathogen when it was isolated from adults with atypical pneumonia syndrome (6, 8). Other causes of this syndrome include adenovirus, *Legionella* species, *Chlamydia pneumoniae*, and *Chlamydia psittaci*. Further investigation demonstrated that *M. pneumoniae* causes respiratory infection in children of all ages, adolescents, and adults in the second through the fourth decades of life. Upper respiratory symptoms are its most common manifestation in children less than 5 years of age (1, 10, 11). Pneumonia due to *M. pneumoniae* has been shown to be responsible for approximately 20% of the lower respiratory tract disease seen in junior high and high school students and up to 50% in college students and young adults (7, 9, 11, 13, 19).

   Community epidemics of *M. pneumoniae* occur in no particular pattern and may persist for months, with low levels of endemic infection underlying the periodic outbreaks (7, 13). Shedding of the organism from the respiratory tract may persist for weeks to months, even in patients with minimal or no symptoms, and even after appropriate antibiotic therapy (27, 29). When initiated within the first 3 to 4 days of illness, antibiotics are beneficial in both adults and children with lower respiratory tract disease (12, 28, 29), though their impact on upper respiratory tract symptoms has not been well studied. Prophylactic oxytetracycline has been shown to protect exposed family members from symptomatic disease (15).

SUSCEPTIBILITY IN VITRO

In vitro susceptibility testing demonstrates that *M. pneumoniae* is most sensitive to the macrolides and tetracyclines (Table 1). MICs are lower for erythromycin than for tetracycline, but erythromycin-resistant strains have been described (3, 20, 30), while tetracycline resistance has not been documented. MICs for clarithromycin and roxithromycin are equivalent to those for erythromycin. The MIC_{90} for azithromycin against clinical isolates from Japan was over 30 times lower than that for erythromycin, clarithromycin, and roxithromycin.

   In vitro data regarding the sensitivity of *M. pneumoniae* to the fluoroquinolones are limited. MICs for sparfloxacin, levofloxacin, and ofloxacin against clinical isolates were 0.031 to 0.063, 0.25 to 0.5, and 0.5 to 1 mg/L, respectively (16). Though several quinolones have been shown to have activity against *M. pneumoniae* at low concentrations, in vitro studies indicate that they are not as effective as the macrolides (4, 5, 22, 31).

ANTIMICROBIAL THERAPY

Early studies in adults indicated that erythromycin and tetracycline were more effective than placebo (18) or penicillin (23, 27) in reducing duration of symptoms, hospitalization, and abnormal chest x-rays in young adults (military recruits and college students) with *M. pneumoniae* pneumonia. Etiology was documented by culture and/or paired antimycoplasmal antibody response in these studies. In children, less impressive benefits from antibiotic therapy have been demonstrated (12, 24), and at least in children and adolescents, initiation of therapy within the first 5 days of illness was important for maximal benefit.

   Treatment of *M. pneumoniae* pneumonia with clarithromycin or azithromycin results in clinical benefit equal to that seen with erythromycin therapy (2, 4, 25, 26), and a 3-day regimen of azithromycin appears to be as effective as 5 days (25). Microbiologic cure has not been carefully compared in these studies, but because the clinical significance of bacteriologic persistence is not known, eradication may not be an appropriate measure for effectiveness. Treatment of *M. pneumoniae* pneumonia with roxithromycin resulted in good-to-excellent results in 12 of 13 patients and eradication of the organism in 4 of the 6 patients cultured (16).

   Little clinical experience is reported regarding fluoroquinolone treatment of documented *M. pneumoniae* infection. In one study, clinical response to ofloxacin therapy was equivalent to physician-determined "standard therapy" for patients with community-acquired pneumonia due to *L. pneumophila*, *C. pneumoniae*, or *M. pneumoniae* (21). In vitro and in vivo testing of sparfloxacin indicates that it may be useful in treating *M. pneumoniae* infection as well (17). Fluoroquinolones are not licensed for use in children.

   Though effective in reducing symptoms, antibiotic therapy does not reliably eradicate shedding of *M. pneumoniae*. Cultures may remain positive for weeks to months, even after a full 7 to 10 days of appropriate antimicrobial therapy and even after symptoms have resolved.

Laboratory diagnosis of *M. pneumoniae* and other causes of atypical pneumonia (*Chlamydia pneumoniae, Legionella pneumoniae, Chlamydia psittaci*) is usually not available. Presumptive antibiotic therapy should be effective against these pathogens as well as the typical bacterial causes of pneumonia (*Streptococcus pneumoniae, Moraxella catarrhalis, Haemophilus influenzae*). The macrolide antibiotics, including erythromycin, clarithromycin, and azithromycin, are the most effective of the single agents available to treat all these causes of community-acquired pneumonia.

Recommended antibiotic doses are listed in Table 2.

Nonpulmonary Disease

Extrapulmonary manifestations of disease ascribed to *M. pneumoniae* infection include enanthem/exanthem, hemolysis, arthritis, central nervous system manifestations, cardiac involvement, hepatitis, pancreatitis, and ocular disease. Most reports are anecdotal, and disease is attributed to *M. pneumoniae* on the basis of antibody testing alone, but isolation of the organism from blood, cerebrospinal fluid, synovial fluid, and skin lesions in some patients attests to the fact that dissemination can occur. Some manifestations, particularly hemolytic disease, are felt to be immune mediated. The role of antibiotic therapy in treatment of nonpulmonary *M. pneumoniae* disease

has not been well studied. Though immune mechanisms are purported to have a role in hemolysis, central nervous system involvement, and arthritis, corticosteroid therapy has not been shown to be of benefit.

REFERENCES

1. Alexander ER, Foy JM, Kenny GE, Kronmal RA, McMahan R, Clarke ER, MacColl WA, Grayston JT. Pneumonia due to *Mycoplasma pneumoniae:* its incidence in the membership of a co-operative medical group. N Engl J Med 1967;275:131–136.
2. Block S, Hedrick J, Hammerschlag MR, Cassell GH, Craft JC. *Mycoplasma pneumoniae* and *Chlamydia pneumoniae* in pediatric community-acquired pneumonia: comparative efficacy and safety of clarithromycin vs. erythromycin ethylsuccinate. Pediatr Infect Dis J 1995;14:471–477.
3. Brunner H, Weidner W. Chemotherapy of human mycoplasma diseases. Isr J Med Sci 1981;17:656–660.
4. Cassell GH, Drnec J, Waites KB, Pate MS, Duffy LB, Watson HL, McIntosh JC. Efficacy of clarithromycin against *Mycoplasma pneumoniae.* J Antimicrob Chem 1991;27(Suppl A):47–59.
5. Cassell GH, Waites KB, Pate MS, Canupp KC, Duffy LB. Comparative susceptibility of *Mycoplasma pneumoniae* to erythromycin, ciprofloxacin, and lomefloxacin. Diagn Microbiol Infect Dis 1989;12:433–435.
6. Chanock RM, Hayflick L, Barile MF. Growth on artificial medium of an agent associated with atypical pneumonia and its identification as a PPLO. Proc Nat Acad Sci USA 1962;48:41–49.
7. Denny FW, Clyde WA Jr, Glezen WP. *Mycoplasma pneumoniae* disease: clinical spectrum, pathophysiology, epidemiology, and control. J Infect Dis 1971;123:74–92.
8. Eaton MD, Meiklejohn G, van Herick W. Studies on the etiology of primary atypical pneumonia. J Exp Med 1944;79:649–668.
9. Evans AS, Allen V, Sueltmann S. *Mycoplasma pneumoniae* infections in University of Wisconsin students. Am Rev Respir Dis 1967;96:237–244.
10. Fernald GW, Collier AM, Clyde WA Jr. Respiratory infections due to *Mycoplasma pneumoniae* in infants and children. Pediatrics 1975;55:327–335.
11. Foy HM, Grayston JT, Kenny GE, Alexander ER, McMahan R. Epidemiology of *Mycoplasma pneumoniae* infection in families. JAMA 1967;197:137–144.
12. Foy HM, Kenny GE, McMahan, Mansy AM, Grayston JT. *Mycoplasma pneumoniae* in an urban area. Five years of surveillance. JAMA 1970;214:1666–1672.

TABLE 1 • Comparative Activity of Antimicrobial Agents against *Mycoplasma pneumoniae*

Antibiotic	MIC$_{90}$ (µg/mL)	MIC$_{50}$ (µg/mL)	Range (µg/mL)
Macrolides			
Erythromycin	≤0.004	≤0.004	≤0.004–0.063
Clarithromycin	≤0.031	≤0.004	≤0.004–0.125
Azithromycin	≤0.0027	0.002	≤0.002–0.0027
Roxithromycin	0.0625	0.0313	0.0156–0.0625
Tetracyclines			
Tetracycline		0.2	0.06–0.4
Chlortetracycline		3.8	0.8–25.0
Oxytetracycline		1.0	0.3–6.3
Doxycycline	0.4	0.4	0.1–1.2
Fluoroquinolones			
Ofloxacin	1.0		0.5–1.0
Sparfloxacin	0.063		0.031–0.063

TABLE 2 • Dose and Duration of Recommended Antimicrobial Therapy for *Mycoplasma pneumoniae* Pneumonia

Antibiotic	Dose	Duration
Erythromycin	Adults: 1–2 g/day divided q.i.d.	10 days
	Children: 40 mg/kg/day divided q.i.d.	10 days
Clarithromycin	Adults: 250–500 mg/day divided b.i.d.	10 days
	Children: 15 mg/kg/day divided b.i.d.	10 days
Azithromycin	Adults: 500 mg/day divided b.i.d. × 1 day followed by 250 mg/day × 5 days	5 days total
	OR 500 mg/day	3 days total
	Children: 10 mg/kg/day divided b.i.d. × day, followed by 5 mg/kg/day × 4 days	5 days total
Tetracycline	1–2 g/day divided q.i.d.	10 days
Doxycycline	200 mg/day divided b.i.d.	10 days

13. Foy HM, Kenny GE, Cooney MK, Allan ID. Long-term epidemiology of infections with *Mycoplasma pneumoniae*. J Infect Dis 1979;39:681–687

14. Ishida K, Kaku M, Irifune K, Mizukane R, Takemura H, Yoshida R, Tanaka H, Usui T, Suyama N, Tomono K. In vitro and in vivo activities of macrolides against *Mycoplasma pneumoniae*. Antimicrob Agents Chemother 1994;38:790–798.

15. Jensen KJ, Senterfit LB, Scully WE, Conway TJ, West RF, Drummy WW. *Mycoplasma pneumoniae* infections in children. An epidemiologic appraisal in families treated with oxytetracycline. Am J Epidemiol 1867;86:419–432.

16. Kaku M, Kohno S, Koga H, Ishida K, Hara K. Efficacy of roxithromycin in the treatment of mycoplasma pneumonia. Chemotherapy 1995;41:149–152.

17. Kaku M, Ishida K, Kohno S, Koga H, Hara K, Usui T. Experimental and clinical studies of sparfloxacin in *Mycoplasma pneumoniae* infection. Drugs 1995;49:412–413.

18. Kingston JR, Chanock RM, Mufson MA, Hellman LP, James WD, Fox HH, Manko MA, Boyers J. Eaton agent pneumonia. JAMA 1961;176:118–123.

19. Mogabgab WJ. *Mycoplasma pneumoniae* and adenovirus respiratory illnesses in military and university personnel 1959–66. Am Rev Respir Dis 1968;97:345–358.

20. Niitu Y, Hasegawa S, Seutaka T, Kubota H, Komatsu S, Horikawa M. Resistance of *Mycoplasma pneumoniae* to erythromycin and other antibiotics. J Pediatr 1970;76:438–443.

21. Plouffe JF, Herbert MT, File TM, Baird I, Parsons JN, Kahn JB, Rielly-Gauvin KT, and the Pneumonia Study Group. Ofloxacin versus standard therapy in treatment of community-acquired pneumonia requiring hospitalization. Antimicrob Agents Chemother 1996;40:1175–1179.

22. Osada Y and Ogawa H. Antimycoplasmal activity of ofloxacin (DL-8280). Antimicrob Agents Chemother 1983;23:509–511.

23. Rasch JR, Mogabgab WJ. Therapeutic effect of erythromycin on Mycoplasma pneumoniae pneumonia. Antimicrob Agents Chemother 1965;5:693–698.

24. Sabato AR, Martin AJ, Marmion BP, Kok TW, Cooper DM. *Mycoplasma pneumoniae:* acute illness, antibiotics and subsequent pulmonary function. Arch Dis Child 1984;59:1034–1037.

25. Schonwald S, Skerk V, Petricevic I, Car V, Majerus-Misic LJ, Gunjaca M. Comparison of three-day and five-day courses of azithromycin in the treatment of atypical pneumonia. Eur J Clin Microbiol Infect Dis 1991;10:877–880.

26. Schonwald S, Gunjaca M, Kolacny-Babic L, Car V, Gosev M. Comparison of azithromycin and erythromycin in the treatment of atypical pneumonias. J Antimicrob Chemo 1990;25(Suppl A):123–126.

27. Shames JM, George RB, Holliday, WB, Rasch JR, Mogabgab WJ. Comparison of antibiotics in the treatment of mycoplasmal pneumonia. Arch Intern Med 1970;125:680–684.

28. Slotkin RI, Clyde WA Jr, Denny RW. The effect of antibiotics on *Mycoplasma pneumoniae* in vitro and in vivo. Am J Epidemiol 1967;86:225–237.

29. Smith CB, Chanock RM, Friedewald WT, Alford RH. Mycoplasma infection in volunteers. Ann NY Acad Sci 1967;143:471–483.

30. Stopler T, Gerichter CB, Branski D. Antibiotic-resistant mutants of *Mycoplasma pneumoniae*. Isr J Med Sci 1980;16:169–173.

31. Waites KB, Cassell GH, Canupp KC, Fernandes PB. In vitro susceptibilities of mycoplasmas and ureaplasmas to new macrolides and aryl-fluoroquinolones. Antimicrob Agents Chemother 1988;32:1500–1502.

Mycoplasma Species

●

Christiane Bébéar and Michel Dupon

Mycoplasmas are frequently present as commensals in the oropharynx or the genital tract of healthy subjects. Of the 16 species found in humans, only a few are clearly pathogenic. Besides *Mycoplasma pneumoniae,* an agent of atypical pneumonia and other respiratory diseases, three genital mycoplasmas, *M. hominis, M. genitalium,* and *Ureaplasma urealyticum,* have been associated with a large variety of illnesses but have been demonstrated as causal for only a few clinical conditions (30). A possible pathogenic role has been proposed for *M. fermentans,* a genital mycoplasma, both in immunocompetent and immunosuppressed patients, but without definitive argument. Other mycoplasma species are usually simple commensals and may exceptionally be involved in infections occurring in immunodeficient patients. The significance of *M. penetrans* detection in human immunodeficiency virus (HIV)-

seropositive patients is still unknown (8). Exceptional cases of human infections due to animal mycoplasmas *M. arginini* (34) and *M. felis* (9) have been reported in immunocompromised patients. The antibiotic therapy of infections related to *M. hominis* and *M. genitalium* only are considered here. Possible developments linked to a better knowledge of the role of *M. fermentans* are mentioned.

GENERAL DESCRIPTION
Mycoplasma hominis

M. hominis belongs to the commensal flora of the lower genital tract of about 10% of healthy women and probably more during pregnancy. It has been associated with various pathologic conditions. The most frequent are genital infections in women but not in men. *M. hominis* is one of the organisms that proliferate during the course of bacterial vaginosis, associated with *Gardnerella vaginalis* and anaerobes, but its contribution to the pathologic process is unknown. The treatment of bacterial vaginosis, when indicated, is not specifically directed against *M. hominis* but, rather, against other microorganisms. However, the high concentration of *M. hominis* in that condition can lead to invasion of the endometria and the upper genital tract.

Pelvic inflammatory disease (PID) is usually considered to be a multibacterial infection in which *M. hominis* can be involved, probably as a secondary agent. The exact proportion of cases of PID related to *M. hominis* infection is not known (30) and is certainly lower than that due to *Chlamydia trachomatis*.

M. hominis is responsible for infections related to pregnancy. It has been isolated from amniotic fluid of women with chorioamnionitis, and there is strong evidence of involvement in postpartum or postabortum fever (22), generally secondary to endometritis. This mycoplasma has also been found in blood cultures and cerebrospinal fluid (CSF) of newborns (33), resulting from in utero infections or mainly from colonization at birth. In most cases, no inflammatory signs can be found in the CSF, and recovery does not require specific treatment. However, in some cases, severe infections with clinical and biologic signs of meningitis have been observed (1), mainly in premature babies born to high-risk mothers.

M. hominis has also been associated with extragenital infections (19, 20, 21). Its frequency is probably underestimated because it is not frequently detected in these specimens. However, it has been demonstrated as responsible for a number of cases including pyelonephritis, bacteremia, vascular infections, wound infections (especially sternal wound infections associated with mediastinitis after thoracic surgery), central nervous system (CNS) infections, joint infections (12), renal and liver abscesses, and respiratory infections. These types of infection appear to be linked to immunosuppression (cell-mediated immunity and/or hypogammaglobulinemia) (21).

Mycoplasma genitalium

A very fastidious mycoplasma, first isolated in the 1980s from patients with nongonococcal urethritis (NGU), *M. genitalium* is now recognized on the basis of its detection by polymerase chain reaction (PCR) as being strongly associated with this clinical condition, independently of other microorganisms such as *C. trachomatis* (14). It has also been found by PCR in the urethras of men with persistent or recurrent disease following acute NGU (29).

The possible role of *M. genitalium* in PID is supported by the presence of antibodies. However this is not yet clear because of antigenic cross-reactivity between *M. pneumoniae* and *M. genitalium* and the lack of isolation caused by the very fastidious growth requirements of mycoplasma.

Exceptionally, *M. genitalium* has been isolated, associated with *M. pneumoniae,* from respiratory (3) and articular specimens (31).

Mycoplasma fermentans

The relationship of *M. fermentans* with rheumatoid arthritis has been debated for a long time. Antibiotic trials have demonstrated the efficacy of tetracyclines, although this efficacy might be due to their antiinflammatory effects. Recently, we isolated seven strains of *M. fermentans* from the synovial fluid or tissues of patients with various rheumatic disorders and detected this organism by PCR in a number of cases (28). *M. fermentans* has also been detected in a small number of immunocompetent adults developing fatal respiratory distress syndrome (17). Erythromycin therapy (which is not active against *M. fermentans*) did not cure the patients. One patient was cured by tetracycline treatment. Except for these last exceptional cases, there is no clear indication for therapy directed against *M. fermentans*.

SUSCEPTIBILITY
In Vitro

Some original features explain the innate resistance of mycoplasmas to certain antibiotics. Because they lack peptidoglycan and penicillin-binding proteins, they are resistant to all the antibiotics inhibiting peptidoglycan biosynthesis, such as β-lactams. They are resistant to rifampin because of the particular structure of their RNA polymerase and also to polymyxins, nalidixic acid, sulfonamides, and trimethoprim.

The antibiotics potentially active include tetracyclines, macrolides-lincosamides-streptogramins (MLS group), aminosides, chloramphenicol, and fluoroquinolones. Some differences are observed according to the species, mainly for the MLS group, and acquired resistance has been described. The antibiotics used for the treatment of human infections are tetracyclines, the MLS group, and fluoroquinolones. Besides their in vitro activity, these drugs achieve high cellular concentrations. This is of interest because of the intracellular location demonstrated for several mycoplasma species. In vitro susceptibility of *M. hominis*, *M. genitalium*, and *M. fermentans* to a range of antibiotics, summarized from a large number of references, is shown in Table 1.

Globally, *M. genitalium* is highly susceptible to tetracyclines, all macrolides, azalide, ketolides, pristinamycin (26), and quinupristin/dalfopristin (4) but less susceptible to lincomycin and clindamycin. The most recent fluoroquinolones such as sparfloxacin, levofloxacin, grepafloxacin, and Bay 12–8039 (23–25) are active. No acquired resistance has been reported, but the number of strains tested is still very low.

M. hominis and *M. fermentans* present globally the same susceptibility profile. Both are naturally susceptible to tetracyclines. However, acquired resistance to tetracyclines has been reported relatively frequently for *M. hominis* (3–30% of cases, depending on the country). This resistance is associated with acquisition of the *tet M* determinant present in many bacteria of the genital tract (27). New tetracycline derivatives, glycylcyclines, have been shown to be active against *M. hominis* strains resistant to other tetracyclines (15).

Drugs in the MLS group have similar activity against *M. hominis* and *M. fermentans*. Both species are resistant to erythromycin, all macrolides with a 14-membered ring (roxithromycin, clarithromycin, dirithromycin, flurithromycin), and azithromycin but are sensitive to josamycin, a 16-membered ring drug. Lincosamides and pristinamycin are very active (5).

TABLE 1 • MICs of Various Antibiotics against Mycoplasmas (μg/mL)[a]

Antibiotics	M. hominis MIC Range	MIC$_{50}$	MIC$_{90}$	M. genitalium MIC Range	M. fermentans MIC Range
Doxycycline	0.02–0.05[b]	0.05[b]	0.05[b]	≤0.01–0.05	0.03–0.1
Minocycline	0.02–0.1[b]	0.05[b]	0.1[b]	≤0.01–0.02	ND[c]
Erythromycin	≥128	≥128	≥128	≤0.01	≥64
Roxithromycin	>16	>16	>16	≤0.01	ND
Clarithromycin	16–≥128	32	64	≤0.01	≥32
Azithromycin	4–64	16	32	≤0.01	≥32
Josamycin	0.1–0.5	0.1	0.2	0.02	0.2–0.5
Lincomycin	0.2–1	0.5	1	1–8	0.1–0.2
Clindamycin	0.02–0.05	0.05	0.05	0.2–1	0.1–0.2
Pristinamycin	0.1–0.5	0.2	0.5	≤0.01–0.02	0.02–0.05
Quinupristin-Dalfopristin	0.5–2	2	2	0.05	0.1–0.5
HMR 3004	0.5–2 2	2	#0.01 0.5–1		
Ofloxacin	0.25–1	1	1	0.5–1	0.05–0.2
Ciprofloxacin	0.125–0.5	0.25	0.5	2	0.05–0.2
Sparfloxacin	0.03–0.12	0.03	0.06	0.05–0.1	≤0.01–0.03
Bay 12-8039	0.06	0.06	0.06	0.03	≤0.01–0.06
Levofloxacin	0.1–0.5	0.2	0.2	0.5–1	0.05
Grepafloxacin	0.03–0.5	0.12	0.12	0.05–0.1	0.02–0.1
Trovafloxacin	0.03–0.06	0.06	0.06	ND	ND
Chloramphenicol	0.5–0.8	—	—	0.5–4	3

[a]Only the MIC range is indicated for *M. genitalium* and *M. fermentans* because of the small number of strains tested.

[b]Tetracycline-susceptible strains.

[c]ND, not determined.

Ketolides (HMR 3004) and quinupristin/dalfopristin have relatively low MICs (4, 7).

Of the fluoroquinolones, sparfloxacin is more active than ofloxacin and ciprofloxacin against all mycoplasma species. The new products levofloxacin (23), trovafloxacin (16), and Bay 12–8039 (24) are promising. Fluoroquinolones have been shown to have bactericidal activity against mycoplasmas. Resistance of *M. hominis* to fluoroquinolones has been associated with mutations in the *gyrA* gene (6), as for other bacterial species, in laboratory strains and clinical isolates.

Resistance to aminoglycosides has been observed in *M. fermentans* strains isolated from cell cultures in which such antibiotics had been used. Chloramphenicol is active against all species studied.

No study concerning the in vitro effect of combinations of drugs against mycoplasmas has been reported.

In Vivo

To our knowledge, there has been no clear evaluation of the in vivo activity of antibiotics in infections due to mycoplasmas other than *M. pneumoniae,* except in rare cases. Very few experimental models are available. However, since most antimicrobial agents active against mycoplasmas are only bacteriostatic, eradicating mycoplasmas depends on the efficacy of the host immune system.

ANTIMICROBIAL THERAPY
Drug of Choice

The drugs of choice are tetracyclines, macrolides and related antibiotics, and fluoroquinolones. However, different situa-

tions occur, depending on the mycoplasma and the clinical setting. Some infections may be treated by a single antibiotic (e.g., NGU or superficial wound infections). In other instances, a combination of drugs is indicated (e.g., polymicrobial infections such as PID). Guidelines are available (10). In other cases such as severe *M. hominis* infections occurring in immunocompromised patients, combination of drugs usually active against the mycoplasmas (e.g., clindamycin and doxycycline (20) or a fluoroquinolone and doxycycline (12)) have been recommended. In those cases, rules for optimal therapy remain to be established. Current therapeutic considerations are based only upon case reports.

Diffusion in some tissues or sites also requires special consideration to obtain sufficient local antibiotic concentration. For example, chloramphenicol may be of interest in CNS infections, and recent fluoroquinolones appear promising for the treatment of some infections (32).

Special Situations

Except for the case of NGU, *M. hominis* is involved in most of the cases reported below.

Nongonococcal Urethritis

M. genitalium is demonstrated only very exceptionally in clinical situations. Empirical antibiotic treatment covering other pathogens involved in NGU (*C. trachomatis, U. urealyticum*) should be given. Theoretically, treatment with a tetracycline (e.g., doxycycline 100 mg twice daily orally for 7 days) will be effective against *M. genitalium*. Documented recurrent urethritis has been reported after one or several courses of treatment; patients were cured by erythromycin (0.5 g four times a day for 7 days). There has been no clinical evaluation of the efficacy of azithromycin and fluoroquinolones for treatment of *M. genitalium* infections. However, because of the slow growth rate of *M. genitalium,* treatment probably requires sufficient duration for mycoplasma cure.

Genital Infections in Women

With infections related to *M. hominis,* one must always keep in mind the possibility of tetracycline-resistant strains. The treatment of some infections in which *M. hominis* may play a role is not directed only against this organism. The treatment of PID, a polymicrobial condition, must be active against several pathogens, such as *C. trachomatis, Neisseria gonorrhoeae, M. hominis,* and Gram-negative aerobes and anaerobes. Several antibiotic combinations can be used. All include an antibiotic potentially active against *M. hominis*—doxycycline (100 mg twice daily), ofloxacin (200–400 mg twice daily), or clindamycin (300–450 mg four times a day). Different regimens have been proposed depending on the severity of the infection (10, 11). The choice of drug depends on possible adverse reactions or contraindications in treatment of infection during pregnancy. Treatment must be reevaluated after 72 h, and its total duration is usually 14 days.

With postpartum or postabortum fever, some of the patients recover uneventfully without antibiotic treatment. Treatment of these infections is directed against *M. hominis* only if mycoplasma is suspected (e.g., persistant fever in spite of β-lactam therapy) and if laboratory tests have demonstrated the presence of this organism. Recommended antibiotics include doxycycline, or in the case of resistance, a 16-membered ring macrolide or a fluoroquinolone. No information is currently available concerning the efficacy of streptogramins in these patients.

Extragenital Infections

Because of the large variety of possible extragenital infections, some examples are considered here, and the main drugs indicated in these cases are only mentioned. For wound infections or other abscesses, antimicrobial agents (doxycycline, clindamycin, ofloxacin, or ciprofloxacin) for at least 2 weeks are added to surgical debridement and drainage of purulent collections. Successful management of joint infection requires a long treatment. Duration of therapy for *M. hominis* arthritis reported in a recent review (18) ranged from 2 weeks to 7 months. The antibiotics used were either doxycycline or clindamycin. Replacement of bone prosthesis may be warranted. Doxycycline-impregnated cement has been used (9). Fluoroquinolones have good bone penetration. Little information is available for treatment of infection in the CSF. Chloramphenicol and fluoroquinolones have good penetration into the CSF. Doxycycline might be added to the treatment (13).

Mycoplasma Infections in Immunosuppressed Patients

Treatment of mycoplasma infections in immunosuppressed patients requires not only antibiotic therapy active against mycoplasmas but also management of the immunosuppression. In hypogammaglobulinemic patients, administration of immunoglobulin can play a role despite a low level of antibodies against mycoplasmas. Discontinuation or reduction of immunosuppressive drugs might also be useful.

Newborn Infections

Treatment of mycoplasma infections in newborns is a very difficult problem because the antibiotics potentially active against mycoplasmas (e.g., tetracyclines, fluoroquinolones, or chloramphenicol) are contraindicated in newborns. However, in very severe infections, such as meningitis due to *M. hominis,* doxycycline has been used at a dosage of 2 to 4 mg/kg/day (2) for 14 days. Because no injectable form of 16-membered macrolide is available for pediatric usage, an alternative could be thiamphenicol (30–50 mg/kg/day) or eventually ciprofloxacin (30 mg/kg/day). In less severe cases, such as respiratory infections, the drug of choice is josamycin (30–50 mg/kg/day) given orally.

ENDPOINTS FOR MONITORING

The route of administration of therapy and its duration depend on the location and severity of the infection. However, because tetracyclines and macrolides have only bacteriostatic activity against mycoplasmas, the course of treatment must be sufficiently long. Clinical improvement is the first element to evaluate. Clearing of mycoplasmas is a valid criterion only for normally sterile sites. Eradication is essential for infections occurring in immunodepressed subjects but can be difficult to obtain.

COMMENTS

The first point concerning mycoplasmas is to think about their possible role in infections. Clinicians should be aware of the possibility of mycoplasma infections in such specific situations as PID, infections related to pregnancy, neonatal infections in premature low-birth-weight newborns, wound infections after thoracic or abdominal surgery, joint infections in patients with prostheses, or various infections in immunosuppressed patients. An additional hint is failure of β-lactam treatment.

Another problem is the difficulty of diagnosing mycoplasma infections. *M. hominis* can be detected accidentally because it can grow on blood agar. This is not the case for other mycoplasma species that are very fastidious. With *M. genitalium,* only PCR can be used, but it is not currently available because of the lack of commercial kits. For all these species, serology has not been evaluated and is not recommended. The major problem concerning mycoplasmas is determining if they are the cause of the infection. For example, isolation of *M. hominis* from sites in which it may be only a commensal, such as the lower genital tract of women or respiratory specimens of neonates, is difficult to interpret. When isolated from normally sterile sites, its presence is more likely to be related to infection. Then, antibiotic susceptibility testing is necessary, but it is not well standardized.

Finally, even when mycoplasmas are detected and considered responsible for infection, it is still necessary to determine whether specific treatment is required. Most postpartum fevers or neonate infections improve without specific therapy, as demonstrated by clinical observations with antibiotics ineffective against mycoplasmas. The clinical course of infection, such as duration of fever and symptoms, is the major indication for specific therapy.

The situation is totally different in mycoplasma infections occurring in immunodeficient patients. In these instances, it is necessary but sometimes difficult to eradicate mycoplasma.

REFERENCES

1. Alonso-Vega C, Wauters N, Vermeylen D, Muller MF, Serruys E. A fatal case of *Mycoplasma hominis* meningoencephalitis in a full term newborn. J Clin Microbiol 1997;35:286–287.
2. Apéré H, Sarlangue J, Renaudin H, Billeaud C, Bébéar C, Sandler B. Infection materno-foetale à mycoplasmes génitaux. Pédiatrie 1993;48:297–299.
3. Baseman JB, Dallo SF, Tully JG, Rose DC. Isolation and characterization of *Mycoplasma genitalium* strains from the human respiratory tract. J Clin Microbiol 1988;26:2266–2269.
4. Bébéar C, Bouanchaud D. A review of the in vitro activity of quinupristin-dalfopristin against intracellular pathogens and mycoplasmas. J Antimicrob Chemother 1997;39(Suppl A):59–62.
5. Bébéar C, Renaudin H, Maugein J, de Barbeyrac B, Clerc M. Pristinamycin and human mycoplasmas: in vitro activity compared with macrolides and lincosamides. In vivo efficacy in *Mycoplasma pneumoniae* experimental infection. Zentralbl Bakteriol 1990;(Suppl 20):77–82.
6. Bébéar CM, Bové JM, Bébéar C, Renaudin J. Characterization of *Mycoplasma hominis* mutations involved in resistance to fluoroquinolones. Antimicrob Agents Chemother 1997;41:269–273.
7. Bébéar CM, Renaudin H, Aydin MD, Chantot JF, Bébéar C. In vitro activity of ketolides against mycoplasmas. J Antimicrob Chemother 1997;39:669–670.
8. Blanchard A, Montagnier L. AIDS-associated mycoplasmas. Annu Rev Microbiol 1994;48:687–712.
9. Bonilla HF, Chenoweth CE, Tully JG, Blythe LK, Robertson JA, Ognenovski VM, Kauffman CA. *Mycoplasma felis* arthritis in a patient with hypogammaglobulinemia. Clin Infect Dis 1997;24:222–225.
10. Centers for Disease Control and Prevention. Pelvic inflammatory disease: guidelines for prevention and management. MMWR 1991;40:1–25.
11. Centers for Disease Control and Prevention. Sexually transmitted diseases treatment guidelines. MMWR 1993;40:75–81.
12. Clough V, Cassell GH, Duffy LB, Rinaldi LZ, Bluestone R, Morgan MA, Meyer RD. Septic arthritis and bacteremia due to mycoplasma resistant to antimicrobial therapy in a patient with systemic lupus erythematosus. Clin Infect Dis 1992;15:402–407.
13. Cohen M, Kubak B. *Mycoplasma hominis* meningitis complicating head trauma: case report and review. Clin Infect Dis 1997;24:272–273.
14. Horner PJ, Gilroy CB, Thomas BJ, Naidoo Ro, Taylor-Robinson D. Association of *Mycoplasma genitalium* with acute nongonococcal urethritis. Lancet 1993;342:582–585.
15. Kenny GE, Cartwright FD. Susceptibility of *Mycoplasma hominis*, *Mycoplasma pneumoniae* and *Ureaplasma urealyticum* to new glycylcyclines in comparison with those of older tetracyclines. Antimicrob Agents Chemother 1994;38:2628–2632.
16. Kenny GE, Cartwright FD. Susceptibilities of *Mycoplasma pneumoniae*, *Mycoplasma hominis* and *Ureaplasma urealyticum*

17. to a new quinolone, trovafloxacin (CP-99,219). Antimicrob Agents Chemother 1996;40:1048–1049.
17. Lo SC, Wear DJ, Green SL, Jones PG, Legier JF. Adult respiratory distress syndrome with or without systemic disease associated with infections due to *Mycoplasma fermentans*. Clin Infect Dis 1993;17(Suppl 1):S259–263.
18. Luttrell LM, Kanj SS, Corey GR, Lins RE, Spinner RJ, Mallon WJ, Sexton DJ. *Mycoplasma hominis* septic arthritis: two case reports and review. Clin Infect Dis 1994;19:1067–1070.
19. Madoff S, Hooper DC. Non-genitourinary infections caused by *Mycoplasma hominis* in adults. Rev Infect Dis 1988;10:602–613.
20. McMahon DK, Dummer JS, Pasculle AW, Cassell GH. Extragenital *Mycoplasma hominis* infections in adults. Am J Med 1990;89:275–277.
21. Meyer RD, Clough W. Extragenital *Mycoplasma hominis* infections in adults: emphasis on immunosuppression. Clin Infect Dis 1993;17(Suppl 1):S243–249.
22. Neman-Simha V, Renaudin H, de Barbeyrac B, Leng JJ, Horovitz J, Dallay D, Billeaud C, Bébéar C. Isolation of genital mycoplasmas from blood of febrile obstetrical gynecologic patients and neonates. Scand J Infect Dis 1992;24:317–321.
23. Renaudin H, Bébéar CM, Aydin MD, Bryskier A, Bébéar C. In vitro activity of levofloxacin against mycoplasmas [Abstract G28]. Abstracts of the 96th general meeting of the American Society for Microbiology, New Orleans, LA, 1996:286.
24. Renaudin H, Bébéar CM, Boudjadja A, Bébéar C. In vitro activity of Bay 12–8039, a new fluoroquinolone against mycoplasmas [Abstract F9]. 36th ICAAC, New Orleans, LA, 1996:101.
25. Renaudin H, Bébéar CM, Schaeverbeke T, Leblanc F, Bébéar C. In vitro activity of grepafloxacin against mycoplasmas [Abstract E159]. 37th ICAAC, Toronto, Canada 1997:143.
26. Renaudin H, Tully JG, Bébéar C. In vitro susceptibility of *Mycoplasma genitalium* to antibiotics. Antimicrob Agents Chemother 1992;36:870–872.
27. Roberts MC. Characterization of the *tet(M)* determinants in urogenital and respiratory bacteria. Antimicrob Agents Chemother 1990;34:476–478.
28. Schaeverbeke T, Renaudin H, Clerc M, Lequen L, Vernhes JP, de Barbeyrac B, Bannwarth B, Bébéar C, Dehais J. Systematic detection of mycoplasmas by culture and polymerase chain reaction (PCR) procedures in 209 synovial fluid samples. Br J Rheumatol 1997;36:310–314.
29. Taylor-Robinson D. The history and role of *Mycoplasma genitalium* in sexually transmitted diseases. Genitourin Med 1995;71:1–8.
30. Taylor-Robinson D. Infections due to species of *Mycoplasma* and *Ureaplasma*. An update. Clin Infect Dis 1996;23:671–684.
31. Tully JG, Rose DL, Baseman JB, Dallo SF, Lazzell AL, Davis CP. *Mycoplasma pneumoniae* and *Mycoplasma genitalium* mixture in synovial fluid isolate. J Clin Microbiol 1995;33:1851–1855.
32. Waites KB, Cassell GH. Clinical applications of fluoroquinolones for genital mycoplasma infections. Infect Med 1994;11:71–88.
33. Waites KB, Rudd PT, Crouse DT, Canupp KC, Nelson KG, Ramsey C, Cassell GH. Chronic *Ureaplasma urealyticum* and *Mycoplasma hominis* infections of central nervous system in preterm infants. Lancet 1988;1:17–21.
34. Yechouron A, Lefebvre J, Robson HG, Rose DL, Tully JG. Fatal septicemia due to *Mycoplasma arginini:* a new human zoonosis. Clin Infect Dis 1992;15:434–438.

Toxoplasma gondii

●

Jacques Couvreur and Catherine Leport

GENERAL DESCRIPTION
Parasitology

Toxoplasma gondii, an obligately intracellular protozoan parasite is a coccidium that exists in three forms. The *tachyzoite* is a rapidly proliferative form that characterizes the acute stage of infection. It is the form that is susceptible to appropriate drugs. The *cyst* is formed within the host cell and is demonstrable on approximately the 8th day of infection. It contains thousands of *bradyzoites* and can persist as a viable parasite throughout the life of the host. The cyst wall protects it against drugs. The bradyzoite replicates more slowly than the tachyzoite and probably does not have the same susceptibility to drugs. *Oocysts* are result from an intraepithelial stage leading to gametogony and sporogony that is exclusively observed in the intestine of cats infected by the oral route. They are eliminated by millions in the feces of this animal from the 5th to the 20th day following ingestion of infective material and sporulate 1 to 5 days after excretion into infectious forms known as sporozoites. These are highly infectious when they are ingested. Oocysts can remain viable in warm moist soil for a year or more. Sporulation cannot occur below 4°C or above 37°C.

Transmission

Humans acquire *Toxoplasma* infection by ingestion of oocysts excreted by cats or by eating undercooked meat containing cysts. All mammalian cells can be invaded following hematogenous and lymphogenous dissemination, with ensuing inflammation and necrosis of the involved tissues. Infection of the fetus is the result of hematogenous and placental transmission of tachyzoites following acute acquired maternal infection during pregnancy.

Immunity

Protection against *T. gondii* infection is influenced by parasite strain, and its antigenic components (48), inoculum size, route of infection, host genetics, host age, host immunity, and sex hormones. The response to *Toxoplasma* infection is of the delayed type of hypersensitivity. The CD4:CD8 ratio is reduced or even inverted. *T. gondii*–specific cytotoxic T lymphocytes have been demonstrated. Macrophages play an important protective role. They are stimulated by interferon-γ, which appears to be the most active lymphokine in mediating resistance against the parasite. Thus immunodeficient patients—AIDS patients, transplant patients and fetuses—are at risk of a patent infection.

SUSCEPTIBILITY IN VITRO AND IN VIVO
Single Drugs
Pyrimethamine

Pyrimethamine (Daraprim), a substituted phenylpyrimidine antimicrobial drug, is a folic acid antagonist that inhibits dihydrofolate reductase (DHFR), a major enzyme in the purine pathway of the parasite (59). Its parasitostatic and cytopathogenic effects were clearly demonstrated by in vitro studies (28, 34, 82, 103). Its activity was documented long ago in animal experiments (91). It can cure acute murine toxoplasmosis but cannot eradicate cysts in chronic infection.

Sulfonamides

The activity of sulfonamides on *T. gondii* was established long ago in animal experiments and more recently by in vitro studies (2, 74). This activity is rather parasitostatic. No cytopathogenic effect on parasites was observed on inhibitory concentrations. The main effect of sulfonamides is inhibition of another enzyme essential in the purine pathway of the parasite, dihydrofolate synthetase.

Spiramycin

Spiramycin, a macrolide antibiotic has favorable effects in vitro and in experimental murine toxoplasmosis. It acts by inhibiting protein synthesis of *T. gondii*. However, its antiparasitic activity appears lower than that of other macrolides.

Clindamycin

The effect of clindamycin on *T. gondii* has been assessed in vitro with variable results: no effect in the study by Harris et al. (44) and an IC_{50} of 0.15 mg/L in the study by Derouin (Derouin, personal communication) (Table 1). Results from animal models suggest a partial response to clindamycin alone in acute or chronic infection and some activity when combined with sulfonamides (68). The drug seems to be unable to eradicate the spread of infection and to have suppressive, rather than curative, activity.

Other Drugs (Alternative Regimens)

The synergistic combination pyrimethamine-sulfonamide remains a mainstay in the treatment of human toxoplasmosis. The frequency of untoward effects (particularly in immunocompromised patients) led investigators to test a number of new drugs against *T. gondii* (Table 2).

Other Macrolides.   The inhibitory activity of macrolides has been shown in vitro. This inhibitory effect increases pro-

TABLE 1 • **In Vitro Activity of Drugs against *T. gondii* Cultivated on MRC5 Fibroblasts[a]**

Drug	IC$_{50}$ (μg/mL)
Macrolides (MLS)	
Erythromycin	3
Spiramycin	12
Roxithromycin	2
Josamycin	1.7
Clindamycin	0.15
Azithromycin	1.2
Clarithromycin	0.8
Sulfa drugs/sulfones	
Sulfadiazine	2.5
Sulfamethoxazole	1.1
Sulfadoxine	42
Dapsone	0.5
Sulfizoxazole	6.4
Inhibitors of dehydrofolate reductase	
Pyrimethamine	0.04
Trimethoprim	2.3
Trimetrexate	0.16×10^{-3}
Piritrexim	6.9×10^{-3}
Quinolones[b]	
Pefloxacin	18
Sparfloxacin	22
Ciprofloxacin	52
Ofloxacin	48

[a]Duration of culture, 72 h; quantification using ELISA techniques. From references 27, 28, 31 and Derouin, personal communication.

[b]Unpublished data.

gressively with the concentration, so that the maximal effect is observed with very high concentrations. IC$_{50}$s are between 0.8 and 12 mg/L (Table 1). The mechanism of action is unknown. The effect has been studied in animal models, in which the macrolides seem poorly effective except when used in high concentrations. Partial protection has been achieved with spiramycin, roxithromycin, clarithromycin, and azithromycin. The newer macrolides discussed below seem to have some pharmacokinetic advantages over the older ones, such as concentration in phagocytes (106).

Roxithromycin is protective for mice with acute toxoplasmosis, even with the highly virulent RH strain of *Toxoplasma*, but does not prevent cyst formation in the brain (9, 18). Azithromycin given orally in a dose of 200 mg/kg/day for 10 days protects mice infected with a highly virulent strain of *Toxoplasma*. It is distinguished by its long serum half-life (5–11 h) and its slow elimination from the body (3, 6). Clarithromycin is active in vitro and in vivo (8). It is protective in acute lethal murine toxoplasmosis at a dosage of 300 mg/kg/day given orally for 9 days (19). Prolonged treatment in chronically infected mice leads to a significant reduction in the number of parasitic cysts in the brain.

Tetracyclines. Doxycycline (300 mg/kg/day for 10 days) or minocycline (100 mg/kg/day for 10 days) protects mice against death following infection with the highly virulent RH strain of *T. gondii*. Minocycline (50 mg/kg/day for 3 weeks) significantly reduces the number of cysts in the brain (16, 17).

Rifamycin Derivatives. One hundred percent of mice infected with a lethal inoculum of trophozoites or cysts of *T. gondii* are protected by rifabutin alone at a dosage of 300 mg/kg/day for 10 days. Rifapentin inhibits intracellular replication of the parasite in vitro. At a dosage of 200 mg/kg/day for 10 days it protects infected mice against death as well as atovaquone and better than rifabutine (5).

Hydroxynaphthoquinones. Atovaquone (566 C 80) is the best documented and the most promising agent in this class (49, 50). It is active in vitro and in vivo (99) and may be the most active compound against cysts. A dose of 100 mg/kg/day for 10 days is protective for 100% of mice inoculated with a lethal dose of the most virulent strains or given a lethal dose of cysts by the oral route. A dose of 50 mg/kg/day for 30 days completely eradicated the parasite. Protection can be achieved even if treatment is started on the 10th day after infection, when there are overt signs of toxoplasmosis (7). In vitro studies revealed a loss of cyst viability with 100 μg/mL of atovaquone (51). Mice treated 5 weeks after infection with 200 mg/kg/day for 12 weeks showed a steady and significant decline in the number of cysts in the brain and a tendency to normalization of brain tissue. The association of the combination pyrimethamine/sulfadiazine with atovaquone is synergistic.

Trovafloxacin. Trovafloxacin is active in vitro. At a dosage of 100 to 200 mg/kg/day, it protects infected mice against death (57).

Other Folate Inhibitors. The mechanism of action of other folate inhibitors is similar to that of pyrimethamine, with inhibition of DHFR. Their activity has been shown in vitro and on the purified enzyme. The most active compounds are trimetrexate and piritrexime, which are 1 to 100 times more potent than pyrimethamine. Trimethoprim has an activity 10 to 50 times lower than that of pyrimethamine (Table 1); it has excellent in vitro activity (28) but is not protective in infected mice. Piritrexim (20 mg/kg/day) combined with sulfadiazine (400 mg/kg/day) and given for 10 days begining 24 h after infection showed significant protection in acute mouse toxoplasmosis (4). Trimetrexate had greater activity on *Toxoplasma* than pyrimethamine and trimethoprim (28, 60).

Miscellaneous Drugs. Arprinocid, a purine analogue used in veterinary medicine as an anticoccidial agent, protects mice remarkably well against lethal toxoplasmic infection at a dose of 100 μg/mouse/day for 4 weeks (9, 70). It has excellent in vitro activity against cysts (51). Dapsone is active in vitro and in vivo. The combination of dapsone (100 mg/kg/day) with pyrimethamine (18.5 mg/kg/day) protected 100% of infected mice with no relapses after discontinuation of the treatment (31). Pentamidine has in vitro activity against *Toxoplasma* (67). Qinghaosu, a drug extracted from a Chinese herb and its derivatives showed in vitro activity against trophozoites of *Toxoplasma* (9) as well as malaria parasites. The inhibitory effect of trioxans could be related to a similar mode of action.

Immunomodulators. The role of cellular immunity in the defense against *T. gondii* has been clearly established. Reinforcement of immunity with interferon-γ has been shown in animal models. It has a synergistic effect with antiparasitic drugs.

TABLE 2 • Assessment of Drugs against *T. gondii* Other Than Pyrimethamine, Sulfonamides, and Clindamycin

Drugs	Activity in Vitro	Activity in Vivo Protection against Lethal Infection	Protection against Cyst Formation in the Brain	Synergistic Activity with Other Drugs	Trials in Humans	References
Macrolides						
Roxithromycin	0	+	0	Interferon-γ	Yes, prophylaxis	18
Azithromycin	+	0 (↑ + sulfadiazine)		Sulfadiazine	Yes, curative	3–6, 106
Clarithromycin	+	± (↑ with pyrimeth-amine or with sulfa-diazine)	+ (alone and with minocycline)	Minocycline, pyrimethamine, sulfadiazine	Yes, curative	34 8
Cyclines						
Doxycycline	+	+		Pyrimethamine, sulfadiazine	Yes, curative	16
Minocycline	+	+	+		Yes, curative	17
Rifamycin derivatives						
Rifabutine	+	+	+ (with atovaquone)	Atovaquone, pyrimethamine, sulfadiazine		10–11, 98
Rifapentine	+	+				5
Naphthoquinones						
Atovaquone	+	+	+	Pyrimethamine, sulfadiazine	Yes, curative, prophylaxis	7, 49 59, 110
Quinolones						
Trovafloxacine	+	+				57
Folate inhibitors						
Trimethoprim	+	+		Sulfamethoxazole	Yes, prophylaxis	28, 8
Piritrexim	±	0 (↑ with sulfadiazine)		Sulfadiazine		
Trimetrexate	+	±		Sulfadiazine	Yes, curative	60, 28
Others						
Arprinocid	+	+				51
Dapsone	+	+		Pyrimethamine, sulfadiazine, sulfamethoxazole	Yes, prophylaxis	31–70, 8
Pentamidine	+	+				67

Interferon-γ is highly effective in vitro and moderately so in vivo. It may act by activating macrophages and stimulating natural killer cells and humoral responses (80) and by interfering in the metabolism of *Toxoplasma*. It showed remarkable decrease in toxoplasmic encephalitis in mice chronically infected (107). Favorable synergistic effects were obtained with the combination interferon/roxythromycin in murine encephalitis (45). Interferon-γ protects mice against lethal infection (9).

Recombinant interleukin-2 significantly decreases mortality in mice with lethal infection and lowers the number of cysts in their brains (102).

Combination Drugs

Pyrimethamine-Sulfonamides

The activity of pyrimethamine is increased 6- to 8-fold by combination with sulfonamide drugs (109). Consequently, this is a combination of choice for synergistic activity against trophozoites. In vitro studies with cultures on fibro-blasts revealed that this activity is important with pyrimethamine at 0.02 μg/mL and sulfadiazine at 0.1 μg/mL (27), while the inhibitory concentration (IC_{50}) of sulfadiazine alone is 2.5 μg/mL. Sulfadiazine is widely used. Sulfapyrazine, sulfamer-

azine, and sulfadimidine are about as effective. Trisulfapyrimidine combination (sulfadimidine, sulfamerazine, and sulfadiazine) can be used. The activity of all other sulfa drugs (e.g., sulfamethoxazole, sulfafuroxazole) is lower, and they are not widely used for curative purpose. Antiparasitic activity of the metabolites of sulfonamide drugs is not documented. The combination pyrimethamine-sulfadoxine is synergistic and proved effective in murine toxoplasmosis (74). Parasitologic eradication was 100% with immediate treatment following inoculation and 32% when it was delayed 72 h.

Other Combinations

Combination of clarithromycin and sulfadiazine is highly synergistic (8). Both combination of rifabutine/atovaquone for 30 days or rifabutine/clindamycin for 15 days gave remarkable results in toxoplasmic encephalitis of mice, with significant lessening of inflammation of the brain (10). It is synergistic, results in prolongation of survival in mice, but does not prevent relapses (98). These promising results warrant clinical trials with prolonged duration of therapy (98). The combinations rifabutine-pyrimethamine and rifabutine/sulfadiazine did not reduce brain inflammation significantly compared with each drug alone (11). The combination trimethoprim-sulfamethoxazole in murine toxoplasmosis gave variable results (42). In mice with acute toxoplasmosis, a 93% survival rate was reached only with the combination trimetrexate (37 mg/kg/day) and sulfadiazine (375 mg/kg/day) (28). The combination of dapsone with sulfamethazine 100 mg/kg/day is active in vivo; this effect is additive, not synergistic.

ANTIPARASITIC THERAPY
Drugs Of Choice

Pyrimethamine

The activity of pyrimethamine in toxoplasmosis has been confirmed in humans. It appears late on low dosage, which favors the hypothesis of the necessity for tissue accumulation to obtain active inhibitory titers (28). This activity is limited to the time of its administration. The possibility of relapses following discontinuation of the drug in immunosuppressed patients warrants prolonged treatment following the acute phase of the infection. With respect to concentrations in body fluids, pyrimethamine in immunocompetent adults at a daily dose of 25 mg (0.3 mg/kg) leads to serum concentrations of 0.9 to 1.7 µg/mL. In human immunodeficiency virus (HIV) patients, a dose of 50 to 75 mg/day yields serum concentrations of 1 to 4.5 µg/mL; peak levels occur at 3.3 ± 1.98 h; and half-life is 114 ± 42 h (58, 76). It has been suggested that a minimal serum concentration of 0.75 µg/mL in the presence of sulfonamide and 3.0 µg/mL in the absence of sulfonamide may be necessary to treat toxoplasmic encephalitis in HIV-infected patients (114).

In infants, the mean serum level at 4 h after a daily dose of 1 mg/kg was 1.3 ± 0.5 µg/mL. It was 0.7 ± 0.3 µg/mL at 4 h when the same dose was given every other day (82). It seems that in a given individual, serum levels remain relatively stable at steady state over weeks on an identical dosage. In infants less than 1 month of age, serum levels did not differ from values obtained in older children on the same dosage. In vitro studies revealed that levels of pyrimethamine achieved in infant sera with standard dosages, alone or in conjunction with sulfadiazine, had good inhibitory effect on most virulent strains, including the RH strain (82).

Spinal fluid concentrations of pyrimethamine range from 10 to 25% of serum levels in patients with leukemia or AIDS patients with toxoplasmic encephalitis (114). Its penetration through the blood/spinal fluid barrier remains to be established. In infants on a daily dose of 1 mg/kg, ventricular fluid concentrations were 0.04 to 0.11 µg/mL at 4 to 54 h postdose—approximately 10 to 25% of serum levels (82). Diffusion of pyrimethamine in brain tissue was quantified in patients undergoing neurosurgery (64): 12 h following a 100-mg dose, the mean level in brain tissue was 0.9 ± 0.33 µg/g. By the 24th hour, it increased to a maximum of 1.56 ± 0.84 µg/g. At the 48th hour, it was 1.02 ± 0.28 µg/gr. The brain tissue:serum level ratio was 2.5, 5.2, and 4.1 at 12, 24, and 48 h, respectively. Half-life of the drug was 40 h in brain tissue and 28 h in serum, which means that a dose of 50 to 100 mg every other day is convenient for prophylactic therapy in AIDS. Daily administration is compulsory for curative treatment in acute infection.

There is no parenteral form of the drug. Pyrimethamine is metabolized in liver, and its pharmacokinetics is not altered by renal insufficiency. The lack of correlation between serum levels and dosage and varying pharmacokinetics between patients suggest genetic differences in metabolizing the drug. Consequently, monitoring serum concentrations of pyrimethamine can be useful. The possibility of interaction between pyrimethamine and other drugs affecting hepatic enzymes including phenobarbital must always be considered. Metabolism of pyrimethamine can be altered in liver disease.

Side effects can be minor as nausea and headaches. More important are the effects related to the antifolinic activity of the drug. It can cause gradual but reversible depression of bone marrow: neutropenia, thrombocytopenia, megaloblastic anemia. These side effects can be prevented by routine oral administration of folinic acid (calcium leucovorin) 5 to 10 mg three times a week in infants and up to 50 mg daily in HIV-infected patients. In contrast to folic acid, folinic acid does not inhibit the activity of the parasite except in in vitro studies at very high concentrations. Indeed *T. gondii* is unable to assimilate exogenous folates, folic and folinic acid, and has to synthesize them from a precursor, *p*-aminobenzoic acid.

During treatment, the neutrophil count must be monitored twice a week, and platelets and hematocrit levels once monthly (78) or more frequently in HIV-infected patients. When the neutrophil count is below 1000/mm^3 or platelets are below 90000/mm^3, increasing the dosage of leucovorin is mandatory. Withdrawal of the drug can be considered if this treatment fails. The phenomenon is reversible as a rule. In infants, there is no close correlation between high pyrimethamine levels and neutropenia, but high serum concentrations require a higher dosage of leucovorin and, more often, withdrawal of the medication. Leucovorin must be given for an additional week following discontinuation of pyrimethamine. High dosages of pyrimethamine can result in seizures. Patients with a serum level of 5 µg/mL or more are at risk. A loading dose of 2 mg/kg in older children weighing 25 kg or more is excessive (82). Intoxication with pyrimethamine can warrant exchange transfusion.

Sulfonamides

Sulfadiazine is currently used. Its loading dose is 100 mg/kg/day, not exceeding 4 to 6 g/day, by the oral route in 3 or 4 divided doses, followed by 50 mg/kg/day for one to several weeks. The serum half-life of sulfadiazine is 5 h. Diffusion into cerebrospinal fluid (CSF) is good.

Monitoring the treatment includes attention to urine output, water metabolism, and blood counts and light microscopy of urine for crystalluria and creatininemia. Nephrolithiasis is treated by discontinuation of the drug and prevented by hydration and alkalinization of the urine. Trisulfamides can then be substituted for sulfadiazine, since the risk of urologic complications is reduced.

Combination of Pyrimethamine and Sulfonamides

The synergistic combination of pyrimethamine and sulfonamides remains a mainstay in the treatment of human toxoplasmosis, but its untoward effects led to use of other drugs.

The combination pyrimethamine-sulfadoxine can be used for protracted treatment. It is available in tablets (pyrimethamine 25 mg/sulfadoxine 500 mg (Fansidar)) and for injection (pyrimethamine 20 mg/sulfadoxine 400 mg). The dosage is one tablet/20 kg every 7 to 10 days because of the half-life of sulfadoxine. Rash following the first doses imposes permanent contraindication. This combination is uncommonly used in immunocompromised patients. Yet it is the only form of pyrimethamine available for injection.

Clindamycin

Clindamycin is completely absorbed following oral administration, with peak levels of 4 and 8 μg/mL after ingestion of 300 and 600 mg, respectively. The half-life is approximately 2.7 h. The drug is excreted in urine and bile and partially metabolized in active and inactive metabolites. Approximately 90% is bound to plasma proteins. The drug is widely distributed, with adequate levels in the iris, choroid, and retina. Diffusion in CSF and brain tissue is uncertain. The most frequent adverse reactions are gastrointestinal manifestations, possibly due to pseudomembranous colitis induced by *Clostridium difficile*. Other adverse effects seen in AIDS patients (most often treated with a combination of clindamycin and pyrimethamine) were rash, liver function test abnormalities, neutropenia, and thrombopenia.

Spiramycin

Spiramycin is now exclusively used to prevent maternofetal transmission of the parasite. In pregnant women treated with a daily dose of 3 g, a comparison study of concentrations in maternal serum, cord blood, and placental tissue revealed average levels of 1.9 μg/mL, 0.78 μg/mL and 6.2 μg/g, respectively (39). The serum fetomaternal ratio is 0.47 in the 21st to 24th weeks of pregnancy and 0.74 at birth (37). Administration of spiramycin to infected women during pregnancy is associated with a significant decrease in the risk of placental infection (32) and reduces by half the risk of maternofetal transmission of the parasite (32). The in vivo effects of spiramycin are explained by its rapid uptake from serum and its high concentrations and exceptional persistence in tissues, especially in placenta.

No curative activity of spiramycin on postnatally treated congenital toxoplasmosis or in acquired toxoplasmosis has been demonstrated. It failed to protect AIDS patients against neurotoxoplasmosis (66). Its indication is the prevention of fetopathy in women with acquired toxoplasmosis during pregnancy. The usual dosage is 3 g/day orally in 2 or 3 divided doses. Apart from occasional slight digestive discomfort, there is no real toxicity, and treatment can be maintained for months.

Clarithromycin

A combination of clarithromycin (200 mg) and pyrimethamine (75 mg) with daily oral administration has been used in humans (35).

Trimethoprim

Combined with sulfamethoxazole, trimethoprim might be useful as primary prophylaxis for toxoplasmic encephalitis in AIDS patients (9).

Special Situations

Acute Acquired Infection in the Immunocompetent Host

Acute acquired toxoplasmosis is subclinical in about 90% of immunocompetent humans. The most common sign is cervical lymphadenopathy, often persisting for months. This condition does not require routine therapy (81). Indications for treatment are pregnancy, systemic marked or prolonged symptoms, evidence of organ involvement (i.e., myocarditis, encephalitis, uveitis), possibility of a laboratory-acquired infection or of contamination through transfusion of blood products, and a setting of other, more severe cases in the neighborhood causing massive contamination. In such instances, the immune status of the patient should be checked, including HIV testing. Pyrimethamine (50 mg/day) and sulfadiazine (3–6 g/day) should be given for 1 or 2 months, depending on the clinical severity.

Acquired Acute Infection in the Immunocompetent Pregnant Woman

In pregnant women, acute toxoplasmosis is usually subclinical and is recognized through routine serologic examination of the pregnant population with careful serologic follow-up of seronegative women. Management of seroconverters is determined by the risk of maternofetal transplacental transmission of *Toxoplasma*. The average risk is 40%. It is reduced by about one-half with spiramycin treatment. The date of maternal infection is of definite importance in this risk. There is practically no risk when infection occurred before conception in an immunocompetent mother. The later the infection occurs during pregnancy, the higher the risk (32). Fetal infection is exceptional when maternal infection occurs during the first 2 weeks of pregnancy. Among women with seroconversion, the incidence of maternofetal transmission increases as the pregnancy progresses in women treated with spiramycin; the incidence of fetal infection goes from 2% when maternal infection occurred between 3 to 10 weeks to over 30% when maternal infection occurred after 31 weeks (46). It reaches 90% in infections during the last weeks. A reverse pattern is observed as far as the clinical pattern is concerned. The earlier the maternal infection occurred during pregnancy, the higher the risk of patent disease and brain injury. The 26th week is a milestone; for maternal infections after this date, most fetal infections are subclinical.

Isolation of *Toxoplasma* from the placenta is regularly associated with toxoplasmic fetopathy, while its research can turn negative in a proportion of infected infants. This proportion varies, depending on the treatment given during pregnancy. The examination is negative in 10% with no treatment, in 25% with spiramycin treatment, and in 50% when the mother received, alternatively, spiramycin and the pyrimethamine/sulfadiazine combination (21).

Since spiramycin alone has no activity on fetopathy, it is mandatory to determine whether or not a fetus at risk is infected. Diagnosis of fetal infection, which was done by parasitologic and serologic study of fetal blood and amniotic fluid taken after the 21st week of pregnancy (33) can now be performed on amniotic fluid taken after the 18th week, using a polymerase chain reaction (PCR) (46). The method is safe. Results are obtained in less than 24 h, with 97.4% sensitivity and 98.8% specificity. When PCR is negative, it is recommended that spiramycin treatment be continued until delivery, since delayed transmission of the parasite can occur. When the in utero diagnosis is positive, serial (twice a month) ultrasound examination of the fetus is necessary to detect signs of patent fetopathy. A negative examination result does not exclude fetopathy.

Termination of the fetus can be discussed in instances of obvious injury to the fetus. Otherwise, in utero treatment with pyrimethamine (50 mg/day) and sulfadiazine (3 g/day) can be given up to the time of delivery with hematologic monitoring. Both drugs can freely cross the placenta. This treatment has significant activity on biologic signs of the disease: reduction of the incidence of positive *Toxoplasma* isolation from the placenta from 77 to 42%; tapering of antibody synthesis in the newborns, with reduction of the number of those with specific IgM from 69 to 17%; and cutting the mean specific IgG titer in half. The clinical pattern of 52 newborns whose mothers were treated appeared satisfactory taking into account a selection bias (fetuses with severe fetopathy were terminated (24)).

Treatment with pyrimethamine and sulfadiazine in mothers requires written consent of the parents, since pharmacokinetics and effects of these drugs on the fetuses have not been specifically studied during pregnancy. However, despite widespread use for prophylaxis of malaria, no teratogenic effect of pyrimethamine has ever been demonstrated (1). It seems wise, however, to avoid this treatment before the 18th week of pregnancy.

Azithromycin was given to 17 pregnant women with primary infection (500 mg once daily for 3 days a week for 1 to 4 weeks). Concentrations in placental tissue were 10-fold or more higher than those in amniotic fluid or maternal or cord blood (106).

Congenital Toxoplasmosis

The possibility of early, secondary, or late complications of congenital toxoplasmosis warrants treatment in any case (94). The clinical pattern of congenital toxoplasmosis has been determined through prospective studies with detection of seroconverting women and study of their offspring (32). The proportion of infected newborns was 61% when the mother was not treated and 23% in the group whose mothers received spiramycin. Congenital toxoplasmosis presents in three forms: subclinical infection in about 75% of cases, mild infection without neurologic injury in 15%, and severe disease with neurologic signs in 10% of the cases (22).

Congenital toxoplasmosis, even subclinical, can be complicated by secondary flare-ups of retinochoroiditis that can occur in up to 80% of patients, particularly during puberty and adolescence (115), and which can be prevented to some extent by early treatment of the patients. This means that any patient with congenital toxoplasmosis must be treated through the first year of life, regardless of the presence or absence of overt disease. The aim of this treatment is twofold: to treat active disease when it is present and to prevent secondary complications. Treatment of the infant is indicated only for confirmed cases.

The combination of pyrimethamine/sulfadiazine is the basis of all the regimens proposed. Initially, the regimen included pyrimethamine (1 mg/kg/day) plus sulfadiazine (50 mg/kg/day) for 21 days. Three to four such courses with spiramycin in the intervals were advocated during the first year. This regimen gave encouraging results, with a trend toward limiting the frequency of ocular recurrences (20). Since 1994, the Chicago Collaborative Treatment Trial (78) recommended continuous treatment during the first 12 months. Spiramycin is not used since its curative activity has not been confirmed in AIDS (66). Pyrimethamine is given with a loading dose of 2 mg/kg/day for 2 days, then 1 mg/kg/day for 6 months and then 1 mg/kg three times a week for the next 6 months. The dosage of sulfadiazine for the whole year is 100 mg/kg/day in two divided doses. Calcium leucovorin is given at a dosage of 5 mg three times a week, increased to 10 mg at 1 month of age or when the weight reaches 4.5 kg. It is increased to 5 to 20 mg daily with neutropenia. An alternative to this regimen is a lower dose of pyrimethamine: 1 mg/kg/day for 2 months and then three times a week for 10 months.

The results of this regimen were fairly good. In overt disease, acute signs when present (e.g., active retinochoroidal disease) became quiescent within 2 weeks or less following the institution of therapy. Visual loss did not occur or worsen in most patients. Almost all infants without hydrocephaly had intellectual development within the normal range (IQ, 85–140). Half of the patients with hydrocephaly who underwent a shunting procedure developed normally (78, 97, 108). Ocular recurrences were reduced. In infants treated early after birth, intracranial calcifications had diminished or resolved in 75% by 1 year of age (89).

The commonest side effect of pyrimethamine in this study was neutropenia. Blood counts with platelets and hematocrit must be performed twice a week in the first months of treatment. Later, the neutrophil count can be checked once a week, hematocrit and platelets every 2 to 4 weeks. A neutrophil count below 1000/mm³ warrants increasing the calcium leucovorin dosage to 10 to 20 mg three times a week. A count below 500 implies temporarily interruption of pyrimethamine. Rash and pancytopenia may be ascribed to sulfadiazine and can warrant its permanent withdrawal.

Compliance with the treatment must be carefully checked. It is improved by comprehensive compounding and simplifying the route of administration of the drugs (78). It is important to take in account possible coadministration of phenobarbital and to avoid any other drugs combined with sulfonamides. Prednisone (initial dose 1 mg/kg/day oral route in two divided doses) can be used to treat an inflammatory process such as high CSF protein content or severe uveitis. The dose must be progressively tapered once the process has subsided, with close follow-up to avoid possible recurrence.

Ocular Toxoplasmosis

Retinochoroiditis is the most common complication of *Toxoplasma* infection. Ocular toxoplasmosis is more often related to congenital infection but it can also complicate acquired toxoplasmosis in immunocompetent children or adults (23, 84,

87). Due to particular epidemiologic conditions, it reaches an exceptional prevalence of 21% in an adult community of southern Brazil. In immunocompromising conditions and particularly in AIDS, it signals relapse of a formerly acquired infection. However for unknown reasons, it occurs less frequently than cerebral toxoplasmosis in AIDS patients. In immunodeficient patients, retinal lesions can be multiple, active, atypical, large, and bilateral (86).

Ocular toxoplasmosis, either primary or relapsing, is an emergency condition requiring immediate antiparasitic treatment. In adults, pyrimethamine is given in a loading dose of 200 mg for 2 days and 50 mg/day on the following days with sulfadiazine 3 to 6 g/day in 2 or 3 divided doses and calcium leucovorin 50 mg twice a week. The treatment must be continued for at least 15 days following the disappearance of the inflammatory process on ophthalmoscopy and possibly angiographic examination. This means a treatment of 6 to 8 weeks' duration. In children, the dosage is pyrimethamine 1 mg/kg/day and sulfadiazine 50 to 100 mg/kg/day. To interrupt a devastating inflammatory process promptly and also to treat a possible allergic component, corticosteroid treatment can be given (prednisone or methylprednisone, 80 mg/day in adults and 1.5 mg/kg/day in children). The treatment is continued until the inflammatory process has subsided. The dosage is then progressively tapered to avoid a rebound phenomenon. Steroids cannot be used without antiparasitic treatment, which must be continued at least 2 weeks following their discontinuation.

Antiparasitic treatment is highly effective, especially in congenital toxoplasmosis in older children. Active lesions resolve within less than 14 days, with appearance of a quiescent scar and no further visual loss (83). Repeated exacerbations raise the question of prolonged prophylactic treatment. The pyrimethamine-sulfadoxine combination (1 tablet for 20 kg every 10 days for 6 to 12 months or more) can be used under strict clinical and hematologic follow-up.

Infection in the Immunocompromised Host

In immunosuppressed patients, treatment of an acute episode of toxoplasmosis is mandatory. The modalities and duration of therapy depend upon several factors: clinical presentation, possibility of oral administration, and cause, degree, and duration of the immunosuppression. Most of the trials have been conducted in HIV-infected patients (71, 73, 96). Before the AIDS epidemic, not more than 50 cases had been reported in other immunosuppressed patients in the literature (53, 100). At the present time, the marked reduction of the number of cases of toxoplasmosis in HIV-infected patients (primarily due to the wide use of cotrimoxazole as primary prophylaxis effective for both pneumocystosis and toxoplasmosis) makes the design of new therapeutic trials in this field difficult.

Curative Treatment of Infection in AIDS

Acute-Stage Therapy.   The regimen of choice is the combination of pyrimethamine and sulfadiazine. After a loading dose of 200 mg/day during the first 48 h, pyrimethamine is given orally at a dose of 1 to 1.25 mg/kg/day. The dose of sulfadiazine is 100 mg/kg/day up to 8 g, in four divided doses. Folinic acid,

10 to 20 mg/day is systematically added to prevent the hematologic toxicity of pyrimethamine (38, 85, 112). Its dose can be increased up to 50 mg/day in case of cytopenia. The duration of acute-stage therapy is not less than 3 weeks. If a complete clinical and radiologic response is obtained at week 3, therapy can be ended. Otherwise the treatment is continued up to week 6 to achieve maximal recovery (65, 113, 116).

A partial or complete clinical response to this combination is achieved in 70 to 75% of patients with toxoplasmic encephalitis in AIDS, and the probability of survival after an acute episode is 90 to 95% (25). Although no study has really addressed the issue, the response rate is expected to be similar in other localizations of the infection, such as ocular disease, provided the hematogenous dissemination of the parasite has not progressed to a pseudo–septic shock presentation, in which the prognosis becomes very severe (69).

The rate of adverse effects from the pyrimethamine-sulfadiazine combination is approximately 50%, and they require discontinuation of one or both drugs in 20 to 25% of cases. The most frequent are blood cytopenias, rashes, and fever. To determine which of the two drugs is responsible, each drug should be discontinued or reintroduced separately.

Treatment is usually initiated upon suspicion of toxoplasmic encephalitis, based on the occurrence of febrile neurologic manifestations and suggestive lesions on brain computed tomography (CT) scan or magnetic resonance imaging (MRI). Favorable response to specific empirical therapy retrospectively suggests the diagnosis. The diagnosis of toxoplasmic encephalitis is improbable in HIV-infected patients with negative *Toxoplasma* serology and/or in those who are taking cotrimoxazole for primary prophylaxis against pneumocystosis.

Maintenance Therapy.   The requirement for maintenance therapy to prevent relapse has been well established in AIDS patients (65). In fact, the relapse rate was approximately 30% (26). Introduction of zidovudine therapy did not reduce this rate. Maintenance therapy is based on the same combination of drugs with doses reduced by half: 25 to 50 mg/day pyrimethamine and 2 to 4 g/day sulfadiazine. This combination has been shown to be more effective than the pyrimethamine-clindamycin alternative combination in preventing relapse; the rate of relapse was 6% patient-years with sulfadiazine versus 23% patient-years with clindamycin in the European study (56). Maintenance therapy must be continued lifelong, since the immune deficiency progresses in AIDS patients (90). Whether the introduction of the new protease inhibitors will allow discontinuation of maintenance therapy in patients with a previous episode of toxoplasmic encephalitis is unknown.

Alternative Regimens for Curative Treatment

Pyrimethamine-Clindamycin.   The alternative regimen for acute therapy in patients who are unable to tolerate sulfadiazine is the combination of pyrimethamine and clindamycin (95). Clindamycin has been given intravenously in doses from 1.2 to 4.8 g/day. It has been assessed at a dose of 2.4 g/day orally. The response rate is approximately 70%, and in one study, 86% of the patients who had a favorable response improved by day 7 of therapy (70). Early improvement was strongly associated with a favorable response at week 6. Patients who failed to respond or did not have toxoplasmic encephalitis had generally progressed by day 12 of therapy when checked by a quantifiable neurologic assessment. The rate of adverse effects due to the pyrimethamine-clindamycin combination is 30 to 50%, requiring discontinuation of the ongoing regimen in 20% of cases. These are primarily gastrointestinal disorders, with a risk of *C. difficile*–related pseudomembranous colitis in a few instances. The combination can be used for maintenance therapy, with a lower success rate than the conventional regimen (56).

Combinations of Pyrimethamine and Macrolides. Owing to the high rate of adverse events with the two previous combinations, there have been attempts to find other active regimens for AIDS patients who did not tolerate sulfadiazine and clindamycin. Limited studies have suggested that the combination of pyrimethamine with clarithromcyin (2 g/day) or azithromycin (500 mg/day) might be effective (35). The rate of adverse effects requiring discontinuation was approximately 20% in the two studies. Increased serum transaminase levels and hearing loss were reported.

Other Regimens Using Pyrimethamine. Pyrimethamine has been used in monotherapy in some situations when other drugs were not available. Although it has some activity, it is probably less effective than in combination for acute and maintenance therapy. Pyrimethamine in combination with atovaquone is currently being investigated in ACTG237-ANRS 039 collaborative trial.

Other Regimens without Pyrimethamine. Although pyrimethamine has long been considered the reference drug for treatment of toxoplasmic encephalitis in AIDS patients, it may induce specific side effects, especially hematologic effects and rashes, which may require discontinuation of the drug. In these situations, drugs used as monotherapy—clindamycin, sulfonamides, macrolides, trimetrexate, or atovaquone—have not been found sufficiently effective.

The use of cotrimoxazole for acute and maintenance therapy has been reported in a few patients. One of the advantages of cotrimoxazole is its availability for intravenous administration (which pyrimethamine is not). Thus, it might be helpful for initiating therapy in patients with coma, until they can take pyrimethamine orally. The appropriate doses of cotrimoxazole have not been determined.

A potential benefit of the clarithromycin-minocycline combination has been suggested in a very limited number of patients (61).

Trials in humans with AIDS and toxoplasmic encephalitis who did not tolerate sulfa drugs revealed that trimetrexate alone gave immediate but transient clinical improvement (93). The efficacy of atovaquone as salvage therapy appeared to be related to plasma concentrations (110).

Infections in the Transplant Patient

Among all organ transplantations, those of heart or heart-lung carry the greatest risk of toxoplasmosis (29, 47, 72, 88, 105, 117). Toxoplasmosis is often severe, with multivisceral foci; interstitial pneumonia is possible. Overt infection is associated with seroconversion in seronegative patients. A subclin-ical serologic reactivation can be observed in seropositive recipients (13). Serologic diagnosis can be difficult if the antibody titer is low or stable. Parasitologic diagnosis relies on isolation of *Toxoplasma* from blood, CSF, bronchoalveolar lavage, and cardiac or cerebral biopsy specimens. Corticosteroids administered in rejections increase the risk of toxoplasmosis. Conversely, cyclosporine proved through in vitro and animal experiments to have antiparasitic properties and should be preferred for treating rejection (79).

For organ transplant patients, acute therapy with a regimen similar to that in AIDS is recommended (104). The requirement for maintenance therapy has to be modulated depending on the intensity and duration of the immune suppression. It can probably be discontinued when the therapeutic immune defect is reduced, depending on the type of drugs that are necessary to allow the transplant to be tolerated. Prophylaxis for toxoplasmosis in heart transplant patients is indicated for high-risk patients.

PROPHYLAXIS
Prevention: Hygienic Rules

Seronegative patients at risk, pregnant women, and immunocompromised persons should avoid acquisition of the parasite. They should have no contact with cat feces. Cat litter must be changed daily by somebody else, because the oocysts sporulate after 4 to 5 days. Gloves should be worn and hands washed after handling potentially contaminated material such as garden soil, sandboxes, or raw meat. Fruits and vegetables should be washed. Meat must be well cooked or deep frozen.

AIDS

The high prevalence of toxoplasmic encephalitis in HIV-infected patients, particularly in some European countries (30–40%), and the mortality rate of approximately 20% prompted efforts to prevent reactivation in patients who are seropositive for *T. gondii* (52). In fact, in seronegative patients, the risk of primary infection is low, approximately 2% patient-years (14). For these patients, prophylactic measures are recommended (see above). *T. gondii* serology should be monitored once or twice a year, especially in countries where the seroprevalence is high.

In patients who are seropositive for *T. gondii,* research has developed in two directions: (*a*) attempting to determine the efficacy and safety of drugs that could be used for chemoprophylaxis (54) and (*b*) defining as accurately as possible the risk factors for occurrence of toxoplasmic encephalitis, to identify the population of patients who should be given prophylaxis (12, 41, 62).

Risk Factors in Patients Seropositive for *T. gondii*

The severity of the immune defect is one of the major factors (62). CDC stage B or C clinical manifestations and a CD4 cell count below 100/mm^3 are independently associated with increased risk of toxoplasmic encephalitis (63). The probability of toxoplasmic encephalitis at 1 year reaches 24% in patients with CDC stage C manifestations and 20% in patients with CD4 below 50/mm^3. Furthermore, in that study, the IgG anti–*T. gondii* antibody titer determined by enzyme-linked immunosorbent assay (ELISA) at baseline was a good independent prognostic marker for risk of toxoplasmic encephalitis (30). The risk in patients with titers above 150 IU/mL was 3.3 times that of patients with titers below 150 IU/mL.

Regimens for Primary Prophylaxis

Although no trial specifically designed for this purpose has currently been published, it was clear in 1993 that patients who had been given cotrimoxazole for primary or secondary prophylaxis of pneumocystosis had a very low incidence of toxoplasmic encephalitis (15, 43, 75, 77, 92, 101). Cotrimoxazole is the drug of choice for toxoplasmic encephalitis prophylaxis (111, 111a). A prospective randomized trial, ANRS 040, is ongoing in France to determine the most convenient dose of cotrimoxazole for this indication: one single-strength tablet per day or one double-strength tablet per day. Some authors propose every-other-day administration.

The pyrimethamine-dapsone combination has been shown effective in preventing toxoplasmic encephalitis (40). However the rate of cross-intolerance between dapsone and cotrimoxazole is approximately 40% (55).

ANRS 005–ACTG 154 was an international, double-blind, placebo-controlled study to assess pyrimethamine (50 mg thrice weekly) for primary prophylaxis of toxoplasmic encephalitis. The incidence of toxoplasmic encephalitis was not different (13% patient-years) in the two arms. Rash was the only adverse effect that was significantly more frequent in the pyrimethamine arm. In the on-treatment analysis, the incidence of toxoplasmic encephalitis was lower in the pyrimethamine arm (4%) than in the placebo arm (12%). In patients who are intolerant to cotrimoxazole, a trial has been designed in France and Spain comparing the efficacy of a strategy starting with pyrimethamine (50 mg three times a week) with a strategy starting with atovaquone suspension (1500 mg/day).

Thus, at the present time, HIV-infected patients who are given cotrimoxazole for prophylaxis of pneumocystosis have minimal risk of toxoplasmic encephalitis. For those intolerant to cotrimoxazole, no simple solution is available. The indications for prophylaxis have to be individualized by estimating the risk from the clinical stage of HIV infection, the CD4 cell count, and the *T. gondii* antibody titer.

Other Immunosuppressed Hosts

In heart or heart and lung recipients who are seronegative for the parasite and who are transplanted with a heart from a donor who is seropositive for *T. gondii*, pyrimethamine 50 mg/day has markedly reduced the risk of toxoplasmosis (72, 117). Cotrimoxazole is a possible alternative that has not been widely assessed. In bone-marrow recipients, the risk of toxoplasmosis is the highest in those who are seropositive for the parasite and receive bone-marrow from a donor who is seronegative for *T. gondii* (36). The pyrimethamine-sulfadoxine combination or cotrimoxazole has been proposed for children.

In these transplant patients, the duration of chemoprophy-laxis depends upon the duration of immunosuppressive therapy. Limited data are available for other causes of immunosuppression. It has been suggested that patients with a cellular immune defect, such as long-term corticosteroid therapy, should be considered for prophylaxis of toxoplasmosis when the CD4 cell count is below 100/mm^3 (63). Pyrimethamine or cotrimoxazole is recommended as long as the immune defect persists.

Vaccine

Experimental data support the concept that a successful human *T. gondii* vaccine may be feasible. However no vaccine is available at the present time.

REFERENCES

1. Anonymous. Pyrimethamine combination in pregnancy [Editorial]. Lancet 1983;2:1005–1007.
2. Allegra CJ, Boarna D, Kovacs JA, Morrison P, Beaver J. Interaction of sulfonamide and sulfone compounds with *Toxoplasma gondii* dihydropropteroate synthetase. J Clin Invest 1990;85:371–379.
3. Araujo FG, Guptill DR, Remington JS. Azithromycin: a macrolide antibiotic with potent activity against *Toxoplasma gondii*. Antimicrob Agents Chemother 1988;32:755–757.
4. Araujo FG, Guptill DR, Remington JS. In vivo activity of piritrexim against *Toxoplasma gondii*. J Infect Dis 1987;156:828–830.
5. Araujo FG, Khan AA, Remington JS. Rifapentine is active in vitro and in vivo against *Toxoplasma gondii*. Antimicrob Agents Chemother 1996;40:1335–1337.
6. Araujo FG, Lin T, Remington JS. Synergistic combination of azithromycin and sulfadiazine for treatment of toxoplasmosis in mice. Eur J Clin Microbiol Infect Dis 1992;11:71–73.
7. Araujo FG, Lin T, Remington JS. The activity of atovaquone (566C80) in murine toxoplasmosis is markedly augmented when used in combination with pyrimethamine or sulfadiazine. J Infect Dis 1993;167:494–497.
8. Araujo FG, Prokocimer P, Lin T, Remington JS. Activity of clarithromycin alone or in combination with other drugs for treatment of murine toxoplasmosis. Antimicrob Agents Chemother 1992;36:2454–2457.
9. Araujo FG, Remington JS. Recent advances in the search for new drugs for treatment of toxoplasmosis. Int J Antimicrob Agents 1992;1:153–164.
10. Araujo FG, Slifer T, Remington JS. Rifabutin is active in murine models for toxoplasmosis. Antimicrob Agents Chemother 1994;38:570–575.
11. Araujo FG, Suzuki Y, Remington JS. Use of rifabutin in combination with atovaquone, clindamycin, pyrimethamine, or sulfadiazine for treatment of toxoplasmic encephalitis in mice. Eur J Clin Microbiol Infect Dis 1996;15:394–397.
12. Beaman MH, Luft BJ, Remington JS. Prophylaxis for toxoplasmosis in AIDS. Ann Intern Med 1992;117:163–164.
13. Bouree P, Romand S, Majoube A. Toxoplasmose et transplantation hépatique: surveillance de 34 patients par deux techniques sérologiques. Bull Soc Fr Parasitol 1995;13:155–160.
14. Candolfi E, Partisani ML, De Mautort E, Bethencourt S, Frantz M, Kien T, Lang JM. Séroprévalence de la toxoplasmose chez 346 sujets infectés par le VIH dans l'est de la France: suivi

sérologique des sujets non contaminés par *Toxoplasma gondii.* Presse Med 1992;21:394–395.

15. Carr A, Tindall B, Brew BJ, Marriott DJ, Harkness JL, Penny R, Cooper DA. Low-dose trimethoprim-sulfamethoxazole prophylaxis for toxoplasmic encephalitis in patients with AIDS. Ann Intern Med 1992;117:106–111.

16. Chang HR, Comte R, Péchère JC. In vitro and in vivo effects of doxycycline on *Toxoplasma gondii.* Antimicrob Agents Chemother 1990;34:775–780.

17. Chang HR, Comte R, Piguet PF, Péchère JC. Activity of minocycline against *Toxoplasma gondii* in mice. J Antimicrob Chemother 1991;27:639–645.

18. Chang HR, Pechère JC. Effects of roxithromycin on acute toxoplasmosis in mice. Antimicrob Agents Chemother 1987;31: 1147–1149.

19. Chang HR, Rudareanu FC, Pechère JC. Activity of A-56268(TE-031), a new macrolide, against *Toxoplasma gondii* in mice. J Antimicrob Chemother 1988;22:359–361.

20. Couvreur J, Desmonts G, Aron-Rosa D. Le pronostic oculaire de la toxoplasmose congénitale: role du traitement. Ann Pediatr (Paris) 1984;31:855–858.

21. Couvreur J, Desmonts G, Thulliez P. Prophylaxis of congenital toxoplasmosis. Effects of spiramycin on placental infection. J Antimicrob Chemother 1988;22:193–200.

22. Couvreur J, Desmonts G, Tournier G, Szusterkac M. Etude d'une série homogène de 210 cas de toxoplasmose congénitale chez des nourrissons âgés de 0 à 12 mois et dépistés de façon prospective. Ann Pediatr (Paris) 1984;31:815–819.

23. Couvreur J, Thulliez P. Toxoplasmose acquise à localisation oculaire ou neurologique. Etude de 49 cas. Presse Med 1996;25: 438–442.

24. Couvreur J, Thulliez P, Daffos F, Aufrant C, Bompard Y, Gesquiere A, Desmonts G. Foetopathie toxoplasmique: traitement in utero par l'association pyrimethamine-sulfamides. Arch Fr Pediatr 1991;48:397–403.

25. Dannemann B, McCutchan JA, Israelski D, Antoniskis D, Leport C, Luft B, Nussbaum J, Clumeck N, Morlat P, Chiu J, Vilde JL, Orellana M, Feigal D, Bartok A, Heseltine P, Leedom J, Remington JS, and the California Collaborative Treatment Group. Treatment of toxoplasmic encephalitis in patients with AIDS: a randomized trial comparing pyrimethamine plus clindamycin to pyrimethamine plus sulfadiazine. Ann Intern Med 1992;116:33–43.

26. De Gans J, Portegies P, Reiss P, Troost D, Van Gool T, Lange JMA. Pyrimethamine alone as maintenance therapy for central nervous system toxoplasmosis in 38 patients with AIDS. J Acquir Immune Defic Syndr 1992;5:137–142.

27. Derouin F, Chastang C. Enzyme immunoassay to assess effect of antimicrobial agents on *Toxoplasma gondii* in tissue culture. Antimicrob Agents Chemother 1988;36:1204–1210.

28. Derouin F, Chastang C. In vitro effects of folate inhibitors on *Toxoplasma gondii.* Antimicrob Agents Chemother 1989;33: 1753–1759.

29. Derouin F, Devergie A, Auber P, Gluckman E, Beauvais B, Garin YJF, Larivière M. Toxoplasmosis in bone marrow-transplant recipients: report of seven cases and review. Clin Infect Dis 1992;15:267–270.

30. Derouin F, Leport C, Pueyo S, Morlat P, Letrillart B, Chêne G, Ecobichon JL, Luft B, Aubertin J, Hafner R, Vildé JL and ANRS 005/ACTG 154 Trial Group. Predictive value of *Toxoplasma gondii* antibody titres on the occurrence of toxoplasmic encephalitis in HIV-infected patients. AIDS 1996;10:1521–1527.

31. Derouin F, Piketty C, Chastang C, Chau F, Rouveix R, Pocidalo JJ. Anti-toxoplasma effects of dapsone alone and combined with pyrimethamine. Antimicrob Agents Chemother 1991;35: 352–355.

32. Desmonts G, Couvreur J. Congenital toxoplasmosis: a prospective study of 378 pregnancies. N Engl J Med 1974;290:1110–1116.

33. Desmonts G, Forestier F, Capella-Pavlowsky M, Thulliez P, Daffos F, Chartier M. Prenatal diagnosis of congenital toxoplasmosis. Lancet 1985;1:500–504.

34. Eyles DE, Coleman N. Synergistic effect of sulfadiazine and Daraprim against experimental toxoplasmosis in the mouse. Antibiot Chemother 1953;3:483–490.

35. Fernandez-Martin J, Leport C, Morlat P, Meyohas MC, Chauvin JP, Vilde JL. Pyrimethamine-clarithromycin combination for therapy of acute *Toxoplasma* encephalitis in patients with AIDS. Antimicrob Agents Chemother 1991;35:2049–2052.

36. Foot ABM, Garin YJF, Ribaud P, Devergie A, Derouin F, Gluckman E. Prophylaxis of toxoplasmosis infection with pyrimethamine/sulfadoxine (Fansidar) in bone marrow transplant recipients. Bone Marrow Transplant 1994;14:241–245.

37. Forestier F, Daffos F, Rainaut M, Desnotte JF, Gaschard JC. Suivi thérapeutique foeto-maternel de la spiramycine au cours de la grossesse. Arch Franç Pediatr 1987;44:539–544.

38. Frenkel JK, Hitchings GH. Relative reversal by vitamins (p-aminobenzoic, folic and folinic acids) of the effects of sulfadiazine and pyrimethamine on *Toxoplasma* in mouse and man. Antibiot Chemother 1957;7:630–638.

39. Garin JP, Pellerat J, Maillard MA, Woehrle J. Bases théoriques de la prévention par la spiramycine de la toxoplasmose congénitale chez la femme enceinte. Presse Med 1968;76:2266.

40. Girard PM, Landman R, Gaudebout C, Olivares R, Saimot AG, Jelasko P, Certain A, Boue F, Bouvet E, Lecompte T, Coulard JP, and the PRIO Study Group. Dapsone-pyrimethamine compared with aerosolized pentamidine as primary prophylaxis against *Pneumocystis carinii* pneumonia and toxoplasmosis in HIV infection. N Engl J Med 1993;328:1514–1520.

41. Grant IH, Gold JWM, Rosenblum M, Niedzwiecki D, Armstrong D. *Toxoplasma gondii* serology in HIV-infected patients: the development of central nervous system toxoplasmosis in AIDS. AIDS 1990;4:519–521.

42. Grossman PL, Remington JS. The effect of trimethoprim plus sulfamethoxazole on *Toxoplasma gondii* in vitro and in vivo. Am J Trop Med Hyg 1979;28:445–455.

43. Hardy WD, Feinberg J, Finkelstein DM, Power ME, He W, Kaczka C, Frame PT, Holmes M, Waskin H, Fass RJ. A controlled trial of trimethoprim-sulfamethoxazole or aerosolized pentamidine for secondary prophylaxis of *Pneumocystis carinii* pneumonia in patients with the acquired immunodeficiency syndrome. N Engl J Med 1992;327:1842–1848.

44. Harris C, Salgo MP, Tanowizt HB, Wittner M. In vitro assessment of antimicrobial agents against *Toxoplasma gondii.* J Infect Dis 1988;157:14–22.

45. Hofflin JM, Remington JS. In vivo synergism of roxithromycin (RU 965) and interferon against *Toxoplasma gondii.* Antimicrob Agents Chemother 1987;81:346–348.

46. Hohlfeld P, Daffos F, Costa JM, Thulliez P, Forestier F, Vidaud M. Prenatal diagnosis of congenital toxoplasmosis with a polymerase-chain-reaction test on amniotic fluid. N Engl J Med 1994;331:695–699.

47. Holliman RE, Johnson JD, Adams S, Pepper JR. Toxoplasmosis and heart transplantation. J Heart Lung Transplant 1991;10: 608–610.

48. Howe DK, Sibley LD. *Toxoplasma gondii* comprises three clonal lineages: correlations of parasite genotype with human disease. Infect Dis 1995;172:1561–1566.

49. Hudson AT, Randall AW, Ginger CD, Hill B, Latter VS, Mc Hardy N, Williams RB. Novel antimalarial hydroxynaphthoquinones with potent broad spectrum antiprotozoal activity. Parasitology 1985;90:45–55.

50. Hughes WT, Kennedy W, Shenep J, Flynn PM, Hetherington G, Fullen G, Lancaster DJ, Stein DS, Palte S, Rosenbaum D, Liao SA, Blum MR, Rogers MD. Safety and pharmacokinetics of 566C80, a hydroxynaphthoquinone with anti-*Pneumocystis carinii* activity: a phase 1 study in human deficiency virus (HIV) infected men. J Infect Dis 1991;163:843–848.

51. Huskinson-Mark J, Araujo FG, Remington JS. Evaluation of the effect of drugs on the cyst form of *Toxoplasma gondii*. J Infect Dis 1991;164:170–177.

52. Israelski DM, Chmiel JS, Poggensee L, Phair JP, Remington JS. Prevalence of *Toxoplasma* infection in a cohort of homosexual men at risk of AIDS and toxoplasmic encephalitis. J Acquir Immune Defic Syndr 1993;6:414–418.

53. Israelski DM, Remington JS. Toxoplasmosis in patients with cancer. Clin Infect Dis 1993;17(Suppl):423–435.

54. Jacobson MA, Besch CL, Child C, Hafner R, Matts JP, Muth K, Wentworth DN, Neaton JD, Abrams D, Rimland D, Perez G, Grant IH, Saravolatz LD, Brown LS, Deyton L, and the Terry Beirn Community Programs for Clinical Research on AIDS. Prophylaxis with pyrimethamine for toxoplasmic encephalitis in patients with advanced HIV disease: results of a randomized trial. J Infect Dis 1994;169:384–394.

55. Jorde UP, Horowitz HW, Wormser GP. Utility of dapsone for prophylaxis of *Pneumocystis carinii* pneumonia in trimethoprim-sulfamethoxazole-intolerant, HIV-infected individuals. AIDS 1993;7:355–359.

56. Katlama C, De Wit S, O'Doherty E, Van Glabeke M, Clumeck N, and the European Network for Treatment of AIDS Toxoplasmosis Study Group. Pyrimethamine-clindamycin vs. pyrimethamine-sulfadiazine as acute and long term therapy for toxoplasmic encephalitis in patients with AIDS. Clin Infect Dis 1996;22:268–275.

57. Khan AA, Slifer T, Araujo FG, Remington JS. Trovafloxacin is active against *Toxoplasma gondii* [Abstract E74]. 36th Interscience Conference on Antimicrobial Agents and Chemotherapy. New Orleans, 1996.

58. Klinker H, Langmann P, Richter E. Plasma pyrimethamine concentrations during long-term treatment for cerebral toxoplasmosis in patients with AIDS. Antimicrob Agents Chemother 1996;40:1623–1627.

59. Kovacs JA, Allegra CJ, Beaver J, Boarman D, Lewis M, Parillo JE, Chabner B, Masur H. Characterization of de novo folate synthesis in *Pneumocystis carinii* and *Toxoplasma gondii:* potential for screening therapeutic agents. J Infect Dis 1989;160:312–320.

60. Kovacs JA, Allegra CJ, Chabner BA, Swan JC, Drake J, Lunde M, Parillo JE, Masur H. Potent effect of trimetrexate, a lipid soluble antifolate, on *Toxoplasma gondii*. J Infect Dis 1987;155:1027–1032.

61. Lacassin F, Schaffo D, Perronne C, Longuet P, Leport C, Vildé J-L. Clarithromycin-minocycline combination as salvage therapy for toxoplasmosis in patients infected with human immunodeficiency virus. Antimicrob Agents Chemother 1995;39:76–277.

62. Leport C, Ambroise-Thomas P, Bazin C, Chêne G, Derouin F, Katlama C, Mayaud C, Pelloux H, Raffi F, Vildé JL. Les facteurs de risque de survenue d'une toxoplasmose cérébrale chez les patients infectés par le VIH. Presse Med 1996;25:519–521.

63. Leport C, Chêne G, Morlat P, Luft BJ, Rousseau F, Pueyo S, Hafner R, Miro J, Aubertin J, Salamon R, Vilde JL, and ANRS OO5-ACTG 154 Group Members. Pyrimethamine for primary prophylaxis of toxoplasmic encephalitis in patients with human immunodeficiency virus infection: a double-blind, randomized trial. J Infect Dis 1996;173:91–97.

64. Leport C, Meulemans A, Robine D, Dameron G, Vilde JL. Levels of pyrimethamine in serum and penetration into brain tissue in humans. AIDS 1992;6:1040–1041.

65. Leport C, Raffi F, Matheron S, Katlama C, Regnier B, Saimot AG, Marche C, Vedrenne C, Vilde JL. Treatment of central nervous system toxoplasmosis with pyrimethamine/sulfadiazine combination in 35 patients with the acquired immunodeficiency syndrome. Efficacy of long-term continuous therapy. Am J Med 1988;84:94–100.

66. Leport C, Vildé J, Katlama C, Regnier B, Matheron S, Saimot AG. Failure of spiramycin to prevent neurotoxoplasmosis in immunosuppressed patients [Letter]. JAMA 1986;255:2289.

67. Lindsay DS, Blagburn BL, Hall JE, Tidwell RE. Activity of pentamidine and pentamidine analogs against *Toxoplasma gondii* in cell cultures. Antimicrob Agents Chemother 1991;35:1914–1916.

68. Longuet P, Leport C. Clindamycin treatment of toxoplasmosis in immunocompromised patients. Rev Contemp Pharmacother 1992;3:313–320.

69. Lucet JC, Bailly MP, Bedos JP, Wolff M, Gachot B, Vachon F. Septic shock due to toxoplasmosis in patients infected with the human immunodeficiency virus. Chest 1993;104:1054–1058.

70. Luft B, Hafner R, Korzun A, Leport C, Antoniskis D, Bosler EM, Bourland DD, Uttamchandani R, Fuhrer J, Jacobson J, Morlat P, Vildé JL, Remington JS, and members of the ACTG 077 P/ANRS 009 Study Team. Toxoplasmic encephalitis in patients with the acquired immunodeficiency syndrome. N Engl J Med 1993;329:995–1000.

71. Luft BJ, Conley FK, Remington JS. Outbreak of central nervous system toxoplasmosis in Western Europe and North America. Lancet 1983;1:781–783.

72. Luft BJ, Naot Y, Araujo FG, Stinson EB, Remington JS. Primary and reactivated toxoplasma infection in patients with cardiac transplants. Ann Intern Med 1983;99:27–31.

73. Luft BJ, Remington JS. Toxoplasmic encephalitis in AIDS. Clin Infect Dis 1992;15:211–222.

74. Mack DG, McLeod R. New micromethod to study the effect of antimicrobial agents on *Toxoplasma gondii:* comparison of sulfadoxine and sulfadiazine individually and in combination with pyrimethamine and study of clindamycin, metronidazole and cyclosporine A. Antimicrob Agents Chemother 1984;26:26–30.

75. Mallolas J, Zamora L, Gatell JM, Miro JM, Vernet E, Valls ME, Soriano E, SanMiguel JG. Primary prophylaxis for *Pneumocystis carinii* pneumonia: a randomized trial comparing cotrimoxazole, aerosolized pentamidine and dapsone plus pyrimethamine. AIDS 1993;7:59–64.

76. Mansor SM, Navaratnam V. Single dose kinetic study of the triple combination mefloquine/sulphadoxine/pyrimethamine (Fansimel) in healthy male volunteers. Br J Clin Pharmacol 1989;27:381–386.

77. May T, Beuscart C, Reynes J, Marchou B, Leclercq P, Borsa Lebas F, Saba J, Micoud M, Mouton Y, Canton P. Trimethroprim-sulfamethoxazole versus aerosolized pentamidine for primary prophylaxis of *Pneumocystis carinii* pneumonia: a prospective,

randomized, controlled, clinical trial. J Acquir Immune Defic Syndr 1994;7:457–462.

78. McAuley J, Boyer K, Patel D, Mets M, Swisher C, Roizen N, Wolters W, Stein L, Stein M, Schey W, Remington J, Meir P, Johnson D, Heydeman P, Holfels E, Withers S, Mack D, Brown C, Patton D, McLeod R. Early and longitudinal evaluations of treated infants and children and untreated historical patients with congenital toxoplasmosis: the Chicago collaborative treatment trial. Clin Infect Dis 1994;18:38–72.

79. McCabe RE, Luft BJ, Remington JS. The effects of cyclosporine in *Toxoplasma gondii* in vivo and in vitro. Transplantation 1986;41:611–615.

80. McCabe RE, Luft BJ, Remington JS. Effect of murine interferon gamma on murine toxoplasmosis. J Infect Dis 1984;150: 961–962.

81. McCabe RE, Oster S. Current recommendations and future prospects in the treatment of toxoplasmosis. Drugs 1989;38:973–987.

82. McLeod R, Mack D, Foss R, Boyer K, Withers SE, Levon S, Hubbe J, and the Toxoplasmosis Study Group. Levels of pyrimethamine in sera and cerebrospinal and ventricular fluid from infants treated for congenital toxoplasmosis. Antimicrob Agents Chemother 1992;36:1040–1048.

83. Mets MB, Holfels E, Boyer KM. Eye manifestations of congenital toxoplasmosis. Am J Ophthalmol 1996;122:309–324.

84. Montoya JG, Remington JS. Toxoplasmic chorioretinitis in the setting of acute acquired toxoplasmosis. Clin Infect Dis 1996;23:277–282.

85. Niyongabo T, Leport C, Vildé JL. Utilité de l'acide folinique dans les cytopénies induites par les médicaments antiparasitaires au cours du SIDA. Presse Med 1991;34:1677–1681.

86. Nussenblatt RB, Belfort R. Ocular toxoplasmosis. An old disease revisited. JAMA 1994;271:304–307.

87. Nussenblatt RB, Mittal KK, Fuhrman S. Lymphocyte proliferative response of patients with acute ocular toxoplasmosis to the parasite and retinal antigens. Am J Ophthalmol 1989;107:632–641.

88. O'Driscoll JC, Holliman RE. Toxoplasmosis and bone marrow transplantation. Rev Med Microbiol 1991;2:215–222.

89. Patel DV, Holfels EM, Vogel NP, Boyer KM, Mets MB, Swisher CN, Roizen NJ, Stein LK, Stein MA, Hopkins J, Withers SE, Mack DG, Luciano RA, Meier P, Remington JS, McLeod R. Resolution of intracranial calcifications in infants with treated congenital toxoplasmosis. Radiology 1996;199:433–440.

90. Pedrol E, Gonzalez-Clemente JM, Gatell JM Mallolas J, Miro JM, Graus F, Alvarez R, Mercader JM, Berenger J, Jimenez de Anta MT. Central nervous system toxoplasmosis in AIDS patients: efficacy of an intermittent maintenance therapy. AIDS 1990;4:511–517.

91. Piketty C, Derouin F, Rouveix B, Pocidalo JJ. In vivo assessment of antimicrobial agents against *Toxoplasma gondii* by quantification of parasites in the blood, lungs and brain of infected mice. Antimicrob Agents Chemother 1990;34: 1467–1472.

92. Podzamczer D, Santin M, Jimenez J, Casanova A, Bolao F, Gudiol GRF. Thrice-weekly cotrixomazole is better than weekly dapsone-pyrimethamine for the primary prevention of *Pneumocystis carinii* in HIV-infected patients. AIDS 1993;7:501–506.

93. Polis MA, Masur H, Tuazon C. Salvage trial of trimetrexate-leucovorin for treatment of cerebral toxoplasmosis in AIDS patients. Clin Res 1989;37:47.

94. Remington JS, McLeod R, Desmonts G. Toxoplasmosis. In: Remington JS, Klein JO, eds. Infectious diseases of the fetus and newborn infant. 4th ed. Philadelphia; WB Saunders, 1995:140–267.

95. Remington JS, Vildé JL. Clindamycin for *Toxoplasma* encephalitis in AIDS. Lancet 1991;338:1142–1143.

96. Renold C, Sugar A, Chave JP, Perrin L, Delavelle J, Pizzolato G, Burkhard P, Gabriel V, Hirschel B. *Toxoplasma* encephalitis in patients with the acquired immunodeficiency syndrome. Medicine 1992;71:224–239.

97. Roizen N, Swisher CN, Stein MA, Hopkins J, Boyer KM, Holfels E, Mets MB, Stein L, Pattet D, Meier P, Withers SE, Remington JS, Mack D, Heydemann P, Patton D, McLeod R. Neurologic and developmental outcome in treated congenital toxoplasmosis. Pediatrics 1995;95:11–20.

98. Romand S, Della-Bruna C, Farinotti R, Derouin F. In vitro and in vivo effects of rifabutine alone or combined with atovaquone against *Toxoplasma gondii*. Antimicrob Agents Chemother 1996;40:2015–2020.

99. Romand S, Pudney M, Derouin F. In vitro and in vivo activities of the hydroxynaphtholoquinolone atovaquone alone or combined with pyrimethamine, sulfadiazine, clarithromycin and minocycline against *Toxoplasma gondii*. Antimicrob Agents Chemother 1993;37:2371–2378.

100. Ruskin J, Remington JS. Toxoplasmosis in the compromised host. Ann Intern Med 1976;84:193–199.

101. Schneider MME, Hoepelman AIM, Eeftinck Schattenkerdk JK, Nielsen TL, van der Graaf Y, Frissen JP, van der Ende IM, Kolsters AF, Borleffs JC. A controlled trial of aerosolized pentamidine or trimethoprim-sulfamethoxazole as primary prophylaxis against *Pneumocystis carinii* pneumonia in patients with human immunodeficiency virus infection. N Engl J Med 1992;327:1836–1841.

102. Sharma SD, Hofflin JM, Remington JS. In vivo recombinant interleukin 2 administration enhances survival against a lethal challenge with *Toxoplasma gondii*. J Immunol 1985;135:4160–4163.

103. Sheffield HG, Melton ML. Effect of pyrimethamine and sulfadiazine on the fine structure and multiplication of *Toxoplasma gondii* in cell culture. J Parasitol 1975;61:704–712.

104. Slavin MA, Meyers JD, Remington JS, Hackman RC. *Toxoplasma gondii* infection in marrow transplant recipients: a 20 years experience. Bone Marrow Transplant 1994;13:549–557.

105. Speirs GE, Hakim TG, Calne RY, Wreghitt TG. Relative risk of donor acquired *Toxoplasma gondii* in heart, liver and kidney transplant recipients. Clin Transplant 1988;2:257–260.

106. Stray-Pederson B, and the European Research Network on Congenital Toxoplasmosis. Azithromycin levels in placental tissue, amniotic fluid and blood (Abstract A68). Program and abstracts of the 36th Interscience Conference on Antimicrobial Agents and Chemotherapy, New Orleans, Sept 15–18th, 1996. Washington, DC: American Society for Microbiology, 1996.

107. Suzuki Y, Conley FK, Remington JS. Treatment of toxoplasmic encephalitis in mice with recombinant gamma interferon. Infect Immunol 1990;58:3050–3055.

108. Swisher CN, Boyer KM, McLeod R, the Toxoplasmosis Study Group. Congenital toxoplasmosis. Semin Pediatr Neurol 1994;1:4–25.

109. Thiermann E, Apt W, Atias A, Lorca M, Olguin J. A comparative study of some combined treatment regimens in acute toxoplasmosis in mice. Am J Trop Med Hyg 1978;27:747–750.

110. Torres RA, Weinberg W, Stansell J, Leoung G, Kovacs J, Rogers M, Scott J, and the Atovaquone/Toxoplasmic En-

cephalitis Study Group. Atovaquone for salvage treatment and suppression of toxoplasmic encephalitis in patients with AIDS. Clin Infect Dis 1997;24:422–429.

111. USPHS/IDSA Prevention of opportunistic infections working group: USPHS/IDSA guidelines for the prevention of opportunistic infections in persons infected with human immunodeficiency virus: disease-specific recommendations. Clin Infect Dis 1995;21(Suppl 1):S32–S43.

111a. USPHS/IDSA: guidelines for the prevention of opportunistic infections in persons infected with human immunodeficiency virus. MMWR 1997;46:6.

112. Van Delden C, Hirschel B. Folinic acid supplements to pyrimethamine-sulfadiazine for *Toxoplasma* encephalitis are associated with better outcome. J Infect Dis 1996;173:1294–1295.

113. Wanke C, Tuazon CU, Kovacs A, Dina T, Davis DO, Barton N, Katz B, Lunde M, Levy C. *Toxoplasma* encephalitis in patients

with acquired immune deficiency syndrome: diagnosis and response to therapy. Am J Trop Med Hyg 1987;36:509–516.

114. Weiss LM, Harris C, Berger M. Pyri-methamine concentrations in serum and cerebrospinal fluid during treatment of acute *Toxoplasma* encephalitis in patients with AIDS. J Infect Dis 1988;157:580–583.

115. Wilson CB, Remington JS, Stagno S, Reynolds DW. Development of children born with subclinical congenital *Toxoplasma* infection. Pediatrics 1980;66:767–774.

116. Wong B, Gold JW, Brown AE, Lange M, Fried R, Grieco M, Mildvan D, Giron J, Tapper ML, Lenner CW. Central-nervous-system toxoplasmosis in homosexual men and parenteral drug abusers. Ann Intern Med 1984;100:36–42.

117. Wreghitt TG, Hakim M, Gray JJ, Balfour AH, Stovin PGI, Stewart S, Scott J, English TAH, Allwork JW. Toxoplasmosis in heart and heart and lung transplant recipients. J Clin Pathol 1989;42:194–199.

Trichomonas vaginalis

●

Joseph G. Pastorek II

GENERAL DESCRIPTION

Trichomonas vaginalis is a flagellated protozoan that commonly causes sexually transmitted illness in humans. Discovered in 1836 (8) but only determined to be a human pathogen in the middle of this century (18, 22), *T. vaginalis* is now known to cause more than simply urethritis and vaginitis.

In men, *T. vaginalis* is primarily responsible for urethritis; colonization by the organism results in an uncomfortable, inflammatory urethral discharge (19). However, sites other than the urethra may be involved (e.g., seminal vesicles); prolonged asymptomatic carriage is common, and spontaneous resolution of urethral colonization may occur in up to a third of infected individuals (20). Rarely, infection may be more parenchymal in location, as in trichomoniasis of the median raphe of the penis (36). Asymptomatic carriage predisposes to ongoing sexual transmission, since the lack of symptoms precludes seeking medical care.

Trichomoniasis in women is primarily thought of as an inflammatory vaginitis, although up to half of women harboring the organism may be asymptomatic (32). Characteristic clinical findings include yellow vaginal discharge, vulvar pruritus, vulvar erythema, and vaginal erythema (42). In pregnant women, trichomoniasis is significantly associated with a yellow, green, or bloody vaginal or cervical discharge; abnormal odor after addition of KOH (positive "whiff test"); vaginal pH over 5.0; and friability of the cervix (30). In addition, trichomoniasis during pregnancy has been associated with low birth weight and prematurity (4, 15, 26) as well as respiratory

disease and vaginitis in the neonate born to a gravida colonized with *Trichomonas* (5, 25).

Besides prematurity and neonatal infection, trichomoniasis has been shown to increase intrauterine transmission of cytomegalovirus (12). In addition, infection with *T. vaginalis* increases the risk of transmission of human immunodeficiency virus (21). Human trichomoniasis is now recognized as a more important disease than previously thought.

SUSCEPTIBILITY IN VITRO

T. vaginalis is not susceptible to many of the usual antibiotic medications, as one would expect of a protozoan (35). However, the nitroimidazole family of drugs, which are active against a number of bacteria, protozoa, and helminths, offers many compounds that are useful now, or show promise for the future, in the treatment of human trichomoniasis.

The mechanism of action of the nitroimidazoles compounds against trichomonads depends upon the anaerobic metabolism of the organism. Initially, the parent compound passively diffuses into the cell. Then, the drug is reduced at the nitro group by anaerobic cellular metabolism. In the presence of molecular oxygen, this reduction would be reversed, since oxygen is a ready electron acceptor. Thus, anaerobic metabolism is needed for significant cell damage. The reduced nitro group damages DNA, causing strand breakage and cell death; disrupts electron flow; and increases the gradient of unreduced drug, thus facilitating more passive diffusion of the compound into the cell (10).

The standard nitroimidazole agent used for trichomoniasis for many years has been metronidazole. Susceptibility of *Trichomonas* to metronidazole can be determined under aerobic or anaerobic conditions. Generally, the presence of oxygen causes higher minimum lethal concentrations (MLCs), since the presence of oxygen prevents the reduced nitro group from causing cellular damage. In fact, one suspected mechanism of resistance of the organism to the nitroimidazoles is tolerance to oxygen, that is, allowing higher concentrations of oxygen within the cell, providing more electron sinks to prevent reduction of the parent drug (11). Thus, one measure of clinically significant metronidazole resistance is an elevated *aerobic* MLC or, more specifically, an elevated aerobic/anaerobic MLC ratio (23, 27).

Most strains of *T. vaginalis* are clinically susceptible, with MLCs in the range of 0.5 to 32 µg/mL, based upon aerobic testing conditions (6). However, since 1962, metronidazole resistance has been demonstrated among trichomonads (33). Based upon in vitro testing under aerobic conditions, the resistance of *Trichomonas* to metronidazole has been classified as follows (24):

- Susceptible   MLC < 50 µg/mL
- Marginal resistance   MLC = 50 µg/mL
- Mild resistance   MLC = 100 µg/mL
- Moderate resistance   MLC = 200 µg/mL
- Severe resistance   MLC > 200 µg/mL

One caveat, however, is that these measured MLCs, based upon aerobic in vitro testing, do not indicate blood or tissue levels of drug necessary for clinical efficacy, as is generally understood for bacterial minimum inhibitory concentrations (MICs) used in determining dosing of an antibiotic. Much of the dosing knowledge of metronidazole has been determined empirically, accumulated as the "collected wisdom" of those experienced in treating human trichomoniasis.

Other nitroimidazole compounds have been shown to be active against *T. vaginalis*. Tinidazole appears to be about as active, with "sensitive" aerobic MLCs of 25 µg/mL or less. However, metronidazole-resistant strains are generally resistant to tinidazole as well, with MLCs of 50 µg/mL or above (28), though some metronidazole-resistant strains respond clinically to tinidazole (17). Ornidazole, a nitroimidazole with pharmacokinetic parameters that allow single-dose (1.5 g oral) administration, has been shown to be effective in human trichomoniasis (13), as has nimorazole (4.0 g in divided doses) (3). Other compounds with activity similar to that of metronidazole are under investigation (9).

Older imidazole drugs that have been developed in topical form for such maladies as vaginal candidiasis have some activity against trichomonads, though the MLCs are somewhat higher than that of metronidazole. However, topical application of such drugs as clotrimazole has been used to augment the activity of systemic metronidazole, to achieve synergistic activity against metronidazole-resistant strains (6).

Some alternative chemical species have been investigated for trichomoniasis, especially in view of the existence of resistant organisms. The nitrofuran drug furazolidone was shown to be active against *T. vaginalis*, with MLCs in the range of 0.8 to 3.1

µg/mL, even for organisms with metronidazole and tinidazole MLCs in excess of 200 mg/mL (28). Another drug, purpuromycin, a naphtharazin-isocoumarin compound, as well as some of its semisynthetic derivatives, were shown to be active (MLC ≤ 25 µg/mL) in vitro against *T. vaginalis* (14). Clinical efficacy was demonstrated with the aminocyclitol paromomycin, given as a vaginal cream to a patient with nitroimidazole-resistant trichomoniasis (29). And, a rather archaic therapy, arsenic, was used successfully to treat resistant trichomoniasis. Arsenicals were used for *Trichomonas* infection before the availability of the nitroimidazole drugs. Thus, it is not surprising that arsenical pessaries would be efficacious in the therapy of vaginitis due to highly nitroimidazole resistant *Trichomonas* (41).

Not only does *T. vaginalis* develop resistance to the various antiprotozoal compounds by becoming more tolerant to oxygen and hence less anaerobic and less sensitive to the nitroimidazole drugs, but the organism, being motile, may actually "run away" from toxic chemicals. *Trichomonas* displays chemorepulsion activity very shortly after exposure to various toxic agents, allowing the organism to avoid cidal concentrations of drug (39). In fact, the more toxic the compound, the more evasive the chemotaxis exhibited by the protozoan. This would explain the inability of topical preparations (e.g., clotrimazole vaginal cream) to effect much more than symptomatic relief in patients with trichomonal vaginitis. It would also explain the poor efficacy observed when topical metronidazole is compared with systemic administration of the drug (40).

ANTIMICROBIAL THERAPY

Metronidazole is the drug of choice for the treatment of human trichomoniasis. It is the only antitrichomonal medication available in the United States, though other nitroimidazoles, such as tinidazole, are available in Canada and Europe. Metronidazole has essentially 100% bioavailability when given orally, and it is readily distributed throughout most of the body. The major toxicity of metronidazole is its disulfuram-like effect, consisting of tachycardia, flushing, nausea, and vomiting, when taken with ethanol. As well, metronidazole and disulfuram taken together may induce an acute psychosis. At higher dosages, such as those over 2 g/day used when treating nitroimidazole-resistant strains of *T. vaginalis,* metronidazole may cause gastrointestinal upset, metallic taste in the mouth, and peripheral neuropathy. The urine may become darkly colored (34).

Several metronidazole dosing regimens are recommended for treatment of uncomplicated trichomoniasis caused by metronidazole-sensitive organisms. The current recommendation by the Centers for Disease Control (CDC) (2) is metronidazole 2 g orally in a single dose, with metronidazole 500 mg orally twice daily for 7 days as an alternate. An older, slightly different regimen (metronidazole 250 mg orally thrice daily for 7 days) has also been used, with efficacy similar to the single-dose regimen (16). Recently, the lowest effective single dose of metronidazole was shown to be 1.5 g orally, given once (38). Recently, the U.S. Food and Drug Administration has approved metronidazole 375 mg orally twice a day for 7 days, though clinical studies of the regimen are lacking (2).

Patients being treated for trichomoniasis should be instructed to avoid sexual intercourse until they and their partners are cured, although such barrier methods as the female condom have been shown to prevent transmission of the organism (37). Simultaneous treatment of the partner is recommended to prevent reinfection. If this is accomplished, all of these regimens are said to be 85 to 95% effective.

Treatment with vaginal metronidazole gel, while effective for the therapy of bacterial vaginosis, is not recommended for trichomoniasis (2, 40).

ENDPOINTS FOR MONITORING THERAPY

According to the CDC, patients who become asymptomatic following treatment need no follow-up. However, if symptoms persist or there is any other reason to suspect relapse or reinfection, reexamination is recommended and retreatment with the 7-day regimen. The practitioner should be wary, however, of the possibility of a metronidazole-resistant or tolerant strain of *Trichomonas*. In fact, in cases such as this, the CDC recommends consultation with an expert and performance of metronidazole susceptibility studies (2).

SPECIAL CONSIDERATIONS
Metronidazole Resistance

Should the practitioner suspect metronidazole resistance or tolerance, several metronidazole dosing alterations are available. The CDC recommends metronidazole at an oral dose of 2 g daily for 3 to 5 days (2). One alternative, which attempts to achieve higher blood and tissue levels than oral administration, is intravenous metronidazole given as a 2-g loading dose and 1 g intravenously every 6 h for 24 h, followed by an increase to 2 g orally every 6 hours for 36 h. In the patient treated by this protocol, a serum level of 110 µg/mL was reached, significantly higher than the 40 µg/mL attained by an oral 2-g dose (7). The shortcoming of this strategy is the adverse symptoms with high blood levels of drug (although this patient only demonstrated mild nausea).

Other therapeutic strategies include simultaneous use of oral and vaginal metronidazole, use of an imidazole cream vaginally along with oral metronidazole, or the use of another of the nitroimidazole medications (e.g., tinidazole), though none of these strategies is well studied, and no other drugs have been approved in the United States for the treatment of trichomoniasis.

Metronidazole Allergy

If a patient with trichomoniasis is allergic to metronidazole, the CDC offers no alternative therapy (2). Other appropriate drugs would be hard to find, since true allergy to any one of the nitroimidazoles would probably mean a high degree of cross-allergenicity (e.g., to tinidazole). However, there has been at least one attempt at desensitizing patients with metronidazole allergy that shows promise. Women were treated with gradually increasing doses in the microgram range over a period of several hours, followed by increasing doses of oral tablets, culminating in a 2-g dose. No ill effects were noted, and the patients were cured of infestation (31).

Trichomoniasis in Pregnancy

Since pregnancy can be adversely affected by trichomoniasis, the general trend in recent years has been treatment of trichomoniasis during pregnancy whenever it is discovered. The theoretical drawback to the use of metronidazole during pregnancy has been the threat of teratogenicity, since metronidazole was shown to be mutagenic in bacterial experimental systems and carcinogenic and tumorigenic when given to rats and mice at high doses. However, this has not been found to be a problem in humans (34). A recent meta-analysis confirms that the entire human experience with metronidazole in pregnancy has been relatively uneventful (1).

Even so, the CDC recommends withholding metronidazole during the first trimester, to obviate the need for worry about possible effects on the infant. Thereafter, they recommend the 2-g single dose of metronidazole (2). However, there are arguments for and against the 2-g single dose. To minimize the amount of metronidazole crossing the placenta, should the patient be given one large dose, with its attendant higher blood level but shorter duration, or a lower dose of longer duration? The question has not been addressed. In the author's experience, the 7-day course of 500 mg twice a day is often preferred by obstetricians. Further research is needed to adequately address this conundrum.

REFERENCES

1. Burtin P, Taddio A, Ariburnu O, Einarson TR, Koren G. Safety of metronidazole in pregnancy: a meta-analysis. Am J Obstet Gynecol 1995;172:525–529.
2. Centers for Disease Control and Prevention. 1998 Guidelines for the treatment of sexually transmitted diseases. MMWR 1998;47(no. RR-1):74–75.
3. Chunge CN, Kangethe S, Pamba HO, Owate J. Treatment of symptomatic trichomoniasis among adult women using oral nitroimidazoles. East Afr Med J 1992;69:398–401.
4. Cotch MF, Pastorek JG, Nugent RP, Hillier SL, Gibbs RS, Martin DH, Eschenbach DA, Edelman R, Carey JC, Regan JA, Krohn MA, Klebanoff MA, Rao AV, Rhoads GG. *Trichomonas vaginalis* associated with low birth weight and preterm delivery. Sex Transm Dis 1997;24:1–8.
5. Danesh IS, Stephen JM, Gorbach J. Neonatal *Trichomonas vaginalis* infection. J Emerg Med 1995;13:51–54.
6. Debbia EA, Campora U, Massaro S, Boldrini E, Schito GC. In vitro activity of metronidazole alone and in combination with clotrimazole against clinical isolates of *Trichomonas vaginalis*. J Chemother 1996;8:96–101.
7. Dombrowski MP, Sokol RJ, Brown WJ, Bronsteen RA. Intravenous therapy of metronidazole-resistant *Trichomonas vaginalis*. Obstet Gynecol 1987;69:524–525.
8. Donné MA. Animalcules observes dans les matienes purulentes et le produit des secretions des organes genitaux de l'homme et de la femme extrait d'une lettre. Acad Sci (Paris) 1836;3:385–386.
9. Dubini F, Riviera L, Cocuzza C, Bellotti MG. Antibacterial, antimycotic and trichomonicidal activity of a new nitroimidazole (EU 11100). J Chemother 1992;4:342–346.
10. Edwards DI. Nitroimidazole drugs—action and resistance mechanisms I. Mechanisms of action. J Antimicrob Chemother 1993;34:9–20.
11. Edwards DI. Nitroimidazole drugs—action and resistance mechanisms II. Mechanisms of resistance. J Antimicrob Chemother 1993;34:204–210.

12. Fowler KB, Pass RF. Sexually transmitted diseases in mothers of neonates with congenital cytomegalovirus infection. J Infect Dis 1991;164:259–264.

13. Fugere P, Verschelden G, Caron M. Single oral dose of ornidazole in women with vaginal trichomoniasis. Obstet Gynecol 1983;62:502–505.

14. Goldstein BP, King A, Ripamonti F, Trani A, Phillips I. In-vitro activity of purpuromycin and MDL 63,604 against microorganisms that cause vaginitis and vaginosis. J Antimicrob Chemother 1995;36:1061–1065.

15. Grice AC. Vaginal infection causing spontaneous rupture of the membranes and premature labor. Aust NZ J Obstet Gynecol 1974;14:156–158.

16. Hager WD, Brown ST, Kraus SJ, Kleris GS, Perkins GJ, Henderson M. Metronidazole for vaginal trichomoniasis. JAMA 1990;244:1219–1220.

17. Hamed KA, Studemeister AE. Successful response of metronidazole-resistant trichomonal vaginitis to tinidazole. A case report. Sex Transm Dis 1992;19:339–340.

18. Hesseltine HC, Wolters SL, Campbell A. Experimental human vaginal trichomoniasis. J Infect Dis 142;71:127–130.

19. Krieger JN, Jenny C, Verdon M, Siegel N, Springwater R, Critchlow CW, Holmes KK. Clinical manifestations of trichomoniasis in men. Ann Intern Med 1993;118:844–849.

20. Krieger JN, Verdon M, Siegel N, Holmes KK. Natural history of urogenital trichomoniasis in men. J Urol 1993;149:1455–1458.

21. Laga M, Manoka A, Kivuvu M, Malele B, Tuliza M, Nzola N, Goeman J, Behets F, Batter V, Alary M, Heyward WL, Ryder RW, Piot P. Non-ulcerative sexually transmitted diseases as risk factors for HIV-1 transmission in women: results of a cohort study. AIDS 1993;7:95–102.

22. Lancely F, MacEntgart MC. Trichomonas vaginalis in the male: the experimental infection of a few volunteers. Lancet 1953;4:668–671.

23. Lossick JG, Müller M, Gorrell TE. In vitro drug susceptibility and doses of metronidazole required for cure in cases of refractory vaginal trichomoniasis. J Infect Dis 1986;153:948–955.

24. Lossick J. Chemotherapy of nitroimidazole-resistant vaginal trichomoniasis. Acta Univ Carol Biol 1988;30:533–545.

25. McLaren LC, Davis LE, Healy GR, James CG. Isolation of Trichomonas vaginalis from the respiratory tract of infants with respiratory disease. Pediatrics 1983;71:888–890.

26. Minkoff H, Grunebaum AN, Schwarz RH, Feldman J, Cummings M, Crombleholme W, Clark L, Pringle G, McCormack WM. Risk factors for prematurity and premature rupture of membranes: a prospective study of the vaginal flora in pregnancy. Am J Obstet Gynecol 1984;150:965–972.

27. Müller M, Lossick JG, Gorrell TE. In vitro susceptibility of Trichomonas vaginalis to metronidazole and treatment outcome in vaginal trichomoniasis. Sex Transm Dis 1988;15:17–24.

28. Narcisi EM, Secor WE. In vitro effect of tinidazole and furazolidone on metronidazole-resistant Trichomonas vaginalis. Antimicrob Agents Chemother 1996;40:1121–1125.

29. Nyirjesy P, Weitz MV, Gelone SP, Fekete T. Paromomycin for nitroimidazole-resistant trichomonosis. Lancet 1995;346:1710.

30. Pastorek JG, Cotch MF, Martin DH, Eschenbach DA. Clinical and microbiological correlates of vaginal trichomoniasis during pregnancy. Clin Infect Dis 1996;23:1075–1080.

31. Pearlman MD, Yashar C, Ernst S, Solomon W. An incremental dosing protocol for women with severe vaginal trichomoniasis and adverse reactions to metronidazole. Am J Obstet Gynecol 1996;174:934–936.

32. Rein MF, Müller M. Trichomonas vaginalis and trichomoniasis. In: Holmes KK, Mårdh P-A, Sparling PF, Wiesner PJ, Cates W, Lemon SM, Stamm WE, eds. Sexually transmitted diseases. 2nd ed. New York: McGraw-Hill, 1990:481–492.

33. Robinson SC. Trichomonal vaginitis resistant to metronidazole. Can Med Assoc J 1962;86:665.

34. Schwebke JR. Metronidazole: utilization in obstetric and gynecologic patients. Sex Transm Dis 1995;22:370–375.

35. Sears SD, O'Hare J. In vitro susceptibility of Trichomonas vaginalis to 50 antimicrobial agents. Antimicrob Agents Chemother 1988;32:144–146.

36. Soendjojo A, Pindha S. Trichomonas vaginalis infection of the median raphe of the penis. Sex Transm Dis 1981;8:255–257.

37. Soper DE, Shoupe D, Shangold GA, Shangold MM, Gutmann J, Mercer L. Prevention of vaginal trichomoniasis by compliant use of the female condom. Sex Transm Dis 1993;20:137–139.

38. Spence MR, Harwell TD, Davies MC, Smith JL. The minimum single oral metronidazole dose for treating trichomoniasis: a randomized, blinded study. Obstet Gynecol 1997;89:699–703.

39. Sugarman B, Mummaw N. Effects of antimicrobial agents on growth and chemotaxis of Trichomona vaginalis. Antimicrob Agents Chemother 1988;32:1323–1326.

40. Tidwell BH, Lushbaugh WB, Laughlin MD, Gleary JD, Finley RW. A double-blind placebo-controlled trial of single-dose intravaginal versus single-dose oral metronidazole in the treatment of trichomonal vaginitis. J Infect Dis 1994;170:242–246.

41. Watson PG, Pattman RS. Arsenical pessaries in the successful elimination of metronidazole-resistant Trichomonas vaginalis. Int J STD AIDS 1996;7:296–297.

42. Wølner-Hanssen P, Drieger JN, Stevens CE, Kiviat NB, Koutsky L, Critchlow C, DeRouen T, Hillier S, Holmes KK. Clinical Manifestations of vaginal trichomoniasis. JAMA 1989;261:571–576.

Tropheryma whippelii (Whipple's Disease)

David N. Fredricks and David A. Relman

GENERAL DESCRIPTION

Whipple's disease is a rare, chronic, systemic illness first described in a 36-year-old physician by George Whipple in 1907 (30). Whipple's disease primarily affects the small intestine, although disease may be found in almost any organ, including brain, lymph node, heart, lung, eye, liver, spleen, and synovium (12). Patients often have migratory arthritis or arthralgia that precedes other symptoms by years. Eventually, patients may develop diarrhea, malabsorption, weight loss, malaise, fever, or abdominal pain. Signs of cachexia, lymphadenopathy, skin hyperpigmentation, abdominal tenderness, peripheral edema, and fever may be apparent. Laboratory abnormalities may include anemia, thrombocytosis, hypoalbuminemia, electrolyte disturbances, and increased stool fat content.

George Whipple named the disorder "intestinal lipodystrophy," based on his belief that altered fat metabolism played a role in its pathogenesis (30). He also noted numerous rod-shaped organisms resembling *Mycobacterium tuberculosis* in a silver-stained lymph node from his 1907 patient. Empirical trials of antibiotics demonstrated that patients could be cured of this usually fatal disease. Electron microscopy revealed the presence of unique bacillary structures within tissues from patients with Whipple's disease. Clinical response to antibiotics was associated with disappearance of bacilli. Reappearance of bacilli heralded clinical relapse (27). Despite the accumulated evidence of a bacterial etiology for Whipple's disease, no organism was reproducibly cultured from tissues of affected patients. Without an isolated organism, Koch's postulates for establishing microbial disease causation, as originally constructed, cannot be fulfilled.

Further characterization of the Whipple bacillus became possible through application of nucleic acid amplification technology and molecular phylogenetic analysis. A portion of a bacterial 16S ribosomal RNA gene was amplified with the polymerase chain reaction (PCR) directly from human Whipple's disease tissues, using primers directed against highly conserved regions of the bacterial gene (21, 31). A phylogenetic tree with inferred evolutionary relationships was created from a set of aligned 16S rDNA sequences that included the amplified Whipple's bacillus sequence. The Whipple bacillus was assigned to the actinomycete group of bacteria. The name *Tropheryma whippelii* was proposed, derived from the Greek words "trophe" for nourishment and "eryma" for barrier, and "whippelii" in honor of George Whipple.

Microbiology

Attempts to propagate *T. whippelii* in culture media, cell culture, and animal hosts have not met with reproducible success.

Knowledge of this organism is therefore limited to histologic (light and electron microscopy) and molecular (rRNA sequence) data. There is no known natural reservoir or animal host for this bacterium other than man.

The Whipple bacillus measures 0.20 microns in diameter and 1.5 to 2.5 microns in length (5). No flagella are apparent. A 20-nm-thick cell wall lies external to a cytoplasmic membrane and contains peptidoglycan. A second phospholipid membrane is external to the cell wall. Although an outer membrane is typical of Gram-negative bacilli, the symmetric appearance and lack of lipopolysaccharide in the *T. whippelii* outer membrane and the thickness of the cell wall distinguish this bacterium from the Gram-negative group.

The histologic hallmark of Whipple's disease is periodic acid–Schiff (PAS)-reactive vacuoles in macrophages within the lamina propria of the small bowel. The magenta stain indicates carbohydrate within these vacuoles. It is believed that PAS reagent reacts with intact and partially degraded bacterial cell wall polysaccharide remnants. The reactivity of Whipple's disease tissue persists after treatment with diastase, indicating that a nonstarch polysaccharide is present. PAS-positive, diastase-resistant macrophages found in tissues other than the small bowel (e.g., colon, brain) are not specific for Whipple's disease (12). The Whipple bacillus can be visualized with Giemsa stain and some silver stain methods (e.g., Gomori) but not with acid-fast staining procedures. Tissues with PAS-positive macrophages should be subjected to acid-fast staining to exclude mycobacteria (e.g., *Mycobacterium avium* complex), which may also be PAS reactive (13). *T. whippelii* stains weakly Gram positive.

Another tool for diagnosis of Whipple's disease is the PCR. Primers directed against a region of the *T. whippelii* 16S rRNA gene can be used in a PCR assay to amplify bacterial DNA directly from infected tissue. Sometimes patients with clinical evidence of Whipple's disease fail to have convincing histologic evidence of disease, yet *T. whippelii* 16S rDNA can be detected in tissue samples by PCR (22).

SUSCEPTIBILITY IN VITRO

Since *T. whippelii* has not been reproducibly cultivated to date in vitro, no antibiotic susceptibility data exist. Likewise, attempts to propagate *T. whippelii* in nonhuman hosts have been unsuccessful, preventing in vivo drug efficacy studies. A recent report describes the laboratory propagation of *T. whippelii* within macrophages treated with interleukin-4 (24). If reproducible cultivation is achieved in cell culture, then antibiotic susceptibility testing may be feasible in the near future.

The absence of any known close phylogenetic relationship with a bacterium having well-characterized drug sensitivities prevents one from making accurate inferences about susceptibilities of the Whipple bacillus.

ANTIMICROBIAL THERAPY

General

Given the lack of in vitro and animal data, retrospective studies of antibiotic treatment of Whipple's disease in humans constitute the only data on which to base antimicrobial therapy. Prospective controlled trials of antibiotic therapy have been impractical because of the low incidence of disease and the long follow-up period required to monitor relapse rates.

The first successful use of antibiotics in Whipple's disease was reported in 1952 by Paulley who used chloramphenicol (16). Subsequent reports have noted successful responses to penicillin, penicillin plus streptomycin, ampicillin, amoxicillin (2), ceftriaxone (1, 25), cefixime (3, 17), gentamicin, tetracyclines (tetracycline, doxycycline), sulfonamides, trimethoprim, trimethoprim/sulfamethoxazole (TMP-SMX), erythromycin, neomycin, rifampin plus other antibiotics, and salicylazosulfapyridine (10). The optimal duration of antibiotic treatment is not known. The most commonly used regimens have included 2 weeks of parenteral antibiotics followed by months to years of oral antibiotic therapy (20).

Whipple's disease has a propensity to relapse. While many antibiotics have initial efficacy, the therapeutic challenge is to effect a complete and sustained cure. In their retrospective review of antibiotic treatment outcome in 88 patients with Whipple's disease, Keinath et al. (10) found that 31 patients relapsed (35%), with a mean time to relapse of 4.2 years. The 13 patients with central nervous system (CNS) relapses (42% of all relapses) had dismal outcomes, whereas patients with non-CNS relapses had excellent outcomes. Relapse rates were correlated with antibiotic treatment, revealing that 21 of 49 patients (43%) treated with a tetracycline alone experienced a relapse. Three of 8 patients (37.5%) treated with penicillin alone relapsed. Two of 5 patients (40%) treated with parenteral penicillin plus streptomycin relapsed. In contrast, only 2 of 15 patients (13%) relapsed when treated with parenteral penicillin/streptomycin followed by oral tetracycline (the Duke regimen (12)), and both of these patients received only 2 weeks of tetracycline. None of the 15 patients treated with the Duke regimen experienced a CNS relapse. Three patients were treated with oral TMP-SMX, and none relapsed. Based on this large collection of patients, the authors recommended an antibiotic regimen of parenteral penicillin (1.2 million units/day procaine penicillin) plus streptomycin (1.0 g/day) for 10 to 14 days followed by TMP-SMX (one double-strength tablet twice daily) for 1 year. An alternative regimen proposed was oral trimethoprim-sulfamethoxazole alone for 1 year. A higher dose of TMP-SMX (one double-strength tablet three times a day) was offered as an alternative for the first 2 weeks of treatment. Penicillin or tetracycline alone were not suggested. Although these recommendations were based on trends in their data, the authors acknowledged that statistical confirmation of significant differences between treatment groups was lacking.

Durand et al. (6) reported relapse rates for 52 patients with Whipple's disease from France. Five of 28 patients (18%) treated with tetracycline relapsed, compared with none of 7 patients treated with penicillin-streptomycin, and none of 12 patients treated with trimethoprim-sulfamethoxazole.

Fleming et al. (8) described outcomes in 25 patients with Whipple's disease treated with antibiotics and followed at the Mayo Clinic. Relapse occurred in 2 of the 25 patients, and both of these patients were treated with tetracycline alone, one for 9 months, one for 18 months. On the other hand, one patient remained free of clinically apparent disease for at least 26 years after receiving only 5 days of penicillin! The authors argue that selection of an antibiotic that crosses the blood-brain barrier may be more important in preventing CNS relapses than duration of antibiotic therapy. Nevertheless, they also recommend a regimen of parenteral penicillin plus streptomycin for 2 weeks followed by a year of oral TMP-SMX. The numbers of patients in each treatment group were again too small for meaningful statistical analysis.

von Herbay and Otto reported 22 patients with Whipple's disease diagnosed in Germany at the University of Hamburg (29). Two patients with CNS disease were treated successfully with intravenous ampicillin and chloramphenicol. Seventeen patients without CNS disease but with long-term follow up received tetracycline, usually for 2 to 3 years. Two of these patients (12%) relapsed after 2 years of treatment, neither with apparent CNS disease. The authors suggest that prolonged antibiotic therapy may compensate for the poor CNS penetration of tetracycline.

Geboes et al. described 16 patients followed at the University Hospital of Leuven, Belgium (9). Twelve patients were treated with tetracycline, 3 of whom also received an initial course of penicillin plus streptomycin. There were 4 relapses among those treated with tetracycline alone, and 1 relapse in the combination group. Four patients were treated with TMP-SMX for 1 year, with no relapses noted, although patient follow-up was not as long as in the tetracycline-treated group.

Feurle and Marth (7) provide a retrospective, nonrandomized comparison of 30 patients, involving 22 treatment courses with tetracyclines versus 13 courses with TMP-SMX. Most patients in the tetracycline group received 100 mg/day of doxycycline, while a double-strength TMP-SMX tablet was prescribed twice daily in the other group. Initial remission was induced with 13 of 22 tetracycline courses (59%) versus 12 of 13 TMP-SMX courses (92%), a significant difference ($P < .05$), although one must recognize the limitations of the study design. Relapses occurred in 8 patients, 5 of whom were noncompliant with medication or stopped antibiotic treatment outright. Three patients developed CNS Whipple's disease while on antimicrobial treatment, 2 of whom took tetracycline and 1 who took TMP-SMX. The patient who experienced CNS disease on TMP-SMX was documented to have resolution of intestinal disease on therapy. The authors point out that even a drug such as TMP-SMX, which can penetrate the CNS, may not be sufficient to eradicate T. whippelii from the brain despite 14 months of treatment.

Recognizing the significant limitations of the above data, we recommend an antibiotic regimen of parenteral penicillin, at least 1.2 million units per day intravenously or intramuscularly, concurrent with streptomycin (1.0 g/day for 10–14 days), followed by oral TMP/SMX, one double-strength tablet twice daily for 1 year (Table 1). A reasonable alternative is an all oral regimen of TMP-SMX, one double-strength tablet by mouth twice daily for 1 year. Although a year of antimicrobial therapy is probably curative in most patients, clinical judgment may dictate longer courses of treatment. Patients who are slow to respond to antibiotics or who have CNS disease may benefit from extended treatment courses. For the patient who is intolerant of TMP-SMX, doxycycline (100 mg orally twice daily) or penicillin VK (500 mg orally four times a day) may be used for consolidation oral treatment after parenteral penicillin plus streptomycin. We suggest using the higher doxycycline dose of 100 mg twice daily for at least 1 year because of the higher relapse rates found in some studies when lower doses of tetracyclines were used. For the penicillin-allergic patient, consider using ceftriaxone if the allergy is mild (i.e., rash) or chloramphenicol in the setting of previous anaphylaxis.

Is combination therapy superior to monotherapy in Whipple's disease? Few data exist at the present time to suggest that combination therapy improves outcome, reduces the relapse rate, or shortens the duration of therapy required to effect a cure. The lack of rigorous data does not stop us from recommending initial combination therapy with penicillin and streptomycin based on the success of this regimen in retrospective reviews when it is followed with a prolonged course of an appropriate oral antibiotic.

Special Situations

Patients with uveitis should be treated with antibiotics that are expected to achieve high intraocular concentrations, such as TMP-SMX, chloramphenicol, or third-generation cephalosporins, although patients have also responded to erythromycin and doxycycline. Patients with meningitis should probably be started on parenteral therapy, preferably with high-dose penicillin, ceftriaxone, or chloramphenicol, and have clinical improvement documented before changing to oral therapy. Options for oral therapy in CNS disease include TMP-SMX, chloramphenicol, and cefixime. High-dose oral penicillin (e.g., 0.5–1 g every 6 h) in conjunction with oral probenecid would be a reasonable alternative therapy for the patient who is intolerant of other therapies, although this regimen is not well tested. No data exist on the efficacy of intrathecal antibiotics for CNS Whipple's disease. Few data exist to guide the therapy of endocarditis with *T. whippelii,* but the initial selection of parenteral, presumably bactericidal, antibiotics such as penicillin plus gentamicin or streptomycin would be reasonable.

Alternative Therapy

For the patient who fails, or is intolerant of, first-line antibiotic treatment (e.g., penicillin/streptomycin, TMP-SMX, tetracyclines, chloramphenicol, third-generation cephalosporins) there are several less well studied alternatives. Erythromycin or rifampin show some evidence of efficacy. Antimycobacterial agents have shown some success when used in combination, including isoniazid, *p*-aminosalicylic acid, streptomycin, and rifampin (14). Vancomycin is untested but would be reasonable to try in the refractory patient on the basis of the Gram-positive characteristics of *T. whippelii.* Other untested antibiotics may be effective on the basis of phylogenetic similarity between *T. whippelii* and the actinomycetes. Such potentially useful but untried antibiotics include clindamycin, amikacin, imipenem, dapsone, clofazimine, azithromycin, clarithromycin, and the fluoroquinolones.

ENDPOINTS FOR MONITORING THERAPY

Clinical response to antibiotics is usually observed in the first days to week of therapy. Cessation of diarrhea and fever are usually the first objective signs of improvement. Within 1 month, significant weight gain usually occurs, and arthralgias resolve. Correction of laboratory and histologic abnormalities lags behind the clinical gains. Intestinal epithelial cells begin to normalize within days of treatment, and extracellular bacilli disappear within the first few weeks (15). However, the architecture of the intestinal mucosa usually remains abnormal for many months. PAS-staining macrophages may persist in the lamina propria for years after successful treatment. Laboratory abnormalities usually resolve within 6 to 18 months. A Herxheimer-type reaction has been described with initiation of antibiotics, marked by brief clinical deterioration (fever, hypotension) and a rise in acute-phase reactants (19, 26).

How can one best monitor the response to antibiotic therapy in the patient with Whipple's disease? The lack of many objective indicators of disease regression during initial treatment forces one to rely on more subjective indicators. Patients who experience decreased diarrhea, abdominal pain, arthralgias, fever, night sweats, edema, and malaise with an increased sense of well-being are likely on the right course. Obviously one must follow the presenting symptoms and signs of the individual patient (e.g., altered mental status and supranuclear ophthalmoplegia in a patient with CNS disease). If the patient is improving clinically, there is no need for frequent intestinal

TABLE 1 • Recommended Antimicrobial Regimens for Whipple's Disease	
Induction (10–14 days)	**Consolidation (1 year)**
Procaine penicillin 1.2 million units i.m. q.d. or penicillin G 6–24 million units i.v. q.d. + streptomycin 1 g i.m. q.d.	TMP/SMX[a] 160 mg/800 mg p.o. b.i.d.
TMP/SMX 160 mg/800 mg i.v. or p.o. b.i.d.	Doxycycline 100 mg p.o. b.i.d.
Chloramphenicol 50 mg/kg/day i.v., i.m., or p.o. divided q. 6 h	Chloramphenicol 250–500 mg p.o. q.i.d.
Ceftriaxone 1–2 g i.v. q.d.	Cefixime 400 mg p.o. b.i.d.
	Penicillin VK 500 mg p.o. q.i.d.

[a]TMP-SMX, trimethoprim-sulfamethoxazole.

biopsies, since most histologic abnormalities persist for months. It is reasonable to perform an intestinal biopsy in the patient with gastrointestinal disease just prior to terminating antibiotic treatment (e.g., at 1 year of antibiotics). The histologic picture observed at this time can serve as a new baseline for comparison with future specimens obtained when disease relapse is a concern. The presence of PAS-positive macrophages in the lamina propria at termination of treatment does not by itself indicate persistent disease. On the contrary, these abnormal macrophages continue to be found in most patients for years, albeit in decreasing numbers.

What should be done with the patient who fails to improve clinically or who improves initially but subsequently deteriorates while on antibiotic therapy? Before switching to second-line antibiotics, one should first address the question of patient compliance. Patients may not feel compelled to take their antibiotics month after month once they feel healthy. The degree of compliance with antibiotic treatment should be sought through discussions with the patient, the family, and the pharmacist (e.g., record of refills). If the patient is not reliable, one should consider using parenteral antibiotics such as daily intramuscular procaine penicillin or intravenous ceftriaxone, at least during the initial weeks of therapy.

If the patient is thought to be compliant but fails to improve, one should consider a repeat biopsy. In the patient with gastrointestinal disease who is receiving effective therapy, epithelial cells should be normal in hematoxylin and eosin–stained sections after 3 to 4 weeks. Extracellular bacilli, as assessed by electron microscopy, should be absent or markedly reduced after 1 to 2 months of antibiotics (4). Persistence of these abnormalities suggests antibiotic failure. Although laboratory and histological abnormalities may persist for months, a trend toward normalization should be evident with effective treatment. Patients who show evidence of worsening laboratory studies such as anemia, hypoalbuminemia, rising ESR, or steatorrhea should have their treatment plans reevaluated. For whatever reason, some patients fail to respond to one antibiotic regimen but respond rapidly to another.

A particularly worrisome scenario may occur when a patient with Whipple's disease appears to respond to treatment but develops neurologic symptoms and signs, either while on antibiotics or after therapy is completed (11). Patients have had clinical and histologic improvement of gastrointestinal disease while receiving tetracycline yet have developed CNS disease that then required treatment with chloramphenicol, penicillin, or TMP-SMX. The relatively high incidence of CNS relapse has been attributed to early dissemination of the Whipple bacillus, with subclinical seeding of the brain. The CNS may be a sanctuary for *T. whippelii,* especially when antibiotics are used that have poor CNS penetration. The rationale for using TMP-SMX instead of tetracycline as standard oral therapy is based on the high levels of TMP and SMX achievable in the CNS and the belief that the rate of CNS relapse will be reduced (23).

Recent studies suggest that a PCR-based assay for *T. whippelii* may be useful for diagnosing Whipple's disease and monitoring response to antibiotics (18). Although *T.*

whippelii DNA may persist in intestinal tissue for weeks or months after initiation of antibiotics, microbial DNA disappears from tissues more rapidly than histologic abnormalities resolve (28). Most probably, persistence of *T. whippelii* DNA in tissues after 4 to 6 months of treatment is evidence of antibiotic failure. One caveat is that eradication of *T. whippelii* DNA from intestinal tissue does not exclude the possibility of ongoing CNS disease. A PCR-based assay of cerebrospinal fluid may be used to diagnose CNS Whipple's disease.

FUTURE DIRECTIONS

A prospective controlled study of antibiotic therapy in Whipple's disease has yet to be published. To determine the optimal antibiotic regimen, a multicenter trial of selected antibiotics and combinations would likely be necessary. However, even if such a trial were funded, many years of follow-up would be required to determine accurate relapse rates for each treatment arm. Several questions are worthy of further investigation. Does streptomycin provide any additional benefit when used in combination with penicillin? Should Whipple's disease be treated like tuberculosis (another actinomycete infection), using combinations of antibiotics to prevent emergence of resistant organisms? Is clinical relapse explained by emergence of such resistant clones? Is treatment with parenteral penicillin/streptomycin necessary prior to long-term oral antibiotics? What is the optimal duration of oral and parenteral antibiotic therapy? What are the best oral antibiotics in terms of initial response rate, relapse rate (especially of the CNS), cost-effectiveness, and long-term side effect profile? Answers to many of these questions are not imminent. Hope for rapid but indirect answers to some of these questions may arise from successful propagation of *T. whippelii* in the laboratory with determination of antibiotic susceptibilities and/or the development of an appropriate animal model of disease.

REFERENCES

1. Adler CH, Galetta SL. Oculo-facial-skeletal myorhythmia in Whipple disease: treatment with ceftriaxone. Ann Intern Med 1990;112:467–469.
2. Bai JC, Crosetti EE, Maurino EC, Martinez CA, Sambuelli A, Boerr LA. Short-term antibiotic treatment in Whipple's disease. J Clin Gastroenterol 1991;13:303–307.
3. Cooper GS, Blades EW, Remler BF, Salata RA, Bennert KW, Jacobs GH. Central nervous system Whipple's disease: relapse during therapy with trimethoprim-sulfamethoxazole and remission with cefixime. Gastroenterology 1994;106:782–786.
4. Denholm RB, Mills PR, More IA. Electron microscopy in the long-term follow-up of Whipple's disease. Effect of antibiotics. Am J Surg Pathol 1981;5:507–516.
5. Dobbins W3, Kawanishi H. Bacillary characteristics in Whipple's disease: an electron microscopic study. Gastroenterology 1981;80:1468–1475.
6. Durand DV, Lecomte C, Cathebras P, Rousset H, Godeau P. Whipple disease. Clinical review of 52 cases. The SNFMI Research Group on Whipple Disease. Societe Nationale Francaise de Medecine Interne. Medicine (Baltimore) 1997;76:170–184.
7. Feurle GE, Marth T. An evaluation of antimicrobial treatment

for Whipple's Disease. Tetracycline versus trimethoprim-sulfamethoxazole. Dig Dis Sci 1994;39:1642–1648.

8. Fleming JL, Wiesner RH, Shorter RG. Whipple's disease: clinical, biochemical, and histopathologic features and assessment of treatment in 29 patients. Mayo Clin Proc 1988;63:539–551.

9. Geboes K, Ectors N, Heidbuchel H, Rutgeerts P, Desmet V, Vantrappen G. Whipple's disease: endoscopic aspects before and after therapy. Gastrointest Endosc 1990;36:247–252.

10. Keinath RD, Merrell DE, Vlietstra R, Dobbins W3. Antibiotic treatment and relapse in Whipple's disease. Long-term follow-up of 88 patients. Gastroenterology 1985;88:1867–1873.

11. Knox DL, Bayless TM, Pittman FE. Neurologic disease in patients with treated Whipple's disease. Medicine (Baltimore) 1976;55:467–476.

12. Maizel H, Ruffin JM, Dobbins W 3. Whipple's disease: a review of 19 patients from one hospital and a review of the literature since 1950. Medicine (Baltimore) 1970;49:175–205.

13. Maliha GM, Hepps KS, Maia DM, Gentry KR, Fraire AE, Goodgame RW. Whipple's disease can mimic chronic AIDS enteropathy. Am J Gastroenterol 1991;86:79–81.

14. Maxwell JD, Ferguson A, McKay AM, Imrie RC, Watson WC. Lymphocytes in Whipple's disease. Lancet 1968;1:887–889.

15. Miksche LW, Blumcke S, Fritsche D, Kuchemann K, Schuler HW, Grozinger KH. Whipple's disease: etiopathogenesis, treatment, diagnosis, and clinical course. Case report and review of the world literature. Acta Hepatogastroenterol (Stuttg) 1974; 21:307–326.

16. Paulley JW. A case of Whipple's disease (intestinal lipodystrophy). Gastroenterology 1952;22:128–133.

17. Peters FP, Elbrecht EA, Wouters RS, Engels LG, Stockbrugger RW. Whipple's disease: a difficult diagnosis? Neth J Med 1996;49:106–111.

18. Ramzan NN, Loftus EJ, Burgart LJ, Rooney M, Batts KP, Wiesner RH, Fredricks DN, Relman DA, Persing DH. Diagnosis and monitoring of Whipple disease by polymerase chain reaction. Ann Intern Med 1997;126:520–527.

19. Reed JI, Sipe JD, Wohlgethan JR, Doos WG, Canoso JJ. Response of the acute-phase reactants, C-reactive protein and serum amyloid A protein, to antibiotic treatment of Whipple's disease. Arthritis Rheum 1985;28:352–355.

20. Relman DA. Whipple's disease. In: Blaser MJ, Smith PD, Ravdin JI, Greenberg HB, Guerrant RL, ed. Infections of the gastrointestinal tract. New York: Raven Press, 1995:919–936.

21. Relman DA, Schmidt TM, MacDermott RP, Falkow S. Identification of the uncultured bacillus of Whipple's disease [see comments]. N Engl J Med 1992;327:293–301.

22. Rickman LS, Freeman WR, Green WR, Feldman ST, Sullivan J, Russack V, Relman DA. Brief report: uveitis caused by Tropheryma whippelii (Whipple's bacillus) [see comments]. N Engl J Med 1995;332:363–366.

23. Ryser RJ, Locksley RM, Eng SC, Dobbins W3, Schoenknecht FD, Rubin CE. Reversal of dementia associated with Whipple's disease by trimethoprim-sulfamethoxazole, drugs that penetrate the blood-brain barrier. Gastroenterology 1984;86: 745–752.

24. Schoedon G, Goldenberger D, Forrer R, Gunz A, Dutly F, Hochli M, Altwegg M, Schaffner A. Deactivation of macrophages with interleukin-4 is the key to the isloation of Tropheryma whippelii. J Infect Dis 1997;176:672–677.

25. Simpson DA, Wishnow R, Gargulinski RB, Pawlak AM. Oculo-facial-skeletal myorhythmia in central nervous system Whipple's disease: additional case and review of the literature. Move Disord 1995;10:195–200.

26. Tauris P, Moesner J. Whipple's disease. Clinical and histopathological changes during treatment with sulphamethoxazole-trimethoprim. Acta Med Scand 1978;204:423–427.

27. Trier JS, Phelps PC, Eidelman S, Rubin CE. Whipple's disease: light and electron microscopic correlation of jejunal mucosal histology with antibiotic treatment and clinical status. Gastroenterology 1965;48:684–707.

28. von Herbay A, Ditton HJ, Maiwald M. Diagnostic application of a polymerase chain reaction assay for the Whipple's disease bacterium to intestinal biopsies. Gastroenterology 1996;110: 1735–1743.

29. von Herbay A, Otto HF. Whipple's disease: a report of 22 patients. Klin Wochenschr 1988;66:533–539.

30. Whipple GH. A hitherto undescribed disease characterized anatomically by deposits of fat and fatty acids in the intestinal and mesenteric lymphatic tissues. Johns Hopkins Hosp Bull 1907;18:382–391.

31. Wilson KH, Blitchington R, Frothingham R, Wilson JA. Phylogeny of the Whipple's-disease-associated bacterium. Lancet 1991;338:474–475.

PART E

Antibacterial Agents

Aminoglycosides

David P. Nicolau and Richard Quintiliani, Jr.

Despite the introduction of numerous antimicrobials over the past five decades, aminoglycosides have remained an important therapeutic modality for the management of a variety of infectious processes. Since the introduction of this class of agents into clinical practice, the major obstacle that has curtailed their use is the potential for drug-related toxicity, most notably oto- and nephrotoxicity. However, over the last several years, information has become available relating to the development of toxicity and optimization of their bactericidal effects. As a result, parenteral aminoglycoside dosing techniques have been modified in an attempt to minimize toxicity and to maximize their therapeutic potential. Application of these new principles in addition to these agents' sustained in vitro activity, synergistic potential, rapid bactericidal activity, longstanding clinical efficacy, and relative insusceptibility to the emergence of resistance, support the continued use of aminoglycosides for the treatment of serious infections.

BACKGROUND

The aminoglycosides include an important group of compounds, natural and semisynthetic, that are particularly active against aerobic Gram-negative bacilli and Gram-positive cocci. Streptomycin, the first parenterally administered aminoglycoside was introduced in 1944. Streptomycin and neomycin, kanamycin, tobramycin, and paromomycin (used for its amebicidal and antihelminthic activities) are all natural occurring compounds that were isolated from *Streptomyces* spp. Gentamicin and sisomicin (not available in the U.S.) are produced from *Micromonospora* spp., while amikacin and netilmicin are semisynthetic derivatives of kanamycin and sisomicin, respectively. Isepamicin (not available in the U.S.) is a semisynthetic derivative of gentamicin B. The suffixes "mycin" and "micin" indicate that the compound was isolated directly or indirectly from *Streptomyces* spp. or *Micromonospora* spp., respectively.

CLASS

Structurally, aminoglycosides consist of a six-membered, amino-group-containing ring called an aminocyclitol that is linked to two or more sugars (Fig. 1). The aminocyclitol ring of streptomycin is a streptidine; for the other aminoglycosides, it is 2-deoxystreptamine (Fig. 1). Although discussions of aminoglycosides frequently include spectinomycin (a pure aminocyclitol used principally for anogenital infections due to

Neisseria gonorrhoeae), it is not, strictly speaking, an aminoglycoside, since it does not contain aminosugars or glycosidic bonds (Fig. 1). Thus, the complete group of compounds is more correctly termed *aminoglycoside-aminocyclitols*.

Two groups of 2-deoxystreptamine-containing aminoglycosides can be distinguished on the basis of the position (4,5 and 4,6) of their substituents on the 2-deoxystreptamine ring. By convention, this ring (labeled *A* in Fig. 1) is numbered 1 to 6 in a counterclockwise manner. The 4,5-disubstituted deoxystreptamines (neomycin family) include neomycin and paromomycin, and the 4,6-disubstituted deoxystreptamines, kanamycin, tobramycin, amikacin (kanamycin family), and gentamicin, sisomicin, and netilmicin (gentamicin family). The sugar molecules linked to the aminocyclitol are numbered in a clockwise manner, 1' to 6' for the aminosugar substituent at the 4-position and 1" to 6" for sugar substituents at either the 5- or 6-positions. Neomycin and paromomycin are distinguished by inclusion of a pentose ring at the 5-position of the 2-deoxystreptamine in addition to two aminohexoses. For streptomycin, the substituted streptidine is numbered in a clockwise fashion 1 to 6, and subsequent rings 1' to 6' and 1" to 6" (Fig. 1).

As marketed commercially, kanamycin consists of 95% kanamycin A and 5% kanamycin B (Fig. 2). Tobramycin is 3'-deoxykanamycin B, while amikacin is derived from kanamycin A following a 2-hydroxy-4-aminobutyric acid semisynthetic addition to the amino group at position 1 of the aminocyclitol. Gentamicin as used clinically is the gentamicin C complex, which consists of roughly equal mixtures of the closely related compounds C1, C1a, and C2 (Fig. 2). Sisomicin is the dehydro analogue of gentamicin C1a, while netilmicin is derived from sisomicin after ethylation of its 1-amino group.

MECHANISM OF ACTION

The mechanism of action of aminoglycosides has been generally believed to result from inhibition of protein biosynthesis by irreversible binding of the aminoglycoside to the bacterial ribosome. The intact bacterial ribosome is a 70S particle consisting of two subunits (50S and 30S) that are assembled from three species of rRNA (5S, 16S, and 23S) and 52 ribosomal proteins. The smaller 30S ribosomal subunit, which contains the 16S rRNA (see below), has been identified as a primary target for aminoglycoside-aminocyclitol antibiotics. Although

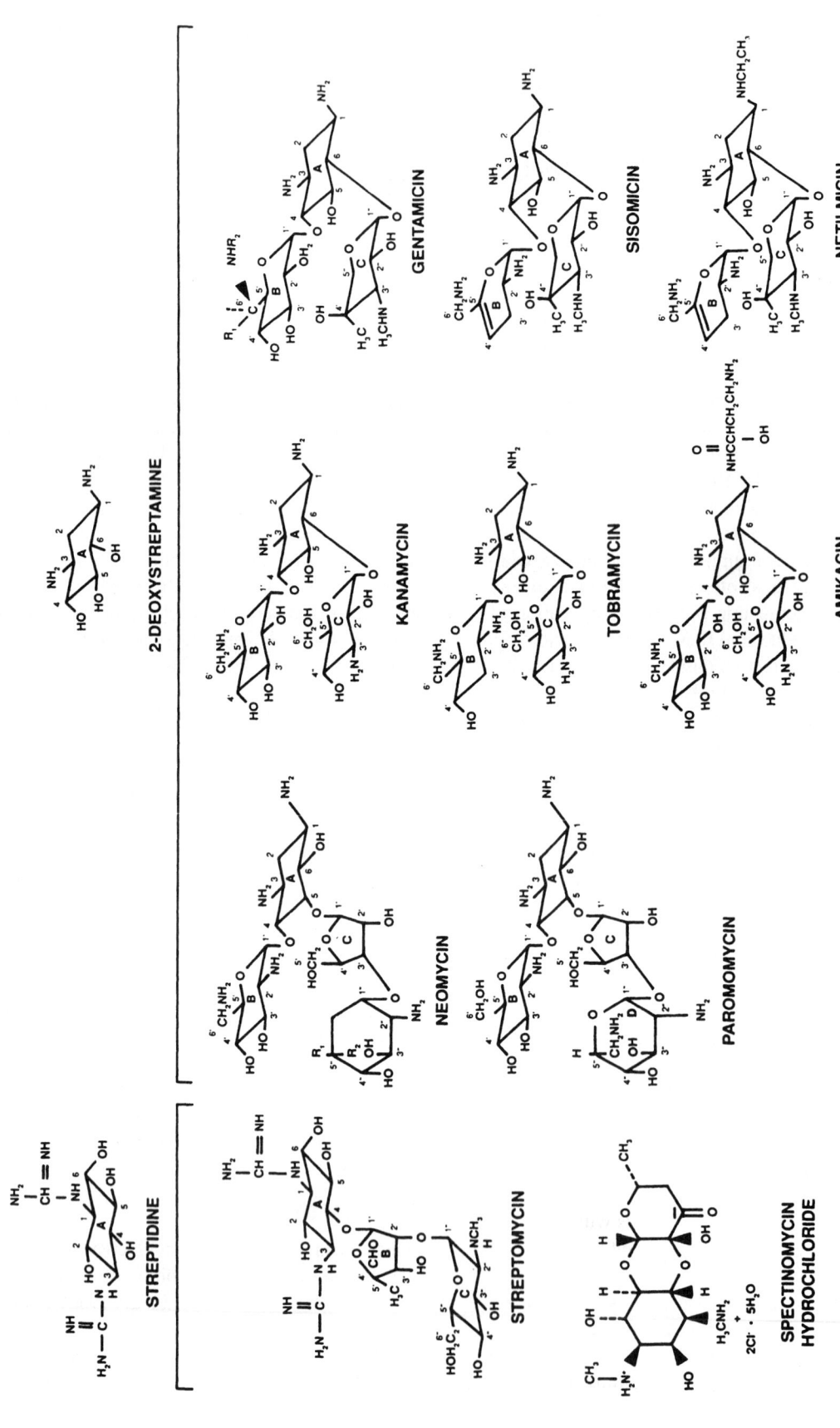

FIGURE 1. Chemical structure of the aminoglycosides and spectinomycin. Neomycin contains approximately equal amounts of neomycin B (R_1 = H; R_2 = CH_2NH_2) and neomycin C (R_1 = CH_2NH_2; R_2 = H). Kanamycin is principally kanamycin A, as shown. Gentamicin is gentamicin C complex with roughly equal amounts of C1 (R_1 = R_2 = CH_3), C1a (R_1 = R_2 = H), and C2 (R_1 = CH_3; R_2 = H). (Modified from Gilbert DN. Aminoglycosides. In: Mandell GL, Bennett JE, Dolin R, eds. Principles and practice of infectious diseases. New York: Churchill Livingstone, 1995:281.)

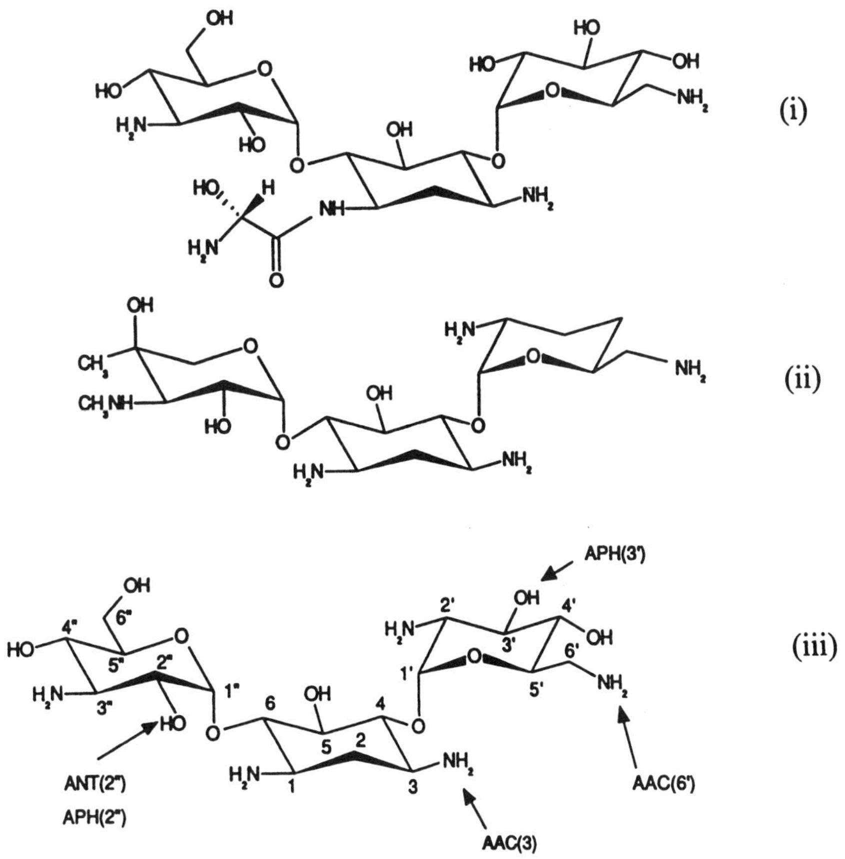

FIGURE 2. Structures of amikacin (*i*), gentamicin C1a (*ii*), and kanamycin B (*iii*). *Arrows* indicate sites of modification by resistance enzymes. Tobramycin is 3'-deoxykanamycin B.

aminoglycoside with the ribosome may vary, all aminoglycosides induce mistranslation on prokaryotic ribosomes (21, 24). Aminoglycosides of the gentamicin, kanamycin, and neomycin families induce misreading of mRNA codons during translation as well as inhibit translocation of mRNA (46). Streptomycin induces misreading of the genetic code in addition to inhibiting translational initiation (28, 46, 53, 112). By contrast, spectinomycin, a pure aminocyclitol with only bacteriostatic activity, does not cause translation errors but inhibits translocation. These findings support the notion that translational misreading is at least partly responsible for the bactericidal activity characteristic of aminoglycosides (see below). Studies in which aminoglycosides bound to ribosomes protect specific rRNA residues from chemical attack indicate that aminoglycosides make important contacts with a number of highly conserved and functionally significant nucleotides in 16S ribosomal RNA (87). Genetic analysis of acterial strains resistant to aminoglycosides obtained in vitro revealed mutations in rRNA that disrupt antibiotic-RNA interactions.

The numerous ribosomal proteins found in the intact ribosome can also affect the capacity of aminoglycosides to bind to rRNA. For example, the ribosomal protein S12, which makes several important contacts with 16S rRNA, is modified in streptomycin-resistant *Escherichia coli* mutants. Mutations

in many other ribosomal proteins may also contribute to streptomycin resistance (119). The aminoglycoside-resistance mutations lead to single amino acid substitutions in ribosomal proteins which result in lowered binding affinity for the drug (17). Such mutations are not confined to streptomycin, since similar mutations are responsible for resistance to other aminoglycosides, as well as to spectinomycin.

However, although the ribosome has been identified as a primary target for these agents, the precise mechanism by which aminoglycosides exert their bactericidal activity remains elusive, since these drugs manifest pleiotropic effects on bacterial cells. Among others, these effects include disruption of the outer membrane, irreversible uptake of the antibiotic, and blockade of initiation of DNA replication (83). Inhibition of protein biosynthesis and codon misreading alone do not adequately account for their bactericidal activity. For instance, chloramphenicol and most other inhibitors of ribosomal function, including spectinomycin, have only a bacteriostatic effect. Moreover, the amino acid ethionine, which is a strong inducer of codon misreading, is not bactericidal (105). Although, as yet, there is no completely satisfactory biochemical explanation for their bactericidal activity, to a large extent, rapid action at the outer membrane, irreversible binding to the ribosome, and incorporation of mistranslated proteins, as detailed below, can account for this activity. The various aminoglycosides also affect protein synthesis differently, and a "consensus" mechanism of action is unlikely.

To reach their cytoplasmic ribosomal target, aminoglycosides must initially cross the outer membrane (in Gram-negative organisms) and the cytoplasmic membrane (in Gram-negative and Gram-positive bacteria). In Gram-negative bacteria, the initial step involves ionic binding of the highly positively charged aminoglycosides to negatively charged phosphates, mainly in lipopolysaccharides (LPS) on the outer membrane surface. Much evidence from studies of *Pseudomonas aeruginosa* and *E. coli* indicate that uptake across the outer membrane may be due to a "self-promoted uptake" mechanism, analogous to that previously described for polycationic detergents such as polymyxin (56, 58). The divalent cations Ca^{2+} and Mg^{2+} function as salt bridges between adjacent LPS and phospholipids by serving as counterions for their phosphoryl groups (42, 104, 128). This arrangement appears to be essential for outer membrane integrity (78). The cationic aminoglycosides may act by competitively displacing the divalent cations that cross-bridge adjacent LPS molecules, thus making the outer membrane permeable and facilitating entry of the antibiotic (56, 66, 93). The rapid initial binding of the aminoglycosides to the cell may account for the rapid kinetics of killing and the fact that bacterial killing is a direct function of the aminoglycoside concentration in the growth medium. This characteristic of concentration- or dose-dependent killing explains the recent attention to giving the entire dose of aminoglycoside on a once-daily basis to maximize bacterial killing (49, 51, 94).

Aminoglycoside uptake across the cytoplasmic membrane in Gram-positive and Gram-negative organisms takes place in three steps. First, aminoglycosides bind electrostatically to the polar heads of phospholipids. In the case of Gram-positive bacteria, teichoic acids are also bound (73). Two not completely understood energy-dependent steps follow: a slow phase termed EDP-I followed by a more rapid phase, EDP-II. During EDP-I, the cellular transmembrane electrical potential is thought to furnish the driving force for aminoglycoside entry (13, 124). Thus, inhibitors of electron transport and oxidative phosphorylation can block EDP-I. EDP-II is characterized by rapid binding to the ribosome and accelerated aminoglycoside uptake across the cytoplasmic membrane (17, 124). EDP-II requires aminoglycoside-sensitive ribosomes engaged in active protein synthesis. A unifying theory of aminoglycoside uptake and bactericidal killing suggests that the increase in cell membrane permeability associated with EDP-II results from incorporation of mistranslated (nonsense) proteins into the cytoplasmic membrane due to aminoglycoside-induced codon misreading. These altered proteins may function as nonspecific channels that facilitate further aminoglycoside uptake (25–27). As a consequence, the ribosome is inhibited further, more aberrant proteins are incorporated, and so on. In fact, the presence of mistranslated proteins in the cell has been correlated with an increase in cell membrane permeability (16).

In short, although the bactericidal activity of aminoglycosides remains to be satisfactorily elucidated, a number of features seem to be required, including irreversible inhibition of the bacterial ribosome, codon misreading, incorporation of mistranslated proteins, and their direct disruptive action at the cell surface.

ANTIMICROBIAL ACTIVITY

As a group, the currently available agents of this class are primarily active against a variety of Gram-negative pathogens such as: *Acinetobacter* spp., *Citrobacter* spp., *Enterobacter* spp., *E. coli, Klebsiella* spp., *Serratia* spp., *Proteus* spp., *Morganella* spp. and *P. aeruginosa* and Gram-positive pathogens such as *Staphylococcus aureus*. However, significant differences in antimicrobial activity exist among the various aminoglycosides.

Although streptomycin has been used extensively for many years, emergence of resistance in *Mycobacterium tuberculosis* and aerobic Gram-negative bacilli as well as the relatively frequent occurrence of vestibular toxicity and the availability of less toxic antibiotics has greatly diminished its clinical utility. While the microbiologic activity of this agent is generally considered poor, it maintains adequate activity against *M. tuberculosis, Francisella tularensis, Yersinia pestis,* and *Brucella* spp. Among the aminoglycosides, streptomycin has the greatest in vitro activity against *M. tuberculosis.*

The development of kanamycin provided a broader spectrum of activity against Gram-negative bacilli, including streptomycin-resistant strains, but it is not active against *P. aeruginosa.* As with streptomycin, extensive use of kanamycin quickly led to emergence and widespread dissemination of kanamycin resistance among Enterobacteriaceae. The development of gentamicin, tobramycin, netilmicin, and amikacin further expanded the spectrum of antimicrobial activity of this class to cover many kanamycin-resistant strains, including *P. aeruginosa.*

Even though the antimicrobial spectra of gentamicin and tobramycin are quite similar, tobramycin is generally more active in vitro against *P. aeruginosa,* whereas gentamicin is more active against *Serratia.* However, these differences are probably not clinically significant. For the most part, the aminoglycoside-modifying enzymes that confer resistance to gentamicin and tobramycin (see "Mechanisms of Resistance") are similar. Since amikacin is usually a poor substrate for these enzymes, it is often active against Enterobacteriaceae resistant to gentamicin and tobramycin and is therefore often used when resistance to these aminoglycosides is prevalent. Amikacin is also active against many *Mycobacterium* spp. In addition, the aminoglycosides are also active against *Salmonella* and *Shigella* spp. and only moderately active against *N. gonorrhoeae* and *Haemophilus influenzae;* however, these antimicrobials are not recommended for infections caused by these species because of the availability of more effective and less toxic drugs.

Although aminoglycosides are generally active against staphylococci, they are not advocated as single agents for the treatment of staphylococcal infections. An aminoglycoside, usually gentamicin, is frequently administered in combination with a cell wall–active agent such as a β-lactam or vancomycin to provide synergy in the treatment of serious infections due to staphylococci, enterococci, and viridans streptococci.

While generalizations can be made concerning the antimicrobial spectrum of the aminoglycosides, wide variations in activity may be observed from institution to institution. As a result, an institutional-specific aminoglycoside antibiogram may be useful for selection of the optimal therapeutic agent.

MECHANISMS OF RESISTANCE

At least three mechanisms can confer resistance to the aminoglycosides: impaired drug uptake, mutations of the ribosome, and enzymatic modification of the drug. Intrinsic resistance is often due to impaired uptake, while acquired resistance usually results from acquisition of transposon- and plasmid-encoded modifying enzymes. Evidence suggests that the enzymes have arisen from both antibiotic-producing organisms and by mutation of resident host genes. Acquired resistance can also result from chromosomal mutations that lead to reduced drug affinity for the ribosomal target or decreased antibiotic uptake.

Decreased Aminoglycoside Uptake

Resistance secondary to decreased uptake can be either intrinsic to the species or acquired by chromosomal mutation. Resistance due to decreased uptake generally confers low-level, cross-resistance to all aminoglycosides. As mentioned, aminoglycoside uptake depends on the cell's electrical potential, which is established by the cell's electron transport system. This may explain the relative inherent resistance characteristic of electron-transport-deficient anaerobic organisms and the diminished susceptibility of facultative anaerobes such as enterococci, streptococci, and members of the family *Enterobacteriaceae* when grown anaerobically (12, 118). This may also explain why aminoglycoside efficacy is reduced in the anaerobic, low pH environment that exists in an infectious abscess. Acquired resistance to all aminoglycosides in bacteria with a variety of "energy deficiencies" is also probably due to decreased uptake (11). These strains frequently have impaired growth rates and grow as small colonies. Such strains may therefore be less pathogenic (11).

Since disruption of the outer membrane appears to be a prominent feature of their bactericidal activity, intrinsic differences in aminoglycoside activity among various species may, at least partly, be due to differences in the composition of their outer membranes. Chromosomal mutations may also confer resistance. For example, decreased gentamicin binding was demonstrated in an *E. coli* strain with a mutation in LPS phosphates (104). Furthermore, acquired resistance in *P. aeruginosa* has been associated with overproduction of the major outer membrane protein, H1. This protein may inhibit "self-promoted uptake" by substituting for Mg^{2+} (56, 59, 93).

Ribosomal Target Modification

As mentioned previously, genetic mutations that result in altered ribosomal protein S12 have been shown to determine high-level resistance to streptomycin (12). Although rare, streptomycin resistance due to ribosomal modification has been reported in clinical isolates of *N. gonorrhoeae* (81), *S. aureus* (74), *P. aeruginosa* (126), and *Enterococcus faecalis* (38). Mutational alterations in 16S rRNA and in ribosomal protein S12 have also been shown in streptomycin-resistant strains of *M. tuberculosis* (43).

Aminoglycoside-Modifying Enzymes

There are three classes of aminoglycoside-modifying enzymes: acetyltransferases (AACs), adenyltransferases/nucleotidyltransferases (ANTs), and phosphotransferases (APHs) (for a review, see reference 122). AAC enzymes acetylate amino groups; ANT and APH enzymes adenylylate and phosphorylate hydroxyl groups, respectively. The structures of typical aminoglycosides and their sites of enzymatic modification are shown in Figure 2. In general, only phosphorylating enzymes confer very high levels of resistance. The individual enzymes of a particular class are further divided into subclasses depending upon which hydroxyl or amino group substituents of an aminoglycoside they are capable of modifying. For example, the acetyltransferase class consists of three subclasses. Members of each subclass can acetylate amino groups at either the 3, 2', or 6' position: AAC(3), AAC(2'), and AAC(6'). A specific enzyme subclass consists of various enzyme types, each of which confers a different resistance phenotype. A Roman numeral designates each enzyme type. For example, AAC(3)-I determines resistance to gentamicin, AAC(3)-II determines resistance to gentamicin, netilmicin, and tobramycin, and AAC(3)-III determines resistance to gentamicin, tobramycin, and kanamycin. Finally, unique proteins (isoenzymes) that are functionally identical and confer identical resistance phenotypes are designated by an a, b, etc. (e.g., AAC(6')-Ia and AAC(6')-Ib).

A detailed description of the numerous aminoglycoside-modifying enzymes is beyond the scope of this chapter (for a review, see reference 122). Their epidemiology has become increasingly complicated because of the increasing complexity of aminoglycoside resistance mechanisms themselves in addition to often significant differences among different geographic regions and hospitals (for a review, see reference 86). A brief description of some of the more widespread enzymes is given below. While only a few aminoglycosides are used clinically, complete characterization of an aminoglycoside resistance phenotype (not considered below) requires testing the enzyme against a variety of aminoglycosides, a number of which are experimental and available only in the laboratory. At least five distinct AAC(3) resistance profiles have been characterized: the AAC(3)-I and II (see above) and more recently AAC(3)-VI (gentamicin, tobramycin, and netilmicin) (86). Among *Enterobacteriaceae*, AAC(3)-II (gentamicin, tobramycin, netilmicin) frequently occurs in combination with AAC(6')-I (tobramycin, netilmicin, kanamycin, and amikacin, see below), and therefore strains harboring the combination are resistant to gentamicin, tobramycin, netilmicin, kanamycin, and amikacin.

The AAC(6') enzymes, which are capable of modifying clinically important aminoglycosides are common but vary among different Gram-negative bacteria. The common AAC(6')-I enzyme determines resistance to tobramycin, netilmicin, kanamycin, and amikacin, but not to gentamicin.

At least nine different genes that encode type-I AAC(6′) enzymes (a-i) have been cloned. Depending on the geographic region, AAC(6′)-I can be found alone or, more commonly, combined with a gentamicin-modifying enzyme, particularly AAC(3)-II and ANT(2″)-I (86). ANT(2″)-I confers resistance to gentamicin, tobramycin, and kanamycin and is the principal mechanism observed in U.S. isolates of *Enterobacteriaceae*. Of particular note, the *aac(6′)-Ie* gene that is found in strains of *Staphylococcus* and *Enterococcus* encodes the amino-terminal portion of the bifunctional enzyme AAC(6′) + APH(2″). The bifunctional enzyme comprises an amino terminus that acetylates 6′-amino groups and a carboxy terminus that phosphorylates 2″-hydroxyl groups (111). The APH(2″) portion of this enzyme has much the same substrate profile as ANT(2″)-I, namely gentamicin, tobramycin, and kanamycin are modified, whereas the AAC(6′) enzyme has a spectrum of activity similar to the type-I AAC(6′) enzymes of Gram-negative bacteria. This explains why no aminoglycoside (except streptomycin in strains without high-level resistance to streptomycin) can be used against enterococci and staphylococci highly resistant to gentamicin. The bifunctional enzyme AAC(6′) + APH(2″) is the most common aminoglycoside-modifying enzyme in Gram-positive bacteria. In a recent survey of 898 aminoglycoside-resistant staphylococci, 42% of isolates had this enzyme as the sole cause of resistance, and 49% had it combined with one or more enzymes (86). *Enterococcus faecium* is unique among enterococci in that all strains examined produce a chromosomally encoded AAC(6′)-I enzyme (19). In these strains, the aminoglycosides are modified at a rate insufficient to confer high-level resistance, but sufficient to result in the loss of synergy between the aminoglycoside and cell wall inhibitors such as β-lactams and vancomycin.

The APH(3′) enzymes confer resistance to kanamycin and neomycin. At least seven APH(3′) enzymes have been identified and can be distinguished by the bacteria in which they are found. APH(3′)-I and II are found in many Gram-negative bacteria, APH(3′)-III in Gram-positive bacteria, APH(3′)-IV and V in *Bacillus* and *Streptomyces,* respectively. APH(3′)-VI occurs frequently in *Acinetobacter,* and APH(3′)-VII in *Campylobacter.* Although APH(3′)-I and II of Gram-negative bacteria can also modify the 3′-hydroxyl group of amikacin, it is not modified sufficiently to confer resistance in bacteria with normal aminoglycoside permeability. Susceptibility to amikacin is due to a significantly higher K_m of the enzyme for amikacin than for kanamycin or neomycin. Thus, an enzyme's catalytic efficiency for a particular substrate plays an important role in determining the resistance phenotype. By contrast, the APH(3′)-VI enzyme, which is seen primarily in *Acinetobacter* spp., confers resistance to amikacin (as well as kanamycin and neomycin) (86). The APH(3′)-III enzyme of Gram-positive bacteria also modifies kanamycin, neomycin, and amikacin. However, it does not always confer high-level resistance, especially to amikacin, and strains harboring this enzyme may test susceptible to this drug by standard susceptibility testing, resulting in a misleading resistance phenotype. Thus, in *S. aureus* and *Enterococcus* spp., although APH(3′)-III does not determine resistance to amikacin, synergy with β-lactams or vancomycin is abolished (23, 76).

Determining the enzyme content of a cell on the basis of the resistance phenotype can be difficult. As discussed, the fact that an antibiotic is a substrate for an enzyme in vitro does not necessarily imply that a bacterial strain producing that enzyme is resistant to the antibiotic. Furthermore, the level of resistance often depends significantly on the bacterial host. Enzymes that determine resistance to gentamicin or tobramycin in *P. aeruginosa* may not confer detectable resistance in *E. coli* (69). Such species-related phenotypic differences may be due to differences in gene copy number or expression or physiologic differences in membrane structure and antibiotic uptake (69). Finally, the resistance phenotype can also be complicated because strains can harbor multiple plasmids, with each plasmid encoding various enzymes with overlapping substrate ranges.

The genes that encode aminoglycoside-modifying enzymes are often carried on mobile genetic elements such as transposons and self-transferable plasmids that facilitate horizontal transfer among diverse genera. In addition, many of these genes can be located in so-called integrons, which assist in their dissemination. Integrons consist of an insertion site and an integrase gene that encodes a system for site-specific integration of one or more antibiotic resistance genes (18, 54, 123). The capacity of integrons to acquire multiple resistance determinants may partly explain the increased prevalence of multiply-aminoglycoside-resistant strains (109).

PHARMACOKINETIC DISPOSITION

Aminoglycosides are highly polar cations that are poorly absorbed from the gastrointestinal tract when administered orally. Although these agents are considered to have low oral bioavailability, prolonged use of large oral doses in patients with altered renal function may result in detectable aminoglycoside serum concentrations and development of toxicity. Aminoglycosides penetrate poorly through intact skin; however, when used as a topical antibacterial for large areas of denuded skin (i.e., burns) substantial systemic absorption may occur. Similarly, the use of aminoglycosides for local irrigation of closed body cavities may result in considerable systemic accumulation and potential toxicity. To achieve a consistent serum concentration profile, aminoglycosides must be given either intramuscularly or intravenously. Although the intramuscular route is well tolerated and results in essentially complete absorption, the intravenous route is preferred because of the rapid attainment and predictability of the concentration-versus-time profile.

The aminoglycosides are weakly bound to serum proteins and, therefore, freely distribute into the interstitial or extracellular fluid. The apparent volume of distribution of this class of agents is approximately 25% of the total body weight that corresponds to the estimated extracellular fluid volume. However, their volume of distribution, generally approximated at 0.25 to 0.3 L/kg, may be altered significantly in patients who are malnourished, obese, or pregnant, have ascites, or are in an intensive care unit (35, 134, 135, 138). In these patients, adjustment of the aminoglycoside dosage may be required. In general, the concentrations of the aminoglycosides attained in tissue and body fluids are lower than that obtained in serum, with the notable exceptions of the kidney, perilymph of the inner ear, and urine. Approximately 20 to 50% of the serum concentration can be achieved in bronchial fluid, sputum, pleural fluid, synovial fluid, and unobstructed bile. While excellent penetration has been noted in pulmonary tissue, prostate and bone penetration is poor. Penetration of aminoglycosides into cerebral spinal fluid in the presence of inflammation or in the fluid of the eye is inadequate and variable, therefore direct instillation is required to provide therapeutic concentrations for infection at these sites. In addition, since aminoglycosides cross the placenta, the potential risk to both the fetus and mother must be considered prior to use. Although low aminoglycoside bronchial fluid levels may be considered suboptimal, use of once-daily dosing substantially improves drug penetration into this fluid and reduces drug accumulation in the renal tissue, compared with conventional administration techniques (30, 113, 129).

The aminoglycosides are not metabolized, and biliary excretion is minimal. The kidneys, via glomerular filtration, are responsible for essentially all aminoglycoside elimination from the body. As a result, aminoglycoside clearance is proportional to glomerular filtration rate (139). This relationship not only assists with aminoglycoside dosage adjustments but may be useful in accurately estimating the glomerular filtration rate for adjustment of other therapeutic agents for which therapeutic drug monitoring is not routinely undertaken. In adults and children older than 6 months with normal renal function, the elimination half-life is approximately 2 to 3 h. In premature, low-birth-weight infants and those less than 1 week old, the half-life is 8 to 12 h; the half-life decreases to 5 h for neonates whose birth weight exceeds 2 kg. Since aminoglycosides are eliminated primarily by the renal route, substantial increases in the half-life should be expected in patients with renal dysfunction. As a result, the dosing regimen must be altered to minimize potentially toxic effects. Aminoglycosides can be removed from the systemic circulation by hemodialysis, peritoneal dialysis, or continuous hemofiltration techniques.

PHARMACODYNAMIC EFFECTS

Bactericidal Activity

Over the last decade much has been learned about the complex interactions involving the pathogen-drug-host triad (97). Much of this focus has revolved around a more complete understanding of the influence of drug concentration on bacterial cell death. The pharmacodynamic properties or the correlation of drug concentration and clinical effect (e.g., bacterial killing) of a specific antibiotic class are, therefore, an integration of two related areas—microbiologic activity and pharmacokinetics. A distinct pharmacodynamic profile exists for all antimicrobials, since the influence of drug concentration on the rate and extent of bactericidal activity differs among the various classes of drugs. A general pharmacodynamic division among antimicrobials occurs between the aminoglycosides and fluoroquinolones, whose bactericidal activity depends upon drug concentration, and the β-lactams, whose bactericidal activity is independent of drug concentration when the

concentration exceeds four times the minimum inhibitory concentration (MIC) (3, 20, 33, 34). This principle is illustrated in Figure 3, in which bacteria are exposed to various multiples of the MIC in vitro. In the case of ticarcillin, little difference in the rate of bactericidal activity is noted when its concentration exceeds four times the MIC. Therefore, this type of killing, which is characteristic of β-lactams, is termed nonconcentration or dose-independent bactericidal activity.

By contrast, when the same multiples of the MIC are studied with tobramycin and ciprofloxacin, the number of organisms decreases more rapidly with each rise in MIC interval. Since these agents eliminate bacteria more rapidly when their concentrations are appreciably above the MIC of the organism, their killing activity is referred to as concentration- or dose-dependent bactericidal activity. For the aminoglycosides, optimum bactericidal activity is achieved when the peak concentration is approximately 10 times the MIC (3, 25, 36, 70, 88).

Postantibiotic Effect

The postantibiotic effect (PAE) is characterized by continued suppression of bacterial growth after limited exposure of the bacteria to an antimicrobial agent. The aminoglycosides exhibit a PAE for both Gram-positive and Gram-negative bacteria; however, the duration is variable (0.5–7.5 h) and depends greatly on the study conditions (e.g., organism, duration of exposure) (3, 14, 22, 48, 61, 132, 140). Like bactericidal activity, the PAE of the aminoglycosides increases with increasing exposure concentrations (61, 132, 140).

Immunomodulation

Although much of the scientific focus on the pathogen-drug-host triad has been centered on either the pathogen-host or pathogen-drug interaction, antimicrobials may also directly interact with the immune system (60, 72, 130). Recently, Van Vlem et al. (129) reviewed the immunomodulating effects of numerous antimicrobials. Of the contemporary parenteral aminoglycosides, only gentamicin had sufficient data for determining an immunoregulatory profile. Although gentamicin

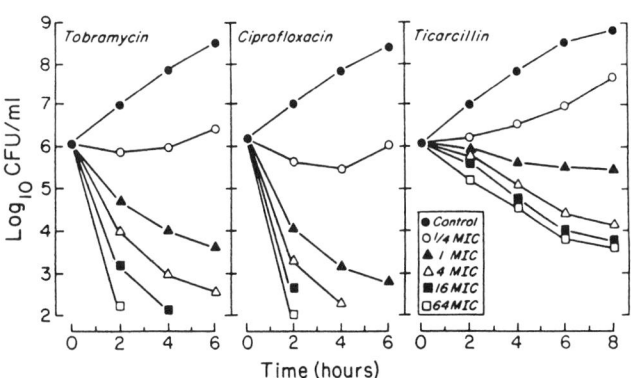

FIGURE 3. Influence of drug concentration on the bactericidal activity of tobramycin, ciprofloxacin and ticarcillin. (Reprinted from Craig WA, Ebert SC. Killing and regrowth of bacteria in vitro: a review. Scand J Infect Dis 1991;74(Suppl):63–70. With permission.)

had an apparent negative effect on phagocytosis, lymphocyte proliferation, delayed hypersensitivity, and natural killer-cell activity, the vast majority of the compiled studies were conducted in vitro, making extrapolation of these findings to clinical practice a matter of debate.

Correlation with Clinical Outcomes

Antimicrobial activity in vivo is a complex and multifactorial process. The antimicrobial must reach the target site, maintain adequate concentrations there, and remain long enough to interrupt the normal functions of the cell. This description of the antimicrobial's microbiologic activity is further integrated in the host by the drug disposition or pharmacokinetic profile (Figure 4). As a result of the complex interactions occurring among the pathogen, drug, and host, basing drug selection solely on microbiologic activity or pharmacokinetics often leads to an incorrect conclusion and inappropriate antimicrobial selection. Rather, pharmacodynamic integration of microbiologic activity and pharmacokinetics better defines an antibiotic's efficacy.

Since we cannot yet measure drug concentrations at the site of action (i.e., ribosome for the aminoglycosides), we commonly employ a microbiologic parameter such as the MIC or minimum bactericidal concentration (MBC) of the organism as the critical value in the interpretation of these pharmacodynamic relationships. When integrating the microbiologic activity and pharmacokinetics of an antimicrobial, several parameters appear to be significant constituents of drug efficacy. The pharmacokinetic parameter of AUC (area under the concentration-time curve), maximum observed concentration (C_{max} or peak), and half-life are often integrated with the MIC of the pathogen to produce pharmacodynamic parameters such as the AUC/MIC, peak:MIC ratio, and the time that the drug concentration remains above the MIC (time > MIC). For the aminoglycosides, the AUC/MIC, peak:MIC ratio, and time > MIC are all pharmacodynamic correlates of efficacy (3, 77). It is not surprising that several pharmacodynamic parameters have been related to efficacy with these agents since these parameters are all interrelated. Since the amount of drug delivered against the pathogen is proportional to the amount of drug delivered to the host (AUC), the AUC is the primary pharmacokinetic parameter associated with efficacy. However, since the AUC is a product of concentration and time under certain conditions, the influence of concentration appears to be a predominant factor, whereas under a different set of conditions, the exposure to the drug or the time > MIC may assume a larger role in bacterial eradication. For the aminoglycosides, which exhibit concentration-dependent killing and a relatively long PAE, the influence of the time > MIC is small compared with the influence of peak concentration.

As stated above, the aminoglycosides' rate and extent of bacterial killing depend more on the concentration of aminoglycoside than on length of exposure, and optimal bactericidal activity is achieved when the peak concentration is approximately 10 times the MIC. In addition, peak:MIC ratios of this magnitude may also diminish the likelihood of emergence of resistant organisms (10). Aminoglycoside peak:MIC ratios above 8 have been associated with treatment success (88–90). One study examined a total of 236 patients with Gram-negative bacterial infections. The maximal peak concentration (C_{max}) was defined as the highest concentration determined during therapy, and the mean peak concentration was calculated as the average of all values. Of the 188 patients who had a clinical response to therapy, the C_{max}/MIC average value was 8.5 ± 5.0 µg/mL, whereas the 48 nonresponders had a ratio of 5.5 ± 4.6 µg/mL ($P < .00001$). The average values for the mean peak:MIC ratios were 6.6 ± 3.9 µg/mL and 4.6 ± 3.6 µg/mL ($P < .0001$), respectively. Although these studies used fixed 8-h dosing intervals and were not originally designed to assess pharmacodynamic parameters and their relationship to outcome, these data provide the backbone for our commitment to the peak:MIC ratio in clinical practice. In another study by Keating et al. (70), response rates of 57, 67, and 85% were observed in neutropenic patients with mean serum aminoglycoside concentration:MIC ratios of 1:4, 4:10, and greater than 10, respectively. Other investigators have also shown a beneficial correlation between pharmacodynamic parameters and therapeutic outcomes in patients treated with aminoglycosides (1, 31, 68, 99).

TOXICITY
General

Since the introduction of the class into clinical practice, the major obstacle limiting their use is the potential for drug-related oto- and nephrotoxicity. Like many therapeutic agents, the aminoglycosides have been associated with a variety of adverse events (i.e., gastrointestinal, central nervous system, and hepatobiliary), which for the most part are mild and resolve upon discontinuation of therapy. The aminoglycosides rarely produce hypersensitivity reactions and are generally well tolerated at the site of administration when given by the intravenous, intramuscular, aerosol, or topical route. Although direct injection into the central nervous system and the eye is required to ensure adequate concentrations at the site of infection, these administration techniques have not been associated with local adverse events (i.e., seizures, hypersensitivity reaction).

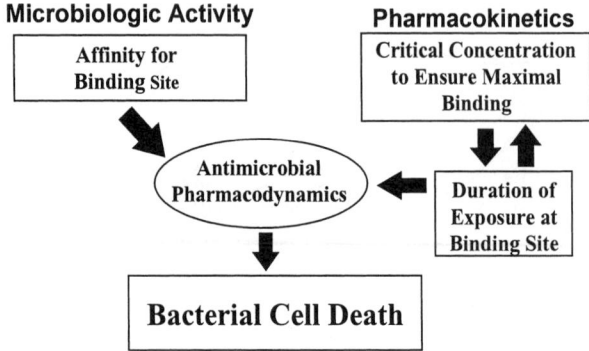

FIGURE 4. Antimicrobial pharmacodynamics: an integration of microbiologic activity and pharmacokinetics.

Neuromuscular Blockade

Although infrequent in contemporary clinical practice, the aminoglycosides have the potential to cause or exacerbate neuromuscular blockade. For this reason, it is recommended that parenteral agents be administered over at least 15 to 30 min and that direct instillation of highly concentrated aminoglycoside-containing solutions be avoided in the peritoneal cavity. Despite the concern for increased risk with administration of the high doses routinely used in once-daily dosing protocols, this adverse event has not been observed (49, 94). The risk of neuromuscular blockade may be increased in patients receiving concurrent neuromuscular blockers or calcium channel blockers or in those with myasthenia gravis, hypocalcemia, or hypomagnesium (64, 102). Neuromuscular blockade can usually be reversed by administration of calcium gluconate.

Ototoxicity

Although ototoxicity has long been recognized as a potential complication of aminoglycoside therapy, the precise mechanism of injury, delineation of risk factors, and a universally accepted definition remain elusive. As a result of discrepancies in both definition and sensitivity of testing, the reported incidence of ototoxicity has spanned a wide range (2–25%). Two distinct forms of ototoxicity, auditory and vestibular, have been reported and may occur alone or simultaneously. Ototoxicity is generally considered irreversible; however, hearing loss may be reversible if detected in the early stages of injury. Notwithstanding differences in clinical presentation, ototoxicity is believed to develop after destruction of the sensory hair cells in the cochlea and the vestibular labyrinth and is related to aminoglycoside-induced mitochondrial dysfunction (65).

Auditory toxicity often occurs at higher frequencies than those required for conversation (40). Consequently, patients are unlikely to complain of hearing loss until considerable auditory damage has been done. Auditory deficits may be preceded by tinnitus or a feeling of fullness in the ear; however, as described, toxicity can occur in the absence of clinical signs. Auditory toxicity is often bilateral, though unilateral disease does occur. Although early higher-frequency hearing impairment can be detected with audiometry and the progression to perceivable hearing loss may be avoided, practical application of this technique is often limited in the hospitalized patient because it is not easily employed at bedside (40). In addition, the lack of comparative baseline studies obtained prior to initiation of therapy and a universally accepted definition further complicate detection of drug-induced toxicity.

As with hearing loss, the initial symptoms of vestibular toxicity usually go unrecognized. Typical symptoms include nausea, vomiting, cold sweats, nystagmus, vertigo, and dizziness (41). Because of the nonspecific nature of its initial presentation, vestibular toxicity is often difficult to diagnose in the debilitated patient. However, vestibular dysfunction may progress to a severely disabling disorder in which the patient can neither walk nor stand unsupported (29). While considered to occur less frequently than hearing loss, vestibular toxicity is usually irreversible and may have a profound impact on the daily functional status of the affected patient.

While some studies suggest that a particular aminoglycoside may preferentially result in one form of ototoxicity rather than another, the lack of well-controlled comparative trials with sufficient power to detect such differences and the lack of analysis of risk factors for toxicity suggest that inherent differences among patients and treatment regimens are more likely determinants of toxicity than the specific agent (15, 67, 91).

Although serum concentration determinations may be useful for maintaining therapeutic concentrations, these data can only poorly predict development of ototoxicity. Moreover, significant toxicity can occur despite therapeutic concentrations. Despite these apparent difficulties, several investigators have reported that elevated trough concentrations are associated with ototoxicity (79, 80, 100). In addition, more-recent data obtained in an animal model suggest that ototoxicity is related to drug accumulation within the ear, not peak concentrations (2). These data suggest that a saturable transport system exists; therefore, higher peak concentrations should not result in increased ototoxicity. Thus, once-daily administration techniques may minimize drug accumulation and therefore drug-related toxicity. Although limited comparative data are available in humans that evaluate the vestibular effects of once-daily versus thrice-daily administration, Proctor et al. (108) reported no significant difference in risk between the two regimens.

Nephrotoxicity

Nephrotoxicity has been reported to occur in up to 60% of patients receiving aminoglycosides; however, the broad range of definitions used to define toxicity and the often-used requirement of 5 days of therapy prior to assessibility make the actual incidence difficult, if not impossible, to determine. In addition, since a rise in serum creatinine or a change in creatinine clearance are often used to determine toxicity, patients with these changes are considered to have aminoglycoside-induced toxicity, even though there may be a variety of additional causes of toxicity in these patients. This is particularly important when toxicity is defined by alterations in serum creatinine that occur within 3 days of initiation of therapy.

Although aminoglycoside-induced nephrotoxicity has been generally considered a severe adverse event, it is usually mild and reversible and rarely progresses to kidney dysfunction requiring dialysis (47). When dialysis has been required, multiple risk factors for severe renal failure have been present. Even though the nephrotoxic effects of this class have been widely described because of the availability of surrogate makers of toxicity (i.e. serum creatinine), the exact mechanism of toxicity is complex and not completely understood. Aminoglycosides are believed to accumulate in the lysosomes of the renal proximal tubule cells and, once in this acid environment, bind to the phospholipid bilayer and ultimately impair the activity of lysosomal phospholipidases (127). The reduced lysosomal function triggers a series of cascading effects that ultimately result in necrosis of the tubular cells and the clinical presentation of acute tubular necrosis manifested by nonoliguric renal failure after 5 to 7 days of therapy.

Several investigators have described risk factors for aminoglycoside-associated toxicity in a multiple-dose regimen.

These include advanced age, preexisting renal dysfunction, hypovolemia, shock, liver dysfunction, obesity, duration of therapy, use of concurrent nephrotoxic agents, and elevated peak/trough aminoglycoside concentrations (92, 117, 136). More recently, Bertino et al. (7) reported the incidence of, and risk factors for, toxicity in patients receiving pharmacokinetically individualized multiple-dose regimens. The overall incidence of toxicity in the study population of 1489 was 7.9%, despite modification of the dosing regimen on the basis of patient-specific pharmacokinetic parameters. In addition, multiple logistic regression revealed that trough concentration, duration of therapy, advanced age, leukemia, male gender, decreased albumin, ascites, and concurrent clindamycin, vancomycin, piperacillin, or cephalosporins were independent risk factors for nephrotoxicity. An assessment of risk factors for nephrotoxicity in patients receiving once-daily aminoglycosides revealed findings similar to those noted above, further reinforcing the notion that toxicity is a multifactorial process (98).

Like development of ototoxicity, development of nephrotoxicity is more likely due to intrinsic differences in patients, concurrent nephrotoxins, and duration of therapy than to a specific aminoglycoside (92). In addition, a saturable aminoglycoside transport system has been used to described the uptake of drug in the kidney. Therefore, less-frequent administration of aminoglycosides may minimize renal accumulation and nephrotoxicity (30, 131).

Although the possibility of aminoglycoside-induced oto- or nephrotoxicity cannot be completely eliminated, dosing regimens that minimize drug accumulation, therapeutic monitoring, recognition of risk factors, and moderate duration of therapy will lead to optimal therapeutic outcomes and minimize toxicity.

DOSAGE REGIMENS

At present, two parenteral aminoglycoside administration techniques are being used. The first (considered the conventional, or multiple-dose method) requires administration of multiple doses, usually every 8 to 12 h. The second method (the so-called once-daily, single-daily, or extended-interval dosing method) appears to be gaining routine acceptance for the treatment of patients requiring aminoglycoside therapy (120). Regardless of the dosing methodology used, the standard dosing regimen must be modified in patients exhibiting renal dysfunction. In addition, although the aminoglycosides undergo no biotransformation by the liver, severe liver disease as manifested by ascites results in markedly increased volumes of distribution and lower peak concentrations (135). Although higher dosages are generally required to achieve the desired concentrations, substantial changes in the intravascular volume status of the patient with liver disease make dosage adjustment difficult and often predispose such patients to drug-induced toxicities. Therefore, although the aminoglycosides are useful therapeutic agents in this population, the selection of potentially less toxic agents is advocated when possible.

Obesity may also alter the disposition of aminoglycosides, since they are distributed into the additional body water that accompanies adipose tissue. Therefore, dosage modification is required in this patient group because a dosing protocol based solely on ideal body weight would generally result in inadequate concentrations. Although dosing weight may be individualized for each patient, dosing is usually based on actual body weight unless the patient is obese (i.e., >20% over ideal body weight (IBW)). IBW is calculated by the following formulas:

$$IBW_{male} = 50 \text{ kg} + 2.3 \text{ kg for every inch over 5 feet}$$
$$IBW_{female} = 45.5 \text{ kg} + 2.3 \text{ kg for every inch over 5 feet}$$

For the obese patient, a dosing weight can be calculated using the following (121):

$$\text{Obese dosing weight} = IBW + 0.4$$
$$(\text{actual body weight} - IBW)$$

In pregnant patients, aminoglycosides generally have a greater volume of distribution and more rapid clearance; therefore, with standard regimens (Table 1), drug concentrations tend to be lower (35). However, despite lower concentrations, treatment outcomes are usually excellent because the pathogenic bacteria of the urogenital tract which are usually responsible for infection are highly susceptible, and as a result, dosage increases are not generally required. However, dosage adjustment may be required for infections caused by less-susceptible pathogens.

Multiple-Dose Regimens

Although guidelines have been established to assist in determining appropriate aminoglycoside dosage, several recent reviews have questioned the validity of conventional therapeutic drug monitoring protocols and the presently accepted therapeutic range (Table 1) on the basis of our current under-

---

TABLE 1 • Therapeutic Range and Dosage for Patients with Normal Renal Function Receiving Conventional Aminoglycoside Multiple-Dose Regimens

	Aminoglycoside Therapeutic Range (μg/mL)		
	Peak	Trough	Dosage for Normal Renal Function
Gentamicin	6–10	<2	1.7–2 mg/kg every 8 h
Tobramycin	6–10	<2	1.7–2 mg/kg every 8 h
Netilmicin	6–10	<2	1.7–2 mg/kg every 8 h
Amikacin	15–30	<5	5 mg/kg every 8 h or 7.5 mg/kg every 12 h
Streptomycin	15–30	<5	Generally 1.0 g every 24 h (range, 0.5–2.0 g)

TABLE 2 • Selection of Aminoglycoside Maintenance Dosing Using the Method of Sarubbi and Hull (1978)				
Creatinine Clearance (mL/min)	Half-life (h)	8-h Dose Interval	12-h Dose Interval	24-h Dose Interval
90	3.1	84%	—	—
80	3.4	80	91%	—
70	3.9	76	88	—
60	4.5	71	84	—
50	5.3	65	79	—
40	6.5	57	72	92%
30	8.4	48	63	86
25	9.9	43	57	81
20	11.9	37	50	75
17	13.6	33	46	70
15	15.1	31	42	67
12	17.9	27	37	61
10	20.4	24	34	56
7	25.9	19	28	47
5	31.5	16	23	41
2	46.8	11	16	30
0	69.3	8	11	21

standing of these agents (37, 84). Notwithstanding, adherence to these therapeutic ranges has become the standard of practice. Maintaining drug concentrations within these ranges requires dosage adjustment for patients with renal dysfunction, which can be accomplished either by the use of nomograms based on estimated creatinine clearance or by individualized pharmacokinetic dosing methods based on aminoglycoside disposition.

When aminoglycoside concentrations are not readily available, a variety of protocols that incorporate estimates of creatinine clearance can be used. Of these, the method of Sarubbi and Hull appears to have gained the widest acceptance (114). In this method, a loading dose of gentamicin or tobramycin (1–2 mg/kg) and amikacin (5–7.5 mg/kg) based on the IBW is given to adults with renal impairment. Once the loading dose has been calculated, the maintenance dose is a percentage of the chosen loading dose, depending on the desired dosing interval and the estimated creatinine clearance of the patient (Table 2). Creatinine clearance (Ccr) is estimated as follows:

$$Ccr_{male} = (140 - age)/serum\ creatinine$$
$$Ccr_{female} = 0.85 \times Ccr_{male}$$

Alternatively, one-half of the loading dose may be given at intervals equal to the estimated half-life. In addition, although the authors provide dosage adjustments for a Ccr as low as zero, it has been suggested that serum concentrations be used to assist with dosage adjustment in patients with an estimated Ccr below 10 mL/min.

When aminoglycoside concentration determinations are readily available, the preferred method of dosage adjustment is to individualize the regimen using the standard pharmacokinetic dosing principles described by Sawchuk et al. (115, 116).

Once-Daily Regimens

Although the clinical utility of once-daily dosing was recognized more than a decade ago, this approach was generally reserved for the treatment of urologic infections (75). However, with our current understanding of antimicrobial pharmacodynamics and a more precise knowledge of aminoglycoside-induced toxicity, once-daily dosing is now being used in the treatment of infectious processes other than urinary tract infections. This new methodology differs from conventional multiple-dose administration techniques in that the drug is administered in a single dose rather than in divided doses over a 24-h period (Figure 5). As shown in Figure 5, the body is presented with high peak serum concentrations that decline to provide a drug-free interval at the end of the dosing interval. As mentioned above, this new regimen enhances concentration-dependent killing and PAE by maximizing the peak concentration: MIC ratio for the infecting organism (see "Pharmacodynamic Effects"). In addition, this dosing approach may also reduce the occurrence of aminoglycoside-induced toxicity, because the drug-free interval minimizes drug accumulation (see "Toxicity").

Although many publications have reported apparently good clinical and toxicological outcomes using this new administration technique since the early 1990s (see reviews, references 32, 44, 49, 103, 106), considerable debate remains regarding the appropriateness of this approach (8, 51). Despite this controversy, many institutions have already initiated once-daily aminoglycoside protocols for adults (120). At present, the strategy for once-daily dosing is not consistent in the literature, as doses for gentamicin, tobramycin, and netilmicin have ranged from 3 to 7 mg/kg, whereas, the usual amikacin dose is 15 to 20 mg/kg. Dosing regimens that use doses below 6 mg/kg for gentamicin, tobramycin, and netilmicin base have converted the conventional mg/kg dose to once-daily administration. An alternative method of dosage determination has

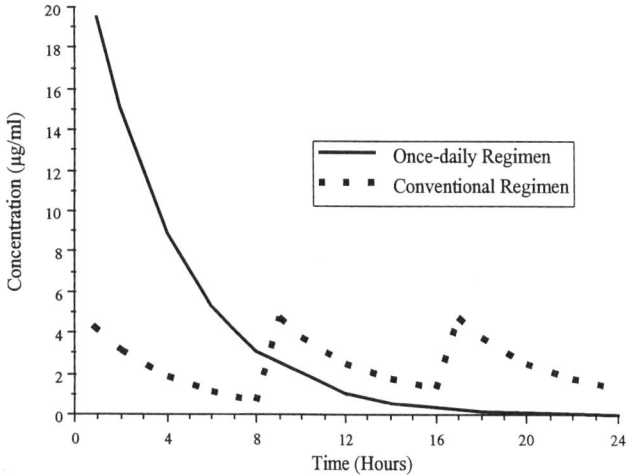

FIGURE 5. Simulated concentration versus time profile for once-daily (7 mg/kg q. 24 h) and conventional (1.5 mg/kg q. 8 h) regimens in patients with normal renal function.

been proposed, based on the pharmacokinetic and pharmacodynamic profile of these agents. In this method, intended to optimize the peak:MIC ratio in most clinical situations, a dose of 7 mg/kg of either gentamicin or tobramycin is given (94).

Like conventional regimens, once-daily protocols also require modification for patients with renal dysfunction. The Hartford Hospital program (Hartford, CT) uses a fixed dose with dosing-interval adjustments for patients with impaired renal function (94). The fixed dose is advocated because if reductions are made in the dose as a result of poor renal function, the subsequent serum concentrations would also be lower, ultimately resulting in a peak:MIC ratio that is less than optimal and quite possibly no better than conventional dosing regimens. Because of the high peak concentrations obtained and the drug-free period at the end of the dosing interval, standard peak and trough samples are no longer necessary. In this program, monitoring of the once-daily regimen is completed by obtaining a single random blood sample between 6 to 14 h after the start of the aminoglycoside infusion. This single serum concentration is used to determine the dosing interval, using a nomogram for once-daily dosing (Figure 6). If the level falls in the area designated *q24h,* the dosing interval is q24h (the same applies for the areas designated *q36h* and *q48h*). If the point is near the line, the longer interval is chosen to avoid drug accumulation and provide a sufficient drug-free period. If the random serum concentration is off (i.e., above) the nomogram between the 6 to 14 h time points, the scheduled therapy is stopped, and serial serum concentrations are followed to determine the appropriate time for the next dose (i.e., concentration < 1 μg/mL).

As a result of low toxicity, the short duration of therapy, and the excellent renal function of most patients, the initial random concentration (after the first or second dose) is not determined in patients (*a*) receiving 24-h dosing, (*b*) without concurrently administered nephrotoxic agents (e.g., amphotericin, cyclosporine, vancomycin), (*c*) without exposure to contrast media, (*d*) not quadriplegic nor amputee, (*e*) not in the intensive care unit, and (*f*) under 60 years of age. Although the initial random concentration may not be determined in eligible patients, the serum creatinine level should be monitored at 2- to 3-day intervals throughout the course of therapy. For patients who continue on the once-daily regimen (5 days), a random concentration is determined for the fifth day, and weekly thereafter. Even though an initial random concentration may no longer be necessary in many patients, it is necessary to obtain several samples from patients with changing creatinine clearances or those with significantly reduced creatinine clearance.

In addition to this method, Gilbert (49, 50, 52) also suggested a protocol for once-daily therapy in clinical practice. This protocol uses a 5 mg/kg gentamicin or tobramycin dose in patients without renal dysfunction. If dosage adjustment is required to compensate for diminished renal function, the dose and/or dosing interval may be modified to optimize therapy and minimize drug accumulation (Table 3). A similar modification in the daily dose was advocated by Prins et al. (107) for patients with renal dysfunction. Lastly, Begg et al. (4) suggested two methods to optimize once-daily dosing. The first, for patients with normal renal function, uses a graphical approach with target AUC values. The second method, for patients with renal dysfunction, uses two aminoglycoside serum concentrations and a target AUC value based on the 24-h AUC that would result from multiple-dose regimens for dosage modifications. Although these methods vary somewhat with regard to dose and/or interval for any given degree of renal failure, all of them reflect the need for dosage modification in the patient with renal disease. As yet, no method has been shown to be superior. Our current understanding of aminoglycoside-induced toxicity indicates that concern about the extended intervals and possible risk of increased toxicity in patients with reduced drug clearance should be no greater than that encountered with conventional dosing.

Even though once-daily regimens to date have used fixed mg/kg doses, dosage requirements may be guided by individualized pharmacokinetic methods similar to that for conventional dosing. While limited data exist, this individualized approach has not been shown to improve outcomes or toxicity in a small population of elderly patients (71); however, additional data are required to evaluate this individualized approach objectively.

At present, the once-daily approach has been used to treat a variety of infectious processes that would be amenable to therapy with traditional multiple-dose therapy (32, 44, 49, 103, 106). Although this approach has been used successfully in combination treatment of infective endocarditis due to streptococci and staphylococci (45, 94), it does not appear to be optimal for treatment of enterococcal endocarditis and should be avoided for this indication (82). In addition, although limited data exist with regard to once-daily dosing in the pediatric population, preliminary studies indicate that this approach is well tolerated and provides outcomes similar to those obtained by conventional dosing (96). In addition to op-

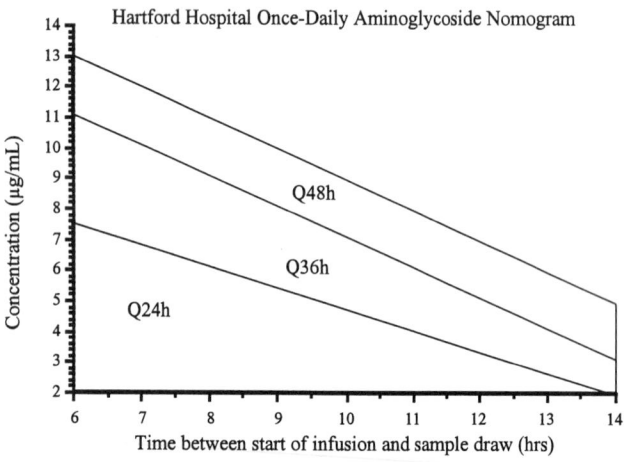

FIGURE 6. Once-daily aminoglycoside nomogram for the assessment of dosing interval using a mg/kg dose of gentamicin or tobramycin. (Reprinted from Nicolau DP, Freeman CD, Belliveau PP, Nightingale CH, Ross JW, Quintiliani R. Experience with a once-daily aminoglycoside program administered to 2,184 adult patients. Antimicrob Agents Chemother 1995;39:650–655. With permission.)

TABLE 3 • Suggested Once-Daily Dosage Requirements for Patients with Altered Renal Function			
Aminoglycoside	Creatinine Clearance (mL/min)	Dosage Interval (h)	Dose (mg/kg)
Gentamicin/ Tobramycin	>80	24	5.0
	70	24	4.0
	60	24	4.0
	50	24	3.5
	40	24	2.5
	30	24	2.5
	20	48	4.0
	10	48	3.0
	Hemodialysis[a]	48	2.0
Amikacin	>80	24	15
	70	24	12
	50	24	7.5
	30	24	4.0
	20	48	7.5
	10	48	4.0
	Hemodialysis[a]	48	5.0

Adapted from Gilbert DN, Bennett WM. Use of antimicrobial agents in renal failure. Infect Dis Clin North Am 1989;3:517–531.

[a]Administer posthemodialysis.

timizing the pharmacodynamic profile of the aminoglycosides and reducing the potential for drug-related toxicity, once-daily dosing may also have substantial potential economic advantages over traditional dosing techniques (63, 95, 103).

Dialysis Regimens

Since the aminoglycosides are removed during hemodialysis, a supplemental dose (1–2 mg/kg for gentamicin, tobramycin, and netilmicin; amikacin 5–7 mg/kg) is required after dialysis. Aminoglycosides are also cleared by continuous arteriovenous hemofiltration, a dialytic support technique used in critically ill patients (137). However, because of the instability of the critically ill patient and changing hemofiltration flow rates, multiple aminoglycoside concentration determinations are necessary for accurate determination of drug clearance and dosage requirements. Aminoglycosides may also be added to the peritoneal dialysis fluid of patients who develop peritonitis. These agents may be added to each peritoneal dialysis exchange (4–8 mg/L for gentamicin, tobramycin, and netilmicin; 6–12 mg/L for amikacin) or higher doses may be added to a single exchange per day (20 mg/L for gentamicin, tobramycin, and netilmicin; 60 mg/L for amikacin).

DRUG INTERACTIONS
Potentiation of Toxicity

Since the toxic effects of the aminoglycosides may be additive, concurrent or sequential administration of these agents in combination with other neuro-, oto-, or nephrotoxic agents (i.e., acyclovir, amphotericin B, vancomycin) should be avoided whenever possible. Because of the additive toxic potential of aminoglycosides, concurrent administration of other ototoxic agents such as ethacrynic acid, furosemide, urea, and mannitol

should also be avoided. In addition, concurrent use of an aminoglycoside and neuromuscular blockers, general anesthetics, or calcium channel blockers may potentiate neuromuscular blockade.

Aminoglycoside Deactivation

Although aminoglycosides are often administered with a β-lactam, the combination can potentially lead to inactivation of both drugs. The reaction is time- and concentration-dependent and occurs by nucleophilic opening of the β-lactam ring and acylation of an amino group of the aminoglycoside, resulting in a biologically inactive amide (5, 133). Of the aminoglycosides, gentamicin and tobramycin may be most susceptible to this effect. Clinically, this phenomenon is probably relevant only in situations where β-lactams accumulate to very high concentrations, as in patients with severe renal failure (9, 39, 110, 125). Additionally, in vivo degradation was not noted after administration of 7 mg/kg once-daily gentamicin and piperacillin/tazobactam given as either intermittent 4.5-g bolus doses at a 6- and 8-h dosing interval or 9.0 g continuously infused over 24 h in healthy subjects with normal renal function (62).

Owing to this interaction, aminoglycosides should never be mixed with β-lactams prior to systemic infusion or in peritoneal dialysis solutions. Likewise, serum samples taken for aminoglycoside concentration determinations should be assayed immediately or frozen to minimize deactivation and improve the accuracy of therapeutic drug monitoring.

Synergistic Combinations

Aminoglycosides exhibit synergistic bactericidal activity when given in combination with cell wall–active agents such as β-lactams and vancomycin. For example, enterococcal endocarditis should be treated with a combination of an aminoglycoside plus a penicillin or vancomycin, because by themselves, neither agent is bactericidal. However, when combination therapy is advocated to achieve synergy for Gram-negative organisms, maximally effective doses of both agents should be maintained because synergy does not occur universally for all pathogens to all β-lactam plus aminoglycoside combinations (55, 101).

CLINICAL INDICATIONS

The parenteral aminoglycosides, particularly gentamicin, tobramycin, and amikacin, have long been used empirically for treatment of febrile neutropenic patients or patients with serious nosocomial infection because of their broad spectrum of bactericidal activity against common and unusual *Enterobacteriaceae, P. aeruginosa,* and staphylococci. In addition, because of the widespread use of broad-spectrum β-lactam antibiotics and fluoroquinolones there has been a significant increase in the emergence of multiresistant bacteria, such as *Burkholderia cepacia, Stenotrophomonas maltophilia,* and enterococci, which often require treatment with a synergistic combination of an aminoglycoside with another antibiotic.

It is also apparent that the antipseudomonal β-lactams should not be given alone to treat systemic pseudomonal infections, since this organism often develops resistance under therapy. Thus, a well-established empirical approach to the febrile neutropenic patient remains an aminoglycoside given in combination with an antpseudomonal penicillin (e.g., ticarcillin, piperacillin, mezlocillin, ticarcillin/clavulanate, pipericillin/tazobactam) or cephalosporin (ceftazadime, cefepime). Although aminoglycosides are usually not used alone to treat staphylococcal infections because of the availability of less toxic agents, the fact that aminoglycosides have appreciable activity against staphylococci at least partly explains the frequent exclusion of a purely antistaphylococcal agent such as vancomycin to the initial empirical regimen for treatment of the febrile neutropenic patient. By contrast, in serious staphylococcal infections, a β-lactam or vancomycin is often combined with an aminoglycoside to take advantage of synergy and increased rates of killing. As mentioned above, although tobramycin is somewhat more active in vitro against *P. aeruginosa,* and gentamicin more active against *Serratia,* these differences are probably not clinically meaningful.

Aminoglycosides are commonly used in combination with a cell wall–active agent such as β-lactams and vancomycin in therapy for enterococcal endocarditis. Historically, although perhaps a third of patients were cured with penicillin alone, it became evident that significantly better clinical outcomes were achieved when an aminoglycoside was added to penicillin. The improved efficacy of combination therapy is due to bactericidal synergism between the two classes of antibiotics. Synergy is usually observed despite the fact that enterococci are inherently resistant to low levels of β-lactams and aminoglycosides. A notable exception is *E. faecium* which harbors a chromosomally encoded AAC(6′) aminoglycoside-modifying enzyme (see "Aminoglycoside-Modifying Enzymes"). Thus, only gentamicin or streptomycin can be considered for treatment of infections due to this species.

Enterococci resistant to high levels (MIC ≥ 2000 µg/mL) of aminoglycosides and concomitantly to synergism have unfortunately become increasingly common. Enterococci with high-level resistance (HLR) to gentamicin usually contain the bifunctional aminoglycoside-modifying enzyme AAC(6′)-APH(2″). This "fusion" enzyme abolishes synergy with all aminoglycosides except streptomycin. Although the bifunctional enzyme modifies amikacin and abolishes synergism with β-lactams and vancomycin, the modification does not confer an apparent resistant phenotype. For these reasons, amikacin should not be used against enterococci with HLR to gentamicin even if the strain is reported susceptible to amikacin. To avoid this pitfall, clinical microbiology laboratories often do not report amikacin susceptibilities for this genus. Thus, streptomycin (assuming no HLR to streptomycin) remains the only alternative aminoglycoside for strains highly resistant to gentamicin.

Aminoglycosides are often used for treatment of tuberculosis. Among the aminoglycosides, streptomycin has the greatest in vitro activity against *M. tuberculosis* and is considered among the first-line agents. The second-line agents kanamycin and amikacin are sometimes used in multidrug-resistant tuberculosis, which has become an extremely important health care concern worldwide, including the United States. *Mycobacterium avium* complex infections and other mycobacterioses other than tuberculosis also often include amikacin or streptomycin as part of a multidrug therapeutic regimen.

Paromomycin is an aminoglycoside that is too toxic to be administered intravenously and is not absorbed following oral administration. This agent has amebicidal and antihelminthic activities and is used to treat intestinal amebiasis and tapeworm infections. Paromomycin may also provide some benefit to AIDS patients with cryptosporidiosis.

Like paromomycin, neomycin is too toxic to be administered intravenously. It has been mostly used orally for the treatment of hepatic encephalopathy or along with erythromycin as a prophylactic regimen during colonic surgery. Streptomycin is also used alone for exotic infections due to *Francisella tularensis* (tularemia) and *Yersinia pestis* (plague) and in combination with a tetracycline for infections due to *Brucella* spp. (brucellosis).

REFERENCES

1. Anderson ET, Young LS, Hewitt WL. Simultaneous antibiotic levels in "breakthrough" gram-negative rod bacteremia. Am J Med 1976;61:493–497.
2. Beaubien AR, Ormsby E, Bayne A, Carrier K, Crossfield G, Downes M, Henri R, Hodgen M. Evidence that amikacin ototoxicity is related to total perilymph area under the concentration-time curve regardless of concentration. Antimicrob Agents Chemother 1991;35:1070–1074.
3. Begg EJ, Peddie BA, Chambers ST, Boswell DR. Comparison of gentamicin dosing regimens using an in-vitro model. J Antimicrob Chemother 1992;29:427–433.
4. Begg EJ, Barclay ML, Duffull SB. A suggested approach to once-daily aminoglycoside dosing. Br J Clin Pharmacol 1995;39:605–609.
5. Benveniste R, Davies J. Structure-activity relationships among the aminoglycoside antibiotics: role of hydroxyl and amino groups. Antimicrob Agents Chemother 1973;4:402–409.
6. Berk DP, Chalmers T. Deafness complicating antibiotic therapy of hepatic encephalopathy. Ann Intern Med 1970;73:393–396.
7. Bertino JS Jr, Booker LA, Franck PA, Jenkins PL, Nafziger AN. Incidence and significant risk factors for aminoglycoside-associated nephrotoxicity in patients dosed by using individualized pharmacokinetic monitoring. J Infect Dis 1993;167:173–179.
8. Bertino JS Jr, Rotschafer JC. Editorial response: single daily dosing of aminoglycosides—a concept whose time has not yet come. Clin Infect Dis 1997;24:820–823.
9. Blair DC, Duggan DO, Schroeder ET. Inactivation of amikacin and gentamicin by carbenicillin in patients with end-stage renal failure. Antimicrob Agents Chemother 1982;22:376–379.
10. Blaser J, Stone BB, Groner MC, Zinner SH. Comparative study with enoxacin and netilmicin in a pharmacodynamic model to determine importance of ratio of antibiotic peak concentration to MIC for bacterial activity and emergence of resistance. Antimicrob Agents Chemother 1987;31:1054–1060.
11. Bryan LE. Aminoglycoside resistance. In: Bryan LE, ed. Microbial resistance to drugs. Berlin: Springer-Verlag, 1989:35–57.
12. Bryan LE, Kowand SK, Van den Elzen HM. Mechanism of aminoglycoside antibiotic resistance in anaerobic bacteria: *Clostridium perfringens* and *Bacteroides fragilis*. Antimicrob Agents Chemother 1979;15:7–13.

13. Bryan LE, Van den Elzen HM. Effects of membrane energy mutations and cations on streptomycin and gentamicin accumulation by bacteria: a model for entry of streptomycin and gentamicin in susceptible and resistant bacteria. Antimicrob Agents Chemother 1977;12:163–177.

14. Bundtzen RW, Gerber AU, Cohn DL, Craig WA. Postantibiotic suppression of bacterial growth. Rev Infect Dis 1981;3:28–37.

15. Buring JE, Evans DA, Mayrent SL, Rosner B, Colton T, Hennekens CH. Randomized trials of aminoglycoside antibiotics: quantitative overview. Rev Infect Dis 1988;10:951–957.

16. Busse HJ, Wöstmann C, Bakker E. The bactericidal action of streptomycin: membrane permeabilization caused by the insertion of mistranslated proteins into the cytoplasmic membrane of *Escherichia coli* and subsequent caging of the antibiotic inside the cells due to degradation of these proteins. J Gen Microbiol 1992;138:551–561.

17. Chang, FN, Flaks JG. Binding of dihydrostreptomycin to *Escherichia coli* ribosomes: characteristics and equilibrium of the reaction. Antimicrob Agents Chemother 1972;2:294–307.

18. Collis CM, Hall R. Site-specific deletion and rearrangement of integron insert genes catalyzed by the integron DNA integrase. J Bacteriol 1992;174:1574–1585.

19. Costa Y, Galimand M, Leclercq R, Duval J, Courvalin P. Characterization of the chromosomal aac(6')-Ii gene specific for *Enterococcus faecium*. Antimicrob Agents Chemother 1993;37:1896–1903.

20. Craig WA, Ebert SC. Killing and regrowth of bacteria in vitro: a review. Scand J Infect Dis 1991;74(Suppl):63–70.

21. Cundliffe E. Antibiotics and prokaryotic ribosomes: action, interaction and resistance. In: Hill WE, Dahlberg A, Garrett RA, Moore PB, Schlessinger D, Warner JR, eds. Ribosomes. Washington, DC: American Society for Microbiology, 1990:479–490.

22. Daikos GL, Jackson GG, Lolans VT, Livermore DM. Adaptive resistance to aminoglycoside antibiotics from first-exposure down-regulation. J Infect Dis 1990;162:414–420.

23. Davies J. Aminoglycoside-aminocyclitol antibiotics and their modifying enzymes. In: Lorian V, ed. Antibiotics in laboratory medicine. Baltimore: Williams & Wilkens, 1991:691–713.

24. Davies JE. Resistance to aminoglycosides: mechanisms and frequency. Rev Infect Dis 1983;5:S261–266.

25. Davis BD. Mechanism of the bactericidal action of the aminoglycosides. Microbiol Rev 1987;51:341–350.

26. Davis BD. The lethal action of aminoglycosides. J Antimicrob Chemother 1988;22:1–3.

27. Davis BD, Chen L, Tai PC. Misread protein creates membrane channels: an essential step in the bactericidal action of aminoglycosides. Proc Natl Acad Sci USA 1986;83:6164–6168.

28. Davis BD, Tai PC, Wallace BJ. Complex interactions of antibiotics with the ribosome. In: Nomura M, Tissieres A, Lengyel P, eds. Ribosomes. New York: Cold Spring Harbor Laboratory, 1974:771–789.

29. Dayal VS, Smith EL, McCain WG. Cochlear and vestibular gentamicin toxicity. Arch Otolaryngol 1974;100:338–340.

30. De Broe ME, Verbist L, Verpooten GA. Influence of dosage schedule on renal cortical accumulation of amikacin and tobramycin in man. J Antimicrob Chemother 1991;27(Suppl C):41–47.

31. Deziel-Evans LM, Murphy JE, Martin LJ. Correlation of pharmacokinetic indices with therapeutic outcome in patients receiving aminoglycosides. Clin Pharm 1986;5:319–324.

32. Dew RB, Susla GM. Once-daily aminoglycoside treatment. Infect Dis Clin Pract 1996;5:12–24.

33. Drusano GL, Johnson DE, Rosen M, Standiford HC. Pharmacodynamics of a fluoroquinolone antimicrobial agent in a neutropenic rat model of Pseudomonas sepsis. Antimicrob Agents Chemother 1993;37:483–490.

34. Dudley MN. Pharmacodynamics and pharmacokinetics of antibiotics with special reference to the fluoroquinolones. Am J Med 1991;91(Suppl 6A):45S–50S.

35. Duff P. The aminoglycosides. Obstet Gynecol Clin North Am 1992;19:511–517.

36. Ebert SC, Craig WA. Pharmacodynamic properties of antibiotic: application to drug monitoring and dosage regimen design. Infect Control Hosp Epidemiol 1990;11:319–326.

37. Edwards DJ. Therapeutic drug monitoring of aminoglycosides and vancomycin: guidelines and controversies. J Pharm Pract 1991;4:211–224.

38. Eliopoulos GM, Farber BF, Murray BE, Wennersten C, Moellering RC Jr. Ribosomal resistance of clinical enterococcal isolates to streptomycin. Antimicrob Agents Chemother 1984;25: 398–399.

39. Ervin TR, Bullock WE, Nuttall CE. Inactivation of gentamicin by penicillins in patients with renal failure. Antimicrob Agents Chemother 1976;9:1004–1011.

40. Fausti SA, Henry JA, Scheffer HI, Olson DJ, Frey RH, McDonald WJ. High-frequency audiometric monitoring for early detection of aminoglycoside ototoxicity. J Infect Dis 1992;165: 1026–1032.

41. Federspil P. Drug-induced sudden hearing loss and vestibular disturbances. Adv Otorhinolaryngol 1981;27:144–158.

42. Ferris FG, Beveridge T. Physiochemical roles of soluble metal cations in the outer membrane of Escherichia coli K-12 lipopolysaccharide. Can J Microbiol 1986;32:52–55.

43. Finken M, Kirschner P, Meir A, Wrede A, Böttger EC. Molecular basis of streptomycin resistance in *Mycobacterium tuberculosis:* alterations of the ribosomal protein S12 gene and point mutations within a functional 16S ribosomal RNA pseudoknot. Mol Microbiol 1993;9:1239–1246.

44. Freeman CD, Nicolau DP, Belliveau PP, Nightingale CH. Oncedaily aminoglycosides: review and recommendations for clinical practice. J Antimicrob Chemother 1997;39:677–686.

45. Francioli P, Ruch W, Stamboulian D, International Infective Endocarditis Study Group. Treatment of streptococcal endocarditis with a single daily dose of ceftriaxone and netilmicin for 14 days: a prospective multicenter study. Clin Infect Dis 1995;21: 1406–1410.

46. Gale EF, Cundliffe E, Reynolds PE, Richmond MH, Waring MJ. The molecular basis of antibiotic action. London: John Wiley & Sons, 1981.

47. Garrison MW, Zaske DE, Rotschafer JC. Aminoglycosides: another perspective. DICP, Ann Pharmacother 1990;24:267–272.

48. Gerber AU, Wiprachtiger P, Stettler-Spichiger U, Lebek G. Constant infusion vs. intermittent doses of gentamicin against *Pseudomonas aeruginosa* in vitro. J Infect Dis 1982;145:554–560.

49. Gilbert DN. Once-daily aminoglycoside therapy. Antimicrob Agents Chemother 1991;35:399–405.

50. Gilbert DN. Aminoglycosides. In: Mandell GL, Bennett JE, Dolin R, eds. Principles and practice of infectious diseases. New York: Churchill Livingstone, 1995:281.

51. Gilbert DN. Editorial response: meta-analyses are no longer required for determining the efficacy of single daily dosing of aminoglycosides. Clin Infect Dis 1997;24:816–819.

52. Gilbert DN, Bennett WM. Use of antimicrobial agents in renal failure. Infect Dis Clin North Am 1989;3:517–531.

53. Gorini L. Streptomycin and misreading of the genetic code. In:

Nomura M, Tissieres A, Lengyel P, eds. Ribosomes. New York: Cold Spring Harbor Laboratory, 1974:791–803.

54. Hall RM, Brooks DE, Stokes HW. Site-specific insertion of genes into integrons: role of the 59-base element and determination of the recombination cross-over point. Mol Microbiol 1991; 5:1941–1959.

55. Hallander HO, Donrbusch K, Gezelius L, Jacobson K, Karlsson I. Synergism between aminoglycosides and cephalosporins with anti-pseudomonal activity: interaction index and killing curve method. Antimicrob Agents Chemother 1982;22:743–752.

56. Hancock REW. Aminoglycoside uptake and mode of action—with special reference to streptomycin and gentamicin. J Antimicrob Chemother 1981;8:249–276.

57. Hancock REW. Alterations in outer membrane permeability. Ann Rev Microbiol 1984;38:237–264.

58. Hancock REW, Farmer SW, Li Z, Poole K. Interaction of aminoglycosides with the outer membranes and purified lipopolysaccharide and OmpF porin of Escherichia coli. Antimicrob Agents Chemother 1991;35:1309–1314.

59. Hancock REW, Raffle VJ, Nicas TI. Involvement of the outer membrane in gentamicin and streptomycin uptake and killing in Pseudomonas aeruginosa. Antimicrob Agents Chemother 1981; 19:777–785.

60. Hauser WE, Remington JS. Effect of antibiotics on the immune response. Am J Med 1982;72:711–716.

61. Hessen MT, Pistsakis PG, Levison ME. Postantibiotic effect of penicillin plus gentamicin versus Enterococcus faecalis in vitro and in vivo. Antimicrob Agents Chemother 1989;33: 608–611.

62. Hitt CM, Patel KB, Nicolau DP, Zhu Z, Nightingale CH. Influence of piperacillin/tazobactam on the pharmacokinetics of once-daily gentamicin. Am J Health Syst Pharm 1997; 54:2704–2708.

63. Hitt CM, Klepser ME, Nightingale CH, Quintiliani R, Nicolau DP. Pharmacoeconomic impact of a once-daily aminoglycoside administration. Pharmacotherapy 1997;17:810–814.

64. Hokkanen E. The aggravating effect of some antibiotics on the neuromuscular blockade in myasthenia gravis. Acta Neurol Scand 1964;40:346–352.

65. Hutchin T, Cortopassi G. Proposed molecular and cellular mechanism for aminoglycoside ototoxicity. Antimicrob Agents Chemother 1994;38:2517–2520.

66. Kadurugamuwa JL, Clarke AJ, Beveridge TJ. Surface action of gentamicin on Pseudomonas aeruginosa. J Bacteriol 1993;175: 5798–5805.

67. Kahlmeter G, Dahlager JI. Aminoglycoside toxicity—a review of clinical studies published between 1975 and 1982. J Antimicrob Chemother 1984;13(Suppl A):9–22.

68. Kashuba ADM, Nafziger AN, Drusano GL, Bertino JS. Early optimization of aminoglycoside pharmacokinetic goals reduces time to therapeutic response in Gram-negative pneumonia [Abstract]. In: Program and abstracts of the 36th ICAAC Conference of the American Society for Microbiology, New Orleans, LA, Sep 15–18, 1996. Washington, DC: American Society for Microbiology, 1996:A-100.

69. Kato T, Sato Y, Iyobe S, Mitsuhashi S. Plasmid-mediated gentamicin resistance of Pseudomonas aeruginosa and its lack of expression in Escherichia coli. Antimicrob Agents Chemother 1982;22:358–363.

70. Keating MF, Bodey GP, Valdivieso M, Rodriguez V. A randomized comparative trial of three aminoglycosides—comparison of continuous infusions of gentamicin, amikacin, and sisomicin com-

bined with carbenicillin in the treatment of infections in neutropenic patients with malignancies. Medicine 1979;58:159–170.

71. Koo J, Tight R, Rajkumar V, Hawa Z. Comparison of once-daily versus pharmacokinetic dosing of aminoglycosides in elderly patients. Am J Med 1996;101:177–183.

72. Korzeniowski OM. Effects of antibiotics on the mammalian immune system. Infect Dis Clin North Am 1989;3:469–478.

73. Kusser W, Zimmer K, Fiedler F. Characteristics of the binding of aminoglycoside antibiotics to teichoic acids. Eur J Biochem 1985;151:601–605.

74. Lacey RW, Chopra I. Evidence for mutation to streptomycin resistance in clinical strains of Staphylococcus aureus. J Gen Microbiol 1972;73:175–180.

75. Landes RR. Single daily doses of tobramycin in therapy of urinary tract infections. J Infect Dis 1976;134(Suppl):S142–S145.

76. Leclercq R, Dutka-Malen S, Brisson-Noël A, Molinas C, Derlot E, Arthur M, Duval J, Courvalin P. Resistance of enterococci to aminoglycosides and glycopeptides. Clin Infect Dis 1992;15: 495–501.

77. Leggett JE, Ebert S, Fantin B, Craig WA. Comparative dose-effect relationships at several dosing intervals for β-lactam, aminoglycoside and quinolone antibiotics against gram-negative bacilli in murine thigh-infection and pneumonitis models. Scand J Infect Dis 1991;74:179–184.

78. Leive L. The barrier function of the gram-negative cell envelope. Ann NY Acad Sci 1974;235:109–127.

79. Lerner SA, Schmitt BA, Seligsohn R, Matz GJ. Comparative study of ototoxicity and nephrotoxicity in patients randomly assigned to treatment with amikacin or gentamicin. Am J Med 1986;80(Suppl 6B):98–104.

80. Line DH, Poole GW, Waterworth PM. Serum streptomycin levels and dizziness. Tubercle 1970;51:76–81.

81. Maness MJ, Foster GC, Sparling PF. Ribosomal resistance to streptomycin and spectinomycin in Neisseria gonorrhoeae. J Bacteriol 1974;120:1293–1299.

82. Marangos MN, Nicolau DP, Quintiliani R, Nightingale CH. Influence of gentamicin dosing interval on the efficacy of penicillin containing regimens in experimental Enterococcus faecalis endocarditis. J Antimicrob Chemother 1997;39:519–522.

83. Matsunaga K, Yamaki H, Nishimura T, Tanaka N. Inhibition of DNA replication initiation by aminoglycoside antibiotics. Antimicrob Agents Chemother 1986;30:468–474.

84. McCormack JP, Jewesson PJ. A critical reevaluation of the therapeutic range of aminoglycosides. Clin Infect Dis 1992;14: 320–329.

85. Miller GH, Aminoglycoside Resistance Study Groups. Increasing complexity of aminoglycoside resistance mechanisms in gram-negative bacteria. APUA Newslett 1994;Summer:12.

86. Miller GH, Sabatelli FJ, Hare RS, Glupczynski Y, Mackey P, Shlaes D, Shimizu K, Shaw KJ, Aminoglycoside Resistance Study Groups. The most frequent aminoglycoside resistance mechanisms—changes with time and geographic area: a reflection of aminoglycoside usage patterns. Clin Infect Dis 1997;24(Suppl 1): S46–S62.

87. Moazed D, Noller HF. Interaction of antibiotics with functional sites in 16S ribosomal RNA. Nature 1987;327:389–394.

88. Moore RD, Lietman PS, Smith CR. Clinical response to aminoglycoside therapy: importance of the ratio of peak concentration to minimal inhibitory concentration. J Infect Dis 1987;155:93–99.

89. Moore RD, Smith CR, Lietman PS. Association of aminoglycoside plasma levels with therapeutic outcome in gram-negative pneumonia. Am J Med 1984;77:657–662.

90. Moore RD, Smith CR, Lietman PS. The association of aminoglycoside plasma levels with mortality in patients with gram-negative bacteremia. J Infect Dis 1984;149:443–448.

91. Moore RD, Smith CR, Lietman PS. Risk factors for the development of auditory toxicity in patients receiving. J Infect Dis 1984;149:23–30.

92. Moore RD, Smith CR, Lipsky JJ, Mellitis ED, Lietman PS. Risk factors for nephrotoxicity in patients treated with aminoglycosides. Ann Intern Med 1984;100:352–357.

93. Nicas TI, Hancock REW. Outer membrane protein H1 of *Pseudomonas aeruginosa:* involvement in adaptive and mutational resistance to ethylenediaminetetraacetate, polymixin B, and gentamicin. J Bacteriol 1980;143:872–878.

94. Nicolau DP, Freeman CD, Belliveau PP, Nightingale CH, Ross JW, Quintiliani R. Experience with a once-daily aminoglycoside program administered to 2,184 adult patients. Antimicrob Agents Chemother 1995;39:650–655.

95. Nicolau DP, Wu AHB, Finocchiaro S, Udeh E, Chow MSS, Quintiliani R, Nightingale CH. Once-daily aminoglycoside dosing: impact on requests for therapeutic drug monitoring. Ther Drug Monit 1996;18:263–266.

96. Nicolau DP, Quintiliani R, Nightingale CH. Once-a-day aminoglycoside therapy. Rep Pediatr Infect Dis 1997;7:28.

97. Nightingale CH, Quintiliani R, Nicolau DP. Intelligent dosing of antimicrobials. In: Remington JS, Swartz MN, eds. Current clinical topics in infectious diseases. Cambridge, MA: Blackwell Scientific 1994;14:252–265.

98. Nodoushani M, Nicolau DP, Hitt CH, Quintiliani R, Nightingale CH. Evaluation of nephrotoxicity associated with once-daily aminoglycoside administration. J Pharm Tech 1997;131:258–262.

99. Noone P, Parsons TMC, Pattison JR, Slack RCB, Garfield-Davies D, Hughes K. Experience in monitoring gentamicin therapy during treatment of serious gram-negative sepsis. Br Med J 1974;1:477–481.

100. Nordström L, Banck G, Belfrage S, Juhlin I, Tjernström O, Toremalm NG. Prospective study of the ototoxicity of gentamicin. Acta Pathol Microbiol Scand [B] Microbiol Immunol 1973;81(Suppl 241):58–61.

101. Owens RC Jr, Banevicius MA, Nicolau DP, Nightingale CH, Quintiliani R. Synergistic activity between tobramycin and selected β-lactams against 75 Gram-negative nosocomial isolates. Antimicrob Agents Chemother 1997;41:2586–2588.

102. Paradelis AG, Triantaphyllidis CJ, Mironidou M, Crassaris LG, Karachalios DN, Giala MM. Interaction of aminoglycoside antibiotics and calcium channel blockers at the neuromuscular junction. Methods Find Exp Clin Pharmacol 1988;10:687–690.

103. Parker SE, Davey PG. Once-daily aminoglycoside administration in gram-negative sepsis: economic and practical aspects. PharmacoEconomics 1995;7:393–402.

104. Peterson AA, Fesik SW, McGroaty EJ. Decreased binding of antibiotics to lipopolysaccharides from polymyxin-resistant strains of *Escherichia coli* and *Salmonella typhimurium.* Antimicrob Agents Chemother 1987;31:230–237.

105. Pine MJ. Comparative physiological effects of incorporated amino acid analogs in *Escherichia coli.* Antimicrob Agents Chemother 1978;13:676–685.

106. Preston SL, Briceland LL. Single daily dosing of aminoglycosides. Pharmacother 1995;15:297–316.

107. Prins JM, Koopmans RP, Buller HR, Kuijper EJ, Speelman P. Easier monitoring of aminoglycoside therapy with once-daily dosing schedules. Eur J Clin Microbiol Infect Dis 1995;14:531–535.

108. Proctor L, Petty B, Lietman P, Thakor R, Glackin R, Shimizu H. A study of potential vestibulotoxicity effects of once daily versus thrice daily administration of tobramycin. Laryngoscope 1987;97:1443–1449.

109. Rather PN, Mann P, Hare RS, Miller GH, Sabatelli FJ, Mierzwa R, Shaw K. Characterization and DNA sequence analysis of an AAC(3)-VI gene from *Enterobacter cloacae.* 30th Interscience Conference Antimicrobial Agents and Chemotherapy, Atlanta, GA, 1990.

110. Riff L, Jackson GG. Laboratory and clinical conditions for gentamicin inactivation by carbenicillin. Ann Intern Med 1972;130:887–891.

111. Rouch PN, Byrne ME, Kong YC, Skurray RA. The aacA-aphD gentamicin and kanamycin resistance determinant of Tn 4001 from *Staphylococcus aureus:* expression and nucleotide sequence analysis. J Gen Microbiol 1987;133:3039–3052.

112. Ruusala T, Kurland CG. Streptomycin preferentially perturbs ribosomal proofreading. Mol Genet 1984;198:100–104.

113. Santre C, Georges H, Jacquier JM, Leroy O, Beuscart C, Buguin D, Beaucaire G. Amikacin levels in bronchial secretions of 10 pneumonia patients with respiratory support treated once daily versus twice daily. Antimicrob Agents Chemother 1995;39:264–267.

114. Sarubbi FA Jr, Hull JH. Amikacin serum concentrations: prediction of levels and dosage guidelines. Ann Intern Med 1978;89:612–618.

115. Sawchuk RJ, Zaske DE. Pharmacokinetics of dosing regimens which utilize multiple intravenous infusions: gentamicin in burn patients. J Pharmacokinet Biopharm 1976;4:183–195.

116. Sawchuk RJ, Zaske DE, Cipolle RJ, Wargin WA, Strate RG. Kinetic model for gentamicin dosing with the use of individual patient parameters. Clin Pharmacol Ther 1977;21:362–369.

117. Sawyers CL, Moore RD, Lerner SA, Smith CR. A model for predicting nephrotoxicity with aminoglycosides. J Infect Dis 1986;153:1062–1068.

118. Schlessinger D. Failure of aminoglycoside antibiotics to kill anaerobic, low-pH, and resistant cultures. Clin Microbiol Rev 1988;1:54–59.

119. Schreiner G, Nierhaus KH. Protein involved in the binding of dihydrostreptomycin to ribosomes of *Escherichia coli.* J Mol Biol 1973;81:71–82.

120. Schumock GT, Raber SR, Crawford SY, Naderer OJ, Rodvold KA. National survey of once-daily dosing of aminoglycoside antibiotics. Pharmacotherapy 1995;15:201–209.

121. Schwartz SN, Pazin GJ, Lyon JA, Ho M, Pasculle AW. A controlled investigation of the pharmacokinetics of gentamicin and tobramycin in obese subjects. J Infect Dis 1978;138:499–505

122. Shaw KJ, Rather PN, Hare RS, Miller GH. Molecular genetics of aminoglycoside resistance genes and familial relationships of the aminoglycoside-modifying enzymes. Microbiol Rev 1993;57:138–163.

123. Stokes HW, Hall RM. A novel family of potentially mobile DNA elements encoding site-specific gene-integration functions: integrons. Mol Microbiol 1989;3:1669–1683.

123a.Taber HW, Mueller JP, Miller PF, Arrow AS. Bacterial uptake of aminoglycoside antibiotics. Microbiol Rev 1987;51:439–457.

124. Thompson MIB, Russo ME, Saxon BJ, Atkinthor E, Matsen MJ. Gentamicin inactivation by piperacillin or carbenicillin in patients with end-stage renal disease. Antimicrob Agents Chemother 1982;21:268–273.

125. Tseng, JL, Bryan LE, Van Den Elzen HM. Mechanisms and spectrum of streptomycin resistance in a natural population of

Pseudomonas aeruginosa. Antimicrob Agents Chemother 1972;2:136–141.

126. Tulkens PM. Experimental studies on the nephrotoxicity of aminoglycosides at low doses: mechanisms and perspectives. Am J Med 1986;80(Suppl 6B):105–114.

127. Vaara M. Agents that increase the permeability of the cell envelope of *Pseudomonas aeruginosa.* Microbiol Rev 1992;56: 395–411.

128. Valcke YJ, Vogelaers DP, Colardyn FA, Pauwels RA. Penetration of netilmicin in the lower respiratory tract after once-daily dosing. Chest 1992;101:1028–1032.

129. Van Vlem B, Vanholder R, De Paepe P, Vogelaers D, Ringoir S. Immunomodulating effects of antibiotics: literature review. Infect 1996;24:275–290.

130. Verpooten GA, Giuliano RA, Verbist L, Eestermans G, De Broe ME. Once daily dosing decreases the accumulation of gentamicin and netilmicin. Clin Pharmacol Ther 1989;45: 22–27.

131. Vogelman B, Gudmundsson S, Turnidge J, Leggett J, Craig WA. In vivo postantibiotic effect in a thigh infection model in neutropenic mice. J Infect Dis 1988;157:287–298.

132. Waitz JA, Drube CG, Moss EL Jr, Oden EM, Bailey JV, Wagman GH, Weinstein MJ. Biological aspects of the interaction

between gentamicin and carbenicillin. J Antibiot 1972;25: 219–225.

133. Watling SM, Dasta JF. Aminoglycoside dosing considerations in intensive care unit patients. Ann Pharmacother 1993;27:351–357.

134. Westphal JF, Brogard JM. Clinical pharmacokinetics of newer antibacterial agents in liver disease. Clin Pharmacokinet 1993; 24:46–58.

136. Whelton A. Therapeutic initiatives for avoidance of aminoglycoside toxicity. J Clin Pharmacol 1985;25:67–81.

137. Zarowitz BJ, Anandan JV, Dumler F, Jayashankar J, Levin N. Continuous arteriovenous hemofiltration of aminoglycoside antibiotics in critically ill patients. J Clin Pharmacol 1986; 26:686–689.

138. Zarowitz BJ, Pilla AM, Popovich J Jr. Expanded gentamicin volume of distribution in patients with indicators of malnutrition. Clin Pharm 1990;9:40–44.

139. Zarowitz BJ, Robert S, Peterson EL. Prediction of glomerular filtration rate using aminoglycoside clearance in critically ill medical patients. Ann Pharmacother 1992;26:1205–1210.

140. Zhanel GG, Hoban DJ, Harding GKM. The postantibiotic effect: a review of in-vitro and in-vivo data. Ann Pharmacother 1991;25:153–163.

Antimycobacterial Agents: Cycloserine

Shaun E. Berning and Charles A. Peloquin

Chemical Structure

Cycloserine was isolated both from *Streptomyces orchidaceus* by Harned and Kropp and from *Streptomyces garyphalus* by Harris and colleagues in 1955 (10, 18, 24, 32). It is a white crystalline powder with a chemical structure of D-4-amino-*s*-isoxazolidone or D-4-aminoisoxalidine-3-one. It is highly soluble in water and has a low molecular weight of 102.09. These properties allow cycloserine to diffuse readily into body tissues (10, 32). Cycloserine is unstable in an acid or neutral environment but stable in an alkaline environment.

Terizidone, an agent not available in the United States, is formed by reaction of two cycloserine molecules with terephthalaldehyde(24). Terizidone is similar to cycloserine in antibacterial activity and toxicity profile.

Structure-Activity Relationships

Cycloserine is a structural analogue of D-alanine. Many analogues have been synthesized, but these were either inactive or less active than cycloserine (35, 36).

ANTIMICROBIAL ACTIVITY
Spectrum

Cycloserine's greatest in vitro activity is against *Mycobacterium tuberculosis,* with minimal inhibitory concentrations

(MICs) of 6.2 to 25 μg/mL in liquid media and Lowenstein-Jensen medium. Cycloserine is also active against other species of mycobacteria such as *M. kansasii, M. intracellulare,* and *M. avium;* 31% of *M. avium* strains are susceptible to cycloserine 30 μg/mL by the proportion method in 7H11 agar plates (15, 18).

Cycloserine possesses marginal activity against other organisms such as *Staphylococcus aureus* and some Gram-negative bacilli, such as *Escherichia coli.* Although the MIC of cycloserine to *E. coli* often exceeds 50 μg/mL, concentrations higher than this are achieved in the urine at standard doses. Thus, it has been used effectively in the treatment of urinary tract infections (18, 32). *Proteus, Pseudomonas,* and *Klebsiella* species are more resistant to cycloserine.

Pharmacodynamic Effects
Bactericidal Effects

Cycloserine is generally bacteriostatic (33). Bactericidal activity is possible only with concentrations 50 to 1000 times the MIC. Because the chemical structure of cycloserine is similar to that of D-alanine, the presence of D-alanine in the culture medium will interfere with cycloserine's antimicrobial activity, sometimes causing intensified growth (13, 33, 35, 36). Heating or autoclaving the test media often releases D-alanine, exacerbating the problem. This has made evaluation of cycloserine's bactericidal activity technically difficult in liquid media, and contributed to disparities in MICs determined with different media. Cycloserine's activity in vitro is optimal in neutral to slightly acidic pH (6.4–7.0) (33). Vitamin B_6 complexes with cycloserine, and this can negate in vitro activity. Similar effects can be seen with various elements, including Cu, Zn, Co, Fe, as well as citrate, phosphate, and oxalate (33). Thus, in vitro testing requires careful control of the media. Cycloserine appears to act slowly, with its effect becoming evident over 96 h.

Postantibiotic Effects (PAE)

Pulse exposures of cycloserine for 24 h at 100 μg/mL produced a 1-day delay in regrowth of mycobacteria. Because the pharmacokinetics of the drug do not allow maximum concentrations of cycloserine to be maintained for this time period, this effect cannot be considered a PAE (15).

Effects of Subinhibitory Concentrations

No specific activity has been attributed to subinhibitory concentrations of cycloserine. In vitro, subinhibitory concentrations may enhance the ability to isolate resistant subpopulations (33). It is not known if subinhibitory concentrations of cycloserine contribute to multidrug therapy in vivo.

Effects on Host Immunity

Cycloserine has no known direct effects on host immunity.

Pharmacodynamic Correlates with Outcome

In vitro, sustained concentrations above the MIC appear to be required, as activity is not evident for several days (33). Increasing the concentration within the achievable clinical range (20–35 μg/mL) does not produce bactericidal activity in vitro. In animals, the pharmacokinetics of cycloserine are considerably altered, with much shorter half-lives, resulting in poor activity in most models (33). In man, approximately 7 mg/kg/day is generally recognized as the minimum dose.

Cycloserine disrupts D-alanine incorporation into peptidoglycan during bacterial cell wall synthesis. Thus, it is natural to compare cycloserine with the β-lactams (33, 35, 36, 38). If the drugs act in an analogous fashion, time above MIC would be the most important parameter. This is consistent with cycloserine's reduced activity in animals that rapidly clear the drug and consistent with the extended time required to demonstrate in vitro activity. Fortunately, cycloserine has a long serum half-life in humans, making it relatively easy to achieve extended time > MIC values.

MECHANISM OF ACTION

Cycloserine, a structural analogue of D-alanine, inhibits bacterial cell wall synthesis by competitively inhibiting the enzymes that link D-alanine molecules into peptidoglycan in the bacterial cell wall (18, 33, 35, 36, 38). Cycloserine produces a loss of acid-fastness in mycobacteria (38). The unique susceptibility of mycobacteria to cycloserine may reflect a special transport mechanism that allows cytoplasmic accumulation of cycloserine (35, 36). Alternatively, mycobacteria may have

relatively low D-alanine content in the cytoplasm, making the threshold for inhibition lower.

MECHANISMS OF RESISTANCE
Commonly Resistant Organisms

Typically, cycloserine is used only against mycobacteria, as superior agents exist for Gram-negative urinary tract infections. Therefore, resistance among bacteria is rarely assessed. Cycloserine-resistant isolates of *M. tuberculosis* remain uncommon, largely because of limited use of cycloserine. Among the other mycobacteria, *M. africanum* may be naturally resistant. Cross-resistance with the other antimycobacterial drugs has not been demonstrated (18, 32). The incidence of primary resistance of *M. tuberculosis* to cycloserine in the United States from 1975 to 1982 was less than 1% (18).

Mechanisms of Resistance

As with other antimycobacterial agents, previously susceptible organisms may develop resistance rapidly, both in vivo and in vitro, when cycloserine is used as a single agent in the treatment of tuberculosis (33, 38). This appears to be due to naturally occurring resistant mutants present in a population of mycobacteria. Under the selective pressure of a single drug, all organisms are eliminated except the resistant subpopulation, which continues to multiply, eventually becoming the dominant population. The precise defect that allows survival of the mutants has not been described. Resistance to cycloserine in some bacteria may be due to reduced uptake of the drug into the cell, much like resistance to tetracyclines (18).

Methods to Overcome and Prevent Resistance

Acquired resistance to cycloserine may be prevented by using it in combination with at least one or two other antimycobacterial drugs (18, 28). Higher doses of cycloserine as monotherapy are not tolerated and do not prevent emergence of resistance. In vitro, subinhibitory concentrations enhance selection of resistant organisms (33). It is not known if this also occurs in vivo, although the possibility exists. Therefore, it appears desirable to achieve serum concentrations above the MIC of the isolate.

PHARMACOKINETICS
Absorption

The pharmacokinetics of cycloserine were studied extensively when it was first developed for clinical use (2, 7, 12, 21–23, 26, 37, 40). Cycloserine is rapidly absorbed from the gastrointestinal tract, appearing in the blood as early as 1 h after 250- to 500-mg doses (7, 12, 21, 22, 26, 40). The time to maximum concentration is usually 2 to 3 h postdose following 250- to 500-mg doses. Two subjects who received both oral and intramuscular doses showed almost identical urinary excretion of cycloserine, consistent with nearly complete absorption from the gastrointestinal tract (7). However, according to Iwainsky, oral administration produces lower serum concentrations than parenteral administration (17). The parenteral route used and the percentage difference between the routes of administration was not stated. Plasma concentrations achieved after a 250-mg dose ranged from 4 to 8 μg/mL following a single dose, increasing to 15 μg/mL with chronic daily administration (22, 40). Concentrations following a 500-mg dose were higher, with concentrations of 6 to 14 μg/mL following a single dose and up to 28 μg/mL with chronic daily administration.

This is consistent with our experience at National Jewish Medical and Research Center, where we often see increases in serum concentrations over the first 2 weeks of therapy with no change in daily dose. Concentrations following higher doses of 750 to 1000 mg demonstrate concentrations only slightly higher (14–17 μg/mL), although these differences may, in part, be attributed to different study conditions (37, 40). The potential for saturable absorption or nonlinear elimination of cycloserine has not been adequately studied. Food taken with cycloserine reportedly reduces and delays the drug's absorption (17).

Distribution

The combination of cycloserine's water solubility and its low molecular weight allow it to diffuse readily into many body compartments and tissues (7, 21, 26). In addition, cycloserine appears to have very low protein binding (17). Cycloserine concentrations near that of plasma concentrations can be found in ascitic fluid, pleural fluid, and human breast milk (7, 21, 26). Cerebrospinal fluid concentrations 54 to 79% of plasma cycloserine concentrations have been reported. Measurable cycloserine concentrations, some higher than plasma concentrations, have been found in sputum, lung tissue, and lymph nodes (22). No significant amount of cycloserine has been found in feces, while urine cycloserine concentrations greatly exceed those of the serum (26, 37). Cycloserine concentrations as high as 52 to 1138 μg/mL have been found in urine (21, 22, 37).

Metabolism and Excretion

Cycloserine is primarily eliminated by urinary excretion (26). It can be found in the urine as soon as 2 h after a 250-mg dose. Forty-seven to 80% of the total amount of cycloserine eliminated occurs within 24 h following standard doses (7, 17). The percentage of cycloserine excreted varies greatly among individuals (12, 26, 40). At 24 h after a dose, the percentage of cycloserine excreted ranges from 38.8 to 92% of standard doses. In general, elderly patients or those with diminished renal function have slower excretion rates. At 30 h following a 500-mg dose, a group of young patients (mean age, 29 years) showed 49.1% of the dose being excreted, while elderly patients (mean age, 67 years) only showed 28.9% of the dose being excreted (40). This was attributed to differences in renal and hepatic function and perhaps also absorption. As expected with such variations in urinary excretion, the serum half-life of cycloserine also varies greatly. The reported serum half-life ranges from 8 to 25 h following standard doses (7, 40). While there appears to be great variation in the urinary excretion among individuals, there is not as much variation across the standard doses (250–750 mg) of cycloserine (37, 40). Probenecid reportedly does not alter cycloserine's renal elimination, suggesting that tubular secretion is not an important excretory route (17).

DOSAGE REGIMENS

Normal

The usual dose of cycloserine ranges from 250 to 750 mg/day, typically divided every 12 h. Occasionally, doses as high as 1000 mg/day are necessary to achieve adequate serum concentrations. However, because of the risk of central nervous system (CNS) toxicity, dose increases to this range should be undertaken only with the guidance of serum concentrations. Doses of 250 mg produce concentrations of 8 to 20 μg/mL (26). Higher doses generally produce proportionally higher concentrations, although some reports show that concentrations following doses greater than 500 mg do not produce proportionally higher doses (26, 40). As noted above, some studies have shown that cycloserine accumulates over the first 3 days of therapy with no change in dose (7). Our experience at National Jewish Medical and Research Center has shown that cycloserine concentrations may increase over the first 2 weeks of therapy with no change in dose or renal function. Given that cycloserine is typically dosed at intervals approximating its half-life, accumulation over the first 5 to 7 doses would be expected.

Pediatric doses of 10 to 20 mg/kg/day (maximum, 1000 mg) in two equally divided doses have been used. Serum concentrations should be monitored, as experience in this population is limited.

Therapeutic Drug Monitoring

Therapeutic drug monitoring (TDM) of cycloserine is our standard of practice at National Jewish Medical and Research Center for a number of reasons (26, 28). The patients requiring cycloserine in their regimens are generally harboring very resistant organisms, making adequate serum concentrations of the utmost importance. Also, because cycloserine is associated with concentration-related toxicities and its clearance is affected by changing renal function, TDM is necessary to ensure safe use of the medication. We measure 2- and 10-h postdose cycloserine concentrations on our patients weekly until stable serum concentrations in the normal range are obtained. Thereafter, patients are monitored periodically, particularly if they experience a change in renal function. The 2-h concentration provides us with the maximum concentration, while the 10-h concentration yields information on clearance of the drug (28). When indicated, more-frequent time points are obtained. Also, if a patient is exhibiting signs of CNS toxicity, we often determine serum concentrations at that time to determine if the CNS symptoms are indeed related to excessive cycloserine concentrations (28).

Renal Failure

Cycloserine dosages need to be adjusted in renal impairment (18, 20, 26). Depending upon the degree of impairment, usual doses given once daily or every other day should be used initially (26). Cycloserine serum concentrations should be checked after 1 to 2 weeks on the medication to evaluate the patient's clearance of the drug; dosages can then be individually adjusted (26, 28). Patients on hemodialysis should receive the drug less frequently (two to three times per week, after hemodialysis sessions), and their serum concentrations should be monitored closely. Because the CNS toxicity of cycloserine appears to be closely related to serum concentrations of the drug, the use of cycloserine in renal impairment should be avoided if alternative agents exist (18, 20).

Hepatic Failure

Unless ascites exists, dosage adjustment in hepatic failure is usually unnecessary.

Obesity, Ascites, and Edema

Because cycloserine is hydrophilic, it distributes into ascites and edema (7, 21, 22). Given these larger volumes of distribution, larger doses may be necessary; dosages should be adjusted according to serum concentrations.

No dosage adjustment is necessary in obesity; however serum concentrations of cycloserine should be monitored to ensure that adequate concentrations are being achieved.

Pregnancy

Although no prospective studies exist regarding the use of cycloserine in pregnant women, it has been used safely (14, 18, 20, 26, 34). As with most drugs, cycloserine should be avoided during the first trimester if possible. Studies in rats have revealed no teratogenicity at dosages up to 100 mg/kg/day. It should be used with caution in nursing mothers because of the risk of adverse effects to the infant.

ADVERSE EFFECTS

The primary adverse effect of cycloserine is CNS toxicity. As mentioned above, the chemical structure and properties of cycloserine allow it to cross the blood-brain barrier easily (7, 21, 22). In addition, cycloserine inhibits the enzyme glutamic decarboxylase, which is necessary to form γ-aminobutyric acid (GABA) (5, 8). The resulting reduced production of GABA is thought to contribute to cycloserine's neurotoxicity, as GABA regulates neural activity. The neurotoxicity of cycloserine may be exhibited in many ways, including hyperexcitability, dizziness, lethargy, depression (including suicidal tendencies), anxiety, confusion, memory loss, and both focal and grand mal seizures (1, 3, 5, 13, 16, 18, 19, 25, 31). There are conflicting reports about whether these changes are associated with electroencephalograph (EEG) changes (5, 13, 16, 25). Although these effects are usually associated with elevated serum cycloserine concentrations (>35 μg/mL) and larger doses (750–1500 mg/day), some CNS disturbances are often seen at "normal" concentrations (1, 3, 19, 25, 29). In our experience, patients may complain of difficulty concentrating even though their serum concentrations are normal.

DRUG INTERACTIONS

The fluoroquinolones are now being used for treatment of multidrug-resistant tuberculosis. This has led to a recent report of increased neurologic symptoms seen when ofloxacin and cycloserine were given together (39). We suspect that this occurred recently with one of our patients. However, a retrospective review of our experience did not reveal either a significant increase in CNS effects nor an apparent pharmacokinetic interaction between cycloserine and ofloxacin (4, 27). Clearly, prospective studies are needed. It is thought that the coadministration of pyridoxine (vitamin B_6) at doses of 50 to 60 mg/day may prevent some of the CNS effects of cycloserine, and there is no clear evidence that this antagonizes cycloserine's action in vivo (5, 16, 31). Other rare side effects reported include gastrointestinal disturbances, rash, drug fever, and cardiac arrhythmias (13, 16, 18, 20).

CLINICAL INDICATIONS

Cycloserine's primary clinical application is in the treatment of *M. tuberculosis*. Because cycloserine is bacteriostatic and is associated with toxicities at achievable serum concentrations, it is usually reserved as a second-line agent (6, 9, 15, 18, 30, 32). Although it was initially used with isoniazid alone to treat some patients with refractory tuberculosis, it is now being used in combination with two or more other second-line antituberculosis agents, such as *p*-aminosalicylic acid (PAS), ethionamide, and ofloxacin, for the treatment of multidrug-resistant tuberculosis (1, 6, 9, 11, 29). Cycloserine is used occasionally in the treatment of *M. avium-intracellulare* infections (15, 18).

Historically, cycloserine was used to treat urinary tract infections caused by Gram-negative bacteria, but superior agents are now available. Because cycloserine has direct effects upon the CNS, it is being studied as either a probe or a potential therapeutic agent for several noninfectious disease indications, including seizure disorders, Alzheimer's disease, and other memory disorders, and the effects of ethanol on the CNS.

REFERENCES

1. Aceto JN, Covert DF. Observations on cycloserine-isoniazid in pulmonary tuberculosis. Antibiot Med Clin Ther 1960;7: 705–712.
2. Anderson RC, Worth HM, Welles JS, et al. Pharmacology and toxicology of cycloserine. Antibiot Chemother 1956;6:360–368.
3. Baroni V, Foddai G, Lukinovig N, Pontiggia P. Clinical evaluation of intolerance to cycloserine. Scand J Respir Dis Suppl 1970;71:217–219.
4. Berning SE, Madsen L, Iseman MD, Peloquin CA. Long-term safety of ofloxacin and ciprofloxacin in the treatment of Mycobacterial infections. Am J Respir Crit Care Med 1995;151: 2006–2009.
5. Bucco T, Meligrana G, DeLuca V. Neurotoxic effects of cycloserine therapy in pulmonary tuberculosis of adolescents and young adults. Scand J Respir Dis Suppl 1970;71:259–265.
6. Craig JW, Williams H, Alston JM. Cycloserine treatment of outpatients with chronic drug-resistant pulmonary tuberculosis. Tubercle 1961;42:7–13.
7. Conzelman GM. The physiologic disposition of cycloserine in the human subject. Am Rev Tuberc 1956;74:739–746.
8. Curci C. Pharmacological considerations on cycloserine. Scand J Respir Dis Suppl 1970;71:51–60.
9. DeLeon AR, Lopez AB. Cycloserine in the treatment of advanced pulmonary tuberculosis. J Philipp Med Assoc 1958;34: 721–728.
10. Desmeules R, Dorval C, Dion R, Montminy L, et al. Considérations sur la cylcosérine dans le traitement de la tuberculose pulmonaire. Laval Med 1957;24:157–167.

11. Epstein IG, Nair KGS, Boyd LJ. Cycloserine, a new antibiotic, in the treatment of human pulmonary tuberculosis: a preliminary report. Antibiotic Med 1955;1:80–93.
12. Georgescu P, Savuleanu E, Daniello I. The rhythm of absorption and elimination of cycloserine as studied with the chromatographic technique. Scand J Respir Dis Suppl 1970;71:61–63.
13. Goble M, Iseman MD, Madsen LA, Waite D, Ackerson L, Horsburgh CR. Treatment of 171 patients with pulmonary tuberculosis resistant to isoniazid and rifampin. N Engl J Med 1993;328:527–532.
14. Hamadeh MA, Glassroth J. Tuberculosis and pregnancy. Chest 1992;101:1114–1120.
15. Heifets LB. Antituberculosis drugs: antimicrobial activity in vitro. In: Heifets LB, ed. Drug susceptibility in the chemotherapy of mycobacterial infections. Boca Raton, FL: CRC Press, 1991:27–41.
16. Helmy B. Side effects of cycloserine. Scand J Respir Dis Suppl 1970;71:220–225.
17. Iwainsky H. Mode of action, biotransformation and pharmacokinetics of antituberculosis drugs in animals and man. In: Bartmann K, ed. Antituberculosis drugs. Berlin: Springer-Verlag, 1988:399–553.
18. Kucers A, Bennett N McK, eds. The use of antibiotics. 4th ed. Philadelphia: JB Lippencott, 1988:1418.
19. Mattila MJ, Nieminen E, Thiitinen H. Serum levels, urinary excretion, and side-effects of cycloserine in the presence of isoniazid and p-aminosalicylic acid. Scand J Respir Dis 1969;50:291–300.
20. McEvoy GK, ed. AHFS drug information. Bethesda, MD: American Society of Health-Systems Pharmacists, 1996:406–408.
21. Morton RF, McKenna MH, Charles E. Studies on the absorption, diffusion, and excretion of cycloserine in man. Antibiot Ann 1955;6:169–171.
22. Nair KGS, Epstein IG, Baron H, Mulinos MG. Absorption, distribution and excretion of cycloserine in man. Antibiot Ann 1955;6:136–139.
23. Niemesto M. The influence of sustained release effect on cycloserine concentration in serum. Scand J Respir Dis Suppl 1970;64–67.
24. Offe HA. Historical introduction and chemical characteristics of antituberculosis drugs. In: Bartmann K, ed. Antituberculosis drugs. Berlin: Springer-Verlag, 1988:1–save30.
25. Pasargiklian M, Biondi L. Neurologic and behavioural reactions of tuberculous patients treated with cycloserine. Scand J Respir Dis Suppl 1970;71:201–208.
26. Peloquin CA. Antituberculosis drugs: pharmacokinetics. In: Heifets LB, ed. Drug susceptibility in the chemotherapy of mycobacterial infections. Boca Raton, FL: CRC Press 1991:89–122.
27. Peloquin CA, Berning SE, Madsen L, Iseman MD. Ofloxacin and ciprofloxacin in the treatment of mycobacterial infections: development of resistance and drug interactions. J Infect Dis Pharmacother 1995;1:45–65.
28. Peloquin CA. Using therapeutic drug monitoring to dose the antimycobacterial drugs. Clin Chest Med 1997;18:79–87.
29. Perfeito JB. Clinical activity of cycloserine in the treatment of tuberculosis. Int Symp Cycloserine 1970:180–188.
30. Renzetti AD, Wright KW, Edling JH, Bunn PH. Clinical, bacteriologic, and pharmacologic observations upon cycloserine. Am Rev Tuberc 1956;74:128–135.
31. Riska N. Tolerance to cycloserine. Scand J Respir Dis Suppl 1970;71:209–214.
32. Storey PB, McLean RL. A current appraisal of cycloserine. Antibiot Med Clin Ther 1957;4:223–232.
33. Trnka L, Mison P, Bartmann K, Otten H. Experimental evaluation of efficacy. In: Bartmann K, ed. Antituberculosis drugs. Berlin: Springer-Verlag, 1988:31–232.
34. Vallejo JG, Starke JR. Tuberculosis and pregnancy. Clin Chest Med 1992;13:693–707.
35. Verbist L. Mode of action of antituberculous drugs (part I). Medicon Int 1974;3:11–23.
36. Verbist L. Mode of action of antituberculous drugs (part II). Medicon Int 1974;3:3–17.
37. Welch H, Putnam LE, Randall WA. Antibacterial activity and blood and urine concentrations of cycloserine, a new antibiotic, following oral administration. Antibiot Med 1955;1:72–79.
38. Winder FG. Mode of action of the antimycobacterial agents and associated aspects of the molecular biology of the mycobacteria, In: Ratledge C, Stanford J, eds. The biology of mycobacteria, vol 1—physiology, identification, and classification. London: Academic Press, 1982:353–438.
39. Yew WW, Wong CF, Wong PC, Lee J, Chow CH. Adverse neurological reactions in patients with multidrug-resistant pulmonary tuberculosis after coadministration of cycloserine and ofloxacin. Clin Infect Dis 1993;17:288–289.
40. Zitkova L, Tousek J. Pharmacokinetics of cycloserine and terizidone. Chemotherapy 1974;20:18–28.

Antimycobacterial Agents: Ethambutol

●

Milena L. Lewis

CLASS: N-SUBSTITUTED ETHYLENEDIAMINE
Chemistry

Ethambutol was discovered as the result of a systematic search for new antituberculous agents by scientists at the Lederle Laboratories. During screening of randomly selected compounds they observed that N,N'-diisopropyl ethylenediamine had in vitro and in vivo antituberculous activity in mice infected with *Mycobacterium tuberculosis* H37Rv (74). This prompted a systematic evaluation of analogues of N-substituted ethylenediamine. Changing the length of the alkylene chain or substitution on the chain led to loss of activity, as did substitutions at only one end of the molecule. Similarly, variations in the extent of substitutions on the amino nitrogens resulted in loss of activity (68).

All active compounds required the presence of two basic centers and had the characteristics of chelating agents. The investigators postulated that branched-alkyl substituents on the nitrogen would result in a relatively open chelate and addition of a hydroxyl group would result in a stable chelate consisting of three five-membered rings. This reasoning led to them to synthesize 2,2'-ethylenediimino-di-1-butanol, which has the following formula:

$$C_2H_5-CH-NH-CH_2-CH_2-NH-CH-C_2H_5$$
$$\underset{CH_2OH}{\vert} \qquad\qquad\qquad\qquad \underset{CH_2OH}{\vert}$$

The dextro isomer of this compound proved to have 110 times the in vivo activity (calculated as the ratio of oral dosage) of N,N'-diisopropyl ethylenediamine in mice infected with *M. tuberculosis* H37Rv. The levo isomer had no antimycobacterial activity (74). Ethambutol was released for general use in 1963. Only the dextro isomer is used therapeutically and marketed as ethambutol.

ANTIMICROBIAL ACTIVITY
Spectrum

Ethambutol is active only against mycobacteria. The compound has no activity against Gram-positive or Gram-negative organisms or fungi (74). Many strains of *Staphylococcus aureus*, *Coli-aeruginosa*, *Proteus*, and *Pseudomonas* species were found resistant to more than 100 µg/mL in culture (37).

In Vitro Studies

In 170 strains of *M. tuberculosis,* 23 strains of *M. bovis,* and 10 strains of photochromogens (*M. kansasii*) tested, growth was completely inhibited in vitro at ethambutol concentrations of 1 to 5 µg/mL (37). However, species in Runyon group II

and group III, which include *M. avium-intracellulare* complex, generally required higher concentrations of the drug, with some strains resistant to 10 µg/mL. Reports from France and Japan confirmed minimum inhibitory concentrations (MICs) from 0.5 to 2.5 µg/mL for *M. tuberculosis*. MICs were 1 to 2 µg/mL for H37Rv as well as several wild strains; only 2 of 16 wild strains had MICs of 4 to 8 µg/mL. In these 2 strains MICs appeared to vary slightly with the culture medium used (63).

Significant differences in MICs were found comparing growth on 7H10 with Lowenstein-Jensen (L-J) medium. Of 323 clinical specimens cultured on 7H10, MICs of 2 µg/mL ethambutol were observed in only 22%, and more than 60% showed MICs of 4 to 8 µg/mL. Comparison of further specimens of wild-type *M. tuberculosis* grown on both L-J and 7H10 media demonstrated significantly lower MICs on L-J than on 7H10. Growth was inhibited by 1 µg/mL in 89% of cultures grown on L-J medium but in only 1% of cultures grown on 7H10. This difference was ascribed to the difference in ionic content of the artificial media (24).

Using an elegant in vitro "man model" in which drug dialyzes away from the culture, Gangadharam et al. reported the effects on *M. tuberculosis* H37Rv of daily exposure to 1.0, 3.0, and 10 µg/mL of ethambutol. At 1 µg/mL, growth was the same as control. However with 3.0 and 10 µg/mL, sterilization was achieved by 6 to 7 days; after that time, development of resistance was noted (25). The authors concluded that ethambutol is bactericidal for sensitive organisms.

Ethambutol also exhibited in vitro activity against certain nontuberculous mycobacteria. Among 18 strains of *M. kansasii* (13 isolated in the United States) evaluated by Kuze et al., 60% were inactivated by 0.78 µg/mL of ethambutol; 90% of 15 isolates of *M. scrofulaceum* were sensitive to this concentration (42). Yates and Collins evaluated sensitivities of 1176 patient-related isolates of atypical mycobacteria in vitro, using a resistance ratio (RR) method. Of 246 strains of *M. kansasii,* 93% were sensitive to ethambutol (RR < 2); 96% of 293 strains of scotochromogens (*M. gordonae*) were sensitive, as were all 4 strains of *M. marinum*. In contrast only 24% of 399 strains of *M. xenopi* and 9% of 130 strains of *M. avium-intercellulare* were sensitive to ethambutol. All 118 strains of *M. fortuitum* and *M. chelonae* were highly resistant (RR > 4) (85).

Tsukumura reported that a concentration of 3.13 µg/mL of ethambutol, sufficient to inhibit growth in several strains of *M. tuberculosis,* also inhibited 100% of *M. szulgai,* 90% of *M. gordonae,* 88% of *M. marinum,* and 77% of *M. kansasii* strains obtained from patient material (76).

Using the BACTEC method, Heifets et al. demonstrated that ethambutol inhibited growth in several clinical strains of *M. avium,* with MICs in a range consistent with blood levels attainable at usual ethambutol dosage. The MICs observed in liquid medium were significantly lower than those determined by the agar dilution method (32).

In Vivo Studies

When mice infected with *M. tuberculosis* H37Rv were treated orally with 200 to 800 mg/kg/day of ethambutol racemate (50% D-isomer) 100% survived for 60 days after infection, whereas 100% of untreated infected mice died within 26 days (74). Of 10 control guinea pigs infected with H37Rv strain, 90% were dead or moribund by the 60th day, whereas only 20% of animals treated orally with 50 mg racemate/day (days 21–60 after infection), and 0% of animals treated subcutaneously with 50 mg racemate/day died (38). Less satisfactory results were seen in guinea pigs given a daily dose 45 mg/kg ethambutol from day 21 to day 98 after infection—only 42% survived (19).

Ethambutol was given in a single daily dose by stomach tube to rhesus monkeys infected intratracheally with a single strain of *M. tuberculosis* starting on the 30th day after infection. Of 11 animals treated with 25 mg/kg/day, 4 died, and culture revealed *M. tuberculosis* in the lungs of 4 others at autopsy. Of 10 animals treated at a dose of 50 mg/kg/day, only 1 died, but 4 others were culture positive for *M. tuberculosis.* Nine animals received 100 mg/kg/day, and all survived for 22 weeks, but two remained culture positive for *M. tuberculosis* (66).

Serum levels of ethambutol were determined in two monkeys at each dosing level from 25 to 400 mg/kg/day, over several months. Highest serum levels were observed 2 h after ingestion. While among certain pairs there were twofold differences in serum levels, mean values at 2 h at a dose of 25 mg/kg/day were 1.9 μg/mL; at a dose of 50 μg/mL, 3.4 μg/mL; and at a dose of 100 mg/kg/day, 7 μg/mL.

The search for new antimycobacterial agents, initiated several years after the effectiveness of isoniazid was established, was prompted by the rising incidence of multidrug-resistant tuberculosis. The consensus that single-drug therapy was inappropriate in tuberculosis was already established. Thus minimal data exist concerning the efficacy of ethambutol administered as a single agent, and that only in patients with multidrug-resistant organisms.

In their initial clinical study, the Lederle group reported on five patients with multidrug-resistant *M. tuberculosis,* given ethambutol at a dose of 50 mg/kg/day for 2 months, followed by ethambutol at 25/mg/kg for another 7 weeks. Prompt clinical improvement was noted, and in most, sputum became negative by culture. Roentgenographic improvement was noted in a significant number of patients (55).

Bobrowitz et al. reported the results of treatment with ethambutol as the single new agent in nine patients who remained sputum positive after treatment with isoniazid, streptomycin, and PAS for 2 years. Prompt improvement was seen in constitutional symptoms such as fever, cough, and volume of sputum. Of five patients treated with ethambutol 25 mg/kg/day for at least 6 months, two became culture negative, but three remained culture positive. Of these five patients, three showed some radiologic improvement. Of four patients who had been on single-drug ethambutol treatment for less than 6 months, only one was culture negative (9). A follow-up report from this institution of 18 patients who had had at least 4 months of ethambutol as the single new drug administered showed similar results: 8 patients converted their sputum, but all eventually became sputum positive again (10).

A multihospital trial in Japan reporting on 47 retreatment patients given ethambutol as the only new drug, at a dose of 1 g/day, found that 20 (42.5%) were culture negative at the end of a 6-month course; thereafter, bacteriologic relapse was observed in a small number of patients (20). In 23 retreatment patients treated with ethambutol alone for at least 6 months, 11 were culture negative at the end of this period, but the long-term outcome is unclear. Five retreatment patients had sufficient improvement to permit resectional surgery (57, 58).

Among atypical mycobacteria, *M. kansasii* frequently shows some resistance to isoniazid. The organism is sensitive to rifampin, and most strains are also sensitive to ethambutol; clinical studies indicate a good response to a three-drug regimen that includes these two drugs (1). Even patients with AIDS (CD4 counts < 200/mL) with pulmonary *M. kansasii* infection generally respond both clinically and bacteriologically to antituberculous regimens that include isoniazid, rifampin, and ethambutol (45).

Prior to the recognition of HIV infection, pulmonary disease due to *M. avium-intracellulare* was not uncommon in certain endemic areas (81). Despite apparent in vitro resistance to most antituberculous drugs, successful treatment with multiple drug regimens was reported in 31 to 85% of cases. This variability might reflect definition of infection as well as variability in regimens. Using a standard four-drug regimen that included isoniazid, rifampin, ethambutol, and streptomycin for the first 6 months, sputum conversion was obtained in 91% of 46 patients. Of 12 patients who completed a 24-month course and 10 who completed an 18-month course, only 4 (18%) relapsed after termination of therapy (2).

Since multiple serovars are included in the classification *M. avium* complex, variation in response to antituberculous drugs may reflect differences in susceptibility (64, 75). However, using probit analysis of different concentration combinations, Heifets reported synergism between rifampin, streptomycin, ethionamide, and ethambutol in vitro against serovar 8 of *M. avium* complex (33). Subsequently, synergism was found between rifampin and ethambutol in 12 of 16 serovars and between rifabutin and ethambutol in 13 of serovars of *M. avium* complex (31, 32).

Synergy has been found in vitro between ethambutol and other antimycobacterial drugs, presumably resulting from its effect on the integrity of mycobacterial cell wall. Viable cell counts of *M. tuberculosis* H37Rv fall significantly more rapidly with exposure to the combination of rifampin and ethambutol in the culture medium than with exposure to rifampin alone (35). Synergism between rifampin and ethambutol was found against several serovars of *M. avium* (31–33). In vitro synergism was also found between clarithromycin and ethambutol against several strains of *M. avium* and for ethambutol and the quinolones against *M. tuberculosis* (60–62).

MECHANISMS OF ACTION

The Lederle group found that ethambutol (1 μg/mL) inhibited multiplication and eventually caused death of *M. smegmatis*. Larger amounts of drug appeared to have no greater inhibitory effect than the MIC. Inhibition was not seen immediately but became apparent only after 3 to 4 h of apparent growth, as measured by turbidity in liquid medium. If subcultured during this initial period, inhibited organisms showed impaired oxygen uptake. In contrast, ethambutol had no effect on the survival of nonproliferating cells of *M. smegmatis,* even at a concentration of 1 mg/mL, and no apparent effect on the endogenous metabolism of nonproliferating organisms. Both proliferating and nonproliferating organisms took up ^{14}C-labeled ethambutol, indicating that the effect on growth was not due to a difference in binding and that binding was passive. Even an ethambutol-resistant strain of *M. smegmatis* took up the drug to an equal degree. Uptake was rapid, with about equal amounts of activity in cells exposed for 15 min as in those exposed for 24 h. However, uptake was inhibited by ions such as sodium or potassium chloride or phosphates in the medium (21).

Further work using *M. tuberculosis* H37Rv confirmed that length of exposure was not a factor in binding, since washed cells exposed for 2 h contained as much activity as those exposed to ethambutol for 96 h. In *M. tuberculosis* H37Rv, growth inhibition was not manifest until 1 to 2 days after addition of ethambutol. As with *M. smegmatis,* the early effects of the drug are reversible; when resuspended in drug-free medium, inhibited *M. tuberculosis* cells resumed growth after a lag (22).

M. smegmatis inhibited by ethambutol became deficient in RNA; RNA production slowed, and after 3 h of exposure, total cellular RNA decreased. Production of protein also decreased over 3 h and then ceased. Production of DNA continued in the first 3 h but then slowed markedly. Addition of spermidine and magnesium ions to drug-free subcultures aided recovery of *M. smegmatis* inhibited by ethambutol and also counteracted growth inhibition by ethambutol when added simultaneously to the medium. Although ionic solutions affect ethambutol binding, the investigators concluded that magnesium had a specific effect unrelated to binding, since both MgCl$_2$ and MgSO$_4$ counteracted ethambutol, whereas equimolar concentrations of NaCl or Na$_2$SO$_4$ did not. They postulated that the chelating properties of ethambutol might have activity against metal-containing enzyme systems essential to bacterial metabolism and thus explain its bactericidal activity (23).

However, Beggs and Andrews determined that binding inhibition was related to ionic strength rather than concentration, since 80 mM NaCl and 27 mM Na$_2$SO$_4$ had an effect equivalent to that of 20 mM MgSO$_4$. They concluded that the effect of magnesium ion on protection from ethambutol was nonspecific. They further observed a protective effect on cell mul-

tiplication when 20 mM MgSO$_4$ or 80 mM NaCl was added to the medium up to 90 min after initial exposure to ethambutol, with a resultant marked decrease in cell-bound ^{14}C activity, indicating that bound ethambutol could be displaced (6, 7).

Similar, but weaker, effects on binding and protection were noted with 2 mM spermidine trihydrochloride added up to 90 min after exposure to ethambutol. Since spermidine was effective at much lower molar and ionic strength than 20 mM MgSO$_4$, its effect may reflect competition with ethambutol, either on the basis of its cationic nature or its structural similarity. In 1985, Paulin, Brander, and Pösö reported that ethambutol inhibits spermidine biosynthesis in mycobacteria, providing a possible locus of ethambutol action. Spermidine is a constituent of many bacteria and is related to RNA synthesis (51).

In 1977, Kilburn and Greenberg noted that for several hours after initial exposure to ethambutol, the rate of rise of CFUs of *M. smegmatis,* determined by serial dilution, was significantly greater that in untreated cultures. At a concentration of ethambutol of 0.1 μg/mL, growth was identical to control. At concentrations between 0.25 and 3.0 μg/mL, an early rapid rise in CFUs was observed and maintained for the 4 h; thereafter, the number of CFUs fell. The rapid rise in CFUs was observed only in multiplying cells; there was no increase in CFUs of cells exposed to ethambutol 3 μg/mL while maintained at 4°C. Concentrations of ethambutol between 1.5 and 3.0 μg/mL ultimately led to cell death. However, in cultures exposed to 0.25 to 0.5 μg/mL, the number of CFUs began to rise again after 24 h, suggesting that the effects of low-dose ethambutol could be repaired by the organism (39).

The early rapid rise in bacterial counts could not be explained by cell division, since incorporation of ^{3}H-thymidine did not increase during this time. Under electron microscopy, ethambutol-treated cells appeared wider and shorter than controls, with decreased surface area. Filtration through a 5 μ membrane permitted 10% of untreated cells to pass, whereas 25% of cells treated for 4 h with ethambutol passed through the filter. Coulter counts revealed that treated cells had a definite shift to a lower volume range than those in untreated cultures. The authors postulated that the changes in shape, surface area, and decreased clustering after ethambutol exposure reflected an effect on cell wall properties.

In further studies using ^{14}C-acetate as precursor, a decrease in cell wall mycolic acid content was demonstrated within 15 to 30 min after exposure to ethambutol. Within 1 min of exposure to 3.0 μg/mL of ethambutol, cellular levels of trehalose monomycolate increased, followed by an increase in dimycolate and free mycolic acid. After 30 min, these substances began to leak out of the cells (72). In agreement with prior observations by Winder et al. (80), the authors found no effect of ethambutol on the synthesis of mycolic acids per se. Rather, when *M. smegmatis* was cultured with various ^{14}C-labeled monosaccharides and exposed to 3.0 μg/mL ethambutol, transfer of labeled glucose into the arabinogalactan and arabinomannan residues of the cell wall was immediately inhibited (40, 73).

Subsequently, McNeil and Brennan demonstrated that ethambutol inhibits arabinotransferases involved in the biosynthetic pathway of mycobacterial cell wall (47). Several arabinotransferases have been found in mycobacteria, with differing affinities for ethambutol, but the principal, and most rapid, antimycobacterial effect of ethambutol is on the type III enzyme involved in polymerization of arabinofuranose, a step required for synthesis of arabinogalactan (48). Disruption of the mycobacterial cell wall complex, permitting passage of other antimycobacterial drugs, can explain the well-known synergy between ethambutol and other antimycobacterial drugs such as rifampicin. Ethambutol also has an inhibitory effect on the polymerization of arabinofuranose into lipoarabinomannan, but this occurs more slowly, requiring longer exposure of mycobacteria to the drug, and presumably involving arabinotransferases other than type III.

Using a genomic library from an ethambutol-resistant strain of *M. avium,* these investigators transferred resistance to a previously ethambutol-sensitive strain of *M. smegmatis* by means of a plasmid. The resistance region contains three open reading frames, two of which, designated *embA* and *embB,* are coupled and essential for transfer of ethambutol resistance (8).

The resistance region defined in *M. avium* was found to be ubiquitous in many mycobacteria, including *M. tuberculosis* H37Rv. This resistance region from *M. avium* has been sequenced, and its G-C content determined to be 70.4%, consistent with mycobacterial DNA. Thus, the region does not confer resistance per se. Rather, in transfected resistant clones of *M. smegmatis,* the degree of resistance to ethambutol correlated with the number of copies of the transferred genetic material. The investigators postulate that *embAB* encodes for arabinosyl transferase III. The fact that the level of ethambutol resistance is related to gene copy number, indicating higher production of arabinosyl transferase, supports the conclusion that the primary target of ethambutol is arabinosyl transferase III. Increased production of the transferase would overcome the inhibitory effect of the drug, permitting formation of arabinogalactan.

RESISTANCE

Resistance of *M. tuberculosis* to ethambutol is the result of random spontaneous genetic mutation, as indicated by the fluctuation analysis of Luria and Delbrück (46). Applying this method, the mutation rate to resistance to ethambutol (5 μg/mL) was calculated to be 10^{-7}, or 1 mutation/10^7 organisms/generation (17). Resistance may be determined by the number of copies of the genes responsible for production of adenosyl transferase III, hence of the quantity of the enzyme produced (8) (see "Mechanisms of Action").

The first survey of primary resistance to ethambutol, initiated in July 1968, revealed that 5.3% of 153 samples were resistant to 10 μg/mL (34). In subsequent years, primary resistance rates were 15.8% for 1968–69, only 1.6% for 1970–71 and 2.2% for 1971–72, but 9.7% for 1972–73 (36). By contrast, a survey of primary drug resistance conducted by the Centers for Disease Control, covering 1975 to 1977, reported only 0.7% resistance to 5.0 μg/mL ethambutol among 3100 cultures (41). All survey samples were cultured on 7H10 medium, which may affect ethambutol binding, but the wide fluctuations in apparent primary resistance to ethambutol

among wild-type *M. tuberculosis* must reflect other differences in methodology. More recently, a primary resistance rate to ethambutol of 0.2% and an acquired resistance rate of 0.3% were reported from the Medical Research Council center in the Western Cape, S. Africa (78). This group also noted a marked decrease in both initial and acquired resistance to all antituberculosis drugs over a 25-year period, as treatment modalities improved (79). However, in areas such as New York City, where tuberculosis control measures had been allowed to fall into abeyance, a rate of resistance to ethambutol as high as 14% has been reported (49).

PHARMACOKINETICS

In 10 normal volunteers administered a single oral dose of 25 mg/kg first in a fasting state and then in a nonfasting state, mean values at 1, 2, 4, and 8 h were 2.1, 3.9, 2.0, and 0.8 μg/mL after dosing in the fasting state and slightly higher when nonfasting. By 24 h, serum levels were undetectable and approximately 50% of the dose had been excreted in the urine (55). In 17 patients treated with ethambutol 25/mg/kg/day, Bobrowitz et al. reported peak serum levels ranging from 2.3 to 6.7 μg/mL. They noted that most patients who remained sputum positive had average maximum blood levels below 5 μg/mL (9).

Using ^{14}C-labeled ethambutol, the Lederle investigators evaluated metabolism in three patients with tuberculosis. Following an oral dose of 25 mg/kg, peak serum concentrations of 4 to 5 μg/mL were reached at about 4 h, with levels falling below 1 μg/mL at 24 h. Over the first 48 h, 60 to 67% of activity was recovered from urine and 12 to 19% from feces. Over 5 days, about 20% was recovered from feces, compared with only 1% after an intravenous dose (tested in one patient), indicating that ethambutol is not completely absorbed from the gut. The major radiolabeled product in urine was unchanged ethambutol; two minor metabolites, identified as the aldehyde of ethambutol and 2,2'-ethylenediimino-di-butyric acid, constituted 8% and 7% of drug excreted in the first 24 h (52). In the single patient who received 10 mg of ^{14}C-ethambutol injected intravenously, the drug accumulated in erythrocytes.

Lee et al. reported that in six normal volunteers, peak levels following a single oral dose of 15 mg/kg ethambutol ranged from 3.25 to 5.6 μg/mL, and on average 61% of the drug was excreted unchanged in the urine (43). Following intravenous infusion, peak plasma levels were significantly higher (11.6–15.4 μg/mL), with subsequent multiphasic decay. Ultimately, approximately 80% of the dose was excreted unchanged, with renal clearance ranging from 6 to 8.5 mL/min/kg, indicating active tubular secretion (44).

DOSAGE REGIMENS

In individuals who were not immunosuppressed, a 6-month course of antituberculosis chemotherapy proved adequate for cure. In areas where the prevalence of isoniazid resistance is above 4%, the accepted course of initial treatment is a four-drug regimen (isoniazid, rifampin, pyrazinamide, and ethambutol) for 2 months, followed by 4 months of isoniazid and rifampin if initial cultures indicate sensitivity to both. The recommended dosage of ethambutol is 15 mg/kg/day, given in a single daily dose. Pending information regarding the sensitivity of the organism, a dose of 25 mg/kg may be used in retreatment cases. The drug is supplied in 100-mg and 400-mg tablets. Absorption is not significantly affected by food, but decreased absorption has been reported if the drug is taken with antacids (5, 13, 29).

Directly observed administration is currently recommended for all treatment regimens. Several intermittent treatment options have also been evaluated. The above four-drug regimen may be given daily for 2 weeks, followed by the same regimen twice-weekly under direct observation for 6 weeks. Dosage for a twice-weekly four-drug regimen is 50 mg/kg of ethambutol (in combination with isoniazid 15 mg/kg, rifampin 10 mg/kg, and pyrazinamide 50 mg/kg). Subsequent twice-weekly therapy depends on sensitivity of the organism (5). Ethambutol is not recommended for routine treatment of tuberculosis in children. However, the American Academy of Pediatrics accepts the above daily and twice-weekly dosages when there is a risk of infection with an isoniazid-resistant organism (3, 4). Ethambutol should not be used in children less than 6 years old, too young to undergo valid visual testing.

Essentially the same dosage schemes are recommended for extrapulmonary tuberculosis, with the continuation phase possibly extended to 9 months (4). Ethambutol does not cross the blood-brain barrier well; even at a dose of 25 mg/kg, cerebrospinal fluid (CSF) levels of only 1 to 2 μg/mL were reported (4). For this reason, the British Thoracic Society does not recommend ethambutol for treatment of tuberculous meningitis (50).

Since ethambutol is principally excreted unchanged by the kidneys, use in patients with significant renal disease should be avoided unless infection with resistant organisms is suspected. The drug is cleared by dialysis. In patients with renal failure, on dialysis, a daily dose of 5 mg/kg or 1.5 mg/kg every 8 h has been suggested, with testing of serum ethambutol levels and visual acuity (14).

On the basis of plasma levels observed following an intravenous infusion of ethambutol in a group of 13 patients with renal failure, Varughese et al. reported average renal clearance to be 0.3 mL/min/kg, markedly lower than reported in normal individuals. However, renal clearance contributed to no more than 26% of the dose, indicating significantly higher metabolism of the drug than observed in normal persons. Mean effective clearance of ethambutol was 4.2 mL/min/kg. On this basis, the authors recommend a daily dose of 7.2 mg/kg in anephric patients and 10.8 mg/kg in patients with 50% compromised renal function (77).

Dosage of ethambutol does not have to be altered in the presence of hepatic disease. While there is a single well-studied case of cholestatic jaundice in an individual receiving ethambutol as a single drug (see "Adverse Effects"), 67 patients with coexisting viral hepatitis and tuberculosis treated with streptomycin, isoniazid, and ethambutol were observed closely for 15 days. In most, serum bilirubin and alanine transferase decreased, and none developed fulminant hepatitis (18).

Administration of ethambutol during pregnancy is considered safe, when clearly indicated (11). Reviewing the world literature in 1980, Snider et al. found reports on 655 pregnancies during which ethambutol was administered in addition to other antituberculous drugs. Among these there were 592 normal-term infants, 20 elective terminations, 1 spontaneous abortion, 26 premature births, 5 stillbirths, and 14 fetuses or infants with various abnormalities, but no ocular injuries were reported. The results cannot be strictly compared with usual rates of undesirable pregnancy outcome; nevertheless, only the incidence of fetal abnormalities associated with streptomycin administration appeared to be exceptionally high (69).

Information regarding the effects on infants of nursing mothers who take ethambutol is virtually nonexistent. However, considering the worldwide use of ethambutol and the extensive surveillance by agencies concerned with tuberculosis, it is reasonable to suppose that significant adverse effects would have been reported. Bobrowitz observed ethambutol levels of 1.5 and 4.6 mg/L in the milk of two women, levels similar to the range usually observed in serum. Using this information, Snider and Powell calculated that a 3.5-kg infant would ingest 0.5 to 0.9 mg/kg/day (70). This dose is not likely to be toxic, although there is no body of data on toxicity of ethambutol in neonates.

A single study of blood levels of ethambutol in an obese patient weighing 166 kg (ideal body weight, 87 kg) was reported (27). At a dosing regimen of 27.5 mg/kg of ideal body weight, given in three divided doses, peak and trough levels were slightly higher than those reported by Place et al. for a single dose of 25 mg/kg administered to 10 normal volunteers (54). The authors suggested that dosage should be calculated on ideal body weight to obviate increased risk of toxicity.

ADVERSE EFFECTS

At a dose of 15 mg/kg/day, adverse effects of ethambutol are uncommon. At higher dosage, the most important adverse reaction is retrobulbar neuropathy, manifested by decreasing visual acuity, color blindness, and restriction of visual fields. While optic neuritis is virtually unreported at the standard dose, preexisting ophthalmologic disease may predispose to ethambutol toxicity (4). Therefore, prior to initiating ethambutol therapy, patients should be questioned about visual problems and have color vision tested with Ishihara plates. If visual problems are reported, patients may be referred to an ophthalmologist for further assessment. Ethambutol should not be given to patients with optic neuritis, and some authorities recommend that ethambutol not be administered to any patients with visual difficulties, since this could confound recognition of ethambutol toxicity. After initial testing, patients should be questioned about visual symptoms at each visit, since optic neuritis has been related to duration of therapy. Visual acuity may be assessed with a standard Snellen chart, with the drug discontinued if a significant decrease is confirmed pending more extensive testing of color vision and visual fields. The optic neuritis is usually reversed weeks to months after ethambutol is discontinued (4). Since ethambutol is principally excreted by the kidneys, patients with renal insufficiency may be at increased risk of developing optic neuritis.

Renal clearance of urates is decreased by ethambutol in a significant proportion of normal patients, and acute attacks of gout have been precipitated in patients at risk (56, 67).

A case of cholestatic jaundice was reported in a patient receiving ethambutol as a single drug (30). The patient developed evidence of hepatitis while receiving isoniazid and ethambutol. All drugs were discontinued for 10 days, and ethambutol was restarted alone. After 6 days, alkaline phosphatase and aspartate transaminase serum levels increased significantly. Ethambutol was discontinued, and liver function improved. Four days after initiation of a second trial of ethambutol, enzyme levels again increased.

There are five case reports of interstitial nephritis developing in patients receiving ethambutol as part of a multidrug regimen; renal biopsies were performed in four. In two patients, both isoniazid and ethambutol were discontinued, and other drugs substituted, implicating either ethambutol or isoniazid as the cause of nephritis. In three patients, renal function returned toward normal when ethambutol was discontinued; in one of these, isoniazid dosage was maintained, and in two others, isoniazid was reintroduced without further renal complications (15, 26, 71).

Isolated cases of thrombocytopenia, epidermal necrolysis, eosinophilia and neutropenia, and eosinophilic pneumonia have also been attributed to ethambutol (53, 59, 83, 84).

DRUG INTERACTIONS

Aluminum hydroxide is reported to affect absorption of ethambutol (29). No other significant adverse interactions between other classes of drugs and ethambutol have been reported. Since ethambutol is principally excreted unchanged in the urine, it presumably produces little enzyme induction, such as seen with rifampin.

INDICATIONS

Ethambutol is indicated solely for the treatment of mycobacterial infections in a multidrug regimen. It is indicated in the management of *M. tuberculosis* infection as part of the primary treatment in areas where there is a significant prevalence of drug resistance and as part of a secondary regimen when drug susceptibility has been determined.

Ethambutol is also indicated in infection with *M. avium-intracellulare* complex, both endemic type and in immunocompromised hosts. However, in HIV-infected patients with disseminated *M. avium* infection treated with normal recommended dosage regimens, low plasma levels of several antituberculous drugs, including ethambutol, have been observed (28).

As indicated by in vitro susceptibility testing, ethambutol may also be used as part of a multidrug regimen for other atypical mycobacterioses, since it primarily inhibits formation of arabinogalactan, which is a component of all mycobacterial cell walls (12).

REFERENCES

1. Ahn CH, Lowell JR, Ahn SS, Ahn S, Hurst GA. Chemotherapy for Pulmonary disease due to Mycobacterium kansasii: efficacies of some individual drugs. Rev Infect Dis 1981;3:1028–1034.
2. Ahn CH, Ahn SS, Anderson RA, Murphy DT, Mammo A. A four-drug regimen for initial treatment of cavitary disease caused by Mycobacterium avium complex. Am Rev Respir Dis 1986;134:438–441.
3. American Academy of Pediatrics Committee on Infectious Diseases. Chemotherapy of tuberculosis in infants and children. Pediatrics 1992;89:161–165.
4. American Thoracic Society and Centers for Disease Control. Treatment of tuberculosis infection in adults and children. Am Rev Respir Dis 1986;134:355–363.
5. American Thoracic Society. Treatment of tuberculosis and tuberculosis infection in adults and children. Am J Respir Crit Care Med 1994;140:1359–1374.
6. Beggs WH, Andrews FA. Nonspecific ionic inhibition of ethambutol binding by Mycobacterium smegmatis. Antimicrob Agents Chemother 1973;4:115–119.
7. Beggs WH, Andrews FA. Uptake of ethambutol by Mycobacterium smegmatis and its relation to growth inhibition. Am Rev Respir Dis 1973;108:691–693.
8. Belanger AE, Besra GS, Ford ME, Mikusova K, Belisle JT, Brennan PJ, Inamine JM. The embAB genes of Mycobacterium avium encode an arabinosyl transferase involved in cell wall arabinan biosynthesis that is the target for the antimycobacterial drug ethambutol. Proc Natl Acad Sci USA 1996;93:11919–11924.
9. Bobrowitz ID, Garber M, Sukumalchantra Y. The use of ethambutol in pulmonary tuberculosis: a preliminary report. Trans 22nd Res Conf Pulm Dis. Washington, DC: Veterans Administration Department of Medicine and Surgery, 1963:254–261.
10. Bobrowitz ID. Ethambutol in the retreatment of pulmonary tuberculosis. Ann NY Acad Sci 1966;135:796–822.
11. Bobrowitz ID. Ethambutol in pregnancy. Chest 1974;66:20–26.
12. Brennan PJ, Nikaido H. The envelope of mycobacteria. Annu Rev Biochem 1995;64:29–63.
13. Centers for Disease Control and Prevention. Initial therapy for tuberculosis in the era of multidrug resistance. Recommendations of the Advisory Council for the Elimination of Tuberculosis. MMWR 1993;42(No. RR-7):2–7.
14. Christopher TG, Blair A, Forrey A, Cutler RE. Kinetics of ethambutol elimination in renal disease. Proc Dial Transplant Forum 1973;3:96–101.
15. Collier J, Joekes AM. Two cases of ethambutol nephrotoxicity. Br Med J 1976;2:1105–1106.
16. Daffe M, Brennan PJ, McNeil M. Predominant structural features of the cell wall arabinogalactan of Mycobacterium tuberculosis as revealed through characterization of oligoglycosyl alditol fragments by gas chromatography/mass spectrometry and by ^{1}H and ^{13}C NMR analyses. J Biol Chem 1990;265:6734–6743.
17. David HL. Probability distribution of drug-resistant mutants in unselected populations of Mycobacterium tuberculosis. Appl Microbiol 1970;20:810–814.
18. Deshpande DV, Nachne D, Koyande D, Rodrigues CJ. Antitubercular treatment in patients with hepatitis. J Assoc Physicians India 1991;39:599–601.
19. Dickinson JM, Mitchison DA. Bactericidal activity in vitro and in the guinea-pig of isoniazid, rifampicin and ethambutol. Tubercle 1976;57:251–258.
20. Donomae I, Yamamoto K. Clinical evaluation of ethambutol in pulmonary tuberculosis. Ann NY Acad Sci 1966;135:849–881.
21. Forbes M, Peets EA, Kuck NA. Effect of ethambutol on mycobacteria. Ann NY Acad Sci 1966;135:726–731.
22. Forbes M, Kuck NA, Peets EA. Modes of action of ethambutol. J Bacteriol 1962;84:1099–1103.

23. Forbes M, Kuck NA, Peets EA. Effects of ethambutol on nucleic acid metabolism in Mycobacterium smegmatis and its reversal by polyamines and divalent cations. J Bacteriol 1965;89:1299–1305.

24. Gangadharam PR, Gonzales ER. Influence of the medium on the in-vitro susceptibility of Mycobacterium tuberculosis to ethambutol. Am Rev Respir Dis 1970;102:653–655.

25. Gangadharam PRJ, Pratt PF, Perumal VK, Iseman MD. The effects of exposure time, drug concentration, and temperature on the activity of ethambutol versus Mycobacterium tuberculosis. Am Rev Respir Dis 1990;141:1478–1482.

26. Garcia-Martin F, Mampaso F, de Arriba G, Moldenhauer F, Martin-Escobar E, Saiz F. Acute interstitial nephritis induced by ethambutol. Nephron 1991;59:679–680.

27. Geisler JP, Manis RD, Maddux MS. Dosage of antituberculous drugs in obese patients. Am Rev Respir Dis 1985;131:944–946.

28. Gordon SM, Horsburgh CR Jr, Peloquin CA, Havlik JA, Metchock B, Heifets L, McGowan JE Jr, Thompson SE III. Low serum levels of oral antimycobacterial agents in patients with disseminated Mycobacterium avium complex disease. J Infect Dis 1993;168:1559–62.

29. Gugler R, Allgayer H. Effects of antacids on the clinical pharmacokinetics of drugs. Clin Pharmacokinet 1990;18:210–219.

30. Gulliford M, Mackay AD, Prowse K. Cholestatic jaundice caused by ethambutol. Br Med J 1986;292:866.

31. Heifets LB, Iseman MD, Lindholm-Levy PJ. Combinations of rifampin or rifabutine plus ethambutol against Mycobacterium avium complex. Am Rev Respir Dis 1988;137:711–715.

32. Heifets LB, Iseman MD, Lindholm-Levy PJ. Ethambutol MICs and MBCs for Mycobacterium avium complex and Mycobacterium tuberculosis. Antimicrob Agents Chemother 1986;30:927–932.

33. Heifets LB. Synergistic effects of rifampin, streptomycin, ethionamide, and ethambutol on Mycobacterium intracellulare. Am Rev Respir Dis 1982;125:43–48.

34. Hobby GL, Johnson PM, Boytar-Papirnik V, Wilber J. Primary drug resistance: a continuing study of tubercle bacilli in a veteran population within the United States. Am Rev Respir Dis 1969;99:777–779.

35. Hobby GL, Lenert TF. Observations on the action of rifampin and ethambutol alone and in combination with other antituberculous drugs. Am Rev Respir Dis 1972;105:292–295.

36. Hobby GL, Johnson PM, Boytar-Papirnik V. Primary drug resistance: a continuing study of drug resistance in tuberculosis in a veteran population within the United States. Am Rev Respir Dis 1974;110:95–98.

37. Karlson AG. The in vitro activity of ethambutol (dextro-2,2′[ethylenediimino]di-1-butanol) against tubercle bacilli and other microorganisms. Am Rev Respir Dis 1961;83:905–906.

38. Karlson AG. The combined use of ethambutol (dextro-2,2′[ethylene-diimino]di-1-butanol) and isoniazid in experimental tuberculosis of guinea pigs. Am Rev Respir Dis 1962;86:439–441.

39. Kilburn JO, Greenberg J. Effect of ethambutol on the viable cell count in Mycobacterium smegmatis. Antimicrob Agents Chemother 1977;11:534–540.

40. Kilburn JO, Takayama K. Effects of ethambutol on accumulation and secretion of trehalose mycolates and free mycolic acid in Mycobacterium smegmatis. Antimicrob Agents Chemother 1981;20:401–404.

41. Kopanoff DE, Kilburn JO, Glassroth JL, Snider DE, Farer LS, Good RC. A continuing survey of tuberculosis primary drug resistance in United States: March 1975 to November 1977. Am Rev Respir Dis 1978;118:835–842.

42. Kuze F, Kurasawa T, Bando K, Lee K, Mackawa N. In vitro and in vivo susceptibility of atypical mycobacteria to various drugs. Rev Infect Dis 1981;3:885–897.

43. Lee CS, Gambertoglio JG, Brater DC, Benet LZ. Kinetics of oral ethambutol in the normal subject. Clin Pharmacokinet Ther 1977;22:615–621.

44. Lee CS, Brater DC, Gambertoglio JG, Benet LZ. Disposition kinetics of ethambutol in man. J Pharmacokinet Biopharm 1980;8:335–346.

45. Levine B, Chaisson RE. Mycobacterium kansasii: a cause of treatable pulmonary disease associated with advanced human immunodeficiency virus (HIV) infection. Ann Intern Med 1991;114:861–868.

46. Luria SE, Delbrück M. Mutations of bacteria from virus sensitivity to virus resistance. Genetics 1943;28:491–511.

47. McNeil MR, Brennan PJ. Structure, function and biogenesis of the cell envelope of mycobacteria in relation to bacterial physiology, pathogenesis and drug resistance; some thoughts and possibilities arising from recent structural information. Res Microbiol 1991;142:451–463.

48. Mikusova K, Slayden RA, Besra GS, Brennan PJ. Biogenesis of the mycobacterial cell wall and the site of action of ethambutol. Antimicrob Agents Chemother 1995;39:2484–2489

49. Neville K, Bromberg A, Bromberg R, Bonk S, Hanna BA, Rom WN. The third epidemic multidrug-resistant tuberculosis. Chest 1994;105:45–48.

50. Ormerod LP. Chemotherapy and management of the Joint Tuberculosis Committee of the British Thoracic Society. Thorax 1990;45:403–408.

51. Paulin LG, Brander EE, Poso HJ. Specific inhibition of spermidine synthesis in mycobacteria spp. by the dextro isomer of ethambutol. Antimicrob Ag Chemother 1985;28:157–159.

52. Peets EA, Sweeney WM, Place VA, Buyske DA. The absorption, excretion and metabolic fate of ethambutol in man. Am Rev Respir Dis 1965;91:51–58.

53. Pegram PS, Mountz JD, O'Bar PT. Ethambutol-induced toxic epidermal necrolysis. Arch Intern Med 1981;141:1877–1878.

54. Place VA, Peets EA, Buyske DA. Metabolic and special studies of ethambutol in normal volunteers and tuberculous patients. Ann NY Acad Sci 1966;135:775–795.

55. Place VA, Thomas JP. Clinical pharmacology of ethambutol. Am Rev Respir Dis 1963;87:901–904.

56. Postlethwaite AE, Kelley WN. Studies on the mechanism of ethambutol-induced hyperuricemia. Arthritis Rheum 1972;15:403–409.

57. Pyle MM, Pfuetze KH, Pearlman MD, de la Huerga J, Hubble RH. A four-year clinical investigation of ethambutol in initial and re-treatment cases of tuberculosis. Am Rev Respir Dis 1966;93:428–441.

58. Pyle MM. Ethambutol in the retreatment and primary treatment of tuberculosis: a four year clinical investigation. Ann NY Acad Sci 1966;135:835–845.

59. Prasad R, Mukerji. Ethambutol-induced thrombocytopenia. Tubercle 1989;70:211–212.

60. Rastogi N, Blom-Potar MC. Intracellular bactericidal activity of ciprofloxacin and ofloxacin against Mycobacterium tuberculosis H37Rv multiplying in the J-774 macrophage cell line. Zentralbl Bakteriol 1990;273:195–199.

61. Rastogi N, Labrousse V. Extracellular and intracellular activities of clarithromycin used alone and in association with ethambutol and rifampin against Mycobacterium avium complex. Antimicrob Agents Chemother 1991;35:462–470.

62. Rastogi N, Goh KS, Bryskier A, Devallois A. In vitro activities of levofloxacin used alone and in combination with first- and second-line antituberculous drugs against Mycobacterium tuberculosis. Antimicrob Agents Chemother 1996;40:1610–1616.

63. Robinson LB, Wichelhausen RH. In vitro studies on two recently developed antituberculous agents: ethambutol and capreomycin. Trans 21st Res Conf Pulm Dis. Washington, DC: Veterans Administration Dept of Medicine and Surgery, 1962: 351–355.

64. Schaefer WB. Incidence of the serotypes of Mycobacterium avium and atypical mycobacteria in human and animal diseases. Am Rev Respir Dis 1968;97:18–23.

65. Schmidt LH, Lang J, Good RC, Hoffman R. Experimental studies on the toxicity and antituberculosis activity of ethambutol. Trans 21st Res Conf Pulm Dis. Washington, DC: Veterans Administration Dept of Medicine and Surgery, 1962:355–366.

66. Schmidt LH, Good RC, Mack HP, Zeek-Minning P, Schmidt IG. An experimental appraisal of the therapeutic potentialities of ethambutol. Trans 22nd Res Conf Pulm Dis. Washington, DC: Veterans Administration Dept of Medicine and Surgery, 1963: 262–275.

67. Self TH, Fountain FF, Taylor WJ Jr, Sutliff W. Acute gouty arthritis associated with the use of ethambutol. Chest 1977;71: 561–562.

68. Shepherd RG, Baughn CO, Cantrall ML, Goodstein B, Thomas JP, Wilkinson RG. Structure-activity studies leading to ethambutol, a new type of antituberculous compound. Ann NY Acad Sci 1966;135:686–710.

69. Snider DE, Layde PM, Johnson MW, Lyle MA. Treatment of tuberculosis during pregnancy. Am Rev Respir Dis 1980;122: 65–79.

70. Snider DE, Powell KE. Should women taking antituberculosis drugs breast-feed? Arch Intern Med 1984;144:589–90

71. Stone WJ, Waldron JA, Dixon JH, Primm RK, Horn RG. Acute diffuse interstitial nephritis related to chemotherapy of tuberculosis. Antimicrob Agents Chemother 1976;10:164–172.

72. Takayama K, Armstrong EL, Kunugi KA, Kilburn JO. Inhibition by ethambutol of mycolic acid transfer into the cell wall of Mycobacterium smegmatis. Antimicrob Agents Chemother 1979;16:240–242.

73. Takayama K, Kilburn JO. Inhibition of synthesis of arabinogalactan by ethambutol in Mycobacterium smegmatis. Antimicrob Agents Chemoth 1989;33:1493–1499.

74. Thomas JP, Baughn CO, Wilkinson RG, Shepherd RG. A new synthetic compound with antituberculous activity in mice: ethambutol (dextro-2,2′-(ethylenediimino)-di-1-butanol). Am Rev Respir Dis 1961;83:891–893.

75. Tsukamura M, Miyachi T. Correlations among naturally occurring resistances to antituberculous drugs in Mycobacterium avium complex strains. Am Rev Respir Dis 1989;139:1033–1035.

76. Tsukamura M. Evaluation of clinical efficacy of isoniazid and ethambutol in the treatment of nontuberculous mycobacterioses based on in vitro susceptibility testing. Kekkaku 1989;64:511–518.

77. Varughese A, Brater DC, Benet LZ, Lee CC. Ethambutol kinetics in patients with impaired renal function. Am Rev Respir Dis 1986;134:34–38.

78. Weyer K, Kleeberg HH. Primary and acquired drug resistance in adult black patients with tuberculosis in South Africa: results of a continuous national drug resistance surveillance program involvement. Tuberc Lung Dis 1992;73:106–112.

79. Weyer K, Groenewald P, Zwarenstein M, Lombard CJ. Tuberculosis drug resistance in the Western Cape. S Afr Med J 1995; 85:499–504.

80. Winder FG, Collins P B, Whelan D. Effects of ethionamide and isoxyl on mycolic acid synthesis in Mycobacterium tuberculosis BCG. J Gen Microbiol 1971;66:3379–3380.

81. Wolinsky E. State of the art. Nontuberculous mycobacteria and associated diseases. Am Rev Respir Dis 1979;119:107–159.

82. Wolucka BA, McNeil MR, de Hoffman E, Chojnacki T, Brennan PJ. Recognition of the lipid intermediate for arabinogalactan/arabinomannan biosynthesis and its relation to the mode of action of ethambutol on mycobacteria. J Biol Chem 1994;269: 23328–23335.

83. Wong CF, Yew WW. Ethambutol-induced neutropenia and eosinophilia. Chest 1994;106:1638–1639.

84. Wong PC, Yew WW, Wong CF, Choi HY. Ethambutol-induced pulmonary infiltrates with eosinophilia and skin involvement. Eur Respir J 1995;8:866–868.

85. Yates MD, Collins CH. Sensitivity of opportunist mycobacteria to rifampin and ethambutol. Tubercle 1981;62:117–121.

Antimycobacterial Agents: Ethionamide

Shaun E. Berning and Charles A. Peloquin

CLASS: THIOAMIDES
Chemical Structure

Ethionamide (ETA, 2-ethylisothionicotinamide, 2-ethyl-4-pyridinecarbothioamide) was first synthesized in 1956 (9, 11). Subsequently, prothionamide, the *n*-propyl derivative of ethionamide, was synthesized. This compound, which is felt to

be equivalent in activity to ethionamide, is considered by some to be better tolerated than ethionamide (1, 9).

Ethionamide is a bright yellow powder with a slight sulfur-like odor. It is slightly soluble in water, less so in alcohol (10, 19), and readily soluble in organic solvents. Ethionamide shares structural features with two other antimycobacterial agents, isonicotinic acid hydrazide (isoniazid) and, more distantly, thiacetazone (10, 16, 19).

Structure-Activity Relationships

Experiments showed that the free carbothionamide group is essential for activity (21, 22). This group is also found on thiacetazone. The pyridine ring of ethionamide also appears to have a special role in its mechanisms of action. The pyridine ring is also found in isoniazid.

ANTIMICROBIAL ACTIVITY
Spectrum

Ethionamide is a very specific agent only active against organisms of the genus *Mycobacterium* (5, 19, 21–23). Although it has activity against organisms such as *M. bovis* and *M. kansasii,* it is most often used to treat infections due to *M. tuberculosis, M. avium-intracellulare,* and *M. leprae.* The minimum inhibitory concentrations (MICs) of ethionamide versus *M. tuberculosis* vary depending upon the media in which they were tested. In 7H12 broth, MICs range from 0.3 to 1.2 μg/mL and in 7H11 agar, 2.5 to 10 μg/mL. The inhibitory effect of ethionamide against *M. avium* strains is similar to its effect against *M. tuberculosis,* with MICs of 0.3 to more than 15 μg/mL in 7H12 broth and 2.5 to 15 μg/mL in 7H10 agar (5). Ethionamide is very active against *M. leprae,* with MICs estimated to be 0.05 μg/mL (1, 9, 18). The drug was found more effective when administered to mice daily than once or twice weekly.

When considering in vitro activity, one must take into account the potential for degradation of ethionamide within the test media, which can approach 50% loss of drug over several days (19). Under certain conditions, heavy metal salts can have an inactivating effect. Increasing alkalization and increasing protein concentrations in the test media also may decrease ethionamide's apparent activity (19).

Pharmacodynamic Effects

Bactericidal Effects

The MBCs (minimal bactericidal concentrations) of ethionamide in 7H12 broth are 2.5 to 5.0 μg/mL, giving MBC:MIC ratios of 2 to 4 (4, 5, 19). Ethionamide doses of 500 mg may produce serum concentrations in vivo above the MBC (12). The bactericidal activity against *M. avium* is poor, with MBCs of 80 μg/mL, producing MBC:MIC ratios of 16 to 64. These MBCs are much higher than achievable serum or tissue ethionamide concentrations (5, 12, 19). The drug was bactericidal against *M. leprae* in mice at dietary doses of 0.01% but only bacteriostatic at dietary doses of 0.003% (1, 18).

Postantibiotic Effects (PAEs)

Although a 3- to 17-day delay in regrowth of mycobacteria was reported following pulse exposures to ethionamide at concentrations of 50 μg/mL, this cannot be considered to indicate a true PAE. These concentrations are well above attainable maximum serum ethionamide concentrations, and the delay was partially due to the killing effect of the drug (4).

Like many antimycobacterial drugs, ethionamide retains some activity when given to animals once or twice weekly (19). It is not clear if this represents an in vivo PAE or simply reflects the fact the mycobacteria grow relatively slowly, with regrowth taking time to become apparent.

Effects of Subinhibitory Concentrations

No specific activity has been attributed to subinhibitory concentrations of ethionamide. In vitro, subinhibitory concentrations may enhance the ability to isolate resistant subpopulations (19). It is not known if subinhibitory concentrations of ethionamide contribute to multidrug therapy in vivo.

Effects on Host Immunity

Ethionamide has no known direct effects on host immunity.

Pharmacodynamic Correlates with Outcome

In animals and in man, 10 mg/kg is generally recognized as the threshold dose for activity (19). In vitro, sustained concentrations above the MIC appear to be more effective than widely fluctuating concentrations (19). Increasing the concentration from 4 to 16 μg/mL did not potentiate the short-term bactericidal activity of ethionamide (4 days of incubation), although the higher concentrations were more effective during longer incubation periods (19).

Because ethionamide is potentially bactericidal and because its affects appear to be directed at cell wall synthesis, it is tempting to make comparisons with the β-lactams. Under this scenario, time above MIC would be the most important parameter. However, unlike the β-lactams, ethionamide may have indirect cell-wall activity involving disruption of synthesis of mycolic acids that are subsequently incorporated into the mycobacterial cell wall. Thus, ethionamide's action may resemble, in some ways, that of other intracellular poisons such as the aminoglycosides, for which the C_{max}:MIC ratio appears more important.

Further complicating the analysis is the fact that mycobacteria grow very slowly relative to the serum concentration-versus-time curve of most antimycobacterial drugs. In addition, mycobacteria appear to exist in different subpopulations in vivo, and these subpopulations may vary in their responses to antimycobacterial drugs (4). *M. tuberculosis* is capable of remaining dormant for long periods of time in vivo, and these dormant bacteria appear relatively impervious to the short-term effects of antimycobacterial drugs. Therefore, it is difficult to draw inclusive and conclusive pharmacodynamic correlates for ethionamide. From a practical standpoint, most patients cannot tolerate individual doses larger than 500 mg, and these doses produce C_{max} of 5 μg/mL or less in most patients. This, combined with ethionamide's short serum half-life, has led to the common practice of twice-daily dosing.

MECHANISM OF ACTION

Although the mechanism of action of ethionamide is not fully understood, it appears to share some aspects of activity with isoniazid and with thiacetazone. In fact, ethionamide shows some cross-resistance with thiacetazone (5, 19, 21–23). Ethionamide was once thought to work through inhibition of protein synthesis or disruption of ATP-controlled metabolism (19, 20, 23). However, more-recent work suggests that like isoniazid, ethionamide disrupts mycolic acid synthesis (21–23). When added to cultures of actively multiplying mycobacteria, ethionamide can induce a rapid loss of acid fastness. Ethionamide is active against both extra- and intracellular mycobacteria in monocytes (5, 19, 21–23).

Still, there are differences between isoniazid and ethionamide that remain unresolved (17). A clear-cut relationship was not established between ethionamide susceptibility and mycolic acid biosynthesis, given the great variability in the behaviors of the different mycobacterial species tested. Quémard et al. (17) postulated that ethionamide selectively alters formation of oxygenated mycolic acids early in the synthetic pathway. This contrasts with isoniazid, which acts at a very early step of mycolic acid synthesis, resulting in complete inhibition of all types of mycolic acid synthesis. Consistent with these differences in mechanisms of action is the frequently observed lack of cross-resistance between isoniazid and ethionamide when mycobacterial isolates are tested in vitro.

MECHANISMS OF RESISTANCE
Commonly Resistant Organisms

As mentioned above, ethionamide is effective only against organisms of the genus *Mycobacterium*. Among the mycobacteria, *M. africanum* may be resistant (9, 17). Although ethionamide does not show cross-resistance with any agents commercially available in the United States, it does show cross-resistance with thiosemicarbazones (e.g., thiacetazone) and diphenylthioureas, namely, thiocarlide (DATC) (5, 9, 19–23).

Primary drug resistance of antituberculosis medications was monitored in the United States from 1975 to 1982 (9). Overall resistance to ethionamide was reported at 1.1% and was reported higher in certain ethnic groups such as Hispanics and Asians. It was also higher in certain areas such as the U.S.-Mexico border region and Chicago (9).

Mechanisms of Resistance

As with other antimycobacterial agents, resistance in previously susceptible organisms may develop rapidly both in vivo and in vitro when ethionamide is used as a single agent in the treatment of tuberculosis (5, 9, 19, 21–23). This appears to be due to naturally occurring resistant mutants present in a population of mycobacteria. Under the selective pressure of a single drug, all organisms are eliminated except the resistant subpopulation, which continues to multiply, eventually becoming the dominant population.

Methods to Overcome and Prevent Resistance

Acquired resistance to ethionamide may be prevented by using the drug in combination with at least one or two other antimycobacterial drugs (9, 10). Higher doses of ethionamide as monotherapy do not prevent emergence of resistance (19). In vitro, subinhibitory concentrations enhance the selection of resistant organisms (19). It is not known if this also occurs in vivo, although the possibility exists. Thus, it appears desirable to achieve serum concentrations above the MIC of the isolate.

PHARMACOKINETICS
Absorption

Although the absolute bioavailability of ethionamide has not been determined, the available data suggest that its absorption is nearly complete (6–8, 12, 13). The time to maximum concentration (T_{max}) following 500-mg oral doses is 1.75 ± 0.75 h, with maximum concentrations (C_{max}) of 2.24 ± 0.82 µg/mL. The $AUC_{0-\infty}$ following 500-mg doses in 12 healthy volunteers was reported to be 10.34 µg/h/mL (13).

When administered as a 500-mg rectal dose in 12 normal volunteers, the bioavailability of ethionamide was 57.3% of that after oral administration, based on the area under the serum-concentration-versus-time curve, or AUC (13). Maximum serum concentrations following these rectal doses were 33% of those from oral doses, and T_{max} occurred 3 to 5 h after the rectal doses.

Distribution

Ethionamide is widely distributed into most body tissues and fluids (5, 12). An estimated 10 to 30% of the drug is protein bound. The drug readily crosses both normal and inflamed meninges, with cerebrospinal fluid concentrations reported to be equal to those in the plasma. Ethionamide readily crosses the placenta; it is unknown if it is distributed into human breast milk (9, 12). Given that ethionamide is of similar size and chemical structure as isoniazid, it is likely that some ethionamide passes into breast milk.

Metabolism and Excretion

Ethionamide is extensively metabolized by sulfoxidation, desulfuration, and deamination, followed by methylation. Metabolism most likely occurs in the liver, producing both active and inactive metabolites (6, 8, 9, 12, 16). The sulfoxide metabolite appears to have comparable activity to the parent compound, and interconversion between the two compounds has been described in animals and in humans (6, 8, 16). The serum concentration profile of the sulfoxide metabolite parallels that of ethionamide, at slightly lower concentrations (6). Limited amounts (≤5% of the dose) are excreted in the urine as unchanged drug and as ethionamide sulfoxide, its principal metabolite (5, 9, 12, 13). The serum elimination half-life of ethionamide ranges from 1.5 to 3.0 h. Renal elimination of ethionamide is generally complete at 13 h (6).

DOSAGE REGIMENS
Normal

The usual dose of ethionamide ranges from 250 to 1000 mg/day. Most patients tolerate doses of 250 to 500 mg every 12 h (9, 10). Ethionamide may also be dosed at 15 to 20 mg/kg/day, with a maximum dose of 30 mg/kg or 1000 mg (10). Doses above 500 mg at one time are not usually tolerated (2).

Therapeutic Drug Monitoring

At National Jewish Medical and Research Center, where therapeutic drug monitoring (TDM) of antimycobacterial drugs is standard practice, samples for serum ethionamide determinations are drawn at 2 and 6 h postdose (15). The 2-h value provides information on the maximum concentrations, while the 6-h value gives information on the rate and completeness of absorption and on clearance of the drug (15). Previously reported wide variations of serum concentrations were probably due to problems with enteric-coated tablets, which are no longer used (3, 9). At National Jewish, we use 1 to 5 μg/mL as our serum concentration "normal range" for doses of 250 to 500 mg (2). When treating leprosy, lower doses of 250 to 375 mg (5–10 mg/kg) daily may be used (9).

Although the manufacturer states that the optimum pediatric dose has not been established, doses have been reported at 15 to 20 mg/kg/day, with a 1000-mg maximum (10, 14).

Renal Failure

No dosage adjustment is necessary in renal impairment (12).

Hepatic Failure

Some references state that ethionamide is relatively contraindicated in patients with severe hepatic impairment (10). This clearly depends on the availability of therapeutic alternatives. We are unaware of data showing enhanced ethionamide toxicity in the face of hepatic impairment. Because the elimination of ethionamide may be compromised in patients with severe hepatic impairment, serum concentration monitoring of ethionamide would be indicated in such patients (12, 15).

Obesity, Ascites, and Edema

Ethionamide is fairly lipophilic, and it appears to be distributed into most body tissues and fluids (5, 10, 12). It has not been studied in obese patients or those with ascites or edema, so it is not known if larger doses should be used in such patients. Serum concentration monitoring is indicated in these settings.

Pregnancy

Although the drug has been used safely on occasion in pregnant women, the safe use of ethionamide in pregnancy has not been established. Its use during pregnancy has been associated with premature delivery, congenital deformities, and Down's syndrome. The drug has also caused teratogenic effects in animals at high doses. Because of these factors, ethionamide should generally be avoided in women who are pregnant, provided therapeutic alternatives are available (10, 12).

ADVERSE EFFECTS

The most significant adverse effect of ethionamide is gastrointestinal (GI) intolerance, primarily nausea or vomiting (2, 3, 9, 10). This may occur at any dose of ethionamide and is reported to occur more frequently in females than males. It has also been reported that when it occurs at low doses of ethionamide, it may not necessarily occur at higher doses (2); however, given the narrow range of tolerated doses, intolerance at lower doses does not typically lead to attempts to use higher doses.

Because GI intolerance is so common and at times severe, the potential benefit of enteric-coated tablets was studied. Unfortunately, these did not offer any significant reduction in GI symptoms, and they caused erratic absorption of the drug (3). These findings led the authors to conclude that GI intolerance to ethionamide was due more to toxicity of the drug than to irritation of the gastric mucosa. GI intolerance with ethionamide has also been reported with intravenous administration, suggesting that the mechanism of this reaction is centrally mediated. However, ethionamide accumulates in gastric fluids even after intravenous doses, so local irritation remains a potential sole cause of this toxicity (5). Ethionamide suppositories, alone or combined with smaller oral doses, have been used successfully in some patients to circumvent GI toxicity.

Ethionamide has been administered with food or prior to bedtime to minimize GI intolerance (9). Because data are not available regarding the effect of food on the absorption of ethionamide, minimal amounts of simple carbohydrates should be considered if food must be given with ethionamide.

Hepatocellular injury is possible with ethionamide (2, 9, 10). It is usually manifested as a rise in AST and ALT, with occasional increases in the total bilirubin as well. It is not known if this hepatotoxicity is due to a direct toxic effect or to a hypersensitivity reaction. In our experience, the duration of the biochemical abnormalities with ethionamide hepatitis may be considerably longer (4–6 weeks) than that seen with isoniazid or rifampin (1–2 weeks). Concomitant use of rifampin has been reported to increase the risk of hepatotoxicity, although data appear sparse (9).

Ethionamide may cause central nervous system (CNS) toxicity (2, 9, 10). Various CNS effects such as headache, drowsiness, giddiness, depression, psychosis, peripheral neuritis, and visual disturbances have been reported during treatment with ethionamide (2, 9, 10). Of course ethionamide is generally used with other drugs, so isolating the toxicity to ethionamide may not have been possible. Although some reports indicate that use of a B-complex vitamin may reduce or prevent these effects, others found that these vitamins offered no benefit in reducing these symptoms (2, 9, 10).

Other adverse effects reported with ethionamide include goiter (with or without hypothyroidism), gynecomastia, alopecia, impotence, menorrhagia, photodermatitis, acne, and arthritis (9, 10). The management of diabetes may also be more difficult in patients receiving ethionamide. It is not known how ethionamide interferes with hormonal regulation to produce some of these effects.

DRUG INTERACTIONS

There are some reports that the incidence of CNS effects may be increased when ethionamide is used in combination with isoniazid or cycloserine. Therefore caution should be taken when these drug combinations are used (10).

We have observed that the incidence of hypothyroidism is increased when ethionamide is used in combination with p-aminosalicylic acid (PAS). Therefore, we recommend checking the thyroid-stimulating hormone (TSH) concentrations every 1 to 2 months.

As stated above, because data are not available regarding the effect of food on the absorption of ethionamide, minimal amounts of simple carbohydrates should be considered if food must be given with ethionamide. Antacids should be avoided, as these have been shown to inhibit the absorption of chemically related isoniazid (12).

CLINICAL INDICATIONS

Ethionamide is generally reserved for patients with multidrug-resistant tuberculosis (MDR-TB) or patients intolerant of first-line agents such as isoniazid and rifampin. It frequently causes GI intolerance; therefore, doses should be gradually increased over several days. Patients typically require counseling and encouragement to complete regimens that contain ethionamide.

REFERENCES

1. Closton MJ, Ellard GA, Gammon PT. Drugs for combined therapy: experimental studies on the antileprosy activity of ethionamide and prothionamide, and a general review. Lepr Rev 1978;49:115–126.
2. Fox W, Robinson DK, Tall R, Mitchison DA, Kent PW, Macfadyen DM. A study of acute intolerance to ethionamide, including a comparison with prothionamide, and of the influence of a vitamin B-complex additive in prophylaxis. Tubercle 1969;50:125–143.
3. Gronroos JA, Toivanen A. Blood ethionamide levels after enteric-coated and uncoated tablets. Curr Ther Res 1964;6:105–114.
4. Heifets LB. Antituberculosis drugs: antimicrobial activity in vitro. In: Heifets LB, ed. Drug susceptibility in the chemotherapy of mycobacterial infections. Boca Raton, FL: CRC Press, 1991:13–57.
5. Iwainsky H. Mode of action, biotransformation and pharmacokinetics of antituberculosis drugs in animals and man. In: Bartmann K, ed. Antituberculosis drugs. Berlin: Springer-Verlag, 1988:399–553.
6. Jenner PJ, Ellard GA, Gruer PJK, Aber VR. A comparison of the blood levels and urinary excretion or ethionamide and prothionamide in man. J Antimicrob Chemother 1984;13:267–277.
7. Jenner PJ, Smith SE. Plasma levels of ethionamide and prothionamide in a volunteer following intravenous and oral dosages. Lepr Rev 1987;58:31–37.
8. Johnston JP, Kane PO, Kibby MR. The metabolism of ethionamide and its sulphoxide. J Pharm Pharmacol 1967;19:1–9.
9. Kucers A, Bennett N McK, eds. The use of antibiotics. 4th ed. Philadelphia: JB Lippencott, 1988:1418.
10. McEvoy GK, ed. AHFS drug information. Bethesda, MD: American Soc Health-Systems Pharmacists, 1996:406–408.
11. Offe HA. Historical introduction and chemical characteristics of antituberculosis drugs. In: Bartmann K, ed. Antituberculosis drugs. Berlin: Springer-Verlag, 1988:1–30.
12. Peloquin CA. Antituberculosis drugs: pharmacokinetics. In: Heifets LB, ed. Drug susceptibility in the chemotherapy of mycobacterial infections. Boca Raton, FL: CRC Press, 1991: 89–122.
13. Peloquin CA, James GT, McCarthy E, Goble M. Pharmacokinetic evaluation of ethionamide suppositories. Pharmacotherapy 1991;11:359–363.
14. Peloquin CA, Berning SE. Tuberculosis and multi-drug resistant tuberculosis in children. Pediatr Nurs 1995;21:566–572.
15. Peloquin CA. Using therapeutic drug monitoring to dose the antimycobacterial drugs. Clin Chest Med 1997;18:79–87.
16. Prema K, Gopinathan KP. Metabolism of ethionamide, a second-line antitubercular drug. J Ind Inst Sci 1976;58:16–27.
17. Quémard A, Lanéelle G, Lacave C. Mycolic acid synthesis: a target for ethionamide in mycobacteria? Antimicrob Agent Chemother 1992;36:1316–1321.
18. Shepard CC, Jenner PJ, Ellard GA, Lancaster RD. An experimental study of the antileprosy activity of a series of thioamides in the mouse. Int J Lepr 1985;53(4):587–594.
19. Trnka L, Mison P, Bartmann K, Otten H. Experimental evaluation of efficacy. In: Bartmann K, ed. Antituberculosis drugs. Berlin: Springer-Verlag, 1988:31–232.
20. Tsukamura M, Tsukamura S, Mizuno S, Nakano E. The mechanism of action of ethionamide. Am Rev Respir Dis 1964;89: 933–935.
21. Verbist L. Mode of action of antituberculous drugs (part I). Medicon Intl 1974;3:11–23.
22. Verbist L. Mode of action of antituberculous drugs (part II). Medicon Intl 1974;3:3–17.
23. Winder FG. Mode of action of the antimycobacterial agents and associated aspects of the molecular biology of the mycobacteria. In: Ratledge C, Stanford J, eds. The biology of mycobacteria: vol 1—Physiology, identification, and classification. London: Academic Press, 1982:353–438.

Antimycobacterial Agents: Isoniazid

Shaun E. Berning and Charles A. Peloquin

CLASS: ISONICOTINIC ACID HYDRAZIDE
Chemical Structure

Isoniazid (INH, isonicotinic acid hydrazide, isonicotinoylhydrazine, pyridine-4-carboxylic acid hydrazide) is a synthetic agent with the chemical formula $C_6H_7N_3O$ and a molecular weight of 137.15 (56). It is a white crystalline powder with a solubility of 125 mg/mL in water and 20 mg/mL in alcohol (40, 46, 56). INH displays varying stability in solutions: aqueous solutions are said to be stable for up to a week at 37°C (76). However, INH decays fairly rapidly in serum or plasma left at room temperature. Work from our laboratory indicates that degradation is measurable as early as 1 hour (unpublished data).

Structure-Activity Relationships

Both the pyridine nucleus and the carboxylic acid hydrazide moiety appear to be key functional groups on the isoniazid molecule (78, 79). Conversion to the acetylated form by hepatic *N*-acetyltransferase, for example, renders INH inactive. Other monosubstitutions on the terminal nitrogen yield less active or inactive compounds (78, 79).

ANTIMICROBIAL ACTIVITY
Spectrum

INH is highly specific; it is active only against mycobacteria. Its minimum inhibitory concentration (MIC) against *Mycobacterium tuberculosis* is 0.01 to 0.25 μg/mL (76, 78, 79). Most nontuberculous mycobacteria (NTM) are resistant to INH. Among the NTM, *M. kansasii* and *M. xenopi* are the most susceptible to INH (73, 76, 78, 79).

Pharmacodynamic Effects
Bactericidal Effects

INH is generally considered bactericidal. It has been reported to kill mycobacteria at concentrations at or very near the MIC. The MICs vary slightly, depending upon the medium. MICs in 7H12 broth were reported to be 0.025 to 0.05 μg/mL and 0.1 to 0.2 μg/mL in 7H10 or 7H11 agar (31). The minimum bactericidal concentrations (MBCs) in 7H12 broth were equivalent to the MICs (0.05 μg/mL), confirming INH's high bactericidal activity. Upon exposure to 0.5 μg/mL of INH, *M. tuberculosis* cells begin to lose their ability to synthesize mycolic acid immediately. Complete loss occurs as early as 60 min. The antimycobacterial effects of INH become irreversible after about 12 h of exposure (76, 78, 79, 84). Any cells remaining viable at that time gradually die within 2 h (73). INH's activity in vitro is relatively insensitive to the size of the inoculum, but its activity is abolished under anaerobic conditions. Mycobacteria undergoing logarithmic-phase growth are most susceptible; older cultures and slower-growing organisms show slower INH killing kinetics. Dormant organisms are not susceptible to INH, as uptake of INH is an active process (76, 78, 79, 84).

Postantibiotic Effects (PAEs)

There have been discrepancies reported regarding the effect of the exposure time of INH. Beggs and Jenne found that cells of *M. tuberculosis* exposed to 0.5 μg/h of INH for 6 days showed 25% growth inhibition, whereas cells exposed to 1 μg/h for the same time showed 50% inhibition (9). The findings of Awaness and Mitchison differed slightly (6). They found INH to be more active given as successive short exposures than given as single short or prolonged exposures. According to their analysis, INH's activity was related more to the total period of exposure than to the time-concentration product. The lag period before regrowth after these successive exposures was 5 days. Additional work by these investigators showed that 24-h exposure of the H37Rv strain of tuberculosis to 1 μg/mL of INH produced a growth delay of 2.5 to 6.9 days (76). Exposure to 96 h produced a delay of 6.2 to 19 days. Exposure periods of 2 to 12 h did not slow the lag phase at all (76, 84). The differences

between these studies may be explained, in part, by differences in the physiologic state of the organisms (6).

Of course, animals and humans are not the same as in vitro systems, since INH is actively removed from the body even as it is being absorbed from the gastrointestinal (GI) tract. Still, repeated short exposures to the drug (i.e., daily doses) can produce bactericidal effects and markedly delay resumption of tuberculosis multiplication (76, 78, 79, 84). These effects form the basis for intermittent therapy with INH. An important factor related to intermittent therapy is that mycobacteria grow slowly even in the absence of drug, with doubling times of approximately 24 h.

Effects of Subinhibitory Concentrations

No specific activity has been attributed to subinhibitory concentrations of INH. In vitro, subinhibitory concentrations may enhance the ability to isolate resistant subpopulations (76). It is not known if subinhibitory concentrations of INH contribute to multidrug therapy in vivo. Conversely, it has been shown that even low levels of in vitro resistance (MIC, 0.2–1.0 μg/mL) involve an elevated risk of therapeutic failure, even with combined therapy. If bacilli are completely resistant to 0.1 μg/mL or partly resistant to 1 μg/mL of INH, the efficacy of even high doses of INH (20–75 mg/kg/day) is reduced. INH-dependent mycobacteria have not been described (76).

Effects on Host Immunity

INH has no known direct effects on host immunity.

Pharmacodynamic Correlates with Outcome

In vitro, 1 μg/mL of INH generally produces the maximum killing effect on organisms with an MIC of 0.06 μg/mL (76). Further increases in INH concentration do not increase its effect. The C_{max}:MIC ratio at 1 μg/mL is about 17:1.

In guinea pigs, rabbits, and monkeys, 10 mg/kg generally produces optimal results (76). Because of their more rapid acetylation of INH, rats require higher doses. Single doses appear to be slightly better than divided doses in these animal models. Comparison of animal versus human serum and tissue concentrations suggests that similar efficacy should be seen in man at 5 mg/kg. In rodent models, shorter intervals between doses produced better results (daily > every 3 days > every 7 or 10 days).

Because INH is potentially bactericidal and because its effects appear to be directed at cell wall synthesis, it is tempting to make comparisons with the β-lactams. Under this scenario, time above MIC would be the most important parameter. However, unlike the β-lactams, INH's cell wall activity may be indirect, involving disruption of synthesis of mycolic acids that are subsequently incorporated into the mycobacterial cell wall. Thus INH's action may resemble, in some ways, that of other intracellular poisons such as the aminoglycosides, for which the C_{max}:MIC ratio appears to be more important.

To further complicate the analysis, mycobacteria grow very slowly relative to the serum concentration-versus-time curve of most antimycobacterial drugs. In addition, mycobacteria appear to exist in different subpopulations in vivo, and these subpopulations may vary in their responses to antimycobacterial drugs (31). One proposed population of mycobacteria is capable of remaining dormant for long periods of time in vivo, and these dormant bacteria appear relatively impervious to the short-term effects of antimycobacterial drugs. Thus it is difficult to draw inclusive and conclusive pharmacodynamic correlates for INH. From a practical standpoint, intermittent regimens (INH given at higher doses two to three times per week) have been effective in humans (described below).

MECHANISM OF ACTION

Although the mechanism of action of INH is not fully understood, the drug appears to act by inhibiting mycolic acid synthesis, which results in loss of acid fastness and disruption of the cell wall (31, 40, 46, 76, 78, 79, 84). Mycolic acids are primary components of mycobacterial cell walls, conferring a permeability barrier to hydrophilic solutes (13). Disruption of their synthesis leads to cellular deformities in *M. tuberculosis* (6, 73, 76, 78, 79). INH specifically inhibits synthesis of unsaturated fatty acids containing 26 carbons or more (13, 47, 79).

Recent investigations using newer genetic techniques suggest that INH is a prodrug, activated within *M. tuberculosis* by the endogenous enzyme katG (37, 47, 89). Activated INH then appears to attack the enzyme(s) involved in production of an unsaturated 24-carbon fatty acid required for mycolic acid synthesis (47). The *katG* gene encodes for mycobacterial catalase-peroxidase (13). Most isolates highly resistant to INH do not synthesize catalase or peroxidase (13, 79). Further research has shown that about 50% of INH-resistant clinical isolates of *M. tuberculosis* have deletions or missense mutations in the *katG* gene (13).

In *M. smegmatis,* hyperexpression of the protein InhA confers resistance to INH. InhA, however, does not match the profile of the 24-carbon fatty acid denaturase described above (47). Mdluli et al. have shown that the precise target for the action of INH in *M. smegmatis* appears to differ from that found in *M. tuberculosis.* This suggests that future research on the mechanism of action of INH should be conducted in *M. tuberculosis,* despite the greater difficulty of working with a potential pathogen.

Other mechanisms, including depletion of nicotinamide-adenine-dinucleotide (NAD), had been considered as possible mechanisms for INH's action; however, these have given way to a mechanism in which INH is activated within *M. tuberculosis* and subsequently disrupts mycolic acid synthesis (6, 73, 79).

MECHANISMS OF RESISTANCE
Commonly Resistant Organisms

As mentioned above, INH is active primarily against *M. tuberculosis;* it has moderate activity against some other mycobacteria species such as *M. kansasii* and *M. bovis* (31, 40, 46, 76, 79, 84). *M. avium-intracellulare* is resistant to INH; MICs of *M. avium* in 7H12 broth or 7H10 agar are 1.25 to more than 10 μg/mL (31).

Mechanisms of Resistance

As with other antimycobacterial agents, resistance in previously susceptible organisms may develop rapidly both in vivo

and in vitro when ethionamide is used as a single agent in the treatment of tuberculosis (6, 40, 46, 76, 79). This appears to be due to naturally occurring resistant mutants present in a population of mycobacteria. Under the selective pressure of a single drug, all organisms are eliminated except the resistant subpopulation, which continues to multiply, eventually becoming the entire population.

INH-resistant isolates may display lower virulence than fully susceptible isolates, as demonstrated in various animal models (76). However, INH-resistant isolates are still quite capable of causing human disease, and in this host, reduced virulence has not been clearly demonstrated.

Although inhibition of mycolic acid synthesis is believed to be the mechanism of action for INH, the exact target of action has not been identified. Activity of the catalase-peroxidase may normally produce an INH intermediate that then targets a step in mycolic acid synthesis. As described above, mutations in the *katG* gene can lead to loss of catalase-peroxidase activity and to INH resistance (13, 37, 47, 89). Other mechanisms of resistance remain possible.

The protein InhA has also been identified as a possible target of action for INH and therefore may be related to its resistance (4, 8, 13, 47, 66). However, this mechanism may be more specific to *M. smegmatis* than *M. tuberculosis* (47).

Primary resistance to INH, which occurs with inhalation of INH-resistant strains, is a recent concern in the United States. In 1991, the Centers for Disease Control and Prevention (CDC) found that 14.4% of recurrent infections were resistant to at least one drug, most often INH, and 3.3% were resistant to both INH and rifampin. Among recurrent cases, the incidence of resistance to INH and rifampin doubled from 3.0% in 1982–86 to 6.9% in 1991 (15). The overall incidence of INH plus rifampin resistance is higher in certain ethnic groups such as African Americans, Mexican Americans, and Indochinese refugees (15, 40). Recent outbreaks of multidrug-resistant tuberculosis (MDR-TB) have occurred in institutional settings, such as health-care facilities and correctional facilities. Other factors contributing to MDR-TB include human immunodeficiency virus (HIV) seropositivity, drug abuse, homelessness, mental illness, and poor socioeconomic conditions (15). Primary drug resistance to INH also occurs more frequently in developing countries such as those in Southeast Asia, Africa, and Latin America (40).

Cross-resistance between INH and other antimycobacterial drugs generally does not occur (76). Highly resistant isolates may show reduced sensitivity to ethionamide, which may be related to some overlap in their mechanisms of action (13, 76).

Mechanisms to Overcome and Prevent Resistance

Acquired resistance to INH may be prevented by using it in combination with at least one or two other antimycobacterial drugs (46, 76). Higher doses of INH as monotherapy do not prevent emergence of resistance (76). In vitro, subinhibitory concentrations enhance selection of resistant organisms. It is not known if this also occurs in vivo, although the possibility exists. Thus, it appears desirable to achieve serum concentrations above the MIC of the isolate.

PHARMACOKINETICS
Absorption

INH is readily absorbed from the GI tract and from intramuscular injection sites (40, 46, 57). Its oral absorption may be affected by the presence of food, especially after meals high in carbohydrates (44, 57, 88). This may be due to the ability of INH to react readily with glucose, aldehydes, and ketones present in food (56). Antacids may also reduce INH's absorption (44, 57). Maximum serum concentrations are obtained within 0.5 to 2 h after oral doses (57, 58, 63). Maximum concentrations of 3 to 6 µg/mL are achieved after a 300-mg dose and 9 to 18 µg/mL after a 900-mg dose. Concentrations may be somewhat lower in fast acetylators because of greater first-pass metabolism (57, 58, 63). Absorption of INH does not vary with the various combination oral products (i.e., INH plus rifampin (Rifamate, Hoechst Marion Roussel) or INH, rifampin, and pyrazinamide (Rifater, Hoechst Marion Roussel) (46).

Distribution

INH is widely distributed into most body tissues and fluids, with a volume of distribution (Vd) of 0.6 to 1.2 L/kg and somewhat larger volumes for fast acetylators after oral doses (57, 58, 63), which probably reflects lower bioavailability due to greater first-pass clearance in fast acetylators. Because the calculation of volume following oral doses assumes complete bioavailability, a falsely larger Vd is seen. There is probably no significant difference in Vd between slow and fast acetylators.

INH penetrates the cerebrospinal fluid (CSF), even in the absence of inflammation (57). CSF concentrations have been reported at 20 to 100% of serum concentrations and are generally well above the typical MIC for *M. tuberculosis*. INH is therefore a key agent in treating tuberculosis infections of the central nervous system (57). INH readily crosses the placenta and is excreted in human breast milk at concentrations nearly equal to serum concentrations. Protein binding of INH has been reported to be 0 to 10% (57). INH penetrates the macrophage and therefore acts intracellularly against mycobacteria (35, 40, 76).

Metabolism/Excretion

INH is extensively metabolized in the liver to a number of compounds, mostly by acetylation and dehydrazination (14, 25, 35, 57, 58, 82). Hepatic and (potentially) intestinal *N*-acetyltransferase form the principle metabolite, acetylisoniazid. This is further metabolized to form mono- and diacetylhydrazine. Isonicotinyl glycine and isonicotinic acid are additional potential metabolites (35, 57, 58). All of the metabolites are biologically inactive (35). Although acetylisoniazid could be cleaved to reform active isoniazid, this has not been demonstrated in humans. INH may also be directly conjugated to form acid-labile hydrazones of pyruvic or α-ketoglutaric acid; these hydrazones are readily cleaved back to INH. Finally, INH may directly form isonicotinic acid and hydrazine, although the contribution of this pathway in human metabolism is not clear (40, 46, 57).

The rate at which humans acetylate INH is genetically determined. Slow acetylation is an autosomal recessive trait that results from *N*-acetyltransferase deficiency (35, 57, 58). Rapid acetylators are heterozygous or homozygous dominants. The distribution of acetylator status is racially dependent; approximately 50% of whites and blacks are slow acetylators, and 80 to 90% of Asians and Eskimos are rapid acetylators (25, 35, 40, 46, 57).

Rapid acetylators form more acetylisoniazid and thus more monoacetylhydrazine, which appears to be related to INH's hepatotoxicity (25, 35, 57, 58). Metabolism of this compound potentially forms reactive intermediates that may include hydrazine, acetyldiazine, acetylonium ion, acetyl radical, or ketene. These compounds may then bind to hepatic macromolecules and cause hepatic necrosis (42, 58, 64, 75). Because of this, rapid acetylators were thought to perhaps be at increased risk of hepatotoxicity. However, rapid acetylators not only form more monoacetylhydrazine, they also acetylate this compound more rapidly to diacetylhydrazine, which is not toxic (24, 30, 42, 58, 75). It has been proposed that slow acetylators may be at increased risk of hepatotoxicity (42). However, clinical trials show the association of acetylator status and risk of hepatotoxicity to be weak (24, 30, 35, 58).

The serum half-life of INH ranges from 1.0 to 1.8 h in most rapid acetylators and 3.0 to 4.0 h in most slow acetylators (14, 25, 57, 58, 82). Approximately 75 to 96% of INH is excreted in the urine in 24 h as unchanged drug or metabolites. Fast acetylators excrete roughly 10% of the dose as unchanged INH, about 50% as acetylisoniazid, about 18% as diacetylhydrazine, and only trace amounts as monoacetylhydrazine. In contrast, slow acetylators excrete 30 to 35% of the dose as unchanged INH, about 50% as acetylisoniazid, and only trace amounts as mono- and diacetylhydrazine (57, 58).

DOSAGE REGIMENS
Normal

INH is used both to prevent tuberculosis disease in those exposed to active cases and to treat active disease. INH preventive therapy (IPT), also known as chemoprophylaxis or treatment of tuberculosis infection without active disease, reduces the risk of future tuberculosis by reducing the small bacterial population present in new infections and healed lesions (5, 40). The use of IPT is controversial, primarily because of its risk of hepatitis, which is discussed in greater detail below (18, 34, 71).

Because of this controversy, the American Thoracic Society (ATS) and CDC have prepared specific guidelines for who should be given IPT. The usual criterion for tuberculosis infection, based upon the Mantoux skin test (purified protein derivative, or PPD), depends upon the population being tested (5, 16, 59, 60). For HIV-infected children and adults, close contacts of infectious cases, and those with fibrotic lesions on the chest radiograph, 5 mm or more of induration is considered positive. For other at-risk adults, infants, and children, 10 mm induration or more is considered positive. In persons with no risk factors, 15 mm induration or more is considered positive (5).

Persons with the following risk factors and a positive PPD reaction should be considered for IPT regardless of age: HIV-infected persons (especially those in contact with infectious tuberculosis patients), persons at risk for HIV infection, close contacts of newly diagnosed sputum smear–positive tuberculosis patients, and recent skin-test converters (5). Persons with concurrent disease states known to increase the risk of tuberculosis should also be considered, such as those with diabetes mellitus, end-stage renal disease, diseases requiring the use of adrenocorticosteroids, intravenous drug abuse, malignancies, and chronic malnutrition. IPT should be considered for persons without the above risk factors but from high-risk groups, such as those from countries with high tuberculosis prevalence, those from medically underserved high-risk populations (i.e., Hispanics and Native Americans), and residents of long-term care facilities (e.g. nursing homes, prisons) (5).

For prevention of tuberculosis, the usual daily dose of INH is 300 mg once daily orally or (rarely) intramuscularly (5). When used for preventive therapy, INH is given as the sole agent when drug resistance is not suspected. When INH resistance is suspected, rifampin alone, or rifampin plus one other agent may be given as preventive therapy. The recommended length of preventive therapy is 12 months in the presence of HIV infection and other forms of immune suppression, and at least 6 months in persons without HIV infection.

When nonadherence is a potential problem, it has been suggested that IPT may also be administered as a twice-weekly dose of INH 15 mg/kg up to 900 mg orally or intramuscularly under directly observed therapy (DOT). Oral doses should be given 1 h before or 2 h after a meal (5, 46, 57).

Although it is not labeled for intravenous use, the intramuscular preparation can be administered intravenously (19, 35). A short-bolus injection of up to 300 mg/day should be administered over 5 to 10 min. Intermittent elevated serum INH concentrations have been associated with a greater risk of adverse neurologic effects, but this effect has not been established with intravenous administration of INH (19).

For treatment of active tuberculosis, the usual recommended dose of INH is 3 to 5 mg/kg up to 300 mg orally or intramuscularly once daily, 1 h before or 2 h after a meal (5, 16, 59, 60). It should be given in combination with one or more other antituberculous agents. INH may also be given intermittently two to three times per week in combination with various other antituberculous agents at a dose of 15 mg/kg up to 900 mg orally or intramuscularly. For the treatment of uncomplicated pulmonary tuberculosis the CDC/ATS currently recommend one of the following three short-course regimens.

1. INH, rifampin, and pyrazinamide daily for 8 weeks, followed by INH and rifampin daily or two to three times per week for 16 more weeks (24 weeks total). When the reported INH resistance is 4% or above, ethambutol or streptomycin should be added until INH and rifampin susceptibility can be demonstrated. This regimen should continue for at least 6 months and 3 months beyond culture conversion.
2. INH, rifampin, pyrazinamide, and streptomycin or ethambutol daily for 2 weeks, followed by the same medications twice weekly for 6 weeks (subtotal of 8 weeks), followed by INH and rifampin twice weekly for 16 more weeks (24 weeks total).
3. INH, rifampin, pyrazinamide, and streptomycin or ethambutol three times weekly for 8 weeks, followed by INH and

rifampin three times per week for 16 more weeks (24 weeks total).

All doses in the above regimens should be administered by DOT, especially those being given intermittently. Missed doses from intermittent therapy may seriously compromise treatment efficacy. Also, the above regimens *only* apply to isolates that prove to be susceptible to all of the drugs listed.

When treating tuberculosis in patients coinfected with HIV, the same regimens may be followed for 9 months, and 6 months after culture negativity (5, 16). When using the combination product Rifater (INH 50 mg, rifampin 120 mg, and pyrazinamide 300 mg per tablet), the daily dose is 4 tablets (INH 200 mg) for persons weighing less than 44 kg, 5 tablets (INH 250 mg) for persons weighing 44 to 54 kg, or 6 tablets (INH 300 mg) for persons weighing 55 kg or more (40).

The pediatric dose of INH is larger than that of adults. The ATS/CDC/American Academy of Pediatrics (AAP) recommend a dose of 10 to 20 mg/kg/day up to 300 mg once daily for treatment and prevention of tuberculosis. The reasons for higher doses appear to include more rapid clearance of the drug by children, excellent tolerance, and the fact that young children are more susceptible to severe forms of tuberculosis, including meningitis and miliary tuberculosis.

When treating tuberculosis with intermittent regimens, the recommended dose is 20 to 40 mg/kg twice or thrice weekly. Regimens used in adults may also be used in children with uncomplicated pulmonary tuberculosis and most cases of extrapulmonary tuberculosis (5, 16, 59, 60).

INH should be administered with pyridoxine (vitamin B_6) in both adults and children to reduce the risk of peripheral neuritis in high-risk patients such as pregnant women, the malnourished, alcoholics, cancer patients, and those predisposed to neuritis. Ten to 20 mg daily appears to be sufficient (29, 40, 46).

At National Jewish Medical and Research Center, therapeutic drug monitoring (TDM) of antimycobacterial drugs is standard practice (61, 62). Samples for serum INH concentration determinations are drawn at 2 and 6 h postdose. The 2-h concentration provides information on the maximum concentrations, while the 6-h concentration lends information on the rate and completeness of absorption and on the clearance of the drug. A 300-mg dose generally produces concentrations of 3 to 6 μg/mL at 1 to 2 h postdose, while intermittent doses of 900 mg produce concentrations of 9 to 18 μg/mL.

The acetylator status of a patient has no effect on the efficacy of INH administered daily or two to three times per week. However, rapid acetylators receiving the drug only once-weekly have shown a reduced response (26, 35).

Renal Failure

Little or no dosage adjustment of INH is necessary in most patients with renal impairment (57). Rarely, such patients may experience adverse effects related to the nervous system; for these patients, the dose can be reduced to 300 mg every other day or three times weekly, perhaps with 100 mg of pyridoxine (40, 69). INH should be administered after dialysis, because both hemodialysis and peritoneal dialysis remove some of the parent drug (46, 57). Reduced hepatic N-acetylation and reduced renal excretion of INH has been reported in chronic renal failure, leading to reduced clearance of INH, although this appears to be relatively uncommon (38).

Hepatic Failure

INH relies on the liver for most of its elimination and therefore should be used with caution in the face of hepatic failure, especially in those with ascites (see below) (57). Although INH should be used with caution in daily users of alcohol, studies have shown that its use in these patients in combination with other antimycobacterial agents does not necessarily contribute to an increased incidence of hepatotoxic effects (20, 23, 35). This group of patients may show an increased incidence of elevated transaminases; however clinical hepatitis is not common, and cessation of the drug may not be required.

Obesity

INH is a hydrophilic drug and probably does not distribute significantly into adipose tissue. In obese patients, initial dosing should be based upon ideal body weight (IBW). Serum concentrations should then be monitored to confirm adequate concentrations (57).

Ascites and Edema

Because INH is hydrophilic, it will likely distribute into ascites. Serum concentrations should thus be monitored to ensure appropriate serum concentrations are being attained (57). Although not reported, the same could be assumed for patients with significant edema.

Pregnancy

INH has been used frequently in pregnancy and is reportedly safe. As with any drug during pregnancy, the potential risks and benefits should be weighed carefully. Active tuberculosis disease needs to be treated in pregnant women. Therapy may be delayed until the second trimester if possible. The ATS, CDC, and AAP currently recommend that INH be given to pregnant women recently infected or those with other high-risk medical conditions (e.g., HIV) who are exposed to active cases of tuberculosis or shown by PPD to be infected (5, 16, 59, 60). They recommend that in patients without the above risk factors, INH preventive treatment should be withheld until after delivery. These women should be monitored carefully, as they may be at greater risk of hepatotoxicity (34). If INH is used during pregnancy, supplementation with pyridoxine is recommended (40, 46, 57).

INH does cross the placenta and is present in breast milk; therefore close monitoring of neonates and breast-fed infants for adverse effects is recommended (35, 46, 57). Typically, the dose of INH delivered to the infant is very small, and toxicity is rare.

ADVERSE EFFECTS
Hepatotoxicity

INH causes hepatitis, both alone and when used in combination with other agents (35, 46, 57). Hepatocellular damage, necrosis, and inflammation result and are indistinguishable from changes seen in viral hepatitis (12, 43, 50). Although some evidence suggests a possible hypersensitivity reaction, it is now believed that this is not the case, because peripheral eosinophilia, rash, and other markers of hypersensitivity are usually absent (80). Also, the toxicity often does not recur on rechallenge. On the other hand, hepatotoxicity does not appear to result from a direct toxic effect, as its incidence is not related to serum drug concentrations (12, 40, 72). As discussed above under metabolism, debate remains about which compound is responsible for INH-induced hepatitis. Monoacetyl-hydrazine degradation products appear most likely to be associated with the hepatotoxicity (41, 49, 68, 72, 74).

Subclinical hepatitis is often present in patients on INH, with asymptomatic mild transaminase elevation occurring in approximately 10% of persons on the drug (12, 40, 43). When clinical hepatitis is present, the symptoms usually consist of anorexia, nausea, vomiting, abdominal pain, and weight loss. Laboratory changes usually consist of elevations in AST, ALT, and occasionally bilirubin. Onset of the adverse effect usually occurs within the first few months of therapy (39, 40).

Risk factors for developing INH-induced hepatitis include age above 35 years, chronic alcohol intake, preexisting hepatic disease, and concurrent hepatotoxic agents (5, 39). In a study of 13,838 patients on INH preventative therapy, the incidence of clinical hepatitis for patients aged 0 to 34 years was 0 to 0.3%, and for patients over 35 years, 1.2 to 2.3% (39). A review by Snider and Caras in 1992 showed that the overall rate of death in patients receiving INH preventative therapy in the United States was 23.2 per 100,000 persons completing preventative therapy (71). The incidence was higher in women (69% of cases), particularly postpartum women. Some 40% of cases involved non-Hispanic white persons, and 38% were black. A retrospective meta-analysis by Steele et al. (72) looking at all reports from 1966 to 1989 of hepatitis due to regimens containing INH and/or rifampin showed that the incidence of hepatitis due to INH without rifampin was 1.3% in adults; the incidence of hepatitis in patients on regimens containing both INH and rifampin was 2.7%. This increased incidence in combination with rifampin was additive, not synergistic as once thought. The incidence of hepatitis in children on regimens with only INH was 1%; it rose to 4.7% in children on both INH and rifampin.

With the onset of clinical hepatitis, INH should be stopped immediately, because its continuation can lead to severe hepatitis or death. Serum liver function tests (LFTs) usually return to normal and symptoms subside within a short period of time (39, 40, 46, 50). Although routine monitoring of LFTs has been suggested, the often benign transient increase in transaminases makes this confusing. Routine monitoring of symptoms appears to be more important, with patients being checked monthly (5, 39). For persons over 35 years of age, baseline hepatic enzyme values should be obtained and checked monthly throughout treatment. Should enzymes reach five times the high end of the normal range, then INH should be discontinued until the enzymes approach normal. Some more-conservative guidelines suggest three to five times normal. These patients should also be monitored for symptoms of hepatitis. More careful monitoring of hepatic enzymes should be considered in high-risk groups such as chronic users of alcohol, those with chronic liver disease, and injection drug abusers. Some evidence has also shown African-American, Hispanic, and postpartum women to be at higher risk for hepatitis (5, 34).

Neurotoxicity

INH causes pyridoxine deficiency by forming hydrazones that inhibit the conversion of pyridoxine to its active form, pyridoxal phosphate. This alteration of pyridoxine metabolism leads to a variety of neuropathic events (40).

The most benign neuropathy is peripheral neuritis (28, 46). It may start as a mild paresthesia of the feet. Left untreated, this can progress to the knees and hands in a stocking-glove pattern. Muscle weakness, pain, and ataxia are occasionally seen. Patients most at risk for developing this are those deficient in pyridoxine such as malnourished patients, pregnant women, alcoholics, cancer patients, chronically ill patients, and those predisposed to neuritis, such as AIDS patients and diabetics (28, 29). Slow acetylators of INH have also been reported to be at a higher risk of developing peripheral neuritis because of their overall higher concentrations of INH (29).

Although peripheral neuritis may be seen with any dose, its incidence is much higher with daily doses of 8 mg/kg or above (10, 11, 22). Daily doses of that size are no longer used. The neuritis usually reverses within a few weeks upon prompt discontinuation of the drug. If INH is continued for more than a few weeks beyond the initial onset of symptoms, the neuritis may linger for an extended time (10, 29). Minor effects such as muscle twitching, restlessness, insomnia, and lethargy may occur at normal doses (40, 46).

Supplementation with pyridoxine at low doses (6 to 50 mg/day) in those patients at risk may prevent the onset of peripheral neuritis (29, 40, 46). Larger doses (100 to 200 mg/day) may be used to treat the neuropathy should it develop (40). The use of large doses of pyridoxine has been controversial, as some feel that they may reduce the effect of INH by competitive antagonism. This effect has not been proven (10, 40, 56).

INH has also been associated with other central nervous system (CNS) effects such as psychosis, delirium, euphoria, somnolence, coma, seizures, and death (28, 32). These are usually associated with elevated serum concentrations, in particular, intentional INH overdoses. Patients with a pyridoxine deficiency or other CNS problems may be at an increased risk of developing these CNS effects. It has also been suggested that patients on both INH and *p*-aminosalicylic acid (PAS) are at an increased risk of CNS changes (2, 3). Supplementation of pyridoxine at the lower dose may benefit these patients. Withdrawal of INH will also reduce the symptoms if caught early (11, 29, 36, 46). The more serious effects are often seen with greatly elevated concentrations as a result of accidental or intentional overdose. Prompt removal of the drug and treatment with pyridoxine doses equal to the INH dose ingested is recommended (1–4 g of pyridoxine intravenously followed by 1 g intramuscularly every 30 min until the entire dose is given) (46). Some of these effects may linger after INH is stopped and treatment is given (32).

Pellagra may occur and may be very difficult to treat in patients receiving INH. Supplementation with pyridoxine and a diet with sufficient niacin (nicotinic acid) have been recommended. It is suggested that INH be withheld until the pellagra is under control (45, 85).

Other

INH-induced rheumatic complications have been reported (29, 40, 65). Symptoms consist of arthralgias of the fingers, elbows, wrists, shoulders, hips and spine and fever and occasional edema. These symptoms have occurred from 5 days to several weeks into therapy. Symptoms may appear in otherwise healthy patients, with or without a rheumatic history. Although some patients have improved with salicylate administration while remaining on INH, it is generally recommended that INH be withdrawn as soon as possible to prevent permanent damage. Symptoms usually abate soon after withdrawal of the drug.

INH is known to cause drug-induced lupus syndrome. Approximately 20% of patients on INH may experience a positive antinuclear antibody test with no symptoms; a small percentage of these may go on to develop overt systemic lupus erythematosus (SLE) (29, 67). As with native SLE, females seem more prone to developing overt SLE; no racial predilection has been determined. Slow acetylators of INH appear more likely to develop overt SLE. Symptoms of INH-induced SLE have consisted of fever, arthralgia, pleural effusion, and mild leukopenia (29, 40). Prompt withdrawal of the drug has alleviated symptoms and is therefore recommended.

Other INH-induced adverse reactions include fever in the absence of rheumatic symptoms, optic neuritis, keratitis, lactic acidosis, and a variety of hematologic effects (17, 21, 29, 40, 54), including hemolytic anemia, pyridoxine-responsive anemia, agranulocytosis, and rare reports of red cell aplasia.

DRUG INTERACTIONS

INH is a potential inhibitor of cytochrome P-450 (81, 87). Therefore, compounds cleared through these pathways may be affected (7). Some of the more prominent interactions include those with antiepileptic medications. Both Murray and Miller et al. found clinically significant interactions in their combined total of 661 patients receiving both INH and phenytoin (48, 53). They found that 11 to 27% of these patients experienced an increased incidence of CNS effects (confusion, drowsiness, psychosis) when on the two medications. Although neither reported serum phenytoin concentrations, Miller et al. reported the need to reduce phenytoin doses to alleviate the CNS effects. Murray found that the CNS effects decreased when both medications were discontinued. He also found the incidence of CNS effects to be higher than it was in patients on INH alone. Monitoring of serum phenytoin concentrations is recommended when phenytoin and INH are used concurrently (7).

Similar reports have occurred for INH used in combination with carbamazepine (7). Patients on the two medications have experienced symptoms of carbamazepine toxicity (headache, blurred vision, stupor). One patient showed an increase in serum carbamazepine concentration from 5 to 8 μg/mL before INH to 18 to 22 μg/mL with INH. Monitoring the serum concentration of carbamazepine is recommended when the two agents are used concurrently (7, 86). Conversely, carbamazepine is known to induce hepatic metabolism and is thought to have contributed to INH hepatotoxicity in at least one patient.

INH inhibits not only pathways used to metabolize drugs but also some used for foods. INH is a potential inhibitor of monamine oxidase (MAO) and diamine oxidase (histaminase) and is chemically related to iproniazid (7). There have been several reports of flushing, hypertension, headache, nausea, vomiting, and palpitations in patients on INH who have ingested tyramine-containing foods such as aged cheese, red wine, and beer. This is thought to result from inhibition of MAO by INH (7, 70). Histaminase inhibition by INH has led to similar reports in patients on INH who ingested foods high in histamine, such as skipjack, tuna, and other fish (77). Patients on INH should be aware of these potential food/drug interactions.

Although INH is most notably an inhibitor of cytochrome P-450 enzymes, it has also been reported to induce cytochrome P450IIE1 enzymes (81, 87). Acetaminophen is one important medication that may be affected by this. Several recent reports of hepatotoxicity are consistent with acetaminophen toxicity in patients on INH alone and in combination with rifampin (51, 52, 55). Interestingly, some of these reports involved patients who had received smaller doses of acetaminophen (4.5–6 g) than are usually associated with acetaminophen toxicity (12–14 g). These effects are thought to result from INH (and rifampin) inducing metabolism of acetaminophen to toxic metabolites. Patients receiving INH with or without other antimycobacterial agents should be warned about the risks of acetaminophen ingestion.

Other noteworthy drug interactions include a possible increased risk of CNS toxicity in patients receiving both INH and disulfiram. This is thought to result from altered metabolism of brain catecholamines (83). Administration of food or aluminum hydroxide may reduce the absorption of INH, so INH should be given 1 to 2 h before food or antacids (7, 33). Serum ketoconazole concentrations may be significantly reduced by concurrent INH-containing regimens, although this may be largely due to the enzyme-inducing effects of the rifampin component of these regimens (27). There have been conflicting reports on the effect of INH on warfarin metabolism. Some have reported an increased warfarin effect, whereas others have noted no change. Monitoring of prothrombin time or international normalized ratio (INR) may be worthwhile in these patients (7). Finally, the other antituberculosis drugs, including rifampin, do not appear to significantly affect the pharmacokinetics of INH (1, 46, 57).

CLINICAL INDICATIONS

INH and rifampin form the core of all modern short-course regimens. INH is extremely potent against *M. tuberculosis* and should be used whenever possible for the treatment of tuberculosis, regardless of the patient's age. Twice-weekly regimens are both convenient and well tolerated and lend themselves to DOT.

INH is proven effective for the treatment of infection with *M. tuberculosis, without* active disease (chemoprophylaxis), and should be used with confidence for most recent converters to a positive PPD skin test. It certainly should be used for all children who are recent converters when the index case is known or suspected to harbor INH-susceptible organisms.

Hepatotoxicity is the primary toxicity limiting the use of INH. This is rare in children, and is not a major consideration in patients under 35 years of age. Older patients may still benefit from the drug for both treatment of disease and chemoprophylaxis, but they may require additional monitoring for increased liver enzymes.

REFERENCES

1. Acocella G, Bonollo L, Garimoldi M, Mainardi M, Tenconi LT, Nicolis FB. Kinetics of rifampicin and isoniazid administered alone and in combination to normal subjects and patients with liver disease. Gut 1972;13:47–53.
2. Adams BG, Davies BM. Neurological changes associated with PAS and INAH therapy. J Ment Sci 1961;107:943–947.
3. Adams P, White C. Isoniazid-induced encephalopathy. Lancet 1965:680–682.
4. Ahern H. Insights into molecular mechanism of drug-resistant tuberculosis. ASM News 1993;59:593–594.
5. American Thoracic Society. Treatment of tuberculosis and tuberculosis infection in adults and children. Am J Respir Crit Care Med 1994;149:1359–1374.
6. Awaness AM, Mitchison DA. Cumulative effects of pulsed exposures of Mycobacterium tuberculosis to isoniazid. Tubercle 1973;54:153–158.
7. Baciewicz AM, Self TH. Isoniazid interactions. South Med J 1985;78:714–718.
8. Banerjee, Dubnau E, Quemard A, Balasubramanian V, Um KS, Wilson T, Collins D, de Lisle G, Jacobs WR Jr. InhA, a gene encoding a target for isoniazid and ethionamide in *Mycobacterium tuberculosis*. Science 1994;263:227–230.
9. Beggs WH, Jenne JW. Isoniazid uptake and growth inhibition of mycobacterium tuberculosis in relation to time and concentration of pulsed drug exposures. Tubercle 1969;50:377–385.
10. Biehl JP, Vilter RW. Effects of isoniazid on pyridoxine metabolism. JAMA 1954;156:1549–1552.
11. Biehl JP, Nimitz HJ. Studies on the use of a high dose of isoniazid. Am Rev Tuberc 1954;70:430–441.
12. Black M. Isoniazid and the liver. Am Rev Respir Dis 1974; 110:1–3.
13. Blanchard JS. Molecular mechanisms of drug resistance in Mycobacterium tuberculosis. Annu Rev Biochem 1996;65: 215–239.
14. Boxenbaum HG, Riegelman S. Pharmacokinetics of isoniazid and some metabolites in man. J Pharmacokinet Biopharm 1976;4:287–325.
15. Centers for Disease Control. National action plan to combat multidrug-resistant tuberculosis. MMWR 1992;41(RR-11):5–48.
16. Centers for Disease Control. Initial therapy for tuberculosis in the era of multidrug resistance—recommendations of the advisory council for the elimination of tuberculosis. MMWR 1993; 42(RR-7):1–8.
17. Claiborne RA, Dutt AK. Isoniazid-induced pure red cell aplasia. Am Rev Respir Dis 1985;131:947–949.
18. Comstock GW. Evaluating isoniazid preventive therapy: the need for more data. Ann Intern Med 1981;94:817–819.
19. Crabbe SJ. Intravenous isoniazid. P & T 1990;15:1483–1484.

20. Cross FS, Long MW, Banner AS, Snider DE. Rifampin-isoniazid therapy of alcoholic and nonalcoholic tuberculosis patients in a US Public Health Service cooperative therapy trial. Am Rev Respir Dis 1980;122:349–353.

21. Dasta JF, Prior JA, Kurzrok S. Isoniazid-induced fever. Chest 1979;75:196–197.

22. Devadatta S, Gangadharam PRJ, Andrews RH, Fox W, Ramakrishnan CV, Selkon JB, Velu S. Peripheral neuritis due to isoniazid. Bull WHO 1960;23:587–598.

23. Dossing M, Wilcke JT, Askgaard DS, Nybo B. Liver injury during antituberculosis treatment: an 11-year study. Tubercle Lung Dis 1996;77:335–340.

24. Ellard GA, Gammon PT. Pharmacokinetics of isoniazid metabolism in man. J Pharmacokinet Biopharm 1976;4:83–113

25. Ellard GA, Gammon PT. Acetylator phenotyping of tuberculosis patients using matrix isoniazid or sulphadimidine and its prognostic significance for treatment with several intermittent isoniazid-containing regimens. Br J Clin Pharmacol 1977;4: 5–14.

26. Ellard GA. The potential clinical significance of the isoniazid acetylator phenotype in the treatment of pulmonary tuberculosis. Tubercle 1984;65:211–227.

27. Engelhard D, Stutman HR, Marks MI. Interaction of ketoconazole with rifampin and isoniazid. N Engl J Med 1984;311: 1681–1682.

28. Girling DJ. Adverse effects of antituberculosis drugs. Drugs 1982;23:56–74.

29. Goldman AL, Braman SS. Isoniazid: a review with emphasis on adverse effects. Chest 1972;62:71–77.

30. Gurmurthy P, Krishnamurthy MS, Nazareth O, Parthasarathy R, Raghupati Sarma G, Somasundaram PR, Tripathy SP, Ellard GA. Lack of relationship between hepatic toxicity and acetylator phenotype in three thousand South Indian patients during treatment with isoniazid for tuberculosis. Am Rev Respir Dis 1984;129:58–61.

31. Heifets LB. Antituberculosis drugs: Antimicrobial activity in vitro. In: Heifets LB, ed. Drug susceptibility in the chemotherapy of mycobacterial infections. Boca Raton, FL: CRC Press, 1991:13–57.

32. Hunter RA. Confusional psychosis with residual organic cerebral impairment following isoniazid therapy. Lancet 1952:960–962.

33. Hurwitz A, Schlozman DL. Effects of antacids on gastrointestinal absorption of isoniazid in rat and man. Am Rev Respir Dis 1974;109:41–47.

34. Israel HL, Gottlieb JE, Maddrey WC. Perspective: preventive isoniazid therapy and the liver. Chest 1992;101:1298–1301.

35. Iwainsky H. Mode of action, biotransformation and pharmacokinetics of antituberculosis drugs in animals and man. In: Bartmann K, ed. Antituberculosis drugs. Berlin: Springer-Verlag, Berlin, 1988:399–553.

36. Jackson SLO. Psychosis due to isoniazid. Br Med J 1957: 743–746.

37. Johnsson K, Schultz PG. Mechanistic studies of the oxidation of isoniazid by the catalase peroxidase from Mycobacterium tuberculosis. J Am Chem Soc 1994;116:7425–7426.

38. Kim Y, Shin J, Shin S, Jang I, Kim S, Lee J, Han J, Cha Y. Decreased acetylation of isoniazid in chronic renal failure. Clin Pharmacol Ther 1993;54:612–620.

39. Kopanoff DE, Snider DE, Caras GJ. Isoniazid-related hepatitis—a US Public Health Service cooperative surveillance study. Am Rev Respir Dis 1978;117:991–1001.

40. Kucers A, Bennett NM. The use of antibiotics. 4th ed. Philadelphia: JB Lippincott, 1987.

41. Kumar A, Misra PK, Mehotra R, Govil YC, Rana GS. Hepatotoxicity of rifampin and isoniazid—is it all drug-induced hepatitis? Am Rev Respir Dis 1991;143:1350–1352.

42. Lauterburg BH, Smith CV, Todd EL, Mitchell JR. Pharmacokinetics of the toxic hydrazino metabolites formed from isoniazid in humans. J Pharmacol Exp Ther 1985;235:566–570.

43. Maddrey WC, Boitnott JK. Isoniazid hepatitis. Ann Intern Med 1973;79:1–12.

44. Mannisto P, Mantyla R, Klinge E, Nykanen S, Koponen A, Lamminsivu U. Influence of various diets on the bioavailability of isoniazid. J Antimicrob Chemother 1982;10:427–434.

45. McConnell RB, Cheetham HD. Acute pellagra during isoniazid therapy. Lancet 1952:959–960.

46. McEvoy GK, ed. AHFS drug information. Bethesda, MD: American Soc Health-Systems Pharmacists, 1996:423–428.

47. Mdluli K, Sherman DR, Hickey MJ, Kreiswirth BN, Morris S, Stover CK, Barry CE. Biochemical and genetic data suggest that InhA is not the primary target for activated isoniazid in Mycobacterium tuberculosis. J Infect Dis 1996;174:1085–1090.

48. Miller RR, Porter J, Greenblatt DJ. Clinical importance of the interaction of phenytoin and isoniazid. Chest 1979;75:356–358.

49. Mitchell JR, Thorgeirsson UP, Black M, Timbrell JA, Snodgrass WR, Potter WZ, Jollow DJ, Keiser HR. Increased incidence of isoniazid hepatitis in rapid acetylators: possible relation to hydrazine metabolites. Clin Pharmacol Ther 1975;18:70–79.

50. Mitchell JR, Zimmerman HJ. Ishak KG, Thorgeirsson UP, Timbrell JA, Snodgrass WR, Nelson SD. Isoniazid liver injury: clinical spectrum, pathology, and probable pathogenesis. Ann Intern Med 1976;84:181–192.

51. Moulding TS, Redeker AG, Kanel GC. Acetaminophen, isoniazid, and hepatic toxicity. Ann Intern Med 1991;114:431.

52. Murphy R, Swartz R, Watkins PB. Severe acetaminophen toxicity in a patient receiving isoniazid. Ann Intern Ned 1990;113: 799–800.

53. Murray FJ. Outbreak of unexpected reactions among epileptics taking isoniazid. Am Rev Respir Dis 1962;86:729–732.

54. Neff TA. Isoniazid toxicity: reports of lactic acidosis and keratitis. Chest 1971;59:245–248.

55. Nolan CM, Sadblom RE, Thummel KE, Slattery JT, Nelson SD. Hepatotoxicity associated with acetaminophen usage in patients receiving multiple drug therapy for tuberculosis. Chest 1994; 105:408–411.

56. Offe HA. Historical introduction and chemical characteristics of antituberculosis drugs. In: Bartmann K, ed. Antituberculosis drugs. Berlin: Springer-Verlag, 1988:1–30.

57. Peloquin CA. Antituberculosis drugs: pharmacokinetics. In: Heifets LB, ed. Drug susceptibility in the chemotherapy of mycobacterial infections. Boca Raton, FL: CRC Press, 1991:89–122.

58. Peloquin CA, James GT, Craig LD, Kim M, McCarthy EA, Iklé DN, Iseman MD. Pharmacokinetic evaluation of aconiazide, a potentially less toxic isoniazid pro-drug. Pharmacotherapy 1994;14:415–423.

59. Peloquin CA, Berning SE. Infections due to Mycobacterium tuberculosis. Ann Pharmacother 1994;28:72–84.

60. Peloquin CA, Berning SE. Tuberculosis and multi-drug resistant tuberculosis in children. Pediatr Nurs 1995;21:566–572.

61. Peloquin CA. Therapeutic drug monitoring of the antimycobacterial drugs. Clin Lab Med 1996;16:717–729.

62. Peloquin CA. Using therapeutic drug monitoring to dose the antimycobacterial drugs. Clin Chest Med 1997;18:79–87.

63. Peloquin CA, Jaresko GS, Yong CL, Keung ACF, Bulpitt AE, Jelliffe RW. Population pharmacokinetic modeling of isoniazid,

rifampin, and pyrazinamide. Antimicrob Agents Chemother 1997;41:2670–2679.

64. Peretti E, Karlaganis G, Lauterburg B. Acetylation of acetylhydrazine, the toxic metabolite of isoniazid, in humans. Inhibition by concomitant administration of isoniazid. J Pharmacol Exp Ther 1987;243:686–689.

65. Periman P, Venkataramani TK. Acute arthritis induced by isoniazid. Ann Intern Med 1975;83:667–668.

66. Ristow M, Mohlig M, Rifal M, Schatz H, Feldman K, Pfeiffer A. New isoniazid/ethionamide resistance gene mutation and screening for multidrug-resistant *Mycobacterium tuberculosis* strains. Lancet 1995;346;502–503.

67. Rothfield NF, Bierer WF, Garfield JW. Isoniazid induction of antinuclear antibodies—a prospective study. Ann Intern Med 1978;88:650–652.

68. Sarma GR, Immanuel C, Kailasam S, Narayana ASL, Venkatesan P. Rifampin-induced release of hydrazine from isoniazid—a possible cause of hepatitis during treatment of tuberculosis with regimens containing isoniazid and rifampin. Am Rev Respir Dis 1986;133:1072–1075.

69. Siskind MS, Thienemann D, Kirlin L. Isoniazid-induced neurotoxicity in chronic dialysis patients: report of three cases and a review of the literature. Nephron 1993;64:303–306.

70. Smith CK, Durack DT. Isoniazid and reaction to cheese. Ann Intern Med 1978;88:520–521.

71. Snider DI, Caras GJ. Isoniazid-associated hepatitis deaths: a review of available information. Am Rev Respir Dis 1992;145:494–497.

72. Steel MA, Burk RF, DesPrez RM. Toxic hepatitis with isoniazid and rifampin: a meta-analysis. Chest 1991;99:465–71.

73. Takayama K, Wang L, David HL. Effect of isoniazid on the in vivo mycolic acid synthesis, cell growth, and viability of *Mycobacterium tuberculosis*. Antimicrob Agents Chemother 1972;2:29–35.

74. Timbrell JA, Mitchell JR, Snodgrass WR, Nelson SD. Isoniazid hepatotoxicity: the relationship between covalent binding and metabolism in vivo. J Pharmacol Exp Ther 1980;213:364–369.

75. Timbrell JA, Wright JM. Urinary metabolic profile of isoniazid in patients who develop isoniazid-related liver damage. Hum Toxicol 1984;3:485–495.

76. Trnka L, Mison P, Bartmann K, and Otten H. Experimental evaluation of efficacy. In: Bartmann K, ed. Antituberculosis drugs. Berlin: Springer-Verlag, 1988:31–232.

77. Uragoda CG. Histamine poisoning in tuberculous patients after ingestion of tuna fish. Am Rev Respir Dis 1980;121:157–159.

78. Verbist L. Mode of action of antituberculous drugs (part I). Medicon Int 1974;3:11–23.

79. Verbist L. Mode of action of antituberculous drugs (part II). Medicon Int 1974;3:3–17.

80. Warrington RF, Tse KS, Gorske BA, Schwenk R, Sehon AH. Evaluation of isoniazid-associated hepatitis by immunological tests. Clin Exp Immunol 1978;32:97–104.

81. Watkins Paul B. Drug metabolism by cytochromes P450 in the liver and small bowel. Gastroenterol Clin North Am 1992;21:511–526.

82. Weber WW, Hein DW. Clinical pharmacokinetics of isoniazid. Clin Pharmacokinet 1979;4:401–422.

83. Whittington HG, Grey L. Possible interaction between disulfiram and isoniazid. Am J Psychiatry 1969;125:1725–1729.

84. Winder FG. Mode of action of the antimycobacterial agents and associated aspects of the molecular biology of the mycobacteria, In: Ratledge C, Stanford J, eds. The biology of mycobacteria: vol 1—Physiology, identification, and classification. London: Academic Press, 1982:353–438.

85. Wood MM. Central nervous system complications during INH treatment of pulmonary tuberculosis. Br J Tuberc Dis Chest 1954:20–29.

86. Wright JM, Stokes EF, Sweeney VP. Isoniazid induced carbamazepine toxicity and vice versa. 1982;307:1325–1327.

87. Zand R, Nelson SD, Slattery JT, Thummel KE, Kalhorn TF, Adams SP, Wright JM. Inhibition and induction of cytochrome P4502E1-catalyzed oxidation by isoniazid in humans. Clin Pharmacol Ther 1993;54:142–149.

88. Zent C, Smith P. Study of the effect of concomitant food on the bioavailability of rifampicin, isoniazid and pyrazinamide. Tuberc Lung Dis 1995;76:109–113.

89. Zhang Y, Heym B, Allen B, Young D, Cole S. The catalase-peroxidase gene and isoniazid resistance of *Mycobacterium tuberculosis*. Nature 1992;358:591–593.

Antimycobacterial Agents: *p*-Aminosalicylic Acid

Shaun E. Berning and Charles A. Peloquin

Chemical Structure

p-Aminosalicylic acid (PAS) is a synthetic structural analogue of aminobenzoic acid (27, 17). It was discovered in the mid-1940s by Lehmann as a result of a deliberate search for new antituberculosis agents.

PAS is a white powder, with a slight odor of acetic acid. It is slightly soluble in water and is soluble in alcohol. It has a pK$_a$ of 3.2. Aminosalicylate sodium, which is no longer available in the United States, contains 4.7 meq of sodium per gram of the compound (27).

Structure-Activity Relationships

PAS is unique among salicylic acid derivatives in its ability to inhibit the growth of *Mycobacterium tuberculosis*. Most alterations of the structure to chemically related compounds abolish antimycobacterial activity (42, 43).

ANTIMICROBIAL ACTIVITY
Spectrum

PAS is specifically active only against acid-fast organisms, with clinically useful activity primarily against *M. tuberculosis* and *M. bovis* (39–41, 44). PAS does not have sufficient in vitro activity against *M. avium* and most other atypical mycobacteria to warrant its use (5, 10, 11, 39–41, 44). The minimal inhibitory concentrations (MICs) of PAS against *M. tuberculosis* vary, depending upon both the media and the inoculum size (11). Susceptible strains with MICs of 0.5 to 2.0 μg/mL or 1 to 10 μg/mL have been reported (11, 16). It is important to note that MICs reported with PAS often do not represent complete (>90%) inhibition (11).

Pharmacodynamic Effects
Bactericidal Effects

PAS is not bactericidal (11, 40, 41). It does not penetrate well into mammalian cells, and it does not appear to inhibit the growth of *M. tuberculosis* within macrophages, based on current data (11). PAS solutions may be light sensitive, and heat (>80°C) can rapidly destroy the drug in solution (39). *p*-Aminobenzoic acid (PABA) competitively antagonizes the action of PAS in vitro, but neither folic acid nor folinic acid appears to antagonize PAS action (39–41, 44). Plasma or serum does not appear to interfere with PAS activity in vitro (39).

Postantibiotic Effects (PAEs)

No postantibiotic effect has been reported with PAS.

Effects of Subinhibitory Concentrations

Subinhibitory concentrations of PAS do not seem to exert a significant beneficial effect; they may be associated with selection of resistant isolates in vitro (39). It is not known if subinhibitory concentrations of PAS contribute to multidrug therapy in vivo.

Effects on Host Immunity

PAS has no known direct effects on host immunity.

Pharmacodynamic Correlates with Outcome

There appears to be a linear relationship between PAS concentration in vitro and growth of mycobacteria, producing 50 to 95% inhibition (39). PAS is fairly slow to act, taking more than 24 h to show inhibition, even at high concentrations (39). There also appears to be a significant inoculum effect with PAS; large inocula yield nonlinear decreases in the in vitro activity of PAS (39).

The question of whether PAS works optimally with continuous serum concentrations or intermittent high serum concentrations has been raised. Animal studies appeared to show a threshold dose (125 mg per guinea pig per day, or ~210 mg/kg) required for efficacy (39). Further increases up to 500 mg per animal per day did not improve outcome. Additional studies showed no difference among doses of 100 mg twice

daily, 200 mg once daily, and 200 mg twice daily. Thus, daily doses above the threshold appear to suffice in guinea pigs. Separate studies showed that dosing PAS three times weekly was less effective than daily doses (39).

A controlled, prospective study compared the outcomes of patients receiving self-administered isoniazid (INH) (4.7 mg/kg/day) plus PAS (0.2 g/kg) every day, each as two equally divided doses, with directly observed INH (15 mg/kg/day) and PAS (0.2 g/kg) twice weekly, each as single oral doses (38). All patients received 14 days of an initial intensive regimen of daily directly observed INH, streptomycin, and PAS. Of the evaluable patients, favorable bacteriologic responses were obtained in 79 of 90 (88%) twice-weekly patients and in 72 of 83 (87%) of the daily patients. Exceptions to the favorable responses in the twice-weekly group included those resistant to INH and those with advanced disease. The twice-weekly regimen was better tolerated. Although the differences were not large, they do indicate that future studies into varying dose regimens of PAS may be warranted (24).

MECHANISM OF ACTION

Varying theories exist on the mechanism of action of PAS. Initially PAS was thought to inhibit the synthesis of folic acid (11, 39–41, 44). Based on the proposal of Seydel et al., Verbist has suggested that PAS acts at an early stage of coenzyme F biosynthesis in the folic acid pathway (40, 41). PAS does not show cross resistance with sulfonamides for the few organisms that are susceptible to both. Others have suggested that the action of PAS lies in its ability to interfere with the uptake and use of salicylic acid, thus altering iron transfer (5, 11, 39–41, 44). Whether PAS can interfere with mycobactin synthesis has been debated. Thus, the mechanism of action of PAS remains elusive.

MECHANISMS OF RESISTANCE
Commonly Resistant Organisms

As mentioned above, PAS is generally only used to treat *M. tuberculosis*. *M. avium* is considered naturally resistant to PAS (11, 39–41, 44).

Mechanisms of Resistance

Resistance to PAS may be natural or acquired. As with other antimycobacterial agents, resistance in previously susceptible organisms may develop rapidly both in vivo and in vitro when PAS is used as a single agent in the treatment of tuberculosis (16, 23, 39). This appears to be due to naturally occurring resistant mutants present in a population of mycobacteria. Under the selective pressure of a single drug, all organisms are eliminated except the resistant subpopulation, which continues to multiply, eventually becoming the dominant population. It was found that 17.2% of patients previously treated with PAS acquired resistance; this was more profound in those receiving PAS monotherapy (16). Acquired resistance may be prevented by using PAS in combination with at least one or two other antimycobacterial drugs (23, 24).

Although primary drug resistance to PAS is possible, it is much less common in developed countries. In 1963, Britain reported an incidence of 0.8% primary resistance, while Australia reported 0.7 to 1.0% from 1972 to 1977 (16). An incidence of PAS primary resistance below 1% was reported from 1975 to 1982 in the United States, with some geographic and ethnic variance. The incidence is higher in developing countries and in Southeast Asia.

PAS does not show cross-resistance with any other antituberculosis agents currently available in the United States, but it has shown cross-resistance with thiacetazone (16). Strains of *M. tuberculosis* that were resistant to high concentrations of PAS were also resistant to thiacetazone, but thiacetazone-resistant strains were susceptible to PAS (40). This cross-resistance would not be predicted on the basis of structure or known mechanisms of action, and its mechanism is not known.

Methods to Overcome and Prevent Resistance

Acquired resistance to PAS may be prevented by using it in combination with at least one or two other antimycobacterial drugs (23, 24). Higher doses of PAS as monotherapy do not prevent emergence of resistance. In vitro, subinhibitory concentrations enhance selection of resistant organisms (39). It is not known if this also occurs in vivo, although the possibility exists. Thus, it appears desirable to achieve serum concentrations above the MIC of the isolate.

PHARMACOKINETICS
Absorption

Oral PAS tablets are no longer available in the United States, but they are available elsewhere. PAS and its sodium salt are both readily and extensively absorbed from the gastrointestinal (GI) tract, with the absorption of the sodium salt being more rapid and complete (23, 29, 32). PAS doses of 4 g produce maximum concentrations (C_{max}) of 70 to 80 μg/mL within 1 to 2 h (29, 42). Recovery of the drug in the urine is high—80 to 88% of the drug is recovered in the urine within 24 h.

In the United States, PAS is now available as sustained-release tablets (Paser, Jacobus Pharmaceuticals). In a phase I study in 12 healthy volunteers, PAS 4-g granules given with food produced a median C_{max} of 15.25 μg/mL (11 evaluable subjects) (30). The time to maximum concentration (T_{max}) of this sustained-release dosage form was longer than that for plain tablets, occurring at a median 6 h postdose. A summary of the absorption characteristics of six different PAS forms, including area under the curve (AUC) estimates, is shown in Table 1 (30).

Distribution

PAS is widely distributed in most body tissues; highest concentrations are found in the kidney, lung, and liver (29, 42). PAS is not well distributed to the central nervous system (CNS). The volume of distribution of PAS has been reported to be 98 L/kg in normal volunteers. PAS is reported to be 50 to 73% bound to plasma protein (14, 29, 30, 42).

Metabolism and Excretion

The serum half-life of PAS is reported to be 45 to 60 min following oral tablets (14, 29, 30, 44). PAS is rapidly metabolized

TABLE 1 • **Summary of Absorption Characteristics of Different PAS Forms, Including Area under the Curve (AUC) Estimates**

	Dose (g)	C_{max} (μg/mL)	T_{max} (h)	$AUC_{(0-\infty)}$ (μg · h/mL)
PAS	4.0	49.98	3.54	209.07
Na$^+$ PAS	2.8	155.44	0.83	313.22
Ca^{2+} PAS	2.6	139.51	1.02	326.83
K$^+$ PAS	2.6	121.09	1.10	313.22
PAS resin	4.0	78.0	2.1	—
Paser	4.0	20.23	7.95	107.92

starting in the GI tract and then in the liver. It is acetylated to two main metabolites, *N*-acetyl-PAS, and *p*-aminosalicyluric acid, neither of which are active against *M. tuberculosis* (29, 40, 41, 43). The *N*-acetyl-PAS metabolite is thought to contribute to some of the nonantimicrobial pharmacologic properties of the drug. Acetylation of PAS is a saturable process; 100 μg/mL of unchanged PAS is found in the urine after a 4-g dose, and more than 500 μg/mL after an 8-g dose. Glycine conjugates of PAS are also formed; this process is proportional to the PAS dose (14, 29, 43). Although most of the drug is excreted as metabolites, the parent drug is also recovered in the urine. As mentioned above, approximately 80 to 88% of the drug is excreted renally, via both glomerular filtration and tubular secretion.

In the study by Peloquin et al., the new sustained-release granules have a longer median apparent serum half-life of 1.6 h (30). This likely reflects overlapping absorption, distribution, and elimination phases of the granules. PAS concentrations above 100 μg/mL were found in the urine after a 4-g dose. As with the tablets, *N*-acetyl-PAS was the primary metabolite of the granular form. Most PAS was recovered in the urine, either as parent drug or *N*-acetyl-PAS (2607 mg of a 4000-mg dose), giving an estimate of bioavailability of 65.2%. *N*-Acetyl-PAS was found in the serum prior to PAS, which is consistent with first-pass metabolism of PAS. Previous work showed that metabolism of PAS begins in the gut (14).

DOSAGE REGIMENS
Normal

As noted above, PAS should not be given alone; it must be given with at least one to three other antimycobacterial agents. The usual adult dose of PAS granules recommended by the manufacturer is 12 g/day in three divided doses, based upon initial pharmacokinetic studies (23, 30). Preliminary pharmacokinetic studies have been performed on this dosage form given once daily and twice daily to patients with *M. tuberculosis*. Both dosage regimens produced adequate maximum concentrations of 20 to 60 μg/mL (6/6 twice-daily patients; 5/6 daily patients). The twice-daily regimen maintained concentrations above 5 μg/mL throughout the dosing interval (6/6 patients); however, the once-daily regimen failed to do so in 6/6 patients (Peloquin and Berning, unpublished data). Based upon these findings, at National Jewish Medical and Research Center we regularly administer PAS granules at 4 g twice daily, with occasional increases to 5 to 6 g twice daily. The American Thoracic Society (ATS) and Centers for Disease Control and Prevention (CDC) recommend a PAS dose of 150 mg/kg daily in adults and children, with a maximum daily dose of 12 g (1). To date, these recommendations have not been changed with the introduction of the PAS granules. The granules have an acid-resistant coating that dissolves within 1 min at neutral pH, such as that found in the small intestine or in neutral foods. They must therefore be administered in an acidic food or beverage (e.g., applesauce, yogurt, and various fruit juices). The granules should not be chewed (Paser package insert).

Other dosage forms not currently available in the United States have similar daily dose ranges. The aminosalicylate sodium recommended dose is 150 mg/kg/day (10–15 g) in two to four equally divided doses (Paser package insert). Pediatric doses have ranged from 150 to 360 mg/kg daily in equally divided doses.

Therapeutic Drug Monitoring

At National Jewish Medical and Research Center, where therapeutic drug monitoring (TDM) of the antimycobacterial drugs is standard practice, samples for serum PAS determinations are drawn 6 and 10 h after a granule dose (31). The 6-h concentration provides information on the maximum concentrations, while the 10-h concentration lends information on the rate and completeness of absorption and on clearance of the drug. The 10-h concentration also allows us to determine whether adequate concentrations are being maintained throughout the dosing interval. We use 20 to 60 μg/mL as our "normal range" for maximum (peak) concentrations and aim to maintain concentrations above 5 μg/mL throughout the dosing interval to optimize this bacteriostatic drug.

Renal Failure

PAS granules are generally avoided in severe renal disease, unless no therapeutic alternative exists. Although the serum half-life of the parent compound, PAS, is not altered in renal disease, that of the metabolites is prolonged 6-fold (13). Because deacetylation is not significant, accumulation of the acetyl metabolite is likely. This may add to uremic GI symptoms and potentiate acidosis (29). Although no specific guidelines exist with the granule dosage form, dose adjustments for the previous dosage forms recommended extending an 8-h dosing interval to 12 h in patients with a glomerular filtration rate (GFR) of 10 to 50 mL/min. PAS should be avoided in patients with a GFR below 10 mL/min, if possible (2). It seems reasonable to extend the dosing interval for the granule dosage form in the presence of renal dysfunction.

Hepatic Failure

Although some reports show no alteration of the drug in patients with liver disease, compared with normal volunteers, PAS should be used with caution in patients with hepatic impairment, as these patients may not tolerate PAS as well as patients without liver disease (13, 23).

Obesity, Ascites, and Edema

No recommendations for dose adjustments in obesity have been made. PAS is a hydrophilic drug, and therefore, larger than usual doses may be required in patients with ascites or edema. This can be determined by measuring serum concentrations.

Pregnancy

Although PAS has been used safely in pregnant women, a complete safety profile in pregnant women has not been established (21, 23, 29). The primary adverse effect may be increased nausea in these patients. As with any medication, PAS should be avoided in the first trimester of pregnancy if possible.

ADVERSE EFFECTS

GI disturbances from PAS are the most common adverse effects. With the older dosage forms, nausea, vomiting, abdominal pain, and diarrhea were very common (16, 23). The new Paser granules offer significant relief from the nausea, vomiting, and abdominal pain; however, diarrhea remains a significant problem. This diarrhea is usually self-limited, with symptoms improving after the first 1 to 2 weeks of therapy. The empty granules appear in the stool (30).

Various types of malabsorption with PAS are common. Steatorrhea, both at high and normal doses of PAS, has been reported. The symptoms of steatorrhea may occur early or late in therapy and may take up to 2 months to subside after discontinuation of the drug. The mechanism of this effect is unknown (18–20). These effects have not been clearly documented with the new granule dosage form.

Malabsorption of vitamin B_{12}, folate, xylose, and iron has also been reported (20). The mechanism of vitamin B_{12} malabsorption also has not been determined. Abnormal Schilling tests occur 2 to 6 weeks into therapy (12, 20). No abnormality in the production of intrinsic factor (IF) or its binding has been found, nor is malabsorption of vitamin B_{12} corrected by coadministration of IF (12, 27). Megaloblastic anemia has not been reported. Malabsorption of folate, which is structurally similar to PAS, results from competitive inhibition. It had been thought that absorption of vitamin B_{12} depended upon folate and could be overcome by coadministration of folate; this has since been disproved (20, 28). Hypocholesterolemia found in patients taking PAS may be due to reduced serum folate levels, rather than steatorrhea.

Hypersensitivity reactions with common manifestations of fever, conjunctivitis, and rash may occur in up to 5 to 10% of patients on PAS, usually within the first 5 weeks of therapy (16, 23). Less common manifestations include vasculitis, arthralgias, eosinophilia, leukopenia, thrombocytopenia, hepatitis, and a lymphoma-like syndrome consisting of lymphadenopathy, rash, and hepatomegaly (16, 23, 25). Desensitization to PAS hypersensitivity is not recommended.

PAS-induced hepatitis differs from that of other antimycobacterial drugs. The most common initial symptom is rash, followed by fever, anorexia, and diarrhea. Once hepatitis is diagnosed, other findings may include lymphadenopathy, leukocytosis, eosinophilia, hepatomegaly, and exfoliative dermatitis. Early recognition of the initial symptoms is of utmost importance, as the mortality associated with PAS-induced hepatitis may be as high as 21%. This reaction usually occurs within the first 90 days of therapy, with recovery likely if the drug is discontinued (8, 36). Monitoring of liver function tests may be helpful; however because this reaction is so rapid, it is more important that both health care professionals and patients be aware of any new rash early in therapy.

PAS may cause a positive direct Coombs' test. Also, patients with glucose-6-phosphate dehydrogenase deficiency may experience hemolytic anemia (9, 16, 23). PAS-induced hemolytic anemia has been reported to cause acute renal failure. Other rare blood dyscrasias occurring with PAS include neutropenia, agranulocytosis, and thrombocytopenia.

PAS is known to produce goiter, with or without myxedema. This is thought to be caused by inhibition of thyroid synthesis rather than inhibition of iodide incorporation. It can be prevented or treated with thyroxine (7, 16, 23). In our experience, it occurs more frequently with concomitant ethionamide therapy.

Sodium overload was a problem with the sodium-PAS tablets, which contain 4.7 meq of sodium per gram. This is no longer a problem in the United States because Paser granules do not contain any sodium. Hypoglycemia has been reported rarely with PAS (6).

DRUG INTERACTIONS

Many drug interactions of varying significance have been reported with PAS. Previous dosage forms of PAS that contained bentonite reportedly reduced serum rifampin concentrations; this is not a problem with the new granules (3, 23). PAS reduces the rate of acetylation of INH in rapid acetylators, presumably by competing with INH for N-acetyltransferase; these reactions with INH are of little clinical significance (15, 22, 23, 37). Also, at PAS serum concentrations of 100 μg/mL, a modest increase in serum INH concentrations is possible due to displacement of INH from serum proteins (37). Although it has not been studied, this reaction is unlikely with the new granules, which usually do not produce serum concentrations this high (30) (Paser package insert).

Conflicting reports exist on the interaction with the renal tubular blocking agent probenecid. Because PAS is excreted by glomerular filtration and tubular secretion, it is reasonable to expect this to occur (39). However, it has not been reported to be clinically significant (23, 33–35).

Diphenhydramine has been reported to reduce absorption of PAS; however, the effect is so transient that it is of little significance (17, 23). Reduced serum digoxin concentrations were reported once in 2 of 10 patients treated and has not been reported since (4, 23). Other reported interactions include enhancement of the hypoprothrombinemic effect of oral anticoagulants and an increased probability of crystalluria with ammonium chloride (23). Ammonium chloride should not be used with PAS.

CLINICAL INDICATIONS

PAS was once a first-line drug for tuberculosis, along with INH and streptomycin. Regimens of 18 to 24 months duration were common. PAS is now a second-line antituberculosis drug, generally reserved for patients with multidrug-resistant tuberculosis (MDR-TB) or patients intolerant of such first-line agents as INH and rifampin. Empirical treatment for tuberculosis pending susceptibility data generally includes INH, rifampin, pyrazinamide (PZA), and either streptomycin or ethambutol. Although PAS is somewhat more potent than ethambutol, the latter drug is used more frequently because it is better tolerated than plain PAS tablets. With the availability of the better-tolerated PAS granules, it may be reasonable to reconsider the role of PAS in empirical regimens. PAS is rarely used for infections caused by other mycobacteria.

REFERENCES

1. American Thoracic Society/American Academy of Pediatrics/Centers for Disease Control/Infectious Disease Society of America. Joint statement: diagnostic standards and classification of tuberculosis. Am Rev Respir Dis 1990;142:725–735.
2. Bennett WM, Singer I, Golper T, Feig P, Coggins CJ. Guidelines for drug therapy in renal failure. Ann Intern Med 1977;86:754–783.
3. Boman G, Lundren P, Stjernstrom G. Mechanism of the inhibitory effect of PAS granules on the absorption of rifampicin: adsorption of rifampicin by an excipient, bentonite. Eur J Clin Pharmacol 1975;8:293–299.
4. Brown DD, Juhl RP, Warner SL. Decreased bioavailability of digoxin due to hypocholesterolemic interventions. Circulation 1978;58:164–172.
5. Brown KA, Ratledge C. The effect of p-aminosalicylic acid on iron transport and assimilation in mycobacteria. Biochim Biophys Acta 1975;385:207–220.
6. Dandona P, Beckett AG, Greenbury E. Para-aminosalicylic acid-induced hypoglycemia in a patient with diabetic nephropathy. Postgrad Med J 1980;56:135–136.
7. Edwards DAW, Rowlands EN, Trotter WR. The mechanism of the goitrogenic action of p-aminosalicylic acid. Lancet 1954: 1051–1052.
8. Fulkerson LL, Husen LA, Lieberman P, Stein E. Hyper-sensitivity, misdiagnosis, and death in tuberculosis treated with para-aminosalicylic acid. NY State J Med 1968;3045–3046.
9. Hansten PD. Drugs in the production of direct Coombs' test positivity. Am J Hosp Pharm 1971;28:629–632.
10. Heifets LB. Choice of antimicrobial agents for *M. avium* disease based on quantitative test of drug susceptibility. N Engl J Med 1990;323:419–420.
11. Heifets LB. Antituberculosis drugs: antimicrobial activity in vitro. In: Heifets LB, ed. Drug susceptibility in the chemotherapy of mycobacterial infections. Boca Raton, FL: CRC Press, 1991:13–57.
12. Heinvaara O, Palva IP. Malabsorption and deficiency of vitamin B$_{12}$ caused by treatment of para-aminosalicylic acid. Acta Med Scand 1965;177:337–341.
13. Held H, Fried F. Elimination of para-aminosalicylic acid in patients with liver disease and renal insufficiency. Chemotherapy 1977;23:405–415.
14. Iwainsky H. Mode of action, biotransformation and pharmacokinetics of antituberculosis drugs in animals and man. In: Bartmann K, ed. Antituberculosis drugs. Berlin: Springer-Verlag, 1988:399–553.
15. Kreukniet J, van Assendelft PMB, Mouton RP, Tasman A, Bangma PJ. The influence of para-aminosalicylic acid on isonicotinic acid hydrazide blood levels after oral and intravenous administration. Scand J Respir Dis 1967;47:236–243.

16. Kucers A, Bennett NM. The use of antibiotics. 4th ed. Philadelphia: JB Lippincott, 1987.

17. Lavigne JG, Marchand C. Inhibition of the gastrointestinal absorption of p-aminosalicylate (PAS) in rats and humans by diphenhydramine. Clin Pharmacol Ther 1972;14:404–412.

18. Levine RA. Steatorrhea induced by para-aminosalicylic acid. Ann Intern Med 1968;68:1265–1270.

19. Longstreth GF, Newcomer AD, Westbrook PR. Para-aminosalicylic acid-induced malabsorption. Dig Dis 1972;17:731–734.

20. Longstreth GF, Newcomer AD. Drug-induced malabsorption. Mayo Clin Proc 1975;50:284–293.

21. Lowe CR. Congenital defects among children born to women under supervision of treatment for pulmonary tuberculosis. Br J Prev Soc Med 1964;18:14–16.

22. Mandel W, Cohn ML, Russell WF and Middlebrook G. Effect of para-aminosalicylic acid on serum isoniazid levels in man. Proc Soc Expl Biol Med 1956;91:409–411.

23. McEvoy GK. AHFS drug information. Bethesda, MD: American Society of Health-System Pharmacists, 1996:399–401.

24. Mitchison DA. Basic mechanisms of chemotherapy. Chest 1979;76(Suppl):771–781.

25. Nagaratnam N, Jiffry AJ, Bhuvanendran N, Ramachandra V. Lymphoma-like syndrome following para-aminosalicylic acid. Postgrad Med J 1982;58:729–730.

26. Offe HA. Historical introduction and chemical characteristics of antituberculosis drugs. In: Bartmann K, ed. Antituberculosis drugs. Berlin: Springer-Verlag, 1988:1–30.

27. Palva IP, Heinvaara O. Drug-induced malabsorption of vitamin B_{12} in vitro studies using the dialysis technique. Scand J Haematol 1966;3:33–37.

28. Palva IP, Heinvaara O, Mattila M. Drug-induced malabsorption of vitamin B_{12}. III. Interference of PAS and folic acid in the absorption of vitamin B_{12}. Scand J Haematol 1966;3:149–153.

29. Peloquin CA. Antituberculosis drugs: pharmacokinetics. In: Heifets LB, ed. Drug susceptibility in the chemotherapy of mycobacterial infections. Boca Raton, FL: CRC Press, 1991:89–122.

30. Peloquin CA, Henshaw TL, Huitt GA, Berning, SE, Nitta AT, James GT. Pharmacokinetic evaluation of p-aminosalicylic acid granules. Pharmacotherapy 1994;14:40–46 [correction: Pharmacotherapy 1994;14:P-2].

31. Peloquin CA. Using therapeutic drug monitoring to dose the antimycobacterial drugs. Clin Chest Med 1997;18:79–87.

32. Pentikainen P, Wan SH, Azarnoff DL. Bioavailability studies on p-aminosalicylic acid and its various salts in man. I: Absorption from solution and suspension. J Pharmacol Biopharm 1974;2:1–12.

33. Rekola J. On the effect of benemid on the concentration of aminosalyl in the blood. Acta Tuberc Scand 1953;28:113–116.

34. Rieber CW, Saline M, Friedman MM. Plasma concentrations of para-aminosalicylic acid (PAS) after oral and rectal administration as influenced by p-(di-n-propylsulfamyl) benzoic acid (Benemid). Am Rev Tuberc 1951;64:448–452.

35. Riley C, Clowater RA, Shane SJ. Failure of p-(di-n-propylsulfamyl) benzoic acid (Benemid) to influence p-aminosalicylic acid blood levels. Dis Chest 1953;23:90–93.

36. Rossouw JE, Saunders SJ. Hepatic complication of antituberculous therapy. Q J Med 1975;XLIV:1–16.

37. Tiitinen H. Modification by para-aminosalicylic acid and sulfamethazine of the isoniazid inactivation in man. Scand J Resp Dis 1969;50:281–290.

38. Tuberculosis Chemotherapy Centre, Madras. Controlled comparison of oral twice-weekly and oral daily isoniazid plus PAS in newly diagnosed pulmonary tuberculosis. Br Med J 1973;2:7–11.

39. Trnka L, Mison P, Bartmann K, Otten H. Experimental evaluation of efficacy. In: Bartmann K, ed. Antituberculosis drugs. Berlin: Springer-Verlag, 1988:31–232.

40. Verbist L. Mode of action of antimycobacterial drugs (part I). Medicon Int 1974;3:11–23.

41. Verbist L. Mode of action of antituberculous drugs (part II). Medicon Int 1974;3:3–17.

42. Way EL, Smith PK, Howie DL, Weiss R, Swanson R. The absorption, distribution, excretion and fate of para-aminosalicylic acid. Proc Am Soc Pharmacol Exp Ther 1948:368–382.

43. Way EL, Pent C, Allawala N, Daniels TC. The metabolism of p-aminosalicylic acid (PAS) in man. J Am Pharm Assoc 1955;XLIV:65–69.

44. Winder FG. Mode of action of the antimycobacterial agents and associated aspects of the molecular biology of the mycobacteria, In: Ratledge C, Stanford J, eds: The biology of mycobacteria: vol 1—Physiology, identification, and classification. London: Academic Press, 1982:353–438.

Antimycobacterial Agents: Pyrazinamide

Leonid B. Heifets

CLASS PYRAZINES, NICOTINAMIDE ANALOGUES
Chemical Structure

Pyrazinamide (PZA) is a pyrazinoic acid amide (carboxyamide-2-pyrazine), $C_5H_5N_3O$. The chemical structures of pyrazinamide and related compounds are shown in Figure 1. The discovery that nicotinamide had some antituberculosis activity (17, 58, 70) led to further search for antituberculosis drugs among similar compounds and, particularly, to synthesis of pyrazinamide as a pyrazine analogue of nicotinamide (59), though this structure was known before (21, 42).

Pyrazinamide is a white crystalline powder, usually manufactured in tablets containing 500 mg of the drug (33). It has a

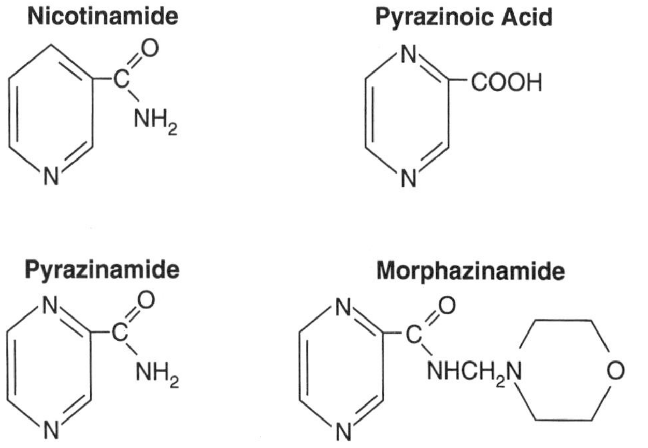

Nicotinamide

Pyrazinoic Acid

Pyrazinamide

Morphazinamide

FIGURE 1. Chemical structure of nicotinamide, pyrazinoic acid, pyrazinamide, and morphazinamide.

pK$_a$ of 0.5 and molecular weight of 123.11. Solubility in water or methanol is limited to 15 and 13.8 mg/mL, respectively, and it is less soluble in absolute ethanol or chloroform (5.7 and 7.4 mg/mL). Morphazinamide, or *N*-morpholinomethyl pyrazinamide, is a more water soluble analog of pyrazinamide (333 mg/mL).

Mode of Action and Structure-Activity Relationships

PZA is an antituberculosis drug active only against *Mycobacterium tuberculosis* and *M. africanum;* it does not exhibit any antimicrobial activity against *M. bovis* or any of the nontuberculous mycobacteria. Based on the correlation between antimicrobial activity of PZA and pyrazinamidase production by the *M. tuberculosis* strains susceptible to PZA, the mode of action of this agent was associated with pyrazinoic acid (POA), an enzyme-generated product considered the active moiety of PZA (57). The validity of this hypothesis has been questioned because of very low activity of POA against *M. tuberculosis* in vitro (45) and because other mycobacteria producing pyrazinamidase are not susceptible to PZA (44, 57). On the other hand, *M. bovis,* which does not have pyrazinamidase, is resistant to PZA but susceptible to POA.

It was postulated that not only PZA but also pyrazinoic acid esters might serve as prodrugs by being hydrolyzed by a variety of enzymes and thus circumvent the requirement for activation by an amidase (20). After synthesizing a number of such esters, this group of authors found that *n*-propyl pyrazinoate had the highest activity in vitro among them against both susceptible and PZA-resistant *M. tuberculosis* strains (95). In another study, a search among 39 synthesized PZA analogues led to selection of four compounds active against both *M. tuberculosis* and *M. avium-intracellulare:* pyrazine thiocarboxamide, *N*-hydroxymethyl pyrazine thiocarboxamide, pyrazinoic acid *n*-ostil ester, and pyrazinoic acid pivaloyloxymethyl ester (110). These studies point a new direction in the search for new antituberculosis drugs.

ANTIMICROBIAL ACTIVITY
Activity in Vitro in Cell-Free Media

As stated above, PZA is active against *M. tuberculosis* and *M. africanum* only. Its inhibitory activity in vitro was reported to be low and variable in early studies using normal pH standard culture media (22, 94, 99, 103). Experiments using acidic media have yielded more consistent results. The MIC of PZA at pH 5.5 in liquid medium containing Tween-80 was 16 μg/mL (67). The MIC in a high citrate medium at pH 5.6 without Tween-80 ranged from 8 to 16 μg/mL, and a concentration of 50 μg/mL produced even some decrease in the number of viable bacteria if the inoculum was relatively small (24). In 7H12 broth, at pH 5.5 to 5.6, the MICs ranged from 6.2 to 60 μg/mL (46, 47, 83).

No postantibiotic effect of PZA has been reported, and the bactericidal activity of PZA in vitro has been considered relatively low. The minimum bactericidal concentration (MBC) has never been reported, and only some decline in the number of the bacteria occurred at low pH in broth cultures (25, 46). Killing of 33 to 57% of the bacterial population took place in the presence of concentrations twice the MIC, but further increases in the concentrations, up to 500 and 1000 μg/mL, resulted in killing no more than 74% (46). Only when a large bacterial inoculum was maintained in liquid medium at pH 4.8 to 5.0 (in which case the number of bacteria in drug-free controls did not increase) 50 μg/mL of PZA led to a sharp, more than 1000-fold decline in the number of viable bacteria (48). This phenomenon was described as an in vitro sterilizing effect against the semidormant population versus very limited bactericidal activity against actively multiplying tubercle bacilli (48).

Activity against Intracellular *M. tuberculosis*

The data on antimicrobial activity of PZA against intracellular *M. tuberculosis* are quite controversial. Multiplication of strain H$_{37}$Rv within normal rabbit peritoneal macrophages was completely inhibited at a concentration of 12.5 μg/mL of PZA, with some bactericidal activity (66–75% decline in the number of viable bacteria) after exposure to 25 μg/mL for 72 h (69). These results were obtained with infected monocytes exposed to PZA-containing agar medium with streptomycin (1 μg/mL) added to prevent growth of contaminants. A substantial rate of killing, up to 93%, has been reported in experiments with mouse peritoneal macrophages exposed to 30 μg/mL of PZA for 24 h (14). However, the number of viable bacteria within macrophages increased during the second and third days of cultivation.

Bacteriostatic and even some bactericidal activity of PZA has been reported in human monocyte-derived macrophages (18). The data indicate, however, that 40 μg/mL produced only an inhibitory effect and only for the first 4 days, and in the presence of 20 μg/mL, growth was only partially inhibited. Concentrations of 80 and 160 μg/mL produced some bactericidal effect with a decline in the number of bacteria (by about 0.3 log$_{10}$) within the first 4 days of cultivation. Subsequent studies showed that none of the PZA concentrations completely inhibited growth, and even 800 μg/mL was only bacteriostatic, inhibiting up to 96.6% of the bacterial population

(85). Data from a more recent observation using the same model indicate that 40 μg/mL of PZA only partially inhibited intracellular growth (87). Experiments with J774 macrophages infected with *M. tuberculosis* detected neither inhibition nor bactericidal activity of PZA (80).

Antimicrobial Activity in Animal Experiments

Data from animal experiments led to the introduction of PZA into clinical use. This work was inspired by the finding that nicotinamide was effective in treating murine tuberculosis although it showed no antimycobacterial activity in vitro when tested at normal pH (17, 70). The first encouraging evidence of PZA activity in vivo, reported in 1952, showed that this agent, administered subcutaneously, significantly prolonged the life of mice intravenously infected with *M. tuberculosis* and was more effective than PAS and less effective than streptomycin (62, 94). Guinea pig experiments showed a similar result but with much lower PZA activity (23). A controversy arose after very limited PZA activity was reported, even in mice, but subsequently, the same authors showed that a better response could have been achieved with larger doses of PZA (99).

Combined Effect of PZA with Other Drugs in Experimental Models

The data on the effect of combination of PZA with other antituberculosis drugs in various experimental models is no less controversial than any other information on this agent. Simultaneous administration of PZA and isoniazid was reported to produce a sterilizing effect in infected mice that was not achievable by either drug alone (64). At the same time, under certain conditions, PZA increased the bactericidal effect of isoniazid against tubercle bacilli multiplying in rabbit macrophages during only the first 30 h of cultivation (69). Further studies of this sterilizing activity, reported 10 years later, showed that after a 90-day drug-free interval, *M. tuberculosis* was recovered in one-third of previously treated mice, indicating that the sterilizing effect of PZA was not complete (65, 66). Furthermore, PZA produced an antagonism with isoniazid when tested in cell-free liquid medium (25) and mouse experiments (40). In subsequent mouse experiments, combination of PZA with rifampin for preventive therapy was superior to combination with isoniazid or treatment with rifampin alone (41). In human monocyte-derived macrophages, PZA diminished the bactericidal effect of rifampin if the infected cells were treated with PZA 2 days prior to their exposure to rifampin (86). In the same experimental model, the very limited inhibitory effects of PZA and oflotoxin used singly in concentrations attainable in vivo, were slightly increased in a combination, but PZA enhanced the bactericidal effect of higher concentrations of ofloxacin (87).

Efficacy of PZA in Tuberculosis Patients

The first observation (in 1949 to 1951, on 43 patients) indicated that monotherapy with PZA (up to 700 mg four times per day for 33–42 days) resulted in improved clinical condition and a good bacteriologic response in most patients, depending on the severity of tuberculosis (111). In patients with a favorable response to therapy, the improvements occurred much faster than previously observed by the same authors for streptomycin or PAS. In a subsequent study, a group of 21 patients with advanced cavitary tuberculosis, who failed treatment with streptomycin and PAS, were treated for 18 months with a combination of isoniazid and PZA (12, 13). Stable sputum conversion occurred in 19 of them after 2 to 4 months of therapy. In the 2 remaining patients, who failed to respond, the isolates were found to be resistant to isoniazid.

In another clinical observation, treatment with PZA plus isoniazid was found to be more effective than use of PZA alone or in combination with streptomycin or PAS and equal to use of the combination of isoniazid, streptomycin, and PAS (88). Other early clinical observations of that period on the effectiveness of PZA in tuberculosis patients were tainted with controversy and doubts regarding its usefulness. Unlike the studies cited above, others reported that response to therapy with PZA alone or in combination with other drugs was favorable in new cases of tuberculosis, but not in those who failed previous therapy with streptomycin and had streptomycin-resistant organisms (78). Confirming the superiority of isoniazid plus PZA over other treatment regimens evaluated in patients and in the animal experiments, the authors of this extensive study concluded, nevertheless, that this combination of two drugs in doses used at that time (daily PZA 50 mg/kg and isoniazid total 5 mg) is "inadvisable as a treatment" because of the high incidence of hepatitis caused by this regimen (68). So, this period of initial studies was colored by reservations about the potential use of PZA because of either inconsistent data on the clinical efficacy, rapid emergence of drug resistance, or the high probability of side effects, particularly hepatotoxicity.

The attitude toward PZA changed after a series of controlled clinical trials demonstrated that PZA played a unique role in accelerating the sterilizing effect of isoniazid and rifampin (26–29, 53, 54, 92). This allowed reducing the duration of therapy from 9 to 6 months, the basis for modern short-course therapy regimens (8, 37, 38, 73, 74, 93). Currently, PZA is considered the third most important drug in tuberculosis therapy and should be included in the standard treatment regimen for the first 2 months of therapy (4, 39, 56, 73, 113).

MECHANISMS OF ACTION

Less is known about the mode of action of PZA than about that of any other antimycobacterial agent. In peak concentrations attainable in vivo (30–40 μg/mL), PZA is active only in acidic environments, at pH 5.5 to 5.6 (57, 67), and it has been suggested that the effect of PZA in vivo takes place in the acidic intracellular environment of the macrophages (69). This could explain why PZA is more effective in the mouse than in the guinea pig, which have different types of lesions—tubercle bacilli are almost exclusively intracellular in the mouse and necrosis predominates in the guinea pig (69). The problem, both in the early studies and today, is that there is no clear evidence that the pH is actually 5.5 to 5.6 in the compartments of the macrophages where PZA and tubercle bacilli interact. On one hand, there are reports that in the vicinity of the phagocytosed tubercle bacilli the pH could be as low as 4.7 (75, 96).

On the other hand, the presence of live tubercle bacilli in the phagosome prevents its fusion with lysosomes, which supposedly keeps the intraphagosomal environment neutral or at only slightly acidic pH (5, 36). More recently, direct evidence has been obtained that in human monocyte-derived macrophages, tubercle bacilli persisted at neutral pH (19). Conditions under which the tubercle bacilli–containing phagosomes are acidified remain unclear; some data indicate that such acidification, if occurring under certain conditions, does not go below pH 6.3 (102). Another explanation of the activity of PZA in vivo is that it interacts with tubercle bacilli in the acidic early inflammation sites, affecting the semidormant part of the bacterial population persisting in this acidic environment (73).

It is assumed that in an acidic environment, pyrazinamidase produced by the *M. tuberculosis* strains susceptible to PZA convert PZA into POA, which specifically affects tubercle bacilli (57). The actual target of either PZA or POA in *M. tuberculosis* remains unknown; however, resistance of tubercle bacilli to PZA was associated with the loss of pyramidase and nicotinamidase activity (57). Recently, this activity was shown to be controlled by the *pncA* gene, in which mutations presumably cause PZA resistance (89).

RESISTANCE TO PYRAZINAMIDE

Rapid emergence of resistance of *M. tuberculosis* to PZA was reported in the first clinical study, with 42 patients given PZA as monotherapy for 33 to 42 days (111). In this study, resistance to PZA appeared more rapidly in patients with large cavities and large quantities of sputum with high bacterial content and was accompanied by failure to respond to continued therapy with PZA. Subsequently, PZA has been used only in combination with other antituberculosis drugs. The recommendation for the last decade has been to use PZA for the first 2 months of therapy only, in combination with isoniazid and rifampin or, for some patients, in a four-drug regimen that also includes ethambutol or streptomycin (39, 77).

Under these circumstances, there have been no recent reports on monoresistance to PZA and most often resistance to this agent appears along with, and usually after, development of resistance to isoniazid or to isoniazid and rifampin. No cross-resistance with other antituberculosis drugs has been reported. Emergence of resistance to PZA, part of the multidrug-resistance problem in tuberculosis patients (MDR-TB), results from improper treatment management or nonadherence to the treatment regimen (56). For example, resistance to PZA develops rapidly if this drug is added alone to a failing regimen, when the patient's bacterial population is already resistant to the other drugs (61).

Resistance to PZA in *M. tuberculosis* is associated with loss of pyrazinamidase/nicotinamidase activity, which in susceptible strains hydrolyzes PZA to POA (7, 57, 63, 104). This enzyme was recently reported to be controlled by the *pncA* gene (89). The identified mutations are dispersed along the *pncA* gene, with some clustering in the regions *Gly*132–*Thr*142, *Pro*69–*Leu*85, *Ile*5–*Asp*12 (90). These findings indicate that mutation in the *pncA* gene is probably the major cause of development of PZA resistance in *M. tuberculosis*. The natural resistance of *M. bovis*, which does not have pyrazinamidase, is probably associated with a single characteristic mutation at nucleotide position 169, changing C to G, which causes substitution of histamine for aspartic acid at amino acid position 57 (89). The mechanism of natural PZA resistance in nontuberculous mycobacteria is unknown.

Detection of PZA resistance in *M. tuberculosis* clinical isolates by in vitro testing is difficult because of the poor growth of *M. tuberculosis* in the acidic environment required for detection of PZA activity (100). Therefore, the pyrazinamidase test, proposed originally as a taxonomic test (106), has been used in some clinical laboratories to detect resistance to PZA (57, 63). This method may cause false susceptible reports due to insufficient growth of some isolates.

An attempt was made to improve growth of *M. tuberculosis* at pH 5.5 for a PZA susceptibility test by changing the composition of 7H10 agar (9, 10), but about 10% of isolates did not grow at all at this medium, and the growth of other isolates was partially inhibited, with delayed appearance of colonies and a substantial reduction in colony size. Using an excessive inoculum to overcome the problem of poor growth can lead to local pH neutralization by the bacterial mass (67, 100), which may increase the probability of false resistance. To counteract the problem, a radiometric BACTEC susceptibility test was developed with initial cultivation in standard (pH 6.8) 7H12 broth followed by addition of the PZA solution and lowering the pH to 5.5 with phosphoric acid solution after the culture reaches the exponential growth phase (43). This method worked accurately, but it was too laborious, and some isolates did not grow in drug-free controls after the pH was lowered to 5.5.

The correlation between the degree of acidity of the medium and the PZA concentrations needed to inhibit growth of susceptible *M. tuberculosis* strains has been known since the 1950s (67). After confirming the validity of this correlation for 7H12 broth conditions, an improvement in the radiometric susceptibility test was suggested using pH 6.0 instead of 5.5, with an eightfold increase in PZA concentration: 400 μg/mL at pH 6.0 versus 50 μg/mL at pH 5.5 (83). The radiometric test was further modified, adding 100 μg/mL of PZA at the beginning of cultivation instead of a few days after the vial was inoculated with the culture (84). This technique was adopted by the BACTEC manufacturer (91). This test is supposed to identify the isolate as PZA resistant if the bacterial population contains more than 10% resistant bacteria, based on comparison (>11%) of the radiometric growth indices (GIs) in the presence of 100 μg PZA and in the drug-free control.

Substantial discordance in results between this and other methods was observed by some laboratories testing strains isolated during outbreaks of MDR-TB (15). Controversy arose after the same isolates were submitted to different laboratories (50). A study with participation of the BACTEC manufacturer showed that 3.5% of the tested isolates did not grow enough to provide interpretable results (72). The insufficient growth was attributed to the presence of polyoxyethylene stearite (POES) in the medium, and exclusion of this ingredient improved the growth at pH 6.0 but yielded a greater proportion of false resistance than in the presence of POES. It has been reported that the isolates that gave questionable or false-resistant results at pH 6.0 with 100 μg/mL were completely inhibited by 300 μg/mL (47). Therefore, the National Jewish Medical and Research Center in Denver currently determines MICs with a quantitative test using three PZA concentrations: 100 μg or below as the susceptible breakpoint; 300 μg as moderately susceptible (or intermediate); and 900 μg or above as resistant (49). Current experience at the National Jewish in Denver confirms the validity of the suggestion that the single-concentration qualitative test would give more reliable and reproducible results if the PZA concentration were increased to the originally suggested 300 or 400 μg/mL, with or without POES in the medium.

PHARMACOKINETIC DISPOSITION
Absorption

Based on a lack of detectable PZA in feces, absorption of PZA is considered complete. Studies in laboratory animals and man showed that administration of 20 mg/kg resulted in a C_{max} of 65 μg/mL within 1 to 4 h (101). Following a single oral dose of 1.5 g of PZA in healthy adults, the plasma peak concentration (C_{max}) after 2 h ranged from 30 to 40 μg/mL (30). The concentration attainable in blood is dose dependent, and C_{max} can be 9 to 12 μg/mL after a dose of 0.5 g, 45 μg/mL after 1 g, and 60 to 70 μg/mL after a 3 g (11, 30).

Distribution

The time to the peak serum concentration of PZA is usually within 2 h after its oral administration, and the half-life ($t_{1/2}$) is about 9 to 10 h in individuals with normal renal and hepatic function (30). Actual V_d and protein binding of PZA are not known, but on the basis of its structural similarity with isoniazid, PZA diffusion into the extravascular fluid was suggested to be about 0.6 to 0.7 L/kg (76). PZA is well distributed in lungs, liver, kidneys, but was not detected in skeletal muscle, spleen, brain, or bone marrow in rabbits given one oral dose (101). Concentrations of PZA in cerebrospinal fluid can reach 39 to 52 μg/mL after 2 h of oral administration of 41 mg/kg (mean dose) and were equal to those in serum after 5 h (32, 34). PZA rapidly penetrates into macrophages, and its intracellular concentration is about the same as that in the extracellular fluid (1).

Metabolism and Excretion

PZA is converted (mostly in liver) to POA by the microsomal pyrazinamide deaminidase, and POA is then oxidized to 5-hydroxypyrazinoic acid (30, 82, 107, 112). Along with these major products, additional metabolites (e.g., 5-hydroxypyrazinamide and pyrazinuric acid) may also appear (6, 51, 60, 79, 81, 109). Only a very small amount of unchanged PZA, about 3 to 14%, is excreted in urine within 24 h, primarily via glomerular filtration; most is reabsorbed by the renal tubules (30, 101, 107). Up to 70% of PZA is excreted in urine as the major metabolites mentioned above. The rate of POA excretion reaches its maximum at 2 h, and 32 and 40% of it is excreted at 24 and 48 h, respectively (30).

DOSAGE REGIMENS
Normal

PZA is an essential part of the initial treatment of tuberculosis and is administered in combination with other antituberculosis drugs for the first 8 weeks. It should not be used for monotherapy. There are three basic options in the currently recommended short course 6-months therapy (4, 56). In option 1, PZA is administered daily for children and adults in doses of 15 to 30 mg/kg, not exceeding 2 g/day, for 8 weeks, along with isoniazid and rifampin, followed by 16 weeks of daily administration of isoniazid and rifampin without PZA. In option 2, with directly observed therapy (DOT), four drugs (isoniazid, rifampin, PZA, and streptomycin or ethambutol) are administered daily for 2 weeks followed by twice-weekly administration of the same drugs for 6 weeks, followed by twice-weekly administration of only isoniazid and rifampin for 16 weeks. In this regimen the doses of PZA are 50 to 70 mg/kg, not exceeding 4 g/day. In option 3, also DOT, the same drugs are administered three times per week, and PZA is given in doses of 50 to 70 mg/kg without exceeding 3 g/day.

Renal Failure

As mentioned above, PZA is excreted in urine in the form of its major metabolites POA and 5-hydroxypyrazinoic acid (30, 107). In patients with renal failure, the $t_{1/2}$ of PZA and its metabolites is extended, but hemodialysis can shorten it with high clearance of both PZA and POA (31, 60, 97, 108). Impaired renal function does not contraindicate PZA administration, but reduction of doses may be considered. In patients undergoing dialysis, PZA can be administered after each dialysis session, along with other drugs (e.g., under the provisions of a thrice-weekly regimen).

Hepatic Failure

In patients with hepatic failure, PZA metabolism can be affected, which may result in a high accumulation of the drug in blood (101). All patients should be tested for liver function before PZA administration and every 2 to 3 weeks thereafter. PZA is contraindicated in patients with severe hepatic damage (76).

Obesity

Dosage of PZA, as well as other hydrophilic drugs likely to have low V_ds, should be based on ideal body weight (35).

Pregnancy

PZA has not been studied during pregnancy, but its similarity to isoniazid suggests that it probably can cross the placenta (76). The potential teratogenicity of PZA is not known, and it should be given to pregnant women with caution (51). PZA should also be given to nursing mothers with caution, since it has been found in small amounts in milk (52).

ADVERSE EFFECTS

Hepatotoxicity and other toxic effects of PZA were reported in the first clinical study, in which PZA was administered in doses of 50 mg/kg (2, 68, 71), but subsequent studies with doses of 20 to 30 mg/kg have shown that PZA toxicity is not a major problem (26, 105). Nevertheless, hepatotoxicity is the most frequent adverse effect of PZA, and it is usually dose related, affecting up to 15% of patients receiving 3 g daily. The frequency of hepatotoxicity in patients who received PZA in doses of 25 to 35 mg/kg along with isoniazid and rifampin was the same as that among patients who received these two drugs without PZA. The most frequent manifestations of hepatotoxicity are a transient increase in serum aminotransferase concentration, jaundice, liver tenderness, splenomegaly, anemia, and malaise. Some authors recommend checking the levels of serum glutamic oxaloacetic transaminase (SGOT) before and during therapy and discontinuing PZA if the SGOT concentration is rising rapidly or exceeds twice the upper limit of normal (51).

Other adverse effects of PZA include nausea, anorexia, nongouty polyarthralgia in about 40% of patients (related to the increased concentrations of uric acid in blood), gouty arthritis, maculopapular rash, urticaria and other hypersensitivity reactions, thrombocytopenia and sideroblastic anemia, vacuolation of erythrocytes, and increased iron concentrations in serum.

DRUG INTERACTIONS

There are no reports of patients with undesirable interactions between PZA and any other drugs, including other antituberculosis drugs and agents currently used in HIV-infected individuals. Data on interactions between PZA and other antituberculosis drugs in experimental models are described above.

CLINICAL INDICATIONS

PZA is an essential part of initial therapy for any form of tuberculosis, including meningitis (32). It should be excluded from therapy if the isolate identified by one of the rapid methods as *M. tuberculosis* complex is *M. bovis*. The recommended treatment regimens for children do not differ from those for adults, and a twice-weekly dose of 18 to 40 mg/kg (up to 2 g/day) is recommended (3, 98).

For adults with HIV infection, the recommended antituberculosis regimen under DOT conditions includes isoniazid 300 mg/day, rifampin 600 mg/day (450 mg for persons weighing less than 50 kg), ethambutol 15 mg/kg/day, and PZA 20 to 30 mg/kg/day for the first 2 months of therapy, followed by at least 4 months of therapy without PZA (55). Under DOT, the drugs can be given twice or thrice weekly after an initial phase of daily treatment (16). For patients who have isolates resistant to isoniazid and rifampin and for those who cannot tolerate these drugs (e.g., some HIV-infected persons), other treatment regimens should be administered for 9, 12, 18, or 24 months depending on the situation (55, 56).

PZA is under consideration for combined preventive therapy in cases of suspected isoniazid resistance, particularly in combination with rifampin or one of other rifamycins, shown to be superior to rifampin alone in mouse experiments (41). When MDR-TB is a suspected source of infection, another al-

ternative preventive therapy regimen is combination of PZA with one of the quinolones, especially for HIV-infected patients, but no clinical data on such regimens are available (41).

COMMENTS

The history of PZA use in therapy for tuberculosis is full of controversy (113). The early observations when PZA was used for monotherapy in small groups of patients are of great value, since for ethical reasons such studies became impossible after the antituberculosis activity of PZA was confirmed and multidrug regimens were introduced for tuberculosis therapy. These observations showed clear antituberculosis activity of PZA in patients, certain limitations to its potential use, inevitable emergence of PZA resistance under monotherapy, and hence the clinical predictability of in vitro susceptibility tests. Among the questions that remain unanswered for PZA are its actual mode of action and target in the bacterial cell. It is also unclear whether the predominant interaction between PZA and bacteria is taking place intracellularly in macrophages or extracellularly in the acidic environment of the early inflammation sites. Most likely, PZA has only bacteriostatic activity in concentrations attainable in vivo. Nevertheless, PZA is among the first-line drugs, and it became an essential element of the modern treatment regimens by shortening the course of tuberculosis therapy from 9 to 6 months when used in combination with isoniazid and rifampin. PZA will likely be recommended for preventive therapy in combination with rifampin or one of the quinolones when resistance to isoniazid is suspected.

REFERENCES
1. Acocella G, Carlone NA, Cuffini AM, Cavallo G. The penetration of rifampicin, pyrazinamide, and pyrazinoic acid into macrophages. Am Rev Respir Dis 1985;132:1268–1273.
2. Allison ST. Pyrazinamide-isoniazid in low dosage in treatment of pulmonary tuberculosis. Am Rev Tuberc 1956;74:400–401.
3. American Academy of Pediatrics. Chemotherapy for tuberculosis in infants and children. Pediatrics 1992;89:161–165.
4. American Thoracic Society. Treatment of tuberculosis and tuberculous infection in adults and children. Am J Respir Crit Care Med 1994;149:1359–1374.
5. Armstrong JA, D'Arcy Hart P. Response of cultured macrophages to *M. tuberculosis* with observations on fusion of lysosomes with phagosomes. J Exp Med 1971;134:713–740.
6. Auscher C, Pasquier C, Pehuet P, Delbarre F. Study of urinary pyrazinamide metabolites and their action on the renal excretion of xanthine and hypoxanthine in a xanthinuric patient. Biomedicine 1978;28:129–133.
7. Brander E. A simple way of detecting pyrazinamide resistance. Tubercle 1972;53:128–131.
8. British Thoracic Association. A controlled trial of six months chemotherapy in pulmonary tuberculosis. Final report: results during the 36 months after the end of chemotherapy and beyond. Br J Dis Chest 1984;78:330–336.
9. Butler WR, Kilburn JO. Improved method for testing susceptibility of Mycobacterium tuberculosis to pyrazinamide. J Clin Microbiol 1982;16:1106–1109.

10. Butler WR, Kilburn JO. Susceptibility of *Mycobacterium tuberculosis* to pyrazinamide and its relationship to pyrazinamidase activity. Antimicrob Agents Chemother 1983;24:600–601.

11. Caccia PA. Spectrophotometric determination of pyrazinamide blood concentrations and excretion through the kidneys. Am Rev Respir Dis 1957;75:105–112.

12. Campagna M, Calix AA, Hauser G. Observations on the combined use of pyrazinamide (Aldinamide) and isoniazid in the treatment of pulmonary tuberculosis. Am Rev Tuberc 1954;69: 334–350.

13. Campagna M, Hauser G, Greenberg HB. The eradication of *Mycobacterium tuberculosis* from the sputum of patients treated with pyrazinamide and isoniazid. Am Rev Respir Dis 1962; 86:636–639.

14. Carlone NA, Acocella G, Guffini AM, Forno-Pizzogio M. Killing of macrophage-ingested mycobacteria by rifampin, pyrazinamide, and pyrazinoic acid alone and in combination. Am Rev Respir Dis 1985;132:1274–1277.

15. Centers for Disease Control and Prevention. Nosocomial transmission of multidrug-resistant tuberculosis among HIV-infected persons—Florida and New York 1988–1991. MMWR 1991;40: 585–591.

16. Chaisson RE, Clermont HC, Holt EA. Six-months supervised intermittent tuberculosis therapy in Haitian patients with and without chemotherapy. Am J Respir Crit Care Med 1996;154: 1034–1038.

17. Chorine MV. Action of nicotinamide on bacillus of the species *Mycobacterium*. C R Acad Sci 1945;220:150–156.

18. Crowle AJ, Sbarbaro JA, May MH. Inhibition by pyrazinamide of tubercle bacilli within cultured human macrophages. Am Rev Respir Dis 1986;134:1052–1055.

19. Crowle AJ, Dahl R, Ross E, May MH. Evidence that vesicles containing living virulent *M. tuberculosis* or *M. avium* in cultured human macrophages are not acidic. Infect Immun 1991; 59:1823–1831.

20. Cynamon MH, Klemens SP, Chou TS, Gimi RH, Welch JT. Antimycobacterial activity of a series of pyrazinoic acid esters. J Med Chem 1992;35:1212–1215.

21. Dalmer O, Walter E. German patent no. 362257,1936.

22. Dessau FI, Burger T, Yager RL, Kulish M. A method for the determination of in vitro sensitivity of tubercle bacilli to pyrazinamide (Aldinamide). Am Rev Tuberc 1952;65:635–636.

23. Dessau FI, Yager RL, Burger FJ, Williams JN. Pyrazinamide (Aldinamide) in experimental tuberculosis in the guinea pig. Am Rev Tuberc 1952;65:519–522.

24. Dickinson JM, Mitchison DA. Observations in vitro on the suitability of pyrazinamide for intermittent chemotherapy of tuberculosis. Tubercle 1970;51:389–396.

25. Dickinson JM, Aber VR, Mitchison DA. Bactericidal activity of streptomycin, isoniazid, rifampin, ethambutol, and pyrazinamide alone and in combination against *Mycobacterium tuberculosis*. Am Rev Respir Dis 1979;116:627–635.

26. East African/British Medical Research Council. Controlled clinical trial of four short course (6 months) regimens of chemotherapy for treatment of pulmonary tuberculosis. Lancet 1973;2: 237–240.

27. East African/British Medical Research Council. Controlled trial of four short-course (6-month) regimens of chemotherapy for treatment of pulmonary tuberculosis. Third report. Lancet 1974;2:237–240.

28. East African/British Medical Research Council. Controlled clinical trial of four short-course (6-month) regimens of chemotherapy for treatment of pulmonary tuberculosis. Second East African/British Medical Research Council study. Lancet 1974; 2:1100–1106.

29. East African/British Medical Research Council. Fifth collaborative study. Controlled clinical trial of 4 short-course regimens of chemotherapy (three 6-months and one 8-months) for pulmonary tuberculosis. Final report. Tubercle 1986;67:5–15.

30. Ellard CA. Absorption, metabolism and excretion of pyrazinamide in man. Tubercle 1969;50:144–158.

31. Ellard GA, Haslam RM. Observations on the reduction of the renal elimination of urite in man caused by the administration of pyrazinamide. Tubercle 1976;57:97–103.

32. Ellard GA, Humphries MY, Gabriel M, Teoh R. Penetration of pyrazinamide into the cerebrospinal fluid in tuberculous meningitis. Br Med J 1987;294:284–285.

33. Feldner E, Pitre D. Pyrazinamide. In: Florey K, ed. Analytical profiles of drug substances. New York: Academic Press, 1983:12:433–462.

34. Forgan-Smith R, Ellard GA, Newton D, Mitchison DA. Pyrazinamide and other drugs in tuberculous meningitis. Lancet 1973;2:374–375.

35. Geiseler PJ, Manis RD, Maddux MS. Dosage of antituberculosis drugs in obese patients. Am Rev Respir Dis 1985;131:944–946.

36. Goren MB. Phagocyte lysosomes: interaction with infectious agents, phagosomes and experimental perturbation in function. Annu Rev Microbiol 1977;31:507–533.

37. Grosset J. Sterilizing value of rifampicin and pyrazinamide in experimental short-course chemotherapy. Tubercle 1978;59: 287–289.

38. Grosset J. Bacteriologic basis of short-course chemotherapy for tuberculosis. Clin Chest Med 1980;1:231–241.

39. Grosset JH. Present status on chemotherapy of tuberculosis. Rev Infect Dis 1989;11(Suppl 2):S347–S352.

40. Grosset J, Truffot-Pernot C, Lavoix C, Ji B. Antagonism between isoniazid and the combination pyrazinamide-rifampin against tuberculosis infection in mice. Antimicrob Agents Chemother 1992;36:548–555.

41. Grosset JH, O'Brien RJ. Advances in tuberculosis preventive therapy. In: LB Heifets, ed. Tuberculosis, seminars in respiratory and critical care medicine. New York: Thieme Medical Publishers, Inc., 1997;18:449–457.

42. Hall SA, Spoerri PE. Synthesis in the pyrazine series: preparation and properties of amino-pyrazine. J Am Chem Soc 1940; 62:664–665.

43. Heifets LB, Iseman MD. Radiometric method for testing susceptibility of mycobacteria to pyrazinamide in 7H12 broth. J Clin Microbiol 1985;21:200–204.

44. Heifets LB, Iseman MD, Crowle AJ, Lindholm-Levy PJ. Pyrazinamide is not active in vitro against *Mycobacterium avium* complex. Am Rev Respir Dis 1986;134:1287–1288.

45. Heifets LB, Flory MA, Lindholm-Levy PJ. Does pyrazinoic acid as an active moiety of pyrazinamide have specific activity against *Mycobacterium tuberculosis*? Antimicrob Agents Chemother 1989;33:1252–1254.

46. Heifets LB, Lindholm-Levy PJ. Is pyrazinamide bactericidal against *M. tuberculsos*? Am Rev Respir Dis 1990;141:250–252.

47. Heifets LB. Drug susceptibility tests in the management of chemotherapy of tuberculosis. In: Heifets LB, ed. Drug susceptibility in the chemotherapy of mycobacterial infections. Boca Raton: CRC Press, 1991:89–122.

48. Heifets L, Lindholm-Levy P. Pyrazinamide sterilizing activity in vitro against semi-dormant *M. tuberculosis* bacterial population. Am Rev Respir Dis 1992;145:1223–1225.

49. Heifets LB. Drug susceptibility testing. In: LB Heifets, ed. Clinical mycobacteriology, clinics in laboratory medicine. Philadelphia: WB Saunders, 1996;16:641–656.

50. Hewlett D, Horn D, Alfalla C. Drug-resistant tuberculosis: inconsistent results of pyrazinamide susceptibility testing [Letter]. JAMA 1995;273:916–917.

51. Holdiness MR. Clinical pharmacokinetics of the antituberculosis drugs. Clin Pharmacokinet 1984;9:511–544.

52. Holdiness M. Antituberculosis drugs in breast-feeding. Arch Intern Med 1984;144:1888–1889.

53. Hong Kong Tuberculosis Treatment Service/British Medical Research Council. Controlled trial of 6- and 9-month regimens daily and intermittent streptomycin plus isoniazid plus pyrazinamide for pulmonary tuberculosis in Hong Kong. Tubercle 1975;56:81–96.

54. Hong Kong Chest Service/British Medical Research Council. Controlled trial of four thrice-weekly regimens and a daily regimen all given for 6 months for pulmonary tuberculosis. Lancet 1981;1:171–174.

55. Hopewell PC. Tuberculosis in persons with human immunodeficiency virus infection: clinical and public health aspects. In: LB Heifets, ed. Seminars in respiratory and critical care medicine. New York: Thieme Medical Publishers, Inc.,1997;18:471–483.

56. Iseman MD. Treatment of multidrug-resistant tuberculosis. N Engl J Med 1993;329:784–791.

57. Konno K, Feldman FM, McDermott W. Pyrazinamide susceptibility and amidase activity of tubercle bacilli. Am Rev Respir Dis 1967;95:461–469.

58. Kushner S, Dalalian H, Cassell RT, Sanjurjo JL, McKenzie D, Subbarow Y. Experimental chemotherapy of tuberculosis. I. Substituted nicotinamides. J Org Chem 1948;13:834–836.

59. Kushner S, Dalalian H, Sanjurjo JL, Bach FL, Safir SR, Smith VK, Williams JH. Experimental chemotherapy of tuberculosis. II. Synthesis of pyrazinamide and related compounds. JAMA 1952;74:3617–3621.

60. Lacroix C, Hoang TP, Nouveau J, Guyonnaud C, Laine G, Dewoos H, Lafont O. Pharmacokinetics of pyrazinamide and its metabolites in healthy subjects. Eur J Clin Pharmacol 1989;36:394–400.

61. Mahmoudi A, Iseman MD. Pitfalls in the care of patients with tuberculosis: common errors and their association with the acquisition of drug resistance. JAMA 1993;270:65–68.

62. Malone L, Schurr A, Lindth H, McKenzie D, Kiser JS, Williams JH. The effect of pyrazinamide (Aldinamide) on experimental tuberculosis in mice. Am Rev Tuberc 1952;65:511–518.

63. McClatchy JK, Tsang AY, Cernich MS. Use of pyrazinamidase activity in *Mycobacterium tuberculosis* as a rapid method for determination of pyrazinamide susceptibility. Antimicrob Agents Chemother 1981;20:556–557.

64. McCune RM, Tompsett R, McDermott W. The fate of *M. tuberculosis* in mouse tissue as determined by the microbial enumeration technique. II. The conversion of tuberculosis infection to the latent state by the administration of pyrazinamide and a companion drug. J Exp Med 1956;104:763–802.

65. McCune RM, Feldman FM, Lambert HP, McDermott W. Microbial persistence. I. The capacity of tubercle bacilli to survive sterilization in mouse tissues. J Exp Med 1966;123:445–468.

66. McCune RM, Feldman FM, McDermott W. Microbial persistence. II. Characteristics of the sterile state of tubercle bacilli. J Exp Med 1966;123:469–486.

67. McDermott W, Tomsett R. Activation of pyrazinamide and nicotinamide in acidic environments in vitro. Am Rev Tuberc 1954;70:748–754.

68. McDermott W, Ormond L, Muschenheim C, Deuschle K, McCune RM, Tompsett R. Pyrazinomide-isoniazid in tuberculosis. Am Rev Tuberc 1954;69:319–333.

69. McKaness GB. The intracellular activation of pyrazinamide and nicotinamide. Am Rev Tuberc 1956;74:718–728.

70. McKenzie D, Malone L, Kushner S, Oleson JJ, Subbarow Y. The effect of nicotinic acid amide on the experimental tuberculosis in white mice. J Lab Clin Med 1948;33:1249–1253.

71. McLeod HM, Hay D, Stewart SM. The use of pyrazinamide plus isoniazid in the treatment of pulmonary tuberculosis. Tubercle 1959;40:14–20.

72. Miller MA, Thibert L, Desjardins F, Siddiqi SH, Dascal A. Growth inhibition of *M. tuberculosis* by polyoxyethilene sterite present in the BACTEC pyrazinamide susceptibility test. J Clin Microbiol 1996;34:84–86.

73. Mitchison DA. The action of antituberculosis drugs in short-course chemotherapy. Tubercle 1985;66:219–225.

74. O'Brien RJ, Snider DE. Tuberculosis drugs—old and new [Editorial]. Am Rev Respir Dis 1985;131:309–311.

75. Pavlov EP, Tushov EG, Konyaev GA. The effect of pyrazinamide on pH of cytoplasma areas surrounding phagocytized mycobacteria. Probl Tuberk 1974;1:77–79.

76. Peloquin CA. Antituberculosis drugs: pharmacokinetics. In: LB Heifets, ed. Drug susceptibility in the chemotherapy of mycobacterial infections. Boca Raton, FL: CRC Press, 1991:59–89.

77. Perez-Stable EJ, Hopewell PC. Current tuberculosis regimens: choosing the right one for your patient. In: DE Snider, ed. Clinics in chest medicine. Philadelphia: WB Saunders, 1989;10:323–339.

78. Phillips S, Larkin JC, Litzenberger WL, Horton GE, Haimsohn JS. Observations on pyrazinamide (Aldinamide) in pulmonary tuberculosis. Am Rev Tuberc 1954;69:443–450.

79. Pitre D, Facino RM, Carini M, Carlo A. In vitro biotransformation of pyrazinamide by rat liver: identification of a new metabolite. Pharmacol Res Commun 1981;13:351–362.

80. Rastogi N, Potar MC, David HL. Pyrazinamide is not effective against intracellularly growing *M. tuberculosis*. Antimicrob Agents Chemother 1988;32:287–288.

81. Ratti B, Toselli A, Beretta E, Bernareggi A. HPLC assay of pyrazinoic acid in human plasma in the presence of pyrazinamide and other antituberculosis drugs using automatic sampler. Farmaco 1982;37:226–234.

82. Roboz J, Suzuki R, Yu TF. Mass fragmentographic determination of pyrazinamide and its metabolites in serum and urine. J Chromatogr 1978;147:333–347.

83. Salfinger M, Heifets LB. Determination of pyrazinamide MIC for *M. tuberculosis* at different pHs by the radiometric method. Antimicrob Agents Chemother 1988;32:1002–1004.

84. Salfinger M, Reller LB, Demchuk B, Johnson ZT. Rapid radiometric methods for pyrazinamide susceptibility testing of *Mycobacterium tuberculosis*. Res Microbiol 1989;140:301–309.

85. Salfinger M, Crowle AJ, Reller LB. Pyrazinamide and pyrazinoic acid activity against tubercle bacilli in cultured human macrophages and in the BACTEC system. J Infect Dis 1990;162:201–207.

86. Sbarbaro JA, Iseman MD, Crowle AJ. Synergism of rifampin and pyrazinamide within the human macrophages. Am Rev Respir Dis 1992;146:1448–1451.

87. Sbarbaro JA, Iseman MD, Crowle AJ. Combined effect of pyrazinamide and ofloxacin within the human macrophage. Tuberc Lung Dis 1996;77:491–495.

88. Schwartz WS, Moyer RE. The chemotherapy of pulmonary tuberculosis with pyrazinamide alone or in combination with streptomycin, PAS or isoniazid. Am Rev Tuberc 1954;70:413–422.

89. Scorpio A, Zhang Y. Mutations in *pncA*, a gene encoding pyrazinamidase/nicotinamidase, cause resistance to the antituberculous drug pyrazinamide in tubercle bacilli. Nature Med 1996;2:662–667.

90. Scorpio A, Lindholm-Levy P, Heifets L, Gilman R, Siddiqi S, Cynamon M, Zhang Y. Characterization of *pncA* mutations in pyrazinamide-resistant *Mycobacterium tuberculosis*. Antimicrob Agents Chemother 1997;41:540–543.

91. Siddiqi S. Radiometric (BACTEC) tests for slowly growing mycobacteria. In: Isenberg H, ed. Clinical microbiology procedures handbook. Washington, DC: American Society for Microbiology 1992;5.14:1–25.

92. Singapore Tuberculosis Service/British Medical Research Council. Clinical trial of six-month and four-month regimens of chemotherapy in the treatment of pulmonary tuberculosis: the results up to 30 months. Tubercle 1981;62:95–102.

93. Snider DE, Rogowski J, Zierski M, Bek E, Long MW. Successful intermittent treatment of smear-positive pulmonary tuberculosis in six months: a cooperative study in Poland. Am Rev Respir Dis 1982;125:265–267.

94. Solotorovsky M, Gregory FJ, Ironson EJ, Bagie EJ, O'Neil RC, Pfister K. Pyrazinoic acid amide—an agent active against experimental murine tuberculosis. Proc Soc Exp Biol Med 1952;79:563–565.

95. Speirs RJ, Welch JT, Cynamon MH. Activity of n-propyl pyrazinoate against pyrazinamide-resistant *M. tuberculosis:* investigation into mechanism of action and of mechanism of resistance to pyrazinamide. Antimicrob Agents Chemother 1995;39:1269–1271.

96. Sprick MG, Pathogenesis of *M. tuberculosis* and *M. smegmatis* stained with indicator dyes. Am Rev Tuberc 1956;74:552–565.

97. Stamathakis G, Montes C, Trouvin JH, Faronotti R, Fessi R, Kenouch S, Mary JP. Pyrazinamide and pyrazinoic acid pharmacokinetics in patients with chronic renal failure. Clin Nephrol 1980;30:230–234.

98. Starke JR. Multidrug therapy for tuberculosis in children. Pediatr Infect Dis J 1990;9:785–793.

99. Steenken W, Wolinsky E. The antituberculosis activity of pyrazinamide in vitro and in the guinea pig. Am Rev Tuberc 1954;70:367–369.

100. Stottmeier KD, Beam RE, Kubica GP. Determination of drug susceptibility of mycobacteria to pyrazinamide in 7H10 agar. Am Rev Respir Dis 1967;96:1072–1075.

101. Stottmeier KD, Beam RE, Kubica CP. The absorption and excretion of pyrazinamide. Am Rev Respir Dis 1968;98:70–74.

102. Sturgill-Koszycki SP, Schlesinger P, Chakrabotry P, Haddix PL, Collins HL, Fok AK, Allen RD, Gluck SL, Henser J, Russel DG. Lack of acidification in *Mycobacterium* phagosomes produced by exclusion of the vesicular proton ATPase. Science 1994;263:678–681.

103. Tarshis MS, Weed WA. Lack of significant in vitro sensitivity of *M. tuberculosis* to pyrazinamide in three different solid media. Am Rev Tuberc 1953;67:391–395.

104. Tatar J. Sensitivity of tubercle bacilli to pyrazinamide determined on the basis of their sensitivity to nicotinamide and their pyrazinamidase and nicotinamidase activities. Gruzlica 1974;42:773–777.

105. Velu S, Dawson JJY, Devadatta S, Fox W, Kulkurni KG, Mohan K, Ramakrishnan CV, Scott H. A controlled comparison of streptomycin plus pyrazinamide and streptomycin plus PAS in the treatment of patients excreting isoniazid-resistant organisms. Tubercle 1964;45:144–159.

106. Wayne LG. Simple pyrazinamidase and urease tests for routine identification of mycobacteria. Am Rev Respir Dis 1974;109:147–151.

107. Weiner IM, Tinker JP. Pharmacology of pyrazinamide: metabolic and renal function studies related to the mechanism of drug-induced urate retention. J Pharmacol Exp Ther 1972;180:411–434.

108. Woo J, Leung A, Chan K, Lai KN, Teoh R. Pyrazinamide and rifampin regimens for patients on maintenance dialysis. Int J Artif Organs 1988;11:181–185.

109. Yamamoto T, Moriwaki Y, Takahashi S, Hada T, Higashino K. 5-Hydroxypyrazinamide, a human metabolite of pyrazinamide. Biochem Pharmacol 1987;36:2415–2416.

110. Yamamoto S, Toida I, Watanabe N, Ura T. In vitro antimycobacterial activities of pyrazinamide analogs. Antimicrob Agents Chemother 1995;39:2088–2091.

111. Yeager RL, Monroe WGC, Dessau F. Pyrazinamide (Aldinamide) in the treatment of pulmonary tuberculosis. Am Rev Tuberc 1952;65:523–534.

112. Yu TF, Berger L, Stone DJ, Wolf J, Gutman AB. Effect of pyrazinamide and pyrazinoic acid on urate clearance and other discrete renal functions. Proc. Soc. Exp. Biol 1957;96:264–267.

113. Zierski M. Pharmakologie, Toxikologie und Klinische Anwendung von Pyrazinamid. Prax Klin Pneumol 1981;35:1075–1105.

β-Lactam and β-Lactamase Inhibitor Combinations

Peggy S. McKinnon, Collin Freeman, and Wladimir Sougakoff

EVOLUTION OF β-LACTAMASE INHIBITORS

In 1940, penicillin resistance secondary to enzymatic inactivation of penicillin was reported, even though penicillin was not yet widely used. The enzyme, first isolated from *Escherichia coli* by Abraham and Chain, was called penicillinase (1). Soon after this discovery, penicillinase was also described in other organisms including *Staphylococcus aureus,* which by the mid-1940s was widely resistant to penicillin. Following the introduction of penicillin for general use in the 1950s, most isolates of *S. aureus* isolated in hospitals produced penicillinase.

Many unsuccessful attempts to find an inhibitor of this enzyme were made, as early as the 1950s. It was initially discovered that some semisynthetic penicillins, such as oxacillin, could function in vitro as β-lactamase inhibitors, however none proved clinically useful. The olivanic acids and clavulanic acid were discovered as part of a large-scale screening of compounds which began in the mid-1960s. In 1981, clavulanic acid became the first β-lactamase inhibitor introduced into clinical practice, when a formulation that combined it with amoxicillin became available. Since that time, clavulanic acid has been formulated in combination with other broad-spectrum penicillins (e.g., ticarcillin), and other β-lactamase inhibitors, including sulbactam and tazobactam, have been developed. These antibiotic combinations have significantly enhanced spectrums of activity compared with the β-lactam component alone. Resistance due to β-lactamase production occurs in strains of many common organisms such as *S. aureus, Haemophilus influenzae,* and *Bacteroides fragilis.* These agents provide additional therapeutic alternatives for increasingly resistant pathogens.

STRUCTURE-ACTIVITY RELATIONSHIPS FOR β-LACTAMASE INHIBITORS
Chemical Structure of β-Lactamase Inhibitors

β-Lactamases are enzymes that catalyze the hydrolysis of β-lactam antibiotics. On the basis of their structures and catalytic mechanisms, β-lactamases have been divided into four major groups. Class A β-lactamases such as the TEM and SHV enzymes are mainly plasma mediated and are widely spread among Gram-negative bacteria. Generally, class A β-lactamases are considered "penicillinases" because they display higher activity with penicillins than with cephalosporins. Class B β-lactamases are metalloenzymes that require a Zn^{2+} ion for activity. Class C β-lactamases are the so-called cephalosporinases that are chromosomally encoded in many Gram-negative bacteria. Finally, class D β-lactamases exhibit original substrate profiles by hydrolyzing oxacillin.

β-Lactamase inhibitors are β-lactam compounds that lack significant antibacterial activity but potentiate the activity of classical β-lactamase-sensitive antibiotics by protecting them from the hydrolytic activity of β-lactamases. They include clavulanic acid, the penam sulfones sulbactam and tazobactam, and new compounds such as BRL 42715 (Fig. 1). Clavulanic acid is characterized by an oxazolidine ring and the absence of an acylamino side chain in position C6. Sulbactam is a penicillanic sulfone obtained by oxidation of the thiazolidine sulfur of penicillanic acid, whereas tazobactam is a triazolyl-substituted penicillanic sulfone. Finally, BRL42715 belongs to a novel class of inhibitors, the 6-[substituted methylene] penems (29). Of these compounds, clavulanic acid, sulbactam, and tazobactam are currently in clinical use; e.g., clavulanic acid with amoxicillin (Augmentin) and ticarcillin (Timentin), sulbactam with ampicillin (Unasyn), and tazobactam with

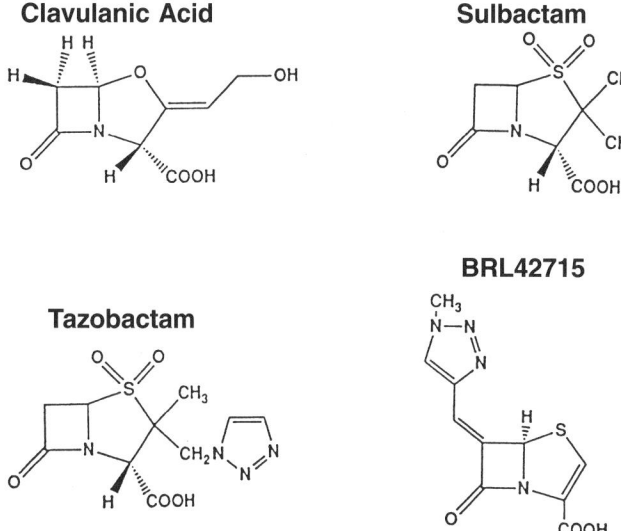

FIGURE 1. Chemical structures of β-lactamase inhibitors.

piperacillin (Tazocillin, Zosyn). Both clavulanic acid and the two penam sulfones are more inhibitory to class A than class C β-lactamases. BRL42715 is an excellent inhibitor of both enzyme classes, but development of this inhibitor as a therapeutic agent has now ceased. To date, no inhibitors of class B β-lactamases are available other than the metal chelators.

Inhibiting Activity of β-Lactamase Inhibitors

The inhibitor concentration that causes a 50% reduction in β-lactamase activity (IC_{50}) has been determined for various β-lactamases and is summarized in Table 1 (22). For class A β-lactamases, clavulanic acid and tazobactam display similar activities against TEM-1, TEM-2, and the *S. aureus* enzymes. Conversely, clavulanic acid is more active than tazobactam against the so-called extended-spectrum β-lactamases such as TEM-9 and TEM-10. Compared with clavulanic acid and tazobactam, sulbactam is a less potent inhibitor of class A enzymes, particularly SHV-1. Regarding class C β-lactamases, the penam sulfones sulbactam and tazobactam are more potent than clavulanic acid, which is a very poor inhibitor of the P99 chromosomal enzyme. Finally, the inhibitory potency of clavulanic acid, sulbactam, and tazobactam is lower against class D β-lactamases than against class A enzymes, and the OXA-type enzymes are not as well inhibited as TEM-1 by the three inhibitors (Table 1).

Mechanism of Action of β-Lactamase Inhibitors

Most β-lactamase inhibitors developed to date are mechanism-based inhibitors or "suicide" inhibitors of β-lactamases. These compounds, initially recognized as normal substrates by the β-lactamase, eventually form covalent bonds with various amino acid residues within the active site, thus leading to irreversible inactivation of the enzymatic activity. Clavulanic acid was one of the first β-lactamase inhibitors for which a convincing catalytic scheme was proposed (33). Nowadays, it is generally recognized that inactivation of class A β-lactamases by suicide inactivators occurs via a complex mechanism, and various schemes have been proposed to describe the interactions of a given compound with the class A β-lactamases (17, 22, 47, 58, 69).

Despite the diversity of the mechanisms reported so far, the general scheme depicted in Figure 2 is now generally accepted because it accounts for the kinetic data reported for inactivation of various β-lactamases by suicide inhibitors. According to this scheme, the active-site serine hydroxyl group first attacks the β-lactam carbonyl to form acyl-enzyme B. This intermediate can then undergo three competing hydrolytic events. First, the inhibitor is hydrolyzed, yielding the intermediate product C in which the β-lactam ring is opened, and then it spontaneously hydrolyzes to give smaller products. Secondly, the inhibitor forms a reversible intermediate (product D) that constitutes a transiently inhibited form of the enzyme. During the course of inhibition, more than 90% of the enzyme can be present in the transiently inhibited form that corresponds to the enamine tautomer of acyl-enzyme B. Finally, interaction of the inhibitor with the enzyme leads to formation of product E, in which the degraded inhibitor is covalently bound to the β-lactamase active site, resulting in irreversible inhibition.

Such a model seems to apply to interactions between clavulanic acid or sulbactam and the TEM-2 penicillinase (33,47) but not to inactivation of the β-lactamase from *S. aureus* by clavulanic acid nor that of class A β-lactamases by BRL 42715. For the latter inhibitor, the general interaction model shown below has been proposed (29, 69):

$$E + C \rightleftharpoons EC \rightleftharpoons EC^* \rightarrow E + P$$
$$\uparrow\downarrow$$
$$ECi \rightarrow E + P$$

where C is BRL 42715, and E, the enzyme. In this model, the acyl-enzyme, EC^*, in which the enzyme and inhibitor are covalently bound, can undergo both hydrolysis and rapid rearrangement to a very stable intermediate (ECi). However, this intermediate was shown to be a transiently inhibited species that can slowly hydrolyze to regenerate active enzyme E and release reaction product P (a dihydrothiazepine molecule) (69).

TABLE 1 • IC$_{50}$ Values for Inhibition of Various β-Lactamases by Commercially Available β-Lactamase Inhibitors

	IC$_{50}$ (μM)		
Enzyme	Clavulanic Acid	Sulbactam	Tazobactam
Class A			
S.aureus PC1	0.03	0.08	0.03
TEM-1	0.09	0.9	0.1
TEM-2	0.02	2.4	0.02
TEM-9	0.009	0.27	0.08
TEM-10	0.005	0.94	0.09
SHV-1	0.012	12	0.15
Class C			
P99	>100	5.6	0.008
Class D			
OXA-1	1.8	4.7	1.4

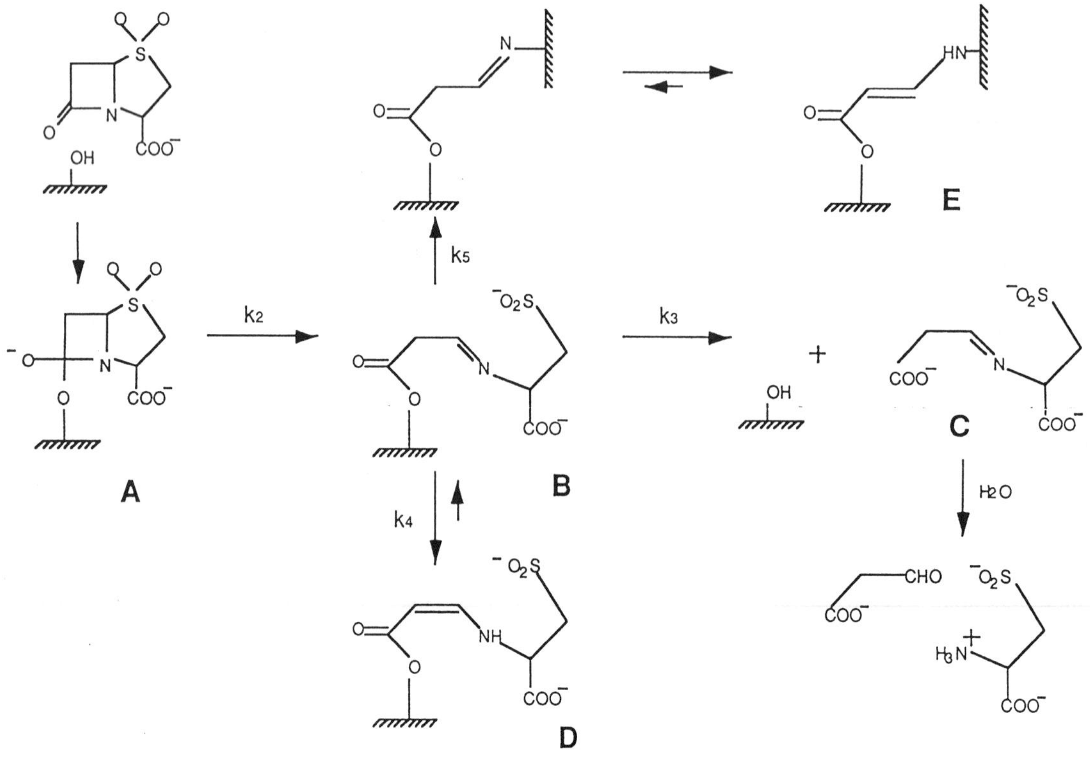

FIGURE 2. General scheme for the mechanism-based inhibitors of class A β-lactamases.

ANTIMICROBIAL ACTIVITY OF β-LACTAMASE INHIBITORS
Spectrum

In general, β-lactamase inhibitors have very little antimicrobial activity themselves but rather, typically restore antimicrobial activity to other β-lactams such as amoxicillin, ticarcillin, ampicillin, and piperacillin. For example, *Streptococcus pneumoniae, H. influenzae,* and *E. coli* have MICs to clavulanic acid of 64, 128, and 16 μg/mL, respectively (21, 95). Similarly, high MICs are observed when these and other bacteria are tested with sulbactam or tazobactam (20, 21, 23). Also, it is clear that the amount of β-lactamase inhibitor that is tested against a particular bacteria makes a difference in the final MIC results (49, 73, 104). The National Committee for Clinical Laboratory Standards (NCCLS) breakpoints for these three β-lactamase inhibitors alone and in combination with their respective penicillin combinations are given in Tables 2 and 3 for a variety of organisms.

Pharmacodynamic Effects

β-lactamase inhibitor activity involves irreversible binding with most β-lactamases. Although β-lactamase inhibitors have poor antibacterial activity by themselves, they apparently exhibit synergy when combined with β-lactam antibiotics (55). Combining these agents with penicillin-β-lactams increases the antibacterial activity approximately 4- to 32-fold (8, 20, 23, 49, 62, 76, 81, 102). Purposed mechanisms involve direct antibacterial activity at penicillin-binding proteins in addition to inhibition of hydrolyzing enzymes produced by the bacteria (21).

β-Lactamase inhibitory activity varies to some extent between these three agents. The Richmond-Sykes (R-S) classification of β-lactamases can be useful in distinguishing these different β-lactam-hydrolyzing enzymes, but it contains some inconsistencies (21, 49). R-S class I β-lactamases are not typically inhibited by the current β-lactamase inhibitors because of poor affinity between the drug molecule and the β-lactamase

TABLE 2 • Activities of the β-Lactamase Inhibitors against Selected Bacteria

Organism	Type of β-Lactamase (gene abbreviation)	Clavulanic Acid MIC (μg/mL)	Sulbactam MIC (μg/mL)	Tazobactam MIC (μg/mL)
Staphylococcus aureus[a]	Pencillinases	16–32	≥128	32
Klebsiella pneumoniae	Broad spectrum (SHV)	16–64	32–128	≥128
Proteus mirabilis	Penicillinase	32–128	≥128	>128
Escherichia coli	Broad spectrum (OXA, TEM, SHV)	16–64	16->128	≥128
Pseudomonas aeruginosa	Penicillinase (PSE)	≥128	>128	8.0–32
Moraxella catarrhalis	Broad spectrum (TEM)	4.0	16–128	≤0.5–16
Haemophilus influenzae	Broad spectrum (TEM)	8.0–128	128	0.5–128
Bacteroides fragilis	Penicillinases	16–≥64	32–≥128	8.0–128

Compiled from references 21, 23, 30, 61, 81, 95.

[a] Methicillin sensitive.

TABLE 3 • NCCLS MIC Breakpoints (μg/mL) for β-Lactamase Inhibitor/β-Lactam Combinations

Antibiotic	Susceptible	Intermediate	Resistant
Amoxicillin/clavulanic acid (2:1 ratio)			
when testing staphylococci	≤4/2	–	≥8/4
when testing other organisms	≤8/4	16/8	≥32/16
Ampicillin/sulbactam (2:1 ratio)			
when testing Gram-negative enterics and staphylococci	≤8/4	16/8	≥32/16
Piperacillin/tazobactam (8:1 ratio)			
when testing *P. aeruginosa*	≤64/4	–	≥128/4
when testing other Gram-negative organisms	≤16/4	32/4–64/4	≥128/4
when testing staphylococci	≤8/4	–	≥16/4
Ticarcillin/clavulanic acid (30:1 ratio)			
when testing *P. aeruginosa*	≤64/2	–	≥128/2
when testing other gram-negative organisms	≤16/2	32/2–64/2	≥128/2
when testing staphylococci	≤8/2	–	≤16/2

From NCCLS Table 2-M7-A4 (M100-S7), minimum inhibitory concentration (MIC) interpretive standards (μg/mL) for organisms other than *Haemophilus* spp., *Neisseria gonorrhoeae,* and *Streptococcus* spp. Villanova, PA: National Committee for Clinical Laboratory Standards, 1997;17.

(20, 23, 49, 82). However, the β-lactamase inhibitors are particularly effective in inhibiting enzymes in R-S classes II–V, including most of the enzymes produced by bacteria containing the TEM, PSE, or SHV genes (21, 49). On the basis of a weight-to-weight comparison and the IC_{50} values, clavulanic acid appears to be more potent than tazobactam, which is more potent than sulbactam (61, 76). Clavulanic acid, sulbactam, and tazobactam can inhibit both plasmid and chromosomal β-lactamases belonging to R-S classes II, III, IV, and V (20, 23, 82). Tazobactam has excellent inhibitory activity against R-S types II, III, IV, and V β-lactamases and the Ic β-lactamases but not the other type I enzymes.

Like their β-lactam counterparts, β-lactamase inhibitors are subject to an "inoculum effect." In this phenomenon, as the inoculum size increases from 10^5 organisms to 10^7 or more, the effectiveness of the β-lactam/β-lactamase inhibitor combination antibiotics decreases (20, 52, 55). The inoculum effect often appears in MIC/MBC susceptibility testing, increasing MIC results with increased inoculum size.

Finally, β-lactamase inhibitors can paradoxically induce increased production of β-lactamases from the bacteria they encounter. Various studies have shown greater production of β-lactamases when the bacteria have been exposed to β-lactamase inhibitors (3, 99, 103). The relative ability of the β-lactamase inhibitors to induce β-lactamase production is in the following order, from greatest to least: clavulanic acid > sulbactam > tazobactam.

MECHANISMS OF RESISTANCE TO β-LACTAMASE INHIBITORS

In the last decade, the clinical usefulness of β-lactamase inhibitors has been compromised by emergence of isolates resistant to clavulanic acid. It was previously shown that resistance to the combination of a penicillin plus clavulanate could result from mutations in the chromosomally encoded class C β-lactamases (80). More recently, several reports demonstrated that clavulanate resistance in *E. coli* is increasingly associated with overproduction of the wild-type class A penicillinases TEM-1 and TEM-2 or with production of class A β-lactamases showing low sensitivity to β-lactamase inhibitors, e.g., the IRT and the OXA enzymes (80, 106).

Resistance to amoxicillin-clavulanate in clinical isolates producing inhibitor-resistant TEM (IRT) enzymes results from point mutations that alter the region of the bla_{TEM} genes encoding penicillinases TEM-1 and TEM-2 (9, 24, 101). Such substitutions, initially described in *E. coli,* have been reported recently in *Klebsiella pneumoniae* and *Proteus mirabilis* (15, 64). The mutations (summarized in Table 4) are located in or near the active site of the enzyme. In the standard amino acid numbering of class A β-lactamases (5), mutations identified in the IRT enzymes are found in positions 69, 165, 182, 244, 275, and 276 (24). Among them, substitutions altering amino acids Met-69 and Asn-276 are frequently encountered and are associated with resistance to β-lactamase inhibitors. By contrast, the amino acid changes identified in positions 165 and 182 are infrequent and seem not to be involved in clavulanate resistance (11, 44). At the molecular level, mutations in positions 69, 244, 275, and 276 of the TEM-related β-lactamases might deform the active-site pocket such that β-lactam binding would be impaired (59). Accordingly, the IRT enzymes harboring such mutations are characterized by decreased affinity for β-lactam antibiotics, especially for suicide inhibitors such as clavulanic acid for which binding relies in part on an attractive interaction with the amino acid residue at position 244 (14, 19, 83). Finally, resistance to clavulanic acid has been described recently in a clinical isolate of *E. coli* that produces an SHV-5 variant characterized by a Ser-130 → Gly mutation (78). How such a mutation can confer lower sensitivity to clavulanate inhibition remains to be elucidated.

As mentioned above, hyperproduction of wild-type TEM-1 or TEM-2 penicillinases is a frequent mechanism of resistance to β-lactamase inhibitors in clinical isolates (24, 80). This mechanism causes resistance not only to combinations of amoxicillin and clavulanic acid but also to ampicillin/sulbac-

---

TABLE 4 • **Comparison of Residues Found in Positions ABL 69, 165, 182, 244, 275, and 276 in the Amino Acid Sequences of β-Lactamases TEM-1 and IRT-1 to IRT-10**

β-Lactamase	Amino Acid Position					
	69	165	182	244	275	276
TEM-1	Met	Trp	Met	Arg	Arg	Asn
IRT-1 (TEM-31)[a]				Cys		
IRT-2 (TEM-30)[b]				Ser		
IRT-3 (TEM-32)	Ileu		Thr			
IRT-4 (TEM-35)	Leu					Asp
IRT-5 (TEM-33)	Leu					
IRT-6 (TEM-34)	Val					
IRT-7 (TEM-36)	Val					Asp
IRT-8 (TEM-37)	Ileu					Asp
IRT-9 (TEM-38)	Val				Leu	
IRT-10 (TEM-39)	Leu	Arg				Asp
IRT-14 (TEM-45)	Leu				Gln	

[a] recently reported in *Klebsiella pneumoniae* (64).

[b] recently reported in *Proteus mirabilis* (15).

tam, amoxicillin/tazobactam and piperacillin/tazobactam (80). At the molecular level, β-lactamase overproduction is generally caused by a point mutation in the nucleotide at position 162 in the promoter region of the bla_{TEM} gene (24). Indeed, this position is located within the -10 consensus sequence forming the Pribnow box of the *bla* promoter. Therefore, presence of a T instead of a G at this position increases the efficiency of the promoter, thus leading to enough overproduction of the enzyme to bypass the inhibiting effect of clavulanate. Finally, overproduction of β-lactamases can also result from an increased number of copies of the plasmid harboring the *bla* gene in the bacterial cell (80).

Resistance to the amoxicillin-clavulanate combination has also been described in clinical isolates of *E. coli* with no mutations in the promoter and coding regions of the bla_{TEM} genes, suggesting that other mechanisms can also confer resistance to β-lactamase inhibitors (80). For example, mutations in the genes involved in porin synthesis can alter the permeability of the outer membrane. Uptake of β-lactamase inhibitors into the bacterial cell, which is likely affected by outer membrane permeability, is then limited, and the antibacterial potency of β-lactams combined with β-lactamase inhibitors is lowered. Also, a synergistic effect between β-lactamase overproduction and decreased permeability has been suggested, and the two mechanisms are frequently associated in an individual clinical isolate (45, 80).

PHARMACOKINETIC DISPOSITION

Summary data of the key pharmacokinetic parameters for the β-lactamase inhibitors are presented in Table 5.

Absorption

Clavulanic acid was initially reported to have an oral bioavailability of 64 to 75% (13, 27) but, more recently, more-accurate pharmacokinetic modeling of data has demonstrated that clavulanic acid is absorbed in a three-phase process, with a resulting bioavailability of 89 to 97% (4, 41). After a 125-mg dose of clavulanic acid administered orally in combination with amoxicillin 500 mg, a C_{max} of 2.1 µg/mL with a T_{max} of 1.0 h was reported for eight normal volunteers (31).

Unlike clavulanic acid, sulbactam is not well absorbed by the oral route (23), but it has been formulated as a double-ester prodrug in combination with ampicillin, called sultamicillin (23). The sultamicillin formulation increases the oral bioavailability of sulbactam to 68% (41). Sulbactam peak concentrations after a 0.5 g dose are approximately 20 to 43 µg/mL (23, 35).

Tazobactam is not absorbed to an appreciable extent by the oral route. The C_{max} of a 0.375-g dose of tazobactam is approximately 29 µg/mL (92).

Distribution

Clavulanic acid has a volume of distribution at steady-state (Vd_{ss}) of 0.16 to 0.25 L/kg in normal healthy adults (13, 27, 41, 46). Approximately 20% of clavulanic acid is bound by serum proteins (10). Animal studies have determined that clavulanic acid penetrates best into liver and kidney tissue (50). Concentration in human lymph node tissue is approximately 79% of that in serum, and blister fluid concentrations are also high (50). Other fluids and tissues that have clavulanic acid peak concentrations similar to those in serum are bile, bone, and synovial fluid (86). Patients with bacterial meningitis have clavulanic acid concentrations in cerebrospinal fluid (CSF) that are 8.4% of those in plasma or serum (7). Clavulanic acid concentrations in peritoneal fluid are approximately 67% of those in serum (68).

The mean Vd_{ss} for sulbactam ranges from 0.16 to 0.50 L/kg in different trials involving healthy adult and pediatric subjects (12, 23, 41, 71, 85). Serum protein binding is approximately 38% (56). Sulbactam penetrates into such fluids and tissues as intraperitoneal fluid (60%), sputum (12–14%), CSF in inflamed meninges (11–34%), intestinal mucosa (0.7–0.8%), and myometrium (64%) (23, 34).

Tazobactam was reported to have a mean Vd_{ss} of 0.18 to 0.33 L/kg in healthy adult volunteers (90). Serum protein binding for tazobactam is 20 to 23% (90). The penetration of tazobactam into cortical and cancellous bone tissues is approximately 22 to 26% (48). Tazobactam's penetration into bronchial secretions is approximately 78% (51). Other tissues and fluids investigated for tazobactam penetration include fat (14%), muscle (46%), omentum (9%), intestinal mucosa (>200%), lung (78%), appendix (114%), skin (93%), prostate (29%), and gallbladder (42%) (92).

Metabolism/Excretion

Clavulanic acid undergoes some hepatic metabolism. The two major metabolites have been identified as 2,5-dihydro-4-(2-hydroxyethyl)-5-oxo-1*H*-pyrrole-3-carboxylic acid and 1-amino-4-hydroxybutan-2-one, which make up 23 and 13% of the dose, respectively (13). These metabolites are renally eliminated and do not appear to possess antimicrobial or β-lactamase-inhibiting qualities. Approximately 40 to 75% of clavulanic acid is excreted in the urine as unchanged drug (13, 41, 46, 50, 86). A smaller percentage (8%) is excreted in the feces (13). The terminal half-life for clavulanic acid is approximately 0.70 to 1.3 h in adults who have normal renal function (13, 31, 41, 46, 50, 86). A study performed in 15 severely ill pediatric patients found a large variation in clavulanic acid half-lives because of variations in plasma clearance (55).

TABLE 5 • **Pharmacokinetics of Clavulanic Acid, Sulbactam, and Tazobactam Administered Intravenously in Normal Adults**

Pharmacokinetic Parameter	Clavulanic Acid (200 mg)	Sulbactam (500 mg)	Tazobactam (375 mg)
C_{max} (µg/mL)	8.5–14.3	20–43	29
Vd_{ss} (L/kg)	0.16–0.25	0.16–0.50	0.18–0.33
Protein binding (%)	20	38	20–23
$AUC_{0-\infty}$ (µg · h/mL)	15–21	44	24
Elimination $T_{1/2}$ (h)	0.7–1.3	1.0–1.7	0.35–0.94
Cl_{renal} (mL/min)	87–93	177–200	104–297
Cl_{total} (mL/min)	116–227	200–270	202–418

Compiled from references 10, 12, 20, 23, 34, 46, 56, 71, 86, 90.

Clavulanic acid has decreased elimination in patients with renal insufficiency, although nonrenal clearance allows greater clearance than for coadministered β-lactams whose clearance is entirely renal (86). In renal insufficiency, the AUC for ticarcillin is increased more than that of clavulanate because of the additional nonrenal mechanisms of clearance available for clavulanic acid. The disproportionally prolonged half-life of ticarcillin may allow time periods during the dosing interval when concentrations of the β-lactamase inhibitor are inadequate for significant enhancement of the effect of ticarcillin alone (42). The clinical significance of this effect is unknown.

Clavulanic acid is cleared to some extent by hemodialysis; one study reported a mean clearance of 93 mL/min from dialysis and a total clearance of 136 mL/min in six patients (28). Removal of approximately one-third of a dose of ticarcillin during hemodialysis has led to the recommendation that supplemental doses be given after hemodialysis (see dosing).

Sulbactam does not undergo any appreciable metabolism in humans. Excretion occurs via the renal route, with 75% of the dose recovered in the urine in the first 8 to 12 h (23, 34). A small portion of a given dose appears to be excreted in the bile (56). Sulbactam's terminal half-life is approximately 1.0 to 1.7 h in healthy young adults (12, 23, 34, 71). Urinary excretion of sulbactam in newborn infants varies widely, from 7 to 91% in a 12-h period (96).

Clearance of sulbactam is greatly decreased in patients with renal impairment (12, 23). In contrast to the disproportionate concentrations that result in renal failure with ticarcillin/clavulanate in patients with renal insufficiency, ampicillin and sulbactam appear to maintain the 2:1 concentration ratio throughout the entire dosing interval (42). A 4-h dialysis period in four patients removed approximately 45% of a 500-mg sulbactam dose in one study (12). Dialysis clearance for sulbactam in this study was 87 mL/min. As with ticarcillin/clavulanate, supplemental doses of ampicillin/sulbactam are recommended after dialysis.

Tazobactam is primarily excreted in the urine, increasing from 60 to 77% as the dose is increased, but renal clearance remains unchanged (90). Nonrenal clearance is accounted for by biliary excretion and hepatic metabolism, with the clearance rate decreasing as the dose increases (90). One of the more common metabolites, referred to as M_1, is formed by hydrolysis of the β-lactam ring and further breakdown to a butanoic acid derivative (40, 90). Renal clearance of tazobactam appears to be inhibited to an appreciable extent (~43%) by piperacillin, which inhibits renal tubular secretion of tazobactam, resulting in higher tazobactam serum concentrations (60, 90). The serum half-life of tazobactam varies from 0.35 to 0.94 h in healthy adults (90, 92).

Clearance of tazobactam varies with renal function. Patients with a creatinine clearance (CrCl) below 20 mL/min typically have a 4- to 5-fold increase in the total AUC of tazobactam (90). Nonrenal clearance is also decreased in patients with CrCl below 20 mL/min. Because reduced CrCL has a greater effect on reduction of tazobactam clearance than on clearance of piperacillin, the resulting tazobactam concentrations are disproportionally higher than those of piperacillin. This allows effective β-lactamase inhibition throughout the dosing interval. Patients receiving hemodialysis reportedly have a mean tazobactam clearance of 25 mL/min (53). A 3.2-h dialysis removed approximately 39% of a 0.375-g tazobactam dose at a dialysis clearance of 95 mL/min (53), necessitating supplemental dosing after hemodialysis. Patients with hepatic cirrhosis are reported to have a tazobactam clearance approximately 25% lower and an AUC 23% higher than normal subjects (63).

AVAILABILITY AND DOSAGE REGIMENS

Formulations of β-lactam/β-lactamase antimicrobials available in the United States are listed in Table 6. Relative costs (1997 $US) per dose and per day of treatment for usual maximal doses of each agent are compared in Table 7.

Amoxicillin/Clavulanic Acid

Amoxicillin/clavulanate is available in tablets and liquid formulations that contain varying proportions of amoxicillin and clavulanic acid. Different-strength tablet formulations of Augmentin do not contain the same relative amounts of each component. Similarly, the 250-mg chewable tablets contain different amounts of clavulanate from the regular tablets (Table 6). Because of these differences, amoxicillin equivalents may not be used to create equivalent total doses of the various products or different strengths of the same product. Adult doses of 250 to 500 mg have traditionally been given three times a day; however, recent studies support treatment with doses of 500 to 875 mg twice daily. Amoxicillin/clavulanate is indicated for pediatric infections. Of the available formulations, the suspension and chewable tablets are recommended for children weighing less than 40 kg, as they contain less clavulanic acid than the regular (adult) tablets. For recommended pediatric dosing see Table 8.

Ampicillin/Sulbactam

Ampicillin/sulbactam is available parenterally as a combination of ampicillin and the β-lactamase inhibitor sulbactam, both as the sodium salts, combined in a 2:1 ratio. This product may be administered either intravenously or intramuscularly. The usual dose is 1.5 (1 g of ampicillin and 500 mg of sulbactam) to 3.0 g (2 g of ampicillin and 1 g of sulbactam), generally given every 6 or 8 h to patients with normal renal function. Ampicillin/sulbactam may be given intramuscularly in the same dose recommended for intravenous administration; however, pain is often reported at the injection site. A lower dose (1.5 g intravenously every 6 h) is effective in surgical prophylaxis, skin and soft-tissue infections, and respiratory tract infections. Only the 3.0-g dose given either every 6 or every 8 h has been proven effective in intraabdominal infections; 3.0-g doses should also be used when penetration of the drugs may be questionable (e.g., diabetic foot infections or abscesses). Early in 1997, the use of ampicillin/sulbactam in children more than 1 year old was approved for treatment of skin and soft-tissue infections. The usual dose of 150–300 mg/kg/day is divided every 6 hours. Prior to this, its use in children under 12 years of age had been studied but was not FDA approved.

TABLE 6 • **Available Formulations of β-Lactam/β-Lactamase Inhibitor Combinations**

Drug	Trade Name	Availability	
Amoxicillin/ clavulanate	Augmentin (SK Beecham)	(Amoxicillin trihydrate/ clavulanic acid)	
		Tablets:	250 mg/125 mg
			500 mg/125 mg
			875 mg/125 mg
		Chewable Tablet:	125 mg 31.25 mg
			200 mg/28.5 mg
			250 mg/62.5 mg
			400 mg/57 mg
		Powder for Oral Suspension (per 5 mL):	125 mg/31.25 mg
			200 mg/28.5 mg
			250 mg/62.5 mg
			400 mg/57 mg
Ampicillin/ sulbactam	Unasyn (Pfizer)	(Ampicillin/sulbactam)	
		Powder for Injection:	1.0 g/0.5 g
			2.0 g/1.0 g
Piperacillin/ tazobactam	Zosyn (Wyeth-Ayerst)	(Piperacillin/tazobactam)	
		Powder for Injection:	2.0 g/0.25 g
			3.0 g/0.375 g
			4.0 g/0.5 g
Ticarcillin/ clavulanate	Timentin (SK-Beecham)	(Ticarcillin/clauvulanic acid)	
		Powder for Injection:	3.0 g/0.1 g

TABLE 7 • **Cost per Dose and per Day of Usual Maximal Doses of the β-Lactam/β-Lactamase Inhibitor Combinations**

	Maximum Adult Dosing (Cost in $US, 1997)		
Drug	Dose	Cost/Dose	Cost[a]/Day
Amoxicillin/clavulanate	875 mg p.o. q. 12 h	4.30	8.60
Ampicillin/sulbactam	3.0 g i.v. q. 6 h	10.60	42.40
Ticarcillin/clavulanate	3.1 g i.v. q. 4 h	10.20	61.20
Piperacillin/tazobactam	3.375 i.v. q. 4 h	11.60	69.90

[a] Cost includes drug acquisition costs only (79). Costs of preparation and administration of multiple doses are not considered.

Ticarcillin/Clavulanate

Ticarcillin/clavulanate is available parenterally as a combination of ticarcillin sodium and clavulanate potassium in a 30:1 ratio that contains 14.7 meq of sodium/3.1-g dose. The most frequently used dose is 3.1 g intravenously every 4 to 6 h, with the more frequent interval used for serious or *Pseudomonas* infections. While ticarcillin/clavulanate is not indicated in children under 12 years of age, the doses used in neonatal trials have ranged from 150 to 225 mg/kg/day divided every 6 to 8 h, and in pediatric trials, 200 to 400 mg/kg/day. Pediatric doses based on milligrams per kilogram should not exceed the usual adult doses.

Piperacillin/Tazobactam

Piperacillin/tazobactam is available parenterally as a combination of piperacillin and tazobactam, both as monosodium salts, which contains 7.0 meq of sodium per 3.375-g dose. The

usual dose of piperacillin/tazobactam is 3.375 g (3 g piperacillin/375 mg tazobactam) every 4 to 6 h, with the more frequent interval recommended for serious *Pseudomonas* infections. Piperacillin/tazobactam is not indicated for treatment of infections in children under 12 years of age.

Dosing in Renal and Hepatic Insufficiency

Recommended doses of β-lactam/β-lactamase antimicrobials for patients with renal impairment are summarized in Table 9. Although the half-lives of these agents may be moderately increased in patients with severe hepatic disease, no specific recommendations are included for adjusting doses, with the exception of ticarcillin/clavulanate, for which dosage adjustment is recommended for patients with combined hepatic and renal insufficiency as shown in Table 9.

Dosage in Patients Requiring Hemodialysis

Manufacturer's recommendations for maintenance doses in patients receiving hemodialysis are the same as those for the lowest indicated creatinine clearances, as shown on Table 9. Supplemental doses are recommended after dialysis for all agents. For piperacillin/tazobactam, a dose approximately 1/3 the normal dose has been recommended following dialysis. For all other agents, it is recommended that a full supplemental dose be administered after hemodialysis, or preferably, one of the daily doses be given following dialysis so that no additional dose is required.

Pregnancy

All available agents are in FDA pregnancy category B. No specific dosing recommendations are made for pregnant patients.

TABLE 8 • Usual Adult and Pediatric Doses for Mild-Moderate, and Severe Infections

Drug	Adult Dosing		Pediatric Dosing	
	Mild/Moderate	Severe	Mild/Moderate	Severe
Amoxicillin/clavulanate	250–500 mg q. 8 h	875 mg q. 12 h	20–25 mg/kg/day divided q. 8 h	40–45 mg/kg/day divided q. 8 h
Ampicillin/sulbactam	1.5 g q. 6–8 h	3.0 g q. 6 h	150–300 mg/kg/day divided q. 6 h	
Ticarcillin/clavulanate	3.1 g q. 6 h	3.1 g q. 4 h	Not indicated in children <12 years	
Piperacillin/tazobactam	2.25–3.375 g q. 6 h	3.375 g q. 4 h–4.5 g q. 6 h	Not indicated in children <12 years	

TABLE 9 • Manufacturer-Recommended Doses of β-Lactam/β-Lactamase Inhibitor Combinations in Adult Patients with Various Degrees of Renal Dysfunction

Drug	CrCL (mL/min)	Dose
Amoxicillin/clavulanate	>30	500 mg q. 8–12 h or 875 mg q. 12 h
	10–30	250–500 mg q. 12 h
	<10	250–500 mg q. 24 h
Ampicillin/sulbactam	>30	1.5–3.0 g q. 6–8 h
	15–29	1.5–3.0 g q. 8–12 h
	5–14	1.5–3.0 g q. 12–24 h
Ticarcillin/clavulanate	>60	3.1 g q. 4 h
	30–60	2.0 g q. 4 h
	10–30	2.0 g q. 4 h
	<10	2.0 g q. 12 h (q. 24 h with hepatic dysfunction)
Piperacillin/tazobactam	>40	3.375 g q. 4–6 h
	20–40	2.25 g q. 6 h
	<20	2.25 g q. 8 h

ADVERSE EFFECTS

No new or major adverse events result from addition of a β-lactamase inhibitor to ampicillin, amoxicillin, ticarcillin, or piperacillin. Adverse effects are minimal and not unlike those seen with other β-lactam antimicrobials. The major adverse effects associated with β-lactam/β-lactamase inhibitor combinations are hypersensitivity reactions and gastrointestinal tract effects such as nausea and diarrhea. Oral clavulanate given in doses of 125 to 250 mg three times a day is associated with diarrhea. Intravenous administration of clavulanic acid, sulbactam, and tazobactam shows no increase in gastrointestinal side effects over the β-lactam component given alone. Pain at the injection site has been reported for ampicillin/sulbactam given intramuscularly; this may be prevented by adding 0.5 to 2.0% lidocaine. Elevated transaminase levels have been occasionally reported with all agents, and a positive Coombs' test with either piperacillin/tazobactam or ticarcillin/clavulanate was reported in less than 10% of patients.

DRUG INTERACTIONS

The drug interaction profiles for the β-lactamase inhibitor combinations are best described by evaluating the potential in-teractions of the individual components. While concurrent probenecid administration may have a pronounced effect on the concentrations of ampicillin, amoxicillin, and piperacillin, increasing serum concentrations by as much as 30%, this effect is not consistent between the β-lactamase inhibitors. Sulbactam renal tubular secretion is inhibited by probenecid, and the resulting serum half-life may be increased by 18 to 45%, but Staniforth et al. documented a lack of interaction between probenecid and clavulanic acid (93).

Aminoglycosides

The physical and chemical incompatibility of penicillins and aminoglycosides also occurs with β-lactam/β-lactamase inhibitor combinations. Each of the β-lactams contained in these combinations has been implicated in aminoglycoside inactivation in vitro. This effect has also been described in patients with renal impairment. At concentrations higher than are generally achievable clinically, sulbactam causes in vitro inactivation of tobramycin. The clinical relevance of this effect is unknown.

CLINICAL APPLICATIONS

Amoxicillin/clavulanate, ampicillin/sulbactam, ticarcillin/clavulanate and piperacillin/tazobactam have been studied extensively in clinical trials in the United States and abroad. Based on the broad spectrum of activity of these agents, their use has primarily been evaluated for treatment of polymicrobial infections. The controlled clinical trials that have been published in peer-reviewed journals are the primary focus of this review.

Ampicillin/sulbactam, ticarcillin/clavulanate, and piperacillin/tazobactam have been evaluated as intravenous therapy primarily for treatment of mixed infections due to Gram-positive, Gram-negative, and anaerobic organisms. Infections for which the most utility has been demonstrated include intraabdominal, skin and soft-tissue, gynecologic, and upper and lower respiratory tract infections. A summary of clinical trials comparing β-lactamase inhibitor combinations with conventional therapies is presented in Table 10. While large, randomized multicenter clinical trials are lacking for many indications, most trials have used the standardized FDA guidelines for definitions and diagnostic criteria. One important criterion required by many comparative protocols was that for inclusion, all isolated pathogens had to be susceptible to both treatment regimens. This may falsely minimize any true differences between agents and negate a potential advantage that may exist for the antibiotic with the broader spectrum of activity.

TABLE 10 • **Clinical and Bacterial Cure Rates of Standard Therapy Compared with β-Lactamase Inhibitor Combinations for Treatment of Various Infections**

Authors	Study Drug vs. Comparator Regimen	Patients (N)	Clinical Response (%)	Bacteriologic Cure (%)
Intraabdominal infections				
SGIA (84)	Ampicillin/sulbactam	46	78	87
	Clindamycin + gentamicin	37	89	96
Yellin et al. (105)	Ampicillin/sulbactam	67	76	NR
	Clindamycin + gentamicin	38	87	NR
Polk et al. (77)	Piperacillin/tazobactam	104	88	86
	Clindamycin + gentamicin	43	77	75
Brismar et al. (16)	Piperacillin/tazobactam	69	91	93
	Imipenem/cilastatin	65	70	73
Gynecologic infections				
Senft et al. (87)	Ampicillin/sulbactam	39	87	83
	Cefoxitin	36	91	59
Pastorek et al. (75)	Ticarcillin/clavulanate	47	93	NR
	Cefoxitin	46	84	NR
Sweet et al. (97)	Piperacillin/tazobactam	196	78	77
	Clindamycin/gentamicin	103	82	79
Skin and soft-tissue infections				
Stromberg et al. (94)	Ampicillin/sulbactam	31	93	67
	Clindamycin and tobramycin	29	81	35
Tan et al. (98)	Piperacillin/tazobactam	153	76	77
	Ticarcillin/clavulanate	98	77	79
Grayson et al. (38)	Ampicillin/sulbactam	48	81	67
	Imipenem/cilastatin	48	85	75
Respiratory tract infections				
Shlaes et al. (88)	Piperacillin/tazobactam	177	81	84
	Ticarcillin/clavulanate	122	68	64

Most published clinical trials demonstrate relatively equal efficacy for the β-lactam/β-lactamase inhibitors and the comparator agents. When differences are demonstrated between the compared treatments, they appear most often to be due to a difference in coverage of an infecting pathogen. Often the overall clinical outcomes are similar, but when subgroup analyses are performed and the results evaluated for a given pathogen or specific diagnosis, differences are detected.

Intraabdominal and Gynecologic Infections

Most intraabdominal infections are mixed aerobic and anaerobic infections. Optimal treatment requires coverage of both Gram-negative and anaerobic organisms. Because of the broad spectrum of activity of the β-lactam/β-lactamase inhibitors, these agents have been extensively studied in the treatment of intraabdominal infections, and clinically, they have been used extensively in this area. Intraabdominal infections included in most of the published trials include peritonitis, appendicitis, abdominal abscess, cholecystitis, and penetrating abdominal trauma. The published comparisons almost always resulted in equivalent or similar clinical cure rates for the study agents tested and the comparator regimen. A review of these clinical trials reveals an overall success rate of 78 to 96% for most regimens, with primary differences in outcomes attributed to varying severity of illness.

In one study, (105), clinical success rates were significantly higher for clindamycin and gentamicin than for ampicillin/ sulbactam (3 g intravenously every 6 h). This study included 105 patients (67 ampicillin/sulbactam; 38 clindamycin/ gentamicin) with perforated or gangrenous appendicitis, and overall clinical cure was observed in 88 and 100% of patients, respectively. Infection due to *Pseudomonas aeruginosa* in a subgroup of patients with a perforated appendix was cited as the primary reason for this difference. Of note, a greater percentage of patients treated with ampicillin/sulbactam (76% vs. 60% of clindamycin/gentamicin-treated patients) were diagnosed with a perforated appendix. In all other studies comparing β-lactam/β-lactamase inhibitors with the "gold standard" of clindamycin plus gentamicin, the clinical outcomes observed have been similar.

In one study of 134 patients with appendicitis, peritonitis, or intraabdominal abscess, the clinical efficacy of piperacillin/ tazobactam (4.5 g intravenously every 8 h) was statistically superior to results achieved with imipenem/cilastatin (500 mg intravenously every 8 h) ($P = .005$). The greater efficacy observed with piperacillin/tazobactam may be partially attributed to the dose of imipenem/cilastatin used, which is lower than that usually recommended for patients with normal renal function (500 mg intravenously every 6 h) (16). No documented difference in microbiologic results or outcomes and no development of imipenem resistance were reported in this study. Other studies have reported that imipenem/cilastatin yields clinical outcomes similar to those with the β-lactam/ β-lactamase inhibitor combinations and clindamycin plus gentamicin therapy (84, 89). From the available data, it seems that most trials would support considering the above-reviewed regimens to be equivalent for treatment of intraabdominal infections.

Gynecologic Infections

Most gynecologic infections are polymicrobial. The most frequently isolated organisms include enteric Gram-negative organisms and anaerobes. Additionally, in pelvic inflammatory disease, the sexually transmitted organisms *Neisseria gonorrhoeae* and *Chlamydia trachomatis* are often isolated. Clinical studies in gynecologic infections are most often performed in young healthy women who subsequently develop acute pelvic inflammatory disease, tuboovarian abscesses, vaginal cuff cellulitis, or pelvic soft-tissue diseases. In the clinical studies reviewed comparing ampicillin/sulbactam, ticarcillin/clavulanate, or piperacillin/tazobactam with regimens of cefoxitin, clindamycin plus gentamicin, or ampicillin, metronidazole, and gentamicin, no significant differences were found in clinical outcomes (18, 26, 39, 43, 87, 97) (Table 10). All agents provide excellent activity against the most frequently isolated organisms, and clinical efficacy rates range from 81 to 100% with all regimens studied.

Hemsell reported summary data on 168 women treated with ampicillin/sulbactam (3 g intravenously every 6–8 h) in clinical trials for a variety of acute polymicrobial pelvic infections. Infections studied included endomyometritis after caesarean section, acute pelvic inflammatory disease, pelvic cellulitis after hysterectomy, and postoperative wound infections. Comparator regimens studied in 116 patients included cefoxitin, clindamycin and gentamicin or metronidazole and gentamicin. Overall clinical efficacy in the women treated with ampicillin/sulbactam was 92.4%, compared with 95.1% combined efficacy in women given comparative regimens. With all agents studied, overall efficacy rates have been consistently above 85%. No significant differences in failure rates by either drug regimen, infecting pathogen, or specific diagnosis could be identified.

Surgical Prophylaxis

Studies of surgical prophylaxis in appendectomy and colorectal, genitourinary, and gynecologic surgery have demonstrated that ampicillin/sulbactam is more effective than placebo and is equal in efficacy to cefoxitin or ampicillin plus metronidazole or metronidazole plus cefotaxime (56). Ticarcillin/clavulanate was evaluated and compared with cefamandole for surgical prophylaxis of thoracic and vascular surgery and compared with clindamycin plus an aminoglycoside for biliary tract surgery. In both cases, equal clinical outcomes were reported (37, 57).

Skin and Soft-Tissue Infections

Mild skin infections are most often monomicrobial, with Gram-positive organisms such as *S. aureus* or β-hemolytic streptococcus most commonly isolated. More-complicated infections are often associated with underlying conditions such as postoperative wounds, human or animal bites, and pressure

or diabetic foot ulcers. These are more frequently caused by mixed aerobic and anaerobic pathogens and often require surgical debridement for curative therapy. Clinical trials of β-lactam/β-lactamase inhibitors for treatment of skin and soft-tissue infections have most often included cellulitis, decubitus ulcers, diabetic foot infections, abscesses, and postoperative wound infections (32, 66, 74, 94). In general, local wound care and surgical debridement are appropriately included as part of the treatment protocols. Most frequently, results have demonstrated no significant differences between study agents and comparator regimens.

Diabetics with foot infections often present with complicated infection due to underlying ischemia and neuropathy, which may delay identification of infection. The type of organisms isolated is related in part to the severity of the disease, with infections characterized as "limb-threatening" most often being polymicrobial. Ampicillin/sulbactam (3 g intravenously every 6 h) was compared with imipenem/cilastatin (500 mg intravenously every 6 h) in 96 episodes of limb-threatening diabetic foot infection. Clinical success rates did not differ between the two treatment groups (38). Subsequent economic analysis of this study revealed that because of the lower drug costs and less frequent adverse events reported in the ampicillin/sulbactam-treated patients, ampicillin/sulbactam, while equally effective clinically, was more cost-effective than imipenem/cilastatin.

Human and animal bite wound infections are potentially serious and have unique bacteriology that must be considered when selecting antibiotic therapy. Human bites are usually more serious and prone to more infections and complications than animal bites. Human bites often include *S. aureus,* and β-lactamase-producing mouth anaerobes, and *Eikenella corrodens* may be isolated in up to 25% of cases. Although no clinical studies have been performed with the β-lactam/β-lactamase inhibitors in human bites and animal bites, their use is widely recommended. Based on the spectrum of activity and likely organisms, the most commonly recommended agents for bite infections are ampicillin/sulbactam and amoxicillin/clavulanate.

Respiratory Tract Infections

Amoxicillin/clavulanate is commonly used for the treatment of community-acquired upper and lower respiratory tract infections, which are often caused by β-lactamase-producing strains of *H. influenzae,* or *Moraxella catarrhalis*. Ampicillin, sulbactam, piperacillin, tazobactam, and ticarcillin/clavulanate are commonly used for these indications, and also offer intravenously available alternatives for more severe infections, and those due to mixed organisms. The most frequent respiratory tract infections involving mixed organisms include aspiration pneumonia, sinusitis, and lung abscess. Aspiration pneumonia (particularly when nosocomially acquired) may be polymicrobial, including Gram-negative organisms as well as anaerobes. Many small open-label or noncomparative studies have demonstrated good clinical outcomes with ampicillin/sulbactam (32), ticarcillin/clavulanate (72) and piperacillin/tazobactam. Although few clinical data from large-scale, randomized clinical trials exist to evaluate these agents (88), the spectrum of activity is consistent with the suspected pathogens of the above infections. When any of the above agents are used for empirical treatment of nosocomially acquired respiratory tract infections, addition of an aminoglycoside should be considered.

In small reports, patients treated for nosocomial pneumonia due to *Acinetobacter baumanii* resistant to multiple other antibiotics had good clinical outcomes when treated with ampicillin/sulbactam (100). In one series of 10 intensive care unit patients treated with ampicillin/sulbactam, all 10 improved clinically, however only 6 of 10 demonstrated eradication of *Acinetobacter* from the site of infection. This is likely due to the high rate of colonization frequently seen with this organism.

Immunocompromised Patients

Empirical management of febrile neutropenic patients has been evaluated for multiple monotherapy and combination therapy regimens. Coverage of Gram-negative organisms including *P. aeruginosa* is necessary, and some studies have demonstrated the benefits of early Gram-positive coverage. Piperacillin/tazobactam plus amikacin was compared with ceftazidime plus amikacin as empirical therapy in 858 febrile episodes in neutropenic patients (25). Antibiotic treatment was successful in 61% of patients treated with piperacillin/tazobactam plus amikacin and 54% of those treated with ceftazidime plus amikacin (P = .05). This study included 185 febrile episodes in pediatric patients, and while this subpopulation was not analyzed separately, no significant differences in adverse events or toxicities were reported. Ticarcillin/clavulanic acid plus tobramycin has also been shown to be as effective as piperacillin plus tobramycin, with success rates of approximately 70% for both treatment regimens (67).

REFERENCES

1. Abraham EP, Chain E. Enzymes from bacteria able to destroy penicillin. Nature 1940;146:837–845.
2. Acar JF, Gutmann L, Kitzis MD. β-Lactamses in clinical isolates: spectrum implications of sulbactam/ampicillin. Drugs 1988;35(Suppl 7):12–16.
3. Akova M, Yang Y, Livermore DM. Interactions of tazobactam and clavulanate with inducibly- and constitutively-expressed class I β-lactamases. J Antimicrob Chemother 1990;25:199–208.
4. Allen GD, Coates PE, Davies BE. On the absorption of clavulanic acid. Biopharm Drug Dispos 1988;9:127–136.
5. Ambler RP, Coulson AFW, Frère J-M, Ghuysen J-M, Joris B, Forsman M, Levesque RC, Tiraby G, Waley SG. A standard numbering scheme for the class A β-lactamases. Biochem J 1991;276:269–272.
6. Anonymous. Minimum inhibitory concentration (MIC) interpretive standards (μg/mL) for organisms other than *Haemophilus* spp., *Neiserria gonorrhoeae,* and *Streptococcus* spp. (Table 2). NCCLS, document M100-S7 (for use with M7-A4; aerobic dilution). Villanova, PA: National Committee for Clinical Laboratory Standards, 1997;17.
7. Bakken JS, Bruun JN, Gaustad P, Tasker TCG. Penetration of amoxicillin and potassium clavulanate into the cerebrospinal fluid of patients with inflamed meninges. Antimicrob Agents Chemother 1986;30:481–484.
8. Bansal MB, Chuah SK, Thadepalli H. In vitro activity and in vivo evaluation of ticarcillin plus clavulanic acid against aerobic and anaerobic bacteria. Am J Med 1985;79(Suppl 5B):33–38.
9. Belaaouaj A, Lapoumeroulie C, Caniça MM, Vedel G, Névot P, Krishnamoorthy R, Paul G. Nucleotide sequences of the genes coding for the TEM-like β-lactamases IRT-1 and IRT-2 (formerly called TRI-1 and TRI-2). FEMS Microbiol Lett 1994;120: 75–80.
10. Bergan T, Olszewski W, Engeset A. Penetration to peripheral human lymph of clavulanic acid and ticarcillin. J Antimicrob Chemother 1986:17:97–103.
11. Blazquez J, Baquero MR, Canton R, Alos I, Baquero F. Characterization of a new TEM-type β-lactamase resistant to clavulanate, sulbactam, and tazobactam in a clinical isolate of *Escherichia coli*. Antimicrob Agents Chemother 1993;37:2059–2063.
12. Blum RA, Kohli RK, Harrison NJ, Schentag JJ. Pharmacokinetics of ampicillin (2.0 grams) and sulbactam (1.0 gram) coadministered to subjects with normal and abnormal renal function and with end-stage renal disease on hemodialysis. Antimicrob Agents Chemother 1989;33:1470–1476.
13. Bolton GC, Allen GD, Davies BE, Filer CW, Jeffery DJ. The disposition of clavulanic acid in man. Xenobiotica 1986;16: 853–863.
14. Bonomo RA, Dawes CG, Knox JR, Shlaes DM. β-Lactamase mutations far from the active site influence inhibitor binding. Biochim Biophys Acta 1995;1247:121–125.
15. Bret L, Chanal C, Sirot D, Labia R, Sirot J. Characterization of an inhibitor-resistant enzyme IRT-2 derived from TEM-2 β-lactamase produced by *Proteus mirabilis* strains. J Antimicrob Chemother 1996;38:183–191.
16. Brismar B, Malmborg AS, Tunevall G, Wretlind B, Bergman L, Mentzing LO, Nystrom PO, Kihlstrom E, Backstrand B, Skau T, Kasholm-Tengve B, Sjoberg L, Olsson-Liljequist B, Tally FP, Gatenbeck L, Eklund AE, Nord CE. Piperacillin-tazobactam versus imipenem-cilastatin for treatment of intra-abdominal infections. Antimicrob Agents Chemother 1992;36:2766–2773.
17. Brown RPA, Aplin RT, Schofield CJ. Inhibition of TEM-2 β-lactamase from *Escherichia coli* by clavulanic acid: observation of intermediates by electrospray ionization mass spectrometry. Biochemistry 1996;5:12421–12432.
18. Bruhat MA, Pouly JL, Le Boedec G, Mage G. Treatment of acute salpingitis with sulbactam/ampicillin. Comparison with cefoxitin. Drugs 1986;31(Suppl 2):7–10.
19. Brun T, Péduzzi J, Caniça MM, Paul G, Névot P, Barthélémy M, Labia R. Characterization and amino acid sequence of IRT-4, a novel TEM-type enzyme with a decreased susceptibility to β-lactamase inhibitors. FEMS Microbiol Lett 1994;120:111–118.
20. Bryson HM, Brogden RN. Piperacillin/tazobactam: a review of its antibacterial activity, pharmacokinetic properties and therapeutic potential. Drugs 1994;47:506–535.
21. Bush K. β-Lactmase inhibitors. Clin Microbiol Rev 1988;1: 109–123.
22. Bush K, Macalintal C, Rasmussen BA, Lee VJ, Yang Y. Kinetic interactions of tazobactam with β-lactamases from all major structural classes. Antimicrob Agents Chemother 1993;37: 851–858.
23. Campoli-Richards D, Brogden RN. Sulbactam/ampicillin. Drugs 1987;33:577–609.
24. Caniça MMM, Lu CY, Krishnamoorthy R, Paul GC. Molecular diversity and evolution of *bla*TEM genes encoding β-lactamases resistant to clavulanic acid in clinical *E. coli*. J Mol Evol 1997;44:57–65.
25. Cometta A, Zinner S, de Bock R, Calandra T, Gaya H, Klastersky J, Langanaeken J, Paesmans M, Viscoli C, Glauser MP. Piperacillin-tazobactam plus amikacin versus ceftazidime plus amikacin as empiric therapy for fever in granulocytopenic patients with cancer. Antimicrob Agents Chemother 1995;39: 445–452.

26. Crobleholme W, Landers D, Ohm-Smith M, Robbie MO, Hadley WK, DeKay V, Dahrouge, Sweet RL. Sulbactam/ampicillin vs. metronidazole/gentamicin in the treatment of severe pelvic infections. Drugs 1986;31(Suppl 2);11–13.

27. Davies BE, Coates PE, Clarke JGN, Thawley AR, Sutton JA. Bioavailability and pharmacokinetics of clavulanic acid in healthy subjects. Int J Clin Pharmacol Ther Toxicol 1985;23:70–73.

28. Davies BE, Boon R, Horton R, Reubi FC, Descoeudres CE. Pharmacokinetics of amoxycillin and clavulanic acid in haemodialysis patients following intravenous administration of Augmentin. Br J Clin Pharmacol 1988;26:385–390.

29. Farmer TH, Page JW, Payne DJ, Knowles DJC. Kinetic and physical studies of β-lactamase inhibition by a novel penem, BRL 42715. Biochem J 1994;303:825–830.

30. Fass RJ, Prior RB. Comparative in vitro activities of piperacillin-tazobactam and ticarcillin-clavulanate. Antimicrob Agents Chemother 1989;33:1268–1274.

31. Ferslew K, Daignaeault EA, Aten EM, Roseman JM. Pharmacokinetics and urinary excretion of clavulanic acid after oral administration of amoxicillin and potassium clavulanate. J Clin Pharmacol 1984;24:452–456.

32. File TM, Tan J. Treatment of skin and soft-tissue infections. Am J Surg 1995;169:27S–33S.

33. Fisher J, Charnas RL, Knowles JR. Kinetic studies on the inactivation of Escherichia coli RTEM β-lactamase by clavulanic acid. Biochemistry 1978;17:2180–2184.

34. Foulds G. Pharmacokinetics of sulbactam/ampicillin in humans: a review. Rev Infect Dis 1986;8(Suppl 5):S503–S511.

35. Foulds G, McBride TJ, Knirsch AK, Rodriguez WJ, Khan WN. Penetration of sulbactam and ampicillin into cerebrospinal fluid of infants and young children with meningitis. Antimicrob Agents Chemother 1987;31:1703–1705.

36. Fuchs PC, Barry L, Jones RN. In vitro activity and disk susceptibility of Timentin: current status. Am J Med 1985;79(Suppl 5B):25–32.

37. Gagic N, Rennie R, Kiss Z, Menon G, Thornley JH. A blinded investigator comparison of ticarcillin-clavulanic acid vs. netilmicin-metronidazole as prophylaxis in surgery for acute cholecystitis. Curr Ther Res 1989;45:460–468.

38. Grayson ML, Gibbons GW, Habershaw GM, Greeman DV, Pomposelli FB, Rosenblum BI, Levin E, Karchmer AW. Use of ampicillin/sulbactam versus imipenem/cilastatin in the treatment of limb-threatening foot infections in diabetic patients. Clin Infect Dis 1994;18:683–693.

39. Gunning J. A comparison of parenteral sulbactam/ampicillin vs. clindamycin/gentamicin in the treatment of pelvic inflammatory disease. Drugs 1986;31(Suppl 2);14–17.

40. Halstenstein CE, Wong MO, Johnson CA, Zimmerman SW, Onorato JJ, Keane WF, Doepner M, Sia L, Tantillo K, Bansai S, Kuye O, Yacobi A, Faulkner R, Lathia CD. Pharmacokinetics of tazobactam M1 metabolite after administration of piperacillin/tazobactam in subjects with renal impairment. J Clin Pharmacol 1994;34:1208–1217.

41. Hampel B, Lode H, Bruckner G, Koeppe P. Comparative pharmacokinetics of sulbactam/ampicillin and clavulanic acid/amoxycillin in human volunteers. Drugs 1988;35(Suppl 7):29–33.

42. Hardin TC, Butler SC, Ross S, Wakeford JH, Jorgensen JH. Comparison of ampicillin sulbactam and ticarcillin clavulanic acid in patients with chronic renal failure: effects of differential pharmacokinetics on serum bactericidal activity. Pharmacotherapy 1994;14:147–152.

43. Hemsell DL. Sulbactam/ampicillin for treatment of polymicrobial pelvic infections. Drugs 1986;31(Suppl 2);22–25.

44. Henquell C, Chanal C, Sirot D, Labia R, Sirot J. Molecular characterization of nine different types of mutants among 107 inhibitor-resistant TEM β-lactamases from clinical isolates of Escherichia coli. Antimicrob Agents Chemother 1995;39:427–430.

45. Hiraoka M, Okamoto R, Inoue M, Mitsuhashi S. Effects of β-lactamases and omp mutation on susceptibility to β-lactam antibiotics in Escherichia coli. Antimicrob Agents Chemother 1989;3:382–386.

46. Höffken G, Tetzel H, Koeppe P, Lode H. The pharmacokinetics of ticarcillin, clavulanic acid and their combination. J Antimicrob Chemother 1986;17(Suppl C):47–55.

47. Imtiaz U, Manavathu EK, Mobashery S, Lerner S. Reversal of clavulanate resistance conferred by a ser-244 mutant of TEM-1 β-lactamase as a result of a second mutation (arg to ser at position 164) that enhances activity against ceftazidime. Antimicrob Agents Chemother 1994;38:1134–1139.

48. Incavo SJ, Ronchetti PJ, Choi JH, Wu H, Kinzig M, S'rgel F. Penetration of piperacillin-tazobactam into cancellous and cortical bone tissues. Antimicrob Agents Chemother 1994;38:905–907.

49. Itokazu GS, Danziger LH. Ampicillin-sulbactam and ticarcillin-clavulanic acid: a comparison of their in-vitro activity and review of their clinical efficacy. Pharmacotherapy 1991;11:382–414.

50. Jackson D, Cockburn A, Cooper DL, Langley PF, Tasker TCG, White DJ. Clinical pharmacology and safety evaluation of Timentin. Am J Med 1985;79(Suppl 5B):44–55.

51. Jehl F, Muller-Serieys C, de Larminat V, Monteil H, Bergogne-Berezin E. Penetration of piperacillin-tazobactam into bronchial secretions after multiple doses to intensive care patients. Antimicrob Agents Chemother 1994;38:2780–2784.

52. Jett BD, Ritchie DJ, Reichley R, Bailey TC, Sahm DF. In vitro activities of various β-lactam antimicrobial agents against clinical isolates of Escherichia coli and Klebsiella spp. resistant to oxyimino cephalosporins. Antimicrob Agents Chemother 1995;39:1187–1190.

53. Johnson CA, Halstenstein CE, Kelloway JS, Shapiro BE, Zimmerman SW, Tonelli A, Faulkner R, Dutta A, Haynes J, Green DS, Kuye O. Single-dose pharmacokinetics of piperacillin and tazobactam in patients with renal disease. Clin Pharmacol Ther 1992;51:32–41.

54. Jones AE, Barnes ND, Tasker TCG, Horton R. Pharmacokinetics of intravenous amoxycillin and potassium clavulanate in seriously ill children. J Antimicrob Chemother 1990;25:269–274.

55. Jones RN. In vitro evaluations of aminopenicillin/β-lactamase inhibitor combinations. Drugs 1988;35(Suppl 7):17–26.

56. Kager L, Liljeqvist L, Malmborg AS, Nord CE, Pieper R. Effects of ampicillin plus sulbactam on bowel flora in patients undergoing colorectal surgery. Antimicrob Agents Chemother 1982;22:208–212.

57. Kitzis M, Andreassian B, Branger C. Prophylactic Timentin in patients undergoing thoracic or vascular surgery. J Antimicrob Chemother 1986;17:183–187.

58. Knowles JR. Penicillin resistance: the chemistry of β-lactamase inhibition. Acc Chem Res 1985;18:97–104.

59. Knox JR. Extended-spectrum and inhibitor-resistant TEM-type β-lactamases: mutations, specificity, and three-dimensional structure. Antimicrob Agents Chemother 1995;39:2593–2601.

60. Komuro M, Maeda T, Kakuo H, Matsushita H, Shimada J. Inhi-

bition of the renal excretion of tazobactam by piperacillin. J Antimicrob Chemother 1994;34:555–564.

61. Kuck NA, Jacobus NV, Petersen PJ, Weiss WJ, Testa RT. Comparative in vitro and in vivo activities of piperacillin combined with the β-lactamase inhibitors tazobactam, clavulanic acid, and sulbactam. Antimicrob Agents Chemother 1989;33:1964–1969.

62. Labia R, Morand A, Lelievre V, Mattioni D, Kazmierczak A. Sulbactam: biochemical factors involved in its synergy with ampicillin. Rev Infect Dis 1986;8(Suppl 5):S496–S502.

63. Lathia C, Sia L, Greene D, Kuye O, Batra V, et al. Pharmacokinetics (PK) of piperacillin/tazobactam combination (pip/taz) IV in normal and cirrhotic subjects [Abstract PPDM8309]. Pharm Res 1991;8:S303.

64. Lemozy J, Sirot D, Chanal C, Huc C, Labia R, Dabernat H, Sirot J. First characterization of inhibitor-resistant TEM (IRT) β-lactamases in *Klebsiella pneumoniae* strains. Antimicrob Agents Chemother 1995;33:2580–2582.

65. Livermore DM. Evolution of β-lactamase inhibitors. Intensive Care Med 1994;20:S10–13.

66. Loffler L, Bauernfeind A, Keyl W, Hoffstedt B, Piergies A, Lenz W. An open comparative study of sulbactam plus ampicillin vs. cefotaxime as initial therapy for serious soft tissue and bone and joint infections. Rev Infect Dis 1986;8:S593–598.

67. Mackie MJ, Reilly JT, Purohit S, Bartzokas CA. A randomized trial of Timentin and tobramycin versus piperacillin and tobramycin in febrile neutropenic patients. J Antimicrob Chemother 1986;17:219–224.

68. Manek N, Wise R, Donovan IA. Intraperitoneal penetration of ticarcillin/clavulanic acid (Timentin). J Antimicrob Chemother 1987;19:363–366.

69. Matagne A, Ledent P, Monnaie D, Felici A, Jamin M, Raquet X, Galleni M, Klein D, François I, Frère JM. Kinetic study of interaction between BRL 42715, β-lactamases, and D-alanyl-D-alanine peptidases. Antimicrob Agents Chemother 1995;39:227–231.

70. McKinnon PS, Paladino JA, Grayson ML, Gibbons GW, Karchmer AW. Cost-effectiveness of ampicillin/sulbactam vs. imipenem/cilastatin in the treatment of limb-threatening foot infections in diabetic patients. Clin Infect Dis 1997;24:57–63.

71. Meyers BR, Wilkinson P, Mendelson MH, Walsh S, Bournazos C, Hirschman SZ. Pharmacokinetics of ampicillin-sulbactam in healthy elderly and young volunteers. Antimicrob Agents Chemother 1991;35:2098–2101.

72. Mostow SR, Obrien RF. Safety and effectiveness of ticarcillin plus clavulanate potassium in treatment of lower respiratory tract infections. Am J Med 1985;79(Suppl 5B):78–80.

73. Muratani T, Yokota E, Nakane T, Inoue E, Mitsuhashi S. In-vitro evaluation of the four β-lactamase inhibitors: BRL42715, clavulanic acid, sulbactam, and tazobactam. J Antimicrob Chemother 1993;32:421–429.

74. Nichols RL, Smith JW, Adinolfi MF, Galli R, Vivoda LM. Inhibition of β-lactamase induced resistance in soft-tissue infections. Arch Surg 1985;120:36–42.

75. Pastorek JG, Aldridge KE, Cunningham GL Garo S, Graffeo S, McNeely GS, Tan JS. Comparison of ticarcillin plus clavulanic acid with cefoxitin in the treatment of female pelvic infection. Am J Med 1985;79:161–163.

76. Pfaller M, Barry A, Fuchs P, Gerlach E, Hardy D. McLaughlin J. Relative efficacy of tazobactam, sulbactam and clavulanic acid in enhancing the potency of ampicillin against clinical isolates of *Enterobacteriaceae*. Eur J Clin Microbiol Infect Dis 1993;12:200–205.

77. Polk HC Jr, Fink MP, Laverdiere M, Wilson SE, Garber GE, Barie PS, Herbert JC, Cheadle J. Prospective randomized study of piperacillin/tazobactam therapy of surgically treated intraabdominal infections. Am Surg 1993;59:598–605.

78. Prinarakis EE, Miriagou V, Tzelepi E, Gazouli M, Tzouvelekis LS. Emergence of an inhibitor-resistant β-lactamase (SHV-10) derived from an SHV-5 variant. Antimicrob Agents Chemother 1997;41:838–840.

79. Red Book. Montvale, NJ: Medical Economics, 1994.

80. Reguera JA, Baquero F, Pérez-Diaz JC, Martinez JL. Factors determining resistance to β-lactam combined with β-lactamase inhibitors in *Escherichia coli*. J Antimicrob Chemother 1991;27:569–575.

81. Retsema JA, English AR, Girard A, Lynch JE, Anderson M, Brennan L, Cimochowski C, Faiella J, Norcia W, Sawyer P. Sulbactam/ampicillin: in vitro spectrum, potency, and activity in models of acute infection. Rev Infect Dis 1986;8(Suppl 5):S528–S534.

82. Rolinson GN. Evolution of β-lactamase inhibitors. Rev Infect Dis 1991;13(Suppl 9):S727–S732.

83. Saves I, Burlet-Schiltz O, Swarén P, Lefèvre F, Masson JM, Promé JC, Samama JP. The asparagine to aspartic acid substitution at position 276 of TEM-35 and TEM-36 is involved in the β-lactamase resistance to clavulanic acid. J Biol Chem 1995;270:18240–18245.

84. Scandinavian Study Group. Imipenem/cilastatin versus gentamicin/clindamycin for treatment of serious bacterial infections. Lancet 1984;i:868–871.

85. Schaad UB, Guenin K, Straehl P. Single-dose pharmacokinetics of intravenous sulbactam in pediatric patients. Rev Infect Dis 1986;8(Suppl 5):S512–S517.

86. Scully BE Chin NX, Neu HC. Pharmacology of ticarcillin combined with clavulanic acid in humans. Am J Med 1985;79(Suppl 5B):39–43.

87. Senft HH, Stiglmayer R, Eibach HW, Koerner H. Sulbactam/ampicillin vs. cefoxitin in the treatment of obstetric and gynaecological infections. Drugs 1986;31(Suppl 2):18–21.

88. Shlaes DM, Baughman R, Boylen CT, Chan JC, Gharan NB, Cormier YC, Erickson A, Grossman R, Kirmani N, Suh B. Piperacillin/tazobactam compared with ticarcillin/clavulanate in community acquired lower respiratory tract infection. J Antimicrob Chemother 1994;34:565–577.

89. Solomkin JS, Dellinger EP, Christou NV, Busuttil RW. Results of a multicenter trial comparing imipenem/cilastatin to tobramycin/clindamycin for intra-abdominal infections. Ann Surg 1990;212:581–591.

90. Sörgel F, Kinzig M. The chemistry, pharmacokinetics and tissue distribution of piperacillin/tazobactam. J Antimicrob Chemother 1993;31(Suppl A):39–60.

91. Sörgel F, Kinzig M. Pharmacokinetics and tissue and penetration of piperacillin/tazobactam with particular reference to its potential in abdominal and soft tissue infections. Eur J Surg 1994;573(Suppl):39–44.

92. Sörgel F, Kinzig M. Pharmacokinetic characteristics of piperacillin/tazobactam. Intensive Care Med 1994;20:S14–S20.

93. Staniforth DH, Jackson D, Clarke HL. Amoxicillin/clavulanic acid: the effect of probenecid. J Antimicrob Chemother 1983;12:273.

94. Stromberg BV, Reines HD, Hunt P. Comparative clinical study of sulbactam and ampicillin and clindamycin and tobramycin in infections of soft tissues. Surg Gynecol Obstet 1986;162:575–578.

95. Sutherland R, Beale AS, Boon RJ, Griffin KE, Slocombe B, Stokes DH, White AR. Antibacterial activity of ticarcillin in the presence of clavulanate potassium. Am J Med 1985;79(Suppl 5B):13–24.

96. Sutton AM, Turner TL, Cockburn E, McAllister TA. Pharmacokinetic study of sulbactam and ampicillin administered concomitantly by intraarterial or intravenous infusion in the newborn. Rev Infect Dis 1986;8(Suppl 8):S518–S522.

97. Sweet RL, Roy S, Faro S, O'Brien, Sanfilippo JS, Seidlin M, and the Piperacillin/Tazobactam Study Group. Piperacillin and tazobactam versus clindamycin and gentamicin in the treatment of hospitalized women with pelvic infection. Obstet Gynecol 1994;83:280–285.

98. Tan JS, Wishnow RM, Talan DA, Duncanson FP, Norden CW. Treatment of hospitalized patients with complicated skin and skin structure infections: double-blind, randomized, multicenter study of piperacillin-tazobactam vs ticarcillin-clavulanate. Antimicrob Agents Chemother 1993;37:1580–1586.

99. Thomson KS, Weber DA, Sanders CC, Sanders WE Jr. Beta-lactamase production in members of the family *Enterobacteriaceae* and resistance to β-lactam-enzyme inhibitor combinations. Antimicrob Agents Chemother 1990;34:622–627.

100. Urban C, Go E, Mariano N, Berger BJ, Avraham I, Rubin D, Rahal JJ. Effect of sulbactam on infections caused by imipenem resistant Acinetobacter calcoaceticus biotype anitratus. J Infect Dis 1993;167;448–451.

101. Vedel G, Belaaouaj A, Gilly L, Labia R, Philippon A, Névot P, Paul G. Clinical isolates of *Escherichia coli* producing TRI β-lactamases: novel TEM-enzymes conferring resistance to β-lactamase inhibitors. J Antimicrob Chemother 1992;30:449–462.

102. Verbist L, Verhaegen J. Susceptibility of ticarcillin-resistant gram-negative bacilli to different combinations of ticarcillin and clavulanic acid. J Antimicrob Chemother 1986;17(Suppl C):7–15.

103. Weber DA, Sanders CC. Diverse potential of β-lactamase inhibitors to induce class I enzymes. Antimicrob Agents Chemother 1990;34:156–158.

104. Wexler HM, Molitoris E, Finegold SM. Effect of beta-lactamase inhibitors on the activities of various beta-lactam agents against anaerobic bacteria. Antimicrob Agents Chemother 1991;35:1219–1224.

105. Yellin AE, Heseltine PNR, Berne TV, Appleman MD, Gill MA, Riggio CE, Chenella FC. The role of *Pseudomonas* species in patients treated with ampicillin and sulbactam for gangrenous and perforated appendicitis. Surg Gynecol Obstet 1985;161:303–307.

106. Zhou XY, Bordon F, Sirot D, Kitzis MD, Gutmann L. Emergence of clinical isolates of *Escherichia coli* producing TEM-1 derivatives or an OXA-1 β-lactamase conferring resistance to β-lactamase inhibitors. Antimicrob Agents Chemother 1994;38:1085–1089.

Carbapenems

●

Douglas N. Fish

CLASS

The thienamycins are a group of bicyclic β-lactam compounds that share a common carbapenem nucleus. These naturally occurring antibiotics are produced by the soil organism *Streptomyces cattleya* and were first discovered in the mid-1970s. Thienamycin was noted to be stable to β-lactamase hydrolysis and to have a broad spectrum of antimicrobial activity; however, it was chemically unstable in concentrated solution. Imipenem, a semisynthetic *N*-formimidoyl derivative of thienamycin, was developed to overcome the chemical instability of the parent compound but was subsequently found to be extensively metabolized by human renal dehydropeptidase I (DHP-I). This enzyme, found in the brush border of the proximal renal tubular cells, substantially decreased renal excretion of unchanged imipenem and limited the antimicrobial activity of imipenem in urine (97). Nephrotoxic imipenem metabolites resulting from DHP-I action were also implicated as the cause of proximal tubular necrosis seen in animals during preclinical studies (62). Cilastatin, a competitive inhibitor of DHP-I with a pharmacokinetic profile similar to that of imipenem, was then developed

and combined with imipenem in a 1:1 ratio. This combination of imipenem and cilastatin has been available in the United States since 1986 and has proven extremely useful in clinical practice.

Meropenem, also a semisynthetic derivative of thienamycin, is the second carbapenem agent available in the United States and was approved for use in 1996. Meropenem was developed after chemical modification of thienamycin to provide greater resistance to DHP-I metabolism. The DHP-I stability of meropenem is such that it eliminates the need for coadministration of a dehydropeptidase inhibitor (44, 135). A third carbapenem agent, panipenem, is in clinical use in Japan but not available in the United States.

Chemical Structure

Imipenem and meropenem are semisynthetic β-lactam antibiotics that share the carbapenem nucleus. There are two main structural differences between carbapenem and penicillin antibiotics: the substitution of a carbon atom for the sulfur atom at position 1 of the 4:5 fused thiazolidine ring structure, and the presence of an unsaturated bond between C-2 and C-3. The chemical structures of meropenem and imipenem are shown in Figure 1.

Structure-Activity Relationships

The carbapenems possess a 6-*trans*-hydroxyethyl group that confers relative stability to a wide variety of bacterial β-lactamases. Meropenem differs from imipenem by the addition of a methyl group substitution at C-1 and a dimethylcarbamylpyrrolidinethio side chain at C-2. The introduction of the methyl group at C-1 confers resistance to degradation by human renal DHP-I (44, 53). The substituent chain at C-2 probably accounts for the increased activity of meropenem against Gram-negative organisms compared with imipenem (26, 88). The difference in side chains at C-2 is also thought to account for the comparatively lower epileptogenic activity of meropenem (26, 31).

ANTIMICROBIAL ACTIVITY
Spectrum

The carbapenems as a class exhibit the broadest antimicrobial spectrum of any β-lactam antibiotics available to date. They possess excellent activity against both aerobic and anaerobic Gram-positive and Gram-negative bacteria. Representative in vitro susceptibilities of various organisms for imipenem and carbapenem are given in Table 1 (3, 9, 21, 47, 54, 59, 61, 63, 65, 72, 73, 78, 89, 95, 111, 113, 116, 120, 122, 130, 133, 138).

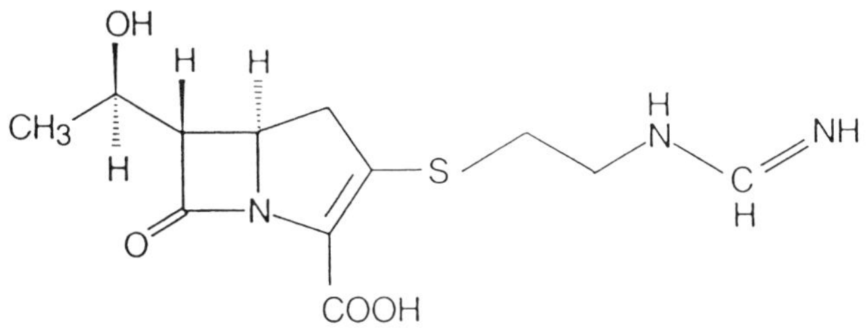

Imipenem

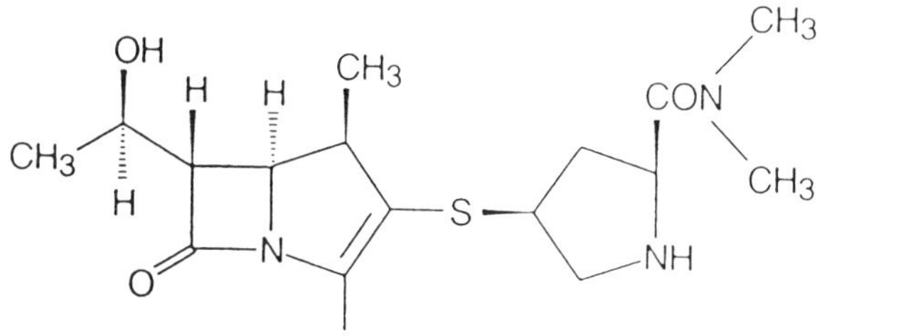

Meropenem

FIGURE 1. Chemical structures of imipenem and meropenem.

In vitro minimum inhibitory concentration (MIC) breakpoints for susceptibility have been approved by the National Committee on Clinical Laboratory Standards (NCCLS) and are similar for imipenem and meropenem when using standard agar or broth microdilutional techniques for clinical isolates. The breakpoints for most Gram-negative and Gram-positive organisms are as follows (37):

Susceptible, MIC ≤4 mg/L (≥14-mm zone of inhibition)
Moderately susceptible, MIC >4 to <16 mg/L (12- to 13-mm zone of inhibition)
Resistant, ≥16 mg/L (≤11-mm zone of inhibition)

The breakpoint for susceptibility to meropenem is 0.5 mg/L or below for *Haemophilus* spp. and viridans streptococci and 0.12 mg/L or below for *S. pneumoniae* (105).

Among Gram-positive aerobes, the carbapenems are active against most strains of methicillin-susceptible *Staphylococcus aureus* and coagulase-negative staphylococci. Aerobic hemolytic streptococci of Lancefield groups A, B, C, and G are also highly susceptible, as is *Listeria monocytogenes* (37, 59, 63). Strains of *Streptococcus pneumoniae* with intermediate- or high-level resistance to penicillin are usually susceptible to carbapenems; however, these strains are usually four- to eightfold less susceptible than fully penicillin-susceptible strains (37, 73). Activity of the carbapenems against enterococci varies considerably between species. Most strains of *Enterococcus faecalis, E. avium* and *E. liquefaciens* are susceptible or moderately susceptible, while most strains of *E. faecium* are resistant (9, 21, 37, 54, 59, 111). Approximately 50 to 60% of *Rhodococcus equi* and *Nocardia asteroides* strains are susceptible to the carbapenems (96, 137). Meropenem is generally similar to, or slightly less active than, imipenem against Gram-positive aerobic bacteria (9, 37, 63, 65, 111, 116, 122, 130). However, these differences in relative activities against Gram-positive organisms are not likely to be clinically significant in most cases.

Carbapenems exhibit excellent in vitro activity against Gram-negative aerobic bacteria (9, 17, 21, 37, 54, 59, 61, 63, 65, 72, 78, 95, 111, 113, 116, 122, 130, 133, 138). Meropenem is generally slightly more active than imipenem against Gram-negative clinical isolates. Both imipenem and meropenem have often shown excellent efficacy against clinical isolates of *Enterobacteriaceae* resistant to other β-lactam agents including second- and third-generation cephalosporins (i.e., ceftazidime, cefotaxime, and ceftriaxone) (78, 113, 116). Meropenem may be somewhat more active than imipenem in vitro against cephalosporin-resistant *Enterobacteriaceae,* and may in some cases be active against imipenem-resistant isolates as well (113, 116). The carbapenems are extremely active against both β-lactamase-positive and -negative strains of *Neisseria gonorrhoeae* and *Haemophilus influenzae,* including ampicillin-resistant β-lactamase-negative *Haemophilus* strains (61, 138).

Meropenem and imipenem appear relatively similar in in vitro activity against clinical isolates of *Pseudomonas aeruginosa,* although 1- to 2-fold lower MIC90s have been demonstrated with meropenem (59, 116, 122, 133). Clinical isolates of *Acinetobacter* spp. are usually quite susceptible to the carbapenems (9, 21, 37, 59, 113).

TABLE 1 • Antibacterial Activity (MIC$_{90}$) of Meropenem and Comparator Antibiotics against Gram-Positive and Gram-Negative Aerobic Bacteria.

Organism[a]	Imipenem			Meropenem		
	MIC$_{50}$	MIC$_{90}$	Range	MIC$_{50}$	MIC$_{90}$	Range
Gram-positive aerobes						
Staphylococcus aureus (MS)	0.06	0.06	0.03–0.06	0.12	0.25	0.06–0.25
Staphylococcus epidermidis (MS)	0.01	0.12	≤0.008–0.12	0.06	0.5	0.06–0.5
Staphylococcus saprophyticus	0.06	0.06	0.016–0.06	0.25	0.5	0.06–0.5
Streptococcus pyogenes	≤0.015	≤0.015	≤0.015	0.008	0.008	0.008
Streptococcus pneumoniae (PS)[b]	≤0.015	≤0.015	≤0.015	0.015	0.015	0.008–0.015
Streptococcus pneumoniae (PR)[b]	0.03	0.12	≤0.015–0.25	0.12	0.25	0.06–0.5
Enterococcus faecalis		1	0.5–2	4	4	0.5–8
Enterococcus faecium	32	>128	1–>128	32	128	4–>128
Listeria monocytogenes	0.12	0.25	0.03–0.12	0.12	0.25	0.06–0.25
Gram-negative aerobes						
Nutritionally fastidious organisms						
Legionella pneumophila	0.12	0.25	0.06–0.5	0.03	0.06	0.01–0.25
Haemophilus influenzae[c, d]	0.12	1	0.06–1	0.12	0.5	0.008–1
Neisseria gonorrhoeae (PS)	0.12	0.5	0.03–1	0.015	0.03	≤0.008–0.06
Neisseria gonorrhoeae (PR)	0.25	0.25	0.06–0.5	0.015	0.5	≤0.008–0.5
Neisseria meningitidis	0.03	0.03	≤0.015–0.03	≤0.004	0.015	0.004–0.015
Moraxella catarrhalis	<0.015	0.03	≤0.015–0.03	<0.03	<0.03	<0.03
Gardnerella vaginalis	0.06	0.12	0.03–0.12	0.016	0.03	0.004–0.12
Campylobacter jejuni	0.06	0.12	0.03–0.25	0.008	0.03	0.004–0.06
Helicobacter pylori	0.13	0.25	0.13–0.25	0.06	0.25	0.06–0.25
Enterobacteriaceae and other lactose-fermenting organisms						
Escherichia coli	0.12	0.25	0.03–0.25	0.01	0.03	0.008–0.06
Citrobacter freundii	0.25	2	0.12–2	0.03	0.06	0.01–0.12
Salmonella spp.	0.12	0.12	0.12–0.5	0.03	0.03	0.015–0.03
Shigella sonnei	0.12	0.25	0.03–0.5	0.03	0.06	0.015–0.06
Klebsiella pneumoniae	0.12	0.25	0.12–0.5	0.03	0.06	0.01–0.12
Klebsiella oxytoca	0.25	0.5	0.12–0.5	0.03	0.03	0.01–0.03
Enterobacter cloacae	0.5	0.5	0.12–1	0.03	0.06	≤0.008–0.12
Enterobacter aerogenes	0.5	0.5	0.12–2	0.03	0.06	0.008–1
Serratia marcescens	0.5	1	0.25–1	0.06	0.25	0.03–1
Hafnia alvei	0.25	0.5	0.25–0.5	0.016	0.03	0.016–0.03
Proteus mirabilis	0.5	2	0.12–4	0.06	0.06	0.01–0.06
Proteus vulgaris		4	0.25–8	0.06	0.06	0.03–0.25
Morganella morganii		2	1–4	0.12	0.25	0.06–0.25
Providencia rettgeri		1	0.5–2	0.03	0.12	0.015–0.12
Providencia stuartii		2	0.5–2	0.06	0.06	0.03–0.12
Yersinia enterocolitica	0.25	0.25	0.12–0.5	0.03	0.06	0.03–0.06
Aeromonas hydrophilia	0.25	0.25	0.06–0.5	0.016	0.03	0.008–0.25
Non-lactose-fermenting organisms						
Acinetobacter calcoaceticus		2	0.5–2	1	2	0.25–2
Pseudomonas aeruginosa		2	0.12–>8	0.5	2	0.06–16
Pseudomonas fluorescens		16	2–16	2	4	0.5–4
Burkholderia cepacia		8	4–8	2	2	2
Gram-positive anaerobes						
Veillonella parvula	0.25	0.5	0.12–1	0.06	0.13	0.06–1
Eubacterium lentum	0.5	1	0.5–1	0.5	0.5	0.25–0.5
Peptococcus magnus	0.25	1	0.25–2	0.12	0.25	≤0.06–2
Clostridium perfringens	0.03	0.03	0.01–0.03	≤0.008	<0.06	≤0.008–0.06
Clostridium difficile	4	8	1–>8	1	2	1–2
Gram-negative anaerobes						
Bacteroides fragilis	0.06	0.5	0.03–2	0.12	1	0.06–4
Bacteroides vulgatus	0.5	1	0.25–8	0.5	0.5	0.25–8
Bacteroides distasonis	0.12	1	0.06–4	0.25	1	0.12–4
Bacteroides thetaiotaomicron	0.25	0.5	0.25–0.5	0.5	0.5	0.25–0.5
Bacteroides ovatus	0.25	1	0.25–1	0.5	0.5	0.5–1
Bacteroides uniformis	0.12	1	0.12–2	0.25	0.5	0.25–0.5

continued

TABLE 1 • Antibacterial Activity (MIC$_{90}$) of Meropenem and Comparator Antibiotics against Gram-Positive and Gram-Negative Aerobic Bacteria.

Organism[a]	Imipenem			Meropenem		
	MIC$_{50}$	MIC$_{90}$	Range	MIC$_{50}$	MIC$_{90}$	Range
Prevotella bivia	0.25	0.5	0.25–1	0.25	0.5	0.25–1
Fusobacterium nucleatum	0.03	0.06	0.008–0.06	0.008	0.016	0.002–0.016

[a] NCCLS-recommended susceptibility breakpoints for most Gram-negative and Gram-positive organisms: susceptible, MIC ≤4 mg/L; intermediate, MIC >4–<16 mg/L; resistant, ≥16 mg/L. MS, methicillin susceptible; PS, penicillin susceptible; PR, penicillin resistant; NT, not tested.

[b] NCCLS-recommended meropenem susceptibility breakpoints for *S. pneumoniae* are 0.5 mg/L.

[c] Includes β-lactamase positive and ampicillin-resistant non-β-lactamase-positive strains.

[d] NCCLS-recommended meropenem susceptibility breakpoints for *Haemophilus* spp. and viridans streptococci are 0.12 mg/L.

The carbapenems are also active against most strains of clinically significant anaerobes (3, 37, 47, 89, 95, 120). Imipenem and meropenem appear to be similar in activity against both Gram-negative and Gram-positive anaerobes and more active in vitro (based on MICs) than other antianaerobic agents such as metronidazole, clindamycin, cefoxitin, or piperacillin/tazobactam (3, 37, 47, 89, 95). In addition to the organisms shown in Table 1, carbapenems also have excellent activity against clinical isolates of *Peptostreptococcus* spp., *Propionibacterium acnes*, *Actinomyces* spp., and *Actinobacillus* spp. (3, 89, 95, 120).

Carbapenems have variable activity in vitro against some mycobacteria including *M. fortuitum*, *M. chelonae*, *M. fallax*, and some strains of *M. avium* complex (56).

Organisms commonly considered to be minimally susceptible or resistant to the carbapenems include methicillin-resistant staphylococci, *E. faecium*, *Stenotrophomonas* (*Xanthomonas*) *maltophilia*, and *Flavobacterium meningosepticum*. Atypical bacteria such as *Mycoplasma* and *Chlamydia* are also resistant to the carbapenems.

Pharmacodynamic Effects

Bactericidal Effects

The minimum bactericidal concentration (MBC) of carbapenems is usually similar to or only two- to fourfold greater than the MIC for most aerobic and anaerobic bacteria (23, 37). Like other β-lactam antibiotics, carbapenems exhibit lower bactericidal activity during static and slow bacterial growth phases than under study conditions providing optimal bacterial growth. Bactericidal effects on *H. influenzae*, *Proteus mirabilis* and *P. aeruginosa* are reportedly delayed for 1 to 2 h when these organisms are exposed to drug at concentrations 2 to 32 times the MIC (140, 141).

Most in vitro susceptibility studies of carbapenems were conducted using inoculum sizes of 10^4 to 10^5 colony-forming units (CFU)/mL of clinical bacterial isolates at physiologic pH. Increasing inoculum sizes to 10^6 or 10^7 CFU/mL has little effect on carbapenem MICs for *Enterobacteriaceae* or Gram-positive organisms (9, 21, 37, 60). However, further increasing the inoculum size to 10^8 CFU/mL may increase the MIC of imipenem 4- to 16-fold against strains of *Klebsiella*, *Enterobacter*, *Citrobacter* and *Proteus* (94).

Choice of agar media generally has little effect on results of in vitro carbapenem susceptibility testing. Although carbapenems are inactivated in growth media containing cysteine, standard agars such as Mueller-Hinton, Wilkins-Chalgren, and supplemented brain-heart infusion agar appear to produce comparable and consistent susceptibility results (51, 60). The addition of 20 or 50% human serum to the medium may increase MIC values for *Enterobacteriaceae*, *P. aeruginosa*, and *S. aureus* by 2- to 4-fold (45). Carbapenem activity is substantially decreased when the pH of the culture media is above 7 and to a lesser extent at acidic pH (11). Although concentrations of magnesium or calcium ions in culture media have generally not been associated with alterations in susceptibility test results, increased concentrations of zinc ions markedly increase MICs for both imipenem and meropenem (24, 25).

Postantibiotic Effects

Carbapenems have been reported to produce a postantibiotic effect (PAE) lasting 1 to 2 h against many strains of *Enterobacteriaceae*, *P. aeruginosa*, *Burkholderia cepacia*, *B. fragilis*, *S. aureus*, and *E. faecalis* (70, 79, 90, 91, 100). Against strains of *P. aeruginosa*, meropenem has been shown to have a slightly longer and less variable PAE than imipenem (1.2–2.5 h vs. 0.8–2.0 h, respectively). The PAEs with *S. aureus* are reportedly similar for imipenem and meropenem, 1.8 and 1.7 h, respectively (90).

Effects of Subinhibitory Concentrations

Subinhibitory concentrations of imipenem produced an initial bactericidal effect and a subsequent delay of bacterial growth that lasted a mean of 12 h when *P. aeruginosa* was exposed in vitro to drug at concentrations 0.5 times the MIC (80). Subinhibitory concentrations of imipenem may also enhance in vitro killing of *E. coli* by polymorphonuclear cells as well as enhance the complement-mediated bactericidal effects of human serum against *P. aeruginosa* (30, 82, 100). The significance of these effects in vivo is unknown.

Important Effects on Host Immunity

Carbapenems are rapidly taken up and extensively accumulated within macrophages. Exposure of human macrophages to meropenem 1.0 mg/L for 3 h resulted in an intracellular:extracellular concentration ratio of 12.6 (28). Meropenem has also been demonstrated to enhance the rate and extent of phagocytosis and intracellular killing of *S. aureus, Serratia marcescens,* and *E. coli,* compared with antibiotic-free controls (28). In addition to subinhibitory effects, clinically relevant concentrations of imipenem have been shown to enhance the in vitro chemotaxis, adherence, phagocytosis, and opsonization functions of human neutrophils and to stimulate synthesis of complement C3b receptors (8, 36, 101, 109).

Pharmacodynamic Correlates with Outcome

Like those of other β-lactam antibiotics, the bactericidal effects of the carbapenems are time dependent rather than concentration dependent. Thus the pharmacodynamic parameter that appears most predictive of optimal bactericidal effects and clinical outcome is the time during which drug concentrations remain in excess of the MIC, or time > MIC. The importance of time > MIC has been demonstrated for other β-lactams agents in a number of animal models and human studies (34, 115, 131). However, the only data specifically related to carbapenems comes from animal models in which the bactericidal effect of imipenem against *P. aeruginosa* and *E. coli* was shown to depend on time > MIC rather than peak plasma concentrations (43).

MECHANISMS OF ACTION

The carbapenems cause rapid bacterial cell death by covalently binding to penicillin-binding proteins (PBPs) involved in the biosynthesis of mucopeptides in bacterial cell walls. The actions of carbapenems result in bactericidal effects through inhibition of cellular growth and division and loss of cell wall integrity, eventually causing cell lysis. The binding affinity of carbapenems for specific PBPs is genus specific and differs slightly between various agents (87).

The primary target, with highest binding affinity for both imipenem and meropenem in tested strains of *E. coli* and *P. aeruginosa,* is PBP 2. Carbapenems also inhibit the peptidase activities of PBPs 1A, 1B, 3, 4, and 5 to lesser degrees in various organisms. Meropenem has a higher binding affinity than imipenem for both PBP 2 and 3 of *P. aeruginosa* as well as for PBP 3 of *E. coli* (66, 81). This may perhaps account for the slightly greater activity of meropenem against many Gram-negative aerobes. The relative PBP binding affinities of meropenem and imipenem are quite similar in strains of *S. aureus,* both agents demonstrating high affinity for PBPs 1, 2, and 4 (123).

MECHANISMS OF ANTIMICROBIAL RESISTANCE
Commonly Resistant Organisms

As with other β-lactam antibiotics, carbapenems are not reliably active against methicillin-resistant *S. aureus* or *S. epidermidis* (37). Most strains of *E. faecium* are also resistant to carbapenems, with MIC$_{90}$s often 128 mg/L or above. Clinical isolates of *Corynebacterium jeikeium* are uniformly resistant to all carbapenems (37). Although up to 80 to 90% of *N. asteroides* strains are susceptible to carbapenems, most strains of other *Nocardia* species are usually resistant (96, 137). Among

Gram-negative aerobes, *B. cepacia* is usually either moderately susceptible or resistant in vitro to both meropenem and imipenem (72, 122). *S. maltophilia* is also routinely resistant to available carbapenems (17, 54, 111, 122). Most strains of *Flavobacterium meningosepticum* are considered resistant as well. Neither meropenem nor imipenem are routinely active against *M. avium* complex in vitro (56).

Mechanisms of Resistance
Alterations in Penicillin-Binding Proteins

Decreased PBP affinity is an important mechanism of intrinsic resistance to the carbapenems, particularly related to decreased activity against Gram-positive organisms. Carbapenems, like other β-lactam antibiotics, are not active against methicillin-resistant strains of *S. aureus* or coagulase-negative staphylococci that produce PBPs with decreased binding affinity for these agents (75). Some PBPs, particularly PBPs 4 and 5 produced by *E. faecium,* have decreased affinity for all currently available β-lactam antibiotics including the carbapenems. Alterations in PBP binding affinities have also been associated with resistance in Gram-negative bacteria including *P. mirabilis, P. aeruginosa,* and *Acinetobacter baumanii* (92).

β-Lactamases

Carbapenems are not highly susceptible to hydrolysis by most plasmid-mediated β-lactamases, including extended-spectrum β-lactamases produced by *Enterobacteriaceae* and *P. aeruginosa.* Studies have demonstrated that MICs were unchanged when various strains of these bacteria, either producers or nonproducers of plasmid-mediated β-lactamases, were exposed to carbapenems in vitro (17, 112).

Carbapenems are strong inducers of chromosomally mediated β-lactamase production, meropenem having slightly less potential for induction of these enzymes than imipenem. However, unlike other inducers such as cefoxitin and cefotetan, enzyme induction does not alter the activity of the carbapenems, because of their resistance to β-lactamase degradation (69, 112). Carbapenems are not likely to select for stably derepressed Richmond-Sykes class I mutants or be significantly hydrolyzed by β-lactamase enzymes produced by them (140). In fact, both imipenem and meropenem can reversibly deactivate these β-lactamase enzymes (76, 83, 121). Carbapenems are also highly resistant to hydrolysis by the extended-spectrum TEM- and SHV-type β-lactamase enzymes (Richmond-Sykes class III) that possess activity against many β-lactam antibiotics, including third-generation cephalosporins (121). With the exception of *S. maltophilia,* production of type I chromosomally mediated β-lactamases produces little cross-resistance between carbapenems and other β-lactams. *S. maltophilia* resistance is usually due to high-level expression of zinc metallo-β-lactamases with activity against both meropenem and imipenem (112). Zinc metalloenzymes with activity against carbapenems have also been described in some strains of *B. fragilis, S. marcescens, Bacillus cereus,* and *Flavobacterium odoratum* (27, 57, 69).

Chromosomally or plasmid-mediated β-lactamase production has been demonstrated to be involved in resistance of *P. aeruginosa* to meropenem (112, 114). Membrane passage of carbapenems is apparently associated with outer membrane porin D2 (OprD), a novel porin not used by other β-lactam agents (46, 74). *P. aeruginosa* strains with high-level resistance to meropenem tend to have both high-level chromosomal β-lactamase production and altered permeability due to loss of OprD (74).

Impermeability

Carbapenems rapidly penetrate OprD porins of *Enterobacteriaceae* and other Gram-negative organisms because of their low molecular weight and zwitterionic nature (48). Carbapenem-resistant *P. aeruginosa* mutants lack OprD (107, 114, 127). However, such resistant mutants often remain susceptible to these agents (83, 103). Impermeability-related resistance is a clinical problem with *P. aeruginosa* and Gram-negative bacteria, but impermeability rarely causes high-level carbapenem resistance in and of itself (75, 136). Resistance to meropenem among some strains of *E. cloacae* and *P. aeruginosa* is due to synergism between altered membrane permeability caused by a decreased quantity of OprD plus slow hydrolytic inactivation by chromosomal β-lactamase enzymes (76, 107). Resistance among *E. aerogenes* isolates may also be related to alterations in certain outer membrane lipopolysaccharides. Finally, membrane-associated active efflux mechanisms may play a role in carbapenem resistance in *P. aeruginosa,* especially when combined with altered membrane permeability (76).

Methods to Overcome and Prevent Resistance

The most common methods to either prevent or overcome carbapenem resistance are adequate drug dosing to optimize time > MIC and combination therapy to provide additive or synergistic antibacterial activity. Synergy has been demonstrated against methicillin-resistant *S. aureus* with combinations of carbapenems plus teicoplanin, vancomycin, piperacillin, ampicillin, cefazolin, cefotiam, cefpiramide, and cefmetazole (11, 41, 135, 136). Imipenem plus an aminoglycoside has been shown to be synergistic against most strains of *E. faecalis, E. faecium,* and *Listeria monocytogenes* (38). The combination of carbapenem plus gentamicin or amikacin may also be synergistic against *P. aeruginosa,* including up to 72% of aminoglycoside-resistant strains (11, 135). Imipenem plus amikacin may be additive or synergistic against imipenem-resistant *P. aeruginosa* as well, although this is not consistent (14, 86). Additive or indifferent effects (FIC index > 0.5–1.0) are usually seen with combinations of meropenem plus amikacin or gentamicin against *Enterobacteriaceae* (41). Combinations of carbapenems plus fluoroquinolones have variable synergy against *P. aeruginosa* and *Enterobacter,* although the three-drug combination of imipenem, ciprofloxacin, and rifampin was reportedly synergistic against 75% of tobramycin-resistant *B. cepacia* strains tested (11).

PHARMACOKINETICS
Absorption

The pharmacokinetics of imipenem and carbapenem are quite similar; these are summarized in Table 2. The pharmacokinet-

TABLE 2 • Mean Pharmacokinetic Parameters of Carbapenems in Healthy Male Volunteers at Steady State after Intravenous Infusions

Drug	Imipenem	Meropenem
Dose	1.0 g	1.0 g
C_{max} (mg/L)	69.9	61.6
$t_{1/2}$ (h)	1.11	0.98
$t_{1/2}$ renal failure (h)	3–4	7–10
% serum protein binding	15	2
V (L)	14.4	12.5
AUC (mg • hr/L)	92.5	90.8
Renal clearance (ml/min/1.73 m²)	130	176
Urinary excretion (%)	70	75

ics of carbapenems in children appear to be very similar to those in adults. Carbapenems are not absorbed after oral administration. Short intravenous infusion of 15 to 30 minutes' duration is the most common method of administration. The carbapenems exhibit linear pharmacokinetics, with peak serum concentrations increasing predictably in relation to increased doses. Peak serum concentrations of imipenem are approximately 35 and 69 mg/L following the administration of single 30-min intravenous infusions of 500 and 1000 mg doses, respectively (11). Peak concentrations following 500 and 1000 mg doses of meropenem are approximately 28 and 62 mg/L, respectively (93). Minimum plasma concentrations following repeated administration of imipenem 1 g every 6 h are approximately 3 mg/L and are approximately 0.25 mg/L following repeated administration of meropenem 1 g every 8 h (33, 35).

Imipenem may also be administered intramuscularly with a commercially available suspension formulation. Imipenem is incompletely absorbed following intramuscular administration, with approximately 60 to 75% of each dose being ultimately absorbed over a total period of 6 to 8 h. Peak plasma concentrations occur at 2 h and average approximately 10 mg/L following a 500-mg intramuscular dose (119).

Distribution

The carbapenems are widely distributed into most body tissues and fluids (Table 3) (11, 42). The apparent volumes of distribution (Vd) of carbapenems are similar and average approximately 0.25 L/kg (11, 35, 64). This Vd, similar to that of most other β-lactam drugs, indicates that distribution of carbapenems in the body is primarily extracellular. The degree of protein binding of the carbapenems is low, approximately 15% for imipenem and 2% for meropenem (33, 35). Penetration of carbapenems into the cerebrospinal fluid (CSF) is highly variable and depends to some degree on whether the meninges are intact or inflamed. Drug concentrations range from less than 1% to 10% of simultaneous plasma concentrations in patients with intact uninflamed meninges. In patients with meningitis, CSF concentrations of imipenem may reach approximately 14 to 16% of plasma concentrations, while concentrations of meropenem may reach as high as 42 to 52% of simultaneous plasma concentrations (11, 29). Although penetration into the

TABLE 3 • **Concentration of Carbapenems in Body Fluids and Tissues after Single 500-mg Intravenous Doses**

Body Tissue or Fluid	Sample Times (h)	Meropenem		Imipenem	
		Concentration (mg/L)[a]	Tissue/Fluid:Serum Ratio	Concentration (mg/L)[a]	Tissue/Fluid:Serum Ratio
CSF (infected)	1.5–3.5	0.33–6.5[b]	2–52%	1.1–2.3[b]	4–16%
CSF (uninfected)	1.5–3.5	0.10–0.18[b]	—	0.62–0.9[b]	2–5%
Tonsil	0.5–1.5	0.6	5.3%	2.2	15%
Maxillary sinus mucosa	0.5–2.5	—	7–40%	10.7	32%
Aqueous humor	5–35 min	0.52	3%	1.6	6%
Sputum	1–1.5	2.2	8%	1.6–2.7[b]	6–11%
Lung	0.5–3.5	2.86–4.83[b]	40%	13.0	29%
Peritoneal exudate	2.5–3.5	6.84	—	12.9	43%
Peritoneal fluid	1.5–2.5	14.3	—	6.0	—
Bile	0.5–2.5	—	0.2–16%	3.0–5.3[b]	10–26%
Gall bladder	0.5–3.5	0.92–3.93[b]	—	1.8	11%
Colon	0.5–3.5	2.07–2.57[b]	—	8.1	12%
Prostate	0.5–2.5	2.3	16%	5.3	28%
Ovary	0.5–4.5	1.23–2.76[b]	—	13.2	20%
Myometrium	0.5–3.5	1.28–3.76[b]	—	10.1	16%
Endometrium	0.5–3.5	0.99–4.16[b]	—	2.2–3.8[b]	7–13%
Joint tissue & fluid	1–2.5	—	>50%	7.9–20.4[b]	64–105%
Skin	1–2	3.97	10%	4.3	7%
Blister fluid	3.5–4.5	1.36	85%	>1.0	>40%

[a] Mean concentration.

[b] Reported as range of actual concentrations rather than mean value.

CSF varies considerably, both imipenem and meropenem have been used successfully in the treatment of severe central nervous system infections.

Metabolism and Excretion

The elimination half-lives of the carbapenems are approximately 1 h. The major route of elimination of these agents is urinary excretion of unchanged drug. Approximately 50 to 70% of imipenem is eliminated in the urine unchanged when the drug is administered concurrently with cilastatin, compared with only 5 to 38% of each dose in the absence of cilastatin (12, 97). Renal elimination of unchanged drug accounts for 58 to 83% of each meropenem dose (10, 12, 50). Glomerular filtration is responsible for most carbapenem renal clearance, although tubular secretion is also involved to some degree (10). Approximately 1 to 2% of each dose of imipenem or meropenem is excreted in feces (35, 98).

DOSAGE AND ADMINISTRATION
Normal

The carbapenems are usually administered by short (20–30 min) intravenous infusion. Intramuscular injections may also be used. Intramuscular administration of imipenem requires use of the suspension formulation, which should be reconstituted with 1% lidocaine hydrochloride (without epinephrine), because of pain on injection.

The usual adult dose of imipenem/cilastatin for the treatment of mild infections due to susceptible bacteria is 250 mg intravenously every 6 h (Table 4). For moderately severe infections or mild infections caused by pathogens with intermediate susceptibility, the usual dose is 500 mg every 6 h (2

g/day). Up to 1 g every 6 h (4 g/day) may be administered in the treatment of severe life-threatening infections. When administered by intramuscular injection, the usual adult dose of imipenem/cilastatin is 500 to 750 mg every 12 h because of the sustained-release characteristics following intramuscular injection of the drug (119). Although not currently approved in the United States for use in children, doses of imipenem/cilastatin 15 to 25 mg/kg every 6 h have been successful.

The usual recommended adult dose of meropenem is 1 g intravenously every 8 h. Doses of 40 mg/kg (up to 6 g/day) have been used successfully in adult patients with acute bacterial meningitis. Meropenem may also be used for treatment of infections in pediatric patients, including acute bacterial meningitis (children 3 months of age or older have been studied). The recommended dose for pediatric meningitis is 40 mg/kg intravenously every 8 h (maximum dose, 2 g every 8 h); the dosage for other types of infections is 20 mg/kg every 8 h. Pediatric patients weighing more than 50 kg should receive the same doses as adults, i.e., 1 to 2 g every 8 h, depending on the site of infection (108).

The pharmacokinetics of imipenem and meropenem in elderly patients (over 65 years of age) appear to be similar to those in younger patients when age-related changes in glomerular filtration rate are taken into account. Therefore dosage adjustments of these agents in elderly patients should be based on renal function (77, 126).

Renal Failure

The dosage of both imipenem and meropenem should be reduced in patients with renal insufficiency, because of the predominantly renal clearance of these drugs (Table 4). Dosage

TABLE 4 • **Dosage in Patients with Normal Renal Function and Renal Insufficiency**			
CrCL[a] (mL/min)	Imipenem Adult	Meropenem Adult	Pediatric[b]
>70	0.25–1.0 g every 6 h	1 g every 8 h	20–40 mg/kg every 8 h
50–70	250–500 mg every 6–8 h	1 g every 8 h	20–40 mg/kg every 8 h
26–50	250–500 mg every 8–12 h	1 g every 12 h	20–40 mg/kg every 12 h
10–25	250–500 mg every 12 h	500 mg every 12 h	10–20 mg/kg every 12 h
<10	250–500 mg every 12 h	500 mg every 24 h	10–20 mg/kg every 24 h

[a] CrCL, creatinine clearance.

[b] Recommended for children ≥3 months of age.

adjustments are also recommended to reduce drug accumulation and enhanced potential for neurotoxicity, particularly with imipenem (2, 19, 20, 67). The significance of cilastatin accumulation in patients with renal dysfunction is currently unknown (11). There are currently no recommendations for adjustment of dosage in pediatric patients with renal impairment; carbapenems should be used with caution in these patients, and drug dosage be adjusted on the basis of recommendations for adults.

Carbapenams are effectively removed by hemodialysis and intermittent hemofiltration; half-lives of imipenem and meropenem in patients undergoing these procedures have reportedly been reduced from 3.3 to 1.4 h and from 7 to 2.2 h, respectively (2, 19, 20, 67). Administration of meropenem after hemodialysis is recommended because of effective dialytic clearance of the drug. Imipenem should also be administered following hemodialysis and every 12 h thereafter. Imipenem has been studied in patients receiving continuous arteriovenous hemofiltration (CAVH), continuous artiovenous hemodiafiltration (CAVHD), and continuous venovenous hemofiltration (CVVH); daily doses recommended for patients with creatinine clearance below 25 mL/min appear to be appropriate in these patients also (132).

Hepatic Failure

The pharmacokinetics of carbapenems are not significantly altered in patients with hepatic impairment; therefore no dosage adjustments are necessary (35, 110, 125).

Obesity

The pharmacokinetics of the carbapenems have not been studied in the obese population. No formal dosage recommendations are currently available for patients weighing substantially more than 70 kg.

Ascites/Edema

Imipenem has been shown to distribute extensively into ascitic fluid; the ratio of ascitic fluid:plasma concentrations ranged from 85 to 166% following a single 500-mg intravenous dose. The half-life of imipenem in ascitic fluid was also significantly prolonged to approximately 14 h (110). However, the presence of ascites or other edema fluid does not appear to alter the systemic disposition of carbapenems significantly, and no dosage modifications are recommended.

Pregnancy

Carbapenems are U.S. FDA pregnancy risk category C. Imipenem concentrations in human fetal blood are approximately 33% of simultaneous maternal blood concentrations (52). Both the Vd and total clearance of imipenem are 2- to 3-fold higher in late pregnancy, resulting in decreased peak serum concentrations and a relatively unchanged drug half-life (52). Small animal studies with imipenem dosed at 10 to 33 times the normal human dose (300–1000 mg/kg) failed to reveal evidence of teratogenicity. However, there are no adequate well-controlled studies of carbapenems demonstrating drug safety in pregnant women. With known pharmacokinetic alterations and an absence of safety data or dosage recommendations, these drugs should be used only when the potential benefits outweigh possible risks to the fetus.

ADVERSE EFFECTS
Neurotoxicity

Induction of convulsive seizures has been associated with carbapenem therapy. The mechanism of toxicity is thought to involve inhibition of γ-aminobutyric acid (GABA) receptors and resultant decreased inhibitory neurotransmission in the central nervous system (CNS) (124). Imipenem has been associated with seizures in as many as 7% of patients, although the true incidence of seizures during imipenem therapy is probably closer to 1% (15, 16, 39, 71, 102, 104, 117). Although meropenem also appears to be associated with the occurrence of seizures, the overall incidence and potential risk are probably lower than with imipenem. Animal models have shown imipenem to have 4.4 times more epileptogenic potency than meropenem and have demonstrated that meropenem has a significantly lower potential to induce seizures (31, 32, 102). The incidence of seizures reported during actual clinical use of meropenem is approximately 0.1% (42, 99). Differences in neurotoxicity among carbapenems may be explained by differences in in vitro drug-specific receptor binding affinities or lipophilicity (31). The difference in side chains at the C-2 position is thought to account for the comparatively lower epileptogenic activity of meropenem (26).

Risk factors for carbapenem-induced seizures appear to include impaired renal function, failure to adjust drug doses for renal impairment and/or weight, advanced age, and previous CNS conditions such as head trauma, cerebrovascular accident, meningitis, or other CNS pathology (17, 32, 117). Concomitant administration of certain other medications (e.g., theophylline, ganciclovir, cyclosporine A) has also been associated with seizures in patients receiving carbapenems (7). Animal models have shown the epileptogenic potential of the carbapenems to be related to drug concentration (124). This would explain the apparently higher incidence of seizures in patients at risk for excessive drug accumulation because of failure to adjust doses properly for renal impairment or patient weight. Although a higher incidence of seizures has been reported in elderly patients, this probably reflects age-related changes in renal function and a higher prevalence of CNS risk factors in this population (17). The carbapenems do not appear to be associated with long-term neurotoxicities.

Withdrawal of carbapenem therapy is the treatment of choice for drug-induced seizures. Although administration of intravenous benzodiazepines or phenytoin has reportedly been effective in the treatment of carbapenem-induced seizures, this is usually unnecessary if carbapenem therapy can be discontinued (32). Prevention of neurotoxicity is aimed at limiting carbapenem use in patients with identified risk factors. If the benefits of drug use outweigh the potential risks, drug doses must be appropriately adjusted for weight and/or renal impairment. Meropenem may be the agent of choice in patients with underlying CNS disorders or other risk factors in whom use of a carbapenem is indicated. Meropenem has been associated with a very low incidence of seizures even during high-dose treatment of patients with bacterial meningitis or other risk factors for neurotoxicity (39, 42, 71, 102).

Gastrointestinal

Nausea, vomiting, and diarrhea, the most commonly reported adverse effects during carbapenem therapy, occur in approximately 2 to 6% of patients. Slowing the rate of intravenous drug infusion may decrease the severity of nausea and vomiting in some patients (142). Cholestasis has also been reported during imipenem/cilastatin therapy (118). Carbapenem therapy is associated with alterations in gastrointestinal flora, particularly increasing numbers of enterococci and *Candida* spp. (128). Pseudomembranous colitis occurs in approximately 0.1% of patients receiving carbapenem therapy (16, 99).

Other

Phlebitis, thrombophlebitis, and erythema and/or pain at the infusion site occur in approximately 3% of patients receiving intravenous carbapenems. Pain may also occur with intramuscular injection and may be decreased by administering the drugs with 1% lidocaine hydrochloride. Hypersensitivity reactions manifest as rash, drug fever, and/or urticaria in approximately 2 to 3% of patients. Use of carbapenems should be avoided in patients with severe allergic reactions to other β-lactam drugs, since cross-sensitivity does occur (16, 99). Rare hematologic adverse events include eosinophila, thrombocytopenia, neutropenia, and aplastic anemia (40, 99). Biochemical abnormalities seen during carbapenem therapy include increased hepatic transaminase and alkaline phosphatase concentrations in 2 to 7% of patients (16, 99). A positive Coombs' test has also been reported in approximately 2% of patients receiving imipenem/cilastatin (16).

Superinfection reportedly occurs in up to 5 to 7% of patients receiving full courses of carbapenem therapy. The most common pathogens causing these infections are Gram-positive aerobes (particularly enterococci), *P. aeruginosa, S. maltophilia,* and *Candida* spp. (15, 42, 49, 99).

DRUG INTERACTIONS

Probenecid competes with carbapenems for active renal tubular secretion. In the presence of probenecid, renal clearance of meropenem was reduced by 36%, and the plasma half-life increased by 33% (10). The manufacturer recommends that meropenem and probenecid not be administered concurrently to avoid excessive drug accumulation and potential for increased adverse effects (105). In contrast, concomitant administration of imipenem and probenecid results in only minimal increases in imipenem half-life or serum concentrations (106).

CLINICAL INDICATIONS

The carbapenems have been evaluated in a wide range of bacterial infections because of their extremely broad spectrum of antimicrobial activity and stability to β-lactamase-mediated resistance that often renders other β-lactam antibiotics ineffective. The carbapenems have been shown to be clinically useful, either as a single agent or in combination therapy, in the treatment of lower respiratory tract, CNS, skin and soft-tissue, complicated urinary tract, bone and joint, intraabdominal, and obstetric/gynecologic infections. In addition, the carbapenems are clinically useful in the treatment of endocarditis, bacteremia, and infections in cystic fibrosis and febrile neutropenic patients (7, 42). The carbapenems have found widespread use in the treatment of mixed infections because of their excellent activity against both anaerobic and aerobic bacteria. However, clinical studies have generally shown the carbapenems to be equivalent to, rather than superior to, less expensive and equally efficacious comparator regimens. Thus the carbapenems are considered the agents of choice in few infections.

The carbapenems are most appropriately used in the treatment of infections due to cephalosporin-resistant *Enterobacteriaceae,* particularly those caused by *Citrobacter freundii* and *Enterobacter* spp. The carbapenems are also useful in the treatment of infections due to cephalosporin-resistant *P. aeruginosa.* The use of imipenem as a single agent for the treatment of *P. aeruginosa* infections in cystic fibrosis patients or serious systemic infections in non–cystic fibrosis patients has been associated with development of carbapenem resistance and clinical treatment failures (1, 68, 83, 134, 142). The carbapenems should thus not be used alone in the treatment of serious pseudomonal infections but rather should be combined with agents such as the aminoglycosides.

The carbapenems may be considered as empirical therapy in the treatment of severe systemic infections in patients previously exposed to multiple courses of antibiotics. The risk of cephalosporin-resistant pathogens is increased in these patients, and the initial use of carbapenems may be justified. The carbapenems have also recently been recommended as monotherapy in the empirical treatment of febrile neutropenic patients, although monotherapy with antipseudomonal cephalosporins such as ceftazidime and cefepime may also be appropriate in this setting (55). The use of carbapenems may also be considered when therapy with traditional aminoglycoside-based combination regimens may place patients at high risk for nephrotoxicity or other undesirable adverse events. The carbapenems have reportedly been efficacious in the treatment of infections due to penicillin-resistant *S. pneumoniae,* including meningitis infections in children (4, 5). However, their optimal role in infections of this type has yet to be defined.

Imipenem/cilastatin and meropenem appear equally efficacious in the treatment of most bacterial infections. Meropenem may be favored over imipenem/cilastatin for the treatment of CNS infections because of the potential for less neurotoxicity. Meropenem may also be favored in the treatment of certain infections (e.g., cystic fibrosis) in which pathogens may be resistant to imipenem yet still susceptible to meropenem (113, 116, 133). However, imipenem/cilastatin and meropenem are considered equally safe and efficacious in most situations in which a carbapenem would be considered for use.

In addition to infections caused by more typical bacterial pathogens, the carbapenems have also been reported to be efficacious in the treatment of infections due to *N. asteroides* and *Nocardia novus* (13, 129), *R. equi* (58, 84), and *M. chelonae* and *M. fortuitum* (139).

REFERENCES

1. Acar JF. Therapy for lower respiratory tract infections with imipenem/cilastatin: a review of worldwide experience. Rev Infect Dis 1995;7(Suppl 3):S513–517.
2. Alarabi AA, Cars O, Danielson BG, Salmonson T, Wikstrom B. Pharmacokinetics of intravenous imipenem/cilastatin during intermittent haemofiltration. J Antimicrob Chemother 1990;26:91–98.
3. Appelbaum PC, Spangler SK, Jacobs MR. Susceptibilities of 394 *Bacteroides fragilis,* non-*B. fragilis* group *Bacteroides* species, and *Fusobacterium* species to newer antimicrobial agents. Antimicrob Agents Chemother 1991;35:1214–1218.
4. Arrieta A. Use of meropenem in the treatment of serious infections in children: review of the current literature. Clin Infect Dis 1997;24(Suppl 2):S207–212.
5. Asensi F, Otero MC, Perez-Tamarit D, Rodriguez-Escribano I, Cabedo JL, Gresa S, Canton E. Risk/benefit in the treatment of children with imipenem-cilastatin for meningitis caused by penicillin-resistant pneumococcus. J Chemother 1993;5:133–134.
6. Asensi V, Carton JA, Maradona JA, Asensi JM, Perez F, Redondo P, Lopez A, Arribas JM. Imipenem therapy of brain abscess. Eur J Clin Microbiol Infect Dis 1996;15:653–657.
7. Balfour JA, Bryson MB, Brogden RN. Imipenem/cilastatin. An update of its antibacterial activity, pharmacokinetics and therapeutic efficacy in the treatment of serious infections. Drugs 1996;51:99–136.
8. Barriga C, Muriel E, Benitez P, de la Fuente M. Effects of imipenem and cefmetazol on lymphocyte receptors CD2, Fc and C3b of complement. Comp Immunol Microbiol Infect Dis 1991;14:297–302.
9. Bauernfeind A, Jungwirth R, Schweighart S. In-vitro activity of meropenem, the penem HRE-664 and ceftazidime against clinical isolates from West Germany. J Antimicrob Chemother 1989;24(Suppl A):73–84.

10. Bax RP, Bastain W, Featherstone A, Wilkinson DM, Hutchison M, Haworth SJ. The pharmacokinetics of meropenem in volunteers. J Antimicrob Chemother 1989;24(Suppl A):311–320.
11. Buckley MM, Brogden RN, Barradell LB, Goa KL. Imipenem/cilastatin: a reappraisal of its antibacterial activity, pharmacokinetic properties and therapeutic efficacy. Drugs 1992;44:408–444.
12. Burman IA, Nilsson-Ehle I, Hutchison M, Haworth EJ, Norrby SR. Pharmacokinetics of meropenem and its metabolite ICI 213,689 in healthy subjects with known renal metabolism of imipenem. J Antimicrob Chemother 1991;27:219–224.
13. Burucoa C, Breton I, Ramassamy A, Soyer J, Becq-Giraudon B, Fauchere JL. Western blot monitoring of disseminated *Nocardia nova* infection treated with clarithromycin, imipenem, and surgical drainage. Eur J Clin Microbiol Infect Dis 1996;15:943–947.
14. Bustamante CI, Drusano GL, Wharton RC, Wade JC. Synergism of the combinations of imipenem plus ciprofloxacin and imipenem plus amikacin against *Pseudomonas aeruginosa* and other bacterial pathogens. Antimicrob Agents Chemother 1987;31:632–634.
15. Calandra GB, Brown KR, Grad LC, Ahonkhai VI, Wang C, Aziz MA. Review of adverse experiences and tolerability in the first 2516 patients treated with imipenem/cilastatin. Am J Med 1985;78(Suppl 6A):73–78.
16. Calandra G, Lydick E, Carrigan J, Weiss L, Guess H. Factors predisposing to seizures in seriously ill infected patients receiving antibiotics: experience with imipenem/cilastatin. Am J Med 1988;84:911–918.
17. Calandra GB, Ricci FM, Wang C, Brown KR. The efficacy results and safety profile of imipenem/cilastatin from the clinical research trials. J Clin Pharmacol 1988;28:120–127.
18. Chanal C, Sirot D, Chanal M, Cluzel M, Sirot J, Cluzel R. Comparative in-vitro activity of meropenem against clinical isolates including Enterobacteriaceae with expanded-spectrum beta-lactamases. J Antimicrob Chemother 1989;24(Suppl A):133–141.
19. Chimata M, Nagase M, Suzuki Y, Shimomura M, Kakuta S. Pharmacokinetics of meropenem in patients with various degrees of renal function, including patients with end-stage renal disease. Antimicrob Agents Chemother 1993;37:229–233.
20. Christensson BA, Nilsson-Ehle I, Hutchison M, Haworth SJ, Oqvist B, Norrby SR. Pharmacokinetics of meropenem in subjects with various degrees of renal impairment. Antimicrob Agents Chemother 1992;36:1532–1537.
21. Clarke AM, Zemcov SJV. In-vitro activity of meropenem against clinical isolates obtained in Canada. J Antimicrob Chemother 1989;24(Suppl A):47–55.
22. Clissold SP, Todd PA, Campoli-Richards DM. Imipenem/cilastatin. A review of its antibacterial activity, pharmacokinetic properties and therapeutic efficacy. Drugs 1987;33:183–241.
23. Cohn DL, Reimer LG, Reller B. Comparative in vitro activity of MK0787 (*N*-formimidoyl thienamycin) against 540 blood culture isolates. J Antimicrob Chemother 1982;9:183–194.
24. Cooke P, Heritage J, Kerr K, Hawkey PM, Newton KE. Different effects of zinc ions on in vitro susceptibilities of *Stenotrophomonas maltophilia* to imipenem and meropenem. Antimicrob Agents Chemother 1996;40:2909–2910.
25. Cooper GL, Louie A, Baltch AL, Chu RC, Smith RP, Ritz WJ, Michelsen P. Influence of zinc on *Pseudomonas aeruginosa* susceptibilities to imipenem. J Clin Microbiol 1993;31:2366–2370.
26. Craig WA. The pharmacology of meropenem, a new carbapenem antibiotic. Clin Infect Dis 1997;24(Suppl 2):S266–275.
27. Cuchural GJ, Malamy MH, Tally FP. β-Lactamase-mediated

imepenem resistance in *Bacteroides fragilis*. Antimicrob Agents Chemother 1986;30:645–648.

28. Cuffini AM, Tullio V, Allocco A, Giachino F, Fazari S, Carlone NA. The entry of meropenem into human macrophages and its immunomodulating activity. J Antimicrob Chemother 1993;32: 695–703.

29. Dagan R, Velghe L, Rodda JL. Penetration of meropenem into the cerebrospinal fluid of patients with inflamed meninges. J Antimicrob Chemother 1994;34:175–179.

30. Darveau RP, Cunningham MD. Influence of subinhibitory concentrations of cephalosporins on the serum sensitivity of *Pseudomonas aeruginosa*. J Infect Dis 1990;162:914–921.

31. De Sarro A, Ammendola D, Zappala M, Grasso S, De Sarro GB. Relationship between structure and convulsant properties of some B-lactam antibiotics following intracerebroventricular microinjection in rats. Antimicrob Agents Chemother 1995;39: 232–237.

32. Del Favero A. Clinically important aspects of carbapenem safety. Curr Opin Infect Dis 1994;7(Suppl 1):S38–42.

33. Drusano GL, Standiford HC, Bustamante C, Forrest A, Rivera G, Leslie J, Tatem B, Delaportas D, MacGregor RR, Schimpff SC. Multiple-dose pharmacokinetics of imipenem-cilastatin. Antimicrob Agents Chemother 1984;26:715–721.

34. Drusano GL. Role of pharmacokinetics in the outcome of infections. Antimicrob Agents Chemother 1988;32:289–297.

35. Drusano GL, Hutchison M. The pharmacokinetics of meropenem. Scand J Infect Dis 1995;96(Suppl):11–16.

36. Easmon CSF. Interaction of meropenem with humoral and phagocytic defenses. J Antimicrob Chemother 1989;24(Suppl A):259–264.

37. Edwards JR. Meropenem: a microbiological overview. J Antimicrob Chemother 1995;36(Suppl A):1–17.

38. Eliopoulos GM, Moellering RC Jr. Susceptibility of enterococci and *Listeria monocytogenes* to N-formimidoyl thienamycin alone and in combination with an aminoglycoside. Antimicrob Agents Chemother 1981;19:789–796.

39. Eng RHK, Munsif AN, Yangco BG, Smith SM, Chmel H. Seizure propensity with imipenem. Arch Intern Med 1989;149: 1881–1883.

40. Farinas MC, de Vega T, Garmendia J, Gonzales-Macias J. Severe neutropenia in a patient treated with imipenem/cilastatin. Eur J Clin Microbiol Infect Dis 1993;12:303–304.

41. Ferrara A, Grassi G, Grassi FA, Piccioni PD, Gialdroni Grassi G. Bactericidal activity of meropenem and interactions with other antibiotics. J Antimicrob Chemother 1989;24(Suppl A): 239–250.

42. Fish DN, Singletary TJ. Meropenem: a new carbapenem antibiotic. Pharmacotherapy 1997;17:644–669.

43. Flueckiger U, Segessenmann C, Gerber AU. Integration of pharmacokinetics and pharmacodynamics of imipenem in a human-adapted mouse model. Antimicrob Agents Chemother 1991;35: 1905–1910.

44. Fukasawa M, Sumita Y, Harabe ET, Tanio T, Nouda H, Kohzuki T, Okuda T, Matsumura H, Sunagawa M. Stability of meropenem and effect of 1 beta-methyl substitution on its stability in the presence of renal dehydropeptidase I. Antimicrob Agents Chemother 1992;36:1577–1579.

45. Fukasawa M, Sumita Y, Tada E. In vitro antibacterial activity of meropenem. Chemotherapy 1992;40(Suppl 1):74–89.

46. Gimeno C, Navarro D, Savall F, Millas E, Farga MA, Garau J, Cisterna R, Garcia-de-Lomas J. Relationship between outer membrane protein profiles and resistance to ceftazidime, imipenem,

and ciprofloxacin in *Pseudomonas aeruginosa* isolates from bacteremic patients. Eur J Clin Microbiol Infect Dis 1996;15:82–85.

47. Goldstein EJC, Citron DM, Cherubin CE, Hillier SL. Comparative susceptibility of the *Bacteroides fragilis* group species and other anaerobic bacteria to meropenem, imipenem, piperacillin, cefoxitin, ampicillin/sulbactam, clindamycin and metronidazole. J Antimicrob Chemother 1993;31:363–372.

48. Gotoh N, Tanaka S, Nishino T. Permeability of the outer membrane of *Moraxella catarrhalis* for β-lactam antibiotics. J Antimicrob Chemother 1992;29:279–285.

49. Gray JW, Pedler SJ, Kernahan J, Pearson AD, Craft AW. Enterococcal superinfection in paediatric oncology patients treated with imipenem. Lancet 1992;339:1487–1488.

50. Harrison MP, Moss SR, Featherstone A, Fowkes AG, Sanders AM, Case DE. The disposition and metabolism of meropenem in laboratory animals and man. J Antimicrob Chemother 1989; 24(Suppl A):265–277.

51. Hecht DW, Lederer L. Effect of choice of medium on the results of in vitro susceptibility testing of eight antibiotics against the *Bacteroides fragilis* group. Clin Infect Dis 1995;20(Suppl 2): S346–349.

52. Heikkila A, Renkonen OV, Erkkola R. Pharmacokinetics and transplacental passage of imipenem during pregnancy. Antimicrob Agents Chemother 1992;36:2652–2655.

53. Hikida M, Kawashima K, Yoshida M, Mitsuhashi S. Inactivation of new carbapenem antibiotics by dehydropeptidase-I from porcine and human renal cortex. J Antimicrob Chemother 1992; 30:129–134.

54. Hoban DJ, Jones RN, Yamane N, Frei R, Trilla A, Pignatari AC. In vitro activity of three carbapenem antibiotics. Comparative studies with biapenem (L-627), imipenem, and meropenem against aerobic pathogens isolated worldwide. Diagn Microbiol Infect Dis 1993;17:299–305.

55. Hughes WT, Armstrong D, Bodey GP, Brown AE, Edwards JE, Feld R, Pizzo P, Rolston KVI, Shenep JL, Young LS. 1997 Guidelines for the use of antimicrobial agents in neutropenic patients with unexplained fever. Clin Infect Dis 1997;25:551–573.

56. Inderlied CB, Lancero MG, Young LS. Bacteriostatic and bactericidal in-vitro activity of meropenem against clinical isolates, including *Mycobacterium avium* complex. J Antimicrob Chemother 1989;24(Suppl A):85–99.

57. Ito H, Arakawa Y, Ohsuka S, Wacharotayankun R, Kato N, Ohta M. Plasmid-mediated dissemination of the metallo-beta-lactamase gene blaIMP among clinically isolated strains of *Serratia marcescens*. Antimicrob Agents Chemother 1995;39:824–829.

58. Javaloyas M, Garcia D, Ruffi G. Recurrent abscess of the lung caused by *Rhodococcus equi* in an HIV-positive patient: response to the combination imipenem/vancomycin. Med Clin 1993;100:759.

59. Jones RN, Barry AL, Thornsberry C. In-vitro studies of meropenem. J Antimicrob Chemother 1989;24(Suppl A):9–24.

60. Jones RN, Gardiner RV. Stability of SM-7338, a new carbapenem in mediums recommended for the susceptibility testing of anaerobic bacteria and gonococci. Diagn Microbiol Infect Dis 1989;12:271–273.

61. Jorgensen JH, Maher LA, Howell AW. Activity of a new carbapenem antibiotic, meropenem, against *Haemophilus influenzae* strains with beta-lactamase and non-enzyme mediated resistance to ampicillin. Antimicrob Agents Chemother 1991;35: 600–602.

62. Kahan FM, Kropp H, Sundelof JG, Birnbaum J. Thienamycin: development of imipenem-cilastatin. J Antimicrob Chemother 1983;12(Suppl D):1–35.

63. Kayser FH, Morenzoni G, Strassle A, Hadorn K. Activity of meropenem, against gram-positive bacteria. J Antimicrob Chemother 1989;24(Suppl A):101–112.

64. Kelly HC, Hutchison M, Haworth SJ. A comparison of the pharmacokinetics of meropenem after administration by intravenous injection over 5 min and intravenous infusion over 30 min. J Antimicrob Chemother 1995;36(Suppl A):35–42.

65. King A, Boothman C, Phillips I. Comparative in-vitro activity of meropenem on clinical isolates from the United Kingdom. J Antimicrob Chemother 1989;24(Suppl A):31–45.

66. Kitzis MD, Acar JF, Gutman L. Antibacterial activity of meropenem against gram-negative bacteria with a permeability defect and against staphylococci. J Antimicrob Chemother 1989;24 (Suppl A):125–132.

67. Konishi K, Suzuki H, Saruta T, Hayashi M, Deguchi N, Tazaki H, Hisaka A. Removal of imipenem and cilastatin by hemodialysis in patients with end-stage renal failure. Antimicrob Agents Chemother 1991;35:16–20.

68. Krilov LR, Blumer JL, Stern RC, Hartstein AI, Iglewski BN, Goldmann DA. Imipenem/cilastatin in acute pulmonary exacerbations of cystic fibrosis. Rev Infect Dis 1985;7(Suppl 3):S482–489.

69. Kropp H, Gerckens L, Sundelof JG, Kahan FM. Antibacterial activity of imipenem: the first thienamycin antibiotic. Rev Infect Dis 1985;7(Suppl 3):S389–410.

70. Kumar A, Hay MB, Maier GA, Dyke JW. Post-antibiotic effect of ceftazidime, ciprofloxacin, imipenem, piperacillin and tobramycin for *Pseudomonas cepacia*. J Antimicrob Chemother 1992;30:597–602.

71. Leo RJ, Ballow CH. Seizure activity associated with imipenem use: clinical case reports and review of the literature. Ann Pharmacother 1991;25:351–353.

72. Lewin C, Doherty C, Govan J. In vitro activities of meropenem, PD 127391, PD 131628, ceftazidime, chloramphenicol, cotrimoxazole, and ciprofloxacin against *Pseudomonas cepacia*. Antimicrob Agents Chemother 1993;37:123–125.

73. Linares J, Alonso T, Perez JL, Ayats J, Dominguez MA, Pallares R, Martin R. Decreased susceptibility of penicillin-resistant pneumococci to twenty-four beta-lactam antibiotics. J Antimicrob Chemother 1992;30:279–288.

74. Livermore DM, Yang Y. Comparative activity of meropenem against *Pseudomonas aeruginosa* strains with well-characterized resistance mechanisms. J Antimicrob Chemother 1989;24(Suppl A):149–159.

75. Livermore DM. Mechanisms of resistance to β-lactam antibiotics. Scand J Infect Dis 1991;78(Suppl):7–16.

76. Livermore DM. Interplay of impermeability and chromosomal beta-lactamase activity in imipenem-resistant *Pseudomonas aeruginosa*. Antimicrob Agents Chemother 1992;36:2046–2048.

77. Ljungberg B, Nilsson-Ehle I. Pharmacokinetics of meropenem and its metabolite in young and elderly healthy men. Antimicrob Agents Chemother 1992;36:1437–1440.

78. MacGowan AP, Bowker KE, Bedford KA, Holt HA, Reeves DS, Hedges A. The comparative inhibitory and bactericidal activities of meropenem and imipenem against *Acinetobacter* spp and Enterobacteriaceae resistant to second generation cephalosporins. J Antimicrob Chemother 1995;35:333–337.

79. MacKenzie FM, Gould IM, Chapman DG, Jason D. Postantibiotic effect of meropenem on members of the family Enterobacteriaceae determined by five methods. Antimicrob Agents Chemother 1994;38:2583–2589.

80. Maggiolo F, Taras A, Frontespezi S, Legnani MC, Silanos MA, Pravettoni G, Suter F. Pharmacodynamic effects of subinhibitory concentrations of imipenem on *Pseudomonas aeruginosa* in an in vitro pharmacodynamic model. Antimicrob Agents Chemother 1994;38:1416–1418.

81. Majcherczyk PA, Livermore DM. Penicillin-binding protein (PBP) 2 and the post-antibiotic effect of carbapenems. J Antimicrob Chemother 1990;26:593–594.

82. Mandell LA, Afnan M. Mechanisms of interaction among subinhibitory concentrations of antibiotics, human polymorphonuclear neutrophils, and gram-negative bacilli. Antimicrob Agents Chemother 1991;35:1291–1297.

83. Margaret BS, Drusano GL, Standiford HC. Emergence of resistance to carbapenem antibiotics in Pseudomonas aeruginosa. J Antimicrob Chemother 1989;24(Suppl A):161–167.

84. Mascellino MT, Iona E, Ponzo R, Mastroianni CM, Delia S. Infections due to *Rhodococcus equi* in three HIV-infected patients: microbiological findings and antibiotic susceptibility. Int J Clin Pharmacol Res 1994;14:157–163.

85. Margaret BS, Drusano GL, Standiford HC. Emergence of resistance to carbapenem antibiotics in *Pseudomonas aeruginosa*. J Antimicrob Chemother 1989;24(Suppl A):161–7.

86. McGrath BJ, Lamp KC, Rybak MJ. Pharmacodynamic effects of extended dosing intervals of imipenem alone and in combination with amikacin against *Pseudomonas aeruginosa* in an in vitro model. Antimicrob Agents Chemother 1993;37:1931–1937.

87. Moellering RC, Eliopoulos GM, Sentochnik DE. The carbapenems: new broad spectrum beta-lactam antibiotics. J Antimicrob Chemother 1989;24 (Suppl A):1–7.

88. Mouton JW, van den Anker JN. Meropenem clinical pharmacokinetics. Clin Pharmacokinet 1995;28:275–286.

89. Murray PR, Niles AC. In vitro activity of meropenem (SM-7338), imipenem, and five other antibiotics against anaerobic clinical isolates. Diagn Microbiol Infect Dis 1990;13:57–61.

90. Nadler HL, Pitkin DH, Sheikh W. The postantibiotic effect of meropenem and imipenem against selected bacteria. J Antimicrob Chemother 1989;24(Suppl A):225–231.

91. Nadler HL, Sheik W. A comparison of the in vitro post-antibiotic effect of meropenem and imipenem versus selected enterobacteriaceae and other pathogens. Diagn Microbiol Infect Dis 1993;17:71–73.

92. Neuwirth C, Siebor E, Duez JM, Pechinot A, Kazmierczak A. Imipenem resistance in clinical isolates of proteus mirabilis associated with alterations in penicillin-binding proteins. J Antimicrob Chemother 1995;36:335–342.

93. Nilsson-Ehle I, Hutchison M, Haworth SJ, Norrby SR. Pharmacokinetics of meropenem compared to imipenem-cilastatin in young healthy males. Eur J Clin Microbiol Infect Dis 1991;10:85–88.

94. Nishino T, Fukuoka T, Honmura T. In vitro and in vivo antibacterial activity of panipenem/betamipron, a new carbapenem antibiotic. Chemotherapy 1991;39(Suppl 3):55–74.

95. Nord CE, Lindmark A, Persson I. Susceptibility of anaerobic bacteria to meropenem. J Antimicrob Chemother 1989;24(Suppl A):113–117.

96. Nordmann P, Ronco E. In-vitro antimicrobial susceptibility of *Rhodococcus equi*. J Antimicrob Chemother 1992;29:383–393.

97. Norrby SR, Alestig K, Bjornegard B, Burman LA, Ferber F, Huber JL, Jones KH, Kahan FM, Kahan JS, Kropp H, Meisinger MA, Sundelof JG. Urinary recovery of N-formididoyl thienamycin (MK0787) as affected by coadministration of N-formididoyl thienamycin dehydropeptidase inhibitors. Antimicrob Agents Chemother 1983;23:300–307.

98. Norrby SR, Rogers JD, Ferber F, Jones KH, Zacchei AG, Weidner LL, Demetriades JL, Gravallese DA, Hsien JY. Disposition of radiolabeled imipenem and cilastatin in normal human volunteers. Antimicrob Agents Chemother 1984;26: 707–714.

99. Norrby SR, Newell PA, Faulkner KL, Lesky W. Safety profile of meropenem: international clinical experience based on the first 3125 patients treated with meropenem. J Antimicrob Chemother 1995;36(Suppl A):207–223.

100. Odenholt-Tornqvist I. Studies on the postantibiotic effect and the postantibiotic sub-MIC effect of meropenem. J Antimicrob Chemother 1993;31:881–892.

101. Pasqui AL, Di Renzo M, Bruni F, Fanetti G, Campoccia G, Auteri A. Imipenem and immune response: in vitro and in vivo studies. Drugs Exp Clin Res 1995;21:17–22.

102. Patel J, Giles RE. Meropenem: evidence of lack of proconvulsive tendency in mice. J Antimicrob Chemother 1989;24(Suppl A):307–309.

103. Perez FJ, Gimeno C, Navarro D, Garcia-de-Lomas J. Membrane permeation through the outer membrane of *Pseudomonas aeruginosa* can involve pathways other than the OprD porin channel. Chemotherapy 1996;42:210–214.

104. Pestotnik SL, Classen DC, Evans RS, Stevens LE, Burke JP. Prospective surveillance of imipenem/cilastatin use and associated seizures using a hospital information system. Ann Pharmacother 1993;27:497–501.

105. Product Information: Merrem, meropenem. Wilmington, DE: Zeneca Pharmaceuticals, 1996.

106. Product Information: Primaxin, imipenem/cilastatin. West Point, PA: Merck & Co., 1995.

107. Raimondi A, Traverso A, Nikaido H. Imipenem- and meropenem-resistant mutants of *Enterobacter cloacae* and *Proteus rettgeri* lack porins. Antimicrob Agents Chemother 1991; 35:1174–1180.

108. Reed M, Kearns G, Jacobs R, Yamashita T, Thompson S, Gooch W III, Yogev R, Williams K, Blumer J. Dose ranging and pharmacokinetic evaluation of meropenem in infants and children [Abstract]. Presented at the 32nd Interscience Conference on Antimicrobial Agents and Chemotherapy, Anaheim, CA, Oct 11–14, 1992.

109. Rodriguez AB, Barriga C, de la Fuente M. Phagocytic function and antibody-dependent cellular cytotoxicity of human neutrophils in the presence of N-formimidoyl thienamycin. Agents Actions 1990;31:86–95.

110. Rolando N, Wade JJ, Philpott-Howard JN, Casewell MW, Williams R. The penetration of imipenem-cilastatin into ascitic fluid in patients with chronic liver disease. J Antimicrob Chemother 1994;33:163–167.

111. Sader HS, Jones RN. Antimicrobial activity of the new carbapenem biapenem compared to imipenem, meropenem and other broad-spectrum beta-lactam drugs. Eur J Clin Microbiol Infect Dis 1993;12:384–391.

112. Sanders CC, Sanders WE, Thomson KS, Iaconis JP. Meropenem activity against resistant gram-negative bacteria and interactions with beta-lactamases. J Antimicrob Chemother 1989;24(Suppl A):187–196.

113. Sarubbi F, Franzus B, Verghese A. Comparative activity of meropenem (SM-7338) against major respiratory pathogens and amikacin-resistant nosocomial isolates. Eur J Clin Microbiol Infect Dis 1992;11:65–68.

114. Satake S, Yoneyama H, Nakae T. Role of OmpD2 and chromosomal beta-lactamase in carbapenem resistance in clinical isolates of *Pseudomonas aeruginosa*. J Antimicrob Chemother 1991;28:199–207.

115. Schentag JJ, Smith IL, Swanson DJ, DeAngelis C, Fracasso JE, Vari A, Vance JW. Role for dual individualization with cefmenoxime. Am J Med 1984;77(Suppl 6a):43–50.

116. Schito GC, Sanna A, Chezzi C, Ravizzola G, Leone F, Molinari G, Menozzi MG, Pirali F. In-vitro activity of meropenem against clinical isolates in a multi-center study in Italy. J Antimicrob Chemother 1989;24(Suppl A):57–72.

117. Schliamser SE, Cars O, Norrby SR. Neurotoxicity of B-lactam antibiotics: predisposing factors and pathogenesis. J Antimicrob Chemother 1991;27:405–425.

118. Schreiber C, May B. Cholestasis in imipenem/cilastatin treatment. Z Gastroenterol 1993;31(Suppl 2):76–77.

119. Sexton DJ, Wlodaver CG, Tobey LE, Yangco BG, Graziani AL, MacGregor RR. Twice daily intramuscular imipenem/cilastatin in the treatment of skin and soft tissue infections. Chemotherapy 1991;37(Suppl 2):26–30.

120. Sheikh W, Pitkin DH, Nadler H. Antibacterial activity of meropenem and selected comparative agents against anaerobic bacteria at seven North American centers. Clin Infect Dis 1993;16(Suppl 4):361–366.

121. Sirot D. Expanded-spectrum plasmid-mediated β-lactamases. J Antimicrob Chemother 1995;36(Suppl A):19–34.

122. Sumita Y, Inoue M, Mitsuhashi S. In vitro antibacterial activity and beta-lactamase stability of the new carbapenem SM-7338. Eur J Clin Microbiol 1989;8:908–916.

123. Sumita Y, Fukasawa M, Okuda T. Comparison of two carbapenems, SM-7338 and imipenem: affinities for penicillin-binding proteins and morphological changes. J Antibiot (Tokyo) 1990; 43:314–320.

124. Sunagawa M, Matsumura H, Sumita Y, Nouda H. Structural features resulting in convulsive activity of carbapenem compounds: effect of C-2 side chain. J Antibiot 1995;48: 408–416.

125. Thyrum PT, Yeh C, Birmingham B, Lasseter K. Pharmacokinetics of meropenem in patients with liver disease. Clin Infect Dis 1997;24(Suppl 2):S184–190.

126. Toon S, Hopkins KJ, Garstang FM, Aarons L, Rowland M. Pharmacokinetics of imipenem and cilastatin after their simultaneous administration to the elderly. Br J Clin Pharmacol 1987;23:143–149.

127. Trias J, Nikaido H. Outer membrane protein D2 catalyzes facilitated diffusion of carbapenems and penems through the outer membrane of *Pseudomonas aeruginosa*. Antimicrob Agents Chemother 1990;34:52–57.

128. Van der Leur JJ, Thunnissen PL, Clasener HA, Muller NF, Dofferhoff AS. Effects of imipenem, cefotaxime and cotrimoxazole on aerobic microbial colonization of the digestive tract. Scand J Infect Dis 1993;25:473–478.

129. Vassallo J, Galizia AC, Cuschieri P. Mixed pulmonary infection with *Nocardia, Candida,* methicillin-resistant *Staphylococcus aureus,* and group D *Streptococcus* species. Postgrad Med J 1996;15:82–85.

130. Visser MR, Hoepelman IM, Beumer H, Rozenberg-Arska M, Verhoef J. Comparative in vitro antibacterial activity of the new carbapenem meropenem (SM-7338). Eur J Clin Microbiol Infect Dis 1989;8:1061–1064.

131. Vogelman B, Gudmundsson S, Leggett J, Turnidge J, Ebert S, Craig WA. Correlation of antimicrobial pharmacokinetic parameters with therapeutic efficacy in an animal model. J Infect Dis 1988;158:831–847.

132. Vos MC, Vincent HH, Yzerman EP. Clearance of imipenem/cilastatin in acute renal failure patients treated by continuous hemodiafiltration. Intensive Care Med 1992;18: 282–285.

133. Voutsinas D, Mavroudis T, Avlamis A, Giamarellou H. In-vitro activity of meropenem, a new carbapenem, against multiresistant *Pseudomonas aeruginosa* compared with that of other antipseudomonal antimicrobials. J Antimicrob Chemother 1989; 24(Suppl A):143–147.

134. Winston DJ, McGrattan MA, Busuttil RW. Imipenem therapy of Pseudomonas aeruginosa and other serious bacterial infections. Antimicrob Agents Chemother 1984;26:673–677.

135. Wise R, Ashby JP, Andrews JM. The antibacterial activity of meropenem in combination with gentamicin or vancomycin. J Antimicrob Chemother 1989;24(Suppl A):233–238.

136. Wiseman LR, Wagstaff AJ, Brogden RN, Bryson HM. Meropenem: a review of its antibacterial activity, pharmacokinetic properties and clinical efficacy. Drugs 1995;50: 73–101.

137. Yazawa K, Mikami Y, Ohashi S, Miyaji M, Ichihara Y, Nishimura C. In-vitro activity of new carbapenem antibiotics: comparative studies with meropenem, L-627 and imipenem against pathogenic *Nocardia* spp. J Antimicrob Chemother 1992;29:169–172.

138. Yeo S-F, Livermore DM. Comparative in-vitro activity of biapenem and other carbapenems against *Haemophilus influenzae* isolates with known resistance mechanisms to ampicillin. J Antimicrob Chemother 1994;33:861–865.

139. Yew WW, Lau KS, Tse WK, Wong CF. Imipenem in the treatment of lung infections due to *Mycobacterium fortuitum* and *Mycobacterium chelonae:* further experience. Clin Infect Dis 1992;15:1046–1047.

140. Yourassowsky E, Van der Linden MP, Lismont MJ, Crokaert F, Glupczynski Y. Bactericidal activity of meropenem against *Pseudomonas aeruginosa.* J Antimicrob Chemother 1989; 24 (Suppl A):169–174.

141. Yourassowsky E, van der LMP, Crokaert F. Antibacterial effect of meropenem and imipenem on *Proteus mirabilis.* J Antimicrob Chemother 1990;26:185–192.

142. Zajac BA, Fisher MA, Gibson GA, MacGregor RR. Safety and efficacy of high-dose treatment with imipenem-cilastatin in seriously ill patients. Antimicrob Agents Chemother 1985;27: 745–749.

Cephalosporins: Oral

●

André J. Bryskier and Suzanne R. Belfiglio

Few families of oral antibacterials are available for physicians. The most important are penicillins, cephalosporins, macrolides, and fluoroquinolones and to a lesser extent, cyclines and lincosamides. Within this category of antibacterials, cephalosporins are considered safe drugs, acid stable, with a broad antibacterial spectrum that covers the common pathogens encountered in everyday clinical practice. A diversity of antibacterials are needed to overcome intrinsic or acquired bacterial resistance (e.g., *Haemophilus influenzae* producing β-lactamase).

The first parenteral cephalosporin resulted from chemical modification of cephalosporin C (especially 7ACA), which was isolated from the fermentation broth of *Cephalosporicum acremonium,* now named *Acremonium cryseogenum.* Cephalosporins are acid stable but are poorly absorbed. Modification of the side chain at the C-7 position of the cephem nucleus by fixing a D-phenylglycine moiety gave cephalexin in 1967 (333). Since then, many series of compounds bearing a 7-D-phenylglycine residue were synthesized, but only few of them were introduced into clinical practice.

The aim with the Ó-aminocephalosporins was to improve the pharmacokinetic profile to reduce the number of daily doses. This goal was reached with cefadroxil, which differs from cephalexin by a *p*-hydroxyphenyl moiety instead of a phenyl, allowing one to two administrations per day. Some esters were also prepared, such as cephaloglycin or cephalexin esters. The second target was to enhance the antibacterial activity. The first wave of oral cephalosporins was directed against penicillinase-producing strains of *Staphylococcus aureus.* The second wave was oriented against Gram-negative bacilli. Polar groups were appended at the C-3 position. One widely used compound was introduced in clinical practice, cefaclor.

In the development of parenteral third-generation cephalosporins, much effort was directed toward obtaining absorbable compounds, first with existing parenteral compounds. Efforts were unsuccessful with cefotaxime and ceftriaxone. Some success was realized with ceftizoxime (KY020), but the absorption rate was too moderate to allow clinical development. Two compounds were esterified and are widely used, cefuroxime-axetil and cefotiam-hexetil. Ó-Aminocephalosporin compounds that have been developed include cefprozil and an Ó-aminocarbacephem, loracarbef, which is similar to cefaclor.

Among the 2-amino-5-thiazolyl derivatives, two types of compounds were developed, esterified and nonesterified. Nonesterified cephems possess a hydroxy (cefdinir) or an acetoxy (cefixime) residue on the oxime group. Other groups have been added instead of the oxime ring (ceftibuten). Many of the new oral cephems are prodrugs, with a cleavable ester at C-4 (carboxylic group). They differ in their C-3 side chain and ester chain. The main compounds are cefpodoxime-proxetil, cefetamet-pivoxil, cefcamate-pivoxil, and cefditoren-pivoxil. Research in this field continues with the goal of extending the antibacterial spectrum and enhancing antibacterial activity.

This chapter reviews the main characteristics of available oral cephems introduced in clinical practice or under clinical development (phase III).

CLASSIFICATION OF ORAL CEPHALOSPORINS

Two classifications can be described, the most reliable chemical classification and the vernacular microbiologic classification.

Microbiologic Classification

The microbiologic classification could mimic the parenteral cephalosporin classification (48). Compounds can be divided into three groups according to their antibacterial spectrum and in vitro activity. However, it is difficult to insert some compounds that have an intermediate antibacterial activity (Fig. 1).

The first group (limited spectrum) is divided into two subgroups I_A and I_B. Group I_A is composed of most of the Ó-amino cephalosporins, with differences between compounds. All of them display good in vitro activity against Gram-positive

cocci. They are less active against isolates of *S. aureus* producing penicillinase, and they are inactive against *E. faecalis*. Cefaclor and to a lesser extent cefatrizine and cefprozil are active against enteric bacilli (especially methicillin-susceptible *S. aureus*), but other derivatives exhibit weak antibacterial activity against Gram-negative bacilli.

Group II contains only one available drug, cefuroxime-axetil, and one compound, cefcanel-daloxil, which was only developed up to phase III. Parenteral cefuroxime is more active than cefaclor in covering Gram-negative bacilli, *H. influenzae,* and Gram-positive cocci, but it is less active than compounds in group III.

Group III compounds, which have an extended antibacterial spectrum among the oral cephalosporins, can be divided into two groups, III_A and III_B, according to their in vitro activity against Gram-positive cocci, mainly *S. aureus*. Compounds in group III_B are inactive against *S. aureus* and are poorly active against *Streptococcus pneumoniae*.

Chemical Classification

On the basis of chemical structure, oral cephalosporins can be divided into seven groups. Groups I and II contain Ó-amino-

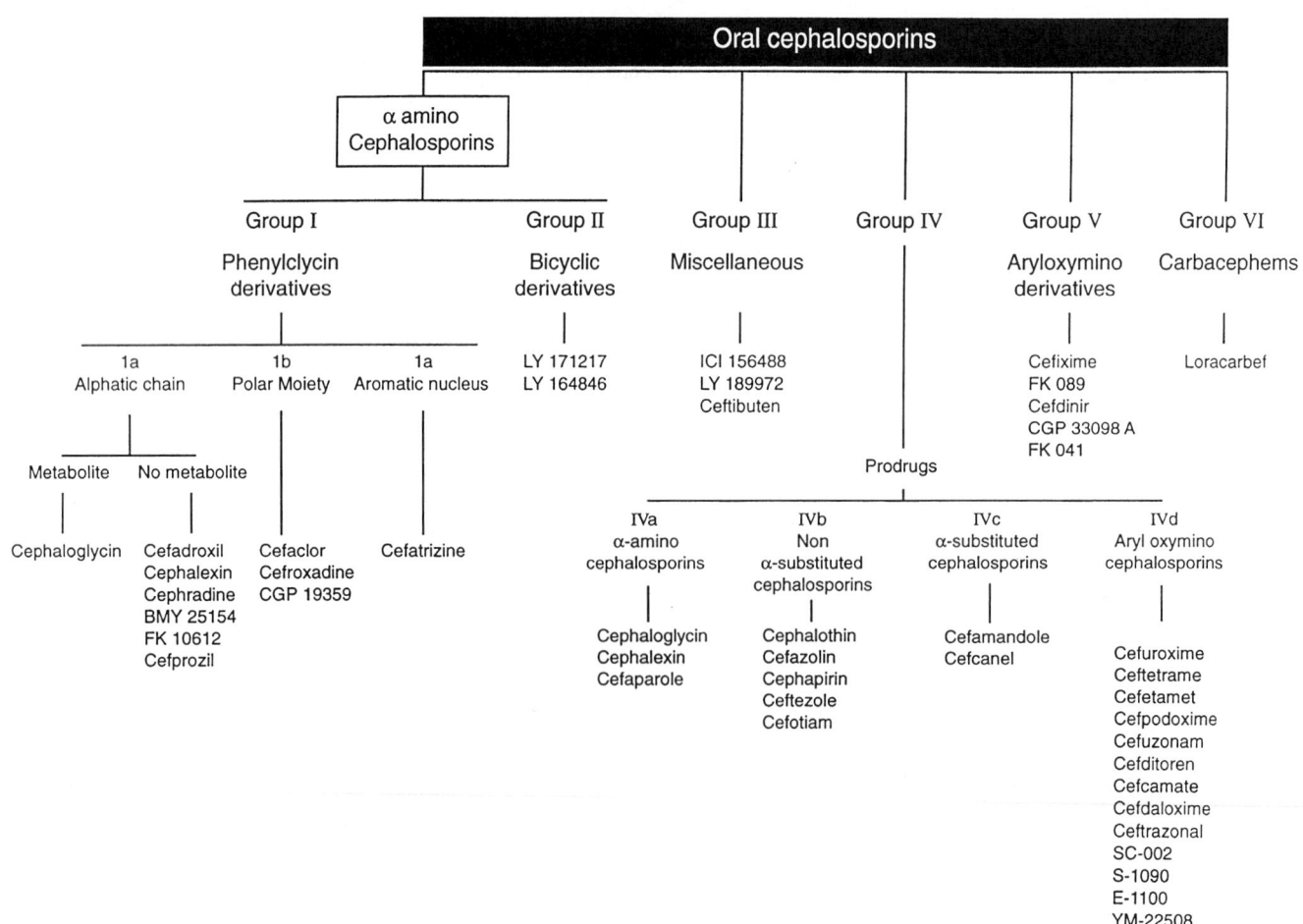

FIGURE 1. Oral cephalosporins.

cephalosporins. Group I contains most of the common old cephalosporins, which are divided into three subgroups according to their C-3 side chain. In subgroup I_A, only one compound was introduced, cephaloglycin. However, among the compounds with a C-3 aliphatic side chain, four drugs are currently used in clinical practice, cefadroxil, cephalexin, cephradine and cefprozil (Fig. 2). Only two compounds with a polar side chain are available for clinical use, cefaclor and cefroxadine, and one with an aromatic nucleus, cefatrizine (Fig. 3).

Group III is composed of miscellaneous derivatives such as ceftibuten. Group IV is more complex, composed of oral cephalosporin prodrugs. Group V is subdivided into four subgroups. The most important one, considering the clinical use, is group IV_C with at least four compounds introduced for human clinical use, cefuroxime, cefetamet, cefpodoxime, and cefteterame (Japan), and one under clinical development, cefditoren-pivoxil (Fig. 4). Group V, the aryloxiimino derivative nonesterified compounds, contains two main drugs, cefixime and cefdinir (Fig. 5). Group VI is composed of carbacephems. Loracarbef is the only member of this group at the present time.

The available chemicophysical data for esterified and nonesterified compounds are listed in (Tables 1 and 2).

These compounds (ester or nonester) are colorless (cefaclor, cefuroxime-axetil) to slightly yellowish (cefixime, cefprozil, ceftibuten, cefuroxime-axetil, cefditoren) or brownish (cefpodoxime-proxetil) crystalline powder.

Cefprozil is a 9:1 mixture of its *cis* and *trans*-isomers and cefuroxime-axetil and cefpodoxime-proxetil are mixtures of diastereoisomers in almost equal proportions. Ceftibuten is formulated as the pure active *cis*-isomer, but it is partially converted (up to 20 %) to the less active *trans*-isomer in serum

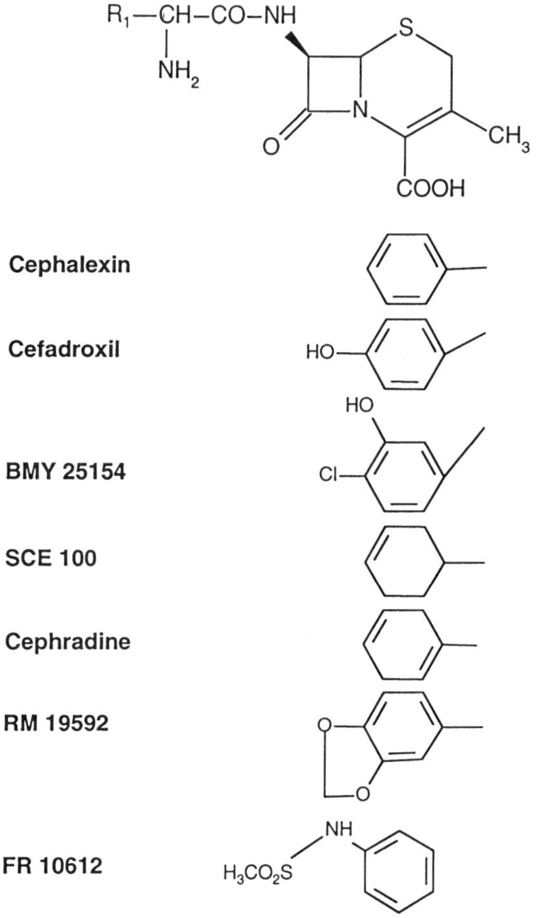
R1—CH-CO-NH
NH2
S
N
O
CH3
COOH
Cephalexin
Cefadroxil
HO
BMY 25154
Cl
SCE 100
Cephradine
RM 19592
O
FR 10612
NH
H3CO2S

FIGURE 2. 3-Methyl cephem (group Ia).

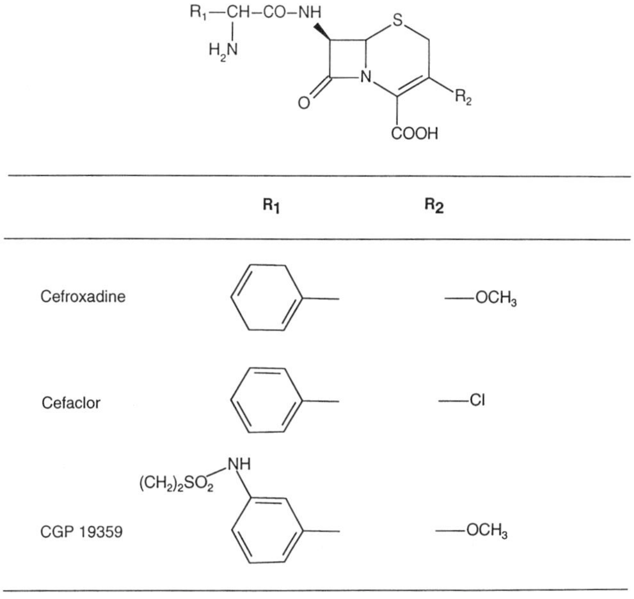
R1—CH-CO-NH
H2N
S
N
O
R2
COOH
R1
R2
Cefroxadine
—OCH3
Cefaclor
—Cl
(CH2)2SO2
NH
CGP 19359
—OCH3

FIGURE 3. Oral cephalosporin (group Ib).

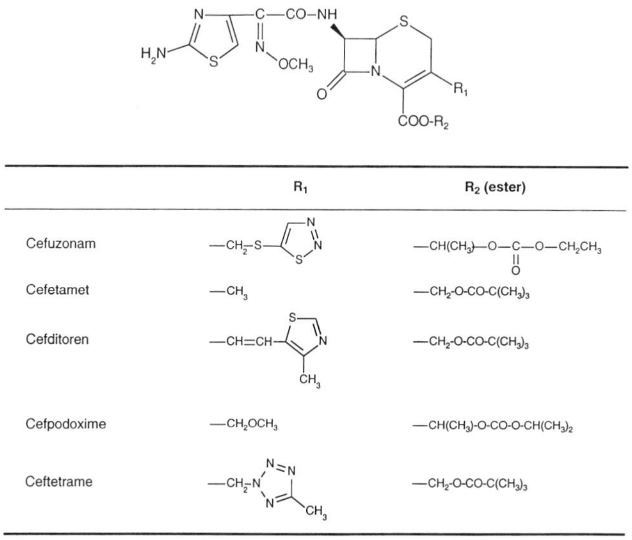
N
C—CO-NH
H2N
S
N
OCH3
S
N
O
R1
COO-R2
R1
R2 (ester)
Cefuzonam
—CH2-S—
—CH(CH3)—O—C—O—CH2CH3
Cefetamet
—CH3
—CH2-O-CO-C(CH3)3
Cefditoren
—CH=CH—
CH3
—CH2-O-CO-C(CH3)3
Cefpodoxime
—CH2OCH3
—CH(CH3)-O-CO-O-CH(CH3)2
Ceftetrame
—CH2-N
CH3
—CH2-O-CO-C(CH3)3

FIGURE 4. Oral cephalosporin (group IV c).

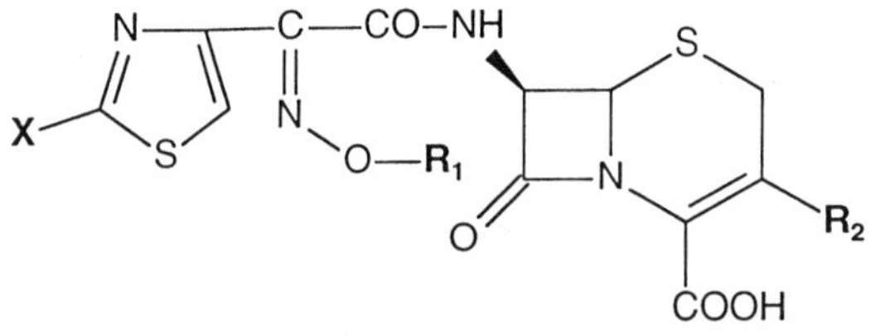

	X	R₁	R₂
Cefixime	—NH₂	—CH₂COOH	—CH=CH₂
FK 089	—H	—CH₂COOH	—H
Cefdinir	—NH₂	—OH	—CH=CH₂
CGP 33098A	—NH₂	—CH₂COOH	S—CH₂CH₂NH₂

FIGURE 5. Oral cephalosporin (group V).

TABLE 1 • Chemicophysical Properties of α-Aminocephalosporins

Generic Name	Empirical Formula	Molceular Weight	pKa1	pKa2	pKa3	Degradation Half-life pH 1, 35°C (min)	Group (oral)
Cephalexin	$C_{16}H_{17}N_3O_4S$	347.40	2.67	6.96	–	36,000	I
Cefadroxil	$C_{16}H_{17}N_3O_5S$	381.41	2.69	7.22	–	44,000	I
Cephaloglycin	$C_{18}H_{19}N_3O_6S$	405.44	2.03	6.89	–	2,100	I
Cephradine	$C_{16}H_{19}N_3O_4S$	349.41	2.63	7.35	–	38,000	I
Cefaclor	$C_{15}H_{14}ClN_3O_3S$	367.82	1.5	7.17	–	–	II
Cefatrizine	$C_{18}H_{18}N_6O_5S_2$	462.50	2.62	6.99	–	19,000	I
Cefroxadine	$C_{16}H_{19}N_3O_5S$	365.40	–	–	–	–	II
Loracarbef	$C_{16}H_{16}ClN_3O_4$	349.57	–	–	–	–	VI
Cefprozil	$C_{18}H_{19}N_3O_5S$	407.5	2.8	7.3	9.7	–	II

TABLE 2 • Chemicophysical Properties of Non-α-Amino Oral Cephems

Generic Name	Empirical Formula	Molecular Weight	Dissociation Constant pKa1/pKa2	Oral	Parenteral
Cefpodoxime	$C_{15}H_{17}N_5O_6S_2$	427.5	2.01, 3.17	IVd	–
Cefpodoxime proxetil	$C_{21}H_{27}N_5O_9S_2$	557.6	3.2	IVd	–
Cefuroxime	$C_{16}H_{16}N_4O_8S$	424.4	2.2	–	II
Cefuroxime axetil	$C_{20}H_{22}N_4O_{10}S$	510.5	–	IVd	–
Cefetamet	$C_{14}H_{15}N_5O_5S_2$	397.4	2.6, 3.6	IVd	–
Cefetamet-pivoxil	$C_{20}H_{25}N_5O_7S_2$	511.17	3.1	IVd	–
Cefditoren-pivoxil	$C_{25}H_{28}N_6O_7S_3$	620.73	–	IVd	–
Cefditoren	$C_{19}H_{18}N_6O_5S_3$	506.59	–	IVd	–
Ceftibuten	$C_{15}H_{14}N_4O_6S_2$	410.43	2.3, 3.2, 4.5	III	–
Cefdinir	$C_{14}H_{13}N_5O_5S_2$	395.4	1.9, 3.3, 9.9	V	–
Cefixime	$C_{16}H_{15}N_5O_7S_2$	453.5	2.1, 2.7, 3.7	V	–
Cefotiam	$C_{18}H_{23}N_9O_4S_2$	598.5	2.6, 4.6, 7.0	–	IIIa
Cefotiam-hexetil	$C_{27}H_{37}N_9O_7S_3$	768.77	4.6, 7.2	IVb	–

and liver. With the ester prodrugs, there is no difference in antibacterial activity, since the asymmetric center is located in the ester side chain. The *cis-trans* isomers of cefprozil differ in their antibacterial activity. The *trans*-isomer is 6 to 8 times less active against *Escherichia coli, Klebsiella pneumoniae, Neisseria gonorrhoeae,* and *H. influenzae.*

Another common characteristic of the cephem prodrug ester is its bitter taste. Cefaclor and loracarbef differ in the substituent in position 1, a sulfur atom (cefaclor) and a methylene (loracarbef). The carbacephem is chemically stable compared with its cephalosporin analogue (cefaclor).

ANTIMICROBIAL ACTIVITY

The in vitro activity of oral cephalosporins is well documented. In general, studies using more than 10 isolates and broth or agar dilution methods with bacterial inocula of 10^4 to 10^6 CFU/mL are considered in this review. The natural antibacterial spectrum of oral cephalosporins covers Gram-positive cocci, Gram-negative cocci, and some Gram-negative bacilli. Numerous studies have been conducted to determine the in vitro activity of oral cephalosporins against common pathogens.

Gram-Positive Bacteria

Oral cephalosporins are inactive against *Listeria monocytogenes* and *Corynebacterium jeikeium.* Among staphylococci, they are inactive against methicillin-resistant isolates. Among *S. aureus* susceptible or resistant to penicillin G, two kinds of oral cephems can be described. One subgroup is inactive against *S. aureus* such as cefixime (MIC_{50} = 16 mg/L), cefetamet (MIC > 64 mg/L), and ceftibuten (MIC_{50} > 64 mg/L). Loracarbef and cefaclor are less active against penicillin G–resistant isolates, showing some susceptibility to hydrolysis by penicillinases produced by *S. aureus.* Among other cephems, the most active compound is cefdinir ($MIC_{50/90}$, 0.5 mg/L), whatever the strains, because of its chemical structure (hydroxyimino residue at C-7 position) (Table 3).

Against *Staphylococcus epidermidis,* ceftibuten, cefetamet, and cefixime are inactive. Other cephalosporins exhibit good activity. However, against isolates of *S. epidermidis* resistant to

penicillin G, cefprozil, cefaclor, and loracarbef are less active, with two populations, one susceptible and one resistant. Against coagulase-negative staphylococci, cefetamet, ceftibuten, and cefixime are inactive. The most active compound is cefdinir. Other compounds show the same activity (Table 4).

All cephalosporins are inactive against *Enterococcus faecalis, Enterococcus faecium,* and *Enterococcus liquefaciens* (MIC = 64 mg/L).

Against β-hemolytic streptococci (Lancefield groups A, B, C, and G), all compounds show good in vitro activity except ceftibuten, which is inactive against *Streptococcus agalactiae* (group B) (Table 5). Against viridans streptococci, cefetamet, ceftibuten, cefaclor and cefadroxil are weakly active or inactive. Cefixime ($MIC_{50/90}$, 0.5/4 mg/L) and loracarbef ($MIC_{50/90}$, 1/4 mg/L) are less active than other compounds ($MIC_{50/90}$, 0.03–0.25 mg/L)(Tables 6–8).

Against *S. pneumoniae,* Baquero and Loza (16) defined three subgroups of cephalosporins against penicillin-susceptible isolates (Fig. 6). Cefixime, ceftibuten, and cefetamet are less active compounds. One of the most active is cefditoren (Table 9).

TABLE 3 • In Vitro Activity of Oral Cephems against *S. aureus*

| | MIC (mg/L) | | | |
| | *S. aureus* Peni-S | | *S. aureus* Peni-R | |
	50	90	50	90
Cefadroxil	2	4	4	8
Cefaclor	2	4	8	16
Loracarbef	1	2	4	16
Cefprozil	0.5	0.5	1	4
Cefuroxime	1	2	2	2
Cefpodoxime	2	4	4	4
Cefixime	16	32	16	32
Cefetamet	>64	>64	>64	>64
Ceftibuten	>64	>64	>64	>64
Cefdinir	0.5	0.5	0.5	0.5
Cefditoren	–	–	0.5	1

From references 25, 94.

TABLE 4 • In Vitro Activity of Oral Cephalosporins Against Coagulase-Negative Staphylococci

| | $MIC_{50/90}$ (mg/L) | | | | | |
	S. epidermidis	*S. haemolyticus*	*S. simulans*	*S. hominis*	*S. saprophyticus*	*S. cohnii*
Cefadroxil	2 / 2	2 / 4	2 / 4	2 / 4	2 / 4	8 / 8
Cefaclor	1 / 2	1 / 2	1 / 2	0.5 / 4	1 / 8	4 / 8
Loracarbef	1 / 1	1 / 2	2 / 2	1 / 4	2 / 4	2 / 8
Cefprozil	0.5 / 0.5	0.5 / 2	0.5 / 0.5	1 / 2	1 / 1	2 / 2
Cefuroxime	0.5 / 1	1 / 2	0.5 / 1	0.25 / 1	2 / 4	2 / 4
Cefpodoxime	1 / 1	2 / 4	1 / 2	1 / 2	4 / 8	8 / 8
Cefixime	4 / 8	16 / 32	8 / 16	4 / 8	32 / 64	64 / >64
Cefetamet	8 / 16	16 / >64	16 / 32	8 / 32	64 / >64	>64 / >64
Ceftibuten	16 / 32	64 / >64	64 / >64	8 / >64	>64 / >64	>64 / >64
Cefdinir	0.06 / 0.1	0.1 / 0.5	0.06 / 0.1	0.06 / 0.1	0.25 / 0.25	0.25 / 1

From reference 25.

TABLE 5 • In Vitro Activity of Oral Cephalosporins against Group B Streptococci (*S. agalactiae*)

	MIC (mg/L)		
	50	90	Range
Ceftetrame	0.125	0.25	≤0.015–2
Cefetamet	1	1	0.5–2
Cephalexin	1	8	0.125–8
Cefaclor	0.5	8	0.125–8
Cefpodoxime	0.06	0.25	0.03–0.25
Cefixime	1.0	2.0	0.5–2
Cefdinir	0.016	0.03	0.008–0.03
Ceftibuten	16	16	16
Cefprozil	0.03	0.06	0.016–0.13
Cefadroxil	0.25	0.25	0.06–0.25
Loracarbef	0.06	0.5	0.06–0.5
Cefdaloxime	0.03	0.06	0.016–0.13
Cefuroxime	0.03	0.06	0.016–0.13
Cefditoren	0.016	0.03	0.016–0.06
Cefcamate	0.03	0.06	0.03–0.03
Cefotiam	0.5	0.25	0.125–0.25

From references 25, 163, 221.

TABLE 7 • In Vitro Activity of Oral Cephalosporins against Group G Streptococci

	MIC (mg/L)		
	50	90	Range
Ceftetrame	0.25	2	≤0.015–4
Cefetamet	0.13	0.5	0.13–0.5
Cephalexin	1	8	0.125–8
Cefaclor	0.06	0.25	0.016–0.25
Cefpodoxime	0.03	0.06	0.016–0.06
Cefixime	0.13	0.25	0.13–0.5
Cefdinir	0.016	0.016	0.008–0.03
Ceftibuten	1.0	1.0	0.5–1
Cefprozil	0.03	0.06	0.016–0.12
Cefadroxil	0.13	0.25	0.06–0.25
Loracarbef	0.13	0.13	0.06–0.25
Cefdaloxime	0.03	0.03	0.016–0.06
Cefuroxime	0.03	0.06	0.016–0.13
Cefotiam	0.03	0.06	<0.015–0.06

From references 25, 163, 221.

TABLE 6 • In Vitro Activity of Oral Cephalosporins against Group A Streptococci (*S. pyogenes*)

	MIC (mg/L)		
	50	90	Range
Ceftetrame	≤0.015	0.25	≤0.015–0.25
Cefetamet	0.03	0.5	≤0.15–1
Cephalexin	0.25	4	0.06–4
Cefaclor	≤0.06	2	0.06–4
Cefpodoxime	0.03	0.06	0.016–0.06
Cefixime	0.13	0.25	0.13–0.5
Cefdinir	0.016	0.03	0.008–0.06
Ceftibuten	1	1	0.25–4
Cefprozil	0.03	0.06	0.016–0.13
Cefadroxil	0.13	0.25	0.06–0.25
Loracarbef	0.13	0.13	0.06–0.5
Cefdaloxime	0.016	0.06	0.016–0.06
Cefuroxime	0.03	0.06	0.016–0.25
Cefditoren	≤0.025	≤0.025	≤0.025
Cefcamate	0.008	0.008	0.008–0.016
Cefotiam	0.03	0.06	<0.015–0.06

From references 25, 163, 221, 303.

TABLE 8 • In Vitro Activity of Oral Cephalosporins against Group C Streptococci

	MIC (mg/L)		
	50	90	Range
Ceftetrame	0.25	2	≤0.015–4
Cefetamet	0.13	0.5	0.03–0.5
Cephalexin	1	8	0.125–8
Cefaclor	0.03	0.13	0.016–0.13
Cefpodoxime	0.5	0.5	0.03–0.5
Cefixime	0.5	1	0.25–1
Cefdinir	0.008	0.016	0.008–0.016
Ceftibuten	1.0	1.0	0.5–1
Cefprozil	0.016	0.03	0.016–0.03
Cefadroxil	0.06	0.13	0.06–0.13
Loracarbef	0.06	0.13	0.06–0.13
Cefdaloxime	0.016	0.03	0.016–0.03
Cefuroxime	1.0	1.0	0.016–1

From references 25, 221.

Gram-Negative Bacteria

Against *Proteus* and *Providencia* spp., there are two groups of oral cephems, those that are poorly active (cefuroxime) or inactive (cefadroxil, loracarbef, cefaclor, or cefprozil) and those that display good in vitro activity such as cefpodoxime, cefixime, cefetamet, ceftibuten, and cefdinir. However, cefdinir is poorly active against *Proteus vulgaris* (Table 10).

Against *Enterobacteriaceae* that are known to produce type 1 β-lactamases, such as *Enterobacter cloacae, Serratia marcescens, Citrobacter freundii,* and *Morganella morganii,* oral cephems can also be divided into two groups: compounds

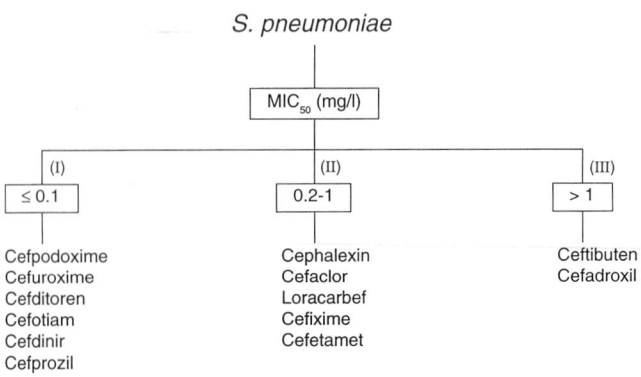

FIGURE 6. *S. pneumoniae.*

totally inactive, cefadroxil, cefaclor, loracarbef, cefprozil, cefuroxime, and to a lesser extent cefdinir and those that display bimodal activity, such as ceftibuten, cefixime and cefpodoxime. Cefetamet is inactive against *E. cloacae* and *M. morganii* but remains active against *S. marcescens*. The four later compounds showed good activity against *C. freundii* (Table 11).

TABLE 9 • In Vitro Activity of Oral Cephalosporins against *S. pneumoniae*

| | \multicolumn{6}{c}{MIC (mg/L)} | | | | | |
| | \multicolumn{2}{c}{Pen-S} | \multicolumn{2}{c}{Pen-I} | \multicolumn{2}{c}{Pen-R} |
	50%	90%	50%	90%	50%	90%
Penicillin G	0.015	0.03	0.5	1.0	2.0	4.0
Cefdinir	≤0.06	0.125	0.25	2.0	4.0	8.0
Cefuroxime	0.03	0.03	0.5	4.0	4.0	8.0
Cefpodoxime	0.03	0.06	0.5	2.0	4.0	4.0
Cefaclor	0.5	1.0	4.0	64	64	128
Cefixime	0.25	0.25	4.0	32	32	32
Cefditoren	0.01	0.01	0.25	0.5	1.0	1.0
Cefprozil	0.03	0.125	0.5	4.0	4.0	16.0
Cefetamet	0.25	1.0	4.0	>32.0	4.0	>32.0
Loracarbef	1.0	2.0	4.0	32	≥32	≥32
Cefotiam	0.125	0.25	1.0	4.0	4.0	16

From references 23, 102, 177, 276, 284, 285, 344.

TABLE 10 • In Vitro Activity of Oral Cephems against *Proteus* spp. and *Providencia* spp.

| | \multicolumn{4}{c}{MIC$_{50/90}$ (mg/L)} | | | |
	P. mirabilis	*P. vulgaris*	*P. rettgeri*	*P. stuartii*
Cefadroxil	8/8	>64/>64	>64/>64	32/>64
Cefaclor	4/4	>64/>64	>64/>64	>64/>64
Loracarbef	2/2	>64/>64	64/>64	32/>64
Cefprozil	8/16	>64/>64	16/>64	64/>64
Cefuroxime	4/4	>64/>64	2/8	2/4
Cefpodoxime	0.06/0.1	0.13/1.0	0.06/0.5	0.06/0.5
Cefixime	0.01/0.06	0.01/0.03	0.01/0.1	0.01/0.1
Cefetamet	0.06/0.1	0.12/0.25	0.06/0.25	0.03/0.15
Ceftibuten	0.03/0.03	0.03/0.06	0.008/0.12	0.01/0.06
Cefdinir	0.13/0.5	8/32	0.06/0.25	0.06/2

Cefadroxil is poorly active against *E. coli* isolates. Cefaclor and cefprozil are weakly active against *E. coli* resistant to ampicillin. Cefuroxime is also moderately active against *E. coli* whatever the susceptibility to ampicillin. The 2-amino-5-thiazolyl derivatives, cefixime, cefpodoxime, cefetamet, and ceftibuten, display identical in vitro activity against *E. coli*.

Cefadroxil, cefprozil, and to a lesser extent cefuroxime are poorly active against *K. pneumoniae* and *Klebsiella oxytoca;* other compounds show good in vitro activity. Cefpodoxime, cefixime, cefetamet, cefdinir, and ceftibuten show bimodal activity against *Enterobacter aerogenes* and *Streptococcus liquefaciens*. Other compounds are inactive against these two microorganisms (Table 12). Except for ceftibuten (MIC$_{50/90}$, 0.5/8 mg/L), other compounds are inactive (MIC > 64 mg/L) or moderately active with two populations, cefpodoxime, cefixime (MIC$_{50}$, 4 mg/L) and cefdinir (MIC$_{50}$, 2 mg/L), with MIC$_{90}$ values above 32 mg/L against *Hafnia alvei*.

Except cefixime (MIC$_{50}$, 4/8 mg/L), the 2-amino-5-thiazolyl cephalosporins show good in vitro activity against *Yersinia enterocolitica*. Cefuroxime and cefixime are poorly active. Other compounds are inactive. Cefadroxil and cefuroxime are inactive or poorly active against *Salmonella* and *Shigella* spp. Other compounds show good activity against these microorganisms, except cefixime, which is weakly active against *Shigella* spp. (MIC$_{50/90}$, 2/2 mg/L) (Table 13).

All available oral cephalosporins are inactive against *Pseudomonas aeruginosa* (MIC > 64 mg/L), *Pseudomonas* spp., *Stenotrophomonas maltophilia,* and *Burkholderia cepacia* and *Acinetobacter baumannii*. They are also inactive against *Bordetella pertussis* (MIC > 64 mg/L).

Against *H. influenzae*, some compounds are inactive (cefadroxil, cephalexin), some poorly active (cefprozil and loracarbef).

In vitro activity of cefpodoxime, cefuroxime, and cephalexin was tested against *Klebsiella rhinoscleromatis*. MIC$_{50/90}$s for cefuroxime and cefpodoxime were 0.06/0.5 mg/L and 0.03/0.06 mg/L, respectively. *K. rhinoscleromatis* is a nonobligate intracellular pathogen (Mikulicz cells) that is responsible for rhinoscleroma, a chronic granulomatous infection of the upper airway (237).

Other compounds display good activity against *H. influenzae*

TABLE 11 • In Vitro Activity of Oral Cephalosporins against *E. cloacae, S. marcescens, C. freundii* and *M. morganii*.

| | \multicolumn{4}{c}{MIC$_{50/90}$ (mg/L)} | | | |
	E. cloacae	*S. marcescens*	*C. freundii*	*M. morganii*
Cefadroxil	>64/>64	>64/>64	>64/>64	>64/>64
Cefaclor	>64/>64	>64/>64	32/>64	>64/>64
Loracarbef	32/>64	>64/>64	8/32	32/64
Cefprozil	>64/>64	>64/>64	64/64	>64/>64
Cefuroxime	>64/>64	>64/>64	4/64	>64/>64
Cefpodoxime	0.5/64	4/64	1/8	0.5/64
Cefixime	2/64	1/16	1/8	2/64
Cefetamet	16/64	2/64	1/2	16/64
Ceftibuten	0.25/32	0.25/2	0.5/4	0.25/32
Cefdinir	16/32	8/64	0.5/16	16/32

From reference 25.

TABLE 12 • In Vitro Activity of Oral Cephalosporins against *Enterobacteriaceae*

	MIC$_{50/90}$ (mg/L)					
	E. coli ampi-R	*E. coli* ampi-S	*K. pneumoniae*	*K. oxytoca*	*E. aerogenes*	*S. liquefaciens*
Cefadroxil	8/8	8/8	8/16	8/8	>64/>64	>64/>64
Cefaclor	4/8	1/2	0.5/8	0.5/1	>64/>64	>64/>64
Loracarbef	0.5/1	0.5/1	0.5/1	0.5/2	32/>64	>64/>64
Cefprozil	2/8	1/2	4/8	4/8	>64/>64	>64/>64
Cefuroxime	2/4	2/4	2/8	2/8	8/64	>64/>64
Cefpodoxime	0.5/0.5	0.25/0.5	0.1/0.5	0.1/1	1/64	2/64
Cefixime	0.25/0.5	0.25/0.25	0.06/0.25	0.03/0.5	1/64	2/32
Cefetamet	0.25/1	0.25/0.5	0.25/0.5	0.1/0.5	0.5/32	0.5/16
Ceftibuten	0.1/0.25	0.1/0.25	0.06/0.1	0.06/0.1	0.5/64	0.25/8
Cefdinir	0.25/0.5	0.25/0.5	0.1/0.5	0.1/0.25	1/>64	4/>64

TABLE 13 • In Vitro Activity of Oral Cephalosporins against Enteric Pathogens

	MIC$_{50/90}$ (mg/L)		
	Salmonella spp.	*Shigella* spp.	*Yersinia enterocolitica*
Cefadroxil	8/8	4/8	16/32
Cefaclor	2/8	1/1	16/16
Loracarbef	0.05/1	0.5/1	16/64
Cefprozil	0.5/1	2/8	16/32
Cefuroxime	8/16	2/4	4/4
Cefpodoxime	0.25/0.5	0.25/0.25	1/2
Cefixime	0.03/0.1	2/2	4/8
Cefetamet	0.5/1	0.5/0.5	0.25/2
Ceftibuten	0.03/0.06	0.1/0.25	0.1/0.25
Cefdinir	0.1/0.5	0.1/0.25	0.5/1
Cefditoren	0.5/0.5	0.25/4	–

From reference 173.

isolates, β-lactamase producing or not. However, they are slightly less active or poorly active against *H. influenzae* isolates resistant to "ampicillin" by a nonenzymatic mechanism (Table 14).

New oral cephem derivatives show good activity against *Moraxella (Branhamella)* isolates whether or not they produce β-lactamases (Table 15).

MECHANISM OF ACTION

β-Lactam antibiotics inhibit peptidoglycan synthesis. Their targets are biosynthetic enzymes, transpeptidases, carboxypeptidases, and endopeptidases. Penicillin-sensitive enzymes have been identified as penicillin-binding proteins (PBP$_S$) located in the outer part of the inner membrane in Gram-negative bacteria and on the outer side of the membrane in Gram-positive organisms. Each bacterial species possesses a characteristic set of PBP$_S$, with different affinity to β-lactams. The differences between oral cephalosporins are related to their affinity for PBP$_S$. *E. coli* possesses 8 PBP$_S$. The major target for available oral cephalosporins is PBP$_S$ 3. To a lesser extent, these compounds show a good affinity to PBP 1a, 1b and 2. Affinities (I$_{50}$) for the different PBP$_S$ of oral cephems are listed in Table 16.

Inhibition of PBP 2 and PBP 3 is required for antistaphylo-

coccal activity. Cefuroxime has good affinity for PBP 2 and 3 of *S. aureus*. Cefdinir has a high affinity for PBP$_S$ 1, 2, and 3 of *S. aureus* 209 PJC, with I$_{50}$s of 0.54, 0.06, and 0.07 mg/L, respectively (MIC, 0.2 mg/L) (126). The lack of activity of cefixime against *S. aureus* and coagulase-negative staphylococci is due to poor binding to PBP 2 (265). Cefetamet exhibits poor affinity for the PBP$_S$ of *S. aureus* (I$_{50}$, 52->100 mg/L, for PBP1 to PBP4) (67).

Cefpodoxime has a strong affinity for PBPs 1, 3, and 4 of *S. aureus* FDA 209 PCJ-I (Table 17) compared with cefaclor and cephalexin (321).

Cefdinir affinity for *Streptococcus pyogenes* C-203 PBP$_S$ 1 to 6 is high. I$_{50}$ values ranged from less than 0.04 mg/L for PBP$_S$ 1, 2, and 3 to 0.53 mg/L for PBP 5 (MIC, 0.012 mg/L) (126).

New oral cephalosporins showed good affinity for PBP 2, 4, and 5 of *H. influenzae* (197) (Table 18).

In *Moraxella catarrhalis* N-5, nine major PBP$_S$ were detected. Cefpodoxime showed affinities for PBP$_S$ 3 and 4, with respective I$_{50}$s of 3.7 and 2.1 mg/L; 50% saturation of the other 7 PBP$_S$ required concentrations in excess of 400 mg/L, the highest concentration tested. I$_{50}$ for PBP 3 of *M. catarrhalis* N-5 for cephalexin is 3.7 mg/L; for other PBP$_S$, I$_{50}$s are above 100 mg/L (301).

PBP$_S$ 4 and 5 of *H. influenzae* are known to be involved in cell wall synthesis and appear to have transpeptidase activity, which, coupled with the affinity, implicates them as important targets for cephalosporins (185).

Against *E. cloacae* 9085, cefetamet exhibits strong affinity for PBP 3 (I$_{50}$, 1.3 mg/L) and PBP 1 (I$_{50}$, 0.3 mg/L) (306).

MECHANISM OF RESISTANCE
Epidemiology of Resistance

Doern et al. (77) in an epidemiologic survey between November 1994 and April 1995, collected 1527 clinical isolates of *S. pneumoniae* in 30 different U.S. medical centers. Cephalosporins with high intrinsic activity against penicillin-susceptible isolates (i.e., cefotaxime, ceftriaxone, cefpodoxime, cefuroxime) were tested as well as other cephem derivatives. Among these isolates, 216 (14.1%) were intermediately susceptible to penicillin G, and 145 (9.5%) were resistant to penicillin G. The

TABLE 14 • In Vitro Activities of Oral β-Lactams against *Haemophilus influenzae*

| | MIC (mg/L) | | | | | |
| | Ampi-S | | Ampi-R β+ | | Ampi-R-β− | |
	50%	90%	50%	90%	50%	90%
Amoxicillin	0.5	1	8	128	16	32
Co-amoxiclav	0.5	1	0.5	2	8	16
Cefadroxil						
Cefaclor	4	16	4	32	32	64
Cefuroxime	1	2	1	4	2	8
Cefixime	0.12	0.12	0.03	0.12	0.12	1
Cefdinir	0.12	0.25	0.12	0.25	1	1
Cefotiam	0.5	1.0	0.5	1.0	−	−
Cefpodoxime	0.06	0.125	0.06	0.125	0.125	0.125
Cefprozil	2.0	16	16	≥32	−	−
Cefetamet	0.12	0.25	0.25	0.5	0.5	1.0
Loracarbef	2	4	2	8	8	32
Cefditoren	0.015	0.015	0.008	0.015	−	−
Ceftibuten	0.06	0.06	0.06	0.06	2	4
Sanfetrinem	0.06	0.125	0.06	0.125	0.25	0.50

From references 42, 69, 71, 94, 130, 148, 276, 337.

TABLE 15 • In Vitro Activity of Oral β-Lactams against *M. catarrhalis*

| | MIC (mg/L) | | | |
| | β-Lactamase− | | β-Lactamase+ | |
	50%	90%	50%	90%
Amoxicillin	0.25	0.5	32	64
Co-amoxiclav	0.06	0.25	0.12	1.0
Cefaclor	0.5	1.0	1.0	4.0
Cefuroxime	0.5	1.0	1.0	2.0
Cefixime	0.06	0.25	0.25	0.5
Cefpodoxime	0.06	0.12	0.25	0.5
Ceftibuten	0.12	2.0	1.0	4.0
Cefprozil				
Cefetamet	0.5	0.5	1.0	1.0
Cefdinir	0.03	0.06	0.06	0.12
Loracarbef	≤0.25	≤0.25	1.0	2.0
Cefadroxil	2.0	4.0	4.0	4.0
Cephalexin	2.0	4.0	2.0	4.0
Cefroxadine	2.0	2.0	4.0	16
Ceftetrame	0.03	0.5	0.12	1.0
Cephradine	2.0	2.0	4.0	8.0
Cefditoren	0.03	0.03	0.5	1.0

Adapted from 24, 28, 41, 42, 56, 68, 80, 148, 172, 219, 256, 276, 293.

percentage of strains not susceptible to penicillin G varied from 2.1 to 52.9% (Miami). Among the oral cephalosporins, cefpodoxime = cefuroxime > cefprozil = cefixime, > cefaclor = loracarbef > cefadroxil = cephalexin.

MIC values of cefpodoxime are summarized in Table 19. No breakpoints for *S. pneumoniae* have been given for cefpodoxime by the National Committee for Clinical Laboratory Standards (NCCLS) subcommittee. Breakpoints were given only for cefotaxime, ceftriaxone, and cefuroxime (resistant MIC = 2 mg/L). In this study, about 12% of the isolates were resistant to cefuroxime.

Some 723 isolates of *M. catarrhalis* were collected from outpatients in 30 U.S. medical centers between November 1994 and May 1995. The overall rate of β-lactamase producing strains was 95.3% (n = 689). NCCLS breakpoints for *H. influenzae* were applied in this study. The percentage of isolates susceptible to cefpodoxime was 99%, compared with 98.5% for cefuroxime and 99.3% for cefixime(80). MIC values obtained for cefpodoxime are summarized in Table 20.

A recent national surveillance study in the United States recovered 1537 isolates of *H. influenzae;* 36.4% produced β-lactamases; 39 strains were intermediately resistant or resistant to ampicillin, and 17 β-lactamase-producing strains were also resistant to co-amoxiclav (modal MIC, 32 mg/L). Modal MICs for oral cephems are higher than those for β-lactamase-producing strains (76).

Consecutive isolates of *H. influenzae* were collected by the Public Health Laboratory, Bath (U.K.) between June 1992 and June 1993. Of 379 isolates, 40 strains (10.6%) were β-lactamase producers. The overall resistance rate for cefpodoxime was 0.3% (142) (Table 21).

Some 352 blood culture isolates of viridans group streptococci obtained from 43 U.S. medical centers during 1993 and 1994 were characterized. High levels of penicillin resistance were noted in 13.4% of the strains; for 42.9% of the strains, penicillin MIC$_S$ were 0.25 to 2 mg/L (intermediately susceptible isolates).

Among the cephalosporins tested, the rank order of activity for five cephalosporins versus viridans group streptococci was cefpodoxime = ceftriaxone > cefprozil = cefuroxime > cephalexin. The percentages of isolates resistant (MIC = 2 mg/L) were 15, 17, 18, 20, and 96%, respectively. *Streptococcus mitis* was the most resistant, and *Streptococcus milleri* was the most susceptible (79) (Table 22).

The MIC$_S$ of *S. pyogenes*, *S. pneumoniae*, *H. influenzae*, *M. catarrhalis*, *S. aureus*, *E. coli*, *K. pneumoniae*, *P. mirabilis*, and *Staphylococcus saprophyticus* collected during 1992 were determined against a broad set of antibacterials including cef-

TABLE 16 • Affinities of Oral Cephalosporin for PBP$_s$ of *E. coli*

| | MIC (mg/L) | PBP$_s$ | \multicolumn{7}{c}{I$_{50}$ (mg/L)} |
			1a	1b	2	3	4	5	6
Cephalexin	8		4	240	>250	8	30	>100	>100
Cefaclor	3.2		1	4.4	130	2	22	>100	>100
Cefuroxime	2		0.12	1.6	13.7	0.09	200	>250	>180
Cefixime	0.05		<0.2	<0.2	16	<0.2	>125	>125	12
Ceftibuten	0.5		>4	>4	>4	1	–	–	–
Cefetamet	0.5		8	2	>50	0.5	–	–	–
Cefpodoxime	2		0.6	0.5	2.2	0.4	13	>100	>100
Cefdinir	0.2		0.09	2.3	1.6	0.07	1.1	>125	>125

TABLE 17 • Affinities for PBP$_s$ of *S. aureus* 209P

| | \multicolumn{4}{c}{I$_{50}$ (mg/L)} |
	1	2	3	4
Cefpodoxime	0.3	2.4	0.9	0.1
Cefaclor	0.6	8.4	0.2	0.1
Cephalexin	0.8	3.2	0.2	0.9

podoxime (100). β-Lactamase production was found in 10% of *H. influenzae* and 80 to 90% of *S. aureus* and *M. catarrhalis*. Among *H. influenzae* isolates, resistance to ampicillin by a nonenzymatic mechanism was recorded in 3% of the isolates. Decreased susceptibility to penicillin G by *S. pneumoniae* was detected in 11% of isolates. Decreased susceptibility to erythromycin A for *S. pyogenes* was 9% in 1992 (Table 23). All isolates of *S. pyogenes* including those resistant to erythromycin A (9%) were fully susceptible to cefpodoxime. Eleven strains showed decreased susceptibility to penicillin G. Six of them were resistant to cotrimoxazole. One strain was resistant to penicillin G (MIC, 2 mg/L), and cefpodoxime had an MIC of 2 mg/L against this isolate. Cefpodoxime was stable to hydrolysis by TEM-1 β-lactamase of *H. influenzae*. MIC$_s$ values reached 4 mg/L against *H. influenzae* resistant to ampicillin by a nonenzymatic mechanism.

In a recent survey (59), 282 respiratory tract isolates and 431 isolates from severe or invasive diseases of group A streptococci were tested against 11 oral antibiotics including oral cephalosporins. Approximately 83% of the 282 pharyngeal isolates could be serologically characterized; 21 different M types were identified. Over half of these isolates were M types 1, 2, 3, 4, or 12. The isolates from severe group A streptococcal infections were predominantly M types 1 and 3. The MIC$_{90}$ for penicillin G was 0.012 mg/L; only one isolate had an MIC of 0.024 mg/L. All of 325 isolates were inhibited by a cephalothin concentration of 0.25 mg/L or less (MIC$_{90}$, 0.1 mg/L). At a concentration of 1 mg/L, cefaclor inhibited 282 isolates (MIC$_{90}$, 0.5 mg/L). MIC$_{90}$ for cefixime was 0.5 mg/L; however 6% of the isolates (16 of 282 strains) demonstrated MICs above the NCCLS breakpoints. Cefpodoxime MIC$_{90}$ was 0.016 mg/L. Eight (2.8%) of the isolates showed an MIC of 0.5 mg/L or above for macrolides (erythromycin A, cla-

rithromycin, and azithromycin). These eight isolates were susceptible to clindamycin. An efflux mechanism of resistance could be involved. Some 9.8% of the 325 isolates were resistant to tetracycline (MIC = 4 mg/L). MIC$_{90}$s for ciprofloxacin were 0.5 mg/L. Slightly more than 9% of the isolates tested showed an MIC of 1 mg/L or above for ciprofloxacin. There are numerous reports of an increased prevalence of group A streptococci resistant to erythromycin A, an agent long considered the alternative for patients allergic to penicillin G.

Cephalosporins showed considerable variation in their in vitro activity against group A streptococci. Cefaclor and cefixime are the less active. Cefixime and cefaclor required 30-fold higher concentrations than cefpodoxime.

β-Lactamase Interactions

Kinetics of Oral Cephem Hydrolysis by β-Lactamases

The rate of hydrolysis (V$_{max}$) is a measure of the ability of an enzyme to hydrolyze a compound bound to its active site. It only measures the activity of the enzyme once the compound has bound. K$_m$ values establish the affinity of the substrate bound to the enzyme; the higher the value, the lower the affinity.

Among the Ó-amino-cephalosporins, cefatrizine and cephradine are more stable to β-lactamases hydrolysis than cefaclor. They are poorly hydrolyzed by TEM-1, TEM-2, OXA-2, OXA-3, and SHV-1. Like cefaclor, they are partially hydrolyzed by *S. aureus* penicillinase. Against *M. catarrhalis* enzyme, cephradine and cefatrizine are partially hydrolyzed, while cefaclor is totally hydrolyzed. They are partially hydrolyzed by P-99 and K-1 enzymes (220). Cefuroxime, cefetamet, cefixime, and cefpodoxime showed poor affinity for TEM-2 and OXA-1 enzymes. Enzyme produced by *K. oxytoca* hydrolyzed cefaclor and cefpodoxime to some extent, whereas breakdown of cefixime and cefetamet was undetectable. All compounds tested exhibited a high affinity for *E. cloacae* chromosomally encoded enzyme. Cefixime, cefetamet, and cefpodoxime were poor substrates for the enzyme of *Proteus vulgaris* 4917 (66).

Ceftibuten is not hydrolyzed by TEM-3, SHV-2 and SHV-3 enzymes, while cefotaxime, ceftazidime and aztreonam are affected. All these compounds are good substrates for SHV-4 and SHV-5 (305). Cefdinir is highly hydrolyzed by TEM-3 compared with cefixime and cefuroxime. Cefuroxime and cefdinir are hydrolyzed identically by TEM-5. They display

TABLE 18 • Affinities for PBP_s of *H. influenzae* MAP

	IC_{50} (mg/L)							
	1	**2**	**3**	**4**	**5**	**6**	**7**	**8**
Cefpodoxime	0.3	0.01	0.20	0.04	0.12	ND	>4.0	0.18
Cefixime	0.4	0.09	0.48	0.009	0.02	ND	>4.0	ND
Ceftibuten	2.37	0.016	ND	0.038	0.023	ND	>4.0	0.47
Cefotaxime	0.2	0.037	0.28	0.0008	0.002	ND	>8.0	0.02

TABLE 19 • Activity of Cefpodoxime against *S. pneumoniae* (National Surveillance, U.S.)

	MIC (mg/L)			
Penicillin G	**N**	**50**	**90**	**Range**
Susceptible	1165	0.03	0.03	≤0.015–4
Intermediate	216	0.5	2	0.06–>16
Resistant	145	4	16	1–>16

Adapted from reference 77.

TABLE 20 • Susceptibility of *M. catarrhalis* to Cefpodoxime

	MIC (mg/L)			
M. catarrhalis	**N**	**50**	**90**	**Range**
β-Lactamase+	689	1.0	2.0	0.6–8
β-Lactamase−	34	0.12	0.25	0.06–1

From reference 78.

TABLE 21 • Activity of Cefpodoxime against *H. influenzae* (U.K. Survey)

	MIC (mg/L)				
Organisms	**N**	**50**	**90**	**Range**	**% Resistant**
β-lactamase−	399	0.07	0.18	<0.03–6.6	0.3
β-lactamase+	40	0.07	0.23	<0.03–0.37	0

From reference 142.

higher stability to TEM-4 than cefixime (308). Cefdinir is not hydrolyzed by *S. aureus* PC-1. Cefprozil is hydrolyzed more slowly by *S. aureus* penicillinase than cefaclor. Cefixime is slightly less stable than cefdinir and cefuroxime to TEM-10 enzyme (235). In direct enzyme hydrolysis studies, cefpodoxime has been shown to be resistant to hydrolysis by the following β-lactamases: type I, Ia, most I_C (J20), II, IIa, IV, IVb, IV (Kc), and V (PSE-1) (318). Compared with cefaclor and cefotaxime, cefpodoxime is stable to β-lactamase hydrolysis of Ia, IIa, IV, and V enzyme (Table 24) (149). These data agree with those of Wise et al. (339, 341).

Cefpodoxime is not a good substrate for BRO-1 of *M. catarrhalis*. The β-lactamase of *M. catarrhalis* belongs to group 2C of the Busch classification. This enzyme hydrolyzes carbenicillin and is inhibited by clavulanic acid. Cefpodoxime is less hydrolyzed by BRO-1 than cefaclor but slightly more than

ceftetrame. However, the affinity for the enzyme is higher for ceftetrame (301) (Table 25).

In Vitro Activity of Oral Cephems against Isolates Producing β-Lactamases

Kitzis et al. (160) tested the in vitro activity of 15 β-lactams against *K. pneumoniae* and isogenic *E. coli* harboring extended-spectrum β-lactamases (ESBLs). All β-lactams were affected by SHV-4 and SHV-5 (Table 26) as well as TEM-3 and TEM-4. Ó-Aminocephems were less affected by TEM-1 and TEM-7. Cefuroxime is not affected by TEM-7; it is poorly active against *E. coli* BM684 harboring SHV-4 to SHV-5.

All of the 2-amino-5-thiazolyl cephalosporins are affected by TEM-3 and TEM-5. They are slightly less active against isolates harboring SHV-1 enzyme, except cefixime. Decreased activity was noted for SHV-2 and SHV-3. *E. coli* harboring SHV-5 enzymes are less susceptible to oral cephalosporins except for cefetamet. These results were confirmed in another study (25). In addition, other compounds were included and other enzymes were inserted in the panel (*E. coli* CF694 TEM-5, *E. coli* HB 80–251 TEM-6, and *K. pneumoniae* CHO CMY-1 (Table 27). Except cefdinir, ceftibuten, and cefetamet, all compounds tested are inactive against *E. coli* CF 604 (TEM-5) and *E. coli* HB 80–251 (TEM-6). Cefetamet and ceftibuten display good activity against *K. pneumoniae* CF-104 (TEM-3) compared with other oral cephems. All oral cephems tested are inactive against *K. pneumoniae* CHO (CMY-1). Cefaclor, cefixime, and cefuroxime are less active than cefdinir against *E. coli* 2639E (TEM-9) (308).

Induction of β-Lactamases

Induction of β-lactamases is an important mechanism of antibiotic resistance in species such as *E. cloacae, E. aerogenes, S. marcescens, M. morganii, C. freundii,* and *P. aeruginosa* (178). The most effective inducers are those that stimulate β-lactamase production at concentrations below the MIC of the inducer for a given strain. Ceftibuten can be classified as a weak inducer of the class I β-lactamases of *E. cloacae, E. aerogenes,* and *S. marcescens,* such as cefotaxime (233). Cefetamet is a poor inducer of β-lactamase from a selected strain of *E. cloacae* (P99 enzyme), the *M. morganii* enzyme, the *K. oxytoca* K-1 enzyme, and the inducible β-lactamases of *P. aeruginosa* (222). Ceftibuten was identified as a potent inhibitor of class-Ia β-lactamase (147); ceftibuten is a weak inducer of class Ia enzyme (233).

Cefpodoxime inhibits the hydrolytic action of β-lactamases from certain strains of *C. freundii, E. cloacae, M. morganii,*

TABLE 22 • In Vitro Activity of Oral Cephems against *H. influenzae* Isolates Producing β-Lactamases and Co-amoxiclav-Resistant

	Modal MIC (mg/L)			
	Ampi-S 977	Ampi-R β+ 560	Ampi-R 17 (β+) Co-amoxiclav-R (MIC ≥ 8 mg/L)	Ampi-R-β−29
Amoxicillin	≤1	32	≥128	≥2
Co-amoxiclav	≤1	≤2	≥8	4
Cefpodoxime	0.06–0.12	0.06	0.06–0.12	0.25–0.5
Cefaclor	4	4	4	16–32
Loracarbef	2–4	4	2–4	16
Cefprozil	4	8	4	32
Cefuroxime	1.0	1	1	4–8
Cefixime	0.03	–	0.03	0.06

From reference 76.

TABLE 23 • Activity of Cefpodoxime in Swedish Epidemiologic Surveillance

	MIC (mg/L)				
Organism	N	50	90	Range	Breakpoint (mg/L)
S. pyogenes	100	0.015	0.015	0.015–0.03	1
S. pneumoniae	100	0.015	0.12	0.015–2	1
H. influenzae	100	0.12	0.12	0.06–4	1
M. catarrhalis	100	1	2	0.25–4	1
E. coli	100	0.5	0.5	0.12–4	1
Klebsiella spp.	100	0.12	0.5	0.06–2	1
E. cloacae	100	1	4	0.12–≥32	1
P. mirabilis	100	0.06	0.12	0.03–0.25	1
S. aureus	100	4	4	2–4	1
S. saprophyticus	100	8	8	4–≥32	1

From reference 100.

TABLE 24 • Relative Hydrolysis Rate of Cefpodoxime vs. Cephaloridin (100%)

		Relative Hydrolysis Rate		
Organism	β-Lactamase Type	Cefpodoxime	Cefaclor	Cefotaxime
E. cloacae	Ia (P99)	4.7	108	<1.0
E. coli	IIIa (TEM-1)	2.9	122	3.2
K. oxytoca	IV (K–1)	3.7	44	3.2
E. coli	V (CARB-2)	2.5	67	<1.0
E. coli	V (OXA-1)	11.7	339	10.5

Adapted from reference 150.

TABLE 25 • Hydrolysis of Oral Cephalosporins by β-Lactamases of *M. catarrhalis*

	Relative V_{max}	K_m (μM)
Cefpodoxime	19	72
Cephalexin	30	41
Cefadroxil	22	35
Cefaclor	216	76
Ceftetrame	10	32

and *Proteus inconstans* but does not inhibit β-lactamase from other Gram-negative bacteria (312). Induction of synthesis of chromosomal β-lactamases in *E. cloacae, P. aeruginosa,* indol-positive *Proteus, S. marcescens,* and *C. freundii* with cefpodoxime increased enzyme activity 0.8 to 2.3-fold. The corresponding figures after induction with cefoxitin ranged from 24- to 270-fold (292) (Table 28).

Outer Membrane Impermeability

Cefetamet demonstrated a better penetration rate across the outer membrane of *P. vulgaris* and *S. marcescens* than cefixime, cefaclor, and cefuroxime (184). The ability of cefdinir to penetrate the outer membrane of *E. coli* was one order of magnitude lower than that of cefaclor and cephalexin, but twice that of cefixime (202). Penetration through the ompF porin of *E. coli* is faster for cefixime than for ceftetrame and cefditoren; penetration rates relative to that of cefazolin are 0.11, 0.31, and 0.36, respectively (154).

Debbia et al. (71) studied the in vitro activity of ceftibuten against an *E. coli* mutant with outer membrane protein alterations. An *omp*F⁻ alteration usually increased the ceftibuten MIC 8-fold, compared with nil or 2-fold changes of *omp*A or *omp*C, respectively (Table 29).

Alterations of PBP_S

Resistance due to alteration of PBP_S is far more common in Gram-positive than in Gram-negative bacteria. *S. pneumoniae* possesses six PBP_Ss (1a, 1b, 2a, 2b, 2x, and 3). The affinity of β-lactams for PBP_S 1a, 2x, 2b, and 2a decreased in penicillin- and cephalosporin-resistant isolates. Altered forms of PBP 1a and 2x with low affinity for 2-amino-5 thiazolylcephalosporins are present in *S. pneumoniae* strains (205). This phenomenon has been observed in *N. meningitidis, N. gonorrhoeae,* and *H. influenzae* (240).

PHARMICOKINETICS AND DOSAGE REGIMENS
Kinetics in Young Adult Volunteers

Single Oral Doses
Among the Ó-aminocephalosporins, highest peak levels after a single oral dose of 500-mg were achieved with cephalexin (C_{max}, 20.7 mg/L), and the lowest with cefroxadin (C_{max}, 4.9

TABLE 26 • In Vitro Activity of Oral Cephalosporins against *E. coli* BM 684 Harboring Various β-Lactamases

	MIC (mg/L)										
	E. coli BM 684	TEM-1	TEM-2	TEM-3	TEM-4	TEM-7	SHV-1	SHV-2	SHV-3	SHV-4	SHV-5
Cephalexin	4	8	8	16	16	8	8	32	256	32	128
Cephradin	8	16	16	32	16	16	16	32	128	32	128
Cefadroxil	8	8	8	16	16	8	8	32	64	32	128
Cefaclor	1	4	8	32	32	2	64	32	128	32	128
Cefatrizine	1	8	32	64	64	8	64	64	128	64	256
Cefprozil	2	4	64	64	64	4	64	>256	256	64	256
Cefuroxime	4	4	4	64	64	4	16	16	32	8	128
Cefotiam	0.25	0.25	0.5	2	2	0.5	1	8	16	2	8
Cefpodoxime	0.25	0.5	0.5	64	32	1	8	8	32	8	32
Cefixime	0.25	0.25	0.25	4	8	0.25	0.25	1	1	8	32
Cefetamet	0.25	0.25	0.25	4	8	0.25	1	1	2	1	2
Cefotaxime	0.06	0.06	0.06	8	4	0.12	0.06	4	4	1	4
Ceftazidine	0.12	0.25	0.50	16	8	8	4	4	8	16	64
Aztreonam	0.06	0.06	0.2	4	4	0.25	0.12	2	2	32	128

TABLE 27 • In Vitro Activity of Oral Cephems against *Enterobacteriaceae* Isolates Harboring TEM-, SHV- and CMY-1 Enzymes

Strains Enzymes	MIC (mg/L)					*K. pneumoniae*		
	K. pneumoniae CF-104 TEM-3	*E. coli* CF604 TEM-5	*E. coli* HB 80-251 TEM-6	*E. coli* TEM-7	SH122 SHV-2	197 SHV-4	160 SHV-5	CHO CMY-1
Cefadroxil	16	36	16	8	64	>64	>64	>64
Cefaclor	32	32	8	4	16	>64	>64	>64
Cefprozil	64	64	16	16	8	>64	>64	>64
Loracarbef	16	64	4	2	1	>64	>64	>64
Cefuroxime	64	16	16	8	16	64	64	>64
Cefdinir	4	8	1	0.5	8	8	16	64
Cefetamet	0.5	2	4	0.5	0.5	4	8	>64
Cefpodoxime	3.2	16	16	16	64	64	64	>64
Ceftibuten	0.25	1	1	0.12	0.25	8	8	>64
Cefixime	8	32	2	0.5	0.25	>64	>64	>64
Cefotaxime	32	2	2	0.25	32	32	32	128
Ceftazidime	32	128	256	32	16	32	32	4
Cefoxitin	16	16	4	8	8	8	8	512

mg/L). Peak serum level of cefprozil (C_{max}, 10.2 mg/L) is lower than those of cephardine (C_{max}, 17.7 mg/L) and cefaclor (C_{max}, 17.3 mg/L). After a 400-mg dose, the C_{max} of loracarbef is lower than that of cefaclor after a 500-mg dose (12 mg/L vs. 17.3 mg/L) but equivalent to that after a 250-mg single dose of cefaclor. After a 400-mg dose of cefpodoxime-proxetil, the peak serum concentration was higher than that of cefotiam-hexetil (C_{max}, 4.5 mg/L vs. 3.4 mg/L), and identical to those achieved after 500 mg of cefetamet-pivoxil or cefuroxime-axetil.

Among the nonesterified cephalosporins, cefdinir has a lower peak concentration after a 400-mg single oral dose (C_{max}, 2.15 mg/L) than ceftibuten (C_{max}, 6.9 mg/L). Cefixime has a C_{max} of 3.6 mg/L after a 400-mg single dose, close to that of cefpodoxime-proxetil, cefuroxime-axetil, or cefotiam-hexetil.

The time taken to achieve C_{max} values (T_{max}) for the new oral cephems range from 1.0 h for loracarbef to above 4.0 h for cefetamet-pivoxil and cefixime. The T_{max} of most oral

TABLE 28 • Fold Increase in Specific β-Lactamase Activity after Induction with Cefpodoxime and Cefoxitin

Organism	N	Cefpodoxime	Cefoxitin
E. cloacae	3	0.9–1.3	90–272
P. aeruginosa	3	1.1–1.6	60–260
Indole + Ve *Proteus*	3	1.0–1.2	25–41
S. marcescens	3	0.8–1.1	13–140
C. freundii	1	0.8	24

cephems is independent of the dose. For cefixime, T_{max} increases with increased dose; T_{max} is 2.7 h for 50 mg and 8.9 h for 2000 mg.

Nonlinearity in the relationship between ascending single oral doses and $AUC_{0-ÿ}$ has been noted for most nonesterified cephalosporins and prodrug ester cephalosporins. For cefpodoxime-proxetil, dose-normalized AUC decreased about 25%

TABLE 29 • In Vitro Activity of Ceftibuten against *E. coli* *omp* Mutants

| | MIC (mg/L) | |
	Ceftibuten	Cefaclor
Control	0.125	1.0
*omp*A[a]	0.125	0.25
*omp*C	0.25	2.0
*omp*F	1.0	4.0

[a]*omp* mutant.

over the dose range of 100 to 800 mg (38). For cefixime, 35% decreases have been noted comparing AUC after 50 mg and 400 mg (45). For cefetamet-pivoxil, dose-normalized AUC decreased 12% with doses between 500 and 2000 mg (302). A linear relationship between AUC and oral doses has been reported for cefprozil (250–1000 mg) (18, 19), ceftibuten (25–200 mg) (212), and cefuroxime-axetil (125–1000 mg) (99).

Among the new oral cephalosporins, the percentage of protein binding of cefpodoxime is the lowest (21–33%), while cefditoren displays the highest degree of protein binding, with about 91.5% of the total serum concentration being protein bound.

Ceftibuten undergoes substantial (about 10%) conversion to the *trans* isomer. The cefprozil parent compound consists of *cis* and *trans* isomers at the propenyl side chain at position 3 of the cephem nucleus in approximately a 90:10 ratio.

These oral β-lactams are eliminated mainly by the renal route. The two carboxymethyl derivatives, ceftibuten and cefixime are partly eliminated by bile (332). For these two drugs, only 40 and 60% of the absorbed drug is recovered in urine. Renal clearance of the free drug ranges between 150 and 100 mL/min for cefpodoxime-proxetil, cefetamet-pivoxil, and ceftibuten. Renal clearances are higher for cefuroxime axetil (Clr, 360 mL/min) and cefprozil (Clr, 230 mL/min). Renal elimination is primarily by glomerular filtration in the first group and by glomerular filtration and tubular secretion in the second. Cefixime shows low renal clearance (80 mL/min) but displays a high hepatic clearance of 60%.

Cefpodoxime-proxetil is an equal mixture of a pair of diasteroisomers (A and B) that possesses optical activity in their ester moiety. Twenty healthy male volunteers received 100 mg cefpodoxime proxetil of each form A and B as a solution in a cross-over design. The mean values of the kinetic parameters are listed in Table 30. There was no significant difference between the three forms in T_{max}, AUC, and MRT. C_{max} and AUC were higher for compound A than for the racemate (+18.7% and +15.7%, respectively; $P < .05$). There was no significant difference between the racemate and compound B. However, considering the slight difference between compound A and racemate, use of the latter is fully justified (175).

Repeated Doses

The pharmacokinetics of cefixime was determined after repeated 200 mg twice-a-day (group I; n = 14) or 400 mg once-a-day (group II; n = 13) dosing for 15 days (Tables 31 and 32). The pharmacokinetics of cefixime after repeated dosing to steady state were similar to the drug profile after single dosing. There was no accumulation of the drug in serum or urine after a multiple-dose regimen for 15 days (90, 93). Given the relative short apparent elimination half-lives of the oral cephalosporins (1–3 h) and dosing intervals, significant accumulations were not seen by comparing $AUC_{0-\acute{y}}$ after the first dose and the last dose of the repeated dosing regimen. The main kinetic parameters after multiple doses are listed in Table 33.

Specific Populations

Renally Impaired Patients

Renal Dysfunction. For all compounds mainly eliminated by the kidney, changes in the pharmacokinetic parameters in relation to the degree of renal impairment have been recorded. Peak concentrations, T_{max}, AUC, and apparent elimination half-life increased and urinary elimination decreased. For all compounds, but cefixime and cefetamet, body clearance and renal clearance are closely related to creatinine clearance. For ceftibuten and cefixime, dose adjustments are recommended only for patients with severe renal impairment (CrCl 3/4 10–20 mL/min). The apparent elimination half-life of cephalexin increases particularly when the creatinine clearance is below 30 mL/min (12).

Hemodialysis. Hemodialysis is warranted in patients with end-stage renal failure. This procedure is typically implemented three times a week, and each dialysis lasts about 3 h. Hemodialysis removed about 22% of a cefpodoxime-proxetil dose (39). Hemodialysis clearance of cefpodoxime was 120 ± 31 mL/min. Cefprozil is removed by hemodialysis; the Cl_{HB} is 87 mL/min. Approximately 55% of cefprozil is removed during the 3-h hemodialysis procedure (273). During a 6- to 8-h hemodialysis session, cefadroxil concentrations decreased by 75% (136). Approximately one-third of a cefaclor dose was recovered in the dialysate (29). For cephalexin, the mean serum concentration at the end of hemodialysis was 3.3 mg/L, compared with 14.7 mg/L at the beginning. The clearance of cephalexin was 25 mL/min (12).

Continuous Ambulatory Peritoneal Dialysis (CAPD). Eight noninfected patients and eight healthy volunteers received a single oral dose of 200-mg cefpodoxime proxetil (145). Only 5.74 ± 3.1% of the dose was recovered from the dialysate. In healthy volunteers, 24.2 ± 13% of the administered dose was recovered from urine, in contrast to only 5.5 ± 6.9% for the five nonanuric CAPD patients. Peak dialysate cefpodoxime levels occurred on the average of 14.8 ± 6 h, with a mean C_{max} of 1.06 ± 0.4 mg/L.

TABLE 30 • Bioavailability of Diastereoisomers of Cefpodoxime Proxetil

	C_{max} (mg/L)	T_{max} (h)	$AUC_{0-\infty}$ (mg.h/l)	Cl_R (L/h)	MRT (h)
Racemate	1.34	2.08	7.0	6.4	4.2
Isomer A	1.59	2.17	8.1	6.1	4.3
Isomer B	1.19	2.38	6.5	6.1	4.3

TABLE 31 • Pharmacokinetics of Oral Cephalosporins after a Single Oral Dose to Young Healthy Volunteers

Generic Name	Dose (mg)	N	C_{max} (mg/L)	T_{max} (h)	$AUC_{0-\infty}$ (mg.h/L)	$T_{1/2}$ (h)	Urinary Elimination (%)	Protein Binding (%)	Reference
Ceftibuten	200	18	9.85	1.75	42.07	2.01	–		20
	400	18	16.99	2.00	79.18	2.29	–	63	20
	800	18	23.34	1.96	117.55	2.25	–		20
Loracarbef	200	10	6.0	1.0	10.6	1.02	–		279
	400	10	12.0	2.0	27.8	1.02	–	25	279
Cefpodoxime-proxetil	100	12	1.4	2.4	7.03	2.1	40.0		314
	200	12	2.6	2.4	14.5	2.3	39.2		314
	400	12	4.5	8.5	26.5	2.4	23.8	21–3	314
	800	12	6.9	2.9	46.4	2.9	27.9		314
Cefotiam-hexetil	200	12	2.16	1.55	4.16	1.0	34.75		
	400	12	3.43	2.26	8.52	0.9	31.92	40	
Cefixime	200	12	2.5	4.3	21.4	3.9	–		90
	400	12	3.6	3.7	25.7	3.1	–		90
	800	12	4.9	4.4	37.7	3.7	–		90
	1600	12	7.8	4.3	56.4	3.5	–	69	90
	2000	12	8.9	3.8	67.0	3.4	–		90
Ceftetram-pivoxil	400	6	4.2	1.5	14.2	1.2	–	74.6	234
	800	6	7.0	1.9	24.8	1.2	–		
	1200	6	8.3	1.8	27.3	1.2	–		
Cefditoren-pivoxil	100	5	1.7	1.4	3.7	0.8	19.9		267
	200	5	3.4	2.0	10.0	1.1	19.6	91.5	
	300	5	4.4	2.0	13.7	1.1	21.7		
Cephradine	500	12	17.7	0.8	27.5	0.61	~90		262
	1000	10	27.7	1.1	4	1.1	84	10–20	239
	2000	5	44.9	1.4	102.5	0.86	89.7		57
Cefprozil cis	500	8	10.2	1.7	29.7	1.33	71		273
Cefprozil trans	500	8	1.2	1.6	3.2	1.33	65		273
Cefprozil cis	1000	6	12.3	2.1	45.9	1.7	56.9		274
Cefprozil trans	1000	6	1.1	1.7	4.3	1.9	37.6	36	274
Cefprozil cis	250	12	6.1	1.5	16.1	1.4	69.2		17, 18
Cefprozil trans	500	12	11.2	1.4	32.0	1.3	62.1		
Cefaclor	250	12	10.6	0.5	8.7	0.5	66.5		17, 18
	500	12	17.3	0.7	17.5	0.6	78.9		17, 18
	1000	6	34.6	1.1	74.5	0.7	52.7	25	181
Cephalexin	250	16	9.3	0.9	14.0	0.5	~80		239
	500	12	20.7	0.7	29.0	0.6	~80	18–2	239
	IND	9	28.5	1.2	61.8	0.8	89.6		98
	2000	5	50.5	1.4	116.3	0.86	91.9		57
Cefadroxil	300	16	9.8	1.2	26.8	1.05	~80		239
	500	12	16.2	1.9	47.4	1.3	~80		239
	1000	6	33.0	1.7	108.5	1.6	89.6	18–2	181
Cefatrizine	250	10	4.1	1.6	15.9	1.9	63.6	63	190
	500	10	7.1	1.6	27.7	2.9	62.9		190
	500	12	7.37	1.79	24.38	1.5	–		61
Cefroxadin	250	–	9.7	1.0	13.4	0.7	97.6	10	343
	1000	6	23.0	1.0	70.1	0.9	78.9		181
Cefuroxime-axetil	250	12	4.8	–	12	–	32	50	123
	500	12	4.9	2.3	19	–	32		99
	1000	6	7.3	1.5	23	–	30		283
	1000	23	9.9	2.1	36	–	30		338
Cefetamet-pivoxil	500	16	4.1	4.0	24.6	2.3	51.3	22	302
	1000	16	7.2	4.23	45.3	2.4	47.4		302
	1500	16	9.4	4.6	64.6	2.5	44.6		302
	2000	16	11.4	4.9	88.3	2.8	44.9		302
Cefdinir	200	16	1.0	3.31	4.08	1.43	23.0	73	249
	300	16	1.55	3.20	6.53	1.46	17.7		249
	400	16	2.15	3.0	8.83	1.43	17.3		249
	600	16	2.35	3.22	9.84	1.50	12.7		249

At 6 and 24 h, mean dialysate cefpodoxime levels were 0.6 ± 0.4 and 0.37 ± 0.4 mg/L, respectively. The cefpodoxime clearance in dialysate was 0.03 mL/min/kg. Main kinetics parameters are listed in Table 34.

Hepatic Impairment

Cefprozil is almost completely absorbed by the gastrointestinal tract. The urinary excretion data show that approximately 40% is cleared through nonrenal mechanism. A study conducted by Shyu et al. (274) showed that the pharmacokinetics of the two isomers of cefprozil are not significantly modified in patients with hepatic impairment. The bioavailability of cefotiam-hexetil is not significantly altered in impaired hepatic patients, AUC is about twofold greater than in healthy volunteers, and the apparent elimination half-life is twice as long as in healthy volunteers.

Cefixime was given in a 200-mg oral single dose to volunteers and nine patients with impaired hepatic function (Pugh index range, 7–12) (245). Peak serum concentrations and AUC were similar for both populations. Apparent elimination half-life was twice that of the controls, as an effect of increased volume of distribution (V/F, 0.51 ± 0.05 vs. 1.05 ± 0.2 L/kg). However, no change in dosing is required in these patients (278) (Table 36).

Elderly Subjects

Several factors that influence pharmacokinetic parameters, such as glomerular filtration, body protein stores, metabolic capacity, and hepatic and renal blood flow, are reduced in the elderly. Age-related alterations in renal function appear to have the greatest potential influence on the pharmacokinetics of oral cephalosporins. These compounds are not highly protein bound nor do they undergo significant hepatic metabolism. A decrease of about 35% in the glomerular filtration rate occurs after age 65 years. Increased apparent elimination half-life and AUC values have been reported for elderly subjects (Table 37).

Bioavailability values for cefetamet-pivoxil and cefpodoxime proxetil in young volunteers were comparable to those in elderly patients. The apparent elimination half-lives for both compounds are significantly prolonged in the elderly as a result of age-related impaired renal function. The AUC of cefixime was significantly higher in the elderly than in the young, whereas C_{max} and urinary recovery values did not differ significantly with age.

The pharmacokinetics of cefprozil in young and aged persons (41–60 years and 61–80 years) were determined (335). The apparent elimination half-lives were greater in the elderly persons than in the younger subjects. After intravenous infusion of cefetamet sodium salt (500 mg) to 12 elderly patients (69 ± 4 years) and 12 young volunteers (29 ± 5 years), the total body clearance was 22% lower in the elderly on average (119 vs. 155 mL/min), which could be due to reduced renal clearance (88 vs. 119 mL/min) in the aged group.

Cephradine was administered to young and elderly subjects either intravenously (5 min) or orally. After a 1-g dose, the total body clearance was reduced by 45% in elderly patients (4.81 vs. 2.64 mL/min/kg), resulting in corresponding 53% increases in mean AUC and apparent elimination half-life. Renal clearance was reduced (4.11 vs. 2.38 mL/min/kg), while the relative bioavailability remained unchanged (94 vs. 94.8%).

Pediatric Patients

The plasma concentrations of ceftibuten (C_{max}) are similar in children and adults. The apparent elimination half-life is constant and independent of age (Table 38). Kearns et al. (157) suggested that there is significant nonrenal clearance in infants (aged 6 to 26 months) of 1.3 ± 0.6 mL/min/kg, compared with renal clearance of 1.0 ± 10.5 mL/min/kg. In adults, nonrenal clearance is estimated to 10 to 20% of the total body clearance.

TABLE 32 • **Kinetics of Repeated Oral Doses of Cefixime in Healthy Volunteers**

	Day 1		Day 8		Day 15	
	I	II	I	II	I	II
C_{max} (mg/L)	1.7	2.8	1.8	3.0	1.9	2.7
T_{max} (h)	4.3	4.4	3.1	4.0	3.3	4.0
$AUC_{0-\infty}$ (mg.h/L)	13.6	24.0	11.9	24.2	12.6	21.6
$T_{1/2}$ (h)	3.4	3.7	3.4	3.7	3.3	4.0
Urinary elimination (%)	14.5	12.4	12.5	11.7	11.9	9.9

TABLE 33 • **Pharmacokinetic Parameters of Oral Cephalosporin after Multiple Doses**

	Dose (mg)	N	Day	C_{max} (mg/L)	T_{max} (h)	$AUC_{0-\infty}$ (mg.h/L)	T1/2 β (h)	Reference
Cefprozil	500		1	11.5	2.3	33.3	0.97	179
	500		8	9.3	1.7	27.5	0.91	179
Ceftibuten	200		1	10.6	–	45.7	18.8	212
	200		14	10.9	–	49.7	2.2	212
Cefixime	400		1	2.76	–	24.6	3.7	90
	400		15	2.67	–	19.9	4.0	90
Cefpodoxime-proxetil	200		1	2.2	3.1	11.8	2.7	314
	200		5	2.3	2.3	11.8	2.3	314
Cefuroxime-axetil	500		1	8.6	2.4	30.3	–	283
	500		21	9.0	1.8	28.6	–	283
Cefetamet pivoxil	1000		1	7.4	4.0	45.7	2.3	168
	1000		10	6.0	4.3	42.5	2.8	168

The ratio of *trans*-ceftibuten in pediatric subjects was 20%, compared with 6 to 7% in adults. The fraction of drug absorbed decreases with decreasing age.

A single oral dose of cefixime (8 mg/kg) was given to 12 infants (aged 2–22 months). The peak serum concentration of cefixime ranged from 0.85 to 6.2 mg/L and occurred at 2 to 8 h after dosing. The area under the serum concentration-time curve (AUC) ranged from 5.3 to 28.04 mg·h/L, and the apparent elimination half-life ranged from 2.6 to 5.6 h (208). Variability in urine elimination values is due to the difficulty of collecting urine in infants.

Eighteen pediatric patients (aged 8 months to 8 years) received a single oral dose of cefprozil (15 or 30 mg/kg). Cefprozil consists of *cis* and *trans* isomers in approximately a 90:10 ratio. The mean apparent elimination half-lives were 1.77 and 2.14 h, and the mean AUCs were 28.05 and 45.28 mg·h/L for 15 and 30 mg/kg body weight, respectively. The peak plasma concentration for the *cis* and *trans* isomers were 12.09 and 1.16 mg/L and 18.04 and 1.63 mg/L for 15 and 30 mg/kg, respectively. In those pediatric patients, the mean peak plasma concentrations and the mean apparent elimination half-lives were slightly higher and longer than those found in studies of healthy adults. The ratio between *cis* and *trans* isomers is equivalent to those described in adult kinetics (252). The pharmacokinetics of cefetamet were determined after intravenous administration (cefetamet sodium) and oral cefetamet-pivoxil syrup to 18 pediatric patients (aged 3 to 12 years). The

TABLE 34 • Kinetics of Cefpodoxime in CAPD Patients

	C_{max} (mg/L)	T_{max} (h)	T_{lag} (h)	$AUC_{0-\infty}$ (mg.h/L)	$T_{1/2}$ (h)	Urinary Recovery (%)
Healthy	1.88	2.44	0.21	10.2	1.98	24.2
CAPD	3.25	12.0	0.56	10.7	24.4	5.5

TABLE 35 • Kinetics of Oral Cephalosporins in Renally Impaired Patients after a Single Oral Dose

Generic Name	Creatinine Clearance (mL/min)	Dose (mg)	N	C_{max} (mg/L)	T_{max} (h)	$AUC_{0-\infty}$ (mg.h/L)	$T_{1/2}\beta$ (h)	Urinary Recovery (%)	Reference
Ceftibuten	≥100	300	6	11.7	2.67	65.6	2.7	67.7	158
	50–80	300	6	13.9	2.83	94.1	3.85	52.6	
	30–49	300	6	13.0	3.17	167.7	7.07	41.1	
	5–29	300	6	19.5	3.0	472.2	22.28	18.0	
Cefdinir	≥100	100	3	0.49	2.0	2.76	1.66	17.7	224
	51–70	100	1	1.49	2.0	10.74	2.41	28.9	
	31–50	100	3	0.73	4	7.48	2.92	10.9	
	≤30	100	2	1.59	8	16.94	4.06	14.25	
Cefprozil cis	>90	1000	6	12.3	2.1	45.9	1.7	56.9	272
trans	>90	1000	6	1.1	1.7	4.3	1.9	37.6	
cis	61–90	1000	6	16.1	1.8	71.9	2.1	53.4	
trans	61–90	1000	6	1.4	1.7	5.4	1.9	30.1	
cis	31–60	1000	6	22.6	2.7	117.0	3.4	46.0	
trans	31–60	1000	6	1.8	2.9	8.3	1.8	25.1	
cis	≤30	1000	6	30.4	3.7	260.0	5.2	23.8	
trans	≤30	1000	6	2.2	3.7	16.1	3.4	10.5	
Cefpodoxime-proxetil	>90	200	6	2.34	2.50	14.8	3.55	32.2	287
	50–80	200	6	3.53	2.58	26.6	3.53	36.2	
	30–49	200	6	3.03	3.67	33.3	5.90	26.2	
	5–29	200	6	3.71	3.75	63.5	9.80	21.7	
Cefixime	>100		6	2.49	2.83	22.0	3.82	27.6	75
	40–80		6	4.65	4.25	71.1	6.60	22.1	75
	20–39		8	5.83	3.68	99.5	8.44	9.2	75
	5–19		6	6.67	4.33	152	13.8	7.1	75
Cefatrizine	>100	500	15	6.9	1.8		1.5	–	60
	10–50	500	15	10.7	2.8	–	2.6	–	60
Cefeamet-pivoxil	>80	1000*	9	5.9	3.9	41.6	2.6	38	162
	40–79	1000	12	7.8	4.1	77.0	4.4	34	162
	10–39	1000	15	12.3	4.9	248	10.6	23	162
	<10	1000	11	41.7	8.4	613	28.8	11	162
Cefuroxime-axetil	>85	250	6	5.2	3.0	21.6	1.4	42	165
	50–84	250	6	5.5	3.0	28.5	2.4	33	165
	15–49	250	7	8.6	3.9	89.0	4.6	34	165
	<15	250	9	10.7	6.3	258	16.8	22	165
Loracarbef	>90	400	10	15.4	1.2	32.0	1.29	94.3	307
	75–90	400	5	18.0	1.5	41.8	1.52	76.2	307
	50–75	400	7	21.6	1.4	67.5	2.45	81.7	307
	10–49	400	10	24.7	1.3	168.8	5.62	49.9	307
	<10	400	8	23.0	3.7	1 085.0	31.6	–	307

TABLE 36 • Kinetics of Oral Cephalosporins in Hepatically Impaired Patients

Generic Name			Dose (mg)	N	C_max (mg/L)	T_max (h)	AUC_{0-∞} (mg.h/L)	T_{1/2} β (h)	Urinary Recovery (%)	Reference
Cefprozil	N	cis	1000	12	16.7	1.8	62.7	1.6	65.8	274
		trans	1000	12	1.8	2.0	5.7	1.2	54.0	
Cefprozil	HP[a]	cis	1000	12	15.8	1.9	70.7	2.2	61.2	
		trans	1000	12	1.7	2.0	6.7	1.5	50.0	
Cefpodoxime-proxetil	N		200	8	2.6	8.4	14.5	2.3	39.2	314
	HP		200	8	1.7	2.6	10.79	2.68	35.0	314
Cefotiam hexetil	N		200	12	2.2	1.6	4.2	1.0	–	
	HP		200	12	2.7	3.0	11.0	2.7	–	
Cefixime	N		200	ND	3.9	3.6	32.2	3.5	16.0	278
	HP		200	9	3.7	5.2	36.2	6.4	43.0	

[a]HP, hepatic impairment.

TABLE 37 • Kinetics of Oral Cephalosporins in Elderly Persons

		Age (years)	N	Dose (mg)	C_max (mg/L)	T_max (h)	AUC (mg.h/L)	T_{1/2} β (h)	F (%)	Ref.
Cefpodoxime-proxetil	Y	31.7 ± 2.2	15	100	1.3	2.7	7.3	2.4	–	314
	E	70.8 ± 1.0	9	100	1.4	3.1	9.0	2.9	–	131
Cefetamet-pivoxil	Y	29.5 ± 5	12	1000	6.2	4.0	39.7	2.2	51.0	32
	E	69 ± 4	12	1000	6.8	4.2	47.2	2.8	46.5	32
Cefuroxime-axetil	Y	–	10	500	11.1	1.8	36.4	1.4		123
	E	65–83 Y	10	500	10.3	2.8	59.4	2.4		324
Cefixime	Y	20–32 Y	12	400	3.9	3.7	28.6	3.2		92
	E	65–74 Y	12	400	4.9	4.2	41.0	3.9		
Cephradine	Y	–	10	1000	27.7	1.1	–	1.1		
	E		9	1000	35.1	1.1	–	1.7		
Cefdinir	E	74–77 Y	3	100	0.85	3.0	4.2	1.8		264
	E	74–77 Y	2	200	1.15	3.5	6.6	1.9		

mean oral bioavailabilities of cefetamet-pivoxil were 49.3% in 3- to 7-year-old children who received a 500-mg dose and 37.9% in 8- to 12-year-old children who received a 1000-mg dose. These values did not differ from those observed in the adult group after two 500-mg tablets (127).

Metabolism

The nonesterified oral cephalosporins are not metabolized, except ceftibuten. The esterified oral cephalosporins are metabolized (isomerization), and the ester side chain is removed by esterases in the intestinal mucosa during enteral absorption and then metabolized.

Ceftibuten Metabolism

Formation of metabolites after oral administration of ceftibuten was investigated using HPLC and thin-layer chromatography. The olefinic isomer of ceftibuten (*trans*-isomer) has been recovered in urine and plasma from healthy and renally impaired patients. After a single oral dose of 200 mg of ceftibuten, urine recovery of the *trans*-isomer ranged from 7.3 to 9.8% of the administered dose, and up to 12.6% after repeated doses (211) (Table 39).

Isomerization of ceftibuten to *trans*-ceftibuten occurred in human serum, but not in protein-free human filtrate, suggesting that human serum protein might contribute to isomerization of ceftibuten. The albumin fraction was found to accelerate isomerization (266). Wise et al. (341) found that the peak levels of the *trans*-isomer in plasma were 4.8 to 7% of the peak *cis*-isomer levels. Of the total amount of ceftibuten, Shiba (263) found 4.3 to 4.5% of the isomer in plasma and 7.2 to 9.2% in urine. In renally impaired patients, renal clearance of the *trans* isomer decreased and the AUC increased (158) (Table 40).

Trans-ceftibuten is an active metabolite, but it is at least eight times less active than ceftibuten (215) (Table 41).

Isomerization of Oral Cephalosporin Esters

The esterified oral cephalosporins undergo reversible isomerization of the Δ3-double bond to give a mixture of Δ3 cephems and Δ2-unsaturated ester. The cephalosporin free acid does not isomerize under the same conditions. By hydrolysis, Δ2 cephalosporin esters yield Δ2 cephalosporins that are bacteriologically inactive.

In the proposed mechanism of the isomerization, a proton in the 2-position is abstracted by a base. The resulting ambident carbanion can be reprotonated in the 4 position, giving

TABLE 38 • Kinetics of Oral Cephalosporins in Pediatric Patients

	Age (years)	N		Dose (mg/kg)	C_{max} (mg/L)	T_{max} (h)	AUC (mg.h/L)	Urinary Elimination (%)	$T_{1/2}\,\beta$ (h)	Ref.
Loracarbef	4.6–16.7	8		7.5	10.6	0.78	21.4	32–94	1.23	209
	0.5–16.6	10		15	18.0	0.83	35.6	26–93	1.13	209
Cefpodoxime-proxetil	1.0–17.2	30		2.7–5	2.24	2.55	11.4	1.45		47.1	156, 204
Cefpodoxime-proxetil	8–11	3		3	2.0	2.0	10.85	44.7	2.03	204
		3		6	4.27	2.0	21.80	43.5	2.23	204
Ceftibuten	0.5–4	20	cis	9	16.2	2.2	72.7	2.38	–	22
			trans	9	3.2	2.5	13.9	–	–	22
			cis	13.5	23.2	2.6	114.8	2.44	–	22
			trans	13.5	3.9	2.6	20.1	–	–	22)
	0.5–3	4	cis	4.5	5.3	–	19.4	1.5	45.7	22
	3–5	6	cis	4.5	8.3	–	28.6	1.8	51.3	22
	6–11	6	cis	4.5	9.1	–	33.6	2.1	38.6	22
	12–17	9	cis	4.5	8.1	–	37.1	2.2	50.3	22
	0.5–3	15	cis	9.0	9.0	–	38.7	1.9	45.6	22
	3–5	15	cis	9.0	9.0	–	38.7	1.9	45.6	22
	6–11	9	cis	9.0	16.2	–	69.1	2.0	54.2	22
	12–17	5	cis	9.0	16.3	–	78.4	2.5	56.9	22
Cefprozil	8 months–8 years	9	cis	15	11.6	1.2	28.0	1.8	–	254
	8 months–8 years	9	trans	15	11.6	1.2	2.9	1.7		254
	8 months–8 years	9	cis	30	15.1	1.6	44.1	2.1		254
	8 months–8 years	9	trans	30	1.6	1.7	4.3	1.6		254
Cefuroxime-axetil	1 month–11 years	11		12	3.9	–	11.3	–	–	111
	11–68 months	22		15	4.6	–	12.6	–	–	111
				20	5.1	–	18.5	–	–	111
Cefixime	2–22 months	12		8	3.1	4.5	15.1	4.3	–	208
	1–13 years	3		6	2.4	6.0	–	5.0	26.0	297
	5–12 years	6		7	5.0	4.0	–	4.8	23.5	297
Cefadroxil	1.1–11 years	16		15	3.7	1.0	0.4	1.3	–	110
Cephradine	13 months–8 years	15		15	21.3	0.5	0.3	0.8	–	110
Cephalexin	2 months–6 years	11		15	23.4	0.5	40	1.0	–	110
Cefaclor	4 months–4 years	10		15	13.1	0.5	20	0.6	–	110
Cefaclor	34 months	7		10	10.8	0.5	15	1.0		192
Cefetamet-pivoxil	3–17 years	9		500 mg[a]	5.2	4.8	37.8	2.8	38.1	127
	8–12 years	4		1000 mg[b]	6.1	4.7	42.6	2.1	29.9	127
Cefdinir	0.5–2 years	6		7	2.04	2.0	6.79	–	1.3	119
		6		15	4.11	2.3	13.0	–	1.2	119
	2–12 years	6		7	2.56	2.3	9.83	–	1.5	119
		6		15	3.60	1.7	13.7	–	1.5	119

[a] 340 mg free acid.

[b] 680 mg free acid.

a $\Delta 2$ ester (250). $\Delta 2$ Isomerization was well studied for cefotiam-hexetil. $\Delta 2$ Cefotiam represents 1.4% of the administered dose in plasma. Peak concentration of 0.06 mg/L (200 mg) and 0.11 mg/L (400 mg) was achieved 2.5 h after dosing. The apparent elimination half-life of $\Delta 2$ cefotiam is 1.3 h.

Metabolism of the Ester Side Chain

Different side chains have been placed on the C-4 carboxylic group. They are released in the intestinal cell wall by esterase and metabolized.

Acetoxymethyl Side Chain (e.g., Cefuroxime Axetil). The acetoxymethyl side chain is fixed on the C-4 carboxylic group of cefuroxime axetil and is metabolized to acetaldehyde and acetic acid. The acetaldehyde is rapidly converted into acetic acid.

Isopropyloxycarbonyloxyethyl Group (e.g., Cefpodoxime Proxetil). The isopropyloxycarbonyloxyethyl side chain is

TABLE 39 • Urinary Recovery of *trans*-Ceftibuten

Ceftibuten	N	Dose (mg)	Urinary Recovery (%)	
			Ceftibuten	*trans*-Isomer
Fasted	6	200 SD	67.4±7.1	9.8±1.7
Fed	6	200 SD	60.4±4.0	7.3±1.3
1st dose	6	200 MD	72.6±11.0	9.2±2.9
15th dose	6	200 MD	84.0±6.0	10.5±2.5
27th dose	6	200 MD	84.8±4.8	12.6±2.4

fixed on the C-4 carboxylic group of cefpodoxime. This side chain is mainly metabolized to isopropanol, carbon dioxide, and acetaldehyde (210).

Pivaloyloxymethyl. Numerous oral cephalosporins bear

TABLE 40 • Kinetics of *trans*-Ceftibuten in Renally Impaired Patients

Creatinine Clearance (mL/min)	C_{max} (mg/L)	T_{max} (h)	$AUC_{0-\infty}$ (mg.h/L)	$T_{1/2}\beta$ (h)	Cl_R (mL/min)	Urinary Elimination (%)
≥100	2.12	3.5	14.12	2.63	49.89	9.8
50–80	1.18	4.3	19.62	5.37	43.03	15.3
30–49	1.71	6.7	52.20	14.29	15.06	14.7
5–29	2.68	11.3	111.68	19.46	6.51	8.7

TABLE 41 • In Vitro Activity of the *trans* Isomer of Ceftibuten

	MIC (mg/L)	
	cis	*trans*
S. pyogenes C-23	0.2	1.6
S. pneumoniae I	3.1	25
E. coli EC-14	0.05	0.4
K. pneumoniae SR-1	0.012	0.1
P. mirabilis PR-4	0.025	0.2
P. vulgaris CN 329	0.025	0.2
S. marcescens ATCC 13880	0.1	0.78
H. influenzae SR 3508	0.1	0.78

the pivaloyloxymethyl (POM) side chain on the C-4 carboxylic group, (e.g., cefetamet, cefditoren, cefcamate). Metabolism of this ester side chain has been studied in detail for cefcamate-pivoxil (213, 269, 313). Metabolism of the pivaloyloxymethyl side chain gave two components, formaldehyle and pivalic acid. The formaldehyde liberated from POM has been hypothesized to be metabolized to carbon dioxide via the C_1 metabolic cycle.

The main metabolite recovered in urine from POM is pivaloylcarnitine (325). Carnitine is an essential cofactor in fatty acid β-oxidation, which takes place mainly in the mitochondrial matrix. Carnitine acts as a carrier of acyl groups to transport fatty acids into the mitochondrion inner membrane, which is otherwise impermeable to coenzyme A compounds, and plays an important role in detoxification of xenobiotics with carboxylic acid in animals and humans.

Three subjects were given 100- or 200-mg tablets of cefcamate-pivoxil 0.5 h after a standard meal. Plasma and urine concentrations of cefcamate, pivalic acid (PA) and pivaloylcarnitine (PC) were assayed. After repeated doses, the free carnitine concentrations in plasma were reduced to 65% of the control levels, and plasma pivaloylcarnitine increased, but all returned to normal 3 to 5 days after completion of the treatment (Table 42).

Other metabolites in humans are glucuronide and glycine conjugates (195). Conjugation with glycine could be a minor route of excretion pivalic acid.

Cyclohexyloxycarbonylethoxy Side Chain (e.g., Cefotiam-Hexetil). The side chain of cefotiam-hexetil is metabolized to cyclohexanol, and then three different metabolites, (1–4), (1–3), and (1–2) cyclohexanediol, are synthesized in the liver.

All these metabolites are detectable in plasma and urine (Table 43). However, cyclohexanol levels remain low. After repeated doses of 400 mg every 8 h for 7 days, cyclohexanol could be detected between 1 and 3 h after dosing. The peak serum level of cyclohexanol is 0.13 mg/L, reached 1.7 h after dosing. The elimination half-life is 1.7 h, for an AUC of 0.42 mg·h/L. It accounts for less than 1.0% of the administered dose in urine. (1–2) Cyclohexanediol (CH) accounts for 36% and (1–3 plus 1–4) for 18% of the administered dose. The elimination half-lives are long, about 17 h. In plasma, the peak concentrations of (1–2) CH and (1–3 plus 1–4) CH are 0.72 and 0.26 mg/L and 1.3 and 0.5 mg/L after administration of 200 mg and 400 mg of cefotiam-hexetil. These peaks are reached after an average of 4.5 h for all metabolites. In severe renal impairment, both compounds accumulate.

Gastrointestinal Absorption

Absolute Bioavailability

All the oral cephalosporin prodrugs exhibit incomplete bioavailability but they are comparable (Table 44). The absolute bioavailability was reported to be 50% for cefpodoxime-proxetil (314), 55 to 58% for cefetamet-pivoxil (294), and 52% for cefuroxime-axetil (99). The cefuroxime-axetil suspension had 10 to 20% less bioavailability than a tablet (81), and the bioavailability of cefetamet-pivoxil syrup is about 30% lower than that of tablets (83). The absolute bioavailability of cefprozil is 89% (273). Absolute bioavailability was not determined for cefaclor and ceftibuten; however, recovery of unchanged drug accounted for 90 to 95% of the administered cefaclor (286) and 75 to 90% of ceftibuten (20). The absolute bioavailability of cefixime is less than 50% (95). Urinary recovery of cefdinir after oral administration is about 36% (268). The absolute bioavailability of cefotiam-hexetil is 45% after oral and intravenous doses of 400 mg. The absolute bioavailability of cephradine is 94% (262). The bioavailability of cefpodoxime proxetil tablets was 82% of that of the oral solution, as determined from AUC ratios (38). Based on serum AUC values, the absolute bioavailability of cefixime was 52.9%, 47.9%, and 40.2% after a 200-mg oral solution, a 200-mg capsule, and a 400-mg capsule, respectively (92).

Mechanisms of Gastrointestinal Absorption

Nonesterified Cephalosporins. Many studies have been conducted to determine mechanisms involved in the oral absorption of β-lactams.

TABLE 42 • Pharmacokinetics of Pivalic Acid and Pivaloylcarnitine (Plasma)

	Dose (mg)	N	C_{max} (mg/L)	T_{max} (h)	$T_{1/2}\beta$ (h)	$AUC_{0-\infty}$ (mg.h/L)	Urinary Recovery (%)
Cefcamate	100	3	0.83	4.3	2.24	5.28	93.7
PA	100	3	0.44	3.7	6.07	2.66	92.5
PC	100	3	0.94	4.3	2.64	7.62	89.1
Cefcamate	200	3	2.06	2.3	1.53	10.08	41.3
PA	200	3	1.0	2.3	4.16	5.10	92.5
PC	200	3	2.07	2.3	3.01	13.69	93.8

TABLE 43 • Kinetics of Cefotiam-Hexetil Metabolites

	(1–2) Normal	CU Renal Imp.	(1–3, 1–4) CH Normal	(1–3, 1–4) CH Renal Imp.
C_{max} (mg/L)	0.72	1.8	0.26	1.1
T_{max} (h)	4.5	6.0	4.4	9.0
$AUC_{0-\infty}$ (mg.h/L)	–	33	–	50
$T_{1/2}$ (h)	15.5	20	16.7	44
Urinary elimination (%)	36	28	18	9.0

Transport System. Oral β-lactams are structural analogues of tripeptides that contain a β-lactam ring, two peptide bonds, and a free carboxylic acid group. The transporter takes up cephalosporins that exist as zwitterions, such as Ó-amino cephalosporins, as well as those that exist as anions (cefixime, ceftibuten). The cephem molecules are discriminated by the membrane protein, and the structure of the side chain is very important for recognition of oral antibiotics as tripeptides. Transport of ceftibuten and cephalexin is stereospecific, depending on the isomerism of the side chain at the 7 position. The *cis* isomer of ceftibuten and D-cephalexin are absorbed, while *trans*-ceftibuten and L-cephalexin are not taken up.

Muranushi et al. (206) showed that there are at least three different transport carriers for oral cephems, depending on the N-terminal amino acid of the carrier and the structure of the 7 side chain of the molecules. The first transport system, exemplified by cefaclor (an Ó-aminocephalosporin), carries aromatic (hydrophobic) peptides such as Phe-Ala-Ala. The side chains of Ó-aminocephems are D-phenylglycine. Depending on the orientation of the D-phenyl of cefaclor, it could be taken for L-Phe.

The second carrier is the concentrative transport system, relatively hydrophilic, that transports an aliphatic peptide such as Gly-Gly or Glu-Ala-Ala. Ceftibuten could use this carrier system. Ceftibuten has a structure similar to the side chain of glutamic acid, and the nitrogen of the thiazole ring is located at the position of the amino group of glutamic acid.

The third carrier is a transport system for peptides with a heterocyclic amino acid (tryptophan or histidine) at the N terminus. S-1090 is mainly absorbed through the oligopeptide, which recognizes a peptide with histidine as the N-terminal amino acid.

Transport through the Basolateral Membrane. Once concentrated within intestinal enterocytes, cephalosporins must go through the basolateral membrane to the bloodstream. A peptide carrier (glycylsarcosine) seems to be located in the basolateral membrane surface and is proton dependent. Cephalexin, cephradine, and loracarbef use a specific basolateral transporter (134, 139).

Esterified Cephalosporins. Cefuroxime, cefpodoxime, cefetamet, and cefditoren are not absorbed by the intestinal mucosa. The C-4 ester increases the lipophilicity of the molecule, which diffuses passively through the intestinal mucosa. Using luminal washing and crude mucosal homogenate, it was observed that hydrolysis of the ester leads to the release of free cefpodoxime. The enzyme involved is a choline esterase. It seems that the luminal cefpodoxime proxetil esterase has a broader specificity than the mucosal one (65). A carboxylesterase seems to be involved in the release of cefuroxime (50). The bioavailability of these compounds could be related to the hydrolysis of the ester chain by esterase within the lumen of the intestine.

CLINICAL INDICATIONS
Upper Respiratory Tract Infections
Acute Otitis Media (AOM)

Otitis media is the most commonly diagnosed disease in infants sand children in Western countries (35). The impact of otitis media is substantial, since it affects most children at least once. Only 20% of the pediatric population do not experience an episode of AOM in the first 3 years of life while almost 50 % experience 3 or more episodes (304).

The use of antibacterial agents for AOM and otitis media with effusion has become a mainstay of medical management for these disorders.

Although it is recognized that 20% of episodes of AOM are caused by viruses, nearly all children with AOM are treated with an antibiotic. Reasons for this decision include the difficulty of identifying the etiologic pathogen at the time of diagnosis and the possibility that AOM can be complicated by superimposed bacterial infections. The third reason for routine use of an antibacterial agent in this infection is the belief that antibiotic therapy eradicates the middle-ear pathogen, shortens the period of morbidity, and prevents suppurative complications. Howie and Poussard (133) demonstrated that antimicrobial therapy was superior to placebo in sterilizing the middle ear fluid (MEF).

Effective treatment of AOM in infants, children, and adults should be based on a knowledge of the bacterial etiology. Amox-

TABLE 44 • Absolute Bioavailability of Oral Cephalosporins

		N	Doses (mg)	C_{max} (mg/L)	Co (mg/L)	T_{max} (h)	$AUC_{0-\infty}$ (mg.h/L)	$T_{1/2}\,\beta$ (h)	Cl_R (mL/min)	Cl_P (mL/min)	Urinary Elimination (%)	F (%)	Ref.
Cephradine	oral	10	1000	27.7	–	1.12	–	1.12	–	–	84	94	(262)
	IV	10	1000	–	57.75	0.08	–	1.12	(4.1 (kg))	4.8 (kg)			(262)
Cefprozil	oral *cis*	8	500	10.2	–	1.7	29.7	1.33	–	–	71	89	(273)
	trans	8	500	1.2	–	1.6	3.2	1.33	–	–	65	103	(273)
	IV *cis*	8	500	–	26	0.5	31.4	1.45	2.4	3.1	76	–	(273)
	trans	8	500	–	2.7	0.5	3.5	1.29	1.9 (kg)	2.8 (kg)	63	–	–
Cefpodoxime-proxetil	oral	12	100	0.96	–	2.3	4.75	2.4	–	–	40.2	50	(314)
	IV	12	100	–	2.97	2.0	10.3	2.3	8.1 (kg)	9.9 (l/h)	80.5	–	(314)
Cefixime	solution	16	200	3.22	–	3.1	26.0	3.3	–	–	21.3	52.13	(92)
	capsule	16	200	2.92	–	3.8	23.6	3.4	–	–	18.0	41.9	(92)
	IV	16	200	–	30.5	0.08	47.0	3.2	29	73	40.8	–	(92)
	capsule	16	400	4.84	–	3.8	39.4	3.5	–	–	18.0	40.2	(92)
Cefotiam-hexetil	IV	400	12	–	–	–	19.6	1.3	24.6	345	70	–	
	oral	400	12	3.3	–	2.5	8.8	1.0	–	–	29	45	

icillin has been considered the drug of choice, however recent microbiologic research demonstrated an increasing prevalence of β-lactamase-producing strains of *H. influenzae* and *M. catarrhalis* from children with AOM. In areas where β-lactamase-producing strains are frequently encountered, the oral cephems and amoxicillin-clavulanate should be considered.

Etiology of AOM. The bacteriology of AOM has been studied extensively. Although some minor variations exist, *S. pneumoniae* is still the most common single isolate. Its contribution to the etiology of AOM has fallen substantially from 10 to 20 years ago, when approximately two-thirds of AOM episodes were due to pneumococci. *S. pneumoniae* and *H. influenzae* have predominated in many studies. *S. pneumoniae* is found in an average of 39% of AOM patients. *H. influenzae* accounts for about 27% of cases; 90% are nontypeable and 10% are type b. The third most common pathogen is now *M. catarrhalis,* which is found in about 10% of cases overall (16, 161).

Group A streptococci have been isolated less frequently in recent years and now account for only 3% of middle ear infections. The overall contribution of *S. pyogenes* to the etiology of AOM varies with the season. In midwinter, *S. pyogenes* can represent up to 10% of isolates. This microorganism is frequently isolated in Scandinavian countries and Japan. *S. aureus* (2%) and Gram-negative bacilli are less common. Infections with more than one pathogen can occur, the most frequent combination being *S. pneumoniae* and *H. influenzae* (4%).

The published bacteriologic data on adult AOM are difficult to analyse for a variety of reasons. Most data include children, and patients with chronic otitis media (in which *P. aeruginosa* is prevalent) are not always excluded. In adults, *H. influenzae* is an important pathogen not only in adult sinusitis, pneumonia, and epiglottis (328) but also in AOM (53) (Table 45).

Penetration of Oral Cephems into Middle Ear Fluid. As highlighted by Bluestone (35), adequate penetration of new drugs into the MEF of patients with otitis media should be demonstrated. After a 25-mg/kg dose of oral cephalexin, the average serum level achieved at 90 min was 25 mg/L, and MEF levels were 5 mg/L (range, 3.1–6.5 mg/L). Concentra-

TABLE 45 • Bacteriology of Middle Ear Aspirates from Adults

	Number of Patients	%
H. influenzae	9	26
S. pneumoniae	7	21
M. catarrhalis	1	3
S. pyogenes	1	3
S. aureus	1	3
Other	9	20
No growth	9	26

Adapted from reference 531.

tions in MEF were lower in younger patients (1–24 months) than in older patients (193).

A single oral dose of cefpodoxime proxetil suspension (4 mg/kg) was administered 2, 3, 4, or 6 h before planned MEF collection. All samples were assayed microbiologically (*Micrococcus luteus,* 0.5–16 mg/L; *Proteus rettgeri,* 0.015–0.5 mg/L). Twenty-four children whose ages ranged from 5 months to 9 years received cefpodoxime-proxetil (Table 46) (322). Van Dyk et al. (322) found that the concentrations of cefpodoxime reached in the MEF at 6 h exceeded the $MIC_{50/90}$ of penicillin-susceptible *S. pneumoniae* (MIC $\leq$ 0.06 mg/L) and *H. influenzae* (MIC $\leq$ 0.06 mg/L) independent of any production of β-lactamase. In addition, MIC_{50} values for intermediately susceptible *S. pneumoniae* and *M. catarrhalis* (MIC_{50}, 0.25 mg/L) were under MEF values at 6 h. However, cefpodoxime levels did not reach the MIC value for *S. pneumoniae* isolates resistant to penicillin G (MIC $\geq$ 2 mg/L). These data were confirmed in an experimental chinchilla model (37). After 5 and 10 mg/kg body weight of cefpodoxime-proxetil, the mean peak MEF levels were 0.20 and 0.24 mg/L respectively (216).

MEF values from studies with cefaclor are summarized in Table 47. In one kinetic study (25 children with serous otitis media) (169) no cefaclor was detected in plasma and MEF 2 h after dosing (15 mg/kg) (Table 48).

Penetration of cefprozil into the MEF was investigated in patients with chronic otitis media. A total of 89 patients ranging from 7 months to 11 years old were enrolled in this study. MEF was removed at times ranging from 0.38 to 5.97 h after oral administration of a single dose of 15 or 20 mg/kg of body weight. Concentrations of cefprozil in plasma were assayed by HPLC and in MEF by microbiologic assay (*M. luteus* A 24959). Lower limits of quantification were 0.1 and 0.02 mg/L for plasma and MEF, respectively. Penetration of cefprozil in MEF was rapid, 0.17 to 3.0 mg/L at 0.5 h after dosing. At 5 h after dosing, MEF levels ranged from 0.18 to 0.59 mg/L (271). Similar results were obtained by Kafetzis (152). After a 15 mg/kg twice-daily dose of cefprozil, 2 mg/L was reached at 2 h in MEF, and the trough level at 8 h was 0.1 mg/L (Tables 49 and 50).

Two studies evaluated the penetration of ceftibuten into MEF in patients with AOM (21). In the first study, 30 pediatric patients received a single oral dose of 9 mg/kg of ceftibuten. Ceftibuten reached a maximum of 4 mg/L within 4 h of dosing. At 12 h, the ceftibuten concentration was 0.52 mg/L. In the second study, ceftibuten levels were higher, mainly due to different methodology. The peak level in MEF was delayed to 2 h from C_{max} in plasma (Table 51).

MEF values for cefixime after administration of a single oral dose of 8 mg/kg, although varying considerably, average 14% of serum values ($\leq$ 0.06–0.12 mg/L), which range from 0.76 to 33 mg/L (334). MEF levels of cefixime (3–5 h after an 8-mg/kg single dose) from AOM and otitis media externa (OME) were 1.32 (0.35–2.86 mg/L) and 1.51 mg/L (0.32–5.69 mg/L), respectively, with serum concentrations of 2.51 mg/L and 4.21 mg/L, respectively, in each group (125).

Loracarbef MEF concentrations, 2 h after a single oral dose of 7.5 mg/kg were 2 $\pm$ 2.6 mg/L and 3.9 $\pm$ 2.6 mg/L after oral administration of 15 mg/kg (171). At 2 h after administration of a 750-mg dose of cefuroxime, MEF levels were 0.73 to 1.7 mg/L (189). At 2 to 5 h after a single 250-mg dose of cefuroxime axetil, MEF levels of cefuroxime were 0.20 to 4.85 mg/L (122). After a single oral dose of 500 mg of cefatrizine, MEF levels were 9.5 and 3.7 mg/L at 3 and 6 h after dosing, respectively, for plasma concentrations of 6.2 and 2.9 mg/L (255). Four to 6 h after a single oral dose of 200 mg of cefdinir, the concentration in the MEF was 0.02 mg/L, and the plasma level, 0.16 mg/L (154).

Pharmacodynamics. The major determinant of efficacy with oral cephalosporins is the time at which drug concentrations at the site of infection exceed the MIC for the pathogen. With both Gram-positive and Gram-negative bacteria, killing occurs when serum concentrations exceed the MIC for only 40 to 50% of the dosing interval. Maximal killing is found when values exceed the MIC for 60 to 70% of the dosing interval. These results were also found with cefpodoxime-proxetil and *S. pneumoniae* (319) (Table 52). Craig and Andes (64) demonstrated that an MEF:MIC ratio between 3.2 and 6.3 correlates with 80 to 85% bacterial eradication, and maximal efficacy is seen when MEF:MIC ratio exceeds 10. It is difficult to evaluate time above MIC in MEF because of methodology problems in collecting and assaying MEF.

Clinical Experience in AOM. Bacterial etiology and antibacterial susceptibility information from recent comparative trials for AOM in children, conducted across the United States, showed that antibiotic resistance in pneumococci was not encountered commonly but was increasing (153, 216). In France, in the Paris area, children with AOM unresponsive to oral antibiotics after 48 h of therapy were referred to an ENT specialist for tympanocentesis and culture of MEF. The mean age of 171 children studied was 16 months. *S. pneumoniae* was recovered from 49 children. 38 isolates were penicillin resistant, and 41 isolates were resistant to erythromycin A; 34 isolates of *H. influenzae* were detected, and about 50% were β-lactamase producers (58).

Clinical outcome is a less sensitive way to demonstrate differences between two or more antibacterial agents than bacte-

TABLE 46 • MEF Levels of Cefpodoxime

Time of Sampling (h)	N	Serum conc. (mg/L)	MEF conc. (mg/L)
2	6	2.64±0.51	0.87±0.67
3	8	2.48±0.75	0.82±0.61
4	7	2.01±0.45	0.49±0.25
6	7	1.01±0.46	0.52±0.24

TABLE 47 • Cefaclor Levels in Middle Ear Fluid

Dose (mg/kg)	Sampling Time (h)	Serum (c) (mg/L)	Sampling Time (h)	Mef (c) (mg/L)	Reference
13.3 b.i.d.	2	3.6	2	1.0	152
	4	0.6	4	0.5	121
15	0.5	7	2	1.1	217
15	1.5–2	6.9	1.5–2	1.3	169
20	1.5–2	13	1.5–2	2.8	85
20 MD	1.5–2	15.5	1.5–2	4.6	87
20	1.5–2	12.3	1.5–2	2.9	87
40	1.5–2	33	1.5–2	4.8	85
40	1.5–2	31.7	1.5–2	5.9	87
40	ND	ND	1.5–2	2.1	30
40	2	3.63	2	0.96	21
	4	0.69	4	0.49	21
	6	–	6	–	21

TABLE 48 • Kinetics of Cefaclor Penetration in MEF

Time of Sampling (h)	Serum (c) (mg/L)	MEF (c) (mg/L)
0–0.5	12.8±6.7	3.8±2.8
0.5–1	16.8±6.5	2.8±2.1
1–1.5	11.2±3.6	2.3±1.3
1.5–2	6.9±2.6	1.3±0.3
2–3	ND	ND
3–4	ND	ND

TABLE 49 • Cefprozil Levels in MEF (Chronic Otitis)

Dose (mg/kg)	Plasma (c) (mg/L)	MEF (c) (mg/L)
15	0.38–15.97	0.06–4.44
20	1.28–21.47	0.17–8.67

TABLE 50 • Kinetics of Cefprozil and Cefaclor Penetration in MEF

Time of Sampling (h)	Cefprozil (15 mg/kg b.i.d.) Serum	Cefprozil (15 mg/kg b.i.d.) MEF	Cefaclor (13.3 mg/kg b.i.d.) Serum	Cefaclor (13.3 mg/kg b.i.d.) MEF
2	5.5	2.0	3.6	1.0
4	4.4	1.6	0.6	0.5
6	1.5	1.0	–	–
8	1.0	0.1	–	–

TABLE 51 • MEF Levels of Ceftibuten

Time of Sampling (h)	Study 1 Serum	Study 1 MEF	Study 2 Serum	Study 2 MEF
2	6.73	0.85	14.48	4.41
4	5.93	4.03	10.02	14.27
6	3.15	1.28	2.72	0.81
8	1.56	0.62		–
12	0.8	0.52	1.28	1.29

riologic outcome (186). However, studies of AOM are difficult to conduct because microbiologic specimens are hard to obtain and symptoms resolve spontaneously in 65% of patients and improve in a further 15% with treatment. In about half of AOM caused by *S. pneumoniae,* the organism persists without treatment, while *H. influenzae* tends to be eliminated spontaneously by endogenous immune mechanisms.

When the bacteriologic failure rate is used as an endpoint, amoxicillin (3%) and cotrimoxazole (12%) are superior to cefaclor (18%) and cefixime (26%) in eradicating *S. pneumoniae,* while cefixime (3%) is superior to amoxicillin with or without clavulanate (20%), cotrimoxazole (19%), and cefaclor (33%) in eradicating *H. influenzae* (132, 161). Cefprozil (15 mg/kg twice daily) was compared with amoxicillin (40 mg/kg)/clavulanate (10 mg/kg) in three divided doses in the treatment of AOM for 10 days in 530 pediatric patients. Clinical response rates were similar (84% for cefprozil vs. 78% for co-amoxiclav). However, cefprozil eradicated the most common pathogens (91% vs. 84% for co-amoxiclav). The eradication rates for *H. influenzae* and *M. catarrhalis* were similar (7).

A randomized multicenter study compared cefprozil (15 mg/kg twice daily) with both cefaclor (40 mg/kg/day in 3 divided doses) and cefixime (8 mg/kg/daily) for 10 days in 394 pediatric patients with AOM (244). Similar clinical response rates were recorded between groups—85% (cefprozil), 89% (cefaclor), and 85% (cefixime). There were significantly more diarrheal episodes in the cefixime-treated group (15.7%) than in patients treated with cefprozil (3.1%) or cefaclor (3.1%). After a follow-up of 14 days, relapse rates were similar for the three drugs: 20.2% (cefprozil) vs. 17.7% (cefixime) vs. 13.3% (cefaclor).

Cefpodoxime-proxetil (5 mg/kg twice daily) and co-amoxiclav (40 mg/kg twice daily) were administered to 143 children with AOM for 14 days. Clinical cure or improvement occurred in 91% of the cefpodoxime-proxetil group and 88% of co-amoxiclav group (196).

Cefetamet-pivoxil efficacy was investigated at two dosages (10 and 20 mg/kg twice daily) in the treatment of AOM in children. In six randomized comparative studies, the efficacy rates of cefetamet-pivoxil and cefaclor (13.5 mg/kg twice daily) were comparable with a 7-day course. In one study, 71 children who were bacteriologically assessable showed the predominant pathogen to be *S. pneumoniae* (25.4%). Bacterio-

TABLE 52 • Time above MIC for Oral Cephalosporin against *S. pneumoniae, H. influenzae* and *M. catarrhalis*

		S. pneumoniae Peni-S MIC₉₀	Peni-S T>MIC	Peni-I MIC₉₀	Peni-I T>MIC	Peni-R MIC₉₀	Peni-R T>MIC	H. influenzae MIC₉₀	H. influenzae T>MIC	M. catarrhalis MIC₉₀	M. catarrhalis T>MIC
	Doses	MIC₉₀	T>MIC	MIC₉₀	T>MIC	MIC₉₀	T>MIC	MIC₉₀	T>MIC	MIC₉₀	T>MIC
Cefaclor	13.3 mg/kg tid	0.5	44	8–16	0	16–32	0	8	0	2	35
Cefuroxime	250 mg bid	0.12	73	0.5–2	55–33	4–8	23–0	2	33	2	33
Cefixime	8 mg/kg gd	0.5	48	4–16	0	32–64	0	0.06	88	0.5	48
Cefpodoxime	5 mg/kg bid	0.25	62	0.25–2	54–0	2–4	0	0.12	82	1	37
Cefprozil	15 mg/kg bid	0.25	78	0.5–4	66–28	4–16	28–0	8	16	2	41
Loracarbef	7.5 mg/kg bid	0.5	42	2–16	26–0	16	0	8	9	2	26

Adapted from reference 64.

logic eradication was achieved by the end of the 7-day treatment period with cefetamet-pivoxil in 28 of 30 patients (2 failures: *S. aureus* and *P. aeruginosa*). In the cefaclor group, 7 of 41 assessable children failed to have a successful bacteriologic outcome (246).

An NCCLS subcommittee recently approved the following breakpoints for cefuroxime (axetil): susceptible, 0.5 mg/L or below; intermediately susceptible, 1 mg/L; and resistant, 2 mg/L or above. No breakpoints are yet approved for other oral β-lactams. Dagan et al. (70) showed good clinical and microbiologic correlation between these breakpoints and the success rate with cefuroxime-axetil in AOM due to *S. pneumoniae* intermediately susceptible to penicillin G.

An investigator-blinded randomized multicenter study compared the efficacy and safety of two dosage regimens of cefdinir (14 mg/kg daily and 7 mg/kg twice daily) with that of co-amoxiclav in the treatment of AOM in pediatric patients. In intend-to-treat analysis, among the 752 patients recruited, clinical cure rates in the three treatment groups were equivalent (85% in cefdinir daily, 84% in cefdinir twice daily, and 81% in co-amoxiclav). No microbiologic evaluation was done (3).

To date, there have been no published reports of cefditoren in the treatment of acute otitis media in humans. In a chinchilla model, ceftibuten, cefixime, and ampicillin were administered every 8 h intramuscularly. No significant differences were noted in the time required to sterilize the MEF (251). Two randomized multicenter studies compared ceftibuten (9 mg/kg daily, 10 days) with co-amoxiclav (40 mg/kg twice daily) or cefaclor (40 mg/kg twice daily) in pediatric patients with AOM. Clinical cure rates were similar in ceftibuten and cefaclor-treated patients, with 88% eradication (36, 193).

Acute Purulent Rhinitis

The diagnosis and management of acute purulent rhinitis of short duration (3/43 days) is one of the most common reasons for a child to be brought to a pediatrician or family physician. There is a controversy concerning antibiotic therapy for the management of rhinitis, which is considered a benign, self-limited infection (260). After 10 days without spontaneous improvement or resolution of symptoms, antibacterials are recommended because of the high probability of bacterial infection of the paranasal sinuses (327). A double-blind controlled study comparing cephalexin with placebo for acute nasopharyngitis showed no significant improvement or resolution of symptoms (311).

Pharyngitis/Tonsillitis

In the early 1950s, the classic studies of Denny et al. (73) and Wannamaker et al. (329) showed that treatment with penicillin G for a minimum of 10 days was necessary to eradicate group A β-hemolytic streptococci (GABHS) from patients with streptococcal pharyngitis and that this regimen prevented rheumatic fever. In 1951, intramuscular benzathine penicillin G was introduced, and it was the reference therapy for streptococcal pharyngitis until the 1970s, when oral penicillin V was introduced. Numerous studies have established that the optimum regimen is 250 mg three times daily with phenoxymethylpenicillin (penicillin V). Erythromycin A (estolate or ethylsuccinate) is considered the first alternative to penicillin V. Increasing erythromycin-A-resistant isolates are being recorded in many countries. A failure rate as high as 15% and common gastrointestinal adverse events have been noted with erythromycin A.

Rationale for Oral Cephems.   In the 1950s and 1960s, bacteriologic failure rates after penicillin G fell below 10%. In the last decade, a disturbing trend toward increased penicillin failures was recorded. Recent studies have documented bacteriologic failure rates of 30% or more in penicillin-treated children (241). Bacteriologic and clinical failures may be caused by the same serotype of GABHS that caused the first infection (relapse) or be due to infection with a different serologic type (recurrences). Prescription of penicillin G for clinical relapse and/or recurrent infection is widely debated.

Several explanations have been proposed to account for the increasing failure of penicillin G in clinical studies: lack of compliance, copathogenicity, or immunologic parameters. Penicillin G may not eradicate β-lactamase-producing organisms from the pharynx (*H. influenzae, M. catarrhalis, S. aureus, H. parainfluenzae*). Penicillin G is inactivated by the lactamase produced by these microorganisms. Repeated penicillin G administration shifts the oral microflora, with selection of β-lactamase-producing strains.

Pichichero and Margolis (243) completed a statistical meta-analysis of all published trials in the English language literature from 1970 until 1990. They compare the bacteriologic and clinical efficacy of cephalosporins with that of penicillin G in the treatment of pharyngitis/tonsillitis due to GABHS. In the 19 studies analyzed, oral cephalosporins had a statistically superior bacteriologic cure rate (92 vs. 84%). Oral cephalosporins reduce the bacteriologic failure rate to 5 to 10% (200). Today, successful treatment of GABHS tonsillopharyngitis has taken on special significance because of the resurgence of serious complications of streptococcal disease.

Bacterial Etiology.   Streptococcal pharyngitis is one of the most common bacterial infections in children and adolescents. It has been estimated that 11% of all school-age children visit the physician annually for streptococcal tonsillitis/pharyngitis (107). Until 10 years ago, it was assumed that group A streptococci were responsible for 30% of pharyngitis cases, viruses accounted for 40%, and the cause remained unknown in 30%. More recently, attention was drawn to group C and G streptococci and *N. gonorrhoeae* (~1%). Streptococci in groups B and F could also cause pharyngitis. The role of copathogens such as staphylococci, *H. influenzae, M. catarrhalis, S. pneumoniae, Prevotella melaninogenica,* and anaerobes in general has been highlighted. Controversy still exists about the role of staphylococci, *Chlamydia,* and *Mycoplasma* (124).

Vincent's angina is due to a combination of two anaerobic bacteria, *Fusobacterium necrophorum* and *Borrelia vincenti.* However, fusospirochetal association represents about 1 to 2% of the normal buccal flora and is especially abundant at the gingival border.

The pharynx and tonsils present the appropriate anatomy (crypts) for deep-seated colonization by difficult-to-treat anaerobes. Peptostreptococci are frequently cultured in tonsillopharyngitis; *P. anaerobius* (40%) and *P. asaccharolyticus* (10%) resistant to penicillin G have been isolated in Spain.

Clostridium haemolyticum, which causes an exudative tonsillitis, or *C. ulcerans* are a rare cause of pharyngitis (201).

In a prospective study, Brook and Gober (46) showed that among the β-lactamase-producing bacteria isolated from childrens pharynx were pigmented *Prevotella, H. influenzae* nontypeable, *M. catarrhalis, Fusobacterium* species, and *S. aureus.* These isolates were recovered from 34 to 37% of the patients. This 2-year study showed a monthly variation in the recovery rate of aerobic and anaerobic β-lactamase-producing

isolates and of *S. pneumoniae* resistant to penicillin G. Maximum recovery of these organisms occurred during winter, when the rate of β-lactamase-producing bacteria reached a peak of 63 to 67%. In contrast, during the summer and fall, the rate declined to a low of 10 to 13%.

Oral Cephem Concentrations in Tonsils and Adenoids.
Concentrations of oral cephalosporins in tonsils are listed in Table 53.

Clinical Efficacy of Oral Cephems

Ten-Day Therapy. Stillerman et al. (291) were the first to report higher bacteriologic cure rates in GABHS pharyngitis patients treated with cephalexin than in those treated with

TABLE 53 • Oral Cephalosporin Concentrations in Tonsils

	N	Dose (mg)	Sample Time (h)	Tissues C (mg/kg)	Plasma C (mg/L)	Reference
Cefpodoxime-proxetil	11	100 SD	4	0.24	1.25	106
			7	0.09	0.39	106
	12	5.0	3	0.06	1.39	13
	12		6	0.05	0.66	13
	12		12	0.05	0.11	13
Cefuroxime-axetil	16	500 SD	1–7	0.5		72
	2	15 mg/kg	0–2	0.15	1.42	143
	5	15 mg/kg	2–3	0.65	1.83	
	3	15 mg/kg	3–4	0.54	2.91	
	3	15 mg/kg	4–5	0.92	3.50	
	6	15 mg/kg	5–6	0.67	2.28	
Cefetamet-pivoxil	25	1000 SD	2	0.82	–	34
			4	1.2	–	34
			6	0.5	–	34
			12	0.3	–	34
Cefprozil	15	7.5 mg/kg	0.7–3.2	0.48–2.42		
Cefaclor	30	500	2	5.2–6	6.1–6.1	141
Cefixime	4	100	3	0.32–0.72	0.9–1.7	103
	1	200	3	0.95	2.5	
	21	4 mg/kg MD	5.3	0.5–0.7	1.2	27
Cephalexin	6	1000	2.5	1.1	24	1
	10	1000	3.5	0.9	ND	1
	5	1000	2.0	2.6	23.9	1
	13	1000	2.0	1.8	11.9	1
	10	1000	5	0.1	ND	1
	15	1000 × 4	2	2.0	16.2	131
			4	2.4	15.9	131
Cefadroxil	10	1000	2.5	3.5	20.6	1
	10	1000	3.5	1.9	ND	1
	10	1000	5	1.6	ND	1
	10	1000 × 2	2	2.0	16.2	131
	5	1000 × 2	4	2.4	15.9	131
Cefatrizine	3	500	3	10.7	7.8	255
	3	500	6	4.2	2.6	257
Ceftibuten	5	400	2.3	2.3	14.1	257
	5	400	4.4	5.3	7.4	257
	5	400	8.3	1.9	2.8	257
	5	400	12.4	1.0	1.3	257
	5	400	24.6	0.3	0.15	257
Cefdinir	2	100	2	0.06–0.3	0.5–1	155
	2	100	4	0.2	0.7–1	155
	2	100	5	0.1	0.4	155
Cefditoren-pivoxil	13	200	1.5–4	0.1–0.09	0.5–2	225
Cefotiam-hexetil	6	200	1	0.5	2.2	203
	6	200	2	0.3	2.2	203
	6	200	2.5	0.1	0.8	203

penicillin. Eight of the clinical trials included in the meta-analysis of Pichichero et al. compared cephalexin with penicillin G or V. In seven of them, the bacteriologic cure rate was higher with cephalexin than with penicillin. In the remaining trial, the cure rates were identical.

Cefadroxil produced high bacteriologic cure rates ranging from 90 to 98% in children with acute streptococcal pharyngitis treated once daily. Cefaclor efficacy was compared with that of penicillin V in 104 children with acute GABHS pharyngitis. Bacteriologic failure rates of 30 and 14% were recorded in penicillin- and cefaclor-treated patients (288). Another trial compared cefaclor with cefadroxil; among the 250 children enrolled, the failure rate was 21.1% with cefaclor and 4.6% with cefadroxil (248). Cefuroxime-axetil (6 mg/kg/daily, in two doses) was as effective as penicillin V (thrice daily) in 93 children. In another study, the bacteriologic cure rate obtained with cefuroxime-axetil in 115 children was 92%, compared with 77% with penicillin V (117). In a comparative clinical trial with amoxicillin, cefixime showed a 93% bacteriologic eradication rate (159).

A total of 348 patients with culture-documented GABHS pharyngitis were randomized to receive 10-day treatment with 20 mg/kg of cefprozil (500 mg/day) or cefaclor (250 mg thrice daily); cefprozil gave a better bacteriologic response (82). Three other comparative studies have been conducted with erythromycin ethylsuccinate (30 mg/kg/day; max. 1600 mg/day in four doses) or penicillin V (191). Bacteriologic cure rates were always better with cefprozil. Five clinical trials compared cefetamet-pivoxil with phenoxymethylpenicillin for 10 days (20 mg/kg daily in children or 1000 mg in adults twice a day). Clinical and bacteriologic outcomes were at least as good as those with penicillin V (236). Most oral cephalosporins have demonstrated better activity than phenoxymethylpenicillin or penicillin G in the treatment of GABHS pharyngitis, including even the oldest ones such as cephalexin, cefatrizine (289), cefadroxil, and cephaloglycin (290).

Five-Day Therapy.   Schwartz et al. (261) and Gerber et al. (108) have shown that shortened courses of oral penicillin or injectable penicillin G produce a bacteriologic eradication rate inferior to that achieved with 10-day therapy. However, since symptomatic improvement is generally achieved within 24 to 48 h of starting therapy, parental or patient motivation to complete a recommended 10-day course of therapy diminished rapidly after 2 to 3 days (242). In 1991, Milatovic found no significative statistical difference between a 10- or a 5-day course therapy with cefadroxil (200). Recent trials evaluating shorter courses (4 to 7 days) of therapy for GABHS tonsillopharyngitis with new cephalosporins demonstrated bacteriologic rates equivalent to those with a 10-day course of therapy.

A prospective, randomized, observer-blind, multicenter study, compared the clinical and bacteriologic efficacy of cefpodoxime-proxetil (10 mg/kg twice daily or once daily) for 5 or 10 days versus penicillin V (40 mg/kg/day, thrice daily) administered to 484 children with signs and symptoms of acute tonsillopharyngitis. Bacteriologic efficacy was evaluated at the end of therapy (4 to 8 days after the completion of treatment) and at long-term follow-up (32 to 38 days after the start of treatment). At the end of treatment, 112 (95%) of 118 assessable patients who were treated with cefpodoxime-proxetil for 10 days and 113 of 125 (90%) who were treated with cefpodoxime-proxetil for 5 days showed eradication of the original infecting strain, compared with 101 of 129 (78%) patients who were treated with penicillin V. At the end of therapy, bacteriologic efficacy for the cefpodoxime-proxetil 10-day and 5-day regimens was 17% and 12% higher, respectively, than that of penicillin V treatment (242).

Acute Maxillary Sinusitis

Acute sinusitis is a complication of upper respiratory infections in 0.5 to 5% of children and adults (326). Amoxicillin is considered the antibiotic of reference in the treatment of uncomplicated acute maxillary sinusitis, with a cure rate of about 80%. Spontaneous recovery occurs in 40 to 45% of all cases, and the bacteriologic outcome is often missed. Aspiration is important for demonstration of secretion in the sinus and for identification of the etiologic agent. Failure to improve with amoxicillin or recurrent sinusitis suggests use of a broader-spectrum antibacterial therapy, including β-lactamase-stable agents.

Etiology of Acute Sinusitis.   The endogenous bacterial flora of the nose of adults contains S. aureus (25–40%) in the nasal vestibule. The posterior nasopharynx usually contains S. pneumoniae (15–25%), H. influenzae (6–40%), S. pyogenes (6%), and S. aureus (12%) (121). Acute maxillary sinusitis usually complicates the common cold or other viral infections of the upper respiratory tract. Culture of sinus aspirates has been used during the past four decades to investigate the bacterial etiology of acute community-acquired sinusitis (120) (Table 54). S. pneumoniae and nonencapsulated strains of H. influenzae are the most frequently isolated pathogens, although M. catarrhalis is being recovered with increasing frequency. S. pyogenes, S. aureus, and other Gram-negative bacilli are occasional pathogens, and sinusitis caused by anaerobic bacteria tends to occur in patients with dental disease (183). Mycoplasma spp. have not been implicated in acute sinusitis and are an unlikely cause of disease. Chlamydia pneumoniae is a more likely candidate, but is not a proven cause at this time.

TABLE 54 • Acute Sinusitis in Adults: Percentages of Respiratory Pathogens in Puncture Aspirate of the Maxillary Antrum

	%[a]	%[b]
S. pneumoniae	20–41	21
H. influenzae	6–50	52
S. pneumoniae + H. influenzae	1–9	–
Anaerobic bacteria	0–10	9
M. catarrhalis	2–4	2
S. pyogenes	1–8	6
Other streptococci spp.	2	2
S. aureus	0–8	1
Coagulase-negative staphylococci	–	6

[a]Adapted from reference 120.

[b]Adapted from reference 151.

However, as aspiration of the sinuses is not undertaken routinely, antibiotics are almost always given empirically. The incidence and relative importance of bacteria causing acute sinusitis in the community has not been changed since the early studies in the 1950s, but their antibacterial susceptibilities have changed and are continuing to evolve.

Other studies have shown a difference between adults and children (299, 326). *S. pneumoniae* and *M. catarrhalis* seem to be more frequent in adults, while *H. influenzae* is less frequent (299).

Concentrations of oral cephems in sinus mucosa are listed in Table 55.

Clinical Efficacy.   Several oral cephalosporins, such as cefaclor, cefuroxime-axetil, cefprozil, cefpodoxime-proxetil, and cefixime were investigated in a few clinical trials, both in children and adults, and were found comparable to amoxicillin.

Lower Respiratory Tract Infections

Lower respiratory tract infections (LRTIs) are the most common infectious disease throughout the world, with an estimated morbidity of 5.5%, including both community-acquired and nosocomial infections, among which LRTIs represent 45 and 25%, respectively. LRTIs can be divided into two pathologic entities: parenchymal and nonparenchymal respiratory infections. In LRTIs, a relevant therapeutic problem arises because the failure to identify the causative pathogen in most cases, both in hospitalized patients and in those with community-acquired infections, means that therapy needs to be chosen with empirical criteria. Empirical treatment of LRTIs requires antibacterial drugs endowed with high efficacy against the three main respiratory pathogens, including β-lactamase-producing strains (*H. influenzae* or *M. catarrhalis*), good pharmacokinetics, and optimal penetration into the tissues of the respiratory tract.

Etiology of Community-Acquired Pneumonia (CAP)

CAP continues to be worrisome because of recent changes in its clinical and epidemiologic characteristics and its association with mortality, ranging from 2 to 21% (96, 188). Prior inappropriate antibiotic treatment is significantly related to a poor clinical course (323). CAP continues to challenge physicians. The causative agents of pneumonia are established in only about 50% of cases. Termed "Captain of the men death" in 1901 by W. Osler, lobar pneumonia was a dreaded disease in the early years of the century, with a case fatality rate from untreated illness of about 30 to 35% (129).

Treatment of pneumococcal pneumonia underwent profound changes after 1944 with the report by Tillet et al. (310) of the treatment of pneumococcal pneumonia with penicillin G. *S. pneumoniae* accounted for over 80% of cases of CAP in the prepenicillin era. The incidence rates of pneumococcal pneumonia vary between 46% (Sweden) and 8% (Canada) and might be related to the use of pneumococcal polysaccharide capsular antigen in some studies and not in others (180).

S. pneumoniae, and microorganisms associated with atypical pneumonia (*Mycoplasma pneumoniae, C. pneumoniae,* and *Legionella pneumophila*) have been identified as the most common causes of CAP in patients who do not have a previous history of aspiration or an underlying risk factor for either tracheobronchial colonization by *H. influenzae* or respiratory tract infections caused by aerobic Gram-negative bacilli. The etiology has been always a source of controversy, with figures such as 0 to 21% of *Legionella* isolates or 0.5 to 75% of *S. pneumoniae* isolates in CAP. Acquired resistance of *S. pneumoniae* isolates to β-lactams and other antibacterials represent a therapeutic challenge and emphasize the need for alternative drugs, especially when oral administration is feasible.

In the 1996 report by Gomez et al. (116), 35 and 23% of *S. pneumoniae* isolates were resistant to penicillin G and erythromycin A, respectively. In other studies, the resistance rates were lower (116), with resistance rates to penicillin G and erythromycin A of 20 to 24% and 10 to 12%, respectively. In France, 35% of *S. pneumoniae* isolates from blood cultures are resistant to penicillin G and 40% are resistant to macrolides in patients suffering with pneumonia (109).

C. pneumoniae is responsible for 6 (31) to 34% (6) of CAP. The proportion of pneumonia due to *H. influenzae* ranged between 8 and 20% (8, 26, 188). Approximately 10% of cases of CAP that occur in an endemic period and up to 50% of cases that occur in epidemic periods are caused by *M. pneumoniae* (101). *S. pyogenes* and other streptococci (viridans streptococci and Lancefield groups C and G) cause pneumonia rarely.

TABLE 55 • **Concentrations of Oral Cephalosporins into Sinus Mucosa**

	Dose (mg)	N	Time of Sampling (h)	Plasma Concentration (mg/L)	Tissue Concentration (mg/kg)	Reference
Cephalexin	500	19	2	19	3.1	164
Cefpodoxime-proxetil	100	3	3		0.34	270
	200	2	1	1.79	0.24	
Cefetamet-pivoxil	500 MD	13	2	ND	0.8–4.5	294
Cefixime	100	4	3	1.4–2.3	<0.01–1.0	103
Cefotiam hexetil	100	4	1–5	<0.1–0.7	<0.1–0.5	104
	200	16	1–6.5	<0.1–0.7	<0.1–0.6	104
Cefditoren-pivoxil	200	13	2–3.5	0.74–3.19	0.11–0.48	225
Cefdinir	100	1	4	0.82	0.32	155
	100	2	4.5	0.76	0.20	155
	100	1	5	0.92	0.55	155

Lancefield group B streptococci are important etiologic agents of pneumonia in neonates and have caused rare cases in adults (89). Two studies have questioned the role of *K. pneumoniae* in CAP (51, 167). *M. catarrhalis* is responsible for CAP in a very small percentage (~1%) (88). Psittacosis and *Coxiella burnetii* pneumonia are unusual infections and occurred in epidemics. Table 56 summarizes the global incidence of different microorganisms in CAP.

These differences may be due to patient characteristics, and they emphasize the need to investigate epidemiologic factors specific to different regions that represent the major basis for the choice of initial empirical treatment. Interest has been renewed in the fluoroquinolone agents, which exhibit activity against a wide range of respiratory pathogens, including those which are not susceptible to the β-lactam or macrolide antibiotics.

Etiology of Acute Exacerbation of Chronic Bronchitis

Since the 1950s, evidence has suggested that bacterial infections are a cause of acute exacerbations of chronic bronchitis (AECB). Bacteria can be primary invaders of the airways, resulting in initial colonization and subsequent infection, or can invade after initial viral or mycoplasma infections. Antibacterial therapy for bacterial causes of AECB has been controversial.

Nontypeable *H. influenzae* (207, 280) is the pathogen most commonly implicated in acute purulent exacerbations of chronic bronchitis, followed by *S. pneumoniae*. Nontypeable *M. catarrhalis*, an emerging pathogen, has been isolated with increasing frequency from patients with AECB. Often these pathogens are associated and are coresponsible. *M. pneumoniae* also seems to be a frequent cause of acute respiratory infections in patients with chronic bronchitis (281).

These microbiologic data emphasize the need for drugs with a wider spectrum than β-lactams.

Tissue Penetration of Oral Cephalosporins

Concentrations in lung tissue, pleural fluid, and the bronchial mucosa have been studied for the different oral cephalosporins. The data are listed in Table 57.

Clinical Efficacy of Oral Cephalosporins

Clinical diagnosis of CAP is based on the presence of fever, cough, dyspnea, sputum abnormalities, abnormal breath sounds, general impaired conditions, leukocytosis, and atyp-

ical chest x-rays. Acute bacterial exacerbations of chronic bronchitis are defined on the basis of an increase in volume and purulence of tracheobronchial secretions and other symptoms.

The efficacy of an antibacterial drug is mainly based on the clinical outcome. The evaluation of the potential antibacterial agents is rarely reported, as well as the microbiologic etiology.

In LRTIs, the clinical efficacy of cefpodoxime-proxetil was compared with that of many different β-lactams (amoxicillin, cefuroxime-axetil, co-amoxiclav). Cefpodoxime-proxetil (100 mg twice daily) and amoxicillin (250 mg thrice daily) are similarly effective in acute exacerbation of chronic bronchitis (174). In a double-blind comparative design study, cefpodoxime-proxetil (200 mg twice daily) is as effective as amoxicillin (250 mg three times a day) in CAP (176).

Studies comparing cefuroxime axetil with other oral antibiotics (amoxicillin, cefaclor, co-amoxiclav, doxycycline) have been carried out in a non-double-blind design. However, it was shown that the bacteriologic efficacy is dose dependent, no effect was seen with a daily dose is below 1 g. Many investigations have involved cefetamet-pivoxil. Cefetamet-pivoxil (500 or 1000 mg twice daily in adults or 10–20 mg/kg twice daily in children) was compared with amoxicillin and cefaclor. With a treatment duration of 7 to 10 days, the clinical efficacies were identical.

Ceftibuten (200–400 mg twice daily) has been compared with cefaclor, but only one was a double-blind study. The two drugs were equivalent in bacteriologic and clinical efficacy. Cefixime was administered in doses of 200 mg twice daily or 400 mg once a day for 8 days. A double-blind trial demonstrated equivalent efficacy and tolerability for the different regimens.

Studies compared amoxicillin (250–500 mg three times a day or 1000 mg twice daily), cephalexin (250 mg four times a day or 1000 mg twice daily), cefaclor (250–500 mg three times a day), and co-amoxiclav (625 mg three times a day). In three double-blind trials with amoxicillin or co-amoxiclav, cefixime was at least as effective.

Acute bronchitis is usually self-limited, and management of fever and cough is the mainstay of therapy. The use of antibacterials remains unclear. Given the self-limited nature of acute bronchitis, studies comparing antibacterials without a placebo are difficult to interpret (259). Randomized, double- or single-blind trials in patients with acute bronchitis compared loracarbef or cefixime with co-amoxiclav or cefaclor. None of these studies included a placebo arm. In two trials, the clinical and bacteriologic outcomes (=91%) were identical, whatever the drug. In a comparative study of cefixime versus co-amoxiclav, clinical efficacy rates were lower (71 vs. 74%).

Skin and Skin Structure Infections (SSSIs)

The resident flora of the skin generally is low in virulence, stable in number, and a frequent cause of skin disease. When the integrity of the skin is disturbed, transient organisms are able to cause primary or secondary SSSIs. Uncomplicated SSSIs, including impetigo, cellulitis, and other pyodermas such as folliculitis are frequent among children and represent a common reason (up to 18%) for visits to pediatric outpatient clinics.

TABLE 56 • Incidence Rates of Respiratory Pathogens in CAP

	%
S. pneumoniae	8–76
M. pneumoniae	0–18
H. influenzae	0–12
M. catarrhalis	~1
C. pneumoniae	6–34
L. pneumophila	1–15
S. aureus	1–9
C. psittaci	0–6
C. burnetii	0.8–3

TABLE 57 • **Oral Cephalosporins in Respiratory Tissues**

	Tissue or Fluid	Subject (n)	Dose (mg)	Sampling Time (h)	Tissue Fluid Levels (mg/kg or mg/L)	Plasma Concentration (mg/L)	Ref.
Cephradine	Lung		500	ND	2.6		
Cefadroxil	Lung	22	500	2–4	7.4±0.7	11.5±1.3	247
	Pleural Fluid	4	1000	3–5	11.4±3.0	9.4±2.5	247
Cefixime	Bronchial mucosa	10	200 MD	3.8	1.5	3.9	339
		10	400 MD	4.3	2.4	6.6	
	Lung	9	200 MD	4	0.78	2.76	105
				7.8	0.32	1.29	105
		14	400 MD	3.7	1.52	3.76	105
				8.4	1.31	2.76	105
Cefetamet-pivoxil	Lung	6	1000 SD	5	0.96		34
				8	1.3		
		6	2000 SD	5	3.2		
				8	2.0		
Cefaclor	Bronchial mucosa	8	500 MD	0.75–1	4.4		187
		6	1000 MD	0.75–1	7.7		
	Lung		500	3	0.12	1.68	138
		ND	500	5	0.29	0.45	
Cefpodoxime-proxetil	Lung	6	200 SD	3	0.63	1.05	62
		6		6	0.52	0.91	
		6		12	0.52	0.36	
	Pleural fluid	18	200 SD	3	0.6	2.7	84
				6	1.9	2.7	
				12	0.78	0.7	
	Bronchial mucosa	13	200 SD	1–5	0.9	1.9	15
Cefuroxime-axetil	Bronchial mucosa	19	500 SD	1–6	1.8	3.9	14
Cefotiam-hexetil	Lung	6	400 MD	3–4	0.25	0.54	199
	Lung	6	800 MD	3–4	0.35	0.69	
	Lung	6	1600 MD	5–6	0.29	0.58	
Cefatrizine	Lung	4	500 SD	2.0	0.9–1.4	7.5–9.6	198
	Lung	4	500 SD	3.0	1.2–1.6	6.5–7.5	198
	Bronchial mucosa	4	500 SD	3.0	9.4–11.4	7.0–8.0	198
		4	500 SD	6.0	3.4–4.5	2.1–3.1	198

Epidemiology of SSSI

Uncomplicated SSSI.   The most common pathogenic bacteria are *S. aureus* and *S. pyogenes*. The next most common organisms from SSSIs are *S. epidermidis* (1.6% in children, up to 16.5% in adults) and *E. coli* (~1% in children, up to 16% in adults).

Bite Wounds.   Dog, cat, and human bites frequently harbor Ó-, β- and nonhemolytic streptococci, *S. aureus*, coagulase-negative staphylococci, anaerobes, and *Corynebacteria* spp. *Pasteurella multocida* is a frequent pathogen in dog and cat bites, whereas human bites may become infected with *Eikenella corrodens* as well as a variety of fastidious aerobic and anaerobic veterinary species (Table 58).

Cefprozil, loracarbef, and cefpodoxime are more active than cefadroxil, cephalexin, and penicillin G against many aerobic bite wound isolates, including *P. multocida* (except cefpodoxime). In vitro activity against *E. corrodens* remains low except for cefpodoxime. Cefprozil and loracarbef are poorly active against peptostreptococci. While some clinicians advocate the use of cephalexin and cefadroxil for bite wounds (49), clinical failures are currently reported. Weber et al. (330) noted that cephalexin and cefaclor do not achieve high enough levels in blood to treat *P. multocida* infections. Some new oral

cephalosporins could be alternative treatments, depending on the origin of the bite wounds.

Complicated SSSI.   *P. aeruginosa* is a common pathogen in puncture wounds of the foot (e.g., the diabetic foot).

Pharmacodynamics

Skin Blister Concentrations.   Cephalosporins exhibit time-dependent killing. Thus, the length of time that the drug concentration at its site of action (e.g., skin blister fluid (SBF)) is above the MIC for a given pathogen is most closely correlated with ability to kill and clinical outcome. Concentrations achieved in skin blisters with different techniques are listed in Table 59. The drug concentration of oral cephalosporins in normal skin is summarized in Table 60.

Pharmacodynamics.   Oral cephalosporins that achieve concentrations above the MIC$_{90}$ of *S. aureus* methicillin-susceptible isolates for 50 to 90% of their dosing interval include cefuroxime (axetil), cephalexin, and cefadroxil. The level of activity against *S. pyogenes* in SSSIs is reached by most of the oral cephalosporins: cephalexin, cefadroxil, cefaclor, cefprozil, cefuroxime (axetil), loracarbef, and cefpodoxime (proxetil). Stone et al. (295) showed that the SBF concentration of cefixime remained above 0.1 mg/L at 24 h. MIC$_{50/90}$ for *S.*

TABLE 58 • In Vitro Activity of Oral Cephems against Bite Wound Isolates

	MIC$_{50/90}$ (mg/L)					
	Cephalexin	Cefadroxil	Loracarbef	Cefprozil	Cefuroxime	Cefpodoxime
Pasteurella spp.	2.0/2.0	4.0/4.0	0.25/0.25	0.25/0.25	0.12/0.25	0.03/0.06
EF-4	4.0/8.0	8.0/8.0	0.5/1.0	0.5/1.0	0.5/16	0.06/0.12
E. corrodens	>64/>64	>64/>64	4.0/4.0	8.0/4.0	8.0/8.0	0.12/2
Fusobacterium spp.	0.25/1.0	0.12/0.5	0.06/2.0	0.12/1.0	0.25/0.5	–
Prevotella, Phorphyromonas and *Bacteroides* spp.	1.0/4.0	1.0/4.0	0.25/8.0	0.25/2.0	0.06/8.0	–
Miscellaneous Gram-negative bacteria	4.0/8.0	8/16	0.25/1.0	1.0/4.0	0.25/2.0	0.5/0.5
Peptostreptococcus spp.	16/64	16/64	2.0/16	2.0/64	0.5/4.0	–
Actinomyces spp.	–	–	–	–	–	0.06/0.06

From references 9, 112–114.

TABLE 59 • Skin Concentrations of Oral Cephalosporins

	Dose (mg)	N	Time (h)	Concentrations		Ref.
				Plasma (mg/L)	Skin Tissue (mg/kg)	
Cefpodoxime-proxetil	100 MD	14	2–3	2.07	0.43	345
Cefditoren-pivoxil	200	5	0.5	5.42	0.35	5
	200	5	1.0	14.94	1.06	5
	200	5	2.0	22.16	1.57	5
	200	5	4.0	22.94	2.25	5
	200	5	6.0	17.20	1.41	5
Cefdinir	100	1	3.0	0.77	0.37	226

TABLE 60 • Oral Cephalosporin Concentrations in Blister Fluid

	Subject (n)	Dose (mg)	C$_{max}$ (mg/L)		T$_{max}$ (h)		T$_{1/2}$(h)		Ref.
			Plasma	SBF	Plasma	SBF	β Plasma	SBF	
Cefpodoxime-proxetil									
Cantharidin blister	6	200 SD	2.1	1.7	2.9	3.5	2.6	3.6	
Suction blister	8	200 SD	2.2	1.6	3.1	4.7	2.7	3.0	40
	8	200 MD	2.3	1.6	2.3	3.5	2.6	2.3	40
	8	400 SD	4.2	2.9	2.9	4.3	2.6	2.7	40
	8	400 MD	4.1	2.8	2.4	3.5	2.7	3.2	40
Cefetamet-pivoxil									
Cantharidin blister	9	500 MD	5.1	4.8	2.8	3.9	2.3	3.1	294
Cefixime (cantharidin blister)	6	400 SD	3.7	3.2	3.7	6.7	3.8	4.1	295
Ceftibuten (canthuridin blister)	6	200 MD	10.9	9.2	1.8	3.7	2.5	1.1	341
Cefprozil									
Cantharidin blister	6	500 SD	9.6	4.9	1.9	3.5	1.4	1.4	232
Suction blister	12	250 SD	6.1	3.0	1.5	2.4	1.4	2.4	18
	12	500 SD	11.2	5.8	1.4	2.5	1.3	2.2	18
Cefaclor	12	250 SD	10.6	3.6	0.5	1.1	0.5	1.5	18
	12	500 SD	17.3	6.5	0.7	1.0	0.6	1.4	18
Cefuroxime axetil		600 SD	6.4	4.1	2.5	3.3	1.1	1.9	
Cefotiam-hexetil									
Cantharidin blister	6	400 SD	2.6	0.9	2.1	3.5	0.8	2.6	166
Suction blister	6	400 SD	2.6	0.9	2.1	3.3	0.8	4.6	166
Cefdinir		200	1.0	0.5	3.3	4.9	1.4	3.4	249
		300	1.6	0.7	3.2	4.9	1.5	3.7	249
		400	2.2	0.9	3.0	4.8	1.4	3.9	249
		600	2.4	1.1	3.2	4.8	1.5	3.7	249

pyogenes is 0.1 mg/L or less, but MIC$_{50/90}$ is above the peak SBF concentration (C$_{max}$, 3.2 ± 1.0 mg/L) for methicillin-sensitive *S. aureus*. Concentrations of cefprozil in SBF are above the MIC$_{50/90}$ of *S. pyogenes* up to 8 h (C$_{8h}$, 0.3–1 mg/L) but remain above the MIC$_{50/90}$ against *S. aureus* up to 3 to 4 h (C$_{4h}$, 3.2–6.9 mg/L) (232). After 200 or 400 mg, single or multiple dose, SBF levels remain above the MIC$_{50/90}$ of *S. pyogenes* up to 24 h.

Clinical Efficacy of Oral Cephalosporins

Standard therapies during the past three decades for treatment of uncomplicated SSSIs have been erythromycin A, dicloxacillin, and cephalexin. Clindamycin has been used for such SSSIs as furunculosis due to *S. aureus*. The major limitations of erythromycin A are gastrointestinal intolerance and emergence of erythromycin A–resistant isolates of *S. pyogenes* and *S. aureus*. Dicloxacillin is unpalatable for children. Before 1990, cefadroxil, cefaclor, and cephradine were approved for treatment of uncomplicated SSSIs, but they were used as second-line therapy.

The focus when treating uncomplicated SSSI in children must be therapy that is effective against both *S. aureus* and *S. pyogenes*. Although treatment with an antibiotic decreases the healing time of lesions of impetigo from about 2 weeks to 7 to 10 days; it does not appear to prevent acute poststreptococcal glomerulonephritis. However, prompt treatment can decrease the risk of bacteria and prevent the spread of nephritogenic strains of *S. pyogenes*.

A series of randomized, multicenter studies compared the efficacy and safety of cefpodoxime-proxetil, loracarbef, cefdinir (300), and cefprozil with those of co-amoxiclav for the treatment of such SSSIs as cellulitis, impetigo, pyoderma, furunculosis, infected wounds, and subcutaneous abscesses. Study methodologies were identical for all studies, but most of the evaluable trials contain methodology problems, including poor blinding methods, broad diagnostic categories, small sample sizes, and dropped patients (failed to incorporate in intention-to-treat analysis).

With all drugs tested, clinical and microbiologic responses were both favorable in 85 to 100% of patients evaluated. In one study, recurrent bacterial infections were documented (loracarbef vs. cefaclor). The incidence was 5 and 3% for loracarbef and cefaclor, respectively.

Sexually Transmitted Diseases

Sexually transmitted diseases (STD) are mainly due to *N. gonorrhoeae*, *Treponema pallidum* (syphilis), *Haemophilus ducreyi* (chancroid), *Gardnerella vaginalis*, and atypical microorganisms, *Chlamydia trachomatis* and *Ureaplasma urealyticum* (nongonococcal urethritis). β-Lactam antibiotics could be used for the treatment of gonorrhea, chancroid, or syphilis. However, cephalosporins are mainly recommended for gonorrhea. A progressive decrease in susceptibility of *N. gonorrhoeae* to penicillin G and the rapid spread of penicillinase-producing *N. gonorrhoeae* (PPNG) as well as increased resistance to spectinomycin have led to the search for alternative treatment for gonorrhea.

In Vitro Activity of Oral Cephalosporins against STD Pathogens

Neisseria gonorrhoeae. New oral cephalosporins are very active in vitro against *N. gonorrhoeae* producing penicillinase. However, Ó-amino-cephalosporins, such as cefadroxil, cefaclor, cefprozil, cefroxadine, and cephradine are less active than the new cephem derivatives such as cefpodoxime or cefixime (Table 61). MIC values for those compounds depend on the level of resistance to penicillin G. However, cefixime, cefpodoxime and other new derivatives are slightly less active against PPNG.

Against chromosomally resistant (CMRNG) isolates and spectinomycin-resistant isolates (SPRNG), cefpodoxime and cefuroxime display good in vitro activity. However, they are less active against CMRNG strains than against susceptible ones (Table 62) (258).

Haemophilus ducreyi. The in vitro efficacy of cefetamet, ceftetrame, cefpodoxime and ceftriaxone was tested against 100 isolates of *H. ducreyi* (Table 63) (115). Ceftriaxone is more active than oral cephalosporins tested against *H. ducreyi*.

Gardnerella vaginalis. MIC$_{50}$ values against *G. vaginalis* are 0.5 mg/L and 2 mg/L for cefpodoxime and cefetamet, respectively.

Clinical Efficacy of Oral Cephalosporins

With the emergence of PPNG isolates as well as spectinomycin-resistant strains, the efficacy of oral cephalosporins as an oral alternative treatment for gonococcal infection was assessed. More recently, concern has been raised about the emergence of clinical isolates with decreased susceptibility to fluoroquinolones in certain parts of the world. Discouraging results were obtained with cephalexin (336). Cefaclor was effective at a single oral dose of 3 g in the treatment of uncomplicated gonococcal infections, even those due to PPNG (170, 316). A total of 43 male patients with acute gonococcal urethritis were treated with a single 400-mg oral dose of cefixime. Good bacteriologic cure rates were recorded at follow-up 17 days after dosing (11).

A total of 832 patients received a single oral dose of cefuroxime-axetil (1000 mg) or ciprofloxacin (500 mg) for the treatment of uncomplicated gonorrhea due to PPNG. The design was a randomized, multicenter, investigator-blind trial. *N. gonorrhoeae* was eradicated from the cervix in 114 of 118 (99%) and 118 of 119 (99%) bacteriologically evaluable females treated with cefuroxime axetil and ciprofloxacin, respectively, and from the urethra in 154 of 166 (93%) and 171 of 171 (100%) bacteriologically evaluable male patients treated with cefuroxime-axetil and ciprofloxacin, respectively (P < .001). Both treatments were effective in eradicating PPNG in females with rectal infections (29 of 30 in the cefuroxime-axetil group vs. 24 of 25 in the ciprofloxacin group). In small numbers of patients, cefuroxime-axetil was less effective than ciprofloxacin in treating males with pharyngeal infections (4 of 10 in the cefuroxime-axetil group versus 8 of 8 patients in the ciprofloxacin-treated group) (309).

Cefpodoxime-proxetil efficacy was tested in an open-labeled uncontrolled study in uncomplicated gonorrhea in

TABLE 61 • In Vitro Activity of Oral Cephems against *N. gonorrhoeae*

| | MIC (mg/L) | | | |
| | Penicillin-S | | Penicillin-R (MIC : 64 mg/L) | |
	50	90	50	90
Cefpodoxime	0.008	0.03	0.03	0.06
Cefixime	0.008	0.01	0.01	0.03
Cefuroxime	0.06	0.125	0.25	1.0
Cefetamet	0.01	0.06	0.03	0.06
Ceftetrame	≤0.025	0.05	–	–
Cefditoren	≤0.004	0.008	0.008	0.006
Cefdinir	0.008	0.03	0.01	0.06
Ceftibuten	0.06	0.25	0.1	0.50
Cefadroxil	8.0	64	16	64
Cefaclor	8.0	32	>16	>64
Loracarbef	0.5	2.0	1.0	4.0
Cefprozil	8.0	32	16	>64

From references 25, 94, 223, 303.

TABLE 62 • In Vitro Activity of Cefpodoxime and Cefuroxime against CMRNG and SPRNG Isolates

| | MIC (mg/L) | | | |
| | CMRNG | | SPRNG | |
	50	90	50	90
Cefpodoxime	0.03	0.125	≤0.008	0.015
Cefuroxime	0.25	1.0	0.015	0.125
Ceftriaxone	≤0.008	0.03	≤0.008	≤0.008
Spectinomycin	–	–	>256	>256

TABLE 63 • In Vitro Activity of Cefetamet against *H. ducreyi*

| | MIC (mg/L) | |
	50	90
Cefetamet	0.25	0.50
Ceftetrame	0.015	0.03
Ceftriaxone	0.004	0.004
Cefpodoxime	0.03	0.06

males at a single oral dose of 50, 100, 200, 400, or 600 mg. *N. gonorrhoeae* was eradicated (100%) in every evaluable patients in each dosage group (230). The Centers for Disease Control (CDC) (U.S.) (54) in 1993 recommended ceftriaxone (intramuscular administration), ciprofloxacin, ofloxacin, and cefixime (oral administration) as the single-dose regimen of choice in the treatment of uncomplicated gonorrhea.

Urinary Tract Infections (UTIs)

Urinary tract infections are the second most common bacterial (296) infections encountered in medical practice, after up-

per respiratory tract infections. Infections may involve the upper tract (pyelonephritis) or be limited to the lower tract. They are more frequent in women than in men until age 60.

Epidemiology

In uncomplicated community-acquired UTIs, the most common pathogen is *E. coli* (70–85%). Other uropathogens include *Klebsiella* spp., *Enterobacter* spp. (6–9%), *P. mirabilis* (0–4%), coagulase-negative staphylococci (4–14%), and *Enterococcus* spp. (0–2%). Nosocomial UTIs and catheter-associated UTIs have a different uropathogenic spectrum. While *E. coli* is still a frequent isolate (32%), there is an increased incidence of resistant Gram-negative isolates, including *Klebsiella* spp. (8%), *Enterobacter* spp. (4%), *P. aeruginosa* (13%), and enterococci (15%). Many clinical isolates of *E. coli* are resistant to ampicillin.

Urinary Elimination of Oral Cephalosporin

The new oral cephalosporins combine high concentration in urine (Table 64) with a broad antibacterial spectrum that includes isolates producing TEM-1 β-lactamase. When an oral cephalosporin must be given, in uncomplicated UTIs as well as in pyelonephritis, the natural spectrum of the compound has to be considered (e.g., susceptibility of non–*E. coli* Enterobacteriaceae) before the susceptibility of the involved microorganisms is available.

Clinical Efficacy

Cephalexin was the only early oral cephalosporin that was adequately compared in clinical trials with other urinary antibacterials. In one study, it was significantly less effective than cotrimoxazole in a 7-day course. In seven comparative studies (six of them double-blinded) of uncomplicated UTIs, comparing cefixime (200–400 mg daily) with cotrimoxazole or amoxicillin, showed, at the end of the follow-up, identical bacteriologic cure rates (75–95% in cefixime-treated patients, 78–98% in cotrimoxazole-treated patients, and 84–92% in the amoxicillin group) (140). Numerous studies were published using cefuroxime-axetil in the treatment of cystitis in women. In uncomplicated UTIs, cefetamet-pivoxil was proven superior to cefadroxil (90% vs. 77% cure rates). Few studies have been done with ceftibuten and cefprozil.

TABLE 64 • Urinary Recovery of Oral Cephalosporins

	Urinary Elimination (%)	Dose (mg)
Cefixime	21.2±7.4	400
Cefdinir	12.7±6.2 to 23.0±6.8	200 to 600
Cefpodoxime-proxetil	39.7±7.6	200
Cefetamet-pivoxil	51.3±6.3	1,500
Cefuroxime-axetil	26–52	500
Ceftibuten	67.5±5	200
Cefprozil	63.6±8.2	500
Loracarbef	85.3±7.8	400
Cefditoren-pivoxil	19.6	200
Cefotiam-hexetil	31	400

Cox et al. (63), in two randomized 2:1 double-blind trials, compared cefpodoxime proxetil (100 mg twice daily for 7 days) with cefaclor (250 mg three times a day) or amoxicillin (250 mg three times a day) in the treatment of 463 patients with uncomplicated UTIs. All three compounds were equally active in both clinical cure rates (79 vs. 79 vs. 72%) and bacteriologic eradication rates (80 vs. 82 vs. 70%).

In uncomplicated UTI studies, loracarbef (200 mg thrice daily) for 7 days was compared with cefaclor (250 mg thrice daily), norfloxacin (400 mg twice daily). In two double-blind studies, loracarbef was as effective as norfloxacin and cefaclor in the treatment of uncomplicated pyelonephritis due to *E. coli* in 85% of the patients; bacteriologic cure rates were 86.8, 80, and 88.4% for loracarbef, cefaclor, and norfloxacin, respectively. The late bacteriologic eradications were 79.6, 60, and 88.9%, respectively (137).

The new oral cephalosporins could be used to permit hospitalized patients to be discharged from the hospital.

ADVERSE EFFECTS AND DRUG INTERACTIONS
General Tolerance of Oral Cephalosporins

Oral cephalosporins generally cause few side effects. Hypersensitivity reactions have been reported in less than 5% of patients treated with oral cephems. Pruritus, urticaria, or other skin manifestations have been reported. Central nervous system complaints such as reversible hyperactivity, nervousness, insomnia, confusion, dizziness, and somnolence have been reported infrequently.

Other Clinical Indications
Bone Infections

There are important differences between bone infections in children and adults. *S. aureus* is responsible for bone infections in almost 90% of cases. Cefadroxil was administered orally in a dose of 1000 mg, 24, 12, and 2 h prior to the collection of fluid or tissue; the levels in different fluid and tissue are listed in Table 65 (247). In another study, after a simple oral dose of 1000 mg, 4 to 5 h prior to sampling bone (n = 10) and muscle (n = 11), the bone and muscle concentrations were 4.2 and 3.0 mg/kg, respectively, while simultaneous serum levels were 11 to 12 mg/L (247).

Cefadroxil (25 mg/kg every 12 h) was given to 28 children, including 22 who had undergone orthopaedic surgery. *S. aureus* susceptible to cefadroxil was isolated from all patients. Of the 28 treated children, 23 had good clinical, bacteriologic, and radiologic outcomes (144).

Lyme Disease

Lyme disease is a tick-transmitted spirochetal infection caused by *Borrelia burgdorferi* (today separated into three genospecies) (238).

In Vitro Activity of Oral Cephems. Agger et al. (4) determined the in vitro activity of cephalexin, cefadroxil, cefaclor, cefixime, and cefuroxime against eight isolates of *B. burgdorferi*. MIC$_s$ values (geometric mean) for *B. burgdorferi* 297 were 23, 45, 91, 0.12, and 0.8 mg/L for cephalexin, cefadroxil, cefaclor, cefixime, and cefuroxime, respectively. The MIC of ceftriaxone was 0.02 mg/L. The good in vitro activity of cefuroxime was confirmed in vivo in infected Syrian hamsters; the CD$_{50}$ of cefuroxime sodium was 28.6 mg/kg (15.34–53.14 mg/kg) (146). The MIC of cefpodoxime for the three genospecies is 2 mg/L (238).

Clinical Efficacy. A randomized, multicenter, investigator-blinded clinical trial was carried out to compare the efficacy of cefuroxime-axetil (500 mg twice daily) and doxycycline (100 mg three times a day) for 20 days in erythema migrans; 232 patients were enrolled. At 1 month posttreatment, a satisfactory clinical response was obtained in 90 and 94% of evaluable patients, in the cefuroxime-axetil and doxycycline groups, respectively; 7 and 4 patients failed to respond in the cefuroxime-axetil and doxycycline groups, respectively (182).

Alterations of Microflora

Gastrointestinal disturbances are the most common adverse events reported with oral cephalosporins—nausea, vomiting, and diarrhea. The microflora can be influenced by antimicrobial agents because of incomplete absorption of orally administered drugs, high elimination by bile, and strong activity against microorganisms of the flora. Cefuroxime-axetil (600 mg dose every 8 h for 3 days) decreased *Enterobacteriaceae* in three volunteers who developed diarrhea. *Bacteroides* spp. and anaerobic cocci decreased significantly, but not clostridia (340).

Cefixime (200 mg twice daily for 7 days) was administered to 10 healthy volunteers. Cefixime was detectable in the feces (237–912 mg/kg feces) from day 1 to day 7. The number of *Enterobacteriaceae* and the anaerobic flora decreased markedly. *Clostridium difficile* was isolated from five volunteers. Cytotoxin was detected in only one subject. The intestinal microflora normalized within 2 weeks after treatment was stopped (229).

Cefpodoxime-proxetil was given for 10 days. Cefpodoxime was measured in the feces (0 to 3.65 units of cefpodoxime/g of feces). *C. difficile* was detected (55). The same results were obtained with cefprozil (500 mg twice daily for 8 days) (179), ceftibuten (400 mg/day for 10 days) (43). With cefetamet-pivoxil in one study (500 mg twice daily for 10 days), no *C. difficile* was detected (231) (Table 66).

Drug Interactions

Patients usually receive numerous drugs simultaneously, which can lead to possible drug interaction.

Interaction with Absorption

Absorption of oral cephems given concomitantly with other drugs could be affected.

TABLE 65 • Bone and Synovial Levels of Cefadroxil

Specimen	N	Tissue/Fluid Concentrations (mg/kg or mg/L)	Serum Concentrations (mg/L)
Bone	14	5.0±0.9	21.5±2.8
Muscle	12	6.5±0.9	20.7±2.9
Synovial capsule	21	7.8±1.5	20.5±3.1
Synovial fluid	13	11.0±1.7	25.5±2.0

TABLE 66 • **Alteration of the Intestinal Microflora by Oral Cephalosporin**

	Dose (mg/day)	Days of Administration	N	Enterobacteriaceae	Gram-positive Cocci	Anaerobic Bacteria	C. difficile	C. albicans	Ref.
				Impact on			**Overgrowth of Resistant Strains**		
Cefaclor	250 × 3	14	6	−	−	−	+	−	97
	250 × 3	7	10	−	−	−	−	−	228
	250 × 3	7	40	−	↓	−	−	+	298
Cephradine	1000 × 2	7	6	−	−	−	−	−	47
Loracarbef	200 × 2	7	20	−	−	−			227
Cefprozil	500 × 2	8	8	↓	↑	−	−	−	179
Cefixime	400 × 1	14	6	↓	↑	↓	+	−	97
	200 × 2	7	10	↓	↑	↓↓	+		229
Ceftibuten	400 × 1	10	14	↓	↑	−	+	+	43
Cefuroxime axetil	600 × 3	3	6	↓	↓	↓	−	+	340
	250 × 2	10	10	−	↑	−	+	+	86
Cefpodoxime proxetil	200 × 2	7	10	↓↓	↑↓	↓	+	+	44
Cefetamet pivoxil	500 × 2	10	18	−	−	−	+	+	231
Cefadroxil	500 × 2	10	20	−	−	−	−	−	2

Anti–H2 Receptors and Antacid Drugs. The effect of antacids and anti–H2 receptors on the bioavailability of oral prodrug cephalosporins is important, since the solubility of these compounds is pH dependent (Table 67). Little or no information exists on the potential interaction of cephalexin, cephradine, cefadroxil, cefaclor, cephaloglycin, and antacids or H2-receptor antagonists. Extensive data have been published for cefpodoxime-proxetil and to a lesser extent for cefuroxime-axetil, cefprozil, and cefixime. Agents that increase gastric pH (e.g. cimetidine, ranitidine, famotidine, sodium carbonate) could potentially reduce the dissolution of the prodrug cephalosporins, resulting in impaired bioavailability.

Hughes et al. (135) found that pretreatment with ranitidine sodium carbonate reduced the bioavailability of cefpodoxime-proxetil by 30% (Table 68). Saathoff et al. (253) showed that the relative bioavailability of cefpodoxime-proxetil is reduced by 60% after pretreatment with famotidine and Maalox. After pentagastrin stimulation (Table 68), the relative bioavailability of cefpodoxime-proxetil increased. These differences could be due in part to better dissolution of cefpodoxime tablets under acidic conditions and also due to better solubility of the drug at low pH. After oral doses of ranitidine (300 mg) and sodium bicarbonate (4 g), the peak plasma concentration (C_{max}) and AUC for cefuroxime-axetil are reduced by 19 and 43%, respectively (282, 283).

Antacids seem to have no effect on the relative bioavailability of cefixime (128), cefprozil (275), ceftibuten (335), and cefetamet-pivoxil (33). The pharmacokinetic parameters of cefpodoxime were not affected by metoclopramide and anisotropine methylbromide (317). The bioavailability of cefetamet-pivoxil (33) and cefotiam hexetil are slightly affected by either ranitidine or Maalox.

Food Interactions. Various studies investigating the effect of food on the relative bioavailability of oral cephalosporins showed a delay (T_{max}) in the absorption of most of the drugs. The absorption of cefetamet-pivoxil (32), cefuroxime

TABLE 67 • **Solubility of Oral Cephalosporins at Various pHs**

	pH	Solubility (mg/mL)
Cefpodoxime-proxetil	1.5	11.4
	6.8	0.4
Cefuroxime axetil	<1	1.0
Cefetamet pivoxil	1.0	21
	4.0	0.18
	6.8	0.14
Cefixime	2.0	0.34
	4.4	491
Cefprozil	1.8	40
	5 (cis)	6.18
	5 (trans)	1.0

TABLE 68 • **Effect of Various Drugs Modifying Gastric pH on Pharmacokinetics of Cefpodoxime (200 mg to 17 volunteers)**

Cefpodoxime-proxetil	C_{max} (mg/L)	T_{max} (h)	$AUC_{0-\infty}$ mg.h/L	Urinary Elimination (%)
Alone (fast)	2.24	2.44	13.40	32.4
+ ranitidine	1.5	3.65	9.21	23.9
+ pentagastrin	2.61	2.68	15.30	36.4
+ sodium bicarbonate	1.31	2.50	8.76	25.8
+ aluminium hydroxide	1.70	2.50	9.58	27.0

axetil (338) and cefpodoxime-proxetil is delayed when administered with food (135) (Table 69).

Effect of the Diet on Absorption. Food produces many complex effects on gastrointestinal function. Sixteen healthy nonsmoking adults participated in a study of food interaction with cefpodoxime-proxetil (200-mg) (135). Five different diets were given: (a) normal diet, (b) high-protein diet, (c) low-protein diet, (d) high-fat diet, and (e) low-fat diet. The kinetic parameters are

TABLE 69 • Oral Cephalosporin Kinetics—Food Effects

		Dose (mg)	N	C_{max} (mg/L)	T_{max} (h)	$AUC_{0-\infty}$ (mg.h/L)	Reference
Cefetamet-pivoxil	Fasted	1500	6	7.4	3.0	45.8	168
	Fed	1500	6	9.7	4.8	64.7	
Cefuroxime axetil	Fasted	1000	6	1.5	7.3	23.4	282
	Fed	1000	6	1.5	13.6	39.8	282
Cefditoren-pivoxil	Fasted	200	6	2.3	1.4	6.28	267
	Fed	200	6	3.4	2.0	10.02	
Ceftetram-pivoxil	Fasted	400	5	7.4	1.9	24.8	234
	Fed	400	5	6.3	2.2	25.3	234
Cefixime	Fasted	400		4.24	3.8	32.02	93
	Fed	400		4.22	4.8	30.78	93
Cefotiam-hexetil	Fasted	400	12	4.8	1.4	9.1	74
	Fed	400	12	4.4	1.9	10.0	74
Cefprozil	Fasted	250	12	6.13	1.2	15.0	19
	Fed	250	12	8.70	0.6	8.6	19
Ceftibuten	Fasted	100	6	6.10	2.6	24.2	211
	Fed	100	6	5.10	3.2	23.2	211
Loracarbef	Fasted	400	12	19.2	1.1	33.04	252
	Fed	400	12	13.64	2.4	35.38	252
Cefdinir	Fasted	100	6	1.25	3.5	6.16	268
	Fed	100	6	0.79	4.3	4.04	268
Cefaclor	Fasted	250	12	8.7	0.6	8.60	19
	Fed	250	12	4.29	1.3	7.59	19
Cephalexin	Fasted	1000	6	38.8	0.9	93	181
	Fed	1000	6	23.1	1.8	70	181
Cefadroxil	Fasted	500	16	14.7	0.5	43.3	239
	Fed	500	16	16.3	0.6	45.1	239

listed in Table 70. Statistically significant differences in mean values were determined for the $AUC_{0-\acute{y}}$ among the six diets. Fasted subjects had a significantly lower AUC ($\acute{y}$) than subjects receiving any of the diets. Absorption of a meal increases the overall absorption of cefpodoxime. Composition of the meal does not appear to influence the overall extent of absorption. Food may increase the C_{max} relative to maximum drug concentrations obtained under fasting conditions.

Iron Interactions. Cefdinir is a hydroxyiminocephalosporin which complexes iron ion. When cefdinir (200 mg) and ferrous sulfate (105 mg) are given concomitantly, the bioavailability of cefdinir decreases. When ferrous sulfate is given 3 h after cefdinir intake, the relative bioavailability of cefdinir remains unchanged (Table 71) (319).

Other Drug Interactions

Administration of an oral dose of 200 mg of ceftibuten every 12 h does not alter the systemic clearance of theophylline given in a single intravenous dose (10). Ceftibuten, like some other β-lactams (ticarcillin, latamoxef, carbenicillin) possesses a carboxylic group at C-7; tested in humans and animals, ceftibuten did not affect platelet function and blood coagulation (214).

Coexistence with warfarin reduced both the percentage of protein binding and the isomerization rate constant of ceftibuten (266). It is suggested that ceftibuten is isomerized at the warfarin binding site on albumin.

After pretreatment with a single oral dose of either 200 or

TABLE 70 • Kinetics of Cefpodoxime-proxetil (200 mg) with Different Diet Meals

Diet	C_{max} (mg/L)	Lagtime (h)	T_{max} (h)	$AUC_{0-\infty}$ (mg.h/L)	Urinary Elimination (%)
Fasted	2.62	0.40	2.75	13.5	41.0
(a)	3.11	0.81	3.25	17.6	51.8
(b)	3.19	0.85	3.78	16.9	64.1
(c)	3.14	0.82	3.38	17.0	52.2
(d)	3.02	0.62	3.22	16.3	54.0
(e)	3.25	0.69	3.47	18.0	55.4

TABLE 71 • Interaction of Cefdinir and Ferrous Ion

	Dose (mg)	N	C_{max} (mg/L)	T_{max} (h)	$AUC_{0-\infty}$ (mg.h/L)
Cefdinir alone	200	6	1.71	4.2	10.3
Cefdinir + iron	200	6	0.16	1.8	0.78
Cefdinir + iron 3 h after	200	6	1.28	3.3	6.55

400 mg of cefixime, no impairment in the metabolism of vitamin K_1 could be detected in healthy volunteers (315).

REFERENCES

1. Adam D, Kreutle O. Investigation on the diffusion of cefadroxil and cephalexin into tonsil tissue. Infection 1980;8(Suppl 5): 580–583.

2. Adamson I, Edlund C, Sjöstedt S, Nord CE. Comparative effects of cefadroxil and phenoxypenicillin on the normal oropharyngeal and intestinal microflora. Infection 1997;25:154–158.

3. Adler M, McDonald PJ, Trostmann U, Keyserling C, Tack K. Cefdinir versus amoxicillin/clavulanic acid in the treatment of suppurative acute otitis media in children. Eur J Clin Microb Infect Dis 1997;16:214–219.

4. Agger WA, Callister SM, Jobe DA. In vitro susceptibilities of *Borrelia burgdorferi* to five oral cephalosporins and ceftriaxone. Antimicrob Agents Chemother 1992;36:1788–1790.

5. Akiyama H, Torigoe R, Yamada T. ME 1207 in the field of dermatology. Chemotherapy (Japan) 1992;40(Suppl 2):619–623.

6. Almirall J, Morato I, Riera F, Verdaquer A, Priu R, Coll P, Vidal J, Murgai I, Vallas F, Catalan F. Incidence of community acquired pneumonia and *Chlamydia pneumoniae* infection: a prospective multicenter study. Eur Respir J 1993;6:14–18.

7. Aronovitz GH, Doyle CA, Durham SJ. Cefprozil vs amoxicillin-clavulanate in the treatment of otitis media. Infect Med 1992;9(Suppl C):19–32.

8. Ausina V, Coll P, Sambeat M, Paig J, Condom J, Luquin M, Ballester F, Prats G. Prospective study on the etiology of community-acquired pneumonia in children and adults in Spain. Eur J Clin Microb Infect Dis 1988;7:342–347.

9. Avril JL, Mesnard R, Donnio PY. In vitro activity of penicillin, amoxycillin and certain cephalosporins, including cefpodoxime, against human isolates of *Pasteurella multocida*. J Antimicrob Chemother 1991;473–474.

10. Bachman K, Schwartz J, Janregui L, Martin M, Nunlee M. Failure of ceftibuten to alter single dose theophylline clearance. J Clin Pharmacol 1990;30:444–448.

11. Backhaus A, Tinz J. Cefixim Therapie bei Patienten mit nachgewiesener Gonorrhoe. Infection 1990;18(Suppl 3: 145–146.

12. Bailey RR, Gower PEC, Dash CH. The effect of impairment of renal function and hemodialysis on serum and urine levels of cephalexin. Postgrad Med J 1970;46:60–64.

13. Bairamis TN, Nikolopoulos T, Kafetzis DA. Concentrations of cefpodoxime in plasma, adenoid and tonsillar tissue after repeated administration of cefpodoxime proxetil in children. J Antimicrob Chemother 37:1996;821–824.

14. Baldwin DR, Andrews JM, Wise R, Honeybourne D. Bronchealveolar distribution of cefuroxime axetil and in vitro efficacy of observed concentrations against respiratory pathogens. J Antimicrob Chemother 1992;30:377–385.

15. Baldwin DR, Wise R, Andrews JM, Honeybourne D. Concentrations of cefpodoxime in serum and bronchial mucosa biopsies. J Antimicrob Chemother 1992;30:67–71.

16. Baquero F, Loza E. Antibiotic resistance of micro-organisms involved in ear, nose and throat infections. Pediatr Infect Dis J 1994;13:S9–14.

17. Barbhaiya RH, Gleason GR, Shyu WC, Wilber RC, Martin RR, Pittman KA. Phase I study of single-dose BMY 28100, a new oral cephalosporin. Antimicrob Agents Chemother 1990;34:202–205.

18. Barbhaiya RH, Shukla UA, Gleason CR, Shyu WC, Wilber RB, Pittman KA. Comparison of cefprozil and cefaclor pharmacokinetics and tissue penetration. Antimicrob Agents Chemother 1990;34:1204–1209.

19. Barbhaiya RH, Shulka UA, Gleason CR. Comparison of the effects of food on the pharmacokinetics of cefprozil and cefaclor. Antimicrob Agents Chemother 1990;34:1210–1213.

20. Barr W, Lin CC, Radwanski E, Lim J, Symchovicz S, Affrime M. The pharmacokinetics of ceftibuten in humans. Diagn Microbiol Infect Dis 1991;14:93–100.

21. Barr WH, Affrime M, Lin CC, Batra V. Pharmacokinetics of ceftibuten in children. Pediatr Infect Dis J 1995;14:S93–101.

22. Barr WH, Affrime M, Lin CC, Batra V. Pharmacokinetics of ceftibuten in children. Pediatr Infect Dis J 1993;12:S55–S63.

23. Barry A. Antipneumococcal activity of a ketolide (HMR 3647) and seven related drugs in vitro. 37th Intersci Conf Antimicrob Agents Chemother, Toronto, 1997.

24. Bauernfeind A. Comparative in-vitro activities of the new quinolone, Bay y 3118, and ciprofloxacin, sparfloxacin, tosufloxacin, CI-960 and CI-990. J Antimicrob Chemother 1993;31: 505–522.

25. Bauernfeind A, Jungwirth R. Antibacterial activity of cefpodoxime in comparison with cefixime, cefdinir, cefetamet, ceftibuten, loracarbef, cefprozil, BAY 3522, cefuroxime, cefaclor and cefadroxil. Infection 1991;19:353–362.

26. Beam TR Jr, Gilbert DN, Kunin CM. General guidelines for the clinical evaluation of anti-infectives drug products. Clin Infect Dis 1992;15(Suppl 1:5–32.

27. Bégué P, Garabédian N, Quinet B, Baron S. Diffusion amygdalienne du cefixime chez l'enfant. Presse Med 1989;18: 1593–1595.

28. Berk SL, Kalbfleisch JH and the Alexander Project Group. Antibiotic susceptibility patterns of community-acquired respiratory isolates of *M. catarrhalis* in Western Europe and in the USA. J Antimicrob Chemother 1996;38(Suppl A):85–96.

29. Berman SJ, Boughton WH, Sugihara JG, Wong EGC, Sato MM, Siemsen AW. Pharmacokinetics of cefaclor in patients with end stage renal disease and during hemodialysis. Antimicrob Agents Chemother 1978;14:281–283.

30. Bessaguet MF, Champy R, Chassagnac F, Defaye P, Dumont Y, Renaudie P, Servole JP, Denis F, Mounier M. Concentrations de céfaclor dans l'oreille moyenne chez l'enfant. Med Mal Infect 1994;24:719–722.

31. Blasi F, Cosentini R, Legnani D, Denti F, Allegra L. Incidence of community acquired pneumonia caused by *Chlamydia pneumoniae* in Italian patients. Eur J Clin Microbiol Infect Dis 1993; 12:696–699.

32. Blouin RA, Kneer J. Stoeckel K. Pharmacokinetics of intravenous cefetamet (Ro 15–8074) and oral cefetamet pivoxil (Ro 15–8075) in young and elderly subjects. Antimicrob Agents Chemother 1989;33:291–296.

33. Blouin RA, Kneer J, Ambros RJ, Stoeckel K. Influence of antacid and ranitidine on the pharmacokinetics of oral cefetamet pivoxil. Antimicrob Agents Chemother 1990;34:1744–1748.

34. Blouin RA, Stoeckel K. Cefetamet pivoxil clinical pharmacokinetics. Clin Pharmacokinet 1993;25:172–188.

35. Bluestone CD. Current therapy for otitis media and criteria for evaluation of new antimicrobial agents. Clin Infect Dis 1992; 14(Suppl 2):S197–203.

36. Blummer JL, McLinn SE, Deabate CA, Kafetzis DA, Perrotta RJ, Salgado O. Multinational multicenter controlled trial comparing ceftibuten with cefaclor for the treatment of acute otitis media. Pediatr Infect Dis J 1995;14:S115–120.

37. Bolduc GR, Tam PG, Pelton S. Therapeutic approaches to experimental otitis media due to penicillin resistant *Streptococcus pneumoniae*. Recent Advances in Otitis Media 1996;518–519.

38. Borin MT, Forbes KK, Hughes GS. The bioavailability of cefpodoxime proxetil tablets relative to an oral solution. Biopharm Drug Dispos 1995;16:295–302.

39. Borin MT, Hughes GS, Kelloway JS, Shapiro BE, Halstenson CE. Disposition of cefpodoxime proxetil in hemodialysis patients. J Clin Pharmacol 1992;92:1038–1044.

40. Borin MT, Hughes GS, Spillers CR, Patel RK. Pharmacokinetics of cefpodoxime in plasma and skin blister fluid following oral dosing of cefpodoxime proxetil. Antimicrob Agents Chemother 1990;34:1094–1099.

41. Brenwald N, Andrews J, Baswell F, Wise R. CG 5501 in vitro study against clinical isolates including *Chlamydia* spp and *Mycobacterium tuberculosis* [Abstract F54]. Program and Abstracts of 36th Intersci Conf Antimicrob Agents Chemother New Orleans, 1996.

42. Briggs BM, Jones RN, Erwin ME, Barrett MS, Johnson DM. In vitro activity evaluation of cefdinir (FK 482, CI-983 and PD 1314393)—a novel orally administered cephalosporin. Diagn Microbiol Infect Dis 1991;14:424–425.

43. Brismar B, Edlund C, Nord CE. Effect of ceftibuten on the normal intestinal microflora. Infection 1993;21:373–375.

44. Brismar B, Edlund C, Nord CE. Impact of cefpodoxime proxetil and amoxicillin on the normal oral and intestinal microflora with special emphasis on β-lactamase production. Eur J Clin Microbiol Infect Dis 1993;12(9):714–719.

45. Brittain DC, Scully BE, Hirose T, Neu HC. The pharmacokinetic and bactericidal characteristics of oral cefixime. Clin Pharmacol Ther 1985;38:590–594.

46. Brook I, Gober AE. Monthly changes in the rate of recovery of penicillin-resistant organisms from children. Pediatr Infect Dis J 1997;16:255–257.

47. Brumfitt W, Franklin I, Grady D, Hamilton JMT. Effect of amoxicillin-clavulanic and cephradine on the fecal flora of healthy volunteers not exposed to a hospital environment. Antimicrob Agents Chemother 1986;30:335–337.

48. Bryskier A, Aszodi J, Chantot JF. Parenteral cephalosporin classification. Exp Opin Invest Drug 1994;3:145–171.

49. Callaham M. Prophylatic antibiotics in common dog bite wounds: a controlled study. Ann Emerg Med 1980;9:410–414.

50. Campbell CJ, Chantrell LJ, Eastmond R. Purification and partial characterisation of rat intestinal cefuroxime axetil esterase. Biochem Pharmacol 1987;36:2317–2324.

51. Carpentier JL. Klebsiella pulmonary infections: occurrence at one medical center and review. Rev Infect Dis 1990;12:672–682.

52. Carson JWK, Watters K, Taylor MRH, Keane CT. Clinical trial of cefuroxime axetil in children. J Antimicrob Chemother 1987;19:109–112.

53. Celin SE, Bluestone CD, Stephenson JY, Imag HM, Collins JF. Bacteriology of acute otitis media in adults. JAMA 1991;266:2249–2252.

54. Centers for Disease Control. 1993 Sexually transmitted diseases treatment guideline. MMWR 1993;42(RR-14):56–59.

55. Chachaty E, Depitre C, Mario N. Presence of *Clostridium difficile* and β-lactamase activities in feces of volunteers treated with oral cefixime, oral cefpodoxime-proxetil or placebo. Antimicrob Agents Chemother 1992;36:2009–2013.

56. Chaïbi EB, Mugnier P, Kitzis MD, Goldstein FW, Acar JF. β-Lactamases de *Branhamella catarrhalis* et leurs implications phénotypiques. Res Microbiol 1995;146:761–771.

57. Chow M, Quintilliani R, Cunha BA, Thompson M, Finkelstein E, Nightingale CH. Pharmacokinetics of high-dose oral cephalosporins. J Clin Pharmacol 1979;19:185–194.

58. Cohen R, Roque F, Dort C. High rates of penicillin-resistant *S. pneumoniae* in otitis media unresponsive to initial antibiotherapy. 33rd Intersci Conf Antimicrob Agents Chemother, 1993:337.

59. Coonan KM, Kaplan EL. In vitro susceptibilities of recent North America group A streptococcal isolates to eleven oral antibiotics. Pediatr Infect Dis J 1994;13:630–635.

60. Couet W, Fauvet JP, Laville M, Pozet N, Fourtillan JB. Pharmacokinetics of oral cefatrizine in patients with impaired renal function. Int J Clin Pharmacol Ther Toxicol 1991;29:213–217.

61. Couet W, Reigner BG, Lefebvre MA, Bizouard J, Fourtillan JB. Pharmacocinétique de la céfatrizine administrée en doses répétées. Pathol Biol 1988;36:513–516.

62. Couraud L, Andrews JM, Lecoeur H, Sultan E, Lenfant B. Concentrations of cefpodoxime in plasma and lung tissue after a single oral dose of cefpodoxime proxetil. J Antimicrob Chemother 1990;26(Suppl E):35–40.

63. Cox CE, Graveline JF, Luongo JM. Review of clinical experience in the United States with cefpodoxime-proxetil in adults with uncomplicated urinary tract infections. Drugs 1991;42 (Suppl 3):41–50.

64. Craig W, Andes D. Pharmacokinetics and pharmacodynamics of antibiotics in otitis media. Pediatr Infect Dis J 1996;15:255–259.

65. Crauste-Manciet S, Huneau JF, Decroix MO, Tomé D, Farinotti R, Chaumeil JC. Cefpodoxime proxetil esterase activity in rabbit small intestine: a role in the partial cefpodoxime absorption. Int J Pharm 1997;149:241–249.

66. Cullmann W, Dick W. Cefpodoxime: comparable evaluation with other orally available cephalosporins: with a note on the role of β-lactamases. Int J Med Microbiol 1990;273:501–517.

67. Cullmann W, Then RL. Cefetamet. Its in vitro activity and interaction with β-lactamases and penicillin-binding proteins. Drug Invest 1991;3:299–307.

68. Dabernat H, Avril JL, Boussougant Y. In vitro activity of cefpodoxime against pathogens responsible for community-acquired respiratory tract infections. J Antimicrob Chemother 1990;26 (Suppl E):1–6.

69. Dabernat H, Delmas C, Lareng MB. Infections respiratoires à *Haemophilus influenzae* intérêt du céfuroxime axétil. Med Mal Infect 1991;21(Hors série):22–26.

70. Dagan R, Abramson O, Leibovitz E, Lang R, Gosben S, Greenberg D, Yagupsky P, Liberman A, Fliss DM. Impaired bacteriologic response to oral cephalosporins in acute otitis media caused by pneumococci with intermediate resistance to penicillin. Pediatr Infect Dis J 1996;15:980–985.

71. Debbia EA, Schito GC, Pesce A. Antibacterial activity of ceftibuten, a new oral third generation cephalosporin. J Chemother 1991;3:209–225.

72. Dellamonica P. Cefuroxime axetil. Int J Antimicrob Agents 1994;23–26.

73. Denny FW, Wannamaker LW, Brink WR. Prevention of rheumatic fever: treatment of the preceding streptococci infection. JAMA 1950;142:151–153.

74. Deppermann KM, Garbe C, Hasse K. Comparative pharmacokinetics of cefotiam hexetil, cefuroxime, cefixime, cephalexin and effect of H2 blocker, standard breakfast and antacids on the bioavailability of cefotiam hexetil [Abstract 1223]. 29th Intersci Conf Antimicrob Agents Chemother, Houston, TX, 1989.

75. Dhib M, Moulin B, Leroy A, Hammeau B, Godin M, Johannides R, Fillastre JP. Relationship between renal function and disposition of oral cefixime. Eur J Clin Pharmacol 1991;41:579–583.

76. Doern G, Brueggeman AB, Pierce G, Halley HP Jr, Rauch A. Antibiotic resistance among clinical isolates of *H. influenzae* in the United States in 1994 and 1995 and detection of β-lactamase-positive strains resistant to amoxicillin-clavulanate: results of a national multicenter surveillance study. Antimicrob Agents Chemother 1997;41:292–297.

77. Doern G, Brueggemann A, Halley HP Jr, Rauch AM. Antimicrobial resistance of *S. pneumoniae* recovered from outpatients in the United States during the winter months of 1991 to 1995: results of a 30-center national surveillance study. Antimicrob Agents Chemother 1996;40:1208–1213.

78. Doern G, Brueggemann AB, Pierce G, Hogan T, Halley HP Jr, Rauch A. Prevalence of antimicrobial resistance among 723 outpatients clinical isolates of *M. catarrhalis* in the United States in 1994 and 1995: results of a 30-center national surveillance study. Antimicrob Agents Chemother 1996;40:2884–2886.

79. Doern G, Ferraro MJ, Brueggemann AB, Ruoff KL. Emergence of high rates of antimicrobial resistance among viridans group streptococci in the United States. Antimicrob Agents Chemother 1996;40:891–894.

80. Doern GV, Vautour R, Parker D, Tubert T, Torres B. In vitro activity of loracarbef (LY 163892), a new oral carbacephem antibacterial agent, against respiratory isolates of *H. influenzae* and *M. catarrhalis*. Antimicrob Agents Chemother 1991;35:1504–1507.

81. Donn KH, James NC, Powell JR. Bioavailability of cefuroxime axetil formulations. J Pharm Sci 1994;83:842–844.

82. Doyle CA, Durham JJ, Hamilton HA. Cefprozil vs. cefaclor in the treatment of pharyngitis and tonsillitis in adults. Infect Med 1992;9(Suppl E):66–67.

83. Ducharme MP, Edwards DJ, McNamara PJ, Stoeckel K. Bioavailability of syrup and tablet formulations of cefetamet pivoxil. Antimicrob Agents Chemother 1993;37:2706–2709.

84. Dumont R, Andrews JM, Guetat F, Sultan E, Lenfant B. Concentrations of cefpodoxime in plasma and pleural fluid after a single oral dose of cefpodoxime-proxetil. J Antimicrob Chemother 1990;26(Suppl E):41–46.

85. Eden T, Amari M, Emston S. Penetration of cefaclor to adenoid tissue and middle ear fluid in secretory otitis media. Scand J Infect Dis 1983;39(Suppl):48–52.

86. Edlund C, Brismar B, Sakamoto H, Nord CE. Impact of cefuroxime axetil on the normal intestinal microflora. Microb Ecol Health Dis 1993;12(9):714–719.

87. Emston S, Amari M, Eden T. Penetration of cefaclor to adenoid tissue and middle ear fluid effusion in chronic OME. Acta Otolaryngol 1985;424:7–12.

88. Fang GD, Fise M, Orloff J, Arisumi D, Yu VL, Kapoor WA, Grayston JT, Pin Wang S, Kholer R, Muder RR, Yee YC, Rihs JD, Vickers RM. New and emerging etiologies for community-acquired pneumonia with implications for therapy. A prospective multicenter study of 359 cases. Medicine 1990;69:307–315.

89. Farr BM, Mandell GL Gram-positive pneumonia. In Pennington JF, ed. Respiratory infections—diagnosis and management. 3rd ed. New York: Raven Press, 1994:349–367.

90. Faulkner RD, Bohaychuk W, Desjardins RE. Pharmacokinetics of cefixime after once-a-day and twice-a-day dosing to steady state. J Clin Pharmacol 1987;27:807–812.

91. Faulkner RD, Bohaydruk W, Lanc RA. Pharmacokinetics of cefixime in the young and elderly. J Antimicrob Chemother 1988;21:787–794.

92. Faulkner RD, Fernandez PB, Laurence G. Absolute bioavailability of cefixime in man. Clin Pharmacol 1988;28:700–705.

93. Faulkner RD, Yacobi A, Barone JS, Kaplan SA, Silber BM. Pharmacokinetic profile of cefixime in man. Pediatr Infect Dis J 1987;6:963–970.

94. Felmingham D, Robbins MJ, Ghosh G, Bhogal H, Mehta MD, Leakey A, Clark S, Dencer CA, Ridgway GL, Grüneberg RN. An in vitro characterization of cefditoren, a new oral cephalosporin. Drugs Exp Clin Res 1994;20:127–147.

95. Fernandez P, Laurence G, Sia LL, Falkowski AJ. Absolute bioavailability of cefixime in man. J Clin Pharmacol 1988;28:700–706.

96. File JM Jr. Aetiology and incidence of community-acquired pneumonia. Infect Dis Clin Pract 1996;5(Suppl 4):S127–135 .

97. Finegold SM, Ingram-Drake L, Gee R. Bowel flora changes in human receiving cefixime (CL 248:635) or cefaclor. Antimicrob Agents Chemother 1987;31:443–446.

98. Finkelstein E, Quintiliani R, Lee R, Bracci A, Nightingale CH. Pharmacokinetics of oral cephalosporins: cephradine and cephalexin. J Pharm Sci 1978;67:1447–1450.

99. Finn A, Straughn A, Meyer M, Chubb J. Effect of dose and food on the bioavailability of cefuroxime axetil. Biopharm Drug Dispos 1987;8:519–526.

100. Forsgren A, Walder M. Antimicrobial susceptibility of bacterial isolates in south Sweden including a 13-year follow-up study of some respiratory pathogens. APMIS 1994;102:227–235.

101. Foy HM, Kenny GE, Cooney MK, Allan ID. Long-term epidemiology of infection with *Mycoplasma pneumoniae*. J Infect Dis 1979;139:681–687.

102. Frémaux A, Sissia G, Brumpt I, Geslin P. Cefditoren (ME 1206), a new cephalosporin: in vitro activity against penicillin-susceptible and resistant pneumococci [Abstract 998]. 18th Int Congr ChemoTher, Stockholm, 1993..

103. Fujimaki Y, Kawamura S, Watanabe H, Itabashi T. Clinical and experimental studies of FK027 for otorhinolaryngological infections. 13th Int Congr ChemoTher, Tokyo, 1985.

104. Furuta S, Tsurumaru H, Fukami S. Cefotiam-hexetil in the field of otorhinolaryngology. Chemotherapy (Tokyo) 1988;36(Suppl 6):843–857.

105. Gallet J, Couraud L, Saux MC, Roche G. Diffusion pulmonaire du cefixime chez l'homme. Presse Med. 1989;18:1589–1592.

106. Gehanno P, Andrews JM, Ichou F, Sultan E, Lenfant B. Concentrations of cefpodoxime in plasma and tonsillar tissue after a single oral dose of cefpodoxime-proxetil. J Antimicrob Chemother 1990;26(Suppl E):47–51.

107. Gerber MA, Markowitz M. Management of streptococcal pharyngitis reconsidered. Pediatr Infect Dis 1985;4:518–526.

108. Gerber MA, Randolph MF, Chanatry J, Wright LL, DeMeo K, Kaplan EL. Five vs. ten-days of penicillin V therapy for streptococcal pharyngitis. Am J Dis Child 1987;141:224–227.

109. Geslin P, Frémaux A, Sissia G, Spicq C, Aberrane S. Rapport du Centre National de référence des pneumocoques années 1994–1995. Créteil 1996.

110. Ginsburg CM. Comparative pharmacokinetics of cefadroxil, cefaclor, cephalexin and cephradine in infants and children. J Antimicrob Chemother 1982;10(Suppl B):27–31.

111. Ginsburg CM, McCracken GH, Petruska M, Olson K. Pharmacokinetics and bactericidal activity of cefuroxime axetil. Antimicrob Agents Chemother 1985;28:504–507.

112. Goldstein EJ, Citron DM. Comparative activities of cefuroxime, amoxicillin-clavulanic acid, ciprofloxacin, enoxacin, and ofloxacin against aerobic and anaerobic bacteria isolated form bite wounds. Antimicrob Agents Chemother 1988;32:1143–1148.

113. Goldstein EJ, Nesbit CA, Citron DM. Comparative in vitro activities of azithromycin, Bay Y 3118, levofloxacin, sparfloxacin, and 11 other oral antimicrobial agents against 194 aerobic and anaerobic bite wound isolates. Antimicrob Agent Chemother 1995;39:1097–1100.

114. Goldstein EJC, Citron DM, Gerardo SH, Hudspeth M, Merriam CV. Comparative in vitro activity of HMR 3004, a new ketolide, with azithromycin (AZ), clarithromycin (CL), roxithromycin (RX) and erythromycin (ERY) against 311 aerobic and anaerobic bacteria isolated from human and animal bite wound infections [Abstract F-123]. 37th Intersci Conf Antimicrob Agents Chemother, Toronto, 1997:167.

115. Goldstein F, Kitzis MD, Gutmann L, Acar JF. Comparative activity of oral cephalosporins against β-lactamases producing pathogens. Med Mal Infect 1992;22:535–543.

116. Gomez J, Branos V, Ruiz-Gomez J, Soto MC, Munoz L, Nunez ML, Canteras M, Valdès M. Prospective study of epidemiology and pronostic factors in community-acquired pneumonia. Eur J Clin Microb Infect Dis 1996;15:556–560.

117. Gooch WM III, Swenson E, Highbee MD, Cocchito M, Evan EC. Cefuroxime-axetil and penicillin V compared in the treatment of group A beta-hemolytic streptococcal pharyngitis. Clin Ther 1987;9:670–677.

118. Guay DRP, Meatherall RC, Harding GK, Brown GR. Pharmacokinetics of cefixime in healthy subjects and patients with renal insufficiency. Antimicrob Agents Chemother 1986;30:485–490.

119. Guttendorf R, Koup I, Misiak P, Hawking P, Olson S. Pharmacokinetics of cefdinir (CI-983-FK482) in children—NON-MEM analysis dose selection and body size factors [Abstract 1227]. 32nd Intersci Conf Antimicrob Agents Chemother, Annheim, 1992:315.

120. Gwaltney JM Jr. Sinusitis. In: Mandell GI, Bennett JE, Dolin R eds. Principles and practice of infectious diseases. 4th ed. New York: Churchill Livingstone, 1995:585–590.

121. Gwaltney JM Jr, Hayden FG. In: Proctor DF, Anderson I, eds. The nose, upper airway physiology and the atmospheric environment. Amsterdam: Elsevier Biomedical Press, 1982:399–423.

122. Haddad J Jr, Isaacson G, Respler DS, Hart RW, Yilmaz HM, Collins JJ, Bluestone CD. Concentration of cefuroxime in serum and middle-ear effusion after single dose treatment with cefuroxime-axetil. Pediatr Infect Dis J 1991;10:294–298.

123. Harding SM, Williams PE, Ayrton J. Pharmacology of cefuroxime as the 1-acetoxyethyl ester in volunteers. Antimicrob Agents Chemother 1984;25:78–82.

124. Harrison HR, Magder LS, Boyce WT. Acute *Chlamydia trachomatis* respiratory tract infections in childhood—serologic evidence. Am J Dis Child 1986;140:1067–1071.

125. Harrisson CJ, Chartrand SA, Rodriguez W. Middle-ear fluid (MEF) concentrations of cefixime in acute otitis media and otitis media with effusion. 34th Intersci Conf Antimicrob Agent Chemother, Orlando 1994:A67.

126. Hatano K, Nishino T. Morphological alterations of *Staphylococcus aureus* and *Streptococcus pyogenes* exposed to cefdinir, a new oral broad-spectrum cephalosporin. Chemotherapy 1994;40:73–79.

127. Hayton WL, Walstad RA, Thurmann-Nielsen E. Pharmacokinetics of intravenous cefetamet and oral cefetamet pivoxil in children. Antimicrob Agents Chemother 1991;35:720–725.

128. Healy DP, Sahai JV, Sterling LP, Rachat EM. Influence of an antacid containing aluminium and magnesium on the pharmacokinetics of cefixime. Antimicrob Agents Chemother 1989;33:1994–1997.

129. Heffron R. Pneumonia: with special reference to pneumococcus lobar pneumonia. Cambridge: Harvard University Press, 1979:656–663.

130. Herrington JA, Federici JA, Painter BG, Remy JM, Barbiero ML, Thurberg BE. In vitro activity of Bay 12–8039, a new 8-methoxy quinolone [Abstract F004]. Program and Abstract 36th Intersci Conf Antimicrob Agents Chemother New Orleans, 1996..

131. Holm SE, Ekedahl C. Comparative study of the penetration of penicillin V and cefadroxil into tonsils in man. J Antimicrob Chemother 1982;10(Suppl B):121–123.

132. Howie VM, Owen MJ. Bacteriology and clinical efficacy of cefixime compared with amoxicillin in acute otitis media. Pediatr Infect Dis J 1987;6:989–991.

133. Howie VM, Poussard JH. Efficacy of fixed combination antibiotics versus separate components in otitis media. Clin Pediatr 1972;11:205–214.

134. Hu M, Chen J, Zhu Y, Dantzig AH, Strafford RE Jr, Kuhfeld MT. Mechanism and kinetics of transcellular transport of a new β-lactam antibiotic loracarbef across an intestinal epithelial membrane model system (CaCO$_2$). Pharm Res 1994;11:1405–1413.

135. Hughes GS, Heald DL, Barker KB. The effects of gastric pH and food on the pharmacokinetics of a new oral cephalosporin, cefpodoxime proxetil. Clin Pharmacol Ther 1989;46:674–685.

136. Humber G, Leroy A, Fillastre JP, Godin M. Pharmacokinetics of cefadroxil in normal subjects and in patients with renal insufficiency. Chemotherapy 1979;25:189–195.

137. Hyslop D, Bischoff W. Loracarbef versus cefaclor and norfloxacin in the treatment of uncomplicated pyelonephritis. Am J Med 1992;92(Suppl 6A):86–94.

138. Imaizumi M, Kajita M, Fujita K. Clinical studies on the concentration of cefaclor in sera and lung tissues of patients with respiratory diseases. Jpn J Antibiot 1986;39:2754–2760.

139. Inui KI, Yamamoto M, Saito H. Transepithelial transport of oral cephalosporins by monolayers of intestinal epithelial cell line CaCO$_2$; specific transport systems in apical and basolateral membranes. J Pharmacol Exp Ther 1992;261:195–201.

140. Iravani A, Richard GA. A double-blind multicenter comparative study of the safety and efficacy of cefixime versus amoxicillin in the treatment of acute urinary tract infections in adult patients. Am J Med 1988;85(Suppl 3A):17–23.

141. Iwasawa T. Fundamental and clinical studies on cefaclor in the otorhino-laryngologic field. Chemotherapy (Japan) 1979;696.

142. James PA, Lewis DA, Zordens JZ, Gribb J, Dawson SJ, Murray SA. The incidence and epidemiology of β-lactam resistance in *H. influenzae*. J Antimicrob Chemother 1996;37:737–746.

143. Jetlund O, Walstad RA, Thurmann-Nielsen E. Comparison of the serum and tissue concentrations of cefuroxime from cefuroxime axetil and phenoxymethylpenicillin in patients undergoing tonsillectomy. Int J Clin Pharmacol Res 1991;11:1–6.

144. Jimenez-Shebab M, Barrogan A. Oral cefadroxil in the treatment of bone and joint infections in children and adults. J Antimicrob Chemother 1982;10(Suppl B):149–152.

145. Johnson CA, Ateshkadi A, Zimmerman SW. Pharmacokinetics and ex-vivo susceptibility of cefpodoxime proxetil in patients receiving continuous ambulatory peritoneal dialysis. Antimicrob Agents Chemother 1993;37:2650–2655.

146. Johnson RC, Kodner CB, Jurkovich PJ, Collins JJ. Comparative in vitro and in vivo susceptibilities of the Lyme disease spirochete *Borrelia burgdorferi* to cefuroxime and other antimicrobial agents. Antimicrob Agents Chemother 1990;34:2131–2136.

147. Jones AN, Barry AL. Ceftibuten (7432-S, SCH 39720): comparative antimicrobial activity against 4735 clinical isolates,

beta-lactamase stability and broth microdilution quality control guidelines. Eur J Clin Microbiol Infect Dis 1988;7:802–807.

148. Jones RN. Ceftibuten: a review of antimicrobial activity, spectrum and other microbiologic features. Pediatr Infect Dis J 1993;12:S37–44.

149. Jones RN, Barry AL. In vitro evaluation of U-76,252 (CS-807): antimicrobial spectrum, beta-lactamase stability and enzyme inhibition. Diagn Microbiol Infect Dis 1987;8:245–249.

150. Jones RN, Barry AL, Pfaller M, Allen SD, Ayers LW, Fuchs PC. Antimicrobial activity of U-76,252 (CS-807), a new orally administered cephalosporin ester, including recommendations for MIC quality control. Diagn Microbiol Infect Dis 1988;9: 59–63.

151. Jousimies-Somer HR, Savolainen S, Ylikoski JS. Bacteriological findings of acute maxillary sinusitis in young adults. J Clin Microbiol 1988;26:1919–1925.

152. Kafetzis DA. Multi-investigator evaluation of the efficacy and safety of cefprozil, amoxicillin-clavulanate, cefixime and cefaclor in the treatment of acute otitis media. Eur J Clin Microb Infect Dis 1994;13:857–865.

153. Kaplan SL, Mason EO Jr. Antimicrobial agents: resistance patterns of common pathogens. Pediatr Infect Dis J 1994;15: 1050–1053.

154. Kawaharajo K, Miyata A, Kakinuma K. In vitro and in vivo antibacterial activity of ME1207, a new oral cephalosporin. Chemotherapy (Tokyo) 1992;40(Suppl 2):51–58.

155. Kawamura S, Ichikawa GI, Watanabe I. Fundamental and clinical studies on cefdinir in otorhinolaryngological infection. Chemotherapy (Tokyo) 1989;37(Suppl 2):1041–1052.

156. Kearns GL, Darville T, Wells TG, Jacobs RF, Hughes GS, Borin MT. Single dose pharmacokinetics of cefpodoxime proxetil in infants and children. Drug Invest 1994;7:221–233.

157. Kearns GL, Reed MD, Jacob RF, Ardite M, Yogen RD, Blumer JL. Single-dose pharmacokinetics of ceftibuten (SCH 39720) in infants and children. Antimicrob Agents Chemother 1991;35: 2078–2084.

158. Kelloway JS, Awni WM, Lin CC. Pharmacokinetics of ceftibuten-*cis* and its *trans* metabolites in healthy volunteers and in patients with chronic renal insufficiency. Antimicrob Agents Chemother 1991;35:2267–2274.

159. Kiani R, Johnson D, Nelson B. Comparative, multicenter studies of cefixime and amoxicillin in the treatment of respiratory tract infections. Am J Med 1988;85(Suppl 3A):6–13.

160. Kitzis MD, Liassine N, Ferré B, Gutmann L, Acar JF, Goldstein F. In vitro activities of 15 oral β-lactams against *K. pneumoniae* harbouring new extended-spectrum β-lactamases. Antimicrobial Agent Chemother 1990;34:1783–1786.

161. Klein JO. Selection of oral antimicrobial agents for otitis media and pharyngitis. Infect Dis Clin Pract 1994;3:151–157.

162. Kneer J, Tam YK, Blouin RA, Frey FJ, Keller E, Stathakis C, Lunginbuehl B, Stoeckel K. Pharmacokinetics of intravenous cefetamet and oral cefetamet pivoxil in patients with renal insufficiency. Antimicrob Agents Chemother 1989;33: 1952–1957.

163. Knothe H, Shah PM, Eckardt O. Cefpodoxime: comparative antibacterial activity, influence of growth conditions and bactericidal activity. Infection 1991;19:370–376.

164. Kohonen A, Paavolainen M, Renkonen OV. Concentration of cephalexin in maxillary sinus mucosa and secretions. Ann Clin Res 1975;7:50–53.

165. Konishi K, Suzuki H, Hayashi M, Saruta T. Pharmacokinetics of cefuroxime axetil in patients with normal and impaired renal function. J Antimicrob Chemother 1993;31:413–420.

166. Korting HC, Schäfer-Korting M, Kees F, Lukacs A, Grobecker H. Skin tissue fluid levels of cefotiam in healthy man following oral cefotiam hexetil. Eur J Clin Pharmacol 1990;39:33–36.

167. Korvick JA, Hackett AK, Yu VL, Muder RR. *Klebsiella pneumoniae* in the modern era: clinicoradiographic correlations. South Med J 1991;84:200–204.

168. Koup JR, Dubach UC, Brandt R, Wyss R, Stoeckel K. Pharmacokinetics of cefetamet (Ro15–8076) and cefetamet-pivoxil (Ro-15–8075) after intravenous and oral doses in humans. Antimicrob Agents Chemother 1988;32:573–579.

169. Krause PJ, Owen NJ, Nightingale CH, Klimek JJ, Lehmann WB, Quintiliani R. Penetration of amoxicillin, cefaclor, erythromycin-sulfixazole and trimethoprim-sulfamethoxazole into the middle ear fluid of patients with chronic serous otitis media. J Infect Dis 1982;145:815–821.

170. Kuhlwein A, Nies RA. Efficacy and safety of a single 400 mg oral dose of cefixime in the treatment of uncomplicated gonorrhoea. Eur J Clin Microb Infect Dis 1989;8:261–262.

171. Kusmiesz H, Shelton S, Brown O, Manning S, Nelson JD. Loracarbef concentrations in the middle ear fluid. Antimicrob Agent Chemother 1990;34:2030–2031.

172. Laurans G, Orfila J. *Moraxella (Branhamella) catarrhalis* dans les infections respiratoires activité in vitro de la cefuroxime. Med Mal Infect 1991;21(hors série):34–40.

173. Le Noc P, Croizé J, Bryskier A, Le Noc D. Activité antibactérienne de quatre céphalosporines à forme orale sur 338 souches de bactéries entéropathogènes. Réunion Interdisc Chemother Anti-infect 1990:48/P5.

174. Leigh DA, Fraser S, Hannington J, Mason T. Comparative trial of the efficacy and tolerance of cefpodoxime-proxetil and amoxicillin in the treatment of acute and actue-on-chronic bronchitis. Int Congr Chemother, Berlin, 1991.

175. Lenfant B, Molinier P, Gigliotti G, Coussedière D, Dupront A, Tremblay D. Bioavailability of the two diastereoisomers of cefpodoxime proxetil in healthy volunteers [Abstract P305–05]. Vth World Conf Clin Pharmacol Ther, Yokohama, Japan, 1992:248.

176. Léophonte P, Rouquet R, Gustin M. Cefpodoxime-proxetil vs amoxicillin in the treatment of community-acquired pneumonia in adult patients [Abstract 32]. Int Congr Infect Dis, Montréal, 1990..

177. Linares J Tubau FE, Alcaide F, Ardany C, Garcia A, Martin R. Antimicrobial resistance of *S. pneumoniae*: comparison of the in vitro activity of 16 antibiotics. Curr Ther Res 1996;57(Suppl A):57–64.

178. Livermore DM. Clinical significance of β-lactams induction and stable derepression in Gram-negative rods. Eur J Clin Microbiol 1987;6:439–445.

179. Lode H, Müller C, Borner K, Nord CE, Koeppe P. Multiple-dose pharmacokinetics of cefprozil and its impact on intestinal flora of volunteers. Antimicrob Agents Chemother 1992;36: 144–149.

180. Lode H, Schaberg T, Mauch H. Management of community-acquired pneumonia. Curr Opin Infect Dis 1996;9:367–371.

181. Lode H, Stahlmann R, Koeppe P. Comparative pharmacokinetics of cephalexin, cefaclor, cefadroxil and CGP 9000. Antimicrob Agents Chemother 1979;16:1–6.

182. Luger SW, Paparone P, Wormsmer GP. Comparison of cefuroxime axetil and doxycycline in treatment of patients with early Lyme disease associated with erythema migrans. Antimicrob Agents Chemother 1995;39:661–667.

183. Lundberg C, Carenfelt C, Engquist S, Nord CE. Anaerobic bacteria in maxillary sinusitis. Scand J Infect Dis 1979;(Suppl 19): 74–76.

184. Mancini R, Massida O, Satta G. Rate of penetration of cefetamet, cefixime, cefuroxime and cefaclor in different strains of *Enterobacteriaceae*. Med Mal Infect 1992;22:544–547.

185. Mandelman PM, Chaffin DO. Penicillin binding proteins 4 and 5 of *H. influenzae* are involved in cell wall incorporation. FEMS Microbiol Lett 1987;239–242.

186. Marchant CD, Shurin PA. Antibacterial therapy for acute otitis media: a critical analysis. Rev Infect Dis 1982;4:506–510.

187. Marlin GE, Nicholls AJ, Funnell GR, Bradbury R. Penetration of cefaclor into bronchial mucosa. Thorax 1984;39:813–817.

188. Marrie TJ, Durant H, Yates L. community-acquired pneumonia requiring hospitalization: 5 years prospective study. Rev Infect Dis 1989;11:586–599.

189. Martini A, Xerri L. Study of diffusion of cefuroxime into middle ear effusions of patients with chronic purulent otitis media. J Antimicrob Chemother 1982;10:197–198.

190. Mastrandrea V, Ripa S, La Rosa F, Ghezzi A. Pharmacokinetics of cefatrizine after oral administration in human volunteers. Int J Clin Pharm Res 1985;5:319–323.

191. McCarthy JM. Comparative efficacy and safety of cefprozil versus penicillin, cefaclor and erythromycin in the treatment of streptococcal pharyngitis and tonsillitis. Eur J Clin Microbiol Infect Dis 1994;13:846–850.

192. McCracken GH, Ginsburg CM, Clahsen JC, Thomas ML. Pharmacokinetics of cefaclor in infants and children. J Antimicrob Chemother 1978;4:515–521.

193. McLinn SE. Serum and middle ear levels of cephalexin, a new cephalosporin in acute otitis media. Prog 8th Int Congr Chemother, Athens, 1973;1:305–310.

194. McLinn SE, McCarty JM, Perrotta R, Pichichero ME, Reidenberg BE. Multicenter controlled trial comparing ceftibuten with amoxicillin-clavulanate in the empiric treatment of acute otitis media. Pediatr Infect Dis J 1995;14:S108–114.

195. Melegh B, Kerner J, Bieber LL. Pivampicillin-promoted excretion of pivaloylcarnitine in humans. Biochem Pharmacol 1987; 20:3405–3409.

196. Mendelman PM, Del Beccaco MA, McLin SE, Todd WM. Cefpodoxime-proxetil compared with amoxicillin-clavulanate for the treatment of otitis media. J Pediatr 1992;12:459–465.

197. Mendelman PM, Henzitzy LL, Chaffin DO. In vitro activities and targets of three cephem antibiotics against *Haemophilus influenzae*. Antimicrob Agents Chemother 1989;33:1878–1882.

198. Mignini F, Magni A, Dainelli D, Patrizi L. Determinations of tissue levels of cefatrizine in blood, lungs and bronchi. Drugs Exp Clin Res 1985;11:457–460.

199. Mignot A, Millerioux L, Couraud L, Durgeat S, Joubert M. Distribution of cefotiam in human lung tissue after multiple oral administration of cefotiam-hexetil. Eur J Clin Pharmacol 1994; 46:383–384.

200. Milatovic D. Evaluation of cefadroxil, penicillin and erythromycin in the treatment of streptococcal tonsillopharyngitis. Pediatr Infect Dis J 1991;10(Suppl 10):S61–63.

201. Miller RA, Brancato F, Holmes KK. *Corynebacterium haemolyticum* as a cause of pharyngitis and scarlatiniform rash in young adults. Ann Intern Med 1986;105:867–872.

202. Mine Y, Watanabe Y, Matsumoto Y. Mechanism of action of cefdinir, a new orally active cephalosporin. Chemotherapy (Tokyo) 1989;37(Suppl 2):122–134.

203. Mori Y, Baba S, Suzuki K, Shimada J, Inagaki M, Soyano K,

Kobayashi T, Maruo T, Kinoshita H, Yamamoto S, Wada M. Cefotiam-hexetil in the otorhinolaryngological field. Chemotherapy (Tokyo) 1988;36(Suppl 6):813–821.

204. Motohiro T, Maruoka T, Nagai K. Pharmacokinetic and clinical studies of cefpodoxime proxetil dry syrup in the field of pediatrics. Jpn J Antibiot 1989:42:1629–1666.

205. Munoz R. Genetics of resistance to third generation cephalosporins in clinical isolates of *Streptococcus pneumoniae*. Mol Microbiol 1992;6:2461–2465.

206. Muranushi N, Hashimoto N, Hirano K. Transport characteristics of S-1090, a new oral cephem in rat intestinal brush-border membrane vesicles. Pharm Res 1995;10:1488–1492.

207. Murphy TF, Apicella MA. Non typeable *H. influenzae:* a review of clinical aspects, surface antigens and the human response to infection. Rev Infect Dis 1987;9:1–15.

208. Nahata MC, Kolbrenner VM, Barson WJ. Pharmacokinetics and cerebral fluid concentrations of cefixime in infants and young children. Chemotherapy 1993;39:1–5.

209. Nahata MC, Koranyi KI. Pharmacokinetics of loracarbef in pediatric patients. Eur J Drug Metabol Pharmacokinet 1992;17: 201–204.

210. Nakao H, Ide J, Yanagisawa H, Iwata M, Komai T, Masuda H, Hirasawa T. Cefpodoxime proxetil (CS 807), a new orally active cephalosporin. Sankyo Kenkyusho Nempo 1987;39:1–44.

211. Nakashima M, Ida M, Yoshida T, Kitagawa T, Oguma T, Ishii H. Pharmacokinetics and safety of 7432-S in healthy volunteers [Abstract 591]. 26th Intersci Conf Antimicrob Agents Chemother, New Orleans, 1986.

212. Nakashima M, Uematsu T, Takiguchi Y. Phase I clinical studies of 7432-S, a new oral cephalosporin: safety and pharmacokinetics. J Clin Pharmacol 1988;28:246–252.

213. Nakashima M, Uematsu T, Oguma T. Phase I clinical studies of S-1108: safety and pharmacokinetics in a multiple-administration study with special emphasis on the influence on carnitine body stores. Antimicrob Agents Chemother 1992;36:762–768.

214. Nakashima M, Uematsu T, Takiguchi Y, Mizuno A, Uchida K, Matsubara T. Phase I clinical studies of 7432-S: effect of 7432-S on platelet aggregation and blood coagulation. J Clin Pharmacol 1988;28:253–258.

215. Nakashima M, Uematsu Y, Takiguchi Y. Phase I studies of 7432-S, a new oral cephem antibiotic. Chemotherapy (Tokyo) 1989;37(Suppl 1):78–109.

216. Nelson CT, Mason EO, Kaplan SL. Activity of oral antibiotics in middle-ear and sinus infections caused by penicillin-resistant *Streptococcus pneumoniae:* implications for treatment. Pediatr Infect Dis J 1994;13:585–589.

217. Nelson JD, Ginsburg CM, Mac Leland O. Concentration of antimicrobial agents in middle ear fluid, saliva and tears. Int J Pediatr Otorhinolaryngol 1981;3:327–334.

218. Nelson JD, Shelton S, Kusmiesz H. Pharmacokinetics of LY 163892 in infants and children. Antimicrob Agents Chemother 1988;32:1738–1739.

219. Neu HC, Chin NX. In vitro activity of the new fluoroquinolones CP99,219. Antimicrob Agents Chemother 1994;38:2615–2622.

220. Neu HC, Chin NX, Labthavikul P. Comparative in vitro activity and β-lactamases stability of FR 17027, a new orally active cephalosporin. Antimicrob Agents Chemother 1984;26: 174–180.

221. Neu HC, Chin NX, Labtkavikul P. In vitro activity and β-lactamase stability of two oral cephalosporins, ceftetrame (Ro 19–5247) and cefetamet (Ro 15–8074). Antimicrob Agents Chemother 1986;30:423–428.

222. Neu HC, Saha G, Chin NX. Comparative in vitro activity and β-lactamases stability of FK 482, a new oral cephalosporin. Antimicrob Agent Chemother 1989;33:1795–1800.

223. Ng WS, Chan PY, Leung YK, Wong PCL. In vitro activity of Ro 15–8074, a new oral cephalosporin against *Neisseria gonorrhoeae*. Antimicrob Agents Chemother 1985;28:461–463.

224. Nishitani Y, Yamada D, Hayata S. Basic and clinical studies on cefdinir in urology. Chemotherapy (Tokyo) 1989;37(Suppl 2):823–840.

225. Nishizono H, Uchiazono A, Shima T. Basic and clinical studies on ME 1207 for the infectious disease in the field of otorhinolaryngology. Chemotherapy (Japan) 1992;40(Suppl 2):643–650.

226. Nogita T, Iozumi K, Shimozuma M. Skin tissue concentration and clinical evaluation of cefdinir in dermatology. Chemotherapy (Tokyo) 1989;37(Suppl 2):955–969.

227. Nord CE, Grahnen A, Eckernäs SA. Effect of loracarbef on the normal oropharyngeal and intestinal microflora. Scand J Infect Dis 1991;23:255–260.

228. Nord CE, Heimdahl A, Lundberg C, Marklund G. Impact of cefaclor on the normal human oropharyngeal and intestinal microflora. Scand J Infect Dis 1987;19:681–685.

229. Nord CE, Movin F, Stalberg D. Impact of cefixime on the normal intestinal microflora. Scand J Infect Dis 1988;20:547–552.

230. Novak E, Paxton LM, Tubbs HJ, Turner LF, Keck CW, Yatsu J. Orally administered cefpodoxime proxetil for treatment of uncomplicated gonococcal urethritis in males: a dose response study. Antimicrob Agents Chemother 1992;36:1764–1765.

231. Novelli A, Mazzei T, Nicoletti P. Intestinal flora changes in patients treated with cefetamet-pivoxil, cefixime and cefuroxime-axetil. J Chemother 1994.

232. Nye K, O'Neill P, Andrews JM, Wise R. Pharmacokinetics and tissue penetration of cefprozil. J Antimicrob Chemother 1990;25:831–835.

233. Papanicolaou GA, Medeiros AA. Ability of ceftibuten to induce the class I beta-lactamase of *E. cloacae, S. marcescens* and *E. aerogenes*. Diagn Microbiol Infect Dis 1991;14:85–85.

234. Patel IH, Chang DH, Gustavson L, Reele S. Dose proportionality and food effect on Ro 19–5248/T2588 absorption in humans [Abstract 2027]. 26th Intersci Conf Antimicrob Agents Chemother, New Orleans, LA, 1986.

235. Payne DJ, Amyes GB. Stability of cefdinir (CI-983, FK 482) to extended spectrum plasmid-mediated β-lactamases. J Med Microbiol 1993;38:114–117.

236. Peixoto E, Ramet J Kissling M. Cefetamet pivoxil in pharyngotonsillitis due to group A beta-haemolytic streptococci. Curr Ther Res 1993;53:694–706.

237. Perkins BA, Hamill RH, Musher DM, O'Hara C. In vitro activities of streptomycin and 11 oral antimicrobial agents against clinical isolates of *Klebsiella rhinoscleromatis*. Antimicrob Agents Chemother 1992;36:1785–1787.

238. Péter O, Bretz AG. In vitro susceptibility of *Borrelia burgdorferi, Borrelia garinii* and *Borrelia afzelii* to 7 antimicrobial agents. VI Int Conference on Lyme Borreliosis, Bologne, 1994.

239. Pfeffer M, Jackson A, Ximenes J, Perche de Menezes J. Comparative human oral clinical pharmacology of cefadroxil, cephalexin and cephradine. Antimicrob Agents Chemother 1977;11:331–338.

240. Philpot-Howard J. Antibiotic resistance and *Haemophilus influenzae*. J Antimicrob Chemother 1984;13:199–208.

241. Pichichero ME. The rising incidence of penicillin treatment failure in group A streptococcal pharyngitis: an emerging role for the cephalosporins. Pediatr Infect Dis J 1991;10:S50–55.

242. Pichichero ME, Gooch WM, Rodriguez W, Blumer JL, Aronoff SC, Jacobs RF, Musser JM. Effective short-course treatment of acute group A β-haemolytic streptococcal tonsillo-pharyngitis. Arch Pediatr Adolesc Med 1994;148:1053–1060.

243. Pichichero ME, Margolis PA. A comparison of cephalosporins and penicillins in the treatment of group A β-haemolytic streptococcal pharyngitis: a meta-analysis supporting the concept of microbial co-pathogenialy. Pediatr Infect Dis J 1991;10:275–281.

244. Poole JM, Rosenberg R, Aronovitz GH. Cefprozil vs cefixime and cefaclor in otitis media in children. Infect Med 1992;9(Suppl C):21–32.

245. Pugh RNH, Murray LIM, Dawon JL, Pietroni MC, Williams R. Transection of the oesophagus for bleeding oesophageal varices. Br J Surg 1973;60:646–649.

246. Pukander JS, Paloheim SH, Sipilä MM. Cefetamet-pivoxil in pediatric otitis media. Chemotherapy (Tokyo) 1992;38(Suppl 2):25–28.

247. Quintiliani R. A review of the penetration of cefadroxil into human tissue. J Antimicrob Chemother 1982;10(Suppl B):33–38.

248. Randolph MF. Clinical comparison of once-daily cefadroxil and thrice-daily cefaclor in the treatment of streptococcal pharyngitis. Chemotherapy (Basel) 1988;34:512–518.

249. Richer M, Allard S, Manseau L, Vallée F, Pak R, Le Bel M. Suction-induced blister fluid penetration of cefdinir in healthy volunteers following ascending doses. Antimicrob Agents Chemother 1995;39:1082–1086.

250. Richter WF, Chong YH, Stella VJ. On the mechanism of isomerization of cephalosporin esters. J Pharm Sci 1990;79:185–186.

251. Rosenfeld RM, Doyle WJ, Swarts DJ, Seroky J, Perez Pinero B. Third generation cephalosporin in the treatment of acute pneumococcal otitis media—an animal study. Arch Otolaryngol Head Neck Surg 1992;118:49–52.

252. Rotter S, Lode H, Stelzer I. Pharmacokinetics of loracarbef and interaction with acetylcysteine. Eur J Clin Microbiol Infect Dis 1992;11:851–855.

253. Saathoff N, Lode H, Neider K, Depperman KM, Borner K, Koeppe P. Pharmacokinetics of cefpodoxime proxetil and interactions with antacid and an H2 receptor antagonist. Antimicrob Agents Chemother 1992;36:796–800.

254. Saez-Lorens X, Shyu WC, Shelton S, Kumiesz H, Nelson J. Pharmacokinetics of cefprozil in infants and children. Antimicrob Agents Chemother 1990;34:2152–2155.

255. Santacroce F, Dainelli B, Mignini F, Fasanella L, Marangoni F, Ripa S. Determination of cefatrizine levels in blood, tonsils, paranasal sinuses and middle-ear fluid. Drugs Exp Clin Res 1985;11:453–456.

256. Sarubbi FA, Verghese A, Caggiano C, Holtsclaw-Berk S, Berk SL. In vitro activity of cefpodoxime proxetil (U-76,252, CS 807) against clinical isolates of *Branhamella catarrhalis*. Antimicrob Agents Chemother 1989;33:113–114.

257. Scaglione F, Pintucci JP, Demartini G, Dugnani S. Ceftibuten concentrations in human tonsillar tissue. Eur J Clin Microbiol Infect Dis 1996;15:940–943.

258. Schaadt RD, Yagi BH, Zurenko GE. In vitro activity of cefpodoxime proxetil (U-76:252, CS 807) against *N. gonorrhoeae*. Antimicrob Agents Chemother 1990;34:371–172.

259. Schatz B, Karavokiros KT, Tauebel MA, Itokazu GS. Comparison of cefprozil, cefpodoxime proxetil, loracarbef, cefixime and ceftibuten. Ann Pharmacother 1996;30:258–268.

260. Schwartz RH, Freij BJ, Ziai M, Sheridan MJ. Antimicrobial prescribing for acute purulent rhinitis in children: a survey of

pediatricians and family practitioners. Pediatr Infect Dis J 1997; 16:185–190.

261. Schwartz RH, Wientzen RI Jr, Pedrera F. Penicillin V for group A streptococcal pharyngitis: a randomized trial of seven versus ten day therapy. JAMA 1981;246:1790–1795.

262. Schwinghammer TL, Norden CW, Gill E. Pharmacokinetics of cephradine administered intravenously and orally to young and elderly subjects. J Clin Pharmacol 1990;30:893–899.

263. Shiba K. Pharmacokinetic evaluation of ceftibuten (7432-S) [Abstract 452]. 28th Intersci Conf Antimicrob Agents Chemother, Los Angeles, 1988.

264. Shiba K, Saito A, Shimada J. Clinical studies on cefdinir. Chemotherapy (Tokyo) 1989;37(Suppl 2):345–352.

265. Shigi Y, Matsumoto Y, Kaizu M, Fujishita Y, Koyo H. Mechanisms of action of the new orally active cephalosporin FK027. Jpn J Antibiot 1984;37:790–796.

266. Shimada J, Hori S, Oguma T, Yoshikawa T, Yamamoto S, Nishikawa T, Yamada H. Effects of protein binding on the isomerization of ceftibuten. J Pharm Sci 1993;82:461–465.

267. Shimada K, Kobayashi Y, Shinkai S, Komiya I, Matsumoto T. Phase I clinical studies on a novel orally active cephem antibiotic, ME1207 [Abstract 366]. 29th Intersci Conf Antimicrob Agents Chemother, Houston, Texas, 1989.

268. Shimada K, Soejima R. FK482, a new orally active cephalosporin: pharmacokinetics and tolerance in healthy volunteers [Abstract 655]. 27th Intersci Conf Antimicrob Agents Chemother, New York, 1987.

269. Shimizu K, Saito A, Shimada J. Carnitine studies and safety after oral administration of S-1108, a new oral cephem, to patients. Antimicrob Agents Chemother 1993;37:1043–1049.

270. Shinikawa A, Tamura Y, Shimizu K, Miyake H. CS-807 in otorhinolaryngological infections. Chemotherapy (Tokyo) 1988;36(Suppl 1):1046–1055.

271. Shyu WC, Haddad J, Reilly J, Khan WN, Campbell DA, Tsai Y, Barbhaiya KH. Penetration of cefprozil into middle ear fluid of patients with otitis media. Antimicrob Agent Chemother 1994;38:2210–2212.

272. Shyu WC, Pittman KA, Wilber RB, Matzke GR, Barbhaiya RH. Pharmacokinetics of cefprozil in healthy subjects and patients with renal impairment. J Clin Pharmacol 1991;31:362–371.

273. Shyu WC, Shah WR, Campbell DA, Wilber RB, Pittman KA, Barbhaiya RH. Oral absolute bioavailability and intravenous dose-proportionality of cefprozil in humans. J Clin Pharmacol 1992:32:789–803.

274. Shyu WC, Wilber RB, Pittman KA, Gorg DC, Barbhaiya RH. Pharmacokinetics of cefprozil in healthy subjects and patients with hepatic impairment. J Clin Pharmacol 1991:31:372–376.

275. Shyu WC, Wilber RD, Pittman K, Barbhaiya RH. Effect of antacid on the bioavailability of cefprozil. Antimicrob Agents Chemother 1992:36:962–965.

276. Sifaoui F, Duval F, Boucot I, Leblanc F, Gutmann L, Berche P. In vitro activity of sanfetrinem (GV 104326) against bacterial isolates from acute otitis media in children [Abstract F151]. Program and Abstract 36th Intersci Conf Antimicrob Agents Chemother New Orleans, 1996.

277. Sifaoui F, Kitzis MD, Gutmann L. In vitro selection of one-step mutants of *Streptococcus pneumoniae* resistant to different oral β-lactam antibiotics is associated with alterations of PBP2x. Antimicrob Agents Chemother 1996;40:152–156.

278. Singlas E, Lebrec D, Gaudin C, Montay G, Roche G, Taburet AM. Influence de l'insuffisance hépatique sur la pharmacocinétique du cefixime. Presse Med 1989;18:1587–1588.

279. Sitar D, Hoban DJ, Aoki FY. Pharmacokinetic disposition of loracarbef in healthy young men and women at steady state. J Clin Pharmacol 1994;34:924–929.

280. Smith CB, Golden C, Kanner RE, Renzetti AD. *H. influenzae* and *H. parainfluenzae* in chronic obstructive pulmonary disease. Lancet 1976;1:1253–1255.

281. Smith CB, Golden CA, Kanner RE, Renzetti AD. Association of viral and *Mycoplasma pneumoniae* infections with acute respiratory illness in patients with chronic obstructive pulmonary diseases. Am Rev Respir Dis 1980;121:225–232.

282. Sommers DEK, Van Wyk M, Moncrieff J, Schoeman HS. Influence of food and reduced gastric acidity on the bioavailability of bacampicillin and cefuroxime axetil. Br J Clin Pharmacol 1984;18:535–539.

283. Sommers DK, Van Wyk M, Williams PEO, Harding SM. Pharmacokinetics and tolerance of cefuroxime axetil in volunteers during repeated dosing. Antimicrob Agents Chemother 1984; 25:344–347.

284. Spangler SK, Jacobs MR, Appelbaum PC. Activities of RPR 106972 (a new oral streptogramin), cefditoren (a new oral cephalosporin), two new oxazolidinone (U 100592 and U 100766) and other oral and parenteral agents against 203 penicillin-susceptible and -resistant pneumococci. Antimicrob Agents Chemother 1996;40:481–484.

285. Spangler SK, Jacobs MR, Appelbaum PC. In vitro susceptibility of 185 penicillin-susceptible and -resistant pneumococci to WY-49605 (SUN/SY5555), a new oral penem, compared with those to penicillin G, amoxicillin, amoxicillin-clavulanate, cefixime, cefaclor, cefpodoxime, cefuroxime and cefdinir. Antimicrob Agents Chemother 1994;38:2902–2904.

286. Spyker DA, Thomas BL, Sande MA, Bolton WK. Pharmacokinetics of cefaclor and cephalexin: dosages normograms for impaired renal function. Antimicrob Agents Chemother 1978;14: 172–177.

287. St Peter J, Borin MT, Hughes G, Kelloway J, Shapiro B, Halstentson C. Disposition of cefpodoxime proxetil in healthy volunteers and patients with impaired renal function. Antimicrob Agents Chemother 1992;36:126–131.

288. Stillerman M. Comparison of oral cephalosporins with penicillin therapy for group A streptococcal pharyngitis. Pediatr Infect Dis J 1986;5:649–654.

289. Stillerman M. Cefatrizine and potassium phenoxymethylpenicillin on group A streptococcal pharyngitis. Antimicrob Agent Chemother 1976;16:185.

290. Stillerman M. Comparison of cephaloglycin and penicillin in streptococcal pharyngitis. Clin Pharmacol Ther 1969;11: 205–213.

291. Stillerman M, Isenberg HD, Moody M. Streptococcal pharyngitis therapy: comparison of cephalexin, phenoxymethylpenicillin and ampicillin. Am J Dis Child 1972;123:457–461.

292. Stobberingh EE, Houbon AW, Philips JH. In vitro activity of cefpodoxime, a new oral cephalosporin. Eur J Clin Microb Infect Dis 1989;8:656–658.

293. Stobberingh EE, Winderink M, Philips M, Houben A. *Branhamella catarrhalis*: β-lactamase production and sensitivity to oral antibiotics, including new cephalosporins. J Antimicrob Chemother 1987;20:765–766.

294. Stoeckel K, Hayton WL, Edwards DJ. Clinical pharmacokinetic or oral cephalosporins. Antibiot Chemother 1995;47: 34–71.

295. Stone JW, Linong G, Andrews JM, Wise R. Cefixime, in-vitro activity, pharmacokinetics and tissue penetration. J Antimicrob Chemother 1989;23:221–228.

296. Straffon RA. Urinary tract infection: problems in diagnosis and management. Med Clin North Am 1974:545–554.

297. Sunakawa K, Iwata S. Clinical evaluation of cefixime in pediatrics. Jpn J Antibiot 1986;39:1035–1054.

298. Swedish Study Group (Christensson). A randomized multicenter trial to compare the influence of cefaclor and amoxycillin on the colonization resistance of the digestive tract in patients with lower respiratory tract infections. Infection 1991;19:208–215.

299. Sydnor A, Gwaltney JM Jr, Cochetto DM, Scheld WM. Comparative evaluation of cefuroxime-axetil and cefaclor for treatment of acute bacterial maxillary sinusitis. Arch Otolaryngol Head Neck Surg 1989;115:1430–1433.

300. Tack K, Keyserling CH, McCarty J, Heddrick JA. Study of use of cefdinir versus cephalexin for the treatment of skin infections in pediatric patients. Antimicrob Agents Chemother 1997;41:739–742.

301. Takenouchi T, Nishino T. Antibacterial activity of cefpodoxime against *Branhamella catarrhalis*. Microbiol Immunol 1991;35:1059–1071.

302. Tam YK, Kneer J, Dubach UC, Stoeckel K. Pharmacokinetics of cefetamet pivoxil (Ro 15–8075) with ascending oral doses in normal healthy volunteers. Antimicrob Agents Chemother 1989;33:957–959.

303. Tamura A, Okamoto R, Yoshida T, Yamamoto H, Kondo S, Inoue M, Mistuhashi S. In vitro and in vivo antibacterial activity of ME 1207, a new oral cephalosporin. Antimicrob Agent Chemother 1988;32:1421–1426.

304. Teele D.W, Klein JO, Rosner B. Epidemiology of otitis media during the first seven years of life in children in Greater Boston: a prospective, cohort study. J Infect Dis 1989;160:83–94.

305. Thabaut A, Meyran M, Sofer L, Morand A, Labia R. Interactions of ceftibuten with extended beta-lactamases. A bacteriological and enzyme analysis. Drugs Exp Clin Res 1994;20: 49–54.

306. Then RL. Ability of new-β-lactam antibiotics to induce β-lactamase production in *Enterobacter cloacae*. Eur J Clin Microbiol 1987;6:451–455.

307. Therasse DG, Farlow DS, Davidson RL. Effects of renal dysfunction on the pharmacokinetics of loracarbef. Clin Pharmacol Ther 1993;54:311–316.

308. Thornber D, Wise R, Andrews JM, O'Sullivan N. The in vitro activity and β-lactamase stability of cefdinir (CI-983, KFK 482): a new oral cephalosporin. 17th Int Congr Chemother, Berlin, 1991.

309. Thorpe EM Jr, Schwerbke JR, Hook EW III. Comparison of single-dose cefuroxime axetil with ciprofloxacin in treatment of uncomplicated gonorrhoea caused by penicillinase-producing and non-penicillinase-producing *Neisseria gonorrhoeae* strains. Antimicrob Agents Chemother 1996;40:2275–2280.

310. Tillett WS, Cambier MJ, MacCormack JE. The treatment of lobar pneumonia and pneumococcal empyema with penicillin. Bull NY Acad Med 1944;20:142–178.

311. Todd JK, Todd N, Damato J, Todd WA. Bacteriology and treatment of purulent nasopharyngitis a double-blind, placebo controlled evaluation. Pediatr Infect Dis J 1984;3:226–232.

312. Todd WM. Cefpodoxime proxetil: a comprehensive review. Int J Antimicrob Agent 1994;4:37–67.

313. Totsuka K, Shimizu K, Konishi M, Yamamoto S. Metabolism of S-1108, a new oral cephem antibiotic, and metabolic profiles of its metabolites in humans. Antimicrob Agents Chemother 1992;32:757–761.

314. Tremblay D, Dupont A, Ho C, Coussedière D, Lenfant B. Pharmacokinetics of cefpodoxime in young and elderly volunteers after single doses. J Antimicrob Chemother 1990;26:(Suppl E):21–28.

315. Trenk D, Wagner F, Bechtold H, Nier B, Jähnchen E. Lack of effect of cefixime on the metabolism of vitamin K1. J Clin Pharmacol 1990;30:737–742.

316. Tupasi TE, Calubiran OV, Torres CA. Single oral dose of cefaclor for the treatment of infections with penicillinase-producing strains of *Neisseria gonorrhoeae*. Br J Vener Dis 1982;58:176–179.

317. Uchida E, Kobayashi S, Kamijo Y. The effects of ranitidine, metoclopramide and anisotropine methylbromide on the availability of cefpodoxime proxetil in Japanese healthy subjects. IVe Word Conf Clin Pharmacol Ther 1989, Mannheim-Heidelberg. Eur J Clin Pharmacol 1989;36(Suppl):11–33.

318. Ueda Y, Okubo H, Ida Y, Yanezu S, Sakakibara Y, Yasunaga K. Laboratory and clinical study on CS-807. Chemotherapy (Tokyo) 1988;36(Suppl 1):502–511.

319. Ueno K, Kazahiko T, Tsujimura K. Impairment of cefdinir absorption by iron ion. Clin Pharmacol Ther 1993;54:473–475.

320. Urban A, Andes D, Craig WA. In vivo activity of cefpodoxime against penicillin-resistant pneumococci. 19th Int Congr Chemother, Montreal, 1995.

321. Utsui Y, Inoue M, Mitsuhashi S. Antibacterial activity of CS-807, a new oral cephalosporin. Chemotherapy (Tokyo) 1988; 36(Suppl 1):1–15.

322. Van Dyk JC, Terespolsky SA, Meyer CS, Van Niekerk CH, Klugman K. Penetration of cefpodoxime into middle ear fluid in paediatric patients with acute otitis media. Pediatr Infect Dis J 1997;16:79–81.

323. Venkatesan P, Mac Farlane JT. Epidemiology and pathogenesis of prevention of pneumonia. Curr Opin Infect Dis 1991;4:154–159.

324. Veyssier P, Darchis JP, Devillers A. Pharmacocinétique du céfuroxime—axétil administré par voie orale chez le sujet âgé. Therapie 1988;43:355–359.

325. Vickers S, Ducan CAH, White SD. Carnitine and glucuronic acid conjugates of pivalic acid. Xenobiotics 1985;15:453–458.

326. Wald ER. Epidemiology, pathophysiology and etiology of sinusitis. Pediatr Infect Dis 1985;4:S51–S54.

327. Wald ER. Purulent nasal discharge. Pediatr Infect Dis J 1991;10:329–333.

328. Wallace RJ Jr, Masher DM, Martin PR. *Haemophilus influenzae* in adults. Am J Med 1978;64:87–93.

329. Wannamaker LW, Rammelkermp CR Jr, Denny FW. Prophylaxis of acute rheumatic fever by treatment of the preceding streptococcal infection with various amounts of depot penicillin. Am J Med 1951;10:673–695.

330. Weber DJ, Wolfson JS, Swartz MN, Hooper DC. *Pasteurella multocida* infections: report of 34 cases and review of the literature. Medicine 1984;63:133–154.

331. Westbloom TU, Gudipati S, Midkiff BR. In vitro susceptibility of *Helicobacter pylori* to the new oral cephalosporins cefpodoxime, ceftibuten and cefixime. Eur J Clin Microbiol Infect Dis 1990;9:691–693.

332. Westphal JF, Jehl F, Brogard JM. Cinétique de la clairance biliaire du céfixime chez des patients cholécystectomisés. Therapie 1994;49:35–39.

333. Wick WE. Cephalexin, a new orally absorbed cephalosporin antibiotic. Appl Microbiol 1967;15:765–769.

334. Wiederman BL, Schwartz RH. Effect of blood contamination on the interpretation of antibiotics concentrations in the middle ear fluid. Pediatr Infect Dis J 1992;11:244–245.

335. Wieseman LR, Benfield P. Cefprozil, a review of its antibacterial activity, pharmacokinetic properties and therapeutic potential. Drugs 1993;45:295–317.

336. Wilcox RR, Woodcook KS. Cephalexin in the oral treatment of gonorrhoea by a double-blind method. Postgrad Med J 1970;46(Suppl):103–106.

337. Williams JD, Powell M, Fah Ys, Seymour A, Yuan M. In vitro susceptibility of *Haemophilus influenzae* to cefaclor, cefixime, cefetamet and loracarbef. Eur J Clin Microb Infect Dis 1992;11: 748–751.

338. Williams PO, Harding SM. The absolute bioavailability or oral cefuroxime axetil in male and female volunteers after fasting and after food. J Antimicrob Chemother 1984;13:191–196.

339. Wise R, Andrews JM, Ashby JP, Thornsber D. The in vitro activity of cefpodoxime: a comparison with other oral cephalosporins. J Antimicrob Chemother 1990;25:541–550.

340. Wise R, Bennet SA, Dent J. The pharmacokinetics of orally absorbed cefuroxime compared with amoxycillin/clavulanic acid. J Antimicrob Chemother 1984;13:603–610.

341. Wise R, Nye K, O'Neill P, Wastenholme M, Andrews JM. Pharmacokinetics and tissue penetration of ceftibuten. Antimicrob Agents Chemother 1990;34:1053–1055.

342. Wiseman LR, Balfour JA. Ceftibuten: a review of its antibacterial activity, pharmacokinetic properties and clinical efficacy. Drugs 1994;47:784–808.

343. Yamasaku F, Suzuki Y, Uno K. Comparative study of pharmacokinetics of cefdinir and cefroxadine in the same healthy volunteers. Chemotherapy (Tokyo) 1989;37(Suppl 2):441–446.

344. Yee YC, Thornsberry C. Penicillin-resistant *Streptococcus pneumoniae* on the rise in the United States: its effect on oral cephalosporines. Antimicrob Infect Dis Newslett 1994;13: 49–57.

345. Zolfino I, Senesi S, Campa M. Human skin disposition of cefpodoxime after oral administration of its proxetil ester. J Antimicrob Chemother 1992;30:731–733.

Cephalosporins: Parenteral

●

Suzanne R. Belfiglio and André J. Bryskier

Since the 1940s, remarkable growth in the number of clinically useful antibacterial agents has occurred. The cephalosporins account for a large proportion of the new antibiotics introduced since the mid-1970s and today are among the most widely prescribed agents (10).

The first cephalosporin antibiotic was isolated in 1948 from a fungus, *Cephalosporium acremonium,* near a sewer outlet off the Sardinian coast, by Guiseppe Brotzu. Brotzu had speculated that antibiotic-producing microorganisms were responsible for the good health of recreational bathers on heavily polluted beaches. He subsequently used the extracts of his mold with apparent success to treat a variety of infections, including typhoid fever (9, 10).

Cephalosporin C was discovered by Abraham and Newton in 1953 while they were studying the antibiotics of a strain of *C. acremonium.* Cephalosporin C was found to have several remarkable properties, being active against *Escherichia coli, Salmonella typhi,* and the Oxford strain of *Staphylococcus aureus* but resistant to penicillinase from *Bacillus subtilis* (10). Removal of a side chain from this molecule yielded a nucleus, 7-aminocephalosporanic acid, from which all subsequent cephalosporins have been derived as semisynthetic compounds (9). In 1964, cephalothin and cephaloridine were introduced into medicine and were followed by cefazolin. These antibiotics were active against penicillinase-producing *S. aureus,* and unlike methicillin, they also showed significant activity against a number of Gram-negative bacilli. None of the early cephalosporins were absorbed through the gut, despite their relative acid stability. Cephalexin, the desacetoxy cephalosporin, was the first cephem to be absorbed when given orally (10).

In the early 1970s, another family of β-lactam antibiotics was discovered, the cephamycins. Similar to the cephalosporins, these compounds differ in having a methoxy group in the 7-position of the β-lactam ring and being produced naturally by actinomycetes rather than fungi. The cephamycins were associated with high resistance to hydrolysis by most β-lactamases. However, like the cephalosporins, the cephamycins lend themselves to removal of a side-chain to provide a nucleus from which semisynthetic derivatives can be obtained (9, 10).

Thousands of structural modifications have been made to virtually every position on the cephem nucleus. The search for new substituents at C-3' led to the discovery of quanternary ammonium cephems (cefpirome, cefepime, cefclidin, cefprozan, etc.) (10).

CLASSIFICATION

Numerous classifications of cephalosporins have been published based on chemical, biologic, microbiologic, pharmacologic, and immunologic criteria. The pharmacokinetic and microbiologic classifications seem to be the most suitable for the therapeutic setting (10). Categorizing these agents into chemically similar groups is not useful because the antimicrobial spectrum is generally not closely associated with chemical structure (61).

No classification has been entirely suitable; nevertheless, the somewhat arbitrary system that is most widely used combines the parenteral and oral cephalosporins into generations on the basis of their antibacterial activity and spectrum of microbiologic activity. Cephems are traditionally divided into first-, second-, third-, and now fourth-generation cephalosporins. The distinction, originally used as a marketing point, is clinically more useful. However, considerable differences in antibacterial spectrum have been noted among cephalosporins of a given generation, together with overlapping activity among compounds belonging to different generations. Use of the word *generation*, as applied to groups of new cephems, has served to reinforce the implication that each new wave provides general advances in all areas rather than fairly specific modifications to one or more properties (10).

The first-generation compounds have a relatively narrow spectrum of activity focused primarily on Gram-positive cocci. Second-generation cephalosporins have variable activity against Gram-positive cocci but have increased activity against Gram- negative bacteria. In spite of relatively increased potency against Gram-negative aerobic and anaerobic bacilli, the cephamycins are included in the second generation. Those cephalosporins with very marked activity against the Gram- negative bacteria are grouped in a third generation; some of these compounds have limited activity against Gram-positive cocci, particularly methacillin-susceptible *S. aureus* (38). Only ceftazidime and cefoperazone have clinically useful activity against *Pseudomonas aeruginosa*. The newest cephalosporins represent attempts to maintain activity against Gram-positive and Gram-negative organisms, including *P. aeruginosa* and many of the *Enterobacteriaceae,* and avoid many of the problems of resistance that have affected other antimicrobial compounds. Such agents have been termed fouth-generation cephalosporins (38, 61).

STRUCTURE-ACTIVITY RELATIONSHIP

The basic cephalosporin structure consists of a dihydro-thiazine ring fused to a β-lactam ring (Fig. 1). Structural manipulation of the cephalosporin nucleus has primarily involved two sites: (*a*) the 7-acyl group of the β-lactam ring with the resultant change in the antibacterial spectrum and (*b*) substitution in the third position on the dihydrothiazine ring, which changes the pharmacokinetic properties of the drug (9), although some change in antibacterial activity can also result from substitutions at this position. Substitution of different

acyl side chains has significantly advanced the spectrum of more recent cephalosporins as well as increasing their intrinsic β- lactamase stability.

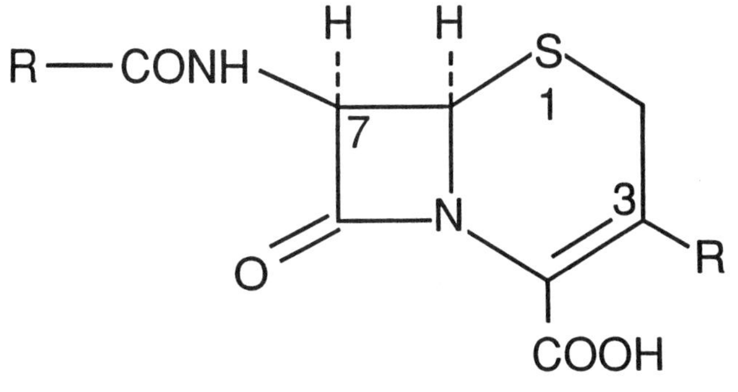

A significant advance in the chemistry of cephalosporins was the introduction of the 2-amino-5-thiazolyl nucleus. Merger of this moiety with the *syn* (Z)-methoxyimino chain found in cefuroxime yielded the new third-generation cephalosporins of which cefotaxime was the leading compound (12). Introduction of the 2-amino-5-thiazolyl moiety greatly enhances antibacterial activity against Gram-negative bacilli. Addition of the *syn* (Z)-methoxyimino residue enhanced the stability to broad-spectrum β-lactamase hydrolysis.

After the discovery of cefotaxime, one of the aims of research in the field of cephalosporins was to modify the 3- hetero-cyclic moiety to affect the plasma half-life. This goal was reached with ceftriaxone (65). Many of the earlier compounds have an *N*-methyltetrazol thio at the C-3 position of the cephem nucleus, which was found to give rise to disulfiram-like reactions and coagulation abnormalities in humans.

Another goal of research in the field of cephalosporins was to improve the antibacterial activity against *P. aeruginosa, S. aureus,* and Gram-negative bacilli producing type 1 β- lactamases. Cefsulodin and ceftazidime were the first cephalosporins with improved activity against *P. aeruginosa* and used in this clinical setting. They bear a 1-pyridinium group at the C-3 position. This observation prompted researchers to prepare a new series of cephalosporins with a 2-amino-5- thiazolyloxi-imino chain at the 7-β position and a positively charged group at C-3 (azolium group). Most C-3 quaternary ammonium cephems have a condensed azolium moiety, except ceflupre-nam (Fig. 2). All of these derivatives are zwitterionic compounds, and they have no net anionic charge, since the negative charge of the carboxylic acid group is (internally) neutralized (compensated) by a positive charge of the 3-quaternary ammonium group.

Ceftazidime is an earlier oxiimino-2-amino-5-thiazolyl quaternary ammonium cephalosporin. Other cephalosporins contain a C-3 pyridium, but none possess a 2-amino-5-thiazolyl moiety. Ceftazidime is a dianionic cephalosporin, in contrast to other compounds (e.g., cefpirome, cefepime), which are zwitterionic derivatives. Ceftazidime contains a carboxypropyloxiimino substituent attached to the α-acetyl chain. The additional carboxylic group provides acidic (negative charge) properties to this compound. The carboxylate anion of the cephem ring is neutralized by the positively charged quaternary ammonium group. The extra negative charge strongly influences the biologic properties of ceftazidime (Figure 3). The 2-amino-5-thiazolyl ring was modified also. Substitution of the thiazolyl ring with a chlorine atom increased the antibacterial activity against *P. aeruginosa*, whereas activity against other Gram-negative bacilli decreased. Introduction of a 5-amino-2-thiadiazolyl nucleus instead of a 2-amino-5-thiazolyl ring enhanced the antipseudomonal activity but slightly decreased activity against the *Enterobacteriaceae* (78). Analogues bearing a hydroxyimino residue exhibit higher activity against *S. aureus* but are less active against Gram-negative bacteria than their methoxyimino counter-

FIGURE 1. Cephalosporin structure.

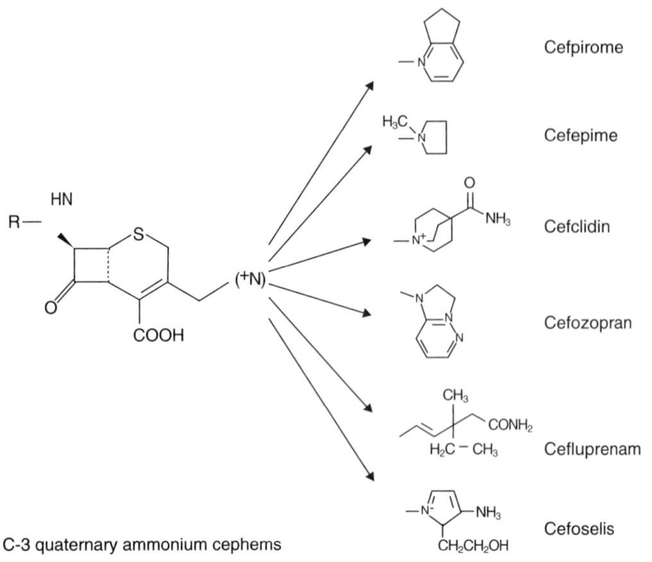

Cefpirome

Cefepime

Cefclidin

Cefozopran

Cefluprenam

Cefoselis

C-3 quaternary ammonium cephems

FIGURE 2. C-3′ quaternary ammonium cephems.

parts. Introduction of a monofluoromethoxyimino group at the 7-position led to a twofold increase in activity against most bacteria, compared with the methoxyimono counterpart.

Among all of the C-3 quaternary ammonium cephems, research continues into overcoming production of extended-spectrum β- lactamases by *Enterobacteriaceae,* increasing antipseudomonal activity, and trying to obtain compounds active against methicillin-resistant isolates of *S. aureus.*

Extended-spectrum β-lactamases are recognized for their ability to provide resistance to cefotaxime, ceftriaxone, ceftazidime, and aztreonam and, to some extent, to C-3 quaternary ammonium cephalosporins. However, MICs for cefpirome or cefepime to *Enterobacteriaceae* producing TEM-type enzymes are 8 mg/L or less, but these compounds are less stable to hydrolysis by SHV-type enzymes (MICs ≥ 16 mg/L) except for SHV-5 (MIC, 2–4 mg/L) (34). Substitution with catechol or pridone moieties yielded a new wave of cephalosporins that are stable to hydrolysis by these enzymes, such as RU 59863 (3).

ANTIMICROBIAL ACTIVITY

First-generation cephalosporins are very active against Gram-positive cocci and have moderate activity against community-acquired *Moraxella catarrhalis, E. coli, Proteus mirabilis* (indole negative), *Klebsiella pneumoniae, Salmonella* spp., and *Shigella* spp. (Tables 1 and 2). The antibacterial activity of these agents for other *Enterobacteriaceae* is unpredictable and should not be assumed (32). While active against most of the penicillin-susceptible oral cavity anaerobes, the *Bacteroides fragilis* group is resistant. First-generation cephalosporins have poor activity against *Haemophilus influenzae* and are not active against methicillin-resistant staphylococci, penicillin-resistant pneumococci, and enterococci. Even when in vitro susceptibility tests suggest that cephalosporins are likely to be effective against methicillin-resistant staphylococci, these agents are not effective therapeutically (38).

Second-generation cephalosporins should be considered in two groups: the true cephalosporins and the cephamycins (cefoxitin, cefotetan, cefmetazole). The true cephalosporins in this group provide greater activity against staphylococci and nonenterococcal streptococci than the first-generation group. In addition, they have significantly improved activity against *H. influenzae, M. catarrhalis, Neisseria meningitidis,* and *Neisseria gonorrhoeae.* Compared with the first-generation compounds and the second-generation true cephalosporins, cephamycins have inferior activity against staphylococci and streptococci, but they (particularly cefotetan) have an enhanced antibacterial effect against selected *Enterobacteriaceae.* They are noteworthy as the cephems most active against *Bacteroides* spp., particularly *B. fragilis* (38, 62).

Third-generation cephalosporins are commonly viewed as the most potent cephalosporins against facultative Gram-negative bacilli. In addition, however, they have superior antimicrobial activity against *Streptococcus pneumoniae* (including those with relative penicillin resistance), *S. pyogenes,* and other streptococci. Most have modest activity against *S. aureus,* with the exception of ceftazidime. They also have excellent activity against *H. influenzae, N. meningitidis, N. gonorrhoeae,* and *Moraxella* spp. In spite of wide use, these agents have retained a high degree of activity against *E. coli, Klebsiella, P. mirabilis, Providencia,* and *Serratia* (38, 40).

Third-generation cephalosporins may be subdivided on the basis of their activity against *P. aeruginosa;* ceftizoxime, ceftriaxone, moxalactam (an oxacephem), cefixime, and cefpodoxime lack activity against *P. aeruginosa.* Antipseudomonal activity is found in cefoperazone, ceftazidime, and the newer fourth-generation agents, cefsulodin, cefepime, cefpirome, and cefpiramide.

Third-generation cephalosporins, like all of the compounds based on the cephem nucleus, lack activity against *Enterococcus* spp., methicillin-resistant staphylococci, highly penicillin-resistant *S. pneumoniae, Listeria,* and *Xanthomonas.* They have variable activity against *Acinetobacter.* The superior broad activity of these agents against *Enterobacteriaceae*

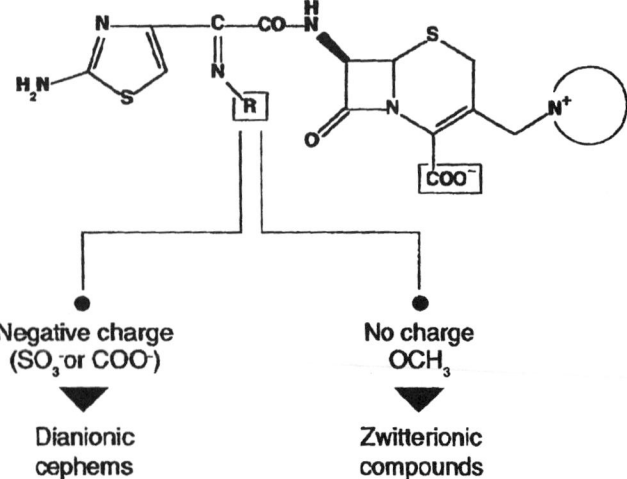

FIGURE 3. Structure of dianionic and zwitterionic cephalosporins.

TABLE 1 • **In Vitro Antimicrobial Activity against Common Gram-Positive Pathogens**

Species	Antimicrobial Agent	MIC Range	MIC$_{50}$	MIC$_{90}$	References
Methicillin-sensitive *S. aureus*	Cefazolin		0.32	1.2	28
	Cephalothin		0.2	1	28, 76
	Cefamandole		0.5	1	28, 76
	Cefotetan				
	Cefoxitin		2.3	3.1	28, 76
	Cefuroxime		1.1	2.2	28, 76
	Cefixime				
	Cefoperazone		2	4	28
	Cefotaxime	1–4	1.6	3.1	5, 28, 70
	Cefpodoxime				
	Ceftazidime	6–28.5	6.7	12.5	5, 28, 70
	Ceftizoxime		0.6	8	20, 28
	Ceftriaxone		3.3	5.5	20, 28
	Cefepime	0.5–16	2.1	2.8	5, 60, 68, 70
Methicillin-resistant *S. aureus*	Cefazolin				
	Cephalothin			32	76
	Cefamandole			8	6, 76
	Cefotetan				
	Cefoxitin			6.3	76
	Cefuroxime			0.2	76
	Cefixime				
	Cefoperazone			>256	6, 20
	Cefotaxime			128	6, 20
	Cefpodoxime				
	Ceftazidime			128	5, 6
	Ceftizoxime			>256	20
	Ceftriaxone			256	20
	Cefepime			8–256	5, 60
S. pneumoniae	Cefazolin				
	Cephalothin			0.12	76
	Cefamandole			0.25	6, 76
	Cefotetan				
	Cefoxitin			2	76
	Cefuroxime		0.01	0.015	35, 76
	Cefixime		0.5		35
	Cefoperazone			0.25	35
	Cefotaxime	0.02	0.02	<0.09	5, 35, 70
	Cefpodoxime		0.03	0.06	20, 35
	Ceftazidime	0.12–0.5	0.27	0.33	5, 20, 70
	Ceftizoxime			0.25	20
	Ceftriaxone			0.5	20
	Cefepime	0.01–0.25	0.03	<0.25	5, 61, 68, 70
S. pyogenes	Cefazolin				
	Cephalothin			<0.25	6
	Cefamandole			<0.25	6
	Cefotetan				
	Cefoxitin				
	Cefuroxime		0.008		35
	Cefixime		0.05		35
	Cefoperazone			0.12	6, 20
	Cefotaxime		0.03	0.06	6, 20, 35
	Cefpodoxime		0.008		35
	Ceftazidime	0.1		0.4	5, 20
	Ceftizoxime			<0.01	20
	Ceftriaxone			0.03	20
	Cefepime	<0.015–0.25		0.1	5, 61

has recently been challenged by β-lactamase and plasmid-mediated resistance, representing a widening threat to the utility of third-generation cephalosporins (38, 53).

Cefpirome, a fourth-generation cephalosporin, has superior activity against streptococci, *S. aureus, Neisseria* spp., *H. influenzae,* and the *Enterobacteriaceae.* It is less active than ceftazidime against *P. aeruginosa.* Cefepime, like cefpirome, a fourth-generation cephalosporin, has exceptionally broad an-

TABLE 2 • In Vitro Antimicrobial Activity against Common Gram-Negative Pathogens

Species	Antimicrobial Agent	MIC Range	MIC$_{50}$	MIC$_{90}$	Reference
B. fragilis	Cefazolin		64	>128	28
	Cephalothin		128	>128	28
	Cefamandole		16	128	28
	Cefotetan				
	Cefoxitin		8	16	28
	Cefuroxime		32	>100	28
	Cefixime				
	Cefoperazone		32	>128	28
	Cefotaxime		4–32	60–>128	28, 77
	Cefpodoxime				
	Ceftazidime		20	94	28
	Ceftizoxime		24	54	28
	Ceftriaxone		22	100	28
	Cefepime				
C. freundii	Cefazolin	16–>128	14	>128	14
	Cephalothin				
	Cefamandole				
	Cefotetan	0.03–64	0.25	64	14
	Cefoxitin				
	Cefuroxime				
	Cefixime				
	Cefoperazone				
	Cefotaxime	0.06–32	0.12	16	14
	Cefpodoxime				
	Ceftazidime	0.25–64	0.5	64	14
	Ceftizoxime	0.06–32	0.25	32	14
	Ceftriaxone				
	Cefepime	0.015–0.12	0.03	0.6–4	14, 73
E. cloacae	Cefazolin	128–>128	>128	>128	14
	Cephalothin	32–>32	>32	>32	8
	Cefamandole				
	Cefotetan	0.06–>128	32	>128	14
	Cefoxitin				
	Cefuroxime	1–>132	16	>32	8
	Cefixime				
	Cefoperazone				
	Cefotaxime	0.06–>128	0.25	2–128	14, 44
	Cefpodoxime			>32	41
	Ceftazidime	0.1–>32	1	32	8, 14
	Ceftizoxime	0.06–128	0.25	128	14
	Ceftriaxone	≤0.1–>64	0.3	16	8
	Cefepime	0.015–8	0.06	0.5–8	14. 41. 73
E. coli	Cefazolin	0.3–>32	1	8	8, 14, 28
	Cephalothin		1.4	5	28
	Cefamandole		≤0.5	4	28
	Cefotetan	0.015–0.5	0.06	0.25	14
	Cefoxitin		4.5	8.2	28
	Cefuroxime	1–128	4	8	8, 28
	Cefixime				
	Cefoperazone		0.74	43	28
	Cefotaxime	0.03–8	0.06	0.125–0.5	14, 28, 77
	Cefpodoxime			2	41
	Ceftazidime	≤0.1–32	0.3	0.5–1	8, 14, 28
	Ceftizoxime	0.015–4	0.06	0.25	14, 28
	Ceftriaxone	≤0.1–4	≤0.1	0.1–.89	8, 28
	Cefepime	0.015–2	0.03	0.12	14, 41, 73
	Cefpirome	≤0.1–2	≤0.1	≤0.1	8
H. influenzae	Cefazolin		8	16	72
	Cephalothin				
	Cefamandole		0.8	2	72
	Cefotetan	0.6	1.2		72
	Cefoxitin		4.5	8.2	28, 72
	Cefuroxime			0.5	41

continued

TABLE 2 • **In Vitro Antimicrobial Activity against Common Gram-Negative Pathogens**

Species	Antimicrobial Agent	MIC Range	MIC$_{50}$	MIC$_{90}$	Reference
	Cefixime			≤0.06	41
	Cefoperazone		0.1	0.1	72
	Cefotaxime	<0.12–0.5	≤0.12	≤0.12	25, 77
	Cefpodoxime			0.13	41
	Ceftazidime	<0.12–0.5	≤0.12	≤0.12	25, 77
	Ceftizoxime	<0.12–0.5	≤0.12	0.25	25, 28
	Ceftriaxone	<0.12–0.5	0.07	0.89	25, 28
	Cefepime	≤0.016–1	≤0.016–0.06	0.12	41, 60, 73
K. pneumoniae	Cefazolin	0.12–>128	0.5	>128	14
	Cephalothin	≤0.1–>32	1–8	2–32	8, 14
	Cefamandole		1	8	28
	Cefotetan	0.03–64	0.06	0.25	14
	Cefoxitin		2.5	5.1	28
	Cefuroxime	≤0.1–>32	2	8	8, 28
	Cefixime				
	Cefoperazone		≤0.25	2–8	28, 72
	Cefotaxime	<0.008–64	0.06	0.6–0.8	14, 44, 77
	Cefpodoxime				
	Ceftazidime	≤0.1–8	0.3	1–4	8, 14
	Ceftizoxime	<0.008–8	0.015	4	14
	Ceftriaxone	≤0.1–0.3	≤0.1	≤0.1	8
	Cefepime	<0.008–2	0.03	0.12–1	14, 41, 73
P. mirabilis	Cefazolin	1–>32	4	8–128	8, 14, 72
	Cephalothin				
	Cefamandole		1.6	8	72
	Cefotetan	0.06–0.12	0.12	0.12–8	14, 72
	Cefoxitin				
	Cefuroxime	≤0.1–16	1	2	8
	Cefixime				
	Cefoperazone		0.5	1	72
	Cefotaxime	≤0.008–0.06	0.03	0.03	14
	Cefpodoxime				
	Ceftazidime	≤0.1–2	≤0.1	0.5	8, 14
	Ceftizoxime	≤0.008–0.015	≤0.008	≤0.008	14
	Ceftriaxone	≤0.1	≤0.1	≤0.1	8
	Cefepime	0.06–0.12	0.06	<0.006–0.06	14, 73
M. morganii	Cefazolin	32–>128	128	>128	14
	Cephalothin				
	Cefamandole				
	Cefotetan	0.25–64	1	8	14
	Cefoxitin				
	Cefuroxime				
	Cefixime				
	Cefoperazone				
	Cefotaxime	0.015–32	0.25	16	14
	Cefpodoxime				
	Ceftazidime	0.06–64	0.25	16	14
	Ceftizoxime	0.015–64	1	32	14
	Ceftriaxone				
	Cefepime	0.015–0.25	0.03	0.06	14
	Cefpirome				
N. gonorrhoea	Cefazolin		0.6	1.7	28
	Cephalothin		0.8	4.6	28
	Cefamandole		0.027	3.1	28
	Cefotetan				
	Cefoxitin		0.8	1.6	28
	Cefuroxime		0.015	0.25	28
	Cefixime				
	Cefoperazone		0.008	0.06	28
	Cefotaxime		<0.025	<0.12	28
	Cefpodoxime				
	Ceftazidime		0.015	0.12	28
	Ceftizoxime			0.007	28

continued

TABLE 2 • In Vitro Antimicrobial Activity against Common Gram-Negative Pathogens

Species	Antimicrobial Agent	MIC Range	MIC$_{50}$	MIC$_{90}$	Reference
	Ceftriaxone		<0.025	0.04	28
	Cefepime	≤0.03–0.5	0.06–0.2	≤0.12–0.5	60
P. aeruginosa	Cefazolin	>32	>32	>32	8
	Cephalothin				
	Cefamandole		>100	>100	28
	Cefotetan	128–>128	>128	>128	14
	Cefoxitin		>100	>100	28
	Cefuroxime	>32	>32	>32	8
	Cefixime				
	Cefoperazone		4	16	72
	Cefotaxime	8–>128	64	>128	14
	Cefpodoxime				
	Ceftazidime	0.5–>32	4	16	8, 14
	Ceftizoxime	16–>128	128	>128	14
	Ceftriaxone	4–>64	32	>64	8
	Cefepime	1–32	8	32	14
S. marcescens	Cefazolin	>32	>32	>32	8
	Cephalothin		>100	>100	28
	Cefamandole		100	>100	28
	Cefotetan		128	256	72
	Cefoxitin		25	>64	28
	Cefuroxime	32–>32	>32	>32	8
	Cefixime				
	Cefoperazone		6.5	26.3	28
	Cefotaxime		3.6–16	9.5–64	28, 72
	Cefpodoxime				
	Ceftazidime	0.1–8	0.5	4	8
	Ceftizoxime	1.6–32	3.7–64		28, 72
	Ceftriaxone	<0.1–16	0.3–16	2–64	8, 28, 72
	Cefepime	≤0.016–32	0.031–0.5	0.063–1	60
Salmonella spp.	Cefazolin	1–8	2	4	14
	Cephalothin				
	Cefamandole	0.19–200			75
	Cefotetan	0.06–0.12	0.06	0.12	14
	Cefoxitin				
	Cefuroxime	0.02–1.6			75
	Cefixime				
	Cefoperazone	<0.125–38			75
	Cefotaxime	0.03–0.25	0.12	0.25	14, 75
	Cefpodoxime				
	Ceftazidime	0.12–0.25	0.25	0.5	14
	Ceftizoxime	0.015–0.25	0.03	0.06	14, 75
	Ceftriaxone	0.07–0.19			75
	Cefepime	0.03–0.5	0.06	0.12	14, 75

tibacterial activity against *S. pneumoniae, S. pyogenes, S. aureus, H. influenzae, Neisseria* spp., and the *Enterobacteriaceae*. Fifty percent of *P. aeruginosa* strains are inhibited by cefepime at concentrations less than 8 µg/mL (70).

Pharmacodynamics

The pharmacology of antimicrobial therapy can be separated into two distinct components. The first is pharmacokinetics, which deals with the absorption, distribution, and elimination of antimicrobials. These factors determine the time course of antimicrobial concentrations in serum and tissues for a given dosing regimen. Pharmacodynamics, the second component, is concerned with the relationship between concentration and antimicrobial effect. The time course of antimicrobial therapy reflects the interrelationship between pharmacokinetics and pharmacodynamics.

The minimum inhibitory and minimum bactericidal concentrations (MIC and MBC) are major parameters used to quantify the activity of an antimicrobial against the infecting pathogen. However, these parameters do not provide information about the activity of higher drug concentrations or the antimicrobial effects that can persist after drug exposure. Persistent suppression of bacterial growth after short exposure to an antimicrobial is called the *postantibiotic effect* (PAE). The effect of increasing concentrations on the bactericidal activity of antimicrobials and the presence or absence of a PAE give a much better description of the time course of antimicrobial activity than is provided by the MIC and MBC.

Two major patterns of bactericidal activity are observed with increasing drug concentrations. The first pattern is characterized by marked concentration-dependent killing over a wide range of concentrations. The higher the drug concentration, the greater the extent and rate of bactericidal activity. This pattern is observed with the aminoglycosides and fluoroquinolones (17, 38).

The second pattern is characterized by a saturation of the rate of killing at concentrations near the MIC. Thus, high concentrations do not kill the organism faster or more extensively than low concentrations. Duration of exposure, rather than concentration, is the major determinant of the extent of killing. This pattern of bactericidal activity, also called time-dependent killing, is seen with the β-lactams, including cephalosporins, vancomycin, macrolides, and clindamycin (17).

All antimicrobials appear to be capable of producing prolonged PAEs with Gram-positive cocci (19), and drugs that inhibit protein or nucleic acid synthesis also induce PAEs with Gram-negative bacilli. β-Lactam antibiotics produce short or no PAEs with Gram-negative bacilli. The presence of neutrophils does not markedly enhance the in vivo PAEs observed with cephalosporins (18).

Because β-lactams, including cephalosporins, exhibit time-dependent killing and produce prolonged PAEs only with staphylococci, the goal of dosing with these agents is to optimize the duration of exposure. The length of time that concentrations exceed the MIC should be the pharmacodynamic parameter that best correlates with therapeutic efficacy of β-lactam antibiotics (77).

Because most infections occur in tissues and the common bacterial pathogens are extracellular, interstitial fluid concentrations at the site of infection are the prime determinants of efficacy. Although some studies suggest that the tissue concentration of broad-spectrum cephalosporins such as cefotaxime may be lower than that in serum (59), most tissue sites within the body can be described as having a large capillary surface area across which antimicrobials diffuse into a relatively small volume of interstitial fluid. Drug concentrations at these sites show little lag and are very close to serum concentrations. This has been demonstrated for the broad-spectrum cephalosporins in humans (42, 67). Thus, for most suseptible organisms, levels will exceed the MIC for a longer time in sites with a low surface area:volume ratio than in serum (17).

MECHANISMS OF ACTION

Like other β-lactam agents, cephalosporins interfere with the later stages of bacterial cell wall synthesis by inhibiting peptidoglycan cross-linkage and by binding to and inactivating one or more of the seven penicillin-binding proteins (PBPs) of the bacterial cell wall (40). Thus, the intrinsic activity of a cephalosporin depends upon the ability of the antibiotic to penetrate the cell surface and its binding affinity to protein receptor molecules. The multiplicity of PBPs and the observation that most β-lactam antibiotics bind to only one or two proteins suggests that β-lactams that bind to different proteins may act synergistically when used in combination (9). The effectiveness of cephalosporins against Gram-negative bacilli

is due to a combination of their ability to penetrate the outer membrane, their stability to β-lactamase hydrolysis in the periplasmic space, and their affinity for penicillin-binding proteins.

Nikaido et al., using proteoliposome, demonstrated that cefclidin, cefpirome, and cefepime penetrated the porin channel of *E. coli* and *Enterobacter cloacae* more rapidly than ceftazidime (56). Yoshimura and Nikaido showed that the C-7-β-methoxyimino residue on the O-carbon of the 7-β substituent could decrease the rate of penetration of monoanionic cephalosporins through the outer membrane into *E. coli* OmpF porin by a factor of 10 or more (79). Non-2-amino-5-thiazolyl quanternary ammonium cephalosporins are hydrolyzed at low concentrations (<10 μM) of type 1 β-lactamases (45). Type 1 β-lactamases hydrolyze these cephalosporins (cefpirome, cefepime, cefclidin) more slowly than the earlier compounds at low substrate concentrations.

Cefpirome, cefepime, and cefclidin share low affinities or high K_m values for type 1 β-lactamases and can be expected to be hydrolyzed slowly in vivo (33, 71). Cefpirome, cefepime, cefclidin, and ceftazidime share a high affinity for PBP3 of *E. coli* K-12 (62).

MECHANISMS OF RESISTANCE

A microorganism may have either intrinsic or acquired resistance to an antimicrobial. Intrinsic resistance is a stable genetic property encoded in the chromosomal DNA and shared by all members of the genus. Acquired resistance occurs when there is a change in the bacterial DNA so that a new phenotype trait can be expressed. Bacteria can acquire resistance through a mutation in the host's chromosomal DNA or by acquisition of new DNA, of either chromosomal or extrachromosomal origin, that carries information for resistance. Enterococci are intrinsically resistant to all clinically available cephalosporins (50).

Microorganisms resist the antibacterial activity of the cephalosporins by several acquired mechanisms acting alone or in combination. One major mechanism of resistance to this group of β-lactams is by inhibiting uptake. Gram-negative bacteria are surrounded by an outer phospholipid membrane that retards entry of various substrates, including cephalosporins. A second mechanism for resistance is the production of β-lactamases, a group of enzymes that hydrolyze the β-lactam ring of the cepahalosporins and render the antibiotic ineffective. In general, Gram-negative microorganisms produce β-lactamase that is more effective than that produced by Gram-positive organisms. Different cephalosporins vary in their sensitivity to hydrolysis by these enzymes. The antibacterial properties of the various cephalosporins depend on a combination of factors acting simultaneously, including the ability of the antibiotic to penetrate the bacteria and gain access to the target site, the affinity to bind to the proteins involved in the cell wall synthesis, and the degree of resistance to β-lactamases (9, 11).

β-Lactam antimicrobials may be strong or weak inducers of β-lactamase expression and may be stable against, or very labile to, the induced enzyme. An antimicrobial's efficacy thus depends on a combination of characteristics. If an antimicrobial is both labile and a strong inducer, it causes its own destruction. This is seen with the early cephalosporins, which lack activity against β-lactamase- inducible species because they are potent inducers and good substrates for these enzymes. Most later- generation cephalosporins are labile to these enzymes but are weak inducers, so they do not cause their own hydrolysis and thus retain activity against β-lactamase-inducible organisms.

Another therapeutic consideration is the amount of β-lactamase that is produced and the associated phenomenon of stable derepression, which, along with reversible derepression, is seen in class 1 chromosomal β-lactamases. In stable derepression, a bacterial mutation in the repressor gene causes irreversible genetic regulation of class 1 β-lactamase expression, and the enzyme is secreted steadily and copiously. Strong inducers (stable or otherwise) are not very selective, and they provide no advantage to β-lactamase-derepressed bacteria in relation to bacteria in which the enzyme is induced. Once selected, the derepressed class 1 mutants are cross-resistant to most penicillins, including pipercillin and ticarcillin, as well as to expanded-spectrum cephalosporins such as cefotaxime and ceftazidime. In general, carbapenems, cefpirome, and cefepime remain active, although with increasing use, their efficacy is expected to diminish.

Of the plasmid-mediated β-lactamases, the most important are staphylococcal penicillinase and the TEM and SHV enzymes of Gram-negative bacilli. Staphylococcal β-lactamase is an inducible penicillinase with very poor activity against cephalosporins. However, methicillin-resistant *S. aureus* (MRSA) is resistant to cephalosporins. The plasmid-mediated β-lactamases of Gram-negative bacteria are not inducible, unlike those of Gram-positive bacteria. Many of these plasmids are conjugative, and the spread of resistance among Gram-negative bacteria is a major problem.

Historically, most bacteria produced only trace amounts of chromosomally mediated β-lactamases, but with the widespread use of β-lactam antimicrobials, bacterial strains that secrete the enzyme copiously and those that produce enzymes that attack an extended range of β-lactam substrates have been favored by natural selection. These evolutionary processes have been accelerated by the spread of β-lactamase genes to plasmids; the potential for spreading is further exaggerated by superimposing transposition on existing conjugative and other exchange mechanisms (50).

PHARMACOKINETIC DISPOSITION
Absorption

Most cephalosporins, especially the third-generation agents, are either inactivated by stomach acid or are not significantly absorbed from the intestine (7). Absorption from the gastrointestinal tract occurs for cephalexin, cephradine, and cefadroxil among first-generation agents, for cefaclor, cefuroxime axetil, cefpodoxime, cefprozil, and loracarbef among second-generation agents, and for cefixime and ceftibuten among third-generation agents. These are acid stable (38).

Absorption of cefuroxime and cefpodoxime is facilitated by their formulation as esters, or prodrugs. The compounds are cleaved to active drug by intestinal mucosal esterases during absorption. Absorption of esterified cephalosporins is enhanced by administration with food, apparently because of the more-prolonged contact with the gastric mucosa due to food-associated delay in gastric emptying (52). Gastrointestinal absorption of other oral cephalosporins is delayed in the presence of food in the stomach, resulting in lower and delayed peak serum concentrations, although the total amount of drug absorbed is not affected (57).

Generally, cephalosporins are well absorbed when administered intramuscularly; peak serum concentrations appear after 0.5 to 1.0 h. The modest discomfort of intramuscular cephalosporin administration is reduced by adding 1% lidocaine solution to the diluent. This does not interfere with absorption of the cephalosporin. However, absorption from an intramuscular site is unpredictable in seriously ill patients, and they should receive intravenous drug administration (7).

Protein Binding

In the blood, cephalosporins bind reversibly to serum proteins, primarily albumin. The percentage of drug bound to proteins is characteristic of each compound (Table 3). Only unbound drug can leave the vascular compartment and penetrate tissues (52). Binding ranges from 10% for a few oral cephalosporins to approximately 95% for cefonicid and ceftriaxone. Serum protein binding is easily dissociated and the bound cephalosporin represents a temporary pool of the drug, which partly explains the long serum half- life of cefotetan, cefonicid, and ceftriaxone (7). These agents also display concentration-dependent protein binding; the extent of protein binding decreases at higher serum concentrations because of saturation of the binding sites (52). Except for the influence on serum half-life, even when binding approaches 95%, it is of questionable significance. The high degree of protein binding associated with ceftriaxone does not prevent penetration into the cerebrospinal fluid. None of the cephalosporins is bound to the extent that displacement of highly protein-bound drugs results in clinically significant drug interactions (15, 20, 52).

Distribution

Cephalosporins penetrate well into most tissues and body fluids (40, 52). The first-generation cephalosporins achieve therapeutic concentrations in the pericardial, pleural, and synovial fluids, and in most tissue spaces except the central nervous system. Only cefuroxime and the third-generation cephalosporins penetrate the cerebrospinal fluid in high enough concentrations to treat meningitis caused by a susceptible organism (52). All second-generation cephalosporins penetrate osseous tissue and attain bone levels significantly higher than those of first-generation agents (57). Penetration of cephalosporins into the aqueous humor of the eye may be sufficient with high-dose parenteral therapy to allow effective treatment of anterior chamber infection caused by susceptible bacteria, although cephalosporins do not achieve significant concentrations in the posterior chamber vitreous humor (38).

Biliary concentrations of cephalosporins are in the therapeutic range if biliary obstruction is not present. Due to significant biliary excretion, cefoperazone and ceftriaxone attain

TABLE 3 • Pharmacokinetic Parameters of Parenteral Cephalosporins

Cephalosporin	Protein Binding (%)	Peak Conc. (mg/L)(g)	Elim. Half-life (h)	Apparent Vd (L)	CL(Tot) (mL/min)	CL(Ren) (mL/min)	Urinary Excretion (%)	Biliary Excretion	CSF Concentration Range (mg/L)	Reference
First-generation										
Cefazolin	86	189(1)	1.8	10	64	64	80 +/- 16	yes		27, 32, 47
Cephalothin	70	64(1)	0.6	18.5	470	268	52	yes		27, 32, 47
Cephapirin	54	73(1)	0.7	16		342	48 +/- 7	yes		27, 32, 47
Second-generation										
Cefamandole	70	139(1)	0.8	17	250	257	96 +/- 3	yes		27, 32, 47
Cefmetazole	85	140(2)	1–1.5	10	90–165	90–110	75	yes		38, 80
Cefonicid	98	260(2)	4.4	9		270	88 +/- 6	yes		29, 32, 38, 47
Cefoxitin	73	64(1)	0.7	8	268		78	yes		29, 32, 38, 47
Cefotetan	90		3.3	11	33–46	25–30	61 +/- 1	no		29, 32, 38, 47, 80
Cefuroxime	33	40–130(0.75)	1.7	13	128	123	96 +/- 10	yes	1.1–17	29, 32, 38, 47
Third-generation										
Cefoperazone	87	74–152 (1)	2.1	11	80	18	29 +/- 4	yes		29, 32, 38, 47, 80
Cefotaxime	30	102(1)	1.1	14	260–326	154	50 +/- 5	yes	5.6–44	29, 32, 38, 47, 80
Ceftazidime	17	83(1)	1.8	13.6	78–144	72–130	84 +/- 4	yes	0.5–30	29, 32, 38, 47, 80
Ceftizoxime	31	84(1)	1.8	28	155	89–110	93 +/- 8	yes	0.5–29	29, 32, 38, 47, 80
Ceftriaxone	95	110(0.5)	8	10.7	17.6	6	46 +/- 7	yes	1.2–39	29, 32, 38, 47, 80
Fourth-generation										
Cefepime	16	130(2)	2–2.3	20.5	122–131	103–110	84	no		32, 80

very high biliary concentrations (52). Cefuroxime also attains high biliary levels with patent or obstructed cystic ducts, suggesting that the drug may diffuse in the gall bladder and bile from the bloodstream (57).

Cephalosporins readily cross the placenta, and fetal serum concentrations may be 10% or more of the maternal serum concentration. Cephalosporins distribute into breast milk in low concentrations.

Metabolism

Metabolism is a factor in the elimination of cephalothin, cephapirin, and cefotaxime. For these agents, 20 to 30% of the administered dose is metabolized in the liver to desacetyl derivatives that have some synergistic antibacterial activity and are excreted by the kidneys (52). Desacetylcefotaxime has considerable antimicrobial activity and good penetration into extravascular tissue (40). Biotransformation partially accounts for the short half-lives of cephalothin and cephapirin (7).

Elimination

Most cephalosporins are excreted primarily by the kidneys in an active unchanged form; hence they achieve very high urine concentrations. This excess urine concentration relative to the MIC of the usual urinary tract pathogen often allows effective treatment of urinary tract infection with reduced doses of cephalosporins. Moderate-to-severe renal dysfunction necessitates dosage adjustment of most cephalosporins (38, 57). Biliary excretion plays a significant role in the elimination of cefoperazone, ceftriaxone, and cefixime. Approximately 70% of cefoperazone and approximately 40% of ceftriaxone is excreted unchanged in the bile. These agents do not require dosage adjustment in renal insufficiency. The half-life of cefotaxime is not significantly increased with renal failure; however, its desacetyl and other metabolites accumulate significantly. Thus, reduced cefotaxime dosing is warranted with severe azotemia (52).

All first- and second-generation cephalosporins except cefaclor and cefonicid are removed by hemodialysis. Peritoneal dialysis enhances the elimination of cephalothin, cephalexin, and cephradrine (57). Cefoperazone and ceftriaxone are not removed by hemodialysis and do not require additional dosing after dialysis (58). Severe hepatic disease can alter the pharmacokinetics of cefoperazone and cefotaxime but has little impact on ceftriaxone. Compensatory renal excretion generally occurs in that setting. Accumulation of cefoperazone, ceftriaxone, and cefotaxime is likely to occur in the setting of combined hepatic and renal failure, and dose adjustment is likely to be required (38).

DOSAGE REGIMENS

Cephalosporins in appropriate forms may be administered orally, intravenously via deep intramuscular injection, or intraperitoneally. In general, orally administered cephalosporins should not be relied on for treatment of the initial phase of severe infections or in patients with nausea or vomiting. Cephalosporins should be given intravenously to patients with septicemia or other severe or life-threatening infections. Intra-

muscular injections should be made in the vastus lateralis or deltoid muscles to ensure maximal absorption rates (49). Cephalosporins have also been administered by regional perfusion, subconjunctivally, intraventricularly, or intrathecally, but the risk of CNS toxicity must be considered with the latter route.

The duration of cephalosporin therapy depends on the type of infection. Generally, therapy should be continued for a minimum of 48 to 72 h after the patient becomes asymptomatic or evidence of eradication of the infection has been obtained. In infections caused by β-hemolytic streptococci, therapy should be continued for at least 10 days. At least 4 to 6 weeks of therapy may be required for serious infections such as septicemia, endocarditis, or osteomyelitis. Perioperative prophylaxis is generally discontinued within 24 h after surgery. Many clinicians believe that postoperative prophylaxis is usually unnecessary for clean or clean-contaminated procedures (47).

Patients with impaired renal function may require decreased doses and/or frequency of administration of cephalosporins; these should be based on the degree of renal impairment, severity of the infection, susceptibility of the causative organism, and serum concentrations of the cephalosporin (Table 4). The dosage of ceftriaxone and cefoperazone needs adjustment only if hepatic failure is also a factor (80).

Maximal daily doses for life-threatening infections or infections of the central nervous system in which high drug concentrations are difficult to obtain are listed in Table 5. For mild-to-moderate infections with highly sensitive microorganisms, lower dosages and less frequent administration may be warranted (32).

Physiologic changes with aging include change in body composition (i.e., decreased lean body mass and increased body fat), reduced protein binding, and diminished elimination capacity. Pharmacokinetic studies of ceftazidime and ceftizoxime conducted in the elderly population show a doubling of the serum half-life by age 70, indicating the need for dosage reduction for renally eliminated cephalosporins in this age group. Dosage adjustment in the elderly is not indicated for cefmetazole, cefixime, or ceftriaxone if renal function remains normal other than the usual decline in creatinine clearance with aging.

Pharmacokinetics in pediatric patients is more complex. In general, administration at less frequent intervals is recommended for neonates; dosages (on a milligram per kilogram basis) for infants and children approach those for adults (Table 5) (80).

ADVERSE EFFECTS

The cephalosporins are a remarkably safe class of antibiotics, that produce few side effects and have a highly favorable toxicity profile compared with other antibiotics. With a few exceptions, the adverse effects caused by cephalosporins are similar across the group (Table 6).

Hypersensitivity reactions to cephalosporins are the most common side effect, and there is no evidence that any single cephalosporin is more or less likely to cause such reaction. The reactions seem to be identical to those caused by the penicillins, which may be related to the shared β-lactam structure of both groups. Infrequently, immediate reactions such as anaphylaxis,

TABLE 4 • Cephalosporin Dosing in Patients with Renal Insufficiency

Cephalosporin	Maintenance 90–50	Dose (g) / Dosing GFR (mL/min) 50–10	Interval (h) <10	Adult Dosing during Dialysis	
				Hemodialysis	CAPD
First-generation					
Cefazolin	usual	0.5–1 / 8–12	0.5–1 / 24	0.5–1 g	0.5 g q. 12 h
Cephapirin	usual	2 / 8	2 / 12	2 g	2 g q. 12 h
Second-generation					
Cefamandole	usual	2/ 8	1 / 12	1 g	1 g q. 12 h
Cefmetazole					
Cefonicid	usual	1 / 24	1 / 72	none	1 g q. 72 h
Cefotetan	usual	2 / 24	2 / 48	1 g	1 g q. 24 h
Cefoxitin	2 / 8	2 / 12	1 / 12	2 g	1 g q. 24 h
Cefuroxime	usual	1.5 / 12	0.75 / 24	1.5 g	0.75 g q. 24 h
Third-generation					
Cefoperazone	usual	usual	usual	usual	usual
Cefotaxime	usual	2 / 12	2 / 24	1 g	1 g q. 24 h
Ceftazidime	usual	1 / 12	1 / 24	1 g	0.5 g q. 24 h
Ceftizoxime	usual	1 / 12	0.5 / 12	1 g	0.5 g q. 24 h
Ceftriaxone	usual	usual	usual	usual	usual
Fourth-generation					
Cefepime	usual	1 / 12–24	0.25–1 / 24	0.25 g	1–2 g q. 48 h

From references 5, 38, 47.

TABLE 5 • Parenteral Cephalosporins and Dosing Ranges

Cephalosporin	Usual Adult Dose in Serious Infection	Adult Daily Dose, Serious Infection	Children (mg/kg/day) / Interval
First-generation			
Cefazolin	1 g q. 8 h	3–6 g	50–100 / q. 6–8 h
Cephalothin	0.5–2 g q. 6 h	6–12 g	75–125 / q. 4–6 h
Cephapirin	2 g q. 6 h	6–12 g	40–80 / q. 4–6 h
Second-generation			
Cefamandole	2 g q. 6 h	6–12 g	100–150 / q. 4–8 h
Cefmetazole	2 g q. 6–12 h	8 g	
Cefonicid	2 g q. 24 h	2 g	40 / q. 24 h
Cefotetan	2 g q. 12 h	4–6 g	40–80 / q. 12 h
Cefoxitin	2 g q. 6 h	6–12 g	80–160 / q. 4–6 h
Cefuroxime	1.5 g q. 8 h	4.5–6 g	100–240 / q. 6–8 h
Third-generation			
Cefoperazone	2 g q. 12 h	6–12 g	100–150 / q. 8–12 h
Cefotaxime	2 g q. 6–8 h	6–12 g	100–180 / q. 4–6 h
Ceftazidime	2 g q. 8 h	6 g	90–150 / q. 8 h
Ceftizoxime	2 g q. 8 h	6–12 g	100–200 / q. 6–8 h
Ceftriaxone	1–2 g q. 12 h	2–4 g	50–100 / q. 12–24 h
Fourth-generation			
Cefepime	2 g q. 12 h	4–6 g	50 / q. 8 h

From references 38, 47.

bronchospasm, and urticaria can occur. More commonly, maculopapular rash develops, usually after several days of therapy, and can be accompanied by fever and eosinophilia.

Because of the similarity in structure of the cephalosporins and penicillins, patients who are allergic to one class may manifest cross-reactivity when an agent of the other class is administered. Clinical studies indicate an approximately 1% frequency of such reactions (47). In general, cephalosporins can be administered safely to patients who had developed a rash, but not anaphylaxis, to penicillin. There are no convincing studies to indicate that cephalosporins can be given routinely to patients with type 1 anaphylaxis to penicillins (55).

TABLE 6 • Adverse Events Associated with Cephalosporins

	Frequency (%)
Thrombophlebitis	1–5
Hypersensitivity reactions	
Maculopapular rash	1–3
Urticaria	1–3
Pruritis	
Anaphylaxis / angioedema	rare
Serum sickness (↑ with cefaclor)	
Eosinophilia	1–7
Hemotologic reactions	
Reversible neutropenia	< 1
Leukopenia	0.5–5
Thrombocytosis	2–5
Thrombocytopenia	0.5–5
Coombs' test positive (hemolysis is rare)	1–5
Coagulation abnormalities	
Hypoprothrombinemia (related to cefamandole, cefotetan, cefoperazone—MTT group)	
Gastrointestinal reactions	
Abnormal liver function tests (mild)	1–7
Diarrhea, nonspecific; C. difficile–related	2–5
Biliary sludge (ceftriaxone - dose related)	20–45
Nephrotoxicity	
Interstitial nephritis	rare
Decrease in GFR	1–6

From references 4, 20, 38, 47, 55.

No test systems reliably predict who is at risk for an allergic reaction to cephalosporins (38).

Antibiotics can cause a variety of hematologic reactions. Hemolytic anemia, caused by some of the early cephalosporins, is currently quite rare. Neutropenia, as seen with cephalexin and with virtually all antimicrobials including cefotaxime, ceftazidime, ceftriaxone, is also very rare. Agranulocytosis, thrombocytosis, and thrombocytopenia have been noted in association with cephalosporins. A serum sickness–like reaction does occur, although infrequently, in children treated orally with cefaclor (55).

Some cephalosporins can alter hemostasis mechanisms. Although antibiotic therapy may inhibit the synthesis and absorption of vitamin K by inhibition of gut flora, hypoprothrombinemia has been associated with competitive inhibition of vitamin K–dependent clotting factors II, VII, IX, and X by the MTT group that occupies position 3 in cefomandole, cefoperazone, cefotetan, and cefmetazole. Like warfarin, this group may also inhibit vitamin K 2,3-epoxide reductase, which converts vitamin K to its active form. Hypoprothrombinemia in patients receiving these agents is variable and is markedly enhanced by poor nutritional status, debilitation, recent surgery, and renal failure. Vitamin K treatment restores the prothrombin time to normal over 24 to 36 h. Weekly prophylaxis with vitamin K has been recommended when MTT-bearing cephalosporins are administered to patients at risk for hypoprothrombinemia (38). Disulfiram-like reactions have been noted when alcohol was ingested within 48 to 72 h after administration of cephalosporins that contain the MTT side chain—cefamandole, cefotetan, and

cefoperazone. The reactions appear to result from accumulation of acetaldehydes and do not occur if alcohol is ingested prior to the first dose of the antibiotic (49).

The most frequent adverse reactions to orally administered cephalosporins are nausea, vomiting and diarrhea. These are usually mild and transient but may be severe enough to require discontinuation of the drug. Adverse gastrointestinal effects can also occur with intramuscular or intravenous cephalosporins. The frequency of nonspecific antibiotic-associated diarrhea is 2 to 5% with cephalosporins. Diarrhea is thought to be more frequent with cefoperazone and ceftriaxone as a consequence of biliary excretion, which raises intraintestinal concentrations and subsequently affects the gastrointestinal flora. Ceftriaxone has also been associated with formation of sonographically identifiable sludge in the gallbladder and common bile duct. While commonly asymptomatic, the sludge may form in 20 to 45% of patients receiving ceftriaxone 2 g daily (38, 55).

The cephalosporins have been implicated as potentially nephrotoxic agents. Renal tubular necrosis has followed administration of early cephalosporins. Currently available cephalosporins are much less toxic and rarely produce significant renal toxicity when used alone in recommended doses (47). Acute tubular necrosis has occasionally been attributed to extremely high doses of cephalothin or to standard high-dose therapy in the elderly. Interstitial nephritis occurs as an apparent hypersensitivity response to cephalosporins.

Thrombophlebitis, a common complication with intravenous administration of medications, occurs in 1 to 5% of cephalosporin recipients and is not uniquely associated with a specific agent. Pain at the site of intramuscular injection is not uncommon and can be alleviated by adding lidocaine to the diluent (38).

DRUG INTERACTIONS

As mentioned above, alcoholic beverages consumed concurrently with or up to 72 h after cefamandole, cefoperazone, or cefotetan may produce acute alcohol intolerance (disulfiram-like reaction). These cephalosporins possess a methyltetrazolethiol side chain that may inhibit aldehyde dehydrogenase. The reaction begins 30 min after alcohol ingestion and may subside 30 min to several hours afterward. The reaction may occur up to 3 days after the last dose of the antibiotic (4).

Nephrotoxicity of the aminoglycosides may be potentiated by concurrent use of some cephalosporins, specifically cephalothin. Renal function should be monitored closely.

Probenecid may increase and prolong cephalosporin plasma levels by competitive inhibition of renal tubular secretion. This interaction is most significant for cephalosporins eliminated primarily by tubular secretion.

Unlike the fluoroquinolones, antacids do not have considerable influence on absorption of oral cephalosporin antibiotics with one exception, absorption of cefpodoxime proxetil was significantly reduced by coadministration of both H2-antagonists and antacids (46). This decrease may be due to incomplete dissolution of the drug in the stomach at increased gastric pH.

Bioavailability of the ester cephalosporins is enhanced by administration after food intake. This effect is not related to a change in gastric pH, since gastric alkalinity induced by H2-antagonists or antacids did not increase enteral absorption of these drugs. One possible explanation for the effect of food is prolonged contact between the ester cephalosporin and the esterases of the intestinal mucosa because of delayed gastric emptying (22).

CLINICAL INDICATIONS
Febrile Neutropenia

Enterobacteriaceae and *P. aeruginosa* are the most prevalent Gram-negative bacteria responsible for febrile neutropenic infections in cancer patients, which are often rapidly fatal (26). Combinations of third-generation cephalosporins, particularly ceftazidime and an aminoglycoside, were, until recently, standard therapy for empirical treatment of febrile episodes in neutropenic patients. This approach provided optimal coverage against Gram-negative bacteria. More recently, the prevalence of Gram-positive bacteria has increased (30). In 1994, the incidence of bacteremia due to Gram-positive cocci rose to 89% (26). In response to this, vancomycin was used empirically in combination with the broad-spectrum antibiotics. This addition has neither improved morbidity or mortality nor reduced time to defervescence. Alternatives to third-generation cephalosporins should be carbapenems, pipercillin-tazobactam, or a fourth-generation cephalosporin.

Because of geographic variations, the epidemiology of resistance in a given center must be considered when choosing a regimen. Recent clinical trials in febrile neutropenia patients support considering fourth-generation cephalosporins as first-line agents in this setting, at least as effective as ceftazidime. In addition, their specific activity against Gram-positive pathogens fully supports their empirical use, especially in patients at high risk for streptococcal bacteremia, which is increasing in neutropenic patients (16, 21, 30).

Bacterial Meningitis

Acute bacterial meningitis is a life-threatening infection needing urgent empirical treatment. Community-acquired pathogens such as *N. meningitidis, H. influenzae,* and *S. pneumoniae* are the predominant causes, accounting for 75% of cases, followed by nosocomial pathogens such as Gram-negative bacilli, *S. aureus,* and *Listeria monocytogenes* (26).

At present, the third-generation cephalosporins cefotaxime and ceftriaxone are the preferred antibiotics for initial empirical therapy for suspected pneumococcal meningitis. Most penicillin-resistant strains are inhibited by a maximum MIC of 2 mg/L (43). The emergence of penicillin-resistant and multidrug-resistant *S. pneumoniae* has severely limited the available therapeutic options. Recent reports of therapeutic failures with some third-generation cephalosporins have further complicated the matter (36, 66, 74). Failure of cephalosporin treatment is increasingly reported with strains having MIC values of 2 mg/L or above, and cefotaxime or ceftriaxone should not be used alone to treat resistant cases. For resistant strains, vancomycin or rifampin should be used in addition to a third-generation cephalosporin (43). All other cephalosporins, with the exception of the fourth-generation cephalosporins, almost uniformly fail to penetrate into noninflamed meninges, and often, penetration through inflamed meninges is not adequate to be useful in the treatment of meningitis and other CNS infections (63).

The fourth-generation cephalosporins, cefpirome and cefepime, have excellent in vitro activity against the pathogens likely to cause meningitis (except *L. monocytogenes*), and with their excellent penetration in the CSF, they offer considerable therapeutic potential. A number of studies found that the MICs and MBCs of cefpirome for penicillin-resistant pneumococci are generally one- to twofold lower than those for cefotaxime, ceftriaxone, or cefepime (24, 43, 48). Although small, such differences may be critical in the treatment of meningitis, when the CSF cephalosporin concentration is similar to the MIC. Preliminary results in studies using cefpirome in the treatment of bacterial meningitis are encouraging, although additional studies are required to support the use of fourth- generation cephalosporins in this setting (26).

Nosocomial and Community-Acquired Pneumonia

Nosocomial pneumonia may be caused by a a number of diverse pathogens including methicillin-resistant *S. aureus* (MRSA), *Legionella pneumophila, Enterobacteriaceae,* or *P. aeruginosa* (23). Third-generation cephalosporins, especially those with antipseudomonal activity, are often used as empirical therapy for nosocomial pneumonia. These agents cover *Enterobacteriaceae* that are often resistant to the extended-spectrum penicillins and second-generation cephalosporins. They also cover commensal flora of the oral cavity including *S. pneumoniae* and *H. influenzae*. Other antibiotics are often added to cover common nosocomial pathogens such as methicillin-resistant *S. aureus* or *Legionella* spp. Aminoglycosides are often added to provide synergistic coverage against resistant Gram-negative rods, minimizing emergence of resistant bacteria, or for double coverage against *P. aeruginosa*.

The common, "typical" pathogens in community-acquired pneumonia are *H. influenzae, M. catarrhalis, S. aureus,* and *S. pneumoniae* (64). Second-generation cephalosporins (e.g., cefuroxime), often in combination with a macrolide, are preferred agents for empirical therapy of community-acquired pneumonia (1, 13). Ceftriaxone can be justified on economic grounds because of its once-daily dosing regimen.

Bacteremia/Septicemia

Morbidity and mortality from bacteremia can be a serious problem in the young, the elderly, and immunocompromised and neutropenic patients. In some studies, mortality associated with bacteremia ranged from 20 to 30% of affected patients and more than 50% in those with severe sepsis of septic shock, although mortality is partly due to underlying disease. Prompt recognition of the infection and empirical antibiotic treatment before microbiologic results are available are essential to avoid complications such as septic shock and multisystem organ failure. The predominant microorganisms responsible for bacteremia include *S. aureus,* coagulase-negative staphylococci, *Enter-*

obacteriaceae (*E. coli*, *Klebsiella* spp., *Enterobacter* spp.), and *P. aeruginosa*. Anaerobes are less likely to be encountered (26).

Gram-positive cocci have now replaced Gram-negative bacilli as the predominant pathogens responsible for single-organism bacteremia (43). Historically, aminoglycosides were used widely in empirical therapy for Gram-negative nosocomial infections, but they have now been replaced by third-generation cephalosporins and fluoroquinolones. Ceftazidime was used frequently as a first-line agent, but the emergence of resistance in up to 50% of strains of *Enterobacteriaceae* has diminished the utility of third-generation cephalosporins in the ICU.

A fourth-generation cephalosporin (e.g., cefpirome or cefepime) with activity against Gram-positive cocci and *Enterobacteriaceae* and stability to β-lactamase may be considered for first-line empirical therapy for these infections before microbiologic results are available, when infections are likely to be polymicrobial, or when there is no information regarding the strains colonizing the patient.

Surgical Prophylaxis

The ability of antibiotics to penetrate tissue is important, especially when they are used to prevent infection; it is generally agreed that protection from infection is provided only when adequate concentrations are present in tissues at the time of the operative procedure. Infection after foreign body surgery is particularly serious, because eradication of the infection is difficult even with a seemingly appropriate antibiotic. Attempts to avoid this problem involve prophylactic administration of antibiotics, usually directed against *S. aureus* and *S. epidermidis,* the organisms implicated in more than 90% of infections after implant surgery.

Studies of the penetration characteristic of cephalosporins into myocardial and pericardial fluid of patients undergoing open-heart operations show that the peak concentrations of all cephalosporins are usually achieved in these tissues about 20 to 40 min after a bolus intravenous injection. True tissue peaks and peak times are not known, but they probably occur within 10 to 30 minutes. If a cephalosporin with a long half-life, such as a cefazolin, is used, the concentration persists above the MICs for staphylococci for about 4 h. Thus, a cephalosporin antibiotic should be administered at the induction of anesthesia, about 20 to 30 min prior to the initial skin incision, for this provides the best antibiotic concentration in tissue during the perioperative period. With shorter-acting cephalosporins, an intraoperative dose may also be necessary, particularly if the operation lasts more than 2 h. Two additional doses of the cephalosporin in the postoperative period are usually recommended, but there is no evidence that continuing cephalosporin beyond 24 h improves protection against infection (63).

Because of its spectrum of action, favorable toxicity profile, relatively long half-life, modest cost, and proven efficacy, cefazolin has been the prophylactic antibiotic of choice for surgical procedures involving foreign body implantation and many clean and clean-contaminated procedures that carry a relatively high risk for infection (2, 37). These include cardiac

surgery, arterial reconstruction, insertion of orthopaedic devices, head and neck surgery that crosses the oropharyngeal mucosa, high-risk gastroduodenal and biliary tract procedures, vaginal and abdominal hysterectomy, high-risk cesarean sections, and procedures on fresh trauma wounds. This first-generation agent is not recommended as prophylaxis for colorectal surgery or appendectomy or when MRSA is a particular threat (47). Despite the widespread use of modern aseptic techniques and perioperative antimicrobial prophylaxis, *S. aureus* wound infections continue to complicate "clean" surgical procedures. Although some *S. aureus* infections are caused by resistant strains, some studies indicate that most wound isolates are susceptible to methicillin. One study found that "prophylaxis failures" may occur because some *S. aureus* isolates can efficiently hydrolyze the cephalosporin used in prophylaxis. Cefazolin is particularly susceptible to degradation by a common variant of staphylococcal β-lactamase (39).

Cefoxitin, cefotetan, and cefmetazole have been shown to be effective and comparable in systemic prophylaxis for surgery performed at various levels of the gastrointestinal tract, for appendectomy, and for selected gynecologic procedures (31, 37). These agents have not been proven superior to cefazolin except in the setting of colorectal surgery and appendectomy and hence are recommended only in these settings. Although in elective colorectal surgery the benefits of systemic prophylaxis in addition to oral erythromycin-neomycin preoperative bowel preparation have not been fully established, it is common practice to use one of these agents in this setting (31).

Major clinical successes of the third-generation cephalosporins have led to dramatically increased use of these agents. These agents and cephamycins are often used for prophylaxis when an antimicrobial with a narrower spectrum would be equally efficacious. Overuse has resulted in relentless selective pressure by β-lactam antibiotics on the *Enterobacteriaceae* flora, yielding a prominent array of β-lactamase-producing organisms that are resistant to many of the most potent and previously reliable antimicrobials (51, 69).

REFERENCES

1. American Thoracic Society Consensus Committee guidelines for the initial management of adults with community-acquired pneumonia: diagnosis, assessment of severity, and initial antimicrobial therapy. Am Rev Respir Dis 1993;148:1418–1426.
2. Anonymous. Antimicrobial prophylaxis in surgery. Med Lett 1993;35:91–94.
3. Aszodi J, Humbert D, Bonnefoy A, Collette P, Mauvais P, Chantot JF. RU 59863, a novel catechol substituted vinylogous cephalosporin: in vitro antibacterial activity. Program and abstracts of 35th Intersci Conf Antimicrob Agents Chemother, San Francisco, 1995:F-99.
4. Balant L, Dayer P, Auckenthaler R. Clinical pharmacokinetics of the third generation cephalosporins. Clin Pharmacokinet 1985;10:101–143.
5. Barradell LB, Bryson HM. Cefepime, a review of its antibacterial activity, pharmacokinetic properties and therapeutic use. Drugs 1994;47:471–505.
6. Barriere SL, Flaherty JF. Third-generation cephalosporins: a critical evaluation. Clin Pharm 1984;3:351–373.

7. Bergan T. Pharmacokinetic properties of the cephalosporins. Drugs 1987;34(Suppl 2):89–104.

8. Bergeron MG, Bernier M. Bactericidal activity of cefpirome (HR 810) against 513 gram-negative bacteria isolates from blood of septicemic patients. Infection 1994;22:299–305.

9. Bertino JS, Speck WT. The cephalosporin antibiotics. Pediatr Clin North Am 1983;30:17–25.

10. Bryskier A, Sszodi J, Chantot JF. Parenteral cephalosporin classification. Expert Opin Invest Drugs 1994;3:145–171.

11. Bryskier A. New concepts in the field of cephalosporins: C- 3′ quaternary ammonium cephems (group IV). Clin Microbiol Infect 1997;(Suppl 1):S1–S20.

12. Bucourt R, Heymes R, Lutz A, Penasse L, Perronet J. Proprietes antibiotiques intendues dans le domaine des cephalosporines. CR Acad Sci Serie D 1977;284:1847–1849.

13. Canadian Community Acquired Pneumonia Consensus Committee. Antimicrobial treatment of community acquired pneumonia in adults: a conference report. Can J Infect Dis 1993;4:25–28.

14. Chong Y, Lee K, Kwon OH. In vitro activities of cefepime against Enterobacter cloacae, Serratia marcescens, Pseudomonas aeruginosa and other aerobic gram-negative bacilli. J Antimicrob Chemother 1993;32(Suppl B):21–29.

15. Christ W. Pharmacological properties of cephalosporins. Infection 1991;19(Suppl 5):S244–S252.

16. Cordonnier C, Herbrecht R, Pico JL, Gardembas M, Delmer A, Delain M, Moreau P, Ladeb S, Nalet V, Rollin C, Greg JJ. Cefepimeamikacin vs. ceftazidime-amikacin as empiric therapy for febrile episodes in neutropenic patients: a comparative study. Clin Infect Dis 1997; 24:41–51.

17. Craig WA. Interrelationship between pharmakokinetics and pharmacodynamics in determining dosage regimens for broad- spectrum cephalosporins. Diagn Microbiol Infect Dis 1995;22: 89–96.

18. Craig WA. Post-antibiotic effects in experimental infection models: relationship to in vitro phenomena and to treatment of infections in man. J Antimicrob Chemother 1993;31(Suppl D): 249–258.

19. Craig WA, Gudmundsson S. The postantibiotic effect. In: Lorian V, ed. Antibiotics in laboratory medicine. 3rd ed. Baltimore: Williams & Wilkins, 1992:403–431.

20. Cunha BA. Third-generation cephalosporins: a review. Clin Ther 1992;14:616–647.

21. Eggimann P, Glauser MP, Aoun M, Meunier F, Calandra T. Cefepime monotherapy for the empiric treatment of fever in granulocytopenic patients. J Antimicrob Chemother 1993:32 (Suppl B):S141–S149.

22. Fassbender M, Lode H, Schaberg T, Borner K, Koeppe P. Pharmacokinetics of new oral cephalosporins, including a carbacephem. Clin Infect Dis 1993;16:646–653.

23. Francioli P, Chastre J, Langer M, Santos JI, Shah PM, Torres A. Ventilator-associated pneumonia—understanding epidemiology and pathogenesis to guide prevention and empiric therapy. Clin Microbiol Infect 1997;3(Suppl 1):S61–S76.

24. Friedland IR, Paris M, Ehrett S, Hickey S, Olsen K, McCracken GH. Evaluation of antimicrobial regimens for treatment of experimental penicillin-cephalosporin resistant pneumococcal meningitis. Antimicrob Agents Chemother 1993;37: 1630–1636.

25. Fuchs PC, Barry AL, Brown SD. Survey of antimicrobial activity of four commonly used third generation cephalosporins tested against recent bacterial isolates from ten American medical centers, and assessment of disk diffusion test performance. Diagn Microbiol Infect Dis 1996;24:213–219.

26. Garau J, Wilson W, Wood M, Carlet J. Fourth-generation cephalosporins: a review of in vitro activity, pharmacokinetics, pharmacodynamics and clinical utility. Clin Microbiol Infect 1997; 3(Suppl 1):S87–S101.

27. Garzone P, Lyon J, Yu VL. Third-generation and investigational cephalosporins: I. Structure-activity relationships and pharmacokinetic review. DICP 1983;17:507–515.

28. Garzone P, Lyon J, Yu VL. Third-generation and investigational cephalosporins: II. microbiologic review and clinical summaries. DICP 1983;17:615–622.

29. Garzone P, Lyon J, Yu VL, Zuravleff J, Diven W, Pasculle W. Steady-state moxalactam kinetics: comparisons with other cephalosporins. Clin Pharmacol Ther 1981;30:86–93.

30. Glauser M, Boogaerts M, Cordonnier C, Palmblad J, Martino P. Empiric therapy of bacterial infections in severe neutropenia. Clin Microbiol Infect 1997;3(Suppl 1):S77–S86.

31. Gorbach SL. The role of cephalosporins in surgical prophylaxis. J Antimicrob Chemother 1989;23(Suppl D):61–70.

32. Gustaferro CA, Streckelberg JM. Cephalosporin antimicrobial agents and related compounds. Mayo Clin Proc 1991;66: 1064–1073.

33. Inoue E, Mitushuhashi S. Interaction of E-1040 with cephalosporinases from C. freundii GN 739. Antimicrob Agent Chemother 1989;33:2157–2159.

34. Jacoby GA, Carreras I. Activities of β-lactam antibiotics against Escherichia coli strains providing extended spectrum β-lactamases. Antimicrob Agent Chemother 1990;34:858–862.

35. Janknegt R, van der Meer JWM. Antimicrobial practice—sequential therapy with intravenous and oral cephalosporins. J Antimicrob Chemother 1994;33:169–177.

36. John CC. Treatment failure with use of third-generation cephalosporin for penicillin-resistant pneumococcal meningitis: case report and review. Clin Infect Dis 1994;18:188–193.

37. Kaiser AB. Antimicrobial prophylaxis in surgery. N Engl J Med 1986;315:1129–1138.

38. Karchmer AW: Cephalosporins. In: Mandell GL, Bennett JE, Dolin R, eds. Principles and practice of infectious diseases. 4th ed. New York: Churchill Livingstone, 1995.

39. Kernodle DS, Classen DC, Burke JP, Kaiser AB. Failure of cephalosporins to prevent Staphylococcus aureus surgical wound infections. JAMA 1990;263:961–966.

40. Klein NC, Cunha BA. Third-generation cephalosporins. Med Clin North Am 1995;79:705–719.

41. Klepser ME, Marangos MN, Patel KB, Nicolau DP, Quintiliani R, Nightingale CH. Clinical pharmacokinetics of newer cephalosporins. Clin Pharmacokinet 1995;28:361–384.

42. Kolger T, Digroves A, Bergan T, Solberg CO. The pharmacokinetics of ceftriaxone in serum, skin blisters and thread fluid. J Antimicrob Chemother 1984;13:479–485.

43. Klugman K, Goldstein F, Kohno S, Baquero F. The role of fourth-generation cephalosporins in the treatment of infections caused by penicillin-resistant streptococci. Clin Microbiol Infect 1997;3(Suppl 1):S48–S60.

44. Lemmen S, Kropec A, Engels I, Busse A, Daschner FD. Serum bactericidal activity after administration of four cephalosporins in healthy volunteers. Eur J Clin Microbiol Infect Dis 1993;12: 856–860.

45. Livermore DM. Kinetics and significance of the activity of the Sabath and Abraham's β-lactamase of P. aeruginosa against cefotaxime and cefsulodin. J Antimicrob Chemother 1983;11:169–179.

46. Lode H, Fassbender M, Schaberg T, Borner K, Koeppe P. Comparative pharmacokinetics of the new oral cephalosporins. Drugs 1994;47(Suppl 3):10–20.

47. Mandell GL, Sande MA. Antimicrobial agents, penicillins, cephalosporins and other beta-lactam antibiotics. In: Gilmann AG, Rall TW, Nies AS, Taylor P, eds. The pharmacological basis of therapeutics. 8th ed. New York: Pergamon Press, 1990.

48. Mason EO, Kaplan SL, Lamberth LB, Tillman J. Increased rate of isolation of penicillin-resistant Streptococcus pneumoniae in a children's hospital and in vitro susceptibilities to antibiotics of potential therapeutic use. Antimicrob Agents Chemother 1992; 36:1703–1707.

49. McEvoy GK, Litvak K, Welsh GH, eds. AHFS drug information. Bethesda, MD: American Society of Hospital Pharmacists, 1994.

50. McManus MC. Mechanisms of bacterial resistance to antimicrobial agents. Am J Health Syst Pharm 1997;54:1420–1433.

51. Medeiros AA. Nosocomial outbreaks of multiresistant bacteria: extended spectrum beta-lactamases have arrived in North America. Ann Intern Med 1993;119:429–439.

52. Molavi A. Cephalosporins: rationale for clinical use. Am Fam Physician 1991;43:937–948.

53. Murray PR, Jones RN, Allen SD, Erwin ME, Fuchs PC, Gerlach EH. Multilaboratory evaluation of the in vitro activity of 13 beta-lactam antibiotics against 1474 clinical isolates of aerobic and anaerobic bacteria. Diagn Microbiol Infect Dis 1993;16:191–203.

54. Neu HC. The place of cephalosporins in antibacterial treatment of infectious diseases. J Antimicrob Chemother 1980;6(Suppl A):1–11.

55. Neu HC. Third generation cephalosporins: safety profiles after 10 years of clinical use. J Clin Pharmacol 1990;30:396–403.

56. Nikaido H, Liu W, Rosenberg EY. Outermembrane permeability and beta-lactamases stability of dipolar ionic cephalosporins containing methoxyimino substituents. Antimicrob Agent Chemother 1990;34:337–342.

57. Norris SM. The cephalosporin antibiotic agents—II. First- and second-generation agents. Infect Control 1984;5:577–581.

58. Norris SM. The cephalosporin antibiotic agents—III. Third-generation cephalosporins. Infect Control 1985;6:78–83.

59. Novick WJ. Levels of cefotaxime in body fluids and tissues: a review. Rev Infect Dis 1982:4(Suppl 4):S346–S353.

60. Okamoto MP, Nakahiro RK, Chin A, Bedikian A. Cefepime clinical pharmacokinetics. Clin Pharmacokinet 1993;25: 88–102.

61. Okamoto MP, Nakahiro RK, Chin A, Bedikian A, Gill MA. Cefepime: a new fourth-generation cephalosporin. Am J Hosp Pharm 1994;51:463–475.

62. Pucci MJ, Sowek JB, Kessler RE, Dougherty TJ. Comparison of cefpirome, cefepime, and cefclidine binding affinities for penicillin binding proteins in E. coli K-12 and P. aeruginosa SC 8329. Antimicrob Agent Chemother 1991;35:2312–2317.

63. Quintiliani R, French M, Nightingale CH. First and second generation cephalosporins. Med Clin North Am 1982;66:183–195.

64. Quintiliani R. Cefixime in the treatment of patients with lower

respiratory tract infections: results of US clinical trials. Clin Ther 1996;18:373–390.

65. Reinert R, Weiss U, Brombacher U, Lanz P, Montavon M, Furlenmeier R, Angehrn P, Probst PJ. RO 13–9904/001, a novel potent long acting parenteral cephalosporin. J Antibiot 1992;45: 1526–1532.

66. Rubinstein E, Rubinovich B. Treatment of severe infections caused by penicillin-resistant pneumococci. Role of third- generation cephalosporins. Infection 1994;22(Suppl 3):S161–S165.

67. Ryan DM, Hodges B, Spencer GR, Harding SM. Simultaneous comparison of three methods for assessing penetration of ceftazidime into extracellular fluid. Antimicrob Agents Chemother 1982;22:995–998.

68. Rybak M. The pharmacokinetic profile of a new generation of parenteral cephalosporin. Am J Med 1996;100(Suppl 6A): 39S–44S.

69. Sanders CC, Sanders E Jr. Beta-lactam resistance in gram- negative bacteria: global trends and clinical impact. Clin Infect Dis 1992;15:824–839.

70. Sanders CC. Cefepime: the next generation? Clin Infect Dis 1993;17:369–379.

71. Satakes S, Hiraoka M, Mitshuhashi S. Interaction of cefpirome and a cephalosporinase from C. freundii GN 7391. Antimicrob Agent Chemother 1989;33:398–399.

72. Schumacher GE. Comparison of antibiotic dosage regimens using pharmacokinetic and microbiologic factors. Clin Pharm 1987;6:59–68.

73. Segreti J, Levin S. Bacteriologic and clinical applications of a new extended-spectrum parenteral cephalosporin. Am J Med 1996;100(Suppl 6A):45S–51S.

74. Sloas MM, Barrett FF, Chesney PJ, English BK, Hill BC, Tenover FC, Leggiadro RJ. Cephalosporin treatment failure in penicillin- and cephalosporin-resistant Streptococcus pneumoniae meningitis. Pediatr Infect Dis J 1992;11: 662–666.

75. Soe GB, Overturf GD. Treatment of typhoid fever and other systemic salmonelloses with cefotaxime, ceftriaxone, cefoperazone, and other newer cephalosporins. Rev Infect Dis 1987;9: 719–736.

76. Tartaglione TA, Polk RE. Review of the new second- generation cephalosporins: cefonicid, ceforanide, and cefuroxime. DICP 1985;19:188–195.

77. Turnidge JD. Pharmacodynamic (kinetic) considerations in the treatment of moderately severe infections with cefotaxime. Diag Microbiol Infect Dis 1995;22:57–69.

78. Watanabe NA, Sugiyama I. Role of the aminothiadiazolyl group in the antipseudomonal activity of cefclidin. J Antibiot 1992;45: 1526–1532.

79. Yoshimura H, Nikaido H. Diffusion of beta-lactam antibiotics through the porin channel of Escherichia coli K-12. Antimicrob Agent Chemother 1985;27:84–92.

80. Yuk-Choi JH, Nightingale CH, Williams TW. Considerations in dosage selection for third generation cephalosporins. Clin Pharmacokinet 1992;22:132–143.

Chloramphenicol

●

Kerstin E. Calia and Frank M. Calia

Chloramphenicol, introduced in 1949, is one of many antibiotics derived from soil organisms of the genus *Streptomyces* (44, 45). The drug has a wide spectrum of antibacterial activity, and is active against both gram- positive and gram-negative bacteria, rickettsiae and some anaerobic bacteria. However, its usefulness is limited today due to the risk of side effects, in particular irreversible aplastic anemia and the gray baby syndrome (23, 83, 85, 145). In selected life-threatening infections when active alternatives are not available, its use should still be considered.

ANTIMICROBIAL ACTIVITY

Chloramphenicol has a broad spectrum of activity. The drug is bacteriostatic for most organisms. Chloramphenicol is active against Gram-positive bacteria including aerobes and anaerobes, with notable exceptions including methicillin-resistant *Staphylococcus aureus, Enterococcus,* and *Nocardia* (54). While chloramphenicol is bacteriostatic for most organisms, it is cidal for *Streptococcus pneumoniae, Haemophilus influenzae* (including those that produce β-lactamase), and *Neisseria meningitidis* (142, 182). β-Lactams and other antibiotics now are being used in many instances in which chloramphenicol had been used previously, due to concerns about chloramphenicol toxicity.

Chloramphenicol has activity against some vancomycin-resistant enterococci (VRE) and is sometimes used to treat VRE infections (130). A recent study of in vitro susceptibilities of clinical isolates of VRE revealed that while many of the isolates were considered susceptible to chloramphenicol, the minimum inhibitory concentrations (MICs) of most were at the breakpoint of 8 μg/mL (49). Resistance to multiple antimicrobial agents, especially β-lactam antibiotics, is currently emerging in viridans group streptococci, but development of resistance to chloramphenicol appears uncommon (41).

The sensitivity of Gram-negative enteric organisms to chloramphenicol is variable. *Escherichia coli* and *Proteus mirabilis* are usually sensitive, and organisms with a reputation for multidrug resistance such as *Klebsiella, Serratia, Morganella,* and *Enterobacter* are somewhat more resistant (10, 55). Chloramphenicol is active against *Brucella* species, *Bordetella pertussis, Salmonella* species including *S. typhi, Shigella* species, and *Vibrio cholerae* (35, 149, 154). Resistance to *S. typhi* and *Shigella* species has been reported around the world, including the United States (6, 15, 31, 105, 121, 122, 124). Most isolates of *Yersinia enterocolitica* are susceptible (141). Most *Pseudomonas* species with the important exception of *P. pseudomallei* are resistant to chloramphenicol (46). Resistance to chloramphenicol in association with resistance to quinolones and tetracyclines is seen in *Stenotrophomonas maltophilia* (4).

Other small Gram- negative bacilli and cocci including *H. influenzae* (β-lactamase positive or negative), *Neisseria gonorrhoeae* and *N. meningitidis* are sensitive (35). Surveillance of moderately penicillin-resistant *N. meningitidis* isolates shows that thus far these organisms remain sensitive to chloramphenicol (16). *Acinetobacter* are generally resistant to chloramphenicol (13).

Most Gram-negative anaerobes including *Bacteroides fragilis* exhibit in vitro sensitivity to chloramphenicol (26, 33, 52). Gram-positive anaerobes such as clostridia species are also inhibited by chloramphenicol (26, 28). The drug is also active against spirochetes, chlamydiae, rickettsiae, ehrlichiae, and some species of mycoplasmas (7, 39, 51, 56, 73, 118, 151). Minimum inhibitory concentrations (MICs) of chloramphenicol required for *Rochalimaea (Bartonella) quintana, Rochalimaea (Bartonella) henselae,* and *Rochalimaea vinsonii* have been somewhat variable but close to maximum clinically achievable serum levels (112).

MECHANISM OF ACTION

Chloramphenicol has a simple chemical structure consisting of a paranitrobenzene ring attached to a propanediol group with a dichloracetamide side chain. The propanediol and dichloracetamide portions of the molecule are required for bacteriostatic activity (71, 139). Chloramphenicol is available as a base and palmitate and succinate esters (64, 116). These esters must be hydrolyzed to yield active drug. An analogue of chloramphenicol, thiamphenicol, is used in Europe and Japan but is not available in the United States.

Chloramphenicol interferes with microbial protein synthesis by binding to the prokaryotic 50S ribosomal subunit. The drug prevents the aminoacyl-tRNA from binding to the ribosome, and polypeptide chain synthesis is terminated (135, 136). Unfortunately, this mechanism may be at the heart of toxicity associated with chloramphenicol. Protein synthesis in mitochondria, organelles thought to have arisen from prokaryotes, is also inhibited by chloramphenicol (58, 110). Prolonged inhibition of bacterial protein synthesis by chloramphenicol alters the ability of some organisms such as *Salmonella typhimurium* and enterohemorrhagic *E. coli* to invade cells, disrupting what may be a significant factor in their pathogenicity (107, 131). The mechanism of chloramphenicol's cidal activity against *S. pneumoniae, H. influenzae,* and *N. meningitidis* has not been determined (142, 182).

MECHANISMS OF RESISTANCE

Organisms become resistant to chloramphenicol by one of two major mechanisms. Acetylation of the drug by the enzyme chloramphenicol acetyltransferase (CAT) yields diacetyl chloramphenicol, which does not have antimicrobial activity. This enzyme is usually plasmid encoded (R plasmids), and its gene can be transferred along with genes conferring resistance to a number of other antibiotics (12, 66, 124). Genes for CAT actually comprise a family of different genes encoding similar enzymes in many different bacteria, which may be chromosomal or associated with a transposon as well as on plasmids (125). Pathogens associated with these resistance plasmids in Gram-negative bacteria include *S. typhi* and *Shigella dysenteriae* and *Pasteurella* species (27, 37, 165, 176). At least one outbreak of plasmid-mediated resistant salmonella has been associated with antibiotic use in cattle feed, and the use of chloramphenicol in raising dairy and beef cattle is not legal in the United States (167).

A second mechanism of resistance is based on loss of a bacterial outer membrane protein. Without this protein, chloramphenicol can no longer penetrate the organism and exert its toxic effects. This mechanism has been found in *E. coli, H. influenzae, P. aeruginosa,* and *Serratia* (20, 62, 79, 174). In *Pseudomonas,* genes responsible for this resistance are encoded by transposable elements on plasmids (21). In *H. influenzae,* this phenomenon is chromosomally encoded (20). An efflux pump, associated with appearance of a new outer membrane protein, appears to be an additional mechanism of resistance in *P. aeruginosa, Rhodococcus fascians, S. maltophilia, Burkholderia cepacia,* and possibly actinomycetes (4, 22, 40, 103, 140). The phenomenon of energy-dependent efflux of chloramphenicol was also recently demonstrated in enterococci and *E. coli* (106, 129). Some strains of *Clostridium* and *Bacteroides* are able to inactivate chloramphenicol through nitroreduction (188). An altered target in the form of a 50S ribosomal subunit less able to bind chloramphenicol was described in *Bacillus subtilis* (132).

PHARMACOKINETICS AND METABOLISM

The pharmacokinetics of chloramphenicol are determined by the chemical form of the drug administered, the dosage, and the route of administration. Chloramphenicol base given orally to adults is well absorbed and produces serum peak levels within 1 to 2 h (8). This form of the drug is bitter and not very water soluble, limiting its use in children. The pediatric oral formulation, the palmitate ester, is more soluble and palatable. The succinate ester is used for intravenous administration. Higher serum levels are achieved with the oral palmitate ester than with the intravenous succinate ester (164). Both esters must be hydrolyzed to be biologically active. Hydrolysis to microbiologically active chloramphenicol base is produced either by pancreatic lipase in the gut or by the liver, kidneys, or lungs (64, 83). Because of variable hydrolysis of the drug, serum levels achieved with the oral palmitate ester are lower than those with similar doses of oral base (156). The succinate ester is rapidly cleared following intravenous administration, approximately two-thirds of it being hydrolyzed to the active base (137). Intramuscular injection of chloramphenicol is not recommended because of variable hydrolysis resulting in subtherapeutic concentrations of active drug (161). It also appears

that when given intravenously rather than intramuscularly, chloramphenicol has a smaller volume of distribution, resulting in higher plasma concentrations (2).

Chloramphenicol has good penetration into most tissues and bodily fluids (synovial, pleural, peritoneal, and pericardial fluid) (11, 116, 143). Low levels of drug are found in the bile (65). Whether or not the meninges are inflamed, approximately 40 to 65% of serum levels crosses the blood-brain barrier into the cerebrospinal fluid (CSF) (61, 116, 144). Concentrations of chloramphenicol in the brain itself can be up to nine times as high as serum levels, because of the lipophilic character of the drug (95). Chloramphenicol appears to penetrate and be concentrated in alveolar macrophages and polymorphonuclear leukocytes (123).

Chloramphenicol in ophthalmic preparations (ointments or solutions) is absorbed into the aqueous humor to produce bacteriostatic concentrations (63). Subconjunctival injections of chloramphenicol do not produce adequate concentrations in the aqueous humor to treat panophthalmitis (119). Topical chloramphenicol should not be used to treat bacterial conjunctivitis because of the risk of aplastic anemia and the availability of other, potentially less toxic, agents (42).

An understanding of the metabolism of chloramphenicol is important to identify conditions under which drug toxicity occurs. Clearance of chloramphenicol depends more on hepatic metabolism than on renal excretion (2). The drug is first conjugated in the liver to chloramphenicol glucuronide. The glucuronide is nontoxic and is inactive against microbes (65). Most of this chloramphenicol glucuronide is secreted by the renal tubule; only 5 to 10% of the active drug is excreted by glomerular filtration (65). In patients with renal failure, there is no need to greatly adjust chloramphenicol dosing because it is the nontoxic glucuronide that accumulates. Hemodialysis and peritoneal dialysis do not affect the serum half-life of chloramphenicol, and dosage adjustment is not necessary (98).

Patients with liver disease do not conjugate chloramphenicol well, and increased levels of active drug may cause myelosuppression (170). If chloramphenicol must be used in a patient with hepatic insufficiency, the dose should be reduced, and the shortest possible course used.

In normal adults, chloramphenicol has a serum half-life of 3 to 4 h and one-quarter to one-half of the drug is protein bound (68, 99). The recommended doses produce serum levels between 5 and 25 μg/mL, and susceptible organisms are defined as those with an MIC of 16 μg/mL or less (47).

Neonates cannot conjugate chloramphenicol to glucuronide efficiently and have a diminished glomerular filtration rate of the active drug. For these reasons, higher concentrations of active drug can easily accumulate in newborns (65). Infants, especially newborns, have a variable rate of hydrolysis of the succinate ester to active chloramphenicol base (184). Therefore, dosages should be reduced, and serum drug levels carefully monitored in any infant receiving chloramphenicol (184) (see below). Chloramphenicol does cross the placenta and is excreted in breast milk. Thus, the drug should be used with caution in pregnant or breast-feeding patients (74).

DOSAGE REGIMENS

See Tables 1 and 2.

ADVERSE EFFECTS

Major adverse drug reactions described with chloramphenicol include gray baby syndrome, hematologic toxicity including aplastic anemia, and neurologic toxicity (particularly, optic neuritis). Gray baby syndrome, described in both premature and full-term infants, consists of vomiting, lethargy, irregular respirations, cyanosis, abdominal distention, hypotension, hypothermia, and death (171). Gray baby syndrome can be seen in older children and adults if the ingested dose of chloramphenicol is high enough (32, 172). Babies manifesting this syndrome accumulate excessive amounts of the active form of the drug because of inadequate conjugation and excretion of chloramphenicol (184). Usually occurring 3 to 4 days into therapy, gray baby syndrome can present initially with metabolic acidosis due to inhibition of oxidation and consequent production of lactic acid (48). Serum chloramphenicol levels are usually above 75 μg/mL, over three times the therapeutic level (23). Administration of bicarbonate does not correct the acidosis. Over the next 6 to 12 h, progressive hypotension ensues, resulting in cyanosis and skin pallor that gives the syndrome its name. This leads to a cycle of tissue hypoperfusion, lactic acidosis, and decreasing ability to conjugate chloramphenicol. The mortality rate approaches 40%. Gray baby syndrome can be reversed if suspected and chloramphenicol is immediately discontinued. Charcoal- column hemoperfusion and

TABLE 1 • Available Preparations of Chloramphenicol

Oral	
Chloramphenicol capsules	250 mg, 500 mg
Chloramphenicol palmitate solution	150 mg/mL
Intravenous	
Chloramphenicol sodium solution	1-g vial
Otic	
Chloramphenicol otic solution	5 mg/mL
Ophthalmic	
Chloramphenicol ophthalmic solution	25-mg vial
Chloramphenicol ophthalmic cream	1%

TABLE 2 • Dosing of Chloramphenicol

Newborns <2 weeks old and premature infants	25 mg/kg/day in 6-h intervals; must assay serum concentration
Infants 2–4 weeks old	25 mg/kg q. 12 h
Older children and adults[a]	50 mg/kg/day in 6-h intervals
Older children and adults with meningitis	100 mg/kg/day in 6-h intervals

[a] Renal insufficiency: dose modification is not necessary. Serum concentration is not altered sufficiently by hemodialysis or peritoneal dialysis to necessitate dose alteration. Hepatic insufficiency: suggested dosing is an initial 1-g loading dose, followed by 500 mg q. 6 h. Limit therapy when possible to 10–14 days, and monitor serum concentration, adjusting as necessary to achieve 10–30 mg/mL.

exchange transfusion may be helpful (88, 111). The incidence of gray syndrome is related to the age of the infant and the quantity of chloramphenicol administered (32, 172).

There are two major types of hematologic toxicity produced by chloramphenicol, a dose-related myelosuppression and a rare idiosyncratic aplastic anemia (145, 190, 191). Myelosuppression results from chloramphenicol inhibiting mitochondrial enzymes, including those needed for heme synthesis (109, 189). Early signs of toxicity include a lowered reticulocyte count and an elevated serum iron concentration due to underuse of iron. This occurs approximately a week into therapy (153, 159). Red cell, white cell, and platelet counts may all be depressed (159). Thrombocytopenia is a late complication, occurring 2 to 3 weeks into therapy. Patients at greater risk of myelosuppression include those with liver disease, those with serum levels of chloramphenicol above 25 μg/mL, and those on doses above 4 g/day (159, 170). Examination of the bone marrow reveals vacuolization of myeloid and erythroid precursors, but this is not pathognomonic of chloramphenicol toxicity (120, 192). If chloramphenicol therapy is discontinued, these toxic effects on the marrow are reversible. Myelosuppression is dose and duration related.

Aplastic anemia is a rare and idiosyncratic form of marrow toxicity, with an incidence estimated to be between 1 in 25,000 to 1 in 200,000 (14, 180). Approximately a quarter of all cases of aplastic anemia are due to chloramphenicol, and this complication is usually fatal (5). The time from initiation of chloramphenicol therapy to the first manifestation of aplasia varies widely and is usually a matter of several weeks but can be months or years (29, 159, 180, 191). This complication is independent of dose and has been reported with topical chloramphenicol as well as oral and intravenous drug (53, 76, 152). The etiology of aplastic anemia is unknown, but evidence in identical twins suggests a genetic predisposition (14, 127). Concurrent intravenous administration of cimetidine noted in two patients suggests that this drug may be an additional risk factor (185). Bone marrow transplantation is the recommended therapy for aplastic anemia due to chloramphenicol (138, 191).

Chloramphenicol has induced hemolysis in patients with the Mediterranean form of glucose-6-phosphate dehydrogenase (G6PD) deficiency (113).

Because of the potential for hematologic toxicity, it is recommended that complete blood counts be monitored at least twice a week in patients receiving chloramphenicol. Development of anemia, leukopenia, or thrombocytopenia dictates immediate discontinuation of therapy. Some cases of late-developing aplasia may be missed with this approach, but early cases as well as dose-related toxicity and G6PD-related hemolysis can be identified (38). Unfortunately, aplastic anemia is usually not reversed by discontinuing chloramphenicol.

Optic neuritis is the major neurologic complication described with chloramphenicol. It has been reported in patients receiving long courses of therapy (78, 179). Red-green color changes, central scotoma, and decreased vision have been described. These effects may be reversible or permanent (30). Other neurotoxicities reported in patients receiving chloramphenicol include headache, ophthalmoplegia, peripheral neuropathy, depression, and acute encephalopathy (102). Hypersensitivity reactions have been described, including exanthems and drug fevers. Topical chloramphenicol has been reported to cause cutaneous allergic reactions, and there is one report of anaphylaxis in a patient who ingested the drug orally after previously receiving it topically (147). Jarisch-Herxheimer reactions have been reported in patients treated for typhoid fever, brucellosis, borreliosis, and syphilis (163, 187). Gastrointestinal complaints including nausea, vomiting, diarrhea, and glossitis occur with high doses (187). Chloramphenicol has demonstrable immunosuppressive effects in animal models; the clinical significance of this in humans is unknown but may be relevant in rare instances of chronic congenital idiopathic neutropenia (36, 50, 183).

DRUG INTERACTIONS

Chloramphenicol inhibits enzymes of the cytochrome P-450 complex (72). Therefore, it prolongs the half-life of drugs metabolized by this mechanism, such as warfarin, phenytoin, tolbutamide and chlorpropamide, and cyclosporine (3, 93, 160, 168). Patients receiving these drugs concurrently with chloramphenicol should have their prothrombin times and serum glucose or phenytoin levels monitored during chloramphenicol therapy. Phenytoin and phenobarbital may decrease the serum half-life of chloramphenicol by increasing conjugation, so chloramphenicol levels should be monitored when the two drugs must be given together (17, 96). Acetaminophen may have the opposite effect, prolonging the half-life by blocking hepatic uptake of chloramphenicol (19, 84). Cimetidine may contribute to the risk of aplastic anemia (185).

CLINICAL INDICATIONS

Major indications for chloramphenicol are limited due to the rare but life-threatening toxicity of the drug. Many other drugs now available share chloramphenicol's broad spectrum (alone or in combination) without carrying the hematologic or neurologic risks. Because of the increasing antibiotic resistance of a variety of organisms and the emergence of previously unappreciated pathogens, use of chloramphenicol should be considered when appropriate. β-Lactam antibiotics have replaced chloramphenicol in most instances because of lower toxicity. For patients with a history of β-lactam-induced anaphylaxis, chloramphenicol remains an alternative. The drug is used in treating serious *H. influenzae* infections, including epiglottitis, osteomyelitis, and septic arthritis in such patients (34). Chloramphenicol's ability to penetrate the blood-brain barrier and produce high concentrations in brain tissue makes it valuable in treating central nervous system infections (95, 144). Septic thrombophlebitis of the head and neck has been treated with penicillin and chloramphenicol (173).

As chloramphenicol is bactericidal for *S. pneumoniae, H. influenzae,* and *N. meningitidis,* it is used in treating meningitis in older children and adults who have life- threatening β-lactam allergies (77, 142, 186). Due to emergence of resistance in a number of pathogens, local antibiotic resistance data may alter usage of chloramphenicol. Chloramphenicol and ampicillin were previously preferred for empiric combination ther-

apy for meningitis in children, because of its excellent penetration into the CSF and its spectrum of activity. This is no longer the case because of risks of toxicity and the rise in chloramphenicol-resistant isolates of *S. pneumoniae* around the world (59, 60, 82, 90, 91, 101, 146). Many penicillin-resistant pneumococci are simultaneously resistant to chloramphenicol (59, 60, 82). Some of these isolates have MBCs substantially higher than the corresponding MICs; this may explain chloramphenicol treatment failures in cases of penicillin-resistant pneumococcal meningitis (59, 60, 146). Chloramphenicol and β-lactam antibiotics can interact in an antagonistic fashion in vitro; the clinical significance of this is unclear (59, 178). *H. influenzae* isolates resistant to both chloramphenicol and ampicillin have also been reported (87). In the United States, third-generation cephalosporins have largely replaced chloramphenicol for treatment of bacterial meningitis (114, 169).

Pneumococcal resistance to penicillin is an increasing problem. A recent survey of pneumococcal isolates from patients with acute otitis media showed many of these organisms to be highly or moderately resistant to chloramphenicol (150). A survey of nasopharyngeal swab and blood isolates from Egypt revealed approximately 20 to 30% resistance to chloramphenicol, respectively (133). Ampicillin resistance in *H. influenzae* type b (Hib) is common, and the use of chloramphenicol in treatment of Hib meningitis has established its efficacy. A comparison of chloramphenicol with cefotaxime for treatment of *H. influenzae* meningitis concluded that the two were equally efficacious with similar incidences of neurologic sequelae (175).

Chloramphenicol is bacteriostatic for most Gram-negative aerobic bacilli and is not considered effective in the treatment of Gram-negative bacillary meningitis (142). The organisms usually implicated in neonatal meningitis, group B streptococci, Gram-negative bacilli including *E. coli,* and *Listeria,* are inhibited but not killed by chloramphenicol (164). Therefore, other antimicrobials are used in this age group.

Chloramphenicol in combination with penicillin is useful in treating pyogenic brain abscesses because of its excellent penetration and activity against anaerobes (18, 65, 95, 134). Chloramphenicol has been used successfully in therapy for subacute meningitis due to *Clostridium* species following head trauma (128). The drug was also useful in therapy for *B. fragilis* arthritis in a patient with sickle-cell disease (92).

Chloramphenicol therapy has been considered first-line therapy (and is still the standard with which other therapeutic agents are compared) for severe salmonella infections, particularly enteric fever (97, 149). Clinicians must be aware, however, that chloramphenicol resistance is rising in many parts of the world, unsurprisingly with higher mortality rates due to infections from resistant *S. typhi* (15, 70, 108, 162). Because of its efficacy and low cost, chloramphenicol is still a major drug used to treat enteric fever in developing countries, but it cannot be the drug of choice in areas of endemic resistance (24). To minimize emergence of resistance, patients with uncomplicated gastroenteritis should receive supportive care, with antimicrobial therapy reserved for those with systemic infection. Some evidence indicates that patients who are carriers of

S. typhi can be treated with quinolones, although some of these patients will relapse (67). Quinolones and ceftriaxone are alternative antimicrobials for therapy of *S. typhi* that is simultaneously resistant to chloramphenicol, trimethoprim-sulfamethoxazole, and ampicillin (43, 80, 89, 100, 121). *S. typhi* resistance to chloramphenicol in a given locale probably varies with antibiotic use patterns (decreases in chloramphenicol resistance are now seen where quinolones are extensively used), so susceptibility data for a given isolate is potentially important (157). Patients with AIDS have been reported to have bacteremia and metastatic abscesses due to *Salmonella* species. Chloramphenicol has been used successfully to treat nontyphoid salmonella subdural empyema in a patient with AIDS (126).

The drug has been useful in therapy of vancomycin-resistant enterococcal infections, particularly those caused by *Enterococcus faecium* (130). Most clinical isolates studied by one institution had MICs at the breakpoint of 8 μg/mL (49). With susceptibility defined as an MIC of 8 to 16 μg/mL and clinically achievable serum levels falling in the range of 5 to 25 μg/mL, the margin between MICs and serum levels may not be great. It is not known how important this observation is clinically.

Chloramphenicol is the drug of choice for treating rickettsial or ehrlichial infections in patients who are allergic to tetracyclines or who are pregnant (86, 97). Treating children less than 9 years of age with tetracycline or chloramphenicol is controversial. The clinician must weigh the risk of tetracycline causing staining of teeth against the low but serious complication of aplastic anemia due to chloramphenicol (104, 158, 177). Tooth discoloration by tetracycline is dose related (69), and the incidence of discoloration with doxycycline, which binds calcium less well, is lower (57). Despite the recommendation of the American Academy of Pediatrics to use chloramphenicol in children under 9 years of age with rickettsial infections to avoid tooth staining, some clinicians choose to avoid it because of the fear of aplastic anemia (1, 158). Either chloramphenicol or a tetracycline should be used to treat ehrlichial disease, as they have been shown to decrease mortality and shorten length of fever and hospital stay when therapy is started early (9, 56). Chloramphenicol is an acceptable alternative to doxycycline in treatment of patients with scrub typhus *(Rickettsia tsutsugamushi);* however, reports of resistance to both agents are emerging in Thailand (181).

Diseases uncommonly seen in the United States for which chloramphenicol is useful include meliodosis, tularemia, and plague. Meliodosis is treated with a combination of chloramphenicol, a tetracycline, and an aminoglycoside. Alternative regimens have been compared with the chloramphenicol-containing regimen. Ceftazidime and trimethoprim-sulfamethoxazole therapy may have lower mortality rates and lower rates of relapse than standard chloramphenicol therapy (25, 166). Although chloramphenicol is bacteriostatic for *Yersinia pestis* and *Francisella tularensis,* the drug can successfully treat plague and tularemia if standard therapy cannot be used (115, 117). Chloramphenicol is an alternative drug for brucellosis and can be considered a second-line agent for *Aeromonas* infections (81,

148). Chloramphenicol has also been used successfully to treat *Streptobacillus moniliformis* sepsis (bacillary rat bite fever) (155). Even though *Bartonella quintana* and *Bartonella henselae* MICs tend to be toward the upper limit of clinically achievable serum levels, patients with trench fever and *B. henselae* infection have been successfully treated with chloramphenicol (112).

Ironically, given its ability to cause several different types of hematologic toxicity, chloramphenicol was used to treat chronic congenital idiopathic neutropenia in two patients (50). The mechanism of action in these cases is unclear but an immunomodulatory effect is postulated.

SERUM ASSAYS

While in some circumstances, assaying serum levels is strongly recommended, this capability may not be readily available at all institutions. Serum levels should be monitored in infants at risk for gray syndrome, patients with hepatic insufficiency, or those on medications that interfere with chloramphenicol metabolism. The therapeutic range is between 5 and 25 μg/mL, and myelosuppression begins to occur above 25 μg/mL (159, 170). Levels of chloramphenicol and its metabolites can be measured by high-performance liquid chromatography (HPLC) (75, 94).

REFERENCES

1. Abramson JS, Givner LB. Should tetracycline be contraindicated for therapy of presumed Rocky Mountain spotted fever in children less than 9 years of age? Pediatrics 1990;86:123.
2. Acharya GP, Davis TME, Ho M, Harris S, Chataut C, Acharya S, Tuhladar N, Kafle KE, Pokhrel B, Nosten F. Factors affecting the pharmacokinetics of parenteral chloramphenicol in enteric fever. J Antimicrob Chemother 1997;40:91–98.
3. Adams HR, Issacson EL, Masters BS. Inhibition of hepatic microsomal enzymes by chloramphenicol. J Pharmacol Exp Ther 1977;203:388–396.
4. Alonso A, Martinez JL. Multiple antibiotic resistance in *Stenotrophomonas maltophilia.* Antimicrob Agents Chemother 1997;41:1140–1142.
5. Alter BP, Potter NU, Li FP. Classification and etiology of the aplastic anemias. Clin Hematol 1978;7:431–465.
6. Ashkenazi S, May-Zahav M, Sulkes J, Zilberberg R, Samra Z. Increasing antimicrobial resistance of *Shigella* isolates in Israel during the period 1984 to 1992. Antimicrob Agents Chemother 1995;39:819–823.
7. Barry AL, Thornsberry C, eds. Susceptibility testing: appendix 2. In: Lennette EH, ed. Manual of clinical microbiology. 3rd ed. Washington, DC: American Society for Microbiology, 1980.
8. Bartelloni PJ, Calia FM, Minchew BH, Beisel WR, Ley HLJ. Absorption and excretion of two chloramphenicol products in humans after oral administration. Am J Med Sci 1969;258:203–208.
9. Barton LL, Rathore MH, Dawson JE. Infection with *Ehrlichia* in childhood. J Pediatr 1992;120:998–1001.
10. Bauernfeind A, Group TAPC. Antibiotic susceptibility patterns of respiratory isolates of *Klebsiella pneumoniae* in Europe and the USA in 1992 and 1993. J Antimicrob Chemother 1996;38 (Suppl A):107–115.
11. Bennett WM, Singer I, Golper T, Feig P, Coggins CJ. Guidelines for drug therapy in renal failure. Ann Intern Med 1977;86:754–83.

12. Benveniste R, Davies J. Mechanisms of antibiotic resistance in bacteria. Annu Rev Biochem 1973;42:471.

13. Bergogne-Berezin E, Joly-Guillou ML. An underestimated nosocomial pathogen, *Acinetobacter calcoaceticus*. J Antimicrob Chemother 1985;16:535–538.

14. Best WK. Chloramphenicol-associated blood dyscrasias. JAMA 1967;201:181.

15. Bhutta ZA, Naqui SA, Razzaz RA, Farooqui BJ. Multi-drug resistant typhoid in children: presentation and clinical features. Rev Infect Dis 1991;13:832–836.

16. Blondeau JM, Yaschuk Y. In vitro activities of ciprofloxacin, cefotaxime, ceftriaxone, chloramphenicol, and rifampin against fully susceptible and moderately penicillin- resistant *Neisseria meningitidis*. Antimicrob Agents Chemother 1995;39:2577–2579.

17. Bloxham RA, Durbin GM, Johnson T. Chloramphenicol and phenobarbitone: a drug interaction. Arch Dis Child 1979;54:76–77.

18. Brewer NS, MacCarty CS, Wellman WE. Brain abscess: a review of recent experience. Ann Intern Med 1975;82:571–576.

19. Buchanan M, Moodley GP. Interaction between chloramphenicol and paracetamol. Br Med J 1979;2:307.

20. Burns JL, Mendelman PM, Levy J, Stull TL, Smith AL. A permeability barrier as a mechanism of chloramphenicol resistance in *Haemophilus influenzae*. Antimicrob Agents Chemother 1985;27:45–46.

21. Burns JL, Rubens CE, Mendelman PM, Smith AL. Cloning and expression in *Escherichia coli* of a gene encoding nonenzymatic chloramphenicol resistance from *Pseudomonas aeruginosa*. Antimicrob Agents Chemother 1986;29:445–450.

22. Burns JL, Wadsworth CD, Barry JJ, Goodall CP. Nucleotide sequence analysis of a gene from *Burkholderia (Pseudomonas) cepacia* encoding an outer membrane lipoprotein involved in multiple antibiotic resistance. Antimicrob Agents Chemother 1996;40:307–313.

23. Burns LE, Hodgman JE, Cass AB. Fatal circulatory collapse in premature infants receiving chloramphenicol. N Engl J Med 1959;261:1319.

24. Chakravorty B, Jain N, Gupta B, Rajvanshi P, Sen MK, Krisha A. Chloramphenicol resistant enteric fever. J Indian Med Assoc 1993;91:10–13.

25. Chaowagul W, Suputtamongkol Y, Dance DAB, Rajchanuvong A, Pattara-arechachai J. Relapse in meliodosis: incidence and risk factors. J Infect Dis 1993;168:1181–1185.

26. Chen SCA, Gottlieb T, Palmer JM, Morris G, Gilbert GL. Antimicrobial susceptibility of anaerobic bacteria in Australia. J Antimicrob Chemother 1992;30:811–820.

27. Cherubin CE, Neu HC, Rahal JJ. Emergence of resistance to chloramphenicol in salmonella. J Infect Dis 1977;135:807.

28. Citron DM, Goldstein EJC, Kenner MA, Burnham LB, Inderlied CB. Activity of ampicillin/sulbactam, ticarcillin/clavulanate, clarithromycin, and eleven other antimicrobial agents against anaerobic bacteria isolated from infections in children. Clin Infect Dis 1995;20(Suppl 2):S356–360.

29. Clarke WTW. Fatal aplastic anemia and chloramphenicol. Can Med Assoc J 1967;97:815.

30. Cocke JG, Brown RE, Geppert LJ. Optic neuritis with prolonged use of chloramphenicol. J Pediatr 1981;68:27.

31. Cohen ML, Tauxe RV. Drug-resistant *Salmonella* in the United States: an epidemiologic perspective. Science 1986;234:964.

32. Craft AW, Brocklebank JT, Hey EN, Jackson RH. The "grey toddler" chloramphenicol toxicity. Arch Dis Child 1974;49:235–237.

33. Cuchural GJ, Tally FP, Jacobus NV, Aldridge K, Cleary T, Finegold SM, Hill G, Iannini P, O'Keefe JP, Pierson C. Susceptibility of the *Bacteroides fragilis* group in the United States: analysis by site of isolation. Antimicrob Agents Chemother 1988;32:717–722.

34. Dajani AS, Asmar BI, Thirumoothi MC. Systemic *Haemophilus influenzae* disease: an overview. J Pediatr 1979;94:355–364.

35. Dajani AS, Kaufman RE. The renaissance of chloramphenicol. Pediatr Clin North Am 1981;28:195.

36. DaMert GJ, Sohle PG. Effect of chloramphenicol on in vitro function of lymphocytes. J Infect Dis 1979;139:220.

37. Datta N, Richards H, Datta C. Salmonella typhi in vivo acquires resistance to both chloramphenicol and co-trimoxazole. Lancet 1981;1:1181–1183.

38. Daum RS, Cohen DL, Smith AL. Fatal aplastic anemia following apparent dose-related chloramphenicol toxicity. J Pediatr 1979;94:403–406.

39. Denny FW, Clyde WAJ, Glezen WP. *Mycoplasma pneumoniae* disease: clinical spectrum, pathophysiology, epidemiology, and control. J Infect Dis 1971;123:74–92.

40. Desomer J, Vereeke D, Crespi M, Van Montagu M. The plasmid-encoded chloramphenicol-resistance protein of *Rhodococcus fascians* is homologous to the transmembrane tetracycline efflux proteins. Mol Microbiol 1992;6:2377–2385.

41. Doern GV, Ferraro MJ, Brueggemann AB, Ruoff KL. Emergence of high rates of antimicrobial resistance among viridans group streptococci in the United States. Antimicrob Agents Chemother 1996;40:891–894.

42. Doona M, Walsh JB. Use of chloramphenicol as topical eye medication: time to cry halt? Br Med J 1995;310:1217–1218.

43. DuPont HL. Quinolones in *Salmonella typhi* infection. Drugs 1993;45(Suppl 3):119.

44. Ehrlich J, Bartz QR, Smith RM. Chloromycetin, a new antibiotic from a soil actinomycete. Science 1947;106:417.

45. Ehrlich J, Gottlieb D, Burkholder RR. *Streptomyces venezuelae*: n. sp., the source of chloromycetin. 1948;56:467.

46. Eickhoff TC, J.V. B, Hayes PS, Feeley J. *Pseudomonas pseudomallei* susceptibility to chemotherapeutic agents. J Infect Dis 1970;73:179–187.

47. Ericsson H, Sherrie JC. Antibiotic sensitivity testing: report on an international collaborative study. Acta Pathol Microbiol Scand 1971;Suppl 271.

48. Evans LS, Kleiman MB. Acidosis as a presenting feature of chloramphenicol toxicity. J Pediatr 1986;108:475.

49. Evans PA, Norden CW, Rhoads S, Deobaldia J, Silber J. In vitro susceptibilities of clinical isolates of vancimycin- resistant enterococci. Antimicrob Agents Chemother 1997;41:1406.

50. Feder HM, Bergstrom SK. Treatment of chronic neutropenia with chloramphenicol. J Pediatr 1994;125:649–651.

51. Feder HMJ, Osier C, Maderazo EG. Chloramphenicol: a review of its uses in clinical practice. Rev Infect Dis 1981;141:597–598.

52. Finegold SM. Therapy for infections due anaerobic bacteria: an overview. J Infect Dis 1977;135(Suppl):S25.

53. Fink TJ, Gump DW. Chloramphenicol: an inpatient study of use and abuse. J Infect Dis 1978;138:690.

54. Finland M. Changing patterns in the susceptibility of common bacterial pathogens to antimicrobial agents. Ann Intern Med 1972;76:1009.

55. Finland M, Garner C, Wilcox C, Sabath LD. Susceptibility of enterobacteria to aminoglycoside antibiotics: comparisons with tetracyclines, polymyxins, chloramphenicol, and spectinomycin. J Infect Dis 1976;134(Suppl):S37–74.

56. Fishbein DB, Dawson JE, Robinson LE. Human ehrlichiosis in the United States, 1985 to 1990. Ann Intern Med 1994;120: 736–743.

57. Forti G, Benincari C. Doxycycline and the teeth [Letter]. Lancet 1969;1:78.

58. Freeman KB. Inhibition of mitochondrial and bacterial protein synthesis by chloramphenicol. Canadian J Biochemistry 1970;48:479.

59. Friedland IR, Klugman KP. Failure of chloramphenicol therapy in penicillin-resistant pneumococcal meningitis. Lancet 1992; 339:405.

60. Friedland IR, Shelton S, McCracken GH. Chloramphenicol in penicillin-resistant pneumococcal meningitis [Letter]. Lancet 1993;342:240–241.

61. Friedman CA, Lovejoy FC, Smith AL. Chloramphenicol disposition in infants and children. J Pediatr 1979;95:1071–1077.

62. Gaffney DF, Cundliffe E, Foster TJ. Chloramphenicol resistance that does not involve chloramphenicol acetyltransferase encoded by plasmids from gram-negative bacteria. J Gen Microbiol 1981;125:113–121.

63. George FJ, Hanna C. Ocular penetration of chloramphenicol. Arch Ophthalmol 1977;93:184.

64. Glazko AJ, Edgerton WH, Dill WA. Chloromycetin palmitate: a synthetic ester of chloromycetin. Antibiot Chemother 1952;2:234.

65. Glazko AJ, Wolf LM, Dill WA. Biochemical studies on chloramphenicol (Chloromycetin). J Pharmacol Exp Ther 1949;96: 445.

66. Goldstein FW, Chumpiatz JC, Guevara JM, Papadopoulou B, Acar JF, Fieu JF. Plasmid-mediated resistance to multiple antibiotics in Salmonella typhi. J Infect Dis 1986;153:261–266.

67. Gotuzzo E, Guerra JG, Benavente L, Palomino JC, Carrillo C, Lopera J, Delgado F, Nalin DR, Sabbaj J. Use of norfloxacin to treat chronic typhoid carrierrs. J Infect Dis 1988;157: 1221–1225.

68. Grafnetterova J, Grafnetter D, Schuck O, Tamkova D, Blaha J. The effects of endogenous compounds isolated from the sera of uremic patients on chloramphenicol binding to proteins. Biochem Pharmacol 1979;28:2923–2928.

69. Grossman ER, Walchek A, Freedman H. Tetracyclines and permanent teeth: the relation between dose and tooth color. Pediatrics 1971;47:567–570.

70. Gupta A. Multidrug resistant typhoid fever in children: epidemiology and therapeutic approach. Pediatr Infect Dis 1994; 13:134.

71. Hahn JE, Gund P. A structured model of the chloramphenicol receptor site. In: Drews J, Hahn FE, eds. Drug receptor interactions in antimicrobial chemotherapy. New York: Springer- Verlag, 1975;245–366.

72. Halpert J. Further studies of suicide inactivation of purified rat liver cytochrome P-450 by chloramphenicol. Mol Pharmacol 1982;21:166.

73. Harrel GT. Treatment of Rocky Mountain spotted fever with antibiotics. Ann NY Acad Sci 1952;55:1027.

74. Havelka J, Hejzlar M, Popov V, Viktorinova D, Prochazka J. Excretion of chloramphenicol in human milk. Chemotherapy 1968;13:204–211.

75. Holt DE, Hurley R, Harvey D. A reappraisal of chloramphenicol metabolism: detection and quantification of metabolites in the sera of children. J Antimicrob Chemother 1995;35:115–127.

76. Holt R. The bacterial degradation of chloramphenicol. Lancet 1967;1:1259.

77. Hornick RB, Gallager LR, Ronald AR. Chloramphenicol treatment of pyogenic myositis. Bull Sch Med Univ Maryland 1966;51:43.

78. Huang NN, Harley RD, Promadhattavedi V, Sproul A. Visual disturbances in cystic fibrosis following chloramphenicol administration. J Pediatr 1966;68:32–44.

79. Irvin JE, Ingram JM. Chloramphenicol-resistant variants of Pseudomonas aeruginosa defective in amino acid transport. Can J Biochem 1980;58:1165.

80. Islam A, Butler T, Kabir I, Alam NH. Treatment of typhoid fever with ceftriaxone for 5 days or chloramphenicol for 14 days: a randomized clinical trial. Antimicrob Agents Chemother 1993; 37:1572–1575.

81. Jones BL, Wilcox MH. Aeromonas infections and their treatment. J Antimicrobial Therapy 1995;35:453–461.

82. Kanakavi S, Karabela S, Marinis E, Legakis NJ. Antibiotic resistance of clinical isolates of Streptococcus pneumoniae in Greece. J Clin Microbiol 1994;32:3056–3058.

83. Kauffman RE, Miceli JN, Strebel L, Buckley JA, Done AK, Dajani AS. Pharmacokinetics of chloramphenicol and chloramphenicol succinate in infants and children. J Pediatr 1981;98: 315–320.

84. Kearns GL, Bocchini JA, Brown RD, Cotter DL, Wilson JT. Absence of a pharmacokinetic interaction between chloramphenicol and acetaminophen in children. J Pediatr 1985;107:134–139.

85. Keiser C, Buchegger U. Hematologic side effects of chloramphenicol and thiampenicol. Helv Med Acta 1973;37:265.

86. Kelsey DS. Rocky Mountain spotted fever. Pediatric Clin North Am 1979;26:369.

87. Kenny JF, Isburg CD, Michaels RH. Meningitis due to Haemophilus influenzae type b resistant to both ampicillin and chloramphenicol. Pediatrics 1980;66:14–16.

88. Kessler DL, Smith AL, Woodrum DE. Chloramphenicol toxicity in a neonate treated with exchange transfusion. J Pediatr 1980;96:140–141.

89. Khan MA, Hayat Z, Sadick A. Ofloxacin in the treatment of typhoid fever resistant to chloramphenicol and amoxicillin. Clin Ther 1994;16:815–818.

90. Klein JO. Report of the task force on diagnosis and management of meningitis. Pediatrics 1986;78(Suppl):959.

91. Klugman KP. Pneumococcal isolates resistant to antibiotics. Clin Microbiol Rev 1990;3:171.

92. Konstantopoulos K, Avlami A, Demarongona K, Sideris G, Rekoumi L, Loukopoulos D. Bacteroides fragilis arthritis in a sickle cell-thalassaemia patient. Scand J Infect Dis 1994;26: 495–497.

93. Koup J, Gibaldi M, McNamara P, Hilligloss DM, Colburn WA, Bruck E. Interaction of chloramphenicol with phenytoin and phenobarbital. Clin Pharmacol Ther 1978;24:571–575.

94. Koup JR, Brodsky B, Lau A, Beam TRJ. High-performance liquid chromatographic assay of chloramphenicol in serum. Antimicrob Agents Chemother 1978;14:439–443.

95. Kramer PW, Griffith RS, Campbell RL. Antibiotic penetration of the brain. J Neurosurg 1969;31:295–302.

96. Krasinski K, Kusmiesz H, Nelson JD. Pharmacologic interactions among chloramphenicol, phenytoin, and phenobarbital. Pediatr Infect Dis 1982;1:232–235.

97. Kucers A. Current position of chloramphenicol therapy. J Antimicrob Chemother 1980;6:1.

98. Kunin CM. A guide to use of antibiotics in patients with renal disease. Ann Intern Med 1967;67:151.

99. Kunin CM, Glazko AJ, Finland M. Persistence of antibiotics in blood of patients with acute renal failure. II. Chloramphenicol

and its metabolism products in the blood of patients with severe renal disease or hepatic cirrhosis. J Clin Invest 1959;38:1498.

100. Lasserre R, Sangalang RP, Santiago L. Three-day treatment of typhoid fever with two different doses of ceftriaxone compared to 14-day therapy with chloramphenicol: a randomized trial. J Antimicrob Chemother 1991;28:765–772.

101. Lee HJ, Park JY, Jang SH. High incidence of resistance of clinical isolates of *Streptococcus pneumoniae* from a university hospital in Korea. Clin Infect Dis 1995;20:826.

102. Levine PH, Regelson W, Holland JF. Chloramphenicol-associated encephalopathy. Clin Pharmacol Ther 1970;11:194–199.

103. Li XZ, Livermans DM, Nikaido H. Role of efflux pump(s) in intrinsic resistance of *Pseudomonas aeruginosa:* resistance to tetracycline, chloramphenicol, and norfloxacin. Antimicrob Agents Chemother 1994;38:1732–1741.

104. Liles WC, Spach DH. Tick-borne diseases [Letter]. N Engl J Med 1994;330:292.

105. Lima AAM, Lima NL, Pinho MC, Barros EA, Teixeira MJ, Martins MCV, Guerrant RL. High frequency of strains multiply resistant to ampicillin, trimethoprim-sulfamethoxazole, streptomycin, chloramphenicol, and tetracycline isolated from patients with shigellosis in northeastern Brazil during the period 1988 to 1993. Antimicrob Agents Chemother 1995;39:256–259.

106. Lynch C, Courvalin P, Nikado H. Active efflux of antimicrobial agents in wild-type strains of enterococci. Antimicrob Agents Chemother 1997;41:869–871.

107. MacBeth KJ, Lee CA. Prolonged inhibition of bacterial protein synthesis abolishes *Salmonella* invasion. Infect Immun 1993;61:1544–1546.

108. Mandal BK. *Salmonella typhi* and other salmonellae. Gut 1994;35:726.

109. Manyan DR, Arimura GK, Yunis AA. Chloramphenicol-induced erythroid suppression and bone marrow ferrochelatase in dogs. J Lab Clin Med 1972;79:137–144.

110. Martelo OJ, Manyan DR, Smith US, Yunis AA. Chloramphenicol and bone marrow mitochondria. J Lab Clin Med 1969;74:927–940.

111. Mauer SM, Chavers BM, Kjellstrand CM. Treatment of an infant with severe chloramphenicol intoxication using charcoal column hemoperfusion. J Pediatr 1980;96:136–139.

112. Maurin M, Raoult D. Antimicrobial susceptibility of *Rochalimaea quintana, Rochalimaea vinsonii* and the newly recognized *Rochalimaea henselae.* J Antimicrob Chemother 1993;32:587–594.

113. McCaffrey RP, Halsted CH, Wahab MFA, Robertson RP. Chloramphenicol-induced hemolysis in Caucasian glucose-6-phosphate dehydrogenase deficiency. Ann Intern Med 1971;74:722–726.

114. McCracken GH Jr, Nelson JD, Kaplan SL. Consensus report: antimicrobial therapy for bacterial meningitis in infants and children. Pediatr Infect Dis J 1987;6:501–505.

115. McCrumb FR, Mercier S, Robic G. Chloramphenicol and terramycin in the treatment of pneumonic plague. Am J Med 1953;14:284.

116. McCrumb FR Jr, Snyder MJ, Hicken WJ. The use of chloramphenicol acid succinate in the treatment of acute infections. Antibiotics Annual 1957–1958. New York: Medical Encyclopedia, 1958:837–841.

117. McCrumb FR, Snyder MJ, Woodward TE. Studies on human infection with *Pasturella tularensis:* comparison of streptomycin and chloramphenicol in the prophylaxis of clinical disease. Trans Assoc Am Physicians 1957;70:74.

118. McLean IWJ, Schwab JH, Hillegas AB. Susceptibility of microorganisms to chloramphenicol (Chloromycetin). J Clin Invest 1948;28:953.

119. McPherson SDJ, Presley GD, Crawford JR. Aqueous humor assays of subconjunctival antibiotics. Am J Ophthalmol 1968;66:430–435.

120. Meissner HC, Smith AL. The current status of chloramphenicol. Pediatrics 1979;64:3348.

121. Mourad AS, Metwally M, Nour El Deen A, Threlfall EJ, Rowe B, Mapes T, Hedstrom R, Bourgeois AL, Murphy JR. Multiple drug- resistant *Salmonella typhi.* Clin Infect Dis 1993;17:134–135.

122. Munoz P, Diaz MD, Rodriguez-Crexiems M, Cercenado E, Pelaez T, Bouza E. Antimicrobial resistance of *Salmonella* isolates in a Spanish hospital. Antimicrob Agents Chemother 1993;37:1200–1202.

123. Murdoch MB, Peterson LR. Antimicrobial penetration into polymorphonuclear leukocytes and alveolar macrophages. Semin Respir Infect 1991;6:112–121.

124. Murray BE. Resistance of *Shigella, Salmonella,* and other selected enteric pathogens to antimicrobial agents. Rev Infect Dis 1986;8(Suppl 2):S172–181.

125. Murray IA, Shaw WV. *O*-Acetyltransferases for chloramphenicol and other natural products. Antimicrob Agents Chemother 1997;41:1–6.

126. Mussini C, Trenti F, Manicardi G, Mongiardo N, Codeluppi M, D'Andrea L, Guaraldi G, Squadrini F, De Rienzo B. Non-typhoidal *Salmonella* subdural empyema in a patient with AIDS. Scand J Infect Dis 1995;27:173–174.

127. Nagao T, Mauer AM. Concordance for drug-induced aplastic anemia in identical twins. N Engl J Med 1969;281:7.

128. Neal GW, Downing EF. Clostridial meningitis as a result of craniocerebral arrow injury. J Trauma 1996;40:476–480.

129. Nilsen IW, Bakke I, Vader A, Olsvik O, El-Gewely MR. Isolation of *cmr,* a novel *Escherichia coli* chloramphenicol resistance gene encoding a putative efflux pump. J Bacteriol 1996;178:3188–3193.

130. Norris AH, Reilly JP, Edelstein PA, Brennan PJ, Schuster MG. Chloramphenicol for the treatment of vancomycin-resistant enterococcal infections. Clin Infect Dis 1995;20:1137–1144.

131. Oelschlaeger TA, Barrett TJ, Kopecko DJ. Some structures and processes of human epithelial cells involve uptake of enterohemorrhagic *Escherichia coli* O157:H7 strains. Infect Immun 1994;62:5142–5150.

132. Osawa S, Takata R, Tanaka K, Tamaki M. Chloramphenicol resistant mutants of *Bacillus subtilis.* Mol Gen Genet 1973;127:157–161.

133. Ostroff SM, Harrison LH, Khallaf N, Assaad M, Guirguis NI, Harrington S, el-Alamy M, Group tARS. Resistance patterns of *Streptococcus pneumoniae* and *Haemophilus influenzae* isolates recovered in Egypt from children with pneumonia. Clin Infect Dis 1996;23:1069–1074.

134. Overturf GD. Pyogenic bacterial infections of the CNS. Neurol Clin 1986;4:69.

135. Pestka S. Studies on formation of transfer ribonucleic acid-ribosome complexes. XI. Antibiotic effects on phenylalanyloligonucleotide binding to ribosomes. Proc Natl Acad Sci USA 1969;64:709.

136. Pestka S. Inhibitors of ribosome functions. Annu Rev Microbiol 1971;25:487.

137. Pickering LK, Hoeker JL, Kramer WG, Kohl S, Cleary TG. Clinical pharmacology of two chloramphenicol preparations in

children: sodium succinate (IV) and palmitate (oral) esters. J Pediatr 1980;96:757–761.

138. Pillow RP, Epstein RB, Buckner CD, Giblett ER, Thomas ED. Treatment of bone marrow failure by isogenic bone marrow infusion. N Engl J Med 1966;275:94–97.

139. Pongs O. Chloramphenicol. In: Hahn FE, ed. Antibiotics, vol 1. New York: Springer-Verlag, 1979.

140. Poole K, Gotoh N, Tsujimoto H, Zhao Q, Wada A, Yamasaki T, Neshat S, Yamagishi J, Li X-Z, Nishino T. Overexpression of the *mexC-mexD-oprJ* efflux operon in *nfxB*-type multidrug-resistant strains of *Pseudomonas aeruginosa*. Mol Microbiol 1996;21:713–724.

141. Preston MA, Brown S, Borczyk AA, Riley G, Krishnan C. Antimicrobial susceptibility of pathogenic *Yersinia enterocolitica* isolated in Canada from 1972 to 1990. Antimicrob Agents Chemother 1994;38:2121–2124.

142. Rahal JJS, Simberkoff MS. Bactericidal and bacteriostatic action of chloramphenicol against meningeal pathogens. Antimicrob Agents Chemother 1979;16:13.

143. Rapp GF, Griffith RS, Hebble WM. The permeability of traumatically inflamed synovial membrane to commonly used antibiotics. J Bone Joint Surg 1966;48A:1534–1540.

144. Rensimer ER, Pickering LK, Ericsson CD, Kramer WG. Sequential CSF concentration of chloramphenicol after administration of oral chloramphenicol palmitate. Lancet 1981;1:165.

145. Rich ML, Ritterhoff RJ, Hoffman RJ. A fatal case of aplastic anemia following chloramphenicol therapy. Ann Intern Med 1950;33:1459.

146. Ridgway EJ, Allen KD, Neal TJ, Lombard M, Rigby A. Penicillin-resistant pneumococcal meningitis [Letter]. Lancet 1992;339:931.

147. Rietschel RL. Dermatologic manifestations of antimicrobial adverse reactions with special emphasis on topical exposure. Infect Dis Clin North Am 1994;8:607–615.

148. Rizzo-Naudi J, Griscti-Soler N, Canado W. Human brucellosis: an evaluation of antibiotics in the treatment of brucellosis. Postgrad Med 1967;43:520–526.

149. Robertson RP, Wahab MFA, Rasch FO. Evaluation of chloramphenicol and ampicillin in *Salmonella enteritis*. N Engl J Med 1968;278:171–176.

150. Rodriguez WJ, Schwartz RH, Akram S, Khan WN. *Streptococcus pneumoniae* resistant to penicillin: incidence and potential therapeutic options. Laryngoscope 1995;105(3 Part 1):300–304.

151. Romansky MJ, Olansky S, Taggart SR. The antitreponemal effect of chloromycetin in 32 cases of early syphilis in man: a preliminary report. Science 1948;110:639.

152. Rosenthal RL, Blackman A. Bone marrow hypoplasia following use of chloramphenicol eyedrops. JAMA 1965;191:136.

153. Rubin D, Weisberger AS, Botti ERE. Changes in iron metabolism in early chloramphenicol toxicity. J Clin Invest 1958;37:1286.

154. Rubinstein E, Shamberg B. In vitro activity of cinoxacin, ampicillin, and chloramphenicol against *Shigella* and non- typhoid *Salmonella*. Antimicrob Agents Chemother 1977;11:577.

155. Rygg M, Foyn Brunn C. Rat bite fever *(Streptobacillus moniliformis)* with septicemia in a child. Scand J Infect Dis 1992;24:535–540.

156. Sack CM, Koup JR, Smith AL. Chloramphenicol pharmacokinetics in infants and young children. Pediatrics 1980;66:579–584.

157. Saha SK, Saha S, Ruhulamin M, Hanif M, Islam M. Decreasing trend of multiresistant *Salmonella typhi* in Bangladesh. J Antimicrob Chemother 1997;39:554–556.

158. Schwartz SN. Tick-borne diseases [Letter]. N Engl J Med 1994;330:292.

159. Scott JL, Finegold SM, Belkin GA. A controlled double blind study of the hematologic toxicity of chloramphenicol. N Engl J Med 1965;272:1137.

160. Serino F, Grevel J, Napoli KL, Kahan BD, Strobel HW. Oxygen radical formation by the cytochrome P-450 system as a cellular mechanism for cyclosporin toxicity. Transplant Proc 1994;26:2916–2917.

161. Shah PN, D'Souza J, Dathani KK. Absorption of chloramphenicol by various routes of administration. Indian J Med Res 1977;65:549–553.

162. Sharma KB, Bhat MB, Pasricha A, Vaze S. Multiple antibiotic resistance among salmonellae in India. J Antimicrob Chemother 1979;5:15–21.

163. Smadel JE. Chloramphenicol (chloromycetin) in the treatment of infectious diseases. Am J Med 1949;7:671.

164. Smith AL, Weber A. Pharmacology of chloramphenicol. Pediatr Clin North Am 1983;30:209.

165. Smith SH, Palumbo PE, Edelson PJ. Salmonella strains resistant to multiple antibiotics: therapeutic implications. Pediatr Infect Dis 1984;3:455–460.

166. Sookpranee M, Paithoon B, Susaengrat W, Bhuripanyo K, Punyagupta S. Multicenter prospective randomized trial comparing ceftazidime plus co-trimoxazole with chloramphenicol plus doxycycline and co-trimoxazole for treatment of severe melioidosis. Antimicrob Agents Chemother 1992;36:158–162.

167. Spika JS, Waterman SH, Soo Hoo GW, St. Louis ME, Pacer RE, James SM, Bissett ML, Mayer LW, Chiu JY, Hall B. Chloramphenicol resistant *Salmonella newport* traced through hamburger to dairy farms. N Engl J Med 1987;316:565–570.

168. Steinfort CL, McConachy KA. Cyclosporin-chloramphenicol drug interaction in a heart-lung transplant recipient. Med J Aust 1994;161:455.

169. Strandberg DA, Jorgenson JH, Drutz DJ. Activities of newer beta-lactam antibiotics against ampicillin, chloramphenicol, or mutiply-resistant *Haemophilus influenzae*. Diagn Microbiol Infect Dis 1984;2:333–337.

170. Suhrland LG, Weisberger AS. Chloramphenicol toxicity in liver and renal disease. Arch Intern Med 1963;112:161.

171. Sutherland JM. Fatal cardiovascular collapse of infants receiving large amount of chloramphenicol. Am J Dis Child 1959;97:761.

172. Thompson WL, Anderson SEJ, Lipsky JJ, Lietman PS. Overdoses of chloramphenicol [Letter]. JAMA 1975;243:149–150.

173. Tovi F, Gatot A. Septic jugular thrombosis with abscess formation. Ann Otol Rhinol Laryngol 1991;100:682.

174. Traub WH, Fukushima PI. Nonspecific resistance of *Serratia marcescens* against antimicrobial drugs. Chemotherapy 1979;25:196.

175. Vallejo JG, Kaplan SL, Mason EOJ. Treatment of meningitis and other infections due to ampicillin-resistant *Haemophilus influenzae* type b in children. Rev Infect Dis 1991;13:197–200.

176. Vassort-Bruneau C, Lesage-Descauses M-C, Martel J-L, Lafont J-P, Chaslus-Dancla E. CAT III chloramphenicol resistance in *Pasteurella haemolytica* and *Pasteurella multocida* isolated from calves. J Antimicrob Chemother 1996;38:205–213.

177. Walker DH. Rocky Mountain spotted fever: a seasonal alert. Clin Infect Dis 1995;20:1111–1117.

178. Wallace JF, Smith RH, Garcia M, Petersdorf RG. Studies on the pathogenesis of meningitis: antagonism between penicillin and

chloramphenicol in experimental pneumococcal meningitis. J Lab Clin Med 1967;70:408–418.

179. Wallenstein L, Snyder J. Neurotoxic reactions to chloromycetin. Ann Intern Med 1952;36:1526.

180. Wallerstein RO, Condit PK, Kasper CK, Brown JW, Morrison FR. Statewide study of chloramphenicol therapy and fatal aplastic anemia. JAMA 1969;208:2045–2050.

181. Watt G, Chouriyagune C, Ruangweerayud R, Watcharapichat P, Phulsuksombati D, Jongsakul K, Teja-Isavadharm P, Bhodhidatta D, Corcoran KD, Dasch GA. Scrub typhus infections poorly responsive to antibiotics in northern Thailand. Lancet 1996;348:86–89.

182. Wehrle PF, Mathies AW, Leedom JM, Ivler D. Bacterial meningitis. Ann NY Acad Sci 1967;145:488–498.

183. Weisberger AS, Daniel TM. Suppression of antibody synthesis by chloramphenicol analogs. Proc Soc Exp Biol Med 1969;131:570.

184. Weiss CF, Glazko AJ, Weston JK. Chloramphenicol in the newborn infant: a physiologic explanation of its toxicity when given in excessive doses. N Engl J Med 1960;262:787.

185. West BC, DeVault GAJ, Clement JC, Williams DM. Aplastic anemia associated with parenteral chloramphenicol: review of 10 cases, including the second case of possible increased risk with cimetidine. Rev Infect Dis 1988;10:1048–1051.

186. Westenfeld GO, Paterson PY. Life-threatening infections: choice of alternate drugs when penicillin cannot be given. JAMA 1969;210:845.

187. Woodward TE, Wisseman CLJ. Chloromycetin (chloramphenicol). New York: Medical Encyclopedia, 1958.

188. Yunis A. Chloramphenicol: relation of structure to activity and toxicity. Annu Rev Pharmacol Toxicol 1988;28:83.

189. Yunis AA. Chloramphenicol-induced bone marrow suppression. Semin Hematol 1973;10:225.

190. Yunis AA. Chloramphenicol toxicity: 25 years of research [Review]. Am J Med 1989;87(3N):44N.

191. Yunis AA, Bloomberg GR. Chloramphenicol toxicity: clinical features and pathogenesis. Prog Hematol 1964;4:138.

192. Yunis AA, Smith US, Restrepo A. Reversible bone marrow suppression from chloramphenicol: a consequence of mitochondrial injury. Arch Intern Med 1970;126:272–275.

Clindamycin

●

Jan Verhoef and Matthew E. Levison

Clindamycin has been in clinical use for almost 30 years; nevertheless, it remains an important antimicrobial agent, highly active against Gram-positive and anaerobic bacteria. Clindamycin was introduced as an orally administered agent, intended primarily for the treatment of staphylococcal and streptococcal infections (52, 55–57, 118). However, because of its excellent activity against anaerobic bacteria, it soon also became the drug of choice for infections caused by these bacteria. The combination of clindamycin and gentamicin emerged later as the standard treatment for mixed aerobic-anaerobic infections (14). Over the years clindamycin has also been considered for some additional indications: acne vulgaris, *Pneumocystis* and *Toxoplasma* infections in patients with acquired immunodeficiency syndrome (AIDS), etc.

During more than 25 years of clindamycin use worldwide, numerous investigators have written about its in vitro activity, its activity in experimental animal infections, and its clinical usefulness. A number of reviews have been published (35, 51, 55–57, 118). The monograph *Clindamycin in the Treatment of Human Infections* published at the 20th anniversary of the worldwide introduction of clindamycin is a valuable source of information (146).

CHEMICAL STRUCTURE AND STRUCTURE-ACTIVITY RELATIONSHIPS

The parent molecule of clindamycin, lincomycin, was discovered by Mason and coworkers in 1961 (79). Lincomycin is produced by a new species of *Streptomyces lincolnensin* var. *lincolnensis,* which was isolated from a soil sample collected in Gering, Nebraska (in the vicinity of Lincoln, Nebraska; hence the name). The compound is active in vitro and in vivo against a variety of Gram-positive bacteria and is well absorbed following oral administration. No cross-resistance was observed in bacteria resistant to other antibiotics known at that time (79).

In 1967, lincomycin was approved for use in human infections and a large program was initiated at the Upjohn company to modify the product chemically to enhance its pharmacokinetic characteristics and to improve its antibacterial activity. Halogenation at the C-7 position in the sugar moiety led to production of very active semisynthetic compounds (12, 73, 77); the best example is clindamycin, the 7(S)-chloro-7-deoxylincomycin derivative (Fig. 1). It has a broader spectrum of antimicrobial activity, greater potency, and better absorption than lincomycin. Thus, clindamycin was developed for clinical studies. Clindamycin subsequently passed the various phases of clinical research and received approval in many countries.

Clindamycin is worldwide available in several forms:

- Capsules for oral administration (clindamycin hydrochloride)
- In solution as a prodrug (clindamycin phosphate, developed to reduce pain on injection, for intramuscular and intravenous administration)

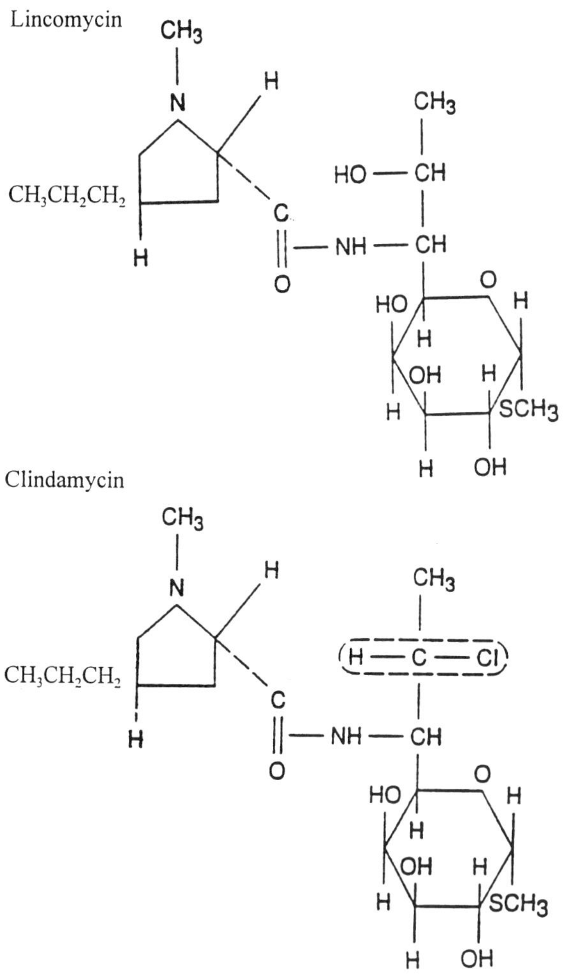

FIGURE 1. The chemical structures of lincomycin and clindamycin. (From Zambrano D, ed. Clindamycin in the treatment of human infections. Kalamazoo, MI: The Upjohn Company, 1992. With permission.)

- An oral liquid pediatric formulation (clindamycin palmitate)
- A topical solution for the treatment of acne vulgaris (clindamycin phosphate)

ANTIMICROBIAL ACTIVITY

The National Committee for Clinical Laboratory Standards (NCCLS) published the breakpoints for clindamycin to define susceptible, intermediately susceptible, and resistant microorganisms (87, 88). Susceptible aerobic bacteria have a breakpoint concentration of clindamycin of 0.50 mg/L or less, intermediately susceptible aerobic bacteria have breakpoint concentrations of 1 to 2 mg/L, and minimal inhibitory concentrations (MICs) of 4 mg/L or more indicate resistant aerobic bacteria. Anaerobic bacteria are considered susceptible when the MIC is 4 mg/L or less and resistant when the MIC is 8 mg/L or more.

Of course, susceptibility to clindamycin can also be determined by disk. The standard disk-diffusion method uses a 2-μg clindamycin disk (89). A 10-μg clindamycin disk was developed for susceptibility testing of anaerobes, using thioglycolate broth containing a disk (133). Results of this assay correlate closely with those of the NCCLS agar dilution method for clindamycin; however, NCCLS has not approved the broth disk method because of quality control problems (88). The antimicrobial activity of clindamycin is summarized in the various tables, using MIC_{90} data (142).

Gram-Positive Aerobic Bacteria

Clindamycin is active against a large variety of Gram-positive aerobic bacteria, such as Gram-positive bacilli, staphylococci (including penicillinase-producing strains), and streptococci (Table 1). *Streptococcus pyogenes, Streptococcus pneumoniae, Streptococcus bovis,* and Lancefield group B, C, and G streptococci are all susceptible to clindamycin, although an increasing number of centers are isolating some clindamycin-resistant group A streptococci together with group A streptococci resistant to erythromycin (11). Penicillin-susceptible viridans streptococci are generally susceptible to clindamycin; penicillin-resistant strains of this group, however, may have reduced susceptibility to clindamycin (31). Some penicillin-resistant pneumococci are resistant to clindamycin; others are susceptible (4, 23, 30, 62, 63). Thus, clindamycin cannot be given empirically when penicillin-resistant pneumococci cannot be ruled out, and laboratory testing is mandatory. Methicillin-susceptible *Staphylococcus aureus* isolates are susceptible to clindamycin as well (102). Although clindamycin is active against some strains of methicillin-resistant staphylococci, an increasing number of staphylococcal strains resistant to methicillin are also resistant to clindamycin. This limits the use of clindamycin for infections due to these organisms (77, 98, 102, 108). Thus, as is the case with penicillin-resistant pneumococci, clindamycin cannot be used empirically to treat infections possibly due to methicillin-resistant *S. aureus* (MRSA).

As with *S. aureus*, most methicillin-resistant strains of coagulase-negative staphylococci are also resistant to clindamycin

TABLE 1 • **In Vitro Activity of Clindamycin against Gram-Positive Aerobic Bacteria**		
Organism	**MIC_{90} Range (mg/L)**	**MIC_{90} (mg/L)**
Bacillus cereus	1	1
Listeria monocytogenes	1 to 8	2.22
Staphylococcus aureus (methicillin susceptible)	0.12 to 2	0.50
Staphylococcus saprophyticus	0.12 to 0.25	0.16
Streptococcus agalactiae	≤0.06 to 0.50	0.15
Streptococcus bovis	0.04	0.04
Streptococcus pneumoniae (penicillin susceptible)	0.03 to 0.25	0.23
Streptococcus pyogenes	0.13 to 0.25	0.19
Streptococcus spp. group B	≤0.12 to 0.25	0.15
Streptococcus spp. group C	≤0.12 to 0.50	0.22
Streptococcus spp. group G	0.06 to 0.50	0.31
Streptococcus species, viridans group (penicillin susceptible)	≤0.06 to 1.6	0.53

Adapted with permission from Zambrano D, ed. Clindamycin in the treatment of human infections. Kalamazoo, MI: The Upjohn Company, 1992.

(5, 37, 102). The urinary tract pathogen *Staphylococcus sapro-phyticus* as well as *Staphylococcus warneri, Staphylococcus capitis,* and *Staphylococcus stimulans* is usually susceptible to clindamycin (38). However, increased resistance among Gram-positive bacteria against a variety of antibiotics dictates proper in vitro susceptibility testing before agents such as clindamycin are used to treat patients with infections due to these microorganisms.

Clindamycin has some activity against various other bacteria, including *Listeria monocytogenes, Bacillus cereus, Bacillus anthracis* (85), and *Corynebacterium diphtheriae,* but the clinical significance of these in vitro observations is not known. Clindamycin is not active against *Enterococcus faecalis* (30, 31, 38), *Enterococcus faecium* (31), and *Nocardia asteroides* (48, 53).

Gram-Negative Aerobic Bacteria

Clindamycin has poor activity against almost all species of Gram-negative aerobic bacteria. Only some activity has been observed against some strains of *Moraxella catarrhalis* (7, 20), *Haemophilus influenzae* (20, 30), *Legionella* (60), and *Neisseria meningitidis* (7), but the clinical value is limited. Clindamycin does have some in vitro activity against *Campylobacter jejuni, Campylobacter fetus, Campylobacter coli, Helicobacter pylori* (138), *Gardnerella vaginalis,* and *Neisseria gonorrhoeae.* However, very few patients with infections caused by these organisms have been treated with clindamycin.

Anaerobic Bacteria

Clindamycin has been widely used against infections caused by anaerobic bacteria because of its broad spectrum of activity. Although resistance rates are slowly increasing, clindamycin has remained one of the drugs of choice in the treatment of infections due to anaerobic Gram-negative bacteria, belonging to the *Bacteroides fragilis* group including *Bacteroides distasonis, Bacteroides fragilis, Bacteroides ovatus, Bacteroides thetaiotamicron,* and *Bacteroides vulgatus.*

Summary data for over 4000 isolates of the *B. fragilis* group and approximately 2000 *B. fragilis* isolates indicate that more than 90% of these strains are susceptible to 2 to 3 mg/L clindamycin. Resistance within the *B. fragilis* group is more likely to be seen in species other than *B. fragilis. B. distasonis, B. ovatus, B. vulgatus,* and *B. thetaiotaomicron* are slightly more resistant (15). *B. fragilis,* the most commonly isolated anaerobic species, has remained relatively susceptible to clindamycin in a number of surveillance studies (0.8 to 5% resistance rates). In a more recent study of 2800 isolates of *B. fragilis,* 14% of the strains were resistant (2). Encapsulated *Bacteroides* strains especially appear to be more resistant (19).

These data underscore the need for continuous monitoring of susceptibility patterns for *Bacteroides. Prevotella melaninogenicus, Prevotella bivia, Prevotella disiens, Fusobacterium* species, and *Veillonella* species are highly susceptible (55, 56). *Eikenella* is usually resistant (48, 66). The in vitro activity of clindamycin against many important Gram-positive anaerobic species is summarized in Table 2. The compound is highly effective in vitro against most strains of actinomycetes, eubacte-

TABLE 2 • In Vitro Activity of Clindamycin against Gram-Positive Anaerobic Bacteria

Organism	MIC$_{90}$ Range (mg/L)	MIC$_{90}$ (mg/L)
Actinomyces species	0.12 to 1	0.8
Clostridium botulinum	4	4
Clostridium difficile	4 to >256	57.7
Clostridium perfringens	0.25 to 8	3.4
Eubacterium species	0.4 to 2	1.1
Lactobacillus species	0.50 to 1	0.8
Peptostreptococcus	0,12 to 4	3
Anaerobic Gram-positive cocci	0.5 to 1	0.9
Propionibacterium acnes	0.10 to 0.25	0.2
Propionibacterium species	0.12 to 0.20	0.16

Adapted with permission from Zambrano D, ed. Clindamycin in the treatment of human infections. Kalamazoo, MI: The Upjohn Company, 1992.

ria, lactobacilli, propionibacteria, and peptostreptococci. Clostridia are often more resistant to clindamycin than most other anaerobes. The activity of clindamycin against *C. difficile,* the cause of pseudomembranous colitis, is highly variable: MIC$_{90}$s range from 4 to more than 256 μg/mL (55).

Clindamycin is also active against *Chlamydia trachomatis.* But *Mycoplasma pneumoniae* and *Ureaplasma* are usually resistant (98). At a concentration of about 2 mg/L, clindamycin inhibits 90% of *C. trachomatis* strains. Often, synergy is observed between an aminoglycoside and clindamycin against *Chlamydia* (95). Therefore, this combination is one of the recommended treatment schedules for patients requiring hospitalization for pelvic inflammatory disease (96).

Protozoa

During the screening of antibiotics against *Plasmodium berghei* infection in rodents, it was found that clindamycin was also active against protozoa such as *Plasmodium, Pneumocystis carinii,* and *Toxoplasma gondii.* In in vitro and human studies, clindamycin is active against both chloroquine-resistant and chloroquine-susceptible malaria. Clindamycin exerts its antiprotozoal activity mainly after 48 to 72 h. Exposure of protozoa to clindamycin for 24 h leads to only 20 to 25% inhibition, independent of dosage; exposure for 72 h leads to 75% inhibition. This time-dependent effect of clindamycin observed in vitro may explain the slow clinical response of *P. falciparum* to clindamycin (105). In vitro, clindamycin has limited activity against *Toxoplasma;* however, in combination with primaquine, it is active in vivo in prophylactic and therapeutic regimens (131). Clindamycin can also be used in combination with pyrimethamine for *Toxoplasma* infections of the central nervous system in AIDS patients.

In vitro, clindamycin alone has a poor activity against *P. carinii* and is ineffective as either prophylaxis or treatment for *P. carinii* pneumonia in animals. On the other hand, primaquine alone has a good in vitro activity against *P. carinii* but is surprisingly ineffective as prophylaxis or treatment. However, the combination of clindamycin and primaquine is active therapeutically and prophylactically.

Influence on Host-Parasite Interactions

At subinhibitory concentrations, clindamycin enhances opsonization and subsequent phagocytosis of *S. pyogenes,* probably because of inhibition of M protein synthesis, and under these conditions, opsonization of *S. aureus* and *Bacteroides* is enhanced (Fig. 2). Opsonization of *S. aureus* is enhanced because synthesis of protein A (an important cell wall component of staphylococci that inhibits phagocytosis) is inhibited by clindamycin. Clindamycin also inhibits capsule production by *S. aureus* (82, 136). Several bacteria produce a glycocalyx that plays a role in adherence of bacteria to foreign bodies and tissues. Glycocalyx produced by staphylococci, *Bacteroides,* and streptococci is an important virulence factor and is implicated in the pathogenesis of osteomyelitis, endocarditis, and catheter-related sepsis (24). Clindamycin concentrations below the MIC decrease glycocalyx production and subsequent adherence of bacteria to cells and foreign bodies (136).

Clindamycin at a concentration one-third of its MIC alters the cell wall of *S. aureus,* increases consumption of complement, and enhances phagocytosis of the strains by polymorphonuclear leukocytes in vitro. Clindamycin reduces fibronectin binding to *S. aureus* at a concentration as low as 1/32 of the MIC, with maximal reduction at 1/16 of that concentration. This may be relevant in that fibronectin possibly plays a role in bacterial adherence to host cells.

MECHANISM OF ACTION

Clindamycin and lincomycin inhibit bacterial protein synthesis by their action at the bacterial ribosome. The antibiotics bind preferentially to the 50S ribosomal subunit and inhibit initiation of peptide chain synthesis (106). Clindamycin may inhibit the binding of aminoacyl-tRNA or inhibit the translocation reaction following amino acid binding on the ribosome

(68). Clindamycin acts at the same ribosomal binding site as erythromycin and chloramphenicol; therefore, the binding of any one of these antibiotics can inhibit the action of the other compounds (140).

At low concentrations, clindamycin strongly inhibits production of toxic-shock-syndrome toxin and other toxins by *S. aureus.* The concentration of clindamycin that interfered with toxin production is of the order of 0.001 to 0.01 μg/mL. Similar observations were made with group A streptococci and clostridia. Clindamycin inhibits erythrogenic toxin production by streptococci (124).

Although clindamycin is regarded primarily as a bacteriostatic agent (47, 48, 68, 86, 115, 120, 135), the drug has a concentration-dependent bactericidal activity against a variety of organisms, including staphylococci (1, 10, 58, 83), streptococci (1, 83), anaerobes (63, 101, 113, 125, 134, 145), and *H. pylori* (49). Clindamycin was bactericidal for *B. fragilis* in a number of studies (63, 101, 113, 145). The activity of clindamycin is not affected by serum or by variation in inoculum size. Clindamycin is more active against Gram-positive aerobic bacteria in an alkaline environment than in an acidic environment. However the pH does not affect the activity of clindamycin against anaerobes. Interestingly, clindamycin can inhibit β-lactamase production by *Enterobacter* and *Pseudomonas* (91) without inhibiting growth (112).

Postantibiotic Effect

Bacterial protein synthesis inhibitors, such as clindamycin, exert a pronounced postantibiotic effect (PAE) against susceptible species (21). This is likely due to persistence of the drug at the ribosomal binding site. Clindamycin demonstrates a prolonged PAE (2.5–5.5 h) for a variety of species, including *S. aureus, S. pyogenes,* and *S. pneumoniae* (21, 67). Animal

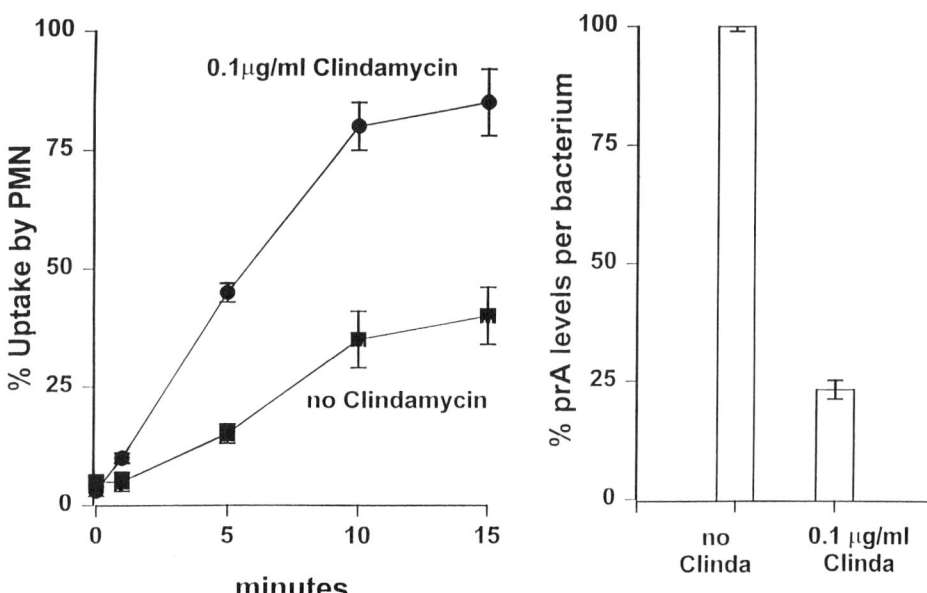

FIGURE 2. Subinhibitory concentrations of clindamycin enhances uptake of *S. aureus* by PMN and decreased protein levels in the cell wall. *PrA,* protein A.

studies have confirmed the in vivo expression of a clindamycin PAE. In experiments with *S. aureus,* the protein synthesis inhibitors clindamycin and erythromycin induced PAEs of 7.1 and 6.8 h, respectively; the cell wall–active β-lactam antibiotics induced PAEs of only 1.2 to 4.6 h (137).

MECHANISMS OF RESISTANCE

Resistance may be due to a chromosomal mutation that results in an altered drug receptor site on the 50S ribosomal protein. A plasmid- or transposon-mediated target modification by methylation of adenine on the 23S ribosomal RNA of the 50S ribosomal subunit may also confer resistance (102, 121). These strains are cross-resistant to all macrolide, lincosamide, and streptogramin B antibiotics (MLS$_B$ phenotype). Expression of MLS$_B$ resistance may be constitutive or inducible (103). Expression of inducible MLS$_B$ resistance differs in staphylococci, streptococci, and enterococci. In staphylococci, 14- and 15-membered macrolides, but not lincosamides or streptogramins, are inducers of the methylase. In streptococci and enterococci, macrolides, lincosamides, and streptogramin B are efficient inducers (36). Strains with inducible resistance can be shown to become resistant to clindamycin when erythromycin is present; in a double-disk induction test, clindamycin distorts the zone of inhibition in the vicinity of erythromycin because of induction of methylase by subinhibitory concentrations of erythromycin. Resistance is not due to reduced drug uptake (127). Rare isolates of staphylococci (121) and some veterinary isolates of streptococci (28) may enzymatically inactivate clindamycin by adenylation. Plasmid-mediated transferable resistance to clindamycin (and erythromycin) was found in *B. fragilis* in 1991 (54).

PHARMICOKINETIC DISPOSITION

Serum Half-Life

Clindamycin phosphate (900 mg intravenously) produces peak levels of 15 μg/mL and trough levels of about 2.0 μg/mL; clindamycin phosphate (600 mg intravenously) gives levels of about 11.0 and 2.0 μg/mL, respectively (55; Fig. 3). Serum half-life is about 3 h.

Absorption

The presence of food can delay absorption, but peak and trough levels are usually not reduced (Fig. 4). Both esters, clindamycin palmitate and clindamycin phosphate, are absorbed as the inactive ester and are readily hydrolyzed in blood to active clindamycin. Intramuscular clindamycin phosphate administration, which is relatively painless, results in slightly lower peak serum levels than equivalent doses administered intravenously. A 600-mg oral dose of clindamycin administered every 8 h is usually bioequivalent to a 450-mg dose given every 6 h, when both regimens are evaluated over a 3-day period.

In normal newborn infants, 5- to 7-mg/kg doses of clindamycin given intravenously and intramuscularly produce peak serum levels of 8 to 10 μg/mL. Premature infants in the first month postpartum display a longer half-life (8.68 h) following clindamycin administration than full-term infants (3.60 h) (see ref. 146 for details).

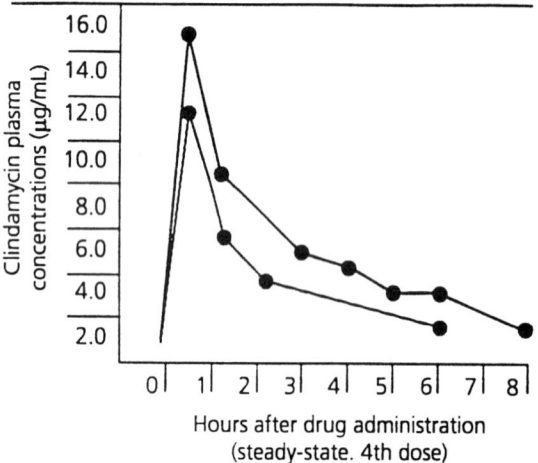

Plasma concentrations, after i.v. clindamycin phosphate injection

● 900 mg clindamycin phosphate (IV)
● 600 mg clindamycin phosphate (IV)

FIGURE 3. Average plasma concentrations of clindamycin obtained for six normal adult male volunteers following i.v. adminstration of 900 mg q. 8 h and 600 mg q. 6 h clindamycin phosphate sterile solution in a crossover study design. (From Zambrano D, ed. Clindamycin in the treatment of human infections. Kalamazoo, MI: The Upjohn Company, 1992. With permission.)

Tissue Penetration

Clindamycin is rapidly and markedly concentrated inside polymorphonuclear leukocytes, reaching an intracellular concentration about 40 times that in the extracellular environment. Patients with chronic granulomatous disease suffer from recurrent infections with catalase-producing organisms, particularly staphylococci. Phagocytosis occurs in chronic granulomatous disease, but the microorganisms survive inside the leukocytes. Clindamycin significantly reduced the number of viable intracellular staphylococci in normal and patient leukocytes tested in vitro. Controlled clinical trials are needed to translate these laboratory findings into applicable therapy (55).

Lincosamides penetrate into choledochal bile, cholecystic bile, and gallbladder and liver tissue. An intravenous dose of 1.5 g of lincomycin results in the following concentrations: serum, 34 μg/mL (at 2 h); choledochal bile, 215 μg/mL (at 3 h 15 min); cholecystic bile, 28 μg/mL (at 3 h 36 min); gallbladder tissue, 28 μg/g (at 2 h, 55 min); and liver tissue, 15.4 μg/g (at 4 h). These concentrations exceed the MICs at which 90% of strains of clinical anaerobic strains are inhibited (MIC$_{90}$) (55).

Distribution

Clindamycin reaches most tissues. In some instances (e.g., tonsils, sputum, bronchi, lungs, pleura, pleural fluid, liver, gallbladder, appendix, and decubitus ulcer), tissue concentrations may exceed serum levels. Higher tissue concentrations offer an advantage when treating skin, intraabdominal, and lower respiratory tract infections. Clindamycin concentrations in bone reach

Plasma concentrations, after i.m. clindamycin
phosphate injection (300 mg; 157)

Plasma concentrations, after oral clindamycin
hydrochloride (300 mg; 157)

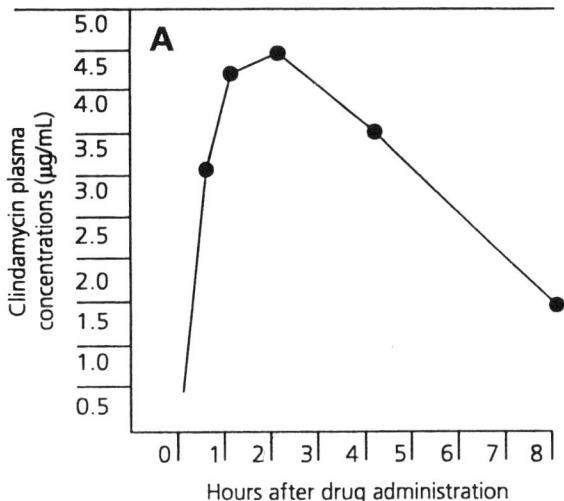
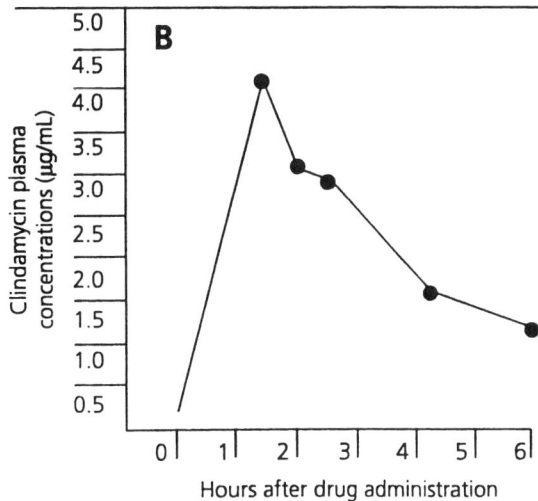

FIGURE 4. ***A.*** Average plasma concentrations of clindamycin obtained for 13 normal adult male volunteers following i.m. administration of 300 mg clindamycin phosphate sterile solution. ***B.*** Average plasma concentrations of clindamycin obtained for 22 normal adult male volunteers following oral administration of 300 mg clindamycin hydrochloride immediately after a meal. (From Zambrano D, ed. Clindamycin in the treatment of human infections. Kalamazoo, MI: The Upjohn Company, 1992. With permission.)

60 to 80% of those attained in serum, suggesting the usefulness of clindamycin treatment for some patients with osteomyelitis. Distribution of clindamycin into the cerebrospinal fluid is limited, even when the meninges are inflamed, and clindamycin concentrations in spinal cord blood reach only half the levels found in serum. As a result, clindamycin is of limited use in treating meningitis. The fact that clindamycin penetrates into abscess tissues, first discovered in an animal model, has been successfully applied to treatment of human abscesses. Clindamycin concentrations in breast milk are variable.

Elimination

Approximately 95% of administered clindamycin or its esters is either excreted unchanged or metabolized in the liver to a mixture of active and inactive metabolites that are excreted chiefly in the feces. Although the half-life of clindamycin is prolonged in patients with moderate-to-severe liver disease, dosage reduction is not considered necessary if the antibiotic is administered every 8 h. Because the half-life of clindamycin may be prolonged in patients with impaired renal function, some clinicians suggest adjusting dosage on the basis of serum drug levels and creatinine clearance time. Other clinicians, however, do not find such adjustment necessary. During hemodialysis or peritoneal dialysis, clindamycin is not lost in the dialysate, so dose adjustment is probably not necessary (see ref. 146 for further detail).

DOSAGE REGIMENS
Normal

Oral Administration

Clindamycin can be administered orally as the hydrated hydrochloride salt (Cleocin HCL) or the palmitate esteric ester (Cleocin Pediatric). Clindamycin hydrochloride is available as a capsule for adults and for children who are able to swallow capsules. The capsules are in the following strengths: 75, 150, and 300 mg. A peak serum level of about 3 µg/mL is achieved 1 to 2 h after oral administration of a dose of 300 mg in an adult, and the peak is doubled by doubling the dose (62). A dosage of 150 to 450 mg every 6 h is recommended for adults, depending on the severity of infection. Similarly, two dosage ranges are recommended for children: 8 to 16 mg/kg daily or 16 to 20 mg/kg daily, each in three or four divided equal doses, depending on the severity of infection. Food does not significantly impair adsorption (81). Higher serum levels are reported after oral administration of clindamycin to patients with Crohn's disease, celiac disease, and jejunal diverticulosis (62).

Clindamycin palmitate hydrochloride is a water-soluble hydrochloride salt of the ester of clindamycin and palmitic acid. The ester is available as granules to be suspended in water for children and adults who are unable to swallow capsules. Each 5 mL contains the equivalent of 75 mg of clindamycin base. The ester is hydrolyzed in vivo to the active base. Dosage of the ester is similar to that of salt, 8 to 25 mg/kg daily in three or four divided equal doses, and serum levels achieved are similar to those achieved with oral administration of clindamycin hydrochloride (22). In children weighing 10 kg or less, the minimal dose should be 37.5 mg every 8 h.

Parenteral Administration

The water-soluble ester, clindamycin-2-phosphate (Cleocin Phosphate) is used for parenteral administration, as the base is too irritating and poorly soluble at neutral pH. The intramuscular dose of clindamycin is 600 to 2700 mg daily in adults, given in two, three, or four divided equal doses. A dose of 300 mg produces a peak serum level of about 5 μg/mL at 2.5 h after intramuscular administration. Lower serum levels are attained in diabetic patients after intramuscular administration (37). A single intramuscular dose of 600 mg or more is not recommended.

Each milliliter contains the equivalent of 150 mg of clindamycin. For intravenous administration, clindamycin-2-phosphate is diluted, 1 part to 25 parts, and infused over 10 to 40 min, depending on the volume. The usual dose is 900 to 2700 mg daily in adults and as much as 4800 mg daily in life-threatening infections in adults, given in two, three, or four divided equal doses. Administration of more than 1200 mg in a single 1-h infusion is not recommended. A 300 mg-dose infused over 30 min produces a peak serum level of about 15 μg/mL in an adult (37).

Parenteral dosage (intramuscular or intravenous) in neonates (≤1 month) is 15 to 20 mg/kg daily in three or four divided equal doses, the lower dose being adequate in premature infants. In children over 1 month of age, the dosage is 20 to 40 mg/kg daily in three or four divided equal doses.

Intravaginal Administration

Clindamycin phosphate is used for intravaginal administration in a semisolid white cream (Cleocin Vaginal Cream 2%) that contains 2% of the drug at a concentration equivalent to 20 mg/g of clindamycin. Each applicatorful of 5 g of vaginal cream contains approximately 100 mg of clindamycin phosphate. The recommended dose is one applicatorful of vaginal cream intravaginally, preferably at bedtime, for 7 consecutive days.

Topical Administration

Clindamycin phosphate is used for topical administration in a solution, lotion, and gel (Cleocin T) at a concentration equivalent to 10 mg/mL of clindamycin. Topical preparations are applied as a thin film twice daily to the affected area of skin.

Renal Failure

Clindamycin is mainly excreted by nonrenal mechanisms. The dose of clindamycin is not necessarily reduced in patients with renal failure, but in severe renal failure accompanied by severe metabolic aberrations, monitoring of serum levels is recommended during high-dose therapy. Clindamycin is not significantly removed by hemodialysis (29) or peritoneal dialysis (78).

Hepatic Failure

The rate of elimination of clindamycin is prolonged in severe hepatic disease but is not consistently correlated with any specific liver functional abnormality (34, 62, 139). The dose of clindamycin is not necessarily reduced in patients with hepatic failure, but in severe hepatic failure accompanied by severe metabolic aberrations, monitoring of serum levels (if available) is recommended during high-dose therapy.

Obesity

The effect of obesity on dosing of clindamycin is unknown.

Ascites/Edema

The effect of ascites or edema on dosing of clindamycin is unknown.

Pregnancy

Safety of clindamycin for use in pregnancy has not been established. Clindamycin is placed in pregnancy category B, drugs for which adequate, well-controlled studies in pregnant patients have not been done but which have shown no evidence of teratogenicity or fetal toxicity in animal or human studies. Thus, clindamycin should be used during pregnancy only if clearly needed.

Nursing Mothers

Clindamycin is reported to appear in breast milk in concentrations of 0.7 to 3.8 μg/mL after doses of 150 mg orally to 600 mg intravenously.

ADVERSE EFFECTS
Diarrhea

Diarrhea occurs in up to 20% of patients receiving clindamycin. In most patients the cause of the diarrhea is unknown, but in up to 20% of patients with clindamycin-associated diarrhea, the stool culture is positive for toxigenic *C. difficile,* and the stool toxin assay is positive. This organism (8, 45) produces inflammation of the colon that spans the spectrum from slight mucosal erythema to pseudomembranous colitis (46, 50, 62, 129). In all patients with pseudomembranous colitis, the stool culture is positive for *C. difficile* and the stool toxin assay is positive. Diarrhea may be mild to severe and is frequently associated with abdominal cramps, fever, and passage of blood or mucus in the stool. The occurrence of pseudomembranous colitis is unrelated to size of the dose; it occurs after either oral, parenteral, or topical administration of clindamycin in 0.01 to 10% of clindamycin-treated patients. Pseudomembranous colitis can occur in association with other antibiotics, but less frequently than with clindamycin. The onset may occur during clindamycin therapy or up to several weeks after stopping. Neutrophilic leukocytosis is common.

Colitis following oral administration may be three to four times more frequent than following parenteral administration. Older patients with significant accompanying underlying illnesses, patients recuperating from abdominal surgery, and patients with a history of gastrointestinal diseases, particularly colitis, may be able to tolerate diarrhea less well than younger patients or those without underlying gastrointestinal disease.

Some patients respond spontaneously when clindamycin is stopped, but many patients require specific therapy. Nevertheless, despite specific antimicrobial therapy with oral or intravenous metronidazole or oral vancomycin, diarrhea may persist or relapse in some patients. The disease may be complicated by dehydration, hypoalbuminemia, hypotension, toxic megacolon, and colonic perforation and is potentially fatal.

Use clindamycin cautiously in patients with previous gastrointestinal disease, particularly colitis. If mild diarrhea occurs, stopping clindamycin may be all that is necessary. Cholestyramine and colestipol resins, which bind the toxin in vitro, may be given orally. In moderate-to-severe cases, fluids and electrolytes, protein supplementation, and treatment for 7 to 10 days with an antimicrobial agent that has specific activity against *C. difficile* (e.g., oral or intravenous metronidazole 500 mg every 4 h, or oral vancomycin, 500–2000 mg/day in three or four divided doses) should be given. If a resin and vancomycin are to be used concurrently, vancomycin should be given either 1 to 2 h before or 4 h after the resin. Although usually not advisable, clindamycin may be continued if absolutely necessary, with the addition of oral vancomycin or metronidazole and close observation of the patient. Relapses, which occur in up to 55% of patients (9), may be treated with repeated courses of the same antibiotic as before or an alternative agent (9). Antiperistaltic agents such as opiates, diphenoxylate with atropine (Lomotil), or loperamide (Imodium) may prolong or worsen the condition (93).

Neuromuscular Blockade

Rare instances have been reported of enhancement of the action of neuromuscular blocking agents by concomitantly administered clindamycin that results in possible profound and severe respiratory depression (6, 40, 109). Patients who receive these combinations should be closely monitored.

Allergy

Allergic reactions may result from hypersensitivity to clindamycin or lincomycin in susceptible individuals. Rash is a frequent adverse reaction to clindamycin, reported in up to 10% of treated patients in one study (43). Rarely, more-severe hypersensitivity reactions, such as Stevens-Johnson syndrome, anaphylaxis, polyarthritis, or blood cell abnormalities may occur (69). Clindamycin is contraindicated in individuals with a history of allergy to clindamycin and lincomycin.

Allergic reactions, including asthma, may occur to yellow dye no. 5 (tartrazine) in the 75- and 150-mg capsules in susceptible individuals. The frequency of tartrazine sensitivity in the general population is low, but it is frequent in patients with preexisting bronchial asthma and aspirin hypersensitivity.

Esophagitis

Esophageal irritation caused by a capsule swallowed without water lodging in the lower esophagus has been reported (126).

Cardiovascular Reaction

Rare instances of hypotension and cardiopulmonary arrest have been reported following too-rapid intravenous infusion of clindamycin. The intravenous dose should infuse over 10 to 40 min, depending on the size of the dose.

"Gasping Syndrome"

Clindamycin phosphate sterile solution contains benzyl alcohol as a preservative, which has been associated with potentially fatal "gasping syndrome" in premature infants, according to the package insert. However, since market introduction, no cases of gasping syndrome have been reported to Pharmacia & Upjohn through their worldwide product safety surveillance unit (personal communication).

Symptomatic Cervicitis/Vaginitis

Symptomatic cervicitis/vaginitis occurs in 16% of patients treated with intravaginal application of clindamycin phosphate 2% vaginal cream. It may be due to local irritation from the topical medication or to overgrowth and subsequent infection by antibiotic-resistant *Candida albicans,* which occurs in 11% of treated patients. Development of symptomatic cervicitis/vaginitis requires discontinuation of clindamycin phosphate use, and if clinically appropriate, antimicrobial treatment specific for *C. albicans* vaginitis.

Condom Breakage

Clindamycin phosphate 2% vaginal cream contains mineral oil, which may weaken latex or rubber products such as condoms or vaginal contraceptive diaphragms. Clindamycin phosphate 2% vaginal cream should be discontinued at least 72 h before use of latex condoms or diaphragms.

Skin Irritation

Skin dryness, erythema, burning, peeling, etc. or contact dermatitis may occur with topical application of clindamycin phosphate solution, gel, or lotion. Overgrowth and subsequent follicular infection with antibiotic-resistant organisms, such as Gram-negative bacilli, may be complicating factors. In addition, the topical solution contains an alcohol base that may be irritating to abraded skin, eyes, or mucous membranes of the mouth. In the event of accidental contact with sensitive surfaces, bathe the surface (e.g., abraded skin, affected eye, or oral mucosa) with copious amounts of cool water.

DRUG INTERACTIONS

Drug/Food

No significant interaction has been reported (81).

Drug/Drug

Antagonism has been demonstrated between clindamycin and erythromycin and other macrolide antimicrobial agents (e.g., azithromycin and clarithromycin) and between clindamycin and lincomycin in vitro by competition for the same bacterial binding site. The clinical significance of the in vitro interactions is unknown.

Concomitant administration of some skeletal muscle relaxants and clindamycin has been reported to result in enhanced neuromuscular blockade. Muscle relaxants include atracrium, baclofen, carisoprodol, cyclobenzaprine, dantrolene, diazepam, doxacurium, meprobamate, methocarbamol, metocurine, pancuronium, quazepam, tubocurarine, and vecuronium. Other drugs that may potentiate neuromuscular blockade include the antimicrobial agents, colistin and aminoglycosides (40). Patients who receive these combinations should be closely monitored and may require a reduction in dosage of the neuromuscular blocking agent. The need for respiratory support should be anticipated.

Concomitant use of anion-exchange resins (e.g., cholestyramine or colestipol) and some antibiotic agents may result in reduced or delayed antibiotic absorption. However, no interaction of colestipol with clindamycin has been found, and interaction of cholestyramine with clindamycin is not documented in the current package insert. In general, it is recommended that if concomitant administration is required, the antibiotic should be given at least 1 h before or 4 h after administration of the resin or kaolin/pectin.

Clindamycin phosphate in solution is incompatible with ampicillin, phenytoin, barbiturates, aminophylline, calcium gluconate, and magnesium sulfate.

Drug/Laboratory

Intramuscular clindamycin injections elevate CPK values in most patients, possibly because of muscle irritation from the intramuscular injection (61).

Clindamycin has been reported to cause transient leukopenia, thrombocytopenia, and eosinophilia (97); agranulocytosis may occur. Reversible mild elevations in transaminase alkaline phosphatase values occur in some patients (37, 69, 144), rarely associated with other evidence of hepatic injury such as jaundice (32, 69). Some of these abnormal laboratory results may be false-positive colorimetric reactions (89). Intramuscular clindamycin injections may elevate SGOT values, possibly because of muscle irritation from the intramuscular injection (37). During prolonged therapy with clindamycin, periodic liver and kidney function tests and blood counts should be monitored.

CLINICAL INDICATIONS

Because clindamycin does not diffuse adequately into cerebrospinal fluid, clindamycin should not be used in the treatment of meningitis. Clindamycin has been reported to be no more effective than placebo in treatment of *M. pneumoniae* pneumonia (118). Because of the risk of clindamycin-associated colitis, use of clindamycin is restricted to serious infection and patients in whom other, less-toxic, alternative antimicrobial therapy is inappropriate. Use clindamycin cautiously in patients with previous gastrointestinal disease, particularly colitis. If mild diarrhea occurs, stopping clindamycin may be all that is necessary.

Actinomycosis

Actinomyces spp., usually *A. israelii,* can produce a chronic necrotizing pulmonary infection that follows aspiration of oral flora into the lower respiratory tract and is characterized by fibrosis and fistulae that cross tissue planes from the lung to pleura, bone, and skin. This infection is frequently polymicrobial and involves, in addition to *Actinomyces* spp., other oral bacteria, including *Actinobacillus actinomycetemcomitans.* Actinomycosis can be treated effectively with clindamycin (37). However, although most members of the oral flora that cause necrotizing pneumonia are sensitive to clindamycin, *A. actinomycetemcomitans* is resistant to this antibiotic. *A. actinomycetemcomitans* is reported to be susceptible to cephalosporins, fluoroquinolones, tetracycline, and azithromycin. Failure of therapy for necrotizing anaerobic pneumonia with clindamycin was reported in one patient to be likely due to this clindamycin-resistant pathogen (84).

Regimens

The usual parenteral dose is 900 to 2700 mg daily in adults, given in two, three, or four divided equal doses for 4 to 6 weeks, and the oral dose is 150 to 450 mg every 6 h in adults, depending on the severity of the infection. The total duration of therapy is 6 to 12 months.

Acne

Clindamycin phosphate as a solution, lotion, or gel for topical administration has been found effective for the treatment of acne (74). *Propionibacterium acne,* the presumed pathogen is susceptible to clindamycin.

Regimens

Clindamycin phosphate in solution, lotion, and gel for topical administration is applied as a thin film twice daily to the affected area of skin until a clinical response results.

Bacterial Vaginosis

Patients with bacterial vaginosis usually complain of a vaginal discharge that has a "fishy" ammonia odor or emits such an odor when mixed with 10% KOH solution. The vaginal discharge has a few or no WBCs, a pH above 4.5, and many "clue cells" (i.e., epithelial cells coated on the surface with tiny bacilli that stain Gram negative). The presumed pathogens, such as *Gardnerella vaginalis* or *Mobiluncus* sp., are susceptible to clindamycin. Clindamycin phosphate vaginal cream 2% has been found effective for the treatment of bacterial vaginosis (3, 114).

Regimens

The dose is one applicatorful of clindamycin phosphate vaginal cream 2% intravaginally, preferably at bedtime, for 7 consecutive days.

Pneumococcal Disease

Clindamycin can be used for serious infections caused by clindamycin-susceptible strains of pneumococci ($\leq$0.5 μg/mL) that involve the respiratory tract, when penicillin is judged to be inappropriate (e.g., the patient has a penicillin allergy) (71).

S. pneumoniae, the most common cause of community-acquired pneumonia, accounts for 30 to 60% of community-acquired bacterial pneumonias. In the United States, this microorganism causes an estimated 500,000 cases of pneumonia annually. *S. pneumoniae* had been almost uniformly susceptible to penicillin; however, a few clones of penicillin-resistant pneumococci emerged under the selective pressure of antibiotic usage. These clones spread throughout the world as a result of human migration and have become established in new areas, again under selective pressure of antibiotic usage over the past several decades (65). Penicillin-resistant strains are more likely to be resistant to other antimicrobial agents, such as clindamycin, macrolides, chloramphenicol, tetracycline, and trimethoprim-sulfamethoxazole. Therefore, excessive use of a number of different antimicrobial agents may select for penicillin resistance.

In many parts of the world, the prevalence of penicillin-resistant *S. Pneumoniae* (MIC $\geq$0.1 μg/mL) has reached 40 to 50% of isolates, and up to half of these strains are highly resistant to penicillin (MIC $\geq$ 2.0 μg/mL). In the contiguous

United States, national surveillance studies revealed a low prevalence of intermediate penicillin-resistance (MIC 0.1–1.0 μg/mL) of 3 to 7% of isolates and very rare recovery of highly penicillin-resistant strains for the years 1979 to 1987. Since 1988–89, however, penicillin resistance has spread rapidly in the United States; in some communities at least 30% of isolates are resistant to penicillin. High-level resistance to penicillin increased more than 60-fold, from 0.02% in 1979 to 1987 to 1.3% in 1992, among isolates from invasive infections (17). Levels of resistance have varied geographically. Resistance has spread rapidly in crowded environments, such as children in day-care centers (23). Vancomycin and rifampin are reliably active against these multidrug-resistant strains (64, 75).

In both South Africa and Spain, clindamycin resistance has been found to parallel erythromycin resistance. However, strains isolated more recently in the United States are commonly reported to be susceptible to clindamycin (41, 90).

Optimal treatment regimens for drug-resistant *S. pneumoniae* infections remain to be defined. Studies have suggested that the cephalosporins, ceftriaxone or cefotaxime, and high-dose penicillin may be effective in patients with nonmeningeal bacteremic infections if the MIC of penicillin is 2.0 μg/mL or less (42, 94, 128). Effectiveness of high-dose intravenous penicillin for pneumonia due to highly resistant strains is unknown, but MICs of cefotaxime and ceftriaxone are usually lower than those of penicillin or ampicillin and most other β-lactam antibiotics for penicillin-resistant strains. Ceftriaxone or cefotaxime may thus be effective when the MIC of penicillin is 1 μg/mL or above and those of ceftriaxone and cefotaxime are 2 μg/mL or less. However, highly cephalosporin-resistant strains have become a problem in certain geographic areas. Since all penicillin-resistant strains are sensitive to vancomycin, initial empirical therapy should include this antibiotic (1 g intravenously every 12 h) for patients with pneumococcal pneumonia who live in regions where highly penicillin- or cephalosporin-resistant strains have become common and who are severely ill or have significant comorbidity. If susceptibility to clindamycin among these strains in the United States is confirmed by reliable assays and the prevalence of clindamycin susceptibility remains high, clindamycin is an option for treatment of pneumonia due to these strains. Clindamycin susceptibility among drug-resistant *S. pneumoniae* needs to be monitored closely at the community level because of the rapid emergence of resistance in other parts of the world.

Regimens

The usual parenteral dose is 900 to 2700 mg daily in adults, given in two, three, or four divided equal doses for 1 to 2 weeks. Oral dosage of 150 to 450 mg every 6 h is recommended for adults, depending on the severity of infection, for 1 to 2 weeks.

Malaria

Clindamycin alone has been found effective for the treatment of falciparum malaria (33).

Regimens

Clindamycin 5 mg/kg twice daily for 5 days is given.

Babesiosis

Clindamycin in combination with quinine has been found effective for the treatment of patients with severe babesiosis (141).

Regimens

Clindamycin is given in a dosage of 20 mg/kg daily in children or 300 to 600 mg parenterally every 6 h in adults plus quinine 25 mg/kg daily in children or 650 mg orally every 6 or 8 h in adults for 7 to 10 days. Quinine is contraindicated in pregnancy.

Toxoplasmosis

Clindamycin in combination with pyrimethamine has been found effective for the treatment of toxoplasmosis of the central nervous system (26, 76, 104). If serum toxoplasma antibody assay is negative or if single lesions are seen on computed tomography (CT) or magnetic resonance imaging (MRI) scans, a biopsy of the brain lesions should be performed to confirm the diagnosis in patients with AIDS. If multiple enhancing ring lesions are seen on CT or MRI scans, cerebral toxoplasmosis may be treated empirically. If no response is seen in symptoms or scans in 14 days, then biopsy of the brain lesion is required to confirm the diagnosis. Folinic acid is used to reduce the bone marrow depressive effects of pyrimethamine without interfering with its antitoxoplasma effects. Maintenance therapy is required, because the relapse rate in untreated patients exceeds 30%. Pyrimethamine is a category C drug (animal studies show toxicity, human studies inadequate, but benefit outweighs risk), but limited studies have shown no teratogenicity in the first trimester of pregnancy.

Regimens

Pyrimethamine 200 g loading dose on day 1, then 50 to 75 mg once daily plus folinic acid 10 mg orally plus clindamycin 600 to 1200 mg orally or intravenously every 6 h for 3 to 6 weeks is given. Suppressive therapy must be continued for life in patients with AIDS to prevent relapse: pyrimethamine 50 to 75 mg/day orally plus folinic acid 10 mg/day orally plus clindamycin 300 mg every 6 h orally.

Pneumocystis carinii Pneumonia

Community-acquired pneumonia in a population with known or suspected HIV infection is likely due to *P. carinii,* especially if chest radiographs reveal diffuse interstitial infiltrates. The combination of clindamycin and primaquine has shown excellent activity against *P. carinii* in vitro and in an experimental rat model (100) and has proven effective for patients with mild-to-severe disease due to this organism in uncontrolled trials (13, 92, 110, 131). One randomized, double-blind trial that compared intravenous clindamycin plus oral primaquine with intravenous or oral trimethoprim/sulfamethoxazole in 49 patients with a first episode of *P. carinii* pneumonia (PCP) and arterial pO$_2$ of 50 mm Hg or above found no difference in clinical response rate (about 90% response rate) or in rate of dose-limiting toxicity between the respective treatment groups (132). Similarly, a recent large multicenter, prospective double-blind, randomized trial of oral trimethoprim/sulfamethoxazole, dapsone/trimethoprim, and clindamycin/primaquine in mild-to-moderate PCP ($pAO_2 - paO_2 \leq 45$ mm Hg at entry) in 181 patients with HIV infection found no statistically significant difference in clinical response, survival, or dose-limiting toxicity among the three treatment groups (111). Toxicity associated with clindamycin/primaquine therapy has included usually mild rash, neutropenia, methemoglobinemia, fever, serum transaminase elevations, diarrhea, and hemolysis. Because hemolytic anemia may occur with primaquine in patients with glucose-6-phosphate dehydrogenase (G6PD) deficiency, determination of G6PD is recommended before starting primaquine. Primaquine is contraindicated in pregnancy.

Regimens

For alternate therapy for patients with severe sulfa hypersensitivity, the dose of clindamycin is 450 to 900 mg orally or intravenously every 6 to 8 h plus primaquine base 15 to 30 mg once daily orally in adults for 3 weeks. Prednisone or prednisolone 40 mg orally or intravenously twice daily for 5 days, then 40 mg orally once daily for 5 days, then 20 mg once daily for 11 days is indicated at the initiation of antipneumocystis therapy if the initial paO_2 is 70 mm Hg or below.

Surgical Prophylaxis

Because of its antimicrobial activity against microflora of the sinuses and oronasopharynx, clindamycin can be used for chemoprophylaxis of clean-contaminated neurosurgery that crosses the sinuses or oronasopharynx or prophylaxis for head and neck surgery that enters the oral cavity.

Regimen

Clindamycin 900 mg intravenously is given in a single dose.

Prophylaxis for Bacterial Endocarditis

Because of its antimicrobial activity against periodontal and upper respiratory tract microflora, clindamycin can be used for chemoprophylaxis of endocarditis in penicillin-allergic patients with significant cardiac lesions (prosthetic cardiac valves, previous endocarditis, most congenital cardiac defects, and rheumatic and other acquired valvular dysfunction, including mitral valve prolapse with valvular insufficiency) who are to undergo certain dental procedures that cause gingival or mucosal bleeding, tonsillectomy and adenoidectomy, bronchoscopy with a rigid bronchoscope, sclerotherapy for esophageal varices, or surgical procedures involving the respiratory mucosa.

Regimens

Clindamycin 600 mg in adults and 20 mg/kg in children (single dose) is given orally (1 h) or intravenously (30 min) before the procedure (25).

Anaerobic Bacterial Infections

Clindamycin can be used to treat infection caused by susceptible anaerobic bacteria (MIC ≤ 4 μg/mL), in particular anaer-

obic Gram-negative bacilli (e.g., *B. fragilis, P. melaninogenica,* and *Fusobacterium nucleatum*), *Peptostreptococcus* sp., *Capnocytophagia ochracea, Clostridium perfringens,* involving the respiratory tract, skin and soft tissue, bone and joint, bloodstream, intraabdominal cavity (including peritonitis and intraperitoneal abscesses), female pelvis, and genital tract. Indeed, most anaerobic pathogens are sensitive to clindamycin. However, these infections are frequently polymicrobial and involve clindamycin-resistant *Enterobacteriaceae* or enterococci, which require additional specific antimicrobial therapy such as a β-lactam or aminoglycoside antibiotic.

Clindamycin offers an advantage over β-lactamase-sensitive β-lactams, because of the frequency of anaerobic pathogens (e.g., 100% of *B. fragilis* and up to 50% of *P. melaninogenica*) that produce β-lactamase (27, 53, 70, 85, 130). Metronidazole, β-lactamase-resistant β-lactam antibiotics (e.g., cefotixin, imipenem, or meropenem), or combinations of β-lactam antibiotics with β-lactamase inhibitors (e.g., ampicilin/sulbactam, amoxicillin/clavulanic acid, piperacillin/tazobactam, or ticarcillin/clavulanic acid) can be used with similar efficacy in place of clindamycin for antianaerobe activity; indeed all the β-lactam antimicrobial agents can be used alone for polymicrobial anaerobic infection because of the additional activity against an aerobic bacterial component (116, 119). Metronidazole must be combined with another antimicrobial agent with activity against aerobes.

Regimens

The usual parenteral dose of clindamycin is 900 to 2700 mg/day in adults, given in two, three, or four divided equal doses for 2 to 4 weeks in combination with an antimicrobial agent active against concomitant aerobic pathogens, such as a third-generation cephalosporin (e.g., ceftriaxone), aminoglycoside, or aztreonam. The oral dose of clindamycin recommended for adults is 150 to 450 mg every 6 h, depending on the severity of infection, for 2 to 4 weeks.

Aerobic Bacterial Infections

Clindamycin can be used to treat infections caused by susceptible aerobic bacteria (MIC ≤ 0.5 μg of clindamycin/mL), such as streptococci (16, 43) and staphylococci that involve, for example, the respiratory tract, bloodstream, skin and soft tissue, and bone.

Streptococcal Infections

Several studies have suggested that β-lactamase-producing *Bacteroides* sp. or *S. aureus* coexisting with group A streptococci may antagonize the activity of β-lactamase-susceptible β-lactam antibiotics such as penicillin in the treatment of group A streptococci pharyngitis and result in persistent or relapsing streptococcal infection, whereas clindamycin has been effective in these circumstances (18, 59). Certain strains of group A streptococci are particularly invasive and may produce toxic shock syndrome because of their M protein, streptococcal pyrogenic exotoxins, and perhaps other virulence factors. High-dose penicillin therapy is the treatment of choice, but penicillin is relatively ineffective in eradicating dense populations of these organisms in tissues, presumably because expression of penicillin-binding proteins in organisms in the stationary phase (the predominant state in maximally dense microbial tissue populations) is lower than that of log-phase organisms. Indeed in the mouse model of streptococcal myositis, survival was better with clindamycin than with penicillin. In addition, clindamycin, an inhibitor of microbial protein synthesis may decrease production of M protein and streptococcal pyrogenic exotoxin. For these reasons, although the clinical benefit of the addition of clindamycin to penicillin therapy is unknown, it is advisable in patients with life-threatening streptococcal disease (123, 124).

Staphylococcal Infections

Most methicillin-sensitive staphylococci are sensitive to clindamycin, but methicillin-resistant staphylococci are variably clindamycin resistant. Clindamycin has been effective in therapy for *S. aureus* infection caused by susceptible strains, especially osteomyelitis and septic arthritis (38, 44, 107).

Regimens

Clindamycin 150 to 300 mg orally every 6 h, or 600 to 2700 mg intravenously daily in two, three, or four divided equal doses is given in adults. Treatment of streptococcal infection should be continued for at least 10 days to prevent subsequent development of acute rheumatic fever.

Diphtheria

Clindamycin orally was found to be as effective as a single injection of benzathine penicillin in eradication of *C. diphtheriae* from the nasopharynx of asymptomatic carriers (80).

Regimen

A 7-day course of clindamycin, 150 mg four times daily, is given.

REFERENCES

1. Ahonkhai VI, Cherubin CE, Shulman MA, Jhagroo M, Bancroft U. In vitro activity of U-57930E, a new clindamycin analog, against aerobic gram-positive bacteria. Antimicrob Agents Chemother 1982;21:902–905.
2. Aldridge KE, Gelfand M, Reller LB, Ayers LW, Pierson CL, Schoenknecht F, Tilton RC, Wilkins J, Henderberg A, Schiro DD. A five-year multicenter study of the susceptibility of the Bacteroides fragilis isolates to cephalosporins, cephamins, penicillins, clindamycin, and metronidazole in the United States. Diagn Microbiol Infect Dis 1994;18:235–241.
3. Andres FJ, Parker R, Hosein I, Benrubi GI. Clindamycin vaginal cream versus oral metronidazole in the treatment of bacterial vaginosis: a prospective double-blind clinical trial. South Med J 1992;85:1077–1080.
4. Appelbaum PC, Spangler SK, Crotty E, Jacobs MR. Susceptibility of penicillin-sensitive and resistant strains of *Streptococcus pneumoniae* to new antimicrobial agents, including daptomycin, teicoplanin, cefpodoxime and quinolones. J Antimicrob Chemother 1989;23:509–516.
5. Arditi M, Yogev R. In vitro interaction between rifampin and clindamycin against pathogenic coagulase-negative staphylococci. Antimicrob Agents Chemother 1989;33:245–247.
6. Avery D, Finn R. Succinylcholine-prolonged apnea associated with clindamycin and abnormal liver liver function tests. Dis Nerv Syst 1977;38:473–475.
7. Barry AL, Jones RN, Thornsberry C. In vitro activities of azithromycin (CP 62,993), clarithromycin (A-56268; TE-031), erythromycin, roxithromycin, and clindamycin. Antimicrob Agents Chemother 1988;32:753–754.
8. Bartlett JG, Chang TW, Onderdonk AB. Will the real Clostridium species responsible for antibiotic associated colitis please step forward. Lancet 1978;i:338.
9. Bartlett JG. Treatment of *Clostridium difficile* colitis. Gastroenterology 1985;89:1192–1195.
10. Baxter R, Chapman J, Drew WL. Comparison of bactericidal activity of five antibiotics against *Staphylococcus aureus*. J Infect Dis 1990;161:1023–1025.
11. Betriu C, Sanchez A, Gomez M, Cruceyra A, Picazo JJ. Antibiotic susceptibility of group A streptococci: a 6-year follow-up study. Antimicrob Agents Chemother 1993;37:1717–1719.
12. Birkenmeyer RD, Kagan F. Lincomycin. XI. Synthesis and structure of clindamycin, a potent antibacterial agent. J Med Chem 1970;13:616–619.
13. Black JR, Feinberg J, Murphy RL, Fass RJ, Finkelstein D, Akil B, Safrin S, Carey JT, Stansell J, Plouffe JF. Clindamycin and primaquine therapy for mild to moderate episodes of *Pneumocystis carinii* pneumonia in patients with AIDS. AIDS Clinical Trials Group 044. Clin Infect Dis 1994;18:905–913.
14. Bohnen JM, Solomkin JS, Dellinger EP, Bjornson HS, Page CP. Guidelines for clinical care: anti-infective agents for intra-abdominal infection. A Surgical Infection Society policy statement. Arch Surg 1992;127:83–89.
15. Bourgault AM, Lamothe F, Hoban DJ, Dalton MT, Kibsey PC, Harding G, Smith JA, Low DE, Gilbert H. Survey of Bacteroides fragilis group susceptibility patterns in Canada. Antimicrob Agents Chemother 1992;36:343–347.
16. Breese BB, Disney FA, Talpey W, Green JL, Tobin J. Streptococcal infections in children. Comparison of the therapeutic effectiveness of erythromycin administered twice daily with erythromycin, penicillin phenoxymethyl, and clindamycin, administered three times daily. Am J Dis Child 1974;128: 457–460.
17. Breiman RF, Butler JC, Tenover FC, Elliott JA, Facklam RR. Emergence of drug-resistant pneumococcal infections in the United States. JAMA 1994;271:1831–1835.
18. Brook L, Hirokawa R. Treatment of patients with a history of recurrent tonsillitis due to group A beta-hemolytic streptococci. A prospective randomized study comparing penicillin, erythromycin and clindamycin. Clin Pediatr 1985;24:331–336.
19. Brook I, Gillmore JD. Increased resistance of encapsulated *Bacteroides fragilis* to clindamycin. Chemotherapy 1994;40:16–20.
20. Brorson J-E, Larsson P, Zackrisson G. Antibiotic susceptibility of bacteria commonly isolated from the upper respiratory tract. Infection 1983;11:59–60.
21. Bundtzen RW, Gerber AU, Cohn DL, Craig WA. Postantibiotic suppression of bacterial growth. Rev Infect Dis 1981;3:28–37.
22. Campbell IW, Hossack DJN, Monro JF. Absorption and urinary excretion of clindamycin palmitate in the elderly. Curr Med Res Opin 1973;1:369–375.
23. CDC Drug-resistant *Streptococcus pneumoniae*—Kentucky and Tennesee, 1993. MMWR 1994;43:23–25.
24. Costerton JW, Lappin-Scott HM. Behavior of bacteria. ASM News 1989;55:649–651.
25. Dajani AS, Taubert KA, Wilson W, Bolger AF, Bayer A, Ferri-

eri P, Gewitz MH, Shulman ST, Nouri S, Newburger JW, Hutto C, Pallasch TJ, Gage TW, Levison ME, Peter G, Zuccaro G Jr. Prevention of bacterial endocarditis. Recommendations by the American Heart Association. Circulation 1997;96:358–366.

26. Dannemann B, McCutchan JA, Israelski D, Antoniskis D, Leport C, Luft B, Nussbaum J, Clumeck N, Morlat P, Chiu J. Treatment of toxoplasmic encephalitis in patients with AIDS. A randomized trial comparing pyrimethamine plus clindamycin to pyrimethamine plus sulfadiazine. The California Collaborative Treatment Group. Ann Intern Med 1992;116:33–43.

27. DiZerega G, Yonekura L, Roy S, Nakamura RM, Ledger WJ. Comparison of clindamycin-gentamicin and penicillin-gentamicinin the treatment of post-cesarian section endomyometritis. Am J Obstet Gynecol 1979;134:238–242.

28. Dutta GN, Devriese LA. Resistance to macrolide, lincosamide and streptogramin antibiotics and degradation of lincosamide antibiotics in streptococci from bovine mastitis. J Antimicrob Chemother 1982;10:403–408.

29. Eastwood JB, Gower PE. A study of the pharmacokinetics of clindamycin in normal subjects and patients with chronic renal failure. Postgrad Med J 1974;50:710–712.

30. Eliopoulos GM, Gardella A, Moellering C. in vitro activity of Sch 29482 in comparison with other oral antibiotics. J Antimicrob Chemother 1982;19(Suppl C):143–152.

31. Eliopoulos GM, Reiszner E, Ferraro MJ, Moellering RC Jr. Comparative in vitro activity of A-56268 (TE-031), a new macrolide antibiotic. J Antimicrob Chemother 1987;20: 671–675.

32. Elmore M, Rissing JP, Rink L, Brooks GF. Clindamycin-associated hepatotoxicity. Am J Med 1974;57:627–630.

33. El Wakeel ES, Homeida MM, Ali HM, Geary TG, Tensen JB. Clindamycin for the treatment of falciparum malaria in Sudan. Am J Trop Med Hyg 1985;34:1065–1068.

34. Eng RHK, Gorski S, Person A, Mangura C, Chmel H. Clindamycin elimination in patients with liver disease. J Antimicrob Chemother 1981;8:277–281.

35. Falagas ME, Gorbach SL. Clindamycin and metronidazol. Med Clin North Am 1995;79:845–867.

36. Fantin B, Leclercq R, Merlé Y, St Julien L, Veyrat C, Duval J, Carbon C. Critical influence of resistance to streptogramin B-type antibiotics on activity of RP 59500 (quinupristin-dalfopristin) in experimental endocarditis due to *Staphylococcus aureus*. Antimicrob Agents Chemother 1995;39:400–405.

37. Fass RJ, Saslaw S. Clindamycin: clinical and laboratory evaluation of parenteral therapy. Am J Med Sci 1972;263:368–382.

38. Fass RJ, Helsel VL, Barnishan J, Ayers LW. In vitro susceptibilities of four species of coagulase-negative staphylococci. Antimicrob Agents Chemother 1986;30:545–552

39. Fernandes CJ, Wilson RD, Ackerman VP. In vitro activity of A-56619 and A-56620 against multi-resistant and routine clinical isolates. Chemotherapy 1988;34:216–228.

40. Fogdall RP, Miller RD. Prolongation of pancuronium-induced neuromuscular blockade by clindamycin. Anesthesiology 1974;41:407–408.

41. Friedland IR, Shelton S, Paris M, Rinderknecht S, Ehrett S, Krisher K, McCracken GH Jr. Dilemmas in diagnosis and management of cephalosporin-resistant *Streptococcus pneumoniae* meningitis. Pediatr Infect Dis J 1993;12:196–200.

42. Garcia-Leoni ME, Cercenado E, Rodeno P, Bernaldo de Quiros JC, Martinez-Hernandez D, Bouza E. Susceptibility of *Streptococcus pneumoniae* to penicillin: a prospective microbiological and clinical study. Clin Infect Dis 1992;14:427–435.

43. Geddes AM, Bridgwater FAJ, Williams DN, Oon J, Grimshaw GJ. Clinical and bacteriological studies with clindamycin. Br Med J 1970:2:703–704.

44. Geddes AM, Dwyer NSJ, Ball AP, Amos RS. Clindamycin in bone and joint infections. J Antimicrob Chemother 1977;3: 501–507.

45. George RH, Symonds JM, Dimock F, Brown JD, Arabi Y, Shinigawa N, Keighley MR, Alexander-Williams J, Burdon DW. Identification of *Clostridium difficile* as a cause of pseudomembranous colitis. Br Med J 1978;1:695.

46. Gibson GF, Rowland R, Hecker R. Diarrhoea and colitis associated with antibiotic treatment. Aust NZ J Med 1975;5:340–347.

47. Glauser MP, Francioli P. Successful prophylaxis against experimental streptococcal endocarditis with bacteriostatic antibiotics. J Infect Dis 1982;146:806–810.

48. Goldstein EJC, Gombert ME, Agyare EO. Effect of atmosphere of incubation and inoculum size on the susceptibility of *Eikenella corrodens*. J Antimicrob Chemother 1982;10:37–42.

49. Goodwin CS, Blake P, Blincow E. The minimum inhibitory and bactericidal concentrations of antibiotics and anti-ulcer agents against *Campylobacter pylori*. J Antimicrob Chemother 1986; 17:309–314.

50. Gorbach SI, Bartlett JG. Pseudomembranous enterocolitis: a review of its diverse forms. J Infect Dis 1977;135(Suppl): S89–S94.

51. Gorbach SI. Current experience with clindamycin in the treatment of abdominal and female pelvic infections. Scand J Infect Dis 1984;43:82–88.

52. Gorbach SL. Antibiotic treatment of anaerobic infections. Clin Infect Dis 1994;18 (Suppl 4):S305–S310.

53. Gudiol F, Manresa F, Pallares R, Dirca J, Rufi G, Boada J, Ariza X, Casanova A, Viladrich PF. Clindamycin vs penicillin for anaerobic lung infections. High rate of penicillin failures associated with penicillin-resistant *Bacteroides melaninogenicus*. Arch Intern Med 1990;130:2525–2529.

54. Hecht DW, Jagielo TJ, Malamy MH. Conjugal transfer of antibiotic resistance factors in *Bacteroides fragilis:* the btgA and btgB genes of plasmid pBFTM10 are required for its transfer from *Bacteroides fragilis* and for its fragilis mobilization by IncP beta plasmid R751 in *Escherichia coli*. J Bacteriol 1991; 173:7471–7480.

55. Hermans PE. Lincosamides. In: Peterson PK, Verhoef J, eds. The antimicrobial agents annual/1. Amsterdam: Elsevier, 1986: 103–114 .

56. Hermans PE. Lincosamides. In: Peterson PK, Verhoef J, eds. The antimicrobial agents annual/2. Amsterdam: Elsevier, 1987: 108–115.

57. Hermans PE. Lincosamides. In: Peterson PK, Verhoef J, eds. The antimicrobial agents annual/3. Amsterdam: Elsevier, 1988: 113–121.

58. Ho JL, Klempner MS. In vitro evaluation of clindamycin, in combination with oxacillin, rifampin, or vancomycin against *Staphylococcus aureus*. Diagn Microbiol lnfect Dis 1986;4: 133–138.

59. Jensen JH, Larsen SB. Treatment of recurrent acute tonsillitis with clindamycin. An alternative to tonsillectomy? Clin Otolaryngol 1991;16:498–500.

60. Johnson DM, Erwin ME, Barrett MS, Gooding B, Jones RN. Antimicrobial activity of ten macrolide, lincosamine, and streptogramin drugs tested against *Legionella* species. Eur J Microbiol Infect Dis 1992;11:751–755.

61. Kauffman RE, Shoeman DW, Suk-Han-Wan, Azarnoff DL. Absorption and excretion of clindamycin-2-phosphate in children after intramuscular injection. Clin Pharmacol Ther 1972;13:704–709

62. Keusch GT, Present DH. Summary of a workshop on clindamycin colitis. J Infect Dis 1976;133:578–587.

63. Klastersky J, Husson M. Bactericidal activity of the combinations of gentamicin with clindamycin or chloramphenicol against species of *Escherichia coli* and *Bacteroides fragilis*. Antimicrob Agents Chemother 1977;12:135–138.

64. Klugman KP, Koornhof HJ. Drug resistance patterns and serogroups or serotypes of pneumococcal isolates from cerebrospinal fluid or blood, 1979–1986. J Infect Dis 1988;158: 956–964.

65. Klugman KP. Pneumococcal resistance to antibiotics. Clin Microbiol Rev:1990;3:171–196.

66. Knudsen TD, Simko EJ. *Eikenella corodens:* an unexpected pathogen causing a persistent peritonsillar abscess. Ear Nose Throat J 1995;74:114–117.

67. Kuenzi B, Segessenmann Ch, Gerber AU. Postantibiotic effect of roxithromycin, erythromycin, and clindamycin against selected gram-positive bacteria and *Haemophilus influenzae*. J Antimicrob Chemother 1987;20(Suppl B):39–46.

68. LeFrock JL, Molavi A, Prince RA. Clindamycin. Antimicrob Ther 1984;235–247.

69. Levison ME, Bran JL, Ries K. Treatment of anaerobic bacterial infections with clindamycin 2 phosphate. Antimicrob Agents Chemother 1974;5:276–280.

70. Levison ME, Mangura CT, Lorber B, Abrutyn E, Pesanti EL, Levy RS, MacGregor RR, Schwartz AR. Clindamycin compared with penicillin for the treatment of anaerobic lung abscess. Ann Intern Med 1983;98:466–471.

71. Levison ME. Clindamycin in the treatment of lower respiratory tract infections. In: Zamboro D, ed. Clindamycin in the treatment of human infections. Kalamazoo, MI: The Upjohn Company, 1992.

72. Lewis C, Clapp HW, Grady JE. In vitro and in vivo evaluation of lincomycin, a new antibiotic. Antimicrob Agents Chemother 1962;570–582.

73. Lewis C. Clinically useful antibiotics obtained by directed chemical modification—lincomycins. Fed Proc 1974;33:2303–2306.

74. Leyden JJ, Shalita AR, Saatjian GD, Sefton J. Erythromycin 2% gel in comparison with clindamycin phosphate 1% solution in acne vulgaris. J Am Acad Dermatol 1987;16:822–827.

75. Linares J, Pallares R, Alonso T, Perez JL, Ayats J, Gudiol F, Viladrich PF, Martin R. Trends in antimicrobial resistance in clinical isolates of *Streptococcus pneumoniae* in Bellvitge Hospital, Barcelona, Spain (1970–1990). Clin Infect Dis 1992;15:99–105.

76. Luft BJ, Hafner R, Korzun AH, et al. Toxoplasmic encephalitis in patients with the acquired immunodeficiency syndrome. N Engl J Med 1993;329:574–580.

77. Magerlein BJ, Birkenmeyer RD, Kagan F. Chemical modification of lincomycin. Antimicrob Agents Chemother 1966;6:727–736.

78. Malacoff RF, Finkelstein FO, Andriole VT. Effect of peritoneal dialysis on serum levels of tobramycin and lincomycin. Antimicrob Agents Chemother 1975;8:574–580.

79. Mason DJ, Dietz A, DeBoer C. Lincomycin, a new antibiotic. Antimicrob Agents Chemother 1963;554–559.

80. McCloskey RV, Green MJ, Eller J, Smilack J. Treatment of diphtheria carriers: benzathine penicillin, erythromycin and clindamycin. Ann Intern Med 1974;81:788–791.

81. McGehee RF Jr, Smith CB, Wilcox C, Finland M. Comparative studies of antibacterial activity in vitro and absorption and excretion of lincomycin and clindamycin. Am J Med Sci 1968;256:279–292.

82. Milatovic D, Braveny IN, Verhoef J. Clindamycin enhances opsonization of *Staphylococcus aureus*. Antimicrob Agents Chemother 1983;24:413–417.

83. Modde H. Die bakteriostatische und bakterizide Wirkung des 7-chlor-7-desoxy-lincomycins gen Staphylokokken, Streptokokken und Pneumokokken. Schweiz Med Wochenschr 1971;101:1629–1631.

84. Morris JM, Sewell DL. Necrotizing pneumonia caused by mixed infection with *Actinobacillus actinomycetemcomitans* and *Actinomyces israelii:* case report and review. Clin Infect Dis 1994;18:451–452.

85. Murray PR, Rosenblatt JE. Penicillin resistance and penicillinase production in clinical isolates of *Bacteroides melaninogenicus*. Antimicrob Agents Chemother 1977;11:605–608.

86. Nastro LJ, Finegold SM. Bactericidal activity of five antimicrobial agents against *Bacteroides fragilis*. J lnfect Dis 1972;126: 104–107.

87. National Committee for Clinical Laboratory Standards (NCCLS). Methods for dilution antimicrobial susceptibility tests for bacteria that grow aerobically. 2nd ed. Villanova, PA: NCCLS, 1990.

88. National Committee for Clinical Laboratory Standards (NCCLS). Methods for antimicrobial susceptibility testing of anaerobic bacteria. 2nd ed. Villanova, PA: NCCLS, 1990.

89. National Committee for Clinical Laboratory Standards (NCCLS). Performance standards for antimicrobial disk susceptibility. 4th ed. Villanova, PA: NCCLS, 1990.

90. Nelson CT, Mason EO, Kaplan SL. Activity of oral antibiotics in middle ear and sinus infections caused by penicillin-resistant *Streptococcus pneumoniae:* implications for treatment. Pediatr Infect Dis J 1994;13:585–589.

91. Nishihata T, Kunieda S, Nakahama C, Soejima R. Inhibitory effect of clindamycin on production of beta-lactamase in beta-lactam-resistant bacteria. Biol Pharm Bull 1994;17:715–720.

92. Noskin GA, Murphy RL, Black JR, Phair JP. Salvage therapy with clindamycin/primaquine for *Pneumocystis carinii* pneumonia. Clin Infect Dis 1992;14:183–188.

93. Novak E, Lee JG, Seekman CE, Phillips JP, DiSanto AR. Unfavourable effect of atropine-diphenoxylate (Lomotil) therapy on lincomycin-caused diarrhea. JAMA 1976;235:1451–1454.

94. Pallares R, Gudiol F, Linares J, Arisa J, Rufi G, Murgui L, Dorca J, Viladrich PF. Risk factors and response to antibiotic therapy in adults with bacteremic pneumonia caused by penicillin-resistant pneumococci. N Engl J Med 1987;317: 18–22.

95. Pearlman MD, Faro S, Riddle GD, Tortolero G. In vitro synergy of clindamycin and aminoglycosides against Chlamydia trachomatis. Antimicrob Agents Chemother 1990;34:1339–1401.

96. Pelvic lnflammatory Disease. In: 1989 Sexually transmitted diseases treatment guidelines. MMWR 1989;38:31–34.

97. Phillips I. Clinical uses and control of rifampin and clindamycin. J Clin Pathol 1971;24:410–418.

98. Poulin SA, Perkins RE, Kundsin RB. Antibiotic susceptibilities of AIDS-associated mycoplasmas. J Clin Microbiol 1994;34: 1101–1103.

99. Qadri SM, Halim M, Ueno Y, Saldin H. Susceptibility of methicillin-resistant Staphylococcus aureus to minocycline and other antimicrobials. Chemotherapy 1994;40:26–29.

100. Queener SF, Bartlett MS, Richardson JD, Durkin MM, Jay MA, Smith JW. Activity of clindanycin with primaquine against *Pneumocystis carinii* in vitro and in vivo. Antimicrob Agents Chemother 1988;32:807–813.

101. Ralph ED, Kirby WMM. Unique bactericidal action of metronidazole against *Bacteroides fragilis* and *Clostridium perfringens*. Antimicrob Agents Chemother 1975;8:409–414.

102. Rasmussen BA, Bush K, Tally FP. Antimicrobial resistance in *Bacteroides*. Clin Infect Dis 1993;16(Suppl 4):S390–S400.

103. Reig M, Fernandez MC, Ballesta JP, Baquero F. Inducible expression of ribosomal clindamycin resistance in *Bacteroides vulgatus*. Antimicrob Agents Chemother 1992;36:639–642.

104. Remington JS, Vilde JL. Clindamycin for toxoplasma encephalitis in AIDS. Lancet 1991;338:1142–1143.

105. Rivera DG, Cabrera BD, Lara NT. Treatment of falciparum malaria with clindamycin. Rev Inst Med Trop Sao Paolo 1982;24(S6):70–81.

106. Reusser F. Effect of lincomycin and clindamycin on peptide chain initiation. Antimicrob Agents Chemother 1975;7:32–37.

107. Rodriguez W, Ross S, Khan W, McKay D, Moskowitz P. Clindamycin in the treatment of osteomyelitis in children. Am J Dis Child 1977;131: 1088–1093.

108. Rolston K, Gooch G, Ho D. In-vitro activity of clarithromycin (A-56268; TE-031) against gram-positive bacteria. J Antimicrob Chemother 1989;23:455–457.

109. Rubbo JT, Gergis SD, Sokoll MD. Comparative neuromuscular effects of lincomycin and clindamycin. Anesth Analg 1977;56:329–332.

110. Ruff B, Pohle HD. Clindamycin/primaquine for *Pneumocystis carinii* pneumonia. Lancet 1989;6:626–627.

111. Safrin S, Finkelstein DM, Feinberg J, Frame P, Simpson G, Wu A, Cheung T, Soeiro R, Hojczyk P, Black JR. Comparison of three regimens for treatment of mild to moderate *Pneumocystis carinii* pneumonia in patients with AIDS. A double-blind, randomized trial of oral trimethoprim-sulfamethoxazole, dapsone-trimethoprim, and clindamycin-primaquine, Ann Intern Med 1996;124:792–802.

112. Sanders CC, Sanders WE Jr, Goering RV. Influence of clindamycin on depression of β-lactamases in *Enterobacter* spp. and *Pseudomonas aeruginosa*. Antimicrob Agents Chemother 1983;24:48–53.

113. Santoro J, Kaye D, Levison ME. In vitro activity of josamycin and rosamicin against *Bacteroides fragilis* compared with clindamycin, erythromycin, and metronidazole. Antimicrob Agents Chemother 1976;10:188–190.

114. Schmitt C, Sobel JD, Meriwether C. Bacterial vaginosis: treatment with clindamycin cream versus oral metronidazole. Obstet Gynecol 1992;79:1020–1023.

115. Shanholtzer CJ, Peterson LR, Mohn ML, Noody JA, Gerding DN. MBCs for *Staphylococcus aureus* as determined by macrodilution and microdilution techniques. Antimicrob Agents Chemother 1984;26:214–219.

116. Sirinek KR, Levine BA. A randomized trial of ticarcillin and clavulanate versus gentamicin and clindamycin in patients with complicated appendicitis. Surg Gynecol Obstet l992;172(Suppl):30–35.

117. Smilack JD, Burgin W.W Jr, Moore WL Jr, Sanford JP. *Mycoplasma pneumoniae* pneumonia and clindamycin therapy. Failure to demonstrate efficacy. JAMA 1974;228:729–731.

118. Smilack JD, Wilson WR, Cockerill FR. Tetracyclines, chloramphenicol, erythromycin, clindamycin, and metronidazole. Mayo Clin Proc 1991;66:1270–1280.

119. Solomkin JS, Dellinger EP, Christou NV, Busuttil RW. Results of a multicenter trial comparing imipenem/cilastatin to tobramycin/clindamycin. For intra-abdominal infections. Ann Surg 1990;212:581–591.

120. Soriano F, Ponte M, Garcia-Hierro P. Bactericidal activity of chloramphenicol, clindamycin, metronidazole and cefoxitin against *Bacteroides fragilis*. J Antimicrob Chemother 1980;6:676–680.

121. Steigbigel NH. Erythromycin, lincomycin, and clindamycin. In: Mandell GL, Douglas RG Jr, Bennett JE, eds. Principles and practice of infectious diseases. 3rd ed. New York: Churchill Livingstone, 1990:312–317.

122. Stevens DL, Gibbons AE, Bergstrom R, et al. The eagle effect revisited: efficacy of clindamycin, erythromycin, and penicillin in the treatment of streptococcal myositis. J Infect Dis 1988;158:23–28.

123. Stevens DL, Yan S, Bryant AE. Penicillin-binding protein expression at different growth stages determines penicillin efficacy in vitro and in vivo: an explanation for the inoculum effect. J Infect Dis 1993;167:1401–1405.

124. Stevens DL, Bryant AE, Hackett SP. Antibiotic effects on bacterial viability, toxin production and host response. Clin Infect Dis 1995;20(Suppl 2):S154–S157.

125. Sutter VL, Finegold SM. Susceptibility of anaerobic bacteria to carbenicillin, cefoxitin, and related drugs. J lnfect Dis 1975;131:417–422.

126. Sutton DR, Gosnold JK. Oesophageal ulceration due to clindamycin. Br J Med 1977;1:1598.

127. Tally FP, Cuchural GJ Jr, Bieluch VM, Jacobus NV, Malamy MH. Clindamycin resistance in anaerobic bacteria. Scand J lnfect Dis Suppl 1984;43:34–43.

128. Tan TQ, Mason EO Jr, Kaplan SL. Systemic infections due to *Streptococcus pneumoniae* relatively resistant to penicillin in a children's hospital: clinical management and outcome. Pediatrics 1992;90:928–933.

129. Tedesco FJ, Barton RW, Alpers DH. Clindamycin-associated colitis. A prospective study. Ann Intern Med 1974;81:429.

130. Thadepalli H, Gorbach S, Broido PW, Norsen J, Nyhus L. Abdominal trauma, anaerobes and antibiotics. Surg Gynecol Obstet 1973;137:270–276.

131. Toma E, Fournier S, Poisson M, Morisset R, Phaneuf D, Vega C. Clindamycin with primaquine for *Pneumocystis carinii* pneumonia. Lancet 1989;1:1046–1048.

132. Toma E, Fournier S, Dumont M, Bolduc P, Deschamps H. Clindamycin/primaquine versus trimethoprim/sulfamethoxazole as primary therapy for *Pneumocystis carinii* pneumonia in AIDS. A randomized, double-blind pilot trial. Clin Infect Dis 1993;17:178–184.

133. Toohey KL, Kurzynski TA, Schell RF, Birk RJ, Zabransky RJ. Evaluation of the 10 μg clindamycin disk for susceptibility testing of anaerobes by the aerobically incubated thioglycolate broth disk method. J Clin Microbiol 1986;23:619–621.

134. Traub WH. Comparative in vitro bactericidal activity of 24 antimicrobial drugs against *Clostridium perfringens*. Chemotherapy 1990;36:127–135.

135. Vanhoof R, Gordts B, Dierickx R, Coignau H, Butzler JP. Bacteriostatic and bactericidal activities of 24 antimicrobial agents against *Campylobacter fetus* subsp. *jejuni*. Antimicrob Agents Chemother 1980;18:118–121.

136. Veringa EM, Ferguson DA Jr, Lambe DW Jr, Verhoef J. The role of glycocalyx in surface phagocytosis of *Bacteroides* spp., in the presence and absence of clindamycin. J Antimicrob Chemother 1989;23:711–720.

137. Vogelman B, Gudmundsson S, Turnidge J, Leggett J, Craig WA. In vivo postantibiotic effect in a thigh infection in neutropenic mice. J Infect Dis 1988;157:287–298.

138. Westblom TU, Midkiff BR, Czinn CJ. In vitro susceptibility of *Helicobacter pylori* to trospectomycin, pirlimycin (U-57930E),

mirincamycin (U-24729A) and N-demethyl clindamycin (U-26767A). Eur J Clin Microbiol Infect Dis 1993;12:560–562.

139. Williams DN, Crossley K, Hollman C, Sabath LD. Parenteral clindamycinn phosphate: pharmacology with normal and abnormal liver function and effect on nasal staphylococci. Antimicrob Agents Chemother 1975;7:153–158.

140. Wilson WR, Cockerill FR. Tetracyclines, chloramphenicol, erythromycin, and clindamycin. Mayo Clin Proc 1987;62: 906–915.

141. Wittner M, Rowin KS, Tanowitz HB, Hobbs JF, Saltzman S, Wenz B. Successful chemotherapy of transfusion babesiosis. Ann Intern Med 1982;96:601–604.

142. Yagi BH, Schaadt RD, Zurenko GE. The bactericidal activity and postantibiotic effect of trospectomycin. Diagn Microbiol Infect Dis 1992;15:417–423.

143. Yancey RJ Jr, Klein LK. In-vitro activity of trospectomycin sulphate against Mycoplasma and Ureaplasma species isolated from humans. J Antimicrob Chemother 1988;21: 731–736.

144. Young GP, Ward PB, Bayley N, Gordon D, Higgins G, Trapani JA, McDonald MI, Labrooy J, Hecker R. Antibiotic-associated colitis due to *Clostridium difficile:* double-blind comparison of vancomycin with bacitracin. Gastroenterology 1985;89: 1038–1045.

145. Zabransky RJ, Johnston JA, Hauser KJ. Bacteriostatic and bactericidal activities of various antibiotics against Bacteroides fragilis. Antimicrob Agents Chemother 1973;3:152–156.

146. Zambrano D, ed. Clindamycin in the treatment of human infections. 2nd ed. Kalamazoo, MI: The Upjohn Company, 1997.

Fosfomycin Tromethamine

●

Gary E. Stein and Daniel H. Havlichek, Jr.

CLASS

Fosfomycin (*cis*-1,2-epoxypropyl phosphonic acid) was first isolated from cultures of *Streptomyces fradiae* (ATCC 21096), *Streptomyces viridochromogenes* (ATCC 21240), and *Streptomyces wedmorensis* (ATCC 21239) in 1969 (35). This antibiotic is a derivative of phosphonic acid (molecular weight, 138) and includes unusual chemical features such as an epoxide ring and a carbon-phosphorus bond (Fig. 1). This compound is highly water soluble, and the most clinically useful oral preparation contains a soluble salt of fosfomycin, fosfomycin tromethamine (Monurol, Zambon Group). A parenteral formulation (disodium fosfomycin) is available in some countries but is not commonly used.

Fosfomycin is bactericidal against Gram-positive and Gram-negative bacteria by blocking an early step in bacterial wall synthesis (31). Unlike penicillin, fosfomycin must first cross the bacterial cell wall to reach its target site. This is accomplished by two main transport systems: the L-α-glycerophosphate transport system and the hexose phosphate uptake system. The latter system is induced by glucose-6-phosphate (G-6-P). Cell wall synthesis is blocked due to inhibition of pyruvyl transferase. Fosfomycin inactivates the transferase by acting as a phosphoenolpyruvate analogue. It attaches to pyruvyl transferase and forms an irreversible complex. Fosfomycin also decreases adherence of bacteria to epithelial surfaces at subinhibitory concentrations (15).

ANTIMICROBIAL ACTIVITY

The in vitro activity of fosfomycin varies with culture media, inoculum size, pH, and the presence of blood or urine (27). The presence of G-6-P in the culture media optimizes transport of fosfomycin into the bacterial cell and is necessary for accurate determination of the in vitro susceptibility of this antibiotic. The presence of urine in the test media or a high bacterial inoculum ($>10^8$ CFU/mL) increases MICs 2- to 8-fold (22). Fosfomycin exhibits its greatest activity at acidic pH.

Fosfomycin possesses antibacterial activity against Gram-negative and Gram-positive bacterial pathogens (5), but the microbiologic potency of this antibiotic limits its clinical use to the urinary tract. Its spectrum of activity includes isolates of *Escherichia coli, Enterobacter* spp., *Citrobacter* spp., *Klebsiella* spp., *Proteus* spp., *Providencia* spp., *Enterococcus* spp., *Staphylococcus* spp., and *Pseudomonas aeruginosa* (Table 1). Uropathogens inhibited by 64 mg/L or less are considered susceptible, and those with an MIC of 256 mg/L or above are categorized as resistant to fosfomycin (4). Bacteria with an MIC of 128 have intermediate sensitivity to fosfomycin. Use of a 200-μg fosfomycin disk supplemented with 50 μg of G-6-P exhibits high correlation with fosfomycin MICs determined in the presence of G-6-P (42). Corresponding zone diameter breakpoints were found to be 16 mm or above and 12 mm or less for susceptible and resistant bacteria, respectively.

Fosfomycin is rapidly bactericidal at concentrations close to the MICs. Time-kill kinetic studies have found 99% kill in a mean time of 2.9 h at twice the MIC against strains of *E. coli, Klebsiella* spp., *Enterobacter cloacae, Citrobacter freundii*, and *Staphylococcus aureus*. At eight times the MIC, the mean kill time was reduced to 2.2 h (45). Models that simulate urinary bladder concentrations of fosfomycin show similar rates of bacterial killing (16).

A number of other antimicrobial properties of fosfomycin have been observed. Exposure of *E. coli* to fosfomycin for 1 h

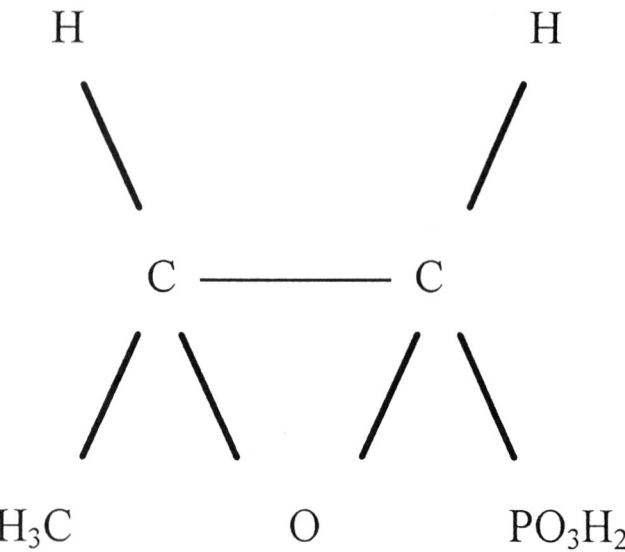

FIGURE 1. Chemical structure of fosfomycin.

TABLE 1 • In Vitro Activity of Fosfomycin (5).

Organism	MIC$_{50}$ (mg/L)	MIC$_{90}$ (mg/L)	MIC Range (mg/L)
Gram-negative bacteria			
E. coli	≤2.0	≤2.0	≤2.0–128
C. freundii	≤2.0	≤2.0	≤2.0–64
E. aerogenes	16	64	≤2.0–512
K. pneumoniae	16	128	≤2.0–>512
P. mirabilis	≤2.0	32	≤2.0–>512
P. stuartii	16	128	≤8.0–>512
P. aeruginosa	32	64	4.0–>512
Gram-positive bacteria			
E. faecium	32	64	16–128
E. faecalis	32	64	16–64
S. saprophyticus	64	>512	≤2.0–>512

Data from Barry AL, Brown SD. Antibacterial spectrum of fosfomycin trometamol. J Antimicrob Chemother 1995;35:228–230.

in Mueller-Hinton broth revealed a postantibiotic effect (PAE) of approximately 3 h. The extent of this PAE appears to correlate with the fosfomycin uptake into bacteria. Fosfomycin has demonstrated intracellular activity in human granulocytes. Incubation with fosfomycin results in a 2 log reduction in intracellular staphylococci within 18 h (56). The effects of fosfomycin on adherence of bacteria to human uroepithelial cells has been tested against *E. coli* and *Proteus mirabilis* (1). After a 1-h exposure to fosfomycin, at concentrations similar to those found in human urine, almost complete inhibition of adhesivness was observed. Fosfomycin also inhibits bacterial adhesion in resistant bacterial strains, as demonstrated by a 50% reduction in adhesiveness of a resistant strain of *P. aeruginosa* to urinary tract cells (26).

The pharmacodymanic potential of fosfomycin has been investigated in urinary bladder models and in experimental mouse and rat models of infection. In an in vitro urinary bladder model, high inocula (10^9 CFU/mL) of bacteria in sterilized urine at pH 6.5 were exposed to drug concentrations similar to those attained in the bladder following a single 3-g dose of fosfomycin. Fosfomycin exhibited more than 99.9% bacterial killing in approximately 4 h against 6 different species, *Enterococcus faecalis, S. aureus, P. aeruginosa, E. coli, Klebsiella pneumoniae,* and *P. mirabilis* (16). In experimentally induced bacterial cystitis and pyelonephritis in the rat, fosfomycin was found to be as effective as norfloxacin, trimethoprim/sulfamethoxazole, and gentamicin (21, 50).

MECHANISMS OF RESISTANCE

Both chromosomal and plasmid-mediated resistance to fosfomycin has been observed. Chromosomal mutations result in reduced fosfomycin uptake into the bacterial cell (30). The L-α-glycerophosphate system, hexose-phosphate transport system, or both can be affected (31). Fosfomycin activity can also be hindered by mutations that decrease pyruvyl transferase affinity for this antibiotic (58). Plasmid-mediated resistance appears less commonly. This form of resistance involves inactivation of fosfomycin by glutathione (2).

The emergence of resistant bacterial strains of fosfomycin depends upon the experimental conditions under study (33). In the presence of high concentrations of fosfomycin (≥500 μg/mL), resistant variants in vitro occur at a low frequency (10^{-7}–10^{-9}). Isolates of *K. pneumoniae,* indole- positive *Proteus,* and *P. aeruginosa* were found more likely to give rise to resistant strains (22). At lower concentrations of fosfomycin, a higher frequency (10^{-6}–10^{-4}) of resistant variants was observed. Isolates of *E. coli* and *P. mirabilis* were less prone to originate resistant variants. Similar findings have been observed in in vitro bladder model studies of *E. coli* (28). Emergence of resistant strains was only observed following low peak fosfomycin concentrations (≤250 μg/mL).

Development of resistant strains during therapy for urinary tract infection (UTI) doesn't appear to be a problem with single-dose oral fosfomycin trometamol. This is in contrast to observations with multiple parenteral doses of fosfomycin in complicated infections (51). Fosfomycin-resistant coliforms have been observed in the fecal flora of healthy volunteers following a single 3-g oral dose; albeit these strains could no longer be recovered after 7 to 14 days (46). Colonization with *Pseudomonas,* yeasts, or *Clostridium difficile* was not observed in these volunteers.

The overall activity of fosfomycin has been studied in a large number urinary pathogens isolated from outpatients and hospitalized patients. In an investigation of 500 isolates, 83% were sensitive to fosfomycin—89% of the outpatient strains and 77% of the inpatient strains (29). Fosfomycin was generally less active against *Klebsiella* spp. than other commonly used drugs to treat urinary infections and exhibited poor activity against *Pseudomonas* spp. A relative lack of cross-resistance to other antibiotics was observed in this study. More than 70% of strains resistant to ampicillin, sulfamethoxazole, or trimethoprim were sensitive to fosfomycin.

PHARMACOKINETICS

The calcium salt of fosfomycin has limited bioavailability (~12%). This is attributable to several factors including the poor solubility of this complex and hydrolysis of fosfomycin in the acid milieu of the stomach (13). The tromethamine salt protects fosfomycin from stomach acid and increases its bioavailability to over three times that observed with the calcium salt (59).

Dose-ranging studies with fosfomycin tromethamine are consistent with linear, non-dose-dependent, serum pharmacokinetics (8) (Table 2). Fosfomycin tromethamine attains maximum serum concentrations (C_{max}) in about 2 h (T_{max}) following a dose of 50 mg/kg to healthy subjects (59). The C_{max} is significantly delayed when fosfomycin is administered with food and in patients with renal insufficiency (10, 25). Following a dose of 50 mg/kg, a mean C_{max} of 26 mg/L (range, 22–32 mg/L) is attained (7, 53, 59). The bioavailability of fosfomycin tromethamine is approximately 40% (7, 59) and is similar in children (14).

Fosfomycin has a large apparent volume of distribution (140 L) and is not significantly bound to plasma proteins (48). Concentrations attained in the prostate, bladder wall, and seminal vesicles are comparable to mean serum concentrations (9). Cerebrospinal fluid levels of fosfomycin in patients with infected meninges were found to be one-third of simultaneously determined serum concentrations (20). Concentrations in breast milk are approximately one-tenth simultaneous serum levels (32). Fetal blood concentrations of fosfomycin are comparable to the serum levels of the mother (24).

Fosfomycin is primarily excreted unchanged in the urine. Biotransformation to active metabolites has not been observed. Clearance of fosfomycin is similar to the glomerular filtration rate, which implies that tubular secretion does not occur (32). The mean renal clearance is approximately 7 L/h. The serum half-life of fosfomycin is about 4 h in young adults (7, 59) and 8 h in the elderly (25). In patients with severe renal failure (CrCl = 7 mL/min), the elimination half-life increases to 50 h (25), and the percentage of fosfomycin excreted in the urine decreases by two-thirds. The pharmacokinetics in children and pregnant women are similar to those of young adults (14, 44).

Urine concentrations of fosfomycin following a 50-mg/kg dose are extremely high. Peak concentrations in the urine occur in 2 to 4 h and range from 3000 to 5000 mg/L in young adults (6,9). Fosfomycin concentrations in the urine parallel serum concentrations. Urine concentrations decrease to a mean of 484 mg/L by 16 to 24 h and 50 mg/L at 36 to 48 h (6). Urine concentrations in the elderly are about 50% of those in young adults. The observed urine levels in young and elderly patients usually suffice to inhibit growth of common uropathogens for at least 24 to 36 h (5, 9).

DOSAGE REGIMENS

Fosfomycin tromethamine is most commonly used in the treatment of women with uncomplicated lower urinary tract infections. A single 3-g dose (approximately 50 mg/kg) is the recommended dosing regimen. The same dose has also been used for antibiotic prophylaxis prior to and after transurethral instrumentation. A 2-g dose has most commonly been used to treat UTIs in children 5 years of age and older (49).

Elderly patients and pregnant women have also received fosfomycin tromethamine in a 3-g single dose. Dosage adjustment in patients with renal or hepatic insufficiency does not appear to be necessary, but the clinical efficacy of fosfomycin in these patient groups is not known.

The single-dose 3-g sachets of fosfomycin tromethamine should be dissolved in 50 to 100 mL of water and can be taken with or without food (12).

ADVERSE EFFECTS

Fosfomycin tromethamine is well tolerated and causes few untoward effects (Table 3). The overall incidence of adverse effects was found to be approximately 6% in women treated with a 3-g dose of fosfomycin tromethamine (36). Common side effects involve the gastrointestinal tract, and diarrhea is most often reported (37). Other side effects have included vaginitis, nausea, headache, dizziness, and dyspepsia. Serious adverse events associated with fosfomycin tromethamine were rarely reported. A similar rate of adverse effects has been observed after a 3-g dose of fosfomycin tromethamine or amoxicillin in patients with uncomplicated UTI (38).

The safety of fosfomycin in pregnant women has been studied in only a small number of patients. Preliminary data in approximately 200 pregnant women treated with single doses of fosfomycin tromethamine showed this drug to be well tolerated during pregnancy (47). In one multicenter study, nausea and epigastric pain were reported by 9% of patients (44). Fosfomycin tromethamine has not been found to be teratogenic in animals (pregnancy category B). Moreover, no teratogenic effects have been associated with the use of fosfomycin tromethamine in clinical studies. Since most safety observations in this patient group were not gathered systematically, there is clearly a need for further information.

Fosfomycin tromethamine also appears safe in children (14, 43). The side effect profile observed in children was similar to that reported in adults. Transient diarrhea, occurring in approximately 5% of patients, was reported most often. Transient rises in serum transaminases were occasionally found.

FOOD AND DRUG INTERACTIONS

Food impairs absorption of fosfomycin tromethamine. Both peak plasma concentration and overall bioavailability were reduced when fosfomycin trometamol was administered with

---

TABLE 2 • **Pharmacokinetic Profile of Fosfomycin Tromethamine (7).**

Parameter	50 mg/kg Single Dose[a]
T_{max} (h)	2.5 ± 0.8
C_{max} (mg/L)	26.2 ± 8.1
AUC (mg h/L)	148 ± 23.2
$T_{1/2}$ (h)	3.6 ± 0.44
Urinary recovery over 48 h (% of dose)	43.3 ± 9.4

Data from Bergan T. Degree of absorption, pharmacokinetics of fosfomycin trometamol and duration of urinary antibacterial activity. Infection 1990;18(Suppl 2):65–69.

[a] Healthy young adults.

TABLE 3 • Adverse Effects Associated with Fosfomycin Tromethamine (37)

Adverse Effect	Incidence (%)
Gastrointestinal	
Diarrhea	3.9
Nausea/vomiting	1.3
Abdominal pain	3.8
Reflux	0.4
Central nervous system	
Dizziness	1.8
Fatigue/drowsiness	2.0
Dermatologic	
Rash	0.8
Pruritis	0.2

Data from Naber KG, Johnson FN. The safety and tolerability of fosfomycin trometamol. Rev Contemp Pharmacother 1995;6:63–70.

food to healthy volunteers (12). A delay in achieving the peak plasma concentration was also observed. Mean urinary concentrations at approximately 2 h after the dose were decreased by approximately 8%.

Few drug-drug interactions with fosfomycin tromethamine have been studied. No significant changes in the pharmacokinetics of fosfomycin tromethamine were observed when it was administered with cimetidine to healthy volunteers (6). In contrast, metoclopramide significantly reduces the absorption and urinary concentrations of fosfomycin (6). Coadministration of fosfomycin tromethamine and metoclopramide should be avoided as well as other prokinetic drugs, such as cisapride.

CLINICAL INDICATIONS

Fosfomycin tromethamine has generally been used as single-dose monotherapy in the treatment and prophylaxis of UTI. Treatment populations have included young women (including pregnant patients), elderly women, and children with acute complicated and uncomplicated lower UTIs. Both men and women have received fosfomycin tromethamine for prophylaxis of UTI.

Adult Women

Fosfomycin tromethamine has been evaluated in over 1000 women in numerous comparative studies of patients with acute uncomplicated UTIs (49). In two large, randomized, double-blind studies, fosfomycin tromethamine (3-g single dose) was compared with 7-day treatment regimens of norfloxacin (11) and nitrofurantoin (57). Clinical and bacteriologic cures were similar in the treatment groups in both studies. Bacteriologic eradication rates posttherapy were between 80 and 90% in these studies. Fosfomycin tromethamine has been compared with single doses of norfloxacin (800 mg), pefloxacin (800 mg), and trimethoprim (200 mg) in double-blind treatment studies (17, 54). No differences in clinical or bacteriologic outcome were observed in these comparative single-dose trials. Similar outcomes were also observed in numerous open, comparative treatment studies (49). Comparative agents have included amoxicillin (single dose), ofloxacin (single

dose), cotrimoxazole (1 and 3 days), amoxicillin-clavulanate (5 days), norfloxacin (3 and 5 days), and cephalexin (5 days).

Children

Comparative studies of fosfomycin tromethamine 2-g single dose (1 g in children under 1 year of age) have been conducted in female and male children with lower uncomplicated and complicated UTIs (49). The largest study involved 131 children randomized to fosfomycin tromethamine or single-dose intramuscular netilmicin (5 mg/kg) (40). Bacteriologic cure was achieved in 2 to 4 days in 90 and 97% with fosfomycin tromethamine and netilmicin, respectively. At 30 days, success rates were similar in the two treatment groups for both complicated and uncomplicated infections. Several small comparative and noncomparative trials in children (1–16 years) have also shown good bacteriologic cure rates with single-dose fosfomycin tromethamine. Bacteriologic efficacies were similar to those observed in adults.

Pregnant Women

The efficacy of fosfomycin tromethamine has been evaluated in pregnant women with asymptomatic and symptomatic bacteriuria (49). In a multicenter, randomized study, single-dose fosfomycin tromethamine was compared with a 7-day course of pipemidic acid in 182 patients (44). Bacteriologic cure was achieved in 94 and 86%, at 1 month posttreatment with fosfomycin tromethamine and pipemidic acid, respectively. Similar results were found in a small study comparing single-dose fosfomycin tromethamine with a 7-day course of nitrofurantoin in 23 pregnant women with asymptomatic bacteriuria (55).

Elderly Patients

In two small randomized studies, a single 3-g dose of fosfomycin tromethamine was compared with norfloxacin, 400 mg twice daily for 7 and 10 days, in elderly patients (23, 39). A total of 53 women and 19 men were studied. Patients with known pathology of the urinary tract were excluded. Clinical and bacteriologic outcomes were similar in the two treatment groups in both studies. Bacteriologic cure at follow-up was seen in 77% of the 30 fosfomycin tromethamine–treated patients and 73% of the 30 norfloxacin-treated patients in the study reported by Ferraro et al. (23).

In two small open studies of hospitalized elderly patients with UTIs, a 3-g single dose of fosfomycin tromethamine produced bacteriologic eradication rates of 65 and 96% 10 days posttreatment (34, 52). Recurrent infections were only observed in patients with previous UTIs in the study reported by Rolandi and Indiereri (52).

Prophylaxis

Over 700 patients undergoing transurethral instrumentation have received prophylactic fosfomycin tromethamine in comparative and open studies (49). In a large, randomized study, 900 males undergoing transurethral resection of the prostate received two doses (3 h before and 24 h after surgery) of either fosfomycin tromethamine (3 g), cotrimoxazole (1.92 g), or amoxicillin (3 g) (41). Significantly fewer patients who received fosfomycin tromethamine (16%) had postoperative bacteriuria within 2 weeks of surgery than patients who received cotrimoxazole (27%) or amoxicillin (25%). Symptomatic infections developed in fewer patients given fosfomycin tromethamine (3%) than in those treated with amoxicillin (8%) or cotrimoxazole (8%).

In a large multicenter open study of 618 patients, fosfomycin tromethamine (3 g) was given 3 h before and 24 h after a variety of transurethral procedures (19). Twenty (3.2%) patients developed UTIs on the second day and 22 (3.6%) on the seventh day after treatment. These results were very similar to those observed in the comparative study reported by Periti et al. (41) and to other smaller trials of prophylactic chemotherapy with fosfomycin tromethamine (3, 18).

COMMENTS

Single-dose fosfomycin tromethamine has been shown to be effective in the treatment of lower UTIs in women and children 5 years of age or older. High success rates have been observed in pregnant women with bacteriuria, and fosfomycin has not been associated with teratogenic effects. Fosfomycin tromethamine is also effective prophylaxis for prevention of urinary infections after transurethral instrumentation. In these studies, prophylactic regimens used 2 doses of fosfomycin tromethamine.

REFERENCES

1. Albini E, Arena E, Belluco G, Marca G. Adhesion of bacteria to human uroepithelial cells and bactericidal activity of fosfomycin trometamol. In: Neu HC, Williams JD, eds. New trends in urinary tract infections. Basel: Karger, 1988:250–254.
2. Arca P, Hardisson C, SuErez, JE. Purification of a glutathione S-transferase that mediates resistance in bacteria. Antimicrob Agents Chemother 1990;34:844–848.
3. Baert L, Billiet I, Vandepitte J. Prophylactic chemotherapy with fosfomycin trometamol versus placebo during transurethral prostatic resection. Infection 1990;18(Suppl 2):103–106.
4. Barry AL, Fuchs PC. In vitro susceptibility testing procedures for fosfomycin tromethamine. Antimicrob Agents Chemother 1991;35:1235–1238.
5. Barry AL, Brown SD. Antibacterial spectrum of fosfomycin trometamol. J Antimicrob Chemother 1995;35:228–230.
6. Bergan T, Mastropaolo G, DiMario F, Naccarato R. Pharmacokinetics of fosfomycin and influence of cimetidine and metoclopramide on the bioavailability of fosfomycin trometamol. In: Neu HC, Williams JD, eds. New trends in urinary tract infections. Basel: Karger, 1988:157–166.
7. Bergan T. Degree of absorption, pharmacokinetics of fosfomycin trometamol and duration of urinary antibacterial activity. Infection 1990;18(Suppl 2):65–69.
8. Bergan T, Thorsteinsson S, Albini E. Pharmacokinetic profile of fosfomycin trometamol. Chemotherapy 1993;39:297–301.
9. Bergan T. Pharmacokinetics of fosfomycin. Rev Contemp Pharmacother 1995;6:55–62.
10. Bergogne-Berezin E, Mulber-Serieys C, Joly-Guillou ML, Dronne N. Trometamol-fosfomycin (Monuril) bioavailability and food-drug interaction. Eur Urol 1987;13(Suppl 1):64–68.
11. Boerema JBJ, Williams FTC. Fosfomycin trometamol in single dose versus norfloxacin for seven days in treatment of uncom-

plicated urinary infections in general practice. Infection 1990;18(Suppl 2):S80–88.
12. Borgia M, Longo A, Lodola E. Relative bioavailability of fosfomycin and of trometamol after administration of single dose by oral route of fosfomycin trometamol in fasting conditions and after a meal. Int J Clin Pharm Ther Toxicol 1989;27:411–417.
13. Bundgaard H. Acid-catalyzed hydrolysis of fosfomycin and its implication in oral absorption of the drug. Int J Pharm 1980; 6:1–9.
14. Careddu P, Borzani M, Varotto F, Garlashi L, Fontana P. Trometamol salt of fosfomycin (Monuril). Preliminary pharmacokinetic study and clinical experience in the treatment of urinary tract infections in children. Eur Urol 1987;13(Suppl 1): 114–118.
15. Carlone NA, Borsotto M, Cuffini AM, Savoia D. Effects of fosfomycin trometamol on bacterial adhesion in comparison with other chemotherapeutic agents. Eur Urol 1987;13(Suppl 1): 86–91.
16. Cornaglia G, Pompei R, Foddis G, Satta G. Antibacterial activity of fosfomycin trometamol in an in vitro model of the urinary bladder. In: Neu HC, Williams JD, eds. New trends in urinary tract infections. Basel: Karger, 1988:255–260.
17. Davis HR, O'Dowd TC, Holmes W, Smail J, Slack RCB. A comparative double-blind randomized study of single dose fosfomycin trometamol with trimethoprim in the treatment of uncomplicated urinary tract infections in general practice. Chemotherapy 1990;36(Suppl 1):34–36.
18. DiSilverio F, Cruciani E, Ferrone G, Principe MG, Lauretti S, Fini D. Evaluation of fosfomycin trometamol in the prevention of urinary tract infection after ESWL and ureteropyeloscopy. In: Neu HC, Williams JD, eds. New trends in urinary tract infections. Basel: Karger, 1988:329–332.
19. DiSilverio F, Ferrone G, Carati L. Prophylactic fosfomycin trometamol during transurethral surgery and urological manoeuvers. Results of a multicenter study. Infection 1990;18 (Suppl 2): 98–102.
20. Drobnic L, Quiles M, Rodriguez A. A study of the levels of fosfomycin in the cerebrospinal fluid in adult meningitis. Chemotherapy 1977;23(Suppl 1):180–188.
21. Dubini F, Riviera L. Treatment of experimental cystitis in the rat with a single dose of fosfomycin trometamol. Chemioterapia 1988;7:24–28.
22. Ferrara A, Migliori GB, Piccioni PD, Grassi FA, Colombo ML, Grassi GG. Influence of experimental conditions on in vitro activity of fosfomycin trometamol and emergence of resistant variants. In: Neu HC, Williams JD, eds. New trends in urinary tract infections. Basel: Karger, 1988:269–283.
23. Ferraro G, Ambrosi G, Bucci L, Palmieri R, Palmieri G. Fosfomycin trometamol versus norfloxacin in the treatment of uncomplicated lower urinary tract infections in the elderly. Chemotherapy 1990;36(Suppl 1):46–49.
24. Ferreres L, Paz M, Martin G, Gobernado M. New studies on placental transfer of fosfomycin. Chemotherapy 1977;23(Suppl 1): 175–179.
25. Fillastre JP, Leroy A, Humbert G, Borsa F, Josse S. Comparative pharmacokinetics of fosfomycin trometamol versus calcium fosfomycin in elderly subjects and uraemic patients. In: Neu HC, Williams JD, eds. New trends in urinary tract infections. Basel: Karger, 1988:143–156.
26. Gismondo MR, Romeo MA, Lobue AM, Chisari G, Nicoletti G. Microbiological basis for the use of fosfomycin as single-dose therapy for simple cystitis. Chemioterapia 1986;5:278–282.

27. Greenwood D, Jones A, Eley A. Factors influencing the activity of the trometamol salt of fosfomycin. Eur J Clin Microbiol 1986;5:29–24.

28. Greenwood D. Activity of the trometamol salt of fosfomycin in an in vitro model of the treatment of bacterial cystitis. Infection 1986;14:186–189.

29. Greenwood D, Edwards R, Brown J, Ridout P. The comparative activity of fosfomycin trometamol against organisms isolated from infected urines. Infection 1992;20(Suppl 4):302–304.

30. Kadner RJ, Winkler HH. Isolation and characterization of mutations affecting the transport of hexose phosphates in *Escherichia coli*. J Bacteriol 1973;113:895–900.

31. Kahan FM, Kahan JS, Cassidy JP, Kropp H. The mechanisms of action of fosfomycin. Ann NY Acad Sci 1974;235:364–386.

32. Kirby WMM. Pharmacokinetics of fosfomycin. Chemotherapy 1977;23(Suppl 1):141–151.

33. Lerner SA, Price S, Kulkarni S. Microbiological studies of fosfomycin trometamol against urinary isolate in vitro. In: Neu HC, Williams JD, eds. New trends in urinary tract infections. Basel: Karger, 1988:121–129.

34. MacGowan AP, Bailey RA, Egner W, Picken DM, Reeves DS. An open study of the efficacy and safety of single dose fosfomycin trometamol treatment of hospitalized patients with urinary tract infection (pilot study). Infection 1990;18(Suppl 2):107–108.

35. Miller AK, Wolf J, Miller TW, Chaist L, Korat FM, Foltz EI, Woodruff HB, Hendlin D, Skiplay EO, Jackson M, Wallick H. Phosphonomycin: a new antibiotic produced by strains of streptomyces. Science 1969;166:122–123.

36. Naber KG. Fosfomycin trometamol in treatment of uncomplicated lower urinary tract infections in adult women—an overview. Infection 1992;20(Suppl 4):S310–311.

37. Naber KG, Johnson FN. The safety and tolerability of fosfomycin trometamol. Rev Contemp Pharmacother 1995;6:63–70.

38. Neu HC. Fosfomycin trometamol versus amoxicillin-single-dose multicenter study of urinary tract infections. Chemotherapy 1990;36(Suppl 1):19–23.

39. Palmieri G, Palmieri R, Ambrosi G, Bucci L, Agratti AM, Ferraro G. A new single-dose antibiotic in urinary tract infection in elderly patients. In: Neu HC, Williams JD, eds. New trends in urinary tract infections. Basel: Karger, 1988:322–324.

40. Peratoner L, Corrias A, Tumbarello R, Bassetti D, Varese LA, Principi N, Del Bono GP, Fontana P. Fosfomycin trometamol versus netilmicin in pediatric urinary tract infection. In: Neu HC, Williams JD, eds. New trends in urinary tract infections. Basel: Karger, 1988:171–177.

41. Periti P, Novelli A, Reali EF, Del Bono GP, Fontana P. Prophylactic chemotherapy with fosfomycin trometamol salt in transurethral prostatectomy. In: Neu HC, Williams JD, eds. New trends in urinary tract infections. Basel: Karger, 1988:207–223.

42. Pfaller MA, Barry AL, Fuchs PC. Evaluation of disk susceptibility testing of fosfomycin tromethamine. Diagn Microbiol Infect Dis 1993;17:67–70.

43. Principi N, Corda R, Bassetti D, Varese LA, Peratoner L. Fosfomycin trometamol versus netilmicin in children's lower urinary tract infections. Chemotherapy 1990;36(Suppl 1):41–45.

44. Ragni N, Pivetta C, Paccagnella F, Foglia G, Del Bono GP, Fontana P. Urinary tract infections in pregnancy. In: Neu HC, Williams JD, eds. New trends in urinary tract infections. Basel: Karger, 1988:197–206.

45. Reeves DS, Holt HA, Bywater MJ. In vitro study of fosfomycin trometamol. In: Neu HC, Williams JD, eds. New trends in urinary tract infections. Basel: Karger, 1988:224–231.

46. Reeves DS, Holt HA, Bywater MJ, Ley D. Effect of fosfomycin trometamol on the faecal flora of eight healthy volunteers. In: Neu HC, Williams JD, eds. New trends in urinary tract infections. Basel: Karger, 1988:292–298.

47. Reeves DS. Treatment of bacteriuria in pregnancy with single dose fosfomycin trometamol: a review. Infection 1992;20(Suppl 4):S313–316.

48. Reeves DS. Fosfomycin trometamol. J Antimicrob Chemother 1994;34:853–858.

49. Reeves DS. Clinical efficacy and safety of fosfomycin trometamol in the prevention and treatment of urinary tract infections. Rev Contemp Pharmacother 1995;6:71–83.

50. Ritzerfeld W. Fosfomycin in the treatment of experimental pyelonephritis. In: Proceedings of the 10th International Congress of Chemotherapy, Zurich, Switzerland. 1977:683–685.

51. Rodriguez A, Gallego A, Olay T, Mata JM. Bacteriological evaluation of fosfomycin in clinical trials. Chemotherapy 1977;23(Suppl 1):247–258.

52. Rolandi E, Indiereri F. Fosfomycin trometamol single-dose therapy in lower urinary tract infections of elderly women. In: Neu HC, Williams JD, eds. New trends in urinary tract infections. Basel: Karger, 1988:319–321.

53. Segre G, Bianchi E, Cataldi A, Zannini G. Pharmacokinetic profile of fosfomycin trometamol (Monuril). Eur Urol 1987;13 (Suppl 1):56–63.

54. Selvaggi FP, Ditonno P, Traficante A, Battaglia M, DiLorenzo V. Fosfomycin trometamol versus norfloxacin in single dose for adult female uncomplicated UTIs. Chemotherapy 1990;36 (Suppl 1):31–33.

55. Thoumsin H, Aghayan M, Lambotte R. Single dose fosfomycin trometamol versus multiple dose nitrofurantoin in pregnant women with bacteriuria: preliminary results. Infection 1990;18 (Suppl 2):94–97.

56. Trautmann M, Meincke C, Vogt K, Ruhnke M, Lajous-Petter AM. Intracellular bactericidal activity of fosfomycin against staphylococci: a comparison with other antibiotics. Infection 1992;20:350–354.

57. Van Pienbroek E, Hermans J, Kaptein AA, Mulder JD. Fosfomycin trometamol in a single dose versus seven days of nitrofurantoin in the treatment of acute uncomplicated urinary tract infections in women. Pharm World Sci 1993;61:257–262.

58. Venkateswaran PS, Wu HC. Isolation and characterization of a phosphonomycin-resistant mutant of *Escherichia coli* K-12. J Bacteriol 1972;110:935–944.

59. Wilson P, Williams JD, Rodandi E. Comparative pharmacokinetics of fosfomycin trometamol, sodium fosfomycin and calcium fosfomycin in humans. In: Neu HC, Williams JD, eds. New trends in urinary tract infections. Basel: Karger, 1988:136–142.

Macrolides

●

Lütfiye Mülazimoglu and Piero Periti

Chemical Structure

Macrolides are a homogenous group of antimicrobial drugs with similar chemical structures, antibacterial spectra, mechanisms of action and resistance but different pharmacokinetic properties (227). The chemical structure of macrolides is characterized by a large lactone ring containing between 12 and 16 atoms, to which one or more sugars are attached via glycosidic bonds. The lactone ring is substituted by hydroxyls of alkyl groups, one ketone at C7 in 12-membered macrolides and at C9 in 14-membered macrolides, and one aldehyde group in the 16-membered compound. The only compound with a 15-membered ring, azithromycin, contains a tertiary amino group. Neutral or basic sugars can substitute one, two, or three hydroxyl groups of the lactone ring, conferring a more or less basic character to the molecule.

Erythromycin, discovered in 1952 as a metabolite of a strain of *Streptomyces erythreus,* is the prototype of all the antimicrobial agents of the macrolide class. A major effort has been made to overcome the problems of this macrolide by converting the base to an acid-stable palatable salt, ester, or salt of an ester (63, 224, 225). Two relatively water-soluble salts of erythromycin, gluceptate and lactobionate, are available for intravenous injection (45, 192). Chemical structures of erythromycin and its ester and salt derivatives for oral use are given in Figure 1 (227).

After the discovery of erythromycin and other natural compounds, much research was devoted to synthesizing derivatives or analogues with improved chemical, biologic, and pharmacokinetic properties. These new macrolides are semisynthetic molecules that differ from the original compounds in their substitution pattern in the lactone ring system (Table 1).

Of the four new semisynthetic agents, three have similar 14-membered lactone nuclei: roxithromycin is identical to erythromycin except for a complex 9-ethyloxime substitution; clarithromycin is 6-*O*-methyl-erythromycin; and dirithromycin is a bis-deoxo-iminomethoxyethoxy derivative of erythromycylamine (Fig. 2). These seemingly minor modifications confer pronounced new properties. The fourth new macrolide, azithromycin, is a semisynthetic compound in which the lactone ring was expanded to a 15-membered structure by insertion of a nitrogen atom and is considered to be the prototype for new macrolide structures termed azalides (Figure 3).

A 3-keto function in place of the L-cladinose moiety gave a new class of semisynthetic 14-membered-ring macrolides, the ketolides, which are very active against streptococci and pneumococci, irrespective of their resistance phenotype. The presence of the neutral sugar in 14- and 15-membered ring macrolides could make a distinct conformation of the macrolactone, explaining

their ability to induce MLS_B resistance. Unlike macrolides, ketolides are noninducers of MLS_B resistance in Gram-positive cocci, at least in staphylococci and streptococci (42).

The chemical and biochemical modifications of 16-membered macrolides have been less successful. Chemical modifications have included acylation of hydroxyl groups in the lactone ring and in the neutral sugar, resulting in miocamycin, the 9,3″-di-*O*-acetyl derivative of midecamycin, and rikamycin (rokitamycin), the 3″-*O*-propionyl derivative of leucomycin A5 (Fig. 4).

Structure-Activity Relationship

Structure-activity studies of macrolide antibiotics were specifically directed toward two goals. The first has been achieved with considerable success, protecting erythromycin from substantial acid-catalyzed degradation and loss of antibiotic activity when passing through the stomach. However in all of these cases involving different esters, salts, and formulations, the active antibiotic ingredient is always erythromycin base (Fig. 1). Studies on the correlation between structure and the activity of macrolides have demonstrated that the most basic compounds are the most active (50). The second goal was synthesis of new derivatives of erythromycin that retain potent antimicrobial activity while offering improved pharmacokinetic properties and inhibiting the relatively facile decomposition due to intramolecular cyclization into the 6,9;9,12-spiroketal. This result was obtained through modification of the functional groups on erythronolide carbon atoms 6–12, namely the ketone at C-9 (roxithromycin, dirithromycin, azithromycin), the proton at C-8, and the diol moiety at C-11 and C-12.

Inhibition of the dehydration step that leads to the erythronolide anhydrohemiketal was another approach to preventing the decomposition of erythromycin. To accomplish this objective, alkylation of the hydroxyl group at C-6, which is involved in the initial cyclization stage, was thoroughly investigated, resulting in synthesis of 6-*O*-methylerythromycin (clarithromycin) (Fig. 2). By the same approach, 8-fluoroerythromycin, flurithromycin, was prepared by using both chemical and bioconversion methods for its synthesis (153).

With only a few exceptions, the new macrolide derivatives are similar to their parent compounds with regard to spectrum of antimicrobial activity, bacteriostatic versus bactericidal effect, profile of antibiotic cross-resistance, and the influence on minimal inhibitory concentrations (MICs) of variables such as pH, presence of serum, size of bacterial inoculum, or bacterial growth medium (154). Nitrogen substitution enhances the activity of azithromycin against Gram-negative species as well as improving the stability of the compound in acid.

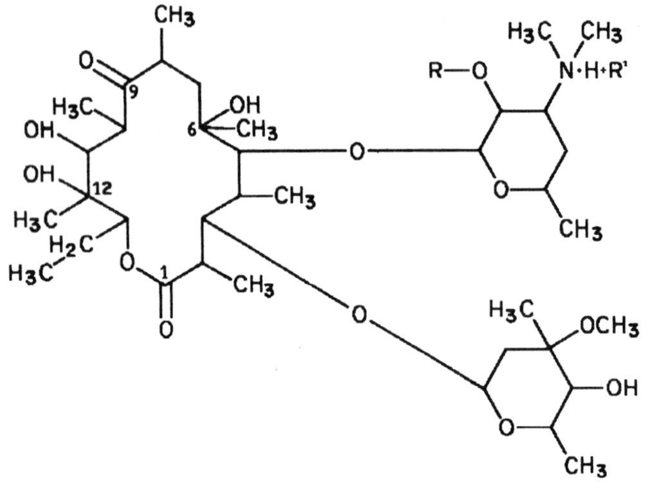

	R	R₁	
Erythromycin	H		(base)
Propionyl erythromycin	$(CH_2)_2CO$		(ester)
Erythromycin ethylsuccinate	$(CH_2)_2OOC(CH_2)_2COO$		(ester)
Erythromycin stearate	H	$C_{17}H_{35}COO$	(salt)
Erythromycin estolate	$(CH_2)_2CO$	$C_{12}H_{25}OSO_3$	(salt of an ester)
Propionyl erythromycin mercaptosuccinate*	$(CH_2)_2CO$	$C_4H_6O_4S$	(salt of an ester)
Propionyl erythromycin N-acetylcysteine*	$(CH_2)_2CO$	$C_5H_9NO_3S$	(salt of an ester)
Erythromycin acistrate	CH_3CO	$CH_{17}H_{35}COO$	(salt of an ester)

*The two salts of propionyl erythromycin combine antibiotic and mucolytic activities in a single agent

FIGURE 1. Chemical structure of erythromycin A and its ester and salt derivatives for oral use.

TABLE 1 • Marketed Macrolide Antibacterials (Numbers in parentheses give the number of ring members in the n-membered aglyone macrolide ring)

Naturally Occurring	Prodrugs	Semisynthetic
Established agents		
Erythromycin (14)	Erythromycin ester[a]	Miocamycin (16)
Oleandomycin (14)	propionyl	Flurithromycin (14)
Spiramycin (16)	ethylsuccinate	
Josamycin (16)	Erythromycin salt	
Midecamycin (16)	stearate	
	Erythromycin salt of an ester	
	estolate	
	propionyl-mercaptosuccinate	
	acetylcysteinate	
	Oleandomycin ester	
	triacetyl-oleandomycin	
Recently developed agents		
	Erythromycin acistrate	Roxithromycin (14)
	acetyl-erythromycin stearate	Clarithromycin (14)
	Rikamycin (rokitamycin) (16)	Dirithromycin (14)
		Azithromycin (15)

[a] Erythromycin and its prodrugs are usually indicated as 'erythromycins'.

ANTIMICROBIAL ACTIVITY
Spectrum

The antimicrobial activity of the different macrolides is listed in Table 2. In general, the macrolides show fairly uniform ac-tivity against streptococci and methicillin- susceptible staphylococci. Clarithromycin is the most active against *Bacteroides* species but the least active against *Haemophilus influenzae;* when clarithromycin is combined with its metabolite, it has

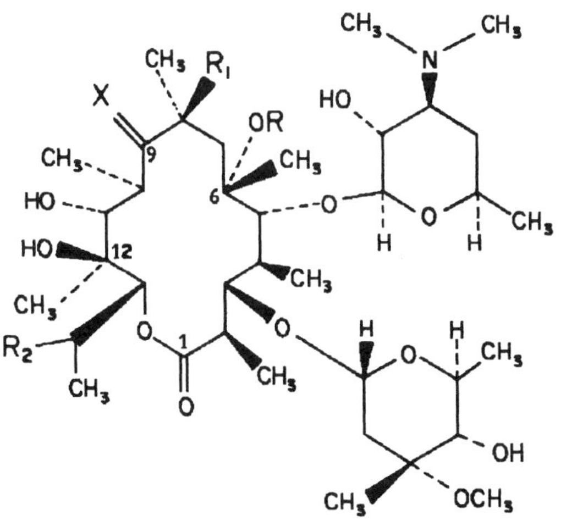

	X	R	R₁	R₂
Erythromycin	O	H	H	H
Erythromycylamine	NH_2	H	H	H
Clarithromycin	O	CH_3	O	H
Flurithromycin	O	H	F	H
Roxithromycin	$NOCH_2O(CH_2)_2OCH_3$	H	H	H
Dirithromycin	$NCHCH_2O(CH_2)_2OCH_3$	H	H	

*Ketolides are a new class of semi-synthetic 14-membered-ring macrolides, characterized by a 3-keto function in place of the L-cladinose moiety, the neutral sugar thought to be essential for antibacterial activity. One of them (RU 64004) was found to be very active against respiratory pathogens, particularly pneumococci, irrespective of their resistance phenotype.[42]

FIGURE 2. Chemical structure of 14-membered macrolide. (From reference 228.)

additive activity against *H. influenzae* (210). Azithromycin is the most active against *H. influenzae, Moraxella catarrhalis, Neisseria gonorrhoeae,* and *Fusobacterium* species (301). All macrolides have excellent activity against *Bordetella pertussis* (133). Clarithromycin has excellent activity against *Mycobacterium avium* complex (47, 72). Azithromycin has excellent activity against *Chlamydia* species (3), *Legionella* species (12), and *Mycoplasma pneumoniae* (138). There is also direct evidence of antipseudomonal activity of macrolides (278).

Pharmacodynamic Effects

Postantibiotic effect (i.e., persistent suppression of regrowth after short exposure of bacteria to the study drug in vitro) has been shown for macrolides, which allows long dosing intervals for macrolides (87, 216).

MECHANISMS OF ACTION

Although the overall mechanism of action of erythromycin and the macrolides has been well known for more than 30 years, many aspects are not yet clear and continue to be controversial. All macrolide compounds bind to the 50S subunit of prokaryotic ribosomes with a specific target in the 23S ribosomal RNA molecule and in various ribosomal proteins.

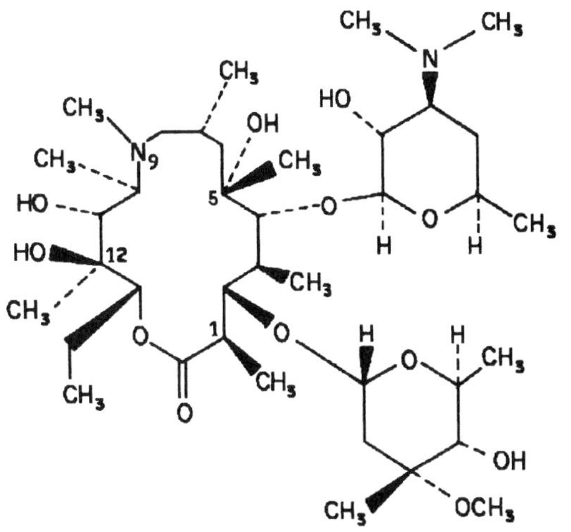

FIGURE 3. Chemical structure of azithromycin (15-membered macrolide). (From reference 228.)

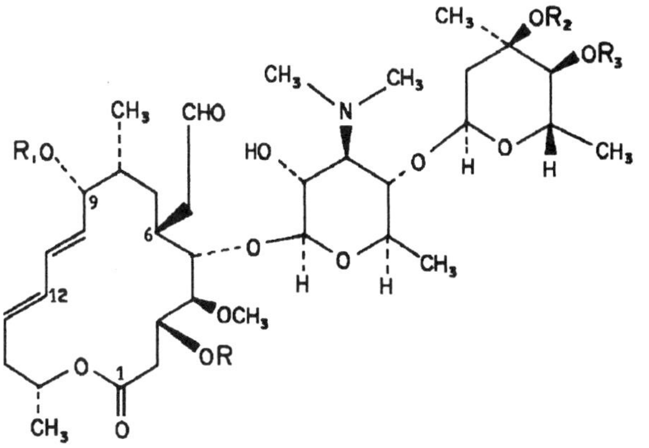

	R	R₁	R₂	R₃
Spiramycin	H	Forosamine	H	H
Leucomycin A₅	H	H	$COCH_2CH_3$	H
Josamycin	$COCH_3$	H	H	$COCH_2CH(CH_3)_2$
Miocamycin	$COCH_2CH_3$	$COCH_3$	$COCH_3$	$COCH_2CH_3$
Midecamycin	$COCH_2CH_3$	H	H	$COCH_2CH_3$
Rokitamycin	H	H	$COCH_2CH_3$	$CO(CH_2)_2CH_3$

FIGURE 4. Chemical structure of 16-membered macrolides. (From reference 228.)

The most recent and credible hypothesis suggests that all macrolides stimulate dissociation of peptidyl-tRNA from the ribosome during the elongation phase, leading to inhibition of protein synthesis (199). The 14-membered compounds inhibit the translocation of peptidyl-tRNA, whereas 16-membered compounds inhibit the peptidyl transferase reaction (188). Direct binding has also been demonstrated between the 14- and 16-membered macrolides and rRNA. Modifications of this

TABLE 2 • **In Vitro Antibacterial Activity**

Organism	Erythromycin		Dirithromycin		Clarithromycin		Azithromycin		Roxithromycin	
	MIC$_{50}$	MIC$_{90}$	MIC$_{50}$	MIC$_{90}$	MIC$_{50}$	MIC$_{90}$	MIC$_{50}$	MIC$_{90}$	MIC$_{50}$	MIC$_{90}$
Gram-positive bacteria										
Staphylococcus aureus (methicillin susceptible)	0.25	0.25	0.25	8	0.25	0.25	0.25	0.25	0.5	0.5
Staphylococcus aureus (methicillin resistant)	>8	>8			>32	>32	32	>32	>64	>64
Staphylococcus epidermidis (methicillin susceptible)	0.25	>8			0.12	>32	0.12	>32	0.25	>64
Staphylococcus epidermidis (methicillin resistant)	>8	>8			>32	>32	>32	>32	>64	>64
Streptococcus pneumoniae (penicillin susceptible)	0.25	0.25	0.25	1	0.25	0.25	0.25	0.25	0.50	1
Streptococcus pneumoniae (penicillin resistant)	0.25	32	0.25	1	0.25	16	0.25	>32	1	2
Streptococcus pyogenes	0.25	0.25	0.25	0.5	0.25	0.25	0.25	0.5	0.25	0.25
Streptococcus agalactiae	0.06	0.12			0.06	0.06	0.12	0.12	0.06	0.06
Enterococcus faecalis	>8				>32	2	>32	8	>64	
Enterococcus faecium	>8	>8	32	>32	32	>32	32	>32	>64	>64
Listeria monocytogenes									0.5	0.5
Clostridium perfringens	4	4			2	4	2	4	2	4
Corynebacterium jeikeium	>64	>64							32	>128
Gram-negative bacteria										
Haemophilus influenzae (β-lactamase negative)	4	16	4	8	8	16	1	2	4	16
Haemophilus influenzae (β-lactamase positive)	4	8	8	16	8	16	1	2	8	16
Neisseria gonorrhoeae	0.25	0.25							0.25	2
Neisseria meningitis										
Morexella catarrhalis (β-lactamase negative)	0.25	0.5	0.25	0.5	0.25	0.5	0.25	0.25	0.125	0.125
Morexella catarrhalis (β-lactamase positive)	0.25	0.5			0.25	0.25	0.25	0.25	0.125	0.25
Bordetella pertussis									0.5	0.5
Helicobacter pylori					0.03	0.06	0.06	0.25	0.25	0.25
Legionella pneumophila	0.5				0.25		0.5		0.0625	
Campylobacter jejuni	1	4			2	4	0.25	0.5	8	16
Bacteroides fragilis	8	>8			1	4	8	16	4	>64
Fusobacterium sp.	>8	>8			16	>32	0.25	16	2	64
Others										
Chlamydia trachomatis	1	1	1	1	0.125	1	0.125	1	0.015	0.06
Chlamydia pneumoniae	0.06	0.125			0.015	0.03	0.06	0.125	0.05	0.0125
Mycobacterium avium					2	4			4	16
Mycoplasma pneumoniae	0.0078	0.0156	0.1	0.1	0.0039	0.0078	0.0001	0.0002	0.015	0.03
Mycoplasma hominis									8	16
Ureaplasma urealyticum	2	>128	4	>128	0.6	>256			0.25	0.25

Data from references 3, 5, 12, 24, 40, 51, 117, 182, 241, 242, 264.

molecule, principally methylation, impede binding and determine cross-resistance between macrolides. This type of binding, however, does not conflict with the binding to ribosomal proteins since both events are possible (44). In addition they interfere with a second cellular process, formation of the 50S ribosomal subunit (58).

MECHANISM OF RESISTANCE

Macrolide antibiotics inhibit protein synthesis by their effect on ribosome function. The metabolic modifications that enable bacteria to cope with the inhibitory action of macrolides as well as those of other antibiotics include (*a*) target site alteration, (*b*) antibiotic modification, and (*c*) altered antibiotic transport (294). Clinically, the predominant form of resistance is an alteration of the 23S rRNA by methylation of adenine, which confers resistance to all macrolides as well as to lincosamide and streptogramin (MLS resistance) by a similar mode of action (167). It is specified by a class of approximately 30 genes named *erm* (erythromycin ribosome methylation). This form of resistance is unrelated to the class of the *erm* determinant. It can have either a chromosomal or a plasmid basis and can be inducible or constitutive (210). Mutations in the 23S rRNA also confer resistance to macrolides (176, 196, 209). Acquisition of new genetic information (macrolide-inactivating enzymes) results in structural modification of macrolides by phosphorylation, glycosylation, and lactone ring cleavage by erythromycin esterase (215, 294, 302). Changes in membrane permeability and active drug efflux are other resistance mechanisms against macrolides (302).

Gram-negative enteric bacteria are intrinsically resistant to macrolides because of the relative impermeability of their outer membrane to these compounds, with few exceptions. Methicillin-resistant *Staphylococcus aureus* is resistant to macrolides (126). Although relative in vitro susceptibilies to different macrolides vary with individual bacteria, bacteria resistant to one macrolide are generally resistant to other macrolides (92).

Furthermore, there is full cross-resistance among all available macrolides, lincosamides, and group B streptogramins, giving rise to the so-called phenotype of MLS$_B$ resistance. In staphylococci, MLS$_B$ resistance can be constitutively expressed. More frequently, it can be induced in the presence of 14- and 15- but not 16-membered ring macrolides. The observed cross- resistance to the three structurally unrelated groups of macrolide antibiotics is explained by their known overlapping binding site in 50S ribosomal subunits. In contrast, the ketolide derivatives that have a 3-keto function in place of the L-cladinose moiety cannot induce MLS$_B$ resistance in various erythromycin-inducible resistant strains (42).

The prevalence of resistance to macrolides varies for different countries. Erythromycin resistance for β-hemolytic group A streptococci was 44% in Finland (258), 3% in Spain (36), 0.5% in Japan (25), and over 70% in southern Taiwan (135). Resistance to erythromycin was not detected in the United States in 187 isolates (149). Resistance of *Streptococcus pneumoniae* was about 20% in Europe (23, 146) and 5 to 23% in the United States (175). *Corynebacterium diphtheria* resistant to erythromycin (210) and one strain of *B. pertussis* resistant to erythromycin (57) have been reported. Erythromycin-resistant *M. pneumoniae* have been isolated (176). Monotherapy of *M. avium* complex or *Helicobacter pylori* with macrolides results in macrolide-resistant strains (75, 196). Nevertheless, at present it is unknown whether combination therapy actually prevents or delays the emergence of macrolide resistance (209).

PHARMACOKINETIC DISPOSITION

Macrolide antibiotics are normally administered orally and are readily absorbed from the intestinal tract, if not inactivated by stomach acids; they have high lipid solubility and good tissue penetration. These antibiotics also achieve high intracellular concentrations, which may contribute to their proven clinical efficacy (227).

The metabolism of macrolides has not been studied extensively; substantial conversion to less active derivatives has, however, been demonstrated for most molecules. Macrolides are excreted in both the urine and bile. Percentages excreted vary, depending on the mode of administration, being higher after intravenous than after oral dosing (15, 114).

Absorption and Bioavailability (Table 3)

Erythromycin and Erythromycins
Erythromycin is only slightly soluble in water and is a weak base with a pK$_a$ of 8.8. It is a bitter crystalline compound, readily inactivated in an acid medium. The active form of the drug is erythromycin base, and originally the drug was available only in this form. Subsequently, a number of modifications were made to improve oral absorption, eliminate the bitter taste, or make it suitable for intravenous use (Table 1).

Erythromycin base is now marketed in an acid-resistant enteric-coated form to retard gastric inactivation and thus improve absorption (224, 225). Erythromycin base is absorbed intact. Excellent bioavailability has been demonstrated for enteric-coated erythromycin base in both fasting and nonfasting states in single- and multiple-dose regimens. Absorption of film-coated erythromycin base tends to be erratic, and administration under fasting conditions is required (45). Erythromycin base administered rectally as a suppository demonstrated satisfactory absorption and therapeutic plasma concentrations for 6 h after a dose similar to that used orally (235).

Erythromycin stearate is less readily destroyed in the stomach than the base and dissociates in the duodenum, liberating the active form, which is absorbed at this site. Serum concentrations achieved with capsules or film-coated tablets are lower than the mean values obtained with the erythromycin base preparations (141, 142). A high loading dose of oral erythromycin stearate has been recommended for antibiotic prophylaxis of endocarditis in susceptible dental patients who are allergic to penicillin (259). Food seems to play a significant

Antibiotic	Dose (mg)	Absorption Orally	C$_{max}$ (mg/L)	T$_{max}$ h	T$_{1/2}$h	AUC mg.h/l	References
Erythromycin	500	Better in fasting state	2.1	1.2	1.6	7.3	147
Roxithromycin	150	Better in fasting state	7.9	1.3–2.2	10.5	91.4	256
Clarithromycin	1200	Better after food	2.66–4.66	2	2.3–6.0	1.67–44.6	64–66
Dirithromycin	500	Better after food	0.1–0.5	4	28	0.86	263
Azithromycin	500	Better in fasting state	0.38	2	11	3.4	100, 260

TABLE 3 • Absorption and Bioavailability

role in the bioavailability; it is best absorbed when taken immediately before meals.

Erythromycin ethylsuccinate ester is well absorbed from the gastrointestinal tract as the esterified molecule and is hydrolyzed to the base in the blood. Absorption is delayed by food (279).

Erythromycin estolate, the dodecyl sulfate salt of the propionyl ester, is more acid stable than the ethylsuccinate and is absorbed from the gastrointestinal tract more completely and mainly as the ester (229). Food does not appreciably alter the absorption of estolate.

Propionyl erythromycin mercaptosuccinate has excellent oral bioavailability administered in the form of enterosoluble tablets. Single- and multiple-dose regimens of 1 g resulted in peak serum concentrations of 5.6 to 6.3 mg/L at 1.6 h (225). However, it is still not clear precisely how much of this erythromycin salt of an ester is hydrolyzed in vivo.

Erythromycin acistrate, the 2'-acetyl ester of erythromycin stearate, was readily and uniformly absorbed after a single oral dose. The total antibiotic concentrations in plasma exceeded the erythromycin levels achieved by equimolar doses of the stearate tablets or erythromycin base enterocapsules. Only a minor part of 2'-acetyl erythromycin seemed to be hydrolyzed to erythromycin in human plasma. When taken before a standard meal, absorption of erythromycin acistrate 400 mg tablets with acid-protected coating is adequate in most persons, although interindividual variation does exist, and absorption can be markedly impaired (283).

Other Natural and Semisynthetic Macrolides

Oleandomycin.   Oleandomycin phosphate can be given orally or by slow intravenous infusion. Oleandomycin is also available in an oral preparation as the triacetyl ester, troleandomycin. The mean peak concentration is about 0.8 mg/L after an oral dose of oleandomycin 500 mg; an identical dose of triacetyloleandomycin produced a C_{max} of 2.0 mg/L (74).

Spiramycin.   Spiramycin is well absorbed from the gastrointestinal tract, and simultaneous administration of food does not affect its bioavailability (145, 296).

Josamycin.   Josamycin is administered only by the oral route and is well absorbed from the gastrointestinal tract. A single dose of 400 mg produces peak concentrations of 0.33 mg/L within 0.77 h (261), and single doses of 500 mg provide peak concentrations of 0.61 to 0.71 mg/L within 1 h (272). Increases in C_{max} were obtained with multiple-dose regimens of 500 mg three times daily, 500 mg four times daily, and 1000 mg three times daily over 3 days (102). A comparative study of josamycin and erythromycin pharmacokinetics conducted in 21 healthy volunteers demonstrated that the two drugs in comparable doses produced similar plasma concentrations (272).

Midecamycin.   Few data are available concerning the pharmacokinetic properties of midecamycin in humans (67).

Miocamycin.   Miocamycin, a semisynthetic derivative of midecamycin bearing 2 acetyl groups at C-9 and C-3″, is rapidly and almost completely absorbed by the gastrointestinal tract. Oral administration of 400 mg of miocamycin

yielded a mean peak serum concentration of 1.65 mg/L; with a dose of 600 mg (tablets or dry syrup) peak serum concentrations obtained within 40 to 60 min range from 1.31 to 3 mg/L on average (104, 108). Absorption of the compound appears not to be influenced by the presence of food in the stomach.

Rosaramicin.   Rosaramicin is rapidly absorbed after oral administration as a tablet or solution, with absorption and disposition kinetics independent of the dosage form (171). There are few published data describing the pharmacokinetics and metabolism of this drug in humans (107).

Roxithromycin.   Roxithromycin is well absorbed from the gastrointestinal tract. A 150-mg oral dose containing 30.7 μCi of ^{14}C- roxithromycin produced peak plasma concentrations of 3.2 mg/L within about 3 h (194). Comparing single doses of 150, 300, and 450 mg of roxithromycin showed that peak plasma concentrations increased in a dose-dependent manner, but T_{max} was not affected (238). AUC also increased, but dose proportionality was not observed. The peak plasma concentrations obtained with roxithromycin were 3.75 times those with erythromycin (6.61 vs. 1.78 mg/L). During multiple dosing, steady-state concentrations were reached by day 4. The trough plasma concentrations of roxithromycin at steady-state (days 4–11) ranged from 3.22 to 3.69 mg/L with 150 mg twice daily and from 2.2 to 2.22 mg/L with 300 mg every day (161). C_{max} after a single 150-mg dose of roxithromycin was 3.3 times that produced by a single 250-mg dose of erythromycin. The AUC produced by roxithromycin was 16.2 times that produced by erythromycin. Similar differences were observed after multiple doses (37). A single dose of roxithromycin (300 mg) produced a higher peak plasma concentration than single 500-mg doses of clarithromycin and azithromycin, when directly compared in volunteers. Food delays the absorption of roxithromycin (256).

Clarithromycin.   Clarithromycin is rapidly absorbed, and its availability after an oral dose of 250 mg is approximately 55%. This is probably due to first-pass metabolism, which produces, in particular, the 14-hydroxy metabolite (65, 106). The maximal serum concentrations following oral administration are dose dependent, and peak blood concentrations are achieved in about 3 h. After multiple doses of clarithromycin (250 mg twice daily for 3.5 days) in Western volunteers, steady-state concentrations were attained after 5 doses. Maximal serum clarithromycin concentrations and concentrations of its 14-hydroxy derivative were 1 mg/L and 0.6 mg/L, respectively. Mean peak plasma concentrations, evaluated by HPLC after repeated doses ranging from 100 to 800 mg every 12 h, ranged from 0.37 to 3.73 mg/L. Clarithromycin showed linear pharmacokinetics between oral doses of 100 and 400 mg in healthy volunteers. Compared with erythromycin, clarithromycin has a favorable pharmacokinetic profile, allowing it to be given twice daily (232). Food intake immediately before administration increases clarithromycin bioavailability by a mean of 25%. Such increases can be considered of little clinical significance with the dosage regimen of 250 mg and 500 mg twice daily (65). In children, clarithromycin suspension appears to be well absorbed after oral administration (113).

Dirithromycin.   A ^{14}C-radiolabeled dirithromycin study was performed in healthy volunteers to assess the absolute oral bioavailability of the drug (43). Following 500 mg oral administration, peak serum concentrations of 0.1 to 0.5 mg/L were observed 4 to 4.5 h after dosing. The linearity of dirithromycin absorption was studied in another group of healthy volunteers who received four single doses of 250, 500, 750, and 1000 mg of the antibiotic orally; peak plasma concentrations were not detected following an oral dose of 250 mg. With oral doses of 500, 750, and 1000 mg, peak plasma concentrations measured, respectively, 0.29 ± 0.21, 0.64 ± 0.44, and 0.41 ± 0.24 mg/L, and the AUCs were 0.86 ± 0.59, 1.84 ± 1.22, and 1.61 ± 1.01 mg · h/L. T_{max} occurred at 4 h and was independent of dose: absorption was linear in the dosage range of 250 to 750 mg, but linearity fell off with a 1000 mg dose.

Following oral administration of the final marketed dirithromycin formulation of 500 mg daily for 10 days, the mean C_{max} was 0.48 ± 0.43 mg/L and the mean trough concentration, 0.09 ± 0.17 mg/L. The AUC was 3.37 (0.39–17.16) mg · h/L. Plasma accumulation was not noted in multiple-dose studies with administration of 500 mg dirithromycin orally daily for either 17 or 21 days. Food does not effect mean C_{max} but prolongs the mean T_{max} and increases the AUC. Calculations based on urinary recovery data indicate that the systemic oral bioavailability of dirithromycin is 6 to 14% of the dose (262).

Azithromycin. Preliminary evaluation of azithromycin in man has shown that after a single 500-mg dose, the oral bioavailability is approximately 37%, with peak concentrations of 0.38 mg/L about 2 h after oral administration. When this loading dose is followed by 250 mg once daily for 4 days, the steady-state peak drug concentration is 0.24 mg/L. Azithromycin is absorbed rapidly, but oral bioavailability is affected significantly by food, decreasing by 43%.

Azithromycin is stable at the low pH of the stomach: this macrolide is 300 times more stable in acid medium than erythromycin (172, 252). The azithromycin oral bioavailability is consequently higher than that of erythromycin, which reaches only 25% (100).

After therapeutic oral azithromycin dosage regimens (including 500 mg on day 1, followed by 250 mg on days 2 to 5), serum concentrations range from a peak of 0.4 mg/L 2 to 3 h postdose to a trough of 0.04 mg/L 24 h after administration. The low serum levels recorded prior to the next dose are thought to reflect slow release of azithromycin from tissues (172).

Distribution (Table 4)

Erythromycin and Erythromycins

Erythromycin. Erythromycin appears to be distributed throughout the total body fluid. The volume of distribution at steady-state reaches about 45 L in adult subjects (193). Erythromycin is highly bound to plasma proteins (65–90%), primarily to α_2-globulin (28, 63). It is usually well distributed into various tissues and fluids. In general, animal studies indicate that tissue concentrations are higher than those in serum and persist longer. In humans, the ratios of tissue or body fluid to contemporaneous serum concentrations vary from 0.1 for saliva, cord serum, and cerebrospinal fluid with meningitis to values of more than 1 for bronchial secretions, lung tissues, breast milk, and bile; other body tissues and fluids have intermediate values (193).

An interesting aspect of erythromycin is its ability to penetrate phagocytes, as measured by microscopic autoradiography with ^{3}H-labeled drug. Compared with extracellular fluid, the intracellular concentration of erythromycin is 9 to 23 times higher in alveolar macrophages, and 4 to 24 times higher in polymorphonuclear leukocytes (53).

Erythromycin Acistrate. After oral dosing of erythromycin acistrate 400 mg acid- protected tablets thrice daily for 5 days, the 2′-acetyl ester of erythromycin is readily absorbed into the blood circulation, where about one-third of the ester is hydrolyzed to erythromycin. Concentrations of erythromycin in suction skin blister fluid, urine, and saliva were

TABLE 4 • Distribution Examples of Macrolides for Different Tissue or Fluids

Antibiotic	Tissue or Fluid	Dose	Sampling Time (h)	Peak Serum Concentration (mg/L)	Tissue(t) or Fluid(f) Concentration (mg/kg or mg/L)	Ratio t/s or f/s	References
Erythromycin	Sinus mucosa	1000 mg	1.5–2	1.60 ± 0.50	1.20 ± 0.4	0.80	39
Erythromycin gluceptate	Plasma	250 mg	0	3.5–10.7	10	1–3	114
Roxithromycin	Pulmonary tissue	300 mg+ 3×150 mg	12h after the last dose	5.85	5.64	1	281
	Tonsils	300 mg	12	2.00 ± 0.28	1.26 ± 0.66	0.26	104
Clarithromycin	Middle ear effusion	7.5 mg/kg daily	2.5 h after 5th dose	1.7 ± 1.2	2.5 ± 2.3	2.5 ± 3.6	274
14-OH-metabolite	Middle ear effusion	7.5 mg/kg daily	2.5 h after 5th dose	0.8 ± 0.3	1.3 ± 1.0	1.7 ± 1.4	274
Dirithromycin	Pulmonary tissue	250 mg	12	0.1	2.03	20	33
	Tonsils	500 mg	15	0.08	1.8	22	33
Azithromycin	Tonsils	500 mg	13	0.03 ± 0.04	4.5 ± 2.6	>150	100
	Prostate	500 mg	96		0.8 to 2.3	>40	173
	Alveolar cells	500 mg	12	0	26.1		68
	Macrophages	0.5 mg/mL	2			>300	222

considerably higher after the erythromycin base (500 mg trice daily). The plasma:saliva concentration ratio ranged from 0.11 to 0.17 after acistrate and 0.17 to 0.22 after the erythromycin base. Penetration of 2′-acetyl erythromycin into the extravascular space is moderate after oral erythromycin acistrate, but concentrations of antimicrobially active erythromycin (0.9–1.5 mg/L in blister fluid) are higher than the MICs for most erythromycin-sensitive bacteria (283). Concentrations of erythromycin and 2′-acetyl erythromycin were analyzed in serum and tonsil tissue after repeated dosage (500 mg thrice daily for 3 days) of oral erythromycin acistrate in young patients; this salt of an ester gives erythromycin levels in circulation and tonsil tissue comparable to those of reference erythromycins. Hydrolysis of 2′-acetyl erythromycin to erythromycin was 23 to 43% higher in tonsil tissue than in the circulation (247).

Other Natural and Semisynthetic Macrolides

Oleandomycin.   Oleandomycin is well distributed in tissues, achieving high concentrations that persist for prolonged periods in various organs or body fluids, including middle-ear exudate, adenoids, bronchial secretions, and skin window fluids (30).

Spiramycin.   Spiramycin penetrates well into tissues such as lung, prostate, and muscle, and into body fluids, persisting for prolonged periods at these sites. It is secreted in saliva, with peaks 1.4 to 4.8 times higher than serum concentrations (145). Tissue concentrations of spiramycin reach a maximum after 7 days of treatment (179). Spiramycin showed good and rapid penetration into bronchial secretions, with levels varying from 2 to 7.3 mg/L (29). Spiramycin does not enter the cerebrospinal fluid, even in meningitis. Protein binding is about 30%.

Josamycin.   The ability of josamycin to penetrate and accumulate in various tissues and body fluids has been well documented. Josamycin showed good penetration into bronchial secretions after both single and repeated doses of 500 mg and 1000 mg (36, 103), into eye fluids (54), into long bones (103), and into prostatic tissue (90). In adult patients undergoing tonsillectomy, administration of josamycin base 500 mg in a single dose produced a mean tonsillar concentration of 13.65 mg/kg with a tissue:serum ratio of 7.54. After administration of the same dose of josamycin propionate in pediatric patients, the mean tonsillar levels were higher at 21.24 mg/kg (54). Josamycin also demonstrated good penetration into middle-ear fluid, sinus secretions, and adenoids (30).

The intracellular accumulation of ^{14}C-labeled josamycin was investigated (299). The ratio of cellular:extracellular concentration (C:E) of josamycin demonstrated significant accumulation of the drug by polymorphonuclear leukocytes and monocytes in vitro.

Midecamycin.   Early observations in humans with oral doses of midecamycin (1000 mg) showed a mean concentration of 0.3 mg/kg in palatine tonsil, compared with an average plasma level of 1.9 mg/L, with a tissue:plasma ratio of 0.16. The compound was detectable only in traces, or not at all, in maxillary sinus mucosa. Nevertheless, relatively high concentrations of the antibiotic were observed in bronchial secretions 4 h after

single or multiple oral administration of 1200 mg, with an average bronchial secretion:plasma ratio of 0.86, confirming good diffusion and tropism for the respiratory tract (67).

Miocamycin.   Binding of miocamycin to serum protein is 47% (107), and the apparent volume of distribution is large, ranging from 228 to 329 L in healthy volunteers (109), indicating extensive extravascular penetration of miocamycin. Miocamycin diffuses rapidly in the extravascular compartment, with tissue concentrations always higher than those in serum in the 6 h after a single or multiple dose of 600 mg. During the 1- to 2-h period following administration, lung and palatine tonsil concentrations ranged from 2.4 to 4 mg/kg, being 1.5 to 3 times higher than corresponding plasma levels, while in larynx and nasal mucosa, miocamycin concentrations 2 h postadministration were 1.0 and 1.4 mg/kg, respectively. After the sixth oral dose of 600 mg every 8 h, miocamycin achieved prostatic concentrations twice the plasma levels (211). Moreover, miocamycin was detected in bronchial secretion and sputum at concentrations ranging from 0.68 to 5.16 mg/L within 2 to 4 h after administration (96).

Miocamycin diffusion into respiratory tract tissues or fluid was also substantial, with the drug achieving concentrations of 1.5 to 5.2 mg/kg after single- or multiple-dose administration. Penetration into bronchial secretions or sputum was particularly extensive; a tissue:fluid penetration ratio of 600% was reached after single-dose administration (96). In gynecologic tissues, miocamycin concentrations ranged from 1.1 to 2.5 mg/kg after multiple-dose administration (110).

Rosaramicin.   The mean serum concentration of rosaramicin at the end of a 1-h infusion of 500 mg was almost 4 mg/L. The disposition kinetics are biexponential, with a rapid distribution phase and a slow elimination half-life (3.28 h). With the same dosage in oral solution or in tablets, mean peak serum concentrations of 0.418 to 0.486 mg/L were achieved within 1.58 to 1.83 h after administration, with mean bioavailabilities of 32% and 39%, respectively, while after oral dosing with ^{14}C-rosaramicin, a mean peak serum concentration of 0.73 mg/L was observed within 56 min. With the oral route, the elimination half-life ranges from 4.4 to 5.01 h, with a cumulative urinary recovery of 6 to 7% (271).

Roxithromycin.   Roxithromycin is preferentially bound to α_1-acid glycoprotein. The binding is strong, specific, and saturable. It is weakly and nonspecifically bound to albumin. Maximum protein binding of roxithromycin is 96.4% at concentrations of 2.5 mg/L (306). Concentrations of roxithromycin in tissue and body fluids are generally higher than MIC_{90}s for susceptible bacteria (227). The mean concentrations of roxithromycin in pulmonary tissue after a 300-mg loading dose followed by 3 doses of 150 mg at 12-h intervals were 5.64 and 3.70 mg/kg, 6 and 12 h after the last dose, respectively; in serum, the levels were 6.26 and 5.85 mg/L at these times. The ratio of lung tissue:serum concentrations was about 1 at both 6 and 12 h (281). In another group of subjects, after 7 doses of 150 mg at 12-h intervals, pulmonary concentrations of roxithromycin were 2.1, 2.1, and 3.2 mg/kg at 3, 6, and 10 h, respectively. The tissue:serum concentration ratio was about 0.3 at all times (201).

Roxithromycin showed good penetration into bronchial secretions (243). Concentrations of roxithromycin were also determined in cells and fluid lining the epithelial surface of the lower respiratory tract. These were obtained by fiberoptic bronchoscopy with bronchoalveolar lavage in patients given 10 300-mg doses at 12-h intervals. At 2 h after the last dose, the mean concentration in epithelial lining fluid was 2.0 mg/L, 17% of the simultaneous mean plasma concentrations (11.4 mg/L). Concentrations of roxithromycin in cells recovered by bronchoalveolar lavage (21 mg/L) were 2 and 10 times higher than those in plasma and epithelial lining fluid, respectively (61).

The mean concentrations of roxithromycin in tonsillar tissue taken during surgery after a 5 mg/kg loading dose followed by 1 and 2 doses of 2.5 mg/kg at 12-h intervals were 2.63 and 1.65 mg/kg of tissue, respectively, at 6 and 12 h after the last dose. Similar results were obtained in children (27). Roxithromycin concentrations in adenoids were high, with median values of 10.25 mg/kg (range, 1.96–62.74) following administration of a single 3-mg/kg dose, and 13.30 mg/kg (range, 3.92–59.91) following multiple administrations of the same dose. These were higher than the concurrent plasma concentrations (144).

Diffusion of roxithromycin in skin blister fluid has been studied following single or multiple doses. Penetration into suction blister fluid was good following a single 150-mg dose, with a mean penetration index (defined as the ratio of blister fluid AUC:plasma AUC) of 36.8% (201). Uptake of roxithromycin into phagocytes was an active process that displayed saturation kinetics characteristic of a carrier-mediated membrane transport system (124). Placental transfer of roxithromycin was good, with an amniotic fluid:serum concentration ratio of about 0.3 to 0.4 (31). Penetration of roxithromycin into cerebrospinal fluid is poor; no detectable concentrations were observed in patients with normal meninges receiving 2 doses of the drug (150 mg at 12-h intervals) (283).

Clarithromycin. Clarithromycin binds predominantly to albumin, ranging from 42 to 50% over a concentration rate of 0.25 to 5 mg/L (81). Clarithromycin achieves tissue concentrations markedly higher than circulating levels, due to its wide distribution. This aspect is relevant for clinical activity. After single oral doses of 250 mg to volunteers, the apparent volume of distribution of clarithromycin was 243 to 266 L, while that of the 14-hydroxy derivative was 304 to 309 L (64). Following repeated oral doses of 250 and 500 mg, clarithromycin gave tissue concentrations (tonsils, skin, nasal mucosa, lung) markedly higher than those in serum and those reached in tissues by other macrolides (106). The drug is actively concentrated in human neutrophils (11).

Dirithromycin. Dirithromycin is about 19% bound to plasma proteins, principally to α_1-acid glycoprotein, and is characterized by a plasma elimination half-life of 44 h (range, 16–65) (262). It is rapidly converted by nonenzymatic hydrolysis during absorption to erythromycylamine, which is microbiologically active. The low C_{max} and AUC values reported are thought to reflect the rapid, extensive distribution of drug from plasma to extravascular tissues. This appears to be confirmed by the large apparent volume of distribution, reported to be 800 L (262).

The concentration of biologically active products (principally erythromycylamine) 12 or 24 h after a 250- or 500-mg tablet in healthy or pathologic lung parenchymal tissue (2.03–3.81 mg/kg), bronchial mucosa (1.3–1.7 mg/kg), or bronchial sections (0.49–1.04 mg/L) was usually about 20 to 40 times the simultaneous value in plasma. At this time, the tissue:plasma concentration ratio for nasal mucosa and tonsillar and prostatic tissue was usually about 20 to 35 (33), and therapeutic dirithromycin concentrations have been shown to persist in pulmonary tissues for 48 to 72 h. In comparison, concentrations of erythromycin in bronchial secretions (0.59 mg/L) and tonsillar (0.05–3.39 mg/kg) and prostatic tissue (0.42 mg/kg) were generally lower than those of dirithromycin and less sustained. Dirithromycin concentrations in alveolar macrophages were 5.6 times higher than those of erythromycin, whereas the converse was true for serum concentrations (26). The ability to concentrate within phagocytes and alveolar macrophages accounts for the high lung tissue concentrations of dirithromycin.

Azithromycin. Azithromycin's serum protein binding is low, with 50% binding observed at a serum concentration of 0.05 mg/L (99). However, it penetrates extensively into tissues, exceeding the serum concentration by 10- to 100-fold, while with erythromycin, tissue concentrations are 0.5 to 5 times that in serum (172). Between 12 and 24 h after a single oral dose of azithromycin 500 mg, the concentration in most tissue is between 1 and 9 mg/kg. At 18 to 36 h after a total oral dose of 500 mg (i.e., 2 doses of 250 mg every 12 h), azithromycin concentrations in prostate (1.2–2.2 mg/kg), tonsils (3.9–4.5 mg/kg), and assorted tissues largely exceeded corresponding serum concentrations. The high concentrations found in the tonsil and prostate were sustained and remained above 2 mg/kg at 12 and 24 h postdose. The average tissue half-life is between 2 and 4 days (172). However, 4 days after a single 500-mg oral dose, the concentration in the prostate was still 0.8 to 2.3 mg/kg, in pulmonary tissue 2.3 to 8.1 mg/kg, and in gynecologic tissue 0.27 to 1.48 mg/kg (98, 204).

After a single 500-mg dose of azithromycin, day 4 concentration in the tonsils was 0.26 to 2.0 mg/L; concentrations remained above detectable levels for over a week after administration. Much lower concentrations (0.2–1.0 mg/kg) were found in muscle, fat, and bone (99, 260); however, all tissue concentrations exceeded those obtained in serum. Following administration of a single oral 500-mg dose approximately 18 h before surgery, azithromycin concentrations in gynecologic tissues (2.7 to 3.5 mg/kg) were higher than those in serum and largely exceeded the MIC_{90} for most relevant pathogens.

The volume of distribution at steady-state was 23 L/kg. The only explanation for this accumulation in extravascular compartments is that azithromycin is actively transported into cells and then slowly released into the extracellular fluid compartments (213). The serum elimination half-life has been estimated to be 41 h between 24 and 72 h after dosing (98, 172, 252), allowing a 5-day once-daily regimen for the treatment of many common infections (160).

Metabolism, Elimination, and Effect of Age and Pathophysiologic States (Table 5)

Erythromycin is concentrated by the liver and excreted into the bile as active drug in high concentrations ranging from 5 to 250 mg/L (10 mg/L in subjects receiving the propionyl ester, and 64 mg/L in those receiving the base). Only about 1.5% of the dose of the base and 0.2% of the estolate appears in the bile in the first 8 h. The bile:serum concentration ratio is approximately 4 for the propionyl ester and 30 for the base; much of the rest is presumably demethylated or otherwise degraded. Up to 4.5% of an oral dose and 15% of a parenteral dose of erythromycin are recoverable in the urine (114). The elimination half-life of erythromycin base in adult patients with normal renal and hepatic function varies between 1.9 and 2.1 h following multiple oral drug administration of 500 mg twice daily or 250 mg four times daily (141, 304).

There is a dearth of adequate information on age-specific pharmacokinetics for erythromycin in children or in the elderly (212). Renal impairment has only a minor impact on the pharmacokinetics of erythromycin (83), while alcoholic liver disease increases the elimination half-life from 2.0 to 3.2 h (120). No dose adjustment of erythromycin in these categories of patients is necessary (212). Erythromycin is not removed by peritoneal dialysis or hemodialysis (266).

Renal clearance of erythromycin is significantly correlated with creatinine clearance, without affecting the elimination half-life and total clearance of the drug (83). In complete renal failure, with large doses (>4 g/day), erythromycin may accumulate and many toxic effects might be seen (45).

Josamycin is metabolized in the liver and excreted mainly in the bile. Less than 20% of the drug is excreted in urine in an active form (137). The metabolic pathway of josamycin in humans leads to 4 metabolites (102). Josamycin pharmacokinetics were impaired in patients with liver cirrhosis and Gilbert's syndrome. Dosage adjustment is indicated when dealing with these patients (217). Comparison of the main pharmacokinetic parameters in aged and young subjects after a single 1000-mg dose showed a significant increase in the half-life in aged subjects (3.4 ± 0.67 h), suggesting lower doses and longer intervals between doses in aged patients (115).

Midecamycin undergoes liver metabolism, and a major metabolite formed by direct 14-hydroxylation, with lower activity (almost 50%) than the parent drug, is detected in human urine.

Miocamycin is excreted as unchanged drug, as fully active metabolites, and as metabolites with reduced biologic activity (almost half that of the parent compound) through hydroxylation in the C-14 position of the lactonic ring or deacetylation in C-4″ of the mycarose molecule. Biliary excretion represents the main elimination route of miocamycin and its derivatives (108).

Rosaramicin undergoes extensive hepatic metabolism, and at least four metabolites are present in urine (171).

Following oral administration of 150 mg of *roxithromycin* containing ^{14}C-radiolabeled drug, 74.2% of the drug was recovered. Most of it was eliminated unchanged, predominantly by fecal excretion (53.4%), followed by pulmonary (13.4%) and urinary (7.4%) excretion. An elimination half-life of about 13 h following oral administration of ^{14}C-radiolabeled roxithromycin 150 mg has been reported (194). Studies of the pharmacokinetics of single 150-, 300-, and 450-mg doses, showed that the elimination half-life of the drug was not affected by dose variations, but the amount of drug excreted in the urine increased as a function of dose (238, 281). In comparative pharmacokinetic studies, the elimination half-life of roxithromycin was found to be 6 to 9 times longer than that of erythromycin (256).

The plasma concentrations observed for infants and children treated with 2.5 mg/kg were lower (4.7 and 5.9 mg/L) than those previously reported for adults receiving the recommended dosage of 150 mg twice daily. In contrast, those recorded for infants receiving 5 mg/kg were higher (14.9 mg/L). It is therefore suggested that the pediatric dosage of roxithromycin should be 2.5 to 5.0 mg/kg twice daily (144).

The pharmacokinetics of a single 300-mg dose of roxithromycin in healthy young and elderly volunteers showed a significantly higher AUC and half-life in the elderly group, compared with the young group (238). The pharmacokinetics of roxithromycin after a single 300-mg oral dose were studied in patients with severe renal insufficiency and healthy volunteers; there was no indication for dose modification in renal insufficiency (238). The pharmacokinetics of roxithromycin have also been assessed in patients with alcoholic cirrhosis (166). After a single dose of 150 mg, the elimination half-life was significantly longer (25.2 h) than that of healthy volunteers. These differences are not considered clinically relevant, and no dose modification is necessary in these patients since the trough plasma concentrations 12 h postadministration do

TABLE 5 • **Metabolism Elimination Effect of Age and Pathophysiologic Status**						
Antibiotic	**Primary Route of Elimination**	**Dosage Adjustment for Renal Failure**	**Dosage Adjustment for Hepatic Failure**	**Removal by Peritoneal Dialysis**	**Removal by Hemodialysis**	**References**
Erythromycin	Bile	Not necessary	Not necessary	No	No	83, 266
Roxithromycin	Bile	Not necessary	Not necessary			194
Clarithromycin	Bile and urine	Yes	Not necessary			210
Dirithromycin	Bile	Not necessary	Yes, if hepatic failure is severe		Negligible amounts	46, 159, 190
Azithromycin	Bile	Not necessary	Not necessary			189

not vary, and the duration of treatment with such a drug is likely to be short (226). Pharmacokinetic parameters in pregnancy showed a lower C_{max} and similar elimination half-life and AUC (31, 32). The amount of roxithromycin cleared from plasma to milk is very small, with no clinically significant effect in breastfeeding infants (238).

Clarithromycin's main metabolite in humans is 14-hydroxy-(R)-clarithromycin, which occurs in much greater quantities than the 14-hydroxy (S) epimer and is endowed with antimicrobial activity (1). The primary metabolic pathways are oxidative N-demethylation and stereospecific hydroxylation at position 14 (95). The pharmacokinetic behavior of clarithromycin is nonlinear. Clarithromycin is excreted in urine and feces in a dose-dependent manner; at low doses, the two fractions are similar, while at high doses, the urinary route predominates (95). The mean elimination half-life of clarithromycin varies with the dose, showing values above 2 h. After repeated 500-mg doses of clarithromycin every 12 h, steady-state half-lives were 3.8 h for unchanged drug and 5.8 h for the 14-OH derivative (65).

Recently, the single- and multiple-dose pharmacokinetics of clarithromycin and its 14-hydroxy metabolite were studied after oral administration under fasting and nonfasting conditions in Western children. Drug absorption appeared rapid after a brief delay in onset. The C_{max} for clarithromycin was reached within 3 h in both conditions, with values of 3.59 and 4.58 mg/L in single-dose fasting and nonfasting patients, respectively. The respective C_{max} values for the metabolite were 1.9 and 1.2 mg/L. These data indicate good absorption and no significant effects of food. No accumulation was apparent from the AUC of C_{max} values in the multiple-dose group (113).

Renal clearance of clarithromycin (500 mg twice a day for 2.5 days) was significantly lower in the elderly and correlated with decreased creatinine clearance and urinary elimination (66). For this reason, once-daily administration is advisable in patients with renal failure. Clarithromycin plasma concentrations must be monitored in patients with creatinine clearance rates below 0.6 L/h. The pharmacokinetics and metabolism of clarithromycin are not significantly affected by mild hepatic impairment.

Dirithromycin is rapidly hydrolyzed to erythromycylamine; 60 to 90% of a dose of the parent drug is converted to the active metabolite within 35 min of intravenous administration (262); 62 to 81% of an oral dose of dirithromycin and 81 to 97% of an intravenous dose were eliminated in the feces, predominantly as erythromycylamine. Urinary recovery accounted for 1.2 to 2.9% of the administered oral dose, mostly within the first 48 h. Following oral administration of a single 500-mg dose of dirithromycin, the mean peak biliary drug concentration (HPLC bioassay) was 139 mg/L (46). Beside total clearance values of 250 to 500 mL/min (15–30 L/h), higher values of 5.51 L/kg/h on day 1 and 1.9 L/kg/h on day 10 with once-daily administration of dirithromycin 500 mg were reported (159). Like total clearance, nonrenal clearance was reduced after 10 days' administration. The elimination half-life of dirithromycin was reported to range from 30 to 44 h in healthy volunteers, but the sampling duration was not stated.

The half-life was significantly longer on day 10 than on day 1 with once-daily oral administration (159, 262).

There was a trend toward increased AUC with increased age, but neither C_{max} nor AUC was significantly increased in elderly volunteers 65 years of age or older (286). Studies in patients with chronic hepatic or biliary diseases associated with mild impairment of liver function (Child-Pugh class A) who received 500 mg of dirithromycin as a single dose or once daily for 10 days revealed few important changes in pharmacokinetic values. Renal and nonrenal clearance was lower in patients with biliary disease than in other patients or healthy volunteers. There were no significant differences in pharmacokinetic values after administration of a single 500-mg dose to patients with Child A or B liver cirrhosis. However, in patients with cirrhosis, dirithromycin C_{max} and half-life were higher and total clearance was lower than values in healthy volunteers (190). These data suggest that no adjustment of dirithromycin dosage is required in patients with mild or moderate hepatic impairment receiving 500 mg once daily for 10 days (159).

A study in 32 patients with various degrees of renal failure who received dirithromycin 500 mg as a single dose or once daily for 10 days, indicated that urinary excretion and clearance of the drug decreased only in patients whose creatinine clearance was 22 mL/min or below ($\leq$1.32 L/h). Negligible amounts of the drug were removed during hemodialysis (46).

Azithromycin remains unmetabolized within the body for most of an absorbed dose. When metabolism does occur, hepatic demethylation is the primary route. The metabolites are not thought to have any significant antimicrobial activity. Although hepatic accumulation of azithromycin occurs and elevates azithromycin demethylase activity, there has been no evidence of hepatic cytochrome P-450 induction or inactivation (252). Biliary concentrations of azithromycin exceed serum concentrations, suggesting biliary excretion. More than 50% of the drug-related material in the bile is unchanged parent drug. The feces are also an important route of elimination. Urinary excretion of the unchanged drug appears to be minor (<6% within 1 week after an oral dose). About 20% of the drug that reaches the systemic circulation is excreted unchanged in the urine. Renal clearance is in the range of 6 to 11.3 L/h (260).

The pharmacokinetics of azithromycin were determined over a 192-h period following oral administration of a single 500-mg dose to healthy volunteers and to cirrhotic patients. Elimination half-lives were 53.5 h in control subjects and 60.6 and 68.1 h in class A and class B cirrhotic patients, respectively. Mean residence time was significantly higher in class B patients, but AUC, apparent volume of distribution, and total and renal drug clearance values appeared to be similar in all groups. The mean urinary recovery of azithromycin at 192 h varied from 11 to 15.7% and did not differ significantly among groups. These results demonstrate that azithromycin pharmacokinetics do not differ consistently in patients with mild or moderate hepatic impairment compared with healthy volunteers; thus no dosage modifications of azithromycin seem to be required for patients with class A or B liver cirrhosis (189).

DOSAGE REGIMENS

Dosages for macrolides are given in Table 6. Dosage reduction (50–75%) is only required for erythromycin and clarithromycin (and possibly dirithromycin) for severe renal failure. A 50% reduction in daily roxithromycin dosage has been recommended for patients with liver cirrhosis but not in the other macrolides. Adjustment of conventional doses is not required in the elderly. Since macrolides are concentrated in extravascular tissues rather than plasma, dosage adjustment is not required in patients with ascites, edema, or obesity. Erythromycin and azithromycin, like penicillins and cephalosporins, are in FDA pregnancy category B, and clarithromycin is in category C (B, animal studies no risk, but human not adequate *or* animal toxicity but human studies no risk; C, animal studies show toxicity, human studies inadequate but benefit of use may exceed risk).

Table 7 lists the principal proprietary names of macrolides on the world market.

TABLE 6 • **Dosages for Macrolides for Oral Administration**

Drug	Adult	Child
Erythromycin	250–1000 mg every 6 h	30–50 mg/kg/day 4 times daily
Roxithromycin	150 mg every 12 h	5–10 mg/kg/day 2 times daily
Clarithromycin	250–500 mg every 12 h	7.5–10 mg/kg/day 2 times daily
Dirithromycin	250–500 mg daily	NA
Azithromycin[a]	250–500 mg daily	5–10 mg/kg daily

[a] Intravenous doses up to 4 g are well tolerated (178).

ADVERSE EFFECTS
Gastrointestinal Adverse Effects

Macrolides are considered among the safest antimicrobial agents, and serious adverse effects are rare. Gastrointestinal adverse effects are the most common. Abdominal pain (16%), nausea and vomiting (14%), and diarrhea are reported with an overall incidence of 30% for erythromycin (88). Erythromycin acts as a motilin receptor agonist in the gastrointestinal tract and stimulates motility. Erythromycin is used as a therapeutic agent in some motility disorders because of this effect. The presence of dimethylamino group on the neutral sugar at C3 of the lactone ring appears necessary for the motor-stimulating activity. Macrolide-induced emesis may be partially due to 5-hydroxytryptamine receptors; this adverse effect is dose dependent and probably structure related (218). Gastrointestinal adverse effects can also occur with parenteral administration (257). The new derivative erythromycin acistrate causes fewer gastrointestinal side effects (7%) than erythromycin base (50%) (303). The newer macrolides have fewer gastrointestinal side effects than erythromycin: 3% for roxithromycin (38), 9% for clarithromycin (126), 10% for azithromycin (132), and 22% for dirithromycin (78).

Hepatotoxicity

Hepatotoxicity is a very rare but serious adverse effect of erythromycin. The incidence of acute symptomatic liver disease resulting in hospitalization after a 10-day course of erythromycin was estimated at 2.3 per million patients (55). The risk of cholestatic jaundice was estimated at 0.4 per million patients (77). Hepatotoxicity occurs most commonly in adults and usually after 1 to 2 weeks of drug administration. Nausea and abdominal pain are initial symptoms followed by fever (50%). Patients have eosinophilia (>500 cells/mm^3; 75%) and

TABLE 7 • **Principal Proprietary Names of Macrolides on the World Market**

Macrolide	Trademark	Manufacturer
Erythromycin	EES[a,e], Eritrocina[a,e,f], ERY[a,e,f], Eryderm[h], Erypelle[e], Erythrocin[a,e,f,g,i], Pediamycin[e]	Abbott
Miocamycin	Mosil[a], Myoxam[a,b,d], Merced[a,b], Miocacin[a,b], Mocamen[a,b,d]	Menarini
Roxithromycin	Assoral[a], Overal[a], Rulid[a], Rulide[a,b], Surlid[a,c]	Hoechst Marion Roussel
Clarithromycin	Abbotic[a], Biaxin[e], Biclar[a,e], Claricid[g], Clarith[a,e], Cyllind[a,e], Klacid[a,e,g], Klaciped[e], Klaricid[a,e], Kofron[a,e], Helillar[a], Macladin[a,e,g], Maclar[a], Mavil[a], Maxy[a], Veclam[a,e,g], Zaclon[a]	Abbott
Dirithromycin	Dinabac[a], Dynabac[a], Nortron[aa], Dimac[a]	Lilly
Azithromycin	Azitrocin[a], Ribotrex[a], Trozocina[a], Zithromax[a], Zitromax[a]	Pfizer

[a] Tablet.

[b] Powder for oral suspension.

[c] Powder for syrup.

[d] Powder in sachets.

[e] Granular.

[f] Intramuscular.

[g] Intravenous.

[h] Ointment.

[i] Drops.

uniformly elevated transaminase levels. Liver function tests revert to normal within days after discontinuation of drug but may recur after rechallenge (86). This toxicity may represent hypersensitivity and toxic reactions resulting from formation of nitrosoalkanes (230). Troleandomycin and erythromycin and its prodrugs form nitrosoalkanes. The semisynthetic macrolides rarely or never form nitrosoalkanes and therefore are unlikely to cause hepatotoxicity (229). Hepatotoxicity can occur with any erythromycin formulation (82, 219), although most initial reports implicated the estolate formulation (86). Elevated liver enzymes were reported with high-dose clarithromycin (2000 mg/day) in elderly patients (47).

Ototoxicity

The incidence of ototoxicity is uncertain, but it is probably underestimated. A prospective case-control study found evidence of ototoxicity in 21% of patients receiving 4 g/day of erythromycin, when audiograms were performed and patients were closely monitored (275). Subjective symptoms begin within the first week of drug administration (275), but are usually reversed within 1 to 30 days after discontinuation of the drug (49). However, irreversible unilateral tinnitus (169) and irreversible hearing loss (16) have been reported with intravenous administration of erythromycin lactobionate 4 and 2 g/day, respectively. Ototoxicity has also been reported with clarithromycin (72) and azithromycin (291).

The mechanism of erythromycin ototoxicity is not known, but it may involve an effect on the central auditory pathway (49) and is probably dose dependent (275). Auditory dysfunction is most common, but vestibular dysfunction may also occur (239). Erythromycin causes low local tinnitus, and hearing loss ranges from bilateral flat to high-frequency sensorineural loss, which can be detected on audiograms at both conventional (0.25–8.0 kHz) and extended high frequencies (8–14 kHz). Ototoxicity can occur with all formulations, including lactobionate and stearate (85). Preexisting hepatic or renal abnormalities, advanced age, high dosages, and concurrent ototoxic medications are predisposing factors (128, 285, 287). Ototoxicity has also been reported in patients without predisposing factors (16).

Other Adverse Reactions

Allergic reactions are rarely reported for all macrolides (229). Erythromycin administered intramuscularly can cause pain at the injection site and when administered intravenously causes thrombophlebitis (4%) (275). Qtc-interval prolongation with intravenous erythromycin use has been reported (143).

DRUG INTERACTIONS

Macrolide antibiotics may interact with several compounds, with possible effects on their pharmacokinetics (228). During the past 25 years, a number of case reports have incriminated macrolide antibiotics as a potential source of clinically severe drug interactions (289). However, some differences were found among the macrolide derivatives, and not all of them are potential sources of drug interactions. Dirithromycin, azithromycin, rokitamycin, and the older compound spiramycin have not been involved in drug interactions to date (116, 228).

Drug/Drug Interaction

Experimental in vitro and in vivo models have shown that macrolides selectively induce forms of cytochrome P-450 belonging to group IIIA, which are also involved in oxidation of other drugs such as theophylline, caffeine, and cyclosporine. The same enzymes are inducible by glucocorticosteroids that could be involved in complex drug interactions when associated with macrolide antibiotics for antimicrobial chemotherapy (228). Several reports indicate drug interaction due to the above mechanisms between erythromycin and other drugs such as natural and semisynthetic ergot alkaloids, oral contraceptives, carbamazepine, theophylline, lovastatin, the benzodiazepines triazolam and midazolam and the benzodiazepine clozapine, the antiarrhythmic agent disopyramide, warfarin, antipyrine, methylprednisolone, cyclosporine, alfentanil and sufentanil, terfenadine and astemizole and quinidine sulfate, rifampicin and rifabutin, zidovudine, antacids, cimetidine, bromocriptine, felodipine, glibenclamide, levodopa, phenytoin, and valproic acid (228, 289). Erythromycin inhibits degradation of digoxine in the gut and may lead to digoxine toxicity. The most frequently encountered interactions as well as rare one and those of dubious clinical importance are listed in Table 8.

In macrolides that have a second sugar attached to the amino sugar, this bulky molecule may prevent, by steric hindrance, close proximity between the tertiary amine and the iron of cytochrome P-450, thus reducing or preventing oxidation of the macrolide substrates and inactivation of the enzyme system. Conversely, the semisynthetic modifications of the

---

TABLE 8 • Clinically Important Drug Interactions with Macrolide Antibiotics[228,289]

Expected and well assessed

Astemizole[a]	Rifampin[b]
Carbamazepine[a]	Rifabutin[b]
Cyclosporin[a]	Terfenadine[a]
Disopyramide[a]	Theophylline[a]
Midazolam[a]	Triazolam[a]
Quinidine[a]	Zidovudine[a]

Rare or dubious

Alfentanil[a]	Felodipine[a]
Antacids (oral)[b]	Glibenclamide[a]
Bromocriptine[a]	Levodopa[b]
Caffeine[a]	Lovastatin[a]
Carbidopa[b]	Methylprednisolone[a]
Cimetidine[b]	Phenazone[a]
Clozapine[a]	Phenytoine[a]
Contraceptives (oral)[b]	Sufentanil[a]
Digoxin[a]	Valproic acid[a]
Ergot alkaloids[a]	Warfarin[a]

Data from references 228 and 289.

[a] Activity increased by macrolides (metabolic interaction).

[b] Interaction resulting in reduced macrolide activity (pharmacokinetic interaction).

aglycone ring can also decrease the macrolide nitrosoalkanes and consequent inhibition of cytochrome P-450.

Importance and Clinical Significance

The following structural features of macrolide antibiotics might be of critical importance in explaining the differences in pharmacokinetic drug interactions: first, the presence of an accessible tertiary amine function $N(CH_3)_2$ and the steric hindrance around this group and second (but no less important), the hydrophobicity of each molecule, which is proportional to its potency as a metabolite–cytochrome P-450 complex precursor (228). Thus, several factors could explain why only some macrolide antibiotics modify the plasma concentrations and therapeutic responses to drugs given in combination with them. In this respect, these antimicrobial drugs can be divided into the three subgroups shown in Figure 5.

Group 1 macrolides should be avoided in patients who must receive other drugs metabolized by cytochrome P-450. The possibility that macrolides in groups 2 and 3 should be avoided in patients simultaneously treated with pharmacologic agents such as theophylline, carbamazepine, ergot alkaloids, oral contraceptives, and methylprednisolone cannot be ruled out at present. It should be emphasized that the four compounds in group 3 (dirithromycin, azithromycin, rokitamycin, and spiramycin) do not form an inhibitory P-450-metabolite complex in vivo, even at very high doses, and the possibility of drug interactions should be extremely low (116, 228).

As a consequence of accelerated metabolism of all macrolides with rifampin and rifabutin, lower serum concentrations are seen. However, concomitant use of rifabutin, clarithromycin, and fluconazole has been associated with increased levels of rifabutin in patients with acquired immunodeficiency syndrome (AIDS), resulting in hypopyon uveitis (246) and arthralgias (35, 119).

CLINICAL INDICATIONS
Skin and Soft-Tissue Infections

In vitro erythromycin, roxithromycin, clarithromycin, dirithromycin, and azithromycin have good activity against most commonly isolated pathogens of skin and soft-tissue infections, namely, methicillin-sensitive *S. aureus,* methicillin-sensitive coagulase-negative staphylococci, *Streptococcus pyogenes,* and other *Streptococcus* species (Table 2). Erythromycin is the drug of choice for treating bacillary angiomatosis in patients with AIDS and treating erythrasma due to *Corynebacterium minitissimum* as well as an alternative drug for soft-tissue infections such as erysipelas and cellulitis due to streptococci.

Comparative studies showed that roxithromycin (150 mg twice daily for up to 14 days) was as effective and as well tolerated as the comparator drugs (doxycycline 200 mg once daily or penicillin 2.5 mU eight times daily intravenously, then 6 mU daily orally) in the treatment of skin and soft tissue infections (4, 34).

A comparative study in pediatric patients on the treatment of mild-to-moderate skin and skin-structure infections showed clarithromycin (7.5 mg/kg twice daily for 10 days) to be as effective and as safe as cefadroxil (15 mg/kg twice daily for 10 days). Equivalent clinical and bacteriologic response rates achieved with both drugs were above 90% (129). A comparative study showed dirithromycin (500 mg once daily for 5–7 days) to be as effective as erythromycin (250 mg four times daily for 7 days) with equivalent clinical and/or bacteriologic response rates in the treatment of subcutaneous abscess, pyoderma, and impetigo (79).

Comparative studies in pediatric patients with skin and/or soft-tissue infections showed azithromycin (10 mg/kg once daily for 3 days) to be as effective and as well tolerated as the comparator drugs (dicloxacillin 12.5–25 mg/kg or flu-

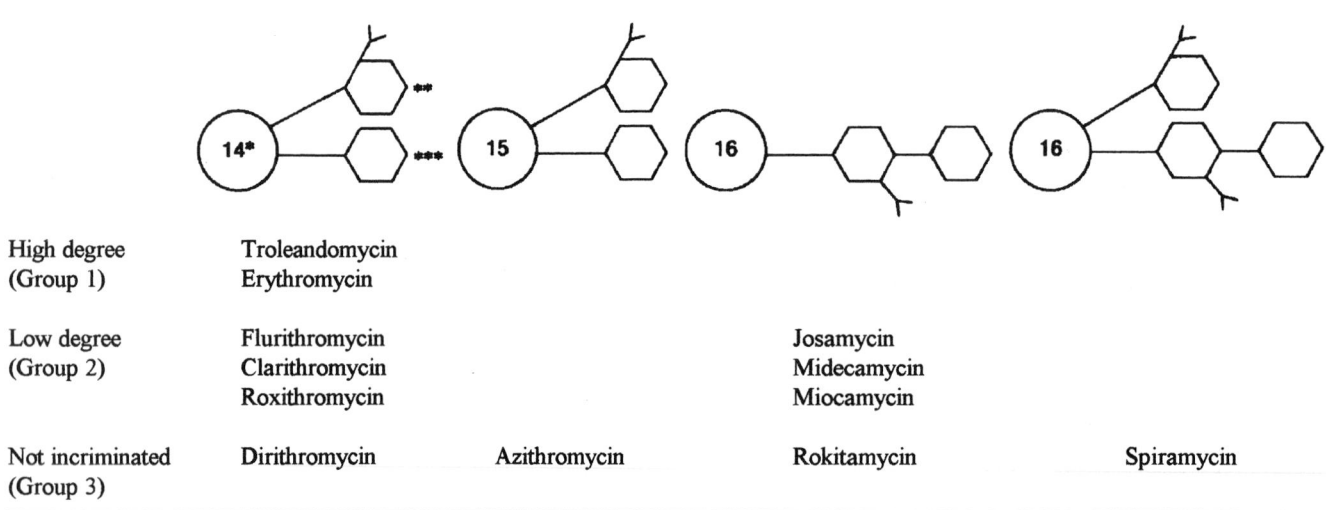

High degree (Group 1)	Troleandomycin Erythromycin			
Low degree (Group 2)	Flurithromycin Clarithromycin Roxithromycin		Josamycin Midecamycin Miocamycin	
Not incriminated (Group 3)	Dirithromycin	Azithromycin	Rokitamycin	Spiramycin

Symbols: * = n-membered aglycone macrolide ring; ** = amino sugar bearing a tertiary amine function; *** = neutral sugar

FIGURE 5. Correlations between the molecular structure and differential degree of drug interaction potential of macrolide antibiotics. (From reference 228.)

cloxacillin 250–2000 mg/day) administered for 7 to 10 days (203, 244). Once-daily (500 mg/day for 3 days) azithromycin appeared as effective and as safe in the treatment of adult skin and skin-structure infections as cephalexin (500 mg twice daily for 10 days) (152, 180) or dicloxacillin (250 mg four times a day for 7 days) (8). Equivalent clinical and bacteriologic response rates above 90% were achieved with all drugs.

Sexually Transmitted Diseases

In vitro erythromycin, roxithromycin, clarithromycin, dirithromycin, and azithromycin have good activity against commonly isolated pathogens of sexually transmitted diseases, namely, *N. gonorrhoeae, Chlamydia trachomatis, Mycoplasma* spp., and *Ureaplasma urealyticum* (Table 2). Erythromycin is the drug of choice in treating chlamydial infections in pregnancy and chancroid caused by *Haemophilus ducreyi.* Roxithromycin (150 mg twice daily for 10 days) was effective in eradicating 97% of the isolates of *C. trachomatis,* 88% of *U. urealyticum,* and 73% of *Mycoplasma hominis* in patients with nongonococcal urethritis (162).

Azithromycin (1-g single dose) was found to be effective in the treatment of clinically diagnosed chancroid, allowing single-visit treatment of genital ulcer disease when combined with a single injection of long-acting penicillin (20). Azithromycin (500 mg twice daily for one day, or 500 mg on day 1 followed by 250 mg on days 2 and 3, or 1000 mg as a single dose) was compared with doxycycline (100 mg twice daily for 7 days) in the treatment of sexually transmitted diseases in which the causative pathogens were *C. trachomatis, N. gonorrhoeae,* and *U. urealyticum.* All three regimens were found as effective as the standard treatment (267, 268, 298). Azithromycin (2-g single dose) was found as effective as ceftriaxone (250-mg single dose) in the treatment of uncomplicated gonorrhea (125). A comparative study in patients with nongonococcal urethritis showed single-dose azithromycin (1 g) to be as effective as doxycycline (100 mg twice daily for 7 days). The clinical response in chlamydia-positive patients was comparable in both treatment groups; the cure rate in chlamydia-negative patients was higher in the azithromycin group (164). However, another study showed comparable cure rates above 75% in the treatment of nongonococcal urethritis syndrome in men with either of the above regimens, regardless of the presence or absence of *Chlamydia* or *Ureaplasma* infection (265). The adverse effects were mild-to-moderate for both drugs in the mentioned studies. Two open noncomparative studies showed azithromycin (1-g single dose) to be effective in the treatment of gonococcal and nongonococcal urethritis (89, 234); all patients with gonococcal, chlamydial, and mixed infections were cured, and all baseline pathogens were eradicated, with only 8% of patients experiencing mild side effects (234).

Azithromycin (1 g in a single dose) was as effective as doxycycline (100 mg twice daily for 7 days) in the treatment of cervical infections caused by *C. trachomatis* in adults (185, 220) and adolescents (122). Azithromycin also might be a valid treatment option for cervical chlamydial infection during pregnancy (52). Limited studies with newer macrolides are available for other sexually transmitted diseases such as

syphilis. The efficacy of oral azithromycin (500 mg daily for 10 days or 500 mg on alternate days for 11 days) was studied in 100 patients with early syphilis and compared with results obtained in patients treated with erythromycin 2 g daily for 15 days or benzylpenicillin or benzathine-penicillin. Chancres like many other symptoms resolved more rapidly in patients treated with azithromycin than in those treated with other regimens. In 3 to 4 years of follow-up, no patient who received azithromycin showed any signs of visceral syphilis or neurosyphilis (186).

Respiratory Tract Infections

Erythromycin is one of the most effective antimicrobial agents for treatment of nonstreptococcal pharyngitis due to *Chlamydia pneumoniae* and *M. pneumoniae* (118, 192). It is very effective for pertussis infection, and decreases transmission in pertussis outbreaks (269). For diphtheria and the carrier state with *C. diphtheriae,* erythromycin is the drug of choice.

Pharyngitis

Erythromycin is the alternative therapy of choice for penicillin-allergic patients with group A β-hemolytic streptococcal pharyngitis (2), the most common bacterial cause of pharyngitis (156). The efficacy of roxithromycin for streptococcal pharyngitis remains uncertain. Two open studies found roxithromycin (300 mg once daily for 9 days or 150 mg twice a day for 7–14 days) effective for the treatment of tonsillopharyngitis, with 100 and 97% clinical success rates, respectively (76, 183). However, one study of 31 available patients (197) showed comparable clinical response (83% for 300 mg daily for 10 days and 100% for 150 mg twice a day for 10 days) but an unacceptable bacteriologic cure rate (33%) for both regimens. This study excluded patients considered to be carriers rather than infected. Tonsil concentrations of roxithromycin are somewhat lower than those of the other macrolides (112).

Comparative studies of clarithromycin (250 mg twice a day for 10 days) versus penicillin V (17, 168) and versus erythromycin (500 mg twice daily for 10 days) (248) in adults showed clinical and bacteriologic cure rates of about 90% without significant differences between the drugs. In children with streptococcal pharyngitis, clarithromycin (7.5 mg/kg twice a day for 10 days) was significantly more likely to produce bacteriologic cure than penicillin V (92 vs. 81%; $P < .004$), although clinical cure rates were identical (96 vs. 94%) (270). Gastrointestinal adverse effects were greater for clarithromycin (14%) than with penicillin V (5%; $P < .001$).

In adults with streptococcal pharyngitis, dirithromycin (500 mg once daily for 10 days) had comparable clinical and bacteriologic response to erythromycin (250 mg four times daily for 10 days) (78, 206). Cure rates were above 79% for both macrolides; gastrointestinal adverse effects were significantly more frequent for erythromycin (54 vs. 44%; $P < .01$) in the first study (78).

Azithromycin (10–12 mg/kg/day for 3 days for children; 500 mg initially, then 250 mg/day for 5 days for adults) was compared with penicillin V (125 or 250 mg three or four times daily for 10 days) and erythromycin (30–50 mg/kg/day for 10 days) in adults and children with streptococcal pharyngitis; efficacy was about 90%, both clinically and bacteriologically, for all drugs (121, 131, 214, 293). Adverse effects, mainly gastrointestinal, were significantly more frequent for azithromycin than for penicillin V in one study in adults (17 vs. 2%; P <.001) (131). However, azithromycin (12 mg/kg/day for 5 days) was statistically superior to penicillin V, both clinically (97 vs. 82%; P < .001) and bacteriologically (95 vs. 69%, P < .001) in a study of children (271), while another study found azithromycin (10/mg/kg once daily for 3 days) clinically as effective as penicillin V (100,000 IU/kg/day in three doses for 10 days) but inferior in eliminating group A β-hemolytic streptococci from the throat (250).

Otitis Media

Erythromycin-sulfisoxazole has long been standard therapy for acute otitis media (290). Long-term erythromycin (erythromycin base 600 mg/day for 4 months) was effective for the treatment of sinobronchial syndrome–associated otitis media with effusion (136). Clarithromycin (7.5 mg/kg twice a day for 10 days) compared with amoxicillin in the treatment of acute otitis media in children showed clinical success rates above 90% for both drugs, with no significant differences between the two drugs (237). Clarithromycin (7.5 mg/kg twice a day for 10 days) and amoxicillin/clavulanate showed clinical response rates above 90% in two comparative studies (14, 191); diarrhea (14, 191) (32 vs. 12%, P < .001; and 40 vs. 12%, P < .001) and diaper rash (14) (12 vs. 1%; P < .004) were significantly more common in patients treated with amoxicillin/clavulanate.

Azithromycin (5–10 mg/day for 3–5 days) compared with amoxicillin (202), amoxicillin/clavulanate (70, 195, 151, 231, 233, 249), or cefaclor (40 mg/kg daily in three divided doses for 10 days) (245) showed comparable clinical success of about 90%. However, a significantly higher incidence of side effects were found in the amoxicillin/clavulanate group in three studies (16 vs. 2.5%, 30.8 vs.8.8%, and 17.1 vs.7.2%; P < .001) (151, 195, 249) in contrast to the low incidence of adverse effects for the other studies mentioned. Azithromycin (10 mg/kg initially, then 5 mg/kg for 4 days) was comparable to amoxicillin/clavulanate in an another study, with 61 and 65% clinical response, respectively. Side effects (mostly diarrhea) were more common in the amoxicillin/clavulanate group (17 vs. 7%; P < .001) (151). Azithromycin (10 mg/kg once daily for 6 months) was found to be a valid alternative to amoxicillin (20 mg/kg once daily for 6 months) in preventing recurrent acute otitis media in children, without substantial modifications of the nasopharyngeal flora (181).

Sinusitis

Clarithromycin (500 mg twice a day for 10–14 days) was comparable to amoxicillin and amoxicillin/clavulanate for therapy of acute maxillary sinusitis in adults (84, 147). Clinical success rates were about 90%, with comparable radiologic and bacteriologic outcomes for all drugs. However, amoxicillin/clavulanate had significantly more gastrointestinal side effects than clarithromycin (38 vs. 21%, P < .001).

Azithromycin (500 mg initially, then 250 mg/day for 5 days) was comparable to amoxicillin for therapy of acute maxillary and frontal sinusitis as defined by radiologic and bacteriologic criteria, with success rates above 70% for both drugs (56, 93). Azithromycin (500 mg daily for 3 days) was comparable to clarithromycin (250 mg twice a day for 10 days) with clinical and bacteriologic response rates above 90% for both drugs for the treatment of adult patients with acute sinusitis (205).

Bronchitis

Roxithromycin (300 mg once daily for 7 days) was comparable to sparfloxacin (400 mg initially, then 200 mg/day for 5 days) for the same indication, with cure rates of 85% for both drugs (157). Clarithromycin (250 mg twice a day for 7–14 days) was comparable to ampicillin (250 mg four times daily for 7–14 days) for the treatment of patients with acute bacterial exacerbations of chronic bronchitis. Clinical success rates were about 90%, with comparable bacteriologic outcomes for all drugs (6). Dirithromycin (500 mg once a day for 5–7 days) compared with erythromycin (250 mg four times daily for 7 days) or clarithromycin (250 mg twice daily) showed clinical and bacteriologic efficacy above 80% for both drugs for the same indication (111, 134, 263). Azithromycin (500 mg once a day for 3 days) was as effective, clinically and microbiologically, as amoxicillin/clavulanate (625 mg thrice daily for 10 days) or amoxicillin (500 mg thrice daily for 5 days) in the treatment of acute lower respiratory tract infections and acute bacterial exacerbations of chronic bronchitis (13, 21, 130, 200).

Pneumonia

Despite the fact that macrolides cover the major pathogens responsible for community-acquired pneumonia (91), including *S. pneumoniae, Legionella* sp., *C. trachomatis, M. pneumoniae,* and *H. influenzae,* only limited studies are available. However the drug of choice for treatment of community-acquired pneumonia is a macrolide (10). Erythromycin (1 g twice daily for 7–14 days) was as effective (85%) as the comparator drugs sparfloxacin (87%) and amoxicillin/clavulanic acid (80%) in the treatment of community-acquired pneumonia (173). Two studies comparing clarithromycin (250 mg twice daily for 14 days for adults and 15 mg/kg/day twice daily for 10 days for children) and erythromycin (500 mg four times a day for 14 days and 40 mg/kg/day twice or thrice daily for 10 days) found clinical success or radiologic response of about 90% for both drugs (11, 40).

Adverse effects were significantly higher in the erythromycin group (19 vs. 4%; P < .01) in the first study (11). Dirithromycin (500 mg once daily for 10–14 days) was as effective as erythromycin (250 mg four times daily for 10–14 days) in the treatment of community-acquired pneumonia (139, 170). Azithromycin (250 mg twice daily on day 1 followed by 250 mg once daily for a total of 3 to 5 days) was found as effective as erythromycin (500 mg four times daily for 10 days) or roxithromycin (150 mg twice daily for 10 days) in the treatment of atypical pneumonias in which causative pathogens were identified serologically (253–255). Azithromycin (500 mg once daily for 3 days) was effective and well tolerated in patients with community-acquired pneumonia in three studies with 89, 96, and 77.5% clinical cure rates (130, 207, 246). The main pathogens were *S. pneumoniae* and *Legionella pneumophila* in the second study (207). The comparator drug was amoxicillin-clavulanic acid (625 mg thrice daily for 10 days), with cure rates of 88 and less than 80.5% in the first and third studies (130, 246).

Azithromycin (500 mg once daily for 3 days) compared with clarithromycin (250 mg twice daily for 10 days) in the treatment of adults with mild-to-moderate community-acquired pneumonia showed clinical response rates of 95% and bacterial eradication rates of 97% for azithromycin and 91% for clarithromycin, with similar adverse effects rates (7 vs. 8%) (214). Azithromycin was as effective as cefuroxime plus erythromycin for hospitalized patients with community-acquired pneumonia (288). A study conducted in the pediatric age group found azithromycin (10 mg/kg day for 3 days) as effective as erythromycin (40–50 mg/kg/day for 10 days) in the treatment of lower respiratory tract infections (7).

Other Infections

Prevention of Bacterial Endocarditis
Updated prophylactic regimens for dental, oral, respiratory tract, or esophageal procedures recommended by the American Heart Association for prevention of bacterial endocarditis in individuals at risk for this disease and penicillin-allergic included clarithromycin for children (15 mg/kg orally 1 h before the procedure) and azithromycin for adults (500 mg orally 1 h before the procedure) (9).

Mycobacterium avium Complex (MAC) Disease
The United States Public Health Service recommended that every regimen for the treatment of MAC disease contain either clarithromycin (500–1000 mg twice daily) or azithromycin (500 mg daily) and preferably ethambutol as a second drug (236). A newer study suggested that not this drug especially but multidrug therapy with or without clarithromycin was essential for the treatment of disseminated MAC disease (155). Once-weekly azithromycin (1200 mg) was found more effective than daily rifabutin for protection against disseminated MAC disease in a trial with 693 HIV-infected patients. Rifabutin plus azithromycin was even more effective but not well tolerated (127). Other prospective controlled clinical trials should clarify the optimal regimen for disseminated MAC disease.

Helicobacter pylori Infections
Clarithromycin (250 mg for 14 days) combined with omeprazole and/or metronidazole eradicated *H. pylori* very effectively (83%), with frequent but mild side effects (62, 174). These regimens were also shown to be more cost-effective in patients with duodenal ulcer disease than episodic therapy with omeprazole or maintenance therapy with ranitidine (140).

Toxoplasmosis
Although pyrimethamine/sulfadiazine is the most effective combination in the treatment of acute toxoplasmosis, limited

in vitro and in vivo studies suggest that azithromycin and clarithromycin may have an important role in the treatment or prophylaxis of toxoplasmosis (60, 80, 94). Spiramycin, although used for prevention of congenital toxoplasmosis during pregnancy, cannot be recommended for eradication of the most severe forms of toxoplasmosis (59).

Trachoma
Two controlled studies showed single-dose azithromycin (20 mg/kg) to be as effective as a 6-week course of topical tetracycline ointment or tetracycline plus erythromycin ointments in the treatment of active trachoma, without any adverse effects. This finding may help establish high compliance in treating trachoma and could contribute to its control (19, 251, 277).

Mediterranean Spotted Fever
Azithromycin (10 mg/kg/day for 3 days) was found as effective as doxycycline (5 mg/kg/day for 5 days) in the treatment of children infected with Mediterranean spotted fever due to *Rickettsia conorii* (208).

Lyme Disease
Clarithromycin (500 mg twice daily for 21 days) was found effective in the treatment of early Lyme disease due to *Borrelia burgdorferi* with 91% complete response of evaluable patients at the end of therapy (71). Azithromycin (500 mg on day 1, followed by 250 mg once a day for 4 days, or 500 mg twice daily on day 1 followed by 500 mg once daily for 4 days) was found as effective as amoxicillin (500 mg), probenecid (500 mg thrice daily for 10 days) and doxycycline (100 mg twice daily for 10 or 14 days) in the treatment of early Lyme disease (187, 273). Six of 19 patients (32%) given amoxicillin/probenecid developed a drug eruption, whereas none of the patients given azithromycin or doxycycline had this complication (187). However, another study enrolling 246 patients showed fewer relapses with a 20-day course of amoxicillin (500 mg three times a day) than with a 7-day course azithromycin (500 mg once daily) (4 vs. 16%; $P < .005$) in the treatment of erythema migrans (177).

Shigellosis
Azithromycin (500 mg on day 1 followed by 250 mg once daily for 4 days) was as effective as ciprofloxacin (500 mg twice daily for 5 days) in the treatment of shigellosis due to multidrug-resistant *Shigella* species. Both azithromycin and ciprofloxacin were less effective in patients infected with *Shigella dysenteriae* type 1 than in patients infected with other *Shigella* species (150).

REFERENCES

1. Adachi T, Morimoto S, Kondoh H, Nagate T, Watanabe Y, Sota K. 14-hydroxy-6-O- methylerythromycins A: active metabolites of 6-O- methylerythromycin A in human. J Antibiot 1988;41:966–975.
2. Adam D, Scholz H, and the Pharyngitis Study Group. Five days of erythromycin estolate versus ten days of penicillin V in the treatment of group A streptococcal tonsillopharyngitis in children. Eur J Clin Microbiol Infect Dis 1996;15:712–717.

3. Agaçfidan A, Moncado J, Schacter J. In vitro activity of azithromycin (CP-62,993) against *Chlamydia trachomatis* and *Chlamydia pneumoniae*. Antimicrobial Agents Chemother 1993; 37:1746–1748.

4. Agache P, Amblard P, Moulin G, Barriere H, Texier L, Beylot C, Bergoend H. Roxithromycin in skin and soft tissue infection. J Antimicrob Chemother 1987;20(Suppl B):153–156.

5. Akalin HE, Pontani D, Washton H, Johnson JL. The Artemis Project: an international antimicrobial susceptibility surveillance study [Abstract 330]. 8th European Congress Infect Dis Clin Microbiol, Lausanne, 1997:270.

6. Aldons PM. A comparison of clarithromycin with ampicillin in the treatment of out-patients with acute bacterial exacerbations of chronic bronchitis. J Antimicrob Chemother 1991;27(Suppl A):101–108.

7. Alimenti A, Franckart G, Waelbrock A, De Mol P, Lewy J. Azithromycin versus erythromycin in the treatment of lower respiratory tract infections in children [Abstract 13.18]. 3rd Int Conference on the macrolides, azalides and streptogramins, Lisbon 1996:91.

8. Amaya-Tapia G, Aguirre-Avalos G, Andrade-Villanueva J, Peredo- Gonzales G, Morfin-Otero R, Esperza-Ahumada S, Rodriguez-Noriega E. Once daily azithromycin in the treatment of adult skin and skin-structure infections. J Antimicrobiol Chemother 1993;(Suppl E):129–135.

9. American Heart Association. Prevention of bacterial endocarditis. JAMA 1997;277:1794–1801.

10. American Thoracic Society. Guidelines for the initial management of adults with community-acquired pneumonia: diagnosis, assessment of severity and initial antimicrobial chemotherapy. Am Rev Respir Dis 1993;148:1418–1426.

11. Anderson G, Esmonde TS, Coles S, Macklin J, Carnegie C. A comparative safety and efficacy of clarithromycin and erythromycin stearate in community acquired pneumonia. J Antimicrob Chemother 1991;27(Suppl A):117–124.

12. Arnold B, Ta A, Stout JE, Yu VL. Erythromycin, dirithromycin, azithromycin, clarithromycin, and roxithromycin activity against *Legionella* by broth dilution and intracellular penetration [Abstract E29]. 34th Intersci Conf Antimicrob Agents Chemother, Orlando, 1994:156.

13. Aronovitz G. A multicenter, open label trial of azithromycin vs. amoxicillin/clavulanate for the management of acute otitis media in children. Pediatr Infect Dis J 1996;15:S15–19.

14. Aspin MM, Hobermann A, McCarty J, et al. Comparative study of the safety and efficacy of clarithromycin and amoxicillin-clavulanate in the treatment of acute otitis media in children. J Pediatr 1994;125:136–141.

15. Auckenthaler RW, Zwahlen A, Waldvogel FA. Macrolides. In Peterson KP, Varholf J, eds. The antimicrobial agents annual/2. Amsterdam: Elsevier, 1987:31–38.

16. Augusti C, Ferran F, Gea J, Picado C. Ototoxic reaction to erythromycin. Arch Intern Med 1991;151:380.

17. Bachand RT Jr. A comparative study of clarythromycin and penicillin VK in the treatment of streptococcal pharyngitis. J Antimicrob Chemother 1991;27:75–82.

18. Bachman K, Jauregui L, Sides G, Sullivan TJ. Steady state pharmacokinetics of theophylline in COPD patients treated with dirithromycin. J Clin Pharmacol 1993;33:861–865.

19. Bailey RL. Randomized controlled trial of single dose-azithromycin in tratment of trachoma. Lancet 1993;342:453–456.

20. Ballard RC, Ye H, Matta A, Dangor Y, Radebe F. Treatment of chancroid with azithromycin. Int J STD AIDS 1996;7(Suppl 1):9–12.

21. Balmes P, Clerc G, Dupont B, Labram C, Pariente R, Poirier R. Comparative study of azithromycin and amoxicillin/clavulanic acid in the treatment of lower respiratory tract infections. Eur J Clin Microbiol Infect Dis 1990;10:437–439.

22. Baohong JI, Lounis N, Truffot-Pernot, Grosset J. Selection of resistant mutants of *Mycobacterium avium* in beige mice by clarithromycin monotherapy. Antimicrob Agents Chemother 1992; 36:2839–2840.

23. Baquero F, Loza E. Antibiotic resistance of microorganisms involved in ear, nose and throat infections. Pediatric Infect Dis J 1994;13:S9–S14.

24. Barry AL, Fuchs PC. In vitro activities of a streptogramin (RP59500), three macrolides, and an azalide against four respiratory tract pathogens. Antimicrob Agents Chemother 1995;39: 238–240.

25. Bass JW, Weisse ME, Plymyer MR, Murphy S, Eberly BJ. Decline of erythromycin resistance of group A beta hemolytic streptococci in Japan: comparison with worldwide reports. Arch Pediatr Adolesc Med 1994;148:67–71.

26. Baughman RP, DeSante KA, Lanier TL, Conforti PM, Sides GD. The penetration of dirithromycin into bronchoalveolar lavage fluid and alveolar macrophages. J Antimicrob Chemother 1994;33:1045–1050.

27. Bégué P, Lacombe H, Cotin G. Diffusion of roxithromycin into tonsillar tissue in children. Br J Clin Pract 1988;42(Suppl 55): 78–79.

28. Bergan T, Engeset A, Olszewski W. Does serum protein binding inhibit tissue penetration of antibiotics? Rev Infect Dis 1987;9: 713–718.

29. Bergogne-Bérézin E, Morel C, Even P, Benard Y, Kafe H, Berthelot G, Pierre J, Lambert-Zechovsky N. Pharmacocinétique des antibiotiques dans les voies respiratoires. Nouv Presse Med 1978;7:2831–2836.

30. Bergogne-Bérézin E. The tissue penetration of macrolides with particular reference to the respiratory tract. In: Butzler JP, Kobayashi H, eds. Macrolides: a review with an outlook on future developments. Amsterdam: Excerpta Medica, 1986:43–53.

31. Bergogne-Bérézin E. Tissue distribution of roxithromycin. J Antimicrob Chemother 1987;20(Suppl B):113–120.

32. Bergogne-Bérézin E, Bertholet G, Uzzan J, Ravina JH. Evaluation of placental transfer of roxithromycin in late pregnancy [Abstract 10977]. 27th ICAAC, New York 1987:285.

33. Bergogne-Bérézin E. Tissue distribution of dirithromycin: comparison with erythromycin. J Antimicrob Chemother 1993;31 (Suppl C):77–87.

34. Bernard P, Plantin P, Roger H. Roxithromycin versus penicillin in the treatment of erysipelas in adults: a comparative study. Br J Dermatol 1992;127:155–159.

35. Berning SE, Peloquin CA. Adverse events associated with high dose rifabutin in macrolide containing regimens for the treatment of Mycobacterium avium complex lung disease [Letter]. Clin Infect Dis 1996;22:885.

36. Betriu C, Sanchez A, Gomez M. Antibiotic susceptibility of group A streptococci. A 6 year follow-up study. Antimicrob Agents Chemother 1993;37:1717–1719.

37. Birkett DJ, Robson RA, Grgurinovich N, Tonkin A. Single oral dose pharmacokinetics of erythromycin and roxithromycin and the effects of chronic dosing. Ther Drug Monit 1990;12:65–71.

38. Blanc F, D'Enfert J, Fiessinger S. An evaluation of tolerance of roxithromycin in adults. J Antimicrob Chemother 1987;20: 179–183.

39. Blenk H, Simm K, Blenk B, Jahnake G. Vergleich von Erythromycin und Sinusgewebe bei Patienten mit Tonsillitis und Sinüsitis. Infektion 1982;10(Suppl 2):108–112.

40. Block S, Hedrick J, Hammerschlag MR, Cassell GH, Craft JC.

Mycoplasma pneumoniae and *Chlamydia pneumoniae* in pediatric community-acquired pneumonia: comparative efficacy and safety of clarithromycin vs. erythromycin ethylsuccinate. Pediatr Infect Dis J 1995:14:471–477.

41. Bohte R, van't Wout JW, Lobatto S, Blusse van Oud Alblas A, Boekhout M, Nauta EH, Hermans J, van den Broek PJ. Efficacy and safety of azithromycin versus benzylpenicillin or erythromycin in community acquired pneumonia. Eur J Clin Microbiol Infect Dis 1995;14:182–187.

42. Bonnefoy A, Girard AM, Agouridas C, Chantot JF. Ketolides lack inducibility properties of MLS$_B$ resistance phenotype. J Antimicrob Chemother 1997;40:85–90.

43. Bozler G, Heinzel G, Lechner U, et al. Pharmacokinetic properties and metabolic behaviour of dirithromycin determine its high tissue penetration in man [Abstract 924]. 28th International Conference on Antimicrobial Agents and Chemotherapy, Los Angeles, 1988:274.

44. Brisson-Nöel A, Trieu-Ccuot P, Courvalin P. Mechanism of action of spiramycin and other macrolides. J Antimicrobiol Chemother 1988;(Suppl B):13–23.

45. Brittain DC. Update on antibiotics I. Erythromycin. Med Clin North Am 1987;71:1147–1154.

46. Brogden RN, Peters DH. Dirithromycin. A review of its antimicrobial activity, pharmacokinetic properties and therapeutic efficacy. Drugs 1994;48:509–616.

47. Brown BA, Wallace RJ Jr, Griffith DE, Girad W. Clarithromycin induced hepatotoxicity [Letter]. Clin Infect Dis 1995;20:1073–1074.

48. Brown BA, Wallace RJ Jr, Only GO. Activities of clarythromycin and other antimicrobial agents against eight slowly growing species of nontuberculous mycobacteria, determined by using a broth microdilution MIC system. Antimicrob Agents Chemother 1992;36:1987–1990.

49. Brummet RE. Ototoxic liability of erythromycin and analogues. Otolaryngol Clin North Am 1993;26:61–68.

50. Bryskier A, Chanton JF, Gasc JC. Classification and structure-activity relationships of macrolides with emphasis on new developments. In: Butzler JP, Kobayashi K, eds. Macrolides: a review with an outlook on future developments. Amsterdam: Excerpta Medica, 1986:7–21.

51. Bryskier A. Roxithromycin: review of its antimicrobial activity. J Antimicrob Chemother 1998;41(suppl B):1–21.

52. Bush MR, Rosa C. Azithromycin and erythromycin in the treatment of cervical chlamydial infection during pregnancy. Obstet Gynecol 1994;84:61–63.

53. Carlier MB, Zenebergh A, Tulkens PM. Cellular uptake and subcellular distribution of roxithromycin and erythromycin in phagocytic cells. J Antimicrob Chemother 1987;20(Suppl B):47–56.

54. Carlone NA, Ciuffini AM, Del Mastro S, Bonino S. Determinazione microbiologica dei livelli tonsillari ed oculari di josamicina in soggetti ospedalizzati. G Ital Chemioter 1982;29(Suppl 1):77–83.

55. Carson JL, Strom BL, Duff A. Acute liver disease associated with erythromycin, sulfonamides, and tetracyclines. Ann Intern Med 1993;119:576–583.

56. Casione RR. Azithromycin and amoxicillin in the treatment of acute maxillary sinusitis. Am J Med 1991;91 Suppl 3A:27S–30S.

57. Centers for Disease Control and Prevention. Erythromycin resistant *Bordetella pertussis*—Yuma County, Arizona, May–October 1994. JAMA 1995;273:13–14.

58. Champney WS, Burdine R. 50S Ribosomal subunit synthesis and translation are equivalent targets for erythromycin inhibition in *Staphylococcus aureus*. Antimicrob Agents Chemother 1996;40:1301–1303.

59. Chang HR, Pechere JCF. Activity of spiramycin against *Toxo-*

60. plasma gondii in vitro, in experimental infections and in human infection. J Antimicrob Chemother 1988;22(Suppl B):87–92.

60. Chang HR. The potential role of azithromycin in the treatment or prophylaxis of toxoplasmosis. Int J STD AIDS 1996;7(Suppl 1):18–22.

61. Chastre J, Brun P, Fourtillan JB, Soler P, Basset G, Manuel C, Trouillet JL, Gibert C. Pulmonary disposition of roxithromycin (RU 28965), a new macroide antibiotic. Antimicrob Agents Chemother 1987;31:1312–1316.

62. Chiba N. Omeprazole and clarithromycin with and without metronidazole for the eradication of Helicobacter pylori. Am J Gastroenterol 1996;91:2139–2143.

63. Chow AW. Erythromycin. In: Rustica AM, Cunha BA, eds. Antimicrobial Chemotherapy. New York: Raven Press, 1984:209–218.

64. Chu SY, Wilson DS, Eason C, Deaton RL. Single and multi-dose pharmacokinetics of clarithromycin [Abstract 759]. 30th Annual Interscience Conference on Antimicrobial Agents and Chemotherapy, Atlanta, GA, October, 1990.

65. Chu SY, Park Y, Locke C, Wilson DS, Cavanaugh C. Drug-food interaction potential of clarithromycin, a new macrolide antimicrobial. J Clin Pharmacol 1992;32:32–36.

66. Chu SY, Wilson DS, Guay DR, Craft C. Clarithromycin pharmacokinetics in healthy young and elderly volunteers. J Clin Pharmacol 1992;32:1045–1049.

67. Clauzel AM, Simeon de Buochberg M, Jars N, Michel FB. Etude du passage de la midécamycine dans les expectorations. Nouv Presse Med 1981;10:1658.

68. Conte JE Jr, Golden J, Duncan S, McKenna E, Lin E, Zurlinden E. Single dose intrapulmoner pharmacokinetics of azithromycin, clarithromycin, ciprofloxacin and cefuroxime in volunteer subjects. Antimicrobial Agents Chemother 1996;40:1617–1622.

69. Daniel R and European Azithromycin Study Group. Azithromycin, erythromycin and cloxacillin in the treatment of infection of skin and associated soft tissues. J Int Med Res 1991;19:433–445.

70. Daniel R. Comparison of azithromycin and co-amoxyclav in the treatment of otitis media in children. J Antimicrob Chemother 1993;31(Suppl E):65–71.

71. Dattwyler RJ, Grünwald E, Luft BJ. Clarithromycin in the treatment of early Lyme disease: a pilot study. Antimicrob Agents Chemother 1996;40:468–469.

72. Dautzenberg B, Saint Marc T, Meyohas MC. Clarithromycin and other antimicrobial agents in the treatment of disseminated *Mycobacterium avium* infections in patients with acquired immuno-deficiency syndrome. Arch Intern Med 1993;153:368–372.

73. Davey PG. The pharmacokinetics of clarithromycin and its 14-0H metabolite. J Hosp Infect 1991;19(Suppl A):29–37.

74. De Louvois J. Factors influencing the assay of antimicrobial drugs in clinical samples by the agar plate diffusion method. J Antimicrob Chemother 1982;9:253.

75. Debets-Ossenkopp YJ, Sparrius M, Kusters JG, Kolkman JJ, Vandenbroucke-Grauls CM. Mechanism of clarithromycin resistance in clinical isolates of *Helicobacter pylori*. FEMS Microbiol Lett 1996;15;142:37–38.

76. de Campora E, Carnaioni A, Leonardi M, Fardella P, Fiaoni M. Comparative efficacy and safety of roxithromycin and clarithromycin in upper respiratory tract infections. Diagn Microbiol Infect Dis 1992;15:119S–122S.

77. Derby LE, Jick H, Henry DA, Dean AD. Erythromycin associated cholestatic hepatitis. Med J Aust 1993;158:600–602.

78. Deriennic M, Conforti PM, Sides GD. Dirithromycin in the treat-

ment of streptococcal pharyngitis. J Antimicrob Chemother 1993;31:89–95.

79. Deriennic M, Escande JP. Dirithromycin in the treatment of skin and skin structure infections. J Antimicrob Chemother 1993;31 (Suppl C):159–168.

80. Derouin F. New pathogens and mode of action of azithromycin: *Toxoplasma gondii*. Pathol Biol Paris 1995;43:561–564.

81. Dette GA, Knothe H, Koulen G. Comparative in vitro activity, serum binding and binding activity interactions of macrolides A-56 258, RU-28965, erythromycin and josamycin. Drugs Exp Clin Res 1987;13:567–576.

82. Diehl AM, Latham P, Boitnott JK. Cholestatic hepatitis from erythromycin ethylsuccinate: report of two cases. Am J Med 1984;76:931–934.

83. Disse B, Gundert-Remy U, Weber E, Andrassy K, Sietzen W, Lang A. Pharmacokinetics of erythromycin in patients with different degrees of renal impairment. Int J Clin Pharmacol Ther Toxicol 1986;24:460–464.

84. Dubois J, Saint-Pierre C, Tremblay C. Efficacy of clarithromycin versus amoxicillin/clavulanate in the treatment of acute maxillary sinusitis. Ear Nose Throat J 1993;72:804–810.

85. Dylewski J. Irreversible sensorineural hearing loss due to erythromycin. Can Med Assoc J 1988;139:230–231.

86. Eichenwald HF. Adverse reactions to erythromycin. Pediatr Infect Dis J 1986;5:147–150.

87. Ellis LC, Benson CA, Koenig GI, Trenholme GM. Postantibiotic effect of clarithromycin alone and combined with ethambutol against *Mycobacterium avium* complex. Antimicrob Agents Chemother 1995;39:2803–2806.

88. Ellsworth AJ, Christensen DB, Volpone-McMahon MT. Prospective comparison of patient tolerance to enteric-coated vs. nonenteric- coated erythromycin. J Fam Pract 1990;31:265–270.

89. Erdogru T, Agacfidan A, Önel M, Badur S, Ang Ö, Tellaloglu S. The treatment of non-gonococcal urethritis with single dose oral azithromycin. J Int Med Res 1995;23:386–393.

90. Fagioli A, Cruciani E, Riario Sforza G, Ferrone G, Di Silverio F. Livelli tissutali prostatici di josamicina. G Ital Chemioter 1982:(Suppl 1):85–87.

91. Fang GD, Fine M, Orloff J, Arisumi D, Yu VL, Kapoor W, Grayston JT, Wang SP, Kohler R, Muder RR; Yee YC, Rihs JD, Vickers RM. New and emerging etiologies for community acquired pneumonia with implication for therapy: a prospective multicenter study of 359 cases. Medicine (Baltimore) 1990;69:307–316.

92. Fass RJ. Erythromycin, clarithromycin and azithromycin: use of frequency distribution curves, scattergrams, and regression analyses to compare in vitro activities and describe cross resistance. Antimicrob Agents Chemother 1993;37:2080–2086.

93. Felstead SJ, Daniel R, and the European Azithromycin Study Group. Short course treatment of sinusitis and other respiratory tract infections with azithromycin. J Int Med Res 1991;19: 363–372.

94. Fernandez-Martin J, Leport C, Morlat P. Pyrimethamine-clarithromycin combination for therapy of acute toxoplasma encephalitis in patients with AIDS. Antimicrob Agents Chemother 1991;35:2049–2052.

95. Ferrero JL, Bopp BA, Marsh KC, Quigley SC, Johnson MJ, Anderson DJ, Lamm JE, Tolman KG, Sanders SW, Cavanaugh JH. Metabolism and disposition of clarithromycin in man. Drug Metab Dispos 1990;18: 441–446.

96. Fioretti M, Bandera M, Rimoldi R. Attività terapeutica e comportamento farmacocinetico della miocamicina a livello dell'apparato respiratorio. G Ital Chemioter 1984;31:145–148.

97. Fish DN, Gotfried MH, Danziger LH, Rodvold KA. Penetration of clarithromycin into lung tissues from patients undergoing lung resection. Antimicrobial Agents Chemother 1994;38: 876–878.

98. Foulds G, Shepard RM, Johnson RB. The pharmacokinetics of azithromycin in human serum and tissues. J Antimicrob Chemother 1990;25(Suppl A):73–82.

99. Foulds G, Madssen P, Cox C, Shepard R, Johnson R. Concentration of azithromycin in human prostatic tissue. Eur J Clin Microbiol Infect Dis 1991;10:868–871.

100. Foulds G, Chan KH, Johnson JT, Shepard RM, Johnson RB. Concentration of azithromycin in human tonsillar tissue. Eur J Clin Microbiol Infect Dis 1991;10:853–856.

101. Fourtillan JB, Lefèbvre MA, Gobin P. Josamycin chemical determination in biological fluids. G Ital Chemioter 1982;29 (Suppl 1):103–108.

102. Fourtillan JB, Lefèbvre MA, Ghanassia JP. Pharmacokinetic handling of josamycin and its metabolites during oral repeated dosing in man. In: Spitzy KH, Karrer S, eds. Proceedings of the 13th International Congress of Chemotherapy, Vienna, 1983, vol 5, Egermann Druckereigesellschaft, 1983:SS 4.4/1–2, 36/11–14.

103. Fraschini F, Braga PC, Gagliardi V, Falchi M, Scaglione F, Scarpazza G, Manganelli V. Farmacocinetica della josamicina nell'uomo e distribuzione in vari compartimenti. G Ital Chemioter 1982;29(Suppl 1):69–76.

104. Fraschini F, Scaglione F, Cantarella Marchi E. Plasma and tissue concentrations of miocamycin in humans. In Ishigami, ed. Recent advances in chemotherapy. Proceedings of the 14th International Congress of Chemotherapy, 23–28 June 1985. Antimicrobial section 2. Tokyo: University of Tokyo Press, 1985:1447–1449.

105. Fraschini F, Scaglione F, Pintucci G, Maccarinelli G, Dugnani S, Demartini G. The diffusion of clarithromycin and roxithromycin into nasal mucosa, tonsil and lung humans. J Antimicrob Chemother 1991;27(Suppl 4):61–65.

106. Fraschini F, Scaglione F, Demartini G. Clarithromycin clinical pharmacokinetics. Clin Pharmacokinet 1993;25:189–204.

107. Fukaya K, Shomura S, Kitai S, Murata S, Umemura K. Absorption, metabolism and excretion of 9,3″-diacetyl-midecamycin (MOM) in humans. Acta Toxicol Ther 1981;2:45–64.

108. Fukaya K, Watanabe S, Fujita M. Absorption and excretion of miocamycin tablets and dry syrup. In: Ishigami J, ed. Recent advances in chemotherapy. Proceedings of the 14th International Congress of Chemotherapy, Kyoto, 23–28 June 1986. Antimicrobial section 2. Tokyo: University of Tokyo Press, 1985: 1450–1451.

109. Furneri PM, Scalia G, Garozzo A, Tempera G. Some pharmacokinetic data on miocamycin I. Serum, urinary and prostatic levels. Drugs Exp Clin Res 1988;14:755–762.

110. Furneri PM, Cianci A, Garozzo A. Some pharmacokinetic data on miocamycin II. Concentrations in gynaecological tissues. Drugs Exp Clin Res 1991;17:181–186.

111. Gaillat J. A multicenter study comparing the safety and efficacy of dirithromycin with erythromycin in the treatment of bronchitis. J Antimicrob Chemother 1993;31(Suppl C):139–151.

112. Galioto GB, Ortisi G, Mevio E, Sassella D, Bartacci F, Privitera G. Roxithromycin disposition in tonsils after single and repeated administration. Antimicrobial Agents Chemother 1988;32:1461–1463.

113. Gan VN, Chu SY, Kusmiesz HT, Craft JC. Pharmacokinetics of a clarithromycin suspension in infants and children. Antimicrob Agents Chemother 1992;36:2478–2480.

114. Garrod LP, Lambert HP, O'Grady F. Macrolides and lincosamides. In: O'Grady FW, Lambert HP, Finch RG, Greenwood D, eds. Antibiotic and chemotherapy. London: Churchill Livingstone, 1981:183–201.

115. Ghanassia JP, Modai J, Fourtillan JB. Pharmacokinetics of josamycin in young adults and geriatric patients. In: Periti P, Gialdroni Grassi G, eds. Current chemotherapy and immunotherapy. Proceedings of the 12th International Congress of Chemotherapy, Florence, 19–24 July 1981, vol II. Washington, DC: American Society for Microbiology, 1985:89–90.

116. Gillum JG, Israel D, Scott B, Climo MW, Polk RE. Effect of combination therapy with ciprofloxacin and clarithromycin on theophylline pharmacokinetics in healthy volunteers. Antimicrobial Agents Chemother 1996;40:1715–1716.

117. Goldstein EJ, Nesbit CA, Citron DM. Comparative in vitro activities of azithromycin, Bay y 3118, levofloxacin, sparfloxacin, and 11 other oral antimicrobial agents against 194 aerobic and anaerobic bite wound isolates. Antimicrob Agents Chemother 1995;39:1097–1100.

118. Grayston JT. *Chlamydia pneumoniae,* strain TWAR: review. Chest 1989;95:664–669.

119. Griffith DE, Brown BA, Girard WM, Wallace RJ Jr. Adverse events associated with high dose rifabutin in macrolide containing regimens for the treatment of *Mycobacterium avium* complex lung disease. Clin Infect Dis 1995;21:594–598.

120. Hall KW, Nightingale CH, Gibaldi M, Nelson E, Bates TR, DiSanto AR. Pharmacokinetics of erythromycin in normal and alcoholic liver disease subjects. J Clin Pharmacol 1982;22:321–325.

121. Hamill J. Multicentre evaluation of azithromycin and penicillin V in the treatment of acute streptococcal pharyngitis and tonsillitis in children. J Antimicrob Chemother 1993;31:74–89.

122. Hammerschlag MR, Golden N, Oh MK, Gelling M, Sturdevant M, Brown PR, Aras Z, Newhoff S, DuMornay W, Roblin PM. Single dose of azithromycin for the treatment of genital chlamydial infections in adolescents. J Pediatr 1993;122:961–965.

123. Hammerschlag MR, Qumei K, Roblin PM. In vitro activities of azithromycin, clarithromycin, L-ofloxacin, and other antibiotics against Chlamydia pneumoniae. Antimicrob Agents Chemother 1992;36:1573–1574.

124. Hand LW, King-Thompson N, Holman JW. Entry of roxithromycin (RU 965), imipenem, cefotaxime trimethoprim, and metronidazole into human polymorphonuclear leukocyte. Antimicrob Agents Chemother 1987;31:1553–1557.

125. Handsfield HH, Dalu ZA, Martin DH, Douglas JM Jr, McCarty JM, Schlossberg D. Multicenter trial of single dose azithromycin vs ceftriaxone in the treatment of uncomplicated gonorrhea. Sex Transm Dis 1994;21(2):107–111.

126. Hardy DJ, Hensey DM, Beyer JM. Comparative in vitro activities of new 14-, 15-, and 16-membered macrolides. Antimicrob Agents Chemother 1988;32:1710–1719.

127. Havlir D, DubeMP, Sattler FR, Forthal DN, Kemper CA, Dunne MW, Parenti DM, Lavelle JP, White AC Jr, Witt MD, Bozzette SA, McCuthan, for the California Collaborative Treatment Group. Prophylaxis against disseminated *Mycobacterium avium* complex with weekly azithromycin, daily rifabutin or both. N Engl J Med 1996;335:392–398.

128. Haydon RC, Thelin JW, Dawis WE. Erythromycin ototoxicity. Analysis and conclusions based on 22 case reports. Otolaryngol Head Neck Surg 1984;92:678–684.

129. Hebert AA, Still GJ, Reuman PD. Comparative safety and efficacy of clarithromycin and cefadroxil suspensions in the treatment of mild to moderate skin and skin structure infections. Pediatr Infect Dis J 1993;12S:112–117.

130. Hoepelman AIM, Möllers MJ, Van Schie MH, Greefhorst APM, Schlösser NJJ, Sinninghe Damate HEJ, Van DE Moosdijk, Dalinghaus WH, Eland ME, Rozenberg-Arska M.

131. Hooton TM. A comparison of azithromycin and penicillin V for the treatment of streptococcal pharyngitis. Am J Med 1991;91: 3S–23S.

132. Hopkins S. Clinical toleration and safety of azithromycin. Am J Med 1991;91:40S–45S.

133. Hoppe JE, Eichhorn A. Activity of new macrolides against *Bordetella pertussis* and *Bordetella parapertussis*. Eur J Clin Microbiol Infect Dis 1989;8:653–654.

134. Hosie J, Quinn P, Smiths P, Sides G. A comparison of 5 days of dirithromycin and 7 days of clarithromycin in acute bacterial exacerbations of chronic bronchitis. J Antimicrob Chemother 1995;36:173–183.

135. Hsueh PR, Chen HM, Huang AH, Wu JJ. Decreased activity of erythromycin against *Streptococcus pyogenes* in Taiwan. Antimicrob Agents Chemother 1995;39:2239–2242.

136. Iiono Y, Sugita K, Toriyama M, Kudo K. Erythromycin therapy for otitis media with effusion in sinobronchial syndrome. Arch Otolarynol Head Neck Surg 1993;119:648–651.

137. Ikeda C, Kikuchi Y, Matsui H, Tahibana A. Effects of food on bioavailability of josamycin and josamycin propionate. In: Ishigami J, ed. Recent advances in chemotherapy. Proceedings of the 14th International Congress of Chemotherapy, Kyoto, 23–28 June 1985. Antimicrobial section 2. Tokyo: University of Tokyo Press, 1986:1483–1484.

138. Ishida K, Kaku M, Irifune K, Mizukane R, Takemura H, Yoshida R, Tanaka H, Usui T, Suyama N, Tomono K, Koga H, Kohno S, Izumikava K, Hara K. In vitro and in vivo activities of macrolides against *Mycoplasma pneumoniae*. Antimicrob Agents Chemother 1994;38:790–798.

139. Jacobson K. Clinical efficacy of dirithromycin in pneumonia. J Antimicrob Chemother 1993;31(Suppl C):121–129.

140. Jonsson B. Cost effectiveness of *Helicobacter pylori* eradication therapy in duodenal ulcer disease. Scand J Gastroenterol Suppl 1996;215:90–95.

141. Josefsson K, Steinbakk M, Bergan T, Midtvedt T, Magni L. Pharmacokinetics of a new, microencapsulated erythromycin base after repeated oral doses. Chemotherapy 1982;28: 176–184.

142. Josefsson K, Graffner C, Magni L. Reproducibility of erythromycin serum levels when given in enteric coated pellets. In: Spitzy KH, Karrer S, eds. Proceedings of the 13th International Congress of Chemotherapy, Vienna 1983;107:15–18.

143. Joslin S, Guay D, Straka R. Qtc-interval prolongation and intravenous erythromycin lactobionate infusions in critically ill patients [Abstract M63]. 34th Intersci Conf Antimicrob Ag Chemother. Washington, DC: American Society for Microbiology 1994:246.

144. Kafetzis DA, Ligatsikas C, Saint-Salvi B, Lenfant B, Blanc F. Concentrations of roxithromycin in tonsil and adenoid tissues after single and repeated administrations to children. Br J Clin Pract 1988;42(Suppl 55):80.

145. Kamme C, Kahlmeter G, Melander A. Evaluation of spiramycin as a therapeutic agent for elimination of nasopharyngeal pathogens. Scand J Infect Dis 1978;10:135–142.

146. Kanavaki S, Karebala S, Marinis E, Legakis NJ. Antibiotic resistance of clinical isolates of *Streptococcus pneumoniae* in Greece. J Clin Microbiol 1994;32:3056–3058.

147. Karma P, Pukander J, Pentilla M. The comparative efficacy and safety of clarithromycin and amoxicillin in the treatment of out-

Azithromycin tablets for 3 days versus 10-day co-amoxiclav in adults with lower respiratory tract infection, effects on long term outcome [Abstract 13.26]. 3rd Int Conference on the macrolides, azalides and streptogramins, Lisbon, 1996:96.

patients with acute maxillary sinusitis. J Antimicrob Chemother 1991;27:83–90.

148. Kees F, Grobecker H, Fourtillan JB, Tremblay D, Saint-Salvi B. Comparative pharmacokinetics of single dose roxithromycin (150 mg) versus erythromycin stearate (500 mg) in healthy volunteers. Br J Clin Pract 1988;42(Suppl 55):51.

149. Kelley R, Langley G, Bates L. Erythromycin: Still a good choice for strep throat. Clin Pediatr 1993;32:744–745.

150. Khan WA, Seas C, Dhar U, Salam MA, Bennish ML. Treatment of shigellosis: a comparison of azithromycin and ciprofloxacin. A double blind, randomized, controlled trial. Ann Intern Med 1997;126:697–703.

151. Khurana CM. A multicenter, randomized, open label comparison of azithromycin and amoxicillin/clavulanate in acute otitis media among children attending day care centers or school. Pediatr Infect Dis J 1996;15:S24–29.

152. Kiani R. Double blind, double dummy comparison of azithromycin and cephalexin in the treatment of skin and skin structure infections. Eur J Clin Microbiol Infect Dis 1991;10: 880–884.

153. Kirst HA, Sides GD. New directions for macrolide antibiotics: structural modifications and in vitro activity. Antimicrob Agents Chemother 1989;33:1413–1418.

154. Kirst HA. Macrolide antibiotics. Ann Rep Med Chem 1989;25: 119–128.

155. Kissinger P, Clark R, Morse A, Brandon W. Comparison of multiple drug regimens for HIV-related disseminated Mycobacterium avium complex disease. J AIDS Hum Retrovir 1995;9:133–137.

156. Klein JR. Current issues in upper respiratory tract infections in infants and children: rationale for antibiotic therapy. Pediatr Infect Dis J 1994;13:S5–8.

157. Köhler D, Kemper P, Möller M, and Study Group. Acute exacerbation of chronic bronchitis in out-patients; sparfloxacin vs. roxithromycin [Abstract]. 8th European Congress of Infect Dis Clin Microbiol, Lausanne, 1997.

158. Kondo Y, Torii K, Itoh Z, Omura S. Erythromycin and its derivatives with motilin like biological activities inhibit the specific binding of 125I-motilin to duodenal muscle. Biochem Biophys Res Commun 1988;150:877–882.

159. LaBrecque D, Johlin F, Janda R. Pharmacokinetics of dirithromycin in patients with impaired hepatic function. J Antimicrob Chemother 1993;32:741–750.

160. Lalak NJ, Morris DL. Azithromycin clinical pharmacokinetics. Clin Pharmacokinet 1993;25:370–374.

161. Lassman HB, Puri SK, Ho I, Sabo R, Barry A. Influence of food on the absorption of RU 28965 (a new macrolide antibiotic) from film-coated tablets in healthy men. In: Butzler, Kobayashi, eds. Macrolides: a review with an outlook on future developments. Amsterdam: Excerpta Medica, 1986:138–142.

162. Lassus A, Seppala A. Roxithromycin in nongonococcal urethritis. J Antimicrob Chemother 1987;20(Suppl B):157–165.

163. Lassus A. Comparative studies of azithromycin in skin and soft tissue infections and sexually transmitted infections by Neisseria and Chlamydia species. J Antimicrob Chemother 1990;25 (Suppl A):115–121.

164. Lauharanta J, Saarinen K, Mustonen MT, Happonen HP. Single dose oral azithromycin versus seven day doxycycline in the treatment of non-gonococcal urethritis in males. J Antimicrob Chemother 1993(Suppl E):177–183.

165. Le Roux Y, Desnottes JF, Frydman AM. Pharmacokinetics of spiramycin after single and multiple administration of a one-

hour 500 mg i.v. infusion in healthy volunteers. In: Ishigami J, ed. Recent advances in chemotherapy, Kyoto, 23–28 June 1985, Antimicrobial section I. Tokyo: University of Tokyo Press, 1986:134–135.

166. Lebrec D, Benhamou JP, Fourtillan JB. Roxithromycin: pharmacokinetics in patients suffering from alcoholic cirrhosis. Br J Clin Pract 1988;42(Suppl 55):63.

167. Leclercq R, Courvalin P. Bacterial resistance to macrolide, lincosamide, and streptogramin antibiotics by target modification. Antimicrob Agents Chemother 1991;35:1267–1272.

168. Levenstein JH. Clarythromycin versus penicillin VK in the treatment of outpatients with streptococcal pharyngitis. J Antimicrob Chemother 1991;27:75–82.

169. Levin G, Behrenth E. Irreversible ototoxic effect of erythromycin. Scand Audiol 1986;15:41–42.

170. Liipio K, Tala E, Puolijoki H, Bruckner OJ, Rodrig J, Smith JP. A comparative study of dirithromycin and erythromycin in bacterial pneumonia. J Infect 1994;28:131–139.

171. Lin CC, Chung M, Gural R, Schuessler D, Kim HK, Radwanski E, Marco A, DiGiore C, Symchowitz S. Pharmacokinetics and metabolism of rosaramicin in humans. Antimicrob Agents Chemother 1984;26:522–526.

172. Lode H. The pharmacokinetics of azithromycin and their clinical significance. Eur J Clin Microbiol Infect Dis 1991;10: 807–812.

173. Lode H, Garau J, Grassi C, Hosie J, Huchon G, Legakis N, Segev S, Wijnands G. Treatment of community acquired pneumonia: a randomized comparison of sparfloxacin, amoxicillin-clavulanic acid and erythromycin. Eur Res J 1995;8:1999–2007.

174. Logan RPH, Bardhan KD, Celestin LR, Theodossi A, Palmer KR, Reed PI, Baron JH, Misiwicz JJ. Eradication of Helicobacter pylori and prevention of recurrence of duodenal ulcer: a randomized, double blind, multi-center trial of omeprazole with or without clarithromycin. Aliment Pharm Ther 1995;9:417–423.

175. Lonks JR, Medeiros AA. High rate of erythromycin and clarythromycin resistance among Streptococcus pneumoniae from blood cultures from Providence, R.I. Antimicrob Agents Chemother 1993;37:1742–1745.

176. Lucier TS, Heitzman K, Liu SK, Hu PC. Transition mutations in the 23S rRNA of erythromycin-resistant isolates of Mycoplasma pneumoniae. Antimicrob Agents Chemother 1995; 39:2770–2773.

177. Luft B, Dattwyler RJ, Johnson RC, Luger S, Bosler E, Rahn DW, Masters EJ, Grünwaldt E, Gadgil SD. Azithromycin compared with amoxicillin in the treatment of erythema migrans. A double blind, randomized, controlled trial. Ann Intern Med 1996;124:785–791.

178. Luke DR, Foulds G, Cohen SF, Levy B. Safety, toleration, and pharmacokinetics of intravenous azithromycin. Antimicrob Agents Chemother 1996;40:2577–2581.

179. MacFarlane JA, Mitchell AAB, Walsh JM, Roverbson JJ. Spiramycin in the prevention of postoperative staphylococcal infections. Lancet 1968;1:1–4.

180. Mallory SB. Azithromycin compared with cephalexin in the treatment of skin and skin structure infections. Am J Med 1991;91(Suppl 3A):36S–39S.

181. Marchioso P, Pirincipi N, Sala E, Lanzoni L, Sorella S, Massimini A. Comparative study of once weekly azithromycin and once daily amoxicillin treatments in prevention of recurrent acute otitis media in children. Antimicrob Agents Chemother 1996;40:2732–2736.

182. Markham A, Faulds D. Roxithromycin: an update on its an-

timicrobial activity, pharmacokinetic properties and therapeutic use. Drugs 1994;48:297–326.

183. Marsac JH. An international clinical trial on the efficacy and safety of roxithromycin in 40000 patients with acute community-acquired respiratory tract infections. Diagn Microbiol Infect Dis 1992;15:81S–84S

184. Martin DH, Mroczkowski TF, Dalu ZA, McCarty J, Jones RB, Hopkins SJ, Johnson RB, and the Azithromycin for Chlamydial Infections Study Group. Controlled trial of a single dose of azithromycin for the treatment of chlamydial urethritis and cervicitis. N Engl J Med 1992;327:921–925.

185. Martin DH, Sargent SJ, Wendel GD Jr, McCormack WM, Spier NA, Johnson RB. Comparison of azithromycin and ceftriaxone for the treatment of chancroid. Clin Infect Dis 1995;21:409–414.

186. Mashkilleyson AL, Gomberg MA, Mahkilleyson N, Kutin SA. Treatment of syphilis with azithromycin. Int J STD AIDS 1996;7(Suppl 1):13–15.

187. Massarotti EM, Luger SW, Rahn DW, Messner R, Wong JB, Johnson RC, Steere AC. Treatment of early Lyme disease. Am J Med 1992;92:3964–3963.

188. Mazzei T, Mini E, Novelli A, Periti P. Chemistry and mode of action of macrolides. J Antimicrob Chemother 1993;31(Suppl C):1–9.

189. Mazzei T, Surrenti C, Novelli A, Crispo A, Fallani S, Carla V, Surrenti E, Periti P. Pharmacokinetics of azithromycin in patients with impaired hepatic function. J Antimicrob Chemother 1993;31(Suppl E):57–63.

190. Mazzei T, Surrenti C, Novelli A, Biagini MR, Surrenti E, Periti P. Pharmacokinetics of dirithromycin in patients with impaired hepatic function. In: Einhorn J, Nord CE, Norrby R, eds. Recent advances in chemotherapy. Proceedings of the 18th International Congress of Chemotherapy, 1993. Stockholm, Sweden: American Society for Microbiology, 1994:410–411.

191. McCarty JM, Philips A, Wilsanen R. Comparative safety and efficacy of clarythromycin and amoxicillin/clavulanate in the treatment of acute otitis media in children. Pediatr Infect Dis J 1993;12:S122–127.

192. McDonald PJ, Tierney WM, Hui Sl. A controlled trial of erythromycin in adults with nonstreptococcal pharyngitis. J Infect Dis 1985;152:1093–1094.

193. McDonald PJ. Macrolide antibiotics—pharmacology and the importance of formulation. In: Butzler JP, Kobayashi H, eds. Macrolides: a review with an outlook on future developments. Amsterdam: Excerpta Medica, 1986:22–29.

194. McLean A, Sutton JA, Salmo J, Chatelet D. Roxithromycin—pharmacokinetic and metabolism study in humans. Br J Clin Pract 1988;42(Suppl 55):52–53.

195. McLinn S. A multicenter, double blind comparison of azithromycin and amoxicillin/clavulanate for the treatment of acute otitis media in children. Pediatr Infect Dis J 1996;15:S20–23.

196. Meier A, Heifets L, Wallace RJ Jr, Zhang Y, Brown BA, Sander P, Böttger EC. Molecular mechanism of clarithromycin resistance in *Mycobacterium avium:* observation of multiple 23S rDNA mutations in a clonal population. J Infect Dis 1996;174:354–360.

197. Melcher GP, Hadfield TL, Gaines JK, Winn RE. Comparative efficacy and toxicity of roxithromycin and erythromycin ethylsuccinate in the treatment of streptococcal pharyngitis in adults. J Antimicrob Chemother 1988;22:549–556.

198. Meloni G. Azithromycin vs. doxycycline for Mediterranean spotted fever. Pediatr Infect Dis J 1996;15:1042–1044.

199. Menninger JR. Functional consequences of binding macrolides to ribosomes. J Antimicrob Chemother 1985;16(Suppl A): 23–24.

200. Mertens JCC, van Barneweld PWC, Asin HRG, Ligtvoet E, Visser MR, Branger T, Hoepelman AIM. Double-blind randomized study comparing the efficacies and safeties of a short (3-day) course of azithromycin and a 5-day course of amoxicillin in patients with acute exacerbations of chronic bronchitis. Antimicrob Agents Chemother 1992;36:1456–1459.

201. Mini E, Mazzei T, Reali EF, Periti P. Penetration of the new macrolide roxithromycin (RU 28965) into lung tissue and suction blister fluid. In: Berkarda B, Kuemmerle JF, eds. Progress in chemotherapy. Proceedings of the 15th International Congress of Chemotherapy, Istanbul, 19–24 July, 1987. Antimicrobial section, vol 1. Landsberg: Comed, 1988:1350–1352.

202. Mohs E, Rodriguez Solares A, Rivas E, El Hoshy Z. A comparative study of azithromycin and amoxicillin in pediatric patients with with acute otitis media. J Antimicrob Chemother 1993;31(Suppl E):73–79.

203. Montero L. A comparative study of the efficacy, safety and tolerability of azithromycin and cefaclor in the treatment of children with acute skin and/or soft tissue infections. J Antimicrob Chemother 1996;37(Suppl C):125–131.

204. Morris DL, De Souza A, Jones JA, Morgan WE. High and prolonged pulmonary tissue concentrations of azithromycin following a single oral dose. Eur J Clin Microbiol Infect Dis 1991;10:859–861.

205. Müller O. Comparison of azithromycin versus clarithromycin in the treatment of patients with upper respiratory tract infections. J Antimicrob Chemother 1993;31(Suppl E):137–146.

206. Müller O, Wettich K. Clinical efficacy of dirithromycin in pharyngitis and tonsillitis. J Antimicrob Chemother 1993;37: 97–102.

207. Myburgh J, Nagel GJ, Petschel E. The efficacy and the tolerance of a three day course of azithromycin in the treatment of community acquired pneumonia. J Antimicrob Chemother 1993;31(Suppl E):163–169.

208. Nahata MC, Koranyi K, Luke D, Foulds G. Pharmocokinetics of azithromycin in pediatric patients with acute otitis media. Antimicrob Agents Chemother 1995;39:1875–1877.

209. Nash KA, Inderlied C. Genetic basis of macrolide resistance in *Mycobacterium avium* isolated from patients with disseminated disease. Antimicrob Agents Chemother 1995;39:2625–2630.

210. Neu HC. The development of macrolides: clarithromycin in perspective. J Antimicrob Chemother 1991;27:1–9.

211. Nicoletti P, Rizzo M, Mazzei T. Aspetti farmacocinetici della miocamicina. Chemioterapia 1983;2(Suppl 3):140–141.

212. Nilsen OG. Comparative pharmacokinetics of macrolides. J Antimicrob Chemother 1987;20(Suppl B):81–88.

213. Norrby SR. Azithromycin: an antibiotic with unusual properties. Eur J Clin Microbiol Infect Dis 1991;10:805–806.

214. O'Doherty B, Müller O, and the Azithromycin Study Group. A randomized, multicenter study to compare the efficacy and the toleration of azithromycin and clarithromycin in the treatment of adult with mild-to-moderate community-acquired pneumonia [Abstract 1281]. 8th European Congress of Infect Dis Clin Microbiol, Lausanne, 1997.

215. O'Hara K, Yamamoto K. Reaction of clarithromycin with macrolide inactivating enzymes from highly erythromycin-resistant *Escherichia coli.* Antimicrob Agents Chemother 1996: 40:1036–1038.

216. Odenholt-Tornqvist I, Lövdin E, Cars O. Postantibiotic effects and postantibiotic sub MIC effects of roxithromycin, cla-

rithromycin and azihtromycin on respiratory tract pathogens. Antimicrob Agents Chemother 1995;39:221–226.

217. Okolicsanyi L, Venuti M, Strazzabosco M, Biral A, Orlando R, Iemmolo RM, Nassuato G, Muraca M, Padrini G, Miglioli PA. Pharmacokinetics of Josamycin in patients with liver cirrhosis and Gilbert's syndrome after repeated doses. Int J Clin Pharmacol 1985;23: 434–438.

218. Omura S, Tsuzuki K, Sunazuka T. Gastrointestinal motor-stimulating activity of macrolide antibiotics and its structure activity relationship. J Antibiot (Tokyo) 1985;38:1631–1632.

219. Ortuno JA, Olaso V, Berenguere J. Cholestatic hepatitis caused by erythromycin propionate [Letter]. Med Clin (Barc) 1984;82: 912.

220. Ossewaarde JM, Plantema FHF, Rieffe M, Nawrocki RP, de Vires A, van Loon AM. Efficacy of single dose azithromycin versus doxycycline in the treatment of cervical infections caused by *Chlamydia trachomatis*. Eur J Clin Microbiol Infect Dis 1992;11:693–697.

221. Pacifico L, Scopetti F, Ranucci A, Pataracchia, Savignoni F, Chiesa C. Comparison of three-day azithromycin versus ten day penicillin V in the treatment of children with streptococcal group A pharyngitis. Antimicrob Agent Chemother 1996;40: 1005–1008.

222. Panteix G, Guillaumond B, Harf R, Desbos A, Sapin V, Leclercq M, Perrin-Fayolle M. In-vitro concentration of azithromycin in human phagocytic cells. J Antimicrob Chemother 1993;31(Suppl E):1–4.

223. Patel KP, Xuan D, Tessier PR, Russomanno JH, Quintiliani R, Nightingale CH. Comparison of bronchopulmonary pharmacokinetics of clarithromycin and azithromycin. Antimicrob Agents Chemother 1996;40:2375–2379.

224. Periti P, Fini-Storchi O, Novelli A. Penetrazione nella mucosa nasale della eritromicina somministrata per via orale sotto forma del sale mercaptosuccinato del propilestere (RV11 Pierrel). Farm Ter 1986;3:194–197.

225. Periti P, Marino C, Novelli A. Valutazione farmacocinetica clinica della eritromicina propionato d,l- mercaptosuccinato (RV11 Pierrel). Farm Ter 1986;3:189–193.

226. Periti P, Mazzei T. Pharmacokinetics of roxithromycin in renal and hepatic failure and drug interactions. J Antimicrob Chemother 1987;20(Suppl B):107–112.

227. Periti P, Mazzei T, Mini E, Novelli A. Clinical pharmacokinetics properties of the macrolide antibiotics. Effects of age and various pathophysiological states (part I). Clin Pharmacokinet 1989;16:193–214.

228. Periti P, Mazzei T, Mini E, Novelli A. Pharmacokinetic drug interactions of macrolides. Clin Pharmacokinet 1992;23:106–131.

229. Periti P, Mazzei T, Mini E, Novelli A. Adverse effects of macrolide antibacterials. Drug Safety 1993;9:346–364.

230. Pessayre D, Larrey D, Funck-Brentono C, Benhamou JP. Drug interactions and hepatitis produced by some macrolides antibiotics. J Antimicrob Chemother 1985;16:181–194.

231. Pestalozza G, Cioce C, Facchini M. Azithromycin in upper respiratory tract infections: a clinical trial in children with otitis media. Scand J Infect Dis 1992;(Suppl 83):22–25.

232. Peters DH, Clissold SP. Clarithromycin: a review of its antimicrobial activity, pharmacokinetic properties and therapeutic potential. Drugs 1992;44:117–164.

233. Pirincipi N. Multicentre comparative study of the efficacy and safety of azithromycin compared with amoxicillin/clavulanic acid in the treatment of paediatric patients with otitis media. Eur J Clin Microbiol Infect Dis 1995;14:669–676.

234. Pontani D, Arevalo C, Gallegos B, Carmona O, Lugo L, Campos O. An open, multicenter, noncomparative study of the safety and efficacy of azithromycin in the treatment of gonococcal and non-gonococcal urethritis. 3rd Int conference on the macrolides, azalides and streptogramins, Lisbon 1996:27.

235. Pozzi E, Ferrara A, Sardi A, Berti MA, Coppi G. Bioavailability studies on erythromycin administered by rectal and oral routes. Curr Ther Res 1982;31:530–535.

236. Public Health Service Task Force on Prophylaxis and Therapy for Mycobacterium avium complex for adults and adolescents infected with human immundeficiency virus. MMWR 1993;42: 17–20.

237. Pukander JS, Jero JP, Kaprio EA, Sorri MJ. Clarithromycin versus amoxicillin suspensions in the treatment of pediatric patients with acute otitis media. Pediatr Infect Dis J 1993;12: S118–121.

238. Puri SK, Lassman HB. Roxithromycin: a pharmacokinetic review of a macrolide. J Antimicrob Chemother 1987;20(Suppl B):89–100.

239. Quinnan GV, McCabe WR. Ototoxicity of erythromycin. Lancet 1978;1:1160–1161.

240. Rastogi N, Goh KS. Effect of pH on radiometric MICs of clarithromycin against 18 species of mycobacteria. Antimicrob Agents Chemother 1992;36:2841–2842.

241. Rastogi N, Bauriaud RM, Bourgoin A, Carbonnelle B, Chippaux C, Gevaudan MJ, Goh KS, Moinard D, Roos P. French multicenter study involving eight test sites for radiometric determination of activities of 10 Antimicrob Agents against *Mycobacterium avium* complex. Antimicrob Agents Chemother 1995;39:683–686.

242. Rice RJ, Bhullar V, Mitchell SH, Bullard J, Knapp JS. Susceptibilities of *Chlamydia trachomatis* isolates causing uncomplicated female genital tract infections and pelvic inflammatory disease. Antimicrob Agents Chemother 1995;39:760–762.

243. Rimoldi R, Mangiarotti P, De Rose V. Penetration of roxithromycin into bronchial secretions. Br J Clin Pract 1988;41(Suppl 55):74–77.

244. Rodriguez-Solares A, Gutierrez-Perez F, Prosperi J, Milgram E, Martin A. A comparative study of efficacy, safety and tolerance of azithromycin, dicloxacillin and flucloxacillin in the treatment of children with acute skin and skin structure infections. J Antimicrob Chemother 1993;31(Suppl E):103–109.

245. Rodriguz AF. An open study to compare azithromycin with cefaclor in the treatment of children with acute otitis media. J Antimicrob Chemother 1996;37(Suppl C):63–69.

246. Rossi M, Ramsberger B, Altwegg M, Gerber AU, and the Swiss Multicenter Study Group on Lower Respiratory Tract Infections. Azithromycin versus co-amoxiclav in patients with lower respiratory tract infections [Abstract 1282]. 8th European Congress of Clinical Microbiology and Infectious Diseases, Lausanne, Switzerland, 1997.

247. Sacristan JA, Soto JA, deCos MA. Erythromycin induced hypoacusis: 11 new cases and literature review. Ann Pharmacother 1993;27:950–955.

248. Scaglione F. Comparison of the clinical and bacteriological efficacy of clarithromycin and erythromycin in the treatment of streptococcal pharyngitis. Curr Med Res Opin 1990;12:25–53.

249. Schaad UB. Multicenter evaluation of azithromycin in comparison with co-amoxiclav for the treatment of acute otitis media in children. J Antimicrob Chemother 1993;31(Suppl E):81–88.

250. Schaad UB, Heynen G, and the Swiss Tonsillopharyngitis Study Group. Evaluation of the efficacy, safety and toleration of azithromycin vs. penicillin V in the treatment of acute streptococcal pharyngitis in children: results of a multicenter, open comparative study. Pediatr Infect Dis J 1996;15:791–795.

251. Schachter J. Azithromycin øn control of trachoma [Abstract 2.10]. 3rd Int conference on the macrolides, azalides and streptogramins, Lisbon, 1996:22.

252. Schentag JJ, Ballow CH. Tissue directed pharmacokinetics. Am J Med 1991;91(Suppl 3A):5S–11S.

253. Schönwald S, Gunjaca M, Kolaeny-Babic L, Car V, Gosev M. Comparison of azithromycin and erythromycin in the treatment of atypical pneumonias. J Antimicrob Chemother 1990;25 (Suppl A):123–126.

254. Schönwald S, Skerk V, Petricevic I, Car V, Majerus-Misic LJ, Gunjaca M. Comparison of three day courses of azithromycin in the treatment of atypical pneumonia. Eur J Clin Microbiol Infect Dis 1991;10:877–880.

255. Schönwald S, Barsic B, Klinar I, Gunjaca M. Three day azithromycin compared with ten day roxithromycin treatment of atypical pneumonia. Scand J Infect Dis 1994;26:706–710.

256. Segre G, Bianchi E, Zanolo G, Bartucci F, Sassella D. Influence of food on the bioavailability of roxithromycin versus erythromycin stearate. Br J Clin Pract 1988;42(Suppl 55):55–57.

257. Seifert CF, Swaney RJ, Bellanger-McCleery RA. Intravenous erythromycin lactobionate-induced severe nausea and vomiting. Ann Pharmocother 1989;23:40–44.

258. Seppala H, Nissinen A, Jarvinen H, Huovinen S, Henriksson T, Herva E, Holm SE, Jahkola M, Katila ML, Klaukka T. Resistance to erythromycin in group A streptococci. N Engl J Med 1992;5: 292–297.

259. Shanson DC, McNabb WR, Ruby K. High dose erythromycin for preventing endocarditis. Lancet 1983;1:299–300.

260. Shepard RM, Falkner FC. Pharmacokinetics of azithromycin in rats and dogs. J Antimicrob Chemother 1990;25(Suppl A):49–60.

261. Shiiki K, Sakamoto H. Penetration of antimicrobial agents into saliva (clinical application as a therapeutic drug monitoring method). Progress in chemotherapy. 15th International Congress of Chemotherapy, Istanbul, 19–24 July, 1987. Antimicrobial section, vol 1. Landsberg: Ecomed, 1987:211–213.

262. Sides GD, Cerimele BJ, Black HR, Busch U, DeSante KA. Pharmacokinetics of dirithromycin in patients with impaired hepatic function. J Antimicrob Chemother 1993;31(Suppl C):65–75.

263. Sides GD. Clinical efficacy of dirithromycin in acute exacerbations of chronic bronchitis. J Antimicrob Chemother 1993;31 (Suppl C):131–138.

264. Sjögren E, Kaijser B, Werner M. Antimicrobial susceptibilities of Campylobacter jejuni and Campylobacter coli isolated in Sweden: a 10-year follow-up report. Antimicrob Agents Chemother 1992;36:2847–2849.

265. Stamm WE, Hicks CB, Martin DH, Leone P, Hook III EW, Cooper RH, Cohen MS, Batteiger BE, Workowski K, McCormack WM, Bolan G, Douglas M, Wong E, Pappas PG, Johnson RB. Azithromycin for empirical treatment of the nongonococcal urethritis syndrome in men. JAMA 1995;274:545–549.

266. Steigbigel NH. Erythromycin, lincomycin and clindamycin. In: Mandell GL, Douglas GR Jr, Bennett JE, eds. Anti-infective therapy. New York: John Wiley & Sons, 1985:197–218.

267. Steingrimsson Ö, Ölafson JH, Thorarinsson H, Ryan RW, Johnson RB, Tilton RC. Azithromycin in the treatment of sexually transmitted disease. J Antimicrob Chemother 1990;25 Suppl A:109–114.

268. Steingrimsson Ö, Ölafson JH, Thorarinsson H, Ryan RW, Johnson RB, Tilton RC. Single dose azithromycin treatment of gonorrhea and infections caused by C. trachomatis and U. urealyticum in men. STD 1992;21:43–46.

269. Steketee RW, Wassilak SGF, Adkins WN, Burstyn DG, Manclark CR, Berg J, Hopfensperger D, Schell WL, Davis JP. Evidence for high attack rate and efficacy of erythromycin prophylaxis in a pertussis outbreak in a facility of for the developmentally disabled. J Infect Dis 1988;157:434–440.

270. Still JG, Hubbard WC, Poole JM, Sheafer CI, Charrand S, Jacobs R. Comparison of clarithromycin and penicillin VK suspensions in the treatment of children with streptococcal pharyngitis and review of currently available alternative antibiotic therapies. Pediatr Infect Dis J 1993;12:S134–141.

271. Stoehr GP, Juhl RP, Veals J, et al. The excretion of rosaramicin in breast milk. J Clin Pharmacol 1985;25:89–94.

272. Strausbaugh LJ, Bolton WK, Dilworth JA, Guerrant RL, Sande MA. Comparative pharmacology of josamycin and erythromycin stearate. Antimicrob Agents Chemother 1976;10:450–456.

273. Strle F, Preac M, Cimperman J, Ruzie E, Maraspin V, Jereb M. Azithromycin versus doxycycline for the treatment of erythema migrans: clinical and microbiological findings. Infection 1993; 21:83–88.

274. Sundberg L, Cederberg A. The diffusion of clarithromycin and its 14-hydroxy metabolite into middle ear effusion in children with secretory otitis media. J Antimicrob Chemother 1994;33: 299–307.

275. Swanson DJ, Sung RJ, Fine JM, Orloff J, Sou YC, Yu VL. Erythromycin ototoxicity: prospective assessment with serum concentrations and audiograms in a study of patient with pneumonia. Am J Med 1992;92:61–68.

276. Swanson DJ, Sung RJ, Fine MJ. Erythromycin ototoxicity: prospective assessment with serum concentrations and audiograms in a study of patients with pneumonia. Am J Med 1992; 92:61–68.

277. Tabbara KF, El-Asrar A, Al-Omar O, Choudhurry AH, Faisal Z. Single dose azithromycin in the treatment of trachoma. A randomized, controlled study. Ophthalmology 1996;103:842–846.

278. Tateda K, Ishii Y, Matsumato T, Furuya N, Nagashima M, Matsunaga T, Ohno A, Miyazaki S, Yamaguchi K. Direct evidence for antipseudomonal activity of macrolides: exposure dependent bactericidal activity and inhibition of protein synthesis by erythromycin, clarithromycin, and azithromycin. Antimicrob Agents Chemother 1996;40:2271–2275.

279. Thomson PJ, Burgess KR, Marlin GE. Influence of food on absorption of erythromycin ethyl succinate. Antimicrob Agents Chemother 1980;18:829–831.

280. Tremblay D, Jaeger H, Fourtillan JB, Manuel C. Pharmacokinetics of three single doses (150, 300, 450 mg) of roxithromycin in young volunteers. Br J Clin Pract 1988;42(Suppl 55):49–50.

281. Tremblay D, Mignot A, Couraud L, Saux MC, Manuel C. Concentrations of roxithromycin in lung tissue after repeat dosing. Br J Clin Pract 1988;42(Suppl 55):73.

282. Truffot-Pernot C, Lounis N, Grosset JH, Ji B. Clarithromycin is inactive against Mycobacterium tuberculosis. Antimicrob Agents Chemother 1995;39:2827–2828.

283. Tuominen RK, Männistö PT, Pohto P, Solkinen A, Vuorela A. Absorption of erythromycin acistrate and erythromycin base in the fasting and non-fasting state. J Antimicrob Chemother 1988;21(Suppl D):45–55.

284. Tyndall MW, Agoki E, Plummer FA, Malisa W, Ndinya-Achola JO, Ronald AR. Single dose azithromycin for the treatment of chancroid: a randomized comparison with erythromycin. Sex Transm Dis 1994;21:231–234.

285. Umstaed GS, Neumann KH. Erythromycin ototoxicity and acute psychotic reaction in cancer patients with hepatic dysfunction. Arch Intern Med 1986;146:897–899.

286. Varanese L. Pharmacokinetics and safety of dirithromycin in the elderly. J Antimicrob Chemother 1993;31(Suppl C): 169–174.
287. Vasquez EM, Maddux MS, Sanchez J, Pollack R. Clinically significant hearing loss in renal allograft recipients treated with intravenous erythromycin. Arch Intern Med 1993;153: 879–882.
288. Vergis EN, Phillips J, Bates JH, File TM, Tan JS, Sarosi GA, Grayston JT, Yu VL. A prospective, randomized, multicenter trial of azithromycin versus cefuroxim plus erythromycin for community acquired pneumonia in hospitalized patients [Abstract]. IDSA, San Francisco, 1997:410.
289. Von Rosentiel N-A, Adam D. Macrolide antibacterials. Drug interactions of clinical significance. Drug Safety 1995;13: 105–122.
290. Wald ER. Antimicrobial therapy of pediatric patients with sinusitis. J Allergy Clin Immunol 1992;90:469–473.
291. Wallace MR, Miller LK, Nguyen MT, Shields AR. Ototoxicity with azithromycin. Lancet 1994;343:241.
292. Wallace RJ Jr, Brown BA, Griffith DE. Drug intolerance to high dose clarithromycin among elderly patients. Diagn Microbiol Infect Dis 1993;16:215–220.
293. Weippl G. Multicentre comparison of azithromycin versus erythromycin in the treatment of paediatric pharyngitis and tonsillitis caused by group A streptococci. J Antimicrob Chemother 1993;31:95–101.
294. Weisblum B. Erythromycin resistance by ribosome modification. Antimicrob Agents Chemother 1995;39:577–585.
295. Weiss K, Laverdiére M, Rivest R. Comparison of antimicrobial susceptibilities of *Corynebacterium* species by broth microdilution and disk diffusion methods. Antimicrob Agents Chemother 1996;40:930–933.
296. Welling PG. Effect of food on bioavailability of drugs. Pharm Int 1980;1:14–18.
297. Welsch L, Gaydos C, Quinn TC. In vitro activities of azithromycin, clarithromycin, erythromycin and tetracycline against 13 strains of *Chlamydia pneumoniae*. Antimicrob Agents Chemother 1996;40:212–214.
298. Whatley JD, Thin RN, Mumtaz G, Ridgway GL. Azithromycin vs doxycycline in the treatment of non-gonococcal urethritis. Int J STD AIDS 1991;2:248–251.
299. Wildfeuer A, Laufen H, Rader K. Activity of josamycin in human tissue and neutrophils. In Ishigami J, ed. Recent advances in chemotherapy. Proceedings of the 14th International Congress of Chemotherapy, Kyoto, 23–28 June, 1986. Antimicrobial section 2. Tokyo: University of Tokyo Press, 1985:1478–1480.
300. Wildfeuer A, Laufen H, Zimmermann T. Uptake of azithromycin by various cells and its intracellular activity under in vivo conditions. Antimicrob Agents Chemother 1996;40:75–79.
301. Williams JD. Spectrum of activity of azithromycin. Eur J Clin Microbiol Infect Dis 1991;10:813–820.
302. Wondrack L, Massa M, Yang BV, Sutcliffe J. Clinical strain of *Staphylococcus aureus* inactivates and causes efflux of macrolides. Antimicrob Agents Chemother 1996;40:992–998.
303. Wuolijoki E, Flygare U, Hilden M. Treatment of respiratory tract infections with erythromycin acistrate and two formulations of erythromycin base. J Antimicrob Chemother 1988;21:107–112.
304. Yakatan GJ, Rasmussen CE, Feis PJ, Wallen S. Bioinequivalence of erythromycin ethylsuccinate and enteric- coated erythromycin pellets following multiple oral doses. J Clin Pharmacol 1985;25:36–42.
305. Yoshii T, Motoji S, Nakasuji K. Basic study on TE-031 (A-56268) in oral surgery. Chemotherapy 1989;37:1085–1089.
306. Zini R, Fournet MP, Barre J. In vitro study of roxithromycin binding to serum proteins and erythrocytes in humans. Br J Clin Pract 1988;42(Suppl 55):54.

Metronidazole

●

Abdolghader Molavi and Craig A. Wood

Metronidazole is a nitroimidazole compound that was synthesized in 1957 at Rhône-Poulenc Research Laboratories in France. Its antiprotozoal activity was recognized first, and it was introduced in 1959 for the treatment of *Trichomonas vaginalis* infections. Shortly thereafter, it was shown to be effective in other protozoal infections, including amebiasis and giardiasis. The activity of metronidazole against anaerobic bacteria was first noted in 1962; however, its clinical implications were not appreciated for a decade until Tally et al. (129) demonstrated that the drug was effective in the treatment of anaerobic infections, including those caused by *Bacteroides fragilis*. More recently, metronidazole has become the treatment of choice for *Clostridium difficile* colitis and has been used in treatment regimens aimed at eradication of *Helicobacter pylori*. After many years of extensive use, metronidazole remains a "gold standard" first-line treatment of a variety of anaerobic and protozoal infections.

Chemically, metronidazole is 1-(β-hydroxyethyl)-2-methyl-5-nitroimidazole. It is the only nitroimidazole antimicrobial available for clinical use in the United States. A related compound, tinidazole, which has a longer elimination half-life, is available for oral administration in Europe.

ANTIMICROBIAL ACTIVITY

Metronidazole is active against anaerobic organisms, both bacteria and protozoa, and a few facultative anaerobes. The approved susceptibility breakpoint for metronidazole is 16 μg/mL. Organisms with an MIC of 16 μg/mL or below are considered fully susceptible to metronidazole; those with an MIC above 16 μg/mL are considered resistant (there is no intermediate susceptibility category for metronidazole). Organisms generally considered routinely susceptible to metronidazole are listed in Table 1.

Gram-Negative Anaerobic Bacilli

Metronidazole is active against nearly all Gram-negative anaerobic bacilli. *Bacteroides* species, including *Bacteroides fragilis* group (*B. fragilis, B. distasonis, B. ovatus, B. thetaiotaomicron,* and *B. vulgatus*), *B. ureolyticus,* and *B. gracilis* are susceptible to metronidazole; nearly 100% of strains are inhibited by 8 μg/mL or less (13, 23, 42, 44, 95, 120, 122, 126). Metronidazole is the most active antimicrobial agent against *Bacteroides* species as judged by time-kill curves. *Prevotella* species, including *P. melaninogenicus, P. intermedia, P. bivia, P. disiens, P. oris, P. oralis,* and *P. buccae,* are uniformly susceptible to metronidazole; almost 100% of strains are inhibited by 8 μg/mL or less (44, 95, 116, 122). *Porphyromonas* species (*P. gingivalis* and *P. endodontalis*) and *Fusobacterium* species (*F. nucleatum, F. necrophorum, F. mortiferum,* and *F. varium*) are highly sensitive to metronidazole; nearly all strains are inhibited by 4 μg/mL or less (95, 116, 122). Metronidazole is active and uniformly bactericidal against *Bilophila wadsworthia* (8).

Gram-Positive Anaerobic Bacilli

Clostridium species, including *C. perfringens, C. septicum, C. tertium, C. bifermentans, C. histolyticum, C. novyi,* and *C. difficile,* are sensitive to metronidazole; nearly all strains are inhibited by 8 μg/mL or less (17, 42, 44, 95, 116, 122). Some strains of *C. ramosum* require higher concentrations for inhibition.

Metronidazole has moderate-to-poor activity against anaerobic, nonsporeforming, Gram-positive bacilli. Approximately 50% of the strains of *Bifidobacterium* and *Eubacterium* are inhibited by 16 μg/mL or less (42). *Actinomyces* species, *Propionibacterium propionica, Propionibacterium acne,* and *Lactobacillus* species are mostly resistant, only 25% of strains are inhibited by 16 μg/mL or less (42, 95, 122). Metronidazole has poor activity against *Mobiluncus* species; *Mobiluncus curtisii* is usually resistant, but over 50% of *Mobiluncus mulieris* strains are sensitive (123).

Anaerobic Cocci

Metronidazole is active against *Peptostreptococcus* species, including *P. magnus, P. anaerobius, P. micros, P. asaccharolyticus,* and *P. prevotii;* 80 to 90% of strains are inhibited by 8 μg/mL or less (23, 95, 116). *Veillonella* species are also sensitive; nearly 100% of strains are inhibited by 16 μg/mL or less (42).

Other Bacteria

Metronidazole is active against *Helicobacter pylori* (microaerophilic); 60 to 90% of strains in Western countries are sensitive to the drug (40, 140, 146). Metronidazole is active against a few facultative anaerobes including *Gardnerella vaginalis* (42), *Actinobacillus actinomycetemcomitans* (96), and *Capnocytophaga* species. The hydroxy metabolite of the drug is two to eight times more active than the parent compound against most *G. vaginalis* strains (7, 31) and *Actinobacillus actinomycetemcomitans* (55). Approximately 70% of strains of *Capnocytophaga* species are inhibited by 8 μg/mL or less, and 93% by 16 μg/mL or less (128). Metronidazole has bactericidal action against dormant cells of *Mycobacterium tuberculosis* in vitro under anaerobic conditions (144).

Protozoa

Metronidazole is active against anaerobic protozoa, including *Trichomonas vaginalis, Entamoeba histolytica, Giardia lamblia, Blastocystis hominis,* and *Balantidium coli.* Resistant strains of *T. vaginalis* have been isolated from patients with refractory trichomoniasis. *T. vaginalis* and *E. histolytica* both generally have metronidazole MICs of 1 μg/mL or less.

PHARMACODYNAMIC EFFECTS

Metronidazole has bactericidal action against anaerobic bacteria (8, 72, 125, 126). The bactericidal concentration of metronidazole is generally at or very close to the MIC for the antibiotic. The bactericidal effect of metronidazole is rapid, and the killing rate is proportional to the drug concentration (125, 126). Similarly, metronidazole exhibits concentration-dependent killing of *T. vaginalis* (91) and *Entamoeba histolytica* (105). Comparison of the bactericidal activity of clindamycin and metronidazole against strains of *B. fragilis* and *C. perfringens* showed metronidazole to have the more rapid killing rate (103). There is no antagonism between metronidazole and various other antibiotics, including clindamycin, rifampin, and ticarcillin, against *B. fragilis* strains (101).

The susceptibility of anaerobic bacteria to metronidazole is affected only slightly by the inoculum size (100). Changes of pH within the range from 5.5 to 8.8 do not significantly affect its activity (100).

MECHANISM OF ACTION

Metronidazole exerts its action on susceptible organisms in four successive stages: entry of the drug into the organism, its reductive activation, interaction of the reduced intermediate products with intracellular targets, and breakdown of the toxic intermediate products (33, 84). Metronidazole has a low molecular weight and diffuses readily into both aerobic and anaerobic

TABLE 1 • Organisms Routinely Susceptible to Metronidazole[a]	
Anaerobic Gram-negative bacilli	*Bacteroides* species
	Bilophila wadsworthia
	Fusobacterium species
	Porphyromonas species
	Prevotella species
Anaerobic Gram-positive bacilli	*Clostridium* species
Anaerobic cocci	*Peptostreptococcus* species
	Veillonella species
Protozoa	*Balantidium coli*
	Blastocystis hominis
	Entamoeba histolytica
	Giardia lamblia
	Trichomonas vaginalis

[a] Nearly all susceptible at MIC ≤ 16 μg/mL.

microorganisms. It is, however, active only against organisms that are capable of anaerobic metabolism.

In obligate anaerobes, reductive activation occurs by the pyruvate:ferredoxin oxidoreductase system. The nitro group of metronidazole acts as an electron sink by capturing electrons from reduced ferredoxin that would normally be donated to hydrogen ions (32, 84). The metabolic source of electrons is the oxidative decarboxylation of pyruvate, which is catalyzed by pyruvate:ferredoxin oxidoreductase is the major route of ATP generation. Reduction plays a dual role. It decreases the intracellular concentration of the unchanged drug and thus maintains a gradient driving the uptake, and it generates short-lived intermediate compounds and free radicals that are toxic to the cell. These toxic transitory products interact with DNA, causing strand breaks and helix destabilization and unwinding, resulting in cell death (134, 135). The cytotoxic intermediate products decompose into inactive end products, including acetamide and N-(2-hydroxyethyl) oxamic acid (41).

Pyruvate:ferredoxin oxidoreductase is found exclusively in obligate anaerobic bacteria. The mechanism of action of metronidazole in H. pylori, G. vaginalis, and other susceptible facultative anaerobic bacteria is different from that in obligate anaerobes and is not well-characterized (33).

MECHANISMS OF RESISTANCE

Acquired resistance to metronidazole is extremely rare in anaerobic bacteria, despite extensive use worldwide (33). The mechanism of resistance is decreased pyruvate:ferredoxin oxidoreductase activity (87), which reduces activation and uptake of the drug. The level of pyruvate:ferredoxin oxidoreductase activity is correlated with the degree of susceptibility of the organism to metronidazole as well as with the rate of drug uptake into the cell (86). Resistant strains have increased levels of lactate dehydrogenase, which appears to compensate for the decreased activity of pyruvate:ferredoxin oxidoreductase.

Resistance to metronidazole is extremely rare among clinical isolates of *Bacteroides* species; only a few strains have been reported. Resistance may be either plasmid-borne or chromosomally mediated (106, 107). The transfer of plasmid-mediated resistance to susceptible strains has been extremely rare over the years.

Resistance to metronidazole is not uncommon in *H. pylori* (40, 140). Furthermore, resistance can develop during therapy (94). The precise mechanism of resistance is not known, but resistant strains accumulate a lesser amount of the drug at a slower rate than sensitive strains (65, 83). Resistance may be due to inability of the strain to achieve a sufficiently low redox potential under microaerophilic conditions to reduce metronidazole (20).

T. vaginalis is an aerotolerant anaerobe that lacks mitochondria; instead, an organelle (hydrogenosome) contains the pyruvate:ferredoxin oxidoreductase system. Fermentative oxidation of pyruvate to acetate as well as ferredoxin-dependent reduction of metronidazole occurs within the hydrogenosomes. Metronidazole resistance is associated with reduced intracellular levels of ferredoxin, secondary to a decrease in transcription of the ferredoxin gene (99) and a concomitant decrease in the pyruvate:ferredoxin oxidoreductase system. Metronidazole-resistant strains exhibit altered carbohydrate metabolism in which oxidation of pyruvate to lactate within hydrogenosomes is abolished, and instead, oxidation to lactate occurs in the cytosol by lactate dehydrogenase (34).

PHARMACOKINETICS

Early pharmacokinetic studies of metronidazole were conducted using microbiologic assays. These assays could not individually measure the concentrations of metronidazole and its bioactive metabolites. Later studies using high-performance liquid chromatography (HPLC) allowed measurement and separation of metronidazole and its major bioactive metabolites (51). An extensive review of the clinical pharmacokinetics of metronidazole has been published (69).

Absorption

Metronidazole administered orally is almost completely absorbed from the intestinal tract, with a bioavailability of approximately 100% (52, 75). Peak serum concentrations are usually attained 0.5 to 2.0 h after administration. Food delays absorption but does not affect bioavailability.

Single doses of 250 and 500 mg administered orally to adults produced mean peak serum concentrations (C_{max}) of 5.1 to 6.2 µg/mL and 11.5 to 13.0 µg/mL, respectively (4, 27, 47, 73, 102). With 1-g and 2-g single doses, the mean C_{max}s were 19.6 and 40.6 µg/mL, respectively (4). At steady state, a regimen of 500 mg administered orally every 8 h produced mean C_{max} and mean trough serum concentrations (C_{min}) of 19.8 and 11.8 µg/mL, respectively (131). With a regimen of 500 mg administered orally every 12 h, mean C_{max} and C_{min} at steady level were 17.4 and 5.5 µg/mL, respectively (30).

A single 500-mg dose infused intravenously to adults over 20 min produced a mean C_{max} of 11.7 to 18.0 µg/mL (38, 47). A single 1-g dose infused over 30 min produced a mean C_{max} of 28.8 µg/mL; the mean serum concentration at 24 h was 4.2 µg/mL. (80). With a regimen of 500 mg infused intravenously every 8 h, the mean C_{max} and C_{min} at steady state were 26 to 27.6 and 12 to 15 µg/mL, respectively (35, 47).

Metronidazole is absorbed slowly when given rectally via suppository. A suppository dose of 500 mg produced a mean C_{max} of 5.5 µg/mL at 4 h (10). With a 1-g suppository dose, the mean C_{max} values were 9.5–11.3 µg/mL (10, 11). The bioavailability of rectal suppositories is 67 to 82%.

Metronidazole administered vaginally in the form of tablet, insert, or suppository is partially absorbed; a 500-mg dose produced a mean C_{max} of 1 to 2 µg/mL (2, 38, 113). A single 5-g dose of vaginal gel (containing 37.5 mg metronidazole) produced a mean C_{max} of 0.237 µg/mL, which is less than 2% of the serum level obtained with a 500 mg oral dose (27).

Distribution

Metronidazole is minimally bound to plasma proteins. Protein binding reported in various studies ranges from 1 to 20%. The absence of significant protein binding and the small size of the molecule favor good distribution throughout the body; the volume of distribution ranges from 0.6 to 0.9 L/kg (60–90% of body weight).

Metronidazole penetrates well into all body tissues and fluids, including vaginal secretions, seminal fluid, and saliva. Therapeutically adequate concentrations are attained in hepatic abscesses and alveolar bone. Adipose tissue concentrations are approximately 20% of the serum levels (59). In patients with a normal biliary tract, the drug enters the bile in concentrations similar to those in serum and is concentrated in the gallbladder (89). In patients with a nonfunctioning gallbladder, gallbladder bile concentrations are lower than those in serum. Metronidazole is secreted in breast milk in concentrations similar to those found in plasma. It also crosses the placenta; fetal concentrations are similar to maternal levels.

Metronidazole penetrates well into the cerebrospinal fluid (CSF). With normal meninges, CSF levels are approximately 50% of the simultaneous serum concentrations (54, 143). In patients with meningitis, CSF levels approximate those in the serum (93, 102). Metronidazole readily penetrates into brain abscesses, where it attains concentrations equal to those in serum (48).

Metabolism and Excretion

Approximately 6 to 18% of administered metronidazole is excreted unchanged in the urine (52, 90). Most of the remainder is metabolized in the liver to oxidative products (2-hydroxy metronidazole and metronidazole-1-acetic acid), and a small proportion is conjugated with glucuronic acid. The hydroxy metabolite is the major metabolite and has 30 to 65% of the bioactivity of the parent compound; it is detectable in plasma in concentrations of up to 5 μg/mL. The metabolites and the glucuronic acid conjugates of metronidazole and its hydroxy metabolite are excreted in the urine.

In healthy volunteers, metronidazole and its hydroxy metabolite are not detectable in feces. However, in patients with *C. difficile* colitis, bactericidal fecal concentrations are obtained (16, 61), most likely because of secretion through inflamed colonic mucosa.

The mean elimination half-life of metronidazole, as reported in studies using HPLC, ranges from 6 to 9 h (average, 8 h), with a total body clearance of 70 to 90 mL/min (69). The renal clearance of the drug is 8 to 12 mL/min in individuals with normal renal function (75). The elimination half-life of the hydroxy metabolite ranges from 9.5 to 19.2 h in patients with normal kidney function (67).

In patients with renal failure, the elimination half-life of metronidazole remains unchanged, but excretion of its metabolites is delayed. These metabolites, however, are removed by hemodialysis. In patients with severe renal insufficiency not on dialysis, the metabolites accumulate, but this has not been associated with any adverse effects. During hemodialysis, the mean elimination half-life of metronidazole is reduced to 2.1 to 3.3 h (69). Peritoneal dialysis has an insignificant effect on metronidazole pharmacokinetics.

In premature neonates, hepatic metabolism of metronidazole is decreased, and the elimination half-life is inversely related to the gestational age. The mean elimination half-lives in

neonates with gestational age 32 to 35 weeks and 36 to 40 weeks were 35.4 h and 24.8 h, respectively (49). Upadhyaya et al. found that the mean elimination half-life in term infants aged 1 to 7 days was approximately twice that in adults (137). The elimination half-life increases with age; in infants more than 8 weeks old, it is similar to that seen in older children and adults (109). In severely malnourished children, metabolic clearance of metronidazole is decreased, and the elimination half-life of the drug is prolonged (66). In elderly patients, the elimination half-life of metronidazole is similar to that in young individuals (76).

Patients with severe liver dysfunction metabolize metronidazole slowly, and the elimination half-life of the drug is prolonged to 18 to 20 h (36, 68). The decreased metabolic clearance of the drug in these patients is due to slower biotransformation to its oxidative metabolites (hydroxy and acid) rather than diminished glucuronidation. The degree of delay in metabolic elimination of metronidazole is proportional to the degree of liver function impairment.

DOSAGE REGIMENS

For anaerobic infections, the package insert recommends a dosage of intravenous metronidazole of 15 mg/kg (1 g for most adults) infused over 1 h followed by 7.5 mg/kg (500 mg for most adults) every 6 h. (Dosage recommendations for indications other than anaerobic infections are in the appropriate sections under "Clinical Indications.") Despite the relatively long elimination half-life of the drug, this 6-hourly dosage schedule has been recommended, with no evidence that such frequent administration is necessary for maintenance of therapeutic concentrations. From a pharmacokinetic perspective, dosing every 8 or 12 h (500 mg every 8 h or 1 g every 12 h) would be a more appropriate regimen to maintain adequate serum concentrations for susceptible organisms. Data suggesting that metronidazole possesses a postantibiotic effect against certain anaerobic bacteria adds further support to lengthening the dosage interval. Currently, the most commonly used dosage in adults for treatment of anaerobic infections is 500 mg every 8 h. Limited data suggest that a dosage of 500 mg every 12 h, or 1 g every 24 h, may also be satisfactory. Since oral therapy provides serum levels comparable to those achieved by the intravenous route, parenteral therapy should be changed to oral therapy when conditions warrant. The maximum daily dose recommended is 4 g.

Patients with renal failure do not require dosage alteration. However, since hemodialysis removes a substantial amount of the drug, it is best to schedule doses so that a dose is administered following dialysis. Patients on chronic ambulatory peritoneal dialysis need not make any adjustments in dosage schedules, as only a small amount of drug is removed this way. In patients with severe hepatic dysfunction, the dosage of metronidazole should be reduced by 50% to avoid drug accumulation and possible toxicity. In preterm infants and term infants less than 4 weeks old, metronidazole dosage should also be reduced.

Metronidazole should be used during pregnancy only if clearly needed and should be avoided during the first trimester.

Since the drug is excreted into breast milk, nursing should be discontinued during, and for 3 days after, metronidazole therapy. The safety of metronidazole in children has not been established.

Metronidazole should be diluted, after reconstitution, to a concentration of 8 mg/mL or less and be neutralized with sodium bicarbonate (5 meq for each 500 mg) to pH 6.0 to 7.0 before intravenous administration. A ready-to-use intravenous preparation (Flagyl IV RTU) that does not require dilution and buffering is available and most commonly used.

ADVERSE EFFECTS

The incidence of adverse effects associated with metronidazole is low. Gastrointestinal symptoms, including abdominal discomfort, anorexia, nausea, and (rarely) vomiting are occasionally experienced. Such effects are frequently reported along with a metallic taste. Furring of the tongue and glossitis may occur. Several cases of acute pancreatitis (21, 24, 114) induced by metronidazole, with documented recurrence following inadvertent reexposure, have been reported. The mean duration of therapy prior to the onset of symptoms was 7 days but can be as short as 1 day. If a patient on metronidazole develops pancreatitis, the drug should be discontinued once other causes of this disease are excluded. Rare cases of hepatitis associated with metronidazole have been reported (5, 45). One case of *C. difficile* colitis associated with metronidazole administration was reported (112); the isolate proved sensitive to the drug at 0.25 μg/mL.

Hypersensitivity reactions, including maculopapular rashes, urticaria, pruritus, bronchospasm, and serum sickness, may occur but are rare (60, 62). Peripheral neuropathy manifested by numbness or paraesthesia has been reported in a few patients after prolonged treatment with metronidazole (usually high doses). Ataxia, confusion, encephalopathy, tremors, and seizures have been reported in association with high doses of the drug (3, 63, 70). One case of recurrent aseptic meningitis associated with metronidazole administration was reported (26). Reversible neutropenia and drug fever has occurred in association with metronidazole administration. Instances of darkened urine secondary to the presence of a metronidazole metabolite have been reported and appear to have no clinical significance.

Metronidazole exhibits mutagenic activity in a number of in vitro bacterial test systems including the Ames *Salmonella typhimurium* system (29). This activity depends on the presence of a nitroreductase system and is due to the drug's reduction products. However, in vitro tests have not implicated metronidazole as a mammalian mutagen (29). Mammalian tissues have very little nitroreductase activity. A concern has been that during metronidazole therapy, the reductive products of the drug might escape from the bacterial cells and act as mutagens on the host tissues. These products, however, are very short-lived and either promptly bind to macromolecules within the bacterial cell or are promptly reduced to inert compounds. A carcinogenic effect of very high doses of metronidazole in rodents has been reported (110, 111), but this effect has not been confirmed in other experimental animals. A

large retrospective study of patients treated with metronidazole did not show an increased incidence of cancer (9).

Reproductive studies in animals have revealed no evidence of harm to the fetus due to metronidazole. The occurrence of congenital defects in infants born to mothers treated with metronidazole during pregnancy has been investigated in a few studies. There was no excess of overall birth defect occurrence in the offspring of exposed women, nor could an excess risk be detected for any category of birth defects (98, 108). A meta-analysis of 7 studies on metronidazole use during pregnancy showed that exposure to the drug during the first trimester was not associated with increased teratogenic risk (18).

DRUG INTERACTIONS

Metronidazole drug interactions are listed in Table 2.

Effect of Metronidazole on Other Drugs

Warfarin

Metronidazole enhances the anticoagulant effect of racemic sodium warfarin (Coumadin) by increasing its plasma half-life. This interaction is stereospecific; metronidazole augments only the effect of $S(-)$-warfarin (levowarfarin) and not that of $R(+)$-warfarin (dextrowarfarin) (92). Metronidazole should be used with caution in patients on Coumadin; prothrombin time should be monitored closely and the dosage of Coumadin adjusted as necessary.

Alcohol

A disulfiram-like effect manifested as flushing, palpitation, tachycardia, nausea, and vomiting may occur with concomitant use of alcohol and metronidazole. This is possibly due to inhibition of aldehyde dehydrogenase in the central nervous system (141). Patients taking metronidazole should be warned of potential side effects with consumption of alcohol.

Disulfiram

An acute psychotic or confusional state may occur if metronidazole is administered to patients receiving disulfiram. The mechanism of this interaction is unknown.

TABLE 2 • Metronidazole Drug Interactions

Drug	Interaction
Warfarin	Increased anticoagulant effect
Alcohol	Disulfiram reaction
Disulfiram	Acute psychotic or confusional state
Phenytoin	Increased phenytoin concentration, decreased metronidazole concentration
Lithium	Increased lithium concentration
Phenobarbital	Decreased metronidazole concentration
Prednisone	Decreased metronidazole concentration
Rifampin	Decreased metronidazole concentration
Cimetidine	Increased metronidazole concentration
Antacids (Al/Mg hydroxide)	Decreased bioavailability oral metronidazole
Cholestyramine	Decreased bioavailability oral metronidazole

Phenytoin

Metronidazole decreases the clearance of phenytoin by 15% (15) by interfering with the hepatic metabolism of the drug. The clinical significance of the interaction is unknown.

Lithium

Metronidazole may enhance renal retention of lithium, resulting in lithium intoxication. The dosage of lithium should be reduced temporarily when metronidazole is used concurrently.

Interference with Chemical Assays

Metronidazole may interfere with chemical determinations of aspartate aminotransferase (AST), alanine aminotransferase (ALT), lactate dehydrogenase (LDH), and triglycerides, resulting in falsely low values. These assays involve enzymatic coupling to oxidation-reduction of nicotine adenine dinucleotide (NAD+ ↔ NADH); interference is due to the similarity in absorbance peaks of NADH and metronidazole.

Effect of Other Drugs on Metronidazole

Phenobarbital

Phenobarbital induces microsomal liver enzymes and enhances the hepatic metabolism of metronidazole. When used concurrently, the body clearance of metronidazole is increased by 1.5-fold, and the elimination half-life decreased to 67% of normal (77). This can potentially result in treatment failure. In patients taking phenobarbital, a higher dose of metronidazole should be used, especially if the patient fails to respond to metronidazole treatment.

Phenytoin

Phenytoin induces microsomal liver enzymes and accelerates metabolic clearance of the drug, resulting in reduced plasma levels.

Prednisone

Prednisone enhances metabolism and body clearance of metronidazole when both agents are coadministered.

Rifampin

Rifampin enhances hepatic metabolism of metronidazole, increasing its clearance by 44% (28).

Cimetidine

Cimetidine decreases microsomal liver enzyme activity, thus decreasing plasma clearance and prolonging the elimination half-life of metronidazole.

Absorbing Agents

Antacids containing aluminum and magnesium hydroxide decrease the bioavailability of oral metronidazole by a mean of 14.5%. Similarly, the bioavailability of metronidazole is decreased by 21.3% when administered with cholestyramine (82).

CLINICAL INDICATIONS

The major clinical indications for metronidazole use are listed in Table 3.

TABLE 3 • Clinical Indications for Metronidazole

Anaerobic infections	Intraabdominal
	Gynecologic
	Central nervous system
	Endocarditis
	Bone and joint
	Skin and soft tissue
	Bacteremia
Clostridium difficile colitis	
Helicobacter pylori infection	
Bacterial vaginosis	
Protozoal infections	Trichomoniasis
	Amebiasis
	Giardiasis
	Blastocystis hominis

Anaerobic Infections

Metronidazole is an effective agent for a variety of anaerobic infections, particularly those caused by *Bacteroides* species. The notable exception is infections caused by nonsporeforming anaerobic Gram-positive rods (including actinomycosis) and some of the more aerotolerant peptostreptococci. Since most anaerobic infections are polymicrobial, involving aerobes as well as anaerobes, metronidazole is usually combined with an agent active against aerobic organisms.

Metronidazole combined with an aminoglycoside, a third-generation cephalosporin, or a quinolone is an effective empirical regimen for treatment of intraabdominal infections (88, 115, 121). Most of these infections also require appropriate surgical drainage. Several prospective randomized clinical studies showed metronidazole and clindamycin to be equivalent agents for the treatment of intraabdominal infections when either drug was combined with an aminoglycoside (19, 57, 118, 138). Metronidazole combined with an aminoglycoside or a cephalosporin (second- or third-generation) is effective for the treatment of pelvic infections following childbirth or gynecologic surgery. For these infections, a metronidazole-aminoglycoside combination is comparable to clindamycin-aminoglycoside (39).

Because of its bactericidal activity and excellent penetration into the brain, metronidazole is an important component of regimens used to treat brain abscess (48). Since most of these infections are polymicrobial, involving both aerobes and anaerobes, metronidazole is combined with another agent (such as ceftriaxone or penicillin) for the initial empirical therapy (43, 117). Metronidazole is the drug of choice for treatment of *B. fragilis* meningitis.

Use of metronidazole alone for the treatment of anaerobic pleuropulmonary infections has been associated with a significant failure rate. This is not surprising since most of these infections are polymicrobial and include aerobes such as microaerophilic and other streptococci that are resistant to metronidazole.

Metronidazole is effective for the treatment of bacteremia, endocarditis, and septic thrombophlebitis caused by anaerobic Gram-negative bacilli. It is effective in periodontal and gingival infections, anaerobic osteomyelitis in diabetic patients, and tetanus (1). Metronidazole combined with an appropriate agent for aerobes can be used for the treatment of necrotizing skin and soft-tissue infections. The bactericidal activity of metronidazole against *C. perfringens* and other clostridia indicates that it would be of value in the treatment of gas gangrene.

Clostridium difficile Colitis

Metronidazole is an effective alternative to vancomycin for the treatment of *C. difficile* diarrhea (130, 145). There is no significant difference between the two antibiotics in overall response or relapse rates. The usual dose of oral metronidazole is 500 mg three times daily. A concern has been that metronidazole given by mouth is usually undetectable in stool (53). Although this is true for patients with normal intestinal transit time, Bolton and Culshaw showed that bactericidal fecal levels of metronidazole were present in patients with acute *C. difficile* diarrhea who were receiving metronidazole and that levels fell as the diarrhea improved, becoming undetectable after recovery (16). The increase in incidence of vancomycin-resistant enterococcal infection during the last few years has made metronidazole the drug of choice for initial management of *C. difficile* diarrhea. In patients who cannot take oral medications or who have ileus or toxic megacolon, metronidazole can be given intravenously at a dose of 500 mg every 8 h (58).

Helicobacter pylori Infection and Peptic Ulcer Disease

Metronidazole is one of the components of many regimens used to treat duodenal and gastric ulcer. Two-week triple therapy with a bismuth compound, metronidazole, and tetracycline (or amoxicillin) is effective in eradicating *H. pylori* (22, 132, 133), but side effects are common. If the *H. pylori* strain is resistant to metronidazole, the therapy is less effective (104, 139). Currently, 10- to 14-day triple therapy with omeprazole, clarithromycin (or amoxicillin), and metronidazole is most commonly used; it provides cure rates of 80 to 90% (64, 71, 136).

Bacterial Vaginosis

In patients with bacterial vaginosis, the normal *Lactobacillus*-dominated vaginal flora is replaced by other organisms, such as *G. vaginalis, Mobiluncus* species, and other anaerobes, but the exact contribution of these organisms has not been elucidated. Oral metronidazole is currently the treatment of choice for bacterial vaginosis, with reported cure rates of 85 to 90%. The most commonly recommended regimen is 500 mg twice daily for 7 days. A meta-analysis of various oral metronidazole treatment regimens showed no significant differences in cure or in relapse rates between a 2-g single dose and a 7-day or 5-day regimen (79). However, 2 of the 10 studies used in the meta-analysis found a statistically higher cure rate with 7 days of therapy than with the single-dose regimen.

Metronidazole vaginal gel is an effective alternative to oral metronidazole for the treatment of bacterial vaginosis (37, 46, 74), particularly in patients who do not tolerate oral metronidazole. The recommended dose is one applicator full (5 g of gel) intravaginally twice a day for 5 days. Each gram of gel contains 7.5 mg of metronidazole.

Protozoal Infections

Trichomoniasis

Metronidazole is the drug of choice for *T. vaginalis*. A single dose of 2 g orally (recommended regimen) is as effective as 500 mg twice daily for 7 days. Both regimens provide cure rates of 90 to 95%. Low-to-moderate resistance to metronidazole is found in approximately 1 in 200 to 400 cases; these usually respond to higher doses of the drug: 2 g daily in divided doses for 5 to 10 days (78). Patients with high-level resistant strains are refractory to metronidazole therapy.

Amebiasis

Metronidazole is the treatment of choice for symptomatic intestinal amebiasis, amebic liver abscess, and other forms of extraintestinal amebiasis. The recommended dose is 750 mg orally three times daily (in children, 35 to 50 mg/kg daily in 3 divided doses) for 10 days. This regimen gives a cure rate of 92% in amebic dysentery and nearly 100% in amebic liver abscess. In patients unable to take oral medications, the drug can be administered intravenously. Metronidazole does not effectively eradicate cysts in the colon. Treatment, therefore, should be followed by a course of an intraluminal amebicide (paromomycin, diloxanide furoate, or iodoquinol) to eradicate cysts that may persist in the colon after treatment with metronidazole.

Giardiasis

Metronidazole, 250 mg orally tree times daily for 5 days, is as effective as quinacrine for the treatment of *G. lamblia* infection.

Blastocystis hominis

Result of clinical reports and limited in vitro studies make metronidazole the drug of choice for diarrhea caused by *B. hominis* (124). However, the precise pathogenicity of this organism remains to be determined.

Other Therapeutic Uses

Metronidazole appears to have a beneficial effect in Crohn's disease, particularly in patients with perianal lesions (12, 50, 127). Metronidazole gel (0.75%) applied topically and oral metronidazole are both effective for treatment of inflammatory papules and pustules of rosacea. Individual case reports have described successful use of metronidazole to treat lichen planus (142), granulomatous cheilitis (56, 81), eosinophilic pustular folliculitis in individuals infected with human immuno-deficiency virus (119), and Sweet's syndrome (6).

Prophylactic Use

Metronidazole provides effective prophylaxis in surgical operations with a high risk of postoperative anaerobic infection. In patients undergoing elective colonic surgery, preoperative administration of metronidazole combined with an aminoglycoside significantly reduces the incidence of postoperative wound and intraabdominal infections. The recommended dose of metronidazole in adults is 1 g infused over 60 min and completed 1 h before surgery, followed by 500 mg 8 h later. Perioperative administration of metronidazole significantly reduces the incidence of infection after both vaginal and abdominal hysterectomy and cesarean section.

REFERENCES

1. Ahmadsyah I, Salim A. Treatment of tetanus: an open study to compare the efficacy of procaine penicillin and metronidazole. Br Med J 1985;291:648–650.
2. Alper MM, Barwin BN, McLean WM, McGilveray IJ, Sved S. Systemic absorption of metronidazole and its main metabolites by the vaginal route. Obstet Gynecol 1985;65:781–784.
3. Alvarez RS, Richardson DA, Bent AE, Ostergard DR. Central nervous system toxicity related to prolonged metronidazole therapy. Am J Obstet Gynecol 1983;145:640–641.
4. Amon I, Amon K, Huller H. Pharmacokinetics and therapeutic efficacy of metronidazole at different dosages. Int J Clin Pharmacol 1978;16:384–386.
5. Appleby DH, Vogtland HD. Suspected metronidazole hepatotoxicity. Clin Pharmacol 1983;2:373–374.
6. Banet DE, McClave SA, Callen JP. Oral metronidazole, an effective treatment for Sweet's syndrome in a patient with associated inflammatory bowel disease. J Rheumatol 1994;21: 1766–1768.
7. Bannatyne RM, Jackowski J, Cheung R, Briers K. Susceptibility of *Gardnerella vaginalis* to metronidazole, its bioactive metabolites, and tinidazole. Am J Clin Pathol 1986;87:640–641.
8. Baron EJ, Ropers G, Summanen P, Coucol RJ. Bactericidal activity of selected antimicrobial agents against *Bilophila wadsworthia* and *Bacteroides gracilis*. Clin Infect Dis 1993; 16(Suppl 4):S339–343.
9. Beard CM, Noller KL, O'Fallon WM, Kurland LT, Dahlin DC. Cancer after exposure to metronidazole. Mayo Clin Proc 63;1988:147–153.
10. Bergan T, Arnold E. Pharmacokinetics of metronidazole in healthy adult volunteers after tablets and suppositories. Chemotherapy 1980;26:231–241.
11. Bergan T, Leineb O, Blom-Hagen T, Salvesen B. Pharmacokinetics and bioavailability of metronidazole after tablets, suppositories and intravenous administration. Scand J Gastroenterol 1984;19(Suppl 91):45–60.
12. Bernstein CN, Shanahan F. Metronidazole in Crohn's disease: what's the score. Gastroenterology 1992;102:1435–1436.
13. Betriu C, Cabronero C, Gomez M, Picazo JJ. Changes in the susceptibility of *Bacteroides fragilis* group organisms to various antimicrobial agents 1979–1989. Eur J Clin Microbiol Infect Dis 1992;11:352–356.
14. Betriu C, Campos E, Cabronero C, Rodriguez-avial C, Picazo JJ. Susceptibilities of species of the *Bacteroides fragilis* group to 10 antimicrobial agents. Antimicrob Agents Chemother 1990;34: 671–673.
15. Blyden GT, Scavone JM, Greenblatt DJ. Metronidazole impairs clearance of phenytoin but not of alprazolam or lorazepam. J Clin Pharmacol 1988;28:240–245.
16. Bolton RP, Culshaw MA. Fecal Metronidazole concentrations during oral and intravenous therapy for antibiotic associated colitis due to *Clostridium difficile*. Gut 1986;27:1169–1172.
17. Brazier JS, Levett PN, Stannard AJ, Phillips KD, Willis AT. Antibiotic susceptibility of clinical isolates of clostridia. J Antimicrob Chemother 1985;15:181–185.
18. Burtin P, Taddio A, Ariburnu O, Einarson TR, Koren G. Safety of metronidazole in pregnancy: a meta-analysis. Obstet Gynecol 1995;172:525–529.
19. Canadian Metronidazole-Clindamycin Study Group. Prospective, randomized comparison of metronidazole and clindamycin, each with gentamicin, for the treatment of serious intra-abdominal infection. Surgery 1983;93:221–229.
20. Cederbrant G, Kahlmeter G, Ljungh A. Proposed mechanism for metronidazole resistance in *Helicobacter pylori*. J Antimicrob Chemother 1992;29:115–120.
21. Celifarco A, Warschauer C, Burakoff R. Metronidazole-induced pancreatitis. Am J Gastroenterol 1989;84:958–960.
22. Chiba N, Rao BV, Rademaker JW, Hunt RH. Meta-analysis of the efficacy of antibiotic therapy in eradicating *Helicobacter pylori*. Am J Gastroenterol 1992;87:1716–1727.
23. Citron DM, Goldstein EJC, Kenner MA, Burnham LB, Inderlied CB. Activity of ampicillin/sulbactam, ticarcillin/clavulanate, clarithromycin, and eleven other antimicrobial agents against anaerobic bacteria isolated from infections in children. Clin Infect Dis 1995;20(Suppl 2):S356–360.
24. Corey WA, Doebbeling BN, DeJong KJ, Britigan BE. Metronidazole-induced acute pancreatitis. Rev Infect Dis 1991;13: 1213–1215.
25. Cornick NA, Cuchural GJ Jr, Snydman DR, Jacobus NV, Iannini P, Hill G. The antimicrobial susceptibility pattern of the *Bacteroides fragilis* group in the United States. 1987. J Antimicrob Chemother 1990;25:1011–1019.
26. Corson AP, Chretien JH. Metronidazole-associated aseptic meningitis. Clin Infect Dis 1994;19:974.
27. Cunningham FE, Kraus DM, Brubacker L, Fischer JH. Pharmacokinetics of intravaginal metronidazole gel. J Clin Pharmacol 1994;34:1060–1065.
28. Djojosaputro M, Mustofa, Suryawati S, Donatus IA, Santoso B. The effect of doses and pretreatment with rifampicin on the elimination kinetics of metronidazole. Eur J Pharmacol 1990;183: 1870–1871.
29. Dobiás L, Cerná M, Rössner P, Srám R. Genotoxicity and carcinogenicity of metronidazole. Mutation Res 1994;317: 177–194.
30. Earl P, Sisson PR, Ingham HR. Twelve-hourly dosage schedule for oral and intravenous metronidazole. J Antimicrob Chemother 1989;23:619–621.
31. Easmon CS, Ison CA, Kaye CM, Timewell RM, Dawson SG. Pharmacokinetics of metronidazole and its principal metabolites and their activity against *Gardnerella vaginalis*. Br J Vener Dis 1982;58:246–249.
32. Edwards DI. Reduction of nitroimidazoles in vitro and DNA damage. Biochem Pharmacol 1986;35:53–58.
33. Edwards DI. Nitroimidazole drugs—action and resistance mechanisms. I. Mechanisms of action. J Antimicrob Chemother 1993;31:9–20.
34. Edwards DI. Nitroimidazole drugs—action and resistance mechanisms. II. Mechanisms of resistance. J Antimicrob Chemother 1993;31:201–210.
35. Eykyn S, Phillips I. Metronidazole and anaerobic sepsis. Br Med J 1976;2:1418–1421.
36. Farrell G, Baird-Lambert J, Cvejic M, Buchanan N. Disposition and metabolism of metronidazole in patients with liver failure. Hepatology 1984;4:722–726.
37. Ferris DG, Litaker MS, Woodward L, Mathis D, Hendrich J. Treatment of bacterial vaginosis: a comparison of oral metronidazole, metronidazole vaginal gel, and clindamycin vaginal cream. J Fam Pract 1995;41:443–449.
38. Fredricsson B, Hagstrom B, Nord CE, Rand A. Systemic concentrations of metronidazole and its metabolites after intravenous, oral and vaginal administration. Gynecol Obstet Invest 1987;24:200–207.

39. Gall SA, Kohan AP, Ayers OM, Hughes CE, Addison WA, Hill GB. Intravenous metronidazole or clindamycin with tobramycin for therapy of pelvic infection. Obstet Gynecol 1981;57:51–58.

40. Glupczynski Y. Results of a multicenter European survey in 1991 of metronidazole resistance in *Helicobacter pylori*. Eur J Clin Microbiol Infect Dis 1992;11:777–781.

41. Goldman P, Koch RL, Teung T-C, Chrytal EJT, Beaulieu BBJ, McLafferty MA, Sudlow G. Comparing the reduction of nitroimidazoles in bacteria and mammalian tissues and relating it to biological activity. Biochem Pharmacol 1986;35:43–51.

42. Goldstein EJC, Citron DM, Cherubin CE, Hillier SL. Comparative susceptibility of the Bacteroides fragilis group species and other anaerobic bacteria to meropenem, imipenem, piperacillin, cefoxitin, ampicillin/sulbactam, clindamycin and metronidazole. J Antimicrob Chemother 1993;31:363–372.

43. Harris AA, Levin S. Brain abscess. In: Gorbach SL, Bartlett JG, Blacklow NR, eds. Infectious diseases. Philadelphia: WB Saunders, 1992:1197–1206.

44. Hecht DW, Lederer L, Osmolski JR. Susceptibility results for the *Bacteroides fragilis* group: comparison of the broth microdilution and agar dilution methods. Clin Infect Dis 1995;20(Suppl 2):S342–345.

45. Hestin D, Hanesse B, Frimat L, Trechot P, Netter P, Kessler M. Metronidazole-associated hepatotoxicity in a hemodialyzed patient. Nephron 1994;68:286.

46. Hillier S, Lipinski C, Briselden AM, Eschenbach DA. Efficacy of intravaginal 0.75% metronidazole gel for treatment of bacterial vaginosis. Obstet Gynecol 1993;81:963–967.

47. Houghton GW, Thorne PS, Smith J, Tempelton R, Collier J, et al. The pharmacokinetics of intravenous metronidazole (single and multiple dosing). In: Phillips I, Collier J, eds. Metronidazole. Proceedings of the Second International Symposium on Anaerobic Infections, Geneva, April, 1979. London, Royal Society of Medicine and Academic Press, 1979:35–40.

48. Ingham HR, Selkon JB, Roxy CM. Bacteriologic study of otogenic cerebral abscesses: chemotherapeutic role of metronidazole. Br Med J 1977;2:991–993.

49. Jager-Roman E, Doyle PE, Baird-Lambert J, Cvejic M, Buchanan N. Pharmacokinetics and tissue distribution of metronidazole in the newborn infant. J Pediatr 1982;100:651–654.

50. Jakobovitz J, Schuster MM. Metronidazole therapy for Crohn's disease and associated fistulae. Am J Gastroenterol 1984;79:533–540.

51. Jensen JC, Gugler R. Sensitive high-performance liquid chromatographic method for the determination of metronidazole and metabolites. J Chromatography 1983;277:381–384.

52. Jensen JC, Cugler R. Single- and multiple-dose metronidazole kinetics. Clin Pharmacol Ther 1983;34:481–487.

53. Johnson S, Homann SR, Bettin KM, Quick JN, Clabots CR, Peterson LR, Gerding DN. Treatment of asymptomatic *Clostridium difficile* carriers (fecal excretors) with vancomycin or metronidazole. Ann Intern Med 1992;117:297–302.

54. Jokipii AMM, Myllyla VV, Hokhanen E. Penetration of blood-brain barrier by metronidazole and tinidazole. J Antimicrob Chemother 1977;3:237–245.

55. Jousimies-Somer H, Asikainen S, Suomala P, Summanen P. Activity of metronidazole and its hydroxy metabolite against clinical isolates of *Actinobacillus actinomycetemcomitans*. Oral Microbiol Immunol 1988;3:31–34.

56. Kano Y, Shiohara T, Yagita A, Nagashima M. Granulomatous cheilitis and Crohn's disease. Br J Dermatol 1990;123:409–412.

57. Kirkpatrick JR, Anderson BJ, Louie JJ, Stiver HG. Double-blind comparison of metronidazole plus gentamicin and clindamycin plus gentamicin in intra-abdominal infection. Surgery 1983;93:215–216.

58. Kleinfeld DI, Sharpe RJ, Donta ST. Parenteral therapy for antibiotic-associated pseudomembranous colitis. J Infect Dis 1988;157:389.

59. Kling P-R, Burman LG. Serum and tissue pharmacokinetics of intravenous metronidazole in surgical patients. Acta Chir Scand 1989;155:347–350.

60. Knowles S, Choudhury T, Shear NH. Metronidazole hypersensitivity. Ann Pharmacother 1994;28:325–326.

61. Krook A, Lindstrom B, Kjellander J, Jarnerot G, Bodin L. Relation between concentrations of metronidazole and *Bacteroides* spp in feces of patients with Crohn's disease and healthy individuals. J Clin Pathol 1981;34:645–650.

62. Kurohara ML, Kwong FK, Lebherz TB, Klaustermeyer ML. Metronidazole hypersensitivity and oral desensitization. J Allergy Clin Immunol 1991;88:279–280.

63. Kusumi RK, Plouffe JF, Wyatt RH, Fass RJ. Central nervous system toxicity associated with metronidazole therapy. Ann Intern Med 1980;93:59–60.

64. Labenz J, Idstrom JP, Tillenburg B, Peitz U, Adamek RJ, Borsch G. One-week low-dose triple therapy for Helicobacter pylori is sufficient for relief from symptoms and healing of duodenal ulcers. Aliment Pharmacol Ther 1997;11:89–93.

65. Lacey SL, Moss SF, Taylor GW. Metronidazole uptake by sensitive and resistant isolates of *Helicobacter pylori*. J Antimicrob Chemother 1993:32:393–400.

66. Lares-Asseff I, Cravioto J, Santiago P, Perez-Otiz B. Pharmacokinetics of metronidazole in severely malnourished and nutritionally rehabilitated children. Clin Pharmacol Ther 1992;51:42–50.

67. Lau AH, Emmons K, Seligsohn R. Pharmacokinetics of intravenous metronidazole at different dosages in healthy subjects. Int J Clin Pharmacol Ther Toxicol 1991;29:386–390.

68. Lau AH, Evans R, Chang C-W, Seligsohn R. Pharmacokinetics of metronidazole in patients with alcoholic liver disease. Antimicrob Agents Chemother 1987;31:1662–1664.

69. Lau AH, Lam NP, Piscitelli SC, Wilkes L, Danziger LH. Clinical pharmacokinetics of metronidazole and other nitroimidazole anti-infectives. Clin Pharmacokinet 1992;23:328–364.

70. Lawford R, Sorrell TC. Amebic abscess of the spleen complicated by metronidazole-induced neurotoxicity: case report. Clin Infect Dis 1994;19:346–348.

71. Lerang F, Moum B, Haug JB, Tolas P, Breder O, Aubert E, Hoie O, Soberg T, Flaaten B, Farup P, Berg T. Highly effective twice-daily triple therapies for *Helicobacter pylori* infection and peptic ulcer disease; does in vitro metronidazole resistance have any clinical relevance. Am J Gastroenterol 1997;92:248–253.

72. Levett PN. Time-dependent killing of *Clostridium difficile* by metronidazole and vancomycin. J Antimicrob Chemother 1991;27:55–62.

73. Levison ME. Microbiological agar diffusion assay for metronidazole concentrations in serum. Antimicrob Agents Chemother 1974;5:466–468.

74. Livengood CH, McGregor JA, Soper DE, Newton E, Thomason JL. Bacterial vaginosis. Efficacy and safety of intravaginal metronidazole treatment. Am J Obstet Gynecol 1994;170:759–764.

75. Loft S, Dossing M, Poulsen HE, Sonne J, Olesen KL, Simonsen K, Andreason PB. Influence of dose and route of administration

on disposition of metronidazole and its major metabolites. Eur J Clin Pharmacol 1986;30:467–473.

76. Loft S, Egsmose C, Sonne J, Poulsen HE, Dossig M, Andreasen PB. Metronidazole elimination is preserved in the elderly. Hum Exp Toxicol 1990;9:155–159.

77. Loft S, Sonne J, Dossing M, Andreasen PB. Metronidazole pharmacokinetics in patients with hepatic encephalopathy. Scand J Gastroenterol 1987;22:117–123.

78. Lossick JG, Kent HL. Trichomoniasis: trends in diagnosis and management. Am J Obstet Gynecol 1991;195:1217–1222.

79. Lugo-Miro VI, Green M, Mazur L. Comparison of different metronidazole therapeutic regimens for bacterial vaginosis. JAMA 1992;268:92–95.

80. Martin C, Sastre B, Mallet MN, Bruguerolle B, Brun JP, De Micco P, Gouin F. Pharmacokinetics and tissue penetration of a single 1,000-milligram, intravenous dose of metronidazole for antibiotic prophylaxis of colorectal surgery. Antimicrob Agents Chemother;1991;35:2602–2605.

81. Miralles J, Barnadas MA, de Moragas JM. Cheilitis granulomatosa treated with metronidazole. Dermatology 1995;191:252–253.

82. Molokhia AM, Al-Rahman S. Effect of concomitant oral administration of some absorbing drugs on the bioavailability of metronidazole. Drug Dev Ind Pharm 1987;13:1329–1337.

83. Moore RA, Beckthold B, Bryan LE. Metronidazole uptake in *Helicobacter pylori*. Can J Microbiol 1995;41:746–749.

84. Muller M. Reductive activation of nitroimidazoles in anaerobic microorganisms. Biochem Pharmacol 1986;35:37–41.

85. Nagi E, Foldes J. Inactivation of metronidazole by *Enterococcus faecalis*. J Antimicrob Chemother 1991;27:63–70.

86. Narikawa S. Distribution of metronidazole susceptibility factors in obligate anaerobes. J Antimicrob Chemother 1986;18:565–574.

87. Narikawa S, Suzuki T, Yamamoto M, Nakamura M. Lactate dehydrogenase activity as a cause of metronidazole resistance in *Bacteroides fragilis* NCTC 11295. J Antimicrob Chemother 1991;28:47–53.

88. Nicolau DP, Patel KB, Quintiliani R, Nightingale CH. Cephalosporin-metronidazole combinations in the management of intra-abdominal infections. Diagn Microbiol Infect Dis 1995;22:189–194.

89. Nielsen ML, Justesen T. Excretion of metronidazole in human bile. Scand J Gastroenterol 1977;12:1003–1008.

90. Nilsson-Ehle I, Ursing B, Nilsson-Ehle P. Liquid chromatographic assay for metronidazole and tinidazole: pharmacokinetic and metabolic studies in human subjects. Antimicrob Agents Chemother 1981;19:754–760.

91. Nix DE, Tyrrell R, Muller M. Pharmacodynamics of metronidazole determined by a time-kill assay for *Trichomonas vaginalis*. Antimicrob Agents Chemother 1995;39:1848–1852.

92. O'Reilly RA. The stereoselective interaction of warfarin and metronidazole in man. N Engl J Med 1976;295:354–357.

93. O'Grady LR, Ralph ED. Anaerobic meningitis and bacteremia caused by *Fusobacterium* species. Am J Dis Child 1976;130:871–873.

94. Owen RJ, Bell GD, Desai M, Moreno M, Gant PV, Jones PH, Linton D. Biotype and molecular fingerprints of metronidazole-resistant strains of *Helicobacter pylori* from antral gastric mucosa. J Med Microbiol 1993;38:6–12.

95. Pankuch GA, Jacobs MR, Appelbaum PC. Susceptibilities of 428 gram-positive and -negative anaerobic bacteria to Bay y3118 compared with their susceptibilities to ciprofloxacin,

clindamycin, metronidazole, piperacillin, piperacillin- tazobactam, and cefoxitin. Antimicrob Agents Chemother 1993;37:1649–1654.

96. Pavicic MJAMP, van Winkelhoff AJ, Pavicic-Temming YAM, de Graaff J. Metronidazole susceptibility factors in *Actinobacillus actinomycetemcomitans*. J Antimicrob Chemother 1995;35:263–269.

97. Pendland SL, Piscitelli SC, Schreckenberger PC, Danziger LH. In vitro activities of metronidazole and its hydroxy metabolite against *Bacteroides* species. Antimicrob Agents Chemother 1994;38:2106–2110.

98. Piper JM, Mitchel EF, Ray WA. Prenatal use of metronidazole and birth defects: no association. Obstet Gynecol 1993;82:348–352.

99. Quon DVK, d'Oliveira CE, Johnson PJ. Reduced transcription of the ferredoxin gene in metronidazole-resistant *Trichomonas vaginalis*. Proc Natl Acad Sci USA 1992;89:4402–4406.

100. Ralph ED. The bactericidal activity of nitrofurantoin and metronidazole against anaerobic bacteria. J Antimicrob Chemother 1978;4:177–184.

101. Ralph ED, Amatnieks YE. Potentially synergistic antimicrobial combinations with metronidazole against *Bacteroides fragilis*. Antimicrob Agents Chemother 1980;17:379–382.

102. Ralph ED, Clarke JT, Libke RD, Luthy RP, Kirby WMM. Pharmacokinetics of metronidazole as determined by bioassay. Antimicrob Agents Chemother 1974;6:691–696.

103. Ralph ED, Kirby WMM. Unique bactericidal action of metronidazole against *Bacteroides fragilis* and *Clostridium perfringens*. Antimicrob Agents Chemother 1975;8:409–414.

104. Rautelin H, Seppalla K, Renkonen Ov, Vainio U, Kosunen TU. Role of metronidazole resistance in therapy of *Helicobacter pylori* infections. Antimicrob Agents Chemother 1992;36:163–166.

105. Ravdin JI, Skilogiannis J. In vitro susceptibilities of *Entamoeba histolytica* to azithromycin, CP-63,956, erythromycin, and metronidazole. Antimicrob Agents Chemother 1989;33:960–962.

106. Reysset G, Haggoud A, Sebald M. Genetics of resistance of *Bacteroides* species to 5-nitroimidazole. Clin Infect Dis 1993;16 (Suppl 4):S401–403.

107. Reysset G, Haggoud A, Su W-J, Sebald M. Genetics and molecular analysis of pIP417 and pIP419: *Bacteroides* plasmids encoding 5-nitroimidazole resistance. Plasmid 1992;27:181–190.

108. Rosa FW, Baum C, Shaw M. Pregnancy outcomes after first-trimester vaginitis drug therapy. Obstet Gynecol 1987;69:751–755.

109. Rubenson A, Rosetzsky A. Single-dose prophylaxis with metronidazole in infants during abdominal surgery: a pharmacokinetic study. Eur J Clin Phamacol 1986;29:625–628.

110. Rustia M, Shubik P. Induction of lung tumors and malignant lymphomas in mice by metronidazole. J Natl Cancer Inst 1972;48:721–729.

111. Rustia M, Shubik P. Expermental induction of hepatomas, mammary tumors, and other tumors with metronidazole in noninbred Sac:MRC(W1)BR rats. J Natl Cancer Inst 1979;63:863–867.

112. Saginur R, Hawley CR, Bartlett JG. Colitis associated with metronidazole theray. J Infect Dis 1980;141:772–774.

113. Salas-Herrera IG, Lawson M, Johnston A, Turner P, Gott DM, Dennis MJ. Plasma metronidazole concentrations after single and repeated vaginal pessary administration. Br J Clin Pharmacol 1991;32:621–623.

114. Sanford KA, Mayle JE, Dean HA, Greenbaum DS. Metronidazole-associated pancreatitis. Ann Intern Med 1988;109:756–757.

115. Sawyer MD, Dunn DL. Antimicrobial therapy of intra-abdominal sepsis. Infect Dis Clin North Am 1992;6:545–470.

116. Sheikh W, Pitkin DH, Nadler H. Antibacterial activity of meropenem and selected comparative agents against anaerobic bacteria at seven North American centers. Cin Infect Dis 1993;16(Suppl 4):S361–366.

117. Sjolin J, Lilja A, Eriksson N, Arneborn P, Otto C. Treatment of brain abscess with cefotaxime and metronidazole: prospective study on 15 consecutive patients. Clin Infect Dis 1993;17:857–863.

118. Smith JA, Skidmore AG, Forward AD, Clarke AM, Sutherland E. Prospective, randomized, double-blind comparison of metronidazole and tobramycin with clindamycin and tobramycin in the treatment of intraabdominal sepsis. Ann Surg 1980;192:213–220.

119. Smith KJ, Skelton HG, Yeager J, Ruiz N, Wagner KF. Metronidazole for eosinophilic pustular folliculitis in human immunodeficiency virus type 1-positive patients. Arch Dermatol 1995;131:1089–1091.

120. Snydman DR, Cuchural GJ Jr, the National Anaerobic Susceptibility Study Group. Susceptibility variations in *Bacteroides fragilis:* a national survey. Infect Dis Clin Pract 1994;3(Suppl 1):S34–S43.

121. Solomkin JS, Reinhart HH, Dellinger EP, Bohnen JM, Rotstein OD, Vogel SB, Simms HH, Hill CS, Bjornson HS, Haverstock DC, Coulter HO, Echols RM. Results of a randomized trial comparing sequential intravenous/oral treatment with ciprofloxacin plus metronidazole to imipenem/cilastatin for intra-abdominal infections. The Intra-Abdominal Infection Study Group. Ann Surg 1996;223:303–315.

122. Spangler SK, Jacobs MR, Appelbaum PC. Susceptibility of anaerobic bacteria to trovafloxacin: comparison with other quinolones and non-quinolone antibiotics. Infect Dis Clin Pract 1996;5(Suppl3):S101–109.

123. Spiegel CA. Susceptibility of *Mobiluncus* species to 23 antimicrobial agents and 15 other compounds. Antimicrob Agents Chemother 1987;31:249–252.

124. Stenzel DJ, Boreham PFL. *Blastocystis hominis* revisited. Clin Microbiol Rev 1996;9:563–584.

125. Stratton CW, Weeks LS, Aldridge KE. Comparison of the bactericidal activity of clindamycin and metronidazole against cefoxitin-susceptible and cefoxitin-resistant isolates of the *Bacteroides fragilis* group. Diagn Microbiol Infect Dis 1991;14:377–382.

126. Stratton CW, Weeks LS, Aldridge KE. Inhibitory and bactericidal activity of selected beta-lactam agents alone and in combination with beta-lactamase inhibitors compared with that of cefoxitin and metronidazole against cefoxitin-susceptible and cefoxitin-resistant isolates of the *Bacteroides fragilis* group. Diagn Microbiol Infect Dis 1992;15:321–330.

127. Sutherland L, Singleton J, Sessions J, Hanauer S, Krawitt E, Rankin G. Double-blind placebo-controlled trial of metronidazole in Crohn's disease. Gut 1991;32:1071–1075.

128. Sutter VL. In vitro susceptibility of anaerobic and microaerophilic bacteria to metronidazole and its hydroxy metabolite. In: Finegold SM, George WL, Rolfe RD, eds. Proceedings of the First United States Metronidazole Conference. Tarpon Springs, FL, February 1982. New York: Biomedical Information Corp, 1982:61.

129. Tally FP, Sutter VL, Finegold SM. Metronidazole versus anaerobes, in vitro data and initial clinical observations. Calif Med 1972;117:22–26.

130. Teasley DG, Olson MM, Olsen MM, Peterson LR, Gebhard RL, Schwartz MJ, Lee TJ. Jr. Prospective randomized trial of metronidazole versus vancomycin for *Clostridium-difficile*-associated diarrhea and colitis. Lancet 1983;2:1043–1046.

131. Thiercelin JF, Diquet B, Levesque C, Ghesquiere F, Simon P, Viars P. Metronidazole kinetics and bioavailability inpatients undergoing gastrointestinal surgery. Clin Pharmacol Ther 1984;35:510–519.

132. Thijs JC, van Zwet AA, Moolenaar W, Wolfhagen MJHM, Huinink JB. Triple therapy vs amoxicillin plus omeprazole for treatment of *Helicobacter pylori* infection: a multicenter, prospective, randomized, controlled study of efficacy and side effects. Am J Gastroenterol 1996;91:93–96.

133. Thijs JC, van Zwet AA, Oey HB. Efficacy and side effects of a triple drug regimen for eradication of *Helicobacter pylori*. Scand J Gastroenterol 1993;28:934–938.

134. Tocher JH, Edwards DI. The interaction of reduced metronidazole with DNA bases and nucleosides. Int J Radiat Oncol Biol Phys 1992;22:661–663.

135. Tocher JH, Edwards DI. Evidence for the direct interaction of reduced metronidazole derivatives with DNA bases. Biochem Pharmacol 1994;48:1089–1094.

136. Treiber G. The influence of drug dosage on *Helicobacter pylori* eradication: a cost effectiveness analysis. Am J Gastroenterol 1996;91:246–257.

137. Upadhyaya P, Bhatnagar V, Basu N. Pharmacokinetics of intravenous metronidazole in neonates. J Pediatr 1988;23:263–265.

138. van der Auwera P, Collier J, Goris RJA, Saario I, Willis AT. A comparison of metronidazole and clindamycin for the treatment of intra-abdominal anaerobic infection: a multicenter trial. J Antimicrob Chemother 1982;10:57–66.

139. van Zwet AA, Thijs JC, Oom JAJ, Hoogeveen J, Düringshoff BL. Failure to eradicate *Helicobacter pylori* in patients with metronidazole resistant strains. Eur J Gastroenterol Hepatol 1993;5:185–186.

140. van Zwet AA, Thijs JC, Schievink-de Vries W, Schiphuis J, Snijder JAM. In vitro studies on stability and development of metronidazole resistance in *Helicobacter pylori*. Antimicrob Agents Chemother 1994;38:360–362.

141. Vasiliou V, Malamas M, Marselas M. The mechanism of alcohol intolerance produced by various therapeutic agents. Acta Pharmacol Toxicol 1986;58:305–310.

142. Wahba-Yahav AV. Idiopathic lichen planus: treatment with metronidazole. J Am Acad Dermatol 1995;33:301–302.

143. Warner JF, Perkins RL, Cordero L. Metronidazole therapy of anaerobic bacteremia, meningitis and brain abscess. Arch Intern Med 1979;139:167–169.

144. Wayne LG, Sramek HA. Metronidazole is bactericidal to dormant cells of *Mycobacterium tuberculosis*. Antimicrob Agents Chemother 1994;38:2054–2058.

145. Wenisch C, Parschalk B, Hasenhundl M, Hirschl AM. Comparison of vancomycin, teicoplanin, metronidazole, and fusidic acid for the treatment of *Clostridium difficile*-associated diarrhea. Clin Infect Dis 1996;22:813–818.

146. Xia HX, Buckley M, Keane RT, O'Morain CA. Clarithromycin resistance in *Helicobacter pylori:* prevalence in untreated dyspeptic patients and stability in vitro. J Antimicrob Chemother 1996;37:473–481.

Monobactams

●

Patricia Kauffman, Bruce Kreter, and Thomas Fekete

The monobactams (monocyclic bacterially derived β-lactams) are a unique class of β-lactam antibiotics whose central core is composed solely of a four-member β-lactam ring and who differ from penicillins, cephalosporins, and carbapenems in that they lack a five- or six-membered side ring. They were originally discovered in parallel by two groups of scientists working independently; one for Squibb Pharmaceuticals and the other for Takeda Pharmaceuticals (33, 87).

The first monobactams isolated did not exhibit particularly potent antimicrobial activity; however, synthetic side-chain modifications resulted in active compounds with increased potency and β-lactamase stability (84). Aztreonam (originally named azthreonam; also SQ 26,776) was among the first synthetic candidates selected for clinical development (Fig. 1). Since aztreonam is the only representative of its class to be commercially developed, most available information regarding monobactams relates specifically to aztreonam.

MECHANISM OF ACTION

Aztreonam, like other β-lactam antibiotics, interferes with cell wall synthesis by binding to and inactivating penicillin-binding proteins (primarily PBP 3), producing bacterial filamentation, cell lysis, and death (33, 86).

ANTIMICROBIAL ACTIVITY

Aztreonam has potent activity against most aerobic Gram-negative bacteria, including *Pseudomonas aeruginosa*, but is very limited in its activity against Gram-positive bacteria and anaerobes. Its activity against Gram-negative organisms is similar to that of third-generation cephalosporins.

Aztreonam is active against more than 90% of *Enterobacteriaceae*, including some strains that are resistant to other β-lactams and aminoglycosides (35). Susceptibility testing has shown that the in vitro activity of aztreonam against *Escherichia coli, Proteus mirabilis, P. vulgaris, Morganella morganii, Providencia rettgeri*, and *Providencia stuartii, Citrobacter freundii*, and *Klebsiella* species, including *K. pneumoniae*, consistently produces MIC$_{90}$s below 1 mg/L (13, 60, 84). *Acinetobacter* are less susceptible than the *Enterobacteriaceae* to aztreonam, and *Enterobacter aerogenes* and *Enterobacter cloacae*, like *P. aeruginosa*, have widely varying MIC$_{90}$ values. Certain fastidious organisms such as *Neisseria gonorrhoeae* and *Haemophilus influenzae* show greater susceptibility, with MIC$_{90}$s of 0.12 to 0.2 mg/L. MIC$_{90}$s for aerobic Gram-negative pathogens that are generally susceptible to aztreonam are presented in Table 1.

Aztreonam generally exhibits synergistic activity in combination with aminoglycosides and additive or synergistic activity

in combination with other β-lactam antibiotics. Antagonism is rare, except when it is added to antibiotic regimens containing potent inducers of β-lactamase, such as cefoxitin or imipenem.

SUSCEPTIBILITY TO β-LACTAMASES

Aztreonam is active in vitro against most Gram-negative aerobic bacteria because of its resistance to hydrolysis by transferable as well as chromosomal β-lactamases (45, 62). Aztreonam is both a poor inducer and a poor substrate for β-lactamases and can inhibit chromosomal β-lactamases (8, 14, 44, 57, 85, 91). Although overt selection of resistant populations of bacteria during treatment does not tend to occur with β-lactam antibiotics, with the exception of strains that have an inducible β-lactamase (e.g., *Enterobacter* spp., *Citrobacter* spp.), resistant strains may emerge when the drug serves as a suitable substrate. Resistance can occur from intrinsic difficulty passing through the Gram-negative outer membrane, particularly with *P. aeruginosa* (46). This mechanism generally applies to all β-lactam antibiotics, although it is less pronounced with cefepime and other zwitterions.

PHARMACODYNAMIC EFFECTS

Aztreonam exerts its bactericidal action like other β- lactams, i.e., through inhibition of Gram-negative penicillin binding proteins (primarily PBP 3). Aztreonam exhibits a short postantibiotic effect; therefore, the primary pharmacodynamic correlate with outcome is assumed to be maintenance of serum concentrations in excess of the MIC for most of a dosing interval.

PHARMACOKINETICS
Absorption

The pharmacokinetics of aztreonam in adults were extensively reviewed by Mattie (48). Aztreonam is generally administered intravenously, although intramuscular injections are well tolerated, and absorption via this route is almost complete. Oral administration results in absorption of less than 1% of the parent compound.

Distribution

Following intravenous administration, the plasma concentration profile follows a two-compartment open model, with an elimination half-life of 1.7 to 2.0 h. The volume of distribution at steady-state is approximately 0.16 L/kg. Aztreonam is not extensively bound to plasma proteins (approximately 56%), and the protein binding is not concentration dependent.

Aztreonam exhibits linear pharmacokinetics; mean peak serum concentrations of 54, 90, and 204 μg/mL were found in

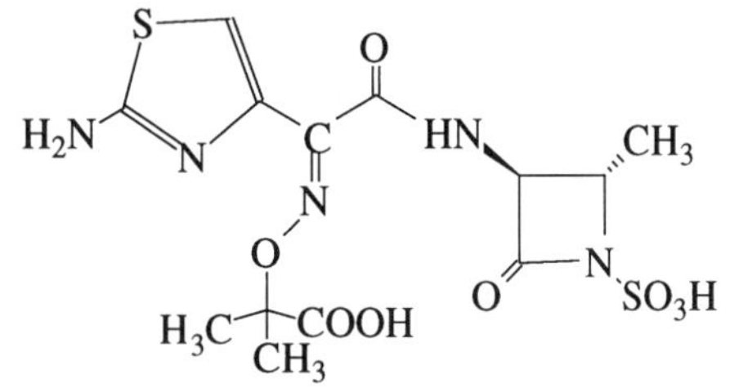

FIGURE 1. Structural formula of aztreonam.

TABLE 1 • **Minimum Inhibitory Concentrations for Aztreonam in 90% of Aerobic Gram-Negative Bacterial Isolates (60, 88)**

Organism	Range of Reported MIC$_{90}$s (mg/L)[a]
Acinetobacter	8–32
Citrobacter freundii	0.7–16
Enterobacter aerogenes	4–16
Enterobacter cloacae	4–16
Escherichia coli	0.2–0.5
Haemophilus influenzae (ampicillin sensitive or resistant)	0.06–0.2
Klebsiella pneumoniae	0.3–0.5
Klebsiella spp.	<1
Morganella morganii	0.6–2
Neisseria gonorrhoeae	0.12–0.2
Proteus mirabilis	<0.1–0.5
Proteus vulgaris	<0.1–2
Providencia rettgeri	<0.1
Providencia stuartii	<0.1
Pseudomonas aeruginosa	8–32
Salmonella spp.	0.3–4
Serratia marcescens	<1–4
Serratia spp.	<1–4

[a] MIC$_{90}$ is the minimal concentration of antibiotic necessary to inhibit 90% of microorganisms.

healthy subjects following single 30-min intravenous infusions of 500 mg, 1 g, and 2 g, respectively. At the end of 8 h, trough serum concentrations were 1, 3, and 6 μg/mL, respectively (12).

Aztreonam has been demonstrated to penetrate well into most tissues. As with other β-lactams, aztreonam penetrates inflamed meninges better than uninflamed meninges. Concentrations in the cerebrospinal fluid (CSF) range from 17 to 33% of concurrent serum values. Low amounts of aztreonam cross the placenta, and low concentrations (<1 μg/mL) are found in breast milk of lactating women (9, 56).

Metabolism and Elimination

Aztreonam is both passively filtered and actively secreted in the kidney, with renal clearance of the parent compound accounting for approximately 60 to 70% of drug elimination in adults. Only 1 to 7% of the parent compound is recovered in the urine as inactive metabolites (83). Probenecid inhibits the active tubular excretion of aztreonam.

In 23 patients studied as part of a clinical trial of penetrating abdominal trauma, the half-life of aztreonam was found to be prolonged in trauma patients (mean, 2.2 h); however no significant differences were observed in the volumes of distribution or total clearance (21). In a group of 10 patients treated with aztreonam for nosocomial pneumonia, the volume of distribution at steady state was increased and the half-life longer than in volunteer studies (50). The authors concluded that standard dosing regimens may result in lower initial concentrations in critically ill patients than were suggested by phase I studies in normal volunteers.

Pediatrics

Peak serum concentrations of approximately 100 and 200 μg/mL are achieved following 30-min infusions of 30 and 50 mg/kg, respectively. The clearance of aztreonam was studied in infants of various birth weights during the first week of life and also during weeks 2 to 4. In very low birth weight infants (<2000g) in their first week of life, the half-life of aztreonam ranged from 5.5 to 9.9 h. In general, the older the infant, the more closely the pharmacokinetics mirror those of the adult. By 1 month of age, the half-life of aztreonam is similar to that in an adult (43). Due to the relatively low plasma protein binding of aztreonam, the drug shows little displacement of bilirubin, even at levels five times those used clinically (78).

In 10 pediatric patients with cystic fibrosis, the volume of distribution was found to be larger and the half-life shorter than in noncystic children (65). As a result, it was estimated that a dose of 50 mg/kg every 6 h would be necessary to maintain serum concentrations above the MIC for most of a dosing interval.

DOSAGE REGIMENS
Adults

In most studies, aztreonam has been administered intravenously to adults in doses of 1 to 2 g every 8 h; however, severe systemic or life-threatening infections, including those caused by *P. aeruginosa,* may require 2 g every 6 h. Due to the extensive renal elimination of the drug, lower doses (0.5–1 g) every 8 to 12 h have proven effective for urinary tract infections (12).

The manufacturer recommends dosage adjustment for patients with significant renal impairment, to avoid accumulation of aztreonam in the bloodstream (12), although no specific adverse events have been described with normal doses of the drug in renally impaired patients. Dosage adjustments are also recommended for patients receiving hemodialysis or continuous ambulatory peritoneal dialysis.

Specific dosing recommendations are not available for pregnant women, obese patients, or those with ascites. Since elderly patients frequently demonstrate diminished renal function, dosage modification based on creatinine clearance is recommended.

Pediatrics

Since the clearance of aztreonam changes with age during the first weeks of life, a dose of 30 mg/kg every 12 h is recommended for infants less than 1 week of age, 30 mg/kg every 8 h for infants 1 to 4 weeks of age, and 30 mg/kg every 6 to 8 h for pediatric patients over 1 month of age (41). Dosing of 50 mg/kg every 6 h may be necessary to maintain serum concentrations above the MIC of *P. aeruginosa* (78). Clinical studies in pediatric patients evaluated aztreonam for the treatment of neonatal sepsis, serious Gram-negative bacterial infections, meningitis, urinary tract infections, and cystic fibrosis (41, 78).

ADVERSE EFFECTS

The clinical safety profile of aztreonam was developed during the registrational trial process from 346 patients who received single doses and 2388 patients who received multiple doses (58). No toxicities are associated with aztreonam that are not recognized for the β-lactams as a class.

Of patients who received multiple doses, 6.8% reported adverse clinical events. The most common were local reactions at the injection site, rash, diarrhea, nausea, and/or vomiting. Laboratory evaluations demonstrated threefold increases in serum aspartate aminotransferase (SGOT) and serum alanine aminotransferase (SGPT) values in 1 and 1.4% of patients, respectively. Aztreonam therapy was discontinued in 2.1% of 2388 patients because of adverse clinical events or abnormal laboratory test values. Superinfections were reported in 2 to 6% of aztreonam-treated patients, similar to what is seen with other antimicrobials used in controlled studies.

Immunology

Despite the β-lactam structure of aztreonam, patients allergic to penicillins or cephalosporins do not generally exhibit cross-allergenicity to aztreonam. A series of studies by Adkinson et al. demonstrated that rabbits made allergic to ceftazidime did not generate IgG or IgM antibodies when exposed to aztreonam, and rabbits made allergic to aztreonam did not generate IgG or IgM antibodies when exposed to ceftazidime (2, 3). Clinical experience with aztreonam has generally supported these findings, and aztreonam is frequently used without incident in patients who describe a history of allergy to a penicillin or cephalosporin (1, 72). It is possible, however, for patients who are allergic specifically to ceftazidime to also exhibit cross- allergenicity to aztreonam because of the 2-aminothiazolyl-iminopropyl-carboxyl side chain common to both compounds.

Nephrotoxicity and Ototoxicity

Aztreonam has frequently been compared with aminoglycosides because of their similar spectra of activity. However, because of its β-lactam structure, aztreonam, unlike aminoglycosides, has negligible effects on renal and auditory function. This was shown in a randomized double-blind clinical trial of 184 patients, in which 15% of 92 patients receiving aminoglycosides developed nephrotoxicity, compared with 1 of 92 patients receiving aztreonam ($P < .004$) (54).

Drug Interactions

No clinically interesting interactions were described between aztreonam and cephradine, clindamycin, gentamicin, metronidazole, nafcillin, probenecid, or furosemide (80).

Safety in Pediatric Patients

Aztreonam therapy was generally well tolerated in pediatric clinical trials (15). The most frequent clinical adverse events were rash, diarrhea, and abdominal pain; the most common laboratory abnormalities were transient elevations in liver function tests, eosinophilia, and thrombocytosis.

One concern with the use of aztreonam in pediatric patients relates to the potential metabolic effects of arginine, which is used as a salt in the commercial preparation (750 mg arginine per gram of aztreonam). Uuay et al. studied the effect of aztreonam infusions on serum chemistry parameters and concluded that although serum arginine and insulin levels rose shortly after infusion of aztreonam, the effect was similar to that seen with infusion of parenteral nutrition (93).

CLINICAL INDICATIONS

Aztreonam is appropriately used in the setting of moderate-to-severe infections that require coverage for aerobic Gram-negative pathogens. Although the narrow spectrum of aztreonam is of potential benefit with regard to minimizing bacteriologic disruption of the host's normal flora, it is generally used in combination with another antibiotic with Gram-positive activity—most commonly clindamycin and vancomycin. Due to its spectrum of activity, most clinicians consider aztreonam an alternative to aminoglycosides in patients at risk of renal or auditory toxicity or an alternative to a third-generation cephalosporin such as ceftazidime.

Adults

Lower Respiratory Tract Infection

Aztreonam was compared with aminoglycosides in five trials of lower respiratory tract infection; clindamycin was used concurrently with both Gram-negative agents in four of the studies (59, 66, 67, 74, 81). Clinical and microbiologic cure rates with aztreonam were superior to those with aminoglycoside in three of the studies. In the largest reported series, the combination of aztreonam plus clindamycin resulted in a 94% clinical cure rate, compared with 79% for tobramycin/clindamycin; bacteriologic successes were similarly different (81). Bjornson et al. reported the results of 84 patients with either Gram-negative bacillary pneumonia or purulent bronchitis who received either aztreonam or aminoglycoside as Gram-negative therapy (10). Other agents, such as intravenous clindamycin, cephalosporins, or penicillins were used for broader coverage of Gram-positive organisms. Clinical response rates of 83% were found in both groups. With the advent of third-generation cephalosporins and aztreonam in the late 1980s, the use of aminoglycosides as primary therapy for hospitalized patients with lower respiratory tract infections fell from favor.

More recently, additional studies have demonstrated the efficacy of aztreonam in nosocomial lower respiratory tract infections. Fekete et al. compared the combination of aztreonam plus cefazolin to ceftazidime for treatment of nosocomial pneumonia in a group of primarily medical patients (22). Of 48 evaluable patients, clinical cure or improvement was found in 90% of aztreonam/cefazolin-treated patients and 86% of ceftazidime-treated patients. Polk et al. compared aztreonam plus vancomycin with imipenem monotherapy in 122 mechanically ventilated trauma patients with pneumonia (63). Although the aztreonam patients were somewhat more severely ill, their clinical and microbiologic responses were somewhat better than those of the imipenem patients (77 vs. 70% microbiologic response), superinfections were less common in the narrowspectrum aztreonam group, and adverse events were also less common in the aztreonam-treated cohort.

Urinary Tract Infection

A large number of comparative trials were conducted in the 1980s (versus either cephalosporins or aminoglycosides) to demonstrate the efficacy of aztreonam for urinary tract infections. Most patients were treated for complicated urinary tract infections, and clinical success in the aztreonam and comparator arms ranged from 80 to 100% (4, 71, 82). Since aztreonam concentrates in urine and the primary organism responsible for most of the urinary tract infections was *E. coli,* such response rates are not surprising.

Septicemia

Prior to the recent development of clear definitions of sepsis, *septicemia* indicated patients with an identifiable primary source of infection and positive concurrent blood cultures. Data from the registrational filing of aztreonam and two comparative trials versus aminoglycosides or ceftazidime generally support the use of aztreonam in patients with positive blood cultures due to Gram-negative aerobic bacteria (31, 40, 75).

Intraabdominal and Penetrating Trauma

Aztreonam has generally been combined with clindamycin for treatment of intraabdominal infections, perforated appendicitis, and penetrating trauma. Most randomized trials have compared aztreonam with an aminoglycoside/clindamycin regimen. A multicenter, randomized trial of aztreonam/clindamycin versus tobramycin/clindamycin in 316 patients with intraabdominal infections found an equivalent clinical response rate but a superior bacteriologic response rate in the aztreonam group (95). When aztreonam was compared with amikacin (each combined with clindamycin) in 62 patients with perforated appendicitis or intraabdominal abscess, Barboza et al. found similar clinical responses, but length of hospitalization was reduced by 1.5 days in the aztreonam-treated patients (7). In a multicenter, prospectively randomized, double-blind trial of 119 patients with penetrating abdominal trauma due to gunshot or stab wounds, Fabian et al. compared aztreonam/clindamycin with gentamicin/clindamycin (21). Seven of eight patients who failed therapy were randomized to the aminoglycoside regimen. In addition, the aztreonam patients required an average of four fewer days of hospitalization.

Recently, the Surgical Infection Society developed guidelines for management of intraabdominal infections (79). For severe infections, the society recommends the use of imipenem/cilastatin or the combination of aztreonam, a thirdgeneration cephalosporin, or an aminoglycoside with clindamycin or metronidazole.

Gynecologic

Aztreonam has commonly been combined with clindamycin in the treatment of gynecologic infections such as postpartum endometritis or pelvic inflammatory disease (17, 26, 29, 32, 47, 61). Comparisons with aminoglycoside/clindamycin regimens generally demonstrate similar outcomes.

Fever/Neutropenia

Aztreonam has been extensively studied in the empirical treatment of neutropenic patients with fever. In most circumstances, the drug is combined with a Gram-positive agent such as vancomycin to provide broader coverage. In hospitals where *P. aeruginosa* is a common pathogen, an aminoglycoside is frequently added for synergy.

Most studies with aztreonam for this indication were conducted at M. D. Anderson Cancer Center in Houston. Some 340 patients with 535 febrile episodes were randomized to receive either aztreonam/vancomycin, aztreonam/amikacin/vancomycin, or moxalactam/ticarcillin (36). The response rates were similar in the three treatment groups; however, the aminoglycoside-containing regimen was somewhat more effective for patients with persistent neutropenia ($<100/mm^3$). Bodey et al. reported equivalent outcomes in 617 febrile episodes with two different dosing regimens of aztreonam plus cefoperazone (11). Raad et al. compared aztreonam/vancomycin with imipenem/vancomycin in 292 febrile episodes; a trend toward better clinical outcomes in the imipenem group was offset by a higher frequency of adverse reactions in this group (64).

Recently, aztreonam has been used to manage low-risk neutropenic outpatients with fever (68). In combination with intravenous clindamycin, it was compared with an oral regimen of ciprofloxacin and clindamycin in 78 cancer patients with 83 episodes of fever. A larger percentage of aztreonam patients responded to therapy (95 vs. 88% of the oral therapy patients). In addition, 6 ciprofloxacin patients required admission to the hospital: 3 had failed to respond to oral treatment, and 3 had developed acute renal failure. No aztreonam patients required admission to the hospital for adverse events or for management of fever.

Gonorrhea

Three comparative studies of almost 500 patients found similar outcomes with a single 1-g intramuscular dose of aztreonam, intramuscular procaine penicillin/oral probenecid, or intramuscular spectinomycin for the treatment of gonorrhea (28, 52, 53). Three noncomparative studies of almost 300 patients further supported use of single 1-g intramuscular infusions of aztreonam for gonorrhea (20, 77, 90).

Aztreonam was found effective in the treatment of urethritis produced by both penicillin-sensitive and penicillin-resistant strains of gonococci. Rare failures tended to occur in oropharyngeal or rectal infection.

Meningitis

Aztreonam was shown to penetrate inflamed meninges and effectively treat rabbits with experimental meningitis induced by *H. influenzae* or *E. coli* (49, 70, 73). The penetration of aztreonam into purulent rabbit CSF fluid was estimated to be 23%. Penetration into human CSF was subsequently confirmed (19, 30, 51), and clinical trials in humans were undertaken. Girgis et al. studied the efficacy of intramuscular aztreonam 50 mg/kg every 8 h in 13 children with *H. influenzae* meningitis (27). All children recovered quickly, except 2 infants who were comatose and died within 24 h of starting therapy.

Ayroza-Galvao found good outcomes in 21 of 22 young patients treated with 50-mg/kg doses of aztreonam every 6 h for meningitis caused by *H. influenzae* or *Salmonella heidelberg* (one patient) (6).

Feris described results in 41 children with Gram-negative meningitis due to *H. influenzae, Salmonella* spp., *Neisseria meningitidis,* or *Serratia marcescens, K. pneumoniae, P. vulgaris,* and *P. aeruginosa* (23).

A total 122 patients were treated with aztreonam for presumptive or confirmed Gram-negative bacillary meningitis in an open, multinational study (42); 77 patients had microbiologically confirmed Gram-negative meningitis due to an aztreonam-susceptible organism (*H. influenzae, Enterobacteriaceae, N. meningitidis,* and *Pseudomonas* species). All but four patients were microbiologically cured.

Finally, a series of 10 patients with Gram-negative meningitis due to *Pseudomonas, Proteus, Salmonella,* and *Klebsiella* spp. were treated effectively with aztreonam (38).

Although aztreonam has demonstrated activity against Gram-negative meningitis, the virtual eradication of *Haemophilus* meningitis in countries with Hib immunization and the lack of activity against streptococci limits its practical use, except when the etiologic agent of meningitis has been isolated.

Pediatric Patients

Clinical studies of aztreonam in pediatric patients have focused on the treatment of neonatal sepsis, serious Gram-negative bacterial infections, meningitis, urinary tract infections, and cystic fibrosis (41, 78). Although most studies used an open-label, noncomparative design, the response rates of 88 to 100% observed with aztreonam were generally in the range expected for parenteral antibacterial agents.

Sklavunu-Tsurutsoglu et al. studied aztreonam for the treatment of sepsis in 55 neonates in an open trial (76); 52 of 55 neonates were cured with the combination of aztreonam and penicillin G (including 46 of 48 neonates with positive blood cultures). Umana et al. described the results of a comparative trial of aztreonam plus ampicillin versus amikacin plus ampicillin in 147 neonates (92). Of the 60 evaluable patients, there was a significantly greater proportion of failures among the amikacin patients than the aztreonam patients (28 vs. 7%, respectively); however, there were significantly more neonates with shock or infection caused by *P. aeruginosa* in the amikacin group.

Summary of Clinical Use

In most hospitals, aztreonam is used as an alternative agent for treatment of Gram-negative infections (Table 2). In many institutions, it takes the place of ceftazidime when pseudomonal

TABLE 2 • Indications and Uses of Aztreonam

FDA-Approved Indications	Nonapproved Uses
Lower respiratory tract infections	Meningitis
Septicemia	Gonorrhea
Skin and skin-structure infections	Neonatal sepsis
Intra-abdominal infections	Neutropenic fever
Urinary tract infections	Exacerbations of lower
Gynecologic infections	respiratory tract
Moderate-to-severe pediatric	infections in patients
infections	with cystic fibrosis

activity is not an issue; in others, it takes the place of an aminoglycoside in combination therapies with a Gram-positive and/or anaerobic agent. Finally, aztreonam is generally recognized as being safe in patients with a history of penicillin or cephalosporin allergy.

Recently, the spread of type I cephalosporinase–producing organisms (particularly *Acinetobacter, Citrobacter,* and *Enterobacter* species) in the intensive care unit environment has limited the empirical use of aztreonam, since these β-lactamases confer aztreonam and cephalosporin resistance to the organism. Susceptibility testing is recommended prior to the use of aztreonam if the local hospital or an individual ICU is known to contain these multiresistant pathogens.

OTHER MONOBACTAMS

Although aztreonam is the best known member of its class, it is not the only monobactam to have been synthesized. Following further structural modification, Squibb Pharmaceuticals studied two additional monobactams. The first, pirazmonam (SQ 83,360), was similar to aztreonam with regard to activity against members of the *Enterobacteriaceae* family but was also highly active against *P. aeruginosa.* Also, significant gains were made with pirazmonam in activity against *Pseudomonas* and *Acinetobacter* spp. (89).

The second Squibb compound, tigemonam (SQ 30,836), was an oral monobactam that demonstrated bactericidal activity in vitro (MIC ≤ 1 μg/mL) against members of the *Enterobacteriaceae* family, *H. influenzae, Moraxella catarrhalis,* and *N. gonorrhoeae,* including those producing β-lactamase. It did not inhibit *Pseudomonas* spp. or *Acinetobacter* spp., and Gram-positive organisms demonstrated in vitro resistance to tigemonam (16, 24, 69).

Carumonam (AMA-1080, RO 17–2301), another injectable monobactam, was developed by Roche Laboratories at about the same time as aztreonam. Carumonam was highly active in vitro against Gram-negative *Enterobacteriaceae, P. aeruginosa,* and *H. influenzae,* weakly active against *Streptococcus pneumoniae,* and inactive against *Staphylococcus aureus.* Carumonam exhibited resistance to hydrolysis by plasmid-mediated and chromosomal β-lactamases, with more stability than aztreonam to the extended-spectrum β-lactamases expressed by *K. pneumoniae* and *E. cloacae;* however, its activity against *P. aeruginosa* was intermediate between aztreonam and ceftazidime (5, 25, 34, 37). Carumonam underwent limited clinical development in the late 1980s for treatment of urinary tract infections, septicemia, and severe sepsis (18, 39, 55, 94).

REFERENCES

1. Adkinson N Jr. Immunogenicity and cross-allergenicity of aztreonam. Am J Med 1990;88:12S–15S.
2. Adkinson N Jr, Saxon A, Spence M, Swabb E. Cross-allergenicity and immunogenicity of aztreonam. Rev Infect Dis 1985;7(Suppl 4):S613–S621.
3. Adkinson N Jr, Swabb E, Sugerman A. Immunology of the monobactam aztreonam. Antimicrob Agents Chemother 1984; 25:93–97.
4. Albertazzi A, Bonadio M, Fusaroli M, Lotti T, Miano L, Salvia G, Sasdelli M, Villa G, Zucchelli P, Ventriglia L. Multicenter comparative study of aztreonam and gentamicin in the treatment of renal and urinary tract infections. Chemotherapy 1989;35 (Suppl 1):77–80.
5. Angehrn P. Antibacterial properties of carumonam (Ro 17–2301, AMA-1080), a new sulfonated monocyclic beta-lactam antibiotic. Chemotherapy 1985;31:440–450.
6. Ayroza-Galvao PA, Milstein-Kuschnaroff TM, Mimica IM, Maassen S, Barbosa SP Jr, Cavalcante NJ, Lorenco R, Mimica LM, Martino MD. Aztreonam in the treatment of bacterial meningitis. Chemotherapy 1989;35(Suppl 1):39–44.
7. Barboza E, del Castillo M, Yi A, Gotuzzo E. Clindamycin plus amikacin versus clindamycin plus aztreonam in established intraabdominal infections. Surgery 1994;116:28–35.
8. Barry A, Thornsberry C, Jones R, Gavan T. Aztreonam: antibacterial activity, β-lactamase stability, and interpretive standards and quality control guidelines for disk-diffusion susceptibility tests. Rev Infect Dis 1985;7(Suppl 4):S594–S604.
9. Berthelot G, Bergogne BE, Vernant D, Ravina J. [Diffusion of aztreonam in the tissues and biological fluids of the female genital tract]. Pathol Biol (Paris) 1986;34:339–341.
10. Bjornson H, Ramirez-Ronda C, Saavedra S, Rivera-Vazquez C, Liu C, Hinthorn D. Comparison of empiric aztreonam and aminoglycoside regimens in the treatment of serious gram-negative lower respiratory infections. Clin Ther 1993;15:65–78.
11. Bodey G, Reuben A, Elting L, Kantarjian H, Keating M, Hagemeister F, Koller C, Velasquez W, Papadopoulos N. Comparison of two schedules of cefoperazone plus aztreonam in the treatment of neutropenic patients with fever. Eur J Clin Microbiol Infect Dis 1991;10:551–558.
12. Bristol-Myers Squibb Company. Azactam package insert. 1997.
13. Brogden RN, Heel RC. Aztreonam. A review of its antibacterial activity, pharmacokinetic properties and therapeutic use. Drugs 1986;31:96–130.
14. Bush K, Freudenberger J, Sykes R. Interaction of azthreonam and related monobactams with beta-lactamases from gram-negative bacteria. Antimicrob Agents Chemother 1982;22:414–420.
15. Chartrand S. Safety and toxicity profile of aztreonam. Pediatr Infect Dis J 1989;8:S120–S123.
16. Chin NX, Neu HC. Tigemonam, an oral monobactam. Antimicrob Agents Chemother 1988;32:84–91.
17. Dodson M, Faro S, Gentry L. Treatment of acute pelvic inflammatory disease with aztreonam, a new monocyclic beta-lactam antibiotic, and clindamycin. Obstet Gynecol 1986;67:657–662.
18. Drabu YJ, Mehtar S, Blakemore PH. Clinical efficacy of carumonam. Drugs Exp Clin Res 1988;14:665–667.
19. Duma RJ, Berry AJ, Smith SM, Baggett JW, Swabb EA, Platt TB. Penetration of aztreonam into cerebrospinal fluid of patients with and without inflamed meninges. Antimicrob Agents Chemother 1984;26:730–733.
20. Evans DT, Crooks AJ, Jones C, Holman RA, Price SW. Treatment of uncomplicated gonorrhoea with single dose aztreonam. Genitourin Med 1986;62:318–320.
21. Fabian T, Hess M, Croce M, Wilson R, Wilson S, Charland S, Rodman J, Boucher B. Superiority of aztreonam/clindamycin compared with gentamicin/clindamycin in patients with penetrating abdominal trauma. Am J Surg 1994;167:291–296.
22. Fekete T, Castellano M, Ramirez J, Siefkin A, Martin M, Redington J, North D, Krumpe P, Javaheri S, Jones R, Gagnon S. A randomised comparative trial of aztreonam plus cefazolin versus ceftazidime for the treatment of nosocomial pneumonia. Drug Invest 1994;7:117–126.
23. Feris J, Moledina N, Rodriguez W, Khan W, Puig J, Wiedermann B, Ahmad S. Aztreonam in the treatment of gram-negative meningitis and other gram-negative infections. Chemotherapy 1989;35(Suppl 1):31–38.
24. Fuchs PC, Jones RN, Barry AL. In vitro antimicrobial activity of tigemonam, a new orally administered monobactam. Antimicrob Agents Chemother 1988;32:346–349.
25. Fuchs PC, Jones RN, Barry AL, Ayers LW, Gavan TL, Gerlach EH. In vitro activity of carumonam (RO 17–2301), BMY-28142, aztreonam, and ceftazidime against 7,620 consecutive clinical bacterial isolates. Diagn Microbiol Infect Dis 1986;5:345–349.
26. Gibbs R, Blanco J, Lipscomb K, St Clair P. Aztreonam versus gentamicin, each with clindamycin, in the treatment of endometritis. Obstet Gynecol 1985;65:825–829.
27. Girgis NI, Abu el Ella AH, Farid Z, Woody JN, Haberberger RLJ, el Messidy M, Dessouky A. Parenteral aztreonam in the treatment of Haemophilus influenzae type b meningitis in Egyptian children. Scand J Infect Dis 1988;20:111–112.
28. Gottlieb A, Mills J. Effectiveness of aztreonam for the treatment of gonorrhea. Antimicrob Agents Chemother 1985;27:270–271.
29. Greenberg RN, Reilly PM, Weinandt WJ, Wilson KM, Bollinger M, Ojile JM. Comparison trial of clindamycin with aztreonam or gentamicin in the treatment of postpartum endometritis. Clin Ther 1987;10:36–39.
30. Greenman RL, Arcey SM, Dickinson GM, Mokhbat JE, Sabath LD, Platt TB, Friedhoff LT. Penetration of aztreonam into human cerebrospinal fluid in the presence of meningeal inflammation. J Antimicrob Chemother 1985;15:637–640.
31. Gudiol F, Pallares R, Ariza X, Fernandez-Viladrich P, Rufi G, Linares J. Comparative clinical evaluation of aztreonam versus aminoglycosides in gram-negative septicaemia. J Antimicrob Chemother 1986;17:661–671.
32. Henry S. Overall clinical experience with aztreonam in the treatment of obstetric-gynecologic infections. Rev Infect Dis 1985; 7(Suppl 4):S703–S708.
33. Imada A, Kitano K, Kintaka K, Muroi M, Asai M. Sulfazecin and isosulfazecin, novel β-lactam antibiotics of bacterial origin. Nature 1981;289:590–591.
34. Imada A, Kondo M, Okonogi K, Yukishige K, Kuno M. In vitro and in vivo antibacterial activities of carumonam (AMA-1080), a new N-sulfonated monocyclic beta-lactam antibiotic. Antimicrob Agents Chemother 1985;27:821–827.
35. Jacobus N, Ferreira M, Barza M. In vitro activity of azthreonam, a monobactam antibiotic. Antimicrob Agents Chemother 1982; 22:832–838.
36. Jones PG, Rolston KV, Fainstein V, Elting L, Walters RS, Bodey

GP. Aztreonam therapy in neutropenic patients with cancer. Am J Med 1986;81:243–248.

37. Jones RN, Barry AL, Thornsberry C, Fuchs PC, Packer RR. The anti-microbial activity, beta-lactamase stability, and disk diffusion susceptibility testing of carumonam (RO 17–2301, AMA-1080), a new monobactam. Am J Clin Pathol 1986;86:608–618.

38. Kilpatrick M, Girgis N, Farid Z, Bishay E. Aztreonam for treating meningitis caused by gram-negative rods. Scand J Infect Dis 1991;23:125–126.

39. Kotilainen P, Huovinen P, Hanninen P. Carumonam in the treatment of severe and complicated urinary tract infections. Chemioterapia 1987;6(Suppl 2):514–515.

40. Lagast H, Klastersky J, Kains J, van der Auwera P, Meunier F, Woussen F, Thijs J. Empiric antimicrobial therapy with aztreonam or ceftazidime in gram-negative septicemia. Am J Med 1986;80(Suppl 5C):79–84.

41. Lebel M, McCracken G Jr. Aztreonam: review of the clinical experience and potential uses in pediatrics. Pediatr Infect Dis J 1988;7:331–339.

42. Lentnek AL, Williams RR. Aztreonam in the treatment of gram-negative bacterial meningitis. Rev Infect Dis 1991;13(Suppl 7):S586–S590.

43. Likitnukul S, McCracken G Jr, Threlkeld N, Darabi A, Olsen K. Pharmacokinetics and plasma bactericidal activity of aztreonam in low-birth-weight infants. Antimicrob Agents Chemother 1987;31:81–83.

44. Livermore D. Resistance mechanisms of *Pseudomonas aeruginosa* to antibiotics (Thesis). University of London, 1983.

45. Livermore D, Williams J. In-vitro activity of the monobactam, SQ 26,776, against gram-negative bacteria and its stability to their beta-lactamases. J Antimicrob Chemother 1981;8(Suppl E):29–37.

46. Livermore D, Williams R, Williams J. In vitro activity of MK 0787 (N-formimidoyl thienamycin) against Pseudomonas aeruginosa and other gram-negative rods and its stability to their beta- lactamases. J Antimicrob Chemother 1981;8:351–353.

47. Mangioni C, Bianchi L, Bolis P, Lomeo A, Mazzeo F, Ventriglia L, Scalambrino S. Multicenter trial of prophylaxis with clindamycin plus aztreonam or cefotaxime in gynecologic surgery. Rev Infect Dis 1991;13(Suppl 7):S621–S625.

48. Mattie H. Clinical pharmacokinetics of aztreonam. Clin Pharmacokinet 1988;14:148–155.

49. McCracken GH Jr, Sakata Y, Olsen KD. Aztreonam therapy in experimental meningitis due to Haemophilus influenzae type b and Escherichia coli K1. Antimicrob Agents Chemother 1985;27:655–656.

50. McKindley DS, Boucher BA, Hess MM, Croce MA, Fabian TC. Pharmacokinetics of aztreonam and imipenem in critically ill patients with pneumonia. Pharmacotherapy 1996;16:924–931.

51. Modai J, Vittecoq D, Decazes JM, Wolff M, Meulemans A. Penetration of aztreonam into cerebrospinal fluid of patients with bacterial meningitis. Antimicrob Agents Chemother 1986;29:281–283.

52. Mohanty KC, Deighton Fimls R, Strachan RG. A comparative study of aztreonam and procaine penicillin/probenecid in the treatment of uncomplicated gonorrhoea. Scand J Infect Dis 1988;20:33–36.

53. Mohanty KC, Deighton R, Strachan RG. Single intramuscular injection of aztreonam in the treatment of uncomplicated gonorrhoea in women. Curr Med Res Opin 1987;10:634–637.

54. Moore R, Lerner S, Levine D. Nephrotoxicity and ototoxicity of aztreonam versus aminoglycoside therapy in seriously ill nonneutropenic patients. J Infect Dis 1992;165:683–688.

55. Naber K, Kees F, Denk K, Bauernfeind A, Grobecker H. Carumonam versus ceftazidime: in vitro activity, pharmacokinetics in elderly patients, safety and therapeutic efficacy in the treatment of complicated urinary tract infections. Chemioterapia 1987;6(Suppl 2):517–518.

56. Nau H. Clinical pharmacokinetics in pregnancy and perinatology. II. Penicillins. Dev Pharmacol Ther 1987;10:174–198.

57. Neu H, Labthavikul P. In vitro activity and beta-lactamase stability of a monobactam, SQ 26,917, compared with those of aztreonam and other agents. Antimicrob Agents Chemother 1983;24:227–232.

58. Newman TJ, Dreslinski GR, Tadros SS. Safety profile of aztreonam in clinical trials. Rev Infect Dis 1985;7(Suppl 4):S648–S655.

59. Nolen T, Phillips H, Hall H. Comparison of aztreonam and tobramycin in the treatment of lower respiratory tract infections caused by gram-negative bacilli. Rev Infect Dis 1985;7(Suppl 4):S666–S668.

60. Parry M. Aztreonam susceptibility testing. A retrospective analysis. Am J Med 1990;88:7S–11S.

61. Pastorek J 2d, Cole C, Aldridge K, Crapanzano J. Aztreonam plus clindamycin as therapy for pelvic infections in women. Am J Med 1985;78(Suppl 2A):47–50.

62. Phillips I, King A, Shannon K, Warren C. SQ 26,776: in-vitro antibacterial activity and susceptibility to beta-lactamases. J Antimicrob Chemother 1981;8(Suppl E):103–110.

63. Polk H Jr, Livingston D, Fry D, Malangoni M, Fabian T, Trachtenberg L, Gardner S, Kesterson L, Cheadle W. Treatment of pneumonia in mechanically ventilated trauma patients: results of a prospective trial. Arch Surg 1997;132:1086–1092.

64. Raad I, Whimbey E, Rolston K, Abi-Said D, Hachem R, Pandya R, Ghaddar H, Karl C, Bodey G. A comparison of aztreonam plus vancomycin and imipenem plus vancomycin as initial therapy for febrile neutropenic cancer patients. Cancer 1996;77:1386–1394.

65. Reed M, Aronoff S, Stern R, Yamashita T, Myers C, Friedhoff L, Blumer J. Single-dose pharmacokinetics of aztreonam in children with cystic fibrosis. Pediatr Pulmonol 1986;2:282–286.

66. Rivera-Vazquez C, Ramirez-Ronda C, Rodriguez J, Saavedra S. A comparative analysis of aztreonam + clindamycin versus tobramycin + clindamycin or amikacin + mezlocillin in the treatment of gram- negative lower respiratory tract infections. Chemotherapy 1989;35(Suppl 1):89–100.

67. Rodriguez J, Ramirez-Ronda C. Efficacy and safety of aztreonam versus tobramycin for aerobic gram-negative bacilli lower respiratory tract infections. Am J Med 1985;78(Suppl 2A):42–43.

68. Rubenstein E, Rolston K, Benjamin R, Loewy J, Escalante C, Manzullo E, Hughes P, Moreland B, Fender A, Kennedy K, Holmes F, Elting L, Bodey G. Outpatient treatment of febrile episodes in low-risk neutropenic patients with cancer. Cancer 1993;71:3640–3646.

69. Rylander M, Gezelius L, Norrby SR. Comparative in-vitro activity of tigemonam, a new monobactam. J Antimicrob Chemother 1988;22:307–313.

70. San Joaquin VH, Stutman HR, Marks MI. Hemophilus influenzae type b meningitis in infant rabbits. Pathogenesis and therapy. Am J Dis Child 1984;138:455–458.

71. Sattler FR, Moyer JE, Schramm M, Lombard JS, Appelbaum PC. Aztreonam compared with gentamicin for treatment of serious urinary tract infections. Lancet 1984;1:1315–1318.

72. Saxon A. Aztreonam in the management of gram-negative

infections in penicillin-allergic patients: a review. Pediatr Infect Dis J 1989;8(Suppl 9):S124–S132.

73. Scheld WM, Brodeur JP, Gratz JC, Foresman P, Rodeheaver G. Evaluation of aztreonam in experimental bacterial meningitis and cerebritis. Antimicrob Agents Chemother 1983;24: 682–688.

74. Schentag J, Vari A, Winslade N, Swanson D, Smith I, Simons G, Vigano A. Treatment with aztreonam or tobramycin in critical care patients with nosocomial gram-negative pneumonia. Am J Med 1985;78(Suppl 2A):34–41.

75. Scully B, Henry S. Clinical experience with aztreonam in the treatment of gram-negative bacteremia. Rev Infect Dis 1985; 7(Suppl 4):S789–S793.

76. Sklavunu-Tsurutsoglu S, Gatzola-Karaveli M, Hatziioannidis K, Tsurutsoglu G. Efficacy of aztreonam in the treatment of neonatal sepsis. Rev Infect Dis 1991;13(Suppl 7):S591–S593.

77. Spencer RC, Talbot MD. The use of aztreonam in the treatment of uncomplicated gonorrhoea. Curr Med Res Opin 1985;9: 591–593.

78. Stutman H. Clinical experience with aztreonam for treatment of infections in children. Rev Infect Dis 1991;13 (Suppl 7): S582–585.

79. Surgical Infection Society. Guidelines for clinical care: anti-infective agents for intra-abdominal infection. Arch Surg 1992; 127:83–9.

80. Swabb E. Clinical pharmacology of aztreonam in healthy recipients and patients: a review. Rev Infect Dis 1985;7(Suppl 4): S605–S612.

81. Swabb E, Cone C, Muir J. Summary of worldwide clinical trials of aztreonam in patients with lower respiratory tract infections. Rev Infect Dis 1985;7(Suppl 4):S675–S678.

82. Swabb E, Jenkins S, Muir J. Summary of worldwide clinical trials of aztreonam in patients with urinary tract infections. Rev Infect Dis 1985;7(Suppl 4):S772–S777.

83. Swabb E, Singhvi S, Leitz M, Frantz M, Sugerman A. Metabolism and pharmacokinetics of aztreonam in healthy subjects. Antimicrob Agents Chemother 1983;24:394–400.

84. Sykes R, Bonner D. Discovery and development of the monobactams. Rev Infect Dis 1985;7(Suppl 4):S579–S593.

85. Sykes R, Bonner D, Bush K, Georgopapadakou N. Azthreonam (SQ 26,776), a synthetic monobactam specifically active against aerobic gram-negative bacteria. Antimicrob Agents Chemother 1982;21:85–92.

86. Sykes R, Bonner D, Bush K, Georgopapadakou N, Wells J. Monobactams—monocyclic beta-lactam antibiotics produced by bacteria. J Antimicrob Chemother 1981;8(Suppl E):1–16.

87. Sykes R, Cimarusti C, Bonner D, Bush K, Floyd D, Georggopapadakou N, Koster W, Liu W, Parker W, Principe P, Rathnum M, Slusarchyk W, Trejo W, Wells J. Monocyclic β-lactams produced by bacteria. Nature 1981;291:489–491.

88. Sykes RB, Bonner DP. Aztreonam: the first monobactam. Am J Med 1985;78(Suppl 2A):2–10.

89. Sykes RB, Koster WH, Bonner DP. The new monobactams: chemistry and biology. J Clin Pharmacol 1988;28:113–119.

90. Tait IB, Winning J, Sleigh JD. Single dose aztreonam in treating gonorrhoea. Genitourin Med 1987;63:13–15.

91. Then RL. Interaction of Ro 17–2301 (AMA-1080) with beta-lactamases. Chemotherapy 1984;30:398–407.

92. Umana MA, Odio CM, Castro E, Salas JL, McCracken GH Jr. Evaluation of aztreonam and ampicillin vs. amikacin and ampicillin for treatment of neonatal bacterial infections. Pediatr Infect Dis J 1990;9:175–180.

93. Uuay R, Mize C, Argyle C, McCracken G Jr. Metabolic tolerance to arginine: implications for the safe use of arginine salt-aztreonam combination in the neonatal period. J Pediatr 1991; 18:965–970.

94. Westenfelder M, Frankenschmidt A, Pelz K. Carumonam and cefotiam in the treatment of complicated urinary tract infection (UTI): a randomized study. Chemioterapia 1987;6(Suppl 2): 515–516.

95. Williams R, Hotchkin D. Aztreonam plus clindamycin versus tobramycin plus clindamycin in the treatment of intraabdominal infections. Rev Infect Dis 1991;13 (Suppl 7):S629–S633.

Mupirocin

●

Suzanne F. Bradley

CLASS

In 1887, it was recognized that extracts from cultures of *Pseudomonas fluorescens* inhibited the growth of bacteria (33). Four monoxycarbolic acids, pseudomonic acids A-D, were subsequently isolated that were responsible for the antimicrobial activity of *P. fluorescens* (NCIB 10586) (59). A new name, mupirocin, was applied to the major metabolite pseudomonic acid A, by the World Health Organization, British Pharmacopoeia, and the United States Adopted Names Committee because of concern that the original name implied

activity against *Pseudomonas* (33, 101). The structure of mupirocin [$(CH_2)_8CO_2H$] has been called unique because of a short fatty acid side chain, 9-hydroxynonanoic acid. This side chain is linked to a larger molecule, monic acid, by an ester linkage (59, 101, 103).

ANTIMICROBIAL ACTIVITY

Mupirocin is very active against methicillin-susceptible *Staphylococcus aureus* (MSSA) (0.04–0.32 µg/mL) and methicillin-resistant *S. aureus* (MRSA) (0.04–0.25 µg/mL) as well as

Streptococcus pyogenes (0.03–0.5 µg/mL), *Streptococcus galactiae* (0.5 µg/mL), *Streptococcus viridans* (0.25–2 µg/mL), *Streptococcus pneumoniae* (0.12 µg/mL), and some Gram-negative bacteria including *Hemophilus influenzae* (0.12 µg/mL), *Moraxella catarrhalis, Neisseria* spp. (0.05 µg/mL), *Bordetella pertussis* (0.02 µg/mL), and *Pasturella multocida* (0.25 µg/mL). Mupirocin is less active against other Gram-positive bacteria including *Corynebacterium* sp. (>128 µg/mL), *Micrococcus luteus* (>128 µg/mL), *Listeria monocytogenes* (8 µg/mL), *Erysipelothrix rhusiopathiae, Enterococcus* spp., and anaerobes. Mupirocin has no appreciable activity against fungi or *Chlamydia trachomatis* (1, 5, 58, 103, 124, 126, 130, 136).

Susceptibility to mupirocin is defined as an MIC below 2.0 µg/mL by microdilution methods and a zone of inhibition exceeding 14 mm for the 5-µg disk (Beecham Laboratories, Bristol, TN) and exceeding 16 mm for the 10-µg disk (Clinical Microbiology Institute, Tualatin, OR) (58). Correlation between agar dilution methods and E-test strips (AB Biodisk, Solna, Sweden) have been described as excellent for staphylococci and *H. influenzae,* with somewhat lower correlations with streptococci and *M. catarrhalis* (120).

The antimicrobial activity of mupirocin is very pH dependent. The antistaphylococcal activity of the drug is greatest in a slightly acidic environment (pH 6.0), a level approaching that of human skin. Media composition has little influence upon mupirocin susceptibilities (31). Decreased mupirocin activity has been described when inocula of *S. aureus* exceeded 10^6 CFU (31).

In general, mupirocin is considered a bacteriostatic agent. In vitro, the MBCs for mupirocin are 8- to 100-fold higher than the MICs for strains of *S. aureus*. In addition, mupirocin did not demonstrate significant bactericidal activity against MRSA strains by time-kill assays (35). However in vivo, concentrations achieved locally in skin (20,000 µg/mL) are bactericidal for *S. aureus*.

MECHANISMS OF ACTION

Mupirocin enters bacterial cells by passive diffusion (28). The 9-hydroxynonoic acid component of mupirocin is structurally similar to L-isoleucine. 9-Hydroxynonoic acid competes for two hydrophobic portions of the enzyme isoleucyl-tRNA synthetase that normally bind methyl and ethyl groups of L-isoleucine (76). The reversible binding of mupirocin to isoleucyl-tRNA synthetase inhibits isoleucine incorporation, depletes isoleucine-charged tRNA, and inhibits the production of protein and RNA (76, 101, 103). It has been suggested that the monic acid portion of the mupirocin molecule may further inhibit isoleucyl-tRNA synthetase by binding to its ATP binding site (137). Mupirocin is toxic to bacteria, but not to mammalian cells, because of its low affinity for mammalian isoleucyl-tRNA synthetase (101).

MECHANISMS OF RESISTANCE

Many bacteria are intrinsically resistant to the effects of mupirocin because the drug cannnot bind effectively with their isoleucyl synthetase (28). Mupirocin resistance is not due to alterations in drug transport or to increased destruction by bac-

terial products (28, 39, 55). Mupirocin resistance has been assessed primarily in staphylococci, and it has emerged mostly in patient populations in whom use was common and prolonged (22, 36, 50, 80, 83, 84, 96, 109). Mupirocin resistance has been reportedly most commonly in MRSA isolates, but resistance has also been described in MSSA and coagulase-negative staphylococci (29, 38, 80, 83, 84, 86, 99, 109, 114). No single antibiotic susceptibility pattern, phage type, or plasmid profile has been associated specifically with emergence of mupirocin resistance (38, 83, 84, 108, 109).

S. aureus variants resistant to mupirocin (MIC > 4 µg/mL) have been described in nature at a frequency of 1 to 4×10^{-9} (31). Mupirocin-susceptible isolates of *S. aureus* serially subcultured onto agar containing 0.01 to 40 µg/mL of drug eventually developed MICs of 25 to 40 µg/mL (31). This low-level resistance (MIC < 100 µg/mL) has emerged slowly and is stable, nontransferable, and chromosomally mediated (22). Despite emergence of low-level mupirocin resistance, microbiologic treatment failures were uncommon, presumably because of the high concentrations of drug (20,000 µg/mL) present in the ointment. In contrast, isolation of high-level mupirocin-resistant (MIC > 500 µg/mL) staphylococcal strains has been associated with microbiologic and clinical failures (80, 83, 84, 109). High-level mupirocin-resistant staphylococcal strains contain conjugative plasmids of varying size that are capable of transferring mupirocin resistance (38, 53, 79, 97, 100, 108–110).

Mupirocin-resistant plasmids contain the gene *ileS*-2 or *mup*A, which encodes for a modified isoleucyl tRNA synthetase with reduced ability to bind mupirocin (55, 61, 72). High-level mupirocin-resistant strains contain both the novel and native isoleucyl tRNA synthetase, while low-level mupirocin-resistant and mupirocin-susceptible strains contain only a single enzyme (61). The activity of the enzyme in the low-level mupirocin resistant strains is reduced (61). In addition, the *mup*A gene has been identified on the chromosome of some low-level resistant strains (111).

The structure of the modified isoleucyl tRNA synthetase differs markedly from the native enzyme, indicating that perhaps more than random mutation occurred (61, 72). It has been suggested that bacteria more intrinsically resistant to mupirocin such as coagulase-negative staphylococci, enterococci, or Gram-negative bacilli might have served as a reservoir for resistance genes that ultimately were transferred to *S. aureus* (38, 40, 61, 72, 79, 121).

PHARMACOKINETIC DISPOSITION

Mupirocin is 95% protein bound in human serum. The serum half-life of mupirocin (20–35 min) is so short that systemic use of the drug is not practical. After oral or intravenous dosing in humans, mupirocin undergoes rapid hydrolysis by renal esterases to the inactive metabolite monic acid, and approximately 90% of that metabolite is eliminated by renal excretion within 6 to 12 h. Elimination of mupirocin by hepatic esterases was suggested by animal studies but has not been studied in humans (33, 101, 103, 130).

In skin, hydrolysis of mupirocin to monic acid occurs slowly, with less than 3 to 27% conversion by 48 h, depending upon whether studies of human or animal skin were done. Studies of topical administration of ^{14}C-labeled mupirocin on intact skin in humans, with or without occlusive dressings, found no detectable drug in urine, feces, or blood (103, 130).

FORMULATIONS AND DOSAGE REGIMENS

There are two formulations of mupirocin ointment. The original formulation (Bactroban, SmithKline Beecham, Philadelphia, PA) contained 2% mupirocin in a polyethylene glycol vehicle (polyethylene glycol 400/polyethylene glycol 3350). This drug has been approved for the treatment of impetigo. The newer formulation (Bactroban Nasal) has been approved for decolonization of nasal carriers during outbreaks of MRSA infection. For impetigo, thrice-daily treatment is recommended, with reassessment in 3 to 5 days. For nasal carriage, twice-daily treatment for 5 days has been recommended. However, the doses actually used in many studies of mupirocin have varied widely in frequency (from one to four times daily or one to three times weekly) and in duration (from 5 days to months) (see "Clinical Indications"). No dosage adjustment is required for size or medical condition.

ADVERSE EFFECTS

Mupirocin is not teratogenic or mutagenic. Photosensitization does not occur with mupirocin therapy, and contact sensitization has been reported rarely (54). Local irritation is the most common adverse event ascribed to mupirocin ointment applied topically in the nares. These symptoms, occurring in 1.5 to 3% of patients treated, have been attributed to the polyethylene glycol vehicle rather than mupirocin itself (130). Erythema, pruritus, burning, rhinorrhea, bad taste, and others have been described with mupirocin (2%) polyethylene glycol ointment. Concerns were also raised about using polyethylene glycol on mucous membranes or abraded skin, especially in neonates, leading to development of calcium mupirocin (2%) ointment. Despite the new formulation, local symptoms related to topical application (rhinitis, alterations in taste, pharyngitis) have been reported in 17% of adults treated (product insert).

Because higher concentrations of mupirocin might affect the isoleucyl transferases of mammalian cells, the effect of mupirocin on wound healing has been evaluated. Mupirocin at concentrations below 100 μg/mL has not been cytotoxic to human keratinocytes or fibroblasts in vitro, but concentrations of 700 μg/mL have inhibited the growth of human fibroblasts (4,20). Thus, while higher levels of mupirocin might achieve bactericidal levels in skin, impairment of wound healing is possible.

Concern has also been raised regarding systemic absorption of the polyethylene glycol vehicle (polyethylene glycol 400/ polyethylene glycol 3500). A syndrome of increased serum calcium, high anion gap metabolic acidosis, and renal failure has been described in burn patients and in animal models treated with topical antimicrobial agents in polyethylene glycol base (26, 37, 65). While mupirocin (2%) in polyethylene glycol has been used successfully in patients with burns of less than 20%, it has been suggested that the drug be avoided in persons with more extensive burns because of potential toxic-

ity (117). There have been anecdotal reports of the polyethylene glycol formulation causing structural defects in peritoneal catheters (132), but this rare event has not been observed in our experience or in the published literature (8) to our knowledge.

DRUG INTERACTIONS

The stability of mupirocin (2%) in polyethylene glycol has been assessed in combination with other topical agents (78). More than 90% of initial mupirocin levels persisted following mixture with a variety of disinfectants, glucocorticoids, and antifungal agents formulated as creams, lotions, or ointments. Some physical separation occurred over time when some topical agents were mixed with mupirocin, but the activity of mupirocin was not affected. Only Valisone and Lotrimin (Schering, Kenilworth, NJ) lotions were physically incompatible with mupirocin ointment.

CLINICAL INDICATIONS
Approved Indications

Treatment of Impetigo/Primary Skin Infections
Mupirocin 2% polyethylene glycol has been shown to be more effective than the polyethylene glycol vehicle alone in eradicating the bacteria that cause impetigo. However, because impetigo is a mild, sometimes self-limited disease, demonstration of significant differences in clinical outcomes has been difficult. In clinical trials, mupirocin applied thrice daily for 5 to 10 days was as effective in the treatment of impetigo as oral ampicillin (133), dicloxacillin (2), and erythromycin (7, 24, 45, 52, 62, 64, 92, 95, 115). In some trials, mupirocin yielded better microbiologic cure and a trend toward better clinical cure than topical fusidic acid (18).

The increasing frequency with which *S. aureus* has been implicated as a cause of impetigo, increasing frequency of staphylococci resistant to oral antibiotics, and the side effects of oral antibiotics have made mupirocin an attractive agent for the treatment of impetigo (45, 77, 88). Evidence suggests that other localized primary skin infections due to *S. aureus* or *S. pyogenes,* such as furunculosis and folliculitis (74), localized cellulitis (93), and vaginitis (41) may be successfully treated with mupirocin.

Control of Epidemic MRSA Infection
S. aureus carriage by health care workers may play an important role in transmission of the organism from patient to patient. Double-blinded placebo-controlled trials of the efficacy of calcium mupirocin ointment have been performed primarily in this cohort (27, 30, 48, 49, 56, 57, 113, 119). Mupirocin or its vehicle was applied to the nares of persons persistently colonized with MSSA two to four times daily for 5 days (27, 30, 49, 56, 57, 113, 119). At the completion of therapy, eradication of nasal carriage was achieved in 74 to 100% of persons treated (30, 49, 56, 119). Significant reductions in carriage of MSSA on hands was also seen (113). However, nares were recolonized in approximately 50% of patients treated with mupirocin by 6 months (49, 56). Health care workers who became recolonized were equally likely to relapse with their original strain or acquire a new strain (49). Many investigators suggest that health care workers can remain on the job while

being treated with mupirocin, as most clear their nasal carriage within 48 h of initiating therapy (32, 70, 71).

On the basis of studies in health care workers and anecdotal use during epidemics, calcium mupirocin ointment has been recommended as adjunctive therapy to treat patients and health care workers colonized with MRSA in nares during outbreaks of infection (21). It has been recommended that therapy be limited to treatment in nares twice daily for 5 days, to prevent emergence of resistance. During outbreak situations, many different strategies are used to limit the spread of MRSA, including cohorting patients and use of other topical disinfectants and systemic antibiotics; thus assessment of the efficacy of mupirocin alone is difficult (21, 63). Successful initial eradication of nasal carriage has been achieved in 90 to 100% of those treated (10, 44, 46, 67, 70, 104, 114). Termination of outbreaks has been attributed to the use of mupirocin in several studies (6, 47, 51, 91, 94, 118, 125, 128), but failure of mupirocin to terminate epidemics has also been described (3, 25, 60). Mupirocin failure in those circumstances was attributed to the facts that all MRSA-colonized patients were not identified and that treatment of nasal colonization did not eliminate MRSA from other colonized sites.

Nonapproved Indications

Treatment of Secondary Skin Infections

Mupirocin 2% polyethylene ointment treatment of secondary infection of abraded skin with *S. aureus* or group A β-hemolytic streptococci has been assessed in patients with atopic dermatitis (23, 64, 86, 87, 89), epidermolysis bullosa (98, 106), acne (135), and venous stasis ulcers (102). Patients with atopic dermatitis treated with mupirocin or placebo for 7 to 14 days showed clinical improvement and significant reduction in colonization with *S. aureus* (23, 86). Patients with epidermolysis bullosa treated with twice-daily mupirocin for up to 4 years exhibited rapid healing of large wounds without side effects (98). However, high-level mupirocin resistance developed in 12% of patients, with associated lack of clinical response. In patients with venous stasis ulcers, use of mupirocin ointment significantly reduced, but did not eliminate, staphylococci, compared with polyethylene glycol alone; the clinical appearance of the ulcers did not improve.

In vitro studies have shown that mupirocin has better antimicrobial activity against clinical isolates of Gram-positive cocci than other topical agents (silver sulfadiazine, bacitracin/neomycin/polymyxin B, mafenide acetate) used to treat burn wounds (122, 129). Mupirocin effectively penetrates scar tissue and significantly reduces the MRSA bacterial burden (116, 122). In one study, 59 burn patients who had failed therapy with 1% silver sulfadiazine and 0.2% chlorhexidine attained microbiologic cure following treatment with mupirocin (2%) polyethylene glycol ointment twice daily for 5 days (117).

Prevention of Infection in Hemodialysis Patients

S. aureus is the most common cause of serious infection in hemodialysis patients (12). Approximately 30 to 70% of hemodialysis patients are persistently colonized with *S. aureus* (11), and it has been estimated that 75% of *S. aureus* infections

are associated with antecedent nasal colonization (16). The efficacy of mupirocin porphylaxis has been assessed primarily in persistent carriers of MSSA, rather than MRSA.

MSSA colonization in nares was almost completely eradicated after initial twice- or thrice-daily treatment with calcium mupirocin ointment for 5 to 14 days (11, 13, 73). However, following a single course of therapy, most patients became recolonized by 3 months, generally with their original strain (11, 14, 73). After initial therapy, once-weekly therapy is as effective as thrice-weekly mupirocin in preventing recolonization and bacteremia (14, 15).

Reduction of infection may be due to reduction in *S. aureus* skin colonization associated with eradication of the nasal carrier state (16, 17). Following therapy, 67% of mupirocin-treated persons had *S. aureus* eradicated from the skin (17). However, a single course of mupirocin intranasal therapy does not permanently eradicate *S. aureus* skin carriage in most patients. Bommer et al. found that 4 months following discontinuation of therapy, only 44% of patients remained free of *S. aureus* skin colonization (17). Persistent elimination of *S. aureus* skin colonization can be obtained by weekly mupirocin maintenance therapy and concommitent use of chlorhexidine body scrubs (16, 131).

Mupirocin prophylaxis and eradication of MSSA carriage has been associated with a significant reduction in *S. aureus* bacteremia, although most studies have used historical controls (11–13, 73, 81). It has been suggested that more than $1,000,000 per 1000 hemodialysis patients could be saved if all patients were given mupirocin prophylaxis whether they were *S. aureus* carriers or not (9).

Prevention of *S. aureus* Infection in Peritoneal Dialysis Patients

Patients undergoing continuous ambulatory peritoneal dialysis (CAPD) who are *S. aureus* carriers are at increased risk of exit-site infection, peritonitis, and catheter loss (66, 107). Perez-Fontan et al. noted that intranasal mupirocin three times daily for 7 days cleared all patients of *S. aureus* colonization, but recolonization occurred in 75% by 1 year (105). Comparing the mupirocin treatment group with historical controls showed a trend toward an increase in exit-site infections due to other Gram-positive bacteria and an increase in peritonitis and exit-site infections due to Gram-negative bacilli. Topical prophylaxis of the catheter exit site has also been studied (8). In *S. aureus* carriers, topical mupirocin applied to the exit site was as effective as oral rifampin given for 5 days every 3 months in reducing exit-site infection, peritonitis, or catheter loss due to *S. aureus*. Side effects occurred more often in the rifampin group than in the mupirocin group (12 vs. 0%).

Prevention of Postoperative Wound Infection

S. aureus carriers undergoing surgical procedures and those with burn wounds are at increased risk of infection with their colonizing strain (19, 75, 134). In one study, burn patients (>30% area) who received oral selective decontamination plus nasal mupirocin (four times daily for 5 days then weekly thereafter) were compared with matched historical controls who only received the same oral decontamination regimen. A significant decline in *S. aureus* colonization of wounds, gastric aspirates, and sputum was seen in the mupirocin-treated group over 4 weeks of follow-up (90).

When all patients admitted to surgical and cardiothoracic intensive care units were treated with mupirocin twice daily for 5 to 7 days, colonization and infection with *S. aureus* was significantly lower than in historical controls (82, 123). In the cardiothoracic intensive care unit, more than $16,000 was saved per surgical-site infection (127). Postoperative infections were also significantly reduced when mupirocin three times daily was given 2 days prior to resection of skin cancers (42, 43).

Prevention of Intravenous Catheter Colonization

The effect of topical mupirocin applied to the insertion site was compared with no treatment in preventing infections in cardiothoracic surgery patients requiring short-term internal jugular catheter placement (48 h). Mupirocin significantly reduced the number of catheters colonized, and Gram-negative superinfection did not ensue (69, 70). In contrast, a neonatal intensive care unit where mupirocin application to catheter insertion sites had been a standard of care for more than 5 years, had frequent colonization with high-level mupirocin- resistant coagulase-negative staphylococcal skin flora (138). The incidence of mupirocin resistance declined with discontinuation of the drug. No clinical benefit was noted in reducing the number of colonized catheters during the time mupirocin was in use.

Prevention of Infection in Long-Term Care

While the actual incidence of *S. aureus* infection in long-term care is unknown, mupirocin (2%) polyethylene glycol ointment has been used in an attempt to eradicate colonization in the hope of preventing infection (34, 80). Treatment of persistent nasal carriers with mupirocin twice daily for 7 days led to initial eradication in 91% of patients treated (34). However, within 8 weeks after stopping therapy, 44% of residents were recolonized. More intensive continuous therapy, similar to the regimens used for hemodialysis patients, was attempted for persistent eradication of MRSA colonization (80). At the end of 7 days of daily therapy, MRSA was initially eradicated in 83% of patients treated in nares alone and 95% of residents treated in both nares and wounds. Unlike the hemodialysis population, recurrence of colonization on maintenance therapy was common (38–47%) when the dosing regimens were reduced from once-daily to thrice- or once-weekly dosing. The overall rate of MRSA colonization in the nursing home was significantly reduced (22 vs. 11%), but only if both nares and colonized wounds were treated. Mupirocin resistance developed in 11% of patients. MRSA infections were few, and no reduction in rates resulted from mupirocin use.

Prevention of Recurrent Staphylococcal Infection in Immunocompetent Hosts

Patients with recurrent *S. aureus* infection and persistent nasal carriage showed significant reductions in nasal colonization and infection when they were treated on an intermittent basis; mupirocin resistance was demonstrated in only one patient

(112). In families with recurrent staphylococcal infection, twice-daily calcium mupirocin was more effective than chlorhexidine 0.1%/neomycin ointment in eradicating *S. aureus* nasal colonization and preventing recurrence for up to 3 months (85). Fewer infections developed in patients and their families treated with mupirocin.

REFERENCES

1. Aldridge KE. In vitro antistaphylococcal activities of two investigative fluoroquinolones, CI-960 and WIN 57273, compared with those of ciprofloxacin, mupirocin (pseudomonic acid), and peptide-class antimicrobial agents. Antimicrob Agents Chemother 1992;36:851–853.

2. Arredondo JL. Efficacy and tolerance of topical mupirocin compared with oral dicloxacillin in the treatment of primary skin infections. Curr Ther Res 1987;41:121–127.

3. Back NA, Linnemann CC, Staneck JL, et al. Control of methicillin-resistant *Staphylococcus aureus* in a neonatal intensive-care unit: use of intensive microbiologic surveillance and mupirocin. Infect Control Hosp Epidemiol 1996;17:227–231.

4. Balin AK, Leong I, Carter DM. Effect of mupirocin on the growth and lifespan of human fibroblasts. J Invest Dermatol 1987;88:736–740.

5. Barry AL, Pfaller MA, Fuchs PC. Ramoplanin susceptibility testing criteria. J Clin Microbiol 1993;31:1932–1935.

6. Barrett SP. The value of nasal mupirocin in containing an outbreak of methicillin-resistant *Staphylococcus aureus* in an orthopedic unit. J Hosp Infect 1990;15:137–142.

7. Barton LL, Friedman AD, Sharkey AM, et al. Impetigo contagiosa III. Comparative efficacy of oral erythromycin and topical mupirocin. Pediatr Dermatol 1989;6:134–138.

8. Bernardini J, Piraino B, Holley J, Johnston JR, Lutes R. A randomized trial of *Staphylococcus aureus* prophylaxis in peritoneal dialysis patients: mupirocin calcium ointment 2% applied to the exit site versus cyclic rifampin. Am J Kidney Dis 1996;27:695–700.

9. Bloom BS, Fendrick AM, Chernew ME, Patel P. Clinical and economic effects of mupirocin calcium on preventing *Staphylococcus aureus* infection in hemodialysis patients: a decision analysis. Am J Kidney Dis 1996;27:687–694.

10. Blumberg LH, Klugman KP. Control of methicillin-resistant *Staphylococcus aureus* bacteraemia in high-risk areas. Eur J Clin Microbiol Infect Dis 1994;13:82–85.

11. Boelaert JR. *Staphylococcus aureus* infection in haemodialysis patients. Mupirocin as a topical strategy against nasal carriage: a review. J Chemother 1994;6:19S–24S.

12. Boelaert JR, De Baere YA, Geernaert MA, Godard CA, Van Landuyt HW. The use of nasal mupirocin ointment to prevent *Staphylococcus aureus* bacteraemias in haemodialysis patients: an analysis of cost-effectiveness. J Hosp Infect 1991;19B:41–46.

13. Boelaert JR, DeSmedt RA, De Baere YA, Godard CA, Matthys EG, Schurgers ML, Daneels RF, Gordts BZ, Van Landuyt HW. The influence of calcium mupirocin nasal ointment on the incidence of *Staphylococcus aureus* infections in haemodialysis patients. Nephrol Dial Transplant 1989;4:278–281.

14. Boelaert JR, Van Landuyt HW, De Baere YA, Gheyle DW, Daneels RF, Schurgers ML, Matthys EG, Gordts BZ. Epidemiologie et prevention des infections a *Staphylococcus aureus* en hemodialyse. Nephrologie 1994;15:157–161.

15. Boelaert JR, Van Landuyt HW, Godard CA, Daneels RF, Schurgers ML, Matthys EG, DeBaere YA, Gheyle DW, Gordts

BZ, Herwaldt LA. Nasal mupirocin ointment decreases the incidence of *Staphylococcus aureus* bacteraemias in haemodialysis patients. Nephrol Dial Transplant 1993;8:235–239.

16. Boelaert JR, Van Landuyt HW, Gordts BZ, De Baere YA, Messer SA, Herwaldt LA. Nasal and cutaneous carriage of *Staphylococcus aureus* in hemodialysis patients: the effect of nasal mupirocin. Infect Control Hosp Epidemiol 1996;17:809–811.

17. Bommer J, Vergetis W, Andrassy K, Hingst V, Borneff M, Huber W. Elimination of *Staphylococcus aureus* in hemodialysis patients. ASAIO J 1995;41:127–131.

18. Booth JH, Benrimoj SI. Mupirocin in the treatment of impetigo. Int J Dermatol 1992;31:1–9.

19. Boyce JM. Preventing staphylococcal infections by eradicating nasal carriage of *Staphylococcus aureus:* proceeding with caution. Infect Control Hosp Epidemiol 1996;17:775–779.

20. Boyce ST, Warden GD, Holder IA. Cytotoxicity testing of topical antimicrobial agents on human keratinocytes and fibroblasts for cultured skin grafts. J Burn Care Rehabil 1995;16:97–103.

21. Bradley SF. Effectiveness of mupirocin in the control of methicillin-resistant *Staphylococcus aureus*. Infect Med 1993;10:23–31.

22. Bradley SF, Ramsey MA, Morton TM, Kauffman CA. Mupirocin resistance: clinical and molecular epidemiology. Infect Control Hosp Epidemiol 1995;16:354–358.

23. Breneman DL. Use of mupirocin ointment in the treatment of secondarily infected dermatoses. J Am Acad Dermatol 1990;22:886–892.

24. Britton JW, Fajardo JE, Krafte-Jacobs B. Comparison of mupirocin and erythromycin in the treatment of impetigo. J Pediatr 1990;117:827–829.

25. Brun-Buisson C, Legrand P. Can topical and nonabsorbable antimicrobials prevent cross-transmission of resistant strains in ICUs? Infect Control Hosp Epidemiol 1994;15:447–455.

26. Bruns DE, Herold DA, Rodeheaver GT, Edlich RF. Polyethylene glycol intoxication in burn patients. Burns 1982;9:49–52.

27. Bulanda M, Gruszka M, Heczko B. Effect of mupirocin on nasal carriage of *Staphylococcus aureus*. J Hosp Infect 1989;14:117–124.

28. Capobianco JO, Doran CC, Goldman RC. Mechanisms of mupirocin transport into sensitive and resistant bacteria. Antimicrob Agents Chemother 1989;33:156–163.

29. Casewell MW. New threats to the control of methicillin-resistant *Staphylococcus aureus*. J Hosp Infect 1995;30:465–471.

30. Casewell MW, Hill RLR. Elimination of nasal carriage of *Staphylococcus aureus* with mupirocin ('pseudomonic acid')—a controlled trial. J Antimicrob Chemother 1986;17:365–372.

31. Casewell MW, Hill RLR. In-vitro activity of mupirocin ('pseudomonic acid') against clinical isolates of *Staphylococcus aureus*. J Antimicrob Chemother 1985;15:523–531.

32. Casewell MW, Hill RLR. Minimal dose requirements for nasal mupirocin and its role in the control of epidemic MRSA. J Hosp Infect 1991;19B:35–40.

33. Casewell MW, Hill RLR. Mupirocin ('pseudomonic acid')—a promising new topical antimicrobial agent. J Antimicrob Chemother 1987;19:1–5.

34. Cederna JE, Terpenning MS, Ensberg M, Bradley SF, Kauffman CA. *Staphylococcus aureus* nasal colonization in a nursing home: eradication with mupirocin. Infect Control Hosp Epidemiol 1990;11:13–16.

35. Chapnick EK, Gradon JD, Kreiswirth B, Lutwick LI, Schaffer BC, Schiano TD, Levi MH. Comparative killing kinetics of methicillin-resistant *Staphylococcus aureus* by bacitracin or mupirocin. Infect Control Hosp Epidemiol 1996;17:178–180.

36. Chatfield CA, O'Neill WA, Cooke RPD, McGhee KJ, Issack M, Rahman M, Noble WC. Mupirocin-resistant *Staphylococcus aureus* in a specialist school population. J Hosp Infect 1994;26:273–278.

37. Chirife J, Herszage L, Joseph A, Bozzini JP, Leardini N, Kohn ES. In vitro antibacterial activity of concentrated polyethylene glycol 400 solutions. Antimicrob Agents Chemother 1983;24:409–412.

38. Connolly S, Noble WC, Phillips I. Mupirocin resistance in coagulase-negative staphylococci. J Med Microbiol 1993;39:450–453.

39. Cookson B. Failure of mupirocin-resistant staphylococci to inactivate mupirocin. Eur J Clin Microbiol Infect Dis 1989;8:1038–1040.

40. Cookson BD. Mupirocin resistance in staphylococci. J Antimicrob Chemother 1990;25:497–503.

41. Cool-Foley AA, Nathan C, O'Donovan C III, Simon D. Eradication of methicillin-resistant *Staphylococcus aureus* vaginitis with mupirocin. DICP Ann Pharmacother 1991;25:1331–1333.

42. Czarnecki D, Meehan C, Nash C. Prevention of post-excisional wound infections: a comparison of oral cephalexin with topical mupirocin and topical cetrimide-chlorhexidine cream. Int J Dermatol 1992;31:359–360.

43. Czarnecki DB, Nash CG, Bohl TG. The use of mupirocin before skin surgery. Int J Dermatol 1991;30:218–219.

44. Dacre J, Emmerson AM, Jenner EA. Gentamicin-methicillin-resistant *Staphylococcus aureus:* epidemiology and containment of an outbreak. J Hosp Infect 1986;7:130–136.

45. Dagan R, Bar-David Y. Double-blind study comparing erythromycin and mupirocin for treatment of impetigo in children: implications of a high prevalence of erythromycin-resistant *Staphylococcus aureus* strains. Antimicrob Agents Chemother 1992;36:287–290.

46. Darouiche R, Wright C, Hamill R, Koza M, Lewis D, Markowski J. Eradication of colonization by methicillin-resistant *Staphylococcus aureus* by using oral minocycline-rifampin and topical mupirocin. Antimicrob Agents Chemother 1991;35:1612–1615.

47. Davies EA, Emmerson AM, Hogg EM, Patterson MF, Shields MD. An outbreak of infection with a methicillin-resistant *Staphylococcus aureus* in a special care baby unit: value of topical mupirocin and of traditional methods of infection control. J Hosp Infect 1987;10:120–128.

48. Doebbling DN, Breneman DL, Neu HC, Aly R, Yangco BG, Holley HP, Marsh RJ, Pfaller MA, McGowan JE, Scully BE, Reagen DR, Wenzel RP, and the Mupirocin Collaborative Study Group. Elimination of *Staphylococcus aureus* nasal carriage in health care workers: analysis of six clinical trials with calcium mupirocin ointment. Clin Infect Dis 1993;17:466–474.

49. Doebbling BN, Reagen DR, Pfaller MA, Houston AK, Hollis RJ, Wenzel RP. Long-term efficacy of intranasal mupirocin ointment. A prospective cohort study of *Staphylococcus aureus* carriage. Arch Intern Med 1994;154:1505–1508.

50. Dos Santos KRN, De Souza LF, Filho PPG. Emergence of high-level mupirocin resistance in methicillin-resistant *Staphylococcus aureus* isolated from Brazilian university hospitals. Infect Control Hosp Epidemiol 1996;17:813–816.

51. Duckworth GJ, Lothian JLE, Williams JD. Methicillin-resistant *Staphylococcus aureus:* report of an outbreak in a London teaching hospital. J Hosp Infect 1988;11:1–15.

52. Dux PH, Fields L, Pollock D. 2% Topical mupirocin versus systemic erythromycin and cloxacillin in primary and secondary skin infections. Curr Ther Res 1986;40:933–940.

53. Dyke KGH, Curnock SP, Golding M, Noble WC. Cloning of the gene conferring resistance to mupirocin in *Staphylococcus aureus*. FEMS Microbiol Lettr 1991;77:195–198.

54. Eedy DJ. Mupirocin allergy in the setting of venous ulceration. Contact Dermatitis 1995;32:240–241.

55. Farmer TH, Gilbart J, Elson SW. Biochemical basis of mupirocin resistance in strains of *Staphylococcus aureus*. J Antimicrob Chemother 1992;30:587–596.

56. Fernandez C, Gaspar C, Torrellas A, Vindel A, Saez-Nieto JA, Cruzet F, Aguilar L. A double-blind, randomized, placebo-controlled clinical trial to evaluate the safety and efficacy of mupirocin calcium ointment for eliminating nasal carriage of *Staphylococcus aureus* among hospital personnel. J Antimicrob Chemother 1995;35:399–408.

57. Frank U, Lenz W, Damrath E, Kappstein I, Daschner FD. Nasal carriage of *Staphylococcus aureus* treated with topical mupirocin (pseudomonic acid) in a children's hospital. J Hosp Infect 1989;13:117–120.

58. Fuchs PC, Jones RN, Barry AL. Interpretive criteria for disk diffusion susceptibility testing of mupirocin, a topical antibiotic. J Clin Microbiol 1990;28:608–609.

59. Fuller AT, Banks GT, Mellows G, Barrow KD, Woolford M, Chain EB. Pseudomonic acid: an antibiotic produced by Pseudomonas fluorescens. Nature 1971;234:416–417.

60. Gaspar MC, Sanchez P, Uribe P, Coello R, Arroyo P, Cruzet F. Mupirocin susceptibility in vitro and nasal eradication of epidemic methicillin-resistant *Staphylococcus aureus*. J Hosp Infect 1993;24:237–238.

61. Gilbart J, Perry CR, Slocombe B. High-level mupirocin resistance in *Staphylococcus aureus:* evidence for two distinct isoleucyl-tRNA synthetases. Antimicrob Agents Chemother 1993;37:32–38.

62. Goldfarb J, Crenshaw D, O'Horo J, Lemon E, Blumer JL. Randomized clinical trial of topical mupirocin versus oral erythromycin for impetigo. Antimicrob Agents Chemother 1988;32:1780–1783.

63. Gordon J. Clinical significance of methicillin-sensitive and methicillin-resistant *Staphylococcus aureus* in UK hospitals and the relevance of povidone-iodine in their control. Postgrad Med J 1993;69:S106–S116.

64. Gratton D. Topical mupirocin versus oral erythromycin in the treatment of primary and secondary skin infections. Int J Dermatol 1987;26:472–473.

65. Herold DA, Rodeheaver GT, Bellamy WT, Fitton LA, Bruns DE, Edlich RF. Toxicity of topical polyethylene glycol. Toxicol Appl Pharmacol 1982;65:329–335.

66. Herwaldt LA. *Staphylococcus aureus* nasal carriage: role in continuous ambulatory peritoneal dialysis-associated infections. Periton Dial Int 1992;13:S301–S305.

67. Hill RLR, Duckworth GJ, Casewell MW. Elimination of nasal carriage of methicillin-resistant *Staphylococcus aureus* with mupirocin during a hospital outbreak. J Antimicrob Chemother 1988;22:377–384.

68. Hill RLR, Casewell MW. Nasal carriage of MRSA: the role of mupirocin and outlook for resistance. Drugs Exp Clin Res 1990;16:397–402.

69. Hill RLR, Casewell MW. Reduction in the colonization of central venous cannulae by mupirocin. J Hosp Infect 1991;19:47–57.

70. Hill RLR, Fisher AP, Ware RJ, Wilson S, Casewell MW. Mupirocin for the reduction of colonization of internal jugular cannulae—a randomized controlled trial. J Hosp Infect 1990;15:311–321.

71. Hill S. Intranasal mupirocin. J Hosp Infect 1994;28:235.

72. Hodgson JE, Curnock SP, Dyke KGH, Morris R, Sylvester DR, Gross MS. Molecular characterization of the gene encoding high-level mupirocin resistance in *Staphylococcus aureus* J2870. Antimicrob Agents Chemother 1994;38:1205–1208.

73. Holton DL, Nicolle LE, Diley D, Bernstein K. Efficacy of mupirocin nasal ointment in eradicating *Staphylococcus aureus* nasal carriage in chronic hemodialysis patients. J Hosp Infect 1991;17:133–137.

74. Hoss DM, Feder HM. Addition of rifampin to conventional therapy for recurrent furunculosis. Arch Dermatol 1995;131:647–648.

75. Hudson IRB. The efficacy of intranasal mupirocin in the prevention of staphylococcal infections: a review of recent experience. J Hosp Infect 1994;27:81–98.

76. Hughes J, Mellows G. On the mode of action of pseudomonic acid: inhibition of protein synthesis in *Staphylococcus aureus*. J Antibiot 1978;31:330–335.

77. Infectious Diseases and Immunization Committee, Canadian Pediatric Society. Mupirocin in the treatment of impetigo. Can Med Assoc J 1990;142:543–544.

78. Jagota NK, Stewart JT, Warren FW, John PM. Stability of mupirocin ointment (Bactroban) admixed with other proprietary dermatological products. J Clin Pharm Ther 1992;17:181–184.

79. Janssen DA, Zarins LT, Schaberg DR, Bradley SF, Terpenning MS, Kauffman CA. Detection and characterization of mupirocin resistance in *Staphylococcus aureus*. Antimicrob Agents Chemother 1993;37:2003–2006.

80. Kauffman CA, Terpenning MS, He X, Zarins LT, Ramsey MA, Jorgensen KA, Sottile WS, Bradley SF. Attempts to eradicate methicillin-resistant *Staphylococcus aureus* from a long-term care facility with the use of mupirocin ointment. Am J Med 1993;94:371–378.

81. Kluytmans JAJ, Manders M-J, Van Bommel E, Verbrugh H. Elimination of nasal carriage of *Staphylococcus aureus* in hemodialysis patients. Infect Control Hosp Epidemiol 1996;17:793–797.

82. Kluytmans JAJ, Mouton JW, VandenBergh MFQ, Manders M-J AAJ, Maat APWM, Wagenvoort JHT, Michel MF, Verbrugh HA. Reduction of surgical-site infections in cardiothoracic surgery by elimination of nasal carriage of *Staphylococcus aureus*. Infect Control Hosp Epidemiol 1996;17:780–785.

83. Layton MC, Perez M, Heald P, Patterson JE. An outbreak of mupirocin-resistant *Staphylococcus aureus* on a dermatology ward associated with an environmental reservoir. Infect Control Hosp Epidemiol 1993;14:369–375.

84. Layton MC, Patterson JE. Mupirocin resistance among consecutive isolates of oxacillin-resistant and borderline oxacillin-resistant *Staphylococcus aureus* at university hospital. Antimicrob Agents Chemother 1994;38:1664–1667.

85. Leigh DA, Joy G. Treatment of familial staphylococcal infection—comparison of mupirocin nasal ointment and chlorhexidine/neomycin (Naseptin) cream in eradication of nasal carriage. J Antimicrob Chemother 1993;31:909–917.

86. Lever R, Hadley K, Downey D, Mackie R. Staphylococcal colonization in atopic dermatitis and the effect of topical mupirocin therapy. Br J Dermatol 1988;119:189–198.

87. Leyden JJ. Mupirocin: a new topical antibiotic. J Am Acad Dermatol 1990;22:879–883.

88. Leyden JJ. Review of mupirocin ointment in the treatment of impetigo. Clin Pediatr 1992;31:549–553.

89. Luber H, Amornsiripanitch S, Lucky AW. Mupirocin and the eradication of *Staphylococcus aureus* in atopic dermatitis. Arch Dermatol 1988;124:853.

90. Mackie DP, van Hertum WAJ, Schumberg TH, Kuijper EC, Knape P, Massaro F. Reduction in *Staphylococcus aureus* wound colonization using nasal mupirocin and selective decontamination of the digestive tract in extensive burns. Burns 1994;20:S14–S18.

91. Mayall B, Martin R, Keenan AM, Irving L, Leeson P, Lamb K. Blanket use of intranasal mupirocin for outbreak control and long-term prophylaxis of endemic methicillin-resistant *Staphylococcus aureus* in an open ward. J Hosp Infect 1996;32:257–266.

92. McLinn S. A bacteriologically controlled, randomized study comparing the efficacy of 2% mupirocin ointment (Bactroban) with oral erythromycin in the treatment of patients with impetigo. J Am Acad Dermatol 1990;22:883–885.

93. Medina S, Gomez MI, de Misa RF, Ledo A. Perianal streptococcal cellulitis: treatment with mupirocin. Dermatology 1992;185:219.

94. Meier PA, Carter CD, Wallace SE, Hollis RJ, Pfaller MA, Herwaldt LA. A prolonged outbreak of methicillin-resistant *Staphylococcus aureus* in the burn unit of a tertiary medical center. Infect Control Hosp Epidemiol 1996;17:798–802.

95. Mertz PM, Marshall DA, Eaglstein WH, Piovanetti Y, Montalvo J. Topical mupirocin treatment of impetigo is equal to oral erythromycin therapy. Arch Dermatol 1989;125:1069–1073.

96. Miller MA, Dascal A, Portnoy J, Mendelson J. Development of mupirocin resistance among methicillin-resistant *Staphylococcus aureus* after widespread use of nasal mupirocin ointment. Infect Control Hosp Epidemiol 1996;17:811–813.

97. Morton TM, Johnston JL, Patterson J, Archer GL. Characterization of a conjugative staphylococcal mupirocin resistance plasmid. Antimicrob Agents Chemother 1995;39:1272–1280.

98. Moy JA, Caldwell-Brown D, Lin AN, Pappa KA, Carter DM. Mupirocin-resistant *Staphylococcus aureus* after long-term treatment of patients with epidermolysis bullosa. J Am Acad Dermatol 1990;22:893–895.

99. Naguib MH, Naguib MT, Flournoy DJ. Mupirocin resistance in methicillin-resistant *Staphylococcus aureus* from a veterans hospital. Chemotherapy 1993;39:400–404.

100. Noble WC, Rahman M, Cookson B, Phillips I. Transferable mupirocin-resistance. J Antimicrob Chemother 1988;22:771–776.

101. Pappa KA. The clinical development of mupirocin. J Am Acad Dermatol 1990;22:873–879.

102. Pardes JB, Carson PA, Eaglstein WH, Falanga V. Mupirocin treatment of exudative ulcers. J Am Acad Dermatol 1993;29:497–498.

103. Parenti MA, Hatfield SM, Leyden JJ. Mupirocin: a topical antibiotic with a unique structure and mechanism of action. Clin Pharm 1987;6:761–770.

104. Parras F, Del Carmen Guerrero M, Bouza E, Blazquez MJ, Moreno S, Menarguez MC, Cercenado E. Comparative study of mupirocin and oral co-trimoxazole plus topical fusidic acid in eradication of nasal carriage of methicillin-resistant *Staphylococcus aureus*. Antimicrob Agents Chemother 1995; 39:175–179.

105. Perez-Fontan M, Garcia-Falcon T, Rosales M, Rodriguez-Carmona A, Adeva M, Rodriguez-Lozano I, Moncalian J. Treatment of *Staphylococcus aureus* nasal carriers in continuous ambula-

tory peritoneal dialysis with mupirocin: long-term results. Am J Kidney Dis 1993;22:708–712.

106. Petersen S, Brocks K, Weismann K, Kobayasi T, Thomsen HK. Pretibial epidermolysis bullosa with vulvar involvement. Acta Derm Venereol 1996;76:80–81.

107. Piraino B. *S. aureus* nasal carriage: importance and approaches. Periton Dial Int 1995;15:301–302.

108. Rahman M, Connolly S, Noble WC, Cookson B, Phillips I. Diversity of staphylococci exhibiting high-level resistance to mupirocin. J Med Microbiol 1990;33:97–100.

109. Rahman M, Noble WC, Cookson B. Transmissable mupirocin resistance in *Staphylococcus aureus*. Epidemiol Infect 1989;102:261–270.

110. Rahman M, Noble WC, Dyke KGH. Probes for the study of mupirocin resistance in staphylococci. J Med Microbiol 1993;39:446–449.

111. Ramsey MA, Bradley SF, Kauffman CA, Morton TM. Identification of chromosomal location of *mup*A gene, encoding low-level mupirocin resistance in staphylococcal isolates. Antimicrob Agents Chemother 1997;40:2820–2823.

112. Raz R, Miron D, Colodner R, Staler Z, Samara Z, Keness Y. A 1-year trial of nasal mupirocin in the prevention of recurrent staphylococcal nasal colonization and skin infection. Arch Intern Med 1996;156:1109–1112.

113. Reagen DR, Doebbling BN, Pfaller MA, Sheetz CT, Houston AK, Hollis RJ, Wenzel RP. Elimination of coincident *Staphylococcus aureus* nasal and hand carriage with intranasal application of mupirocin calcium ointment. Ann Intern Med 1991; 114:101–106.

114. Redhead RJ, Lamb YJ, Rowsell RB. The efficacy of calcium mupirocin in the eradication of nasal *Staphylococcus aureus* carriage. Br J Clin Pract 1991;45:252–254.

115. Rice TD, Duggan AK, DeAngelis C. Cost-effectiveness of erythromycin versus mupirocin for the treatment of impetigo in children. Pediatrics 1992;89:210–214.

116. Rode H, De Wet PM, Millar AJW, Cywes S. Bactericidal efficacy of mupirocin in multi-antibiotic resistant *Staphylococcus aureus* burn wound infection. J Antimicrob Chemother 1988; 21:589–595.

117. Rode H, Hanslo D, De Wet PM, Millar AJW, Cywes S. Efficacy of mupirocin in methicillin-resistant *Staphylococcus aureus* burn wound infection. Antimicrob Agents Chemother 1989;33:1358–1361.

118. Rumbak MJ, Cancio MR. Significant reduction in methicillin-resistant *Staphylococcus aureus* ventilator-associated pneumonia associated with the institution of prevention protocol. Crit Care Med 1995;23:1200–1203.

119. Scully BE, Briones F, Gu J-W, Neu HC. Mupirocin treatment of nasal staphylococcal colonization. Arch Intern Med 1992;152:353–356.

120. Simpson IN, Gisby J, Hemingway CP, Durodie J, Macpherson I. Evaluation of mupirocin E-test for determination of isolate susceptibility: comparison with standard agar dilution techniques. J Clin Microbiol 1995;33:2254–2259.

121. Slocombe B, Perry C. The antimicrobial activity of mupirocin — an update on resistance. J Hosp Infect 1991;19B:19–25.

122. Strock LL, Lee MM, Rutan RL, Desai MH, Robson MC, Herndon DM, Heggers JP. Topical Bactroban (mupirocin): efficacy in treating burn wounds infected with methicillin-resistant staphylococci. J Burn Care Rehabil 1990;11:454–459.

123. Talon D, Rouget C, Cailleaux V, Bailly P, Thouverez M, Barale F, Michel-Briand Y. Nasal carriage of *Staphylococcus au-*

reus and cross-contamination in a surgical intensive care unit: efficacy of mupirocin ointment. J Hosp Infect 1995;30:39–49.

124. Utrup LJ, Finlay JE, Rittenhouse SF, Poupard JA. Comparison of mupirocin susceptibility of nasal and nonnasal *Staphylococcus aureus* isolates. Diagn Microbiol Infect Dis 1994;20: 171–174.

125. Valls V, Gomez-Herruz P, Gonzalez-Palacios R, Cuadros JA, Romanyk JP, Ena J. Long-term efficacy of a program to control methicillin-resistant *Staphylococcus aureus*. Eur J Clin Microbiol Infect Dis 1994;13:90–95.

126. Van Der Auwera P, Godard C, Denis C, De Maeyer S, Vanhoof R. In vitro activities of new antimicrobial agents against multiresistant *Staphylococcus aureus* isolated from septicemic patients during a Belgian national survey from 1983 to 1985. Antimicrob Agents Chemother 1990;34:2260–2262.

127. VandenBergh MFQ, Kluytmans JAJW, Van Hout VA, Maat APWM, Seerden RJ, McDonnel J, Verbrugh HA. Cost-effectiveness of perioperative mupirocin nasal ointment in cardiothoracic surgery. Infect Control Hosp Epidemiol 1996;17: 786–792.

128. Vandenbroucke-Grauls CM, Frenay HME, van Klingeren B, Savelkoul TF, Verhoef J. Control of epidemic methicillin-resistant *Staphylococcus aureus* in a Dutch university Hospital. Eur J Clin Microbiol Infect Dis 1991;10:6–11.

129. Vizcaino-Alcaide MJ, Herruzo-Cabrera R, Rey-Calero J. Efficacy of a broad-spectrum antibiotic (mupirocin) in an in vitro model of infected skin. Burns 1993;19:392–395.

130. Ward A, Campoli-Richards DM. Mupirocin: a review of its antibacterial activity, pharmacokinetic properties and therapeutic use. Drugs 1986;32:425–444.

131. Watanakunakorn C, Brandt J, Durkin P, Santore S, Bota B, Stahl C. The efficacy of mupirocin ointment and chlorohexadine body scrubs in the eradication of nasal carriage of *Staphylococcus aureus* among patients undergoing long-term hemodialysis. Am J Infect Control 1992;20:138–141.

132. Weaver NE, Dumbeck DC. Mupirocin causes permanent structural changes in peritoneal catheters. Abstracts of the 14th Annual Conference on Peritoneal Dialysis, 1994.

133. Welsh O, Saenz C. Topical mupirocin compared with ampicillin in the treatment of primary and secondary skin infections. Curr Ther Res 1987;41:114–120.

134. Wenzel RP, Perl TM. The significance of nasal carriage of *Staphylococcus aureus* and the incidence of postoperative wound infection. J Hosp Infect 1995;31:13–24.

135. Williams REA, Doherty VR, Perkins W, Aitchison TC, Mackie RM. *Staphylococcus aureus* and intra-nasal mupirocin in patients receiving isotretinoin for acne. Br J Dermatol 1992;126: 362–366.

136. Witte W, Klare I. Sensitivity to mupirocin of staphylococci isolated from colonized or infected patients in Germany. Eur J Clin Microbiol Infect Dis 1993;12:476–478.

137. Yanagisawa T, Lee JT, Wu HC, Kawakami M. Relationship of protein structure of isoleucyl-tRNA synthetase with pseudomonic acid resistance of *Escherichia coli*. J Biol Chem 1994;269:24304–24309.

138. Zakrzewska-Bode A, Muytjens HL, Liem KD, Hoogkamp-Korstanje JAA. Mupirocin resistance in coagulase-negative staphylococci, after topical prophylaxis for the reduction of colonization of central venous catheters. J Hosp Infect 1995;31: 189–193.

Nitrofurantoin

●

Gary E. Stein and Daniel H. Havlichek, Jr.

CLASS

Nitrofurantoin [1-(5-nitro-2-furanyl) methylene amino-2,4-imidazolidinedione] is a synthetic nitrofuran compound (MW = 238) with limited water solubility (Fig. 1). This drug has been marketed for over 40 years for the treatment of urinary tract infections (UTIs). Because of a high rate of nausea associated with the crystalline formulation (Furadantin), this product has been replaced by macrocrystals of nitrofurantoin (Macrodantin, Proctor & Gamble Pharmaceuticals). A slow-release formulation is also available (Macrobid, Proctor & Gamble Pharmaceuticals).

The mechanism of action of nitrofurantoin is unusual among antimicrobials. Reductases in bacteria are able to reduce nitrofurantoin to reactive metabolites and an inverse correlation exists between reductase levels and nitrofurantoin MICs (23). These electrophilic intermediates react with nucleophilic sites on bacterial macromolecules and inhibit enzymes of the citric acid cycle as well as DNA, RNA, and protein synthesis. At low concentrations, nitrofurantoin inhibits the synthesis of inducible enzymes β-galactosidase and galactokinase without affecting total protein synthesis (15). A recent observation suggests that nitrofurantoin can also exert antibacterial activity in the absence of reductive activation (23).

ANTIMICROBIAL ACTIVITY

Nitrofurantoin is active in vitro against uropathogens such as *Escherichia coli, Citrobacter* spp., *Staphylococcus saprophyticus,* and *Enterococcus faecalis* (1). More than 90% of these organisms remain sensitive to this drug. Strains of *Klebsiella* spp., *Proteus* spp., and *Enterobacter* spp. are usually resistant. Nitrofurantoin has no activity against *Pseudomonas aeruginosa* (Table 1).

Bacteria with an MIC below 32 μg/mL are considered susceptible to nitrofurantoin in urine. In a study of patients with

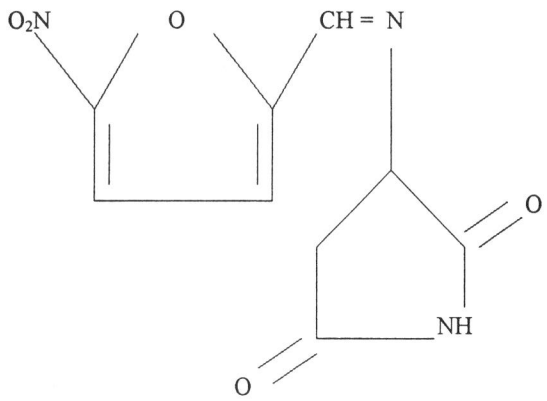

FIGURE 1. Structure of nitrofurantoin.

TABLE 1 • Microbiological Activity of Nitrofurantoin (1)		
Organism (No. tested)	MIC$_{50}$ (μg/mL)	Range (μg/mL)
Gram-negative bacteria		
E. coli (22)	≤8.0	≤8–>128
Klebsiella spp. (25)	64	16–256
Citrobacter spp. (35)	16	≤8–64
Enterobacter spp. (60)	64	16–256
Proteus spp. (74)	64	32–256
Pseudomonas spp. (57)	>256	256–>256
Gram-positive bacteria		
S. saprophyticus (4)	≤8.0	≤8.0–128
E. faecalis (10)	≤8.0	≤8.0–64

chronic or recurrent UTIs, this inhibitory breakpoint concentration was found to correlate with clinical success (42). Urinary infections with organisms that had MICs above 32 μg/mL persisted or relapsed shortly after treatment. The activity of nitrofurantoin is increased in acidic urine (4); for example, nitrofurantoin activity against *E. coli* was observed to increase twentyfold when the pH was changed from 8 to 5. Bactericidal activity in urine can be achieved with therapeutic doses of nitrofurantoin.

MECHANISMS OF RESISTANCE

The multiple mechanisms and sites of action for nitrofurantoin appear to reduce the ability of bacteria to develop resistance to this drug (23). Reduced nitrofuran reductase activity has been observed in nitrofurantoin-resistant strains of *E. coli* (3). These resistance genes have been found on chromosomes as well as R plasmids. Resistance also appears mediated by changes in cell wall permeability to nitrofurantoin. Permeabilization by EDTA of nitrofurantoin-resistant *E. coli* strains has been reported to dramatically decrease the MIC of nitrofurantoin, even in strains with little nitroreductase activity (27).

No clinically significant increase in resistance to nitrofurantoin has been reported. In a 20-year study of urinary pathogens collected in London from 1971 to 1992, approximately 85% of uropathogens isolated from patients seen by general practitioners remained sensitive to nitrofurantoin (12). Of these, over 90% of *E. coli* were still fully sensitive to this drug. Moreover, cross-resistance between nitrofurantoin and other antibacterial agents is uncommon (26).

PHARMACOKINETICS

Nitrofurantoin is well absorbed from the gastrointestinal tract and has an absolute bioavailability of about 90% (16). Peak plasma levels of about 0.4 μg/mL occur approximately 2 h after a 50-mg dose. Absorption occurs more slowly when nitrofurantoin is taken with food or given in a macrocrystalline formulation.

Nitrofurantoin is rapidly distributed in the body, but therapeutically active concentrations are not achieved in blood or tissues (13). This drug has a volume of distribution of 40 L, and approximately 60% of nitrofurantoin is bound to plasma protein (16). Maximum urine concentrations average 132 μg/mL after a single 50-mg dose in normal subjects.

About one-third of a dose of nitrofurantoin is excreted unchanged in the urine (16). The drug is eliminated by glomerular filtration as well as tubular secretion. Renal clearance of nitrofurantoin is approximately 245 mL/min (13). Tubular reabsorption is enhanced in acidic urine and decreased in alkaline urine (44). Nitrofurantoin accumulates in the serum of patients with impaired renal function. Urinary recovery of nitrofurantoin decreases in a linear relationship to the fall in creatinine clearance (33). Serum levels as high as 6.5 μg/mL have been observed in severe uremia. These patients excrete only small amounts of nitrofurantoin in the urine. Inactivation of nitrofurantoin appears to take place in many body tissues, especially the liver. The effects of liver disease on excretion are unknown.

The elimination half-life of nitrofurantoin in patients with normal renal function is about 1 h (16). Effective urine concentrations (>32 μg/mL) average 90 min following a single 50-mg dose in normal subjects.

DOSAGE REGIMENS

The oral dose is identical for the crystalline and macrocrystalline preparations. For acute UTI in adults, the dosage is 50 to 100 mg four times daily. Children should receive 5 to 7 mg/kg/day, given in four divided doses. Macrobid (75 mg nitrofurantoin monohydrate/25 mg macrocrystals) is dosed every 12 h. All formulations of nitrofurantoin should be taken with food to improve absorption and tolerance. Therapy for cystitis should be continued for 1 week. For long-term suppressive therapy in adults, 50 to 100 mg of nitrofurantoin is given at bedtime. Pediatric patients should receive 2 mg/kg.

Patients with elevated serum creatinine or a creatinine clearance below 60 mL/min should not receive nitrofurantoin. Nitrofurantoin is also contraindicated in newborns and nursing mothers. There are no well-controlled studies in pregnant women, but nitrofurantoin does not appear to be teratogenic at therapeutic dosages (pregnancy category B). Nitrofurantoin is contraindicated in pregnant women at term (>38 weeks) because of the possibility of precipitating hemolytic anemia in the newborn.

ADVERSE EFFECTS

Numerous organ systems can be affected by nitrofurantoin, and a large number of side effects are associated with use of this drug (17). The most frequent adverse effects involve the gastrointestinal tract. Nausea and vomiting are reported commonly and appear to be related to the dose and rate of absorption of nitrofurantoin. Dose reduction, slow-release formulations, and administration with food have been used to decrease the incidence of nausea (21). Nitrofurantoin has also been associated with inducing parotitis and pancreatitis (25, 28).

Dermatologic reactions are also commonly associated with nitrofurantoin administration (17). Common manifestations include rashes, eosinophilia and fever, and urticaria.

A variety of central nervous system reactions, including headache, dizziness, and confusion, have been reported by patients receiving nitrofurantoin (29). Peripheral neuritis is a rare but serious complication of nitrofurantoin therapy (8). It usually occurs in the elderly or patients with renal insufficiency who develop toxic blood levels of nitrofurantoin or its metabolites (9). Symptoms usually begin within 45 days of starting treatment, and the clinical course is one of ascending motor and sensory polyneuropathy (41).

A number of other rare but significant untoward effects are associated with nitrofurantoin use (8). Three types of pulmonary reactions have been reported with nitrofurantoin therapy. Acute pneumonitis, usually evident within days of beginning treatment, is characterized by cough, fever, and dyspnea (20). Respiratory infection or pulmonary edema are secondary complications. This pneumonitis is probably allergic in nature and is often accompanied by eosinophilia. Clinical symptoms usually subside within 2 days after the drug is discontinued. Subacute pneumonitis has also been described (36). Chronic pulmonary reactions are of great concern because patients can develop interstitial fibrosis, which has led to death (31). This insidious reaction is associated with long-term nitrofurantoin therapy, and patients usually have limited recovery. Chronic pulmonary infiltration appears to be due to a different immunologic mechanism than the acute form of pneumonitis, and eosinophilia does not occur. A toxic effect of the drug may also occur through oxidant mechanisms (34).

Nitrofurantoin has been associated with both hepatocellular damage and cholestatic jaundice (11). These toxic reactions are usually self-limiting and associated with short-term use. Chronic active hepatitis or granulomatous reaction has been observed with long-term use of nitrofurantoin. Continued use of the drug after the onset of jaundice can lead to massive necrosis and death (35). The mechanism of injury suggests an immunologically mediated reaction. An association between HLA-B8 antigen and nitrofurantoin-induced chronic active hepatitis has been observed and may be a marker of enhanced immunoresponsiveness (40).

Nitrofurantoin is associated with several types of blood disorders (8). It can precipitate acute hemolysis in patients with glucose-6-phosphate dehydrogenase deficiency (10). The drug, therefore, should be used with caution in patients of Mediterranean origin and avoided in infants under 1 month of age. Nitrofurantoin has also been reported to cause megaloblastic anemia due to folate deficiency, leukopenia, thrombocytopenia, agranulocytosis, and aplastic anemia.

DRUG AND FOOD INTERACTIONS

Food may increase the bioavailability of nitrofurantoin and prolong the duration of therapeutic urinary concentrations (2). Unlike other nitrofurans, nitrofurantoin does not appear to cause a "disulfuram-like" interaction with alcohol (8). An increase in the metabolism of phenytoin by nitrofurantoin was suggested in one reported case, but this finding has not been confirmed by additional cases or studies (14). Concomitant administration of magnesium trisilicate antacids can reduce both the rate and extent of nitrofurantoin absorption (24). Probenecid can inhibit tubular secretion of nitrofurantoin, which could decrease urinary levels and therapeutic efficacy.

Nitrofurantoin in combination with quinolone antibiotics has been shown to be antagonistic in vitro (43). The clinical significance of this finding is unknown.

CLINICAL INDICATIONS
Acute Infection

Nitrofurantoin is best suited for the treatment of acute uncomplicated lower urinary infections. It has remained an effective agent with continued activity in urine against common uropathogens such as E. coli and S. saprophyticus (19). Nitrofurantoin is also effective in eradication of vaginal E. coli in women with cystitis.

Nitrofurantoin was shown to be effective in a 3-day treatment regimen (22, 32). However, a randomized comparative study of 3-day regimens found trimethoprim-sulfamethoxazole to be superior to nitrofurantoin for uncomplicated cystitis in women (18). A 7-day treatment course of nitrofurantoin appears to be optimal in the treatment of lower UTIs (37).

Nitrofurantoin can be effective for renal infection because renal medullary and urinary concentrations are similar (38). However, this antimicrobial should not be used in severely ill patients because of the low systemic levels that are achieved. Nitrofurantoin concentrations in prostatic fluid are low, and consequently it is not recommended for treatment of acute prostatitis. Nitrofurantoin is also contraindicated in patients with impaired renal function.

Prophylaxis

Nitrofurantoin has been helpful as long-term suppressive therapy in patients with chronic bacteriuria. It is highly effective in preventing bacteriuria and rarely induces resistant coliforms in fecal flora (5, 6, 39). However, side effects are common and often lead to drug discontinuation (5, 6, 30). Of greatest concern are the chronic changes that may occur in the liver and lungs with long-term nitrofurantoin therapy (17).

COMMENTS

Nitrofurantoin continues to be a useful antimicrobial agent for the treatment of acute uncomplicated UTI (7). One-week regimens of macrocrystalline formulations are generally safe and well tolerated. Nitrofurantoin has been widely used during pregnancy without being implicated as a cause of congenital abnormalities. Prophylactic use of nitrofurantoin is useful for prevention of recurrent UTIs, but long-term therapy should be carefully monitored because of the risk of severe toxicity, especially in the elderly.

REFERENCES

1. Barry AL, Jones RN. Reassessment of nitrofurantoin disk susceptibility test criteria. Report to the National Committee for Clinical Laboratory Standards. December 21, 1988.
2. Bates TR, Sequeira JA, Tembo AV. Effect of food on nitrofurantoin absorption. Clin Pharmacol Ther 1974;16:63–68.
3. Breeze AS, Obaseiki-Ebor EE. Nitrofuran reductase activity in nitrofurantoin-resistant strains of *Escherichia coli* K12: some with chromosomally determined resistance and others carrying R-plasmids. J Antimicrob Chemother 1983;12:543–547.
4. Brumfitt W, Percival A. Laboratory control of antibiotic therapy in urinary tract infection. Ann NY Acad Sci 1967;145:329–343.
5. Brumfitt W, Smith GW, Hamilton-Miller JMT, Gargan RA. A clinical comparison between macrodantin and trimethoprim for prophylaxis in women with recurrent urinary infections. J Antimicrob Chemother 1985;16:111–220.
6. Brumfitt W, Hamilton-Miller JMT. A comparative trial of low dose cefaclor and macrocrystalline nitrofurantoin in the prevention of recurrent urinary tract infection. Infection 1995;23:98–102.
7. Cunha BA. Nitrofurantoin—current concepts. Urology 1988;32:67–71.
8. D'Arcy PF. Nitrofurantoin. Drug Intell Clin Pharm 1985;19:540–547.
9. Ellis FG. Acute polyneuritis after nitrofurantoin therapy. Lancet 1962;2:1136–1138.
10. Gait JE. Hemolytic reactions to nitrofurantoin in patients with glucose-6-phosphate dehydrogenase deficiency: theory and practice. DICP Ann Pharmacother 1990;24:1210–1213.
11. Goldstein LI, Ishak KG, Burns W. Hepatic injury associated with nitrofurantoin therapy. Am J Dig Dis 1974;19:987–995.
12. Gruneberg RN. Changes in urinary pathogens and their antibiotic sensitivities, 1971–1992. J Antimicrob Chemother 1994;33 (Suppl A):1–8.
13. Guelen PJM, Boerema JBJ, Vree TB. Comparative human bioavailability study of macrocrystalline nitrofurantoin and two prolonged-action hydroxymethyl-nitrofurantoin preparations. Drug Intell Clin Pharm 1988;22:959–964.
14. Heipertz R, Pilz H. Interaction of nitrofurantoin with diphenylhydantoin. J Neurol 1978;218:297–301.
15. Herrlich P, Schweiger M. Nitrofurans, a group of synthetic antibiotics, with a new mode of action: discrimination of specific messenger RNA classes. Proc Nat Acad Sci USA 1976;73:3386–3390.
16. Hoener BA, Patterson SE. Nitrofurantoin disposition. Clin Pharmacol Ther 1981;29:808–816.
17. Holmberg L, Boman G, Bottiger LE, Eriksson B, Spross R, Wessling A. Adverse reactions to nitrofurantoin. Am J Med 1980;69:733–738.
18. Hooton TM, Winter C, Tiu F, Stamm WE. Randomized comparative trial and cost analysis of 3-day antimicrobial regimens for treatment of acute cystitis in women. JAMA 1995;273:41–45.
19. Iravani A, Richard GA, Baer H. Trimethoprim once daily vs. nitrofurantoin in treatment of acute urinary tract infections in young women, with special reference to periurethral, vaginal, and fecal flora. Rev Infect Dis 1982;4:378–387.
20. Israel HL, Diamond P. Recurrent pulmonary infiltration and pleural effusion due to nitrofurantoin sensitivity. N Engl J Med 1962;266:1024–1026.
21. Kalowski S, Radford N, Kincaid-Smith P. Crystalline and macrocrystalline nitrofurantoin in the treatment of urinary-tract infection. N Engl J Med 1974;290:385–387.
22. Lohr JA, Hayden GF, Kesler RW. Three-day therapy of lower urinary tract infections with nitrofurantoin macrocrystals: a randomized clinical trial. J Pediatr 1981;99:980–983.
23. McOsker CC, Fitzpatrick PM. Nitrofurantoin: mechanism of action and implications for resistance development in common uropathogens. J Antimicrob Chemother 1994;33(Suppl A):23–30.
24. Naggar VF, Khalil SA. Effect of magnesium trisilicate on nitrofurantoin absorption. Clin Pharmacol Ther 1979;25:857–863.
25. Nelis GF. Nitrofurantoin-induced pancreatitis: report of a case. Gastroenterology 1984;84:1032–1034.
26. Obaseiki-Ebor EE. Cross-resistance to nitrofurans of aminoglycoside-aminocyclitol resistant strains of *Escherichia coli*. J Antimicrob Chemother 1983;11:485–487.
27. Obaseiki-Ebor EE. Enhanced *Escherichia coli* susceptibility to nitrofurantoin by EDTA and multiple aminoglycoside antibiotics resistance mutation. Chemotherapy 1984;30:88–91.
28. Pellinen TJ, Kalske J. Nitrofurantoin-induced parotitis. Br Med J 1982;285:344.
29. Penn RG, Griffin JP. Adverse reactions to nitrofurantoin in the United Kingdom, Sweden, and Holland. Br Med J 1982;284:1440–1442.
30. Raz R, Boger S. Long-term prophylaxis with norfloxacin versus nitrofurantoin in women with recurrent urinary tract infection. Antimicrob Agent Chemother 1991;35:1241–1242.
31. Rosenow EC, Deremee RA, Dines DE. Chronic nitrofurantoin pulmonary reaction. N Engl J Med 1968;279:1258–1262.
32. Ruberto U, D'Eufemia P, Ferretti L, Giardini O. Effect of 3- versus 10-day treatment of urinary tract infections. J Pediatr 1984;104:483–484.
33. Sachs J, Geer T, Noell P, Kunin CM. Effect of renal function on urinary recovery of orally administered nitrofurantoin. N Engl J Med 1968;278:1032–1035.
34. Sasame HA, Boyd MR. Superoxide and hydrogen peroxide production and NADPH oxidation stimulated by nitrofurantoin in lung microsomes. Possible implications for toxicity. Life Sci 1979;24:1091–1096.
35. Sharp JR, Ishak KG, Zimmerman HJ. Chronic active hepatitis and severe hepatic necrosis associated with nitrofurantoin. Ann Intern Med 1980;92:14–19.
36. Sovijaervi ARA, Lemola M, Stenius B, Idaenpaeaen-heikkilae J. Nitrofurantoin-induced acute, subacute and chronic pulmonary reactions. A report of 66 cases. Scand J Respir Dis 1977;58:41–50.
37. Spencer RC, Moseley DJ, Greensmith MJ. Nitrofurantoin modified release versus trimethoprim or co-trimoxazole in the treatment of uncomplicated urinary tract infection in general practice. J Antimicrob Chemother 1994;33(Suppl A):121–129.
38. Stamey TA, Govan DE, Palmer JM. The localization and treatment of urinary tract infections: the role of bactericidal urine levels as opposed to serum levels. Medicine 1965;44:1–36.
39. Stamey TA, Condy M, Mihara G. Prophylactic efficacy of nitrofurantoin macrocrystals and trimethoprim-sulfamethoxazole in urinary infections. N Engl J Med 1977;296:780–783.
40. Tolman KG. Nitrofurantoin and chronic active hepatitis. Ann Intern Med 1980;92:119–120.

41. Toole JF, Parrish ML. Nitrofurantoin polyneuropathy. Neurology 1973;23:554–559.
42. Turck M, Ronald AR, Petersdorf RG. Susceptibility of Enterobacteriaceae to nitrofurantoin correlated with eradication of bacteriuria. Antimicrob Agents Chemother - 1966. 1967: 446–452.
43. Westwood GPC, Hooper WL. Antagonism of oxolinic acid by nitrofurantoin. Lancet 1975;1:460.
44. Woodruff MW, Malvin RL, Thompson IM. The renal transport of nitrofurantoin. Effect of acid-base balance upon its excretion. JAMA 1961;175:1132–1135.

Penicillins

●

Sandra L. Preston and George L. Drusano

In 1929, Alexander Fleming isolated penicillin from a strain of *Penicillium notatum* (76). By 1941, benzylpenicillin could be produced in sufficient quantity to treat several infected patients. Clinical trials with the agent, conducted by Florey and colleagues, were successful, and during World War II, benzylpenicillin was used to treat patients with streptococcal, gonococcal, and treponemal infections. Shortages of the agent continued until the late 1940s when production of large amounts of drug became possible by a deep-fermentation procedure (77). Since then, many synthetic penicillins have been developed, but resistance to the agents has increased. Despite the emergence of resistance to penicillins and the development of other classes of antiinfective agents, the penicillins remain one of the most important antiinfective classes of drugs well into the nineties. In fact, penicillin G is still the drug of choice for many types of infections, including syphilis and certain types of endocarditis.

CLASS
Chemical Structure

The basic chemical structure of all penicillins consists of a β-lactam ring, a thiazolidine ring, and a side chain (6-aminopenicillanic acid). The antibacterial activity of the penicillins lies within the β-lactam ring. Any alteration in this ring structure forms penicilloic acid, and the antibacterial activity of the compound is lost. The side chain varies with each penicillin compound and generally determines the spectrum of activity as well as the pharmacokinetic properties of the compound. There are several natural penicillins (penicillin dihydro F, X, and K), of which benzylpenicillin (penicillin G) is the most active and the only natural penicillin used clinically (153).

Structure-Activity Relationships

Manipulations of the side chain have produced compounds that are stable against certain bacteria, such as *Staphylococcus aureus,* which produce β-lactamase enzymes (penicillinase). The side chain sterically inhibits β-lactamase hydrolysis of the β-lactam ring. Other penicillin compounds have side chains that are stable against β-lactamases produced by Gram-nega-

tive rods. Side chain changes can also increase the bacterial permeability of the compound and can result in increased oral absorption from the intestinal tract by rendering oral agents more stable to gastric acid breakdown (155, 173).

ANTIMICROBIAL ACTIVITY
Classification of Penicillins and Spectrum of Activity

The penicillin compounds can be divided into categories based upon their spectrum of activity (Table 1). Minimum inhibitory concentration (MIC) data for 50% and 90% of specific organisms are located in Tables 2 and 3 (10, 62, 139, 215, 232, 242, 243, 247). For Gram-negative organisms and anaerobes, resistance in up to 15% of strains is possible, therefore $MIC_{90}s$ must be interpreted cautiously.

Natural Penicillins

Penicillin G is a natural penicillin that is produced directly from fermentation of *Penicillium crysogenum.* Penicillin V is a derivative of penicillin G and, because of similarities in spectrum of activity, is considered a natural penicillin. The natural penicillins have activity against non-β-lactamase-producing Gram-positive cocci, including viridans streptococci, group A streptococci, *Streptococcus pneumoniae,* and anaerobic streptococcus (*Peptostreptococcus, Peptococcus* spp.). *Enterococcus* spp. are most susceptible to the natural penicillins. Other potential organisms with susceptibility include non-penicillinase-producing strains of *S. aureus* and coagulase-negative *Staphylococcus;* however, because of the high likelihood of resistance, it is inappropriate to use natural penicillins as empirical treatment for a suspected staphylococcal infection unless the organism's susceptibility is known. The natural penicillins have activity against *Clostridium* spp. (excluding *Clostridium difficile*) and *Actinomyces* spp. Activity against Gram-negative cocci is limited and includes *Neisseria meningitidis,* non-penicillinase-producing *Neisseria gonorrhoeae,* and *Pasteurella multocida.* As with staphylococcal infection, natural penicillins should not be used for treatment of gonorrhea due to the increased potential of a resistant organism and subsequent treatment failure. The anaerobic coverage of peni-

TABLE 3 • **Minimal Inhibitory Concentrations (MIC$_{90}$) of Specific Organisms**

Organism	MIC$_{90}$ (μg/mL)				
	Penicillin G	Oxacillin	Ampicillin/Amoxicillin	Ticarcillin	Mezlocillin/Piperacillin
Gram-Positive aerobes					
Enterococcus sp.	2.0	>100	4	128	4
Staphylococcus aureus					
(non-penicillinase-producing)	0.03	3.1	0.125	1.0	0.06
(penicillinase-producing)	>32	6.3	>32	32	32
Staphylococcus epidermidis				1.0	1.0
Streptococcus pneumoniae	0.03	0.8	0.02	1	0.02
Viridans streptococci				8	0.25
Streptococcus pyogenes	0.015	0.4	0.03	0.25	0.125
Listeria monocytogenes	0.5	>4	0.5	4	0.5
Gram-negative aerobes					
Neisseria gonorrhoeae[a]	0.5	12.5	0.06	0.03	0.015
Neisseria meningitidis	0.06	6.3	0.25	0.03	0.03
Escherichia coli	64	>128	>256	>256	256
Proteus mirabilis	32	>128	>256	128	16
Indole+ *P. mirabilis*	>500	>128	>256	>256	64
Haemophilus influenzae[a]	4	100	0.5	0.25	0.5
Salmonella sp.	16	>128	>256	>256	>256
Shigella sp.	32				
Serratia marcescens	>128	>128	>128	>256	128
Klebsiella sp.	>128	>128	>128	500	16
Enterobacter sp.	>128	>128	>128	>256	128
Citrobacter sp.	>128	>128	128	256	8
Acinetobacter sp.	>128	>128	64	64	128
Pseudomonas aeruginosa	>128	>128	>128	128	32
Anaerobes					
Peptostreptococcus	1.0	>32	8.0	2.0	4.0
Fusobacterium nucleatum	1.0	>64	16.0	0.5	0.5
Clostridium perfringens	0.5	>64	<0.1[b]	0.5	0.5
Bacteroides fragilis	>64	>64	>64	128	128

[a] Non-β-lactamase-producing strains.

[b] Amoxicillin's MIC$_{90}$ is 0.5.

Pharmacodynamic Effects

When choosing an antimicrobial agent and designing appropriate dosing regimens for the drug, it is important to consider spectrum of activity but also incorporate known pharmacodynamic principles about the drug. In this manner, efficacy can potentially be maximized while toxicity can be minimized. Some excellent reviews on these concepts have been published (63, 68). Pharmacodynamic variables to consider for the penicillins include concentration-independent bactericidal activity, the postantibiotic effect (PAE), and the duration of the dosing interval that drug serum concentrations are above the organism's MIC (time > MIC).

Bactericidal Effects

All β-lactam drugs (including the penicillins) exert relatively concentration-independent bactericidal activity; that is, the concentration of drug does not appreciably affect its antibacterial effect (21, 196). This assumes, however, a level that exceeds the organism's MIC. Theoretically, the bactericidal rate at twice the MIC or four times the MIC would be the same. However, once the drug concentration falls below the MIC and the PAE has

ceased, the kill rate diminishes. Time > MIC is therefore the important determinant of outcome for these drugs.

A paradoxical phenomena of decreased effect with higher drug concentrations, known as the "Eagle effect," has been described with some strains of streptococci and staphylococci (102). This effect, however, does not appear to be clinically significant; very limited data support decreased bactericidal activity in vivo because of high serum concentrations.

Another factor that may influence bactericidal activity is bacterial inoculum size. Generally, the denser the bacterial population (i.e., the older the infection), the more likely are resistant variants of the organism. This may be the case with nosocomial Gram-negative pneumonias or other serious infections. Treatment with a penicillin as monotherapy may result in a relapse after completion of therapy when the resistant subvariants are no longer suppressed and begin to regrow. This scenario is not unique to the penicillins and in fact may occur with other antibiotics used as monotherapy.

The bactericidal activity of the penicillins does not appear to be affected by changes in pH or oxygen tension. The location of the organism is important, however, as in vitro efficacy may not correspond to in vivo efficacy. Penicillins and other β-lactams do not penetrate well into phagocytes (95), which limits their ability to kill intracellular pathogens. In addition, penicillins only exert their bactericidal effect on bacteria that are actively replicating.

Synergistic Bactericidal Activity

Some organisms are killed most effectively by combinations of a β-lactam plus another agent, such as an aminoglycoside. In these cases, antibacterial synergy occurs. Synergy is defined as an effect (e.g., bactericidal activity) that is significantly greater with the combination than the sum of the two agents used alone. The mechanism of this effect with penicillins and aminoglycosides may be cell wall disruption by the penicillin facilitating increased entry of the aminoglycoside into the bacteria (147). Enterococcal endocarditis is an example; penicillin monotherapy results in bacteriostatic activity and very high relapse rates after treatment (138), while the combination of penicillin plus an aminoglycoside is bactericidal (146).

Other organisms for which synergy seems to be important with regard to the penicillins include *P. aeruginosa*. Again, combined therapy with an antipseudomonal penicillin and an aminoglycoside may increase bactericidal activity. This has been demonstrated in vitro and animal studies (5, 69, 108), but there are limited data in humans to support these findings. In vitro synergy between the extended-spectrum penicillins (azlocillin, mezlocillin) and ciprofloxacin has also been demonstrated (142, 165, 212). Immunocompromised patients may benefit the most from antipseudomonal synergy. Data suggest that synergistic combination therapy results in better survival than nonsynergistic combinations of drugs (114, 120, 191).

Antagonism of Antibacterial Combinations

Antibacterial antagonism is defined as an effect that is significantly less with a combination than with either of the two drugs used as monotherapy. Antagonism was demonstrated with the penicillins in combination with chlortetracycline; in patients with pneumococcal meningitis, penicillin monotherapy was more effective than the combination of agents (123). Combinations of penicillin plus chloramphenicol have in vitro antagonism against pneumococci (175); clinically, this may be of little importance, since the combination only diminishes penicillin's bactericidal activity (resulting in bacteriostatic activity), and chloramphenicol retains its antibacterial effect. Also, the use of chloramphenicol has decreased dramatically in the last decade because of the availability of newer agents that are equally effective and less toxic.

Antagonism can also occur because of physical incompatibility and inactivation between two drugs when infused together. This can occur with carbenicillin or ticarcillin with an aminoglycoside. These drugs should therefore not be mixed in the same infusion.

Postantibiotic Effect (PAE)

PAE is defined as persistent suppression of bacterial growth after effective exposure to an antimicrobial agent, when serum concentrations of the drug have fallen below the MIC. This ef-

fect differs between infecting organisms and between drugs. The mechanism of the PAE is not entirely clear, but may involve persistent binding of the penicillin to penicillin-binding proteins (PBPs) and the time necessary for the organism to resynthesize new PBPs (205).

PAE was first noted with penicillin G and *S. aureus* (166); for a short period of time, bacterial regrowth did not occur after exposure to the drug. Subsequently, this phenomena was described with the penicillins for other Gram-positive organisms (38, 99), including *S. pneumoniae* and *Enterococcus faecalis*. The length of the PAE can range from 0 to 6 h (Table 4), depending upon the penicillin.

As stated previously, the type of organism can effect the PAE. Penicillins do not exhibit an appreciable PAE against Gram-negative organisms. Also, combinations of antimicrobial agents can result in a synergistic PAE. Combinations of penicillins plus various aminoglycosides have resulted in synergistic or additive PAEs for *E. faecalis* and *Enterococcus faecium* (78, 99), along with *S. aureus* (91).

Models of Antibacterial Outcome Determination

Bactericidal activity of penicillins and other β-lactams appears to be related to the time > MIC, as demonstrated in several in vitro models. A number of studies of β-lactam agents demonstrated that increased half-life and not peak concentration influenced bactericidal activity (88, 115, 241, 257). This implies that longer drug exposure above the MIC would be more predictive of positive outcome than higher drug doses and subsequent increased peak concentrations.

Data from animal models supports time > MIC as the primary determinant of efficacy for β-lactam agents (67, 234). In a neutropenic mouse model infected with *P. aeruginosa,* the impact of different dosing intervals of ticarcillin was studied. Equivalent daily doses were administered every hour or every 3 h. The mice that received drug every hour (a lower dose administered more frequently) had a greater antibacterial effect (80).

These findings were also supported by studies of *Klebsiella pneumoniae* pneumonia in rats (184), *K. pneumoniae* lung and thigh infections in neutropenic mice (122), *P. aeruginosa* infection in neutropenic rats (148), *S. aureus* in rats recovering from hemorrhagic shock (132), and enterococcal endocarditis (218). Additional data (234) demonstrated that for Gram-negative infections, time > MIC of 100% of the dosing interval was most closely associated with outcome, whereas for Gram-positive organisms, a time > MIC of approximately 50% was all that was needed to be effective. For Gram-negative infec-

TABLE 4 •	In Vitro Postantibiotic Effect of Selected Penicillins		
	S. aureus	*S. pneumoniae*	*E. faecalis*
Penicillin G	2–3.5 h	2.5–3.5 h	2.5–3.5 h
Ampicillin	2–2.5 h	2–6 h	0.5–2.5 h
Nafcillin	1.5–2 h	ND	ND
Piperacillin	≤0.5 h	ND	≤0.5 h

a ND, no data.

tions, continuous infusion of the penicillin may be most appropriate to maintain serum concentrations above the MIC for the entire dosing interval.

Clinical trials examining the impact of time $>$ MIC for β-lactams on outcome are limited. One study examined combinations of carbenicillin plus continuous-infusion cefamandole, carbenicillin plus intermittent cefamandole, and carbenicillin plus continuous-infusion tobramycin in febrile neutropenic cancer patients (28). The most effective regimen was carbenicillin plus continuous-infusion cefamandole. Although actual times $>$ MIC were not calculated, the most effective regimen most likely had the greatest time $>$ MIC, as the carbenicillin was administered every 4 h, effectively providing serum concentrations that would remain above the MIC throughout the dosing interval.

A study of cefmenoxime in 14 critically ill patients examined bacterial eradication rates as a function of time $>$ MIC (190) and found a relationship between increased time $>$ MIC and increased eradication rates of Gram-negative pathogens.

Continuous Infusion of Penicillins

In vitro data support more frequent administration of piperacillin in suppression of microbial growth (158). As previously stated, data comparing continuous infusion with intermittent dosing in humans are limited. The study by Bodey et al. appears to support such dosing; however, some small studies did not demonstrate any differences in response rates (119, 255). The study by Zeisler et al. (255) was not randomized, and the study by Lagast et al. (119) only included 45 patients and most likely lacked sufficient power to detect a statistical difference.

The advantage of continuous infusion is the potential maximization of efficacy and potentially decreased costs (255). Disadvantages, however, include patient inconvenience with a continually infusing solution, lack of knowledge about proper dosing, and compatibility issues with other necessary intravenous drugs (235). Many of these concerns may be addressed by educational efforts. Other concerns include adequate tissue penetration with continuous infusion. Some studies have demonstrated good penetration of continuous-infusion β-lactams into extravascular space (168, 231). Other data appear to indicate that intermittent injections result in increased tissue penetration, as seen in models of rabbit fibrin clots (14, 121); however, the concentrations achieved with continuous infusion may be enough above the organism MIC to treat the infection. However, in this model, the clots are implanted in the rabbit's back and may not be an appropriate representation of physiology.

Continuous infusion may be most beneficial in patients with impaired host defenses or in life-threatening infections. In these cases, patient convenience is less of an issue, and the potential benefit from maximizing efficacy is greatest. Dosing by continuous infusion can be accomplished by use of nomograms (233) or by monitoring a steady-state serum concentration (after 4 to 5 half-lives or approximately 4 to 5 h into the infusion for most penicillins) and adjusting the dose in relation to the serum concentration and the organism MIC. A bolus dose may be used to bring the serum concentrations to a therapeutic level quickly.

MECHANISMS OF ACTION

Penicillins are bactericidal agents that inhibit bacterial cell wall synthesis and induce a bacterial autolytic effect.

Inhibition of Bacterial Cell Wall Synthesis

Penicillins exert their bactericidal activity primarily by inhibiting bacterial cell wall synthesis. Though the exact mechanism of action is not fully elucidated, it appears that penicillins bind to penicillin-binding proteins (PBPs), which are enzymes (transpeptidases, carboxypeptidases, and endopeptidases) that play an important role in formation and maintenance of the cell wall structure. The cell wall is made up of peptidoglycan, or murein sacculus, a polymeric component consisting of long polysaccharide chains of N-acetylglucosamine and N-acetylmuramic acid cross-linked by shorter peptide chains. Peptidoglycan is formed in three stages: precursor formation in the cytoplasm, linkage of precursor products into a long polymer, and finally cross-linking by transpeptidation. It is the final transpeptidation process that is inhibited by penicillins acting as structural analogues of acyl-D-alanyl-D-alanine (the substrate of the enzyme) and acylating the transpeptidase enzyme. The peptidoglycan structure, and therefore the cell wall structure, is weakened, leading to cell death (221, 223, 252).

Other mechanisms of cell death are also possible. Binding to PBPs 1A, 1B, 2, and 3 results in a bactericidal effect (206); however, binding to PBPs 4, 5, and 6 is not lethal. Also, PBPs differ between Gram-positive and Gram-negative bacteria, and penicillins differ in affinity to various PBPs. These differences can affect the spectrum of activity.

Penicillin-Induced Bacterial Autolytic Effect

Several PBPs are inactivated simultaneously by penicillins. Inhibition of certain PBPs may be related to a bacterial autolytic process activated by inactivation of endogenous inhibitors of autolysins or murein hydrolases (222). These enzymes cleave parts of the cell wall to make room for peptidoglycan synthesis for cell wall expansion (100). With inhibition of cell wall synthesis, bacterial lysis can result from increased osmotic pressure. This autolysis may be cell-cycle dependent, that is, be most likely to occur while the cell is dividing (136). Certain "tolerant" species of staphylococci and streptococci are autolysin deficient. These organisms are inhibited, but not killed, by penicillins (220).

MECHANISMS OF RESISTANCE

Clinical use of penicillins is limited by the emergence of resistant organisms. Antimicrobial resistance can arise during therapy by selective pressure or can be present in a naturally resistant strain. A classic example of penicillin resistance is the case of S. aureus, which was susceptible to penicillin G when the compound was first discovered (around 1941). Since then, more than 95% of strains have become resistant, leading to the necessity of using such alternative compounds as the antistaphylococcal penicillins or vancomycin. Resistance of other Gram-positive and Gram-negative organisms also occurs, which can make treatment of active infection challenging. Resistance rates for different organisms vary by geographic location and are summarized in Table 5 (84, 107, 149, 156, 187, 193). Of particular concern in the United States is the emergence of penicillin-resistant (and multidrug resistant) pneumococci and methicillin-resistant staphylococci, as treatment options in these scenarios are limited (8, 224).

There are three main mechanisms of resistance to penicillins: (*a*) enzymatic degradation of the penicillin, (*b*) inability of the penicillin to penetrate the cell membrane to reach its target site, and (*c*) alteration of the PBP target site.

Enzymatic Degradation

Inactivation by β-lactamase enzymes is the most common mechanism of resistance to the β-lactam agents. β-Lactamase hydrolyzes the β-lactam bond, forming acidic derivatives, with subsequent loss of antibacterial activity. There are several classification schemes for the numerous β-lactamases, including those of Jack and Richmond (106), Richmond and Sykes (178), and Bush (40, 41). The Bush scheme classifies according to substrate preference and susceptibility to clavulanate inhibition. However, these schemes can be confusing because of their numerous codes and abbreviations (130). Both Gram-positive and Gram-negative organisms produce β-lactamases, mediated by either plasmids or chromosomes. An important difference is that Gram-positive organisms generally produce more enzyme because it must be excreted into the extracellular space for the antibiotic to be inactivated, while Gram-negative bacterial enzymes are located in their periplasmic space.

Gram-positive bacteria that produce β-lactamases (particularly staphylococci) can transfer resistance through plasmids

or transposons. Plasmids are extrachromosomal genetic entities that are autonomous, are self-reproducing, and can conjugate. By conjugation, the genetic information is transferred to other *Staphylococcus* species, including *S. aureus* and *S. epidermidis*. Transposons are DNA elements that can move from one part of the bacterial chromosome to another. Genetic information can be transferred to other bacteria through movement of the transposon to a plasmid or by direct transfer to another bacteria's chromosome—conjugative transposons (203). β-Lactamases of *Staphylococcus* can be induced by β-lactam antibiotics; that is, after exposure to a β-lactam agent, the organism can greatly increase β-lactamase production. Inducible production generally ceases after the β-lactam inducer is removed (160).

As stated above, Gram-negative bacteria secrete β-lactamases into the periplasmic space and are effective in protecting the PBPs located on the bacterial inner membrane from the antibiotic. These enzymes can be either chromosomally encoded or plasmid encoded (214). They are either constitutive (a constant amount of β-lactamase is produced regardless of exposure to β-lactam agents) or inducible, and they can affect β-lactam compounds in different ways. Some agents are quickly destroyed; others are destroyed more slowly and thus exert increased antibacterial activity.

Emergence of stably derepressed mutants is a concern during therapy with β-lactam agents that are weak inducers of β-lactamase production, such as extended-spectrum and third-generation cephalosporins. These mutants produce increased quantities of β-lactamases (hyperproduction) despite removal of the inducible antibiotic. This is most likely to occur with the chromosomally mediated Bush group I enzymes for which the preferred substrate is cephalosporins. Resistance can emerge rapidly in this circumstance, particularly in infections caused by *P. aeruginosa* or *Enterobacter cloacae* (44, 131), because of selection of the mutants after the more susceptible organisms are killed during treatment. In this instance, the mutants can proliferate and become the predominant infecting organism. The only effective β-lactam would be a carbapenem, as class I β-lactamases can hydrolyze all other types of β-lactam agents.

Extended-spectrum β-lactamases (ESBLs) are plasmid mediated with a wide substrate profile. These enzymes are a relatively recent problem, affecting some strains of *Klebsiella* spp. as well as some strains of *Enterobacter* and *E. coli*. The emergence of ESBL-producing organisms has been linked to the widespread use of extended-spectrum cephalosporins (143, 177). A carbapenem is the drug of choice against these organisms, and β-lactamase inhibitor combinations may also be effective (84).

Reduced Penetration of the Penicillin

It is easier for penicillins to acetylate the PBPs in Gram-positive bacteria because these bacteria have only a thick cell wall layer protecting the PBPs on the inner membrane. Gram-negative bacteria have an outer membrane composed of a lipopolysaccharide and phospholipid bilayer, with a periplasmic space between the layers. An inner membrane is com-

TABLE 5 • Prevalence of Resistance of Organisms to Penicillins	
Organism	**Prevalence**
Gram-positive	
Streptococcus pneumoniae[a]	Intermediate pcn resistance 14%; highly pcn resistant 9.5%
Staphylococcus aureus	Pcn resistant >95%; methicillin resistant (nosocomial) 23–38%
Gram-negative	
Haemophilus influenzae	Ampicillin 1–64%
Moraxella catarrhalis	Up to 85%
Escherichia coli	Ampicillin 30–50%
Neisseria gonorrhoeae	1.2–38%
Neisseria meningitidis	Up to 20%
Extended-spectrum β-lactamase producers	
Klebsiella pneumoniae	Up to 24%
Pseudomonas aeruginosa	Piperacillin 5–30%

[a] Intermediate resistant strains have MICs of 0.12–1.0 μg/mL, highly resistant strains have MICs of ≥2.0 μg/mL.

posed of peptidoglycan. Another space separates the inner membrane from the cytoplasmic membrane. PBPs are located in the cytoplasmic membrane and are protected by β-lactamases. In the outer membrane, proteins known as porins act as channels for nutrients and waste products into and out of the bacteria. Penicillins may enter Gram-negative bacteria by this route. Porin permeability to penicillins depends upon the molecules's size, hydrophilicity, and electric charge (253). Decreases in the number of porin channels has been reported to be a mechanism of resistance to β-lactam agents (96). Most research has been conducted with the outer-membrane proteins (Omp) of *E. coli*. Omp F and Omp C are the two main porins, with Omp F being most permeable to β-lactam agents. Some mutants that lack Omp F porins are resistant to β-lactams because of decreased and slower penetration through the remaining porins (Omp C) and subsequent increased β-lactamase degradation (58).

Alteration of the PBP Target Site

The penicillin must bind to the PBP to exert its antibacterial effect. Natural differences exist in the affinity for a penicillin to a PBP. For instance, the enterococcal PBP has a very low affinity for the antistaphylococcal penicillins and a high affinity for penicillin G or ampicillin, which explains the resistance of enterococci to oxacillin.

Mutations can change the susceptibility of an organism that is "normally" susceptible to a particular penicillin, usually by producing PBPs with a decreased affinity for the penicillin. An alteration from PBP2 to PBP2a by *Staphylococcus* results in methicillin resistance, as PBP2a exhibits decreased affinity for methicillin and most other β-lactam agents (93). With *S. aureus* (228), production of PBPs with decreased affinity for the penicillin is induced by exposure to the agent, resulting in decreased susceptibility to low concentrations of the drug.

An important example of bacteria developing mutations that confer resistance is *S. pneumoniae* that is penicillin resistant. The resistance mutation is genetically coded with "mosaics" made up of native pneumococcal DNA and DNA that is presumably from another streptococcal species, such as viridans streptococci, more resistant to penicillin (84, 117). The genes that appear to be most affected are PBP 2b and 2x.

Methods of Overcoming and Preventing Resistance

Preventive measures are needed because of the emergence of infectious organisms resistant to standard therapies. Infection control practices should be followed, including hand washing and changing gloves between patient examinations. These methods can limit dissemination of a resistant organism in a hospital environment (86). Unfortunately, such practices are not routinely followed by health care providers despite educational efforts (85, 60).

Optimization of antimicrobial use in hospitals is desirable, because use (and overuse) of broad-spectrum antimicrobials is associated with emergence of resistant organisms (44, 236), particularly ESBL-producing organisms (143, 177), and is suspected with penicillin- and vancomycin-resistant enterococci. Antibiotic control programs have been implemented in

many institutions with some success (71, 250). However, successful policies can be time and labor intensive, and they require a full institutional commitment in the form of adequate personnel for implementation and medical staff support for the program.

Pharmacologically, there are strategies to overcome and prevent resistance. The use of combination antimicrobial therapy provides adequate coverage against suspected organisms (11). Animal model data suggest that synergistic combination chemotherapy may prevent emergence of resistance (81, 108). However, clinical data are limited.

PHARMACOKINETIC DISPOSITION

The pharmacokinetics of the penicillins vary among compounds. Absorption of oral agents varies greatly; amoxicillin and dicloxacillin produce adequate serum concentrations, while penicillin G and carbenicillin produce very low serum concentrations. The penicillins are widely distributed in the body, with adequate levels achieved in serum, tissues, bile, and synovial fluid. Penetration into the cerebrospinal fluid (CSF) in patients with uninflamed meninges is relatively poor, with only 0.5 to 2% of serum concentration attained (162). When the meninges are inflamed, however, penetration increases to approximately 5 to 20% of serum concentration, as demonstrated in rabbit models (189, 216). The primary route of elimination for most penicillins is renal, with some hepatic metabolism; however, some compounds are primarily eliminated by the hepatic route.

Absorption, distribution, metabolism, and excretion are described below for each class of penicillins. Pharmacokinetic properties for the penicillins are summarized in Table 6.

Natural Penicillins

Aqueous crystalline penicillin G, or benzylpenicillin, administered intravenously is the most commonly used formulation in this class of penicillins. This route of administration is preferred in ill patients because higher serum concentrations are achieved than with oral or intramuscular administration of penicillin G or other natural penicillins. The drug is widely distributed, with an apparent volume of distribution (V_d) of 0.35 L/kg. Distribution into the CSF is minimal with uninflamed meninges but increases with inflammation. CSF concentrations can reach approximately 5% of serum concentrations (192). Elimination is primarily (90%) renal (10% by glomerular filtration, 90% by tubular secretion) (36, 65), with some hepatic elimination. The pharmacokinetic advantage to this drug is that high serum concentrations are achieved rapidly; but the half-life is approximately 30 min, necessitating redosing every 4 to 6 h.

Penicillin G is poorly absorbed orally, with a bioavailability of 15 to 30%. Absorption is decreased by gastric acid breakdown in the stomach. In hypochlorhydric patients, such as the elderly, oral penicillin G has increased absorption due to increased gastric pH. Penicillin V administered orally has greater absorption than penicillin G because of its increased acid stability (nearly double the peak serum concentrations). Low concentrations are attained in tissues. Concurrent admin-

TABLE 6 • Pharmacokinetic Properties of Penicillins

Drug	Dose	Peak Serum Conc.[a]	% Bioavailability	Half-Life(h)	% ppb[b]
Natural penicillins					
Benzylpenicillin	2 g	20 μg/mL	na	0.5	50–60
Penicillin G oral	400,000 u	0.3 μg/mL	15–30	0.5	
Penicillin VK	250 mg	3 μg/mL	60	0.5	75–85
Procaine pen G i.m.	300,000 u	0.9 μg/mL			
Benzathine pen G i.m.	1.2 mu	0.09 μg/mL			
Penicillinase-resistant penicillins					
Nafcillin i.v.	1 g	20 μg/mL	na	0.5–1.0	90
Oxacillin i.v.	500 mg	52–63 μg/mL	na	0.5–0.7	94
Oxacillin oral	500 mg	5–7 μg/mL	30–35%	0.5–0.7	
Cloxacillin oral	500 mg	7.5–14 μg/mL	50	0.5	95
Dicloxacillin oral	500 mg	10–17 μg/mL	37	0.8	98
Aminopenicillins					
Ampicillin i.v.	1 g	40 μg/mL	na	1–1.3	20
Ampicillin oral	1 g	3 μg/mL	30–50	1–1.3	
Amoxicillin oral	1 g	7.5 μg/mL	80	1–1.3	20
Extended-spectrum penicillins					
Carbenicillin i.v.	3 g	223 μg/mL	na	1.1	50
Carbenicillin oral	1 g	9 μg/mL	30		
Ticarcillin	3.5 g	210 μg/mL	na	1.2	45
Mezlocillin	3 g	263 μg/mL	na	0.8	16–42
Piperacillin	4 g	240 μg/mL	na	1.0	16

[a] Data complied from product package information and reference 62.

[b] Percentage plasma protein bound.

istration of food can decrease absorption of the oral natural penicillins, most likely because the penicillin is bound onto food particles. Because of poor absorption and limited clinical utility, oral penicillin G is no longer available in the United States.

Procaine penicillin G (PPG) and benzathine penicillin G (BPG) are repository forms of penicillin administered intramuscularly, with prolonged absorption and subsequent extended serum concentrations of penicillin G. PPG serum concentration can last up to 24 h, while low-level BPG serum concentrations (0.10–0.15 units/mL) can last up to 3 to 4 weeks. The advantage of these long-acting agents is that dosing can be less frequent if the organism is susceptible to the lower levels achieved; for example, with BPG and *T. pallidum,* the causative agent of syphilis, for which MICs are usually 0.03 units/mL. PPB contains 120 mg procaine for every 300,000 units of penicillin G. Patients who are hypersensitive to procaine may experience adverse reactions, particularly when high doses (e.g., 4.8 million units PPG) are used.

Penicillinase-Resistant Penicillins

Methicillin is not orally absorbed and is therefore only given by the intravenous route. Nafcillin has poor oral absorption and its use is generally limited to intravenous or intramuscular routes. Oxacillin, cloxacillin, and dicloxacillin can be administered orally; however, oral oxacillin produces a peak serum concentration about one-fourth that of dicloxacillin.

Penetration into the CSF with inflamed meninges is variable because of increased protein binding (50–92%). Penetra-

tion into the bile is highest with nafcillin—approximately 4000% of the serum concentration (153). Methicillin is eliminated primarily through the kidney by glomerular filtration or tubular secretion. Oxacillin is both eliminated renally and metabolized hepatically. Nafcillin is primarily metabolized hepatically, thus dosage adjustment in renally impaired patients is not necessary.

Aminopenicillins

Unlike the natural penicillins, aminopenicillins exhibit increased stability to gastric acid hydrolysis. Amoxicillin has greater bioavailability than ampicillin (75–90% with amoxicillin vs. 30–50% with ampicillin). Because of this difference, oral ampicillin has been favored for treatment of localized *Shigella* infection when lack of absorption is desirable. However, the incidence of diarrhea is increased with this agent because of its effect on normal flora of the gastrointestinal tract. Food delays absorption of ampicillin and amoxicillin, but the extent of absorption is decreased only for ampicillin.

Ampicillin penetrates into the CSF in patients with inflamed meninges, with CSF concentrations reaching approximately 1.5 μg/mL after a single 1-g dose. Elimination of the drug is primarily renal, but about 10% of the drug is metabolized hepatically. Both drugs are removed by hemodialysis (30–40%).

Bacampicillin is a prodrug of ampicillin and is hydrolyzed to ampicillin by esterases during absorption and distribution. Increased serum concentrations of ampicillin are seen because of increased absorption (bioavailability, 80–95%).

Extended-Spectrum Penicillins

Absorption of carbenicillin (the only orally available extended-spectrum penicillin) is poor, with a bioavailability of 30 to 40%. Serum concentrations achieved are inadequate for appropriate treatment of systemic infection; thus its clinical use is limited to urinary tract infection and, in some instances, prostatitis. However, use of this drug has decreased since orally administered quinolones became available for these indications.

Ticarcillin, mezlocillin, and piperacillin penetrate fairly well into the CSF in patients with inflamed meninges. Continuous-infusion piperacillin in four meningitis patients receiving 325 to 425 mg/kg/day attained a mean CSF level of 23 μg/mL (60). They also distribute well into bile, with concentrations of piperacillin nearly 50 times that in serum (83, 186). Penetration into diseased biliary tracts (e.g., cholecystitis) is limited, and adequate concentrations may not be achieved in this setting. Elimination of these compounds is by both renal and non-renal routes.

Effects of Renal Impairment and Dialysis on Clearance of Penicillins

Because many penicillins are renally excreted, impaired renal function can prolong half-lives and subsequently increase serum concentrations of drug (14) and the propensity for adverse effects. Thus doses or dosing intervals must be adjusted for many penicillins in these patients (Table 7). Penicillin G is excreted renally, and its clearance can be related to creatinine clearance (CrCL) by the equation penicillin clearance in mL/min = 35.5 + 3.35 × CrCL in mL/min. The daily dose of penicillin G can be calculated by the equation dose (in million units per day) = 3.2 + CrCL/7 (36). Other penicillins, including mezlocillin and piperacillin (20, 57) should also have their dosing regimens adjusted in renal impairment. However, these drugs also have biliary excretion, so serum concentrations are proportional to the degree of renal impairment. Oxacillin, cloxacillin, and dicloxacillin are partially renally excreted but have only moderately increased half-lives (1.5- to 2-fold) in anuric patients (18, 37, 244); therefore, dosage adjustment is probably necessary only with severe renal impairment. Carbenicillin should be avoided in patients with renal impairment and renal failure, because urinary concentrations are inadequate for treatment of urinary tract infection (the drug's only clinical indication).

Many penicillins are cleared during hemodialysis (50–90% of serum concentrations) (18, 69); therefore, a supplemental dose after dialysis is recommended for penicillin G, ampicillin, piperacillin, ticarcillin, and mezlocillin. Nafcillin and oxacillin are not appreciably cleared by hemodialysis, so supplemental dosing is not necessary. Since peritoneal dialysis does not significantly remove any of the penicillins, supplemental dosing is not necessary.

Effects of Hepatic Insufficiency

Most penicillins are primarily renally eliminated and do not require dosage adjustment for hepatic impairment. Because of the nonspecific nature of liver function tests (ALT, AST, GGT,

etc.) and the fact that increases in these markers may not correlate with intrinsic hepatocellular activity, it is difficult to recommend precise dosage adjustments for hepatically eliminated drugs. Some penicillins that may warrant dosage adjustment in hepatic impairment include nafcillin and mezlocillin. Reducing the dose of nafcillin up to 50% may be appropriate in patients with a combination of renal and hepatic insufficiency. Mezlocillin dosage may be reduced by half or the dosing interval be doubled in patients with severe hepatic impairment (39, 144).

Effects of Pregnancy

V_d increases in pregnant patients, which may decrease the serum concentrations of drugs. This has been demonstrated with piperacillin (97) and ampicillin (116) and may occur with other penicillins as well. In a comparative study with piperacillin and mezlocillin, shorter half-lives and greater clearance were seen in postpartum patients receiving piperacillin than in nonpregnant patients; but this was not seen in postpartum women receiving mezlocillin (141). These data imply that dosage increases may be more important in postpartum patients given piperacillin, as this drug may be more affected by the physiologic changes induced by pregnancy.

DOSAGE REGIMENS AND AVAILABILITY

A summary of common adult and pediatric dosage regimens for the penicillins is shown in Table 7 (145). Many pediatric dosages are specified on a per kilogram basis. It is important to keep in mind that the pediatric dosage should not exceed the usual adult dose when using this method of dosing, particularly in a large child. Available formulations are listed in Table 1 and costs for typical courses of therapy are shown in Table 8.

Natural Penicillins

Penicillin G dosages are usually described in units. One unit is defined as the concentration of drug that produces a certain size zone of growth inhibition around an Oxford strain of *S. aureus*. One unit is equivalent to 0.6 μg of crystalline sodium salt of penicillin G; therefore, 250 mg equals 400,000 units. Aqueous crystalline penicillin G is administered intravenously at dosages of 6 to 20 million units daily, either in 4 to 6 divided doses or by continuous infusion.

Benzylpenicillin is available as a sodium or potassium salt, either providing 20 meq of sodium or 1.7 meq potassium per 1 million units. The potassium salt is most often used clinically, except in patients with severe renal failure, when the sodium salt may be more appropriate.

BPG and PPG should not be administered subcutaneously because of severe pain and induration at the injection site. In adults, injection should be into the gluteus maximus or mid-lateral thigh. Intravenous injection may result in severe neurotoxicity and should be avoided.

Penicillinase-Resistant Penicillins and Aminopenicillins

The penicillinase-resistant penicillins are available as sodium salts. Dosages for methicillin are expressed as methicillin sodium, while the other agents in this class have their dosages

TABLE 7 • **Guidelines for Adult and Pediatric Dosing of Penicillins**

Drug	Normal Adult Dose[a]	Normal Pediatric Dose[a]	Dosage Adjustment in Renal Impairment[b,c]
Natural penicillins			
Benzylpenicillin (penicillin G)	Enterococcal endocarditis: 4–6 mu[d] i.v. q. 4 h	≤1 week and >2 kg: 20,000–50,000 u/kg i.v. q. 8 h	CrCL 10–50 mL/min: increase dosing interval to q. 6–8 h
Benzathine penicillin G	Streptococcal meningitis: 2–3 mu i.v. q. 4 h	≤1 week and ≤2 kg: 20,000–50,000 u/kg i.v. q. 12 h	CrCL < 10 mL/min: increase dosing interval to q. 12 h
	Streptococcal infection: 2 mu i.v. q. 4–6 h	>1 week and ≤2 kg: 25,000–65,000 u/kg i.v. q. 8 h	
		>1 week and >2 kg: 25,000–65,000 u/kg i.v. q. 6 h	
		>1 month and <12 years, severe infection: 40,000–60,000 u/kg i.v. q. 4–6 h	
		>12 years: usual adult dose	
Penicillin VK	Streptococcal pharyngitis: 500 mg p.o. b.i.d.-t.i.d. for 10 days	>1 month: 15–50 mg/kg/day p.o. in 3–6 divided doses	Few data available; adjust dose if CrCL < 10 mL/min
	Lyme disease: 250–500 mg p.o. q.i.d. for 10–30 days	Lyme disease and <9 years: 25–50 mg/kgday p.o. in 3 divided doses for 10–30 days	
Procaine penicillin G (PPG)	Streptococcal infection: 600,000–1.2 mu i.m. q.d. for 10 days	Neonates: 50,000 u/kg/day i.m. >1 month and <12 years: 25,000–50,000 u/kg/day i.m.	Not necessary
		≥12 years: usual adult dose	
Benzathine penicillin G (BPG)	Early syphilis: 2.4 mu i.m. Group A streptococcus infection and prophylaxis of recurrent rheumatic fever: 1.2 mu i.m.	<27 kg: 300,000–600,000 u i.m. ≥27 kg: 1.2 mu i.m.	Not necessary
Penicillinase-resistant penicillins			
Methicillin	1 g i.v. q. 4–6 h	>1 month: 150–400 mg/kg/day i.v. in 4–6 divided doses	CrCL < 10 mL/min: extend dosage interval to q. 8–12 h
Nafcillin	500 mg–1 g p.o. q. 4–6 h	>1 month: 50–100 mg/kg/day p.o. in 3–4 divided doses	CrCL < 10 mL/min: extend dosage interval to q. 8–12 h
	1–2 g i.v. q. 4–6 h	>1 month: i.v. data limited, 100–200 mg/kg/day in 4–6 divided doses	
Oxacillin	500 mg–1 g p.o. q. 4–6 h	>1 month and <40 kg: 50–100 mg/kg/day p.o. or i.v. in 4 divided doses	CrCL < 10 mL/min: use lower range of usual dose
	1–2 g i.v. q. 4–6 h	≥40 kg: usual adult dose	
Cloxacillin	250–500 mg po q. 6 h	>1 month and <20 kg: 50–100 mg/kg/day p.o. in 4 divided doses	
		≥20 kg: usual adult dose	
Dicloxacillin	125–250 mg p.o. q. 6 h	>1 month and <40 kg: 12.5–25 mg/kg/day p.o. in 4 divided doses	Not necessary
		≥40 kg: usual adult dose staphylococcal osteomyelitis: 50–100 mg/kg/day in 4 divided doses	
Aminopenicillins			
Ampicillin	250–500 mg p.o. q. 6 h 1–2 g i.v. q. 4 h	≥1 month and <40 kg: 50–200 mg/kg/day i.v. in 4–6 divided doses	CrCL 10–50 mL/min: extend dosing interval to q. 6–8 h
		<1 week: 25 mg/kg i.v./i.m. q 8–12 h	CrCL < 10 mL/min: extend dosing interval to q. 8–12 h
		≥1 week and <1 month: 25 mg/kg i.v./i.m. q. 6–8 h	
		>40 kg: usual adult dose	
Amoxicillin	250–500 mg p.o. q. 8 h	>1 month and <20 kg: 20–40 mg/kg/day in 3 divided doses	CrCL 10–50 mL/min: consider extending dosing interval to q. 12 h
		>20 kg: usual adult dose	CrCL < 10 mL/min: extend dosing interval to q. 12–24 h
Bacampicillin	400–800 mg p.o. q. 12 h	<25 kg: 12.5–25 mg/kg p.o. q. 12 h	Same as with ampicillin
		≥25 kg: usual adult dose	

continued

TABLE 7 • Guidelines for Adult and Pediatric Dosing of Penicillins

Drug	Normal Adult Dose[a]	Normal Pediatric Dose[a]	Dosage Adjustment in Renal Impairment[b,c]
Extended-spectrum penicillins			
Carbenicillin	382–764 mg p.o. q.i.d.	No data	No data
Ticarcillin	3 g i.v. q. 4 h	>1 month and <40 kg: 100–300 mg/kg/day in 4–6 divided doses ≥40 kg: usual adult dose	CrCL 30–60 mL/min: 2 g q. 4 h CrCL 10–30 mL/min: 2 g q. 8 h CrCL < 10 mL/min: 2 g q. 12 h Supplement after HD[e]: 3 g
Mezlocillin	3–4 g i.v. q. 4–6 h	<1 week: 75 mg/kg q. 12 h ≥1 week and <1 month: 75 mg/kg q. 6–8 h ≥1 month and <12 years: 50–75 mg/kg q. 4 h ≥12 years: usual adult dose	CrCL 10–50 mL/min: 1.5–3 g q. 6–8 h CrCL < 10 mL/min: 1.5–2 g q. 8 h Supplement after HD: 3–4 g
Piperacillin	3–4 g i.v. q. 4–6 h	1 month–12 years: 50 mg/kg q. 4 h	CrCL 20–40 mL/min: 3–4 g q. 8 h CrCL < 20 mL/min: 3–4 g q. 12 h Supplement after HD: 1 g

[a] These dosages are ranges of acceptable doses. The lower range of usual dose is generally used for mild infection, upper range for severe infection (e.g., meningitis, endocarditis). Higher dosages than recommended may be used in certain circumstances. Clinical judgment should be used when dosing, and prescribing information for the specific drugs should be consulted for more information.

[b] Clinical judgment should be used when making decisions regarding dosage adjustment in renally impaired patients, taking into account severity of renal impairment, site of infection, expected length of therapy, organism isolated, etc.

[c] Data complied using McEvoy 1997 AHFS Drug Information and product package inserts

[d] mu, million units.

[e] HD, hemodialysis.

TABLE 8 • Cost of Typical Therapeutic Regimens of Selected Penicillins

Drug	Dosing Regimen	Cost[a]
Oral agents		
Ampicillin	500 mg p.o. q. 6 h × 10 days	$5.00
Penicillin VK	500 mg p.o. q. 8 h × 10 days	$4.66
Amoxicillin	500 mg p.o. q. 8 h × 10 days	$3.48
Long-acting agents		
Procaine penicillin G	1.2 mu i.m. × 1	$11.46
Benzathine penicillin G	2.4 mu i.m. × 1	$22.95
Intravenous agents		
Ampicillin	2 g i.v. q. 4 h × 10 days	$46.20
Penicillin G potassium	2 mu i.v. q. 4 h × 10 days	$31.63
Penicillin G sodium	2 mu i.v. q. 4 h × 10 days	$135.46
Oxacillin	1 g i.v. q. 6 h × 10 days	$38.82
Ticarcillin	3 g i.v. q. 4 h × 10 days	$446.70
Mezlocillin	4 g i.v. q. 6 h × 10 days	$368.80
Piperacillin	4 g i.v. q. 6 h × 10 days	$448.00

[a] Drug acquisition costs for Albany Medical Center Hospital, Albany, New York, a participant in the University Health Consortium.

---

expressed as the base compound (e.g., 1 g methicillin sodium = 900 mg methicillin). With the aminopenicillins, 400 mg of bacampicillin is equivalent to 280 mg of ampicillin.

Extended-Spectrum Penicillins

Extended-spectrum penicillins are available as disodium salts and contain a significant amount of sodium with each dose. Ticarcillin sodium has the highest sodium load, 5.2 meq/g (120 mg/g). Carbenicillin (intravenous form), carbenicillin in-

danyl (oral form), mezlocillin, and piperacillin contain 4.7, 2.6, 1.85, and 1.85 meq/g, respectively. This increased sodium load can be problematic in patients with congestive heart failure and renal impairment.

PENICILLIN HYPERSENSITIVITY
Incidence

Allergy to penicillin is estimated to occur in 1 to 10% of patients receiving the drug (58). Manifestations can range from a maculopapular rash to an anaphylactic reaction. While anaphylaxis is relatively rare (0.004 – 0.015% of patients (104)), the reaction can be potentially fatal, with rates of approximately 3 to 9% in such patients (104, 188).

Mechanism and Types of Allergic Reactions

Penicillin is degraded into several products including benzylpenicilloyl, the major determinant, which makes up 95% of the breakdown products. The remaining 5%, the minor determinants, include a mixture of benzylpenicillin, benzylpenicilloate, and benzylpenilloate. Benzylpenicilloylamine may also be included as a minor determinant, though its clinical relevance is questionable (16). Antibodies can exist to the major and minor determinants, and an immune response can be elicited when these determinants bind to tissue proteins to form a hapten-protein complex and, hence, a complete antigen (125). Antibodies to the major determinant can include IgE, IgG, and IgA. Only IgE antibodies have been demonstrated to the minor determinants. Sensitivity to the β-lactam ring or the side chain of semisynthetic penicillins may also elicit an immune response.

A type I, or immediate anaphylactic reaction, can occur, usually within 2 to 20 min of drug administration. When contact is made with the antigen, IgE antibodies cause mast cells and basophils to degranulate, releasing various mediators, including histamine, prostaglandins, leukotrienes and others. Histamine release increases capillary permeability and stimulates bronchial smooth muscle and nerve endings. Bronchoconstriction, laryngeal edema, and urticaria occur, along with hypotension (27, 164). While sensitivity to the major determinant can cause an anaphylactic reaction, sensitivity to the minor determinants are more closely associated with that allergic manifestation (125). This may be explained by the high affinity of the minor determinant to IgE. With exposure to the major determinant, IgG is also produced, which may compete for binding to the antigen. Minor determinants do not elicit IgG; thus there is no competition for antigen binding (125, 126).

Type II reactions are cytotoxic reactions that can result from exposure to the major determinant and are mediated by IgG reacting with penicillin adsorbed on red cells. Manifestations include a Coombs-positive nonacute hemolytic anemia that usually occurs in a small percentage of patients receiving increased doses of intravenous penicillin for a prolonged period of time (179). The anemia is reversed upon drug discontinuation.

Type III hypersensitivity to penicillin can result from circulating antigen-antibody complexes that can deposit in the skin, kidneys, and blood vessels and cause tissue damage via activation of complement. This type of reaction is usually due to IgG or IgM antibodies, although IgE may enhance complex deposition (167). A serum sickness–like syndrome can occur 1 to 3 weeks after the start of penicillin therapy or even after drug discontinuation and can manifest as rash, fever, arthralgia, and lymphadenopathy (197). The syndrome diminishes when the drug is completely cleared from the body.

Delayed hypersensitivity, or type IV reactions, can also occur with exposure to penicillin. Lymphocytes and macrophages are believed to mediate these reactions, which can manifest a number of ways. Contact dermatitis can occur secondary to skin exposure. Acute interstitial nephritis can occur with any penicillin but is most commonly associated with methicillin and is believed to be caused by a type IV reaction. Renal insufficiency can occur, along with hematuria, eosinophilia, eosinophiluria, and proteinuria. This effect is usually reversed by drug discontinuation (129).

Risk Factors

Though allergy can occur at any age, patients between 20 and 49 years of age are at increased risk for anaphylaxis (104). Reactions may be more frequent and severe with parenteral formulations of drug. It is believed that up to 85% of patients who reacted to penicillin may not react upon a second exposure if the time interval from the last exposure is prolonged (101, 197). However, discerning the 15% of patients who will indeed have an allergic reaction upon rechallenge may be difficult without skin testing. Traditionally, atopic individuals were believed to be predisposed to development of a penicillin allergy. The data suggest, however, that there is no relationship (89). Family history of allergy is also not a risk factor.

Diagnosis

There are many indications for which a penicillin is a drug of choice or the drug of choice. Patients with a label of "penicillin allergy" have an alternative therapy prescribed or need to be desensitized to the agent. Alternative therapies can be less effective (e.g., enterococcal endocarditis) and desensitization can be time consuming. Therefore, accurate diagnosis is important. Methods of diagnosis include patient history and skin testing.

A detailed history about the allergic reaction is important for distinguishing a true allergy from simple gastrointestinal (GI) intolerance. Nearly 20% of patients with a penicillin allergy label described symptoms of GI intolerance when a detailed history was obtained (172). Those patients could potentially receive a penicillin if necessary, despite the allergy label. Patient histories can be unreliable, however, and some may have been too young to remember the reaction fully. Reliance on history alone can result in overdiagnosis of allergy.

Skin testing for allergy may also be used to detect a propensity for a type I reaction. Positive skin tests have been observed in 7 to 19% of patients with a positive history for allergy (42, 79, 198). Approximately 0.02 to 0.03 mL is injected intradermally, and wheal size is measured 10 to 20 min after injection. A wheal size 3 to 5 mm greater than a saline control at 10 to 20 min is considered a positive result. The major determinant, benzylpenicilloyl poly-L-lysine, is commercially available as Pre-Pen at a concentration of 10^{-6} M. Alone, this detects 90% of allergic patients. To increase this percentage, the minor determinant mixture (MDM) must also be used, as up to 10% of patients react only to these determinants (79, 229), and patients sensitive to the MDM are at highest risk of a type I reaction (126). Even the combination of the major determinant mixture and benzylpenicillin (a minor determinant) can result in false-negative results in 3% of patients (89). In fact, it may be that side-chain-specific reagents are necessary to truly exclude the possibility of allergy in patients with a clinical history (198).

There are several disadvantages and limitations to routine skin testing of all patients with a history of penicillin allergy. First, the MDM must be compounded freshly, as a commercial preparation is not available (176), which can be time consuming and costly. Second, skin testing can precipitate an anaphylactic reaction in sensitized individuals; however this is rare and may be avoided by performing a scratch test and observing for a wheal and flare reaction. Third, skin testing does not identify patients at risk for type II to IV reactions, though these are generally not immediately life-threatening effects in the way anaphylaxis is. Lastly, a negative skin test result is only valid for 48 h prior to administration of the penicillin. When an acceptable therapeutic alternative is available, a substitution may be more appropriate than skin testing. Skin testing is an alternative in patients with a positive history of allergy with an infection for which a penicillin is a drug of choice. A patient with a positive skin test has a 67% chance of an allergic reaction to penicillin exposure (33); therefore, a therapeutic alternative should be used or desensitization to the penicillin compound should be instituted before treatment with the drug.

Desensitization

In instances such as enterococcal endocarditis, neurosyphilis, and infections with organisms resistant to other antibiotics, desensitization should be considered when there is a likelihood of a type I allergic reaction (desensitization is not effective in preventing type II–IV reactions). Administering gradually increasing doses of the agent every 15 min can increase the threshold of IgE-induced mast cell degranulation (151). The procedure should be continuously supervised (intensive care setting preferred), and epinephrine should be available. Intravenous, subcutaneous, or oral routes may be used for the procedure. The oral route is shorter and may possibly be safer, although in one study, 5 of 25 patients receiving oral penicillin desensitization acutely developed urticaria, pruritus, and angioedema (207). Once the desensitization protocol has been completed, treatment doses may be initiated. Interruption of penicillin treatment by more than 48 h is an indication for repeat desensitization (197).

Cross-Reactivity with Other β-Lactams and Related Compounds

There is a concern about the potential for allergy to other β-lactam compounds, such as cephalosporins, aztreonam, and the carbapenems, in patients allergic to penicillin. Estimates of cross-reactivity with cephalosporins range from 2 to 10% (169, 182), although there are data to suggest that the incidence is much lower (6). No major or minor determinants exist with cephalosporins, which could account for the low cross-reaction potential. Cross-reaction with the carbapenems may also occur; however, the monobactams (aztreonam) appear to have a low propensity for eliciting an immune response and have not shown a cross-reaction with penicillin antibodies when tested in vitro (1). The bulky side chain, rather than the β-lactam ring, may be the site of immunologic reactivity. In vitro studies (1, 188) also demonstrated cross-reaction between aztreonam and ceftazidime, which is expected, since the two compounds have identical side chains. Though the risk of cross-reactivity appears low, it may be prudent to avoid the use of cephalosporins in patients with a history of severe allergy, because good therapeutic alternatives are available.

The potential for a cross-reaction with penicillamine has also been explored, as penicillamine is a metabolite of penicillin degradation. A study examined 40 patients with a positive history of penicillin allergy; 16 patients had positive skin testing results with penicillin only, and 1 patient had a positive result with penicillamine (17). These data suggest that the incidence of cross-reaction is low but that penicillamine should be administered with caution to these patients.

ADVERSE EFFECTS

The penicillins are associated with several adverse effects. They are discussed below according to the body system affected.

Gastrointestinal Effects

Gastrointestinal effects are perhaps the most common adverse reaction to orally administered penicillins. Diarrhea occurs in up to 20% and 5% of patients receiving oral ampicillin and amoxicillin, respectively. The incidence may be increased up to 40% in children. Other effects, such as nausea, vomiting, and epigastric distress may also occur. Diarrhea has also been reported in patients receiving intravenous penicillins (approximately 3%).

Antibiotic-associated pseudomembranous colitis caused by *C. difficile* may occur during or immediately after therapy with a penicillin, because of changes in normal bowel flora from broad-spectrum coverage and overgrowth of this organism. While *C. difficile* is "sensitive" to ampicillin and amoxicillin, it produces spores that survive. In the scenario of diarrhea associated with *C. difficile,* depending upon the severity of illness, appropriate treatment with metronidazole or oral vancomycin should be considered.

Skin Effects

Rash may occur with administration of any penicillin. Patients are more than twice as likely to develop a rash while receiving ampicillin or amoxicillin (5–10%) than with the other penicillins (2%) (128). The ampicillin rash is maculopapular and is often self-limited. Patients who have infectious mononucleosis, cytomegalovirus infection, or chronic lymphocytic leukemia, or who are on concurrent allopurinol are at increased risk of developing such a rash.

Hematologic Effects

Neutropenia can occur with administration of any penicillin, with an estimated incidence of 3 to 8%. Risk factors include high doses for a prolonged (>10 days) period of time (154, 163) and hepatic impairment (199). The mechanism may involve immune-complex deposition on the neutrophil cell membranes (185). Patients receiving prolonged treatment courses should be monitored for this adverse effect.

Platelet aggregation can be inhibited because of alterations in adenosine diphosphate responses, particularly with ticarcillin and carbenicillin. Prolonged bleeding times can result, along with actual bleeding (2, 4, 74, 213). Patients with thrombocytopenia and/or azotemia appear to be at increased risk. Increased bleeding times were seen in a study of 156 patients receiving either ticarcillin (73%), piperacillin (43%), mezlocillin (25%), or cefotaxime (17%). Though some patients were receiving chemotherapy (which could confound results), the trend remained after those patients were removed from the analysis. Bleeding occurred in 34, 17, and 2% of patients receiving ticarcillin, piperacillin, and mezlocillin, respectively (74). This effect generally reverses upon drug discontinuation.

CNS Effects

Increased doses and resultant serum concentrations of penicillin G have been associated with encephalopathy, particularly in patients with severe renal impairment (26). Seizures can also be induced with elevated CSF concentrations of any penicillin (195). Predisposing factors include renal impairment, a history of a seizure disorder, meningitis, or intraventricular antibiotic administration (12). If neurologic symptoms develop, the dose of penicillin should be reduced or discontinued. If seizures develop, benzodiazepines may be effective as treatment.

Metabolic Effects

Hypokalemia has been reported with the penicillins (35), possibly due to effects on renal tubules and subsequent potassium loss. This effect is more common with the carboxypenicillins. Hyperkalemia can result from use of penicillin G potassium, and deaths have been reported (227). Hypernatremia may also occur with the carboxypenicillins because of the increased sodium content in their formulations. Patients with renal impairment should be monitored for potential electrolyte disturbances.

Hepatic Effects

Transient increases in transaminases can occur. Hepatitis or cholestasis can occur with high-dose oxacillin and is generally reversed by drug discontinuation (34).

Thrombophlebitis

Intravenous administration of penicillin G, nafcillin, oxacillin, and methicillin can cause thrombophlebitis. Tissue necrosis can occur with extravasation of nafcillin. If extravasation occurs, hyaluronidase can be used as a local antidote at the site of injury.

Jarisch-Herxheimer Reaction

A Jarisch-Herxheimer reaction occurs in patients being treated with a penicillin (usually penicillin G) for a spirochetal infection (usually syphilis, but can include leptospirosis, Lyme disease, and others) and results from release of pyrogens from infecting organisms (254). The incidence is 50% in patients with primary syphilis and rises to 75% in those with secondary syphilis. The reaction usually begins within 2 h of initiating syphilis treatment and consists of fever, chills, sweating, tachycardia, hyperventilation, flushing, and myalgia. It lasts about 1 day, and it can be treated with aspirin or prednisone (225).

Miscellaneous

When procaine penicillin G is given intramuscularly, less than 1% of patients experience a procaine reaction consisting of dizziness; auditory, visual, and/or taste disturbances; neuromuscular twitching; and a fear of imminent death. This reaction has been associated with doses of 4.8 mu and typically lasts up to 10 min (90).

DRUG INTERACTIONS

The penicillins are associated with relatively few drug interactions, compared with other drugs such as some quinolones and protease inhibitors. Notable interactions are listed below.

Aminoglycosides

Inactivation of aminoglycosides by the penicillins has been documented in vitro (171, 180) and can be a particular problem if the penicillin and aminoglycoside are mixed in the same infusion solution and allowed to sit for 30 min or more. Clinically, this interaction can occur in patients with severe renal impairment, in whom drug elimination and serum concentrations are prolonged, increasing the time that the drugs are in contact with one another (24, 71, 94). Amikacin appears to be the most stable aminoglycoside to penicillin-induced inactivation (110); therefore this aminoglycoside may be preferred in patients with end-stage renal disease who require a combination of a penicillin and aminoglycoside for treatment.

Probenecid

Probenecid competitively inhibits renal tubular secretion of penicillins and so increases serum concentrations of the penicillins (82, 239). Studies with piperacillin demonstrated that probenecid increases the peak concentration by 30% and decreases the volume of distribution by 20% (219). This interaction has been used clinically in patients receiving procaine penicillin G for treatment of gonorrhea to increase serum concentrations of the penicillin.

Mezlocillin and Oxacillin

Oxacillin clearance was decreased by 38% when administered concomitantly with mezlocillin (111). Therefore decreasing the dose of oxacillin by 50% is recommended in severely renally impaired patients receiving this combination.

Penicillin VK and Neomycin

Absorption of penicillin VK is decreased by nearly 50% when administered with neomycin (43). Concomitant use of these drugs should be avoided.

CLINICAL INDICATIONS
Bone and Joint Infections

The most common pathogen causing infectious arthritis is *S. aureus*. Other causative organisms include *N. gonorrhoeae,* streptococci, and Gram-negative bacilli. It is recommended that empirical therapy be based upon synovial fluid Gram stain results, patient age, and sexual activity (200, 201). A penicillinase-resistant penicillin (e.g., nafcillin 2 g intravenously every 6 h) can be used to treat staphylococcal arthritis; however, if *N. gonorrhoeae* is suspected, ceftriaxone or another third-generation cephalosporin is recommended. Streptococcal arthritis does not respond well to the penicillinase-resistant penicillins, so penicillin G (2 mu intravenously every 4 h) or clindamycin should be used (200, 201). Length of therapy ranges from 1 to 4 weeks, with the longer duration for staphylococcal disease.

Osteomyelitis may be caused by a number of different organisms, including *S. aureus* (most common), Gram-negative rods, group A streptococci, *P. aeruginosa,* and anaerobes (particularly with direct extension osteomyelitis). Penicillins are recommended as treatments of choice for several types of osteomyelitis, including penicillin G (4 mu every 6 h) for penicillin-sensitive *S. aureus,* nafcillin or oxacillin (2 g every 6 h) for penicillin-resistant *S. aureus,* and penicillin G (4 mu every 6 h) for streptococcal infection (127). Duration of therapy should be 4 to 6 weeks. Children with staphylococcal osteomyelitis have been treated successfully with oral antibiotics and may be switched to oral therapy (with dicloxacillin or cephalexin) after 2 weeks of a positive response to intravenous therapy (217). For staphylococcal osteomyelitis, rifampin may be used in combination with the penicillin to enhance the antimicrobial response (159).

Central Nervous System Infections

Acute bacterial meningitis is caused by a number of different organisms, usually depending upon the age of the patient. In young adults and children, *N. meningitidis* is a common pathogen for which intravenous penicillin G is the drug of choice. Reduced susceptibility (MICs, 0.1–1.0 µg/mL) has been reported in certain areas (109, 230, 249), but penicillin G may still be effective against these organisms (109).

Another common pathogen causing meningitis is *S. pneumoniae.* Traditionally, intravenous penicillin G or ampicillin have been drugs of choice for penicillin-susceptible strains. Strains with intermediate resistance (MIC, 0.1–1.0 µg/mL) and high-level resistance (MIC ≥ 1.0 µg/mL) are becoming more common, and CSF fluid levels achieved with penicillin G may not exceed the MIC or MBC of these organisms (174). In other body sites of infection, pneumococcal penicillin resistance can be overcome by increasing the penicillin dose; however in meningitis, neurotoxicity may result. Empirically, vancomycin plus a cephalosporin is recommended as treatment for Gram-positive coccal meningitis or pneumococcal meningitis until susceptibility to penicillin G is determined (174).

H. influenzae produces β-lactamase in approximately 32% of cases of acute meningitis in which it is the causative pathogen (240). Use of penicillins is therefore limited in these infections, and alternatives (e.g., third-generation cephalosporins) should be chosen for empirical treatment. If the strain is β-lactamase negative, therapy can be changed to ampicillin.

Other pathogens that can cause meningitis for which penicillin G or ampicillin are drugs of choice include *L. monocytogenes* and *Streptococcus agalactiae.* When treating listerial meningitis, gentamicin is often used in combination with ampicillin because of in vitro synergy, though adequate evidence of this in humans has not been demonstrated (181).

Brain abscess may be caused by streptococci, microaerophilic streptococci *(Streptococcus milleri),* or anaerobes such as *Bacteroides* spp., as well as other organisms. High-dose penicillin G (4 mu intravenously every 4 h) in combination with metronidazole is often used empirically for treatment (54, 248) for at least 4 to 6 weeks. Penicillin G has acceptable penetration into brain abscess fluid but may be degraded by enzymes in the abscess (53, 251).

Endocarditis

Endocarditis is a serious infection of the endocardial surface of the heart. The most common organisms causing endocarditis include viridans streptococci, enterococci, and *Staphylococcus* spp. Intravenous penicillin G is the drug of choice for treatment of viridans streptococcal and *Streptococcus bovis* endocarditis. Several regimens can be used for treatment of organisms with an MIC of 0.1 µg/mL or less, including a 4-week course of penicillin G 10 to 20 mu/day continuously or in 6 divided doses (112, 137) or a 4-week course of penicillin G plus a 2-week course of an aminoglycoside (streptomycin or gentamicin). A 2-week course of the combination of penicillin G at the above doses plus an aminoglycoside may also be used, and successful use of PPG (1.2 mu intramuscularly every 6 h) with streptomycin for 2 weeks in uncomplicated cases has been reported (245, 246). In patients with organisms with MICs between 0.1 µg/mL and 0.5 µg/mL or with nutritionally deficient streptococci, the combination of 4 weeks of penicillin G at the higher dose with a 2-week course of an aminoglycoside is recommended (22), as animal models suggest that the combination is superior to penicillin alone in reducing nutritionally deficient streptococci colony counts (98).

Enterococcal infections should always be treated with a combination of a penicillin plus an aminoglycoside, as neither agent alone is bactericidal against this organism and the combination is synergistic (147, 237). A 4- to 6-week course of intravenous penicillin G (20–30 mu/day continuously or in 6 divided doses) or ampicillin (12 g/day continuously or in 6 divided doses) plus gentamicin or streptomycin is recommended (22).

To treat staphylococcal endocarditis appropriately, one must know whether prosthetic material is involved and if the organism is methicillin susceptible. If methicillin resistant, vancomycin with rifampin and gentamicin should be used. For patients with methicillin-susceptible staphylococci and no prosthetic material, an antistaphylococcal penicillin (intravenous nafcillin or oxacillin) can be used; the dosage is 1.5 to 2 g every 4 h for 4 to 6 weeks. Gentamicin may be added for the first 3 to 5 days of therapy.

If prosthetic material is involved, the causative organism is more likely to be a coagulase-negative staphylococcus (usually methicillin-resistant). Treatment is more prolonged (≥6 weeks), gentamicin is utilized for the first 2 weeks of the regimen, and rifampin 300mg every 8h orally is used for the entire treatment course. If methicillin susceptible, nafcillin or oxacillin can be used; if methicillin resistant, vancomycin must be used (22).

Penicillins are often used for prophylaxis of infective endocarditis in certain at-risk patients (e.g., prosthetic valve in place or congenital heart anomaly) undergoing dental procedures/surgery or minor gastrointestinal or genitourinary procedures. The prophylaxis is believed to treat the bacteremia that occurs during these procedures, which could cause endocarditis. While no prospective study has proved the effectiveness of such prophylaxis, oral amoxicillin 3.0 g given 1 h prior to the procedure and 1.5 g 6 h later has traditionally been a standard recommended regimen (64). A 2.0-g dose yielded adequate serum concentrations in a normal volunteer study and may result in decreased gastrointestinal adverse effects (48). The most recent recommendations therefore include an initial 2.0-g dose with no follow-up antibiotic dose (47). In penicillin-allergic patients, clindamycin, cefadroxil, or azithromycin may be substituted.

Intraabdominal Infection

Infections in the abdomen are often caused by mixed flora, including anaerobes and facultative aerobes. *Bacteroides fragilis* must be adequately covered empirically, and it is typically resistant to the penicillins except for β-lactam/β-lactamase-inhibitor combinations. A combination of β-lactam/β-lactamase inhibitor or a cephalosporin with activity against *B. fragilis* is recommended for mild-to-moderate community-acquired infections. Imipenem monotherapy or combinations of aztreonam, metronidazole, and aminoglycoside may be used for severe infections (29).

Obstetrics and Gynecologic Infections

Penicillin has been studied as prophylaxis for infectious complications of premature rupture of the membranes. Patients received either intravenous penicillin G 1 mu every 4 h with oral penicillin VK as follow-up or placebo. Significantly fewer infections occurred in patients receiving penicillin (70).

Penicillin and ampicillin administered intrapartum have been studied as prophylaxis for group B streptococcal infection in infants of mothers with birth canal colonization. Bactericidal concentrations of ampicillin are achieved in the amniotic fluid within 5 min of a 2-g infusion (25). A meta-analysis demonstrated an apparent benefit of such prophylaxis, but appropriate timing of therapy and methods of determining vaginal colonization are not yet known (3). Oral ampicillin (1000 mg every 8 h for 7 days) also gave positive results (152).

Postpartum endomyometritis, often caused by anaerobes, can be treated effectively with ampicillin or mezlocillin, unless the causative organism is *B. fragilis*. Response rates of 80 to 90% were seen in one prospective study of these agents (204).

Respiratory Tract Infections

Pharyngitis is commonly caused by *Streptococcus pyogenes* and should be treated to prevent rheumatic fever and complications such as sinusitis and otitis media (92). Penicillin is the treatment of choice since it is cost-effective and has a narrow spectrum of activity and resistance is not currently a widespread problem (49). Adults can be treated with oral penicillin VK 250 to 500 mg four times daily for 10 days. Alternatively, benzathine penicillin can be used if compliance is considered a problem (56).

Acute otitis media, an infection of the middle ear, commonly occurs in children and can be caused by a number of organisms, including *S. pneumoniae* (40%), *H. influenzae* (30%), and *M. catarrhalis* (10%). Treatment is complicated by the fact that *H. influenzae* and *M. catarrhalis* produce β-lactamase 30 to 90% of the time, and ear fluid from needle aspiration is not often cultured, so a culture and sensitivity report is rare. Amoxicillin is considered a drug of choice for treatment of this infection, particularly in children with their first episode of otitis media, because this agent has activity against the likely infecting organisms and the cost of the agent is relatively low. Since amoxicillin is not effective against β-lactamase-producing organisms, patients should be monitored for improvement in signs and symptoms of infection within 48 to 72 h. If treatment failure occurs, an alternative agent with activity against β-lactamase-producing organisms (e.g., the combination of amoxicillin-clavulanic acid or a cephalosporin) should be used.

Sinusitis is commonly caused by *S. pneumoniae* and β-lactamase-producing *H. influenzae*. Because of the prevalence of resistance to the penicillins, they are not recommended as treatment (except for penicillin/β-lactamase-inhibitor combinations) for sinusitis.

Treatment of acute exacerbation of chronic bronchitis is controversial; however, amoxicillin (500 mg four times daily) or a combination of amoxicillin/clavulanic acid may be used for this indication.

Pneumonia can be divided into community-acquired pneumonia and nosocomial pneumonia. Community-acquired pneumonia is often treated empirically to cover the most likely organisms, including *S. pneumoniae, H. influenzae,* and atypical pneumonia (*Mycoplasma pneumoniae* and *Legionella pneumophila*) (13). Recommendations for drugs of choice vary among experts and include amoxicillin (500 mg three times daily), a macrolide, or doxycycline for uncomplicated pneumonia. Recent data suggest that azithromycin is more effective clinically and radiologically than intravenous penicillin G for suspected pneumococcal community-acquired pneumonia (30); however, optimal therapy in patients with pneumococcal bacteremia is not known. In hospitalized patients, second- or third-generation cephalosporins or β-lactam/β-lactamase-inhibitor combinations are among the recommended agents (13, 32, 157). In patients with documented pneumococcal pneumonia that requires hospitalization, intravenous penicillin G may be used for 7 to 14 days (31). Nosocomial pneumonia is often due to Gram-negative rods and may be treated with an extended-spectrum penicillin plus an aminoglycoside in certain circumstances. Resistance patterns may vary between institutions, so treatment strategies should be individualized.

Sexually Transmitted Diseases

N. gonorrhoeae, the causative organism of gonorrhea, was once universally susceptible to penicillin. Now, penicillinase-producing gonococci are prevalent worldwide (194). Because of difficulties in determining susceptibility and the need to have a quick and effective method of treatment available, ceftriaxone, cefixime, or an oral quinolone are now the recommended treatments.

Penicillin G is considered the drug of choice for treatment of syphilis, caused by *T. pallidum*. In patients with primary or secondary syphilis, BPG 2.4 mu intramuscularly each week for 2 to 3 weeks is effective. Oral amoxicillin (3 g twice daily) in combination with probenecid (1 g) for 14 days is another alternative (150). In patients with tertiary or neurosyphilis, or in those with HIV infection, penicillin G (2–4 mu intravenously every 4 h for 10 days) should be used. Penicillin is most effective against *T.pallidum* if serum concentrations are above 0.03 μg/mL for at least 7 days (105). If serum concentrations fall below the MIC for 18 to 24 h, spirochetal regrowth occurs (66). There is concern that BPG does not achieve adequate concentrations in the CSF to eradicate *T. pallidum;* therefore the CNS would not be treated appropriately (134, 226). However, the treponemal burden may be low early in the disease process in immunocompetent patients, so treatment with BPG may suffice (105, 256). Some clinicians may wish to use more aggressive therapy, however. Patients with HIV infection and early syphilis may fail treatment with BPG and develop neurosyphilis (87); thus these patients should be treated as if they had neurosyphilis, particularly in the later stages of HIV infection. In patients with neurosyphilis, high-dose penicillin may fail (87).

Infants with congenital syphilis may be treated with either intravenous penicillin G or PPG. The data suggest, however, that CSF concentrations achieved with intravenous penicillin G are significantly higher than those achieved with PPG (9); thus intravenous penicillin G may be preferred.

Skin and Soft-Tissue Infections

Penicillins are commonly used to treat skin and soft-tissue infections. Impetigo is commonly caused by either group A streptococci or *S. aureus* and can occasionally result in acute glomerulonephritis. BPG (1.2 mu in adults), penicillin VK, or amoxicillin have been used as treatment, but treatment may fail if the causative organism is *S. aureus* (55). A penicillinase-resistant oral penicillin (e.g., dicloxacillin) is an effective alternative (23). Bullous impetigo, usually caused by *S. aureus,* may be treated with an oral penicillinase-resistant penicillin. Staphylococcal scalded skin syndrome should be treated with an intravenous penicillinase-resistant penicillin.

Erysipelas, commonly caused by group A streptococci, is a type of superficial cellulitis that may be treated successfully with oral penicillin VK (250–500 mg every 6 h) (23). If the infection is more severe, intravenous penicillin G may be used. Cellulitis is a more extensive infection that may be due to a number of different streptococci or *S. aureus*. A penicillinase-resistant penicillin should be used empirically, either orally or intravenously, depending upon the severity of infection.

More-severe skin infections, including necrotizing fasciitis, can be caused by group A streptococci (streptococcal gangrene) along with other organisms such as anaerobes and Gram-negative rods. Skin infections caused by streptococci have been associated with morbidity and mortality despite aggressive therapy with penicillin G (23). It is thought that the high organism inoculum seen in these infections indicates an increased number of organisms that are not actively replicating, against which penicillin is less effective (211). Experimental data suggest that penicillin in combination with clindamycin may be more effective, since clindamycin's mechanism of action is cell-cycle independent (210, 211).

Gas gangrene is a complication of a surgical or traumatic wound that can result in severe pain, skin discoloration, and edema. *Clostridium perfringens* and other clostridial species are the common causative organisms. While surgical debridement is a cornerstone of therapy, antibiotic treatment is essential. The drug of choice is penicillin G (intravenously 10 to 24 mu daily in divided doses) (50). Decreased susceptibility of *C. perfringens* has been seen in vitro, however (140), and some animal model studies have demonstrated poorer results in penicillin-treated animals than in animals that received other antibiotics such as metronidazole or clindamycin (209). The clinical significance of these findings is unclear, but some clinicians are using combinations of penicillin G and another agent to treat this serious infection.

Cutaneous anthrax, caused by *Bacillus anthracis* spores, can occur in patients exposed to wool (118). Intravenous penicillin G (1 mu every 4–6 h) has resulted in negative cultures of previously positive blister fluid (183) and is considered the treatment of choice.

Oral penicillin VK is often used in patients who receive an animal bite, particularly a cat bite. Antimicrobial prophylaxis is often indicated after such bites, as the infection rate is high, and *P. multocida* is often causative (133). Penicillin VK has good coverage against this organism, and a dosage of 250 to 500 mg every 6 h for 10 days is often used. The oral flora of a cat or dog can also include *S. aureus* and anaerobes; therefore some clinicians may choose amoxicillin/clavulanic acid to cover other possible organisms adequately. Human oral flora includes *S. aureus, Eikenella corrodens,* and anaerobes; thus human bites should be treated with amoxicillin/clavulanic acid.

Other traumatic wounds may require antimicrobial prophylaxis as well. In a study of 599 patients with traumatic wounds of the hands or feet with underlying bone, tendon, or joint lesions, a penicillin G injection was compared with 6 days of oral penicillin VK or no treatment. Patients receiving intravenous penicillin G were significantly less likely to develop infection than those who received no treatment, and patients receiving oral therapy had more gastrointestinal complaints. A single dose of penicillin G may be a useful alternative for prophylaxis in these patients (135).

Urinary Tract Infections

Treatment of acute pyelonephritis depends upon urinary Gram-stain and culture results. Amoxicillin may be used to treat enterococcal infection, but cephalosporins are probably a better choice for coverage of staphylococci (e.g., *S. saprophyticus*). In the past, ampicillin and amoxicillin were drugs of choice for treatment of *E. coli* infection; however, 25 to 35% of isolates are now reported to be resistant (103). If use of a penicillin compound is desired, a combination β-lactam/β-lactamase inhibitor can be used (either orally or intravenously).

Lower urinary tract infection can be treated with single-dose therapy; amoxicillin 3 g has been used (161), but because of increasing resistance, other agents may be more desirable. Some experts suggest that with single-dose or a 3-day course of therapy, the β-lactams are inferior to other agents such as trimethoprim-sulfamethoxazole at early and late follow-up (202).

Miscellaneous

In infants and young children with sickle cell disease, oral penicillin VK is recommended as prophylaxis against pneumococcal infection at a dose of 125 mg twice daily, starting before the child is 4 months of age. Oral penicillin VK is also recommended for children with functional or anatomic asplenia (7).

Yaws, caused by *T. pallidum* subspecies *pertenue,* affects persons in tropical or subtropical areas and is characterized by skin and bone lesions. Treatment of choice is a single dose of BPG 1.2 mu for individuals aged 10 or over and 600,000 u for younger children. Other treponemal diseases include pinta (which manifests as unsightly skin lesions) and bejel, or endemic syphilis (which causes lesions of skin and bone and is not transmitted by sexual contact). BPG 1.2 mu as a single dose is effective for both these diseases (45).

Leptospirosis, transmitted from animals and caused by the spirochete *Leptospira interrogans,* can manifest in a self-limited form (anicteric) or a more severe form of multiorgan dysfunction (icteric). Mild disease can be treated with oral ampicillin (500–750 mg every 6 h), amoxicillin (500 mg every 6 h), or doxycycline (73). In moderate-to-severe disease, intravenous penicillin G (1.5 mu every 6 h) has improved symptoms and shortened hospital stay (238). For prophylaxis, doxycycline (but not penicillin) is recommended (73).

Lyme disease, caused by *Borrelia burgdorferi,* is treated with amoxicillin 500 mg four times daily or doxycycline (52). Length of therapy is usually 10 days for mild (localized) infection and 20 to 30 days for disseminated disease (e.g., arthritis). In patients with objective neurologic abnormalities or high-degree atrioventricular heart block, intravenous therapy with penicillin G (5 mu four times daily), ceftriaxone, or cefotaxime may be used (51, 170, 208). Doses of intravenous penicillin G (3 g every 6 h) given to patients with neuroborreliosis yielded concentrations of 0.5 μg/mL in the CSF 2 to 3 h after dosing. This concentration was determined appropriate to treat neuroborreliosis (113).

Enteritis necroticans is caused by *C. perfringens* type C and manifests as severe abdominal pain and bloody stools. Transmural necrosis of the small bowel occurs with this infection, and surgery may be indicated. Penicillin G is the drug of choice; alternative antibiotics include metronidazole, clindamycin, or chloramphenicol.

Actinomycosis can manifest as a disease of the oral-cervicofacial or thoracic area or as abdominal disease. *Actinomyces* species are causative organisms, particularly *Actinomyces israelii*. It is important to treat this infection with high doses for a prolonged period of time because of decreased antimicrobial penetration into scarred areas. Penicillin G intravenously at doses of 18 to 24 mu daily for 2 to 6 weeks is the treatment of choice for most actinomycosis infections, followed by oral penicillin VK or amoxicillin for 6 to 12 months. In vitro susceptibility of *Actinomyces* spp. to oxacillin and dicloxacillin is poor, so these drugs should be avoided (124).

SUMMARY

Penicillins are important agents in the therapeutic armamentarium of antimicrobial agents, being efficacious with relatively limited toxicity profiles. While penicillins remain the drug of choice for many infections, resistance in certain organisms is increasing, so their utility in certain infections may change.

REFERENCES

1. Adkinson NF Jr, Swabb EA, Sugerman AA. Immunology of the monobactam aztreonam. Antimicrob Agents Chemother 1984; 25:933–937.
2. Alexander DP, Russo ME, Fohrman DE, Rothstein G. Nafcillin-induced platelet dysfunction and bleeding. Antimicrob Agents Chemother 1983;23:59–62.
3. Allen UD, Navas L, King SM. Effectiveness of intrapartum penicillin prophylaxis in preventing early-onset group B streptococcal infection: results of a meta-analysis. Can Med Assoc J 1993;149:1659–1665.
4. Andrassy K, Weischedel E, Ritz E, Andrassy T. Bleeding in uremic patients after carbenicillin. Thromb Haemost 1976;36: 115–126.
5. Andriole VT. Antibiotic synergy in experimental infection with *Pseudomonas.* II. The effect of carbenicillin, cephalothin, or cephanone combined with tobramycin or gentamicin. J Infect Dis 1974;129:124–133.
6. Anne S, Reisman RE. Risk of administering cephalosporin antibiotics to patients with histories of penicillin allergy. Ann Allergy Asthma Immunol 1995;74:167–170.
7. Anonymous. MMWR 1997;46:1–24.
8. Ayliffe GAJ. The progressive intercontinental spread of methicillin-resistant *Staphylococcus aureus.* Clin Infect Dis 1997; 24(Suppl 1):S74–79.
9. Azimi PH, Janner D, Berne P, Fulroth R, Lvoff V, Franklin L, Berman SM. Concentrations of procaine and aqueous penicillin in the cerebrospinal fluid of infants treated for congenital syphilis. J Pediatr 1994;124:649–653.
10. Barber M, Waterworth PM. Antibacterial activity of the penicillins. Br Med J 1962;1:1159–1164.
11. Barriere SL. Bacterial resistance to β-lactams, and its prevention with combination antimicrobial therapy. Pharmacotherapy 1992; 12:397–402.
12. Barrons RW, Murray KM, Richey RM. Populations at risk for penicillin-induced seizures. Ann Pharmacother 1992;26:26–29.
13. Bartlett JG, Mundy LM. Community-acquired pneumonia. N Engl J Med 1995;333:1618–1624.
14. Barza M, Weinstein L. Pharmacokinetics of the penicillins in man. Clin Pharmacokinet 1976;1:297–308.
15. Basker MJ, Edmondson RA, Sutherland R. Comparative antibacterial activity of azlocillin, mezlocillin, carbenicillin, and ticarcillin and relative stability to beta-lactamases of *Pseudomonas aeruginosa* and *Klebsiella aerogenes.* Infection 1979;7:67–73.
16. Beall GN. Penicillins. In: Saxon A, moderator. Immediate hypersensitivity reactions to beta-lactam antibiotics. Ann Intern Med 1987;107:205–209.

17. Bell CL, Graziano FM. The safety of administration of penicillamine to penicillin-sensitive individuals. Arthritis Rheum 1983; 26:801–803.

18. Bennett JV, Gravenkemper CF, Brodie JL, Kirby WMM. Dicloxacillin, a new antibiotic: clinical studies and laboratory comparisons with oxacillin and cloxacillin. Antimicrob Agents Chemother 1964;257–262.

19. Bennett WM, Aronoff GR, Morrison G, Golper TA, Pulliam J, Wolfson M, Singer I. Drug prescribing in renal failure: dosing guidelines for adults. Am J Kidney Dis 1983;3:155–193.

20. Bergen T, Brodwall EK, Wilk-Larsen E. Mezlocillin pharmacokinetics in patients with normal and impaired renal functions. Antimicrob Agents Chemother 1979;16:651–654.

21. Bergen T, Carlsen IB. Bacterial kill rates of amoxicillin and ampicillin at exponentially diminishing concentrations simulation in vivo conditions. Infection 1980;8:S103–108.

22. Bisno AL, Dismukes WE, Durack DT, Kaplan EL, Karchmer AW, Kaye D, Rahimtoola SH, Sande MA, Sanford JP, Watanakunakorn C, Wilson WR. Antimicrobial treatment of infective endocarditis due to viridans streptococci, enterococci, and staphylococci. JAMA 1989;261:1471–1477.

23. Bisno AL, Stevens DL. Streptococcal infections of skin and soft tissues. N Engl J Med 1996;334:240–245.

24. Blair DC, Duggan DO, Schroeder ET. Inactivation of amikacin and gentamicin by carbenicillin in patients with end-stage renal failure. Antimicrob Agents Chemother 1982;22:376–9.37

25. Bloom SL, Cox SM, Bawdon RE, Gilstrap RC. Ampicillin for neonatal group B streptococcal prophylaxis: how rapidly can bactericidal concentrations be achieved? Am J Obstet Gynecol 1996;175:974–976.

26. Bloomer HA, Barton LJ, Maddock RJ Jr. Penicillin-induced encephalopathy in uremic patients. JAMA 1967;200:121–123.

27. Bochner BS, Lichtenstein LM. Anaphylaxis. N Engl J Med 1991;324:1785–1790.

28. Bodey GP, Ketchel SJ, Rodriguez V. A randomized study of carbenicillin plus cefamandole or tobramycin in the treatment of febrile episodes in cancer patients. Am J Med 1979;67: 608–616.

29. Bohnen JMA, Solomkin JS, Dellinger EP, Bjornson HS, Page CP. Guidelines for clinical care: anti-infective agents for intra-abdominal infection. A surgical infection society policy statement. Arch Surg 1992;127:83–89.

30. Bohte R, van't Wout JW, Lobatto S, Blusse van Oud, Alblas A, Boekhout M, Nauta EH, Hermans J, van den Broek PJ. Efficacy and safety of azithromycin versus benzylpenicillin or erythromycin in community-acquired pneumonia. Eur J Clin Microbiol Infect Dis 1995;14:182–187.

31. Brewin A, Arango L, Hadley WK, Murray JF. High-dose penicillin therapy and pneumococcal pneumonia. JAMA 1974;230: 409–413.

32. The British Thoracic Society, Public Health Laboratory Service. Community-acquired pneumonia in adults in British hospitals in 1982–1983: a survey of aetiology, mortality, prognostic factors, and outcome. Q J Med 1987;62:195–220.

33. Brown BC, Price EV, Moore MB Jr. Penicilloyl-polylysine as an intradermal test of penicillin sensitivity. JAMA 1964;189: 599–604.

34. Bruckstein AH, Attia AA. Oxacillin hepatitis. Am J Med 1978;64:519–522.

35. Brunner FP, Erick PG. Hypokalemia, metabolic acidosis, and hypernatremia due to massive sodium penicillin therapy. Br Med J 1968;4:550–552.

36. Bryan CS, Stone WJ. "Comparably massive" penicillin G therapy in renal failure. Ann Intern Med 1975;82:189–195.

37. Bulger RJ, Lindholm DD, Murray JS, Kirby WMM. Effect of uremia on methicillin and oxacillin blood levels. JAMA 1964; 187:319–322.

38. Bundtzen RW, Gerber AU, Cohn DL, Craig WA. Postantibiotic suppression of bacterial growth. Rev Infect Dis 1981;3:28–37.

39. Bunke CM, Aronoff GR, Brier ME, Sloan RS, Luft FC. Mezlocillin kinetics in hepatic insufficiency. Clin Pharmacol Ther 1983;33:73–76.

40. Bush K. Characterization of β-lactamases. Antimicrob Agents Chemother 1989;33:259–276.

41. Bush K, Jacoby GA, Medeiros AA. A functional classification scheme for β-lactamases and its correlation with molecular structures. Antimicrob Agents Chemother 1995;39:1211–1233.

42. Chandra RK, Joglekar SA, Tomas E. Penicillin allergy: antipenicillin IgE antibodies and immediate hypersensitivity skin reactions employing major and minor determinants of penicillin. Arch Dis Child 1980;55:857–860.

43. Cheng SH, White A. Effect of orally administered neomycin on the absorption of penicillin V. N Engl J Med 1962;267: 1296–1297.

44. Chow JW, Fine MJ, Shlaes DM, Quinn JP, Hooper DC, Johnson MP, Pamphal R, Wagener MM, Miyashiro DK, Yu VL. Enterobacter bacteremia: clinical features and emergence of antibiotic resistance during therapy. Ann Intern Med 1991;115:650–651.

45. Chulay JD. Treponema species (yaws, pinta, bejel). In: Mandell GL, Bennett JE, Dolin R, eds. Principles and practice of infectious diseases. New York: Churchill Livingstone, 1995:2133–2137.

46. Coppens L, Klastersky J. Comparative study of anti-*Pseudomonas* activity of azlocillin, mezlocillin, piperacillin, and ticarcillin, alone and in combination with an aminoglycoside. Antimicrob Agents Chemother 1979;15:396–399.

47. Dajani AS, Taubert KA, Wilson W, Bolger AF, Bayer A, Ferrieri P, Gewitz MH, Shulman ST, Nouri S, Newburger JW, Pallasch TJ, Gage TW, Levison ME, Peter G, Zuccaro G Jr. Prevention of bacterial endocarditis. Recommendations by the American Heart Association. JAMA 1997;277:1794–1801.

48. Dajani AS, Bawdon RE, Berry MC. Oral amoxicillin as prophylaxis for endocarditis: what is the optimal dose? Clin Infect Dis 1994;18:157–160.

49. Dajani A, Taubert K, Ferrieri P, Peter G, Shulman S. Treatment of acute streptococcal pharyngitis and prevention of rheumatic fever: a statement for health professionals. Pediatrics 1995;96: 758–764.

50. Darke SG, King AM, Slack WK. Gas gangrene and related infection: classification. Clinical features and etiology, management and mortality. A report of 88 cases. Br J Surg 1977;64:104–112.

51. Dattwyler RJ, Halperin JJ, Volkman DJ, Luft BJ. Treatment of late Lyme borreliosis—randomized comparison of ceftriaxone and penicillin. Lancet 1988;1:1191–1194.

52. Dattwyler RJ, Volkman DJ, Conaty SM, Platkin SP, Luft BJ. Amoxycillin plus probenecid versus doxycycline for treatment of erythema migrans borreliosis. Lancet 1990;336:1404–1406.

53. de Louvois J, Hurley R. Inactivation of penicillin by purulent exudates. Br Med J 1977;1:998–1000.

54. de Louvois J. The bacteriology and chemotherapy of brain abscess. J Antimicrob Chemother 1978;4:395–413.

55. Demidovich CW, Wittler RR, Ruff ME, Bass JW, Browning WC. Impetigo: current etiology and comparison of penicillin, erythromycin, and cephalexin therapies. Am J Dis Child 1990; 144:1313–1315.

56. Denny FW. Current management of streptococcal pharyngitis. J Fam Pract 1992;35:619–620.

57. DeSchepper PJ, Tjandramaga TB, Mullie A, Verbesselt R, Van Hecken A, Verberckmoes R, Verbist L. Comparative pharmacokinetics of piperacillin in normals and in patients with renal failure. J Antimicrob Chemother 1982;9(Suppl B):49–57.

58. Deswarte RD. Drug allergy-problems and strategies. J Allergy Clin Immunol 1984;74:209–221.

59. Dever LA, Dermody TS. Mechanisms of bacterial resistance to antibiotics. Arch Intern Med 1991;151:886–895.

60. Dickinson GM, Droller DG, Greenman RL, Hoffman TA. Clinical evaluation of piperacillin with observations on penetrability into cerebrospinal fluid. Antimicrob Agents Chemother 1981; 20:481–486.

61. Doebbeling BN, Stanley GL, Sheetz CT, Pfaller MA, Houston AK, Annis L, Li N, Wenzel RP. Comparative efficacy of alternative hand-washing agents in reducing nosocomial infections in intensive care units. N Engl J Med 1992;327:88–93.

62. Donowitz GR, Mandell GL. Beta-lactam antibiotics. N Engl J Med 1988;318:419–426.

63. Drusano GL. Role of pharmacokinetics in the outcome of infections. Antimicrob Agents Chemother 1988;32:289–297.

64. Durack DT. Prevention of infective endocarditis. N Engl J Med 1995;332:38–44.

65. Eagle H, Newman E. Renal clearance of penicillin F, G, K, and X in rabbits and man. J Clin Invest 1947;26:903–918.

66. Eagle H. Therapeutic significance of penicillin blood levels. Ann Intern Med 1948;28:260.

67. Eagle H, Fleischman R, Musselman AD. Effect of schedule of administration on the therapeutic efficacy of penicillin. Am J Med 1950;9:280–299.

68. Ebert SC, Crain WA. Pharmacodynamic properties of antibiotics: application to drug monitoring and dosage regimen design. Infect Control Hosp Epidemiol 1990;11:319–326.

69. Eliopoulos GM, Moellering RC Jr. Azlocillin, mezlocillin, and piperacillin: new broad-spectrum penicillins. Ann Intern Med 1982;97:755–760.

70. Ernest JM, Givner LB. A prospective, randomized, placebo-controlled trial of penicillin in preterm premature rupture of membranes. Am J Obstet Gynecol 1994;170:516–521.

71. Ervin FR, Bullock WE Jr, Nuttal CE. Inactivation of gentamicin by penicillins in patients with renal failure. Antimicrob Agents Chemother 1976;9:1004–1011.

72. Evans RS, Pestotnik SL, Burke JP, Gardner RM, Larsen RA, Classen DC. Reducing the duration of prophylactic antibiotic use through computer monitoring of surgical patients. DICP 1990;24:351–354.

73. Farr RW. Leptospirosis. Clin Infect Dis 1995;21:1–8.

74. Fass RJ, Copelan EA, Brandt JT, Moeschberger ML, Ashton JJ. Platelet-mediated bleeding caused by broad-spectrum penicillins. J Infect Dis 1987;155:1242–1248.

75. Finland M, Garner C, Wilcox C, Sabath LD. Susceptibility of pneumococci and *Haemophilus influenzae* to antibacterial agents. Antimicrob Agents Chemother 1976;9:274–287.

76. Fleming A. On the antibacterial action of cultures of a penicillium, with special reference to their use in the isolation of *B. influenzae*. Br J Exp Pathol 1929;10:226.

77. Fleming A. History and development of penicillin. In: Fleming A, ed. Penicillin: its practical application. Philadelphia: Blakiston, 1946:1–33.

78. Fuursted K. Comparative killing activity and postantibiotic effect of streptomycin combined with ampicillin, ciprofloxacin, imipenem, piperacillin, or vancomycin against strains of *Streptococcus faecalis* and *Streptococcus faecium*. Chemotherapy 1988;34:229–234.

79. Gadde J, Spence M, Wheeler B, Adkinson F. Clinical experience with penicillin skin testing in a large inner-city STD clinic. JAMA 1993;270:2456–2463.

80. Gerber AU, Craig WA, Brugger HP, Feller C, Vastada AP, Brandel J. Impact of dosing intervals on activity of gentamicin and ticarcillin against *Pseudomonas aeruginosa* in granulocytopenic mice. J Infect Dis 1983;147:910–917.

81. Gerber AU, Vastola AP, Brandel J, Craig WA. Selection of aminoglycoside-resistant variants of *Pseudomonas aeruginosa* in an in vivo model. J Infect Dis 1982;146:691–697.

82. Gibaldi M, Schwartz MA. Apparent effect of probenecid on the distribution of penicillin in man. Clin Pharmacol Ther 1968;9: 345–349.

83. Giron JA, Meyers BR, Hirshman SZ. Biliary concentration of piperacillin in patients undergoing cholecystectomy. Antimicrob Agents Chemother 1981;19:309–311.

84. Gold HS, Moellering RC Jr. Antimicrobial drug resistance. N Engl J Med 1996;335:1445–1453.

85. Goldmann DA. Hand-washing and nosocomial infections. N Engl J Med 1992;327:120–122.

86. Goldmann DA, Weinstein RA, Wenzel, RP, Tablan OC, Duma RJ, Gaynes RP, Schlosser J, Martone WJ. Strategies to prevent and control the emergence and spread of antimicrobial-resistant microorganisms in hospitals. A challenge to hospital leadership. JAMA 1996;275:234–240.

87. Gordon SM, Eaton ME, George R, Larsen S, Lukehart SA, Kuypers J, Marra CM, Thompson S. The response of symptomatic neurosyphilis to high-dose intravenous penicillin G in patients with human immunodeficiency virus infection. N Engl J Med 1994;331:1469–1473.

88. Grasso S, Menardi G, De Carneri I, Tamassia V. New in vitro model to study the effect of antibiotic concentration and rate of elimination on antibacterial activity. Antimicrob Agents Chemother 1978;13:570–576.

89. Green GR, Rosenblum A. Report of the penicillin study group—American Academy of Allergy. J Allergy Clin Immunol 1971; 48:331–343.

90. Green RL, Lewis JE, Kraus SJ, Fredrickson EL. Elevated plasma procaine concentrations after administration of procaine penicillin G. N Engl J Med 1974;291:223–226.

91. Gudmundsson S, Erlendsdottir H, Gottfredsson M, Gudmundsson A. The postantibiotic effect induced by antimicrobial combinations. Scand J Infect Dis 1991;74(Suppl):63–70.

92. Gwaltney JM Jr. Pharyngitis. In: Mandell GL, Bennett JE, Dolin R, eds. Principles and practice of infectious diseases. New York: Churchill Livingstone, 1995:566–572.

93. Hackbarth CJ, Chambers HF. Methicillin-resistant staphylococci: genetics and mechanisms of resistance. Antimicrob Agents Chemother 1989;33:991–994.

94. Halstenson CE, Wong MO, Herman CS, Heim-Duthoy KL, Teal MA, Affrime MB, Kelloway JH, Keane WF, Awni WM. Effect of concomitant administration of piperacillin on the dispositions of insepamicin and gentamicin in patients with end-stage renal disease. Antimicrob Agents Chemother 1992;36: 1832–1836.

95. Hand WL, King-Thompson N, Holman JW. Entry of roxithromycin (RU 965), imipenem, cefotaxime, trimethoprim, and metronidazole into human polymorphonuclear leukocytes. Antimicrob Agents Chemother 1987;31:1553–1557.

96. Harder KJ, Nikaido H, Matsuhasi M. Mutants of *Escherichia coli* that are resistant to certain beta-lactam compounds that lack ompF porin. Antimicrob Agents Chemother 1981;20:549–552.

97. Heikkila A, Erkkola R. Pharmacokinetics of piperacillin during pregnancy. J Antimicrob Chemother 1991;28:419–423.

98. Henry NK, Wilson WR, Roberts RB, Acar JF, Geraci JE. Antimicrobial therapy of experimental endocarditis caused by nutritionally variant viridans group streptococci. Antimicrob Agents Chemother 1986;30:465–467.

99. Hessen MT, Pitsakis PG, Levison ME. Postantibiotic effect of penicillin plus gentamicin versus *Enterococcus faecalis* in vitro and in vivo. Antimicrob Agents Chemother 1989;33:608–611.

100. Higgins ML, Shockman GD. Procaryotic cell division with respect to wall and membranes. CRC Crit Rev Microbiol 1971; 1:29–72.

101. Holgate ST. Penicillin allergy: how to diagnose and when to treat [Letter]. Br Med J 1988;296:1213–1214.

102. Holm SE, Tornqvist IO, Cars O. Paradoxical effects of antibiotics. Scand J Infect Dis 1991;74(Suppl):113–117.

103. Hooten TM, Stamm WE. Management of acute uncomplicated urinary tract infection in adults. Med Clin North Am 1991; 75:339–357.

104. Idsoe O, Guthe T, Wilcox RR, Weck AL. Nature and extent of penicillin side reactions with particular reference to fatalities from anaphylactic shock. Bull WHO 1968;38:159–188.

105. Idsoe O, Guthe T, Wilcox RR. Penicillin in the treatment of syphilis. The experience of three decades. Bull WHO 1972; 47(Suppl):1–68.

106. Jack GW, Richmond MH. A comparative study of eight distinct β-lactamases synthesized by gram-negative bacteria. J Gen Microbiol 1970;61:43–61.

107. James PA, Lewis DA, Jordens JZ, Cribb J, Dawson SJ, Murray SA. The incidence and epidemiology of β-lactam resistance in *Haemophilus influenzae*. J Antimicrob Chemother 1996;36: 737–746.

108. Johnson DE, Thompson B, Calia FM. Comparative activities of piperacillin, ceftazidime, and amikacin, alone and in all possible combinations, against experimental *Pseudomonas aeruginosa* infections in neutropenic rats. Antimicrob Agents Chemother 1985;27:735–739.

109. Jones DM, Sutcliffe EM. Meningococci with reduced susceptibility to penicillin. Lancet 1990;335:863–864.

110. Jorgenson JH, Crawford SA. Selective inactivation of aminoglycosides by newer beta-lactam agents. Curr Ther Res Clin Exp 1982;32:25–35.

111. Kampf D. Effects of mezlocillin on the pharmacokinetics of oxacillin and dicloxacillin. J Antimcrob Chemother 1983;11 (Suppl C):25–32.

112. Karchmer AW, Moellering RC Jr, Maki DG, Swartz MN. Single-antibiotic therapy for streptococcal endocarditis. JAMA 1979;241:1801–1806.

113. Karlsson M, Hammers S, Nilsson-Ehle I, Malmborg AS, Wretlind B. Concentrations of doxycycline and penicillin G in sera and cerebrospinal fluid of patients treated for neuroborreliosis. Antimicrob Agents Chemother 1996;40:1104–1107.

114. Klastersky J, Hensgens C, Meunier-Carpentier F. Comparative effectiveness of combinations of amikacin with penicillin G and amikacin with carbenicillin in gram-negative septicemia: double-blind clinical trial. J Infect Dis 1976;134(Suppl): S433–440.

115. Klaus U, Henninger W, Jacobi P, Wiedemann B. Bacterial elimination and therapeutic effectiveness under different sched-

ules of amoxicillin administration. Chemotherapy 1981;27: 200–208.

116. Kubacka RT, Johnstone HE, Tan HSI, Reeme PD, Myre SA. Intravenous ampicillin pharmacokinetics in the third trimester of pregnancy. Ther Drug Monit 1983;5:55–60.

117. Labile G, Spratt BG, Hakenbeck R. Interspecies recombinational events during the evolution of altered PBP 2x genes in penicillin-resistant clinical isolates of *Streptococcus pneumoniae*. Mol Microbiol 1991;5:1993–2002.

118. LaForce FM. Anthrax. Clin Infect Dis 1994;19:1009–1014.

119. Lagast H, Meunier-Carpentier F, Klastersky J. Treatment of gram-negative bacillary septicemia with cefoperazone. Eur J Clin Microbiol 1983;2:554–558.

120. Lau WK, Young LS, Black RE, Winston DJ, Linne SR, Weinstein RJ, Hewitt WL. Comparative efficacy and toxicity of amikacin/carbenicillin versus gentamicin/carbenicillin in leukopenic patients. Am J Med 1977;62:959–966.

121. Lavoie GY, Bergeron MG. Influence of four modes of administration on penetration of aztreonam, cefuroxime, and ampicillin into interstitial fibrin clots and on in vivo efficacy against *Haemophilus influenzae*. Antimicrob Agents Chemother 1985; 28:404–412.

122. Leggett JE, Fantin B, Ebert S, Totsuka K, Vogelman B, Calame W, Mattie H, Craig WA. Comparative antibiotic dose-effect relationship at several dosing intervals in murine pneumonitis and thigh-infection models. J Infect Dis 1989;159:281–292.

123. Lepper MH, Dowling HF. Treatment of pneumococcic meningitis with penicillin compared with penicillin plus aureomycin. Arch Intern Med 1951;88:489–494.

124. Lerner PI. Susceptibility of pathogenic Actinomycetes to antimicrobial compounds. Antimicrob Agents Chemother 1974; 5:302–309.

125. Levine BB. Immunologic mechanisms of penicillin allergy. A haptenic model system for the study of allergic diseases in man. N Engl J Med 1966;275:1115–1125.

126. Levine BB, Zolov DM. Prediction of penicillin allergy by immunological tests. J Allergy 1969;43:231–244.

127. Lew DP, Waldvogel FA. Osteomyelitis. N Engl J Med 1997; 336:999–1007.

128. Lieberman R, Erffmeyer JE, Treadwell G. Drug reactions. In: Lockey RF, Buknatz SC, eds. Principles of immunology and allergy. Philadelphia: WB Saunders, 1987:111–137.

129. Linton AL, Clark WF, Driedger AA, Turnbull I, Lindsay RM. Acute interstitial nephritis due to drugs. Ann Intern Med 1980; 93:735.

130. Livermore DM. β-lactamases in laboratory and clinical resistance. Clin Microbiol Rev 1995;8:557–584.

131. Livermore DM. Clinical significance of beta-lactamase induction and stable derepression in gram-negative rods. Eur J Clin Microbiol 1987;6:439–445.

132. Livingston DH, Wang MT. Continuous infusion of cefazolin is superior to intermittent dosing in decreasing infection after hemorrhagic shock. Am J Surg 1993;165:203–207.

133. Lucas GL, Bartlett DH. *Pasteurella multocida* infection in the hand. Plast Reconstr Surg 1981;67:49–53.

134. Lukehart S, Hook EW, Baker-Zander SH, Collier AC, Critchlow CW, Hansfield HH. Invasion of the central nervous system by Treponema pallidum. Implications for diagnosis and therapy. Ann Intern Med 1988;109:855–862.

135. Madsen MS, Neumann L, Andersen JA. Penicillin prophylaxis in complicated wounds of hands and feet: a randomized, double-blind trial. Injury 1996;27:275–278.

136. Maidhof H, Johannsen L, Labischinski H, Giesbrecht P. Onset of penicillin-induced bacteriolysis in staphylococci is cell cycle dependent. J Bacteriol 1989;171:2252–2257.

137. Malacoff RF, Frank E, Andriole VT. Streptococcal endocarditis (nonenterococcal, non-group A): single vs. combination therapy. JAMA 1979;241:1807–1810.

138. Mandell GL, Kaye D, Levison ME, Hook EW. Enterococcal endocarditis. An analysis of 38 patients observed at the New York Hospital-Cornell Medical Center. Arch Intern Med 1970;125:258–264.

139. Marcy SM, Klein JO. The isoxazolyl penicillins: oxacillin, cloxacillin, and dicloxacillin. Med Clin North Am 1970;54:1127–1143.

140. Marrie TJ, Haldane EV, Swantee CA, Kerr EA. Susceptibility of anaerobic bacteria to nine antimicrobial agents and demonstration of decreased susceptibility of *Clostridium perfringens* to penicillin. Antimicrob Agents Chemother 1981;19:51–55.

141. Martens MG, Faro S, Feldman S, Cotton DB, Dorman K, Riddle GD. Pharmacokinetics of the acylureidopenicillins piperacillin and mezlocillin in the postpartum patient. Antimicrob Agents Chemother 1987;31:2015–2017.

142. Meyer RD, Liu S. In vitro synergy with ciprofloxacin and selected beta-lactam agents and aminoglycosides against multidrug resistant *Pseudomonas aeruginosa*. Diagn Microbiol Infect Dis 1988;11:151–157.

143. Meyer KS, Urban C, Eagan JA, Berger BJ, Rahal JJ. Nosocomial outbreak of *Klebsiella* infection resistant to late-generation cephalosporins. Ann Intern Med 1993;119:353–358.

144. Meyers BR, Srulevitch ES, Sacks HS, Hirschman SZ, Worner TM, Wormser GP, Jacobson J. Pharmacokinetics of mezlocillin in patients with hepatobiliary dysfunction. J Antimicrob Chemother 1986;18:709–713.

145. McEvoy GK, ed. AHFS drug information 1997. Bethesda, MD: American Society of Health-System Pharmacists, 1997.

146. Moellering RC Jr, Wennersten C, Weinberg AN. Studies on antibiotic synergism against enterococci: I. Bacteriologic studies. J Lab Clin Med 1971;77:821–828.

147. Moellering RC JR, Weinberg AN. Studies on antibiotic synergism against enterococci. II. Effect of various antibiotics on the uptake of ^{14}C-labelled streptomycin by enterococci. J Clin Invest 1971;50:2580–2584.

148. Mordenti JJ, Quintiliani R, Nightingale CH. Combination antibiotic therapy: comparison of constant infusion and intermittent bolus dosing in an experimental animal model. J Antimicrob Chemother 1985;15(Suppl A):313–321.

149. Moreira BM, Daum RS. Antibiotic-resistant pneumococci. Pediatr Clin North Am 1995;42:519–537.

150. Morrison E, Harrison S, Tramont EC. Oral amoxicillin, an alternative treatment of neurosyphilis. Genitourin Med 1985;61:359–362.

151. Naclerio R, Mizrahi ED, Adkinson NF Jr. Immunologic observations during desensitization and maintenance of clinical tolerance to pencillin. J Allergy Clin Immunol 1983;71:294–301.

152. Nadisauskiene R, Bergstrom S, Kilda A. Ampicillin in the treatment of preterm labor: a randomized, placebo-controlled study. Gynecol Obstet Invest 1996;41:89–92.

153. Nathwani D, Wood MJ. Penicillins. A current review of their clinical pharmacology and therapeutic use. Drugs 1993;45: 866–894.

154. Neftel KA, Hauser SP, Muller MR. Inhibition of granulopoiesis in vivo and vitro by beta-lactam antibiotics. J Infect Dis 1985;152:90–98.

155. Neu HC. Relation of structural properties of beta-lactam antibiotics to antibacterial activity. Am J Med 1985;79(Suppl 2A):2–13.

156. Neu HC. The crisis in antibiotic resistance. Science 1992;257:1064–1073.

157. Niederman MS, Bass JB Jr, Campbell GD, Fein AM, Grossman RF, Mandell LA, Marrie TJ, Sarosi GA, Torres A, Yu VL. Guidelines for the initial management of adults with community acquired penumonia: diagnosis, assessment of severity, and initial antimicrobial therapy. Am Rev Respir Dis 1993;148:1418–1426.

158. Nolting A, Dalla Costa T, Rand KH, Derendorf H. Pharmacokinetic-pharmacodynamic modeling of the antibiotic effect of piperacillin in vitro. Pharm Res 1996;13:91–96.

159. Norden CW, Bryant R, Palmer D, Montgomerie JZ, Wheat J. Chronic osteomyelitis caused by Staphylococcus aureus: controlled clinical trial of nafcillin therapy and nafcillin-rifampin therapy. South Med J 1986;79:947–951.

160. Nordstrom K, Sykes RB. Induction kinetics of β-lactamase biosynthesis in *Pseudomonas aeruginosa*. Antimicrob Agents Chemother 1974;6:734–740.

161. Norrby SR. Short-term treatment of uncomplicated lower urinary tract infections in women. Rev Infect Dis 1990;12:458–467.

162. Norrby R. A review of the penetration of antibiotics into CSF and its clinical significance. Scand J Infect Dis 1978;14 (Suppl):296–309.

163. Olaison L, Alestig K. A prospective study of neutropenia induced by high doses of beta-lactam antibiotics. J Antimicrob Chemother 1990;25:449–453.

164. O'Leary MR, Smith MS. Penicillin anaphylaxis. Am J Emerg Med 1986;4:241–247.

165. Orlando PL, Barriere SL, Hindler JA, Frost RW. Serum bactericidal activity from intravenous ciprofloxacin and azlocillin given alone and in combination to healthy subjects. Diagn Microbiol Infect Dis 1990;13:93–97.

166. Parker RF, Marsh HC. The action of penicillin on staphylococcus. J Bacteriol 1946;51:181–186.

167. Patterson R, Anderson J. Allergic reactions to drugs and biologic agents. JAMA 1982;248:2637–2645.

168. Peterson LR, Gerding DN, Fasching CE. Effects of antibiotic administration on extravascular penetration: cross-over study of cefazolin given by intermittent injection or constant infusion. J Antimicrob Chemother 1981;7:71–79.

169. Petz LD. Immunologic cross-reactivity between penicillins and cephalosporins: a review. J Infect Dis 1978;137(Suppl):74–79.

170. Pfister HW, Preac-Mursic V, Wilske B, Schielke E, Sorgel F, Einhaupl KM. Randomized comparison of ceftriaxone and cefotaxime in Lyme neuroborreliosis. J Infect Dis 1991;163:311–318.

171. Pickering LK, Gearhart P. Effect of time and concentration upon interaction between gentamicin, tobramycin, netilmicin, or amikacin and carbenicillin or ticarcillin. Antimicrob Agents Chemother 1979;15:592–596.

172. Preston SL, Briceland LL, Lesar TL. Accuracy of penicillin allergy reporting. Am J Hosp Pharm 1994;51:79–84.

173. Price KE, Gourevitch A, Cheney LC. Biological properties of semisynthetic penicillins: structure-activity relationships. Antimicrob Agents Chemother 1966;13:670–708.

174. Quagliarello VJ, Scheld WM. Treatment of bacterial meningitis. N Engl J Med 1997;336:708–716.

175. Rahal JJ Jr. Antibiotic combinations: the clinical relevance of synergy and antagonism. Medicine (Baltimore) 1978;57:179–195.

176. Ressler C, Neag PM, Mendelson LM. A liquid chromatographic study of the minor determinants of penicillin allergy: a stable minor determinant mixture skin test preparation. J Pharm Sci 1985;74:448–454.

177. Rice LB, Willey SH, Papanicolaou GA, Medeiros AA, Eliopoulous GM, Moellering RC Jr, Jacoby GA. Outbreak of ceftazidime resistance caused by extended-spectrum β-lactamases at a Massachusetts chronic care facility. Antimicrob Agents Chemother 1990;34:2193–2199.

178. Richmond MH, Sykes RB. The β-lactamases of gram-negative bacteria and their possible physiological role. Adv Microb Physiol 1973;9:31–88.

179. Ries CA, Rosenbaum TJ, Garratty G, Petz LD, Fudenberg HH. Penicillin-induced immune hemolytic anemia. JAMA 1975; 233:432–435.

180. Riff LJ, Jackson GG. Laboratory and clinical conditions for gentamicin inactivation by carbenicillin. Arch Intern Med 1972;130:887–891.

181. Rockowitz J, Tunkel AR. Bacterial meningitis. Practical guidelines and management. Drugs 1995;50:838–853.

182. Rohr ES. Cephalosporins. In: Saxon A, moderator. Immediate hypersensitivity reactions to beta lactam antibiotics. Ann Intern Med 1987;107:204–215.

183. Ronaghy HA, Azadeh B, Kohout E, Dutz W. Penicillin therapy of human cutaneous anthrax. Curr Ther Res Clin Exp 1972;14: 721–725.

184. Roosendaal R, Bakker-Woudenberg IAJM, van den Berghe JC, Michel MF. Therapeutic efficacy of continuous versus intermittent administration of ceftazidime in an experimental *Klebsiella pneumoniae* pneumonia in rats. J Infect Dis 1985;152: 373–378.

185. Rouveix B, Lassoued K, Vittecoq D, Regnier B. Neutropenia due to beta-lactamine antibodies. Br Med J 1983;287: 1832–1834.

186. Saito T, Yamada Y. Excretion in bile and clinical study of T-1220 (piperacillin) in biliary tract diseases. Jpn J Antibiot 1977; 30:835–839.

187. Sanders CC, Sanders WE Jr. β-lactam resistance in gram-negative bacteria: global trends and clinical impact. Clin Infect Dis 1992;15:824–829.

188. Saxon A, Swabb E, Adkinson NF Jr. Investigation into the immunologic cross-reactivity of aztreonam with other beta-lactam antibodies. Am J Med 1985;78:19–26.

189. Scheld WM, Brodeur JP, Sande MA, Allegro GM. Comparison of cefoperazone with penicillin, ampicillin, gentamicin, and chloramphenicol in the therapy of experimental meningitis. Antimicrob Agents Chemother 1982;22:652–656.

190. Schentag JJ, Smith IL, Swanson DJ, DeAngelis C, Fracasso JE, Vari A, Vance JW. Role for dual individualization with cefmenoxime. Am J Med 1984;77(Suppl 6A):43–50.

191. Schimpff S, Satterlee W, Young VM, Serpick A. Empiric therapy with carbenicillin and gentamicin for febrile patients with cancer and granulocytopenia. N Engl J Med 1971;284: 1061–1065.

192. Schoth PE, Walters EC. Penicillin concentrations in serum and CSF during high dose intravenous treatment for neurosyphilis. Neurology 1987;37:1214–1216.

193. Schreiber JR, Jacobs MR. Antibiotic-resistant pneumococci. Pediatr Clin North Am 1995;42:519–537.

194. Schwarcz SK, Zenilamn JM, Schnell D, Knapp JS, Hook EW, Thompson S, Judson FN, Holmes KK, and the Gonococcal Isolate Surveillance Project. National surveillance of antimicrobial resistance in *Neisseria gonorrhoeae*. JAMA 1990;264: 1413–1417.

195. Seamans KB, Gloor P, Dorbell RAR, Wyant JD. Penicillin-induced seizures during cardiopulmonary bypass—a clinical and electroencephalographic study. N Engl J Med 1968;278:861–868.

196. Shah PM, Ghahremani M, Gorres FJ, Stille W. Bactericidal activity of antimicrobials in the dynamic kill-curve model. J Drug Dev 1988;1(Suppl 3):35–47.

197. Sher TH. Penicillin hypersensitivity—a review. Pediatr Clin North Am 1983;30:161–176.

198. Silviu-Dan F, McPhillips S, Warrington RJ. The frequency of skin test reactions to side-chain penicillin determinants. J Allergy Clin Immunol 1993;91:694–701.

199. Singh N, Yu VL, Mieles LA, Wagener MM. Beta-lactam antibiotic-induced leukopenia in severe hepatic dysfunction: risk factors and implications for dosing in patients with liver disease. Am J Med 1993;94:251–256.

200. Smith JW, Piercy EA. Infectious arthritis. Clin Infect Dis 1995;20:225–231.

201. Smith JW, Piercy EA. Infectious arthritis. In: Mandell GL, Bennett JE, Dolin R, eds. Principles and practice of infectious diseases. New York: Churchill Livingstone, 1995:1032–1039.

202. Sobel JD, Kaye D. Urinary tract infections. In: Mandell GL, Bennett JE, Dolin R, eds. Principles and practice of infectious diseases. New York: Churchill Livingstone, 1995:662–690.

203. Solth NE, Allignet J, Bismuth R, Buret B, Fouace JM. Conjugative transfer of staphylococcal antibiotic resistance markers in the absence of detectable plasmid DNA. Antimicrob Agents Chemother 1986;30:161–169.

204. Sorrell TC, Marshall JR, Yoshimori R, Chow AW. Antimicrobial therapy of postpartum endomyometritis. II. Prospective, randomized trial of mezlocillin vs. ampicillin. Am J Obstet Gynecol 1981;141:246–251.

205. Spivey JM. The postantibiotic effect. Clin Pharm 1992;11: 865–875.

206. Spratt BG. Biochemical and genetical approaches to the mechanism of action of penicillin. Philos Trans R Soc Lond 1980;289:27–283.

207. Stark BJ, Earl HS, Gross GN, Lumry WR, Goodman EL, Sullivan TJ. Acute and chronic desensitization of penicillin-allergic patients using oral penicillin. J Allergy Clin Immunol 1987;79:523–532.

208. Steere AC, Pachner AR, Malawsita SE. Neurologic abnormalities of Lyme disease: successful treatment with high-dose intravenous penicillin. Ann Intern Med 1983;99:767.

209. Stevens DL, Maier KA, Laine BM, Mitten JE. Comparison of clindamycin, rifampin, tetracycline, metronidazole, and penicillin for efficacy in prevention of experimental gas gangrene due to *Clostridium perfringens*. J Infect Dis 1987;155:220–228.

210. Stevens DL, Gibbons AE, Bergstron R, Winn V. The Eagle effect revisited: efficacy of clindamycin, erythromycin, and penicillin in the treatment of streptococcal myositis. J Infect Dis 1988;158:23–28.

211. Stevens DL, Yan S, Bryant AE. Penicillin-binding protein expression at different growth stages determines penicillin efficacy in vitro and in vivo: an explanation for the inoculum effect. J Infect Dis 1993;167:1401–1405.

212. Stratton CW, Francke JJ, Weeks LS, Manion FA. Comparison of the bactericidal activity of ciprofloxacin alone and in combination with selected antipseudomonal beta-lactam agents against clinical isolates of Pseudomonas aeruginosa. Diagn Microbiol Infect Dis 1988;11:41–52.

213. Stuart JJ. Ticarcillin-induced hemorrhage in a patient with thrombocytosis. South Med J 1980;73:1084–1085.

214. Sykes RB, Matthew M. The β-lactamases of gram-negative bacteria and their role in resistance to β-lactam agents. J Antimicrob Chemother 1976;2:115–157.

215. Sutter VL, Finegold SM. Susceptibility of anaerobic bacterial to 23 antimicrobial agents. Antimicrob Agents Chemother 1976;10:736–752.

216. Tauber MG, Doroshow CA, Hackbarth CJ, Rusrak MG, Drake TA, Sande MA. Antibacterial activity of beta-lactam antibiotics in experimental meningitis due to Streptococcus pneumoniae. J Infect Dis 1984;149:568–574.

217. Tetzloff TR, McCracken GH, Nelson FD. Oral antibiotic therapy for skeletal infections in children. II. Therapy of osteomyelitis and suppurative arthritis. J Pediatr 1978;92: 485–490.

218. Thauvin C, Eliopoulos GM, Willey S, Wennersten C, Moellering RC. Continuous-infusion ampicillin therapy of enterococcal endocarditis in rats. Antimicrob Agents Chemother 1987; 31:139–143.

219. Tjandramaga TP, Mullie A, Verbesselt R, DeSchepper PJ, Verbist L. Piperacillin: human pharmacokinetics after intravenous and intramuscular administration. Antimicrob Agents Chemother 1978;14:829–837.

220. Tomasz A, Albino A, Zanati E. Multiple antibiotic resistance in a bacterium with suppressed autolytic system. Nature 1970; 227:138–150.

221. Tomasz A. The mechanism of the irreversible antimicrobial effects of penicillin: how the beta-lactam antibiotics kill and lyse bacteria. Annu Rev Microbiol 1979;33:113–137.

222. Tomasz A. From penicillin-binding proteins to the lysis and death of bacteria: a 1979 view. Rev Infect Dis 1979;1:434–467.

223. Tomasz A. Penicillin-binding proteins and the antibacterial effectiveness of the beta-lactam antibiotics. Rev Infect Dis 1986; 8(Suppl 3):S270–278.

224. Tomasz A. Antibiotic resistance in Streptococcus pneumoniae. Clin Infect Dis 1997;24(Suppl 1):S85–88.

225. Tramont EC. Treponema pallidum (syphilis). In: Mandell GL, Bennett JE, Dolin R, eds. Principles and practice of infectious diseases. New York: Churchill Livingstone, 1995:2117–2132.

226. Tramont EC. Persistence of Treponema pallidum following penicillin G therapy. JAMA 1976;236:2206–2207.

227. Tullett GL. Sudden death occurring during "massive-dose" potassium penicillin G therapy. Wisconsin Med J 1970;69: 216–217.

228. Ubukata K, Yamashita N, Konno M. Occurrence of a beta-lactam inducible penicillin-binding protein in methicillin-resistant staphylococci. Antimicrob Agents Chemother 1985; 27:851–857.

229. Van Arsdel PP, Martonick GJ, Johnson LE, Sprenger JD, Altman LC, Henderson WR. The value of skin testing for penicillin allergy diagnosis. West J Med 1986;144:311–314.

230. Van Esso D, Fontanals D, Uriz S, Morera MA, Juncosa T, Latorre C, Duran M. Neisseria meningitidis with reduced susceptibility to penicillin. Pediatr Infect Dis 1987;6:438–439.

231. Van Etta LL, Kravitz GR, Russ TE, Fasching CE, Gerding DN, Peterson LR. Effect of method of administration on extravascular penetration of four antibiotics. Antimicrob Agents Chemother 1982;21:873–880.

232. Verbist L. Comparison of the activities of the new ureidopenicillins piperacillin, mezlocillin, azlocillin, and Bay k 4999 against gram-negative organisms. Antimicrob Agents Chemother 1979;16:115–119.

233. Visser LG, Arnouts P, van Furth R, Mattie H, van den Broek PJ. Clinical pharmacokinetics of continuous intravenous administration of penicillins. Clin Infect Dis 1993;17:491–495.

234. Vogelman B, Gudmundsson S, Leggett J, Turnidge J, Ebert S, Craig WA. Correlation of antimicrobial pharmacokinetic parameters with therapeutic efficacy in an animal model. J Infect Dis 1988;158:831–847.

235. Vondracek TG. Beta-lactam antibiotics: is continuous infusion the preferred method of administration? Ann Pharmacother 1995;29:415–424.

236. Walder M, Haeggman S, Tullus K, Burman LG. A hospital outbreak of high-level beta-lactam resistant Enterobacter spp.: association more with ampicillin and cephalosporin therapy than with nosocomial transmission. Scand J Infect Dis 1996;28: 293–296.

237. Wantanakunakorn C, Glotzbecker C. Synergism with aminoglycosides of penicillin, ampicillin, and vancomycin against nonenterococcal group D streptococci and viridans streptococci. J Med Microbiol 1977;10:133–138.

238. Watt G, Padre LP, Tuazon ML, Calubaquib C, Santiago E, Ranoa CP, Laughlin LW. Placebo-controlled trial of intravenous penicillin for severe and late leptospirosis. Lancet 1988;1: 433–435.

239. Weiner IM, Washington JA, Mudge GH. On the mechanism of action of probenecid on renal tubular secretion. Bull Johns Hopkins Hosp 1960;106:333–346.

240. Wenger JD, Hightower AW, Facklam RR, Gaventa S, Broome CV, Bacterial Meningitis Study Group. Bacterial meningitis in the United States 1986: report of a multistate surveillance study. J Infect Dis 1990;162:1316–1323.

241. White CA, Toothaker RD. Influence of ampicillin elimination half-life on in vitro bactericidal effect. J Antimicrob Chemother 1985;15(Suppl A):257–260.

242. White GW, Malow JB, Zimelis VM, Pahlavanzadeh H, Panwalker AP, Jackson GG. Comparative in vitro activity of azlocillin, ampicillin, mezlocillin, piperacillin, and ticarcillin, alone and in combination with an aminoglycoside. Antimicrob Agents Chemother 1979;15:540–543.

243. Wiggins GL, Albritton WL, Feeley JC. Antibiotic susceptibility of clinical isolates of Listeria monocytogenes. Antimicrob Agents Chemother 1978;13:854–860.

244. Williams TW Jr, Lawson SA, Brook MI, Ory EM, Morgen RO. Effect of hemodialysis on dicloxacillin concentration in plasma. Antimicrob Agents Chemother 1967;7:767–769.

245. Wilson WR, Geraci JE, Wilkowske CJ, Washington JA 2d. Short-term intramuscular therapy with procaine penicillin plus streptomycin for infective endocarditis due to viridans streptococci. Circulation 1978;57:1158–1161.

246. Wilson WR, Thompson RL, Wilkowske CJ, Washington JA 2d, Giuliani ER, Geraci JE. Short-term therapy for streptococcal infective endocarditis: combined intramuscular administration of penicillin and streptomycin. JAMA 1981;245:360–363.

247. Wise R, Gillett AP, Andrews JM, Bedford KA. Activity of azlocillin and mezlocillin against gram-negative organisms: comparison to other penicillins. Antimicrob Agents Chemother 1978;13:559–565.

248. Wispelwey B, Scheld WM. Brain abscess. Clin Neuropharmacol 1987;10:483–510.

249. Woods CR, Smith AL, Wasilauskas BL, Campos J, Givner LB. Invasive disease caused by Neisseria meningitidis relatively resistant to penicillin in North Carolina. J Infect Dis 1994;170: 453–456.

250. Woodward RS, Medoff G, Smith MD, Gray JL. Antibiotic cost savings from formulary restrictions and physician monitoring in a medical-school affiliated hospital. Am J Med 1987; 83: 817–823.

251. Yamamoto M, Jimbo M, Ide M, Tanaka N, Umebara Y, Hagiwara S. Penetration of intravenous antibiotics into brain abscesses. Neurosurgery 1993;33:44–49.

252. Yocum RR, Waxman DW, Strominger JL. The mechanism of action of penicillin. J Biol Chem 1980;255:3977–3986.

253. Yoshimura F, Nikaido H. Diffusion of β-lactam antibiotics through the porin channels of *Escherichia coli* K-12. Antimicrob Agents Chemother 1985;27:84–92.

254. Young EJ, Weingarten NM, Baughn RE, Duncan WC. Studies on the pathogenesis of the Jarisch-Herxheimer reaction. J Infect Dis 1982;146:606–615.

255. Zeisler JA, McCarty JD, Richelieu WA, Nichol MB. Cefuroxime by continuous infusion: a new standard of care? Infect Med 1992;9:54–60.

256. Zenker PN, Rolfs RT. Treatment of syphilis. Rev Infect Dis 1989;(Suppl 6):90–96.

257. Zinner SH, Dudley MN, Gilbert D, Bassignani M. Effect of dose and schedule on cefoperazone pharmacodynamics in an in vitro model of infection in a neutropenic host. Am J Med 1988; 85(Suppl 1A):56–58.

Quinolones

•

Jerome J. Schentag and Brian E. Scully

Structure-Activity Relationships

The quinolones have contributed an increasingly important chapter to the evolution of antimicrobials, and their value is still expanding. The story of the quinolones begins in 1962 with the discovery of nalidixic acid, the prototype 4-quinolone antibiotic (84). Nalidixic acid had adequate activity against Gram-negative aerobes, but its modest serum and tissue concentrations and its relatively high minimal inhibitory concentrations (MICs) removed the opportunity to treat systemic infections. Analogues were not much different from the prototype, and development of the class proceeded very slowly for about 15 years, waiting for a structural breakthrough that would either increase their antibacterial activity or improve their suboptimal pharmacokinetics.

Structures of the quinolones are shown in Figure 1. Much was learned by studying the promising structure-activity relationships in the early 4-quinolones: the 3-carboxyl group and the 4-oxo group were linked to antimicrobial activity, and many quinoline, naphthylidine, cinnoline, and pyridopyrimidine derivatives with the 3-carboxy and the 4-oxo units were synthesized. Some examples include cinoxacin, pipemidic acid, flumequine, miloxacin, and rosoxacin. Many of these were toxic, but cinoxacin and pipemidic acid were considered improvements over nalidixic acid. They were metabolically stable and had sufficient clinical efficacy, considering the other contemporary antibiotics. Pipemidic acid penetrated into tissues very well and was used to treat otitis media and sinusitis. Pipemidic acid was also moderately active against *Pseudomonas aeruginosa,* an organism resistant to most available antibiotics. Pipemidic acid held the key to the antipseudomonal activity of the piperazinyl group at position 7 of the ring. Ten years later, this structural characteristic was used to enhance the activity of the norfloxacin molecule and the other 6-fluoroquinolones.

All of the new fluoroquinolones contain 6-fluoro substituents, which greatly broadens the spectrum of activity against both Gram-negative and Gram-positive pathogens, possibly by improving tissue penetration and binding to the DNA gyrase enzyme. Fluorine at this position provides greater activity than any other halogen or any other substituent (27, 58, 112, 135, 140, 148). Structural modifications have been made primarily on ring positions 1, 2, 5, 7, and 8 (27, 58, 112, 135, 140, 148). Norfloxacin, having both the 6-fluoro group and the 7-piperazinyl group, was discovered in 1978. This fluoroquinolone compound was an order of magnitude more potent than the old quinolones in antibacterial activity, and its antibacterial spectrum included some Gram-positive bacteria. Furthermore, norfloxacin was metabolically stable and penetrated well into tissues. Its oral absorption was poor, and its activity against Gram-positive bacteria and pseudomonads was only modest. Norfloxacin was only suitable for treatment of urinary tract infections. Enoxacin and pefloxacin, reported in 1979, and ofloxacin, first reported in 1981, had antibacterial activity similar to that of norfloxacin but better oral absorption. Ciprofloxacin, discovered in 1981 and marketed in the United States in 1987, possessed considerably more potent antibacterial activity than earlier fluoroquinolones. It featured a cyclopropyl group on position 1 of the quinolone ring structure. The cyclopropyl group became a component of compounds such as grepafloxacin, sparfloxacin, gatifloxacin, and others, as seen in Figure 1.

The main fluoroquinolone nucleus is a nitrogen-containing, 8-membered heterocyclic aromatic quinoline ring. Analogues that feature an additional nitrogen at the position 8 are called naphthyridines. With extensive chemical modification of the

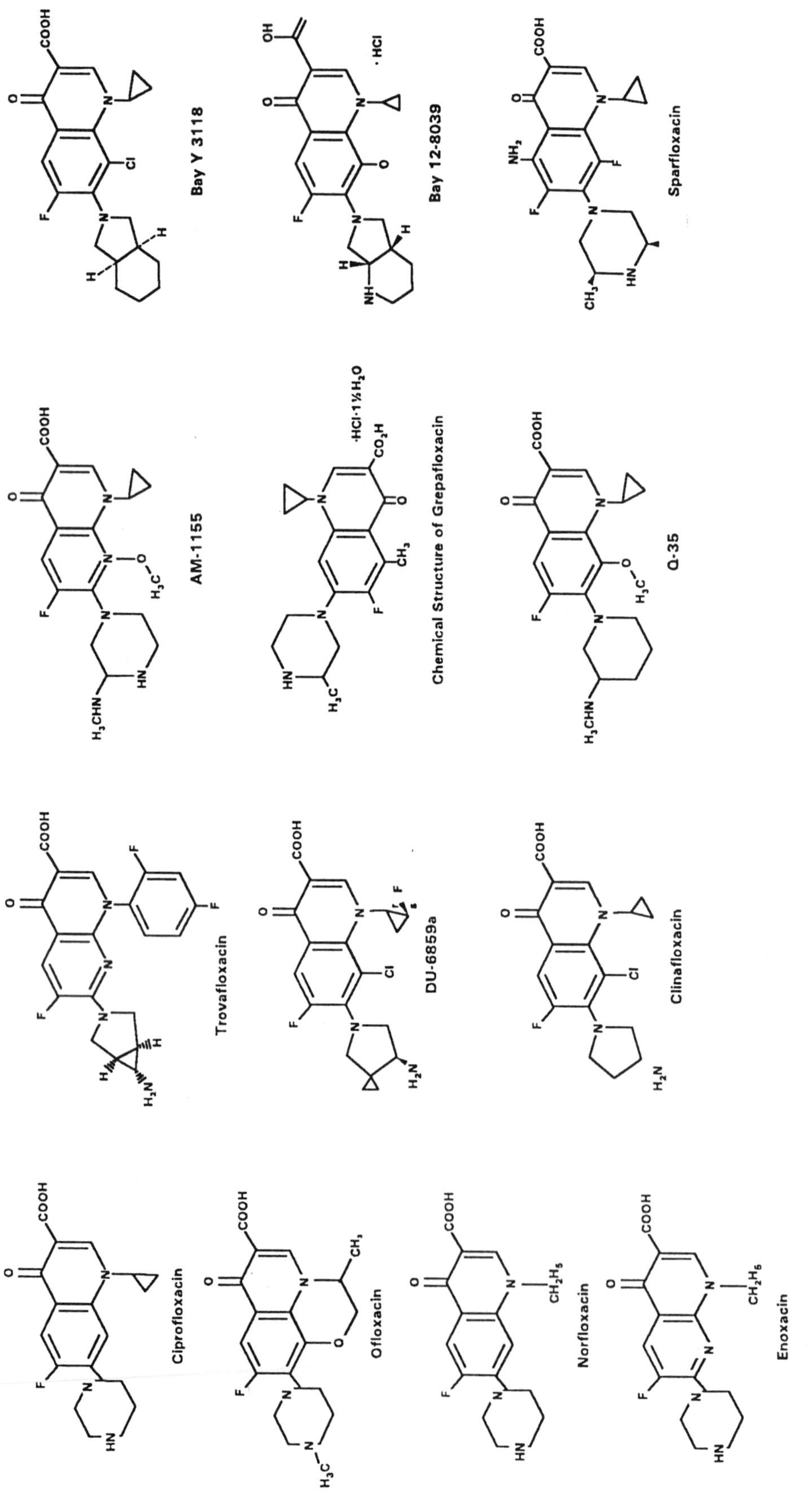

FIGURE 1. Structures of the fluoroquinolones.

main structure, the resultant group of fluoroquinolones have an improved antibacterial spectrum, favorable pharmacokinetic parameters (including absorption by the oral route and better tissue penetration), lower toxicity profiles, and a reduced tendency to develop bacterial resistance.

Recent structural modifications among the fluoroquinolones include additional fluorine atoms at position 8 and substituents other than piperazine on position 7. These new compounds enhanced the Gram-positive activity of this class at the expense of activity against pseudomonads. Fluorine or chlorine atoms at position 8 seem to enhance the phototoxicity of these compounds (27). A methoxy group in place of fluorine or chlorine at position 8 appears to remove the risk of phototoxicity, as was discovered by the manufacturers of moxifloxacin (Bay 12–8039) and gatifloxacin (AM 1155). Moxifloxacin (10, 22, 177) and gatifloxacin (58, 178) have some interesting pharmacokinetic properties and are discussed in more detail below.

MECHANISM OF ACTION

Nalidixic acid selectively inhibits bacterial DNA synthesis in the presence of competent RNA and protein synthesis. Additionally, nalidixic acid exhibited dose-dependent inhibition of RNA synthesis, resulting in the paradoxical effect of decreased killing at higher concentrations in some species. Subsequently, the discovery of topoisomerase II (also called DNA gyrase) further elucidated the mechanism by which nalidixic acid exerted its effect (44). DNA gyrase belongs to a group of related enzymes known as DNA topoisomerases found in every organism. Only the topoisomerase type II DNA gyrase enzyme from bacteria uniquely inserts negative supercoils into DNA, which may explain the actions of the quinolones on bacterial DNA synthesis without effects on mammalian DNA. Since DNA gyrase maintains the chromosome in a supercoiled state and repairs small single-strand breaks in DNA that occur during replication, its inhibition provides a possible explanation for the bactericidal activity of these agents. This does not explain why the fluoroquinolones kill bacteria so rapidly, but it has been suggested that some additional protein synthesis mechanisms are important to the rapidity of the fluoroquinolone effect (176).

When viewed by electron microscopy, the tetromeric DNA gyrase takes on a heart-shaped configuration, with the upper portion of the heart formed by the A_2 dimer and the B subunit attached below the A unit. The gyr A protein has a molecular weight of approximately 105,000 and is the specific target of the fluoroquinolones. The A subunit is involved in breakage and reunion of DNA, while the B subunit is the site of ATP hydrolysis and conformational changes in the complete enzyme to allow DNA strand passage as new molecules are produced (135).

Fluoroquinolones bind to complexes of DNA gyrase and linear DNA in the presence of ATP. It is postulated that quinolone molecules are stacked within the DNA molecules and form hydrogen bonds between the 2-carboxyl and 3-carbonyl groups of the quinolone molecules and the duplex DNA created by the ATP-promoted DNA gyrase action. Fluoroquinolones presumably interfere with the DNA breakage-reunion activity of the complex, mediated by the A subunit (58).

In Gram-positive bacteria, fluoroquinolones readily pass through the outer areas of the cell membrane and enter the cytoplasm to reach the enzyme. In these organisms, the binding affinity to DNA gyrase appears to be critical to their antibacterial activity. In contrast, Gram-negative bacteria have outer cell wall lipopolysaccharide components and porin channels for entry of molecules. There appear to be three mechanisms for the uptake of fluoroquinolones by Gram-negative bacteria. The first is simple diffusion through the outer wall and the cytoplasmic membrane. Fluoroquinolones bind to the cell surface and rapidly diffuse through both components to produce an intracellular pool in the periplasmic space and subsequently within the cell. Fluoroquinolones can also enter cells via outer membrane protein porins, particularly OmpF. Finally, it appears that fluoroquinolones chelate magnesium, causing stripping of lipopolysaccharide due to the carbonyl groups at C-3 and C-4. This creates hydrophobic patches, exposing the outer membrane. Thus, the hydrophobicity of a specific fluoroquinolone is important in its activity against some Gram-negative organisms. There are indications of an active efflux mechanism that removes quinolones from the inside of both Gram-positive and Gram-negative bacterial cells.

ANTIMICROBIAL ACTIVITY
Spectrum and MIC Tables

Fluoroquinolones have excellent in vitro activity against a wide range of both Gram-negative and Gram-positive organisms. A selected group of pathogens and the concentrations required to inhibit 90% of the strains studied (minimum inhibitory concentration; MIC_{90}) are assembled in Tables 1 and 2 (7, 28, 58, 76, 95, 97, 148, 176). Table 1 presents the data for the earlier fluoroquinolones and Table 2 for newer compounds of this class. The data in these tables come from multiple sources. No single investigator has tested all of these agents against all of these organisms. Thus the data were assembled in an attempt to provide relative differences in activity as they are noted using reference compounds, such as ciprofloxacin, within the class.

Quinolones are considered bactericidal agents, as minimum bactericidal concentrations (MBCs) are typically no more than one to two serial dilution steps higher than MICs. Fluoroquinolones, as a rule, possess excellent activity against members of the family *Enterobacteriaceae* and other Gram-negative organisms, such as *Haemophilus influenzae, Neisseria gonorrhoeae, Neisseria meningitides,* and *Moraxella (Branhamella) catarrhalis.* They also exhibit good activity against methicillin-susceptible *Staphylococcus aureus* and *Staphylococcus epidermidis.* Although quinolones had some activity against methicillin-resistant *S. aureus* (MRSA) when they first became available in the mid-1980s, none of them (even the newer Gram positive–active compounds) can be assumed to be useful at the present time. The quinolones in Table 1 are less active against streptococcal species, including *Streptococcus pyogenes, Streptococcus pneumoniae,* and viridans streptococci, and their activity against *Enterococcus* is vari-

TABLE 1 • In Vitro Activity Profiles of the Fluoroquinolones (MIC$_{50}$–MIC$_{90}$)

Organism	Nalidixic Acid	Norfloxacin	Ofloxacin	Levofloxacin	Lomefloxacin	Ciprofloxacin
Escherichia coli	4	0.12	0.12	0.05	0.2	0.01–0.25
Klebsiella pneumoniae	8–16	0.5	0.25	0.25–3.13	1.0	0.02–0.25
Salmonella/Shigella	2–4	0.06	0.12–0.25	0.12	0.25	0.01–0.06
Acinetobacter spp.	>32	>8	0.25–1.0	0.5–16	4.0	0.25–2.0
Proteus mirabilis	8	0.1	0.5	0.25	0.5–1.0	0.06
Enterobacter cloacae	8	0.25–2	0.25	0.12–0.78	0.5	0.03–0.25
Serratia marcescens	>100	1.0	1.0	0.25–12.5	2.0	0.5–1.0
Neisseria gonorrhoea	1.0	0.6	0.06	0.15–0.1	0.12	0.008–0.12
Haemophilis influenzae	1.0	0.6	0.06	0.015	0.06–0.12	<0.01
Moraxella catarrhalis	2.0	0.4	0.06	0.06	0.1–1.0	0.01–0.03
Pseudomonas aeruginosa	16	4.0	4.0	2–8	4.0	0.25–1.0
Staphylococcus aureus	>100	2.0	0.5	0.25–0.5	2.0	0.5–2.0
MR *Staphylococcus aureus*	>100	>16	>16	>8	>16	>16
Streptococcus pneumoniae	>100	16	2–4	1–3.13	8	1–8
Streptococcus faecalis	>64	8.0	4.0	1–3.13	8	0.5–4.0
Streptococcus gp A,B	>64	16.0	4.0	0.5–2	8	1–4
Enterococcus faecium	>64	>12.5	6.0	3.13	8	2–8
Bacteroides fragilis	512	>128	2–12.5	2–6.25	8–64	8.0
Clostridium spp.	256	2	1–8	0.25–3.13	16	>1
Mycobacterium tuberculosis		8	0.8–1.3	0.5	4	0.5–1.0
Mycoplasma pneumoniae		12	0.8–2.0		4–8	2.0
Chlamydia pneumoniae			1.0		4.0	1–2
Legionella pneumophila	1.0		0.19			0.38
Ureaplasma urealyticum			2.0			8–16

TABLE 2 • In Vitro Activity Profiles of the Fluoroquinolones (MIC$_{50}$–MIC$_{90}$)

Organism	Levofloxacin	Sparfloxacin	Grepafloxacin	Gatifloxacin	Moxifloxacin	Trovafloxacin
Escherichia coli	0.05	0.03–0.12	0.06–0.12	0.05–0.1	0.01–0.25	0.03–0.5
Klebsiella pneumoniae	0.25–3.13	0.06–0.25	0.12–0.25	0.1–0.39	0.02–0.25	0.06–0.12
Salmonella/Shigella	0.12	0.02–0.06	0.03–0.12	0.125	0.01–0.06	0.02–0.12
Acinetobacter spp.	0.5–16	0.12–0.25	0.4–4.0	0.1	0.25–2.0	0.03–8.0
Proteus mirabilis	0.25	0.5–1.0			0.06	
Enterobacter cloacae	0.12–0.78	0.06–1–0.12	0.12–0.25	0.5–0.25	0.03–0.25	0.06–0.5
Serratia marcescens	0.25–12.5	2.0	1–25	0.5–12.5	0.5–1.0	0.5–1.0
Neisseria gonorrhoea	0.15–0.1	0.008–0.12	0.006–0.06	0.01–0.03	0.008–0.12	0.002–0.25
Haemophilis influenzae	0.015	0.01–0.12	>0.06	0.25	<0.01	>0.02
Moraxella catarrhalis	0.06	0.02–0.03	0.02–0.06	0.06	0.01–0.03	0.02–0.06
Pseudomonas aeruginosa	2–8	2–8	1–8	3–16	1–4	1–4
Staphylococcus aureus	0.25–0.5	0.125–0.25	0.1–0.25	0.1–0.25	0.125–0.25	0.125–0.5
MR *Staphylococcus aureus*	>8	>4	>8	>4	>16	1–8
Streptococcus pneumoniae	1–3.13	0.12–0.25	0.25–0.5	0.39–0.78	0.125–0.25	0.12–0.25
Streptococcus faecalis	1–3.13	0.5–2.0	0.4–4.0	0.4–16	0.5–4.0	0.5–2.0
Streptococcus gp A,B	0.5–2	0.25–1.0	0.25–0.5	0.39–0.78	0.25–0.5	0.06–0.5
Enterococcus faecium	3.13	0.5–2.0	4–12	0.78–12.5	0.5–2.0	1–4
Bacteroides fragilis	2–6.25	1–4	2–12	1.56–3.13	4	0.25–2
Clostridium spp.	0.25–3.13	0.25–8	1–6	0.39–1.56	>1	0.1–1.0
Mycobacterium tuberculosis	0.5	0.5–1.0			0.5–1.0	
Mycoplasma pneumoniae		0.01–0.12	0.06–0.25		>1	0.06–0.25
Chlamydia pneumoniae		0.25			1–2	
Legionella pneumophila		0.19	0.06		0.6	0.19
Ureaplasma urealyticum		0.5	0.1–2.0			0.125

able to poor. These quinolones are also inactive against anaerobic bacteria. The newer agents listed in Table 2 correct this problem, but the tradeoff is lower antipseudomonal activity than ciprofloxacin.

Antimicrobial Activity In Vitro

Gram-Negative Organisms. All of the commercially available 6-fluoroquinolones have excellent in vitro activity against *Enterobacteriaceae*, fastidious Gram-negative species such as

H. influenzae and other *Haemophilus* species, *N. gonorrhoeae, N. meningitides,* and *M. catarrhalis* (Tables 1 and 2). In 1988, virtually 99% of strains of the aforementioned organisms were susceptible to less than 2.0 μg/mL. However by 1991, resistance was building among *Klebsiella* species, *Enterobacter* species, *Serratia marcescens,* and occasional *Providencia* species. There are increasing reports that even *Escherichia coli* is losing susceptibility to these compounds. Currently 90% of community isolates of *Enterobacteriaceae* would be inhibited by concentrations below 2 μg/mL (a typical laboratory breakpoint, but also an MIC that typically is associated with failure to eradicate the organism in seriously ill patients).

Among the commercially available quinolones, ciprofloxacin is the most active agent against pseudomonads and most Gram-negative organisms. Ciprofloxacin has long been the most active agent, and prior to 1988, it inhibited 90% of *P. aeruginosa* at concentrations below 0.25 μg/mL. Sparfloxacin is the most active agent against most Gram-positive and atypical organisms. With the exception of pseudomonads, for which it is considerably less active, levofloxacin has activity similar to that of ciprofloxacin. Ofloxacin, sparfloxacin, and enoxacin have activity profiles similar to that of ciprofloxacin against the *Enterobacteriaceae,* but they are also less active against pseudomonads. Overall, norfloxacin, lomefloxacin, pefloxacin, and fleroxacin have limited antimicrobial profiles; sparfloxacin, levofloxacin, trovafloxacin, and ciprofloxacin are far more active agents.

Most fluoroquinolones inhibit *P. aeruginosa* at concentrations achievable in urine. Recently, increasing numbers of urinary *P. aeruginosa* isolates show ciprofloxacin MICs in the range of 0.5 to 1.0 μg/mL. Agents such as norfloxacin, enoxacin, ofloxacin, lomefloxacin, grepafloxacin, sparfloxacin, and trovafloxacin inhibit these urinary ciprofloxacin-susceptible *P. aeruginosa* at concentrations of 2 to 8 μg/mL, with most inhibited at 4 μg/mL. Among the newly marketed fluoroquinolones, trovafloxacin, sparfloxacin, and grepafloxacin have generally similar antipseudomonal activity, slightly less than that of ciprofloxacin (Table 2).

In contrast to *P. aeruginosa,* the activity of fluoroquinolones against other *Pseudomonas* species is extremely variable. Organisms such as *Pseudomonas cepacia* often have MICs in the range of 1 to 8 μg/mL for ciprofloxacin, whereas some of the newer compounds such as sparfloxacin, trovafloxacin, and tosufloxacin are slightly more active. Fluoroquinolones inhibit *Xanthomonas maltophilia* at MICs in the range of 1 to 8 μg/mL, but for some agents, MICs are as high as 32 μg/mL. The activity of fluoroquinolones against *Acinetobacter calcoaceticus* is also extremely variable, but many strains are inhibited by fluoroquinolone concentrations between 0.25 and 4 μg/mL. *Aeromonas hydrophila* is inhibited by 0.015 μg/mL. *Campylobacter jejuni* is usually very susceptible. In contrast, *Helicobacter pylori* is inhibited by concentrations ranging from 1 to 8 μg/mL. Trovafloxacin, tosufloxacin, grepafloxacin, and ciprofloxacin appear to be the most active compounds against *H. pylori.*

Fluoroquinolones have excellent activity against organisms involved in genital infections. Virtually all of the agents inhibit *N. gonorrhoeae* at concentrations below 0.1 μg/mL, and

Haemophilus ducreyii is inhibited at even lower concentrations. In contrast, *Gardnerella vaginalis* is resistant, poorly inhibited at concentrations of 2 to 16 μg/mL, and *Chlamydia trachomatis* activity depends on the quinolone under discussion. Most *Ureaplasma urealyticum* strains require concentrations of 4 to 16 μg/mL and should therefore be considered a marginal organism for all but trovafloxacin.

Gram-Positive Organisms. As shown in Table 1, most of the older fluorinated compounds are moderately active against methicillin-susceptible *S. aureus* (MSSA), and all are considerably more active against this pathogen than nalidixic acid. Ciprofloxacin, levofloxacin, and ofloxacin have MIC$_{90}$s against both enterococci and pneumococci that approach their achievable peak serum concentrations. This limits their utility in treating serious infections caused by these organisms. In the mid 1980s, the MICs of fluoroquinolones against staphylococci, including methicillin-resistant staphylococci, ranged from 0.25 to 2.0 μg/mL. Since 1989, MRSA resistant to fluoroquinolones have been encountered throughout the United States and the rest of the world. These strains now have MICs in the range of 4 to 32 μg/mL.

The newest fluoroquinolones such as sparfloxacin and trovafloxacin have very good activity against MSSA, and at the moment, their spectrum includes some of the coagulase-negative staphylococci. This includes *S. epidermidis, Staphylococcus haemolyticus,* and the urinary pathogen *Staphylococcus saprophyticus.* As is apparent in Table 2, compounds such as trovafloxacin and sparfloxacin inhibit staphylococci at lower concentrations (i.e., 0.125 μg/mL) and will inhibit some, but not many, MRSA resistant to ciprofloxacin.

A number of the older fluoroquinolones do not have clinically effective activity against streptococci such as *S. pyogenes, Streptococcus agalactiae,* and *S. pneumoniae.* As shown in Table 1, enoxacin, lomefloxacin, ofloxacin, and norfloxacin, as well as pefloxacin and fleroxacin have MICs for these species in the range of 4 to 16 μg/mL. Ciprofloxacin, ofloxacin, trovafloxacin, grepafloxacin, gatifloxacin, levofloxacin, and sparfloxacin all inhibit streptococcal species, with the greatest activity being seen with sparfloxacin, moxifloxacin, and trovafloxacin. Penicillin-susceptible and penicillin-resistant strains of pneumococci have similar MICs to these new fluoroquinolones.

The activity of fluoroquinolones against enterococcal species is variable, although many strains are inhibited by 2 μg/mL of ofloxacin, levofloxacin, sparfloxacin, ciprofloxacin, and trovafloxacin. Gatifloxacin and sparfloxacin are generally the most active. *Listeria monocytogenes* is inhibited by the new fluoroquinolones but not by the fluoroquinolones with poor activity against other streptococcal species.

Anaerobic Organisms. Most of the commercially available fluoroquinolones do not have adequate activity against anaerobic species such as *Bacteroides fragilis* group organisms, oral *Bacteroides* species, and *Clostridium* species. Trovafloxacin, tosufloxacin, and sparfloxacin inhibit anaerobic species at concentrations that may be obtainable in humans. Several of these have proved efficacious in animal models of anaerobic infection. Except for trovafloxacin, which achieved labeling for use against anaerobic infections, there have been no clinical studies to demonstrate that these agents are effective. Trovafloxacin appears to be clinically effective in human abdominal infections. The relationship between antianaerobic activity and colonization resistance has not been studied for any of the fluoroquinolones.

Mycobacteria. The fluoroquinolones have variable activity against mycobacteria. In general, they are more active against *Mycobacterium tuberculosis* than against other mycobacteria, and the data are shown in Tables 1 and 2. Sparfloxacin is the most active agent. Agents such as sparfloxacin, ofloxacin, and ciprofloxacin have been used to treat mycobacterial infections. Concentrations of 2.0 μg/mL inhibit some *M. tuberculosis* and *Mycobacterium avium*. Organisms causing cutaneous infections such as *Mycobacterium chelonei* or *Mycobacterium chelonei-abscessus* have shown quinolone MICs between 0.25 and 16 μg/mL.

Other Pathogens. Fluoroquinolones inhibit organisms such as *Legionella pneumophila* and other *Legionella* species at concentrations that can be readily achieved in serum and alveolar macrophages. Fewer data are available on their activity against *Chlamydia pneumoniae,* although they do appear to be active. *Bordetella pertussis* is inhibited. *Mycoplasma* is inhibited. *Brucella* species are inhibited at concentrations of 1 to 2 μg/mL. *Treponema pallidum* is usually resistant, and the MICs against *Borrelia burgdorferi* are 4 to 8 μg/mL, also resistant. In keeping with their early history as antimalarials, recent studies have suggested that fluoroquinolones may inhibit proliferation of some *Plasmodium* species, such as *Plasmodium falciparum;* however, these activity profiles are modest, at best. Data suggest that some fluoroquinolones may have activity against *Leishmania* and inhibit amastigotes of *Trypanosoma cruzi* in hamster models of infection. Fluoroquinolones are not active against *Toxoplasma gondii*.

Pharmacodynamic Effects

Bactericidal Effects

A number of factors markedly affect the in vitro activity of the new fluoroquinolones. Fluoroquinolones are most active at alkaline or neutral pH and have significantly less activity at an acid pH of 6.0 or lower. This is particularly true for organisms such as *P. aeruginosa*. The activity of fluoroquinolones is markedly decreased by high concentrations of magnesium and, to a lesser degree, high concentrations of calcium and iron. In general, quinolones are less active in urine, but normal human serum has no effect on their activity. Their MBCs are similar to MICs for most bacteria, and there are minimal differences in MICs as the inoculum size is increased, with the exception of activity against pseudomonads.

In Vitro Pharmacodynamics. Fluoroquinolones kill bacteria in a concentration-dependent fashion. The MICs or MBCs and serum bactericidal titers (SBTs) are the pharmacodynamic parameters that express these in vitro concentration-dependent fluoroquinolone actions on the bacteria. Bactericidal rates are pharmacodynamic expressions of bacterial killing versus time, although these rates of bacterial killing also exhibit marked dependence on quinolone concentration in the biophase. Many time-kill (cidal rate) studies have been performed to analyze the pharmacodynamics of the fluoro-

quinolones. In a time-killing study, bacterial killing usually begins just as concentrations of the drug approach the MIC of the organism and then increases in rate until the concentration:MIC ratio reaches its maximum at 15 to 20 times the MIC. Not surprisingly, the quinolone killing rate plateaus at multiples above 20 times the MIC.

Most of the newer fluoroquinolones produce different bacterial killing actions than nalidixic acid. Whereas nalidixic acid was bacteriostatic at high concentrations, the 6-fluoro compounds are bactericidal over a wide range of therapeutically achievable concentrations. Concomitant administration of rifampin and nalidixic acid is bacteriostatic, while addition of rifampin to either ciprofloxacin or ofloxacin does not interfere with the agent's bactericidal activity. The combination does slow the rate of bacterial killing.

Because killing rate depends on concentration with quinolones, in vitro evaluation of bacterial killing rate should use a concentration-time profile that mimics the serum concentration decline observed after a dose is given to humans. In vitro models can be used to mimic these changing serum concentrations. Comprehensive studies using these models have been conducted by Blaser et al. (8), Dudley et al. (31), and others (93). Quinolones kill bacteria rapidly at peak serum concentrations in these models, and they continue to kill bacteria as long as concentrations exceed the MIC, showing the influence of time above MIC. Most of these workers argue for quinolone dosing regimens that divide the daily dose in a manner that produces high peak concentrations in patients, but some of these regimens put considerable time between doses, which can present problems, since fluoroquinolone peaks are generally low and half-lives are long with this class of antibiotics.

Pharmacodynamics of Resistance. The other relevant in vitro observation in these models is the emergence of an initially small population ($<10^3$) of resistant organisms, which becomes the dominant flora after 24 h of antibiotic exposure. High peak concentrations prolong the time before this emergence, presumably by killing even greater numbers (those with the highest MICs) of the small minority population of highly resistant microbes. This argument has been used to support dosing regimens that provide high peak concentrations and high doses for quinolones, and it also supports the arguments favoring high peak concentrations for aminoglycosides.

In vitro models that study resistance in relationship to concentrations have direct clinical relevance. There is a strong relationship between the in vitro and in vivo AUC:MIC ratios (an index called the AUIC) and emergence of resistance in patients with LRTI. In vitro data demonstrate emergence of resistance at AUC:MIC ratios below 100 (94). Unfortunately, such low exposure conditions are all too common in the nosocomial pneumonia patient (159). When the same conditions are reproduced in animal models, resistance also results, presumably because of low killing power and the resulting selective pressure (101).

Postantibiotic Effects

Fluoroquinolones in vitro demonstrate a 3- to 6-h postantibiotic effect on staphylococci, *Enterobacteriaceae,* and *P. aeru-*

ginosa. Organisms that are killed very rapidly, such as *Haemophilus* spp., *E. coli,* and *Klebsiella* spp., have shown almost no in vitro PAE, and the PAE for *E. faecalis* is considerably shorter than that of other organisms such as pseudomonads. A modest in vivo PAE can also be demonstrated in animal models, ranging from 2 to 6 h, depending on the bacteria. The significance of PAE for dosing regimen design in humans remains largely unknown. Indeed, the PAE may not be clinically important. Objective evidence from LRTI studies shows that therapy fails to eradicate the organism when more than 20% of the time between doses falls below the organism's MIC (47). This finding would ordinarily rule out a significant PAE in humans and would favor concentrations above MIC in vivo for most of the dosing interval. Thus the MIC of the pathogen and how well the regimen maintains concentrations above the MIC may be more important than the duration of an in vivo PAE.

Effects of Subinhibitory Concentrations

At least a portion of the argument for PAE, in fact, may be confusion caused by the effects of sub-MIC concentrations in vivo. For example, the long half-life of most quinolones, even in animal models, ensures that serum and tissue concentrations remain measurable for 3 to 6 h after they fall below the MIC of the organism. It could easily be the residual effects of these concentrations that are perceived as an in vivo PAE. Further, it is assumed that sub-MIC concentrations are part of the story in selection of resistant subpopulations, an intrinsic mechanism of resistance in the patient care setting.

Important Effects on Host Immunity (Positive or Negative)

Fluoroquinolones do not exert much effect on the host immune system, either positive or negative, beyond the observation that patients without host defense are more difficult to cure and more often develop antimicrobial resistance. This is especially true when dosing does not exceed the MIC of the organism more than 80% of the dosing interval (159). These drugs prevent liberation of endotoxin in vitro, even though they kill bacteria quite rapidly. This may result in less risk of sepsis (and thus a lesser effect on host response to bacterial challenge).

Pharmacodynamic Correlates with Outcome

Pharmacodynamics refers to drug action versus serum concentrations and should be related to the patient's time course of serum concentrations. Then, quinolone pharmacodynamics can be expressed in terms of their in vivo concentration versus bacterial-killing capabilities as well as concentration (or dose) relationships to bacterial resistance (also a pharmacodynamic effect). The preferred way to express these relationships is to define the interaction of a pharmacokinetic parameter such as AUC or peak concentration and an index of organism susceptibility such as MIC (141). The genesis of the relationship between these parameters was a study conducted in 1985 by Barriere et al. (5).

An overall integration of serum concentrations with bacterial MICs is shown for ciprofloxacin in Figure 2. The AUC of 64 for the regimen shown, in relationship to an MIC of 0.25 μg/mL, yields an AUIC of 256. This corresponds to a peak:MIC

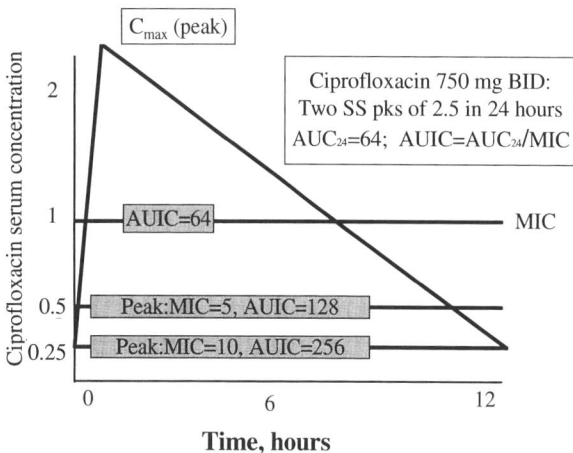

FIGURE 2. Relationship between serum concentrations of ciprofloxacin and selected MIC values. At each value of MIC, the AUIC and peak to MIC ratio is calculated. Values are based on a 750-mg dose given twice daily.

ratio of 10:1. A peak:MIC ratio of 5:1 is approximately equal to an AUC:MIC ratio of 125 (66, 93). Thus there is a strong concordance among the PK/PD parameters that describe this class of antibiotics (30, 126, 142).

Bacterial killing rates are usually expressed as a change in colony forming units (CFUs) over a period of time. Time to sterile cultures is a useful descriptor of this process for clinical trials, as it is readily applied to patient data. In vitro, the quinolones kill bacteria more rapidly than β-lactam antibiotics. In most cases, these cidal rates are similar to the killing rates of aminoglycosides. The mechanism for the rapid action of aminoglycosides and quinolones is largely unknown, but rapid bacterial killing may confer a clinical advantage on quinolones and aminoglycosides over β-lactams in the form of a shorter duration of therapy. It is relatively easy to show more rapid bacterial killing effects in patients with the fluoroquinolones. An example of these comparative studies is shown in Figure 3, which compares data from ciprofloxacin with data on a third-generation cephalosporin, cefmenoxime (59). For both agents, we monitored bacterial killing rates in vivo, using daily cultures. These data show that in patients with nosocomial pneumonia, the killing rate of ciprofloxacin at the same AUC:MIC ratio is considerably faster, even though both agents killed the same number of organisms by the end of therapy (59).

Clinical cure of infection is also a relevant pharmacodynamic endpoint, in that clinical cure is a composite parameter. The components of a clinical cure are bacterial killing versus concentration, and the rates of host repair and resolution of inflammation. The relative importance of these two factors differs with the type of infection. For this reason, it is more enlightening to model antibiotic concentration versus bacterial killing than versus clinical cure. These parameters also correlate, but to a different degree in different types of infections. Respiratory tract infections show good agreement between organism eradication and clinical cure, a condition termed *antibiotic responsive.*

In Vitro MICs as Pharmacodynamic Predictors of Outcome.
Although the in vitro pharmacodynamic models yield mechanistic information on the killing rates of these antibiotics versus one or two organisms, most of the available information regarding fluoroquinolone pharmacodynamics must be gleaned from in vitro studies of organism MICs. While low MICs do indicate greater in vitro potency, MIC data must be interpreted from the perspective of achievable quinolone concentrations in vivo. The peak serum concentrations for most fluoroquinolones exceed the MICs for *Haemophilus, Neisseria, Moraxella,* and *Enterobacteriaceae* for 4 to 6 h. Newer agents with long half-lives (e.g., trovafloxacin, grepafloxacin, and sparfloxacin) have serum levels above the MICs of Gram-positive organisms for 24 h. Until recently, the peak plasma concentrations of many quinolones did not exceed the MICs of streptococci and *S. pneumoniae,* ex-

cept for higher doses of ciprofloxacin (i.e., 750 mg orally twice daily) and for levofloxacin, trovafloxacin, sparfloxacin, gatifloxacin, and grepafloxacin.

Integration of MIC and Antibiotic Concentration. Pharmacokinetics and pharmacodynamics can be simultaneously considered by integrating these endpoints to form activity indices during comparative evaluation of the fluoroquinolones. An example of this process is pictured in Figure 2, the derivation of AUIC. In the exercises that follow, we use the 24-h AUC value for each of the quinolones, as shown in Figure 4. In Table 3, we used ciprofloxacin MIC values from Millard Fillmore Hospital, along with that agent's in vivo pharmacokinetics (AUC values from Fig. 4) to calculate the AUICs. Our primary index of beneficial effect has been achieving a 24-h AUIC above 125, a value associated with cure and prevention of resistance (47, 141). These data illustrate why an intravenous dose of 400 mg every 8 h of ciprofloxacin is needed to treat *S. aureus* and *P. aeruginosa,* while lower doses of this antibiotic work very well against organisms with lower MICs (144).

The 24-h AUIC:MIC$_{90}$ ratios were used to compare the pharmacodynamics of the quinolones and, via the calculated AUICs, evaluate the dosage for each of these agents for patients with different infecting organisms (141). The 24-h AUCs for the various quinolones were used, because the usual doses of these agents are known. These data are found in Tables 4 and 5 and illustrated in Figure 4.

The AUIC data in Tables 4 and 5 are used to determine the highest MIC that can be covered and still reach an AUIC of 125. Then, this value is compared with the MIC$_{90}$s in the last column of Table 4 (CCr, 100 mL/min) and Table 5 (CCr, 50 mL/min). For this exercise, we selected four organisms: *P. aeruginosa, S. aureus, E. coli,* and *S. pneumoniae.* The exercise can be carried out with other organisms as well, using their MICs and the 24-h AUC data. However, if a different dose is chosen in a 24-h period, Figure 4 also contains the AUC values for a 100-mg dose. These data can be used to construct AUIC

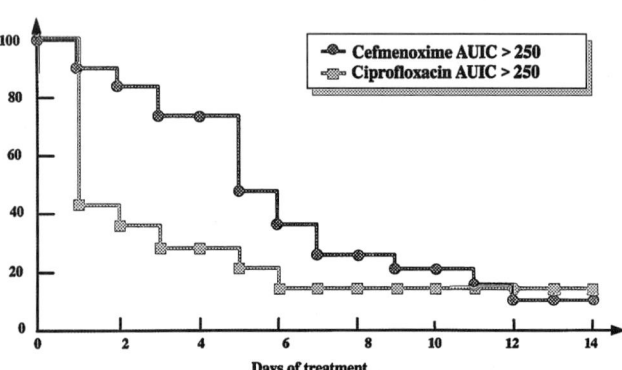

FIGURE 3. Relationship between the day of bacterial eradication and AUIC values above 250 for cefmenoxime (●) and ciprofloxacin (■). At the same AUIC range above 250, ciprofloxacin eradicates bacteria earlier in therapy. (Modified from reference 59.)

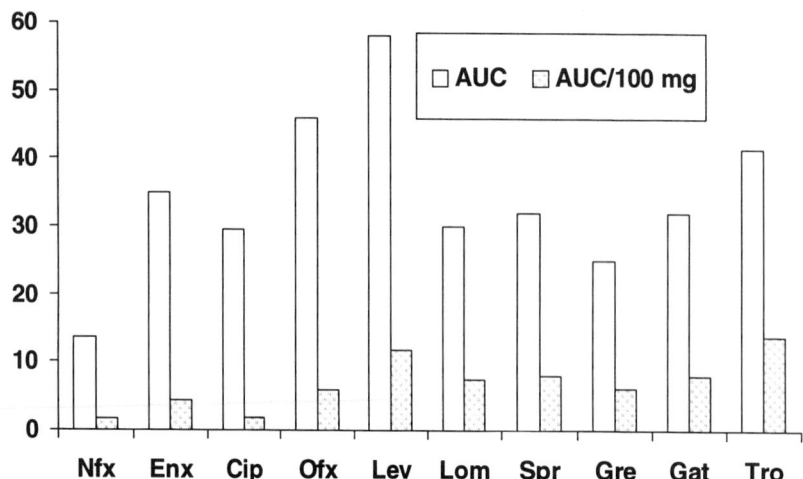

FIGURE 4. Area under the curve (AUC) values for the fluoroquinolones. AUC values are provided for the usual dose and for 100-mg doses. *Nfx,* norfloxacin, *Enx,* enoxacin, *Cip,* ciprofloxacin, *Ofx,* ofloxacin, *Lev,* levofloxacin, *Lom,* lomefloxacin, *Spr,* sparfloxacin, *Gre,* grepafloxacin, *Gat,* gatifloxacin, *Tro,* trovafloxacin. (Modified from reference 144.)

TABLE 3 • Susceptibility of Pathogenic Organisms to Ciprofloxacin, and Anticipated AUIC Profiles for IV Dosages of 200 mg q. 12 h to 400 mg q. 8 h, in Patients with Creatinine Clearances of 50 mL/min

Organism	MIC µg/mL	200 mg q. 12 h	400 mg q. 12 h	400 mg q. 8h
H. influenzae	0.01	2050	4100	6200
B. catarrhalis	0.12	171	341	517
E. coli	0.2	103	205	310
Klebsiella spp.	0.12	171	341	517
E. cloacae	0.25	82	164	256
Legionella spp.	0.06	266	532	1033
P. aeruginosa	0.5	41	82	128
S. pneumoniae	1.0	20	41	64
S. aureus	0.5	41	82	128

TABLE 4 • Breakpoint AUIC and MIC for Fluoroquinolones in Normal Volunteers with 100 mL/min Creatinine Clearance

Fluoroquinolone	Oral Dose (mg/24 h)	AUC_{24} (mg·h/L)	Breakpoint MIC for AUIC of 125	P. aeruginosa MIC_{90}	S. aureus MIC_{90}	E. coli MIC_{90}	S. pneumoniae MIC_{90}
Norfloxacin	800	13.6	0.10	2.0	6.3	0.125	8.0
Ciprofloxacin	1500	29.6	0.25	0.5	0.5	0.01	2.0
Ofloxacin	800	46.6	0.30	2.0	0.5	0.125	2.0
Levofloxacin	500	58	0.5	2.0	0.5	0.05	1.0
Enoxacin	800	35.6	0.30	4.0	2.0	0.25	4.0
Lomefloxacin	400	30	0.25	12.5	4.0	0.50	4.0
Fleroxacin	400	48	0.4	2.0	0.5	0.125	4.0
Pefloxacin	800	108	0.80	1.0	0.5	0.125	4.0
Sparfloxacin	400	32	0.25	2.0	0.5	0.12	0.25
Grepafloxacin	400	26	0.25	4.0	0.25	0.06	0.25
Gatifloxacin	400	32	0.25	4.0	0.12	0.06	0.5
Trovafloxacin	200	27	0.21	2.0	0.25	0.06	0.25
Moxifloxacin	400	25	0.25	2.0	0.25	0.06	0.25

TABLE 5 • Breakpoint AUIC and MIC for Fluoroquinolones in Normal Volunteers with 50 mL/min Creatinine Clearance

Fluoroquinolone	Oral Dose (mg/24 h)	AUC_{24} (mg·h/L)	Breakpoint MIC for AUIC of 125	P. aeruginosa MIC_{90}	S. aureus MIC_{90}	E. coli MIC_{90}	S. pneumoniae MIC_{90}
Norfloxacin	800	14	0.125	2.0	6.3	0.125	8.0
Ciprofloxacin	1500	64	0.5	0.5	0.5	0.01	2.0
Ofloxacin	800	133	1.0	2.0	0.25	0.125	2.0
Levofloxacin	500	138	1.0	2.0	0.5	0.05	1.0
Enoxacin	800	38	0.30	4.0	2.0	0.25	4.0
Lomefloxacin	400	75	0.60	12.5	4.0	0.50	4.0
Fleroxacin	400	170	1.25	2.0	0.5	0.125	4.0
Pefloxacin	800	108	0.80	1.0	0.5	0.125	4.0
Sparfloxacin	400	45	0.5	2.0	0.5	0.125	0.25
Grepafloxacin	400	40	0.25	4.0	0.25	0.06	0.25
Gatifloxacin	400	80	0.5	4.0	0.12	0.06	0.25
Trovafloxacin	200	27	0.21	2.0	0.25	0.06	0.25
Moxifloxacin	400	32	0.25	2.0	0.25	0.06	0.25

values for any alternate dosing regimens being evaluated. Of the marketed drugs, only sparfloxacin can typically cover *S. pneumoniae* with their typical dosing regimens if the target AUIC is 125. Trovafloxacin should also cover the MIC, depending on the dose. Grepafloxacin and gatifloxacin will be close to the 125 target, while levofloxacin and ciprofloxacin are similar but too low if the target is covering the MIC_{90}.

In Tables 4 and 5, the derived AUIC values used reflect steady-state quinolone concentrations for patients with and without renal or hepatic disease. Clearly, some renal insufficiency improves the patient's ratio of 24-h AUC:MIC, particularly against organisms harder to eradicate, such as *S. pneumoniae, P. aeruginosa,* and *S. aureus.* The advantages of the newer fluoroquinolones with Gram-positive actions (e.g., sparfloxacin, trovafloxacin, and grepafloxacin) are apparent from the information in these two tables. The data show good coverage when the organism has an MIC at or below 0.25. This means that serum concentration profiles for ciprofloxacin interact with MIC values of this agent, as shown in Figure 2. Coverage is achieved when peak:MIC ratios are approximately 6:1, which is also associated with AUIC values of 128 in this case. Peak to MIC multiples of 10 to 1 are associated with an AUIC value of 250, which in the case of intravenous ciprofloxacin was capable of killing LRTI pathogens on the first day of therapy. Thus, quinolones are acting similarly in the in vitro models and in vivo with respect to the relationships between their concentrations and the rate at which they kill bacteria. When dosages are normalized to those that produce an AUIC of 125 to 250, all of these quinolones should be useful for treating infections, because their peak:MIC ratios exceed 5:1. However, the peak concentration:MIC ratio is below 5 when typical doses of any of these agents (except ciprofloxacin) is used to treat patients infected with *P. aeruginosa*. At its recommended dose of 1500 mg/day, only ciprofloxacin fulfills this 5:1 ratio criterion for *Pseudomonas*. On the Gram-positive side, sparfloxacin, grepafloxacin, and trovafloxacin are the most active, often having peak:MIC ratios above 10 for *S. pneumoniae* and MSSA.

For specific bacteria, quinolones can be determined to be either overdosed or underdosed by using the criterion of AUIC above 125. An AUIC target of 125 was chosen because at this value, concentrations of quinolones in serum remain in excess of the MIC_{90} for about 80% of the dosing interval. This target has been shown to be necessary for quinolone antibacterial action. These drugs also work in many cases (126). One potential explanation is the difference between the MIC_{90} and the true MIC of the *S. pneumoniae* infecting the patient. If the true MIC is lower than the MIC_{90}, this worst-case analysis may explain why patients who are treated with ciprofloxacin and levofloxacin improve in spite of the inability to exceed an AUIC of 125. There is little evidence for the existence of a PAE in our studies, which clearly demonstrate that either time or AUIC less than 80% above the MIC of the organism is predictive of clinical failure.

Human Pharmacodynamics. A large body of human pharmacokinetic data has been accumulated during studies of the various quinolones. A pharmacodynamic perspective on these kinetic data comes from attempts to correlate either microbiologic or clinical endpoints to these kinetic indices. To the extent that this has not yet been done, a consequence has been a high degree of uncertainty over the proper dosage for these drugs in patients. A similar problem dominates clinical trials of the β-lactams, vancomycin, and the macrolides, for the same reason. For most of these antibiotics, there are often only vague notions of the effective concentration in vivo. For reasons explained above, the effective concentration in vivo is considered to be the serum concentration for all of these classes of antibiotics, including the fluoroquinolones.

The key factor in conducting and interpreting successful human pharmacodynamic studies is the chosen endpoint of drug effect. The typical clinical trial endpoints of cure and fail-

ure have some clinical relevance but are too insensitive to detect any but the most dramatic changes in the time course of antibacterial effects. In an attempt to identify more sensitive endpoints of effect for pharmacodynamic analysis, we have been exploring the time course of bacterial eradication from the infection site, using serial cultures. The site most amenable to serial cultures is the respiratory tract, particularly in nosocomial settings in which intubated patients offer ready access to suctioned endotracheal secretions. This site is highly amenable to PK/PD model development. Relevance to these models can be established by correlating the derived PK/PD relationships with both bacterial eradication and clinical cure, and we have recently conducted such an analysis using ciprofloxacin (47), and in acute exacerbation of chronic bronchitis (AECB), grepafloxacin (48). Other fluoroquinolones have not yet been studied, and it is unknown whether our findings with ciprofloxacin and grepafloxacin apply to other fluoroquinolones, although we have suggested that the other quinolones should behave similarly. In normal volunteers, these findings apply to ciprofloxacin and piperacillin (143) and to ofloxacin with cefotaxime (115).

Thus far, ciprofloxacin and grepafloxacin show good correlation between pharmacodynamics and microbiologic outcomes. The most useful parameter describing these relationships was AUIC. The AUIC mathematical relationship has its roots in the bactericidal titer and the concept of area under the bactericidal titer curve. To discriminate these relationships during conduct of the usual fixed-dose clinical trials, it is necessary to measure MIC and blood levels and determine AUC, then calculate AUIC for each study patient. We then measure day of eradication via serial culturing of the site of infection and correlate day of eradication with AUIC.

These three procedures must be done in each patient, because there is tremendous variability between patients in their AUC (even if the dose is the same) and their organism MIC (even if the organism is the same). The AUIC of ciprofloxacin in our study ranged from 6 to over 5500 (47). A range of this magnitude occurs in any patient population, which explains why clinical studies that do not directly measure AUIC or another index of the interaction between pharmacokinetics and pharmacodynamics cannot possibly differentiate between two doses of the same antibiotic or between two different antibiotics.

However, all of these indices give the same answer if the pharmacokinetics of the drugs being compared are similar (142). We prefer AUIC primarily because it offers the same target regardless of the antibiotic being used. This latter feature facilitates its use in computerized assessment strategies of drug exposure versus outcomes. Secondly, AUICs are additive, allowing ease in working with antibiotics alone as well as in combination (115, 144).

The calculations of microbiological breakpoints in Tables 4 and 5 clearly show that overall antibacterial actions (i.e., pharmacodynamics) are determined for each quinolone only when both MIC and pharmacokinetics are considered. Defects in either pharmacokinetics (low AUC) or in potency (high MIC) may partially compensate for defects in the other. Of course, one could compensate for either problem by raising the dosage and making any fluoroquinolone more active. This happens naturally in some patient populations. For example, even mild renal insufficiency greatly improves the potency of most quinolones by increasing AUC, and renal failure helps those quinolones that are renally excreted (levofloxacin, ofloxacin, lomefloxacin, gatifloxacin, fleroxacin) more than two-pathway drugs such as ciprofloxacin, norfloxacin, sparfloxacin, and enoxacin. This is probably the most important message of the AUIC data, given the current marketing-based strategy of using once-daily regimens of quinolones with marginal activity but long half-lives.

Whether raising the dosage or shortening the dosing interval for selected patients would increase microbiologic cure rates remains a question for further study, as does the question of applicability of these results to infection sites beyond nosocomial pneumonia or AECB. We believe that actions of all fluoroquinolones can be mathematically described by indices such as AUIC, even though only ciprofloxacin and grepafloxacin have been studied to date. This must also be confirmed by further study. Finally, our data thus far also correlate development of bacterial resistance with low AUC, high MIC, and troughs below MIC. Although this is largely consistent with the results of in vitro animal and human studies, it is hardly proven at this early stage and must have further study. However, a propensity to resistance development as bacteria are exposed to low AUIC or troughs below MIC may become the single greatest reason to resist the marketing-driven attempts to lower quinolone dosages or to further prolong dosing intervals. If a pharmacodynamic perspective can be used to prolong the time that we have useful and microbiologically active fluoroquinolones, then its purpose has been well served.

METHODS OF OVERCOMING AND PREVENTING RESISTANCE

Although it is possible in the laboratory to select single-step mutants to all of the fluoroquinolones by exposing the organisms to increasing concentrations over a period of time, the frequency of single-step resistance is exceedingly low ($<10^{-9}$). In spite of in vitro predictions, resistance has been found clinically, particularly with MRSA and *P. aeruginosa*. Furthermore, with extensive worldwide use of the fluoroquinolones, resistance is now being seen in *Enterobacteriaceae,* including *E. coli* and *Klebsiella* species. Most recently, *N. gonorrhoeae* is becoming resistant to ciprofloxacin and other quinolones.

Resistance to the newer fluoroquinolones as a result of spontaneous single-step mutation occurs less frequently ($>10^{-9}$–10^{-11}) than following exposure to nalidixic acid (10^{-6}–10^{-8}). Stepwise increase in resistance to quinolones follows serial exposure of bacteria to subinhibitory drug concentrations. The resulting strains often exhibit cross-resistance to the other fluorinated quinolones. Resistance appears to result from reduced quinolone affinity to gyr A subunit or alteration in cell wall permeability because of a loss of outer membrane proteins.

The mechanism of resistance appears to be both alteration of the DNA gyr A subunit and, in the case of Gram-negatives,

outer membrane proteins and/or changes in lipopolysaccharide. A change in a single amino acid in the DNA gyrase due to mutation in the gyr A gene has been shown to be associated with resistance. Mutants isolated from patients have had changes in the serine residue. In general, changes in the gyr A gene produce an 8- to 16-fold increase in the concentration of a fluoroquinolone required to inhibit or kill bacteria.

Plasmid-mediated resistance to fluoroquinolones has not been clearly established and appears less likely because fluoroquinolones inhibit transfer of large plasmids. Thus, interference by quinolones with DNA gyrase activity necessary for plasmid replication may promote loss of plasmids and inhibit transfer of R-factor-mediated resistance. However, reports of resistance of *S. aureus* and *P. aeruginosa* to ciprofloxacin have appeared. The mechanism by which this resistance develops was not well characterized. A Japanese group has tentatively reported plasmid-mediated quinolone resistance in MRSA. In Gram-negative organisms, the gyr A gene that confers susceptibility to fluoroquinolones appears to be dominant over gyr A resistance genes so that resistance does not occur through genetic transfer.

Resistance to quinolones can also result from changes in permeability. Yoshida et al. (181) described decreased expression of OmpF because of changes in the *nfxB and cfxB* genes that prevented fluoroquinolone accumulation in cells, as normally occurs in an energy-dependent fashion. Permeation and DNA gyrase mutations have been described in *P. aeruginosa* and *Citrobacter freundii*.

Although cross-resistance occurs among the fluoroquinolones, cross-resistance of fluoroquinolone-resistant strains to nonquinolone antimicrobials develops infrequently. Colonization resistance is generally maintained with the fluoroquinolones. They lack antianaerobic activity and thus produce only minor alterations in salivary and fecal microflora. The number of *Neisseria* (including *Moraxella*) recovered from saliva decreases, and aerobic enteric bacteria are rapidly eliminated from stool, with little or no reduction in most anaerobic species during therapy. The flora has completely returned to normal by 1 to 2 weeks following discontinuation of ciprofloxacin and norfloxacin; pefloxacin causes a more protracted alteration of normal flora. Resistant enteric bacteria or *Pseudomonas* uncommonly emerge, and replacement of normal flora with inherently resistant microorganisms, such as fungi, occurs infrequently.

PHARMACOKINETIC DISPOSITION

The fluoroquinolones are characterized by rapid oral absorption, blood and urine concentrations that markedly exceed the MICs for many common bacterial pathogens, wide distribution into body tissues, with serum and tissue concentrations above the MIC for most Gram-negative and many Gram-positive aerobic organisms, and half-lives sufficiently long to permit dosing every 12 to 24 h. The pharmacokinetic parameters of the newer fluoroquinolones have many similarities, although there are differences in half-life, degree of absorption, metabolism, and elimination. In general, quinolones exhibit linear pharmacokinetics, with increases in serum concentrations directly proportional to dose size, and pharmacokinetic properties (serum half-life, total body clearance, etc.) independent of dose.

Renal clearance mechanisms are the most important for removal of ofloxacin, lomefloxacin, levofloxacin, gatifloxacin, and fleroxacin. Renal excretion of these compounds is via both tubular secretion and glomerular filtration, with glomerular filtration as the major component. Hepatic mechanisms of elimination are more important for removal of pefloxacin, grepafloxacin, and trovafloxacin; both hepatic and renal mechanisms are used by norfloxacin, ciprofloxacin, enoxacin, tosufloxacin, and sparfloxacin. Fluoroquinolones are excreted across the bowel wall into the intestinal lumen, which also explains their efficacy in diarrheal diseases. Clinically relevant basic pharmacokinetic parameters of quinolones are summarized in Table 6 (58, 112, 114, 144, 148).

Absorption

The excellent bioavailability of the quinolones, which defines the extent of drug absorbed into the systemic circulation, allows oral dosing in place of the more traditional parenteral administration. With most of the new fluoroquinolones, oral absorption is sufficient to achieve adequate serum bactericidal activity for systemic infections (103, 106, 114, 144, 157, 165, 172). This is not the case with nalidixic acid, cinoxacin, or norfloxacin. Nalidixic acid and the other older quinolones are less completely absorbed and are more rapidly cleared from the body than their fluorinated progeny (39), but the real problem is the high MICs of modern bacteria. Fluoroquinolones are absorbed primarily in the duodenum and the proximal jejunum. They do not require acidity or an alkaline environment and are absorbed to a similar extent in a fasting state or ingested with a meal (81, 114, 182). The absolute bioavailability of many of these compounds has not been characterized because intravenous dosage forms are not available for human studies.

Approximately 96% of an oral dose of nalidixic acid is absorbed (125). Bioavailability is good (probably above 80%) for enoxacin and pefloxacin and probably in excess of 90% for ofloxacin, levofloxacin (25,43), trovafloxacin (157), lome-

floxacin (110), and sparfloxacin (106, 149). Oral bioavailability of ciprofloxacin in one study ranged from 75% for a 500-mg dose to 54% for a 750-mg dose(63). Subsequent investigations suggest that the bioavailability of ciprofloxacin is not dose dependent because the areas under the plasma concentration-time curve are proportional to administered oral doses. Consequently, the bioavailability of ciprofloxacin is about 75 to 80% (80, 85, 114, 144). This is also true in patients (46, 150, 182). The bioavailability of grepafloxacin is lower, in the range of 40% (48).

In contrast, the fluoroquinolones are rapidly absorbed after oral dosing, reaching peak serum concentrations in 1 to 2 h. Peak plasma levels differ for each drug, as shown in Table 6. After 400-mg doses, there were peak levels of 1.5 μg/mL for norfloxacin, 4 μg/mL for pefloxacin, and 3 μg/mL for enoxacin. A 500-mg dose of ciprofloxacin produces a blood level of approximately 2.5 μg/mL, and a 750-mg dose produces a blood level of 3.5 μg/mL. Doses of 400 mg of ofloxacin, lomefloxacin, levofloxacin, and fleroxacin produce peak plasma levels in the range of 3.0 to 4.0 μg/mL (16). A 400-mg dose of sparfloxacin yields a peak plasma level of 1.6 μg/mL (106, 149). Figure 5 compares these maximal serum concentrations for the quinolones (144). For comparison purposes, all values were normalized to a 500-mg oral dose, making the assumption that serum peak concentrations and AUC are proportional to dose. Nalidixic acid, ofloxacin/levofloxacin, fleroxacin, and gatifloxacin reach the highest peak values; norfloxacin, enoxacin, sparfloxacin, grepafloxacin, trovafloxacin, pefloxacin, and ciprofloxacin are lower (58, 114, 144). These latter compounds have larger steady-state volumes of distribution (Table 6) (16, 81, 103, 106, 110, 114, 144, 149, 157, 165, 172, 173, 182).

After oral dosing, peak serum concentrations occur in 1 to 2 h. Elderly and critically ill individuals absorb the drugs normally, but peak concentrations in these individuals are generally delayed and are usually higher, since such patients frequently have a concomitant decrease in renal function.

The 24-h areas under the serum concentration-time curve (AUC) for typical doses of each new quinolone agent are

TABLE 6 • Pharmacokinetic Parameters of the Fluoroquinolones

Parameter	Norfloxacin	Ciprofloxacin	Enoxacin	Ofx/Levo	Lomefloxacin	Sparfloxacin	Grepafloxacin	Gatifloxacin	Trovafloxacin
Dose (mg)	400	750	400	400/500	400	400	400	400	300
Peak (mg/mL)	1.5	3.5	2.6	4.0/6.0	3.0	1.6	1.3	3.4	4.0
Peak from 500 mg dose	1.9	2.3	3.25	5.0/6.0	3.75	2.0	1.63	4.25	6.6
Protein bound (%)	15	25	30	25	30	45	50	18	70
VDss (L/kg)	1.7	3.2	1.8	1.45	4.4	3.6	1.8	1.7	1.1
$t^{1/2}$ (h), (CCr 100 mL/min)	3.3	4.0	4.9	6.0	8.0	18	10.3	8.4	10.0
$t^{1/2}$ (h), (CCr 10 mL/min)	8.0	10.0	9.4	30.0	25.0	45	NA	>40	12
AUC (mg·h/mL)	13.6	29	16.2	38/58	30	32	25	32	41.4
AUC/100-mg dose	1.7	1.9	4.3	11.7	7.26	8	6.2	8	13.8
Cl_{renal} (mL/min)	234	250	193	190	189	190	NA	NA	10
% Nonrenal	60	40	53	5	30	50	95	10	90
% Renal	40	60	47	95	70	50	5	90	10

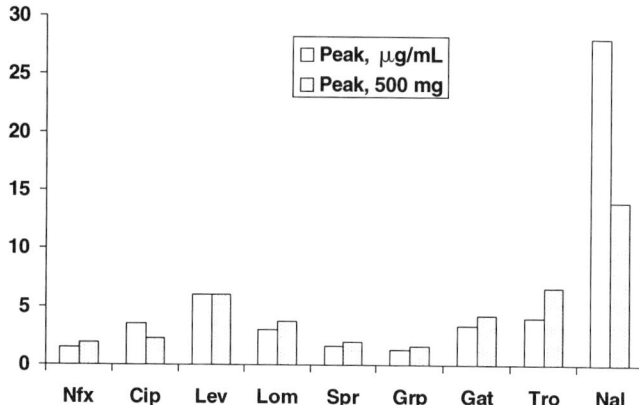

FIGURE 5. Peak serum concentrations of the fluoroquinolones following usual dosing and also normalized to 500 mg in each case. *Nfx,* norfloxacin, *Cip,* ciprofloxacin, *Lev,* levofloxacin, *Lom,* lomefloxacin, *Spr,* sparfloxacin, *Grp,* grepafloxacin, *Gat,* gatifloxacin, *Tro,* trovafloxacin, *Nal,* nalidixic acid. (Modified from references 114 and 144.)

shown in Figure 4 (58, 114, 144, 148). This figure also presents the data normalized to a 100-mg oral dose. In addition to nalidixic acid and ofloxacin/levofloxacin, sparfloxacin shows a large AUC, chiefly because of its longer half-life. For comparison purposes, all values were normalized to a 100-mg oral dose, assuming that serum peak concentrations and AUC are proportional to dose. In some studies, peak concentration or AUC changed out of proportion to dose; however, the deviations from linearity were not substantial. The potential clinical significance of the large differences between compounds in peak serum concentrations and AUC will be addressed as these AUC values are integrated with relative antimicrobial potency.

Distribution

Fluoroquinolones have a large volume of distribution, ranging from 1 to more than 4 L/kg. Values are provided for each of these agents in Table 6 (11, 58, 112, 114, 135, 144, 148, 172). Clearly, the apparent volume of distribution of all fluoroquinolones exceeds the 0.6 L/kg that corresponds to total body water. However, the derived values in the literature vary considerably, even for the same quinolone, presumably because few studies use the intravenous forms of these drugs to determine precise volumes of distribution. The accuracy of the derived value depends upon knowing bioavailability accurately enough to factored it out. For example, after intravenous administration of ciprofloxacin, the apparent volume of distribution was 2.2 to 2.7 L/kg. If an oral dose were used to assess this parameter, it would appear to be higher (in the range of 3.2 L/kg). Adjustment with a bioavailability of 70 to 85% corrects the derived volume parameter. This effect deserves attention because most of the fluoroquinolones that appear to have larger distribution volumes actually have incomplete bioavailability.

All of the newer fluoroquinolones are widely distributed throughout the body, and they are widely distributed within body tissues and fluids. Table 7 summarizes some of the extracellular site concentrations in relation to the simultaneous serum concentrations (3, 14–16, 18, 24, 36, 79, 96, 98, 99, 108, 109, 119, 120, 136, 144, 154, 156, 169).

Interstitial fluid concentrations range from 50 to 100% of peak plasma levels after 2 h, and between 4 and 24 h they generally exceed serum concentrations. These quinolones reach appreciable concentrations in salivary and lacrimal secretions, nasal mucosa, bronchial epithelium, and sputum. They also reach high concentrations inside many cells. Fluoroquinolones enter polymorphonuclear cells, alveolar macrophages, peritoneal macrophages, and phagocytic cells within the liver, producing concentrations ranging from 3 to 10 μg/mL (145, 175, 178). An anionic transport mechanism removes the compounds from white blood cells (58, 114, 148).

Concentrations significantly above those in serum are attained in the kidney, prostate, liver, and lung; levels in saliva, bronchial secretions, and prostatic fluid are lower than those in serum (58, 114, 144, 148). Tissue concentrations are always higher in infected tissues than in uninfected tissues, because of WBC accumulation. There are more WBCs in infected tissue, and these compounds are probably present intracellularly in concentrations higher than those in extracellular fluids, although the degree of antimicrobial activity of these drugs at intracellular sites has not been well studied. Figure 6 gives the concentrations and tissue:serum concentration ratios for one of these compounds (sparfloxacin) in lung tissue and at pulmonary sites (144, 174). The ratios reported in Figure 6 were obtained at steady-state after chronic dosing. In the few studies conducted thus far, no significant tissue accumulation was noted from the first dose to steady state on chronic dosing. Tissue concentrations of these fluoroquinolones invariably exceed plasma concentrations except in brain tissue.

Urine drug concentrations are high and remain above the MICs of common urinary pathogens; in most instances, they exceed inhibitory levels for urinary pathogens for a full 24 h. Urinary concentrations above 10 μg/mL often can be detected up to 48 h after ingestion of a single dose. The lowest concentrations of fluoroquinolones in urine are seen with tosufloxacin, grepafloxacin (14), trovafloxacin (23, 157, 158), and sparfloxacin (72, 107, 133, 149). The highest urinary concentrations are noted with lomefloxacin (110), fleroxacin (165), gatifloxacin (58, 67), and levofloxacin (15, 25, 43), because these compounds are well absorbed and are excreted completely unchanged. Most fluoroquinolones continue to produce adequate therapeutic concentrations in the urine, even when renal function is greatly reduced.

Consistent with transintestinal elimination (133, 134, 152), the fecal levels of most quinolones are sufficient to inhibit most gastrointestinal bacterial pathogens. The cerebrospinal fluid levels of ciprofloxacin and ofloxacin in patients with inflamed meninges are 40 to 90% of the serum concentrations. The levels of ciprofloxacin and ofloxacin in human aqueous humor range from 3.8 to 25% and 44 to 88% of serum levels, respectively. Depending on the quinolone under study, biliary concentrations are five to eight times the simultaneous serum levels.

TABLE 7 • **Tissue Penetration of the Fluoroquinolones**

Site	Dose	Route	Frequency	Time to Ct	Conc, Tissue (mg/L)	Time to Cp	Conc., Plasma (mg/L)	Reference
Ciprofloxacin								
Bile	500 mg	p.o.	b.i.d. × 6	25–26 h	4.5	4 h	2.5	36
Blister, suction	500 mg		1 ×		84.70%		2.26	37
Lung, parenchyma	200 mg	i.v.	1 ×		3.4 μg/g		0.6	24
Lung, pleura	200 mg	i.v.	1 ×		1.7 μg/g		0.6	24
Muscle, heart valve	750 mg	p.o.	q. 12 h × 4	1–3 h	8.3/3.1 μg/g		11.59/3.95	98
Muscle, myocardium	400 mg	i.v.	1 ×	1 h	31.6/25 μg/g		6.19/1.73	98
Prostate, TURP	200 mg	p.o.	t.i.d. × 9		1.32/0.64 (5.5 h)		0.65/0.31 (5.5 h)	109
Enoxacin								
Prostate, TURP	200 mg	p.o.	t.i.d. × 5		5.81/2.95 (2.99–7.92) Intraoperative		4.87/1.39 (3.13–7.44) 30 mins preop	179
Fleroxacin								
Blister, suction	400 mg	p.o.	q.d. × 5		5.7/0.9		6.7	119
Tonsil	200 mg	p.o.	1 ×	1–2 h	3.27 mg/kg	1–2 h	2.84	3
Grepafloxacin								
Blister, cantharides	400 mg	p.o.	1 ×	4.8 h	1.1	2.0 h	1.5	14
Mucosa, Lung	400 mg	p.o.	q.d. × 4		3.13 mucosa % plasma ratio		1.2	18
Levofloxacin								
Bile	100 mg	p.o.	1 ×	2–6 h	0.49–5.63	2–6 h	0.55–1.63	156
Lomefloxacin								
Blister, cantharides	400 mg		1 ×	2.7 h	3.5	1 h	4.7	154
Prostate, TURP	200 mg	p.o.	t.i.d. × 9	17 h	3.31/1.16 μg/g	17 h	1.70/0.56	108
Norfloxacin								
Prostate, TURP	200 mg	p.o.	t.i.d. × 5		4.42/1.94 (2.45–7.76) Intraoperative		2.89/2.34 (0.87–8.33) 30 mins preop	179
Ofloxacin								
Blister	400 mg	p.o.	1 ×		2.8		3.9	136
Bone	300 mg	p.o.	1 ×	1 h	1.58/0.06 μg/g	1 h	2.61/0.17	120
Lung, parenchyma	600 mg	p.o.	1 ×	2 h	17.7/9.2 μg/g	2 h	8.7/4.2	169
Muscle, myocardium	400 mg	i.v.	1 ×	1 h	8.89/2.16		15.9/2.5	99
Prostate, TURP	200 mg	p.o.	t.i.d. × 5		5.51/1.79 (3.62–7.19) Intraoperative		5.36/1.28 (3.12–8.24) 30 mins preop	179

Adapted from reference 144.

All fluoroquinolones studied distribute extensively in body fluids and tissues. The total areas under the blister fluid concentration curves exceed serum levels by 120% for ciprofloxacin, enoxacin, norfloxacin, and ofloxacin (172, 173). Ciprofloxacin and norfloxacin levels in lung, gallbladder tissue, skeletal muscle, prostate, and uterus exceed serum levels. Distribution into bone, skin, saliva, and cerebrospinal fluid results in concentrations below simultaneously measured serum levels (21, 161).

Ciprofloxacin, enoxacin, ofloxacin, and other quinolones appear to penetrate into prostate tissue and seminal fluid, reaching concentrations exceeding those achieved in serum. Biliary concentrations also exceed those in serum (36). After a single 200-mg intravenous dose, concentrations of cipro-floxacin in cortical bone and cancellous bone were 6.9 and 9.7 μg/g. Other quinolones also appear to penetrate bone. However, these values should be interpreted cautiously, because tissue:serum ratios change in relation to time after administration, and study designs differed. Bone marrow tissue concentrations are excellent and, in almost every case, exceed the MICs for infecting bacteria (98, 114, 144).

Protein binding has been measured for most of these compounds, and values are reported in Table 6 (58, 114, 117, 144, 148). Nalidixic acid is the highest, with more than 90% of circulating nalidixic acid bound to plasma proteins. In sharp contrast to nalidixic acid, most of the fluoroquinolones have relatively low protein binding, 14 to 45% (117). Thus, any compromise of antimicrobial activity by the presence of serum

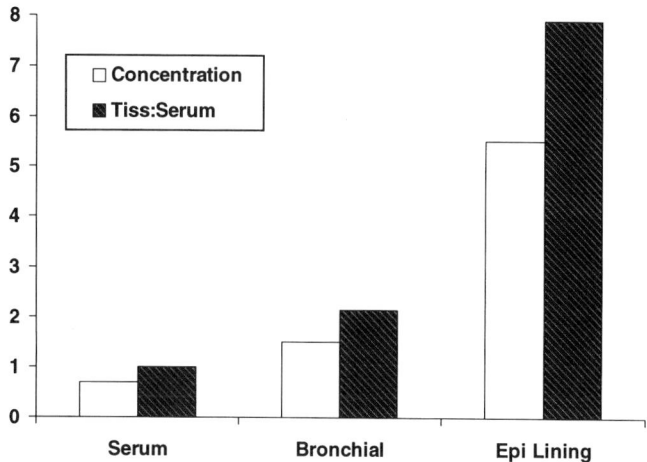

FIGURE 6. Site concentrations, tissue:serum ratios, and the serum concentration for sparfloxacin at a 400-mg dose. (Adapted from reference 144.)

protein should be minimal. The protein binding of trovafloxacin is 65 to 70% (157, 158), which is high for a member of this class of compounds. Sparfloxacin approaches 45% (106, 149). Ciprofloxacin, pefloxacin (106), enoxacin, levofloxacin, gatifloxacin (67), and ofloxacin are 10 to 25% protein bound (114, 117). Grepafloxacin is 50% bound (14, 164).

Metabolism

Hepatic metabolism is essential for clearance of several fluoroquinolones. Nalidixic acid is rapidly metabolized to hydroxynalidixic acid (microbiologically active) and inactive glucuronide conjugates in the liver. The site of nalidixic acid glucuronidation is most likely the carboxy group at position 3 on all quinolone antimicrobials. Approximately one-third of the active drug in plasma is hydroxy metabolite and two-thirds is parent drug. In urine, 85% of an oral dose is recovered as inactive glucuronide conjugates; and the remainder is recovered as hydroxynalidixic acid (125).

In the case of fluoroquinolones such as pefloxacin, norfloxacin, and ciprofloxacin, most metabolism occurs at the piperazine substituent on ring position 7 (Figure 7). Norfloxacin, "oxo-norfloxacin," and "oxo-pefloxacin" are active metabolites of pefloxacin, but the N-oxide is not active. The 55 to 60% recovery of parent drug and metabolites in urine is as oxo metabolites. Traces of pefloxacin glucuronide are also found in urine. Pefloxacin and known metabolites found in urine account for only 58.9% of an 800-mg oral dose. The remainder of the dose is probably excreted in feces, either as parent drug or as a glucuronide conjugate (104).

At least four metabolites have been identified in urine after ciprofloxacin administration. As with most oxoquinolone metabolites, the oxo metabolite of ciprofloxacin is active, although less so than ciprofloxacin. In urine, 36% of a 500-mg dose is recovered as unchanged ciprofloxacin, 9.6% as the oxo metabolite, 2 to 4% as the dioxo metabolite, and less than 2% as other metabolites (157). In animal studies using ^{14}C-labeled

ciprofloxacin, all of the radiolabeled drug can be accounted for in the combined collections of urine and stool. In rats, 90% of a 10-mg/kg oral dose and 48% of an equal intravenous dose was recovered in stool. The remainder was recovered in urine as unchanged drug and metabolites (63, 80, 134).

Extensive data on the metabolism of many of the newest fluoroquinolones are not yet available. However, gatifloxacin appears to have little metabolic conversion, and trovafloxacin and grepafloxacin clearly are mostly metabolized and have very little renal excretion. Sparfloxacin provides an example of balanced and dual elimination: 50% of the dose is excreted in feces, and the other 50% in urine (106, 149). Representative of some of the newest fluoroquinolones, sparfloxacin has little metabolic attack on the position 7 ring structure (149).

The sparfloxacin metabolite is the acylglucuronide formed by metabolic attack on position 3 (106, 149). This pathway appears to also be quite important for lomefloxacin and grepafloxacin. Their metabolism, targeted to position 3, also results in formation of glucuronides. Because of the larger molecular weight of fluoroquinolone glucuronides, biliary elimination is important, and this is how they reach the feces. Urinary elimination of these conjugates would be low, consistent with the available data on urinary glucuronide metabolites of fluoroquinolones. Slow formation of position 3 glucuronides would explain the longer half-lives of some newer fluoroquinolones, such as sparfloxacin, trovafloxacin, and grepafloxacin.

In contrast to the pathway for the earlier quinolone compounds, metabolic alteration of the newer fluoroquinolones does not typically occur on the position 7 ring. Whereas the metabolic products of earlier quinolones had antimicrobial activity, glucuronides formed at position 3 are clearly inactive, because this part of the molecule is essential for antimicrobial activity.

Ciprofloxacin Metabolism and Excretion

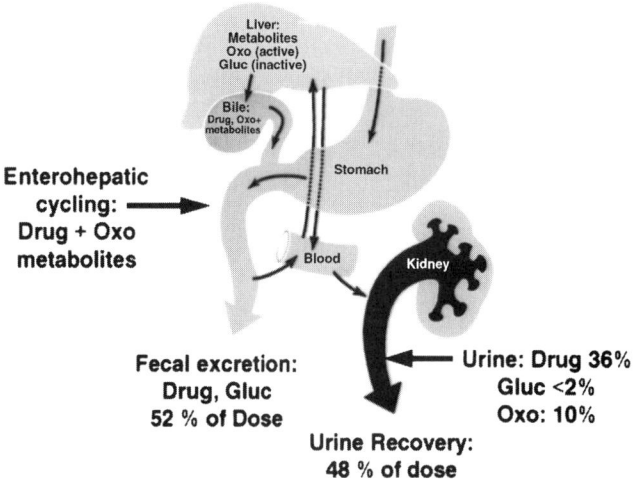

FIGURE 7. Metabolic and renal excretion pathways for ciprofloxacin, a fluoroquinolone with balanced renal and metabolic elimination. *oxo* refers to oxo and dioxo metabolites (partially active); *gluc* refers to glucuronides (inactive). (Modified from references 114 and 144.)

To some extent, all fluoroquinolones are excreted in bile, unchanged and as metabolites. Enoxacin, ciprofloxacin, and ofloxacin all achieve biliary concentrations eight to ten times their peak serum concentrations (12, 45, 114, 144, 155). In studies of biliary ciprofloxacin concentrations during cholecystectomy, concentrations ranged from 21.7 to 79.6 mg/L (12, 155); 24-h collection of T-tube drainage, after a 500-mg oral dose, yielded only 1.6 mg of ciprofloxacin (123). This would be expected, given the relatively small total amount of bile produced by humans. Bile concentrations were significantly lower if there was biliary obstruction.

For reasons detailed above, hepatic disease in the presence of normal renal function does not produce major changes in the serum half-life of dual-pathway quinolones such as ciprofloxacin or sparfloxacin or for the renally excreted agents ofloxacin, levofloxacin, and gatifloxacin (167). Little is known about the disposition of the hepatically cleared fluoroquinolones such as grepafloxacin and trovafloxacin in patients with hepatic disease. Dramatic changes in half-life, similar to those occurring for renally excreted fluoroquinolones in renal failure, would be anticipated for these agents. In the case of pefloxacin, an earlier-generation metabolized quinolone, the half-life was 219% higher in patients with hepatic cirrhosis than in normal volunteers (102). In contrast, no significant changes in the pharmacokinetics of norfloxacin were observed when patients with acute hepatitis B were compared with normal volunteers (34). The cirrhosis patient is a better predictor of alterations in metabolism than is the patient with acute hepatitis B, because hepatitis does not routinely alter drug metabolism. Two-pathway compounds such as sparfloxacin, enoxacin, pefloxacin, and ciprofloxacin would shift rapidly to renal excretory pathways in the event of biliary obstruction (105, 149). Quantitative metabolic studies in patients with severe hepatic disease are rare, and detailed studies should be conducted to determine whether the predicted interpathway shift actually occurs.

Renal Elimination

Quinolones are eliminated by renal mechanisms, including glomerular filtration and tubular secretion, as well as by nonrenal routes, such as hepatic metabolism and transintestinal transportation (134). The terminal half-lives of the fluoroquinolones range from 3.5 to 20 h (Table 6). Ciprofloxacin, enoxacin, and norfloxacin have terminal half-lives of approximately 4 h; ofloxacin and levofloxacin, 5 to 6 h; pefloxacin, lomefloxacin, gatifloxacin, and fleroxacin (151), 8 to 10 h. Trovafloxacin and grepafloxacin are both in the range of 10 to 12 h (157, 164, 175). Sparfloxacin has a terminal half-life of 20 h (106, 149). Since the elimination of the compounds is different, terminal half-lives increase to varying degrees, depending on the degree of elimination via renal and hepatic function. Fluoroquinolones excreted primarily by hepatic metabolism (pefloxacin, tosufloxacin, grepafloxacin, trovafloxacin) have longer half-lives in many cases (23, 58, 157, 158) than quinolones excreted primarily by renal mechanisms, and especially longer than quinolones excreted by both pathways (58, 114, 144).

Renal clearance usually exceeds the glomerular filtration rate, suggesting that tubular secretion plays a major role. The fact that most of these antibiotics interact with probenecid (114, 144, 149, 153) is further evidence of renal tubular secretion. Renal clearance of the fluoroquinolones ranges from 140 to 425 mL/min in patients with normal renal function. Administration of probenecid reduced the renal clearance of ciprofloxacin by 50% and total urine recovery by 24% (70). Probenecid also reduces the renal excretion rate of norfloxacin and sparfloxacin (114, 144, 153).

In renal disease, many of the quinolones show altered disposition. In Figure 8, the serum half-lives of eight of these compounds are compared in patients with normal renal function and patients with severe renal insufficiency. These compounds are moderately affected by renal disease, with levofloxacin, ofloxacin, gatifloxacin, lomefloxacin, sparfloxacin (150), and nalidixic acid showing the greatest sensitivity (41). For nalidixic acid, however, the metabolite, hydroxynalidixic acid, accumulates in the serum of patients who have renal dysfunction. In anuric patients (creatinine clearance < 10 mL/min) serum half-lives increase to 8 to 10 h for ciprofloxacin and norfloxacin; 11 to 15 h for pefloxacin; 40 h for enoxacin; and 25 to 45 h for ofloxacin, levofloxacin, lomefloxacin, fleroxacin, gatifloxacin, and sparfloxacin (Table 6) (42, 104, 114, 149).

The half-life of fluoroquinolones is decreased approximately 50% by hemodialysis during the 4-h procedure, but this removes minimal amounts of these drugs. Accordingly, patients undergoing hemodialysis should receive the same reduced doses that would normally be given to patients with endstage renal function (114, 144). Supplemental doses are not needed between dialyses in patients with anuria. In most cases, once-daily smaller doses would be used in patients whose creatinine clearance is below 20 mL/min, whether or not they are undergoing dialysis. Renal function reduced to this degree significantly prolongs most quinolone elimination, necessitating

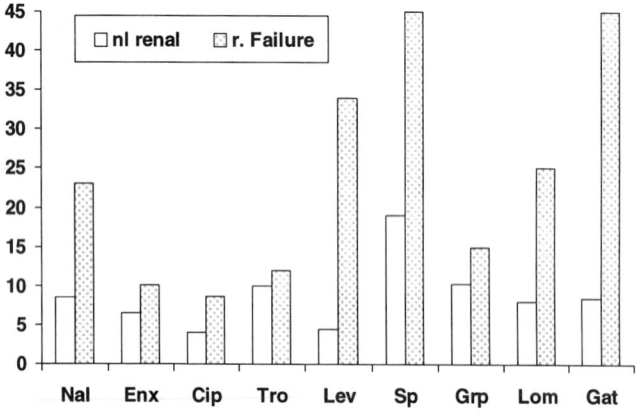

FIGURE 8. Serum half-lives of the quinolones in normal renal function and in patients with renal failure. *Nal,* nalidixic acid, *Enx,* enoxacin, *Cip,* ciprofloxacin, *Tro,* trovafloxacin, *Lev,* levofloxacin, *Sp,* sparfloxacin, *Grp,* grepafloxacin, *Lom,* lomefloxacin, *Gat,* gatifloxacin. (Modified from references 114 and 144.)

dosage adjustments. Grepafloxacin (164) and trovafloxacin (23) are probable exceptions, given their dependence on hepatic metabolism.

Most likely, alternate pathways account for excretion of the drug in patients with renal failure, because the serum half-life only doubles for most (41, 114, 144). Thus, for many of the compounds in Table 6, only modest dose reductions are required for the two-pathway quinolones, even for patients with severe renal dysfunction. Ofloxacin, levofloxacin, and gatifloxacin are exceptions, because their half-lives can increase three- to fivefold in severe renal dysfunction. Renal impairment does not markedly affect trovafloxacin, pefloxacin, and grepafloxacin, because these compounds are primarily metabolized. However, the metabolite of pefloxacin is norfloxacin, which is cleared by both renal and nonrenal pathways.

In Figure 9, total and renal clearance for eight of these compounds is shown for normal subjects and for patients with severe renal insufficiency. Clearly, renal clearance of unchanged compound accounts for a substantial percentage of the total clearance in normal volunteers. Nalidixic acid is omitted from these figures because renal excretion is not an important route of elimination for the unchanged drug, as is the case with pefloxacin, trovafloxacin, and grepafloxacin.

Renal failure reduces renal clearance to very small fractions of the renal clearance values typical of normal volunteers (Fig. 9), yet the serum half-life data in Figure 8 indicates only moderate increases in the half-life of many of these compounds in renal failure. Drug metabolism occurs to the greatest extent with pefloxacin, which is metabolized primarily to norfloxacin (104), grepafloxacin (14), and trovafloxacin (23, 157, 158), and less so for the other quinolones. Metabolites constitute between 15 and 30% of norfloxacin, enoxacin, and ciprofloxacin recoverable from urine. As shown in Table 6, the total clearance of these compounds is only modestly altered by renal

dysfunction. This comparison verifies a shift in the excretion pattern of these drugs in patients with renal failure, for more of the compound is metabolized or excreted in bile. Thus, two-pathway behavior confers an advantage on the dosing of ciprofloxacin, pefloxacin, norfloxacin, and enoxacin. As with all drugs subject to excretion by combinations of renal and metabolic pathways, patients with multiple organ failure and resulting impairment of both pathways would show extreme prolongations of serum half-life. In this case, neither elimination pathway can compensate for failure of the other, and marked accumulation would occur. Severe hepatic disease also would be expected to prolong the serum half-lives of trovafloxacin, grepafloxacin, norfloxacin, and pefloxacin (52, 105). In fact, ciprofloxacin and norfloxacin may accumulate in patients with hepatic failure (51), particularly with concomitant renal impairment (50, 167).

ADVERSE EFFECTS

The most frequent adverse effects experienced by quinolone recipients include nausea, upper gastrointestinal tract (GI) discomfort, and central nervous system (CNS) effects such as headache, insomnia, agitation, dizziness, and phototoxicity (4, 116, 135). However, unlike the aminoglycosides and other antibiotics of the past, the adverse events associated with the quinolones are typically milder, are self-limited, and only rarely require discontinuation of treatment. Each quinolone tends to produce a characteristic profile of adverse effects. The frequency of these various effects has not been subjected to comparative studies between the members of the fluoroquinolone class, because the clinical trials conducted for registration purposes usually study comparators from other antibiotic classes. While there has never been head-to-head study, from reference points of clinical trials against the same or similar comparators, the relative frequency of the more common events was compiled from a large body of literature and rank ordered in Table 8.

Corrado et al. recently summarized tolerability data from clinical trials involving 1540 norfloxacin-treated patients (19). From this patient population the investigators identified 63 adverse drug events as probably or possibly related to norfloxacin therapy. Adverse drug events required discontinuation of therapy in approximately 1% of patients and were considered serious in less than 1% of patients. The most frequently reported symptoms included nausea (1.9%), headache (1.8%), dizziness (1.2%), and abdominal pain, dyspepsia, constipation, and flatulence (0.3% each).

Arcieri et al. (2) analyzed safety data for 2829 ciprofloxacin recipients. The attending physician determined that an adverse drug event was either probably or possibly related to ciprofloxacin therapy in approximately 16% of the patients; 8% complained of signs or symptoms associated with the GI tract (primarily nausea, vomiting, or diarrhea), and 3.3% experienced CNS abnormalities (most notably dizziness, headache, tremors, and restlessness).

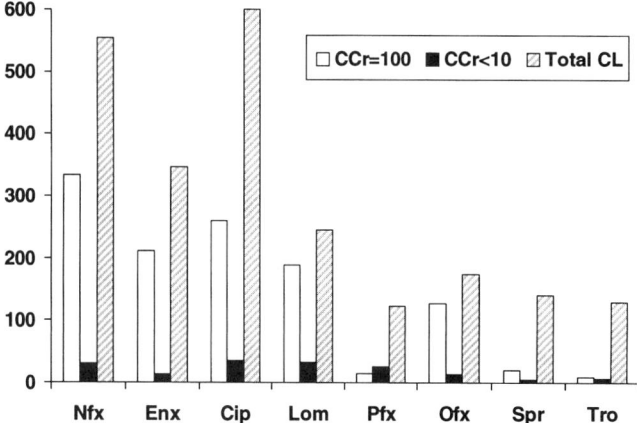

FIGURE 9. Quinolone total and renal clearance values for the fluoroquinolones in normal renal function (CCr = 100 mL/min) and in renal failure (CCr < 10 mL/min). *Nfx*, norfloxacin; *Enx*, enoxacin; *Cip*, ciprofloxacin; *Lom*, lomefloxacin; *Pfx*, pefloxacin; *Ofx*, Ofloxacin; *Spr*, sparfloxacin; *Tro*, trovafloxacin. (Modified from references 114 and 144.)

Articular Damage

Clinical experience with the quinolones in the pediatric population is limited because routine use in this age group is currently

TABLE 8 • Side Effect Profile of the Fluoroquinolones[a]

Parameter	Norfloxacin	Ciprofloxacin	Ofx/Levo	Lomefloxacin	Sparfloxacin	Grepafloxacin	Gatifloxacin	Trovafloxacin
GI upset	+2	+1	+1	+1	+1	+3	?	+1
Photosensitivity	0	0	+1	+4	+4	0	?	0
CNS effects	+1	+1	+2	+1	+1	+1	?	+2
Theophylline interaction	+1	+2	+1	0	0	+4	0	0
Antacid interaction	+4	+4	+4	+4	+ 4	+4	+4	+4

[a]Codes: 0, none; +4, maximum among comparators. For theophylline interactions: 0, none; +1, 5–10% change; +2, 11–25% change; +3, 26–40% change; +4, >40% change. For GI upset and photosensitivity: 0, none; +1, 1–2%; +2, 2–3%; +3, 3–5%; +4, >5%.

not approved. This restriction is based primarily on arthropathies observed in young experimental animals, especially beagle dogs. Dogs are clearly the most sensitive species to this effect, and the damage is worsened if the dog is ambulatory. Articular damage is almost nonexistent if the dogs are not allowed to put weight on the joints being tested.

A moderate number of pediatric patients (probably more than 2500) have received ciprofloxacin, with no definite arthropathy attributable to this antibiotic. It may be that doses are not high enough or exposures are not long enough in humans to reproduce the injury patterns of the toxicologic experiments. The lack of a reliable early marker for articular damage in pediatric patients and the uncertain causal relationship between the use of the newer fluoroquinolones (as opposed to nalidixic acid) may further complicate the question of risk-benefit for many years. While this is being sorted out, the long-term risks to juveniles, however, make use of quinolones in pediatric patients a matter of assessing risk vs benefit. Currently, no quinolone antibiotic is approved for pediatric use in the United States. In carefully selected pediatric patients, the use of quinolones with close monitoring has been justified. We suggest that ambulation be limited if these agents are being used.

Renal Injury

Animal studies suggest the possibility of interstitial inflammatory reactions associated with precipitation of quinolone complexes within the kidney's tubular walls. Human volunteers have occasionally developed crystalluria in phase I trials of new fluoroquinolones. Animals with distinct crystalluria have subsequently developed obstructive uropathy. The dose producing nephropathy always exceeded the doses that produced crystalluria, and doses for both of these events are well above the human therapeutic range. Acute renal failure, interstitial nephritis, and nonspecific nephritis were each reported once in the 2829 ciprofloxacin recipients reviewed by Arcieri et al. (2), even though causality can be very difficult to establish in these complicated clinical settings.

Ocular Damage

Several quinolones (e.g., pefloxacin, rosoxacin, and nalidixic acid) induce ocular damage in animals given high doses. Problems noted include subcapsular cataracts, retinal morphologic changes, and altered visual acuity. In limited studies, neither ciprofloxacin nor norfloxacin had any effect on electroretino-

graphic findings or on the fundus. No significant drug-associated ocular changes were noted in over 800 ciprofloxacin-treated patients evaluated by ophthalmologic examinations. Once again, this may simply illustrate the outcomes when very high doses are used in animals in the course of toxicology studies. The relevance of these findings to the lower doses actually used in humans needs to be established. None of the recently marketed quinolones have been associated with ocular toxicity during their clinical trials.

Central Nervous System

A number of the fluoroquinolones demonstrate a propensity for mild but detectable CNS effects. In particular, ofloxacin and trovafloxacin appear to cause occasional CNS events. Levofloxacin, the *l*-isomer of ofloxacin, has decreased the amount of ofloxacin by 50% and appears to have reduced the frequency of CNS events. Many patients reporting CNS symptoms in the early studies of fluoroquinolones had received concomitant theophylline or caffeine. Enoxacin and also ciprofloxacin, pefloxacin, and grepafloxacin significantly increase peak and trough serum theophylline concentrations. In 30% of patients experiencing increased theophylline concentrations, theophylline concentrations were clearly in the toxic range. In a recent study that was uncontrolled for theophylline administration, enoxacin (400–600 mg twice daily) was associated with a 42.3% incidence of nausea and dizziness and a 15.4% incidence of CNS symptomatology, compared with 6.3 and 2.5% incidences, respectively, for ciprofloxacin (500–1000 mg twice daily) and 4 and 0% for pefloxacin (400 mg twice daily), respectively, and no reactions for 30 ofloxacin patients given 400 mg once or twice daily (168). These results follow the rank order of potency of these fluoroquinolones in inhibiting the theophylline-metabolizing isozyme.

Photosensitivity

Varying frequencies of photosensitization have been reported with the quinolones. Of the older quinolones, nalidixic acid is well known to cause occasional phototoxic skin reactions, and on the basis of previous reactions to this agent, the potential for phototoxicity in the newer fluoroquinolones was predicted. This side effect is dose related and can be avoided or prevented by avoiding exposure to sunlight or ultraviolet radiation.

The potential for phototoxicity associated with ciprofloxacin, ofloxacin, trovafloxacin, grepafloxacin, and levofloxacin appears similar and lower than that of lomefloxacin, sparfloxacin, enoxacin, and nalidixic acid (163). Indeed, photosensitivity has been reported significantly more often with lomefloxacin than with other fluoroquinolones. In an analysis by the Food and Drug Administration (FDA) of spontaneous reports, lomefloxacin phototoxicity occurred in 70 per 100,000 prescriptions, compared with less than 0.1 per 100,000 for ciprofloxacin and 0.4 per 100,000 for ofloxacin (35). By March 1993, 182 confirmed reports of lomefloxacin-induced phototoxicity had been received by the FDA, 7 of which required hospital admission, leading to circulation of a letter to U.S. doctors warning of possible phototoxic reactions to this fluoroquinolone. Patients given these more definitively phototoxic fluoroquinolones should be cautioned to avoid exposure to sunlight.

Treatment and Prevention

At the moment, nine fluoroquinolones are approved by the FDA for human use in the United States: norfloxacin, ciprofloxacin, ofloxacin, levofloxacin, lomefloxacin, sparfloxacin, grepafloxacin, trovafloxacin, and enoxacin. Fleroxacin has also been approved but will not be marketed. This discussion focuses mainly on these compounds, with emphasis on clinical utility in the adult population.

DRUG INTERACTIONS

The important drug interactions and adverse drug reactions of the quinolones are summarized in Table 8. As with the adverse events, there is no head-to-head comparative study, and the rank ordering is by inference on the basis of noncomparative reports and studies against the same or similar nonquinolone comparator antibiotics (69). Some significant and potentially significant interactions are summarized below.

NSAIDs

Enoxacin, when used together with the nonsteroidal antiinflammatory agent (NSAID) fenbufen, has been associated with development of seizures. Similar problems have not been observed with other quinolones. Fenbufen is not marketed in the United States, and there is no evidence that other marketed NSAIDs similarly augment risk.

Anticoagulants

Studies on the interactions between quinolones and warfarin demonstrate that enoxacin prolongs the elimination half-life of (R)-warfarin, while not affecting (S)-warfarin. Because the (R)-enantiomer is five to eight times less active than the (S)-isomer, the overall enoxacin-warfarin interaction should be of little clinical significance. However, several anecdotal cases have implied clinically significant interactions between warfarin and quinolones. Any patient receiving a quinolone along with warfarin anticoagulation should have prothrombin times closely monitored.

Antacids

Fluoroquinolones interact with multiple drugs to result in reduced quinolone absorption from the gastrointestinal tract. Therapeutic failures can result. Fluoroquinolones form chelates with divalent cations, particularly aluminum and magnesium and, to a lesser degree, iron, zinc, and calcium. Thus, coadministration of fluoroquinolones with antacids or agents such as sucralfate reduces bioavailability as much as 85%. Iron preparations behave similarly to antacids, and adequate time should be allowed between doses. Multivitamin preparations that contain minerals should be avoided as well. Allowing a 4- to 6-h interval between the administration of antacids or sucralfate and fluoroquinolones could avoid the interaction, but this is not always a suitable alternative for patients on long-term antacid treatment. H_2 antagonists do not affect the oral absorption of fluoroquinolones and can be used for acid control when the quinolones must be used in the presence of acidity.

Theophylline, Caffeine, and the Xanthines

Clearance of theophylline and caffeine is inhibited by some of the quinolones, in approximately the rank order shown in Table 8. Given the different affinity for the cytochrome P-450 isozyme IA-2, the fluoroquinolones vary in their relative degree of interaction with theophylline. Interactions are strongest with enoxacin, lesser with grepafloxacin, ciprofloxacin, and pefloxacin, and virtually nonexistent with ofloxacin, fleroxacin, trovafloxacin, sparfloxacin, gatifloxacin, and lomefloxacin. Coadministration of enoxacin with theophylline results in an approximate doubling of theophylline levels. Norfloxacin and ciprofloxacin interact with theophylline similarly, although to a lesser extent, and raise the serum concentration of theophylline by 2 to5 µg/mL. In some studies, ofloxacin showed detectable interaction with theophylline, which may not be strong enough to have clinical significance. Caffeine, a chemical analogue of theophylline, interacts similarly when coadministered with quinolones. Patients receiving certain fluoroquinolones should be advised against excessive caffeine intake, and if CNS effects develop, they should be instructed to cease caffeine intake.

Probenecid

Probenecid administration increases peak plasma concentrations and prolongs the half-life of agents primarily excreted by the renal route, such as ciprofloxacin, lomefloxacin, ofloxacin, levofloxacin, sparfloxacin, gatifloxacin, and fleroxacin. The mechanism of this effect is inhibition of renal tubular secretion. Accordingly, trovafloxacin and grepafloxacin would be expected to be less affected, since they are excreted primarily by hepatic clearance mechanisms.

CLINICAL INDICATIONS
Respiratory Tract Infections

The quinolones have been extensively studied as therapy for community and nosocomially acquired pneumonia, bronchitis, sinusitis, and exacerbations of cystic fibrosis. Some of the indications along with quinolones of choice and dosages are listed in Table 9. In general, the fluoroquinolones have been found equivalent or superior to such comparator drugs as β-lactams or β-lactam/macrolide combinations (49, 91, 113, 138). The spectrum of ofloxacin or levofloxacin, trovafloxacin, and sparfloxacin makes these drugs attractive for community-acquired infections (40, 160). Ciprofloxacin with its stronger Gram-negative spectrum is most suitable for nosocomial

TABLE 9 • Clinical Indications for the Fluoroquinolones and Dosage Regimens		
Indication		**Regimen**
Respiratory infections		
Acute community-acquired pneumonia	Ofloxacin	300–400 mg q. 12 h
	Levofloxacin	500 mg daily
	Sparfloxacin	400 mg × 1, then 200 mg q.d.
	Trovafloxacin	200 mg daily
Exacerbations of chronic lung disease	Ciprofloxacin	750 mg q 12 h.
	Ofloxacin	as per pneumonia
	Levofloxacin	" "
	Sparfloxacin	" "
Exacerbations of cystic fibrosis associated with *Pseudomonas aeruginosa*	Ciprofloxacin	750 mg p.o. q. 8–12 h
Nosocomial pneumonia	Ciprofloxacin ± another agent	400 mg i.v. q. 8–12 h
	Trovafloxacin ± another agent	300 mg i.v. q. 24 h
Urinary Tract Infections		
Simple cystitis	Norfloxacin	400 mg p.o. b.i.d.
	Ofloxacin	200 mg p.o. b.i.d.
	Ciprofloxacin	250–500 mg p.o. b.i.d.
	Levofloxacin	250 mg p.o. daily
	Enoxacin	300 mg p.o. b.i.d.
Pyelonephritis	Ciprofloxacin	i.v. or oral
	Ofloxacin	i.v. or oral
Prostatitis	Levofloxacin	400 mg daily
	Ofloxacin	400 mg p.o. q. 12 h
Venereal diseases		
Urethritis	Ofloxacin	300 mg q. 12 h
Chancroid	Fleroxacin	400 mg × 1
	Ciprofloxacin	500 mg q. 12 h × 3 days
Osteomyelitis		
Gram-negative osteomyelitis	Ciprofloxacin	500–750 mg q. 12 h
	Ofloxacin	300 to 400 mg q. 12 h
Unknown organism	As above but consider additional agent for *S. aureus* or anaerobes.	
Abdominal infections		
Gastroenteritis	Ciprofloxacin	500 mg q. 12 h × 3–5 days
	Ofloxacin	300 mg q. 12 h × 3–5 days
Travelers' diarrhea	Ciprofloxacin	500 mg q. 12 h × 3 days
	Ofloxacin	300 mg q. 12 h × 3 days
	Norfloxacin	400 mg q. 12 h × 3 days
	Fleroxacin	400 mg daily × 3 days

infections and exacerbations of cystic fibrosis (71, 90, 121, 139, 146, 147). A modest literature supports the use of these drugs in *Legionella* infections and in atypical pneumonia (49, 64, 171).

Synergy or additive effects between the quinolones and β-lactams such as piperacillin and ceftazidime against *P. aeruginosa* and other Gram-negatives argues in favor of combinations in certain clinical situations. *S. aureus* and *P. aeruginosa* often develop resistance to quinolones used in therapy, particularly in patients who are intubated or have cystic fibrosis (146). These events are typically associated with low serum concentration:MIC ratios (121), low AUICs (159), or both.

Tuberculosis

Many fluoroquinolones have good activity against *M. tuberculosis,* especially sparfloxacin, levofloxacin, and ofloxacin.

Experience with ofloxacin has been the most extensive (6, 180). Results have been favorable, and the drugs are becoming established as second-line antituberculosis agents. When used for tuberculosis they are best given as single daily doses (e.g., ofloxacin 600–800 mg or levofloxacin 500–750 mg) in the morning. Resistance has been described particularly when the quinolone is the only active drug in a regimen or when extensive cavitary disease is present (111). Ofloxacin has been used in combination with imipenem to treat pulmonary disease due to *Mycobacterium fortuitum* and *M. chelonae* (180).

Urinary Tract Infections

All available fluoroquinolones achieve high concentrations in renal tissue and urine, and many achieve good levels in the prostate. Concentrations in urine are generally above 100 μg/mL, even 12 h after dosing. This is more than adequate to treat most Gram-negative pathogens and even susceptible enterococci. Prostatic levels (e.g., 4–6 mg/g for ofloxacin or ciprofloxacin) suffice to treat the *Enterobacteriaceae* but may not suffice to treat *P. aeruginosa* or enterococci. Although the usual serum concentrations of trovafloxacin are in the range of 2 μg/mL, these concentrations might be effective against enterococci in the prostate, given the considerably lower MIC of this organism.

The quinolones have been effective in simple and complicated urinary tract infections. In both situations, they are as effective as trimethoprim-sulfamethoxazole (T/S) and more effective than the β-lactams (65, 74, 122, 137). Though effective in simple cystitis, many effective narrower-spectrum and less expensive drugs are available, leaving the quinolones for the more difficult cases.

Both ciprofloxacin and ofloxacin have been effective in chronic bacterial prostatitis due to enterobacteriaceae (17,20,128,166). Cure rates of 60 to 80% are possible with 4 to 6 weeks of therapy. This compares favorably to T/S. Infections due to *P. aeruginosa* and enterococci are much more difficult to eradicate. Suppression followed by relapse appear to be the rule when these drugs are used as single agents. Resistance is a risk, and might be anticipated if the MIC of the isolate is high at baseline.

Sexually Transmitted Diseases

Most quinolones have good activity against *N. gonorrhoeae, H. ducreyii, C. trachomatis,* and the genital mycoplasmas and ureaplasmas. Excellent results have been obtained with single-dose therapy of gonorrhea using ciprofloxacin, ofloxacin, enoxacin, fleroxacin, norfloxacin, or pefloxacin (1, 13, 78, 92, 118). The quinolone of choice for chlamydia infections is ofloxacin, which achieves 90% cure rates with a 7-day course of therapy (132). Data are very limited in ureaplasma and mycoplasma infections. Ofloxacin appears similar in efficacy to erythromycin, about 80%. For chancroid, single doses of fleroxacin or two doses of ciprofloxacin daily for 1 to 3 days are highly effective (9). Combinations of quinolones with agents effective against anaerobes have been very successful in pelvic inflammatory disease (162).

Skin and Soft-Tissue Infections

Ofloxacin and ciprofloxacin have been extensively studied for therapy for soft tissue infections. When compared with third-generation cephalosporins in difficult-to-treat infections, they have both fared well (38, 53, 54). Reservations abound because of their marginal activity against β-hemolytic streptococci and staphylococci. Ofloxacin is preferable to ciprofloxacin in this regard, and the newer agents trovafloxacin, sparfloxacin, and levofloxacin are promising (89). Resistance may occur during therapy, especially when there are large wounds with necrotic tissue and organisms with high MICs at baseline.

Osteomyelitis

Ciprofloxacin and ofloxacin are effective therapy for osteomyelitis due to Gram-negative organisms (55–57). Cure rates of 70 to 80% at least in the short term can be expected. Success has also been seen with *S. aureus*. In general, higher doses should be used. Ofloxacin in combination with rifampin was used successfully in one study of infected hip prostheses (29). Ciprofloxacin is very effective in malignant otitis externa (62, 86). Published data on trovafloxacin, sparfloxacin, and other fluoroquinolones with a Gram-positive spectrum are very limited. All of these could be effective against osteomyelitis due to Gram-positive pathogens.

Gastrointestinal Infections

Gastroenteritis has been a major area of quinolone usage. The major pathogens—*Salmonella, Shigella, E. coli, Aeromonas, Campylobacter*—are all very susceptible. Ciprofloxacin and ofloxacin given for 5 days are drugs of choice for travelers' diarrhea (32, 37). Typhoid fever has been well treated with 10- to 14-day courses of ciprofloxacin, pefloxacin, or ofloxacin (60, 129). *Campylobacter* infections are more problematic, as persistence may develop rapidly (130).

Hepatobiliary infections and a variety of intraabdominal infections can also be treated with ciprofloxacin or ofloxacin, often in combination with a drug such as metronidazole or clindamycin, effective against anaerobes. The anaerobic spectrum of trovafloxacin makes it a promising agent as sole therapy in these situations, but published data are lacking thus far.

Neutropenia

The fluoroquinolones, because of their excellent Gram-negative activity but poor anaerobic activity, are effective in eradicating Gram-negative bacteria from the intestinal flora without disrupting colonization resistance to new organisms. They are thus attractive candidates for prophylaxis of infection in the neutropenic host. Norfloxacin, ciprofloxacin, and ofloxacin have all been effective in this situation (26, 87, 170). Gram-negative infections are essentially eliminated in treated patients; however, infections due to Gram-positive organisms may be more frequent.

Ciprofloxacin has also been used to treat febrile episodes in neutropenic patients, either alone or in combination with an aminoglycoside. Used at doses of 400 mg every 8 to 12 h, it has been as effective as comparator β-lactam-aminoglycoside regimens (73, 75, 88, 124). Gram-positive superinfections may occur (100) and resistance may develop in *Pseudomonas* and some other Gram-negative organisms if dosages are too low or baseline MICs are elevated. Ciprofloxacin in combination with a ureidopenicillin has also been used successfully (61).

Nasal Carriage of *Neisseria meningitides*

Ciprofloxacin achieves concentrations of 0.1 to 0.4 μg/mL in nasal secretions, which are well above the 0.004 μg/mL required to inhibit *N. meningitides*. Single doses of 750 mg or 500 mg twice daily are very effective in eradicating meningococcal carriage for 2 days (33, 127, 131).

Eye Infections

Norfloxacin, ciprofloxacin, and ofloxacin ophthalmic solutions contain 3 to 5 mg/mL of the quinolone. They have been used very successfully to treat conjunctivitis and keratitis due to *S. aureus, H. influenzae, S. pneumoniae,* and *P. aeruginosa* (68, 82, 83). Systemic norfloxacin (1200 mg as a single dose) has been very successful in the treatment of gonococcal conjunctivitis (77).

REFERENCES

1. Albrecht LM, Rybak MJ, Schubiner HH, Weiner LM. Single dose enoxacin for the treatment of uncomplicated urogenital gonorrhea. Sex Transm Dis 1989;16:114–117.

2. Arcieri GM, Becker N, Esposito B, Griffith E, Heyd A, Neumann C, O'Brien B, Schacht P. Safety of intravenous ciprofloxacin. Am J Med 1989;87(5A):92S–97S.

3. Baba S, Mori Y, Maruo T. Penetration of fleroxacin into maxillary sinus mucosa and palatine tonsil. J Antimicrob Chemother 1988;22(Suppl D):195–197.

4. Ball P, Tillotson G. Tolerability of fluoroquinolone antibiotics. Drug Safety 1995;13:343–358.

5. Barriere SL, Ely E, Kapusnik JE, Gambertoglio JG. Analysis of a new method for assessing activity of combinations of antimicrobials. Area under the bactericidal activity curve. J Antimicrob Chemother 1985;16:49–59.

6. Besozzi G, Colombo F, Montellini PV, Miradoli A. Use of ofloxacin in mycobacterial lung infections. Am Rev Respir Dis 1991;143:119.

7. Biedenbach DL, Marco F, Jones RN. Antimicrobial activity of trovafloxacin compared to seven other compounds against Legionella spp including validation of E test [Abstract D-40]. 37th Interscience Conference on Antimicrobial Agents and Chemotherapy, Toronto, Ontario, Sept 28–Oct 1, 1997.

8. Blaser J, Stone BB, Groner MC, Zinner SH. Comparative study with enoxacin and netilmicin in a pharmacodynamic model to determine the importance of ratio of antibiotic peak concentration to MIC for bactericidal activity and emergence of resistance. Antimicrob Agents Chemother 1987;31:1054–1060

9. Bodhidatta L, Taylor DN, Chitwarakorn A, Kuvanont K, Echeverria P. Evaluation of 500- and 1,000-mg doses of ciprofloxacin for the treatment of chancroid. Antimicrob Agents Chemother 1988;32:723–725.

10. Boswell FJ, Andrews JM, Wise R. Pharmacodynamic properties of BAY 12–8039 on gram-positive and gram-negative organisms as demonstrated by studies of time-kill kinetics and postantibiotic effect. Antimicrob Agents Chemother 1997;41:1377–1379.

11. Bressolle F, Goncalves F, Gouby A, Galtier M. Pefloxacin and clinical pharmacokinetics. Clin Pharmacokinet 1994;27:418–446.

12. Brogard JM, Jehl F, Monteil H, Adloff M, Blickle JF, Levy P. Comparison of high-performance liquid chromatography and microbiological assay for the determination of biliary elimination of ciprofloxacin in humans. Antimicrob Agents Chemother 1985;28:311–314.

13. Bryan JP, Hira SK, Brady W, Luo N, Mwale C, Mpoko G, Krieg R, Siwiwaliondo E, Reichart C, Waters C, Perine PL. Oral ciprofloxacin versus ceftriaxone for the treatment of urethritis from resistant *Neisseria gonorrhoeae* in Zambia. Antimicrob Agents Chemother 1990;34:819–822.

14. Child J, Andrews JM, Wise R. Pharmacokinetics and tissue penetration of the new fluoroquinolone grepafloxacin. Antimicrob Agents Chemother 1995;39:513–515.

15. Child J, Mortiboy D, Andrews JM, Chow AT, Wise R. Open-la-

bel crossover study to determine pharmacokinetics and penetration of two dose regimens of levofloxacin into inflammatory fluid. Antimicrob Agents Chemother 1995;39:2749–2751.

16. Deleted.

17. Childs SJ. Ciprofloxacin in treatment of chronic bacterial prostatitis. Urology 1990;35(Suppl 1):15–18.

18. Cook PJ, Andrews JM, Wise R, Honeybourne D, Moudgil H. Concentrations of OPC-17116, a new fluoroquinolone antibacterial, in serum and lung compartments. J Antimicrob Chemother 1995;35:317–326.

19. Corrado ML, Struble WE, Peter C. Norfloxacin: review of safety studies. Am J Med 1987;82(Suppl 6B):22–26.

20. Corrado ML. Worldwide clinical experience with ofloxacin in urological cases. Urology 1991;27(Suppl):28–32.

21. Cutler NR, Vincent J, Jhee SS, Teng R, Wardle T, Lucas G, Dogolo LC, Sramek JJ. Penetration of trovafloxacin into cerebrospinal fluid in humans following intravenous infusion of alatrofloxacin. Antimicrob Agents Chemother 1997;41:1298–1300.

22. Dalhoff A, Petersen U, Endermann R. In vitro activity of BAY 12–8039, a new 8-methoxyquinolone. Chemotherapy 1996;42:410–425.

23. Dalvie DK, Khosla N, Vincent J. Excretion and metabolism of trovafloxacin in humans. Drug Metab Dispos 1997;25:423–427.

24. Dan M, Torossian K, Weissberg D, Kitzes R. The penetration of ciprofloxacin into bronchial mucosa, lung parenchyma, pleural tissue after intravenous administration. Eur J Clin Pharmacol 1993;44:101–102.

25. Davis R, Bryson HM. Levofloxacin. A review of its antibacterial activity, pharmacokinetics and therapeutic efficacy. Drugs 1994;47:677–700.

26. Dekker AW, Rozenberg-Arska M, Verhoef J. Infection prophylaxis in acute leukemia: a comparison of ciprofloxacin with trimethoprim-sulfamethoxazole and colistin. Ann Intern Med 1987;106:7–12.

27. Domagala JM. Structure-activity and structure-side-effect relationships for the quinolone anti-bacterials. J Antimicrob Chemother 1994;33:685–706.

28. Dowzicky M, Nadler H, Dorr MB, Acusta A, Talbott G. The in vitro activity and pathogen responses of sparfloxacin versus comparative therapy for the treatment of respiratory tract, urinary tract, and skin and skin structure infections in North American clinical trials [Abstract]. 36th Interscience Conference on Antimicrobial Agents and Chemotherapy, New Orleans, LA, Sept 15–18, 1996.

29. Drancourt M, Stein A, Argenson NJ, Zannier A, Curvale G, Raoult D. Oral rifampin plus ofloxacin for treatment of *Staphylococcus*-infected orthopedic implants. Antimicrob Agents Chemother 1993;37:1214–1218.

30. Drusano GL. Minireview: role of pharmacokinetics in the outcome of infections. Antimicrob Agents Chemother 1988;32:289–297.

31. Dudley MN, Blaser J, Gilbert D, Zinner SH. Bactericidal activity of ciprofloxacin against P aeruginosa and other bacteria in an in-vitro two compartment capillary model. Rev Infect Dis 1988;10(Suppl):S34–S35.

32. DuPont HL, Ericsson CD, Mathewson JJ, DuPont MW. Five versus three days of ofloxacin therapy for traveler's diarrhea: a placebo-controlled study. Antimicrob Agents Chemother 1992;36:87–91.

33. Dworzack DL, Sanders CC, Horowitz EA, Allais J, Sookpranee M, Sanders WE, Ferraro FM. Evaluation of single-dose cipro-

floxacin in the eradication of *Neisseria meningitides* from nasopharyngeal carriers. Antimicrob Agents Chemother 1988;32:1740–1741.

34. Eandi M, Viano I, Di Nola F, Leone L, Genazzani E. Pharmacokinetics of norfloxacin in healthy volunteers and patients with renal and hepatic damage. Eur J Clin Microbiol 1983;2:253–259.

35. Echols RM, Oliver MK. (Abstract) 18th International Congress of Chemotherapy, Washington, DC, Jun 27–Jul 2, 1993.

36. Edmiston CE Jr, Suarez EC, Walker AP, Demeure MP, Frantzides CT, Schulte WJ, Wilson SD. Penetration of ciprofloxacin and fleroxacin into biliary tract. Antimicrob Agents Chemother 1996;40:787–791.

37. Ericsson CD, Johnson PC, DuPont HL, Morgan DR, Bitsura JA, Cabada FJ. Ciprofloxacin or trimethoprim/sulfamethoxazole as initial therapy for acute traveler's diarrhea. Ann Intern Med 1987;106:216–220.

38. Fass RJ, Plouffe JF, Russell JA. Intravenous/oral ciprofloxacin versus ceftazidime in the treatment of serious infections. Am J Med 1989;87(Suppl 5A):164–168.

39. Ferry N, Cuisinaud G. Pozet N. Nalidixic acid kinetics after single and repeated oral doses. Clin Pharmacol Ther 1981;29:695–698.

40. File TM, Segreti J, Dunbar L, Player R, Kohler R, Williams RR, Kojak C, Rubin A. A multicenter randomized study comparing the efficacy and safety of intravenous and/or oral levofloxacin versus ceftriaxone and/or cefuroxime axetil in treatment of adults with community acquired pneumonia. Antimicrob Agents Chemother 1997;41:1965–1972.

41. Fillastre JP, Leroy A, Moulin B, Dhib M, Borsa-Lebas F, Humbert G. Pharmacokinetics of quinolones in renal insufficiency. J Antimicrob Chemother 1990;26:51–60.

42. Fillastre JP, Montay G, Bruno R, Etienne I, Dhib M, Vivier N, Le Roux Y, Guimart C, Gay G, Schott D. Pharmacokinetics of sparfloxacin in patients with renal impairment. Antimicrob Agents Chemother 1994;38:733–737.

43. Fish DN, Chow AT. The clinical pharmacokinetics of levofloxacin. Clin Pharmacokinet 1997;32:101–119.

44. Fisher LM, Mizuuchi K, O'Dea MH, Ohmori H, Gellert M. Site specific interaction of DNA gyrase with DNA. Proc Natl Acad Sci USA 1981;78:4165–4169.

45. Flowerdew A, Walker E, Karran SJ. Evaluation of biliary pharmacokinetics of oral enoxacin, a new quinolone antibiotic. Proceedings of the 14th Interscience Congress of Chemotherapy, Kyoto, Japan, 1985:1739–1740.

46. Forrest A, Ballow CH, Nix DE, Birmingham MC, Schentag JJ. Development of a population pharmacokinetic model and optimal sampling strategies for intravenous ciprofloxacin. Antimicrob Agents Chemother 1993;37:1065–1072.

47. Forrest A, Nix DE, Ballow CH, Goss TF, Birmingham MC, Schentag JJ. The pharmacodynamics of intravenous ciprofloxacin in seriously ill patients. Antimicrob Agents Chemother 1993;37:1073–1081.

48. Forrest A, Chodosh S, Amantea MA, Collins DA, Schentag JJ. Pharmacokinetics and pharmacodynamics of oral grepafloxacin in patients with acute bacterial exacerbations of chronic bronchitis. J Antimicrob Chemother 1997;40(Suppl A):45–57.

49. Forsberg P, Maller R, Nilsson L. Comparative study of oral ofloxacin and erythromycin in the treatment of pneumonia. Rev Infect Dis 1989;11(Suppl 5):S1229–S1230.

50. Fraise AP, Smith SP. Ciprofloxacin in combined renal and hepatic impairment [Letter to editor]. J Antimicrob Chemother 1990;25:297–303.

51. Galante D, Esposito S, Barba D, Giusti G. Ciprofloxacin in the treatment of urinary and respiratory tract infections in patients with chronic liver disease. Chemioterapia 1986;5:322–326.

52. Galtier M, Bressolle F, de la Coussaye JE, Gomeni R, Joubert P, Geny F, Dubois A, Raffanel C, Saisii G, Eledjam JJ. Multiple-dose pharmacokinetics of pefloxacin in patients with hepatocellular deficiency. Clin Pharmacokinet 1993;25:415–423.

53. Gentry LO, Rodriguez-Gomez G, Zeluff BJ, Khoshdel A, Price M. A comparative evaluation of oral ofloxacin versus intravenous cefotaxime therapy for serious skin and skin structure infection. Am J Med 1989;87(Suppl 6C):57–60.

54. Gentry LO, Ramirez-Ronda CH, Rodriguez-Noriega E, Thadepalli H, del Rosal PL, Ramirez C. Oral ciprofloxacin vs. parenteral cefotaxime in the treatment of difficult skin and skin structure infections: a multicenter trial. Arch Intern Med 1989;149:2579–2583.

55. Gentry LO, Rodriguez GG. Oral ciprofloxacin compared with parenteral antibiotics in the treatment of osteomyelitis. Antimicrob Agents Chemother 1990;34:40–43.

56. Gentry LO, Rodriguez-Gomez G. Ofloxacin versus parenteral therapy for chronic osteomyelitis. Antimicrob Agents Chemother 1991;35:538–541.

57. Gentry LO. Oral antimicrobial therapy for osteomyelitis [Editorial]. Ann Intern Med 1991;114:986–987.

58. Gootz TD, Brighty KE. Fluoroquinolone anti-bacterials: SAR, mechanism of action, resistance, and clinical aspects. Med Res Rev 1996;16:433–486.

59. Goss TF, Forrest A, Nix DE, Ballow CH, Birmingham MC, Cumbo TJ, Schentag JJ. Mathematical examination of dual individualization principles (II): the rate of bacterial eradication at the same area under the inhibitory curve (AUIC) is more rapid for ciprofloxacin than for cefmenoxime. Ann Pharmacother 1994;28:863–868.

60. Hajji M, Mdaghri NE, Benbachir M, El Filali KM, Himmich H. Prospective randomized comparative trial of pefloxacin versus cotrimoxazole in the treatment of typhoid fever in adults. Eur J Clin Microbiol Infect 1988;7:361–363.

61. Hebrecht R, Liu KL, Ortiz S, Jehl F, Bergerat JP, Dufour P, Duclos B, Maloisel F, Giron C, Oberling F. [Abstract 107]. Program Abstr. 6th Int. Symp. Infect Immunocompromised Host, 1990.

62. Hickey SA, Ford GR, Fitzgerald O'Connor AF, Eykyn SJ, Sonksen PH. Treating malignant otitis with oral ciprofloxacin. Br Med J 1989;299:550–551.

63. Hoffken G, Lode H, Prinzing C, Borner K, Koeppe P. Pharmacokinetics of ciprofloxacin after oral and parenteral administration. Antimicrob Agents Chemother 1985;27:375–379.

64. Hooper TL, Gould FK, Swinburn CR, Featherstone G, Odom NJ, Corris PA, Freeman R, McGregor CGA. Ciprofloxacin: a preferred treatment for Legionella infections in patients receiving cyclosporin. Antimicrob Chemother 1988;22:952–953.

65. Hooton TM, Latham RH, Wong ES, Johnson C, Roberts PL, Stamm WE. Ofloxacin versus trimethoprim-sulfamethoxazole for treatment of acute cystitis. Antimicrob Agents Chemother 1989;33:1308–1312.

66. Hyatt JM, McKinnon PS, Zimmer GS, Schentag JJ. The importance of pharmacokinetic/pharmacodynamic surrogate markers to outcome. Clin Pharmacokinet 1995;28:143–160.

67. Investigator brochure. Gatifloxacin. Bristol Myers Squibb Co. 1996:39.

68. Jacobson JA, Call NB, Kasworm EM, Dirks MS, Turner RB. Safety and efficacy of topical norfloxacin versus tobramycin in

the treatment of external ocular infections. Antimicrob Agents Chemother 1988;32:1820–2824.

69. Jacobus RB, Brouwers J. Drug Interactions with quinolone antibiotics. Drug Safety 1992;7:268–281.

70. Jaehde U, Sörgel F, Reiter A, Sigl G, Naber KG, Schunack W. Effect of probenecid on the distribution and elimination of ciprofloxacin in humans. Clin Pharmacol Ther 1995;58:532–541.

71. Jensen T, Pedersen SS, Hoiby N, Koch C. Efficacy of oral fluoroquinolones versus conventional intravenous antipseudomonal chemotherapy in treatment of cystic fibrosis. Eur J Clin Microbiol 1987;6:618–622.

72. Johnson JH, Cooper MA, Andrews JM, Wise R. Pharmacokinetics and inflammatory fluid penetration of sparfloxacin. Antimicrob Agents Chemother 1992;36:2444–2446.

73. Johnson PRE, Leu Yin JA, Tooth JA. [Abstract 70] 16th Int Congr Chemother, 1989.

74. Jonsson M, Englund G, Nörgard K. Norfloxacin versus pivmecillinam in the treatment of uncomplicated lower urinary tract infections in hospitalized elderly patients. Scand J Infect Dis 1990;22:339–344.

75. Kelsey SM, Wood ME, Shaw E, Jenkins GC, Newland AC. A comparative study of intravenous ciprofloxacin and benzylpenicillin versus netilmicin and piperacillin for the empirical treatment of fever in neutropenic patients. J Antimicrob Chemother 1990;25:149–157.

76. Kenny GE, Cartwright FD. Susceptibilities of *Mycoplasma pneumoniae, Mycoplasma hominis,* and *Ureaplasma urealyticum* to a new quinolone: CP 99219 [Abstract]. 35th Interscience Conference on Antimicrobial Agents and Chemotherapy, San Francisco, CA, Sept 17–20, 1995.

77. Kestelyn P, Bogaerts J, Stevens AM, Piot P, Meheus A. Treatment of adult gonococcal keratoconjunctivitis with oral norfloxacin. Am J Ophthalmol 1989;108:515–523.

78. Lassus A, Renkonen OV, Ellmen J. Fleroxacin versus standard therapy in gonococcal urethritis. J Antimicrob Chemother 1988;22(Suppl D):223–225.

79. LeBel M. Vallee F, Bergeron MG. Tissue penetration of ciprofloxacin after single and multiple doses. Antimicrob Agents Chemother 1986;29:501–505.

80. LeBel M. Ciprofloxacin: chemistry, mechanism of action, resistance, antimicrobial spectrum, pharmacokinetics, clinical trials, and adverse reactions. Pharmacotherapy 1988;8:3–33.

81. Ledergerber B, Bettex J-D, Joos B, Flepp M, Luthy R. Effect of standard breakfast on drug absorption and multiple-dose pharmacokinetics of ciprofloxacin. Antimicrob Agents Chemother 1985;27:350–352.

82. Leibowitz HM. Antibacterial effectiveness of ciprofloxacin 0.3% ophthalmic solution in the treatment of bacterial conjunctivitis. Am J Ophthalmol 1991;112:29S–33S.

83. Leibowitz HM. Clinical evaluation of ciprofloxacin 0.3% ophthalmic solution for treatment of bacterial keratitis. Am J Ophthalmol 1991;112:34S–47S.

84. Lesher GY, Froelich EJ, Gruetton D. 1,8 Napthyridine derivative. A new class of chemotherapeutic agents. J Med Pharmacol Chem 1962;5:1063–1068.

85. Lettieri JT, Rogge MC, Kaiser L, Echols RM, Heller AH. Pharmacokinetic profiles of ciprofloxacin after single intravenous and oral doses. Antimicrob Agents Chemother 1992;36:993–996.

86. Levenson MJ, Parisier SC, Dolitsky J, Bindra G. Ciprofloxacin: drug of choice in the treatment of malignant external otitis (MEO). Laryngoscope 1991;101:821–824.

87. Liang RHS, Yung RWH, Chau TK, Chan PY, Lam WK, So SY, Todd P. Ofloxacin versus co-trimoxazole for prevention of infection in neutropenic patients following cytotoxic chemotherapy. Antimicrob Agents Chemother 1990;34:215–218.

88. Lims SH, Smith MP, Goldstone AH, Machin SJ. A randomized prospective study of ceftazidime and ciprofloxacin with or without teicoplanin as an empiric antibiotic regimen for febrile neutropenic patients. Br J Haematol 1990;76(Suppl 2):41–44.

89. Lipsky BA for the Sparfloxacin Multicenter SSSI Study Group. 36th ICAAC 1996 [Abstract LM 11].

90. Lode H, Wiley R, Höffken G, Wagner J, Borner K. Prospective, randomized, controlled study of ciprofloxacin versus imipenem-cilastatin in severe clinical infections. Antimicrob Agents Chemother 1987;31:1491–1496.

91. Lode H, Gara J, Grassi C. Treatment of community acquired pneumonia: a randomized comparison of sparfloxacin amoxycillin-clavulanate and erythromycin. Eur Respir J 1996;8:1999–2007.

92. Lutz FB Jr. Single-dose efficacy of ofloxacin in uncomplicated gonorrhea. Am J Med 1989;87:69S–74S.

93. Madaras-Kelly KJ, Ostergaaard BE, Hovde LB, Rotschafer JC. Twenty-four-hour area under the concentration-time curve/MIC ratio as a generic predictor of fluoroquinolone antimicrobial effect by using three strains of *Pseudomonas aeruginosa* and an in vitro pharmacodynamic model. Antimicrob Agents Chemother 1996;40:627–632.

94. Madaras-Kelly KJ, Moody J, Larsson A, Baeker Hovde L, Rotschafer JC. Chemotherapy 1997;43:108–117.

95. Mandell GL, Douglas GV, Bennett J. Principles and practice of infectious diseases. 4th ed. New York: Churchill Livingstone, 1995:268.

96. Maruyama K, Tanimura H, Kobavashi N. Efficacy of ofloxacin on biliary tract infections compared with other drugs. Proceedings of the 14th Interscience Congress of Chemotherapy. Kyoto, Japan, 1985:1811–1812.

97. Matsumara SO, Pong-Porter S, Trpeski L, Deazanedo J, Low DE. The in vitro activity of recently developed antimicrobials against *S. pneumoniae* [Abstract]. 37th Interscience Conference on Antimicrobial Agents and Chemotherapy, Toronto, Ontario, Sept 28–Oct 1, 1997.

98. Mertes PM, Voiriot P, Dopff C, Scholl H, Clavey M, Villemot JP, Canton P, Dureux JB. Penetration of ciprofloxacin into heart valves, myocardium, mediastinal fat, and sternal bone marrow in humans. Antimicrob Agents Chemother 1990;34:398–401.

99. Mertes PM, Jehl F, Burtin P, Dopff C, Pinelli G, Villemot JP, Monteil H, Dureux JB. Penetration of ofloxacin into heart valves, myocardium, mediastinal fat, and sternal bone marrow in humans. Antimicrob Agents Chemother 1992;36:2493–2496.

100. Meunier F, Zinner SH, Gaya H, Calandra T, Viscoli C, Klastersky J, Glauser M, and EORTC International Antimicrobial Therapy Cooperative Group. Prospective randomized evaluation of ciprofloxacin versus piperacillin plus amikacin for empiric antibiotic therapy of febrile granulocytopenic cancer patients with lymphomas and solid tumors. Antimicrob Agents Chemother 1991;35:873–878.

101. Michéa-Hamzehpour M, Auckenthaler R, Regamey P, Pechere JC. Resistance occurring after fluoroquinolone therapy of experimental *Pseudomonas aeruginosa* peritonitis. Antimicrob Agents Chemother 1987;31:1803–1808.

102. Montay G, Bariety J, Jacquot C. Pharmacokinetics of the antibacterial pefloxacin in hepatic and renal disease. Proceedings

of the 4th Mediterranean Congress on Chemotherapy, Rhodes, Greece, 1984:501–502.

103. Montay G, Goueffon Y. Roquet F. Absorption, distribution, metabolic fate, and elimination of pefloxacin mesylate in mice, rats, dogs, monkeys, and humans. Antimicrob Agents Chemother 1984;25:463–472.

104. Montay G, Jacquot C, Bariety J, Cunci R. Pharmacokinetics of pefloxacin in renal insufficiency. Eur J Clin Pharmacol 1985; 29:345–349.

105. Montay G, Gaillot J. Pharmacokinetics of fluoroquinolones in hepatic failure. J Antimicrob Chemother 1990;26:61–67.

106. Montay G, Bruno R, Vergniol JC, Ebmeier M, Roux YL, Guimart C, Frydman A, Chassard D, Thebault JJ. Pharmacokinetics of sparfloxacin in humans after single oral administration at doses of 200, 400, 600 and 800 mg. J Clin Pharmacol 1994;34:1071–1076.

107. Montay G. Pharmacokinetics of sparfloxacin in healthy volunteers and patients: a review. J Antimicrob Chemother 1996;37: 27–39.

108. Morita M, Hatakeyama T, Suzuki K. [Lomefloxacin concentration in human prostatic tissue following 3-day administration]. [Japanese] Hinyokika Kiyo 1993;39:97–99.

109. Morita M, Nakagawa H, Suzuki K. [Ciprofloxacin concentration in human prostatic tissue following 3 days' administration]. [Japanese] Hinyokika Kiyo 1991;37:563–566.

110. Morrison PJ, Mant TGK, Norman GT, Robinson J, Kunka RL. Pharmacokinetics and tolerance of lomefloxacin after sequentially increasing oral doses. Antimicrob Agents Chemother 1988;32:1503–1507.

111. Nakae I, Nakatani K, Inoue S, Takahasi K, Ikeda N, Matsumoto T, Ozawa S, Sakatani M, Kita N, Tanaka S. Therapeutic effect of ofloxacin on intractable pulmonary tuberculosis and ofloxacin resistance of tubercle bacilli isolated from the patients. Kekkaku 1991;66:299–307.

112. Neuman M. Clinical pharmacokinetics of the newer antibacterial 4-quinolones. Clin Pharmacokinet 1988;14;96–121.

113. Niederman M, Traub W, Ellison WT, Hopkins DW, and the Trovafloxacin Pneumonia Study Group. [Abstract M72] 37 ICAAC, 1997.

114. Nix DE, Schentag JJ. The quinolones: an overview and comparative appraisal of their pharmacokinetics and pharmacodynamics. J Clin Pharmacol 1988;28:169–178.

115. Nix DE, Wilton JH, Hyatt JC, Thomas J, Strenkoski-Nix LC, Forrest A, Schentag JJ. Pharmacodynamic modeling of the in vitro interaction between cefotaxime and ofloxacin using serum inhibitory titers. Antimicrob Agents Chemother 1997;41: 1108–1114.

116. Norrby SR. Side effects of quinolones: comparisons between quinolones and other antibiotics. Eur J Clin Microbiol Infect Dis 1991;10:378–383.

117. Okezaki E, Terasaki T, Nakamura M, Nagata O, Kato H, Tsuji A. Serum protein binding of lomefloxacin, a new antimicrobial agent, and its related quinolones. J Pharm Sci 1989;78:504–507.

118. Panikabutra K, Lee CT, Ho B, Bamberg P. Single dose oral norfloxacin or intramuscular spectinomycin to treat gonorrhea (PPNG and non-PPNG infections): analysis of efficacy and patient preference. Genitourin Med 1988;64:235–240.

119. Panneton AC, Bergeron MG, LeBel M. Pharmacokinetics and tissue penetration of fleroxacin after single and multiple 400- and 800-mg-dosage regimens. Antimicrob Agents Chemother 1988;32:1515–1520.

120. Pappalardo G, Bianchi A, Scire Scappuzzo G, Mirone M, Salomone S. Preliminary pharmacokinetic and clinical evaluation of ofloxacin in dental and oral cavity diseases. Int J Clin Pharmacol Res 1989;9:229–232.

121. Peloquin CA, Cumbo TJ, Nix DE, Sands MF, Schentag JJ. Evaluation of intravenous ciprofloxacin in patients with nosocomial lower respiratory tract infections. Arch Intern Med 1989;149:2269–2273.

122. Peters HJ. Comparison of intravenous ciprofloxacin and mezlocillin in treatment of complicated urinary tract infections. In: Neu HC, Reeves DS, eds. Current topics. 1986:124–126.

123. Petrikkos G, Giamarellou H, Kavouklis M, Makrakis G. A study of ciprofloxacin kinetics in various body-fluid compartments. Proceedings of the 14th Interscience Congress of Chemotherapy, Kyoto, Japan, 1985:1593–1594.

124. Philpott-Howard JN, Barker KF, Wade JJ, Kaczmarski RS, Smedley JC, Mufti GJ. Randomized multicenter study of ciprofloxacin and azlocillin versus gentamicin and azlocillin in the treatment of febrile neutropenic patients. J Antimicrob Chemother 1990;26(Suppl F):89–99.

125. Portmann GA, McChesney EW, Stander H, Molre WE. Pharmacokinetic model for nalidixic acid in man. II. Parameters for absorption, metabolism and elimination. J Pharm Sci 1966;55: 72–78.

126. Preston SL, Drusano GL, Berman AL, Fowler CL, Chow AT, Dornseif B, Reichl V, Natarajan J, Corrado M. Pharmacodynamics of levofloxacin: a new paradigm for early clinical trials. JAMA 1998;279(2):125–129.

127. Pugsley MP, Dworzack DL, Roccaforte J, Sanders CC, Bakken J, Sanders WE. An open study of the efficacy of a single dose of ciprofloxacin in eliminating the chronic nasopharyngeal carriage of Neisseria meningitidis. J Infect Dis 1988;157:852–853.

128. Pust RA, Ackenheil-Koppe HR, Gilbert P, Weidner W. Clinical efficacy of ofloxacin (Tarivid) in patients with chronic bacterial prostatitis: preliminary results. J Chemother 1989;1 (Suppl 4):469–471.

129. Ramirez CA, Bran JL, Mejia CR, Garca JF. Open, prospective study of the clinical efficacy of ciprofloxacin. Antimicrob Agents Chemother 1985;28:128–132.

130. Rautelin H, Renkonen O, Kosunen TU. Emergence of fluoroquinolone resistance in Campylobacter jejuni and Campylobacter coli in subjects from Finland. J Antimicrob Chemother 1991;35:2065–2069.

131. Renkonen O, Sivonen A, Visakorpi R. Effect of ciprofloxacin on carrier rate of Neisseria meningitidis in army recruits in Finland. Antimicrob Agents Chemother 1987;31:962–963.

132. Richmond SJ, Bhattacharyya MN, Maiti H, Chowdhury FH, Stirland RM, Tooth JA. The efficacy of ofloxacin against infection caused by Neisseria gonorrhoeae and Chlamydia trachomatis. J Antimicrob Chemother 1988;22(Suppl C):149–153.

133. Ritz M, Lode H, Fassbender M, Borner K, Koeppe P, Nord CE. Multiple-dose pharmacokinetics of sparfloxacin and its influence on fecal flora. Antimicrob Agents Chemother 1994;39: 455–459.

134. Rohwedder RW, Bergan T, Thorsteinsson SB, Scholl H. Transintestinal elimination of ciprofloxacin. Diagn Microbiol Infect Dis 1990;13:127–133.

135. Rosen T. The fluoroquinolone antibacterial agents. Prog Med Chem 1990;27:235–295.

136. Sanchez Navarro A, Martinez Lanao J, Sanchez Recio MM, Dominguez-Gil Hurle A, Tabernero Romo JM, Gomez Sanchez JC, Terreiro Delgado MM. Effect of renal impairment on distribution of ofloxacin. Antimicrob Agents Chemother 1990;34: 455–459.

137. Sandberg T, Englund G, Lincoln K, Nilsson LG. Randomized double-blind study of norfloxacin and cefadroxil in the treatment of acute pyelonephritis. Eur J Clin Microbiol Infect Dis 1990;9:317–323.

138. Sanders WE, Alessi P, Madres AT, McCloskey RV, Iannini P, Bittner MJ. Oral ofloxacin for the treatment of acute bacterial pneumonia. Use of a non-traditional protocol to compare experimental therapy with "usual care" in a multicenter clinical trial. Am J Med 1991;91:261–266.

139. Schaad UB, Wedgwood-Krucko J, Guenin K, Buchlmann U, Kraemer R. Anti-pseudomonal therapy in cystic fibrosis: aztreonam and amikacin vs ceftazidime and amikacin administered intravenously, followed by oral ciprofloxacin. Eur J Clin Microbiol Infect Dis 1989;8:858–865.

140. Schentag JJ, Domagala JM. Structure activity relationships with the quinolone antibiotics. Res Clin Forum 1984;7:9–14.

141. Schentag JJ, Nix DE, Adelman MH. Mathematical examination of dual individualization principles (I). Relationships between AUC above MIC and area under the inhibitory curve for cefmenoxime, ciprofloxacin, and tobramycin. DICP, Ann Pharmacother 1991;25:1050–1057.

142. Schentag JJ, Nix DE, Forrest A, Adelman MH. AUIC—the universal parameter within the constraint of a reasonable dosing interval. Ann Pharmacother 1997;30:1029–1031

143. Schentag JJ, Strenkoski-Nix LC, Nix DE, Forrest A. Pharmacodynamic interactions of antibiotics alone and in combination. Clin Infect Dis 1997, in press.

144. Schentag JJ, Turnak MR. Pharmacokinetics and pharmacodynamics of the fluoroquinolone antibiotics. J Clin Pharmacol 1998, in press.

145. Schuler P, Zemper K, Borner K, Koeppe P, Schaberg, Lode H. Penetration of sparfloxacin and ciprofloxacin into alveolar macrophages, epithelial lining fluid, and polymorphonuclear leukocytes. Eur Respir J 1997;10:1130–1136.

146. Scully BE, Parry MF, Neu HC, Mandell W. Oral ciprofloxacin therapy of infections due to Pseudomonas aeruginosa. Lancet 1986;1:819–822.

147. Scully BE, Nakatomi M, Ores C, Davison S, Neu HC. Ciprofloxacin therapy of cystic fibrosis. Am J Med 1987;82(Suppl 4A):196–201.

148. Sharma AK, Khosla R, Kela AK, Mehta VL. The fluoroquinolones: antimicrobial agents of the 1990s. Can J Pharmacol 1994;26:249–261.

149. Shimada J, Nogita T, Ishibashi Y. Clinical pharmacokinetics of sparfloxacin. Clin Pharmacokinet 1993;25:358–369.

150. Silverman SH, Johnson M, Burdon DW, Keighley MRB. Pharmacokinetics of single dose intravenous ciprofloxacin in patients undergoing gastrointestinal surgery. J Antimicrob Chemother 1986;18:107–112.

151. Sörgel F, Seelmann R, Naber K, Metz R, Muth P. Metabolism of fleroxacin in man. J Antimicrob Chemother 1988;22:169–178.

152. Sörgel F, Naber KG, Jaehde U, Reiter A, Seelmann R, Sigl G. Brief report: gastrointestinal secretion of ciprofloxacin. Am J Med 1989;87:62S–65S.

153. Stein GE. Drug interactions with fluoroquinolones. Am J Med 1991;91:81S–86S.

154. Stone JW, Andrews JM, Ashby JP, Griggs D, Wise R. Pharmacokinetics and tissue penetration of orally administered lomefloxacin. Antimicrob Agents Chemother 1988;32:1508–1510.

155. Strachan CJL, Thom BT. Excretion of intravenous and oral ciprofloxacin in biliary disease. Proceedings of the 14th International Congress of Chemotherapy. Kyoto, Japan, 1985:1591–1592.

156. Tanimura H, Ohnishi H, Okamura T, Uenishi M, Ichimiya G, Kobayashi Y, Aoki Y, Oka S, Yamamoto S, Shimada K. [Chemotherapy of biliary tract infections (XXXVII). Excretion into bile and gallbladder tissue levels of levofloxacin and its clinical effect in biliary tract infections]. [Japanese] Jpn J Antibiot 1992;45:557–568.

157. Teng R, Harris SC, Nix DE, Schentag JJ, Foulds G, Liston TE. Pharmacokinetics and safety of trovafloxacin (CP-99,219), a new quinolone antibiotic, following administration of single oral doses to healthy male volunteers. J Antimicrob Chemother 1995;36:385–394.

158. Teng R, Liston TE, Harris SC. Multiple-dose pharmacokinetics and safety of trovafloxacin in healthy volunteers. J Antimicrob Chemother 1996;37:955–963.

159. Thomas JK, Forrest A, Bhavnani SM, Hyatt JM, Cheng A, Ballow CH, Schentag JJ. Pharmacodynamic evaluation of factors associated with the development of bacterial resistance in acutely ill patients during therapy. Antimicrob Agents Chemother 1998;42(3):521–527.

160. Unertl KE, Lenhart FP, Forst H, Vogler G, Wilm V, Ehret W, Ruckdeschel G. Brief report: ciprofloxacin in the treatment of legionellosis in critically-ill patients, including those cases unresponsive to erythromycin. Am J Med 1989;87(Suppl 5A):128–131.

161. Valainis G, Thomas D, Pankey G. Penetration of ciprofloxacin into cerebrospinal fluid. Eur J Clin Microbiol 1986;5:206–207.

162. Verhoest P, Fernandez H, Boulanger JC, Orfila J, Papiernik E. Use of ofloxacin plus amoxicillin-clavulanic acid for the treatment of acute genital tract infections. Rev Infect Dis 1989;11(Suppl 5):S1307.

163. Wagai N, Tawara K. Possible reasons for differences in phototoxic potential of 5 quinolone antibacterial agents: generation of toxic oxygen. Free Radic Res Commun 1992;17:387–398.

164. Wagstaff AJ, Balfour JA. Grepafloxacin. Drugs 1997;53:817–824.

165. Weidekamm E, Portmann R, Partos C, Dell D. Single and multiple dose pharmacokinetics of fleroxacin. J Antimicrob Chemother 1988;22:145–154.

166. Weidner W, Schiefer HG, Dalhoff A. Treatment of chronic bacterial prostatitis with ciprofloxacin. Results of a one-year follow-up study. Am J Med 1987;82(Suppl 4A):280–283.

167. Westphal JF, Brogard JM. Clinical pharmacokinetics of newer antibacterial agents in liver disease. Clin Pharmacokinet 1993;24:46–58.

168. Wijnands WJ, Vree TB, van Herwarrden CLA. Quinolones increase plasma theophylline levels in patients with COLD. Br J Clin Pharmacol 1986;22:677–683.

169. Wijnands WJ, Vree TB, Baars AM, Hafkenscheid JC, Kohler BE, van Herwaarden CL. The penetration of ofloxacin into lung tissue. J Antimicrob Chemother 1988;22(Suppl C):85.

170. Winston DJ, Ho WG, Nakao SL, Gale RP, Champlin RE. Norfloxacin versus vancomycin/polymyxin for prevention of infections in granulocytopenic patients. Am J Med 1986;80:884–890.

171. Winter JH, McCartney C, Bingham J, Telfer M, White LO, Fallon RJ. Ciprofloxacin in the treatment of severe Legionnaire's disease. Rev Infect Dis 1988;10(Suppl 1):218–219.

172. Wise R, Lister C, McNulty CAM, Griggs D, Andrews JM. The comparative pharmacokinetics of five quinolones. J Antimicrob Chemother 1986;18:71–81.

173. Wise R, Lister D, McNulty CAM, Griggs D, Andrews JM. The comparative pharmacokinetics and tissue penetration of four quinolones including intravenously administered enoxacin. Infection 1986;14:S196–S202.

174. Wise R, Honeybourne D. A review of the penetration of sparfloxacin into the lower respiratory tract and sinuses. J Antimicrob Chemother 1996;37:57–63.

175. Wise R, Mortiboy D, Child J, Andrews JM. Pharmacokinetics and penetration into inflammatory fluid of trovafloxacin (CP-99,219). Antimicrob Agents Chemother 1996;40:47–49.

176. Wolfson JS, Hooper DC. The fluoroquinolones: structures, mechanisms of action and resistance, and spectra of activity in vitro. Antimicrob Agents Chemother 1985;28:581–586.

177. Woodcock JM, Andrews JM, Boswell FJ, Brenwald NP, Wise R. In vitro activity of BAY 12–8039, a new fluoroquinolone. Antimicrob Agents Chemother 1997;41:101–106.

178. Yamamoto T, Kusajima H, Hosaka M, Fukuda H, Oomori Y, Shinoda H. Uptake and intracellular activity of AM-1155 in phagocytic cells. Antimicrob Agents Chemother 1996;40: 2756–1759.

179. Yasumoto R, Asakawa M. [Comparison of enoxacin, ofloxacin, and norfloxacin concentration in human benign prostatic tissue]. [Japanese] Hinyokika Kiyo 1988;34:1519–1521.

180. Yew WW, Kwan SYL, Ma WK, Khin MA, Chau PK. In-vitro activity of ofloxacin against *Mycobacterium tuberculosis* and its clinical efficacy in multiply-resistant pulmonary tuberculosis. J Antimicrob Chemother 1990;26:227–236.

181. Yoshida T, Muratani T, Iyobe S, Mitsuhashi S. Mechanisms of high level resistance to quinolones in urinary tract isolates of *Pseudomonas aeruginosa*. Antimicrob Agents Chemother 1994;38:1466–1469.

182. Yuk JH, Nightingale CH, Sweeney KR, Quintiliani R, Lettieri JT, Frost RW. Relative bioavailability in healthy volunteers of ciprofloxacin administered through a nasogastric tube with and without enteral feeding. Antimicrob Agents Chemother 1989; 33:1118–1120.

Rifamycins

●

Anne B. Morris, Thomas P. Kanyok, James Scott, Charles A. Peloquin, and Shaun E. Berning

CLASS

Rifamycins are a class of macrocyclic antibiotics derived from *Amycolatopsis mediterranei,* previously known as *Streptomyces mediterranei.* First described in the 1960s as a treatment for Gram-positive and Gram-negative infections, rifampicin (the first of the rifamycins) has become one of the first-line agents for the treatment of *Mycobacterium tuberculosis.* Multiple different rifamycin derivatives demonstrate broad activity against many microorganisms. Extensive data are presented below on rifampicin (rifampin), rifabutin, and rifaximin, the agents currently available commercially in different countries. Limited information on other derivatives such as rifapentine, reprimun, and as yet unnamed compounds like KRM-1648 and KRM-1657 is included. In vitro, in vivo, and clinical data on the different agents against microorganisms and data on noninfectious uses are presented in this chapter.

The chemical structures of the currently available rifamycins are shown in Figures 1 to 3. The rifamycins contain two chromophore rings and a closed ansa chain, with varying substituents that identify the individual members of this group.

ANTIMICROBIAL ACTIVITY
Spectrum

In vitro data including MIC_{50}s, MIC_{90}s, and ranges of rifampicin, rifabutin, and rifaximin against microorganisms are found in Tables 1, 2, and 3. In vitro synergy and antibiotic combination studies are found in Table 4, and a summary of the noninfectious uses of rifamycins is found in Table 5. These data are from multiple sources and include multiple methodologies. Additionally, the in vitro susceptibility of rifampicin depends on the culture media used, so data must be interpreted within the context of the study (483). Available in vivo animal data are presented in this section for Gram-positive bacilli, Gram-positive cocci, Gram-negative cocci, Gram-negative bacilli, mycobacteria, chlamydia, rickettsia, fungi, parasites, mycoplasma, spirochetes, and viruses.

Gram-Positive Bacilli
Clostridium difficile. In a hamster model of antibiotic-associated colitis, animals that received rifampicin before receiving clindamycin lived longer than those who did not, suggesting a protective effect. Later, large numbers of animals that had received only rifampicin died of cecitis, with resistant *C. difficile* isolated (529).

Listeria monocytogenes. Some in vitro data on the use of rifampicin against *L. monocytogenes* have shown conflicting results. Combination therapy with low-dose rifampicin combinations was bactericidal, compared with high-dose regimens (730), though in a review of the data, others concluded that rifampicin was generally bacteriostatic (491, 641). Rifampicin was found efficacious in the treatment of *Listeria* infections in both mice and rabbits (640, 762).

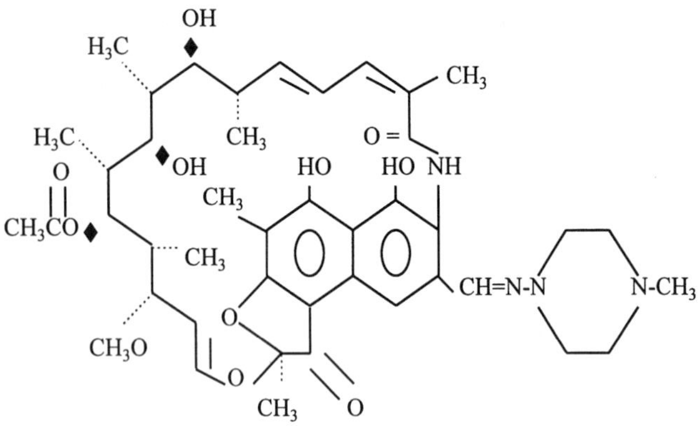

FIGURE 1. Rifampicin.

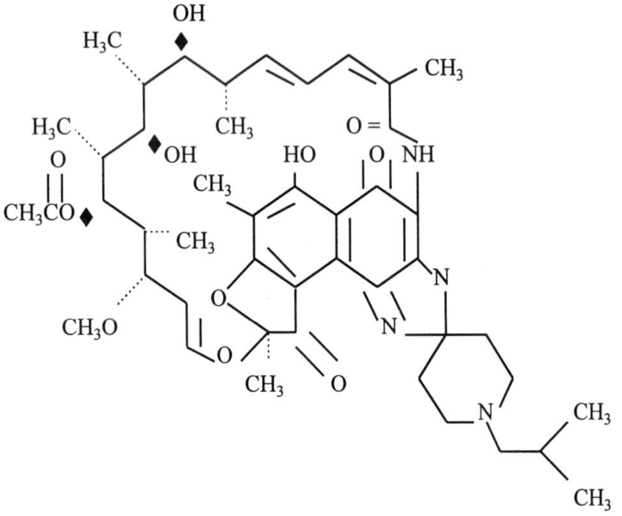

FIGURE 2. Rifabutin.

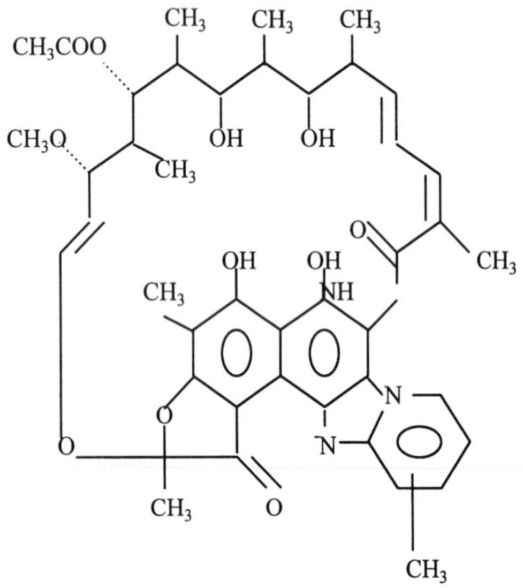

FIGURE 3. Rifaximin.

Rhodococcus equi, Rhodococcus rubropertinctus. In a retrospective review of *R. equi* pneumonia in 48 foals, 10 of the 20 surviving foals were treated with a combination of erythromycin and rifampicin. Three other surviving foals had either rifampicin or erythromycin in their treatment regimens (691). In another series of 57 foals, 50 (88%) recovered from their disease after treatment with rifampicin combined with erythromycin (334). This combination was also effective in nude mice, as was rifampicin plus minocycline (526).

Gram-Positive Cocci

Enterococcus faecalis. In a report evaluating the activity of several rifampicin combinations in a mouse pyelonephritis model, rifampicin plus ampicillin, gentamicin, vancomycin, or cephacetrile was superior to monotherapy regimens (408).

Enterococcus faecium. In an experimental rat model of endocarditis with a resistant strain, rats that received the combination of rifampicin, ciprofloxacin, and gentamicin had higher survival rates than those treated with non-rifampicin-containing regimens, although resistance to rifampicin was detected in some animals (784).

Staphylococcus aureus. In a rabbit model of experimental *S. aureus* endocarditis, rifampicin monotherapy resulted in premature death in 45 to 64% of the animals infected with two different strains. The combination of ciprofloxacin plus rifampicin, vancomycin, and ciprofloxacin alone showed equal efficacy in reducing bacterial counts in the spleens and kidneys of the infected rabbits for both strains tested. Combination therapy was superior in reducing the bacterial counts in vegetations in animals infected with one strain but was inferior to ciprofloxacin alone for the other strain, so no conclusions regarding efficacy could be drawn (383). In another experimental rabbit model of endocarditis, the combination of rifampicin plus cloxacillin produced antagonism, indifference, and synergy, depending on the dosages of the two agents (815). In an in vivo rat model of chronic staphylococcal foreign-body infection, the combination regimens of fleroxacin plus rifampicin or vancomycin-fleroxacin plus rifampicin were superior to monotherapy for treating methicillin-resistant staphylococcal (MRSA) chronic foreign-body infections (148). Despite inconsistent in vitro results, rifampicin combination regimens were beneficial in a rabbit model of chronic osteomyelitis (525). In vivo studies evaluating combination therapy for chronic osteomyelitis due to MRSA have also shown efficacy of rifampicin-quinolone combinations (220, 329). Oral administration of rifaximin, which is poorly absorbed, to mice with experimental *S. aureus* infection demonstrated no therapeutic activity until the highest dose (10 mg/kg) was used (752).

Staphylococcus epidermidis. In one rabbit model of experimental endocarditis with *S. epidermidis,* the combinations of vancomycin, gentamicin plus rifampicin, and vancomycin plus rifampicin were more effective than vancomycin alone (402). In another report, resistance developed in vivo in 2 of 17 rabbits with initially susceptible isolates from vegetations with experimental endocarditis with *S. epidermidis.* Overall, however, rifampicin was one of the most effective antibiotics in re-

TABLE 1 • Summary Table of Susceptibilities to Rifampicin

Organism	No. of Isolates	MIC$_{50}$ μg/mL	MIC$_{90}$ μg/mL	Range or (MIC, unspecified) μg/mL	Reference
Gram-positive bacilli					
Anaerobic Gram-positive rods[a]	20	0.5	16	≤0.06–16	567
Arcanobacterium hemolyticum–Actinomyces pyogenes	12	≤0.003	0.007	≤0.003–0.007	678
Bacillus subtilis	1			0.0313	259
	1			≤0.2	801
Bifidobacterium species	6	0.8	6.2	0.1–5.0	228
Brevibacterium casei	50	≤0.03	≤0.03	≤0.03	261
Clostridium beijerinckij	2			0.05	228
Clostridium botulinium A	1			0.0625	259
Clostridium botulinium B	1			0.0039	259
Clostridium difficile	56	1.56	>100	0.10->100	606
	4	0.2	0.4	0.1–0.4	228
	20			(≤0.2)	529
	15			(≤0.2)	242
	55		0.002[b]	0.002[b]	48
Clostridium histolyticum	1			(0.125)	259
Clostridium perfringens	1			0.0039	259
	15			(0.125)	426
	2			0.1	228
	34		0.13	0.13–1	785
Clostridium species[c]	26	0.2	50	0.0125->100	228
Clostridium species	17	<0.125	<0.125	<0.125	817
Corynebacterium amycolatum	101	≤0.03	>64	≤0.03->64	261
Corynebacterium auris	48	≤0.03	0.06	≤0.03–0.06	261
Corynebacterium diphtheriae	83		≤0.06	≤0.06->2.0	460
Corynebacterium glucuronolyticum	86	≤0.03	≤0.03	≤0.03	261
Corynebacterium jeikeium	43	≤0.003	64	≤0.003->256	678
Corynebacterium JK	102	≤0.25	≤0.25	≤0.25->64	785
Corynebacterium minutissimum	20	≤0.003	256	≤0.003->256	678
Corynebacterium pseudodiphtheriticum	12	≤0.003	≤0.003	≤0.003	678
Corynebacterium pseudotuberculosis	9		0.0156	0.008–0.0156	787
Corynebacterium striatum	11	2	>256	≤0.003->256	678
	86	>128	>128	>128	468
Corynebacterium urealyticum (*Corynebacterium* group D2)	94	0.06	0.06	0.06–8	269
	63	0.015	4	≤0.003->256	678
	65	≤0.008	8	≤0.008->128	270
	30	4	8	≤0.25–512[d]	629
	30	128	>1024	≤0.25->1024[e]	629
Corynebacterium xerosis	20	≤0.003	4	≤0.003–32	678
	1			≤0.2	801
Corynebacterium species[f]	20	≤0.003	0.007	≤0.003–0.015	678
Dermabacter hominis	49	≤0.03	≤0.03	≤0.03–32	261
Erysipelothrix rhusiopathiae	5	128		64–256	678
Eubacterium aerofaciens	1			0.125	259
Eubacterium lentim	1			0.001	259
Eubacterium limosum	1			0.001	259
Eubacterium species	14	0.1	0.4	0.0125–6.2	228
Gordonna terrae	3			≤1.0–4.0	213
Lactobacillus confusus	11			16–32	692
Lactobacillus species	2	32	32	16–32	692
Listeria monocytogenes	40	≤0.12	0.25	≤0.12–0.25	714
	16	≤0.003	0.125	≤0.003–0.125	678
	10		0.06	0.06	788
	10		0.12	0.12	492

continued

TABLE 1 • Summary Table of Susceptibilities to Rifampicin

Organism	No. of Isolates	MIC$_{50}$ μg/mL	MIC$_{90}$ μg/mL	Range or (MIC, unspecified) μg/mL	Reference
Nocardia asteroides	37	>50	400	≤0.39–400	801
	52	128	>256	0.5->256	201
	12	32	≥256	2–≥256	309
Nocardia brasiliensis	45	400	400	12.5–400	801
Nocardia farcinica	38	400	400	≤0.39–400	801
Nocardia nova	21	>200	400	0.78–400	801
Nocardia otitidiscaviarum	19	400	400	50–400	801
Oerskovia xanthineolytica	1			4	384
Oerskovia species	4	≤0.003		≤0.003–2	678
Propionibacterium acnes	2			0.05	228
Propionibacterium species	10	0.025	12.5	0.0125–12.5	228
Rhodococcus equi	N/A	0.06	0.06	0.008–0.25	576
	18		0.125	0.0156–0.25	787
	7		≤0.25		321
	8			0.14–0.20	214
	3			0.02–<0.1	469
	8	0.30		0.030–0.06	678
Turicella otitidis	146	≤0.03	≤0.03	≤0.03	261
Gram-positive cocci					
Aerococcus urinae	56	0.031		<0.004->32	672
	43	0.008	0.012		377
Enterococcus species	202	2.85	10.25	<0.03->16	62
	35			0.01–12.5	245
Enterococcus avium	16	2	4	0.5–4	241
Enterococcus durans	17	2	>8	≤0.03–≥1	241
Enterococcus faecalis	12	2.0	8.0	1.0–8	714
	30	2.0	8.0	≤0.015–≥0.5	241
	15	2	8	0.25–8	817
	17	2	4	1–8	152
	44	3	14.8	0.032–64	598
Enterococcus faecium	30	2	>8	≤0.13–≥2	241
	10	8	16	0.015–16	152
	9	12	32	0.023–64	598
Enterococcus faecium, vancomycin resistant	12	8	8	0.008–16	152
	1			0.1	784
Leuconostoc citreum	12			1–2	692
Leuconostoc dextranicum	1			0.06	692
Leuconostoc lactis	2			1–8	692
Leuconostoc mesenteroides	18			0.5–8	692
	2			0.12–0.25	796
Leuconostoc paramesenteroides	1			64	692
Leuconostoc pseudomesenteroides	4			1–2	692
Leuconostoc species	7	1	8	0.06–64	692
Micrococcus luteus	1			0.0078	259
	1			≤0.2	801
Micrococcus species	188	≤0.031	≤0.031	<0.031–0.063	763
Pediococcus acidilactici	20			0.12–4	692
Pediococcus pentosaceus	3			1–2	692
Pediococcus species[g]	24	0.5	2	0.12–4	692
Pediococcus species[h,i]	36	2[d]	4[d]	0.5–8[d]	705
	21	0.25[g]	1[g]	0.06–2[g]	796
Peptococcus niger	4	2		0.5–4	567
Peptococcus species	19	0.1	3.1	0.025->100	228
Peptostreptococcus anaerobius	1			0.0005	259
Peptostreptococcus asaccharolyticus	1			0.001	259
Peptostreptococcus magnus	1			0.25	259
Peptostreptococcus species	28	0.05	25	0.0125->100	228
Peptostreptococcus species[j]	35	1	32	≤0.06–32	567
Staphylococcus aureus	26	0.015	0.015	0.008–0.015	714
	15	0.015	0.015	≤0.008–0.015	817

continued

TABLE 1 • Summary Table of Susceptibilities to Rifampicin

Organism	No. of Isolates	MIC$_{50}$ µg/mL	MIC$_{90}$ µg/mL	Range or (MIC, unspecified) µg/mL	Reference
Staphylococcus aureus	30	≤0.015	≤0.015	≤0.015	241
methicillin sensitive	55	<0.03	1	<0.003->16	62
	20	0.0039	0.0078	0.002–0.0625	259
	63	0.01	0.08	0.005->10.24	753
Staphylococcus aureus	52	>16	>16	<0.003->14	62
methicillin resistant	20	0.0078	0.078	0.0039–0.016	259
	30	≤0.015	≤0.015	≤0.015->8	241
	10	1	2	≤0.008–4	817
	49	0.01	>10.24	0.005->10.24	753
Staphylococcus aureus methicillin- and quinolone-resistant	16	0.0078	1	0.0039–1	259
Staphylococcus epidermidis	25	0.015	0.015	0.004–0.015	714
	20	0.0078	0.016	0.002–0.0625	259
	50	0.015	0.015	0.03–0.5	415
Staphylococcus epidermidis	37	<0.03	0.03	<0.03->16	62
methicillin sensitive	30	≤0.015	≤0.015	≤0.015	241
	52	0.01	0.64	0.0012–2.56	753
Staphylococcus epidermidis	24	<0.03	4.0	<0.03->16	62
methicillin resistant	30	≤0.015	≤0.015	≤0.03->4	241
	10		≤0.008^b	≤0.008^b	817
	40	0.64	>10.24	0.0025->10.24	753
Staphylococcus haemolyticus	30	≤0.015	≤0.015	≤0.015	241
Staphylococcus haemolyticus	9	<0.03	<0.03		62
methicillin sensitive	47	≤0.06	≤0.06	≤0.06–0.5	362
Staphylococcus haemolyticus	7	<0.3	2.85	0.03->16	62
methicillin resistant	49	≤0.06	≤0.06	≤0.06–2	362
Staphylococcus hominis methicillin sensitive	30	≤0.015	≤0.015	≤0.015–0.03	241
Staphylococcus hominis methicillin resistant	6	≤0.015	≤0.015		241
Staphylococcus lugdunensis	52		≤0.03	≤0.03–0.13	330
Staphylococcus saprophyticus	30	≤0.015	0.03	≤0.015–0.03	241
	34	0.0075	0.0075	≤0.037–0.0075	522
Coagulase-negative *Staphylococcus*^{k} methicillin sensitive	18	<0.03	0.59	<0.03–2	62
Coagulase-negative *Staphylococcus*^{l} methicillin resistant	8	>16	>16		62
Coagulase-negative *Staphylococcus*^{m} methicillin sensitive	73	0.02	1.28	0.005–2.56	753
Coagulase-negative *Staphylococcus*^{m} methicillin resistant	36	0.04	10.24	0.005->10.24	753
Stomatococcus mucilaginosus	63	≤0.031	≤0.031	≤0.031	763
	1			0.06	348
Streptococcus agalactiae	25	1.0	1.0	0.25–1.0	714
	30	0.13	0.25	0.06–0.25	241
	88	0.12	0.25	0.03–0.5	456
	20	0.30	0.60	0.15–0.60	676
	9	0.125	0.35	0.032–0.5	598
	145	0.5	1	0.125–2	723
Streptococcus anginosus	7	0.032	0.064	0.016–0.064	598
Streptococcus bovis	19	0.13	0.25	≤0.015–0.25	241
	13	0.125	0.354	0.032–0.75	598
Streptococcus equi	10		0.0625	0.008–0.0625	787
Streptococcus equisimilis	6		0.125	0.0625–0.125	787
Streptococcus mitis	27	0.039	0.055	0.016–0.38	598
Streptococcus mutans	5	0.032	0.047	0.016–0.047	598
Streptococcus oralis	6	0.079	0.11	0.047–0.125	598

continued

TABLE 1 • Summary Table of Susceptibilities to Rifampicin

Organism	No. of Isolates	MIC$_{50}$ μg/mL	MIC$_{90}$ μg/mL	Range or (MIC, unspecified) μg/mL	Reference
Streptococcus pneumoniae	28	0.12	4.0	0.06–32	714
	20	0.016	0.25	0.016–2	259
	30	0.03	0.06	≤0.015–0.13	241
	18	0.06	0.125	0.03–0.25	817
	1165	0.03	0.06	≤0.015–>32	205
	66	0.016	0.023	0.003–0.047	598
Streptococcus pneumoniae, penicillin intermediate	216	0.03	0.06	≤0.015–>32	205
Streptococcus pneumoniae, penicillin resistant	145	0.03	0.06	≤0.015–8	205
Streptococcus pyogenes	20	0.0313	0.0625	0.0078–0.0625	259
	30	0.13	0.13	≤0.015–0.13	241
	25	0.12	0.12	0.03–0.12	714
	36	0.047	0.094	0.016–0.19	598
	63	0.5	0.5	≤0.003–0.5	723
Streptococcus salivarius	4	0.109	0.125	0.094–0.125	598
Streptococcus sanguis	16	0.056	0.094	0.023–0.19	598
Streptococcus species group A, B, C, G	26	0.125	0.125	≤0.008–8	817
Streptococcus species, group C	6	0.0275	0.532	0.016–1	598
Streptococcus species, group G	29	0.023	0.032	0.016–0.047	598
Streptococcus species, group C, F, G	104	0.125	0.5	≤0.03–1	723
Streptococcus suis	21		10[b]	10[b]	775
Streptococcus zooepidemicus	10		0.0625	0.0156–0.0625	787
Viridans group streptococci	34	0.06	0.12	0.03–8	714
	30	0.06	0.13	≤0.25–2	241
α- and nonhemolytic streptococci[n]	278	0.125	0.25	≤0.03–≥64	724
Gram-negative cocci					
Acidaminococcus fermentens	7	2		≤0.06–32	567
Branhamella catarrhalis, β-lactamase positive (Moraxella catarrhalis)	58	0.03	0.03	0.007–0.06	206
Branhamella catarrhalis, β-lactamase negative (Moraxella catarrhalis)	16	0.03	0.03	0.007–0.25	206
Megasphaera elsdenii	20	1	8	≤0.06–16	567
Neisseria gonorrhoeae	11			>0.125–0.5	44
	29	0.25	0.5	0.06–2	714
	44		0.2	≤0.006–0.78	259
Neisseria meningitidis	26	0.03	0.5	0.015–1	714
	68	0.016	0.032	0.004–0.25	92
	102	0.032	0.19	≤0.016–>256	355
Veillonella parvula	1			2	259
Veillonella species	13			0.13–2	785
Gram-negative bacilli					
Acinetobacter species	15	8	8	4–16	714
	15	2	4	0.06–8	817
Acinetobacter calcoaceticus	17			0.4–12.5	245
	1			2	259
Actinobacillus actinomycetemcomitans	24		1.6	0.1–3.12	808
	14			0.2–0.8	341
	1			0.39	637
	1			0.04	425
Actinobacillus equuli	5		2	1–2	787
Actinobacillus suis species	14	1	4	1–4	787
Aeromonas hydrophila	41			≤300[o]	136
Aeromonas sobria	32		≤300		136

continued

TABLE 1 • Summary Table of Susceptibilities to Rifampicin

Organism	No. of Isolates	MIC$_{50}$ µg/mL	MIC$_{90}$ µg/mL	Range or (MIC, unspecified) µg/mL	Reference
Bacteroides distasonis	1			0.025	228
Bacteroides fragilis	1			0.0313	259
	14	0.05	12.5	0.025–>100	228
	13	0.25	0.25	<0.125–0.5	817
	75			≤0.06–<64	426
	34			0.26^o	388
Bacteroides ovatus	3			0.4	228
Bacteroides thetaiotaomicron	2			0.4	228
Bacteroides vulgatus	1			0.025	228
	1			0.0625	259
Bacteroides species	17^p			0.06^p	426
	59	0.05	50	0.025–>100	228
Bordetella avium	10		1	0.5–1	504
Bordetella bronchiseptica	9			0.125–>16	787
	48		2	0.06–2	504
	11	>128	>128	64–>128	422
Bordetella parapertussis	46	8	16	4–64	422
Bordetella pertussis	75	0.5	1	0.12–8	422
Brucella abortus	54	0.31	1.25	0.018–2.5	167
Brucella canis	4	0.62		0.15–5.0	167
Brucella melitensis	N/A		0.50	0.03–1.0	11
	81		1	0.5–2	37
Brucella neotomae	1			0.31	167
Brucella ovis	3		0.075^b	0.075^b	167
Brucella suis	24	1.25	5.0^b	0.31–5.0	167
Brucella species^q	27	0.3			313
	62	0.5	1.0	0.1–4	271
Campylobacter coli	10	32	64	32–64	274
Campylobacter hyointestinalis	10	32	64	32–64	274
Campylobacter jejuni	54	12.5	>100^b	1.56–>100	606
Campylobacter pyloridis (*Helicobacter pylori*)	12	0.5	0.5	0.5–2	740
	50	1	1	0.5–2	427
Campylobacter sputorum subsp. *mucosalis*	10	16	32	2–32	274
Citrobacter freundii	4	32	32	32	714
Citrobacter diversus	4	32	32	32	714
Citrobacter species	2			12.25	194
	4			>25	752
DF-2 (*Capnocytophaga canimorsus*)	8			(0.06)	756
Eikenella corrodens	40	0.5	2	≤0.5–2	29
Enterobacter species	31			12.5–25	245
	6			12.84^o	194
	6			6–25	752
Enterobacter aerogenes	15	32	64	16–64	714
	25	32	64	16–64	510
Enterobacter agglomerans	14	32	64	8–64	714
	27	32	64	8–128	510
Enterobacter amnigenus	11	16	32	8–32	510
Enterobacter cloacae	13	64	64	16–64	714
	15	16	>16	8–>16	817
	29	32	32	16–32	510
Enterobacter gergoviae	11	16	16	8–32	510
Enterobacter intermedium	10	16	16	8–32	510
Enterobacter sakazakii	195	8	8	2–16	510
Enterobacter taylorae	10	16	32	8–32	510
Escherichia coli	15	8	16	8–16	714
	35			3.1–25	245
	15	8	>16	0.06–>16	817
	71			5.3^o	109, 388

continued

TABLE 1 • Summary Table of Susceptibilities to Rifampicin

Organism	No. of Isolates	MIC$_{50}$ μg/mL	MIC$_{90}$ μg/mL	Range or (MIC, unspecified) μg/mL	Reference
Flavobacterium	3			0.625–1.25	434
meningosepticum	1			0.25	338
	1			0.39	135
	11	0.6		0.6–1.25	17
Flavobacterium species	28	1		0.25–2	2
Fusobacterium mortiferum	1			>32	259
Fusobacterium nucleatum	1			1	259
Fusobacterium varium	1			≥32	259
Fusobacterium species	10	0.4	50	0.025–>100	228
Gardnerella vaginalis	93	1.0	2.0		392
Haemophilus ducreyi	103	0.004	0.008	0.0001–1.0	88
	38	0.016	0.03	0.008–0.03	1
	122	0.004	0.03	≤0.0001–0.125	180
Haemophilus influenzae	26	1.0	1.0	0.5–64	714
	20	0.25	0.25	0.0625–1	259
	18	0.25	0.5	0.125–0.5	817
	20			0.2–0.4	292
	20			0.12–0.5	371
Haemophilus influenzae, β-lactamase negative	977	0.25	0.25	≤0.03–≥64	207
Haemophilus influenzae, β-lactamase positive	560	0.25	0.25	≤0.03–16	207
Helicobacter pylori	N/A		0.5		421
Klebsiella aerogenes	57			11.9^o	388
Klebsiella pneumoniae	14	32	32	16–32	714
	35			6.3–50	245
	15	>16	>16	8–32	817
	57			(11.9)	109, 388
Klebsiella rhinoscleromatis	23	2	4	0.5–4	560
Klebsiella species	9			15.37^o	194
Legionella bozemanii	4			0.038^o	714
	2			<0.0625	544
	1			≤0.002	139
Legionella dumoffii	2			0.06^o	714
Legionella gormanii	1			0.03	714
	1			<0.0625	544
Legionella jordanis	1			0.03	714
Legionella longbeachae	5			0.25^o	714
	2			≤0.002–0.004	139
Legionella micdadei	4			0.026^o	714
	1			0.031	511
	5			<0.0625–0.125	544
	2			0.008	139
	1			0.018	733
Legionella oakridgensis	8			0.12^o	714
Legionella pneumophila	22			0.015–0.03	714
	22			0.027^o	714
	14			(≤0.05)	630
	33		0.125^b	0.125^b	221
	20			0.002–0.004	496
	30			0.002–0.004	139
	56	≤0.004	≤0.004	≤0.004–0.008	49
	98		0.015	0.007–0.015	532
	32	0.06	0.12	0.03–0.25	556
Legionella wadsworthii	1			0.022	224
Legionella species^r	11	0.12	0.5	0.03–0.5	556
Mobiluncus curtisii	12	≤0.004	≤0.004	≤0.004	680
Mobiluncus mulieris	10	≤0.004	≤0.004	≤0.004	680
Morganella morganii	15	16	32	8–32	714
	15	8	16	4–>16	817
Pasteurella species	7			0.125–4	787

continued

TABLE 1 • Summary Table of Susceptibilities to Rifampicin

Organism	No. of Isolates	MIC$_{50}$ μg/mL	MIC$_{90}$ μg/mL	Range or (MIC, unspecified) μg/mL	Reference
Proteus species	34[s]			3.1–25[s]	245
	9			4–16	787
	9			6.97[o]	194
	26	6.25–12.5	25–50	1.56–>50	752
Proteus mirabilis	15	4	8	4–8	714
	15	4	4	>16	817
	33			3.85[o]	817
Proteus morganii	15			11.4[o]	109, 388
Proteus rettgeri	15			5.8[b]	109, 388
Proteus vulgaris	17	16	32	8–32	714
	15	4	8	4–8	817
	18			4.28[o]	109, 388
Providencia rettgeri	15	16	32	8–64	714
Providencia stuartii	15	8	16	4–16	714
	34			3.1–12.5	245
	15	8	16	4–16	817
Pseudomonas aeruginosa	17	32	64	32–>64	714
	35			1.6–25	245
	15	8	>16	8–32	817
	32	16	32	2–32	738
	33		15.6	15.6–31.3	821
	21			19.95[o]	109, 388
Pseudomonas cepacia	16		≥400		417
Pseudomonas inconstans	1			2.5	194
Pseudomonas pseudomallei	97	25	25	3.13–25	794
	64	25	50	6.3–100	246
	8			35–55	409
Pseudomonas species	12	8	32	4–>64	714
Salmonella agona	2		>256		457
Salmonella enteriditis	3		>256		457
Salmonella infantis	6		>256		457
Salmonella typhi	18		12	12–25	662
Salmonella typhimurinum	1			4	259
	1			16	259
	64		>256		457
	9			0.01–10	736
	25			7.16[o]	109, 388
Salmonella species	56	3.12–6.25	6.25–12.5	0.78–>25	752
Serratia marcescens	15	64	64	32–64	714
	35			25–100	245
	15	>16	>16	16–>16	817
Serratia species	10		20–50	12–>50	752
Shigella species	10			(2.5)	44
Tissierella praeacuta	30	1	64	≤0.06–64	567
Xanthomonas maltophila	14			<1–31.3	243
	14	7.8		0.5–31.3	812
Yersinia enterocolitica	74		12.5	0.20–25	606
Yersinia frederiksensii	2		3.12[b]	3.12[b]	606
Yersinia intermedia	2		6.25[b]	3.12–6.25	606
Yersinia kristensensii	12		12.5[b]	0.78–12.5	606
Yersinia pestis	78	4	8	2–8	674
	100	2.0	8.0	<0.03–8.0	253
Yersinia pseudotuberculosis	1		3.12		606
Mycobacteria					
Mycobacterium abscessus	1			>20	621
Mycobacterium acapulcensis	1			2.5	621
Mycobacterium asiaticum	10			>1	290
Mycobacterium aurum	1			10	621

continued

TABLE 1 • Summary Table of Susceptibilities to Rifampicin

Organism	No. of Isolates	MIC$_{50}$ μg/mL	MIC$_{90}$ μg/mL	Range or (MIC, unspecified) μg/mL	Reference
Mycobacterium avium-	35	≤0.12	2	≤0.12–4	347
intracellulare complex	52	6.25	50	0.78->100	624
	523	10			325
	16	2.0	8.0	0.25–16	326
Mycobacterium borstelense	1			>20	621
Mycobacterium bovis	38		1		290
Mycobacterium bovis-BCG	22		1		290
Mycobacterium celatum	2			128–256	719
Mycobacterium chelonae	15	>64	>64	>64	714
	60		>5		325
	16	64		0.25–≥256	242
Mycobacterium chelonae	1			50	178
subsp. abscessus	20	>100	>100	50->100	624
Mycobacterium chelonae	20	>100	>100	25->100	624
subsp. chelonae					
Mycobacterium	5	>16		0.25->16	347
chelonae-fortuitum					
Mycobacterium chitae	2			10–20	621
Mycobacterium diernhoferi	1			20	621
Mycobacterium fallax	10	≤0.25	4	≤0.25–16	454
Mycobacterium flavescens	1			25	178
	15			≥1	290
Mycobacterium fortuitum	18	>64	>64	16->64	714
	17	5	>20		734
	10			>16	628
	30	>10			325
	9	>8		>8	735
	28	64		0.125–≥256	242
	20	50	100	12.5–100	624
Mycobacterium gastri	4	1			290
Mycobacterium gordonae	32		1[b]	1[b]	325
	141	1			290
Mycobacterium haemophilum	17	0.5	1.0	0.5–2.0	83
	3			0.25–1	43
Mycobacterium intracellulare	20	0.5	2		766
Mycobacterium kansasii	6			0.1–0.5	480
	10	1.25	1.25		734
	13	≤0.25	0.5		766
	32		1[b]	1[b]	325
	8	1			163
	1			1	280
	10	0.25		0.125–0.5	735
	19	0.2	3.13	0.025–3.13	624
	71	1.0			290
Mycobacterium leprae	N/A			(<1)	115
Mycobacterium malmoense	1			1	816
	47	1			290
Mycobacterium marinum	17	0.5	1		766
	12		1[b]	1[b]	325
	10			0.4–1.6	795
	1			1.25	792
	28			(1)	746
	10			(1.56)	625
	11			1.25–2.5	621
	5	0.25		0.25–0.5	735
	10	0.2	0.39	0.1–0.39	624
	33		1.0[b]	1.0[b]	290
Mycobacterium microti	1			0.0025–0.040	202
Mycobacterium parafortuitum	1			10	621
	1			50	178
Mycobacterium phlei	12		≤0.32		621
Mycobacterium runyonii	1			>20	621

continued

TABLE 1 • Summary Table of Susceptibilities to Rifampicin

Organism	No. of Isolates	MIC$_{50}$ μg/mL	MIC$_{90}$ μg/mL	Range or (MIC, unspecified) μg/mL	Reference
Mycobacterium scrofulaceum	19	1.56	12.5		625
	19	0.78	6.25	0.1–6.25	624
	51			≥1	290
Mycobacterium simiae	3		>10[b]	>10[b]	325
	2			>25	412
	28			(>1)	290
Mycobacterium smegmatis	1			17	418
	27	>16	>16	4–>16	765
	2			50	178
Mycobacterium szulgai	23	1			290
	9		5.0[b]	5.0[b]	638
	1		1.0[b]	1.0[b]	185
Mycobacterium terrae	7		5	1–5	325
	64			≥1	290
Mycobacterium thermoresistibile	1			1	517
	1			1	779
	1			1	791
Mycobacterium trivale	2		1[b]	1[b]	290
Mycobacterium tuberculosis rifampicin sensitive	16	0.1	0.2	0.025–0.2	624
Mycobacterium tuberculosis rifampicin resistant	6	100	100	50–100	624
Mycobacterium ulcerans	N/A			(0.005–0.2)	240
Mycobacterium vaccae	1			2.5	621
	1			6.25	178
Mycobacterium xenopi	3		1[b]	1[b]	325
	34	1			163
	1			<1[t], 1.5[u]	594
	25		1		290
	40			0.5–2	720
	7			1	667

Rickettsia

Organism	No. of Isolates	MIC$_{50}$ μg/mL	MIC$_{90}$ μg/mL	Range or (MIC, unspecified) μg/mL	Reference
Afipia felis	3			4	474
Bartonella elizabethae	1			0.03	477
Bartonella henselae	1			<0.125	475
	3			0.03–0.06	477
Bartonella quintana	1			<0.125	475
	2	0.008–0.016	0.022–0.028		512
	9	0.12	0.25	0.06–0.25	477
Bartonella vinsonii	1			<0.125	475
	1			0.12	477
Coxiella burnetii	1			0.5	803
Coxiella burnetii, "S" isolate	1	0.02	0.05		805
Coxiella burnetii, Nine Mile isolate	1	0.08	0.3		805
Ehrlichia chaffeensis	1			0.125	107
Ehrlichia risticii	1			0.5	106
Ehrlichia sennetsu	1			0.5	106
Agent of human granulocytic ehrlichiosis (HGE)	3			0.5	401
Rickettsia azadi	1			0.25–0.5	588
Rickettsia conorii	1			0.25	591
Rickettsia prowazekii	1			0.008	790
	1			>0.001–≤0.01	790
Rickettsia rickettsii	1			0.5	591

Other

Organism	No. of Isolates	MIC$_{50}$ μg/mL	MIC$_{90}$ μg/mL	Range or (MIC, unspecified) μg/mL	Reference
Chlamydia trachomatis	2			0.005–0.007	378
	22		0.125	(0.060–500)	237
	1			0.008	725
	N/A			(0.008)	100

continued

TABLE 1 • Summary Table of Susceptibilities to Rifampicin

Organism	No. of Isolates	MIC$_{50}$ μg/mL	MIC$_{90}$ μg/mL	Range or (MIC, unspecified) μg/mL	Reference
Mycoplasma genitalium	7			32–64	597
Mycoplasma hominis	N/A			1.6–>100	785
Mycoplasma pneumoniae	3			64–128	597
	11	64	128	≤0.06–128	785
Treponema denticola	1			>20	585
Treponema socranskii	N/A			(>20)	585
Treponema vincentii	N/A			(>20)	585
Ureaplasma urealyticum	20	≥128	≥128	≥128	785
Fungi					
Aspergillus flavus	9	≥1000	>1000	≥1000	353
	3	≥1000		500–1000	399
Aspergillus fumigatus	17	≥1000	≥1000	≥1000	353
	3			1000[b]	399
Aspergilllus niger	5		≥1000	≥1000	353
Blastomyces dermatitidis	1			12.5	400
Fusarium proliferatum	1			500–1000	696
Histoplasma capsulatum	1			80	403
	1			>100	400
Trichosporon beigelii (*T. cutaneum*)	1			>50	463
Parasites					
Acanthamoeba castellani	1			>10	361
Leishmania aethiopica	1			100	231
Leishmania donovani	1			500	231
	1			20	39
Leishmania tropica major	1			500	231
Leishmania tropica minor	1			500	231
Naegleria fowleri	1			>50	652

N/A, not available.

Note: Methodologies and media vary between reports.

[a] Includes 4 *Clostridium malenominatum*, 2 *C. scatogenes*, 1 *C. sporogenes*, 1 *C. tyrobutyricum*, 4 *Eubacterium combesii*, 2 *E. brachy*, 1 *E. nitritogenes*, and 1 *Propionibacterium acidiopropionici*.

[b] MIC$_{100}$.

[c] Includes *Clostridium perfringens* and *C. beijerinckij*.

[d] pH = 7.4.

[e] pH = 8.5.

[f] Includes 4 *Corynebacterium aquaticum*, 2 *C. diphtheriae*, 6 *C. ulcerans*, 4 *C. pseudotuberculosis*, and 4 *C. renale*.

[g] Includes 20 *Pediococcus acidilactici* and 3 *P. pentosaceus*.

[h] Includes *Pediococcus acidilactici, P. pentosaceus, P. urinaeequi*.

[i] Includes 14 *Pediococcus acidilactici* and 7 *P. pentosaceus*.

[j] Includes 26 *Peptostreptococcus anaerobius*, 4 *P. asaccharolyticus*, and 5 *P. prevotii*.

[k] Includes *Staphylococcus saprophyticus, S. hominis, S. warneri, S. simulans, S. scuri, S. capitis*, and *S. cohnii*.

[l] Includes *Staphylococcus simulans, S. hominis, S. saprophyticus*.

[m] Includes *Staphylococcus capitus, S. cohnii, S. haemolyticus, S. hominus, S. saprophyticus, S. simulans, S. warneri*, and *S. xylosus*.

[n] Includes 127 *Streptococcus mitis*, 41 *S. sanguis* II, 17 *S. sanguis*, 52 *S. salivarius*, 9 *S. oralis*, 4 *S. milleri*, 22 *S. sanguis* I, 2 *S. intermedius*, 2 *S. milleri*, 1 *S. anginosus*, and 1 *S. equinus*.

[o] Geometric mean MIC.

[p] Includes *Bacteroides eggerthii, B. melaninogenicus, B. oralis, B. ruminicola, B. uniformis*.

[q] Includes *Brucella abortus, B. canis, B. melitensis, B. neotomae, B. ovis*, and *B. suis*.

[r] Includes 3 *Legionella bozemanii*, 3 *L. longbeachae*, 2 *L. dumoffii*, 1 *L. gormanii*, 1 *L. erythra*, and 1 *L. micadei*.

[s] Includes 15 *Proteus mirabilis*, 11 *P. morganii*, 6 *P. rettgeri*, and 3 *P. vulgaris*.

[t] 7H9 broth.

[u] 7H11 agar.

TABLE 2 • Summary Table of Susceptibilities to Rifabutin

Organism	No. of Isolates	MIC$_{50}$ μg/mL	MIC$_{90}$ μg/mL	Range or (MIC, unspecified) μg/mL	Reference
Gram-positive bacilli					
Bacillus subtilis	1			0.016	259
Clostridium botulinum A	1			0.0313	259
Clostridium botulinum B	1			0.0078	259
Clostridium histolyticum	1			0.016	259
Clostridium perfringens	1			0.007	194
	1			0.016	259
Eubacterium aerofaciens	1			0.0078	259
Eubacterium lentum	1			≤0.00003	259
Eubacterium limosum	1			≤0.00003	259
Gram-positive cocci					
Enterococcus faecalis	1			2.5	194
	1			0.125	259
Micrococcus luteus	1			0.0039	259
Peptostreptococcus anaerobis	1			0.0005	259
Peptostreptococcus asaccharolyticus	1			≤0.00003	259
Peptostreptococcus magnus	1			0.0078	259
Staphylococcus aureus	1			0.005	194
Staphylococcus aureus methicillin susceptible	20	0.016	0.0313	0.002–0.0625	259
Staphylococcus aureus methicillin resistant	20	0.0313	0.0625	0.0313–0.0625	259
Staphylococcus aureus methicillin and quinolone resistant	16	0.0313	2	0.016–2	259
Staphylococcus epidermidis	20	0.0313	0.0625	0.016–0.0625	259
Staphylococcus haemolyticus	1			0.075	194
Streptococcus pneumoniae	20	0.0039	0.0313	0.005–0.25	259
Streptococcus pyogenes	20	0.016	0.016	0.002–0.0313	259
Gram-negative cocci					
Neisseria gonorrhoeae non-penicillinase-producing	31	0.78	0.78	0.2–1.56	259
Neisseria gonorrhoeae penicillinase producing	13	0.78	1.56	0.39–3.13	259
Veillonella parvula	1			1	259
Gram-negative bacilli					
Acinetobacter calcoaceticus	1			4	259
Bacteroides fragilis	1			0.0313	259
	1			0.075	194
Bacteroides vulgatus	1			0.0078	259
Campylobacter jejuni	200	0.31	0.62	0.31–0.62	743
Citrobacter species	2			10	194
Enterobacter cloacae	2			25	421
Enterobacter species	6			14.10[a]	194
Escherichia coli	1			16	259
	3			6.25–25	421
	10			0.01–10	736
	9			5.95[a]	194
Fusobacterium mortiferum	1			>32	259
Fusobacterium nucleatum	1			2	259
Fusobacterium varium	1			>32	259
Haemophilus ducreyi	38	0.08	0.016	0.004–0.016	1
Haemophilus influenzae	20	0.5	0.5	0.125–2	259
	1			0.62	194
Helicobacter pylori	49		0.0078		421
Klebsiella pneumoniae	1			16	259
	2			25	421
	1			10	194
Klebsiella species	9			15.42[a]	194
Legionella micdadei	1			0.078	733

continued

TABLE 2 • **Summary Table of Susceptibilities to Rifabutin**

Organism	No. of Isolates	MIC$_{50}$ μg/mL	MIC$_{90}$ μg/mL	Range or (MIC, unspecified) μg/mL	Reference
Legionella pneumophila	12		0.078		733
Proteus vulgaris	1			5	194
Proteus species	9			22.45[a]	194
Pseudomonas aerugnosa	1			20	194
	1			16	259
	3			0.01–30	736
Pseudomonas inconstans	1			2.5	194
Pseudomonas species	5			>20[a]	194
Salmonella typhimurium	1			4	259
	1			16	259
	10			0.01–10	736
Serratia marcescens	1			32	259
Mycobacteria					
Mycobacterium avium complex	52	0.39	1.56	0.025–100	624
	523		2.0		325
	21	0.5	2	0.25–64	386
	16	0.5	1.0	0.063–2.0	326
Mycobacterium bovis	N/A			(<2)	421
Mycobacterium celatum	2			0.5	719
	2			8	470
Mycobacterium chelonae	18	32	64	2–64	454
	N/A			(32)	421
	N/A			(>5)	587
	60		(>2.0)		325
Mycobacterium chelonae subsp. *abscessus*	20	12.5	25	3.13–25	624
Mycobacterium chelonae subsp. *chelonae*	20	12.5	50	3.13–50	624
Mycobacterium fallax	10	≤0.25	1	≤0.25–1	454
	N/A			(<2)	421
Mycobacterium flavescens	N/A			(>5)	587
Mycobacterium fortuitum	17	1.25	2.5		734
	28	1	8	≤0.25–8	454
	N/A			(>5)	587
	20	3.13	6.25	1.56–6.25	624
	30	>2.0			325
Mycobacterium gastri	N/A			(≤1)	587
Mycobacterium gordonae	32		0.5[b]	0.5[b]	325
	N/A			(≤1)	587
Mycobacterium haemophilum	17	≤0.03	≤0.03	≤0.03–0.06	83
	3			0.25–1	43
Mycobacterium intracellulare	20	0.25	1		766
Mycobacterium kansasii	10	0.075	0.075		734
	13	≤0.25	≤0.25		766
	21			0.25[b]	339
	32			0.5[b]	325
	19	0.025	0.1	≤0.0125–0.2	624
Mycobacterium malmoense	1			0.12	816
Mycobacterium marinum	17	≤0.25	≤0.25		766
	12			0.5[b]	325
	N/A			(≤1)	587
	10	0.1	0.1	0.025–0.2	624
Mycobacterium microti	N/A			(<2)	421
	1			0.0015–0.026	202
Mycobacterium paratuberculosis	8	0.06		0.03–0.25	143, 144
Mycobacterium phlei	N/A			(<2)	421
Mycobacterium scrofulaceum	N/A			(<2)	421
	N/A			(≤1)	421
	19	0.2	1.56	0.025–100	624

continued

TABLE 2 • Summary Table of Susceptibilities to Rifabutin

Organism	No. of Isolates	MIC$_{50}$ µg/mL	MIC$_{90}$ µg/mL	Range or (MIC, unspecified) µg/mL	Reference
Mycobacterium simiae	3			>2[b]	325
	N/A			(>5)	587
	1			0.5	470
	1			8	405
Mycobacterium smegmatis	27	4	8	1–8	765
Mycobacterium szulgai	N/A			(>5)	587
Mycobacterium terrae	7		1.0[b]	(0.5[c])	325
	N/A			(≤1)	587
Mycobacterium thermoresistible	1			2.0	791
	1			0.5	517
Mycobacterium triviale	N/A			(≤1)	587
Mycobacterium tuberculosis rifampicin sensitive	16	0.025	0.5	0.025–0.05	624
	180			0.5[b]	325
Mycobacterium tuberculosis rifampicin resistant	6	12.5	12.5	6.25–12.5	624
	122	2.0			325
Mycobacterium ulcerans	N/A			(<2)	421
Mycobacterium xenopi	3			0.5[b]	325
	N/A			(≤1)	587
	40		0.5	0.5–2	720
	1			0.5	470
	1			0.1[d], 0.25[e]	594
Rickettsia					
Agent of human granulocytic ehrlichiosis (HGE)	3			(≤0.125)	401
Other					
Chlamydia trachomatis	1			0.009	725
	21			0.007–0.030	237
Toxoplasma gondii	1	1.68		1.63–1.71	612
	1	26.5			531

N/A, not available.

Note: Methodologies and media vary between reports.

[a] Geometric mean.

[b] 100% of isolates susceptible.

[c] 71.4% of isolates susceptible.

[d] 7H9 broth.

[e] 7H11 agar.

ducing bacterial totals in vegetations and in early sterilization of vegetations (748). The combination of rifampicin plus a β-lactam antibiotic did not prevent emergence of resistance in vivo in an experimental model of endocarditis in rabbits (33).

Streptococcus pneumoniae. In experimental pneumococcal meningitis in rabbits, addition of rifampicin to ofloxacin resulted in indifference, with a trend toward reduced activity (516).

Gram-Negative Bacilli
Bacteroides fragilis. In a mouse model, rifampicin was superior to clindamycin in eradicating *B. fragilis* from experimentally induced abscesses and in reducing the incidence of abscess formation. Rifampicin achieved higher levels in the abscess fluid, with a longer half-life than clindamycin (257). A subsequent study also demonstrated the efficacy of

rifampicin against mixed intraabdominal infections with *B. fragilis* and *Pseudomonas aeruginosa* (258).

Brucella melitensis, Brucella abortus, Brucella Species. In an experimental model of murine brucellosis with *B. melitensis,* both intraperitoneal and oral rifampicin were effective in curing splenic infections. Given orally, rifampicin (20 and 25 mg/kg/day for 21 days) cured all animals, although lower cure rates were seen when it was given for 14 days (663). In another murine model, synergy was demonstrated with the combination of streptomycin plus rifampicin. Synergy was also seen in time-kill experiments (428).

Campylobacter Species. Selective media designed to grow *Campylobacter* species contain a number of antibiotics including rifampicin. When the inhibition of aerotolerant *Campylobacter* species by these antibiotics was assessed, 59% of 64 isolates of *C. butzleri* tested were susceptible to

TABLE 3 • **Summary Table of Susceptibilities to Rifaximin**

Organism	No. of Isolates	MIC$_{50}$ μg/mL	MIC$_{90}$ μg/mL	Range or (MIC, unspecified) μg/mL	Reference
Gram-positive bacilli					
Bacillus cereus	7	0.06		0.03–0.12	347
Bifidobacterium species	6	0.8	6.2	0.4–50	228
Clostridium beijerinckij	2			0.05–0.1	228
Clostridium difficile	4	0.2	0.8	0.2–0.8	228
	56	0.39	100	0.10–>100	606
Clostridium perfringens	15		0.25[a]	0.25[a]	426
	2		0.1		228
Clostridium species	26	0.4	50	0.0125–>100	228
Eubacterium species	14	0.2	0.4	0.05–6.2	228
Lactobacillus species	31	0.12	0.5	≤0.03–1	347
Propionibacterium acnes	2			0.05	228
Propionibacterium species	10	0.2	12.5	0.025–12.5	228
Gram-positive cocci					
Enterococcus faecalis	21	2	8	0.5–>8	347
Enterococcus faecium	11	2	>8	<0.015–>8	347
Enterococcus species[b]	10	0.25	2	≤0.015–>4	347
Peptococcus species	19	0.1	3.1	0.025–>100	228
Peptostreptococcus species	28	0.2	25	0.025–>100	228
Staphylococcus aureus	30	0.022–0.045	0.7–1.5	≤0.005–3	752
Staphylococcus aureus oxacillin susceptible	40	0.015	≤0.015	≤0.015–0.03	347
Staphylococcus aureus oxacillin resistant	11	≤0.015	>8	0.015–>8	347
Staphylococcus epidermidis	20	≤0.015	≤0.015	≤0.015	347
Staphylococcus haemolyticus	10	≤0.015	≤0.015	≤0.015–>8	347
Staphylococcus species coagulase negative[c]	20	≤0.015	≤0.015	≤0.015	347
Streptococcus agalactiae	20	0.12	0.25	0.06–0.25	347
Streptococcus species Groups C, F, and G	14	≤0.03	0.06	≤0.03–0.5	347
Streptococcus pneumoniae	30	≤0.03	0.06	≤0.03–>4	347
Streptococcus pyogenes	19	0.12	0.25	≤0.03–0.25	347
Gram-negative cocci					
Moraxella catarrhalis	20	≤0.03	≤0.03	≤0.03–0.06	347
Neisseria species[d]	16	0.5	2	≤0.03–2	347
Neisseria gonorrhoeae penicillin susceptible	35	0.25	16	0.12–>16	347
Neisseria gonorrhoeae penicillin resistant (PPNG[e])	14	0.25	8	0.12–16	347
Neisseria gonorrhoeae penicillin resistant (CMRNG[f])	11	0.25	0.25	0.25–1	347
Gram-negative bacilli					
Acinetobacter species	10	2	4	0.06–4	347
Bacteroides bivius-disiens	*40*	*0.12*	*0.25*	≤0.03–0.5	347
Bacteroides distasonis	1			0.0125	228
Bacteroides fragilis	75			≤0.06–<64	426
	14	0.1	12.5	0.025–>100	228
Bacteroides ovatus	3			0.1–0.4	228
Bacteroides thetaiotaomicron	2			0.05–0.8	228
Bacteroides vulgatus	1			0.05	228
Bacteroides species[g]	17		0.5[a]	0.5[a]	426
Bacteroides species[h]	59	0.1	50	0.025–>100	228
Campylobacter jejuni	54	≥6.25	>100	0.78–>100	606
Citrobacter amalonatica	2			4–>8	347
Citrobacter diversus	10	>8	>8	4–>8	347
Citrobacter freundii	20	>8	>8	>8	347
Citrobacter species	4			12.5–>25	752
Enterobacter aerogenes	20	>8	>8	4–>8	347
Enterobacter agglomerans	10	4	8	1–8	347

continued

TABLE 3 • Summary Table of Susceptibilities to Rifaximin

Organism	No. of Isolates	MIC$_{50}$ μg/mL	MIC$_{90}$ μg/mL	Range or (MIC, unspecified) μg/mL	Reference
Enterobacter cloacae	20	>8	>8	0.25->8	347
Enterobacter sakazakii	2			4->8	347
Enterobacter taylorae	1			4->8	347
Enterobacter species	6		12–50[a]	12–50	752
Escherichia coli	20	8	>8	2->8	347
	15	3.12–6.25	12.5–25	0.7->25	752
Fusobacterium species	10	0.4	50	0.05->100	228
Gardnerella vaginalis	23	0.5	1	0.25–1	347
Haemophilus ducreyi	25	0.25	0.5	0.03–0.5	347
Haemophilus influenzae	58	0.25	2	≤0.03–2	347
Hafnia alvei	2			4->8	347
Helicobacter pylori	29	8	16	2–64	347
	40	4	8	4–16	345
Klebsiella oxytoca	10	>8	>8	8->8	347
Klebsiella ozaenae	2			4->8	347
Klebsiella pneumoniae	20	>≥8	>8	8->8	347
Mobiluncus species	13	≤0.03	≤003	≤0.03	347
Morganella morganii	10	>8	>8	4->8	347
Proteus mirabilis	20	4	4	1–4	347
Proteus vulgaris	10	4	4	2->8	347
Proteus species	26	6.25–12.5	12.5–25	3.12->50	752
Providencia rettgeri	10	8	>8	2->8	347
Providencia stuartii	10	4	4	2–4	347
Pseudomonas aeruginosa	28	8	>8	4->8	347
Salmonella enteritidis	10	2	8	2->8	347
Salmonella paratyphi	1			6	461
Salmonella species	56	3.12–6.25	6.25–12.5	0.78->25	752
Serratia liquefaciens	1			4->8	347
Serratia marcescens	20	>8	>8	4->8	347
Serratia species	10	25–50		12->50	752
Shigella species	10	4	8	2->8	347
Xanthomonas maltophilia	10	8	<8	≤0.015-<8	347
Yersinia enterocolitica	10	8	>8	4->8	347
	74		12.5[a]	0.20–12.5	606
Yersinia frederiksenii	2		3.12[a]	3.12[a]	606
Yersinia intermedia	2		3.12[a]	1.56–3.12	606
Yersinia kristensenii	12		12.5[a]	0.39–12.5	606
Yersinia pseudotuberculosis	1		6.25		606
Mycobacteria					
Mycobacterium avium-intracellulare complex	35	0.5	1	≤0.12–2	347
Mycobacterium chelonae-fortuitum	5	8		2–16	347
Other					
Candida species[i]	23	>5000	>5000	>5000	347
Chlamydia trachomatis	7			25–30	574
Herpes virus	10	>512	>512	>512	347
Mycoplasma hominis	20	64	>64	64->64	347
Trichomonas vaginalis	10	>256	>256	>256	347
Ureaplasma urealyticum	25	>64	>64	32->64	347

Note: Methodologies and media vary between reports.

[a] MIC$_{100}$.

[b] Includes 2 Enterococcus gallinarum, 2 E. casselifavus, 2 E. raffinosus, 1 E. mundtii, 1 E. durans, 1 E. avium, 1 E. hirae.

[c] Includes Staphylococcus warneri, S. simulans, S. saprophyticus, S. hominis, and S. xylosus.

[d] Includes Neisseria meningitidis, N. mucosa, N. sicca, and N. subflava.

[e] PPNG, penicillinase-producing N. gonorrhoeae.

[f] CMRNG, chromosomally resistant N. gonorrhoeae.

[g] Includes Bacteroides eggerthii, B. melaninogenicus, B. oralis, B. ruminicola, B. uniformis.

[h] Includes Bacteroides ovatus, B. distasonis, B. vulgatus, B. thetaiotaomicron, Bacteroides group 3452 A.

[i] Candida albicans, C. glabrata (now known as Torulopsis glabrata), C. krusei, C. parapsilosis, and C. tropicalis.

TABLE 4 • In Vitro Synergy/Combination Studies with Rifamycins

Organism	RMP[a]	RBT[b]	Other Antibiotics[c]	Result[d]	Reference
Gram-positive bacilli					
Clostridium difficile	x		Bacitracin	S	48
	x		Vancomycin	S, AD	48
	x		Metronidazole	S, AD	48
Clostridium species	x		Fleroxacin	I, AD	817
Corynebacterium bovis	x		Erythromycin	PNS	97
Listeria monocytogenes	x		Penicillin	I	640
	x		Ampicillin	A	788
	x		Levofloxacin	A	492
	x		Sparfloxacin	A	492
	x		Clinafloxacin	A	492
Rhodococcus equi	x		Erythromycin	S	577
	x		Gentamicin	A	577
	x		Erythromycin	I	527
Gram-positive cocci					
Enterococcus species	x		Penicillin	I	495
	x		Vancomycin	I	495
	x		Fleroxacin	I	817
	x		Ampicillin	A	364
Enterococcus faecalis	x		Gentamicin	I	495
Enterococcus faecium	x		Gentamicin	I	495
	x		Gentamicin, ciprofloxacin	PNS	442
	x		Novobiocin	A	255
Staphylococcus aureus	x		Fleroxacin	I	817
	x		Oxacillin	S, A, I	741
	x		Nafcillin	S	731
	x		Vancomycin	S	731
	x		Vancomycin	A	776
	x		Trimethoprim	A	109
Staphylococcus aureus, methicillin sensitive	x		Fleroxacin	AD	817
	x		Minocycline	S	650
	x		Cephalothin	I	524
	x		Trimethoprim	A	524
Staphylococcus aureus, methicillin resistant	x		Minocycline	S	650
	x		Fleroxacin	I	610
Staphylococcus epidermidis	x		Vancomycin, gentamicin	S	811
	x		Vancomycin	A	811
	x		Gentamicin	S, I	811
	x		Dicloxacillin	S, I	811
	x		Fusidic acid	S, I	811
	x		Dicloxacillin, fusidic acid	S, I	811
	x		Fleroxacin	A, S, I	415
	x		Cephazolin	A, I	415
Staphylococcus epidermidis, methicillin resistant	x		Fleroxacin	I	817
	x		Nafcillin	S, A, I	33
	x		Gentamicin, vancomycin, cephalothin	A, I, AD	33
Coagulase-negative staphylococci[e], methicillin sensitive	x		Minocycline	S	650
Coagulase-negative staphylococci[e], methicillin resistant	x		Minocycline	S	650
Streptococcus agalatiae	x		Penicillin	S, A, I	456
	x		Ampicillin	A	676
	x		Fleroxacin	S, A, I	817
Streptococcus pneumoniae	x		Fleroxacin	I	817
	x		Penicillin	A	286
	x		Ceftriaxone	A	286
	x		L-ofloxacin	A	286
Streptococcus pyogenes	x		Trimethoprim	S	109
Groups A, B, C, and G streptococci	x		Fleroxacin	I, AD	817

continued

TABLE 4 • In Vitro Synergy/Combination Studies with Rifamycins

Organism	RMP[a]	RBT[b]	Other Antibiotics[c]	Result[d]	Reference
Gram-negative cocci					
Neisseria gonorrhoeae	x		Trimethoprim	A	109
Gram-negative bacilli					
Acinetobacter species	x		Fleroxacin	S	817
Actinobacillus	x		Penicillin	S, AD, A, I	808
actinomycemcomitans	x		Ceftriaxone	S, AD, I	808
	x		Cephapirin	AD, A, I	808
	x		Fleroxacin	I	817
Bacteroides fragilis	x		Trimethoprim	S	109, 388
Enterobacter cloacae	x		Fleroxacin	I	817
Enterobacter species	x		Trimethoprim	S	109
	x		Imipenem	S, AD, I	141
	x		Imipenem, ciprofloxacin	S	141
Escherichia coli	x		Fleroxacin	I	817
	x		Trimethoprim	S, AD	109
Haemophilus influenzae	x		Cefuroxime	S	292
	x		Ceftazidime	S	292
	x		Ceftriaxone	S	292
	x		Cefotaxime	S	292
	x		Fleroxacin	S	817
	x		Trimethoprim	S	109
	x		Ampicillin	AD, I	371
	x		Chloramphenicol	AD, I	371
Helicobacter pylori	x		Bismuth subcitrate	S	740
Klebsiella pneumoniae	x		Trimethoprim	S	109
	x		Fleroxacin	AD, I	817
Legionella pneumophila	x		Erythromycin	S	496
	x		Ciprofloxacin	I	496
	x		Ofloxacin	S	49
	x		Levofloaxacin	S	49
	x		Erythromycin	I	571
	x		Cefoxitin	I	571
	x		Fleroxacin	I	571
	x		RPR 106972[f]	AD, I	556
Legionella species[g]	x		RPR 106972[f]	AD, I	556
Morganella morganii	x		Fleroxacin	I	817
Proteus mirabilis	x		Fleroxacin	S	817
	x		Trimethoprim	S	109
Proteus morganii	x		Trimethoprim	S	109
Proteus rettgeri	x		Trimethoprim	S	109
Proteus vulgaris	x		Fleroxacin	S	817
	x		Trimethoprim	S	109, 388
Providencia stuartii	x		Trimethoprim	AD	109
	x		Fleroxacin	I	817
Pseudomonas aeruginosa	x		Trimethoprim	S	109, 388
	x		Fleroxacin	AD, I	817
	x		Imipenem	S, AD, I	141
	x		Imipenem, ciprofloxacin	S	141
	x		Ceftazidime, gentamicin	S, AD, I, A	738
	x		Ceftazidime, tobramycin	S, AD, I, A	738
	x		Ceftazidime, amikacin	S, AD, I, A	738
	x		Cefpirome, gentamicin	S, AD, I, A	738
	x		Cefpirome, tobramycin	S, AD, I, A	738
	x		Cefpirome, amikacin	S, AD, I, A	738
	x		Ticarcillin, tobramycin	S	821
Pseudomonas cepacia	x		Imipenem	S	417
	x		Ticarcillin, imipenem	S	417
	x		Tobramycin, imipenem	S	417
	x		Tobrmycin, imipenem	S	417
Salmonella typhi	x		Novobicin	S	662
Salmonella typhimurium	x		Trimethoprim	AD	109, 388

continued

TABLE 4   •   In Vitro Synergy/Combination Studies with Rifamycins

Organism	RMP[a]	RBT[b]	Other Antibiotics[c]	Result[d]	Reference
Serratia marcescens	x		Fleroxacin	I	817
	x		Trimethoprim	S	109
	x		Imipenem	AD, I	141
	x		Imipenem, Ciprofloxacin	S	141
Pseudoonas maltophila	x		TMP/SMX, carbenicillin	S	812
	x		Gentamicin, carbenicillin	S	812
Mycobacteria					
Mycobacterium		x	Ethambutol	S, AD	326, 386
avium-intracellulare	x		Ethambutol	S, AD	326
		x	Clarithromycin	S, AD, I	386
		x	Ciprofloxacin	AD, I, A	386
		x	Amikacin	AD, I, A	386
Mycobacterium kansasii	x		Ethambutol	S	339
		x	Ethambutol	S, AD	339
Mycobacterium malmoense	x		Ethambutol	S, AD	343
		x	Ethambutol	S, AD	343
	x		Ethambutol	S	55
	x		Streptomycin	AD	55
Mycobacterium paratuberculosis		x	Cefazolin	S	143
		x	Cefazolin, ethambutol	S	143
		x	Cefazolin, streptomycin	S	143
Mycobacterium xenopi	x		Ethambutol	S	55
	x		Streptomycin	AD	55
Rickettsia					
Coxiella burnetii,	x		Ciprofloxacin	S	804
Priscilla isolate					
Fungi					
Aspergillus fumigatus	x		Amphotericin B	S	353, 399, 686
Aspergillus flavus	x		Amphotericin B	S	353, 399
Aspergillus niger	x		Amphotericin B	S	353, 686
Aspergillus species	x		Amphotericin B	S, I	198
Candida species	x		Amphotericin B	S	25, 72, 73, 227, 686
Candida albicans	x		Amphotericin B	S	73, 451, 686
				S, A	227
	x		Miconazole	S	498
	x		Miconazole nitrate	S	498
	x		Ketoconazole	I	498
				A	490
	x		Fluconazole	S, I	687
	x		Amphotericin B,	AD	295
			ketoconazole		
Candida guilliermondii	x		Amphotericin B	S, A	227
				S	73
Candida krusei	x		Amphotericin B	S	73, 686
	x		Miconazole	S	498
	x		Miconazole nitrate	S	498
	x		Ketoconazole	I	498
Candida parapsilosis	x		Amphotericin B	S	73, 686
				S, A	227
Candida pseudotropicalis	x		Amphotericin B	S	73
	x		Ketoconazole	A	490
Candida stellatoidea	x		Amphotericin B	S, A	227
				S	73
	x		Ketoconazole	A	490
Candida tropicalis	x		Amphotericin B	S, A	227
	x		Miconazole	S	498
	x		Miconazole nitrate	S	498
	x		Ketoconazole	I	498
				A	490

continued

TABLE 4 • In Vitro Synergy/Combination Studies with Rifamycins

Organism	RMP[a]	RBT[b]	Other Antibiotics[c]	Result[d]	Reference
Coccidioides immitis	x		Itraconzaole	S	732
	x		Amphotericin B	S	603
				I	363
Cryptococcus neoformans	x		Amphotericin B	S	260, 797
	x		Fluconazole	S	687
	x		Itraconazole	S	732
Fusarium solani	x		Amphotericin B	S	686
	x		Natamycin	S	686
Histoplasma capsulatum	x		Amphotericin B	S	403, 486
Malassezia furfur	x		Itraconazole	I	732
Paecilomyces lilacinus	x		Amphotericin B	I	686
Penicillium species	x		Amphotericin B	S	686
Rhizopus arrhyzus	x		Amphotericin B	S	686
Rhizopus oryzae	x		Amphotericin B	S	686
Rhizopus species	x		Amphotericin B	S	332
Rhodotorula species	x		Amphotericin B	S	686
Saccharomyces brevicaulis	x		Amphotericin B	I	686
Saccharomyces cerevisiae	x		Amphotericin B	S	67, 487
Torulopsis glabrata	x		Miconazole	S	498
	x		Miconazole nitrate	S	498
	x		Ketoconazole	I	498
Trichosporon beigelii	x		Amphotericin B	S	463
Parasites					
Leishmania tropica	x		Amphotericin B	S	232
Toxoplasma gondii		x	Atovaquone	S	612

Note: Definition of synergy and methodologies vary among studies, and all effects of the combinations were not included in all reports.

[a] RMP, rifampicin.

[b] RBT, rifabutin.

[c] TMP/SMX, trimethoprim/sulfamethoxazole.

[d] S, synergy; A, antagonism; I, indifference; AD, additive; V, variable; NS, precise result not specified; PNS, positive effect, but precise result not specified.

[e] Includes *Staphylococcus hominis* and *S. haemolyticus.*

[f] RPR 106972 is a new oral streptogramin.

[g] Includes 3 *Legionella bozemanii,* 3 *L. longbeachae,* 2 *L. dumoffii,* 1 *L. gormanii,* 1 *L. erythra,* and 1 *L. micadei.*

rifampicin at a concentration of 10 U/mL, the concentration found in some media, and 50 and 17% of two groups of *C. cryaerophila* were susceptible (394).

Legionella pneumophila, Legionella Species. Intracellular inhibition of *Legionella* by rifampicin has been reported in human macrophages (759) and in peripheral human monocytes (323). Intracellular concentrations of rifampicin of 0.005 μg/mL in guinea pig alveolar phagocytes inhibit *L. pneumophila* (247). Administration of rifampicin by small-particle aerosol was an effective treatment in a guinea pig pneumonia model (248). Prophylactic rifampicin at a minimum dose of 0.02 mg was effective in preventing deaths with *L. pneumophila* in embryonated eggs. Rifampicin also proved very effective in treatment of infection in this model (438). In the guinea pig animal model, rifampicin was considered to be at least additive and possibly synergistic with erythromycin against *L. pneumophila* (252). In another report using a guinea pig model, no differences were seen between rifampicin, ciprofloxacin, or the combination of the two agents (324). Rifampicin attains fairly high concentrations in lung tissue and was correlated with reduced lung bacterial counts and decreased histologic sequelae of pneumonia in a guinea pig model (222). Resistance has not been demonstrated in this model (222, 223). Rifampicin-resistant mutants have been demonstrated in other studies and were more rapidly killed with the combination of rifampicin-erythromycin than erythromycin alone (58). The same positive therapeutic results were reported with *L. micdadei* pneumonia in the guinea pig model (543).

Pseudomonas aeruginosa. In neutropenic mice, the combination of rifampicin-ticarcillin-tobramycin was as efficacious as rifampicin alone in the inhibition of *P. aeruginosa*. Both were superior to ticarcillin-tobramycin. Unlike monotherapy, resistant mutants rarely emerged with triple combination therapy (822). Also in a leukopenic mouse model, addition of rifampicin did not improve the survival over cefpirome alone (739).

Pseudomonas pseudomallei. In a mouse model of infection, 67% of mice treated with rifampicin survived. Of these, 75% cultured negative (246). Similar results were seen in a third study, in which rifampicin (35–55 μg/mL) proved very effec-

TABLE 5 • Reports of Noninfectious Uses of Rifamycins	
Disease	**Reference**
Alzheimer's disease	716
Antitumor	6, 118, 239, 352, 609, 614, 626, 649, 737, 780, 799
Crohn's disease	145, 314, 407, 564, 619, 646, 657, 711, 772, 789
Dermatomyositis	547
Diverticulitis	166, 277, 539
Folliculitis decalvans	108
Hemolytic anemia	547
Henoch-Schönlein purpura	395
Hepatic encephalopathy	112, 197, 203, 244, 279, 471, 540, 550, 710
Kaposi sarcoma	547
Periarteritis nodosum	547
Pruritis	46, 47, 177, 276, 340, 570
Psoriasis	613, 760
Rheumatoid arthritis	99, 125, 126, 127, 128, 173, 263, 440, 481
Sarcoidosis	548
Thrombocytopenia	547
Silicosis	547
Systemic lupus erythematosus	547
Ulcerative colitis	564

tive in eliminating the organism from the hearts, lungs, livers, spleens, and kidneys of experimentally infected mice (409).

Yersinia pestis. In one report, rifampicin was efficacious for treatment and prophylaxis of plaque in albino mice (459).

Mycobacteria

Mycobacterium africanum. Investigators have characterized the genetic mutations involved in resistant strains of mycobacteria. Rifampicin-resistant strains of *Mycobacterium africanum* contained mutations in the *rpoB* gene, similar to that in *M. tuberculosis* (786).

Mycobacterium bovis. An in vivo animal model used to evaluate single and combination therapy with steroids in the treatment of BCG *(Mycobacterium bovis)* sepsis in mice showed a survival advantage in mice treated with steroids plus combination antimycobacterial therapy including rifampicin. Due to a significant hypersensitivity component, the advantage was lost without steroids (191, 411).

Mycobacterium haemophilum. Monotherapy with rifabutin significantly reduced the splenic burden of *M. haemophilum* in a murine animal model of disseminated infection. Combination therapy with rifabutin and clarithromycin was even more effective in this model (43).

Mycobacterium kansasii. In one study of in vivo infection with *M. kansasii* in mice, rifampicin plus streptomycin was the most effective regimen, although rifampicin plus isoniazid (INH) and monotherapy with rifampicin were also effective (665). Resistance to rifampicin was demonstrated in clinical isolates from two patients who received rifampicin in combination with ineffective agents. One of the initial isolates

was sensitive to 1.0 μg/mL of rifampicin with the subsequent isolate being resistant at 10 μg/mL (184).

Mycobacterium malmoense. In vitro sensitivities of 36 clinical isolates showed only 15 to be susceptible to rifampicin; 7 had borderline sensitivities, 12 were resistant, and 2 were not tested. MICs were not reported (54).

Mycobacterium marinum. In vivo rifampicin was effective in a mouse model (51).

Mycobacterium paratuberculosis. In a rabbit model, the combination of rifampicin and levamisole led to complete elimination of *M. paratuberculosis* from the feces, intestines, lymph nodes, spleen, kidneys, lungs, and liver. The characteristic lesions of paratuberculosis in the visceral organs were also absent in animals treated with this regimen (497). In a mouse model, monotherapy with rifabutin (50 mg/kg) significantly reduced the level of infection but did not yield complete bacterial clearance (142). Stumptail macaques infected with *M. paratuberculosis* responded well to treatment with rifabutin in another series; the isolates were reported to be sensitive to both rifampicin and rifabutin (485).

Mycobacterium smegmatis. A clinical isolate of *M. smegmatis* from a patient with disseminated disease was found to be resistant to both rifampicin and rifabutin (565).

Mycobacterium ulcerans. In one report, most isolates of *M. ulcerans* were found to be sensitive to rifampicin, which proved useful for in vivo infection in mice, with improvement at 1 month and apparent cure at 10 weeks. Sulfadoxine plus pyrimethamine or clofazimine was ineffective, and combinations of these with rifampicin were no more effective than rifampicin alone (681). In another report, both rifampicin alone and combinations of rifampicin plus heat and rifampicin plus both heat and hyperbaric oxygen were effective in treating *M. ulcerans* infections in mice (414).

Mycobacterium xenopi. In a large series of clinical isolates, 18 of 47 isolates were susceptible to rifampicin, 16 were resistant, and 13 were borderline, though specific concentrations were not given (53). One study found discrepancies between MICs observed in test-tube-grown *M. xenopi* and intracellular inhibition in macrophages. The MICs of rifampicin in agar and broth were 1.5 and less than 1.0 μg/mL, and for rif-abutin, 0.25 and 0.1 μg/mL, respectively. In macrophages, rifampicin was only moderately active, while rifabutin was only growth inhibiting (594).

Chlamydia

Chlamydia trachomatis, Chlamydia psittaci. Rifamycins exhibited good activity (71); however, resistance emerged rapidly, and *Chlamydia* was passaged in subinhibitory levels of rifampicin (378, 389, 725). Emergence of resistance can be prevented with subinhibitory concentrations of erythromycin and oxytetracycline (378). Rifabutin had good activity, and resistance after passaging in subinhibitory levels of the drug has not been demonstrated (725). Rifampicin was effective in vivo in embryonated eggs and in baboon eyes experimentally infected with trachoma. Higher levels of rifampicin were needed to inhibit the agent of psittacosis (as it was described at that time) (71).

Rickettsia

Coxiella burnetii. Rifamycins have activity against several rickettsial species. In a chick embryo model, rifampicin was highly effective in suppressing infection with *C. burnetii* in the five strains tested (679), although a subsequent in vitro study did not find significant bactericidal activity of rifampicin against *C. burnetii* (473). In a different report 13 different isolates were all susceptible to rifampicin when tested by the shell-vial technique (590).

Ehrlichia risticii. The combination of erythromycin and rifampicin was efficacious in treating experimentally induced colitis with *E. risticii* in ponies (537). In a murine model of Potomac horse fever, rifampicin produced some improvement of symptoms; however, *E. risticii* was reisolated from the spleens of the rifampicin-treated mice (605).

Rickettsia azadi. In a rat model of experimental infection, the duration of rickettsemia was shorter with rifampicin treatment than in the control (588).

Rickettsia rickettsii, Rickettsia typhi. Rifampicin was highly effective in suppressing infection with *R. rickettsii* and *R. typhi* in a chick embryo model (679).

Fungi

***Aspergillus* Species.** In a murine model of aspergillosis, the combination of rifampicin and amphotericin B was synergistic, with prolonged survival in the mice; however, infections were not completely eliminated from the kidneys (40).

Blastomyces dermatitidis. In a murine model of infection with *B. dermatitidis,* the combination of amphotericin B with rifampicin significantly increased survival (80%) compared with either agent alone. Following therapy, however, all surviving animals died and had positive splenic cultures for *B. dermititidis*. The fungicidal level reported was above 100 μg/mL, with an MIC of 12.5 μg/mL (400).

Candida albicans. Addition of rifampicin did not increase amphotericin B activity in experimental candidiasis with *C. albicans* in guinea pigs (235). Activity was potentiated by combination of rifampicin with both amphotericin B and ketoconazole in one report, but this did not translate into increased clinical efficacy in a murine model of candidiasis (295).

Coccidioides immitis. In vitro synergy was seen between rifampicin and itraconazole against the mycelial phase of *C. immitis,* with somewhat less synergy seen against the spherule/endospore phase (732). Synergy existed with the combination of amphotericin B and rifampicin against the arthroconidia of *C. immitis* (603) but not against the spherule phase or in vivo in mice (363).

Cryptococcus neoformans. In a mouse model of systemic cryptococcosis, the combination of fluconazole plus rifabutin provided no advantage over fluconazole alone (151).

Histoplasma capsulatum. When added to both rifampicin and rifamycin SV, subtherapeutic levels of amphotericin B potentiated the effects of these agents against *H. capsulatum* (403, 404). Synergy was demonstrated in vitro with the combination of amphotericin B and rifampicin as well as in vivo in mice (486). Others found that while treatment of *H. capsula-*

tum infection in mice was unsuccessful with either amphotericin B or rifampicin alone, the combination of the two agents proved successful. All animals were alive and clinically well 4 weeks after therapy was discontinued; however, upon sacrifice, their spleens still had viable *H. capsulatum* (400).

Pneumocystis carinii. In a SCID mouse model of *P. carinii* pneumonia, one study evaluating the prophylactic efficacy of rifabutin alone (200 mg/kg/day) found a small, but nonsignificant reduction in the infection score. At 100 mg/kg/day, no effect was seen; however, the combination of rifabutin plus atovaquone had a pronounced synergistic effect (159). In another animal model using rats, rifabutin (200 mg/kg/day) was active against *P. carinii;* the combination of atovaquone plus rifabutin did not demonstrate synergy, only enhanced effects (770). In a corticosteroid-treated rat model of *P. carinii* pneumonia, rifampicin was ineffective for both prophylaxis and treatment (354).

***Rhizopus* Species.** Medoff has postulated that the avid binding of amphotericin to the fungal cell wall alters the permeability barrier, allowing entry of rifampicin into the cell to have a direct effect on the DNA-dependent RNA polymerases (487).

Parasites

***Acanthamoeba* Species.** Infection with *Acanthamoeba* species in the central nervous system of mice generally progresses rapidly. In a small, placebo-controlled study, prophylactic rifampicin protected fully against infection with *A. culbertsoni,* at doses of 75 and 100 mg/kg. These two doses also cured most mice (5 of 6 and 7 of 8, respectively) experimentally infected with the parasite (183).

Naegleria fowleri. In a murine model of infection with *N. fowleri,* the combination of tetracycline and either amphotericin or rifampicin decreased mortality over that with monotherapy (288). Decreased mortality was also seen in mice with a combination of amphotericin and rifamycin (713). In vitro suppression of *N. fowleri* in culture by rifamycin (10 and 100 μg/mL) was reported (712). In contrast, in another report, rifampicin at concentrations of 1, 10, and 50 μg/mL did not inhibit growth of *N. fowleri,* although the patient survived following a regimen that included rifampicin (652).

Entamoeba histolytica. The activity of rifampicin against *E. histolytica* was reported. Rifampicin did not inhibit trophozoites, but a 40% decrease in cyst production was seen (651).

***Leishmania* Species.** Limited in vitro data exist on the efficacy of rifamycins against *Leishmania* species. In one in vitro study using *L. tropica,* both rifampicin and amphotericin B alone inhibited growth. Synergistic inhibition was seen with the combination (232). Potentiation of INH and rifampicin was seen against *L. mexicana amazonensis* in mice (562). Another study showed a reduction in the size of lesions due to *L. amazonensis* in experimentally infected mice treated with rifampicin (212). On a molecular level, rifampicin inhibits transcription of 9S and 12S RNA of *L. tarentolae* (668).

***Plasmodium* Species.** In vitro data exist for rifamycins against various *Plasmodium* species. Rifampicin acted rapidly against all stages of *P. falciparum* erythrocytic cell cycle with a IC_{50} of 2.19–2.5 μM (273, 688). Rifampicin significantly reduced parasitemia in the murine model of malaria with *P. chabaudi*, although there was recrudescence after the drug was redrawn (688). In a mouse model of *P. berghei* infection, rifampicin treatment prolonged life, but did not yield clinical cure. It was postulated that this was due to the insolubility of the formulation that was used (12). In another study, rifampicin exhibited poor activity in the rhesus monkey against *P. cynomolgi*, although this may have been due to the low dose of drug used (5.0 and 20 mg/kg body weight) (643).

Toxoplasma gondii. *T. gondii* has emerged as a significant pathogen in persons with cell-mediated immune deficiencies. Rifampicin at concentrations of 50 $\mu g/mL$ or above inhibits the growth of toxoplasma in L cell culture, but it also inhibits the growth of L cells at that concentration. Rifampicin has not shown efficacy against this sporozoan parasite in vivo in a mouse model (596); however, efficacy was demonstrated with rifabutin in vitro and in mice (31, 531, 612). The IC_{50} of rifabutin was 26.5 $\mu g/mL$. Rifabutin treatment increased survival significantly in the murine model of acute toxoplasmosis, versus untreated mice, with an ED_{50} of 160.5 mg/kg/day. Survival was further improved by the combination of clarithromycin and rifabutin (531). In another report, the IC_{50} of rifabutin was 1.68 $\mu g/mL$, with a range of 1.63 to 1.71 $\mu g/mL$. Rifabutin also effectively eradicated parasites and prolonged survival in experimentally infected mice. Synergy was noted both in vitro and in vivo with the combination of rifabutin and atovaquone (612). In another study of murine toxoplasmosis, enhanced efficacy was seen when rifabutin was combined with pyrimethamine, sulfadiazine, clindamycin, or atovaquone (31). In addition, rifapentine was shown to be active against *T. gondii* in vitro and more active than rifabutin in vivo in a mouse model (32).

Viruses

The effect of rifamycins on viral replication has also been studied. Rifampicin inhibited growth of vaccinia, cowpox, and adenovirus type 1 in one study. Development of partial resistance was seen with vaccinia (694). The vaccination response was inhibited in half the human volunteers receiving the DV strain of vaccinia virus in an arm pretreated with topical rifampicin in a 10% ointment or 15% cream (505). Various rifampicin derivatives with modified aminopiperazine side chains inhibited the DNA polymerase activity of several viruses, including murine sarcoma virus (MSV), feline leukemia virus, and avian myeloblastosis virus. Rifampicin did not show activity (307, 308). Another rifampicin derivative (dimethyl-benzyl rifampicin) also showed activity against MSV (311). Rauscher murine leukemia virus reverse transcriptase was also inhibited by rifamycin derivatives (799), and activity was again demonstrated against the retroviral reverse transcriptase of several leukemia viruses and human immunodeficiency virus (HIV)-1 at concentrations higher than that required for bacterial inhibition (63). Rifampicin inhibited formation of polyhedral inclusion bodies of group A *Baculoviridae* (nuclear polyhedrosis virus) (210). Rifabutin was reported to inhibit HIV at concentrations above 5 to 10 $\mu g/mL$

and to cross the blood-brain barrier (187). Rifamycin SV exhibits weak inhibition of the reverse transcriptase of Rous sarcoma virus (IC_{50}, 14 μM) (140). Rifazone-8$_2$, a rifamycin derivative, has much more antiviral activity against Rous sarcoma virus and decreases the infectivity of progeny virus by 95 to 99% (697). In an embryonated chicken egg system, rifampicin inhibited the growth of one strain of influenza A (315). One report exists of the use of rifampicin for treatment of experimentally induced rabies in albino mice; survival rates were higher in those treated with rifampicin than in controls (820). In an experimental model of tumors induced by adenoviruses in male hampsters, rifampicin decreased the incidence of tumors (718).

Noninfectious Uses of Rifamycins

In vitro and animal studies have demonstrated antitumor activity for several rifamycins. Tamoxifen and rifampicin showed an additive interaction against human biliary tract carcinoma cells (780). Rifampicin enhances cellular vinblastine retention in both rat hepatocytes and human multidrug-resistant leukemia cells, thereby acting as a chemosensitizing agent. It also decreased doxorubicin resistance in some cells. Rifamycin SV had only a weak effect, and rifamycin B had no effect (239). Rifampicin and two rifamycin derivatives (dimethylbenzyldesmethylrifampicin and rifazone-8$_2$) had an inhibitory effect on adenocarcinoma TA3 ascites tumors in mice when given via the intraperitoneal route (352). Rifampicin also showed antitumor activity against Walker 256 carcinosarcoma (7). Derivatives of rifamycins inhibit the DNA polymerases of certain human leukemic cells (799). In the chick fibroblast model, cells transformed by Rous sarcoma virus lost their viability when treated with rifampicin (737). The possibility that rifamycins may actually enhance tumor growth via their immune suppressive effects has been explored. Mice pretreated with rifampicin prior to implantation of tumor cells showed increased tumor growth and an increased number of metastases (614).

Pharmacodynamic Effects

Bactericidal Effects

Rifampicin shows bactericidal activity against *M. tuberculosis* and several other mycobacterial species, including *M. bovis* and *M. kansasii*. Other nontuberculous mycobacteria (NTM), including *M. avium* complex, show variable susceptibility to rifampicin (726). The activity of rifampicin appears to pass from bacteriostatic to bactericidal as its concentration is increased during continued drug exposure (726).

The inhibitory activity of rifampicin in vitro against *M. tuberculosis* depends upon the medium used. Its activity is highest in Dubos Tween-Albumin liquid media and lowest in Lowenstein-Jensen and may be affected by inoculum size (327, 726). Bactericidal activity against *M. tuberculosis* was demonstrated when 1 Ag/mL of rifampicin in Dubos Tween-Albumin liquid media sterilized cultures in 7 in 9 days (327). Its bactericidal potency against *M. tuberculosis* has been estimated to equal that of INH under conditions of continuous drug exposure. The activity of rifampicin against *M. avium* strains in vitro is lower in agar medium than in 7H12 liquid broth. This lower activity is attributed to degradation of the drug during the prolonged incubation period required for cultivation in agar medium. The MICs of rifampicin versus *M. avium* strains were not adversely affected by reducing the pH to 5.0, indicating that rifampicin may be active in phagolysosomes of macrophages, where the pH arguably may be that low (327). Rifampicin shows excellent sterilizing activity in vivo against semidormant *M. tuberculosis*. According to Mitchison's theory, this is due to rifampicin's rapid onset of action, which catches organisms during their occasional bursts of metabolism (327, 726). Rifampicin displays activity against *M. tuberculosis* multiplying at a reduced rate at both acidic and neutral pH, the latter attribute being unique to rifampicin among antimycobacterial drugs (726).

Postantibiotic Effects (PAE)

A 2-h exposure of 0.2 Ag/mL of rifampicin delayed regrowth of mycobacteria for 1.8 days, but this may be due to the rapid bactericidal activity of rifampicin. Because of rapid bactericidal activity, regrowth was delayed after the bacterial population was reduced by the initial exposure (327). Other investigators have shown a relatively short lag in regrowth of *M. tuberculosis* under various conditions (726).

Effects of Subinhibitory Concentrations

No specific activity has been attributed to subinhibitory concentrations of rifampicin, particularly when used alone. In vitro, subinhibitory concentrations may enhance the ability to isolate resistant subpopulations (726). Rifampicin alone at 0.9 Ag/mL in Dubos Tween-Albumin liquid medium initially reduced the population of *M. tuberculosis* by 5 log10 colony forming units (CFUs), but at 21 days of incubation, only rifampicin-resistant organisms were present (726). It is not known if subinhibitory concentrations of rifampicin contribute to multidrug therapy in vivo. Rifampicin-dependent mycobacteria have not been described.

Effects on Host Immunity

Reports on the effect of rifampicin on cellular and humoral activity have varied. Suppression of lymphocyte responses in vitro in tuberculosis (TB) patients after 8 to 16 weeks of therapy has been reported; however, there is no evidence of suppression of cellular or humoral immunity in TB patients receiving rifampicin at standard doses (358, 416). Rifampicin is able to concentrate within monocytes and macrophages (726).

Pharmacodynamic Correlates with Outcome

Because rifampicin targets intracellular processes, its activity is probably enhanced by maximizing the peak serum concentration:MIC ratio (551). High C_{max}:MIC ratios, which typically covary with high area under the concentration versus time curve above the MIC (AUC>MIC), are key variables for other intracellular poisons such as aminoglycosides and quinolones (432, 551). In vitro studies have shown that 5 Ag/mL of rifampicin for 7 to 9 days of exposure has complete bactericidal activity. Increasing the concentration to 40 Ag/mL shortens the required exposure time to 5 to 7 days. Concentrations below 5 Ag/mL, on the other hand, show only partial bactericidal activity (726). In mouse models, rifampicin's activity is strongly dose dependent (726). Large weekly doses reduce the number of culturable bacilli more effectively than the same dose divided daily in mice. However, weekly combinations of INH and rifampicin were less effective than twice-weekly or more frequent regimens at sterilizing infected animals. Sterilization of infected animals also depends on the number of months of treatment (726). As mentioned above, rifampicin is able to concentrate within monocytes and macrophages, where it can kill intracellular *M. tuberculosis* (726).

MECHANISMS OF ACTION

The macrocyclic ring is considered the active area that binds to the β-subunit of the prokaryotic DNA-dependent RNA polymerase and prevents all types of RNA production. Although binding actually occurs at the β-subunit, the binding affinity increases when some combination of the remaining subunits (α_2, β', σ, and/or ω) are combined to form the complete polymerase molecule (264, 319, 656). The size of the β-subunit varies from one species to another and correlates with differing binding affinities, which could account for differences in activity from species to species and a lack of activity against eukaryotic cells (319). Rifamycins prevent initiation of RNA production but cannot stop production once it has started, as is shown by a short lag time during which RNA continues to be synthesized after exposure to the drug (264). The binding site of rifamycins is not the active site of RNA replication on the RNA-polymerase. It is about 30 Å from the first active site of the enzyme and about 17 to 20 Å from the second site required for enzyme function. This results in noncompetitive inhibition of the enzyme (i.e., addition of more nucleic acid will not render the rifamycin inactive) (419).

Some recent reports indicate that rifamycins can indirectly cause DNA damage in the presence of electron-accepting molecules (e.g., metallic ions). The reactions cause the formation of hydroxy radicals that damage DNA. The reactions occur as follows:

$$RifH_2 \text{ (reduced)} + 2\,O_2 \rightarrow Rif \text{ (oxidized)} + 2\,O_2^- + 2\,H^+$$
$$RifH_2 \text{ (reduced)} + 2\,Cu_2^+ \rightarrow Rif \text{ (oxidized)} + 2\,Cu^+ + 2\,H^+$$
$$2\,O_2^- + 2H^+ \rightarrow H_2O_2 + O_2$$
$$Cu^+ + H_2O_2 \rightarrow Cu_2^+ + OH^- + \cdot OH$$
$$\text{(Adapted from 586)}$$

This hydroxy radical damages the deoxyribose and causes formation of 8-hydroxy-2′-deoxyguanosine (8-OHdG), which is a mutagen (507). Glutathione decreases the formation of hydroxy radicals by acting as a free radical scavenger (622). The clinical significance of these findings has not been fully elucidated.

Bartolucci et al. reported on the use of rifamycins to inhibit HIV-1 reverse transcriptase (RT). They concluded that the mechanism of action is binding of the chromophore rings (at the benzofurane site) to the RT (64).

MECHANISMS OF RESISTANCE
Commonly Resistant Organisms

Rifampicin has been shown effective against many mycobacteria and Gram-positive organisms and some Gram-negatives. It was once touted as comparable to penicillin (764). Resistance of microorganisms to rifampicin has been reported since at least 1968, when McCabe and Lorian reported rapid development of resistance in strains of *S. aureus*, the organism against which its use was being proposed at the time. They cautioned against using it as monotherapy in infections caused by these organisms (479). Gram-negative species that may be resistant include species of *Enterobacteriaceae*, *Acinetobacter*, and *Pseudomonas* (368). Resistant strains of *M. kansasii*, *M. africanum*, *M. avium*, and *M. leprae* have been reported (416, 482, 726). Clinical failures due to resistance to rifampicin were reported with isolates of *Proteus*, *E. coli*, and *Pseudomonas* sp. when prior isolates were sensitive (44). In addition, recolonization with resistant mutants can occur following short-course chemoprophylaxis with rifampicin and can persist (137).

Mechanisms of Resistance

Resistance in most mycobacteria probably results from modification of the RNA polymerase β subunit, which decreases the binding affinity of the drug for its active site. It is usually a one base-pair change in the *rpo*B gene that codes for the polymerase, although the base pair may change from species to species and within a species (154). Single amino acid substitutions in this β subunit alter rifampicin binding, and the degree of resistance varies greatly, depending on the location and nature of the amino acid substitution (708, 777, 786). This has also been shown for *Neisseria meningitidis* (124) but not for *M. avium* or *M. intracellulare* (302). High-level resistance to rifampicin by a laboratory mutant of *P. aeruginosa* was also shown to be due to a mutation in *rpoB*, but some mutants may also have a natural permeability barrier (806). Since the rifamycin binding site is not an enzymatically active site, the base pair change does not affect the functioning of the RNA polymerase (419). Similar mutations have been shown to occur in resistance to rifabutin (509). Cross resistance between rifampicin-resistant *M. tuberculosis* and rifabutin or rifapentine depends on the area of the RNA-polymerase that has the mutation. Thus, clinical use of rifabutin or rifapentine may be an option with some rifampicin-resistant clinical isolates (94). Although several authors have supported these findings (194, 281, 578), others (346) as well as general clinical practicians do not recommend the regular use of rifabutin for tuberculosis when strains are resistant to rifampicin. Mixed data have been published on cross-resistance of rifampicin and rifabutin against *M. leprae* (807). Although MICs of rifapentine against *M. tuberculosis* are generally lower than that of rifampicin (336, 375, 499), data are not yet sufficient to support the use of rifapentine in the treatment of tuberculosis.

The spontaneous rate of resistance to rifampicin in *M. tuberculosis* is estimated to be 1 in 10^8 organisms. The mutation leading to this resistance occurs at a rate of 10^8 in *E. coli*, 10^7 in *S. aureus*, *Streptococcus* species and *Meningococcus* species (89, 132, 240, 777). This mutation may occur rapidly and in one step, especially when rifampicin is used alone for the treatment of both bacterial and mycobacterial infections (416). No plasmids or transposons have been shown to carry resistance. The cell wall does not appear to affect susceptibility of *M. tuberculosis* to rifampicin (154). According to Baohong, resistance does not develop on an organism-specific basis (57). Rather, naturally occurring organisms are selected during therapy (and potentially conveyed to other patients).

Although primary resistance in tuberculosis to rifampicin alone remains uncommon, the incidence of rifampicin resistance is increasing, especially in the context of concurrent INH resistance. From March 1975 to September 1982, the incidence of rifampicin resistance in the United States was less than 1%. This incidence is much higher in developing countries where rifampicin is used (132). The incidence of rifampicin plus INH resistance (multidrug-resistant tuberculosis, or MDR-TB) in the United States is also much higher. In 1991, 6.9% of TB patients in the United States were resistant to both INH and rifampicin, while this rate was only 0.5% from 1982 to 1986. In New York City in 1991, the rate was 33% (132, 133). The overall incidence of INH plus rifampicin resistance is higher in certain ethnic groups such as African Americans, Mexican Americans, and Indochinese refugees (132, 133, 416). Recent outbreaks of MDR-TB have occurred in institutional settings, such as health care and correctional facilities. Other factors contributing to MDR-TB include HIV seropositivity, drug abuse, homelessness, mental illness, and poor socioeconomic conditions (132, 133).

Della Bruna et al. showed that natural resistance of *M. tuberculosis* to rifabutin was less common than to rifampicin and that exposure to subinhibitory concentrations led to development of less resistance to rifabutin than to rifampicin (195). This does not, however, contradict Baohong's work, because it did not show that resistance developed in previously uniformly sensitive organisms.

Some mycobacteria that are inherently resistant to rifamycins have been postulated to have other mechanisms of resistance. Hui et al. showed that one strain of *M. intracellulare* had a graduating level of resistance depending on rifampicin concentration (which is not consistent with the one-base substitution mentioned above, which would code for resistance or susceptibility with no gradations). The RNA polymerase was susceptible to rifampicin, indicating that either impermeability to rifampicin or inaccessibility to the RNA-polymerase conferred resistance. This was confirmed when addition of Tween 80 (which acts as a cell wall solubilizer) increased the killing efficacy of rifampicin (356).

In atypical mycobacteria, ethambutol (which interferes with cell wall synthesis) increases the susceptibility of *M. avium* to antimycobacterial agents that were previously not effective (344). Additionally, *E. coli* is more resistant to rifampicin than its RNA polymerase when its cell wall is intact; changing the cell wall structure confers susceptibility (607).

Methods to Overcome Resistance

Use of multiple drugs has been advocated to delay or prevent emergence of resistance in the treatment of tuberculosis (110,

344). Accordingly, current recommendations for the treatment of tuberculosis and other mycobacteria mandate multidrug therapy (23). Other medications such as trimethoprim or vancomycin have been used to prevent resistance to *Staphylococcus* species (416). Higher doses of rifampicin as monotherapy do not prevent the emergence of resistance (726). In vitro, subinhibitory concentrations enhance the selection of resistant organisms (726). It is not known if this also occurs in vivo, although the possibility exists. Therefore, it appears desirable to achieve serum concentrations well above the MIC of the isolate.

PHARMACOKINETIC DISPOSITION
Absorption

Rifampicin is almost completely absorbed after oral administration. Giving it on an empty stomach slightly increases peak levels (4). This difference is greater with lower doses. An acidic pH increases absorption, and rifampicin undergoes first-pass metabolism (4). Patients with AIDS do not absorb rifampicin normally. Several studies have shown that patients may display incomplete absorption, possibly leading to treatment failure and selection of drug-resistant *M. tuberculosis*. Measurement of rifampicin serum concentration should be considered in patients with known gastrointestinal (GI) problems (e.g., cystic fibrosis, advanced diabetes mellitus, AIDS, or a history of GI surgery) (84, 546, 552, 553).

Rifabutin was only 20% absorbed in early, symptomatic, HIV-infected individuals upon initiation of therapy. This decreased to 12% by day 28 (671). However, it was 85% absorbed in normal healthy volunteers (513). This discrepancy was not discussed by either set of authors nor in the scientific literature. It takes 3.3 h to reach maximal concentrations (671). Food decreases the rate, but not the extent, of absorption (513).

Rifaximin is not absorbed, topically or orally (82, 200). Animal data show recovery of 53.4 to 78.8% of rifaximin in feces after 1 to 72 h (283).

Rifapentine pharmacokinetic data are only available in the United States in animal models. Absorption is rapid, with a bioavailability of 65 to 84%, with high doses being absorbed to a lesser extent (41).

Distribution

Rifampicin distributes into most body tissues and fluids, including cerebrospinal fluid (CSF) (482). It is 80% (8–96%) protein bound, enters breast milk (4), and crosses the placenta (482). The volume of distribution (Vd) is about 1 L/kg (90). Rifampicin concentrates in healthy, human polymorphonuclear leukocytes (PMNs) at a concentration approximately 4 to 5 times the extracellular concentration (5–6 times for PMNs infected with *S. aureus*) (316, 744, 798). Bile concentrations of 150 mg/L have been seen after a 300- to 450-mg dose (4).

Rifabutin's Vd is 9.3 L/kg on day 1 and decreases to 8.2 L/kg by day 28 of therapy. Protein binding was 71% (671). It concentrates intracellularly, 9 to 15 times the extracellular concentrations (734, 744). Rifabutin is more lipid soluble and distributes more into tissues than rifampicin, possibly contributing to the decreased levels and extended half-life (90) compared with

rifampicin. Lowest tissue concentrations of rifabutin were found in the brain, the highest in the liver. It enters both the placenta and uterus, but distribution was minimal into the amniotic fluid and fetus of rats. Excretion is presumed to occur through the urinary and biliary tracts (66). Biliary concentrations 3 to 5 times the plasma level are reached after a 150-mg dose (90).

Rifaximin achieves biliary concentrations of 4.5 to 15.6 mg/L after oral administration of 400-mg doses, four times a day for 2 days (755).

Rifapentine is well distributed into many tissue sites. The average Vds for the three animals tested were 0.44 L/kg for the rabbit, 0.59 L/kg for the rat, and 1.29 L/kg for the mouse (41). Rifapentine achieved intracellular concentrations 40.8 times the extracellular concentrations in one in vitro study (542). Table 6 summarizes the tissue penetration data available for rifampicin, rifabutin and rifapentine.

Metabolism/Elimination

The elimination half-life of rifampicin is about 3 h (4). It is metabolized in the liver to an active deacetylated derivative, 25-desacetylrifampicin. It is also metabolized to 3-formyl-25-desacetylrifamycin SV and 3-formyl rifamycin SV. 25-Desacetylrifamycin is primarily removed through the bile (366). Yazawa et al. have isolated two glycosylated metabolites (RIP-1 and RIP-2) of rifampicin from *Nocardia brasiliensis* and two phosphorylated metabolites (RIP-3 and RIP-4) from *Nocardia otitidiscaviarum*. None of these four metabolites was as microbiologically active as rifampicin (801, 802). Dabbs et al. showed that two ribosylated metabolites (RIP-Ma and RIP-Mb) that were produced by *M. smegmatis* were also inactive (178).

Rifabutin's elimination half-life is 38 h in HIV patients and 45 h in healthy adults. It is cleared primarily by the liver and excreted via renal and biliary routes (65, 671). The primary metabolite is a 31-hydroxylated derivative (65). Dose reduction may be needed in patients with severe hepatic impairment because of increased area under the curve (AUC) (90, 727). It is not dialyzed (482).

TABLE 6 • Tissue: Plasma Ratio (6–12 h/postdose)

Tissue	Rifampicin	Rifabutin	Rifapentine
Lung	>1	1.4–8.6	>1
Muscle	1	0.22–0.43	>1
Bile	<1	320–505	>1
Gallbladder	<1	2–4.3	NA
Ileum	NA	54	NA
Jejunum	NA	93	NA
Stomach wall	>1	NA	NA
Skin	1	>1	NA
Liver	<1	>1	>1
Fat	>1	>1	>1
Breast milk	>1	NA	NA
CNS, brain	<1	<1	<1
Aqueous humor	<1	NA	NA
Spleen	1	>1	>1

Data from references 4, 41, 66, 90, 515, 534.

After oral administration, 0.023 to 0.001% of the rifaximin dose was recovered from the urine (200).

Rifapentine, like rifampicin, is metabolized to the 25-deacyl derivative. Its elimination half-life ranged from 14.4 to 22.8 h for the rat and mouse models and was approximately 2 h in the rabbit model (41).

All probably undergo a significant amount of enterohepatic recirculation, as is seen by elevated levels in the bile. Increased levels of rifampicin, and possibly other rifamycins, may lead to hyperbilirubinemia because of competitive biliary excretion (727).

DOSAGE REGIMENS

(Specific doses depend on indication; see "Clinical Indications," below.)

Rifampicin

The normal adult dose is 600 to 1200 mg/day orally or intravenously (10–20 mg/kg/day). Persons weighing less than 50 kg may take 450 mg once daily (416). Oral doses should be given 1 h before or 2 h after a meal. Rifampicin may be given intravenously over 30 min to patients unable to take rifampicin orally. The normal pediatric dose is 10 to 20 mg/kg/day (children).

Renal failure does not require dose adjustment, because rifampicin is primarily cleared by the liver (416, 483). Plasma concentrations are not significantly affected by hemodialysis or peritoneal dialysis (483).

Rifampicin should be used in patients with impaired hepatic function only if medically necessary, when no alternatives are available, and with close medical supervision, including monitoring liver function tests every 2 to 4 weeks. Although there are no clear dosing guidelines for its use in hepatic failure, higher rifampicin concentrations have been reported in cirrhotic patients, albeit without adverse effects (5, 6). Because smaller doses may produce lower C_{max}:MIC ratios, it may be better to give the usual dose at longer intervals to patients with severe hepatic impairments. Because elimination of rifampicin may be compromised, serum concentration monitoring of rifampicin is indicated in such patients (554).

Although rifampicin is a lipophilic drug, it displays a relatively small Vd and does not distribute into adipose tissue (554). Because of this, for obese patients, rifampicin should be dosed on the basis of ideal (lean) body weight (275, 554).

Rifampicin does distribute into ascites, therefore individualization of such patients is recommended (482, 554). Although not reported, the same could be assumed for patients with edema.

Rifampicin is classified as category C. The effects on the fetus are unknown. It should be used only if the potential benefits outweigh the risks to the fetus. In the last few weeks of pregnancy, it can cause postnatal hemorrhages in both mother and infant, necessitating the use of vitamin K. An increased incidence of spina bifida and cleft palate has occurred in the offspring of mice and rats receiving 150 to 250 mg/kg/day during pregnancy (482). Rifampicin does cross the human placenta, and on rare occasions, fetal malformations have occurred

(482, 554). The use of rifampicin in pregnancy should be reserved for more advanced cases, and the risk:benefit ratio should always be determined (482, 554).

Rifampicin is distributed in the milk; however, it is considered to carry a very low risk of adverse effects. The American Academy of Pediatrics considers this agent to be compatible with breastfeeding (161).

Rifabutin

The normal adult dose is 300 mg/day orally (patients with a propensity toward nausea or GI upset, may be given 150 mg twice daily). No pediatric indication exists; however, the manufacturer states that there is no evidence that dosages above 5 mg/kg are required. Doses averaging 18.5 mg/kg (up to 25 mg/kg) or 8.6 mg/kg (up to 18.6 mg/kg) have been used for active treatment of infants 1 year of age and children 2 to 10 years of age, respectively.

No adjustment is necessary for renal failure or hepatic failure.

Rifabutin should be used in pregnancy only when the potential benefits justify the possible risk to the fetus.

It is not known whether rifabutin is distributed in the milk.

Rifaximin

The normal dose for adults and children over 12 years of age is 10 to 15 mg/kg/day of 5% cream topically. The normal pediatric dose is 20 to 30 mg/kg/day of 5% cream topically.

No adjustment is necessary for renal failure or hepatic failure.

Although no significant systemic absorption occurs, the drug should be used in pregnancy only when the potential benefits justify the possible risk to the fetus.

Although no significant systemic absorption occurs, the drug should be used in nursing mothers only when the potential benefits justify the possible risks.

ADVERSE EFFECTS

A report from the U.S. Public Health Service reviewing three regimens of rifampicin and INH in the treatment of tuberculosis noted that 3.3% of patients discontinued treatment because of side effects (448). Dutt et al. reported that 22 of 814 (2.7%) patients treated for tuberculosis with rifampicin and INH therapy discontinued rifampicin therapy because of adverse events (219). A complete listing of adverse reactions to the rifamycins is available with the individual drugs' company literature. This section includes only frequent or severe adverse reactions.

Mild reactions seen with rifampicin include GI distress (e.g., nausea, vomiting, diarrhea), headache, fever, dizziness (and other typical CNS effects), and cutaneous reactions (including rash, itching, and flushing). GI bleeding caused by rifampicin (and confirmed by rechallenge) was reported (814). Ulcerative colitis was reported in a patient receiving rifampicin therapy (700). Although it is not a true adverse event, it is important for patients to know that bodily fluids (e.g., sweat, saliva, tears) will very likely change color, ranging from orange to brown or, commonly, red.

Anaphylactic reactions to rifampicin have been reported. Cardot et al. reported a systemic hypersensitivity reaction to a locally applied rifamycin derivative (122). Pujet et al. reported on their patients who developed intolerance to rifampicin. Testing revealed antibodies to rifampicin for up to 16 months after discontinuation of therapy (582). A flulike illness has been reported (219, 582) and may be due to an immune reaction. Miscellaneous reports of fever associated with rifampicin have been published (523). A serum sickness–like reaction has also been reported (541). One case report exists of a fixed drug eruption in a previously healthy patient receiving rifampicin for prophylaxis following exposure to a patient with meningococcemia (494).

Hematologic reactions include primarily thrombocytopenia. Company literature states that it first appears as purpura. Cerebral hemorrhages and fatalities have been described when rifampicin therapy was not discontinued. A recent report (488) discussed three cases of rifampicin-induced thrombocytopenia. All three patients had antiplatelet antibodies, and antibody binding increased in the presence of rifampicin. A case report described one patient who experienced subclinical disseminated intravascular coagulopathy (along with leukocytosis, flulike illness, intravascular hemolysis, and acute renal failure) (365).

Altered renal status is a widely reported adverse effect of rifampicin. Although it is a rare event, Nessi et al. reported on 37 cases and Cohn et al. reported on 83 cases. Length of rifampicin therapy prior to the event ranged from 13 days to 1 year, and severity ranged from mild and reversible to severe, requiring dialysis and/or causing death (153, 518). Cohn et al. speculated that intermittent or interrupted therapy was a possible risk factor for development of renal insufficiency, and the data of Nessi et al. appear to support this assumption (153, 518). However, Kumar et al. reported two patients who developed light-chain proteinurea with reversible renal failure after receiving daily, uninterrupted, or recently initiated therapy (420). Hirsch et al. reported a patient who developed rapid glomerulonephritis that began 3 weeks after initiation of rifampicin therapy, while Warrington et al. reported light-chain proteinuria with an insidious onset of renal failure (337, 773). Bansal et al. described a patient with rifampicin-induced renal failure and noted the presence of immune globulins in the tubules and glomeruli of the kidneys (56). In summary, serum creatinine and urinary protein should be checked in all patients receiving prolonged therapy with rifampicin.

Several reviews have discussed hepatitis caused by rifampicin (284, 299, 545, 781). Despite early reports indicating rifampicin as the probable sole cause of the hepatitis (642), the consensus now appears to be that rifampicin rarely causes hep-atitis without some other intervening, or predisposing, factor. When used to treat tuberculosis, rifampicin is associated with a variety of effects that may not be seen with other therapies. Used alone, rifampicin is known to cause hepatotoxicity (267, 482, 684), and the risk of this may be increased by combination with other antimycobacterial agents, particularly INH (209, 267, 684). Concern over a possible drug-drug interaction leading to a synergistic increase in hepatotoxicity led Steele et al. to perform a meta-analysis to evaluate this issue. They reviewed all reports from 1966 to 1989 of hepatitis due to regimens containing INH without rifampicin, INH plus rifampicin, and rifampicin without INH. Their findings showed an increase in clinical hepatotoxicity when the two agents were used together; however, this incidence was additive, occurring at the expected rate of 2.55%. Reports on the mechanism of a possible interaction between these two medications are varied, and it has not been fully determined which toxic metabolite may be causing the hepatitis (267, 684). Rifampicin has also been associated with an increased risk of hepatitis when used in combination with ethionamide and prothionamide (299, 416). Risk factors associated with rifampicin-induced hepatitis include advanced age, alcohol consumption, diabetes, and concomitant hepatotoxic agents (209, 299, 684).

Rifampicin has induced early-phase hyperglycemia in patients taking the agent for tuberculosis, while it was not noticed in the healthy controls, patients with tuberculosis but not being treated, or in patients being treated for tuberculosis without rifampicin (701). A patient who had insulin-dependent diabetes required an increased dose of insulin while on rifampicin (42). Immune dysfunction has also been noted with rifampicin. Humber et al. noted decreased albumin, increased immune globulins, and decreased T cell counts in patients receiving rifampicin therapy for treatment or prophylaxis of tuberculosis. These irregularities returned to baseline within 6 weeks while on therapy (358). Gupta et al. also found a decrease in T cell counts that returned to baseline within 2 weeks after discontinuation of rifampicin therapy (306). Shah et al. reported osteomalacia in a patient receiving prolonged rifampicin therapy. They postulated that the hepatic metabolism of vitamin D results in a deficiency of that vitamin (as can happen with some anticonvulsants) (660).

Some of the adverse effects associated with rifampicin in treating tuberculosis arise from its use in intermittent regimens. These effects include thrombocytopenia, hemolytic anemia, acute renal failure, the "respiratory syndrome," and the "flu syndrome." These reactions were more frequent with higher intermittent rifampicin doses (900–1200 mg twice weekly or 1200–1800 mg once weekly) (28, 219, 250, 285, 299, 416, 436). Many of these reactions are thought to be immunologically related because rifampicin-dependent antibodies of the IgM or IgG type have been observed in the serum of patients receiving intermittent therapy (299, 436). These reactions may occasionally be seen with daily therapy, especially in patients who are nonadherent to therapy (250, 435, 436, 615). These reactions can be avoided by using the usual daily dose (600 mg) during intermittent therapy (23, 132, 416) and by avoiding rifampicin use in nonadherent patients or properly educating patients about these effects (250, 436).

Since it is a much newer drug than rifampicin, the full array of side effects associated with rifabutin are yet to be elucidated. Common, minor side effects include GI discomfort, abdominal pain, fever, myalgia, and rash. Blood dyscrasias, such as anemia and neutropenia, were more common with rifabutin than with placebo and caused withdrawal of 2% of patients being treated with rifabutin in clinical trials.

Uveitis is the best-known adverse effect associated with rifabutin. It is rare, dose-related, and usually reversible. Uveitis is an inflammation of the eyes, involving the choroid, ciliary body, and/or the iris. It is characterized by decreased vision and eye pain. Although originally seen with higher doses (1200 mg/day) during dose-escalation studies (666), it has recently been described at normal therapeutic doses (300–600 mg/day) (728). It occurred in 23 of 119 patients receiving 600 mg/day of rifabutin as well as 1 g of clarithromycin and 15 mg/kg of ethambutol (659). Concurrent ritonavir administration increased the incidence of uveitis (690). It is assumed that drugs that may increase the AUC of rifabutin may increase the incidence of uveitis.

Arthritis and arthralgias were reported in most patients who received doses above 1050 mg/day in a dose-escalation study (666). The skin of these patients turned orange-tan as a result of the medication. This is supported also by a case report of a patient who experienced arthralgias, myalgias, and ageusia (loss of the sense of taste) while on rifabutin. The symptoms subsided upon discontinuation and resumed on rechallenge (502). Ritonavir significantly increases the incidence of arthralgias and joint stiffness (690).

Rifaximin adverse events center mostly around GI intolerance (abdominal pain, nausea, vomiting), but even these are rare. Skin reactions and urticarial rash have been described in patients on high doses or receiving rifaximin for a prolonged period. In general, rifaximin is well tolerated.

DRUG INTERACTIONS

Rifampicin has long been known as a potent inducer of drug metabolism and, hence, a leading cause of drug interactions. Rifampicin causes proliferation of smooth endoplasmic reticulum, which is assumed to cause the enzyme induction (374). Rifampicin induces the cytochrome P-450 enzyme system (96), specifically, P450–3A (77) and, to a lesser extent, P450–2C8 and P450–2C9 (294). For this reason, it primarily causes decreased levels of drugs metabolized by these enzyme systems. Rifabutin induces similar enzyme systems but to a lesser extent. Therefore, drug interactions attributed to rifampicin may also exist to a lesser extent with rifabutin. Both drugs also induce their own metabolism (77). Table 7 lists drugs whose levels are decreased by the inductive effects of either rifampicin or rifabutin. The clinical significance varies from drug to drug depending on the degree of metabolism by the P450–3A enzyme and alternate routes of metabolism or elimination. More information is available for rifampicin, since it has been available longer. (For a more thorough review of pharmacokinetic interactions involving rifampicin see reference 751.) Rifabutin probably interacts with similar drugs but to a lesser degree.

In addition to the interactions listed in Table 7, several other interactions are of interest. Rifampicin levels are decreased by *p*-aminosalicylic acid (PAS), presumably by inhibition of absorption (98). This can be clinically important because PAS is a second-line drug in the treatment of tuberculosis, especially multidrug-resistant tuberculosis (186). However, this effect was most likely due to bentonite, an excipient found in dosage

TABLE 7 • Drug Interactions

Affected Drug	Causative Drug	Reference
Antiarrhythmics[a]	Rifampicin	10, 129, 439, 478, 557, 602, 647, 689
Antifungals[b]	Rifampicin	27, 204, 217, 722, 732
Benzodiazepines[c]	Rifampicin	103, 528
β-Blockers[d]	Rifampicin	78, 398, 661
Bunazosin	Rifampicin	13
Ca channel blockers[e]	Rifampicin	218, 589, 699, 729
Chloramphenicol	Rifampicin	580
Clarithromycin	Rifampicin	768
	Rifabutin	282
Clofibrate	Rifampicin	350
Corticosteroids	Rifampicin	113, 429, 458,
Dapsone	Rifampicin	566
Digoxin	Rifampicin	272, 819
Doxycycline	Rifampicin	158
Fluoroquinolones[f]	Rifampicin	359, 644
Haloperidol	Rifampicin	702
Hexobarbital	Rifampicin	818
Hypoglycemics[g]	Rifampicin	654, 751, 818
Immune suppressants[h]	Rifampicin	262, 294, 429
Narcotic analgesics[i]	Rifampicin	413, 472
Nortriptyline	Rifampicin	69
Oral contraceptives	Rifampicin	96, 379
	Rifabutin	483
Phenytoin	Rifampicin	294
Quinine	Rifampicin	10, 683
Sulfasalazine	Rifampicin	658
Theophylline, caffeine	Rifampicin	608, 778
Warfarin	Rifampicin	328
Zidovudine	Rifampicin	117
	Rifabutin	282

[a] Disopyramide, lorcainide, mexiletine, pirmenol, propafenone, quinidine, tocainide, lidocaine.

[b] Fluconazole, itraconazole, ketoconazole.

[c] Diazepam, temazepam.

[d] Metoprolol, propanolol, bisprolol.

[e] Verapamil, diltiazem, nifedipine.

[f] Pefloxacin, fleroxacin.

[g] Glyburide, tolbutamide, chlorpropamide.

[h] Cyclosporine, tacrolimus, azathioprine.

[i] May precipitate withdrawal in susceptible patients, including those on methadone.

forms of PAS that are no longer available in the United States (482), and it is no longer an issue with the new PASER granules of PAS. Probenecid increases rifampicin serum levels, most likely because of competition for hepatic metabolism (387).

Sulfamethoxazole-trimethoprim may increase the levels and half-life of rifampicin (87). However, conflicting data are seen with trimethoprim alone combined with rifampicin. While one group found decreased levels and half-lives of both drugs (116), another saw trimethoprim clearance decrease (234), and a third saw no change in levels (5). Conflicting data also exist with ciprofloxacin. Animal data show a significant increase in ciprofloxacin clearance (59), while Chandler et al. found that neither ciprofloxacin nor rifampicin pharmacokinetic parameters changed significantly when administered together (134).

Protease inhibitors interact with both rifampicin and rifabutin. Ritonavir increased the minimum and maximum concentrations and the 24-h AUC for rifabutin (130). Saquinavir levels were decreased by 80% when administered with rifampicin, and by 40% when administered with rifabutin (company literature). Current information regarding the use of indinavir and rifabutin together states that concurrent use of rifabutin (150 mg/day) and indinavir at recommended doses is acceptable (500). Current recommendations for the treatment of tuberculosis with rifampicin (as part of the normal regimen for tuberculosis) in patients being treated for HIV infection with a protease inhibitor offer three options: *(a)* discontinue the protease inhibitor for the duration of the tuberculosis therapy; *(b)* discontinue the protease for the duration of rifampicin therapy, but modify the tuberculosis regimen by using rifampicin for the first 2 months and use a 16-month continuation phase that does not include rifampicin (assuming the patient becomes culture negative for *M. tuberculosis* after the initial 2 months); or *(3)* use rifabutin (150 mg/day) instead of rifampicin. The third option is only for patients receiving indinavir therapy; patients receiving either saquinavir or ritonavir should be switched to indinavir before starting this option (500).

Pharmacokinetic interactions are not the only type of interactions seen with rifampicin. As discussed in the section on adverse events, rifampicin has been known to cause hepatitis. This adverse reaction may be potentiated by other possibly hepatotoxic drugs. Either INH (298, 445) or halothane (506) combined with rifampicin increases the incidence of hepatic damage over that with either rifampicin, INH, or halothane alone. The mechanism of these reactions are not known, but Gronhagen-Riska et al. state that the rifampicin-INH hepatotoxic reaction appears to be a caused by a different mechanism than the toxicity of either drug alone (298).

Fluconazole was shown to increase the plasma levels of rifabutin by 82% (722). Rifampicin and, to a lesser extent, rifabutin decrease plasma levels of clarithromycin (768). This is clinically important, as clarithromycin and rifabutin are commonly used together in treatment of *M. avium* complex (MAC).

Drug interactions have been noted with the combination of rifampicin and clarithromycin because of hepatic metabolism of clarithromycin, a mainstay in the treatment of MAC infection (85, 769). In 45 patients receiving clarithromycin but not rifampicin or rifabutin who underwent therapeutic drug monitoring at the Infectious Disease Pharmacokinetic Laboratory (IDPL) at National Jewish Medical and Research Center in Denver, the median maximum concentration was 4.59 Ag/mL after 1.5 to 4.5 h. This median maximum concentration fell to 0.60 Ag/mL in 25 others receiving both clarithromycin and rifampicin. The concentration of the principle metabolite, 14-OH clarithromycin, was 1.63 Ag/mL in the 45 patients on clarithromycin alone and 2.02 Ag/mL in the 25 patients on clarithromycin and rifampicin. This interaction is of concern,

given the frequency of their combined use against MAC. Proper dosing of these medications may be facilitated by therapeutic drug monitoring (85).

Special note should be made of the interaction between the rifamycins and estrogen-containing oral contraceptive agents. Rifampicin and, to a lesser extent, rifabutin decrease the effectiveness of these agents and may cause a high incidence of menstrual disorders such as breakthrough bleeding. Women should be advised to use alternative forms of contraception (483).

CLINICAL INDICATIONS
Rifamycin

The following clinical indications include those in which rifamycins are used as the standard of care or noted authorities have suggested their use as an option. For greater detail, refer to the individual chapters on specific organisms or processes. Other diseases with reports of rifamycin usage are discussed below.

Gram-Positive Bacilli
Clostridium difficile

• Vancomycin, bacitracin (oral), cholestyramine, lactobacilli, ± rifampicin (61)

In one clinical series of seven patients with relapses of *C. difficile* colitis despite vancomycin therapy, clinical improvement was seen with the combination of rifampicin plus vancomycin. All stool cultures became negative, although they subsequently reverted to positive despite the patients remaining asymptomatic (114).

Gram-Positive Cocci
Staphylococcus aureus

• Penicillin or vancomycin ± rifampicin 600 mg/day (61)

The clinical utility of combination therapy with rifampicin plus oxacillin or vancomycin was prospectively evaluated in 27 patients in a randomized study. Despite a reduction in the bactericidal activity of serum with high oxacillin concentrations, a beneficial effect was seen in patients treated with the combination (742). In a series of 28 patients with chronic staphylococcal osteomyelitis, 70% had an apparent cure with rifampicin-containing combination regimens (525). In a retrospective review of 10 patients with *S. aureus* meningitis, all 6 treated with a semisynthetic penicillin plus rifampicin were cured, while 3 of the 4 treated with other combinations died (291). One report described 10 neonates who had persistent bacteremia with *Staphylococcus* species including methicillin-susceptible and resistant *S. aureus* and coagulase-negative staphylococci despite therapy with vancomycin with or without aminoglycosides; 8 had sterile blood cultures within 24 h of rifampicin addition, 1 within 48 h, and 1 within 5 days (703). Rifampicin or the combination of rifampicin plus cloxacillin effectively eradicated nasal carriage of coagulase-positive staphylococci in 70 and 80% of subjects in two different studies (782).

Colonization with MRSA remains a serious clinical problem. Rifampicin has been used in a variety of regimens with variable success. The combination of oral minocycline and rifampicin for 2 weeks (plus nasal mupirocin if nasal colonization was present) cleared 10 of 11 (91%) patients and 20 of 21 (95%) sites of MRSA (182). Short-course therapy with novobiocin plus rifampicin for 5 days cleared MRSA in 79% of patients and 81% of sites in another study (30). The combination of rifampicin plus trimethoprim/sulfamethoxazole showed limited success in eradicating MRSA in colonized patients. Clearance was seen in some patients, although persistent colonization and relapse were also noted (230). One report described resolution with rifampicin of chronic suppurative lymphadenitis due to *S. aureus* infection in a patient with chronic granulomatous disease (449). Rifampicin has also been useful in the treatment of *Staphylococcus*-infected orthopaedic implants, including *S. aureus* and coagulase-negative staphylococci. In one series, patients were prospectively treated with the combination of rifampicin plus ofloxacin; 62% were cured without implant removal (215). In a series involving infected orthopaedic implants, rifampicin plus fusidic acid was effective in 55% of those treated (216).

Gram-Negative Cocci
Neisseria meningitidis prophylaxis

- Rifampicin 10 mg/kg twice daily (maximum, 600 mg/dose) for 2 days

Outbreaks of *N. meningitidis* meningitis remain a serious problem. Rifampicin continues to be the main agent used in prophylaxis following exposure to the organism. The recommended regimen is 10 mg/kg (maximum dose, 600 mg) orally every 12 h, for a total of four doses. Prophylaxis is indicated for household contacts, child-care center and nursery school contacts, and persons who have come in contact with the patient's oral secretions through sharing food or drink and kissing (21).

Rifampicin is the standard antimicrobial recommended for prophylaxis for contacts of persons with *N. meningitidis,* as well as for eradication of nasopharyngeal carriage in the index case (424). Its efficacy in reducing nasal staphylococcal carriage and preventing secondary cases during an outbreak was documented in a large trial of military recruits. Resistance to rifampicin was documented in persons who failed to clear initially, relapsed, or acquired the organism after discontinuing prophylaxis (68). In another large trial of prophylaxis, after an initial decrease in the carriage rate from 60 to 13%, the rate then rose to 30% 4 weeks after discontinuation of medication. This may have been due to recolonization (670). Invasive meningococcal disease has been documented in persons who received prophylaxis because of antimicrobial resistance or new exposure to an untreated carrier (81, 164, 393).

Gram-Negative Bacilli
Brucella Species

- Rifampicin 600 mg/day plus doxycycline (61)

In one prospective, open trial of brucellosis, 16 of 16 patients treated with rifampicin plus cotrimoxazole and 24 of 24 treated with rifampicin plus tetracycline were cured. Only 8 of 10 treated with rifampicin monotherapy were cured (664). Several randomized, double-blind studies of rifampicin plus

doxycycline versus streptomycin-doxycycline in the treatment of infections due to *B. melitensis* have been reported. In one trial in which therapy was continued for 30 days, the relapse rate in the rifampicin-containing arm was 38.8%, compared with 7.1% in the other (36). In a 45-day trial, excluding patients with spondylitis, the different regimens were equally effective, with failure rates of 4.9 and 4.3% in the two arms. In patients with spondylitis, the failure or relapse rate was higher in the rifampicin group, although it was not statistically significant (37). In a third trial, patients in the rifampicin arm had a cure rate of 86.5%, compared with 91.6% in the other arm (157). A subsequent randomized, open, controlled trial using the same drugs showed the rifampicin-containing therapy to be significantly less effective when initial lack of therapeutic efficacy and relapse were considered together (677). Another prospective, randomized trial compared 6 weeks of ofloxacin-rifampicin with doxycycline-rifampicin for treatment of *B. melitensis*. The two regimens were equally effective, though more side effects were observed with the doxycycline regimen (11). One small open study using rifampicin as monotherapy for *B. melitensis* infection showed an 85% cure rate (446). One case report exists of successful treatment of aortic valve endocarditis due to *B. abortus* with a valve replacement and rifampicin plus trimethoprim-sulfamethoxazole for 3 months (369). Another patient with *B. melitensis* aortic valve endocarditis was successfully treated with rifampicin, tetracycline, and streptomycin after a valve replacement (575). Three other patients with endocarditis due to *Brucella* species were treated successfully with rifampicin plus cotrimoxazole for 6 months following their valve replacements (373). A 6-week course of this combination was successful in a fourth patient (3). Rifampicin, tetracycline, and streptomycin for 6 weeks was used successfully in five of six patients with *Brucella* endocarditis. One patient did not require surgery, and the sixth patient died prior to surgery (14, 15). Success has also been reported in treating neurobrucellosis with the combination of doxycycline and rifampicin plus steroids (558).

Haemophilus influenzae Type b Prophylaxis

- Rifampicin 600 mg/day orally for 4 days (adults)
- Rifampicin 20 mg/kg/day (maximum dose, 600 mg) orally for 4 days (children under 12 years)

Although immunization has decreased the incidence of invasive disease due to *H. influenzae* type b, the need for appropriate postexposure prophylaxis still exists. All members of a household (children and adults) with a child in the susceptible age group (less than 4 years of age) should receive prophylaxis. Rifampicin remains the standard agent (20 mg/kg/day for children under age 12 years and 600 mg/day orally for adults for 4 days). Previously vaccinated childhood contacts should receive prophylaxis as well as susceptible, unvaccinated children. Whether prophylaxis should be administered to nonhousehold contacts should be determined on a case-by-case basis, depending on the type and duration of exposure (20).

Rifampicin has been evaluated for the chemoprophylaxis of intimate contacts of patients with invasive *H. influenzae* type B in many randomized trials. In one large multicenter, prospective, blinded, randomized trial of rifampicin versus placebo in close contacts of patients with systemic invasive *Haemophilus* disease, 4 days of rifampicin prophylaxis (20 mg/kg/day) significantly reduced carriage of *H. influenzae* type b as well as the risk of secondary disease. Recommendations for rifampicin prophylaxis for contacts were based primarily on this study (50). A 2-day regimen of rifampicin (10 mg/kg/day) plus trimethoprim was less effective than the standard 4-day course (287). A later study found a 2-day course of rifampicin to be as effective as a 4-day course in eradicating pharyngeal colonization with *H. influenzae* (296).

Legionella pneumophila

- Erythromycin ± rifampicin 600 mg intravenously or orally every 12 h (61, 22, 813)

Serious infections due to *L. pneumophila* are often refractory to therapy. Clinical data support the recommendation for combination therapy with erythromycin and rifampicin in these cases. Case reports of serious disease due to *Legionella* species have shown a benefit in patients treated with the combination of erythromycin and rifampicin (165, 303). Although data from large prospective human studies treating *Legionella* infections with rifamycins are lacking, reviews of the disease suggest a role for rifampicin in combination with other agents on the basis of in vitro and animal studies (390). In one series of compromised patients, two of six received rifampicin in addition to intravenous erythromycin, with further improvement noted (631). Combinations of erythromycin and rifampicin were superior to erythromycin alone in another retrospective review, although other regimens including pefloxacin may offer additional benefit (211). For severe infection due to *L. pneumophila,* combination therapy with erythromycin and rifampicin is generally recommended (304, 521, 611, 813). Seven patients were reported with endocarditis due to *Legionella* species: two had *L. pneumophila* isolated from the blood of valves; three had *L. dumoffii;* and one had both *L. pneumophila* and *L. dumoffii* diagnosed serologically. Six of the seven were clinically and microbiologically cured with the combination of erythromycin and rifampicin. The seventh patient had a similar positive outcome with the combination of ciprofloxacin and rifampicin (717). The combination of erythromycin and rifampicin was used successfully in one patient with community-acquired pneumonia due to *L. gormanii* (721) as well as in an immunosuppressed patient with pneumonia due to *L. dumoffii* (225). The combination of trimethoprim-sulfamethoxazole plus rifampicin resulted in clinical cure of a patient with pneumonia due to *L. micdadei* (618). *L. wadsworthii* was the causative agent in a patient with pneumonia who began to respond clinically when rifampicin was added to his therapeutic regimen, which included erythromycin (224).

Mycobacteria
Mycobacterium avium complex

- Rifabutin 300 mg/day for prophylaxis (see other chapter for recommendations including rifabutin) (104)
- Rifabutin 300 to 600 mg/day or rifampicin 600 mg/day in combination with at least two other anti-MAC agents (104, 767) (see chapter on *Mycobacterium avium* complex)

Mycobacterium fortuitum

- Rifampicin 600 mg/day as well as other agents (61)

Limited clinical data exist on the use of rifampicin in infections due to *M. fortuitum*. In one report, 10 patients received rifampicin as part of their therapeutic regimens, but limited details are provided. Two of 3 with pulmonary disease had good clinical responses, although one remained culture positive after 2 years. Three of 3 patients with pleural disease had positive responses. One each with disseminated disease, sternal osteitis, and adenitis responded to rifampicin-containing regimens. A single patient with a subarachnoid abscess died (467).

Mycobacterium kansasii

- Rifampicin 600 mg/day combined with isoniazid plus ethambutol (61, 767, 793)

Rifampicin has been considered an important component of treatment regimens for *M. kansasii* for many years (8, 52, 317, 349, 563). In one retrospective review of 135 patients, 100% of those treated initially with a rifampicin-containing regimen were culture negative at the fourth and fifth months. Of those not treated with rifampicin, 80% were culture negative by 6 months (563). A second retrospective review of 256 patients also found 100% sputum conversion in those given rifampicin-containing regimens, versus 90% of those without rifampicin (8). A prospective study of 40 patients found 12 months of therapy to be effective for initial treatment of *M. kansasii* pulmonary disease (9). A randomized trial of 28 patients that also examined duration of treatment found 12 months of therapy with INH, rifampicin, and ethambutol (first 6 months only) to be as effective as an 18-month course of the same regimen (634). In a larger, open study, 173 patients with pulmonary disease were treated with the combination of ethambutol and rifampicin for 9 months. Of the 15 (9.7%) patients who relapsed after termination of chemotherapy, 8 had factors predisposing to relapse. The investigators concluded that a 9-month course was adequate for patients without predisposing factors (121, 599).

M. kansasii infection in HIV-infected patients has been reviewed. In one report those with disease limited to the lung seemed to have an adequate response to chemotherapy including rifampicin, although the optimal duration is not known. Those with disseminated disease did poorly despite therapy that included rifampicin (123). In three other case reports of *M. kansasii* disease in patients with AIDS, two patients treated with rifampicin-containing regimens died of the infection (381, 335); one survived (370). One case report exists of INH and rifampicin successfully treating *M. kansasii* peritonitis secondary to continuous ambulatory peritoneal dialysis (280).

Mycobacterium leprae

- Rifampicin combined with dapsone ± clofazimine (61) (see chapter on *M. leprae*)

Mycobacterium malmoense

- Rifampicin 600 mg/day combined with ethambutol, isoniazid, plus streptomycin or amikacin (767, 793)

One patient with AIDS was reported with pulmonary and disseminated infection with *M. malmoense*. He was successfully treated with a combination of rifabutin, clofazamine, and INH (816). Two other patients without AIDS had positive clinical responses to the combination of rifabutin, ethambutol, and amikacin, with no evidence of disease in the 2- to 4-year follow-up period (331). Another HIV-infected patient with pulmonary disease had a clinical response and clearing of his sputum when ethambutol was added to his rifampicin-containing regimen, but approximately a year later, *M. malmoense* was isolated from his stools (150). Another patient who had a coinfection with *P. carinii* did not respond to a rifampicin-containing regimen (174). A single patient with hairy cell leukemia and disseminated *M. malmoense* infection responded well to 16 months of a multidrug regimen that included rifampicin (102). Thirty-four patients were treated for pulmonary disease in one series: 5 of 5 patients who received INH, ethambutol, and rifampicin for 18 months did well; 3 of the 5 who received this combination for less time relapsed. Those treated with only two drugs (INH and rifampicin) generally did not respond satisfactorily; nor did those who received second-line agents (54). Rifampicin was part of the successful multidrug regimen in 20 patients from Scotland, though only 60% of the isolates were sensitive. All patients had an initial clinical response, although five patients treated with less than 5 months of ethambutol relapsed. All responded to a second, longer course of therapy (251). In a review of cases of disseminated disease reported in the literature, two persons died despite therapy that included rifampicin, one improved, and one progressed on regimens including rifampicin. Rifampicin was also part of the treatment regimens for several patients with tenosynovitis and lymphadenitis due to *M. malmoense,* though limited data exist on which to base conclusions regarding efficacy (816). A patient with a cold abscess due to *M. malmoense* on the hand and one with carpal tunnel syndrome responded well to a combination of rifampicin, INH, pyrazinamide, and ethambutol in the second case (233, 579). A patient with cutaneous disease did not respond to INH and rifampicin, to which the organism was subsequently found resistant (268).

Mycobacterium marinum

- Rifampicin 600 mg/day combined with ethambutol (61, 767, 793)

The mainstay of treatment for *M. marinum* infections has been a combination of ethambutol and rifampicin. Case reports generally show success when this regimen is given over many weeks (45, 305, 746, 749, 792). One retrospective review of 31 patients with skin infections showed a clinical response in five of five patients treated with ethambutol and rifampicin. Treatment failures occurred in 18% of those receiving tetracyclines (226). Four patients were reported who failed tetracycline therapy and then responded to rifampicin-containing regimens, including two who received rifampicin as monotherapy (208). Another patient failed doxycycline and then responded to an 8-month course of rifampicin and ethambutol (444). An additional patient was described who had a clinical response with rifampicin monotherapy (581). Rare reports exist describing the failure of rifampicin-containing regimens for *M. marinum* infections (360).

Mycobacterium scrofulaceum

- Rifampicin 600 mg/day combined with others, including ethambutol and streptomycin (767, 793)

Two patients with adenitis and one with pulmonary disease due to *M. scrofulaceum* were treated with rifampicin-containing regimens with clinical success (467). An immunocompetent patient with disseminated disease was treated successfully with a multidrug regimen that included rifampicin (351).

Mycobacterium simae

- Rifampicin 600 mg/day combined with ethambutol, INH, plus streptomycin or amikacin (767, 793)

One series reported patients from whom *M. simae* was isolated. The details of therapeutic regimens were not included, although one patient did fail a rifampicin-containing regimen; the isolates were resistant to all conventional antituberculous agents (74). A patient with AIDS and disseminated disease due to *M. simae* improved with the combination of clarithromycin plus rifabutin (405).

Mycobacterium szulgai

- Rifampicin 600 mg/day combined with INH plus ethambutol (767, 793)

M. szulgai infection in humans is uncommonly reported in the literature. One patient with slowly progressive pulmonary disease had a good clinical response to prolonged treatment with a rifampicin-containing regimen (185). Three patients in another series received rifampicin in their regimens with good clinical outcomes (638). An earlier paper reported one patient with a good clinical response to a rifampicin-containing regimen and another who apparently progressed while on rifampicin (465).

Mycobacterium tuberculosis

- Rifampicin 600 mg/day combined with INH, pyrazinamide ± ethambutol (61)
- Rifabutin 300 to 600 mg/day in combination with at least two other antituberculous agents (104) (see chapter on *M. tuberculosis*)

Mycobacterium xenopi

- Rifampicin 600 mg/day combined with others including INH, ethambutol, and streptomycin (767, 793)

M. xenopi typically causes disease in patients with altered host defenses. Case reports exist for two patients who responded to combination therapy including rifampicin (709). Three of 19 patients in one series were treated with rifampicin-containing regimens; two improved, and one showed no change at the time of the report. Sixteen of 20 isolates in this series were resistant to 1.0 μg of rifampicin (169). In a third report, one patient had a positive clinical response to a rifampicin-containing regimen, while another did not, although both patients' isolates were sensitive to 5 to 20 μg/mL of rifampicin (95). In another series, five of seven patients with isolates sensitive to rifampicin responded to rifampicin-containing regimens (675). One patient with discitis due to *M. xenopi* progressed on 2 months of rifampicin, INH, and pyrazinamide (256). The largest review included 47 patients with pulmonary disease due to *M. xenopi*. Response to therapy was generally unpredictable, although the best drug regimen seemed to be the combination of rifampicin, INH, and either streptomycin or ethambutol (53). In a smaller series, eight of the nine patients were on multidrug regimens that included rifampicin, but only one improved. The others died or relapsed (667).

Other
Coxiella burnetii

- Rifampicin plus doxycycline (592)

Effective therapy of Q fever endocarditis requires an initial high level of suspicion for accurate diagnosis, followed by long-term therapy. While no controlled trials exists, the data support the use of doxycycline plus rifampicin for a prolonged period. Several reports described successful treatment of Q fever endocarditis from *C. burnetii* with a combination of a tetracycline and rifampicin (396, 592), although others did not report success (695). Additionally, one report exists of successful treatment of chronic Q fever during pregnancy. Rifampicin/doxycycline and rifampicin/erythromycin followed by rifampicin/doxycycline were used (80).

Infectious Diarrhea, Including Traveler's Diarrhea (283, 535)

- Rifaximin 200 mg every 6 h for 5 to 7 days (adults)
- Rifaximin 100 to 200 mg every 6 h (ages 6–12 years)
- Rifaximin 100 mg every 6 h (ages 2–6 years)

Rifaximin has been used in many trials evaluating the treatment for infectious enterocolitis. In one open label trial of patients who were seriously disabled by infectious enterocolitis and unable to take oral alimentation, the use of rifaximin significantly improved symptoms, including lessening the number of stools, rectal tenesmus, abdominal pain, nausea and vomiting, and general malaise (18). In another open study, rifaximin effectively treated acute diarrheal enteritis in 20 patients, including one with *Yersinia* species, 4 with *Shigella* species, 4 with group b *Salmonella,* and 11 with enteropathogenic *E. coli* (455). In four double-blind trials, two comparing rifaximin with neomycin and the other two comparing rifaximin with placebo in the treatment of infectious diarrhea, rifaximin demonstrated efficacy in reducing symptoms and complications, including dehydration (19, 196, 278, 761).

With increased use of rifaximin, concern exists about the possible emergence of resistant organisms. In one study in healthy volunteers, colonization of resistant bacteria was monitored during and after cessation of rifaximin. Thirty to 90% of bacterial strains initially isolated were resistant, but these disappeared rapidly after the drug was stopped (193).

Pre- and Postoperative Prophylaxis in Gastrointestinal Surgery (283, 535)

- Rifaximin 400 mg every 12 h for 3 days preoperatively (adults and children over 12 years)
- Rifaximin 200 to 400 mg every 12 h (ages 6–12 years)
- Rifaximin 100 to 200 mg every 12 h (ages 2–6 hours)

Rifaximin is used in the preparation of the bowel prior to surgery. In one report, both 600 and 800 mg/day for 3 days prior to surgery significantly lowered the intestinal bacterial counts (635). One small randomized trial compared rifaximin with paromomycin for this indication. Lower bacterial counts of aerobic and anaerobic bacteria and fewer postoperative complications were seen in the rifaximin group (754). In another randomized study, preoperative rifaximin, perioperative gentamicin, and combination of the two were compared. Both aerobic and anaerobic bacteria counts were lower in the rifaximin-containing arms, although no difference was seen in the incidence of postoperative complications in the three groups (300).

Hepatic Encephalopathy Due to Elevated Ammonia (283, 535)

- Rifaximin 400 mg every 8 h for 7 to 21 days (adults and children over 12 years)
- Rifaximin 200 to 300 mg every 8 h (ages 6–12 years)
- Rifaximin 100–200 mg every 8 hours (ages 2–6 years)

Rifaximin, a nonabsorbable rifamycin derivative, has been used successfully in several GI processes. In randomized trials of rifaximin versus neomycin (244, 550), rifaximin versus paromomycin (197, 710), and rifaximin versus lactulose (112, 244, 279, 471) for hepatic encephalopathy, ammonia levels in patients on the rifaximin arms were reduced significantly faster than levels with comparator agents. In addition, patients experienced a notable lack of side effects with rifaximin in all studies. Rifaximin and paromomycin showed equal efficacy (540). In another small study, patients receiving rifaximin plus lactulose had a more favorable response than those receiving neomycin plus lactulose (203).

Monitoring

With rifampicin, complete blood cell counts and serum concentrations of AST (SGOT), ALT (SGPT), and bilirubin should be determined prior to initiation of therapy and monitored during therapy. With rifabutin, hematologic status should be monitored throughout therapy. No specific monitoring is indicated for patients on rifaximin because there is no significant systemic absorption.

At National Jewish Medical and Research Center, where therapeutic drug monitoring (TDM) of antimycobacterial drugs is the standard of treatment, samples for serum rifampicin concentration determination are drawn 2 and 6 h postdose. The 2-h concentrations provide information about the maximum concentrations, while the 6-h concentration lends information on the rate and completeness of absorption and on clearance of the drug (555). A 600-mg dose generally produces concentrations of 8 to 16 Ag/mL, with a few patients showing concentrations as high as 24 Ag/mL; 8 to 24 Ag/mL is used as the "normal range" following usual doses of 450 to 600 mg (554, 555).

Other Diseases with Reported Rifamycin Usage

Gram-Positive Bacilli
Actinomyces meyeri, Actinomyces **Species**. One patient with septic discitis due to *A. meyeri* was successfully treated with a combination of pefloxacin and rifampicin (466). A patient with *A. meyerii* and *A. actinomycetemcomitans* who had been treated for 14 weeks with INH and rifampicin for a presumed atypical mycobacterium had resolution of his cervicofacial disease on

this regimen (79). A third patient with pulmonary actinomycosis showed improvement on a 2-week course of antimycobacterial therapy prior to identification of the organism as *Actinomyces* species and a change to penicillin (397). Two additional patients with pulmonary actinomycosis were treated successfully with rifampicin alone (503).

Corynebacterium bovis.   One patient with a ventriculo-jugular shunt infection and bacteremia with *C. bovis* was reported to have responded to medical therapy without shunt removal. The patient initially relapsed after a course of penicillin, but then responded to erythromycin and rifampicin (97).

Gordonna terrae.   One patient receiving antineoplastic chemotherapy was successfully treated with the combination of imipenem and rifampicin for a brain abscess due to *G. terrae* (213).

Oerskovia xanthineolytica.   One patient with a ventriculoperitoneal shunt who developed meningitis due to *O. xanthineolytica* was successfully treated with shunt removal and 10 days of rifampicin plus penicillin (384).

Rhodococcus equi, Rhodococcus rubropertinctus.   The clinical utility of rifamycins in the treatment of human infections due to *Rhodococcus equi* is somewhat difficult to determine. The literature on rifampicin-containing regimens for treatment is primarily from individual case reports, usually involving patients with compromised immune systems such as leukemia and HIV syndrome and coinfection with other opportunistic organisms (16, 119, 214, 238, 321, 469, 627, 632, 673, 757). While clinical responses reported are variable, most patients with successful outcomes were treated with prolonged combination regimens (16, 119, 214, 238, 333, 431, 469, 616, 627, 632, 636, 673, 757). Rifabutin was used unsuccessfully in one case report (469). A single patient was reported to have responded clinically to antituberculous therapy including rifampicin for treatment of *R. rubropertinctus* pneumonia (320).

Gram-Positive Cocci

Enterococcus faecium.   Limited human data exist on the use of rifampicin for infections due to *Enterococcus* species. One patient with enterococcal meningitis was treated successfully with a combination of rifampicin and intrathecal vancomycin, although the exact contribution of rifampicin is unknown (620). Another patient with multiply-resistant *E. faecium* meningitis was treated successfully with intrathecal teicoplanin plus intravenous clindamycin, rifampicin, and ampicillin (450).

Staphylococcus epidermidis.   One trial of rifampicin prophylaxis in cardiac surgery patients resulted in a significant number of patients (75%) developing rifampicin-resistant coagulase-negative staphylococci as part of their skin flora (34, 35). Rifampicin was used successfully in combination with other agents in one case report of prosthetic valve endocarditis with *S. epidermidis* and in another with *Micrococcus* species (155). In a retrospective review of prosthetic valve endocarditis with *S. epidermidis*, cure rates were higher in patients treated with vancomycin plus rifampicin than in those treated with vancomycin alone. Addition of rifampicin to β-lactams did not improve the response over β-lactams alone (385). Two case reports exist of successful use of oral rifampicin in the treatment of *S. epidermidis* ventriculitis (682).

Stomatococcus mucilaginosus.   Infection due to *S. mucilaginosus* is uncommon and usually seen in compromised patients. One report exists of successful treatment of a lower respiratory tract infection with rifampicin in a patient with AIDS. The patient had a relapse 8 months later and subsequently received prophylaxis with rifampicin (175). Another patient with prosthetic valve endocarditis died despite multidrug therapy that included rifampicin; cultures of the vegetation at autopsy were negative (171).

Streptococcus morbillorum.   One patient with endocarditis due to *S. morbillorum* had an apparent cure with 6 weeks of intravenous penicillin and oral rifampicin, followed by 16 weeks of oral penicillin and rifampicin. He had previously failed both 4 weeks of intravenous penicillin and later 5 weeks of penicillin plus amikacin (170).

Streptococcus pneumoniae.   Two case reports (101, 376) and a retrospective review of seven patients with penicillin-resistant pneumococcal meningitis suggested that children with highly penicillin-resistant disease may be best treated initially with a combination of vancomycin and rifampicin until the MICs of third-generation cephalosporins are known (376).

Streptococcus pyogenes.   Rifampicin was evaluated in a few clinical studies of *S. pyogenes*. Penicillin plus rifampicin for the last 4 days of therapy had better clinical and bacteriologic efficacy than penicillin alone in one randomized trial of treatment of group A *Streptococcus* pharyngitis (138). Whether this was due to synergistic or additive interaction between the two drugs or to eradication of β-lactamase-producing organisms remains unclear (105). In another study, pharyngeal carriage was eliminated more effectively with a combination of benzathine penicillin plus rifampicin than with penicillin alone or no therapy (706); however, a subsequent study showed clindamycin to be superior to penicillin plus rifampicin (707). Short-course therapy with rifampicin once daily for 4 days did not eradicate group A streptococci effectively in persons with pharyngeal colonization, with only 38% clearance of bacteria (188). One case report describes a health care worker who had anal colonization with group A *Streptococcus*. The organism was eradicated with a course of penicillin, rifampicin, and hexachlorophene showers. When he became recolonized 14 months later, a regimen of oral vancomycin plus rifampicin was used successfully (758). An association between psoriasis and streptococcal infections has been reported. One report found clinical improvement in psoriasis with addition of rifampicin to penicillin or erythromycin (613); a later report did not find benefit (760).

Gram-Negative Cocci

Moraxella lacunata.   Rifampicin successfully eradicated *M. lacunata* from 10 of 11 patients with conjunctivitis and all 17 nasal carriers of this organism. During the next 11 months, 26% of this group developed conjunctivitis, as did 26% of those who received education concerning risk factors but no systemic therapy, while 76% of controls who received neither education nor antimicrobials developed conjunctivitis with *M. lacunata* (648).

Neisseria gonorrhoeae.   The combination of erythromycin and rifampicin has been used successfully to treat *N.*

gonorrhoeae infections, including those due to penicillinase-producing strains (93, 533, 538). Urogenital, rectal, and pharyngeal infections were effectively cured with this regimen (93). Monotherapy with rifampicin has also been used (76).

Neisseria Species. In one report, administration of two doses of rifampicin to healthy volunteers decreased the bacterial counts of their oral flora. There was a 68.9% decrease in *Neisseria* species, including *N. meningitidis, N. sicca,* and *N. lactamica* (26).

Gram-Negative Bacilli

Actinobacillus actinomycetemcomitans. Two patients with endocarditis due to *A. actinomycetemcomitans* were treated successfully with rifampicin-containing regimens. One received a 6-week course of rifampicin plus streptomycin (637). The other had rifampicin added to penicillin plus gentamicin for the second half of a 6-week course of therapy (425). As discussed above, one patient with both *A. actinomycetemcomitans* and *A. meyerii* responded to treatment with rifampicin and isoniazid for 14 weeks (79).

Bacteroides Species, Capnocytophaga Species, Leptotrichia Species. Two doses of rifampicin given to healthy volunteers significantly decreased the bacterial counts of their oral flora. For *Bacteroides* species, including *B. ureolyticus, B. melaninogenicus/intermedius, B. oralis,* and *B. fragilis,* and *Capnocytophaga* species including *C. ochracea,* and *Leptotrichia* species, there was a 94.5% reduction (26).

Campylobacter Species. In a retrospective review of the incidence of campylobacter infections in 90 patients participating in a prospective trial of rifabutin prophylaxis against MAC, those receiving rifabutin had a significantly lower incidence than those on placebo, suggesting a possible protective effect (584).

Escherichia coli. Monotherapy with rifampicin for urinary tract infections due to *E. coli* and other organisms was generally not successful in one report. All of those who had an initial response relapsed within a few weeks (508). Combination therapy with trimethoprim and rifampicin in patients with recurrent urinary tract infections produced cure rates at 2 and 6 weeks of 81% and 67%, respectively (109).

Flavobacterium meningosepticum. Neonatal meningitis due to *F. meningosepticum* generally carries a high mortality risk. Three cases were reported in which systemic and intraventricular rifamycin resulted in clinical cures (434). In other cases, rifampicin use resulted in clinical cures in 5 of 6 infants with meningitis due to *F. meningosepticum* (135, 162, 715). One neutropenic adult with acute leukemia and *F. meningosepticum* bacteremia responded clinically when rifampicin was added to her antibiotic regimen (338).

Fusobacterium naviforme, Fusobacterium nucleatum. Short-course rifampicin in healthy volunteers resulted in 78.6% inhibition of *F. naviforme* and *F. nucleatum* (26).

Haemophilus ducreyi. A 3-day course of rifampicin alone or rifampicin plus trimethoprim resulted in clinical cures and was effective in eradicating *H. ducreyi* from genital ulcers in one randomized, controlled trial. An uncontrolled, open study also saw good results with a single dose of rifampicin plus trimethoprim (569).

Haemophilus influenzae biogroup aegyptius. Rifampicin was effective in eliminating the Brazilian purpuric fever (BPF) clone from the conjunctivas of children with conjunctivitis due to *H. influenzae* biogroup *aegyptius*. The sample size was too small to determine if rifampicin was effective in preventing Brazilian purpuric fever (559).

Klebsiella rhinoscleromatis. Local application of rifampicin resulted in complete cure of rhinoscleroma, a chronic granulomatous disease caused by *K. rhinoscleromatis,* in 70% of the atrophic cases and 50% of the granulomatous cases (265). Systemic rifampicin has also been successful (266).

Proteus Species. Monotherapy with rifampicin for urinary tract infections due to *Proteus* species was not successful. Combination therapy with rifampicin and trimethoprim did prove useful in patients with recurrent disease (109).

Pseudomonas aeruginosa. Limited data exist on the use of rifamycins in the treatment of *P. aeruginosa* infections. In one report, four patients with serious pseudomonal disease had positive clinical and bacteriologic responses with addition of rifampicin to carboxypenicillin-aminoglycoside regimens (809). One prospective, randomized trial found that bacteriologic cure in patients with bacteremia was significantly more likely in patients randomized to standard therapy with an antipseudomonal penicillin and aminoglycoside plus rifampicin than in those who did not receive rifampicin. However, no difference was seen in survival in this trial (410). In an uncontrolled trial of oral ciprofloxacin plus rifampicin for malignant otitis externa due to *P. aeruginosa,* 10 of the 11 had bacteriologic and clinical cures (617).

Pseudomonas pseudomallei. The presumptive diagnosis of *P. pseudomallei* meningitis was made in a Vietnam War veteran on the basis of a fourfold rise in serum antibody titers. He was successfully treated with a rifampicin-containing regimen (70).

Mycobacteria

Mycobacterium bovis. Acute sepsis from intravesical bacillus Calmette-Guérin (BCG) therapy for bladder cancer has been reported. In one series, four of the five patients received therapy including rifampicin; two died. No steroids were administered (595). One patient with hepatic and pulmonary disease from BCG therapy was successfully treated with INH, rifampicin, and steroids (685). Progressive infection due to *M. bovis* from a BCG vaccination was reported in an HIV positive patient. He was successfully treated with INH, ethambutol, and rifampicin for 9 months (453). One patient with BCG-induced lupus vulgaris was successfully treated with rifampicin monotherapy for 14 weeks (367). Reports also exist of success with prolonged combination therapy including rifampicin for vertebral osteomyelitis due to *M. bovis* following intravesical BCG (149, 501). One patient with HIV infection died with disseminated *M. bovis* (non-BCG vaccine strain) while on therapy with INH, rifampicin, and pyrazinamide. His isolate was later found to be multiply resistant, including to both rifampicin and rifabutin (645).

Mycobacterium chelonae subspecies abscessus. Limited details were presented on one patient with urinary disease due to *M. chelonae* subspecies *abscessus* who responded to a combination of rifampicin, INH, and ethambutol (467).

Mycobacterium gordonae.   One case report describes successful treatment of a cavitary lung disease due to *M. gordonae* with a rifabutin-containing regimen. The patient was initially treated with a four-drug regimen including rifampicin for 9 months without success. The subsequent positive clinical response was attributed to addition of rifabutin (514). Rifabutin was given to a patient known to have many years of progressive disease with *M. gordonae* resistant to multiple agents including rifampicin. His sputum cultures became negative for the first time, although no long-term follow-up was reported (301). Two years of therapy with INH, ethambutol, and rifampicin for *M. gordonae* prosthetic valve endocarditis resulted in an apparent cure in one patient (447). Infection due to *M. gordonae* was reported in one patient each with a thyroid abscess, maxilar osteitis, and pulmonary disease. Each responded clinically to rifampicin-containing regimens, although the patient with pulmonary disease remained culture positive (467). A patient on peritoneal dialysis with multiple abdominal abscesses due to *M. gordonae* had a poor clinical response to antimicrobial therapy including rifampicin (318).

Mycobacterium haemophilum.   Limited details are included in one report of two patients with *Mycobacterium haemophilum*. Both patients were treated with rifamycin-containing regimens. One patient whose therapy including rifampicin was on hold because of elevated liver function test results developed disseminated disease. At autopsy, isolates from the lymph nodes and adrenals showed sensitivities similar to those of his initial isolates; however, isolates from his spleen demonstrated significant rifamycin resistance. The other patient, initially treated with a rifampicin-containing regimen and later with rifabutin in his therapy, also developed resistant organisms (83). Another report describes successful treatment of two patients with AIDS and osteomyelitis due to *M. haemophilum* with rifampicin-containing regimens for 14 and 17 months. In vitro susceptibility testing showed one patient's isolate to be sensitive and the other's to be resistant (800). One cardiac transplant patient with osteomyelitis due to *M. haemophilum* was successfully treated with clarithromycin plus rifampicin (568). In a large literature review of disease due to *M. haemophilum,* approximately three quarters of the 37 patients on rifampicin-containing regimens had positive responses; 10 had persistent disease (633).

Mycobacterium thermoresistibile.   Human infection with *M. thermoresistibile* is exceedingly rare. One case report involves successful treatment of a breast abscess with rifampicin and ethambutol for 16 months (791). Two patients with pulmonary disease due to *M. thermoresistibile* responded to the combination of rifampicin, ethambutol, and streptomycin (441, 779). A third report describes successful and prolonged use of ethambutol, rifampicin, and INH to treat a cutaneous infection following a cardiac transplant (517).

Mycobacterium ulcerans.   A combination of surgery and an antimicrobial regimen that included rifampicin was successful in one patient with *M. ulcerans* panniculitis, but not in another with a chronic ulcer (293). A multidrug regimen including rifampicin was successful in one HIV-infected patient with an ulcerating skin lesion (192).

Mycobacterium vaccae.   Previously not considered to be a human pathogen, the rapidly growing organism *M. vaccae* has now been reported to have caused diseases in four patients. The isolate from one patient was reported susceptible to rifampicin. No rifampicin susceptibilities were noted for the other isolates. One patient was briefly treated with a rifampicin-containing regimen prior to final successful treatment with doxycycline and ciprofloxacin (310).

While a definitive cause has not been determined; erythema induratum of Bazin is assumed to be associated with mycobacteria. Case reports describe successful treatment of this skin disease with antimycobacterial chemotherapy including rifampicin (156, 190).

Chlamydia

Chlamydia trachomatis, Chlamydia psittaci.   Rifampicin was effective in the treatment of nongonococcal urethritis due to *C. trachomatis* in one study. Only 1 of 53 with the organism isolated initially failed to achieve microbiologic cure, although all had clinical responses (172). In a study of eye infections due to *C. trachomatis,* 1% rifampicin eye ointment yielded a clinical cure rate of 75% and a microbiologic cure rate of 86% (181). In another report of topical agents, efficacy of rifampicin equaled that of tetracycline at 5 weeks but was lower at 19 weeks (189). One small series showed clinical efficacy in 8 patients with lymphogranuloma venereum treated with rifampicin (489). One report describes a patient with serologically diagnosed *C. psittaci* endocarditis who failed treatment with tetracycline but responded well to rifampicin (372).

Rickettsia

Afipia felis.   A large retrospective review of 202 cases considered due to *A. felis* assessed the clinical efficacy of the multiple different antibiotics used. Rifampicin was the most efficacious (87%) in achieving absence or decrease in symptoms within 3 to 10 days (462).

Bartonella henselae.   Cat scratch disease has variably been ascribed to different rickettsial organisms. Two children diagnosed with hepatosplenic cat scratch disease with high antibody titers to *Rochalimaea henselae* (now known as *Bartonella henselae*) were treated successfully with 10 to 20 days of rifampicin (289). In another report, two siblings with hepatosplenic disease due to *B. henselae* responded to 2 weeks of rifampicin (704). Another child with disease due to *R. henselae* confirmed by PCR responded to rifampicin after failing a 10-day course of trimethoprim-sulphamethoxazole and 10 days of oxacillin (160). Earlier reports describe four patients with HIV infection and cutaneous infection due to cat scratch bacillus who had complete resolution with rifampicin-containing regimens. Two had regimens that included erythromycin (312, 406, 433).

Bartonella quintana, Bartonella Species.   In one series of 22 patients with endocarditis due to *B. quintana* and other *Bartonella* species, 6 received rifampicin-containing regimens, resulting in a cure in 3 patients, death in 1, and unknown outcomes in 2 (593).

Rickettsia conorii.   Rifampicin has been studied prospectively in the treatment of *R. conorii,* the causative agent of Mediterranean spotted fever. A randomized trial evaluated two doses of doxycycline versus 5 days of rifampicin in 32 consecutive patients. While all patients ultimately did well, defervescence and disappearance of symptoms took longer in the rifampicin group, but rifampicin may still have a role in patients for whom tetracyclines are contraindicated (75).

Fungi

***Aspergillus* Species.**   Data on the use of rifampicin in human fungal infections are primarily derived from case reports. The combination of amphotericin B and rifampicin was successful in treating infections due to *Aspergillus* species in two leukemic patients with pulmonary aspergillosis (86, 601), a leukemic patient with osteomyelitis (249), and a patient with disseminated aspergillosis and chronic granulomatous disease (430). Based on in vitro studies demonstrating synergy, a child with chronic granulomatous disease and *A. fumigatus* infection of the ribs, lung, and pleura was treated successfully with amphotericin B and rifampicin (168). Primary aspergillosis of the spine in an otherwise healthy patient responded well to the same combination therapy (484). One patient with necrotizing otitis externa due to *A. fumigatus* had an apparent response to a radical mastoidectomy, amphotericin B, and rifampicin (176). Another patient with sinoorbital aspergillosis had a clinical response to the addition of rifampicin and flucytosine following progressive neurologic disease after receiving amphotericin and surgical debridement (810). A subsequent patient with sinusitis due to *A. flavus* did not respond to the combination of amphotericin B, rifampicin, and granulocyte transfusions (693). Other failures using amphotericin B and rifampicin occurred in a patient with a brain abscess due to *A. fumigatus* (561), one with pulmonary and central nervous system disease due to *A. terreus* (549), a leukemic patient with disseminated *A. niger* (452), and a leukemic patient with *A. flavus* endocarditis (493). In all cases, fungi were cultured from postmortem specimens. A patient with cavernous sinus thrombosis due to *A. fumigatus* who did not respond to a rifampicin-containing regimen, subsequently responded to amphotericin B and flucytosine (653). One neonate with *A. fumigatus* infection of the brain was cured with the combination of amphotericin B, rifampicin, and drainage (600). Two renal transplant patients diagnosed with pulmonary aspergillosis responded to the combination of amphotericin B and rifampicin, although one was receiving rifampicin for empiric treatment of tuberculosis (423). A diabetic patient on steroids with bilateral renal aspergillosis had a clinical response to this combination regimen (774). Retrospective assessment of 26 cases of invasive aspergillosis treated with the combination of amphotericin B and rifampicin demonstrated a 65% overall response rate; among the neutropenic patients in this group, only 44% responded, compared with 65% of those treated with amphotericin B alone (199).

Candida albicans.   One report describes successful treatment of *C. albicans* endophthalmitis with amphotericin B plus rifampicin. This combination demonstrated synergy in vitro against the strain isolated from the patient (451).

Candida tropicalis.   A retrospective review of *C. tropicalis* infections in children with leukemia in one center revealed 12 cases. Two children were treated with the combination of amphotericin B and rifampicin, and five received the triple combination of amphotericin B, rifampicin, and flucytosine. Six of these seven survived (464).

Coccidioides immitis.   Two patients with coccidiomycosis treated simultaneously with itraconazole and rifampicin did not fare well on the combination. One patient improved after rifampicin was stopped; the other developed a pulmonary aspergilloma during rifampicin therapy (732).

Cryptococcus neoformans.   Five patients with disease due to *C. neoformans* who were treated with itraconazole and concurrent rifampicin for other processes had serum levels of the azole that were either undetectable or markedly reduced from the levels seen with itraconazole alone. Despite this, four of the five responded clinically, possibly because of synergy that has been demonstrated in vitro (732).

***Fusarium* Species.**   Like many fungal infections, infections with *Fusarium* species usually occur in profoundly neutropenic patients who have been on prolonged therapy with broad-spectrum antibiotics. The synergistic combination of amphotericin B and rifampicin successfully treated disseminated disease in one child following a bone marrow transplant (60), but the combination was unsuccessful in many other patients with acute leukemias or malignancies (24, 91, 696, 750). One allogenic bone marrow transplant patient had progressive *F. moniliforme* infection and died despite addition of rifampicin and an increased dose of amphotericin B (382).

Histoplasma capsulatum.   Rare case reports describe the use of rifampicin in the treatment of *H. capsulatum*. One patient with esophageal obstruction due to *Histoplasma* granulomas was successfully treated with a combination of amphotericin B and rifampicin (357). A patient with cutaneous and lymphatic disease due to *H. capsulatum* var. *duboisii* was treated successfully with 4.5 months of this combination (519). Two children with disseminated disease due to *H. capsulatum* who had failed amphotericin B plus trimethoprim-sulfamethoxazole responded clinically after addition of rifampicin (655). A patient with disseminated disease was given 6 weeks of amphotericin B plus three antituberculous agents including rifampicin; 10 months later he had no clinical evidence of histoplasmosis (179).

Malassezia furfur.   The course of seborrheic dermatitis thought to be due to *M. furfur* seemed to be adversely affected by the concomitant use of itraconazole and rifampicin in two patients being treated for other fungal diseases (732).

Pneumocystis carinii.   Several anecdotal reports described clinical responses in the treatment of *P. carinii* infections with rifampicin (669, 698). One case report described a patient coinfected with *P. carinii* and *M. malmoense* who did not respond to a rifampicin-containing regimen (174).

***Rhizopus* Species.**   Zygomycoses are generally devastating infections with a high mortality rate. Several case reports describe successful treatment of such infections with a combination of amphotericin B and rifampicin. Two involved pulmonary disease due to *R. oryzae* (147, 437), another sinusitis due to *Cunninghamella bertholletiae* (520), and another unspecified disease with *Rhizopus* species in a child with acute lymphoblastic leukemia (38). Two neutropenic patients with a *Rhizopus* infection limited to the skin improved on a regimen of amphotericin B and rifampicin (332, 391).

Parasites

***Acanthamoeba* Species, *Naegleria fowleri*.** In one case report, an *Acanthamoeba* sp. isolate was not sensitive to rifampicin by vitro sensitivity testing, although the patient showed evidence of a clinical response on a regimen of 5-fluorocytosine and rifampicin for treatment of her cerebral abscess (322). Amebic meningoencephalitis in humans is usually fatal; only seven instances of survival have been reported. In four of these, rifampicin was used in combination with other agents including amphotericin B against *Naegleria* species (146, 573, 652, 771). In a case of cerebral abscess with *Acanthamoeba* species, treatment with rifampicin and 5-fluorocytosine yielded a clinical and radiographic response, although the patient later succumbed to other causes (322). One case report describes a patient with AIDS and cutaneous infection due to *Acanthamoeba castellani* (see above) who had an initial clinical response to amphotericin B, 5-fluorocytosine, and rifampicin. The organism was resistant to rifampicin, and the patient subsequently relapsed and died with active disease (361). A patient with AIDS and skin and sinus infections due to *Acanthamoeba* species responded clinically to the combination of rifampicin, amphotericin B, and ketoconazole (572).

***Leishmania* Species.** Conflicting results have been reported in the treatment of leishmaniasis with rifampicin. Several anecdotal and small-scale studies have shown benefit of rifampicin therapy for leishmanial infections. In one early report, 41 of an original 46 patients with cutaneous leishmaniasis completed a full course of rifampicin (1200 mg/day) and were cured (229). A single patient with *L. mexicana amazonensis* was reported to have had a clinical response to the combination of rifampicin and INH (562). One patient with post–kala azar dermal leishmaniasis thought to be due to *L. donovani* also responded to rifampicin therapy (623). While other anecdotal reports of successful treatment with rifampicin exist (297, 747), several reports describe rifampicin failures (120, 783). Six of eight patients with cutaneous leishmaniasis in one series responded to rifampicin; the strain was only specified in one patient from whom *L. tropica* was isolated (236). An 80% cure rate was achieved in another small study using rifampicin to treat *L. major* (380). In a series of 39 patients with cutaneous disease, the combination of rifampicin plus INH was only slightly more effective than rifampicin alone (443). Five of 6 patients with cutaneous disease due to *L. aethiopica* did not respond to a combination of rifampicin and isoniazid (745). In another series, none of 34 patients with cutaneous ulcerative leishmaniasis due to *L. braziliensis* showed any response to a 30-day course of rifampicin (212).

***Plasmodium* Species.** The antimalarial effects of rifampicin were examined prospectively in a trial comparing rifampicin alone, rifampicin followed by primaquine, and chloroquine followed by primaquine against *Plasmodium vivax* in 60 adults. All patients cleared their parasitemia; however, those on monotherapy with rifampicin all relapsed. Additionally, defervescence took significantly longer in the rifampicin-primaquine group than the chloroquine-primaquine group. Parasitemia reduction rates were also lower in both rifampicin-containing arms (583). In a preliminary report, the combination of rifampicin, INH, sulfamethoxazole, and trimethoprim was considered useful in both treatment and prophylaxis of malaria (254). While rifampicin does have relatively slow and weak antimalarial effects, it may have a role in children and pregnant women for whom some other agents are contraindicated.

Mycoplasma

***Mycoplasma hominis, Ureaplasma urealyticum*.** One double-blind trial compared rifampicin with minocycline for nongonococcal urethritis; 55 of 68 patients with initial positive cultures for *U. urealyticum* failed to achieve a microbiologic cure with rifampicin. Of the 26 patients with *M. hominis* isolates, 20 did not achieve a microbiologic cure (172).

Spirochetes

***Borrelia burgdorferi*.** Clinical data on the use of rifamycins in viral and spirochetal diseases in humans is limited to one report of a patient coinfected with *B. burgdorferi* and tick-borne encephalitis virus. The patient was unsuccessfully treated with a combination of antibiotics that included rifampicin (530).

Miscellaneous Infectious Uses of Rifamycins

Rifaximin cream 5% has been used topically without systemic absorption (82). A single blinded study demonstrated efficacy in treating pyogenic skin infections with more rapid regression than with oxytetracycline (536).

Noninfectious Uses of Rifamycins

Limited human data exist on the possible antitumor effects of the rifamycins. One study showed a delay in relapse of patients with acute myelogenous leukemia who were receiving rifampicin (118). In another report, seven patients with unresectable cholangiocarcinoma treated with rifampicin had a mean survival of 26 months compared with the expected survival of 8 months, and two patients were alive at the time of the report at 30 and 48 months (626). Several reports of patients who actually had an increase in tumors or tumor growth while on rifampicin for other reasons have raised concerns over the possibility that the agent actually facilitates tumor growth (609, 649).

In vitro rifampicin inhibited the aggregation of amyloid β protein that is a major component of senile plaques in Alzheimer's disease. It also inhibits the neurotoxicity induced by amyloid β protein on rat pheochromocytoma cells (716).

The noninfectious uses of rifamycins are expanding, with immunomodulatory effects proposed as the possible mechanism in some of these processes. Pruritus is a serious problem in patients with cholestatic liver disease, especially primary biliary cirrhosis. In several studies including one small randomized, placebo crossover study, rifampicin was effective in the relief of pruritic symptoms (46, 47, 276, 340, 570). In one long-term study the alkaline phosphatase level was significantly reduced, suggesting that rifampicin may actually affect the disease process (47). Relief from pruritus was seen in children with cholestatic liver disease treated with rifampicin in a double-blind, crossover trial (177).

Another report involving the possible utility of rifampicin's immune suppressive effects showed decreased intensity and extent of immune deposits in five of seven patients with Henoch-Schönlein purpura with the use of rifampicin. Additionally, proteinuria resolved in each of the children receiving rifampicin (395).

Studies of the treatment of Crohn's disease with antimycobacterial agents including rifamycins have yielded mixed results. One placebo-controlled trial showed fewer relapses in patients on a rifampicin-containing regimen (407), whereas another found no difference between rifampicin plus ethambutol and placebo (657). Several smaller studies and case reports have reported benefit from antimycobacterial therapy including rifampicin in the treatment of Crohn's disease (314, 564, 646, 772, 789). Six patients with refractory Crohn's disease were treated successfully with the combination of streptomycin and rifabutin for 2 to 4 months (711). The combination of rifabutin and ethambutol for 6 to 12 months did not benefit 15 patients with disease of the neoterminal ileum (619). A comprehensive review of the possible links between Crohn's disease and mycobacterioses and treatment with antimycobacterial agents reached no definitive conclusions and made no specific recommendations (145).

One case report describes a patient with ulcerative colitis who had an apparent initial clinical response to treatment with antimycobacterial therapy including rifampicin. The patient subsequently relapsed on therapy (564).

Rifampicin resulted in a clinical response of at least 1 year's duration in one patient with folliculitis decalvans who had been unresponsive to previous therapies. The cause of this unusual inflammatory response of the scalp is unknown, although a bacterial etiology has been postulated (108).

Rifaximin was evaluated for the treatment of diverticular disease. In one double-blind, placebo-controlled trial, rifaximin gave better symptomatic relief than fiber supplementation alone (539). Cyclic use of rifaximin also proved useful in controlling symptoms and averting complications in one series of 79 patients with stenosis of the sigmoid colon following diverticulitis (277). In a small series of patients with bacterial overgrowth, rifaximin resulted in significant improvement in 10 of 12 patients (166).

Reprimun was evaluated in the treatment of five patients with thrombocytopenia and one with hemolytic anemia refractory to steroid therapy. Platelets and hemoglobin levels increased in the respective cases (547).

The efficacy of reprimun in the treatment of sarcoidosis was also evaluated. Reprimun alone or reprimun plus prednisone produced lasting remissions in 89% of 112 patients reported in one series (548). The same author refers to successful treatment of a variety of other processes with reprimun including dermatomyositis, Kaposi's sarcoma, systemic lupus erythematosus, periarteritis nodosum, and silicosis, but no specifics were provided (547).

The efficacy of rifamycins in the treatment of rheumatoid disease and ankylosing spondylitis seems to depend on the route of administration. In an open study, oral administration of rifampicin in patients with ankylosing spondylitis showed no benefit, whereas intraarticular infiltration of rifamycin SV in large peripheral joints yielded significant laboratory and clinical improvement, including a positive response in axial symptoms (125). All 15 patients with rheumatoid knee synovitis treated with intraarticular rifamycin SV in a double-blind placebo-controlled trial had their effusions disappear and showed clinical improvement (126). Similar positive responses were seen in early rheumatoid arthritis and pauci- or polyarticular juvenile rheumatoid arthritis treated with intraarticular rifamycin SV (127, 128). In another series, arthroscopy before and after administration of intraarticular rifamycin SV demonstrated an antiinflammatory effect; however, a local chemical synovitis developed after repeated injections (440). Although in one report, 7 of 20 patients treated with oral rifampicin with or without INH improved clinically and by laboratory parameters (481), subsequent reports have not demonstrated benefit in the treatment of rheumatoid disease from oral rifampicin or rifampicin plus INH (99, 173, 263).

REFERENCES

1. Abeck D, Johnson AP, Dangor Y, Ballard RC. Antibiotic susceptibilities and plasmid profiles of *Haemophilus ducreyi* isolates from southern Africa. J Antimicrob Chemother 1988;22:437–444.
2. Aber RC, Wennersten C, Moellering RC Jr. Antimicrobial susceptibility of flavobacteria. Antimicrob Agents Chemother 1978;14:483–487.
3. Abu Romeh SH, Kozma GN, Johny KV, Sabha M. *Brucella* endocarditis causing acute renal failure. Nephron 1987;46:388–389.
4. Acocella G. Clinical pharmacokinetics of rifampicin. Clin Pharmacokinet 1978;3:108–127.
5. Acocella G, Scotti R. Kinetic studies on the combination rifampicin-trimethoprim in man. J Antimicrob Chemother 1976;2:271–277.
6. Acocella G, Bonollo L, Garimoldi M, Mainardi M, Tenconi LT, Nicolis FB. Kinetics of rifampin and isoniazid administered alone and in combination to normal subjects and patients with liver disease. Gut 1972;13:47–53.
7. Adamson RH. Antitumor activity of two antiviral drugs—rifampicin and tilorone [Letter]. Lancet 1971;1:398.
8. Ahn CH, Lowell JR, Ahn SS. Chemotherapy for pulmonary disease due to *Mycobacterium kansasii:* efficacies of some individual drugs. Rev Infect Dis 1981;3:1028–1034.
9. Ahn CH, Lowell JR, Ahn SS, Hurst GA. Short course chemotherapy for pulmonary disease caused by *Mycobacterium kansasii*. Am Rev Respir Dis 1983;128:1048–1050.
10. Aitio ML, Mansury L, Tala E, Haataja M, Aitio A. The effect of enzyme induction on the metabolism of disopyramide in man. Br J Clin Pharmacol 1981;11:279–285.
11. Akova M, Uzon O, Akalin HE, Hayran M, Ünal S, Gür D. Quinolones in treatment of human brucellosis: comparative trial of ofloxacin-rifampin versus doxycycline-rifampin. Antimicrob Agents Chemother 1993;37:1831–1834.
12. Alger NE, Spira DT, Silverman PH. Inhibition of rodent malaria in mice by rifampicin. Nature 1970;227:381–382.

13. Al-Hamdan Y, Otto U, Kirch W. Interaction of rifampicin with bunazosin, an alpha$_1$-adrenoreceptor antagonist [Abstract]. J Clin Pharmacol 1993;33:998.

14. Al-Harthi SS. Association of brucella endocarditis with intracerebral haemorrhage. Int J Cardiol 1987;16:214–216.

15. Al-Harthi SS. The morbidity and mortality pattern of *Brucella* endocarditis. Int J Cardiol 1089;25:321–324.

16. Allen UD, Niec A, Kerem E, Greenberg M, Gold R. *Rhodococcus equi* pneumonia in a child with leukemia. Pediatr Infect Dis J 1989;8:656–658.

17. Altmann G, Bogokovsky B. In-vitro sensitivity of *Flavobacterium meningosepticum* to antimicrobial agents. J Med Microbiol 1971;4:296–299.

18. Alvisi V, D'Ambrosi A, Loponte A, Pazzi P, Greco A, Zangirolami A, Palazzini E. Rifaximin, a rifamycin derivative for use in the treatment of intestinal bacterial infections in seriously disabled patients. J Int Med Res 1987;15:49–56.

19. Alvisi V, D'Ambrosi A, Onofri W, Catellani M. Treatment of secretory diarrhoeas. A double-blind trial of the effectiveness of rifaximin (L 105) and neomycin. Clin Trials J 1984;21:215–223.

20. American Academy of Pediatrics. *Haemophilus influenzae* infections. In: Peter G, ed, 1994 red book: report of the Committee on Infectious Diseases. 23rd ed. Elk Grove Village, IL: American Academy of Pediatrics, 1994:203–216.

21. American Academy of Pediatrics. Meningococcal infections. In: Peter G, ed, 1994 red book: report of the Committee on Infectious Diseases. 23rd ed. Elk Grove Village, IL: American Academy of Pediatrics, 1994:323–326.

22. American Academy of Pediatrics. *Legionella pneumophila* infections. In: Peter G, ed, 1994 red book: report of the Committee on Infectious Diseases. 23rd ed. Elk Grove Village, IL: American Academy of Pediatrics, 1994:287–288.

23. American Thoracic Society. Treatment of tuberculosis infection in adults and children. Am J Res Crit Care Med 1994;149:1359–1374.

24. Anaissie E, Kantarjian H, Jones P, Barlogie B, Luna M, Lopez-Berestein G, Bodey GP. *Fusarium*. A newly recognized fungal pathogen in immunosuppressed patients. Cancer 1986;57:2141–2145.

25. Ånséhn S, Granström S, Höjer H, Nilsson L, Åkesson E, Lundin L, Thore A. In-vitro effects on *Candida albicans* of amphotericin B combined with other antibiotics. Scand J Infect Dis 1976;9(Suppl).62–66.

26. Appelbaum PC, Spangler SK, Potter CR, Sattler FR. Reduction of oral flora with rifampin in healthy volunteers. Antimicrob Agents Chemother 1986;29:576–578.

27. Apseloff G, Hilligoss DM, Gardner MJ, Henry EB, Inskeep PB, Gerber N, Lazar JD. Induction of fluconazole metabolism by rifampin: in vivo study in humans. J Clin Pharmacol 1991;31:358–361.

28. Aquinas SM, Allan WGL, Horsfall PAL, Jenkins PK, Hung-yan W, Girling D, Tall R, Fox W. Adverse reactions to daily and intermittent rifampicin regimens for pulmonary tuberculosis in Hong Kong. Br Med J 1972;1:765–771.

29. Aracil B, Gomez-Garces JL, Alos JI, Balas D. Susceptibility of *Eikenella corrodens* to newer and older oral antimicrobial agents [Abstract E099]. 36th ICAAC, Annual Meeting of the American Society for Microbiology, New Orleans, September 15–18, 1996.

30. Arathoon EG, Hamilton JR, Hench CE, Stevens DA. Efficacy of short courses of oral novobiocin-rifampin in eradicating carrier state of methicillin-resistant *Staphylococcus aureus* and in vitro killing studies of clinical isolates. Antimicrob Agents Chemother 1990;34:1655–1659.

31. Araujo FG, Slifer T, Remington JS. Rifabutin is active in murine models of toxoplasmosis. Antimicrob Agents Chemother 1994;38:570–575.

32. Araujo FG, Khan AA, Remington JS. Rifapentine is active in vitro and in vivo against *Toxoplasma gondii*. Antimicrob Agents Chemother 1996;40:1335–1337.

33. Archer GL, Johnston L, Vazquez GJ, Haywood HB III. Efficacy of antibiotic combinations including rifampin against methicillin-resistant *Staphylococcus epidermidis:* in vitro and in vivo studies. Rev Infect Dis 1983;5:S538–542.

34. Archer GL, Armstrong BC. Alteration of staphylococcal flora in cardiac surgery patients receiving antibiotic prophylaxis. J Infect Dis 1983;147:642–649.

35. Archer GL, Climo MW. Antimicrobial susceptibility of coagulase-negative staphylococci. Antimicrob Agents Chemother 1994;38:2231–2237.

36. Ariza J, Gudiol F, Pallares R, Rufi G, Fernandez-Viladrich P. Comparative trial of rifampin-doxycycline versus tetracycline-streptomycin in the therapy of human brucellosis. Antimicrob Agents Chemother 1985;28:548–551.

37. Ariza J, Gudiol F, Pallares R, Viladrich PF, Rufi G, Corredoira J, Miravitlles MR. Treatment of human brucellosis with doxycycline plus rifampin or doxycycline plus streptomycin. Ann Intern Med 1992;117:25–30.

38. Armstrong D. Problems in management of opportunistic fungal diseases. Rev Infect Dis 1989;11(Suppl):S1591–599.

39. Arora SK, Singha R, Sehgal S. Use of in vitro method to assess different brands of anti-leishmanial drugs. Med Microbiol Immunol 1991;180:21–27.

40. Arroyo J, Medoff G, Kobayashi GS. Therapy of murine aspergillosis with amphotericin B in combination with rifampin or 5-fluorocytosine. Antimicrob Agents Chemother 1977;11: 21–25.

41. Assandri A, Ratti B, Cristina T. Pharmacokinetics of rifapentine, a new long lasting rifamycin, in the rat, the mouse, and the rabbit. J Antibiot 1984;37(9):1066–1075.

42. Atkin SL, Masson EA, Bodmer CW, Walker BA, White MC. Increased insulin requirement in a patient with type 1 diabetes on rifampicin. Diabetic Med 1993;10:392.

43. Atkinson BA, Bocanegra JR, Graybill JR. Treatment of *Mycobacterium haemophilum* infection in a murine model with clarithromycin, rifabutin, and ciprofloxacin. Antimicrob Agents Chemother 1995;39:2316–2319.

44. Atlas E, Turck M. Laboratory and clinical evaluation of rifampicin. Am J Med Sci 1968;256:247–254.

45. Aubrey M, Fam AG. A case of clinically unsuspected *Mycobacterium marinum* infection. Arthritis Rheum 1987;30:1317–1318.

46. Bachs L, Pares A, Elena M, Piera C, Rodes J. Comparison of rifampicin with phenobarbitone for treatment of primary biliary cirrhosis. Lancet 1989;1:574–576.

47. Bachs L, Parés A, Elena M, Piera C, Rodés J. Effects of long-term rifampicin administration in primary biliary cirrhosis. Gastroenterology 1992;102:2077–2080.

48. Bacon AE, McGrath S, Fekety R, Holloway WJ. In vitro synergy studies with *Clostridia difficile*. Antimicrob Agents Chemother 1991;35:582–583.

49. Baltch AL, Smith RP, Ritz W. Inhibitory and bactericidal activities of lovofloxacin, ofloxacin, erythromycin, and rifampin used singly and in combination against *Legionella pneumophila*. Antimicrob Agents Chemother 1995;39:1661–1666.

50. Band JD, Fraser DW, Ajello G, Hemophilus Influenzae Study Group. Prevention of *Haemophilus influenzae* type b disease. JAMA 1984;251:2381–2386.

51. Banerjee DK, Holmes IB. In vitro and in vivo studies of the action of rifampicin, clofazamine, and B1912 on *Mycobacterium marinum*. Chemotherapy 1976;22:242–252.

52. Banks J, Hunter AM, Campbell IA, Jenkins PA, Smith AP. Pulmonary infection with *Mycobacterium kansasii* in Wales, 1970–1979: review of treatment and response. Thorax 1983;38:271–274.

53. Banks J, Hunter AM, Campbell IA, Jenkins PA, Smith AP. Pulmonary infection with *Mycobacterium xenopi:* review of treatment and response. Thorax 1984;39:376.

54. Banks J, Jenkins PA, Smith AP. Pulmonary infection with *Mycobacterium malmoense*—a review of treatment and response. Tubercle 1985;66:197–203.

55. Banks J, Jenkins W. Combined versus single antituberculosis drugs on the in vitro sensitivity patterns of non-tuberculous mycobacteria. Thorax 1987;42:838–842.

56. Bansal VK, Bennett D, Molnar Z. Prolonged renal failure after rifampin. Am Rev Respir Dis 1977;116:137–140.

57. Baohong J. Drug resistance in leprosy—a review. Lepr Rev 1985;56:265–278.

58. Barker JE, Farrell ID. The effects of single and combined antibiotics on the growth of *Legionella pneumophila* using time-kill studies. J Antimicrob Chemother 1990;26:45–53.

59. Barriere SL, Kaatz GW, Seo SM. Enhanced elimination of ciprofloxacin after multiple-dose administration of rifampin to rabbits. Antimicrob Agents Chemother 1989;33:589–590.

60. Barrios NJ, Kirkpatrick DV, Murciano A, Stine K, Van Dyke RB, Humbert JR. Successful treatment of disseminated *Fusarium* infection in an immunocompromised child. Am J Pediatr Hematol Oncol 1990;12:319–324.

61. Bartlett JG. Tables of Antimicrobial Agents. In: Gorbach SL, Bartlett JG, Blacklow NR, eds. Infectious diseases. Philadelphia: WB Saunders, 1992:361–366.

62. Bartoloni A, Gracia Colao M, Orsi A, Dei R, Giganti E, Parenti F. In-vitro activity of vancomycin, teicoplanin, daptomycin, ramoplanin, MDL 62873 and other agents against staphylococci, enterococci and *Clostridia difficile*. J Antimicrob Chemother 1990;26:627–633.

63. Bartolucci C, Cellai L, Di Filippo P, Segre A, Brufani M, Filocamo L, Bianco AD, Guiso M, Brizzi V, Benedetto A, Di Caro A, Giuliano E. Rifamycins as inhibitors of retroviral reverse transcriptase from M-MULV, RAV-2, and HIV-1. Il Farmaco 1992;47:1367–1383.

64. Bartolucci C, Cellai L, Marzano M, Segre A, Brufani M, Filocamo L, Bianco AD, Guiso M, Brizzi V, Benedetto A, DiCaro A. Structure-activity relationships in open ansa-chain rifamycin S derivatives as inhibitors of HIV-1 reverse transcriptase. Il Farmaco 1995;50:587–593.

65. Battaglia R, Pianazzola E, Salgrollo G, Zini G, Benedetti MS. Absorption, disposition and preliminary metabolic pathway of ^{14}C-rifabutin in animals and man. J Antimicrob Chemother 1990;26:813–822.

66. Battaglia R, Salgarollo G, Zini G, Montesanti L, Benedetti MS. Absorption, disposition and urinary metabolism of ^{14}C-rifabutin in rats. Antimicrob Agents Chemother 1991;35:1391–1396.

67. Battaner E, Kumar BV. Rifampin: inhibition of ribonucleic acid synthesis after potentiation by amphotericin B in *Saccharomyces cerevisiae*. Antimicrob Agents Chemother 1974;5:371–376.

68. Beaty HN. Rifampin and minocycline in meningococcal disease. Rev Infect Dis 1983;5:S451–458.

69. Bebchuk JM, Stewart DE. Drug interaction between rifampin and nortriptyline: a case report. Int J Psychiatry Med 1991;21:183–187.

70. Beck RW, Janssen RS, Smiley L, Schatz NJ, Savino PJ, Rubin DH. Melioidosis and bilateral third-nerve palsies. Neurology 1984;34:105–107.

71. Becker Y, Asher Y, Himmel N, Zakay-Rones Z. Rifampicin inhibition of trachoma agent in vivo. Nature 1969;224:33–34.

72. Beggs WH, Sarosi GA, Andrews FA. Synergistic action of amphotericin B and rifampin on *Candida albicans*. Am Rev Respir Dis 1974;110:671–673.

73. Beggs WH, Sarosi GA, Walker MI. Synergistic action of amphotericin B and rifampin against *Candida* species. J Infect Dis 1976;133:206–209.

74. Bell RC, Higuchi JH, Donovan WN, Krasnow I, Johanson WG Jr. *Mycobacterium simiae*. Clinical features and follow-up of twenty-four patients. Am Rev Respir Dis 1983;127:35–38.

75. Bella F, Espejo E, Uriz J, Serrano JA, Alegre D, Tort J. Randomized trial of 5-day rifampin versus 1-day doxycycline therapy for Mediterranean spotted fever [Letter]. J Infect Dis 1991;164:433–434.

76. Belli L, Ambrona MS, Gennaro EA, Isola EH, Gonzalez Reseigno GR. Acute gonococcal urethritis: treatment with a single dose of rifampicin. J Int Med Res 1983;11:32–37.

77. Benedetti MS, Dostert P. Induction and autoinduction properties of rifamycin derivatives: a review of animal and human studies. Environ Health Perspect 1994;102(Suppl 9):101–105.

78. Bennett PN, John VA, Whitmarsh VB. Effect of rifampicin on metoprolol and antipyrine kinetics. Br J Clin Pharmacol 1982;13:387–391.

79. Bennhoff DF. Actinomycosis: diagnostic and therapeutic considerations and a review of 32 cases. Laryngoscope 1984;94:1198–1217.

80. Bental T, Fejgin M, Keysary A, Rzotkiewicz S, Oron C, Nachum R, Beyth Y, Lang R. Chronic Q fever of pregnancy presenting as *Coxiella burnetii* placentitis: successful outcome following therapy with erythromycin and rifampin. Clin Infect Dis 1995;21:1318–1321.

81. Berkey PK, Rolson K, Zukiwski A, Gooch G, Bodey GP. Rifampin-resistant meningococcal infection in a patient given rifampin chemoprophylaxis. Am J Infect Control 1988;16:250–252.

82. Bërlo JA, Debruyne HJ, Gortz JP. A prospective study in healthy volunteers of the topical absorption of a 5% rifaximin cream. Drugs Exp Clin Res 1994;20:205–208.

83. Bernard EM, Edwards FF, Kiehn TE, Brown ST, Armstrong D. Activities of antimicrobial agents against clinical isolates of *Mycobacterium haemophilum*. Antimicrob Agents Chemother 1993;37:2323–2326.

84. Berning SE, Huitt GA, Iseman MD, Peloquin CA. Malabsorption of antituberculosis medications by a patient with AIDS. N Engl J Med 1992;327:1817–1818.

85. Berning SE, Peloquin. Clarithromycin (CLAR) and 14-OH clarithromycin serum concentrations in patients with mycobacterial infections with or without rifampin (RIF). Abstract presented at American Thoracic Society 1997 International Conference, San Francisco, May 16–21, 1997.

86. Beyt BE Jr, Cannon RO III, Tuteur PG. Successful treatment of invasive pulmonary aspergillosis in the immunocompromised host. South Med J 1978;71:1164–1166.

87. Bhatia RS, Uppal R, Malhi R, Behera D, Jindal SK. Drug interaction between rifampicin and cotrimoxazole in patients with tuberculosis. Hum Exp Toxic 1991;10:419–421.

88. Bilgeri YR, Ballard RC, Duncan MO, Mauff AC, Koornhof HJ. Antimicrobial susceptibility of 103 strains of *Haemophilus ducreyi* isolated in Johannesburg. Antimicrob Agents Chemother 1982;22:686–688.

89. Blanchard JS. Molecular mechanisms of drug resistance in *Mycobacterium tuberculosis*. Annu Rev Biochem 1996;65: 215–239.

90. Blaschke TF, Skinner MH. The clinical pharmacokinetics of rifabutin. Clin Infect Dis 1996;22(Suppl 1):S15–22.

91. Blazar BR, Hurd DD, Snover DC, Alexander JW, McGlave PB. Invasive *Fusarium* infections in bone marrow transplant recipients. Am J Med 1984;77:645–651.

92. Blondeau JM, Yaschuk Y. In vitro activities of ciprofloxacin, cefotaxime, ceftriaxone, chloramphenicol, and rifampin against fully susceptible and moderately penicillin-resistant *Neisseria meningitidis*. Antimicrob Agents Chemother 1995;39: 2577–2579.

93. Boakes AJ, Loo PSL, Ridgway GL, Tovey S, Oriel JD. Treatment of uncomplicated gonorrhea in women with a combination of rifampicin and erythromycin. Br J Vener Dis 1984;60:309–311.

94. Bodmer T, Zurcher G, Imboden P, Telenti A. Mutation position and type of substitution in the b-subunit of the RNA polymerase influence in-vitro activity of rifamycins in rifampin-resistant *Mycobacterium tuberculosis*. J Antimicrob Chemother 1995; 35:345–348.

95. Bogaerts Y, Elinck W, van Renterghem D, Pauwels R, van der Straeten. Pulmonary disease due to *Mycobacterium xenopi:* report of two cases. Eur J Respir Dis 1982;63:298–304.

96. Bolt HM, Kappus H, Bolt M. Effect of rifampicin-treatment on the metabolism of oestadiol and 17O-ethinyloestradiol by human liver microsomes. Eur J Clin Pharmacol 1975;8:301–307.

97. Bolton WK, Sande MA, Normansell DE, Sturgill BC, Westervelt FB Jr. Ventriculojugular shunt nephritis with *Corynebacterium bovis*. Am J Med 1975;59:417–423.

98. Boman G, Hanngren A, Malmboro AS, Borga O, Sjoqvist F. Drug interaction: decreased serum concentrations of rifampicin when given with P.A.S. Lancet 1971:800.

99. Borg AA, Davis MJ, Fowler PD, Shadforth MF, Dawes PT. Rifampicin in early rheumatoid arthritis. Scand J Rheumatol 1993;22:39–42.

100. Bowie WR, Lee CK, Alexander ER. Prediction of the efficacy of antimicrobial agents in the treatment of infections due to *Chlamydia trachomatis*. J Infect Dis 1978;138:655–677.

101. Bradley JS, Connor JD. Ceftriaxone failure in meningitis caused by *Streptococcus pneumoniae* with reduced susceptibility to β-lactam antibiotics. Pediatr Infect Dis 1991;10:871–873.

102. Brinch L, Rostad H, Mehl A, Blichfeldt P, Eng J. Hairy cell leukemia and *Mycobacterium malmoense* infection. Tidsskr Nor Laegeforen 1990;110:835–836.

103. Brockmeyer NH, Mertins L, Klimer K, Goos M, Ohnhaus EE. Comparative effects of rifampin and/or probenecid on the pharmacokinetics of temazepam and nitrazepam. Int J Clin Pharmacol Ther Toxicol 1990;28:387–393.

104. Brogden RN, Fitton A. Rifabutin. a review of its antimicrobial activity, pharmacokinetic properties and therapeutic efficacy. Drugs 1994;47:983–1009.

105. Brook I. Penicillin V and rifampin for streptococcal pharyngitis [Letter]. J Pediatr 1985;107:825.

106. Brouqui P, Raoult D. In vitro susceptibility of *Ehrlichia sennetsu* to antibiotics. Antimicrob Agents Chemother 1990;34: 1593–1596.

107. Brouqui P, Raoult D. In vitro susceptibility of the newly recognized agent of ehrlichiosis in humans, *Ehrlichia chafeensis*. Antimicrob Agents Chemother 1992;36:2799–2803.

108. Brozena SJ, Cohen LE, Fenske NA. Folliculitis decalvans—response to rifampin. Cutis 1988;42:512–515.

109. Brumfitt W, Dixson S, Hamilton-Miller JMT. Use of rifampin in urinary tract infections. Rev Infect Dis 1983;5:S573–582.

110. Brumfitt W, Hamilton-Miller JMT. Use of trimethoprim alone or in combination with drugs other than sulfonamides. Rev Infect Dis 1982;4:402–409.

111. Brunfani M, Cellai L, Cerrini S, Fedeli W, Marchi E, Segre A, Vaciago A. X-ray crystal structure of 4-deoxy-3′-bromopyridol[1′,2′-1,2]imidazo[5,4-c]rifamycin S. J Antibiot 1984;37: 1623–1627.

112. Bucci L, Palmieri GC. Double-blind, double-dummy comparison between treatment with rifaximin and lactulose in patients with medium to severe degree hepatic encephalopathy. Curr Med Res Opin 1993;13:109–118.

113. Buffington GA, Dominguez JH, Piering WF, Herbert LA, Kauffman HM, Lemann J. Interaction of rifampin and glucocorticoids. JAMA 1976;236:1958–1960.

114. Buggy BP, Fekety R, Silva J Jr. Therapy of relapsing *Clostridium difficile*-associated diarrhea and colitis with the combination of vancomycin and rifampin. J Clin Gastroenterol 1987;9: 155–159.

115. Bullock WE. Rifampin in the treatment of leprosy. Rev Infect Dis 1983;5:S606–613.

116. Buniva G, Palminteri R, Berti M. Kinetics of a rifampicin-trimethoprim combination. Int J Clin Pharmacol Toxicol Ther 1979;17:256–259.

117. Burger DM, Meenhorst PL, Koks CHW, Beijnen JH. Pharmacokinetic interaction between rifampin and zidovudine. Antimicrob Agents Chemother 1993;37:1426–1431.

118. Burghouts J, Haanen C. A possible role of rifampicin in prolonging remission duration in acute myelogenous leukaemia. Scand J Haematol 1986;36:376–378.

119. Byard RW, Thorner PS, Edwards V, Greenberg M. Pulmonary malacoplakia in a child. Pediatr Pathol 1990;10:417–424.

120. Bygbjerg IC, Knudsen L, Kieffer M. Failure of rifampicin therapy to cure leishmaniasis [Letter]. Arch Dermatol 1980; 116:988.

121. Campbell IA. BTS study of the treatment of *Mycobacterium kansasii* pulmonary disease. Thorax 1993;48:423.

122. Cardot E, Tillie-Leblonde I, Jeanin P, et al. Anaphylactic reaction to local administration of rifamycin SV. J Allergy Clin Immunol 1995;95:1–7.

123. Carpenter JL, Parks JM. *Mycobacterium kansasii* infections in patients positive for human immunodeficiency virus. Rev Infect Dis 1991;13:789–796.

124. Carter PE, Abadi FJR, Yakubu DE, Pennington TH. Molecular characterization of rifampin-resistant *Neisseria meningitidis*. Antimicrob Agents Chemother 1994;38:1256–1261.

125. Caruso I, Cazzola M, Santandrea S. Clinical improvement in ankylosing spondylitis with rifamycin SV infiltrations of peripheral joints. J Int Med Res 1992;20:171–181.

126. Caruso I, Montrone F, Fumagalli M, Patrono C, Santandrea S, Gandini MC. Rheumatoid knee synovitis successfully treated with intra-articular rifamycin SV. Ann Rheum Dis 1982;41: 232–236.

127. Caruso I, Santandrea S, Sarzi Puttini P, Montreone F, Boccassini L, Azzolini V, Cazzola M, Dell'Acqua D. Prevention of appearance of radiological lesions in early rheumatoid arthritis: a randomized, single-blind study comparing intra-articular rifamycin with auranofin. J Int Med Res 1992;20:61–77.

128. Caruso I, Principi N, D'Urbino G, Santandrea S, Boccassini L, Montrone F, Sarzi Puttini PC, Bombaci A, Bozzato, A, Azzolini V, Dell'Acqua D. Rifamycin SV administered by intra-articular infiltrations shows disease modifying activity in patients with pauci- or polyarticular juvenile rheumatoid arthritis. J Int Med Res 1993;21:243–256.

129. Castel JP, Cappiello E, Leopaldi D, Latini R. Rifampicin lowers plasma concentrations of propafenone and its antiarrhythmic effect. Br J Clin Pharmacol 1990;30:155–156.

130. Cato A, Cavanaugh JH, Shi H, Hsu A, Granneman GR, Leonard J. Assessment of multiple doses of ritonavir on the pharmacokinetics of rifabutin [Abstract no. B.1199]. Presented at XI International Conference on AIDS. Vancouver, July 8, 1996.

131. Cavalleri B, Turconi M, Tamborini G, Occelli E, Cietto G, Pallanza R, Scotti R, Berti M, Romano G, Parenti F. Synthesis and biological activity of some derivatives of rifamycin P. J Med Chem 1990;33:1470–1476.

132. Centers for Disease Control and Prevention. Initial therapy for tuberculosis in the era of multidrug resistance. Recommendations of the Advisory Council for the Elimination of Tuberculosis. MMWR 1993;42(RR-7):1–8.

133. Centers for Disease Control and Prevention. National action plan to combat multidrug-resistant tuberculosis. MMWR 1992;41(RR-11):5–48.

134. Chandler MHH, Toler SM, Rapp RP, Muder RR, Korvick JA. Multiple-dose pharmacokinetics of concurrent oral ciprofloxacin and rifampin therapy in elderly patients. Antimicrob Agents Chemother 1990;34:442–447.

135. Chandrika T, Adler SP. A case of neonatal meningitis due to *Flavobacterium meningosepticum* successfully treated with rifampin. Pediatr Infect Dis 1982;1:40–41.

136. Chang BJ, Bolton SM. Plasmids and resistance to antimicrobial agents in *Aeromonas sobria* and *Aeromonas hydrophila* clinical isolates. Antimicrob Agents Chemother 1987;31: 1281–1282.

137. Chapalain J, Dusseau J, Perrier-Gros-Claude J, Rouby Y, Bartoli M. Effect of rifampicin chemoprophylaxis on the aerobic bacterial flora of the oropharynx. J Antimicrob Chemother 1994;33:151–155.

138. Chaudhary S, Bilinsky SA, Hennessy JL, Soler SM, Wallace SE, Schacht CM, Bisno AL. Penicillin V and rifampin for the treatment of group A streptococcal pharyngitis: a randomized trial of 10 days penicillin vs 10 days penicillin with rifampin during the final 4 days of therapy. J Pediatr 1985;106:481–486.

139. Chen SCA, Paul ML, Gilbert GL. Susceptibility of *Legionella* species to antimicrobial agents. Pathology 1993;25:180–183.

140. Chernov AP, Mel'nikov AA, Fodor II. Recombinant reverse transcriptase of Rous sarcoma virus: characterization of DNA polymerase and RNAase activities. Biomed Sci 1991;2:49–53.

141. Chin N, Neu HC. Synergy of imipenem—a novel carbapenam, and rifampin and ciprofloxacin against *Pseudomonas aeruginosa, Serratia marcescens* and *Enterobacter* species. Chemotherapy 1987;33:183–188.

142. Chiodini RJ, Kreeger JM, Thayer WR. Use of rifabutin in treatment of systemic *Mycobacterium paratuberculosis* infection in mice. Antimicrob Agents Chemother 1993;37:1645–1648.

143. Chiodini RJ. Antimicrobial activity of rifabutin in combination with two and three other antimicrobial agents against strains of *Mycobacterium paratuberculosis*. Antimicrob Agents Chemother 1991;27:171–176.

144. Chiodini RJ. Bactericidal activities of various antimicrobial agents against human and animal isolates of *Mycobacterium paratuberculosis*. Antimicrob Agents Chemother 1990;34:366–367.

145. Chiodini RJ. Crohn's disease and the mycobacterioses: a review and comparison of two disease entities. Clin Microbiol Rev 1989;2:90–117.

146. Chotmongkol V, Pipitgool V, Khempila J. Eosinophilic cerebrospinal fluid pleocytosis and primary amebic meningoencephalitis. Southeast Asian J Trop Med Public Health 1993;24: 399–401.

147. Christenson JC, Shalit I, Welch DF, Guruswamy A, Marks MI. Synergistic action of amphotericin B and rifampin against *Rhizopus* species. Antimicrob Agents Chemother 1987;31: 1775–1778.

148. Chuard C, Herrmann M, Vaudaux P, Waldvogel FA, Lew DP. Successful therapy of experimental chronic foreign-body infection due to methicillin-resistant *Staphylococcus aureus* by antimicrobial combinations. Antimicrob Agents Chemother 1991;35:2611–2616.

149. Civen R, Berlin G, Panosian C. Vertebral osteomyelitis after intravesical administration of bacille Calmette-Guérin. Clin Infect Dis 1994;18:1013–1014.

150. Claydon EJ, Coker RJ, Harris JRW. *Mycobacterium malmoense* infection in HIV positive patients. J Infect 1991;23: 191–194.

151. Clemens KV, Minn AY, Aristizabal BH, Stevens DA. Efficacy of fluconazole (FCZ) alone or in combination with azithromycin (AZI) or rifabutin (RIF) against systemic murine cryptococcosis [Abstract B050]. 36th ICAAC, Annual Meeting of the American Society for Microbiology, New Orleans, Sep 15–18, 1996.

152. Cohen MA, Yoder SL, Huband MD, Roland GE, Courtney CL. In vitro and in vivo activities of clinafloxacin, CI-990 (PD 131112), and PD 138312 versus enterococci. Antimicrob Agents Chemother 1995;39:2123–2127.

153. Cohn JR, Fye DL, Sills JM, Francos GC. Rifampicin-induced renal failure. Tubercle 1985;66:289–293.

154. Cole ST. Rifamycin resistance in mycobacteria. Res Microbiol 1996:147:48–52.

155. Colebunders R, Ursi JP, Pattyn S, Snoeck J. Prosthetic valve endocarditis due to methicillin-resistant *Staphylococcus epidermidis* and *Micrococcus* species successfully treated with rifampicin combined with other antibiotics. J Infect 1985;11:35–39.

156. Collins P, Clancy L, Barnes L. Erythema induratum (Bazin's disease). Ir Med J 1991;84:96–98.

157. Colmenero Castillo JD, Marquez SH, Iglesias JMR, Franquelo FC, Diaz FR, Alonzo A. Comparative trial of doxycycline plus streptomycin versus doxycycline plus rifampin for the therapy of human brucellosis. Chemotherapy 1989;35:146–152.

158. Colmenero JD, Fernandez-Gallardo LC, Agundez JAG, Sedeno J, Benitez J, Valverde E. Possible implications of doxycycline-rifampin interaction for treatment of brucellosis. Antimicrob Agents Chemother 1994;38:2798–2802.

159. Comley JC, Sterling AM. Effect of atovaquone and atovaquone drug combinations on prophylaxis of *Pneumocystis carinii* pneumonia in SCID mice. Antimicrob Agents Chemother 1995;39:806–811.

160. Commare MC, Dauga C, Sednaoui P, Ronco E, Nordmann P. Diagnostic and therapeutic problems due to cat scratch disease. J Infect 1995;30:1834–1835.

161. Committee on Drugs, American Academy of Pediatrics. The transfer of drugs and other chemicals into human milk. Pediatrics 1994;93:137–150.

162. Conti R, Parenti F. Rifampin therapy for brucellosis, flavobacterium meningitis, and cutaneous leishmaniasis. Rev Infect Dis 1983;5:S600–605.

163. Contreras MH, Cheung OT, Sanders DE, Goldstein RS. Pulmonary infection with nontuberculous mycobacteria. Am Rev Respir Dis 1988;137:149–152.

164. Cooper ER, Ellison III RT, Smith GS, Blaser MJ, Reller LB, Paisley JW. Rifampin-resistant meningococcal disease in a contact patient given prophylactic rifampin. J Pediatr 1986;108:93–96.

165. Copeland J, Wieden M, Feinberg W, Salomon N, Hager D, Galgiani J. Legionnaires' disease description following cardiac transplantation. Chest 1981;79:669–671.

166. Corazza BR, Ventucci M, Strocchi A, Sorge M, Pranzo, Pezzilli R, Gasharrini G. Treatment of small intestine bacterial overgrowth with rifaximin, a non-absorbable rifamycin. J Int Med Res 1988;16:312–316.

167. Corbel MJ. Determination of the in vitro susceptibility of *Brucella* strains to rifampicin. Br Vet J 1976;132:266–275.

168. Corrado ML, Cleri D, Fikrig SM, Phillips JC, Ahonkhai VI. Aspergillosis in chronic granulomatous disease: therapeutic considerations. Am J Dis Child 1980;134:1092–1094.

169. Costrini AM, Mahler DA, Gross WH, Hawkins JE, Yesner R, D'Esopo ND. Clinical and roentgenographic features of nosocomial pulmonary disease due to *Mycobacterium xenopi*. Am Rev Respir Dis 1981;123:104–109.

170. Coto H, Berk SL. Endocarditis caused by *Streptococcus morbillorum*. Am J Med Sci 1984;287:54–58.

171. Coudron PE, Markowitz SM, Mohanty LB, Schatzki PF, Payne JF. Isolation of *Stomatococcus mucilaginosus* from drug user with endocarditis. J Clin Microbiol 1987;25:1359–1363.

172. Coufalik ED, Taylor-Robinson D, Csonka GW. Treatment of nongonococcal urethritis with rifampicin as a means of defining the role of *Ureaplasma urealyticum*. Br J Vener Dis 1979;55:36–43.

173. Cox NL, Prowse MV, Maddison MC, Maddison PJ. Treatment of early rheumatoid arthritis with rifampicin. Ann Rheum Dis 1992;51:32–34.

174. Crellin EJ, Owen JR. Disseminated *Mycobacterium malmoense* infection. Br Med J 1984;289:734.

175. Cunniffe JG, Mallia C, Alcock PA. *Stomatococcus mucilaginosus* lower respiratory tract infection in a patient with AIDS. J Infect 1994;29:327–330.

176. Cunningham M, Yu VL, Turner J, Curtin H. Necrotizing otitis externa due to *Aspergillus* in an immunocompetent patient. Arch Otolaryngol Head Neck Surg 1988;114:554–556.

177. Cynamon HA, Andres JM, Iafrate RP. Rifampin relieves pruritus in children with cholestatic liver disease. Gastroenterology 1990;98:1013–1016.

178. Dabbs ER, Yazawa K, Mikami Y, Miyaji M, Morisaki N, Iwasaki S, Furihata K. Ribosylation by mycobacterial strains as a new mechanism of rifampin inactivation. Antimicrob Agents Chemother 1995;39:1007–1009.

179. Daly VV, Damania RF, Hung CH, Trubowitz S, Ayvazian LF. Transient plasma cell dyscrasia in disseminated histoplasmosis. J Med Soc NJ 1975;72:737–741.

180. Dangor Y, Miller SD, Esposito F da L, Koornhof HJ. Antimicrobial susceptibilities of southern African isolates of *Haemophilus ducreyi*. Antimicrob Agents Chemother 1988;32:1458–1460.

181. Darougar S, Viswalingham N, El-Sheikh H, Hunter PA, Yearsley P. A double-blind comparison of topical therapy of chlamydial ocular infection (TRIC infection) with rifampicin or chlortetracycline. Br J Ophthalmol 1981;65:549–552.

182. Darouiche R, Wright C, Hamill R, Koza M, Lewis D, Markowski J. Eradication of colonization by methicillin-resistant *Staphylococcus aureus* by using minocycline-rifampin and topical mupirocin. Antimicrob Agents Chemother 1991;35:1612–1615.

183. Das SR, Asiri S, El-Soofi A, Baer HP. Protective and curative effects of rifampicin in *Acanthamoeba* meningitis of the mouse. J Infect Dis 1991;163:916–917.

184. Davidson PT, Waggoner R. Acquired resistance of rifampicin by *Mycobacterium kansasii*. Tubercle 1976;52:271–273.

185. Davidson PT. *Mycobacterium szulgai*. A new pathogen causing infection of the lung. Chest 1976;69:799–801.

186. Davidson PT, Le HQ. Drug treatment of tuberculosis—1992. Drugs 1992;43:651–673.

187. Davidson BP, Siegal FP, Reife RA, Gehan K, Burger H, Weiser B, Anand R. Ansamycin (rifabutin), an inhibitor of HIV in vitro, crosses the blood brain barrier [Abstract THP.228]. 3rd International Conference on AIDS. Washington, DC, June 1–5, 1987.

188. Davies HD, Low DE, Schwartz B, Scriver S, Fletcher A, O'Rourke K, Ipp M, Goldbach M, Lloyd D, Saunders NR, Greenberg S, Farber R, Tannenbaum DW, Talbot J, the Ontario GAS Study Group, McGeer A. Evaluation of short-course therapy with cefixime or rifampin for eradication of pharyngeally carried group A streptococci. Clin Infect Dis 1995;21:1294–1296.

189. Dawson CR, Hoshiwara I, Daghfous T, Messadi M, Vastine DW, Schachter J. Topical tetracycline and rifampin therapy of endemic trachoma in Tunesia. Am J Ophthalmol 1975;79:803–811.

190. Degitz K, Messer G, Schirren H, Classen V, Meurer M. Successful treatment of erythema induratum of Bazin following rapid detection of mycobacterial DNA by polymerase chain reaction. Arch Dermatol 1993;129:1619–1620.

191. DeHaven JL, Traynellis C, Riggs DR, Ting E, Lamm DL. Antibiotic and steroid therapy of massive systemic bacillus Calmette-Guérin toxicity. J Urol 1992;147:738–742.

192. Delaporte E, Alfandari S, Piette F. *Mycobacterium ulcerans* associated with infection due to the human immunodeficiency virus. Clin Infect Dis 1994;18:839.

193. De Leo C, Eftimiadi C, Schito GC. Rapid disappearance from the intestinal tract of bacteria resistant to rifaximin. Drugs Exp Clin Res 1986;12:979–981.

194. Della Bruna C, Schioppacassi G, Ungheri D, Jabès D, Morvillo E, Sanfilippo A. LM 427, a new spiropiperidylrifamycin: in vitro and in vivo studies. J Antibiot 1983;36:1502–1506.

195. Della Bruna C, Jabes D, Rossi R, Olliaro P. *Mycobacterium tuberculosis* (MTB): natural resistance and effect of prolonged exposure to rifabutin (RBT) and rifampicin (RMP) [Abstract P0-B07–1181]. Ninth Int Conf on AIDS 1993.

196. Della Marchina M, Renzi G, Palazzini E. Infectious diarrhea in the aged: controlled clinical trial of rifaximin. Chemioterpia 1988;7:336–340.

197. De Marco F, Amato PS, D'Arienzo A. Rifaximin in collateral treatment of portal-systemic encephalopathy: a preliminary report. Curr Ther Res 1984;36:668–674.

198. Denning DW, Hanson LH, Perlman AM, Stevens DA. In vitro susceptibility and synergy studies of *Aspergillus* species to con-

ventional and new agents. Diagn Microbiol Infect Dis 1992;15: 21–34.

199. Denning DW, Stevens DA. Antifungal and surgical treatment of invasive aspergillosis: review of 2121 published cases. Rev Infect Dis 1990;12:1147–1201.

200. Descombe JJ, Dubourg D, Picard M, Palazzini E. Pharmacokinetic study of rifamixin after oral administration in healthy volunteers. Int J Clin Pharmacol Res 1994;14:51–56.

201. Dewsnup DH, Wright DN. In vitro susceptibility of *Nocardia asteroides* to 25 antimicrobial agents. Antimicrob Agents Chemother 1984;25:165–167.

202. Dhillon J, Mitchison DA. Activity in vitro of rifabutin, FCE 22807, rifapentine, and rifampin against *Mycobacterium microti* and *M. tuberculosis* and their penetration into mouse peritoneal macrophages. Am Rev Respir Dis 1992;145:212–214.

203. DiPiazza S, Filippazzo MG, Valenza LM, Morello S, Pastore L, Conti A, Cottone S, Pagliaro L. Rifaximine versus neomycin in the treatment of portosystemic encephalopathy. Ital J Gastroenterol 1991;23:403–407.

204. Doble N, Shaw R, Rowland-Hill C, Lush M, Warnock DW, Keal EE. Pharmacokinetic study of the interaction between rifampicin and ketoconazole. J Antimicrob Chemother 1988;21: 633–635.

205. Doern GV, Brueggemann A, Holley HP Jr, Rauch AM. Antimicrobial resistance of *Streptococcus pneumoniae* recovered from outpatients in the United States during the winter months of 1994 to 1995: results of a 30-center national surveillance study. Antimicrob Agents Chemother 1996;40:1208–1213.

206. Doern GV, Tubert TA. In vitro activities of 39 antimicrobial agents for *Branhamella catarrhalis* and comparison of results with different quantitative susceptibility test methods. Antimicrob Agents Chemother 1988;32:259–261.

207. Doern GV, Brueggemann A, Pierce G, Holley HP Jr, Rauch A. Antibiotic resistance among clinical isolates of *Haemophilus influenzae* in the United States in 1994 and 1995 and detection of β-lactamase-positive strains resistant to amoxicillin-clavulanate: results of a national multicenter surveillance study. Antimicrob Agents Chemother 1997;41:292–297.

208. Donta S, Smith P, Levitz R, Quintiliani R. Therapy of *Mycobacterium marinum* infections. Use of tetracycline versus rifampin. Arch Intern Med 1986;146:902–904.

209. Dossing M, Wilcke JT, Askgaard DS, Nybo B. Liver injury during antituberculosis treatment: an 11-year study. Tuberc Lung Dis 1996;77:335–340.

210. Dougherty EM, Weiner RM, Vaughn JL, Reichelderfer CF. Rifampin inhibition of the occluded virus form of a nuclear polyhedrosis virus. Antimicrob Agents Chemother 1982;22:527–530.

211. Dournon E, Mayaud Ch, Wolff M, Schlemmer B, Samuel D, Sollet JP, Levasseur-Rajagopalan P. Comparison of the activity of three antibiotic regimens in severe Legionnaires' disease. J Antimicrob Chemother 1990;26:129–139.

212. Do Valle TZ, Oliveira Neto MP, Schubach A, Lagrange PH, Gonçalves Da Costa SC. New World tegumenter leishmaniasis: chemotherapeutic activity of rifampicin in human and experimental murine model. Pathol Biol (Paris) 1995;43:618–621.

213. Drancourt M, McNeil MM, Brown JM, Lasker BA, Maurin M,Choux M, Raoult D. Brain abscess due to *Gordonna terrae* in an immunocompromised child: case report and review of infections caused by *G. terrae*. Clin Infect Dis 1994;19:258–262.

214. Drancourt M, Bonnet E, Gallais H, Peloux Y, Raoult D. *Rhodococcus equi* infection in patients with AIDS. J Infect 1992;24:123–131.

215. Drancourt M, Stein A, Argenson JN, Zannier A, Curvale G,

216. Drancourt M, Stein A, Argenson JN, Roiron R, Groulier P, Raoult D. Oral treatment of *Staphylococcus* spp. infected orthopaedic implants with fusidic acid or ofloxacin in combination with rifampicin. J Antimicrob Chemother 1997;39:235–240.

217. Drayton J, Dickinson G, Rinaldi MG. Coadministration of rifampin and itraconazole leads to undetectable levels of serum itraconazole. Clin Infect Dis 1994;18:266.

218. Drda KD, Bastian TL, Self TH, Lawson J, Lanman RC, Bunew BS, Lalonde RL. Effects of debrisoquine hydroxylation phenotype and enzyme induction with rifampin on diltiazem pharmacokinetics and pharmacodynamics [Abstract]. Pharmacotherapy 1991;11:278.

219. Dutt AK, Moers D, Stead WW. Undesirable side effects of isoniazid and rifampin in largely twice-weekly short-course chemotherapy for tuberculosis. Am Rev Respir Dis 1983;128: 419–424.

220. Dworkin R, Modin G, Kunz S, Rich R, Zak O, Sande M. Comparative efficacies of ciprofloxacin, pefloxacin, and vancomycin in combination with rifampin in a rat model of methicillin-resistant *Staphylococcus aureus* chronic osteomyelitis. Antimicrob Agents Chemother 1990;34:1014–1016.

221. Edelstein PH, Meyer RD. Susceptibility of *Legionella pneumophila* to twenty antimicrobial agents. Antimicrob Agents Chemother 1980;18:403–408.

222. Edelstein PH, Calarco K, Yasui VK. Antimicrobial therapy of experimentally induced legionnaires' disease in guinea pigs. Am Rev Respir Dis 1984;130:849–856.

223. Edelstein PH. Rifampin resistance of *Legionella pneumophila* is not increased during therapy for experimental Legionnaires' disease: study of rifampin resistance using a guinea pig model of Legionnaires' disease. Antimicrob Agents Chemotherapy 1991;35:5–9.

224. Edelstein PH, Brenner DJ, Moss CW, Steigerwalt AG, Francis EM, George WL. *Legionella wadsworthii* species nova: a cause of human pneumonia. Ann Intern Med 1982;97:809–813.

225. Edelstein PH, Pryor EP. A new biotype of *Legionella dumoffii*. J Clin Microbiol 1985;21:641–642.

226. Edelstein H. *Mycobacterium marinum* skin infections. Report of 31 cases and review of the literature. Arch Intern Med 1994;154:1359–1364.

227. Edwards JE Jr, Morrison J, Henderson DK, Montgomerie JZ. Combined effect of amphotericin B and rifampin on *Candida* species. Antimicrob Agents Chemother 1980;17:484–487.

228. Eftimiadi C, Deleo C, Schito GC. Treatment of hepatic encephalopathy with L/105, a new non-absorbable rifamycin. Drugs Exp Clin Res 1984;10:691–696.

229. El-Din Salim MM, Kandil E. Rifampicin in the treatment of cutaneous leishmaniasis. J Kuwait Med Assoc 1972;6:159–166.

230. Ellison RT III, Judson FN, Peterson LC, Cohn DL, Ehret JM. Oral rifampin and trimethoprim/sulfamethoxazole therapy in asymptomatic carriers of methicillin-resistant *Staphylococcus aureus* infections. West J Med 1984;140:735–740.

231. El-On J, Pearlman E, Schnur LF, Greenblatt CL. Chemotherapeutic activity of rifampicin on leishmanial amastigotes and promastigotes in vitro. Isr J Med Sci 1983;19:240–245.

232. El-On J, Messer G, Greenblatt CL. Growth inhibition of *Leishmania tropica* amastigotes in vitro by rifampicin combined with amphotericin B. Ann Trop Med Parasitol 1984;78:93–98.

233. Elston RA. Missed diagnosis of mycobacterial infection [Letter]. Lancet 1989;1:1144.

234. Emmerson AM, Gruneberg RN, Johnson ES. The pharmacokinetics in man of a combination of rifampicin and trimethoprim. J Antimicrob Chemother 1978;4:523–531.

235. Ernst JD, Rusnak M, Sande MA. Combination antifungal chemotherapy for experimental disseminated candidiasis: lack of correlation between in vitro and in vivo observations with amphotericin B and rifampin. Rev Infect Dis 1983;5:S626–630.

236. Even-Paz Z, Weinrauch L, Livshin R, El-On J, Greenblatt CL. Rifampicin treatment of cutaneous leishmaniasis. Int J Dermatol 1982;21:110–112.

237. Fadda G, Zanetti S. Antimicrobial activity of rifabutine and rifampicin against Chlamydia trachomatis isolates in cell culture. In; Berkarda B, ed. Progress in antimicrobial and anticancer chemotherapy. Istanbul: Ecomed, 1987:347–349.

238. Fairley CK, Yung A. Rhodococcus equi and HIV infection. Aust NZ J Med 1990;20:99.

239. Fardel O, Lecureur V, Loyer P, Guillouzo A. Rifampicin enhances anti-cancer drug accumulation and activity in multidrug-resistant cells. Biochem Pharmacol 1995;49:1255–1260.

240. Farr B, Mandell GL. Rifampin. Med Clin North Am 1982;66:157–168.

241. Fass RJ. In vitro activity of RP 59500, a semisynthetic injectable pristinamycin, against staphylococci, streptococci, and enterococci. Antimicrob Agents Chemother 1991;35:553–559.

242. Fekety R, Silva J, Toshniwal R, Allo M, Armstrong J, Browne R, Ebright J, Rifkin G. Antibiotic-associated colitis: effects of antibiotics on Clostridium difficile and the disease in hamsters. Rev Infect Dis 1979;1:386–396.

243. Felegie TP, Yu VL, Rumans LW, Yee RB. Susceptibility of Pseudomonas maltophilia to antimicrobial agents, singly and in combination. Antimicrob Agents Chemother 1979;16:833–837.

244. Festi D, Mazzella G, Orsini M, Sotilli S, Sangermano A, Li Bassi S, Parini P, Ferrieri A, Falcucci M, Grossi L, Marzio L, Roda E. Rifaximin in the treatment of chronic hepatic encephalopathy; results of a multicenter study of efficacy and safety. Curr Ther Res 1993;54:598–609.

245. Finland M, Garner C, Wilcox C, Sabath LD. Susceptibility of "enterobacteria" to penicillins, cephalosporins, lincomycins, erythromycin, and rifampin. J Infect Dis 1976;134(Suppl):S75–96.

246. Fisher MW, Hillegas AB, Nazeeri PL. Susceptibility in vitro and in vivo of Pseudomonas pseudomallei to rifampin and tetracyclines. Appl Microbiol 1971;22:13–16.

247. Fitzgeorge RB. The effect of antibiotics on the growth of Legionella pneumophila in guinea-pig alveolar phagocytes infected in vivo by an aerosol. J Infect 1985;10:189–193.

248. Fitzgeorge RB, Baskerville A, Featherstone ASR. Treatment of experimental Legionnaires' disease by aerosol administration of rifampicin, ciprofloxacin, and erythromycin. Lancet 1986;1:502–503.

249. Flynn PM, Magill L, Jenkins JJ III, Pearson T, Crist WM, Hughes WT. Aspergillus osteomyelitis in a child treated for acute lymphoblastic leukemia. Pediatr Infect Dis J 1990;9:733–736.

250. Flynn CT, Rainford DJ, Hope E. Acute renal failure and rifampicin: danger of unsuspected intermittent dosage. Br Med J 1974;8:482.

251. France AJ, McLeod DT, Calder MA, Seaton A. Mycobacterium malmoense infections in Scotland: an increasing problem. Thorax 1987;42:593–595.

252. Frazer DW, Wachsmuth IK, Bopp C, Feeley JC, Tsai TF. Antibiotic treatment of guinea-pigs infected with agent of Legionnaires' disease. Lancet 1978;1:175–177.

253. Frean JA, Arntzen L, Capper T, Bryskier A, Klugman KP. In vitro activities of 14 antibiotics against 100 human isolates of Yersinia pestis from a southern African plague focus. Antimicrob Agents Chemother 1996;40:2646–2647.

254. Freerksen E, Kanthumkumwa EW, Kholowa ARK. Malaria therapy and prophylaxis with cotrifazid, a multiple complex combination consisting of rifampicin + isoniazid + sulfamethoxazole + trimethoprim. Chemotherapy 1995;41:396–398.

255. French P, Venuti E, Fraimow HS. In vitro activity of novobiocin against multiresistant strains of Enterococcus faecium. Antimicrob Agents Chemother 1993;37:2736–2739.

256. Froideveaux D, Claudepierre P, Brugières P, Larget-Piet B, Chevalier X. Iatrogenically induced spondylodiskitis due to Mycobacterium xenopi in an immunocompetent patient. Clin Infect Dis 1996;22:723–724.

257. Fu KP, Lasinski ER, Zogonas HC, Kimble EF, Konopka EA. Therapeutic efficacy and pharmacokinetic properties of rifampicin in a Bacteroides fragilis intra-abdominal abscess. J Antimicrob Chemother 1984;14:633–640.

258. Fu KP, Lasinski ER, Zogonas HC, Kimble EF, Konopka EA. Efficacy of rifampicin in experimental Bacteroides fragilis and Pseudomonas aeruginosa mixed infections. J Antimicrob Chemother 1985;15:579–585.

259. Fujii K, Tsuji A, Miyazaki S, Yamaguchi K, Goto S. In vitro and in vivo antibacterial activities of KRM-1648 and KRM-1657, new rifamycin derivatives. Antimicrob Agents Chemother 1994;38:1118–1122.

260. Fujita NK, Edwards JE Jr. Combined in vitro effect of amphotericin B and rifampin on Cryptococcus neoformans. Antimicrob Agents Chemother 1981;19:196–198.

261. Funke G, Pünter V, von Graevenitz A. Antimicrobial susceptibility patterns of some recently established coryneform bacteria. Antimicrob Agents Chemother 1996;40:2874–2878.

262. Furlan V, Perello L, Jacquemin E, Debray D, Taburet AM. Interactions between FK506 and rifampicin or erythromycin in pediatric liver recipients. Transplant 1995;59:1217–1218.

263. Gabriel SE, Conn DL, Luthra H. Rifampin therapy in rheumatoid arthritis. J Rheumatol 1990;17:163–166.

264. Gale EF, Cundliffe E, Reynolds PE, Richmond MH, Waring MJ, eds. The molecular basis of antibiotic action, 2nd ed. New York: John Wiley & Sons, 1981:370–401.

265. Gamea AM. Local rifampicin in treatment of rhinoscleroma. J Laryngol Otol 1988;102:319–321.

266. Gamea AM, El-Tatawi AY. The effect of rifampicin on rhinoscleroma: an electron microscopic study. J Laryngol Otol 1990;104:772–777.

267. Gangadharam PRJ. Isoniazid, rifampin, and hepatotoxicity. Am Rev Respir Dis 1986;133:963–965.

268. Gannon M, Otridge B, Hone R, Dervan P, O'Loughlin S. Cutaneous Mycobacterium malmoense infection in an immunocompromised patient. Int J Dermatol 1990;29:149–150.

269. Garcia-Bravo M, Aguado JM, Morales JM, Noriega AR. Influence of external factors in resistance of Corynebacterium urealyticum to antimicrobial agents. Antimicrobial Agents Chemother 1996;40:497–499.

270. García-Rodríguez JA, García Sánchez JE, Muñoz Bellido JL, Nebreda Mayoral T, García Sánchez E, García García I. In vitro activity of 79 antimicrobial agents against Corynebacterium group D2. Antimicrob Agents Chemother 1991;35:2140–2143.

271. García-Rodríguez JA, Muñoz Bellido JL, Fresnadillo MJ, Trujillano I. In vitro activities of new macrolides and rifapentine against *Brucella* spp. Antimicrob Agents Chemother 1993;37: 911–913.

272. Gault H, Longerich L, Dawe M, Fine A. Digoxin-rifampin interaction. Clin Pharmacol Ther 1984;35:750–754.

273. Geary TG, Jensen JB. Effects of antibiotics on *Plasmodium falciparum* in vitro. Am J Trop Med Hyg 1983;32:221–225.

274. Gebhart CJ, Ward GE, Kurtz HJ. In vitro activities of 47 antimicrobial agents against three *Campylobacter* spp. from pigs. Antimicrob Agents Chemother 1985;27:55–59.

275. Geisler PJ, Manis RD, Maddux MS. Dosage of antituberculous drugs in obese patients. Am Rev Respir Dis 1985;131:944–946.

276. Ghent CN, Carruthers SG. Treatment of pruritus in primary biliary cirrhosis with rifampin. Gastroenterology 1988;94:488–493.

277. Giaccari S, Tronci S, Falconieri M, Ferrieri A. Long-term treatment with rifaximin and lactobacilli in post-diverticular stenoses of the colon. Eur Rev Med Pharmacol Sci 1993;15: 29–34.

278. Giacometti A, Ferrieri A, Cirioni O, Siquini FM, Petroni S, Scalise G. Treatment of diarrhea in AIDS patients: double-blind clinical trial. Farmaci Terapia 1993;10:107–109.

279. Giacomo F, Francesco A, Michele N, Oronzo S, Antonella F. Rifaximin in the treatment of hepatic encephalopathy. Eur J Clin Res 1993;4:57–66.

280. Giladi M, Lee E, Berlin OGW, Panosian CB. Peritonitis caused by *Mycobacterium kansasii* in a patient undergoing continuous ambulatory peritoneal dialysis. Am J Kidney Dis 1992;19: 597–599.

281. Gillespie SH, Baskerville AJ, Davidson RN, Felmingham D, Bryceson ADM. The serum rifabutin concentrations in a patient successfully treated for multi-resistant *Mycobacterium tuberculosis* infection. J Antimicrob Chemother 1990;25:490–491.

282. Gillim JG, Israel DS, Polk RE. Pharmacokinetic drug interactions with antimicrobial agents. Clin Pharmacokinet 1993;25: 450–482.

283. Gillis JC, Brogden RN. Rifaximin. a review of its antibacterial activity, pharmacokinetic properties and therapeutic potential in conditions mediated by gastrointestinal bacteria. Drugs 1995;49:467–484.

284. Girling DJ. Adverse reactions to rifampicin in antituberculosis regimens. J Antimicrob Chemother 1977;3:115–132.

285. Girling DJ, Hitze KL. Adverse reactions to rifampicin. Bull WHO 1979;57:45–49.

286. Giron KP, Gross ME, Musher DM, Williams TW Jr, Tharappel RA. In vitro antimicrobial effect against *Streptococcus pneumoniae* of adding rifampin to penicillin, ceftriaxone, or 1-ofloxacin. Antimicrob Agents Chemother 1995;39:2798–2800.

287. Glode MP, Daum RS, Halsey NA, Johansen TL, Goldmann DA, Ambrosino D, Boies E, Granoff DM. Rifampin alone and in combination with trimethoprim in chemoprophylaxis for infections due to *Haemophilus influenzae* type b. Rev Infect Dis 1983;5:S549–555.

288. Gogate A, Dadkar V. Effect of some antimicrobial agents in primary amoebic meningoencephalitis in mice. Indian J Med Res 1986;83:148–151.

289. Golden SE. Hepatosplenic cat-scratch disease associated with elevated anti-*Rochalimaea* antibody titers. Pediatr Infect Dis 1993;12:868–871.

290. Good RC, Silcox VA, Kilburn JO, Plikaytis BD. Identification and drug susceptibility test results for *Mycobacterium* spp. Clin Microbiol Newslett 1985;7:133–136.

291. Gordon JJ, Harter DH, Phair JP. Meningitis due to *Staphylococcus aureus*. Am J Med 1985;78:965–970.

292. Gordon RC, Wofford-McQueen R, Shu K. In vitro synergism of rifampin-cephalosporin combinations against *Haemophilus influenzae* type b. Eur J Clin Microb Infect Dis 1990;9:201–205.

293. Goutzamanis JJ, Gilbert GL. *Mycobacterium ulcerans* infection in Australian children: report of eight cases and review. Clin Infect Dis 1995;21:1186–1192.

294. Grange JM, Winstanley PA, Davies PDO. Clinically significant drug interactions with antituberculosis agents. Drug Safety 1994;11:242–251.

295. Graybill JR, Ahrens J. Interaction of rifampin with other antifungal agents in experimental murine candidiasis. Rev Infect Dis 1983;5:S620–625.

296. Green M, Li KI, Wald ER, Guerra N, Byers C. Duration of rifampin chemoprophylaxis for contacts of patients infected with *Haemophilus influenzae* type B. Antimicrob Agents Chemother 1992;36:545–547.

297. Griffiths WAD. Use of metronidazole in cutaneous leishmaniasis [Letter]. Arch Dermatol 1976;112:1791.

298. Gronhagen-Riska C, Hellstrom PE, Froseth B. Predisposing factors in hepatitis induced by isoniazid-rifampin treatment of tuberculosis. Am Rev Respir Dis 1978;118:461–466.

299. Grosset J, Leventis S. Adverse effects of rifampin. Rev Infect Dis 1983;5(Suppl 3):S440–S450.

300. Gruttadauria G, LaBarbera F, Cutaia G, Salanitri G. Prevention of infection in colonic surgery by rifaximin. a controlled, prospective, randomized trial. Eur Rev Med Pharmacol Sci 1987;9:101–105.

301. Guarderas J, Alvarez S, Berk SL. Progressive pulmonary disease caused by *Mycobacterium gordonae*. South Med J 1986;79:505–507.

302. Guerrero C, Stockman L, Marchesi F, Bodmer T, Roberts GD, Telenti A. Evaluation of the *rpoB* gene in rifampicin-susceptible and -resistant *Mycobacterium avium* and *Mycobacterium intracellulare*. J Antimicrob Chemother 1994;33:661–663.

303. Gump DW, Frank RO, Winn WC Jr, Foster RS Jr, Broome CV, Cherry WB. Legionnaires' disease in patients with associated serious disease. Ann Intern Med 1979;90:538–542.

304. Gump DW, Keegan M. Pulmonary infections due to *Legionella* in immunocompromised patients. Semin Respir Infect 1986:1: 151–159.

305. Gunther SF, Levy CS. Mycobacterial infections. Hand Clin 1989;5:591–598.

306. Gupta S, Grieco MH, Siegel I. Suppression of T-lymphocyte rosettes by rifampin. Ann Intern Med 1975;82:484–488.

307. Gurgo C, Ray RK, Thiry L, Green M. Inhibitors of the RNA and DNA dependent polymerase activities of RNA tumour viruses. Nature New Biol 1971;229:111–114.

308. Gurgo C, Ray R, Green M. Rifamycin derivatives strongly inhibiting RNA-DNA polymerase (reverse transcriptase) of murine sarcoma virus. J Natl Cancer Inst 1972;49:61–79.

309. Gutmann L, Goldstein FW, Kitzis MD, Hautefort B, Darmon C, Acar JF. Susceptibility of *Nocardia asteroides* to 46 antibiotics, including 22 β-lactams. Antimicrob Agents Chemother 1983;23:248–251.

310. Hachem R, Raad I, Rolston KVI, Whimbey E, Katz R, Tarrand J, Libshitz H. Cutaneous and pulmonary infections caused by *Mycobacterium vaccae*. Clin Infect Dis 1996;23:173–175.

311. Hackett AJ, Owens RB, Calvin M, Joss U. Inhibition of MSV viral function by rifampicin derivatives. Medicine 1972;51: 175–180.

312. Hall, AV, Roberts CM, Maurice PD, McLean KA, Shousha S. Cat-scratch disease in a patient with AIDS: atypical skin manifestation. Lancet 1988;2:453–454.

313. Hall WH, Manion RE. In vitro susceptibility of *Brucella* to various antibiotics. Appl Microbiol 1970;20:600–604.

314. Hampson SJ, Parker MC, Saverymuttu SSH, Joseph AE, McFadden J-JP, Hermon-Taylor J. Quadruple anti-mycobacterial chemotherapy in Crohn's disease; results at 9 months of a pilot study in 20 patients. Aliment Pharm Ther 1989;3:343–352.

315. Hamzehei M, Ledinko N. Inhibition of influenza A virus replication by rifampicin and selenocystamine. J Med Virol 1980;6:169–174.

316. Hand WL, King-Thompson NL. Contrasts between phagocyte antibiotic uptake and subsequent intracellular bactericidal activity. Antimicrob Agents Chemother 1986;29:135–140.

317. Harris GD, Johanson WG Jr, Nicholson DP. Response to chemotherapy of pulmonary infection due to *Mycobacterium kansasii*. Am Rev Respir Dis 1975:112:31–36.

318. Harro C, Braden GL, Morris AB, Lipkowitz GS, Madden RL. Failure to cure *Mycobacterium gordonae* peritonitis associated with continuous ambulatory peritoneal dialysis. Clin Infect Dis 1997;24:955–957.

319. Harshey RM, Ramakrishnan T. Purification and properties of DNA-dependent RNA polymerase from *Mycobacterium tuberculosis* H$_{37}$R$_v$. Biochim Biophys Acta 1976;432:49–59.

320. Hart DHL, Peel MM, Andrew JH, Burdon JGW. Lung infection caused by *Rhodococcus*. Aust NZ J Med 1988;18:790–791.

321. Harvey RL, Sunstrum JC. *Rhodococcus equi* infection in patients with and without human immunodeficiency virus syndrome. Rev Infect Dis 1991;13:139–145.

322. Harwood CR, Rich GE, McAleer R, Cherian G. Isolation of *Acanthameba* from a cerebral abscess. Med J Aust 1988;148:47–49.

323. Havlichek D, Saravolatz L, Pohlod D. Effects of 4 quinolones, erythromycin, cefoxitin, and rifampicin on the extra- and intracellular growth of virulent *Legionella pneumophila* [Abstract]. 86th annual meeting, American Society for Microbiology, Washington, DC, 1986;226:365.

324. Havlichek D, Pohlod D, Saravolatz L. Comparison of ciprofloxacin and rifampicin in experimental *Legionella pneumophila* pneumonia. J Antimicrob Chemother 1987;20:875–881.

325. Heifets LB, Iseman MD. Determination of in vitro susceptibility of mycobacteria to ansamycin. Am Rev Respir Dis 1985;132:710–711.

326. Heifets LB, Iseman MD, Lindholm-Levy J. Combinations of rifampin or rifabutine plus ethambutol against *Mycobacterium avium* complex. Am Rev Respir Dis 1988;137:711–715.

327. Heifets LB. Antituberculosis drugs: antimicrobial activity in vitro. In: Heifets LB, ed. Drug susceptibility in the chemotherapy of mycobacterial infections. Boca Raton, FL: CRC Press, 1991:13–57.

328. Heimark LD, Gibaldi M, Trager WF, O'Reilly RA, Goulart DA. The mechanism of the warfarin-rifampin drug interactions in humans. Clin Pharmacol Ther 1987;42:388–394.

329. Henry NK, Rouse MS, Whitesell AL, McConnell ME, Wilson WR. Treatment of methicillin-resistant *Staphylococcus aureus* experimental osteomyelitis with ciprofloxacin or vancomycin alone or in combination with rifampin. Am J Med 1987;82(Suppl 4A):73–75.

330. Herchline TE, Barnishan J, Ayers LW, Fass RJ. Penicillinase production and in vitro susceptibilities of *Staphylococcus lugdunensis*. Antimicrob Agents Chemother 1990;34:2434–2435.

331. Heurlin N, Petrini B. Treatment of non-tuberculous mycobacterial infections in patients without AIDS. Scand J Infect Dis 1993;25:619–623.

332. Hicks WL, Nowels K, Troxel J. Primary cutaneous mucormycosis. Am J Otolaryngol 1995;16:265–268.

333. Hillerdal G, Riesenfeldt-Örn I, Pedersen A, Ivanicova E. Infection with *Rhodococcus equi* in a patient with sarcoidosis treated with corticosteroids. Scand J Infect Dis 1988;20:673–677.

334. Hillidge CJ. Use of erythromycin-rifampin combination in treatment of *Rhodococcus equi* pneumonia. Vet Microbiol 1987;14:337–342.

335. Hirasuna JD. Disseminated *Mycobacterium kansasii* infection in the acquired immunodeficiency syndrome (AIDS) [Letter]. Ann Intern Med 1987;107:784.

336. Hirata T, Saito H, Tomioka H, Sato K, Jidoi J, Hosoe K, Hidaka T. In-vitro and in-vivo activities of the benzoxazinorifamycin KRM-1648 against *Mycobacterium tuberculosis*. Antimicrob Agents Chemother 1995;39:2295–2303.

337. Hirsch DJ, Bia FJ, Kashgarian M, Bia MJ. Rapidly progressive glomerulonephritis during antituberculosis therapy. Am J Nephrol 1983;3:7–10.

338. Hirsh BE, Wong B, Kiehn TE, Gee T, Armstrong D. *Flavobacterium meningosepticum* bacteremia in an adult with acute leukemia. Diagn Microbiol Infect Dis 1986;4:65–69.

339. Hjelm C, Kaustová J, Kubín M, Hoffner SE. Susceptibility of *Mycobacterium kansasii* to ethambutol and its combination with rifamycins, ciprofloxacin and isoniazid. Eur J Clin Microbiol Infect Dis 1992;11:51–54.

340. Hoensch HP, Balzer K, Dylewizc P, Kirch W, Goebell H, Ohnhaus EE. Effect of rifampicin treatment on hepatic drug metabolism and serum bile acids in patients with primary biliary cirrhosis. Eur J Clin Pharmacol 1985;28:475–477.

341. Höffler U, Niederau W, Pulverer G. Susceptibility of *Bacterium actinomycetemcomitans* to 45 antibiotics. Antimicrob Agents Chemother 1980;17:943–946.

342. Hoffner SE, Klintz L, Olsson-Liljequist B, Bolmström A. Evaluation of Etest for rapid susceptibility testing of *Mycobacterium chelonae* and *M. fortuitum*. J Clin Microbiol 1994;32:1846–1849.

343. Hoffner SE, Hjelm U, Källenius G. Susceptibility of *Mycobacterium malmoense* to antibacterial drugs and drug combinations. Antimicrob Agents Chemother 1993;37:1285–1288.

344. Hoffner SE, Svenson SB. Studies on the role of the mycobacterial cell envelope in the multiple drug resistance of atypical mycobacteria. Res Microbiol 1991:142:448–451.

345. Holton J, Vaira D, Menegatti M, Barbara L. The susceptibility of *Helicobacter pylori* to the rifamycin, rifaximin. J Antimicrob Chemother 1995;35:545–549.

346. Hong Kong Chest Service/British Medical Council. A controlled study of rifabutin and an uncontrolled study of ofloxacin in the retreatment of patients with pulmonary tuberculosis resistant to isoniazid, streptomycin and rifampicin. Tuberc Lung Dis 1992;73:59–67.

347. Hoover WW, Gerlach EH, Hoban DJ, Eliopoulos GM, Pfaller MA, Jones RN. Antimicrobial activity and spectrum of rifaximin, a new topical rifamycin derivative. Diagn Microbiol Infect Dis 1993;16:111–118.

348. Hopkins RJ, Schwalbe RS, Donnenberg M. Infections due to *Stomatococcus mucilaginosus*: report of two new cases and review. Clin Infect Dis 1992;14:1264.

349. Hornick DB, Dayton CS, Bedell GN, Fick RB Jr. Nontubercu-

lous mycobacterial lung disease. substantiation of a less aggressive approach. Chest 1988;93:550–555.

350. Houin G, Tillement JP. Clofibrate and enzyme induction in man. Int J Clin Pharmacol 1978;16:150–154.

351. Hsueh P, Hsiue T, Jarn J, Ho S, Hsieh W. Disseminated infection due to *Mycobacterium scrofulaceum* in an immunocompetent host. Clin Infect Dis 1996;22:159–161.

352. Hughes AM, Tenforde TS, Calvin M, Bissell MJ, Tischler AN, Bennett EL. Inhibition of adenocarcinoma TA3 ascites tumor growth by rifamycin derivatives. Oncology 1978;35:76–82.

353. Hughes CE, Harris C, Moody JA, Peterson LR, Gerding DN. In vitro activities of amphotericin B in combination with four antifungal agents and rifampin against *Aspergillus* spp. Antimicrob Agents Chemother 1984;25:560–562.

354. Hughes WT. Rifampicin for *Pneumocystis carinii* pneumonia [Letter]. Lancet 1983;2:162.

355. Hughes JH, Biedenbach DJ, Erwin ME, Jones RN. E test as susceptibility test and epidemiologic tool for evaluation of *Neisseria meningitidis* isolates. J Clin Microbiol 1993;31:3255–3259.

356. Hui J, Gordon N, Kajioka R. Permeability to rifampin in mycobacteria. Antimicrob Agents Chemother 1977;11:773–779.

357. Hull PR. Systemic histoplasmosis with oesophageal obstruction due to *Histoplasma* granulomas. S Afr Med J 1979;55:639–640.

358. Humber DP, Nsanzumuhire H, Aluoch JA, Webster ADB, Aber VR, Mitchison DA, Girling DJ, Nunn AJ. Controlled double-blind study of the effect of rifampin on humoral and cellular immune responses in patients with pulmonary tuberculosis and in tuberculosis contacts. Am Rev Respir Dis 1980;122:425–436.

359. Humbert G, Brumpt I, Montay G, LeLiboux A, Frydman A, Borsa-Lebas F, Moore N. Influence of rifampin on the pharmacokinetics of pefloxacin. Clin Pharmacol Ther 1991;50:682–687.

360. Huminer D, Pitlik SD, Block C, Kaufman L, Amit S, Rosenfeld JB. Aquarium-borne *Mycobacterium marinum* skin infection. Arch Dermatol 1986;122:698–703.

361. Hunt SJ, Reed SL, Matthews WC, Torian B. Cutaneous *Acanthamoeba* infection in the acquired immunodeficiency syndrome: response to multidrug therapy. Cutis 1995;56:285–287.

362. Hunter PR, George RC, Griffiths JW. Mathematical modeling of antimicrobial susceptibility data of *Staphylococcus haemolyticus* for 11 antimicrobial agents, including three experimental glycopeptides and an experimental lipoglycopeptide. Antimicrob Agents Chemother 1990;34:1769–1772.

363. Huppert M, Pappagianis D, Sun SH, Gleason-Jordan I, Collins MS, Vukovich KR. Effect of amphotericin B and rifampin against *Coccidioides immitis* in vitro and in vivo. Antimicrob Agents Chemother 1976;9:406–413.

364. Iannini PB, Ehret J, Eickhoff TC. Effects of ampicillin-amikacin and ampicillin-rifampin on enterococci. Antimicrob Agents Chemother 1976;9:448–451.

365. Ip M, Cheng KP, Cheung WC. Disseminated intravascular coagulopathy associated with rifampicin. Tubercle 1991;72:291–293.

366. Ishii M, Ogata H. Determination of rifampicin and its main metabolites in human plasma by high-performance liquid chromatography. J Chromatogr 1988;426:412–416.

367. Izumi AK, Matsunaga J. BCG vaccine-induced lupus vulgaris. Arch Dermatol 1982;118:171–172.

368. Jackson GG. Session I: summary. Rev Infect Dis 1983;5:S447–450.

369. Jacobs F, Abramowicz D, Vereerstraeten P, Le Clerc JL, Zech

F, Thys JP. Brucella endocarditis: the role of combined medical and surgical treatment. Rev Infect Dis 1990;12:740–744.

370. Jacobson MA, Isenberg WM. *Mycobacterium kansasii* diffuse pulmonary infection in a patient with acquired immune deficiency syndrome. Am J Clin Pathol 1989;91:236–238.

371. Jadavji T, Prober CG, Cheung R. In vitro interactions between rifampin and ampicillin or chloramphenicol against *Haemophilus influenzae*. Antimicrob Agents Chemother 1984;26:91–93.

372. Jariwalla AG, Davies BH, White J. Infective endocarditis complicating psittacosis; response to rifampicin. Br Med J 1980;280:155.

373. Jeroudi MO, Halim MA, Harder EJ, Al-Siba'l MB, Ziady G, Mercer EN. Brucella endocarditis. Br Heart J 1987;58:279–283.

374. Jezequel AM, Orlandi F, Tenconi LT. Changes of the smooth endoplasmic reticulum induced by rifampicin in human and guinea-pig hepatocytes. Gut 1971;12:984–987.

375. Ji B, Truffot-Pernot C, Lacroix C, Raviglione MC, O'Brien RJ, Olliaro P, Roscigno G, Grosset J. Effectiveness of rifampin, rifabutin, and rifapentine for preventative therapy of tuberculosis in mice. Am Rev Respir Dis 1993;148:1541–1546.

376. John CC. Treatment failure with use of a third-generation cephalosporin for penicillin-resistant pneumococcal meningitis: case report and review. Clin Infect Dis 1994;18:188–193.

377. Jones R, Master R, Powell D. Antimicrobial susceptibility testing of *Aerococcus urinae* [Abstract E058]. 36th ICAAC, annual meeting of the American Society for Microbiology, New Orleans, Sept 15–18, 1996.

378. Jones RB, Ridgway GL, Boulding S, Hunley KL. In vitro activity of rifamycin alone and in combination with other antibiotics against *C. trachomatis*. Rev Infect Dis 1983;5(Suppl 3):556–561.

379. Joshi JV, Joshi UM, Sankolli GM, Gupta K, Rao AP, Hazari K, Sheth UK, Saxena BN. A study of interaction of a low-dose combination oral contraceptive with anti-tubercular drugs. Contraception 1980;21:617–629.

380. Joshi RK, Nambiar PMK. Dermal leishmaniasis and rifampicin. Int J Dermatol 1989;28:612–614.

381. Jost PM, Hodges GR. *Mycobacterium kansasii* infection in a patient with AIDS. South Med J 1991;84:1501–1504.

382. June CH, Beatty PG, Shulman HM, Rinaldi MG. Disseminated *Fusarium moniliforme* infection after allogenic marrow transplantation. South Med J 1986;79:513–515.

383. Kaatz GW, Seo SM, Barriere SL, Albrecht LM, Rybak M. Ciprofloxacin and rifampin, alone and in combination, for therapy of experimental *Staphylococcus aureus* endocarditis. Antimicrob Agents Chemother 1989;33:1184–1187.

384. Kailath EJ, Goldstein E, Wagner FH. Case report: meningitis caused by *Oerskovia xanthineolytica*. Am J Med Sci 1988;295:216–217.

385. Karchmer AW, Archer GL, Dismukes WE. Rifampin treatment of prosthetic valve endocarditis due to *Staphylococcus epidermidis*. Rev Infect Dis 1983;5:S543–S548.

386. Kent RJ, Bakhtiar M, Shanson DC. The in-vitro bactericidal activities of combinations of antimicrobial agents against clinical isolates of *Mycobacterium avium-intrcellulare*. J Antimicrob Chemother 1992;30:643–650.

387. Kenwright S, Levi AJ. Impairment of hepatic uptake of rifamycin antibiotics by probenecid, and its therapeutic implications. Lancet 1973;2:1401–1405.

388. Kerry DW, Hamilton-Miller JMT, Brumfitt W. Trimethoprim

and rifampicin: in vitro activities separately and in combination. J Antimicrob Chemother 1975;1:417–427.

389. Keshishyan H, Hanna L, Jawetz E. Emergence of rifampin-resistance in *Chlamydia trachomatis*. Nature 1972;244:173–174.

390. Keys TF. Therapeutic considerations in the treatment of *Legionella* infections. Semin Respir Infect 1987;2:270–273.

391. Khardori N, Hayat S, Rolston K, Bodey GP. Cutaneous *Rhizopus* and *Aspergillus* infections in five patients with cancer. Arch Dermatol 1989;125:952–956.

392. Kharsany ABM, Hoosen AA, van den Ende J. Antimicrobial susceptibilities of *Gardnerella vaginalis*. Antimicrob Agents Chemother 1993;37:2733–2735.

393. Khuri-Bulos N. Meningococcal meningitis following rifampin prophylaxis. Am J Dis Child 1973;126:689–691.

394. Kiehlbauch JA, Baker CN, Wachsmuth IK. In vitro susceptibilities of aerotolerant *Campylobacter* isolates to 22 antimicrobial agents. Antimicrob Agents Chemother 1992;36:717–722.

395. Kim PK, Kim KS, Lee JK, Lee JS, Jeong HJ, Choi IJ. Rifampin therapy in Henoch-Schönlein purpura nephritis accompanied by nephrotic syndrome. Child Nephrol Urol 1988;89:50–56.

396. Kimbrough RC III, Ormsbee RA, Peacock MG. Q fever endocarditis: a three and one-half year follow-up. In Burgdorfer W, Anacker RL, eds. Rickettsiae and rickettsial diseases. New York: Academic Press, 1981:125–132.

397. King JW, White MC. Pulmonary actinomycosis: rapid improvement with isoniazid and rifampin. Arch Intern Med 1981;141:1234–1235.

398. Kirch W, Rose I, Klingmann I, Pabst J, Ohnhaus EE. Interaction of bisprolol with cimetidine and rifampicin. Eur J Clin Pharmacol 1986;31:59–62.

399. Kitahara M, Seth VK, Medoff G, Kobayashi GS. Activity of amphotericin B, 5-fluorocytosine, and rifampin against six clinical isolates of *Aspergillus*. Antimicrob Agents Chemother 1976;9:915–919.

400. Kitahara M, Kobayashi GS, Medoff G. Enhanced efficacy of amphotericin B and rifampin combined in treatment of murine histoplasmosis and blastomycosis. J Infect Dis 1976;133:663–668.

401. Klein MB, Nelson CM, Goodman JL. Antibiotic susceptibility of the newly cultivated agent of human granulocytic ehrlichiosis: promising activity of quinolones and rifamycins. Antimicrob Agents Chemother 1997;41:76–79.

402. Kobasa WD, Kaye KL, Shipiro T, Kaye D. Therapy for experimental endocarditis due to *Staphylococcus epidermidis*. Rev Infect Dis 1983;5:S533–S537.

403. Kobayashi GS, Medoff G, Schlessinger D, Kwan CN, Musser WE. Amphotericin B potentiation of rifampin as an antifungal agent against the yeast phase of *Histoplasma capsulatum*. Science 1972;177:709–710.

404. Kobayashi GS, Cheung SC, Schlessinger D, Medoff G. Effects of rifamycins derivatives, alone and in combination with amphotericin B, against *Histoplasma capsulatum*. Antimicrob Agents Chemother 1974;5:16–18.

405. Koeck JL, Debord T, Fabre M, Vincent V, Cavallo JD, Le Vagueresse R. Disseminated *Mycobacterium simae* infection in a patient with AIDS: clinical features and treatment. Clin Infect Dis 1996;23:832–833.

406. Koehler JE, LeBoit PE, Egbert BM, Berger TG. Cutaneous vascular lesions and disseminated cat-scratch disease in patients with the acquired immunodeficiency syndrome (AIDS) and AIDS-related complex. Ann Intern Med 1988;109:449–455.

407. Kohn A, Prantera C, Mangiarotti R, Luzi C, Andreoli A. Antimycobacterial therapy and Crohn's disease; a randomized, placebo controlled trial. Gastroenterology 1992;102:A647.

408. Konopka EA, Zoganas H, Kimble E, Coldreck R, Lasinski E. Activity of rifampin combinations in an enterococcal pyelonephritis in mice. In: Nelson JD, Grassi C, eds. Current chemotherapy, vol 2. Washington, DC: American Society for Microbiology, 1980:1288–1290.

409. Konopka EA, Jones SC, Stieglitz A, Zogonas HC. Laboratory evaluation of rifampin and other antimicrobial agents against selected strains of *Pseudomonas pseudomallei*. Antimicrob Agents Chemother 1970;10:503–508.

410. Korvick JA, Peacock JE Jr, Muder RR, Wheeler RR, Yu VL. Addition of rifampin to combination antibiotic therapy for *Pseudomonas aeruginosa* bacteremia: prospective trial using the Zelen protocol. Antimicrob Agents Chemother 1992;36:620–625.

411. Koukol SC, DeHaven JI, Riggs DR, Lamm DL. Drug therapy of bacillus Calmette-Guérin sepsis. Urol Res 1995;22:373–376.

412. Krasnow I, Gross W. *Mycobacterium simiae* infection in the United States. Am Rev Respir Dis 1975;111:357–360.

413. Kreek MJ, Garfield JW, Gutjahr CL, Giusti LM. Rifampin-induced methadone withdrawal. N Engl J Med 1976;294:1104–1106.

414. Krieg RE, Wolcott JH, Meyers WM. *Mycobacterium ulcerans* infection: treatment with rifampin, hyperbaric oxygenation, and heat. Aviat Space Environ Med 1979;50:888–892.

415. Kropec A, Daschner F. In vitro activity of fleroxacin and 14 other antimicrobials against slime- and non-slime-producing *Staphylococcus epidermidis*. Chemotherapy 1989;35:351–354.

416. Kucers A, Bennett NMcK. The use of antibiotics. 4th ed. Philadelphia: JB Lippincott, 1987.

417. Kumar A, Wofford-McQueen R, Gordon RC. In vitro activity of multiple antimicrobial combinations against *Pseudomonas cepacia* isolates. Chemotherapy 1989;35:246–253.

418. Kumar S, Ganguly NK, Kohli KK. Interaction of rifampicin with nonprotein thiols in *Mycobacterium smegmatis*. Biochem Int 1991;23:1041–1047.

419. Kumar KP, Reddy PS, Chatterji D. Proximity relationship between the active site of *Escherichia coli* RNA polymerase and rifampicin binding domain: a resonance energy-transfer study. Biochemistry 1992;31:7519–7526.

420. Kumar S, Mehta JA, Trivedi HL. Light-chain proteinuria and reversible renal failure in rifampin-treated patients with tuberculosis. Chest 1974;70:564–565.

421. Kunin CM. Antimicrobial activity of rifabutin. Clin Infect Dis 1996;22(Suppl 1):S3–14.

422. Kurzynski TA, Boehm DM, Rott-Petri JA, Schell RF, Allison PE. Antimicrobial susceptibilities of *Bordetella* species isolated in a multicenter pertussis surveillance project. Antimicrob Agents Chemother 1988;32:137–140.

423. Kyriakides GK, Zinneman HH, Hall WH, Arora VK, Lifton J, DeWolf WC, Miller J. Immunologic monitoring and aspergillosis in renal transplant patients. Am J Surg 1976;131:246–252.

424. Laboratory Centre for Disease Control. Guidelines for control of meningococcal disease. Can Med Assoc J 1994;150:1825–1831.

425. Lalonde G, Hand R. Infective endocarditis due to *Actinobacillus actinomycetemcomitans* in a patient with a porcine prosthetic mitral valve. Can Med Assoc J 1980;122:316–319.

426. Lamanna A, Orsi A. In vitro activity of rifaximin and rifampicin

against some anaerobic bacteria. Chemoterapia 1984;3: 365–367.

427. Lambert T, Mégraud F, Gerbaud G, Courvalin P. Susceptibility of *Campylobacter pyloridis* to 20 antimicrobial agents. Antimicrob Agents Chemother 1986;30:510–511.

428. Lang R, Shasha B, Rubinstein E. Therapy of experimental murine brucellosis with streptomycin alone and in combination with ciprofloxacin, doxycycline, and rifampin. Antimicrob Agents Chemother 1993;37:2333–2336.

429. Langhoff E, Madsen S. Rapid metabolism of cyclosporin and prednisone in kidney transplant patient receiving tuberculostatic treatment. Lancet 1983;2:1031.

430. Lazzarin A, Grassi F, Tortorano AM. Disseminated aspergillosis [Letter]. Am J Dis Child 1982;136:654.

431. LeBar WD, Pensler MI. Pleural effusion due to *Rhodococcus equi* [Letter]. J Infect Dis 1986;154:919–920.

432. LeBel M, Spino M. Pulse dosing versus continuous infusion of antibiotics. Clin Pharmacokinet 1988;14:71–95.

433. LeBoit PE, Berger TG, Egbert BM, Yen TSB, Stoler MH, Bonfiglio TA, Strauchen JA, English CK, Wear DJ. Epithelioid haemangioma-like vascular proliferation in AIDS: manifestation of cat scratch disease bacillus infection? Lancet 1988;1: 960–963.

434. Lee EL, Robinson MJ, Thong ML, Puthucheary SD. Rifamycin in neonatal flavobacterial meningitis. Arch Dis Child 1976;51:209.

435. Lee CH, Lee CJ. Thrombocytopenia—a rare but potentially serious side effect of initial daily and interrupted use of rifampicin. Chest 1989;96:202–203.

436. Levine M, Collin K, Kassen BO. Acute hemolysis and renal failure following discontinuous use of rifampin. DICP Ann Pharmacother 1991;25:743–744.

437. Levy H, Sacho H, Feldman C, Naude GE, Peskin J, Stead KJ, Kallenbach JM. Pulmonary mucormycosis presenting with Horner's syndrome. S Afr Med J 1986;70:363–365.

438. Lewis VJ, Thacker WL, Shepard CC, McDade JE. In vivo susceptibility of the Legionnaires' disease bacterium to ten antimicrobial agents. Antimicrob Agents Chemother 1978;13: 419–422.

439. Li AP, Rasmussen A, Xu L,Kaminski DL. Rifampicin induction of lidocaine metabolism in cultured human hepatocytes. J Pharmacol Exp Ther 1995;274:673–677.

440. Lindblad S, Hedfors E, Malmborg A. Rifamycin SV in local treatment of synovitis—a clinical, arthroscopic and pharmacologic evaluation. J Rheumatol 1985;12:900–903.

441. Liu F, Andrews D, Wright DN. *Mycobacterium thermoresistibile* infection in an immunocompromised host. J Clin Microbiol 1984;19:546–547.

442. Livornese LL, Dias S, Samel C, Romanowski B, Taylor S, May P, Pitsakis P, Woods G, Kaye D, Levison ME, Johnson CC. Hospital-acquired infection with vancomycin-resistant *Enterococcus faecium* transmitted by electronic thermometers. Ann Intern Med 1992;117:112–116.

443. Livshin R, Weinrauch L, Even-Paz Z, El-On J. Efficacy of rifampicin and isoniazid in cutaneous leishmaniasis. Int J Dermatol 1987;26:55–59.

444. Ljungberg B, Christensson B, Grubb R. Failure of doxycycline treatment in aquarium-associated *Mycobacterium marinum* infections. Scand J Infect Dis 1987;19:539–543.

445. Llorens J, Serrano RJ, Sanchez R. Pharmacodynamic interference between rifampicin and isoniazid. Chemotherapy 1978; 24:97–103.

446. Llorens-Terol J, Busquets RM. Brucellosis treated with rifampicin. Arch Dis Child 1980;55:486–488.

447. Lohr DC, Goeken JA, Doty DB, Donta ST. *Mycobacterium gordonae* infection of a prosthetic valve. JAMA 1978;239: 1528–1530.

448. Long MW, Snider DE, Farer LS. U.S. Public Health Service Cooperative trial of three rifampin-isoniazid regimens in treatment of pulmonary tuberculosis. Am Rev Respir Dis 1979;119: 879–894.

449. Lorber B. Rifampin in chronic granulomatous disease [Letter]. N Engl J Med 1980;303:111.

450. Losonsky GA, Wolf A, Schwalbe RS, Nataro J, Gibson CB, Lewis EW. Successful treatment of meningitis due to multiply resistant *Enterococcus faecium* with a combination of intrathecal teicoplanin and intravenous antimicrobial agents. Clin Infect Dis 1994;19:163–165.

451. Lou P, Kazdan J, Bannaatayne RM, Cheung R. Successful treatment of *Candida* endophthalmitis with a synergistic combination of amphotericin B and rifampin. Am J Ophthalmol 1977;83:12–15.

452. Luce JM, Ostenson RC, Springmeyer SC, Hudson LD. Invasive aspergillosis presenting as pericarditis and cardiac tamponade. Chest 1979;76:703–705.

453. Lumb R, Shaw D. *Mycobacterium bovis* (BCG) vaccination. Med J Aust 1992;156:286–287.

454. Luquin M, Mirelis B, Ausina V, Condom MAJ, Matas L. Susceptibility of rapidly growing mycobacteria to 21 antimicrobial agents. In Casal M, ed. Mycobacteria of clinical interest. New York: Elsevier Science Publishers, 1986:188–191.

455. Luttichau U, Arcangeli P, Sinapi S. The use of rifaximin in the treatment of acute diarrhoeal enteritis: open study. Panminerva Med 1985;27:129–132.

456. Maduri-Traczewski M, Szymczak EG, Goldmann DA. In vitro activity of penicillin and rifampin against group B streptococci. Rev Infect Dis 1983;5:S586–592.

457. Maiorini E, Lopez EL, Morrow AL, Ramirez F, Procopio A, Furmanski S, Woloj GM, Miller G, Cleary TG. Multiply resistant nontyphoidal *Salmonella* gastroenteritis in children. Pediatr Infect Dis 1993;12:139–145.

458. Maisey DL, Brown RC, Day JL. Rifampicin and cortisone replacement therapy. Lancet 1974;2:896.

459. Makarovskaya LN, Shcherbanyuk AI, Bugaeva OK. Rifampicin efficacy in experimental plague infection. Antibiot Khimioter 1993;38:34–36.

460. Maple PAC, Efstratiou A, Tseneva G, Rikushin Y, Deshevoi S, Jahkola M, Vuopio-Varkila J, George RC. The in-vitro susceptibilities of toxigenic strains of *Corynebacterium diphtheriae* isolated in northwestern Russia and surrounding areas to ten antibiotics. J Antimicrob Chemother 1994;34: 1037–1040.

461. Marchi E, Montecchi L, Venturini AP, Mascellani G, Brufani M, Cellai L. 4-Deoxypyrido[1',2':1,2]imidazo[5,4-c]rifamycin SV derivatives. a new series of semisynthetic rifamycins with high antibacterial activity and low gastroenteric absorption. J Med Chem 1985;28:960–963.

462. Margileth AM. Antibiotic therapy for cat-scratch disease: clinical study of therapeutic outcome in 268 patients and a review of the literature. Pediatr Infect Dis 1992;11:474–478.

463. Marier RT, Zakhireh B, Downs J, Wynne B, Hammond GL, Andriole VT. *Trichosporon cutaneum* endocarditis. Scand J Infect Dis 1978;10:255–256.

464. Marina NM, Flynn PM, Rivera GK, Hughes WT. *Candida*

tropicalis and *Candida albicans* fungemia in children with leukemia. Cancer 1991;68:594–599.

465. Marks J, Jenkins PA, Tzukamura M. *Mycobacterium szulgai—* a new pathogen. Tubercle 1972;53:210–214.

466. Marquet-Van Der Mee N, Goupille P. Isolation of *Actinomyces meyeri* from percutaneous disc biopsy specimens following 453ar disc surgery. Eur J Clin Microbiol Infect Dis 1994;13: 278–279.

467. Martin Casabona R, González Fuente T, Pla RV, Reina Prieto J, De Gracia Roldan J. Clinical significance of environmental mycobacteria (1975–1984). In: Casal M, ed. Mycobacteria of clinical interest. New York: Elsevier Science Publishers, 1986: 282–285.

468. Martínez-Martínez L, Pascual A, Bernard K, Suárez AI. Antimicrobial susceptibility pattern of *Corynebacterium striatum.* Antimicrob Agents Chemother 1996;40:2671–2672.

469. Mascellino MT, Iona E, Ponzo R, Mastroianni CM, Delia S. Infections due to *Rhodococcus equi* in three HIV-infected patients: microbiological findings and antibiotic susceptibility. Int J Clin Pharmacol Res 1995;14:157–163.

470. Maslo C, Buré-Rossier A, Girard PM, Gholizadeh Y, Lebrette MG, Rozenbaum W. Clinical and bacteriologic impact of rifabutin prophylaxis for *Mycobacterium avium* complex in patients with human immunodeficiency infection. Clin Infect Dis 1997;24:344–349.

471. Massa P, Vallerino E, Dodero M. Treatment of hepatic encephalopathy with rifaximin: double blind, double dummy study versus lactulose. Eur J Clin Res 1993;4:7–18.

472. Maurer PM, Bartkowski RR. Drug interactions of clinical significance with opioid analgesics. Drug Safety 1993;8:30–48.

473. Maurin M, Benoliel AM, Bongrand P, Raoult D. Phagosomal alkalinization and the bactericidal effect of antibiotics: the *Coxiella burnetti* paradigm. J Infect Dis 1992;166:1097–1102.

474. Maurin M, Lepocher H, Mallet D, Raoult D. Antibiotic susceptibilities of *Afipia felis* in axenic medium and in cells. Antimicrob Agents Chemother 1993;37:1410–1413.

475. Maurin M, Raoult D. Antimicrobial susceptibility of *Rochalimaea quintana, Rochalimaea vinsonii,* and the newly recognized *Rochalimaea henselae.* J Antimicrob Chemother 1993; 168:1034–1036.

476. Maurin M, Raoult D. *Bartonella (Rochalimaea) quintana* infections. Clin Microbiol Rev 1996;9:273–292.

477. Maurin M, Gasquet S, Ducco C, Raoult D. MICs of 28 antibiotic compounds for 14 *Bartonella* (formerly *Rochalimaea*) isolates. Antimicrob Agents Chemother 1995;39:2387–2391.

478. Mauro VF, Somani P, Temesy-Armos PN. Drug interaction between lorcainide and rifampicin. Eur J Clin Pharmacol 1987;31:737–738.

479. McCabe WR, Lorian V. Comparison of the antibacterial activity of rifampicin and other antibiotics. Am J Med Sci 1968;256:255–265.

480. McClatchy JK, Waggoner RF, Lester W. In vitro susceptibility of mycobacteria to rifampin. Am Rev Respir Dis 1969;100: 234–236.

481. McConkey B, Situnayake RD. Effects of rifampicin with and without isoniazid in rheumatoid arthritis. J Rheumatol 1988;15: 46–50.

482. McEvoy GK, ed. AHFS (American Hospital Formulary Service) drug information. Bethesda, MD: American Society of Health-Systems Pharmacists, 1996:417–423.

483. McEvoy GK, ed. AHFS (American Hospital Formulary Service) drug information. Bethesda, MD: American Society of Health-Systems Pharmacists, 1997:430–439.

484. McKee DF, Barr WM, Bryan CS, Lunceford EM Jr. Primary aspergillosis of the spine mimicking Pott's paraplegia. J Bone Joint Surg 1984;66-A:1481–1483.

485. McLure HM, Chiodini RJ, Anderson DC, Swenson RB, Thayer WR, Contu JA. *Mycobacterium paratuberculosis* infection in a colony of stumptail macaques *(Macaca artoides).* J Infect Dis 1987;155:1011–1019.

486. Medoff G. Antifungal action of rifampin. Rev Infect Dis 1983; 5:S614–619.

487. Medoff G, Kobayashi GS, Kwan CN, Schlessinger D, Venkov P. Potentiation of rifampicin and 5-fluorocytosine as antifungal antibiotics by amphotericin B. Proc Natl Acad Sci USA 1972;69:196–199.

488. Mehta YS, Jijina FF, Badakere SS, Pathare AV, Mohanty D. Rifampicin-induced immune thrombocytopenia. Tuberc Lung Dis 1996;77:558–562.

489. Menke HE, Schuller JL, Stolz E, Niemel PLA, Michel MF. Treatment of lymphogranuloma venereum with rifampicin [Letter]. Br J Vener Dis 1979;55:379.

490. Meunier F. Serum fungistatic and fungicidal activity in volunteers receiving antifungal agents. Eur J Clin Microbiol 1986;5:103–109.

491. Michelet C, Avril JL, Cartier F, Berche P. Inhibition of intracellular growth of *Listeria monocytogenes* by antibiotics. Antimicrob Agents Chemother 1994;38:438–446.

492. Michelet C, Avril JL, Arvieux C, Jacquelinet C, Vu N, Cartier F. Comparative activities of new fluoroquinolones, alone or in combination with amoxicillin, trimethoprim-sulfamethoxazole, or rifampin against intracellular *Listeria monocytogenes.* Antimicrob Agents Chemother 1997;41:60–65.

493. Mikulski SM, Love LJ, Berquist EJ, Haragadon MT, Applefield MM, Mergner W. *Aspergillus* vegetative endocarditis and complete heart block in a patient with acute leukemia. Chest 1979;76:4736.

494. Mimouni A, Hodak E, Mimouni M. Fixed drug eruption following rifampin treatment. Ann Pharmacother 1990;24: 947–948.

495. Moellering RC, Wennersten C. Therapeutic potential of rifampin in enterococcal infections. Rev Infect Dis 1983;5(Suppl): S528–532.

496. Moffie BG, Mouton RP. Sensitivity and resistance of *Legionella pneumophila* to some antibiotics and combinations of antibiotics. J Antimicrob Chemother 1988;22:457–462.

497. Mondal D, Sinha RP, Gupta MK. Effect of combination therapy in *Mycobacterium paratuberculosis* infected rabbits. Indian J Exp Biol 1994;32:318–323.

498. Moody MR, Young VM, Morris MJ, Schimpff SC. In vitro activities of miconazole, miconazole nitrate, and ketoconazole alone and combined with rifampin against *Candida* spp. and *Torulopsis glabrata* recovered from cancer patients. Antimicrob Agents Chemother 1980;17:871–875.

499. Mor N, Simon B, Mezo N, Heifets L. Comparison of activities of rifapentine and rifampin against *Mycobacterium tuberculosis* residing in human macrophages. Antimicrob Agents Chemother 1995;39:2073–2077.

500. MMWR 1996;45:921–925.

501. Morgan MB, Iseman MD. *Mycobacterium bovis* vertebral osteomyelitis as a complication of intravesical administration of Bacille Calmette-Guérin. Am J Med 1996;100:372–373.

502. Morris JT, Kelly JW. Rifabutin-induced ageusa. Ann Intern Med 1993;119:171–172.

503. Morrone N, De Castro Pereira CA, Saito M, Dourado AM,

Pereira da Silva Mendes ES. Treatment of pulmonary actino-mycosis with rifampin. G Ital Chemioter 1982;29:121–124.

504. Mortensen JE, Brumbach A, Shryock TR. Antimicrobial susceptibility of *Bordetella avium* and *Bordetella bronchiseptica* isolates. Antimicrob Agents Chemother 1989;33:771–772.

505. Moshkowitz A, Goldblum N, Heller E. Studies in the antiviral effect of rifampicin in volunteers. Nature 1971:229:422–424.

506. Most JA, Markel GB. A nearly fatal hepatotoxic reaction to rifampin after halothane anesthesia. Am J Surg 1974;127:593.

507. Muniz P, Valls V, Perez-Broseta C, Iradi A, Climent JV, Oliva MR, Saez GT. The role of 8-hydroxy-2'-deoxyguanosine in rifamycin-induced DNA damage. Free Rad Biol Med 1995; 18:747–755.

508. Murdoch JM, Speirs CF, Wright N, Wallace ET. Rifampicin [Letter]. Lancet 1969;1:1094.

509. Musser JM. Antimicrobial agent resistance in mycobacteria: molecular genetic insights. Clin Microbiol Rev 1995;8: 496–514.

510. Muytjens HL, van der Ros-van de Repe J. Comparative in vitro susceptibilities of eight *Enterobacter* species, with special reference to *Enterobacter sakazakii*. Antimicrob Agents Chemother 1986;29:367–370.

511. Myerowitz RL, Pasculle W, Dowling JN, Pazin GJ, Puerzer M, Yee RB, Rinaldo CR Jr, Hakala TR. Opportunistic lung infection due to "Pittsburgh pneumonia agent." N Engl J Med 1979;301:953–958.

512. Myers WF, Grossman DM, Wisseman CL Jr. Antibiotic susceptibility patterns in *Rochalimaea quintana,* the agent of trench fever. Antimicrob Agents Chemother 1984;25:690–693.

513. Narang PK, Lewis RC, Bianchine JR. Rifabutin absorption in humans: relative bioavailability and food effect. Clin Pharmacol Ther 1992;52:335–341.

514. Nathan V, Mehta JB, Dralle W. Rifabutin in the treatment of cavitary lung disease due to *Mycobacterium gordonae*. South Med J 1993;86:839–841.

515. Nau R, Prange HW, Menck S, Kolenda H, Visser K, Seydel JK. Penetration of rifampicin into the cerebrospinal fluid of adults with uninflamed meninges. J Antimicrob Chemother 1992;29: 719–724.

516. Nau R, Kaye K, Sachdeva M, Sande ER, Täuber MG. Rifampin for therapy of experimental pneumococcal meningitis in rabbits. Antimicrob Agents Chemother 1994;38:1186–1189.

517. Neeley SP, Denning DW. Cutaneous *Mycobacterium thermoresistibile* infection in a heart transplant recipient. Rev Infect Dis 1989;11:608–611.

518. Nessi R, Bonoldi GL, Redaelli B, DiFilippo G. Acute renal failure after rifampicin: a case report and survey of the literature. Nephron 1976;16:148–159.

519. Nethercott JR, Schachter RK, Givan KF, Ryder DE. Histoplasmosis due to *Histoplasma capsulatum* var *duboisii* in a Canadian Immigrant. Arch Dermatol 1978;114:595–598.

520. Ng TTC, Campbell CK, Rothera M, Houghton JB, Hughes D, Denning DW. Successful treatment of sinusitis caused by *Cunninghamella bertholletiae*. Clin Infect Dis 1994;19:313–316.

521. Nguyen MH, Stout JE, Yu VL. Legionellosis. Infect Dis Clin North Am 1991;5:561–584.

522. Nicolle LE, Harding GKM. Susceptibility of clinical isolates of *Staphylococcus saprophyticus* to fifteen commonly used antimicrobial agents. Antimicrob Agents Chemother 1982;22: 895–896.

523. Nolan RL, Cleary JD, Chapman SW. Fever associated with daily rifampin therapy. Clin Pharm 1990;9:57–58.

524. Norden CW. Experimental chronic staphylococcal osteomyelitis in rabbits: treatment with rifampin alone and in combination with other antimicrobial agents. Rev Infect Dis 1983;5:S491–494.

525. Norden CW, Fierer J, Bryant RE, Chronic Staphylococcal Osteomyelitis Study Group. Chronic staphylococcal osteomyelitis: treatment with regimens containing rifampin. Rev Infect Dis 1983;5:S495–501.

526. Nordmann P, Kerestedjian JJ, Ronco E. Therapy of *Rhodococcus equi* disseminated infections in nude mice. Antimicrob Agents Chemother 1992;36:1244–1248.

527. Novak RM, Polisky EL, Janda WM, Libertin CR. Osteomyelitis caused by *Rhodococcus equi* in a renal transplant patient. Infection 1988;16:186–188.

528. Ochs HR, Greenblatt DJ, Roberts GM, Dengler HJ. Diazepam interaction with antituberculosis drugs. Clin Pharmacol Ther 1981;29:671–678.

529. O'Connor RP, Silva J, Fekety R. Rifampicin and antibiotic-associated colitis. Lancet 1981;1:499.

530. Oksi J, Viljanen M, Kalimo H, Peltonen R, Marttila R, Salomaa P, Nikoskelainen J, Budka H, Halonen P. Fatal encephalitis caused by concomitant infection with tick-borne encephalitis virus and *Borrelia burgdorferi*. Clin Infect Dis 1993;16: 392–396.

531. Olliaro P, Gorini G, Jabes D, Regazzetti A, Rossi R, Marchetti A, Tinelli C, Della Bruna C. In-vitro and in-vivo activity of rifabutin against *Toxoplasma gondii*. J Antimicrob Chemother 1994;34:649–657.

532. Onody C, Matsiota-Bernard P, Nauciel C. Lack of resistance to erythromycin, rifampicin and ciprofloxacin in 98 clinical isolates of *Legionella pneumophila*. J Antimicrob Chemother 1997;39:815–816.

533. Oriel JD, Ridgway GL, Goldmeir D, Felmingham D. Treatment of gonococcal urethritis in men with a rifampicin-erythromycin combination. Sex Transm Dis 1982;9:208–211.

534. Outman WR, Levitz RE, Hill DA, Nightingale CH. Intraocular penetration of rifampin in humans. Antimicrob Agents Chemother 1992;36:1575–1576.

535. Palazzini E. [Personal communication] Alfa Wasserman S.p.A. part IB. Summary of product characteristics. 1996:1–6.

536. Palazzini E, Palmerio B. Treatment of pyogenic skin infections with rifaximin cream. Eur Rev Med Pharmacol Sci 1993; 15:87–92.

537. Palmer JE, Benson CE. Effect of treatment with erythromycin and rifampin during the acute stages of experimentally induced ehrlichial colitis in ponies. Am J Vet Res 1992;53:2071–2076.

538. Panikabutra K, Ariyarit C, Chitwarakorn A, Wongba C. The combination of erythromycin-rifampin in the treatment of gonococcal urethritis in men. J Med Assoc Thai 1985;68: 579–582.

539. Papi C, Ciaco A, Koch M, Capurso L. Efficacy of rifaximin in the treatment of symptomatic diverticular disease of the colon. A multicentre double-blind placebo-controlled trial. Aliment Pharmacol Ther 1995;9:33–39.

540. Parini P, Cipolla A, Ronchi M, Salzetta A, Mazzella G, Roda E. Effect of rifaximin and paromomycin in the treatment of portal-systemic encephalopathy. Curr Ther Res 1992;51:1–6.

541. Parra FM, Perez-Elias MJ, Cuevas M, Ferreira A. Serum sickness-like illness associated with rifampicin. Ann Allergy 1994;73:123–125.

542. Pascual A, Tsukayama D, Kovarik J, Gekker G, Peterson P. Uptake and activity of rifapentine in human peritoneal macrophages

and polymorphonuclear leukocytes. Eur J Clin Microbiol 1987;6:152–157.

543. Pasculle AW, Dowling JN, Frola FN, McDevitt DA, Levi MA. Antimicrobial therapy of experimental *Legionella micdadei* pneumonia in guinea pigs. Antimicrob Agents Chemother 1985;28:730–734.

544. Pasculle AW, Dowling JN, Weyant RS, Sniffen JM, Cordes LG, Gorman GM, Feeley JC. Susceptibility of Pittsburgh pneumonia agent *(Legionella micdadei)* and other newly recognized members of the genus *Legionella* to nineteen antimicrobial agents. Antimicrob Agents Chemother 1981;20:793–799.

545. Patel AN, McKeon J. Avoidance and management of adverse reactions to antituberculosis drugs. Drug Safety 1995;12:1–25.

546. Patel KB, Belmonte R, Crowe HM. Drug malabsorption and resistant tuberculosis in HIV-infected patients [Letter]. N Engl J Med 1995;332:336–337.

547. Paunescu E. Reprimun—an antibiotic with large spectrum and immunomodulatory properties. Pneumoftiziologia 1994;43: 189–195.

548. Paunescu E, Didilescu C, Mihaltan FL, Udrea S, Serbescu A, Danalache-Dumitrescu M, Smarandache M, Stoinescu M, Zaharescu C, Petre A, Oprisiu G. Advantages of treatment with reprimun in sarcoidosis. Rev Roum Med (Internal Medicine) 1989;23:225–228.

549. Peacock JE Jr, McGinnis MR, Cohen MS. Persistent neutrophilic meningitis. Report of four cases and review of the literature. Medicine 1984;63:379–395.

550. Pedretti G, Calzetti C, Missale G, Fiaccadori F. Rifaximin versus neomycin on hyperbilirubinemia in chronic portal systemic encephalopathy of cirrhotics: a double-blind, randomized trial. Ital J Gastroenterol 1991;23:175–178.

551. Peloquin CA. Using therapeutic drug monitoring to dose the antimycobacterial drugs. Clin Chest Med 1997;18:79–87.

552. Peloquin CA, MacPhee AA, Berning SE. Malabsorption of antimycobacterial medications. N Engl J Med 1993;329: 1122–1123.

553. Peloquin CA, Nitta AT, Burman WJ, Brudney KF, Miranda-Massari JR, McGuinness ME, Berning SE, Gerena GT. Incidence of low anti-tuberculosis drug concentrations in patients with AIDS. Ann Pharmacother 1996;30:919–925.

554. Peloquin CA. Antituberculosis drugs: pharmacokinetics. In: Heifets LB, ed. Drug susceptibility in the chemotherapy of mycobacterial infections. Boca Raton, FL: CRC Press, 1991: 59–88.

555. Peloquin CA. Therapeutic drug monitoring of the antimycobacterial drugs. Clin Lab Med 1996;16:717–729.

556. Pendland SL, Killian AD, Woodward JG, Rodvold KA. In-vitro activity of a new oral streptogramin, RPR 106972, alone and in combination with rifampicin or ciprofloxacin against *Legionella* spp. J Antimicrob Chemother 1997;39:651–653.

557. Pentikainen PJ, Koivula IH, Hiltunen HA. Effect of rifampicin treatment on the kinetics of mexiletine. Eur J Clin Pharmacol 1982;23:261–266.

558. Pérez MAH, Rodriguez BA, Garcia AF, Diez-Tejedor E, Tella PB. Treatment of nervous system brucellosis with rifampin and doxycycline. Neurology 1986;36:1408–1409.

559. Perkins BA, Tondella ML, Bortolottto IM, Takano OA, Da Silva GA, Irino K, Brandileone MC, Harrison LH, Wenger JD, Broome CV, the Brazilian Purpuric Fever Study Group. Comparative efficacy of oral rifampin and topical chloramphenicol in eradicating conjunctival carriage of *Haemophilus influenzae* biogroup *aegyptius*. Pediatr Infect Dis 1992;11:717–721.

560. Perkins BA, Hamill RJ, Musher DM, O'Hara C. In vitro activities of streptomycin and 11 oral antimicrobial agents against clinical isolates of *Klebsiella rhinoscleromatis*. Antimicrob Agents Chemother 1992;36:1785–1787.

561. Perlmutter I, Perlmutter D, Hyams PJ. Fungal infection of the brain: an increasing threat. South Med J 1980;73:499–501.

562. Peters W, Lainson R, Shaw JJ, Robinson BL, Franca Leao A. Potentiating action of rifampicin and isoniazid against *Leishmania mexicana amazonensis*. Lancet 1981;1:1122–1123.

563. Pezzia W, Raleigh JW, Bailey MC, Toth EA, Silverblatt J. Treatment of disease due to *Mycobacterium kansasii*: recent experience with rifampicin. Rev Infect Dis 1981;3:1035–1039.

564. Picciotto A, Gesu GP, Schito GC, Testa R, Varagona G, Celle G. Antimycobacterial chemotherapy in 2 cases of inflammatory bowel disease. Lancet 1988;2:536–537.

565. Pierre-Audigier C, Jouanguy E, Lamhamedi S, Altare F, Rauzier J, Vincent V, Canioni D, Emile J, Fisher A, Blanche S, Gaillard J, Casanova J. Fatal disseminated *Mycobacterium smegmatis* infection in a child with inherited interferon-p receptor deficiency. Clin Infect Dis 1997;24:982–984.

566. Pieters FAJM, Woonink F, Zuidema J. Influence of once-monthly rifampicin and daily clofazimine on the pharmacokinetics of dapsone in leprosy patients in Nigeria. Eur J Clin Pharmacol 1988;34:73–76.

567. Piriz S, Cuenca R, Valle J, Vadillo S. Susceptibilities of anaerobic bacteria isolated from animals with ovine foot rot to 28 antimicrobial agents. Antimicrob Agents Chemother 1992;36: 198–201.

568. Plemmons RM, McAllister CK, Garces MC, Ward RL. Osteomyelitis due to *Mycobacterium haemophilum* in a cardiac transplant patient: case report and analysis of interactions among clarithromycin, rifampin, and cyclosporine. Clin Infect Dis 1997;24:995–997.

569. Plummer FA, Nsanze H, D'Costa LJ, Maggwa ABN, Girouard Y, Karasira P, Albritton WL, Ronald AR. Short-course and single-dose antimicrobial therapy for chancroid in Kenya: studies with rifampin alone and in combination with trimethoprim. Rev Infect Dis 1983;5:S565–572.

570. Podesta A, Lopez P, Terg R, Villamil F, Flores D, Mastai R, Udaondo CB, Companc JP. Treatment of pruritus of primary biliary cirrhosis with rifampin. Diagn Dis Sci 1991;36: 216–220.

571. Pohlad DJ, Saravolatz LD, Somerville MM. Inhibition of *Legionella pneumophila* multiplication within human macrophages by fleroxacin. J Antimicrob Chemother 1988;22(Suppl D): 49–54.

572. Portnoy BL, Micheletti GA Jr. *Acanthamoeba* infection of skin and sinuses in an AIDS patient, diagnosis and treatment [Abstract PuB7450). International Conference on AIDS 1992;8: 124.

573. Poungvarin N, Jariya P. The fifth nonlethal case of primary amoebic meningoencephalitis. J Med Assoc Thai 1991;74: 112–115.

574. Prasad ES, Wenman WM. In vitro activity of rifaximin, a topical rifamycin derivative, against *Chlamydia trachomatis*. Diagn Microbiol Infect Dis 1993;16:135–136.

575. Pratt DS, Tenney JH, Bjork CM, Reller LB. Successful treatment of *Brucella melitensis* endocarditis. Am J Med 1978;64:897–900.

576. Prescott JF. *Rhodococcus equi:* an animal and human pathogen. Clin Microbiol Rev 1991;4:20–34.

577. Prescott JF, Nicholson VM. The effects of combinations of se-

lected antibiotics on the growth of *Corynebacterium equi*. J Vet Pharmacol Ther 1984;7:61–64.

578. Pretet S, Lebeaut A, Parrot R, Truffot C, Grosset J, Dinh-Xuan AT, G.E.T.I.M. Combined chemotherapy including rifabutin for rifampicin and isoniazid resistant pulmonary tuberculosis. Eur Respir J 1992;5:680–684.

579. Prince H, Ispahani P, Baker M. A *Mycobacterium malmoense* infection of the hand presenting as carpal tunnel syndrome. J Hand Surg (Br) 1988;13-B:328–330.

580. Prober CG. Effect of rifampin on chloramphenicol levels. N Engl J Med 1985;312:788–789.

581. Puiatti P, Alberico G, Cotilli G, Salvai M, Goitre M. Sporotrichoid infection: two cases. G Ital Dermatol Venereol 1990;125: 349–352.

582. Pujet JC, Homberg JC, Decroix G. Sensitivity to rifampicin: incidence, mechanism and prevention. Br Med J 1974;2: 415–418.

583. Pukrittayakamee S, Viravan C, Charoenlarp P, Yeamput C, Wilson RJM, White NJ. Antimalarial effects of rifampin in *Plasmodium vivax* malaria. Antimicrob Agents Chemother 1994; 38:511–514.

584. Pulik M, Leterdu F, Lionnet F, Genet P, Petitdidier C, Touahri T. Rifabutin prevents campylobacter infection in patients with AIDS. Clin Infect Dis 1996;23:1197–1198.

585. Qiu YS, Klitorinos A, Rahal MD, Siboo R, Chan ECS. Enumeration of viable oral spirochetes from periodontal pockets. Oral Microbiol Immunol 1994;9:301–304.

586. Quinlan GJ, Gutteridge MC. DNA base damage by β-lactacm, tetracycline, bacitracin and rifamycin antibacterial antibiotics. Biochem Pharmacol 1991;42:1595–1599.

587. Quraishi MAH, Soeiro R, Boma L. In vitro activity of ansamycin (LM-427) vs. fifteen different species of mycobacteria [Abstract U55]. In: Program and abstracts of the 85th Annual Meeting of the American Society for Microbiology, Washington, DC: American Society for Microbiology, 1985.

588. Radulovic S, Higgins JA, Jaworski DC, Azad AF. In vitro and in vivo antibiotic susceptibilities of ELB rickettsiae. Antimicrob Agents Chemother 1995;39:2564–2566.

589. Rahn KH, Mooy J, Bohm R, Van der Vet A. Reduction of bioavailability of verapamil by rifampin. N Engl J Med 1985; 312:920–921.

590. Raoult D, Torres H, Drancourt M. Shell-vial assay: evaluation of a new technique for determining antibiotic susceptibility, tested in 13 isolates of *Coxiella burnetii*. Antimicrob Agents Chemother 1991;35:2070–2077.

591. Raoult D, Roussellier P, Vestris G, Tamalet J. In vitro antibiotic susceptibility of *Rickettsia rickettsia* and *Rickettsia conorii:* plaque assay and microplaque colorimetric assay. J Infect Dis 1987;155:1059–1062.

592. Raoult D, Etienne J, Massip P, Iaocono S, Prince MA, Beaurain P, Benichou S, Auvergnat JC, Mathieu P, Bachet Ph, Serradimigni A. Q fever endocarditis in the south of France. J Infect Dis 1987;155:570–573.

593. Raoult D, Fournier PE, Drancourt M, Marrie TJ, Etienne J, Cosserat J, Cacoub P, Poinsignon Y, Leclercq P, Sefton AM. Diagnosis of 22 new cases of *Bartonella* endocarditis. Ann Intern Med 1996;125:646–652.

594. Rastogi N, Blom-Potar M-C, David HL. Drug action against intracellularly growing *Mycobacterium xenopi*. Curr Microbiol 1989;19:83–89.

595. Rawls WH, Lamm DL, Lowe BA, Crawford ED, Sarosdy MF, Montie JE, Grossman HB, Scardino PT. Fatal sepsis following intravesical bacillus Calmette-Guérin administration for bladder cancer. J Urol 1990;144:1328.

596. Remington JS, Yagura T, Robinson WS. The effect of rifampin on *Toxoplasma gondii*. Proceedings of the Society for Experimental Biology and Medicine 1970;135:167–172.

597. Renaudin H, Tully JG, Bebear C. In vitro susceptibilities of *Mycoplasma genitalium* to antibiotics. Antimicrob Agents Chemother 1992;36:870–872.

598. Renneberg J, Niemann LL, Gutschik E. Antimicrobial susceptibility of 278 streptococcal blood isolates to seven antimicrobial agents. J Antimicrob Chemother 1997;39:135–140.

599. Research Committee, British Thoracic Society. *Mycobacterium kansasii* pulmonary infection: a prospective study of the results of nine months of treatment with rifampicin and ethambutol. Thorax 1994;49:442–445.

600. Rhine WD, Arvin AM, Stevenson DK. Neonatal aspergillosis. a case report and review of the literature. Clin Pediatr (Phila) 1986;25:400–403.

601. Ribner B, Keusch GT, Hanna BA, Perloff M. Combination amphotericin B-rifampin therapy for pulmonary aspergillosis in a leukemic patient. Chest 1976;70:681–683.

602. Rice TL, Patterson JH, Celestin C, Foster JR, Powell JR. Influence of rifampin on tocainide pharmacokinetics in humans. Clin Pharm 1989;8:200–205.

603. Rifkind D, Crowder ED, Hyland RN. In vitro inhibition of *Coccidioides immitis* strains with amphotericin B plus rifampin. Antimicrob Agents Chemother 1974;6:783–784.

604. Rikihisa Y, Jiang BM. In vitro susceptibility of *Ehrlichia risticii* to eight antibiotics. Antimicrob Agents Chemother 1988;32:986–991.

605. Rikihasa Y, Jiang BM. Effect of antibiotics on clinical, pathologic and immunologic responses in murine Potomac horse fever: protective effects of doxycycline. Vet Microbiol 1989;19:253–262.

606. Ripa S, Mignini F, Prenna M, Falcioni E. In vitro antibacterial activity of rifaximin against *Clostridium difficile, Campylobacter jejuni* and *Yersinia* spp. Drugs Exp Clin Res 1987;13: 483–488.

607. Riva S, Silvestri LG. Rifamycins: a general view. Annu Rev Microbiol 1972;26:199–224.

608. Robson RA, Miners JO, Wing MH, Birkett JD. Theophylline-rifampicin interaction: non-selective induction of theophylline metabolic pathways. Br J Clin Pharmacol 1984;18:445–448.

609. Rodescu D, Abeles H, Zelefsky MN, Williams MH Jr. Accelerated growth of lung cancer in association with rifampicin administration for tuberculosis. Lancet 1981;1:983.

610. Rohner P, Herter C, Auckenthaler R, Pechère JC, Waldvogel FA, Lew DP. Synergistic effect of quinolones and oxacillin on methicillin-resistant *Staphylococcus* species. Antimicrob Agents Chemother 1989;33:2037–2041.

611. Roig J, Carreres A, Domingo C. Treatment of Legionnaires' disease: current recommendations. Drugs 1993;46:63–79.

612. Romand S, Della Bruna C, Farinotti R, Derouin F. In vitro and in vivo effects of rifabutin alone or combined with atovaquone against *Toxoplasma gondii*. Antimicrob Agents Chemother 1996;40:2015–2020.

613. Rosenberg EW, Noah PW, Zanolli MD, Skinner RB, Bond MJ, Crutcher N. Use of rifampin with penicillin and erythromycin in the treatment of psoriasis. J Am Acad Dermatol 1986;14: 761–764.

614. Roszkowski W, Lipinska R, Roszkowski K, Jeljaszewicz J, Pulverer G. Rifampicin-induced suppression of antitumor immunity. Med Microbiol Immunol 1984;172:197–205.

615. Rothwell DL, Richmond DE. Hepatorenal failure with self-initiated intermittent rifampicin therapy. Br Med J 1974;2:481–482.

616. Rouquet RM, Clave D, Massip P, Moatti N, Leophonte P. Imipenem/vancomycin for *Rhodococcus equi* pulmonary infection in HIV-positive patient [Letter]. Lancet 1991;337:375.

617. Rubin J, Stoehr G, Yu VL, Muder RR, Matador A, Kamerer DB. Efficacy of oral ciprofloxacin plus rifampin for the treatment of malignant otitis externa. Arch Otolaryngol Head Neck Surg 1989;115:1063–1069.

618. Rudin JE, Evans TL, Wing EJ. Failure of erythromycin in treatment of *Legionella micdadei* pneumonia. Am J Med 1984;76:318–320.

619. Rutgeerts P, Geboes K, Vantrappen G, Van Isveldt J, Peeters M, Penninckx F, Hiele M. Rifabutin and ethambutol do not help recurrent Crohn's disease in the neoterminal ileum. J Clin Gastroenterol 1992;15:24–28.

620. Ryan JL, Pachner A, Andriole VT, Root RK. Enterococcal meningitis, combined vancomycin and rifampin therapy. Am J Med 1980;68:449–451.

621. Rynearson TK, Shronts JS, Wolinsky E. Rifampin: in vitro effect on atypical mycobacteria. Am Rev Respir Dis 1971;104:272–274.

622. Saez GT, Valls V, Muniz P, Perez-Broseta C, Iradi A, Oliva MR, Bannister JV, Bannister WH. The role of glutathione in protection against DNA damage induced by rifamycin SV and copper (II) ions. Free Rad Res Commun 1993;19:81–92.

623. Saha SK. Dermal leishmaniasis after kala-azar infection: successful treatment with rifampicin. Cutis 1985;36:81–82.

624. Saito H, Sato K, Tomioka H. Comparative in vitro and in vivo activity of rifabutin and rifampicin against *Mycobacterium avium* complex. Tubercle 1988;69:187–192.

625. Saito H, Tomioka H, Sato K, Emori M, Yamane T, Yamashita K. In vitro antimycobacterial activities of newly synthesized benzoxazinorifamycins. Antimicrob Agents Chemother 1991;35:542–547.

626. Sali A, McQuillan T, Read A, Kune G. Rifampicin as cytotoxic agent for cholangiocarcinoma: preliminary report of seven cases. J Cancer Res Clin Oncol 1991;117:503–504.

627. Samies JH, Hathaway BN, Echols RM, Veazey JM Jr, Pilon VA. Lung abscess due to *Corynebacterium equi:* report of the first case in a patient with acquired immune deficiency syndrome. Am J Med 1986;80:685–688.

628. Sanders WE Jr, Hartwig EC, Schneider NJ, Cacciatore R, Valdez H. Susceptibility of organisms in the *Mycobacterium fortuitum* complex to antituberculous and other antimicrobial agents. Antimicrob Agents Chemother 1977;12:295–297.

629. Santamaría M, Ponte C, Wilhelmi I, Soriano F. Antimicrobial susceptibility of *Corynebacterium* group D2. Antimicrob Agents Chemother 1985;28:845–846.

630. Saravolatz LD, Pohlod DJ, Quinn EL. In vitro susceptibility of *Legionella pneumophila,* serogroups I-IV. J Infect Dis 1979;140:251.

631. Saravolatz LD, Burch KH, Fisher E, Madhavan T, Kiani D, Neblett T, Quinn EL. The compromised host and Legionnaires' disease. Ann Intern Med 1979;90:533–537.

632. Sasal M, Roig J, Cervantes M, Matas L, Segura F. Good response to antibiotic treatment of lung infection due to *Rhodococcus equi* in a patient infected with human immunodeficiency virus. Clin Infect Dis 1992;15:747–748.

633. Saubolle MA, Kiehn TE, White MH, Rudinsky MF, Armstrong D. *Mycobacterium haemophilum:* microbiology and expanding clinical and geographic spectra of disease in humans. Clin Microbiol Rev 1996;9:435–447.

634. Sauret J, Hernándaz-Flix S, Castro E, Hernández L, Ausina V, Coll P. Treatment of pulmonary disease caused by *Mycobacterium kansasii:* results of 18 vs 12 months' chemotherapy. Tuberc Lung Dis 1995;76:104–108.

635. Scalco GB, Rossi MR, Rubbini M, Cirelli C. Rifaximin: a new rifamycin for the prophylaxis of the septic complications in large bowel surgery. Policlinico Sez Chir 1987;94:41–45.

636. Scannell KA, Portoni EJ, Finkle HI, Rice M. Pulmonary malacoplakia and *Rhodococcus equi* infection in a patient with AIDS. Chest 1990;97:1000–1001.

637. Schack SH, Smith PW, Penn RG, Rapoport JM. Endocarditis caused by *Actinobacillus actinomycetemcomitans*. J Clin Microbiol 1984;20:579–581.

638. Schaefer WB, Wolinsky E, Jenkins PA, Marks J. *Mycobacterium szulgai*—a new pathogen: serologic identification and report of five new cases. Am Rev Respir Dis 1973;108:1320–1326.

639. Schaumann RF, Shah PM. Effect of amphotericin B alone and in combination with rifampicin on phagocytosis of *Candida* species by human polymorphonuclear leukocytes. Methods Find Exp Clin Pharmacol 1992;14:753–758.

640. Scheld WM, Fletcher DD, Fink FN, Sande MA. Response to therapy in an experimental rabbit model of meningitis due to *Listeria monocytogenes*. J Infect Dis 1979;140:287–294.

641. Scheld WM. Evaluation of rifampin and other antibiotics against *Listeria monocytogenes* in vitro and in vivo. Rev Infect Dis 1983;5:S562–564.

642. Scheuer PJ, Summerfield JA, Lal S, Sherlock S. Rifampicin hepatitis. Lancet 1974;7855:421–425.

643. Schmidt LH. Appraisals of compounds of diverse chemical classes for capacities to cure infections with sporozoites of *Plasmodium cynomolgi*. Am J Trop Med Hyg 1983;32:231–257.

644. Schrenzel J, Dayer P, Leemann T, Weidekamm E, Portmann R, Lew DP. Influence of rifampin on fleroxacin pharmacokinetics. Antimicrob Agents Chemother 1993;37:2132–2138.

645. Schultsz C, Kuijper EJ, van Soolingen D, Prins JM. Disseminated infection due to multidrug-resistant *Mycobacterium bovis* in a patient who was seropositive for human immunodeficiency virus. Clin Infect Dis 1996;23:841–843.

646. Schultz MG, Rieder HL, Hersh T, Riepe S. Remission of Crohn's disease with antimycobacterial chemotherapy. Lancet 1987;2:1391–1392.

647. Schwartz A, Brown JR. Quinidine-rifampin interaction. Am Heart J 1984;107:789–790.

648. Schwartz B, Harrison LH, Motter JS, Motter RN, Hightower AW, Broome CV. Investigation of an outbreak of *Moraxella* conjunctivitis at a Navajo boarding school. Am J Ophthalmol 1989;107:341–347.

649. Sebba L, Beamis JF, Webb-Johnson DC. Lung cancer in patient taking rifampicin. Lancet 1982;1:105.

650. Segreti J, Gvazdinskas LC, Trenholme GM. In vitro activity of minocycline and rifampin against staphylococci. Diagn Microbiol Infect Dis 1989;12:253–255.

651. Segura JJ, Calzado-Flores C, Gonzalez-Cisneros F. Inhibition of *E. invadens* cysts induced by the addition of rifampicin. Proc West Pharmacol Soc 1991;34:369–371.

652. Seidel JS, Harmatz P, Visvesvara GS, Cohen A, Edwards J, Turner J. Successful treatment of primary amoebic meningoencephalitis. N Engl J Med 1982;306:346–348.

653. Sekhar LN, Dujovny M, Rao GR. Carotid-cavernous sinus thrombosis caused by *Aspergillus fumigatus:* case report. J Neurosurg 1980;52:120–125.

654. Self TH, Tsiu SJ, Bould WF, Fowler JW. Interaction of rifampin and glyburide. Chest 1989;96:1443–1444.

655. Seriki O, Aderele WI, Johnson A, Smith JA. Disseminated histoplasmosis due to *Histoplasma capsulatum* in two Nigerian children. J Trop Med Hyg 1975;78:248–255.

656. Sethi VS. Structure and function of DNA-dependent RNA-polymerase. Prog Biophys Mol Biol 1971;23:67–101.

657. Shaffer JL, Turnberg LA. Does antituberculous chemotherapy for Crohn's disease provide long term benefit? A five year follow up study. Gut 1989;30:A1480.

658. Shaffer JL, Houston JB. The effect of rifampicin on sulphapyridine plasma concentrations following sulphasalazine administration. Br J Clin Pharmacol 1985;19:526–528.

659. Shafran SD, Deschenes J, Miller M, Phillips P, Toma E. Uveitis and pseudojaundice during a regimen of clarithromycin, rifabutin, and ethambutol. N Engl J Med 1994;330:439–440.

660. Shah SC, Sharma RK, Hemangini, Chitle AR. Rifampicin induced osetomalacia. Tubercle 1981;62:207–209.

661. Shaheen O, Biollaz J, Koshakji RP, Wilkinson GR, Wood AJJ. Influence of debrisoquin phenotype on the inducibility of propranolol metabolism. Clin Pharmacol Ther 1989;45:439–443.

662. Shanson DC, Leung T. Susceptibility of *Salmonella typhi* to rifamycins and novobiocin. J Antimicrob Chemother 1976;2:81–86.

663. Shasha B, Lang R, Rubinstein E. Therapy of experimental murine brucellosis with streptomycin, co-trimoxazole, ciprofloxacin, ofloxacin, pefloxacin, doxycycline, and rifampin. Antimicrob Agents Chemother 1992;36:973–976.

664. Shehabi A, Shakir K, El-Khateeb M, Qubain H, Fararjeh N, Shamat ARA. Diagnosis and treatment of 106 cases of human brucellosis. J Infect 1990;20:5–10.

665. Shronts JS, Rynearson TK, Wolinsky E. Rifampin alone and combined with other drugs in *Mycobacterium kansasii* and *Mycobacterium intracellulare* infections in mice. Am Rev Respir Dis 1971;104:728–741.

666. Siegal FP, Eilbott D, Burger H, Gehan K, Davidson B, Kaell AT, Weiser B. Dose-limiting toxicity of rifabutin in AIDS-related complex: syndrome of arthralgia/arthritis. AIDS 1990;4:433–441.

667. Simor AE, Salit IE, Vellend H. The role of *Mycobacterium xenopi* in human disease. Am Rev Respir Dis 1984;129:435–438.

668. Simpson L, Simpson AM. Kinetoplast RNA of *Leishmania tarentolae.* Cell 1978;14:169–178.

669. Singh B, Jones RS. Treatment with rifampicin for *Pneumocystis carinii* pneumonia. Ann Trop Paediatr 1984;4:49–50.

670. Sivonen A, Renkonen O, Weckström P, Koshenvuo K, Raunio V, Mäkelä PH. The effect of chemoprophylactic use of rifampin and minocycline on rates of carriage of *Neisseria meningitidis* in army recruits in Finland. J Infect Dis 1978;137:238–244.

671. Skinner MH, Hsieh M, Torseth J, Pauloin D, Bhatia G, Harkonen S, Merigan TC, Blaschke TF. Pharmacokinetics of rifabutin. Antimicrob Agents Chemother 1989;33:1237–1241.

672. Skov R, Christensen JJ, Busch-Sorensen C, Korner B, Facklam RR, Frimodt-Moller N, Espersen F. In vitro antimicrobial susceptibility of *Aerococcus urinae* to 10 antibiotics [Abstract E057]. 36th ICAAC, annual meeting of the American Society for Microbiology, New Orleans, Sept 15–18, 1996.

673. Sladek GG, Frame JN. *Rhodococcus equi* causing bacteremia in an adult with acute leukemia. South Med J 1993;86:244–246.

674. Smith MD, Vinh DX, Hoa NTT, Wain J, Thung D, White NJ. In vitro antimicrobial susceptibilities of strains of *Yersinia pestis.* Antimicrob Agents Chemother 1995;39:2153–2154.

675. Smith MJ, Citron KM. Clinical review of disease caused by *Mycobacterium xenopi.* Thorax 1983;38:373–377.

676. Smith SM, Eng RHK, Landesman S. Effect of rifampin on ampicillin killing of group B streptococci. Antimicrob Agents Chemother 1982;22:522–524.

677. Solera J, Rodríguez-Zapata M, Geijo P, Largo J, Paulino J, Sáez L, Martínez-Alfaro E, Sánchez L, Sepulveda M, Ruiz-Ribó M, the Gecmei Group. Doxycycline-rifampin versus doxycycline-streptomycin in treatment of human brucellosis due to *Brucella melitensis.* Antimicrob Agents Chemother 1995;39:2061–2067.

678. Soriano F, Zapardiel J, Nieto E. Antimicrobial susceptibilities of *Corynebacterium* species and other non-spore-forming gram-positive bacilli to 18 antimicrobial agents. Antimicrob Agents Chemother 1995;39:208–214.

679. Spicer AJ, Peacock MG, Williams JC. Effectiveness of several antibiotics in suppressing chick embryo lethality during experimental infections by *Coxiella burnetii, Rickettsia typhi,* and *R. rickettsii.* In: Burgdorfer W, Anacker RL, eds. Rickettsiae and rickettsial diseases. New York: Academic Press, 1981:375–383.

680. Spiegel CA. Susceptibility of *Mobiluncus* species to 23 antimicrobial agents and 15 other compounds. Antimicrob Agents Chemother 1987;31:249–252.

681. Stanford JL, Phillips I. Rifampicin in experimental *Mycobacterium ulcerans* infection. J Med Microbiol 1972;5:39.

682. Stanley TV, Balakrishnan V. Rifampicin in neonatal ventriculitis. Aust Paediatr J 1982;18:200–201.

683. Staum JM. Enzyme induction: rifampin-disopyramide interaction. Ann Pharmacother 1990;24:701–702.

684. Steele MA, Burk RF, DesPrez RM. Toxic hepatitis with isoniazid and rifampin. Chest 1991;99:465–471.

685. Steg A, Leleu C, Debré B, Boccon-Gibod L, Sicard D. Systemic bacillus Calmette-Guérin infection, 'BCGitis', in patients treated by intravesical bacillus Calmette-Guérin therapy for bladder cancer. Eur Urol 1989;16:161–164.

686. Stern GA. In vitro antibiotic synergism against ocular fungal isolates. Am J Ophthalmol 1978;86:359–367.

687. Stevens DA. Antifungal interaction in vitro between fluconazole, rifabutin, and azithromycin [Abstract 89]. 1994 Infectious Disease Society of America annual meeting. Clin Infect Dis 1994;19:578.

688. Strath M, Scott-Finnigan T, Gardner M, Williamson D, Wilson I. Antimalarial activity of rifampicin in vitro and in rodent models. Trans R Soc Trop Med Hyg 1993;87:211–216.

689. Stringer KA, Cetnarowski AB, Goldfarb A, Lebsack ME, Chang T, Sedman AJ. Enhanced pirmenol elimination by rifampin. J Clin Pharmacol 1988;28:1094–1097.

690. Sun E, Heath-Chiozzi M, Cameron DW, Hsu A, Granneman RG, Maurath CJ, Leonard JM. Concurrent ritonavir and rifabutin increases risk of rifabutin-associated adverse events [Abstract B.171]. Presented at XI International Conference on AIDS, Vancouver, Jul 8, 1996.

691. Sweeney CR, Sweeney RW, Divers TJ. *Rhodococcus equi* pneumonia in 48 foals: response to antimicrobial therapy. Vet Microbiol 1987;14:329.

692. Swenson JM, Facklam RR, Thornsberry C. Antimicrobial sus-

ceptibility of vancomycin-resistant *Leuconostoc, Pediococcus,* and *Lactobacillus* species. Antimicrob Agents Chemother 1990;34:543–549.

693. Swerdlow B, Deresinski S. Development of aspergillus sinusitis in a patient receiving amphotericin B. Treatment with granulocyte transfusions. Am J Med 1984;76:162–166.

694. Subak-Sharpe JH, Timbury MC, Williams JF. Rifampicin inhibits the growth of some mammalian viruses. Nature 1969; 222:341–345.

695. Subramanya NI, Wright JS, Khan MAR. Failure of rifampicin and co-trimazole in Q fever endocarditis. Br Med J 1982;285:343–344.

696. Summerbell RC, Richardson SE, Kane J. *Fusarium proliferatum* as an agent of disseminated infection in an immunosuppressed patient. J Clin Microbiol 1988;26:82–87.

697. Szabo C, Bissell MJ, Calvin M. Inhibition of infectious Rous sarcoma virus production by a rifamycin derivative. J Virol 1976;18:445–453.

698. Szychowska Z, Prandota-Schoepp A, Chabudzinska S. Rifampicin for *Pneumocystis carinii* pneumonia [Letter]. Lancet 1983;1:935.

699. Tada Y, Tsuda Y, Otsuka T, Nagasawa K, Kimura H, Kusaba T, Sakata T. Case report: nifedipine-rifampicin interaction attenuates the effect on blood pressure in a patient with essential hypertension. Am J Med Sci 1992;303:25–27.

700. Tajima A, Mine T, Ogata E. Rifampicin-associated ulcerative colitis. Ann Intern Med 1992;116:778–779.

701. Takasu N, Yamada T, Miura H, Sakamoto S, Korenaga M, Nakajima K, Kanayama M. Rifampicin-induced early phase hyperglycemia in humans. Am Rev Respir Dis 1982;125: 23–27.

702. Takeda M, Nishinuma K, Yamashita S, Matsubayashi T, Tanino S, Nishimura T. Serum haloperidol levels of schizophrenics receiving treatment for tuberculosis. Clin Neuropharmacol 1986;9:386–397.

703. Tan TQ, Mason EO, Ou C, Kaplan SL. Use of intravenous rifampin in neonates with persistent staphylococcal bacteremia. Antimicrob Agents Chemother 1993;37:2401–2406.

704. Tan TQ, Wagner ML, Kaplan SL. *Bartonella (Rochalimaea) henselae* hepatosplenic infection occurring simultaneously in two siblings. Clin Infect Dis 1996;22:721–722.

705. Tankovic J, Leclercq R, Duval J. Antimicrobial susceptibility of *Pediococcus* spp. and genetic basis of macrolide resistance in *Pediococcus acidilactici* HM3020. Antimicrob Agents Chemother 1993;37:789–792.

706. Tanz RR, Shulman ST, Barthel MJ, Willert C, Yogev R. Penicillin plus rifampin eradicates pharyngeal carriage of group A streptococci. J Pediatr 1985;106:876–880.

707. Tanz RR, Poncher JR, Corydon KE, Kabat K, Yogev R, Shulman ST. Clindamycin treatment of chronic pharyngeal carriage of group A streptococci. J Pediatr 1991;119:123–128.

708. Telenti A, Imboden P, Marchesi F, Schmidheini T, Bodmer T. Direct, automated detection of rifampin-resistant *Mycobacterium tuberculosis* by polymerase chain reaction and single-strand conformation polymorphism analysis. Antimicrob Agents Chemother 1993;37:2054–2058.

709. Terashima T, Sakamaki F, Hasegawa N, Kanazawa M, Kawashiro T. Pulmonary infection due to *Mycobacterium xenopi*. Intern Med 1994;33:536–539.

710. Testa R, Eftimiadi C, Sukkar GS, De Leo C, Rovida S, Schito GC, Celle G. A non-absorbable rifamycin for treatment of hepatic encephalopathy. Drugs Exp Clin Res 1985;11:387–392.

711. Thayer WR, Coutu JA, Chiodini RJ, Van Kruiningen HJ. Use of rifabutin and streptomycin in the therapy of Crohn's disease. Gastroenterology 1988;94:A458.

712. Thong YH. Growth inhibition of *Naegleria fowleri* by tetracycline, rifamycin, and miconazole [Letter]. Lancet 1977;2:1976.

713. Thong YH, Rowan-Kelly B, Ferrante A. Treatment of experimental *Naegleria* meningoencephalitis with a combination of amphotericin B and rifamycin. Scand J Infect Dis 1979;11: 151–153.

714. Thornsberry C, Hill BC, Swenson JM, McDougal LK. Rifampin: spectrum of antibacterial activity. Rev Infect Dis 1983;5 (Suppl):S412–417.

715. Tizer KB, Cervia JS, Dunn AM, Stovola JJ, Noel GJ. Successful combination vancomycin and rifampin therapy in a newborn with community-acquired *Flavobacterium meningosepticum* neonatal meningitis. Pediatr Infect Dis J 1995;14:916–917.

716. Tomiyama T, Asano S, Suwa Y, Morita T, Kataoka K, Mori H, Endo N. Rifampicin prevents the aggregation and neurotoxicity of amyloid β protein in vitro. Biochem Biophys Res Commun 1994;204:76–83.

717. Tompkins LD, Roessler BJ, Redd SC, Markowitz LE, Cohen ML. Legionella prosthetic-valve endocarditis. N Engl J Med 1988;318:530–535.

718. Toolan HW, Ledinko N. Effect of rifampicin on the development of tumours induced by adenovirus in male hampsters. Nature New Biol 1972;237:200–202.

719. Tortoli E, Piersimoni C, Bacosi D, Bartoloni A, Betti F, Bono L, Burrini C, De Sio G, Lacchini C, Mantella A, Orsi PG, Penati V, Simonetti MT, Böttger EC. Isolation of the newly described species *Mycobacterium celatum* from AIDS patients. J Clin Microbiol 1995;33:137–140.

720. Tortoli E, Simonetti MT. Radiometric susceptibility testing of *Mycobacterium xenopi*. J Chemother 1995;7:114–117.

721. Towns ML, Fisher D, Moore J. Community-acquired pneumonia due to *Legionella gormanii*. Clin Infect Dis 1994;18: 265–266.

722. Trapnell CB, Narang PK, Li R, Lavelle JP. Increased plasma rifabutin levels with concomitant fluconazole therapy in HIV-infected patients. Ann Intern Med 1996;124:573–576.

723. Traub WH, Leonhard B. Comparative susceptibility of clinical group A, B, C, F, and G β-hemolytic streptococcal isolates to 24 antimicrobial agents. Chemother 1997;43:10–20.

724. Traub WH, Leonhard B. Antibiotic susceptibility of O- and nonhemolytic streptococci from patients and healthy adults to 24 antimicrobial agents. Chemotherapy 1997;43:123–131.

725. Treharne JD, Yearsley PJ, Ballard RC. In vitro studies of *Chlamydia trachomatis* susceptibility and resistance to rifampin and rifabutin. Antimicrob Agents Chemother 1989;33: 1393–1394.

726. Trnka L, Mison P, Bartmann K, Otten H. Experimental evaluation of efficacy. In: Bartmann K, ed. Antituberculosis drugs. Berlin: Springer-Verlag, 1988:31–232.

727. Tschida SJ, Vance-Bryan K, Zaske DE. Anti-infective agents and hepatic disease. Med Clin North Am 1995;79:895–917.

728. Tseng AL, Walmsley SL. Rifabutin-associated uveitis. Ann Pharmacother 1995;29:1149–1155.

729. Tsuchihashi K, Fukami K, Kishimoto H, Sumiyoshi T, Haze K, Saito M, Hiramori K. A case of variant angina exacerbated by administration of rifampicin. Heart Vessels 1988;3:214–217.

730. Tuazon CU, Shamsuddin D, Miller H. Antibiotic susceptibility and synergy of clinical isolates of *Listeria monocytogenes*. Antimicrob Agents Chemother 1982;21:525–527.

731. Tuazon CU, Lin MY, Sheagren JN. In vitro activity of rifampin alone and in combination with nafcillin and vancomycin against pathogenic strains of *Staphylococcus aureus*. Antimicrob Agents Chemother 1978;13:759–761.

732. Tucker RM, Denning DW, Hanson LH, Rinaldi MG, Graybill JR, Sharkey PK, Pappagianis D, Stevens DA. Interaction azoles with rifampin, phenytoin, and carbamazepine: in vitro and clinical observations. Clin Infect Dis 1992;14:165–174.

733. Ungheri D, Sanfilippo A. Activity of LM 427 on *Legionella* spp: in vitro study and intracellular killing. In: Ishigami J, ed. Recent advances in chemotherapy. Tokyo: Tokyo Press, 1986:1919–1920.

734. Ungheri D, Penati V, Giobbi A. Rifabutine (LM 427): in vitro and in vivo activity against rifampicin-resistant and atypical mycobacteria. In: Casal M, ed. Mycobacteria of clinical interest. New York: Elsevier Science Publishers, 1986:184–187.

735. Utrup LJ, Moore TD, Actor P, Poupard JA. Susceptibilities of nontuberculous mycobacterial species to amoxicillin-clavulanic acid alone and in combination with antimycobacterial agents. Antimicrob Agents Chemother 1995;39:1454–1457.

736. Vaara M. Comparative activity of rifabutin and rifampicin against gram-negative bacteria that have damaged or defective outer membranes. J Antimicrob Chemother 1993;31:799–801.

737. Vaheri A, Hanafusa H. Effect of rifampicin and a derivative on cells transformed by Rous sarcoma virus. Cancer Res 1971;31:2032–2036.

738. Valdes JM, Baltch AL, Smith RP, Hammer MC, Ritz WJ. The effect of rifampicin on the in-vitro activity of cefpirome or ceftazidime in combination with aminoglycosides against *Pseudomonas aeruginosa*. J Antimicrob Chemother 1990;25:575–584.

739. Valdes JM, Baltch AL, Smith RP, Franke M, Ritz WJ, Williams S, Michelsen P, Singh J. Comparative therapy with cefpirome alone and in combination with rifampin and/or gentamicin against *Pseudomonas aeruginosa* infection in leukopenic mice. J Infect Dis 1990;162:1112–1117.

740. Van Caekenberghe DL, Breyssens J. In vitro synergistic activity between bismuth subcitrate and various antimicrobial agents against *Campylobacter pyloridis (C. pylori)*. Antimicrob Agents Chemother 1987;31:1429–1430.

741. Van Der Auwera P, Klastersky J. In vitro study of the combination of rifampin with oxacillin against *Staphylococcus aureus*. Rev Infect Dis 1983;5:S509–514.

742. Van Der Auwera P, Meunier-Carpentier F, Klastersky J. Clinical study of combination therapy with oxacillin and rifampin for staphylococcal infections. Rev Infect Dis 1983;5:S515–522.

743. Van Der Auwera P, Scorneaux B. In vitro susceptibility of *Campylobacter jejuni* to 27 antimicrobial agents and various combinations of β-lactams with clavulanic acid or sulbactam. Antimicrob Agents Chemother 1985;28:37–40.

744. Van Der Auwera P, Matsumoto T, Husson M. Intraphagocytic penetration of antibiotics. J Antimicrob Chemother 1988;22:185–192.

745. Van Der Meulen J, Mock B, Fekete E, Serojini PA. Limited therapeutic action of rifampicin/isoniazid against *Leishmania aethiopica* [Letter]. Lancet 1981;2:197–198.

746. Van Dyke JJ, Lake KB. Chemotherapy for aquarium granuloma. JAMA 1975;233:1380–1381.

747. Vásquez FR. Rifampin in leishmaniasis [Letter]. Arch Dermatol 1977;113:1610–1611.

748. Vazquez GJ, Archer GL. Antibiotic therapy of experimental *Staphylococcus epidermidis* endocarditis. Antimicrob Agents Chemother 1980;17:280–285.

749. Vazquez JA, Sobel JD. A case of disseminated *Mycobacterium marinum* infection in an immunocompetent patient. Eur J Clin Microbiol Infect Dis 1992;11:908–911.

750. Veglia KS, Marks VJ. *Fusarium* as a pathogen. A case report of *Fusarium* sepsis and review of the literature. J Am Acad Dermatol 1987;16:260–263.

751. Venkatesan K. Pharmacokinetic drug interactions with rifampicin. Clin Pharmacokinet 1992;22:47–65.

752. Venturini AP, Marchi E. In vitro and in vivo evaluation of L/105, a new topical intestinal rifamycin. Chemioterapia 1986;5:257–262.

753. Varaldo PE, Debbia E, Schito GC. In vitro activities of rifapentine and rifampin, alone and in combination with six other antibiotics, against methicillin-susceptible and methicillin-resistant staphylococci of different species. Antimicrob Agents Chemother 1985;27:615–618.

754. Verardi S, Verardi V, Fusillo M. Rifaximin effectiveness evaluation in the preparation of large intestine to surgery. Eur Rev Med Pharmacol Sci 1986;8:267–270.

755. Verardi S, Verardi V. Bile rifamixin concentration after oral administration in patients undergoing cholecystectomy. Farmaco 1990;45:131–135.

756. Verghese A, Hamati F, Berk S, Franzus, Berk S, Smith JK. Susceptibility of dygonic fermenter 2 to antimicrobial agents in vitro. Antimicrob Agents Chemother 1988;32:78–80.

757. Vestbo J, Lundgren JD, Gaub J, Ryder B, Gutschik E. Severe *Rhodococcus equi* pneumonia: case report and literature review. Eur J Clin Microbiol Infect Dis 1991;10:762–768.

758. Viglionese A, Nottebart VF, Bodman HA, Platt R. Recurrent group A streptococcal carriage in a health care worker associated with widely separated nosocomial outbreaks. Am J Med 1991;91(Suppl 3B):329S–333S.

759. Vilde JL, Dournon E, Rajagopalan P. Inhibition of *Legionella pneumophila* multiplication within human macrophages by antimicrobial agents. Antimicrob Agents Chemother 1986;30:743–748.

760. Vincent F, Ross JB, Dalton M, Wort AJ. A therapeutic trial of the use of penicillin V or erythromycin with or without rifampin in the treatment of psoriasis. J Am Acad Dermatol 1992;26:458–461.

761. Vinci M, Gatto A, Giglio A, Raciti T, D'Avola G, Di Stefano B, Salanitri G, Di Stefano B. Double-blind clinical trial on infectious diarrhoea therapy: rifaximin versus placebo. Curr Ther Res 1984;36:92–99.

762. Vischer WA, Rominger C. Rifampicin against experimental listeriosis in the mouse. Chemotherapy 1978;24:104–111.

763. von Eiff C, Herrmann M, Peters G. Antimicrobial susceptibilities of *Stomatococcus mucilaginosus* and *Micrococcus* spp. Antimicrob Agents Chemother 1995;39:268–270.

764. Walker AE, Frenk E, Smith AJ. Therapeutics XVII: "reserve" drugs in the treatment of tuberculosis. Br J Dermatol 1972;86:210–214.

765. Wallace RJ Jr, Nash DR, Tsukamura M, Blacklock ZM, Silcox VA. Human disease due to *Mycobacterium smegmatis*. J Infect Dis 1988;158:52–59.

766. Wallace RJ Jr, Nash DR, Steele LC, Steingrube V. Susceptibility testing of slowly growing mycobacteria by a microdilution MIC method with 7H9 broth. J Clin Microbiol 1986;24:976–981.

767. Wallace RJ Jr, O'Brien R, Glassroth J, Raleigh J, Dutt A. Diagnosis and treatment of disease caused by non-tuberculous mycobacteria. Am Rev Respir Dis 1990;142:940–952.

768. Wallace RJ Jr, Brown BA, Griffith DE, Girard W, Tenaka K. Reduced serum levels of clarithromycin in patients treated with multidrug regimens including rifampin or rifabutin for *Mycobacterium avium-M. intracellulare* infection. J Infect Dis 1995;171:747–750.

769. Deleted.

770. Walzer PD, Runck J, Orr S, Foy J, Steele P, White M. Clinically used antimicrobial drugs against experimental pneumocystosis, singly and in combination: analysis of drug interactions and efficacies. Antimicrob Agents Chemother 1997;41:242–250.

771. Wang A, Kay R, Poon WS, Ng HK. Successful treatment of amoebic meningoencephalitis in a Chinese living in Hong Kong. Clin Neurol Neurosurg 1993;95:249–252.

772. Warren JB, Rees HC, Cox TM. Remission of Crohn's disease with tuberculous chemotherapy [Letter]. N Engl J Med 1986;314:182.

773. Warrington RJ, Hogg GR, Paraskevas F, Tse KS. Insidious rifampin-associated renal failure with light-chain proteinuria. Arch Intern Med 1977;137:927–930.

774. Warshawsky AS, Keiller D, Gittes RF. Bilateral renal aspergillosis. J Urol 1975;113:8–11.

775. Wasteson Y, HYie S, Roberts MC. Characterization of antibiotic resistance in *Streptococcus suis*. Vet Microbiol 1994;41: 41–49.

776. Watanakunakorn C, Guerriero JC. Interaction between vancomycin and rifampin against *Staphylococcus aureus*. Antimicrob Agents Chemother 1981;19:1089–1091.

777. Wehrli W. Rifampin: mechanisms of action and resistance. Rev Infect Dis 1983;5(S3):S407–S411.

778. Weitholtz H, Zysset T, Marshall HU, Generet K, Matern S. The influence of rifampin treatment on caffeine clearance in healthy man. J Hepatol 1995;22:78–81.

779. Weitzman I, Osadczyi D, Corrado ML, Karp D. *Mycobacterium thermoresistibile:* a new pathogen for humans. J Clin Microbiol 1981;14:593–595.

780. West CML, Reeves SJ, Brough W. Additive interaction between tamoxifen and rifampicin in human biliary tract carcinoma cells. Cancer Lett 1990;55:159–163.

781. Westphal JF, Vetter D, Brogard JM. Hepatic side-effects of antibiotics. J Antimicrob Chemother 1994;33:387–401.

782. Wheat LJ, Kohler RB, Luft FC, White A. Long-term studies of the effect of rifampin on nasal carriage of coagulase-positive staphylococci. Rev Infect Dis 1983;5:S459–S462.

783. White SW, Hendricks LD, Chulay JD. Leishmaniasis: a case history and treatment failure with rifampin [Letter]. Arch Dermatol 1980;116:620–621.

784. Whitman MS, Pitsakis PG, Zausner A, Livernese LL, Osborne AJ, Johnson CC, Levison ME. Antibiotic treatment of experimental endocarditis due to vancomycin- and ampicillin-resistant *Enterococcus faecium*. Antimicrob Agents Chemother 1993;37:2069–2073.

785. Wiedemann B, Grimm H. Susceptibility to antibiotics: species incidence and trends. In: Lorian V, ed. Antibiotics in laboratory medicine. 4th ed. Baltimore: Williams & Wilkins, 1996:900–1168.

786. Williams DL, Waguespack C, Eisenach K, Crawford JT, Portaels F, Salfinger M, Nolan CM, Abe C, Sticht-Groh V, Gillis TP. Characterization of rifampin resistance in pathogenic mycobacteria. Antimicrob Agents Chemother 1994;38: 2380–2386.

787. Wilson WD, Spensley MS, Baggot JD, Hietala SK. Pharmaco-

788. Winslow DL, Damme J, Dieckman E. Delayed bactericidal activity of β-lactam antibiotics against *Listeria monocytogenes:* antagonism of chloramphenicol and rifampin. Antimicrob Agents Chemother 1983;23:555–558.

789. Wirostko E, Johnson L, Wirostko B. Crohn's disease: rifampin treatment of the ocular and gut disease. Hepatogastroenterology 1987;34:90–93.

790. Wisseman CL Jr, Waddell AD, Walsh WT. In vitro studies of the action of antibiotics on *Rickettsia prowaseki* by two basic methods of cell culture. J Infect Dis 1974;130:564–574.

791. Wolfe JM, Moore DF. Isolation of *Mycobacterium thermoresistibile* following augmentation mammaplasty. J Clin Microbiol 1992;30:1036–1038.

792. Wolinsky E, Gomez F, Zimpfer F. Sporotrichoid *Mycobacterium marinum* infection treated with rifampin-ethambutol. Am Rev Respir Dis 1972;105:964–967.

793. Wolinsky E. Mycobacterial diseases other than tuberculosis. Clin Infect Dis 1992;15:1–12.

794. Yamamoto T, Naigowit P, Dejsirilert S, Chiewsilp D, Kondo E, Yokota T, Kanai K. In vitro susceptibilities of *Pseudomonas pseudomallei* to 27 antimicrobial agents. Antimicrob Agents Chemother 1990;34:2027–2029.

795. Yamamoto Y, Saito H, Tomioka H, Sato K, Yamane T, Yamashita K, Hosoe K, Hidaka T. In vitro and in vivo activities of KRM-1648, a newly synthesized benzoxazinorifamycin, against *Mycobacterium marinum*. Zentralbl Bakteriol 1992; 277:204–209.

796. Yamane N, Jones RN. In vitro activity of 43 antimicrobial agents tested against ampicillin-resistant enterococci and gram-positive species resistant to vancomycin. Diagn Microbiol Infect Dis 1991;14:337–345.

797. Yamane N, Behiry IK, Eduardo MV. Determination of in vitro synergy when amphotericin B is combined with various antimicrobial agents against yeasts by using colorimetric microdilution checkerboard [Abstract E052]. 36th ICAAC, Annual Meeting of the American Society for Microbiology, New Orleans, Sept 15–18, 1996.

798. Yancey RJ, Sanchez MS, Ford CW. Activity of antibiotics against *Staphylococcus aureus* within polymorphonuclear neutrophils. Eur J Clin Microbiol Infect Dis 1991;10:107–113.

799. Yang SS, Herrera FM, Smith RG, Reitz MS, Lancini G, Ting RC, Gallo RC. Rifamycin antibiotics: inhibitors of Rauscher murine leukemia virus reverse transcriptase and of purified DNA polymerases from human normal and leukemic lymphoblasts. J Natl Cancer Inst 1972;49:7–25.

800. Yarrish RL, Shay W, LaBombardi VJ, Meyerson M, Miller DK, Larone D. Osteomyelitis caused by *Mycobacterium haemophilum:* successful therapy in two patients with AIDS. AIDS 1992;6:557–561.

801. Yazawa K, Mikami Y, Maeda A, Akao M, Morisaki N, Iwasaki S. Inactivation of rifampin by *Nocardia brasiliensis*. Antimicrob Agents Chemother 1993;37:1313–1317.

802. Yazawa K, Mikami Y, Maeda A, Morisaki N, Iwasaki S. Phosphorylative inactivation of rifampicin by *Nocardia otitidiscaviarum*. J Antimicrob Chemother 1994;33:1127–1135.

803. Yeaman MR, Mitscher LA, Baca OG. In vitro susceptibility of *Coxiella burnetii* to antibiotics, including several quinolones. Antimicrob Agents Chemother 1987;31:1079–1084.

804. Yeaman MR, Roman MJ, Baca OG. Antibiotic susceptibilities

of two *Coxiella burnetii* isolates implicated in distinct clinical syndromes. Antimicrob Agents Chemother 1989;33: 1052–1057.

805. Yeaman MR, Baca OG. Unexpected antibiotic susceptibility of a chronic isolate of *Coxiella burnetii*. Ann NY Acad Sci 1990; 590:297–305.

806. Yee YC, Kisslinger B, Yu VL, Jin DJ. A mechanism of rifamycin inhibition and resistance in *Pseudomonas aeruginosa*. J Antimicrob Chemother 1996;38:133–137.

807. Yoder LJ, Jacobson RR, Hastings RC. The activity of rifabutin against *Mycobacterium leprae*. Lepr Rev 1991;62:280–287.

808. Yogev R, Shulman D, Shulman ST, Glogowski WG. In vitro activity of antibiotics alone and in combination against *Actinobacillus actinomycetemcomitans*. Antimicrob Agents Chemother 1986;29:179–181.

809. Yu VL, Zuravleff JJ, Peacock JE, DeHertogh D, Tashjian L. Addition of rifampin to carboxypenicillin-aminoglycoside combination for the treatment of *Pseudomonas aeruginosa* infection: clinical experience with four patients. Antimicrob Agents Chemother 1984;26:575–577.

810. Yu VL, Wagner GE, Shadomy S. Sino-orbital aspergillosis treated with combination antifungal therapy. JAMA 1980;244:814–815.

811. Yu VL, Zuravleff JL, Bornholm J, Archer G. In-vitro synergy testing of triple antibiotic combinations against *Staphylococcus epidermidis* isolates from patients with endocarditis. J Antimicrob Chemother 1984;14:359–366.

812. Yu VL, Felegie TP, Yee RB, Pasculle AW, Taylor FH. Synergistic interaction in vitro with use of three antibiotics simultaneously against *Pseudomonas maltophilia*. J Infect Dis 1980; 142:602–607.

813. Yu VL. Legionella pneumophila (Legionnaires'disease). In:

Mandell GL, Bennett JE, Dolin R, eds. Principles and practice of infectious diseases. 4th ed. New York: Churchill Livingstone, 1995:2087–2097.

814. Zargar SA, Thapa BR, Sahni A, Mehta S. Rifampicin-induced upper gastrointestinal bleeding. Postgrad Med J 1990;66: 310–311.

815. Zak O, Scheld WM, Sande MA. Rifampin in experimental endocarditis due to *Staphylococcus aureus* in rabbits. Rev Infect Dis 1983;5:S481–S490.

816. Zaugg M, Salfinger M, Opravil M, Luthy R. Extrapulmonary and disseminated infections due to *Mycobacterium malmoense:* case report and review. Clin Infect Dis 1993;16:540–549.

817. Zhang YX, Neu HC. Fleroxacin combined with rifampin. Diagn Microbiol Infect Dis 1991;14:23–27.

818. Zilly W, Breimer DD, Richter E. Induction of drug metabolism in man after rifampicin treatment measured by increased hexobarbital and tolbutamide clearance. Eur J Clin Pharmacol 1975; 9:219–227.

819. Zilly W, Breimer DD, Richter E. Pharmacokinetic interactions with rifampicin. Clin Pharmacokinet 1977;2:21–70.

820. Zubovich JJ, Votyakov VI, Mishaeva NP, Samoilova TI. Rifampicin protective action in experimental rabies infection of albino mice. Antibiot Khimioter 1989;34:123–125.

821. Zuravleff JJ, Yu VL, Yee RB. Ticarcillin-tobramycin-rifampin: in vitro synergy of the triple combination against *Pseudomonas aeruginosa*. J Lab Clin Med 1983;101:896–902.

822. Zuravleff JJ, Chervenick P, Yu VL, Muder RR, Diven WF. Addition of rifampin to ticarcillin-tobramycin combination for the treatment of *Pseudomonas aeruginosa* infections: assessment in a neutropenic mouse model. J Lab Clin Med 1984;103: 878–875.

Streptogramin

●

Michael J. Rybak and Jeffrey R. Aeschlimann

CLASS

Streptogramins are a unique class of naturally occurring antibiotics derived from Streptomyces pristinaspiralis (5). Related antibiotics that make up the streptogramin family include the mikamycins, pristinamycins, ostreomycins, and virginiamycins (39). Pristinamycin has been available for approximately 30 years in the European market as an oral antistaphylococcal antibiotic. However, because of its poor water solubility, an injectable product has not been available. This has limited overall clinical experience with the drug and restricted its use to non-life-threatening infections.

Pristinamycin is made up of two primary components: pristinamycin I_A and pristinamycin II_A. Pristinamycin I_A is a peptidic macrolactone that belongs to the group B streptogramin family and pristinamycin II_A is a polyunsaturated macrolactone that belongs to the group A streptogramin family. The molecular weights of these compounds are approximately 500 for group A streptogramins and 800 for group B streptogramin agents. These compounds are bacteriostatic individually but synergistically bactericidal in combination. Optimum synergy between the two components occurs at ratios between 1:9 and 9:1 for pristinamycin I_A and II_A, respectively (47).

Modifications to pristinamycin derivatives by introduction of an amino-containing functional group at the 5δ-position of pristinamycin I_A and at the 26-position of pristinamycin II_A yields forms of these compounds that are acid-salt soluble in water. The semisynthetic derivative RP 59500 (Synercid; Rhone-Poulenc Rorer) was selected from a group of these water-soluble pristinamycin derivatives on the basis of biologic, toxicologic, and chemical criteria, and represents the first parenteral formulation of these antibiotics. RP 59500 (Fig. 1) consists of quinupristin (RP 57669, a pristinamycin I_A)

and dalfopristin (RP 54476, a pristinamycin II_A) in a 30:70 ratio (w/w) (8) . An oral pristinamycin derivative combination is also under development in the United States (RP 106972) and consists of pristinamycin I (RP 112808) and pristinamycin II (RP 106950) in a 45:50 ratio (w/w) (68).

MECHANISM OF ACTION

Group A and B streptogramin compounds sequentially bind to different sites on the 50S subunit of bacterial ribosomes, effectively inhibiting translation of messenger RNA at the elongation step (6). Group A streptogramins such as dalfopristin bind tightly to proteins of the 50S subunit region, blocking substrate attachment to the donor and acceptor sites of the peptidyltransferase center (74). This binding also effects a ribosomal conformational change that increases the binding affinity constant of group B streptogramins such as quinupristin. As a consequence, a stable group A and B streptogramin–ribosomal ternary complex is formed that constricts the protein exit channel, effectively preventing extrusion of newly synthesized proteins. The substantial inhibition of ribosomal function ultimately results in bacterial cell death (6).

ANTIMICROBIAL ACTIVITY

Streptogramins are active against a variety of Gram-positive and Gram-negative pathogens. The combination streptogramin product quinupristin/dalfopristin has activity against methicillin-susceptible and -resistant *Staphylococcus*

aureus, coagulase-negative staphylococci, streptococci (including penicillin- and macrolide-resistant strains of *S. pneumoniae*) and vancomycin-sensitive and -resistant enterococci. Quinupristin/ dalfopristin also has activity against a variety of Gram-negative and intracellular pathogens commonly associated with upper respiratory infections including *Neisseria meningitidis, Haemophilus influenzae, Moraxella catarrhalis, Legionella* spp., *Mycoplasma pneumoniae* and *Chlamydia* spp. In addition, quinupristin/dalfopristin displays excellent in vitro activity against a variety of Gram-positive and Gram-negative anaerobic organisms from the *Bacteroides, Prevotella, Fusobacterium, Clostridium, Actinomyces, Peptostreptococcus,* and *Lactobacillus* genera. The results of various in vitro susceptibility studies are summarized in Table 1.

Since there are more limited antimicrobial choices for methicillin-resistant staphylococci, penicillin- and macrolide-resistant *S. pneumomiae,* and vancomycin-resistant enterococci, streptogramins such as quinupristin/dalfopristin will probably have their greatest use against these problematic pathogens. In general, quinupristin/dalfopristin MICs against *S. aureus* are comparable to those of vancomycin. Consistent inhibitory activity is maintained against *S. aureus* strains that are both inducibly and constitutively resistant to erythromycin (MIC_{90} range, 0.25–2.0 μg/mL). Against streptococci, including *S. pneumoniae,* quinupristin/dalfopristin has an MIC profile comparable to that of such macrolide compounds as azithromycin

---

TABLE 1 • In Vitro Activities of Quinupristin/Dalfopristin

Organism	MIC_{90}[a] (μg/mL)	Range (μg/mL)
Staphylococcus aureus		
Methicillin-sensitive	0.6	0.03–16.0
Methicillin-resistant	0.7	0.03–4.0
Coagulase-negative Staphylococci including MS[b] and MR	0.5	0.03–4.0
Streptococcus pneumoniae including PCN[c] and eryth resistant	0.8	0.125–4.0
Streptococci including viridans streptococci, Streptococcus pyogenes, Streptococcus agalactiae	0.6	0.03–4.0
Enterococcus faecium includes ampicillin- and vancomycin-resistant strains	3.2	0.25–8.0
Enterococcus faecalis includes ampicillin- and vancomycin-resistant strains	8.3	0.25–32.0
Neisseria spp.	0.3	0.015–8.0
Moraxella catarrhalis	0.5	0.015->16.0
Haemophilus influenzae	6.3	1.0–8.0
Legionella spp.	0.2	0.008–2.0
Listeria monocytogenes	1.6	0.06–16.0
Bacteroides fragilis	5.6	2.0–8.0
Clostridium spp.	0.25	≤0.012–0.25

[a] MIC_{90}, minimum inhibitory concentration for 90% of the strains. When applicable, this value represents a geometric mean MIC_{90} calculated from the various references listed in this review, if a specific MIC_{90} value was reported (20, 31, 39, 64, 65, 72, 75).

[b] MR, methicillin resistant; MS, methicillin susceptible.

[c] PCN, penicillin; eryth, erythromycin.

and clarithromycin (MIC_{90} range, 0.015–2.0 μg/mL) and retains activity against erythromycin-resistant strains. Quinupristin/dalfopristin has susceptibility patterns similar to that of vancomycin against *Enterococcus faecium,* but has the advantage of also inhibiting strains that are vancomycin resistant at achievable serum concentrations. However, it is considerably less active against most strains of *Enterococcus faecalis.*

The minimum bactericidal concentration (MBC) of quinupristin/dalfopristin is within a 1- to 4-fold dilution of the MIC against most Gram-positive pathogens. Some strains of *S. aureus* with constitutive macrolide-lincosamide-group B streptogramin resistance (MLS_B resistance) may have MBCs reported as high as 8 μg/mL or above. The clinical significance of this finding is unknown (47). Like other classes of compounds such as the β-lactams and glycopeptides, quinupristin/dalfopristin is not bactericidal against enterococci (18, 36, 44, 66).

The oral pristinamycin combination product (RP 106972) has a spectrum of activity similar to that of quinupristin/dalfopristin (43). Limited data suggest that adequate concentrations are achieved in serum; the drug was effective in a mouse model of *S. pneumoniae* infection (10). Serum concentrations achieved after oral administration in humans suggest that the drug may be useful for treatment of community-acquired respiratory, cutaneous, and genital infections (68).

The effect of combining quinupristin/dalfopristin with other antimicrobials has been evaluated against a variety of pathogens. Quinupristin/dalfopristin had no effect on the activity of cefotaxime, ciprofloxacin, or gentamicin against Gram-negative pathogens such as *Escherichia coli, Klebsiella pneumoniae, Enterobacter cloacae, Serratia marcescens,* and *Pseudomonas aeruginosa.* Quinupristin/dalfopristin had a minor effect on the MICs of ciprofloxacin or gentamicin against *Bacteroides* spp. but did not affect the activity of these agents against staphylococci (61). Synergy and/or additive effects have been reported with the combination of quinupristin/dalfopristin and vancomycin, clinafloxacin, tetracycline, doxycycline, or LY333328 (an investigational glycopeptide) against vancomycin-sensitive and -resistant *E. faecium* and methicillin-sensitive and -resistant *S. aureus* (41, 42, 52, 55, 66, 76, 77). However, antagonism was reported when quinupristin/dalfopristin was combined with gentamicin or oxacillin against *S. aureus* or with ampicillin against *E. faecalis* (29).

PHARMACODYNAMICS

Quinupristin/dalfopristin has demonstrated consistent bactericidal activity, predominantly independent of concentration once above four times the MIC for *S. aureus, Staphylococcus epidermidis, Streptococcus pyogenes,* and *S. pneumoniae* (34, 38, 41). The activity of quinupristin/dalfopristin is not affected by inoculum size or changes in pH (41, 61). However, Boswell et al. (13) reported that the combination of high inoculum and stationary growth phase reduced the bactericidal activity of quinupristin/dalfopristin against two strains of *S. aureus.* Human serum slightly diminished the activity of quinupristin/dalfopristin against *S. aureus, S. pyogenes, S. pneumoniae,* and *E. faecium* (37, 61). In time-kill studies, quinupristin/dalfopristin

is rapidly bactericidal against most strains of *S. pneumoniae, S. aureus,* and *S. epidermidis,* including penicillin- and methicillin-resistant isolates. In general, the bactericidal action of quinupristin/dalfopristin against these strains is equal to, or more effective than, that of oxacillin or vancomycin (38, 41, 42).

Quinupristin/dalfopristin shows bactericidal activity against *S. aureus* with both constitutive and inducible MLS_B resistance. However, recent investigations indicate that both the in vitro and in vivo bactericidal activity can be modified by expression of constitutive MLS_B resistance (23, 26, 70). Fantin et al. (26) examined the effects of quinupristin/dalfopristin on inducibly and constitutively MLS_B-resistant strains of *S. aureus* using in vitro time-kill studies and a rabbit endocarditis model. Of the 19 *S. aureus* strains examined by time-kill studies, quinupristin/dalfopristin was bactericidal against 6 of 6 erythromycin-susceptible strains but only 7 of 13 constitutive MLS_B-resistant strains. The observed differences in killing activity appeared to correlate with higher MBC:MIC ratios for the constitutive MLS_B-resistant organisms. In the animal endocarditis model experiments, quinupristin/dalfopristin was as effective as vancomycin against erythromycin-susceptible and inducible MLS_B-resistant strains. In contrast, quinupristin/dalfopristin was significantly less effective than vancomycin against the strains that expressed constitutive MLS_B resistance, which also confers resistance to quinupristin. Stepwise multilinear regression analysis of pharmacokinetic and pharmacodynamic parameters indicated that the $AUC_{quinupristin/dalfopristin}/MBC_{quinupristin/dalfopristin}$ was a significant ($P = .02$) predictor of in vivo outcome, but the correlation was poor ($r = 0.37$). The parameter $AUC_{quinupristin/dalfopristin}/MIC_{quinupristin}$ correlated much more strongly with in vivo efficacy ($r = 0.55$, $P = .0001$), emphasizing the therapeutic importance of elevated group B streptogramin MICs in constitutive MLS_B-resistant organisms. The investigators further noted that no parameter involving in vitro susceptibility of the combined product quinupristin/dalfopristin is likely to predict in vivo outcome accurately.

In an *S. aureus* rat endocarditis model that simulated human quinupristin/dalfopristin pharmacokinetics and dosage regimens of 7 mg/kg every 12 h, Entenza et al. (23) found quinupristin/dalfopristin to be as effective as vancomycin against erythromycin-susceptible strains of *S. aureus* but inferior to vancomycin against constitutive MLS_B-resistant organisms (quinupristin MICs > 64 μg/mL). Vegetation bacterial titer increased despite quinupristin/dalfopristin therapy in 18 of 21 (86%) rats infected with constitutive MLS_B-resistant *S. aureus.* Pharmacokinetic evaluations of serum concentrations indicated that the concentrations of quinupristin and dalfopristin fluctuated disproportionately; dalfopristin serum concentrations became unmeasurable 2 h after a dose, while quinupristin serum concentrations were detectable up to 6 h after the dose. Thus, synergism between the group A and group B streptogramin was absent for much of the 12-h dosage interval. When the experiments were repeated with artificially sustained dalfopristin serum concentrations via administration of a second bolus of the drug or by continuous infusion over 6 or 12 h, efficacy against the constitutively resistant strains improved and was similar to that achieved with vancomycin. The authors concluded that maintaining adequate dalfopristin concentrations was critical for efficacy against these strains and that administration of quinupristin/dalfopristin three times daily might therefore be more efficacious. Furthermore, like Fantin (26), these authors concluded that quinupristin/dalfopristin's total susceptibility pattern was not sufficient to predict in vivo efficacy (23).

In a recent investigation, Rybak et al. (70) examined the activity of quinupristin/dalfopristin against an erythromycin- and methicillin-susceptible strain of *S. aureus* and an MLS$_B$-resistant strain of methicillin-resistant *S. aureus* at high inocula in simulated endocardial vegetations. The experiments were performed over 72 h, using an in vitro infection model that can simulate human drug pharmacokinetics. Quinupristin/dalfopristin was administered at doses of 7.5 mg/kg every 6, 8, and 12 h and as a continuous infusion. Quinupristin/dalfopristin had bactericidal activity against both strains, compared with controls. Against the erythromycin-susceptible isolate, quinupristin/dalfopristin reduced organism density by more than three $\log_{10}$s over 72 h. No difference in killing for this isolate was detected between any of the dosing regimens, despite differences in the AUC$_{24}$/MIC and or T > MIC. However, against the MLS$_B$-resistant strain, quinupristin/dalfopristin's activity was significantly lower ($P \leq$ .01) than against the erythromycin-sensitive isolate. A relationship between the dosing interval and its corresponding AUC$_{24}$ with reduction in bacterial density favored the more frequent dosing intervals over dosing every 12 h. As in other studies, bactericidal activity did not correlate with quinupristin/dalfopristin's total MIC or MBC values (70).

Pharmacodynamic parameters that predict efficacy against vancomycin-resistant *E. faecium* have not been as well characterized. However, Aeschlimann et al. (1) characterized the activity of quinupristin/dalfopristin against 23 strains of vancomycin-resistant *E. faecium* via time-kill curve analysis. Quinupristin/dalfopristin activity was correlated with either the quinupristin MIC (R = 0.74, P = .008) or the quinupristin/dalfopristin MBC (R = 0.98, P < .0001). In a rabbit endocarditis model, Fantin et al. (28) reported that quinupristin/dalfopristin activity was lower than that of amoxicillin and was significantly lower for two strains of *E. faecium* with inducible MLS$_B$ resistance than for a strain that was susceptible to MLS$_B$ antibiotics. Interestingly, combination of quinupristin/dalfopristin with amoxicillin yielded better results than amoxicillin alone. The authors emphasized the importance of adequate dalfopristin concentrations at the site of infection to maintain synergistic activity against strains expressing MLS$_B$ resistance.

Quinupristin/dalfopristin has an in vitro postantibiotic effect (PAE) of approximately 2 to 4 h (53, 62, 70). Using more sensitive methods such as examination of cellular structure or cell diameters after exposure to quinupristin/dalfopristin, Lorian et al. (54) reported PAEs as long as 8 h. The PAE of quinupristin/dalfopristin appears to depend on both concentration and duration of exposure. At 1, 2, and 4 times the MIC, the PAE against four strains of *S. aureus* increased from 15 min to 1.3 h. The PAE increased to five h when the organisms were exposed for a minimum of 80 min at four times the MIC (62). Brumfitt et al. (14) reported an average PAE of 2.4 h for quinupristin/dalfopristin against erythromycin-sensitive, -inducible, and -constitutive MLS$_B$-resistant strains of *S. aureus* and resistant enterococci. The PAE was concentration dependent, and its duration could be extended to 4.4 h at three times the MIC and to 5.5 h at 10 times the MIC. This appears to be consistent with data reported by other investigators (52, 68). Data from Aeschlimann et al. (1) indicated that the PAE against vancomycin-resistant *E. faecium* (VREF) ranges from 0.15 to 3.2 h and may depend on the organism's MBC.

There is some evidence that the PAE for quinupristin/dalfopristin is prolonged in clinical settings. In a murine infection model, the in vivo PAE was reported to be as long as 10 h for *S. aureus* and 9.1 h for *S. pneumoniae* (19). Boswell et al. (12) reported that the PAE of quinupristin/dalfopristin against three clinical strains of *S.aureus* was 1.9 h when the test was performed in broth media but increased to 2.9 h in the presence of human serum. The PAE is an important contributing factor to the overall activity of quinupristin/dalfopristin, since quinupristin/dalfopristin maintains activity at a dosing interval of every 8 to 12 h, even though drug concentrations may fall below the MIC during this time (23, 70).

In summary, the quinupristin MIC may be the most important microbiologic parameter to consider when evaluating the potential for combined streptogramin activity in vivo, as this value reveals the presence or absence of constitutive MLS$_B$-resistant organisms. In situations of constitutive MLS$_B$ resistance, more-frequent dosing of quinupristin/dalfopristin or continuous infusion may become therapeutic options, based on promising results from both in vivo (23, 25–27, 78) and in vitro (70) infection models. Additionally, combination therapy (which has always been necessary in serious enterococcal infections) can also be considered on the basis of initial in vitro studies.

MECHANISMS OF STREPTOGRAMIN RESISTANCE

Intrinsic resistance to streptogramin antibiotics in Gram-negative bacilli such as *Pseudomonas* and *Enterobacteriaceae* is likely related to the impermeability of these organism's outer cellular membrane to the large hydrophobic streptogramin molecules, as macrolides such as erythromycin can bind to *E. coli* ribosomes in cellular systems devoid of cell walls (45, 46).

Since MLS antibiotics share a similar site of action (the 50S ribosomal subunit), the potential exists for antibiotic cross-resistance. The most common type of resistance to streptogramin antibiotics is associated with the *erm* (erythromycin resistance methylase) gene family and is termed MLS$_B$ (47). These genes encode for an enzyme that N6-dimethylates an adenine residue on 23S rRNA, decreasing binding of antibiotics such as erythromycin, clindamycin, and group B streptogramins. MLS$_B$ resistance in Gram-positive organisms such as staphylococci can be either constitutive or inducible. Organisms that express inducible MLS$_B$ resistance usually remain sensitive to group B streptogramins, while expression of constitutive MLS$_B$ resistance causes resistance to group B streptogramins, as well as to all other macrolides and lincosamides (47). Activity of group A streptogramins is not altered by the ribosomal changes in constitutive MLS$_B$-resistant organisms, and synergistic activity between the two combined streptogramin components is retained. Leclercq et al. (47) reported that the modal MIC for quinupristin exceeded 128 μg/mL for constitutive MLS$_B$-resistant strains of *S. aureus*. When quinupristin was combined with dalfopristin (which had a modal MIC of 4 μg/mL alone) to form quinupristin/dalfopristin, the modal MIC was reduced to 0.5 μg/mL.

The clinical relevance of inducible or constitutive MLS$_B$ resistance is currently controversial. Based on available in vitro susceptibility data, the presence of either type of MLS$_B$ resistance appears to be of minimal importance, since all currently available streptogramin antibiotics contain both group A and group B streptogramin components. Although quinupristin alone can select for constitutive MLS$_B$-resistant mutants of *S. aureus* in vitro, its combination with dalfopristin eliminates this selection potential (47). As discussed above in Pharmacodynamics, both in vitro and in vivo bactericidal activity of the streptogramins appears to be significantly affected by the presence of constitutive MLS$_B$ resistance.

Other types of resistance to streptogramins have also been identified and characterized (46, 47). Enzymatic modification of both group A and group B streptogramins (causing resistance to the combination) was first described in *S. aureus* in 1975 (48, 49). Resistant strains contained a plasmid with the genes *saa* (streptogramin A acetyltransferase) and *sbh* (streptogramin B hydrolase). Other genes such as *vat* or *vatB* (in staphylococci) and *sat* (in enterococci) encode for acetyltransferases that inactivate group A streptogramins (3). Additionally, a chromosomal resistance determinant termed *lsa* that causes resistance to group A streptogramins and lincosamides has been discovered in *S. aureus;* the mechanism of this resistance remains to be determined (22). Combined streptogramin antibiotic activity is usually retained when either group A or group B streptogramin inactivating enzymes are present. Resistance to combined streptogramin antibiotics has been observed only with resistance to the group A streptogramin present (51). The current importance of inactivating enzymes in clinical isolates is minimal, as less than 5% of isolates from a French hospital modified streptogramin antibiotics (21), and 1% or less of isolates in most French hospitals are reported to be resistant to pristinamycin (51).

Active efflux of group B streptogramins has been described in strains of *S. epidermidis* (46) and appears to be due to the *msrA* (macrolide streptogramin resistance) gene, which encodes for a membrane-bound ATP-binding protein. This efflux mechanism also appears to be induced by erythromycin (69). The staphylococcal plasmid gene *vga* also results in production of an efflux protein, but it appears to be specific for group A streptogramin and related compounds (4). The clinical significance of these efflux mechanisms is unknown, since isolates that display these resistance patterns are currently rare.

EPIDEMIOLOGY OF MLS$_B$ AND STREPTOGRAMIN RESISTANCE

MLS$_B$ resistance was first described in staphylococci in France only a few years after the introduction of erythromycin into clinical practice (15, 40). Since these initial reports, MLS$_B$ resistance has spread throughout the world and has been described in numerous aerobic and anaerobic Gram-positive and Gram-negative organisms (Table 2). Epidemiologic studies have provided estimates of the prevalence of MLS$_B$ resistance in clinical isolates of bacteria that commonly cause infections. Most investigations have reported that 15 to 45% of clinical isolates of staphylococci display either inducible or constitutive MLS$_B$ resistance (21, 71). MLS$_B$ resistance may be as high as 90% in strains of methicillin-resistant *S. aureus* isolated in some countries (57).

Unfortunately, a number recent reports describe development of streptogramin resistance during compassionate therapy for VREF-infected patients with quinupristin/dalfopristin (16, 67, 80). A 54-year-old female with VREF intraabdominal abscess (unknown MLS$_B$ resistance profile) was treated with a prolonged course of quinupristin/dalfopristin (>4 weeks). Initial isolates displayed MICs in the range of 0.4 to 0.8 μg/mL, but over a 17-day period, isolate MIC values increased to 1.6 μg/mL and finally to 6.25 μg/mL. All isolates were analyzed microbiologically and appeared to be the same strain (67). Chow et al. (16) described an HIV-infected patient with VREF (constitutive MLS$_B$ resistance) bacteremia that was treated with quinupristin/dalfopristin (7.5 mg/kg intravenously every 8 h). Blood cultures from day 3 of therapy were negative, and the patient received 10 days of therapy. Seven days after the drug was stopped, VREF was again isolated from blood cultures. The MIC of quinupristin/dalfopristin had increased from 0.25 μg/mL to 2.0 μg/mL; DNA analysis indicated that both isolates were from the same clone. Finally, Wood et al. (80) reported that resistance to RP 59500 was observed in 3 of 24 patients treated for VREF infections; MICs in the resistant organisms were as high as 8.0 μg/mL. Pulsed-field gel electrophoresis analysis indicated that resistance developed either by selection of resistant subpopulations or by development of mutant strains.

In summary, administration of quinupristin/dalfopristin twice or thrice daily at the currently investigated 7.5-mg/kg dose could result in development or emergence of streptogramin-resistant

---

TABLE 2 • Organisms Expressing the Macrolide-Lincosamide-Streptogramin B Resistance Phenotype

Aerobic Organisms	Anaerobic Organisms
Gram positive	Gram positive
Staphylococcus spp.	*Clostridium* spp.
Streptococcus spp.	*Lactobacillus* spp.
Enterococcus spp.	*Propionibacterium* spp.
Corynebacterium diphtheriae	
Bacillus spp.	
Gram negative	Gram negative
Enterobacteriaceae	*Bacteroides* spp.
Campylobacter spp.	
	Other Organisms
	Mycoplasma pneumoniae

Data from Leclercq R, Courvalin P. Intrinsic and unusual resistance to macrolide, lincosamide, and streptogramin antibiotics in bacteria. Antimicrob Agents Chemother 1991;35:1273–1276.

organisms, potentially causing treatment failures in patients with serious infections caused by constitutive MLS_B-resistant organisms. As discussed in the Pharmacodynamics section, dosage regimen modification (continuous infusion of quinupristin/dalfopristin or dalfopristin) is a potential means of preventing or overcoming resistance to streptogramins during therapy. Combination therapy also appears to be effective in preventing/overcoming streptogramin resistance. The combination of quinupristin/dalfopristin and vancomycin prevented emergence of Q/D-resistant strains of *S. aureus* (MSSA and MRSA) that occurred when the drug was administered as monotherapy in an in vitro infection model with simulated endocardial vegetations (41). Thal et al. (73) evaluated the effect of various antibiotic combinations with quinupristin/dalfopristin on in vitro development of resistance in *E. faecium*. When *E. faecium* was plated onto agar containing 4 times the MIC of RP 59500, resistant mutants were isolated after 48 h of incubation. When the bacteria were plated onto agar containing RP 59500 in combination with either tetracycline, clinafloxacin, or trovafloxacin, no resistant mutants were detected. Unpublished data from an in vitro pharmacodynamic infection model suggests that combination of quinupristin/dalfopristin with doxycycline may prevent or diminish emergence of resistance to quinupristin/dalfopristin in VREF (2). Further study of these combinations is needed to evaluate optimal strategies for the treatment of infections due to resistant Gram-positive organisms. One hopes that these strategies can further improve streptogramin efficacy and prevent or lessen development of streptogramin resistance in the clinical setting.

PHARMACOKINETICS

Information is limited on the pharmacokinetics of streptogramin antibiotics because of assay difficulties related to *(a)* poor water solubility, *(b)* rapid degradation at physiologic pH (especially in whole blood samples), *(c)* cellular binding and/or degradation, and *(d)* different elimination rates for the individual streptogramin components (17, 44, 63). Additionally, different streptogramin concentration results are obtained depending on the assay technique used (microbiologic assay versus HPLC). Early animal studies indicated that streptogramins distributed evenly throughout the blood and organs. Minimal penetration through the hematoencephalic barrier and high bone concentrations were also noted in these experiments (7, 17, 59). Protein-binding experiments in mice indicated reversible binding of the group A streptogramin (80%) and group B streptogramin (40%) components to serum proteins (17). Excretion of radiolabeled streptogramins was rapid and occurred through the urine, bile, and feces.

The pharmacokinetic behavior of quinupristin/dalfopristin was evaluated in 26 healthy male volunteers in a double-blind, placebo-controlled, phase I trial (24). Doses were administered over 1 h and ranged from 1.4 to 29.4 mg/kg. The peak concentrations obtained at the end of the infusion ranged from 0.95 ± 0.22 mg/L (for the 1.4-mg/kg dose) to 24.20 ± 8.82 mg/L (for the 29.4-mg/kg dose). The mean serum $t_{1/2}$ of quinupristin/dalfopristin (measured by bioassay) ranged from 1.27 ± 0.32 h (16.8 mg/kg dose) to 1.53 ± 0.55 h (22.4-mg/kg dose). The $t_{1/2}$ of quinupristin ranged from only 0.56 to 0.61 h;

the $t_{1/2}$ of dalfopristin was not measurable because of its rapid transformation into RP 12536, its active metabolite. The $t_{1/2}$ of RP 12536 ranged from 0.75 to 0.95 h.

Single-dose pharmacokinetics of quinupristin/dalfopristin (5, 10, or 15 mg/kg) were evaluated in 18 healthy male volunteers, using a crossover design (60). The mean Cp_{max} of quinupristin and dalfopristin for the three dosage regimens were 1.3, 2.4, 3.31 μg/mL and 5.1, 7.1, 8.5 μg/mL, respectively. The $t_{1/2}$s for quinupristin and dalfopristin were 0.6 to 1 h and 0.3 to 0.4 h. The apparent volume of distribution (Vd) was 1 L/kg for quinupristin and 0.6 L/kg for dalfopristin, suggesting extensive distribution throughout the body. Plasma concentrations of the active metabolite of dalfopristin were 20 to 45% of those of the parent drug; this percentage increased as a function of dose administered.

Pharmacokinetics of a single 12-mg/kg dose of RP 59500 and its penetration into suction blister fluid were studied in six healthy male volunteers (9). The mean Cp_{max} was 8.65 μg/mL, the plasma $t_{1/2}$ was 1.48 h, and the $AUC_{0-6 h}$ was 11.11 mg·h/L. The mean blister fluid C_{max} was 2.41 μg/mL, and the $AUC_{0-6 h}$ was 9.19 mg·h/L. Percentage penetration (measured as the ratio of suction blister fluid AUC:serum AUC) was 82.49%. These data indicate that the drug achieves adequate concentrations in tissues commonly infected by streptogramin-sensitive organisms.

Disposition of radiolabeled quinupristin/dalfopristin was studied in six healthy male volunteers (33). An average 75% of quinupristin and 77% of dalfopristin radioactivity was recovered in the feces, while only 15 and 19% of radioactivity was recovered in urine over the first 3 h of administration, respectively. Dalfopristin appeared to be extensively metabolized, as only small amounts of the parent drug were recovered in the feces. Dalfopristin was metabolized to two active compounds (RP 12536 and RP 100391); the contribution of these metabolites to overall in vivo activity is currently not clear. Protein binding of quinupristin and dalfopristin in humans was estimated to be 23 to 32% and 50 to 56%, respectively (low/moderate protein binding).

The pharmacokinetics and disposition of RPR 106972, a new oral streptogramin, were evaluated in animals and in healthy young volunteers (68). Maximal plasma concentrations were observed 0.75 to 2 h after administration of a single dose of the drug to healthy volunteers. No changes in pharmacokinetic parameters were noted when doses were given over 10 days. The presence of food did not appear to affect absorption of the drug significantly. The achievable serum concentrations after oral or intravenous administration and the consistent microbiologic activity of pristinamycin/streptogramin compounds over a wide range of concentration ratios suggest that these agents should maintain their activity against most organisms, despite differences in distribution, metabolism, and elimination of the two components.

DOSAGE REGIMENS

Since the activities of the metabolites of quinupristin/dalfopristin appear to contribute to the overall activity of the drug and because the drug has a significant PAE, a twice- to thrice-daily regimen has been recommended (24). The current dose of 7.5 mg/kg given every 8 to 12 h (used in ongoing clinical trials) provides peak serum drug concentrations substantially above the MIC and MBC for most staphylococci, streptococci, and *E. faecium.* Although adequate data are not yet available, dosage adjustment should not be necessary in the presence of renal dysfunction, as renal clearance of the drug appeared to be minimal in the animal and human studies discussed above. Dosage reduction is likely in the setting of severe hepatic dysfunction, as this appears to be the primary route of elimination of streptogramin antibiotics in animals and humans. Specific guidelines are not yet available. Doses should probably be based on actual patient body weight, as drug distribution is quite extensive. Adjustment of dosage for low serum albumin or for coadministration with highly protein-bound drugs is probably not necessary, since neither component is highly protein bound.

ADVERSE EFFECTS

During the quinupristin/dalfopristin phase I pharmacokinetic study described above (24), mild-to-moderate erythema, itching, pain, and/or burning at the infusion site was observed during 19 of 53 (36%) infusions of active drug. Three patients who received quinupristin/dalfopristin reported diarrhea compared with one who received placebo. There were no significant changes in any hematologic or biochemical indices.

Analysis of preliminary data from 234 patients treated with quinupristin/dalfopristin in a compassionate use protocol indicated that therapy was well tolerated; arthralgias/myalgias, venous intolerance, and liver function abnormalities resulted in drug discontinuation in 17 (7.3%) patients (30). Blumberg et al. (11) reported that 11 of 19 (58%) patients treated with quinupristin/dalfopristin for VREF infections experienced adverse events "possibly related" to therapy. Arthralgias, myalgias, and/or weakness occurred in 6 (32%) patients; in all of them, symptoms resolved after therapy was stopped.

The adverse effects of RPR 106792 have been evaluated in single- and multiple-dose phase I studies (68). Overall, the drug was well tolerated, with mild diarrhea, abdominal pain, flatulence, and headache most commonly reported. One patient who received multiple doses had a significant elevation in AST that resolved upon discontinuation of the drug. The safety of streptogramins in pregnancy has not been fully evaluated; use of these agents probably should be avoided in pregnant patients until additional data are available.

DRUG INTERACTIONS

Limited data are available describing the drug interaction potential of streptogramins. Liver weight and microsomal protein content in rats administered the streptogramins RP54476, RP57669, RP59500, or RP7293 did not differ statistically from those of control animals (58). P-450 metabolite complex was not detectable, and P-450 enzyme activities were not modified by the streptogramins in this study. A case report in the literature describing the effect of pristinamycin on cyclosporine concentrations in bone marrow transplantation patients (35) suggests possible CYP3A4 isoenzyme inhibition,

but data from ongoing drug interaction studies are needed to elucidate the effects of streptogramin antibiotics on drug-metabolizing enzymes in humans.

CLINICAL INDICATIONS

At this time, quinupristin/dalfopristin appear to be an option for infections caused by staphylococci, *E. faecium,* and streptococci, especially when these organisms are resistant to more commonly used antibiotics, or when more commonly used agents are contraindicated because of allergy (30). A number of reports have described initial experience with quinupristin/dalfopristin in compassionate usage protocols (11, 32, 50, 56, 79). Furlong and Bompart (32) described a case of *E. faecium* prosthetic valve endocarditis in a patient with chronic renal failure. The patient had failed intravenous teicoplanin therapy, remaining bacteremic for 4 months. Ten weeks of quinupristin/dalfopristin (5 mg/kg intravenously every 12 h) resulted in both microbiologic and clinical cure of the infection. Lynn et al. (56) described the treatment of three patients with CAPD-associated peritonitis due to VREF. Quinupristin/dalfopristin administered intravenously (10–20 mg/kg intravenously every 12 h) and as an intraperitoneal dwell resulted in rapid, complete response in two patients; the third patient responded after two courses of quinupristin/dalfopristin and removal of the CAPD cannula.

Linden et al. (50) described nine patients with VREF infections treated with quinupristin/dalfopristin at a dose of 7.5 mg/kg intravenously every 8 h. Each patient had fever and serious abdominal infection; five patients also had bacteremia and six were in septic shock. The duration of therapy ranged from 12 to 31 days, and each patient also underwent surgical drainage. Bacteremia cleared in four of five patients, and fever subsided in five of nine patients. VREF recovered at the primary site of infection in four patients despite therapy sustained sensitivity to quinupristin/dalfopristin. Five patients expired; in two of these patients, death was directly attributable to VREF. The investigators concluded that quinupristin/dalfopristin appeared effective in suppressing bloodstream infections and fecal carriage of VREF but that activity in areas of high inoculum or difficult penetration was marginal. This is generally true for all antibiotics, not just streptogramins.

The efficacy of quinupristin/dalfopristin was evaluated in 19 patients with VREF infections (11). Most patients had bacteremia (n = 10) or intraabdominal infection (n = 5), and nearly half of them were neutropenic leukemia patients. The median duration of therapy was 14 days; clinical cure was obtained in 11 (58%) patients, improvement in 5 (26%), and 3 patients had indeterminant responses. Microbiologic cure was documented in 7 patients and was presumptive in 10. Twelve patients became colonized with quinupristin/dalfopristin-resistant organisms (9, VR *E. faecalis;* 2, VR *E. faecium;* and 1, coagulase-negative *Staphylococcus*). Thus, while quinupristin/ dalfopristin appeared efficacious for the treatment of VREF infections, there is a potential for selection of colonizing organisms with resistance to quinupristin/dalfopristin. It is unknown whether superinfection with these organisms will become a significant problem with streptogramin therapy.

Currently, RPR 106972 is being investigated for the treatment of community-acquired lower respiratory tract infections as well as for sinusitis (68). The results from these studies will dictate the clinical utility of this oral streptogramin.

Overall, the streptogramin class of antibiotics are unique compounds that offer a broad spectrum of activity with little risk of serious side effects. The combination of the two streptogramin components is bactericidal against many different pathogens, including methicillin-resistant *S. aureus*. Widespread clinical use will further define the role of the streptogramin class, but prudent use is important to maintain the viability of these agents for the future.

REFERENCES

1. Aeschlimann JR, Rebuck J, Rybak MJ. Pharmacodynamic analysis of quinupristin/dalfopristin (Q/D) versus vancomycin-resistant *Enterococcus faecium* (VREF with differing MBCs using time-kill curve (KC) and post-antibiotic effect (PAE) methods [Abstract E-136]. 37th Interscience Conference on Antimicrobial Agents and Chemotherapy; 1997 Sept 28–Oct 1, Toronto, Ontario, Canada.

2. Aeschlimann JR. Personal communication. September 18, 1997.

3. Allignet J, El Solh N. Diversity among the gram-positive acetyltransferases inactivating streptogramin A and structurally related compounds and characterization of a new staphylococcal determinant, vatB. Antimicrob Agents Chemother 1995;39:2027–2036.

4. Allignet J, Loncle V, El Solh N. Sequence of a staphylococcal plasmid gene, vga, encoding a putative ATP-binding protein involved in resistance to virginiamycin A-like antibiotics. Gene 1992;117:45–51.

5. Archer GL, Auger P, Dorn GV, Ferraro J, Fuchs PC, Jorgensen JH, Low DE, Murray PR, Reller LB, Stratton CW, Wennersten CB, Moellering RC. RP 59500, a new streptogramin highly active against recent isolates of north American staphylococci. Diagn Microbiol Infect Dis 1993;16:223–226.

6. Aumercier M, Boulhallab S, Capmau ML, Le Goffie F. RP 59500: a proposed mechanism for its bactericidal activity. J Antimicrob Chemother 1992;30(Suppl A):9–14.

7. Aumercier M, Capmau ML, Marland M, Le Goffic F. Autoradiography of tissue distribution of the IIA constituent of the pristinamycins. J Antimicrob Chemother 1985;16(Suppl A):201–204.

8. Barriere JC, Bouanchaud DH, Paris JM, Rolin O, Harris NV, Smith C. Antimicrobial activity against *Staphylococcus aureus* of semisynthetic injectable streptogramins: RP 59500 and related compounds. J Antimicrob Chemother 1992;30(Suppl A):1–8.

9. Bernard E, Bensoussan M, Bensoussan F, Etienne S, Cazenave I, Dellamonica P. Pharmacokinetics and suction blister fluid penetration of a semisynthetic injectable streptogramin RP 59500 (RP 57669/RP 54476). Eur J Clin Microbiol Infect Dis 1994;13:768–771.

10. Berthaud N, Huet Y, Bourgues A, Bussiere M, Sautede M, Selingue M, Desnottes JF. In vivo bactericidal activity of RPR 106972, a new oral streptogramin, in *Streptococcus pneumoniae* mouse pneumonia [Abstract B042]. 36th Interscience Conference on Antimicrobial Agents and Chemotherapy; 1996 Sept. 15–18; New Orleans, LA.

11. Blumberg EA, Mandler HD, Fuchs AE. Efficacy and toxicity of quinupristin/dalfopristin for vancomycin-resistant *Enterococcus faecium* infections [Abstract LM32]. 36th Interscience Conference on Antimicrobial Agents and Chemotherapy; 1996 Sept. 15–18; New Orleans, LA.

12. Boswell FJ, Andrews JM, Wise R. The postantibiotic effect of RP 59500 (quinupristin/dalfopristin) on staphylococci in the presence of serum. 34th Interscience Conference on Antimicrobial Agents and Chemotherapy, 1994 October 17–20, Orlando, FL.

13. Boswell FJ, Sunderland J, Andrews JM, Wise R. Time-kill kinetics of quinupristin/dalfopristin on Staphylococcus aureus with and without a raised MBC evaluated by two methods. J Antimicrobial Chemother 1997;39(Suppl A):29–32.

14. Brumfitt W, Hamilton-Miller JMT, Shah S. In-vitro activity of RP 59500, a new semisynthetic streptogramin antibiotic against Gram-positive bacteria. J Antimicrob Chemother 1992;30 (Suppl A):29–37.

15. Chabbert YA. Antagonisme in vitro entre l'erythromycine et la spiramycine. Ann Inst Pasteur (Paris) 1965;90:787–790.

16. Chow JW, Donabedian S, Zervos MJ. Development of increased resistance to quinupristin/dalfopristin during therapy for enterococcus faecium bacteremia. Clin Infect Dis 1997;24:90–91.

17. Cocito C. Antibiotics of the virginiamycin family, inhibitors which contain synergistic components. Microbiol Rev 1979;43: 145–198.

18. Collins LA, Malanoski GJ, Eliopooulos GM, Wennersten CB, Ferraro J, Moellering RC. In vitro activity of RP 59500, an injectable streptogramin antibiotic, against vancomycin-resistant gram-positive organisms. Antimicrob Agents Chemother 1993; 37:598–601.

19. Craig W, Ebert S. Pharmacodynamic activities of RP 59500 in an animal infection model. 33rd Interscience Conference on Antimicrobial Agents and Chemotherapy, October 17–20, New Orleans, LA. 1993.

20. Dubois J, Joly JR. In-vitro activity of RP 59500, a new synergic antibacterial agent, against *Legionella* spp. J Antimicrob Chemother 1992;30(Suppl A):77–81.

21. Duval J. Evolution and epidemiology of MLS resistance. J Antimicrob Chemother 1985;16(Suppl A):137–149.

22. El Sohl N, Bismuth R, Allignet J, Fouace JM. Resistance a la pristinamycine (ou virginiamycine) des souches de *Staphylococcus aureus*. Pathol Biol 1984;32:362–368.

23. Entenza JM, Drugeon H, Glauser MP, Moreillon P. Treatment of experimental endocarditis due to erythromycin-susceptible or -resistant methicillin-resistant *Staphylococcus aureus* with RP 59500. Antimicrob Agents Chemother 1995;39(7):1419–1424.

24. Etienne SD, Montay G, Le Liboux A, Frydman A, Garaud JJ. A phase I, double-blind, placebo-controlled study of the tolerance and pharmacokinetic behaviour of RP 59500. J Antimicrob Chemother 1992;30(Suppl A):123–131.

25. Fantin B, Leclercq R, Garry L, Carbon C. Activity of RP 59500 (quinupristin/dalfopristin) against Enterococcus faecium in vitro and in experimental endocarditis [Abstract B6]. 36th Interscience Conference on Antimicrobial Agents and Chemotherapy; 1996 Sept. 15–18; New Orleans, LA.

26. Fantin B, Leclercq R, Merle Y, et al. Critical influence of resistance to streptogramin B-type antibiotics on activity of RP 59500 (quinupristin-dalfopristin) in experimental endocarditis due to *Staphylococcus aureus*. Antimicrob Agents Chemother 1995;39:400–405.

27. Fantin B, Leclercq R, Ottaviani M, Vallois JM, Maziere B, Duval J, Pocidalo JJ, Carbon C. In vivo activities and penetration of the two components of the streptogramin RP 59500 in cardiac vegetations of experimental endocarditis. Antimicrob Agents Chemother 1994:38;432–437.

28. Fantin B, LeClercq R, Garry L, Carbon C. Influence of inducible cross-resistance to macrolides, lincosamides, and streptogramin

B-type antibiotics in *Enterococcus faecium* on activity of quin-upristin-dalfopristin in vitro and in rabbits with experimental endocarditis. Antimicrob Agents Chemother 1997;41:931–935.

29. Fass RJ. In vitro activity of RP 59500, a semisynthetic injectable pristinamycin, against staphylococci, streptococci and enterococci. Antimicrob Agents Chemother 1991;35:553–559.

30. Finch RG, Rubinstein E. Questions and answers. Drugs 1996; 51(Suppl 1):43–45.

31. Fremaux A, Sissia G, Cohen R, Geslin P. In-vitro antibacterial activity of RP 59500, a semisynthetic streptogramin, against *Streptococcus pneumoniae*. J Antimicrob Chemother 1992;30(Suppl A):19–23.

32. Furlong WB and Bompart F. Therapy for enterococci with Van A/Van B resistance patterns using RP 59500 (quinupristin/dalfopristin) [Abstract M66]. 34th Interscience Conference on Antimicrobial Agents and Chemotherapy; 1994 Oct 4–7; Orlando, FL.

33. Gaillard C, Van Cantfort J, Montay G. Disposition of the radiolabeled streptogramin RP 59500 in healthy male volunteers [Abstract]. 32nd Interscience Conference on Antimicrobial Agents and Chemotherapy; 1992 Oct 12–15; Anaheim, CA.

34. Goto S, Miyazaki S, Kaneko V. The in-vitro activity of RP 59500 against Gram-positive cocci. J Antimicrob Chemother 1992;30(Suppl A):25–28.

35. Herbrecht R, Garcia JJ, Bergerat JP, Oberling F. Effect of pristinamycin on cyclosporin levels in bone marrow transplant recipients. Bone Marrow Transplant 1989;4:457–458.

36. Hill RLR, Smith CT, Casewell MW. Bactericidal and inhibitory activity of RP9500 (quinuprisitin/dalfopristin) and its components against vancomycin- and gentamicin-resistant *Enterococcus faecium*. 35th Interscience Conference on Antimicrobial Agents and Chemotherapy, September 17–20, San Francisco, CA. 1995.

37. Hill RLR, Smith CT, Seyed-Akhavani M, Casewell MW. Bactericidal and inhibitory activity of quinuprisitin/dalfopristin against vancomycin- and gentamicin-resistant *Enterococcus faecium*. J Antimicrobial Chemother 1997;39(Suppl A):23–28.

38. Hoban DJ, Weshnoweski B, Palatnick L, Zhanel G, Davidson RJ. In-vitro activity of streptogramin RP 59500 against staphylococci, including bactericidal kinetic studies. J Antimicrob Chemother 1992;30(Suppl A):69–75.

39. Inoue M, Okamoto R, Okubo T, Inoue K, Misuhashi S. Comparative in-vitro activity of RP 59500 against clinical bacterial isolates. J Antimicrob Chemother 1992;30(Suppl A):45–51.

40. Jones WF, Nichols RL, Finland M. Development of resistance and cross-resistance in vitro to erythromycin, carbomycin, oleandomycin, and streptogramin. Proc Soc Exp Biol Med 1966;93:388–393.

41. Kang SL, Rybak MJ. Pharmacodynamics of RP 59500 alone and in combination with vancomycin against *S. aureus* in an in vitro infected fibrin clot model. Antimicrob Agents Chemother 1995;39:1505–1511.

42. Kang SL, Rybak MJ. In vitro bactericidal activity of RP 59500 (quinupristin/dalfopristin) alone and in combinations against resistant strains of Enterococcus species and *Staphylococcus aureus*. J Antimicrob Chemother 1997;39(Suppl A):33–39.

43. King A, May J, Phillips I. In vitro activity of RP57669/RP54776 (Synercid), a parenteral streptogramin, and RPR 106972, an oral streptogramin, against resistant Gram-positive cocci [Abstract F226]. 36th Interscience Conference on Antimicrobial Agents and Chemotherapy; 1996 Sept 15–18; New Orleans, LA.

44. Koechlin C, Kempf JF, Jehl F, Monteil H. Single oral dose pharmacokinetics of the two main components of pristinamycin in humans. J Antimicrob Chemother 1990;25:651–656.

45. Leclercq R, Courvalin P. Bacterial resistance to macrolide, lincosamide, and streptogramin antibiotics by target modification. Antimicrob Agents Chemother 1991;35:1267–1272.

46. Leclercq R, Courvalin P. Intrinsic and unusual resistance to macrolide, lincosamide, and streptogramin antibiotics in bacteria. Antimicrob Agents Chemother 1991;35:1273–1276.

47. Leclercq R, Nantas L, Soussy CJ, Duval J. Activity of RP 59500, a new parenteral semisynthetic streptogramin, against staphylococci with various mechanisms of resistance to macrolide-lincosamide-streptogramin antibiotics. J Antimicrob Chemother 1992;30(Suppl A):67–75.

48. Le Goffic F, Capmau ML, Abbe J, Cerceau C, Dublanchet A, Duval J. Plasmid mediated pristinamycin resistance: PH 1A, a pristinamycin 1A hydrolase. Ann Inst Pasteur (Paris) 1977;30:471–474.

49. Le Goffic F, Capmau ML, Bonnet ML. Plasmid-mediated pristinamycin resistance: PACIIA, a new enzyme which modifies pristinamycin IIA. J Antibiot 1977;30:665–669.

50. Linden P, Pasculle AW, Riddler S. Quinupristin/dalfopristin (RP 59500) for the treatment of serious infection due to high level vancomycin resistant Enterococcus faecium (VREF) [Abstract M68]. 34th Interscience Conference on Antimicrobial Agents and Chemotherapy; 1994 Oct 4–7; Orlando, FL.

51. Loncle V, Casetta A, Buu-Hoi A, El Solh N. Analysis of pristinamycin-resistant Staphylococcus epidermidis isolates responsible for an outbreak in a Parisian hospital. Antimicrob Agents Chemother 1993;37:2159–2165.

52. Lorian V, Fernandes E. Synergistic activity of injectable streptogramin RP 59500-vancomycin combination [Abstract E150]. 35th Interscience Conference on Antimicrobial Agents and Chemotherapy; 1995 Sept 17–20; San Francisco, CA.

53. Lorian V, Esanu Y, Amaral L. Ultrastructure alterations of *Staphylococcus aureus* exposed to RP 59500. J Antimicrob Chemother 1994;33:625–628.

54. Lorian V, Amaral L, Fernandes F. RP 59500 postantibiotic effect defined by bacterial ultrastructure. Drugs Exp Clin Res 1995;21:125–128.

55. Lorian V and Fernandes F. Synergic activity of vancomycin-quinupristin/dalfopristin combination against *Enterococcus faecium*. J Antimicrobial Chemother 1997;39(Suppl A):63–66.

56. Lynn WA, Clutterbuck E, Want S, Markides V, Lacey S, Rogers TR, Cohen J. Treatment of CAPD-peritonitis due to vancomycin-resistant Enterococcus faecium with quinupristin/dalfopristin. Lancet 1994;344:1025–1026.

57. Maple PAC, Hamilton-Miller JMT, Brumfitt W. World-wide antibiotic resistance in methicillin-resistant *Staphylococcus aureus*. Lancet 1989;i:537–539.

58. Martinet M, Vedrine Y, Piguet V, Frydman A. Lack of effect of streptogramins on hepatic drug metabolism enzymes in the rat. Drug Metab Dispos 1992;20:490–495.

59. Modai J. Comparative evaluation of macrolides, lincosamides, and streptogramins in staphylococcal infections. J Antimicrob Chemother 1985;16(Suppl A):195–197.

60. Montay G, Le Liboux A, Etienne S, Panis R. RP 59500 pharmacokinetics after single dose administration in healthy volunteers [Abstract A20]. 34th Interscience Conference on Antimicrobial Agents and Chemotherapy; 1994 Oct 4–7; Orlando, FL, 1994.

61. Neu HC, Chin N, Gu J. The in-vitro activity of new streptogramins, RP 59500, RP 57669 and RP 54476, alone and in combination. J Antimicrob Chemother 1992;30(Suppl A): 83–84.

62. Nougayrede A, Berthaud N, Bouanchaud DH. Post-antibiotic effects of RP 59500 with *Staphylococcus aureus*. J Antimicrob Chemother 1992;30(Suppl A):101–106.

63. Osono T, Umezawa H. Pharmacokinetics of macrolides, lincosamides, and streptogramins. J Antimicrob Chemother 1985; 16(Suppl A):151–166.

64. Pechere JC. Streptogramins: a unique class of antibiotics. Drugs 1996;51(Suppl 1):13–19.

65. Pechere JC. In-vitro activity of RP 59500, a semisynthetic streptogramin, against staphylococci and streptococci. J Antimicrob Chemother 1992;30(Suppl A):15–18.

66. Penzak SR, Mercier RC, Rybak MJ. In vitro activity of investigational antibiotics alone and in combinations against two strains of vancomycin-resistant *Enterococcus faecium*. 36th Interscience Conference on Antimicrobial Agents and Chemotherapy, Sept 15–18, New Orleans, 1996.

67. Piper J, Steele-Moore L, Berg D. Acquired resistance to quinupristin/dalfopristin (Synercid) during successful antimicrobial therapy of vancomycin-resistant enterococcus (VRE) [Abstract A109]. 96th general meeting of the American Society for Microbiology; 1996 May 19–23; New Orleans, LA.

68. Rhone-Poulenc Rorer. RPR 106972 investigator's brochure. July 19, 1995.

69. Ross JI, Eady EA, Cove JH, Cunliffe WJ, Baumberg S, Wootton JC. Inducible erythromycin resistance in staphylococci is encoded by a member of the ATP binding transport super-gene family. Mol Microbiol 1990;4: 1207–1214.

70. Rybak MJ, Houlihan HH, Mercier RC, Kaatz GW. Pharmacodynamics of RP 59500 (quinupristin-dalfopristin) administered by intermittent versus continuous infusion against *Staphylococcus aureus*-infected fibrin-platelet clots in an in vitro infection model. Antimicrobial Agents Chemother 1997;41:1359–1363.

71. Sanchez ML, Flint KK, Jones RN. Occurrence of macrolide-lincosamide-streptogramin resistances among staphylococcal clinical isolates at a university medical center. Diagn Microbiol Infect Dis 1993:16:205–213.

72. Soussy CJ, Acar JF, Cluzel R, Courvalin P, Duval J, Fleurette J, Megraud F, Meyran M, Thabaut A. A collaborative study of the in-vitro sensitivity of RP 59500 of bacteria isolated in seven hospitals in France. J Antimicrob Chemother 1992;30(Suppl A):53–58.

73. Thal LA, Davison A, Chow J, Zervos M. In vitro evaluation of the development of Synercid resistant mutants in *Enterococcus faecium*. Abstracts of the 34th annual meeting of the Infectious Diseases Society of America; 1996 September: New Orleans, LA.

74. Vannuffel P, Cocito C. Mechanism of action of streptogramins and macrolides. Drugs 1996;51(Suppl 1):20–30.

75. Verbist L, Verhaegen J. Comparative in-vitro activity of RP 59500. J Antimicrob Chemother 1992;30(Suppl A):39–44.

76. Vouillamoz J, Entenza JM, Giddey M, et al. In vitro efficacy of Synercid (quinupristin/dalfopristin) (SYN) combined with other classes of antibiotics against methicillin-susceptible and -resistant *Staphylococcus aureus* (MSSA and MRSA) [Abstract E007]. 36th Interscience Conference on Antimicrobial Agents and Chemotherapy; 1996 Sept 15–18; New Orleans, LA.

77. Vouillamoz J, Entenza JM, Giddey M. In vitro activity of Synercid (quinupristin/dalfopristin) (SYN) combined with other classes of antibiotics against vancomycin-susceptible (VS) E. faecalis and vancomycin-susceptible or -resistant (VR) E. faecium (VSEF and VREF) [Abstract E008]. 36th Interscience Conference on Antimicrobial Agents and Chemotherapy; 1996 Sept 15–18; New Orleans, LA.

78. Vouillamoz J, Entenza JM, Glauser MP, Moreillon P. Synercid (quinupristin/dalfopristin) (SYN) treatment of experimental endocarditis (EE) due to erythromycin-susceptible (ERY-S) and constitutively-resistant (ERY-R) methicillin-susceptible *Staphylococcus aureus* (MSSA) [Abstract B8]. 36th Interscience Conference on Antimicrobial Agents and Chemotherapy; 1996 Sept 15–18; New Orleans, LA.

79. Wade J, Baillie L, Rolando N, Casewell M. Pristinamyin for Enterococcus faecium resistant to vancomycin and gentamicin. Lancet 1992:339:312–313.

80. Wood CA, Mandler HD, Fry-Arrighy BE. Resistance to quinupristin/dalfopristin encountered during treatment of infections caused by vancomycin-resistant Enterococcus faecium [Abstract LB13]. 36th Interscience Conference on Antimicrobial Agents and Chemotherapy; 1996 Sept 15–18; New Orleans, LA.

Sulfonamides

●

Daniel H. Havlichek, Jr. and Gary E. Stein

In 1932, Gerhard Domagk discovered that the dye prontosil rubrum (sulfachrysoidine) was protective in murine streptococcal infections (27). The discovery of antibacterial properties of prontosil rubrum heralded the antimicrobial era. In 1933, a boy with staphylococcal septicemia was cured with prontosil, and in 1935, it was the first antibiotic given in the United States in an unsuccessful attempt to treat a late case of *Haemophilus influenzae* meningitis.

In vivo studies found that prontosil rubrum worked by breakdown of the parent compound to an inactive dye and sulfanilamide. Multiple chemical modifications to sulfanilamide have created the class of antimicrobials known as sulfonamides. These compounds have had a long and important role in patient care; however, development of microbial resistance severely limits their current use as single agents. As part of their physiologic effects, sulfonamides were found to have the potential to cause metabolic acidosis and induce diuresis. This has led to development of other important compounds such as furosemide, tolbutamide, and acetazolamide (24).

CLASS

Sulfanilamide (*p*-aminobenzene sulfonamide) is the parent compound of the sulfonamide class (Fig. 1). It is similar in structure to *p*-aminobenzoic acid (PABA), which is a necessary for folic acid synthesis. Modifications of the sulfanilamide structure produce compounds with differing antimicrobial activity, pharmacokinetics, and safety properties. A free amino group at position 4 is associated with the greatest antibacterial activity and improved absorption from the gastrointestinal tract. The effectiveness of PABA inhibition is also influenced by substitutions on the SO_2 group of sulfanilamide.

Folic acid is necessary for one-carbon transfers for synthesis of thymidine, methionine, glycine, adenine, and guanine in both bacterial and mammalian cells. Since most bacteria cannot use exogenous folate and mammalian cells require exogenous folate, sulfonamides selectively inhibit bacterial growth by competitively inhibiting incorporation of PABA into tetrahydropteroic acid. This inhibits microbial folic acid production and ultimately decreases DNA synthesis. Some binding of sulfonamide with pteridine also occurs, and decreased intracellular pteridine concentrations have been reported. By this mechanism, sulfonamides are considered bacteriostatic.

ANTIMICROBIAL ACTIVITY

Sulfonamides can have in vitro activity against a wide range of Gram-positive and Gram-negative bacteria including *Enterobacteriaceae, Haemophilus, Neisseria, Actinomyces, No-cardia,* staphylococci, and streptococci. Since sensitivity cannot reliably be predicted, testing should be performed before initiating therapy with sulfonamides as single agents. In vitro susceptibility testing of sulfonamides is strongly influenced by extracellular folate, thymidine, and PABA in the media. Sulfonamide effects can be largely reversed by addition of thymidine, methionine, and serine. Large inocula also decrease reported MICs. The optimum pH for sensitivity testing is 7.3.

The effect of subtherapeutic sulfonamide concentrations on bacteria has been incompletely studied. Exposing *E. coli* to sulfadiazine, sulfamethoxazole, or sulfathiazole at concentrations 1/2 to 1/8 the MIC, decreases hemagglutination and adherence to human buccal epithelial cells (41). The importance of this in human disease is uncertain.

Gram-Negative Bacteria

Sulfonamide activity against the *Enterobacteriaceae* has been steadily decreasing over time. These compounds continue to remain active against many pathogenic strains of *Haemophilus* (including ampicillin-resistant isolates) and *Neisseria. Haemophilus ducreyi* is variably sensitive to sulfonamides, depending on the geographic location (18). Sulfonamides have variable activity against *Legionella,* and non-*aeruginosa* strains of *Pseudomonas.* The combination of trimethoprim with sulfamethoxazole is the agent of choice for many non-*aeruginosa* pseudomonal, *Stenotrophomonas,* and *Burkholderia* infections. Anaerobic activity of sulfonamides depends

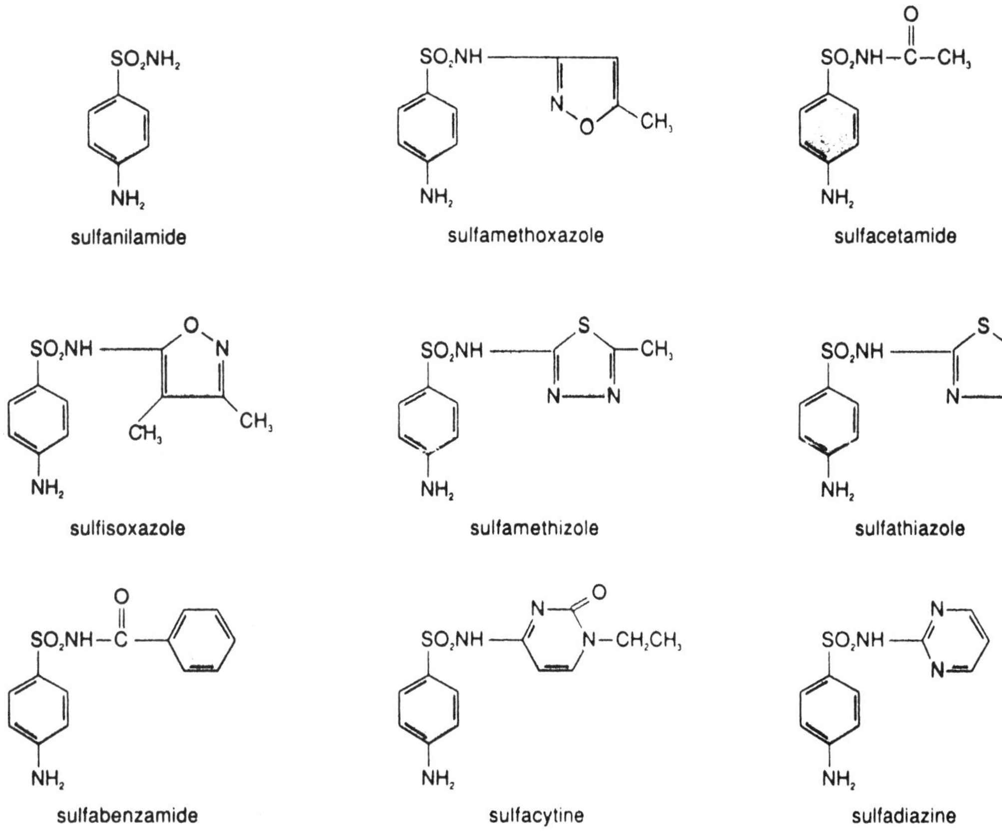

FIGURE 1. Structures of clinically useful sulfonamides.

significantly on the testing methodology used (28). Non-*fragilis* species of *Bacteroides* and *Gardnerella* have been reported to be resistant to low concentrations of sulfonamides; however, at concentrations comparable to those with topical therapy, activity was noted (16).

Gram-Positive Bacteria

Susceptibility of *Staphylococcus aureus* and streptococci is variable, although the combination sulfamethoxazole/trimethoprim often demonstrates activity against *S. aureus,* including those that are methicillin resistant. The combination has been used successfully to treat some cases of staphylococcal endocarditis. The sensitivity of *Listeria monocytogenes* to sulfamethoxazole is variable (45). Actinomycetes and *Nocardia* are usually sensitive to sulfonamides. Inoculum size is an important factor in determining sulfonamide susceptibility. If low inocula are used, isolates of *Nocardia asteroides* are reported sensitive to sulfamethoxazole (42).

Mycobacteria

Sulfonamides have also shown variable in vitro activity against nontuberculous mycobacterial species. Sulfamethoxypyridazine and the sulfone diaminodiphenylsulfone have activity against *M. leprae. M. fortuitum, M. smegmatus,* and *M. mucogenicum* have been reported sensitive to sulfonamides (42), while *M. chelonei* is usually resistant to sulfamethoxazole (37). There have been no controlled clinical studies testing effectiveness of these agents.

Other Microorganisms

Spirochetes, mycoplasmas, rickettsiae and *Chlamydia psittaci* are commonly sulfonamide resistant. *Chlamydia trachomatis* is usually sensitive to sulfonamides. When combined with other folate antagonists, sulfonamides can demonstrate activity against many protozoa including plasmodia, *Toxoplasma, Pneumocystis,* and possibly *Acanthamoeba* spp. (3). Sulfonamides may also exhibit activity against *Histoplasma capsulatum* and *Paracoccidioides brasiliensis* (9, 30).

MECHANISMS OF RESISTANCE

Resistance to sulfonamides occurs commonly and was reported frequently during World War II in United States civilian and military populations (8, 13). Worldwide resistance to this class of antimicrobials has increased dramatically since their introduction. In Sudan between 1979 and 1981, resistance of salmonellae increased from 6 to 71%. Resistance fell, presumably after antimicrobial use practices changed. Some 89% of *Shigella* isolates were also resistant during this time (14). Additionally, 90% of *Enterobacteriaceae* isolates from Sudanese children have been found resistant to sulfonamides (35). A survey in Israel that ended in 1979 demonstrated 50 to 90% sulfadiazine resistance in *E. coli, Klebsiella,* and *Enterobacter* species. Resistance was greater among inpatient services than outpatient clinics (26). Resistance of *H. influenzae* in Ireland to sulfonamides in 1989 was only 2 to 3% (15); however, resistance to sulfonamides alone is commonly seen in the United States.

The most common mechanism of resistance to sulfonamides is by alterations in dihydropteroate synthetase. This resistance can develop while patients are receiving therapy. Single mutations suffice to alter affinity for sulfonamides and confer resistance. Mutations can be chromosomal or on transferable plasmids. Multiple plasmids have been described, and they may carry resistance to other antibiotics as well (5, 12). Plasmid-mediated resistance occurs in vivo and in vitro and is most common with the *Enterobacteriaceae.*

Overproduction of PABA in *Neisseria gonorrhoeae* and *S. aureus* has been reported, but this appears to be a relatively uncommon mechanism of sulfonamide resistance. *Streptococcus pneumoniae* isolates with slightly reduced dihydropteroate synthetase affinity for PABA and markedly reduced affinity for sulfonamides have also been reported. Resistance in *Pasteurella multocida* was documented in 65% of isolates, although 25% did not contain any plasmids (6). Reduced sulfonamide uptake has also been reported. Sulfonamide resistance can occur by more than one mechanism.

PHARMACOKINETIC DISPOSITION

Sulfonamides are generally well absorbed from the stomach and small intestine (70–90%). There is minimal sulfonamide absorption from topical preparations. Sulfonamides have variable affinity for noncovalent binding to albumin (35–95%), depending on the preparation. Sulfonamides penetrate into cerebrospinal fluid, pleural fluid, and synovial fluid reasonably well, with concentrations about 30 to 80% that of serum. Transplacental transfer occurs readily, and significant sulfonamide concentrations are present in fetal blood and amniotic fluid.

Sulfonamides are eliminated from the body by glomerular filtration and metabolism. Between 15 and 70% of unconjugated sulfonamide may be found in the urine, depending on the preparation (2). Metabolism in the liver to inactive compounds is primarily by acetylation and less commonly by glucuronidation. These metabolites are inactive against bacteria and are excreted in the urine by glomerular filtration. Some metabolites, however, may exhibit toxic properties to healthy host cells (34). The low pK_as of sulfamethizole, sulfamethoxizole, and sulfisoxizole increase their urinary excretion. Sulfonamides may precipitate in urine, and this is more common if the urine is acidic (sulfadiazine and sulfathiazole). For most sulfonamides, only about 1% of parent drug appears in the bile, and only about 5% of metabolites are present in bile. Sulfamethoxazole is an exception and may achieve 40 to 60% of serum levels in bile, with concentrations increasing after multiple doses (25). The half-lives of sulfonamides vary widely from a few hours up to 10 days (Table 1).

Although variable pharmacokinetic properties in the elderly have been reported for individual sulfonamides, total absorption, bioavailability, and peak concentrations are generally not significantly influenced by age. Pharmacokinetics in the elderly are primarily influenced by the decreased glomerular filtration that occurs with age (19, 36, 38). Protein binding of sulfonamides is not different in the elderly (42).

TABLE 1 • Pharmacokinetic Characteristics of Several Sulfonamides

Sulfonamide	Adult Dose	Peak Level (μg/mL)	T$_{1/2}$	Protein Binding	Risk of Crystalluria
Sulfisoxazole	4–8 g/day	120–200	4–6 h	85%	Low
Sulfamethoxazole	2–3 g/day	60–80	5–15 h	65%	Low
Sulfadiazine	2–4 g/day	50–100	6–16 h	55%	Moderate
Sulfadoxine	500 mg/week	50–75	5–10 day	95%	Low
Sulfasalazine	2–4 g/day	10–25	4–7 h	See sulfapyridine	Low
Sulfapyridine	See sulfasalazine	15–45	6–9 h	25%	High

DOSAGE REGIMENS

Sulfonamide dosing is based primarily on achieving a peak free sulfonamide level between 50 and 150 μg/mL. When treating serious infections, levels of 200 μg/mL may be advisable, but in this situation, levels should be checked periodically, since the occurrence of side effects increases dramatically when sulfonamide levels exceed 200 μg/mL.

Sulfonamides are not recommended in patients with renal failure because of unpredictable excretion at creatinine clearances below 15 mL/min. Individual drugs should be used at reduced dose and decreased frequency when the creatinine clearance falls below approximately 30 mL/min. Little is known about use of these medications in hepatic insufficiency.

Sulfonamides are classified as pregnancy category C by the FDA. When tested in rats at doses 7 to 9 times the highest recommended daily human dose, sulfisoxazole showed teratogenic potential. Sulfonamides should not be given during the last 4 weeks of pregnancy, since they may displace bilirubin from albumin binding sites. The placenta may be unable to compensate for the increased fetal bilirubin level and kernicterus may ensue. Also, late in pregnancy, fetal red cells may be glutathione deficient, and sulfonamides could cause hemolytic anemia. For these reasons, sulfonamides should not be used in the third trimester and used cautiously in the second, if needed.

ADVERSE EFFECTS

The list of adverse effects that have been associated with sulfonamide use is long and varied, and the cumulative rate of adverse events is approximately 5% (43). The most common adverse events include rash (2–3%), fever (1–4%), and diarrhea. Severe reactions such as toxic epidermal necrolysis/Stevens-Johnson syndrome, agranulocytosis, and vasculitis are uncommon but always of concern. Severe reactions have been reported with all sulfonamides but reported more commonly when longer-acting preparations (sulfadoxine or sulfadiazine) are used or when sulfonamides were used in young children. The use of topical sulfonamides usually results in absorption of some of the parent compound and severe adverse reactions have been reported. Although rare, severe reactions have also been reported with the use of sulfonamide-containing ophthalmic drops (10).

Sulfonamides were the most common cause of rash from 1971 to 1980 (17). In a related study, sulfamethoxazole/trimethoprim caused rash in 3.7% of drug recipients and was second to amoxicillin/ampicillin as a cause of drug rash (1). Rashes frequently occur 1 to 2 weeks after starting therapy.

Nausea, vomiting, and headache occur rarely and were more common with the earlier sulfonamides.

Development of renal crystals was more common when the earlier, less-soluble sulfonamides (sulfapyridine and sulfathiazole) were used. In an attempt to lessen this problem, multiple sulfonamides, at lower doses, would be used concomitantly. This decreased the chance of developing renal stones and had little influence on clinical effectiveness. Hypoalbuminemia has also been postulated to increase risk of developing renal stones (32). Alkalinization of the urine and adequate fluid intake are also recommended to decrease the chance of crystalluria.

Sulfonamides are oxidants, and hemolytic anemia can occur in persons with glucose-6-phosphate dehydrogenase (G6PD) deficiency. This usually occurs during the first week of therapy. Hemolytic anemia not associated with G6PD deficiency, thrombocytopenia, leukopenia, aplastic anemia, and agranulocytosis have all been reported with sulfonamide use. These risks increase significantly when sulfamethoxazole plus trimethoprim is used. In one study, the risk of developing agranulocytosis did increase when sulfonamides were used alone (20). Agranulocytosis may be severe and take several weeks to resolve. Systemic illnesses including anaphylaxis, serum sickness, erythema nodosum, erythema multiforme, fixed drug eruption, vasculitis similar to that occurring in periarteritis nodosa, and lupus have been reported.

In a case-control study, sulfonamides had the greatest risk for associated Stevens-Johnson syndrome of any drug class (4.5 cases per million users per week), with sulfamethoxazole/trimethoprim the sulfonamide preparation most commonly used by case patients (31). Sulfamethoxazole/trimethoprim was also the drug most commonly associated with toxic epidermal necrolysis (11). Sulfadoxine in combination with pyrimethamine carries about a 1:20,000 risk of fatal Stevens-Johnson syndrome in persons receiving the medication for malaria prophylaxis (4). Risk of Stevens-Johnson syndrome is lower with short-acting sulfonamides. Individuals who have previously experienced severe reactions to sulfonamides will exhibit the same reaction upon rechallenge. Individuals allergic to sulfonamides should not receive topical sulfonamide preparations, as Stevens-Johnson syndrome has occurred following the use of sulfonamide-containing eye drops (10). Cross-sensitivity to all sulfonamides usually occurs, and a different sulfonamide should not be given to anyone with prior sensitivity, unless clearly required.

Some adverse reactions to sulfonamides may be related to their acetylation. *N*-Acetyltransferase is a polymorphic enzyme, and individuals are either slow or fast acetylators. All six children who experienced a variety of severe reactions to sulfonamides were found to be slow acetylators. All exhibited lymphocyte sensitivity to sulfonamide metabolites, and all exhibited no toxicity to the parent compounds (34).

DRUG INTERACTIONS

Sulfonamides can potentiate the effects of many drugs including sulfonylurea hypoglycemic agents, Coumadin, phenytoin, and methotrexate by displacement of bound drug from albumin or by decreased metabolism in the liver (21, 29).

CLINICAL INDICATIONS

Sulfonamides have been used to treat a variety of infectious processes including urinary tract infections, gastroenteritis, and meningitis. The use of sulfonamides as single agents is now significantly limited by frequent bacterial resistance and the availability of alternative antimicrobials. Many sulfonamides that were previously important in the management of human disease are no longer manufactured because of their limited usefulness or toxicity (e.g., sulfapyridine).

Sulfisoxazole and sulfamethoxazole may be used alone to treat acute, recurrent, or chronic urinary tract infections caused by susceptible bacteria. Their current activity against common urinary pathogens is limited; many strains of *E. coli* and *Proteus mirabilis* are resistant (33).

Sulfadiazine and sulfisoxazole have been shown effective as single agents in human and animal nocardiosis. Serum levels of 100 to 150 µg/mL should be sought, but these levels can be associated with crystalluria. The importance of combination therapy in nocardiosis is unclear at this time; however, intravenous sulfamethoxazole/trimethoprim is commonly used in management of this infection.

Sulfasalazine is poorly absorbed. This compound is broken down in the colon to release 5-aminosalicylic acid and sulfapyridine. Only about 1/3 of the parent compound is absorbed; however, all of the sulfapyridine that is generated is absorbed, resulting in a mean peak blood level of about 20 µg/mL. Sulfasalazine is indicated in the management of mild-to-moderate ulcerative colitis. Current opinion holds that the 5-aminosalicylic acid moiety is the active component in management of colitis (7).

Topical sulfonamide preparations have been used in management of acne vulgaris, acne rosacea, and seborrheic dermatitis and as antibacterial ophthalmic drops (sulfacetamide). Other uses include management of bacterial vaginosis as a triple sulfa cream or intravaginal tablets (sulfacetamide, sulfathiazole, and sulfabenzamide) and as adjunctive therapy for second- and third-degree burns (silver sulfadiazine, mafenate). In the management of burns, it has been shown that the sulfadiazine component is not required for in vitro antibacterial activity (23). Reactions are more frequent with mafenate than with silver sulfadiazine, and use of mafenate can cause metabolic acidosis.

Because of the limited spectrum of activity and resistance problems, sulfonamides are usually combined with other antimicrobials to make them more effective. Effectiveness is augmented by addition of an agent that inhibits the same metabolic pathway, such as trimethoprim or pyrimethamine. Sometimes a sulfonamide is combined with an unrelated antibiotic, such as erythromycin, to broaden coverage (otitis media). When these agents are used in combination, many previously resistant Gram-positive and Gram-negative bacteria and parasites respond to therapy. These drug combinations (e.g., sulfamethoxazole-trimethoprim) are the agents of choice for management of most uncomplicated urinary tract infections, *Pneumocystis carinii* pneumonia, toxoplasmosis, and some infections caused by resistant Gram-negative bacilli, among others. They may also be used as second-line agents in cases of malaria and in infections caused by resistant Gram-negative rods (e.g., *Enterobacter*) or methicillin-resistant *S. aureus* (22).

Sulfonamides are used commonly in veterinary medicine, often in combination with other agents. In a study of bob veal calves, sulfonamides (usually sulfamethazine) were found in 2 to 3% of specimens taken (44). The use of these agents in domestic livestock raises concern about further development of bacterial resistance and the possibility of further sensitization of humans to sulfonamides.

CONCLUSIONS

Previously, sulfonamides were widely used and were mainstays in the management of many important infectious processes. With the advent of more-effective and safer compounds, their use as single agents has significantly decreased. Sulfonamides are now used primarily in combination with other agents to improve their effectiveness; however, bacterial resistance and the possibility of adverse reactions still significantly influence the decision to use these compounds.

REFERENCES

1. Bigby M, Stern R, Arndt K. Allergic cutaneous reactions to drugs. Prim Care 1989;16:713–727.
2. Bullowa J, Ratish H. A therapeutic and pharmacological study of sulfadiazine, monomethylsulfadiazine, and dimethylsulfadiazine in lobar pneumonia. J Clin Invest 1944;23:676–681.
3. Carter R, Cullity G, Ojeda V, Silberstein P, Willaert E. A fatal case of meningoencephalitis due to a free-living amoebae of uncertain identity—probably Acanthamoeba sp. Pathology 1981;13:51.
4. CDC, Center for Infectious Diseases. Revised recommendations for preventing malaria in travelers to areas with chloroquine-resistant Plasmodium falciparum. MMWR 1985;34:185–190.
5. Chinault C, Blakesley V, Roessler E, Willis D, Smith C, Cook R, Fenwick R. Characterization of transferable plasmids from Shigella flexneri 2a that confer resistance to trimethoprim, streptomycin, and sulfonamides. Plasmid 1986;15:119–131.
6. Cote S, Harel J, Higgins R, Jacques M. Resistance to antimicrobial agents and prevalence of R plasmids in Pasteurella multocida from swine. Am J Vet Res 1991;52:1653–1657.
7. Das K. Sulfasalazine therapy in inflammatory bowel disease. Gastroenterol Clin North Am 1989;18:1–21.
8. Delameter E, Jennings R, Wallace A. Preliminary report of an outbreak of streptococcal disease caused by a sulfadiazine-resistant group A hemolytic streptococcus. JAMA 1946;78:118–127.

9. Goodwin R, Shapiro J, Thurmans G, Desprez R. Disseminated histoplasmosis: clinical and pathologic correlations. Medicine 1980;59:1–33.

10. Gottschalk H, Stone O. Stevens-Johnson syndrome from ophthalmic sulfonamide. Arch Dermatol 1976;112:513.

11. Guillaume JC, Roujeau JC, Revuz J, Penso D, Touraine R. The culprit drugs in 87 cases of toxic epidermal necrolysis (Lyell's syndrome). Arch Dermatol 1987;123:1166–1170.

12. Hall R, Vockler C. The region of the IncN plasmid R46 coding for resistance to B-lactam antibiotics, streptomycin/spectinomycin and sulfonamides is closely related to antibiotic segments found in IncW plasmids and in Tn21-like transposons. Nucleic Acids Res 1987;15:7491–7501.

13. Hamburger M, Mattman C, Grosch D, Hurst V. Susceptibility to sulfadiazine of hemolytic streptococci recovered in army camps. Am J Med 1946;1:23–27.

14. Hassan H. Sensitivity a of Salmonella and Shigella to antibiotics and chemotherapeutic agents in Sudan. J Trop Med Hyg 1985;88:243–247.

15. Howard A, Williams H. The prevalence of antibiotic resistance in *Haemophilus influenzae* in Ireland. J Antimicrob Chemother 1989;24:963–971.

16. Jones B, Kinghorn G, Geary I. In vitro susceptibility of Gardnerella vaginalis and Bacteroides organisms, associated with non-specific vaginitis, to sulfonamide preparations. Antimicrob Agents Chemother 1982;21:870–872.

17. Kauppinen K, Stubb S. Drug eruptions: causative agents and clinical types, a series of in-patients during a 10 year period. Acta Dermatol Vener (Stockh) 1984;64:320–324.

18. Kraus S, Kaufman H, Albriton W, Albritton W, Thornsberry C, Biddle J. Chancroid therapy: a review of cases confirmed by culture. Rev Infect Dis 1982;4(Suppl):848.

19. Ljungberg B, Nilsson-Ehle I. Pharmacokinetics of antimicrobial agents in the elderly. Rev Infect Dis 1987;9:250–264.

20. Levy M, Slone D, Shapiro S, Kaufman D, Anderson T. Anti-infective drug use in relation to the risk of agranulocytosis and aplastic anemia, a report from the International Agranulocytosis and Aplastic Anemia Study. Arch Intern Med 1989;149:1036–1040.

21. Lumholtz B, Siersbaek-Nielsen K, Skovsted L, Kampmann J, Hansen J. Sulfamethizole induced inhibition of diphenylhydantoin, tolbutamide, and warfarin metabolism. Clin Pharmacol Ther 1975;17:731–734.

22. Markowitz N, Quinn E, Saravolatz L. Trimethoprim-sulfamethoxazole compared with vancomycin for the treatment of *Staphylococcus aureus* infection. Ann Intern Med 1992;117:390–398.

23. McManus A, Denton C, Mason A. Mechanisms of in vitro sensitivity to sulfadiazine silver. Arch Surg 1983;118:161–166.

24. Mitchard M. Sulfur compounds used in medicine. Drug Metab Drug Interact 1988;6:183–202.

25. Nagar H, Berger S. The excretion of antibiotics by the biliary tract. Surg Gynecol Obstet 1984;158:601–607.

26. Nitzan Y, Maayan M, Wajsman C, Drucker M. Isr J Med Sci 1983;19:1039–1045.

27. Otten H. Domagk and the development of the sulphonamides. J Antimicrob Chemother 1986;17:689–696.

28. Phillips I, Warren C. Activity of sulfamethoxazole and trimethoprim against Bacteroides fragilis. Antimicrob Agents Chemother 1976;9:736–740.

29. Raasch R. Interactions of oral antibiotics and common chronic medications. Geriatrics 1987;42:69–74.

30. Restrepo A, Arango M. In vitro susceptibility testing of Paracoccidioides brasiliensis to sulfonamides. Antimicrob Agents Chemother 1980;18:190–194.

31. Roujeau JC, Kelly J, Naldi L, Berthold R, Stern R. Medication use and the risk of Stevens-Johnson syndrome or toxic epidermal necrolysis. N Engl J Med 1995;333:1600–1607.

32. Sahai J, Heimberger T, Collins K, Kaplowitz L, Polk R. Sulfadiazine-induced crystaluria in a patient with the acquired immunodeficiency syndrome: a reminder. Am J Med 1988;84:791–792.

33. Sawyer D, Mandell G. New antimicrobial treatment of urinary tract infections and prostatitis. Semin Urol 1985;4:281–286.

34. Shear N, Spielberg S, Grant D, Tang K, Kalow W. Differences in metabolism of sulfonamides predisposing to idiosyncratic toxicity. Ann Intern Med 1986;105:179–184.

35. Shears P, Suliman G, Hart C. Occurrence of multiple antibiotic resistance and R plasmids in Enterobacteriaceae isolated from children in the Sudan. Epidemiol Infect 1988;100:73–81.

36. Simon C, Malerczyk V, Tenschert B, Mohlenbeck J. Die geriatrische pharmakologie von cefazolin, cefradin und sulfisomidin. Arzneimittelforschung 1976;26:1377–1382.

37. Swenson J, Wallace R, Silcox V, Thornsberry C. Antimicrobial susceptibility of five subgroups of Mycobacterium fortuitum and Mycobacterium chelonae. Antimicrob Agents Chemother 1985;28:807.

38. Triggs E, Nation R, Long A, Ashley J. Pharmacokinetics in the elderly. Eur J Clin Pharmacol 1975;8:55–62.

39. Wallace R. Treatment of infections caused by rapidly growing mycobacteria in the era of the newer macrolides. 13th Forum in Microbiology 1995;30–35.

40. Wallace R, Steele L, Sumpter G, Smith J. Antimicrobial susceptibility patterns of Nocardia asteroides. Antimicrob Agents Chemother 1988;32:1776–1779.

41. Vaisanen V, Lounatmaa K, Korhonen T. Effects of sublethal concentrations of antimicrobial agents on the hemagglutination, adhesion, and ultrastructure of pyelonephritogenic *Escherichia coli* strains. Antimicrob Agents Chemother 1982;22:120–127.

42. Wallace S, Whiting B, Runcie J. Factors affecting drug binding in plasma of elderly patients. Br J Clin Pharmacol 1976;3:327–330.

43. Weinstein L, Madoff M, Samet C. The sulfonamides. N Engl J Med 1960;263:793–800.

44. Wilson D, Franti C, Norman B. Antibiotic and sulfonamide agents in bob veal calf muscle, liver, and kidney. Am J Vet Res 1991;8:1383–1387.

45. Winslow D, Pankey G. In vitro activities of trimethoprim and sulfamethoxazole against Listeria monocytogenes. Antimicrob Agents Chemother 1982;22:51–54.

Teicoplanin

●

Sara G. Monroe and Ron Polk

Teicoplanin (formerly known as Teichomycin A2) is a glycopeptide antibiotic derived from the actinomycete *Actinoplanes teichomyceticus*. It is structurally similar to vancomycin and has comparable activity but differs in its pharmacologic properties. Teicoplanin is not approved for use in the United States but has been extensively used in Europe. Teicoplanin may offer advantages over vancomycin: it has a longer elimination half-life, can be administered by intramuscular injection, and has a more favorable side-effect profile. However, concerns about efficacy in the treatment of serious infections may limit its usefulness.

STRUCTURE AND MECHANISM OF ACTION

Teicoplanin, a complex of five closely related glycopeptides, is structurally similar to vancomycin. It differs from vancomycin in the composition of its carbohydrate components and the presence of an acyl (fatty acid) moiety (25, 41). The fatty acid component causes teicoplanin to be more lipophilic, resulting in greater tissue and cellular penetration (25). Like other glycopeptides, teicoplanin inhibits cell wall synthesis in susceptible bacteria. It inhibits polymerization of peptidoglycan in bacterial cell walls by binding to the terminal D-alanyl-D-alanine precursor, which fits into a cleft in the teicoplanin molecule (25, 29, 41).

ANTIMICROBIAL ACTIVITY AND RESISTANCE

The antibacterial activity of teicoplanin is limited to Gram-positive bacteria. It is bactericidal for most organisms but is bacteriostatic for enterococci and listeria with MBCs above achievable serum concentrations. Activity against both methicillin-susceptible and -resistant *Staphylococcus aureus* (MRSA) is comparable to that of vancomycin, with a mean MIC_{90} of 0.2 to 1.5 g/L (34). The susceptibility of coagulase-negative staphylococci is more variable with MICs of 2 to 4 mg/L, and some strains of *Staphylococcus epidermidis* and *Staphylococcus hemolyticus* are resistant (1, 12). In vitro, teicoplanin is more active than vancomycin against most streptococcal species including enterococci. MIC_{90} values for nonenterococcal streptococci are approximately half those of vancomycin: values for *Enterococcus faecalis* range from 0.2 to 3.1 g/L, versus 1.56 to 4.0 g/L for vancomycin (34). Like vancomycin, teicoplanin is bacteriostatic for enterococci, but bactericidal activity can be achieved with addition of an aminoglycoside (38). Teicoplanin is active against other aerobic and anaerobic Gram-positive bacteria including corynebacteria, clostridia (including *C. difficile*), *Bacillus* spp., *Listeria monocytogenes,* and *Propionibacterium acnes* and has MIC_{90} values 2 to 4 times lower than vancomycin for many of these species (34). Teicoplanin is not active against Gram-negative bacteria because it is a large polar molecule that cannot penetrate the lipid membrane. At equivalent concentrations, the postantibiotic effect of teicoplanin exceeds that of vancomycin for MRSA and *E. faecalis* (7).

Resistance to teicoplanin has been reported in *S. aureus* (15), coagulase-negative staphylococci (1, 12), and enterococci (especially *E. faecium*) (14, 18). Enterococci with the VanA phenotype have transferable plasmid-mediated resistance to both vancomycin and teicoplanin. Inducible resistance to teicoplanin has also been reported in an isolate of *E. faecium* with the VanB phenotype (14). Kaatz et al. reported development of constitutive, non-plasmid-mediated resistance in serial isolates of *S. aureus* from a patient being treated for endocarditis (15).

PHARMACOKINETICS

Teicoplanin is poorly absorbed from the gastrointestinal tract, and 40% of an orally administered dose can be found in the stool (22). Intravenous administration of 3 and 6 mg/kg in healthy volunteers resulted in peak plasma levels of 53.5 and 111.8 mg/L, respectively, with concentrations of 2.1 and 4.2 mg/L at 24 h (40). After intravenous administration, teicoplanin has an elimination half-life of 40 to 70 h in patients with normal kidney function. This prolonged half-life is likely due to its high degree of protein binding (90%) and slow renal clearance (25). Unlike vancomycin, teicoplanin can be given by intramuscular injection with 90% bioavailability (30), and peak plasma levels occur 2 h after injection (40). Penetration into body fluids and tissues has not been studied extensively. Therapeutic levels have been found in the heart (3, 44) and blister and peritoneal fluid (45), but cerebrospinal fluid penetration is poor, even in the presence of inflamed meninges (37).

Teicoplanin is excreted almost completely by the kidney, without significant metabolism (5). Elimination half-life is prolonged in patients with renal insufficiency, and dosage adjustments are necessary as renal function declines (10). Clearance of teicoplanin declines as renal function decreases and is correlated linearly with creatinine clearance (10, 16). As with vancomycin, a nomogram is useful for estimating the dose of teicoplanin in patients with renal insufficiency (Fig. 1). Measurement of serum concentrations may help in determining the appropriate dose and dosing interval.

DOSAGE REGIMENS

Due to its prolonged terminal half-life, teicoplanin can be administered less frequently than vancomycin in most patients. Unlike vancomycin, dosage adjustments are made on the ba-

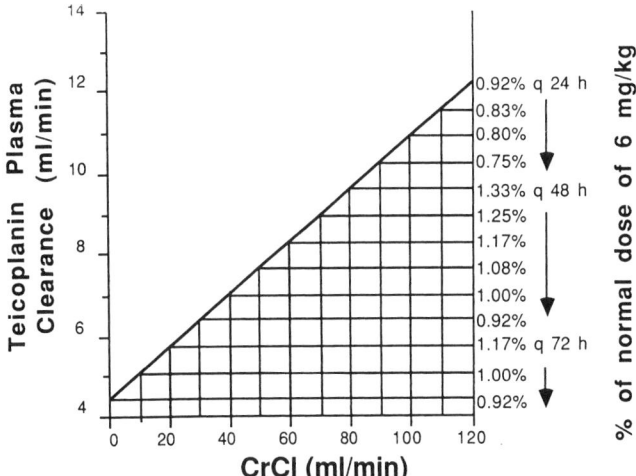

FIGURE 1. Teicoplanin dosage nomogram. (From Lam YWF, Kapusnik-Uner JE, Sachdeva M, Hackbarth C, Gambertoglio JG, Sande ME. The pharmacokinetics of teicoplanin in varying degrees of renal function. Clin Pharmacol Ther 1990;47:655–661.)

sis of the severity of infection as well as renal function. There is no established range for therapeutic serum concentrations of teicoplanin, but it has been suggested that trough levels of at least 10 mg/L are necessary for treatment of severe infections (43). To achieve adequate serum levels rapidly, a loading dose of 400 mg (6 mg/kg) on the first day is recommended. For less serious infections such as those involving the urinary tract, skin and soft tissue, and lower respiratory tract, the usual maintenance dose is 200 mg (3 mg/kg) daily. Treatment of serious Gram-positive infections such as septicemia, endocarditis, and osteomyelitis requires a higher loading dose of 400 to 800 mg (6–12 mg/kg) every 12 h for two to three doses, followed by a maintenance dose of 400 to 800 mg (4, 34). Therapy for endocarditis with teicoplanin as a single agent has been problematic (11), and maintenance of trough levels of 20 to 60 mg/L is recommended (27). Concentrations of 20 to 60 mg/L can be achieved by administration of a loading dose of 2 g (30 mg/kg) every 12 h for two doses, followed by the same dose given daily for maintenance (34). However, at these high doses, the toxicity of teicoplanin may be increased (26).

In patients with moderate renal failure (CrCl, 40–60 mL/min) the usual dose of teicoplanin is administered for 4 days after which half the normal dose (200–400 mg) is given every 1 to 2 days for maintenance. If CrCl is below 40 mL/min, usual doses are given for 4 days followed by maintenance doses of 1/3 the normal dose. Alternatively, higher maintenance doses (6 mg/kg) can be given at less frequent intervals (every 2–3 days). Nomograms and serum drug monitoring may be useful in determining the appropriate dose of teicoplanin in patients with renal failure.

Patients on hemodialysis are generally treated with a loading dose of 800 mg followed by 400 mg weekly (2). However, treatment of more serious infections may require more frequent doses. Teicoplanin does not penetrate well into peritoneal fluid in patients on CAPD when administered intra-

venously but has been effective in the treatment of Gram-positive peritonitis when given intraperitoneally (22).

Oral teicoplanin may be an effective alternative treatment for colitis caused by *C. difficile*. No dosage regimen has been established for therapy of *C. difficile* colitis, but doses of 400 to 600 mg/day for 10 days have been used effectively (9).

ADVERSE EFFECTS

Teicoplanin is generally well tolerated and may have fewer adverse effects than does vancomycin. Unlike with vancomycin, thrombophlebitis during intravenous administration is unusual, and pain with intramuscular injection is minimal. In a large multicenter open trial of teicoplanin in Gram-positive infections, Lewis et al. found side effects in 13.2% of patients (19). The most common adverse events were "nonspecific" (5.1%), hypersensitivity (5%), and biochemical abnormalities (4.7%). Hematologic abnormalities (2.2%), nephrotoxicity (0.35%), and ototoxicity (0.28%) occurred rarely. In a meta-analysis of 11 comparative clinical trials, adverse events occurred significantly more often with vancomycin (21.9%) than with teicoplanin (13.9%) (47). Nephrotoxicity occurred in 4.8% of patients treated with teicoplanin, compared with 10.7% of those who received vancomycin. The use of nephrotoxic drugs was similar in both populations. The incidence of ototoxicity associated with teicoplanin is extremely low, although both auditory and vestibular toxicity have been reported (4, 20). Red man syndrome with rapid administration of teicoplanin intravenously is unusual (31, 34), and histamine release does not occur (31).

There is controversy about the potential for allergic cross-reactivity between vancomycin and teicoplanin. Some have reported allergic reactions in patients with a history of vancomycin hypersensitivity who were given teicoplanin (8, 13, 21), but not others (32, 35). Since uncertainty exists about cross-reactivity and because of its long half-life, teicoplanin should probably not be administered to patients with serious hypersensitivity reactions to vancomycin.

CLINICAL INDICATIONS

In many situations, teicoplanin may be a safe and effective alternative to vancomycin, and indications for use of the two drugs are similar. Teicoplanin can be used in the treatment of many Gram-positive infections including those caused by MRSA and coagulase-negative staphylococci. It is a safe alternative for prophylaxis and therapy of infections in the patient with serious allergic reactions to β-lactam antibiotics.

Two large, open, multicenter studies have evaluated the efficacy of teicoplanin in the treatment of a variety of Gram-positive infections including bone and joint, skin and soft tissue, lung, and endocarditis (17, 19). In these studies, clinical efficacy was 87 to 92%, and bacteriologic efficacy was 79 to 85%. Eleven trials comparing the efficacy of vancomycin and teicoplanin in the treatment of Gram-positive infections in various patient populations have been recently reviewed by meta-analysis (47). Clinical response rates for teicoplanin varied from 54 to 92% and for vancomycin, from 60 to 93%. In no study did the clinical or bacteriologic response rates for vancomycin and teicoplanin differ significantly. Analysis of clinical cure rates in patients with deep-seated infections involving bone and joint, mediastinum, central venous catheters, and pacemaker wires also showed no significant difference between vancomycin and teicoplanin (6, 36, 39).

Teicoplanin has been used effectively in the treatment of staphylococcal, streptococcal, and enterococcal endocarditis (combined with an aminoglycoside) (27). However, substantial failure rates have been seen in the treatment of *S. aureus* endocarditis and other deep-seated infections, especially when lower doses of drug (200 mg/day) are used (11). This problem may be partially overcome by using higher maintenance doses (12–30 mg/kg/day) (27, 43) or by addition of aminoglycosides (33).

Oral teicoplanin is a possible alternative for treatment of *C. difficile* colitis. In a prospective trial, teicoplanin (100 mg orally twice a day) was as effective as oral vancomycin (500 mg four times a day) and was associated with lower relapse rates (9). However, Wistrom et al. reported a cure rate of only 70% and a relapse rate of 35% using the same dose (46). More comparative studies are needed before recommendations can be made about the utility of teicoplanin in the treatment of *C. difficile* colitis.

REFERENCES

1. Bannerman TL, Wadiak DL, Kloos WE. Susceptibility of Staphylococcus species and subspecies to teicoplanin. Antimicrob Agents Chemother 1991;35:1919–1922.
2. Beckers B, Broderson HP, Stolpmann RM, Jansen G, Larbig D. Efficacy and pharmacokinetics of teicoplanin in hemodialysis patients. Infection 1993;21:71–74.
3. Bergeron MG, Saginur R, Desaulniers D, Trottier S, Goldstein W, Faucault P, Cessard C. Concentration of teicoplanin in serum and atrial appendages of patients undergoing cardiac surgery. Antimicrob Agents Chemother 1990;34:1699–1702.
4. Bibler MR, Frame PT, Hagler DN, Bode RB, Stanek JL, Thamlikitkul V, Harris JE, Haregewoin A, Bullock WE Jr. Clinical evaluation of efficacy, pharmacokinetics, and safety of teichoplanin for serious gram-positive infections. Antimicrob Agents Chemother 1987;31:207–212.
5. Carver PL, Nightingale CH, Quintiliani R, Sweeney K, Stevens RC, Maderazo E. Pharmacokinetics of single- and multiple-dose teicoplanin in healthy volunteers. Antimicrob Agents Chemother 1989;33:82–86.
6. Charbonneau P, Harding I, Garraud JJ, Aubertin J, Brunet F, Domart Y. Teicoplanin: a well tolerated and easily administered alternative to vancomycin for gram-positive infections in intensive care patients. Intensive Care Med 1994;20(Suppl 4):35–42.
7. Cooper MA, Jin Y-F, Ashby JP, Andrews JM, Wise R. In-vitro comparison of the post antibiotic effect of vancomycin and teicoplanin. J Antimicrob Chemother 1990;26:203–207.
8. Davenport A. Allergic cross-reactivity to teicoplanin and vancomycin [letter]. Nephron 1993;63:482.
9. deLalla F, Privitera G, Rinaldi E, Ortisi G, Santoro D, Rizzardini G. Treatment of Clostridium difficile-associated disease with teicoplanin. Antimicrob Agents Chemother 1989;33:1125–1127.
10. Falcoz C, Ferry N, Pozet N, Cuisinaud G, Zech PY, Sassard J. Pharmacokinetics of teicoplanin in renal failure. Antimicrob Agents Chemother 1987;31:1255–1262.
11. Galanakis N, Giamarellou H, Vlachogiannis N, Dendrinos C, Daikos GK. Poor efficacy of teicoplanin in the treatment of deep-seated staphylococcal infections. Eur J Clin Microbiol Infect Dis 1988;7:130–134.
12. Greenwood D. Microbiological properties of teicoplanin. J Antimicrob Chemother 1988;21(Suppl A):1–13.
13. Grek V, Andrien F, Collignon J, Fillet G. Allergic cross-reaction of teicoplanin and vancomycin [Letter]. J Antimicrob Chemother 1991;28:476–477.
14. Hayden MK, Trenholme GM, Schultz JE, Sahm DF. In vivo development of teicoplanin resistance in a VanB Enterococcus faecium isolate. J Infect Dis 1993;167:1224–1227.
15. Kaatz GW, Seo S, Dorman NJ, Lerner SA. Emergence of teicoplanin resistance during therapy of Staphylococcus aureus endocarditis. J Infect Dis 1990;162:103–108.
16. Lam YWK, Kapusnik-Uner JE, Sachdeva M, Hackbarth C, Gambertoglio JG, Sande ME. The pharmacokinetics of teicoplanin in varying degrees of renal function. Clin Pharmacol Ther 1990;47:655–661.
17. Lang E, Schafer V, Schaaf B, Dennhardt R. Comparison of efficacy and safety of teicoplanin in gram-positive infections: a multicentre study. Scand J Infect Dis 1990;72(Suppl):54–60.
18. Leclercq R, Derlot E, Duval J, Courvalin P. Plasmid-mediated resistance to vancomycin and teicoplanin in Enterococcus faecium. N Engl J Med 1988;319:157–161.
19. Lewis P, Garaud J, Parenti F. A multicentre open clinical trial of teicoplanin in infections caused by gram-positive bacteria. J Antimicrob Chemother 1988;21(Suppl A):61–67.
20. Maher ER, Hollman A, Gruneberg RN. Teicoplanin-induced ototoxicity in Down's syndrome [Letter]. Lancet 1986;1:613.
21. McElrath MJ, Goldberg D, Neu HC. Allergic cross-reactivity of teicoplanin and vancomycin [Letter]. Lancet 1986;1:47.
22. Neville LO, Baillod RA, Brumfitt W, Hamilton-Miller JMR. Efficacy and safety of teicoplanin in gram-positive peritonitis in patients on peritoneal dialysis. J Antimicrob Chemother 1988;21(Suppl A):123–131.
23. Neville LO, Baillod R, Grady D, Brumfitt W, Hamilton-Miller JM. Teicoplanin in patients with chronic renal failure in dialysis: microbiological and pharmacokinetic aspects. Int J Clin Pharm Res 1987;7:485–490.
24. Parenti F. Glycopeptide antibiotics. J Clin Pharmacol 1988;28:136–140.
25. Parenti F. Structure, and mechanism of action of teicoplanin. J Hosp Infect 1986;7(Suppl):79–83.
26. Phillips G, Golledge CL. Vancomycin and teicoplanin: something old, something new. Med J Aust 1992;156:53–57.
27. Presterl E, Graninger W, Georgopoalos A. The efficacy of teicoplanin in the treatment of endocarditis caused by gram-positive bacteria. J Antimicrob Chemother 1993;31:755–766.
28. Pullanza R, Berti M, Goldstein BP, et al. Teicoplanin: in vitro and in vivo evaluation and comparison to other antibiotics. J Antimicrob Chemother 1983;11:419–423.
29. Reynolds PE. Structure, biochemistry and mechanism of action of glycopeptide antibiotics. Eur J Clin Microbiol Infect Dis 1989;8:943–950.
30. Ripa S, Ferrante L, Miguini F, Falcioni E. Pharmacokinetics of teicoplanin. Chemotherapy 1988;34:178–184.
31. Sahai J, Healy DP, Shelton MJ Miller JS, Ruberg SJ, Polk R. Comparison of vancomycin- and teicoplanin-induced histamine release and "red man syndrome." Antimicrob Agents Chemother 1990;34:765–769.
32. Schlemmer B, Falkman H, Boudjadja A, Jacob L, LeGall JR.

Teicoplanin for patients allergic to vancomycin [Letter]. N Engl J Med 1988;318:1127–1128.

33. Schmit JL. Efficacy of teicoplanin for enterococcal infections: 63 cases and review. Clin Infect Dis 1992;15:302–306.

34. Shea KW, Cunha BA. Teicoplanin. Med Clin North Am 1995; 79:833–844.

35. Smith SR, Cheesbrough JS, Makins M, Davies JM. Teicoplanin administration in patients experiencing reactions to vancomycin [Letter]. J Antimicrob Chemother 1989;23:810–812.

36. Smith SR, Cheesbrough J, Spearing R, Davies JM. Randomized prospective study comparing vancomycin with teicoplanin in the treatment of infections associated with Hickman catheters. Antimicrob Agent Chemother 1989;33:1193–1197.

37. Stahl JP, Croize J, Wolff M, Garaud JJ, Leclercq P, Vachan F, Micoud M. Poor penetration of teicoplanin into cerebrospinal fluid in patients with bacterial meningitis. J Antimicrob Chemother 1987;20:141–142.

38. Van der Auwera P, Klastersky J. Bactericidal activity and killing rate of serum in volunteers receiving vancomycin or teicoplanin with and without amikacin given intravenously. J Antimicrob Chemother 1987;19:623–635.

39. Van Laethem Y, Hermans P, DeWit S, Goosene H, Charneck N. Teicoplanin compared with vanc in methicillin-resistant *Staphylococcus aureus* infections: preliminary results. J Antimicrob Chemother 1988;21(Suppl A):81–87.

40. Verbist L, Tjandramaga B, Hendrick B, Van Hecken P, Van Melle R, Verbesselt J, Verhaegen J, De Schepper PJ. In vitro activity and human pharmacokinetics of teicoplanin. Antimicrob Agents Chemother 1984;26:881–886.

41. Williams AH, Grüneberg RN. Teichoplanin. J Antmicrob Chemother 1984;14:441–445.

42. Wilson APR, Grüneberg RN, Neu H. A critical review of the dosage of teicoplanin in Europe and the USA. Int J Antimicrob Agents 1994;4(Suppl 1):1–30.

43. Wilson APR, Grüneberg RN, Neu H. Dosage recommendations for teicoplanin. J Antimicrob Chemother 1993;32: 792–796.

44. Wilson APR, Taylor B, Treasure T, Grüneberg RN, Sturridge MF, Ross DN. Antibiotic prophylaxis in cardiac surgery: serum and tissue levels of teicoplanin, flucloxacillin and tobramycin. J Antimicrob Chemother 1988;21:201–212.

45. Wise R, Donovan IA, McNaulty CA, Waldron R, Andrews JM. Teicoplanin, its pharmacokinetics, blister and peritoneal fluid penetration. J Hosp Infect 1986;7(Suppl A):47–55.

46. Wistrom J, Lundholm R, Prag M, et al. Treatment of Clostridium difficile associated diarrhea and colitis with an oral preparation of teicoplanin; a dose finding study. Scand J Infect Dis 1994;26:309–312.

47. Wood MJ. The comparative efficacy and safety of teicoplanin and vancomycin. J Antimicrob Chemother 1996;37:209–222.

Tetracyclines

•

Beulah E. Perdue and Harold C. Standiford

CLASS

The first tetracycline, chlortetracycline, was discovered in 1948 by the mycologist Benjamin M. Duggar while screening organisms obtained from the soil for antimicrobial properties. Because of the golden yellow colony formed by the organism, it was designated *Streptomyces aureofaciens*. The second compound, oxytetracycline, was isolated from *Streptomyces rimosus* in 1950. Tetracycline was produced as the result of the catalytic dehalogenation of chlortetracycline in 1953. The tetracyclines were found effective against a wide variety of organisms, including Gram-positive and Gram-negative bacteria, rickettsiae, and chlamydial species and became the first class of antimicrobial agents to be known as "broad spectrum." Doxycycline and minocycline were then derived semisynthetically in 1967 and 1972, respectively. The tetracyclines can be conveniently divided into short-, intermediate-, and long-acting agents on the basis of pharmacokinetic parameters (150). Those available in the United States for systemic use are listed in Table 1.

To combat the problem of resistance to tetracyclines, several derivatives have been developed. Two of these agents called glycylcyclines have been studied thus far: the *N,N*-dimethylglycylamido derivative of minocycline (DMG-MINO) and the *N,N*-dimethylglycylamido derivative of 6-demethyl-6-deoxytetracycline (DMG-DMDOT). These new agents appear to be effective against a variety of tetracycline-resistant bacteria that obtain resistance by either efflux or ribosomal protection mechanisms. Currently, these agents are not available in the United States (156).

The basic tetracycline structure consists of a hydronaphthacene nucleus. Substitutions at carbons 5, 6, and 7 of the four-ring carbocyclic structure result in variations in pharmacokinetic properties. These variations include alterations in gastrointestinal absorption, affinity for multivalent cations, and protein binding, as well as some differences in antimicrobial activity.

ANTIMICROBIAL ACTIVITY
Spectrum

Tetracyclines exhibit a broad spectrum of activity, which includes many aerobic and anaerobic Gram-positive and Gram-negative bacteria. They also possess activity against other microbes such as *rickettsiae spp.*, *Coxiella burnetii*, *Borrelia*

TABLE 1 • Tetracyclines

Agent	Brand Name	Dosage Forms and Strength
Short acting		
Tetracycline	Sumycin	Suspension: 125 mg/5 mL
Tetracycline HCl	Various generic, Achromycin V, Ala-Tet, Nor-Tet, Panmycin, Robitet Robicaps, Sumycin, Teline, Tetracap, Tetralan, Tetram, Tetracycline	Capsules: 100, 250, 500 mg Tablets: 250, 500 mg
	Various generic	Suspensions: 125 mg/5 mL
	Achromycin IM	Powder for i.m. injection: 100, 250 mg
	Achromycin IV	Powder for i.v. injection: 250, 500 mg
Oxytetracycline HCl	Various generic, E.P. Mycin, Terramycin, Uri-Tet	Capsules: 250 mg
	Terramycin IM	Injection: 50, 125 mg with 2% lidocaine
Intermediate acting		
Demeclocycline	Declomycin	Capsules: 150 mg Tablets: 150, 300 mg
Long acting		
Doxycycline hyclate	Various generic, Doxychel Hyclate, Doxy Caps, Doryx, Doxy 100, 200, Vibra-Tabs, Vibramycin	Capsules: 50, 100 mg Tablets: 50, 100 mg Powder for injection: 100, 200 mg
Doxycycline calcium	Vibramycin	Syrup: 50 mg/5 mL
Doxycycline monohydrate	Vibramycin	Powder for oral suspension: 25 mg/5 mL
Minocycline	Minocin IV	Powder for injection: 100 mg
Minocycline HCl	Minocin	Capsule: 50, 100 mg Tablet: 50, 100 mg Oral suspension: 50 mg/5 mL

recurrentis, *Borrelia burgdorferi, Treponema pallidum, Treponema pertenue, Chlamydia* spp., *Mycoplasma pneumoniae, Plasmodium* spp., *Entamoeba histolytica,* and *Mycobacterium marinum.* Tetracyclines have negligible activity against fungi and viruses (75).

Doxycycline and minocycline are considered the most active of the tetracyclines, followed by tetracycline. When dilution susceptibility testing is performed, most bacteria are considered susceptible when the minimum inhibitory concentration (MIC) of tetracycline is 4 μg/mL or less. Moderate susceptibility is defined at 8 μg/mL, and resistance is defined at 16 μg/mL or above. *Haemophilus influenzae* and *Streptococcus pneumoniae* are considered susceptible at MICs of 2 μg/mL or less, intermediately susceptible at 4 μg/mL, and resistant at 8 μg/mL or more. *Neisseria gonorrhoeae* is considered susceptible at an MIC of 0.25 μg/mL, intermediate at 0.5 to 1 μg/mL, and resistant at 2 μg/mL or more (107). In vitro susceptibilities for tetracycline and doxycycline are given in Table 2.

Pharmacodynamic Effects

Tetracycline has been reported to exhibit a postantibiotic effect of approximately 3 h against *Staphylococcus aureus* exposed to the antibiotics for 2 h at approximately five times the MIC (94). This effect, exhibited by tetracycline and other bacteriostatic agents that bind reversibly to ribosomes, has been proposed to be secondary to residual amounts of the drug remaining within the cell for a short period of time.

Concomitant administration of tetracycline with ampicillin or amoxicillin has been reported to mask the bactericidal effect of the penicillin. Clinically, the combination of chlortetracycline and penicillin used for the treatment of pneumococcal meningitis has been shown to be inferior to penicillin alone. Also, the combination of tetracycline and penicillin for group A hemolytic streptococcal pharyngitis appears to have a clinically significant negative interaction (58, 71–72, 74). If this combination is necessary, the penicillin should be given several hours before the tetracycline, and therapeutic doses of each are required.

MECHANISMS OF ACTION

Tetracyclines penetrate the bacterial cell wall presumably by two processes. Penetration through hydrophilic pores in the outer cell membrane occurs by passive diffusion. Further penetration through the inner cytoplasmic membrane occurs by an energy-dependent active transport system. However, this may simply represent diffusion by a pH-dependent process. Once inside the cell, the tetracycline binds reversibly to the 30S ribosomal subunit, thereby reducing the affinity of the aminoacyl-tRNA for the mRNA-ribosome complex. This ultimately inhibits protein synthesis, which is responsible for the bacteriostatic action. Tetracyclines also inhibit protein synthesis in mammalian cells at high concentrations. However, currently recommended doses do not achieve the necessary concentrations under normal conditions for clinically apparent toxicity (28, 137).

TABLE 2 • In Vitro Susceptibilities[a]

Organism	Tetracycline			Doxycycline		
	MIC$_{50}$	MIC$_{90}$	Range	MIC$_{50}$	MIC$_{90}$	Range
Gram-positive aerobes						
Staphylococcus aureus	3.1	>25	0.8->25	1.6	>25	0.4->25
Streptococcus pneumonia	0.8	8	0.125->128	0.4	0.4	0.4
Streptococcus pyogenes	0.8	6.3	0.4->25	0.4	0.8	0.4-25
Streptococcus agalacticae	1.6	>25	1.6->25	0.8	25	0.8-25
Enterococcus spp.	>25	>25	6.3->25	>25	>25	6.3->25
Gram-negative aerobes						
Campylobacter jejuni	0.8	>25	0.4->25	0.4	12.5	0.4->25
Enterobacter spp.	3.1	25	0.8->25	25	>25	6.3->25
Escherichia coli	12.5	>25	3.1->25	12.5	>25	3.1->25
Haemophilus influenzae	6.3	12.5	3.1-12.5	1.6	3.1	1.6-6.3
Klebsiella pneumoniae	>25	>25	6.3->25	>25	>25	6.3->25
Neisseria gonorrhoeae	0.8	6.3	0.4-6.3	0.4	6.3	0.4-6.3
Neisseria meningitidis	0.8	3.1	0.8-3.1	1.6	6.3	1.6-6.3
Proteus mirabilis	>25	>25	>25	>25	>25	>25
Proteus spp. (indole +)	>25	>25	>25	>25	>25	>25
Pseudomonas aeruginosa	>25	>25	>25	>25	>25	>25
Pseudomonas pseudomallei	1.6	3.1	1.6-3.1			
Shigella spp.	3.1	>25	0.8->25			
Gram-positive anaerobes						
Clostridium perfringens	2.0	>32	0.5->32	0.5	16	0.5-16
Peptococcus	16	32	0.5->32	4.0	8.0	0.5-32
Peptostreptococcus	4.0	32	0.5->32	2.0	8.0	0.5-16
Gram-negative anaerobes						
Bacteroides fragilis	16	>32	0.5->32	2.0	16	0.5-32
Bacteroides melaninogenicus	0.5	8.0	0.5->32	0.5	2.0	0.5->32

[a] MIC$_{50}$ and MIC$_{90}$, MICs at which 50 and 90% of strains are inhibited, respectively. Most bacterial organisms: susceptible MIC ≤ 4 μg/mL; intermediate MIC, 8 μg/mL; resistant MIC ≥ 16 μg/mL. Haemophilus influenzae and Streptococcus pneumoniae: susceptible MIC ≤ 2 μg/mL; intermediate MIC, 4 μg/mL; resistant MIC ≥ 8 μg/mL. Neisseria gonorrhoeae: susceptible MIC ≤ 0.25 μg/mL, intermediate MIC, 0.5-1.0 μg/mL; resistant MIC ≥ 2 μg/mL.

MECHANISMS OF RESISTANCE
Commonly Resistant Organisms

Although the tetracyclines have a broad spectrum of activity, they are no longer the drugs of choice for many Gram-positive and Gram-negative bacterial organisms. More-effective agents are now available for the treatment of many of these bacterial infections. Of the Gram-positive bacteria, only 10% of enterococcal strains are susceptible to tetracycline, while only 50% of group B streptococci and 65% of S. aureus are susceptible. With the growth of penicillin-resistant S. pneumoniae has come resistance to the tetracyclines. Of those strains that are susceptible to penicillin, 90% are susceptible to tetracycline; 77% of penicillin-intermediate strains are susceptible to tetracycline, and only 21% that are penicillin resistant are inhibited by tetracycline (127). Some questions have been raised regarding tetracycline and doxycycline for treatment of pneumococcus. Doxycycline may be more effective against penicillin-resistant pneumococcus than tetracycline (141). Therefore, both agents should be tested for susceptibility when penicillin resistance is suspected. N. gonorrhoeae tends to be resistant to tetracycline when resistant to penicillin. In 1995, the Centers for Disease Control and Prevention reported 31.6% of N. gonorrhoeae were resistant to both tetracycline and penicillin (39). Chromosomally mediated resistance of N. gonor-

rhoeae to tetracycline was reported at 15.4% in 1995 (39). Of the Gram-negative bacteria, many Enterobacteriaceae are resistant, although the degree of resistance of many E. coli strains may be overcome by achievable concentrations in the urine. Pseudomonas aeruginosa are resistant.

Mechanisms of Resistance

Once microorganisms develop resistance to one tetracycline, this typically confers resistance to the class of drugs. However, there are differences in the extent of resistance among various species. Resistance may be mediated by decreased accumulation of the tetracycline inside the cell or production of proteins that may protect the ribosome to which they bind (149).

Most commonly, resistance occurs when less tetracycline accumulates within the cell. This may occur in two ways. Influx of tetracycline into the cell may decrease or, more likely, efflux of tetracycline from the cell may increase. Tetracycline influx is altered by chromosomal mutations that change the outer membrane pore through which tetracycline diffuses. This alteration also confers low-level resistance to β-lactams, chloramphenicol, and quinolones. Then, when the organism is exposed to tetracycline or chloramphenicol, there is selection for mutations that confer high-level resistance to tetracycline or chloramphenicol, as well as structurally unrelated drugs such as the penicillins, cephalosporins, and quinolones. For tetracycline, high-level resistance is accomplished by antibiotic efflux, mediated by the Tet membrane proteins, resulting in energy-dependent pumping of the drug from the cell. Thus, tetracycline is prevented from accumulating inside the cell, which ultimately protects the ribosome from inhibition (32, 59, 96).

Another mechanism, which has been poorly elucidated, is the biologic or chemical inactivation of tetracyclines by resistant bacteria. Bacteria produce proteins that interact with the ribosome so that protein synthesis may continue despite the presence of tetracycline within the cell. Tetracycline continues to bind to the ribosome but does not appear to inhibit protein synthesis. The mechanism by which this occurs has not been clearly elucidated (21, 93). Most acquired resistance is plasmid mediated and is an inducible trait. It has been common practice to add tetracyclines to animal feed, which may be linked to selective antibiotic pressure for the spread of plasmid-mediated resistance (137, 149).

Methods to Overcome and Prevent Resistance

Approximately 60% of an oral dose of tetracycline is excreted in the urine. Therefore, urinary tract infections with moderately resistant organisms may be adequately treated with usual doses of tetracycline.

PHARMACOKINETIC DISPOSITION (TABLE 3)
Absorption

Absorption of tetracyclines from the gastrointestinal tract ranges from 60 to 80% with demeclocycline and tetracycline to 95% with doxycycline and up to 100% with minocycline. Absorption occurs primarily in the stomach and upper small intestine. In general, the proportion of tetracycline that is not absorbed increases with increasing doses (8, 92, 109).

Food Effects

Doxycycline and minocycline appear to be adequately absorbed in fasting and nonfasting states. The other derivatives, however, have the greatest absorption when taken on an empty stomach. Absorption decreases by 50% or more for tetracycline and demeclocycline taken with food. Doxycycline and minocycline absorption decreases by less than 20%, which does not appear to be clinically relevant (87, 91). In fact, patients are often instructed to take doxycycline with food or milk to decrease gastrointestinal discomfort associated with the drug.

Multivalent Cations

Tetracyclines chelate with multivalent cations (i.e., aluminum, calcium, iron, magnesium), resulting in decreased absorption. Leyden (87) compared the absorption of tetracycline and minocycline given with iron and found an 81 and 77% decrease, respectively. Demeclocycline has the highest affinity for calcium ions, resulting in a decrease in absorption of at least 50% when given concurrently with compounds containing calcium or other multivalent cations (95). Thus, concurrent administration of agents containing divalent and trivalent cations (i.e., iron products, antacids, sucralfate, didanosine) should be avoided with all the tetracyclines.

Achlorhydria

Elderly patients with achlorhydria were studied to compare rates of absorption. There appeared to be no difference in rate or extent of absorption of tetracyclines in these patients.

Serum Concentrations

Peak serum concentrations of the tetracyclines occur within 1 to 4 h of oral administration and within 30 min of intravenous administration. The wide variation in oral absorption of tetracyclines is presumably due to differences in individual rates of gastrointestinal absorption. A single oral tetracycline dose of 500 mg achieves peak serum concentrations of 3 to 4 μg/mL (152). A single oral 200-mg dose of doxycycline or minocycline achieves peak serum concentrations of approximately 1.5 to 2.5 μg/mL. A single 200-mg intravenous loading dose of doxycycline or minocycline produces peak serum concentrations of approximately 4 to 10 μg/mL (4). Serum concentrations for doxycycline appear to be slightly higher in geriatric patients than in younger patients. This difference probably reflects decreased renal function in the elderly (158). Serum concentrations for both oral and intravenous administration may increase slightly with continued administration.

TABLE 3 • Pharmacokinetic Parameters

Drug	% GI Absorption (fasting)	C_{max} (serum) (μg/mL)	T_{max} (h)	$T_{1/2}$ (h)	$t_{1/2}$ (renal failure) (h)	% Serum Protein Binding	Apparent Volume of Distribution (L/kg)	Renal Clearance (mL/min/1.73 m²)	% Urinary Recovery	% Fecal Recovery
Tetracycline	75–80	1.5–5[a]	2–4	6–12	57–120	20–65	108	74	48–60	
Demeclocycline	60–80	0.9–1.7[b]	3–4	10–17	42–68	36–91	121	35	44	31
Doxycycline	90–100	1.5–3.6[c] 4–10[d]	1.5–4	14–24	18–30	60–95	50	20	20–42	20–40
Minocycline	90–100	2–3.5[e]	1–4	11–26	12–30	55–76	60	9	4–19	20–34

[a] 500 mg oral dose.

[b] 300 mg oral dose.

[c] 200 mg oral dose.

[d] 200 mg intravenous dose.

[e] 200 mg oral dose.

Distribution

Protein binding differs among the various compounds. Doxycycline has the highest (90%) protein binding, followed by minocycline (76%), demeclocycline (70%), then tetracycline (65%). Tetracyclines penetrate well into many tissues and body fluids. Penetration differs depending on the lipid solubility of each compound. Doxycycline is 5 times more lipophilic and minocycline is 10 times more lipophilic than tetracycline (46, 92). Bocker et al. (16) evaluated tissue penetration of doxycycline in the elderly and concluded that it was not affected by age.

Tetracyclines readily accumulate in the reticuloendothelial cells of the spleen, liver, and bone marrow. They are also found in bone and teeth, which may result in toxicity. Tetracyclines are believed to be sequestered by the liver. This results in an apparent volume of distribution that generally exceeds extracellular body water. Tetracyclines are distributed in the bile and undergo enterohepatic circulation, resulting in concentrations in bile 2 to 32 times that of serum (46).

Minocycline crosses the blood-brain barrier to the greatest extent, followed by doxycycline and tetracycline. Penetration depends upon lipid solubility. Cerebrospinal fluid concentrations of tetracyclines are approximately 10 to 26% of that in the serum and increase with inflammation of the meninges (3).

Doxycycline and minocycline penetrate and persist in secretions of the respiratory tract and prostate (18, 106, 144). Due to minocycline's high lipid solubility, it can reach high enough concentrations in tears and saliva to eradicate carriage of meningococcus, a characteristic that is not shared by other members of this class (68). Concentrations of these drugs in the maxillary sinus, gynecologic tissues, and synovial fluid approximate that of serum (41, 89, 164). Tetracyclines also penetrate aqueous humor and seminal fluid at adequate inhibitory concentrations (60, 79). Periodontal and gingival tissue concentrations approach that in the serum (31, 142).

These agents cross the placenta, achieving concentrations in the umbilical-cord plasma of 60% and the amniotic fluid of 20% of that in the maternal circulation. This results in accumulation in fetal bone and teeth (19). Tetracyclines are also found in relatively high concentrations in human breast milk.

However, concentrations in the infant are below the lower level of detectable in the breast-fed infant. Some clinicians attribute this to chelation of tetracycline by calcium present in high concentrations in breast milk (19, 104).

Metabolism and Excretion

The primary route of elimination for tetracycline is the kidney via glomerular filtration. Approximately 60% of an oral dose of tetracycline is excreted in urine; therefore, it should be avoided in patients with renal insufficiency. Demeclocycline is renally cleared at a rate about half that of tetracycline. The primary route of elimination for doxycycline is the intestinal tract. Up to 90% of an oral dose of doxycycline is excreted in feces as a result of inactivation by chelate formation (92). Only 19 to 23% is eliminated through the kidneys by glomerular filtration. Minocycline is metabolized to a considerable extent by the liver to form at least six inactive metabolites. The parent compound is found in low concentrations in feces, and only 4 to 9% of a dose is excreted via the kidneys (75, 92). Doxycycline appears to be safe to use in patients with hepatic or renal insufficiency, but caution should be exercised since it can cause hepatic damage.

DOSAGE REGIMENS

The tetracyclines may be given orally, intravenously, or intramuscularly. The intramuscular route of administration is rarely indicated; it is extremely painful and produces lower serum concentrations than the oral route. Oral administration is preferred. Tetracycline is no longer recommended for intravenous therapy. The injection form of tetracycline is still commercially available but should only be used as a sclerosing preparation. Doxycycline and possibly minocycline may be given intravenously when oral administration is not possible (95).

Normal (Table 4)

Tetracyclines should not be used during the period of tooth development (up to age 8 years) because of the possibility of permanent tooth discoloration. The tetracyclines have also been associated with retardation of bone development during this period. The degree of damage appears to be dose and duration

TABLE 4 • Standard Doses		
Drug	**Adult Range**	**Pediatric Range (children above 8 years of age)**[a]
Tetracycline	1–2 g/day in 2–4 divided doses 500 mg for sclerosing	25–50 mg/kg/day in 2–4 divided doses or 0.6–1.2 mg/m² in 2–4 divided doses
Demeclocycline	150 mg every 6 h 300 mg every 12 h SIADH—600–1200 mg/day in 3–4 divided doses	 6.6–13.2 mg/kg/day in 2–4 divided doses or 300 mg/m² in 2–4 divided doses
Doxycycline	100–200 mg/day given in 1–2 divided doses 500 mg for sclerosing	 2.2–4.4 mg/kg/day in 1–2 divided doses
Minocycline	100–200 mg/day in two divided doses or 50 mg every 6 h	 2–4 mg/kg divided every 12 h

[a] Tetracyclines are contraindicated in children less than 8 years of age.

dependent. However, short courses of tetracyclines may be essential for treatment of certain disease states (i.e., Rocky Mountain spotted fever) in this age group. Recommended pediatric doses are generally for children 8 years of age and older (128–130).

Renal Failure (Table 5)

With the exception of doxycycline and possibly minocycline, the tetracyclines should not be used in patients with end-stage renal disease (12). The tetracyclines appear to be toxic at higher serum concentrations, which may occur in patients with renal failure. Doxycycline is eliminated primarily through the gastrointestinal tract in patients with renal failure, reducing this possibility. Neither dose nor frequency of administration of doxycycline requires modification (97, 163).

The tetracyclines are removed to a small degree by hemodialysis. However, removal by hemodialysis does not appear to be clinically relevant; thus, dosage adjustments are not recommended. Similarly no dosage adjustments are necessary with peritoneal dialysis or continuous hemofiltration (12, 85–86).

Hepatic Failure

Tetracycline causes a protein catabolic effect that may require hepatic metabolism to reduce the endogenous nitrogen load. This process may be impaired in patients with hepatic damage. Doxycycline has not been demonstrated to have this catabolic or antianabolic effect. Serum concentrations of the tetracyclines are not known to increase in patients with hepatic disease (55, 70). However, because of the inherent ability of the tetracyclines to cause hepatic damage (159), caution should be exercised when tetracyclines are indicated in patients with pre-existing hepatic damage. If indicated, doxycycline would be the preferred agent.

Obesity

Tetracyclines are lipophilic drugs (95). The degree to which these agents distribute into fat tissue is unclear. Currently, there are no recommendations for alterations in dosages in this patient population.

Malnutrition

Raghuram and Krishnaswamy (132) studied the pharmacokinetic profile of intravenous doxycycline in undernourished men and found a decrease in plasma protein binding, decreased area under the plasma concentration time curve, increased total body clearance, and a shortened plasma half-life.

Despite these pharmacokinetic changes, they concluded that an alteration in dosage was not necessary.

Pregnancy

Tetracyclines are U.S. FDA pregnancy risk category D. They are not recommended for use in pregnant women because of the possibility of fetal toxicity manifested as retardation of skeletal development in the fetus. They also concentrate in the dentin and enamel of developing teeth resulting in permanent discoloration of the teeth (19). A recent report by Czeizel and Rockenbauer (36) attempted to determine the teratogenicity associated with doxycycline. Case-control surveillance from 1980 to 1992 revealed an overall congenital abnormality rate of 0.30% in the study group, compared with 0.19% in the control group ($P = .01$). The difference in congenital abnormality was primarily evident in the first trimester. The analysis did not show a significantly higher rate in the doxycycline-treated group when the drug was given in the second or third trimester. The authors concluded that doxycycline poses little risk to the fetus in the second and third trimesters and, therefore, may be used when necessary during the second or third trimester of pregnancy. We suggest extreme caution when using any tetracycline during pregnancy.

ADVERSE EFFECTS

Gastrointestinal

Tetracyclines produce an irritating effect in the gastrointestinal mucosa of many patients. This effect is most common after oral administration and includes epigastric burning, abdominal discomfort, nausea, vomiting, and anorexia. Gastrointestinal effects appear to depend on dose, with the amount of absorption inversely related to dose. Tetracycline is not as well absorbed as doxycycline and therefore leaves more residual drug in the gut to cause these effects (49, 100). Food may alleviate the symptoms associated with use of tetracycline or demeclocycline but may also decrease absorption by up to 50%. An alternative approach is to give doxycycline, which may be taken with food. This makes it more tolerable and does not significantly decrease serum concentrations of the agent. Alterations in the bowel flora from tetracyclines result in large bulky stools and diarrhea (51, 67, 100). Diarrhea associated with tetracyclines typically subsides when the agent is discontinued. However, diarrhea that continues or diarrhea associated with fever and a rising white blood cell count should be investigated further. The most serious consequences of this may be pseudomembranous colitis caused by *Clostridium difficile* (61). In earlier literature, an overgrowth of *S. aureus* re-

TABLE 5 • Dosage Adjustment in Renal Insufficiency[a]			
Drug	Normal Dose (CrCl >50 mL/min)	CrCl 10–50 mL/min	CrCl < 10 mL/min
Tetracycline	250–500 mg q.i.d.	250–500 mg b.i.d. q.d.	250–500 mg q.d.[b]
Doxycycline	100 mg q.d. b.i.d.	Same	Same
Minocycline	100 mg b.i.d.	Same	Same

[a] CrCl, creatinine clearance.

[b] Tetracycline is not recommended for use in patients with CrCl < 10 mL/min.

sulting in severe diarrhea, dehydration, and possibly circulatory collapse was reported (90).

Esophagitis and esophageal ulcers have been associated with tetracycline, doxycycline, and minocycline use. Capsules, especially those not enteric coated, are more commonly associated with ulcers than the tablet formulation. The severity of ulceration appears also to depend on the salt of the compound. The hydrochloride or hyclate is more acidic than the monohydrate formulation and can cause more severe ulceration. Endoscopy typically reveals one or more esophageal ulcers. Symptoms may occur within the first day to more than a week after initiation of therapy. Patients complain of a substernal or retrosternal burning pain with dysphagia that is exacerbated by swallowing and hiccups. Symptoms are often self-limiting with discontinuation of therapy. If further intervention is needed, patients may be treated with antacids, sucralfate, or H_2 antagonists. Early cases of this phenomenon appeared to occur in patients taking the drug at bedtime with small amounts of water. Therefore, these antibiotics should be taken with plenty of fluids and not immediately before bedtime. They should be used with caution in patients with esophageal obstruction or motility disorders, since these patients may be at increased risk (5, 15, 17, 35, 38, 76, 138).

Candidal superinfections in the anogenital region may result from alteration in bowel flora (150). These superinfections generally occur with prolonged therapy and/or in debilitated patients. Topical antifungal agents may be used to alleviate symptoms. In patients not responding to topical preparations, an oral imidazole agent (i.e., ketoconazole, fluconazole) may be used. Pancreatitis has also been reported with tetracycline use. Onset may be within days to months to years of continued use (42, 115).

Effects on Teeth and Bone

Deposition of tetracyclines in the teeth and bones appears to result from chelate formation of tetracycline with calcium (101). The tetracyclines cause an initial yellow discoloration that eventually leads to a gray-brown permanent discoloration of the teeth. The degree of discoloration appears to be dose related, with longer (>10 days) or frequent courses (>3 g) of tetracyclines causing darker discoloration. This effect is more prominent in the primary teeth than in the larger, thicker, and more opaque permanent teeth. Tetracyclines also cause hypoplasia of the enamel (52, 140). The concern is not only cosmetic. Deposition of tetracycline in the teeth, causing demineralization, may predispose an individual to increased tooth decay. Doxycycline does not bind serum calcium to the extent of tetracycline (19 versus 40%) (77). Therefore, doxycycline may be an alternative when a tetracycline is unavoidable for therapy in children under 8 years of age, such as may be the case when treating a single episode of Rocky Mountain spotted fever. Minocycline has been reported to cause teeth discoloration in adults who were taking the agent for acne. The mechanism is believed to be chelate formation with iron resulting in insoluble complexes (10, 25, 125).

Kucers and Bennett (80) reported deposition of tetracycline in the skeleton of fetuses and young children. They found that

tetracycline use resulted in skeletal growth retardation of as much as 40%, which was reversible when the agent was removed.

Bhagavan (13) reported a woman who died of acute hemorrhagic pancreatitis and disseminated intravascular coagulation during pregnancy. She had reportedly used tetracycline for acne prior to her pregnancy but none during pregnancy. Bone analysis revealed trace quantities of tetracycline, indicating that tetracycline may be stored in the bone indefinitely and released with increased bone turnover as in pregnancy.

Hepatotoxicity

Hepatotoxicity is rare but often fatal when it occurs. Hepatotoxicity occurs more frequently with tetracycline and minocycline and is rarely reported with doxycycline use (159). Tetracycline-induced intrahepatic cholestasis and ductopenia typically have occurred in patients receiving more than 2 g/day, those on intravenous therapy, and/or pregnant women (139, 159, 162). Also, patients receiving other hepatotoxic drugs or those with preexisting hepatic and/or renal disease are at higher risk. Patients with renal failure were found to have increased serum concentrations and subsequent hepatic damage, attributed to the tetracycline (121, 139). Clinical symptoms may occur 4 to 10 days after initiation of therapy and manifest as nausea, vomiting, and abdominal pain. Jaundice typically occurs much later, followed by azotemia, acidosis, and irreversible shock in rare cases. The hepatic damage is due to inhibition of lipid transport from the liver, resulting in a fine droplet fatty metamorphosis in the liver. Therapy should be discontinued at onset of symptoms. Some patients have been treated with steroid therapy (63, 69, 88, 121, 139). Doxycycline does not appear to have the same profile and is considered safe in patients with hepatic or renal insufficiency. Patients also may experience transient increases in liver function tests without hepatic failure, which is reversible upon discontinuation of therapy (98, 159).

Renal Toxicity

Tetracyclines inhibit protein synthesis, thereby causing a catabolic effect on amino acid metabolism that may exacerbate azotemia in patients with preexisting renal dysfunction. Patients may or may not exhibit an increased serum concentration of tetracycline that does not correlate with the increase in BUN (126). Very little doxycycline is eliminated via the kidneys, therefore, this effect is negligible.

Demeclocycline has been used to induce nephrogenic diabetes insipidus and can reverse the syndrome of inappropriate antidiuretic hormone secretion (SIADH). Patients experience polyuria, polydipsia, and weakness. It may take up to 5 days for diuresis to occur, with resolution within 2 to 6 days after discontinuation (95). The drug has little value in patients with acute water intoxication and should only be given to patients with chronic SIADH.

In the past, expired tetracycline has been associated with a Fanconi-like syndrome and renal tubular acidosis. Patients had nausea, vomiting, polydipsia, polyuria, acidosis, proteinuria, glucosuria, hyperphosphaturia, hypercalciuria, and aminoaciduria. Upon discontinuation, symptoms typically resolved within weeks to a year. These effects resulted from toxic effects of the outdated tetracycline on the proximal renal tubules. Analysis revealed formation of three degradation metabolites. Citric acid, an excipient, was found to accelerate deterioration of tetracycline under storage. Current formulations of tetracycline do not contain citric acid (11, 103). Removal of this excipient has virtually eliminated the possibility of this event with current formulations.

Photosensitivity and Hyperpigmentation

Photosensitivity reactions appearing in severity from a red rash to blistering on sun-exposed areas are most common with demeclocycline but may occur with any of the tetracyclines (3, 10, 43, 54). This reaction may occur within minutes to hours of sun exposure and may persist for 1 to 2 days after discontinuation of the drug. Some patients report similar reactions upon reexposure to the sun in the absence of tetracycline use. The drug is phototoxic, and photosensitivity results from accumulation of the drug in the skin. Patients may also experience photoonycholysis (53, 84, 133). These effects may be minimized by avoiding exposure to UV light or wearing protective clothing with appropriate sunscreen if sun exposure is expected. Minocycline and doxycycline also have rarely been associated with increased pigmentation of the nails, skin, and sclera, presumably as a result of minocycline degradation or a drug-hemosiderin complex. Upon discontinuation, pigmented areas should return to normal within 1 to 5 months (9, 22, 118, 120). Blue or blue-black discoloration of the gums has been reported and appears to be secondary to bone pigmentation that is visible through the nonpigmented oral mucosal tissues. This has been described as "black-blue disease." The incidence of discoloration increases with exposure to the agent. The surrounding areas—teeth, gingiva, tongue, bucca mucosa, and skin—do not appear to be affected. The pigmentation, although less intense, is permanent (24, 116, 143).

Hypersensitivity

Skin reactions are not common with tetracyclines but may manifest as urticaria, morbilliform rashes, exfoliative dermatitis, fixed drug eruptions and periorbital edema. The mechanism of action is unknown. Other rare reactions include anaphylaxis, Stevens-Johnson syndrome, exacerbation of lupus erythematosus, polyarthralgia, and serum sickness–like syndrome. Cross-sensitization occurs with this class of antibiotics; therefore, anyone reporting an allergy to one agent should be considered allergic to all tetracyclines (95).

Miscellaneous

Minocycline has been associated with vertigo (21–90%), which appears to be dose related. Patients complain of dizziness, ataxia, tinnitus, nausea, and vomiting. These effects generally begin on the second or third day of therapy and resolve within 24 to 48 h after discontinuation of the drug. Women (70%) more so than men (28%) experience this effect. If patients report similar complaints, the drug should be discontinued immediately (47, 57).

Pseudotumor cerebri, a benign condition in which there is intracranial hypertension and bulging of the fontanels, has been described in young infants (50, 119). This condition rarely occurs in older patients, although it has been noted in young adolescents taking 1 to 2 g/day of tetracycline for acne (78). Patients complain of lethargy, ataxia, headache, diplopia, and photophobia. Eye examination may reveal bilateral papilledema. Symptoms may develop within 2 weeks to 6 months of therapy and usually resolve upon discontinuation of the drug; however, permanent sequelae may occur. If treatment is needed, acetazolamide or dexamethasone may be used (99, 122, 154).

Hematologic effects are rare but may include hemolytic anemia, thrombocytopenia, eosinophilia, and neutropenia (95).

There have been several cases of thyroid discoloration or "thyroid blackening" with the use of doxycycline and minocycline. The mechanism has not been elucidated but is postulated to be secondary to neuromelanin or lipofuscin. This appears to occur after prolonged use and does not seem to affect thyroid function tests (6, 14, 66, 135).

Thrombophlebitis frequently occurs with intravenous administration. To avoid this irritation, administration sites should be rotated, and large volumes of fluid should be used for dilution. In severe cases, administration by central line should be considered. Due to this effect, tetracyclines have also been used as sclerosing agents in patients with malignant pleural effusions, with the drug instilled directly into the pleural space (95).

A Jarisch-Herxheimer reaction may occur in patients being treated for spirochetal infections (*B. recurrentis,* Lyme disease, syphilis) or brucellosis. Patients experiencing headache, fever, chills, malaise, arthralgias, and/or exacerbation of cutaneous lesions within 12 to 24 h of initiation of tetracycline therapy should be instructed to take aspirin and stay in bed until symptoms resolve (95). All patients should be cautioned about these effects and counseled appropriately for resolution of symptoms.

Between 1972 and 1996, at least 33 cases of a systemic lupus erythematous–like syndrome were reported in association with minocycline. These case reports describe patients as having antinuclear antibody arthralgias/arthritis, lupus, lupuslike symptoms, or systemic lupus erythematosus. These patients were all young and had no other reported causes for these symptoms. Symptoms disappear in most patients within 2 days to 3 months. All patients who were rechallenged with minocycline experienced recurrence of their symptoms (23, 63, 108, 146).

DRUG INTERACTIONS (TABLE 6)

Multivalent Cations

Multivalent cations (aluminum, magnesium, calcium, iron, zinc) decrease oral absorption of tetracyclines as a result of chelate formation. Coadministration of these drugs has resulted in a 30 to 90% reduction in serum concentrations of the tetracyclines. Therefore, patients taking compounds containing multivalent cations such as antacids, multivitamins, didanosine, or sucralfate should be cautioned to space administration of the drugs by 2 h (27, 37, 65, 112, 114).

TABLE 6 • **Drug/Drug and Drug/Food Interactions**

Drug	Effect	Recommendation
Antacids, didanosine, sucralfate, multivitamins	Decreased absorption of tetracycline	Space administration by 2 h
Warfarin	Increased warfarin effect	Monitor PT, INR
Kaolin, bismuth subsalicylate	Decreased absorption of tetracycline	Space administration by 2 h
Barbiturates, phenytoin, carbamazepine	Decreased serum concentrations of doxycycline	Use alternative tetracycline
Methoxyflurane anesthesia	Fatal nephrotoxicity	Avoid concomitant therapy
Oral contraceptives	Decreased serum concentrations of oral contraceptive	Use barrier method of birth control during tetracycline therapy
Food	Decreased absorption of tetracycline and demeclocycline	Space administration or use doxycycline
Dairy products (milk)	Decreased absorption of tetracycline, demeclocycline, and minocycline	Space administration or use doxycycline
Ethanol	Decreased serum concentrations of doxycycline	Use alternative tetracycline

Warfarin

Tetracyclines may impair use of prothrombin or decrease vitamin K production by intestinal bacteria, thereby potentiating the effect of warfarin. The effect is delayed, occurring in days to weeks (51, 161). Close monitoring of prothrombin time and international normalized ratios (INRs) is necessary with concomitant therapy. Warfarin dosage may require adjustment to maintain appropriate anticoagulation.

Antidiarrheal Agents

Products containing kaolin and pectin or bismuth subsalicylate may impair absorption of tetracyclines when used concomitantly. This is believed to be due to chelate formation (2, 44). Administration of these agents should be separated by 2 h.

Barbiturates, Phenytoin, Carbamazepine

Barbiturates, phenytoin, and carbamazepine increase hepatic metabolism and decrease the serum half-life of doxycycline, resulting in decreased serum concentrations (110–111). The other tetracyclines do not appear to be affected by these agents; thus, they may be preferred when a tetracycline is indicated.

Methoxyflurane Anesthesia

Concurrent use of tetracyclines and methoxyflurane anesthesia may result in fatal nephrotoxicity. Onset is rapid with oliguria, tachycardia, and dyspnea. Concomitant therapy should be avoided (30, 82).

Oral Contraceptives

Tetracyclines alter intestinal flora, thereby decreasing enterohepatic recirculation of oral contraceptives. Concurrent usage results in lowered plasma concentrations of ethinyl estradiol and norethindrone. Women have reported unintended pregnancies and menstrual irregularities (7, 105, 155, 157). Women should be counseled to use an additional form of birth control (i.e., barrier method) during concomitant therapy.

Food

Food decreases absorption of tetracycline by up to 65% and minocycline by 13% (87). Food has a negligible affect on doxycycline absorption. Patients should be cautioned to take tetracycline and perhaps minocycline on an empty stomach to maximize absorption.

Dairy Products

Milk and other dairy products reduce tetracycline absorption by 50 to 81% and reduce minocycline absorption by 27% (87). Dairy products have little affect on doxycycline absorption. Patients should be counseled to space administration of dairy products and tetracycline or minocycline by 2 h.

Ethanol

The half-life of doxycycline is reduced in long-term alcoholic patients, resulting in decreased serum concentrations. This phenomenon has not been observed with the other tetracyclines. This is postulated to be due to induction of hepatic microsomal enzymes by chronic ingestion of ethanol (113). Doxycycline should not be used in long-term alcoholic patients. An alternative tetracycline should be used in these patients.

CLINICAL INDICATIONS

Because of their broad spectrum, tetracyclines are used for a wide variety of infections encountered in the United States and the world. Additionally, tetracyclines may be used as alternatives when therapy with the drugs of choice is not feasible (i.e., allergy to the β-lactams, sulfas, or quinolones).

Table 7 lists many of the indications for which tetracyclines are the drugs of choice or alternatives. Readers are referred to other chapters for more detail on the various disease states. For the treatment of most diseases, tetracycline and doxycycline are interchangeable. Doxycycline is often the drug of choice for many reasons. Doxycycline is only given twice a day, it has

TABLE 7 • Clinical Indications

Therapy of Choice	Alternative Therapy
Rickettsial infections	*Mycoplasma pneumoniae*
Epidemic (louse-borne) typhus	Spirochetal infections
Brill-Zinsser disease	*Treponemal pallidum* (syphilis)
Scrub typhus	Leptospirosis
Rocky Mountain spotted fever	*Treponema pertenue* (Yaws)
Endemic (murine) Typhus	Pinta
Q Fever	Bejel
Rickettsial pox	*Helicobacter pylori* (tetracycline)
Chlamydial infections	Traveler's diarrhea
Chlamydial trachomatis (uncomplicated)	Enterotoxigenic *E. coli*
Lymphogranuloma venereum	Shigella
Trachoma and inclusion conjunctivitis	Salmonella
Chlamydial psittacosis pneumonia	Campylobacter spp.
Spirochetal infections	*Plasmodium falciparum* (malaria)
Lyme—*Borrelia burgdorferi*	*Mycobacteria marinum* (minocycline)
Tick-borne (endemic) relapsing fever	Gram-negative bacteria
Louse-borne (epidemic) relapsing fever	*Yersinia pestis* (plague)
Leptospirosis (military prophylaxis)	*Francisella tularensis* (tularemia) + streptomycin
Balantidium coli	*Campylobacter fetus*
Gram-negative bacteria	*Leptotrichia buccalis* (Vincent's infection)
Brucellosis (with streptomycin or gentamicin)	Chancroid
Bartonella bacilliformis	*Spirillum minus* (rat-bite fever)
Calymmatobacterium granulomatis	*Streptobacillus moniliformis* (Haverhill fever)
Vibrio cholerae (tetracycline)	*Pasteurella multocida*
Vibrio vulnificus (tetracycline + aminoglycoside)	Pertussis
Pseudomonas pseudomallei	*Legionella pneumophilia*
(meliodosis) ± chloramphenicol	Gram-positive bacteria
Pseudomonas mallei (glanders) + streptomycin	*Listeria monocytogenes* (anthrax)
Neisseria meningitidis prophylaxis (minocycline)	*Clostridium perfringens* and *tetani*
Acne vulgaris	Actinomycosis
Urethral syndrome, acute	Nocardiosis
Epididymitis, acute (sexually transmitted)	Chronic bronchitis
Pelvic inflammatory disease (with cefoxitin or cefotetam)	
Urethritis, nonspecific	

fewer gastrointestinal side effects, and it may be taken with food or milk. It also is the preferred agent for intravenous administration. When a specific tetracycline is preferred, it is indicated in the table.

Rickettsial Infections

The tetracyclines are particularly useful for rickettsial infections (134). As little as a single dose has been effective for epidemic (louse-borne) typhus, Brill-Zinsser disease, and possibly scrub typhus (20, 136, 148, 153). Patients often have a clinical response within a day of initiating therapy for rickettsial infections.

Sexually Transmitted Diseases

Tetracyclines are very effective in the treatment of many chlamydial diseases. The Centers for Disease Control and Prevention (CDC) along with the Public Health Service recommend doxycycline as the drug of choice for lymphogranuloma venereum (LGV); nongonococcal urethritis (commonly caused by *C. trachomatis* or *Ureaplasma urealyticum*); uncomplicated urethral, endocervical, or rectal *C. trachomatis* infections; pelvic inflammatory disease (with cefoxitin or cefotetam); and

epididymitis (with ceftriaxone). Doxycycline may also be used as an alternative to penicillin in patients with syphilis who have an allergy to penicillin. A controversial area of therapy is the use of doxycycline with ceftriaxone and metronidazole as prophylaxis against sexually transmitted diseases in sexual assault victims (26). Some physicians prefer to withhold therapy until there is an obvious indication for treatment.

Spirochetal Infections

Doxycycline is the drug of choice for early Lyme disease *(Borrelia burgdorferi)* and an alternative in later forms of the disease (myocarditis, arthritis) (151). Tetracyclines are the drug of choice for tick-borne (endemic) or louse-borne (epidemic) relapsing fever caused by *Borrelia*. They are alternatives to penicillin for other spirochetal infections such as yaws, pinta, and leptospirosis. Tetracyclines have been used as prophylaxis against leptospirosis in military recruits (29, 48, 73).

Bacillary Infections

Tetracyclines in combination with rifampin or streptomycin/gentamicin is considered the therapy of choice for acute or chronic infections caused by *Brucella* spp. (1, 33, 147). Tetracycline is the drug of choice for treatment of *Vibrio cholerae* (62, 64). Tetracycline in combination with an aminoglycoside is highly effective against *V. vulnificus*. Doxycycline has been used as prophylaxis for traveler's diarrhea caused by *Shigella, Salmonella,* or other *Enterobacteriaceae* (45). However, due to the growing prevalence of resistance to the tetracyclines, this is not typically recommended.

Other Infections

Minocycline has been used to eradicate nasopharynx carriage of *Neisseria meningitidis* (68). Minocycline and tetracycline have been used both topically and orally as therapy for moderate-to-severe inflammatory acne vulgaris (56). Doxycycline in combination with other agents is now being used as an alternative therapy for vancomycin-resistant enterococci (VRE) (102).

Other Indications

The tetracyclines have been used as sclerosing agents to control pleural effusions caused by metastatic tumors and pericardial effusions associated with cardiac tamponade (160). The tetracycline is administered by intracavitary or intrapericardial injections. Administration of the tetracycline into the chest tube is associated with chest pain and fever. Patients should receive opiates for pain control. Lidocaine is often administered into the chest tube along with the tetracycline for further pain control.

Minocycline has been studied in double-blind placebo-controlled trials for palliative therapy for rheumatoid arthritis (117, 123). These studies reported minocycline (100 mg twice daily) to be effective palliative therapy for early (within the first year of disease) seropositive rheumatoid arthritis.

REFERENCES

1. Acocella G, Bertrand A, Beytout J, Durrande JB, Garcia-Rodriguez G, Kosmidis J, Micoud M, Rey M, Rodriguez-Zapata M, Roux J. Comparison of three different regimens in the treatment of acute brucellosis: a multicenter multinational study. J Antimicrob Chemother 1989;23:433–439.
2. Albert KS, Welch RD, DeSante KA, DiSanto AR. Decreased tetracycline bioavailability caused by a bismuth subsalicylate antidiarrheal mixture. J Pharm Sci 1979;68:586–588.
3. Allen JC. Minocycline. Ann Intern Med 1976;85:482–487.
4. Alestig K. Studies on doxycycline during intravenous and oral treatment with reference to renal function. Scand J Infect Dis 1973;5:193–198.
5. Amendola MA, Spera TD. Doxycycline-induced esophagitis. JAMA 1985;253:1009–1011.
6. Attwood HD, Dennett X. A black thyroid and minocycline treatment. Br Med J 1976;2:1109–1110.
7. Back DJ, Breckenridge AM, Crawford FE, Maelver M, Orme ML, Rowe PH. Interindividual variation and drug interactions with hormonal steroid contraceptives. Drugs 1981;21:46–61.
8. Barr WH, Gerbracht LM, Letcher K, Plaut M, Strahl N. Assessment of the biologic availability of tetracycline products in man. Clin Pharmacol Ther 1972;13:97–108.
9. Basler RS. Minocycline-related hyperpigmentation. Arch Dermatol 1985;121:606–608.
10. Beehner ME, Houston GE, Young JD. Oral pigmentation secondary to minocycline therapy. J Oral Maxillofac Surg 1986;44:582–584.
11. Benitz KF, Diermeir HF. Renal toxicity of tetracycline products. Soc Exp Biol Med 1964;115:930–935.
12. Bennett WM, Aronoff GR, Golper TA, Morrison G, Singer I, Brater DC, eds. Drug prescribing in renal failure. 4th ed. Philadelphia: American College of Physicians, 1994.
13. Bhagavan BS, Wenk RE, McCarthy EF, Gebhardt FC, Lustgarten JA. Long-term use of tetracycline [Letter]. JAMA 1982;247:2780.
14. Billano RA, Ward WQ, Little WP. Minocycline and black thyroid. JAMA 1983;249:1887.
15. Biller JA, Flores A, Bule T, Mazor S, Katz AJ. Tetracycline-induced esophagitis in adolescent patients. J Pediatr 1992;120:144–145.
16. Bocker R, Muhlberg W, Platt D, Estler CJ. Serum level, half-life and apparent volume of distribution of doxycycline in geriatric patients. Eur J Clin Pharmacol 1986;30:105–108.
17. Bokey L, Hugh TB. Oesophageal ulceration associated with doxycycline therapy. Med J Aust 1975;1:236–237.
18. Braga PC. Antibiotic penetrability into bronchial mucus: pharmacokinetics and clinical considerations. Curr Ther Res 1991;49: 300–327.
19. Briggs GG, Freeman RK, Yaffe SJ. Drugs in pregnancy and lactation. 4th ed. Baltimore: Williams & Wilkins, 1994:808–811.
20. Brown GW, Saunders JP, Singh S, Huxsoll DL, Shirai A. Single dose doxycycline therapy for scrub typhus. Trans R Soc Trop Med Hyg 1978;72:412–416.
21. Burdett V. Purification and characterization of Tet(M), a protein that renders ribosomes resistant to tetracycline. J Biol Chem 1991;266:2872–2877.
22. Butler JM, Marks R, Sutherland R. Cutaneous and cardiac valvular pigmentation with minocycline. Clin Exp Dermatol 1985;10:432–437.
23. Byrne PAC, Williams BD, Pritchard MH. Minocycline-related lupus. Br J Rheumatol 1994;33:674–676.
24. Cale AE, Freedman PD, Lumerman H. Pigmentation of the jawbones and teeth secondary to minocycline hydrochloride therapy. J Periodontol 1988;59:112–114.
25. Caro I. Discolorations of the teeth related to minocycline therapy for acne. J Am Acad Dermatol 1980;3:317–318.
26. Centers for Disease Control and Prevention. 1993 Guidelines for the treatment of Sexually transmitted diseases. MMWR 1998;47 (No RR-1):27–86.
27. Chin TF, Lach JL. Drug diffusion and bioavailability: tetracycline metallic chelation. Am J Hosp Pharm 1975;32:625–629.
28. Chopra I, Hawkey PM, Hinton M. Tetracyclines, molecular and clinical aspects. J Antimicrob Chemother 1992;29:245–277.
29. Chulay JD. Treponema species (yaws, pinta, bejel). In: Mandell GL, Bennett JE, Dolin R, eds. Mandell, Douglas and Bennett's principles and practice of infectious diseases. New York: Churchill Livingstone, 1995:2133–2137.
30. Churchill D. Persisting renal insufficiency after methoxyflurane anesthesia. Report of two cases and review of literature. Am J Med 1974;56:575–582.
31. Ciancio S, Slots J, Reynolds HS. The effect of short-term administration of minocycline HCl on gingival inflammation and subgingival microflora. J Periodontal 1982;53:557–561.
32. Cohen SP, McMurry LM, Hooper DC, Wolfson JS, Levy SB. Cross-resistance to fluoroquinolones in multiple-antibiotic-resistant (Mar) *Escherichia coli* selected by tetracycline or

chloramphenicol: decreased drug accumulation associated with membrane changes in addition to OmpF reduction. Antimicrob Agents Chemother 1989;33:1318–1325.

33. Colmenero JD, Fernandez-Gallardo LC, Agundez JA, Sedeno J, Benitez J, Valverde E. Possible implications of doxycycline-rifampin interaction for treatment of brucellosis. Antimicrob Agents Chemother 1994;38:2798–2802.

34. Coonan KN, Kaplan EL. In vitro susceptibilities of recent North American group A streptococcal isolates to 11 oral antibiotics. Pediatr Infect Dis J 1995;13:630–635.

35. Crowson TD, Head LH, Ferrante WA. Esophageal ulcers associated with tetracycline therapy. JAMA 1976;235:2747–2748.

36. Czeizel AE, Rockenbauer M. Teratogenic study of doxycycline. Obstet Gynecol 1997;89:524–528.

37. D'Arcy PF, McElnay JC. Drug-antacid interactions: assessment of clinical importance. Drug Intell Clin Pharm 1987;21:607–617.

38. Delpre G, Kadish U. Tetracycline and doxycycline esophageal ulcerations [Letter]. Gastrointest Endosc 1987;33:397–398.

39. Division of STD Prevention. Sexually transmitted disease surveillance, 1995. U.S. Department of Health and Human Services, Public Health Service. Atlanta: Centers for Disease Control and Prevention, September, 1996.

40. Edwards R. Doxycycline and photosensitivity [Letter]. NZ Med J 1987;100:640.

41. Ehrlich GE. Concentrations of tetracycline and minocycline in joint effusions following oral administration. Penn Med 1972; 75:47–49.

42. Elmore MF, Rogge JD. Tetracycline-induced pancreatitis. Gastroenterology 1981;81:1134–1136.

43. Epstein JH, Seibert JS. Porphyria-like cutaneous changes induced by tetracycline hydrochloride photosensitization. Arch Dermatol 1976;112:661–666.

44. Ericsson CD, Feldman S, Pickering LK, Cleary TG. Influence of subsalicylate bismuth on absorption of doxycycline. JAMA 1982;247:2266–2267.

45. Ericsson CD, DuPont HL. Travelers' diarrhea: approaches to prevention and treatment. Clin Infect Dis 1993;16:616–626.

46. Fabre J, Milek ES, Kalfopoulos P, Merier G. The kinetics of tetracycline in man. II. excretion, penetration in normal and inflammatory tissues, behavior in renal insufficiency and hemodialysis. Schweiz Med Wochenschr 1971;101:625–633.

47. Fanning WL, Gump DW, Sofferman RA. Side effects of minocycline: a double-blind study. Antimicrob Agents Chemother 1977;11:712–717.

48. Farrar WE. Leptospira species (leptospirosis). In: Mandell GL, Bennett JE, Dolin R, eds. Mandell, Douglas and Bennett's principles and practice of infectious diseases. New York: Churchill Livingstone, 1995:2137–2141.

49. Fekety FR Jr. Gastrointestinal complications of antibiotic therapy. JAMA 1968;203:21–22.

50. Fields JP. Bulging fontanel: a complication of tetracycline therapy in infants. J Pediatr 1961;58:74.

51. Finegold SM. Interaction of antimicrobial therapy and intestinal flora. Am J Clin Nutr 1970;23:1466–1471.

52. Fleming P, Witkop CJ Jr, Kuhlmann WH. Staining and hypoplasia of enamel caused by tetracycline: case report. Pediatr Dent 1987;9:245–246.

53. Frank SB, Choen HJ, Minkin W. Photo-oncholytic due to tetracycline hydrochloride and doxycycline. Arch Dermatol 1971; 103:520–521.

54. Frost P, Weinstein GD, Gomez EC. Phototoxic potential of minocycline and doxycycline. Arch Dermatol 1972;105:681–683.

55. Gabduza GJ. Some effects of antibiotics on nutrition in man. Arch Intern Med 1958;101:476.

56. Gammon WR, Meyer C, Lantis S, Shenefelt P, Peizner G, Cripps DJ. Comparative efficacy of oral erythromycin versus oral tetracycline in the treatment of acne vulgaris: a double-blind study. J Am Acad Dermatol 1986;14:183–186.

57. Garnier R, Castot A, Louboutin P Muzard D, Conso F. Vestibular-like reactions associated with minocycline. Therapie 1981;36: 313–317.

58. Garrod LP. Causes of failure in antibiotic treatment. Br Med J 1972;4:473–476.

59. George AM, Levy SB. Amplifiable resistance to tetracycline, chloramphenicol, and other antibiotics in *Escherichia coli:* involvement of a non-plasmid-determined efflux of tetracycline. J Bacteriol 1983;155:531–540.

60. Gnarpe H, Friberg J. Mycoplasma and human reproductive failure. II. Concentrations of doxycycline in serum and seminal fluid and the effect on the growth of T-mycoplasms. Am J Obstet Gynecol 1972;114:963–966.

61. Gorbach SL, Bartlett JG. Anaerobic infections. N Engl J Med 1974;290:1289–1294.

62. Gotuzzo E, Seas C, Echevarria J, Carrillo C, Mostorino R, Ruiz R. Ciprofloxacin for the treatment of cholera: a randomized, double-blind, controlled clinical trial of a single daily dose in Peruvian adults. Clin Infect Dis 1995;20:1485–1490.

63. Gough A, Chapman S, Wagstaff K, Emery P, Elias E. Minocycline induced autoimmune hepatitis and systemic lupus erythematosus-like syndrome. Br Med J 1996;312:169–172.

64. Greenough WB III, Gordon RS Jr, Rosenberg IS. Tetracycline in the treatment of cholera. Lancet 1964;1:355–357.

65. Gugler R, Allgayer H. Effects of antacids on the clinical pharmacokinetics of drugs: an update. Clin Pharmacokinet 1990;18: 210–219.

66. Hanzlick R, Wilson R. Minocycline-related black thyroid. Am J Forensic Med & Pathol 1988;9:201–202.

67. Hirsch DC, Burton GC, Clenden DC. Effect of oral tetracycline on the occurrence of tetracycline-resistant strains of *Escherichia coli* in the intestinal tract of humans. Antimicrob Agents Chemother 1973;4:69–71.

68. Hoeprich PD, Warchauer DM. Entry of four tetracyclines into saliva and tears. Antimicrob Agent Chemother 1974;5:330–336.

69. Hunt CM, Washington K. Tetracycline-induced bile duct paucity and prolonged cholestasis. Gastroenterology 1994;107: 1844–1847.

70. Jacobs I. Antibiotics and liver disease. Calif Med 1969;111: 382–387.

71. Jawetz E. The use of combinations of antimicrobial drugs. Annu Rev Pharmacol 1968;8:151–170.

72. Jawetz E. Synergism and antagonism among antimicrobial drugs, a personal perspective. West J Med 1975;123:87–91.

73. Johnson WD Jr. Borrelia species (relapsing fever). In: Mandell GL, Bennett JE, Dolin R, eds. Mandell, Douglas and Bennett's principles and practice of infectious diseases. New York: Churchill Livingstone, 1995:2141–2143.

74. Kabins SA. Interactions among antibiotics and other drugs. JAMA 1972;219:206–212.

75. Kapusnik-Uner JE, Sande MA, Chambers HF. Tetracyclines, chloramphenicol, erythromycin, and miscellaneous antibacterial agents. In: Hardman JG, Limbird LE, Molinoff PB, Ruddon RW, Gilman AG, eds. Goodman & Gilman's the pharmacological basis of therapeutics. New York: McGraw-Hill, 1996:1123–1153.

76. Khera DC, Herschman BR, Sosa F. Tetracycline-induced

esophageal ulcers: report of 2 cases. Postgrad Med 1980;68:113,115.

77. Klein NC, Cunha BA. Tetracyclines. Med Clin North Am 1995;79:789–801.

78. Koch-Weser J, Gilmore EB. Benign intracranial hypertension in adults after tetracycline therapy. JAMA 1967;200:345–347.

79. Krause U, Raunio V, Mustonen E. Aqueous humor penetration of alpha-deoxyoxy-tetracycline (doxycycline) in man. Am J Ophthalmol 1972;74:77–80.

80. Kucers A, Bennett NM. The use of antibiotics, 4th ed. Philadelphia: JB Lippincott, 1987.

81. Kunin CM. A guide to the use of antibiotics in patients with renal disease. Ann Intern Med 1967;67:151–158.

82. Kuzucu EY. Methoxyflurane, tetracycline and renal failure. JAMA 1970;211:1162–1164.

83. Lanza FL. Esophageal ulceration produced by doxycycline. Curr Ther Res 1988;44:475–484.

84. Lasser AE, Steiner MM. Tetracycline photo-oncholysis. Pediatrics 1978;61:98–99.

85. Lee P, Crutch ER, Morrison RB. Doxycycline: studies in normal subjects and patients with renal failure. NZ Med J 1972;75:355–358.

86. Letteri JM, Miraflor F, Tablante V, Siddiqi S. Doxycycline (vibramycin) in chronic renal failure. Nephron 1973;11:318–324.

87. Leyden JJ. Absorption of minocycline hydrochloride and tetracycline hydrochloride: effect of food, milk, and iron. J Am Acad Dermatol 1985;12:308–312.

88. Lloyd-Still JD, Grand RJ, Vowter GF. Tetracycline hepatotoxicity in the differential diagnosis of postoperative jaundice. J Pediatr 1974;84:366–370.

89. Lundberg C. Antibiotics in sinus secretions [Letter]. Lancet 1968;2:107–108.

90. Lundsgaard-Hansen P, Senn A, Roos B. Staphylococcal enteritis: report of six cases with two fatalities after intravenous administration of *N*-(pyrrolidinomethyl) tetracycline. JAMA 1960;173:1008.

91. MacArthur CG, Johnson AJ, Allen ES, Chadwick MV, Wingfield HJ. The absorption and sputum penetration of doxycycline. J Antimicrob Chemother 1978;4:509–514.

92. MacDonald H, Kelly RG, Allen ES, Noble JF, Kanegis LA. Pharmacokinetic studies of minocycline in man. Clin Pharmacol Ther 1973;14:852–861.

93. Manavathu EK, Fernandez CL, Cooperman BS, Taylor DE. Molecular studies on the mechanism of tetracycline resistance mediated by Tet(O). Antimicrob Agents Chemother 1990;34:71–77.

94. McDonald PJ, Craig WA, Kunin CM. Persistent effect of antibiotics on Staphylococcus aureus after exposure for limited periods of time. J Infect Dis 1977;135:217–223.

95. McEvoy GK, Litvak K, Welsh OH Jr, eds. AHFS drug information. Bethesda, MD: American Society of Health-System Pharmacists, 1996.

96. McMurray LM, Petrucci RE, Levy SB. Active efflux of tetracycline encoded by four genetically different tetracycline resistance determinants in *Escherichia coli*. Proc Natl Acad Sci USA 1980;77:3974–3977.

97. Merier G, Laurencet FL, Rudhardt M, Chuit A, Fabre J. Behaviour of doxycycline in renal insufficiency. Helv Med Acta 1969;35:124–134.

98. Min DI, Burke PA, Lewis WD, Jenkins RL. Acute hepatic failure associated with oral minocycline: a case report. Pharmacotherapy 1992;12:68–71.

99. Minutello JS, Dimayuga RG, Carter J. Pseudotumor cerebri, a rare adverse reaction to tetracycline therapy. J Periodontol 1988;59:848–851.

100. Minton NA. The effect of oral tetracycline HCl and doxycycline on the intestinal flora. Curr Ther Res 1970;12:341–352.

101. Moffitt JM, Cooley RO, Olsen ND, Hefferren JJ. Prediction of tetracycline-induced tooth discoloration. J Am Dent Assoc 1974;88:547–552.

102. Montecalvo, MA, Horowitz H, Wormser GP, Seiter K, Carbonaro CA. Effect of novobiocin-containing antimicrobial regimens on infection and colonization with vancomycin-resistant Enterococcus faecium. Antimicrob Agents Chemother 1995;39:794.

103. Montoliu J, Carrera M, Carnell A, Revert L. Lactic acidosis and Fanconi's syndrome due to degraded tetracycline. Br Med J 1981;283:1576–1577.

104. Morganti G, Ceccarelli G, Ciaffi G. Comparative concentrations of a tetracycline antibiotic in serum and maternal milk. Antibiotica 1968;6:216–223.

105. Murphy AA, Zacur HA Charache P, Burkman RT. The effect of tetracycline on levels of oral contraceptives. Am J Obstet Gynecol 1991;164:28–33.

106. Naline E, Sanceaume M, Toty L, Bakdach H, Pays M, Advenier C. Penetration of minocycline into lung tissues. Br J Clin Pharmacol 1991;32:402–404.

107. National Committee for Clinical Laboratory Standards. Sixth informational supplement: performance standards for antimicrobial susceptibility testing: approved standard. NCCLS publ M2-A5, M&-A3, and M11-A3. Villanova, PA: NCCLS, 1995.

108. National Disease and Therapeutic Index. Plymouth Meeting, PA: IMS America LTD, Sept 1996.

109. Neuvonen PJ. Interference of iron with the absorption of tetracycline in man. Br Med J 1970;4:532–534.

110. Neuvonen PJ, Penttila O. Interaction between doxycycline and barbiturates. Br Med J 1974;1:535–536.

111. Neuvonen PJ, Penttila O, Lehtovaara R, Aho K. Effect of antiepileptic drugs on the elimination of various tetracycline derivatives. Eur J Clin Pharmacol 1975;9:147–154.

112. Neuvonen PJ. Interactions with the absorption of tetracyclines. Drugs 1976;11:45–54.

113. Neuvonen PJ, Penttila O, Roos M, Tirkkonen J. Effect of long-term alcohol consumption on the half-life of tetracycline and doxycycline in man. Int J Clin Pharmacol 1976;14:303.

114. Nguyen VX, Nix DE, Gillikin S, Schentag JJ. Effect of oral antacid administration on the pharmacokinetics of intravenous doxycycline. Antimicrob Agents Chemother 1989;33:434–436.

115. Nicolau DP, Mengehoht DE, Kline JJ. Tetracycline-induced pancreatitis. Am J Gastroenterol 1991;86:1669–1671.

116. Odell EW, Hodgson RP, Haskell R. Oral presentation of minocycline-induced black bone disease. Oral Med Oral Pathol Oral Radiol Endod 1995;79:459–461.

117. O'Dell JR, Haure CE, Palmer W, Drymalski W, Weis S, Blakely K, Churchill M, Ecknoff PJ, Weaver A, Doud D, Erickson N, Dietz F, Olson K, Maloley P, Klassen LW, Moore GF. Treatment of early rheumatoid arthritis with minocycline or placebo: results of a randomized, double-blind, placebo-controlled trial. Arthritis Rheum 1997;40:794–796.

118. Okada N, Moriya K, Nishida K, Kitano Y, Kobayashi T, Nishimura H, Aoyama M, Yoshikana K. Skin pigmentation associated with minocycline therapy. Br J Dermatol 1989;121:247–254.

119. Opfer K. The bulging fontanel. Lancet 1963;1:116.

120. Pepine M, Flowers FP, Ramos-Caro FA. Extensive cutaneous hyperpigmentation caused by minocycline. J Am Acad Dermatol 1993;28:292–295.

121. Peters RL, Edmondson HA, Mikkelsen WP, Tatter D. Tetracycline-induced fatty liver in non-pregnant patients. Am J Surg 1967;113:622–632.

122. Pierog SH, Al-Salihi FL, Cinotti D. Pseudotumor cerebri—a complication of tetracycline treatment of acne. J Adolesc Health Care 1986;7:139–140.

123. Pillemer SR, Fowler SE, Tilley BC, Alarcon GS, Heyse SP, Trenham DE, Neuner R, Clegg DO, Leisen JC, Cooper SM, Duncan H, Tuttleman M. Meaningful improvement criteria sets in a rheumatoid arthritis clinical trial. MIRA trial group. Minocycline in rheumatoid arthritis. Arthritis Rheum 1997;40:419–425.

124. Poirier RH, Ellison AC. Ocular penetration of orally administered minocycline. Am Ophthalmol 1979;11/12:1859.

125. Poliak SC, DiGiovanna JJ, Gross EG, Gantt G, Peck GL. Minocycline-associated tooth discoloration in young adults. JAMA 1985;254:2930–2932.

126. Pothier AJ Jr, Anderson EE. Tetracycline-induced azotemia. J Urol 1966;95:16–18.

127. Poulsen RK, Knudsen JC, Petersen MB. In vitro activity of 6 macrolides, clindamycin, and tetracycline on Streptococcus pneumoniae with different penicillin susceptibilities. APMIS 1996;104:227–233.

128. Product information: Achromycin, tetracycline. Pearl River, NY: Lederle Laboratories, 1995.

129. Product information: Minocin, minocycline. Pearl River, NY: Lederle Laboratories, 1995.

130. Product information: Vibramycin, doxycycline. New York: Pfizer Laboratories, 1995.

131. Quintiliani R Jr, Courvalin P. Mechanisms of resistance to antimicrobial agents. In: Murray PR, Baron EJ, Pfaller MA, Tenover FC, Yolken RH, eds. Manual of clinical microbiology. Washington, DC: ASM Press, 1995:1308–1326.

132. Raghuram TC, Krishnaswamy K. Pharmacokinetics and plasma steady state levels of doxycycline in undernutrition. Br J Clin Pharmacol 1982;14:785–789.

133. Ramelli G. Photo-oncholysis following doxycycline hyclate. Cutis 1972;10:155–156.

134. Raoult D, Drancourt M. Antimicrobial therapy of rickettsial diseases. Antimicrob Agents Chemother 1991;35:2457–2462.

135. Reid JD. The black thyroid associated with minocycline therapy: a local manifestation of a drug-induced lysosome/substrate disorder. Am J Clin Pathol 1983;79:738–746.

136. Saah AJ. Rickettsiosis. In: Mandell GL, Bennett JE, Dolin R, eds. Mandell, Douglas and Bennett's principles and practice of infectious diseases. New York: Churchill Livingstone, 1995: 1719–1720.

137. Schnappinger D, Hillen W. Tetracyclines: antibiotic action, uptake, and resistance mechanisms. Arch Microbiol 1996; 165:359–369.

138. Schneider R. Doxycycline esophageal ulcers. Am J Dig Dis 1977;22:805–807.

139. Schultz JC, Adamsden JS Jr, Workman WW. Fatal liver disease after intravenous administration of tetracycline in high dosage. N Engl J Med 1963;269:999–1004.

140. Scopp IW, Kazandjian G. Tetracycline-induced staining of teeth. Postgrad Med 1986;79:202–203.

141. Shea KW, Cunha BA. Doxycycline activity against penicillin-resistant Streptococcus pneumoniae. Chest 1995;108: 1775–1776.

142. Shifer A, Dany S, Schwarzkopf R, Rubinstein E. Concentrations of tetracycline in human gingival tissue in patients with chronic periodontal disease. J Antimicrob Chemother 1989;23: 464–465.

143. Siller GM, Tod MA, Savage NW. Minocycline-induced oral pigmentation. J Am Acad Dermatol 1994;30:350–354.

144. Silvola H, Tourunen E, Mattila MJ. Serum levels of doxycycline during and after thoracic operation. Ann Clin Res 1981;13:22–25.

145. Simon C, Molerczys V, Preuss I, Schmidt K, Grahmann H. Activity in vitro and pharmacokinetics of minocycline. Arzneimittelforschung 1976;26:556–560.

146. Singer SJ, Piazza-Hepp TD, Girardi LS, Moledina NR. Lupuslike reaction associated with minocycline. JAMA 1997;277: 295–296.

147. Solera J, Rodriguez-Zapata M, Geijo P, Largo J, Paulino J, Saez L, Marinez-Alfaro E, Sanchez L, Sepulveda M-A, Ruiz-Ribo M-D, GECMEI Group. Doxycycline-rifampin versus doxycycline-streptomycin in treatment of human brucellosis due to Brucella melitensis. Antimicrob Agents Chemother 1995;39: 2061–2067.

148. Song JH, Lee C, Chang WH, Choi SW, Choi JE, Kim YS, Cho SR, Ryu J, Pai CH. Short-course doxycycline treatment versus conventional tetracycline therapy for scrub typhus: a multicenter randomized trial. Clin Infect Dis 1995;21:506–510.

149. Speer BS, Shoemaker NB, Salyers AA. Bacterial resistance to tetracycline: mechanisms, transfer, and clinical significance. Clin Microbiol Rev 1992;5:387–399.

150. Standiford HC. Tetracyclines and chloramphenicol. In: Mandell GL, Bennett JE, Dolin R, eds. Mandell, Douglas and Bennett's principles and practice of infectious diseases. New York: Churchill Livingstone, 1995:306–317.

151. Steere AC, Levin RE, Molley PJ, Kalish RA, Abruha JH, Liu NY, Schmid CH. Treatment of Lyme arthritis. Arthritis Rheum 1994;37:878–888.

152. Steigbigel NH, Reed CW, Finland M. Absorption and excretion of five tetracycline analogues in normal young men. Am J Med Sci 1968;255:296–312.

153. Strickman D, Sheer T, Salata K, Hershey J, Dasch G, Kelly D, Kuschner R. In vitro effectiveness of azithromycin against doxycycline-resistant and -susceptible strains of Rickettsia tsutsugamushi, etiologic agent of scrub typhus. Antimicrob Agents and Chemother 1995;39:2406–2410.

154. Stuart BIT, Litt IF. Tetracycline-associated intracranial hypertension in an adolescent: a complication of systemic acne therapy. J Pediatr 1978;92:679–680.

155. Szoka PR, Edgren RA. Drug interactions with oral contraceptives: compilation and analysis of an adverse experience report database. Fertil Steril 1988;49(5 Suppl 2):31s–38s.

156. Tally FT, Ellestad GA, Testa RT. Glycylcyclines: a new generation of tetracyclines. J Antimicrob Chemother 1995;35: 449–452.

157. True RJ. Interactions between antibiotics and oral contraceptives [Letter]. JAMA 1982;247:1408.

158. Vartia KD, Leikola L. Serum levels of antibiotics in young and old subjects following administration of dihydrostreptomycin and tetracycline. J Gerontol 1960;18:392.

159. Vial T, Biour M, Descotes J, Trepo C. Antibiotic-associated hepatitis: update from 1990. Ann Pharmacother 1997;31:304–320.

160. Walker-Renard PB, Vaughan LM, Sahn SA. Chemical pleurodesis for malignant pleural effusions. Ann Intern Med 1994; 120:56–64.

161. Westfall LK, Mintzer DL, Wiser TH. Potentiation of warfarin by tetracycline [Letter]. Am J Hosp Pharm 1980;37:1620, 1625.
162. Whalley PJ, Adams RH, Combes B. Tetracycline toxicity in pregnancy. JAMA 1964;189:357–362.

163. Whelton A. Tetracyclines in renal insufficiency: resolution of a therapeutic dilemma. Bull NY Acad Med 1978;54:223–236.
164. Worgan D, Daniel RJE. The penetration of minocycline into human sinus secretions. Scott Med J 1976;21:197–199.

Trimethoprim and Trimethoprim-Sulfamethoxazole (Cotrimoxazole)

Fred W. Goldstein and Gary E. Stein

The combination trimethoprim (TMP)-sulfamethoxazole (SMX) (cotrimoxazole) is an association of two antibacterial agents that act synergistically against a wide spectrum of bacterial species. Other combinations of a different sulfonamide (sulfamoxole, sulfametrole, and sulfadiazine) with trimethoprim or a trimethoprim analogue (tetroxoprim, epiroprim, brodimoprim) (52, 60, 61) have been studied or marketed, but TMP-SMX is by far the most used combination (20, 74) (Fig. 1).

ANTIMICROBIAL ACTIVITY
Spectrum of Activity

TMP-SMX has an extremely wide spectrum of activity including most Gram-positive and Gram-negative bacteria, some mycobacteria, parasites, and a few fungi. This is essentially due to enhanced activity of the SMX moiety of the combination by TMP. The MICs of TMP and SMX against representative pathogens are presented in Tables 1 and 2 (1, 15, 30, 50, 73).

Bactericidal Activity

TMP alone and (especially) SMX have limited bactericidal effects. On the contrary, the association is highly bactericidal against many bacterial species as long as some amino acids (methionine, glycine, lysine) are present in the medium and if the concentration of thymine/thymidine is not too high (1, 6, 34, 65).

MECHANISMS OF ACTION

SMX is a structural analogue of p-aminobenzoic acid (PABA) and a competitor of PABA in the synthesis of dihydropteroic acid, the first step in the synthesis of dihydrofolic acid (Fig. 2) (11, 30). SMX binds to the enzyme dihydropteroate synthetase (DHPS), which catalyses this reaction.

TMP is a structural analogue of dihydrofolic acid (DHF) and binds preferentially to dihydrofolate reductase (DHFR), the enzyme that transforms DHF into tetrahydrofolic acid (THF). The decreased pool of available THF inhibits thymidine synthesis and then DNA synthesis, as shown in Figure 2.

As a consequence of this mode of action, small amounts of thymidine (which can be present in vivo or in media used for susceptibility testing) can reverse the activity of TMP-SMX and be responsible for false resistance (14, 30). Moreover, mutants lacking the enzyme thymidylate synthetase (thymineless mutants) are no more susceptible to the action of TMP-SMX. Such mutants have been isolated in vitro and in vivo (2).

The sequential enzymatic blockade by TMP and SMX is responsible for the very strong synergistic effect observed between the two compounds. Although observed over a wide range of MICs, the synergistic effect is optimal when the compounds are at their MIC ratio. For most Enterobacteriaceae, this ratio is TMP:SMX of 1:20. This is why TMP-SMX is administered at a 5:1 ratio, which yields a 20:1 ratio in the organism (Tables 3 and 4) (1, 11, 15, 34).

For bacteria that have a higher MIC for TMP (e.g., Nocardia or Neisseria), the ratio that gives the best synergy is 1:2 or 1:1, which always correlates with the ratio of their respective MICs. This explains why optimal therapy against such bacteria can be achieved by increasing the amount of TMP administered.

MECHANISMS OF RESISTANCE TO TMP AND SMX
Commonly Resistant Organisms

Naturally resistant bacteria are listed in Table 5. Some bacteria have decreased permeability for TMP-SMX or a target enzyme for which the drugs have a low affinity. In addition, an active efflux mechanism is present in some bacterial species such as Pseudomonas aeruginosa (30, 48). Only a few bacterial species are naturally resistant to SMX: Enterococcus faecalis and lactobacilli. These bacteria are auxotrophic for folic acid and hence cannot be inhibited by SMX.

As a consequence of the synergy between TMP and SMX, bacteria naturally resistant to TMP at low levels and susceptible to SMX can be inhibited by the combination TMP-SMX. This is particularly true of Neisseria, Nocardia, rapid-growing mycobacteria, Stenotrophomonas maltophilia, and Burkholderia pseudomallei (34, 65, 73).

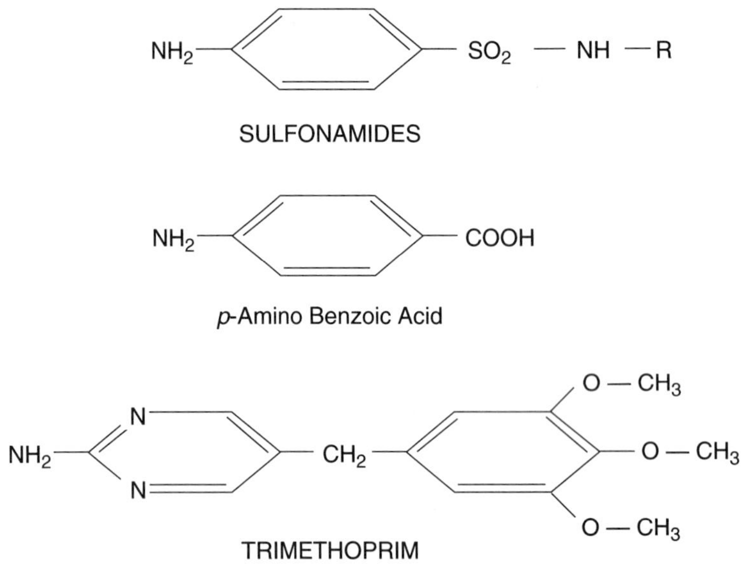

Trimethoprin (2,4-diamino-5 (3'4'5'-trimethoxybenzyl) pyrimidine

FIGURE 1. Sulfonamides, *p*-aminobenzoic acid, and trimethoprim.

TABLE 1 • MIC_{50} of Sulfamethoxazole (SMX) and Trimethoprim (TMP) against Various Gram-Positive Bacterial Pathogens[a]

Bacteria	SMX	TMP
Streptococcus pyogenes	12	0.5
Streptococcus agalactiae	28	5
Streptococcus pneumoniae	28	1.5
Enterococcus faecalis	>1000	0.5
Enterococcus faecium	>1000	1
Staphylococcus aureus	0.2	3
Staphylococcus epidermidis	1	4
Corynebacterium diphtheriae	>100	0.5
Erysipelothrix rhusiopathiae	>100	5
Listeria monocytogenes	2	0.12
Nocardia asteroides	3	15
Mycobacterium tuberculosis	1000	150
Mycobacterium fortuitum	16	64
Clostridium perfringens	28	50

[a] MIC_{50}s represent activity against strains without acquired resistance.

TABLE 2 • MIC_{50} of Sulfamethoxazole (SMX) and Trimethoprim (TMP) against Various Gram-Negative Bacterial Pathogens[a]

Bacteria	SMX	TMP
Escherichia coli	8	0.1
Shigella dysenteriae	4	0.2
Salmonella typhi	2	0.2
Salmonella enteritidis	2	0.2
Klebsiella pneumoniae	16	1
Enterobacter cloacae	16	2
Serratia marcescens	16	2
Proteus mirabilis	8	4
Pseudomonas aeruginosa	32	128
Stenotrophomonas maltophilia	4	32
Burkholderia pseudomallei	4	32
Acinetobacter baumanii	4	16
Haemophilus influenzae	8	0.5
Pasteurella multocida	1	0.1
Bordetella pertussis	50	3
Brucella melitensis	2	16
Neisseria gonorrhoeae	1	16
Neisseria meningitidis	1	16
Bacteroides fragilis	4	32

[a] MIC_{50}s represent activity against strains without acquired resistance.

Bacteria with Acquired Resistance to TMP-SMX

One of the drawbacks of the huge amounts of TMP-SMX used is that resistance to the association has developped in virtually all bacterial species worldwide. Spread of resistance was facilitated by the number of various resistance genes, often present on plasmids and transposons (2, 7, 67). In general, high-level resistance to TMP is due to the presence of transferable plasmids. Important discrepancies in the percentage of resistant strains can be observed for the same bacterial species isolated in different countries (Table 6) (2, 71).

Gram-positive Bacteria

Staphylococci

Resistance to Sulfonamides. Resistance to sulfonamides is extremely common in *Staphylococcus aureus* and coagulase-negative staphylococci all over the world, particularly methicillin-resistant strains. Resistance emerged shortly after the introduction of sulfonamides for clinical use and now

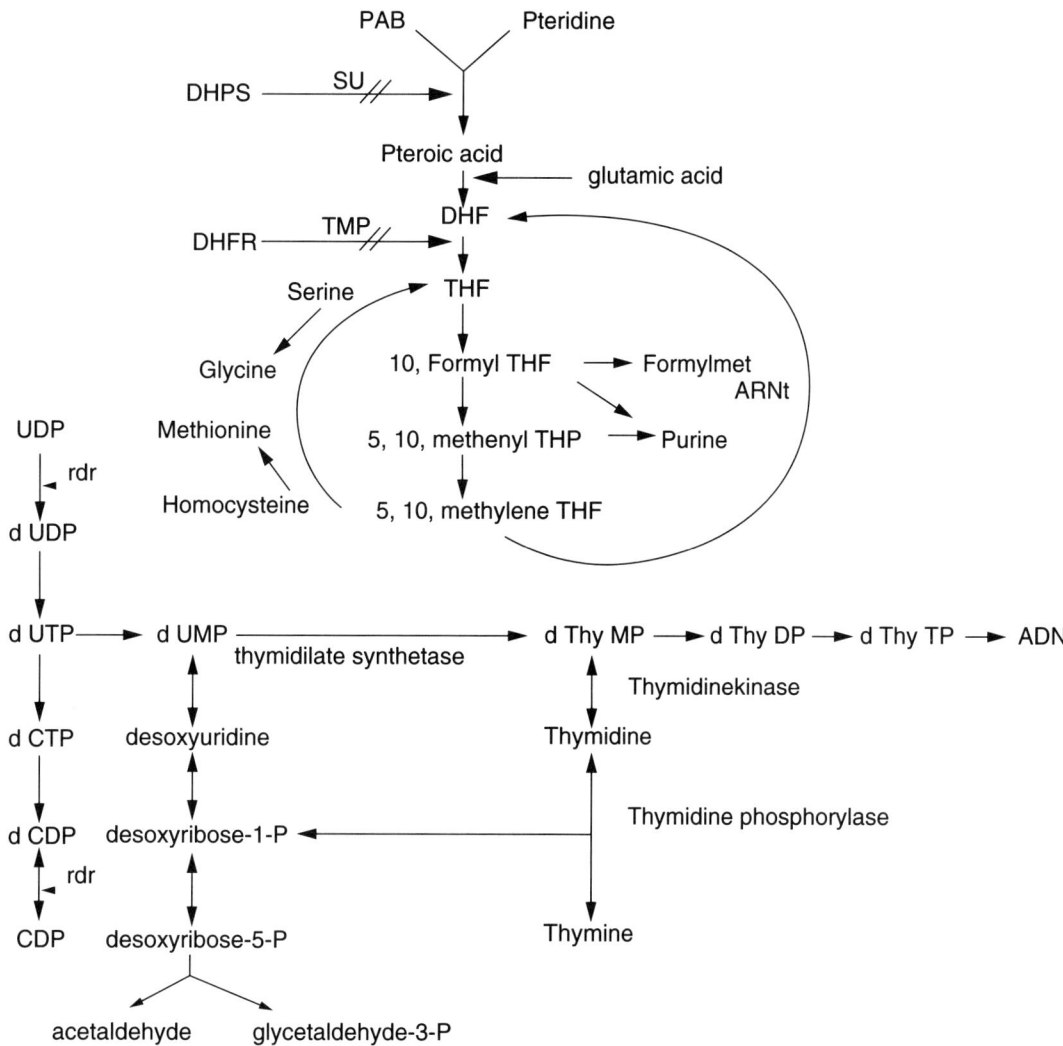

FIGURE 2. Mechanism of action of sulfonamides and trimethoprim.

involves more than 30% of all strains (>80% of methicillin-resistant *S. aureus* (MRSA)) (66, 71).

Despite the frequency of SMX resistance in staphylococci, few studies have dealt with this subject. Several mechanisms have been described: *(a)* hyperproduction of PABA (up to a 70-fold increase) has been described in *S. aureus* and coagulase-negative staphylococci; *(b)* a few thymineless auxotrophic mutants resistant to both SMX and TMP have been found; *(c)* production of an altered DHPS is very likely but has not yet been reported; *(d)* plasmid-mediated SMX resistance, linked to other resistance markers (aminoglycosides, erythromycin) was reported in only one study (21, 30, 66).

Resistance to TMP. Resistance to TMP in *S. aureus* is still uncommon in many countries, with the important exception of Australia and some Southeast Asian countries (69) (Table 6). Resistance is more common in coagulase-negative staphylococci. Some published results clearly overestimate the percentage of resistant strains because of technical problems. For example, the resistance rates in France (8) and Switzerland (75)

TABLE 3 • FIC Index of the Combination Trimethoprim (TMP)-Sulfadiazine (SDZ) *P. vulgaris* MICs: TMP 0.1 μg/mL; SDZ 2

Ratio TMP:SDZ	FIC Index
1:1.24	0.53
1:5	0.31
1:20	0.25
1:83	0.31
1:333	0.53

are 4.5 and 2%, respectively, in contrast to the 67.2! and 47.1% attributed in one study (71). Resistant strains are more often encountered in HIV patients receiving TMP-SMX prophylaxis. Despite the high rate of resistance to sulfonamides, a strong synergistic effect of TMP-SMX is present in nearly all SMX-resistant TMP-susceptible strains (Fig. 3). TMP-SMX is one of

TABLE 4 • Synergistic Effect of SMX-TMP against Selected Pathogens (MICs in μg/mL at the ratio 20:1)

Organism	SMX Alone	SMX + TMP	TMP Alone	TMP + SMX
Streptococcus pyogenes	64	1	1	0.05
Streptococcus pneumoniae	32	2	2	0.1
Staphylococcus aureus	2	0.2	1	0.01
Klebsiella pneumoniae	16	0.3	1	0.01
Escherichia coli	4	1	0.3	0.05
Salmonella typhimurium	8	1	0.3	0.05
Proteus vulgaris	32	2	3	0.15

TABLE 5 • Bacteria Naturally Resistant to Trimethoprim (TMP) (MIC 16–256)

Neisseria sp.	Actinomyces
Acinetobacter	Bacteroides
Moraxella	Clostridium
Branhamella	Brucella sp.
Pseudomonas	Mycobacterium
Stenotrophomonas	Legionella
Burkholderia	Campylobacter
Achromobacter	Mycoplasma
Nocardia	Chlamydia
Treponema	

TABLE 6 • Prevalence of Resistance to TMP-SMX

Streptococci	<10%
S. pneumoniae	10–40%, linked to penicillin resistance
S. aureus	<5% in Europe, U.S.
	>40% in Australia
E. coli	10–20 in Europe, U.S.
Proteus sp.	30–50 in Asia
Klebsiella pneumoniae	
Enterobacter sp.	10–60%, highly dependent on local epidemics
Serratia	
Salmonella	0–50% depending on local epidemics
Shigella	

the few compounds usually effective against MRSA resistant to virtually all antibiotics except glycopeptides (53, 59).

Resistance to TMP is plasmid- or, more frequently, chromosomally mediated (2, 12, 23); low- or intermediate-level resistance (16–25% μg/mL) is usually linked to point mutations in the chromosomal gene for DHFR. The molecular mechanism in all these resistant strains is a substitution of amino acids at the F98Y position which disrupts hydrogen binding with TMP. High-level TMP resistance is linked to an additional TMP-resistant DHFR, DHFR S_1 encoded by transposon Tn 1003, which is very common and present all over the world. Another enzyme, DHFR S_2, has been isolated from a single *S. haemolyticus* strain in Spain. DHFR S_1 is highly homologous (98.1%) to the chromosomal DHFR of *S. epidermidis* and presents the same molecular mechanism of resistance at the F98Y position.

Streptococcus pneumoniae. Resistance to TMP-SMX in *S. pneumoniae* is obviously linked to penicillin resistance (33). The mechanism of this "cross-resistance" is not fully understood, but it seems very likely that it may occur when *S. pneumoniae* are transformed; a gene encoding sulfonamide resistance is linked to the PBP_2x gene, and the gene encoding TMP resistance is linked to the PBP_2b gene (28). This explains the high prevalence of penicillin-resistant *S. pneumoniae* in HIV patients.

Other Gram-Positive Bacteria. Among the other important Gram-positive bacteria, resistance to trimethoprim has been described in *Listeria monocytogenes*. This resistance is due to a new DHFR called dfrD (18).

Enterobacteriaceae

Incidence of Resistance to TMP-SMX. Resistance has been described in all enterobacterial species all over the world. However, the prevalence is extremely variable according to location and bacterial species. The prevalence may be very high in developing countries during outbreaks and epidemics (*Shigella, Salmonella*), in some hospitals and wards (e.g., intensive care units) and for some multiresistant bacterial species such as *Klebsiella, Enterobacter,* or *Serratia* (2, 26, 31, 32, 40, 57).

Resistance to SMX. Resistance to sulfonamides can be due to mutational events or to acquisition of foreign DNA (2, 30, 66). Mechanisms for resistance by mutation include (a) hyperproduction of PABA which directly competes for the active site of the DHPS; (b) altered DHPS with decreased affinity requires more sulfonamide to inhibit bacterial growth; (c) hyperproduction of DHPS, whether normal or altered enzyme; (d) decreased permeability, which is strongly "suggested" when other mechanisms are not obvious, and alteration of some outer membrane proteins may be responsible for a slight increase in the MIC of sulfonamides (35); and (e) in thymineless bacteria—lack of the enzyme thymidylate synthetase—both sulfonamide and TMP are no more effective.

An additional plasmid-encoded sulfonamide-resistant DHPS is the most frequent mechanism of resistance in *Enterobacteriaceae* (2, 30, 40, 57). Resistance to sulfonamide may be associated with other resistance markers. Two different DHPS have been described so far (66).

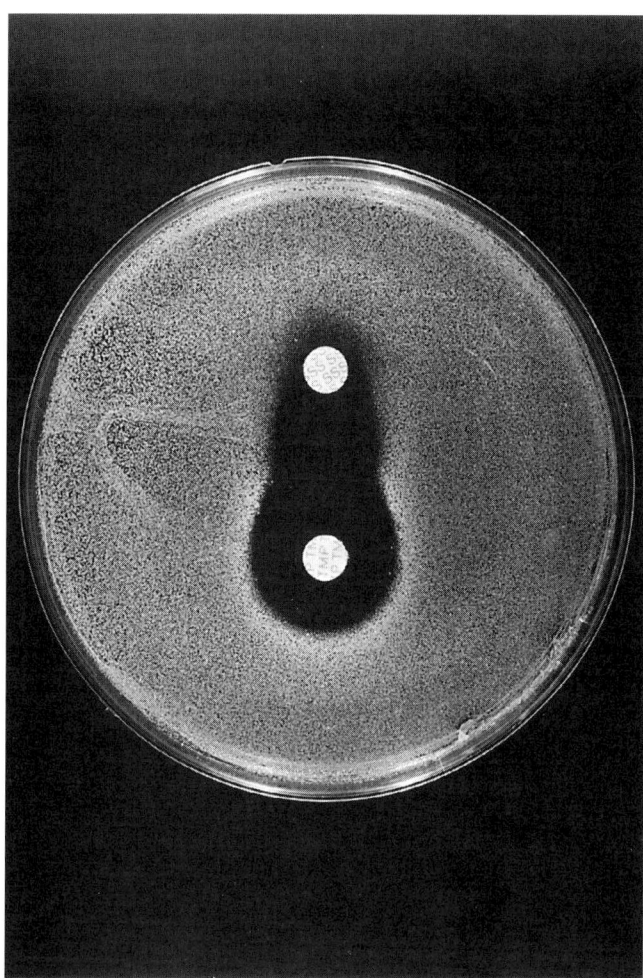

FIGURE 3. Synergistic effect between sulfonamides and trimethoprim against a sulfonamide-resistant (MIC > 1000 μg/mL) *S. aureus.*

Resistance to TMP. Acquired resistance to TMP was documented shortly after the introduction of TMP-SMX for clinical use. As for sulfonamides, resistance can be due to mutational events or to acquisition of foreign DNA (2, 7, 30, 40). Various mechanisms may make bacteria auxotrophic for thymine or thymidine. These bacteria usually lack the enzyme thymidylate synthetase and hence need thymine or thymidine for normal growth. As a consequence, the reactions that precede this step (including that inhibited by TMP) are no longer useful. These bacteria have become resistant to high levels of TMP. A similar effect can be obtained if bacteria lack the enzyme ribonucleoside diphosphate reductase, which belongs to another metabolic chain (Fig. 2) (2, 30, 45).

A decreased affinity of DHFR for TMP is a frequent phenomenon. The mutation rate is about 10^{-10} for *Enterobacteriaceae.* The genes responsible for this altered DHFR are called *fol* A and *fol* B (2).

Hyperproduction of DHFR of 3- to 80-fold has been reported in many species. In some bacteria, hyperproduction can be associated with a DHFR with decreased affinity, explaining high resistance, up to 1000 μg/mL (2).

One-step mutants resistant not only to TMP but also to chloramphenicol, nalidixic acid, and low levels of fluoroquinolones, β-lactams, sulfonamides, and tetracyclines have been isolated in vitro and in vivo from *Klebsiella, Enterobacter,* and *Serratia* (35). The frequency of this mutation is about 10^{-7} in *Klebsiella.* The mechanism responsible for this pleiotropic mutation is a quantitative diminution of one or two porins.

Plasmid-Mediated Resistance to TMP. Since 1972, plasmids mediating resistance to TMP and other antibiotics have been described in all enterobacterial species all over the world and also anecdotally in *P. aeruginosa, Acinetobacter,* and *Pasteurella* (2, 7, 40). These plasmids encode an additional TMP-resistant DHFR. Hence, these bacteria have two DHFRs: the chromosomal susceptible one and an additional one encoded by the plasmid. Type I, discovered in 1974 (5), was followed by the highly resistant type II in 1977 (58). There are more than 15 different types of resistant DHFRs (7). Most but not all encode high-level resistance to TMP.

The DHFR gene may be present on different transposons, integrated in the plasmid, or on the bacterial chromosome. Bacterial species such as *Vibrio cholerae* that usually do not harbor plasmids for long periods may be resistant to TMP because the transposon initially carried by a plasmid has "jumped" onto the bacterial chromosome (32). The most frequent transposon by far is Tn 7, which encodes resistance to TMP and streptomycin and can be easily transposed onto a large variety of plasmids or the chromosome of many bacteria (2, 7, 57).

In Vivo Selection of Resistance

The development of resistant bacteria following treatment with TMP has been studied by several investigators. Resistance of fecal flora was studied in college-aged women following 10 days of therapy with TMP for an acute urinary tract infection (UTI) (42). Initial studies of fecal flora showed that all colonies selected were TMP susceptible. On day 7, 2.7% of isolates were resistant to TMP. In a similar study population, fecal and introital aerobic bacteria were analyzed during and after a 14-day course of therapy with TMP (56). This investigation found no resistant fecal or introital flora during or following TMP administration. An overall analysis of these and other studies indicated that TMP alone does not result in selection of TMP-resistant *Enterobacteriaceae* (55). However, more-recent observations have found increasing TMP resistance in enterobacteria from outpatient urine samples (41). Resistance rates in *Escherichia coli* vary significantly from one region of the world to another (40). Recent surveillance studies found that only 38 to 59% of *E. coli* isolates were susceptible to TMP in Latin America and Asia, compared with 87 to 93% in the United States and Sweden.

PHARMACOKINETIC DISPOSITION (36, 61, 73).
Absorption

After oral administration, 85 to 90% of TMP and 85% of SMX are absorbed during the first 3 h. Plasma peak levels are obtained between 2 and 4 h and reach 1 to 2 μg/mL for TMP and 25 to 60 μg/mL for SMX (active compound). Absorption is not influenced by the intake of other medications (cimetidine) or food or the presence of acute gastroenteritis.

Plasma concentrations above the MICs of most bacteria are maintained up to 6 to 8 h after a single dose. The half-life is 10 to 12 h for both compounds. After repeated intake, an equilibrium is achieved after 3 days, giving 1.3 to 2.8 μg/mL of TMP and 32 to 63 μg/mL of SMX. After intravenous infusion of TMP-SMX, the peak serum levels obtained are 8 to 9.5 μg/mL for TMP and 95 to 115 μg/mL for SMX, twice those obtained after oral intake, but the half-life is 1 to 2 h shorter.

Distribution

TMP-SMX is widely distributed throughout body tissues as indicated in Table 7. Since TMP is more lipophilic, it is more widely distributed than SMX, explaining why the ratio 1:20 observed in serum is often 1:2 to 1:10 in tissues. The apparent volume of distribution is 12 to 18 L for SMX and 100 to 120 L for TMP. One compound does not affect the pharmacokinetics of the other (36).

Metabolism and Excretion

TMP and SMX are excreted mainly by the kidney: about 50% of each compound is eliminated during the first 24 h. About 19% of the ingested SMX is excreted unchanged. The main metabolites are *N*-acetyl SMX (61%) and a glycuronide metabolite (15%). There are three minor metabolites, all with very limited antibacterial activity. About 66% of the ingested TMP is excreted in the urine unchanged. There are four main metabolites with only weak antibacterial activity: TMP-1-oxide and hydroxy-TMP are excreted unconjugated, and two desmethyl metabolites are excreted as glycuronides. Excretion of TMP and SMX is affected by pH variation but in an opposite way: at low pH, reabsorption of SMX is extensive, while excretion of TMP increases. In elderly patients, the half-lives of TMP and SMX are nearly unchanged, with only a small decrease in the clearance of SMX. TMP and SMX are also excreted in the bile and feces.

DOSAGE REGIMENS (20, 73, 74)
Normal Patients

TMP-SMX tablets are presented in several countries with two formulations: the normal tablet or vials for intravenous infusion containing 400 mg SMX/80 mg TMP and the double-strength tablet containing 800 mg SMX/160 mg TMP. For pediatric usage, there is a tablet containing 100 mg SMX/20 mg TMP and a suspension containing 200 mg SMX/400 mg TMP per 5 mL. The usual dosage for adults is 2 low- or 1 high-dose tablet twice daily. For children, the oral dose is TMP 10 mg/SMX 50 mg (1/2 tablet) from 6 weeks to 6 months, 1 to 1 1/2 tablets daily from 6 months to 6 years, and 2 tablets from 6 to 12 years. TMP-SMX is not recommended for infants younger than 6 weeks because the immature hepatic enzyme function results in increased bilirubin levels, with the danger of hyperbilirubinemia.

This daily dose can be considerably increased in severe infections if other therapeutic options are not available: 6 to 8 tablets or vials daily for severe Gram-negative infections and up to 12 tablets or vials daily for pneumocystosis. If oral administration is not feasible, the same doses may be given parenterally.

Renal Failure

Alteration of renal function decreases excretion of TMP and, only marginally, excretion of SMX. Thus, TMP-SMX will achieve effective urinary concentrations even in the presence of renal failure. In patients with severe renal failure, whose creatine clearance is below 20 to 30 mL/min, half of the usual daily dose should be administered. If creatine clearance is below 15 mL/min, serum levels of TMP should be monitored. Patients usually receive an initial loading dose and then a per-

TABLE 7 • Concentration of TMP and SMX in Body Tissues and Fluids

Tissue or Fluid	TMP Level in Tissue/ TMP Level in Serum	SMX Level in Tissue/ SMX Level in Serum	Approximate Ratio TMP:SMX
Saliva	2.0	0.03	3:1
Middle ear fluid	0.75	0.2	1:6
Human breast milk	1.25	0.1	1:2
Prostatic tissue	2.0	0.35	1:3
Seminal fluid	0.5	0.3	1:10
Epididymis	2.0	0.51	1:5
Sputum	1.5	0.2	1:3
Lung parenchyma	3.5	0.3[a] (?)	1:2[a] (?)
Vaginal secretions	1.5	0.01	8:1
Fetal blood	0.6	0.8	1:30
Amniotic fluid	0.8	0.5	1:10
Aqueous humor	0.4	0.25	1:10
Cerebrospinal fluid	0.5	0.4	1:15
Bile	1.0	0.4	1:8
Bone (spongy)	0.67	—	—
Bone (compact)	0.1	—	—
Synovial fluid	1.0	1.0	1:20

[a] Presumptive, based on animal data.

centage of the normal dose more or less equal to the percentage of renal failure (100 − %).

TMP and SMX are dialyzed but not their main metabolites, TMP-1-oxide and *N*-acetyl SMX, which may accumulate and cause crystalluria. Hence, alternative compounds should be used if possible in such patients. Patients who undergo hemodialysis will receive (as above) a normal loading dose after each dialysis and additional doses according to the results of serum assays.

Hepatic Failure and Other Disorders

No modification of dosage regimens is needed in patients with hepatic failure, obesity, or edema.

Pregnancy

Because of its action on DNA synthesis, TMP-SMX should be avoided during pregnancy; the only exception is listeriosis in penicillin-allergic patients. An additional risk of hyperbilirubinemia contraindicates TMP-SMX during the last 3 to 4 weeks.

Dosage Regimens

The usual adult dosage of TMP for treatment of UTI is 100 mg every 12 h. In patients with renal insufficiency (CrCl = 15–30 mL/min), the dose of TMP should be decreased to 50 mg. Use of TMP in patients with a creatinine clearance below 15 mL/min is not recommended. No dose has been established for children under 12 years of age. TMP at bedtime doses of 100 mg has been used as suppressive therapy in women with recurrent UTIs.

ADVERSE EFFECTS
Types

TMP-SMX, widely used for more than 25 years, is generally well tolerated, although a large body of information on adverse effects has become available. As expected, adverse effects are due to the toxicity of the two different compounds (4, 16, 22, 29a,37, 38, 43, 44, 46, 49, 51).

Gastrointestinal Disorders

Reactions are usually very mild; nausea and vomiting in 1 to 4% of patients and diarrhea in 0.6% of patients are attributed to TMP-SMX. However, these effects may be related to the underlying diseases (e.g., salmonellosis). The only real problem with these side effects is that patients may discontinue an effective treatment. A few serious cases of pseudomembranous colitis have been described.

Hematologic Effects

Hematologic effects are the most serious side effects, related to folate deficiency and observed after long-term therapy, particularly in elderly or severely ill patients, alcoholics, and patients with malabsorption or malnutrition. The most common alteration is pancytopenia, fatal in some cases. Other abnormalities linked to SMX and of unknown mechanisms are more frequent, including agranulocytosis, anemia, and thrombocytopenia.

Side effects related to folate deficiency can and must be corrected by preventive and curative administration of folinic acid (but not folic acid). Folinic acid does not antagonize the effect of TMP-SMX on most bacteria, except *E. faecalis*. Thrombocytopenia alone has also been observed and is attributed to the sulfonamide moiety.

Skin Disorders

Serious skin lesions may be observed with TMP-SMX as with sulfonamides alone. A wide spectrum of skin lesions have been attributed to SMX:

- Toxic erythema (a maculopapular eruption with pruritus)
- Erythema nodosum
- Fixed, local eruption
- Erythema multiforme, which may be associated with toxic symptoms, pyrexia, and mucous membrane ulcerations (buccal, genital, conjunctival), referred to as the Stevens-Johnson syndrome
- Lyell's syndrome, the most serious complication due to sulfonamides, varying from mild to fatal—often described as the "scalded skin" syndrome, it is an acute epidermal necrolysis resulting in the peeling of the skin in large sheets
- Exfoliative dermatitis, another serious condition, associated with a toxic syndrome, different from Lyell's syndrome
- Urticaria
- Necrotizing vasculitis
- Photodermatitis
  (The later aspects are much less common and severe)
- Toxic erythema, quite common (1–4%) and usually mild

The incidence of various skin disorders is extremely high in HIV patients receiving TMP-SMX as prophylaxis or therapy for *Pneumocystis carinii* pneumonia; 25 to 50% of these patients experience cutaneous eruptions, maculopapular rash, and pruritus.

Renal Disorders

Most renal disorders are mild and rare. They include
- Transient blood urea and creatinine elevations due to TMP
- Crystalluria due to the sulfonamides, which are metabolized into an acetylated, poorly soluble form
- Acute interstitial nephritis that can be easily avoided with enough water intake

Other Disorders

- Hyperbilirubinemia of the newborn: there is a competition between sulfonamides and bilirubin (unconjugated) for serum albumin; because of immature hepatic enzyme function, the newborn may develop severe kernicterus
- Hepatitis: has been very rarely reported
- Central nervous system effects: headache, confusion, and depression have been rarely reported; aseptic meningitis, fully reversible after cessation of treatment has been reported in several patients (37)
- Metabolic disorders: among the few metabolic disorders observed, hyperkalemia is the must serious because it has been documented with normal TMP-SMX dosages (4)

Management of Adverse Effects

Most adverse effects disappear after cessation of treatment. In some cases (hepatitis, renal damage) corticoids seem to be beneficial; in most others, results of corticoid therapy are controversial. Serious cases need special treatment in intensive care units. Usually, the appearance of serious adverse effects results in immediate discontinuation of the treatment. There is no specific treatment for adverse effects, with the important exception of hematologic effects, which must be treated with folinic acid.

There is one important exception to this approach. Because *Pneumocystis carinii* pneumonia is a life-threatening disease and TMP-SMX is the best available treatment, in most instances, treatment with TMP-SMX can and must continue, despite the presence of skin disorders. Unlike what is observed with β-lactam antibiotics, some patients can be rechallenged once they have recovered without recurrent adverse reactions (46, 72).

Should this approach fail, an alternative is drug desensitization with increasing doses of TMP-SMX; more than 80% of patients can be successfully desensitized (29b). Patients can be desensitized orally within 5 h: they receive hourly a tenfold increased dose of TMP-SMX, starting at 0.004 mg TMP/0.02 mg SMX (i.e., 2 drops! of a solution of ½ normal-strength tablet (80 mg TMP/400 mg SMX) in 1 L of water) up to a double-strength tablet (160 mg TMP/800 mg SMX) at 5 h.

DRUG INTERACTIONS

Other diaminopyrimidines—pyrimethamine, azathioprine, or methotrexate—are potentiated by TMP, resulting in severe leukopenia. Sulfonamides displace warfarin from binding to albumin, thus increasing its serum level. SMX inhibits the clearance of phenytoin, prolonging its half-life. There is a theoretical risk of potentiating the hypoglycemic effect of sulfonylurea by displacing it from serum albumin.

CLINICAL INDICATIONS

The TMP-SMX combination has been used for more than 25 years as curative and prophylactic agent for an ever expanding array of infectious diseases. Today, the clinical indications of TMP-SMX exceed by far the officially "approved" indications in many countries (Table 8). The reasons for the worldwide success of TMP-SMX are excellent clinical results, good tolerance, a wide spectrum of activity, and a low price (50, 73, 74).

Urinary Tract Infections

TMP-SMX has been used successfully for uncomplicated and complicated UTIs in women and men. Although less effective than the modern fluoroquinolones, TMP-SMX is still used in many situations and countries where more expensive compounds such as fluoroquinolones or oral cephalosporins cannot be afforded.

Uncomplicated Lower UTI (Cystitis) in Women

Excellent results are obtained with a 3-day course of TMP-SMX (2 × 800/160 mg) as long as the strains are susceptible to the combination. A body of evidence indicates that even if not approved, a single dose of TMP-SMX (800/160–1600/320) is effective in the treatment of cystitis. Conflicting results have been published for the treatment of enterococcal UTIs. Despite in

TABLE 8 • Approved Indications of TMP-SMX	
Disease	**Comments**
UTI	No indications concerning complicated UTI or prostatitis
Acute otitis media	
Acute exacerbation of chronic bronchitis	Due to *S. pneumoniae* or *H. influenzae*
Shigellosis	Only *S. flexneri* and *S. sonnei* are specified
Pneumocystis carinii pneumonia	
Travelers' diarrhea in adults	Due to enterotoxinogenic *E. coli*

vitro activity, TMP-SMX should no longer be used as a first-line agent. The increasing number of failures observed may be due to the fact that enterococci can incorporate thymine (present in the urine) to a much larger extent than other bacteria (2, 11, 15).

Other UTIs

Acute uncomplicated UTI is probably the only acceptable indication for TMP alone. Even if efficacy of the combination has not been clearly demonstrated in other situations, the reasons for using sulfonamides are very clear: *(a)* the combination of TMP-SMX is highly synergistic in most cases even if the strain is resistant to SMX (Fig. 3); *(b)* SMX decreases the MIC of TMP by 10- to 20-fold; *(c)* the bacteria are present not only in the bladder where the concentration of TMP alone is very high but also in the renal or prostatic parenchyma. In these situations, the concentrations of TMP might often be borderline (usually twice the serum concentration) and the presence of a compound that renders the bacteria 10 or 20 times more susceptible to TMP should be highly beneficial.

Acute Pyelonephritis

A 14-day course of TMP-SMX (2 × 800/160 daily) is highly effective for treatment of pyelonephritis, including bacteremic patients. Since the prevalence of TMP-SMX-resistant *E. coli* now often exceeds 10%, bacteria responsible for complicated UTIs must be tested for in vitro susceptibility to TMP-SMX.

Prostatitis

TMP-SMX is the second-best choice after the fluoroquinolones for treatment of bacterial prostatitis. A 4-week course is a minimum for acute prostatitis. In the treatment of chronic or relapsing prostatitis, 2 to 3 months are often necessary, and cure rates do not exceed 50 to 60%.

UTIs in Children

Since fluoroquinolones are not approved for treatment of non-life-threatening infections in children, TMP-SMX remains, with a few new cephalosporins (cefixime), the preferred antimicrobials, with better activity than ampicillin or first-generation cephalosporins. Because of the propensity for pediatric patients to develop adverse effects to TMP-SMX, careful monitoring of side effects and blood counts is mandatory.

Prophylaxis of UTI with TMP-SMX

Prophylaxis of UTI is indicated in patients prone to frequent recurrences of UTI due to reinfection (i.e., due to different bacteria). A common error is the use of prophylactic agents for bacterial relapse.

TMP-SMX is usually administered 3 times weekly at 400/80 mg or even less for 6 to 9 months. The advantages of TMP-SMX are the low rate of selection of resistant mutants, its persistence in urine, and good tolerance.

Prophylaxis of UTI with TMP alone

Long-term, low-dose TMP has been shown to be an effective prophylactic agent in patients with recurrent UTIs. In a placebo-controlled trial, 290 patients (267 women and 23 men) with a history of three or more infections during the previous year were studied (47). This investigation found that bedtime doses of TMP (100 mg) were superior to nitrofurantoin (75 mg), methenamine hippurate (1 g), and placebo in preventing recurrent UTIs during the following 12 months. In the placebo group, 63% of cases recurred within 1 year, compared with 10% in the TMP group. In a similar study, TMP (100 mg) alone was found comparable to nitrofurantoin (100 mg) and TMP-SMX (40/200 mg) in preventing infections, and all regimens were more effective than placebo (62). During the 6-month study period, no patient developed a UTI caused by TMP-resistant Gram-negative bacilli. In a comparison between nitrofurantoin and TMP for prophylaxis in 72 women with recurrent UTIs, nitrofurantoin was more effective in preventing bacteriuria, albeit more patients receiving TMP had radiologic abnormalities (10). In patients taking TMP, fecal coliforms acquired resistance at a rate of about 5% per month, and breakthrough infections were almost exclusively caused by TMP-resistant coliforms. Side effects were more common in the group taking nitrofurantoin. In summary, numerous clinical studies indicate that prophylaxis with TMP alone is comparable in efficacy to TMP-SMX and other commonly used antimicrobials in preventing recurrent UTIs. A reduction of enterobacteria in the rectal and periurethral flora occurs after long-term TMP treatment, and the emergence of TMP-resistant coliforms is low (64). Low-dose, long-term TMP is also well tolerated.

Genital Infections

Despite wide use of TMP-SMX in genital infections, there are currently few indications in which TMP-SMX can be considered a better therapeutic agent than β-lactams, fluoroquinolones, tetracyclines, or macrolides.

Gonococcal Infections

Neisseria gonorrhoeae is naturally resistant to TMP (MIC, 16–32 µg/mL). Hence, TMP-SMX can only be effective if the strain remains susceptible to SMX and by using high dosages of 6 tablets or more (2400/480 mg/day) for 2 to 5 days, with a cure rate of 80 to 95%. Single-dose treatments with up to 8 to 9 tablets were less effective (70–90%, statistically significant)

than multiday regimens. Better results are obtained with all fluoroquinolones and most cephalosporins.

Chlamydial and *Ureaplasma* Infections

TMP-SMX was more effective than placebo or ampicillin given for gonococcal infection in decreasing postgonococcal urethritis attributed to *Chlamydia.* However, TMP-SMX is not effective against both chlamydial and ureaplasmal infections.

Chancroid

TMP-SMX is highly effective for the treatment of chancroid. Unfortunately, resistant strains have emerged and disseminated in many countries of Southeast Asia and Africa (70).

Ear, Nose, and Throat Infections

TMP-SMX has been used for a long time in the treatment of ear, nose, and throat infections. Interest has clearly diminished for three main reasons: *(a)* infections due to *Haemophilus influenzae,* highly susceptible to TMP-SMX, are much less frequent because of successful vaccination; *(b)* penicillin-resistant *S. pneumoniae,* very frequent in otitis media (>40%) in many centers, are resistant to TMP-SMX; *(c) Streptococcus* A are still susceptible in vitro, but TMP-SMX cannot be considered a first-line treatment.

Bronchitis and Pneumonia

The ratio of TMP:SMX in the sputum is about 1:5, a TMP concentration higher than that in serum. This explains the good activity of TMP-SMX against bacteria with low-level resistance to TMP such as *Nocardia* spp., *Branhamella catarrhalis,* and *Neisseria meningitidis* (39).

Exacerbation of Chronic Bronchitis

TMP-SMX was used heavily in the treatment of exacerbations of chronic bronchitis and remains a valuable compound, although less effective than fluoroquinolones or cephalosporins. The success of TMP-SMX was due to its activity on *H. influenzae* and some other bacteria present in this type of infection such as *Klebsiella, E. coli, S. aureus,* and *B. catarrhalis.*

Pneumonia

Despite several reports showing good activity against pneumococcal pneumonia, TMP-SMX might be used only in cases of infections proven due to Gram-negative bacteria, particularly *H. influenzae.*

Enteric Infections (19)

Typhoid Fever

TMP-SMX has been one of the three effective antibiotics, with chloramphenicol and ampicillin, for the treatment of typhoid fever. The clinical response was similar or better than the one obtained with chloramphenicol, and a 14-day treatment regimen at normal doses was at least as effective. TMP-SMX was more effective than chloramphenicol or ampicillin in eradicating *Salmonella typhi* from healthy carriers. Plasmid-mediated resistance to TMP-SMX has emerged in several countries and was associated with epidemics in Mexico, Vietnam, and Peru (31).

Today, fluoroquinolones are the treatment of choice for typhoid fever, followed by ceftriaxone. These antibiotics can be administered effectively for only 5 days. However, because of the high cost of these antibiotics and the recent emergence of fluoroquinolone-resistant strains, TMP-SMX remains a very valuable and useful drug in developing countries.

Other *Salmonella* Infections
TMP-SMX is effective against all the other *Salmonella* species responsible for diarrhea. A 3-day treatment regimen yields a cure in more than 95% of patients. TMP-SMX is also more effective than chloramphenicol and ampicillin in eradicating *Salmonella* from healthy carriers.

Shigella and *E. coli*
TMP-SMX is effective against all *Shigella* species (including *S. dysenteriae*) and various *E. coli* strains causing diarrhea: enteroinvasive, enterotoxinogenic, enteropathogenic, and those causing the hemolytic-uremic syndrome (E. coli O 157). During outbreaks of *Shigella* infections, an increasing rate of TMP-SMX-resistant *Shigella* has been documented (3).

Vibrio, Aeromonas, Plesiomonas
TMP-SMX is the drug of choice for treatment of enteric infections due to a wide spectrum of bacterial pathogens. Of concern is the recent emergence of TMP-SMX-resistant *V. cholerae* O 139 in Bangladesh.

Bone and Soft-Tissue Infections

Acute and chronic osteomyelitis due to *Salmonella, S. aureus,* or *H. influenzae* responds very favorably to TMP-SMX, which can be considered second-line treatment after the fluoroquinolones. Soft-tissue infections, particularly cellulitis due mainly to *Streptococcus pyogenes* and anaerobes, are not likely to respond to TMP-SMX and should clearly be excluded.

Meningitis

TMP-SMX achieves therapeutic concentrations in the cerebrospinal fluid (CSF), approximately 30 to 40% of serum levels. It has been used successfully in the treatment of meningitis due to *E. coli* in neonates and to *Klebsiella pneumoniae, Salmonella,* staphylococci, and *H. influenzae.* Nowadays, these bacteria are treated with third-generation cephalosporins or fluoroquinolones.

In contrast, TMP-SMX can still be considered a first-line therapeutic agent for the treatment of meningitis due to *L. monocytogenes* (54). Clinical results are similar to those obtained with ampicillin (or better). Best in vitro results are obtained when TMP-SMX and ampicillin or amoxicillin are associated. TMP-SMX must obviously be used at the highest dosage of 20 mg/kg TMP and 100 mg/kg SMX or 12 vials intravenously for an adult.

Nocardiosis

Nocardia spp. are naturally resistant to TMP (low level) but usually susceptible to SMX, with a strong synergistic effect between TMP and SMX. Because of the higher susceptibility to SMX

than to TMP, the ratio TMP:SMX should be higher (i.e. 1:2 instead of 1:5). This can be achieved by adding TMP alone to the usual TMP-SMX regimen: four to six regular tablets/day for 1 month, then not more than four tablets/day for 3 to 6 months.

Treatment outcome with TMP-SMX equals that with most recently used antibiotics (Augmentin, cefuroxime, amikacin, or imipenem). This excellent effect is certainly due to the good diffusion of both compounds, particularly in the brain, since about 30% of patients with nocardiosis have a brain abscess.

Miscellaneous and Unusual Infections

Because of its wide spectrum of activity, TMP-SMX has been used to treat many infectious diseases (13, 20, 24, 50, 63, 73, 74).

Endocarditis
TMP-SMX is useful in some clinical settings where other compounds are not available: endocarditis due to *Stenotrophomonas maltophilia,* usually multiresistant, has been successfully treated with TMP-SMX. Endocarditis due to MRSA has been treated with TMP-SMX when vancomycin could not be used.

Melioidosis
A common disease in Southeast Asia, melioidosis can be successfully treated with TMP-SMX, which is more effective against *Burkholderia pseudomallei* than fluoroquinolones.

Brucellosis
More than 1000 reported cases of brucellosis have been treated with TMP-SMX, with doses ranging from four tablets/day for 15 days to six tablets/day for 2 months in the case of osteomyelitis or endocarditis. Results were generally considered satisfactory, but several studies from Italy, Greece, and Spain showed a poor response or a relapse rate of 30 to 50%.

Legionellosis
TMP-SMX is effective in vitro against *Legionella pneumophila.* Very few patients have been treated successfully, and TMP-SMX appears to be less effective than macrolides, rifampicin, or fluoroquinolones.

Whipple disease
Coxiella infections have been treated; more effective agents are available (25).

Bubonic Plague
Plague is still present in several countries in Asia and Africa and rarely in the United States. TMP-SMX is very effective, but fever seems to be of longer duration than in patients treated with streptomycin.

Acne
TMP-SMX is as effective as tetracycline, since *Propionibacterium acnes* is susceptible to both compounds.

Mycobacteria
Mycobacteria are, like *Nocardia,* susceptible to SMX but resistant to TMP; hence, if TMP-SMX is considered as a thera-

peutic choice, an additional dose of TMP alone should be administered to achieve a 1:2 ratio. Mycobacterial infections due to rapid-growing *Mycobacterium marinum, M. fortuitum,* and *M. chelonei* have been successfully treated with a 3- to 6-month course of TMP-SMX (27).

Mycoses

TMP-SMX is the only antibiotic with some effect against various mycotic infections. *Pneumocystis carinii* was recently classified as a fungus rather than a parasite (17). TMP-SMX is still the best therapeutic agent. TMP-SMX has been used successfully against various disseminated histoplasmoses after initial failure of amphotericin. Treatment regimens used the normal dose for 6 months to 2 years. Several paracoccidioidomycoses due to *Paracoccidioides brasiliensis* have been treated successfully. A few patients with phycomycosis or chromomycosis have been treated successfully with TMP-SMX.

Protozoal Infections

TMP-SMX has been used to treat toxoplasmosis but seems less effective than the macrolides or the combination of pyrimethamine with a long-acting sulfonamide, particularly in patients with life-threating infections. TMP-SMX has been used effectively for treatment of *Plasmodium falciparum* malaria resistant to other drugs. However, TMP-SMX is less effective than combinations of pyrimethamine and a long-acting sulfonamide. Coccidiosis due to *Isospora belli* and *Cyclospora cayetanensis* infections are usually self-limiting diarrheal diseases, but they may persist for longer periods. TMP-SMX at the usual dosage administered for 10 to 15 days is one of the few effective treatments.

Clinical Uses

TMP alone has been used clinically for over 25 years to treat acute UTIs (47). The efficacy of TMP is comparable to that of other antibiotics, including TMP-SMX. This was first demonstrated in a double-blind, comparative study that compared TMP (200 mg twice daily) with ampicillin, cephalexin, and TMP-SMX (9). Overall cure rates were 83% with TMP, 83% with TMP-SMX, 73% with ampicillin, and 69% with cephalexin. Outpatients experienced higher cure rates than inpatients in this study. The cure rates for outpatients were 96% for TMP, 91% for TMP-SMX, 89% for ampicillin, and 62% for cephalexin. Of the patients treated with TMP-SMX, 21% experienced adverse effects, compared with 8% of patients treated with TMP alone. Numerous other studies have observed similar outcomes when TMP was compared with TMP-SMX in patients with acute UTIs (55).

Initial clinical trials with TMP suggested higher response rates with increasing doses (47). These early findings were not substantiated by subsequent clinical trials. The Trimethoprim Study Group (68) conducted a multicentered, double-blind, dose-ranging study and found that 7 days of treatment with 50, 100, or 200 mg TMP twice daily produced similar cure rates after 2 and 6 weeks of treatment. Moreover, the incidence of side effects was similar. A comparative clinical trial of TMP

400 mg/day for 14 days and TMP 200 mg/day for 10 days in women with acute UTIs found no significant difference in recurrence rates (42). In this study, the higher dose of TMP was associated with a higher incidence of maculopapular rash.

REFERENCES

1. Acar JF, Goldstein FW, Chabbert YA. Synergistic activity of trimethoprim-sulphamethoxazole combination in Gram-negative bacilli. Observations in vitro and in vivo. J Infect Dis 1973; 128(Suppl):470–477.
2. Acar JF, Goldstein FW. Resistance: genetics and medical implications. In: Hitchings GH, ed. Handbook of experimental pharmacology, vol 64. Berlin: Springer-Verlag, 1983:243–258.
3. Alam NH, Bardhan PK, Haider R, Mahalanabis D. Trimethoprim-sulphamethoxazole in the treatment of persistent diarrhoea: a double blind placebo controlled clinical trial. Arch Dis Child 1995;72:483–486.
4. Alappan R, Perazella MA, Buller GK. Hyperkalemia in hospitalized patients treated with trimethoprim-sulfamethoxazole. Ann Intern Med 1996;124:316–320.
5. Amyes SGB, Smith JT. R-factor trimethoprim resistance mechanism: an insusceptible target site. Biochem Biophys Res Commun 1974;58:412–418.
6. Amyes SBG. Bactericidal activity of trimethoprim alone and in combination with sulfamethoxazole on susceptible and resistant *Escherichia coli* K12. Antimicrob Agents Chemother 1982;21: 288–293.
7. Amyes SGB, Towner KJ. Trimethoprim resistance; epidemiology and molecular aspects. J Med Microbiol 1990;31:1–19.
8. Branger C, Fournier JM, Loulergue J, Bouvet A, Goullet Ph, Boutonnier A, De Gialluly C, Couetdic G, Chomarat M, Jaffar-Baiyee MC, Mariani P. Epidemiol Infect 1994;112:489–500.
9. Brumfitt W, Pursell R. Double-blind trial to compare ampicillin, cephalexin, co-trimoxazole, and trimethoprim in treatment of urinary infection. Br Med J 1972;2:673–676.
10. Brumfitt W, Smith GW, Hamilton-Miller JMT, Gargan RA. A clinical comparison between Macrodantin and trimethoprim for prophylaxis in women with recurrent urinary infections. J Antimicrob Chemother 1985;16:111–120.
11. Burchall JJ. Mechanisms of action of trimethoprim sulfamethoxazole. II. J Infect Dis 1973;128(Suppl):S437–441.
12. Burdeska A, Ott M, Bannwarth W, Then RL. Identical genes for trimethoprim-resistant dihydrofolate reductase from *Staphylococcus aureus* in Australia and Central Europe. FEBS 1990;266: 159–162.
13. Burlacoff SG, Wong FSH. Wegener's granulomatosis. The great masquerade: a clinical presentation and literature review. J Otolaryngol 1993;22:94–105.
14. Bushby SRM. Sensitivity testing with trimethoprim-sulphamethoxazole. Med J Aust 1973;1(Suppl):10–18.
15. Bushby SRM. Antibacterial activity. In: Hitchings GH, ed. Inhibition of folate metabolism in chemotherapy, vol 64. Berlin: Springer-Verlag, 1983:75–105.
16. Cabanas R, Caballero MT, Vega A, Martin-Esteban M, Pascual C. Anaphylaxis to trimethoprim. J Allergy Clin Immunol 1996; 1:137–138.
17. Cailliez JC, Séguy N, Denis CM, Aliouat EM, Mazars E, Polonelli L, Camus D, Dei-Cas E. *Pneumocystis carinii:* an atypical fungal micro-organism. J Med Vet Mycol 1996;34:227–239.
18. Charpentier E, Courvalin P. Emergence of a new class of trimethoprim resistance gene *dfr*D in *Listeria monocytogenes*

[Abstract C89]. Presented at the 35th Interscience Conference on Antimicrobial Agents and Chemotherapy, San Francisco, Sept 17–20, 1995.

19. Clements ML, Black RE, Levine MM. Treatment of enteric infections and combinations. In: Hitchings GH, ed. Inhibition of folate metabolism in chemotherapy, vol 64. Berlin: Springer-Verlag, 1983:357–378.

20. Cockerill FR III. Trimethoprim-sulfamethoxazole. Mayo Clin Proc 1991;66:1260–1269.

21. Courvalin D, Fiandt M. Aminoglycoside-modifying enzymes of *Staphylococcus aureus,* expression in *Escherichia coli.* Gene 1980;9:247–269.

22. Czeizel A. A case-control analysis of the teratogenic effects of co-trimoxazole. Reprod Toxicol 1990;4:305–313.

23. Dale GE, Langen H, Page MGP, Then RL, Stüber D. Cloning and characterization of a novel, plasmid-encoded trimethoprim-resistant dihydrofolate reductase from *Staphylococcus haemolyticus* MUR313. Antimicrob Agents Chemother 1995;39:1920–1924.

24. Desjardins RE. Treatment of miscellaneous and unusual infections with trimethoprim and trimethoprim-sulfonamide combinations. In: Hitchings GH, ed. Inhibition of folate metabolism in chemotherapy, vol 64. Berlin: Springer-Verlag, 1983:411–440.

25. Feurle GE, Marth T. An evaluation of antimicrobial treatment for Whipple's disease. Tetracycline versus trimethoprim-sulfamethoxazole. Dig Dis Sci 1994;39:1642–1648.

26. Fleming MP, Datta N, Grüneberg RN. Trimethoprim resistance determined by R factors. Br Med J 1972;1:726–728.

27. Fraser I, Macintosh I, Wilkins EG. Prophylactic effect of co-trimoxazole for *Mycobacterium avium* complex infection: a previously unreported benefit. Clin Infect Dis 1994;19:211.

28. Gasc AM, Kauc L, Baraillé P, Sicard M, Goodgal S. Gene localization, size, and physical map of the chromosome of *Streptococcus pneumoniae.* J Bacteriol 1991;173:7361–7367.

29a. Girdwood RH. The nature of possible adverse reactions to co-trimoxazole. Scand J Infect Dis 1976;8(Suppl):10–16.

29b. Gluckstein D, Ruskin J. Rapid oral desensitization to trimethoprim-sulfamethoxazole (TMP-SMZ): use in prophylaxis for *Pneumocystis carinii* pneumonia in patients with AIDS who were previously intolerant to TMP-SMZ. Clin Infect Dis 1995;20:849–853.

30. Goldstein FW. Mécanismes de résistance aux sulfamides et au triméthoprime. Bull Inst Pasteur (Paris) 1977;75:109–139.

31. Goldstein FW, Chumpitaz JC, Guevara JM, Papadopoulou B, Acar JF, Vieu JF. Plasmid-mediated resistance to multiple antibiotics in *Salmonella typhi.* J Infect Dis 1986;153:261–266.

32. Goldstein FW, Gerbaud G, Courvalin P. Transposable resistance to trimethoprim and 0/129 in *Vibrio cholerae.* J Antimicrob Chemother 1986;17:559–569.

33. Goldstein FW, Acar JF, and the Alexander Project Collaborative Group. Antimicrobial resistance among lower respiratory tract isolates of *Streptococcus pneumoniae:* results of a 1992–93 Western Europe and USA collaborative surveillance study. J Antimicrob Chemother 1996;38(Suppl A):71–84.

34. Grüneberg E, de Lorenzo WF. Potentiation of sulfonamides and antibiotics by trimethoprim [(2,4-diamino-5(3,4,5-trimethoxybenzyl) pyrimidine]. Antimicrob Agents Chemother 1966;6:430–433.

35. Gutmann L, Williamson R, Moreau N, Kitzis MD, Collatz E, Acar JF, Goldstein FW. Cross-resistance to nalidixic acid, trimethoprim and chloramphenicol associated with alterations in outer membrane proteins of *Klebsiella, Enterobacter* and *Serratia.* J Infect Dis 1985;151:501–507.

36. Hansen I. Clinical pharmacokinetics of co-trimoxazole. In: Hitchings GH, ed. Inhibition of folate metabolism in chemotherapy, vol 64. Berlin: Springer-Verlag, 1983:229–242.

37. Harrison MS, Simonte SJ, Kauffman CA. Trimethoprim-induced aseptic meningitis in a patient with AIDS: case report and review. Clin Infect Dis 1994;19:431–434.

38. Herrington A, Mahmood A, Berger R. Treatment options in sulfamethoxazole-trimethoprim-induced thrombocytopenic purpura. South Med J 1994;87:948–950.

39. Hughes DTD. Co-trimoxazole in chest infections including in long-term use in chest disease. In: Hitchings GH, ed. Inhibition of folate metabolism in chemotherapy, vol 64. Berlin: Springer-Verlag, 1983:397–410.

40. Huovinen P, Sundstroem L, Swedberg G, Skoeld O. Trimethoprim and sulfonamide resistance. Antimicrob Agents Chemother 1995;39:279–289.

41. Huovinen P. Increase in rates of resistance to trimethoprim. Clin Infect Dis 1997;24(Suppl 1):S63–68.

42. Irvani A, Richard GA, Baer H. Treatment of uncomplicated urinary infections with trimethoprim versus sulfisoxazole, with special reference to antibody-coated bacteria and fecal flora. Antimicrob Agents Chemother 1981;19:842–850.

43. Jick H. Adverse reactions to trimethoprim-sulfamethoxazole in hospitalized patients. Rev Infect Dis 1982;4:426–428.

44. Jick H, Derby LE. Is cotrimoxazole safe? Lancet 1995;345:1118–1119.

45. Johnson JR, Collins GM, Rementer ML, Hall ML. Novel mechanism of resistance to folate analogues: ribonucleoside diphosphate reductase deficiency in bacteriophage T4. Antimicrob Agents Chemother 1976;9:292–300.

46. Jung AC, Paauw DS. Management of adverse reactions to trimethoprim-sulfamethoxazole in human immunodeficiency virus-infected patients. Arch Intern Med 1994;154:2402–2406.

47. Kasanen A, Sundquist H. Trimethoprim alone in the treatment of urinary tract infections: eight years of experience in Finland. Rev Infect Dis 1982;4:358–365.

48. Köhler T, Kok M, Michea-Hamzehpour M, Plesiat P, Gotoh N, Nishino T, Kocjancic Curty L, Péchère JC. Multidrug efflux in intrinsic resistance to trimethoprim and sulfamethoxazole in *Pseudomonas aeruginosa.* Antimicrob Agents Chemother 1996;40:2288–2290.

49. Lawson DH. Adverse effect of co-trimoxazole. In: Hitchings GH, ed. Inhibition of folate metabolism in chemotherapy, vol 64. Berlin: Springer-Verlag, 1983:207–227.

50. Lewis DA, Reeves DS. Antibacterial agents: trimethoprim and cotrimoxazole. Prescriber's J 1995;35:25–31.

51. Lindgren A, Olsson R. Liver reactions from trimethoprim. J Intern Med 1994;236:281–284.

52. Locher HH, Schlunegger H, Hartman PG, Angehrn P, Then RL. Antibacterial activities of epiprim, a new dihydrofolate reductase inhibitor, alone and in combination with dapsone. Antimicrob Agents Chemother 1996;40:1376–1381.

53. Markowitz N, Quinn EL, Saravolatz LD. Trimethoprim-sulfamethoxazole compared with vancomycin for the treatment of *Staphylococcus aureus* infection. Ann Intern Med 1992;117:390–398.

54. Merle-Melet M, Meyer P, Dossou-Gbete L, Weber M, Kuntzburger O, Gerard A. Is amoxicillin-cotrimoxazole the most appropriate antibiotic regimen for *Listeria* meningoencephalitis? Review of 24 cases [Abstract M62]. Presented at the 34th Interscience Conference on Antimicrobial Agents and Chemotherapy, Orlando, FL, Oct 4–7, 1994:260.

55. Neu HC. Trimethoprim alone for treatment of urinary tract infection. Rev Infect Dis 1982;4:366–371.

56. Pancoast SJ, Hyams DM, Neu HC. Effect of trimethoprim and trimethoprim-sulfamethoxazole on development of drug-resistant vaginal and fecal flora. Antimicrob Agents Chemother 1980;17:263–268.

57. Papadopoulou B, Goldstein FW, Acar JF. Etude de l'activité bactériostatique et bactéricide de l'association sulfamethoxazole-triméthoprime sur *Haemophilus* sp. et leur sensibilité in vitro vis-à-vis de 10 antibiotiques. Med Mal Infect 1988;18:367–374.

58. Pattishall KH, Acar JF, Burchall JJ, Goldstein FW, Harvey RJ. Two distinct types of trimethoprim-resistant dihydrofolate reductase specified by R plasmids of different compatibility groups. J Biol Chem 1977;252:2319–2323.

59. Quintiliani R, Levitz R, Nightingale CH. Potential role of trimethoprim-sulfamethoxazole in the treatment of serious hospital-acquired bacterial infections. Rev Infect Dis 1987;9 (Suppl 2):S160–S167.

60. Roth B. Selective inhibitors of bacterial dihydrofolate reductase: structure-activity relationships. In: Hitchings GH, ed. Inhibition of folate metabolism in chemotherapy, vol 64. Berlin: Springer-Verlag, 1983:107–127.

61. Sigel CW. Disposition and metabolism of trimethoprim, tetroxoprim, sulfamethoxazole, and sulfadiazine. In: Hitchings GH, ed. Inhibition of folate metabolism in chemotherapy, vol 64. Berlin: Springer-Verlag, 1983:163–184.

62. Stamm WE, Counts GW, McKevitt M, Turck M, Holmes KK. Urinary prophylaxis with trimethoprim and trimethoprim-sulfamethoxazole: efficacy, influence on the natural history of recurrent bacteriuria, and cost control. Rev Infect Dis 1982;4: 450–455.

63. Stegeman CA, Cohen Tervaert JW, de Jong PE, Kallenberg CG. Prevention of relapses of Wegener's granulomatosis by treatment with trimethoprim-sulfamethoxazole. A multicenter placebo-controlled trial. Kidney Int 1995;48:1367–1368.

64. Svensson R, Larsson P, Lincoln K. Low dose trimethoprim prophylaxis in long term control of chronic recurrent urinary tract infection. Scand J Infect Dis 1982;14:139–142.

65. Then R. Synergism between trimethoprim and sulphamethoxazole. Science 1978;197:1301.

66. Then RL. Resistance to sulfonamides. Reprint from: Bryan LE, ed. Handbook of experimental pharmacology, vol 91. Berlin: Springer-Verlag, 1989.

67. Towner KJ, Slack RCB. Effect of changing selection pressures of trimethoprim resistance in Enterobacteriaceae. Eur J Clin Microbiol 1986;5:502–506.

68. Trimethoprim Study Group. Comparison of trimethoprim at three dosage levels with co-trimoxazole in the treatment of acute urinary tract infection in general practice. J Antimicrob Chemother 1981;7:179–183.

69. Turnidge JP, Nimmo GR, Francis G. Evolution of resistance in *Staphylococcus aureus* in Australian teaching hospitals. Med J Aust 1996;164:68–71.

70. Van Dyck E, Bogaerts J, Smet H, Tello WM, Mukantabana V, Piot P. Emergence of *Haemophilus ducreyi* resistance to trimethoprim-sulfamethoxazole in Rwanda. Antimicrob Agents Chemother 1994;38:1647–1648.

71. Voss A, Milatovic D, Wallrauch-Schwarz C, Rosdahl VT, Braveny I. Methicillin-resistant *Staphylococcus aureus* in Europe. Eur J Clin Microbiol Infect Dis 1994;13:50–55.

72. Waecker NJ, Kelso J, Price B, Robb M. Rapid intravenous trimethoprim-sulfamethoxazole desensitization in an HIV infected infant with *Pneumocystis carinii* [Abstract 184]. Clin Infect Dis 1995;21:750.

73. Williams L. Trimethoprim-sulfamethoxazole. Infect Dis Ther 1994;ser. 9:169–181.

74. Wormser GP. Trimethoprim-sulfamethoxazole II. Clinical studies. NY State J Med 1978;78:2058–2067.

75. Wüst J, Kayser FH. Die Empfindlichkeit von Bakterien gegen Chemotherapeutika. Praxis 1995;84:98–105.

Vancomycin

•

Sara G. Monroe and Ron Polk

Vancomycin is a complex glycopeptide antibiotic isolated in 1956 from a soil sample from Borneo containing a newly discovered actinomycete, *Nocardia orientalis*. In the late 1950s, the incidence of penicillin-resistant strains of *Staphylococcus aureus* was increasing, and interest in alternative effective antimicrobials was high. Initial lots of vancomycin contained large amounts of impurities, and it was termed "Mississippi Mud" because of its brown discoloration. In the early 1960s, interest in vancomycin diminished when various side effects were noted and less-toxic agents such as methicillin and cephalosporins became available. In the past 15 years there has

been a resurgence of interest in vancomycin because of the marked increase in infections caused by β-lactam-resistant Gram-positive bacteria. Usage has also increased because improvements in the manufacturing process have resulted in purer preparations of vancomycin with decreased toxicity. Increased usage, however, has been accompanied by increased resistance, threatening the future utility of these unique drugs.

CHEMISTRY

Vancomycin is a large, complex glycopeptide with a molecular weight of 1449, greater than the molecular weights of any of the penicillins, cephalosporins, tetracyclines, aminoglycosides, or macrolides. It is supplied commercially as a hydrochloride salt and is most soluble at pH 3 to 5. Solubility decreases with increasing pH, and vancomycin is unstable in alkaline solutions. Vancomycin powder is generally reconstituted with sodium chloride or sterile water, and solutions are stable for 14 days at room temperature.

ANTIMICROBIAL ACTIVITY

With rare exceptions, the antibacterial spectrum of vancomycin is limited to Gram-positive aerobic and anaerobic organisms (Table 1). Bacteria inhibited by concentrations of 4 mg/L or less are considered susceptible while, those with minimal inhibitory concentrations (MICs) of 16 or above are resistant (90). Vancomycin is bactericidal against sensitive bacteria, except for the enterococci, which are inhibited but not killed by clinically achievable concentrations. The combination of vancomycin and an aminoglycoside is bactericidal against enterococci unless high-level aminoglycoside resistance (MIC $\geq$ 500 mg/L) is present (59, 126).

More controversy surrounds the efficacy of the combination of vancomycin and rifampin. When used against coagulase-negative staphylococci, vancomycin and rifampin are often synergistic and rarely demonstrate antagonism (42, 76). However, in *S. aureus,* vancomycin-rifampin synergy is found inconsistently (9, 119, 120), and antagonism has been reported (58, 127). In clinical studies of methicillin-resistant *S. aureus* (MRSA) endocarditis, the response to combination therapy has varied. In an experimental model of MRSA endocarditis, Bayer and Lam found vancomycin-rifampin to be more effective in eradicating organisms from the valve and causing clinical cure than vancomycin alone (8). However, in a randomized trial of vancomycin alone versus vancomycin-rifampin

for treatment of MRSA endocarditis in humans, Levine et al. found slow clinical response in both groups, and no advantage to combination treatment (74).

Both methicillin-sensitive and -resistant strains of *S. aureus* and most strains of coagulase-negative staphylococci are highly susceptible to vancomycin and are usually inhibited by concentrations of 0.25 to 4.0 mg/L. However, some strains of *S. aureus* are deficient in autolysins and are tolerant to the bactericidal activity of vancomycin (MBC/MIC $\geq$ 32) (54, 106). Streptococci, including viridans species, anaerobic and microaerophilic strains, and penicillin-sensitive and -resistant pneumococci are susceptible. Most strains of *Listeria monocytogenes* are inhibited by clinically achievable levels of vancomycin, but MBCs may exceed MICs (121), and therapeutic failures have been reported (5, 39).

Nondiphtheroid corynebacteria including *C. jeikeium* are highly susceptible (MICs $\leq$ 1 mg/L) (66). Species of *Lactobacillus, Leuconostoc,* and *Pediococcus* that may be opportunistic pathogens are frequently resistant to vancomycin, with MICs that exceed 256 mg/L (102, 115).

The anaerobic spectrum of vancomycin includes anaerobic and microaerophilic streptococci, and clostridia species, including both *C. perfringens* and *C. difficile.* The susceptibility of actinomycetes is variable (73), and Gram-negative anaerobes such as *Bacteroides* species are resistant. Vancomycin has virtually no activity against Gram-negative organisms including *Enterobacteriaceae,* rickettsiae, chlamydia, and mycobacteria (23).

MECHANISM OF ACTION

Vancomycin acts on the second stage of cell wall synthesis to inhibit formation of peptidoglycan, the major structural polymer of the bacterial cell wall. Penicillins and cephalosporins inhibit

---

TABLE 1 • Antibacterial Spectrum of Vancomycin

Organism	Range (μg/mL)	MIC$_{50}$[a] (μg/mL)	MIC$_{90}$ (μg/mL)
Staphylococcus aureus (methicillin sensitive)	0.25–1	0.5	1
S. aureus (methicillin resistant)	0.3–12.0	1.5	2
Staphylococcus epidermidis (methicillin susceptible)	1–2	2	2
S. epidermidis (methicillin resistant)	1–4	2	4
Streptococcus pyogenes (group A)	0.5	0.5	0.5
Streptococcus agalactiae (group B)	0.03–2	0.5	0.5
Group C and G streptococci	0.25–2	0.5	1
Streptococcus mitis	0.03–2	0.5	1
Streptococcus sanguis	0.03–0.5	0.5	1
Streptococcus bovis	0.25–2	0.25	0.25
Streptococcus pneumoniae (penicillin susceptible)	0.06–0.5	0.25	0.25
S. pneumoniae (penicillin resistant)	0.25–1	0.5	1
Enterococcus faecalis (gentamicin susceptible)	1–4	1	2
E. faecalis (gentamicin resistant)	1–4	1	4
Actinomyces spp.	0.5–2	0.5	2
Bacillus spp.	0.25–4	2	2
Lactobacillus spp.	0.25–32	1	2
Listeria monocytogenes	0.5–2	1	1
Corynebacterium jeikeium (JK diphtheroids)	0.5–1	1	1
Clostridium difficile	0.5–4	1	2

Adapted from Cunha BA. Vancomycin. Med Clin North Am 1995;79:817.

[a]MIC, minimum inhibitory concentration.

the third stage of cell wall synthesis and block cross linkage of peptide side chains. These different sites of action may help explain the lack of cross-resistance between vancomycin and β-lactam antibiotics. Vancomycin also alters the permeability of cytoplasmic membranes of protoplasts and may impair RNA synthesis. The multiple mechanisms of action may partially account for the low incidence of resistance to vancomycin in most Gram-positive bacteria. Vancomycin is bactericidal to multiplying organisms except enterococci and tolerant strains of staphylococci (23). In vitro antibacterial activity continues approximately 2 h after its concentration has fallen below the inhibitory level (postantibiotic effect) (29).

MECHANISMS OF RESISTANCE

Acquired resistance to vancomycin was unusual until the late 1980s, when reports of enterococci resistant to glycopeptides began to occur. This increase in resistance coincided with an explosive increase in the use of vancomycin to treat MRSA and coagulase-negative staphylococcal infections as well as *C. difficile* colitis. As a result of the selective pressure exerted by heavy use of vancomycin and other antibiotics, resistance to glycopeptides developed.

The prevalence of vancomycin-resistant enterococci isolated from intensive care units increased from 0.4% in 1989 to 13.6% in 1993 (19). This pattern of increased resistance has caused concern because of *(a)* the loss of bactericidal activity when glycopeptides are used with aminoglycosides, *(b)* concurrent resistance to multiple antibiotics, *(c)* the potential transfer of vancomycin resistance to other Gram-positive bacteria (72, 97), and *(d)* instances in which no alternative agent(s) may be available. Most vancomycin-resistant enterococcal isolates have been *E. faecium*, but glycopeptide resistance has also been seen in *E. faecalis, E. gallinarum, E. casseliflavus, E. avium, E. durans* (4), *E. hirae, E. mundtii,* and *E. raffinosus* (70).

There are three major glycopeptide resistance types, based on the level, inducibility, and transferability of resistance to vancomycin and teicoplanin (Table 2). VanA is the most common phenotype, and these strains have high-level resistance to both vancomycin and teicoplanin. Normally, glycopeptides inhibit cell wall synthesis by forming complexes with the terminal D-alanine residues of peptidoglycan precursors. VanA resistance is mediated by production of a ligase that results in synthesis of

cell wall precursors that end in the depsipeptide D-alanyl-lactate rather than the dipeptide D-alanyl-D-alanine, the target for vancomycin (4). VanA expression is inducible and may be transferred by plasmids to susceptible enterococci (4) as well as to other Gram-positive organisms. VanA resistance has been found in *E. faecium, E. faecalis, E. avium,* and *E. gallinarum.*

Vancomycin resistance has been transferred to *S. aureus* in vitro (71, 94), and clinical isolates with intermediate susceptibility have been reported recently (20, 63). In Japan, Hiramatsu et al. described the first documented infection caused by *S. aureus* with intermediate-level resistance (MIC, 8 mg/L) to vancomycin (VISA) in a 4-month-old infant with a sternal wound infection (63). This isolate did not carry *vanA* or *vanB* genes, and the mechanism of resistance has not been determined. According to Hiramatsu, 2% of MRSA isolates in his hospital have reduced vancomycin susceptibility. An additional case of VISA was reported from the United States in a chronic ambulatory peritoneal dialysis (CAPD) patient with peritonitis (20). Both VISA isolates were susceptible to other antimicrobials.

VanB strains have lower levels of resistance to vancomycin (MIC, 32–256 mg/L) and are susceptible to teicoplanin, although vancomycin use may induce resistance to teicoplanin. Resistance is inducible and chromosomally mediated but can be transferred by conjugation in some strains (98). VanB resistance has been found in *E. faecium* and *E. faecalis* and was recently described in a clinical isolate of *Streptococcus bovis* (97).

VanC strains have low-level vancomycin resistance (MICs, 8–32 mg/L) and are susceptible to teicoplanin. The *vanC* gene is chromosomal, constitutive, and nontransferable (4). VanC has been described only in *E. gallinarum, E. casseliflavus,* and *E. flavescens.*

Concern that vancomycin use may exert selective pressure that encourages emergence of vancomycin-resistant enterococci (VRE) as well as reports that use is associated with colonization and infection with VRE (21, 67) prompted the Centers for Disease Control and Prevention (CDC) to develop recommendations for prudent use of this antibiotic (21) (Table 3).

PHARMACOKINETIC DISPOSITION

Vancomycin is administered orally or intravenously. Intramuscular injection causes severe pain and is not recommended. Systemic absorption after oral administration is minimal, and serum levels are undetectable in both healthy

TABLE 2 • Glycopeptide Resistance

Resistance Type	MIC (mg/L) Vancomycin	MIC (mg/L) Teicoplanin	Expression	Transferable	Bacterial Species
Acquired					
vanA	64–>1000	16–512	Inducible	Yes	*E. faecium, E. faecalis, E. avium E. durans, E. hirae, E. mundtii, E. raffinosus, E. gallinarium*
vanB	4–1024	0.25–2	Inducible	Yes	*E. casseliflavus, E. faecium, E. faecalis, S. bovis*
Intrinsic					
vanC	2–32	0.12–2	Constitutive	No	*E. gallinarium, E. casseliflavus, E. flavescens*

Adapted from Arthur M, Courvalin P. Genetics and mechanisms of glycopeptide resistance in enterococci. Antimicrob Agents Chemother 1993;37:1563.

Appropriate Use
- Treatment of infections caused by β-lactam-resistant Gram-positive organisms
- Treatment of Gram-positive infections in patients with serious allergies to β-lactam antibiotics
- Treatment of *C. difficile* colitis that has failed to respond to metronidazole or is severe and potentially life threatening
- Endocarditis prophylaxis as recommended by the American Heart Association (34)
- Prophylaxis for implantation of prosthetic devices or materials at institutions with high rates of MRSA or MRSE infection

Inappropriate Use
- Routine surgical prophylaxis
- Empirical therapy for febrile neutropenic patients unless there is evidence of possible Gram-positive infection
- Treatment in response to a single blood culture positive for coagulase-negative staphylococci
- Continued empirical use for presumed infection in the absence of positive cultures
- Prophylaxis for infection or colonization of intravascular catheters
- Selective decontamination of the GI tract
- Eradication of MRSA colonization
- Primary treatment of *C. difficile* colitis
- Routine prophylaxis for very low birth weight infants
- Routine prophylaxis for patients on dialysis
- Treatment chosen for dosing convenience in patients with renal failure
- Topical application or irrigation

Adapted from Recommendations for preventing the spread of vancomycin resistance. MMWR 1995;44:RR-12.

volunteers and anephric patients (15). Inflammation of the gastrointestinal (GI) tract may result in increased absorption, and serum concentrations of 5 mg/L have been measured in patients with *C. difficile* colitis (40). When taken orally, vancomycin is excreted in stool in high concentrations that far exceed the MIC for *C. difficile* (31).

Systemic infections are treated with vancomycin administered by slow (at least 60 min) intravenous infusion to avoid infusion-related events (see "Adverse Effects"). Distribution is a complex process consistent with a two- or three-compartment pharmacokinetic model. An initial distribution half-life of less than 8 min is followed by an intermediate half-life of 30 to 90 min. Elimination half-life varies between 5 and 11 h in normal subjects (87). Vancomycin volume of distribution is approximately 0.9 L/kg, and it penetrates well into most body fluids and tissues (87) (Table 4). With multiple dosing, levels above 75% of those in serum are attainable in ascitic, pericardial, and synovial fluid, 50% in pleural fluid, and 30 to 50% in bile (80). Penetration into aqueous humor (77) and cerebrospinal fluid (CSF) in the absence of inflammation is negligible. Vancomycin penetration into CSF in the presence of inflamed meninges is unpredictable, with reported ranges of 1 to 37% of serum levels (28, 57, 124), and a mean of 2.5 mg/L, or 15% of serum levels (31). This level may be inadequate to treat some organisms, and supplemental intrathecal injection of 3 to 5 mg of vancomycin may be necessary for treatment of meningitis. In animal mod-

els, high tissue levels have been measured in the kidney, liver, and spleen (43), and a preliminary study in humans showed substantial levels in the heart, aorta, kidney, liver, and lung (117). Penetration into bone is more variable, even in patients with osteomyelitis (55). Vancomycin penetrates well into abscess fluid, with levels approximating those found in serum (117). In patients on CAPD, intravenous administration results in peritoneal fluid levels 20 to 25% of concentrations in serum (88).

ELIMINATION

Vancomycin is excreted almost completely by the kidneys, primarily by glomerular filtration. There is no significant metabolism, and 80 to 90% of a dose appears unchanged in urine within 24 h (85). There is a linear relationship between creatinine and vancomycin clearances, with C_{vanc} approximately 70% of C_{cr}. The difference between C_{vanc} and C_{cr} is likely due to by vancomycin-protein binding, since significant renal tubular secretion and absorption have not been reported in humans (28). As renal function declines, the elimination half-life of vancomycin increases, leading to higher levels unless the dosage is reduced. In normal individuals, the elimination half-life is 5 to 11 h; in anephric patients, it may exceed 7 days (87).

DOSAGE REGIMENS

In adults with normal renal function, the usual dose of vancomycin is 1 g (or 15 mg/kg) every 12 h. This dose results in peak serum concentrations of 25 to 40 mg/L 1 h after completion of infusion and trough levels of 5 to 15 mg/L and is unlikely to result in toxicity. Studies in which patients with normal renal function were treated with fixed doses of vancomycin demonstrated clinical efficacy in the treatment of Gram-positive infections (17, 113, 124).

In children with normal renal function, fixed dosage is based on age as follows: <1 week, 15 mg/kg every 12 h; 8 to 30 days, 15 mg/kg every 8 h; >30 days, 10 mg/kg every 6 h (110). Vancomycin doses in premature infants are based on gestational age as follows: <27 weeks, 27 mg/kg every 36 h; 27 to 30 weeks, 24 mg/kg every 24 h; 31 to 36 weeks, 18 mg/kg every 24 h, >37 weeks, 22.5 mg/kg every 12 h (64).

In patients with altered physiology, the dose or dosage interval may need to be altered. Compared with normal individuals, obese patients have larger volumes of distribution and increased rates of glomerular filtration, with shorter a elimination half-life of vancomycin. In obese patients, the dose is 15 mg/kg every 12 h, based on total body weight (12). In burn patients and intravenous drug abusers, the half-life is shorter and dose requirements are higher (49, 105). Elimination half-life is prolonged in patients over 60 years old, possibly as a result of altered tissue binding as well as age-related decreases in GFR, and dosage interval may need to be extended (32). In patients with altered physiology, dosing should be individualized, and measurement of serum vancomycin concentrations may be useful (see below).

Dosing in Renal Failure

Vancomycin is virtually completely eliminated by the kidney, and dose adjustments are needed to prevent accumulation to toxic levels in patients with renal insufficiency. Since van-

TABLE 4 • Penetration of Vancomycin into Body Fluids after Intravenous Administration

Body Fluid	Mean Vancomycin Concentration (mg/dL)	Mean Corresponding Serum Level	Fluid:Serum Ratio
CSF			
Uninflamed meninges	0	6.3	0
Inflamed meninges	2.5[a]–3.9[b]	—	0.18[b]
Bile	2.3	6.4	0.36
Pericardial fluid			
Single dose	2.3	6.2	0.37
Multiple doses	6.7	8.6	0.78
Pleural fluid	2.9	7.3	0.40
Ascitic fluid			
Single dose	2.3	6.2	0.37
Multiple doses	6.7	8.6	0.78
Synovial fluid	5.7	7.0	0.81
Aqueous humor	<0.78	14	<0.06

From Cooper GL, Given DB. Vancomycin: a comprehensive review of 30 years of clinical experience. Park Row Publishers, 1986.

[a]Adults.

[b]Children.

comycin elimination correlates directly with creatinine clearance, measurements of renal function are the best predictors of vancomycin pharmacokinetics. A number of nomograms have been developed to determine the vancomycin dose or dosage interval based on estimates of renal function from creatinine clearance. Creatinine clearance can be estimated with some accuracy on the basis of the patient's age, weight, serum creatinine, and sex, using the following formula (26):

$$CrCl\ (males) = [Wt\ (kg) \times (140 - age)]/[72 \times Scr]$$
$$CrCl\ (females) = 0.85 \times CrCl\ (males)$$

These nomograms are used to predict vancomycin dose for different levels of renal function and are designed to achieve steady-state serum concentrations of 10 to 15 mg/L, peak concentrations of 25 to 40 mg/L, and troughs of 5 to 10 mg/L (85, 93, 100). A disadvantage of these nomograms is that vancomycin is dosed daily, although elimination half-life may be as long as 7 days in patients with end-stage renal disease. Matzke et al. (80) have developed a nomogram designed to take advantage of the favorable pharmacokinetics in patients with abnormal renal function. In Matzke's method, the dose of vancomycin remains constant at 15 mg/kg, but the dosing interval increases with declining renal function (Fig. 1).

Dosing in Dialysis

Vancomycin is not cleared from serum significantly by standard hemodialysis or CAPD (75, 78). The usual dose in patients on dialysis is 1000 mg weekly, since in the average adult, approximately 150 mg/day is removed by nonrenal mechanisms (46). Since clearance with dialysis is minimal, dosing after dialysis is not necessary. Hemodialysis with the newer, more-permeable, high-flux membranes or continuous a-v and v-v hemodialysis results in more rapid vancomycin clearance and more frequent dosing may be necessary (35). In such patients, serum trough level measurement may be useful in determining the appropriate dosing interval.

Vancomycin is not cleared by CAPD, although removal by intermittent peritoneal dialysis is more variable (11). Intravenous administration of vancomycin results in peritoneal fluid levels that are 20 to 25% of serum levels, which may be advantageous in treating peritonitis in patients on CAPD (88). Intraperitoneal administration of 1 g of vancomycin results in high peritoneal fluid concentrations and therapeutic serum levels, although these are achieved slowly (2, 12, 88). The maintenance dose is 10 to 20 mg vancomycin per liter of dialysate, with monitoring of serum trough levels to guide the timing of additional doses.

THERAPEUTIC MONITORING

Many have advocated routine monitoring of vancomycin serum concentrations to ensure therapeutic levels and prevent toxicity. This approach has been questioned because there is little evidence of a correlation between serum vancomycin levels and either clinical efficacy or toxicity (18, 48, 86). Studies confirming a relationship between serum concentrations and clinical outcome are lacking in the literature. In a retrospective chart review, Zimmerman et al. (132) studied clinical outcome (measured by duration of fever and leukocytosis) in patients with Gram-positive bacteremia treated with vancomycin. They concluded that patients with peak levels above 20 mg/L and trough levels above 10 mg/L are more likely to become afebrile and have their white blood cell counts normalize within 24 h. However, their study is limited by the small number of subjects included (31) and retrospective design. In contrast, many studies have demonstrated the efficacy of fixed (empirical) doses of vancomycin in the treatment of Gram-positive infections (18). The pharmacokinetics of vancomycin are sufficiently predictable to allow serum levels above the MIC of most Gram-positive organisms with empirical dosing. There is no evidence that increased serum levels are associated with improved clinical outcome.

The need to monitor vancomycin serum levels to prevent toxicity is also a controversial area. There is little evidence to support the occurrence of ototoxicity, and the incidence of

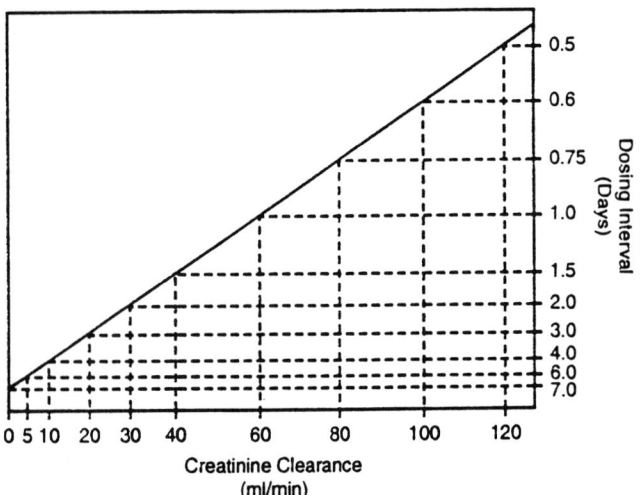

FIGURE 1. Dosage of vancoymcin in patients with varying degrees of renal function. (Adapted from Matzke GR, McGory RW, Halstenson CE, Keane WF. Pharmacokinetics of vancomycin in patients with various degrees of renal function. Antimicrob Agents Chemother 1984;25:433–437.

nephrotoxicity when vancomycin is used alone is approximately 5% (103) (see "Adverse Effects"). A causal relationship between serum concentration and nephrotoxicity has not been proven and there is no evidence that maintaining trough concentrations below a certain level prevents toxicity (25, 103).

Although measurement of serum drug concentrations is not necessary in most cases, monitoring may be useful in the following circumstances (86):

1. Rapidly changing renal function
2. Patients on dialysis receiving infrequent doses for serious systemic infections
3. Patients on CVVH, CAVH, or dialysis with high-flux membranes
4. Use of higher-than-usual doses (i.e., in the treatment of penicillin-resistant *Streptococcus pneumoniae* meningitis, burn patients)

When serum levels are measured, only trough concentrations are needed to determine that adequate levels are being maintained. Peak concentrations are difficult to measure accurately because of rapid distribution of drug (60) and have not been shown to correlate with efficacy or toxicity.

ADVERSE EFFECTS

Shortly after its introduction, vancomycin developed a reputation as a relatively toxic drug. Earlier preparations contained impurities that may have contributed to the frequency of adverse effects (28). Newer formulations are purer, but reports of toxicity continue, and considerable controversy about the toxic potential of vancomycin persists.

Ototoxicity

Reports of hearing loss associated with vancomycin use appeared soon after it was marketed (50). Since then, 53 cases of

tinnitus or hearing loss have been reported in conjunction with vancomycin use; these were recently reviewed by Cantu et al. (18). Of the 53 cases, only 14 occurred without concurrent use of ototoxic drugs or conditions such as meningitis that may cause hearing damage. Vancomycin levels were measured in seven of these patients and ranged from 17 to 62 mg/L, overlapping the accepted therapeutic range. In some cases, ototoxicity has been associated with high serum levels (50, 112, 118) but in others, serum levels have been in the therapeutic range (82). In most reported cases, ototoxicity attributed to vancomycin was reversible.

Ototoxicity due to vancomycin has not been demonstrated in animal models. Gerbils given 80 mg/kg intraperitoneally did not develop abnormal audiograms after 14 days (116). Lutz et al. compared audiometric and histologic findings in guinea pigs treated with vancomycin with those in animals treated with aminoglycosides or placebo. They found no differences between animals given vancomycin and placebo, but animals treated with aminoglycosides developed significant hearing loss and loss of cochlear hair cells. Brummett et al. (14) studied the ototoxicity of gentamicin, vancomycin, and the combination of both drugs. Decreased hearing and loss of cochlear hair cells were seen in animals given gentamicin and were enhanced in animals receiving vancomycin with gentamicin. No audiometric or histologic evidence of ototoxicity was seen in animals given vancomycin alone. These data suggest that vancomycin may augment the ototoxicity of aminoglycosides but has little potential for ototoxicity when used alone.

Studies in humans have yielded similar results. Normal volunteers given vancomycin for 5 days showed no change in audiometry before and after drug administration. Maximum serum concentrations ranged from 40 to 85 mg/L (28). Studies in patients receiving therapeutic vancomycin have shown no evidence of ototoxicity as measured by audiometry. Meyerhoff et al. (83) performed audiometry on 44 patients receiving tobramycin or vancomycin for osteomyelitis. Audiometry was performed at the beginning and end of therapy as well as at biweekly intervals during treatment. Patients treated with vancomycin alone showed no evidence of ototoxicity. van der Hulst et al. (123) examined the ototoxicity of vancomycin or gentamicin administered intraperitoneally to patients on CAPD. Clinical hearing loss developed in 4 of 12 gentamicin-treated patients. One vancomycin-treated patient developed high-frequency hearing loss as measured by audiometry, but clinical ototoxicity did not occur.

The relatively small number of case reports over 40 years of use and the results of animal and human studies suggest that vancomycin ototoxicity is a rare occurrence. In case reports where vancomycin was implicated as the cause of hearing loss, the reaction was reversible when drug was discontinued (18). There is some evidence that vancomycin may potentiate the ototoxicity of other drugs (14), but this remains to be proven.

Nephrotoxicity

In early studies of vancomycin in healthy volunteers, renal abnormalities were unusual (28), but initial clinical trials in patients showed the incidence of nephrotoxicity to be as high as 25% (1). However, most of these studies held other potential causes of renal insufficiency, and the relationship between vancomycin use and nephrotoxicity was not clear. Clinically significant renal toxicity has not been demonstrated in animal models with the use of vancomycin alone (3, 130), but enhancement of aminoglycoside toxicity is reported (130, 131).

Studies of nephrotoxicity in humans are complicated by the number of potentially confounding variables such as concomitant use of nephrotoxic drugs, hypotension, and heart failure. The incidence of nephrotoxicity has been examined in a number of prospective and retrospective studies, and incidence rates range from 0 to 15% (25, 37, 38, 45, 56, 82, 103, 109, 112). This wide range is due to differing definitions of nephrotoxicity and the extent of control for confounding variables. When vancomycin monotherapy is assessed, the incidence of nephrotoxicity is reported as 0 to 14% (25, 37, 38, 45, 56, 103, 109). In studies using monotherapy and excluding patients with confounding variables, the incidence of nephrotoxicity is 5 to 7% (45, 103, 109). Cantu et al. recently reviewed 167 cases of vancomycin nephrotoxicity reported in the literature and found only 3 that occurred without coincident use of aminoglycosides or the presence of other confounding conditions (18). In one study of two 1-g doses of vancomycin administered prophylactically in vascular surgery, the incidence of nephrotoxicity was 14% (65). However, the bulk of the evidence suggests that the nephrotoxic potential of vancomycin is low.

Other variables may affect vancomycin's potential for causing renal damage. In a retrospective study, vancomycin was reported to enhance the nephrotoxicity of aminoglycosides, with incidence rates as high as 35% (45). In prospective and retrospective studies, the rates of nephrotoxicity have been two to five times higher with combined therapy than with aminoglycosides alone (103, 109). However, others have not reported synergistic toxicity with combination therapy (25, 38, 82, 112). Goetz et al. (53) performed a meta-analysis of seven studies comparing rates of nephrotoxicity with vancomycin, aminoglycosides, and the combination. They concluded that the incidence of nephrotoxicity with combination therapy is 13.3% greater than with vancomycin alone and 4.3% greater than with aminoglycosides alone.

The risk of nephrotoxicity may be affected by the patient's age, severity of comorbid disease, use of other nephrotoxic drugs (diuretics, amphotericin B, etc.), and possibly serum levels. A causal relationship between serum vancomycin levels and renal dysfunction has been difficult to prove. Since vancomycin is eliminated by glomerular filtration, as renal function declines vancomycin levels increase, leading to an association between high serum concentrations and renal insufficiency. Some studies have shown an association between elevated trough levels (>10 mg/L) and nephrotoxicity (25, 103). However, nephrotoxicity may occur even if trough levels are maintained in the therapeutic range, and there is no evidence that toxicity can be prevented by keeping serum concentrations below a certain level (18, 25, 103). In animals, endotoxin (*E. coli*) potentiates the nephrotoxicity of the gentamicin/vancomycin combination but not that of vancomycin alone (92).

The significance of this in humans is not certain, but it suggests that other factors may affect the nephrotoxicity of these drugs.

In spite of its reputation as a nephrotoxin, significant renal dysfunction occurs rarely in patients given vancomycin monotherapy. Patients with other risk factors for renal failure, especially concomitant use of aminoglycosides, are more likely to develop nephrotoxicity. High serum levels are not invariably associated with renal failure, and routine monitoring of serum levels to prevent toxicity is not warranted.

"Red Man" Syndrome

Red man syndrome (RMS) is a dose- and infusion rate–dependent, nonimmunologic reaction to vancomycin. It occurs in 80 to 90% of normal volunteers receiving 1 g and 10% receiving 500 mg of vancomycin over 1 h (27, 61, 91, 96). The incidence of RMS in patients is not precisely known but appears to be lower than in normal controls (95, 104). The typical syndrome consists of pruritus and flushing of the head, neck, face, and torso sometimes associated with decreased blood pressure that resolves within minutes of the infusion being stopped. RMS may progress to include dyspnea, throbbing musculoskeletal pain, or muscle spasm in the chest or paraspinal muscles. Symptoms usually begin approximately 10 min after the start of infusion but may follow its completion. Symptoms resolve within 20 min of the infusion being stopped but may persist for several hours (28). RMS occurs primarily with the first dose, and any subsequent reactions are of decreased severity (96).

It has been proposed that RMS is mediated by histamine, since the pharmacologic effects of histamine and the symptoms of RMS are similar. Some studies have shown infusion rate-dependent increases in plasma histamine levels that correlate with the severity of RMS (61, 96, 125). Healy et al. (61) demonstrated that slowing the infusion rate from 1 to 2 h decreased the incidence of RMS and the amount of histamine released. Pretreatment with the H_1 blockers hydroxyzine (107) and diphenhydramine (125) but not the H_2 blocker ranitidine decreases the incidence of RMS. However, histamine levels do not invariably increase in patients with RMS (95), and severe reactions not mediated by histamine have been reported (108). It seems reasonable to conclude that histamine plays a role in the etiology of RMS but may not be the only mediator. Infusion-related symptoms unless severe do not require discontinuation of drug or contraindicate its use in the future. Routine pretreatment with H_1 blockers is not indicated. Patients with a previous episode of RMS should be pretreated with H_1 blockers and receive their infusion over at least 2 h. It may be difficult to distinguish nonallergic, infusion-related RMS from immune-mediated hypersensitivity, but life-threatening allergic reactions to vancomycin are rare (28, 129), and reactions such as rash, urticaria, and drug-related fever occur in only 1 to 8% (45, 51, 112).

Hematologic Toxicity

Thrombocytopenia associated with vancomycin use has been reported rarely. Development of thrombocytopenia and refractoriness to platelet transfusions has been linked to vancomycin-dependent antiplatelet antibodies in patients with leukemia (24).

Neutropenia has been described in up to 2% of patients receiving vancomycin (45). Neutrophil nadir occurs 9 to 30 days after initiation of therapy, and WBC counts return to normal 2 to 3 weeks after drug is discontinued (45). Initially, neutropenia was attributed to impurities in early preparations of vancomycin (33), but the incidence has not decreased with use of purified preparations (45). The cause of vancomycin-associated neutropenia is unknown. An immunologic mechanism has been postulated, but antineutrophil antibodies have been found inconsistently (62, 68, 128).

Other Toxicities

Phlebitis occurs commonly when vancomycin is infused through peripheral veins (45, 112). Drug fever and immunologically mediated rashes have been reported rarely (45, 51, 112). Several cases of severe hypotension and cardiac arrest following bolus administration of vancomycin appear in the literature (52, 81, 84).

DRUG INTERACTIONS

Vancomycin is incompatible in intravenous solution with many drugs, including chloramphenicol, methicillin, corticosteroids, aminophylline, barbiturates, thiazides, diphenylhydantoin, and sodium bicarbonate (31). High concentrations of heparin may inactivate vancomycin and result in persistent bacteremia. Vancomycin should not be given orally with cholestyramine because binding may occur and decrease serum vancomycin concentrations (31).

CLINICAL INDICATIONS

Vancomycin is the drug of choice for treatment of serious infections caused by MRSA. It is also used to treat infections due to methicillin susceptible staphylococci and other Gram-positive organisms in patients who are unable to tolerate β-lactam antibiotics. Most strains of MRSA are susceptible to low concentrations of vancomycin (MICs, 0.06–2.0 mg/L) (129). Recently, clinical isolates with reduced vancomycin susceptibility have been reported (20, 63). However, clinical response to treatment in MRSA endocarditis and septicemia may be slow, and rare isolates show tolerance (MBC > 16 × MIC) (16, 74, 89). Infections caused by methicillin-susceptible *S. aureus* (MSSA) can be treated with vancomycin, but clinical response may be diminished because vancomycin is less rapidly bactericidal than nafcillin in vitro (111). The success rate of vancomycin treatment of MSSA endocarditis is 73 to 93%, compared with 90 to 100% for β-lactam therapy (30). The duration of bacteremia may also be prolonged when vancomycin is used to treat MSSA. Patients treated with vancomycin were bacteremic for 6 to 9 days (74), compared with 2 to 4 days for those given β-lactam antibiotics (69). Because of high failure rates (22), vancomycin cannot be substituted for a penicillin in the short-course (2-week) therapy of right-sided endocarditis in intravenous drug abusers.

Combination therapy has been used to improve the efficacy of vancomycin in the treatment of serious Gram-positive infections. Vancomycin and aminoglycosides are synergistic against many strains of enterococci, viridans streptococci, *S. bovis,*

MRSA, MSSA, and coagulase-negative staphylococci. The combination of rifampin and vancomycin is generally synergistic in the treatment of coagulase-negative staphylococci (42, 76), but the effects against *S. aureus* are more variable, and antagonism has been reported (127). The combination of vancomycin, an aminoglycoside, and rifampin is recommended for treatment of prosthetic valve endocarditis caused by methicillin-resistant coagulase-negative staphylococci. A similar regimen has been recommended for treatment of MRSA endocarditis, although clinical studies have not been performed (10). Addition of an aminoglycoside and/or rifampin should also be considered in patients with persistent staphylococcal bacteremia or no clinical response to vancomycin.

Vancomycin is the drug of choice for infections caused by multiply resistant Gram-positive organisms including corynebacteria and *S. pneumoniae* (129). In patients with penicillin sensitivity, vancomycin may be used as monotherapy for endocarditis due to viridans streptococci or *S. bovis* (10). Vancomycin may be used to treat endocarditis caused by susceptible strains of enterococci in penicillin-allergic patients, but it must be used in combination with an aminoglycoside.

The usefulness of vancomycin in the treatment of central nervous system (CNS) infections is limited by its variable penetration into the CSF, even in the presence of inflamed meninges. Supplemental intrathecal administration of 3 to 5 mg may be necessary to treat meningitis in patients who fail to respond to intravenous therapy (85). Vancomycin has been used successfully to treat CNS shunt infections caused by susceptible organisms. However, removal of hardware and intrathecal administration of drug are generally needed for cure (57, 114). *S. pneumoniae* isolates resistant to penicillin are inhibited by vancomycin, but bactericidal levels may be difficult to achieve in the CSF (Mandel). Nevertheless, vancomycin is considered the drug of choice for meningitis caused by highly penicillin resistant (MIC ≥ 2 mg/L) *S. pneumoniae* (122).

Oral vancomycin is the treatment of choice for refractory or life-threatening episodes of *C. difficile* colitis. Oral administration is used because intraluminal vancomycin is needed to inhibit toxin production (47) and intravenous administration does not yield adequate intraluminal concentrations reliably (47). *C. difficile* rarely penetrates the colonic mucosa so vancomycin is not necessary in serum or tissue. Oral administration of 125 to 250 mg results in luminal levels of 500 to 2000 mg/L, well above the MIC of *C. difficile* (≤16 mg/L) (41). Patients who cannot tolerate oral therapy can be given vancomycin by nasogastric tube with clamping or by enema (solution containing 200 to 500 mg/L).

Vancomycin is recommended as an alternative prophylactic agent for penicillin-allergic patients considered at high risk for bacterial endocarditis undergoing certain dental, oral, or upper respiratory tract procedures (34). It is also recommended in combination with gentamicin as alternative prophylaxis for penicillin-allergic patients undergoing certain GI and genitourinary procedures (34).

Use of vancomycin in initial empirical treatment of febrile neutropenic patients is controversial. Several randomized trials showed no decrease in morbidity or mortality when vancomycin was used as part of initial therapy (44, 99, 101). It should be used if Gram-positive infection is suspected (e.g., purulence at a catheter exit site), especially if there is a high incidence of MRSA in the institution.

Concerns about potential development of vancomycin resistance in enterococci and other Gram-positive organisms prompted the Hospital Infection Control Practices Advisory Committee of the CDC to develop guidelines for prudent use of vancomycin (21) (Table 3). It is hoped that adherence to these guidelines will result in more-rational use of vancomycin and preserve its clinical usefulness.

REFERENCES

1. Alexander MR. A review of vancomycin after 15 years of use. Drug Intell Clin Pharm 1974;8:520–525.
2. Appel GB, Given DB, Levine LR, Cooper GL. Vancomycin and the kidney. Am J Kidney Dis 1986;8:75–80.
3. Aronoff GR, Sloan RS, Dinwiddie CB Jr, Glant MD, Fineberg NS, Luft FC. Effects of vancomycin on renal function in rats. Antimicrob Agents Chemother 1981;19:306–308.
4. Arthur M, Courvalin P. Genetics and mechanisms of glycopeptide resistance in enterococci. Antimicrob Agents Chemother 1993;37:1563–1570.
5. Baldasarre JS, Ingerman MK, Nansteel J, Santoro J. Development of Listeria meningitis during vancomycin therapy: a case report. J Infect Dis 1991;164:221–222.
6. Barg NL, Fekety R, Supena R. Persistent staphylococcal bacteremia in an intravenous drug abuser. Antimicrob Agents Chemother 1986;29:209–211.
7. Barna JCJ, Williams DH. The structure and mode of action of glycopeptide antibiotics of the vancomycin group. Annu Rev Microbiol 1984;38:339–357.
8. Bayer AS, Lam K. Efficacy of vancomycin plus rifampin in experimental aortic-valve endocarditis due to methicillin resistant Staphylococcus aureus: in-vitro-in-vivo correlations. J Infect Dis 1985;151:157–165.
9. Bayer AS, Morrison JO. Disparity between timed-kill and checkerboard methods for determination of in vitro bactericidal interactions of vancomycin plus rifampin versus methicillin-susceptible and -resistant Staphylococcus aureus. Antimicrob Agents Chemother 1984;26:220–226.
10. Bisno AL, Dismukes WE, Durack DT, Kaplan EL, Karchmer AW, Kaye D, Shahbudin HR, Sande MA, Sanford JP, Watanakunakorn C, Wilson WR. Antimicrobial treatment of infective endocarditis due to viridans streptococci, enterococci, and staphylococci. JAMA 1989;261:1471–1477.
11. Blevins RD, Halstenson CE, Salem NG, Matzke GR. Pharmacokinetics of vancomycin in patients undergoing continuous ambulatory peritoneal dialysis. Antimicrob Agents Chemother 1984;25:603–606.
12. Blouin RA, Bauer LA, Miller DD, Record KE, Griffen WO. Vancomycin pharmacokinetics in normal and morbidly obese subjects. Antimicrob Agents Chemother 1982;21:575–580.
13. Boyce NW, Wood C, Thompson NM. Intraperitoneal (IP) vancomycin therapy for CAPD peritonitis—a prospective, randomized comparison of intermittent v. continuous therapy. Am J Kidney Dis 1988;4:304–309.
14. Brummett RE, Fox KE, Jacobs F, Kempton JB, Stokes Z, Richmond AB. Augmented gentamicin ototoxicity in guinea pigs. Arch Otolaryngol Head Neck Surg 1990;116:61–64.
15. Bryan CS, White WL. Safety of oral vancomycin in functionally anephric patients. Antimicrob Agents Chemother 1978;14:634–637.
16. Cafferkey MT, Hone R, Keane CT. Severe staphylococcal infections treated with vancomycin. J Antimicrob Chemother 1982;9:69–74.
17. Cafferky MT, Hone R, Keane CT. Antimicrobial chemotherapy of septicemia due to methicillin-resistant Staphylococcus aureus. Antimicrob Agents Chemother 1985;28:819–825.
18. Cantu TG, Yamanaka-Yuen NA, Lietman PS. Serum vancomycin concentrations: reappraisal of their clinical value. Clin Infect Dis 1994;18:533–543.
19. Centers for Disease Control and Prevention. Nosocomial enterococci. Resistance to vancomycin—United States 1989–1993. MMWR 1993;42:597–600.
20. Centers for Disease Control and Prevention. Staphylococcus aureus with reduced susceptibility to vancomycin—United States, 1997. MMWR 1997;46:765–768.
21. Centers for Disease Control and Prevention. Recommendations for preventing the spread of vancomycin resistance. MMWR 1994;44(RR-12–16).
22. Chambers HF, Miller T, Newman MD. Right sided Staphylococcus aureus endocarditis in intravenous drug abusers: two week combination therapy. Ann Intern Med 1988;109:619–624.
23. Cheung RPF, DiPiro JT. Vancomycin: an update. Pharmacotherapy 1986;6:153–169.
24. Christie DJ, van Buren N, Lennon SS, Putnam JL. Vancomycin-dependent antibodies associated with thrombocytopenia and refractoriness to platelet transfusion in patients with leukemia. Blood 1990;75:518–523.
25. Cimino MA, Rotstein C, Slaughter RL, Emrich LJ. Relationship of serum antibiotic concentrations to nephrotoxicity in cancer patients receiving concurrent aminoglycoside and vancomycin therapy. Am J Med 1987;83:1091–1097.
26. Cockroft DW, Gault MH. Prediction of creatinine clearance from serum creatinine. Nephron 1976;16:31–41.
27. Cook FV, Farrar WE Jr. Vancomycin revisited. Ann Intern Med 1978;88:813–818.
28. Cooper GL, Given DB. Vancomycin: a comprehensive review of 30 years of clinical experience. Park Row Publishers, 1986.
29. Craig WA, Vogelman B. The post-antibiotic effect. Ann Intern Med 1987;106:900–903.
30. Crossley KB, Archer GL, eds. The staphylococci in human disease. New York: Churchill Livingstone, 1997:583–601.
31. Cunha BA. Vancomycin. Med Clin North Am 1995;79:817–831.
32. Cutler NR, Narang PK, Lesko LJ, Ninos M, Power M. Vancomycin disposition: the importance of age. Clin Pharmacol Ther 1984;36:803–810.
33. Dangerfield HG, Hewitt WL, Monzon OT, et al. Clinical use of vancomycin. Antimicrob Agents Ann 1960:428–432.
34. Danjani AS, Taubert KA, Wilson W, Bolger AF, Bayer A, Ferrieri P, Gewitz MH, Shulman ST, Nouri S, Newburger JW, Hutto C, Pallasch TJ, Gage TW, Levison ME, Peter G, Zuccaro G Jr. Prevention of bacterial endocarditis: recommendations by the American Heart Association. JAMA 1997;277:1794–1801.
35. Davies SP, Azadian BS, Kox WJ, Brown EA. Pharmacokinetics of ciprofloxacin and vancomycin in patients with acute renal failure treated by continuous hemodialysis. Nephrol Dial Transplant 1992;7:848–852.
36. De Bock V, Verbeelen D, Maes V, Sennesael J. Pharmacokinetics of vancomycin in patients undergoing haemodialysis and haemofiltration. Nephrol Dial Transplant 1989;4:635–640.

37. Dean RP, Wagner DJ, Tolpin MD. Vancomycin/aminoglycoside nephrotoxicity [Letter]. J Pediatr 1985;106:861.

38. Downs NJ, Neihart RE, Dolezal JM, Hodges GR. Mild nephrotoxicity associated with vancomycin use. Arch Intern Med 1989;149:1777–1781.

39. Dryden MS, Jones NF, Phillips I. Vancomycin therapy failure in Listeria monocytogenes peritonitis in a patient on continuous ambulatory peritoneal dialysis. J Infect Dis 1991;164:1239–1241.

40. Dudley MN et al. Absorption of vancomycin. Ann Intern Med 1984;101:144–148.

41. Dzink J, Bartlett JG. In vitro susceptibility of Clostridium difficile isolates from patients with antibiotic-associated diarrhea or colitis. Antimicrob Agents Chemother 1980;17:695–698.

42. Ein ME, Smith NJ, Aruffo JF, Heerema MS, Bradshaw W, Williams TW Jr. Susceptibility and synergy studies of methicillin-resistant Staphylococcus epidermidis. Antimicrob Agents Chemother 1979;16:655–659.

43. Engineer MS, Ho DW, Bodey GP. Comparison of vancomycin distribution in rats with normal and abnormal renal function. Antimicrob Agents Chemother 1981;20:718–723.

44. European Organization for Research and Treatment of Cancer (EORTC), International Antimicrobial Therapy Cooperative Group and the National Cancer Institute of Canada-Clinical Trials Group. Vancomycin added to empirical combination antibiotic therapy for fever in granulocytopenic cancer patients. J Infect Dis 1991;163:951–958.

45. Farber BF, Moellering RC Jr. Retrospective study of the toxicity of preparations of vancomycin from 1974 to 1981. Antimicrob Agents Chemother 1983;23:138–141.

46. Fekety R. Vancomycin and teicoplanin. In: Mandell GL, Bennett JE, Dolin R, eds. Principles and practice of infectious diseases. New York: Churchill Livingstone, 1995:348–354.

47. Fekety R, Shah AB. Diagnosis and treatment of Clostridium difficile colitis. JAMA 1993;269:71–75.

48. Freeman CD, Quintiliani R, Nightingale CH. Vancomycin therapeutic drug monitoring: is it necessary? Ann Pharmacol 1993;27:594–598.

49. Garrelts JC, Peterie JD. Altered vancomycin dose vs. serum concentration relationship in burn patients. Clin Pharmacol Ther 1988;44:9–13.

50. Geraci JE, Heilman FR, Nichols DR, Wellman WE. Antibiotic therapy of bacterial endocarditis: preliminary report. Mayo Clin Proc 1958;33:172–181.

51. Glew RH, Pavuk RA, Shuster A, Alfred HJ. Vancomycin pharmacokinetics in patients undergoing chronic intermittent peritoneal dialysis. Int J Pharmacol Ther Toxicol 1982;20:559–563.

52. Glicklich D, Figura I. Vancomycin and cardiac arrest [Letter]. Ann Intern Med 1984;101:880.

53. Goetz MB, Sayers J. Nephrotoxicity of vancomycin and aminoglycoside therapy separately and in combination. J Antimicrob Chemother 1993;32:325–334.

54. Gopal V, Bisno AL, Silverblatt FJ. Failure of vancomycin treatment in Staphylococcus aureus endocarditis. In vivo and in vitro observations. JAMA 1976;236:1604–1606.

55. Graziani AL, Lawson LA, Gibson GA. Vancomycin concentrations in infected and noninfected human bone. Antimicrob Agents Chemother 1988;32:1320–1323.

56. Gudmundson GH, Jensen LS. Vancomycin and nephrotoxicity [Letter]. Lancet 1989;1:625.

57. Gump DW,. Vancomycin for treatment of bacterial meningitis. Rev Infect Dis 1981;3(Suppl):S289–292.

58. Hackbarth CJ, Chambers HF. Methicillin-resistant staphylococci: genetics and mechanisms of resistance. Antimicrob Agents Chemother 1989;33:991–996.

59. Harwick HJ, Kalmanson GM, Guze LB. In vitro activity of ampicillin or vancomycin combined with gentamicin or streptomycin against enterococci. Antimicrob Agents Chemother 1973;4:383–387.

60. Healy DP, Polk RE, Garson ML, Rock DT, Comstock TJ. Comparison of steady-state pharmacokinetics of two dosage regimens of vancomycin in normal volunteers. Antimicrob Agents Chemother 1987;31:393–397.

61. Healy DP, Sahai JV, Fuller SH, Polk RE. Vancomycin-induced histamine release and "red man syndrome": comparison of 1- and 2-hour infusions. Antimicrob Agents Chemother 1990;34:550–554.

62. Henry K, Steinberg I, Crossley KB. Vancomycin-induced neutropenia during treatment of osteomyelitis in an out patient. Drug Intell Clin Pharm 1986;20:783–785.

63. Hiramatsu K, Hanaki H, Ino T, Yabuta K, Oguri T, Tenover FC. Methicillin-resistant Staphylococcus aureus clinical strain with reduced vancomycin susceptibility. J Antimicrob Chemother 1997;40:135–136.

64. James A, Koren G, Milliken J, et al. Vancomycin pharmacokinetics and dose recommendations for preterm infants. Antimicrob Agents Chemother 1987;31:52–55.

65. Jensen LJ, Agaard MT, Schifter S. Prophylactic vancomycin versus placebo in arterial prosthetic reconstructions. Thorac Cardiovasc Surg 1985;33:300–303.

66. Judeja L, Fainstein V, LeBlanc B, Bodey GP. Comparative in vitro activity of teichomycin and other antibiotics against JK diphtheroids. Antimicrob Agents Chemother 1983;24:145–146.

67. Karanfil LV, Murphy M, Josephson A, et al. A cluster of vancomycin resistant Enterococcus faecium in an intensive care unit. Infect Control Hosp Epidemiol 1992;13:195–199.

68. Kauffman CA, et al. Neutropenia associated with vancomycin therapy. South Med J 1982;75:1131–1133.

69. Korzeniowski D, Sande MA, and the National Collaborative Endocarditis Study Group. Combination antimicrobial therapy of Staphylococcus aureus endocarditis in parenteral drug addicts and non-addicts. Ann Intern Med 1982;97:496–502.

70. Leclercq R, Courvalin P. Resistance to glycopeptides in enterococci. Clin Infect Dis 1997;24:545–554.

71. Leclercq R, Deriot E, Duval J, Courvalin P. Plasmid-mediated resistance to vancomycin and teicoplanin in Enterococcus faecium. N Engl J Med 1988;319:157–161.

72. Leclercq R, Deroit E, Weber M, Duval J, Courvalin P. Transferable vancomycin and teicoplanin resistance in Enterococcus faecium. Antimicrob Agents Chemother 1989;33:10–15.

73. Lerner PI. Susceptibility of pathogenic actinomycetes to antimicrobial compounds. Antimicrob Agents Chemother 1974;80:302.

74. Levine DP, Fromm BS, Reddy BR. Slow response to vancomycin or vancomycin plus rifampin in methicillin-resistant Staphylococcus aureus endocarditis. Ann Intern Med 1991;115:674–680.

75. Linholm DD, Murray JS. Persistence of vancomycin in the blood during renal failure and its treatment by hemodialysis. N Engl J Med 1966;274:1047–1049.

76. Lowy F, Wexler MA, Steigbigel NH. Therapy of methicillin-resistant Staphylococcus epidermidis experimental endocarditis. J Lab Clin Med 1982;100:94–99.

77. MacIlwaine WA, Sande MA, Mandell GL. Penetration of antistaphylococcal antibiotics into the human eye. Am J Ophthalmol 1979;77:589–592.

78. Magera BE, Arroyo JC, Rosansky SJ, et al. Vancomycin pharmacokinetics in patients with peritonitis on peritoneal dialysis. Antimicrob Agents Chemother 1983;23:710–714.

79. Matzke GR, McGory RW, Halstenson CE, Keane WF. Pharmacokinetics of vancomycin in patients with various degrees of renal function. Antimicrob Agents Chemother 1984;25:433–437.

80. Matzke GR, Zhanel CG, Gway DRP. Clinical pharmacokinetics of vancomycin. Clin Pharmacol 1986;11:257–261.

81. Mayhew JF, Deutsch S. Cardiac arrest following administration of vancomycin. Can Anaesth Soc J 1985;32:65–67.

82. Mellor JA, Kingdom J, Cafferky M, Keane CT. Vancomycin toxicity: a prospective study. J Antimicrob Chemother 1985;15:773–780.

83. Meyerhoff WL, Maale GE, Yellin W, Roland PS. Audiologic threshold monitoring of patients receiving ototoxic drugs. Ann Otorhinolaryngol 1989;98:950–954.

84. Miller R, Tausk HC. Anaphylactoid reaction to vancomycin during anesthesia: a case report. Anesth Analg 1977;56:870–871.

85. Moellering RC Jr, Krogstad DJ, Greenblatt DJ. Vancomycin therapy in patients with impaired renal function: a nomogram for dosage. Ann Intern Med 1981;94:343–346.

86. Moellering RC Jr. Monitoring serum vancomycin levels: climbing the mountain because it is there? [Editorial]. Clin Infect Dis 1994;18:544–546.

87. Moellering RC Jr. Pharmacokinetics of vancomycin. J Antimicrob Chemother 1989;14(Suppl D):43–52.

88. Morse GD, Farolino DF, Apicella MA, Walsh JW. Comparative study of intraperitoneal and intravenous pharmacokinetics during continuous ambulatory peritoneal dialysis. Antimicrob Agents Chemother 1987;31:173–177.

89. Myers JP, Linnemann CC Jr. Bacteremia due to methicillin-resistant Staphylococcus aureus. J Infect Dis 1982;145:532–536.

90. National Committee for Clinical Laboratory Standards. Performance standards for antimicrobial susceptibility testing: third information supplement (NCCLS Document M100-S3). Villanova, PA: NCCLS, 1991.

91. Newfield P, Roizen MF. Hazards of rapid administration of vancomycin. Ann Intern Med 1979;91:581–583.

92. Ngeleka M, Beauchamp D, Tardif D, Auclair P, Gourde Pierrette, Bergeron MG. Endotoxin increases the nephrotoxic potential of gentamicin and vancomycin plus gentamicin. J Infect Dis 1990;161:721–727.

93. Nielsen HE, Hansen HE, Korsager B, Skov PE. Renal excretion of vancomycin in kidney disease. Acta Med Scand 1975;197:261–266.

94. Noble WD, Virani Z, Cree RGA. Co-transfer of vancomycin and other resistance genes from Enterococcus faecalis NCTC 12201 to Staphylococcus aureus. FEMS Microbiol Lett 1992;93:195–199.

95. O'Sullivan TL, Ruffing MJ, Lamp KC, Warbasse LH, Rybak MJ. Prospective evaluation of red man syndrome in patients receiving vancomycin. J Infect Dis 1993;168:773–776.

96. Polk RE, Healy DP, Schwartz LB, Rock WT, Garson ML, Roller K. Vancomycin and the red-man syndrome: pharmacodynamics of histamine release. J Infect Dis 1988;157:502–507.

97. Poyart C, Pierre C, Quesne G, Pron G, Berche P, Trieu-Cuot P. Emergence of vancomycin resistance in the genus streptococcus: characterization of a VanB transferable determinant in Streptococcus bovis. Antimicrob Agents Chemother 1997;41:24–30.

98. Quintiliani R Jr, Evers S, Courvalin P. The vanB gene confers various levels of self-transferable resistance to vancomycin in enterococci. J Infect Dis 1993;167:1220–1223.

99. Ramphal R, Bolger M, Oblon DJ, Sherertz RJ, Malone JD, Rand KH, Gilliom M, Shands JW Jr, Kramer BS. Vancomycin is not an essential component of the initial empiric treatment regime for febrile neutropenic patients receiving ceftazidime: a randomized prospective study. Antimicrob Agents Chemother 1992;36:1062–1067.

100. Rodvold KA, Blum RA, Fischer JH, Zokufa HZ, Rotschafer JC, Crossley KB, Riff LJ. Vancomycin pharmacokinetics in patients with varying degrees of renal function. Antimicrob Agents Chemother 1988;32:848–852.

101. Rubin M, Hathorn JW, Marshall D, Gress J, Steinberg SM, Pizzo PA. Gram-positive infections and the use of vancomycin in 550 episodes of fever and neutropenia. Ann Intern Med 1988;108:30–35.

102. Ruoff KL, Kuritzkes DR, Wolfson JS. Vancomycin-resistant gram positive bacteria isolated from human sources. J Clin Microbiol 1988;26:2064–2068.

103. Rybak MJ, Albrecht LM, Boike SC, Chandrasekar PH. Nephrotoxicity of vancomycin alone and with an aminoglycoside. J Antimicrob Chemother 1990;25:679–687.

104. Rybak MJ, Bailey EM, Warbasse LH. Absence of "red man syndrome" in patients being treated with vancomycin or high dose teicoplanin. Antimicrob Agents Chemother 1992;36:1204–1207.

105. Rybak MJ, Albrecht LM, Berman JR, Warbasse LH, Svensson CK. Vancomycin pharmacokinetics in burn patients and intravenous drug abusers. Antimicrob Agents Chemother 1990;34:792–795.

106. Sabath L, Wheeler N, Laverdiere M. A new type of penicillin resistance in Staphylococcus aureus. Lancet 1977;1:443–447.

107. Sahai J, Healy DP, Garris R, Berry A, Polk RE. Influence of antihistamine pretreatment on vancomycin-induced red-man syndrome. J Infect Dis 1989;160:876–881.

108. Sahai J, Polk RE, Schwartz LB, Healy DP, Westin EH. Severe reaction to vancomycin not mediated by histamine release and documented by rechallenge. J Infect Dis 1988;158:1413–1414.

109. Salama SE, Rotstein C. Prospective assessment of nephrotoxicity with concomitant aminoglycosides and vancomycin therapy. Can J Hosp Pharm 1993;46:53–57.

110. Schaad UB, Nelson JD, McCracken GH Jr. Pharmacology and efficacy of vancomycin for staphylococcal infections in children. Rev Infect Dis 1981;3(Suppl):S282–288.

111. Small PM, Chambers HF. Vancomycin for Staphylococcus aureus endocarditis in intravenous drug users. Antimicrob Agents Chemother 1990;34:1227–1231.

112. Sorrell TC, Collignon PJ. A prospective study of adverse reactions associated with vancomycin therapy. J Antimicrob Chemother 1985;16:235–241.

113. Sorrell TC, Packham DR, Shanker S, et al. Vancomycin therapy for methicillin-resistant Staphylococcus aureus. Ann Intern Med 1982;97:344–350.

114. Swayne RS, Rampling A, Newsom SWB. Intraventricular vancomycin for shunt-associated ventriculitis. J Antimicrob Chemother 1987;19:249–252.

115. Swenson JM, Facklam RR, Thornsberry C. Antimicrobial susceptibility of vancomycin-resistant Leuconostoc, Pediococcus, and Lactobacillus species. Antimicrob Agents Chemother 1990;34:543–549.

116. Tange RA, Keiviet HL, Marle JV. An experimental study of vancomycin-induced cochlear damage. Arch Otorhinolaryngol 1989;246:67–70.

117. Torres JR, Sanders CV, Lewis AC. Vancomycin concentration

in human tissues: preliminary report. J Antimicrob Chemother 1979;5:476–480.

118. Traber PG, Levine DP. Vancomycin ototoxicity in a patient with normal renal function. Ann Intern Med 1981;95:458–460.

119. Tuazon CU, Lin MYC, Sheagren JN. In vitro activity of rifampin alone and in combination with nafcillin and vancomycin against pathogenic strains of Staphylococcus aureus. Antimicrob Agents Chemother 1978;13:759–761.

120. Tuazon CU, Miller H. Comparative in vitro activities of teichomycin and vancomycin alone and in combination with rifampin and aminoglycosides against staphylococci and enterococci. Antimicrob Agents Chemother 1984;25:411–415.

121. Tuazon CU, Shamsuddin D, Miller H. Antibiotic susceptibility and synergy of clinical isolates of Listeria monocytogenes. Antimicrob Agents Chemother 1982;21:525–528.

122. Tunkel AR, Wispelway B, Scheld WM. Bacterial meningitis: recent advances in pathophysiology and treatment. Ann Intern Med 1990;112:610–623.

123. Van der Hulst RJ, Boeschoten EW, Nielsen FW, et al. Ototoxicity monitoring with ultra-high frequency audiometry in peritoneal dialysis patients treated with vancomycin or gentamicin. ORL J Otorhinolaryngol Relat Spec 1991;53:19–22.

124. Viladrich PF, Gudid F, Linares J, et al. Evaluation of vancomycin for therapy of adult pneumococcal meningitis. Antimicrob Agents Chemother 199135:2467–2472.

125. Wallace MR, Mascola JR, Olfield EC III. Red man syndrome: incidence, etiology, and prophylaxis. J Infect Dis 1991;164:1180–1185.

126. Watanakunakorn C, Bakie C. Synergism of vancomycin-gentamicin and vancomycin-streptomycin against enterococci. Antimicrob Agents Chemother 1973;4:120–124.

127. Watanakunakorn C, Guerriero JC. Interaction between vancomycin and rifampin against Staphylococcus aureus. Antimicrob Agents Chemother 1981;19:1089–1091.

128. Weitzman SA, Stossel TP. Drug-induced immunological neutropenia. Lancet 1978;1:1068–1071.

129. Wilhelm MP. Vancomycin. Mayo Clin Proc 1991;66:1165–1170.

130. Wold JS, Turnipseed SA. Toxicity of vancomycin in laboratory animals. Rev Infect Dis 1981;3(Suppl):S224–229.

131. Wood CA, Kohlhepp SJ, Kohnen PW, Houghton DC, Gilbert DN. Vancomycin enhancement of experimental tobramycin nephrotoxicity. Antimicrob Agents Chemother 1986;30:20–24.

132. Zimmerman AE, Katona BG, Plaisance KI. Association of vancomycin serum concentrations with outcomes in patients with gram positive bacteremia. Pharmacotherapy 1995;15:85–91.

SECTION II

Fungi and
Antifungal Agents

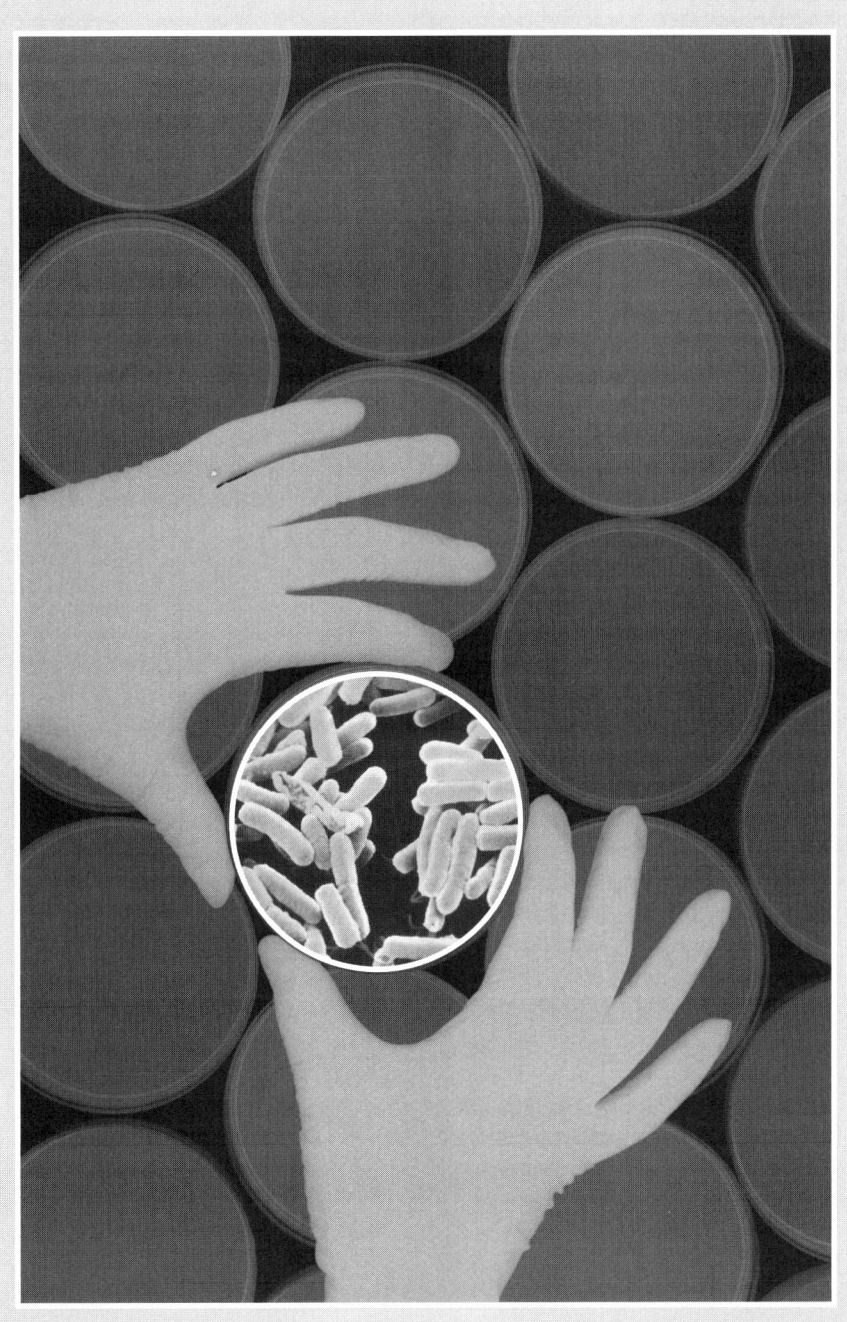

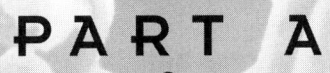

PART A

Fungi

Aspergillus Species

David L. Paterson

GENERAL DESCRIPTION

Mycology

Aspergillus species are ubiquitous molds that can grow in decaying vegetation, soil, and water. In culture, *Aspergillus* species have septate, hyaline, branched hyphae that give rise to upright conidiophores that terminate in a swollen cell (vesicle). *Aspergillus fumigatus* is the most common species to cause serious infections in humans, especially pulmonary infection. *Aspergillus flavus* is a less common cause of pulmonary infection. However, it is responsible for relatively more infections of the sinuses and skin than *A. fumigatus*. *A. niger* is rarely responsible for life-threatening infections, but may produce otitis externa. Species rarely associated with human disease include *A. terreus, A. ustus, A. sydowi, A. nidulans,* and others.

Epidemiology

Direct inoculation from environmental sources occasionally occurs. For example, keratitis after trauma to the cornea is well described. More commonly, serious infection is acquired by inhalation. Primary pulmonary aspergillosis results. In addition to ecologic niches such as vegetation and soil, the organism survives well in the hospital environment. Hospital renovation and construction activities producing bursts of airborne conidia have resulted in numerous clusters of hospital-acquired infections in immunosuppressed patients (12).

Several types of immunosuppression predispose to invasive aspergillosis. Most numerous are patients with prolonged neutropenia and transplant recipients, including both solid organ and bone marrow recipients (313, 351). Corticosteroid use is also a clear risk factor for invasive aspergillosis. Advanced human immunodeficiency virus (HIV) infection, even in the absence of neutropenia or corticosteroid use, may also predispose to serious *Aspergillus* infections (77). Children with chronic granulomatous disease are at significant risk for *Aspergillus* infections (327).

Although *Aspergillus* may be responsible for trivial infections (e.g., otitis externa) or may merely colonize damaged lungs, invasive aspergillosis carries a high mortality. In many immunosuppressed populations, mortality from invasive aspergillosis approaches or even exceeds 90%. Although removal of immunosuppression is often the key to successful resolution of *Aspergillus* infections, choice of antifungal agent is also important. This chapter discusses traditional antifungal therapy as well as new agents for the treatment of invasive aspergillosis.

SUSCEPTIBILITY IN VITRO AND IN VIVO

Interpretation of in vitro susceptibility data for *Aspergillus* species has been difficult because data have been based upon nonstandardized testing methods. The method of testing susceptibility, morphologic variations in the fungus, and differences in growth rates and optimal growth conditions may all influence determination of the susceptibility of the fungi to antifungal drugs. Also, few published data exist that correlate in vitro susceptibility with clinical success in humans. With these caveats, data are presented for recently published studies exploring the susceptibility of *Aspergillus* species to a variety of antifungal agents (Tables 1–3).

As can be seen, the newer azole antifungal agents (itraconazole, voriconazole, SCH-56592) have greater in vitro activity than amphotericin B against most *Aspergillus* isolates. In addition, both itraconazole and voriconazole are active in vitro against laboratory-selected amphotericin-resistant strains of *A. fumigatus* (212). Resistance to itraconazole and voriconazole is occasionally seen, but cross-resistance does not seem to occur. For example, an isolate of *A. fumigatus* had an MIC of 8 mg/L against voriconazole but 0.5 to 1 mg/L against itraconazole (347). Itraconazole resistance has been recently reported in clinical isolates (MIC > 16 μg/mL), but SCH-56592 retains activity against these isolates (MIC, 0.5 μg/mL) (88, 241).

The clinical relevance of itraconazole resistance in *Aspergillus* species remains to be determined. At least two mechanisms of resistance are likely responsible (88). Itraconazole interferes with ergosterol biosynthesis by inhibiting sterol 14α-demethylation. However, itraconazole-resistant isolates may have either increased expression of the sterol 14 α-demethylase or altered affinity of the enzyme for itraconazole. In addition, a reduced intracellular concentration of itraconazole was observed in one of the resistant isolates suggesting altered uptake or efflux mechanisms.

In Vitro Studies Using Combinations of Antifungal Agents

Combinations of amphotericin and azoles have given conflicting results when tested in vitro but do not appear to have a reliable, significant additive effect on each other's activity against *A. fumigatus*. Amphotericin and itraconazole have

1021

TABLE 1 • In Vitro Susceptibility of *Aspergillus fumigatus* to Antifungal Agents

Drug	MIC$_{50}$ (μg/mL)	MIC$_{90}$ (μg/mL)	MIC Range (μg/mL)
Amphotericin B	0.5	2	0.125–2
Fluconazole	>64	>64	>64
Flucytosine	>100	>100	0.5–>64
Itraconazole	0.06	0.5	<0.03–1
Ketoconazole	12.5	25	0.125–>64
Miconazole	4	16	1–>100
Nystatin	—	—	0.5–>50
Rifampin	>1000	>1000	>1000
SCH-56592	0.125	0.25	0.125–4
Terbinafine	1	2	0.02–5
Voriconazole	0.03	0.25	<0.03–0.5

Collated from references 59, 79, 109, 147, 157, 230, 268, 290, 347.

TABLE 2 • In Vitro Susceptibility of *Aspergillus flavus* to Antifungal Agents

Drug	MIC$_{50}$ (μg/mL)	MIC$_{90}$ (μg/mL)	MIC Range (μg/mL)
Amphotericin B	0.5	2	0.25–4
Fluconazole	>64	>64	>64
Flucytosine	>100	>100	10–>100
Itraconazole	0.125	0.25	0.06–0.25
Ketoconazole	6.25	12.5	2–>64
Miconazole	4	16	0.5–>100
Nystatin	—	—	—
Rifampin	>1000	>1000	>1000
SCH-56592	0.25	—	0.125–4
Terbinafine	—	—	0.01–0.5
Voriconazole	0.5	0.5	0.25–0.5

Collated from references 59, 79, 109, 147, 157, 230, 268, 290, 347.

TABLE 3 • In Vitro Susceptibility of *Aspergillus niger* to Antifungal Agents

Drug	MIC$_{50}$ (μg/mL)	MIC$_{90}$ (μg/mL)	MIC Range (μg/mL)
Amphotericin B	0.5	1	0.125–1
Fluconazole	>64	>64	>64
Flucytosine	—	—	0.06–>100
Itraconazole	0.5	1	0.25–2
Ketoconazole	>64	>64	>64
Miconazole	—	—	2–>4
Nystatin	—	—	—
SCH-56592	—	—	—
Terbinafine	—	—	0.005–0.5
Voriconazole	0.25	0.25	0.25–1

Collated from references 59, 79, 109, 147, 157, 230, 268, 290, 347.

been synergistic in 14 to 40% of strains tested, additive in 20 to 26%, but antagonistic in 26% of 15 strains in one series (209) and 0 of 5 strains in another series (79). An isolate from a patient in whom the combination of amphotericin and itraconazole failed showed antagonism between amphotericin and itraconazole (298). Miconazole may be synergistic when combined with amphotericin in up to 60% of strains tested; amphotericin and ketoconazole or fluconazole are rarely syner-

gistic and may be antagonistic combinations in upward of 20% of strains tested against *A. fumigatus* (157, 209).

Combinations of amphotericin and flucytosine, although additive or synergistic in some studies, are more likely to be an indifferent combination in vitro (79, 242). Antagonism was reported in 6 of 26 (23%) strains in one study (79). The combination of voriconazole and flucytosine is indifferent (55).

In contrast, combinations of amphotericin and rifampin or rifabutin are frequently synergistic (58, 59, 79, 157). Addition of rifampin consistently lowers the MICs of amphotericin B by two- to tenfold (157). In 36 of 39 (92%) *Aspergillus* strains from one study, amphotericin and rifampin were synergistic (79). The combination exerts its antifungal effects through inhibition of RNA and protein synthesis (58).

Terbinafine and itraconazole were synergistic in all four strains tested in one small study (290). The combination of terbinafine and amphotericin B was synergistic in one of four and indifferent in three of four strains tested (290).

Indifference or antagonism occurs when two azoles are used together (157, 209).

In Vivo (Animal) Studies Using Amphotericin B Preparations

Amphotericin B Deoxycholate

Amphotericin B deoxycholate ("conventional" amphotericin B, Fungizone, Apothecon, Princeton, NJ) has been widely used in animal models of invasive aspergillosis. The effectiveness of amphotericin B in animal models has varied with its dose and duration, timing of amphotericin B administration relative to time of infection, mode of administration (intravenous, intraperitoneal, or aerosolized), type of animal model used, *Aspergillus* inoculum dose, and site of infection. Early animal studies inoculated *A. fumigatus* intravenously into non-immunocompromised mice. Apart from animal models of *A. fumigatus* endocarditis, in which mortality was universal even with amphotericin B treatment (49, 200), in all other cases, amphotericin B showed some activity (14, 24, 97, 125, 153). However, while in some cases amphotericin B activity was marked, in many it was marginal.

Effectiveness of amphotericin B against *A. fumigatus* appeared to be dose related (341). The comparative effectiveness of higher amphotericin B doses has been assessed more recently in studies of neutropenic rabbits further immunocompromised by use of corticosteroids (113). Amphotericin B at 1.5 mg/kg, but not at 0.5 mg/kg, could sterilize tissues infected with *A. fumigatus* (114). In a separate study with mice given corticosteroids and inoculated intravenously with *A. fumigatus,* all mice died who were given the comparatively low dose of amphotericin B of 0.8 mg/kg/day intraperitoneally (302).

Animal models using amphotericin B in the 1990s for treatment of invasive aspergillosis are summarized in Table 4. As opposed to earlier studies, most more recent studies have used an immunocompromised animal model. Models in which *Aspergillus* is administered intravenously rarely result in development of significant pulmonary disease. Therefore, models of *Aspergillus* pulmonary disease (achieved by instilling *A. fumigatus* intranasally or endotracheally) have been investi-

TABLE 4 • Amphotericin B Use in the Treatment of Experimental Systemic Aspergillosis

Reference	Animal	Type of Immunocompromise	Inoculum
113	New Zealand white rabbits	Neutropenia and corticosteroids	1×10^5–1×10^6 conidia
255	New Zealand white rabbits	Neutropenia and corticosteroids	1×10^6 conidia
114	New Zealand white rabbits	Neutropenia and corticosteroids	1×10^5–1×10^6 conidia
253	New Zealand white rabbits	Neutropenia and corticosteroids	1×10^6 conidia
60	Swiss Webster mice	Corticosteroids	1×10^5–1×10^6 conidia
138	Female CD-1 mice	None	8.3×10^6 conidia
241	Male CD-1	Neutropenic	2×10^6–1×10^7 conidia
78	Female CD-1 No immunocompromise	1×10^7 conidia	
83	Female CD-1 mice No immunocompromise	1×10^7 conidia	
254	New Zealand white rabbits	Neutropenia and corticosteroids	1×10^6 conidia

Ref.	Dose, Route, and Frequency	Time from Infection to Start of Treatment	Treatment Duration	Survival (treated vs. control)
113	0.5 or 1.5 mg/kg i.v. q. 24 h	24 h	5 days	100 vs. 0% ($P < .001$)
255	1.5 mg/kg i.v. q. 24 h	24 h	5 days	90 vs. 20% ($P < .01$)
114	1.5 mg/kg i.v. q. 24 h	24 h	6 days	100 vs. 0% ($P < .01$)
253	1.5 mg/kg i.v. q. 24 h	24 h	5 days	86 vs. 0% ($P < .01$)
60	0.8 mg/kg i.p. q. 24 h	5 h	7 days	0 vs. 0% ($P > .20$)
138	3.3 mg/kg i.p., three times weekly	24 h	14 days	60 vs. 25 ($P < .05$)
241	5 mg/kg i.p. on days 1, 2, 4, 7	18 h	7 days	40–50 vs. 0–10% ($P < .01$)
78	3.3 mg/kg i.p. q. 24 h	24 h	7–14 days	100 vs. 20% ($P < .05$)
83	3.3 mg/kg i.p. every 2nd day	18–24 h	14 days	67–100 vs. 13% ($P < .01$)
254	1.5 mg/kg i.v. q. 24 h	24 h	5 days	90 vs. 0% ($P = .005$)

TABLE 5 • Animal Studies of Amphotericin B in the Treatment of Invasive Pulmonary Aspergillosis

Reference	Animal	Type of Immunocompromise	Inoculum	Site of Inoculation with *Aspergillus*
194	Female R strain albino rats	Neutropenia	1×10^4 conidia	Left main bronchus
106	New Zealand white rabbits	Neutropenia	1.5×10^8 conidia	Trachea
224	Sprague-Dawley rats	Corticosteroids	8×10^3 conidia	Trachea
230	Sprague-Dawley rats	Corticosteroids	1×10^6 conidia	Trachea
78	Female CD-1 mice	Neutropenic	9×10^6 conidia	Nose
357	New Zealand white rabbits	Neutropenic	1.5×10^8 conidia	Trachea

Ref.	Dose, Route, and Frequency	Time from Infection to Start of Treatment	Treatment Duration	Survival (treated vs. control)
194	1 mg/kg i.v. q. 24 h	40 h	10 days	13 vs. 0% ($P > .20$)
106	1 mg/kg i.v. q. 24 h	24 h	10 days	30 vs. 7% ($P = .10$)
224	1 mg/kg i.v. q. 24 h	Immediate	7 days	100 vs. 0% ($P < .05$)
230	4 mg/kg i.p. q. 24 h	Immediate	5 days	100 vs. 37.5% ($P < .02$)
78	3.3 mg/kg i.p.	18 h	10 days	30 vs. 20% ($P > .20$)
357	1 mg/kg i.v. q. 24 h	24 h	10 days	Not stated (pulmonary lesions showed significant improvement compared with untreated controls)

gated (Table 5). Innovative methods such as the use of ultrafast computerized tomography have been used to monitor such infections (357).

Recent studies assessing systemic invasive aspergillosis in immunocompromised animals show that use of amphotericin B delays and/or reduces mortality compared with that in control animals in which no antifungal agents was used (77, 113, 114, 138, 241, 253, 255). Treatment with amphotericin B has also been associated with decreased tissue burden of *Aspergillus* in immunocompromised animal models (113, 253).

In contrast, two studies of invasive pulmonary aspergillosis (Table 5) failed to show that use of amphotericin B was associated with a statistically significant decrease in mortality compared with controls, although mortality was slightly lower in the amphotericin B–treated animals (78, 106, 199). In both of these studies (mirroring what occurs in real-life clinical scenarios), amphotericin B administration was delayed with respect to time of infection. Animal studies of pulmonary aspergillosis in which amphotericin B use was associated with 100% survival were notable for administration of the drug immediately after infection.

Aerosolized Amphotericin B

Inhalation of airborne *Aspergillus* with deposition in the lungs is commonly believed to be the initial step leading to invasive pulmonary aspergillosis. However, as noted in both animal models above and in human studies, intravenous amphotericin B use is associated with poor outcome from invasive pulmonary aspergillosis. It is hypothesized that inhalation of amphotericin B aerosols could maximize local effectiveness of the drug while limiting its systemic toxicity. Hence the aerosolized drug may have particular use as prophylaxis against pulmonary aspergillosis in those at high risk of the disease.

Four studies have examined the use of aersolized amphotericin B in animal models (56, 187, 305), in each case Sprague-Dawley rats immunocompromised by use of cortisone acetate. The animals were infected via the trachea with an inoculum of 10^6 conidia of *A. fumigatus*. This model produces a progressive bronchopulmonary aspergillosis. Death occurs in untreated animals from 48 h after inoculation (305).

In each study, a single dose of aerosolized amphotericin B prior to infection yielded statistically significant improvement in survival compared with that of control animals given neither prophylaxis nor treatment (56, 187). Some 50 to 88.9% of animals given 1.6 mg/kg aerosolized over 15 min, 48 h before infection, survived for at least 10 days, compared with 0 to 30% of control animals (56, 305). In a study in which 0.8 mg/kg of aerosolized amphotericin B was administered 2 h prior to infection, survival at 7 days was 100% in animals given prophylaxis and 20% in controls (187).

While a single dose of aerosolized amphotericin B as prophylaxis was highly effective in decreasing mortality, it did not completely eradicate proliferation of the fungus. When survivors were sacrificed and examined, *Aspergillus* could still be cultured from the lungs of animals given prophylaxis (238). Furthermore, when immunosuppression was recommenced in other survivors, rapid proliferation of aspergilli could be noted within 2 to 3 weeks (238). It seems likely from these results that additional doses of aerosolized amphotericin B may be necessary to prevent reactivation of infection or reinfection from environmental sources.

Aerosolized amphotericin B lipid complex (ABLC), in doses from 0.4 to 1.6 mg/kg, given to rats 2 days before pulmonary infection significantly delayed mortality, compared with that in rats given placebo ($P < .001$) (56). Furthermore, aerosolized ABLC was more effective than an equivalent dose of aerosolized amphotericin B in prolonging survival, with 100% survival at 14 days postinfection in the ABLC group, compared with 62.5% survival in the amphotericin B group. Mean concentrations of amphotericin B in the lungs were 3.7 times higher at day 1 and almost six times higher at day 7 after treatment with aerosolized ABLC (56, 57).

Delivery Systems for Amphotericin B Involving Lipids

A large number of novel delivery systems for amphotericin B, using lipids or liposomes, have been developed and tested in animal models. The premise behind such methods is that incorporating amphotericin B into lipid structures can reduce its toxicity while maintaining its efficacy. This is important, since treatment of aspergillosis requires high-dose therapy for a prolonged duration, often in patients with concomitant renal dysfunction. The various compounds reported have used different lipids, including the presence or absence of sterols (e.g., cholesterol), and particles of different sizes. Some studies have used liposomes (broadly defined as concentric bilayers of lipid material with aqueous-phase material between), whereas others have used unusual lipid structures or aggregates of lipid and amphotericin B that are not liposomes.

The interest in lipid delivery systems for amphotericin B relates to the finding that such formulations are less toxic than amphotericin B deoxycholate for mammalian cells but retain the activity of amphotericin B deoxycholate against fungi (18, 201). For example, marked renal toxicity developed in rabbits treated with amphotericin B deoxycholate at 1 mg/kg/day for 10 days, whereas serum creatinine levels remained normal in rabbits treated with 1 mg/kg/day or 5 mg/kg/day of liposomal amphotericin B (106). Three- to fivefold increases in mean serum urea and creatinine levels occurred, however, in rabbits treated with liposomal amphotericin B at a dose of 10 mg/kg/day (106). The reduction in toxicity is thought to result from differential affinities of the lipids in the lipid carrier to the ergosterol in the fungus membrane (highest affinity) versus the cholesterol in the human cell membrane (lowest affinity). Interaction of the human cell membrane with amphotericin B may be minimized because of selective transfer of amphotericin B from the lipid carrier to the fungus (202). An alternative suggestion is that the reduced nephrotoxicity of lipid preparations results from lower serum and renal levels of drug. For example, levels of amphotericin B in the kidneys of animals given amphotericin B colloidal dispersion (ABCD) were lower than those in animals receiving standard amphotericin B (161).

In view of the expense of commercial lipid-based delivery systems of amphotericin B, some groups have mixed amphotericin B with a parenteral fat emulsion (Intralipid) used in administration of total parenteral nutrition. One small study (performed by the manufacturers of ABLC) showed that amphotericin B–Intralipid emulsion (unlike ABLC) and amphotericin B deoxycholate showed almost toxicity in animals (325). However, the results of this study have been disputed; other experiments show that amphotericin B–Intralipid emulsion (LD_{50} for mice, 4.5 mg/kg) is less toxic than amphotericin B deoxycholate (LD_{50} for mice, 2.5 mg/kg) (53).

Lipid preparations of amphotericin B differ markedly in their organ distribution, compared with amphotericin B deoxycholate. Plasma concentrations of ABLC are actually lower, for example, than the same dose (1 mg/kg) administered as amphotericin B deoxycholate (60). In contrast, concentrations in the liver and spleen are two to five times higher in ABLC-treated mice than they are with the same dose given as amphotericin B deoxycholate (60). When a higher, but still tolerable, dose of ABLC was given, liver and spleen concentrations were 9 to 70 times those achieved with conventional doses of amphotericin B deoxycholate (60, 344). Lung concentrations of amphotericin B after administration of ABLC were considerably lower than liver or spleen concentrations but were still higher than those achieved by the same dose of amphotericin B deoxycholate (60). Use of high-dose ABLC (10 mg/kg) achieved lung concentrations 5 to 15 times those achieved with standard-dose amphotericin B deoxycholate (1 mg/kg). Renal and brain concentrations of amphotericin B were only higher with ABLC administration (compared with amphotericin B deoxycholate) when high doses of ABLC (10 mg/kg) were given (60).

A number of studies comparing the efficacy of lipid formulations of amphotericin B with amphotericin B deoxycholate have been performed in animal models (Table 6). Many of these have shown that if the lipid formulations are used at the same dose as amphotericin B deoxycholate, efficacy is actually inferior to that seen with amphotericin B deoxycholate (111, 194, 195, 357). However, animals with invasive aspergillosis given lipid formulations at doses of 5 to 12.5 mg/kg had better survival than those given amphotericin B deoxycholate at 0.8 to 1 mg/kg (60, 106, 195). Organism burdens in infected tissues were significantly reduced by lipid formulations at doses of 6 to 15 mg/kg but were not reduced by conventional amphotericin B deoxycholate (111, 194, 195, 357).

In Vivo (Animal) Studies Using Azoles

Miconazole

Miconazole had little useful activity in the treatment of aspergillosis in the one animal model in which it was studied (301).

Ketoconazole

In three studies of murine disseminated aspergillosis, ketoconazole use showed little or no survival advantage over no treatment (272, 300). In a rabbit model of *Aspergillus* keratitis, ketoconazole was ineffective when given either topically or orally (179).

Fluconazole

The efficacy of fluconazole is dose related; treated animals were no different from untreated controls at 5 and 20 mg/kg (42, 367) but significantly better than untreated controls at 60 and 120 mg/kg (113). However, fluconazole is clearly inferior to amphotericin B (113, 320), ABLC (60), and itraconzazole (141, 142) in the treatment of experimental invasive aspergillosis.

Itraconazole

Itraconazole administered orally in animal models of invasive aspergillosis resulted in better survival than no treatment or treatment with fluconazole in most (13, 141, 142, 230), but not all (60, 125), studies. Erratic absorption with subsequent low serum levels has been an ongoing problem in studies of orally administered itraconazole, particularly in rodents. However, given intraperitoneally to rabbits with experimental *A. fumigatus* endocarditis, itraconazole was shown to be superior to amphotericin B (200). Intravenous administration of itraconazole (10 or 20 mg/kg/day) resulted in 100% survival of rats immunosuppressed with cortisone acetate and infected intratracheally with *A. fumigatus* (224). Similar survival was seen in

---

TABLE 6 • Animal Studies Using Delivery Systems for Amphotericin B Involving Lipids

Reference	Animal	Type of Immunocompromise	Inoculum	Site of Inoculation with *Aspergillus*
194	Female R strain albino rats	Neutropenia	1×10^4 conidia	Left main bronchus
106	New Zealand white rabbits	Neutropenia	1.5×10^8 conidia	Trachea
260	New Zealand white rabbits	Neutropenia and corticosteroids	10^6 conidia	Intravenous
60	Swiss Webster mice	Corticosteroids	10^5–10^6 conidia	Intravenous
344	Female R-strain rats	Neutropenia	2×10^4 conidia	Inoculation into left lung
357	New Zealand white rabbits	Neutropenic	1.5×10^8 conidia	Trachea

Ref.	Dose, Route, and Frequency	Time from Infection to Start of Treatment	Treatment Duration	Survival (lipid preparations vs. AmB)
194	Liposomal amphotericin (AmBisome) 10 mg/kg i.v. q. 24 h; AmB 1 mg/kg i.v. q. 24 h	40 h	10 days	27 vs. 13% ($P = .75$)
106	Liposomal amphotericin (AmBisome) 5 mg/kg i.v. q. 24 h; AmB 1 mg/kg i.v. q. 24 h	24 h	10 days	100 vs. 30% ($P < .10$)
260	C-AmB 15 mg/kg i.v. q. 24 h; AmB 1.5 mg/kg	24 h	5 days	50 vs. 75% ($P > .20$)
60	ABLC 1 or 10 mg/kg i.v. q. 24 h; AmB 0.8 mg/kg	5 h	7 days	100 vs. 0% ($P < .05$)
357	ABCD (1, 5, 10 mg/kg) i.v. q. 24 h; AmB 1 mg/kg	24 h	10 days	Not stated; ABCD 5–10 mg/kg cleared lesions more rapidly than AmB

AmB, amphotericin deoxycholate; C-AmB, amphotericin B/cholesterol sulfate complex; ABLC, amphotericin B lipid complex; ABCD, amphotericin B colloidal dispersion.

rats given amphotericin B intravenously (1 mg/kg/day), whereas all untreated rats died. All rats given a higher dose of intravenous itraconazole (30 mg/kg and 40 mg/kg) also died, although the mode of toxicity was not investigated (224). An intravenous liposomal formulation of itraconazole has also been developed and used in experimental *Aspergillus* pneumonia in immunocompromised mice (192, 193). It resulted in a significantly improved survival compared that of mice treated with oral itraconazole. Intravenous itraconazole is not yet available for human use in either free or liposomal forms.

Itraconazole Oral Solution (Itraconazole Solubilized in Cyclodextrin)

Absorption in animal models is improved when itraconazole is solubilized in compounds known as cyclodextrins (156). The β-cyclodextrins, naturally occurring cyclic oligosaccharides of seven glucose units, are produced during enzymatic degradation of starch by *Bacillus macerans* (156). Since cyclodextrins contain a hydrophobic interior and hydrophilic exterior, they can carry highly lipophilic drugs such as itraconazole. Solubilization in cyclodextrin allows delivery of high concentrations of itraconazole via an oral route.

Peak serum concentrations of itraconazole in mice (measured 2 h after administration of a 25-mg/kg dose in cyclodextrin) have been as high as 14.5 mg/L (75, 78). In two studies, itraconazole solubilized in cyclodextrin was equivalent in efficacy to amphotericin B (253, 256, 261, 317). In an investigation in immunocompromised rabbits given intravenous *A. fumigatus,* Patterson showed that 9 of 9 rabbits treated with itraconazole oral solution (40 mg/kg/day) survived, compared with 6 of 7 rabbits treated with amphotericin B (256, 259, 261). Both regimens decreased tissue burdens of *Aspergillus* in liver, lungs, and kidney 100- to 1000-fold, compared with controls. Although treatment with itraconazole oral solution (20 mg/kg/day) resulted in 100% survival, tissue burdens were not reduced in lung or brain tissue (256, 259,

261). In contrast, one study of itraconazole oral solution in immunocompromised mice given intranasal *A. fumigatus* showed 100% mortality when doses of 30, 60, and 100 mg/kg were used (5). Serum levels (on average, 9 mg/L) and lung tissue levels (2.5 mg/g) were adequate. It is possible that the high mortality seen in this study reflects an idiosyncratic poor response from itraconazole in this mouse model. Results from itraconazole use in this model have also been poor in other studies (143).

Voriconazole

Voriconazole, a monotriazole antifungal agent, has solubility characteristics that permit both intravenous and oral administration. In animal studies, its efficacy has been compared with that of both itraconazole and amphotericin B. Survival rates in animals with experimental invasive aspergillosis treated with voriconazole have been impressive (Table 7). Studies of experimental *Aspergillus* endocarditis in guinea pigs showed 100% survival when voriconazole was given orally at doses of 5, 7.5, and 10 mg/kg, compared with 0% survival in those treated with itraconazole (10 mg/kg) given orally (214). Although all animals survived in the different voriconazole dose groups, only animals treated with 10 mg/kg had no *Aspergillus* recovered from the heart after treatment (214). In a study of experimental pulmonary aspergillosis in Sprague-Dawley rats, survival was 100% in rats treated with voriconazole (30 mg/kg once daily by gavage) and 75% in rats treated with itraconazole (30 mg/kg once daily by gavage) (230); the difference was not statistically significant. Neither of these two studies used itraconazole solubilized in cyclodextrin (214, 230).

Survival rates have been similar when voriconazole has been compared with amphotericin B (Table 7). Survival rates of 100% were seen in animals treated with voriconazole at a dose of 30 mg/kg/day and animals treated with at least 1.5 mg/kg/day of amphotericin (114, 230). In one study, amphotericin was more effective than voriconazole in reducing tissue burden of *As-*

TABLE 7 • **Animal Studies of Experimental Aspergillosis in Which Voriconazole Was Used**

Reference	Animal	Type of Immunocompromise	Inoculum	Site of Inoculation with *Aspergillus*
114	NZ white rabbits	Cyclophosphamide and triamcinolone	10^5–10^6 conidia	Intravenous
230	Male Sprague-Dawley rats	Cortisone acetate	10^6 conidia	Intratracheal
214	Dunkin-Hartley guinea pigs	None	10^4 conidia	Endocarditis
257	Guinea pigs	Cyclophosphamide and triamcinolone	NS	Intravenous

Reference	Dose, Route, and Frequency	Time from Infection to Start of Treatment	Treatment Duration	Survival (voriconizole vs. controls)
114	VOR p.o. 10–15 mg/kg/day vs. AmB i.v. 1.5 mg/kg/day vs. no treatment	24 h	5 days	100% (VOR) 100% (AmB) 0% (untreated)
230	VOR 30 mg/kg once daily p.o. vs. AmB 4 mg/kg i.p. vs. ITRA 30 mg/kg once daily vs. no treatment	Immediate	5 days	100% (VOR) 100% (AmB) 75% (ITRA) 0% (untreated)
214	VOR 5, 7.5, and 10 mg/kg once daily p.o. vs. ITRA 10 mg/kg once daily p.o.	3 days	7 days	100% (VOR) 0% (ITRA)
257	VOR 10 mg/kg q. 12 h p.o. vs. AmB 1.25 mg/kg i.p. q. 24 h vs. no treatment	24 h	5 days	100% (VOR) 88% (AmB) 0% (untreated)

pergillus in kidneys, liver, and lungs (114), but in another study, voriconazole was more effective than amphotericin (257, 258).

Other Azoles

SCH56592 is a new triazole agent with a broad spectrum of activity in vitro (241). Animal studies have shown its in vivo activity to be as good as, if not better than, that of amphotericin B (96, 241, 256, 259, 261). Oakley et al. (241) showed that SCH 56592 (10 or 25 mg/kg once daily) in a neutropenic murine model of disseminated aspergillosis reduced mortality significantly better than amphotericin B (5 mg/kg once daily by intraperitoneal injection). Furthermore, SCH 56592 (25 mg/kg once daily) was significantly better than amphotericin B in reducing fungal burdens in the lung or kidney (241). SCH 56592 was equivalent to itraconazole in reducing mortality in two studies (96, 241) and more effective than itraconazole in another (256, 259, 261). Oakley (62) showed that SCH 56592 (25 mg/kg/day) was significantly better than itraconazole in reducing fungal burdens in the lung or kidney. Finally, SCH 56592 was effective in treating experimental infection with an itraconazole-resistant isolate of *A. fumigatus* (241).

T-1851 is a new water-soluble triazole antifungal agent that can be administered orally or parenterally (367). It yielded better survival than itraconazole in the two models of systemic aspergillosis that have been studied thus far (367). D0870 is a novel azole compound with moderate in vitro activity against *Aspergillus* (75, 78). Although slightly inferior to amphotericin B and itraconazole in a systemic nonimmunocompromised mouse model, it was superior to both in terms of mortality in a neutropenic mouse respiratory model (75,78). ER-30346, a novel oral thiazole-containing triazole, was at least as effective as itraconazole against experimental murine pulmonary aspergillosis (141, 142).

Saperconazole and SCH 39304 are azoles that reached advanced stages of development, showing excellent efficacy in animal models of invasive aspergillosis (5, 138, 255, 342). Unfortunately, further development of these compounds was curtailed due to concerns about carcinogenicity and toxicity in rodents.

In Vivo (Animal) Studies Involving Other Antifungal Agents

Liposomal Nystatin

Nystatin is a polyene antibiotic derived from *Streptomyces noursei*. Its previous use intravenously in humans was associated with systemic toxicity. In the late 1980s, Lopez-Berestein and coworkers demonstrated that encapsulation of nystatin in liposomes reduced toxicity in mice while preserving efficacy (218). Two recent studies have assessed the efficacy of liposomal nystatin against disseminated or invasive *A. fumigatus* infection (119, 120, 354). Wallace et al. (354), in a study of neutropenic mice given intravenous *A. fumigatus,* showed that treatment with liposomal nystatin (2–8 mg/kg/day) resulted in survival of 59 to 70% of mice, compared with only 19 to 33% of mice in untreated control groups ($P < .0001$). However, survival in liposomal nystatin–treated animals was significantly inferior to the 93% survival seen after treatment with amphotericin B (1 mg/kg/day) ($P < .006$). No renal or hepatic

toxicity was observed in animals treated with liposomal nystatin (354). Gonzalez et al. (119, 120) had similar findings. Although liposomal nystatin was more effective than controls, amphotericin B resulted in significantly greater tissue clearance than liposomal nystatin (119, 120).

Other Antifungal Agents

Pradimicin, a dihydrobenzonaphthacene quinone, and its derivatives have shown good in vitro activity against *A. fumigatus*. Pradimicin showed equivalent efficacy to amphotericin when used against pulmonary aspergillosis in persistently neutropenic rabbits, without producing any nephrotoxicity (119, 120). BMS-181184, a pradimicin derivative, also reduced mortality to the degree seen with amphotericin B in neutropenic rabbits inoculated intravenously with *A. fumigatus* (256, 259, 261). However, BMS-181184 did not reduce the burden of infection in the lungs, whereas amphotericin B did.

Echinocandins, a promising class of antifungal compounds, are potent inhibitors of fungal (1,3)-β-D-glucan synthase, a cell wall polymer vital to the structural integrity of *Aspergillus* (267). Echinocandins studied include LY 303366 (a novel semisynthetic derivative of echinocandin B) and MK-0991 (formerly known as L-743872). LY 303366 was at least as effective as amphotericin B in experimental invasive pulmonary aspergillosis in neutropenic rabbits (267) and in a neutropenic murine model of disseminated aspergillosis (348). The compound was also effective against an isolate of *A. fumigatus* resistant to amphotericin B (348). MK-0991 was shown to be effective in a neutropenic murine model of disseminated aspergillosis (21).

The pneumocandins, cyclic hexapeptides with fatty acyl side chains, are semisynthetic analogues of echinocandins (187). Like the echinocandins, they are potent inhibitors of fungal (1,3)-β-D-glucan synthase. Those studied in animal models of aspergillosis include L-693,989, L-705589, L-731,373, L-733,560, and L-743,872 (1, 2, 187, 316). Each of these compounds has shown efficacy comparable to that of amphotericin B.

A variety of other classes of antifungal agents has been tested in experimental models of aspergillosis, including sordaricin derivatives (GM 237 354) and conjugated styryl ketones (213, 241). Both have shown only modest activity to date (241).

Flucytosine as monotherapy for experimental disseminated aspergillosis in immunosuppressed rabbits had a mortality rate comparable to that with no treatment, even in animals not given a lethal challenge (113).

Although terbinafine shows some activity in vitro against *Aspergillus,* it showed little efficacy in a rat model of experimental pulmonary aspergillosis (304). A possible explanation for the disparity between in vitro and in vivo results is the rapid first-pass hepatic metabolism of terbinafine in rodents, reducing serum levels of the drug. Terbinafine has not been studied in other animal models.

In Vivo (Animal) Studies Using Combinations of Antifungal Agents

In view of the high mortality of human invasive or disseminated aspergillosis when monotherapy is used, combination therapy appears an attractive option. However, only a small number of studies have used combination therapy against experimental aspergillosis. Definitions of synergy, indifference, and antagonism are problematic with reference to animal studies. The subsequent discussion uses the terminology of the original investigators in each study.

There has long been concern about combining amphotericin B with an azole in the treatment of fungal infections. Some of this concern stems from experimental studies that show ketoconazole to be antagonistic to amphotericin B in animal models of disseminated aspergillosis (271, 272, 300). Neither antagonism nor synergy has been observed, however, when amphotericin B is combined with fluconazole (113) or the new triazole SCH 565592 (41). Unfortunately, studies on the most clinically applicable combination, amphotericin B and itraconazole, are very limited. The combination has been synergistic (341), indifferent (125, 271) or antagonistic (11, 271), depending on the study method and strains used.

No conclusion can be drawn from studies of the combination of amphotericin B and flucytosine in experimental aspergillosis. In three studies, the combination was reported to be synergistic (14, 200, 272), but in four studies it was indifferent (49, 113, 200, 272). Similarly, studies on combinations of itraconazole and flucytosine have shown either synergy or indifference (271). Synergy was observed only when the organism was susceptible to flucytosine in vitro and the enhancement of activity was relatively minor (271).

A single study examined the combination of amphotericin B and rifampin (14). Rifampin is not active as monotherapy against aspergillosis, but synergy was observed in the instance reported.

Synergy was observed when amphotericin B was combined with a number of antifungal agents under development in the treatment of experimental aspergillosis. These include a pneumocandin (L-733,560), a fluoroquinolone (DU-6859a), and a synthetic peptide derived from bactericidal/permeability-increasing protein (XMP.391) (8, 187, 235).

ANTIFUNGAL THERAPY
General

The optimal approach to treatment of invasive aspergillosis has yet to be determined. Early initiation of treatment by way of early diagnosis plays an important role, as does reduction of immunosuppression and recovery from neutropenia. Local lesions should be resected if possible. Although published results with itraconazole have been very impressive, these reports have considerable shortcomings, and we consider amphotericin B to remain the antifungal of choice for invasive pulmonary aspergillosis. Treatment should be for at least 6 weeks. A head-to-head randomized comparison of amphotericin deoxycholate (at least 1 mg/kg/day) and lipid preparations of amphotericin is necessary to determine which amphotericin preparation should be initiated as first-line therapy. No evidence, as yet, suggests that lipid formulations increase efficacy, but it is well established that such formulations are less toxic than amphotericin deoxycholate. Lipid preparations of amphotericin should be used in patients intolerant to ampho-

tericin deoxycholate. Flucytosine or rifampin may exhibit synergy when combined with amphotericin, although clinical data on such combination regimens are limited. The primary role of itraconazole is as maintenance therapy following the course of amphotericin. Less invasive forms of aspergillosis may be treatable with itraconazole alone. The role of voriconazole in treatment of invasive pulmonary aspergillosis remains to be determined.

Characteristics of Antifungal Drugs with Reference to Aspergillosis
Amphotericin Deoxycholate

Amphotericin B is relatively unstable and hence is commercially available as a complex with sodium desoxycholate. It is supplied as a 50-mg lyophilized cake that is reconstituted with 10 mL distilled water. It is then diluted in 500 mL of 5% dextrose (pH above 4.2), creating an infusion solution of 0.1 mg/mL. Reasonable animal and human data suggest that doses of amphotericin of 1 to 1.5 mg/kg/day are more efficacious in invasive aspergillosis than the 0.5 to 0.6 mg/kg/day commonly recommended for other systemic fungal infections (113, 341) (39). In patients with life-threatening invasive aspergillosis, 1 mg/kg can be given intravenously on the first day. In the sickest patients, as much as 1.25 or 1.5 mg/kg should be given on the second day. In less severely ill patients, a target dose of 1 mg/kg can be achieved gradually over 3 to 4 days.

Nephrotoxicity, the most important side effect of intravenous amphotericin deoxycholate, is frequently dose limiting during treatment of invasive aspergillosis; 43% of patients treated with amphotericin deoxycholate for at least 7 days for invasive aspergillosis developed nephrotoxicity in one recent study (360). Both animal and human studies suggest that sodium supplementation (e.g., by infusing 500 mL of 0.9% saline before and/or after the amphotericin) may reduce the likelihood of nephrotoxicity in patients who are salt depleted (35, 115, 144). For invasive aspergillosis, the amphotericin deoxycholate dose should not be changed until the serum creatinine concentration rises to three times the upper limit of normal (174). Alternatives at this point are switching to a lipid formulation or discontinuing the drug for 1 day and then resuming at one-half the the previous dosage, followed by a gradual escalation, renal function permitting, over 2 to 3 days until the target dosage is reached (174).

Renal failure is a risk factor for invasive aspergillosis in some patient populations (314). Excretion and serum concentrations of the drug are unaffected by renal failure (29), and hemodialysis does not remove amphotericin (30, 105). Hence in patients with severe renal failure, the usual dosage should be given. In patients with potentially reversible acute renal failure, a lipid preparation of amphotericin may be preferable to amphotericin deoxycholate, to avoid potential insult to the kidneys.

Many patients with invasive aspergillosis are transplant recipients on cyclosporine or tacrolimus. Some data suggest that amphotericin has a synergistic effect on the production of nephrotoxicity by cyclosporine (173, 339, 365). Also, anecdotal reports exist of severe acute renal impairment when intravenous amphotericin was coadministered with tacrolimus

(257, 258). Ideally, immunosuppression should be reduced in transplant patients with invasive aspergillosis.

Amphotericin deoxycholate can also be administered in other modes, depending on the site of infection. Amphotericin B has been instilled directly into the cerebrospinal fluid (CSF) by the intralumbar, intracisternal, or intraventricular routes, in addition to intravenous therapy, in patients with central nervous system (CNS) infection due to *Aspergillus*. The rationale for its use is that following intravenous administration, only 2 to 4% of the simultaneous serum concentration reaches the CSF (70). The dosage range is 0.05 to 0.5 mg/day in 5 mL of 10% glucose (174). Some recommend addition of 5 to 25 mg of hydrocortisone to reduce the incidence of headache, fever, and nausea (190).

Aerosol administration of amphotericin can be used to treat tracheobronchial aspergillosis and for prophylaxis against invasive aspergillosis in certain patient populations (see below). For inhalation, 10 mg of amphotericin deoxycholate is diluted in 5 mL of sterile water and placed in a Respir Grad II nebulizer (26). Others have dissolved 50 mg of amphotericin deoxycholate in 10 mL of sterile water; 1 mL of this solution added to 3 mL of 5% dextrose can be administered via a "Cirrus" nebulizer with a Pall "ultipor" breathing filter over 10 min (63). It has been administered two or three times per day (63, 211). Aerosolized amphotericin is generally well tolerated, although some patients complain of an unpleasant taste and mild nausea (26). Bronchospasm is sometimes observed (94).

Nasally administered amphotericin spray has been used to prevent *Aspergillus* infections in children undergoing bone marrow transplantation (335). Amphotericin deoxycholate in a concentration of 2.5 to 5 mg/mL is added to a sterilized 15-mL plastic reservoir bottle capped with a metered-dose intranasal pump ("Vp7 pump") (335). The dose is age dependent but ranges from 1 to 5 sprays per nostril twice a day. A stinging sensation in the nasal mucosa is common with this therapy. Mixing a small amount of hydrocortisone with the amphotericin spray or using a metered-dose steroid spray just before using the amphotericin spray may reduce the stinging (335).

Intracavitary instillation of amphotericin by percutaneous or bronchoscopic routes has been used as therapy for as-

pergilloma (see below). Both a solution of amphotericin diluted in dextrose water (160) and a paste made by dissolving amphotericin in molten gelatin (116, 229) have been used.

Intravitreal injection of amphotericin deoxycholate has been used to treat *Aspergillus* endophthalmitis. Doses from 0.005 to 5 mg have been used by various authors (72, 92, 126, 128, 185, 191).

Lipid Preparations of Amphotericin

Three lipid preparations of amphotericin are now marketed for clinical use (Table 8): amphotericin liposome for injection (AmBisome, Fujisawa, Deerfield, IL), amphotericin colloidal dispersion (Amphotec, Sequus, Menlo Park, CA), and ABLC (Abelcet, The Lipsome Company, Princeton, NJ). In addition, in-house mixtures of amphotericin and Intralipid have been used as a less expensive alternative to commercial preparations. The nephrotoxicity of amphotericin deoxycholate and high mortality rates for invasive aspergillosis have prompted development of lipid preparations, but high costs and lack of data from randomized controlled trials have limited their use. No randomized controlled trials have been published that compare the efficacy and toxicity of lipid preparations versus amphotericin deoxycholate for the treatment of invasive aspergillosis. However, randomized controlled trials have been published comparing amphotericin liposome for injection (AmBisome), amphotericin deoxycholate for empirical antifungal therapy in febrile neutropenic patients (356), ABLC (Abelcet), and amphotericin deoxycholate in the treatment of invasive and hematogenous candidiasis (10) and amphotericin liposome for injection (AmBisome) and amphotericin deoxycholate for the treatment of cryptococcal meningitis (195). In all of these studies, the lipid preparations were not more likely to result in cure, but they were associated with significantly less nephrotoxicity. Infusion-related reactions may also be less frequent (356), but this has not been well reported in all studies.

Data from reviews of experience with lipid preparations in the treatment of invasive aspergillosis and retrospective comparison with historical controls treated with amphotericin deoxycholate generally support these conclusions (151, 152, 355, 360). Multivariate analyses also suggest that the com-

---

TABLE 8 • Dosages of Antifungal Agents Potentially Useful in Treating Invasive Aspergillosis

Compound	Brand Name	Dose
Amphotericin deoxycholate	Fungizone	1.0–1.5 mg/kg/day i.v.
Amphotericin B liposome for injection	AmBisome	4–5 mg/kg/day i.v.
Amphotericin B colloidal dispersion (ABCD)	Amphocil, Amphotec	4–5 mg/kg/day i.v.
Amphotericin B lipid complex (ABLC)	Abelcet	4–5 mg/kg/day i.v.
Itraconazole capsules	Sporanox	200 mg three times a day for the first 4 days, then 200 mg twice a day (p.o.)
Itraconazole oral solution	Sporanox oral solution	100–150 mg three times a day for the first 4 days, then 100–150 mg twice a day (p.o.)[a]
Voriconazole	—	6 mg/kg every 12 h i.v. for 2 doses, then 3 mg/kg every 12 h i.v. for up to 4 weeks, then 200 mg every 12 h p.o.

[a] Clinical experience with itraconazole oral solution for treatment of invasive aspergillosis is limited. This dose is based on knowledge that area under the plasma concentration versus time curve of itraconazole oral solution is 150% of that obtained with itraconazole capsules.

mercial lipid preparations may be even more efficacious than amphotericin deoxycholate (360). At present, while it may be tempting to use these data to support lipid preparations as first-line therapy for invasive aspergillosis, U.S. Food and Drug Administration (FDA) recommendations for all three commercial preparations are to reserve treatment for infections refractory to amphotericin deoxycholate or for patients with renal impairment or for whom unacceptable toxicity precludes use of amphotericin deoxycholate. Amphotericin liposome for injection (AmBisome) has an additional indication for empirical therapy for presumed fungal infection in febrile, neutropenic patients.

There are currently no data to support use of one commercial lipid preparation over another for treatment of invasive aspergillosis. Dilution of amphotericin in Intralipid, while financially attractive, lacks standardization of preparation procedures and external quality control. Although some preliminary data suggest that lower doses may be successful (98), we recommend using the commercial preparations at 4 to 5 mg/kg/day for invasive aspergillosis.

Itraconazole

Itraconazole (Sporanox, Janssen Pharmaceutica, Titusville, NJ) is an orally administered triazole antifungal agent with marked in vitro activity against *Aspergillus*. It is not yet available in an intravenous formulation. Initial published reports of itraconazole use suggest that complete or partial responses occur in close to 40% of patients treated (80). Unfortunately, only one randomized controlled trial has compared itraconazole with amphotericin B for the treatment of invasive aspergillosis (343). No difference was found in outcome between the two treatment groups, but sample size was small (fewer than 10 in each arm), and the amphotericin dose was only 0.3 to 0.6 mg/kg/day.

Itraconazole has been available for several years as 100-mg capsules. During the first 4 days of therapy for invasive aspergillosis, a loading dose is given: 200 mg three times a day. Thereafter, the usual dose is 200 mg twice daily (80). Absorption of the capsule may be limited in some patients, particularly neutropenic patients who have poor oral intake, since absorption of the capsules improves with food (124). Some transplant patients may also experience suboptimal absorption (256, 259, 261). Serum concentrations of itraconazole may be measured by bioassay approximately 7 days after initiating therapy (at which time steady-state concentrations should be achieved), to demonstrate absorption (80). Although patients may fail itraconazole therapy for aspergillosis with apparently adequate serum itraconazole concentrations, patients who fail are much more likely to lack detectable serum concentrations (80). Some prefer to cover patients with amphotericin as well as itraconazole until itraconazole is detectable in serum (250). There is no clear correlation between a particular serum concentration and outcome (80), but aiming for a level of 5 mg/L or higher seems reasonable (167, 168).

Drug interactions may also reduce the chance of achieving adequate serum itraconazole concentrations. Several patients have had interactions with rifampin and phenytoin that have reduced serum itraconazole levels and led to failure of therapy (80). Concurrent or recent use of carbamazepine and phenobarbitol should also be a contraindication to the use of itraconazole for invasive aspergillosis (338). H2 antagonists may lead to poor absorption of itraconazole, although adequate serum concentrations of itraconazole have been achieved in lung transplant recipients on these drugs (256, 259, 261).

In view of the poor absorption sometimes seen with itraconazole capsules, itraconazole has been solubilized in cyclodextrin to improve absorption. Unlike the itraconazole capsules, it is recommended that the oral solution be administered without food because absorption is slightly higher under fasting conditions (11). The itraconazole capsules and oral solution should not be used interchangeably. Bioavailability of itraconazole oral solution is approximately 150% that of itraconazole capsules (11). The use of itraconazole oral solution has not been widely studied in solid-organ transplant recipients. In a study of itraconazole oral solution for antifungal prophylaxis in 287 neutropenic patients, no *Aspergillus* infections occurred (226). At the time of writing, the FDA indication for itraconazole oral solution is treatment of oropharyngeal and esophageal candidiasis. Although it seems likely that the efficacy of itraconazole oral solution in the treatment of invasive aspergillosis will be just as good as itraconazole capsules, this remains to be determined.

Both itraconazole capsules and oral solution can be predicted to increase the plasma concentrations of a variety of drugs metabolized by the cytochrome P-450 system. Terfenadine, astemizole, oral triazolam, oral midazolam, and cisapride are specifically contraindicated with itraconazole. Lovastatin and simvastatin should be discontinued during itraconazole therapy. Levels of cyclosporine and tacrolimus would be predicted to rise during itraconazole therapy. Solid-organ transplant patients on itraconazole should probably have an immediate cyclosporine or tacrolimus dose reduction followed by frequent monitoring (183, 257, 258). Plasma concentrations of the following drugs may also rise during itracoanzole therapy: warfarin, ritonavir, indinavir, digoxin, vinca alkaloids, and quinidine (11).

Itraconazole has an established role as oral follow-on therapy after a response to amphotericin is established. The question of whether itraconazole should be combined with amphotericin in patients with severe illness is an important one. Unfortunately, current data from animal models (125, 271, 298, 341) and anecdotal human reports (298, 366) are so mixed that no accurate answer can be given.

Voriconazole

Voriconazole is a promising new triazole derivative that is highly active in vitro against *Aspergillus*. Potential advantages over itraconazole include ability to use the drug intravenously and good CNS penetration (163, 307). However, information on its clinical utility is limited at the present time. In an open noncomparative study in immunocompromised patients with acute invasive aspergillosis, 27 of 36 patients (75%) had a favorable clinical response (75); 72% had received previous antifungal treatment with amphotericin or itraconazole. Four of

71 patients (6%) were discontinued from treatment by the investigators: 3 due to liver function test abnormalities and 1 due to rash. Six patients (8%) experienced mild or moderate visual disturbances (enhanced perception of light) that did not lead to study drug withdrawal or result in any residual effects (75). In another clinical study, 11 of 25 patients (44%) reported enhanced perception of light, although in no case did it lead to withdrawal of the drug (95). The drug does not appear to have any appreciable nephrotoxicity.

The exact place of voriconazole in the armamentarium against invasive aspergillosis remains to be determined. At the present time, it should probably be reserved for salvage therapy in patients who have failed, or been intolerant to, other therapies. Most experience has been with a regimen of 6 mg/kg 12-hourly intravenously for two doses, then 3 mg/kg 12-hourly intravenously for up to 4 weeks, followed by 200 mg 12-hourly orally for the remainder of the treatment duration (75).

Flucytosine

The only place for flucytosine in the management of invasive aspergillosis is in combination therapy. *Aspergillus* species are only occasionally susceptible to flucytosine, but synergy with amphotericin has been demonstrated both in vitro and in animal experiments (14, 200, 272). However some strains show in vitro antagonism (81), and some animal studies have shown indifference when the two antifungal agents are used together (49, 113, 200, 272). Nevertheless, anecdotal reports in humans indicate impressive results when amphotericin and flucytosine are used together (39). A small randomized controlled trial failed to show any difference in outcome when amphotericin B alone was compared with the combination of amphotericin B and flucytosine, but sample size was insufficient to definitively determine this (348). The good penetration of flucytosine into most body fluids and tissues make this agent a useful but unproved adjunct to amphotericin. Insufficient data exist to determine whether there is any clinical utility to combining flucytosine and lipid preparations of amphotericin, itraconazole, or voriconazole.

Rifampin

Rifampin has little activity as monotherapy against *Aspergillus,* but anecdotal reports of rifampin use in combination with amphotericin B have appeared (369). An advantage of rifampin is its good penetration into bone, brain, and many other tissues. However, good clinical data on its use in invasive aspergillosis are scarce, and it enhances metabolism of itraconazole, tacrolimus, and cyclosporine, which makes it difficult to establish therapeutic serum levels of these drugs (80, 257, 258) and limit recommendations for its use.

Terbinafine

Terbinafine shows good in vitro activity against *Aspergillus,* especially *A. niger* and *A. flavus* (19). However animal and human data (303, 304) are so limited in the treatment of invasive aspergillosis that it can only be considered as an option if amphotericin, itraconazole, or voriconazole could not be used.

Special Situations

Infections of the Respiratory Tract

Invasive Pulmonary Aspergillosis. Invasive pulmonary aspergillosis is the most common form of invasive aspergillosis. Unfortunately, the frequent occurrence of invasive pulmonary aspergillosis in the immunocompromised host and its characteristic insidious onset contribute to an overall poor outcome, even with treatment (76). Outcome varies in different immunocompromised populations, with heart and renal transplant recipients having the best prognosis and liver transplant and bone marrow transplant recipients having the worst (76). Overall, 80% of immunocompromised patients with invasive pulmonary aspergillosis die (76). In addition to antifungal agents, multiple factors can influence outcome such as recovery from neutropenia, removal of iatrogenic immunosuppression, and presence of extrapulmonary disease. There is little doubt that early diagnosis improves survival (349). Aids to early diagnosis of invasive pulmonary aspergillosis may include use of ultrafast computed tomography even in the absence of abnormalities on chest radiographs (149), bronchoscopy and bronchoalveolar lavage (349), and prospective use of serology in high-risk patients (333).

Although alternative agents are becoming increasingly popular, intravenous amphotericin deoxycholate has long been regarded as standard therapy for invasive pulmonary aspergillosis. Lower doses of the drug (e.g., 0.5–0.7 mg/kg/day) are suboptimal for invasive pulmonary aspergillosis, especially in neutropenic patients (86). Rapid escalation of dose to 1 mg/kg/day is recommended; even higher doses (1.25 or 1.5 mg/kg/day) are recommended if there is no initial response and the therapy is being tolerated (86). Although there is not evidence from well-conducted trials for use of higher doses, animal data (see above), the knowledge that high levels of amphotericin are not easily attained in lung tissue, the relatively high MICs of *Aspergillus* to amphotericin, and limited clinical data all support this practice (39, 76, 86). In one retrospective series, mortality was only 13% (2 of 15) in neutropenic patients with invasive pulmonary aspergillosis who received doses of amphotericin deoxycholate of 1.25 to 1.5 mg/kg/day (39). Other factors may have contributed to the success in this series including strenuous attempts to start treatment early and use of flucytosine in most of the patients.

Since many patients with invasive pulmonary aspergillosis are desperately ill, combination therapy with amphotericin B is often considered. Flucytosine penetrates well into bronchial secretions (263) and achieves tissue levels in the lung that equal or exceed serum levels at the time (154). In animal models, the combination of amphotericin deoxycholate and flucytosine was synergistic or at worst indifferent (14, 49, 113, 200, 272). In the series of high-dose amphotericin deoxycholate mentioned above, 10 of 13 survivors of invasive pulmonary aspergillosis received concomitant flucytosine therapy (39). In all, about two-thirds of reported patients treated with amphotericin deoxycholate and flucytosine have responded (86, 107). A randomized controlled trial compared amphotericin deoxycholate alone with amphotericin deoxycholate plus flucytosine for neutropenic patients with systemic mycoses

(346). Amphotericin doses were between 0.5 and 1.0 mg/kg/day. One of nine patients with invasive pulmonary aspergillosis treated with amphotericin deoxycholate alone survived, compared with two of nine patients treated with the combination therapy. Unfortunately, this study was curtailed (due in part to the poor results observed), and hence the sample size is too small to determine if a true difference between the therapies exists (346). Flucytosine has been associated with fatal cases of bone marrow aplasia (107), often making hematologists reluctant to permit use of the drug in neutropenic patients. However, if peak serum levels are maintained between 40 and 60 μg/mL, duration of granulocytopenia is not prolonged (39, 107).

Although in vitro and animal data on the combination of amphotericin deoxycholate and rifampin are favorable (14), there are few good clinical data on the efficacy of the combination against invasive pulmonary aspergillosis. In a review of the combination for pulmonary aspergillosis in neutropenic patients, 4 of 9 (44%) treated with the combination survived, compared with 45 of 69 (65%) treated with amphotericin deoxycholate alone (86). In addition, rifampin has important interactions with cyclosporine, tacrolimus, and itraconazole that dramatically reduce serum concentrations of these drugs (80, 257, 258).

Lipid preparations of amphotericin are now widely used in the treatment of invasive pulmonary aspergillosis, especially in patients who have been intolerant to amphotericin deoxycholate or whose infections are refractory to amphotericin deoxycholate. At the time of writing, no randomized controlled trials comparing amphotericin deoxycholate and any of the lipid preparations of amphotericin for the treatment of invasive pulmonary aspergillosis have been published. In general, animal studies find relatively high concentrations of amphotericin B in the lung when the lipid preparations are used (60, 243).

ABLC has been compared with amphotericin deoxycholate use in historical controls (355) and has been evaluated in open-label prospective studies (76). These data have the limitations of any nonrandomized comparison. Also, most patients who received ABLC had failed amphotericin deoxycholate or had developed amphotericin deoxycholate–induced nephrotoxicity (152, 217, 355). Of seven neutropenic patients treated for invasive pulmonary aspergillosis with ABLC, four had a complete response, one had a partial response, and two failed treatment (217). Reviews of several hundred patients treated for aspergillosis (predominantly pulmonary) with ABLC in open-label emergency-use protocols show clinical responses in 40 to 60% (152, 355). Most patients received 5 mg/kg. In comparison, only 23% of historical controls treated with amphotericin deoxycholate responded (152). ABLC also appeared to be less nephrotoxic than amphotericin deoxycholate (152, 355).

Amphotericin B colloidal dispersion (ABCD) was evaluated in a phase I study for treatment of invasive fungal infections after bone marrow transplantation (33). The maximum tolerated dose of ABCD was 7.5 mg/kg. Of 14 evaluable patients with A. fumigatus pneumonia, only 5 failed therapy (33). In contrast, failure occurred in 15 of 23 patients (65%) treated with ABCD for invasive pulmonary aspergillosis (244). Fur-

ther data have come from five cancer or transplant centers that evaluated clinical outcome and toxicity of ABCD versus historical controls treated with amphotericin deoxycholate (360). Some 55% of the ABCD-treated group had previously received amphotericin deoxycholate; 82% (66 of 82) of the ABCD treatment group had pulmonary infection. Response rates (48.8%) and survival rates (50%) among ABCD-treated patients were statistically significantly higher than those (23.4 and 28.4%, respectively) among amphotericin deoxycholate–treated controls (360). Renal dysfunction in evaluated patients (those who had received at least 7 days of either therapy) developed less frequently in ABCD recipients (8.2%) than in amphotericin deoxycholate recipients (43.1%). Infusion-related toxicities were not assessed (360).

Liposomal amphotericin (AmBisome) significantly reduces pulmonary Aspergillus loads in animal models of invasive pulmonary aspergillosis (194, 195). The pharmacokinetics of AmBisome appear quite similar in animals and humans (151). No randomized controlled trials comparing the efficacy and toxicity of AmBisome and amphotericin deoxycholate in the treatment of invasive pulmonary aspergillosis in humans have been published. Only small retrospective case series have been presented (221, 236, 279). Analyzing the three studies combined, 48% of patients (31 of 64) had an excellent response to the therapy, and fewer than 10% suffered nephrotoxicity or infusion-related toxicities (221, 236). In one study, 17% of treated patients experienced abnormal hepatic function possibly due to liposomal amphotericin (221). Although most patients in these studies were treated with 5 mg/kg, preliminary data from a randomized multicenter study comparing AmBisome at 1 and 4 mg/kg suggest that outcome and toxicity do not differ at these two doses (98). However, the sample size was insufficient to determine this definitively, and more data are needed to determine whether a low dose is as efficacious as doses of 4 or 5 mg/kg.

As discussed above, amphotericin diluted in lipid emulsion used in total parenteral nutrition (Intralipid) is widely used in some centers as a relatively inexpensive alternative to other lipid preparations. Methods of preparing this mixture have not been standardized, it has not undergone external quality control testing, and it is not approved by the FDA (151, 170). Although amphotericin diluted in Intralipid was evaluated in cryptococcal meningitis and as empirical treatment in neutropenic patients with fever unresponsive to antibiotics (43, 188, 306, 353), there are virtually no data on its use in invasive pulmonary aspergillosis (310). One study has suggested that less nephrotoxicity and infusion-induced chills are seen with amphotericin in Intralipid than with standard amphotericin deoxycholate (43), others have suggested no reduction in adverse effects or even more nephrotoxicity than with amphotericin deoxycholate (164). No studies have evaluated combinations of itraconazole, flucytosine, or rifampin with lipid preparations of amphotericin.

Although negligible amounts of itraconazole have been found in saliva, concentrations in the lung may exceed those in the plasma by up to twofold (124). Itraconazole has been used successfully as monotherapy in treatment of invasive pulmonary aspergillosis in solid organ transplant, bone marrow transplant, and neutropenic patients (52, 80, 81, 84–86, 353). More than 40% of patients showed good responses in these studies, but this rate of response is subject to a number of biases, including publication bias. A randomized controlled trial that compared itraconazole with amphotericin deoxycholate (343) in the treatment of systemic fungal infections in neutropenic patients was far too small to discern any true difference between the regimens. Voriconazole has been studied in a small number of patients with invasive pulmonary aspergillosis thus far. Preliminary results have been encouraging (44, 75).

Itraconazole has also been used successfully in chronic necrotizing pulmonary aspergillosis, a less invasive form of pulmonary aspergillosis (294). Approximately 80% of patients treated with itraconazole responded, compared with less than 40% of patients treated with intravenous amphotericin deoxycholate (294).

Surgery (lobectomy or wedge resection) has been used successfully in conjunction with antifungal agents for treatment of invasive pulmonary aspergillosis. Localized pulmonary lesions have been resected in the acute setting, even when the patient remained neutropenic and thrombocytopenic (134, 280, 364). Support with platelets and if necessary fresh frozen plasma is given before and during the operation with a view to raising platelet counts above 40,000 (134). Postsurgical survival has approached 80% (44, 134, 215, 216, 280, 364). Surgery has been deferred till hematologic recovery in other patients who were facing further chemotherapy or bone marrow transplantation (207, 215, 216, 225, 368). Subsequent recurrence of invasive aspergillosis was prevented in most (215, 216, 225, 368), but not all of these patients (207).

Tracheobronchitis. *Aspergillus* tracheobronchitis is most common in lung transplant recipients but has also been described in other immunocompromised groups (AIDS, hematologic malignancies) and rarely in immunocompetent patients (24, 31, 153, 166, 182). Lung transplant recipients exhibit a spectrum of disease, with ulcerative tracheobronchial aspergillosis at the anastomosis site at the most dangerous end of the spectrum. The disease may also be a precursor to invasive pulmonary aspergillosis. Treatment regimens have been described in retrospective, nonrandomized series that evaluated only a small number of patients. Kramer et al. (182), in the initial description of this entity, treated six patients with itraconazole (200 mg three times a day for 4 days as a loading dose, then 200 mg twice a day) (182). Treatment duration was 4 to 6 months, during which time repeated bronchoscopic examinations were negative (182). Two of the six patients in this report died from invasive or disseminated aspergillosis—both had the course of itraconazole interrupted for a number of days. Other treatment alternatives used successfully include combinations of intravenous amphotericin B and itraconazole (366), aerosolized amphotericin B and oral itraconazole (359), and amphotericin B alone (25, 366). Sequential liposomal amphotericin (1.5–3.5 mg/kg/day, to a mean total dose of 3.1 g) and then itraconazole (400 mg/day) was used successfully in at least four patients (110). A single patient who was intolerant of amphotericin B, liposomal amphotericin, and itracona-

zole was treated successfully with terbinafine (250 mg every 12 h by mouth for 3 months) (139). Finally, surgical resection and stent placement may be necessary in conjunction with antifungal therapy if dehiscence of the anastomosis occurs because of tracheobronchial aspergillosis (28, 155).

Treatment recommendations in patient groups other than lung transplant recipients are based solely on small case series and case reports. Extrapolation from these must recognize reporting bias and the heterogeneity of the clinical illnesses and immunosuppression in the reported patients. Intravenous amphotericin was associated with successful outcome in two of four HIV-infected patients treated (172, 203). Oral itraconazole resulted in a clinical response in three patients, one of whom also received flucytosine and aerosolized amphotericin B (69, 77, 83). Successful treatment of a critically ill immunocompetent female with tracheobronchial aspergillosis with liposomal amphotericin, aerosolized amphotericin, and adjuvant interferon-γ and granulocyte macrophage colony-stimulating factor (GM-CSF) was recently reported (31).

A systemic antifungal agent (amphotericin deoxycholate, lipid preparations of amphotericin, or itraconazole) plus aerosolized amphotericin may be the preferred therapy for tracheobronchial aspergillosis. As the condition is uncommon, randomized controlled trials of different regimens are unlikely to be performed.

Allergic Bronchopulmonary Aspergillosis (ABPA). For many years the only treatment available for ABPA has been steroids. There is increasing evidence that adjunctive therapy of ABPA with itraconazole improves symptoms and pulmonary function, reduces steroid requirements, and occasionally reduces levels of IgG to *A. fumigatus* (87, 247, 321). A recent randomized double-blind study of itraconazole (200 mg twice a day for 16 weeks, then 200 mg once a day for 16 weeks) or placebo for steroid-dependent ABPA showed a significantly greater chance of response in patients given itraconazole (321); 46% of patients treated with itraconazole achieved at least a 50% reduction in steroid dose, 25% showed greater exercise tolerance, and 25% exhibited reduced serum IgE levels. Itraconazole and corticosteroids should now be regarded as the standard of care for most patients with ABPA.

Aspergilloma. Pulmonary aspergillomas results from fungal growth within a preexisting pulmonary cavity. Unfortunately, although the infection is usually localized, erosion of a bronchial artery can lead to life-threatening hemoptysis (171). Systemic administration of antifungal agents is nearly always ineffective (169). Rare successes with oral itraconazole have been described, although significant improvement may require therapy for at least 6 months (20, 46). Early surgical resection (lobectomy) is the treatment of choice in patients with adequate lung function (54, 171). However, because the surgery is technically difficult and associated with significant morbidity and sometimes mortality, and because the underlying lung disease that predisposed to cavity formation is often severe, lobectomy is not a realistic option for some patients.

In patients for whom lobectomy is precluded, a surgical alternative is cavernostomy performed under local or regional anesthesia (100, 171). Intracavitary instillation of antifungal agents, in combination with cavernostomy or as an alternative to surgery, is well described but only occasionally cures aspergillomas (169). Symptomatic relief may be marked, however. Intracavitary instillation of antifungal agents has also been described for management of acute severe hemoptysis (309), although other agents such as sodium or potassium iodide have probably achieved more success (289).

Intracavitary instillation of amphotericin has been by percutaneous or bronchoscopic routes. Both a solution of amphotericin diluted in dextrose water (160) and a paste made by dissolving amphotericin in molten gelatin (116, 229) have been used successfully. The paste (which is injected warm, percutaneously under radiologic control) has the advantage of solidifying at body temperature, which keeps the drug within the cavity and thus precludes the necessity for multiple instillations (229). The optimal dose and number of instillations of the amphotericin/dextrose water solution are unknown. Chest radiographs are an insensitive method of monitoring treatment. In practice, treatment is given until symptoms have fully resolved and then continued for a further arbitrary period (160). Intracavitary ketoconazole and miconazole have also been used successfully (130, 131, 136). It is not certain whether intracavitary administration of antifungal agents is successful because of local irritation and sclerosis or cidal activity against *Aspergillus* (169).

Infections of the Sinuses. Sinus infection by *Aspergillus* takes a variety of forms ranging in severity from fulminant acute invasive sinusitis to allergic sinusitis. Allergic sinusitis due to *Aspergillus* may manifest as chronic, intractable sinusitis and nasal polyposis. There is no evidence at present that antifungal agents are useful in managing this condition. Usual management involves endoscopic removal of polyps and inflammatory material followed by long-term intranasal corticosteroids and short-term systemic corticosteroids (89).

In contrast, fulminant invasive *Aspergillus* infection of the sinuses, particularly in neutropenic patients (including bone marrow transplant recipients) and persons infected with HIV, has a high mortality (295, 345). Survival is often determined by recovery from neutropenia and possibly aggressive debridement of devitalized tissue (89). Although a review in 1990 (82) showed that mortality was higher in those treated with a combination of medical and surgical therapy than in those treated with medical therapy alone, the apparent increase in mortality following surgery may have reflected more severe disease in this group. All of five surviving patients with this condition reported since 1990 have received surgery (usually the Caldwell-Luc procedure) as well as medical therapy (93, 231, 345). In addition, three of the five received granulocyte infusions, emphasizing the importance of neutrophil recovery in resolving this condition. Although amphotericin was given to most patients treated successfully in a previous series (82), four of the five recently reported patients with successfully treated disease had been given amphotericin B colloidal dispersion (231, 345). The fifth patient who responded relapsed after receiving ABLC for 6 weeks; success was achieved with further surgery followed by oral itraconazole and terbinafine in combination (231).

Chronic *Aspergillus* infection in the ethmoid sinus may result in bony erosion toward the orbit or the cavernous sinuses, particularly in patients on systemic corticosteroids or with diabetes mellitus (223). The condition has a poor prognosis and treatment is similar to that for acute invasive sinusitis (89).

A. flavus sometimes produces regional tissue invasion and noncaseating granulomata in immunocompetent persons, primarily from Sudan, India, and Pakistan but also from the United States (127, 222, 293, 358). This produces the curious syndrome known as primary paranasal granuloma. Extension into the orbit, dura, and brain may result. Extensive surgery is indicated, although relapse postoperatively is common. Itraconazole may reduce the postoperative relapse rate (132).

Infections of the Central Nervous System

Aspergillus infection of the CNS is usually manifest as cerebral space-occupying lesions in the context of disseminated disease in immunocompromised patients. Less commonly, cerebral abscesses may be an isolated finding in immunocompromised patients, follow neurosurgical procedures, or result from direct extension from neglected sinus disease. Meningitis and spinal cord involvement are rare.

Optimal management of cerebral aspergillosis is difficult to determine other than reiterating the role of reducing immunosuppression and surgically draining lesions, if possible. Amphotericin remains the treatment of choice. Although unproven in clinical trials, addition of flucytosine to amphotericin appears reasonable on the basis of its good penetration into brain tissue and limited human data (86). It is unclear whether adding rifampin adds any benefit to the above regimen. Lipid preparations of amphotericin in high dose or voriconazole may be useful alternative therapies, but this is based only on animal data and anecdotal human cases.

The difficulties of treating invasive aspergillosis are magnified in patients with infections of the CNS because many drugs have suboptimal penetration of the blood-brain barrier. For amphotericin, CSF levels are 30- to 50-fold lower than simultaneous serum levels (204). In animal studies, amphotericin B could be detected in the brains of mice after administration of 10 mg/kg of ABLC but not 1 mg/kg (60). Liposomal amphotericin also displays a dose-related rise in CSF concentration; a 5-mg/kg dose of liposomal amphotericin B results in a fourfold rise in brain tissue concentration, compared with 1 mg/kg of amphotericin deoxycholate (275). Flucytosine penetrates well into the CSF; levels between 71 and 85% of the concomitant serum level have been obtained (270). Rifampin also penetrates well into the CSF and brain tissue, particularly if the meninges are inflamed (67). Since itraconazole is highly bound to plasma proteins and has a relatively high molecular weight, relatively poor penetration would be expected; 2 to 5% penetration of itraconazole into CSF was observed with uninflamed meninges and 9% penetration with inflamed meninges (74, 264). However, in animal models of disseminated *Aspergillus* infection, itraconazole solubilized in cyclodextrin successfully reduced the tissue burden of *Aspergillus* in the brain (253). Furthermore, itracoanazole as monotherapy has been effective for other fungal meningitides, such as cryptococcosis (84, 85,

337). Studies in guinea pigs have shown that voriconazole has excellent penetration into the CSF and the brain (163). At steady-state, CNS levels were double that found in plasma. CSF levels of voriconazole were approximately half that found in plasma (163). In a recently studied patient with cerebral aspergillosis, CSF levels of voriconazole of 1.36 to 2.65 μg/mL were achieved (307).

Cerebral aspergillosis in the immunocompromised host with disseminated aspergillosis is often not diagnosed until autopsy, but even with treatment, mortality is close to 99% (76, 248). However, 10 case reports have now documented cure in this setting (16, 32, 40, 101, 112, 122, 148, 178, 184, 307). Reduced iatrogenic immunosuppression or recovery from neutropenia appear to play as important a part as antifungal therapy in these successes. In addition, 7 of the 10 patients had cerebral lesions amenable to stereotactic or open drainage. Two patients were given intralesional amphotericin B (148, 307), although in one patient the CNS infection clearly progressed on this therapy (307). The role of local amphotericin B in treating CNS aspergillosis is not certain. A wide variety of systemic antifungal agents was given to the 10 successfully treated patients—5 patients received amphotericin B in combination with either or both flucytosine and rifampin, 2 received amphotericin B alone, and 2 received itraconazole alone (16, 32, 40, 101, 112, 122, 148, 178, 184, 307). One successfully treated patient received initial therapy with amphotericin deoxycholate (1.1 mg/kg) and then liposomal amphotericin B (2.1 mg/kg) before showing clear progression of disease. Subsequent itraconazole and intralesional and intrathecal amphotericin B were unsuccessful, so salvage therapy with voriconazole was attempted (307). The patient was apparently cured of his cerebral and pulmonary aspergillosis, although he died from relapsed leukemia. The dosing schedule of voriconazole was 900 mg intravenously on the first day, then 450 mg intravenously daily for 5 days, then 200 mg orally twice daily for 8 months (307).

An additional 10 immunocompromised patients with cerebral aspergillosis (without evidence of extracerebral disease) have been successfully treated (45, 61, 108, 126, 175, 189, 210, 228, 274, 292). Again, recovery from neutropenia or the ability to reduce iatrogenic immunosuppression has been paramount in managing these patients. In addition, 9 of the 10 patients had open or stereotactic drainage of their cerebral lesions. In some, the fungal mass could be totally extirpated. As with the immunocompromised patients with disseminated disease, a wide variety of antifungal regimens were used including combinations of amphotericin B with flucytosine in four patients. In one patient, the dose of liposomal amphotericin was carefully escalated to 15 mg/kg/day and was combined with itraconazole and extensive surgery with successful result (61). Liposomal amphotericin and ABLC were used in two other successfully treated patients (175, 210). In another successfully treated patient, long-term intracavitary administration of amphotericin B via an Ommaya reservoir was used as an adjunct to radical debridement and systemic antifungal therapy (45).

Cerebral aspergillosis in the nonimmunocompromised patient has a much better prognosis than disease in the immuno-

compromised patient (76). Successful management of disease resulting from invasion from the sinuses has entailed extensive surgical excision and concomitant systemic antifungal therapy (34, 133, 176, 205, 234). Treatment of postneurosurgical *Aspergillus* cerebral infection or meningitis entails removal of any hardware present and addition of systemic antifungal therapy (71, 104, 176, 227). Intrathecal amphotericin was used in two of the successfully treated patients (71, 227). Unfortunately, complications of intrathecal amphotericin have included arachnoiditis, paraparesis, myelopathy, and cranial nerve palsies (48). On the basis of limited clinical data, intravenous amphotericin B plus flucytosine is appropriate first-line therapy.

Reviews of treatment of *Aspergillus* meningitis are based on very few evaluable patients (86). The general principles mentioned above should be followed, including reduction of immunosuppression, surgical removal of infected tissue or neurosurgical hardware (51), and administration of amphotericin B plus flucytosine. Data are insufficient to determine whether lipid preparations of amphotericin hold any advantage over amphotericin deoxycholate for meningitis. Since the treatment duration is likely to be approximately 6 weeks, nephrotoxicity would probably require using a less nephrotoxic agent than amphotericin deoxycholate at some point during the treatment course. Itraconazole as monotherapy (400 mg daily) has been used successfully in the treatment of *Aspergillus* meningitis (220). In this patient, although CSF levels of the drug were not measured, serum levels ranged between 3.2 and 18 mg/mL(220).

Infections of the Eye
Aspergillus is a frequent cause of posttraumatic keratitis (249, 287). Less commonly, endophthalmitis may result from disseminated infection or may occur de novo in intravenous drug abusers or after ophthalmic surgery. Orbital infection can result from invasion from infected sinuses.

Time between injury and recognition of fungal keratitis is a major determinant of success in treatment of *Aspergillus* keratitis. The condition is usually treated empirically with 5% natamycin suspension administered every hour while awake (287). Many clinicians also use a systemic antifungal agent (such as itraconazole) (144), although the benefits of this approach have not been proven. Anecdotal experience suggests that the advent of the azoles has not been paralleled by a decrease in the complications of *Aspergillus* keratitis (287). Indeed, reports of successful outcome with combined topical and systemic therapy in which the systemic agent was ineffective against *Aspergillus* (e.g., ketoconazole) (362) suggest that natamycin is the effective part of the combination rather than the azole. Topical suspensions of amphotericin (at a concentration of 0.15%) have been used successfully as an alternative to topical natamycin (144, 287). Although a topical suspension (1%) of itraconazole has been described, the drug has poor water solubility, and the suspension has not been successful in severe disease (246, 328). As adjunctive therapy, a therapeutic penetrating keratoplasty is sometimes performed for recurrent keratitis in the face of medical therapy (287).

Aspergillus endophthalmitis has a very poor prognosis because of delays in diagnosis and its frequent coexistence with disseminated disease. Only 10 patients have been reported who retained any meaningful sight in the affected eye (72, 92, 128, 135, 185, 191, 219, 286, 311, 340). All 10 were immunocompetent, and none had documented disease elsewhere (although 5 were intravenous drug abusers). A therapeutic vitrectomy performed in 9 of the 10, and 8 eight received intravitreal amphotericin. Although intravitreal injection of amphotericin B is said to be hazardous (17, 319), as much as 5 to 10 mg has been safely injected into the center of the vitreous cavity (127). Most authors have used much smaller doses intravitreally (0.005 mg) (72, 92, 128, 185, 191). Daily administration of subconjunctival amphotericin B (1–2 mg) can follow (286).

The question of concomitant systemic antifungal therapy is vexing. Three of the successfully treated patients received no systemic antifungal therapy or received an azole inactive against *Aspergillus* (72, 128, 135). However one patient was treated with systemic amphotericin alone without vitrectomy (311), and six other successfully treated patients received intravenous amphotericin B in addition to local therapy (92, 185, 191, 219, 286, 340). Three of these patients received amphotericin B for 7 days or fewer. Penetration of amphotericin into the eye is poor; after intravenous administration, levels of amphotericin B in the human aqueous humor remain below 0.5 μg/mL (277). Few data exist on penetration of lipid formulations of amphotericin B into the eye.

In contrast, flucytosine penetrates into the eye reasonably well (165, 277). Levels of 10 to 40 μg/mL were detected in the aqueous humor of patients receiving flucytosine in an oral dose of 200 mg/kg/day (165). Three successfully treated patients were reported who received orally administered flucytosine as an adjunct to local therapy (92, 219, 286). Rifampin in combination with another systemic antifungal agent is another option, since aqueous humor levels up to 1.3 μg/mL can be achieved after a single 600-mg oral dose (245). Yu et al. reported a patient with aggressive eye disease who was treated successfully with a combination of amphotericin, rifampin, and flucytosine (369).

One successfully treated patient received orally administered itraconazole in conjunction with local therapy (185). Itraconazole (80 mg orally) administered to rabbits with inflamed eyes reached levels of 0.92 μg/mL in the aqueous humor and 0.22 μg/mL in the vitreous (296). No data are available on penetration of voriconazole into the eye.

While early pars plana vitrectomy followed by intravitreal and periocular injection of amphotericin B is clearly the cornerstone of successful treatment of *Aspergillus* endophthalmitis, the role of systemic therapy in patients without other foci of disease is uncertain. On the basis of present data, orally administered flucytosine and possibly an active azole are options to consider.

Infections of Skin and Soft Tissue

Aspergillus may involve the skin and soft tissues in the following ways: cutaneous manifestations of systemic disseminated infection, primary cutaneous aspergillosis in the immunocompromised patient, postsurgical or posttraumatic wound infections, burn wound infections, otitis externa (nonin-

vasive), invasive external otitis, and primary cutaneous aspergillosis associated with central venous lines. *A. flavus* is more common than *A. fumigatus* in many of these manifestations (6, 146). *A. niger* may be associated with otitis externa (262). Occasionally, rare species such as *A. ustus* are involved in primary cutaneous infections associated with immunosuppression (322).

Patients with cutaneous manifestations of documented systemic infections have a poor prognosis despite active therapy (146, 192, 193). An exception may be patients with hematologic disorders in which neutropenia may be reversed (86). Successful treatment of primary cutaneous aspergillosis with neutropenia has been associated with reversal of neutropenia by use of G-CSF (146). Cutaneous manifestations may allow early diagnosis and prompt initiation of appropriate therapy (86). Amphotericin B is the preferred initial therapy.

Numerous reports have demonstrated that postsurgical or posttraumatic wound infection requires aggressive surgical intervention in addition to antifungal drugs for successful resolution (47, 118, 146, 297). The surgery may be as aggressive as limb amputation or extensive debridement of the sort used in necrotizing fasciitis (118, 146). Inadequate debridement has resulted in deep invasion into subcutaneous tissue, muscle, and sometimes deep viscera (102). Successful antifungal treatment has included amphotericin deoxycholate (47,297), liposomal amphotericin (71), and itraconazole (250). A number of authors have used local irrigation with amphotericin in addition to systemic antifungal agents (71, 250), although the usefulness of this approach has never been prospectively assessed.

Aspergillus may colonize burn wounds, but true infection is associated with approximately 50% mortality (196). Extensive radical surgery is needed (323) plus systemic antifungal therapy. Burn units with higher than expected numbers of cases of burn wound aspergillosis have routinely irrigated uninfected wounds with mafenide acetate plus nystatin suspension with partial success (196).

Although isolation of *Aspergillus* from an ear canal usually represents saprophytic colonization rather than infection, otitis externa can indeed occur. Thorough cleaning and debridement are the mainstay of management. Boric acid powder, clotrimazole powder or drops, nystatin ointment, or topical flucytosine have all been shown effective (237). Systemic antifungal agents are reserved for only the most refractory cases. Aggressive invasive external otitis is rarely seen but requires early aggressive surgical debridement and excision plus systemic antifungal agents (9, 86). Amphotericin B was used in five previously reported patients (66, 269). Infection recurred in two; one was retreated with amphotericin B (66), while the other was successfully treated with 3 months of itraconazole (269). An additional patient was treated with itraconazole (400 mg daily) alone for 6 months with mycologic cure, although the ear had to be surgically removed because of recurrent breakdown of the wound (66).

Cutaneous infection associated with longstanding central venous access devices (especially Hickman catheters) has been reported in neutropenic patients and patients with HIV infection and is sometimes associated with development of underlying pulmonary aspergillosis (6, 38, 159). Once *As-*

pergillus infection is suspected, the catheter should be removed (6). In the largest series reported, nine patients were treated with intravenous amphotericin (0.75–1.25 mg/kg/day) plus 5-flucytosine (3–8 g/day), and seven of the nine survived (6). The two patients who died did not recover from their neutropenia. These authors chose to defer wide debridement of the eschar until neutropenia had resolved (6). Others have performed immediate extensive chest wall debridement even while the patient was neutropenic (38).

Osteomyelitis

Aspergillus bone infection can be part of disseminated or local disease in immunocompromised patients (including transplant recipients, neutropenic patients, and children with chronic granulomatous disease), can be related to intravenous drug use, trauma, or surgery, or may occur by direct extension from the sinuses or ear. More than 70 cases of bone infection have been reported (7, 15, 22, 27, 37, 50, 64, 65, 68, 73, 86, 103, 123, 137, 145, 158, 177, 180, 181, 251, 266, 291, 318, 324, 326, 352). There appears to be an advantage of surgical therapy in the treatment of bony aspergillosis, with 84% of patients (36 of 43) responding to combined medical and surgical therapy compared with 69% (24 of 35) responding to medical therapy alone (7, 15, 22, 27, 37, 50, 64, 65, 68, 73, 86, 103, 123, 137, 145, 158, 177, 180, 181, 251, 266, 291, 318, 324, 326, 352, 363). One patient was reported to have been cured with surgical treatment only (352).

Surgery may be important because amphotericin B achieves only low concentrations in bone and joint fluid (86, 270). Furthermore, the pathology of aspergillosis involves infarction and necrosis, which results in poor drug delivery to tissues (86). Although not well studied, lipid preparations of amphotericin would not appear to enhance penetration of amphotericin greatly into bone. However, lipid preparations may have an advantage in that their comparative lack of nephrotoxicity allows longer courses to be given, which may be required for treatment of osteomyelitis. Both flucytosine and rifampin penetrate well into bone (107). Tissue concentrations of itraconazole in bone are two to three times those in plasma (150). Entry of voriconazole into bone has not yet been well studied.

More than 90% of reported patients with *Aspergillus* osteomyelitis have been treated with amphotericin deoxycholate. Reports of use of lipid preparations of amphotericin in treatment of *Aspergillus* osteomyelitis have been few (177). The combination of flucytosine with amphotericin was reported successful in 11 of 15 patients (73%), but data are insufficient to determine if this represents an advantage over amphotericin alone (86, 123, 158, 326). In view of the good penetration of flucytosine into bone, this agent would seem a logical addition to a regimen containing amphotericin. Itraconazole has been used successfully as monotherapy in a small number of patients (251, 266, 363), but its major role in successfully treated patients has been as oral follow-on therapy after a prolonged course of amphotericin B. Adjuncts to surgery and antifungal agents have included hyperbaric oxygen (181) and interferon-γ (145, 177, 251). Interferon-γ was only used in children with chronic granulomatous disease.

Infections of the Heart and Vascular System

Aspergillus has been reported to cause endocarditis, myocarditis, pericarditis, mediastinitis, septic thrombophlebitis, and infections of aortic grafts (3, 38, 252, 257, 258). Infection is associated with high mortality despite treatment. In addition, some cases are unsuspected during life and only discovered at autopsy (252, 257, 258). *Aspergillus* endocarditis may occur as part of disseminated disease, as a complication of cardiac surgery, or (rarely) de novo. Early surgical intervention with valve replacement is the cornerstone of successful management (86). Only one patient has been reported who received medical therapy alone and survived (208). Amphotericin B penetrates poorly into cardiac vegetations but nevertheless should probably be used as adjunctive therapy. There is no experience with use of lipid preparations of amphotericin B in the treatment of *Aspergillus* endocarditis. Similarly, there are no clinical data on use of rifampin or flucytosine in conjunction with amphotericin, although it is highly likely that their penetration into vegetations is relatively good.

Both pericarditis and myocarditis are almost always complications of widely disseminated disease. Three patients with pericarditis have been reported to have survived; one was treated with amphotericin B and two with itraconazole.

Septic thrombophlebitis due to *Aspergillus* has been reported in association with infection of longstanding central venous catheters (38). In this patient, histologic examination showed fungal invasion of the vein wall, so the thrombosed veins were resected, in addition to giving the patient amphotericin B in a total dose of 3 g (38).

Eight patients have been reported with *Aspergillus* infections of an aortic graft (six abdominal aortic, two thoracic) (3, 36, 97, 117, 140, 239). Underlying bone involvement was observed in about half of the patients reported (109, 110, 111, 113–115). The infected aortic grafts were excised from all patients with intraabdominal grafts; extraanatomic bypass rather than in situ replacement resulted in a more favorable outcome (3, 36, 117, 239). Both patients with thoracic graft infection had the blood flow rerouted through a clean field and survived (1, 97, 140). Administration of systemic antifungals seems adjunctive to removal of the infected prosthesis. Amphotericin B was used up to 6 weeks in those successfully treated with extraanatomic bypass (3). One patient who had received an interposed abdominal graft relapsed after a course of amphotericin B but improved after receiving an extraanatomic graft plus a prolonged course of itraconazole (3). One patient received flucytosine as monotherapy because renal intolerance precluded amphotericin B (239). His successful outcome appears more likely to be due to excision of the prosthesis and placement of an extraanatomic bypass.

ADJUNCTIVE THERAPY

Host defense against *Aspergillus* involves both macrophages and polymorphonuclear leukocytes (PMNs). Alveolar macrophages provide the first line of defense against airborne infection with *Aspergillus,* inhibiting germination of the conidia (90, 91, 186, 299). After *Aspergillus* germinates and the hyphae invade the pulmonary tissue, PMNs become the main effector cells involved by secreting microbicidal oxidative metabolites that damage the hyphae (90, 91, 186, 299). This illustrates why neutropenia is a risk factor for invasive aspergillosis. Corticosteroids suppress monocyte/macrophage function, including release of both oxidative and nonoxidative metabolites, which decreases damage to the hyphae (281). Transplant recipients are treated with both corticosteroids and either cyclosporine or tacrolimus; both agents inhibit interferon-γ (which is responsible for macrophage activation). Patients with HIV infection can develop invasive aspergillosis in the absence of neutropenia or corticosteroid administration; antifungal activity of PMNs has been shown to be defective in patients with low CD4 lymphocyte counts (282). Finally, patients with chronic granulomatous disease have impaired phagocyte microbicidal activity because of lack of respiratory burst oxidase activity.

Experimental and limited clinical evidence suggests that administration of G-CSF, GM-CSF, and/or interferon-γ may be useful as immunotherapy against Aspergillus infections. The most established indication for immunotherapy is in chronic granulomatous disease (CGD) (327). In a randomized controlled trial, patients with CGD were given either placebo or interferon-γ (50 μg/m² body surface area three times a week) as prophylaxis against infection; 4 of 65 placebo-treated patients developed Aspergillus pneumonia, compared with 1 of 63 given interferon-γ. Adverse effects from interferon-γ included fever, chills, headache, and erythema at the injection site. No serious or life-threatening toxic events occurred, however (327). Recent experimental studies suggest that higher doses of interferon-γ than those used in the randomized controlled trial may further enhance protection against A. fumigatus (4). A small number of clinical reports have described use of interferon-γ as an adjunct to antifungal therapy in children with Aspergillus osteomyelitis who were not previously given interferon-γ as prophylaxis (145, 177, 251).

Although there is considerably less experience with immunotherapy against Aspergillus outside of use in CGD, preliminary reports are encouraging. G-CSF has been shown to not just increase PMN number, but also enhance PMN oxidative burst, thereby enhancing PMN-mediated killing of Aspergillus by fourfold (198, 284). G-CSF also enhances antifungal activity of defective PMNs associated with HIV or corticosteroid use (282, 285). In mice with experimental aspergillosis, G-CSF in combination with antifungal agents enhanced killing (273). GM-CSF also enhances the antifungal activity of normal and dexamethasone-affected elutriated human monocytes (281, 283). Interferon-γ administration has a protective effect against invasive aspergillosis in mice (233). In vitro, the combination of interferon-γ and either G-CSF or GM-CSF may have an additive effect on antifungal activity of PMNs and macrophages, compared with use of either agent alone (283, 285).

Clinical studies in humans are ongoing on the use of G-CSF, GM-CSF, and/or interferon-γ in combination with antifungal agents in the treatment of invasive aspergillosis. At the time of writing, only anecdotal reports of success with interferon-γ and GM-CSF have appeared (31). Immunotherapy certainly appears to be a promising adjunct to traditional therapy of invasive aspergillosis. In addition to direct administration of these immunomodulators to the patient, future options may include transfusion of elutriated human monocytes stimulated by GM-CSF.

CONTROVERSIES AND CAVEATS

Given that the mortality of invasive aspergillosis approaches or exceeds 90% in groups such as bone marrow transplant or liver transplant recipients, there is considerable enthusiasm for strategies that can prevent invasive aspergillosis. Possible approaches include blanket prophylaxis for all transplant recipients or neutropenic patients, targeted prophylaxis in only those immunosuppressed patients with the highest risk, and preemptive treatment based surveillance serologic testing. None of these approaches has been proven effective, but few well-designed studies have been carried out. The available literature is reviewed below.

Fluconazole prophylaxis offers no protection against invasive aspergillosis (99, 121, 206, 315). Itraconazole, which is highly active against Aspergillus in vitro, would appear more suited for prophylaxis against Aspergillus infection. However, few studies have examined its use as prophylaxis. A prospective, randomized, double-blind study of itraconazole versus placebo as prophylaxis in neutropenic patients found no significant reduction in Aspergillus infections (350). Retrospective studies examining lung transplant, bone marrow transplant, and neutropenic patients given itraconazole compared with historical controls receiving no prophylaxis or ketoconazole have shown a reduction in cases of invasive aspergillosis in patients receiving itraconazole (232, 334, 336). However, there are major limitations in accepting data regarding aspergillosis from studies using historical controls. In each of the above-mentioned studies, the incidence of invasive aspergillosis in historical controls was far higher than expected. Aspergillus infections, although usually endemic, may occur in clusters (e.g., related to construction activity); itraconazole prophylaxis may have been introduced after confounding environmental exposure had been reduced in response to an outbreak.

Itraconazole capsules may be suboptmally absorbed in neutropenic patients and liver transplant recipients. The enhanced absorption of itraconazole solubilized in cyclodextrin (itraconazole oral solution) may represent an advance in prophylaxis in high-risk transplant recipients. A large, double-blind, multicenter study evaluating itraconazole oral solution as prophylaxis against invasive aspergillosis was conducted in Europe, but results have not yet been released.

Low-dose intravenous amphotericin deoxycholate (0.1 mg/kg/day) or intravenous amphotericin B liposome (1 mg/kg/day) was evaluated against placebo in four randomized controlled trials in either bone marrow transplant or liver transplant recipients (265, 278, 330–332). None of the studies showed any reduction in Aspergillus infections, but sample sizes were small, control groups had very low rates of invasive aspergillosis, and prophylaxis was given for a limited duration. Numerous anecdotal reports of breakthrough invasive aspergillosis occurring while the patient was on low-dose intravenous amphotericin (197, 240, 288, 308, 312, 361) suggest that at best, this form of prophylaxis is only partially effective.

Since inhalation of airborne conidia with deposition into the lungs is the initial step in the pathogenesis of invasive aspergillosis, several investigators have used inhaled amphotericin (via a nebulizer or nasal spray) as prophylaxis against *Aspergillus* infection. Nebulized amphotericin lacks the systemic toxicity of the intravenous preparation (although it can be associated with bronchospasm). A randomized controlled trial using aerosolized amphotericin for the duration of neutropenia in patients with hematologic malignancies failed to show any reduction in invasive aspergillosis in the treatment arm, compared with placebo (23). However, a number of retrospective analyses comparing bone marrow, heart, and lung transplant recipients given prophylaxis with nebulized amphotericin with historical untreated controls showed a significant reduction in cases of invasive aspergillosis in those given nebulized amphotericin (63, 129, 162, 197, 276, 329, 335). The caveats given above for analysis of studies of prophylaxis against invasive aspergillosis using historical controls apply to these studies too.

Some groups have used inhaled amphotericin plus systemic itraconazole or amphotericin to maximize protection against *Aspergillus* (329, 335). Since the efficacy of prophylaxis against *Aspergillus* has not been established, blanket prophylaxis of all immunosuppressed patients may not be justified. One alternative approach is to offer prophylaxis only to immunosuppressed patients at extraordinarily high risk of developing invasive aspergillosis. Such patients could include allogeneic bone marrow transplant recipients receiving corticosteroids for severe graft-versus-host disease, bone marrow transplant recipients with delayed engraftment, or other patients with prolonged neutropenia, single-lung transplant recipients, and solid organ transplant with poor graft function (particularly those in receipt of OKT3), renal failure requiring hemodialysis, and those with cytomegalovirus infection.

REFERENCES

1. Abruzzo GK, Flattery AM, Gill CJ, Kong L, Smith JG, Krupa D, Pikounis VB, Kropp H, Bartizal K. Evaluation of water-soluble pneumocandin analogs L-733560, L-705589, and L-731373, with mouse models of disseminated aspergillosis, candidiasis, and cryptococcosis. Antimicrob Agents Chemother 1995;39:1077–1081.
2. Abruzzo GK, Flattery AM, Gill CJ, et al. Evaluation of water soluble pneumocandin L-743,872 in mouse models of disseminated aspergillosis, candidiasis, and cryptococcosis [Abstract #F37]. In: Program and Abstracts of 36th Interscience Conference on Antimicrobial Agents and Chemotherapy, New Orleans, 1996.
3. Aguado JM, Valle R, Arjona R, Ferreres JC, Gutierrez JA. Aortic bypass graft infection due to *Aspergillus*: report of a case and review. Clin Infect Dis 1992;14:916–921.
4. Ahlin A, Elinder G, Palmblad J. Dose-dependent enhancements by interferon-gamma on functional responses of neutrophils from chronic granulomatous disease patients. Blood 1997;89:339–401.
5. Allendoerfer R, Loebenberg D, Rinaldi MG, Graybill JR. Evaluation of SCH51048 in an experimental model of pulmonary aspergillosis. Antimicrob Agents Chemother 1995;39:1345–1348.
6. Allo MD, Miller J, Townsend T, Tan C. Primary cutaneous aspergillosis associated with Hickman intravenous catheters. N Engl J Med 1987;317:1105–1108.
7. Alvarez L, Calvo E, Abril C. Articular aspergillosis: case report. Clin Infect Dis 1995;20:457–460.
8. Ammons WS, Aardalen K, Froebel S, et al. Efficacy of a domain III-derived peptide from bactericidal/permeability-increasing protein (BPI) in murine disseminated aspergillosis [Abstract #B-16]. In: Program and Abstracts of 36th Interscience Conference on Antimicrobial Agents and Chemotherapy, Toronto, 1997.
9. Anderson LL, Giandoni MB, Keller RA, Grabski WJ. Surgical wound healing complicated by *Aspergillus* infection in a nonimmunocompromised host. Dermatol Surg 1995;21:799–801.
10. Annaissie EJ, White M, Uzun O. Amphotericin B lipid complex (ABLC) versus amphotericin B (AMB) for treatment of hematogenous and invasive candidiasis: a prospective, randomized, multicenter trial [Abstract # LM-21]. In: Program and abstracts of the 35th Interscience Conference on Antimicrobial Agents and Chemotherapy, San Francisco, 1995.
11. Anonymous. Intraconazole oral solution product information. Janssen Pharmaceuticals, Titusville, NJ, 1997.
12. Arnow PM, Anderson RL, Mainous PD, Smith EJ. Pulmonary aspergillosis during hospital renovation. Am Rev Respir Dis 1978;118:49–53.
13. Arrese JE, Delvenne P, Van Cutsem J, Pierard-Franchimont C, Pierard GE. Experimental aspergillosis in guinea pigs: influence of itraconazole on fungaemia and invasive fungal growth. Mycoses 1994;37:117–122.
14. Arroyo J, Medoff G, Kobayashi GS. Therapy of murine aspergillosis with amphotericin B in combination with rinfampin or 5 fluorocystine. Antimicrobial Agents Chemother 1977;11:21–25.
15. Assaad W, Nuchikat PS, Cohen L, Esguerra JV, Whittier FC. Aspergillus discitis with acute disc abscess. Spine 1994;19:2226–2229.
16. Avet-Loiseau H, Mechinaud-Lacroix F, Cohen JY, Harousseau JL. Probable disseminated cerebral aspergillosis: recovery with medical treatment. Nouv Rev Fr Hematol 1994;36:419–422.
17. Axelrod AJ, Peyman GA, Apple DJ. Toxicity of intravitreal injection of amphotericin B. Am J Ophthalmol 1973;76:578–583.
18. Baker-Woudenberg IAJM, Roerdink FH. Antimicrobial chemotherapy directed by liposomes. J Antimicrob Chemother 1986;17:547–552.
19. Balfour JA, Faulds D. Terbinafine. A review of its pharmacodynamic and pharmacokinetic properties and therapeutic potential in superficial mycoses. Drugs 1992;43:259–284.
20. Barnes M, Burdou J, Harris A. Itraconazole for pulmonary mycetone. Med J Aust 1991:154–160.
21. Bartizal K, Smith JG, Gill CJ, et al. Preclinical efficacy of MK-0991 in pancytopenic mouse models of disseminated candidiasis and aspergillosis [Abstract #F-80]. In: Program and Abstracts of 37th Interscience Conference on Antimicrobial Agents and Chemotherapy, Toronto, 1997.
22. Barzaghi N, Emmi V, Mencherini S, Minzioni G, Marone P, Minoli L. Sternal osteomyelitis due to *Aspergillus fumigatus* after cardiac surgery. Chest 1994;104:1275–1277.
23. Behre GF, Schwartz S, Lenz K, Ludwig WD, Schilling E, Heinemann V, Link H, Boenisch O, Treder W, Siegert W. Aerosol amphotericin B inhalations for prevention of invasive

pulmonary aspergillosis in neutropenic cancer patients. Ann Hematol 1995; 71:287–291.

24. Berlinger NT, Freeman TJ. Acute airway obstruction due to necrotizing tracheobronchial aspergillosis in immunocompromised patients: a new clinical entity. Ann Otol Rhinol Laryngol 1989;98:718–720.

25. Bertocchi M, Thevenet F, Bastien O, Rabodonirina M, Gamonodes JP, Paulus S, Loire R, Piens MA, Celard M, Mornex JF. Fungal infections in lung transplant recipients. Transplant Proc 1995;27:1695.

26. Beyer J, Barzen G, Risse G, Weyer C, Miksits K, Dullenkopf K, Huhn D, Siegert W. Aerosol amphotericin B for prevention of invasive pulmonary aspergillosis. Antimicrob Agents Chemother 1993;37:1367–1369.

27. Bianchi R, Chekikian G, Ciboddo G, Ciceri F, Sbriscia FE, Ruglari C. Primary sternal osteomyelitis by *Aspergillus fumigatus*. Br J Rheumatol 1994;33:994–995.

28. Biggs V, Dummer S, Holsinger FC, Loyd JE, Christman BW, First WH. Successful treatment of invasive bronchial aspergillosis after single-lung transplantation. Clin Infect Dis 1994;18:123–124.

29. Bindschadler DD, Bennett JE. A pharmacologic guide to the clinical use of amphotericin B. J Infect Dis 1969;120:427.

30. Block ER, Bennett JE, Livoti LG. Flucytosine and amphotericin B: hemodialysis effects on the plasma concentration and clearance. Ann Intern Med 1974;80:613.

31. Boots RJ, Paterson DL, Allworth AM, Faoagali JL. Successful treatment of post influenza pseudomembranous necrotising bronchial aspergillosis with liposomal amphotericin, inhaled amphotericin B, gamma interferon and GM-CSF. Thorax 1998, in press.

32. Boriani G, Mirri A, Iacobitti P, Magnani G, Ferretti RM, Gamba A, Mamprin F, Fiocchi R, Ferrazzi P, Binetti G. Cerebral and renal aspergillosis in a patient with orthotopic heart transplant: diagnosis treatment and follow-up. Cardiologia 1989;34:807–811.

33. Bowden RA, Cays M, Gooley T, Mamelok RD, van Burik J. Phase I study of amphotericin B colloidal dispersion for the treatment of invasive fungal infections after marrow transplant. J Infect Dis 1996;173:1208–1215.

34. Bradley SF, McGuire NM, Kauffman CA. Sino-orbital and cerebral aspergillosis: cure with medical therapy. Mykosen 1987;30: 418.

35. Branch RA. Prevention of amphotericin B induced renal impairment. Arch Intern Med 1988;148:2389–2394.

36. Brandt SJ, Thompson RL, Wenzel RP. Mycotic pseudoaneurysm of an aortic bypass graft and contiguous vertebral osteomyelitis due to *Aspergillus fumigatus*. Am J Med 1985;79: 259–262.

37. Bridwell KH, Campbell JW, Barenkamp SJ. Surgical treatment of hematogenous vertebral *Aspergillus* osteomyelitis. Spine 1990;15:281–285.

38. Buescher TM, Moritz DM, Killyon GW. Endobronchial lesions in HIV-infected individuals. Chest 1994;105:1314–1323.

39. Burch PA, Karp JE, Merz WG, Kuhlman JE, Fishman EK. Favorable outcome of invasive aspergillosis in patients with acute leukemia. J Clin Oncol 1987;5:1985–1993.

40. Burton JR, Zachery JB, Bessin R, Rathbun HK. Aspergillosis in four renal transplant recipients. Diagnosis and effective treatment with amphotericin B. Ann Intern Med 1972;77:383–388.

41. Cacciapuoti A, Loebenberg D, Frank D, Moss EL Jr, Mezel F Jr, Michalski M, Norris C, Yaremko B, Hare RS, Miller GH.

Effect of delayed or extended treatment with SCH 56592 or concomitant treatment with amphotericin B, in murine models of pulmonary aspergillosis and systemic candidiasis [Abstract #F-96]. In: Program and Abstracts of 36th Interscience Conference on Antimicrobial Agents and Chemotherapy, New Orleans, 1996.

42. Cacciapuoti A, Loebenberg D, Parmegiani R, Antonacci B, Norris C, Moss EL, Menzel F, Yarosh-Tomaine T, Hare RS, Miller GH. Comparison of SCH 39304, Fluconazole, and Ketoconazole for treatment of systemic infections in mice. Antimicrob Agents Chemother 1992;36:64–67.

43. Caillot D, Reny C, Solary E, Casasnovas O, Chavanet P, Bonnotte B, Perello L, Dumas M, Entezam F, Guy H. A controlled trial of the tolerance of amphotericin B infused in dextrose or in Intralipid in patients with haematogical malignancies. J Antimicrob Chemother 1994;33:603–613.

44. Calliot D, Casasnovas O, Bernard A, Couaillier JF, Durand C, Cuisenier B, Solary E, Piard F, Petrella T, Bonnin A. Improved management of invasive pulmonary aspergillosis in neutropenic patients using early thoracic computed tomographic scan and surgery. J Clin Oncol 1997;15:139–147.

45. Camarata PJ, Dunn DL, Farney AC, Parker RG, Seljeskog EL. Continual intracavitary administration of amphotericin B as an adjunct in the treatment of *Aspergillus* brain abscess:case report and review of the literature. Neurosurgery 1992;31: 575–579.

46. Campbell JH, Winter JH, Richardson MD, Shankland GS, Banham SW. Treatment of pulmonary aspergilloma with itraconazole. Thorax 1991;46:839–841.

47. Carlson GL, Mughal MM, Birch M, Denning DW. *Aspergillus* wound infection following laparostomy. J Infect 1996;33: 119–121.

48. Carnevale NT, Galgiani JN, Stevens DA. Amphotericin B-induced myelopathy. Arch Intern Med 1980;140:1189–1192.

49. Carrizosa J, Kohn C, Levison ME. Experimental *Aspergillus* endocarditis in rabbits. J Lab Clin Med 1975;86:746–753.

50. Cartoni C, Capua A, Damico C, Potente G. *Aspergillus* osteomyelitis of the rib: sonographic diagnosis. J Clin Ultrasound 1992;20:217–220.

51. Casey T, Wilkins P, Uttley D. Aspergillosis infection in neurosurgical practice. Br J Neurosurg 1994;8:31–39.

52. Castelli C, Benazzo F, Minoli L, Marone P, Seghezzi R, Nacari-Carlizzi C. *Aspergillus* infection of the L3-L4 disc space in an immunosuppressed heart transplant patient. Spine 1990;15: 1369–1373.

53. Chavanet P, Caillot D. Lipid-based formulations of amphotericin B. J Antimicrob Chemother 1995;35:711–713.

54. Chen JC, Chang YL, Luh SP, Lee JM, Lee YC. Surgical treatment for pulmonary aspergilloma—a 28 year experience. Thorax 1997;52:810–813.

55. Chin N, Weitzman I, Della-Latta P. In vitro antifungal activity of voriconazole alone and in combination with flucytosine against *Candida* species and other pathogenic fungi [Abstract E-84]. In: Program and Abstracts of 37th Interscience Conference on Antimicrobial Agents and Chemotherapy, Toronto, 1997.

56. Cicogna CE, White MH, Bernard EM, Ishimura T, Sun M, Tong WP, Armstrong D. Efficacy of prophylactic aerosol amphotericin B lipid complex in a rat model of pulmonary aspergillosis. Antimicrob Agents Chemother 1997;41:259–261.

57. Cicogna CE, White MH, Bernard EM, Ishimura T, Sun M, Tong WP, Armstrong D. Efficacy of prophylactic aerosol am-

photericin B lipid complex in a rat model of pulmonary aspergillosis. Antimicrob Agents Chemother 1997;41:259–261.

58. Clancy CJ, Yu YC, Lewin A, Nguyen MH. Inhibition of RNA synthesis as a therapeutic strategy against *Aspergillus* and *Fusarium:* demonstration of in vitro synergy between rifabutin and amphotericin B [Abstract E-80]. In: Program and Abstracts of 37th Interscience Conference on Antimicrobial Agents and Chemotherapy, Toronto, 1997.

59. Clancy CJ, Yu YC, Nguyen MH. Comparison of in vitro activity of voriconazole and amphotericin B against filamentous fungi [Abstract E-89]. In: Program and Abstracts of 37th Interscience Conference on Antimicrobial Agents and Chemotherapy, Toronto, 1997.

60. Clark JM, Whitney RR, Olsen SJ, George RJ, Swerdel MR, Kunselman L, Bonner DP. Amphotericin B lipid complex therapy of experimental fungal infections in mice. Antimicrob Agent Chemother 1991;35:615–621.

61. Coleman JM, Hogg GG, Rosenfeld JV, Waters KD. Invasive central nervous system aspergillosis: cure with liposomal amphotericin B, Itraconazole, and radical surgery—case report and review of the literature. Neurosurgery 1995;36:858–863.

62. Collins LA, Samore MA, Roberts MS, Karchmer A. Risk factors for invasive fungal infections complicating orthotopic liver transplantation. J Infect Dis 1994;170:644–652.

63. Conneally E, Cafferkey MT, Daly PA, Keane CT, McCann SR. Nebulized amphotericin B as prophylaxis against invasive aspergillosis in granulocytopenic patients. Bone Marrow Transplant 1990;5:403–406.

64. Cortet B, Richard R, Deprez X, Lucet L, Flipo RM, LeLoet X, Duquesnoy B, Delcamre B. *Aspergillus* spondylodiscitis: successful conservative treatment in 9 cases. J Rheumotol 1994;21:1287–1291.

65. Cosgarea AJ, Tejani N, Jones NA. Carpal *Aspergillus* osteomyelitis: case report and review of the literature. J Hand Surg 1993;18:722–726.

66. Cunningham M, Yu VL, Turner J, Curtin H. Necrotizing otitis externa due to *Aspergillus* in an immunocompetent patient. Arch Otolaryngol Head Neck Surg 1988;114:554–556.

67. Curi G, Cava FD, Vitalo L. Distribution of rifamycin AMP in blood and cerebrospinal fluid. Minerva Med 1997;60:2399.

68. D'Hoore K, Hoogmartins M. Vertebral aspergillosis. A case report and reivew of the literature. Acta Orthop Belg 1993;59:306–314.

69. Dalconte I, Riva G, Obert R, Lucchini A, Bechis G, Derosa G, Gioannini P. Tracheobronchial aspergillosis in a patient with AIDS treated with aerosolized amphotericin B combined with itraconazole. Mycoses 1996;39:371–374.

70. Danehsmend TK, Warnock DW. Clinical pharmacokinetics of systemic antifungal drugs. Clin Pharmacokinet 1983;8:17.

71. Darrasjoly C, Veber B, Bedos JP, Gachot B, Reginier B, Wolff M. Nosocomial cerebral aspergillosis—a report of 3 cases. Scand J Infect Dis 1996;28:317–319.

72. Das T, Vyas P, Sharma S. *Aspergillus terreus* postoperative endophthalmitis. Br J Ophthalmol 1993;77:386–387.

73. De Vuyst D, Surmont I, Verhaegen J, Vanhaecke J. Tibial osteomyelitis due to *Aspergillus flavus* in a heart transplant patient. Infection 1992;20:48–49.

74. deGans J, Portegies P, Tiessens G. Itraconazole compared with amphotericin B plus flucytosine in AIDS patients with cryptococcal meningitis. AIDS 1992;6:185.

75. Denning D, del Favero A, Gluckman E. UK-109,496, a novel, wide-spectrum triazole derivative for the treatment of fungal infections: clinical efficacy in acute invasive aspergillosis. [Abstract #F-80]. In: Program and Abstracts of 35th Interscience Conference on Antimicrobial Agents and Chemotherapy, San Francisco, 1995.

76. Denning DW. Therapeutic outcome in invasive aspergillosis. Clin Infect Dis 1996;23:608–615.

77. Denning DW, Follansbee SE, Scolaro M, Norris S, Edelstein H, Stevens DA. Pulmonary aspergillosis in the acquired immunodeficiency syndrome. N Engl J Med 1991;324:654–662.

78. Denning DW, Hall L, Jackson M, Hollis S. Efficacy of D0870 compared with those of itraconazole and amphotericin B in two murine models of invasive aspergillosis. Antimicrob Agents Chemother 1995;39:1809–1814.

79. Denning DW, Hanson LH, Perlman AM, Stevens DA. In vitro susceptibility and synergy studies of *Aspergillus* species to conventional and new agents. Diagn Microbiol Infect Dis 1992;15:21–34.

80. Denning DW, Lee JY, Hostetler J, Pappas P, Kauffman CA, Dewsnup DH, Galgiani JN. NIAID Mycoses Study Group multicenter trial of oral itraconazole therapy for invasive aspergillosis. Am J Med 1994;97:135–144.

81. Denning DW, Stepan DE, Blume KG, Stevens DA. Control of invasive pulmonary aspergillosis with oral itraconazole in a bone marrow transplant patient. J Infect 1992;24:73–79.

82. Denning DW, Stevens DA. Antifungal and surgical treatment of invasive aspergillosis: review of 2121 published cases. Rev Infect Dis 1990;12:1147–1201.

83. Denning DW, Stevens DA. Efficacy of cilofungin alone and in combination with amphotericin B in a murine model of disseminated aspergillosis. Antimicrob Agents Chemother 1991;35:1329–1333.

84. Denning DW, Tucker RM, Hanson LH, Hamilton JR, Stevens DA. Itraconazole therapy for cryptococcal meningitis and cryptococcosis. Arch Intern Med 1989;149:2301–2308.

85. Denning DW, Tucker RM, Hanson LH, Stevens DA. Treatment of invasive aspergillosis with itraconazole. Am J Med 1989;86:791–800.

86. Denning DW, Tucker RM, Hanson LH, Stevens DA. Itraconazole in opportunistic mycoses: cryptococcosis and aspergillosis. J Am Acad Dermatol 1990;23:602–607.

87. Denning DW, Van Wye JE, Lewiston NJ, Stevens DA. Adjunctive therapy of allergic bronchopulmonary aspergillosis with itraconazole. Chest 1991;100:813–819.

88. Denning DW, Venkateswaru K, Oakley KL, Anderson MJ, Manning NJ, Stevens DA, Warnock DW, Kelly SL. Itraconazole resistance in *Aspergillus fumigatus*. Antimicrob Agents Chemother 1997;41:1364–1368.

89. Deshazo RD, Chapin K, Swain RE. Fungal sinusitis. N Engl J Med 1997;337:254–259.

90. Diamond RD, Huber E, Haudenschild CC. Mechanisms of destruction of *Aspergillus fumigatus* hyphae mediated by human monocytes. J Infect Dis 1983;147:474–483.

91. Diamond RD, Krzesicki R, Epstein R, Jao W. Damage to hyphal forms of fungi by human leukocytes in vitro: a possible host defense mechanism in aspergillosis and mucormycosis. Am J Clin Pathol 1978;91:313–328.

92. Doft BH, Clarkson JG, Rebell G. Endogenous *Aspergillus* endophthalmitis in drug abusers. Arch Ophthalmol 1980;98:859.

93. Drakos PE, Nagler A, Or R, Naparstek E, Kapelushnik J, Engelhard D, Rahav G, Ne'emean D, Slavin S. Invasive fungal sinusitis in patients undergoing bone marrow transplantation. Bone Marrow Transplant 1993;12:203–208.

94. DuBois J, Bartter T, Gryn J, Pratter MR. The physiologic effects of inhaled amphotericin B. Chest 1995;108:599.

95. Dupont B, Denning D, Lode H, et al. UK-109,496. A novel, wide-spectrum Triazole derivative for the treatment of fungal infections: clinical efficacy in chronic invasive aspergillosis [Abstract #F-81]. In: Program and Abstracts of 35th Interscience Conference on Antimicrobial Agents and Chemotherapy, San Francisco, 1995.

96. Dupont B, Improvisi L, Dromer F. In vitro and in vivo activity of a new antifungal agent SCH56592 [Abstract #F-93]. In: Program and Abstracts of 36th Interscience Conference on Antimicrobial Agents and Chemotherapy, New Orleans, 1996.

97. Echenne B, Brunel D, Astruc J, Perez C. Aspergillose disseminee chez un enfant porteur d'une prosthese aortique. Efficacite du ketoconazole. Med Mal Infect 1980;10:263–266.

98. Ellis M, Meunier SF, Bogaerts M. Randomised multicentre trial of 1 mg/kg versus 4 mg/kg liposomal amphotericin B (AmBisome) in the treatment of invasive aspergillosis [Abstract #LM-39]. In: Program and Abstracts of 36th Interscience Conference on Antimicrobial Agents and Chemotherapy, New Orleans, 1996.

99. Ellis ME, Clink H, Halim MA, Padmos A, Spence D, Kalin M, Hussain QM, Burnie J, Greer W. Controlled study of fluconazole in the prevention of fungal infections in neutropenic patients with haematological malignancies and bone marrow transplant recipients. Eur J Clin Microbiol Infect Dis 1994;13:3–11.

100. Eloakley R, Petrou M, Goldstraw P. Indications and outcome of surgery for pulmonary aspergilloma. Thorax 1997;52:813–815.

101. Epstein NE, Hollingsworth R, Black K, Farmer P. Fungal brain abscesses (aspergillosis/mucormycosis) in two immunosuppressed patients. Surg Neurol 1991;35:286–289.

102. Falsey AR, Goldsticker RD, Ahern MJ. Fatal subcutaneous aspergillosis following necrotizing fasciitis: a case report. Yale J Biol Med 1990;63:9–13.

103. Faure BT, Biondi JX, Flanagan JP, Clarke R. Aspergillar osteomyelitis of the acetabulum. A case report and review of the literature. Orthop Rev 1990;19:58–64.

104. Feely M, Steinberg M. *Aspergillus* infection complicating transphenoidal yttrium-90 pituitary implant. Report of two cases. J Neurosurg 1977;46:530–532.

105. Feldman HA, Hamilton JD, Gutman RA. Amphotericin B therapy in an anephric patient. Antimicrob Agents Chemother 1973;4:302.

106. Francis P, Lee JW, Hoffman A, Peter J, Francesconi A, Bacher J, Shelhamer J, Pizzo PA, Walsh TJ. Efficacy of unilamellar liposomal amphotericin B in treatment of pulmonary aspergillosis in persistently granulocytopenic rabbits: the potential role of bronchoalveolar D-mannitol and serum galactomannan as markers of infection. J Infect Dis 1994;169:356–368.

107. Francis P, Walsh TJ. Evolving role of flucytosine in immunocompromised patients: new insights into safety, pharmacokinetics, and antifungal therapy. Clin Infect Dis 1992;15:1003–1018.

108. Fu YS, Liao WM, Yi ZC, Zhou RX, Sun WG. *Aspergillus* brain abscess. Report of two cases. J West China Univ Med Sci 1988;19:213–216.

109. Fung-Tomc JC, Huczko E, Minassian B, Bonner DP. In vitro activity of a new oral triazole, BMS-207147. Antimicrob Agents Chemother 1998;42:313–318.

110. Gavalda J, Roman A, Bravo C. Liposomal amphotericin B therapy for aspergillosis in lung transplant recipients [Abstract #K-57]. In: Program and Abstracts of 36th Interscience Conference on Antimicrobial Agents and Chemotherapy, New Orleans, 1996.

111. Gavalda J, Roman A, Bravo C. Efficacy of nebulized amphotericin B for prevention of *Aspergillus* infection in lung transplantation [Abstract #LM-54]. In: Program and Abstracts of 37th Interscience Conference on Antimicrobial Agents and Chemotherapy, Toronto, 1997.

112. Gelpi J, Chernoff A, Snydman D, Freeman RB, Rohrer RJ, Haug CE. *Aspergillus* brain abscess after liver transplantation with long-term survival. A case report. Transplantation 1994;57:1669–1672.

113. George D, Kordick D, Miniter P, Patterson TF, Andriole VT. Combination therapy in experimental invasive aspergillosis. J Infect Dis 1993;168:692–698.

114. George D, Miniter P, Andriole VT. Efficacy of UK-109496, a new azole antifungal agent in an experimental model of invasive aspergillosis. Antimicrob Agents Chemother 1996;40:86–91.

115. Gerkens JF, Branch RA. The influence of sodium status and furosemide on canine acute amphotericin B toxicity. J Pharmacol Exp Ther 1980;214:306–311.

116. Giron J, Poey C, Fajadet P, Sans N, Fourcade D, Senac JP, Railhac JJ, Dahan M, Berjaud J, Krempf M. Palliative percutaneous treatment of inoperable pulmonary aspergilloma. Rev Mal Respir 1995;12:593–599.

117. Glotzbach RE. *Aspergillus terreus* infection of pseudoaneurysm of aortofemoral vascular graft with contiguous vertebral osteomyelitis. Am J Clin Pathol 1982;77:224–227.

118. Golladay ES, Baker SB. Invasive aspergillosis in children. J Pediatr Surg 1987;22:504–505.

119. Gonzalez CE, Giri N, Shetty D, Kligys K, Love W, Sein T, Schaufele R, Lyman C, Bacher J, Walsh TJ. Efficacy of a lipid formulation of nystatin against invasive pulmonary aspergillosis [Abstract #B54]. In: Program and Abstracts of 36th Interscience Conference on Antimicrobial Agents and Chemotherapy, New Orleans, 1996.

120. Gonzalez CE, Shetty D, Giri N. Efficacy of Pradimicin against invasive pulmonary aspergillosis [Abstract #F-182]. In: Program and Abstracts of 36th Interscience Conference on Antimicrobial Agents and Chemotherapy, New Orleans, 1996.

121. Goodman JL, Winston DJ, Greenfield PH. A controlled trial of fluconazole to prevent fungal infections in patients undergoing bone marrow transplantation. N Engl J Med 1992;326:845–851.

122. Goodman ML, Coffey RJ. Stereotactic drainage of *Aspergillus* brain abscess with long-term survival: case report and review. Neurosurgery 1989;24:96–109.

123. Govender S, Rajoo R, Goga IE, Charles RW. *Aspergillus* osteomyelitis of the spine. Spine 1991;16:746–749.

124. Grant SM, Clissold SP. Itraconazole—a review of its pharmacodynamic and pharmacokinetic properties, and therapeutic use in superficial and systemic mycoses. Drugs 1989;37:310–344.

125. Graybill JR, Ahrens J. Itraconazole treatment of murine aspergillosis. J Med Vet Mycol 1985;23:219–223.

126. Green M, Wald ER, Tzakis A, Todo S, Starzl TE. Aspergillosis of the CNS in a pediatric liver transplant recipients: case report and review. Rev Infect Dis 1991;13:653–657.

127. Green WR, Font RI, Zimmerman LE. Aspergillosis of the orbit: report of ten cases and review of the literature. Arch Ophthalmol 1969;82:302–313.

128. Gross JG. Endogenous *Aspergillus*-induced endophthalmitis: successful treatment without systemic antifungal medication. Retina 1992;12:341–345.

129. Guillemain R, Lavarde V, Amrein C, Chevalier P, Guinvarch A, Glotz D. Invasive aspergillosis after transplantation. Transplant Proc 1995;27:1307–1309.

130. Guleria R, Gupta D, Jindal SK. Treatment of pulmonary aspergilloma by endoscopic intracavitary instillation of ketoconazole. Chest 1993;103:1301–1302.

131. Guleria R, Pande JN. Endoscopic instillation of fungicide to treat aspergilloma. Lancet 1996;348:621.

132. Gumaa SA, Mahgoub ES, Hay RB. Post-operative responses of paranasal *Aspergillus* granuloma to itraconazole. Trans R Soc Trop Med Hyg 1992;86:93–94.

133. Gupta R, Singh AK, Bishnu P, Mahotra V. Intracranial *Aspergillus* granuloma stimulating meningioma on MR imaging. J Comput Assist Tomogr 1990;14:467–469.

134. Habicht JM, Gratwohl A, Tamm M, Drewe J, Proske M, Stulz P. Diagnostic and therapeutic thoracic surgery in leukemia and severe aplastic anemia. J Thorac Cardiovasc Surg 1997;113:982–988.

135. Halperin LS, Roseman RL. Successful treatment of a subretinal abscess in an intravenous drug abuser. Arch Ophthalmol 1988;106:1651.

136. Hamamoto T, Watanabe K, Ikemoto M. Endobronchial miconazole for pulmonary aspergillosis. Ann Intern Med 1983;98:1030.

137. Hanna E, Hughes G, Eliachar I. Fungal osteomyelitis of the temporal bone: a review of reported cases. Ear Nose Throat J 1993;72:541.

138. Hanson LH, Clemons KV, Denning DW, Stevens DA. Efficacy of oral saperconazole in systemic murine aspergillosis. J Med Vet Mycol 1995;33:311–317.

139. Harari S, Schiraldi GF, De Juli E, Gronda E. Relapsing *Aspergillus* bronchitis in a double lung transplant patient, successfully treated with a new oral antimycotic agent. Chest 1997;111:835–836.

140. Hargrove WC III, Edmunds LH Jr. Management of infected thoracic aortic prosthetic grafts. Ann Thorac Surg 1984;37:72–77.

141. Hata K, Kimura J, Miki H, Toyosawa T, Moriyama M, Kimura S. Efficacy of ER-30346, a novel oral triazole antifungal agent, in experimental models of aspergillosis, candidiasis, and cryptococcosis. Antimicrob Agents Chemother 1996;40:2243–2247.

142. Hata K, Kimura J, Miki H, Toyosawa T, Nakamura T, Katsu K. In vitro and in vivo antifungal activities of ER-30346, a novel oral triazole with a broad antifungal spectrum. Antimicrob Agents Chemother 1996;40:2237–2242.

143. Hector RF, Yee E, Collins MS. Use of DBA/2N mice in models of systemic candidiasis and pulmonary and systemic aspergillosis. Infect Immun 1990;58:1476–1478.

144. Heidemann DG, Dunn SP, Watts JC. *Aspergillus* keratitis after radial keratotomy. Am J Ophthalmol 1995;120:254–256.

145. Heinrich SD, Finney T, Craver R, Yin L, Zembo MM. *Aspergillus* osteomyelitis in patients who have chronic granulomatous disease. Case report. J Bone Joint Surg 1991;73:456–460.

146. Heinz T, Perfect J, Schell W, Ritter E, Ruff G, Serafin D. Soft-tissue fungal infections: surgical management of 12 immunocompromised patients. Plastic Reconstruct Surg 1996;97:1301–1309.

147. Hennequin C, Benailly N, Silly C, Sorin M, Scheinmann P, Lenoir G, Gaillard JL, Berche P. In vitro susceptibilities to amphotericin B, itraconazole and miconazole of filamentous fungi isolated from patients with cystic fibrosis. Antimicrob Agents Chemother 1997;41:2064–2066.

148. Henze G, Alenhoff P, Stephani U, Grosse G, Kazner E, Staib F. Successful treatment of pulmonary and cerebral aspergillosis in an immunosuppressed child. Eur J Pediatr 1982;138:263–265.

149. Heussel CP, Kauczor HU, Heussel G, Fischer B, Mildenberger P, Thelen M. Early detection of pneumonia in febrile patients: use of thin-section CT. AJR 1997;169:1347–1353.

150. Heykants J, Van Peer A, Van de Velde V. The clinical pharmacokinetics of itraconazole: an overview. Mycoses 1989;32:67.

151. Hiemenez JW, Walsh TJ. Lipid formulations of amphotericin B: recent progress and future directions. Clin Infect Dis 1996;22:S133–144.

152. Hiemenz JW, Lister J, Anassie EJ. Emergency-use amphotericin B lipid complex (ABLC) in the treatment of patients with aspergillosis: historical control comparison with amphotericin B [Abstract no 3383]. Blood 1995;86:(Suppl 1)849a.

153. Hines DW, Haber MH, Yaremko L, Britton C, McLawhon RW, Harris AA. Pseudomembranous tracheobronchitis caused by *Aspergillus*. Am Rev Respir Dis 1991;143:1408–1411.

154. Hoeprich PD, Merry JM, Gunther R, Franti CE. Entry of five antifungal agents into the ovine lung. Antimicrob Agents Chemother 1987;31:1234.

155. Horvath J, Dummer S, Loyd J, Walker B, Merrill WH, Frist WH. Infection in the transplanted and native lung after single lung transplantation. Chest 1993;104:681–685.

156. Hostetler JS, Hanson LH, Stevens DA. Effect of cyclodextrin on the pharmacology of antifungal oral azoles. Antimicrob Agents Chemother 1992;33:1391–1392.

157. Hughes CE, Harris C, Moody JA, Peterson LR, Gerding DN. In vitro activities of amphotericin B in combination with four antifungal agents and rifampin against *Aspergillus* species. Antimicrob Agents Chemother 1984;25:560–562.

158. Hummel M, Schuler S, Weber J, Schwertlick G, Hempel S, Theiss D, Rees W, Mueller J, Hetzer R. Aspergillosis with *Aspergillus* osteomyelitis and diskitis after heart transplantation: surgical and medical management. J Heart Lung Transplant 1993;12:599–603.

159. Hunt SJ, Nagi C, Gross KG, Wong DS, Mathews WC. Primary cutaneous aspergillosis near central venous catheters in patients with the acquired immunodeficiency syndrome. Arch Dermatol 1992;128:1229–1232.

160. Jackson M, Flower CD, Shneerson JM. Treatment of symptomatic pulmonary aspergillomas with intracavitary instillation of amphotericin B through an indwelling catheter. Thorax 1993;48:928–930.

161. Janknegt R, deMarie S, Bakker-Woudenberg IA, Crommelin DJ. Liposomal and lipid formulations of amphotericin B: clinical pharmacokinetics. Clin Pharmacokinet 1992;23:279–291.

162. Jeffery GM, Beard MD, Ikram J, Chua J, Allen JR, Heaton DC, Hart DN, Schousboe MI. Intranasal amphotericin B reduces the frequency of invasive aspergillosis in neutropenic patients. Am J Med 1991;90:685–692.

163. Jezequel SG, Clark M, Evans K. UK-109,496, a novel, wide-spectrum triazole derivative for the treatment of fungal infections: disposition in animals [Abstract]. In: Program and Abstracts of 35th Interscience Conference on Antimicrobial Agents and Chemotherapy, San Francisco, 1995.

164. Joly V, Ndayiragide A. Randomized comparison of amphotericin B deoxycholate dissolved in dextrose or intralipid for the treatment of AIDS-associated cryptococcal meningitis. Clin Infect Dis 1996;23:556–562.

165. Jones BR, Clayton YM, Oji EO. Recognition and chemotherapy of oculomycosis. Postgrad Med 1979;55:525.

166. Judson MA, Sahn SA. Endobronchial lesions in HIV-infected individuals. Chest 1994;105:1314–1323.

167. Kanj SS, Tapson V, Davis D, Madden J, Browning I. Infections in patients with cystic fibrosis following lung transplantation. Chest 1997;112:924–930.

168. Kanj SS, Welty-Wolf K, Madden J, Tapson V, Baz MA, David RD, Perfect JR. Fungal infections in lung and heart-lung transplant recipients. Medicine 1996;75:142–156.

169. Kauffman CA. Quandary about treatment of aspergillomas persists. Lancet 1996;347:1640.

170. Kauffman CA, Carver PL. Antifungal agents in the 1990s. Drugs 1997;53:539–549.

171. Kay PH. Surgical management of pulmonary aspergilloma. Thorax 1997;52:753–754.

172. Kemper CA, Hostetler JS, Follansbee SE, Ruane P, Covington D, Leong SS. Ulcerative and plaque-like tracheobronchitis due to infection with Aspergillus in patients with AIDS. Clin Infect Dis 1993;17:344–352.

173. Kennedy MS, Deeg HJ, Siegel M, Crowley JJ, Storb R, Thomas ED. Acute renal toxicity with combined use of amphotericin B and cyclosporine after marrow transplantation. Transplantation 1983;35:211–215.

174. Khoo SH, Bond J, Denning DW. Administering amphotericin B—a practical approach. J Antimicrob Chemother 1994;33: 203–213.

175. Khoury H, Adkins D, Miller G, Goodnough L, Brown R, Dipersio J. Resolution of invasive central nervous system aspergillosis in a transplant recipient. Bone Marrow Transplant 1997;20: 179–180.

176. Kim DG, Hong SC, Kim HJ, Chi JG, Han MH, Choi KS, Han DH. Cerebral aspergillosis in immunologically competent patients. Surg Nephrol 1993;40:326–331.

177. Kline MW, Bocobo FC, Paul ME, Rosenblatt HM, Shearer WT. Successful medical therapy of Aspergillus osteomyelitis of the spine in an 11 year old boy with chronic granulomatous disease. Pediatrics 1994;93:830–835.

178. Kloss S, Schuster A, Schroten H, Lamprecht J, Wahn V. Control of proven pulmonary and suspected CNS Aspergillus infection with itraconazole in a patient with chronic granulomatous disease. Eur J Pediatr 1991;150:483–485.

179. Komadina TG, Wilkes TDI, Shock JP, Ulmer WC, Jackson J, Bradsher RW. Treatment of Aspergillus fumigatus keratitis in rabbits with oral and topical ketoconazole. Am J Ophthalmol 1985;99:476–479.

180. Korovessis P, Repanti M, Katsardis T, Stamatakis M. Anterior decompression and fusion for Aspergillus osteomyelitis of the lumbar spine associated with paraparesis. Spine 1994;19:15–18.

181. Kountakis SE, Kemper JV, Chang CH, DiMaio DJ, Stiernberg CM. Osteomyelitis of the base of the skull secondary to Aspergillus. Am J Otolaryngol 1997;18:19–22.

182. Kramer MR, Denning DW, Marshall SE, Ross DJ, Berry G, Lewiston NJ, Stevens DA, Theodore J. Ulcerative tracheobronchitis after lung transplantation. Am Rev Respir Dis 1991;144: 552–556.

183. Kramer MR, Marshall SE, Denning DW. Drug interactions between cyclosporin and itraconazole in heart-lung and lung transplant recipients with fungal disease. Ann Intern Med 1990;113:327–329.

184. Kreisel W, Kochling G, von Schilling C, Azemar M, Kurzweil B, Dolken G, Lindemann A, Blum U, Windfuhr M, Muller J. Therapy of invasive aspergillosis with itraconazole: improvement of therapeutic efficacy by early diagnosis. Mycoses 1991; 34:385–394.

185. Krzystolik MG, Ciulla TA, Topping TM, Baker S. Exogenous Aspergillus niger endophthalmitis in a patient with a filtering bleb. J Retinal Vitreous Dis 1997;17:461–462.

186. Kullberg BJ. Trends in immunotherapy of fungal infections. Eur J Clin Microbiol Infect Dis 1997;16:51–55.

187. Kurtz MB, Bernard EM, Edwards FF, Marrinan JA, Dropinski J, Douglas CM, Armstrong D. Aerosol and parenteral pneumocandins are effective in a rat model of pulmonary aspergillosis. Antimicrob Agents Chemother 1995;39:1784–1789.

188. Kusne S, Dummer JS, Singh N, Ho M. Infections after liver transplantation, an analysis of 101 consecutive cases. Medicine 1988;67:132–143.

189. Kwong YL, Yu VL, Chan FL, Lam KS, Woo E, Huang CY. High dose ketoconazole in the treatment of cerebral aspergilloma. Clin Neurol Neurosurg 1987;89:193–196.

190. Labadie EL, Hamilton RH. Survival improvement in coccidioidal meningitis by high-dose intrathecal amphotericin B. Arch Intern Med 1986;146:2013.

191. Lance SE, Friberg TR, Kowalski RP. Aspergillus flavus endophthalmitis and retinitis in an intravenous drug abuser: a therapeutic success. Ophthalmology 1988;95:947.

192. Le Conte P, Joly V, Saint-Julien L, Gillardin JM, Carbon C, Yeni P. Tissue distribution and antifungal effect of liposomal itraconazole in experimental cryptococcosis and pulmonary aspergillosis. Am Rev Respir Dis 1992;145:424–429.

193. LeConte P, Blanloeil Y, Michel P, Francois T, Paineau J. Cutaneous aspergillosis in a patient with orthotopic hepatic transplantation. Transplantation 1992;53:1153–1154.

194. Leenders ACAP, de Marie S, ten Kate MT, Bakker-Woudenberg IAJM, Verbrugh HA. Liposomal amphotericin B (AmBisome) reduces dissemination of infection as compared with amphotericin B deoxycholate (Fungizone) in a rat model of pulmonary aspergillosis. J Antimicrob Chemother 1996;38: 215–225.

195. Leenders ACAP, Reiss P, Portegies P, Clezy K, Hop WCJ, de Marie S. A randomized trial of liposomal-amphotericin B (AmBisome) 4 mg/kg vs amphotericin B 0.7 mg/kg for cryptococcal meningitis in HIV-infected patients [Abstract #LM-35]. In: Program and Abstracts of 36th Interscience Conference on Antimicrobial Agents and Chemotherapy, New Orleans, 1996.

196. Levenson C, Wohlford P, Djou J, Evans S, Zawacki B. Preventing postoperative burn wound aspergillosis. J Burn Care Rehabil 1991;12:132–135.

197. Levine MS, Shpiner RB, Waters PF, Kubak BM. Analysis of antifungal prophylaxis in lung transplantation. Am J Respir Crit Care Med 1995;151:A460.

198. Liles WC, Huang JE, van Burik JA, Bowden RA, Dale DC. Granulocyte colony-stimulating factor administered in vivo augments neutrophil-mediated activity against opportunistic fungal pathogens. J Infect Dis 1997;175:1012–1015.

199. Loakley KL, Verweij PE, Morrissey G. In vivo activity of GM237354 in a neutropenic murine model of aspergillosis [Abstract #F-61]. In: Program and Abstracts of 37th Interscience Conference on Antimicrobial Agents and Chemotherapy, Toronto, 1997.

200. Longman LP, Martin MV. A comparison of the efficacy of itraconazole, amphotericin B and 5-fluorocytosine in the treatment of Aspergillus fumigatus endocarditis in the rabbit. J Antimicrob Chemother 1987;20:719–724.

201. Lopez-Berestein G. Liposomal amphotericin B in the treatment of fungal infections. Ann Intern Med 1986;105:130–131.
202. Lopez-Berestein G, Body GP, Fainstein V, Keating M, Frankel B, Zeluff L, Gentry L, Mehta K. Treatment of systemic fungal infections with liposomal amphotericin B. Arch Intern Med 1989;149:2533–2536.
203. Lortholary O, Meyohas MC, Dupont B, Cadranel J, Salmon-Ceron D, Peyramond D, Simonin D. Invasive aspergillosis in patients with acquired immunodeficiency syndrome: report of 33 cases. French Cooperative Study Group on Aspergillosis in AIDS. Am J Med 1993;95:177–187.
204. Louria DB. Some aspects of the absorption, distribution, and excretion of amphotericin B in man. Antibiot Med Clin Ther 1958;5:295.
205. Lucantoni D, Galzio R, Zenobii M, Magliani V, Sciarra G, D'Arrigo C. Right occipital cerebral abscess caused by *Aspergillus fumigatus*. J Neurosurg Sci 1987;31:29–31.
206. Lumbrerase C, Cuervas-Mons V, Jara P, del Palacio A, Turrion VS, Barrios C, Moreno E, Noriega AR, Paya CV. Randomized trial of fluconazole versus nystatin for the prophylaxis of *Candida* infection following liver transplantation. J Infect Dis 1996;174:583–588.
207. Lupinetti FM, Behrendt DM, Giller RH, Trigg ME, deAlarcon P. Pulmonary resection for fungal infection in children undergoing bone marrow transplantation. J Thorac Cardiovasc Surg 1992;104:684–687.
208. Maderazo EG, Hickingbotham N, Cooper B, Murcia A. *Aspergillus* endocarditis: cure without surgical valve replacement. South Med J 1990;83:351–352.
209. Maesaki S, Kohno S, Kaku M, Koga H, Hara K. Effects of antifungal agent combinations administered simultaneously and sequentially against *Aspergillus fumigatus*. Antimicrob Agents Chemother 1994;38:2843–2845.
210. Mahlknecht U, Vonlintig F, Mertelsman R, Lindemann A, Lubbert M. Successful treatment of disseminated central nervous aspergillosis in a patient with acute myelobastic leukemia. Leuk Lymphoma 1997;27:191–194.
211. Mallory GG Jr. Major medical complications of lung transplantation: a pediatric perspective. Semin Thorac Cardiovasc Surg 1997;8:305–312.
212. Manavathu EK, Cutright JL, Chandrasekar PH. A comparative study of the in vitro susceptibility of amphotericin B-resistant isolates of *Aspergillus fumigatus* to voriconazole and itraconazole [Abstract #E-85]. In: Program and Abstracts of 37th Interscience Conference on Antimicrobial Agents and Chemotherapy, Toronto, 1997.
213. Manavathu EK, Cutright JL, Dimmock JR. In vitro and in vivo susceptibility of *Aspergillus fumigatus* to a new conjugated styryl ketone [Abstract #F-103]. In: Program and Abstracts of 37th Interscience Conference on Antimicrobial Agents and Chemotherapy, Toronto, 1997.
214. Martin MV, Yates J, Hitchcock CA. Comparison of voriconazole (UK-109,496) and itraconazole in prevention and treatment of *Aspergillus fumigatus* endocarditis in guinea pigs. Antimicrob Agents Chemother 1997;41:13–16.
215. Massard G, Lioure B, Wihlm JM, Morand G. Resection of mycotic lung sequestra after invasive aspergillosis. Ann Thorac Surg 1993;55:563–564.
216. Massard G, Roeslin N, Wihlm JM, Dumont P, Witz JP, Morand G. Surgical treatment of pulmonary and bronchial aspergilloma. Ann Chir 1993;47:141–151.
217. Mehta J, Kelsey S, Chu P, Powles R, Hazel D, Riley U, Evans C, Newland A, Treleaven J, Singhal S. Amphotericin B lipid complex (ABLC) for the treatment of confirmed or presumed fungal infections in immunocompromised patients with hematologic malignancies. Bone Marrow Transplant 1997;20: 39–43.
218. Mehta RT, Hopfer RL, McQueen T, Juliano RL, Lopez-Berestein G. Toxicity and therapeutic effects in mice of liposome-encapsulated nystatin for systemic fungal infections. Antimicrob Agents Chemother 1987;31:1901–1903.
219. Michelson JB, Freedman SD, Boyden DG. *Aspergillus* endophthalmitis in a drug abuser. Ann Ophthalmol 1982;14:1051.
220. Mikolich DJ, Kinsella LJ, Skowron G, Friedman J, Sugar AM. *Aspergillus* meningitis in an immunocompetent adult successfully treated with itraconazole. Clin Infect Dis 1996;23: 1318–1319.
221. Mills W, Chopra R, Linch DC, Goldstone AH. Liposomal amphotericin B in the treatment of fungal infections in neutropenic patients: a single centre experience of 133 episodes in 116 patients. Br J Haematol 1994;86:754–760.
222. Milose B, el-Mahgoub S, Aal OA, el-Hassan AM. Primary aspergilloma of paranasal sinuses in the Sudan: a review of seventeen cases. Br J Surg 1969;56:132–137.
223. Milroy CM, Blanshard JD, Lucas S, Michaels L. Aspergillosis of the nose and paranasal sinuses. J Clin Pathol 1989;42:123–127.
224. Miyazaki HM, Kohno S, Miyazaki Y, Mitsutake K, Tomono K, Kaku M, Koga H, Hara K. Efficacy of intravenous itraconazole against experimental pulmonary aspergillosis. Antimicrob Agents Chemother 1993;37:2762–2765.
225. Moreau P, Zathar JR, Milpied N. Localized invasive pulmonary aspergillosis in patients with neutropenia—effectiveness of surgical resection. Cancer 1993;72:3223–3226.
226. Morgenstern GR, Prentice AG, Prentice HG. Itraconazole oral solution vs. fluconazole suspension for antifungal prophylaxis in neutropenic patients [Abstract #LM-34]. In: Program and Abstracts of 36th Interscience Conference on Antimicrobial Agents and Chemotherapy, New Orleans, 1996.
227. Morioka T, Tashima T, Nagata S, Fukui M, Hasuo K. Cerebral aspergillosis after burr-hole surgery for chronic subdural hematoma: case report. Neurosurgery 1990;26:232–235.
228. Mrowka C, Heintz B, Weis J, Mayfrank L, Reul J, Sieberth HG. Isolated cerebral aspergilloma—long-term survival of a renal transplant recipient. Clin Nephrol 1997;47:394–396.
229. Munk PL, Vellet AD, Rankin RN, Muller NL, Ahmad D. Intracavitary aspergilloma: transthoracic percutaneous injection of amphotericin gelatin source. Radiology 1993;188:821–823.
230. Murphy M, Bernard EM, Ishimaru T, Armstrong D. Activity of voriconazole (UK-109,496) against clinical isolates of *Aspergillus* species and its effectiveness in an experimental model of invasive pulmonary aspergillosis. Antimicrob Agents Chemother 1997;41:696–698.
231. Mylonakis E, Rich J, Skolnik PR, DeOrchis DF, Flanigan T. Invasive *Aspergillus* sinusitis in patients with human immunodeficiency virus infection. Report of 2 cases and review. Medicine 1997;76:249–255.
232. Nadeem I, Yeldandi V, Sheridan P. Efficacy of itraconazole prophylaxis for aspergillosis in lung transplant recipients [Abstract #341]. In: Program and Abstracts of the 34th Annual Meeting of the Infectious Diseases Society of America, New Orleans, 1996.
233. Nagai H, Guo J, Choi H, Kurup V. Interferon-gamma and tumor necrosis factor-alpha protect mice from invasive aspergillosis. J Infect Dis 1995;172:1540–1560.

234. Naim-Ur-Rahman JA, Jamjoom A, al-Sohaibani MA, Aziz SA. Cranial and intracrancial aspergillosis of sino-nasal origin. Report of nine cases. Acta Neurochir 1996;138:944–950.

235. Nakajima R, Kitamura A, Someya K. In vitro and in vivo antifungal activites of DU-6859a, a fluoroquinolone, in combination with amphotericin B and fluconazole against pathogenic fungi. Antimicrob Agents Chemother 1995;39:1517–1521.

236. Ng TTC, Denning DW. Liposomal amphotericin B (AmBisome) therapy in invasive fungal infections: evaluation of United Kingdom compassionate use data. Arch Intern Med 1995;155:1093–1098.

237. Nguyen MH, Sugar AM. *Aspergillus*. In: Johnson JT, Yu VL, eds. Infectious diseases and antimicrobial therapy of the ears, nose, and throat. Philadelphia: WB Saunders, 1997:221.

238. Niki Y, Bernard EM, Edwards FF, Schmitt HJ, Yu B, Armstrong D. Model of recurrent pulmonary aspergillosis in rats. J Clin Microbiol 1991;29:1317–1322.

239. Nussaume O, Elzaabi M, Icard P, Branger C, Bouttier S, Andreassian B. False aneurysm infected by *Aspergillus fumigatus*: an unusual complication of aortofemoral bypass graft. Ann Thorac Surg 1990;4:388–392.

240. O'Donnell M, Schmidt GM, Tegtmeir BR, Faucett C, Fahey JL, Ito J, Nademanee A, Niland J, Parker P, Smith EP. Prediction of systemic fungal infection in allogeneic marrow recipients: impact of amphotericin prophylaxis in high-risk patients. J Clin Oncol 1994;12:827–834.

241. Oakley KL, Morrissey G, Denning DW. Efficacy of SCH-56592 in a temporarily neutropenic murine model of invasive aspergillosis with an itraconazole-susceptible and an itraconazole-resistant isolate of *Aspergillus fumigatus*. Antimicrob Agents Chemother 1997;41:1504–1507.

242. Odds FC. Interactions among amphotericin B, 5-flucytosine, ketoconazole and miconazole against pathogenic fungi in vitro. Antimicrob Agents Chemother 1982;22:763–770.

243. Olsen SJ, Swerdel MR, Blue B, Clark JM, Bonner DP. Tissue distribution of amphotericin B lipid complex in laboratory animals. J Pharm Pharmacol 1991;43:831–835.

244. Oppenheim BA, Herbrecht R, Kusne S. The safety and efficacy of amphotericin B colloidal dispersion in the treatment of invasive mycoses. Clin Infect Dis 1995;21:1145–1153.

245. Outman WR, Levitz RE, Hill DA, Nightingale CH. Intraocular penetration of rifampin in humans. Antimicrob Agents Chemother 1992;36:1575–1578.

246. Oxford KW, Abbott RL, Fung WE, Ellis DS. *Aspergillus* endophthalmitis after sutureless cataract surgery. Am J Ophthalmol 1995;120:534–535.

247. Pacheco A, Martin JA, Cuevaro M. Serologic response to itraconazole in allergic bronchopulmonary aspergillosis. Chest 1993;103:980–981.

248. Pagano L, Ricci P, Montillo M, Cenacchi A, Nosari A, Tonso A. Localization of aspergillosis to the central nervous system among patients with acute leukemia: report of 14 cases. Clin Infect Dis 1996;23:628–630.

249. Panda A, Sharma N, Das G, Kumar N, Satpathy G. Mycotic keratitis in children: epidemiologic and microbiologic evaluation. Cornea 1997;16:295–299.

250. Paradis IL, Williams P. Infection after lung transplantation. Semin Respir Infect 1993;8:207–215.

251. Pasic S, Abinun M, Pistignjat B, Vlajic B, Rakic J, Sarajanovic L, Ostojic N. *Aspergillus* osteomyelitis in chornic granulomatous disease: treatment with recombinant gamma-interferon and itraconazole. Pediatr Infect Dis J 1996;15:833–834.

252. Paterson DL, Dominguez E, Chang FY, Snydman DR, Singh N. Infective endocarditis in solid organ transplant recipients. Clin Infect Dis 1998;689–694.

253. Patterson TF, Fothergill AW, Rinaldi MG. Efficacy of itraconazole solution in a rabbit model of invasive aspergillosis. Antimicrob Agents Chemother 1993;37:2307–2310.

254. Patterson TF, George D, Ingersoll R, Miniter P, Andriole VT. Efficacy of SCH 39304 in treatment of experimental invasive aspergillosis. Antimicrob Agents Chemother 1991;35:1985–1988.

255. Patterson TF, George D, Miniter P, Andriole VT. Saperconazole therapy in a rabbit model of invasive aspergillosis. Antimicrob Agents Chemother 1992;36:2681–2685.

256. Patterson TF, Kirkpatrick WR, Mcatee RK. The activity of Pradimicin (BMS-181184) in experimental invasive aspergillosis [Abstract #B-51]. In: Program and Abstracts of 36th Interscience Conference on Antimicrobial Agents and Chemotherapy, New Orleans, 1996.

257. Patterson TF, Kirkpatrick WR, Mcatee RK. The efficacy of voriconazole in guinea pig model of disseminated invasive aspergillosis [Abstract #B-14]. In: Program and Abstracts of 37th Interscience Conference on Antimicrobial Agents and Chemotherapy, Toronto, 1997.

258. Patterson TF, Kirkpatrick WR, Mcatee RK. Efficacy of SCH 56592 in a rabbit model of invasive aspergillosis [Abstract #B-48]. In: Program and Abstracts of 37th Interscience Conference on Antimicrobial Agents and Chemotherapy, Toronto, 1997.

259. Patterson TF, Kirkpatrick WR, White M. Therapy of invasive aspergillosis: disease spectrum, treatment practices, and outcomes. [Abstract #LM-38]. In: Program and Abstracts of 36th Interscience Conference on Antimicrobial Agents and Chemotherapy, New Orleans, 1996.

260. Patterson TF, Miniter P, Dijkstra J, Szoka FC, Ryan JL, Andriole VT. Treatment of experimental invasive aspergillosis with novel amphotericin B/cholesterol-sulfate complexes. J Infect Dis 1989;159:717–724.

261. Patterson TF, Peters J, Levine SM, Anzueto A, Bryan CL, Sako EY, Miller OL, Calhoon JH, Rinaldi MG. Systemic availability of itraconazole in lung transplantation. Antimicrob Agents Chemother 1996;40:2217–2220.

262. Paulose KO, Khalifa SA, Shenoy P, Sharma RK. Mycotic infection of ear (otomycosis): a prospective study. J Laryngol Otol 1989;103:30–35.

263. Pennington JE, Block ER, Reynolds HY. 5-Fluorocytosine and amphotericin B in bronchial secretions. Antimicrob Agents Chemother 1974;6:324.

264. Perfect JR, Durack DT. Penetration of imidazole and triazoles into cerebrospinal fluid in rabbits. J Antimicrob Chemother 1985;16:81.

265. Perfect JR, Klotman ME, Gilbert CC, Crawford DD, Rosner GL. Prophylactic intravenous amphotericin B in neutropenic autologous bone marrow transplant recipients. J Infect Dis 1992;165:891–897.

266. Peters-Christodoulou MN, De Beer FC, Bots GTAM, Ottenhoff TMJ, Thompson J, Van't Wout JW. Treatment of postoperative *Aspergillus fumigatus* spondylodiscitis with itraconazole. Scand J Infect Dis 1991;23:373–376.

267. Petraitis V, Petraitiene R, Bell A, Sein T, Schaufele B, Callender DP, Groll A, Candelario M, Lyman CA, Francesconi A. Efficacy of LY303366 against invasive pulmonary aspergillosis [Abstract #720]. In: Programs and abstracts of the 35th annual meeting of the Infectious Diseases Society of America, San Francisco, 1997.

268. Pfaller MA, Messer SA, Marco F, Jones R. Antifungal activity of a new triazole, voriconazole, compared with three other antifungal agents tested against clinical isolates of mould [Abstract #E-83]. In: Program and Abstracts of 37th Interscience Conference on Antimicrobial Agents and Chemotherapy, Toronto, 1997.

269. Phillips P, Bryce G, Shepard J, Mintz D. Invasive external otitis caused by *Aspergillus*. Rev Infect Dis 1990;12:277–281.

270. Polak A. Pharmacokinetics of amphotericin B and flucytosine. Postgrad Med 1979;55:667.

271. Polak A. Combination therapy of experimental candidiasis, cryptococcosis, aspergillosis and wangiellosis in mice. Chemotherapy 1987;33:381–395.

272. Polak A, Scholer HJ, Wall M. Combination therapy of experimental candidiasis, cryptococcosis, and aspergillosis in mice. Chemotherapy 1982;28:461–479.

273. Polak-Wyss A. Protective effect of human granulocyte colony-stimulating factor (hG-CSF) on *Cryptococcus* and *Aspergillus* infections in normal and immunosuppressed mice. Mycoses 1991;34:205–215.

274. Polo JM, Fabrega E, Casefont F, Farinas MC, Salesa R, Vazquez A, Berciano J. Treatment of cerebral aspergillosis after liver transplantation. Neurology 1992;42:1817–1819.

275. Proffitt RT, Satorius A, Chiang SM, Sullivan L, Adler-Moore JP. Pharmacology and toxicology of liposomal formulation of amphotericin B (AmBisome) in rodents. J Antimicrob Chemother 1991;28:49–61.

276. Reichenspurner H, Gamberg P, Nitschke M, Valantine H, Hunt S, Oyer PE, Reitz BA. Significant reduction in the number of fungal infections after lung-, heart-lung, and heart transplantation using aerosolized amphotericin B prophylaxis. Transplant Proc 1997;29:627–628.

277. Richards AB, Jones BR, Whitwell J, Clayton YM. Corneal and intraocular infection by *Candida albicans* treated with 5-fluorocytosine. Trans Ophthalmol Soc UK 1969;29:867.

278. Riley DK, Pavia A, Beatty PG, Petersen FB, Spruance JL, Stokes R, Evans TG. The prophylactic use of low-dose amphotericin B in bone marrow transplant patients. Am J Med 1994; 97:509–514.

279. Ringden O, Meunier F, Tollemar J. Efficacy of amphotericin B encapsulated in liposomes (AmBisome) in the treatment of invasive fungal infections in immunocompromised patients. J Antimicrob Chemother 1991;28:73–82.

280. Robinson LA, Reed EC, Galbraith TA, Alonso A, Moulton AL, Fleming WH. Pulmonary resection for invasive *Aspergillus* infections in immunocompromised patients. J Thorac Cardiovasc Surg 1995;109:1182–1197.

281. Roilides E, Blake C, Holmes A, Pizzo PA, Walsh TJ. Granulocyte-macrophage colony-stimulating factor and interferon-gamma prevent dexamethasone-induced immunosuppression of antifungal monocyte activity against *Aspergillus fumigatus* hyphae. J Med Vet Mycol 1996;34:63–69.

282. Roilides E, Holmes A, Blake C, Pizzo PA, Walsh JJ. Impairment of neutrophil antifungal activity against hyphae of *Aspergillus fumigatus* in children infected with human immunodeficiency virus. J Infect Dis 1993;167:905–911.

283. Roilides E, Holmes A, Blake C, Venzon D, Pizzo PA, Walsh TJ. Antifungal activity of elutriated human monocytes against *Aspergillus fumigatus* hyphae: enhancement by granulocyte-macrophage colony-stimulating factor and interferon-gamma. J Infect Dis 1994;170:894–899.

284. Roilides E, Uhlig K, Venzon D, Pizzo PA, Walsh TJ. Enhance-

ment of oxidative response and damage caused by human neutrophils to *Aspergillus fumigatus* hyphae by granulocyte colony-stimulating factor and gamma interferon. Infect Immun 1993;61:1185–1193.

285. Roilides E, Uhlig K, Venzon D, Pizzo PA, Walsh TJ. Prevention of corticosteroid-induced suppression of human polymorphonuclear leukocyte-induced damage of *Aspergillus fumigatus* hyphae by granulocyte colony-stimulating factor and gamma interferon. Infect Immun 1993;61:4870–4877.

286. Roney P, Barr CC, Chun CH. Endogenous *Aspergillus* endophthalmitis. Rev Infect Dis 1986;8:955.

287. Rosa RH Jr, Miller D, Alfonso EC. The changing spectrum of fungal keratitis in south Florida. Ophthalmology 1994;101: 1005–1013.

288. Rousey SR, Russler S, Gottlieb M, Ash RC. Low-dose amphotericin B prophylaxis against invasive *Aspergillus* infection in allogeneic marrow transplantation. Am J Med 1991:484–492.

289. Rumbak M, Kohler G, Eastrige C, Winermuram H, Gavant M. Topical treatment of life threatening haemoptysis from aspergillomas. Thorax 1996;51:253–255.

290. Ryder NS, Wagner S, Leitner I. In vitro activity of terbinafine against *Aspergillus* in vitro, in combination with amphotericin B or triazoles [Abstract #E-54]. In: Program and Abstracts of 36th Interscience Conference on Antimicrobial Agents and Chemotherapy, New Orleans, 1996.

291. Sachs MK, Paluzzi RG, Moore JH Jr, Fraimow HS, Ost D. Amphotericin-resistant *Aspergillus* osteomyelitis controlled by itraconazole [Letter]. Lancet 1990;335:1475.

292. Sanchez C, Mauri E, Dalmau D, Quintana S, Aparicio A, Carau J. Treatment of cerebral aspergillosis with itraconazole—do high doses improve the prognosis? Clin Infect Dis 1995;21: 1485–1487.

293. Sandisea AT, Gentles JC, Davidson CM, Branko M. Aspergilloma of paranasal sinuses and orbit in northern Sudanese. Sabouraudia 1967;6:57–69.

294. Saraceno JL, Phelps DT, Futerfas R, Schwartz DB. Chronic necrotizing pulmonary aspergilosis. Approach to management. Chest 1997;112:541–548.

295. Savage DG, Taylor P, Blackwell J, Chen F, Szydlo RM, Rule SAJ, Spencer A, Apperley JF, Goldman JM. Paranasal sinusitis following allogeneic bone marrow transplant. Bone Marrow Transplant 1997;19:55–59.

296. Savani DV, Perfect JR, Cobo M, Durack DT. Penetration of new azole compounds into the eye and efficacy in experimental *Candida* endophthalmitis. Antimicrob Agents Chemother 1987;31:6.

297. Sawyer RG, Schenk WG, III, Adams RB, Pruett TL. *Aspergillus flavus* wound infection following repair of a ruptured duodenum in a non-immunocompromised host. Scand J Infect Dis 1992;24:805–809.

298. Schaffner A, Bohler A. Amphotericin B refractory aspergillosis after intraconazole: evidence for significant antagonism. Mycoses 1993;36:421–424.

299. Schaffner A, Douglas H, Braude A. Selective protection against conidia by mononuclear and against mycelia by polymorphonuclear phagocytes in resistance to *Aspergillus*: observations on these two lines of defense in vivo and in vitro with human and mouse phagocytes. J Infect Dis 1982;69:617–631.

300. Schaffner A, Frick PG. The effect of ketoconazole on amphotericin B in a model of disseminated aspergillosis. J Infect Dis 1985;151:902–910.

301. Schar G, Kayser FH, Dupont MC. Antimicrobial activity of

econazole and miconazole in vitro and in experimental candidiasis and aspergillosis. Chemotherapy 1976;22:211–220.

302. Schindler JJ, Warren RP, Allen SD. Immunological effects of amphotericin B and liposomal amphotericin B on splenocytes from immune-normal and immune-compromised mice. Antimicrob Agents Chemother 1993;37:2716–2721.

303. Schiraldi GF, Colombo MD, Harari S, Lo Cicero S, Zilgio G, Ferrarese M, Rossato D, Soresi E. Terbinafine in the treatment of non-immunocompromised compassionate cases of bronchopulmonary aspergillosis. Mycoses 1996;39:5–12.

304. Schmitt HJ, Andrade J, Edwards F. Inactivity of terbinafine in a rat model of pulmonary aspergillosis. Eur J Clin Microb Infect Dis 1990;9:832–835.

305. Schmitt HJ, Bernard EM, Hauser M, Armstrong D. Aerosol amphotericin B is effective for prophylaxis and therapy in a rat model of pulmonary aspergillosis. Antimicrob Agents Chemother 1988;32:1676–1679.

306. Schoffski P, Wunder R, Petersen D. Amphotericin B in Intralipid: no evidence of improved toxicity profile. Results of a randomized phase II-trial in neutropenic patients [Abstract #LM-39]. In: Program and Abstracts of 37th Interscience Conference on Antimicrobial Agents and Chemotherapy, Toronto, 1997.

307. Schwartz S, Milatovic D, Thiel E. Successful therapy of cerebral aspergillosis with a novel triazole (Voriconazole) in a patient with acute leukemia. Br J Haematol 1997;97:663–665.

308. Selby R, Ramirez CB, Singh R, Kleopoulos I, Kusne S, Starzl TE, Fung J. Brain abscess in solid organ transplant recipients receiving cyclosporine-based immunosuppression. Arch Surg 1997;132:304–310.

309. Shapiro MJ, Albelda SM, Mayock RL, McLean GK. Severe hemoptysis associated with pulmonary aspergilloma. Percutaneous intracavitary treatment. Chest 1988;94:1225–1231.

310. Sievers TM, Kubak BM, Wong-Beringer A. Safety and efficacy of Intralipid emulsions of amphotericin B. J Antimicrob Chemother 1996;38:333–347.

311. Sihota R, Agarwal HC, Grover AK. *Aspergillus* endophthalmitis. Br J Ophthalmol 1987;71:611.

312. Singh N, Arnow PM, Bonham A, Dominguez E, Paterson DL, Pankey GA, Wagener MM, Yu VL. Invasive aspergillosis in liver transplant recipients in the 1990s. Transplantation 1997; 64:716–720.

313. Singh N, Bonham A, Dominguez EA, Fukui M, Pankey GA, Paterson DL, Fung JJ. Central nervous system lesions in liver transplant recipients: prospective assessment of indications for biopsy and implications for management [Abstract #J-127]. In: Program and Abstracts of 36th Interscience Conference on Antimicrobial Agents and Chemotherapy, New Orleans, 1996.

314. Singh N, Mieles L, Yu VL, Gayowski T. Invasive aspergillosis in liver transplant recipients: association with candidemia and consumption coagulopathy and failure of prophylaxis with low-dose amphotericin B. Clin Infect Dis 1993;17:906–908.

315. Slavin MA, Osborne B, Adams R, Levenstein MJ, Schoch HG, Feldman AR, Meyers JD, Bowden RA. Efficacy and safety of fluconazole prophylaxis for fungal infections after marrow transplantation—a prospective, randomized, double-blind study. J Infect Dis 1995;171:1545–1552.

316. Smith JG, Abruzzo GK, Gill CJ. Evaluation of pneumocandin L-743872 in neutropenic mouse models of disseminated candidiasis and aspergillosis [Abstract #F-41]. In: Program and Abstracts of 36th Interscience Conference on Antimicrobial Agents and Chemotherapy, New Orleans, 1996.

317. Snydman DR, Werner BG, Dougherty NN, Griffith J, Rubin RH, Dienstag JL. Cytomegalovirus immune globulin prophylaxis in liver transplantation, a randomized, double-blind, placebo controlled trial. Ann Intern Med 1993;119:984–991.

318. Sonin AH, Stern SH, Levi E. Primary *Aspergillus* osteomyelitis in the tibia of an immunosuppressed man. AJR 1996;166: 1277–1279.

319. Souri EN, Green WR. Intravitreal amphotericin B toxicity. Am J Ophthalmol 1974;78:77–81.

320. Spreadbury CL, Cohen J. Invasive aspergillosis: clinical and pathological description of a new animal model, and a comparison of the therapeutic efficacy of amphotericin B and fluconazole [Abstract]. In: Aspergillus and aspergillosis. Antwerp, Belgium: Janssen Pharmaceutica 1987:56–57.

321. Stevens DA, Lee JY, Schwartz HJ, Jerome D, Catanzaro A. Randomized double blind study of itraconazole in allergic bronchopulmonary aspergillosis [Abstract #LB-32]. In: Program and Abstracts of 37th Interscience Conference on Antimicrobial Agents and Chemotherapy, Toronto, 1997.

322. Stiller MJ, Teperman L, Rosenthal SA, Riordan A, Potter J, Shupack JL, Gordon MA. Primary cutaneous infection by *Aspergillus ustus* in a 62-year-old liver transplant recipient. J Am Acad Dermatol 1994;31:344–347.

323. Stone HH, Cuzzell JZ, Kolb LD, Moskowitz MS, McGowan JE. *Aspergillus* infection of the burn wound. J Trauma 1979; 19:765–767.

324. Strauss M, Fine E. *Aspergillus* otomastoiditis in acquired immunodeficiency syndrome. Am J Otol 1991;12:49–53.

325. Swenson CE, Bolsack LE, Perkins WR, Janoff AS. Lipid-based formulations of amphotericin B. J Antimicrob Chemother 1995;35:709–711.

326. Taillandier J, Alemanni M, Cerrina J, Laduri FL, Dartevelle P. *Aspergillus* osteomyelitis after heart-lung transplantation. J Heart Lung Transplant 1997;16:436–438.

327. The International Chronic Granulomatous Disease Cooperative Study Group. A controlled trial of interferon gamma to prevent infection in chronic granulomatous disease. N Engl J Med 1991;324:509–516.

328. Thomas PA. Mycotic keratitis—an underestimated mycosis. J Med Vet Mycol 1994;32:235–256.

329. Todeschini G, Murari GC, Bonesi R, Pizzolo G, Amaddi G, Ambrosetti A, Ceru S, Placentini I, Martini N, Montresor P. Oral itraconazole plus nasal amphotericin B for prophylaxis of invasive aspergillosis in patients with hematological malignancies. Eur J Clin Microb Infect Dis 1993;12:614–618.

330. Tollemar J, Hockerstedt K, Ericzon BG, Jalanko H, Ringden O. Liposomal amphotericin B prevents invasive fungal infections in liver transplant recipients. Transplantation 1995;59:45–50.

331. Tollemar J, Hockerstedt K, Ericzon BG, Jalanko H, Ringden O. Prophylaxis with liposomal amphotericin B (AmBisome) prevents fungal infections in liver transplant recipients: long-term results of a randomized, placebo-controlled trial. Transplant Proc 1995;27:1195–1198.

332. Tollemar J, Ringden O, Anderson S, Sundberg B, Ljungman P, Tyden G. Randomized double-blind study of liposomal amphotericin B (AmBisome) prophylaxis of invasive fungal infections in bone marrow transplant recipients. Bone Marrow Transplant 1993;12:577–582.

333. Tomee JFC, Mannes PM, van der Bij W, van der Werf I, de Boer WJ, Koeter GH, Kauffman HF. Serodiagnosis and monitoring of *Aspergillus* infections after lung transplantation. Ann Intern Med 1996;125:197–201.

334. Tricot G, Joosten E, Boogaerts MA, Vande Pitte J, Cauwenbergh G. Ketoconazole vs. itraconazole for antifungal prophylaxis in patients with severe granulocytopenia: preliminary results of two nonrandomized studies. Rev Infect Dis 1987;9:594–599.

335. Trigg ME, Morgan D, Burns TL, Kook H, Rumelhart SL, Hoida MD, Giller RH. Successful program to prevent *Aspergillus* infections in children undergoing marrow transplantation: use of nasal amphotericin. Bone Marrow Transplant 1997;19:43–47.

336. Troy KM, Cuttner J. Itraconazole prevents invasive fungal disease in patients with acute leukemia undergoing chemotherapy [Abstract]. Blood 1993;82:549a.

337. Tucker RM, Denning DW, Dupont B, Stevens DA. Itraconazole therapy for chronic coccidioidal meningitis. Ann Intern Med 1990;112:1108–1112.

338. Tucker RM, Hanson LH, Denning DW. The interaction of azoles with rifampin, phenytoin and carbamazepine: in vitro and clinical observations. Clin Infect Dis 1992;14:165–174.

339. Tutschka PJ, Beschorner WE, Hesse M, Santos GW. Cyclosporin-A to prevent graft-versus-host disease: a pilot study in 22 patients receiving allogeneic marrow transplants. Blood 1983;61:318–325.

340. Valluri S, Moorthy RS, Liggett PE, Rao NA. Endogenous *Aspergillus* endophthalmitis in an immunocompetent individual. Int Ophthalmol 1993;17:131–135.

341. Van Cutsem J, Janssen PAJ. In vitro and in vivo models to study the activity of antifungals against *Aspergillus*. In: Vanden Bossche H, Mackenzie DWR, Cauwenbergh G, eds. *Aspergillus* and aspergillosis. New York: Plenum Press; 1988:215–217.

342. Van Cutsem J, Ven Gerven F, Janssen PA. Oral and parenteral therapy with saperconazole (R 66905) of invasive aspergillosis in normal and immunocompromised animals. Antimicrob Agents Chemother 1989;33:2063–2068.

343. Van't Wout JW, Novakova I, Verhagen CAH, Fibbe WE, De Pauw BE, Van der Meer JWM. The efficacy of itraconazole against systemic fungal infections in neutropenic patients: a randomized comparative study with amphotericin B. J Infect 1991;22:45–52.

344. Vanetten EWM, ten Kate MT, Bakker-Woudenberg IAJM. Efficacy of a new type of liposomal amphotericin B in severe invasive pulmonary aspergillosis in leukopenic rats [Abstract #B-15]. In: Program and Abstracts of 37th Interscience Conference on Antimicrobial Agents and Chemotherapy, Toronto, 1997.

345. Verscharaegen CF, Vanbesien KW, Dignani C, Hester JP, Andersson BS, Anaissie E. Invasive aspergillus sinusitis during bone marrow transplantation. Scand J Infect Dis 1997;29:436–438.

346. Verweij PE, Donnelly JP, Kullberg BJ, Meis JF, DePauw BE. Amphotericin B versus amphotericin B plus 5-flucytosine: poor results in the treatment of proven systemic mycoses in neutropenic patients. Infection 1994;22:81–85.

347. Verweij PE, Mensink M, Rijs AJ, Donnelly JP, Meis JF, Denning DW. In vitro activity of amphotericin B, itraconazole and voriconazole against 151 clinical and environmental *Aspergillus fumigatus* isolates [Abstract #E-90]. In: Program and Abstracts of 37th Interscience Conference on Antimicrobial Agents and Chemotherapy, Toronto, 1997.

348. Verweij PE, Oakley KL, Morrissey J, et al. Efficacy of LY303,366 against amphotericin B "susceptible" and "resistant" *A. fumigatus* infection in an immunocompromised murine model [Abstract #F-73]. In: Program and Abstracts of 37th Interscience Conference on Antimicrobial Agents and Chemotherapy, Toronto, 1997.

349. von Eiff M, Roos N, Schulten R, Hesse M, Zuhlsdorf M, van de Loo J. Pulmonary aspergillosis: early diagnosis improves survival. Respiration 1995;62:341–347.

350. Vreugdenhil G, Van Dijke BJ, Donnelly JP, Novakova IRO, Raemaekers JMM, Hoogkamp-Korstanje MAA, Koster M, De Pauw BE. Efficacy of itraconazole in the prevention of fungal infections among neutropenic patients with hematologic malignancies and intensive chemotherapy. A double-blind, placebo controlled study. Leuk Lymphoma 1993;11:353–358.

351. Wald A, Leisenring W, van Burik J, Bowden RA. Epidemiology of *Aspergillus* infections in a large cohort of patients undergoing bone marrow transplantation. J Infect Dis 1997;175:1459–1466.

352. Walker WA, Pate JW. Primary *Aspergillus* osteomyelitis of the sternum. Ann Thorac Surg 1991;52:868–870.

353. Wallace TF, Paetznick V, Cossum PA. Nyotran (liposomal nystatin) activity against disseminated *Aspergillus fumigatus* in neutropenic mice [Abstract #B-53]. In: Program and Abstracts of 36th Interscience Conference on Antimicrobial Agents and Chemotherapy, New Orleans, 1996.

354. Wallace TL, Paetznick V, Cossum PA, Lopez-Berestein G, Rex JH, Anaissie E. Activity of liposomal nystatin against disseminated *Aspergillus fumigatus* infection in neutropenic mice. Antimicrob Agents Chemother 1997;41:2238–2243.

355. Walsh JJ, Hiemenz JW, Seibel N. Amphotericin B lipid complex in the treatment of 228 cases of invasive mycosis [Abstract #M-69]. In: Program and Abstracts of 34th Interscience Conference on Antimicrobial Agents and Chemotherapy, Orlando, 1994.

356. Walsh TJ, Bodensteiner D, Hiemenez JW, Thaler S, Greenberg R, Arndt C, Holcenberg J, Schwartz C, Pappas P, Dummer JS. A randomized double-blind trial of AmBisome (liposomal amphotericin B) versus amphotericin B in the empirical treatment of persistently febrile neutropenic patients [Abstract# LM-90]. In: Program and Abstracts of 37th Interscience Conference on Antimicrobial Agents and Chemotherapy, Toronto, 1997.

357. Walsh TJ, Garrett K, Feuerstein E, Girton M, Allende M, Bacher J, Francesconi A, Schaufele R, Pizzo PA. Therapeutic monitoring of experimental invasive pulmonary aspergillosis by ultrafast computerized tomography, a novel, noninvasive method for measuring responses to antifungal therapy. Antimicrob Agents Chemother 1995;39:1065–1069.

358. Washburn RG, Kennedy DW, Begley MG, Henderson DK, Bennett JE. Chronic fungal sinusitis in apparently normal hosts. Medicine 1988;67:231–247.

359. Westney GE, Kesten S, De Hoyos A, Chapparro C, Winton T, Maurer JR. *Aspergillus* infection in single and double lung transplant recipients. Transplantation 1996;61:915–919.

360. White MH, Wingard JR, Gurwith M, Du Mond C, Mamelok RD, Bowden RA. Amphotericin B colloidal dispersion vs. amphotericin B as therapy for invasive aspergillosis. Clin Infect Dis 1997;24:635–642.

361. Wimperis JZ, Baglin TP, Marcus RE, Warren RE. An assessment of the efficacy of antimicrobial prophylaxis in bone marrow autografts. Bone Marrow Transplant 1991;8:363–367.

362. Winchester K, Mathers WD, Sutphin JE. Diagnosis of *Aspergillus* keratitis in vivo with confocal microscopy. Cornea 1997;16:27–31.

363. Witzig RS, Greer DL, Hyslop NE, Jr. *Aspergillus flavus* mycetoma and epidural abscess successfully treated with itraconazole. J Med Vet Mycol 1996;34:133–137.

364. Wong A, Waters CM, Walesby RK. Surgical management of invasive pulmonary aspergillosis in immunocompromised patients. Eur J Cardiothorac Surg 1992;6:138–143.

365. Yee GC, Kennedy MS, Deeg HJ, Leonard TM, Thomas ED, Storb R. Cyclosporine-associated renal dysfunction in marrow transplant recipients. Transplant Proc 1985;17:196–201.

366. Yeldandi V, McCabe MA, Larson R, O'Keefe P, Husalin A, Montoya A, Garrity ER. *Aspergillus* and lung transplantation. J Heart Lung Transplant 1995;14:883–890.

367. Yotsuji A, Shimizu K, Araki J, Fujimaki K, Nishida N, Hori R, Annen N, Yamamoto S, Hayakawa H, Imaizumi H, et al. T-8581, a new orally and parenterally active triazole antifungal

agent: in vitro and in vivo evaluations. Antimicrob Agents Chemother 1997;41:30–34.

368. Young VK, Maghur HA, Luke DA, McGovern EM. Operations for cavitating invasive pulmonary aspergillosis in immuno-compromised patients. Ann Thorac Surg 1992;53:621–624.

369. Yu VL, Wagner GE, Shadomy S. Sino-orbital aspergillosis treated with combination antifungal therapy. Successful therapy after failure with amphotericin B and surgery. JAMA 1980;244:814–815.

Blastomyces dermatitidis

●

Peter G. Pappas

Originally described in 1894 by Gilchrist, blastomycosis is an important pyogranulomatous systemic mycosis caused by *Blastomyces dermatitidis*. While it is now understood that most cases of blastomycosis result from inhalation of infectious spores, early cases were perceived to be a primary dermatologic disorder and not until the early 1950s was the concept of primary pulmonary blastomycosis with secondary dissemination to extrapulmonary sites adopted, largely based on the clinical and pathologic observations of Schwarz and Baum (32).

Blastomycosis is endemic to much of the eastern United States, especially the south central and midwestern regions (9). It also occurs in Canada and has been reported from Central and South America, Western Europe, and Africa (6). The spectrum of disease is quite broad and includes acute self-limited pulmonary infections (30); chronic pulmonary, cutaneous, osseous, or other organ involvement (33); and fulminant, rapidly progressive pulmonary and/or disseminated infections (19).

THE ORGANISM

B. dermatitidis is a thermally dimorphic fungus that grows as a yeast at 37°C and as mycelia at 25°C. The perfect or sexual stage is *Ajellomyces dermatitidis*. In the yeast form, the organism is round, measures 5 to 15 μm in diameter, and has a thick, doubly refractile cell wall. Broad-based budding is characteristic. At room temperature, the imperfect stage of the organism grows as a fluffy white mold on Sabouraud's media, and at 37°C, it grows as a brown folded colony of yeast (15).

EPIDEMIOLOGY

Areas endemic for *B. dermatitidis* in the United States include the south central and midwestern portions of the country, especially the areas around the Great Lakes and the Ohio and Mississippi River valleys. Outside the United States, well-documented cases have been reported most commonly from

central and eastern Canada (29). Fewer well-documented cases have been reported from Central and South America and Western Europe, but the disease seems to be widespread in Africa (15). Current evidence indicates that the organism exists in warm, moist soil enriched by organic debris including decaying vegetation and wood. In endemic areas, small-point-source outbreaks have been associated with recreational and occupational activities occurring in wooded areas along waterways (14). There is a striking male predominance among clinical cases of blastomycosis, and there is usually a recent history of occupational or recreational exposure, especially heavy equipment operation, forestry, farming, or hunting. Because of the lack of sufficiently sensitive and specific screening methods such as skin tests and serology, the actual number of infected individuals is unknown, but the vast majority are likely asymptomatic (29).

Most human infections with *B. dermatitidis* result from inhalation of aerosolized conidia, which leads to either an asymptomatic infection or a self-limited flulike illness in most cases. Primary cutaneous inoculation leading to disease has been reported occasionally, usually from a dog bite or percutaneous exposure in the laboratory or at autopsy (10, 16). Person-to-person transmission rarely, if ever, occurs. Following primary pulmonary infection, most patients develop no significant consequences and do not require therapy. Among patients who develop chronic blastomycosis, most develop pulmonary involvement followed by skin, bone, prostate, and central nervous system (CNS) involvement. Once chronic blastomycosis develops in an individual, the disease does not completely resolve without medical intervention (29).

While most cases of blastomycosis occur in individuals who are living in an endemic area at the time of diagnosis, several clear-cut cases of endogenous reactivation have been documented among patients who had not lived in nor visited an endemic area in several years or even decades (17). Most recent cases of endogenous reactivation blastomycosis have been reported among patients with the acquired immunodeficiency syndrome (AIDS) living in nonendemic areas, a trend that is likely to increase in a highly mobile society (21). These cases provide good evidence that *B. dermatitidis* may reactivate following years of latency.

SUSCEPTIBILITY

While susceptibility testing for dimorphic fungi remains poorly standardized, both in vitro and in vivo data exist regarding the susceptibility of *B. dermatitidis* to various antifungal agents. Among available systemic antifungal agents, all have moderate to excellent activity against *B. dermatitidis* in vitro and in animal models (Table 1). Amphotericin B has the best in vitro activity, consistently demonstrates fungicidal activity in animal models, and is generally regarded as the most active compound. Currently available azoles are less active than amphotericin B, and all are fungistatic. While all three azoles have similar in vitro activity, itraconazole demonstrates the greatest activity in vivo, in both animal models and human trials (7, 12, 13, 35, 36).

ANTIMICROBIAL THERAPY

Currently, four antifungal agents have been proven effective in the treatment of human blastomycosis—amphotericin B, ketoconazole, itraconazole, and fluconazole. Among these agents, only fluconazole is not licensed for treatment of this mycosis. There have been no published therapeutic trials comparing different antifungal agents in blastomycosis; thus our notion of the most effective therapy for this disorder is largely based on small to moderate-sized clinical trials, case reports, retrospective reviews, and anecdotal experience. Historically, amphotericin B has been the mainstay of therapy for all forms of blastomycosis since its availability in 1958. Prior to this time, 2-hydroxystilbamidine was the only useful agent. A clinical trial conducted between 1960 and 1968 comparing these two agents in patients with blastomycosis demonstrated superiority of amphotericin B over 2-hydroxystilbamidine (5).

The published efficacy of amphotericin B in all forms of blastomycosis ranges between 66 and 93%, depending the dose of drug, duration of therapy, underlying illness, and disease severity (2, 5). For mild-to-moderate disease, efficacy generally exceeds 90%. Unfortunately, amphotericin B must be administered by the intravenous route. In addition, it has significant renal, electrolyte, hematologic, and infusion-associated toxicity. Further, it is often given for prolonged periods of weeks to months. Consequently, orally administered

and less toxic azole antifungal agents have been attractive alternatives to traditional therapy with amphotericin B.

Ketoconazole, an orally administered antifungal compound, was the first of the azoles to be extensively studied and widely used for the treatment of non-life-threatening, non-CNS blastomycosis. Experience with miconazole, an intravenous azole, was generally disappointing, and it is no longer used for this purpose. The first large study of ketoconazole for blastomycosis compared different doses (400 and 800 mg daily) in 80 patients and demonstrated a successful outcome in 78 and 100% of patients who received at least 6 months of therapy with 400 mg or 800 mg of ketoconazole daily, respectively (20). A second study evaluated ketoconazole 400 mg daily in 44 patients with blastomycosis and led to a successful outcome in 80% (3). Dose-limiting toxicity due to ketoconazole was seen in both studies and included nausea, vomiting, rash, pruritus, decreased libido, impotence, and gynecomastia (3, 20).

Itraconazole, an orally available antifungal, is the newest of the clinically available triazole agents (1992) and is the drug of choice for most patients with mild-to-moderate blastomycosis that does not involve the CNS. Recently, Dismukes et al. reported the efficacy and toxicity of itraconazole in 48 patients with non-life-threatening non-CNS blastomycosis (8). Initially, patients were randomized to receive either 200 or 400 mg daily, but a favorable response in patients receiving the lower dose led to all patients being started on 200 mg daily. For patients who had persistent or progressive disease at 200 mg daily, the dose could be increased to 300 mg or 400 mg daily. Among 48 evaluable patients, 43 (89%) were successfully treated. Furthermore, 38 of 40 (95%) patients who received at least 2 months of therapy had successful outcomes. These results are similar to the efficacy of amphotericin B for mild-to-moderate disease. The median duration of treatment of successfully treated patients was about 6 months, with follow-up for 12 months off therapy. Itraconazole was well tolerated at both low and higher doses, and only one patient was removed from the study because of drug toxicity. Nausea and vomiting were the most common drug-related toxicities, followed by pedal edema, rash, pruritus, and impotence (8).

Fewer data exist concerning the use of fluconazole for treatment of blastomycosis. Fluconazole was the first orally available triazole antifungal agent (1990) and remains the only approved triazole that can be given intravenously. Its pharmacokinetics are superior to those of the other azoles, in part because of its water solubility. As a result, the drug achieves levels of at least 70% of serum levels in the cerebrospinal fluid and also reaches very high levels in the urine, where it is excreted largely unchanged (12). A recent pilot study of fluconazole in blastomycosis evaluated 200 mg and 400 mg daily in 23 patients with non-life-threatening, non-CNS disease. Overall efficacy in this trial was 65% (15 of 23 patients successfully treated), including 8 of 13 (62%) patients receiving lower-dose and 7 of 10 (70%) receiving higher-dose fluconazole (23). Median duration of therapy was about 6 months, and the drug was well tolerated. Interestingly, six patients who had failed prior antifungal therapy with ketoconazole or amphotericin B all

TABLE 1 • Susceptibility of *Blastomyces dermatitidis* to Antifungal Agents		
	MIC$_{90}$ (μg/mL)	MFC$_{90}$ (μg/mL)
Amphotericin B	0.06–1.0	4.0–6.0
Ketoconazole	1–2	16–>32
Fluconazole	2–4	16–>32
Itraconazole	2–4	16–>32

eventually responded to fluconazole. Because of these encouraging results, a subsequent study was conducted to evaluate higher doses of fluconazole (400 and 800 mg) in patients with mild-to-moderate blastomycosis (24). Overall success in this study was 87%, including 17 of 19 (89%) patients receiving 400 mg daily and 17 of 20 (85%) patients receiving 800 mg daily. Five of six patients who had failed prior antifungal therapy were successfully treated with higher-dose fluconazole. Toxicity leading to removal from study (rash) was seen in only one patient. The efficacy of higher-dose fluconazole in this study approaches that of itraconazole at 200 to 400 mg daily. Further, it equals or exceeds the published efficacy of ketoconazole and is generally much better tolerated. Thus, fluconazole at a daily dose of 400 to 800 mg represents a reasonable alternative for patients who cannot tolerate conventional antifungal therapy or in whom previous therapy has failed.

GENERAL RECOMMENDATIONS

In most clinical settings of mild-to-moderate blastomycosis, initial therapy with itraconazole 200 mg daily is appropriate. In patients with persistent or progressive disease, itraconazole may be increased at monthly intervals by 100 mg increments to a maximum dosage of 400 mg daily (usually given 200 mg twice daily). If absorption is decreased (e.g., secondary to achlorhydria), as demonstrated by low serum itraconazole concentrations (e.g., <1 μg/mL by bioassay), then higher doses can be given. Ketoconazole remains a useful drug, but it is less well tolerated and somewhat less effective than itraconazole; however, it is less expensive. Most experts begin ketoconazole at a dose of 400 mg daily, increasing the dose monthly by 200 mg to a maximum of 800 mg daily in patients with an inadequate response. The role of fluconazole for initial therapy of blastomycosis is unclear. At higher doses (400 to 800 mg/day) fluconazole approaches the efficacy of itraconazole 200 to 400 mg daily and is well tolerated (24). However, it is less effective than itraconazole at comparative doses; thus its role is probably limited to patients who are unable to tolerate itraconazole or in whom conventional therapy with amphotericin B and/or itraconazole has failed or is contraindicated. Regardless of which azole is selected for the therapy of blastomycosis, treatment should be continued for at least 6 months, depending on the clinical, radiographic, and mycologic responses (2, 8).

Amphotericin B is the drug of choice for patients with severe or life-threatening blastomycosis. A cumulative dose of 1.5 to 2.0 g is effective therapy in most cases. Among patients with severe disease, many clinicians administer an induction course of amphotericin B of 500 to 1000 mg to reduce the organism load and to gain control of the disease, followed by therapy with an azole for several months. There is virtually no published experience with the use of the lipid formulations of amphotericin B in the treatment of blastomycosis; however, anecdotally we have treated several patients with severe disease and concomitant chronic renal dysfunction successfully with amphotericin B lipid complex (Abelcet). No clinical data exist concerning combination therapy with amphotericin B plus an azole or flucytosine. Likewise, there are no clinical or experimental data examining combination therapy with the azoles.

SPECIAL CONSIDERATIONS

While most patients with blastomycosis can be treated as described above, several specific aspects of this disorder require special consideration with respect to therapy. Some of the more important circumstances are discussed below.

Acute Pulmonary Blastomycosis

Most primary infections with *B. dermatitidis* are either asymptomatic or are manifest as a self-limited, flulike illness or atypical pneumonia syndrome. Because serologic methods are not routinely used or particularly useful diagnostically and because culture methods may require weeks to isolate *B. dermatitidis,* most patients are misdiagnosed or only diagnosed after they have recovered clinically (6). As most patients improve spontaneously without antifungal therapy (30), many clinicians in the past have elected to observe patients without initiating specific therapy. While there are no compelling data that strongly favor treating all patients with acute pulmonary blastomycosis, most clinicians currently treat these patients with an azole, usually itraconazole, given its safety, patient tolerance, and efficacy. Patients who do not receive systemic antifungal therapy must be followed carefully for evidence of disease activity.

Central Nervous System

The CNS is the fifth most common site of involvement with *B. dermatitidis,* following the lungs, skin and subcutaneous tissue, bones, and prostate gland. CNS involvement occurs in up to 10% of normal hosts (4, 11) and up to 40% of immunocompromised patients (21, 22), and it may be manifest as subacute or chronic meningitis, intracerebral mass lesion(s), or an epidural mass (11, 28). Most patients with proven or suspected CNS involvement should receive aggressive therapy with amphotericin B and should probably receive at least a 2-g cumulative dose. Limited published experience with fluconazole in this setting exists, and it appears to be an effective agent for CNS infection due to *B. dermatitidis* (37), based on these data and our own anecdotal experience. The efficacy of fluconazole in this setting probably relates to its excellent penetration into the cerebrospinal fluid. Fluconazole should be given in higher doses (800 mg/day) for at least 6 months when given for CNS blastomycosis. Ketoconazole and itraconazole have no role in this setting; indeed, there have been several reports of relapsing infection in the CNS following successful treatment of pulmonary and dermatologic blastomycosis with ketoconazole (26, 38).

Ocular

Keratitis, conjunctivitis, and endophthalmitis are rare complications of human infection with *B. dermatitidis* (18). The diagnosis is usually made presumptively in patients with established disease at an extraocular site. Therapy for ocular blastomycosis is not well described but should probably include both systemic and local antifungal therapy. All successfully managed patients have been treated with systemic amphotericin B, although a recent patient also received topical and subconjunctival miconazole and experienced an excellent clinical response (18). The role of the other azoles as adjunctive therapy remains unclear, but fluconazole appears to achieve therapeutic concentrations in the aqueous humor and vitreous body (31) and has been shown effective in the treatment of endophthalmitis due to *Candida* spp. (1).

Immunocompromised Patients

The number of patients with blastomycosis and significant underlying disorders of immune function has increased markedly in recent years, due in part to the large number of solid organ transplant recipients and patients with AIDS, hematologic malignancies, chronic glucocorticosteroid recipients, and other miscellaneous disorders (22, 27, 34). Among these patients, infection with *B. dermatitidis* can be severe, characterized by multiple visceral organ dissemination, frequent involvement of the CNS, and an overall mortality approaching 30% in spite of antifungal therapy (22). Consequently, most immunocompromised patients should receive aggressive initial therapy with amphotericin B, which should be continued until the patient has experienced significant clinical and/or radiographic improvement. Primary therapy with itraconazole or fluconazole should be given only to patients with limited disease and a mild, stable underlying condition associated with immune dysfunction. Among patients who have disorders characterized by ongoing immunosuppression, lifelong suppressive therapy with itraconazole or fluconazole may be necessary to prevent relapsing disease (25).

ENDPOINTS FOR MONITORING THERAPY

For patients with blastomycosis, the efficacy of therapy is generally based on clinical and radiographic (usually pulmonary and bone) findings. Follow-up cultures from involved sites, where available, become negative within 1 month of initiating therapy in most circumstances. Persistently positive cultures after at least 2 months of antifungal therapy indicate an inadequate response to therapy and should prompt strong consideration of changing therapy unless there has been significant clinical and radiographic response. When cultures are unavailable or difficult (e.g., bone involvement, pulmonary nodule), clinical and radiographic evaluation are usually the only means of determining response to therapy. Therapy should be continued for a minimum of 6 months and for at least 1 month after all clinical, radiographic, and laboratory evidence of disease has resolved. There is no current role for serial serologic monitoring for *B. dermatitidis* in the management of blastomycosis.

REFERENCES

1. Akler ME, Vellend H, NcNeely DM, Walmsley SL, Gold WL. Use of fluconazole in the treatment of candidal endophthalmitis. Clin Infect Dis 1995;20:657–664.
2. Bradsher RW. Blastomycosis. Infect Dis Clin North Am 1988;2: 877–898.
3. Bradsher RW, Rice DC, Abernathy RS. Ketoconazole therapy for endemic blastomycosis. Ann Intern Med 1985;103:872–879.
4. Buechner HA, Clawson CM. Blastomycosis of the central nervous system: a report of nine cases from the Veterans Administration Cooperative Study. Am Rev Respir Dis 1966;95: 820–826.
5. Busey JF. Blastomycosis. III. A comparative study of 2-hydroxystilbamidine and amphotericin B therapy. Am Rev Respir Dis 1972;105:812–818.
6. Chapman SW. *Blastomyces dermatitidis*. In: Mandell GL, Bennett JE, Dolin R, eds. Principles and practice of infectious diseases. New York: Churchill Livingstone, 1995:2353–2365.
7. Cutsem JV, Van Gerven FV, Janssen PAJ. Activity of orally, topically, and parenterally administered itraconazole in the treatment of superficial and deep mycoses: animal models. Rev Infect Dis 1987;9(Suppl 1):S15–S32.
8. Dismukes WE, Bradsher RW Jr, Cloud GC, Kauffman CA, Chapman SW, George RB, Stevens DA, Girard WM, Saag MS, Bowles-Patton C, and the Mycoses Study Group. Itraconazole therapy for blastomycosis and histoplasmosis. Am J Med 1992; 93:489–497.
9. Furcolow ML, Chick EW, Busey JF, Menges RW, Chick EW. Prevalence of incidence studies of human and canine blastomycosis I: cases in the United States, 1885–1968. Am Rev Respir Dis 1970;102:60–67.
10. Gnann JW, Bressler GS, Bodet CA, Avent CK. Human blastomycosis after a dog bite. Ann Intern Med 1983;98:48–49.
11. Gonyea RF. The spectrum of primary blastomycotic meningitis: a review of central nervous system blastomycosis. Ann Neurol 1978;3:26–39.
12. Grant SM, Clissold SP. Fluconazole: a review of its pharmacodynamic and pharmacokinetic properties, and therapeutic potential in superficial and systemic mycoses. Drugs 1990;39:877–916.
13. Heel RC, Brogden RN, Carmine A, Morley PA, Speight TM, Avery GS. Ketoconazole: a review of its therapeutic efficacy in superficial and systemic fungal infections. Drugs 1982;23:1–36.
14. Klein BS, Vergeront JM, Weeks RJ, Kamar UN, Mathai G, Varkey B, Kaufman L, Bradsher RW, Stoebig JF, Davis JP. Isolation of *B. dermatitidis* in soil associated with a large outbreak of blastomycosis in Wisconsin. N Engl J Med 1986;314:529–534.
15. Kwon-Chung KJ, Bennett JE, eds. Blastomycosis. In: Medical mycology. Philadelphia: Lea & Febiger, 1992:248–279.
16. Larson EM, Eckman MR, Albec RL. Primary cutaneous (inoculation) blastomycosis: an occupational hazard to pathologists. Am J Clin Pathol 1983;79:253–255.
17. Laskey W, Sarosi GA. Endogenous activation in blastomycosis. Ann Intern Med 1978;88:50–52.
18. Lopez R, Mason JO, Parker JS, Pappas PG. Intraocular blastomycosis: case report and review. Clin Infect Dis 1994;18: 805–807.
19. Meyer KC, McManus EJ, Make DG. Overwhelming pulmonary blastomycosis associated with the adult respiratory distress syndrome. N Engl J Med 1993;329:1231–1236.
20. National Institute of Allergy and Infectious Diseases Mycoses Study Group. Treatment of blastomycosis and histoplasmosis with ketoconazole. Ann Intern Med 1985;103:861–872.
21. Pappas PG, Pottage JC, Powderly WG, Fraser VJ, Stratton CW, McKenzie S, Tapper ML, Chmel H, Bonebrake FC, Blum R, Shafer RW, King C, Dismukes WE. Blastomycosis in patients with the acquired immunodeficiency syndrome. Ann Intern Med 1992;116:847–853.
22. Pappas PG, Threlkeld MG, Bedsole GD, Cleveland KO, Gelfand MS, Dismukes WE. Blastomycosis in immunocompromised patients. Medicine 1993;72:311–325.

23. Pappas PG, Bradsher RW, Chapman SW, Kauffman CA, Dine A, Cloud GA, Dismukes WE. Treatment of blastomycosis with fluconazole: a pilot study. Clin Infect Dis 1995;20: 267–271.

24. Pappas PG, Bradsher RW, Kauffman CA, Cloud GA, Thomas CJ, Campbell GD, Chapman SW, Newman C, Dismukes WE. Treatment of blastomycosis with higher dose fluconazole. Clin Infect Dis 1997;25:200–205.

25. Pappas PG. Blastomycosis in the immunocompromised patient. Semin Respir Infect 1997;12:243–251.

26. Pitrak DL, Andersen BR. Cerebral blastomycoma after ketoconazole therapy for respiratory tract blastomycosis. Am J Med 1989;86:713–714.

27. Recht LD, Davies SF, Eckman MR. Blastomycosis in immunosuppressed patients. Am Rev Respir Dis 1982;125:359–362.

28. Roos KL, Bryan JP, Maggio WW, Jane JA, Scheld WM. Intracranial blastomycoma. Medicine 1987;66:224–235.

29. Sarosi GA, Davies SF. Blastomycosis. Am Rev Respir Dis 1979;120:911–938.

30. Sarosi GA, Davies SF, Phillips JR. Self-limited blastomycosis: a report of 39 cases. Semin Respir Infect 1986;1:40–44.

31. Savani DV, Perfect JR, Cobo LM, Durack DT. Penetration of new azole compounds into the eye and efficacy in experimental

32. *Candida* endophthalmitis. Antimicrob Agents Chemother 1987; 31:6–10.

32. Schwarz J, Baum GL. Blastomycosis. Am J Clin Pathol 1951; 21:999–1029.

33. Schwarz J, Salfelder K. Blastomycosis: a review of 152 cases. Curr Top Pathol 1977;65:165–200.

34. Serody JS, Mill MR, Detterbeck FC, Harris DT, Cohen MS. Blastomycosis in transplant recipients: report of a case review. Clin Infect Dis 1993;16:54–58.

35. Stevens DA, Brummer E, McEwen JG, Perlman AM. Comparison of fluconazole and ketoconazole in experimental murine blastomycosis. Rev Infect Dis 1990;12(Suppl 3):S304–S306.

36. Sugar AM, Liu ZP. In vitro and in vivo activities of SCH 56592 against *Blastomyces dermatitidis*. Antimicrob Agents Chemother 1996;40:1314–1316.

37. Taillan B, Ferrari E, Cosnefroy J, Gari-Toussaint M, Francois Michaels J, Paquis P, Lefichoux Y, Dujardin P. Favorable outcome of blastomycosis of the brain stem with fluconazole and flucytosine treatment. Ann Med 1991;24.71–72.

38. Yancey RW, Perlino CA, Kauffman L. Asymptomatic blastomycosis of the central nervous system with progression in patients given ketoconazole therapy: a report of two cases. J Infect Dis 1991;164:807–810.

Candida Species

●

John H. Rex, Jack D. Sobel, and William G. Powderly

GENERAL DESCRIPTION

The genus *Candida* contains more than 100 different species (162), but only a limited number of these species regularly cause disease in man (Table 1). Morphologically, *Candida* are 4- to 6-μm, thin-walled yeast fungi that reproduce by budding. Candida can also produce hyphae and pseudohyphae in tissues, but this behavior is a function of both species and the involved organ. Identification of the individual species is based on standard sugar assimilation and morphologic techniques. *C. glabrata* is the one species that does not produce hyphae or pseudohyphae, and it has variously been considered to belong to the genus *Candida* and the genus *Torulopsis* (185). However, recent DNA-based data have placed this organism in the genus *Candida* (175).

The major pathogenic species of *Candida* do differ somewhat in their frequency, virulence, and clinical associations (Table 2). *C. albicans* has long been the most frequent cause of all forms of candidiasis and generally appears to be the most virulent of the species. However, recent data from some (1, 187, 191, 200, 226, 267, 315), but not all (161, 312), reports have documented a general reduction in the frequency of *C. albicans* associated with a concomitant increase in the frequency of *C. glabrata, C. tropicalis,* and *C. parapsilosis* infections. Of

these major non-*albicans* species, *C. tropicalis* may be the most virulent. Colonization with this species more often leads to invasive disease (156, 213, 317), and it appears to be especially able to colonize and infect gastrointestinal mucosa that has been compromised by neutropenia, chemotherapy-induced direct damage, and altered bacterial flora (304, 313, 314). After *C. tropicalis, C. glabrata* is either the first or second most common non-*albicans* species found in the blood (Table 2). As *C. glabrata* appears to have relatively low virulence (3, 312), patients infected with it tend to be severely immunocompromised (3, 156), and this may be associated with an increased mortality rate. *C. parapsilosis* is the fourth most common *Candida* sp. found in the blood, and infections due to it are very strongly linked with the presence of intravenous catheters and other prosthetic devices (1, 102, 180, 308, 312). The organism's propensity to grow in glucose-containing solutions such as those used for parenteral hyperalimentation (191, 215, 221, 308, 312) as well as its ability to form a slime that enhances adherence (37, 124, 215) is probably responsible for these associations. *C. parapsilosis* has been generally considered less virulent than *C. albicans* (84), but different isolates of *C. parapsilosis* demonstrate a broad range of pathogenicity (47, 102). *C. krusei,* the fifth most common species, tends to be seen in relatively immunocompromised patients (104, 187), as does *C. lusitaniae,* the sixth most common species (31).

SUSCEPTIBILITY IN VITRO AND IN VIVO
Monotherapy

While additional agents with topical activity are available (see "Nongenital Mucocutaneous Candidiasis," below), the principal systemic agents with anti-*Candida* activity are amphotericin B, ketoconazole, itraconazole, fluconazole, and flucytosine. The activities of these agents against *Candida* are predictable and vary with species (Table 3). *C. albicans* isolates are the most susceptible to all of the antifungal agents. The pattern for *C. tropicalis* and *C. parapsilosis* is quite similar, with just slightly higher MICs for fluconazole. *C. glabrata* tends to have fluconazole MICs that are 16 to 64 times those for *C. albicans*. *C. krusei* isolates have the highest fluconazole

and flucytosine MICs, whereas *C. lusitaniae* isolates frequently have quite elevated amphotericin B MICs.

Interpretation of the MIC results shown in Table 3 is controversial and remains the focus of intensive study. The principal difficulty is that MICs obtained in any in vitro system are arbitrary—variations in methodology can lead to 50,000-fold differences in measured MIC for the same isolate (234). This, along with the many non-drug-related causes of therapeutic failure (e.g., failure to remove a foreign body, drug-drug interactions, reduction in drug availability by protein binding) means that interpretation of MICs is not necessarily as simple as comparing achievable blood levels with measured MICs (233). While studies in animal models can help in correlating MIC differences with therapeutic outcome, translating these results into interpretive breakpoints ultimately requires examining outcomes in therapeutic trials in humans.

To address these overlapping concerns, the National Committee on Clinical Laboratory Standards (NCCLS) established the Subcommittee for Antifungal Susceptibility Testing in 1982. Over many years and in collaboration with numerous workers, a standardized and reproducible method for susceptibility testing of *Candida* and *Cryptococcus* isolates has been developed. This method, known as NCCLS M27 (197), has recently been reviewed in detail (234). This method and its variants have been used in a variety of efforts to correlate outcome with MIC. The most extensive data are available for fluconazole, itraconazole, and flucytosine versus Candida; correlations for other organism-drug combinations are still under development. Tentative interpretive breakpoints for these three drugs when tested by M27 have recently been proposed and are summarized in Table 4. The detailed rationale supporting the fluconazole and itraconazole breakpoints has been described (233).

While an important development, these breakpoints are based on limited data and will require refinement. For fluconazole, the breakpoints are based substantially on experience with *C. albicans* in oropharyngeal candidiasis or in nonneutropenic patients with candidemia. Further, *C. krusei* is presumed to be intrinsically resistant to fluconazole, and its MICs need not be measured and or interpreted with this scale. Itraconazole breakpoints are based entirely on experience with a cyclodextrin-based solution in patients with oropharyngeal candidiasis. For these two drugs, the novel category S-DD implies that susceptibility depends on obtaining the maximal

---

TABLE 1 • Medically Significant *Candida* spp.[a]

Common Species	Less Common Species
C. albicans	*C. guilliermondii*
C. tropicalis	*C. kefyr* (*C. pseudotropicalis*)
C. glabrata (*T. glabrata*)	*C. famata*
C. parapsilosis	*C. haemulonii*
C. krusei	*C. norvegensis*
C. lusitaniae	*C. viswanathii*

[a]While many other species of *Candida* have been isolated from clinical specimens (162), their significance is unclear. The position of the newly described pathogenic species *C. dubliniensis* (280) in this rank order remains to be fully determined.

TABLE 2 • Characteristics of the Major *Candida* spp.

Species	Frequency	Virulence	Clinical Associations
C. albicans	42–65%	High	Most common in all settings
C. tropicalis	14–25%	High	Cancer
C. glabrata	8–15%	Low	Cancer
C. parapsilosis	7–18%	Variable	Plastic devices, hyperalimentation
C. krusei	1–4%	Low	Cancer
C. lusitaniae	1–2%	Low	Cancer

Frequency estimates are from references 1, 95, 201, 230, 312. Virulence and special clinical associations are discussed and cited in the text.

TABLE 3 • Susceptibility (MIC$_{50}$) of *Candida* spp. to Antifungal Agents

	Amphotericin B	Fluconazole	Itraconazole	Flucytosine
C. albicans	0.5	0.5	0.12	≤0.25
C. tropicalis	0.25	1	0.06	≤0.25
C. glabrata	0.5	16	0.25	≤0.25
C. parapsilosis	0.25	1	0.12	≤0.25
C. krusei	0.25	64	0.5	16
C. lusitaniae	≥1	2	0.25	≤0.25

Shown are typical species-specific MIC$_{50}$s (μg/mL) adapted from reports describing recent collections of clinical isolates (179, 214, 231, 232). MICs were obtained by the NCCLS M27 methodology (196) for all drugs but amphotericin B. As this method fails to detect amphotericin B–resistant *Candida* (231), the reported amphotericin B MICs were obtained by a more sensitive method based on use of Antibiotic Medium 3 in a agar-based testing format (306).

TABLE 4 • Interpretive Breakpoints[a] for Antifungal Susceptibility Testing

Antifungal Agent	Susceptible (S)	Susceptible–Dose Dependent (S-DD)	Intermediate (I)	Resistant (R)
Fluconazole	≤8	16–32		≥64
Itraconazole	≤0.125	0.25–0.5		≥1
Flucytosine	≤4		8–16	≥32

[a]Shown are the tentative breakpoints in μg/mL for *Candida* isolates against the indicated antifungal agents (197). See text for a discussion of the S-DD and I categories.

possible drug level. For fluconazole, this implies using doses of 400 mg/day or above in adults with normal renal function; for itraconazole, it implies that measures must be taken to ensure that enough drug is absorbed to produce a measurable blood level, preferably at least 0.5 μg/mL. Large datasets correlating MIC with outcome are not available for flucytosine, a situation further complicated by the fact the drug is rarely used as monotherapy. The interpretive breakpoints for this drug are based on a combination of historical and pharmacokinetic data (197). The intermediate (I) category for this drug differs from the S-DD category for the other two drugs; the designation I implies that insufficient data exist to permit clear categorization of the isolates as either susceptible or resistant. Fortunately, such isolates are uncommon.

Based on these breakpoints, the MICs in Table 3 can now be interpreted. *C. albicans, C. parapsilosis, C. tropicalis,* and *C. lusitaniae* are generally quite susceptible to fluconazole, whereas isolates of *C. glabrata* typically have an MIC that places them in fluconazole's S-DD category. For itraconazole, *C. glabrata, C. krusei,* and *C. lusitaniae* often have MICs in the S-DD category, while the other major species are generally susceptible. Finally, all species but *C. krusei* are generally susceptible to flucytosine.

Measuring meaningful amphotericin B MICs is problematic, and the NCCLS M27 method cannot reliably detect amphotericin B–resistant isolates (231). Recent modifications with use of Antibiotic Medium 3 may help resolve this problem (231), but additional work is required before convincing breakpoints can be established. At present, the available data indicate that isolates with M27 amphotericin B MICs above 1 μg/mL are likely resistant to amphotericin B.

Resistance to Antifungal Agents

Development of resistance to the azole antifungal agents is not uncommon during prolonged therapy of recurrent mucocutaneous disease, is discussed in Section Oropharyngeal and Gastrointestinal Candidiasis, and has been reviewed. Emergence of resistance during therapy in other settings appears uncommon (216a) but has been described in settings other than HIV-infected patients (177a, 194a). Resistance to amphotericin B is relatively uncommon (165b), but has been described for all species. Amphotericin B resistance is most commonly seen in *C. tropicalis, C. lusitaniae, C. parapsilosis* and *C. glabrata* isolates from immunocompromised patients treated extensively with amphotericin B (69, 73, 74, 113, 186, 188, 208, 270). Resistance to amphotericin B appears to be especially

common with *C. lusitaniae.* Resistance to the parent compound of amphotericin B implies that the isolate is also likely to be resistant to the newer lipid-based formulations of amphotericin B (144). Intrinsic or primary resistance to flucytosine may exist in any species of *Candida* (273). More importantly, susceptible isolates commonly acquire resistance during flucytosine monotherapy; thus flucytosine should not be used as monotherapy (222).

Combination Therapy

Combinations of flucytosine with either amphotericin B or an azole have been used, and these combinations often appear at least additive in vitro (24, 223). While rational because these drugs have different mechanisms of action, problems with flucytosine (lack of a widely available intravenous preparation and potential toxicities) have lead to strong interest in combinations of amphotericin B with an azole. Unfortunately, these agents have overlapping mechanisms of action, raising the possibility of antagonism, and the available information does not clarify the relevance of this theoretical possibility. Antagonism is definitely seen under some circumstances, especially when ketoconazole or itraconazole are combined with amphotericin B (246, 247, 249–251). In particular, preincubating the fungus with the azole often raises the apparent MIC to amphotericin B. In addition, modest antagonism can be seen in vitro when the drugs are used simultaneously with both at carefully selected sub-MIC concentrations (100). A recent review of this problem concluded that (*a*) interactions ranging from antagonism to synergy have been reported; (*b*) the interaction depends on the drugs selected, the target organism, and the precise experimental model; and thus (*c*) the available data cannot be generalized to infections in man (279). Relevant to *Candida* infections, antagonism is not seen with simultaneous exposure in vitro or in vivo to therapeutic concentrations of both fluconazole and amphotericin B (100, 277). Based on the accumulated data for this particular combination, intensive efforts to evaluate its clinical utility (including a large, multicenter, randomized trial) are ongoing. Meanwhile, combinations of azole and amphotericin B are not generally recommended outside the setting of a controlled clinical trial.

Clinical Use of Antifungal Susceptibility Testing

Given the problematic nature of antifungal susceptibility testing, routine testing of all isolates is not indicated. Rather, the following approach has been suggested (216):

1. All *Candida* isolates from deep sources should be identified to the species level—this information alone is quite valuable given the usual susceptibilities of *Candida* species (Table 3)
2. Periodic batch testing of hospital-acquired isolates could be used to establish a local antibiogram
3. Testing isolates from patients with oropharyngeal candidiasis refractory to standard doses of fluconazole can be used to differentiate true resistance from other causes of failure (see "Oropharyngeal and Gastrointestinal Candidiasis," below)
4. Testing selected isolates from deep sites may be useful in selecting alternatives to amphotericin B; in particular, determining the fluconazole MIC both provides insight into the likely susceptibility of the isolate to all currently available azole antifungal agents (fluconazole-resistant isolates are often resistant to the other azole antifungal agents) and is useful when considering a possible switch from amphotericin B to an azole

ANTIMICROBIAL THERAPY
General Concepts

Choice of an antifungal agent for a given infection is based on integration of relative drug toxicity, patient status, and microbiologic information. The available information for each particular clinical condition is summarized in the relevant discussion below. Amphotericin B is generally fungicidal in vitro for *Candida* isolates (320). The deoxycholate- and lipid-based derivatives of amphotericin B are similarly active against *Candida* (9, 54, 144), although higher doses of the lipid-based formations are required. The azoles (particularly fluconazole) are generally fungistatic against *Candida* (134).

Antifungal Dosing for *Candida* Infections in Pediatrics

Appropriate dosing regimens in pediatric patients are incompletely defined; appropriate dosing regimens in neonates have been recently reviewed (290). The kinetics of amphotericin B in neonates appear similar to those in adults, and therapy with 0.5 to 1.0 mg/kg/day is usually well tolerated (290). The half-life of flucytosine is variable but tends to be prolonged in neonates. While doses of 50 to 200 mg/kg/day have been used, careful monitoring of serum levels (levels should remain below 100 μg/mL) and consideration of reduced dosing frequency are important. One report found so much variation between patients (including patients with very slow elimination) that the authors recommended initially giving flucytosine every 24 h in newborns with adjustment after checking serum levels (17).

The pharmacokinetics of fluconazole have been studied in several groups of pediatric patients (36, 245, 253). In neonates in particular, the volume of distribution can be 2 to 3 times the 0.7 L/kg figure for adults. However, the volume of distribution is usually below 1 L/kg by 3 months of age. Clearance rates in children are both higher and lower than those seen in adults: neonates have a $t_{1/2}$ of 55 to 90 h, children above the age of 3 months have a $t_{1/2}$ of 21 to 22 h, and adults have a $t_{1/2}$ of approximately 30 h (108). Combining these data with the known progressive changes in renal function in newborns, suggests

that daily doses roughly double those used in adults would be appropriate for most children above 1 month of age. Neonates should be given this doubled dose every 72 h during the first 1 to 2 weeks of life and every 48 h during the remainder of the first month of life (36, 245).

Specific Situations

Nongenital Mucocutaneous Candidiasis

Oropharyngeal and Gastrointestinal Candidiasis. *Candida* is frequently found as an asymptomatic commensal of the human gastrointestinal tract (55, 241). However, compromise of immune and mucosal defenses by human immunodeficiency virus (HIV)-1 infection, chemotherapy-induced neutropenia, or direct mucosal damage permits direct local invasion by *Candida*. Oropharyngeal candidiasis, with or without esophageal involvement, is the most readily appreciated form of disease. Mild infections limited to the oropharynx often respond to topical agents used in a "swish and swallow" or oral troche format. Recognized topical therapies include nystatin (suspension of 100,000 U/mL, 4–6 mL four times daily; one to two flavored pastilles containing 200,000 U, four to five times daily) or clotrimazole (one 10-mg troche five times daily) (57, 254, 322). The nystatin suspension has a bitter taste, and most patients find the flavored nystatin pastilles or clotrimazole troches easier to tolerate. Recent work with a suspension of amphotericin B (68) has led to commercial release of a 100 mg/mL suspension that appears effective when given as 1 mL "swish and swallow" four times daily.

If the oropharyngeal disease is extensive, if the patient has AIDS, or if signs and symptoms of esophageal involvement are present, then systemic therapy is indicated. Ketoconazole (orally, 200–400 mg/day), itraconazole (orally, capsules or solution, 100–200 mg/day), fluconazole (orally, 100–400 mg/day), and amphotericin B (intravenously, 0.4–0.6 mg/kg/day) have all been used (165, 190, 259, 299, 310). Parenteral therapy with amphotericin B is effective but inconvenient and should only be used in extreme circumstances. Ketoconazole and itraconazole can be efficacious, but their bioavailability is unpredictable and may be diminished by lack of gastric acid (especially ketoconazole) or lack of intake with food (itraconazole capsules) (121, 291, 294). Ingestion of ketoconazole with an acidic beverage helps its absorption (52), and the solution of itraconazole in cyclodextrin improves the bioavailability and clinical efficacy of this drug (13, 109, 310). Absorption of the cyclodextrin-based itraconazole solution is further enhanced if it is taken on an empty stomach. On the other hand, fluconazole's ready oral bioavailability makes it attractive under many circumstances, and it is more efficacious than the topical therapies for disease limited to the oropharynx (93, 155, 224) or ketoconazole for *Candida* esophagitis (165). Fluconazole at 100 to 200 mg/day is adequate for disease limited to the oropharynx; 200–400 mg/day is appropriate in patients with esophageal involvement.

Patients with cancer usually experience mucocutaneous candidiasis only while severely immunosuppressed, but patients with advanced AIDS (CD4+ T-cell count < 100/mm³) have a permanent immunosuppression that leads to relapsing episodes of symptomatic oropharyngeal and esophageal disease. The agents discussed above are efficacious in these patients (111), although ketoconazole tends to be poorly absorbed because of frequent gastric atrophy in this setting (38). Patients with AIDS often experience a relapse of the infection, and some require frequent treatment and/or chronic suppressive therapy. Fluconazole is most often used in this setting at doses of 150 mg/week to 100–200 mg/day.

However, prolonged or repeated courses of therapy provide an opportunity for emergence of resistance. This problem has recently been reviewed and is most evident with fluconazole (235). The clinical situation is well understood, and this problem is seen after 1 to 2 years of either continuous or intermittent fluconazole therapy. The resistant infections are almost always due to *C. albicans*. Over time and under antifungal pressure, 5 to 10% of patients develop a mutant strain of *C. albicans* that no longer responds to fluconazole. This pattern (also described with ketoconazole in patients with chronic mucocutaneous candidiasis) is a function of both the underlying disease and the prolonged antifungal pressure in a host with a limited immune response. This problem develops with either intermittent or continuous antifungal therapy, and it is not currently known whether the likelihood of producing resistance differs for the two modes of use. Mutation to resistance can be overcome for a time by increasing the dose of fluconazole stepwise up to 800 mg/day (228). Unfortunately, once begun, this process almost inexorably results in fluconazole becoming completely ineffective (309a). In addition, fluconazole resistance is often (but not always) associated with cross-resistance to the other azole antifungal agents (19, 295). Susceptibility testing and review of the patient's medication history are helpful at this point: noncompliance and/or concomitant use of a medication that lowers the effective level of fluconazole (e.g., rifampin) must be eliminated.

If antifungal resistance seems likely, a variety of second-line strategies can be used. First, azole cross-resistance is not universal, and a trial of itraconazole (200 mg twice daily) is warranted. Second, topical solutions of amphotericin B (68) or azoles (180b) help some patients (68). The topical nystatin preparations may also be tried but anecdotally appear less helpful than amphotericin B solution. Third, parenteral amphotericin B (0.5–0.6 mg/kg/day) is usually, but not always (165a), effective. Flucytosine (50–100 mg/kg/day) is sometimes helpful in combination with amphotericin B. If the patient responds to amphotericin B, suppression may then be attempted with amphotericin B suspension. Other anecdotal remedies include (*a*) a maintenance regimen of amphotericin B (0.5–1 mg/kg) given two to four times weekly for suppression and (*b*) "swish and swallow" three to four times daily with with a 0.1 to 0.5% solution of gentian violet. All these approaches require close clinical observation and dose titration to produce clinical relief without introducing additional side effects. Finally, improvement of immune status is very helpful, and the striking immune recovery that may be seen with initiation of protease inhibitor therapy has been associated with marked clearance of the signs and symptoms of oropharyngeal candidiasis (180a, 325).

Candida overgrowth in the lower gastrointestinal tract has been associated with a variety of ill-defined syndromes; most prominently, persistent diarrhea occurs with heavy colonization of the fecal stream by *Candida* (116, 143, 170). While no firm diagnostic criteria exist, patients with (*a*) persistent diarrhea and (*b*) large numbers of yeast on stool Gram stain sometimes respond to therapy with nystatin (250,000–1,000,000 U three or four times daily) (170).

Candida can produce focal ulcerations in both the small and large bowel that can be associated with invasion of the submucosa (82). This is most common in immunocompromised patients, and therapy follows the principles discussed in the section "Candidemia and Acute Disseminated Candidiasis."

Skin and Nail Candidiasis. Macronodular skin lesions due to disseminated candidiasis can be seen in neutropenic cancer patients (32) but are relatively uncommon and are treated in the context of the disseminated *Candida* infection. In otherwise healthy individuals, *Candida* can affect the glabrous skin, usually in areas compromised by moisture. Thus, intertriginous candidiasis, diaper-related candidiasis, paronychia, and toe or finger web-space candidiasis (also known as erosio interdigitalis blastomycetica) are all well described (137). *Candida* can also cause folliculitis in regions compromised by moisture. Therapy should always begin by promoting local dryness, avoiding occlusion, and providing good local hygiene (12). In conjunction with these local measures, topical antifungal therapy is helpful, and many active agents are available, including the azoles (clotrimazole, econazole, ketoconazole, miconazole, oxiconazole, and sulconazole), ciclopirox olamine, haloprogin, and the polyenes (nystatin, amphotericin B). Of note, tolnaftate-based preparations are active against the dermatophytes but not against *Candida*. Short courses of topical steroids are occasionally needed for severe cases. Systemic therapy with fluconazole, ketoconazole, or itraconazole is rarely appropriate but can be considered for very widespread disease or other difficult situations (e.g., poorly controlled diabetes).

Candida can also cause onychomycosis (82a). General therapy for onychomycosis has long depended on griseofulvin and ketoconazole, but these drugs require prolonged therapy and have cure rates below 50% for toenail infections (237). These drugs have largely been supplanted by terbinafine and the newer azole antifungal agents for onychomycosis caused by a variety of agents (14, 63, 157, 237), but both terbinafine and griseofulvin have minimal in vitro activity against most isolates of *Candida* (23, 212), and neither has been efficacious in *Candida* onychomycosis (237, 239). On the other hand, itraconazole's excellent anti-*Candida* and antidermatophyte activity and its very long half-life in skin and nails have made it very attractive for all forms of onychomycosis (128, 182). In initial studies, it demonstrated excellent activity against *Candida* (100–200 mg/day for 3–6 months) (125). Subsequent studies have taken advantage of the fact that substantial concentrations of itraconazole are present up to 6 to 9 months after cessation of therapy and used pulse regimens of itraconazole in which the drug is given (200 mg twice daily) for 7 days and repeated monthly for 3 to 4 months (64). The nail may not appear completely normal at the end of the third or fourth monthly cycle of therapy because of the time required for new, healthy nail to grow and replace the diseased portions. Fluconazole is also active against *Candida* onychomycosis, but it is not retained by the nail and requires continuous and prolonged therapy (237).

Chronic Mucocutaneous Candidiasis

Because of the associated underlying immune defect, the persistent and recurrent *Candida* infections seen in patients with chronic mucocutaneous candidiasis are difficult to treat and require therapy with a systemic antifungal agent. This situation is analogous to recurrent oropharyngeal candidiasis in patients with advanced AIDS but differs in the universal need for continuous therapy in chronic mucocutaneous candidiasis patients. Therapeutic options are similar to those for patients with AIDS, and ketoconazole, itraconazole, and fluconazole have all been used successfully (43, 150). The required doses are similar and should be adjusted to find the minimal effective dose for each patient. Resistance to these azole antifungal agents can develop (133, 260) (see "Oropharyngeal and Gastrointestinal Candidiasis" above for details). Immunomodulatory approaches have also proven successful in some patients (151).

Genital Candidiasis

Vulvovaginal candidiasis (VVC) affects up to 75% of women during their reproductive years (136, 149). In contrast to oropharyngeal candidiasis, VVC is not an opportunistic infection and affects healthy women, and most attacks occur in the absence of recognizable precipitating factors (263). A small subpopulation of women suffer from recurrent, repeated bouts of VVC, again without known causal factors. This latter group is thought to reflect an immunologic breakdown in local protective mucosal defense mechanisms, and frequent relapse is not due to resistant *Candida* or lack of protective lactobacilli (89). Most (80–95%) infections are caused by *C. albicans* isolates that are predictably susceptible to azole antifungal agents. Some evidence exists of an increased frequency of infections caused by non-*albicans Candida* species, especially *C. glabrata, C. parapsilosis,* and others (132), but the true frequency and epidemiology of this phenomenon is uncertain at present.

An essential part of management of VVC is accurate diagnosis. Millions of women each year receive antifungal agents unnecessarily because of incorrect self- and practitioner-made diagnosis. Topical and systemic therapy is not entirely benign, and local application of azole antifungal agents may induce vulvar contact dermatitis. All treatment regimens should be preceded by microscopic (saline and 10% KOH) confirmation (27). Cultures should be obtained (*a*) from patients with compatible clinical syndromes and negative microscopy and (*b*) to document the rare instances of antifungal resistance.

Treatment of VVC in the 1990s predominantly involves the imidazole and triazole agents available as topical or oral preparations (Table 5). Azoles achieve higher success rates over shorter periods than nystatin vaginal suppositories or creams. Little evidence exists that the choice of formulation of the topical azoles influences cure rates. Topical agents previously prescribed for 7 to 14 days are now available for single-dose or short-course regimens. Topical azoles appropriately prescribed are remarkably free of systemic side effects and toxicity.

The oral azoles used for systemic therapy are ketoconazole, itraconazole, and fluconazole, but only fluconazole (150 mg as a single dose) is approved by the FDA for this indication in the United States. Oral azoles are at least as effective as topical agents and more convenient, popular, and free of local side effects (255, 264). Side effects of fluconazole are rare but include gastrointestinal upset, headache, and rash. More serious hepatotoxicity precludes widespread use of ketoconazole (171).

In selecting an antifungal agent for therapy, it is useful to distinguish uncomplicated and complicated VVC. By far, most episodes of VVC are uncomplicated. These are sporadic, mild-to-moderate infections caused by *C. albicans* that occur

TABLE 5 • Therapy for Vaginal Candidiasis: Topical Agents

Drug	Formulation	Dosage Regimen
[a]Butoconazole	2% cream	5 g/day × 3 days
[a]Clotrimazole	1% cream	5 g/day × 7–14 days
	100 mg vaginal tablet	1 tablet/day × 7 days
	100 mg vaginal tablet	2 tablet/day × 3 days
	500 mg vaginal tablet	1 tablet/day × 1 days
[a]Miconazole	2% cream	5 g/day × 7 days
	100 mg vaginal suppository	1 suppository × 7 days
	200 mg vaginal suppository	1 suppository/day × 3 days
	1200 mg vaginal suppository	1 suppository/day × 1 day
Econazole	150 mg vaginal tablet	1 tablet/day × 3 days
Fenticonazole	2% cream	5 g/day × 7 days
[a]Tioconazole	2% cream	5 g/day × 3 days
	6.5% cream	5 g/day × 1 day
Terconazole	0.4% cream	5 g/day × 7 days
	0.8% cream	5 g/day × 3 days
	80 mg vaginal suppository	80 mg/day × 3 days
Nystatin	100,000 U vaginal tablet	1 tablet/day × 14 days

[a]Available in at least one form in the United States without a prescription.

in normal hosts who lack predisposing factors. Uncomplicated infections can be treated successfully with any of the available topical or oral antifungal agents, including short-course and single-dose regimens. Complicated infections (*a*) have a moderate-to-severe clinical presentation, (*b*) are recurrent (four or more episodes per year), (*c*) are caused by non-*albicans Candida* species, or (*d*) occur in abnormal hosts (e.g., diabetic patients with poor glucose control). Complicated infections are far less likely to respond to abbreviated courses of therapy (264) and should be treated more intensively for 7 to 14 days to achieve clinical and mycologic response. Non-*albicans Candida* species are less sensitive in vitro to azoles and less likely to respond clinically (see "Monotherapy," above). In particular, *C. glabrata* is a vaginal pathogen that frequently fails to respond to azole agents. Encouraging results have been obtained using one 600-mg boric acid capsule vaginally each day for 14 days (these must be prepared in gelatin capsules by a local pharmacy) (265) or topical flucytosine (131).

Recurrent VVC is usually caused by susceptible strains of *C. albicans.* Although more-intensive prolonged induction therapy lasting up to 14 days invariably induces remission, the fungistatic nature of the available agents combined with persistence of the underlying defect makes relapse almost inevitable without a maintenance antifungal regimen. Successful regimens include ketoconazole 100 mg daily (261) or fluconazole 100 mg weekly (262).

Male genital candidiasis presents in two forms. Most commonly, a transient pruritic and erythematous penile cutaneous reaction follows unprotected intercourse with exposure to *Candida* antigens present in the vagina and represents an hypersensitivity reaction. Successful treatment entails eradicating the yeast in the vagina. True superficial penile invasive mycotic infection occurs infrequently, usually in diabetic and uncircumcised males who develop balanoposthitis that responds promptly to topical or systemic azole therapy.

Candidemia and Acute Disseminated Candidiasis

Detection of candidemia is the most specific currently available marker of disseminated or invasive candidiasis. Unfortunately, the term *candidemia* describes a broad range of infections ranging from short-lived catheter-related fungemia in nonneutropenic ICU patients to persistent candidemia of uncertain (but probably gastrointestinal) origin in neutropenic cancer patients. Overall mortality is strongly controlled by the patient's underlying illness (130, 156), but candidemia has been associated with a 38% attributable mortality over and beyond that of the underlying disease (309). Further, an extensive analysis of the impact of microbiological factors on the outcome of nosocomial bloodstream infections found that infection due to *Candida* was the only specific infection that was independently associated with increased mortality in a multivariate analysis (218a).

In the nonneutropenic patient, candidemia is related to the presence of an intravascular catheter in up to 80% of patients (230). In many of the remaining cases, an alternative source (urine, abscess) is apparent. Removal of all intravascular catheters appears to help clear the bloodstream (156, 229), and

some patients have been cured with this simple approach (153). However, even the most benign episodes of candidemia can involve subsequent hematogenous spread, causing such disparate infections as endophthalmitis, osteomyelitis, and brain abscess (see the relevant sections on these infections, below). Indeed, it was observed in a study of *C. glabrata* fungemia that the patients most likely to have a poor outcome were those who had persistent low grade fever (< 102.5 F) in association with a gradually declining clinical course (28a). Thus, all episodes of candidemia are currently believed to merit some form of therapy (76).

Amphotericin B has long been the standard approach (189), and two prospective randomized trials (217, 230) and two recent retrospective reviews (10a, 201) have compared it with fluconazole in this setting. Taken together, these studies showed that amphotericin B (0.5–0.6 mg/kg/day) and fluconazole (400 mg/day), both given for approximately 2 weeks, do not differ significantly as therapy for candidemia in nonneutropenic patients. However, this conclusion applies *only* to nonneutropenic patients and is based largely on *C. albicans* fungemia. The data are less robust for non-*albicans* species, but similar trends hold. However, as noted above, the non-*albicans* species have higher fluconazole MICs in particular, and higher antifungal doses may be required for optimal outcome. This point is especially pertinent to *C. glabrata* and fluconazole, and some clinicians feel that effective treatment of *C. glabrata* isolates with fluconazole requires a minimum of 800 mg/day (12 mg/kg) in adults with normal renal function. A higher dose may be of value even for *C. albicans;* the results of one noncomparative study suggest that 800 mg/day may produce a better response rate than 400 mg/day for *C. albicans* fungemia (107). On a practical basis, detection of fungemia in a nonneutropenic patient should prompt initiation of either amphotericin B (0.6–0.7 mg/kg/day) or fluconazole (800 mg/day). If the isolate is found to be *C. albicans,* then fluconazole (400–800 mg/day) may be continued. Otherwise, high-dose therapy should be continued while awaiting final identification and susceptibility testing of the isolate. Combinations of either fluconazole or amphotericin B with flucytosine (100–150 mg/kg/day) may be useful in some patients, but the precise role of these combinations is not clear. The combination of fluconazole with amphotericin B is intriguing, but the theoretical potential for antagonism between these agents (see "Combination Therapy," above) requires conducting controlled trials of this approach in man. While these studies are under way, this combination is not recommended for general use. The required duration of therapy is not certain, but this form of candidiasis has been treated successfully by giving the selected agent(s) for approximately 2 weeks after the last positive blood culture. With this approach, the rate of subsequent presentation with a recurrent infection at a hematogenously seeded site is about 1% (230).

In the neutropenic patient, candidemia may take a more subacute, but nonetheless deadly, course. Although the gut has on occasion been implicated as the source of fungemia in nonneutropenic patients (28a), it appears likely that the gastrointestinal tract is the most common source of low-grade, persistent candidemia in neutropenic patients. Partial clearance of the blood by the liver and spleen explains the well-known syndrome of hepatosplenic, or chronic disseminated, candidiasis (141). The organism can also spread to virtually every other organ of the body (135).

Therapy for candidemia in the neutropenic patient is less well understood. Removal of intravenous catheters may still be important (166), but the potential for a gastrointestinal source raises the possibility that the therapeutic effect of catheter exchange will not be as striking. One notable exception is a high association of *C. parapsilosis* fungemia with intravascular catheters in cancer patients (102). Recovery of marrow function is critical, and no therapeutic approach is consistently successful in the face of persistent leukopenia. Most experience is with amphotericin B (0.6–1.0 mg/kg/day) until recovery of marrow function. The most appropriate dose of amphotericin B is not certain, but the non-*albicans* species appear to require larger doses (0.8–1.0 mg/kg/day) of amphotericin B. This appears to be especially true of *C. krusei* (104) and *C. glabrata,* the two species that are also least susceptible to fluconazole. Data comparing this approach with fluconazole are limited, but one recent retrospective matched cohort study found that median daily doses of 400 mg for fluconazole and 0.6 mg/kg for amphotericin B yielded similar outcomes in a mixed group of neutropenic and nonneutropenic cancer patients (10). As always, flucytosine has been given to some patients, but its potential for marrow suppression and the lack of a readily available intravenous formulation lessen its attractiveness.

Presumptive Therapy for Disseminated Candidiasis. In neutropenic patients with persistent fever despite several days of broad-spectrum antimicrobial agents, empirical amphotericin B therapy for presumed fungal infections is well accepted (220). Although *Candida* is probably the most common fungus in this situation and fluconazole might well be efficacious, amphotericin B remains the favored agent because of its activity against molds such as *Aspergillus*. Itraconazole might also be considered, but the unpredictable absorption of the capsule form of the drug makes it unattractive.

Disseminated candidiasis in nonneutropenic patients is more poorly understood but probably has a precandidemia phase in at least some patients. The typical setting is a febrile ICU patient with an elevated APACHE II score (154), prolonged use of broad-spectrum antibiotics, parenteral hyperalimentation, central venous catheters, and recent surgery (especially surgery involving the gastrointestinal tract) (156). If alternative explanations for the persistent fever such as pulmonary emboli, cholecystitis, sinusitis, drug allergy, and wound infection are eliminated, the possibility of undetected disseminated candidiasis arises. The most helpful clue in this regard is that colonization with *Candida* at any site definitely increases the likelihood of disseminated candidiasis (219). However, no clear guidelines exist for initiating therapy in this setting. A reasonable approach is to consider use of empirical antifungal therapy in patients with (*a*) several days of unexplained fever, (*b*) at least 7 days of ICU care, (*c*) use of broad-spectrum antibiotics for at least 4 days, (*d*) a nontunneled central venous catheter, and (*e*) colonization with *Candida* in at least one site. If a decision is made to treat such a patient, a full

dose of either fluconazole or amphotericin B should be used. Like all empirical therapies, this approach requires continuous reevaluation of the patient, and therapy should be discontinued after 3 to 4 days if no response is seen.

Chronic Disseminated Candidiasis

Therapy for chronic disseminated or hepatosplenic candidiasis has long depended on prolonged therapy with amphotericin B alone, but this therapy has not been uniformly successful (122). Recent data demonstrate that courses of 0.5 to 1.0 g of amphotericin B followed by a protracted course of fluconazole (200–400 mg/day for 2–14 months) are associated with cure rates above 90% (8, 146). Indeed, use of fluconazole is sometimes successful for this disease when use of amphotericin B was not (8, 146). Lipid-associated amphotericin B has also been used successfully (305b). Provided that the lesions have stabilized, the patient is clinically improved, and antifungal therapy is continued, anti-neoplastic therapies (including those that will induce neutropenia) may be continued (305a).

Neonatal Candidiasis

While critically ill children can develop systemic candidiasis in a pattern just like that seen in adults, two distinct *Candida* syndromes can be defined in neonates, especially in preterm, low-birth-weight neonates. The most serious of these syndromes is neonatal systemic candidiasis. Developing either via ascending infection of the uterine contents prior to birth or from colonization acquired during passage through the birth canal, hematogeneous dissemination of *Candida* presents in the first days or weeks of life with symptoms identical to those of neonatal bacterial sepsis (84, 103, 139, 290). Involvement of the lung, skin, and particularly the central nervous system (83) is common, and involvement of almost all organs has been described. Amphotericin B (0.5–1.0 mg/kg/day to a total of 10–25 mg/kg), with or without flucytosine, has long been the therapy of choice (see introductory discussion above on dosing considerations in the neonate). The excellent penetration of amphotericin B into the cerebrospinal fluid in infants (17) is presumably part of the reason that amphotericin B alone is often successful. The role of the lipid formulations of amphotericin B is unknown in this setting. Fluconazole is also attractive in this setting and has been used successfully at doses of 6 to 12 mg/kg day (296). Given the current data on optimal dosing in adults and the differences in kinetics between children and adults, doses of 12 mg/kg given every 24 to 72 h (see above for a discussion of dosing frequency in pediatrics) appear suitable. Data comparing amphotericin B and fluconazole in this setting are, however, lacking.

Neonatal or congenital cutaneous candidiasis is distinct from the syndrome of neonatal systemic candidiasis. Neonates with congenital cutaneous candidiasis present within a few hours of birth with a diffuse maculopapular, erythematous rash involving almost any part of the skin (40, 103, 140, 142, 243). The rash can evolve to produce pustular or vesicular lesions with subsequent desquamation. Culture and microscopic examination of scrapings of the skin will reveal *Candida* species, usually *C. albicans*. If the affected infant is preterm (<1500 g), systemic involvement is frequent, and the infant should be evaluated repeatedly with blood, urine, and cerebrospinal fluid cultures to rule out neonatal systemic candidiasis (86, 140). On the other hand, this process in full-term infants is usually, but not always (20), limited to the skin and gastrointestinal tract. In this case, topical and oral therapy with agents such as nystatin or an azole antifungal often appears adequate. Systemic therapy as described for neonatal systemic candidiasis would presumably also be efficacious and should certainly be instituted promptly if there is any suspicion of systemic involvement.

Urinary Candidiasis

Urinary candidiasis is manifested by candiduria and involves infection at any of multiple anatomic levels in the urinary tract from kidney to urethra. *Candida* urinary tract infections account for 9% of nosocomial urinary tract infections, and 90% of *Candida* urinary tract infections are related to urinary catheters or instrumentation (268, 307, 319). While numerous host and treatment factors play a role in the pathogenesis of candiduria, a history of present or recent bladder catheterization, other indwelling devices, and use of broad-spectrum antibiotics is found in 85 to 90% of candiduric patients (91, 120, 269). Interpretation of candiduria is difficult, and recent work from an in vivo model has shown that no specific number of CFU/ml can be used to identify true infection (198a). Candiduria in catheterized subjects usually represents catheter or superficial bladder colonization only, is extremely common, almost invariably asymptomatic, and of little clinical significance. Asymptomatic candiduria in this context should not be treated, since ascending or invasive *Candida* infections are rare (11). Asymptomatic candiduria should only be treated in neutropenic patients, in those undergoing elective urinary instrumentation, and following renal transplantation. In contrast to *Candida* infections elsewhere, *C. albicans* is responsible for only 50 to 60% of candiduria episodes, with *C. glabrata* causing 20 to 30%. Other non-*albicans* species also commonly cause *Candida* urinary tract infections, and mixed infection with two or more *Candida* spp. are frequent in catheterized patients.

Symptomatic lower urinary tract infections due to *Candida* are rare and should be treated, especially in noncatheterized patients. Therapeutic options include oral fluconazole (200 mg/day for 7 days) (298), intravenous amphotericin B (0.3 mg/kg single dose) (90), or conventional amphotericin B (0.3 mg/kg for 5–7 days) (87). Topical amphotericin B bladder irrigation (1 L/day of a solution of 50 mg of amphotericin B per liter of sterile water or D5W through a triple-lumen catheter for 7–14 days) is an effective but inconvenient option (242), although shorter courses may prove to be an alternative (168). Ketoconazole and itraconazole achieve poor urinary drug concentrations and produce unreliable therapeutic results (321). Oral flucytosine although effective is rarely indicated because of emergence of resistance.

Ascending pyelonephritis is an uncommon serious infection that may be complicated by candidemia and disseminated infection (11). Therapy consists of relieving any urinary obstruction and use of fluconazole or systemic amphotericin B in doses used for disseminated candidiasis as described above

("Candidemia and Acute Disseminated Candidiasis"). Finally, candiduria may result from renal candidiasis secondary to previous or ongoing candidemia (hematogenous pyelonephritis). Therapy is again identical to that for disseminated candidiasis.

Candida Endophthalmitis

Lesions compatible with *Candida* endophthalmitis were seen in 15% of patients enrolled in a recent candidemia study (230), and other studies have reported values between 9 and 37% (72). The classic lesion is a white, fluffy mass that extends from the retina into the vitreous, but a variety of nonclassic lesions (Roth spots, uveitis, hypopyon, iritis, papillitis, retinal detachment, and ciliary body abscesses) have been described with this infection (77), and the most common lesion is a small, white chorioretinal lesion without extension into the vitreous (72). Progressive endophthalmitis can lead to loss of vision, so examination after pupillary dilatation is a critical part of the evaluation of any patient with candidemia. *Candida* endophthalmitis can also present without a clinically evident episode of candidemia and should be considered in the differential diagnosis of suggestive retinal lesions in patients with recent risk factors for candidemia (207a).

Therapy for lesions compatible with *Candida* endophthalmitis is not standardized. The common small white chorioretinal lesions seen in patients with candidemia appear to respond readily to most available agents (72), but larger lesions or infections that develop following trauma or surgery may require more aggressive and targeted therapy. Penetration of amphotericin B into the eye is variable but generally poor (92, 205). Despite this, courses of at least 1 g of amphotericin B have been curative in more than 90% of infected eyes (77). However, intravenous therapy is not uniformly successful, and intravitreal amphotericin B following vitrectomy has been helpful either as monotherapy or in conjunction with systemic therapy. Intravitreal doses of 5 to 10 mg have been used (39, 46, 129, 211, 271).

Fluconazole diffuses well into all parts of the eye (204, 244, 288), and experience with this agent as therapy for *Candida* endophthalmitis has recently been reviewed (4). Fluconazole given as sole therapy at approximately 200 mg/day for about 2 months cured 15 of 16 infected eyes. Fluconazole was also used effectively following short (~200 mg total dose) courses of amphotericin B. Patients requiring vitrectomy generally have more severe disease, and fluconazole monotherapy was curative in five eyes after vitrectomy when given at approximately 200 mg/day for about 3 months. If present in the infected eye, implant removal appears critical to resolution of the infection (147).

Ketoconazole and itraconazole penetrate the eye less readily than fluconazole in animal models (244). Ketoconazole has been used successfully in a small number of patients, but no meaningful clinical experience with itraconazole has been reported (39, 105).

Candida Endocarditis, Pericarditis, and Suppurative Phlebitis

Candida can cause both native and prosthetic valve endocarditis. Although medical therapy alone is occasionally curative

(85, 118, 324), the inability of even moderately prolonged courses of amphotericin B to cure either form of endocarditis consistently (199, 289) has led to the general recommendation that most patients be treated with a combination of valve replacement and lifelong antifungal therapy (195). The literature on this approach mostly reports use of amphotericin B followed by one of the azoles. While both ketoconazole and itraconazole have been used, fluconazole has been the most frequently used oral agent. Optimal doses of the drugs in combination with surgery are unknown: typical courses are about 2 g of amphotericin B (101) and then an azole (most often fluconazole) at 200 to 400 mg/day (45, 195, 199). Fluconazole has also been used successfully as the sole antifungal therapy in some patients (230). As with other forms of candidiasis, flucytosine is occasionally added to the base regimen, but its overall utility is uncertain. This strategy is applicable to both adults and children (183), although medical therapy alone is often pursued in neonates because of their complicated, overlapping medical problems (85, 183, 324). Late recurrence has been described even several years after the initial episode (140a), emphasizing the need for prolonged followup.

The ready oral availability of fluconazole has made it especially attractive in efforts to use medical therapy alone. Most cases of *Candida* endocarditis are caused by *C. albicans* or *C. parapsilosis,* two species that are generally susceptible to fluconazole. On the basis of in vitro data and some animal models (320), a number of investigators have now successfully used chronic suppressive therapy with fluconazole as part of a medical strategy in selected patients with both native (48, 127, 240) and prosthetic valve endocarditis (48, 300). This long-term suppressive approach has typically followed a course of amphotericin B in patients for whom cardiac surgery is judged unusually risky. The optimal dose and duration of therapy is uncertain; typical courses have been about 2 g of amphotericin B and then fluconazole used indefinitely at 200 to 400 mg/day.

Candida infections of the transvenous portions of cardiac pacemakers have been described and appear to require both surgical removal of the infected device followed by moderately prolonged systemic antifungal therapy (140b).

Purulent *Candida* pericarditis has recently been reviewed (252), and a combination of surgical drainage (pericardiocentesis or pericardiectomy) and prolonged antifungal therapy is required. Most experience is with amphotericin B (81, 112, 252), and the utility of other antifungal agents is unknown.

Persistent candidemia is sometimes due to *Candida* suppurative phlebitis of either central or peripheral veins. In the case of peripheral phlebitis, the involved vein may merely appear thrombosed and is not always tender. Treatment by removal of the catheter; aspiration, resection, or incision and drainage of the vein; and a short course of amphotericin B (total dose of 200–500 mg) is generally effective (28, 286, 301). Surgical resection, aspiration, or drainage often appear to be critical to successful therapy. Fluconazole has been employed successfully in a small number of reported cases (95a).

When a central vein is involved, surgery is not an option, and several authors have reported successful outcomes following amphotericin B to a total of about 30 mg/kg (i.e., about 2 g in a typical adult) (26, 138, 275). Systemic anticoagulation was used in some, but not all, of the described patients.

Candida infections of arteriovenous dialysis fistulas have recently been reviewed (203). These infections are very rare, and effective therapy appears to require both antifungal therapy and removal of the fistula.

Candida Infections of the Peritoneum, Gallbladder, and Pancreas

Candida can cause peritonitis in two settings. First, patients undergoing peritoneal dialysis may develop catheter-related peritonitis. Removal of the dialysis catheter is usually required for successful therapy (79, 192, 193), and some patients have been cured via this maneuver alone (21, 80, 276). Short courses of amphotericin B have been used by both the intravenous and intraperitoneal routes as antifungal therapy. Intraperitoneal therapy with infusate containing amphotericin B (0.5–5 mg/mL) has been recommended but is often associated with significant abdominal pain and development of adhesions (15, 80). Recently, numerous reports have documented the utility of fluconazole, sometimes in combination with flucytosine, as therapy for dialysis catheter-related peritonitis (58, 169, 192, 283). These reports have generally used 100 to 200 mg/day of fluconazole combined with flucytosine given as 15 mg/kg after hemodialysis or 50 to 100 mg/L in the peritoneal dialysate (79, 192).

Candida-related peritonitis is also seen following intraabdominal events such as surgical opening or spontaneous perforation of the bowel. Peritoneal cultures in this setting are often polymicrobial, and the significance of *Candida* in the culture is not always obvious. As described above for involvement of the biliary tree or pancreas, however, the potential for untreated *Candida* to cause disease has been clearly demonstrated (5, 44, 266). While no single set of criteria identify the patients in whom *Candida* is significant, factors such as presence of fungemia, increased severity of illness, multiple operations, pancreatic involvement, and heavy or pure growth of *Candida* from peritoneal cultures strongly suggest that antifungal therapy will be critical to the patient's outcome (5, 44, 227). Examination of biopsy specimens for evidence of tissue invasion has also be used to diagnose and monitor the course of disease (158). As a rule, isolation of *Candida* from patients with non-catheter-related intraabdominal infections should not be ignored. Amphotericin B at widely varying doses (but averaging 0.5–1 g total) has been used to treat this condition (5, 44, 266), as has fluconazole at 200 to 400 mg/day (2, 158, 283). Flucytosine has also been used, but as in other forms of candidiasis, its actual utility is unclear.

Candida may infect the gallbladder, biliary tree, or pancreas (135). It is isolated from bile in up to 2% of cholecystectomies (115), but mere isolation of the organism does not mean that it is pathogenic. However, if the patient has biliary obstruction or gangrenous cholecystitis, then isolation of *Candida* should not be ignored, and systemic therapy with amphotericin B or fluconazole should be given. Amphotericin B achieves bile concentrations that are 2- to 7-fold higher than serum concentrations (1a). There are no meaningful data comparing these agents in this setting. *Candida* fungus balls can obstruct the biliary collecting system and may require surgical removal (115, 176).

Involvement of both the pancreatic parenchyma and pancreatic pseudocysts has recently been reviewed (7, 148). *Candida* is often present in combination with enteric bacteria in these processes, although *Candida* is at times the sole agent isolated (236). In this setting, the relative pathogenic roles of the isolated *Candida* and concomitantly isolated bacteria are not certain, but the accumulated literature makes it clear that initiation of antifungal therapy is sometimes critical. After suitable debridement and/or drainage, amphotericin B at standard systemic doses (0.5–1.0 mg/kg/day to a total of 1–2 g) has been used most commonly. The utility and comparative value of other agents in this setting is unknown.

Candida Osteomyelitis, Arthritis, and Mediastinitis

Candida seems to have a special predilection for causing osteomyelitis. The infection is usually hematogenous (although contiguous infection related to surgical procedures such as median sternotomies is well described), usually involves the vertebral column, and can even occur following reasonable courses of antifungal therapy for presumed or proven candidemia (88, 97, 278). Osteomyelitis is also quite common as part of the widely disseminated disease seen in neonatal systemic candidiasis (see "Neonatal Candidiasis"), and therapy for the systemic disease should be adequate for the bony component. In general, a variety of therapeutic strategies have been successful in adults and children. Surgical debridement can be helpful but is not required (97). Flucytosine monotherapy (78, 96) has occasionally been successful, but most authors have used amphotericin B as the primary agent. Courses of 1 to 1.5 g have usually (6, 78, 88, 94, 97), but not always (88), been successful. A number of authors have followed a course of amphotericin B with 6 to 12 months of ketoconazole (200–600 mg/day) (6, 97) or fluconazole (150 mg/day) (278).

There is also some experience with azoles as sole therapy. Ketoconazole at 50 mg/day for 3 months was used successfully in a 3-year-old boy with phalangeal osteomyelitis (18) and at 400 to 1600 mg/day for 3 to 7 months in adults (71). Fluconazole was successful at 200 to 400 mg/day for 6 to 12 months in three brief reports (126, 278, 282) and at 400 mg/day for 1 month (163). However, fluconazole at 400 mg/day failed as therapy for zygomatic osteomyelitis (16) and as therapy for sternal osteomyelitis in a second patient (62). There is no published experience with itraconazole for *Candida* osteomyelitis, but successful itraconazole therapy for *Aspergillus* osteomyelitis (295a) suggests that it would also likely be efficacious for Candida.

Like osteomyelitis, *Candida* arthritis can develop in adults, children, and neonates (22, 218, 256) and has developed as long as 1 year after an episode of fungemia (281). This topic has recently been reviewed (256). If the infection involves a prosthetic joint, resection arthroplasty is required (287). Amphotericin B has been used intravenously at quite variable doses; as little as 200 mg and as much as 2 g has sometimes been needed (22). Intraarticular amphotericin B has also been used

at variable doses. Typically, 5 to 10 mg is injected at intervals in association with joint aspiration (22). Flucytosine at standard doses has been used with amphotericin B (256). Experience with the azole antifungal agents is limited. Ketoconazole was used successfully at 200 to 800 mg/day (75) but was ineffective at 800 mg/day in another report (145). Fluconazole (200 mg/day) was effective in a patient with prosthetic joint arthritis who had not responded to ketoconazole at 400 mg/day (287). Fluconazole (400 mg/day for 12 weeks) was curative in a patient with native joint arthritis (207). A 7-month course of therapy at 400 mg/day was effective in a second case of native joint arthritis (308a). In this case, simultaneous synovial fluid and blood drug concentrations of 20 mg/mL were reported, thus documenting good drug penetration. Finally, fluconazole was effective at 5 mg/kg/day with 150 mg/kg/day flucytosine in an infant (206) with native joint arthritis.

Mediastinitis due to *Candida* is rare and has recently been reviewed (53a). Based on a small number of cases, surgical debridement followed by either amphotericin B or fluconazole appears suitable.

Candida Meningitis

Three forms of *Candida* meningitis can be identified. First, patients with acute hematogenously disseminated candidiasis may develop involvement of the brain and meninges (67, 174, 209). This occurs most often in neonatal systemic candidiasis (see that section) but can also occur in adults. The available literature on this condition focuses almost entirely on therapy with amphotericin B, often in combination with flucytosine because of the latter agent's ability to penetrate the blood-brain barrier (41, 51, 258). Amphotericin B is usually given intravenously, although occasional patients have required intrathecal therapy, presumably to overcome the poor penetration of amphotericin B into the cerebrospinal fluid. Fluconazole with flucytosine was successful in one case (177), and fluconazole monotherapy was used in another report (116a). Much less commonly, patients with one more risk factors for hematogenous candidiasis present with the clinical picture of a chronic meningitis that otherwise would suggest tuberculosis or one of the endemic mycoses (1, 2). The small number of patients with this form of infection have recently been reviewed, and amphotericin B, sometimes with flucytosine, and sometimes followed by a course of fluconazole were variously used (46a, 297).

Finally, *Candida* can produce meningitis following neurosurgical procedures, especially in association with cerebrospinal fluid devices such as shunts or drains (53, 202). The findings are quite similar to those of bacterial meningitis, and device removal plus antifungal therapy is required. Intravenous amphotericin B is usually effective, but some patients require addition of flucytosine or intrathecal amphotericin B to the regimen. Regimens of amphotericin B (0.5 mg/kg/day) and flucytosine (375 mg/kg/day) for 3 or more weeks have been recommended (202). Both failures and successes have been reported with fluconazole (59, 202), thus precluding any judgment on its utility in this setting. However, the excellent penetration of fluconazole into the cerebrospinal fluid suggests that it might be useful in this setting.

In addition to these forms of *Candida* meningitis, *Candida* brain abscess (30, 42), epidural abscess (33), and intramedullary abscess (173) have been described. Treatment of these rare conditions has been with amphotericin B and flucytosine, sometimes followed by oral azole therapy.

Candida Pneumonia

The most common form of respiratory candidiasis is colonization of the upper airways, especially in intubated patients. Finding *Candida* in cultures of respiratory secretions does not, however, usually mean that the patient has *Candida* pneumonia (80a). Rather, such cultures usually represent only colonization and should be interpreted in the context of the patient's overall status. In afebrile patients, they may be ignored, but they increase the likelihood of disseminated candidiasis in patients with unexplained fever (see "Presumptive Therapy for Disseminated Candidiasis"). Indeed, primary (or bronchogenic) *Candida* pneumonia appears to be quite uncommon and was documented in only 0.2 to 0.4% of patients in two large autopsy series (123, 181). The syndrome of primary *Candida* pneumonia is principally defined on the basis of autopsy results, and little certain knowledge about suitable therapy is available. Since these patients tend to be quite ill, treatment that follows the guidelines for acute disseminated candidiasis would appear suitable.

Candida may also seed the lung during hematogenous dissemination and thus produce pneumonia. This appears to occur most often in neutropenic patients, and therapy follows the general guidelines for treatment of disseminated candidiasis given above ("Candidemia and Acute Disseminated Candidiasis").

Finally, laryngeal candidiasis associated with respiratory stridor has been described. Therapy with amphotericin B (89a, 302a) and fluconazole (305c) has been successful.

Alternative Therapies

Augmentation of host defenses is an intriguing approach to the problem of refractory *Candida* infections, but work in this area is still preliminary at best. Combining such cytokines as interferon-γ (159), granulocyte colony-stimulating factor (G-CSF) (119), and granulocyte macrophage colony-stimulating factor (GM-CSF) (184) with an antifungal agent lessens the course of the infection in animal models of disseminated candidiasis. Experience in animals with M-CSF has been mixed (49). The published experience in man is extremely limited and focuses on use of interferon-γ in patients with chronic granulomatous disease (117). Use of white blood cell transfusions in persistently neutropenic patients has long been of interest for refractory infections of all types. However, problems with obtaining enough cells for transfusion and with transfusion-related side effects diminished interest in this technique (274). Recent work in which white cell donors are treated with G-CSF to augment the number and function of the collected cells is intriguing (70), as are studies showing that ex vivo manipulation of neutrophils with cytokines extends their functional lifetime (152). However, broad application of these tools awaits much additional work. Finally, transfer of *Candida*-specific immunity to pa-

tients with chronic mucocutaneous candidiasis by administration of *Candida*-specific transfer factor has been associated with long-lasting remissions of that disease, which suggests that highly focused manipulation of the immune system may be helpful in specific situations (151).

ENDPOINTS FOR MONITORING THERAPY

Candida is not a fastidious organism and is readily grown from most sites of local infection with any standard culture technique. The notable exception is blood, and it is now clear that blood culture technologies differ in their ability to detect candidemia. Estimates of the sensitivity of blood culture systems have been derived from retrospective analyses of the frequency of fungemia in patients (usually with cancer) proven by other means (often autopsy) to have disseminated candidiasis. These estimates range from 4 to 35% (135). The lysis-centrifugation system (also known as the Isolator system) is clearly superior to older systems and is probably the most sensitive technique currently available (29). However, it is expensive, and the automated BACTEC high-blood-volume fungal media (HBV-FM) was recently shown to be equivalent to lysis-centrifugation for recovery of *Candida* spp. (311). The automated BacT/Alert system also appears to have good sensitivity for candidemia (238).

Unfortunately, even these newer blood culture systems do not detect all patients with disseminated infection. For example, Berenguer et al. demonstrated that while the sensitivity of the lysis-centrifugation on invasive candidiasis rose with the number of organs found to be involved at autopsy, positive cultures were obtained from only 58% of 19 patients with disseminated candidiasis (25). To augment culture-based approaches, much effort has been directed toward developing non-culture-based tools for diagnosis and monitoring. Unfortunately, no simple solution to this problem has emerged. Antibody detection systems have low sensitivity and specificity. While a series of older techniques have failed to achieve widespread acceptance (34, 98, 110), approaches based on new antigens are intriguing (198, 292, 293). Detection of antigens released by the organism works well for other fungi, but while some of the systems developed to date have good specificity, none of them have had the excellent sensitivity seen for other fungal antigen-detection systems (99). Detection of the *Candida* metabolite D-arabinitol is promising, but further work is needed before the method is widely used (305). Finally, PCR for *Candida* DNA has been extensively studied (302), but its place in diagnosis remains uncertain. A system based on detection of fungal glucan may also prove useful (203a). At present, however, use of any of these methods must be regarded as experimental and clinical judgment remains the critical factor in determining the intensity and duration of anti-*Candida* therapy.

PROPHYLAXIS
General Principles

Prophylaxis may refer to prevention of either colonization/asymptomatic infection or symptomatic disease. Since *Candida* spp. are so ubiquitous and often part of the human microbial flora, prevention of colonization is difficult, impractical, and rarely considered. However, in specific circumstances, prevention of acquisition of *Candida* may be important, most notably in nosocomial settings. Aggressive infection control measures (especially hand washing) and, on occasion, selective decontamination of colonized individuals with oral nystatin, have been shown to control outbreaks (61). However, in most circumstances, prophylaxis for *Candida* refers to the use of antifungal agents to protect individual patients from disease, and the remainder of this section focuses on such use.

Specific Situations

HIV-Infected Patients

Although *Candida* infections are the most common opportunistic infection in AIDS, the relatively low morbidity associated with the initial episodes of oropharyngeal candidiasis seen in these patients makes primary prevention unnecessary. Rather, recent work has focused on preventing recurrences in patients who have had several prior episodes of oropharyngeal candidiasis. Most studies have used fluconazole in varying dosages for this purpose, and several have clearly shown that doses ranging from 150 mg once weekly to 100 mg daily are associated with success rates of 60 to 100% in preventing relapses of oropharyngeal candidiasis over short periods (167, 178, 272). However, breakthroughs appear likely during prolonged suppressive therapy. In a recent trial of fluconazole (200 mg/day) as prophylaxis for cryptococcal meningitis, symptomatic oropharyngeal candidiasis occurred during the 3-year study in 15% of patients in the fluconazole group and in almost 50% of patients who took clotrimazole troches regularly (225).

The optimum drug, dose, and dosing frequency for long-term suppression have not been established, nor have clear indications for selecting patients for suppressive therapy. In advanced AIDS, the consequences of recurrent oropharyngeal disease (symptoms may interfere with eating and compound an already poor nutritional state) must be weighed against the risk (usually low) of toxicity or drug interaction, the cost of chronic suppressive therapy, and the approximately 5 to 10% risk of developing azole-resistant disease. Patients with esophageal candidiasis clearly merit long-term suppressive therapy because of the almost 100% risk of recurrence (164). Prophylactic therapy for patients with symptomatic recurrences limited to the oral mucosa should be tailored to the clinical situation, and either intermittent or continuous therapy can be considered. Fluconazole is usually the agent of choice because of its lack of interaction with the other medications commonly used as therapy for advanced AIDS, and doses of 100 to 400 mg/day can be considered.

Neutropenic Patients

Measures to decrease the frequency of *Candida* infections in patients with neutropenia have included local therapy designed to decrease colonization and systemic chemoprophylaxis. In general, oral regimens designed to reduce the amount of *Candida* in the gastrointestinal system by using polyenes (nystatin or amphotericin B) or nonabsorbed azoles such as clotrimazole have had moderate activity in preventing oropharyngeal infection but little or no effect on rates of systemic candidiasis (60, 65). Compliance is a major problem with these regimens.

Fluconazole at dosages of 50 to 400 mg/day has been very effective in preventing oropharyngeal candidiasis and decreasing colonization with *Candida*. At the higher doses, fluconazole decreases systemic candidiasis in adult patients undergoing bone-marrow transplantation and reduces the need for systemic amphotericin B (106, 257). The utility of fluconazole is less clear in other neutropenic patients (248, 318). Because fluconazole is less active against *C. glabrata* and inactive against *C. krusei,* increased colonization and, at some centers, increased infection with these species has resulted from prophylactic use of fluconazole (50, 315, 316). In addition, fluconazole lacks activity against *Aspergillus* species, which may further limit its usefulness in certain high-risk patient groups. Recent data suggest that itraconazole might be able to prevent both *Candida* and *Aspergillus* infections in high-risk patients (194), but its unpredictable absorption makes its use problematic.

Amphotericin B given systemically has also been evaluated as prophylaxis in bone marrow transplant recipients. Low doses of amphotericin B deoxycholate (0.1 mg/kg/day) were reported to reduce the incidence of serious fungal infections (210), but a study that used a lipid-associated amphotericin B preparation (1 mg/kg/day) demonstrated decreased rates of fungal colonization but not of fungal infections (285). By far the greatest experience with amphotericin B in this setting is not as true prophylaxis but rather as early empirical treatment of febrile neutropenic episodes in which the fever persists despite antibacterial agents. Used in this fashion in prospective trials, amphotericin B reduced the incidence and perhaps the morbidity of fungal (especially candidal) infections. Such therapy is generally regarded as standard care in managing patients with prolonged neutropenia with new or persistent fever (303).

Despite these data, selection of patients who should receive antifungal prophylaxis remains somewhat controversial. As a general rule, patients who are likely to be severely neutropenic for 14 or more days would appear to receive the most benefit from prophylaxis. While this would include many bone marrow transplant recipients, it is important to understand that not all antineoplastic regimens are associated with equal levels of risk (302b). Recent data also suggest that the type of chemotherapy is important in predicting the relative risk of invasive candidiasis and thus the likely benefit from prophylaxis, with regimens that produce large amounts of damage to the gastrointestinal mucosa being associated with the highest rates of invasive candidiasis (35). In addition, heavy oral and fecal colonization with *Candida* also predicts increased likelihood of invasive candidiasis, and such patients have benefited from prophylaxis (114).

Solid Organ Transplantation

Certain patients undergoing liver transplantation have been identified as being at high risk for *Candida* infections, especially candidemia (56). Low doses (10–20 mg/day) of amphotericin B deoxycholate, lipid-associated amphotericin B, and fluconazole were evaluated as prophylaxis in this setting and shown to reduce fungal colonization and the risk of serious *Candida* infections (160, 172, 284). However, low-dose amphotericin B therapy may be inadequate to prevent other fungal infections such as aspergillosis. Pancreatic transplant recipients may also be at increased risk for invasive candidiasis and one study has demonstrated a reduced frequency of intraabdominal candidiasis in patients treated post-transplant with fluconazole 400 mg/d (22a). There are no conclusive data on the value of routine antifungal prophylaxis in other groups of solid organ transplant recipients.

Other Settings

Because of the high attributable mortality associated with invasive candidiasis, there has been considerable interest in preventing infection in other high-risk settings such as patients in intensive care units or after abdominal surgery. However, the data to date are inconclusive. Antifungal prophylaxis with oral polyenes was reported to benefit patients after severe burns and patients undergoing continuous ambulatory peritoneal dialysis (66, 323), but data are limited. Well-controlled prospective randomized trials are needed.

REFERENCES

1. Abi-Said D, Anaissie E, Uzun O, Raad I, Pinzcowski H, Vartivarian S. The epidemiology of hematogenous candidiasis caused by different *Candida* species. Clin Infect Dis 1997;24:1122–1128.
1a. Adamson PC, Rinaldi MG, Pizzo PA, Walsh TJ. Amphotericin B in treatment of *Candida* cholecystitis. Pediatr Infect Dis J 1989;8:408–411.
2. Aguado JM, Hidalgo M, Ridriguez-Tudela JL. Successful treatment of candida peritonitis with fluconazole. J Antimicrob Chemother 1994;34:847.
3. Aisner J, Schimpff SC, Sutherland JC, Young VM, Wiernik PH. *Torulopsis glabrata* infections in patients with cancer: increasing incidence and relationship to colonization. Am J Med 1976;61:23–28.
4. Akler ME, Vellend H, McNeely DM, Walmsley SL, Gold WL. Use of fluconazole in the treatment of candidal endophthalmits. Clin Infect Dis 1995;20:657–664.
5. Alden SM, Frank E, Flancbaum L. Abdominal candidiasis in surgical patients. Am Surg 1989;55:45–49.
6. Almekinders LC, Greene WB. Vertebral Candida infections. A case report and review of the literature. Clin Orthop 1991;267:174–178.
7. Aloia T, Solomkin J, Fink AS, Nussbaum MS, Bjornson S, Bell RH, Sewak L, McFadden DW. Candida in pancreatic infection: a clinical experience. Am Surg 1994;60:793–796.
8. Anaissie E, Bodey GP, Kantarjian H, David C, Barnett K, Bow E, Defelice R, Downs N, File T, Karam G, Potts D, Shelton M, Sugar A. Fluconazole therapy for chronic disseminated candidiasis in patients with leukemia and prior amphotericin B therapy. Am J Med 1991;91:142–150.
9. Anaissie E, Paetznick V, Proffitt R, Adler MJ, Bodey GP. Comparison of the in vitro antifungal activity of free and liposome-encapsulated amphotericin B. Eur J Clin Microbiol Infect Dis 1991;10:665–668.
10. Anaissie EJ, Vartivarian SE, Abi-Said D, Uzun O, Pinczowski H, Kontoyiannis D, Khoury P, Pappadakis C, Gardner A, Raad I, Gilbreath J, Bodey GP. Fluconazole versus amphotericin B in

the treatment of hematogenous candidiasis: a matched cohort study. Am J Med 1996;101:170–176.
10a. Anaissie EJ, Rex JH, Uzan Ö, Vartivarian S. Predictors of adverse outcome in cancer patients with candidemia. Am J Med 1998;104:238–245.
11. Ang BSP, Telenti A, King B, Steckelberg JM, Wilson WR. Candidemia from a urinary tract source: microbiological aspects and clinical significance. Clin Infect Dis 1993;17:662–666.
12. Anonymous. Guidelines of care for superficial mycotic infections of the skin: mucocutaneous candidiasis. J Am Acad Dermatol 1996;34:110–115.
13. Anonymous. Sporanox (itraconazole oral solution) product information. Titusville, NJ: Janssen Pharmaceutica, 1997.
14. Arenas R, Dominguez-Cherit J, Fernandez LM. Open randomized comparison of itraconazole versus terbinafine in onychomycosis. Int J Dermatol 1995;34:138–143.
15. Arfania D, Everett ED, Nolph KD, Rubin J. Uncommon causes of peritonitis in patients undergoing peritoneal dialysis. Arch Intern Med 1981;141:61–64.
16. Arranz-Caso JA, Lopez-Pizarro VM, Gomez-Herruz P, Garcia-Altozano J, Martinez-Martinez J. *Candida albicans* osteomyelitis of the zygomatic bone. A distinctive case with a possible peculiar mechanism of infection and therapeutic failure with fluconazole. Diagn Microbiol Infect Dis 1996;24:161–164.
17. Baley JE, Meyers C, Kliegman RM, Jacobs MR, Blumer JL. Pharmacokinetics, outcome of treatment, and toxic effects of amphotericin B and 5-fluorocytosine in neonates. J Pediatr 1990;116:791–797.
18. Bannatyne RM, Clarke HM. Ketoconazole in the treatment of osteomyelitis due to Candida albicans. Can J Surg 1989;32:201–202.
19. Barchiesi F, Colombo AL, McGough DA, Fothergill AW, Rinaldi MG. In vitro activity of itraconazole against fluconazole-susceptible and -resistant *Candida albicans* isolates from oral cavities of patients infected with human immunodeficiency virus. Antimicrob Agents Chemother 1994;38:1530–1533.
20. Barone SR, Krilov LR. Neonatal candidal meningitis in a full-term infant with congenital cutaneous candidiasis. Clin Pediatr 1995;Apr:217–219.
21. Bayer AS, Blumenkrantz MJ, Montgomerie JZ, Galpin JE, Coburn JW, Guze LB. *Candida* peritonitis: report of 22 cases and review of the English literature. Am J Med 1976;61: 832–840.
22. Bayer AS, Guze LB. Fungal arthritis. I. Candida arthritis: diagnostic and prognostic implications and therapeutic considerations. Semin Arthritis Rheum 1978;8:142–150.
22a. Benedetti E, Gruessner AC, Troppmann C, Papalois BE, Sutherland DE, Dunn DL, Gruessner RW. Intra-abdominal fungal infections after pancreatic transplantation: incidence, treatment, and outcome. J Am Coll Surg 1996;183:307–316.
23. Bennett JE. Antimicrobial agents: antifungal agents. In: Gilman AG, Rall TW, Nies AS, Taylor P, eds. Goodman and Gilman's the pharmacological basis of therapeutics. 8th ed. Fairview Park: Pergamon Press, 1990:1165–1181.
24. Bennett JE, Dismukes WE, Duma RJ, Medoff G, Sande MA, Gallis H, Leonard J, Fields BT, Bradshaw M, Haywood H, McGee ZA, Cate TR, Cobbs CG, Warner JF, Alling DW. A comparison of amphotericin B alone and combined with flucytosine in the treatment of cryptococcal meningitis. N Engl J Med 1979;301:126–131.
25. Berenguer J, Buck M, Witebsky F, Stock F, Pizzo PA, Walsh TJ. Lysis-centrifugation blood cultures in the detection of tissue-proven invasive candidiasis. Disseminated versus single-organ infection. Diagn Microbiol Infect Dis 1993;17:103–109.

26. Berg RA, Stein JM. Medical management of fungal suppurative thrombosis of great central veins in a child. Pediatr Infect Dis J 1989;8:469–470.

27. Bergman JJ. Clinical comparison of microscopic and culture techniques in the diagnosis of *Candida* vaginitis. J Fam Pract 1984;18:549–553.

28. Berkowitz FE, Argent AC, Baise T. Suppurative thrombo-phlebitis: a serious nosocomial infection. Pediatr Infect Dis J 1987;6:64–67.

28a. Berkowitz ID, Robboy SJ, Karchmer AW, Kunz LJ. *Torulopsis glabrata* fungemia—a clinical pathological study. Medicine 1979;56:430–440.

29. Bille J, Stockman G, Roberts D, Hortmeier CD, Ilstrup DM. Evaluation of a lysis-centrifugation system for recovery of yeasts and filamentous fungi from blood. J Clin Microbiol 1983; 18:469–471.

30. Black JT. Cerebral candidiasis: case report of brain abscess secondary to *Candida albicans,* and review of literature. J Neurol Neurosurg Psychiatry 1970;33:864–870.

31. Blinkhorn RJ, Adelstein D, Spagnuolo PJ. Emergence of a new opportunistic pathogen, *Candida lusitaniae.* J Clin Microbiol 1989;27:236–240.

32. Bodey GP, Luna M. Skin lesions associated with disseminated candidiasis. JAMA 1974;229.

33. Bonomo RA, Strauss M, Blinkhorn R, Salata RA. *Torulopsis (Candida) glabrata:* a new pathogen found in spinal epidural abscess. Clin Infect Dis 1996;22:588–589.

34. Bougnoux ME, Hill C, Moissente D, de Chauvin MF, Bonnay M, Vicens-Sprauel I, Pietri F, McNeil M, Kaufman L, Dupouy-Camet J, Bohuon C, Andremonti A. Comparison of antibody, antigen, and metabolite assays for hospitalized patients with disseminated or peripheral candidiasis. J Clin Microbiol 1990; 28:905–909.

35. Bow EJ, Loewen R, Cheang MS, Schacter B. Invasive fungal disease in adults undergoing remission-induction therapy for acute myeloid leukemia: the pathogenetic role of the antileukemic regimen. Clin Infect Dis 1995;21:361–369.

36. Brammer KW, Coates PE. Pharmacokinetics of fluconazole in pediatric patients. Eur J Clin Microbiol Infect Dis 1994;13: 325–329.

37. Branchini ML, Pfaller MA, Rhine-Chalberg J, Frempong T, Isenberg HD. Genotypic variation and slime production among blood and catheter isolates of Candida parapsilosis. J Clin Microbiol 1994;32:452–456.

38. British Society for Antimicrobial Chemotherapy Working Party. Antifungal chemotherapy in patients with acquired immunodeficiency syndrome. Lancet 1992;340:648–651.

39. Brod RD, Flynn HW Jr, Clarkson JG, Pflugfelder SC, Culbertson WW, Miller D. Endogenous Candida endophthalmitis. Management without intravenous amphotericin B. Ophthalmol 1990; 97:666–672.

40. Bruner JP, Elliott JP, Kilbride HW, Garite TJ, Knox GE. *Candida* chorioamnionitis diagnosis by amniocentesis with subsequent fetal infection. Am J Perinatol 1986;3:213–218.

41. Buchs S, Pfister P. *Candida* meningitis: course, prognosis and mortality before and after introduction of the new antimycotics. Mykosen 1982;26:73–81.

42. Burgert SJ, Classen DC, Burke JP, Blatter DD. Candidal brain abscess associated with vascular invasion: a devastating complication of vascular catheter-related candidemia. Clin Infect Dis 1995;21:202–205.

43. Burke WA. Use of itraconazole in a patient with chronic mucocutaneous candidiasis. J Am Acad Dermatol 1989;21:1309–1310.

44. Calandra T, Bille J, Schneider R, Mosimann F, Francioli P. Clinical significance of Candida isolated from peritoneum in surgical patients. Lancet 1989;2:1437–1440.

45. Cancelas JA, Lopez J, Cabezudo E, Navas E, Garcia Laraña J, Jimenez Mena M, Diz P, Perez de Oteyza J, Villalon L, Sanchez-Sousa A, Sastre JL, Odriozola J, Navarro JL. Native valve endocarditis due to *Candida parapsilosis:* a late complication after bone marrow transplantation-related fungemia. Bone Marrow Transplant 1994;13:333–334.

46. Cantrill HL, Rodman WP, Ramsay RC, Knobloch WH. Postpartum *Candida* endophthalmitis. JAMA 1980;243:1163–1166.

46a. Casado JL, Quereda C, Oliva J, Navas E, Morenco A, Pintado V, Cobo J, Corral I. Candidal meningitis in HIV-infected patients: analysis of 14 cases. Clin Infect Dis 1997;25:673–676.

47. Cassone A, DeBernardis F, Pontieri E, Carruba G, Girmenia C, Martino P, Fernández-Rodriguez M, Quindós G, Pontón J. Biotype diversity of *Candida parapsilosis* and its relationship to the clinical source and experimental pathogenicity. J Infect Dis 1995;171:967–975.

48. Castiglia M, Smego RA, Sames EL. *Candida* endocarditis and amphotericin B intolerance: potential role for fluconazole. Infect Dis Clin Pract 1994;3:248–253.

49. Cenci E, Bartocci A, Puccetti P, Mocci S, Stanley ER, Bistoni F. Macrophage colony-stimulating factor in murine candidiasis: serum and tissue levels during infection and protective effect of exogenous administration. Infect Immun 1991;59:868–872.

50. Chandrasekar PH, Gatny CM, the Bone Marrow Transplantation Team. The effect of fluconazole prophylaxis on fungal colonization in neutropenic cancer patients. J Antimicrob Chemother 1994;33:309–318.

51. Chesney PJ, Teets KC, Mulvihill JJ, Salit IE, Marks ML. Successful treatment of *Candida* meningitis with amphotericin B and 5-fluorocytosine in combination. J Pediatr 1976;89: 1017–1018.

52. Chin TWF, Loeb M, Fong IW. Effects of an acidic beverage (Coca-Cola) on absorption of ketoconazole. Antimicrob Agents Chemother 1995;39:1671–1675.

53. Chiou C-C, Wong T-T, Lin H-H, Hwang B, Tang R-B, Wu K-G, Lee B-H. Fungal infection of ventriculoperitoneal shunts in children. Clin Infect Dis 1994;19:1049–1053.

53a. Clancy CJ, Nguyen MH, Morris AJ. Candidal mediastinitis: an emerging clinical entity. Clin Infect Dis 1997;25:608–613.

54. Clark JM, Whitney RR, Olsen SJ, George RJ, Swerdel MR, Kunselman L, Bonner DP. Amphotericin B lipid complex therapy of experimental fungal infections in mice. Antimicrob Agents Chemother 1991;35:615–621.

55. Cohen R, Roth FJ, Delgado E, Ahearn DG, Kalser MH. Fungal flora of the normal human small and large intestine. N Engl J Med 1969;280:638–641.

56. Collins LA, Samore MH, Roberts MS, Luzzati R, Jenkins RL, Lewis WD, Karchmer AW. Risk factors for invasive fungal infections complicating orthotopic liver transplantation. J Infect Dis 1994;170:644–652.

57. Conrad D, Lentnek AL. Comparative evaluation of nystatin pastille and clotrimazole troche for the treatment of candidal stomatitis in immunocompromised patients. Curr Ther Res 1990;47: 627–636.

58. Corbella X, Sirvent JM, Carratala J. Fluconazole treatment without catheter removal in *Candida albicans* peritonitis complicating peritoneal dialysis. Am J Med 1991;90:277.

59. Cruciani M, DiPerri G, Molesini M, Vento S, Concia E, Bassetti D. Use of fluconazole in the treatment of *Candida albicans* hy-

drocephalus shunt infection. Eur J Clin Microbiol Infect Dis 1992;11:957.

60. Cuttner J, Troy KM, Fumaro L, Brenden R, Bottone EJ. Clotrimazole treatment for prevention of oral candidiasis in patients with acute leukemia undergoing chemotherapy. Results of a double-blind study. Am J Med 1986;81:771–774.

61. Damjanovic V, Connolly CM, van Saene HK, Cooke RW, Corkill JE, van Belkum A, van Velzen D. Selective decontamination with nystatin for control of a *Candida* outbreak in a neonatal intensive care unit. J Hosp Infect 1993;24:245–259.

62. Dan M, Priel I. Failure of fluconazole therapy for sternal osteomyelitis due to *Candida albicans* [Letter]. Clin Infect Dis 1994;18:126–127.

63. De Doncker P, Decroix J, Pierard GE, Roelant D, Woestenborghs R, Jacqmin P, Odds F, Heremans A, Dockx P, Roseeuw D. Antifungal pulse therapy for onychomycosis. A pharmacokinetic and pharmacodynamic investigation of monthly cycles of 1-week pulse therapy with itraconazole. Arch Dermatol 1996; 132:34–41.

64. de Doncker P, van Lint J, Dockx P, Roseeuw D. Pulse therapy with one-week itraconazole monthly for three or four months in the treatment of onychomycosis. Cutis 1995;56:180–183.

65. DeGregorio MW, Lee WMF, Ries CA. *Candida* infections in patients with acute leukemia: ineffectiveness of nystatin prophylaxis and relationship between oropharyngeal and systemic candidiasis. Cancer 1982;50:2780–2784.

66. Desai MH, Rutan RL, Heggers JP, Herndon DN. *Candida* infection with and without nystatin prophylaxis. An 11-year experience with patients with burn injury. Arch Surg 1992;127: 159–162.

67. DeVita VT, Utz JP, Williams T, Carbone PP. *Candida* meningitis. Arch Intern Med 1966;117:527–535.

68. Dewsnup DH, Stevens DA. Efficacy of oral amphotericin B in AIDS patients with thrush clinically resistant to fluconazole. J Med Vet Mycol 1994;32:389–393.

69. Dick J, Merz W, Saral R. Incidence of polyene-resistant yeasts recovered from clinical specimens. Antimicrob Agents Chemother 1980;18:158–163.

70. Dignani MC, Anaissie EJ, Hester JP, Vartivarian SE, Rex JH, Kantarjian H, Jendiroba DB, Lichtiger B, Andersson BS, Freireich EJ. Treatment of neutropenia-related fungal infections with granulocyte colony-stimulating factor-elicited white blood cell transfusions: a pilot study. Leukemia 1997;11:1621–1630.

71. Dijkmans BAC, Koolen MI, Mouton RP, Falke M, van den Broek PJ, van der Meer JWM. Hematogenous *Candida* vertebral osteomyelitis treated with ketoconazole. Infection 1982;10: 290–292.

72. Donahue SP, Greven CM, Zuravleff JJ, Eller AW, Nguyen MH, Peacock JE, Wagener MM, Yu VL. Intraocular candidiasis in patients with candidemia: clinical implications derived from a prospective multicenter study. Ophthalmology 1994;101: 1302–1309.

73. Drouhet E. Basic mechanisms of antifungal chemotherapy. Mod Treat 1970;7:539–564.

74. Drutz DJ, Lehrer RI. Development of amphotericin B-resistant *Candida tropicalis* in a patient with defective leukocyte function. Am J Med Sci 1978;276:77–92.

75. Duquesnoy B, Fournier E, Berniere L, Delcambre B. Ketoconazole for treatment of Candida arthritis [Letter]. J Rheumatol 1984;11:105–107.

76. Edwards JE. Editorial response: should all patients with candidemia be treated with antifungal agents? Clin Infect Dis 1992; 15:422–423.

77. Edwards JE Jr, Foos RY, Montgomerie JZ, Guze LB. Ocular

manifestations of *Candida* septicemia: review of seventy-six cases of hematogenous *Candida* endophthalmitis. Medicine 1974;53:47–75.

78. Edwards JF Jr, Turkel S, Elder HA, Rand RW, Guze LB. Hematogenous *Candida* osteomyelitis: report of three cases and review of the literature. Am J Med 1975;59:89–94.

79. Eisenberg ES. Intraperitoneal flucytosine in the management of fungal peritonitis in patients on continuous ambulatory peritoneal dialysis. Am J Kidney Dis 1988;11:465–467.

80. Eisenberg ES, Leviton I, Soeiro R. Fungal peritonitis in patients receiving peritoneal dialysis: experience with 11 patients and review of the literature. Rev Infect Dis 1986;8:309–321.

80a. El-Ebiary M, Torres A, Fabrega N, Puig de la Bellacasa J, Gonzalez J, Ramirez J, del Bano D, Hernandez C, Jimenez de Anta MT. Significance of the isolation of *Candida* species from respiratory samples in critically ill, non-neutropenic patients. Am J Respir Crit Care Med 1997;156:583–590

81. Eng RHK, Sen P, Browne K, Louria DB. *Candida* pericarditis. Am J Med 1982;70:867–869.

82. Eras P, Goldstein MJ, Sherlock P. *Candida* infections of the gastrointestinal tract. Medicine 1972;51:367–379.

82a. Evans EGV. Causative pathogens in onychomycosis and the possibility of treatment resistance: a review. J Am Acad Dermatol 1998;38:532–536.

83. Faix RG. Systemic *Candida* infections in infants in intensive care nurseries: high incidence of central nervous system involvement. J Pediatr 1984;105:616–622.

84. Faix RG. Invasive neonatal candidiasis: comparison of albicans and parapsilosis infection. Pediatr Infect Dis J 1992;11:88–93.

85. Faix RG. Nonsurgical treatment of *Candida* endocarditis. J Pediatr 1992;120:665–666.

86. Faix RG, Naglie RA, Barr M Jr. Intrapleural inoculation of Candida in an infant with congenital cutaneous candidiasis. Am J Perinatol 1986;3:119–122.

87. Fan-Havard P, O'Donovan C, Smith SM, Oh J, Bamberger M, Eng RHK. Oral fluconazole versus amphotericin B bladder irrigation for treatment of candidal funguria. Clin Infect Dis 1995;21:960–965.

88. Ferra C, Doebbeling BN, Hollis RJ, Pfaller MA, K LC, Gingrich RD. *Candida tropicalis* vertebral osteomyelitis: a late sequela of fungemia. Clin Infect Dis 1994;19:697–703.

89. Fidel PL Jr, Sobel JD. Immunopathogenesis of recurrent vulvovaginal candidiasis. Clin Microbiol Rev 1996;9:335–348.

89a. Fisher EW, Richards A, Anderson G, Albert DM. Laryngeal candidiasis: a cause of airway obstruction in the immunocompromised child. J Laryngol Otol 1992;106:168–170.

90. Fisher JF, Hicks BC, Dipiro JT, Venable J, Fincher RM. Efficacy of a single intravenous dose of Amphotericin B in urinary tract infections caused by *Candida*. J Infect Dis 1987; 156:685–686.

91. Fisher JF, Newman CL, Sobel JD. Yeast in the urine: solutions for a budding problem. Clin Infect Dis 1995;20:183–189.

92. Fisher JF, Taylor AT, Clark J, Raghunatha R. Penetration of amphotericin B into the human eye. J Infect Dis 1983;147:164.

93. Flynn PM, Cunningham CK, Kerkering T, San Jorge AR, Peters VB, Pitel PA, Harris J, Gilbert G, Catagnaro L, Robinson P, the Multicenter Fluconazole Study Group. Oropharyngeal candidiasis in immunocompromised children: a randomized, multicenter study of orally administered fluconazole suspension versus nystatin. J Pediatr 1995;127:322–328.

94. Fogarty M. Candidal osteomyelitis: a case report. Aust NZ J Surg 1983;53:141–143.

95. Fraser VJ, Jones M, Dunkel J, Storfer S, Medoff G, Dunagan

WC. Candidemia in a tertiary care hospital: epidemiology, risk factors, and predictors of mortality. Clin Infect Dis 1992;15: 414–421.

95a. Friedland IR. Peripheral thrombophlebitis caused by *Candida*. Pediatr Infect Dis J 1996;15:375–377.

96. Gallo WJ, Shapiro DN, Moss M. Suppurative candidiasis: review of the literature and report of case. J Am Dent Assoc 1976; 92:936–939.

97. Gathe JGJ, Harris RL, Garland B, Bradshaw MW, Williams TW. *Candida* osteomyelitis: report of five cases and review of the literature. Am J Med 1987;82:927–937.

98. Gentry LO, McNitt TR, Kaufman L. Use and value of serologic tests for the diagnosis of systemic candidiasis in cancer patients: a prospective study of 146 patients. Curr Microbiol 1978; 1:239–242.

99. Gentry LO, Wilkinson ID, Lea AS, Price MF. Latex agglutination test for detection of *Candida* antigen in patients with disseminated disease. Eur J Clin Microbiol Infect Dis 1983;2:122–128.

100. Ghannoum MA, Fu Y, Ibrahim AS, Mortara LA, Shafiq MC, Edwards JE Jr, Criddle RS. In vitro determination of optimal antifungal combinations against *Cryptococcus neoformans* and *Candida albicans*. Antimicrob Agents Chemother 1995;39: 2459–2465.

101. Gilbert HM, Peters ED, Lang SJ, Hartman BJ. Successful treatment of fungal prosthetic valve endocarditis: case report and review. Clin Infect Dis 1996;22:348–354.

102. Girmenia C, Martino P, De Bernardis F, Gentile G, Boccanera M, Monaco M, Antonucci G, Cassone A. Rising incidence of *C. parapsilosis* fungemia in patients with hematologic malignancies: clinical aspects, predisposing factors, and differential pathogenicity of the causative strains. Clin Infect Dis 1996; 23:506–514.

103. Glassman BD, Muglia JJ. Widespread erythroderma and desquamation in a neonate. Congenital cutaneous candidiasis (CCC). Arch Dermatol 1993;129:899–902.

104. Goldman M, Pottage JC, Weaver DC. *Candida krusei* fungemia. Medicine (Baltimore) 1993;72:143–150.

105. Goodman DF, Stern WH. Oral ketoconazole and intraocular amphotericin B for treatment of postoperative Candida parapsilosis endophthalmitis [Letter]. Arch Ophthalmol 1987;105: 172–173.

106. Goodman JL, Winston DJ, Greenfield RA, Chandrasekar PH, Fox B, Kaizer H, Shadduck FK, Shea TC, Stiff P, Friedman DJ, Powderly WG, Silber JL, Horowitz H, Lichtin A, Wolff SN, Mangan KF, Silver SM, Weisdorf D, Ho WG, Gilbert G, Buell D. A controlled trial of fluconazole to prevent fungal infections in patients undergoing bone marrow transplantation. N Engl J Med 1992;326:845–851.

107. Graninger W, Presteril E, Schneeweiss B, Teleky B, Georgopoulos A. Treatment of *Candida albicans* fungaemia with fluconazole. J Infect 1993;16:133–146.

108. Grant SM, Clissold SP. Fluconazole. A review of its pharmacodynamic and pharmacokinetic properties, and therapeutic potential in superficial and systemic mycoses. Drugs 1990;39: 877–916.

109. Graybill JR, Vazquez J, Darouiche RO, Morhart R, Greenspan D, Tuazon C, Wheat LJ, Carey J, Leviton I, Hewitt RG, MacGregor RR, Valenti W. Restrepo M, Moskovitz BL. Randomized trial of itraconazole oral solution for oropharyngeal candidiasis in HIV/AIDS patients. Am J Med 1998;104:33–39.

110. Greenfield RA, Bussey MJ, Stephens JL, Jones JM. Serial enzyme-linked immunosorbent assays for antibody to *Candida* antigens during induction chemotherapy for acute leukemia. J Infect Dis 1983;148:275–283.

111. Greenspan D. Treatment of oropharyngeal candidiasis in HIV-positive patients. J Am Acad Dermatol 1994;31(Suppl 2):S51–S55.

112. Gronemeyer PS, Weissfeld AS, Sonnenwirth AC. Purulent pericarditis complicating systemic infection with *Candida tropicalis*. Am J Clin Pathol 1982;77:471–475.

113. Guinet R, Chanas J, Goullier A, Bennefoy G, Ambroise-Thomas P. Fatal septicemia due to amphotericin B-resistant *Candida lusitaniae*. J Clin Microbiol 1983;18:443–444.

114. Guiot HFL, Fibbe WE, van't Wout JW. Prevention of invasive candidiasis by fluconazole in patients with malignant hematological disorders and a high grade of Candida. 36th Interscience Conference on Antimicrobial Agents and Chemotherapy. New Orleans, LA, 1996, Abstract No. LM33.

115. Gupta NM, Chaudhary A, Talwar P. Candidal obstruction of the common bile duct. Br J Surg 1985;72:13.

116. Gupta TP, Ehrinpreis MN. *Candida*-associated diarrhea in hospitalized patients. Gastroenterology 1990;98:780–785.

116a. Gurses N, Kalayci AG. Fluconazole monotherapy for candidal meningitis in a premature infant. Clin Infect Dis 1996;23: 645–646.

117. Hague RA, Eastham EJ, Lee RE, Cant AJ. Resolution of hepatic abscess after interferon gamma in chronic granulomatous disease [see comments]. Arch Dis Child 1993;69:443–445.

118. Hallum JL, Williams TW Jr. *Candida* endocarditis. In: Bodey GP, ed. Candidiasis: pathogenesis, diagnosis, and treatment. New York: Raven Press, 1993:357–369.

119. Hamood M, Bluche PF, De Vroey C, Corazza F, Bujan W, Fondu P. Effects of recombinant human granulocyte-colony stimulating factor on neutropenic mice infected with Candida albicans: acceleration of recovery from neutropenia and potentiation of anti-C. albicans resistance. Mycoses 1994;37:93–99.

120. Hamory BH, Wenzel RP. Hospital-associated candiduria: predisposing factors and review of the literature. J Urol 1978;120: 444–448.

121. Hardin TC, Graybill JR, Fetchick R, Woestenborghs R, Rinaldi MG, Kuhn JG. Pharmacokinetics of itraconazole following oral administration to normal volunteers. Antimicrob Agents Chemother 1988;32:1310–1313.

122. Haron E, Feld R, Tuffnell P, Patterson B, Hasselback R, Matlow A. Hepatic candidiasis: an increasing problem in immunocompromised patients. Am J Med 1987;83:17–26.

123. Haron E, Vartivarian S, Anaissie E, Dekmezian R, Bodey GP. Primary *Candida* pneumonia. Medicine 1993;72:137–142.

124. Hawser SP, Douglas LJ. Biofilm formation by Candida species on the surface of catheter materials in vitro. Infect Immun 1994;62:915–921.

125. Hay RJ, Clayton YM, Moore MK, Midgely G. An evaluation of itraconazole in the management of onychomycosis. Br J Dermatol 1988;119:359–366.

126. Hennequin C, Bouree P, Hiesse C, Dupont B, Charpentier B. Spondylodiskitis due to *Candida albicans:* report of two patients who were successfully treated with fluconazole and review of the literature. Clin Infect Dis 1996;23:176–178.

127. Hernández JA, Gonzalez-Moreno M, Llibre JM, Aloy A, Casan JM. Candidal mitral endocarditis and long-term treatment with fluconazole in a patient with human immunodeficiency virus infection. Clin Infect Dis 1992;15:1062–1063.

128. Heykants J, Van Peer A, Van de Velde V, Van Rooy P, Meuldermans W, Kavrijsen K, Woestenborghs R, Van Cutsem J, Cauwenbergh G. The clinical pharmacokinetics of itraconazole: an overview. Mycoses 1989;32(Suppl 1):67–87.

129. Hogeweg M, de Jong PT. Candida endophthalmitis in heroin addicts. Doc Ophthalmol 1983;55:63–71.

130. Horn R, Wong B, Kiehn TE, Armstrong D. Fungemia in a cancer hospital: changing frequency, earlier onset, and results of therapy. Rev Infect Dis 1985;7:646–655.

131. Horowitz BJ. Topical flucytosine therapy for chronic recurrent *Candida tropicalis* infections. J Reprod Med 1996;31:821–824.

132. Horowitz BJ, Biaquista D, Ito S. Evolving pathogenesis of vulvovaginal candidiasis: implications for patient care. J Clin Pharmacol 1992;32:248–255.

133. Horsburgh CR, Kirkpatrick CH. Long-term therapy of chronic mucocutaneous candidiasis with ketoconazole: experience with twenty-one patients. Am J Med 1983;74:23–29.

134. Hughes CE, Beggs WH. Action of fluconazole (UK-49,858) in relation to other systemic antifungal azoles. J Antimicrob Chemother 1987;19:171–174.

135. Hughes JM, Remington JS. Systemic candidiasis: a diagnostic challenge. Calif Med 1972;116:8–17.

136. Hurley R, DeLouvois J. *Candida* vaginitis. Postgrad Med J 1979;55:645–647.

137. Hymes SR, Duvic M. Cutaneous candidiasis. In: Body GP, ed. Candidiasis: pathogenesis, diagnosis, and treatment. New York: Raven Press, 1993:159–166.

138. Jarrett F, Maki DG, Chan C-K. Management of septic thrombosis of the inferior vena cava caused by *Candida*. Arch Surg 1978;113:637–639.

139. Jin Y, Endo A, Shimada M, Minato M, Takada M, Takahashi S, Harada K. Congenital systemic candidiasis. Pediatr Infect Dis J 1995;14:818–820.

140. Johnson DE, Thompson TR, Ferrieri P. Congenital candidiasis. Am J Dis Child 1981;135:273–275.

140a. Johnston P, Lee J, Demanski M, Dressler F, Tucker E, Rothenberg M, Pizzo PA, Walsh TJ. Late recurrent *Candida* endocarditis. Chest 1991;99:1531–1533.

140b. Joly V, Belmatoug N, Leperre A, Robert J, Jault F, Carbon C, Yeni P. Pacemaker endocarditis due to *Candida albicans:* case report and review. Clin Infect Dis 1997;25:1359–1362.

141. Jones JM. Granulomatous hepatitis due to *Candida albicans* in patients with acute leukemia. Ann Intern Med 1981;94:475–477.

142. Kam LA, Giacoia GP. Congenital cutaneous candidiasis. Am J Dis Child 1975;129:1215–1218.

143. Kane JG, Chretien JH, Garagusi VF. Diarrhoea caused by Candida. Lancet 1976;1:335–336.

144. Karyotakis NC, Anaissie EJ. Efficacy of escalating doses of liposomal amphotericin B (AmBisome) against hematogenous *Candida lusitaniae* and *Candida krusei* infection in neutropenic mice. Antimicrob Agents Chemother 1994;38:2660–2662.

145. Katzenstein D. Isolated Candida arthritis: report of a case and definition of a distinct clinical syndrome. Arthritis Rheum 1985;28:1421–1424.

146. Kauffman CA, Bradley SF, Ross SC, Weber DR. Hepatosplenic candidiasis: successful treatment with fluconazole. Am J Med 1991;91:137–141.

147. Kauffman CA, Bradley SF, Vine AK. *Candida* endophthalmitis associated with intraocular lens implantation: efficacy of fluconazole therapy. Mycoses 1993;36:13–17.

148. Keiser P, Keay S. Candidal pancreatic abscesses: report of two cases and review. Clin Infect Dis 1992;14:884–888.

149. Kent HL. Epidemiology of vaginitis. Am J Obstet Gynecol 1991;165:1168–1176.

150. Kirkpatrick CH. Chronic mucocutaneous candidiasis. Eur J Clin Microbiol Infect Dis 1989;8:448–456.

151. Kirkpatrick CH. Chronic mucocutaneous candidiasis. J Am Acad Dermatol 1994;31(Suppl 2):S14–S17.

152. Klebanoff SJ, Ozszowski S, van Voorhis WC, Ledbetter JA, Waltersdorph AM, Schlechte KG. Effects of interferon-gamma on human neutrophils: protection from deterioration on storage. Blood 1992;80:225–234.

153. Klein JJ, Watanakunakorn C. Hospital-acquired fungemia: its natural course and clinical significance. Am J Med 1979;67:51–58.

154. Knaus WA, Draper EA, Wagner DP, Zimmerman JE. APACHE II: a severity of disease classification system. Crit Care Med 1985;13:818–829.

155. Koletar SL, Russell JA, Fass RJ, Plouffe JF. Comparison of oral fluconazole and clotrimazole troches as treatment for oral candidiasis in patients infected with human immunodeficiency virus. Antimicrob Agents Chemother 1990;34:2267–2268.

156. Komshian SV, Uwaydah AK, Sobel JD, Crane LR. Fungemia caused by *Candida* species and *Torulopsis glabrata* in the hospitalized patient: frequency, characteristics, and evaluation of factors influencing outcome. Rev Infect Dis 1989;11:379–390.

157. Korting HC, Schafer-Korting M, Zienicke H, Georgii A, Ollert MW. Treatment of tinea unguium with medium and high doses of ultramicrosize griseofulvin compared with itraconazole. Antimicrob Agents Chemother 1993;37:2064–2068.

158. Kujath P, Lerch K, Dammrich J. Fluconazole monitoring in Candida peritonitis based on histological control. Mycoses 1990;33:441–448.

159. Kullberg BJ, van't Wout JW, Hoogstraten C, van Furth R. Recombinant interferon-gamma enhances resistance to acute disseminated Candida albicans infection in mice. J Infect Dis 1993;168:436–443.

160. Kung N, Fisher N, Gunson B, Hastings M, Mutimer D. Fluconazole prophylaxis for high-risk liver transplant recipients. Lancet 1995;349:1234–1235.

161. Kunová A, Trupl J, Diuholucky S, Galová G, Krcméry V Jr. Use of fluconazole is not associated with a higher incidence of *Candida krusei* and other non-*albicans Candida* species. Clin Infect Dis 1995;21:226–227.

162. Kwon-Chung KJ, Bennett JE. Medical mycology. Philadelphia: Lea & Febiger, 1992.

163. Lafont A, Olive A, Gelman M, Roca-Burniols J, Cots R, Carbonell J. Candida albicans spondylodiscitis and vertebral osteomyelitis in patients with intravenous heroin drug addiction. Report of 3 new cases. J Rheumatol 1994;21:953–956.

164. Laine L. The natural history of esophageal candidiasis after successful treatment in patients with AIDS. Gastroenterology 1994;107:744–746.

165. Laine L, Dretler RH, Conteas CN, Tuazon C, Koster FM, Sattler F, Squires K, Islan MZ. Fluconazole compared with ketoconazole for the treatment of *Candida* esophagitis in AIDS: a randomized trial. Ann Intern Med 1992;117:655–660.

165a. Landman D, Suarina G, Quale JM. Failure of all antifungal therapy for infection due to Candida albicans: a new AIDS-related problem? Clin Infect Dis 1998;26:183–184.

165b. Law D, Moore CB, Denning DW. Amphotericin B resistance testing of *Candida* spp.: a comparison of methods. J Antimicrob Chemother 1997;40:109–112.

166. Lecciones JA, Lee JW, Navarro EE, Witebsky FG, Marshall D, Steinberg SM, Pizzo PA, Walsh TJ. Vascular catheter-associated fungemia in patients with cancer: analysis of 155 episodes. Clin Infect Dis 1992;14:875–883.

167. Leen CL, Dunbar EM, Ellis ME, Mandal BK. Once-weekly fluconazole to prevent recurrence of oropharyngeal candidiasis in patients with AIDS and AIDS-related complex: a double-blind placebo-controlled study. J Infect 1990;21:55–60.

168. Leu H-S, Huang C-T. Clearance of funguria with short-course

antifungal regimens: a prospective, randomized, controlled study. Clin Infect Dis 1995;20:1152–1157.

169. Levine J, Bernard DB, Idelson BA, Farnham H, Saunders C, Sugar AM. Fungal peritonitis complicating continuous ambulatory peritoneal dialysis: successful treatment with fluconazole, a new orally active antifungal agent. Am J Med 1989; 86:825–829.

170. Levine J, Dykoski RK, Janoff EN. *Candida*-associated diarrhea: a syndrome in search of credibility. Clin Infect Dis 1995; 21:881–886.

171. Lewis JH, Zimmerman HJ, Benton GD, Ishak KG. Hepatic injury associated with ketoconazole therapy: analysis of 33 cases. Gastroenterology 1984;86:503–513.

172. Linden P, Kramer DJ, Mazariegos G, Marsh W, Casavilla A, Pinna A, Fung J, Kusen S. Low-dose amphotericin B for the prophylaxis of serious *Candida* infections in high-risk liver recipients [Abstract J47]. 36th Interscience Conference on Antimicrobial Agents and Chemotherapy, 1996.

173. Lindner A, Becker G, Warmuth-Metz M, Schalke BCG, Bogdahn U, Tyoka KV. Magnetic resonance image findings of spinal intramedullary abscess caused by *Candida albicans:* case report. Neurosurgery 1995;36:411–412.

174. Lipton SA, Hickey WF, Morris JH, Loscalzo J. Candidal infection in the central nervous system. Am J Med 1984;76: 101–108.

175. Lott TJ, Kuykendall RJ, Reiss E. Nucleotide sequence analysis of the 5.8S rDNA and adjacent ITS2 region of Candida albicans and related species. Yeast 1993;9:1199–1206.

176. Magnussen CR, Olson JP, Ona FV, Graziani AJ. Candida fungus balls in the common bile duct. Unusual manifestation of disseminated candidiasis. Arch Intern Med 1979;139:821–822.

177. Marr B, Gross S, Cunningham C, Weiner L. Candidal sepsis and meningitis in a very-low-birth-weight infant successfully treated with fluconazole and flucytosine. Clin Infect Dis 1994; 19:795–796.

177a. Marr KA, White TC, van Burik J-AH, Bowden RA. Development of fluconazole resistance in *Candida albicans* causing disseminated infection in a patient undergoing marrow transplantation. Clin Infect Dis 1997;25:908–910.

178. Marriott DJ, Jones PD, Hoy JF, Speed BR, Harkness JL. Fluconazole once a week as secondary prophylaxis against oropharyngeal candidiasis in HIV-infected patients. Med J Aust 1993;158:312–316.

179. Martinez-Suarez JV, Rodriguez-Tudela JL. Patterns of in vitro activity of itraconazole and imidazole antifungal agents against *Candida albicans* with decreased susceptibility to fluconazole from Spain. Antimicrob Agents Chemother 1995;39:1512–1516.

180. Martino P, Girmenia C, Micozzi A, Raccah R, Gentile G, Venditto M, Mandelli F. Fungemia in patients with leukemia. Am J Med Sci 1993;306:225–232.

180a. Martins MD, Lozano-Chiu M, Rex JH. Declining rates of symptomatic oropharyngeal candidiasis, carriage of *Candida albicans*, and fluconazole resistance in HIV patients. 35th Annual Meeting of the Infectious Diseases Society of America, 1997. Abstract No. 138.

180b. Martins MD, Rex JH. Fluconazole suspension for oropharyngeal candidiasis unresponsive to tablets. Ann Intern Med 1997;126:332–333.

181. Masur H, Rosen PP, Armstrong D. Pulmonary disease caused by *Candida* species. Am J Med 1977;63:914–925.

182. Matthieu L, De Doncker P, Cauwenbergh G, Woestenborghs R, van de Velde V, Janssen PA, Dockx P. Itraconazole penetrates the nail via the nail matrix and the nail bed—an investigation in onychomycosis. Clin Exp Dermatol 1991;16:374–376.

183. Mayayo E, Moralejo J, Camps J, Guarro J. Fungal endocarditis in premature infants: case report and review. Clin Infect Dis 1996;22:366–368.

184. Mayer P, Schutze E, Lam C, Kricek F, Liehl E. Recombinant murine granulocyte-macrophage colony-stimulating factor augments neutrophil recovery and enhances resistance to infections in myelosuppressed mice. J Infect Dis 1991;163:584–590.

185. McGinnis MR, Rinaldi MG. Selected medically important fungi and some common synonyms and obsolete names. Clin Infect Dis 1995;21:277–278.

186. Merz WG. *Candida lusitaniae:* frequency of recovery, colonization, infection, and amphotericin B resistance. J Clin Microbiol 1984;20:1194–1195.

187. Merz WG, Karp JE, Schron D, Saral R. Increased incidence of fungemia caused by *Candida krusei*. J Clin Microbiol 1986;24:581–584.

188. Merz WG, Sanford GR. Isolation and characterization of a polyene-resistant variant of *Candida tropicalis*. J Clin Microbiol 1979;9:677–680.

189. Meunier F. Management of candidemia. N Engl J Med 1994; 331:1371–1372.

190. Meunier F, Aoun M, Gerard M. Therapy for oropharyngeal candidiasis in the immunocompromised host: a randomized double-blind study of fluconazole vs. ketoconazole. Rev Infect Dis 1990;12(Suppl 3):S364–S368.

191. Meunier-Carpentier F, Kiehn TE, Armstrong D. Fungemia in the immunocompromised host: changing patterns, antigenemia, high mortality. Am J Med 1981;71:363–370.

192. Michel C, Courdavault L, al Khayat R, Viron B, Roux P, Mignon F. Fungal peritonitis in patients on peritoneal dialysis. Am J Nephrol 1994;14:113–120.

193. Montenegro J, Aguirre R, Gonzalez O, Martinze I, Saracho R. Fluconazole treatment of *Candida* peritonitis with delayed removal of the peritoneal dialysis catheter. Clin Nephrol 1995; 44:60–63.

194. Morgenstern GR, Prentice AG, Prentice HG, Ropner JE, Schey SA, Warnock DW. Itraconazole oral solution vs. fluconazole suspension for antifungal prophylaxis in neutropenic patients [Abstract LM34]. 36th Interscience Conference on Antimicrobial Agents and Chemotherapy, 1996.

194a. Mori T, Matsumura M, Kanamaru Y, Miyano S, Hishikawa T, Irie S, Oshimi K, Saikawa T, Oguri T. Myelofibrosis complicated by infection due to *Candida albicans:* emergence of resistance to antifungal agents during therapy. Clin Infect Dis 1997;25:1470–1471.

195. Muehrcke DD, Lytle BW, Cosgrove DM 3rd. Surgical and long-term antifungal therapy for fungal prosthetic valve endocarditis. Ann Thorac Surg 1995;60:538–543.

196. National Committee for Clinical Laboratory Standards. Reference method for broth dilution antifungal susceptibility testing of yeasts; tentative standard. NCCLS document M27-T. Wayne, PA: National Committee for Clinical Laboratory Standards, 1995.

197. National Committee for Clinical Laboratory Standards. Reference method for broth dilution antifungal susceptibility testing of yeasts; reference standard. NCCLS document M27-A. Villanova, PA: National Committee for Clinical Laboratory Standards, 1997.

198. Navarro D, Monzonis E, Lopez-Ribot JL, Sepulveda P, Casanova M, Nogueira JM, Martinez JP. Diagnosis of systemic candidiasis by enzyme immunoassay detection of specific antibodies to mycelial phase cell wall and cytoplasmic candidal antigens. Eur J Clin Microbiol Infect Dis 1993;12:839–846.

198a. Navarro EE, Almario JS, Schaufele RL, Bacher J, Walsh TJ.

Quantitative urine cultures do not reliably detect renal candidiasis in rabbits. J Clin Microbiol 1997;35:3292–3297.

199. Nguyen MH, Nguyen ML, Yu VL, McMahon D, Keys TF, Amidi M. Candida prosthetic valve endocarditis: prospective study of six cases and review of the literature. Clin Infect Dis 1996;22:262–267.

200. Nguyen MH, Peacock JE Jr, Morris AJ, Tanner DC, Nguyen ML, Snydman DR, Wagener MM, Rinaldi MG, Yu VL. The changing face of candidemia: emergence of non-*C. albicans* species and antifungal resistance. Am J Med 1996;100:617–623.

201. Nguyen MH, Peacock JE Jr, Tanner DC, Morris AJ, Nguyen ML, Snydman DR, Wagener MM, Yu VL. Therapeutic approaches in patients with candidemia. Evaluation in a multicenter, prospective, observational study. Arch Intern Med 1995;155:2429–2435.

202. Nguyen MH, Yu VL. Meningitis caused by *Candida* species: an emerging problem in neurosurgical patients. Clin Infect Dis 1995;21:323–327.

203. Nguyen MH, Yu VL, Morris AJ. *Candida* infection of the arteriovenous fistula used for hemodialysis. Am J Kidney Dis 1996;27:596–598.

203a. Obayashi T, Yoshida M, Mori T, Goto H, Yasuoka A, Iwasaki H, Teshima H, Kohno S, Horiuchi A, Ito A, Yamaguchi H, Shimada K, Kawai T. Plasma (1->3)-beta-D-glucan measurement in diagnosis of invasive deep mycosis and fungal febrile episodes. Lancet 1995;45:17–20.

204. O'Day DM, Foulds G, Williams TE, Robinson RD, Allen RH, Head WS. Ocular uptake of fluconazole following oral administration. Arch Ophthalmol 1990;108:1006–1008.

205. O'Day DM, Head WS, Robinson RD, Stern WH, Freeman JM. Intraocular penetration of systemically administered antifungal agents. Curr Eye Res 1985;4:131–134.

206. Oleinik EM, Della-Latta P, Rinaldi MG, Saiman L. *Candida lusitaniae* osteomyelitis in a premature infant. Am J Perinatol 1993;10:313–315.

207. O'Meeghan T, Varcoe R, Thomas M, Ellis-Pegler R. Fluconazole concentration in joint fluid during successful treatment of Candida albicans septic arthritis [Letter]. J Antimicrob Chemother 1990;26:601–602.

207a. Papanicolaou GA, Meyers BR, Fuchs WS, Guillory SL, Mendelson MH, Sheiner P, Emre S, Miller C. Infectious ocular complications in orthotopic liver transplant patients. Clin Infect Dis 1997;24:1172–1177.

208. Pappagianis D, Collins MS, Hector R, Remington J. Development of resistance to amphotericin B in *Candida lusitaniae* infecting a human. Antimicrob Agents Chemother 1979;16:123–126.

209. Parker JC, McCloskey JJ, Lee RS. The emergence of candidosis: the dominant postmortem cerebral mycosis. Am J Clin Pathol 1978;70:31–36.

210. Perfect JR, Klotman ME, Gilbert CC, Crawford DD, Rosner GL, Wright KA, Peters WP. Prophylactic intravenous amphotericin B in neutropenic autologous bone marrow transplant recipients. J Infect Dis 1992;165:891–897.

211. Perraut LE Jr, Perraut LE, Bleiman B, Lyons J. Successful treatment of Candida albicans endophthalmitis with intravitreal amphotericin B. Arch Ophthalmol 1981;99:1565–1567.

212. Petranyi G, Meingassner JG, Mieth H. Antifungal activity of the allylamine derivative terbinafine in vitro. Antimicrob Agents Chemother 1987;31:1365–1368.

213. Pfaller M, Cabezudo I, Koontz F, Bale M, Gingrich R. Predictive value of surveillance cultures for systemic infection due to

Candida species. Eur J Clin Microbiol Infect Dis 1987;6:628–633.

214. Pfaller MA, Bale MJ, Buschelman B, Rhomberg P. Antifungal activity of a new triazole, D0870, compared with four other antifungal agents tested against clinical isolates of *Candida* and *Torulopsis glabrata*. Diagn Microbiol Infect Dis 1994;19:75–80.

215. Pfaller MA, Messer SA, Hollis RJ. Variations in DNA subtype, antifungal susceptibility, and slime production among clinical isolates of *Candida parapsilosis*. Diagn Microbiol Infect Dis 1995;21:9–14.

216. Pfaller MA, Rex JH, Rinaldi MG. Antifungal susceptibility testing: technical advances and potential clinical applications. Clin Infect Dis 1996;24:776–784.

216a. Pfaller MA., Rhine-Chalberg J, Barry AL, Rex JH, NIAID Mycoses Study Group, the Candidemia Study Group. Strain variation and antifungal susceptibility among bloodstream isolates of *Candida* species from 21 different medical institutions. Clin Infect Dis 1995;21:1507–1509.

217. Phillips P, Shafran S, Garber G, Rotstein C, Smaill F, Fong I, Salit I, Miller M, Williams K, Conley JM, Singer J, Ioannou S. Canadian Candidemia Study Group. Multicenter randomized trial of fluconazole versus amphotericin B for treatment of candidemia in non-neutropenic patients. Eur J Clin Microbiol Infect Dis 1997;16:337–345.

218. Pittard WBI, Thullen JD, Fanaroff AA. Neonatal septic arthritis. J Pediatr 1976;88:621–624.

218a. Pittet D, Li N, Woolson RF, Wenzel RP. Microbiological factors influencing the outcome of nosocomial bloodstream infections: a 6-year validated, population-based model. Clin Infect Dis 1997;24:1068–1078.

219. Pittet D, Monod M, Suter PM, Frenk E, Auckenthaler R. *Candida* colonization and subsequent infections in critically ill surgical patients. Ann Surg 1994;220:751–758.

220. Pizzo PA, Robichaud KJ, Gill FA, Witebsky FG. Empiric antibiotics and antifungal therapy for cancer patients with prolonged fever and granulocytopenia. Am J Med 1982;72: 101–111.

221. Plouffe JF, Brown DG, Silva J, Eck T, Stricof RL, Fekety FR. Nosocomial outbreak of *Candida parapsilosis* fungemia related to intravenous infusions. Arch Intern Med 1977;137: 1686–1689.

222. Polak A. 5-Fluorocytosine—current status with special references to mode of action and drug resistance. Contrib Microbiol Immunol 1977;4:158–167.

223. Polak A. Combination therapy of experimental candidiasis, cryptococcosis, aspergillosis and wangiellosis in mice. Chemotherapy 1987;33:381–395.

224. Pons V, Greenspan D, Lozada-Nur F, McPhail L, Gallant JE, Tunkel A, Johnson CC, McCarty J, Panzer H, Levenstein M, Barranco A, Green S. Oropharyngeal candidiasis in patients with AIDS: randomized comparison of fluconazole versus nystatin oral suspensions. Clin Infect Dis 1997;27:1204–1207.

225. Powderly WG, Finkelstein DM, Feinberg J, Frame P, He W, van der Horst C, Koletar SL, Eyster ME, Carey J, Waskin H, Hooton TM, Hyslop N, Specton SA, Bozzette SA, the NIAID AIDS Clinical Trials Group. A randomized trial comparing fluconazole with clotrimazole troches for the prevention of fungal infections in patients with advanced human immunodeficiency virus infection. N Engl J Med 1995;332:700–705.

226. Price MF, LaRocco MT, Gentry LO. Fluconazole susceptibilities of *Candida* species and distribution of species recovered from blood cultures over a 5-year period. Antimicrob Agents Chemother 1994;38:1422–1424.

227. Rantala A, Lehtonen OP, Kuttila K, Havia T, Niinikoski J. Diagnostic factors for postoperative candidosis in abdominal surgery. Ann Chir Gynaecol 1991;80:323–328.

228. Redding S, Smith J, Farinacci G, Rinaldi M, Fothergill A, Rhine-Chalberg J, Pfaller M. Resistance of *Candida albicans* to fluconazole during treatment of oropharyngeal candidiasis in a patient with AIDS: documentation by in vitro susceptibility testing and DNA subtype analysis. Clin Infect Dis 1994;18:240–242.

229. Rex JH, Bennett JE, Sugar AM, Pappas PG, Serody J, Edwards JE, Washburn RG, the NIAID Mycoses Study Group, the Candidemia Study Group. Intravascular catheter exchanges and the duration of candidemia. Clin Infect Dis 1995;21:994–996.

230. Rex JH, Bennett JE, Sugar AM, Pappas PG, Van der Horst CM, Edwards JE, Washburn RG, Scheld WM, Karchmer AW, Dine AP, Levenstein MJ, Webb CD, the Candidemia Study Group, the NIAID Mycoses Study Group. A randomized trial comparing fluconazole with amphotericin B for the treatment of candidemia in patients without neutropenia. N Engl J Med 1994;331:1325–1330.

231. Rex JH, Cooper CR Jr, Merz WG, Galgiani JN, Anaissie EJ. Detection of amphotericin B-resistant *Candida* isolates in a broth-based system. Antimicrob Agents Chemother 1995;39:906–909.

232. Rex JH, Pfaller MA, Barry AL, Nelson PW, Webb CD, the NIAID Mycoses Study Group and the Candidemia Study Group. Antifungal susceptibility testing of isolates from a randomized, multicenter trial of fluconazole vs. amphotericin B as treatment of non-neutropenic patients with candidemia. Antimicrob Agents Chemother 1995;39:40–44.

233. Rex JH, Pfaller MA, Galgiani JN, Bartlett MS, Espinel-Ingroff A, Ghannoum MA, Lancaster M, Odds FC, Rinaldi MG, Walsh TJ, Barry AL, Subcommittee on Antifungal Susceptibility Testing of the National Committee for Clinical Laboratory Standards. Development of interpretive breakpoints for antifungal susceptibility testing: conceptual framework and analysis of in vitro-in vivo correlation data for fluconazole, itraconazole, and *Candida* infections. Clin Infect Dis 1997;24:235–247.

234. Rex JH, Pfaller MA, Rinaldi MG, Polak A, Galgiani JN. Antifungal susceptibility testing. Clin Microbiol Rev 1993;6:367–381.

235. Rex JH, Rinaldi MG, Pfaller MA. Resistance of *Candida* species to fluconazole. Antimicrob Agents Chemother 1995;39:1–8.

236. Richter JM, Jacoby GA, Schapiro H, Warshaw AL. Pancreatic abscess due to *Candida* albicans. Ann Intern Med 1982;97:221–222.

237. Roberts DT. Oral therapeutic agents in fungal nail disease. J Am Acad Dermatol 1994;31:S78–81.

238. Rohner P, Pepey B, Auckenthaler R. Comparison of BacT/Alert with Signal blood culture system. J Clin Microbiol 1995;33:313–317.

239. Roseeuw D, De Doncker P. New approaches to the treatment of onychomycosis. J Am Acad Dermatol 1993;29:S45–S50.

240. Roupie E, Darmon J-Y, Brochard L, Saada M, Rekik N, Brun-Buisson C. Fluconazole therapy of candidal native valve endocarditis. Eur J Clin Microbiol Infect Dis 1991;10:458–459.

241. Samaranayake LP, Holmstrup P. Oral candidiasis and human immunodeficiency virus infection. J Oral Pathol Med 1989;18:554–564.

242. Sanford JP. The enigma of candiduria: evolution of bladder irrigation with amphotericin B for management—from anecdote to dogma and a lesson from Machiavelli. Clin Infect Dis 1993;16:145–147.

243. Santos JA, Beceiro J, Hernandez R, Salas S, Escriba R, Frias EG, Rodriguez JP, Quero J. Congenital cutaneous candidiasis: report of four cases and review of the literature. Eur J Pediatr 1991;150:336–338.

244. Savani DV, Perfect JR, Cobo LM, Durack DT. Penetration of new azole compounds into the eye and efficacy in experimental *Candida* endophthalmitis. Antimicrob Agents Chemother 1987;31:6–10.

245. Saxen H, Hoppu K, Pohjavuori M. Pharmacokinetics of fluconazole in very low birth weight infants during the first two weeks of life. Clin Pharmacol Ther 1993;54:269–277.

246. Schaffner A, Böhler A. Amphotericin B refractory aspergillosis after itraconazole: evidence for significant antagonism. Mycoses 1993;36:421–424.

247. Schaffner A, Frick PG. The effect of ketoconazole on amphotericin B in a model of disseminated aspergillosis. J Infect Dis 1985;151:902–910.

248. Schaffner A, Schaffner M. Effect of prophylactic fluconazole on the frequency of fungal infections, amphotericin B use, and health care costs in patients undergoing intensive chemotherapy for hematologic neoplasias. J Infect Dis 1995;172:1035–1041.

249. Scheven M, Scheven C, Hahn K, Senf A. Post-antibiotic effect and post-exposure polyene antagonism of azole antimycotics in *Candida albicans:* dependency on lipophilia. Mycoses 1995;38(Suppl 1):14–21.

250. Scheven M, Scheven M-L. Interaction between azoles and amphotericin B in the treatment of candidiasis. Clin Infect Dis 1995;20:1079.

251. Scheven M, Schwegler F. Antagonistic interactions between azoles and amphotericin B with yeasts depend on azole lipophilia for special test conditions in vitro. Antimicrob Agents Chemother 1995;39:1779–1783.

252. Schrank JH Jr, Dooley DP. Purulent pericarditis caused by *Candida* species: case report and review. Clin Infect Dis 1995;21:182–187.

253. Seay RE, Larson TA, Toscano JP, Bostrom BC, O'Leary MC, Uden DL. Pharmacokinetics of fluconazole in immune-compromised children with leukemia or other hematologic disease. Pharmacotherapy 1995;15:52–58.

254. Shechtman LB, Funaro L, Robin T, Bottone EJ, Cuttner J. Clotrimazole treatment of oral candidiasis in patients with neoplastic disease. Am J Med 1984;76:91–94.

255. Silva-Cruz A, Andrade L, Sobral L, Francisca A. Itraconazole versus placebo in the management of vaginal candidiasis. Int J Gynaecol Obstet 1991;36:229–235.

256. Silveira LH, Cuellar ML, Citera G, Cabrera GE, Scopelitis E, Espinoza LR. Candida arthritis. Rheum Dis Clin North Am 1993;19:427–437.

257. Slavin MA, Osborne B, Adams R, Levenstein MJ, Schoch HG, Feldman AR, Meyers JD, Bowden RA. Efficacy and safety of fluconazole prophylaxis for fungal infections after bone marrow transplantation—a prospective, randomized, double-blind study. J Infect Dis 1995;171:1545–1542.

258. Smego RA Jr, Perfect JR, Durack DT. Combined therapy with amphotericin B and 5-fluorocytosine for *Candida* meningitis. Rev Infect Dis 1984;6:791–801.

259. Smith DE, Midgley J, Allan M, Connolly GM, Gazzard BG. Itraconazole versus ketoconazole in the treatment of oral and

oesophageal candidosis in patients infected with HIV. AIDS 1991;5:1367–1371.

260. Smith KJ, Warnock DW, Kennedy CT, Johnson EM, Hopwood V, Van Cutsem J, Vanden Bossche H. Azole resistance in *Candida albicans*. J Med Vet Mycol 1986;24:133–144.

261. Sobel JD. Recurrent vulvovaginal candidiasis. A prospective study of the efficacy of maintenance ketoconazole therapy. N Engl J Med 1986;315:1455–1458.

262. Sobel JD. Treatment of recurrent vulvovaginal candidiasis with maintenance fluconazole. Int J Gynecol Obstet 1992;37:17–34.

263. Sobel JD. Candidal vulvovaginitis. Clin Obstet Gynecol 1993; 36:153–165.

264. Sobel JD, Brooker D, Stein GE, Thomason JL, Wermeling DP, Bradley B, Weinstein L, the Fluconazole Vaginitis Study Group. Single oral dose fluconazole compared with conventional clotrimazole topical therapy of *Candida* vaginitis. Am J Obstet Gynecol 1995;172:1263–1268.

265. Sobel JD, Chaim W. Treatment of *Candida glabrata* vaginitis: a retrospective review of boric acid therapy. Clin Infect Dis 1997;24:649–652.

266. Solomkin JS, Flohr AB, Quie PG, Simmons RL. The role of *Candida* in intraperitoneal infections. Surgery 1980;88:524–530.

267. Solomkin JS, Simmons RL. *Candida* infection in surgical patients. World J Surg 1980;4:381–394.

268. Stamm WE. Catheter-associated urinary tract infections: epidemiology, pathogenesis, and prevention. Am J Med 1991;91 (Suppl 3B):65S–71S.

269. Starfen SP, Medoff G, Fraser VJ, et al. Candiduria: retrospective review in hospitalized patients. Infect Dis Clin Pract 1994;3:23–29.

270. Sterling TR, Gasser RA Jr, Ziegler A. Emergence of resistance to amphotericin B during therapy for *Candida glabrata* infection in an immunocompetent host. Clin Infect Dis 1996;23: 187–188.

271. Stern GA, Fetkenhour CL, O'Grady RB. Intravitreal amphotericin B treatment of Candida endophthalmitis. Arch Ophthalmol 1977;95:89–93.

272. Stevens DA, Greene SI, Lang OS. Thrush can be prevented in patients with acquired immunodeficiency syndrome and the acquired immunodeficiency syndrome–related complex. Randomized, double-blind, placebo-controlled study of 100-mg oral fluconazole daily. Arch Intern Med 1991;151:2458–2464.

273. Stiller RL, Bennett JE, Scholer HJ, Wall M, Polak A, Stevens DA. Susceptibility to 5-fluorocytosine and prevalence of serotype in 402 *Candida albicans* isolates from the United States. Antimicrob Agents Chemother 1982;22:482–487.

274. Strauss RG. Granulocyte transfusion therapy. Hematol Oncol Clin North Am 1994;8:1159–1166.

275. Strinden WD, Helgerson RB, Maki DG. Candida septic thrombosis of the great central veins associated with central catheters. Ann Surg 1985;202:653–658.

276. Sugar AM. Antifungal therapy in CAPD peritonitis—do we have a choice. Semin Dial 1991;4:145–146.

277. Sugar AM, Hitchcock CA, Troke PF, Picard M. Combination therapy of murine invasive candidiasis with fluconazole and amphotericin B. Antimicrob Agents Chemother 1995;39: 598–601.

278. Sugar AM, Saunders C, Diamond RD. Successful treatment of *Candida* osteomyelitis with fluconazole. A noncomparative study of two patients. Diagn Microbiol Infect Dis 1990;13: 517–520.

279. Sugar AS. Use of amphotericin B with azole antifungal drugs: what are we doing? Antimicrob Agents Chemother 1995; 39:1907–1912.

280. Sullivan DJ, Westerneng TJ, Haynes KA, Bennett DE, Coleman DC. Candida dubliniensis sp. nov.: phenotypic and molecular characterization of a novel species associated with oral candidosis in HIV-infected individuals. Microbiology 1995; 141:1507–1521.

281. Swanson H, Hughes PA, Messer SA, Lepow ML, Pfaller MA. *Candida albicans* arthritis one year after successful treatment of fungemia in a healthy infant. J Pediatr 1996;129:688–694.

282. Tang C. Successful treatment of *Candida albicans* osteomyelitis with fluconazole. J Infect 1993;26:89–92.

283. Thomas MG, Ellis-Pegler RB. Fluconazole treatment of Candida glabrata peritonitis [Letter]. J Antimicrob Chemother 1989;24:94–96.

284. Tollemar J, Hockerstedt K, Ericzon BG, Jalanko H, Ringden O. Liposomal amphotericin B prevents invasive fungal infections in liver transplant recipients. A randomized, placebo-controlled study. Transplantation 1995;59:45–50.

285. Tollemar J, Ringden O, Andersson S, Sundberg B, Ljungman P, Tyden G. Randomized double-blind study of liposomal amphotericin B (Ambisome) prophylaxis of invasive fungal infections in bone marrow transplant recipients. Bone Marrow Transplant 1993;12:577–582.

286. Torres-Rojas JR, Stratton CW, Sanders CV, A HT, Hawley HB, Dascomb HE, Vial LJ. Candida suppurative peripheral thrombophlebitis. Ann Intern Med 1982;96:431–435.

287. Tunkel AR, Thomas CY, Wispelwey B. Candida prosthetic arthritis: report of a case treated with fluconazole and review of the literature. Am J Med 1993;94:100–103.

288. Urbak SF, Degn T. Fluconazole in the treatment of Candida albicans endophthalmitis. Acta Ophthalmol 1992;70:528–529.

289. Utley JR, Mills J, Roe BB. The role of valve replacement in the treatment of fungal endocarditis. J Thorac Cardiovasc Surg 1975;69:255–258.

290. van den Anker JN, van Popele NM, Sauer PJ. Antifungal agents in neonatal systemic candidiasis. Antimicrob Agents Chemother 1995;39:1391–1397.

291. van der Merr JWM, Keuning JJ, Scheijgrond HW, Heykants J, van Cutsem J, Brugmans J. The influence of gastric acidity on the bioavailability of ketoconazole. J Antimicrob Chemother 1980;6:552–554.

292. van Deventer AJM, van Vlient HJA, Hop WCJ, Goessens WHF. Diagnostic value of anti-*Candida* enolase antibodies. J Clin Microbiol 1994;32:17–23.

293. van Deventer AJM, van Vliet HJA, Voogd L, Hop WCJ, Goessens WHF. Increased specificity of antibody detection in surgical patients with invasive candidiasis with cytoplasmic antigens depleted of mannan residues. J Clin Microbiol 1993; 31:994–997.

294. Van Peer A, Woestenborghs R, Heykants J, Gasparini R, Gauwenbergh G. The effects of food and dose on the oral systemic availability of itraconzole in healthy subjects. Eur J Clin Pharmacol 1989;36:423–426.

295. Vanden Bossche H, Marichal P, Gorrens J, Bellens D, Moereels H, Janssen AJ. Mutation in cytochrome P-450-dependent 14O-demethylase results in decreased affinity for azole antifungals. Biochem Soc Trans 1990;18:56–59.

295a. Van't Wout JW, Raven EJ, van der Meer JW. Treatment of invasive aspergillosis with itraconazole in a patient with chronic granulomatous disease. J Infect Dis 1990;20:147–150.

296. Viscoli C, Castagnola E, Fioredda F, Ciravegna B, Barigione G, Terragna A. Fluconazole in the treatment of candidiasis in immunocompromised children. Antimicrob Agents Chemother 1991;35:365–367.

297. Voice RA, Bradley SF, Sangeorzan JA, Kauffman CA. Chronic candidal meningitis: an uncommon manifestation of candidiasis. Clin Infect Dis 1994;19:60–66.

298. Voss A, Meis JFGM, Hoogkamp-Korstanje JAA. Fluconazole in the management of fungal urinary tract infections. Infection 1994;4:247–251.

299. Wade J, Schreiber J, Saltzberg D, Bustamante C, Cushing D. Amphotericin B therapy of biopsy-proven *Candida* esophagitis: a double-blind trial [Abstract 740]. 31st Interscience Conference on Antimicrobial Agents and Chemotherapy, 1991.

300. Wallbridge DR, McCartney AC, Richardson MD. Fluconazole in the treatment of *Candida* prosthetic valve endocarditis. Mycoses 1993;36:259–261.

301. Walsh TJ, Bustamente CI, Vlahov D, Standiford HC. Candidal suppurative peripheral thrombophlebitis: recognition, prevention, and management. Infect Control 1986;7:16–22.

302. Walsh TJ, Francesconi A, Kasai M, Chanock SJ. PCR and single-strand conformational polymorphism for recognition of medically important opportunistic fungi. J Clin Microbiol 1995;33:3216–3220.

302a. Walsh TJ, Gray W. *Candida* epiglottitis in immunocompromised patients. Chest 1987;91:482–485.

302b. Walsh TJ, Hiemenz J, Pizzo PA. Editorial response: evolving risk factors for invasive fungal infections—all neutropenic patients are not the same. Clin Infect Dis 1994;18:793–798.

303. Walsh TJ, Lee J, Lecciones J, Rubin M, Butler K, Francis P. Empiric therapy with amphotericin B in febrile granulocytopenic patients. Rev Infect Dis 1991;13:496–503.

304. Walsh TJ, Merz WG. Pathologic features in the human alimentary tract associated with invasiveness of Candida tropicalis. Am J Clin Pathol 1986;85:498–502.

305. Walsh TJ, Merz WG, Lee JW, Schaufele R, Sein T, Whitcomb PO, Ruddel M, Burns W, Wingard JR, Swichenko AC, Goodman T, Pizzo PA. Diagnosis and therapeutic monitoring of invasive candidiasis by rapid enzymatic detection of serum D-arabinitol. Am J Med 1995;99:164–172.

305a. Walsh TJ, Whitcomb PO, Ravankar S, Shannon K, Alish S, Pizzo PA. Successful treatment of hepatosplenic candidiasis through repeated episodes of neutropenia. Cancer 1995;76:2357–2362.

305b. Walsh TJ, Whitcomb PO, Piscitelli S, Figg WD, Hill S, Chanock SJ, Jarosinski P, Gupta R, Pizzo PA. Safety, tolerance, and pharmacokinetics of amphotericin B lipid complex in children with hepatosplenic candidiasis. Antimicrob Agents Chemother 1997;41:1944–1948.

305c. Wang JN, Liu CC, Huang TZ, Huang SS, Wu JM. Laryngeal candidiasis in children. Scand J Infect Dis 1997;29:427–429.

306. Wanger A, Mills K, Nelson PW, Rex JH. Comparison of Etest and National Committee for Clinical Laboratory Standards broth macrodilution method for antifungal susceptibility testing: enhanced ability to detect amphotericin B-resistant *Candida* isolates. Antimicrob Agents Chemother 1995;39:2520–2522.

307. Weber DJ, Rutala WA, Samsa GP, Wilson MB, Hoffmann KK. Relative frequency of nosocomial pathogens at a university hospital during the decade 1980 to 1989. Am J Infect Control 1992;20:192–197.

308. Weems JJ Jr. *Candida parapsilosis:* epidemiology, pathogenicity, clinical manifestations, and antimicrobial susceptibility. Clin Infect Dis 1992;14:756–766.

308a. Weers-Pothoff G, Havermans JF, Kamphuis J, Sinnige HA, Meis JF. *Candida tropicalis* arthritis in a patient with acute myeloid leukemia successfully treated with fluconazole: case report and review of the literature. Infection 1997;25:109–111.

309. Wey SB, Mori M, Pfaller MA, Woolson RF, Wenzel RP. Hospital acquired candidemia: the attributable mortality and excess length of stay. Arch Intern Med 1988;148:2642–2645.

309a. White TC, Marra KA, Bowden RA. Clinical, cellular, and molecular factors that contribute to antifungal drug resistance. Clin Microbiol Rev 1998;11:382–402.

310. Wilcox CM, Darouiche RO, Laine L, Moskovitz BL, Mallegol I, Wu J. A randomized, double-blind comparison of itraconazole oral solution and fluconazole tables in the treatment of esophageal candidiasis. J Infect Dis 1997;176:227–232.

311. Wilson ML, Davis TE, Mirrett S, Reynolds J, Fuller D, Allen SD, Flint KK, Koontz F, Reller LB. Controlled comparison of the BACTEC high-blood-volume fungal medium, BACTEC plus 26 aerobic blood culture bottle, and 10-milliliter isolator blood culture system for detection of fungemia and bacteremia. J Clin Microbiol 1993;31:865–871.

312. Wingard JR. Importance of *Candida* species other than *C. albicans* as pathogens in oncology patients. Clin Infect Dis 1995; 20:115–125.

313. Wingard JR, Dick JD, Merz WG, Sandford GR, Saral R, Burns WH. Pathogenicity of Candida tropicalis and Candida albicans after gastrointestinal inoculation in mice. Infect Immun 1980; 29:808–813.

314. Wingard JR, Dick JD, Merz WG, Sandford GR, Saral R, Burns WH. Differences in virulence of clinical isolates of Candida tropicalis and Candida albicans in mice. Infect Immun 1982; 37:833–836.

315. Wingard JR, Merz WG, Rinaldi MG, Johnson TR, Karp JE, Saral R. Increase in *Candida krusei* infection among patients with bone marrow transplantation and neutropenia treated prophylactically with fluconazole. N Engl J Med 1991;325:1274–1277.

316. Wingard JR, Merz WG, Rinaldi MG, Miller CB, Karp JE, Saral R. Association of *Torulopsis glabrata* infections with fluconazole prophylaxis in neutropenic bone marrow transplant patients. Antimicrob Agents Chemother 1993;37:1847–1849.

317. Wingard JR, Merz WG, Saral R. *Candida tropicalis:* a major pathogen in immunocompromised patients. Ann Intern Med 1979;91:539–543.

318. Winston DJ, Chandrasekar PH, Lazarus HM, Goodman JL, Silber JL, Horowitz H, Shadduck RK, Rosenfeld CS, Ho WG, Islam MZ, et al. Fluconazole prophylaxis of fungal infections in patients with acute leukemia. Results of a randomized placebo-controlled, double-blind, multicenter trial. Ann Intern Med 1993;118:495–503.

319. Wise GJ, Goldberg P, Kozinn PJ. Genitourinary candidiasis: diagnosis and treatment. J Urol 1976;116:778–780.

320. Witt MD, Imhoff T, Li C, Bayer AS. Comparison of fluconazole and amphotericin B for treatment of experimental *Candida* endocarditis caused by non-*C. albicans* strains. Antimicrob Agents Chemother 1993;37:2030–2032.

321. Wong-Beringer A, Jacobs RA, Guglielmo BJ. Treatment of funguria. JAMA 1992;267.

322. Yap BS, Bodey GP. Oropharyngeal candidiasis treated with a troche form of clotrimazole. Arch Intern Med 1979;139:656–657.

323. Zaruba K, Peters J, Jungbluth H. Successful prophylaxis for fungal peritonitis in patients on continuous ambulatory peritoneal dialysis: six years experience. Am J Kidney Dis 1991;17:43–46.

324. Zenker PN, Rosenberg EM, Van Dyke RB, Rabalais GP, Daum RS. Successful medical treatment of presumed *Candida* endocarditis in critically ill infants. J Pediatr 1991;119:472–477.

325. Zingman BS. Resolution of refractory AIDS-related mucosal candidiasis after initiation of didanosine plus saquinavir. N Engl J Med 1996;334:1674–1675.

Coccidioides immitis

Paul L. Williams and Neil M. Ampel

GENERAL DESCRIPTION

Coccidioides immitis, a dimorphic fungus limited to the New World, is the cause of coccidioidomycosis. Its highest prevalence is in the San Joaquin Valley of California and in southwestern Arizona (51). Despite the availability of newer antifungal agents over the past several years, the treatment of coccidioidomycosis, particularly among those with chronic pulmonary infection or extrathoracic disseminated infection, has remained difficult and problematic (59).

Natural History

An understanding of the vagaries of the natural history of symptomatic coccidioidal infection is essential to the managing physician, particularly because no placebo-controlled trials of antifungal therapy for coccidioidomycosis have ever been performed. Approximately 65% of all coccidioidal infections are asymptomatic, recognizable only by a durable delayed-type hypersensitivity reaction after intradermal injection of coccidioidal antigen. The other 35% of infections are symptomatic, generally associated with respiratory symptoms, and almost always self-limited. Chronic illness results in fewer than 5% of all of those infected (28).

Primary pulmonary coccidioidomycosis may present asymptomatically or with nonspecific manifestations (71). Roentgenographic studies during primary coccidioidomycosis usually demonstrate unilateral pulmonary infiltrates that usually resolve within 2 months. In approximately 5% of patients with primary coccidioidomycosis, pulmonary residuae develop, most commonly pulmonary abscesses, which appear radiographically as nodules (6, 7). Nodules can excavate, forming either thin- or thick-wall cavities. Occasionally such cavities become secondarily infected (55). Primary pneumonia with symptoms persisting longer than 6 weeks, termed *chronic progressive pulmonary coccidioidomycosis,* occurs in about 1% of patients (28).

Disseminated coccidioidomycosis, when infection spreads beyond the thoracic cavity, occurs in fewer than 1% of all patients. The most common sites are the skin, soft tissue, bone, joints, central nervous system, or combinations of these. Extrathoracic dissemination almost always occurs within 12 months of the initial pulmonary infection, although the initial infection may have been clinically silent.

Prior to development of specific antifungal therapy, it was recognized that untreated extrathoracic disseminated coccidioidomycosis might follow any one of several clinical courses, including steady progression, persistence without progression, remittence with exacerbation, or spontaneous healing (24). Which course any particular patient might take is unpre-

dictable. These natural history observations imply that one must be careful not to ascribe all clinical improvement in any given case of coccidioidomycosis to antifungal therapy. This is particularly applicable to localized cutaneous disease, where spontaneous improvement is well documented (24).

SUSCEPTIBILITY IN VITRO AND IN VIVO

No standardized method exists for testing the susceptibility of *C. immitis* to antifungal agents in vitro. Similarly, while animal models have been used to assess various therapies after experimental infection with *C. immitis* (12, 23, 47), these in vivo systems were not necessarily predictive of results in humans. Because of this, virtually all information on the treatment of coccidioidomycosis in humans is based on either clinical experience or clinical trials.

ANTIFUNGAL THERAPY

There have been no trials comparing the efficacy of different antifungal therapies for the treatment of coccidioidomycosis. However, given the inconvenience and toxicity of intravenous amphotericin B and the convenience and relatively low toxicity of the currently available oral antifungal agents, we believe that oral azole antifungals, such as fluconazole, itraconazole, and ketoconazole, should be the therapy of choice for most patients with coccidioidomycosis. Intravenous amphotericin B should be reserved for life-threatening nonmeningeal disease or patients who fail to respond to azole therapy.

Amphotericin B

Amphotericin B is a polyene antifungal derived from soil actinomycetes. Originally introduced in 1955 in a colloidal dispersion with deoxycholate (Fungizone), it was the first antifungal agent shown to be clinically effective for the treatment of coccidioidomycosis. It can only be administered intravenously and has numerous toxicities, including fever, phlebitis, hypokalemia, anemia, and renal dysfunction (30). It has been demonstrated to be fungicidal in vitro against *C. immitis* at concentrations of 0.5 μg/mL or less but has never been shown to be more than fungistatic in vivo, either in animal models or in humans.

Although there is consensus that amphotericin B is effective therapy in patients with serious pulmonary or disseminated coccidioidomycosis, no placebo-controlled trial proving its efficacy in coccidioidomycosis has ever been done. The efficacy of amphotericin B in the treatment of coccidioidomycosis was summarized by Hardenbrook and Barriere (37). Of the 103 patients treated with amphotericin B that these authors identified in 34 separate publications, 70% had a favorable clinical response. This summary is complemented by over three decades of unpublished experience supporting the concept that amphotericin B is effective therapy for many cases of serious pulmonary and nonmeningeal disseminated coccidioidomycosis.

There is also consensus that amphotericin B therapy for patients with chronic pulmonary or disseminated coccidioidomycosis should be long enough to achieve symptomatic benefit and a decline in serum complement fixation (IgG) antibody titer to below 1:16, at least. The total dose of amphotericin B required to achieve this effect in any given patient is undefined, but in a study of 11 patients with chronic pulmonary coccidioidomycosis, treatment failure was associated with receiving a total dose of intravenous amphotericin B below 39 mg/kg, or 2.7 g in a 70-kg patient (57). Extrathoracic coccidioidomycosis has generally been treated with total doses of intravenous amphotericin B ranging from 2.5 to 3.0 g. The efficacy of amphotericin B for bone and joint coccidioidomycosis is not fully established. Iger reviewed 112 such cases between 1964 and 1976; of these, only 12 patients were judged to have done well (39). Other investigators have also not been convinced of the efficacy of amphotericin B for bone and joint coccidioidomycosis (69).

Amphotericin B in the management of coccidioidomycosis has had its biggest impact in the treatment of meningitis (22). Combined use of intravenous amphotericin B with direct injection of amphotericin B (1 mg three times weekly) into the cerebrospinal fluid (CSF) has reduced mortality in this disease to between 30 and 50% and even resulted in true cures, defined as a CSF white blood cell concentration below 20 cells/μL with normal protein and glucose concentrations and undetectable complement-fixation antibody (42). Doses as high as 2 mg per injection have been recommended to speed treatment (43), although many patients are unable to tolerate this because of severe headache. Complications of coccidioidal meningitis include obstructive and nonobstructive hydrocephalus, vasculitic events leading to stroke, progressive arachnoiditis, and parenchymal space-occupying brain lesions. These may all occur during therapy (4, 68). In addition, injection of amphotericin B directly into the CSF may also lead to complications. When administered intrathecally by cisternal puncture, brainstem puncture and subarachnoid hemorrhage may occur. When administered through a ventricular, cisternal, or lumbar reservoir, arachnoiditis, secondary bacterial infection, and obstruction may occur. Hence, despite its efficacy, the complications of direct delivery of amphotericin B into the CSF make its use problematic in coccidioidal meningitis.

Because of the dose-limiting toxicity of amphotericin B formulated with deoxycholate, newer alternatives with other lipid formulations that allow higher doses and less toxicity have undergone recent study. However, currently, no peer-reviewed published data exists describing the use of these newer formulations for the treatment of coccidioidomycosis. Two studies have been reported in abstract form, one using lipid-complexed amphotericin B (ABLC, Abelcet) (58), and another using amphotericin B in colloidal dispersion with cholesteryl sulfate (ABCD, Amphotec) (38). Both agents appeared to have efficacy and reasonable safety in the treatment of coccidioidomycosis. However, these unpublished studies are too limited to allow conclusions, and further data are needed before the use of newer amphotericin B formulations can be recommended in the management of coccidioidomycosis (32).

Azole Antifungal Agents

Azole antifungals are synthetic agents that differ significantly in chemistry, site of action, pharmacokinetics, and toxicity from amphotericin B (14). Unlike amphotericin B, the three currently available drugs, fluconazole, itraconazole, and ketoconazole, are all orally absorbable. All are fungistatic against *C. immitis*.

Because of both significant drug interactions and suppression of adrenal and gonadal testosterone synthesis (14, 61), the use of ketoconazole for the treatment of coccidioidomycosis has been supplanted by two newer triazole antifungal agents, fluconazole and itraconazole. Unlike ketoconazole, the triazoles lack significant effects on androgen synthesis (14). Although no comparative trials have been done, the new triazoles appear to have greater efficacy in the treatment of coccidioidomycosis than ketoconazole (28).

Fluconazole, a relatively low molecular weight bis-triazole, is characterized by moderate water solubility, good oral absorption not dependent on gastric acidity, and relatively few drug interactions. In a study of 73 patients with nonmeningeal disseminated coccidioidomycosis, conducted by the Mycoses Study Group, 19 patients had soft-tissue disease, 40 had chronic pulmonary disease, and 14 had skeletal or joint disease. Underlying conditions with immunocompromising characteristics existed in 49 patients, including 7 with HIV infection. Patients initially received 200 mg/day, which was increased to 400 mg/day in those not clinically responding. Overall, there was a 67% response rate, with the best response in those with soft-tissue, skeletal, or joint disease. However, relapses occurred in approximately 30% of patients after fluconazole was discontinued (11).

Fluconazole was also found to be effective therapy for coccidioidal meningitis (29). In another Mycoses Study Group trial, patients were treated with 400 mg of fluconazole daily for up to 4 years. Of the 47 evaluable patients, 37 (75%) responded favorably to treatment, including those with HIV infection. Improvement was maximal within the first 4 to 8 months of therapy. However, most patients responding to therapy continued to demonstrate modest abnormalities in CSF findings after up to 20 months of therapy.

Itraconazole shares structural similarities with ketoconazole and, like it, requires an acidic environment for optimal absorption and has numerous drug interactions (14). A Mycoses Study Group trial examined 49 patients with nonmeningeal chronic coccidioidal pulmonary disease or disseminated disease treated with itraconazole (400 mg/day). Forty-four patients completed a minimum of 6 months of therapy and were evaluable. Of these, 25 (57%) achieved clinical remission, treatment failed in 16 (36%), and 3 (7%) did not complete therapy because of drug toxicity. Of the 25 patients who attained remission, 11 completed at least 1 year of posttreatment follow-up observation and 4 (36%) relapsed. All relapses occurred at the site of primary disease.

Although itraconazole does not achieve significant levels in the CSF, it appears to possess efficacy in treating coccidioidal meningitis. In a small series, Tucker et al. found that four of five patients with coccidioidal meningitis treated with itraconazole (400 mg/day) alone responded to therapy. An additional five patients received concomitant intrathecal amphotericin B with oral itraconazole, and all five responded favorably (63).

Combination Therapy with Amphotericin B and Azoles

The utility of combining amphotericin B with azole antifungal agents for the treatment of fungal diseases has been recently reviewed by Sugar (60). While concern has existed that such a combination might be antagonistic, no clinical evidence supports this contention for most clinical situations. Moreover, the combination of amphotericin B with fluconazole has become a relatively common clinical practice. In the absence of extensive data, Sugar has suggested that combination therapy may be used after careful consideration of the particular clinical situation and with close documentation of the clinical outcome (60).

The combination of amphotericin B and azoles for the treatment of coccidioidomycosis has never been formally studied. However, anecdotal clinical experience and review of specific literature suggests that the combination of amphotericin B and fluconazole in particular may be useful in certain instances. This combination has been most frequently used in the management of recalcitrant coccidioidal meningitis (34, 63, 64) and has often reduced the amount of amphotericin B required to achieve clinical improvement. Hence, the combination of amphotericin B and an azole antifungal, particularly fluconazole, may be considered in any patient with disseminated coccidioidomycosis, particularly meningitis, who clearly lacks a clinical response to single-agent therapy.

SPECIAL SITUATIONS
Primary Focal Pneumonia

Although antifungal therapy is often prescribed for primary focal coccidioidal pneumonia in the nonimmunocompromised patient, there are no data indicating that treatment either shortens the course of the acute disease or prevents later dissemination (28). Based on this, we do not recommend routine antifungal therapy for primary coccidioidal pneumonia in such patients. However, certain factors may mitigate this decision (59). Antifungal therapy may be considered for severely ill patients, patients with high complement-fixation (IgG) serum antibody titers (1:16) or persistently positive tube precipitin (IgM) serum antibodies, high-inoculum exposure (e.g., laboratory accidents or field anthropology infections) (51), or extensive or enlarging pulmonary processes, particularly in the setting of a negative coccidioidal skin test. Underlying conditions that may also prompt initiation of therapy are discussed below.

If antifungal therapy is prescribed, an oral azole is most appropriate, and a dose of at least 400 mg/day should be given. The length of therapy is undefined, but it should continue at least until symptoms have improved. Since dissemination may still occur after a course of therapy, the patient should be followed every 2 to 3 months during the first year after cessation of therapy for signs and symptoms of extrathoracic dissemination.

Residual Coccidioidal Pulmonary Lesions

In general, residual manifestations of pulmonary coccidioidomycosis do not require therapy but occasionally can become management problems, either because of confusion with other diseases or because of complications associated with the lesions themselves.

Nodules

Nodules are one result of primary coccidioidal pneumonia. They are usually single and less than 4 cm in diameter (20). In the coccidioidal endemic area, coccidioidomycosis is the cause of solitary pulmonary nodules in up to 60% of patients (27, 54). They require no therapy but often cannot be differentiated from malignant lesions (50). There are several approaches to their management. First, the nodule can be biopsied. If accessible, percutaneous fine-needle aspiration is a useful technique that yields the diagnosis in up to half of patients. Histologic examination is more sensitive than culture (27). When the nodule is not accessible or definitive diagnosis is not established by needle aspiration even after multiple attempts, either thoracoscopic or open lung biopsy can be performed.

In some patients, it may be reasonable to follow the nodule radiographically over time. Patients who are candidates for this approach are individuals with a low risk for pulmonary malignancy who live in the coccidioidal endemic area and have a positive coccidioidal skin test (70). If the size of the nodule decreases over time in such a patient, it is most likely a coccidioidal nodule.

Cavities

Coccidioidal cavities result from necrosis and excavation of pulmonary nodules. They are usually solitary in the upper lung fields, may either be thin-walled without surrounding infiltration or thick-walled with surrounding infiltration, and are usually less than 4 cm in diameter. In most patients, cavities progressively decrease in size within 2 years, and no therapy is required (20). However, in a small number of patients, cavities may be associated with complications.

Hemoptysis occurs in approximately 15% of patients with cavities and is usually self-limited (20). For such patients, particularly if the sputum culture is positive for *C. immitis,* antifungal therapy is indicated. If the patient is otherwise stable, an oral azole (400 mg/day) is appropriate treatment. Treatment should continue for 3 to 6 months from the time the hemoptysis abates. Occasionally, hemoptysis is massive and life threatening. In these cases, immediate surgical resection of the cavity is indicated, and although there are no data, we would recommend adjunctive antifungal chemotherapy. One approach is to give intravenous amphotericin B to a total dose of 500 to 1000 mg. Alternatively, fluconazole at a daily oral dose of 400 mg could be given. With oral fluconazole, the duration of therapy requires individualization, but we recommend a course of at least 3 months.

Another complication associated with coccidioidal cavities

is secondary infection, generally made apparent by development of a productive cough and an air-fluid level within the cavity. Cavities can be secondarily infected with bacteria or other fungi, especially *Aspergillus* species. Rarely, a coccidioidal mycetoma containing hyphal elements may form within a coccidioidal cavity (55, 62). Management involves empirical antibiotics for cavities secondarily infected with bacteria. For fungal mycetomas, particularly those associated with recurrent hemoptysis, surgical resection is the treatment of choice (10).

Pyopneumothorax results when a subpleural cavity ruptures into the pleural space, causing pneumothorax associated with an exudative pleural fluid. This local complication of coccidioidomycosis does not necessarily indicate dissemination of infection or poor prognosis. Prompt surgical closure of the bronchopleural defect is required (16). Most clinicians would use antifungal therapy adjunctively with surgery, but the type and length of such therapy is not established. We recommend the same approach to antifungal chemotherapy used when surgery is performed for hemoptysis.

Chronic Pulmonary, Diffuse Pulmonary, and Extrathoracic Disseminated Disease

Antifungal therapy is always required for chronic pulmonary, diffuse pulmonary, and extrathoracic disseminated disease. Because no comparative trials of any antifungal agents in coccidioidomycosis exist, there is great latitude in the treatment approach. On the basis of clinical experience, we recommend using amphotericin B as initial therapy for any patient who appears fulminantly ill and requires hospitalization. On the other hand, for less ill patients, an oral azole agent seems a reasonable initial choice. In all cases of azole therapy, the minimum daily starting dose is 400 mg. Many clinicians start at higher doses than this (e.g., 800 mg/day) and reduce the dose to 400 mg/day as the patient responds.

Chronic Progressive Pneumonia

Chronic progressive pneumonia is characterized by pulmonary symptoms for more than 6 weeks, a chest radiograph demonstrating persistent pulmonary parenchymal abnormalities, a positive sputum culture for *C. immitis,* and positive coccidioidal serologic tests (8). All four available chemotherapeutic agents—amphotericin B, ketoconazole, fluconazole, and itraconazole—have shown efficacy in treating chronic, progressive coccidioidal pneumonia. Since most patients with chronic pneumonia do not require hospitalization, initial therapy with an oral azole is a reasonable choice. For all three agents, a daily dosage of at least 400 mg is recommended. Although no comparative trial has been published, review of all the separate trials suggests that ketoconazole is inferior to fluconazole and itraconazole (28). Therefore, we would recommend either fluconazole or itraconazole (400 mg/day orally) as initial therapy (11, 33). If the patient fails to respond over a 1-month period, doses can be increased. A subset of patients will not respond to azole antifungal therapy at any dose. For these patients, amphotericin B should be used.

Some patients with chronic radiographic abnormalities, particularly biapical fibrocavitary changes, have minimal pulmonary symptoms. It is unclear whether these patients benefit from antifungal therapy. A reasonable approach to such patients is close follow-up without therapy. Worsening symptoms with progressive chest radiographic findings (particularly in association with a positive sputum culture for *C. immitis*), rising coccidioidal serologic titers, or systemic symptoms favor initiating antifungal therapy.

Diffuse, Reticulonodular Pneumonia

Diffuse pulmonary involvement is a rare but severe complication of coccidioidal infection. It is usually the initial manifestation of coccidioidomycosis rather than a progression from primary, focal pneumonia. It may mimic bacterial pneumonia with septic shock (48). While the chest radiographic pattern has been described as "miliary" (31), the precise term should be "reticulonodular," since both nodules and interstitial infiltrates are seen. Diffuse pulmonary involvement most commonly occurs in patients with underlying immunosuppressive conditions, such as those with AIDS, those with cancer undergoing chemotherapy, or those on chronic corticosteroid therapy (2), but may be seen in patients without underlying immunosuppression who have been exposed to a large coccidioidal inoculum (45). It is often associated with fungemia and undoubtedly represents a severe form of dissemination (2, 31). Prognosis is grave, with death commonly occurring within 1 month of diagnosis (2).

There are no controlled trials of any form of antifungal therapy for this manifestation of coccidioidomycosis. On the basis of our clinical experience, we recommend beginning intravenous amphotericin B at 1.0 to 1.5 mg/kg/day. Some clinicians combine amphotericin B with a triazole antifungal agent. (Recommendations regarding combining amphotericin B with azoles are discussed above.) If the patient stabilizes with initial therapy, the frequency of infusion of amphotericin B can be reduced to three times per week at the same dosage. Alternatively, if the patient is clinically stable and no longer requires hospitalization, either fluconazole (400–800 mg/day) or itraconazole (400–600 mg/day) can be started. With the 600-mg dose of itraconazole, it is prudent to monitor for gastrointestinal upset, hypertension, hypokalemia, and peripheral edema (14). While on maintenance dosage, the patient must be followed very closely for relapse. The length of therapy is undefined, but it should be lifelong if the patient has an underlying immunosuppressive condition.

Extrathoracic Dissemination

The most common sites of dissemination beyond the thoracic cavity in coccidioidomycosis are the soft tissues, bones, joints, skin, and meninges. Because meningitis requires a unique therapeutic approach, it is discussed separately. All forms of disseminated coccidioidomycosis require antifungal therapy. In severely ill patients with soft-tissue, bone, or joint disease, particularly if it is at multiple sites, we recommend initiating therapy with intravenous amphotericin B (1.0–1.5 mg/kg/day). Once the patient is clinically stable, therapy with an oral azole (≥400 mg/day) should be given. For less severely ill patients, initiation of therapy with fluconazole (400–800 mg/day) or itraconazole (400–600 mg/day) seems reasonable. Patients should be carefully monitored for clinical response and drug toxicity. When higher doses of antifungals are used initially, downward modification within 3 to 6 months is usually possible as the patient responds. In our experience, in rare cases, patients may fail to respond to either fluconazole or itraconazole at high doses but may, paradoxically, respond to ketoconazole.

Meningitis

Coccidioidal meningitis, if untreated, is almost universally fatal (65). Intravenous amphotericin B is ineffective in the treatment of coccidioidal meningitis. However, as mentioned above, repeated direct injection of amphotericin B into the CSF has resulted in improved outcome (22, 43). However, even with careful management, mortality with intrathecal administration of amphotericin B is still 30 to 50% (43), and toxicity is significant. Since they became available, oral azole agents have been tested for efficacy in the treatment of coccidioidal meningitis. Results for ketoconazole have been disappointing. Although some patients may respond to relatively high doses (15), most patients do not (28).

The new triazoles, itraconazole and fluconazole, appear to be major breakthroughs for management of coccidioidal meningitis and have emerged as the initial choices for therapy. However, there are several important caveats regarding their use. First, responses, particularly improvements in CSF param-eters, can be slow. Second, a major complication of coccidioidal meningitis is hydrocephalus. Failure to identify this can lead to significant morbidity despite appropriate antifungal therapy. It is as yet unknown if patients with evidence of continued CSF inflammation during therapy will, over time, be at increased risk for development of hydrocephalus or other complications. Third, there are now compelling data to suggest that treatment for coccidioidal meningitis, at least with azole therapy, should be lifelong (19).

Some patients fail to respond to oral triazole therapy. Recent data suggest that fluconazole doses of 800 mg/day or above may be more clinically effective than 400 mg/day (9). For patients who fail to respond to even high-dose azole therapy, intrathecal amphotericin B is recommended. Many experts continue concomitant azole therapy in doses as high as 1000 to 1200 mg/day in the setting of recalcitrant coccidioidal meningitis. There is no clinical evidence that such a combination is antagonistic (60). We suggest that anyone treating coccidioidal meningitis either have considerable experience themselves or seek advice from someone who does.

Length of Therapy and Relapse

The total length of time a patient with chronic pulmonary or disseminated coccidioidomycosis should receive antifungal therapy is undefined. Relapse occurs in up to one-third of patients with either chronic progressive pneumonia or extrathoracic disseminated disease, once antifungal therapy is discontinued (11, 33). Nonetheless, many clinicians stop therapy when there is no evidence of clinical disease for at least 6 months and coccidioidal serologic test results are significantly improved or negative. Such patients should be monitored closely for evidence of disease recrudescence during the first year after therapy is discontinued. Antifungal therapy should probably be given lifelong to patients with meningitis and to those with underlying cellular immune defects. Lifelong oral azole therapy may also be reasonable for some patients with nonmeningeal disseminated disease, particularly if they have already demonstrated a propensity to relapse, are racially predisposed to severe disease, are skin-test negative, have exhibited multiple sites of dissemination, or have had debilitating disease at one extrathoracic site.

We recommend following patients every 2 to 3 months after therapy is discontinued, for at least 1 year. If treatment is continued, low doses of azole antifungals (<400 mg/day) may be sufficient to prevent relapse. To date, there are no known clinical or serologic parameters that predict which patients are likely to relapse once therapy is discontinued. In addition to a clinical examination focusing particularly on the areas where coccidioidal lesions previously existed, coccidioidal serology should be followed. If the titer of complement fixation (IgG) antibody increases more than twofold, reinitiation of antifungal chemotherapy should be considered, even if the patient is clinically well.

TREATMENT OF SPECIAL HOSTS
HIV

Within the endemic region, coccidioidomycosis is a major cause of opportunistic infection among individuals infected with HIV. Risk of infection is closely associated with degree of immunodeficiency, as reflected by a CD4 lymphocyte count below 250/μL. On the other hand, a prior history of coccidioidomycosis, residence in the coccidioidal endemic area for more than 4 years, and a positive coccidioidal skin test do not predispose HIV-infected patients to develop active coccidioidomycosis (1). These data suggest that development of active coccidioidomycosis in HIV-infected patients in the endemic area is most likely due to new infection, not reactivation of latent disease. Outside the endemic region, coccidioidomycosis among HIV-infected individuals is uncommon (41) and virtually always represents reactivation of a previously clinically quiescent infection.

The presentation of coccidioidomycosis in the vast majority of HIV-infected patients is pulmonary. The most common presentation is a diffuse, reticulonodular pneumonia. As noted above, this presentation indicates overwhelming dissemination with fungemia and is associated with extremely high mortality (1, 25). Although no studies exist regarding therapy for this form of coccidioidomycosis, we recommend amphotericin B at doses of 1.0 to 1.5 mg/kg/day. In patients who survive longer than 1 month, it is reasonable to reduce the administration of amphotericin B to two or three times a week or to place the patient on an oral azole agent (i.e., fluconazole, 400–800 mg/day). Because many patients with HIV infection have relative achlorhydria (44), fluconazole, whose absorption does not depend on gastric acid (72), is preferred to ketoconazole and itraconazole. Patients placed on an oral azole after responding to amphotericin B must be monitored very closely for recrudescence of disease by clinical examination, chest radiograph, and coccidioidal serologic tests.

The second most common presentation of coccidioidomycosis in the HIV-infected patient is focal pulmonary pneumonia. This presentation is clinically indistinguishable from primary coccidioidomycosis in hosts without HIV infection and usually occurs in relatively immunocompetent patients with CD4 lymphocyte counts above 250/μL (25). The course of this form of coccidioidomycosis is usually benign, with prompt response to antifungal therapy. Treatment with an oral azole (400 mg each day) is recommended for all such patients. While there are no studies, we recommend lifelong therapy.

A small subset of HIV-infected patients develop extrathoracic dissemination, particularly meningitis and soft-tissue infection (25). For reasons that are unclear, bone and joint coccidioidomycosis in patients with HIV infection is very uncommon. HIV-infected patients with specific sites of extrathoracic dissemination are generally clinically stable and not profoundly immunosuppressed. They should be managed in the same way as patients without HIV infection, except that therapy should be continued lifelong.

A unique manifestation of coccidioidomycosis among patients with HIV infection is development of positive coccidioidal serologic tests, particularly of the complement-fixation (IgG) type, without evidence of active clinical infection. Analysis of these cases indicates an extremely high risk for development of clinical illness over time (3). Because of this, we recommend treatment with fluconazole (400 mg each day) and close clinical and serologic follow-up of these patients.

Transplantation

Allogeneic organ transplantation is clearly associated with an increased risk for development of active coccidioidomycosis (13, 35, 36). This risk is highest in those who have a prior history of active coccidioidomycosis or positive coccidioidal serologic tests at the time of transplantation, suggesting that most active coccidioidomycosis in these patients is due to reactivation of prior infection (35). Active disease is most likely to occur in the first 6 months after transplantation, when immunosuppressive therapy is greatest. Use of oral azole antifungal therapy in such patients appears to reduce this risk (36).

Based on the above experiences, clearly patients with prior coccidioidomycosis can safely undergo allogeneic organ transplantation. However, coccidioidal serologies should be checked prior to transplantation. A patient with a positive serologic test result or with a prior history of active coccidioidomycosis should be considered for antifungal therapy for at least 4 months posttransplantation (35, 36). While use of oral azoles is reasonable in this situation, they may interfere with the metabolism of cyclosporine. In particular, ketoconazole can result in extraordinary high levels of cyclosporine (14).

Pregnancy

The risk of severe symptomatic coccidioidomycosis increases during pregnancy. The risk of disease and dissemination is particularly high when infection is newly acquired during the second or third trimester (49, 52, 66). Women with a prior history of coccidioidomycosis or stable coccidioidomycosis at the time they become pregnant rarely develop worsening or active disease during pregnancy (5, 67). Infants born of mothers with active coccidioidomycosis are rarely affected.

Mortality from active coccidioidomycosis during pregnancy appears to be significantly reduced by the use of intravenous amphotericin B (52). A review of instances in which amphotericin B was used during pregnancy for a variety of fungal infections revealed no untoward effects in most women or their newborns. However, sustained hypokalemia as well as decreased renal function has been reported in some mothers and infants (17). The safety and teratogenicity of the oral azoles during pregnancy are not known. A study examining repeated low doses of fluconazole for vaginal candidiasis found no increase in adverse events among pregnant women or their offspring (40). However, a case report described congenital malformations in the newborn of a woman who became pregnant while on fluconazole for coccidioidal meningitis and who continued taking fluconazole throughout pregnancy. While the malformations were consistent with an autosomal recessive disorder, they were also similar to some defects in organogenesis seen in animal models studying the effect of fluconazole during pregnancy (46). Subsequently, there have been three more cases of similar congenital anomalies associated with women receiving fluconazole for coccidioidomycosis during pregnancy (53).

On the basis of these data, women who become pregnant who are already on therapy with an oral azole for coccidioidomycosis should be switched to intravenous amphotericin B. Women with histories of previous coccidioidomycosis prior to pregnancy but on no therapy should be followed closely for development of active disease. Therapy with intravenous amphotericin B is recommended for women who acquire primary coccidioidomycosis during pregnancy, particularly if infection occurs during the second or third trimester. If disease is nonmeningeal, we recommend intravenous amphotericin B (0.7–1.0 mg/kg three times weekly) for the remainder of the pregnancy. For meningeal disease, we recommend intravenous combined with intrathecal amphotericin B. After parturition, oral fluconazole or itraconazole may be started, and the amphotericin B discontinued. It is strongly recommended that an infectious diseases consultant knowledgeable in the treatment of coccidioidomycosis be involved in the management of such patients.

Other Conditions

Patients with malignancy undergoing cancer chemotherapy (18, 56) and patients on chronic corticosteroid therapy or other immunosuppressive agents (2, 56) have a very high risk of developing disseminated disease after primary coccidioidal infection. In addition, they have an increased risk of relapsing once antifungal therapy is discontinued. Similarly, patients with chronic renal failure undergoing dialysis, while at no greater risk for acquiring primary coccidioidomycosis, have a very high risk of developing disseminated disease after initial infection (13). We recommend beginning antifungal therapy for primary coccidioidomycosis in all such patients and following them closely for dissemination. Many clinicians would favor continuing antifungal therapy indefinitely once the primary infection cleared.

Genetic factors may place certain patients at a higher risk

for developing severe and disseminated coccidioidomycosis. For example, there are data suggesting that men are far more likely than women to develop both symptomatic and disseminated disease (2, 21, 51). Early studies also demonstrated a propensity for blacks, Filipinos, and Asians to develop disseminated coccidioidomycosis. An increased risk for symptomatic coccidioidomycosis among black men was again noted during an epidemic of coccidioidomycosis that occurred after a windstorm (26). Pappagianis has recommended using particular care in the management of such patients in "anticipation of possible dissemination" (51). We recommend following any such patient with pulmonary coccidioidomycosis very closely for dissemination, especially if that patient is male. Whether early antifungal treatment prevents subsequent dissemination is not known. We have seen several cases where it did not. However, many clinicians would begin oral azole therapy for these patients. The length of such therapy is not known. Whether antifungal therapy is started or not, such patients should be monitored for at least 1 year after the initial presentation to ensure that disseminated or persistent disease has not occurred.

Persons with diabetes mellitus may be at increased risk for more severe pulmonary disease, particularly pulmonary cavitation, but there is no evidence that they are predisposed to disseminated disease (51). Hence, many clinicians begin therapy with an oral azole agent at 400 mg daily in a diabetic patient with primary pulmonary coccidioidomycosis. The length of such therapy and whether it prevents subsequent pulmonary complications are not known.

SURGERY

The role of surgery has diminished since the advent of sensitive imaging technology, such as computed tomography and magnetic resonance imaging, and development of oral antifungal therapy. In the past, management of a large soft-tissue coccidioidal mass would have included immediate surgical drainage. Currently, it is reasonable to use antifungal chemotherapy in a clinically stable patient and follow the size of the mass radiographically. In addition, the aggressiveness of surgical management often depends on the experience and expertise of the local surgeon, which vary from community to community.

Surgical intervention in coccidioidomycosis is clearly indicated under certain circumstances. First, it is required for closure of a bronchopleural fistula associated with pyopneumothorax. CSF shunts, either lumbar or ventricular, are necessary for the patient with coccidioidal meningitis and hydrocephalus. Surgical removal of a cavity is required for the patient with severe hemoptysis or for a cavity that is enlarging during antifungal chemotherapy, particularly if the cavity is adjacent to the pleura. Finally, surgical debridement and drainage may be required for any extrapulmonary site of infection that fails to improve with chemotherapy.

REFERENCES

1. Ampel NM, Dols CL, Galgiani JN. Coccidioidomycosis during human immunodeficiency virus infection: results of a prospective study in a coccidioidal endemic area. Am J Med 1993;94(3):235–240.
2. Ampel NM, Ryan KJ, Carry PJ, Wieden MA, Schifman RB. Fungemia due to *Coccidioides immitis*. Medicine [Baltimore] 1986;65:312–321.
3. Arguinchona HL, Ampel NM, Dols CL, Galgiani JN, Mohler MJ, Fish DG. Persistent coccidioidal seropositivity without clinical evidence of active coccidioidomycosis in patients infected with human immunodeficiency virus. Clin Infect Dis 1995;20(5):1281–1285.
4. Bañuelos AF, Williams PL, Johnson RH, Bibi S, Fredricks DN, Gilroy SA, Bhatti SU, Aguet J, Stevens DA. Central nervous system abscesses due to *Coccidioides* species. Clin Infect Dis 1996;22:240–250.
5. Barbee RA, Hicks MJ, Grosso D, Sandel C. The maternal immune response in coccidioidomycosis. Chest 1991;100:709–715.
6. Bayer AS. Fungal pneumonias: pulmonary coccidioidal syndromes (pt 1). Chest 1981;79:575–583.
7. Bayer AS. Fungal pneumonias: pulmonary coccidioidal syndromes (pt 2). Chest 1981;79:686–691.
8. Bayer AS, Yoshikawa TT, Guze LB. Chronic progressive coccidioidal pneumonitis. Arch Intern Med 1979;139:536–540.
9. Caldwell J, Williams PL, Einstein H, Welch G. Dose response evaluation of fluconazole in coccidioidal meningitis [Abstract 56]. Centennial Conference on Coccidioidomycosis. Stanford, CA, 1994.
10. Catanzaro A. Pulmonary coccidioidomycosis. Med Clin North Am 1980;64:461–473.
11. Catanzaro A, Galgiani JN, Levine BE, Sharkey-Mathis PK, Fierer J, Stevens DA, Chapman SW, Cloud G. Fluconazole in the treatment of chronic pulmonary and nonmeningeal disseminated coccidioidomycosis. Am J Med 1995;98(3):249–256.
12. Clemons KV, Homola ME, Stevens DA. Activities of the triazole SCH 51048 against Coccidioides immitis in vitro and in vivo. Antimicrob Agents Chemother 1995;39:1169–1172.
13. Cohen IM, Galgiani JN, Potter D, Ogden DA. Coccidioidomycosis in renal replacement therapy. Arch Intern Med 1982;142(3):489–494.
14. Como JA, Dismukes WE. Oral azole drugs as systemic antifungal therapy. N Engl J Med 1994;330:263–272.
15. Craven PC, Graybill JR, Jorgensen JH, Dismukes WE, Levine BE. High-dose ketoconazole for treatment of fungal infections of the central nervous system. Ann Intern Med 1983;98:160–167.
16. Cunningham RT, Einstein HE. Coccidioidal pulmonary cavities with rupture. J Thorac Cardiovasc Surg 1982;84:172–177.
17. Dean JL, Wolf JE, Ranzini AC, Laughlin MA. Use of amphotericin B during pregnancy: case report and review. Clin Infect Dis 1994;18:364–368.
18. Deresinski SC, Stevens DA. Coccidioidomycosis in compromised hosts. Experience at Stanford University Hospital. Medicine (Baltimore) 1974;54:377–395.
19. Dewsnup DH, Galgiani JN, Graybill JR, Diaz M, Rendon A, Cloud GA, Stevens DA. Is it ever safe to stop azole therapy for *Coccidioides immitis* meningitis? Ann Intern Med 1996;124:305–310.
20. Drutz DJ, Catanzaro A. Coccidioidomycosis. Part II. Am Rev Respir Dis 1978;117:727–771.
21. Drutz DJ, Huppert M. Coccidioidomycosis: factors affecting the host-parasite interaction. J Infect Dis 1983;147:372–390.
22. Einstein HE, Holeman CW, Sandidge LL, Holden DH. Coccidioidal meningitis. Calif Med 1961;94:339–343.

23. Fierer J, Kirkland T, Finley F. Comparison of fluconazole and SDZ89–485 for therapy of experimental murine coccidioidomycosis. Antimicrob Agents Chemother 1990;34:13–16.

24. Fiese MJ. Coccidioidomycosis. Springfield, IL: Charles C Thomas, 1958.

25. Fish DG, Ampel NM, Galgiani JN, Dols CL, Kelly PC, Johnson CH, Pappagianis D, Edwards JE, Wasserman RB, Clark RJ, Antoniskis D, Larsen RA, Englender SJ, Petersen EA. Coccidioidomycosis during human immunodeficiency virus infection. A review of 77 patients. Medicine (Baltimore) 1990;69(6):384–391.

26. Flynn NM, Hoeprich PD, Kawachi MM, Lee KK, Lawrence RM, Goldstein E, Jordan G, Kundargi RS, Wong GA. An unusual outbreak of windborne coccidioidomycosis. N Engl J Med 1979;301:358–361.

27. Forseth J, Rohwedder JJ, Levine BE, Saubolle MA. Experience with needle biopsy for coccidioidal lung nodules. Arch Intern Med 1986;146:319–320.

28. Galgiani JN. Coccidioidomycosis. West J Med 1993;159(2):153–171.

29. Galgiani JN, Catanzaro A, Cloud GA, Higgs J, Friedman BA, Larsen RA, Graybill JR. Fluconazole therapy for coccidioidal meningitis. The NIAID-Mycoses Study Group. Ann Intern Med 1993;119(1):28–35.

30. Gallis HA, Drew RH, Pickard WW. Amphotericin B: 30 years of clinical experience. Rev Infect Dis 1990;12:308–329.

31. Goldstein E. Miliary and disseminated coccidioidomycosis. Ann Intern Med 1978;89:365–366.

32. Graybill JR. Lipid formulations for amphotericin B: does the emperor need new clothes. Ann Intern Med 1996;124:921–923.

33. Graybill JR, Stevens DA, Galgiani JN, Dismukes WE, Cloud GA. Itraconazole treatment of coccidioidomycosis. Am J Med 1990;89(3):282–290.

34. Graybill JR, Stevens DA, Galgiani JN, Sugar AM, Craven PC, Gregg C, Huppert M, Cloud G, Dismukes WE. Ketoconazole treatment of coccidioidal meningitis. Ann NY Acad Sci 1988;544:488–496.

35. Hall KA, Copeland JG, Zukoski CF, Sethi GK, Galgiani JN. Markers of coccidioidomycosis before cardiac or renal transplantation and the risk of recurrent infection. Transplantation 1993;55(6):1422–1424.

36. Hall KA, Sethi GK, Rosado LJ, Martinez JD, Huston CL, Copeland JG. Coccidioidomycosis and heart transplantation. J Heart Lung Transplant 1993;12:525–526.

37. Hardenbrook MH, Barriere SL. Coccidioidomycosis: evaluation of parameters used to predict outcome with amphotericin B therapy. Mycopathologica 1982;78:65–71.

38. Hotstetler JS, Caldwell JW, Johnson RH, Munoz AD, Einstein HE, Larson RA, Stevens DA. Coccidioidal infections treated with amphotericin B colloid dispersion (Amphocil or ABCD) [Abstract 628]. 32nd Interscience Conference on Antimicrobial Agents and Chemotherapy. Anaheim, CA: American Society for Microbiology, 1992.

39. Iger M. Coccidioidal osteomyelitis. In: Ajello L, ed. Coccidioidomycosis. Current clinical and diagnostic status. Miami, FL: Symposia Specialists, 1977:177–190.

40. Inman W, Pearce G, Wilton L. Safety of fluconazole in the treatment of vaginal candidiasis. Eur J Clin Pharmacol 1994;46:115–118.

41. Jones JL, Fleming PL, Ciesielski CA, Hu DJ, Kaplan JE, Ward JW. Coccidioidomycosis among persons with AIDS in the United States. J Infect Dis 1995;171:961–966.

42. Kelly PC. Coccidioidal meningitis. In: Stevens DA, ed. Coccid-ioidomycosis. A text. New York: Plenum Medical Book Company, 1980:163–194.

43. Labadie EL, Hamilton RH. Survival improvement in coccidioidal meningitis by high-dose intrathecal amphotericin B. Arch Intern Med 1986;146:2013–2018.

44. Lake-Bakaar G, Tom W, Lake-Bakaar D, Gupta N, Beidas S, El-sakr M, Straus E. Gastropathy and ketoconazole malabsorption in the acquired immunodeficiency syndrome (AIDS). Ann Intern Med 1988;109:471–473.

45. Larsen RA, Jacobson JA, Morris AH, Benowitz BA. Acute respiratory failure caused by primary pulmonary coccidioidomycosis. Am Rev Respir Dis 1985;131:797–799.

46. Lee EL, Feinberg M, Abraham JJ, Murthy ARK. Congenital malformations in an infant born to a woman treated with fluconazole. Pediatr Infect Dis J 1992;11:1063–1064.

47. Levine HB. A direct comparison of oral treatments with BAY-n-7133, BAY-1–9139 and ketoconazole in experimental murine coccidioidomycosis. Sabouraudia 1984;22:37–46.

48. Lopez AM, Williams PL, Ampel NM. Acute pulmonary coccidioidomycosis mimicking bacterial pneumonia and septic shock: a report of two cases. Am J Med 1993;95:236–239.

49. McCoy MJ, Ellenberg JF, Killam AP. Coccidioidomycosis complicating pregnancy. Am J Obstet Gynecol 1980;137:739–740.

50. Medeiros AA. Case records of the Massachusetts General Hospital. N Engl J Med 1980;302:218–223.

51. Pappagianis D. Epidemiology of coccidioidomycosis. In: McGinnis M, ed. Current topics in medical mycology, vol 2. New York: Springer-Verlag, 1988:199–238.

52. Peterson CM, Schuppert K, Kelly PC, Pappagianis D. Coccidioidomycosis and pregnancy. Obstet Gynecol Surv 1993;48:149–156.

53. Pursley TJ, Blomquist IK, Abraham J, Andersen HF, Bartley JA. Fluconazole-induced congenital anomalies in three infants. Clin Infect Dis 1996;22:336–340.

54. Read CT. Coin lesion, pulmonary: in the Southwest. (Solitary pulmonary nodules). Ariz Med 1972;29:775–781.

55. Rohatgi PK, Schmitt RG. Pulmonary coccidioidal mycetoma. Am J Med Sci 1984;287:27–30.

56. Rutala PJ, Smith JW. Coccidioidomycosis in potentially compromised hosts: the effect of immunosuppressive therapy in dissemination. Am J Med Sci 1978;275:283–295.

57. Sarosi GA, Parker JD, Doto IL, Tosh FE. Chronic pulmonary coccidioidomycosis. N Engl J Med 1970;283:325–329.

58. Sharkey PK, Lipke R, Renteria A, Galgiani J, Catanzaro A, Diaz M, Kramer M, Whitney R, Gupta R. Amphotericin B lipid complex (ABLC) in treatment (Rx) of coccidioidomycosis (C) [Abstract 742]. 31st Interscience Conference on Antimicrobial Agents and Chemotherapy. Chicago, IL: American Society for Microbiology, 1991.

59. Stevens DA. Coccidioidomycosis. N Engl J Med 1995;332:1077–1082.

60. Sugar AM. Use of amphotericin B with azole antifungal drugs. What are we doing? Antimicrob Agent Chemother 1995;39:1907–1912.

61. Sugar AM, Alsip SG, Galgiani JN, Graybill JR, Dismukes WE, Cloud GA, Craven PC, Stevens DA. Pharmacology and toxicity of high-dose ketoconazole. Antimicrob Agents Chemother 1987;31(12):1874–1888.

62. Thadepalli H, Salem FA, Mandal AK, Einstein HE. Pulmonary mycetoma due to *Coccidioides immitis*. Chest 1977;71:429–430.

63. Tucker RM, Denning DW, Dupont B, Stevens DA. Itraconazole therapy for chronic coccidioidal meningitis. Ann Intern Med 1990;112:108–112.

64. Tucker RM, Galgiani JN, Denning DW, Hanson LH, Graybill JR, Sharkey K, Eckman MR, Salemi C, Libke R, Klein RA, Stevens DA. Treatment of coccidioidal meningitis with fluconazole. Rev Infect Dis 1990;12:S380–389.

65. Vincent T, Galgiani JN, Huppert M, Salkin D. The natural history of coccidioidal meningitis: VA-Armed Forces cooperative studies, 1955–1958. Clin Infect Dis 1993;16:247–254.

66. Wack EE, Ampel NM, Galgiani JN, Bronnimann DA. Coccidioidomycosis during pregnancy. An analysis of ten cases among 47,120 pregnancies. Chest 1988;94:376–379.

67. Walker MPR, Brody CZ, Resnik R. Reactivation of coccidioidomycosis in pregnancy. Obstet Gynecol 1992;79:815–817.

68. Williams PL, Johnson R, Pappagianis D, Einstein H, Slager U, Koster FT, Eron JJ, Morrison J, Aguet J, River ME. Vasculitic

and encephalitic complications associated with Coccidioides immitis infection of the central nervous system in humans: report of 10 cases. Clin Infect Dis 1992;14:673–682.

69. Winter WG Jr, Larson RK, Zettas JP, Libke R. Coccidioidal spondylitis. J Bone Joint Surg Am 1978;60:240–244.

70. Wright EM. The solitary pulmonary nodule [Letter]. JAMA 1980;244:1899.

71. Yozwiak ML, Lundergan LL, Kerrick SS, Galgiani JN. Symptoms and routine laboratory abnormalities associated with coccidioidomycosis. West J Med 1988;148:419–421.

72. Zimmermann T, Yeates RA, Riedel KD, Lach P, Laufen H. The influence of gastric pH on the pharmacokinetics of fluconazole: the effect of omeprazole. Int J Clin Pharmacol Ther 1994;34: 491–496.

Cryptococcus neoformans

M. Hong Nguyen and John R. Graybill

GENERAL DESCRIPTION

Cryptococcus neoformans is currently the second most common cause of fungal infection in the United States. Before the era of amphotericin B, disseminated cryptococcosis was uniformly fatal. Even with amphotericin B, morbidity and mortality still approached 50%. The side effects associated with this drug are tremendous. The new azole agents introduced in the early 1990s offer another approach to this infection, solving the problems of the inconvenience of intravenous dosing and the high rate of adverse reactions associated with amphotericin B.

This chapter reviews the experience with antifungal therapy against cryptococcosis since the introduction of amphotericin B three decades ago. Since the location of infection and the host immune status are of upmost importance in determining outcome, approach to therapy is classified by these factors.

SUSCEPTIBILITY IN VITRO AND IN VIVO

In the last few years, significant progress has been made in antifungal susceptibility testing. Although the method has now been standardized, the task of validating this test remains. Unlike the experience with *Candida,* for which a breakpoint for susceptibility and resistance has been proposed, the correlation between in vitro susceptibility to fluconazole and response to therapy has not been extensively studied for *Cryptococcus.* Using a murine model of cryptococcal meningitis, Nguyen et al. demonstrated a correlation between fluconazole MICs (using the standardized NCCLS method) and in vivo outcome (29). A dose response was demonstrated between the various range of fluconazole MICs and the degree of response to this drug: the isolate exhibiting an MIC of 2 μg/mL responded steadily to fluconazole, the isolate with an MIC of 16 μg/mL responded moderately, and the isolate with an MIC of

32 μg/mL did not respond to fluconazole. These results suggest that in vitro susceptibility testing may be useful in evaluation of fluconazole therapy for cryptococcal meningitis.

In contrast to the findings in animal models, no correlation has been demonstrated between in vitro fluconazole susceptibility results obtained using the NCCLS standard method and outcome of HIV patients with cryptococcal meningitis treated with this drug (55). On the other hand, that study correlated patient outcome with MIC data obtained using a modified susceptibility method (microtiter with Yeast Nitrogen Base as medium and endpoint determined spectrophotometrically). This method of testing must be standardized, reproducible, and validated before it can be advocated for routine use in the clinical setting.

ANITFUNGAL THERAPY

Currently available antifungal agents against *C. neoformans* and their characteristics are listed in Table 1.

Amphotericin B

Amphotericin B has good in vitro activity against *C. neoformans,* although emergence of resistant isolates during prolonged therapy has been reported (35). Amphotericin B is currently the standard therapy against *C. neoformans.* The major limitations of this drug are its toxicity and its poor diffusion into body compartments (including the cerebrospinal fluid (CSF)).

Flucytosine

Flucytosine has good in vitro activity against *C. neoformans* and penetrates well into the CSF. The major limitations of this drug are its toxicity and the development of flucytosine-resistant fungal isolates when the drug is used as monotherapy.

TABLE 1 • Currently Available Antifungal Agents against *Cryptococcus neoformans* and Their Characteristics

Class of Antifungal Agents	Mode of Administration	In Vitro Activity MIC (μg/mL)	Benefits	Limitations
Polyene				
Amphotericin B	i.v., i.t., i.p.	Range: 0.25–1 μg/mL	Standard therapy	—Poor diffusion into body compartment
Liposomal formulations of amphotericin B	i.v.	MIC_{50} = 0.5 μg/mL MIC_{90} = 1 μg/mL		—High toxicity profile
Antimetabolites				
Flucytosine (5-FC)	p.o.	Range: 1–>64 μg/mL MIC_{50} = 4 μg/mL MIC_{90} = 8 μg/mL	Excellent penetration into body compartments, including CSF	—Development of resistance —High toxicity profile
Azoles				
Ketoconazole	p.o.	Range: 0.125–1 μg/mL		—Erractic absorption —Poor CSF penetration —Significant drug-drug interaction
Miconazole	i.v.	Not available		—Short half-life —Serious toxicity profile —Scarce clinical data
Fluconazole	p.o., i.v., i.p.	Range: 0.125–>64 μg/mL MIC_{50} = 4 μg/mL MIC_{90} = 16 μg/mL	Excellent penetration into body compartments, including CSF	—Emergence of resistance
Itraconazole	p.o.	Range: ≤0.03–0.5 μg/mL MIC_{50} = 0.125 μg/mL MIC_{90} = 0.25 μg/mL	High lipophilicity leads to adequate penetration into certain body compartments	—Poor penetration into CSF

Ketoconazole

Ketoconazole has variable in vitro activity against *C. neoformans*. The experience with ketoconazole in cryptococcosis has been limited to a few patients with skin and lung involvement (17). This drug is available only in oral formulation and requires acidic gastric pH for absorption. This property makes it less attractive for treatment of patients with acquired immunodeficiency syndrome (AIDS), since most have achlorhydria. Ketoconazole does not penetrate well into the CSF; dosage of 1200 mg/day or more, which is poorly tolerated, is required to treat coccidioidal meningitis, and failure of this drug was reported in the treatment of cryptococcal meningitis when it was used as monotherapy (32).

Miconazole

Miconazole has variable in vitro activity against *C. neoformans*. Miconazole has been used seldom in the treatment of severe cases of cryptococcosis, and both successes and failures have been reported (48, 54). The lack of clinical information against cryptococcosis, a short half-life, toxicity of the vehicle, and the availability of more potent yet benign new-generation azoles have negated the use of this agent in clinical setting.

Fluconazole

Fluconazole is available for both oral and intravenous administration. Fluconazole has high bioavailability after oral administration. Unlike ketoconazole and itraconazole, its absorption through the gastrointestinal tract is independent of gastric pH. Fluconazole is widely distributed in the body, reaching high concentrations in serum and tissues, including

the CSF. Its long half-life enables once-daily dosing. This drug has been used with success for both acute and suppressive therapy for cryptococcal meningitis in HIV-infected patients. As with *Candida,* fluconazole resistance has been recognized among *Cryptococcus* (3, 28).

Itraconazole

Itraconazole is currently available for oral use only, although an intravenous formulation is being evaluated. Most clinical experience with itraconazole has been with the capsulated form, which depends on the acidic pH of the stomach for absorption. This property makes it less attractive for use in AIDS patients, since they often have achlorhydria. The oral suspension of itraconazole is better absorbed than the capsulated formulation; whether this formulation would provide better efficacy against cryptococcosis is yet to be determined. Another weakness of itraconazole is its poor penetration into the CSF. Several reports of success of this drug in cryptococcal meningitis exist, however (13, 14, 52); its hydrophobicity and accumulation in host cells may target the drug to the site of infection (33). To our knowledge, in vitro itraconazole resistance has not been reported for *Cryptococcus*.

SPECIAL SITUATIONS

CRYPTOCOCCOSIS IN NON-AIDS PATIENTS

Although cryptococcosis has a predilection for patients with impaired cellular immunity, such as those with AIDS, transplant recipients, or those with lymphoreticular malignancy, up to 50% of patients have no obvious immunologic deficiency or underlying diseases (7, 46). Searching for immunodeficiency and underlying disease is important in managing these patients, since these factors often dictate the course of therapy and can adversely affect outcome (18). Studies have shown the mortality rate to be significantly higher for immunocompromised patients (20–85%) or those with serious underlying diseases (100%) than for immunocompetent patients (0–15%) or those with no underlying diseases (67%) (43, 46).

Meningeal Infection

Amphotericin B with or without Flucytosine

Combined amphotericin B and flucytosine is currently the standard therapy for cryptococcal meningitis in non-AIDS patients. In a randomized study of patients with cryptococcal meningitis comparing amphotericin B (0.4 mg/kg/day) with combined amphotericin B (0.3 mg/kg/day) and flucytosine (150 mg/kg/day) for meningitis, mortality was significantly higher for patients treated with amphotericin B alone (47%, 15 of 32) than for patients treated with combination therapy (24%, 8 of 34; $P < .05$) (2). Furthermore, the CSF was sterilized after 10 days of therapy in significantly fewer patients treated with amphotericin B alone (64%, 7 of 11) than in those treated with combination therapy (100%, 16 of 16; $P < .001$). However, the dosage used in the group receiving amphotericin B alone was relatively low (0.4 mg/kg/day); whether higher dosages of amphotericin B given alone (≥ 0.7 mg/kg/day) would be as effective as the combination of amphotericin B and flucytosine in eradicating *Cryptococcus* is not known.

Toxicity was the major problem among the patients receiving combination therapy (2, 18); side effects occurred in 30 to 40% of patients, and in 18% of these patients (6 of 34), flucytosine had to be discontinued because of toxicity. The most common toxicity associated with flucytosine was anemia and leukopenia due to bone marrow suppression. 56% of toxicity appeared during the first 2 weeks of therapy, and 87% during the first 4 weeks. The high flucytosine dosage used in that study (150 mg/kg/day) might explain the high rate of toxicity observed. Recent data show that dosage of 100 mg/kg/day provides adequate blood levels and reduces toxicity (50). If flucytosine is to be used long term (>2 weeks), especially in patients with renal insufficiency, peak levels should be monitored and maintained between 30 and 80 µg/mL; sustained flucytosine levels above 100 µg/mL are associated with bone marrow toxicity.

The duration of therapy for cryptococcal meningitis should be dictated by the immune status and underlying disease of the patients and severity of the infection. Four weeks of therapy is likely not adequate for (*a*) those with immunosuppression, such as those with lymphoreticular cancer or transplant, or those receiving daily corticosteroid dosage above 20 mg of prednisone equivalence after completion of antifungal therapy or (*b*) those with associated poor prognostic factors such as neurologic abnormality, positive cultures for *Cryptococcus* at extraneural sites, pretreatment CSF WBC below 20/mm³ or a pretreatment CSF cryptococcal antigen titer of 1:32 or above, a positive CSF India ink test after 4 weeks of therapy, and serum or CSF cryptococcal Ag titer of 1:8 or above after 4

weeks of therapy (16, 18). All patients who had any of these factors should receive at least 6 weeks of therapy.

Another important adjunct to antifungal therapy is minimizing or discontinuing immunosuppression drugs to optimize the chance of response to therapy.

The role of intraventricular administration of amphotericin B in the therapy of cryptococcal meningitis is unclear. Both success and failure have been reported with this route of administration. Given the complications associated with intraventricular therapy and the lack of extensive evidence of its efficacy in cryptococcal meningitis, this therapeutic modality cannot be advocated for routine use; it should be reserved for patients with refractory infection or those who cannot receive systemic antifungal therapy because of significant side effects (16).

Fluconazole

Due to the significant side effects associated with amphotericin B and flucytosine, the requirement for long-term vascular access and for close monitoring of laboratory values during amphotericin B therapy, alternative therapy has been sought. A randomized comparative study of combined amphotericin B and flucytosine for 2 weeks, followed by fluconazole for 8 weeks versus combined fluconazole and flucytosine for 6 weeks, followed by fluconazole for 4 weeks yielded mortality rates of 80% (4 of 5) for the fluconazole-based regimen and 0% (0 of 9) for the amphotericin B–based regimen. This study was stopped prematurely because of the reluctance of the investigators to enroll severely ill patients in the fluconazole arm (19).

In a pilot study of cryptococcosis in France, fluconazole was as efficacious as amphotericin B for non-AIDS patients afflicted with cryptococcal meningitis (20); the overall cure rate was 74% (26 of 35) for patients treated with amphotericin B and 68% (17 of 25) for those treated with fluconazole. These results should be interpreted with caution, however, given several major limitations of this study. First, this study is a non-randomized comparative trial; thus, allocation of therapy might have been biased in regard to patients' underlying diseases and severity of illness at the onset of cryptococcal infection. For example, patients with lymphoid disorders, those with more severe infections, and those with clinical signs and symptoms associated with poor outcome were more likely to receive amphotericin B. Second, the number of patients assigned to each therapeutic group was small (35 for amphotericin B and 25 for fluconazole); therefore, the study might not have the statistical power to detect a significant difference in outcome between the two groups. Third and most importantly, the patient outcome in each group was not stratified by factors known to independently affect outcome such as dissemination, malignancy, and abnormal mental status examination. For these reasons, this study cannot determine whether fluconazole has any role in the treatment of cryptococcal meningitis in non-AIDS patients.

In summary, the role of fluconazole in the therapy of cryptococcal meningitis in non-AIDS patients is uncertain. Further study is needed before this drug can be recommended as standard therapy in this population.

Other Antifungal Agents

Experience with itraconazole and various liposomal formulations of amphotericin B in the treatment of cryptoccocal meningitis in non-AIDS patients is very limited with regard to appropriate dosage, duration of therapy, and efficacy.

Extraneural Infection

Virtually all organs can be affected by *Cryptococcus*. Lungs are the most common extraneural site of involvement, followed by bladder, prostate, skin, eye, and liver (33). Experience with the therapy of cryptococcal infection at these sites is limited and is based mainly on anecdotal reports. Since lungs are the most common extraneural manifestation of cryptococcosis, this section focuses mainly on therapy for this entity.

Clinical presentations for pulmonary cryptococcosis are broad and depend on the patient's immune status. In patients with normal immune systems, recovery of *C. neoformans* from respiratory samples frequently represents either asymptomatic colonization (often seen in patients with severe underlying lung disease) or self-limited infection. In immunocompromised hosts, infections often disseminate and can be fatal if untreated. Chest radiographic findings are variable and also depend on host's immune status. Hilar adenopathy, interstitial infiltrate, pleural effusions, cavitary lesions, and single or multiple nodules that are indistinguishable from lung tumor have been described (21, 53).

The therapeutic approach ranges from no specific therapy in immunocompetent hosts to aggressive antifungal therapy in immunocompromised hosts. In immunocompetent hosts, the pulmonary process is often self-limited and can resolve spontaneously without antifungal therapy (23, 24). Nevertheless, due to the propensity of *C. neoformans* to disseminate and to affect the CNS, all patients with pulmonary cryptococcosis should have cryptococcal antigen determined in both serum and CSF; a positive antigen titer in either serum or CSF suggests extrapulmonary dissemination, and these patients should be treated with a course of antifungal therapy. The optimal therapy for patients with pulmonary cryptococcosis is unclear, but amphotericin B (with or without flucytosine), ketoconazole, or fluconazole have been used with success (17, 20, 56). The toxicity of amphotericin B and the availability of effective yet benign azole agents mitigate against its use in these patients. The duration of therapy is also unclear, but it is reasonable to treat patients for at least 3 months with azole antifungals. Fluconazole or itraconazole at 400 mg/day would be superior to ketoconazole, in part because of greater potency and in part because of proven efficacy in meningitis.

CRYPTOCOCCAL INFECTION IN PATIENTS WITH AIDS

Amphotericin B, flucytosine (used in combination with other antifungal agents), and fluconazole are the currently acceptable therapy for cryptococcal meningitis in AIDS patients. In contrast with the experience in non-AIDS patients, *Cryptococcus* can rarely be eradicated in AIDS patients. Indeed, the relapse rate for AIDS patients after a successful course of therapy for acute cryptococcal meningitis (acute therapy) is at least 50% (6, 8). This high relapse rate in combination with its associated fatality mandate chronic suppressive therapy (maintenance therapy) for AIDS patients with cryptococcal meningitis (6, 8).

Acute Therapy

Amphotericin B versus Fluconazole

Two prospective, randomized studies have compared fluconazole (400 mg loading dose, followed by 200 mg/day) with amphotericin B (0.3 mg/kg/day) for treatment of cryptococcal meningitis in AIDS patients (Table 2). In both studies, the time required to sterilize the CSF was longer for fluconazole (30–41 days) than for amphotericin B (16 days). In one study, mortality and failure rates were significantly higher for the 14 patients treated with fluconazole at 400 mg/day (14 and 60%, respectively) than for the 6 patients treated with a combination of amphotericin B (0.7 mg/kg/day) and flucytosine (150 mg/kg/day) (0%) (26). In a larger study with 194 patients enrolled, mortality and failure rates did not differ significantly between the amphotericin B (14 and 60%, respectively) and fluconazole groups (18 and 66%, respectively), although there was a trend toward a higher mortality at 2 weeks in the fluconazole group (79%, 19 of 24) than in the amphotericin B group (56%, 5 of 9) (40). The suboptimal outcome of this trial was probably due to use of suboptimal dosages of amphotericin B and fluconazole.

The second study, conducted by the Mycoses Study Group and the AIDS Clinical Trials Groups, assessed the efficacy of amphotericin B at high dose (0.7–0.8 mg/kg/day) either alone or in combination with flucytosine (100 mg/kg/day) for the first 2 weeks of therapy (induction therapy), followed by either

---

TABLE 2 • **Randomized Trials of Amphotericin B versus Fluconazole As Therapy for Cryptococcal Meningitis in AIDS patients.**

Ref.	Amphotericin B				Fluconazole			
	Dose	n	Outcome	Time to (−) Culture	Dose	n	Outcome	Time to (−) Culture
26	0.7 mg/kg/day	6[a]	Mortality = 0% failure = 0%	Mean: 15.6 days	400 mg/day	14	Mortality =29% failure = 71%	Mean: 40.6 days
40	0.3 mg/kg	63[b]	Mortality = 14% failure = 60%	Median: 42 days	200 mg/day	131	Mortality = 18% failure = 66%	Median: 64 days

[a] All 6 patients were treated with combined amphotericin B (0.7 mg/kg) and flucytosine (150 mg/kg/day).

[b] 9 of 63 patients were treated with combined amphotericin B and flucytosine.

fluconazole or itraconazole (400 mg/day) for the following 8 weeks (consolidation therapy) (50). At 2 weeks, 60% of the CSF cultures were sterilized in the combined amphotericin B and flucytosine group versus 51% of those receiving amphotericin B alone ($P = .06$). Mortality rates for both groups were similar (6.1% for the amphotericin B group and 5% for the combined group).

During induction therapy, only 3% of patients required discontinuation of studied drugs because of toxicity. The side effect profile did not differ significantly between the two study groups. This finding was in sharp contrast with the previous observation that up to 53% of patients treated with the combined regimen had to have their medications discontinued because of toxicity (8). The shorter duration of flucytosine and lower daily dose used in the more recent study might explain this difference. Not only was the lower dose and short-term use of flucytosine effective, it also precluded the need to monitor flucytosine levels.

After the initial 2-week course of amphotericin B, patients were randomized to either fluconazole or itraconazole (50). CSF sterilization at 10 weeks was achieved in 70% of the fluconazole group and 60% of the itraconazole group ($P < .05$); the lower response to itraconazole may be attributed to the poor CSF penetration and poor absorption of this drug (most advanced AIDS patients have achlorhydria). However, mortality rates at 10 weeks did not differ for patients treated with fluconazole (1%) or with itraconazole (3%).

The important finding of this study is that the overall mortality rate for AIDS patients treated with this regimen was substantially lower than that of previous studies. The mortality rate decreased from 15 to 5.5% within the first 2 weeks of therapy. Furthermore, sterilization of the CSF was improved from 20 to 50% (50). The significant improvement in the mortality and CSF sterilization rates is most likely due to the use of a higher dosage of amphotericin B. A previous study had shown that amphotericin B (1 mg/kg/day for 2 weeks) followed by fluconazole or itraconazole therapy resulted in a successful outcome in 94%, with no mortality (11). Together, these data indicate that 2 weeks of combined amphotericin B and flucytosine followed by fluconazole therapy should currently be considered the standard treatment for cryptococcal meningitis in AIDS patients.

The use of amphotericin B does not eliminate infusion-associated side effects or the requirement for vascular access for laboratory monitoring of blood urea nitrogen, creatinine, electrolytes, and peripheral blood cell counts. Thus, interest in evaluating alternative therapy to amphotericin B remains. Current options include liposomal formulations of amphotericin B, itraconazole, higher dosage of fluconazole, or combined therapy with various antifungal agents.

Liposomal Formulations of Amphotericin B

In a prospective, randomized, comparative study of amphotericin B lipid complex (ABLC, Abelcet, Liposome Company, Inc., Princeton, NJ) versus amphotericin B for cryptococcal infection in patients with AIDS, ABLC was significantly better tolerated than amphotericin B. The overall clinical and mycologic responses were approximately 69 and 38%, respectively, and did not differ significantly from those in the amphotericin

B (0.7 mg/kg/day) and ABLC groups (1.5 to 5 mg/kg) (44). However, at the end of 4 weeks of therapy, 42% of the ABLC group showed persistent positive CSF cultures, versus 14% in the amphotericin B group. Although this raises the concern that ABLC might not be as potent as amphotericin B or that ABLC might not readily cross the blood-brain barrier, the patients randomized to the ABLC arm were more severely ill than those in the amphotericin B arm; therefore, a fair comparison cannot be made between these two groups.

Experience with another lipid formulation of amphotericin B (AmBisome) in 19 AIDS patients with cryptococcal meningitis was encouraging: the mortality rate was 16%, the clinical cure rate was 63%, the mycologic cure rate was 67%, and the median time to CSF sterilization was 11 days (range, 7–36 days) (9). These rates were comparable to those obtained with the combination of amphotericin B and flucytosine (40). A prospective randomized comparative study of amBisome (4 mg/kg daily) and amphotericin B (0.7 mg/kg daily) for the initial 3 weeks of treatment of cryptococcal meningitis demonstrated that amBisome yielded a significantly earlier CSF sterilization than amphotericin B, had equal clinical efficacy, and was significantly less nephrotoxic (20a).

Itraconazole

A prospective, comparative study of itraconazole (200 mg twice daily) versus combined amphotericin B (0.3 mg/kg/day) and flucytosine (150 mg/kg/day) found combined amphotericin B and flucytosine to be significantly more effective than itraconazole in the therapy for cryptococcal meningitis: 0% of patients (0 of 9) in the combined amphotericin B and flucytosine group and 50% of patients (6 of 12) in the itraconazole group had persistent positive cultures in the CSF despite 6 weeks of therapy (12). Long-term follow-up also demonstrated the superiority of combined amphotericin B and flucytosine over itraconazole: 22% of the combined amphotericin B and flucytosine group (2 of 9), and 58% of the itraconazole group (7 of 12) relapsed, despite itraconazole maintenance therapy (200 mg/day).

A similar result was obtained in a pilot study of itraconazole (200 mg twice daily) in 29 patients with AIDS-associated cryptococcal meningitis (14). Complete response was achieved in 64%, and partial response (improved symptoms but persistently positive CSF cultures) in 22%. Failure was documented in 14%. The median time to sterilization of the CSF was approximately 30 days. Among the responders, recrudescence occurred in 42%; therapeutic serum itraconazole levels were documented at the time of recrudescence. Furthermore, the breakthrough cryptococcal isolates retained their initial in vitro susceptibility pattern to itraconazole.

High-Dose Fluconazole

Although no study has compared amphotericin B with high-dose fluconazole (>400 mg/day), several anecdotal reports of higher dosage of fluconazole have shown this dosage to be not only well tolerated in AIDS patients with cryptococcal meningitis but also efficacious. In one report, fluconazole (800 mg/day) was effective salvage therapy for cryptococcal meningitis for 62% of HIV patients (5 of 8) who had failed a variety of antifungal therapy (4). In another report, six patients were treated with intravenous fluconazole (1600-mg loading dose followed by 800 mg/day oral fluconazole as primary therapy); 83% (5 of 6) had clinical improvement and all six patients attained CSF sterilization by day 82 (median, 21 days) (22). This dosage of fluconazole was well tolerated: nausea occurred in two patients, and liver enzyme tests were mildly elevated in five.

This pilot study was followed by a prospective, randomized study of escalating dosages of fluconazole (800, 1200, 1600, and 2000 mg/day) alone or in combination with flucytosine (150 mg/kg/day) (27). Preliminary data demonstrated no significant difference in the response rate among patients treated with escalating dosage of fluconazole (800 vs. 2000 mg). On the other hand, the patients treated with combined fluconazole and flucytosine had a significantly better response rate than those treated with fluconazole alone (27).

An important part of the management of cryptococcal meningitis is controlling elevated intracranial pressure, which occurs in more than 60% of patients with cryptococcal meningitis. Increased intracranial pressure has been associated with serious sequelae including death (15). In one study, 93% of patients with increased intracranial pressure (13 of 14) died within the first 2 weeks of diagnosis, and an additional 40% died within the ensuing 3 weeks (50). Thus, controlling increased intracranial pressure should be an important part of therapy for cryptococcal meningitis. Patients with increased intracranial pressure should have serial lumbar punctures, with enough CSF removed at each puncture to reduce the pressure to approximately 20 cm water (20b). If serial lumbar punctures do not control the symptoms of increased pressure, placement of a temporary ventriculostomy or lumbar drains can provide acute relief. A small percentage of these patients eventually require permanent shunt placement for chronic control of increased intracranial pressure. Corticosteroid and acetazolamide have questionable effect in controlling pressure and thus should not be routinely administered to patients (41).

Maintenance Therapy

Upward of 50% of AIDS patients who have completed a course of acute therapy for cryptoccocal meningitis are at risk for relapse if chronic suppressive therapy is not administered (6). These relapses represent a failure of the initial therapy to completely eradicate the infection, rather than acquisition of a new infection. Indeed, clinically silent infection with persistently positive culture at the end of primary therapy occurred

in 19% of patients (16 of 84) (34). Prostate and the CNS are potential reservoirs for persistent cryptococcal infection (25).

Given the high fatality rate associated with relapse, several regimens have been evaluated for chronic suppressive therapy. Options include weekly amphotericin B or daily administration of fluconazole or itraconazole. Daily fluconazole (200 mg) was superior to weekly amphotericin B (1 mg/kg) as maintenance therapy for AIDS patients who had achieved culture-negative status after primary treatment for acute cryptococcal meningitis (34); 18% of patients (14 of 78) receiving amphotericin B relapsed, compared with 2% of those receiving fluconazole (2 of 111) (Table 3). In this study, fluconazole was well tolerated. Indeed, the rates of clinical and laboratory toxicity in the fluconazole group did not differ from those in the amphotericin B group. On the other hand, bacterial infections were significantly more frequent in the amphotericin B group (36%) than in the fluconazole group (17%). The higher incidence of bacterial infections in the amphotericin B group was most likely related to the vascular catheters required for chronic amphotericin B administration. This is a major limitation of amphotericin B therapy.

Daily fluconazole (200 mg) was also superior to daily itraconazole (200 mg) as maintenance therapy for cryptococcal meningitis (42). Relapse rates were 4% (2 of 51) with fluconazole and 23% (13 of 57) with itraconazole therapy (Table 3).

Although lack of compliance is the most common cause of relapse, development of drug resistance has also been implicated. Several anecdotal reports have linked failure of fluconazole suppressive therapy to cryptococcal strains exhibiting high fluconazole MICs (Table 4). Also, a gradual increase in fluconazole MICs was documented in serial isolates recovered from patients at the time of initial and relapse infections (5, 10, 30, 31). This finding, along with the demonstration that these serial isolates were clonally related, indicates that fluconazole resistance can develop under the selective pressure of this drug (10, 47).

Most experience with drug resistance has been with fluconazole, but an amphotericin B–resistant cryptococcal isolate was recovered from an AIDS patient receiving long-term amphotericin B prophylaxis (35).

There is no consensus favoring prophylaxis after nonmeningeal cryptococcosis in AIDS patients, but we recommend the same prophylaxis as for meningitis.

Primary Fluconazole Prophylaxis

Several factors influence the decision to implement primary prophylaxis against opportunistic infections: (a) the prevalence of disease, (b) the associated morbidity and mortality, (c) the efficacy of the prophylactic regimen and its impact on outcome, and (d) the cost of the prophylactic regimen (monetary cost, side effects, and emergence of resistant organism).

Prophylaxis against *Pneumocystis* pneumonia (PCP) is standard care in patients with HIV. It occurs in at least 30% of patients with CD4 below 200/mm^3 and carries a high mortality rate. Furthermore, trimethoprim-sulfamethoxazole prophylaxis is very effective in reducing the incidence of PCP (breakthrough infection occurs in <6% of patients) and improving

	Relapse Free at at least 1 Year		
Antifungal	(6)	(34)	(41)
Placebo	63%	—	—
Amphotericin B (1 mg/kg/week)	—	78%	—
Fluconazole (200 mg/day)	97%	97%	96%
Itraconazole (200 mg/kg/day)	—	—	77%

TABLE 3 • Antifungal Therapy for Secondary Prophylaxis

TABLE 4 • **Failure of Fluconazole Chronic Suppressive (Maintenance) Therapy[a]**

Ref.	Age (years)	CD4 Count (/mm³)	Prior Flu Use	Breakthrough Infection Site	Flu MIC Pre/Post Flu Use (μg/mL)	Treatment	Response	Subsequent Treatment	Outcome (duration follow-up)
1	32	20	None	Meningitis, skin	ND/64	Flu 400 mg daily for 9 months	Relapse after 9 months	AmB 3 mg/kg/day + 5-FC; duration: N/A	Alive (no follow-up)
5	28	<30	None	Meningitis	16/128	Flu 800 mg/day for 3 weeks followed by Flu 400 mg/day	Relapse after 6 months	AmB for 6 days, followed by Flu 800 mg/day	Relapse after 3 months[b]
5	45	<30	None	Meningitis	0.25/16	AmB for 2 weeks followed by Flu 400 mg/day	Relapse after 6 months	Ambisome 1 mg/kg/day for 3 weeks, followed by Ambisome 1 mg/kg weekly	Alive (3 months)
31	30	4	None	Meningitis	ND/50	Flu 400 mg/day for 29 days + AmB 1 mg/kg/day × 7 days	Relapse after 29 days	AmB 0.5 mg/kg/day ≥ 6 weeks, followed by AmB 3 times/week	Died (2 years)
30	54	14	None	Meningitis	4/>64	Flu 400 mg/day for 39 days, followed by Flu 100 mg/day for 25 days	Relapse after 25 days	Flu 800 mg for 12 days, followed by AmB 65 mg/day for 6 days, then Flu 800 mg for 18 days, then Flu 400 mg/day for 1 month	Relapsed[c]
10	42	0.1	None	Meningitis	0.25/2.0	AmB 657 mg total, followed by Flu 400 mg/day for 3.5 months	Relapse after 4 months	AmB for 2 weeks, followed by Flu 400 mg daily for 11 months	Died (11 months)

[a] Flu, fluconazole; Am, amphotericin B; ND, not done.

[b] The second relapse was treated with itraconazole 400 mg and 5-FC 6 g daily.

[c] Relapsed after 1 month requiring treatment with Am 1 mg/kg for 26 days, followed by itraconazole 200 mg/day; no long-term follow-up given. Patient was alive at 8 months follow-up.

patient outcome, it is inexpensive, and emergence of resistance has not been documented. This agent also protects against toxoplasmosis, a significant cause of mortality in AIDS patients.

The indication for cryptococcal prophylaxis is not as apparent as that for pneumocystis prophylaxis. The prevalence of cryptococcal infection is between 6 to 10% in the United States and Europe; this prevalence is lower than that of *Pneumocystis*, atypical mycobacterial, and cytomegaloviral infections in patients with AIDS. In a randomized trial of prevention of fungal infection in patients with HIV with CD_4 below 200/mm³, fluconazole (200 mg daily) significantly reduced cryptococcal infection (breakthrough rate, 0.9%, 2 of 217), compared with placebo (breakthrough rate, 7%, 15 of 211)

(37). No survival benefit could be demonstrated, however, as most infections resolved with therapy. Primary prophylaxis with a lower dosage of fluconazole (200 mg thrice weekly) given only to patients with CD_4 of 100/mm³ or below was as efficacious and much less costly (45).

An area of concern is the emergence of fluconazole resistance with prolonged use of fluconazole maintenance therapy. Although fluconazole resistance was not documented in the breakthrough cryptococcal isolate in the study by Singh et al., the follow-up time of 12.1 months was short (45). Contrary to that report, anecdotal reports have linked failure of primary fluconazole prophylaxis to cryptococcal strains exhibiting high fluconazole MICs (Table 5); these reports involved patients with very low CD_4 counts (<25/mm³) who had received

TABLE 5 • **Failure of Primary Fluconazole Prophylaxis**[a]

Ref.	Age (years)	CD$_4$ Count (/mm^3)	Prior Flu Use	Breakthrough Infection Site	Flu MIC (μg/mL)	Treatment	Outcome (duration follow-up)
3	45	14	Flu 100 mg/day for 4 years	Meningitis, cryptococcoma	>32	Am 0.6 mg/kg/day for 3 days, followed by Flu 600 mg/day	Alive (3 months)
3	37	22	Flu 400 mg/day for 17 months	Meningitis	≥16	Am 0.6 mg/kg for 2 weeks + 5-FC, followed by Flu 400 mg/day + 5-FC 1 g/day	Alive (4 months)
51	40	5	Flu 100 mg/day for 4 months	Bacteremia	16	None	Died

[a] Flu, fluconazole; Am, amphotericin B; 5-FC, flucytosine.

primary fluconazole prophylaxis for a prolonged period of time (>12 months) (3). Although the prevalence of fluconazole-resistant *Cryptococcus* among patients receiving primary fluconazole prophylaxis is low, the experience with fluconazole resistance might be a harbinger for the emergence of fluconazole resistance among the cryptococci in the future. Furthermore, the cost of fluconazole prophylaxis is tremendous: it is estimated that 7800 doses of fluconazole would be used to prevent a case of invasive fungal infection (45).

The cost, the risk of emergence of fluconazole resistance, and the lack of impact on survival provide important arguments against primary fluconazole prophylaxis. These issues have led the U.S. Public Health Service/Infectious Diseases Society of America task force to decide that they should not recommend routine antifungal prophylaxis for patients with HIV infection. The incidence of cryptococcal meningitis in HIV-infected patients decreased in 1992–1994, before the era of protease inhibitors; the most likely cause was the rising use of fluconazole for chronic treatment of thrush and candidal esophagitis.

ENDPOINTS FOR MONITORING THERAPY

Detection of cryptococcal polysaccharide capsular antigen is useful in both the diagnosis of infection due to *C. neoformans* and the prediction of prognosis and response to therapy. There are several commercially available latex cryptococcal antigen tests as well as an enzyme-linked immunoassay to detect cryptococcal antigen. These tests are both sensitive (90%) and specific (near 100%). When performed in serum or body fluids (such as CSF, bronchoalveolar fluids, or urine), cryptococcal antigen tests provide a rapid means of diagnosing cryptococcal infection. Both false-positive (due to interfering substances or contamination of syneresis fluids) and false-negative results (due to prozone phenomenon or low cryptococcal antigen concentrations) have been reported, although rarely.

Cryptococcal antigen titres can assist in predicting outcomes. In non-AIDS patients, high antigen titers in both serum and CSF before therapy (baseline titers) predict higher mortality, suboptimal response to therapy, and relapse (2, 16, 18). In AIDS patients, high baseline CSF antigen titers predict mortality in patients with AIDS in some studies (40, 57) but not in

others (8). The discrepancy in findings between these studies might be attributed to the use of a wide variety of uncontrolled antigen test kits between different centers participating in the studies. Indeed, the agreement in titer results between the test kits from different manufacturers was at best 60% (49). Therefore, the prognostic significance assigned to a specific titer should be interpreted with caution.

Cryptococcal antigen titers can also assist in monitoring response during acute therapy and predicting relapse. In non-AIDS patients, rising titers after therapy are associated with relapse; therefore, a longer course of therapy should be contemplated in these cases (16, 18). In AIDS patients, an unchanged or raised cryptococcal antigen titer in the CSF during acute therapy is also associated with a higher likelihood of clinical and microbiologic failure of acute therapy and relapse during maintenance therapy (36, 38). The cryptococcal antigen titer in serum was found to correlate with therapeutic outcome.

Despite the prognostic values of CSF cryptococcal antigen titers in patients with AIDS, we do not think that routine determination of CSF cryptococcal antigen following acute therapy is warranted. First, due to the extremely high relapse rate, all AIDS patients will undergo chronic suppressive (maintenance) therapy. Second, relapse can occur in the setting of improving antigen titers from baseline; in one study, 29% of patients (4 of 14) relapsed despite reductions in CSF cryptococcal antigen titer of fourfold or more (36). Third, subjective symptoms are universally present among patients presenting with relapse (4, 39). For these reasons, routine lumbar puncture is of doubtful value in the management of AIDS patients during maintenance therapy for cryptococcal meningitis. Close monitoring of signs and symptoms of infection is a more rational approach to these patients (36, 39); lumbar puncture should be reserved for situations in which clinical symptoms or signs suggest recurrence of disease.

REFERENCES

1. Amengou A, Porcar C, Marsaro J, Garcia-Bragado F. Possible development of resistance of fluconazole during suppressive therapy for AIDS-associated cryptococcal meningitis. Clin Infect Dis 1996;23:1337–1338.

2. Bennett JE, Dismukes WE, Duma RJ, Medoff G, Sande MA, Gallis H, Leonard J, Fields BT, Bradshaw M, Haywood H, McGee ZA, Cate TR, Cobbs CG, Warner JF, Alling DW. A comparison of amphotericin B alone and combined with flucytosine in the treatment of cryptococcal meningitis. N Engl J Med 1979;301:126–131.

3. Berg J, Clancy CJ, Nguyen MH. The hidden danger of primary fluconazole prophylaxis in patients with acquired immunodeficiency syndrome. Clin Infect Dis 1998;26:231–232.

4. Berry AJ, Rinaldi MG, Graybill JR. Use of high-dose fluconazole as salvage therapy for cryptococcal meningitis in patients with AIDS. Antimicrob Agents Chemother 1992;36:690–692.

5. Birley HDL, Johnson EM, McDonald P, Parry C, Carey PB, Warnock DW. Azole drug resistance as a cause of clinical relapse in AIDS patients with cryptococcal meningitis. Int J STD AIDS 1995;6:353–355.

6. Bozzette SA, Larsen RA, Chiu J, Leal ME, Jacobsen J, Rothman P, Robinson P, Gilbert G, McCutchan JA, Tilles J, Leedom JM, Richman DD, and the California Collaborative Treatment Group. A placebo-controlled trial of maintenance therapy with fluconazole after treatment of cryptococcal meningitis in the acquired immunodeficiency syndrome. N Engl J Med 1991;324: 580–584.

7. Butler WT, Alling DW, Spickard A, Utz JP. Diagnostic and prognostic value of clinical and laboratory findings in cryptococcal meningitis. N Engl J Med 1961;270:59–67.

8. Chuck SL, Sande MA. Infections with *Cryptococcus neoformans* in the acquired immunodeficiency syndrome. N Engl J Med 1989;321:794–799.

9. Coker RJ, Viviani M, Gazzard BG, DuPont B, Pohle HD, Murphy SM, Atouguia J, Champalimaud JL, Harris JRW. Treatment of cryptococcosis with liposomal amphotericin B (AmBisome) in 23 patients with AIDS. AIDS 1993;7:829–835.

10. Currie BP, Ghannoum M, Bessen L, Casadevall A. Decreased fluconazole susceptibility of a relapse *Cryptococcus neoformans* isolated after fluconazole treatment. Infect Dis Clin Pract 1995;48:318–319.

11. De Lalla F, Pellizzer G, Vaglia A, Manfrin V, Franzetti M, Fabris P, Stecca C. Amphotericin B as primary therapy for cryptococcosis in patients with AIDS: reliability of relatively high doses administered over a relatively short period. Clin Infect Dis 1995;20:263–266.

12. De Gans J, Portegies P, Tiessens G, Eeftinck Schattenkerk JKM, van Boxtel CJ, van Ketel RJ, Stam J. Itraconazole compared with amphotericin B plus flucytosine in AIDS patients with cryptococcal meningitis. AIDS 1992;6:185–190.

13. Denning DW, Tucker RM, Hanson LH, Hamilton JR, Stevens DA. Itraconazole therapy for cryptococcal meningitis and cryptococcosis. Arch Intern Med 1989;149:2301–2308.

14. Denning DW, Tucker RM, Hostetler JS, Gill S, Stevens DA. Oral itraconazole therapy of cryptococcal meningitis and cryptococcosis in patients with AIDS. In: H. Vanden Bossche, ed. Mycoses in AIDS patients. New York: Plenem Press, 1990: 305–324.

15. Denning DW, Armstrong RW, Lewis BH, Stevens DA. Elevated cerebrospinal fluid pressures in patients with cryptococcal meningitis and acquired immunodeficiency syndrome. Am J Med 1991;91:267–272.

16. Diamond RD, Bennett JE. Prognostic factors in cryptococcal meningitis. Ann Intern Med 1974;80:176–181.

17. Dismukes WE, Stamm AM, Graybill JR, Craven PC, Stevens DA, Stiller RL, Sarosi GA, Medoff G, Gregg CR, Gallis HA, Fields BT, Marier RL, Kerkering TA, Kaplowitz LG, Cloud G, Bowles C, Shadomy S. Treatment of systemic mycoses with ketoconazole: emphasis on toxicity and clinical response in 52 patients. Ann Intern Med 1983;98:13–20.

18. Dismukes WE, Cloud G, Gallis HA, Kerkering TM, Medoff G, Craven PC, Kaplowitz LG, Fisher JF, Gregg CR, Bowles CA, Shadomy S, Stamm AM, Diasio RB, Kaufman L, Soong SJ, Blackwelder WC, and the National Institute of Allergy and Infectious Diseases Mycoses Study Group. Treatment of cryptococcal meningitis with combination amphotericin B and flucytosine for four as compared with six weeks. N Engl J Med 1987;317:334–341.

19. Dismukes WE. Current recommendations for the treatment of cryptococcosis in non-AIDS patients. 3rd International Conference on *Cryptococcus* and Cryptococcosis, 1996. Paris, France.

20. Dromer F, Mathoulin S, Dupont B, Brugiere O, Letenneur L. Comparison of the efficacy of amphotericin B and fluconazole in the treatment of cryptococcosis in human immunodeficiency virus-negative patients: retrospective analysis of 83 cases. Clin Infect Dis 1996;22(Suppl 2):S154–160.

20a. Leenders ACAP, Reiss P, Portegies P, Clezy K, Hop WCJ, Hoy J, Borleffs JCC, Allworth T, Kauffmann RH, Jones P, Kroon FP, Verbrugh HA, de Marie S. Liposomal amphotericin B (AmBisome) compared with amphotericin B both followed by oral fluconazole in the treatment of AIDS-associated cryptococcal meningitis. AIDS 1997;11:1463–1471.

20b. Fessler RD, Sobel J, Guyot L, Crane L, Vazquez J, Szuba MJ, Diaz FG. Management of elevated intracranial pressure in patients with cryptococcal meningitis. J Acquir Immune Defic Synd Hum Retrovirol 1998;17:137–142.

21. Hammerman KJ, Powell KE, Christianson CS, Huggin PM, Larsh HW, Vivas JR, Tosh FE. Pulmonary cryptococcosis: clinical forms and treatment. Am Respir Dis 1973;108:1116–1123.

22. Haubrich RH, Haghighat D, Bozzette SA, Tilles J, McCutchan JA. High-dose fluconazole for treatment of cryptococcal disease in patients with human immunodeficiency virus infection. J Infect Dis 1994;170:238–242.

23. Houk VN, Moser KM. Pulmonary cryptococcosis. Must all receive amphotericin B? Ann Intern Med 1965;63:583–596.

24. Kerkering TM, Duma RJ, Shadomy S. The evolution of pulmonary cryptococcosis. Ann Intern Med 1981;94:611–616.

25. Larsen RA, Bozzette S, McCutchan JA, Chiu J, Leal, MA, Richman DD, and California Collaborative Treatment Group. Persistent *Cryptococcus neoformans* infection of the prostate after successful treatment of meningitis. Ann Intern Med 1989;111: 125–128.

26. Larsen RA, Leal ME, Chan LS. Fluconazole compared with amphotericin B plus flucytosine for cryptococcal meningitis in AIDS. Ann Intern Med 1990;113:183–187.

27. Larsen RA. Combination therapy for cryptococcosis and speculations for future. 3rd International Conference on Cryptococcus and Cryptococcosis, 1996. Paris, France.

28. Nguyen MH, Barchiesi F, McGough DA, Yu VL, Rinaldi MG. In vitro evaluation of combination of fluconazole and flucytosine against *Cryptococcus neoformans* var. *neoformans*. Antimicrob Agents Chemother 1995;39:1691–1695.

29. Nguyen MH, Najvar LK, Yu CY, Graybill JR. Combination therapy with fluconazole and flucytosine in the murine model of cryptococcal meningitis. Antimicrob Agents Chemother 1997; 41:1120–1123.

30. Paugam A, Dupouy-Camet J, Blanche P, et al. Increased fluconazole resistance of *Cryptococcus neoformans* isolated from a patient with AIDS and recurrent meningitis. Clin Infect Dis 1994;19:975–976.

31. Peetermans W, Bobbaers H, Verhaegen J, Vandepitte J. Flu-

conazole-resistant *Cryptococcus neoformans* var *gattii* in an AIDS patient. Acta Clin Belg 1993;48:405–409.

32. Perfect JR, Durack DT, Hamilton JD, et al. Failure of ketoconazole in cryptococcal meningitis. JAMA 1982;247:3349.

33. Perfect JR, Durack DT, Gallis HA. Cryptococcemia. Medicine 1983;62:98–109.

34. Powderly WG, Saag MS, Cloud GA, Robinson P, Meyer RD, Jackbson JM, Graybill JR, Sugar AM, McAuliffe VJ, Follansbee SE, Tuazon CU, Stern JJ, Feinberg J, Hafner R, Dismukes WE, NIAID AIDS Clinical Trials Group, and the NIAID Mycoses Study Group. A controlled trial of fluconazole or amphotericin B to prevent relapse of cryptococcal meningitis in patients with the acquired immunodeficiency syndrome. N Engl J Med 1992; 326:793–798.

35. Powderly WG, Keath EJ, Sokol-Anderson M, Robinson K, Kitz D, Little JR, Kobayashi G. Amphotericin B-resistant *Cryptococcus neoformans* in a patient with AIDS. Infect Dis Clin Pract 1994;1:314–316.

36. Powderly WG, Cloud GA, Dismukes WE, Saag MS. Measurement of cryptococcal antigen in serum and cerebrospinal fluid: value in the management of AIDS-associated cryptococcal meningitis. Clin Infect Dis 1994;18:789–792.

37. Powderly WG, Finkelstein D, Feinberg J, Frame P, He W, vanderHorst C, Koletar SL, Eyster ME, Carey J, Waskin H. A randomized trial comparing fluconazole with clotrimazole troches for the prevention of fungal infections in patients with advanced human immunodeficiency virus infection. N Engl J Med 1995; 332:700–705.

38. Powderly WG. Use of cryptococcal antigen testing in management of cryptococcosis. 3rd International Conference on Cryptococcus and Cryptococcosis, 1996. Paris, France.

39. Powderly WG. Cryptococcosis: current status of diagnosis and treatment. Cliniguide Fungal Infect 1997;8:1–15.

40. Saag MS, Powderly WG, Cloud GA, Robinson P, Grieco MH, Sharkey PK, Thompson SE, Sugar AM, Tuazon CU, Fisher JF, Hyslop N, Jacobson JM, Hafner R, Dismukes WE, and the NIAID Mycoses Study Group and the AIDS Clinical Trials Group. Comparison of amphotericin B with fluconazole in the treatment of acute AIDS-associated cryptococcal meningitis. N Engl J Med 1992;326:83–89.

41. Saag MS. The treatment of cryptococcal disease in AIDS patients. 3rd International Conference on Cryptococcus and Cryptococcosis, 1996. Paris, France.

42. Saag MS, Cloud GC, Graybill JR, Sobel J, Tuazon C, Wiesinger B, Riser L, Moskovitz BL, Dismukes WE, and the NIAID Mycoses Study Group. Comparison of fluconazole (FLU) versus itraconazole (ITRA) as maintenance therapy of AIDS-associated cryptococcal meningitis [Abstract #I218]. ICAAC, San Francisco, 1995.

43. Sarosi GA, Parker JD, Doto IL, Tosh FE. Amphotericin B in cryptococcal meningitis. Ann Intern Med 1969;71:1079–1087.

44. Sharkey PK, Graybill JR, Johnson ES, Hausrath SG, Pollard RB, Kolokathis A, Mildvan D, Fan-Havard P, Eng RHK, Patterson TF, Pottage JC, Simberkoff MS, Wolf J, Meyer RD, Gupta R, Lee LW, Gordon DS. Amphotericin B lipid complex compared with amphotericin B in the treatment of cryptococcal meningitis in patients with AIDS. Clin Infect Dis 1996; 22:315–321.

45. Singh N, Barnish MJ, Berman S, Bender B, Wagener MM, Rinaldi GM, Yu UL. Low-dose fluconazole as primary prophylaxis for cryptococcal infection in AIDS-patients with CD_4 cell counts of $\leq$ 100/mm^3. Clin Infect Dis 1996; 23: 1282–1286.

46. Spickard A, Butler WT, Andriole V, Utz JP. The improved prognosis of cryptococcal meningitis with amphotericin B therapy. Ann Intern Med 1963;58:66–83.

47. Spitzer ED, Spitzer SG, Freundlich LF, Casadevall A. Persistence of initial infection in recurrent *Cryptococcus neoformans* meningitis. Lancet 1993;341:595–596.

48. Sung JP, Campbell GD, Grendahl JG. Miconazole therapy for fungal meningitis. Arch Neurol 1978;35:443–447.

49. Tanner DC, Weinstein MP, Fedorciw B, Joho KL, Thorpe JJ, Reller LB. Comparison of commercial kits for detection of cryptococcal antigen. J Clin Microbiol 1994;32:1680–1684.

50. Van der Horst CM, Saag MS, Cloud GA, Hamill RJ, Graybill JR, Sobel JD, Hohnson PC, Tuazon CU, Kerkering T, Moskovitz BL, Powderly WG, Dismukes WE. Treatment of cryptococcal meningitis associated with the acquired immunodeficiency syndrome. N Engl J Med 1997;337:15–21.

51. Viard JP, Hennequin C, Fortineau N, Pertuiset N, Rothschild C, Zylberberg H. Fulminant cryptococcal infections in HIV-infected patients on oral fluconazole. Lancet 1995;346:118.

52. Viviani MA, Tortorano AM, Giani PC, Arici C, Goglio A, Crocchiolo P, Almaviva M. Itraconazole for cryptococcal infection in the acquired immunodeficiency syndrome. Ann Intern Med 1987;106:166.

53. Warr W, Bates JH, Stone A. The spectrum of pulmonary cryptococcosis. Ann Intern Med 1968;69:1109–1116.

54. Weinstein L, Jacoby I. Successful treatment of cerebral cryptococcoma and meningitis with miconazole. Ann Intern Med 1908;93:569–571.

55. Witt MD, Lewis RJ, Larsen RA, Milefchik EN, Leal ME, Haubrich RH, Richie JA, Edwards JE Jr, Ghannoum MA. Identification of patients with acute AIDS-associated cryptococcal meningitis who can be effectively treated with fluconazole: the role of antifungal susceptibility testing. Clin Infect Dis 1996;22: 322–328.

56. Yamaguchi H, Ikemoto H, Watanabe K, Ito A, Hara K, Kohno S. Fluconazole monotherapy for cryptococcosis in non-AIDS patients. Eur J Clin Microbiol Infect Dis 1996;15:787–792.

57. Zuger A, Louie E, Holzman RS, Simberkoff MS, Rahal JJ. Cryptococcal disease in patients with the acquired immunodeficiency syndrome. Ann Intern Med 1986;104:234–240.

Dematiaceous Fungi: Chromoblastomycosis, Mycetoma, Subcutaneous and Cutaneous Phaeohyphomycosis, and Noninvasive Sinusitis

Cornelius J. Clancy and Nina Singh

GENERAL DESCRIPTION
Mycology

The dematiaceous (black) fungi are common soil and plant saprophytes grouped together on the basis of their darkly pigmented walls. If the dark walls are visible on hematoxylin and eosin (H&E) staining, a diagnosis is readily established. Frequently, however, the acute-angled branching hyphae of black fungi are indistinguishable from those of filamentous molds such as *Aspergillus* or *Fusarium*. In such cases, the black fungi can identified by the Fontana-Masson stain, which is specific for melanin present in the walls of these organisms. Distinguishing between black fungi and filamentous molds has important therapeutic implications, since the black fungi generally cause localized tissue infections, whereas the filamentous molds are frequently associated with disseminated infections (14, 84). Identification of specific black fungi is based upon morphologic and biochemical characteristics after growth in culture on Sabouraud's, malt extract, or potato dextrose agar.

Clinical Manifestations

The black fungi are increasingly identified as causes of infection in immunocompetent and immunosuppressed hosts (80, 84). These organisms are responsible for three categories of human infections (Table 1). Chromoblastomycosis presents with chronic wartlike or cauliflower-like lesions of the skin and subcutaneous tissue; the pathognomonic histopathologic findings are sclerotic bodies: round, brown, thick-walled forms with intersecting septae within the cells. Mycetoma is characterized by subcutaneous tumefaction (swelling) and draining sinus tracts; the pathognomonic histopathologic findings are granules: dense, tightly packed accumulations of organisms. Mycetoma can be caused by black fungi, other fungi (e.g., *Pseudallescheria*), or bacteria (e.g., *Actinomyces* or *Nocardia*). Chromoblastomycosis and mycetoma are largely diseases of tropical and subtropical regions. Phaeohyphomycosis is a heterogenous collection of conditions, classified as superficial, cutaneous, subcutaneous, or systemic, on the basis of the degree of tissue invasion. On histopathologic examination, black fungi are found in tissue without evidence of sclerotic bodies or granules. Phaeohyphomycoses are encountered worldwide. In addition to these classifications, black fungi cause infections of the central nervous system (cerebral phaeohyphomycosis) and paranasal sinuses (3, 72, 81, 97).

This chapter focuses on therapy of chromoblastomycosis, mycetoma, cutaneous and subcutaneous phaeohyphomycosis, and noninvasive sinusitis. Therapy of invasive sinusitis, and systemic and cerebral phaeohyphomycosis is covered in the chapter "Dematiaceous and Nonpigmented Fungi: Invasive and Systemic Disease."

SUSCEPTIBILITY TESTING IN VITRO AND IN VIVO

Unlike bacterial infections, for which in vitro testing of isolates for susceptibility to antimicrobial agents is useful in guiding therapy, the clinical utility of in vitro antifungal susceptibility testing has not been proven. Until recently, in vitro antifungal susceptibility testing was limited by lack of a standardized testing method, poor reproducibility, and lack of correlation between in vitro results and in vivo outcome. Testing methods proposed by members of the National Committee for Clinical Laboratory Standards (NCCLS) have demonstrated good reproducibility and form the basis for standardized reference methods (29, 30, 67, 68, 73). Although a correlation between in vitro results and in vivo response to therapy has been demonstrated for *Candida* isolates using the NCCLS methods (77), no such correlation has yet been demonstrated for molds, including black fungi. Nevertheless, recent data from animal models of disseminated aspergillosis suggest that the reference method might be able to predict response to therapy for mold infections (24). Given such findings, in vitro antifungal susceptibility testing of black fungi is likely to become clinically relevant in the future and allow physicians to target antifungal therapy more precisely.

ANTIFUNGAL THERAPY

For antifungal agents to be successful, therapy must be prolonged. Clinical response may not become evident for several months, and treatment should be continued for at least 2 to 3 months after apparent clinical and mycologic resolution of infection (10). Although the literature frequently cites good response rates (i.e., clinical improvement) to a number of antifungal regimens, cure rates (i.e., mycologic resolution) are significantly lower. When it is not possible to cure the infection, prolonged suppressive antifungal therapy may be necessary (82). The response to antifungal agents is greater with less extensive infections (74, 76). In addition to the extent of infection, the underlying host immune status also helps determine the response to therapy (14, 82).

TABLE 1 • **Disease Entities Caused by Black Fungi**

Entity	Common Pathogens	Clinical Manifestations	Histopathologic Characteristics	Prognosis
Chromoblastomycosis	*Fonsecaea pedrosi* *Cladosporium carrionii* *F. compacta* *Phialaphora verrucosa* *Rhinocladiella aquaspersa*	Chronic wart- or cauliflower-like lesions of skin and subcutaneous tissue	Sclerotic bodies ("copper pennies")	Limited infections: cure is possible; extensive infections: cure is rare
Mycetoma	*Madurella mycetomatis* *M. grisea* *Curvularia lunata* *Exophiala jeanselmei*	Chronic skin and subcutaneous lesions with swelling and draining sinus tracts	Infectious granules	Worse than chromoblastomycosis; limited infections: cure is possible; extensive infections: cure is very rare
Subcutaneous phaeohyphomycosis	*E. jeanselmei* *Wangiella dermatitidis* *Phialophora* spp. *Bipolaris* spp.	Heterogenous: well-formed cysts; subcutaneous tissue invasion; extensive sinus tracts	Fungi within nonkeratinized tissue beneath the dermal layer; no granules or sclerotic bodies	Cystic form: good; nonencapsulated form: fair, depends on extent of tissue invasion; cures less likely in immunosuppressed patients
Cutaneous phaeohyphomycosis: dermatomycosis and onychomycosis	*Alternaria* spp. *Hendersonula toruloidea* *Phialophora* spp.	Indistinguishable from infections by dermatophytes	Fungi within keratinized tissue with extensive host response and tissue damage	Onychomycosis is difficult to eradicate; dermatomycosis has better prognosis
Cutaneous phaeohyphomycosis: Keratomycosis	*Curvularia* spp. Alternaria spp. *Exophiala jeanselmei* *Exserohilum rostratum*	Nodule progressing to ulcer; feathery, branching pattern in cornea	Superficial or deep fungal invasion of cornea; endophthalmitis rare	Fair: residual visual damage can occur; 25% require penetrating keratoplasty
Sinusitis: allergic sinusitis	*Bipolaris* spp., *Curvularia* spp., *Exserohilum* spp., *Alternaria* spp.	Chronic sinusitis	Sparse fungi; eosinophil-rich mucoid material (allergic mucin); Charcot-Leyden crystals	Cure is rare; frequent relapses
Sinusitis: fungus ball	*Bipolaris* spp., *Curvularia* spp., *Exserohilum* spp., *Alternaria* spp.	Nasal congestion; rhinosinusitis	Fungus ball: abundant fungi within inflammatory mass	Good

Amphotericin B has been ineffective against most infections caused by black fungi (65, 78). The lack of efficacy can be attributed to several factors: potential intrinsic resistance of certain black fungi to the drug (19, 20), poor penetration of the drug into sites of infection (54), the need for high doses and prolonged courses of therapy, and drug toxicity. Local injections of amphotericin B have been effective in some cases (21, 99, 100) but are contraindicated because of pain and the risk of local fibrosis, hemolysis, and thrombosis (7). Experience with liposomal preparations of amphotericin B is too limited to determine whether they have a role against infections caused by these organisms (40).

Itraconazole is increasingly viewed as the drug of choice against most infections caused by black fungi (10, 82, 95). Itraconazole has good in vitro activity against many of these organisms (65, 76), penetrates well into skin and subcutaneous tissue, is available orally, and is well tolerated during long-term therapy. The major limitation of this agent is its erratic absorption, which might be improved by measures to acidify stomach pH or by taking capsules with a high-fat meal. Monitoring serum levels might be useful to document absorption in cases in which the therapeutic response is poor. More-reliable absorption is achieved with a new oral solution formulation of itraconazole, but it is not clear whether the solution can be given for prolonged durations.

Other agents might be effective in selected cases. Ketoconazole has been effective against a variety of infections due to black fungi, particularly mycetoma (28, 40, 62, 91, 96), but toxicity with long-term use is more significant than with itraconazole. Ketoconazole represents front-line therapy against mycetoma, but otherwise is a second-line agent. Miconazole, while also effective in selected cases (98), is associated with greater toxicity than the other azoles and is not routinely recommended. Fluconazole has been largely ineffective against infections caused by black fungi (26) and cannot be recommended because of poor intrinsic activity against molds. Flucytosine has excellent tissue penetration and is initially effective against infections caused by a number of black fungi, but its use as monotherapy is not recommended because of the rapid emergence of resistance (12, 58, 59). The drug remains potentially useful as part of combination regimens with amphotericin B, itraconazole, or ketoconazole.

Therapeutic recommendations for each of the clinical entities caused by black fungi are summarized in Table 2.

TABLE 2 • Recommendations for Therapy of Infections Caused by Black Fungi

Clinical Entity	First-Line Therapy	Second-Line Therapy	Options for Refractory Infections
Chromoblastomycosis	Complete wide- and deep-margin resection combined with itraconazole (200 mg/day) for 2–3 months	Partial surgical resection combined with itraconazole (200–600 mg/day) until 2–3 months after apparent mycologic cure	Repeated surgical resection; itraconazole and flucytosine; amphotericin B and flucytosine; ketoconazole; ketoconazole and flucytosine; terbinafine (500 mg/day)
Mycetoma	Complete wide- and deep-margin resection combined with ketoconazole (300–400 mg/day) or itraconazole (200 mg/day) for 2–3 months	Partial surgical resection combined with ketoconazole (300–400 mg/day) or itraconazole (200–600 mg/day) until 2–3 months after apparent mycologic cure	Repeated surgical resection; amphotericin B; ketoconazole and flucytosine; itraconazole and flucytosine; amphotericin B and flucytosine
Subcutaneous phaeohyphomycosis Immunocompetent hosts	Complete wide- and deep-margin resection combined with itraconazole (200 mg/day) for 2–3 months; if organisms are contained within a cyst, adjunctive antifungal therapy is not needed	Partial surgical resection combined with itraconazole (200–600 mg/day) until 2–3 months after apparent mycologic cure	Repeated surgical resection; amphotericin B; ketoconazole; addition of flucytosine to medical regimen
Immunocompromised hosts	Complete wide- and deep-margin resection combined with itraconazole (200 mg/day), amphotericin B (1 mg/kg/day), or ketoconazole (200–600 mg/day)	Partial surgical resection combined with itraconazole (200–600 mg/day), amphotericin B (1 mg/kg/day), or ketoconazole (300–400 mg/day)	Repeated surgical resection; addition of flucytosine to medical regimen
Cutaneous phaeohyphomycosis Dermatomycosis, onychomycosis	Itraconazole (200 mg/day) until 2–3 months after apparent mycologic cure	Ketoconazole (100–400 mg/day)	Terbinafine
Keratomycosis	Natamycin (5% solution) topically	Amphotericin B drops (0.15%)	Natamycin or amphotericin B combined with flucytosine (1% aqueous solution); topical itraconazole, ketoconazole, or miconazole; oral ketoconazole (400 mg/day); oral itraconazole (400 mg/day); penetrating keratoplasty
Sinusitis Allergic fungal sinusitis	Surgical aeration, drainage, and debridement, combined with postoperative corticosteroids; postoperative nasal saline irrigations and regular surveillance endoscopy		Itraconazole; allergen immunotherapy to decrease IgE production
Fungus ball	Resection of fungus ball, with aeration of sinuses	In cases of local invasion of bone, itraconazole or amphotericin B are indicated as adjunctive therapy	

RECOMMENDED THERAPEUTIC APPROACHES AGAINST SPECIFIC CLINICAL ENTITIES
Chromoblastomycosis

The natural history of chromoblastomycosis is indolent, progressive extension of infection into surrounding cutaneous and subcutaneous tissue. Spontaneous resolution is extremely rare (42), and complications such as elephantiasis and secondary infection occur frequently (32, 53). Therapy is indicated for esthetic reasons, to limit functional impairment, and to prevent complications. Recommended therapy consists of surgical resection combined with antifungal agents. Curettage and desiccation are discouraged because of the frequency of

recurrence and the potential for early lymphatic dissemination (7, 76, 94).

The extent of infection is the major determinant of surgical resectability. In one report, the cure rate following surgical resection was 30% (7 of 23) (5); among patients with limited infections (≤3 lesions), however, the cure rate was 70% (7 of 10), compared with 0% (0 of 13) among patients with more extensive infections (>3 lesions). Indeed, even amputation cannot reliably eradicate extensive infections; stump recurrences have been described (36, 100).

Itraconazole is generally effective against chromoblastomycosis (10, 82, 95). The response rate depends on the extent of the infection. In two studies, itraconazole (100–600 mg/day, administered for periods ranging from 3 months to 3 years) cured 80% of patients with mild infections, 50% with moderate infections, and 0% with severe infections (74, 75). In selected patients with extensive infection for whom cure is not possible, prolonged administration of itraconazole can lead to clinical improvement (10, 51, 57, 74, 75, 82, 85, 95). Ketoconazole (100–400 mg/day) is less effective than itraconazole; clinical improvement with ketoconaozle is noted in 50 to 75% of patients (22, 28, 63, 83, 91), but cure rates are below 50% (22, 28, 91). Thiabendazole (25 mg/kg/day) results in cures for 20 to 40% of patients (6) but is not routinely recommended because of severe toxic/allergic reactions.

In contrast to itraconazole and ketoconazole, amphotericin B is not usually curative in chromoblastomycosis; failure of therapy or relapses following therapy are commonplace (64, 78). However, addition of flucytosine to amphotericin B has been effective. Prior to the introduction of itraconazole, the combination of flucytosine (25 to 50 mg/kg/day) and amphotericin B (25 mg every other day) was the treatment of choice for patients in whom complete surgical resection was not feasible (58, 59). Addition of flucytosine to ketoconazole (28, 83), itraconazole (7, 10, 51), or thiabendazole (7) has also been beneficial in refractory cases. Fluconazole has been useful only in selected cases at high doses (e.g., 800–1200 mg/day).

Terbinafine appears promising against chromoblastomycosis (31), but experience is too limited at present to recommend routine use of this agent. In an open-label study, mycologic cure was reported in over 80% of patients treated with 500 mg/day for 6 to 12 months (31).

Physical measures such as application of heat (40–42°C) (92), cryotherapy with liquid nitrogen (60), and CO_2 laser therapy (55) have been effective in selected cases involving small lesions. In addition, topical heat and cryotherapy have been used successfully in combination with conventional surgery and antifungal agents (51). Topical antifungal agents are ineffective (59).

Mycetoma

In mycetoma, fungi invade more deeply into subcutaneous tissue than in chromoblastomycosis, and it is more difficult to eradicate with surgery and antifungal agents. Unlike chromoblastomycosis, mycetoma can extend into bone or the thoracic or abdominal cavities; these complications are associated with significant morbidity and mortality and are particularly difficult to eradicate (38). Complete surgical resection is possible in only 20 to 30% of mycetoma lesions due to black fungi (8, 33). Recurrence rates following surgery of even localized lesions are high, ranging from 25 to 90% (61, 64, 90).

Ketoconazole (300–400 mg/day) appears to be the most effective antifungal agent, with clinical improvement rates of 70 to 90% (40, 62, 91, 96) and cure rates of approximately 33% (61). These findings have not been consistent, however, and some investigators report little clinical improvement with ketoconazole (7). Itraconazole (200–600 mg/day) appears to be less successful against mycetoma than ketoconazole, although comparative trials have not been performed; improvement

rates of approximately 40% have been reported (10, 40). As with chromoblastomycosis, amphotericin B is largely ineffective (78). Unlike chromoblastomycosis, however, addition of flucytosine to other antifungal agents has not been demonstrated to be effective against mycetoma (7). Fluconazole, griseofulvin, and miconazole are not generally effective and are not recommended (26).

Subcutaneous Phaeohyphomycosis

Infections of subcutaneous tissue are the most common form of phaeohyphomycosis. Subcutaneous phaeohyphomycosis is associated with a range of manifestations. Frequently, the infecting organisms are completely enclosed within a thick-walled fibrous cyst (102). Surgical resection of the cyst is curative, and adjunctive therapy with antifungal agents is not necessary (13). Incision and drainage of cysts, rather than complete resection, does not eradicate infecting organisms and is associated with reaccumulation of pus (27, 44, 89).

In other cases, black fungi might invade the local subcutaneous tissue or lead to development of draining sinus tracts (clinically resembling mycetoma) (4, 35, 70, 71, 72); rarely, extension to surrounding bone (82) or disseminated infection ensues (66). Since surgical resection in these nonencapsulated cases rarely eradicates the infection, adjunctive antifungal therapy is indicated. Itraconazole appears to be the agent of choice in immunocompetent patients; in one study, itraconazole cured all three immunocompetent patients with subcutaneous phaeohyphomycosis who had failed previous antifungal therapy (82). In immunosuppressed patients, no agent has been shown superior. Amphotericin B, itraconazole, and ketoconazole (11, 16, 86, 88) have been anecdotally effective, but failures and relapses have also been documented (43, 50, 101); addition of flucytosine is usually not beneficial (14). Reduction of immunosuppressive medications to the lowest effective doses is an important adjunct to surgery and antifungal agents.

Cutaneous Phaeohyphomycosis

Dermatomycosis and Onychomycosis

The black fungi infrequently cause dermatomycosis or onychomycosis. Both dermatomycosis and onychomycosis are difficult to eradicate and require systemic antifungal therapy; onychomycosis in particular requires prolonged therapy. Itraconazole (100–200 mg/day) and ketoconazole (100–400 mg/day) have been used successfully (56, 93). Amphotericin B, miconazole, and flucytosine have been disappointing. Terbinafine appears effective against superficial dermatophyte and *Candida* infections (46), but experience with dermatomycosis or onychomycosis due to black fungi is too limited to recommend its routine use (2). Griseofulvin is generally not effective (39).

Keratomycosis

Depending on geographic location, black fungi might account for over 10% of cases of keratomycosis (69, 79). Natamycin (5% solution) is the only antifungal agent currently FDA-approved for treatment of keratomycosis. It has been used effectively in superficial keratitis due to black fungi (47, 69). It is applied topically every 30 to 60 min around the clock for the first week and then hourly while awake for a minimum of 12 weeks (1, 34). In cases of deep fungal keratitis, some advocate amphotericin B drops (0.15%) as front-line therapy (34); experience with this agent against black fungi is limited, however, and failures of amphotericin B have been reported (69). The combination of amphotericin B or natamycin and flucytosine (1% aqueous solution) is advocated by some ophthalmologists, although the benefits of this combination are anecdotal (1, 34).

Topical miconazole and ketoconazole have been used successfully against a range of black fungi causing keratitis (69), and topical itraconazole has been effective against other fungi (1). Given the lack of experience, these agents must be considered second-line alternatives.

Systemic therapy with the azoles is reserved for severe or refractory cases. Ketoconazole (400 mg/day) attains high concentrations in the cornea and anterior chamber in animals (41) and has been used effectively in the treatment of patients with keratomycosis (45). Itraconazole (400 mg/day) was effective in 69% of patients with keratomycoses caused by a variety of fungi in one study (1); experience with itraconazole in patients with keratomycosis specifically due to black fungi is limited. Amphotericin B has not been effective when given systemically and is limited by toxicity and poor corneal penetration (69). The use of topical corticosteroids to decrease corneal inflammation is contraindicated (87). If the patient does not respond rapidly to aggressive therapy with antifungal agents, penetrating keratoplasty should be performed before the fungus reaches the limbus or sclera (37).

Noninvasive Sinusitis

Allergic Fungal Sinusitis

Black fungi are now recognized as the most common causes of allergic fungal sinusitis (15). Allergic sinusitis is believed to represent an IgE-mediated hypersensitivity reaction to fungi, rather than an infection of host tissue (48). Surgical aeration, drainage, and debridement of the infected sinus are the key components of therapy (25). Due to frequent recurrences despite surgical intervention, systemic corticosteroids given postoperatively for several weeks appear to be of benefit (52). Thereafter, full-dose, short-acting intranasal corticosteroids are prescribed on a long-term basis (18, 25). Postoperative nasal saline irrigations and regular surveillance endoscopy are advocated to remove synechiae or polyps (25, 53). Antifungal agents are generally not considered necessary (25, 52), although some otolaryngologists suggest they might be useful in patients with repeated relapses (9). Adjunctive itraconazole (400 mg/day) has been shown to be potentially beneficial in patients with allergic bronchopulmonary aspergillosis, an entity that resembles allergic sinusitis pathologically (23). Whether such an approach would improve outcome in allergic sinusitis due to black fungi requires investigation.

Sinus Fungus Balls

Black fungi are also commonly responsible for sinus fungus balls. Therapy consisting of surgical resection of the fungus ball and aeration of the sinus is generally curative. Unless invasion

of the surrounding mucosa or bone is demonstrated, antifungal agents do not appear to be of additional benefit (18, 49).

ADJUNCTIVE THERAPY

Even with prolonged antifungal therapy, infections caused by the black fungi are frequently difficult to eradicate. For this reason, recommended therapeutic approaches combine surgical resection with antifungal therapy (64). Wide-margin surgical resection of infectious lesions can eradicate some, but not all, early-stage infections, without antifungal agents (5, 17). However, even apparently well-circumscribed infections might not be completely resectable and are subject to relapse after surgery (61). Amputation, a common surgical approach in the past, should only be considered in severe cases after other therapeutic options have been exhausted.

REFERENCES

1. Abad J-C, Foster CS. Fungal keratitis. Int Ophthalmol Clin 1996;36:1–15.
2. Abdel-Rahman SM, Nahata MC. Oral terbinafine: a new antifungal agent. Ann Pharmacother 1997;31:445–456.
3. Adam RD, Paquin ML, Petersen EA, Saubolle MA, Rinaldi MG, Corcoran JG, Galgiani JN, Sobonya RE. Phaeohyphomycosis caused by the fungal genera *Bipolaris* and *Exserohilum*. Medicine (Baltimore) 1986;65:203–217.
4. Baker JG, Salkin IF, Forgacs P, Haines JH, Kemna ME. First report of subcutaneous phaeohyphomycosis of the foot caused by *Phoma minutella*. J Clin Microbiol 1987;25:2395–2397.
5. Bansal AS, Prabhakar P. Chromomycosis: a twenty-year-analysis of histologically confirmed cases in Jamaica. Trop Geogr Med 1989;41:222–226.
6. Bayles MAH. Chromomycosis. Arch Derm 1971;104:476–485.
7. Bayles MAH. Tropical mycoses. Chemother 1992;38(Suppl 1):27–34.
8. Bendl BJ, Mackey D, Al-Saati F, Sheth KV, Ofoles SN, Bailey TM. Mycetoma in Saudi Arabia. J Trop Med Hyg 1987;90:51–59.
9. Bent JP III, Kuhn FA. Antifungal activity against allergic fungal sinusitis organisms. Laryngoscope 1996;106:1331–1334.
10. Borelli D. A clinical trial of itraconazole in the treatment of deep mycoses and leishmaniasis. Rev Infect Dis 1987;9:S57–S63.
11. Burges GE, Walls CT, Maize JC. Subcutaneous phaeohyphomycosis caused by *Exserehilum rostratum* in an immunocompetent host. Arch Dermatol 1987;123:1346–1350.
12. Chermsirivathana S, Bunyaratavej K, Pupaibul K. The treatment of chromomycosis with 5-fluorocystine. Int Soc Trop Dermatol 1979;18:377–379.
13. Clancy CJ, Nguyen MH. Subcutaneous phaeohyphomycosis. Clin Infect Dis 1997;25:1065, 1195.
14. Clancy CJ, Wingard JR, Nguyen MH. Subcutaneous phaeohyphomycosis after transplantation influence of host immune system on clinical manifestations, and value of combination antifungal therapy against invasive infection. [Abstract J102] 37th ICAAE. 1997;54: Toronto, Ontario.
15. Cody DT II, Neel HB III, Ferreiro JA, Roberts GD. Allergic fungal sinusitis: the Mayo Clinic experience. Laryngoscope 1994;104:1074–1079.
16. Coldiron BM, et al. Cutaneous phaeohyphomycosis caused by a rare fungal pathogen, *Hormonema dematioides:* successful treatment with ketoconazole. J Am Acad Dermatol 1990;23:363–367.

17. Conway H, Berkeley W. Chromoblastomycosis (mycetoma form) treated by surgical excision. AMA Arch Dermatol Syphil 1952;66:695–702.

18. Corey JP, Delsupehe KG, Ferguson BJ. Allergic fungal sinusitis: allergic, infectious, or both? Otolaryngol Head Neck Surg 1995;113:110–119.

19. Corrado ML, Kramer M, Cummings M, Eng RH. Susceptibility of dematiaceous fungi to amphotericin B, miconazole, ketoconazole, flucytosine and rifampin alone and in combination. Sabouraudia 1982;20:109–113.

20. Corrado ML, Weitzman I, Stanek A, Goetz R, Agyare E. Subcutaneous infection with *Phialophora richardsiae* and its susceptibility to 5-fluorocytosine, amphotericin B and miconazole. Sabouraudia 1980;18:97–104.

21. Costello MJ, DeFeo CP, Littman ML. Chromoblastomycosis treated with local infiltration of amphotericin B solution. AMA Arch Dermatol 1959;100:184–193.

22. Cuce LC, Wroclawski EL, Sampaio SAP. Treatment of paracoccidioidomycosis, candidiasis, chromomycosis, lobomycosis, and mycetoma with ketoconazole. Int J Dermatol 1980;19: 405–408.

23. Denning DW, Van Wye JE, Lewiston NJ, Stevens DA. Adjunctive therapy of allergic bronchopulmonary aspergillosis with itraconazole. Chest 1991;100:813–819.

24. Denning DW, Venkateswarlu K, Oakley KL, Anderson MJ, Manning NJ, Stevens DA, Warnock DW, Kelly SL. Itraconazole resistance in *Aspergillus fumigatus*. Antimicrob Agents Chemother 1997;41:1364–1368.

25. DeShazo RD, Chapin K, Swain RE. Fungal sinusitis. N Engl J Med 1997;337:254–259.

26. Diaz M, Negroni R, Montero-Gei F, Castro LGM, Sampaio SAP, Borelli D, Restrepo A, Franco L, Bran JL, Arathoon EG, Stevens DA, et al. A Pan-American 5-year study of fluconazole therapy for deep mycoses in the immunocompetent host. Clin Infect Dis 1992;14(Suppl 1):S68–S76.

27. Dickinson GM, Cleary TJ, Sanderson T, McGinnis MR. First case of subcutaneous phaeohyphomycosis caused by *Scytalidium lignicola* in a human. J Clin Microbiol 1983;17:155–158.

28. Drouhet E, Dupont B. Laboratory and clinical assessment of ketoconazole in deep-seated mycoses. Am J Med 1983;30–47.

29. Espinel-Ingroff A, Dawson K, Pfaller M, Anaissie E, Breslin B, Dixon D, Fothergill A, Paetznick V, Peter J, Rinaldi M, Walsh T. Comparative and collaborative evaluation of standardization of antifungal susceptibility testing for filamentous fungi. Antimicrob Agents Chemother 1995;39:314–319.

30. Espinel-Ingroff A, Bartlett M, Bowden R, Chin NX, Cooper C Jr, Fothergill A, McGinnis MR, Menezes P, Messer SA, Nelson PW, Odds FC, Pasarell L, Peter J, Pfaller MA, Rex JH, Rinaldi MG, Shankland GS, Walsh TJ, Weitzman I. Multicenter evaluation of proposed standardized procedure for antifungal susceptibility testing of filamentous fungi. J Clin Microbiol 1997;35: 139–143.

31. Esterre P, Inzan CK, Ramercel ER, Andriantsimahavandy A, Ratsioharrana M, Pecarrere JL, Roig P. Treatment of chromomycosis with terbinafine: preliminary results of an open pilot study. Br J Dermatol 1996;134(S46):33–36.

32. Fader RC, McGinnis MR. Infections caused by dematiaceous fungi: chromoblastomycosis and phaeohyphomycosis. Infect Dis Clin North Am 1988;2:925–938.

33. Fahal AH, Hassan MA. Mycetoma. Br J Surg 1992;79: 1138–1141.

34. Foster CS. Fungal keratitis. Infect Dis Clinics North Am 1992; 6:851–857.

35. Gallis HA, Berman RA, Cate TR, Hamilton JD, Gunnells JC, Stickel DL. Fungal infection following renal transplantation. Arch Intern Med 1975;135:1163–1172.

36. Ganer A, Arathoon E, Stevens DA. Initial experience in therapy for progressive mycoses with itraconazole, the first clinically studied triazole. Rev Infect Dis 1987;9:S77–S86.

37. Ghoraishi M, Akova YA, Tugal-Tutkun I, Foster CS. Penetrating keratoplasty in atopic keratoconjunctivitis. Cornea 1995; 14:610–613.

38. Gumaa SA, Mahgoub ES, El Sid MA. Mycetoma of the head and neck. Am J Trop Med Hyg 1986;35:594–600.

39. Haneke E. Fungal infections of the nail. Semin Dermatol 1991; 10:41–53.

40. Hay RJ. Mahgoub ES, Leon G et al. Mycetoma. J Med Vet Mycol 1992;330(Suppl 1):41.

41. Hemady RK, Foster CS. Intraocular penetration of ketoconazole in rabbits. Cornea 1992;11:329–333.

42. Howles JK, Kennedy CB, Garvin WH, Brueck JW, Buddingh GJ. Chromoblastomycosis. AMA Arch Dermatol Syphil 1954;69:83–90.

43. Hsu MM-L, Lee JY-Y. Cutaneous and subcutaneous phaeohyphomycosis caused by *Exserohilum rostratum*. J Am Acad Dermatol 1993;28:340–344.

44. Ikai K, Tomono H, Watanabe S. Phaeohyphomycosis caused by *Phialophora richardsiae*. J Am Acad Dermatol 1988;19: 478–481.

45. Ishibashi Y. Oral ketoconazole therapy for keratomycosis. Am J Ophthalmol 1983;95:342–345.

46. Kagawa S. Clinical efficacy of terbinafine in 629 Japanese patients with dermatomycosis. Clin Exp Dermatol 1989;14: 114–115.

47. Kanungo R, Srinivasan R. Corneal phaeohyphomycosis due to *Exserohilum rostratum*. Acta Ophthalmol Scand 1996;74: 197–199.

48. Katzenstein AL, Sale SR Greenberger PA. Allergic aspergillus sinusitis: a newly recognized form of sinusitis. J Allergy Clin Immunol 1983;72:89–93.

49. Klossek JM, Serrano E, Peloquin L, Percodani J, Fontanel JP, Pessey JJ. Functional endoscopic sinus surgery and 109 mycetomas of paranasal sinuses. Laryngoscope 1997;107:112–117.

50. Kotylo PK, Israel KS, Cohen JS, Bartlett MS. Subcutaneous phaeohyphomycosis of the finger caused by *Exophiala spinifera*. AJCP 1989;91:624–627.

51. Kullavanijaya P, Rojanavanich V. Successful treatment of chromoblastomycosis due to *Fonsecaea pedrosoi* by the combination of itraconazole and cryotherapy. Int J Dermatol 1995;34:804–807.

52. Kupferberg SB, Bent JP III, Kuhn FA. Prognosis for allergic fungal sinusitis. Otolaryng Head Neck Surg 1997;117:35–41.

53. Kwon-Chung KJ, Bennett JE. Chromoblastomycosis. In: Kwan-Cheng KJ, Bennett JE, eds. Medical mycology. Philadelphia: Lea & Febiger, 1992:337–355.

54. Kucers A, Bennett NM. Amphotericin B (AMB) In: Kucers A, Bennett NM, eds. The use of antibiotics. Philadelphia: JB Lippincott, 1987:1441–1477.

55. Kuttner BJ, Siegle RJ. Treatment of chromomycosis with a CO_2 laser. J Dermatol Surg Oncol 1986;12:965–968.

56. Lanigan, SW. Cutaneous *Alternaria* infection treated with itraconazole. Br J Dermatol 1992;127:39–40.

57. Lavalle P, Suchil P, De Ovando F, Raynoso S. Itraconazole for deep mycoses: preliminary experience in Mexico. Rev Infect Dis 1987;9:S64–S70.

58. Lopes CF, Alvarenga RJ, Cisalpino EO, Resende MA, Oliveira LG. Six years' experience in treatment of chromomycosis with 5-fluorocytosine. Int Soc Trop Dermatol 1978;17:414–418.

59. Lopes CF. Recent developments in the therapy of chromoblastomycosis. Bull Pan Am Health Organ 1981;15:58–64.

60. Lubritz RR. Cryosurgery. Clin Dermatol 1987;5:120–127.

61. Lynch JB. Mycetoma in the Sudan. R Coll Surg Engl 1964: 319–340.

62. Mahgoub ES, Gumaa SA. Ketoconazole in the treatment of eumycetoma due to *Madurella mycetomii*. Trans R Soc Trop Med Hyg 1984;78:376–379.

63. McBurney EI. Chromoblastomycosis treatment with ketoconazole. Cutis 1982;30:746–748.

64. McGinnis MR. Mycetoma. Cutaneous Mycol 1996;14:97–104.

65. McGinnis JR, Pasarell L, Cooper CR Jr. In vitro susceptibility of clinical dematiaceous fungal isolates against terbinafine, itraconazole, and amphotericin B [Abstract E75]. 37th ICAAC 1997:127, Toronto, Ontario.

66. Mitchell DM, Fitz-Henley M. A case of disseminated phaeohyphomycosis caused by *Cladosporium devriesii*. West Indian Med J 1990;39:118–123.

67. National Committee for Clinical Laboratory Standards. Reference method for broth dilution antifungal susceptibility testing of yeasts. Proposed standard M27-P. Villanova, PA: National Committee for Clinical Laboratory Standards, 1992.

68. National Committee for Clinical Laboratory Standards. Reference method for broth dilution antifungal susceptibility testing of yeasts. Proposed standard M27-T. Villanova, PA: National Committee for Clinical Laboratory Standards, 1995.

69. O'Day DM. Selection of appropriate antifungal therapy. Cornea 1987;6:238–245.

70. Padhye AA, Helwig WB, Warren NG, Ajello L, Chandler FW, McGinnis MR. Subcutaneous phaeohyphomycosis caused by *Xylohypha emmonsii*. J Clin Microbiol 1988;26:709–712.

71. Padhye AA, Davis MS, Reddick A, Bell MF, Gearhart ED, Von Moll L. *Mycoleptodiscus indicus:* a new etiologic agent of phaeohyphomycosis. J Clin Microbiol 1995;33:2796–2797.

72. Palaoglu S, Sav A, Basak T, Yalcinlar Y, Scheithauer BW. Cerebral phaeohyphomycosis. Neurosurgery 1993;33:894–897.

73. Pfaller MA, Bale M, Buschelman B, et al. Quality control guidelines for National Committee for Clinical Laboratory Standards recommended broth macrodilution testing of amphotericin B, fluconazole, and flucytosine. J Clin Microbiol 1995;33: 1104–1107.

74. Queiroz-Telles F, Purim KS, Fillus JN, Bordignon GF, Lameira RP, Van Cutsem J, Cauwenbergh G. Itraconazole in the treatment of chromoblastomycosis due to *Fonsecaea pedrosoi*. Int J Dermatol 1992;31:805–812.

75. Restrepo A, Gonzalez A, Gomez I, Arango M, DeBedout C. Treatment of chromoblastomycosis with itraconazole. Ann NY Acad Sci 1988;544:504–516.

76. Restrepo A. Treatment of tropical mycoses. J Am Acad Dermatol 1994;31:S91–S102.

77. Rex JH, Pfaller MA, Galgiani JN, Bartlett MS, Espinel-Ingroff A, Ghannoum MA, Lancaster M, Odds FC, Rinaldi MG, Walsh TJ, Barry AL. Development of interpretive breakpoints for antifungal susceptibility testing: conceptual framework and analysis of in vitro-in vivo correlation data for fluconazole, itraconazole, and candida infections. Clin Infect Dis 1997;24:235–247.

78. Rios-Fabra A, Restrepo A, Isturiz RE. Fungal infection in Latin American countries. Infect Dis Clin North Am 1994;8:129.

79. Rosa RH Jr, Miller D, Alfonso EC. The changing spectrum of fungal keratitis in south Florida. Ophthalmology 1994;101: 1005–1013.

80. Rossman SN, Cernoch PL, Davis JR. Dematiaceous fungi are an increasing cause of human disease. Clin Infect Dis 1996;22: 73–80.

81. Salaki JS, Louria DB, Chmel H. Fungal and yeast infections of the central nervous system. A clinical review. Medicine (Baltimore) 1984;63:108–132.

82. Sharkey PK, Graybill JR, Rinaldi MG, Stevens DA, Tucker RM, Peterie JD, Hoeprich PD, et al. Itraconazole treatment of phaeohyphomycosis. J Am Acad Dermatol 1990;23:577–586.

83. Silber JG, Gombert ME, Green KM, Shalita AR. Treatment of chromomycosis with ketoconazole and 5-fluorocytosine. J Am Acad Dermatol 1983;8:236–238.

84. Singh N, Chang FY, Gayowski T, Marino IR. Infections due to dematiaceous fungi in organ transplant recipients: case report and review. Clin Infect Dis 1997;24:369–374.

85. Smith CH, Barker JNWN, Hay RJ. A case of chromoblastomycosis responding to treatment with itraconazole. Br J Dermatol 1993;128:436–439.

86. South DA, Brass C, Stevens DA. Chromohyphomycosis. Arch Dermatol 1981;117:311–312.

87. Stern GA, Buttross M. Use of corticosteroids in combination with antimicrobial drugs in the treatment of infectious corneal disease. Ophthalmology 1991;98:847–853.

88. Stone MS, Rosen T, Clarridge J. Phaeohyphomycosis due to coelomycetes organisms. Int J Dermatol 1988;27:404–405.

89. Sudduth EJ, Crumbley AJ III, Farrar WE. Phaeohyphomycosis due to *Exophiala* species: clinical spectrum of disease in humans. Clin Infect Dis 1992;15:639–644.

90. Suttner JF, Wirth CJ, Wulker N, Seeliger H. Madura foot. A report of two cases. Int Orthop 1990;14:217–219.

91. Symoens J, Moens M, Dom J, Scheijgrond H, Dony J, Schuermans V, Legendre R, Finestine N. An evaluation of two years of clinical experience with ketoconazole. Rev Infect Dis 1980;2: 674–687.

92. Tagami H, Ginoza M, Imaizumi S, Urano-Suehisa S. Successful treatment of chromoblastomycosis with topical heat therapy. J Am Acad Dermatol 1984;10:615–619.

93. Tam M, Freeman S. Phaeohyphomycosis due to *Phialophora richardsiae*. Aust J Dermatol 1989;30:37–40.

94. Tuffanelli L, Milburn PB. Treatment of chromoblastomycosis. J Am Acad Dermatol 1990;23:728–732.

95. Van Cutsem J, Van Gerven F, Janssen PAJ. Activity of orally, topically and parenterally administered itraconazole in the treatment of superficial and deep mycoses: animal models. Rev Infect Dis 1987;9(Suppl 1):S15–S32.

96. Venugopal PV, Venugopal TV. Treatment of eumycetoma with ketoconazole. Aust J Dermatol 1993;34:27.

97. Washburn RG, Kennedy DW, Begley MG, Henderson DK, Bennett JE. Chronic fungal sinusitis in apparently normal hosts. Medicine (Baltimore) 1988;67:231–247.

98. Welsh O. Mycetoma. Int J Dermatol 1991;30:387–398.

99. Whiting DA. Treatment of chromoblastomycosis with high local concentrations of amphotericin B. Br J Dermatol 1967;79: 345–351.

100. Whiting DA, Cloete GNP. Chemotherapy and conservative surgery in the treatment of chromoblastomycosis. S Afr Med J 1968;883–886.

101. Zackheim HS, Halde C, Goodman RS, Marchasin S, Buncke HJ Jr. Phaeohyphomycotic cyst of the skin caused by *Exophiala jeanselmei*. J Am Acad Dermatol 1985;12:207–212.

102. Ziefer A, Connor DH. Phaeomycotic cyst. A clinicopathologic study of twenty-five patients. Am J Trop Med Hyg 1980;29: 901–911.

Dematiaceous and Nonpigmented Fungi: Invasive and Systemic Disease

Elias N. Kiwan and Elias J. Anaissie

GENERAL DESCRIPTION

During the past decade, the invasive mycoses have emerged as common opportunistic infections in immunocompromised patients, particularly in patients with AIDS or those undergoing organ or bone marrow transplantation or cytotoxic chemotherapy (2, 5, 6). Among infections caused by molds, aspergillosis remains the most common (9, 19, 35). However, newly recognized opportunistic molds have emerged as a cause of life-threatening infection (24, 38). These infections can be classified into two categories: those caused by dematiaceous fungi (phaeohyphomycoses) and other mold infections (hyalohyphomycoses) (36, 50). The emergence of these organisms as significant pathogens has important implications for diagnosis and management because of the variable susceptibility of these fungi to currently available antifungal agents (60).

Hyalohyphomycosis

Hyalohyphomycoses are fungal infections caused by molds whose basic tissue form is of hyaline, light-colored, hyphal elements that are branched or unbranched, occasionally toruloid, and without pigment in their wall (Table 1) (41, 43, 47, 57, 61). The number of organisms causing hyalohyphomycosis is increasing and includes important human pathogens such as *Fusarium* spp., *Penicillium* spp., *Scedosporium* spp., *Acremonium* spp., and *Paecilomyces lilacinus* (25, 48, 57).

Fusarium Species

Fusarium spp. may cause localized infections of the skin, nails, and cornea in the normal host. Localized deep *Fusarium* infection is rare but can occur in nonimmunosuppressed individuals following direct inoculation of various body sites including posttraumatic endophthalmitis, osteomyelitis, arthritis, and peritonitis among patients on peritoneal dialysis (1, 4, 7, 12).

Disseminated infections occur most commonly in patients with hematologic malignances and occasionally in patients with extensive burns (16). *Fusarium* species most frequently implicated as a human pathogens include *F. solani, F. oxysporum, F. moniliforme,* and less commonly, *F. proliferatum, F. chlamydosporum,* and *F. anthophilum.* Two likely routes of infection have been identified: respiratory route and breaks in integumentary barriers (especially of the feet) (16, 18, 55). Disseminated infection can involve almost any organ and usually presents as a persistent fever in a profoundly neutropenic cancer patient, although occasionally sinusitis and/or rhinocere-bral infection, endophthalmitis, or pyomyositis may be the presenting manifestation (1, 3, 4, 21).

Three types of cutaneous lesions have been observed: *(a)* multiple erythematous, subcutaneous nodules, suggesting fusarial infection; *(b)* painful erythematous macules and papules with progressive central infection (ecthyma gangrenosum–like lesions); and *(c)* target lesions consisting of ecthyma gangrenosum–like lesions surrounded by a thin rim of erythema. *Fusarium* is the only opportunistic mold that can be easily recovered from the bloodstream. Blood cultures are positive in 60% of cases, which is in sharp contrast to the rare (<5%) isolation of *Aspergillus* spp. from the bloodstream (8, 12, 18, 22).

Penicillium marneffei

Penicillium marneffei is the most important *Penicillium* species in humans. It is restricted in its geographic distribution (Southeast Asia). In recent years, disseminated infection has been reported occasionally in European and North American individuals with human immunodeficiency virus (HIV) infections who had visited Southeast Asia. In certain parts of Southeast Asia, *P. marneffei* is the third most common opportunistic infection in HIV-infected patients (25, 32, 34).

A high index of suspicion should be kept when a susceptible patient has papular molluscum contagiosum–like skin lesions and a nonspecific febrile illness. Diagnosis is based on culture and histopathologic findings (42, 59).

Scedosporium Species

The genus *Scedosporium* is associated with wide spectrum of infections caused by two different species: *(a) Pseudallescheria boydii* (perfect state) and *Scedosporium apiospermum* (imperfect state) and *(b) Scedosporium prolificans (S. inflatum)* (40, 41). There are two portals of entry for these fungal pathogens: respiratory tract and traumatic inoculation through the skin (30, 31, 43). *P. boydii* can cause eumycotic mycetoma and a variety of other infections in the normal host, including infections of the cornea, soft tissue, and bone. Deep-seated infections, such as sinusitis, endophthalmitis, and pneumonia, occur more frequently in the immunocompromised host; these infections appear to be more severe and have a tendency for dissemination and central nervous system involvement (48, 51). Like other agents that cause hyalohyphomycosis, *P. boydii* is histologically similar to *Aspergillus* species; therefore,

TABLE 1 • **Hyalohyphomycosis: Spectrum of Infection**

Pathogen	Normal Host	Immunosuppressed Host
Fusarium spp.	Keratitis Endophthalmitis Bone/joint infection Skin infection Onychomycosis Mycetoma Peritonitis	Mostly disseminated or sinopulmonary infection
Penicillium marneffei	Keratitis/endophthalmitis Bone/joint infection Endocarditis Pulmonary infection	Disseminated infection
Scedosporium spp.	Keratitis Sinusitis Endophthalmitis	Disseminated infection Sinusitis Pneumonia Brain abscess and meningitis
Scopulariopsis spp.	Onychomycosis	Disseminated infection, skin infection, sinusitis, and pneumonia
Paecilomyces lilacinus	Sinusitis Keratitis Onychomycosis Endocarditis Otitis Skin infection	Mostly disseminated infection, pyelonephritis, cellulitis, osteomyelitis, and pneumonia
Acremonium spp.	Keratitis Onychomycosis Osteomyelitis/arthritis Meningitis Endophthalmitis	Peritonitis Cerebritis Disseminated infection Pneumonia Dialysis-access fistula infection

identification of the fungus by culture is important because of the variable susceptibility of these fungi to amphotericin B (52, 62).

Other Species

Members of the genus *Acremonium (Cephalosporium)* have long been recognized as etiologic agents of nail and corneal infection. Occasional deep *Acremonium* infections have been reported in patients with serious underlying medical conditions (41, 48). Other pathogens known to cause opportunistic hyalohyphomycosis include *Scopulariopsis, Paecilomyces lilacinus, Schizophyllum, Chaectoconidium,* and *Coniothyrium* spp. (29, 31, 57).

Phaeohyphomycosis

Phaeohyphomycoses are fungal infections caused by a group of darkly pigmented dematiaceous fungi. In tissue, etiologic agents form either yeastlike cells that are solitary or in short chains, or septate hyphae, often irregularly swollen to toruloid, branched or unbranched, or any combination of the above-mentioned forms, and have a cell wall that contains melanin (2, 7, 27, 29). In tissue, these fungi may be confused with the more common *Aspergillus*. However, after staining with Fontana-Masson, the dematiaceous elements are seen and the correct diagnosis is made (Table 2) (37, 53, 56). Four genera have been most frequently encountered in humans: *Curvalaria* spp., *Bipolaris* spp., *Exserohilum* spp., and *Alternaria* spp.

Other pathogenic fungi include *Exophiala* spp., *Fonsecaea* spp., *Phialophora* spp., and *Negrospora* spp. (38, 39).

Phaeohyphomycosis can be divided into three distinct clinical syndromes: subcutaneous, paranasal sinus, and cerebral infection (40, 46). Subcutaneous infection usually follows traumatic inoculation of the subcutaneous tissue. The principal etiologic agents are *Exophiala jeanselmei, E. spinifera, E. dermatitidis, Phialophora richardsiae,* and *P. parasitica*. The lesions occur mainly on the arms and legs. The initial lesion is a firm, sometimes tender, subcutaneous nodule that may enlarge slowly to form a painless cystic abscess. Unless the cyst ruptures, the overlying skin remains unaffected. In immunosuppressed patients, the lesions are more likely to drain through sinuses (29, 40).

Paranasal sinus infection is usually caused by *Alternaria* spp., *Bipolaris spinifera, B. lawaiiensis, Curvularia lunata,* and *Exserohilum rostratum* (15, 29). The sinuses are filled with thick dark tenacious inspissated mucus. *Alternaria* and *Curvularia* species have occasionally caused necrotic lesions of the nasal septum in patients with leukemia or AIDS (31, 40).

Cerebral phaeohyphomycosis may follow hematogenous dissemination of infection from the lungs or may result from direct spread through the paranasal sinuses. Most infections are due to *Xylohypha bantiana (Cladosporium trichoides), Bipolaris* spp., or *Exophiala dermatitidis* (27, 46, 49).

Less common forms of infection include cutaneous infection, endocarditis following valve insertion or replacement,

TABLE 2 • Invasive Phaeohyphomycosis: Spectrum of Infection

Syndrome/Pathogen	Normal Host	Immunosuppressed Host
Sinusitis *Alternaria* spp. *Bipolaris* spp. *Exophiala* spp. *Curvularia* spp. *Xylohypha* spp.	Localized to the sinuses; rarely extends to adjacent tissues	Severe sinusitis, may extend to brain, and lead to dissemination and/or necrosis of nasal septum
Cerebral *Xylohypha* spp. *Bipolaris* spp. *Dactylaria* spp. *Fonsecaea* spp.	Important in immunocompetent host especially with *Xylohypha bantiana;* the abscess tends to be single and responds to treatment	Multifocal, may disseminate and often difficult to treat
Endocarditis *Curvularia* *Alternaria*	Rare	Rare
Peritonitis *Alternaria* spp.	Rare	Rare
Endophthalmitis *Dactylaria* spp. *Xylohypha* spp.	Rare	Rare
Pneumonia *Xylohypha*	Rare	Rare
Osteomyelitis *Curvularia* *Alternaria*	Rare	Rare

peritonitis in patients on continuous peritoneal dialysis, and posttraumatic osteomyelitis and arthritis (29, 40, 53, 58).

SUSCEPTIBILITY TESTING IN VITRO AND IN VIVO

In vitro antifungal susceptibility testing methods are hampered by the limited correlation of results with clinical outcome. Recent standards have been proposed for testing *Candida* and other yeasts. However, no standards exist for testing the filamentous fungi (40, 44, 46, 59, 60). The results of minimum inhibitory concentration (MIC) determinations with amphotericin B or flucytosine are less subject to test conditions than those obtained with the azoles, particularly fluconazole. Because of the marked variability in the results of in vitro susceptibility testing of molds, a rank order of susceptibility is presented (rather than actual MICs) (Table 3).

ANTIFUNGAL THERAPY
General

Basic understanding and awareness of these emerging opportunistic fungi have become particularly important for clinicians caring for immunocompromised patients. These infections are difficult to diagnose and often refractory to conventional antifungal therapy, particularly when infection has been well established and when the host is continuously immunosuppressed. These infections occur in two settings: in the normal host, where surgery and antifungal therapy may be curative, and in the immunocompromised host, where the critical factor for a favorable outcome is recovery from immunosuppression. Surgery is rarely an option in these throm-

bocytopenic patients (23, 26). Thus, every effort should be made to enhance the status of the patient's immune system including, most importantly, tapering or discontinuing immunosuppressive drugs (such as corticosteroids or cytotoxic agents) and treatment with granulocyte or granulocyte-macrophage colony-stimulating factors (G-CSF, GM-CSF) and CSF-stimulated white blood cell transfusions (investigational) (Table 4). Therapy should continue for 2 weeks after complete eradication of the infection and resolution of myelosuppression (7, 10, 13, 17, 33).

Amphotericin B is commonly used to treat established invasive fungal infection or as empirical treatment in cancer or transplant patients, although therapy of specific infection relies on the pattern of susceptibility of the offending pathogen (14, 28). Successful therapy for fungal infections, especially molds, may require a coordinated medical and surgical approach (Table 5) (45, 49, 51).

Specific Infection

Fusarium Species

Most patients with disseminated fusarial infection in association with persistent profound neutropenia die of progressive infection, despite therapy. The immune status of the host is the single most important factor predicting development and outcome of disseminated infection (6, 9, 12, 16). Disseminated *Fusarium* infection should be treated with amphotericin B at the highest tolerated dose or with one of the lipid formulations of amphotericin B (Table 6) (1, 3, 4, 8). Surgical resection of infected tissue may be useful if the infection is localized. Administration of

TABLE 3 • **In Vitro Antifungal Susceptibility and Drug of Choice**[a]

Pathogen	Amphotericin B	Miconazole	Fluconazole	Itraconazole	Flucytosine	Ketoconazole
Fusarium spp.[d]	I-R	R	R	R	R	R
S. apiospermum	I	S[b]	I-S	S[c]	R	I-S
S. inflatum	R	R	R	R	R	R
P. marneffei	S[b]	I	S	S[c]	I-S	I-S
P. lilacinus	I	S	R	S[b]	I	I-S
Bipolaris spp.	S[b]	S	S	S[c]	S	I
Xylohypha spp.	S[b]	S	S	S[c]	S	NT
Dactylaria spp.	S[b]	NT	NT	S[c]	S	NT
Fonsecaea spp.	S[b]	NT	S	S[c]	NT	NT
Alternaria spp.	S[b]	S	NT	S[c]	S	S
Curvularia spp.	S[b]	S	S	S[c]	I	S
Exophiala spp.	NT	NT	NT	S[c]	NT	S

[a] S, susceptible; I, intermediate; R, resistant; NT, not tested.

[b] Drug of choice in severe infection.

[c] Drug of choice in moderately severe infection or alternative agent.

[d] Topical natamycin useful for fusarial keratitis.

amphotericin B (or a lipid formulation of amphotericin B) to patients with primary fusarial skin lesions who are about to undergo cytotoxic chemotherapy or bone marrow transplantation should be seriously considered (18, 23, 33).

Because of the high rate of relapse and death in patients with a prior history of invasive fusarial infection, clinicians should consider either postponing cytotoxic therapy or using prophylactic G-CSF- or GM-CSF-stimulated granulocyte transfusion if a delay in the underlying cancer is not a viable option (16). We believe that this novel therapy modality should also be considered as early as possible in patients with invasive fusarial infection who are likely to have spontaneous recovery from myelosuppression (20, 28).

Since the skin is frequently the primary source of this life-threatening infection, every attempt to prevent this infection from occurring and/or spreading should be made (13, 21, 26). Hence we recommend that patients with hematologic cancer and onychomycosis and/or a significant break in the integrity of skin surfaces who are about to undergo cytotoxic chemotherapy and/or bone marrow transplantation be evaluated by a dermatologist to ascertain the nature of the onychomycosis or skin breakdown and rule out the presence of fusarial infection (44, 55).

In the presence of cellulitis, a bone scan should be obtained to rule out osteomyelitis and consideration should be given to resection of all infected tissues. In addition, primary skin lesions following a trauma or bite, such as a spider bite, should be considered in these high-risk patients as potentially infected by *Fusarium* species, hence requiring biopsy, culture, and surgical debridement if fusarial origin is confirmed (47, 55).

Penicillium marneffei

Penicilliosis should be suspected in HIV-positive residents of, and travelers to, Southeast Asia who present with an invasive fungal infection (Table 6) (5, 25, 32). Treatment of disseminated penicilliosis in HIV-infected patients with parenteral amphotericin B or itraconazole is relatively effective and safe, but delay in therapy may be fatal. The organism appears to be suscep-

TABLE 4 • **Reversal of Immunosuppression**

- Discontinuation of immunosuppressive drugs (such as corticosteroid, chemotherapy)
- Recombinant cytokines
  Granulocyte colony-stimulating factors (G-CSF)
  Granulocyte-macrophage colony-stimulating factors (GM-CSF)
  Interferon-γ
- Stem cell reconstitution
- Granulocyte transfusion (stimulated with G-CSF or GM-CSF)

TABLE 5 • **Indications for Surgical Removal of Infected Tissue**

- Hemoptysis from a single cavitary lung lesion
- Progressive cavitary lung lesion (always perform a computerized chest scan to rule out multiple lesions)
- Infiltration into the pericardium, great vessels, bone or thoracic soft tissue despite antifungal treatment
- Progressive sinusitis
- Joint/bone infection
- Endophthalmitis
- Skin or nail infection prior to cytotoxic chemotherapy

tible to flucytosine, and some patients have responded to the combination of this drug and amphotericin B. Itraconazole (4–10 mg/kg/day) is the drug of choice for treating moderately severe penicilliosis (33, 34); amphotericin B should be reserved for severe infections (42, 59). Greater detail in treatment is given in Chapter 137.

Scedosporium Species

Scedosporium apiospermum. Like other agents that cause hyalohyphomycosis, *P. boydii* is histologically similar to *Aspergillus* species. Therefore identification of the fungus by culture is important, since *P. boydii* may be somewhat resistant to

TABLE 6 • Management of Selected Invasive Hyalohyphomycosis

Pathogen	Normal Host	Immunosuppressed Host
Fusarium spp.	—Keratitis: topical natamycin 5.0% suspension —Endophthalmitis: vitrectomy, intravitreal amphotericin B, and enucleation in extreme cases —Skin and soft tissue: incision and drainage —Onychomycosis: avulsion of the nail, topical natamycin? —Osteomyelitis: surgical debridement, i.v. amphotericin B.	—Disseminated infection: i.v. amphotericin B, or its lipid formulations —Reversal of immunosuppression —Surgery if the lesion is localized —Catheter-related fungemia (rare): catheter removal and i.v. amphotericin B, or its lipid formulations
P. marneffei	—Itraconazole —Surgery when possible	—Severe infection: amphotericin B —Moderate infections: itraconazole or as maintenance therapy particularly in AIDS patients —Reversal of immunosuppression
S. apiospermum	—Surgery when possible —Miconazole and/or itraconazole —Endophthalmitis: intravitreal injection of amphotericin B —Arthritis: intraarticular injection of amphotericin B	—Surgery when possible —Reversal of immunosuppression —Miconazole or itraconazole
S. inflatum	—Resistant to all antifungal drugs —Surgery whenever possible	—Surgery when possible —Reversal of immunosuppression
P. lilacinus	—Skin infection: debridement —Endophthalmitis: vitrectomy and oral itraconazole	—Severe infection: i.v. amphotericin or its lipid formulations —Reversal of immunosuppression —Moderate infections: itraconazole and as maintenance after initial response (if persistent immunosuppression)

amphotericin B (Table 6) (31, 41, 43). Optimum management of infections caused by these organisms consists of reversal of immunosuppression, surgical resection of localized lesions, and intravenous miconazole (1.2–3.6 g/day) or itraconazole (400–600 mg/day). Intraarticular injections of amphotericin B have proven successful in some cases of trauma-induced arthritis of the knee (48, 51). Surgical resection remains the key to a successful outcome if the lesions are localized (e.g., cavitating lung lesion, sinusitis, arthritis, or osteomyelitis).

The therapeutic outcome is usually poor in the setting of persistent immunosuppression. A combination of interferon-γ and antifungal therapy in a patient with granulomatous disease helped control disseminated infection (51).

Scedosporium prolificans. The spectrum of infection caused by *S. prolificans* resembles pseudallescheriasis. However, this organism is resistant to all antifungal agents, both in vitro and in vivo. Surgical debridement of infected tissue appears to be the major means of halting progression of the infection. Severe and disseminated infections are commonly fatal (3, 52, 62).

Phaeohyphomycosis

These dematiaceous molds have a propensity to involve the brain, so prompt and aggressive therapy is required. Surgical resection of a well-localized lesion is important for both diagnosis and treatment. Relapse following surgery is not uncommon, and therapy with either itraconazole (400–600 mg/day) or flucytosine (50–150 mg/kg/day) is warranted. The choice of

the antifungal agent depends on the susceptibility of the infecting pathogens (Table 7) (11, 14, 37, 39, 40, 49).

ENDPOINTS FOR MONITORING THERAPY

Antifungal therapy should be continued at least 2 weeks after resolution of all clinical and laboratory findings of infection and recovery from immunosuppression (39, 40, 54, 59, 60).

ADJUNCTIVE THERAPY

Adjunctive measures may include reduction of immunosuppressive therapy, addition of synergistic drugs flucytosine or rifampin (investigational), neutrophil transfusions, G-/GM-CSF, removal of indwelling catheters, and treatment of coexisting infections (Tables 4 and 5).

CONTROVERSIES, CAVEATS, AND COMMENTS

New data suggest that these opportunistic fungi are present in water and water systems worldwide, including hospitals caring for severely immunocompromised patients. Thus, infection control measures should be put in place to prevent nosocomial infections in high-risk patients at institutions experiencing such infections. Studies of new antifungal drugs are needed to identify agents that can help reduce the incidence of these emerging mycoses, particularly lipid formulations of amphotericin B, newer triazoles (itraconazole, voriconazole), and the echinocandins. Since impairment of the immune system is the major underlying cause of the high incidence of invasive fungal infections in these patients, future studies should focus on modulating

TABLE 7 • Management of Selected Invasive Phaeohyphomycosis

Syndrome	Normal Host	Immunosuppressed Host
Sinusitis	—Surgical debridement —i.v. amphotericin B or oral itraconazole	—Surgery when possible —i.v. amphotericin B or oral itraconazole
Cerebral	—Surgical resection is the only effective treatment —i.v. amphotericin B or oral itraconazole?	—Same as above
Endophthalmitis	—Vitrectomy and itraconazole and/or i.v. amphotericin B —Intravitreal injection of amphotericin B	—Vitrectomy and/or enucleation —i.v. amphotericin B or oral itraconazole —Intravitreal amphotericin B
Endocarditis	—Surgery and i.v. amphotericin B	—Surgery and i.v. amphotericin B or itraconazole

the immune status of the host such as the use of cytokines or cytokine-stimulated white blood cell transfusions.

REFERENCES

1. Agamanolis DP, Kalwinsky DK, Krill CE, Dasu S, Halasa B, Galloway PG. Meningoencephalitis in a child with acute leukemia. Neuropediatrics 1991;22:110.
2. Ajello L. Hyalohyphomycosis and phaeohyphomycosis two global disease entities of public health importance. Eur J Epidemiol 1986;2:243–251.
3. Alvarez-Franco M, Reyes-Mugica M, Paller AC. Cutaneous Fusarium infection in an adolescent with acute leukemia. Pediatr Dermatol 1992;9:62.
4. Ammari LK, Puck JM, McGowan KL. Catheter related Fusarium solani fungemia and infection in a patient with leukemia in remission. Clin Infect Dis 1993;16:148.
5. Ampel NM. Emerging disease issues and fungal pathogens associated with HIV infection. Emerg Infect Dis 1996;2:109–116.
6. Anaissie EJ. Opportunistic mycoses in immunocompromised host: Experience at a cancer center and review. Clin Infect Dis 1992;14(Suppl):43.
7. Anaissie EJ, Bodey GP, Kantargian H, et al. New spectrum of fungal infections in patients with cancer. Rev Infect Dis 1989;11:369–378.
8. Anaissie EJ, Hachem R, Bodey P. Comparative activities of fluconazole, itraconazole, saperconazole, SCH39304 and amphotericin B against disseminated F. solani infection in mice. Presented at the 30th interscience conference on Antimicrobial Agents and Chemotherapy, Atlanta, GA, October 21–24, 1990.
9. Anaissie EJ, Hachem R, Legrand C, Legenne P, Nelson P, Bodey GP. Lack of activity of amphotericin B in systemic murine fusarial infections. J Infect Dis 1992;165:1155–1157.
10. Anaissie EJ, Kontoyiani SD, Bodey G. SCH 39304 for the treatment of invasive moulds infections in neutropenic cancer patients. Presented at the 30th interscience conference on the Antimicrobial Agents and Chemotherapy, Atlanta, GA, October 21–24, 1990.
11. Anaissie EJ, Kontanyianis DP, Kantargian HM, Vartivarian S, O'Brien, Giralt SA, Anderson BS, Karl S, Champlin RE, Bodey GP. Effectiveness of an oral triazole for opportunistic mould infections in patients with cancer: experience with SCH 39304. Clin Infect Dis 1993;17:1022.
12. Anaissie EJ, Nelson P, Beremond M, et al. Fusarium-caused hyalohyphomycosis: an overview. Curr Top Med Mycol 1992;4:231–249.
13. Anaissie EJ, Ramphal R, Horwith G. Efficacy and safety of amphotericin B lipid complex injection in the treatment of patients with fusariosis. Proceedings of the 38th Annual meeting of the American Society of Hematology, Orlando, FL, Dec 6–10, 1996.
14. Barton K, Miller D, Pflugfelder SC. Corneal chromoblastomycosis. Cornea 1997;16:235–239.
15. Berlanga JJ, Querol S, Gallardo D, Ferra C, Granena A. Successful treatment of Curvularia spp infection in a patient with primarily resistant acute promyelocytic leukemia. Bone Marrow Transplant 1995;16:617–619.
16. Boutati IE, Anaissie EJ. Fusarium a significant emerging pathogen in patients with hematologic malignancy: ten years experience at a cancer center and implication for management. Blood 1997;90:999–1008.
17. Bowden RA, Cays M, Van-Burik JA. Phase one study of amphotericin colloidal dispersion (ABCD, Amphocil) for the treatment of invasive fungal infection after marrow transplant [Abstract 1685]. 35th meeting of the American Society of Hematology, St. Louis, MO, Dec 3–7, 1993.
18. Brint JM, Flynn PM, Pearson TA, Pui CH. Disseminated fusariosis involving bone in an adolescent with leukemia. Pediatr Infect Dis J 1992;11:965.
19. Brown AE. Overview of fungal infections in cancer patients. Semin Oncol 1990;17:2.
20. Bushelman SJ, Callen JP, Roth DN, Cohen LM. Disseminated Fusarium solani infection. J Am Acad Dermatol 1995;32:346.
21. Castagnola E, Garaventa A, Conte M, Barretta A, Faggi E, Viscoli C. Survival after fungemia due to fusarium moniliforme in a child with neuroblastoma. Eur J Clin Microbiol Infect Dis 1993;12:308.
22. Caux F, Aractingi S, Baurmann S, Reygagne P, Dombert H, Rommand S, Dubertret L. Fusarium solani cutaneous infection in a neutropenic patient. Dermatology 1993;186:232.
23. Cofrancesco E, Boshetti C, Vivianni MA, Cortellaro M, Zanussi C. Efficacy of lipisomal amphotericin B in the eradication of Fusarium infection in a leukemic patient. Haematologica 1992;77:280.
24. Denning DW. Epidemiology and pathogenesis of systemic fungal infections in the immunocompromised host. J Antimicrob Chemother 1991;28(Suppl B):1.
25. Duong TA. Infection due to Penicillium marneffei, an emerging pathogen: review of 155 reported cases. Clin Infect Dis 1996;23:125–130.
26. Ellis ME, Clink H, Younge D, Hainau B. Successful combined surgical and medical treatment of Fusarium infection after bone marrow transplantation. Scand J Infect Dis 1994;26:225.

27. Emmens RK, Richardson D, Thomas W, Hunter S, Henningar RA, Wingard JR, Nolte FS. Necrotizing cerebritis in an allogeneic bone marrow transplant recipient due to Cladiophora bantiana. J Clin Microbiol 1996;34:1330–1332.

28. Fleming R, Anaissie EJ, O'Brien S, Kantarjian H, Estey E, Lichtiger B, Jendiroba B, Freireich E. Treatment of neutropenia related fungal infection with G-CSF mobilized granulocytes transfusions. Proceedings of the 38th annual meeting of the American Society of Hematology, Orlando, FL, Dec 6–10, 1996.

29. Fothergill AW. Identification of dematiaceous fungi and their role in human disease. Clin Infect Dis 1996;22S:79–84.

30. Ginter G, De Hoog GS, Pschaid A, Fellinger M, Bogiatzis A, Bergh C, Reich EM, Odds FC. Arthritis without grains caused by Pseudallescharia boydii. Mycoses 1995;38(9–10):369–371.

31. Gucalp R, Carlisle P, Gialanella P, Mitsudo S, McKitrick J, Dutcher J. Paecilomyces sinusitis in an immunocompromised adult patient: case report and review. Clin Infect Dis 1996;23: 391–393.

32. Heath TC, Patel A, Fisher D, Bowden FJ, Currie B. Disseminated Penicillium marneffei: presenting illness of advanced HIV infection; a clinicopathological review, illustrated by a case report. 1995;27:101–105.

33. Hood S, Denning DW. Treatment of fungal infection in AIDS. J Antimicrob Chemother 1996;37S:71–85.

34. Imwidthaya P. Update of penicilliosis marneffei in Thailand. Mycopathology 1994;127:135–137.

35. Isada CM, Kasten BL, Goldman MP, Gray LD, Aberg JA. Infectious diseases handbook. 2nd ed. Ohio: Lexi-Comps, 1997:668.

36. Jantunen E, Ruutu P, Niskanen L, Volin L, Parkkali T, Koukila-Kahkola P, Ruutu T. Incidence and risk factors for invasive fungal infections in allogeneic BMT recipients. Bone Marrow Transplant 1997;19:801–808.

37. Kanungo R, Srinivasan R. Corneal pheohyphomycosis due to Exserohilum rostratum. Acta Ophtalmol Scand 1996;74:197–199.

38. Koll BS, Brown AE. The changing epidemiology of infections at cancer hospitals. Clin Infect Dis 1993;17S:322.

39. Kralovic SM, Rhodes JC. Pheohyphomycosis caused by Dactylaria (human dactylariosis): report of a case with review of the literature. J Infect 1995;31:107–113.

40. Kwon-Chung KJ, Bennett JE. Medical mycology. Philadelphia: Lea & Febiger, 1992:620–677.

41. Kwon-Chung KJ, Bennett JE. Pseudallescheriasis and Scedosporium infection. In: Medical mycology: Philadelphia: Lea & Febiger 1992:678–694/733–767.

42. Lee SS, Lo YC, Wong KH. The first one hundred AIDS cases in Hong-Kong. Chin Med J 1996;109:70–76.

43. Madrigal V, Alonso J, Bureo E, Figols FJ, Salesa R. Fatal meningoencephalitis caused by Scedosporium inflatum in a child with lymphoblastic leukemia. Eur Clin Microbiol Infect Dis 1995;14:601–603.

44. Martino P, Gastaldi R, Raccah R, et al. Clinical pattern of fusarium infections in immunocompromised patients. J Infect 1994;28S:7–15.

45. Migrino RQ, Hall GS, Longworth DL. Deep tissue infections caused by Scopulariopsis brevicaulis: report of a case of prosthetic endocarditis and review. Clin Infect Dis 1995;21: 672–674.

46. Morris A, Shell WA, McDonagh D, Chaffe S, Perfect JR. Pneumonia due to Fonsecaea pedrosoi and cerebral abscess due to Emericella nidulans in a bone marrow transplant recipient. Clin Infect Dis 1995;21:1346–1348.

47. Nelson PE, Dignani MC, Anaissie EJ. Taxonomy, biology, and clinical aspects of Fusarium species, Clin Microbiol Rev 1994; 7:479–504.

48. Nenoff P, Gutz U, Tintelnot K, Bosse-Henk A, Mierzwa M, Hofmann J, Horn LC, Haustein UF. Disseminated mycosis due to Scedosporium prolificans in an AIDS patient with Burkitt lymphoma. Mycoses 1996;39:461–465.

49. Nieto-Rodriguez JA, Kusne S. Successful treatment for cerebral pheohyphomycosis due to Dactylaria gallopova. Clin Infect Dis 1996;23:73–80.

50. Perfect JR, Schell WA. The new fungal opportunists are coming. Clin Infect Dis 1996;22S:112–118.

51. Phillips P, Fobres JC, Speert DP. Disseminated infection with Pseudallescharia boydii in a patient with chronic granulomatous disease: response to gamma-interferon plus antifungal chemotherapy. Pediatr Infect Dis 1991;10:536–539.

52. Pickles RW, Pacey CE, Muir DB, Merrell WH. Experience with infection by Scedosporium prolificans including apparent cure with fluconazole therapy. J Infect 1996;33:193–197.

53. Remon C De la Calle IJ, Vallejo Carrion F, Perez-Ramos S, Fernandez-Ruiz E. Exophiala jeanselmei peritonitis in a patient on CAPD. Perit Dial Int 1996;16:536–538.

54. Richardson MD, Warnock DW. Fungal infection, diagnosis and management. 2nd ed. London: Blackwell Science, 1994:217–222.

55. Rombaux P, Eloy P, Bertrand B, Delos M, Doyen C. Lethal disseminated Fusarium infection with sinus involvement in the immunocompromised host: case report and review of the literature. Rhinology 1996;34:237–241.

56. Rossman SN, Cernoch PL, Davis JR. Dematiaceous fungi are an increasing cause of human disease. Clin Infect Dis 1996;22: 73–80.

57. Shing MM, Li CK, Chik KW, Yuen PM. Paecilomyces variotii fungemia in a bone marrow transplant patient. Bone Marrow Transplant 1996;17:281–283.

58. Shigemori M, Kawakami K, Kitahara T, Ijichi O, Mizota M, Ikarimito N, Miyata K. Hepatosplenic abscess caused by Curvularia boedijn in a patient with acute monocytic leukemia. Pediatr Infect Dis 1996;15:128–129.

59. Supparatpinyo K, Chiewchanvit S, Hirunsri P, Uthammachai C, Nelson KE, Sirisanthana T. Penicillium marneffei infection in patients with human immunodeficiency virus. Clin Infect Dis 1992;14:871–874.

60. Uzun O, Anaissie EJ. Antifungal prophylaxis in patients with hematological malignancies: a reappraisal. Blood 1995;86:2063.

61. Warnock DW, Johnson EM. Clinical manifestations and management of hyalohyphomycosis, phaeohyphomycosis and other uncommon forms of fungal infection in the compromised patient. In: Warnock DW, Richardson MD, eds. Fungal infection in the compromised patient. 2nd ed. West Sussex: John Wiley & Sons, 1991:248–278.

62. Wood GM, McCormack JC, Muir DB, et al. Clinical features of human infection with Scedosporium inflatum. Clin Infect Dis 1992;14:1027–1033.

Histoplasma capsulatum

●

Joseph L. Wheat

GENERAL DESCRIPTION

Histoplasmosis is the most common endemic mycosis and a major cause of morbidity in patients who live in endemic areas. It has emerged as an important opportunistic infection in immunocompromised patients including those with acquired immunodeficiency syndrome (AIDS) or who are taking medications that impair cellular immunity. Exposure to bird or bat guano is an important epidemiologic clue to the diagnosis. Unique clinical manifestations may alert the clinician to consider the diagnosis of histoplasmosis. Serologic tests measuring the antibody response and tests for antigen complement cultural methods for diagnosis. Newer treatment options have improved the outcome of therapy and offer effective and well-tolerated alternatives to amphotericin B.

MYCOLOGY

The mold form grows in soil containing rotted bird or bat guano. Microconidia, the infectious particles of the mold microconidia, are characteristic of the organism. *Histoplasma capsulatum* grows as a yeast above 35°C. The yeast is the pathogenic form of the organism found in tissues of infected individuals. Identification requires conversion of the mold to the yeast, detection of specific antigens by immunologic tests, or genetic verification using nucleic acid probes.

EPIDEMIOLOGY

H. capsulatum is endemic in restricted areas of North and Latin America but can be found throughout the world (Fig. 1) (24). Factors accounting for its geographic distribution are poorly understood but include high humidity, moderate climate, and acidic soil characteristics. Activities that disturb environments containing *H. capsulatum* cause airborne spread of the microconidia, infecting those who are exposed. These environmental sites typically are visibly contaminated by heavy accumulations of bat or bird droppings, but patients often are unaware of any such exposure.

PATHOGENESIS

Infection develops when conidia are inhaled and transform into yeasts in the lungs. Hematogenous dissemination occurs even in healthy individuals but generally is clinically unrecognized (14). Progressive dissemination typically complicates infection in patients with impaired cellular immunity and at the extremes of age but may occur in nonimmunosuppressed individuals (16, 39). Reactivation of old foci of infection may provide a mechanism for infection in immunocompromised individuals, a clinical impression (4) recently supported by genetic analysis of strains from patients with AIDS (20).

Cellular immunity is the primary host defense against *H. capsulatum* (5). A specific cellular immune response occurs during the first month of the infection and coincides with inhibition of growth of the fungus and regression of the infection. Studies using experimental models of histoplasmosis indicate that interferon-γ and other cytokines arm macrophages to kill the fungus and halt progression of the disease.

CLINICAL MANIFESTATIONS

Histoplasmosis usually is asymptomatic or nonprogressive in healthy individuals (27, 45). The common clinical findings of self-limited infection include acute pulmonary histoplasmosis, pericarditis (44), and rheumatologic syndromes (26). Patients present with fever, cough, and chest pain, and chest radiographs show mediastinal lymphadenopathy with infiltrates. Most patients recover in a few weeks, but some experience prolonged fatigue. Heavy exposure causes more-extensive pulmonary involvement, sometimes accompanied by respiratory insufficiency (19). Patients also may experience symptoms caused by obstruction of mediastinal structures by enlarged lymph nodes (21).

Patients with acute histoplasmosis may experience rheumatologic syndromes characterized by arthritis or arthralgia and erythema nodosum or multiforme (26). Pericarditis is another inflammatory complication of acute histoplasmosis (44). Both the pericarditis and rheumatologic syndromes occur in less than 10% of cases (44). Rarely, constrictive pericarditis may develop.

Chronic Pulmonary Histoplasmosis

Patients with emphysema develop chronic pulmonary histoplasmosis characterized by recurrent symptoms, progressive lung infiltrates, fibrosis, and cavitation (15, 45). Upper lobe infiltrates with cavities are present in most cases. While some patients recover spontaneously (15), most progress with cavity enlargement, formation of new cavities, and spread to new areas of the lungs. Rarely, bronchopleural fistula may develop.

Disseminated Histoplasmosis

Hematogenous spread outside the lungs occurs in a high proportion of individuals during the acute infection but rarely is recognized clinically. These patients recover with development of cellular immunity to *H. capsulatum*. Disseminated infection is progressive in about 1 in 2000 acute infections, however (27). Progressive disseminated histoplasmosis is seen most often in patients who are immunosuppressed or at the extremes of age.

Clinical findings of progressive disseminated histoplasmosis are nonspecific. Fever, weight loss, and respiratory symptoms

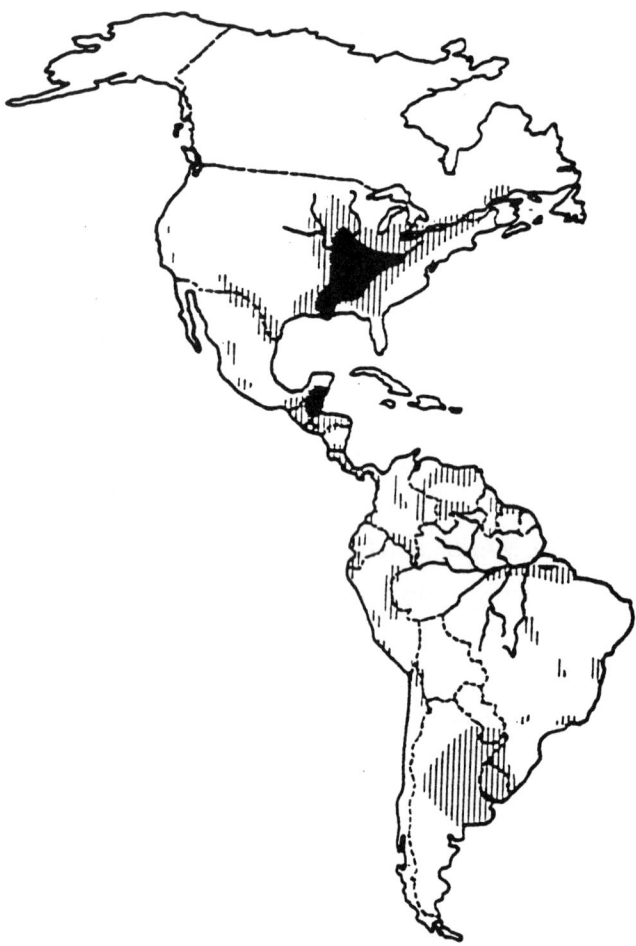

FIGURE 1. Endemic distribution of histoplasmosis in the Americas. The highest incidence is in the *finely stippled area* of North and Central America. (From Rippon JW. Histoplasmosis (Histoplasmosis capsulati). In: Wonsiewicz M, ed. Medical mycology: the pathogenic fungi and the pathogenic actinomycetes. 3rd ed. Philadelphia: WB Saunders, 1988:381, with permission.)

are the most common clinical findings. Examination often reveals hepatomegaly, splenomegaly, or lymphadenopathy; and laboratory tests may show findings of bone marrow suppression and hepatitis. Shock and multiorgan failure may complicate severe cases (39). Chest roentgenograms usually show diffuse infiltrates but may be normal in one-third of cases.

Central nervous system involvement with meningitis, cerebritis, and focal brain or spinal cord lesions complicates about 10% of cases, either as a manifestation of widely disseminated infection or as an isolated manifestation (38). Other frequent sites of dissemination include the oral mucosa, gastrointestinal tract, skin, kidneys, and adrenal glands.

Endocarditis is a rare complication of disseminated histoplasmosis and usually is manifested by systemic emboli in a person with other findings of disseminated disease but may present as isolated culture-negative endocarditis (11, 18). No such cases have been identified during the recurrent outbreaks in Indianapolis, although a single case of a left atrial myxoma infected with *H. capsulatum* was reported from our institution (25).

Broncholithiasis

Calcified mediastinal nodes and pulmonary granulomas may erode into adjacent bronchi (1). Patients may expectorate rock-like particles of tissue and experience hemoptysis, bronchial obstruction, or tracheoesophageal fistula.

Mediastinal Fibrosis

Mediastinal fibrosis, a rare manifestation of histoplasmosis, is felt to represent an abnormal host response to the infection (13, 21). Viable organisms cannot be found in these tissues, supporting the belief that fibrosing mediastinitis represents an exuberant fibrotic reaction to past infection rather than an active, progressive infection. The superior vena cava, airways, pulmonary arteries or veins, or esophagus are most commonly involved, but any mediastinal structure can be trapped in these fibrotic masses (13, 21). Chest radiographs may be normal or show only mediastinal widening, but computed tomography (CT) scans reveal restriction and invasion of mediastinal structures. Calcification is often present. Recurrent hemoptysis is a common symptom, and respiratory failure often ensues.

Pulmonary Histoplasmoma

Rarely, patients may develop a slowly enlarging pulmonary nodule that has been called "enlarging histoplasmoma" (17). Histoplasmomas are usually asymptomatic but often cause concern about malignancy. They range in diameter from 8 to 35 mm and enlarge an average of 2 mm per year, presumably through inflammation and fibrosis in response to antigenic materials released from the central core into the surrounding tissue. Calcification occurs in the core and the periphery of the lesion. Histologically, they are characterized by a necrotic center surrounded by a fibrous capsule. Organisms may be seen in the necrotic center but usually cannot be cultured.

Presumed Ocular Histoplasmosis

Choroiditis involving the macula and causing visual loss has been attributed to histoplasmosis (29, 48), but no scientific basis establishes *H. capsulatum* as its cause. The association has been based on high rates of skin test reactivity rather than demonstration of the fungus in the tissues (30). Identification of patients with similar findings outside the endemic area for histoplasmosis further weakens the association of histoplasmosis with this clinical syndrome (33). However, the eye may be involved in patients with disseminated histoplasmosis (31).

DIAGNOSIS

A battery of diagnostic procedures are needed for diagnosis of histoplasmosis. Serologic tests for antibodies form the basis for diagnosis in most patients with mild infections, while cultures, stains, and tests for antigens are more useful in those with more severe disease.

Serologic Tests

Antibodies to *H. capsulatum* measured by immunodiffusion or complement fixation develop in most patients. H precipitin bands can be demonstrated in less than 25% of patients and clear during the first 6 months following exposure (42, 47). M bands occur in over three-quarters of patients and persist for years in some. Complement fixation titers of 1:8 or more are found in most patients with active histoplasmosis, while those of 1:32 or above are more suggestive of active infection. Both the immunodiffusion and complement fixation tests should be performed to obtain the highest sensitivity for diagnosis. Newer tests for antibodies, using enzyme immunoassay or radioimmunoassay methods, are more difficult to interpret because of higher background positivity rates and have not been validated adequately to replace immunodiffusion and complement fixation (37).

Antibodies require 4 to 8 weeks to develop following acute infection and may be negative when the patient is first seen. Furthermore, serologic tests may have false-negative results in up to one-third of immunocompromised patients (47). Positive results caused by cross-reactions occur in patients with blastomycosis, coccidioidomycosis, and paracoccidioidomycosis (41).

High levels of antibodies, particularly M precipitin bands, and low titers (1:8 or 1:16) of complement-fixing antibodies may require several years to clear after acute infection, occasionally causing confusion in patients with other diseases. Consequently, histoplasmosis may be diagnosed incorrectly in a patient with another illness who has persistent high levels of antibodies to *H. capsulatum* from an earlier episode of histoplasmosis.

Culture

Cultures are most useful in patients with disseminated or chronic pulmonary histoplasmosis. The sensitivity is only l0 to 15% in patients with other forms of histoplasmosis (47). In disseminated histoplasmosis, the highest yield is from bone marrow or blood, positive in over 75% of cases (27, 39). Organisms can be found in sputum or bronchoscopy specimens in 60 to 85% of patients with cavitary histoplasmosis (45).

Antigen Detection

Sensitive methods for rapid diagnosis of histoplasmosis in patients with severe manifestations are essential to allow prompt initiation of therapy. Fungal stain is rapid but insensitive. Detection of antigen offers a valuable approach to rapid diagnosis in severe cases (43, 47). Antigen is found in the blood, urine, and bronchoalveolar lavage fluid of most individuals with disseminated histoplasmosis and in the urine of 75% of those with extensive pneumonitis following heavy acute exposure. Antigen may be found in cerebrospinal fluid (CSF) of 25 to 50% of patients with meningitis caused by histoplasmosis. Cross-reactions may be seen in patients with African histoplasmosis, blastomycosis, paracoccidioidomycosis, and *Penicillium marneffei* infection.

Antigen levels decline during treatment and increase with relapse, providing a tool for monitoring therapy (40). Antigen testing is available at the Histoplasmosis Reference Laboratory.

Histoplasmin Skin Test

Skin tests should not be used diagnostically because of high rates of positivity (50–80%) in endemic areas and false-positive results in patients with other fungal diseases (7). Skin test results also may be falsely negative in patients with disseminated disease. Skin tests increase antibody levels, which confuses the interpretation of serologic tests.

ANTIMICROBIAL THERAPY
Acute Pulmonary Histoplasmosis

Patients with extensive acute pulmonary histoplasmosis benefit from antifungal therapy, and those who are hypoxic should receive adjunctive corticosteroid therapy (Table 1). Patients with acute histoplasmosis who have less extensive disease but who remain symptomatic for a month or more also may benefit from therapy. Amphotericin B (50 mg/day or 0.7 to 1 mg/kg/day) given for 1 to 2 weeks followed by itraconazole (200 mg once or twice daily for 3 months) induces a rapid response and should be used in severely ill patients. Itraconazole (200 mg twice daily for 2 weeks followed by once or twice daily for 3 months) is recommended in patients with milder illnesses and has proven effective in controlled trials in patients with disseminated and chronic pulmonary infection (6, 35).

Itraconazole is highly active against *H. capsulatum,* with MICs below 0.019 µg/mL in most cases. Drug levels of at least 1 µg/mL measured by bioassay should be effective for treatment of histoplasmosis although higher concentrations (4–10 µg/mL) are desirable. Dosages of 200 mg/day achieve peak blood concentrations 2 to 4 h after an oral dose of about 3 µg/mL, while doses of 200 mg twice daily yield concentrations of about 6 µg/mL (35). Dosage could be reduced in patients with concentrations above 10 µg/mL. Itraconazole is better tolerated than ketoconazole and more active than fluconazole against *H. capsulatum* (36).

Chronic Pulmonary Histoplasmosis

Untreated chronic pulmonary histoplasmosis is usually slowly progressive (9, 15). Treatment improves survival, reduces symptoms, promotes radiographic healing, and eradicates *H. capsulatum* from the sputum (32). Most patients with chronic pulmonary histoplasmosis respond well to treatment with itraconazole (6). Amphotericin B (50 mg/day or 0.7 mg/kg/day) may be needed for the first few weeks of therapy in patients with more severe respiratory insufficiency to achieve a more rapid response. Itraconazole (200 mg once or twice daily)

TABLE 1 • Indications for Treatment in Patients with Histoplasmosis

Treatment Indicated	Treatment Usually Not Indicated
Acute pulmonary with hypoxia	Acute self-limited syndromes
Acute pulmonary > 1 month	Acute pulmonary, mildly ill
Disseminated	Rheumatologic
Chronic pulmonary	Pericarditis
Mediastinal granuloma with obstruction or invasion of adjacent tissue	Fibrosing mediastinitis
	Histoplasmoma
	Broncholithiasis
	Presumed ocular

should be continued for at least 18 months and until maximal clinical and radiographic benefit has been achieved. Relapse is common after discontinuation of treatment, emphasizing the need for prolonged follow-up.

Disseminated Histoplasmosis

Disseminated histoplasmosis is usually fatal if untreated (10, 27). Amphotericin B and itraconazole are highly effective therapy, inducing remission in 85 to 90% of patients (27), including those who are immunosuppressed (6, 27, 35, 39). Amphotericin B (50 mg/day or 0.7–1 mg/kg/day) should be given initially in patients who require hospitalization. Treatment can be changed to itraconazole after patients become afebrile, usually in 3 to 7 days. Longer courses of amphotericin B may be required in patients who are severely ill, as indicated by the presence of shock or respiratory failure. Itraconazole 200 mg once or twice daily should be administered for 6 to 12 months in most patients and indefinitely in those with AIDS. Improvement can be expected within 1 week in most patients (27, 35). Relapse is common in patients who are immunosuppressed (27, 39). Levels of *Histoplasma* antigen increase with relapse, providing a useful tool for monitoring the response to therapy (40). Treatment probably should be continued until antigenemia and antigenuria have resolved.

Treatment of meningitis caused by histoplasmosis is unsatisfactory. While 60 to 90% of patients with meningitis caused by *H. capsulatum* respond to treatment with 35 mg/kg of amphotericin B given over 2 to 4 months, half relapse within 2 years (38). Amphotericin B should be given at doses of 0.7 to 1.0 mg/kg/day for total courses of at least 35 mg/kg and until CSF specimens are negative by culture and antigen detection. Fluconazole (100 mg/day typical daily suppressive dose) given concurrently with the amphotericin B and for another year to prevent relapse should be considered. Itraconazole, although more active than fluconazole against *H. capsulatum,* does not enter the CSF, making it a poorer choice for this indication. Resistance to fluconazole may develop during therapy (36), mandating careful follow-up with monitoring of CSF fungal culture and *Histoplasma* antigen levels. Lifelong maintenance therapy with fluconazole (doses as high as 400 mg/day are reported in the literature) or itraconazole (200 mg three times daily) may be needed to maintain remission in patients who relapse. Patients who fail intravenous amphotericin B and oral triazole therapy are candidates for amphotericin B administered directly into the ventricles, cisterna magnum, or lumbar arachnoid space, but such therapy is poorly tolerated because of local inflammatory reactions and bacterial superinfections. Better treatments are needed.

Cerebritis or cerebral histoplasmomas may be more responsive to therapy. Of six such cases in persons without AIDS in the author's series, all responded to amphotericin B therapy, but two relapsed (38). Failure to achieve therapeutic concentrations of the antifungal agent in the CSF appears to be less important than in meningitis. Amphotericin B or itraconazole are reasonable choices for treatment of lesions involving the brain or spinal cord and should be selected on the basis of the severity of the manifestations. More-rapid response can be achieved with amphotericin B than with itraconazole.

The outcome of treatment of fungal endocarditis, including that caused by histoplasmosis, is unsatisfactory (2, 3, 11, 18, 25). Despite treatment with large doses of amphotericin B, mortality is over 50% (11, 18). Aggressive antifungal therapy combined with resection of the infected valve provides the best outcome (18). In that report, 5 of 7 such patients were cured by combined antifungal and surgical therapy, compared with 4 of 9 who received antifungal therapy alone (18). These observations support a recommendation to administer amphotericin B at doses of 50 mg/day or 0.7 mg/kg/day for total courses of at least 35 mg/kg given over 2 to 3 months and to give strong consideration to resection of the infected valve. An additional year of itraconazole 200 mg once or twice daily may reduce the likelihood of relapse, especially in patients who were unable to undergo complete resection of the infected valve and cardiac tissue.

Mediastinal Granuloma

Mediastinal granuloma may produce obstructive symptoms or fistula. Occasional patients with these complications improve following antifungal therapy (28). Itraconazole 200 mg once or twice daily for 6 months is recommended. Other patients have responded favorably to surgical resection of the granuloma (12). Antifungal treatment or resection of granuloma to prevent fibrosing mediastinitis is not indicated because progression of granulomatous mediastinitis to fibrosing mediastinitis has not been documented and must be rare (21).

Mediastinal Fibrosis

Antifungal treatment probably does not influence the course of mediastinal fibrosis (13, 21). However, a few patients showed improvement following treatment with ketoconazole (34). A trial of itraconazole 200 mg once or twice daily for 3 months should be considered in patients with positive serologic tests and elevated sedimentation rates. If a repeat CT at that time shows no improvement, treatment should be stopped. If improvement is demonstrated, itraconazole should be continued for 12 to 18 months. Improvement following resection of the fibrotic tissue has been reported, but the surgical mortality is high (~25%) (23). A conservative approach is recommended, reserving surgery for patients with life-threatening complications including bilateral compression of airways or important vascular structures.

Rheumatologic Syndromes and Pericarditis

Patients with inflammatory manifestations of rheumatologic syndromes and pericarditis usually respond to aspirin or nonsteroidal antiinflammatory agents. Corticosteroids may be required in patients with more severe manifestations or those who do not respond to less aggressive therapy (26, 44). Organisms are not found in the pericardium or joints, and antifungal therapy would not be expected to alter the course in patients with these manifestations of acute histoplasmosis. Nevertheless, itraconazole 200 mg once or twice daily may be appropriate in patients who receive corticosteroids for treatment of pericardial tamponade. Rarely, joints or pericardium are sites of disseminated infection, in which case treatment would be necessary.

Presumed Ocular Histoplasmosis

Presumed ocular histoplasmosis, if indeed caused by *H. capsulatum,* does not represent an active infection and would not be expected to respond to antifungal therapy. Corticosteroids and laser therapy have been used in these patients (8, 22, 29).

New Therapies

Although amphotericin B and itraconazole are highly effective for therapy of histoplasmosis, each has its limitations. Amphotericin B is poorly tolerated and is not effective in nearly half of patients with severe manifestations of histoplasmosis (46). Studies are in progress evaluating AmBisome, a new liposomal preparation of amphotericin B that is better tolerated and can be administered more aggressively because of reduced systemic toxicity or side effects and nephrotoxicity. Newer triazole antifungal agents may overcome the recognized limitations of itraconazole, namely, poor bioavailability and extensive drug interactions.

PREVENTION

Prophylaxis against histoplasmosis in persons with AIDS warrants consideration in endemic regions of the United States and Latin America. A trial comparing itraconazole 200 mg/day with placebo in persons with HIV infection and CD4 counts below 150/mL showed a twofold reduction in the incidence of histoplasmosis in the itraconazole group (2.7% of 149 patients) compared with the placebo group (6.8% of 146 patients) after a median follow-up of 13 months (Drs. David McKinsey and Joseph Wheat for the Mycoses Study Group, unpublished, 1996). Prophylaxis had no impact on survival and failed to prevent recurrent oral candidiasis or esophagitis. Prophylaxis cannot be recommended until its impact on resistance among *Candida* strains and the response of thrush to antifungal therapy is understood.

REFERENCES

1. Arrigoni MG, Bernatz PE, Donoghue FE. Broncholithiasis. J Thorac Cardiovasc Surg 1971;62:231–237.
2. Berman SS, Kazlow GA, Fields BT Jr, Weinberg S. Disseminated histoplasmosis with embolic endovascular complications: a case report. J Vasc Surg 1990;12:577–580.
3. Blair TP, Waugh RA, Pollack M, Ashworth HE, Young NA, Anderson SE, Bem TP. *Histoplasma capsulatum* endocarditis. Am Heart J 1980;99:783–788.
4. Davies SF, Khan M, Sarosi GA. Disseminated histoplasmosis in immunologically suppressed patients. Am J Med 1978;64:94–100.
5. Deepe GS Jr, Bullock WE. Histoplasmosis: a granulomatous inflammatory response. In: Gallin JI, Goldstein IM, Snyderman R, eds. Inflammation: basic principles and clinical correlates. New York: Raven, 1988:733.
6. Dismukes WE, Bradsher RW Jr, Cloud GC, Kauffman CA, Chapman SW, George RB, Stevens DA, Girard WM, Bowles-Patton C, NIAID Mycoses Study Group. Itraconazole therapy for blastomycosis and histoplasmosis. Am J Med 1992;93: 489–497.
7. Edwards LB, Acquaviva FA, Livesay VT, Cross FW, Palmer CE. An atlas of sensitivity to tuberculin, PPD-B and histoplasmin in the United States. Am Rev Respir Dis 1969;99:1–18.
8. Fine SL, Wood WJ, Isernhagen RD, Singerman LJ, Bressler NM, Folk JC, Kimura AE, Fish GE, Maguire MG, Alexander J. Laser treatment for subfoveal neovascular membranes in ocular histoplasmosis syndrome: results of a pilot randomized clinical trial. Arch Ophthalmol 1993;111:19–20.
9. Furcolow ML. Course and prognosis of untreated histoplasmosis. JAMA 1961;177:292–296.
10. Furcolow ML. Comparison of treated and untreated severe histoplasmosis. JAMA 1963;183:121–127.
11. Gaynes RP, Gardner P, Causey W. Prosthetic value endocarditis caused by *Histoplasma capsulatum.* Arch Intern Med 1981; 141:1533–1537.
12. Gilliland MD, Scott LD, Walker WE. Esophageal obstruction caused by mediastinal histoplasmosis: beneficial results of operation. Surgery 1984;95:59–62.
13. Goodwin RA, Nickell JA, des Prez RM. Mediastinal fibrosis complicating healed primary histoplasmosis and tuberculosis. Medicine 1972;51:227–246.
14. Goodwin RA Jr, des Prez RM. Histoplasmosis. Am Rev Respir Dis 1978;117:929–956.
15. Goodwin RA Jr, Owens FT, Snell JD, Hubbard WW, Buchanan RD, Terry RT, des Prez RM. Chronic pulmonary histoplasmosis. Medicine 1976;55:413–452.
16. Goodwin RA Jr, Shapiro JL, Thurman GH, Thurman SS, des Prez RM. Disseminated histoplasmosis: clinical and pathologic correlations. Medicine 1980;59:1–33.
17. Goodwin RA Jr, Snell JD Jr. The enlarging histoplasmoma: concept of a tumor-like phenomenon encompassing the tuberculoma and coccidioidoma. Am Rev Respir Dis 1969;100:1–12.
18. Kanawaty DS, Stalker MJB, Munt PW. Nonsurgical treatment of *Histoplasma* endocarditis involving a bioprosthetic valve. Chest 1991;99:253–256.
19. Kataria YP, Campbell PB, Burlingham BT. Acute pulmonary histoplasmosis presenting as adult respiratory distress syndrome: effect of therapy on clinical and laboratory features. South Med J 1981;74:534–537.
20. Keath EJ, Kobayashi GS, Medoff G. Typing of *Histoplasma capsulatum* by restriction fragment length polymorphisms in a nuclear gene. J Clin Microbiol 1992;30:2104–2107.
21. Loyd JE, Tillman BF, Atkinson JB, des Prez RM. Mediastinal fibrosis complicating histoplasmosis. Medicine 1988;67:295–310.
22. Macular Photocoagulation Study Group. Laser photocoagulation for neovascular lesions nasal to the fovea: results from clinical trials for lesions secondary to ocular histoplasmosis or idiopathic causes. Arch Ophthalmol 1995;113:56–61.
23. Mathisen DJ, Grillo HC. Clinical manifestation of mediastinal fibrosis and histoplasmosis. Soc Thorac Surg 1992;54:1053–1058.
24. Rippon JW. Histoplasmosis (Histoplasmosis capsulati). In: Wonsiewicz M, ed. Medical mycology: the pathogenic fungi and the pathogenic actinomycetes. 3rd ed. Philadelphia: WB Saunders, 1988:381.
25. Rogers EW, Weyman AE, Noble RJ, Bruins SC. Left atrial myxoma infected with *Histoplasma capsulatum.* Am J Med 1978;64:683–690.
26. Rosenthal J, Brandt KD, Wheat LJ, Slama TG. Rheumatologic manifestations of histoplasmosis in the recent Indianapolis epidemic. Arthritis Rheum 1983;26:1065–1070.
27. Sathapatayavongs B, Batteiger BE, Wheat LJ, Slama TG, Wass JL. Clinical and laboratory features of disseminated histoplasmosis during two large urban outbreaks. Medicine 1983;62:263–270.
28. Savides TJ, Gress FG, Wheat LJ, Ikenberry S, Hawes RH. Dysphagia due to mediastinal granulomas: diagnosis with endoscopic ultrasonography. Gastroenterology 1995;109:366–373.

29. Schwarz J. Histoplasmosis of the eye. In: Anonymous. Histoplasmosis. New York: Praeger, 1981:317.

30. Spaeth GL. Presumed *Histoplasma* uveitis: continuing doubts as to its actual cause. In: Ajello L, Chick E, Furcolow M, eds. Histoplasmosis. Springfield, IL: Charles C Thomas, 1971:221.

31. Specht CS, Mitchell KT, Bauman AE, Gupta M. Ocular histoplasmosis with retinitis in a patient with acquired immune deficiency syndrome. Ophthalmology 1991;98:1356–1359.

32. Sutliff WD, Andrews CE, Jones E, Terry RT. Histoplasmosis cooperative study: Veterans Administration–Armed Forces Cooperative Study on histoplasmosis. Am Rev Respir Dis 1964;89:641–650.

33. Suttorp-Schulten MSA, Bollemeijer JG, Bos PJM, Rothova A. Presumed ocular histoplasmosis in the Netherlands—an area without histoplasmosis. Br J Ophthalmol 1997;81:7–11.

34. Urschel HC Jr, Razzuk MA, Netto GJ, Disiere J, Chung SY. Sclerosing mediastinitis: improved management with histoplasmosis titer and ketoconazole. Ann Thorac Surg 1990;50:215–221.

35. Wheat J, Hafner R, Korzun AH, Limjoco MT, Spencer P, Larsen RA, Hecht FM, Powderly W, AIDS Clinical Trial Group. Itraconazole treatment of disseminated histoplasmosis in patients with the acquired immunodeficiency syndrome. Am J Med 1995;98:336–342.

36. Wheat J, Marichal P, Vanden Bossche H, Le Monte A, Connolly P. Hypothesis on the mechanism of resistance to fluconazole in Histoplasma capsulatum. Antimicrob Agents Chemother 1997;41:410–414.

37. Wheat LJ. The role of the serologic diagnostic laboratory and the diagnosis of fungal disease. In: Sarosi GA, Davies SF, eds. Fungal diseases of the lung. 2nd ed. New York: Raven Press, 1993:29.

38. Wheat LJ, Batteiger BE, Sathapatayavongs B. *Histoplasma capsulatum* infections of the central nervous system: a clinical review. Medicine 1990;69:244–260.

39. Wheat LJ, Connolly-Stringfield PA, Baker RL, Curfman MF, Eads ME, Israel KS, Norris SA, Webb DH, Zeckel ML. Disseminated histoplasmosis in the acquired immune deficiency syndrome: clinical findings, diagnosis and treatment, and review of the literature. Medicine 1990;69:361–374.

40. Wheat LJ, Connolly-Stringfield P, Blair R, Connolly K, Garringer T, Katz BP. Histoplasmosis relapse in patients with AIDS: detection using *Histoplasma capsulatum* variety *capsulatum* antigen levels. Ann Intern Med 1991;115:936–941.

41. Wheat LJ, French MLV, Kamel S, Tewari RP. Evaluation of cross-reactions in *Histoplasma capsulatum* serologic tests. J Clin Microbiol 1986;23:493–499.

42. Wheat LJ, French MLV, Kohler RB, Zimmerman SE, Smith WR, Norton JA, Eitzen HE, Smith CD, Slama TG. The diagnostic laboratory tests for histoplasmosis: analysis of experience in a large urban outbreak. Ann Intern Med 1982;97:680–685.

43. Wheat LJ, Kohler RB, Tewari RP. Diagnosis of disseminated histoplasmosis by detection of *Histoplasma capsulatum* antigen in serum and urine specimens. N Engl J Med 1986;314:83–88.

44. Wheat LJ, Stein L, Corya BC, Wass JL, Norton JA, Grider K, Slama TG, French MLV, Kohler RB. Pericarditis as a manifestation of histoplasmosis during two large urban outbreaks. Medicine 1983;62:110–119.

45. Wheat LJ, Wass J, Norton J, Kohler RB, French MLV. Cavitary histoplasmosis occurring during two large urban outbreaks: analysis of clinical, epidemiologic, roentgenographic, and laboratory features. Medicine 1984;63:201–209.

46. Wheat L. Histoplasmosis in the acquired immunodeficiency syndrome. Curr Top Med Mycol 1996;7:7–18.

47. Williams B, Fojtasek M, Connolly-Stringfield P, Wheat J. Diagnosis of histoplasmosis by antigen detection during an outbreak in Indianapolis, Ind. Arch Pathol Lab Med 1994;118:1205–1208.

48. Woods AC, Wahlen HE. The probable role of benign histoplasmosis in the etiology of granulomatous uveitis. Am Heart J 1960;49:205–220.

Mucorales

Laurent Christin and Alan M. Sugar

GENERAL DESCRIPTION
Microbiology

Mucormycosis is a general term referring to infections by fungi of the class *Zygomycetes,* which includes the orders Mucorales and Entomophthorales (30). These fungi are ubiquitous and grow well at room temperature on decaying organic material including food such as bread or fruit. They have no unusual growth requirements; like other microorganisms, they require iron for growth, a characteristic relevant to the increased risk of invasive infection in patients treated with desferrioxamine. Culture on Sabouraud dextrose agar yields large colonies in 2 to 3 days. Presence of broad, somewhat irregular, nonseptate hyphae branching at 90° in addition to the characteristic rhizoids facilitates identification of the fungus.

Clinical Presentation

Human mucormycosis is most frequently caused by *Rhizopus oryzae* and *Rhizopus microsporus* var. *rhizopodiformis, Absidia corymbifera, Apophysomyces elegans, Cunnighamella bertholletiae, Mucor* spp., *Rhizomucor pusillus,* and *Saksenaea vasiformis.* Mucormycosis refers nonspecifically to infections by these fungi. Classically, there are five clinical presentations of mucormycosis: rhinocerebral, pulmonary, gastrointestinal (GI), cutaneous, and disseminated (36, 37). The latter can present with lesions in the skin, GI tract, lung, and other organs, and thus these distinctions do not always strictly apply.

Rhinocerebral mucormycosis is an invasive disease starting in the upper airway mucosa and progressing through surrounding tissues irrespective of anatomic landmarks. Patients at risk for infection include diabetics with ketoacidosis, patients treated with desferrioxamine (dialysis, aplastic anemia, thalassemia, hemochromatosis, etc.), patients on corticosteroids, and those who are immunosuppressed or granulocytopenic.

Pulmonary mucormycosis is frequently a postmortem diagnosis made on a patient who died of progressive pneumonia despite the use of broad-spectrum antibiotics. As with any necrotizing pneumonia, cavitation is common. Isolation of the fungus from the sputum may be disregarded, since these ubiquitous pathogens may colonize abnormal airways. However, recovery of the fungus from patients at risk for mucormycosis is presumptive evidence for invasive infection.

Isolated gastrointestinal mucormycosis is rare and encountered mainly in malnourished children. Complications include bowel perforation, peritonitis, sepsis, and death.

Cutaneous mucormycosis is encountered in immunocompromised patients and most likely follows local inoculation through a puncture wound. It is a serious condition when involving burn wounds; it can spread into underlying tissues and eventually disseminate.

Disseminated mucormycosis is becoming a frequently encountered entity because of increasing numbers of severely immunosuppressed patients following bone marrow transplantation or aggressive chemotherapy. Common sites of dissemination include the brain, spleen, heart, kidney, and sometimes the skin, where biopsy might reveal the diagnosis. Isolated cerebral mucormycosis has been reported in intravenous drug users. Interestingly, helper T-cell deficit as encountered in HIV-infected individuals does not seem to increase risk of the infection unless another of the above-mentioned risk factors is present.

Entomophthoramycosis is caused in humans by *Conidiobolus coronatus* and *Basidiobolus meristosporus* or *B. haptosporus*. In both cases, the infection is limited to the skin and subcutaneous tissues and can be disfiguring through progressive scarring. Lymphatic obstruction can result in lymphedema. Both diseases are rare in temperate climates.

Diagnosis

The diagnosis of mucormycosis is usually made easily by microscopic examination of tissue or secretions. The typical hyphae are readily identified. Final species determination requires culture.

The diagnosis of entomophthoramycosis is usually made on clinical presentation. Culture is more difficult than with agents of mucormycosis, and identification of the typical hyphae on biopsy is frequently hampered by the intense reactive fibrosis.

Treatment

Treatment of invasive mucormycosis includes three essential modalities: *(a)* an attempt to reverse the predisposing condition (e.g., correction of diabetic ketoacidosis), *(b)* surgical re-

moval of infected and necrotic tissue, and *(c)* use of an antifungal agent. Survival and extent of sequelae are closely related to the feasibility of necrotic tissue debridement. Thus, when mucormycosis involves a vital organ (brain, heart) the prognosis worsens significantly. Mucormycosis limited to the skin (cellulitis) usually has a good prognosis.

Treatment of entomophthoramycosis relies essentially on antifungal therapy. Debridement is controversial, since it may accelerate the spread of infection.

ANTIFUNGAL SUSCEPTIBILITY OF MUCORALES

The use of in vitro susceptibility to antifungal agents for clinical purposes is rapidly increasing thanks to better standardization techniques, mainly for *Candida* spp. (28) and *Cryptococcus* spp. (32). Susceptibility testing of the mucorales and other filamentous fungi has only recently been carefully studied (9). No similar data or protocols are available for Mucorales. In vitro susceptibility results should therefore be interpreted with caution.

Sparse data are available on in vitro sensitivity to amphotericin B (8, 27, 33). There are no prospective evaluations of in vitro susceptibility to liposomal or colloidal-dispersion amphotericin B. However, numerous case reports have suggested that these formulations might be effective for treatment of invasive infection (20, 23, 35, 38). The main advantage of these recent formulations is lower toxicity, particularly renal.

Four azole derivatives are currently available for systemic administration: miconazole, ketoconazole, fluconazole, and itraconazole. Because of the usual extremely rapidly destructive pace of invasive mucormycosis and reliable experience with amphotericin B, use of these drugs for first-line therapy has been rare (17, 34). Here again, data on in vitro susceptibility of Mucorales to these antifungal agents are limited and not standardized (8, 27). Mucorales are considered uniformly resistant to 5-fluorocytosine. Synergism of rifampin in combination with amphotericin B has been demonstrated in vitro against clinical isolates of *Rhizopus oryzae* and resulted in a favorable outcome in a patient (4). Other drugs for which in vitro susceptibility of clinical strains is available are nystatin, pimaricin, and naftifine (27), which are either too toxic for systemic use or not available in the United States. Limited in vitro data have suggested that interferon-γ (IFN-γ) might enhance fungicidal activity of murine macrophages (3).

ANTIFUNGAL THERAPY

Antimicrobial therapy of mucormycosis should be considered adjunctive but essential to surgical debridement of infected necrotic tissue. A successful outcome depends heavily upon removal of infected tissue. Involvement of vital organs whose debridement might not be feasible markedly jeopardize the prognosis. Identified predisposing conditions should also be corrected as feasible.

Amphotericin B

Amphotericin B has so far remained the mainstay of antifungal therapy for invasive mucormycosis. It is usually given at 0.8 to 1 mg/kg/day (a 1-mg test dose is optional) in conjunction with extensive surgical debridement as feasible. In critically ill patients, doses up to 1.5 mg/kg/day can be used for the first several days of treatment. Culture and sensitivity to amphotericin B should be routinely requested, since resistance to the drug is encountered. Once the infection seems under control, amphotericin B can be given every other day to minimize toxicity (see below). If responding favorably, the patient should receive a total of 2.5 to 3 g over a 2- to 3-month period or longer.

Severe toxicity despite prophylactic or corrective measures warrants consideration of less-toxic formulations of the drug (liposomal or colloidal dispersion), although experience with these drugs is limited (20, 23, 34, 37). Differences in efficacy between the formulations against mucormycosis has not been prospectively evaluated, but consideration of liposomal preparations of amphotericin B is reasonable for patients intolerant of conventional amphotericin B.

Azole Derivatives

Several case reports of successful treatment of mucormycosis with azole derivatives have been published (1, 31). However, these drugs cannot be recommended for first-line treatment of mucormycosis, with the possible exception of infection limited to the skin. These antifungal agents are also being evaluated for the treatment of the entomophthoramycoses (21).

Rhizopus spp. and *Mucor* spp. tend to be resistant to these drugs in vitro (8, 27) and in animal models (39). Ketoconazole has been used successfully as a single drug to treat cutaneous mucormycosis due to *Absidia corymberifera* (31). Also, it was used successfully in a patient failing therapy with amphotericin B who was infected with *Mucor* sp. resistant to amphotericin B in vitro (MIC = 64 mg/L) (1).

Successful treatment of rhinofacial mucormycosis was achieved with itraconazole (200 mg/day orally) in a patient who failed amphotericin B and ketoconazole (18). Itraconazole has also cured a patient of an entomophthoramycosis (basidiobolomycosis) (21). Because itraconazole absorption can be quite unpredictable, clinical use of this drug is not advisable as first-line therapy for mucormycosis at this time. A serum level of itraconazole should be obtained to assess individual bioavailability, and the patient should be watched closely for treatment failure.

Parenteral fluconazole (300 mg/day for 1 month following a total amphotericin B dose of 295 mg discontinued because of side effects) successfully treated a leukemic patient with pulmonary mucormycosis (13). Other patients with rhinocerebral mucormycosis (17) were cured with fluconazole (200 mg twice daily for 6 weeks to 8 months, followed by oral fluconazole 100 to 200 mg/day for 2 weeks).

These few case reports are difficult to interpret and the role of azoles in treating mucormycosis must be considered experimental. The dose and duration of treatments using azole derivatives have not been standardized, and they should not be used as first-line therapy for mucormycosis.

Rifampin

Rifampin has been used successfully as adjunctive therapy for mucomycosis *(C. bertholletiae)* sinusitis in combination with amphotericin B following surgery in an apparently immunocompetent patient (25). Synergistic efficacy in vitro between amphotericin B and rifampin has correlated with favorable clinical outcome in a limited number of cases (4).

Potassium Iodide

Potassium iodide (10 gtt thrice daily orally) has been used alone for treatment of subcutaneous mucormycosis (40) or in combination with itraconazole for treatment of nasofacial mucormycosis (22).

Hyperbaric Oxygen

Hyperbaric oxygen has been used in several instances for treatment of invasive mucormycosis, always in association with surgery and various drug regimens, usually including amphotericin B. In vitro data show a fungicidal effect of hyperbaric oxygen. Limited clinical data are available, but one study reported a 24% reduction in mortality using 100% O_2 for 2 h every 12 h for 6 to 24 treatments (10). Additional reports have given support to this treatment (6, 7, 26). Lack of access to a hyperbaric chamber might limit its usefulness.

Interferon

In vitro data on an enhancing fungicidal effect on (murine) macrophages by IFN-γ (3) has some clinical correlation. A child with chronic granulomatous disease with disseminated *Pseudallescheria boydii* infection was treated successfully with antifungal therapy and IFN-γ (28). Another patient with extensive intracranial aspergillosis recovered despite failure of amphotericin B, itraconazole, and liposomal amphotericin B with flucytosine (5). IFN-γ was also used successfully as adjunctive therapy in a patient with posttraumatic cutaneous and renal mucormycosis due to *A. elegans* (26). One patient with hairy cell leukemia presented with maxillary mucormycosis and recovered following debridement, amphotericin B, and treatment with IFN-α_2 aimed at the hematologic malignancy (2).

SPECIAL SITUATIONS
Mucormycosis of the Central Nervous System

Isolated central nervous system mucormycosis diagnosed in a patient with non-Hodgkin's lymphoma was successfully treated with topical amphotericin B (19). Abscess enlargement was evident, despite surgical drainage and systemic amphotericin B for 3 weeks. Following a second debridement, an absorbable gelatin sponge impregnated with 30 mg of amphotericin B was left in place and brought full recovery without neurologic deficit.

An intravenous drug abuser with deep cerebral mucormycosis diagnosed by stereotactic biopsy and histology responded without sequela to a total dose of 3.045 g of amphotericin B without surgical intervention (14). HIV status was negative. This favorable outcome might be related to the absence of underlying immunosuppression.

Intrathecal amphotericin B has been used in few patients with evidence of meningeal or parameningeal inflammation (11, 16). Survival has been variable, and definitive benefit has not been demonstrated. Intrathecal amphotericin B is routinely used in meningitis due to *Coccidioides immitis* as a 5-mg weekly injection; complications include arachnoiditis and transverse myelitis.

Mucormycosis in HIV-Infected Individuals

Frazier et al. reported on five HIV-positive patients diagnosed with what appeared as a chronic sinusitis (12). All had AIDS by CD4 criteria and previous opportunistic infections (PCP, histoplasmosis, disseminated *Mycobacterium avium intracellulare* infection, and cytomegalovirus infection). As encountered in other patients, associated risk factors for mucormycosis included periods of neutropenia and use of steroids (nasally and/or systemic) and broad-spectrum antibiotics. Local symptoms (facial pain) and symptoms (necrotic lesions) were present in most patients. Treatment of mucormycosis with amphotericin B following surgical debridement failed in three of five. A favorable contribution of reversal of immune suppression by new antiretroviral agents to improved clinical outcome of mucormycosis awaits confirmation.

ALTERNATIVE THERAPY

No available alternative therapy has proven useful besides that mentioned above.

THERAPEUTIC MONITORING
Side Effects of Treatments

Amphotericin B

Close follow-up of patients receiving intravenous amphotericin B is of paramount importance. Initiation of treatment is frequently associated with mild hemodynamic instability, sometimes temperature elevation, and rarely rigors. Use of acetaminophen (650 mg orally), hydrocortisone (25 mg intravenously) or meperidine (25 mg intravenously) before the infusion may control these symptoms.

Electrolyte abnormalities such as hypokalemia and hypomagnesemia during amphotericin B infusion can be harmful under certain circumstances such as patients on digoxin therapy. Careful monitoring and replacement of potassium and magnesium are required daily. A rise in creatinine concentration is expected with amphotericin B use and can usually be managed with aggressive prehydration. A creatinine level of 3 mg/dL should prompt a change in dosing schedule to every other day. If the creatinine level keeps rising, the dose should be decreased (by 25 to 33%). Most cases of renal dysfunction are reversible upon discontinuation of treatment.

Azole Derivatives

Azole derivatives are usually well tolerated. Ketoconazole requires gastric acidity for absorption and has endocrinologic side effects secondary to inhibition of adrenal steroid synthesis. Hepatitis has also been reported but is rare. Fluconazole has more favorable pharmacokinetic and safety profiles and has few significant drug interactions. Severe hepatotoxicity and cytopenia are rare. It is available for parenteral administration. Itraconazole has rare side effects including gastrointestinal upset and hepatic toxicity. Doses above 400 mg/day may be associated with more toxic side effects. Miconazole infusion is rarely used and is associated with nausea and fever.

Rifampin

Rifampin is an inducer of the hepatic cytochrome P-450 and thus can significantly alter the metabolism and efficacy of other drugs. It enhances metabolic clearance of both fluconazole and itraconazole, which results in lower plasma levels. This is particularly significant with itraconazole. Rifampin also decreases the absorption of ketoconazole.

Monitoring Response to Treatment

Close clinical evaluation is essential in monitoring the response to treatment. The extent of rhinocerebral mucomycosis following surgical debridement is best followed by serial computerized tomography or magnetic resonance imaging studies. No laboratory test is specific, but resolution of leukocytosis, accelerated erythrocyte sedimentation rate, and recovery of organ function (improved gas exchange in the case of pulmonary mucormycosis) suggest a favorable response to the treatment.

COMMENTS

Despite the availability of newer antifungal agents, the treatment and management of invasive mucormycosis has not changed markedly over the last decade. Aggressive surgical debridement associated with antifungal therapy, primarily amphotericin B, has remained the mainstay of treatment. Because of the high mortality associated with these infections, new drugs are urgently needed.

REFERENCES

1. Barnert J, Behr H, Reich H. An amphotericin B-resistant case of rhinocerebral mucormycosis. Infection 1985;13:134–136.
2. Bennett Cl, Westbrook CA, Gruber B, Golomb HM. Hairy cell leukemia and mucormycosis. Treatment with alpha-2 interferon. Am J Med 1986;81:1065–1067.
3. Brummer E, Stevens DA. Activation of pulmonary macrophages for fungicidal activity by gamma-interferon or lymphokines. Clin Exp Immunol 1987;70:520–528.
4. Christenson JC, Shalit I, Welch DF, Guruswamy A, Marks MI. Synergistic action of amphotericin B and rifampin against *Rhizopus* species. Antimicrob Agents Chemother 1987;31:1775–1778.
5. Clancy CJ, Diaz LE, Nguyen MH. Invasive *Aspergillus* sinusitis in normal hosts: value of therapy with interferon-gamma [Abstract 63–215]. 34th annual meeting, Infectious Disease Society of America, New Orleans, Sept 1996.
6. Couch L, Theilen F, Mader JT. Rhinocerebral mucormycosis with cerebral extension successfully treated with adjunctive hyperbaric oxygen therapy. Arch Otolaryngol Head Neck Surg 1988;114:791–794.
7. De La Paz MA, Patrinely JR, Marines HM, Appling WD. Adjunctive hyperbaric oxygen in the treatment of bilateral cerebro-rhino-orbital mucormycosis. Am J Ophthalmol 1992;114:208–211.
8. Eng RHK, Person A, Mangura C, Chmel H, Corrado M. Susceptibility of *Zygomycetes* to amphotericin B, miconazole and ketoconazole. Antimicrob Agents Chemother 1981;20:688–690.
9. Espinel-Ingroff A, Bartlett M, Bowden R, Chin NX, Cooper C Jr, Fothergill A, McGinnis MR, Menezes P, Messer SA, Nelson PW, Odds FC, Pasarell L, Peter J, Pfaller MA, Rex JH, Rinaldi

MG, Shankland GS, Walsh TJ, Weitzman I. Multicenter evaluation of proposed standardized procedure for antifungal susceptibility testing of filamentous fungi. J Clin Microbiol 1997;35: 139–143.

10. Ferguson B, Mitchell TG, Moon R, Camporesi EM, Farmer J. Adjunctive hyperbaric oxygen for treatment of rhinocerebral mucormycosis. Rev Infect Dis 1988;10:551–559.

11. Fong KM, Seneviratne EME, McCormack JG. Mucor cerebral abscess associated with intravenous drug abuse. Aust NZ J Med 1990;20:74–77.

12. Frazier R, Gathe J, Stool E, LeBlanc M, Nichols M, Flaitz C. Head and neck Zygomycete/Aspergillus infections in patients with AIDS [Abstract PO-BO9–1365]. Int Conf AIDS, 1993;9: 363.

13. Funada H, Miyake Y, Kanamori K, Okafudji K, Machi T, Matsuda T. Fluconazole therapy for pulmonary mucormycosis complicating acute leukemia. Jpn J Med 1989;28:228–231.

14. Gollard R, Rabb C, Larsen R, Chandrasoma P. Isolated cerebral mucormycosis: case report and therapeutic considerations. Neurosurgery 1994;34:174–177.

15. Gudewicz TM, Mader JT, Davis CP. Combined effects of hyperbaric oxygen and antifungal agents on the growth of Candida albicans. Aviat Space Environ Med 1987;58:673–678.

16. Hamill R, Oney LA, Crane LR. Successful therapy for rhinocerebral mucormycosis with associated bilateral brain abscess. Arch Intern Med 1983;143:581–583.

17. Kocak R, Tetiker T, Kocak M, Baslamisli F, Zorludemir S, Gonlusen G. Fluconazole in the treatment of three cases of mucormycosis. Eur J Clin Microbiol Infect Dis 1995;14:560–561.

18. Kumar B, Kaur I, Chakrabarti A, Sharma VK. Treatment of deep mycoses with itraconazole. Mycopathologia 1991;115:169–174.

19. Langmayr JJ, Schwarz A, Buchberger W, Hochleitner W, Twerdy K. Local amphotericin for fungal brain abscess. Lancet 1993;342:123.

20. Lim KKT, Potts MJ, Warnoch DW, Ibrahim NBN, Brown EM, Burns-Cox CJ. Another case report of rhinocerebral mucormycosis treated with liposomal amphotericin B and surgery. Clin Infect Dis 1994;18:653–654.

21. Mahe A, Huerre M, Keita S, Traore F, Bobin P. Basidiobolomycose traitée avec succès par l'itraconazole. Ann Dermatol Venerol 1996;123:182–184.

22. Moraes MA, Almeida MM, Veiga RC, Silveira FT. Zigomicose nasofacial. Relato de um caso do estado do Para, Brasil. Rev Inst Med Trop Sao Paulo 1994;36:171–174.

23. Munckhof W, Jones R, Tosolini FA, Marzec A, Angus P, Grayson ML. Cure of Rhizopus sinusitis in a liver transplant recipient with liposomal amphotericin B. Clin Infect Dis 1993; 16:183.

24. Nagy-Agren SE, Peiguo C, Smith GJW, Waskin HA, Altice FL. Zygomycosis (mucormycosis) and HIV infection: report of three cases and review. J Acquired Immune Defic Syndr Hum Retrovirol 1995;10:441–449.

25. Ng TCT, Campbell CK, Rothera M, Houghton JB, Hughes D, Denning DW. Successful treatment of sinusitis caused by Cunninghamella bertholletiae. Clin Infect Dis 1994;13:313–316.

26. Okhuysen PC, Rex JH, Kapusta M, Fife C. Successful treatment of extensive posttraumatic soft-tissue and renal infections due to Apophysomyces elegans. Clin Infect Dis 1994;19:329–331.

27. Otcenasek M, Buchta V. In vitro susceptibility to 9 antifungal agents of 14 strains of Zygomycetes isolated from clinical specimens. Mycopathologia 1994;128:133–137.

28. Phillips P, Forbes JC, Speert DP. Disseminated infection with Pseudallescheria boydii in a patient with chronic granulomatous disease: response to gamma-interferon plus antifungal therapy. Pediatr Infect Dis J 1991;10:536–539.

29. Rex JH, Pfaller MA, Rinaldi MG, Polak A, Galgiani JN. Antifungal susceptibility testing. Clin Microbiol Rev 1993;6: 367–381.

30. Richardson MD, Shankland GS. Rhizopus, Rhizomucor, Absidia and other agents of systemic and cutaneous zygomycoses. In: Murray PR, Baron EJ, Pfaller MA, Tenover FC, Yolken RH, eds. Manual of clinical microbiology. 6th ed. Washington, DC: ASM Press, 1995;66:809–824.

31. Roger H, Biat I, Cambon M, Beyout J, Souteyrand P. Absidia corymbifera cutaneous zygomycosis (mucormycosis), gangrenosum-like ecthyma in a non-diabetic patient. Treatment with ketoconazole. Ann Dermatol Venerol 1989;116:844–846.

32. Sanati H, Messer SA, Pfaller M, Witt M, Larsen R, Espinel-Ingroff A, Ghannoum M. Multicenter evaluation of broth microdilution method for susceptibility testing of Cryptococcus neoformans against fluconazole. J Clin Microbiol 1996;34:1280–1282.

33. Schell WA, Johnson MG, Weitzman I, Crist MY. Zygomycosis caused by Cunnighamella bertholletiae: mycologic aspects. Arch Pathol Lab Med 1982;106:287–291.

34. Selcen D, Secmeer G, Aysun S, Kanra G, Onerci M, Gokoz A, Ecevit Z, Ceyan M, Anlar Y. Mucormycosis in a diabetic child and its treatment with fluconazole: a case report. Turk J Pediatr 1995;37:165–168.

35. Strasser MD, Kennedy RJ, Adam RD, Rhinocerebral mucormycosis therapy with amphotericin B lipid complex. Arch Intern Med 1996;156:337–339.

36. Sugar AM. Agents of mucormycosis and related species. In: Mandell GL, Bennett JE, Dolin R, eds. Principles and practice of infectious diseases. New York: Churchill Livingstone, 1995: 2311–2319.

37. Sugar AM. Mucormycosis. Clin Infect Dis 1992;14(Suppl 1): S126–129.

38. Tkach LS, Kusne S, Eibling D. Successful treatment of zygomycosis of the paranasal sinus with surgical debridment and amphotericin B colloidal dispersion. Am J Otolaryngol 1993;14: 249–253.

39. Van Cutsem J, Van Gerven F, Fransen J, Janssen PA. Treatment of experimental zygomycosis in guinea pigs with azoles and with amphotericin B. Chemotherapy 1989;35:267–272.

40. Verma KK, Pandhi RK. Subcutaneous mucormycosis in a non-immunocompromised patient treated with potassium iodide. Acta Derm Venerol 1994;74:215–216.

41. Vilella JM, Risse JF, Touchard G, Jacquemin JL. Zygomycose (mucormycose) orbitale chez un enfant sain. Traitement par le ketoconazole. J Fr Ophtalmol 1986;9:441–444.

Paracoccidioides brasiliensis

●

Ricardo Negroni

GENERAL DESCRIPTION
Epidemiology

Paracoccidioidomycosis is a systemic mycosis caused by the dimorphic fungus *Paracoccidioides brasiliensis*. It is a granulomatous and suppurative disorder that primarily involves lungs and then disseminates to other organs via lymphatics and the bloodstream (10). Paracoccidioidomycosis has a restricted geographic distribution. It is endemic in humid subtropical areas of Latin America, from Mexico to Argentina and Uruguay (10, 16, 30, 45, 49). It has a high prevalence in Brazil, which accounts for 80% of reported cases, but is also observed in Colombia, Venezuela, Argentina, and Paraguay. The habitat of *P. brasiliensis* is not well known; it probably lives in soil or by rivers or lakes (1, 6, 14, 19, 41). Spontaneous infections of armadillo (39) and squirrel monkey (23) have been reported, but animal-to-human and human-to-human transmission has not been confirmed (28). Several cases outside endemic areas have been reported, but all had visited or lived previously in an endemic area (10).

Primary infection is probably acquired by inhalation of conidia; skin and mucous membranes seem to be very uncommon portals of entry (49). The primary pulmonary infection is often asymptomatic or has mild respiratory manifestations and is self-limited (paracoccidioidomycosis infection). Subclinical infections occur rather frequently in healthy inhabitants of endemic areas as shown by skin reactivity to paracoccidioidin (55). Many surveys with paracoccidioidin skin tests have been carried out, showing that most infections are acquired at an early age (2, 25, 74). *P. brasiliensis* has been found in fibrous or calcified nodules in the lungs or lymph nodes (3, 53). Reactivation of latent pulmonary or lymph node foci yields progressive forms of this mycosis that are always severe (paracoccidioidomycosis disease).

P. brasiliensis antigens elicit a specific immune response that determines antibody production as well as delayed-type hypersensitivity (45, 64). Over 90% of patients with the progressive forms of paracoccidioidomycosis have specific antibodies that may be detected by routine serologic tests: immunodiffusion in agar gel, counterimmunoelectrophoresis, and complement fixation. Titers in these tests are proportional to the severity of disease and generally decline after clinical remission. Enzyme-linked immunosorbent assay (ELISA) discriminates better between progressive and remittent lesions (57).

The paracoccidioidin skin test is a delayed hypersensitivity reaction to *P. brasiliensis* antigens. It shows positive results in healthy individuals who live in endemic areas, but more than 50% of patients with severe paracoccidioidomycosis disease have negative skin tests. These negative reactions revert to positive after treatment, when clinical remission is achieved (45, 66).

Microbiology

P. brasiliensis is a dimorphic fungus. The yeastlike form of *P. brasiliensis* grows well in vitro in brain heart infusion agar, with or without blood, at 37°C (49). The mycelial form of *P. brasiliensis* grows in Sabouraud dextrose-agar, at 25°C. Microscopically, these colonies exhibit branched, septate, hyaline hyphae 2 to 3 μm in diameter, with numerous intercalated or terminal chlamidoconidia (64). Ultrastructure studies have shown that yeast cells of *P. brasiliensis* are multinucleated and septa in the mycelial form are single pore, similar to those of the *Ascomycotina* division, but the sexual state of *P. brasiliensis* is unknown (11, 61).

Diagnosis of paracoccidioidomycosis is confirmed by finding typical yeastlike elements of *P. brasiliensis* in microscopic study of wet-mount preparations of pus, sputum, or tissue specimens. Cultures should be grown on yeast extract agar, Sabouraud dextrose agar, or brain-heart infusion agar with antibacterial antibiotics; these cultures are incubated at 25°C and 37°C for 4 weeks. *P. brasiliensis* grows slowly, and its isolation is often difficult; thus as a diagnostic method, cultures are less sensitive than microscopic examination (49). Clinical specimens can be inoculated intratesticularly in guinea pigs and hamsters; after 2 or 3 weeks, pus from experimental lesions reveals characteristic multiple budding cells of *P. brasiliensis*.

In histologic sections, *P. brasiliensis* is better visualized when special stains such as P.A.S. or Grocott methenamine-silver are used. Direct immunofluorescence with an specific conjugate is not used routinely (45). In severe cases, extensive suppurative areas with necrosis and soft granulomas are observed; conversely, in mild forms, typical compact epithelioid cell granuloma with giant cells and few fungi is seen (43, 67).

Progressive forms of paracoccidioidomycosis usually present with positive serology; specific antibodies can be detected by immunodiffusion in agar gel, counterimmunoelectrophoresis, complement fixation, and ELISA. Metabolic or cytoplasmic antigens as well as a 43-kDa glucoprotein are used in these tests.

Clinical Manifestations

Paracoccidioidomycosis Infection

Paracoccidioidomycosis infection is defined by a positive paracoccidioidin skin test. It is often asymptomatic or subclinical and self-limited. Few cases of acute pulmonary primary infection with spontaneous resolution have been described (49).

Calcifications of the lungs and lymph nodes are infrequent. The asymptomatic latency period between infection and clinical symptoms may last several years (30).

Paracoccidioidomycosis Disease

All clinical cases that do not show a tendency to spontaneous regression are included under this classification.

Subacute Juvenile Form. This clinical entity affects children and adolescents of both sexes and probably results from rapid dissemination of a primary infection due to severe immunologic failure. Its course is subacute with marked deterioration of the overall general condition, with fever, generalized lymphadenopathy, and hepatosplenomegaly. Skin (49), bone, and the gastrointestinal tract (34) can be involved. Mucous membrane and lung involvement are uncommon.

Chronic Adult Form. The chronic adult form affects adults above 30 years of age, mainly men. The infection is subacute with a predominance of respiratory symptoms. In 25% of cases infection is localized to the lung, with manifestations of a chronic pulmonary disease (25, 58). Multifocal presentation is observed in more than 70% of patients, with skin, mucous membranes, larynx (29), lungs, lymph nodes (33), adrenal glands (70), liver (49), spleen (49), bones (49), and central nervous system (CNS) (52) involvement.

SUSCEPTIBILITY IN VITRO AND IN VIVO

Sulfonamide derivatives, amphotericin B, and azoles are active, both in vitro and in vivo, against *P. brasiliensis*. Sulfonamides were introduced in the treatment of paracoccidioidomycosis by Oliveira Ribeiro in 1940. Some years later, several studies showed that these compounds exert a fungostatic effect against *P. brasiliensis* in vitro (24). Sulfadoxine exhibited a good in vitro activity with an MIC between 6.5 and 12.5 µg/mL of culture medium (27). Sulfonamides were also effective in treating experimental paracoccidioidomycosis in guinea pig, but definitive cure depended on the immunologic capacity of the host (56). According to P. Goncalves, sulfonamide serum levels should be maintained at about 50 µg/mL during treatment (36). When sulfonamides are combined with trimethoprim, serum levels of free sulfa should also be monitored, and doses should be adjusted to keep these levels above 50 µg/mL.

Amphotericin B has been used in treating paracoccidioidomycosis since 1958. This polyene antibiotic is very active in vitro against *P. brasiliensis,* with MICs of 0.06 to 0.2 µg/mL (26).

Several azoles have been assayed against *P. brasiliensis:* miconazole, econazole, ketoconazole, itraconazole, fluconazole, saperconazole, and Sch 39.304. All of them are very effective in the treatment of experimental paracoccidioidomycosis in animal models (46, 47, 65, 71).

P. brasiliensis is one of the fungi most susceptible to ketoconazole. Its MIC varies between 0.01 and 0.001 µg/mL, and its minimum fungicidal concentration (MFC), between 0.1 and 0.01 µg/mL; these results are not modified by addition of 10% bovine serum (62). An antagonism of its antifungal action is observed when 40 µg/mL of rifampin is added; con-

versely, combination with amphotericin B is synergistic in vitro (62).

The effectiveness of ketoconazole in the treatment of experimental paracoccidioidomycosis has been demonstrated in mice, rats, hamsters, and guinea pigs (46). In all of these animal models, ketoconazole (80–120 mg/kg/day for approximately 4 weeks) strikingly reduces the number of lesions. Ketoconazole is more effective in guinea pigs and rats than in hamsters (38).

Itraconazole is a triazole very active both in vivo and in vitro against *P. brasiliensis;* MIC for the yeast form of the fungus varies from 0.01 to 0.001 µg/mL, and the mycelial form is 10-fold less susceptible (71). Electron microscope studies have shown that when yeast cells of *P. brasiliensis* are exposed to 70 ng/mL of itraconazole for 24 h, destruction of organelles is observed and development of mycelia is prevented. This triazole is 10 to 100 times more active in vitro than ketoconazole (9). In experimental paracoccidioidomycosis, the efficacy of itraconazole has been shown in mice, rats, and guinea pigs (50). In these two latter experimental models, biologic cure was reached with doses of 8 to 10 mg/kg/day for 3 weeks (47). Itraconazole proved to be significantly more active than fluconazole in a comparative study of the antifungal action of triazoles in experimental paracoccidioidomycosis in Wistar rats. Fluconazole only decreased lesions markedly at doses of 25 mg/kg/day (47). In experimental trials with mice, fluconazole was clearly effective at doses of 100 mg/kg/day (69). This latter bistriazolic compound is known to be minimally active in vitro, even against fungi for which its in vivo antifungal action is very marked; however, both MIC and MFC were approximately 1.6 µg/mL in Sabouraud dextrose medium at pH 7 (47).

In vitro susceptibility tests for antifungal agents against *P. brasiliensis* are not standardized. Espinel-Ingroff et al. (13) used the standard technique for yeastlike fungi to determine MICs for saperconazole, itraconazole, fluconazole, ketoconazole, and amphotericin B in two culture media: buffered (MOPS) RPMI-1640 and synthetic amino acid medium-fungal (SAAMF). A macrodilution test was performed with both the yeast and mycelial forms of 10 isolates of *P. brasiliensis,* and the fungi were incubated at 35°C (yeast form) and 30°C (mycelial form) for 72 h to 7 days. Saperconazole and itraconazole were the most active antimicrobial agents in vitro, showing MIC_{90}s below 0.03 µg/mL for both forms of this fungus; amphotericin B was less active than the azoles — MIC_{90} between 0.12 and 4.0 µg/mL.

Sch 39304 and saperconazole have been shown very effective in the treatment of experimental animal models of paracoccidioidomycosis (65, 72). Saperconazole has also been used in humans with very good results (18). Research with these triazoles has been discontinued because of tumor formation in the later toxicity studies in rats, and they will not be clinically available.

ANTIMICROBIAL THERAPY

The progressive forms of paracoccidioidomycosis are always fatal without specific treatment (42). Treatment of this systemic mycosis should include general measures such as rest, an appropriate diet (usually rich in proteins and calories), vitamin supplementation, suppression of alcohol and tobacco, and treatment of associated diseases. Intestinal parasitosis and tuberculosis are very common in these patients. Parenteral nutrition is rarely indicated in patients with impaired digestive absorption (36).

Treatment of paracoccidioidomycosis usually involves two stages: initial intense antifungal therapy and maintenance treatment to prevent relapses. Azole derivatives, amphotericin B, and sulfonamide have been used for the first part of treatment (36).

Drug of Choice

Itraconazole, first used in 1982 for paracoccidioidomycosis, is now the drug of choice (31, 40, 48, 73). By 1994, 278 patients had received documented treatment. Although therapeutic endpoints varied from study to study, some conclusions can be drawn. Most patients were treated with 50 to 200 mg/day for periods of 2 to 12 months; doses of 200 mg/day were used only rarely. The standard regimen is 100 mg/day orally for 6 months. This drug should be administered once daily after a meal. All but three patients showed clinical improvement, and there were only six clinical relapses (2.1%) after successful treatment courses. Two patients experienced multiple relapses, but both responded favorably to repeated treatment with itraconazole. Twenty-two patients with the acute juvenile form showed therapeutic responses similar to those observed in the chronic adult form (31, 32, 35, 60, 68). Itraconazole seems to be remarkably nontoxic; only subclinical increases in hepatic enzymes were recorded in 14.2% of cases (36). The observed results indicate that maintenance treatment is not necessary in patients who receive itraconazole. Combination therapy is not usually used with itraconazole.

Failures of itraconazole are very rare and are usually due to the lack of digestive absorption in patients with blockage of mesenteric lymph nodes, steatorrhea, and malabsorption. This occurs more frequently in the acute juvenile form (30).

The main problem in paracoccidioidomycosis treatment is that many patients fail to comply with the full course of therapy. These compliance failures are attributable to the cost of treatment and low socioeconomic status and cultural factors in most of these patients (36, 50).

Special Situations

Malabsorption

As mentioned above, when malabsorption of the drug requires administration of an antifungal drug by the intravenous route, amphotericin B and cotrimoxazole are the alternative antimicrobial agents. Good results have been observed with both drugs. Intestinal lesions may occasionally worsen treatment because of the fibrosis that replaces the inflammatory process. These patients should be managed with fractionated oral diet or parenteral nutrition. Patients with intestinal malabsorption usually improve on a low-fat diet (34).

Central Nervous System Involvement

Itraconazole is 99.8% protein bound, which impairs penetration of the blood-brain barrier. Concentrations of the drug in cerebrospinal fluid are negligible. However, itraconazole has been shown to be very effective in some mycoses of the CNS, both experimentally and in humans, probably because of its high affinity for the cerebral parenchyma (36, 50). As stated above, abscessed granulomas are the most frequent clinical manifestations of neuroparacoccidioidomycosis, and in these lesions, itraconazole is very effective. In meningoencephalitis, amphotericin B (0.8 mg/kg/day), cotrimoxazole (2,400 mg/480 mg/day), or fluconazole (400 mg/day), all intravenously, have been used successfully. Amphotericin B and sulfonamide have been used frequently in treating neuroparacoccidioidomycosis with good clinical responses. Nóbrega and Spina-Franca consider the use of sulfonamides to be the first option in the treatment of lesions in the CNS, with amphotericin B reserved for those resistant or intolerant to sulfa (52). Neurosurgical procedures are sometimes indicated. Antifungal drugs must always be used, even when surgery is performed.

Impaired Adrenal Gland Function

Impaired adrenal gland function occurs in more than 30% of patients with disseminated paracocccidioidomycosis. Besides the antifungal therapy, these patients should receive 30 mg/day of hydrocortisone. This substitute hormone treatment is usually administered lifelong (70).

Tuberculosis

Association with tuberculosis is observed in 10 to 12% of patients; its frequency varies among regions. Due to the negative interaction between rifampin and the azoles, this compound is not indicated in this situation. Cotrimoxazole or amphotericin B are usually administered to these patients.

Paracoccidioidomycosis in AIDS Patients

Association of paracoccidioidomycosis and AIDS is rare; only 27 cases had been reported by 1995, all in Brazil (20). In spite of specific therapy, 30% of these patients died. Multiple drug regimens, usually including cotrimoxazole, ketoconazole, and amphotericin B, were administered to most of the patients (33). Itraconazole given to one patient with disseminated disease resulted in a good clinical response. Maintenance treatment with cotrimoxazole or azoles should be administered lifelong (20).

Other

Surgery may be necessary to remove cerebral granulomas and to treat fibrous stenosis of the mouth, larynx, and trachea (49).

Alternative Therapy

Sulfonamide Derivatives

Sulfonamides have fungistatic activity against *P. brasiliensis*. They are inexpensive and, when administered by the oral route, are well tolerated. If these drugs are used at optimal doses, the success rate is over 60% (8). Two types of sulfonamides are distinguished on the basis of their elimination rate and activity: rapidly eliminated drugs (e.g., sulfadiazine) and slowly eliminated drugs (e.g., sulfamethoxypyridazine). Both are administered orally; sulfadiazine is given every 6 h and sulfamethoxypyridazine every 12 h. The daily dose of rapidly eliminated compounds is 3 to 5 g in adults or 0.15 g/kg in children; the slowly eliminated sulfonamides are given at a dose of 1 or 2 g/day (36, 63). Serum sulfonamide levels should be maintained above 50 mg/L. The treatment duration should be 3 years. Early discontinuation of therapy often results in resistance of *P. brasiliensis* to sulfonamides. Side effects are rarely observed; few patients develop crystalluria with hematuria, which can be controlled by increasing the water intake or drinking bicarbonated water. Leukopenia, rash, fever, photosensitization, and digestive disturbances are rarely reported (63).

Combination of sulfamethoxazole with trimethoprim (cotrimoxazole) has proved very effective in the initial treatment of paracoccidioidomycosis (4, 28). This drug can be administered orally or intravenously. The preparation most often used contains 800 mg of sulfamethoxazole and 160 mg of trimethoprim. The usual dose is 1 tablet every 12 h for 1 year. Its therapeutic efficacy does not appear superior to that of sulfonamides, but some patients who are resistant to sulfonamides have improved on cotrimoxazole. A combination of sulfadiazine and trimethoprim (cotrimazine) is used in Brazil, and it has proved very effective in the treatment of neuroparacoccidioidomycosis. Dosages are similar to those of cotrimoxazole (5).

Sulfonamides may be used *(a)* for adult patients suffering chronic unifocal disease, with no previous therapy and in good overall condition; *(b)* when paracoccidioidomycosis is associated with tuberculosis, and *(c)* as maintenance therapy after a course of amphotericin B.

Amphotericin B

The polyene antibiotic amphotericin B was first used to treat paracoccidioidomycosis in 1958. It is useful in the control of this mycosis, although side effects are frequent (12). This drug causes a very rapid regression of all lesions of paracoccidioidomycosis but does not prevent relapses. Therefore, it is usually indicated for use in very severe cases, and once clinical remission is achieved, sulfonamides are given as maintenance therapy.

Amphotericin B is administered intravenously at an initial dose of 0.2 mg/kg/day, increasing up to 0.8 mg/kg/day until a total of 1.5 g is given. Sulfonamides should then be given at the usual dosage for 2 to 3 years. Combination therapy gives better results than administration of amphotericin B alone; relapses have been reduced from 60 to 18% of cases (12, 63).

Amphotericin B combined with rifampin was used in four patients who had not shown clinical improvement with amphotericin B alone. Rifampin was given at a daily dose of 600 mg and amphotericin B was administered at a dose of 25 or 50 mg, three times a week. Clinical remission of the disease was achieved after several months (75).

Amphotericin B should be used with caution, and treatment should be monitored by clinical and laboratory evaluation. The following tests should be done once a week: serum sodium, potassium, and creatinine levels, blood urea nitrogen, and urinalysis; hemogram and electrocardiography may be performed every 15 days (36, 49).

Liposomal amphotericin B has not yet been used in paracoccidioidomycosis.

Ketoconazole

Ketaconazole was first used in paracoccidioidomycosis in 1978 and proved effective. It has very good digestive absorption at acid pH, but its bioavailability decreases in patients who receive medication to reduce gastric acidity. Excellent results have been reported, with over 90% clinical cure after 1 year of therapy. The drug is administered orally at a daily dose of 200 or 400 mg in adults or 5 to 8 mg/kg in children. Peak serum levels of 2 to 4 μg/mL are usually obtained with these doses (51). Relapses were observed in less than 10% of cases; patients who relapse can still be treated successfully with ketoconazole. Treatment failures have been documented in patients with low gastric acidity, those whose digestive absorption is impaired by lymphatic blockage in the acute juvenile type of the disease, and patients who received rifampin (44, 51). Treatment may be interrupted when the patient achieves complete clinical remission, serologic tests become negative or have low titers, and the paracoccidioidin skin test becomes positive in those who displayed negative reactions before treatment.

Ketoconazole is well tolerated; side effects have been registered in less than 10% of patients, and they were usually minor. An asymptomatic increase in hepatic enzyme levels was reported in 8% of cases. Symptomatic hepatitis was unusual in paracoccidioidomycosis patients. Endocrine side effects (e.g., decreased libido and gynecomastia) were rarely observed, and although this drug interferes with corticosteroid synthesis, symptoms of hypoadrenalism were extremely rare. Endocrine effects have been reversible and dose dependent (46). Ketoconazole is considered one of the drugs of choice in the treatment of this mycosis (although it is a bit less effective than itraconazole), and it is the cheapest treatment for paracoccidioidomycosis (59).

Fluconazole

The triazole fluconazole has been used in a few cases of paracoccidioidomycosis. It has excellent and rapid digestive absorption, independent of meals and gastric acidity. Peak serum levels of 6 to 10 μg/mL are frequently obtained 2 h after administration of 200 mg. It may also be given intravenously. Its bioavailability is over 80%. Binding to plasma proteins is low, about 11 to 12%, which allows free circulation of the drug and easy passage through the blood-brain barrier. Levels in cerebrospinal fluid reach 80% of those in blood, but its tissue affinity is lower than that of itraconazole. Over 80% of this triazole is eliminated in its active form in urine and less than 20% is metabolized in the liver, where it is transformed into inactive compounds. Steady state is achieved after 3 to 4 days and is influenced by renal function. With normal renal function, $T_{1/2}$ is approximately 31 h (36).

Fluconazole has been used to treat 37 patients at a daily dose of 200 to 400 mg for at least 6 months. Significant improvement was seen in 34 cases, but one sudden death was observed. There was one failure, and one patient could not be evaluated because of noncompliance. Eight patients received cotrimoxazole as suppressive treatment after achieving clinical remission with fluconazole. Only 25 patients were controlled during more than 6 months after treatment, and only one relapse was observed. No side effects were registered in this group of patients (50).

Both in vitro studies and treatment of experimental paracoccidioidomycosis in animal models have shown fluconazole to be less active than itraconazole against this microorganism. The clinical use of fluconazole has not been as wide as that of itraconazole, nevertheless it has some potential advantages: it can be administered parenterally, it reaches a higher concentration in cerebrospinal fluid and urine, it has more predictable digestive absorption; it presents lower drug interaction, and it produces fewer side effects. Fluconazole should be given in special situations such as renal or brain involvement.

ENDPOINT FOR MONITORING THERAPY

Untreated cases are always fatal after several years (66); death may occur from respiratory failure, malnutrition, or intercurrent infections.

Posttherapeutic latency exists; after successful treatment, clinical cure can be achieved, but lesions remain latent with occasional relapses. The paracoccidioidin skin test is usually positive, and serologic reactions show low titers or negative results. In severe cases, intense fibrosis observed as a consequence of healing lesions may cause tracheal and laryngeal stenosis, buccal atresia, or cardiorespiratory impairment due to pulmonary fibrosis (paradoxical cure) (43).

Criteria for cure of paracoccidioidomycosis include *(a)* clinical remission of all active lesions of at least 6 months duration; *(b)* eradication of *P. brasiliensis* from secretions; *(c)* stabilization of the radiologic pattern of the lungs, and *(d)* immunologic cure, with positive paracoccidioidin skin test and reversion of serologic tests from positive to negative or stable serology that remains at low values. Clinical remission is usually observed after 3 months of treatment; mycologic cure occurs even earlier. Radiologic stabilization often takes more than 6 months, and serologic conversion occurs late, on average, 50 months after the beginning of treatment (36).

Patient follow-up should be continued for at least 2 years after treatment has been completed. Controls should be carried out at 3-month intervals and should include clinical and immunologic evaluations. Patients who exhibit negative paracoccidioidin skin test and positive serology 1 year after ending the initial treatment are at high risk of relapse.

COMMENTS

As mentioned above, cell-mediated immunity is often depressed in severe cases of paracoccidioidomycosis. The use of immunomodulating drugs has been studied in animal models: dialyzable leukocyte extracts, cyclophosphamide, and glucan directly affect the outcome of experimental disease by reducing the number of lesions; interferon-γ improves the activity of azoles activity against paracoccidioidomycosis (7, 22, 36, 54). A β-1.3 glucan extracted from *Saccharomyces cerevisiae* has been administered to a limited number of patients. It was given intravenously or intramuscularly once weekly at a dose of 10 mg for 1 month; then it was administered once a month for 1 year. Treated patients exhibited a better clinical outcome,

faster recovery of cell-mediated immunity, and marked decreases in erythrocyte sedimentation rate and serum levels of specific antibodies. This glucan needs further clinical trials.

No clinical studies have yet assessed the efficacy of interferon-γ for this mycosis.

REFERENCES

1. Albornoz MB de. Isolation of *Paracoccidioides brasiliensis* from rural soil in Venezuela. Proceedings of the Pan American Symposium on Paracoccidioidomycosis. Medellin, Colombia, 1971. Washington, DC: PAHO Scientific Publishers, 1972;254: 71–75.
2. Albornoz MB de. Paracoccidioidomicosis infección. In: Del Negro G, Lacaz C da S, Fiorillo AM, eds. Paracoccidioidomicose (blastomicose sulamericana). Editora da Universidade de Sao Paulo, Sarvier, 1982:91–95.
3. Angulo-Ortega A. Calcifications in paracoccidioidomycosis: are they morphological manifestations of subclinical infections? Proceedings of the Pan American Symposium on Paracoccidioidomycosis. Medellin, Colombia, 1971. Washington, DC: PAHO Scientific Publishers, 1972;254:126–133.
4. Barbosa W, Vasconcelos WMP. Acao da sulfametoxazol associada ao trimetoprim na terapeutica da blastomicose sulamericana. Rev Pat Trop 1973;2:329–345.
5. Barraviera B, Mendes RP, Machado JM, Pereira J, Souza MJ, Meira DA. Evaluation of treatment of paracoccidioidomycosis with cotrimazine (combination of sulfadiazine and trimethoprim). Rev Inst Med Trop Sao Paulo 1989;31:53–55.
6. Batista AC, Shome SK, Santos FM. Pathogenicity of *Paracoccidioides brasiliensis* isolated from soil. Inst Micología de Recife publ no. 373, 1962.
7. Blejer J, Godio CM, Negroni R, Nejamkis MR. Cyclophosphamide effect on paracoccidioidomycosis in rat. Rev Inst Med Trop Sao Paulo 1995;37:219–224.
8. Borelli D. Terapia de la paracoccidioidomicosis. Valor actual de los antigüos tratamientos. Rev Argent Micol 1987;10:13–20.
9. Borgers M, Van de Ven MA. Degenerative changes in fungi after itraconazole treatment. Rev Infect Dis 1987;9(Suppl 1): S33–S36.
10. Brummer E, Castañeda E, Restrepo A. Paracoccidioidomycosis: an update. Clin Microbiol Rev 1993;6:89–117.
11. Carbonell LM. Ultrastructure of *Paracoccidioides brasiliensis* in cultures. Proceedings of the Pan American Symposium on Paracoccidioidomycosis. Medellin, Colombia, 1971. Washington, DC: PAHO Scientific Publishers, 1972;254:21–28.
12. Dillon NL, Marques SA. Vantagens e desvantagens da anfotericina B no tratamento da paracoccidioidomicose. An Bras Dermatol 1990;65:226–227.
13. Espinel-Ingroff A, Kerkering TM, Negroni R, Restrepo A. Susceptibilities of the yeast and mycelial phase of *Paracoccidioides brasiliensis* to five antifungal agents [Abstract]. Rev Argent Micol 1992;15:30.
14. Ferreira MS, Freitas LH, Lacaz C da S, Del Negro GM, Melo NT, García NM, Assis CM, Salebian A, Heins-Vaccari EMH. Isolation and characterization of *Paracoccidioides brasiliensis* strain from a dog food probably contaminated with soil in Uberlandia, Brazil. J Med Vet Mycol 1990;28:253–256.
15. Franco MF, Montenegro MR, Mendes RP, Marques SA, Dillon NL, Mota NGS. Paracoccidioidomycosis: a recently proposed classification of its clinical forms. Rev Soc Bras Med Trop 1987; 20:129–132.

16. Franco MF, Mendes RP, Rezkalla-Iwasso MT, Montenegro MR. Paracoccidioidomycosis. Baillieres Clin Trop Med Commun Dis 1989;4:185–220.

17. Franco MF, Lacaz C da S, Restrepo-Moreno A, Del Negro G, eds. Paracoccidioidomycosis. Boca Raton, FL: CRC Press, 1994.

18. Franco L, Gomez I, Restrepo A. Treatment of subcutaneous and systemic mycoses with a new orally administered triazole, saperconazole R 66905. Int J Dermatol 1992;31:725–729.

19. Gezuele, E. Aislamiento de *Paracoccidioides* sp de heces de pingüinos de la Antártida [Abstract B$_2$]. IVth Encuentro Internacional de Paracoccidioidomicosis. Caracas, Venezuela, 1989.

20. Goldani LZ, Sugar AM. Paracoccidioidomycosis and AIDS: an overview. Clin Infect Dis 1995;21:1275–1281.

21. Grose E, Tamsitt JR. *Paracoccidioides brasiliensis* recovered from intestinal tract of three bats *(Artibeus lituratus)* in Colombia. Sabouraudia 1965;4:124–128.

22. Hostetler JS, Brummer E, Coffman RL, Stevens DA. Efficacy of anti-IL$_4$, INF-gamma and Sch 42427 in chronic paracoccidioidomycosis: IgE predictive of outcome. Clin Exp Immunol 1993;94:11–16.

23. Johnson WD, Lang CM. Paracoccidioidomycosis (South American blastomycosis) in squirrel monkey *(Saimisi sciureus)*. Vet Pathol 1977;14:368–371.

24. Lacaz C da S. Associacao da sulfadiazina e sulfamerazina no tratamento da blastomicose sulamericana. Niveis sanguineos obtidos. Profilaxia dos acidentes sulfamídicos. Hospital (Río de Janeiro) 1950;37:689–697.

25. Lacaz C da S, Passos Filho MCR, Fava Netto C, Macarron B. Contribuicao para o estudo da "blastomicose infeccao." Inquérito com a paracoccidioidina. Estudo serológico e clínicoradiológico dos paracoccidioidino-positivos. Rev Inst Med Trop Sao Paulo 1959;1:245–257.

26. Lacaz C da S, Ulson CM, Sampaio SAP. Acao "in vitro" da anfotericina B sobre o *Paracoccidioides brasiliensis*. Rev Paul Med 1959;54:357–360.

27. Lacaz C da S, Mianmi PS. Acao "in vitro" da sulfamina RO 44393 sobre o *Paracoccidioides brasiliensis*. Resultados preliminares. Hospital (Río de Janeiro) 1963;64:603–612.

28. Lacaz C da S, Porto E, Costa Martins JE. Paracoccidioidomicose. In: Lacaz C da S, Porto E, Costa Martins JE. Micología médica. 8th ed. Sao Paulo, Brazil: Editorial Sarvier, 1991:248–297.

29. Lamartine JP, Lacaz C da S. Oropharyngolaryngeal lesions. In: Franco MF, Lacaz C da S, Restrepo-Moreno A, Del Negro G, eds. Paracoccidioidomycosis. Boca Raton, FL: CRC Press, 1994:267–269.

30. Londero AT. Paracoccidioidomycosis. In: Gatti F, de Vroey CH. Human mycoses in tropical countries. 8 Health cooperation papers. 2nd ed. Bologna: Organizazione per la Cooperazione Sanitaria Internazionale, 1991:187–199.

31. Marcano C, Negroni, R. Paracoccidioidomicosis: aspectos terapéuticos. Interciencias (Venezuela), 1990;15:227–231.

32. Marques SA, Camargo RMP. Clínica [Abstract]. 5th Encuentro Internacional de Paracoccidioidomicosis. Rev Argent Micol 1992;15:15.

33. Marques SA, Shikanai-Yasuda MA. Paracoccidioidomycosis associated with immunosuppression, A.I.D.S. and cancer. In: Franco MF, Lacaz C da S, Restrepo-Moreno A, Del Negro G. Paracoccidioidomycosis. Boca Raton, FL: CRC Press, 1994:393–405.

34. Martinez R. Digestive tract lesions. In: Franco MF, Lacaz C da S, Restrepo-Moreno A, Del Negro G. Paracoccidioidomycosis. Boca Raton, FL: CRC Press, 1994:289–302.

35. Mendes RP, Barraviera B, Souza LR, Pereira PCM, Marcondes-Macado J, Franco MF, Meira DA. Evaluation of Itraconazole in the treatment of paracoccidioidomycosis (PBM) [Abstract]. Rev Argent Micol 1992;15:86.

36. Mendes RP, Negroni R, Arechavala A. Treatment and control of cure. In: Franco MF, Lacaz C da S, Restrepo-Moreno A, Del Negro G. Paracoccidioidomycosis. Boca Raton, FL: CRC Press, 1994:373–392.

37. Montenegro MR. Host parasite relationship in paracoccidioidomycosis. Jpn J Med Mycol 1995;36:209–213.

38. Mota NGS, Viero RM, Rezkallah-Iwasso MT, Peracoli MT, Soares AM, Montenegro MR. The effect of ketoconazole on experimental paracoccidioidomycosis in Siriam hamsters: immunological and histopathological study. Mycopathologia 1984; 88:141–148.

39. Naiff RD, Ferreira LCL, Barrett TV, Naiff MF, Arias J. Paracoccidioidomicose enzoótica em tatus *(Dasypus novencinctus)* no estado de Pará. Rev Inst Med Trop Sao Paulo 1986;28:19–27.

40. Naranjo M, Trujillo M, Munera P, Gomez I, Restrepo A. Treatment of paracoccidioidomycosis with itraconazole. J Med Vet Mycol 1990;28:67–76.

41. Negroni P. *Paracoccidioides brasiliensis* vive saprofíticamente en el suelo argentino. Prensa Med Argent 1966;53:2381–2382.

42. Negroni, P. Blastomicosis Sudamericana. In: Negroni P. Micosis profundas, vol III. Las blastomicosis y coccidioidomicosis. La Plata, Argentina: Comisión de Investigaciones Científicas. Prov. Bs. As., 1968:133–232.

43. Negroni R. Observaciones personales sobre la micosis de Lutz (blastomicosis sudamericana) en la Argentina. Doctora Thesis. Universidad de Buenos Aires, 1969.

44. Negroni R. Estado actual del empleo del ketoconazol en paracoccidioidomicosis (ketoconazol 6 años después). Rev Argent Micol 1987;10:13–20.

45. Negroni R. Paracoccidioidomycosis. In: Balow A, Hauler WJ, Ohasi M, Turano A. eds. Laboratory diagnosis of infectious diseases, principles and practice, vol 1. New York: Springer Verlag, 1988:678–686.

46. Negroni R. Azole derivatives in the treatment of paracoccidioidomycosis. In: St. Georgiev V, ed. Antifungal drugs. Ann NY Acad Sci 1988;544:497–503.

47. Negroni R, Elías Costa MR de, Finquelievich JL, Iovannitti C, Agorio I, Tiraboschi IN. Comparative trials of three triazoles in the treatment of experimental paracoccidioidomycosis in rats. Rev Iberoam Micol 1991;8:8–12.

48. Negroni R. Triazoles en el tratamiento de la paracoccidioidomicosis [Abstract]. Rev Argent Micol 1992;15:16.

49. Negroni R. Paracoccidioidomycosis (South American blastomycosis, Lutz's mycosis). Int J Dermatol 1993;32:847–859.

50. Negroni R. Azoles in the treatment of paracoccidioidomycosis. In: Vanden Bossche H, et al., eds. Dimorphic fungi in biology and medicine. New York: Plenum Press, 1993:391–396.

51. Negroni R. Tratamiento actual de las micosis sistémicas endémicas. Rev Iberoam Micol 1996;13:544–550.

52. Nobrega JP, Spina-Franca NA. Neuroparacoccidioidomycosis. In: Franco MF, Lacaz C da S, Restrepo-Moreno A, Del Negro G. Paracoccidioidomycosis. Boca Raton, FL: CRC Press, 1994: 321–330.

53. Padilha Goncalves A. Lesoes ganglionares. In: Del Negro G, Lacaz C da S, Fiorillo AM. eds. Paracoccidioidomicose (Blastomicose sulamericana). Sao Paulo, Brazil: Editora Sarvier, 1982: 203–210.

54. Peracoli MT, Rezkalla-Iwasso MT, Motta NG, Montenegro MR.

Dialysable leukocyte extracts modify the course of experimental paracoccidioidomycosis in the Syriam hamster. Myco-pathologia 1993;121:149–156.

55. Pereira AJCS, Barbosa W. Inquerito intradérmico para paracoccidioidomicose em Goiania. Rev Pat Trop 1988;17:157–186.

56. Peryassú D. O sistema retículo-endotelial na blastomicose brasileira experimental do cobaio. Sua importancia no tratamento sulfamídico. J Bras Med 1962;6:503–515.

57. Pires de Camargo Z, Taborda CP, Rodrigues EG, Travassos LR. The use of cell-free antigens of *Paracoccidioides brasiliensis* in serological tests. J Med Vet Mycol 1991;29:31–38.

58. Pires de Campos E, Padovani CR, Cataneo AMJ. Pulmonary and radiological studies in 58 paracoccidioidomycosis patients. Rev Inst Med Trop Sao Paulo 1991;33:267–276.

59. Pripas S. Paracoccidioidomicose: atendimento ao nivel de assistencia primaria a saúde. Rev Saude Publica Sao Paulo 1988;22:233–236.

60. Queiroz Telles F, Bendhack L, Hagi NT, Purim KS, Lameira RP, Bordignon GF. Itraconazole in the therapy of paracoccidioidomycosis [Abstract]. Rev Argent Micol 1992;15:85.

61. Queiroz Telles F. *Paracoccidioides brasiliensis*. Ultrastructural findings. In: Franco MF, Lacaz C da S, Restrepo-Moreno A, Del Negro G. Paracoccidioidomycosis. Boca Raton, FL: CRC Press, 1994:27–47.

62. Restrepo MA, Tabares CBAM. "In vitro" susceptibility of *Paracoccidioides brasiliensis* yeast form to antifungal agents. Rev Inst Med Trop Sao Paulo 1984;26:322–331.

63. Restrepo MA. Paracoccidioidomycosis (South American blastomycosis). In: Jacob PA, Nall L, eds. Antifungal drug therapy. A complete guide for practitioners. New York: Marcel Dekker, 1990:181–205.

64. Restrepo MA. Paracoccidioidomycosis. In: Murphy JW, Friedman H, Bendinelli M, eds. Fungal infections and immune response. New York: Plenum Press, 1993:251–276.

65. Rezkalla-Iwasso MT, Villas-Boas MNLF, Soares A, Franco MF, Sugisaki MF, Fecchio D, Peracoli MT. Experimental paracoc-cidioidomycosis of hamsters and mice: treatment with a new triazole Sch 39.304. Rev Iberoam Micol 1992;9:72–75.

66. Robles AM, Arechavala AI, Negroni R, Finquelievich JL. Estudio de algunas pruebas inmunológicas en paracoccidioidomicosis. Rev Argent Micol 1990;13:15–25.

67. Salfelder K. Atlas of fungal pathology. Current histopathology. Dordrecht: Kluwer Academic Publisher Group, 1990:116–126.

68. Shikanai-Yasuda MA, Higaki Y, Del Negro G, Ho Joo S. Randomized therapeutic trial with itraconazole, ketoconazole and sulfadiazine in paracoccidioidomycosis [Abstract]. Rev Argent Micol 1992;15:83.

69. Stevens DA, Brummer E, McEwen, JG, Perlman A. Efficacy of fluconazole, a new oral triazole, in blastomycosis and paracoccidioidomycosis in comparison with ketoconazole [Abstract]. Rev Iber Micol 1988;5(Suppl 1):26.

70. Tendrich M, Wanke B, Del Negro G, Wejchenberg BL. Adrenocortical involvement. In: Franco MF, Lacaz C da S, Restrepo-Moreno A, Del Negro G. Paracoccidioidomycosis. Boca Raton, FL: CRC Press, 1994:303–312.

71. Van Cutsen J, Van Gerven F, Janssen PAJ. In: Fromthing R, ed. Recent trends in discovery, development and evaluation of antifungal agents. Barcelona: J R Prous Scient. Publisher, 1987:177–192.

72. Van Cutsen J, Van Gerven F, Janssen PAJ. Saperconazole, a new potent antifungal triazole: in vitro activity spectrum and therapeutic efficacy. Drug Future 1989;14:1187–1209.

73. Vargas Flores J. El itraconazol en la paracoccidioidomicosis (experiencia en 40 casos bolivianos) [Abstract]. Rev Argent Micol 1992;15:85.

74. Wanke B. Paracoccidioidomicosis. Inquérito intradérmico com a paracoccidioidina em zona urbana do municipio do Río de Janeiro. Doctora Thesis. Fac. Medicina Universidade Federal do Río de Janeiro, 1976.

75. Wanke B, Pedrosa PN, Bretas GS, Seteibal S. Associacao de rifampicina a anfotericina B no tratamento da paracoccidioidomicose. Rev Inst Med Trop Sao Paulo 1984;26:205–208.

Penicillium marneffei

●

Bertrand F. Dupont

GENERAL DESCRIPTION
Microbiology

Penicillium marneffei is a thermally dimorphic fungus belonging to the genus *Penicillium*. The saprophytic phase of the fungus is present in Southeast Asia: Thailand, Vietnam, Indonesia, south China (Guangxi Province), and Hong Kong. The fungus was isolated from soil and from several species of bamboo rats.

Epidemiology

The disease has been recognized since 1973 in native, apparently healthy persons as well as in immunocompromised hosts; 22 cases have been published (3). Since 1988, it has become a major opportunistic infection in acquired immunodeficiency disease (AIDS), occurring at an advanced stage of HIV disease with a CD4 cell count below 50/mm^3. In northern Thailand, in patients infected with HIV, *P. marneffei* infection is the third most common opportunistic infection after tuberculosis and cryptococcosis (13). A case-control study in northern Thailand comparing risk-related behavior and exposures in 80 cases of disseminated infection in patients with AIDS suggests that recent exposure to a potential environmental reservoir of organisms in the soil may be associated with disseminated *P. marneffei* infections (2). Because of the rapid progression of the AIDS epidemic in this part of the world, an increasing number of cases of penicilliosis is expected, warranting prospective studies to establish the best cost-effective curative treatment and a prophylactic approach. Imported cases in Europe, the United States, Canada, and Australia have been described in immunocompromised patients (mainly AIDS) with a past history of traveling in Southeast Asia weeks, months, or years earlier (5).

Clinical Manifestations

The disease is characterized by fever, weight loss, lung infiltrates, cutaneous infectious foci, hepatosplenomegaly, lymphadenopathy, and anemia or pancytopenia (3, 6, 13). The fungus can be detected by direct examination and/or culture of bone marrow aspirate or skin or lymph node biopsy, bronchoalveolar lavage, or blood culture (13). On smear or tissue section, the small nonbudding septate yeasts are characteristic; in culture, the filamentous phase produces a diffusing red pigment and must be differentiated from other species of "red *Penicillium*." The disease is lethal if left untreated, particularly in disseminated infections and in immunocompromised hosts; localized infections can resolve spontaneously.

SUSCEPTIBILITY TESTING IN VITRO AND IN VIVO
In Vitro Studies

Penicillium marneffei is classified as an hazardous microorganism to handle and should be manipulated under a safety cabinet or in a biosafety level 3 laboratory according to national or international regulations.

In vitro testing for susceptibility to antifungal agents is not standardized. Although major progress has been made for yeasts, in vitro testing of filamentous or dimorphic fungi is still controversial with respect to reproducibility and relevance to clinical outcome. When tested in broth, rapid production of red pigment confounds reading results either by the naked eye or by a photometer.

A limited number of studies have tested in vitro susceptibility of isolates of *P. marneffei*. Thirty isolates of *P. marneffei* from clinical specimens were tested in a modified macrobroth dilution bioassay for amphotericin B and 5-fluorocytosine (5-FC), using a microtiter plate with a semisolid growth medium for azoles (12). All isolates were highly susceptible to 5-FC, miconazole, ketoconazole, and itraconazole. Fluconazole was the least active, 20 strains had an MIC of 20 mg/L. Geometric mean of MICs were: amphotericin B, 0.976 mg/L (range, 0.25–4); 5-FC, 0.25 mg/L; miconazole, 0.001 mg/L; itraconazole, 0.009 mg/L; and fluconazole, 7.9 mg/L. Initial therapy failed in 8 of 35 (22.6%) patients treated with amphotericin B, 3 of 12 (25%) patients treated with itraconazole, and 7 of 11 (63.6%) patients treated with fluconazole. Although patients were not randomly assigned to receive therapy with the various antifungal agents, a good correlation was found between in vitro and in vivo data for azoles; results with amphotericin B were more difficult to assess.

We tested 6 isolates from AIDS patients and 4 isolates from non-AIDS patients with amphotericin B, 5-FC, ketoconazole, itraconazole, and fluconazole (5), using Steer's technique on agar plates, with an inoculum of 10^4 spores/mL. Incubation time was 24 h at 35°C. Casitone agar medium was used for amphotericin B and azole derivatives, and yeast morphology agar (YMA), a synthetic medium, was used for 5-FC. There was no difference with respect to the immune status (HIV) of the patients. MICs to amphotericin B were 0.04 mg/L (3 isolates), 0.78 mg/L (3 isolates), and 1.56 mg/L (4 isolates). All isolates had MICs of 0.04 mg/L or below to 5-FC, ketoconazole, and itraconazole, and all isolates had MICs of 50 mg/L or above for fluconazole.

The high MICs to fluconazole may be due to use of an inapropriate medium. Sekhon et al. used different methods to test the susceptibility of mycelial and yeast forms (8). The MIC and minimum fungicidal concentration (MFC) for mycelial forms to amphotericin B were 0.78 to 1.56 and 0.78 to 3.125 mg/L, respectively. MICs of yeast forms were 3.125 to 25 mg/L, and MFCs were one dilution higher. MICs to fluconazole were generally lower for the yeast forms (6.25–25 mg/L) than the mycelial form (25–50 mg/L), while MFCs for mycelial cultures were above 100 mg/L, compared with 6.25 to 100 mg/L for the yeast form. MICs for the mycelial form to 5-FC ranged from less than 0.195 to 0.39 mg/L, and a higher MIC (6.25 mg/L) was recorded for the yeast forms. MFCs to 5-FC for the yeast forms were 25 to 100 mg/L. MICs for the mycelial forms to itraconazole ranged from less than 0.195 to 3.125 mg/L, and higher values (<0.195–50 mg/L) were recorded for the yeastlike forms. MFCs to itraconazole for mycelial and yeast forms ranged from less than 0.195 to 0.39 and 25 to 100 mg/L, respectively (8). MICs to fluconazole tended to be higher for mycelial forms than for yeast forms: 50 versus 25 mg/L (14). In one report, one strain had an MIC to nystatin of 0.65 mg/L in a semisynthetic medium with a reading after 24 h of incubation; the MIC increased to 3.2 mg/L at the 4th day of incubation (5). In other anecdotal reports, one isolate was reported susceptible to amphotericin B, and 3 isolates susceptible to amphotericin B and 5-FC (7).

Boon-Long et al. tested 8 strains to amphotericin B, 5-FC, fluconazole, itraconazole, miconazole, and D 0870—a new triazole antifungal agent—by a microbroth dilution method in RPMI, brain heart infusion, and yeast nitrogen base medium. Although there were differences depending on the medium used, itraconazole had the lowest MICs (range, 0.003–0.016 mg/L), and miconazole and D0870 had similar values (range, 0.013–0.5 mg/L and 0.003–0.1 mg/L, respectively). MICs were amphotericin B, 0.06 to 0.5 mg/L; fluconazole, 2 to 16 mg/L; and flucytosine, 0.25 to 32 mg/L (1).

In the first reported case of natural human infection, the MIC of amphotericin B was 0.78 mg/L (4). For the isolate of the first imported case in Canada, MICs to fluconazole, 5-FC, itraconazole, and miconazole were 12.5, 0.39, less than 0.195, and less than 0.195 mg/L, respectively (9).

In Vivo Studies

Animal studies have shown that in experimentally infected hamsters, nystatin can prolong survival time. Oral itraconazole in immunosuppressed guinea pigs achieved a cure, even at a low dosage (14). In this animal model of infection a good correlation was established between in vitro and in vivo data. These results indicate that polyenes, 5-FC, itraconazole, and ketoconazole are effective in vitro. Limited data are available for fluconazole, which seemed less active than itraconazole.

Antimicobial Therapy

At the current time, the therapy of choice for invasive infection appears to be intravenous amphotericin B followed by oral itraconazole. Three patients were cured by intravenous amphotericin B alone or in combination with oral 5-FC or oral ketoconazole (3, 7). One patient with delayed treatment because of misdiagnosis died despite receiving a combination of amphotericin B and flucytosine for 9 days (7).

In a review of 44 AIDS patients and 44 non-HIV-infected patients (Table 1), all untreated patients and those with disseminated infections died. Amphotericin B, with or without flucytosine and itraconazole, was effective as well as ketoconazole, but only two patients were treated with ketoconazole. Amphotericin B was given at a total cumulative dose of approximately 40 mg/kg. Itraconazole (400 mg/day) was successful. Maintenance therapy was given successfully to a small number of patients (5).

In one AIDS patient, itraconazole appeared to be superior to fluconazole. The MICs of the isolate by serial microdilution tests according to the NCCLS proposed standard were 6.25 mg/L for fluconazole, 0.008 mg/L for itraconazole, and 0.5 mg/L for amphotericin B (11).

Clinical results obtained in patients generally showed a good correlation with in vitro results, as amphotericin B and itraconazole were highly effective. One patient with a subcutaneous finger infection due to a laboratory accident was re-

ported cured with 20 million units of nystatin given orally for 30 days (5). However because of the poor intestinal absorption of this drug, recovery may in fact have been spontaneous. Another patient treated with a low dosage of nystatin (1.5 million units/day) died on the fourth day of treatment (3).

SPECIAL SITUATIONS
Localized Infection in Immunocompetent Hosts

There are no studies comparing treatment with a single agent and with a combination. Some patients obtained good results with amphotericin B and flucytosine. There is no published experience with itraconazole plus flucytosine.

AIDS

The standard treatment for AIDS patients from Thailand is intravenous amphotericin B at a dose of 0.6 mg/kg/day for 2 weeks followed by oral itraconazole 400 mg/day in 2 divided doses for the next 10 weeks. A survival rate of 80% can be expected. Fever and other signs and symptoms resolved within the first 2 weeks. Delayed treatment can result in death. After the initial period of treatment, patients should be given itraconazole 200 mg/day as maintenance for the rest of their lives (10).

No data are available on the treatment of the localized form of the disease in which spontaneous cure can occur, particularly in nonimmunocompromised hosts. In this setting, itraconazole is a logical first-line treatment. If this drug is not available, ketoconazole seems a good alternative, although few patients have been treated with ketoconazole.

PROPHYLAXIS

A prophylaxis trial with itraconazole is scheduled in the Chang Mai (Thailand) area. Due to the severity of the disease and its high incidence, such an approach seems reasonable. Itraconazole prophylaxis could also decrease the incidence of cryptococcosis and histoplasmosis. However, due to the high incidence of tuberculosis, the concomitant use of rifampin is likely to adversely affect the efficacy of itraconazole by accelerating its metabolism.

TABLE 1 •

Treatment[a]	Outcome[b] AIDS (n = 44)				Outcome Non-AIDS (n = 44)			
	n	fav	death	unkn	n	fav	death	unkn
Ampho B	20	16	1	3	5	4	1	
Ampho B + 5-FC	3	3			6	6		
Itraconazole	10	6	1	3				
Ketoconazole	1	1			1	1		
Untreated or nystatin	9		9		24	3[c]	21[d]	
Not specified	1			1	8			8
Total	44	26	11	7	44	14	22	8

[a] n, number; ampho B, amphotericin B; 5-FC, flucytosine.

[b] fav, favorable; unkn, unknown.

[c] Localized infections.

[d] Disseminated infection.

Traveling in an endemic area is not recommended for severely immunocompromised individuals, particularly AIDS patients.

REFERENCES

1. Boon-Long J, Mekha N, Poonwan N, Kusum M, Mikami Y, Yazawa K, Konyama K. In vitro antifungal activity of the new triazole D 0870 against Penicillium marneffei compared with that of amphotericin B, fluconazole, itraconazole, miconazole and flucytosine. Mycoses 1996;39:453–456.
2. Chariyalertsak S, Sirisanthana T, Supparatpinyo K, Praparattanapan J, Nelson KE. Case-control study of risk factors for Penicillium marneffei infection in human immunodeficiency virus-infected patients in northern Thailand. Clin Infect Dis 1997;24:1080–1086.
3. Deng Z, Ribas JL, Gibson DW, Connor DH. Infection caused by Penicillium marneffei in China and Southeast Asia: review of eighteen published cases and report of four more Chinese cases. Rev Infect Dis 1988;10:640–652.
4. Disalvo AF, Fickling AM, Ajello L. Infection caused by Penicillium marneffei: a description of first natural infection in man. Am J Clin Pathol 1973;60:259–263.
5. Drouhet E. Penicilliosis due to Penicillium marneffei: a new emerging systemic mycosis in AIDS patients travelling or living in Southeast Asia. Review of 44 cases reported in HIV infected patients during the last 5 years compared to 44 cases of non AIDS patients reported over 20 years. J Mycol Med 1993;4:195–224.
6. Duong TA. Infection due to Penicillium marneffei, an emerging pathogen: review of 155 reported cases. Clin Infect Dis 1996;23:125–130.
7. Jayanetra P, Nitiyanant P, Ajello L, Padhye AA, Lolekha S, Atichartakarn V, Vathesatogit P, Sathaphatayavongs B, Prajaktam R. Penicilliosis marneffei in Thailand: report of five human cases. Am J Trop Med Hyg 1984;33:637–644.
8. Sekhon AS, Garg AK, Padhye AA, Hamir Z. In vitro susceptibility of mycelial and yeast forms of Penicillium marneffei to amphotericin B, fluconazole, 5-fluorocytosine and itraconazole. Eur J Epidemiol 1993;9:553–558.
9. Sekhon AS, Stein L, Garg AK, Black WA, Glezos JD, Wong C. Pulmonary penicilliosis marneffei: report of the first imported case in Canada. Mycopathologia 1994;128:3–7.
10. Sirisanthana T. Diagnosis and management of Penicillium marneffei infection [Abstract S.132]. Congress of the International Society for Human and Animal Mycology, Parma, Italy, June 8–13, 1997.
11. Sobottka I, Albrecht H, Mack D, Stellbrink HJ, van Lunzen J, Tintelnot K, Laufs R. Systemic Penicillium marneffei infection in a German AIDS patient. Eur J Clin Microbiol Infect Dis 1996;15:256–259.
12. Supparatpinyo K, Nelson KE, Merz WG, Breslin BJ, Cooper CR, Kamwan C, Sirisanthana T. Response to antifungal therapy by human immunodeficiency virus-infected patients with disseminated Penicillium marneffei infection and in vitro susceptibilities of isolates from clinical specimens. Antimicrob Agents Chemother 1993;37:2407–2411.
13. Supparatpinyo K, Khamwan C, Baosoung V, Nelson KE, Sirisanthana T. Disseminated Penicillium marneffei infection in Southeast Asia. Lancet 1994;344:110–113.
14. Van Cutsem J, Van Gerven F. Activité antifongique in vitro de l'itraconazole sur les champignons filamenteux opportunistes. Traitement de la kératomycose et de la pénicilliose expérimentales. J Mycol Med 1991;118:10–15.

Pneumocystis carinii

●

Catherine F. Decker and Henry Masur

GENERAL DESCRIPTION

With the advancement in transplantation and use of immunosuppressive agents over the past several years, *Pneumocystis carinii* has become appreciated as an important cause of pneumonia in the immunocompromised host. A dramatic increase in incidence of *P. carinii* pneumonia occurred as the acquired immunodeficiency syndrome (AIDS) epidemic grew. More recently, the incidence of *P. carinii* pneumonia in HIV-infected patients is declining (71) because of recent advances in prophylaxis, early detection, and aggressive treatment of acute *P. carinii* (50, 58, 71). However, breakthrough cases of *P. carinii* pneumonia will continue to occur even in those receiving prophylaxis, since no regimen is completely effective (109).

While the inability to cultivate *P. carinii* has continued to interfere with development of new drugs, investigators have learned much about the organism's microbiologic characteristics (63, 94). Traditionally considered a protozoan since originally identified by Chagas in 1906, recent applications of molecular techniques demonstrated that the organism shares many characteristics with fungi, leaving its taxonomy in question (10, 22, 104). Based on morphology, the life cycle of *P. carinii* has been divided into three stages: trophozoite, found outside the cyst and believed to be intermediate between the sporozoite and the cyst; cysts, spherical or crescent-shaped forms; and sporozoite or intracystic bodies, found within the cysts (2). Since the organism cannot be cultured, the life cycle has not been fully elucidated, though it has been suggested that replication occurs through binary fission and excystment.

Serologic data in the United States indicate that most humans become subclinically infected with *P. carinii* during childhood and that this infection is usually well contained by an intact immune system (55, 78, 82). Reactivation of latent infection may occur if the host becomes immunosuppressed from illness or drugs, depending on the duration and severity of immunosuppression.

Based on immunologic abnormalities found in patients who develop *P. carinii* pneumonia, including patients with B cell defects, children with severe combined immunodeficiency disease, premature debilitated infants, oncology patients receiving immunosuppressive drugs, and organ transplant patients (9, 46, 80, 98, 105, 108), both humoral and cell-mediated immunity are important host defenses against this infection (87). Corticosteroid use poses a great risk for development *P. carinii* pneumonia.

The depletion of CD4+ lymphocytes caused by HIV-1 infection strongly correlates with the likelihood of developing *P. carinii* pneumonia (7, 64, 81). *P. carinii* pneumonia has been seen primarily in HIV-1-infected patients with recent CD4 counts under 200 cells/mm^3. Most cases occur at CD4 counts below 100 cells/mm^3. Cases are seen in patients with higher CD4 counts (15): about 10 to 15% of patients develop *P. carinii* pneumonia at CD4 cell counts above 200 cells/mm^3 in the absence of protease inhibitor therapy. It is not yet clear at what CD4 count *P. carinii* will occur in patients with a rise in CD4 count due to therapy with a protease inhibitor.

Presenting symptoms in patients infected with *P. carinii* are usually nonspecific and include fever, nonproductive cough, dyspnea, chest tightness, and shortness of breath (24, 57). AIDS patients tend to have a more indolent course with a longer duration of symptoms and less hypoxia than patients treated with cytotoxic chemotherapy or corticosteroids (57). Physical examination is often unrevealing, as is routine laboratory testing except for nonspecific elevations of serum lactate dehydrogenase levels. The typical chest radiograph shows diffuse and symmetric increased interstitial markings, although 20% may be normal (8, 19, 57).

Definitive diagnosis of *P. carinii* disease requires demonstration of cysts or trophozoites within tissue or body fluids, since the organism cannot be cultured. Before the AIDS epidemic, diagnosis of *P. carinii* pneumonia often required an open lung biopsy. With the development of improved diagnostic techniques, diagnoses can now be established by less invasive methods. Virtually all untreated patients can be diagnosed by careful analysis of bronchoalveolar lavage fluid (3, 33, 66). Induced sputum has been shown to be a sensitive, simple, and noninvasive means of diagnosing *P. carinii* pneumonia and often precludes the need for bronchoscopy (4, 49, 54, 73); reported yields for recovery of the organism range from 70 to 95% at various institutions (4, 54, 83). The development of monoclonal antibodies has resulted in a rapid, sensitive, and easily performed immunofluorescence assay that is more sensitive in detecting *P. carinii* in induced sputum specimens than conventional stains (30, 52, 54, 73).

SUSCEPTIBILITY IN VITRO AND IN VIVO

Since *P. carinii* cannot be cultivated, no susceptibility testing has been done.

ANTIMICROBIAL THERAPY
General

The mainstay antimicrobial agents, dating back to the early 1970s, in the treatment of *P. carinii* pneumonia have been trimethoprim-sulfamethoxazole (TMP-SMX) and intravenous pentamidine. Both are efficacious in the treatment of *P. carinii* pneumonia in patients with AIDS and in other immunocompromised hosts. Overall success rates average 80% and are slightly lower for non-AIDS patients (8, 45, 62, 96) (Table 1).

Currently, TMP-SMX is the most effective antimicrobial agent for the treatment of *P. carinii* pneumonia. Intravenous pentamidine is effective but also toxic. Increasing evidence indicates that other regimens have clinical efficacy, including trimethoprim-dapsone (59, 65, 91), primaquine-clindamycin (89, 91, 107), trimetrexate (95), and atovaquone (43).

TMP-SMX remains the agent of choice for initial therapy of acute *P. carinii* pneumonia (7, 43, 62). If a patient has mild disease (PaO$_2$ > 70) and can tolerate oral medications, TMP-SMX may be given in the dosage of two double-strength tablets (160 mg TMP and 800 mg SMX) every 6 to 8 h. The 8-h regimen is preferred by some clinicians, since toxicity would be expected to be lower than with 6-h dosing. Otherwise, with more severe disease or a patient who is unable to tolerate oral medication, intravenous TMP-SMX (total dose, 20 mg/kg/day) should be given. Total duration of therapy is usually 21 days, but there is no concrete evidence that 3 weeks of therapy is more effective than 2 weeks (13). Toxicity associated with TMP-SMX continues to hinder its use in many patients and occurs more frequently in HIV-infected patients than in patients without HIV infection. Treatment-limiting toxicities usually occur between day 6 and day 10 of therapy. Recent trials suggest that approximately 25% of patients are unable to tolerate a full course of TMP-SMX (36, 97).

Pentamidine is one of several alternative agents to TMP-SMX as initial therapy in patients who are sulfa intolerant. The standard dose of pentamidine is 4 mg/kg/day, given intravenously over at least 1 h for a minimum of 14 to 21 days. Some small studies suggest that a lower dose of 3 mg/kg/day may be

TABLE 1 • **Drug Regimens for Treatment of**
P. carinii Pneumonia

Agent	Total Daily Dose	Route	Interval
Trimethoprim/ sulfamethoxazole	15–20 mg/kg 75–100 mg/kg	i.v. or p.o.	6–8 h
Pentamidine isethionate	4 mg/kg	i.v.	24 h
Trimethoprim plus dapsone	15–20 mg/kg 100 mg	p.o. p.o.	8 h 24 h
Clindamycin plus primaquine	1.35–1.8 g 15–30 mg	p.o./i.v. p.o.	8 h 24 h
Atovaquone	1500 mg	p.o.	8 h
Trimetrexate	45 mg/m^2	i.v.	24 h

less toxic (16, 17), but whether the lower dose is equally effective is unknown. Combination therapy with TMP-SMX and pentamidine is no more effective than either agent used alone and may potentially increase risk of toxicities.

Dapsone as a single agent is inadequate for treatment of *P. carinii* pneumonia, with a failure rate of approximately 40% (67, 92). In combination with trimethoprim (20 mg/kg/day), however, its efficacy is comparable to that of TMP-SMX (60). TMP-dapsone is now a commonly used alternative oral regimen in mild-to-moderate disease in patients intolerant of TMP-SMX. This regimen is often well tolerated, even by patients intolerant of TMP-SMX. This regimen can only be given orally and is therefore not suitable for patients with severe disease or gastrointestinal dysfunction.

The combination of clindamycin and primaquine has emerged as another reasonable alternative for treatment of *P. carinii* pneumonia (89, 107). Investigators report success rates of 80% in open noncomparative trials with patients who are intolerant to, or failed, standard treatment and 75% (44 of 55 patients) in patients not previously treated (89, 107). A recently completed randomized trial found the combination to be comparable in efficacy to TMP-SMX or TMP-dapsone in mild-to-moderate disease (91). Clindamycin-primaquine has also been used as a salvage regimen in patients with *Pneumocystis*-induced respiratory failure (75), although many authorities are reluctant to use an oral agent (i.e., primaquine) in this setting. Primaquine base (30 mg) is the usual dose. Clindamycin is given either orally (300–450 mg every 6–8 h) or intravenously (600–900 mg every 6–8 h).

Atovaquone, another approved oral agent for treating *P. carinii* pneumonia, demonstrated more treatment failures and death than TMP-SMX in mild-to-moderate disease (43).

Recently, oral atovaquone and intravenous pentamidine were found to have similar success rates in mild and moderate *P. carinii* pneumonia in patients who were intolerant to TMP-SMX. Atovaquone was better tolerated, but patients receiving atovaquone more frequently failed to respond to therapy; patients receiving pentamidine had more treatment-limiting adverse drug toxicities (20). Low plasma atovaquone levels are associated with a poor response (43) and are in part due to poor bioavailability of the drug. Recently, a new formulation of atovaquone in suspension has replaced the tablet formulation. Whether this improved bioavailability will translate into improved efficacy remains to be determined, but it is not likely to dramatically improve outcomes.

Trimetrexate in combination with leucovorin, assessed in patients with moderate-to-severe disease, was found very effective but was less effective and was associated with more relapses than TMP-SMX. Its role is as an alternative agent for patients intolerant of TMP-SMX who cannot tolerate, or do not respond to, intravenous pentamidine (95).

Other agents that have been evaluated include piritrexim, an orally bioavailable DHFR inhibitor (25), and difluoromethylornithine (DFMO) (33). Neither is currently available for therapy of *P. carinii* pneumonia. Other agents under current investigation include analogues of primaquine, analogues of pentamidine, albendazole, and echinocandins or pneumocandins.

Drug of Choice

After the diagnosis of *P. carinii* is made, outpatient therapy with an oral agent, preferably TMP-SMX, is recommended for mild to moderately severe disease ($PaO_2 > 70$ mm Hg). Other alternatives for oral outpatient therapy include TMP-dapsone, clindamycin-primaquine, and atovaquone. Patients who are more severely ill with moderate-to-severe disease or who cannot tolerate oral medications should be given intravenous TMP-SMX. Intravenous pentamidine should be administered to sulfa-intolerant patients.

Special Situations

The use of corticosteroids in conjunction with antimicrobial agents has become the standard of care in the treatment of moderate-to-severe *P. carinii* pneumonia in AIDS patients (106). Three randomized controlled studies revealed that corticosteroids significantly decreased the frequency of early deterioration in oxygenation and improved survival in patients who had an initial room air PaO_2 below 70 mm Hg (7, 27, 69). Corticosteroid therapy is not recommended unless the diagnosis of *P. carinii* is confirmed promptly (106) (Table 2). Corticosteroid therapy is logical for other immunosuppressed patients as well.

Alternative Therapy

As the host response to *Pneumocystis* infection becomes better defined, interest in immunotherapy or immunoprophylaxis for *P. carinii* has increased, especially with agents such as interferon-γ (99), monoclonal or polyclonal antibodies against *Pneumocystis* (28, 29, 38, 55, 110), and CD4 lymphocyte infusions (39, 79). Agents that interfere with attachment of the organism to the host cells (85) and those that affect the inflammatory response to *P. carinii* (e.g., various cytokines and surfactants) are also being studied (79). These agents are all experimental and currently have no defined role in treating human disease.

ENDPOINTS FOR MONITORING THERAPY

The median time to respond to therapy is 4 to 6 days. Respiratory rate, arterial oxygenation, ventilation, and temperature should be assessed to determine clinical status. Laboratory tests

---

TABLE 2 • Recommendations for the Use of Corticosteroids in the Treatment of *Pneumocystis carinii* Pneumonia

Population
Patients with acute *P. carinii* pneumonia and $PaO_2 < 70$ mm Hg on room air or alveolar-arterial gradient > 35 mm Hg at presentation

Dosage
Prednisone 40 mg p.o. b.i.d. × 5 days, 20 mg p.o. b.i.d. × 5 days, 20 mg p.o. q.d. × 11 days

Timing
Initiate as adjunctive therapy during first 72 h of antipneumocystis therapy

should be done to assess liver, pancreatic, or renal toxicity. A chest radiograph should be repeated during therapy if patients are not improving. Many patients get worse before clinical improvement is observed. This decline has been attributed to dying organisms, which elicit a more intense inflammatory response during the first week of therapy. A decline of 10 to 30 mm Hg in the partial pressure of oxygen has been associated with initiation of therapy in patients with AIDS (69).

Unfortunately, no factors have been demonstrated to distinguish slow responders from treatment failures, and the initial regimen should probably be continued for at least 5 to 10 days (a minimum of 4 days) before considering a therapeutic change. Fluid status should be monitored carefully, because *P. carinii* pneumonia may increase permeability of alveolar capillary membranes, which can lead to accumulation of interstitial and alveolar fluid and respiratory failure. Concomitant congestive heart failure may also occur. In addition, HIV cardiomyopathy may not be evident until the patient is challenged with large volumes of fluids.

Survival from an episode of *P. carinii* pneumonia correlates with several factors; other than the choice of drug, the most important is the pretreatment oxygenation (8, 21). Other factors that influence outcome include number of tachyzoites, degree of chest radiograph abnormality, severity of hypoxia, magnitude of alveolar-arterial oxygen differences, level of LDH elevation, and degree of lymphopenia (8, 47, 57). For those with an initial PaO_2 above 70 mm Hg while breathing room air, expected response rates are at least 60 to 80% for non-AIDS patients and 80 to 95% for patients with AIDS (8, 45, 96).

Evaluation of response to therapy should be based on clinical and radiographic examination. The use of bronchoscopy to assess response to drug therapy is not helpful, because *P. carinii* is present in bronchoscopy specimens for many weeks after initiation of therapy, even in patients who rapidly improve (100).

PROPHYLAXIS
Underlying Disease of Host

Historically, the successful use of TMP-SMX in controlled trials for primary prevention of *P. carinii* pneumonia in pediatric oncology patients (45) has been the model for development of prophylactic strategies in other immunocompromised hosts at risk for *P. carinii* pneumonia, in particular, HIV-infected patients (26). While prophylaxis for *P. carinii* pneumonia has been well defined in the HIV population and shown to decrease morbidity and mortality, definitive recommendations for chemoprophylaxis for other high-risk groups are lacking and generally have been extrapolated from the experience with HIV-infected patients (62, 110). This is in part because the frequency of *P. carinii* pneumonia varies, depending on the underlying disease and the different immunosuppressive therapies used. Most authorities consider it prudent to institute primary prophylaxis to several groups of patients thought to be at high risk, including those with organ transplants (e.g., lung or heart-lung), lymphoreticular malignancies or solid tumors (e.g., brain tumors), and patients with primary immunodeficiencies (35, 41, 62), but there are no standard guidelines for

these groups (110). Secondary prophylaxis should be instituted for all patients who recovered from an episode of *P. carinii* pneumonia. It is generally recommended that prophylaxis be continued as long as immunosuppression continues.

The use of TMP-SMX for *P. carinii* pneumonia prophylaxis in bone marrow transplant patients has virtually eliminated this infection in this population (112). Prophylaxis is given for at least 6 months and longer in patients with ongoing graft-versus-host disease. The precise interval for prophylaxis depends on the type of bone marrow transplant and the immunosuppressive regimens used.

Indications

Recommendations formulated to prevent *P. carinii* pneumonia in HIV-infected patients are based on large databases. Prophylactic agents should be initiated when an HIV-infected patient's absolute CD4 cell count falls below 200 cells/mm³ (109). This threshold is based largely upon results of the prospective Multicenter AIDS Cohort Study (MACS), a natural history study that began following 1665 HIV-infected men at 6-monthly intervals in 1984 (81). The MACS study also suggests that unexplained persistent daily fever above 37.7°C for more than 2 weeks or oropharyngeal candidiasis (unrelated to antibiotic or steroid use) indicates enhanced susceptibility to *P. carinii*, independent of CD4 count. Any patient who develops an opportunistic infection regardless of measured CD4 cell count should also receive *P. carinii* pneumonia prophylaxis (81). Secondary prophylaxis is indicated for patients with a history of *P. carinii* pneumonia, as there is a substantial rate of subsequent episodes without prophylaxis.

In patients with malignancy or organ transplants, observational databases provide data about when to initiate prophylaxis, and how long to continue it.

Drugs of Choice

Regimens for prophylaxis for *P. carinii* pneumonia are given in Table 3. TMP-SMX is the preferred agent in patients who can tolerate it, because it is more effective than any other regimen in preventing *P. carinii* pneumonia in patients with AIDS and in other patient populations (7, 36, 84, 90, 97). The relative efficacy and toxicity of TMP-SMX as primary and secondary prophylactic agents has been assessed in randomized prospective trials. In a European trial evaluating primary prophylaxis, either high-dose (1 DS/day) or low-dose (1 SS/day) TMP-SMX was found significantly more effective in preventing *P. carinii* than aerosolized pentamidine (97). The rate of discontinuation of study drug because of toxicity was higher in the TMP-SMX groups than in the placebo group. The incidence and types of adverse reactions were similar in both TMP-SMX groups, but toxic effects occurred significantly sooner in the group receiving the higher dose. These adverse events may be partially dose related (97).

In a large trial (ACTG 081), 843 patients were randomized to TMP-SMX (1 DS tablet twice daily), dapsone (50 mg twice daily), or aerosolized pentamidine (300 mg once monthly). Fewer episodes of *P. carinii* pneumonia occurred among patients receiving TMP-SMX than in the other two arms when

TABLE 3 • **Drug Regimens for Prophylaxis for *P. carinii* Pneumonia**

Agent	Total Daily Dose	Route	Interval
Trimethoprim/	160/800 mg (DS)	Oral	Daily
sulfamethoxazole	160/800 mg (DS)	Oral	Twice daily
	80/400 mg (SS)	Oral	(3× q.d.) Daily
Pentamidine	300 mg	Aerosol (Respigard)	Monthly
Dapsone	100 mg	Oral	Daily
Pyrimethamine	75 mg	Oral	Weekly
plus dapsone	200 mg	Oral	

patients with CD4+ counts below 100 cells/mm^3 were considered but not when patients with higher CD4+ counts were assessed. In this trial, dapsone appeared more efficacious than aerosolized pentamidine. Dapsone given at doses of 50 mg/day or less was not as effective as 50 mg twice daily (7).

A secondary prophylaxis study in the United States involved 310 patients randomly assigned to administration of aerosolized pentamidine by a Respirgard II nebulizer or to one oral double-strength tablet of TMP-SMX daily (36). When analyzed by the intent-to-treat method, the recurrence rate of *P. carinii* pneumonia was significantly higher among patients assigned to aerosolized pentamidine (18%) than among those that received TMP-SMX (4%). As expected, many patients who received TMP-SMX (27%) experienced sufficient toxicity to discontinue the agent. Most authorities recommended TMP-SMX for both primary and secondary prophylaxis (109).

Although fraught with potential toxicities described above, TMP-SMX has advantages not provided by aerosolized pentamidine, including low cost, oral preparation, and probable protective effect against disseminated *Pneumocystis* infection. In addition, because of its broad spectrum of antimicrobial activity, it offers protection against toxoplasmosis and against *Haemophilus influenzae* and *Streptococcus pneumoniae* (12, 36).

Aerosolized pentamidine delivered by the Fisons (Rochester, NY) hand-held ultrasonic nebulizer at a dose of 60 mg every 2 weeks (after five loading doses) was highly effective for prophylaxis in a prospective, randomized trial (68, 72). Other delivery systems have not been as extensively evaluated and cannot be recommended. Aerosolized pentamidine is usually well tolerated when delivered by the Respirgard II or the Fisons nebulizer in the indicated dosing regimens. Coughing or wheezing occurs in 30 to 40% of patients, but this reaction may be diminished or prevented by administration of a β-adrenergic agonist such as albuterol (18, 59, 68, 72). If aerosolized pentamidine is delivered by the Fisons nebulizer at doses indicated above, it is similarly well tolerated. Bronchospasm rarely necessitates discontinuation of prophylaxis with aerosolized pentamidine treatment. Patients with reactive airway disease or bullous lung disease may not distribute aerosolized pentamidine effectively and thus may not obtain maximum protection. There have been reports of disseminated pneumocystosis in patients receiving aerosolized pentamidine for prophylaxis (37).

There is increasing concern about outbreaks of *Mycobacterium tuberculosis* among health care workers and HIV-infected patients, associated with the coughing induced by aerosol pentamidine. Before administering aerosolized pentamidine, all patients should be screened for tuberculosis, and health care workers should follow guidelines provided by the Centers for Disease Control and Prevention to minimize the risk of spread of tuberculosis to other patients and health care workers (5, 14). Ideally, aerosolized pentamidine should be administered in individual booths or rooms with negative-pressure ventilation and direct exhaust to the outside. After administration of aerosolized pentamidine, patients should not return to common waiting areas until coughing has subsided.

Dapsone has received attention as prophylaxis because it is oral, convenient, and inexpensive. In addition to the data on dapsone alone, weekly doses of dapsone (200 mg) and pyrimethamine (75 mg) demonstrate that the agents are well tolerated but less effective than TMP-SMX (58). Dapsone-pyrimethamine has efficacy as a prophylactic regimen against *P. carinii* pneumonia similar to that of aerosol pentamidine but less effective than TMP-SMX. This has been assessed in a daily regimen (dapsone 50 mg/day orally plus pyrimethamine 75 mg weekly) and in a weekly regimen (dapsone 200 mg plus pyrimethamine 75 mg) (31, 77). It is not clear if pyrimethamine truly adds potency, given the results of the ACTG 081 study mentioned above (7).

Alternative Regimens

Other potential prophylactic agents that have been used empirically or evaluated in small clinical trials include pyrimethamine-sulfadoxine (Fansidar), trimethoprim-dapsone, primaquine-clindamycin, and atovaquone. Although the other agents probably have some efficacy, data dealing with these forms of prophylaxis are limited and do not yet warrant recommending any of these agents, except in patients who require an alternative to TMP-SMX or aerosolized pentamidine.

CONTROVERSIES

Use of TMP-SMX desensitization or, more appropriately, gradual dose escalation has been controversial in terms of prophylaxis or therapy. In uncontrolled studies, some investigators have successfully desensitized patients to TMP-SMX in attempts to reduce the likelihood of adverse reactions in patients with a history of hypersensitivity-like reaction (1, 11, 32, 88). At least two randomized trials assessing desensitization as a method of improving long-term tolerance have been completed in patients with HIV infection. Both suggest that gradual dose escalation is useful on the basis of the fraction of patients still receiving TMP-SMX after several months.

Severe systemic reactions that resemble anaphylaxis or septic shock have been reported in HIV-infected patients who are rechallenged with TMP-SMX after experiencing toxicity within the previous 6 to 8 weeks. Although its mechanism remains unclear, the reaction has features of cytokine-mediated effects that are not IgE mediated (48, 61). Clinicians should be aware that this syndrome may be due to TMP-SMX rather than some other process.

REFERENCES

1. Absar N, Daneshuar H, Beakk G. Desensitization to trimethoprim/sulfamethoxazole in HIV-infected patients. J Allergy Clin Immunol 1994;93:1001–1005.
2. Barton EGJ, Campbell WGJ. *Pneumocystis carinii* in lungs of rats treated with cortisone acetate: ultrastructural observations relating to the life cycle. Am J Pathol 1969;54:209–236.
3. Baughman RP. Current methods of diagnosis. In: Walzer PD, ed. *Pneumocystis carinii* pneumonia. New York: Marcel Dekker, 1994:381–401.
4. Bigby TO, Margolskiii D, Curtis JL, Michael PF, Sheppard D, Hadley WK, Hopewell PC. The usefulness of induced sputum in the diagnosis of *Pneumocystis carinii* pneumonia in patients with the acquired immunodeficiency syndrome. Am Rev Respir Dis 1986;133:515–518.
5. Blumberg HM, Watkins DL, Berschling JD, Antle A, Moore P, White N, Hunter M, Green B, Ray SM, McGowan JE. Preventing the nosocomial transmission of tuberculosis. Ann Intern Med 1995;122:658–663.
6. Blum RN, Laurel LA, Gaggini LC, Cohn DL. Comparative trial of dapsone versus trimethoprim/sulfamethoxazole for primary prophylaxis of *Pneumocystis carinii* pneumonia. J Acquir Immune Defic Syndr 1992;5:341–347.
7. Bozzette SA, Sattler FR, Chiu J, Wu AW, Gluckstein D, Kemper C. A controlled trial of early adjunctive treatment with corticosteroids for *Pneumocystis carinii* pneumonia in acquired immunodeficiency syndrome. N Engl J Med 1990;323:1451–1457.
8. Brenner M, Ognibene FP, Lack EE, Simmons JT, Suffredini AF, Lane HC, Fauci AS, Parrillo JE, Shelhamer JH, Masur H. Prognostic factors and life expectancy of patients with acquired immunodeficiency syndrome and *Pneumocystis carinii* pneumonia. Am Rev Respir Dis 1987;136:1199–1206.
9. Browne MJ. Excess prevalence of *P. carinii* pneumonia in patients treated for lymphoma with combination chemotherapy. Ann Intern Med 1986;104:338–344.
10. Cailliez JC, Seguy N, Denis CM. *Pneumocystis carinii:* an atypical fungal microorganism. J Med Vet Mycol 1996;34:227–239.
11. Carr A, Penny R, Cooper DA. Efficacy and safety of rechallenge with low-dose trimethoprim-sulfamethoxazole in previously hypersensitive HIV-infected patients. AIDS 1993;7:65–71.
12. Carr A, Tindall, Brew BJ, Bruw BJ, Marriott DJ, Harkness JL, Penny R, Cooper DA. Low-dose trimethoprimsulfamethoxazole prophylaxis for toxoplasmic encephalitis in patients with AIDS. Ann Intern Med 1992;117:106–111.
13. Catterall JR, Potasman I, Remington JS. *Pneumocystis carinii* pneumonia in the patient with AIDS. Chest 1985;66:758–762.
14. Centers for Disease Control. Guidelines for preventing the transmission of mycobacterium tuberculosis in health-care settings, with special focus on HIV-related issues. MMWR 1990;39 (RR-17):1–29.
15. Chu Sy, Hanson DL, Ciesielski C, Ward JW. Prophylaxis against *Pneumocystis carinii* pneumonia at higher CD+ T-cell counts [Letter]. JAMA 1995;273:848.
16. Conte JE Jr, Chernoff D, Feigel DW Jr, Joseph P, McDonald C, Golden JA. Intravenous or inhaled pentamidine for treating *Pneumocystis carinii* pneumonia in AIDS. Ann Intern Med 1990;113:203–209.
17. Conte JE Jr, Hollander H. Golden JA. Inhaled pentamidine or reduced dose intravenous pentamidine for *Pneumocystis carinii* pneumonia. A pilot study. Ann Intern Med 1987;107:495–498.
18. Conte JE Jr, Upton RA, Phelps RT, Wofsy CB, Zurlinden E, Lin ET. Use of a specific and sensitive assay to determine pentamidine pharmacokinetics in patients with AIDS. J Infect Dis 1986; 154:923–929.
19. DeLorenzo LJ, Huang CT, Maguire G, Stone DJ. Roentgenographic patterns of *Pneumocystis carinii* pneumonia in 104 patients with AIDS. Chest 1987;91:323–327.
20. Dohn MN, Weinberg WG, Torres RA, Follansbee SE, Caldwell PT, Scott JD, Gathe JC, Haghighat DP, Sampson JH, Spotkov J, Deresinski SC, Meyer RD, Lancaster DJ, and the Atovaquone Study Group. Oral atovaquone compared with intravenous pentamidine for *Pneumocystis carinii* pneumonia in patients with AIDS. Ann Intern Med 1994;121:174–180.
21. Dohn MN, Baughman RP, Vigdorth EM, Frame D. Equal survival rates for first, second and third episodes of *Pneumocystis carinii* pneumonia in patients with AIDS. Arch Intern Med 1992;152:2465–2470.
22. Edman JC, Kovacs JA, Masur H, Santi DV, Elwood HJ, Sogin ML. Ribosomal RNA sequence shows *Pneumocystis carinii* to be a member of the fungi. Nature 1988;334:519–522.
23. Elvin KM, Bjorkman A, Linder E, Heurlin W, Hjerpe A. *Pneumocystis carinii* pneumonia: detection of parasites in sputum and bronchoalveolar lavage fluid by monoclonal antibodies. Br Med J (Clin Res) 1988;297:381–384.
24. Engleberg LA, Lerner CW, Trapper ML. Clinical features of pneumocystis pneumonia in the acquired immune deficiency syndrome. Am Rev Respir Dis 1984;130:669–674.
25. Falloon J, Kovacs J, Allegra C. A pilot study of piritrexim (PIX) with leucovorin (LCV) for the treatment of pneumocystis pneumonia [Abstract THB399]. Presented at the Sixth International Conference on AIDS, San Francisco, 1990.
26. Fischl MA, Dickinson GM, LaVoFe L. Safety and efficacy of sulfamethoxazole and trimethoprim chemoprophylaxis for *Pneumocystis carinii* pneumonia in AIDS. JAMA 1988;259: 1185–1189.
27. Gagnon S, Botta AM, Fischl MA, Daier H. Kirksey OW, La Voie L. Corticosteroids as adjunctive therapy for severe *Pneumocystis carinii* pneumonia in the acquired immunodeficiency syndrome—a double blind, placebo-controlled trial. N Engl J Med 1990;323:1444–1450.
28. Gigliotti F, Hughes WT. Passive immunoprophylaxis with specific monoclonal antibody confers partial protection against *Pneumocystis carinii* pneumonitis in animal models. J Clin Invest 1988;81:1666–1668.
29. Gigliotti F, Stokes DC, Cheatham AB, Davis DS, Hughes WT. Development of murine monoclonal antibodies to *Pneumocystis carinii*. J Infect Dis 1986;145:315–322.
30. Gill VJ, Evans G. Stock F, Parillo JE, Masur H, Kovacs JA. Detection of *Pneumocystis carinii* by fluorescent-antibody stain using a combination of three monoclonal antibodies. J Clin Microbiol 1987;25:1837–1840.
31. Girard PM, Landman R, Gaudebout C, Olivares R, Saimot AG, Jelazko P, Gaudebout C, Certain A, Boue F, Bouvet E, Lecompte T, Coulaud JP, and the PRIO Study Group. Dapsone-pyrimethamine compared with aerosolized pentamidine as primary prophylaxis against *Pneumocystis carinii* pneumonia and toxoplasmosis in HIV infection. N Engl J Med 1993;328:1514–1520.
32. Gluckstein D, Ruskin J. Rapid oral desensitization to trimethoprim-sulfamethoxazole (TMP-SMZ): use in prophylaxis for

Pneumocystis carinii pneumonia in patients with AIDS who were previously intolerant to TMP-SMZ. Clin Infect Dis 1995; 20:849–853.

33. Golden JA, Sjoerdsma A, Santi DV. *Pneumocystis carinii* pneumonia treated with alpha-difluoromethylornithine. West J Med 1984;141:613–623.

34. Goldman JA, Hollander H, Stulberg MS. Bronchoalveolar lavage as the exclusive diagnostic modality in *Pneumocystis carinii* pneumonia. Chest 1986;90:18–22.

35. Gryzan S, Paradis IL, Zeevi A. Unexpectedly high incidence of *Pneumocystis carinii* infection after lung-heart transplantation. Am Rev Respir Dis 1988;137:1268–1274.

36. Hardy WD, Reinberg J, Finkelstein DM, Power ME, He W, Kaczka C, Frame PT, Holmes M, Waskin H, Fass RJ, Powderly WG, Steigbigel RT, Zuger A, Holzman RS, for the AIDS Clinical Trials Group. A controlled trial of trimethoprim-sulfamethoxazole or aerosolized pentamidine for secondary prophylaxis of *Pneumocystis carinii* pneumonia in patients with the acquired immunodeficiency syndrome: AIDS Clinical Trials Group 021. N Engl J Med 1992;327:1842–1848.

37. Hardy WD, Northfelt DW, Drake TA. Fatal disseminated pneumocystosis in patient with acquired immunodeficiency syndrome receiving prophylactic aerosolized pentamidine. Am J Med 1989;87:329–331.

38. Harmsen AG, Chen W, Gigliotti F. Active immunity to *Pneumocystis carinii* reinfection in T-cell-depleted mice. Infect Immun 1995;63:2391–2395.

39. Harmsen AG, Stankiewicz M. Requirement for CD4+ cells in resistance to *Pneumocystis carinii* pneumonia in mice. J Exp Med 1990;172:937–945.

40. Haverkos HW. Assessment of therapy for *Pneumocystis carinii* pneumonia: PCP therapy project group. Am J Med 1984;76: 501–508.

41. Henson JW, Jalaj JK, Walker RW, Stover DE, Fels AOS. *Pneumocystis carinii* pneumonia in patients with primary brain tumors. Arch Neurol 1991;48:406–409.

42. Hirschel B, Lazzarin A, Chopard P, Opravil M, Furrer HJ, Ruttimann S, Vernazza P, Chave JP, Ancarani F, Gabriel V, Heald A, King R, Malinverni, Martin JL, Mermillod B, Nicod L, Simoni L, Vivirito MC, Zerboni R, and the Swiss Group for Clinical Studies on AIDS. A controlled study of inhaled pentamidine for primary prevention of *Pneumocystis carinii* pneumonia. N Engl J Med 1991;324:1079–1083.

43. Hughes WT, Leoung G, Kramer F, Bozzette SA, Safrin S, Frame P, Clumeck N, Masur H, Lancaster D, Chan C, Lavelle J, Rosenstock J, Falloon J, Feinberg H, LaFon S, Rogers M, Sattler F. Comparison of atovaquone (566C80) with trimethoprim-sulfamethoxazole to treat *Pneumocystis carinii* pneumonia in patients with AIDS. N Engl J Med 1993;328:1521–1527.

44. Hughes WT, Smith BL. Efficacy of diaminodiphenylsulfone and other drugs in murine *Pneumocystis carinii* pneumonitis. Antimicrob Agents Chemother 1984;26:436–440.

45. Hughes WT, Kuhn S, Chaudhary S, Feldman S, Verzosa S, Aur RJA, Pratt C, George SL. Successful chemoprophylaxis for *Pneumocystis carinii* pneumonitis. N Engl J Med 1977;297:1419–1426.

46. Hughes WT. Intensity of immunosuppressive treatment and the incidence of *P. carinii* pneumonitis. Cancer 1975;36: 2004–2009.

47. Kales CP, Murren JR, Torres RA, Crocco JA. Early predictors of in hospital mortality for *Pneumocystis carinii* pneumonia in the acquired immunodeficiency syndrome. Arch Intern Med 1987;147:1413–1417.

48. Kelly JW, Dolley DP, Lattuada CP, Smith CE. A severe unusual reaction to trimethoprim-sulfamethoxazole in patients infected with human immunodeficiency virus. Clin Infect Dis 1992;14: 1034–1039.

49. Kirsch CM, Jensen WA, Kagawa FT, Azzi RL. Analysis of induced sputum for the diagnosis of recurrent *Pneumocystis carinii* pneumonia. Chest 1992;102:1152–1154.

50. Kovacs JA, Masur H. Prophylaxis for *Pneumocystis carinii* pneumonia in patients infected with human immunodeficiency virus. Clin Infect Dis 1992;14:1005–1009.

51. Kovacs JA, Allegra CJ, Beaver J, Boar M, Lewis M, Parrillo JE, Chabner B, Masur H. Characterization of de novo folate synthesis in *Pneumocystis carinii* and *Toxoplasma gondii*. Potential utilization for screening therapeutic agents. J Infect Dis 1989; 160:312–320.

52. Kovacs JA, Halpern JL, Lundgren B, Swan JC, Parillo JE, Masur H. Monoclonal antibodies to *Pneumocystis carinii*: identification of specific antigens and characterization of antigenic differences between rat and human isolates. J Infect Dis 1989;159:60–70.

53. Kovacs JA, Masur H (moderator), Lane HC, Allegra CA, Edman JC. Pneumocystis pneumonia: from bench to clinic. Ann Intern Med 1989;111:813–826.

54. Kovacs JA, Ng VL, Masur H, Leoung G, Hadley WK, Evans G, Lane HC, Ognibene FP, Shelhamer J, Parrillo JE, Gill VJ. Diagnosis of *Pneumocystis carinii* pneumonia: improved detection in sputum with use of monoclonal antibodies. N Engl J Med 1988;318:589–593.

55. Kovacs JA, Halpern JL, Swan JC, Moss J, Parillo JE, Masur H. Identification of antigens and antibodies specific for *Pneumocystis carinii*. J Immunol 1988;140:2023–2031.

56. Kovacs JA, Gill V, Swan JC, Ognibene FP, Shelhamer J, Parrillo JE, Masur H. Prospective evaluation of a monoclonal antibody in the diagnosis of *Pneumocystis carinii* pneumonia. Lancet 1986; 2:1–3.

57. Kovacs JA, Hiemenz JW, Macher AM, Stover D, Murray HW, Shelhamer J, Lane HC, Urmacher C, Hong C, Longo DL, Parker MM, Natanson C, Parrillo JE, Fauci AS, Pizzo PA, Masur H. *Pneumocystis carinii* pneumonia: a comparison between patients with the acquired immunodeficiency syndrome and patients with other immunodeficiencies. Ann Intern Med 1984;100:663–671.

58. Lavelle J, Falloon J, Morgan A, Graziani A, Arakaki D, Byrne A, Pierce P, Masur H, MacGregor R. Weekly dapsone and dapsone/pyrimethamine for pneumocystis pneumonia prophylaxis [Abstract 233]. Presented at the VII International conference on AIDS, Florence, Italy, 1991.

59. Leoung GS, Feigel DW Jr, Montgomery AB, Corkery K, Wardlaw L, Adams M, Busch D, Gordon S, Jacobson M, Volkerding P, Abrams D. Aerosolized pentamidine for prophylaxis against *Pneumocystis carinii* pneumonia—the San Francisco community prophylaxis trial. N Engl J Med 1990;323:769–775.

60. Leoung GS, Mills J, Hopewell PC, Hughes W, Wofsy C. Dapsone-trimethoprim for *Pneumocystis carinii* pneumonia in the acquired immunodeficiency syndrome. Ann Intern Med 1986; 105:45–48.

61. Martin GJ, Paparello SF, Decker CF. A severe systemic reaction to trimethoprim-sulfamethoxazole in a patient infected with the human immunodeficiency virus. Clin Infect Dis 1992;16:175–176.

62. Masur H. Drug therapy: prevention and treatment of pneumocystis pneumonia. N Engl J Med 1992;327:1853–1860.

63. Masur H, Lane HC, Kovacs JA, Allegra J, Edman JC. Advances in pneumocystis pneumonia: from bench to clinic. Ann Intern Med 1989;111:813–826.

64. Masur H, Ognibene FP, Yarchoan R, Shelhamer JH, Baird BF, Travis W, Suffredini AF, Deyton L, Kovacs JA, Falloon J, Davey R, Polis M, Metcalf J, Baseler M, Wesly R, Gill VJ, Fauci AS, Lane HC. CD4 counts as predictors of opportunistic pneumonias in human immunodeficiency virus (HIV) infection. Ann Intern Med 1989;111:223–231.

65. Medina I, Mills J, Leoung G, Hopewell PC, Lee B, Modin G, Benowitz, Wofsy CB. Oral therapy for *Pneumocystis carinii* pneumonia in the acquired immunodeficiency syndrome—a controlled trial of trimethoprim-sulfamethoxazole versus trimethoprim-dapsone. N Engl J Med 1990;323:776–782.

66. Meduri GU, Stover DE, Greeno RA, Nash T, Zaman MB. Bilateral bronchoalveolar lavage in the diagnosis of opportunistic pulmonary infections. Chest 1991;100:1272–1276.

67. Mills J, Leoung G, Medina I, Hopewell PC, Hughes WT, Wofsy C. Dapsone treatment of *Pneumocystis carinii* pneumonia in the acquired immunodeficiency syndrome. Antimicrob Agents Chemother 1988;32:1057–1060.

68. Montaner JSG, Lawson LM, Gervais A, Hyland RH, Chan CK, Falutz JM, Renzi PM, McFadden D, Rachlis AR, Fong IW, Garber GE, Simor A, Gilmore N, Fanning M, Taylor D, Martel AY, Schlech WF, Schecter MT. Aerosol pentamidine for secondary prophylaxis of AIDS-related *Pneumocystis carinii* pneumonia: a randomized placebo-controlled study. Ann Intern Med 1991; 114:948–953.

69. Montaner JSG, Lawson LM, Levitt N. Beizberg A, Schechter MT, Ruedy J. Corticosteroids prevent early deterioration in patients with moderately severe *Pneumocystis carinii* pneumonia and the acquired immunodeficiency syndrome (AIDS). Ann Intern Med 1990;113:14–20.

70. Montgomery AB, Eidson RE, Sattler F, Corkery KJ. Aerosolized pentamidine vs. trimethoprim-sulfamethoxazole for acute *Pneumocystis carinii* pneumonia (PCP): a randomized double-blind trial [Abstract ThB395]. Presented at the Sixth International Conference on AIDS, San Francisco, 1990.

71. Moore RD, Chaisson RE. Natural history of opportunistic disease in an HIV-infected urban clinical cohort. Ann Intern Med 1996;124:663–642.

72. Murphy RL, Lavelle JF, Allan JD, Gordin FM, Supliss R, Boswell SL, Waskin HA, Davies SF, Graziano FM, Saag MS, Walter JB, Crane LR, Macdonnell KB, Hodges TL, Pierce PF. Aerosol pentamidine prophylaxis following *Pneumocystis carinii* pneumonia in AIDS patients: results of blinded dose-comparison study using an ultrasonic nebulizer. Am J Med 1991;90:418–426.

73. Ng VL, Virani NA, Chaisson RE, Yaiko DM, Sphar HT, Cabrian K, Rolling Sn Charache P, Krieger M, Hadly K, Hopewell PC. Rapid detection of *Pneumocystis carinii* using a direct fluorescent monoclonal antibody stain. J Clin Microbiol 1990;28: 2228–2233.

74. Ng VL, Garner I, Weymouth LA, Goodman CD, Hopewell PC, Hadley WK. The use of mucolysed induced sputum for the identification of pulmonary pathogens associated with human immunodeficiency virus infection. Arch Pathol Lab Med 1989;113:488–493.

75. Noskin GA, Murphy R, Black JR, Phair JP. Salvage therapy with clindamycin/primaquine for *Pneumocystis carinii* pneumonia. Clin Infect Dis 1992;14:183–188.

76. O'Doherty MJ, Thomas S. Page C, Barlow D, Bradbeer C, Nunan TD, Bateman NA. Differences in relative efficacy of nebulizers for pentamidine administration. Lancet 1988;2:1283–1286.

77. Opravil M, Hirschel B, Lazzarin A, Heald A, Pechere M, Rutti-mann S, Iten A, von Overbeck J, Oertle D, Praz G, Vuitton DA, Mainini F, Luthy R. Once-weekly administration of dapsone/pyrimethamine vs. aerosolized pentamidine as combined prophylaxis for *Pneumocystis carinii* pneumonia and toxoplasmic encephalitis in human immunodeficiency virus-infected patients. Clin Infect Dis 1995;20:531–541.

78. Peglow SL, Smulian AG, Linke MJ, Pogue CL, Nurre S, Crisler J, Phair J, Gold JWM, Armstrong D, Walzer PD. Serologic responses to *Pneumocystis carinii* antigens in health and disease. J Infect Dis 1990;161:296–306.

79. Pesanti EL. Interaction of cytokines and alveolar cells with *Pneumocystis carinii* in vitro. J Infect Dis 1991;163:611–616.

80. Peters SE, Prakash UBS. *Pneumocystis carinii* pneumonia: review of 53 cases. Am J Med 1985;82:73–78.

81. Phair J, Munoz A, Detels R, Kaslow R, Rinaldo C, Saah A, and the Multicenter AIDS Cohort Study Group. The risk of *Pneumocystis carinii* pneumonia among men infected with HIV-1. N Engl J Med 1990;322:1607–1608.

82. Pifer LL, Hughes WT, Stagno S, Wood D. *Pneumocystis carinii* infection: evidence for high prevalence in normal and immunosuppressed children. Pediatrics 1978;61:35–41.

83. Pitchenik AE, Ganjei P, Torres A, Evans DA, Rubin E, Baier H. Sputum examination for the diagnosis of *Pneumocystis carinii* pneumonia in the acquired immunodeficiency syndrome. Am Rev Respir Dis 1986;33:226–229.

84. Podzamczer D, Salazar A, Jiminez J, Consiglio E, Santin M, Casnova A, Rufi G, Gudiol F. Intermittent trimethoprim-sulfamethoxazole compared with dapsone-pyrimethamine for the simultaneous primary prophylaxis of Pneumocystis pneumonia and toxoplasmosis in patients infected with HIV. Ann Intern Med 1995;122:755–761.

85. Pottratz ST, Martin WJ II. Role of fibronectin in *Pneumocystis carinii* attachment to cultured lung cells. J Clin Invest 1990;85: 351–356.

86. Price RA, Hughes WT. Histopathology of *Pneumocystis carinii* infestation and infection in malignant disease in childhood. Hum Pathol 1974;5:737–752.

87. Roths JB, Sidman CL. Single and combined humoral and cell mediated immunotherapy of *Pneumocystis carinii* pneumonia in immunodeficient scid mice. Infect Immun 1993;61:1641–1649.

88. Rubin RH, Iwamoto GK, Richerson HB, Flaherty JP. Trimethoprim-sulfamethoxazole desensitization in the acquired immunodeficiency syndrome [Letter]. Ann Intern Med 1987;106:355.

89. Ruf B, Rohde I, Pohle HD. Efficacy of clindamycin-primaquine vs. trimethoprim-sulfamethoxazole in primary treatment of *Pneumocystis carinii* pneumonia. Eur J Clin Microbiol Infect Dis 1991;10:207–210.

90. Saah AJ, Hoover DR, Peng Y, Phair JP, Visscher B, Kingsley LA, Schrager LK, for the Multicenter AIDS Cohort Study. Predictors for failure of *Pneumocystis carinii* pneumonia prophylaxis. JAMA 1995;273:1197–1202.

91. Safrin S, Finkelstein DM, Feinberg J, Frame P, Simpson G, Wu A, Cheung T, Soeiro R, Hojczk P, Black JR. Comparison of three regimens for treatment of mild to moderate *Pneumocystis carinii* pneumonia in patients with AIDS. A double-blind, randomized, trial of oral trimethoprim-sulfamethoxazole, dapsone-trimethoprim, and clindamycin-primaquine. ACTG 108. Ann Intern Med 1996;124:792–802.

92. Safrin S, Sattler FR, Lee BL, Young T, Bill R, Boylar CT, Mills J. Dapsone as a single agent is suboptimal therapy for *Pneumocystis carinii* pneumonia. J Acquir Immune Defic Syndr 1991;4: 244–249.

93. Salmon D, Saba J, Fontbonne JP, Aboulker JP, Schwartz D, Vilde Anrs JL, and French League for Prevention of Infectious Diseases. Dapsone vs. pentamidine aerosols for secondary prophylaxis for *Pneumocystis carinii* pneumonia (PCP) in AIDS patients [Abstract 1474]. Presented at the Interscience Conference on Antimicrobial Agents and Chemotherapy, Anaheim, California, 1992.

94. Sattler FR, Walzer PD. *Pneumocystis carinii.* Baillieres Clin Infect Dis 1995;2:3.

95. Sattler FR, Frame P, Davis R, Nichols L, Shelton B, Akil B, Baughman R, Hughlett C, Weiss W, Boylen CT, van der Horst C, Black J, Powderly W, Steigbiegel RT, Leedom JM, Masur H, Feinberg J, and the AIDS Clinical Trials Group 029/031 Research Team. Comparison of trimetrexate with leucovorin versus trimethoprim-sulfamethoxazole for moderate to severe episodes of *Pneumocystis carinii* pneumonia in patients with AIDS. J Infect Dis 1994;170:165–172.

96. Sattler FR, Cowan R, Nielsen DM, Ruskin J. Trimethoprim-sulfamethoxazole compared with pentamidine for treatment of *Pneumocystis carinii* pneumonia in the acquired immunodeficiency syndrome: a prospective, noncrossover study. Ann Intern Med 1988;109:280–287.

97. Schneider MME, Hoepelman AIM, Eertlnck Schattenkerk JKM, Nielsen TL, Van Der Graaf Y, Frissen JPHJ, Van Der Ender IME, Kolsters AFP, Borleffs JCC, and the Dutch AIDS Treatment Group. A controlled trial of aerosolized pentamidine or trimethoprim-sulfamethoxazole as primary prophylaxis against *Pneumocystis carinii* pneumonias in patients with human immunodeficiency virus infection. N Engl J Med 1992; 327:1836–1841.

98. Sepkowitz KA, Brown AE, Telzak EE, Gottlieb S, Armstrong D. *Pneumocystis carinii* pneumonia among patients without AIDS at a cancer hospital. JAMA 1992;267:832–837.

99. Shear HL, Valladares G, Narchi MA. Enhanced treatment of *Pneumocystis carinii* pneumonia in rats with interferon-gamma and reduced doses of trimethoprim/sulfamethoxazole. J Acquir Immune Defic Syndr 1990;3:943–948.

100. Shelhamer JH, Ognibene FP, Macher AM, Tuazon C, Steiss R, Longo D, Kovacs JA, Parker MM, Natanson C, Lane HC, Fauci AS, Parrillo JE, Masur H. Persistence of *Pneumocystis carinii* in lung tissue of acquired immunodeficiency syndrome patients treated for pneumocystis pneumonia. Am Rev Respir Dis 1984; 130:1161–1165.

101. Small CB, Harris CA, Friedland GH, Klein RS. The treatment of *Pneumocystis carinii* pneumonia in the acquired immunodeficiency syndrome. Arch Intern Med 1985;145:837–840.

102. Soo Hoo GW, Mohsenifar Z, Meyer RD. Inhaled or intravenous pentamidine therapy for *Pneumocystis carinii* pneumonia in AIDS: a randomized trial. Ann Intern Med 1990;113:199–203.

103. Stover DE, White DA, Romano PA, Gellene RA. Diagnosis of pulmonary disease in acquired immune deficiency syndrome (AIDS): role of bronchoscopy and bronchoalveolar lavage. Am Rev Respir Dis 1984;180:659–662.

104. Stringer SL, Hudson K, Blase MA. Sequence from ribosomal RNA of *Pneumocystis carinii* compared to those of four fungi suggests an ascomycetous affinity. J Protozool 1989;36(Suppl): 1S–16S.

105. Sugimoto H, Uchida H, Akiyama N, Najo T, Tomikawa S, Mita K, Beck Y, Inoune S, Watanabe K, Nakayana Y, Sato K, Otsubs O. Improved survival of renal allograft recipients with *Pneumocystis carinii* pneumonia by early diagnosis and treatment. Transplant Proc 1992;24:1556–1558.

106. The National Institutes of Health–University of California Expert Panel for Corticosteroids as Adjunctive Therapy for Pneumocystis Pneumonia. Consensus statement on the use of corticosteroids as adjunctive therapy for pneumocystis pneumonia in the acquired immunodeficiency syndrome. N Engl J Med 1990;323:1500–1504.

107. Toma E. Clindamycin-primaquine for treatment of *Pneumocystis carinii* pneumonia in AIDS. Eur J Clin Microbiol Infect Dis 1991;10:210–213.

108. Tuan IZ, Dennison D, Weisdorf DJ. *Pneumocystis carinii* pneumonitis following bone marrow transplantation. Bone Marrow Transplant 1992;10:267–272.

109. U.S. Public Health Service (USPHS) and the Infectious Diseases Society of America (IDSA). Guidelines for the prevention of opportunistic infections in persons infected with the human immunodeficiency virus: a summary. MMWR 1997;46(RR):1–12.

110. Walzer PD. Editorial response: *Pneumocystis carinii* pneumonia in patients without human immunodeficiency syndrome. Clin Infect Dis 1997;25:219–220.

111. Wharton JM, Coleman DL, Wofsy CB, Luce J, Blumenfeld W, Hadley W, Ingram-Drake L, Volberding P, Hopewell P. Trimethoprim-sulfamethoxazole or pentamidine for *Pneumocystis carinii* pneumonia in the acquired immunodeficiency syndrome: a prospective randomized trial. Ann Intern Med 1986;105:37–44.

112. Winston DJ. Prophylaxis and treatment of infections in the bone marrow transplant recipient. Curr Clin Top Infect Dis 1993;13: 293–321.

113. Zaman MK, Wootan OJ, Suprahmanya B, Ankobiah W, Finch PJP, Kamholz SL. Rapid noninvasive diagnosis of *Pneumocystis carinii* from the induced liquefied sputum. Ann Intern Med 1988;107:7–10.

Sporothrix schenckii

●

Carol A. Kauffman

GENERAL DESCRIPTION

Sporotrichosis is caused by infection with the dimorphic fungus *Sporothrix schenckii*. The organism is distributed worldwide and is found mostly in soil, decaying vegetable matter, and sphagnum moss (17). Infection occurs primarily by percutaneous inoculation of the conidia of *S. schenckii;* in a much smaller number of patients, inhalation of the conidia leads to pulmonary infection (14). Most infections are sporadic and often associated with scratches from rose bushes, hay, wood splinters, and conifer needles. However, contaminated soil and sphagnum moss used as packing material around plants have been associated with outbreaks of sporotrichosis (8). Infection can also result from scratches or bites from a variety of animals, including armadillos, cats, and rodents (5, 21).

The most common manifestations of sporotrichosis are cutaneous or lymphocutaneous infection of the extremities. Much less common is osteoarticular involvement, which can take the form of osteomyelitis, tenosynovitis, septic arthritis, or bursitis (2). Frequently, multiple joints are involved. Even less common is disseminated sporotrichosis manifested by pulmonary, meningeal, or other visceral infection (20, 27). Dissemination and osteoarticular involvement appear to be more prominent in patients with a history of alcohol abuse and diabetes mellitus. Recently, sporotrichosis has been noted in patients with HIV infection; in this population, infection is usually widely disseminated (3, 16, 19).

Even though sporotrichosis is most commonly a localized infection, resolution rarely occurs unless antifungal therapy is given. The specific treatment and outcome depend on the form of sporotrichosis.

IN VITRO SUSCEPTIBILITY

Susceptibility testing has not been standardized for *S. schenckii*. In fact, a saturated solution of potassium iodide (SSKI), an effective treatment for lymphocutaneous sporotrichosis, does not inhibit growth of *S. schenckii* in vitro (23, 24). Few studies have been done with regard to in vitro testing with amphotericin B or azole agents (17). Clinical experience has been the major determinant for the choice of antifungal therapy for this infection.

ANTIMICROBIAL THERAPY OF SPOROTRICHOSIS
General

Itraconazole has become the drug of choice for lymphocutaneous and cutaneous infection with *S. schenckii*. Response rates of 90 to 100% can be expected with 100 to 200 mg of itraconazole daily for 3 to 6 months (6, 22, 26). Patients unable to take itraconazole because of poor absorption, side effects, or drug interactions, can be given fluconazole at a dosage of 400 mg/day (6, 15).

The response rate for SSKI is also generally over 90%, and the drug is clearly less costly than any of the azoles. The major drawback to the use of SSKI is side effects, which include anorexia, nausea, salivary gland swelling, metallic taste, rash, and fever.

For the occasional patient who may be pregnant or for some other reason cannot take systemic antifungal agents, local application of heat to the lesions can resolve the infection (11, 18).

Special Situations
Osteoarticular Infections

Osteoarticular sporotrichosis is best treated with itraconazole at a total dosage of 400 mg/day, given as two divided doses with food (26, 28). The response rate is approximately 70%, but relapses are common. Therapy should be continued for as long as 1 to 2 years in an attempt to prevent relapse. SSKI is ineffective for osteoarticular infection; fluconazole and ketoconazole have proved less effective than itraconazole (4, 12, 15). However, if itraconazole cannot be tolerated, fluconazole can be tried at a dosage of 800 mg/day. Intravenous amphotericin B is an alternative generally used only after failure of azole therapy. Intraarticular amphotericin B has been used in a few patients but is not recommended as first-line therapy (9).

Pulmonary Infection

Pulmonary sporotrichosis has been the most difficult form of sporotrichosis to treat (14, 20). If the patient is not acutely ill, itraconazole at a dose of 200 mg twice daily can be used; therapy should continue for at least 1 to 2 years. If the patient is acutely ill, amphotericin B should be used; a total dosage of 1 to 2 g should be given. Alternatively, after an initial response to amphotericin B, therapy can be switched to itraconazole in the dosage regimen noted above. Cure rates of only 30 to 40% can be expected with either itraconazole or amphotericin B (14, 20, 26). The response rates to SSKI, ketoconazole, and fluconazole are less than 20% (14, 15, 20). Surgical resection of involved lung tissue is the most definitive therapy for pulmonary sporotrichosis (13, 20), but chronic obstructive pulmonary disease, which is almost always found in these patients, often precludes a surgical procedure.

Disseminated Sporotrichosis

Experience with sporotrichosis that has disseminated to viscera other than the lungs is limited, but most patients have responded to amphotericin B therapy (14, 27). In patients with subacute to chronic illness, itraconazole at a dosage of 200 mg twice daily can be tried (14). At least two reports have documented failure of amphotericin B and success of itraconazole in patients with disseminated sporotrichosis (1, 3).

Meningitis

Sporotrichal meningitis has been treated successfully with amphotericin B, but experience is limited to individual case reports (10). For patients with chronic indolent meningeal disease, itraconazole at a dosage of 200 mg twice daily could be considered for sequential therapy following amphotericin B. However, there is no reported experience for this regimen.

Sporotrichosis in AIDS Patients

Patients with AIDS usually have disseminated infection (3, 16, 19, 25). Initial therapy should be with amphotericin B for those who are acutely ill; for those with less severe disease, itraconazole at a dosage of 200 mg twice daily has been used. Overall, amphotericin B has been only modestly effective (3, 19, 25). Especially problematic has been sporotrichal meningeal involvement in AIDS patients; response of skin lesions with progression of meningitis has been noted in several patients treated with amphotericin B (19, 25). Failures with azoles also have been reported in AIDS patients (3). Patients with AIDS should receive lifelong suppressive therapy with 200 mg itraconazole daily after their acute illness has been treated.

REFERENCES

1. Baker JH, Goodpasture HC, Kuhns HR, Rinaldi MG. Fungemia caused by an amphotericin B resistant isolate of *Sporothrix schenckii*. Successful treatment with itraconazole. Arch Pathol Lab Med 1989;113:1279–1281.
2. Bayer AS, Scott VJ, Guze LB. Fungal arthritis. III. Sporotrichal arthritis. Semin Arthritis Rheum 1979;9:66–74.
3. Bolao F, Podzamczer D, Ventin M, Gudiol F. Efficacy of acute phase and maintenance therapy with itraconazole in an AIDS patient with sporotrichosis. Eur J Clin Microbiol Infect Dis 1994;13:609–612.
4. Calhoun DL, Waskin H, White MP, Bonner JR, Mulholland JH, Rumans LW, Stevens DA, Galgiani JN. Treatment of systemic sporotrichosis with ketoconazole. Rev Infect Dis 1991;13:47–51.
5. Conti Diaz IA. Epidemiology of sporotrichosis in Latin America. Mycopathologia 1989;108:113–116.
6. Conti Diaz IA, Civila E, Gezuele E, Lowinger M, Calegari L, Sanabria D, Fuentes L, De Rosa D, Alzueta G. Treatment of human cutaneous sporotrichosis with itraconazole. Mycoses 1992;35:153–156.
7. Diaz M, Negroni R, Montero-Gei F, Castro LGM, Sampaio SAP, Borelli D, Restrepo A, Franco L, Bran JL, Arathoon EG, Stevens DA, and Fluconazole Pan-American Study Group. A Pan-American 5- year study of fluconazole therapy for deep mycoses in the immunocompetent host. Clin Infect Dis 1992;14(Suppl 1):S68–S76.
8. Dixon DM, Salkin IF, Duncan RA, Hurd NJ, Haines JH, Kemna ME, Coles FB. Isolation and characterization of *Sporothrix*
schenckii from clinical and environmental sources associated with the largest U.S. epidemic of sporotrichosis. J Clin Microbiol 1991;29:1106–1113.
9. Downs NJ, Hinthorn DR, Mhatre VR, Liu C. Intra-articular amphotericin B treatment of *Sporothrix schenckii* arthritis. Arch Intern Med 1989;149:954–955.
10. Ewing BE, Bosl GJ, Peterson PK. *Sporothrix schenckii* meningitis in a farmer with Hodgkin's disease. Am J Med 1980;68:455–457.
11. Hiruma M, Katoh T, Yamamoto I, Kagawa S. Local hyperthermia in the treatment of sporotrichosis. Mykosen 1987;30:315–321.
12. Horsburgh CR, Cannady PB, Kirkpatrick CH. Treatment of fungal infections in the bones and joints with ketoconazole. J Infect Dis 1983;147:1064–1069.
13. Jung JY, Almond CH, Campbell DC, Elkadi A, Tenorio A. Role of surgery in the management of pulmonary sporotrichosis. J Thorac Cardiovasc Surg 1979;77:235–239.
14. Kauffman CA. Old and new therapies for sporotrichosis. Clin Infect Dis 1995;21:981–985.
15. Kauffman CA, Pappas PG, McKinsey DS, Greenfield RA, Perfect JR, Cloud GA, Thomas CJ, Dismukes WE, and the NIAID Mycoses Study Group. Treatment of lymphocutaneous and visceral sporotrichosis with fluconazole. Clin Infect Dis 1996;22:46–50.
16. Keiser P, Whittle D. Sporotrichosis in human immunodeficiency virus-infected patients: report of a case. Rev Infect Dis 1991;13:1027–1028.
17. Kwon-Chung KJ, Bennett JE. Sporotrichosis. In: Medical mycology. Philadelphia: Lee & Febiger, 1992:707–729.
18. Mackinnon JE, Conti Diaz IA. The effect of temperature on sporotrichosis. Sabouraudia 1962;2:56–59.
19. Penn CC, Goldstein E, Bartholomew WR. *Sporothrix schenckii* meningitis in a patient with AIDS. Clin Infect Dis 1992;15:741–743.
20. Pluss JL, Opal SM. Pulmonary sporotrichosis: review of treatment and outcome. Medicine 1986;65:143–153.
21. Reed KD, Moore FM, Geiger GE, Stemper ME. Zoonotic transmission of sporotrichosis: case report and review. Clin Infect Dis 1993;16:384–387.
22. Restrepo A, Robledo J, Gomez I, Tabares AM, Gutierrez R. Itraconazole therapy in lymphangitic and cutaneous sporotrichosis. Arch Dermatol 1986;122:413–417.
23. Rex JH, Bennett JE. Administration of potassium iodide to normal volunteers does not increase killing of *Sporothrix schenckii* by their neutrophils or monocytes. J Med Vet Mycol 1990;28:185–189.
24. Rippon JW. Sporotrichosis. In: Medical mycology. 3rd ed. Philadelphia: WB Saunders, 1988:325–352.
25. Rotz LD, Slater LN, Wack MF, Boyd AL, Scott EN, Greenfield RA. Disseminated sporotrichosis with meningitis in a patient with AIDS. Infect Dis Clin Pract 1996;5:566–568.
26. Sharkey-Mathis PK, Kauffman CA, Graybill JR, Stevens DA, Hostetler JS, Cloud G, Dismukes WE, and the NIAID Mycoses Study Group. Treatment of sporotrichosis with itraconazole. Am J Med 1993;95:279–285.
27. Wilson DE, Mann JJ, Bennett JE, Utz JP. Clinical features of extracutaneous sporotrichosis. Medicine 1967;46:265–279.
28. Winn RE, Anderson J, Piper J, Aronson N, Pluss J. Systemic sporotrichosis treated with itraconazole. Clin Infect Dis 1993;17:210–217.

Amphotericin B

Elizabeth Olek and Alan M. Sugar

CLASS: POLYENE ANTIFUNGALS
Chemical Structure

Amphotericin B is an amphoteric polyene macrolide that occurs as a yellow to orange powder that is insoluble in water. It is produced from a strain of *Streptomyces nodosus*. The chemical formula of amphotericin B is $C_{47}H_{73}NO_{17}$, and its molecular weight is 924.09. Its structure is shown in Figure 1. Amphotericin B is a nonaromatic heptaene, structurally related to the nystatin group of tetraenes. It is a large molecule, characterized by lactone rings containing 7 conjugated carbon-carbon double bonds. Thus the molecule has a polar side and a nonpolar side, leading to the description amphoteric. One sugar moiety is connected to the molecule. The parenteral preparation of amphotericin B for injection (Fungizone) is produced as a lyophilized yellow powder that contains sodium desoxycholate as a solubilizing agent. Once manufactured, air in the vial is replaced with nitrogen. Since the preparation is colloidal once reconstituted, drug may be retained by many filters (88).

Liposomal amphotericin B (AmBisome, Nexstar, San Dimas, CA) is a unilamellar liposomal formulation of amphotericin B. The lipid bilayer is composed of hydrogenated soy phosphatidylcholine, cholesterol, and distearoyl phosphatidylglycerol, which is then combined with amphotericin B in a molar ratio of 2:1:0.8:0.4. The structure consists of small (60–70 nm) unilamellar lipid vesicles of uniform size with amphotericin B inside. The lyophilized powder is rehydrated in sterile water and further diluted in 5% dextrose at the time the drug is administered. The recommended infusion time is 30 to 60 min. In aqueous solution, less than 5% of the drug dissociates from the liposomes over a 72-h period (2). The ability of the liposome to remain intact and not release the amphotericin B is thought to be critical to its decreased toxicity.

Amphotericin B lipid complex injection (Abelcet, ABLC, the Liposome Company) consists of amphotericin B complexed with two phospholipids in a 1:1 drug:lipid molar ratio. The two phospholipids, L-dimyristoylphosphatidylcholine (DMPC) and L-dimyristoylphosphatidylglycerol (DMPG) are present in a 7:3 molar ratio. The structure consists of ribbons of lipid with amphotericin B attached. Each vial of amphotericin B lipid complex injection contains 100 mg of amphotericin B per 20 ml volume. Each milliliter contains 5 mg of amphotericin B, 3.4 mg of DMPC, 1.5 mg of DMPG, and 9 mg of sodium chloride USP. A 5-μm filter needle should be used

to transfer amphotericin B lipid complex into the final infusion apparatus. The compound is opaque yellow with a pH of 5 to 7 (71).

Amphotericin B colloidal dispersion (Amphocil, ABCD, Amphotec, Sequus Pharmaceuticals, Menlo Park, CA) is composed of amphotericin B and cholesteryl sulfate, in discoid structures with amphotericin B attached.

Mechanism of Action

Amphotericin B binds to sterols in the fungal cell membrane. Mammalian cell membranes contain primarily cholesterol, whereas the sterols comprising the fungal cell membrane are ergosterol and other related sterols (59). Amphotericin B has higher affinity for ergosterol and the other fungal sterols than for cholesterol. Nystatin has a higher binding affinity for cholesterol and is consequently toxic to mammalian cells, preventing systemic administration. Both efficacy and toxicity of the polyenes result from binding of the drugs to these components of the cell membrane. Polyene antibiotics are not active against bacteria since bacteria lack sterols.

The major action of amphotericin B is to damage the membrane of fungal cells. Binding to ergosterol causes membrane impairment that results in loss of protons and cations from the cell. The precise mechanism has yet to be explained; however a number of molecular models have been proposed (23, 74). Derangement of the proton gradient results in loss of other cell constituents. Low concentrations of amphotericin B result in loss of small molecules or cations, such as sodium and potassium. Higher concentrations or prolonged incubation results in loss of cell constituents, metabolic disruption, and cell death.

In addition, amphotericin B may act by inducing oxidative damage on the cell (123, 124). The lethal effects of higher concentrations of the drug on *Candida albicans* are not only a consequence of its membrane-permeabilizing effects but also may involve a cascade of oxidative reactions linked to its own oxidation. The actual mechanisms involved remain to be clarified. Amphotericin B has potent immunomodulating effects in the host, also related to oxidation-dependent events (28). Cell-mediated and humoral immunity may be suppressed or stimulated, depending upon drug concentration and timing of its administration (65).

Liposomal amphotericin B contains the same active moiety as amphotericin B and thus has the same mechanism of action.

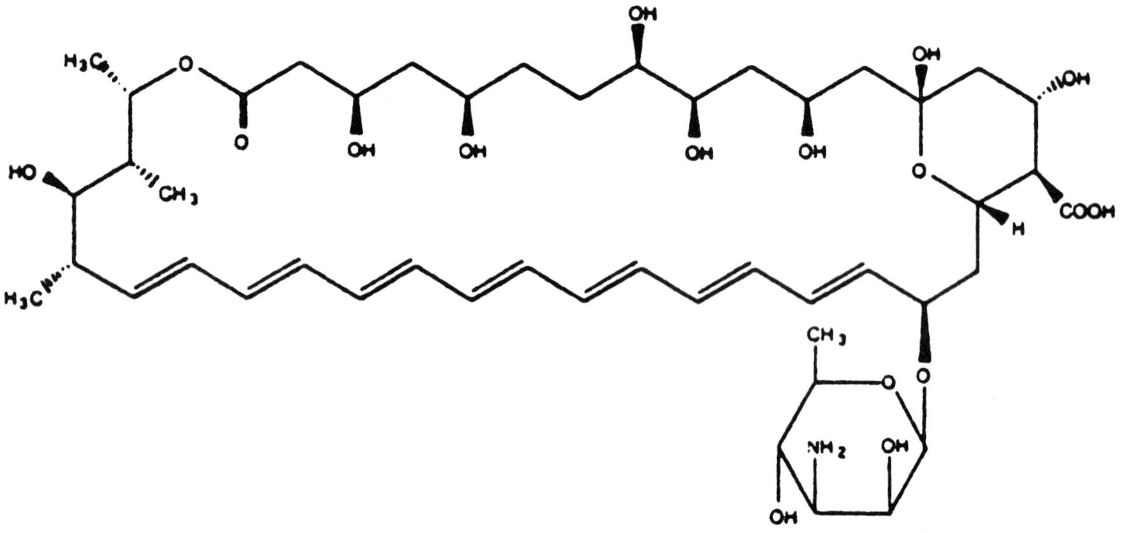

FIGURE 1. Structure of amphotericin B.

In addition, recent data indicate that the lipids constituting the liposomes bind to fungi and are eventually internalized by the fungi if the liposomes contain amphotericin B (1). Fluorescence and electron microscopy show that liposomal amphotericin B and liposomes without drug bind to fungi in vitro. Intact liposomes of either type could be seen attached to the outer surface of the fungal cell wall within 1 h after exposure to the liposomes. Only liposomal amphotericin B was effective in this interaction, resulting in death of the fungi to which the liposomal amphotericin B had bound.

When fluorescently labeled liposomes with or without drug were injected in *Candida*-infected mice, fungal infection was localized with bright fluorescence. The in vitro data suggest that only the liposomal amphotericin B could kill the fungus growing in vivo and that the antifungal efficacy of liposomal amphotericin B was related to its ability to bind to fungi in vivo.

ANTIFUNGAL ACTIVITY
Spectrum of Activity

Amphotericin B has the broadest spectrum of any antifungal compound currently marketed for treatment of invasive fungal infections. This characteristic is what has helped sustain amphotericin B as the "gold standard" of antifungal drugs. Amphotericin B is known to be active against a wide variety of yeasts, yeastlike fungi, and molds. Typical minimum inhibitory concentrations (MICs) are shown in Table 1 and should be interpreted with caution. Most species of *Candida* are inhibited by 2 µg/mL of amphotericin B or less. Most species of *Cryptococcus neoformans* are inhibited by less than 4 µg/mL. Most molds are also inhibited by amphotericin B, but MICs range from 0.1 to more than 100 µg/mL.

Several issues concerning antifungal susceptibility testing remain unresolved, such as reproducibility and correlation of

TABLE 1 • In Vitro Susceptibility of Selected Fungi to Amphotericin B

Organism	MIC Range (µg/mL)
Candida albicans	0.05–4
C. tropicalis	0.04–16
C. parapsilosis	0.025–>6.25
C. krusei	0.05–>6.25
C. lusitaniae	0.39–50
C. guilliermondii	0.02–2
Cryptococcus neoformans	0.04–2.8
Aspergillus fumigatus	0.14–>25
A. flavus	12.5–>25
A. niger	0.12–>25
Absidia corymbifera	0.39–100
Rhizopus oryzae	0.5–>100
R. rhizopodiformis	0.2–>5
Blastomyces dermatitidis	0.05–0.78
Coccidioides immitis	0.15–96
Histoplasma capsulatum	0.001–>100
Paracoccidioides brasiliensis	1.56–>100
Sporothrix schenckii	0.4–>100
Malasezzia furfur	0.3–2.5
Pseudallescheria boydii	1.56–>100

Adapted from George D, Kordick D, Miniter T, et al. Combination therapy in experimental invasive aspergillosis. J Infect Dis 1993;168:692–698.

in vitro results with clinical outcome (56, 117, 118). Therefore little weight should be placed on the absolute value of MICs and maximum fungicidal concentrations (MFCs). Clinical resistance to amphotericin B has been demonstrated in cases of *Candida lusitaniae,* and most experts recommend using alternative therapy for these infections (21, 63, 95, 110). Similar recommendations can be found for *Pseudallascheria boydii,* another fungus usually not clinically responsive to amphotericin B (10, 38, 50, 61). At present, clinical experience is more valuable than the results of laboratory-based in vitro susceptibility testing, especially when interpreting results obtained with methods other than that recommended by the NC-CLS for testing yeasts. Resistance of fungi to amphotericin B has been occasionally described, but de novo appearance of amphotericin B resistance has not been a clinical problem (4, 43, 69, 95, 115, 136).

Liposomal amphotericin B MICs are similar to those obtained with amphotericin B alone (9). Typical MICs obtained with various fungi and liposomal amphotericin B are shown in Table 2. An in vitro study of MICs indicates that little difference between the MICs of liposomal amphotericin B and amphotericin B, with the former leading to growth inhibition, sometimes at lower concentrations than are observed with conventional amphotericin B (9).

Murine animal model investigations suggest that the spectrum of activity of amphotericin B is not altered by incorporation of the drug into liposomes. For example, liposomal amphotericin B was shown to be efficacious in the treatment of murine coccidioidomycosis (5), candidiasis and cryptococcosis (3, 106), aspergillosis (55), blastomycosis (35), candidiasis in leukopenic mice (134), and histoplasmosis (62). In these studies, survival was comparable to that seen with conventional amphotericin B, and fungal colony counts in target organs were decreased as additional proof of efficacy.

Amphotericin B lipid complex demonstrates in vitro activity against *Aspergillus* and *Candida* species. MICs range from 0.1 to more than 10 μg/mL, depending upon the species and strain tested (71). MICs are generally below 1 μg/mL. Animal models of *Aspergillus fumigatus*, *C. albicans*, *C. guillermondi*, *C. stellatoideae*, and *C. tropicalis* demonstrated the beneficial activity of amphotericin B lipid complex, in which endpoints included prolonged survival of infected animals and clearance of fungi from target organs (71). One study of in vitro antifungal activity against *C. albicans*, *C. parapsilosis*, *C. tropicalis*, *C. glabrata*, and *C. krusei* by agar plate dilution revealed the MICs to be the same for amphotericin B lipid complex as for amphotericin B against *C. albicans* (98). MICs increased more than fourfold in 9 of the 20 non-*albicans* strains tested.

Amphotericin B colloidal dispersion tested by broth dilution MIC and MFC for antifungal activity in vitro against conventional amphotericin B shows similar ranges in 41 isolates of 15 pathogenic species (126). The same number of isolates

had lower MICs and MFCs with one drug as with the other. Less than one-third of the isolates demonstrated a large (fourfold or more) increase in MIC for amphotericin B colloidal dispersion compared with conventional amphotericin B.

Animal models of disseminated cryptococcosis (68), *C. albicans* in normal and immunocompromised mice, and *A. fumigatus* in immunocompromised rabbits (7, 107) have shown the efficacy of amphotericin B colloidal dispersion. Amphotericin B colloidal dispersion was compared to conventional amphotericin B in an acute murine model of systemic coccidioidomycosis (34). The agents were not equivalent on a mg/kg basis in clearing *C. immitis* from organs; however a greater therapeutic index for the colloidal dispersion was determined. The amount of amphotericin B colloidal dispersion could be increased per dose to achieve an optimal efficacious level.

Based on this experience, a study using amphotericin B colloidal dispersion in human coccidioidomycosis was undertaken (126) that demonstrated modest response rates at doses starting at 0.5 mg/kg, then 1 mg/kg, to 2 mg/kg three times weekly. Dose escalation was cautious since this was an early study, and safety had not yet been demonstrated for the higher doses. Studies looking at higher doses and longer treatment courses are ongoing.

Case reports describe using amphotericin B colloidal dispersion successfully in the treatment of invasive pulmonary aspergillosis in 1 patient (85), cryptococcal meningitis in 4 patients (133), visceral leishmaniasis in 20 patients (44, 45), invasive fungal infections after bone marrow transplantation (24), paranasal sinus mucormycosis in 1 patient (130), cerebral phaeohyphomycosis due to *Dactylaria gallopava* in 1 patient (135), and chronic disseminated *Geotrichum capitatum* in 1 patient (36). One study of 168 patients with various documented or presumed systemic mycoses who responded incompletely to at least 7 days of conventional amphotericin B treatment showed a 49% response rate in 97 evaluated patients (105).

Pharmacodynamic Effects

Doses of amphotericin B lower than those that induce permeability changes (0.01–0.04 μg/mL) result in immune stimulatory activity, particularly with respect to cells of the immune system (25, 28). This stimulatory effect is manifested by increased DNA and RNA synthesis and increased macrophage oxidative burst activity (80). However as the concentration of amphotericin B increases, toxic effects become apparent, and the stimulatory effect likely diminishes once cellular damage occurs.

Immunomodulatory effects of amphotericin B have been observed in both in vitro and in vivo systems, and the drug's effects on a variety of in vitro assays of phagocyte/lymphocyte functions have been evaluated. Since amphotericin B is known to bind to cell membrane sterols, membrane perturbations following such binding is not surprising, and in cells that can respond to membrane stimulation, a variety of biologic effects should certainly be expected.

Whether the immunomodulatory effects of amphotericin B have any relevance in clinical practice remains controversial. In patients with serious immunocompromise, significant aug-

TABLE 2 • In Vitro Susceptibility of Selected Fungi to AmBisome

Organism	MIC Range (μg/mL)
Candida albicans	0.16–1.25
C. tropicalis	0.16–0.62
C. parapsilosis	0.31–1.25
Cryptococcus neoformans	0.15–1.25
Aspergillus fumigatus	0.31–2.5
Fusarium spp.	1.25–10

Adapted from Hughes CE, Harris C, Moody JA, et al. In vitro activities of amphotericin B in combination with four antifungal agents and rifampin against *Aspergillus* spp. Antimicrob Agents Chemother 1984;25:560–562.

mentation of the immune system is probably not possible. In patients with no definable immune system pathology (e.g., those with endemic mycoses or cryptococcosis) the immunoadjuvant effects of amphotericin B may play a role in the successful outcome of treatment with this agent.

MECHANISMS OF ACTION

Amphotericin B induces membrane permeability by forming complexes with ergosterol located in fungal membranes, leading to intracellular leakage and cell death (89). As mentioned above, mammalian cell membranes contain primarily cholesterol, while the primary sterols in the fungal cell membrane are ergosterol and related sterols. Affinity of amphotericin B for ergosterol is greater than for cholesterol. Polyenes with a higher affinity for cholesterol have correspondingly greater toxicities for mammalian cells (28). Thus, as mentioned above, nystatin is considerably more toxic for mammalian cells than is amphotericin B, reflecting its higher binding affinity for cholesterol. Recent investigations suggest that the interaction of amphotericin B with the cell membrane is probably more complicated and that additional factors are involved (91).

Once amphotericin B is bound to the cell membrane, several events occur. Polyenes typically have concentration-dependent dual effects on cells. At low concentrations (e.g., 0.02–0.1 µg/mL) cells become permeable, which is most easily measured as leakage of potassium into the external environment (123). At higher concentrations (≥0.3 µg/mL), cells lyse and die.

The permeabilizing effects of amphotericin B on cell membranes and lytic effects are presumed to involve different mechanisms. Binding of amphotericin B to membrane sterols causes disorganization of the cell membrane. One result of this is depolarization of the cell and increased permeability of the cell membrane to protons and monovalent cations. In contrast to the lytic effects of amphotericin B, the permeabilizing effects are not thought to involve oxidative mechanisms (123).

There is strong experimental evidence for the role of active oxygen intermediates in mediating the lytic effects of amphotericin B. For example, Brajtburg et al. demonstrated that such amphotericin B–induced cellular injury could be reduced by scavengers of reactive oxygen intermediates or by hypoxic conditions (27). Killing of *C. albicans* or lysis of yeast protoplasts could be inhibited by catalase (123) and augmented by the prooxidant ascorbic acid (26). The precise mechanism involved in formation of reactive oxygen intermediates is not clear but may involve autooxidation of amphotericin B and subsequent formation of free radicals (78).

Catalase has also been implicated in conferring resistance on *C. albicans* to amphotericin B when the antifungal was administered in several smaller doses rather than one large one (124). It was postulated that increased catalase activity in yeast exposed to lower concentrations of amphotericin B decreased amphotericin B–related cellular toxicity, because reactive oxygen intermediates such as hydrogen peroxide were effectively neutralized by the catalase.

Sublethal concentrations of amphotericin B have various effects on *C. albicans* yeast. Cell wall constituents are affected as manifested by a decrease in mannose and an increase in amino acid and glucosamine content (100). In addition, germ tube formation is inhibited, and possibly related to changes in cell wall composition, yeast exposed to sublethal concentrations of amphotericin B adhere less well to serum-coated plastic surfaces and fibrin matrices (103), to human endothelial cells (59), and to rat fibroblasts (93, 94).

MECHANISMS OF RESISTANCE

Clinical isolates of *C. albicans* and *C. neoformans* resistant to amphotericin B have been rarely identified during treatment of human fungal infections. However, resistant strains have been isolated under controlled circumstances, and the lipid composition of the cells in these strains compared with that of the parent strains. Resistance is often associated with alterations in the nature of membrane sterols or in the amount of sterols present. In addition to altered lipid composition, other aspects of cell function may be impaired, and consequently, resistant mutants of *C. albicans* may be less robust and less pathogenic.

Amphotericin B–resistant strains of *C. albicans* and *C. tropicalis* isolated after serial subculture in the presence of increasing concentrations of amphotericin B (13) were found to have reduced ergosterol content. Other investigators also found less ergosterol in mutagen-induced nystatin- and amphotericin B–resistant strains of *C. albicans* (69), and methylated sterols were increased in similar experiments (127). In detailed experiments in mutant strains of *C. albicans,* the higher the amphotericin B concentrations required to inhibit growth, the greater the shift in lipid composition from ergosterol to methylated sterols (111).

Altered sterol content likely does not entirely account for amphotericin B resistance in the strains of *C. albicans* and *C. neoformans* studied. Elevated catalase levels have been detected in several amphotericin B–resistant strains of *C. albicans* (122). This may enhance resistance against oxidative damage to the fungal cell by amphotericin B.

Acquired amphotericin B resistance leading to treatment failure is not common; however, six cases have been documented in which patients had received prolonged therapy. The reports included two patients with *C. tropicalis,* three with *C. lusitaniae,* and one with *C. guilliermondii.* The *C. tropicalis* strains had MICs of 100 µg to 500 µg/L and were each ergosterol deficient (47, 96). Prophylactic treatment with oral nystatin resulted in isolation of one strain of *C. krusei* and one strain of *C. tropicalis* resistant to amphotericin B and nystatin in patients who were followed (119).

MICs of *Candida* spp. from 70 patients who were neutropenic were compared with MICs of similar isolates from control patients (42). None of the 625 strains from the control group were classified as resistant (defined as MIC ≥2.0 µg/L). Six of the 70 neutropenic patients yielded 55 resistant strains, three patients had *C. albicans,* one had *C. tropicalis,* and two had *C. glabrata.* Thus clinical resistance to amphotericin B may be more common than had been suspected.

Amphotericin B-resistant strains identified so far have been non-*albicans* species, including *C. lusitaniae, C. tropicalis, C. guilliermondii,* and *C. parapsilosis,* which shows growth inhibition at concentrations of amphotericin B similar to other species but is much less susceptible to its lethal effects (121). Resistant mutants can be more easily induced in *C. guilliermondii*, a haploid species, than in *C. albicans,* which is diploid (84).

Methods to Overcome and Prevent Resistance

Amphotericin B may interact with other antifungal drugs to produce synergistic, additive, or antagonistic results. The combination of amphotericin B and flucytosine tested against strains of *C. albicans, C. tropicalis,* and *C. neoformans* in vitro showed a synergistic effect, defined as a fourfold or greater reduction in the MIC of flucytosine in the presence of amphotericin B at concentrations below its MIC for each test strain (92). Other investigators have found conflicting results, perhaps reflecting use of different test conditions, strains, and drug concentrations. Likely, the interaction is additive for most strains of *C. albicans* (104). The interaction between amphotericin B and flucytosine against *Aspergillus* spp. in vitro has also varied; early results indicated synergism, which later studies failed to confirm (70, 77, 80).

Combination treatment with amphotericin B and flucytosine in animal models of aspergillosis, candidiasis, and cryptococcosis may be superior to amphotericin B alone (11, 12, 22, 113, 129, 136). However, with the exception of cryptococcal meningitis, there are no results from controlled clinical trials to support use of combination therapy in other fungal infections (19, 136). Combination therapy is not infrequently used in cases of invasive candidiasis and there are anecdotal reports of use in cases of aspergillosis and mucormycosis.

In vitro studies have indicated that combinations of azoles and polyenenes are antagonistic against *C. albicans* (86, 109). This may be related to the action of these agents on the fungal membrane sterol composition. Since amphotericin B binds to sterols in the fungal membrane and azoles inhibit their synthesis, there has been caution in using these drugs together in patients with candidiasis. Although animal models of fungal infections have been used to measure the efficacy of combination therapy, data are conflicting and difficult to interpret because the results depend on the test conditions and drug dosing variations (6, 8, 15, 32, 58, 120, 128).

Investigators in one study found that fluconazole in combination with amphotericin B is not antagonistic in murine invasive candidiasis, regardless of the immune status of the animals, as measured by protection from mortality or a reduced fungal load in tissue (128). The order of administration of fluconazole and amphotericin B did not alter the conclusions drawn, and the results reveal a positive interaction compared with use of fluconazole alone. Other investigators have found no antagonism between fluconazole and amphotericin B in rabbit invasive aspergillosis (58) and in murine cryptococcal meningitis (6). These studies demonstrate that combination therapy is likely beneficial and that clinical studies will likely be needed to demonstrate efficacy.

PHARMACOKINETIC DISPOSITION
Absorption

Amphotericin B is administered parenterally for treatment of invasive fungal infections, through either a peripheral or central venous access site. Peripheral venous administration may predispose patients to develop phlebitis because of the irritant effect of amphotericin B. Central venous administration eliminates the concern about phlebitis. After intravenous infusion of 30 mg of amphotericin B over several hours, the average peak serum concentrations were about 1 μg/mL, and after 50 mg, they were approximately 2 μg/mL (88). The maximum amphotericin B concentration detectable immediately after infusion is only 10% of the administered dose. Average minimum serum concentrations of amphotericin B recorded immediately before the next drug infusion were 0.04 μg/mL after intravenous administration of 30 mg daily or 60 mg every other day.

Dose, frequency, and infusion rate influence serum levels measured after administration of amphotericin B. One report described mean serum concentrations of 1.21, 0.62, and 0.32 μg/mL at 1, 18, and 42 h after intravenous administration of a 50 mg-dose of amphotericin B to 20 subjects (53). Peak levels were obtained within the first hour after a 4- to 6-h infusion and persisted for 6 to 8 h. Another study reported serum levels of 0.14 to 2.39 μg/mL 4 h after infusion of 5 to 70 mg and 1.0 to 2.4 μg/mL after alternate-day dosing of 25 to 105 mg of amphotericin B intravenously (20). Minimum serum concentrations were not affected by the doubled daily dose given every other day. Thus, determination of serum concentrations of amphotericin B has no practical clinical value in the management of patients (51).

A correlation between dose and serum level was reported (116). Investigators report peak levels of 1.2 and 2.4 μg/mL measured 1 h after completed administration after more than 3 days of 0.5- and 1.0-mg/kg doses, respectively. Trough levels of 0.5 and 1.1 μg/mL were obtained 23 h after completed infusion of 0.5- and 1.0-mg/kg doses, respectively. Shorter infusion time may increase the mean serum concentration measured 1 h after completion of infusion, but concentrations did not differ at 18 and 42 h postinfusion (54).

Oral administration results in low and variable blood concentrations. Several studies have demonstrated blood concentrations of amphotericin B from 0.04 to 0.5 μg/mL after oral liquid preparations of amphotericin B were administered (67, 81). When amphotericin B is administered as a lozenge three or four times daily, up to 9% of the oral dose is absorbed in cancer patients (31). Increased absorption of amphotericin B occurs after mucosal damage from cancer chemotherapy. A report of amphotericin B serum concentrations exceeding 0.5 μg/mL in 12 of 17 pediatric recipients of bone marrow transplants who suffered grade two or three mucositis demonstrates the pathway (51).

Intramuscular injection is not feasible, since amphotericin B is too toxic to be given by this route, and absorption from muscle is poor. Therefore, the only reliable method for administration of amphotericin B is intravenously, either through peripheral venous access or through central venous catheters to eliminate phlebitis as a complication.

Various other routes of administration are also used, including intravitreal, intrathecal, intraarticular, intraperitoneal, intravesicular, intracavitary, and by aerosolized solution, depending upon the specific infection being treated. Targeted local therapy is used to achieve higher concentrations of amphotericin B at the site of infection (e.g., the eye, cerebrospinal fluid (CSF), joints, peritoneum, urinary bladder, and bronchial secretions). Clinical outcome after using any of these sites to administer amphotericin B is difficult to assess because many factors intercede, and thus indications for local therapy are not clearly defined (76). Concentrations of drugs at specific sites do not always correlate with clinical response, as is the case with cryptococcal meningitis (19). Observed CSF concentrations of amphotericin B in cryptococcal meningitis are extremely low, and the success of treatment may have more to do with the pathogenesis of the disease than with the specifics of antifungal drug pharmacokinetics. However, certain clinical situations may warrant the use of local amphotericin B injections to treat difficult-to-manage mycoses.

Distribution

Amphotericin B pharmacokinetics are complex and not completely understood. After intravenous administration amphotericin B is approximately 90 to 95% bound to serum proteins, especially β-lipoproteins (25). The distribution of amphotericin B is thought to follow a three-compartment model, with a reported total volume of distribution of 4 L/kg (14). Amphotericin B is delivered into a central compartment (Vc) and rapidly enters the fast compartment (Vf), with more delayed entry into the peripheral slow compartment (Vs), presumably cell membranes throughout the body. The large volumes of distribution within the compartments likely reflect tight cell membrane binding by amphotericin B within the compartments. The exact anatomic identity of the model compartments remains to be elucidated, and it is not known which compartment is most important in obtaining therapeutic concentrations of amphotericin B (14).

Low concentrations of the drug are reportedly attained in aqueous humor and pleural, pericardial, peritoneal, and synovial fluids following intravenous administration of amphotericin B (73, 112). Concentrations in CSF are estimated to be approximately 2 to 4% of simultaneous serum concentrations after intravenous administration to adult subjects (132), but were undetectable in other studies (20, 48, 49). Data from animal models suggest that meningeal levels may be higher than CSF levels (108). Biliary concentrations may be high (39). Amphotericin B reportedly crosses the placental barrier, and cord blood and amnionic fluid levels in one patient were below the measured maternal blood levels (72). Since virtually no amphotericin B is detectable in peritoneal dialysate following intravenous administration of the drug (102), direct intraperitoneal administration of amphotericin B is recommended for treating fungal peritonitis (17).

To achieve fungistatic CSF concentrations, the drug is given intrathecally. In patients with meningitis, intrathecal administration of 0.2 to 0.3 mg of amphotericin B via a subcutaneous reservoir produced peak CSF concentrations of 0.5 to 0.8 μg/mL and, 24 h later, CSF concentrations of 0.11 to 0.29 μg/mL. Amphotericin B is removed from the CSF by arachnoid villi and appears to be stored in the extracellular compartment of the brain, which may act as a reservoir for the drug (88).

Autopsy samples from eight subjects who had received amphotericin B (101–2688 mg intravenously) revealed the highest concentrations of drug in the liver, ranging from 2.2 to 188 μg of amphotericin B per gram of tissue. The spleen had 0.6 to 190 μg/g; kidney, 1.2 to 39 μg/g; lung, 1.2 to 23 μg/g; heart, 0.5 to μg/g; and esophagus, 0.1 to 13 μg/g of amphotericin B, measured by HPLC analysis (33). Most of the total administered dose of amphotericin B remained unaccounted for, with only 16 to 51% of the amphotericin B recovered from the five organs tested.

A similar study of autopsy samples from cancer patients receiving 75 to 1100 mg of amphotericin B revealed the highest concentrations in liver and spleen (37). Biliary excretion ranged from 0.8 to 14.5% of the daily dose of amphotericin B. These studies point out that the tissue levels are most frequently fungistatic, not fungicidal. Presumably, binding of amphotericin B to sterols in mammalian cell membranes prevents the drug from reaching critical targets in the fungal cell. Lipid-based formulations that can be given in higher doses may potentially achieve higher tissue levels.

Metabolism

Amphotericin B metabolism in humans is not well understood. The elimination half-life of amphotericin B in patients with normal renal function prior to therapy is approximately 24 h. One study demonstrated that the elimination rate of amphotericin B decreases after the first 24 h. Cumulative urinary excretion of a single dose of amphotericin B over a 7-day period was approximately 40% of the administered drug. After a course of amphotericin B therapy was instituted, another study demonstrated an elimination half-life of 15 days. Slow release from the peripheral compartment accounted for the long half-life. Only 3% of the total administered dose of amphotericin B is excreted as unchanged drug. After completion of treatment, drug can be detected in blood up to 4 weeks and in urine for 4 to 8 weeks.

Amphotericin B clearance in renal failure is inversely related to creatinine clearance (99). A study of seven patients with renal function ranging from 0 to 100% of normal found that urinary excretion accounted for less than 10% of the administered dose and was lower in patients with abnormal renal function. Increased clearance of amphotericin B in patients with decreased renal function indicates that hepatic clearance of amphotericin B becomes more important in patients with renal insufficiency.

The pharmacokinetics of amphotericin B were evaluated in one patient undergoing hemodialysis for chronic renal failure (52). Since renal excretion of amphotericin B is minimal, and amphotericin B is not appreciably removed by dialysis, the results obtained from this patient are not surprising. The patient received 0.5 mg/kg amphotericin B every 24 to 48 h. Peak serum concentrations were approximately 0.4 μg/mL, and the rate of decline in serum concentrations was slow, so that 8 days after discontinuing amphotericin B, serum concentrations of 0.23 μg/mL were obtained, similar to that obtained approximately 48 h after cessation of drug infusion. These investigators also documented the lack of effect of hemodialysis on amphotericin B serum concentrations. Dosage modifications of amphotericin B are not required in patients with renal insufficiency, in keeping with the low renal excretion of the drug (99).

DOSAGE REGIMENS

In adults, a test dose of intravenous amphotericin B is usually given first to rule out anaphylaxis or other reaction. This may be 1 mg in 50 to 250 mL of 5% dextrose infused over 20 to 30 min or, alternatively, over 2 to 4 h. Patients should not be premedicated prior to administration of the test dose. The patient should be observed for 2 to 4 h for fever, severe rigors, chills, and hypotension, with vital signs monitored 30-min intervals. If there is no reaction to the test dose, premedication is not required before subsequent doses. Amphotericin B can be started at 0.6 mg/kg/day infused over 2 to 3 h. In critically ill patients with severe infections, accelerated increases in dosage are recommended so that the final total daily dose is given within 24 to 36 h of the start of therapy. Alternatively, the amphotericin B dose can be gradually increased over several days, from a dose of 0.25 mg/kg/day up to 0.6 mg/kg/day. If the patient tolerates the initial test dose, this is usually not necessary. Amphotericin B dosage for preterm and newborn infants has not been conclusively determined; however, the doses cited above have been used successfully, with little toxicity.

Dosages may range up to 1 mg/kg/day to 1.5 mg/kg on alternate days. Dosages above 1.5 mg/kg/day are not recommended. If the intended dose is 1.0 to 1.5 mg/kg/day, half of the dose may be given initially on day 1 of therapy, and the remainder 8 h later. Thereafter, the full dose may be given daily. The dose is administered in D5W at a concentration of 0.25 mg/mL or less. The preparation should be discarded if the solution becomes turbid on addition of amphotericin B. Observe for phlebitis if amphotericin B is administered peripherally. For volume-restricted patients, amphotericin B may be double concentrated to 0.5 mg/mL. The duration of therapy depends on the type and extent of the specific fungal infection.

Patients should be assessed for tolerance to sodium loading. If so, infuse 500 mL of normal saline solution over 30 min before administering amphotericin B and 500 mL of normal saline solution after completion of the amphotericin B infusion. Sodium loading in this manner may help prevent drug-induced nephrotoxicity. Serum potassium and magnesium concentrations should be monitored at least twice weekly during amphotericin B administration and frequently for the first 2 to 3 weeks after the drug is discontinued.

If the patient develops an infusion-related adverse reaction to amphotericin B, premedicate one-half hour before the start of the infusion with 650 mg of acetaminophen orally and 25 to 50 mg of meperidine intravenously. Meperidine is recommended rather than corticosteroids to avoid sequelae associated with prolonged corticosteroid use and to minimize the use of steroids. If meperidine administration is not possible, hydrocortisone (25–50 mg) may be given intravenously one-half hour before the start of amphotericin B. In general, unless the patient develops a severe infusion-related adverse reaction, it is not necessary to discontinue therapy.

Amphotericin B has been administered to pregnant women with no unusual clinical side effects, but published experience is limited (87). In one patient treated for candidemia, amphotericin B concentrations in placenta, cord blood, and infant serum were measured 4 weeks after the last dose of amphotericin B (40). Similar concentrations were found in all three sites (0.2 μg/mL), suggesting that amphotericin B is present not only in placenta, which could act as a depot for the drug, but also in the fetus. Indeed, the infant born 1 month after discontinuation of maternal amphotericin B therapy had an elevated serum creatinine at birth. Similar conclusions were reached in three other reports (64, 72, 87).

Amphotericin B lipid complex is usually given as 5 mg/kg/day as a single infusion at a rate of 2.5 mg/kg/h. If the infusion time exceeds 2 h, the contents of infusion bag should be mixed by shaking. Liposomal amphotericin B doses may range from 5 to 7.5 mg/kg/day, and amphotericin B colloidal

TABLE 3 • Lipid Formulations of Amphotericin B					
Preparation	Usual Dosage	Structure	Lipid Composition	Approved in U.S.	Indications
Abelcet (ABLC, amphotericin B lipid complex)	5 mg/kg/day	Ribbons of lipid with amphotericin B attached	Dimyristoylphosphatidyl choline (DMPC); Dimyristoylphosphatidyl glycerol (DMPG)	Yes	Treatment of invasive fungal infections in patients who are refractory to or intolerant of conventional amphotericin B
AmBisome	5–7.5 mg/kg/day	Unilamellar liposomes with amphotericin B inside	Phosphatidylcholine, cholesterol, distearoyl phosphatidylglycerol		
Amphocil (ABCD, amphotericin B colloidal dispersion)	2–7.5 mg/kg/day	Discoid structures with amphotericin B attached	Cholesteryl sulfate		

dispersion doses range from 2 to 7.5 mg/kg/day. Table 3 summarizes dosing of the lipid formulations.

ADVERSE EFFECTS

Amphotericin B toxicity is likely related to nonselective disruption of mammalian cells, despite the differences in affinity of the drug for ergosterol and cholesterol (83). Pediatric patients may generally tolerate amphotericin B better than adult patients when given similar doses on the basis of body weight (125).

Many patients experience several of the following reactions: headache, chills, fever, hypotension, tachypnea, malaise, muscle and joint pain, anorexia, weight loss, dyspepsia, cramping, epigastric pain, and nausea and vomiting. Anaphylaxis can occur rarely. These reactions are largely dose related and diminish with slow infusion or alternate-day dosing. Symptomatic relief is often achieved with antipyretics, antihistamines, and antiemetics.

Fever and chills occur in over half of patients treated with this drug, appearing 1 to 3 h after the start of the intravenous infusion and subsiding within 4 h after discontinuance. The occurrence of this side effect decreases with continued therapy, and if therapy is interrupted, febrile reactions recur. Amphotericin B is a potent inducer of prostaglandin E_2 synthesis in vitro (60). Administration of ibuprofen reduced the rate of occurrence of chills from 87 to 49%. Meperidine and hydrocortisone also reduce the severity of these reactions (30, 131).

Most patients experience some nephrotoxicity, which may occur by several mechanisms. Amphotericin B lowers the glomerular filtration rate and renal blood flow by direct vasoconstriction (29) and impairs proximal and distal tubular reabsorption of electrolytes (46). The main mechanism may involve effects on membrane permeability via lytic action on the cholesterol-rich lysosomal membranes of renal tubular cells. Juxtamedullary glomerulitis and intratubular and interstitial calcium deposits in the distal nephron are found on biopsy. Findings of amphotericin B nephrotoxicity include renal tubular acidosis, casts in the urine, azotemia, oliguria, and magnesium and potassium wasting.

Impaired renal function is generally reversible during the first 2 weeks of therapy and may be reversed by a brief cessation of drug administration or occasionally by use of lower doses. In some patients, reversal may take several months, and irreversible renal damage has been reported rarely. It remains unclear whether irreversible renal damage with amphotericin B administration is dose related or due to individual susceptibility.

Renal tubular acidosis is also generally reversible and occurs with doses of 0.5 to 1 g or more. Hypokalemia is noted within the first 2 weeks of therapy, and systemic acidosis is absent. Patients are predisposed to nephrocalcinosis and potassium wasting. Sodium loading may improve renal function. Patients with underlying disease such as congestive heart failure, cirrhosis with ascites, or renal failure unlikely to tolerate sodium supplementation, which would probably attenuate development of nephrotoxicity. Relationship between the total dose of amphotericin B and nephrotoxicity is lacking

(29). Failure to account for the underlying disease in the population studied, differing follow-up times, and variations in toxicity determinations contribute to varying conclusions from different reports.

Sodium loading may be beneficial for maintaining renal function in some patients (66). Adequate hydration may also reduce the risk of developing nephrotoxicity. The patient's sodium status should be determined and depletion should be corrected. In the absence of complicating underlying disease states such as congestive heart failure, cirrhosis with ascites, or renal failure, sodium loading is undertaken. Close monitoring of clinical and laboratory parameters is necessary to follow sodium status.

Hypomagnesemia may occur, possibly related to a tubular defect in magnesium reabsorption (16). Hypokalemia arises in most patients receiving therapy and may result from enhanced excretion due to infusion-related hyperkalemia or from tubular damage. Serum creatinine may increase and with levels above 3 mg/100 dL, therapy should be interrupted for 24 to 48 h to prevent uremia and allow renal function to stabilize. Therapy may then resume with a reduced dosage or an alternate-day schedule and close monitoring, with daily measurement of potassium, magnesium, and serum creatinine levels.

Normochromic normocytic anemia may occur, usually about 10 weeks into the therapeutic course. This is most likely related to the direct inhibition of erythrocyte and erythropoietin production or may be secondary to renal toxicity (82). There is a lack of data suggesting a dose-related effect, and the hematocrit becomes normal after amphotericin B is discontinued.

Local pain at the injection site, phlebitis, and thrombophlebitis often accompany amphotericin B therapy. The problem is related to repeated and continuous venipunctures for drug administration and can be avoided by using central venous access or by avoiding extravasation by using larger peripheral veins, if possible. Avoiding amphotericin B infusion concentrations exceeding 0.1 mg/mL and infusion times below 4 h may also be of benefit. The addition of heparin may minimize development of thrombophlebitis; however, no controlled data support this use.

Several associated reactions, including nausea, vomiting, anorexia, headache, myalgias, and arthralgias, have occurred during the initiation of amphotericin B therapy (83). Acute allergy reactions including bronchospasm, dyspnea, and tachypnea have been reported and may occur more frequently in patients with a history of asthma or chronic obstructive pulmonary disease (101). Liver function abnormalities have been reported during amphotericin B therapy, but direct association is questionable (18). Intrathecal administration of amphotericin B is associated with headache, nausea and vomiting, urinary retention, radiculopathy, paresthesia, vision changes, arachnoiditis, myelopathy, nerve palsies, and meningitis.

Lipid formulations of amphotericin B attenuate the development of renal insufficiency and infusion-related toxicities (97). In general, the lipid formulations of amphotericin B demonstrate much less systemic and organ-directed toxicity than conventional amphotericin B. However, direct comparisons among the lipid formulations of amphotericin B and amphotericin B deoxycholate have not yet been carried out.

DRUG INTERACTIONS

Multiple drug therapy is often required in patients receiving amphotericin B because of the severity of illness. Thus, these patients are at increased risk for drug interactions. Nephrotoxic effects may be compounded by concurrent use of drugs with similar toxic potential. These include aminoglycosides, cyclosporine, and antineoplastic agents such as cisplatin and the nitrogen mustard compounds. Concomitant use is cautioned, and serum creatinine should be monitored very closely. Hypokalemia induced by amphotericin B therapy may exaggerate the activity of nondepolarizing skeletal muscle relaxants and digitalis glycosides. Corticosteroids may enhance potassium depletion caused by amphotericin B and therefore predicate serum electrolyte and cardiac monitoring.

Leukocyte transfusions may predispose patients receiving amphotericin B therapy to acute dyspnea, hypoxemia, and development of pulmonary infiltrates (137). Avoidance of simultaneous infusion of leukocyte transfusion and slow administration of amphotericin B have been suggested to minimize this interaction.

The additive toxicities of amphotericin B and flucytosine used as combination therapy may be outweighed by the potential for enhanced therapeutic effect and reduced length of amphotericin B therapy. Synergism occurs when amphotericin B binds to sterols in the cell membrane, increasing permeability and allowing greater penetration of flucytosine into the fungal cell. Increased flucytosine cellular penetration or accumulation resulting from amphotericin B–induced renal failure may explain this interaction. Flucytosine concentrations should be checked and dosage adjusted if indicated by high peak serum concentrations. Studies are lacking demonstrating the usefulness of the lipid formulations in combination with flucytosine, but there is no reason to suspect that they would result in a different outcome than with conventional amphotericin B.

Antagonism has been observed in vitro and in animal studies when amphotericin B and the imidazole antifungals are used in combination (109). This has also been observed in vitro with the combination of azole class of antifungals (ketoconazole, fluconazole, and itraconazole) and amphotericin B (86, 128). Such combination therapy should be used with caution, particularly in immunocompromised patients.

CLINICAL INDICATIONS

Indications for amphotericin B treatment include aspergillosis, blastomycosis, disseminated candidiasis, coccidioidomycosis, fungal endocarditis, fungal endophthalmitis, histoplasmosis, intraabdominal infections, American mucocutaneous leishmaniasis, cryptococcal meningitis (treatment and suppression), fungal meningitis, mucormycosis, fungal septicemia, disseminated sporotrichosis, and fungal urinary tract infections. Other accepted uses not included in United States product labeling are treatment of primary amebic meningoencephalitis caused by *Naegleria* and paracoccidioidomycosis. Amphotericin B has also found extensive use in febrile neutropenic

TABLE 4 • Clinical Uses of Amphotericin B as Primary Therapy for Systemic Fungal Infections	
Disease	**General Adult Dosage Guidelines**
Meningitis	
Cryptococcal	1 mg/[kg·day] maximum i.v.; 0.3 mg/[kg·day] amphotericin B with 150 mg/[kg·day] flucytosine for 4–6 weeks
Coccidioidal	Amphotericin B, up to 1.5 mg/dose, with hydrocortisone intrathecally; may be supplemented by i.v. administration in selected patients with refractory disease
Candidal	0.5–1 mg/[kd·day] i.v. alone or with flucytosine
Fungal peritonitis	Total dose of 2–10 mg/kg × 7–14 days i.v.
	Amphotericin B, 1.5–2 mg/L, in peritoneal dialysis fluid, up to a total dose of 1500 mg alone or with flucytosine
Genitourinary infections	50 mg/L in sterile water, instilled by catheter
Ophthalmic mycoses	7.5 mg total subjunctival dose; concomitant systemic therapy usually indicated
Empirical therapy	
Neutropenic cancer patients	0.5 mg/[kg·day]
AIDS patients	0.5 mg/[kg·day]
AML[a] patients	0.5 mg/[kg·day]
Pulmonary infections	
Aspergillus, disseminated	0.5–1 mg/[kg·day] i.v., total 2–4 g (up to 6–8 in resistant forms)
Blastomycosis	0.5–1 mg/[kg·day] i.v., total 1.5–2 g
Coccidioidomycosis	1–1.5 mg/[kg·day] i.v., total 1.5–2 g
Histoplasmosis	0.6 mg/[kg·day] i.v., total 2–2.5 g
Other	
Candidiasis, invasive, life threatening	0.5–1 mg/[kg·day] i.v., total dose 2–4 g
Candidiasis, non-life-threatening	Amphotericin B, 0.5–1 mg/[kg·day] i.v. × 7–14 days plus flucytosine, 150 mg/[kg·day]
Histoplasmosis, disseminated	0.6 mg/[kg·day] i.v., total 2 g
Mucormycosis	1 mg/[kg·day] i.v. × 2–3 mo

[a]Acute myelogenous leukemia.

patients who have not responded to broad-spectrum antibacterial drugs. Table 4 lists the clinical uses of amphotericin B as primary therapy for systemic infections (57).

Amphotericin B is not indicated for treatment of bacterial, rickettsial, or viral infections. Reports of amphotericin B activity against scrapie (41, 90) and hepatitis B virus (75, 114) have appeared in the literature, but there is no clinical experience with amphotericin B in the treatment of these diseases. Amphotericin B is not indicated in the treatment of "common, clinically inapparent fungal infections that show only positive skin or serologic tests."

REFERENCES

1. Adler-Moore J. AmBisome targetings to fungal infections. Bone Marrow Transplant 1994;14(Suppl 5):S3–7.
2. Adler-Moore JP, Profitt RT. Development, characterization, efficacy and mode of action of AmBisome, a unilamellar liposomal formulation of amphotericin B. J Liposome Res 1993;3: 429–450.
3. Adler-Moore JP, Chiang SM, Satorius A, et al. Treatment of murine candidosis and cryptococcosis with a unilamellar liposomal amphotericin B formulation (AmBisome). J Antimicrob Chemother 1991;28(Suppl B):63–71.
4. Ahearn DG, McGlohn MS. In vitro susceptibilities of sucrose-negative Candida tropicalis, Candida lusitaniae, and Candida norvegensis to amphotericin B, 5-fluorocytosine, miconazole, and ketoconazole. J Clin Microbiol 1984;19:412–416.
5. Albert MM, Adams K, Luther MJ, Sun SH, Graybill JR. Efficacy of AmBisome in murine coccidioidomycosis. J Med Vet Mycol 1994;32:467–471.
6. Albert MM, Graybill JR, Rinaldi MG. Treatment of murine cryptococcal meningitis with an SCH 39304-amphotericin B combination. Antimicrob Agents Chemother 1991;35:1721–1725.
7. Allende MC, Lee JW, Francis P, Garrett K, Dollenberg H, Berenguer J. et al. Dose-dependent antifungal activity and nephrotoxicity of amphotericin B colloidal dispersion in experimental pulmonary aspergillosis. Antimicrob Agents Chemother 1994;38:518–522.
8. Allendoefer R, Marquis AJ, Rinaldi MG, Graybill JR. Combined therapy with fluconazole and flucytosine in murine cryptococcal meningitis. Antimicrob Agents Chemother 1991;35:726–729.
9. Anaissie E, Paetznick V, Proffitt R, Adler-Moore J, Bodey GP. Comparison of the in vitro antifungal activity of free and liposome-encapsulated amphotericin B. Eur J Clin Microbiol Infect Dis 1991;10:665–668.
10. Ansari RA, Hindson DA, Stevens DL, Kloss JG. Pseudallescheria boydii arthritis and osteomyelitis in a patient with Cushing's disease. South Med J 1987;80:90–92.
11. Armstrong D. Treatment of opportunistic fungal infections. Clin Infect Dis 1993;16:1–9.
12. Arroyo J, Medoff G, Kobayashi GS. Therapy of murine aspergillosis with amphotericin B in combination with rifampin or 5-fluorocytosine. Antimicrob Agents Chemother 1977;11:21–25.
13. Athar MA, Winner HI. The development of resistance by Candida species to polyene antibiotics in vitro. J Med Microbiol 1971;4:505–517.
14. Atkinson AJ Jr, Bennett JE. Amphotericin B pharmacokinetics in humans. Antimicrob Agents Chemother 1978;13:271–276.
15. Atkinson BA, Bocanegra R, Colombo AL, Graybill JR. Treatment of disseminated Torulopsis glabrata infection with DO870 and amphotericin B. Antimicrob Agents Chemother 1994;38: 1604–1607.
16. Barton CH, Pahl M, Vaziri ND, Cesario T. Renal magnesium wasting associated with amphotericin B therapy. Am J Med 1984;77:471–474.
17. Bayer AS, Blumenkrantz MJ, Montgomerie JZ, Galpin JE, Cobern JW, et al. Candida peritonitis. Report of 22 cases and review of the English literature. Am J Med 1976;61:831–840.
18. Bennett JE. Chemotherapy of systemic mycoses. N Engl J Med 1974;290:30–32.
19. Bennett JE, Dismukes WE, Duma RJ, Medoff G, Sande MA, et al. A comparison of amphotericin B alone and combined with flucytosine in the treatment of cryptococcal meningitis. N Engl J Med 1979;301:126–131.
20. Bindschadler DD, Bennett JE. A pharmacologic guide to the clinical use of amphotericin B. J Infect Dis 1969;120:427–436.
21. Blinkhorn RJ, Adelstein D, Spagnuolo PJ. Emergence of a new opportunistic pathogen, Candida lusitaniae. J Clin Microbiol 1989;27:236–240.
22. Block ER, Bennett JE. The combined effect of 5-fluorocytosine and amphotericin B in the therapy of murine cryptococcosis. Proc Soc Exp Biol Med 1973;142:476–480.
23. Bolard J. How do the polyene macrolide antibiotics affect the cellular membrane properties? Biochim Biophys Acta 1986; 864:257–304.
24. Bowden RA, Cays M. Phase I study of amphotericin B colloidal dispersion for the treatment of invasive fungal infection after marrow transplant [Abstract 56]. Trends in Invasive Fungal Infections, 1993.
25. Brajtburg J, Elberg S, Bolard J, et al. Interaction of plasma proteins and lipoproteins with amphotericin B. J Infect Dis 1984; 149:986–997.
26. Brajtburg J, Elberg S, Kobayashi GS, Medoff G. Effects of ascorbic acid on the antifungal action of amphotericin B. J Antimicrob Chemother 1989;24:333–337.
27. Brajtburg J, Elberg S, Schwartz DR, et al. Involvement of oxidative damage in erythrocyte lysis induced by amphotericin B. Antimicrob Agents Chemother 1985;27:172–176.
28. Brajtburg J, Powderly WG, Kobayashi GS, Medoff G. Amphotericin B: current understanding of mechanisms of action. Antimicrob Agents Chemother 1990;34:183–188.
29. Branch RA. Prevention of amphotericin B-induced renal impairment: a review on the use of sodium supplementation. Arch Intern Med 1988;148:2389–2394.
30. Burks LC, Aisner J, Fortner CL, Wiernik PH. Meperidine for the treatment of shaking chills and fever. Arch Intern Med 1980; 140:483–484.
31. Ching MS, Raymond K, Bury RW, Mashford ML, Morgan DJ. Absorption or orally administered amphotericin B lozenges. Br J Clin Pharmacol 1983;16:106–108.
32. Christenson JC, Shalit I, Welch DF, Guruswamy A, Marks MI. Synergistic action of amphotericin B and rifampin against Rhizopus species. Antimicrob Agents Chemother 1987;31: 1775–1778.
33. Christiansen KJ, Bernard EM, Gold JW, Armstrong D. Distribution and activity of amphotericin B in humans. J Infect Dis 1985;152:1037–1043.
34. Clemons KV, Stevens DA. Comparative efficacy of amphotericin B colloidal dispersion and amphotericin B deoxycholate suspension in treatment of murine coccidioidomycosis. Antimicrob Agents Chemother 1991;35:1829–1833.
35. Clemons KV, Stevens DA. Therapeutic efficacy of a liposomal formulation of amphotericin B (AmBisome) against murine blastomycosis. J Antimicrob Chemother 1993;32:465–472.

36. Cofrancesco E, Viviani MA, Boschetti C, Tortorano AM, Balzani A. et al. Treatment of chronic disseminated *Geotrichum capitatum* infection with high cumulative dose of colloidal amphotericin B and itraconazole in a leukaemia patient. Mycoses 1995;38:377–384.

37. Collette N, van der Auwera P, Lopez AP, Heymans C, Meunier F. Tissue concentrations and bioactivity of amphotericin B in cancer patients treated with amphotericin B-deoxycholate. Antimicrob Agents Chemother 1989;33:362–368.

38. Collignon PJ, Macleod C, Packham DR. Miconazole therapy in *Pseudallescheria boydii* infection. Aust J Dermatol 1985;26:129–132.

39. Daneshmend TK, Warnock DW. Clinical pharmacokinetics of systemic antifungal drugs. Clin Pharmacokinet 1983;8:17–42.

40. Dean JL, Wolf JE, Ranzini AC, Laughlin MA. Use of amphotericin B during pregnancy: case report and review. Clin Infect Dis 1994;18:364–368.

41. Demaimay R, Adjou K, Lasmezas C, et al. Pharmacological studies of a new derivative of amphotericin B, MS-8209, in mouse and hamster scrapie. J Gen Virol 1994;74(Pt 9):2499–2503.

42. Dick JD, Merz WG, Saral R. Incidence of polyene-resistant yeasts recovered from clinical specimens. Antimicrob Agents Chemother 1980;18:158–163.

43. Dick JD, Rosengard BR, Merz WG, Stuart RK, Hutchins GM, Saral R. Fatal disseminated candidiasis due to amphotericin B-resistant *Candida guilliermondii*. Ann Intern Med 1985;102:67–68.

44. Dietze R, Fagundes SM, Brito EF, Milan EP, Feitosa TF, et al. Treatment of kala-azar in Brazil with Amphocil (amphotericin B cholesterol dispersion) for 5 days. Trans R Soc Trop Med Hyg 1995;89:309–311.

45. Dietze R, Milan EP, Berman JD, Grogl M, Falqueto A, et al. Treatment of Brazilian kala-azar with a short course of amphocil (amphotericin B cholesterol dispersion). Clin Infect Dis 1993;17:981–986.

46. Douglas JB, Healy JK. Nephrotoxic effects of amphotericin B, including renal tubular acidosis. Am J Med 1969;46:154–162.

47. Drutz DJ, Lehrer RI. Development of amphotericin B-resistant *Candida tropicalis* in a patient with defective leukocyte function. Am J Med Sci 1978;276:77–92.

48. Drutz DJ, Spickard A, Rogers DE, Koenig MG. Treatment of disseminated mycotic infections. Am J Med 1968;45:405–418.

49. Dugoni B, Guglielmo BJ, Hollander H. Amphotericin B concentrations in cerebrospinal fluid of patients with AIDS and cryptococcal meningitis. Clin Pharm 1989;8:220–221.

50. Dworzack DL, Clark RB, Borkowski WJ Jr, et al. *Pseudallescheria boydii* brain abscess: association with near drowning and efficacy of high-dose, prolonged miconazole therapy in patients with multiple abscesses. Medicine 1989;68:218–224.

51. Emminger W, Lang HRM, Emminger-Schmidmeier W, Peters C, Gadner H. Amphotericin B serum levels in pediatric bone marrow transplant recipients. Bone Marrow Transplant 1991;7:95–99.

52. Feldman HA, Hamilton JD, Gutman RA. Amphotericin B therapy in an anephric patient. Antimicrob Agents Chemother 1973;4:302–305.

53. Fields BT Jr, Bates JH, Abernathy RS. Amphotericin B serum concentrations during therapy. Appl Microbiol 1970;19:955–959.

54. Fields BT Jr, Bates JH, Abernathy RS. Effect of rapid intravenous infusion on serum concentrations of amphotericin B. Appl Microbiol 1971;22:615–617.

55. Francis P, Lee JW, Hoffman A, et al. Efficacy of unilamellar liposomal amphotericin B in treatment of pulmonary aspergillosis in persistently granulocytopenic rabbits: the potential role of bronchoalveolar D-mannitol and serum galactomannan as markers of infection. J Infect Dis 1994;169:356–368.

56. Galgiani JN. Susceptibility testing of fungi: current status of the standardization process. Antimicrob Agents Chemother 1993;37:2517–2521.

57. Gallis HA, Drew RH, Pickard WW. Amphotericin B: 30 years of clinical experience. Rev Infect Dis 1990(12):308–329.

58. George D, Kordick D, Miniter T, Patterson TF, Andriole VT. Combination therapy in experimental invasive aspergillosis. J Infect Dis 1993;168:692–698.

59. Ghannoum MA, Filler SG, Ibrahim AS, Fu Y, Edwards JE Jr. Modulation of interactions of *Candida albicans* and endothelial cells by fluconazole and amphotericin B. Antimicrob Agents Chemother 1992;36:2239–2244.

60. Giglioti F, Shenep JL, Lott L, Thornton D. Induction of prostaglandin synthesis as the mechanism responsible for the chills and fever produced by infusing amphotericin B. J Infect Dis 1987;156:784–789.

61. Goldberg SL, Geha DJ, Marshall WF, Inwards DJ, Hoagland HC. Successful treatment of simultaneous pulmonary *Pseudallescheria boydii* and *Aspergillus terreus* infection with oral itraconazole. Clin Infect Dis 1993;16:802–805.

62. Graybill JR, Bocanegra R. Liposomal amphotericin B therapy of murine histoplasmosis. Antimicrob Agents Chemother 1995;39:1885–1887.

63. Guinet R, Chanas J, Goullier A, Bonnefoy G, Ambroise-Thomas P. Fatal septicemia due to amphotericin B-resistant *Candida lusitaniae*. J Clin Microbiol 1983;18:443–444.

64. Hager H, Welt SI, Cardasis JP, Alvarez S. Disseminated blastomycosis in a pregnant woman successfully treated with amphotericin B. A case report. J Reprod Med 1988;33:485–488.

65. Hauser WE, Remington JS. The effect of antibiotics on the humeral and cell-mediated immune responses. In: Sabath LD, ed. Action of antibiotics in patients. Bern: Huber, 1982:127–147.

66. Heidemann HT, Gerkens JF, Spickard WA, Jackson EK, Branch RA. Amphotericin B nephrotoxicity in humans decreased by salt repletion. Am J Med 1983;75:476–481.

67. Hofstra W, De Vries-Hospers HG, van der Waaij D. Concentrations of amphotericin B in faeces and blood of healthy volunteers after the oral administration of various doses. Infection 1982;10:223–227.

68. Hostetler JS, Clemons KV, Hanson LHH, Stevens DA. Efficacy and safety of amphotericin B colloidal dispersion compared with those of amphotericin B deoxycholate suspension for treatment of disseminated murine cryptococcosis. Antimicrob Agents Chemother 1992;36:2656–2660.

69. HsuChen CC, Feingold DS. Two types of resistance to polyene antibiotics in *Candida albicans*. Nature 1974;251:656–659.

70. Hughes CE, Harris C, Moody JA, Peterson LR, Gerding DN. In vitro activities of amphotericin B in combination with four antifungal agents and rifampin against *Aspergillus* spp. Antimicrob Agents Chemother 1984;25:560–562.

71. Investigator's Brochure. The Liposome Company. Abelcet (amphotericin B lipid complex injection). 1996.

72. Ismail MA, Lerner SA. Disseminated blastomycosis in a pregnant woman. Am Rev Respir Dis 1982;126:350–353.

73. Kerr Cm, Perfect JR, Craven PC, Jorgensen JH, Drutz DJ, et al. Fungal peritonitis in patients on continuous ambulatory peritoneal dialysis. Ann Intern Med 1983;99:334–337.

74. Kerridge D. Mode of action of clinically important antifungal drugs. Adv Microb Physiol 1986;27:1–72.

75. Kessler HA, Dixon J, Howard CR, Tsiquaye K, Zuckerman AJ. Effects of amphotericin B on hepatitis B virus. Antimicrob Agents Chemother 1981;20:826–833.

76. Khoo SH, Bond J, Denning DW. Administering amphotericin B—a practical approach. J Antimicrob Chemother 1994;33: 203–213.

77. Kitahara M, Seth VK, Medoff G, Kobayashi GS. Activity of amphotericin B, 5-fluorocytosine, and rifampin against six clinical isolates of Aspergillus. Antimicrob Agents Chemother 1976;9: 915–919.

78. Lamy-Freund MT, Ferreira VFN, Schreier S. Mechanism of inactivation of the polyene antibiotic amphotericin B: evidence for radical formation in the process of autooxidation. J Antibiot 1985;38:753–757.

79. Lauer BA, Reller LB, Schroter GPJ. Susceptibility of Aspergillus to 5-fluorocytosine and amphotericin B alone and in combination. J Antimicrob Chemother 1979;4:375–380.

80. Little JR, Stein SH, Little KD. Amphotericin B—a model murine immunostimulant. In: Szentuvanyi AFH, Gillissen G, eds. Antibiosis and host immunity. New York: Plenum, 1987: 253–263.

81. Louria DB. Some aspects of the absorption, distribution, and excretion of amphotericin B in man. Antibiot Med Clin Ther 1958;5:295–301.

82. MacGregor RR, Bennett JE, Erslev AJ. Erythropoietin concentration in amphotericin B-induced anemia. Antimicrob Agents Chemother 1978;14:270–273.

83. Maddux MS, Barriere SL. A review of complications of amphotericin B therapy: recommendations for prevention and management. Drug Intell Clin Pharm 1980;14:177–181.

84. Magee BB, Magee PT. Electrophoretic karyotypes and chromosome numbers in Candida species. J Gen Microbiol 1987;133: 425–430.

85. Marks WH, Florence L, Lieberman J, Chapman P, Howard D, et al. Successfully treated invasive pulmonary aspergillosis associated with smoking marijuana in a renal transplant recipient. Transplantation 1996;61:1771–1774.

86. Martin E, Maier F, Bhakdi S. Antagonistic effects of fluconazole and 5-fluorocytosine on candidacidal action of amphotericin B in human serum. Antimicrob Agents Chemother 1994;38: 1331–1338.

87. McCoy MJ, Ellenberg JF, Killam AP. Coccidioidomycosis complicating pregnancy. Am J Obstet Gynecol 1980;137:739–740.

88. McEvoy GK, ed. American Hospital Formulary Service Drug Information. Bethesda: Board of Directors of the American Society of Hospital Pharmacists, 1992.

89. McGinnis MR, Rinaldi MG. Antifungal drugs: mechanisms of action, drug resistance, susceptibility testing and assays of activity in biological fluids. In: Lorian V, ed. Antibiotics in laboratory medicine. 3rd ed. Baltimore: Williams & Wilkins, 1991: 198–257.

90. McKenzie D, Kaczkowski J, Marsh R, Aiken J. Amphotericin B delays both scrapie agent replication and PrP-res accumulation early in infection. J Virol 1994;68:7534–7536.

91. Medoff G, Brajtburg J, Kobayashi GS. Antifungal agents useful in therapy of systemic fungal infections. Annu Rev Pharmacol Toxicol 1983;23:303–330.

92. Medoff G, Comfort M, Kobayashi GS. Synergistic action of amphotericin B and 5-fluorocytosine against yeast-like organisms. Proc Soc Exp Biol Med 1971;138:571–574.

93. Merkel GJ, Phelps CL. The effects of amphotericin B on the interaction of Candida albicans with fibroblast cultures. Can J Microbiol 1989;35:255–259.

94. Merkel GJ, Phelps CL. Conditions affecting the amphotericin B mediated inhibition of Candida albicans attachment to cell cultures. Can J Microbiol 1989;35:260–264.

95. Merz WG. Candida lusitaniae: frequency of recovery, colonization, infection, and amphotericin B resistance. J Clin Microbiol 1984;20:1194–1195.

96. Merz WG, Sandford GR. Isolation and characterization of a polyene-resistant variant of Candida tropicalis. J Clin Microbiol 1979;9:677–680.

97. Meunier F, Prentice HG, Ringden O. Liposomal amphotericin B (AmBisome): safety data from a phase II/III clinical trial. J Antimicrob Chemother 1991;28(Suppl B):83–91.

98. Mitsutake K, Kohno S, Miyazaki Y, Noda T, Miyazaki T, Kaku M, et al. In vitro and in vivo antifungal activities of liposomal amphotericin B, and amphotericin B lipid complex. Mycopathologia 1994;128:13–17.

99. Morgan DJ, Ching MS, Raymond K, et al. Elimination of amphotericin B in impaired renal function. Clin Pharmacol Ther 1983;34:248–253.

100. Mpona-Minga M, Coulon J, Bonaly R. Effects of subinhibitory dose of amphotericin B on cell wall biosynthesis in Candida albicans. Res Microbiol 1989;140:95–105.

101. Murray HW. Allergic reactions to amphotericin B [Letter]. N Engl J Med 1974;290:693.

102. Muther RS, Bennett WM. Peritoneal clearance of amphotericin B and 5-fluorocytosine. West J Med 1980;133:157–160.

103. Nugent KM, Couchot KR. Effects of sublethal concentrations of amphotericin B on Candida albicans. J Infect Dis 1986;154: 665–669.

104. Odds FC. Interactions among amphotericin B, 5-fluorocytosine, ketoconazole, and miconazole against pathogenic fungi in vitro. Antimicrob Agents Chemother 1982;22:763–770.

105. Oppenheim BA, Herbrecht R, Kusne S. The safety and efficacy of amphotericin B colloidal dispersion in the treatment of invasive mycoses. Clin Infect Dis 1995;21:1145–1153.

106. Pahls S, Schaffner A. Comparison of the activity of free and a liposomal amphotericin B in vitro and in a model of systemic and localized murine candidiasis. J Infect Dis 1994;169: 1057–1061.

107. Patterson T, Miniter P, Dijkstra J, Szoka F, Ryan J, Andriole V. Treatment of experimental invasive aspergillosis with novel amphotericin B/cholesterol-sulfate complexes. J Infect Dis 1989;159:717–724.

108. Perfect JR, Durack DT. Comparison of amphotericin B and N-d-ornithyl amphotericin B methyl ester in experimental cryptococcal meningitis and Candida albicans endocarditis with pyelonephritis. Antimicrob Agents Chemother 1985;28:751–755.

109. Petrou MA, Rogers TR. Intractions in vitro between polyenes and imidazoles against yeast. J Antimicrob Chemother 1991; 27:491–506.

110. Pfaller MA, Messer SA, Hollis RJ. Strain delineation and antifungal susceptibilities of epidemiologically related and unrelated isolates of Candida lusitaniae. Diagn Microbiol Infect Dis 1994;20:127–133.

111. Pierce AM, Pierce HD, Unrau AM, Oehlschlager AC. Lipid composition and polyene antibiotic resistance of Candida albicans mutants. Can J Biochem 1978;56:135–142.

112. Polak A. Pharmacokinetics of amphotericin B and flucytosine. Postgrad Med J 1979;55:667–670.

113. Polak A, Scholer HJ, Wall M. Combination therapy of experimental candidiasis, cryptococcosis and aspergillosis in mice. Chemotherapy 1982;28:461–479.

114. Pottage JC Jr, Kessler HA. Inhibition of in vitro HBsAg production by amphotericin B and ketoconazole. J Med Virol 1985;16:275–281.

115. Powderly WGKG, Herzig GP, Medoff G. Amphotericin B-resistant yeast infection in severely immunocompromised patients. Am J Med 1988;84:826–832.

116. Powderly WG, Granich GG, Herzid GP, Krogstad DJ. HPLC measurement of amphotericin B serum levels in cancer patients [Abstract 782]. Program and abstracts of the 27th Interscience Conference on Antimicrobial Agents and Chemotherapy. Washington, DC: American Society for Microbiology, 1987.

117. Rex JHCCJ, Merz WG, Galgiani JG, Anaissie EJ. Detection of amphotericin B-resistant *Candida* isolates in a broth-based system. Antimicrob Agents Chemother 1995;39:906–909.

118. Rex JH, Pfaller MA, Rinaldi MG, Polak A, Galgiani JN. Antifungal susceptibility testing. Clin Microbiol Rev 1993;6:367–381.

119. Safe LM, Safe SH, Subden RE, Morris DC. Sterol content and polyene antibiotic resistance in isolates of *Candida krusei, Candida parakrusei,* and *Candida tropicalis.* Can J Microbiol 1977;23:398–401.

120. Schmitt HJ, Bernard EM, Edwards FF, Armstrong D. Combination therapy in a model of pulmonary aspergillosis. Mycoses 1991;34:281–285.

121. Seidenfeld SM, Cooper BH, Smith JW, Luby JP, Machowiak PA. Amphotericin B tolerance: a characteristic of *Candida parapsilosis* not shared by other *Candida* species. J Infect Dis 1983;147:116–119.

122. Sokol-Anderson M, Sligh JE, Elberg S, Brajtburg JKG, et al. Role of cell defense against oxidative damage in the resistance of *Candida albicans* to the killing effect of amphotericin B. Antimicrob Agents Chemother 1988;32:702–705.

123. Sokol-Anderson MLBJ, Medoff G. Amphotericin B-induced oxidative damage and killing of *Candida albicans.* J Infect Dis 1986;154:76–83.

124. Sokol-Anderson ML, Brajtburg J, Medoff G. Sensitivity of *Candida albicans* to amphotericin B administered as single or fractionated doses. Antimicrob Agents Chemother 1986;29:701–702.

125. Starke JR, Mason EO Jr, Kramer WG, Kaplan SL. Pharmacokinetics of amphotericin B in infants and children. J Infect Dis 1987;155:766–774.

126. Stevens DA. Overview of amphotericin B colloidal dispersion (Amphocil). J Infect 1994;28(Suppl 1):45–49.

127. Subden RE, Safe L, Morris DC, Brown RG, Safe S. Eburicol, lichosterol, ergosterol, and obtusifoliol from polyene antibiotic-resistant mutants of *Candida albicans.* Can J Microbiol 1977;23:751–754.

128. Sugar AM, Hitchcock CA, Troke PF, Picard M. Combination therapy of murine invasive candidiasis with fluconazole and amphotericin B. Antimicrob Agents Chemother 1995;39: 598–601.

129. Titsworth E, Grunberg E. Chemotherapeutic activity of 5-fluorocytosine and amphotericin B against *Candida albicans* in mice. Antimicrob Agents Chemother 1973;4:306–308.

130. Tkatch LS, Kusne S, Eibling D. Successful treatment of zygomycosis of the paranasal sinuses with surgical debridement and amphotericin B colloidal dispersion. Am J Otolaryngol 1993;14:249–253.

131. Tynes BS, Utz JP, Bennett JE, Alling DW. Reducing amphotericin B reactions. A double-blind study. Am Rev Respir Dis 1963;87:264–268.

132. Utz JP, Garriques IL, Sande MA, Warner JF, Mandell GL, et al. Therapy of cryptococcosis with a combination of flucytosine and amphotericin B. J Infect Dis 1975;132:368–373.

133. Valero G, Graybill JR. Successful treatment of cryptococcal meningitis with amphotericin B colloidal dispersion: report of four cases. Antimicrob Agents Chemother 1995;39: 2588–2590.

134. van Etten EW, van den Heuvel-de Groot C, Bakker-Woudenberg IA. Efficacies of amphotericin B-desoxycholate (Fungizone), liposomal amphotericin B (AmBisome) and fluconazole in the treatment of systemic candidosis in immunocompetent and leukopenic mice. J Antimicrob Chemother 1993;32:723–739.

135. Vukmir RB, Kusne S, Linden P, Pasculle W, Fothergill AW. Successful therapy for cerebral phaeohyphomycosis due to *Dactylaria gallopava* in a liver transplant recipient. Clin Infect Dis 1994;19:714–719.

136. Warnock DW. Amphotericin B: an introduction. J Antimicrob Chemother 1991;28(Suppl B):27–38.

137. Wright DG, Robichaud KJ, Pizzo PA, Deisseroth AB. Lethal pulmonary reactions associated with the combined use of amphotericin B and leukocyte transfusions. N Engl J Med 1981; 304:1185–1189.

Azoles: Imidazoles

●

Thomas F. Patterson

ANTIFUNGAL IMIDAZOLES

The azole class of antifungals contains synthetic compounds that have a five-membered ring. The imidazoles contain two nitrogens, while the newer triazoles have three nitrogens in the ring. The triazoles offer increased stability as systemic drugs and have a broader spectrum of activity. In addition, they have greater affinity for fungal target enzymes than for mammalian enzymes so they are associated with decreased toxicity (4, 27).

The advantages of the newer triazoles have significantly reduced the indications for imidazoles in the treatment of systemic fungal infections. However, the imidazoles are used as topical therapy for mucosal fungal infections (oropharyngeal and vaginal infection) and for superficial skin infections, except for tinea capitis (39).

The imidazole compounds have side chains that convey considerable differences in pharmacokinetic properties (Fig. 1). Of these compounds, only ketoconazole is commonly used as an agent for systemic infection. Miconazole was an early azole developed for systemic use, but toxicity of its diluent has limited its use for the most part to topical indications. The lack of a parenteral formulation has also limited the remaining imidazole compounds to topical use for skin and mucosal infections. These agents include clotrimazole, which is used topically for oral, vaginal, and skin indications, and a variety of other topical agents used for vaginal, oral mucosa, and skin infections (3).

Mechanism of Action

The imidazoles are considered fungistatic antifungal agents. They bind to the heme moiety of the fungal cytochrome P-450-dependent enzyme lanosterol 14-α-demethylase. Inhibition of that 14-α-demethylase blocks formation of ergosterol, which leads to the buildup of 14-α-sterols and depletes ergosterol in the cell membrane (75). Both effects serve to inhibit fungal cell growth. With topical use, fungicidal effects against some organisms may be seen because of the extremely high concentrations of antifungal agents that can be achieved with topical preparations (39). When systemically administered, the imidazoles also interact with the mammalian cytochrome P-450 3A enzyme system. Interactions with these mammalian enzymes give these compounds higher hepatic toxicity than the newer triazoles and disrupt mammalian sterol synthesis, which can result in decreased cortisol and testosterone concentrations. The newer triazoles also cause fewer drug interactions with compounds metabolized through the cytochrome P450 CYP3A4 pathway (2, 11).

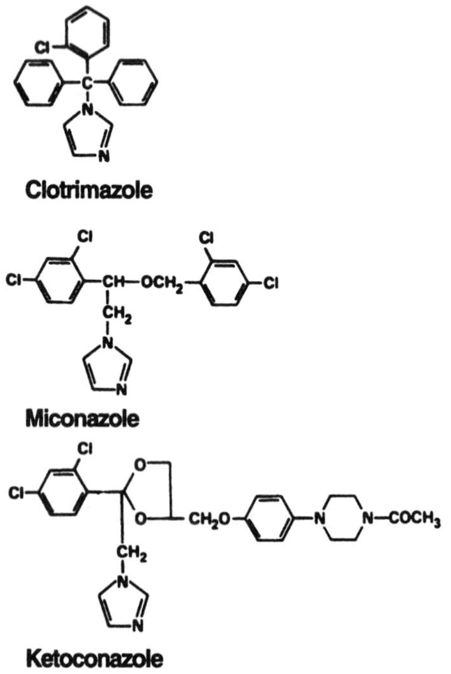

Spectrum of Activity

The imidazoles have a broad spectrum of activity that encompasses many yeasts, dermatophytes, and dimorphic fungi (39) (Table 1). Like the triazole antifungals, ketoconazole and clotrimazole have less activity against some yeasts other than *Candida albicans,* such as *C. glabrata* and *C. krusei* (36). In vitro activity has been demonstrated against some fluconazole-resistant yeasts, although the clinical efficacy of an imidazole in that setting is not established (70). Ketoconazole is the only imidazole that should be used routinely for therapy of systemic infection. Clotrimazole is not well absorbed and undergoes extensive first-pass metabolism; it should be considered topical therapy even when used as oral troches. Miconazole has largely been replaced by the newer triazoles, and its serious toxicity precludes routine use. In addition, the use of ketoconazole in systemic infection should be limited to patients who are immunocompetent and have non-life-threatening extrameningeal infection. Ketoconazole does not possess activity against systemic mold infections such as *Aspergillus* spp. None of these agents has activity against Zygomycetes (39).

Antifungal Resistance

In vitro and clinical resistance to the imidazoles was reported initially in patients with mucocutaneous candidiasis receiving long-term ketoconazole therapy (32). While mycologic resistance to the imidazoles continues to occur, it is significantly less common than with the newer triazole antifungals (21). Whether the increased rate of in vitro resistance for the newer triazoles, particularly fluconazole, is simply due to the widespread use of the newer azoles as therapeutic and prophylactic agents is not clear (15, 35, 46, 57, 58). Molecular mechanisms of resistance include alterations in the target enzyme, decreased permeability of the fungus to the azole, and activation of efflux pumps that decrease intracellular drug concentrations (59, 76, 77). Other potential mechanisms for resistance include alterations in the $\Delta^{5,6}$ desaturase, and decreased ergosterol content in cell wall sterols (30, 80). Fungal resistance may develop from mutations in a single strain or from replacement of the original isolates with inherently less susceptible strains or species (47, 52, 56). It is important to distinguish mycologic from clinical resistance. In many cases, clinical failure relates to the fact that the host is severely immunosuppressed or that the drug has not been delivered effectively to the site of infection (63, 74). Some fungi develop cross-resistance between the newer triazoles and the imidazoles (36, 70).

Another potential cause of antifungal resistance from the use of imidazoles is antagonism between amphotericin B and the azoles. Pretreatment of *Aspergillus* cells in vitro with ketoconazole produced cells that were resistant to amphotericin

FIGURE 1. Chemical structures of imidazole antifungals.

TABLE 1 • **Activity of Imidazoles in Systemic Mycoses: Ketoconazole**

Fungus	Ketoconazole Activity[a]
Opportunistic yeasts	
Candida albicans	+ +
Candida tropicalis	+ +
Candida glabrata	+ +
Candida krusei	+
Cryptococcus neoformans	+ +
Opportunistic molds	
Aspergillus species	0
Fusarium	0
Pseudallescheria boydii	+
Zygomycetes	0
Dimorphic mycoses	
Histoplasma capsulatum	+ + + +
Blastomyces dermatitidis	+ +
Coccidioides immitis	+ +
Sporothrix schenckii	+
Paracoccidioides brasiliensis	+ + +
Penicillium marneffei	+
Agents of phaeohyphomycoses	+

Data from Patterson TF, Graybill JR. Infections caused by fungi. In: Stein J, ed. Internal medicine. 5th ed. St. Louis, MO: CV Mosby, 1997.

[a] Activity: none, 0; + to + + + +, minimal activity to highly active.

B. In vivo resistance was also demonstrated in an animal model of invasive aspergillosis (60). The theoretical mechanism for development of amphotericin B resistance was alteration of cell membrane sterols by the imidazoles, which alters the site of action for amphotericin B. While the newer azoles can also be shown to produce antagonism with amphotericin B (61), other investigators have not demonstrated antagonism (72). The clinical implications of these effects are not well established, but the potential for antagonism with amphotericin B, particularly with ketoconazole, should be considered.

KETOCONAZOLE
Pharmacokinetics

Ketoconazole, a *cis*-1-acetyl-4-[4-[[2-(2,4-dichlorophenyl)-2-(1*H*-imidazole-1-ylmethyl)-1,3-dioxolan-4-yl]methoxyl]phenyl] piperazine, was the first successful oral azole antifungal. Its structure was subsequently modified to produce newer antifungal compounds. Ketoconazole is soluble at a pH of 3. There is no intravenous formulation. Systemic administration is via the oral route as 200-mg tablets; it is also available as a 2% cream or shampoo for topical use (1). Ketoconazole has in vitro activity against many yeasts, including *Candida* spp. and *Cryptococcus,* dermatophytes, dimorphic fungi, and phaeohyphomycetes.

Pharmacokinetic characteristics are summarized in Table 1 in the chapter on triazoles. Following administration of 200 mg of ketoconazole, peak serum levels are generally 1 to 4 mg/mL (12), although significant individual variation occurs. The half-life is generally 7 to 10 h. Absorption is dramatically decreased in patients with decreased gastric acidity, including those receiving antacids, H_2-histaminergic receptor blocking agents (such as cimetidine, ranitidine, or famotidine), or

omeprazole (9). In addition, patients may have achlorhydria following gastric surgery, after chemotherapy, or with advanced HIV infection. Administration of ketoconazole with an acidic solution such as dilute hydrochloric or glutamic acid increases its absorption (6, 40, 43). Administration with a cola beverage (Coca-Cola Classic, which has a pH of 2.5) increased absorption by approximately 65% (7).

The liver metabolizes ketoconazole extensively, with inactive drug excreted mainly in bile. Concentration of active drug in urine is low (2–4% of serum values), and poor central nervous system penetration prohibits its use in meningeal disease (<1% of serum levels) (12). It is highly protein bound (>99%), largely to albumin. Vaginal concentrations are similar to those in plasma (4). Keratinocyte concentrations are also high, and active drug is found in sweat, which may increase its activity in superficial mycoses. Only small concentrations of ketoconazole are found in salivary secretions, which may be why ketoconazole has lower activity than fluconazole in esophageal candidiasis (23).

Dosage Regimens

Ketoconazole is available as 200-mg scored tablets for systemic administration. Use of the topical cream and shampoo formulations for cutaneous mycoses is discussed below. Therapy for mucosal infections (e.g., oropharyngeal candidiasis) and cutaneous infections may be begun at doses of 200 mg/day and be continued for 2 weeks. For more extensive mucosal infection, such as candidal esophagitis, therapy is often begun at a dose of 400 mg/day. When ketoconazole is used for therapy of nonmeningeal non-life-threatening systemic mycoses (e.g., histoplasmosis or blastomycosis in immunocompetent hosts, or paracoccidioidomycosis), therapy is also typically begun at 400 mg/day and continued for an extended course of 6 to 12 months. The dose may be increased to 600 to 800 mg/day or more in patients who fail to respond to initial doses of therapy, but toxicity is greatly increased at those doses, with minimal increase in efficacy (24, 48, 72).

In children over 2 years of age, a single daily dose of 3.3 to 6.6 mg/kg has been used in small numbers of patients. However, it has not been studied extensively, and the drug should not be used in children unless benefits outweigh risks (34). Ketoconazole is a pregnancy class C drug, shown to be teratogenic in rats. Ketoconazole has also been shown to be embryotoxic when given at high doses during the first trimester of gestation; it should be used in pregnancy only if the benefits outweigh risks. Since ketoconazole is probably excreted in breast milk, mothers who are receiving therapy should not breastfeed (4).

The dose of ketoconazole does not need to be adjusted in patients with altered renal function. Dose adjustment is also unnecessary in those with moderate hepatic dysfunction.

Adverse Effects

The side effects associated with ketoconazole are shown in Table 2 in the triazole chapter. The most common side effects of ketoconazole are gastrointestinal, including nausea, vomiting, and anorexia. These side effects are dose dependent, occurring in approximately 20% of patients receiving 400 mg/day and 30% of patients receiving 800 mg/day (71). Better tolerance is achieved with administration with food or, for the higher dose regimens, in divided doses. Rash occurs in less than 5%. Ketoconazole can decrease plasma testosterone concentrations and cause gynecomastia, decreased libido, and impotence (2). In addition, at high doses ketoconazole may interfere with adrenal steroid synthesis and result in decreased plasma cortisol concentrations (24). Adrenal crisis following high-dose ketoconazole therapy has also been reported.

Hepatic abnormalities are common. Approximately 5 to 10% of patients have mild, asymptomatic elevations of liver transaminases, which return to normal without dose adjustment. Symptomatic ketoconazole-induced hepatitis occurs rarely, developing in an estimated 1 in 10,000 patients, but it is potentially fatal (3). Liver function abnormalities are similar to those seen with hepatitis A. The onset of symptoms is usually after a few days of therapy, but may occur after patients have been on therapy for weeks to months; 80% of the cases occur within the first 3 months of therapy (3). Patients should be advised about the possibility of hepatitis, and liver function tests should be performed if symptoms are present.

Drug Interactions

Interactions of ketoconazole with other drugs are substantially more frequent than drug interactions with the newer triazoles, particularly fluconazole (see Table 3 in the triazole chapter) (51). Agents such as rifampicin, and presumably rifabutin, markedly increase ketoconazole clearance through induction of hepatic enzymes (42). Other compounds also increase clearance of ketoconazole including phenytoin and isoniazid. Cyclosporine serum concentrations are markedly increased by use of ketoconazole, presumably because both drugs are metabolized by the cytochrome P-450 enzyme CYP3A4 (26, 67, 68). Ketoconazole is used to raise cyclosporine concentrations, which reduces the daily dose and thus the expense of cyclosporine. A study in heart transplant patients demonstrated significant cost savings, with decreased rejection and fewer episodes of infection using such a strategy (37). An additional impact in transplantation may be the increase in the AUCs for methylprednisolone and prednisone by ketoconazole, through uncertain mechanisms.

Other compounds are also affected by ketoconazole. Ketoconazole elevates terfenadine, astemizole, and cisapride levels and metabolites to toxic concentrations, which can precipitate fatal torsade de pointes by prolonging the QT interval (2, 31). Thus, use of ketoconazole with terfenadine, astemizole, or cisapride is contraindicated. Other effects are less pronounced, including prolongation of the effects of warfarin, increased digoxin levels, and increased activity of oral hypoglycemic agents (42). In addition, ketoconazole increases serum concentrations of midazolam, triazolam, phenytoin, imipramine, and desipramine (69, 73, 76).

Clinical Indications

The indications for ketoconazole are limited because of the increased efficacy and decreased toxicity of the newer azoles (Table 1). Ketoconazole is effective in nonmeningeal endemic mycoses, such as histoplasmosis, blastomycosis, and coccidioidomycosis. However, itraconazole has largely replaced its use in those mycoses. Ketoconazole is also highly active in paracoccidioidomycosis. It is effective for chronic mucocutaneous candidiasis and oral, vaginal, and esophageal candidal infections. However, for serious invasive *Candida* infections, fluconazole has typically replaced ketoconazole for clinical indications in which an azole can be used for therapy (13, 14, 29, 41, 53, 64). For example, a cost-benefit study showed the utility of empirically choosing fluconazole, which is more expensive, over ketoconazole in AIDS patients with *Candida* esophagitis because of the increased efficacy of fluconazole in that setting (55). Other potential indications for ketoconazole include tinea versicolor (due to *Malassezia furfur*) and other superficial dermatoses (20, 78).

MICONAZOLE

Miconazole (1-[2-(2,4-dichlorophenyl) methoxyl] ethyl]-1*H*-imidazole) was the first systemic azole; its serious toxicity and limited efficacy have resulted in its replacement as a clinically useful systemic antifungal agent. It is still available as topical, vaginal, and intravenous preparations (33). The topical and vaginal uses of miconazole are discussed below. The intravenous preparation is no longer marketed in the United States, although it is available in other countries (10). The intravenous preparation is solubilized in a PEG 40 castor oil (Cremophor EL), which is also used to solubilize other drugs such as paclitaxel and cyclosporine. Much of the toxicity of intravenous miconazole is likely due to the solubilizing vehicle (16). Toxicities associated with the vehicle include serious hypersensitivity reactions, hyperlipidemia, anemia, and most importantly, cardiopulmonary arrest secondary to conduction defects (19).

Miconazole has activity against a variety of yeasts, dermatophytes, and selected molds, such as *Pseudallescheria* spp. and other hyalohyphomyetes and phaeohyphomycetes (49, 50). Clinical efficacy is also limited. Recommended doses range from 200 to 2400 mg/day in three divided doses, with the drug diluted in 200 mL of saline and given no more rapidly than 2 h/200 mg (33). Severe, even fatal toxicities have been observed following those guidelines (10). In the past, intravenous miconazole was used in patients intolerant of, or unresponsive to, standard antifungal therapies. However, the availability of the newer triazoles and development of newer antifungals such as liposomal amphotericin have largely reduced the role of miconazole in systemic infection to historical consideration.

TOPICAL ANTIFUNGAL AGENTS

The topical imidazoles are used for treatment of superficial and cutaneous infections including tinea corporis, tinea pedis, tinea cruris, and tinea versicolor, and cutaneous, vaginal, and oral *Candida* infections. They are not useful for tinea capitis. Mycologic resistance to these agents is uncommon in the fungi causing superficial mycoses (4, 45). The topical products are similar in their efficacy and tolerance so that selection of a specific agent should be based on cost, patient preferences, and product availability (1, 5, 81). Many of these agents are available for over-the-counter use (Table 2). In superficial dermatoses that have a

TABLE 2 • Topical Imidazoles for Use As Therapy for Cutaneous Mycoses

Drug	Trade Name	Preparation
Miconazole	Micatin, Monistat-Derm	Cream, lotion, spray, powder
Oxiconazole	Oxistat	Cream
Clotrimazole	Lotrimin, Mycelex	Cream, lotion, spray
Econazole	Spectazole	Cream
Ketoconazole	Nizoral	Cream, spray, shampoo
Sulconazole	Exelderm	Lotion

Data from Bennett JE. Antifungal agents. In: Gilman AG, Hardman JG, Limbird LE, eds. Goodman & Gilman's the pharmacological basis of therapeutics. 9th ed. New York: McGraw-Hill, 1996:1175–1190.

TABLE 3 • Imidazole Compounds for the Treatment of *Candida* Vaginitis

Drug	Trade Name	Preparation	Duration (days)
Miconazole	Monistat 7	Cream, suppository (100 mg)	7
Miconazole	Monistat 3	Suppository (200 mg)	3
Clotrimazole	Gyne-Lotrimin, Mycelex 7	Cream, tablet (100 mg)	7
Clotrimazole	Gyne-Lotrimin, Mycelex G	Tablet (500 mg)	3
Butoconazole	Femstat	Cream	3
Tioconazole	Vagistat	Ointment	1
Terconazole [a]	Terazole 7	Cream	7
Terconazole[a]	Terazole 3	Suppository (80 mg)	3

Data from Bennett JE. Antifungal agents. In: Gilman AG, Hardman JG, Limbird LE, eds. Goodman & Gilman's the pharmacological basis of therapeutics. 9th ed. New York: McGraw-Hill, 1996:1175–1190.

[a] Terconazole is a triazole antifungal.

high likelihood of a fungal etiology, an empirical trial of an inexpensive, but efficacious, over-the-counter product may be the most cost-effective (8). Generally these compounds should be applied twice daily for 3 to 6 weeks.

The imidazoles are also widely used to treat vaginal candidal infections and are available in both over-the-counter and prescription preparations (65). They are available as vaginal creams, tablets, suppositories, and ointments (Table 3). Most are administered once daily at bedtime, generally for 3 to 7 days. Higher-dose preparations of clotrimazole tablet (500 mg) and tioconazole ointment allow single-dose administration. Antifungal resistance of vaginal isolates remains uncommon, but species of yeasts other than *C. albicans* are being increasingly isolated as etiologic agents of vaginitis. Some of these strains, such as *C. glabrata*, respond to topical imidazole therapy (66).

Clotrimazole

The structure of clotrimazole is shown in Figure 1. Clotrimazole is available in oral topical 10-mg troches, 100-mg and 500-mg vaginal tablets and 1% cream, and as a 1% cream, lo-

tion, or solution. Clotrimazole troches are only indicated for treatment of oropharyngeal candidiasis. Clotrimazole administered orally is not effective as systemic therapy and is considered topical therapy. Clotrimazole is well tolerated as an oral agent, with patients sucking on the troches until they dissolve. Serum concentrations following doses of 200 mg/day are 0.2 to 0.35 mg/mL (4). The absorbed drug is hepatically metabolized. Adverse reactions to oral clotrimazole are uncommon, with a mild gastrointestinal irritation in approximately 5% (4).

One problem with patient compliance is that the recommended dosing regimen is for a 10-mg troche to be taken 5 times daily for 14 days. In patients with AIDS and in patients receiving chemotherapy, clotrimazole has been a useful antifungal agent (25, 28, 38, 62). Response rates in some series have approached 100% (53). However, the variability in clotrimazole response rates is likely due to lack of compliance with multiple daily doses. Antifungal resistance has not been extensively evaluated but does not appear to develop commonly (54). However, patients with advanced AIDS and clinically refractory thrush are unlikely to respond to clotrimazole troches as are those with *Candida* esophagitis, which probably reflects tissue invasion by the organisms. The vaginal tablets have been advocated to allow increased doses to be administered less frequently, but they are generally unpalatable for oral use.

Topical clotrimazole is applied to skin twice daily. Vaginal applications can be given for 7 days with the 100-mg vaginal tablets or for one dose with the 500-mg tablet. Clotrimazole cream is given for 7 to 14 days. The major adverse events are minor vaginal and urinary irritation in less than 2% of patients. Overall response rates for cutaneous mycoses to clotrimazole therapy range from 80 to 100% (17, 18), while vaginal response rates are expected to be at least 80%, although relapses are common (4, 22).

Miconazole

In contrast to miconazole intravenous preparations, which have largely been replaced by other compounds, miconazole as a topical spray, powder, cream, or ointment and as a vaginal cream or suppository continues to be a cost-effective therapy for superficial and vaginal mycoses (8). Only a minimal amount of miconazole is absorbed following vaginal or cutaneous administration. It is well tolerated, with adverse events largely limited to local irritation that occurs in less than 5% of recipients. Response rates are similar those with other therapies for topical mycoses. Generally, efficacy rates well above 70% are expected for most superficial and vaginal mycoses. In the treatment of tinea pedis, tinea cruris, and tinea versicolor, response to miconazole may exceed 90% (2). A cost-benefit analysis determined that an empirical course of miconazole as first-line therapy was less expensive than choosing more costly over-the-counter preparations or more expensive therapies requiring a prescription (8). The efficacy rate in vulvovaginal candidiasis may be a little lower, with cure rates ranging from 80 to 95% after 1 month of therapy. Decreased pruritus may be seen after even a single dose of therapy (2).

Ketoconazole

In addition to its availability as an oral, systemic, antifungal agent, ketoconazole is available as a 2% cream or 2% shampoo. It is used for tinea corporis, tinea cruris, and tinea pedis caused by dermatophytes and yeasts (44). It is highly active against tinea versicolor, which is caused by *Malassezia furfur,* and seborrheic dermatitis. The major reaction to this compound has also been skin irritation, which was reported in approximately 5% of patients. Occasionally, allergic reaction may occur.

Econazole

Econazole is a derivative of miconazole. It is used primarily in cutaneous mycoses, with excellent penetration of the skin. As with the other topical imidazoles, its major side effects are local irritation with minimal systemic absorption. It is applied twice daily.

Other Topical Azoles

A number of other topical antifungal agents are available for clinical use, which have similar pharmacokinetic properties, efficacy, and toxicities (4). Tioconazole is marketed for *Candida* vulvovaginitis and is available as an ointment. Tioconazole is given as a single bedtime dose. Butoconazole is an azole similar to clotrimazole. It is used as a 2% vaginal cream for 3 days. Terconazole is technically a triazole antifungal, but it is included here because of its activity in *Candida* vaginal infections. Terconazole is structurally similar to ketoconazole. As with the other topical agents, it can be administered as an 80-mg suppository given at bedtime for 3 days or by using the 0.4% cream, which is continued for 7 days. Its efficacy and tolerance are similar to those of clotrimazole and the other topical imidazoles in vaginal candidiasis. Oxiconazole and sulconazole are both imidazoles that are used for treatment of dermatophyte infections. Oxiconazole is applied as a cream; sulconazole is a solution.

REFERENCES

1. Anonymous. Ketoconazole shampoo for dandruff. Med Lett Drug Ther 1994;36:68.
2. Anonymous. Systemic antifungal drugs. Med Lett Drug Ther 1996;38:10–12.
3. Bennett JE. Antifungal agents. In: Mandell GL, Bennett JE, Dolin R, eds. Mandell, Douglas, and Bennett's principles and practice of infectious diseases. 4th ed. New York: Churchill Livingstone, 1995:401–410.
4. Bennett JE. Antifungal agents. In: Gilman AG, Hardman JG, Limbird LE, eds. Goodman & Gilman's the pharmacological basis of therapeutics. 9th ed. New York: McGraw-Hill, 1996:1175–1190.
5. Bergstresser PR, Elewski B, Hanifin J, Lesher J, Savin R, Shupack J, Stiller M, Tschen E, Zaias N, Birnbaum JE. Topical terbinafine and clotrimazole in interdigital tinea pedis: a multicenter comparison of cure and relapse rates with 1- and 4-week treatment regimens. J Am Acad Dermatol 1993;28:648–651.
6. Blum RA, D Andrea DT, Florentino BM, Wilton JH, Hilligoss DM, Gardner MJ, Henry EB, Goldstein H, Schentag JJ. Increased gastric pH and the bioavailability of fluconazole and ketoconazole. Ann Intern Med 1991;114:755–757.
7. Chin TW, Loeb M, Fong IW. Effects of an acidic beverage (Coca-Cola) on absorption of ketoconazole. Antimicrob Agents Chemother 1995;39:1671–1675.
8. Chren MM, Landefeld CS. A cost analysis of topical drug regimens for dermatophyte infections. JAMA 1995;272:1922–1925.
9. Ciummo PE, Katz NL. Interactions and drug-metabolizing enzymes. Am Pharm 1995;NS35:41–51.
10. Coley KC, Crain JL. Miconazole-induced fatal dysrhythmia. Pharmacotherapy 1997;17:379–382.
11. Como JA, Dismukes WE. Oral azole drugs as systemic antifungal therapy. N Engl J Med 1994;330:263–272.
12. Daneshmend TK, Warnock DW. Clinical pharmacokinetics of ketoconazole. Clin Pharmacokinet 1988;14:13–34.
13. De Repentigny L, Ratelle J. Comparison of itraconazole and ketoconazole in HIV-positive patients with oropharyngeal or esophageal candidiasis. Human Immunodeficiency Virus Itraconazole Ketoconazole Project Group. Chemotherapy 1996;42:374–383.
14. De Wit S, Goossens J, Weerts D, Clumeck N. Comparison of fluconazole and ketoconazole for oropharyngeal candidiasis in AIDS. Lancet 1989;1:746–748.
15. Denning DW. Can we prevent azole resistance in fungi? Lancet 1995;346:454–455.
16. Dorr RT. Pharmacology and toxicity of Cremophor EL diluent. Ann Pharmacother 1994;28:S11–S14.
17. Evans EG, Dodman B, Williamson DM, Brown GJ, Bowen RG. Comparison of terbinafine and clotrimazole in treating tinea pedis. Br Med J 1993;307:645–647.
18. Evans EG. A comparison of terbinafine (Lamisil) 1% cream given for one week with clotrimazole (Canesten) 1% cream given for four weeks, in the treatment of tinea pedis. Br J Dermatol 1994;130(Suppl 43):12–14.
19. Fainstein V, Bodey GP. Cardiorespiratory toxicity due to miconazole. Ann Intern Med 1980;93:432–433.
20. Fernandez-Nava HD, Laya-Cuadra B, Tianco EA. Comparison of single dose 400 mg versus 10-day 200 mg daily dose ketoconazole in the treatment of tinea versicolor. Int J Dermatol 1997;36:64–66.
21. Fong IW, Bannatyne RM, Wong P. Lack of in vitro resistance of *Candida albicans* to ketoconazole, itraconazole and clotrimazole in women treated for recurrent vaginal candidiasis. Genitourin Med 1993;69:44–46.
22. Fong IW. The value of prophylactic (monthly) clotrimazole versus empiric self-treatment in recurrent vaginal candidiasis. Genitourin Med 1994;70:124–126.
23. Force RW, Nahata MC. Salivary concentrations of ketoconazole and fluconazole: implications for drug efficacy in oropharyngeal and esophageal candidiasis. Ann Pharmacother 1995;29:10–15.
24. Galgiani JN, Stevens DA, Graybill JR, Dismukes WE, Cloud GA. Ketconazole therapy of progressive coccidioidomycosis. Comparison of 400- and 800-mg doses and observations at higher doses. Am J Med 1988;84:603–610.
25. Glatt AE. Therapy for oropharyngeal candidiasis in HIV-infected patients. J Acquir Immune Defic Syndr 1993;6:1317–1318.
26. Gomez DY, Wacher VJ, Tomlanovich SJ, Hebert MF, Benet LZ. The effects of ketoconazole on the intestinal metabolism and bioavailability of cyclosporine. Clin Pharm Ther 1995;58:15–19.
27. Graybill JR. The future of antifungal therapy. Clin Infect Dis 1996;22(Suppl 2):S166–S178.
28. Greenspan D. Treatment of oropharyngeal candidiasis in HIV-positive patients. J Am Acad Dermatol 1994;31(3pt2):S51–S55.

29. Hernandez-Sampelayo T. Fluconazole versus ketoconazole in the treatment of oropharyngeal candidiasis in HIV-infected children. Multicenter Study Group. Eur J Clin Microbiol Infect Dis 1994;13:340–344.

30. Hitchcock CA, Barrett-Bee KJ, Russell NJ. The lipid composition and permeability to azole of an azole and polyene resistant mutant of *Candida albicans*. J Med Vet Mycol 1987;25:29–37.

31. Honig PK, Cantilena LR. Ketoconazole and fluconazole drug interactions [Letter, comment]. Arch Intern Med 1994;154:1038, 1041.

32. Hornsburgh CCR, Kirkpatrick CH. Long-term therapy of chronic mucocutaneous candidiasis with ketoconazole: experience with 21 patients. Am J Med 1983;74:23–29.

33. Janssen Pharmaceutica. Monistat i.v. (Miconazole) package insert. Titusville, NJ, 1993.

34. Janssen Pharmaceutica. Nizoral tablets (Ketoconazole) package insert. Titusville, NJ, 1994.

35. Johnson EM, Warnock DW, Luker J, Proter SR, Scully C. Emergence of azole drug resistance in *Candida* species from HIV-infected patients receiving prolonged fluconazole therapy for oral candidosis. J Antimicrob Chemother 1995;35:103–114.

36. Johnson EM, Warnock DW. Azole drug resistance in yeasts. J Antimicrob Chemother 1995;36:751–755.

37. Keogh A, Spratt P, McCosker C, Macdonald P, Mundy J, Kaan A. Ketoconazole to reduce the need for cyclosporine after cardiac transplantation. N Engl J Med 1995;333:628–633.

38. Koletar SL, Russell JA, Fass RJ, Plouffe JF. Comparison of oral fluconazole and clotrimazole troches as treatment for oral candidiasis in patients infected with human immunodeficiency virus. Antimicrob Agents Chemother 1990;34:2267–2268.

39. Kwon-Chung KJ, Bennett JE. Medical mycology. Philadelphia: Lea & Febiger, 1992:81–102.

40. Lake-Bakaar G, Tom W, Lake-Bakaar D, Gupta N, Beidas S, El-sakr M, Straus E. Gastropathy and ketoconazole malabsorption in the acquired immunodeficiency syndrome (AIDS). Ann Intern Med 1988;109:471–473.

41. Laine L, Dretler RH, Conteas CN, Tuazon C, Koster FM, Sattler F, Squired K, Islam MZ. Fluconazole compared with ketoconazole for the treatment of candida esophagitis in AIDS: a randomized trial. Ann Intern Med 1992;117:655–660.

42. Lee YP, Goldman M. The role of azole antifungal agents for systemic antifungal therapy. Cleve Clin J Med 1997;64:99–106.

43. Lelawongs P, Barone JA, Colaizzi JL, Hsuan ATM, Mechlinski W, Legendre R, Guarnieri J. Effect of food and gastric acidity absorption of orally administered ketoconazole. Clin Pharm 1988;7: 228–235.

44. Lester M. Ketoconazole 2 percent cream in the treatment of tinea pedis, tinea cruris, and tinea corporis. Cutis 1995;55: 181–183.

45. Lynch ME, Sobel JD, Fidel PL Jr. Role of antifungal drug resistance in the pathogenesis of recurrent vulvovaginal candidiasis. J Med Vet Mycol 1996;34:337–339.

46. Maenza JR, Keruly JC, Moore RD, Chaisson RE, Merz WG, Gallant JE. Risk factors for fluconazole-resistant candidiasis in human immunodeficiency virus-infected patients. J Infect Dis 1996;173:219–225.

47. Millon L, Manteaux A, Reboux G, Drobacheff C, Monod M, Barale T, Michel-Briand Y. Fluconazole-resistant recurrent oral candidiasis in human immunodeficiency virus-positive patients: persistence of *Candida albicans* strains with the same genotype. J Clin Microbiol 1994;32:1115–1118.

48. NIAID Mycoses Study Group. Treatment of blastomycosis and histoplasmosis with ketoconazole. Results of a prospective randomized clinical trial. Ann Intern Med 1985;103:861–872.

49. Patel R, Gustaferro CA, Krom RAF, Wiesner RH, Roberts GD, Paya CV. Phaeohyphomycosis due to *Scopulariopsis brumptii* in a liver transplant recipient. Clin Infect Dis 1994;19:317–319.

50. Patterson TF, Andriole VT, Zervos MJ, Kauffman CA. The epidemiology of *Pseudallescheria boydii* infections complicating transplantation: community-acquired and nosocomial infection. Mycoses 1990;33:297–302.

51. Patterson TF, Graybill JR. Infections caused by fungi. In: Stein J, ed. Internal medicine. 5th ed. St. Louis, MO: CV Mosby, 1997.

52. Pfaller MA, Rhine-Chalberg J, Redding SW, Smith J, Farinacci G, Fothergill AW, Rinaldi MG. Variations in fluconazole susceptibility and electrophoretic karyotype among oral isolates of *Candida albicans* from patients with AIDS and oral candidiasis. J Clin Microbiol 1994;32:59–64.

53. Pons V, Greenspan D, Debruin M. Therapy for oropharyngeal candidiasis in HIV-infected patients: a randomized, prospective multicenter study of oral fluconazole versus clotrimazole troches. The Multicenter Study Group. J Acquir Immune Defic Syndr 1993;6:1311–1316.

54. Powderly WG, Finkelstein D, Feinberg J, Frame P, He W, van der Horst C, Koletar SL, Eyster ME, Carey J, Waskin H, Hooton TM, Hyslop N, Spector SA, Bozzette SA, NIAID AIDS Clinical Trials Group. A randomized trial comparing fluconazole with clotrimazole troches for the prevention of fungal infections in patients with AIDS. N Engl J Med 1995;332:700–705.

55. Rabeneck L, Laine L. Esophageal candidiasis in patients infected with the human immunodeficiency virus. A decision analysis to assess cost-effectiveness of alternative management strategies. Arch Intern Med 1994;154:2705–2710.

56. Redding S, Smith J, Farinacci G, Rinaldi M, Fothergill A, Rhine-Chalberg J, Pfaller M. Resistance of *Candida albicans* to fluconazole during treatment of oropharyngeal candidiasis in a patients with AIDS: documentation by in vitro susceptibility testing and DNA subtype analysis. Clin Infect Dis 1994;18: 240–242.

57. Revankar SG, Kirkpatrick WR, McAtee R, Dib OP, Fothergill AW, Redding SW, McGough DA, Rinaldi MG, Patterson TF. Detection and significance of fluconazole resistance in oropharyngeal candidiasis in HIV-infected patients. J Infect Dis 1996;174:821–827.

58. Sangeorzan JA, Bradley SF, He X, Zarins LT, Ridenour GL, Tiballi RN, Kauffman CA. Epidemiology of oral candidiasis in HIV-infected patients: colonization, infection, treatment, and emergence of fluconazole resistance. Am J Med 1994;97: 339–346.

59. Sanglard D, Kuchler K, Ischer F, Pagani JL, Monod M, Bille J. Mechanisms of resistance to azole antifungal agents in *Candida albicans* isolates from AIDS patients involve specific multidrug transporters. Antimicrobial Agents Chemother 1995;39: 2378–2386.

60. Schaffner A, Frick PG. The effect of ketoconazole on amphotericin B in a model of disseminated aspergillosis. J Infect Dis 1985;151:902–910.

61. Schaffner A, Bohler A. Amphotericin B refractory aspergillosis after itraconazole: evidence for significant antagonism. Mycoses 1993;36:421–424.

62. Schmidt A. In vitro activity of clotrimazole for *Candida* strains isolated from recent patients' samples. Arzneimittelforschung 1995;45:1338–1340.

63. Silverman S Jr, Gallo JW, McKnight ML, Mayer P, deSanz S,

Tan MM. Clinical characteristics and management responses in 85 HIV-infected patients with oral candidiasis. Oral Surg Oral Med Oral Pathol 1996;82:402–407.

64. Smith DE, Midgley J, Allan M, Connolly GM, Gazzard BG. Itraconazole versus ketoconazole in the treatment of oral and esophageal candidosis in patients infected with HIV. AIDS 1991;5:1367–1371.

65. Sobel JD, Brooker D, Stein GE, Thomason JL, Wemeling DP, Bradley B, Weinstein L. Single oral dose fluconazole compared with conventional clotrimazole topical therapy of *Candida* vaginitis. Am J Obstet Gynecol 1995;172:1263–1268.

66. Sobel JD, Schmitt C, Stein G, Mummaw N, Christensen S. Meriwether C. Initial management of recurrent vulvovaginal candidiasis with oral ketoconazole and topical clotrimazole. J Reprod Med 1994;39:517–520.

67. Sobh M, el-Agroudy A, Moustafa F, Harras F, el-Bedewy M, Ghoneim M. Coadministration of ketoconazole to cyclosporin-treated kidney transplant recipients: a prospective randomized study. Am J Nephrol 1995;15:493–499.

68. Sorenson AL, Lovdahl M, Hewitt JM, Granger DK, Almond PS, Russlie HQ, Barber D, Matas AJ, Canafax DM. Effects of ketoconazole on cyclosporine metabolism in renal allograft recipients. Transplant Proc 1994;26:2822.

69. Spina E, Avenoso A, Campo GM, Scordo MG, Caputi AP, Perucca E. Effect of ketoconazole on the pharmacokinetics of imipramine and desipramine in healthy subjects. Br J Clin Pharm 1997;43:315–318.

70. St-Germain G, Dion C, Espinel-Ingroff A, Ratelle J, de Repentigny L. Ketoconazole and itraconazole susceptibility of *Candida albicans* isolated from patients infected with HIV. J Antimicrob Chemother 1995;36:109–118.

71. Sugar AM, Alsip SG, Galgiani JN, Graybill JR, Dismukes WE, Cloud GA, Craven PC, Stevens DA. Pharmacology and toxicity of high-dose ketoconazole. Antimicrob Agents Chemother 1987;31:1874–1878.

72. Sugar AM, Hitchcock CA, Troke PF, Picard M. Combination therapy of murine invasive candidiasis with fluconazole and amphotericin B. Antimicrob Agents Chemother 1995;39:598–601.

73. Tucker RM, Denning DW, Hanson LH, Rinaldi MG, Graybill JR, Sharkey PK, Pappagianis D, Stevens DA. Interaction of azoles with rifampin, phenytoin, and carbamazepine: in vitro and clinical observations. Clin Infect Dis 1992;14:165–174.

74. Tumbarello M, Caldarola G, Tacconelli E, Morace G, Posterara B, Cauda R, Ortona L. Analysis of the risk factors associated with the emergence of azole resistant oral candidosis in the course of HIV infection. J Antimicrob Chemother 1996;38:691–699.

75. Van den Bossche H. Biochemical targets for antifungal azole derivatives: hypothesis on the mode of action. In: McGinnis M, ed. Current topics in Medical mycology. New York: Springer-Verlag, 1985:313–351.

76. Van den Bossche H, Marichal P, Gorrens J, Bellens D, Moereels H, Janssen PAJ. Mutation in cytochrome P-450 dependent 14-alpha demethylase results in decreased affinity to azole antifungals. Biochem Soc Trans 1990;18:56–59.

77. Van den Bossche H, Marichal P, Odds FC, Le Jeune L, Coone MD. Characterization of an azole resistant *Candida glabrata* isolate. Antimicrob Agents Chemother 1992;36:2602–2610.

78. Van Gerven F, Odds FC. The anti-*Malassezia furfur* activity in vitro and in experimental dermatitis of six imidazole antifungal agents: bifonazole, clotrimazole, flutrimazole, ketoconazole, miconazole, and sertaconazole. Mycoses 1995;38:389–393.

79. Varhe A, Olkkala KT, Neuvonen PJ. Oral triazolam is potentially hazardous to patients receiving systemic antimycotics ketoconazole or itraconazole. Clin Pharmacol Ther 1994;56:601–607.

80. Watson PF, Rose ME, Kelly SL. Isolation and analysis of ketoconazole resistant mutants of *Saccharomyces cerevisiae*. J Med Vet Mycol 1988;26:153–162.

81. Wooley PD, Higgins SP. Comparison of clotrimazole, fluconazole, and itraconazole in vaginal candidiasis. Br J Clin Pract 1995;49:65–66.

Azoles: Triazoles

●

Andreas H. Groll and Thomas J. Walsh

ANTIFUNGAL TRIAZOLES

The antifungal triazoles are stable synthetic compounds with one or more five-membered azole rings containing three nitrogen atoms and—attached to one of the nitrogen atoms—a more- or less-complex side chain. Compared with the antifungal imidazoles, the triazole ring confers improved resistance to metabolic degradation, much greater preferential affinity for fungal than for mammalian targets, increased potency, and an expanded spectrum of antifungal activity (54, 55). Itraconazole and fluconazole are the only licensed systemic antifungal triazoles to date, although several congeners with further expanded antifungal activity are currently undergoing clinical development.

Mechanism of Action

The antifungal azoles are generally considered to be fungistatic against most organisms. They function by inhibition of the fungal cytochrome P-450 3A–dependent enzyme lanosterol 14-α-demethylase, thereby interrupting conversion of lanosterol to ergosterol, which leads to accumulation of 14-α

methylsterols and depletion of ergosterol in the fungal cell wall (Fig. 1). This in turn alters cell membrane properties and function and subsequently increases permeability and inhibits cell growth and replication (146). In addition, azole compounds also inhibit cytochrome P-450 enzyme systems of the fungal respiration chain (141). Other effects include a toxic interaction with fungal membrane phospholipids and inhibition of transformation of yeasts to the mycelial form (29). Interaction with the mammalian cytochrome P-450 3A enzyme system is responsible for most toxicities and drug interactions of this group of compounds.

Spectrum of Activity

The antifungal triazoles fluconazole and itraconazole are principally active against dermatophytes, *Candida albicans*, *Cryptococcus neoformans*, and dimorphic fungi such as *Coccidioides immitis*, *Histoplasma capsulatum*, *Blastomyces dermatidis*, *Paracoccidioides brasiliensis*, and *Sporothrix schenckii* (54, 55). They have less activity against *Candida glabrata* and none against *Candida krusei* (110). Clinically useful activity against *Aspergillus* species and dematiaceous noulds is confined to itraconazole (5, 120), and both fluconazole and itraconazole are quite inactive against *Fusarium* spp. and *Zygomycetes*.

Resistance

A steady stream of reports of treatment failures and improvements in methods of in vitro susceptibility testing has increased discussion of resistance of *Candida* species to azoles, particularly to fluconazole (109). The magnitude of this problem is difficult to assess, and information is essentially limited to fluconazole. In contrast to animal data (4), a clear correlation of MICs and outcome in humans appears to be confined to AIDS patients with chronic oropharyngeal candidiasis (51, 109, 110). In other patient populations, failures and successes were seen with isolates for which MICs are both high and low (108), and factors pertaining to the patients' clinical status, antifungal treatment, and microbiologic data seem pivotal (51, 109). Nevertheless, reproducible antifungal susceptibility testing methods for yeasts are now available that may allow correlation of in vitro susceptibility testing with outcome in vivo and definition of interpretive breakpoints (110).

Acquisition of laboratory and concurrent clinical resistance of *Candida* species to azole compounds was reported in the early 1980s in patients with chronic mucocutaneous candidiasis treated long term with ketoconazole but was quite rare (67). An apparently increased incidence of invasive fungal infections by intrinsically resistant *Candida* species, such as *C. krusei* and *C. glabrata*, through selection in persistently neutropenic patients on fluconazole prophylaxis (159, 160) has not been confirmed in large, prospective, placebo-controlled studies, although breakthrough infections with these species do occur (53, 129, 161). However, acquired resistance to fluconazole is observed in *C. albicans* after long-term suppressive therapy with azoles for chronic or recurrent oropharyngeal candidiasis in patients with advanced stages of AIDS (79, 105, 111).

Molecular typing studies have documented induction of resistance in the original strain (84) or new acquisition of resistant strains during treatment (97), whereby person-to-person transmission between HIV-positive partners may occur (9). On the molecular level, mechanisms of resistance include activated efflux by multidrug transporters (117), increased production of target enzymes (145), mutations of target enzymes (144), mutations in the $\Delta^{5,6}$desaturase (156), or a shift to cell wall sterols other than ergosterol (65). Nevertheless, the extent and degree of fluconazole resistance in *C. albicans* are unclear (109), and fluconazole resistance may not affect susceptibility of the organisms to itraconazole or newer triazoles under clinical development (70, 145).

Acquired fluconazole resistance has been documented in a few patients with *Cr. neoformans* meningitis on maintenance therapy (13, 28, 94). Interestingly, in vitro experiments indicate that exposure of *Aspergillus fumigatus* to subfungicidal concentrations of itraconazole may result in resistance to amphotericin B (118), possibly via depletion of cell wall ergosterol.

FLUCONAZOLE

Fluconazole, (difluoro-2,4-phenyl)-2-bis (1*H*-triazole-1,2)-4-yl-1)-1,3-propanol-2 (Fig. 2), is a low-molecular-weight, water-soluble, fungistatic bis-triazole that possesses very useful clinical efficacy against infections due to dermatophytes, yeasts, and certain dimorphic fungi, in both immunocompetent and immunocompromised hosts. Fluconazole has activity comparable to that of ketoconazole in inhibiting fungal 14-α-demethylase,

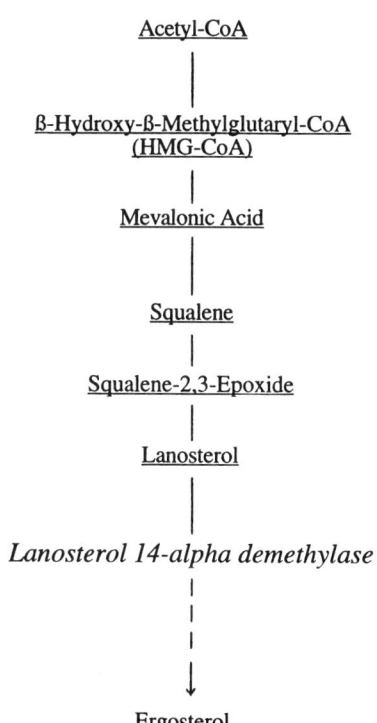

FIGURE 1. Ergosterol biosynthesis and the target of antifungal triazoles.

but it is much less inhibitory toward mammalian demethylases (127).

Pharmacokinetics

Fluconazole is available in oral and intravenous formulations, and its pharmacokinetic properties (Table 1) are independent of both route of administration and formulation (22, 23). Only minor differences appear to exist between healthy and immunocompromised patient populations (52). The drug exhibits linear pharmacokinetics that can be fitted into a two-compartment open model.

Following oral administration, fluconazole is very well absorbed; its absolute bioavailability exceeds 90%. Absorption is not affected by food or intragastric pH, and plasma concentrations peak 1 to 2 h after ingestion. In healthy volunteers, peak plasma concentrations of 2 to 7 µg/mL are obtained after a single oral or parenteral dose of 100 and 400 mg, respectively. Multiple dosing increases peak plasma concentrations 2.5 times of that achieved with single dosing. Steady state is generally reached within 4 to 7 days during once-daily dosing but can be rapidly attained by doubling the dose on the first day (14, 22, 46, 52, 54, 128).

Fluconazole is minimally (12%) bound to serum proteins; most of the compound circulates as free drug. The volume of distribution approximates that of total body water, and the drug penetrates well into virtually all tissue sites (22, 68, 128,

154). Of particular note is the ability of fluconazole to penetrate the central nervous system (CNS) effectively. Several studies, in both laboratory animals and humans, have shown that the cerebrospinal fluid (CSF):serum concentration ratio in healthy subjects is 0.5 to 0.9% (7, 45, 96) and between 0.8 and 0.9 in the setting of meningeal inflammation (140). In addition, excellent penetration into the parenchyma of the brain, vitreous humor, and choroid has been demonstrated (133, 154).

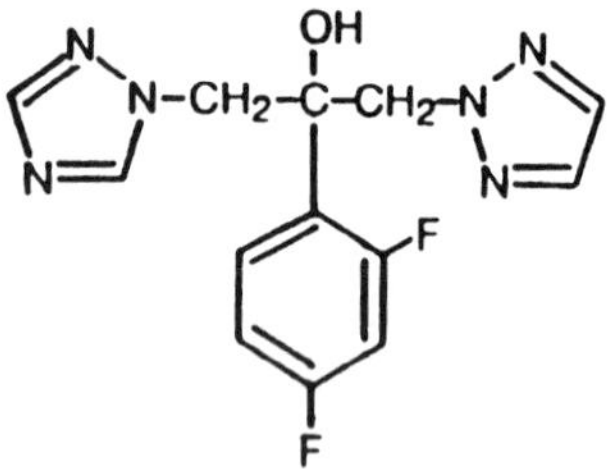

Fluconazole is relatively stable to metabolic conversion. Its terminal half-life ranges from 27 to 37 h. More than 90% of a dose is excreted via the kidneys, with approximately 80% recovered in urine as unchanged, active drug and 11% recovered as inactive metabolites (20, 22, 46).

The pharmacokinetic profile of fluconazole in children older than 3 months is somewhat different and includes an increased volume of distribution, increased plasma clearance, and a considerably shorter half-life of 16 to 20 h (21, 78, 123). The situation is more complex in premature neonates, in whom the volume of distribution may reach up to 2.60 L/kg, and elimination is slow, with mean terminal half-lives ranging from 89 h at birth and 55 h at 2 weeks to 21 h at 3 months (21). No pharmacokinetic data are published for term neonates.

Dose Ranges

The recommended dose range of fluconazole in adults is 100 to 400 mg/day (29, 54), but 800 mg/day may be required for treatment of life-threatening invasive infections. Doses of 3 to 12 mg/kg/day are currently recommended in children between 3 months and 16 years of age (21). For life-threatening fungal infections in children, treatment with 6 mg/kg twice daily has been suggested (152). In premature neonates, a 72-h dosing interval at the same dosage used in older children has been recommended for the first 2 weeks of life, followed by a dosing interval of 48 h during weeks 3 and 4 (21).

Because excretion of fluconazole parallels the glomerular filtration rate, the maintenance dose must be adjusted in patients with renal failure, except when the lower urinary tract is the therapeutic target. A 50% reduction in dosage is recom-

FIGURE 2. Structural formula of fluconazole.

TABLE 1 • **Pharmacokinetic Parameters of Fluconazole, Itraconazole, and Ketoconazole in Healthy Adult Volunteers at Steady State after Oral dosing with 200 mg**

	Fluconazole	Itraconazole	Ketoconazole
Oral bioavailability (%)	>90	55	75[a]
T_{max} (h)	1–2	1.5–4	1–4
C_{max} (µg/mL)	10	10	3–5
AUC_{0-24} (µg·h/L)	170	15.4	12
Protein binding (%)	≤ 12	≥ 95	≥ 85
Vd [L/kg]	0.7–0.8	10.7[b]	1.16
Principal route of elimination	renal	hepatic	hepatic
$T_{1/2} \beta$ (h)	27–37	21–37	6–10
Cl [mL/min·kg]	0.23	3.80	2.75
Unchanged drug in urine (%)	80	<1	2–4
Relative CSF levels (%)	50–90	<1	<10

Data compiled from 15, 20, 31, 52, 54, 55, 62, 64.

[a] Gastric acid–suppressing agents decrease bioavailability to <5%.

[b] Calculated from an intravenous dose of 100 mg.

mended in patients with a creatinine clearance of 50 to 21 mL/min, and a 75% reduction of dose with a creatinine clearance below 21 mL/min (54). The initial loading dose need not be adjusted (12). The drug is removed by hemodialysis, arteriovenous and venovenous hemofiltration, and to a lesser extent by peritoneal dialysis. In patients undergoing regular hemodialysis, 100% of the target dose is given after each dialysis session. In continuous hemofiltration, standard dosing has been suggested. A dose of 150 mg in a single 2-L dialysate bag every second day has been used for continuous ambulatory peritoneal dialysis (34, 54, 89, 121, 134).

Although dose reduction in patients with hepatic insufficiency (liver cirrhosis) appears unnecessary (112), thoughtful use of fluconazole with close monitoring of toxicity is warranted under these circumstances.

No data exist on the pharmacokinetics of fluconazole in obese persons or patients with fluid accumulation in the third space. As the volume of distribution of the drug approximates total body water and no accumulating tissue compartment is known, dosing on a mg/kg basis would be a rational approach in such circumstances.

Fluconazole is teratogenic in rats, and three humans with congenital craniofacial, limb, and cardiac defects after exposure to fluconazole during the first trimester have been described (104). Thus, the drug is contraindicated during pregnancy. Fluconazole is secreted into human milk at concentrations similar to those in plasma and should preferably be avoided in nursing mothers (43).

Adverse Effects

Fluconazole is generally well tolerated at the usual dose range of 100 to 400 mg/day and even at daily doses of up to 1200 mg

(5, 29, 54). Dose escalation to 1600 mg/day resulted mainly in increased hepatotoxicity, and dose-limiting neurotoxicity was observed at 2000 mg/day (5). Data compiled from adult patients who received the drug at dosages of 100 to 400 mg/day over at least 7 days indicate a 16% incidence of possibly related adverse effects overall; significant adverse effects or laboratory abnormalities leading to discontinuation of the drug were noted in 2.8% overall (54). Nausea, vomiting, and other gastrointestinal symptoms are seen in less than 5%, rashes and headaches in less than 2%, and usually reversible, asymptomatic hepatic transaminase elevations in up to 7% of adult patients (29, 54) (Table 2).

In children older than 3 months of age with predominantly cancer or HIV-infection who received fluconazole at doses of 1 to 12 mg/kg/day, related or unrelated clinical side effects or toxicities were observed in 12% overall, with gastrointestinal symptoms and increased hepatic transaminase levels occurring in 5%, and skin reaction in less than 1%. Significant side effects or toxicities led to discontinuation of treatment in 2.4% (58).

Marked increases in hepatic transaminases (to more than 8 times the upper limit of normal) are seen in approximately 1% of patients treated with fluconazole, but more-severe hepatic injury or hepatitis is rare (29, 54, 59). Exfoliative skin reactions have been reported in patients with AIDS; however, the exact role of fluconazole in these reactions is unclear (54). No evidence for myelotoxicity has emerged from studies in the marrow transplant setting (53, 129), although prolonged neutropenia was observed in cancer patients receiving the drug as antifungal prophylaxis during cycles of intensive chemotherapy (119). Finally, in contrast to ketoconazole, fluconazole does not appear to affect the synthesis of steroid hormones at dosages currently in use (29).

TABLE 2 • **Adverse Effects of Fluconazole, Itraconazole, and Ketoconazole in Adults at Usual Dosages (≤400 mg/day)**

	Fluconazole	Itraconazole	Ketoconazole
Gastrointestinal disorders	Nausea, vomiting (<5%) abdominal pain, diarrhea (<2%)	Nausea, vomiting (<5%); diarrhea (3%); abdominal pain (<2%)	Nausea, vomiting (<10%), anorexia, abdominal pain (<2%)
Skin and appendages	Pruritus, rash (<2%), possibly exfoliative	Pruritus, rash (<5%), possibly exfoliative	Pruritus, rash (<5%)
Hepatobiliary	Elevations of hepatic transaminases (<7%); hepatitis (rare)	Elevation of hepatic transaminases (<5%); hepatitis (rare)	Elevation of hepatic transaminases (<5–10%); hepatitis (rare)
Kidney	—	—	—
Bone marrow	Neutropenia, agranulocytosis, thrombocytopenia reported	—	—
Immunologic	Anaphylaxis reported	Anaphylaxis reported	Anaphylaxis reported
Endocrine system	—	Syndrome of mineralocorticoid excess; pedal edema; decreased testosterone synthesis (all rare)	Adrenal insufficiency (<1%); decreased libido, impotence, gynecomastia, menstrual irregularity (all rare)
Nervous system	Headache, seizures	Headache, dizziness	Headache; photophobia
Maximal tolerated dose in clinical trials and limiting events	1200 mg/day Hepatotoxicity CNS toxicity	600–800 mg/day Endocrinologic effects	600–800 mg/day Endocrinologic, gastrointestinal, and hepatic effects

Modified from Como JA, Dismukes WE. Oral azole drugs as systemic antifungal therapy. N Engl J Med 1994;330:263–272.

Drug Interactions

Although drug interactions of fluconazole are generally similar to those of other azoles, the number of relevant interactions reported with fluconazole appears to be substantially lower than with ketoconazole or itraconazole (Table 3). Nevertheless, combination of fluconazole with cisapride and newer antihistaminic drugs such as terfenadine or astemizole can lead to serious cardiac arrhythmias due to inhibition of metabolic pathways of these drugs and is strictly contraindicated (100). By similar mechanisms, fluconazole can precipitate phenytoin toxicity (85), may increase plasma concentrations of cyclosporine, tacrolimus, and all-*trans* retinoic acid (75, 91, 122), and may potentiate the effects of warfarin, sulfonylurea drugs, rifabutin, and benzodiazepines (75, 86, 90). At a small magnitude, fluconazole can decrease plasma clearance of theophylline and zidovudine (72, 116).

On the other hand, drugs notorious for hepatic enzyme induction may decrease fluconazole levels, with therapeutic failure as the ultimate consequence (29, 54). The potential for added hepatotoxicity must also be monitored when fluconazole is given in combination with these compounds (54, 86).

Clinical Indications

Fluconazole is highly effective against superficial infections due to dermatophytes and *Pityrosporum* spp. (60) and has excellent activity in the treatment of vaginal, oropharyngeal, esophageal, and chronic mucocutaneous candidiasis (44, 54, 60, 63, 80). Fluconazole is effective in the treatment of candidemia in nonneutropenic patients who have not received organ transplants and who do not have AIDS (98, 107). Limited data suggest that the compound can be an acceptable alternative to amphotericin B in neutropenic and nonneutropenic cancer patients with acute, presumed, or proven invasive *Candida* infections or chronic disseminated candidiasis (2, 3, 6, 71, 153). The drug has demonstrated useful efficacy in focal *Candida* urinary tract infections and uncomplicated funguria (42, 151) and has been used successfully in *Candida* peritonitis, endocarditis, osteomyelitis, meningitis, and endophthalmitis (1, 29, 152).

Fluconazole is effective for primary (40, 83, 93, 114, 147) and maintenance treatment of cryptococcal meningitis (19, 113), is the current drug of choice in coccidioidal meningitis (49), and, less well evaluated, nonmeningeal coccidioidomycosis (25, 38). Although not as active as itraconazole, fluconazole is effective against paracoccidioidomycosis, blastomycosis, histoplasmosis, and sporotrichiosis (38, 82, 92). High-dose fluconazole in combination with amphotericin B and flucytosine is the current treatment approach for disseminated trichosporonosis in immunocompromised hosts (152).

Given prophylactically, fluconazole has proven effectiveness in decreasing the occurrence of invasive *Candida* infections (53, 129) and reducing crude and excess mortality (129) in patients with acute leukemia or those undergoing bone marrow transplantation. Although the drug is clearly effective in preventing both superficial and invasive fungal infections in HIV-infected patients (101, 132), its role in long-term prophylaxis in this population is controversial due to a lack of survival benefit (101) and the potential emergence of azole resistance (109).

TABLE 3 • Drug-drug Interactions with Fluconazole, Itraconazole, and Ketoconazole

Mechanism and Drug Involved	Triazole/Imiazole Involved[a]	Comment
A. Decreased plasma concentration of triazole		
Decreased absorption of triazole		
—Antacids, H2-antagonists, omeprazole, sucralfate, didanosine	Itra**, Keto**	Take antacids and antifungal agent at least 2 h apart
Increased metabolism of triazole		
—Isoniazid, rifampin, rifabutin, phenytoin, phenobarbital, carbamazepine	Itra**, Flu, Keto**	Potential for therapeutic failure; increased potential for hepatotoxicity
B. Increased plasma concentration of coadministered drug through inhibition of its metabolism by triazole		
—Terfenadine, astemizole, cisapride	Flu†, Itra†, Keto†	Concomitant use prohibited
—Lovastatin, simvastatin	Itra†, Keto†	Concomitant use prohibited
—Phenytoin	Flu**, Itra**, Keto**	Monitor serum levels
—Benzodiazepines	Flu*, Itra*, Keto*	Monitor closely
—Rifampin	Flu*, Itra*	Monitor closely
—Indinavir, ritonavir	Itra*	Monitor closely
—Rifabutin	Flu*	Monitor closely
—Vincristine	Itra*	Avoid concomitant use
—All-*trans* retinoic acid	Flu*	Monitor closely
—Cyclosporine, tacrolimus	Flu, Itra, Keto**	Monitor serum level
—Sulfonylurea drugs, warfarin, prednisolone	Flu, Itra, Keto	Monitor closely
—Digoxin; quinidine	Itra, Keto	Monitor serum levels (dig.)
—Zidovudine; theophylline	Flu	Monitor closely

Modified from references 29 and 100.

[a]**Major, and *, moderate significance; † contraindicated.

ITRACONAZOLE

Itraconazole, $(\pm)$-*cis*-4-[4-[4-[4-[[2-(2,4-dichlorophenyl)-2-(1*H*-1,2,4-triazol-1-ylmethyl)-1,2-dioxolan-4-yl]methoxy]phenyl]-1-piperzinyl]phenyl]-2,4-dihydro-2-(1-methylpropyl)-3*H*-1,2,4-triazole-3-one, is a high-molecular-weight, highly lipophilic, fungistatic bis-triazole (Figure 3). Structurally closely related to ketoconazole, it has a broader spectrum of clinically useful antifungal activity, including superficial infections due to dermatophytes and yeasts, and infections by *Aspergillus* spp. and *Penicillum* spp., various phaeohyphomycetes, and dimorphic fungi, in both normal and immunocompromised hosts. Itraconazole binds more avidly to fungal cytochrome P-450 than does ketoconazole but, unlike the latter, binds only weakly to the mammalian cytochrome P-450 3A enzyme system, which results in relatively less toxicity (55).

Pharmacokinetics

At present, itraconazole is commercially available in an oral capsule formulation and as oral solution. The compound is soluble only at low pH, as prevails in the normal gastric environment. Absorption of the encapsulated formulation is compromised in the fasting state and in patients receiving concurrent treatment with H2-receptor antagonists, omeprazole, or antacids and becomes erratic in granulocytopenic cancer patients or HIV-infected patients with hypochlorhydria (18, 64, 130, 135). Although plasma levels vary widely among individuals, clinically useful bioavailability can be achieved when the capsules are taken with food or an acidic beverage (61, 62, 148).

Both the oral solution and an intravenous formulation that is in advanced stages of clinical development use hydroxypropyl-β-cyclodextrin (HP-β-CD) as vehicle, which increases the solubility of lipophilic compounds in aqueous solutions. Incorporation of itraconazole into a solution of HP-β-CD may enhance bioavailability and thereby improve interindividual variation in absorption, thus expanding the utility of itraconazole to granulocytopenic cancer patients and—not yet approved—also to infants and children (33, 47, 57, 102, 103). The intravenous formulation in HP-β-CD appears to be well tolerated and may offer similar advantages through improved delivery of the drug to the site of action (17, 30, 162). A lipid formulation of the compound has shown promising distribution and efficacy in animal models of invasive fungal infections (76).

Following administration of either the encapsulated formulation or the oral solution, peak plasma concentrations in both healthy and immunocompromised adults are attained within 1.5 to 4 h; with once-daily dosing, steady state is achieved after 7 to 14 days, and peak plasma levels at steady state are two to five times higher than after a single dose (55, 64, 102). Steady state can be reached more rapidly by oral loading (200 mg thrice daily for 3 days) (29) or, under clinical investigation, by intravenous loading (17, 162).

Measured by high-pressure liquic chromotography (HPLC), under steady-state conditions in healthy volunteers, a single daily 200-mg capsule taken orally yielded a mean peak plasma level (C_{max}) of 1.0 and a mean trough level (C_{min}) of 0.4 mg/mL (62); with dosing at 200 mg twice daily, the mean C_{max} was 1.9 to 2.2, and mean C_{min} 1.4 to 1.8 µg/mL, respectively (10, 62). In cancer patients receiving 5 mg/kg in two divided doses as oral solution, mean peak plasma levels of 1.2 µg/mL and trough levels of 0.8 µg/mL were observed at steady state (102). After administration of 200 mg itraconazole twice daily intravenously for 2 days and once daily for 5 more days, steady state through concentrations of 0.5 to 0.8 µg/mL can be obtained and be maintained by continuing treatment with 200 mg twice daily as an oral suspension in patients with hematologic malignancies and advanced HIV infection (17, 162). Attaining adequate plasma concentrations (through levels of 0.5 µg/mL itraconazole or above; by HPLC) appears critical for clinical efficacy, and monitoring plasma levels is highly recommended in treating invasive mycoses (31, 152). This recommendation is based on studies in experimental invasive pulmonary aspergillosis in persistently neutropenic rabbits. Antifungal activity of itraconazole approximated that of amphotericin B only when peak plasma levels above 6 µg/mL (by bioassay) were achieved, and this pharmacodynamic relationship correlated strongly with an inhibitory sigmoid maximum-effect model (11).

Itraconazole exhibits dose-dependent pharmacokinetics over its therapeutic dose range, implying saturable metabolic processes. Incremental increases in dosage from 1.5 to 5.0 mg/kg/day result in nonlinear hyperproportional increases in the area under the concentration-versus-time curve (AUC) (55), and similarly, twice-daily dosing results in a greater AUC than the same amount of the drug given in a single dose (102).

In whole blood, itraconazole is highly (95%) protein bound, and only 0.2% is available as free drug, with the remainder bound to blood cells (Table 1) (64). The compound is extensively distributed throughout the body (31, 64). Whereas concentrations in body fluids equivalent to body water, such as saliva, eye fluids, or CSF, are low to negligible, tissue concentrations in many organs, including the brain, exceed corresponding plasma levels by 2 to 10 times (27, 64), which explains the therapeutic efficacy of the drug despite low plasma concentrations (143). However, no evidence for significant tissue accumulation has derived from chronic toxicity studies in dogs (64).

Itraconazole is extensively metabolized in the liver and is excreted as inactive metabolites almost exclusively into bile and urine (55). Among the more than 30 metabolites identified so far, only one, hydroxy-itraconazole, possesses antifungal

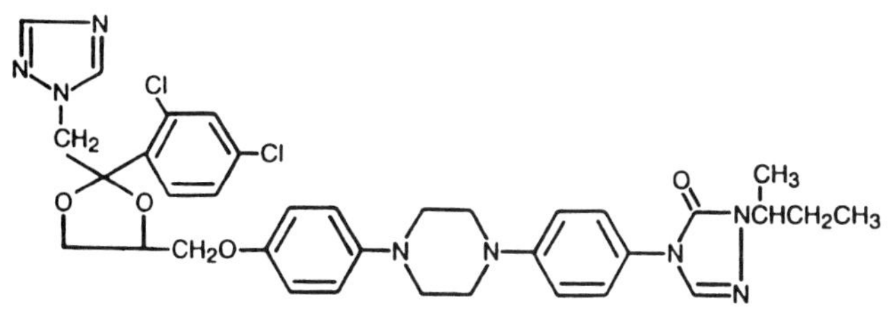

FIGURE 3. Structural formula of itraconazole.

activity. It is eliminated more rapidly than itraconazole, but its plasma concentrations at steady state are 1.5 to 2 times higher than those of the parent compound (29). Plasma concentrations of itraconazole measured by bioassay are thus approximately 3.5 times higher than those determined by HPLC (155). Elimination of systemically administered itraconazole from plasma follows a biexponential pattern. In healthy volunteers, itraconazole has an elimination half-life of 15 to 25 h after single dosing, and 34 to 41 h after repeated dosing with 100 to 400 mg/day, reflecting the dose-dependent kinetic behavior of the drug (62).

Dosage Regimens

The recommended dose range of itraconazole in adults is 100 to 400 mg/day (31). These dosages, however, may be associated with a relatively high failure rate in immunocompromised patients with invasive aspergillosis. Based on the pharmacodynamic relationship between plasma concentrations and antifungal efficacy (11), more aggressive dosage is recommended for life-threatening infections. For such conditions in adults, we recommend a loading dose of 600 to 800 mg/day for 3 days followed by a maintenance dose of 400 to 600 mg/day, respectively, and monitoring of adequate serum concentrations.

The efficacy and safety of itraconazole in neonates and children have not been established. The investigational liquid formulation in HP-β-CD was safe and relatively well tolerated in children older than 6 months of age, and the available data would suggest a daily dose of 5 mg/kg for children weighing less than 30 kg (31, 33). However, the drug should not be used in these patients unless the potential benefit outweighs the potential risks.

Metabolism of itraconazole is not altered by renal dysfunction, hemodialysis, or continuous ambulatory peritoneal dialysis, and no modification of the dosage regimen is needed in these settings (15). The pharmacokinetics and safety of the compound in patients with significant hepatic dysfunction, fluid accumulation in third spaces, or marked obesity have not been systematically studied.

While information in humans is lacking, itraconazole was embryotoxic and teratogenic in rodents (142). The drug is therefore contraindicated in pregnancy except for life-threatening fungal infection with no therapeutic alternative. Itraconazole is excreted into human milk and expected benefits for the mother should be weighed against the unknown risks to the infant.

Adverse Effects

Itraconazole is usually well tolerated, and few limiting adverse effects have been noted in patients receiving doses of up to 400 mg for various periods of time (Table 2) (26, 139). In 189 patients treated for systemic mycoses with doses of 50 to 400 mg/day for a median of 5 months, the overall rate of possibly related adverse reactions was 39%; most of the observed reactions were transient, and included nausea and vomiting (<10%), hypertriglyceridemia (9%), hypokalemia (6%), elevated liver transaminases (5%), rash and/or pruritus (2%), headache or dizziness (<2%), and pedal edema (1%). In 4%

of patients, toxicity led to discontinuation of the drug. No deaths were attributable to itraconazole toxicity (139). Only a few cases of more severe hepatic injury or hepatitis have been described (74).

At doses of up to 400 mg/day, the compound is almost devoid of effects on mammalian steroidogenesis (125, 139, 142). However, a Conn syndrome–like combination of mild hypertension and hypokalemia observed in four and reversible adrenal insufficiency in one of eight patients receiving 600 mg daily for refractory invasive fungal infections over a mean duration of 5.5 months indicates that 600 mg/day is approaching the upper limit of tolerability for long-term treatment (125).

Drug Interactions

There are several clinically important and unpredictable interactions between itraconazole and other drugs (Table 3). Itraconazole-induced inhibition of cytochrome P-450 enzyme systems may lead to increased and potentially toxic concentrations of coadministered drugs. Most important, coadministration of cisapride, terfenadine, and astemizole with itraconazole can lead to serious cardiac arrhythmias and is thus strictly contraindicated (66, 100). Similarly contraindicated is coadministration of cholesterol-lowering agents such as lovastatin or simvastatin, which has been associated with rhabdomyolysis (88). Potentially toxic levels of the coadministered drug can also be reached when itraconazole is given along with phenytoin, benzodiazepines, cyclosporine, tacrolimus, methylprednisolone, digoxin, quinidine, warfarin, sulfonylurea compounds, rifampin, rifabutin, ritonavir, indinavir, and vincristine (16, 69, 73, 90, 100, 115, 149).

Increased metabolism of itraconazole, resulting in decreased plasma levels, can be induced by rifampin, rifabutin, isoniazid, carbamazepine, phenobarbital, and phenytoin (100, 138). As a consequence, patients who receive itraconazole along with one of the listed drugs should be followed closely, and ideally, plasma concentrations of both compounds as well as hepatic function should be monitored carefully.

Clinical Indications

Itraconazole has useful clinical activity against dermatophytic infections and pityriasis versicolor (55), acute and chronic vaginal candidiasis (26, 95, 131), and HIV-associated oral and esophageal candidiasis (8, 24, 47, 48, 50, 57, 77, 99). The clinical efficacy of itraconazole in candidemia and deeply invasive *Candida* infections has not been systematically investigated.

Experience with oral itraconazole in the primary treatment of cryptococcal meningitis is scant (32, 37, 150); however, the drug has demonstrated effectiveness for consolidation or maintenance treatment of this condition (113, 147).

Itraconazole is active in the treatment of invasive aspergillosis (35, 36, 41, 150) and phaeohyphomycoses (124, 125). Itraconazole is currently the preferred agent for treatment of lymphocutaneous sporotrichosis (106, 126) and nonmeningeal, non-life-threatening histoplasmosis, blastomycosis, and paracoccidioidomycosis (39, 87, 157, 158). The drug also appears effective against meningeal and nonmeningeal coccidioidomycosis (56, 136, 137).

Itraconazole was effective as primary prophylaxis in reducing systemic fungal infections in patients with advanced HIV infection who resided in areas where histoplasmosis is endemic (81). No randomized controlled studies have been conducted on prevention of fungal infections in granulocytopenic cancer patients.

REFERENCES

1. Akler ME, Vellend H, McNeely DM, Walmsley SL, Gold WL. Use of fluconazole in the treatment of candidal endophthalmitis. Clin Infect Dis 1995;20:657–664.
2. Anaissie E, Bodey GP, Kantarjian H, David C, Barnett K, Bow E, Defelice R, Downs N, File T, Karam G. Fluconazole therapy for chronic disseminated candidiasis in patients with leukemia and prior amphotericin B therapy. Am J Med 1991;91:142–150.
3. Anaissie EJ, Darouiche RO, Abi-Said D, Uzun O, Mera J, Gentry LO, Williams T, Kontoyannis DP, Karl CL, Bodey GP. Management of invasive candidal infections: results of a prospective, randomized, multicenter study of fluconazole versus amphotericin B and review of the literature. Clin Infect Dis 1996;23:964–972.
4. Anaissie EJ, Karyotakis NC, Hachem R, Dignani MC, Rex JH, Paetznick V. Correlation between in vitro and in vivo activity of antifungal agents against Candida species. J Infect Dis 1994;170:384–389.
5. Anaissie EJ, Kontoyiannis DP, Huls C, Vartivarian SE, Karl C, Prince RA, Basso J, Bodey GP. Safety, plasma concentrations, and efficacy of high-dose fluconazole in invasive mold infections. J Infect Dis 1995;172:599–602.
6. Anaissie EJ, Vartivarian SE, Abi-Said D, Uzun O, Pinczowski H, Kontoyiannis DP, Khoury P, Papadakis K, Gardner A, Raad II, Gilbreath J, Bodey GP. Fluconazole versus amphotericin B in the treatment of hematogenous candidiasis: a matched cohort study. Am J Med 1996;101:170–176.
7. Arndt CAS, Walsh TJ, McCully CL, Balis FM, Pizzo PA, Poplack DG. Fluconazole penetration into cerebrospinal fluid. Implications for treating fungal infections of the central nervous system. J Infect Dis 1988;157:178–180.
8. Barchiesi F, Colombo AL, McGough DA, Fothergill AW, Rinaldi MG. In vitro activity of itraconazole against fluconazole-susceptible and -resistant Candida albicans isolates from oral cavities of patients infected with human immunodeficiency virus. Antimicrobial Agents Chemother 1994;38:1530–1533.
9. Barchiesi F, Hollis RJ, Del Poeta M, McGough DA, Scalise G, Rinaldi MG, Pfaller MA. Transmission of fluconazole-resistant Candida albicans between patients with AIDS and oropharyngeal candidiasis documented by pulsed-field gel electrophoresis. Clin Infect Dis 1995;21:561–564.
10. Barone JA, Koh JG, Bierman RH, Colaizzi JL, Swanson KA, Gaffar MC, Moscovitz BL, Mechlinski W, Van de Welde V. Food interaction and steady-state pharmacokinetics of itraconazole capsules in healthy male volunteers. Antimicrob Agents Chemother 1993;37:778–784.
11. Berenguer J, Ali N, Allende MC, Lee JW, Garrett K, Battaglia S, Piscitelli SC, Rinaldi MG, Pizzo PA, Walsh TJ. Itraconazole in experimental pulmonary aspergillosis: comparison with amphotericin B, interaction with cyclosporin A, and correlation between therapeutic response and itraconazole plasma concentrations. Antimicrob Agents Chemother 1994;38:1303–1308.
12. Berl T, Wilner KD, Gardner M, Hansen RA, Farmer B, Baris BA, Henrich WL. Pharmacokinetics of fluconazole in renal failure. J Am Soc Nephrol 1995;6:242–247.
13. Birley HD, Johnson EM, McDonald P, Parry C, Carey PB, Warnock DW. Azole drug resistance as a cause of clinical relapse in AIDS patients with cryptococcal meningitis. Int J STD AIDS 1995;6:353–355.
14. Blum RA, D'Andrea DT, Florentino BM, Wilton JH, Hilligoss DM, Gardner MJ, Henry EB, Goldstein H, Schentag JJ. Increased gastric pH and the bioavailability of fluconazole and ketoconazole. Ann Intern Med 1991;114:755–757.
15. Boelaert J, Schurgers M, Matthys E, Daneels R, Van Peer A, De Beule K, Woestenborghs R, Heykants J. Itraconazole pharmacokinetics in patients with renal dysfunction. Antimicrob Agents Chemother 1988;32:1595–1597.
16. Bohme A, Ganser A, Hoelzer D. Aggravation of vincristine-induced neurotoxicity by itraconazole in the treatment of adult ALL. Ann Hematol 1995;71:311–312.
17. Boogaerts M, Michaux JL, Bosly A, van Hoof A, Jacqmin P, van Peer A, Woestenborghs R, Stoffels P, Groen K, De Beule K. Pharmacokinetics and safety of seven days intravenous itraconazole followed by two weeks oral itraconazole solution in patients with hematological malignancies [Abstract A87]. Abstracts of the 36th Interscience Conference on Antimicrobial Agents and Chemotherapy, 1996:17.
18. Boogaerts MA, Verhoef GE, Zachee P, Demuynck H, Verbist L, De Beule K. Antifungal prophylaxis with itraconazole in prolonged neutropenia: correlation with plasma levels. Mycoses 1989;32(Suppl 1):103–108.
19. Bozzette SA, Larsen RA, Chiu J, Leal MA, Jacobsen J, Rothman P, Robinson P, Gilbert G, McCutchan JA, Tilles J. A placebo-controlled trial of maintenance therapy with fluconazole after treatment of cryptococcal meningitis in the acquired immunodeficiency syndrome. N Engl J Med 1991;324:580–584.
20. Brammer KW, Coakley AJ, Jezequel SG, Trabit MH. The disposition and metabolism of [14C] fluconazole in humans. Drug Metab Dispos 1991;19:764–767.
21. Brammer KW, Coates PE. Pharmacokinetics of fluconazole in pediatric patients. Eur J Clin Microbiol Infect Dis 1994;13:325–329.
22. Brammer KW, Farrow PR, Faulkner JK. Pharmacokinetics and tissue penetration of fluconazole in humans. Rev Infect Dis 1990;12(Suppl 3):S318–S326.
23. Brammer KW, Tarbit MH. A review of the pharmacokinetics of fluconazole (UK-49,858) in laboratory animals and man. In: Fromtling RA, ed. Recent trends in the discovery, development and evaluation of antifungal agents. Barcelona: JR Prous Science Publishers, 1987:141–149.
24. Cartledge JD, Midgley J, Youle M, Gazzard BG. Itraconazole cyclodextrine solution—effective treatment for HIV-related candidosis unresponsive to other azole therapy. J Antimicrob Chemother 1994;33:1071–1073.
25. Catanzaro A, Galgiani JN, Levine BE, Sharkey-Mathis PK, Fierer J, Stevens DA, Chapman SW, Cloud G. Fluconazole in the treatment of chronic pulmonary and non-meningeal disseminated coccidioidomycosis. Am J Med 1995;98:249–256.
26. Cauwenbergh G, DeDoncker P, Stoops K, DeDier AM, Goyvaerts H, Schuermans V. Itraconazole in the treatment of human mycoses. Review of three years of clinical experience. Rev Infect Dis 1987;9(Suppl 1):S146–S152.
27. Cauwenbergh G, Degreef H, Heykants J, Woestenborghs R, vanRooy P, Haeverans K. Pharmacokinetic profile of orally administered itraconazole in human skin. J Am Acad Dermatol 1988;18:263–268.
28. Coker RJ, Harris JRW. Failure of fluconazole treatment in cryp-

tococcal meningitis despite adequate csf levels. J Infect 1991; 23:101–103.

29. Como JA, Dismukes WE. Oral azole drugs as systemic antifungal therapy. N Engl J Med 1994;330:263–272.

30. De Beule K, Jacqim P, van Peer A, Woestenborghs R, Stoffels P, Heykants J. The pharmacokinetic rationale behind intravenous itraconazole [Abstract A75]. Abstracts of the 35th Interscience Conference on Antimicrobial Agents and Chemotherapy, 1995:14.

31. De Beule K. Itraconazole: pharmacology, clinical experience and future development. Int J Antimicrob Agents 1996;6:175–181.

32. De Gans J, Portegies P, Tiessens G, Eeftinck-Schattenkerk JK, van Baxtel CJ, van Ketel RJ, Stam J. Itraconazole compared with amphotericin B plus flucytosine in AIDS patients with cryptococcal meningitis. AIDS 1992;6:185–190.

33. De Repentigny L, Ratelle J, Leclerc JM, Cornu G, Sokal E, Jacqmin P, de Beule K. Repeated dose pharmacokinetics of itraconazole in oral solution, 5 mg/kg once daily for two weeks, in infants and children [Abstract A72]. Abstracts of the 36th Interscience Conference on Antimicrobial Agents and Chemotherapy, 1996:14.

34. Debruyne D, Ryckelynck JP. Clinical pharmacokinetics of fluconazole. Clin Pharmacokinet 1993;24:10–27.

35. Denning DW, Lee JY, Hostetler JS, Pappas P, Kauffman CA, Dewsnup DH, Galgiani JN, Graybill JR, Sugar AM, Catanzaro A. NIAID Mycoses Study Group Multicenter trial of oral itraconazole therapy for invasive aspergillosis. Am J Med 1994;97:135–144.

36. Denning DW, Tucker RM, Hanson LH, Stevens DA. Treatment of invasive aspergillosis with itraconazole. Am J Med 1989;86: 791–800.

37. Denning DW, Tucker RM, Hostetler JS, Gill S, Stevens DA. Oral itraconazole therapy of cryptococcal meningitis and cryptococcosis in patients with AIDS. In: VandenBosche H, Mackenzie DWR, Cauwenbergh G, VanCutsem J, Drouhet E, Dupont B, eds. Mycoses in AIDS Patients. New York: Plenum Press: 1990:305–324.

38. Diaz M, Negroni R, Montero-Gei F, Castro LG, Sampaio SA, Borelli D, Restrepo A, Franco L, Bran JL, Arathoon EG. A Pan-American 5-year study of fluconazole therapy for deep mycoses in the immunocompetent host. Clin Infect Dis 1992;14(Suppl 1):S68–S76.

39. Dismukes WE, Bradsher RW, Cloud GC, Kauffman CA, Chapman SW, George RB, Stevens DA, Girard WM, Saag MS, Bowles-Patton C. Itraconazole therapy for blastomycosis and histoplasmosis. Am J Med 1992;93:489–497.

40. Dromer F, Mathoulin S, Dupont B, Brugiere O, Letenneur L. Comparison of the efficacy of amphotericin B and fluconazole in the treatment of cryptococcosis in human immunodeficiency virus-negative patients: retrospective analysis of 83 cases. Clin Infect Dis 1996;22(Suppl 2):S154–S160.

41. Dupont B. Itraconazole therapy in aspergillosis: study in 49 patients. J Am Acad Dermatol 1990;23:607–614.

42. Fisher JF, Newman CL, Sobel JD. Yeast in the urine: solutions for a budding problem. Clin Infect Dis 1995;20:183–189.

43. Fluconazole (diflucan) product monograph. New York: Pfizer Roerig, 1996.

44. Flynn PM, Cunningham CK, Kerkering T, San Jorge AR, Peters VB, Pitel PA, Harris J, Gilbert G, Castagnaro L, Robinson P. Oropharyngeal candidiasis in immunocompromised children: a randomized, multicenter study of orally administered fluconazole suspension versus nystatin. J Pediatr 1995;127:322–328.

45. Foulds G, Brennan DR, Wajszczuk C, Catanzaro A, Carg DC, Knopf W, Rinaldi M, Weidler DJ. Fluconazole penetration into cerebrospinal fluid in humans. J Clin Pharmacol 1988;28: 363–366.

46. Foulds G, Wajszczuk C, Weidler DJ, Garg DJ, Gibson P. Steady state parenteral kinetics of fluconazole in man. Ann NY Acad Sci 1988;544:427–430.

47. Frechette G, deBeule K, Weinke W, Tchamouroff S, Stoffels P. Effects of itraconazole in the treatment of oral candidosis in HIV patients, a double blind double dummy, randomized comparison with fluconazole [Abstract I 219]. Abstracts of the 35th Interscience Conference on Antimicrobial Agents and Chemotherapy, 1995:244.

48. Gaenger G, Just-Nuebling G, Eichel M, Hoika R, Stille W. Itraconazole solution in patients with non-response to fluconazole [Abstract 1394]. Abstracts of the IXth International Conference on AIDS, 1993.

49. Galgiani JN, Catanzaro A, Cloud GA, Higgs J, Friedman BA, Larsen RA, Graybill JR. Fluconazole therapy for coccidioidal meningitis. Ann Intern Med 1993;119:28–35.

50. Gazzard B, Vandercam B, Cartier F, Mathiesen L, Stoffels P, DeBeule K. Effect of itraconazole in the treament of oral candidosis and candida esophagitis in HIV positive patients. A double blind, double dummy, randomized comparison with fluconazole [Abstract 0 242]. Abstracts of the 19th International Congress of Chemotherapy, 1995.

51. Ghanoum MA. Is antifungal susceptibility testing useful in guiding fluconazole therapy? Clin Infect Dis 1996;22(Suppl 2): S161–S165.

52. Goa KL, Barradell LB. Fluconazole. An update of its pharmacodynamic and pharmacokinetic properties and therapeutic use in major superficial and systemic mycoses in immunocompromised patients. Drugs 1995;50:558–590.

53. Goodman JL Winston DJ, Greenfield RA, Chandrasekar PH, Fox B, Kaizer H, Shadduck RK, Shea TC, Stiff P, Friedman DJ. A controlled trial of fluconazole to prevent fungal infections in patients undergoing bone marrow transplantation. N Engl J Med 1992;326:845–851.

54. Grant SM, Clissold SP. Fluconazole: a review of its pharmacodynamic and pharmacokinetic properties, and therapeutic potential in superficial and systemic mycoses. Drugs 1990;39: 877–916.

55. Grant SM, Clissold SP. Itraconazole: a review of its pharmacodynamic and pharmacokinetic properties, and therapeutic use in superficial and systemic mycoses. Drugs 1989;37:310–344.

56. Graybill JR, Stevens DA, Galgiani JN, Dismukes WE, Cloud GA. Itraconazole treatment of coccidioidomycosis. Am J Med 1990;89:282–290.

57. Graybill JR, Vazquez J, Darouiche RO, Morhart R, Moskovitz BL, Mallegol I. Itraconazole oral solution versus fluconazole treatment of oropharyngeal candidiasis [Abstract I 220]. Abstracts of the 35th Interscience Conference on Antimicrobial Agents and Chemotherapy, 1995.

58. Groll AH, Just-Nuebling G, Kurz M, Mueller C, Nowak-Goettl U, Schwabe D, Shah PM, Kornhuber B. Fluconazole vs. nystatin in the prevention of *Candida* infections in children and adolescents undergoing remission induction or consolidation chemotherapy for cancer. J Antimicrob Chemother 1997;40:855–862.

59. Guillaume MP, De Prez C, Cogan E. Subacute mitochondrial liver disease in a patient with AIDS: possible relationship to prolonged fluconazole administration. Am J Gastroenterol 1996;91: 165–168.

60. Gupta AK, Sauder DN, Shear NH. Antifungal agents: an overview. J Am Acad Dermatol 1994;30:677–698, 911–933.

61. Hardin J, Lange D, Heykants J, Ding C, VanDeVelde V, Slusser C, Klausner M. The effect of co-administration of a cola beverage on the bioavailability of itraconazole in AIDS-patients [Abstract A29]. Abstracts of the 35th Interscience Conference on Antimicrobial Agents and Chemotherapy, 1995:6.

62. Hardin TC, Graybill JR, Fetchick R, Woestenborghs R, Rinaldi MG, Kuhn JG. Pharmacokinetics of itraconazole following oral administration to normal volunteers. Antimicrob Agents Chemother 1988;32:1310–1313.

63. Hernandez-Sempelayo T. Fluconazole vs. ketoconazole in the treatment of oropharyngeal candidiasis in HIV-infected children. Eur J Clin Microbiol Infect Dis 1994;13:340–344.

64. Heykants J, Michiels M, Meuldermans W, Monbaliu J, Lavrijsen K, van Peer A, Levron JC, Woestenborghs R, Cauwenbergh G. The pharmacokinetics of itraconazole in animals and man: an overview. In Fromtling RA, ed. Recent trends in the discovery, development and evaluation of antifungal agents. Barcelona: JR Prous Science Publishers, 1987:223–249.

65. Hitchcock CA, Barrett-Bee KJ, Russell NJ. The lipid composition and permeability to azole of an azole and polyene resistant mutant of Candida albicans. J Med Vet Mycol 1987;25:29–37.

66. Honig PK, Wortham DC, Hull R, Zamani K, Smith JE, Cantilena LR. Itraconazole affects single-dose terfenadine pharmacokinetics and cardiac repolarization pharmacodynamics. J Clin Pharmacol 1993;33:1201–1206.

67. Horsburgh CR, Kirkpatrick CH. Long term therapy of chronic muco-cutaneous candidiasis with ketoconazole: experience with 21 patients. Am J Med 1983;74:23–29.

68. Humphrey MJ, Jevons S, Tarbit MH. Pharmacokinetic evaluation of UK49858, a metabolically stable triazole antifungal drug, in animals and humans. Antimicrob Agents Chemother 1985;28: 648–653.

69. Itraconazole (sporanox) product monograph. Titusville, NJ: Janssen Pharmaceutica, 1996.

70. Johnson EM, Warnock DW, Luker J, Porter SR, Scully C. Emergence of azole drug resistance in Candida species from HIV-infected patients receiving prolonged fluconazole therapy for oral candidosis. J Antimicrob Chemother 1995;5:103–114.

71. Kauffman CA, Bradley SF, Ross SC, Weber DR. Hepatosplenic candidiasis: successful treatment with fluconazole. Am J Med 1991;91:137–141.

72. Konishi H, Morita K, Yamaji A. Effect of fluconazole on theophylline disposition in humans. Eur J Clin Pharmacol 1994;46: 309–312.

73. Kramer MR, Marshall SE, Denning DW, Keogh AM, Tucker RM, Galgiani JM, Lewiston, NJ, Stevens DA, Theodore AJ. Cyclosporine and itraconazole interaction in heart and lung transplant recipients. Ann Intern Med 1990;113:327–329.

74. Lavrijsen APM, Balmus KJ, Nugteren-Huyning WM, Roldaan AC, Van't Wout JW, Sricker BHC. Hepatic injury associated with itraconazole. Lancet 1992;340:251–252.

75. Lazar JD, Wilner KD. Drug interactions with fluconazole. Rev Infect Dis 1990;12(Suppl 3):S327–S333.

76. Le Conte P, Joly V, Saint-Julien L, Gillardin JM, Carbon D, Yeni P. Tissue distribution and antifungal effect of liposomal itraconazole in experimental cryptococcosis and pulmonary aspergillosis. Am Rev Respir Dis 1992;145:424–429.

77. Le Guennec R, Reynes J, Mallie M, Pujol C, Janbon F, Bastide JM. Fluconazole and itraconazole resistant Candida albicans strains from AIDS patients: multilocus enzyme electrophoresis analysis and antifungal susceptibilities. J Clin Microbiol 1995; 33:2732–2737.

78. Lee JW, Seibel NL, Amantea M, Whitcomb P, Pizzo PA, Walsh TJ. Safety, tolerance, and pharmacokinetics of fluconazole in children with neoplastic diseases. J Pediatr 1992;120:987–993.

79. Maenza JR, Keruly JC, Moore RD, Chaisson RE, Merz WG, Gallant JE. Risk factors for fluconazole-resistant candidiasis in human immunodeficiency virus-infected patients. J Infect Dis 1996;173:219–225.

80. Marchisio P, Principi N. Treatment of oropharyngeal candidiasis in HIV-infected children with oral fluconazole. Eur J Clin Microbiol Infect Dis 1994;13:338–340.

81. McKinsey D, Wheat J, Cloud G, Gutsch H, Thomas C, Wiesinger B, Moscovitz B, Bamberger D, Slama T, Pierce M, Lancaster L, Lancaster D, Threlkeld M, Dismukes W, Kauffman C. Itraconazole is effective in the primary prophylaxis against systemic fungal infections in patients with advanced AIDS [Abstract LB9]. Late Breaker Abstracts of the 36th Interscience Conference on Antimicrobial Agents and Chemotherapy, 1996:9.

82. McKinsey DS, Kauffman CA, Pappas PG, Cloud GA, Girard WM, Sharkey PK, Hamill RJ, Thomas CJ, Dismukes WE. Fluconazole therapy for histoplasmosis. Clin Infect Dis 1996;23: 996–1001.

83. Menichetti F, Fiorio M, Tosti A, Gatti G, Bruna Pasticci M, Miletich F, Marrani M, Bassetti D, Pauluzzi S. High-dose fluconazole therapy for cryptococcal meningitis in patients with AIDS. Clin Infect Dis 1996;22:838–840.

84. Millon L, Manteaux A, Reboux G, Drobacheff C, Monod M, Barale T, Michel-Briand Y. Fluconazole-resistant recurrent oral candidiasis in human immunodeficiency virus-positive patients: persistence of Candida albicans strains with the same genotype. J Clin Microbiol 1994;32:1115–1118.

85. Mitchell AS, Holland JT. Fluconazole and phenytoin: a predictable interaction. Br Med J 1989;298:1315.

86. Narang PK, Trapnell CB, Schoenfelder JR, Lavelle JP, Bianchine JR. Fluconazole and enhanced effect of rifabutin prophylaxis. N Engl J Med 1994;330:1316–1317.

87. Naranjo MS, Trujillo M, Munera MI, Restrepo P, Gomez I, Restrepo A. Treatment of paracoccidioidomycosis with itraconazole. J Med Vet Mycol 1990;28:67–76.

88. Neuvonen PJ, Jalava KM. Itraconazole drastically increases plasma concentrations of lovastatin and lovastatin acid. Clin Pharmacol Ther 1996;60:54–61.

89. Nicolau DP, Crowe H, Nightingale CH, Quintiliani R. Effect of continuous arteriovenous hemofiltration on the pharmacokinetics of fluconazole. Pharmacotherapy 1994;14:502–505.

90. Olkkola KT, Ahonen J, Neuvonen PJ. The effects of the systemic antimycotics, itraconazole and fluconazole, on the pharmacokinetics and pharmacodynamics of intravenous and oral midazolam. Anesth Analg 1996;82:511–516.

91. Osowski CL, Dix SP, Lin LS, Mullins RE, Geller RB, Wingard JR. Evaluation of the drug interaction between intravenous high-dose fluconazole and cyclosporine or tacrolimus in bone marrow transplant patients. Transplantation 1996;61:1268–1272.

92. Pappas PG, Bradsher RW, Chapman SW, Kauffman CA, Dine A, Cloud GA, Dismukes WE. Treatment of blastomycosis with fluconazole: a pilot study. Clin Infect Dis 1995;20:267–271.

93. Pappas PG, Hamill RJ, Kauffman CA, Bradsher RWQ, McKinsey DS, Cloud GW, Dismukes WE. Treatment of cryptococcal meningitis in non-HIV infected patients: a randomized comparative trial [Abstract 73]. Abstracts of the 34th Meeting of the Infectious Disease Society of America, 1994:49.

94. Paugam A, Dupouy-Camet J, Blanche P, Gangneux JP, Tourte-Schaefer C, Sicard D. Increased fluconazole resistance of *Cryptococcus neoformans* isolated from a patient with AIDS and recurrent meningitis. Clin Infect Dis 1994;19:975–976.

95. Peeters F, van der Pas H, Proost J, Janssens D, Snauwaert E. Itraconazole, a new orally active triazole derivative for treatment of vaginal candidosis. Curr Ther Res 1986;39:496–504.

96. Perfect JR, Durack DT. Penetration of imidazoles and triazoles into cerebrospinal fluid in rabbits. J Antimicrob Chemother 1985;16:81–86.

97. Pfaller MA, Rhine-Chalberg J, Redding SW, Smith J, Farinacci G, Fothergil AW, Rinaldi MG. Variations in fluconazole susceptibility and electrophoretic karyotype among oral isolates of *Candida albicans* from patients with AIDS and oral candidiasis. J Clin Microbiol 1994;32:59–64.

98. Phillips P, Shafran S, Garber G, Rotstein C, Smaill F, Williams K, Singer J, Ioannou S. Fluconazole vs. amphotericin B for candidemia in non-neutropenic patients: a multicenter randomized trial [Abstract LM20]. Abstracts of the 35th Interscience Conference on Antimicrobial Agents and Chemotherapy, 1995:330.

99. Phillips P, Zemcov J, Mahmood W, Montaner JSG, Craib K, Clarke AM. Itraconazole cyclodextrine solution for fluconazole-refractory oropharyngeal candidiasis in AIDS [Abstract 2146]. Abstracts of the 19th International Congress of Chemotherapy, 1995.

100. Piscitelli SC, Flexner C, Minor JR, Polis MA, Masur H. Drug interactions in patients infected with human immunodeficiency virus. Clin Infect Dis 1996;23:685–693.

101. Powderly WG, Finkelstein D, Feinberg J, Frame P, He W, van der Horst C, Koletar SL, Eyster ME, Carey J, Waskin H. A randomized trial comparing fluconazole with clotrimazole troches for the prevention of fungal infections in patients with AIDS. N Engl J Med 1995;332:700–705.

102. Prentice AG, Warnock DW, Johnson SA, Phillips MJ, Oliver DA. Multiple dose pharmacokinetics of an oral solution of itraconazole in autologous bone marrow transplant recipients. J Antimicrob Chemother 1994;34:247–252.

103. Prentice AG, Warnock DW, Johnson SA, Taylor PC, Oliver DA. Multiple dose pharmacokinetics of an oral solution of itraconazole in patients receiving chemotherapy for acute myeloid leukaemia. J Antimicrob Chemother 1995;36:657–663.

104. Pursley TJ, Blomquist IK, Abraham J, Andersen HF, Bartley JA. Fluconazole-induced congenital anomalies in three infants. Clin Infect Dis 1996;22:336–340.

105. Redding S, Smith J, Farinacci G, Rinaldi M, Fothergil A, Rhine-Chalberg J, Pfaller M. Resistance of *Candida albicans* to fluconazole during treatment of oropharyngeal candidiasis in patients with AIDS: documentation of in vitro susceptibility testing and DNA-subtype analysis. Clin Infect Dis 1994;18:240–242.

106. Restrepo A, Robledo J, Gomez I, Tabares AM, Gutierrez R. Itraconazole therapy in lymphangitic and cutaneous sporotrichosis. Arch Dermatol 1986;122:413–417.

107. Rex JH, Bennett JE, Sugar AM, Pappas PG, van der Horst CM, Edwards JE, Washburn RG, Scheld WM, Karchmer AW, Dine AP. A randomized trial comparing fluconazole with amphotericin B for the treatment of candidemia in patients without neutropenia. N Engl J Med 1994;331:1325–1330.

108. Rex JH, Pfaller MA, Barry AL, Nelson PW, Webb CD. Antifungal susceptibility testing of isolates from a randomized, multicenter trial of fluconazole versus amphotericin B as treatment of nonneutropenic patients with candidemia. Antimicrob Agents Chemother 1995;39:40–44.

109. Rex JH, Rinaldi MG, Pfaller MA. Resistance of *Candida* species to fluconazole. Antimicrob Agents Chemother 1995;39:1–8

110. Rex JR, Pfaller MA, Galgiani JN, Bartlett MS, Espinel-Ingroff A, Ghannoum MA, Lancaster M, Odds FC, Rinaldi MG, Walsh TJ, Barry AL. Development of interpretive breakpoints for antifungal susceptibility testing: conceptual framework and analysis of in vitro-in vivo correlation data for fluconazole, itraconazole, and *Candida* infections. Clin Infect Dis 1997;24:235–247.

111. Ruhnke M, Eigler A, Tennagen I, Geiseler B, Engelmann E, Trautmann M. Emergence of fluconazole-resistant strains of *Candida albicans* in patients with recurrent oropharyngeal candidosis and human immunodeficiency virus infection. J Clin Microbiol 1994;32:2092–2098.

112. Ruhnke M, Yeates RA, Pfaff G, Sarnow E, Hartmann A, Trautmann M. Single-dose pharmacokinetics of fluconazole in patients with liver cirrhosis. J Antimicrob Chemother 1995;35:641–647.

113. Saag M, Cloud GC, Graybill JR, Sobel J, Tuazon C, Wiesinger R, Riser L, Moskovitz BL, Dismukes WE. Comparison of fluconazole vs. itraconazole as maintenance therapy of AIDS-associated cryptococcal meningitis [Abstract I 218]. Abstracts of the 35th Interscience Conference on Antimicrobial Agents and Chemotherapy, 1995.

114. Saag MS, Powderly WG, Cloud GA, Robinson P, Grieco MH, Sharkey PK, Thompson SE, Sugar AM, Tuazon CU, Fisher JF. Comparison of amphotericin B with fluconazole in the treatment of acute AIDS-associated cryptococcal meningitis. N Engl J Med 1992;326:83–89.

115. Sachs MK, Blanchard LM, Green PJ. Interaction of itraconazole and digoxin. Clin Infect Dis 1993;16:400–403.

116. Sahai J, Gallicano K, Pakuts A, Cameron DW. Effect of fluconazole on zidovudine pharmacokinetics in patients infected with human immuno-deficiency virus. J Infect Dis 1994;169:1103–1107.

117. Sanglard D, Kuchler K, Ischer F, Pagani JL, Monod M, Bille J. Mechanisms of resistance to azole antifungal agents in *Candida albicans* isolates from AIDS patients involve specific multidrug transporters. Antimicrob Agents Chemother 1995;39:2378–2386.

118. Schaffner A, Bohler A. Amphotericin B refractory aspergillosis after itraconazole: evidence for significant antagonism. Mycoses 1993;36:421–424.

119. Schaffner A, Schaffner M. Effect of prophylactic fluconazole on the frequency of fungal infections, amphotericin B use, and health care costs in patients undergoing intensive chemotherapy for hematologic neoplasias. J Infect Dis 1995;172:1035–1041.

120. Schmitt HJ, Edwards F, Andrade J, Niki Y, Armstrong D. Comparison of azoles against aspergilli in vitro and in an experimental model of pulmonary aspergillosis. Chemotherapy 1992;38:118–126.

121. Scholz J, Schulz M, Steinfath M, Hover S, Bause H. Fluconazole is removed by continuous venovenous hemofiltration in a liver transplant patient. J Mol Med 1995;73:145–147.

122. Schwartz EL, Hallam S, Gallagher RE, Wiernik PH. Inhibition of all-trans-retinoic acid metabolism by fluconazole in vitro and in patients with acute promyelocytic leukemia. Biochem Pharmacol 1995;50:923–928.

123. Seay RE, Larson TA, Toscano JP, Bostrom BC, O'Leary MC, Uden DL. Pharmacokinetics of fluconazole in immunocompromised children with leukemia or other hematologic diseases. Pharmacotherapy 1995;15:52–58.

124. Sharkey PA, Graybill JR, Rinaldi MG, Stevens DA, Tucker RM, Peterie JD, Hoeprich PD, Greer DL, Frenkel L, Counts GW. Itraconazole treatment of phaeohyphomycosis. J Am Acad Dermatol 1990;23:577–586.

125. Sharkey PK, Rinaldi MG, Dunn JF, Hardin TC, Fetchick R, Graybill JR. High dose itraconazole in the treatment of severe mycoses. Antimicrob Agents Chemother 1991;35:707–713.

126. Sharkey-Mathis PK, Kauffman CA, Graybill JR, Stevens DA, Hostetler JS, Cloud G, Dismukes WE. Treatment of sporotrichosis with itraconazole. NIAID Mycoses Study Group. Am J Med 1993;95:279–285.

127. Shaw JTB, Tarbit MH, Troke PF. Cytochrome P450 mediated sterol synthesis and metabolism: differences in sensitivity to fluconazole and other azoles. In: Fromtling RA, ed. Recent trends in the discovery, development and evaluation of antifungal agents. Barcelona: JR Prous Publishers, 1987:125–139.

128. Shiba K, Saito A, Miyahara T. Pharmacokinetic evaluation of fluconazole in healthy volunteers. Jpn J Antibiot 1989;42: 17–30.

129. Slavin MA, Osborne B, Adams R, Levenstein MJ, Schoch HG, Feldman AR, Meyers JD, Bowden RA. Efficacy and safety of fluconazole prophylaxis for fungal infections after marrow transplantation—a prospective, randomized, double-blind study. J Infect Dis 1995;171:1545–1552.

130. Smith D, VanDeVelde V, Woestenborghs R, Gazzard BG. The pharmacokinetics of oral itraconazole in AIDS patients. J Pharm Pharmacol 1992;44:618–619.

131. Stein GE, Mummaw N. Placebo-controlled trial of itraconazole for treatment of acute vaginal candidiasis. Antimicrob Agents Chemother 1993;37:89–92.

132. Stevens DA, Greene SI, Lang OS. Thrush can be prevented in patients with acquired immunodeficiency syndrome and the acquired immunodeficiency syndrome-related complex. Randomized, double-blind, placebo-controlled study of 100-mg oral fluconazole daily. Arch Intern Med 1991;151:2458–2464.

133. Thaler F, Bernard B, Tod M, Jedynak CP, Petitjean O, Derome P, Loirat P. Fluconazole penetration in cerebral parenchyma in humans at steady state. Antimicrob Agents Chemother 1995; 39:1154–1156.

134. Toon S, Ross CE, Gokal R, Rowland M. An assessment of the effects of impaired renal function and haemodialysis on the pharmacokinetics of fluconazole. Br J Clin Pharmacol 1990; 29:221–226.

135. Tricot G, Joosten E, Boogaerts MA, Vande Pitte J, Cauwenbergh G. Ketoconazole vs. itraconazole for antifungal prophylaxis in patients with severe granulocytopenia: preliminary results of two nonrandomized studies. Rev Infect Dis 1987; 9(Suppl 1):93–99.

136. Tucker RM, Denning DW, Arathoon EG, Rinaldi MG, Stevens DA. Itraconazole therapy for nonmeningeal coccidioidomycosis: clinical and laboratory observations. J Am Acad Dermatol 1990;23:593–601.

137. Tucker RM, Denning DW, Dupont B, Stevens DA. Itraconazole therapy for chronic coccidioidal meningitis. Ann Intern Med 1990;112:108–112.

138. Tucker RM, Denning DW, Hanson LH, Rinaldi MG, Graybill JR, Sharkey PK, Pappagiannis D, Stevens DA. Interaction of azoles with rifampin, phenytoin, and carbamazepine: in vitro and clinical observations. Clin Infect Dis 1992;14:165–174.

139. Tucker RM, Haq Y, Denning DW, Stevens DA. Adverse events associated with itraconazole in 189 patients on chronic therapy. J Antimicrob Chemother 1990;26:561–566.

140. Tucker RM, Williams PL, Arathoon KG, Levine BE, Hartstein AI, Hanson LH, Stevens DA. Pharmacokinetics of fluconazole in cerebrospinal fluid and serum in human coccidioidal meningitis. Antimicrob Agents Chemother 1988;32:369–373.

141. Uno J, Shigematsu ML, Arai T. Primary site of action of ketoconazole on *Candida albicans*. Antimicrob Agents Chemother 1982;21:912–918.

142. Van Cauteren H, Heykants J, DeCoster R, Cauwenbergh G. Itraconazole: pharmacologic studies in animals and humans. Rev Infect Dis 1987;9:S43–S46.

143. Van Cutsem J, Van Gerven F, Janssen PAJ. Activity of orally, topically, and parenterally administered itraconazole in the treatment of superficial and deep mycoses: animal models. Rev Infect Dis 1987;9:S15–S32.

144. van den Bosche H, Marichal P, Gorrens J, Bellens D, Moereels H, Jansen PAJ. Mutation in cytochrome P-450 dependent 14alpha-demethylase results in decreased affinity fo azole antifungals. Biochim Soc Trans 1990;18:56–59.

145. van den Bosche H, Marichal P, Odds FC, Le Jeune L, Coone MC. Characterization of an azole resistant *Candida glabrata* isolate. Antimicrob Agents Chemother 1992;36:2602–2610.

146. van den Bosche H. Biochemical targets for antifungal azole derivatives: hypothesis on the mode of action. In: McGinnis M, ed. Current topics in medical mycology. New York: Springer-Verlag, 1985:313–351.

147. van der Horst CM, Saag MS, Cloud GA, Hamill RJ, Graybill JR, Sobel JD, Johnson PC, Tuazon CU, Kerkering T, Moskovitz BL, Powderly WG, Dismukes WE. Treatment of cryptococcal meningitis associated with the acquired immunodeficiency syndrome. N Engl J Med 1997;337:15–21.

148. van Peer A, Woestenborhs R, Heykants J, Gasprini R, Cauwenbergh G. The effects of food and dose on the oral systemic availability of itraconazole in healthy subjects. Eur J Clin Pharmacol 1989;36:423–426.

149. Varhe A, Olkkola KT, Neuvonen PJ. Oral triazolam is potentially hazardous to patients receiving systemic antimycotics ketoconazole or itraconazole. Clin Pharmacol Ther 1994;56: 601–607.

150. Viviani MA, Tortorano AM, Pagano A, Vigevani GM, Gubertini G, Cristina S, Anaisso ML, Suter F, Farina C, Minetti B. European experience with itraconazole in systemic mycoses. J Am Acad Dermatol 1990;23:587–593.

151. Voss A, Meis JF, Hoogkamp-Korstanje JA. Fluconazole in the management of fungal urinary tract infections. Infection 1994; 22:247–251.

152. Walsh TJ, Gonzalez C, Lyman CA, Chanock SJ, Pizzo PA. Invasive fungal infections in children: recent advances in diagnosis and treatment. Adv Pediatr Infect Dis 1996;11:187–290.

153. Walsh TJ, Whitcomb PO, Revankar SG, Pizzo PA. Successful treatment of hepatosplenic candidiasis through repeated cycles of chemotherapy and neutropenia. Cancer 1995;76:2357–2362.

154. Walsh, TJ, Foulds G, Pizzo PA. Pharmacokinetics and tissue penetration of fluconazole in rabbits. Antimicrob Agents Chemother 1989;33:467–469.

155. Warnock DW, Turner A, Burke J. Comparison of high performance liquid chromatography and microbiological methods for determination of itraconazole. J Antimicrob Chemother 1988; 21:93–100.

156. Watson PF, Rose ME, Kelly SL. Isolation and analysis of ketoconazole resistant mutants of Saccharomyces cerevisiae. J Med Vet Mycol 1988;26:153–162.

157. Wheat J, Hafner R, Korzun AH, Limjoco MT, Spencer P,

Larsen RA, Hecht FM, Powderly W. Itraconazole treatment of disseminated histoplasmosis in patients with the acquired immunodeficiency syndrome. Am J Med 1995;98:336–342.

158. Wheat J, Hafner R, Wulfsohn M, Spencer P, Squires K, Powderly W, Wong B, Rinaldi M, Saag M, Hamill R. Prevention of relapse of histoplasmosis with itraconazole in patients with the acquired immunodeficiency syndrome. Ann Intern Med 1993; 118:610–616.

159. Wingard JR, Merz WG, Rinaldi MG, Johnson TR, Karp JE, Saral R. Increase in *Candida krusei* infection among patients with bone marrow transplantation and neutropenia treated prophylactically with fluconazole. N Engl J Med 1991;325: 1274–1277.

160. Wingard JR, Merz WG, Rinaldi MG, Miller CB, Karp JE, Saral

R. Association of *Torulopsis glabrata* infections with fluconazole prophylaxis in neutropenic bone marrow transplant patients. Antimicrob Agents Chemother 1993;37:1847–1849.

161. Winston DJ, Chandrasekar PH, Lazarus HM, Goodman JL, Silber JL, Horowitz H, Shadduck RK, Rosenfeld CS, Ho WG, Islam MZ. Fluconazole prophylaxis of fungal infections in patients with acute leukemia. Results of a randomized placebo-controlled, double-blind, multicenter trial. Ann Intern Med 1993;118:495–503.

162. Zhou H, Lee P, Moore LRC, Wu J, Woestenborghs R, Hassell AE, Sachdev OP, Moscovitz BL. Pharmacokinetic study of itraconazole in patients with advanced HIV-infection [Abstract A54]. Abstracts of the 36th Interscience Conference on Antimicrobial Agents and Chemotherapy, 1996:11.

Flucytosine

Richard H. Drew and John R. Perfect

Flucytosine (R-flucytosine, 5-fluorocytosine, RO-2–9915, 5-FC, Ancobon-Roche) is an agent with a unique place in antifungal therapy. Although originally developed in 1957 by Roche Laboratories as an antimetabolite for leukemia, reports of its use in humans as an antifungal to treat candidiasis and cryptococcus were not published until 1968. Flucytosine also demonstrates activity in vitro against selected pathogens causing chromomycosis. While monotherapy is reported in selected infections (primarily in chromomycosis and susceptible, nondisseminated, non-life-threatening candidal infections), combination therapy with other antifungals is most often used in invasive fungal infections because of concern about primary and secondary flucytosine resistance. Such combination therapy (usually with amphotericin B) may give better clinical outcomes than monotherapy with amphotericin B alone and is likely to shorten treatment schedules (16). The role of flucytosine as part of combination therapy with azole antifungals is less clear, but it is gaining some popularity, primarily in the treatment of disseminated cryptococcal infections. A major concern with the use of flucytosine is its hematologic and gastrointestinal side effect profile. Pharmacokinetic monitoring and dose adjustment for renal dysfunction may be critical in reducing the potential for such toxicity.

CHEMICAL CLASS

Flucytosine ($C_4H_4FN_3O$) is a water-soluble, fluorinated pyrimidine structurally related to fluorouracil. Chemically, it is 4-amino-5-fluoropyrimidin-2(1H)-one with a molecular weight of 129 (175). It is sparingly soluble in water and slightly soluble in alcohol (175).

ANTIMICROBIAL ACTIVITY

Standardized in vitro susceptibility testing of flucytosine must be carefully performed. Results may vary with culture media, serum, buffering agents, inoculum, temperature, and incubation time (14, 26, 59, 106). Extreme interlaboratory variability in susceptibility testing has also been reported (26). Despite these limitations, investigators have explored the utility of different in vitro testing methods for flucytosine. Early disk diffusion methods appeared to have limited value for flucytosine (179). Although small agar disk diffusion zone sizes may correlate with poor 5-FC susceptibility, their ability to predict tube dilution MICs was reported to be limited (168). However, data regarding utility of the E-test for flucytosine testing were more promising (51–53). Recently, standards have been approved by the National Committee for Clinical Laboratory Standards (NCCLS) using macrodilution broth techniques for flucytosine and other antifungal agents (132). Other investigators have now advocated adapting these techniques to a microdilution broth procedure, which is reliable and may be easier to perform (147). Traditionally, interpretive criteria applied to isolates tested against flucytosine considered organisms with MICs below 6.25 μg/mL after 48 h of incubation as highly sensitive, and those with MICs above 25 μg/mL were considered resistant (109). Breakpoints from the M27 guidelines propose MICs of 4 μg/mL or below as susceptible, 8.0 to 16 μg/mL as intermediate, and 32 μg/mL or above as resistant for *Candida* spp. Highly resistant organisms can have MICs exceeding 1000 μg/mL. In addition to the complex nature of in vitro susceptibility testing for single agents, in vitro evaluation of antifungal combinations is also highly complex (60).

Despite variations in in vitro testing methods, in vitro test results correlate reliably with in vivo activity in animal models for *Candida albicans* and *Cryptococcus neoformans* and with clinical experience (5, 169). Rising MICs observed in cryptococcal isolates correlated with clinical relapse when flucytosine was used in earlier studies as monotherapy for treatment of cryptococcal meningitis (180, 181). Clinical resistance was also confirmed by in vitro testing for pulmonary cryptococcal infections (88, 181). Some case reports of clinical failures or relapse for other fungi have shown MICs indicating that the fungus was more resistant than the initial isolate. Recent data also suggest a correlation of in vivo failures and in vitro resistance in non-*albicans* strains of *Candida* (3).

The epidemiology of flucytosine susceptibility has been studied. In vitro susceptibility for *Candida* spp. to flucytosine may vary with geographic location, serotype, and species involved (6). The overall incidence of primary resistance of *C. albicans* to flucytosine has been reported to range between 11.5 and 15.5% (14, 168, 169). However, the prevalence and susceptibility of different serotypes of *C. albicans* are also known to vary. *C. albicans* isolates from 402 patients with no prior history of treatment with flucytosine were collected at five U.S. medical centers (168). Serotypes A and B accounted for 50.7 and 49.3%, respectively, of the isolates typed (n = 398). While a total of 60% of these isolates had MICs of 12.5 μg/mL or below after 7 days, serotype A was the most prevalent in this group (74%). Other investigators have confirmed that serotype B is much less susceptible to flucytosine, although the prevalence of this serotype varies with geographic location (6).

Non-*albicans* species of *Candida* are generally considered less susceptible to flucytosine than *C. albicans* (195). For example, the MIC_{50} and MIC_{90} for *Candida krusei* to flucytosine were reported to be 16 and 32 μg/mL, respectively (18). Others have confirmed that *C. krusei* is less susceptible to flucytosine (99, 124, 126). On the other hand, *C. glabrata* may actually demonstrate excellent susceptibility to flucytosine, in contrast to the relatively poor activity of the triazoles against this pathogen (124, 155, 203). In fact, one investigator reported excellent in vitro activity in 15 of 15 isolates of *C. glabrata* tested (124). *C. lusitaniae* has also been reported susceptible to flucytosine, with MIC_{90} reported by one investigator to be below 0.125 μg/mL against 27 clinical isolates (43).

In vitro activities of flucytosine in combination with amphotericin B against *Candida* spp. have been reported. Some form of synergy with amphotericin B (40% static, 45% cidal) were reported in 35 of 40 (85%) *Candida* spp. (113). Fungicidal synergistic activity with amphotericin B may be more common in flucytosine-sensitive organisms, while antagonism may occur in flucytosine-resistant isolates (63). However, antagonism of amphotericin B with flucytosine for *Candida* is infrequent, and synergy appears to depend on methodology and the flucytosine susceptibility of strains of *Candida* tested.

In general, most cryptococcal isolates are initially susceptible to flucytosine (56). In one report, 99% of 93 isolates of *C. neoformans* were susceptible at MICs below 5 μg/mL (14). However, primary resistance rates of *C. neoformans* have ranged from 4 to 24.5%, depending on methodology (30, 159). One investigator reported that in vitro susceptibilities were lower in B/C serotypes of *C. neoformans* than in A/C serotypes (159). Others have observed no difference in susceptibility based on serotypes (57). MICs for non-*C. neoformans* species were noted to be higher than those for *C. neoformans* strains (10).

In vitro activity of the combination of flucytosine with amphotericin B against cryptococcal isolates has given conflicting results, including synergistic, additive, no effect, or antagonistic effects. These results may be influenced by the pretreatment sensitivity to flucytosine, since flucytosine-sensitive isolates more frequently demonstrate at least additive effects, while antagonism is more commonly observed in flucytosine-resistant isolates (63). In addition, flucytosine combined with fluconazole has also been tested in vitro. Synergy was observed in 62% of the 50 clinical strains isolated; antagonism was not reported (121). The combination still showed beneficial effects, even in the absence of true synergy. For example, flucytosine MICs for cryptococcal isolates were markedly reduced in the presence of fluconazole. In contrast, flucytosine failed to enhance the in vitro activity of fluconazole-resistant isolates (i.e., fluconazole MICs ≥ 8 μg/mL).

Flucytosine has inhibitory activity for a group of relatively less pathogenic fungi. Organisms responsible for chromomycoses are generally considered susceptible to flucytosine in vitro. *Cladosporium* spp. and *Phialophora* spp. appear sensitive (22, 107); flucytosine is generally considered fungistatic against these pathogens (62). Similarly, an MIC_{90} of 0.2 μg/mL was reported for 31 isolates of *Saccharomyces cerevisiae* obtained from 19 patients (173).

In vitro inhibitory activity of flucytosine against *Aspergillus* spp. is generally weak, and this fungal pathogen is usually considered moderately or highly resistant to flucytosine (72). However, as with combinations with amphotericin B against other pathogens, conflicting results of additive (125) or indifferent (76, 98) effects have been reported for *Aspergillus* species. Dimorphic fungal pathogens such as *Blastomyces dermatitidis, Paracoccidioides brasiliensis, Sporothrix schenckii, Histoplasma capsulatum,* and *Coccidioides immitis* and most dermatophytes are generally considered resistant (14). *Fusarium* species are generally resistant to flucytosine in vitro (140). Finally, flucytosine has no activity in vitro against any fungi that cause zygomycosis (109).

MECHANISM OF ACTION

Flucytosine penetrates the fungal cell wall with the aid of cytosine permease (114). Once inside the cell, flucytosine is deaminated to 5-fluorouracil (5-FU) by cytosine deaminase (197). This enzyme is not present in mammalian cells, which gives this drug its fungus-selective toxicity. Fluorouracil incorporates into fungal RNA in place of uracil to interrupt protein synthesis (135, 189). The 5-FU is then converted to 5-fluorodeoxyuridylic acid monophosphate, a noncompetitive inhibitor of thymidylate synthetase, which interferes with DNA synthesis (44, 135, 188). However, based on evidence obtained in selected strains of *C. albicans,* incorporation of 5-FU into RNA and 5-fluorodeoxyuridine monophosphate into DNA may be independent of one another (190). The resultant antifungal activity may be fungistatic or fungicidal, depending upon such conditions in vitro as drug concentration and time of incubation (109).

MECHANISMS OF RESISTANCE

As stated above, resistance to flucytosine is common and may be either primary or secondary. The rate of primary resistance has remained steady despite years of use and is reasonably well described in the published literature (184). The incidence of secondary resistance has not been quantified.

Several mechanisms for flucytosine resistance have been proposed. Acquired resistance may be due to a block or deficiency of cytosine deaminase (70, 135). Other mechanisms (namely, defects in UMP pyrophosphorylase (UMPP) and cytosine permease) have also been proposed (114, 188, 192, 199). Of these mechanisms, UMPP defect is thought to be most common (192). Among 29 clinical isolates with relative or absolute resistance to flucytosine, no instance of cytosine permease deficiency was found (135). However, the mechanism may depend upon the fungal pathogen. For example, in *Aspergillus,* susceptibility to flucytosine is independent of drug uptake (135). *Aspergillus* spp. may also be able to use cytosine as a nitrogen source, and this is suggested as a possible mechanism for drug resistance (188). *C. albicans* isolates have demonstrated both decreased UMPP activity and decreased cytosine deaminase activity (199).

The genetic basis of susceptibility to flucytosine has been described in *C. albicans* (41, 199) and accounts largely for the relative resistance previously described (135). Resistance traits (FCY1 and FCY2) are both homozygous and heterozygous. Isolates demonstrating heterozygous resistance traits are only slightly resistant but occur at a significant frequency among clinical strains. It is postulated that after a single-step mutation, drug exposure selects for homozygous progeny; thus demonstrating secondary resistance and accounting for treatment failures (199). However, isolates with heterozygous resistance genes have also been reported to exhibit high-level resistance (41).

Strategies to overcome or prevent emergence of flucytosine-resistant isolates during therapy have generally focused on maintaining sufficient drug concentrations at the infection site, performing sequential isolate susceptibility testing, and combining flucytosine with other antifungal agents. For example, susceptibility testing of fungal pathogens for flucytosine can be done in clinical practice, using the standardized testing methods recently proposed by the NCCLS (132). Combination therapy with other antifungal agents is frequently used to prevent emergence of secondary resistance. Traditional antifungal drug combinations with flucytosine usually include amphotericin B, since isolates with secondary flucytosine resistance due to single-step mutation may be amphotericin B sensitive (14). Other antifungal combinations have also been examined with flucytosine. In vitro, flucytosine and ketoconazole were reported synergistic in 22 of 57 yeast isolates (primarily *Candida*) resistant to flucytosine (13).

PHARMACODYNAMIC EFFECTS

As mentioned above, the in vitro activity of flucytosine depends highly on laboratory test conditions. Therefore, investigating the pharmacodynamic effects of this agent (alone or in combination with other antifungals) is complex (60). For example, preexposure to another antifungal may alter flucytosine activity. In one study, yeasts preincubated for 20 h with flucytosine became less susceptible to killing by amphotericin B (106). On the other hand, it has been hypothesized that amphotericin B may decrease intracellular uptake of flucytosine (13). These authors proposed a theory of sequential drug action, with amphotericin acting alone until it approaches depletion, followed by inhibitory effects due to flucytosine.

Flucytosine possesses postantifungal effect (PAFE) in vitro, similar to the postantibiotic effect (PAE) demonstrated by certain antibacterial agents (153). The length of the PAFE against *C. albicans* was found to depend upon both the concentration of flucytosine and duration of exposure. PAFEs ranged from 0 to 4.2 h after a 0.5-h exposure and extended beyond 10 h after the exposure times were increased to 1 to 2 h. Other investigators have observed similar effects in *Candida* spp. and *C. neoformans,* ranging from 0.8 to 7.4 h and 2.4 to 5.4 h, respectively (177).

The effect of combination therapy of fluconazole with flucytosine on PAFE on *C. albicans* has also been studied in vitro (111, 154). A synergistic PAFE was demonstrated with flucytosine plus fluconazole at concentrations well below the individual MICs. PAFEs in one study ranged from 3.8 to 10.5 h and persisted 1.2 to 2.5 h longer than those achieved with either agent separately (154). The concentrations of each agent required to produce the optimal PAFE varied with the strain tested. Combinations of flucytosine and amphotericin B have also been tested for PAFE against *C. albicans.* A synergistic PAFE was evidenced with combinations of the two drugs at concentrations below their individual MICs (152). Combination PAFEs ranged from 6.3 to 21.8 h and persisted longer than those achieved by the drugs tested separately.

The effects of flucytosine on various aspects of cellular and humoral immunity have been investigated. Flucytosine treatment had no effect on cellular immunity in a guinea pig model (17, 148). The effect of flucytosine with amphotericin B on neutrophil antifungal activity against *C. albicans* was studied in vitro (144). Exposure of yeast isolates to amphotericin B and flucytosine significantly enhanced the ability of neutrophils to kill the pretreated viable yeast cells intracellularly. Combination with immunoglobulin therapy may represent a new use of flucytosine. The efficacy of flucytosine in combination with an IgG1 monoclonal antibody to *C. neoformans* capsular glucuronoxylomannan was studied in vitro and in a murine animal model of cryptococcal infection (54). The combination of flucytosine and IgG1 was more effective than either agent alone in reducing the numbers of *C. neoformans* colony-forming units (CFUs) in the model.

Effects of continuous infusions of flucytosine have been compared with effects of similar doses given intermittently in the hematogenous murine candidiasis model using *C. lusitaniae* (85). Fungal titers in kidneys of mice treated with continuous infusions were significantly lower than those observed with bolus injections given once or three times daily. The clinical significance of these findings, however, is not clear.

PHARMACOKINETICS

Approximately 80 to 90% of a dose of flucytosine is absorbed following oral administration (39). After a single oral dose of 150 mg/kg, peak levels of 30 to 45 μg/mL occur 1 to 2 h postadministration (20, 39). Peak serum concentrations may be delayed in patients with renal insufficiency, but the clinical significance is not known (20). In addition, a case of flucytosine malabsorption was reported in a pediatric patient with Schwachmann syndrome (64). A significant increase in serum concentrations of flucytosine was noted when the drug was administered in a lipophilic vehicle (64). Systemic absorption of flucytosine may also result from intraperitoneal administration (50, 71). Continuous 5-day peritoneal lavage containing flucytosine has maintained serum concentrations above 50 μg/mL (71).

The protein binding at serum concentrations between 2 and 55 μg/mL is low, approximately 4% (38). Consequently, flucytosine is widely distributed in body water, with a volume of distribution ranging from 0.6 to 0.9 L/kg (38). Similar volumes of distribution have been reported in patients receiving continuous hemofiltration (80).

Penetration of flucytosine into various tissues and body fluids has been investigated in both animal models and humans. Flucytosine penetrates into bone (58), vertebral disks (58), and synovial fluid (101, 198). For example, a premature infant receiving flucytosine orally at a dose of 25 mg/kg four times daily had simultaneous serum and synovial fluid levels of 47.5 μg/mL and 39.6 μg/mL, respectively (198). Flucytosine achieved therapeutic levels in both the vitreous and aqueous humor after oral and subconjunctival administration in a rabbit model (123, 191). Drug levels achieved in the spleen, heart, liver, kidney, and lung equal those found in serum (38).

Because of the potential clinical applications of flucytosine, penetration of flucytosine into the central nervous system (CNS), urine, peritoneal fluid, and respiratory tract has particular interest. Flucytosine levels in the cerebrospinal fluid (CSF) are approximately 80% of simultaneous serum levels (134). CSF concentrations range from 17 to 62 μg/mL following a single dose of 1.5 to 2 g (20). Significant peritoneal fluid concentrations have also been documented in most patients studied during treatment (117). Flucytosine levels in respiratory secretions have been investigated (24, 66). Mean maximal concentrations of 7.76 ± 7 μg/mL were obtained in bronchial secretions from 14 patients with chronic respiratory disease at the end of a single 25-mg/kg intravenous perfusion over 30 min (24). However, flucytosine was undetectable in bronchial secretions in four patients, despite serum concentrations of 21.5 ± 5 μg/mL. Other investigators report serum and bronchoalveolar lavage (BAL) fluid levels of flucytosine ranging from less than 0.2 to 9.3 μg/mL and less than 0.4 to 1.5 μg/mL, respectively, after oral administration of 4.5 to 6.0 g/day (66). Flucytosine urine levels may actually be many times simultaneous serum levels (39). Flucytosine may also cross the placental barrier and has been found in amniotic fluid at concentrations of 168 μg/mL 4 h after a 2-g dose (166).

Most of a flucytosine dose does not undergo extensive metabolism; as much as 96% of the total dose may be eliminated as

unchanged drug (186). However, several metabolites of flucytosine have been discovered. Flucytosine can undergo deamination by intestinal microflora to 5-fluorouracil (44, 65, 104, 188). The enzyme or enzymes responsible for this deamination can be induced by chronic exposure to flucytosine (65) or altered in production by effects of broad-spectrum antibacterials on gut flora (104). Other metabolites identified include 5-fluorodeoxyuridine monophosphate (5-FC-UMP) and fluor-oorotic acid (188). α-Fluoro-β-alanine (FBAL)], 5-hydroxy-5-fluorocytosine, O-2-β-glucuronide, 6-hydroxy-5-fluorocytosine (6OHFC), and fluoride ion (F⁻) have been reported in urine (33, 186, 202).

The primary route of flucytosine elimination is renal. Up to 60 to 95% of the dose is eliminated by glomerular filtration without significant tubular reabsorption (37, 39). In one study, total urinary excretion accounted for 100% of the injected dose, and unchanged flucytosine was the major excretory product, accounting for 96.1% of that dose (186).

The elimination half-life of flucytosine ranges from 3 to 8 h, with an average value of 6 h (39, 156). However, this may be extended to 60 to 250 h in patients with end-stage renal disease (39, 156). Renal clearance of flucytosine is reported to be about 75% of creatinine clearance (20, 39).

Elimination of flucytosine by various forms of dialysis has been reported. The serum half-life in patients undergoing continuous hemofiltration has been reported to range between 15.9 and 37.2 h following an intravenous dose of 2.5 g (80). Such removal may depend on ultrafiltration flow rate, serum drug concentration, and hemofilter type (80, 97). For example, mean clearance observed with polysulfone and polyacrylonitrile membranes was 77.0 ± 15.6% (SD) and 51.0 ± 5.7% (SD) of the ultrafiltrate flow rate, respectively (97). Between 2.54 and 22.56 mg of flucytosine was removed from the patient per hour when the serum drug concentrations were 21.1 to 126.5 mg/L. Thus, continuous hemofiltration can remove an appreciable quantity of flucytosine, especially when the ultrafiltrate flow rate is high. Similarly, hemodialysis removes significant amounts of flucytosine (21). As in continuous hemofiltration, flucytosine removal increases with increasing flow rates. A dialysate clearance ratio of approximately 70% was observed with respect to creatinine (21, 142).

Flucytosine is also removed during peritoneal dialysis (71, 116). A serum half-life of 34 h was reported in a patient with C. albicans peritonitis receiving 5 days of continous peritoneal lavage with flucytosine (71). Peritoneal clearance of flucytosine was 7.5 mL/min at a peritoneal dialysis flow rate of 1.2 L/h.

DOSING AND ADMINISTRATION

The usual oral dose is 50 to 150 mg/kg/day in 4 equally divided doses at 6-h intervals. Although the use of higher doses (up to 250 mg/kg/day) have been suggested by some to prevent emergence of resistant strains and/or to treat severe infections, this approach may be limited by dose-related toxicity and should not be undertaken without appropriate serum level monitoring. In fact, recommended doses of 150 mg/kg/day for cryptococcal meningitis are probably too high in most cases, and 100 mg/kg/day is recommended as the initial daily dosage for patients with normal renal function. Because a 500-mg capsule is commercially available, individual oral doses are usually rounded to the nearest 500-mg increments in adult patients.

Monitoring serum levels of flucytosine may minimize toxicity and avoid concentrations outside the "therapeutic range" (131). A variety of methods of analysis have been used, including bioassay (23, 86), fluorometric methods (145), high pressure liquid chromatography (HPLC) (77, 120, 165), enzymatic methods (75, 161, 194), and gas chromatography (196). A reasonable goal is to avoid levels below 25 µg/mL and above 100 µg/mL. Others suggest a range of 50 to 100 µg/mL (49, 167). However, clinical data supporting this range in terms of efficacy are lacking. In contrast, clinical studies have established association of flucytosine toxicity and peak serum flucytosine levels of 100 µg/mL or more during 2 or more weeks of therapy (167). While some authors recommend determining serum levels 2 h after and immediately before a dose (15, 193), others have found minimal difference between such levels (55). Since flucytosine assays may not be routinely available in all institutions and relatively difficult to obtain in some cases, a 2-h postdose level should be determined after 3 to 5 doses have been administered, to ensure that the 2-h postdrug levels are below 100 µg/mL. It is reasonable to monitor all patients receiving high doses of drug for prolonged periods of time. Assays may be repeated on a weekly basis, especially if changes in renal function indicate the potential for altered flucytosine clearance (167). Because of concern about hematologic toxicity and the relative difficulty in obtaining flucytosine levels in many institutions, periodic blood counts may be a more practical way to screen for excessive flucytosine levels.

Combination therapy with amphotericin B has been recommended for treatment of invasive fungal infections such as cryptococcal meningitis. However, consideration should be given to potential alterations in clearance and the subsequent need for dosage reduction in the presence of amphotericin B–induced azotemia. Doses of flucytosine used in clinical trials in combination with amphotericin B range from 100 to 150 mg/kg/day. Doses generally do not exceed 100 mg/kg/day in this population, who may already have bone marrow–depressive illnesses such as HIV infection or cancer (138, 139).

Pediatric patients exhibit extreme interpatient variability in half-life, volume of distribution, and clearance of flucytosine, reinforcing the need for serum drug concentration monitoring (8). The oral pediatric dose of flucytosine on a weight basis is the same as the adult dose (1).

Animal model data indicate that flucytosine doses may be reduced when used in combination with other antifungal agents (45, 94). For example, in the murine cryptococcal meningitis model, decreased doses of flucytosine were required for similar efficacy with increasing fluconazole doses (45, 94). However, limited clinical data are available to support this recommendation. In one randomized study in 60 patients with hematologic malignancies, flucytosine monotherapy was compared with combination therapy with fluconazole plus flucytosine at reduced doses (118). The efficacy of the combination therapy was 60.0% (18 of 30) and that of flucytosine alone was 65.5% (19 of 29). Others, investigating a small number of patients, expressed preliminary concern about the combination of fluconazole plus flucytosine for the treatment of cryptococcal meningitis in patients without acquired immunodeficiency syndrome (AIDS) (128), despite successful use of combination therapy in AIDS patients using "traditional" (i.e. 150 mg/kg/day) doses of flucytosine (95). Thus, reduced doses of flucytosine in combination with azoles must be individually tailored and monitored for each patient.

Patients with renal dysfunction require adjustment of flucytosine dosage (14, 21, 37, 39, 55). Several authors have proposed methods of modifying flucytosine dosing on the basis of creatinine clearance (Table 1). In patients receiving dialysis, flucytosine dosing may require further adjustment postdialysis on the basis of serum concentrations (97, 142). In patients receiving continuous hemofiltration, guidelines have been proposed based on the filtration rate (80). Similarly, for patients undergoing hemo- or peritoneal dialysis, giving a supplemental dose of 25 to 50 mg/kg after dialysis is recommended (14, 21). No evidence indicates a need for dosing adjustment in patients with hepatic insufficiency (19). On the basis of a case report of a patient with morbid obesity, use of ideal body weight for dosing may be best (61).

Alternate formulations of flucytosine have been described. Intravenous preparations are available in select countries outside the United States. A 1% solution can be infused intravenously over 20 to 40 min (1). A stable compounded liquid formulation for oral administration has been published (205). Two 500-mg capsules are added to sufficient distilled water to yield a volume of 100 mL, and pH is adjusted with dilute sodium hydroxide to 5 to 6.5. The resultant formulation of 10 mg/mL was stable for 70 days in glass or plastic prescription bottles kept at 4 or 25°C. An alternate formulation uses a medium-chain

TABLE 1 • Dosage Adjustment of 5-Flucytosine in Patients with Renal Dysfunction

Creatinine Clearance (ml/min)	Reference		
	(14)	(88)	(55)
>50	Full dose q6h	Full dose q6h	37.5 mg/kg q6h
41–50	q12–24h	Full dose q6h	37.5 mg/kg q6h
31–40	q12–24h	One-half dose q6h or full dose q12h	37.5 mg/kg q12h
21–30	q12–24h	One-half dose q6h or full dose q12h	37.5 mg/kg q12h
11–20	q.12–24h	One-fourth dose or full dose q24h	37.5 mg/kg q24h
≤10	q24–48h	One-fourth dose or full dose q24h	37.5 mg/kg q24h

triglyceride oil to produce a flucytosine suspension. This was thought to have better absorption than the water-based slurry in a patient with Schwachmann syndrome (64).

Other routes of administration of flucytosine have been investigated. For example, rabbits were give intravitreal injections of 100 μg of flucytosine for treatment of experimental *Candida* endophthalmitis (209). No ocular injury was reported. Intraperitoneal administration was reported in patients with peritonitis undergoing peritoneal dialysis (71). Vaginitis was successfully treated with flucytosine in a topical vaginal cream (74). Others cite the use of vaginal tablets containing flucytosine (1000 mg) plus candicidin (5 mg) for this indication (90).

ADVERSE EFFECTS

Adverse effects associated with flucytosine therapy that are considered dose limiting are predominantly hematologic, gastric, and hepatic toxicities (55). Often, concomitant therapy makes it difficult to determine the true incidence of such reactions. Although definitive mechanisms are unclear, most toxicities associated with flucytosine (primarily the hematologic reactions) are thought to result from conversion of flucytosine to 5-fluorouracil in vivo (65). The enzyme(s) responsible for this conversion is thought to be induced by chronic exposure to flucytosine; hence longer therapy would increase the risk. However, flucytosine toxicity is frequently seen in the first 2 weeks of treatment. In addition, persistent serum levels in excess of 100 μg/mL have also been associated with increased bone marrow toxicity (48, 55, 87, 167). It is generally thought that amphotericin B–induced azotemia may lead to flucytosine accumulation and contribute to dose-related toxicity. However, one study reported that amphotericin B toxicity preceded flucytosine toxicity in only 11% of patients (167).

Hematologic toxicity resulting from flucytosine therapy may limit its application in many patients at increased risk for such effects. The most common reactions are leukopenia and thrombocytopenia, which are thought to occur more frequently in patients with serum levels exceeding 100 to 125 μg/mL (55, 87, 167). Therefore, serum levels should be monitored to minimize the risk of such reactions. Life-threatening bone marrow aplasia has been reported occasionally in patients receiving flucytosine (25, 110). Hiddemann et al. (68) even reported the delay of recovery of normal hematopoietic cells following intensive cytostatic therapy in patients receiving combination antifungal therapy with amphotericin B plus flucytosine (68). Hematologic effects of flucytosine are also common in patients with AIDS receiving high doses of this drug. In one retrospective report, flucytosine had to be discontinued in over half of patients because of cytopenias (34). Other reports indicate discontinuation rates of 28% in AIDS patients receiving flucytosine concomitantly with fluconazole (95).

Gastrointestinal complaints resulting from flucytosine therapy may occur in up to 6% of patients. However, whether toxicity is correlated with serum levels is less certain than is the case with hematologic toxicity. For example, one group of investigators reported elevated liver enzyme levels, nausea, and diarrhea in patients with mean flucytosine levels below 100

μg/mL (55). Most commonly, this group of adverse side effects includes nausea, vomiting, and diarrhea. Case reports of gastrointestinal side effects from flucytosine include intestinal perforation and peritonitis (146), severe diarrhea, and ulcerating enterocolitis (200). Hepatotoxicity (including hepatic necrosis) may result from flucytosine administration (78, 143) and may be most carefully considered in those with prior liver dysfunction. Approximately 5% of patients receiving flucytosine may have abnormal transaminases or alkaline phosphatase (14).

Cutaneous reactions have been reported in patients receiving flucytosine. In one case report, a patient treated for sporotrichosis received 6 months of flucytosine (8 g/day) plus amphotericin B, followed by continued flucytosine therapy for an additional 6 months (160). A significant photosensitivity reaction was associated with this flucytosine therapy.

Although elevations in BUN have been reported in patients receiving monotherapy, significant nephrotoxicity has not been frequently associated with flucytosine therapy. In fact, flucytosine possesses renal vasodilatory properties in the rat model (67). A nephroprotective effect was observed in models when the drug was administered parenterally in combination with amphotericin B (67). This may have been due in part to coadministration of sodium chloride. A case of urinary crystalluria was reported in a patient being treated with flucytosine (201). Reduction in the flucytosine dosage markedly decreased the excretion of urinary gravel. The sediment was determined to be a coprecipitate of flucytosine and uric acid. Reports of flucytosine nephrotoxicity may be due in part to the interference of the drug with selected laboratory methods used to determine serum creatinine (112). Creatinine values determined by the EKTACHEM method can be falsely elevated in patients with flucytosine serum levels within the therapeutic range. The DuPont ACA and Technicon SMAC are thought to be reasonable alternatives (112).

Despite years of clinical use, flucytosine has rarely been associated with allergic reactions. However, in the first report, anaphylaxis to flucytosine occurred on two occasions in a patient with AIDS (92). CNS reactions such as headache, drowsiness, vertigo, confusion, and hallucinations are also infrequently associated with flucytosine administration.

Because of the conversion of flucytosine to the antineoplastic agent 5-fluorouracil and the resultant teratogenicity (demonstrated in animal models), it is considered contraindicated in pregnancy. Although suspected of producing congenital anomalies in humans, isolated reports of flucytosine use during pregnancy have indicated normal pregnancy with delivery of normal infants (32, 36, 129, 133, 157). In one report, a patient receiving 2 g four times daily for a total dose of 52.6 g during her first and second trimesters delivered an infant with normal growth and development for 7 months (157). Others reported a patient receiving flucytosine in combination with amphotericin B for cryptococcal meningitis during the third trimester who delivered a normal infant without apparent complications (28).

In addition to monitoring serum levels, other methods of minimizing flucytosine-related toxicity have been explored.

Inhibition of granulocyte-monocyte and erythroid precursor cells was reversed by uracil in one investigation (91). Other investigators proposed using allopurinol to reduce 5-fluorouracil anabolism, thus potentially reducing myelosuppression without altering the mycotic activity of flucytosine (89). However, no published data are available in humans to support administration of either uracil or allopurinol in patients receiving flucytosine.

Although amphotericin B administration does not reduce the toxicity associated with flucytosine, the opposite may not be true. The combination of intravenous flucytosine in 0.9% saline and amphotericin B was associated with less nephrotoxicity than amphotericin B alone in the rat model (67).

DRUG INTERACTIONS

The effect of flucytosine on the activity of other antifungal agents has been previously reviewed. Such interactions are often influenced by both their absolute and relative concentrations as well as other laboratory conditions (60). However, the effect of flucytosine on the pharmacodynamics or pharmacokinetics of other agents has not been well studied.

Concomitant aluminum hydroxide/magnesium hydroxide may delay absorption of flucytosine (38). The effects of other antacids, as well as drugs altering gastric pH (such as histamine-2 antagonists) have not been published. Flucytosine is not known to affect the hepatic cytochrome P-450 system, according to in vitro testing. Although the product information states that cytarabine may inactivate the antifungal activity of flucytosine, published data (either in vitro or in vivo) to support this statement are lacking (1, 204). Any reports that implicate such interaction would have to account for stable renal function.

Concomitant administration of agents with toxicities similar to those of flucytosine requires caution. This may often be the case in treating cryptococcal meningitis in AIDS patients receiving concomitant zidovudine, ganciclovir, and/or trimethoprim-sulfamethoxazole, which may also have hematologic toxicities. However, one investigator failed to show an effect of flucytosine on the glucuronidation of zidovudine (151). Caution is also advised in concomitant administration of agents with hepatotoxic properties or those known to have gastrointestinal toxicities. In addition, drugs known to cause renal dysfunction (such as amphotericin B and foscarnet) may alter the elimination of flucytosine and predispose the patient to toxicities related to excessive flucytosine levels.

CLINICAL APPLICATIONS
Candidiasis

Extensive animal model experiments have assessed the efficacy of flucytosine (alone or in combination with other antifungals) in the treatment of infections caused by *Candida* spp. Combination with amphotericin B usually demonstrates synergism in these models (125, 136, 141, 174). However, the inability of flucytosine (alone and in combination with amphotericin B) to eradicate fungi incorporated in blood clots and fibrin clots may help explain the relative lack of efficacy in the treatment of fungal endocarditis (149).

The treatment of candiduria with flucytosine is perhaps the best-studied use of monotherapy in humans (127). In one report, flucytosine was successful in treating 212 of 225 patients (94%) with genitourinary candidiasis caused by strains sensitive in vitro (206). Thirteen patients (6%) subsequently received supplemental therapy with systemic or bladder irrigations of amphotericin B due to failure or relapse. Other investigators have also reported their experience in treating candidal urinary tract infections with flucytosine (176, 208). In the first reports, 7 of 9 patients with candiduria caused by *C. albicans* (n = 6), *Candida tropicalis* (n = 2), and *Candida parapsilosis* (n = 1) were successfully treated with 1500 mg/day of flucytosine for 2 weeks. However, recurrence was seen in 3 of the 7 (208). Others reported on 52 patients who received 20 to 150 mg/kg/day for a mean duration of 11 days (176); 47 of 51 *Candida* spp. (*C. albicans,* 28; *C. glabrata,* 10; *C. tropicalis,* 4; and other specied, 9) and 6 of 6 isolates of *T. beigelii* were eradicated, giving an overall eradication rate of 89.5%. Overall clinical response was 84.4%. Case reports have also been published on the treatment of urinary obstruction caused by fungal bezoars in neonates treated by surgical intervention and flucytosine (either alone or in combination with other antifungal agents) (7, 69).

Flucytosine has also been used in the treatment of patients with *Candida* peritonitis (50, 71, 100, 170). One case report described intraperitoneal administration for treatment of *C. albicans* (71), while another used oral therapy in combination with intravenous miconazole to treat peritonitis caused by *C. parapsilosis* in patients undergoing continuous ambulatory peritoneal dialysis (CAPD) (100). However, other investigators report a high rate of relapse with subsequent removal of the dialysate catheter after intraperitoneal flucytosine administration despite an initial response (50, 137). With its high peritoneal fluid penetration, flucytosine may be helpful as adjunctive therapy with other antifungal agents, along with catheter removal, for fungal peritonitis.

Mucocutaneous forms of candidiasis have also been successfully treated with flucytosine, either systemically or locally. One example is treatment of vulvovaginal candidiasis (74, 90, 150, 158). In one published report, 14 of 15 women with culture-proven *C. tropicalis* vaginitis unresponsive to miconazole or clotrimazole cream topically or ketoconazole orally were successfully treated with flucytosine in a topical vaginal cream applied nightly for 7 nights (74). Vaginal tablets containing flucytosine (1000 mg) plus candicidin (5 mg) produced a mycologic cure in 72 of 96 patients, with 1 or 2 doses (90). This regimen was superior to clotrimazole.

Another form of mucocutaneous candidiasis treated with flucytosine monotherapy is esophageal candidiasis. A double-blind study evaluated the efficacy and cost:benefit ratio of flucytosine compared with fluconazole and placebo in the treatment of the first episode of esophageal candidiasis in 60 patients with AIDS (9). Flucytosine was administered in a dose of 100 mg/kg/daily to 20 patients in a randomized study. Those assigned to receive placebo were crossed over (in a blinded manner) to later receive fluconazole (n = 8) or flucytosine (n = 9). Endoscopic and clinical cure was observed in

19 patients (70%) and 21 patients (77.7%) in the fluconazole group, respectively. Nine patients (33%) and 17 patients (63%) receiving flucytosine were endoscopically and clinically cured, respectively. Side effects were not statistically significantly different in active treatments, compared with placebo.

The role of flucytosine in the treatment of hematogenous candidiasis has recently been discussed in the medical literature (49, 182). Uzun and Anaissie identify high-risk patients for treatment failure with candidiasis (i.e., patients with significant underlying disease, neutropenia, candidemia for more than 48 h, fungal endocarditis, septic thrombophlebitis, endophthalmitis, and high APACHE II scores) (182). Their recommendations include consideration of flucytosine in combination with amphotericin B in these and other patients known, or suspected, to have infections caused by *C. krusei* or *C. glabrata,* and hemodynamically unstable patients whose organism is unknown. One particular patient population who may meet such criteria are those who have received immunosuppressive chemotherapy for hematologic or solid malignancies and prophylactic therapy with an azole antifungal agent (203). A recent international conference for consensus development also discussed the role of flucytosine in the treatment of severe candidal infections (49). Many investigators identified a role for flucytosine (in combination with amphotericin B) in unstable patients and/or those with deep-organ candidal infections.

Additional case reports describe use of flucytosine (primarily in combination with other antifungal agents) in such invasive candidal infections as endocarditis, septic thrombosis, spondylodiscitis, meningitis, disseminated hepatosplenic candidiasis, and ocular infections. In select reports, patients failed previous monotherapy with amphotericin B. However, previous and concomitant antifungal therapy and the small number of patients reported make the role of flucytosine in these infections difficult to determine in most cases. Combination with amphotericin B is generally considered in the more invasive candidal infections because of the potential synergism and protection against primary and secondary flucytosine resistance (47, 193). Therefore, flucytosine is used with amphotericin B for hematogenous candidal endophthalmitis, CNS, renal, hepatosplenic, and thrombophlebitis of the great veins, especially in granulocytopenic cancer patients (47, 193).

Despite such combination therapy, treatment outcome of invasive fungal infections in immunocompromised patients may be poor. A randomized trial in 28 neutropenic patients with microbiologically or histologically documented systemic mycoses in which amphotericin B alone was compared with combination therapy of amphotericin B with flucytosine failed to demonstrate a benefit of combination therapy and reported low survival rates in patients with advanced disease and persistent neutropenia (185). However, in one retrospective study, *C. tropicalis* fungemia in neutropenic patients was successfully controlled in some patients receiving a combination of amphotericin plus flucytosine (5 of 9), but fewer (4 of 25) of those receiving amphotericin B alone (73). No patient died who received combination therapy and whose neutropenia re-

solved, compared with 7 of 11 with amphotericin B alone. Additional data demonstrate the usefulness of flucytosine in combination with amphotericin B in the treatment of *Candida* meningitis (163, 164).

Limited information is available for comparison of the effectiveness of flucytosine in combination with amphotericin B with azole antifungals in the treatment of candidal infections. One open-labeled, prospective, randomized study compared the efficacy of fluconazole (300 mg/day after a one-time dose of 400 mg) with that of combination therapy (amphotericin B plus flucytosine) in the treatment of 40 surgical patients with deep-seated mycoses (93). *C. albicans* was most frequently detected mycologically (n = 34). Microbiologic cure was demonstrated in 12 patients in the fluconazole group and 14 patients in the combination group. Patients receiving the combination therapy showed earlier eradication of the fungal pathogen than patients on monotherapy, without a significant difference in cure rates.

Cryptococcosis

Various animal models of cryptococcal infections have been used to examine the role of flucytosine in the treatment of these infections, alone or in combination with other antifungals. Most of these models examine efficacy in the treatment of cryptococcal meningitis. The standard combination of amphotericin B and flucytosine generally demonstrated an additive effect in these models (35, 130), but data on combination therapy with azoles in the animal model of cryptococcal meningitis are conflicting. Combination of flucytosine with ketoconazole produced results superior to those of either agent used alone (35). Others reported no synergy between ketoconazole and flucytosine and found such combinations to be less effective than combination therapy with flucytosine and amphotericin B (130). While some investigators report increased survival and decreased CFUs with flucytosine combined with fluconazole (2, 45, 46, 122), others demonstrated no in vivo synergism with fluconazole and flucytosine (84). One group of investigators proposed that the severity of infection might influence the response, since animals with more severe meningitis had better responses than those with less-severe disease (46). Other animal models of disseminated disease showed a benefit with flucytosine treatment, but no benefit of combination therapy with fluconazole (11). In contrast, in an experimental model of cryptococcosis in hamsters, combination therapy with itraconazole was less effective than therapy with the drugs separately (79).

Clinical trials with flucytosine for serious infections have generally centered on combination therapy because of relapses with resistant organisms when flucytosine was used alone. Combination therapy with amphotericin B (0.3 mg/kg/day) plus flucytosine (150 mg/kg/day) was compared with monotherapy with amphotericin B (0.4 mg/kg/day) for cryptococcal meningitis in patients without AIDS (16). The combination regimen administered for 6 weeks had similar efficacy (16 vs. 11 cured or improved) and fewer failures or relapses (3 vs. 11) than amphotericin B alone for 10 weeks. In addition, statistical differences were demonstrated; the combination reduced the time to CSF sterilization and produced less nephrotoxicity than amphotericin B alone. In fact, all patients with the combination had sterile CSFs after 2 weeks of treatment. Further investigations comparing amphotericin B plus flucytosine for 4 or 6 weeks in a randomized study of 91 patients led the investigators to conclude that 4-week regimens were associated with higher relapse rates and that the combination regimen should be reserved for patients with good prognostic factors who have (a) no neurologic complications, underlying disease, or immunosuppressive therapy; (b) pretreatment CSF white cell counts above 20/mm³ *and* a serum cryptococcal antigen titer below 1:32; and (c) negative CSF India ink *and* serum and CSF cryptococcal antigen titers below 1:8 after 4 weeks of therapy (48).

Limited data are available regarding combination of flucytosine with triazoles (e.g., fluconazole or itraconazole) in the treatment of cryptococcal meningitis in patients without AIDS. One noncomparative study used itraconazole in combination with flucytosine (150 mg/kg/day) in 10 patients (31); 8 of the patients were considered responders after 8 weeks of treatment (cure, 4; improved, 4). No patients required termination of medication due to toxicity. A recent attempt to study the combination of fluconazole plus flucytosine in this patient population was terminated prematurely because of progression of disease in some patients and difficulty in patient accrual. Therefore, the role of flucytosine in combination with azoles for treatment of cryptococcal meningitis in these patients is unclear.

The data regarding the use of flucytosine in acute treatment of cryptococcal meningitis in patients with AIDS are less clear (139). Amphotericin B with or without flucytosine was investigated in a retrospective study of 106 AIDS patients with cryptococcal infections (34). Among the 89 patients with cryptococcal meningitis confirmed by culture, survival did not differ significantly between those treated with amphotericin plus flucytosine (n = 49) and those treated with amphotericin alone (n = 40). Flucytosine serum levels were not routinely monitored in these patients. More recently, a prospective comparative trial examined the use of amphotericin B (0.7 mg/kg/day) with or without flucytosine (100 mg/kg/day) for 2 weeks, followed by either itraconazole or fluconazole therapy for 8 weeks (183). At 2 weeks, 179 patients (51%) on amphotericin B alone had sterile CSF cultures, compared with 202 patients (60%) on combination therapy. The clinical outcomes of both treatment groups were similar. A multivariate analysis showed addition of flucytosine to be independently associated with increased sterilization at 2 weeks. The authors concluded that flucytosine in combination with this dose of amphotericin B resulted in higher rates of CSF sterilization and lower mortality than had been previously observed in this patient population; it is thus likely that this regimen will become a standard induction regimen for treatment of cryptococcal meningitis.

Amphotericin B (0.7 mg/kg/day) plus flucytosine (150 mg/kg/day) was compared with oral fluconazole (400 mg/day) in a randomized study of 21 AIDS patients (96). While 8 of 14 (57%) patients failed fluconazole therapy, none

of the 6 patients receiving amphotericin B plus flucytosine failed. CSF cultures remained positive for a mean of 40.6 ± 5.4 days in patients receiving fluconazole. In contrast, patients receiving the combination therapy had a significantly shorter time to negative CSF cultures (15.6 ± 6.6 days). These authors concluded that amphotericin B in combination with flucytosine was superior to fluconazole alone for initial treatment of cryptococcal meningitis in patients with AIDS. Combination therapy with amphotericin B plus flucytosine was also superior to therapy with itraconazole for acute infections in this patient population (40).

Combination therapy of fluconazole with or without flucytosine has also been reported in a retrospective study of 76 AIDS patients with acute cryptococcal meningitis (207). The lack of flucytosine therapy was among factors associated with treatment failure. A noncomparative study in 32 AIDS patients examined flucytosine (150 mg/kg/day) in combination with fluconazole (400 mg/day) and reported an overall microbiologic efficacy rate of 75% at 10 weeks, a rate generally superior to that with either drug alone in this patient population (95). CSF cultures became negative at a rate comparable to those observed in studies of amphotericin B plus flucytosine. In addition to combination therapy with fluconazole, combination with itraconazole may also have benefit in treatment of cryptococcal infections in patients with AIDS (187). Excellent success was reported with amphotericin B, flucytosine, and fluconazole in triple therapy for cryptococcal meningitis (82).

As with case reports of flucytosine-containing regimens used to treat disseminated forms of candidiasis, several case reports describe a benefit of flucytosine in combination with other antifungals in various forms of disseminated cryptococcal infections, including osteomyelitis, pneumonia, and prostatitis. However, as with candidiasis, most of these reports involved prior and/or concomitant therapy with other antifungal agents, usually amphotericin B. Flucytosine can be used occasionally in pulmonary cryptococcal infections, but the availability of safe triazoles make use of flucytosine alone at this site less attractive.

Aspergillosis

The combination of itraconazole and flucytosine for treatment of disseminated aspergillosis was studied in animal models and showed at least additive effects in most animals. Combination therapy with ketoconazole yielded weakly additive or indifferent effects (136). Combination therapy with amphotericin B was also been studied (4, 136), and a weakly additive or indifferent effect was reported with this combination.

Amphotericin B plus flucytosine was examined as prophylaxis against recurrent invasive aspergillosis in nine patients with previously documented infection who received 13 subsequent courses of myelosuppressive chemotherapy for leukemia (83). Prophylaxis was initiated at least 48 h prior to chemotherapy and continued until granulocyte recovery. While all patients survived, transient radiographic evidence of invasive aspergillosis reactivation occurred during 2 of the 13 chemotherapy courses. One patient who did not receive such prophylaxis died, with clinical and radiographic evidence of reactivation. The investigators concluded that the prophylaxis was successful in preventing clinically significant reactivation of invasive aspergillosis without irreversible nephrotoxicity, prolonged marrow suppression, alteration of antileukemia treatment, or negative impact on clinical outcome, but the relative impact of flucytosine and amphotericin B is uncertain.

Case reports demonstrate a potential role of flucytosine in selected cases of disseminated aspergillosis, including meningitis, pulmonary infections, and endocarditis. As in other infections, however, relapses or drug resistance during therapy have been demonstrated. Therefore, amphotericin B remains the drug of choice for treatment of severe, life-threatening aspergillosis. Itraconazole is considered alternate therapy. Combination therapy with amphotericin B and flucytosine is generally reserved for severe life-threatening infections with a sensitive isolate and/or clinical situations in which amphotericin B therapy failed to eradicate the infection (42, 108, 171); however, its actual clinical benefit remains uncertain.

Chromomycoses

Flucytosine is perhaps the drug of choice for the treatment of certain chromomycoses (29, 103). This chronic infection of the skin and subcutaneous tissue is caused by a variety of fungi. Successful treatment of this disease by flucytosine has been reported for many of the pathogens known to cause it, including *Cladosporium carrionii* (81) and *Fonsecaea pedrosoi* (178). Combination therapy with ketoconazole and flucytosine was successful in one patient after treatment with ketoconazole alone had failed (162). One investigator recommends routine susceptibility testing of isolates prior to therapy (62) with the realization that drug resistant relapse can occur.

Other Mycotic Infections

Isolated case reports of flucytosine-containing combinations successfully used in the treatment of various fungal infections, including disseminated sporotrichosis (12, 160), *Rhodoturula* (105, 119), *Blastomyces* (172), *Penicillium* (102), and *Paecilomyces* (27) can be found in the medical literature. These cases are too few to allow any treatment recommendations with these fungi and can only be used for help in unique treatment decisions.

Amebiasis

The published literature regarding application of flucytosine for infections other than mycotic disease is limited. A recent publication cites the use of flucytosine in combination with other therapies (including pentamidine, fluconazole, and sulfadiazine) in five AIDS patients with disseminated acanthamebiasis without CNS involvement (115). Determining the efficacy and role of flucytosine in such infections, however, is difficult.

REFERENCES

1. Anonymous. Ancobon® product information. Physician's desk reference 1994. Montvale, NJ: Medical Economics Data Production Company, 1994.

2. Allendoerfer R, Marquis AJ, Rinaldi MG, Graybill JR. Combined therapy with fluconazole and flucytosine in murine cryptococcal meningitis. Antimicrob Agents Chemother 1991;35:726–729.

3. Anaissie EJ, Karyotakis NC, Hachem R, et al. Correlation between in vitro and in vivo activity of antifungal agents against Candida species. J Infect Dis 1994;170:384–389.

4. Arroyo J, Medoff G, Kobayashi GS. Therapy of murine aspergillosis with amphotericin B in combination with rifampin of 5-fluorocytosine. Antimicrob Agents Chemother 1977;11:21–25.

5. Atkinson BA, Bouthet C, Bocanegra R, Correa A, Luther MF, Graybill JR. Comparison of fluconazole, amphotericin B and flucytosine in treatment of a murine model of disseminated infection with Candida glabrata in immunocompromised mice. J Antimicrob Chemother 1995;35:631–640.

6. Auger P, Dumas C, Joly J. A study of 666 strains of Candida albicans: correlation between serotype and susceptibility to 5-fluorocytosine. J Infect Dis 1979;139:590–594.

7. Babut JM, Coeurdacier P, Bawab F, Treguier C, Fremond B. Urinary fungal bezoars in children—report of two cases. Eur J Pediatr Surg 1995;5:248–252.

8. Baley JE, Meyers C, Kliegman RM, Jacobs MR, Blumer JL. Pharmacokinetics, outcome of treatment, and toxic effects of amphotericin B and 5-fluorocytosine in neonates. J Pediatr 1990;116:791–797.

9. Barbaro G, Barbarini G, Dilorenzo G. Fluconazole vs flucytosine in the treatment of esophageal candidiasis in AIDS patients–a double-blind, placebo-controlled study. Endoscopy 1995;27:377–383.

10. Bava AJ, Negroni R. In vitro susceptibility of Cryptococcus strains to 5 antifungal drugs. Rev Inst Med Trop Sao Paulo 1989;31:346–350.

11. Bava AJ, Negroni R. Flucytosine plus fluconazole association in the treatment of a murine experimental model of cryptococcosis. Rev Inst Med Trop Sao Paulo 1994;36:551–554.

12. Beardmore GL. Recalcitrant sporotrichosis: a report of a patient treated with various therapies including oral miconazole and 5-fluorocytosine. Aust J Dermatol 1979;20:10–13.

13. Beggs WH, Sarosi GA. Further evidence for sequential action of amphotericin B and 5-fluorocytosine against Candida albicans. Chemotherapy 1982;28:341–344.

14. Bennett JE. Flucytosine. Ann Intern Med 1977;86:319–321.

15. Bennett JE. Antifungal agents. In: Mandell GL, Bennett JE, Dolin R, eds. Principles and practice of infectious diseases. New York: Churchill Livingstone, 1995:401–410.

16. Bennett JE, Dismukes WE, Duma RJ, et al. A comparison of amphotericin B alone and combined with flucytosine in the treatment of cryptococcal meningitis. N Engl J Med 1979;301:126–131.

17. Berenbaum MC. The immunosuppressive effects of 5-fluorocytosine and 5-fluorouracil. Chemotherapy 1979;25:54–59.

18. Berenguer J, Fernandez-Baca V, Sanchez R, Bouza E. In vitro activity of amphotericin B, flucytosine and fluconazole against yeasts causing bloodstream infections. Eur J Clin Microbiol Infect Dis 1995;14:362–365.

19. Block ER. Effect of hepatic insufficiency on 5-fluorocytosine concentrations in serum. Antimicrob Agents Chemother 1973;3:141–142.

20. Block ER, Bennett JE. Pharmacological studies with 5-fluorocytosine. Antimicrob Agents Chemother 1972;1:476–482.

21. Block ER, Bennett JE, Livoti LG, et al. Flucytosine and amphotericin B: hemodialysis effects on the plasma concentration and clearance. Studies in man. Ann Intern Med 1974;80:613–617.

22. Block ER, Jennings AE, Bennett JE. Experimental therapy of cladosporiosis and sporotrichosis with 5-fluorocytosine. Antimicrob Agents Chemother 1973;3:95–98.

23. Bodet CA 3d, Jorgensen JH, Drutz DJ. Simplified bioassay method for measurement of flucytosine or ketoconazole. J Clin Microbiol 1985;22:157–160.

24. Brasseur P, Bonmarchand G, Caron F, Lecomte F, Leroy J, Humbert G. Diffusion of 5-fluorocytosine in bronchial secretions in patients with respiratory insufficiency. Ann Biol Clin (Paris). 1987;45:685–688.

25. Bryan CS, McFarland JA. Cryptococcal meningitis. Fatal marrow aplasia from combined therapy. JAMA 1978;239:1068–1069.

26. Calhoun DL, Roberts GD, Galgiani JN, et al. Results of a survey of antifungal susceptibility tests in the United States and interlaboratory comparison of broth dilution testing of flucytosine and amphotericin B. J Clin Microbiol 1986;23:298–301.

27. Chan TH, Koehler A, Li PKT. Paecilomyces varioti peritonitis in patients on continuous ambulatory peritoneal dialysis. Am J Kidney Dis 1996;27:138–142.

28. Chen CP, Wang KG. Cryptococcal meningitis in pregnancy. Am J Perinatol 1996;13:35–36.

29. Chermsirivathana S, Bunyaratavej K, Pupaibul K. The treatment of chromomycosis with 5-fluorocystine. Int J Dermatol 1979;18:377–379.

30. Chin CS, Cheong YM, Wong YH. 5-Fluorocytosine resistance in clinical isolates of Cryptococcus neoformans. Med J Malaysia 1989;44:194–198.

31. Chotmongkol V, Jitpimolmard S. Treatment of cryptococcal meningitis with combination itraconazole and flucytosine. J Med Assoc Thai 1994;77:253–256.

32. Chotmongkol V, Siricharoensang S. Cryptococcal meningitis in pregnancy: a case report. J Med Assoc Thai 1991;74:421–422.

33. Chouinilalanne N, Maletmartino MC, Gilard V, Ader JC, Martino R. Structural determination of a glucuronide conjugate of flucytosine in humans. Drug Metab Dispos 1995;23:813–817.

34. Chuck SL, Sande MA. Infections with Cryptococcus neoformans in the acquired immunodeficiency syndrome. N Engl J Med 1989;321:794–799.

35. Craven PC, Graybill JR. Combination of oral flucytosine and ketoconazole as therapy for experimental cryptococcal meningitis. J Infect Dis 1984;149:584–590.

36. Curole DN. Cryptococcal meningitis in pregnancy. J Reprod Med 1981;26:317–319.

37. Cutler RE, Blair AD, Kelly MR. Flucytosine kinetics in subjects with normal and impaired renal function. Clin Pharmacol Ther 1978;24:333–342.

38. Daneshmend TK, Warnock DW. Clinical pharmacokinetics of systemic antifungal drugs. Clin Pharmacokinet 1983;8:17–42.

39. Dawborn JK, Page MD, Schiavone DJ. Use of 5-fluorocytosine in patients with impaired renal function. Br Med J 1973;4:382–384.

40. de Gans J, Portegies P, Tiessens G, et al. Itraconazole compared with amphotericin B plus flucytosine in AIDS patients with cryptococcal meningitis. AIDS 1992;6:185–190.

41. Defever KS, Whelan WL, Rogers AL, Beneke ES, Veselenak JM, Soll DR. Candida albicans resistance to 5-fluorocytosine: frequency of partially resistant strains among clinical isolates. Antimicrob Agents Chemother 1982;22:810–815.

42. Denning DW. Treatment of invasive aspergillosis [Review]. J Infect 1994;28(Suppl)1:25–33.

43. Diagnani MC, Karyotakis NC, Paetznick V, Anaissie E. Candida lusitaniae: in vitro susceptibility and in vivo correlation in experimental murine candidiasis [Abstract A23]. Programs and Abstracts of the Conference on Candida and Candidiasis: Biology, Pathogenesis and Management, Baltimore, 1993.

44. Diasio RB, Lakings DE, Bennett JE. Evidence for conversion of 5-fluorocytosine to 5-fluorouracil in humans: possible factor in 5-fluorocytosine clinical toxicity. Antimicrob Agents Chemother 1978;14:903–908.

45. Ding J, Leal MA, Johnson D, Diamond D, Bauer M, Larsen RA. Effect of fluconazole on fungicidal activity of flucytosine is independent of initial severity of illness in muring cryptococcal meningitis [Abstract]. 34th Infectious Diseases Society of America, 1996.

46. Ding JC, Bauer M, Diamond DM, et al. Effect of severity of meningitis on fungicidal activity of flucytosine combined with fluconazole in a murine model of cryptococcal meningitis. Antimicrob Agents Chemother 1997;41:1589–1593.

47. Dismukes WE. Combination therapy with amphotericin B and flucytosine for selected systemic mycoses. In: Holmberg K, Meyer RD, eds. Diagnosis and therapy of systemic fungal infections. New York: Raven Press, 1989:121–132.

48. Dismukes WE, Cloud G, Gallis HA, et al. Treatment of cryptococcal meningitis with combination amphotericin B and flucytosine for four as compared with six weeks. N Engl J Med 1987;317:334–341.

49. Edwards JE, Body GP, Bowden RA, et al. International conference for the development of a consensus on the management and prevention of severe candidal infections. Clin Infect Dis 1997;25:43–59.

50. Eisenberg ES. Intraperitoneal flucytosine in the management of fungal peritonitis in patients on continuous ambulatory peritoneal dialysis. Am J Kidney Dis 1988;11:465–467.

51. Espinel-Ingroff A. E-test for antifungal susceptibility testing of yeasts. Diagn Microbiol Infect Dis 1994;19:217–220.

52. Espinel-Ingroff A, Pfaller M, Erwin ME, Jones RN. Interlaboratory evaluation of E-test method for testing antifungal susceptibilities of pathogenic yeasts to five antifungal agents by using casitone agar and solidified rpmi 1640 medium with 2-percent glucose. J Clin Microbiol 1996;34:848–852.

53. Favel A, Michelnguyen A, Chastin C, Trousson F, Penaud A, Regli P. In-vitro susceptibility pattern of Candida lusitaniae and evaluation of the E-test method. J Antimicrob Chemother 1997;39:591–596.

54. Feldmesser M, Mukherjee J, Casadevall A. Combination of 5-flucytosine and capsule-binding monoclonal antibody in the treatment of murine cryptococcus neoformans infections and in vitro. J Antimicrob Chemother 1996;37:617–622.

55. Francis P, Walsh TJ. Evolving role of flucytosine in immunocompromised patients: new insights into safety, pharmacokinetics, and antifungal therapy [Review]. Clin Infect Dis 1992;15:1003–1018.

56. Franzot SP, Hamdan JS. In vitro susceptibilities of clinical and environmental isolates of Cryptococcus neoformans to five antifungal drugs. Antimicrob Agents Chemother 1996;40:822–824.

57. Fromtling RA, Abruzzo GK, Bulmer GS. Cryptococcus neoformans: comparisons of in vitro antifungal susceptibilities of serotypes AD and BC. Mycopathologia 1986;94:27–30.

58. Fuzibet JG, Squara P, Verdier JM, et al. Candida albicans spondylitis. Review of the literature apropos of a case with study of bone penetration of 5-fluorocytosine [French]. Ann Med Interne (Paris) 1982;133:410–415.

59. Gehrt A, Peter J, Pizzo PA, Walsh TJ. Effect of increasing inoculum sizes of pathogenic filamentous fungi on MICs of anti-

fungal agents by broth microdilution method. J Clin Microbiol 1995;33:1302–1307.

60. Ghannoum MA, Fu Y, Ibrahim AS, Mortara LA, Shafiq MC, Edwards JE. In vitro determination of optimal antifungal combinations against Cryptococcus neoformans and Candida albicans. Antimicrob Agents Chemother 1995;39:2459–2465.

61. Gillum JG, Johnson M, Lavoie S, Venitz J. Flucytosine dosing in an obese patient with extrameningeal cryptococcal infection. Pharmacotherapy 1995;15:251–253.

62. Gonzaga de Oliveira L, Aparecida de Rezende M, Osorio Cisalpino E, Peixoto de Figueiredo Y, Ferreira Lopes C. In vitro sensitivity to 5-fluorocytosine of strains isolated from patients under treatment for chromomycosis. Int J Dermatol 1975;14:141–143.

63. Hamilton JD, Elliott DM. Combined activity of amphotericin B and 5-fluorocytosine against Cryptococcus neoformans in vitro and in vivo in mice. J Infect Dis 1975;131:129–137.

64. Harper KJ, Sawyer WT. Malabsorption of flucytosine in a pediatric patient with Schwachmann syndrome. Drug Intell Clin Pharm 1989;23:782–783.

65. Harris BE, Manning BW, Federle TW, Diasio RB. Conversion of 5-fluorocytosine to 5-fluorouracil by human intestinal microflora. Antimicrob Agents Chemother 1986;29:44–48.

66. Hayashi Y, Asano T, Ito G, Yamada Y. Study of serial bronchoalveolar lavage in patients with aspergilloma: cell reaction at the affected sites and penetration of miconazole and flucytosine into the lesion. Kansenshogaku Zasshi 1995;69:517–523.

67. Heidemann HT, Brune KH, Sabra R, Branch RA. Acute and chronic effects of flucytosine on amphotericin B nephrotoxicity in rats. Antimicrob Agents Chemother 1992;36:2670–2675.

68. Hiddemann W, Essink ME, Fegeler W, et al. Antifungal treatment by amphotericin B and 5-fluorocytosine delays the recovery of normal hematopoietic cells after intensive cytostatic therapy for acute myeloid leukemia. Cancer 1991;68:9–14.

69. Hitchcock RJ, Pallett A, Hall MA, Malone PS. Urinary tract candidiasis in neonates and infants. Br J Urol 1995;76:252–256.

70. Hoeprich PD, Ingraham JL, Kleker E, Winship MJ. Development of resistance to 5-fluorocytosine in Candida parapsilosis during therapy. J Infect Dis 1974;130:112–118.

71. Holdsworth SR, Atkins RC, Scott DF, Jackson R. Management of Candida peritonitis by prolonged peritoneal lavage containing 5-fluorocytosine. Clin Nephrol 1975;4:157–159.

72. Holt RJ. Recent developments in antimycotic chemotherapy [Review]. Infection 1974;2:95–107.

73. Horn R, Wong B, Kiehn TE, Armstrong D. Fungemia in a cancer hospital: changing frequency, earlier onset, and results of therapy. Rev Infect Dis 1985;7:646–655.

74. Horowitz BJ. Topical flucytosine therapy for chronic recurrent Candida tropicalis infections. J Reprod Med 1986;31:821–824.

75. Huang CM, Kroll MH, Ruddel M, Washburn RG, Bennett JE. An enzymatic method for 5-fluorocytosine. Clin Chem 1988; 34:59–62.

76. Hughes CE, Harris C, Moody JA, Peterson LR, Gerding DN. In vitro activities of amphotericin B in combination with four antifungal agents and rifampin against Aspergillus spp. Antimicrob Agents Chemother 1984;25:560–562.

77. Hulsewede JW. Comparison of high-performance liquid chromatography and bioassay for the determination of 5-fluorocytosine in serum. Int J Med Microbiol Virol Parasitol Infect Dis 1994;281:513–518.

78. Inselmann G, Holzlohner U, Heidemann HT. Effect of 5-fluorocytosine and 5-fluorouracil on human and rat hepatic cytochrome P 450. Mycoses 1989;32:638–643.

79. Iovannitti C, Negroni R, Bava J, Finquelievich J, Kral M. Itraconazole and flucytosine plus itraconazole combination in the treatment of experimental cryptococcosis in hamsters. Mycoses 1995;38:449–452.

80. Ittel TH, Legler UF, Polak A, Glockner WM, Sieberth HG. 5-Fluorocytosine kinetics in patients with acute renal failure undergoing continuous hemofiltration. Chemotherapy 1987;33: 77–84.

81. Jacyk WK. Chromomycosis due to Cladosporium carrionii treated with 5-fluorocytosine. A case report from northern Nigeria. Cutis 1979;23:649–650.

82. Just-Nobling G. Initial triple combination in AIDS patients with cryptococcal meningitis [Abstract]. Third International Conference on Cryptococcus and Cryptococcosis, 1996.

83. Karp JE, Burch PA, Merz WG. An approach to intensive antileukemia therapy in patients with previous invasive aspergillosis. Am J Med 1988;85:203–206.

84. Kartalija M, Kaye K, Tureen JH, et al. Treatment of experimental cryptococcal meningitis with fluconazole—impact of dose and addition of flucytosine on mycologic and pathophysiologic outcome. J Infect Dis 1996;173:1216–1221.

85. Karyotakis NC, Anaissie EJ. Efficacy of continuous flucytosine infusion against Candida lusitaniae in experimental hematogenous murine candidiasis. Antimicrob Agents Chemother 1996;40:2907–2908.

86. Kaspar RL, Drutz DJ. Rapid, simple bioassay for 5-fluorocytosine in the presence of amphotericin B. Antimicrob Agents Chemother 1975;7:462–465.

87. Kauffman CA, Frame PT. Bone marrow toxicity associated with 5-fluorocytosine therapy. Antimicrob Agents Chemother 1977; 11:244–247.

88. Kerkering TM, Duma RJ, Shadomy S. The evolution of pulmonary cryptococcosis: clinical implications from a study of 41 patients with and without compromising host factors. Ann Intern Med 1981;94:611–614.

89. Kerkering TM, Schwartz PM, Espinel-Ingroff A, Turek PJ, Diasio RB. 5-Fluorocytosine susceptibility of pathogenic fungi in the presence of allopurinol: potential for improving the therapeutic index of 5-fluorocytosine. Antimicrob Agents Chemother 1983;24:448–449.

90. Kivinen S, Tarkkila T, Laakso L, Laakso K. Short-term topical treatment of vulvovaginal candidiasis with the combination of 5-fluorocytosine and candicidin. Curr Med Res Opin 1979;6: 88–92.

91. Koeffler HP, Golde DW. 5-Fluorocytosine: inhibition of hematopoiesis in vitro and reversal of inhibition by uracil. J Infect Dis 1979;139:438–443.

92. Kotani S, Hirose S, Niiya K, Kubonishi I, Miyoshi I. Anaphylaxis to flucytosine in a patient with AIDS [Letter]. JAMA 1988;260:3275–3276.

93. Kujath P, Lerch K, Kochendorfer P, Boos C. Comparative study of the efficacy of fluconazole versus amphotericin B/flucytosine in surgical patients with systemic mycoses. Infection 1993;21: 376–382.

94. Larsen RA, Bauer M, Weiner JM, et al. Effect of fluconazole on fungicidal activity of flucytosine in murine cryptococcal meningitis. Antimicrob Agents Chemother 1996;40:2178–2182.

95. Larsen RA, Bozzette SA, Jones BE, et al. Fluconazole combined with flucytosine for treatment of cryptococcal meningitis in patients with AIDS. Clin Infect Dis 1994;19:741–745.

96. Larsen RA, Leal MA, Chan LS. Fluconazole compared with amphotericin B plus flucytosine for cryptococcal meningitis

in AIDS. A randomized trial. Ann Intern Med 1990;113:183–187.

97. Lau AH, Kronfol NO. Elimination of flucytosine by continuous hemofiltration. Am J Nephrol 1995;15:327–331.

98. Lauer BA, Reller LB, Schroter GP. Susceptibility of Aspergillus to 5-fluorocytosine and amphotericin B alone and in combination. J Antimicrob Chemother 1978;4:375–380.

99. Lee J, Cooper I, Postelnick M, Stosor V, Weitzman S, Peterson LR. Nosocomial transmission of *Candida krusei* between oncology patients [Abstract]. 36th Interscience Conference on Antimicrobial Agents and Chemotherapy, 1996.

100. Lempert KD, Jones JM. Flucytosine-miconazole treatment of Candida peritonitis. Its use during continuous ambulatory peritoneal dialysis. Arch Intern Med 1982;142:577–578.

101. Levinson DJ, Silcox DC, Rippon JW, Thomsen S. Septic arthritis due to nonencapsulated Cryptococcus neoformans with coexisting sarcoidosis. Arthritis Rheum 1974;17:1037–1047.

102. Lo CY, Chan DTM, Yuen KY, Li FK, Cheng KP. Penicillium marneffei infection in a patient with SLE. Lupus 1995;4:229–231.

103. Lopes CF, Alvarenga RJ, Cisalpino EO, Resende MA, Oliveira LG. Six years' experience in treatment of chromomycosis with 5-fluorocytosine. Int J Dermatol 1978;17:414–418.

104. Malet-Martino MC, Martino R, de Forni M, Andremont A, Hartmann O, Armand JP. Flucytosine conversion to fluorouracil in humans: does a correlation with gut flora status exist? A report of two cases using fluorine-19 magnetic resonance spectroscopy. Infection 1991;19:178–180.

105. Marinova I, Szabadosova V, Brandeburova O, Krcmery V Jr. Rhodotorula spp. fungemia in an immunocompromised boy after neurosurgery successfully treated with miconazole and 5-flucytosine: case report and review of the literature. Chemotherapy 1994;40:287–289.

106. Martin E, Maier F, Bhakdi S. Antagonistic effects of fluconazole and 5-fluorocytosine on candidacidal action of amphotericin B in human serum. Antimicrob Agents Chemother 1994;38:1331–1338.

107. Mauceri AA, Cullen SI, Vandevelde AG, Johnson JE 3d. Flucytosine. An effective oral treatment for chromomycosis. Arch Dermatol 1974;109:873–876.

108. Mazzoni A, Ferrarese M, Manfredi R, Facchini A, Sturani C, Nanetti A. Primary lymph node invasive aspergillosis. Infection 1996;24:37–42.

109. Medoff G, Kobayashi GS. Strategies in the treatment of systemic fungal infections. N Engl J Med 1980;302:145–155.

110. Meyer R, Axelrod JL. Fatal aplastic anemia resulting from flucytosine. JAMA 1974;228:1573.

111. Mikami Y, Scalarone GM, Kurita N, Yazawa K, Uno J, Miyaji M. Synergistic postantifungal effect of flucytosine and fluconazole on Candida albicans. J Med Vet Mycol 1992;30:197–206.

112. Mitchell RT, Marshall LH, Lefkowitz LB Jr, Stratton CW. Falsely elevated serum creatinine levels secondary to the presence of 5-fluorocytosine. Am J Clin Pathol 1985;84:251–253.

113. Montgomerie JZ, Edwards JE Jr, Guze LB. Synergism of amphotericin B and 5-fluorocytosine for Candida species. J Infect Dis 1975;132:82–86.

114. Montplaisir S, Drouhet E, Mercier-Soucy L. Sensitivity and resistance of pathogenic yeasts to 5-fluoropyrimidines. II. Mechanisms of resistance to 5-fluorocytosine (5-FC) and 5-fluorouracil (5-FU). Ann Microbiol (Paris) 1975;126B:41–49.

115. Murakawa GJ, Mccalmont T, Altman J, Hoffman MD, Kantor GR, Berger TG. Disseminated acanthamebiasis in patients with AIDS—a report of five cases and a review of the literature. Arch Dermatol 1995;131:1291–1296.

116. Muther RS, Bennett WM. Clearance of amphotericin B and 5-fluorocytosine by peritoneal dialysis. Proc Clin Dial Transplant Forum 1979;9:100–101.

117. Muther RS, Bennett WM. Peritoneal clearance of amphotericin B and 5-fluorocytosine. West J Med 1980;133:157–160.

118. Naito K, Murate T, Hotta T. A comparative clinical study on flucytosine alone and in combination with fluconazole in hematological malignancies: a multicenter study using the envelope method. Jpn J Antibiot 1994;47:1413–1420.

119. Naveh Y, Friedman A, Merzbach D, Hashman N. Endocarditis caused by Rhodotorula successfully treated with 5-fluorocytosine. Br Heart J 1975;37:101–104.

120. Ng TKC, Chan RCY, Adeyemidoro FAB, Cheung SW, Cheng AFB. Rapid high performance liquid chromatographic assay for antifungal agents in human sera. J Antimicrob Chemother 1996;37:465–472.

121. Nguyen MH, Barchiesi F, Mcgough DA, Yu VL, Rinaldi MG. In vitro evaluation of combination of fluconazole and flucytosine against Cryptococcus neoformans var neoformans. Antimicrob Agents Chemother 1995;39:1691–1695.

122. Nguyen MH, Najvar LK, Yu CY, Graybill JR. Combination therapy with fluconazole and flucytosine in the murine model of cryptococcal meningitis. Antimicrob Agents Chemother 1997;41:1120–1123.

123. O'Day DM. Studies in experimental keratomycosis. Curr Eye Res 1985;4:243–252.

124. Obias AA, Boschman CR, Noskin GA, et al. Surveillance of inpatient transplant and oncology patients for resistance to antifungal agents in yeast isolates [Abstract]. 36th Interscience Conference on Antimicrobial Agents and Chemotherapy, 1996.

125. Odds FC. Interactions among amphotericin B, 5-fluorocytosine, ketoconazole, and miconazole against pathogenic fungi in vitro. Antimicrob Agents Chemother 1982;22:763–770.

126. Odds FC, Vranckx L, Woestenborghs F. Antifungal susceptibility testing of yeasts—evaluation of technical variables for test automation. Antimicrob Agents Chemother 1995;39:2051–2060.

127. Paladino JA, Crass RE. Amphotericin B and flucytosine in the treatment of candidal cystitis. Clin Pharm 1982;1:349–352.

128. Pappas PG, Hamill RJ, Kauffman CA, et al. Treatment of cryptococcal meningitis in non-HIV infected patients—a randomized comparative trial [Abstract]. 34th Infectious Diseases Society of America, 1996.

129. Pereira CA, Fischman O, Colombo AL, Moron AF, Pignatari AC. Cryptococcal meningitis in pregnancy. Review of the literature. Report of 2 cases. Rev Inst Med Trop Sao Paulo 1993;35:367–371.

130. Perfect JR, Durack DT. Treatment of experimental cryptococcal meningitis with amphotericin B, 5-fluorocytosine, and ketoconazole. J Infect Dis 1982;146:429–435.

131. Petersen D, Demertzis S, Freund M, Schumann G, Oellerich M. Individualization of 5-fluorocytosine therapy. Chemotherapy 1994;40:149–156.

132. Pfaller MA, Bale M, Buschelman B, et al. Quality control guidelines for National Committee for Clinical Laboratory Standards recommended broth macrodilution testing of amphotericin B, fluconazole, and flucytosine. J Clin Microbiol 1995;33:1104–1107.

133. Philpot CR, Lo D. Cryptococcal meningitis in pregnancy. Med J Aust 1972;2:1005–1007.

134. Polak A. Pharmacokinetics of amphotericin B and flucytosine. Postgrad Med J 1979;55:667–670.

135. Polak A, Scholer HJ. Mode of action of 5-fluorocytosine and mechanisms of resistance. Chemotherapy 1975;21:113–130.

136. Polak A, Scholer HJ, Wall M. Combination therapy of experimental candidiasis, cryptococcosis and aspergillosis in mice. Chemotherapy 1982;28:461–479.

137. Pomeranz A, Reichenberg Y, Mor J, Drukker A. Candida peritonitis—inefficacy of amphotericin-B and 5-fluorocytosine treatment. Int J Pediatr Nephrol 1983;4:127–128.

138. Powderly WG. Therapy for cryptococcal meningitis in patients with AIDS [Review]. Clin Infect Dis 1992;14(Suppl 1):S54–S59.

139. Powderly WG. Recent advances in the management of cryptococcal meningitis in patients with AIDS. Clin Infect Dis 1996; 22:S119–S123.

140. Pujol I, Guarro J, Gene J, Sala J. In-vitro antifungal susceptibility of clinical and environmental Fusarium spp. strains. J Antimicrob Chemother 1997;39:163–167.

141. Rabinovich S, Shaw BD, Bryant T, Donta ST. Effect of 5-fluorocytosine and amphotericin B on Candida albicans infection in mice. J Infect Dis 1974;130:28–31.

142. Rault RM, Hulme B, Davies RR. 5-Fluorocytosine treatment of candidiasis on a patient receiving regular hemodialysis. Clin Nephrol 1975;3:225–227.

143. Record CO, Skinner JM, Sleight P, Speller DC. Candida endocarditis treated with 5-fluorocytosine. Br Med J 1971;1: 262–264.

144. Richardson MD, Paton M, Shankland GS. Intracellular killing of Candida albicans by human neutrophils is potentiated by exposure to combinations of amphotericin B and 5-fluorocytosine. Mycoses 1991;34:201–204.

145. Richardson RA. Rapid fluorimetric determination of 5-fluorocytosine in serum. Clin Chim Acta 1975;63:109–114.

146. Robertson DM, Riley FC, Hermans PE. Endogenous Candida oculomycosis. Report of two patients treated with flucytosine. Arch Ophthalmol 1974;91:33–38.

147. Rodrigueztudela JL, Berenguer J, Martinezsuarez JV, Sanchez R. Comparison of a spectrophotometric microdilution method with rpmi-2-percent glucose with the National Committee for Clinical Laboratory Standards reference macrodilution method m27-p for in vitro susceptibility testing of amphotericin B, flucytosine, and fluconazole against Candida albicans. Antimicrob Agents Chemother 1996;40:1998–2003.

148. Roselle GA, Kauffman CA. Amphotericin B and 5-fluorocytosine: effects on cell-mediated immunity. Clin Exp Immunol 1980;40:186–192.

149. Rubinstein E. Amphotericin B and 5-fluorocytosine penetration into blood and fibrin clots. Chemotherapy 1979;25:249–253.

150. Rubio-Lotvin B, Gonzalez Ansorena R, Bolio Arista R, Ruiz Moreno JA. Treatment of vaginal candidiasis with 5-fluorocytosine [Spanish]. Ginecol Obstet Mex 1975;37:23–25.

151. Sampol E, Lacarelle B, Rajaonarison JF, Catalin J, Durand A. Comparative effects of antifungal agents on zidovudine glucuronidation by human liver microsomes. Br J Clin Pharmacol 1995;40:83–86.

152. Scalarone GM, Mikami Y, Kurita N, Yazawa K, Miyaji M. Comparative studies on the postantifungal effect produced by the synergistic interaction of flucytosine and amphotericin B on Candida albicans. Mycopathologia 1992;120:133–138.

153. Scalarone GM, Mikami Y, Kurita N, Yazawa K, Miyaji M. The postantifungal effect of 5-fluorocytosine on Candida albicans. J Antimicrob Chemother 1992;29:129–136.

154. Scalarone GM, Mikami Y, Kurita N, Yazawa K, Uno J, Miyaji M. In vitro comparative evaluations of the postantifungal effect: synergistic interaction between flucytosine and fluconazole against Candida albicans. Mycoses 1991;34:405–410.

155. Schonebeck J, Ansehn S. 5-Fluorocytosine resistance in candida spp. and Torulopsis glabrata. Sabouraudia 1973;11:10–20.

156. Schonebeck J, Polak A, Fernex M, Scholer HJ. Pharmacokinetic studies on the oral antimycotic agent 5-fluorocytosine in individuals with normal and impaired kidney function. Chemotherapy 1973;18:321–336.

157. Schonebeck J, Segerbrand E. Candida albicans septicaemia during first half of pregnancy successfully treated with 5-fluorocytosine. Br Med J 1973;4:337–338.

158. Seligman SA. Letter: treatment of vulval candidiasis with 5-fluorocytosine. Br Med J 1974;3:173–174.

159. Shadomy HJ, Wood-Helie S, Shadomy S, Dismukes WE, Chau RY. Biochemical serogrouping of clinical isolates of Cryptococcus neoformans [published erratum appears in Diagn Microbiol Infect Dis 1987;7:159]. Diagn Microbiol Infect Dis 1987;6:131–138.

160. Shelley WB, Sica PA Jr. Disseminate sporotrichosis of skin and bone cured with 5-fluorocytosine: photosensitivity as a complication. J Am Acad Dermatol 1983;8:229–235.

161. Shivji A, Bernstein M, Noble MA. Enzyme rate assay for 5-fluorocytosine. Am J Clin Pathol 1993;100:299–300.

162. Silber JG, Gombert ME, Green KM, Shalita AR. Treatment of chromomycosis with ketoconazole and 5-flurocytosine. J Am Acad Dermatol 1983;8:236–238.

163. Smego RA Jr, Devoe PW, Sampson HA, et al. Candida meningitis in two children with severe combined immunodeficiency. J Pediatr 1984;104:902–904.

164. Smego RA Jr, Perfect JR, Durack DT. Combined therapy with amphotericin B and 5-fluorocytosine for Candida meningitis. Rev Infect Dis 1984;6:791–801.

165. St. Germain G, Lapierre S, Tessier D. Performance characteristics of two bioassays and high-performance liquid chromatography for determination of flucytosine in serum. Antimicrob Agents Chemother 1989;33:1403–1405.

166. Stafford CR, Fisher JF, Fadel HE, Espinel-Ingroff AV, Shadomy S, Hamby M. Cryptococcal meningitis in pregnancy. Obstet Gynecol 1983;62:35s–37s.

167. Stamm AM, Diasio RB, Dismukes WE, et al. Toxicity of amphotericin B plus flucytosine in 194 patients with cryptococcal meningitis. Am J Med 1987;83:236–242.

168. Stiller RL, Bennett JE, Scholer HJ, Wall M, Polak A, Stevens DA. Susceptibility to 5-fluorocytosine and prevalence of serotype in 402 Candida albicans isolates from the United States. Antimicrob Agents Chemother 1982;22:482–487.

169. Stiller RL, Bennett JE, Scholer HJ, Wall M, Polak A, Stevens DA. Correlation of in vitro susceptibility test results with in vivo response: flucytosine therapy in a systemic candidiasis model. J Infect Dis 1983;147:1070–1077.

170. Struijk DG, Krediet RT, Boeschoten EW, Rietra PJ, Arisz L. Antifungal treatment of Candida peritonitis in continuous ambulatory peritoneal dialysis patients. Am J Kidney Dis 1987;9: 66–70.

171. Symonds RP, Robertson AG, Stewart LM, Boyd G. Fungal lung infections treated by 5 flucytosine. Scott Med J 1982;27:244–246.

172. Taillan B, Ferrari E, Cosnefroy JY, et al. Favourable outcome of blastomycosis of the brain stem with fluconazole and flucytosine treatment. Ann Med 1992;24:71–72.

173. Tiballi RN, Spiegel JE, Zarins LT, Kauffman CA. Saccharomyces cerevisiae infections and antifungal susceptibility studies by colorimetric and broth macrodilution methods. Diagn Microbiol Infect Dis 1995;23:135–140.

174. Titsworth E, Grunberg E. Chemotherapeutic activity of 5-fluorocytosine and amphotericin B against Candida albicans in mice. Antimicrob Agents Chemother 1973;4:306–308.

175. Reynolds JEF, ed. Martindale: The Extra Pharmacopoeia. 28th ed. London: The Pharmaceotical Press, 1982.

176. Tokunaga S, Ohkawa M, Nakashima T, et al. Clinical evaluation of flucytosine in patients with urinary fungal infections [Japanese]. Jpn J Antibiot 1992;45:1060–1064.

177. Turnidge JD, Gudmundsson S, Vogelman B, Craig WA. The postantibiotic effect of antifungal agents against common pathogenic yeasts. J Antimicrob Chemother 1994;34:83–92.

178. Uitto J, Santa-Cruz DJ, Eisen AZ, Kobayashi GS. Chromomycosis. Successful treatment with 5-fluorocytosine. J Cutan Pathol 1979;6:77–84.

179. Utz CJ, Shadomy S. Anitfungal acitvity of 5-fluorocytosine as measured by disk diffusion susceptibility testing. J Infect Dis 1977;135:970–974.

180. Utz JP. Flucytosine. N Engl J Med 1972;286:777–778.

181. Utz JP, Shadomy S, McGehee KF. Flucytosine: experience in patients with pulmonary and other forms of cryptococcosis. Ann Rev Respir Dis 1969;99:975–979.

182. Uzun O, Anaissie EJ. Problems and controversies in the management of hematogenous candidiasis. Clin Infect Dis 1996;22:95s–101S.

183. van der Horst CM, Saag MS, Cloud GA, et al. Treatment of cryptococcal meningitis associated with the acquired immunodeficiency syndrome. National Institute of Allergy and Infectious Diseases Mycoses Study Group and AIDS Clinical Trials Group. N Engl J Med 1997;337:15–21.

184. Vantwout JW. Fungal infections and antifungal drugs—has the age of antifungal resistance dawned. Curr Opin Infect Dis 1996;9:63–66.

185. Verweij PE, Donnelly JP, Kullberg BJ, Meis JF, De Pauw BE. Amphotericin B versus amphotericin B plus 5-flucytosine: poor results in the treatment of proven systemic mycoses in neutropenic patients. Infection 1994;22:81–85.

186. Vialaneix JP, Malet-Martino MC, Hoffmann JS, Pris J, Martino R. Direct detection of new flucytosine metabolites in human biofluids by 19F nuclear magnetic resonance. Drug Metab Dispos 1987;15:718–724.

187. Viviani MA. Cryptococcal meningitis—diagnosis and treatment. Int J Antimicrob Agents 1996;6:169–173.

188. Wagner GE, Shadomy S. Studies on the mode of action of 5-fluorocytosine in Aspergillus species. Chemotherapy 1979;25:61–69.

189. Wain WH, Polak A. The effect of flucytosine on the germination of Candida albicans. Postgrad Med J 1979;55:671–673.

190. Waldorf AR, Polak A. Mechanisms of action of 5-fluorocytosine. Antimicrob Agents Chemother 1983;23:79–85.

191. Walsh A, Haft DA, Miller MH, Loran MR, Friedman AH. Ocular penetration of 5-fluorocytosine. Invest Ophthalmol Vis Sci 1978;17:691–694.

192. Walsh TJ. Mechanisms of antifungal drug resistance: what we know and what we do not know [Abstract]. 36th Interscience Conference on Antimicrobial Agents and Chemotherapy, 1996.

193. Walsh TJ, Pizzo PA. Fungal infections in granulocytopenic patients: current approaches to classification, diagnosis and treatment. In: Holmberg K, Meyer RD, eds. Diagnosis and therapy of systemic fungal infections. New York: Raven Press, 1989:47–70.

194. Washburn RG, Klym DM, Kroll MH, Bennett JE. Rapid enzymatic method for measurement of serum flucytosine levels. J Antimicrob Chemother 1986;17:673–677.

195. Weber S, Polak A. Susceptibility of yeast isolates from defined German patient groups to 5-fluorocytosine. Mycoses 1992;35:163–171.

196. Wee SH, Anhalt JP. Gas chromatographic determination of 5-fluorocytosine: a modified extraction method. Antimicrob Agents Chemother 1977;11:914–915.

197. Wei K, Huber BE. Cytosine deaminase gene as a positive selection marker. J Biol Chem 1996;271:3812–3816.

198. Weisse ME, Person DA, Berkenbaugh JT Jr. Treatment of Candida arthritis with flucytosine and amphotericin. J Perinatol 1993;13:402–404.

199. Whelan WL. The genetic basis of resistance to 5-fluorocytosine in Candida species and Cryptococcus neoformans. Crit Rev Microbiol 1987;15:45–56.

200. White CA, Traube J. Ulcerating enteritis associated with flucytosine therapy. Gastroenterology 1982;83:1127–1129.

201. Williams KM, Chinwah PM, Cobcroft R. Crystalluria during flucytosine therapy. Med J Aust 1979;2:617.

202. Williams KM, Duffield AM, Christopher RK, Finlayson PJ. Identification of minor metabolites of 5-fluorocytosine in man by chemical ionization gas chromatography mass spectrometry. Biomed Mass Spectrom 1981;8:179–182.

203. Wingard JR, Merz WG, Rinaldi MG, Miller CB, Karp JE, Saral R. Association of Torulopsis glabrata infections with fluconazole prophylaxis in neutropenic bone marrow transplant patients. Antimicrob Agents Chemother 1993;37:1847–1849.

204. Wingfield HJ. Absence of fungistatic antagonism between flucytosine and cytarabine in vitro and in vivo. J Antimicrob Chemother 1987;20:523–527.

205. Wintermeyer SM, Nahata MC. Stability of flucytosine in an extemporaneously compounded oral liquid. Am J Health Syst Pharm 1996;53:407–409.

206. Wise GJ, Kozinn PJ, Goldberg P. Flucytosine in the management of genitourinary candidiasis: 5 years of experience. J Urol 1980;124:70–72.

207. Witt MD, Lewis RJ, Larsen RA, et al. Identification of patients with acute AIDS-associated cryptococcal meningitis who can be effectively treated with fluconazole—the role of antifungal susceptibility testing. Clin Infect Dis 1996;22:322–328.

208. Yasumoto R, Asakawa M, Umeda M. Clinical efficacy of flucytosine on urinary candidiasis. Hinyokika Kiyo 1988;34:1679–1682.

209. Yoshizumi MO, Silverman C. Experimental intravitreal 5-fluorocytosine. Ann Ophthalmol 1985;17:58–61.

Nystatin

●

Thomas L. Wallace and Gabriel Lopez-Berestein

CLASS
Structure-Activity Relationships

Nystatin (Fig. 1) is in the class of polyene antifungals. Approximately 100 polyene antifungals have been isolated, but only nystatin, amphotericin B, natamycin, hamycin, trichomycin and candicidin have been used clinically (55). The polyenes are characterized by common structural features, including a macrolide ring of carbon atoms closed by an ester or lactone, a large number of hydroxyls on the macrolide ring on alternate carbon atoms, an extensive double-bond system, and an amino sugar. No extensive structure-activity studies of nystatin derivatives have been performed. Methyl, ethyl, propyl, and butyl esters of nystatin have been synthesized but showed no distinctive advantages over nystatin (11) and were never used clinically.

Nyotram™ (Aronex Pharmaceuticals, The Woodlands, Texas) is a liposomal formulation of nystatin (liposomal nystatin) that contains nystatin, dimyristoyl phosphatidyl choline and dimyristoyl phosphatidyl glycerol in a ratio (by weight) of 1:7:3. Formulation of nystatin into liposomes by Lopez-Berestein and coworkers in the 1980s established that nystatin could be administered intravenously to mice with good evidence of activity and reduced toxicity (56, 57). An intravenous liposomal formulation of nystatin is currently in phase III clinical trials for the treatment of systemic fungal infections and is not commercially available.

Mechanisms of Action

Polyene antifungals bind to ergosterol in the fungal membrane, resulting in altered membrane permeability that allows release of K^+, sugars, and metabolites (82). Disruption of the membrane is believed to be responsible for fungal death (see "Mechanisms of Action," below).

ANTIMICROBIAL ACTIVITY
Spectrum

In Vitro

Nystatin is active against a broad spectrum of fungi in vitro, including yeast and molds (31, 77, 79). Its in vitro spectrum of antifungal activity is much broader than those of azole antifungals and flucytosine. Nystatin has been reported to be active in vitro against HIV (73). Table 1 shows the minimum inhibitory concentration (MIC) range of nystatin and liposomal nystatin against 507 clinical fungal isolates obtained in Europe and the United States (57, and unpublished data). In vitro activities of nystatin and liposomal nystatin are similar, except that in some cases, the MIC for liposomal nystatin is one dilu-

tion lower. In vitro MICs of nystatin and liposomal nystatin are also similar to those of amphotericin B desoxycholate (Fungizone), amphotericin B lipid complex (Abelcet), and liposomal amphotericin B (AmBisome) against clinical fungal isolates. However, nystatin and liposomal nystatin are active against all fluconazole-, all flucytosine- and certain amphotericin B–resistant clinical isolates.

In Vivo

Nystatin has demonstrated antifungal activity against *Candida albicans* (10, 32, 56, 76), *Cryptococcus neoformans* (76), *Histoplasma capsulatum* (12, 18), and *Coccidioides immitis* (18, 24) in animals. Liposomal nystatin has been reported to be active against *C. albicans* in mice (56), and *Aspergillus fumigatus* in mice (86) and rabbits (22).

In addition to its antifungal activity in vitro and in animals, nystatin has been shown effective against a variety of fungi in humans, including *Candida* (54), *Aspergillus* (81), *Histoplasma* (67), and *Coccidioides* (61). Nystatin has demonstrated antifungal activity in humans via different routes of administration, including oral (13, 71), pleural (48, 63), inhalation (22, 74, 78, 85), and topical routes (43, 64, 81). Nystatin has been used since the 1950s, mainly for treatment of cutaneous, vaginal, and oral candidiasis (5). Liposomal nystatin has antifungal activity similar to that of amphotericin B desoxycholate in candidemia in humans but reduced toxicity (24). Liposomal nystatin is active in some patients who have failed therapy with amphotericin B (7).

Pharmacodynamic Effects
Fungicidal Effects

Nystatin and liposomal nystatin are active in a wide variety of media and methods, including the National Committee for Clinical Laboratory Standards (NCCLS) assay. Susceptibility of fungi to nystatin has been reported to increase with growth rate, lower culture temperature, and lower pH (39).

Postantibiotic Effects

There have been no reports of postantibiotic effects with nystatin or liposomal nystatin.

Effects of Subinhibitory Concentrations

Subinhibitory concentrations of nystatin have been reported to block adherence of *Candida* species to human vaginal (8) and buccal (1) cells in vitro and to reduce the concentration of peptidomannans in *C. albicans* (6). Subinhibitory concentrations have been used to develop fungi resistant to nystatin (2), although with great difficulty.

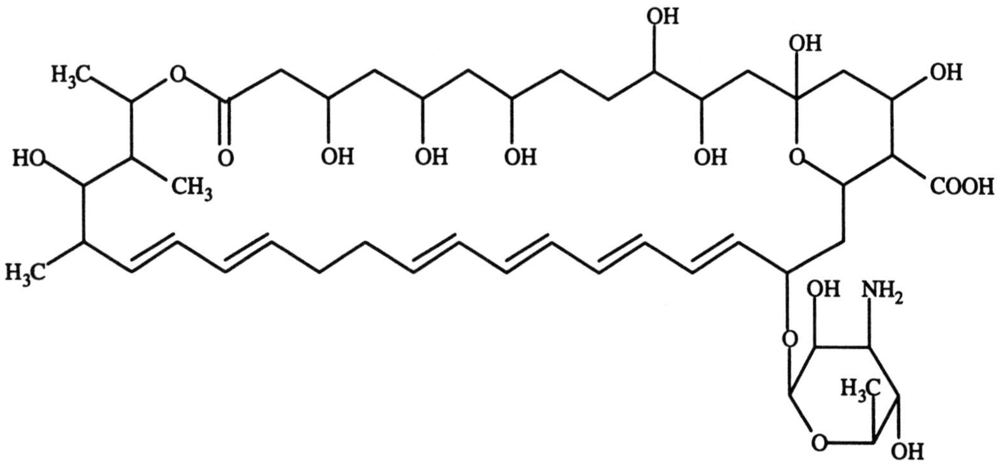

FIGURE 1. Nystatin A$_1$ (MW, 926.13).

TABLE 1 • Activity of Nystatin and Liposomal Nystatin against Clinical Fungal Isolates

	MIC Range in μg/mL (no. isolates tested)[a]		
Fungal Species	**Geographic Source**	**Nystatin**	**Liposomal Nystatin**
Allescheria sp.	US	nd	16 (1)
Alternaria sp.	US	nd	1 (1)
Aspergillus flavus	US, Europe	2–8 (14)	0.5–4 (15)
Aspergillus fumigatus	US, Europe	2–8 (35)	1–8 (36)
Aspergillus niger	US, Europe	2 (1)	2 (2)
Beauvaria sp.	US	2 (1)	2 (1)
Bipolaris sp.	US	0.5 (1)	0.25 (1)
Candida albicans	US, Europe	0.078–10 (139)	0.25–4 (149)
Candida famata	Europe	0.312 (1)	1.25 (1)
Candida glabrata	US, Europe	0.156–8 (41)	0.5–5 (45)
Candida guilliermondii	US, Europe	0.156–2 (10)	0.625–1 (10)
Candida kefyr	Europe	0.312–8 (11)	1–4 (11)
Candida krusei	US, Europe	0.156–8 (37)	0.5–4 (37)
Candida lusitaniae	US, Europe	0.5–8 (15)	0.5–2 (15)
Candida parapsilosis	US, Europe	0.125–4 (59)	0.25–2.5 (63)
Candida rugosa	Europe	0.23 (1)	0.625 (1)
Candida tropicalis	US, Europe	0.156–16 (38)	0.019–8 (42)
Candida wiswanathii	Europe	0.39 (1)	0.625–1.25 (2)
Chryosporium sp.	US	nd	0.5 (1)
Cladosporium sp.	US	1 (1)	1 (1)
Cryptococcus leurentii	Europe	0.312 (1)	0.625 (1)
Cryptococcus neoformans	US, Europe	0.019–8 (45)	0.12–4 (47)
Cunninghamella elegans	US	nd	1 (1)
Curvularia sp.	US	nd	0.5 (1)
Fonsecaea sp.	US	0.5 (1)	0.5 (1)
Fusarium sp.	US	4 (1)	2 (2)
Geotrichum sp.	US	2 (1)	1 (1)
Hansenula anomala	Europe	0.5 (1)	0.5 (1)
Issatchenikia orientalis	US	2.5 (1)	1.25 (1)
Mucor sp.	US	1 (1)	1 (1)
Penicillium sp.	US	0.25 (1)	0.25 (1)
Rhizopus sp.	US	4 (1)	2 (1)
Rhodotorula rubra	Europe	0.312 (2)	0.312–0.625 (2)
Sporothrix sp.	US	2 (1)	1 (1)
Trichosporon sp.	US, Europe	0.156–2 (10)	0.25–1.25 (10)

[a] nd, not determined.

Important Effects on Host Immunity (Positive or Negative)

Nystatin has been reported to stimulate thymus-independent B cells and polyclonal antibody synthesis in vitro (29, 38), but there have been no reports of an effect of nystatin or liposomal nystatin on immune function in humans.

Pharmacodynamic Correlates with Outcome

There are no published studies on the pharmacodynamics or pharmacokinetics of nystatin, because nystatin has very poor absorption after oral administration. Insufficient pharmacokinetic data are available to analyze the pharmacodynamic/pharmacokinetic relationship of liposomal nystatin.

MECHANISMS OF ACTION

The activity of nystatin has been attributed to binding to ergosterol in the fungal membrane, resulting in altered membrane permeability that allows release of K^+, sugars, and metabolites (82). Ergosterol is the main sterol in fungi but is not found in human cells; cholesterol is the main sterol in mammalian cells. Nystatin has been shown to have greater affinity for ergosterol than for cholesterol (45) and to bind directly to ergosterol in the fungal membrane in an essentially irreversible manner (44). Exogenously added sterol can block the antifungal effect of nystatin (26). In nystatin-resistant, ergosterol-deficient *C. albicans* and *Candida krusei* isolates obtained from human patients, addition of ergosterol to the culture medium restored nystatin-induced K^+ leakage (51). Similarly, in ergosterol-deficient *Saccharomyces cerevisiae*, there was a direct correlation between the amount of ergosterol replaced in the fungus and sensitivity to nystatin (69). When ergosterol was replaced in ergosterol-deficient *S. cerevisiae* by cholesterol or cholestanol, sensitivity to nystatin was markedly decreased (69). Disruption of the membrane by nystatin results in fungal death, although it is not clear if ionic changes are responsible for membrane disruption (14).

Despite the close structural resemblance of nystatin to amphotericin B, there are data indicating that nystatin and amphotericin B have different biologic properties. *(a)* The rate at which nystatin causes K^+ release (i.e., membrane disruption) from *C. albicans* in vitro is much faster than that of amphotericin, but fungal death occurs at a faster rate with amphotericin B than with nystatin (14). However, in 24-h susceptibility assays, the two drugs have nearly identical MICs. *(b)* Nystatin has been reported to be markedly less toxic to mammalian cells than amphotericin at equimolar concentrations (82). Kinsky (42) reported that amphotericin B (5 µg/mL) produced 78% lysis in human red blood cells in 40 min, while nystatin (5 µg/mL) produced no lysis in 40 min. Hemolytic activity is known to correlate approximately with mammalian toxicity (30). *(c)* K^+ or NH_4^+ reverses amphotericin B inhibition of fungal glycolysis but does not reverse nystatin inhibition of fungal glycolysis (30). Inhibition of glycolysis is a sequela to polyene-induced K^+ leakage. *(d)* Nystatin and amphotericin B differ in their ability to inhibit ATPase (82). *(e)* Amphotericin B–resistant fungi are sometimes not cross-resistant to nystatin. Hebeka and Solotorovsky (33) developed two *C. albicans* strains with 50-fold increased resistance to amphotericin B but normal sensitivity to nystatin. Broughton et al. (9) reported isolation of a *C. albicans* strain that was resistant to amphotericin B but not to nystatin. On the basis of these data, the mechanisms of action of nystatin and amphotericin B may differ in certain fungal isolates or strains. This suggests that nystatin may be useful in clinical situations in which amphotericin B has failed.

It is assumed that the in vitro and in vivo antifungal mechanism of action of liposomal nystatin and nystatin are the same, since nystatin is the active ingredient in liposomal nystatin. In vivo, it is believed that the liposome encapsulation of liposomal nystatin is responsible for directing the drug toward the cells of the reticuloendothelial system (e.g., macrophages) that localize in inflammatory areas and away from the kidney, which is the primary organ of toxicity. The mechanism by which nystatin is released from the liposomes in vitro or in vivo is not understood but may involve fusion of the liposomes containing nystatin with the fungal cell or transfer of the nystatin from the liposome to the fungi because of the greater affinity of nystatin for ergosterol in the fungal cell. A stability study conducted in vitro in human serum at 37°C showed that 75% of nystatin is retained in liposomes after 4 h, 65% after 24 h, and 30% after 72 h of incubation (57).

MECHANISMS OF RESISTANCE
Commonly Resistant Organisms

Although nystatin-resistant fungi have been created in the laboratory, resistance to nystatin in humans is rare and is not clinically significant. However, resistance has been reported in a small number of clinical cases. See Table 2. Fungi resistant to amphotericin B are not always resistant to nystatin (see "Mechanisms of Action," above), but there are many cases of cross-resistance between amphotericin B and nystatin (88). Although a strain of *C. albicans* obtained in the laboratory was reported to be cross-resistant to azoles and polyenes (34), no cross-resistance between these classes of antifungals has been reported in humans. Resistance to molds has not been reported for nystatin. There are no published data on possible cross-resistance of nystatin to amphotericin B–resistant molds.

Mechanisms of Resistance

There are probably several mechanisms of resistance to nystatin (35) (Table 3). A major contributor to resistance appears

TABLE 2 • Clinical Fungal Isolates Reported to Be Resistant to Nystatin

Organism	Reference
C. tropicalis	88
C. krusei, C. parakrusei, C. tropicalis	72
C. tropicalis	58
C. albicans, C. krusei	50
C. albicans, C. tropicalis, T. glabrata	17
C. albicans	49
T. glabrata	62

TABLE 3 • **Proposed Mechanisms of Fungal Resistance to Nystatin**

Mechanism of Resistance	Organism	Reference
Ergosterol deficient	*Saccharomyces cerevisiae*	83
Decrease in ergosterol and appearance of other sterols	*Saccharomyces cerevisiae*	87
Unknown; no change in ergosterol	*Candida*	21
Decrease in ergosterol and alteration of fatty acids	*Torulopsis glabrata*	46
C-14 demethylation mutation	*Saccharomyces cerevisiae*	84
C-14 demethylation defect	*Candida albicans*	65
$\Delta^8-\Delta^7$ isomerase blocked; Increase in sterol content and change in sterol composition	*Candida albicans*	66
Defects in $\Delta^8-\Delta^7$ isomerase, 24(28) hydrogenase or C-24 methyl transferase in separate mutants	*Neurospora crassa*	27
Increase in fatty acids; unaltered sterol content	*Saccharomyces cerevisiae*	59
Decrease in sterol content and alteration in fatty acid composition	*Candida tropicalis*	16
Blocked ergosterol synthesis	*Rhodotorula gracilis*	36
Δ^{22} Desaturation defect	*Saccharomyces cerevisiae*	28
Lanosterol C-14 demethylase and 5,6-desaturase mutations		80
Δ^{24} Sterol methyltransferase mutation	*Saccharomyces cerevisiae*	53
C-14 Demethylation mutation	*Saccharomyces cerevisiae*	41
Cell wall amino acid and fatty acid changes	*Saccharomyces cerevisiae*	4
Δ^5-Desaturation, $(^8-(^7$ isomerization, and C-24 transmethylation defects	*Saccharomyces cerevisiae*	60
Cytochrome P-450 deficient	*C. albicans*	3
Decrease in ergosterol and appearance of other sterols	*Candida albicans*	34
Decrease in sterol content	*Aspergillus niger*	52
$\Delta^{14,15}$-reductase mutation (*erg-3* gene)	*Neurospora crassa*	19
$\Delta^8-\Delta^7$ isomerase mutation	*Candida albicans*	9
C-14 Sterol reductase mutation (*erg24–1* gene)	*Saccharomyces cerevisiae*	47
C-22 Sterol desaturase gene (*erg5–1*)	*Saccharomyces cerevisiae*	75
Unrelated to ergosterol biosynthesis	*Ustilago maydis*	40

to be reduction in ergosterol content of fungi, although some nystatin-resistant fungi do not have reduced ergosterol content. A reduction in ergosterol molecules would decrease binding sites for nystatin. The mechanism by which nystatin causes a decrease in ergosterol content is probably by mutation of one or more enzymes involved in ergosterol biosynthesis. Mutations in demethylase, desaturase, and isomerase biosynthetic enzymes in various isolates have been associated with resistance. Most of the resistance studies have been conducted in fungal mutants created in vitro in the laboratory. It is not clear if the mechanism of resistance to nystatin in vitro is the same as that seen clinically.

Methods of Overcoming and Preventing Resistance

Other antifungals are available with different mechanisms of action (e.g., azoles) for treatment of nystatin-resistant fungi.

PHARMACOKINETIC DISPOSITION
Absorption

Nystatin is not absorbed to any significant extent following oral, cutaneous, or vaginal administration. The drug is excreted in the feces following oral therapy. Nystatin has been measured in feces and saliva following oral administration, and most nystatin is excreted unchanged. In one study, the concentration of nystatin in feces following oral administration of 3 to 6×10^6 USP

international units (IU) was approximately 70, 200, 200, and 250 IU (37). The concentration of nystatin in the saliva of patients who received 2×10^5 IU of nystatin using a mucosal oral delivery system was 279, 654, and 532 μg/mL at 0.5, 1, or 2 h (20). Other pharmacokinetic information is not available for this drug. Absorption is not applicable to liposomal nystatin, which is administered as an intravenous infusion.

Distribution

No distribution studies have been published on nystatin. The pharmacokinetics of liposomal nystatin in blood have been determined in humans (15). Liposomal nystatin was administered as an intravenous infusion at 2 mL/min every other day at doses of 1, 2, 3, 4, 5, or 7 mg/kg to HIV-infected patients. Blood concentration versus time profiles were generated after the first administration of liposomal nystatin at doses of 2, 3, 4, or 5 mg/kg to three to four patients per dose group. The concentration at the end of infusion (C_o) and blood AUC values increased with increasing dose. Maximal blood concentrations were 4.8, 9.5, 24.3 and 24.1 μg/mL for doses of 2, 3, 4, or 5 mg/kg, respectively. Therapeutic blood levels (in vitro MIC = 1 μg/mL) were maintained for several hours following single doses of liposomal nystatin as low as 2 mg/kg. Following repeated doses of liposomal nystatin every other day, little or no nystatin accumulated in the blood at doses up to 5 mg/kg.

Metabolism

No data are available on the metabolism of nystatin or liposomal nystatin in vitro, in animals, or in humans. No metabolites have been found in the blood of humans following administration of liposomal nystatin.

DOSAGE REGIMENS
Normal (Adult and Pediatric)

Topical Nystatin

Nystatin (Mycostatin) is available as a cream, ointment, and powder, containing 100,000 USP units/g for topical use in adults and children in treatment of local forms of candidiasis. It is also available (Mytrex) as a cream and ointment in combination with the corticosteroid triamcinolone. It is applied liberally several times per day.

Oral Nystatin

An oral suspension of nystatin for thrush contains 100,000 USP units/mL and is given four times per day to adults. Premature and low-birth-weight neonates are given 1 mL, infants are given 2 mL, and children or adults are given 4- to 6-mL doses. A pastille formulation for thrush contains 200,000 USP units of nystatin. One to two pastilles are given 4 to 5 times daily.

Intravenous Nystatin

Following reconstitution of lyophilized powder with sterile saline, each vial of liposomal nystatin contains 1 mg/mL of nystatin. Liposomal nystatin is being given intravenously once daily in clinical trials at 2 to 6 mg/kg for the treatment of systemic fungal infections.

Other

No data are available on use of nystatin with renal failure, hepatic failure, obesity, ascites/edema, or pregnancy.

ADVERSE EFFECTS

Topical nystatin is virtually nontoxic. Nausea, vomiting, diarrhea, and gastrointestinal distress are occasional side effects of oral nystatin; allergic reactions are very uncommon. No data are available for intravenous nystatin (liposomal nystatin).

DRUG INTERACTIONS

None are known.

CLINICAL INDICATIONS

Topical nystatin is indicated for local forms of candidiasis. Oral nystatin is used for treatment of thrush. Intravenous nystatin (liposomal nystatin) is in clinical trials for systemic fungal infections.

REFERENCES

1. Abu-el TK, Ghannoum M, Stretton RJ. Effects of sub-inhibitory concentrations of antifungal agents on adherence of *Candida* spp to buccal epithelial cells in vitro. Mycoses 1989;32:551–562.
2. Ahmed KA, Woods RA. A genetic analysis of resistance to nystatin in *Saccharomyces cerevisiae*. Genet Res 1967;9:179–193.
3. Bard M, Lees ND, Barbuch RJ, Sanglard D. Characterization of a cytochrome P450 deficient mutant of *Candida albicans*. Biochem Biophys Res Commun 1987;147:794–800.
4. Beezer AE, Miles RJ, Park WB, Smith AR, Brain AR. A nystatin-resistant mutant of *Saccharomyces cerevisiae*: isolation and characterization by electron microscopy and chemical analysis of whole cells, cell-walls and protoplasts. Microbios 1986;47:117–126.
5. Bennett JE. Antifungal agents. In: Gilman AG, Rall TW, Nies AS, Taylor P, eds. Goodman and Gilman, the pharmacological basis of therapeutics. 8th ed. New York: McGraw-Hill 1994:1165–1181.
6. Bonaly R, Dari L, Kubiak C, Lejeune C, Poulain D. Changes in the cell wall of *Candida albicans* cultivated in the presence of sublethal doses of nystatin. Ann Inst Pasteur Microbiol 1985;136B:181–193.
7. Boutati E, Maltezou HC, Lopez-Berestein G, Vartivarian SE, Anaissie EJ. Phase I study of maximum tolerated dose of intravenous liposomal nystatin for the treatment of refractory febrile neutropenia (RFN) in patients with hematological malignancies [Abstract]. Interscience Conference on Antimicrob Agents Chemother, 1995.
8. Braga PC, Maci S, Dal Sasso M, Bohn M. Experimental evidences for a role of subinhibitory concentrations of rilopirox, nystatin and fluconazole on adherence of *Candida* spp to vaginal epithelial cells. Chemotherapy 1996;42:259–265.
9. Broughton MC, Bard M, Lees ND. Polyene resistance in ergosterol producing strains of *Candida albicans*. Mycoses 1991;34:75–83.
10. Brown R, Hazen EL, Mason A. Effect of fungicidin (nystatin) in mice injected with lethal mixtures of Aureomycin and *Candida albicans*. Science 1953;117:609–610.
11. Bruzzese T, Cambieri M, Recusani F. Synthesis and biological properties of alkyl esters of polyene antibiotics. J Pharm Sci 1975;64:462–463.
12. Campbell CC, O'Dell ET, Hill GB. Therapeutic activity of nystatin in experimental systemic mycotic infections. In: Welch H, Marti-Ibanez F, eds. Antibiotics annual 1954–1955. New York: Medical Encyclopedia, 1955:858–862.
13. Cahill KM, Mofty AM, Kawaguchi TP. Primary cutaneous aspergillosis. Arch Dermatol 1967;96:545–547.
14. Chen WC, Chou D-L, and Feingold DS, Dissociation between ion permeability and the lethal action of polyene antibiotics on *Candida albicans*. Antimicrob Agents Chemother 1978;13:914–917.
15. Cossum PA, Wyse J, Simmons V, Wallace TL, Rios A. Pharmacokinetics of liposomal nystatin (Liposomal nystatin) in human patients [Abstract #A88]. Interscience Conference on Antimicrob Agents Chemother, 1996.
16. Danilenko II, Stepanyuk VV. Ultrastructure, composition of neutral lipids and their fatty acids of *Candida tropicalis* strain D-2 mutants resistant to the polyene antibiotic nystatin. 1982;691:201–210.
17. Dick JD, Merz WG, Saral R. Incidence of polyene-resistant yeasts recovered from clinical specimens. Antimicrob Agents Chemother 1980;18:158–163.
18. Drouchet E, Schwarz J, Bingham E. Evaluation of the action of nystatin on *Histoplasma capsulatum* in vitro and in hamsters and mice. Antibiotics Chemother 1956;6:23–35.
19. Ellis SW, Rose ME, Grindle M. Identification of a sterol mutant of *Neurospora crassa* deficient in Δ^{1415}-reductase activity. J Gen Microbiol 1991;137:2627–2630.

20. Encarnacion M, Chin I. Salivary nystatin concentrations after administration of an osmotic controlled release tablet and a pastille. Eur J Clin Pharmacol 1994;46:533–535.

21. Fryberg M, Oehlschager AC, Unrau AM. Sterol biosynthesis in antibiotic-resistant yeast: nystatin. Arch Biochem Biophys 1974; 160:83–89.

22. Gero S, Szekely J. Pulmonary moniliasis treated with nystatin aerosol. Lancet 1958:1229–1230.

23. Gonzalez CE, Giri N, Shetty D, Kligys K, Love W, Sein T, Schaufele R, Lyman C, Bacher J, Walsh TJ. Efficacy of a lipid formulation of nystatin against invasive pulmonary aspergillosis [Abstract #B54]. Interscience Conference on Antimicrob Agents Chemother, New Orleans, LA, 1996.

24. Gordon D, Baird I, Darouiche R, Fainstein V, Juaregui L, Levy C, Lewis P. Liposomal nystatin versus amphotericin B for candidemia in non-neutropenic patients: a historical comparison. Infectious Diseases Society of America, 35th Annual Meeting, 1997.

25. Gordon LE, Smith CE, Wedin DS. Nystatin (Mycostatin) therapy in experimental coccidioidomycosis. Am Rev Tuberc 1955; 72:64–70.

26. Gottlieb D, Carter HF, Sloneker JH, Ammann A. Protection of fungi against polyene antibiotics by sterols. Science 1958;128: 361.

27. Grindle M, Farrow R. Sterol content and enzyme defects of nystatin-resistant mutants of *Neurospora crassa*. Mol Gen Genet 1978;165:305–308.

28. Hata S, Oda Y, Nishino T, et al. Characterization of a *Saccharomyces cerevisiae* mutant N22 defective in ergosterol synthesis and preparation of [28-^{14}C]ergosta-57-dien-3(-ol with the mutant. J Biochem 1983;94:501–510.

29. Hammarstrom L, Smith E. Mitogenic properties of polyene antibiotics for murine B cells. Scand J Immunol 1976;5:37–43.

30. Hammond SM. Biological activity of polyene antibiotics. In: Ellisa GP. West GB, eds. Progress in medicinal chemistry, vol 14. Amsterdam: Elsevier/North Holland Biomedical Press 1977: 106–179.

31. Hazen EL, Brown R. Fungicidin, an antibiotic produced by a soil actinomycete. Proc Soc Exp Biol Med 1951;76:93–97.

32. Hazen EL, Brown R, Mason A. Protective action of fungicidin (nystatin) in mice against virulence enhancing activity of oxytetracycline on *Candida albicans*. Antibiot Chemother 1953;3: 1125–1128.

33. Hebeka E, Solotorovsky M, Development of resistance to polyene antibiotics in *Candida albicans*. J Bacteriol 1965;89: 1533–1539.

34. Hitchcock CA, Russell NJ, Barrett-Bee KJ. Sterols in *Candida albicans* mutants resistant to polyene or azole antifungals and of a double mutant *C albicans* 6.4. CRC Crit Rev Microbiol 1987; 15:111–115.

35. Hitchcock CA, Barrett-Bee KJ, Russell NJ. The lipid composition and permeability to azole of an azole- and polyene-resistant mutant of *Candida albicans*. J Med Vet Mycol 1987;25:29–37.

36. Höfer M. Thiele OW, Huh H, Hunneman DH, Mracek M. A nystatin-resistant mutant of *Rhodotorula gracilis*. Transport properties and sterol content. Arch Microbiol 1982;132:313–316.

37. Hofstra W, de Vries-Hospers HG, van der Waaij D. Concentrations of nystatin in faeces after oral administration of various doses of nystatin. Infection 1979;7:166–170.

38. Ishikawa H, Narimatsu H, Saito K. Mechanisms of the adjuvant effect of nystatin on in vitro antibody response of mouse spleen cell: indication of nystatin as a B-cell mitogen and as a stimulant for polyclonal antibody synthesis in B cells. Microbiol Immunol 1977;21:137–152.

39. Johnson B, White RJ, Williamson GM. Factors Influencing the susceptibility of *Candida albicans* to the polyenoic antibiotics nystatin and amphotericin B. J Gen Microbiol 1978;104: 325–333.

40. Joseph-Horne T, Manning N, Holoman D, Kelly S. Nonsterol related resistance in *Ustilago maydis* to the polyene antifungals, amphotericin B and nystatin. Phytochemistry 1996;42:637–639.

41. King DJ, Wiseman A, Kelly DE, Kelly SL. Differences in the cytochrome P-450 enzymes of sterol C-14 demethylase mutants of *Saccharomyces cerevisiae*. Curr Genet 1985;10:261–267.

42. Kinsky SC. Comparative responses of mammalian erythrocytes and microbial protoplasts to polyene antibiotics and vitamin A. Arch Biochem 1963;102:180–188.

43. Kozinn PJ, Taschdjian CL, Dragutsky D, Minsky A. Treatment of cutaneous candidiasis in infancy and childhood with nystatin and amphotericin B. In: Welch H, Marti-Ibanez F. Antibiotics annual 1956–1957. New York: Medical Encyclopedia, 1957:128–134.

44. Lampen JO, Arnow PM, Borowska Z, Laskin AI. Location and role of sterol at nystatin-binding sites. J Bacteriol 1962;84: 1152–1160.

45. Lampen JO, Arnow PM, Saffermen RS. Mechanism of protection by sterols against polyene antibiotics. J Bacteriol 1960; 80:200–206.

46. Lomb M, Fryberg M, Oehlschlager AC, Unrau AM. Sterol and fatty acid composition of polyene macrolide antibiotic resistant *Torulopsis glabrata*. Can J Biochem 1975;53:1309–1315.

47. Lorenz RT, Parks LW. Cloning sequencing and disruption of the gene encoding sterol C-14 reductase in *Saccharomyces cerevisiae*. DNA Cell Biol 1992;11:685–692.

48. Manning LK, Robertston L. Medical memorandum; a case of aspergillosis treated with nystatin. Br Med J 1959;1:345–346.

49. Martin MV, Dinsdale RCW. Nystatin-resistance of *Candida albicans* isolates from two cases of oral candidiasis. Br J Oral Surg 1982;20:294–298.

50. Mas J, Pina E. Disappearance of nystatin resistance in *Candida* mediated by ergosterol. J Gen Microbiol 1980;117:249–252.

51. Mas J, Pina E. Candida resistant to nystatin becomes sensitive upon culture with ergosterol. Arch Invest Med (Mex) 1985;16: 145–155.

52. Mazumder C, Basu J, Manikuntala K, Chakrabarti P. Changes in membrane lipids and amino acid transport in a nystatin-resistant *Aspergillus niger*. Can J Microbiol 1990;36:435–437.

53. McCammon MT, Hartmann M-A, Bottema CDK, Parks LW. Sterol methylation in *Saccharomyces cerevisiae*. J Bacteriol 1984;157:475–483.

54. Meade RH. Drug therapy reviews: clinical pharmacology and therapeutic use of antimycotic drugs. Am J Hosp Pharm 1979; 36:1326–1334.

55. Medoff G, Kobayashi GA. The polyenes. In: Speller DCE, ed. Antifungal chemotherapy. New York: John Wiley & Sons, 1980:3–33.

56. Mehta RT, Hopfer RL, McQueen T, Juliano RL, Lopez-Berestein G. Toxicity and therapeutic effects in mice of liposome-encapsulated nystatin for systemic fungal infections. Antimicrob Agents Chemother 1987;31:1901–1903.

57. Mehta RT, Hopfer RL, Gunner LA, Juliano RL, Lopez-Berestein G. Formulation toxicity and antifungal activity in vitro of liposome-encapsulated nystatin as therapeutic agent for systemic candidiasis. Antimicrob Agents Chemother 1987;31: 1897–1900.

58. Merz WG, Sandford GR. Isolation and characterization of a polyene-resistant variant of *Candida tropicalis*. J Clin Microb 1979;9:677–680.

59. Nagai J, Yokoe S, Tanaka M, Hibasami H, Ikeda T. Increased proportion of medium chain fatty acids in nystatin-resistant yeast mutants. Lipids 1981;16:411–417.

60. Nakanishi S, Nishino T, Nagai J, Katsuki H. Characterization of nystatin-resistant mutants of *Saccharomyces cerevisiae* and preparation of sterol intermediates using the mutants. J Biochem 1987;101:535–544.

61. Newcomer VD, Wright ET, Sternberg TH, Graham JH, Wier RH, Egeberg RO. Evaluation of nystatin in the treatment of coccidioidomycosis in man. In: Sternberg TH, Newcomer VD, eds. Therapy of fungus diseases. Boston: Little, Brown and Co, 1955:260–267.

62. Nobre G, Sobral T, Ferreira AF. In vitro susceptibility to 5-fluorocytosine and nystatin of common clinical yeast isolates. Mycopathologia 1981;73:39–41.

63. Oehling A, Giron M, Subira M-L. Aerosol chemotherapy in bronchopulmonary candidiasis. Respiration 1975;32:179–184.

64. Pace HR, Schantz SI. Nystatin (Mycostatin) in the treatment of monilial and nonmonilial vaginitis. J Am Med Assoc 1956;22:268–271.

65. Pierce AM, Mueller RB, Unrau AM, Oehlschlager AC. Metabolism of (24-sterols by yeast mutants blocked in removal of the C-14 methyl group. Can J Biochem 1978;56:794–800.

66. Pierce AM, Pierce HD Jr, Unrau AM, Oehlschlager AC. Lipid composition and polyene antibiotic resistance of *Candida albicans* mutants. Can J Biochem 1978;56:135–142.

67. Plotnick H, Cerri S. Treatment of oral histoplasmosis by local injection with nystatin. J Am Med Assoc 1957;28:346–348.

68. Procknow JJ, Loosli CG. Treatment of deep mycoses. Arch Intern Med 1958;101:765–802.

69. Richman-Boytas CM, Parks LW. Effects of sterol alterations on nystatin sensitivity in *Saccharomyces cerevisiae*. Microbios 1989;59:101–111.

70. Rios A, Rosenblum M, Crofoot G, Lenk RP, Hayman A, Lopez-Berestein G. Pharmacokinetics of liposomal nystatin in patients with human immunodeficiency virus infection. J Infect Dis 1993;163:253–254.

71. Robinson RCV. Systemic moniliasis treated with mycostatin. J Invest Dermatol 1957;24:375.

72. Safe LM, Safe SH, Subden RE, Morris DC. Sterol content and polyene antibiotic resistance in isolates of *Candida krusei, Candida parakrusei,* and *Candida tropicalis*. Can J Microbiol 1977;23:398–401.

73. Selvam MP, Blay RA, Geyer S, Buck SM, Pollock L, Mayner RE, Epstein JS. Inhibition of HIV-1 replication in H9 cells by nystatin-A compared with other antiviral agents. AIDS Res Hum Retrovirus 1993;9:475–481.

74. Sinclair AJ, Rossof AH, Coltman CA. Recognition and successful management in pulmonary aspergillosis in leukemia. Cancer 1978;42:2019–2024.

75. Skaggs BA, Alexander JF, Pierson CA, Schweitzer KS, Chun KT, Koegel C, Barbuch R, Bard M. Cloning and characterization of the *Saccharomyces cerevisiae* C-22 sterol desaturase gene, encoding a second cytochrome P-450 involved in ergosterol biosynthesis. Gene 1996;169:105–109.

76. Solotorovsky M, Quabeck G, Winsten S. Antifungal activity of Candidin, nystatin, euclin, and stilbamidine against experimental infections in the mouse. Antibiot Chemother 1958;8:364–371.

77. Stanley VC, English MP. Some effects of nystatin on the growth of four *Aspergillus* species. J Gen Microbiol 1965;40:107–118.

78. Stark JE. Allergic pulmonary *Aspergillus* successfully treated with inhalations of nystatin. Dis Chest 1967;51:96–99.

79. Stern JC, Shah MK, Lucente FE. In vitro effectiveness of 13 agents in otomycosis and review of the literature. Laryngoscope 1988;98:1173–1177.

80. Taylor FR, Rodriguez RJ, Parks LW. Requirement for a second sterol biosynthetic mutation for viability of a sterol C-14 demethylation defect in *Saccharomyces cerevisiae*. J Bacteriol 1983;155:64–68.

81. Than KM, Naing KS, Min M. Otomycosis in Burma and its treatment. Am J Trop Med Hyg 1980;29:620–623.

82. Thomas AH. Suggested mechanisms for the antimycotic activity of the polyene antibiotics and the N-substituted imidazoles. J Antimicrob Chemother 1986;17:269–279.

83. Thompson ED, Starr PR, Parks LW. Sterol accumulation in a mutant of *Saccharomyces cerevisiae* defective in ergosterol production. Biochem Biophys Res Commun 1971;43:1304–1309.

84. Trocha PJ, Jasne SJ, Sprinson DB. Yeast mutants blocked in removing the methyl group of lanosterol at C-14: separation of sterols by high-pressure liquid chromatography. Biochemistry 1977;16:4721–4726.

85. Vedder JS, Schorr WF. Primary disseminated pulmonary aspergillosis with metastatic skin nodules. J Am Med Assoc 1969;209:1191–1195.

86. Wallace TL, Paetznick V, Cossum PA, Lopez-Bernstein G, Rex JH, Anaissie E. Activtiy of liposomal nystatin against disseminated *Aspergillus fumigatus* in neutropenic mice. Antimicrob Agents Chemother 1997;41:2238–2243.

87. Woods RA. Nystatin-resistant mutants of yeast: alterations in sterol content. J Bacteriol 1971;108:69–73.

88. Woods RA, Bard M, Jackson IE, Drutz DJ. Resistance to polyene antibiotics and correlated sterol changes in two isolates of *Candida tropicalis* from a patient with an amphotericin B-resistant funguria. J Infect Dis 1974;129:53–58.

SECTION III

Viruses and Antiviral Agents

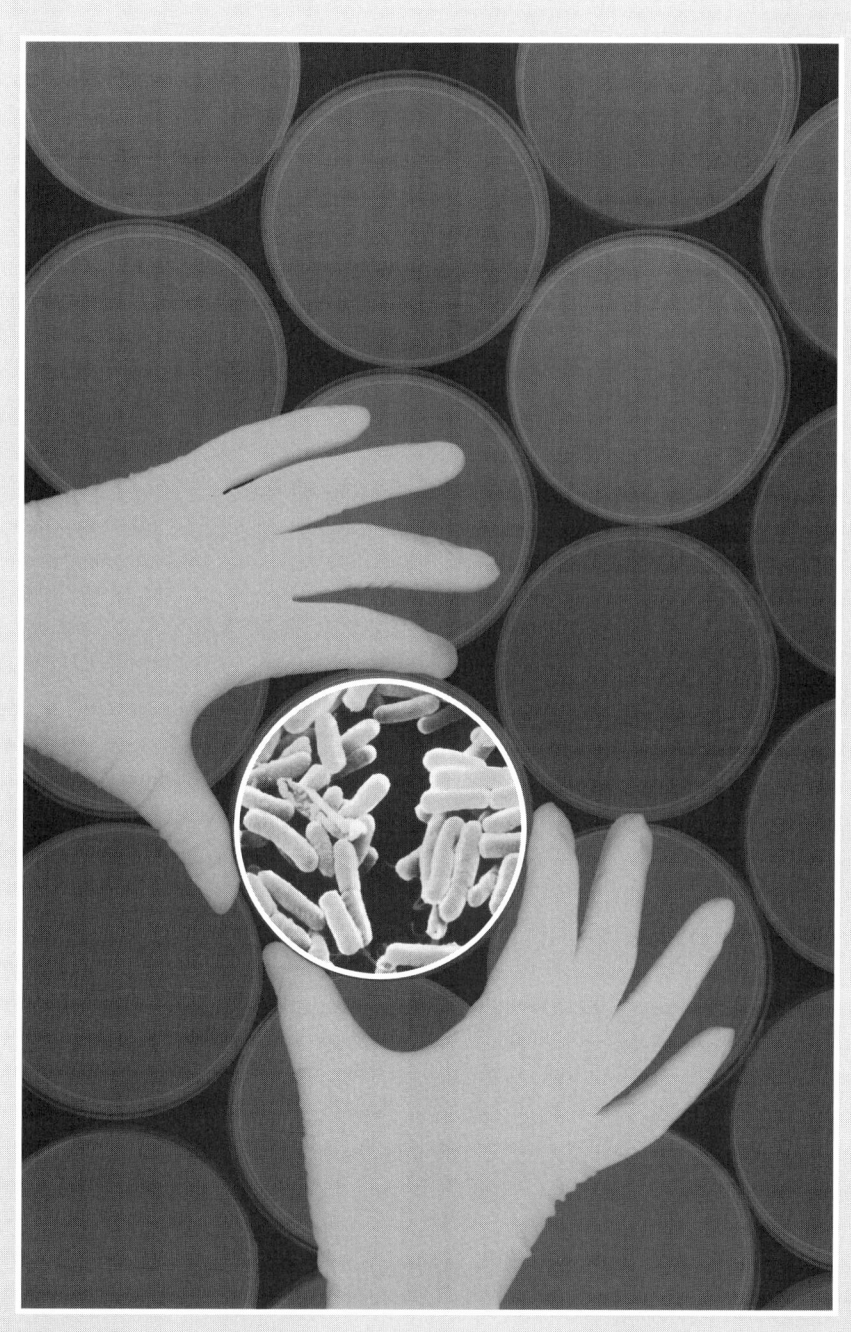

Adenovirus: Enteric

Jason Rosé and Harry Greenberg

GENERAL DESCRIPTION
Virology

The *Adenoviridae* comprise 47 known serotypes and are mainly associated with respiratory diseases. Adenoviruses are classical icosahedral viruses with a distinct 20-triangular-face morphology. The outer capsid encloses a double-stranded DNA genome of approximately 36 kb. Although all adenoviruses appear to be able to replicate in the intestine, only serotypes 40 and 41 (subgroup F) have been associated with pathogenic effects that result in diarrheal illness (9). Unlike most other adenoviruses, the enteric adenoviruses grow poorly in many tissue culture systems. This "fastidious" growth requirement has been used as part of the diagnosis of serotype 40 and 41 adenoviruses.

Epidemiology

Adenoviruses represent the second or third most important viral cause of diarrhea in the developed world, having been identified in 4 to 10% of hospitalized patients (1, 10). In a recent article by Palombo and Bishop, adenovirus-associated diarrhea accounted for approximately 4% of hospitalized patients in Australia (8). Data exist suggesting that these viruses play a less important role in the developing world, where only 2 to 5% of hospitalized diarrheal cases have been diagnosed as due to enteric adenovirus (4). As with rotavirus, most infections with enteric adenoviruses occur in children under the age of 2 years. The infection appears to be spread via the fecal-oral route as a result of person-to-person contact, and no other mechanism of transmission has been confirmed (6). Unlike rotavirus infections, however, adenovirus infections occur in a nonseasonal fashion, probably contributing to a constant low level of gastroenteritis in children. Although adenoviruses have been detected in the stools of HIV-infected patients, no direct correlation has been made between diarrheal illness and enteric adenoviruses in AIDS patients (3).

Pathogenesis

Enteric adenoviruses cause a disease very similar to that caused by rotavirus, although the symptoms are generally milder. Although fever is detected, it is not as commonly seen as in rotavirus-infected patients. While diarrheal symptoms are less severe than those observed with rotavirus, they appear to be more protracted. One distinguishing feature of adenoviral illness is the rather long incubation period (mean, 7 days) and protracted viral shedding after resolution of clinical symptoms (average, 14 days).

Little is known about the pathologic changes induced by adenovirus infection. The virus appears capable of high levels of replication in the intestine, with as many as 10^{11} particles detectable per gram of stool. Enteric adenovirus infection has been linked to malabsorption and prolonged lactose intolerance in some cases (7, 10), which may be the result of damage induced by extensive viral replication.

Diagnosis

Identification of adenovirus infection is fairly straightforward using electron microscopy techniques. However, many adenoviruses can replicate in the intestine without causing disease, so the presence of viruses by electron microscopy is not definitive. Frequently, the inability to culture adenoviruses after detection in the stool is used to indicate the presence of enteric adenovirus (2). Recently, a convenient immunoassay was developed that is specific for serotype 40 and 41 adenovirus and was used for evaluation in outbreaks of diarrheal illness (11). Such assays are now commercially available.

SUSCEPTIBILITY IN VIVO

At the present time, no animal models exist for studying the pathogenesis of enteric adenoviruses. Because of this deficit, no clear therapeutic strategy has been defined for adenovirus-associated diarrhea.

THERAPY

Due to the relative mildness of the illness, the necessity for antiviral therapy is questionable. In a young bone marrow transplant patient with adenovirus-associated gastroenteritis, administration of ribavirin appeared to improve the patient's condition significantly (5). Administration of virus-specific immunoglobulin (as has been performed with other diarrheal viruses) had no observable effect on the course of the illness.

REFERENCES

1. Brandt CD, Kim HW, Rodriguez WJ, Arrobio JO, Jeffries BC, Stallings EP, Lewis C, Miles AJ, Gardner MK, Parrott RH. Adenoviruses and pediatric gastroenteritis. J Infect Dis 1985;151: 437–443.

2. Brandt CD, Rodriguez WJ, Kim HW, Arrobio JO, Jeffries BC, Parrott RH. Rapid presumptive recognition of diarrhea-associated adenoviruses. J Clin Microbiol 1984;20:1008–1009.

3. Durepaire N, Ranger-Rogez S, Gandji JA, Weinbreck P, Rogez JP, Denis F. Enteric prevalence of adenovirus in human immunodeficiency virus seropositive patients. J Med Virol 1995;45:56–60.

4. Herrmann JE, Blacklow NR, Peron-Henry DM, Clements E, Taylor DN, Echeverria P. Incidence of enteric adenoviruses among children in Thailand and the significance of these viruses in gastroenteritis. J Clin Microbiol 1988;26:1783–1786.

5. Kapelushnik J, Or R, Delukina M, Nagler A, Livni N, Engelhard D. Intravenous ribavirin therapy for adenovirus gastroenteritis after bone marrow transplantation. J Pediatr Gastroenterol Nutr 1995;21:110–112.

6. LeBaron CW, Furutan NP, Lew JF, Allen JR, Gouvea V, Moe C, Monroe SS. Viral agents of gastroenteritis. Public health importance and outbreak management. MMWR 1990;39(RR-5):1–24.

7. Mavromichalis J, Evans N, McNeish AS, Bryden AS, Davis HA, Flewett TH. Intestinal damage in rotavirus and adenovirus gastroenteritis assessed by D-xylose malabsorption. Arch Dis Child 1977;52:589–591.

8. Palombo EA, Bishop RF. Annual incidence, serotype distribution, and genetic diversity of human astrovirus isolates from hospitalized children in Melbourne, Australia. J Clin Microbiol 1996;34:1750–1753.

9. Shenk T. *Adenoviridae:* the viruses and their replication. In: Fields BN, Knipe DM, Howley PM, eds. Fields virology, vol 2. Philadelphia: Lippincott-Raven, 1996:2111–2148.

10. Unhoo I, Wadell G, Svenson L, Johansson ME. Importance of enteric adenoviruses 40 and 41 in acute gastroenteritis in infants and young children. J Clin Microbiol 1984;20:365–372.

11. Wood DJ, Dijlsma K, deJong JC, Tonkin C. Evaluation of a commercial monoclonal antibody-based enzyme immunoassay for detection of adenovirus types 40 and 41 in stool specimens. J Clin Microbiol 1989;27:1155–1158.

Astroviruses

Jason Rosé and Harry Greenberg

GENERAL DESCRIPTION
Virology

Astrovirus was recently assigned to its own family, the *Astroviridae,* despite its apparent similarity to Norwalk and other caliciviruses. Like Norwalk virus, astroviruses form 27-nm particles that contain a single positive-stranded, polyadenylated, genomic RNA. Approximately 10% of particles in stool display a characteristic solid five- or six-pointed star by electron microscopy (EM), which contrasts with the hollow-centered stars often seen on caliciviruses. Astroviruses contain three major structural proteins and can be grown in tissue culture under conditions similar to those used for propagating rotaviruses. Recent immunologic studies have identified seven distinct serotypes of human astrovirus, all of which appear to cause diarrheal illness.

Epidemiology

Astrovirus has been found to be a significant pathogen in young children with diarrhea (4, 7, 8) and appears to predominantly infect children between 6 months and 2 years of age. Astrovirus has also been associated with foodborne outbreaks of gastroenteritis in Japanese adults and school children (11). The incidence of astrovirus appears to vary from 4 to 8.6%, depending on geographic location. Infections occur primarily in the winter in temperate climates and in the rainy season in tropical climates, as has been reported for rotavirus. Recent studies have shown that astrovirus can cause sporadic outbreaks of diarrhea in elderly patients and that it is significantly associated with diarrheal illness in immunocompromised AIDS patients (5) and bone marrow transplant recipients (3).

Pathogenesis

Astrovirus pathogenesis has not been well studied in humans. Viral particles have been visualized by EM in intestinal epithelial cells and in epithelial cells located in the lower part of the villus, suggesting that the intestine is the site of replication (9). Other pathologic studies have been conducted in lambs and calves and are discussed below.

Clinical Manifestations

The clinical illness caused by astrovirus in children is similar to that caused by rotavirus, with a high incidence of fever and diarrhea. The illness is considered milder, however, and causes less dehydration than rotavirus infection. The range of symptoms also seems to vary from location to location; an outbreak in Guatemala was characterized by a lower frequency of vomiting and fever than an outbreak in Thailand (2, 4). Astrovirus illness is considerably less pathogenic in young adult volunteers, with only 5% of infected individuals developing clinical symptoms. The increased incidence of astrovirus illness in elderly patients suggests that immunity is acquired in childhood and wanes later in life.

Laboratory Diagnosis

Both EM and immunoelectron microscopy (IEM) have been used to diagnose astrovirus infection, because of the high levels of viral shedding in feces (10^{10} particles/mL). Misclassification of astrovirus as calicivirus is common using these methods, because morphology is typical in only 10% of particles, and microscopists may not be experienced enough to detect it. Noncommercial enzyme-linked immunosorbent assays (ELISA) have been developed that are highly specific for astrovirus and have been used in diagnosis of children with diarrheal illness (6, 7). RNA probes and polymerase chain reaction (PCR) methods have also been developed and have proven useful for confirmation of ELISA results (10). Diagnostic tests for astroviruses are not yet widely available.

IN VIVO SUSCEPTIBILITY

Astrovirus pathogenesis has been studied in lambs and calves, using ovine and bovine astrovirus isolates, respectively. Infection of lambs induces a mild transient diarrhea that occurs 2 days after infection and lasts approximately 2 days. Infection of calves with at least one strain of bovine astrovirus did not induce diarrheal illness, although the infection was associated with sloughing of infected villus cells. Several attempts to infect small laboratory animals with human astrovirus isolates have been unsuccessful.

THERAPY

Very few published reports exist on the use of directed therapeutic efforts for the treatment of astrovirus-associated gastroenteritis. Many of the same strategies that have been attempted for treating rotavirus gastroenteritis are also being attempted for astrovirus, though with limited success. In one case, a patient with Waldenström's macroglobulinemia who developed astrovirus diarrhea during a course of cytoreductive therapy responded to treatment with intravenous immunoglobulin (1). Although treatment eliminated diarrheal symptoms, viral shedding continued for more than 2 weeks after therapy was initiated. Possibly, as the study of these viruses continues, we will improve our ability to make specific antibodies and be able to conduct further tests on their therapeutic efficacy.

REFERENCES

1. Björkholm M, Celsing F, Runarsson G, Waldenström J. Successful intravenous therapy for severe and persistent astrovirus gastroenteritis after fludarabine treatment in a patient with Waldenström's macroglobulinemia. J Hematol 1995;62:117–120.
2. Blacklow NR, Herrmann JE. Astrovirus gastroenteritis. Trans Am Clin Climatol Assoc 1994;106:58–66.
3. Cox GJ, Matsui SM, Lo RS, Hinds MH, Bowden RA, Hackman RC, Meyer WG, Mori M, Tarr PI, Oshiro LS, Ludert JE, Meyers JD, McDonald GB. Etiology and outcome of diarrhea after marrow transplantation: a prospective study. Gastroenterology 1994;107:1398–1407.
4. Cruz JR, Bartlett AV, Herrmann JE, Cáceres P, Blacklow NR, Cano F. Astrovirus-associated diarrhea among Guatemalan ambulatory rural children. J Clin Microbiol 1992;30:1140–1144.
5. Grohmann GS, Glass RI, Pereira HG, Monroe SS, Hightower AW, Weber R, Bryan RT. Enteric viruses and diarrhea in HIV-infected patients. N Engl J Med 1993;329:14–20.
6. Herrmann JE, Nowak NA, Perron-Henry DM, Hudson RW, Cubitt WD, Blacklow NR. Diagnosis of astrovirus gastroenteritis by antigen detection with monoclonal antibodies. J Infect Dis 1989;161:226–229.
7. Herrmann JE, Taylor DN, Cheverria P, Blacklow NR. Astroviruses as a cause of gastroenteritis in children. N Engl J Med 1991;324:1757–1760.
8. Kapikian AZ. Viral gastroenteritis. JAMA 1993;269:627–630.
9. Matsui SM, Greenberg HB. Astroviruses. In: Fields BN, Knipe DM, Howley PM, eds. Fields virology, vol 2. Philadelphia: Lippincott-Raven, 1996:811–824.
10. Moe CL, Allen JR, Monroe SS, Gary HEJ, Humphrey CD, Herrmann JE, Blacklow NR, Carcamo C, Koch M, Kim KH, et al. Detection of astrovirus in pediatric stool samples by immunoassay and RNA probe. J Clin Microbiol 1991;29:2390–2395.
11. Oishi I, Yamazaki K, Kimoto T, Minekawa Y, Utagawa E, Yamazak IS, Inouye S, Grohmann GS, Monroe SS, Stine SE, et al. A large outbreak of acute gastroenteritis associated with astrovirus among students and teachers in Osaka, Japan. J Infect Dis 1994;170:439–443.

Cytomegalovirus

●

Monto Ho

GENERAL DESCRIPTION
Microbiology and Pathogenesis

Human cytomegalovirus (CMV) is a herpesvirus. All herpesviruses are large, double-stranded DNA viruses that contain 162 capsomeres, a tegument between the capsid and envelope, and an envelope containing lipids and glycoproteins that is sensitive to lipid solvents and detergents (134). Characteristically, after infection, all herpesviruses are incurable by host defenses and remain latent in specific cells and tissues of the host. Latent herpesvirus infections may reactivate, for example, when host immune defenses are compromised following an infection with HIV or after transplantation.

Latency-associated genes have not been clearly identified in CMV, nor is it clear that cells in which CMV genome persists can multiply. What is known is that the CMV genome can persist in cells for extended periods of time without viral DNA replication or late gene expression. While leukocytes in the bloodstream are known to carry the CMV genome in this manner, it is by no means clear that they are the only cells that can. Circumstantial evidence that organs from seropositive donors are extremely efficient in transmitting CMV to a seronegative organ or nonimmune recipient suggests that cells in tissues other than blood may be important in carrying the virus.

It is also unclear at the molecular level how a cell that is carrying the virus genome but not actively reproducing can switch to a productive, or "lytic," cycle. This happens in 50 to 100% of seropositive transplant recipients, whose latent CMV infections are activated after transplantation, and when a seronegative recipient becomes infected, primarily or de novo, especially if they have a seropositive CMV-carrying donor (70).

Once primary or reactivated CMV infection takes place in a host, it is also not clear why or how specific organs become affected or diseased. After transplantation, the transplanted organ often becomes diseased with CMV. The degree of immunosuppression plays an important role. Involvement of the central nervous system by CMV is relatively uncommon after transplantation but is common in the late stages of acquired immunodeficiency syndrome (AIDS). CMV retinitis, a devastating, disabling illness, is a hallmark of such late stages. What specific compromised immunologic factor accounts for this is unclear.

Diagnostics Including Susceptibility

Generally there are two requirements for the diagnosis of CMV disease: first, infection by CMV must be demonstrated, and second, evidence must be obtained for specific organ involvement. Even so, satisfying these two necessary conditions may not suffice. Coexistence or preexistence of an alternate etiology may explain a disease picture better than CMV.

CMV infection is relatively common and readily demonstrated, while CMV disease, which requires demonstration of specific organ involvement, is much rarer. Infection of an immunocompromised host by CMV is relatively common and easy to show by demonstrating the virus in body fluids such as throat washings, urine, or blood. The virus can be propagated by inoculating human fibroblast cell cultures and observing for cytopathic effect. This classical method takes anywhere from 3 to 6 weeks. The lag time needed for virus demonstration was shortened after a monoclonal antibody against immediate early antigen of the virus became available (144). The new, more rapid, method of demonstrating CMV is the so-called cytospin method, in which virus from the inoculum is centrifuged onto slide cultures of human fibroblasts. After overnight incubation, the cultures are stained with monoclonal antibody and counterstained for fluorescent or cytochemical demonstration. The immediate early antigens

of CMV are synthesized within hours of infection and hence are demonstrable after overnight incubation of inoculated cultures; this reduces the time required until cultures can be read from 6 weeks to 24 h.

Specific involvement of an organ with CMV is rarely demonstrable on clinical grounds alone. Specific changes due to CMV infection in organs must be demonstrated. This is done by looking for either (a) evidence of viral infection within the tissue or (b) specific histologic changes attributable to CMV infection in such tissues (71). In a biopsy specimen, these objectives may be met by demonstrating CMV infection of cells by staining for specific CMV antigens or by demonstrating specific CMV DNA by in situ hybridization or polymerase chain reaction (PCR). Histologic changes characteristic of CMV include cytomegaly and Cowdry type A intranuclear inclusions.

Gross pathologic changes due to CMV are helpful in diagnosis but are rarely specific. This applies to changes seen directly or indirectly by instrumentation (e.g., by endoscopy, radiology, or scanning). The one possible exception is CMV retinitis in AIDS patients, which can be diagnosed by ophthalmoscopy. Demonstrating the presence of virus in a tissue sample without identifying it in cells may not be adequate because such samples may be contaminated with virus from other sites such as blood or saliva.

In recent years there has been a search for a laboratory method of diagnosing or predicting CMV disease in a patient without necessarily demonstrating it in tissues. Such a method would be especially useful for the institution of prophylactic measures against development of CMV disease. While no such method has yet been universally accepted, there is currently a great deal of interest in using the degree of antigenemia or in developing quantitative PCR methods. Antigenemia, particularly above 50 per 2×10^5 PMNL, is correlated with symptomatic disease in both transplant (59) and HIV/AIDS patients (105). PCR is less well standardized as a prognostic method. It too has been quantitated for monitoring disease in blood, plasma (58), or serum (51, 123); the common denominator that predicts disease in both cases appears to be virus load. Virus load is expressed either as the concentration of late viral antigen (e.g., pp65 tegument antigen) in blood polymorphonuclear leukocytes or as the concentration of CMV DNA in blood, plasma, or serum.

SUSCEPTIBILITY IN VITRO
Single-Drug Susceptibility

At present two drugs are licensed for specific systemic treatment of CMV: ganciclovir and foscarnet. Intravitreal cidofovir has been licensed for CMV retinitis. They all inhibit viral DNA synthesis and act by inhibiting viral DNA polymerase.

Ganciclovir

Ganciclovir ((9-(1,3-dihydroxy-2-propoxy)methyl)-guanine; DHPG), a nucleoside synthesized in 1982, is an important inhibitor of *Herpesviridae* (6, 50). Ganciclovir is an analogue of acyclovir. The effective inhibitory concentration (IC_{50}) of ganciclovir for human CMV ranges from 0.3 to 10 μM/L (4 μM/L equals 1 μg/μL). Most isolates have an IC_{50} of 1.5 μM or higher. Peak plasma concentration of ganciclovir after a dose of 5 mg/kg given as a 1-h intravenous infusion is 6.6 μg/mL. Trough levels were 1 μg/mL after 11 h (156). The usual dose of ganciclovir for intravenous induction is 5 mg/kg twice daily for 2 to 3 weeks. Maintenance dose, if needed, is 5 mg/kg over daily 5 to 7 days per week.

The difference between ganciclovir and acyclovir may be illustrated by the difference in susceptibility to CMV and herpes simplex virus (HSV). Both ganciclovir and acyclovir must be phosphorylated to be active against either virus. Phosphorylation of acyclovir is facilitated by a specific herpes simplex virus–coded thymidine kinase that is absent in CMV. This explains the relative resistance of CMV to acyclovir.

Foscarnet

IC_{50}s in micromoles for CMV, HSV-1 and HSV-2, varicellazoster virus (VZV), and Epstein-Barr virus (EBV) are respectively 50 to 800, 10 to 130, 48 to 90, and less than 500. Foscarnet penetrates the blood–cerebrospinal fluid (CSF) barrier with a coefficient of 0.05 to 0.72. After a single intravenous infusion of 80 mg/kg, plasma levels in 26 subjects were 990 to 5920, with a mean of 2527 μM (1 μM equals 0.3 mg/mL). Corresponding CSF levels were 190 to 750 μM (65).

Cidofovir (HPMPC)

HPMPC $((S)$-1-(3-hydroxy-2-(phosphonylmethoxy)propyl) cytosine (cidofovir)) was identified in the laboratory of E. DeClercq as the most potent and selective anti-CMV compound described so far. It is 10 times more effective than ganciclovir, and it is also endowed with a unique long-lasting antiviral effect (30). The ID_{50} is 0.5 to 2.8 μM for wild isolates (package insert). Cidofovir is a nucleotide (phosphorylated nucleoside) rather than a nucleoside analogue such as ganciclovir or acyclovir. It contains a phosphonate group, absent in nucleosides, that enables it to mimic a nucleotide and bypass initial virus-dependent enzymatic phosphorylation. Cellular enzymes are responsible for serial conversion to the diphosphate form, the active intracellular antimetabolite (69). The diphosphate form has a long intracellular half-life, exceeding 48 h (19).

Acyclovir

While the ID_{50} of acyclovir for HSV-1 and HSV-2 in cell culture is between 0.1 and 0.2 μM, the ID_{50} for human CMV is about 100 μM (98, 118) (1 μg/mL acyclovir is equivalent to 4.4 μM). This is too high for usual doses to reach inhibitory levels in body fluids. The highly selective efficacy of acyclovir against HSV, VZV, and EBV is based on phosphorylation of the compound by a potent thymidine kinase encoded by these viruses. Of the human herpesviruses, CMV does not code for a thymidine kinase.

The high ID_{50} of acyclovir for CMV precludes its use for therapy of CMV infections clinically. However, it has been used for prophylaxis against CMV disease in renal transplant recipients (see antivirals in solid organ recipients in "Prophylactic Strategies," below).

Combination Drugs in Vitro

No data are available.

ANTIVIRAL THERAPY
Drug of Choice

Ganciclovir

The drug of choice against CMV at this time is ganciclovir. This does not mean that it is an ideal drug. Like all antivirals, ganciclovir is virustatic and not virucidal. Therapy requires induction with daily intravenous doses. Neutropenia is a severe possible complication that requires monitoring (see "Endpoints for Monitoring Therapy," below).

In a direct comparison between ganciclovir and foscarnet in the treatment of CMV retinitis in AIDS patients, foscarnet was as effective as ganciclovir, and patients on foscarnet had lower mortality (151, 152), but foscarnet had more toxic reactions.

(Dosages for intravenous ganciclovir are discussed in "Special Clinical Situations," below.)

Oral Ganciclovir

From 1989 to 1994, ganciclovir was available only for intravenous administration. In 1994, the FDA released the oral preparation. Unfortunately, this did not mean that oral forms could supplant intravenous administration. The absolute bioavailability averaged only 9% after daily oral administration of 3000 mg (500 mg six times daily, taken with food) or more. However, 3000 mg/day given in 3 or 6 divided doses produced serum ganciclovir concentrations that exceeded 0.5 μg/mL (2 μM), which is sufficient to inhibit most strains of CMV in vitro. Doses up to 6000 mg of oral ganciclovir are tolerated. Oral ganciclovir reduces virus shedding in urine and semen but still produces neutropenia, particularly in the higher doses (4, 157).

Since high peak titers of ganciclovir cannot be attained with the oral preparation, it is not used for induction treatment. Its first uses have been in maintenance therapy against CMV, particularly in AIDS patients, and in prophylaxis against CMV disease. Controlled studies (described below) have been conducted in maintenance therapy of CMV retinitis and prophylaxis against CMV retinitis in AIDS patients and in prophylaxis against CMV disease in transplant recipients.

Alternative Therapy

Foscarnet

Foscarnet sodium differs chemically from the nucleoside antivirals. It is phosphonoformic acid, trisodium salt. Foscarnet is an analogue of inorganic pyrophosphate that inhibits replication of all herpesviruses by selective inhibition at the pyrophosphate binding site on virus-specific DNA polymerase and reverse transcriptase at concentrations that do not affect cellular DNA polymerase. Unlike some nucleosides, foscarnet does not require activation by phosphorylation by thymidine kinase or other viral or cellular kinases.

At the moment, foscarnet is the only licensed alternative to ganciclovir for systemic treatment of CMV disease. Like ganciclovir, it requires intravenous induction, and it has a high rate of serious complications. However, in a comparative clinical trial, it was found to be as effective in the treatment of CMV retinitis (152).

The recommended dosage for CMV retinitis, approved by the FDA in 1991, is presumably applicable to other CMV diseases in HIV-infected patients. In patients without HIV infection, the necessity for, or duration of, maintenance therapy may vary. Induction treatment consists of 50 mg/kg (minimum 1-h intravenous infusion) every 8 h over 2 to 3 weeks. An infusion pump must be used to control the rate of infusion. Following induction, the maintenance dose is 90 to 120 mg/kg/day given over 2 h. The superiority of 120 mg/kg/day seems established in controlled trials (ACTG 915) (82, 74). The dose administered should be adjusted by creatinine clearance. A table is contained in the package insert. For example, when the creatinine clearance is decreased from more than 1.4 mL/min/kg in 24 h to 0.6 mL/min/kg, the 90-mg/kg dose is reduced to 57 mg/kg.

Cidofovir

Cidofovir is a potent anti-CMV nucleotide with little therapeutic margin for systemic treatment. It has the merit of a long half-life so that doses can be administered weekly. Preclinical studies show the major toxicity of cidofovir to be a dose-dependent nephrotoxicity characterized by degeneration and necrosis of cells of the proximal convoluted renal tubules (96). Probenecid, which is thought to compete with cidofovir uptake in proximal tubular cells, protects against nephotoxocity in animal models. It appears that 5 mg/kg weekly, given intravenously, is the maximum tolerated dose (126). This dose is used once weekly for 2 weeks for induction and once every 2 weeks for maintenance. Probenecid (2 g) must be given orally 3 h before each intravenous administration. Isolates resistant to ganciclovir (usually due to a mutation at UL97) remain susceptible to cidofivir (161). Isolates resistant to ganciclovir because of mutations in the DNA polymerase genes may show resistance to cidofovir (164, 165). Cidofovir has been approved by the FDA only for CMV retinitis in AIDS patients (package insert).

Combinations of Antiviral Agents

In controlled clinical trials, combination of ganciclovir and foscarnet has been shown to be effective in AIDS patients with CMV retinitis who have failed monotherapy with either drug but who have not developed resistance (see below). This combination has also been given anecdotally in other CMV diseases, for example, CMV gastrointestinal disease in AIDS patients.

Special Clinical Situations

CMV Retinitis

Involvement of the retina by CMV is a serious and special disease. Prior to the discovery of AIDS, CMV retinitis was only rarely described in immunocompetent patients. Cases were unusual in adults (53), but it was well recognized as part of congenital cytomegalic inclusion disease (24). Following institution of transplantation and inevitable concurrent immunosuppression, CMV retinitis has been sporadically described in different transplantation centers (44, 127). With the recogni-

tion of AIDS, CMV retinitis became a relatively common medical problem (73).

CMV disease occurs in 21 to 44% of patients with AIDS, of whom 85% have CMV retinitis, especially when their CD4 counts are below $50/mm^3$ (56, 151). Of patients with counts below 100, 21% developed retinitis in 2 years. The natural history of CMV retinitis may have been altered by combination highly active antiretroviral therapy (HAART) in 1996 to 1997, so that CMV retinitis may now appear when CD4 counts are higher (85; see also "Prophylaxis in AIDS Patients," below).

CMV retinitis can be diagnosed by its appearance on clinical ophthalmoscopy: characteristically, fluffy white retinal infiltrates with retinal hemorrhages. Without treatment, retinitis progresses to retinal necrosis and permanent loss of vision, especially when it involves the macula and optic nerve.

Patients with CMV retinitis may have floaters, flashes of light, blurred vision, or blind spots in addition to loss of vision. Mild anterior uveitis, vitritis, and retinal vasculitis may occur. Retinal detachment may be difficult to repair and is associated with poor visual prognosis (54, 120).

With treatment, CMV retinitis may be arrested or contained but not cured. The time to progression of retinal lesions may be prolonged from a median of about 3 weeks to 50 days or longer (151), as long as maintenance therapy is continued. The four different FDA-approved treatment modalities (intravenous ganciclovir, foscarnet, and cidofovir, and intravitreal ganciclovir) are described below (81). In addition, with the availability of oral ganciclovir, measures are now in place to prevent CMV retinitis in patients at risk (see "Prophylaxis in AIDS Patients," below).

Intravenous Ganciclovir. One of the most gratifying findings in antiviral therapy was the discovery of the relative efficacy of ganciclovir against CMV retinitis in patients with AIDS (10, 48), so much so that a controlled study demonstrating its efficacy could not be carried out before it was licensed in 1989 by the FDA (47). In anecdotal reports prior to approval, Masur et al. (103) used 7.5 to 15 mg/kg/day intravenously in 3 divided doses. Holland et al. (75, 76) treated CMV retinitis in 40 patients with AIDS with 7.5 to 10 mg/kg/day for 14 to 20 days; 31 had objective evidence of improvement. However, the common experience was that the disease reoccurred after cessation of treatment and that maintenance treatment was necessary for an indefinite period of time. To prevent relapses, most authors administered single maintenance doses of 5 to 6 mg/kg/day for 5 to 7 days/week (112).

Spector et al. (159) demonstrated the efficacy of intravenous ganciclovir therapy for CMV retinitis in a randomized controlled trial approval of the drug. Patients with peripheral retinitis, whose central vision was not threatened, were selected. They were randomly assigned to receive either immediate intravenous ganciclovir induction therapy (5 mg/kg twice daily for 14 days followed by 5 mg/kg once daily for 14 weeks) or deferred ganciclovir treatment when the retinitis progressed. During the 16-week follow-up, retinitis progressed in most of the patients; that is, in 10 of 13 randomized to immediate treatment and 20 of 22 randomized to deferred treatment. The median time to progression in the immediate treatment group was 49.5 days, compared with 13.5 days for deferred treatment. These data showed conclusively that ganciclovir delayed progression of CMV retinitis.

Intravenous Foscarnet.   In view of the limitations of ganciclovir, there was a pressing need for another primary anti-CMV drug. In anecdotal reports, foscarnet seemed effective in slowing progression of CMV retinitis. It did not produce neutropenia, and it did not interfere with coadministration of zidovudine in AIDS patients.

Palestine et al. (122) conducted a randomized controlled trial in 24 previously untreated patients with AIDS and peripheral CMV retinitis. Treatment consisted of 3 weeks of induction therapy (60 mg/kg every 8 h) followed by maintenance therapy of 90 mg/kg/day. The 11 control patients received no treatment until they reached an endpoint, such as progression of retinitis. Progression was evaluated using retinal photographs. The mean time to progression was 3.2 weeks in the control group and 13.3 weeks in the treatment group. This study showed conclusively that intravenous foscarnet was effective in delaying progression of CMV retinitis in AIDS patients.

On the basis of the limitations of ganciclovir and the favorable reports on foscarnet, in 1992, the Studies of Ocular Complications of AIDS (SOCA) Research Group in collaboration with the AIDS Clinical Trials Group (ACTG) sponsored by the NIH undertook a comparison study of intravenous foscarnet and ganciclovir for initial treatment of cytomegalovirus retinitis (151). Of 234 patients with AIDS and CMV retinitis, 127 were assigned to ganciclovir and 107 to foscarnet. The induction dose of foscarnet was 60 mg/kg of body weight given 3 times/day (i.e., 180 mg/kg/day) for 14 days. The maintenance dose was 90 or 120 mg/kg/day after repeat induction therapy for relapse of retinitis. The induction dose of ganciclovir was 5 mg/kg given twice a day for 14 days, and the maintenance dose was 5 mg/kg/day. The median follow-up time was 9 months per patient. The two groups had similar rates of progression of retinitis. The median time to disease progression was 56 days in the ganciclovir group and 59 days in the foscarnet group. Visual acuity outcomes were also similar (152). These results showed the two drugs to be equally effective against CMV retinitis.

One of the striking results of this trial was the lower mortality of the patients on foscarnet. Mortality in the ganciclovir group was 77% higher than that in the foscarnet group. Median survival times were 5 months in the ganciclovir group and 12.5 months in the foscarnet group. It was thought possible that foscarnet exerted a beneficial antiviral effect against the HIV virus or that it had an additive or synergistic effect with antiviral therapy being given concomitantly. The higher CD4 lymphocyte counts observed 4 and 12 weeks after treatment in the foscarnet group are consistent with this interpretation.

In the SOCA trial comparing intravenous ganciclovir with foscarnet for CMV retinitis, neutropenia was more common in patients who received ganciclovir (34 vs. 14%). Patients assigned to foscarnet reported more infusion-related symptoms (58 vs. 24%) and, in male patients, more genital urinary symptoms (36 vs. 16%). They also experienced more nephrotoxic (elevated serum creatine) effects and electrolyte abnormalities (13 vs. 6%). Patients assigned to foscarnet were more likely to switch to alternative treatment (46 vs. 11%), because of toxic reactions. The incidence of seizures was similar in both groups (9–12%). Toxic effects were reversible, and no permanent disability or death resulted (153).

In conclusion, intravenous foscarnet was as effective as intravenous ganciclovir in arresting CMV retinitis, but foscarnet produced more toxic side reactions necessitating a switch in therapy because of intolerance. The foscarnet-treated group had longer survival. In most centers, when intravenous therapy is initially considered for CMV retinitis, ganciclovir still seems to be preferred.

Intravenous Cidofovir.   Two controlled trials form the basis of approval of cidofovir for CMV retinitis (97, 155). In both, intravenous cidofovir was used with probenecid at 5 mg/kg once weekly for 2 weeks for induction and once every other week for maintenance.

Lalezari et al. (97) randomly assigned 48 previously untreated AIDS patients with peripheral CMV retinitis to either immediate or deferred treatment. Median time to progression of retinitis (measured by retinal photography) was 22 days in the deferred treatment group and 120 days in the immediately treated group ($P < .001$). Treatment was discontinued in 24% of patients because of development of 2+ proteinuria or creatinine levels of 2 g/dL or above.

In the SOCA cidofovir trial (155), 64 patients similar to those in the Lalezari study were randomized to deferred treatment or a high- (5 mg/kg once weekly) or low-dose (3 mg/kg once weekly) group. Induction of all treatment was 5 mg/kg once weekly for 2 weeks. Median time to progression was 20 to 21 days in the deferred treatment group and 64 days in the low-dose group. The median time to progression was not reached in the high maintenance group.

In conclusion, both studies show the median time to first progression to be significantly longer in cidofovir-treated patients than in similar patients treated with either ganciclovir or foscarnet (152, 159). Cidofovir is administered less frequently and does not require a permanent access device. However, more patients discontinued treatment with cidofovir before progression because of toxicity than with ganciclovir or foscarnet.

Combination of Ganciclovir and Foscarnet.   For reasons not entirely understood, without development of antiviral-resistant CMV strains, patients may cease to respond to repeated induction treatment with ganciclovir or foscarnet (95, 167).

The SOCA Study of 1996 (154) was a controlled study of combination foscarnet and ganciclovir in 279 patients with AIDS who had persistently active or relapsed CMV retinitis. Three different treatment groups were defined by different maintenance regimens: *(a)* foscarnet-120, who received a maintenance dose of 120 mg/day, *(b)* ganciclovir-10 who received 10 mg/kg/day of ganciclovir intravenously, and *(c)* combination-90/5, who received 90 mg/kg of foscarnet and 5 mg/kg of ganciclovir. Survival rates were similar in the three groups, unlike the first SOCA Comparison Trial (151), in which patients who received foscarnet survived longer. Time to progression (evaluated in a masked fashion with photographs) was 1.3 months in the foscarnet group, 2.0 months in the ganciclovir group, and 4.3 months in the combination group. Interestingly, patients who remained on monotherapy but whose treatment was switched showed no apparent benefit in time to first progression compared with patients who were not switched. These data support the concept that drug resistance did not account for all relapsed CMV retinitis, although no data on resistance were presented.

The combination group also had the lowest rate of change in retinal area involved by CMV and visual field loss. Combination therapy was clearly superior and was not associated with more toxic effects than either monotherapy. On the other hand, combination therapy had the greatest negative impact on quality-of-life measures. It was associated with more-frequent treatment changes and longer infusion times than the monotherapies.

In conclusion, this study demonstrates a probable synergistic effect of combination therapy with foscarnet and ganciclovir compared with monotherapy for maintenance. The disadvantages are greater inconvenience, higher cost, and probably less-tolerable toxicity.

Oral Ganciclovir as Maintenance Treatment. With the availability of oral ganciclovir, two similar studies compared the efficacy and safety of oral ganciclovir with that of intravenous ganciclovir for maintenance treatment of CMV retinitis in patients with AIDS (39, 121) (Table 1). AIDS patients with CMV retinitis who had been induced with intravenous ganciclovir were randomized. The mean number of days to progression of retinitis during a 20-week follow-up period were similar (compared in both studies by masked assessment of photographs). However, on the basis of funduscopy by ophthalmologists openly aware of the treatment assignments, the mean times to progression differed significantly in both studies. The groups on intravenous maintenance had longer times to progression. Despite this evidence of superiority of intravenous administration, both studies concluded that oral ganciclovir is an effective and safe alternative to intravenous ganciclovir as maintenance therapy for stable retinitis in persons with AIDS. Oral ganciclovir offers greater ease of administration and convenience, an advantage thought to outweigh the small differences in efficacy. Diarrhea and neutropenia were common adverse events in both groups.

Intraocular Administration of Drugs. Intravenous therapy with currently approved drugs against CMV retinitis is complicated by a high frequency of side effects, the inconvenience of intravenous administration, and cost. Experience with local therapy has accumulated since intraocular injection of ganciclovir was first reported in 1987 (66). In 1995, Engstron and Holland summarized 11 reports describing intravitreous ganciclovir injections (46). Most commonly, an injection of 200 μg of ganciclovir was given 2 or 3 times/week for 2 or 3 weeks as induction therapy followed by weekly injections as maintenance therapy. Times to disease progression varied from 8 to 15 weeks.

A recent technical advance was the placement of intravitreal devices consisting of diffusion cells lined by permeable polyvinyl/alcohol membranes and containing ganciclovir. In three studies using this device, CMV retinitis was successfully controlled, although retinal detachment and bacterial endophalmitis did occur. Mean time to progression of retinitis was prolonged to 133 days. In one study, 33% of patients reactivated retinitis once the drug was exhausted (3). Average time before a second implant was needed was 6 months (3, 114, 147).

In the first controlled trial of intraocular devices, Martin et al. (101) studied 26 patients with untreated CMV peripheral retinitis. They were randomized to receive an intraocular device that delivered ganciclovir at 1 μg/h or have therapy deferred until disease progression. Time to disease progression in the treated group was 226 days, compared with 15 days in the group with deferred therapy. This delay of time to progression was significantly longer than that after intravenous ganciclovir or foscarnet for the treatment of the initial CMV retinitis (151).

Musch et al. (115) compared the effect of implants that delivered 1 or 2 μg of ganciclovir with intravenous ganciclovir in 188 AIDS patients with newly diagnosed CMV retinitis. Median times to progression of retinitis in the three groups were 221, 191, and 71 days, respectively. The risk of progression was almost three times as great in those treated with intravenous ganciclovir (risk ratio, 2.8). However, the risk of developing retinitis in the uninvolved eye was lower in that group as was the risk of developing extraocular CMV disease.

Intravitreal cidofovir has been given to patients with HIV disease and CMV retinitis (93). After a single injection of 20 mg, medium time to retinitis progression in 17 patients was 55 days. After 8 repeat injections, it was still 63 days. Although uncontrolled, this study seems to show efficacy, as the time to progression of retinitis compares favorably with systemic treatment with either ganciclovir or foscarnet (151). Mild-to-

---

TABLE 1 • Comparison of Oral vs. Intravenous Ganciclovir for Maintenance Therapy of CMV Retinitis

Study[a]	Group	No. Patients	% Progressed in 20 Weeks		Days to Progression	
			By Photo	By Fundoscopy	By Photo	By Fundoscopy
1	Oral	112	72%	59%	51	86[b]
1	i.v.	47	76%	43%	59	109[b]
2	Oral	63			57	68[b]
2	i.v.	60			62	96[b]

[a] Study 1 is described in reference 121; study 2 is in reference 39. Oral maintenance dose was 3000 mg/day, i.v. dose was 5 mg/day.

[b] Comparison of oral vs. i.v. group, $P < .05$.

moderate iritis developed in 24% of the eyes. Decreased intraocular pressure observed at both 2- and 4-week visits after each injection was thought to be due to cidofovir. Probenecid was used in this trial to counteract such a toxic effect. Efficacy seems to be maintained after second and subsequent injections. Intravitreal cidofovir has not yet been approved by the FDA.

In summary, intraocular administration of antivirals is clearly effective in controlling CMV retinitis. This is better done by placing an intraocular device. The advantage is that a high concentration of drug is delivered locally while avoiding the toxicity of intravenous drug therapy and the inconvenience of intravenous catheters. The disadvantages of local treatment are that the treatment does not prevent development of retinitis in the other eye or of CMV disease elsewhere in the body. Now that there are ways to deal with the neutropenia caused by ganciclovir, the precise indication of intraocular therapy remains to be defined. Perhaps it could be used in conjunction with oral ganciclovir therapy in maintenance therapy.

Central Nervous System Infections
CMV is associated with other clear and distinct disease syndromes of the central nervous system in patients with AIDS besides retinitis (106). As in the case of CMV retinitis, these syndromes are more common in advanced AIDS, when the CD4 lymphocyte count is below 50/mm^3.

Lumbosacral Polyadiculopathy and Myelitis. Of the various syndromes that involve CMV in the central nervous system besides retinitis, CMV polyradiculopathy is the most frequent and characteristic. Patients experience a subacute onset of weakness, loss of reflexes, and variable sensory loss, usually in the legs, in association with bladder and anal sphincter dysfunction. Pathologically, there is CMV infection of the ventral and dorsal roots of the cauda equina and often the adjacent spinal cord, with severe inflammation and axonal necrosis. CSF examination typically shows pleocytosis, often with a preponderance of polymorphonuclear leukocytes and hypoglycorrhachia (27). Although there have been no controlled trials, clinical improvement has been reported after induction and maintenance therapy with intravenous ganciclovir (27, 29, 92). Cohen et al. (27) treated 16 patients of 31, of whom 6 responded with clinical improvement and stabilization. Factors associated with lack of response to therapy were persistence of polymorphonuclear leukocytes, low glucose levels in the CSF, and severe paraparesis (29). Patients who developed polyradiculopathy while on anti-CMV therapy also frequently did not respond. Lack of response is possibly related to irreversible damage in the nervous system.

CMV Encephalitis. There are two types of CMV encephalitis in patients with AIDS. The first is a diffuse, multifocal, micronodular CMV encephalitis that is difficult to distinguish from dementia complex caused by HIV (5). In a retrospective autopsy study, Holland et al. (77) reported that of 220 autopsies done on patients with AIDS, 14 showed CMV encephalitis and 17 showed HIV dementia without involvement of CMV in the central nervous system. Both disorders exhibit cognitive and motor disturbances such as confusion, forgetfulness, apathy and withdrawal, unsteadiness, impaired memory, and diffuse hyperreflexia. CMV encephalitis was not associated with typical abnormalities or positive cultures for CMV in the spinal fluid. Only one-third of CSF samples were PCR positive for CMV. CMV dementia was frequently associated with serum hyponatremia and signs of Addison's disease. There was no response to anti-CMV therapy, and two strains of CMV tested were sensitive to ganciclovir. Fiala et al. (49) did a longitudinal study of 10 AIDS patients with AIDS encephalopathy complicated by CMV infection in the central nervous system; 7 had both HIV and CMV encephalopathy. Such patients had HIV p24 antigenemia as well as elevated HIV and CMV antibodies in the spinal fluid. Patients with the combined disorder had a more rapid course (<6 months) than patients with only HIV encephalopathy. Because of the difficulty in diagnosis of diffuse CMV encephalitis, there is no good documentation of the effectiveness of treatment.

The second type of CMV encephalitis is CMV ventriculoencephalitis. These patients often have a characteristic ventriculitis demonstrable by magnetic resonance imaging (MRI) with gadolinium enhancement of the periventricular areas (89, 129). Ventriculitis is associated with ependymal and subependymal necrosis. Patients are usually in advanced stages of AIDS, with CD4 counts below 50/μL. They have acute onset of apathy, disorientation, cranial nerve palsies, and nystagmus, and usually go rapidly downhill. Ventricular enlargement is usually seen. CSF is usually abnormal, often with neutrophils predominating, but the profile is variable. Treatment with ganciclovir has resulted in radiologic improvement of ventriculitis and conversion of positive CMV cultures but little objective clinical neurologic improvement (129). Salazar et al. (138) reported four autopsy-proven cases of CMV ventriculitis and the clinical and radiologic responses to treatment. Three patients received ganciclovir and two foscarnet. One patient showed marked neurologic improvement and radiologic resolution by MRI after 4 weeks of ganciclovir therapy. Two other patients on ganciclovir and two on foscarnet deteriorated and died. It is not uncommon to develop CMV encephalitis while on maintenance ganciclovir or foscarnet therapy for CMV retinitis, even when retinitis is being controlled (13).

Mononeuritis Multiplex. CMV mononeuritis, the least common of the disorders described above, results from focal necrotizing vasculitis of epineural arteries, characterized by polymorphonuclear leukocytic infiltration. Patients present with multifocal or asymmetric sensory and motor deficits in major peripheral or cranial nerves in a setting of severe immunosuppression. Laryngeal nerves may be especially involved (146). This syndrome may coexist with CMV retinitis, polyradiculitis, or encephalitis. Electrophysiologic studies may show axonal neuropathy. PCR may detect CMV DNA in CSF. Temporary relapse or improvement of symptoms may follow ganciclovir or foscarnet therapy (137).

Cytomegalovirus Pneumonia. The lung is one of the most common targets of CMV disease. CMV pneumonia may result from different mechanisms of pathogenesis. Hence the treatment of CMV pneumonias differs, depending upon the type of patient. Table 2 summarizes four different types of CMV

TABLE 2 • Types of CMV Pneumonias and Their Treatment

Type of Patient with Pneumonia	Mortality (%) Untreated	Treatment Antiviral	Immune Globulin	Immune Pathology
Immunocompetent	0	±	0	0
Bone marrow recipient	70–85	+	+	+
Solid organ recipient	40–70	+	±	+
HIV/AIDS?	+	0	0?	

pneumonia. CMV pneumonia has been described rarely in immunocompetent patients, in association with CMV mononucleosis (100). The mortality of this condition is negligible, and antiviral therapy is highly effective.

The most severe type of pneumonia with the highest mortality occurs in bone marrow recipients. Untreated, the mortality is 70 to 85% (111). Used alone, ganciclovir suppresses the virus but is not effective in reducing morbidity or mortality. Combination therapy of ganciclovir with specific immune globulin is now used widely (45, 131). Reed et al. (131) reported that mortality was reduced to 30% in 10 patients who received ganciclovir (2.5 mg/kg 3 times daily for 20 days) and intravenous immune globulin (500 mg/kg every other day for 10 doses). None of the 11 patients treated with either ganciclovir or intravenous immune globulin alone survived. The course of the patient may be complicated: some resolve after 14 days of treatment, others remain symptomatic and require maintenance treatment, and still others may have a relapse after remission that requires reinduction. Repeated treatment with ganciclovir is limited by the onset of neutropenia, which develops in 67% of patients who receive ganciclovir for at least 14 days (130, 131).

Even so, this treatment remains somewhat controversial, as the European group reported a less favorable result with the combination (99). In a retrospective study of 49 allogeneic bone marrow transplant recipients treated with ganciclovir and intravenous immune globulin using various schedules, only 35% of the patients responded to treatment. Thirty days after diagnosis, the mortality was 69%. The difference between the American and European studies may reflect incomparable data.

In conclusion, CMV pneumonia in marrow recipients is highly fatal if left untreated. Neither ganciclovir or immune globulin alone is effective treatment. Mortality has been reduced by the combination but is still significant.

In solid organ transplantation, the course and treatment of CMV pneumonia is less well documented. Mortality seems to vary in different types of organ recipients, from 48% in an early series of renal recipients (125) to 75% in heart and heart-lung recipients (41). More recent data suggest that mortality associated with CMV pneumonia is generally lower in solid organ recipients than in bone marrow recipients (143, 87). Although there are no controlled studies, some evidence suggests that antiviral therapy is more effective in solid organ recipients than in bone marrow recipients. Duncan et al. (43) reported that 48% of a group of 124 lung recipients developed CMV pulmonary infections. The ganciclovir-treated group had a significantly higher 1-year survival than the untreated group (86 vs. 38%). However, survivors had clinically significant chronic complications, compared with those who did not have CMV pulmonary infection.

The need for immune globulin addition has not been documented in solid organ recipients, although the combination has been reported effective in anecdotal reports (28, 57). For example, clearly death attributed to CMV pneumonia is often due to other causes, such as cardiac dysfunction in heart transplant recipients (87). We conclude that CMV pneumonia after solid organ transplantation may represent either a group of heterogenous entities that differs in pathogenic mechanisms, including the participation of immunopathologic factors, or in outcomes depending upon the underlying patient substrate. Antiviral treatment is at least partly effective.

CMV pneumonia in patients with HIV/AIDS seems to represent yet another variation. Most patients with HIV or AIDS, like transplant recipients, are infected with CMV. The virus is also frequently present in the lungs of persons with AIDS, but its pathogenicity in that organ has been questioned, especially when CMV coexists with other pulmonary pathogens, such as *Pneumocystis*. Treatment of the latter organism alone frequently produces satisfactory clinical remission without any regard to the CMV (18, 86).

However, there are well-documented cases of CMV pneumonia in persons with AIDS reported in the literature (8, 60, 161, 166). CMV pneumonia seems to increase in importance as cases of *Pneumocystis* pneumonia are reduced by prophylaxis. Dore et al. (37) described four such cases in an autopsy series of 25 AIDS patients. None was diagnosed during life. We assume that there is no immunopathologic component to CMV pneumonia in AIDS patients, although there is a report of pulmonary vasculitis and alveolar hemorrhage associated with CMV in AIDS patients (67). Possibly, extreme immunodeficiency precludes the participation of any immunopathologic component (113). McGuinness et al. (107) also emphasized the importance of recognizing and treating CMV pneumonia, particularly in patients who have had repeated *Pneumocystis* pneumonia in the past and who are on prophylaxis for that agent. CMV pneumonia may present as nodular consolidations and may be associated with CMV disease elsewhere or with Kaposi's sarcoma. Jensen et al. (88) suggest in a study of 148 cases of *Pneumocystis* pneumonia that patients who received adjuvant steroid therapy for low pO$_2$ and had coinfection with CMV had a higher mortality than those who did not.

Gastrointestinal Disease
Any part of the gastrointestinal tract from the mouth, esophagus, stomach, small intestines, colon, to the rectum maybe in-

volved with CMV disease in immunosuppressed patients (61). The two most common types of patients are transplant recipients and patients with HIV/AIDS. As pointed out in the section on diagnosis, CMV disease at these sites requires demonstration of the virus as well as local histologic evidence of lesions specific for CMV.

Manifestations of CMV include painful erosions or ulcers of the mouth, epiglottis, or pharynx. Odynophagia is a common symptom. The esophagus may be involved with a solitary ulcer or diffuse esophagitis associated with upper gastrointestinal bleeding. Esophageal strictures may occur after healing. Stomach ulcers may cause bleeding, gastric obstruction, or perforation. Involvement of the small bowel includes progressive diarrhea associated with ulcerated necrosis that may be complicated by perforation. Terminal ileal disease may mimic Crohn's disease clinically. Massive gastrointestinal bleeding may occur. Patients who have colonic disease may have diarrhea, hematochezia, spasms, and abdominal pain associated with constitutional symptoms such as fever, anorexia, and weight loss. Massive acute bleeding has been reported, especially from cecal ulcers in transplant patients. The colon may show diffuse ulcerations, focal ulcerations with skip areas, or less commonly pseudopolyps and pseudomembranes.

The most common site of gastrointestinal involvement in AIDS patients is the colon, particularly in the rectosigmoid region (36). Hematochezia is seen in AIDS patients, but in a minority of patients (32, 36). In an anecdotal report of ganciclovir treatment in 41 AIDS patients with gastrointestinal involvement, Chachoua et al. (23) reported clinical improvement in 30 and virologic response in 32.

In a randomized placebo-controlled trial, 30 AIDS patients with CMV colitis treated with ganciclovir (10 mg/kg daily for 14 days) were compared with 32 in the placebo group. Dieterich et al. (33) reported a significant reduction of CMV-positive colon and urine cultures in the treated group. Further, 63% of those treated showed significant improvement in colonoscopy score versus 33% of the placebo group. The treated group maintained body weight, but the placebo group lost weight. Diarrhea improved equally in both groups.

In anecdotal reports, AIDS patients with CMV gastrointestinal disease who failed ganciclovir therapy (defined as progression of CMV disease) have benefited from foscarnet. Dieterich et al. (34) gave foscarnet (60 mg/kg every 8 h for 14 days) to 19 such patients and observed histopathologic improvement in 67% and clinical improvement in 74%. Another method is to give combined ganciclovir and foscarnet to such patients (35). Until the basis for the lack of response is known (i.e., whether or not resistant mutants of CMV are responsible), it is difficult to justify one or the other approach.

Blanshard et al. (14) undertook a randomized comparison of foscarnet and ganciclovir in AIDS patients with associated gastrointestinal CMV infection; 22 patients received open-label ganciclovir, and 26 received foscarnet. The most frequent sites of involvement in the two groups were (in decreasing order) rectum, esophagus, and colon. In each treatment group, 74% had a complete or good clinical response. Eighty-three percent of the foscarnet-treated and 85% of the ganciclovir-treated patients showed response by endoscopy, and inclusion bodies disappeared from follow-up biopsy specimens in 73% of these. Most patients (35 of 58) developed further evidence of CMV disease during follow-up. Survival in both treatment groups was less than 40 weeks and was unaffected by maintenance treatment therapy. Thus either ganciclovir or foscarnet was effective as first-line treatment for gastrointestinal CMV disease. Maintenance therapy did not prevent progression of the disease.

The frequency of CMV disease of the gastrointestinal tract in transplant recipients varies from 2 to 15% in various reports (21). It probably varies with the frequency of CMV disease in general, of which one determinant is the type of transplantation (70). In kidney and liver recipients, the frequency varies from 2 to 6% (78, 90, 104, 125). In heart and heart-lung recipients, it is 3 to 16% (90, 104, 108). The frequency is even higher in marrow recipients, although specific diagnosis is not always possible because of coexisting graft-versus-host disease (21).

In anecdotal trials, ganciclovir therapy resulted in symptomatic improvement of gastrointestinal CMV disease in as many as 93 to 100% of solid organ transplant recipients (104, 90). Mayoral et al. (104) used ganciclovir to treat 14 solid organ transplant recipients with gastrointestinal CMV disease (all but one endoscopically proven); 13 improved, but 4 required additional treatment for recurring disease.

Kaplan et al. (90) reported that gastrointestinal disease was the most common infection in heart and heart-lung transplant recipients. An incidence of 9.9% included gastritis, 9; gastric ulceration, 4; duodenitis, 3; esophagitis, 1; pyloric perforation, 1; and celomic hemorrhage, 1. They were treated with 5 mg/kg twice daily for 2 to 8 weeks. Relapses occurred in 4 of 9 patients who were followed for a median of 18 months.

Reed et al. (132) conducted the only controlled trial in marrow recipients who had gastrointestinal CMV disease; 14 patients were treated with ganciclovir and 19 received placebo. The most common involvement was the esophagus. Ganciclovir was given at a dosage of 2.5 mg/kg every 8 h for 14 days. No patient had resolution of all symptoms after treatment with ganciclovir. Partial improvement was observed in both treated and placebo control groups. The only significant difference was virtual elimination of the virus from both systemic and local cultures in the treated group; 73% of the treated and 79% of the placebo group showed some improvement. This study showed no clear advantage of treatment and reemphasizes the importance of controlled trials in evaluating therapeutic interventions.

Congenital CMV Infection

About 1% of newborns in the United States, or 30,000 to 40,000 infants, are born with congenitally acquired CMV infection. About 5% of these are symptomatic at birth or have cytomegalic inclusion disease (CID) and usually suffer severe neurologic sequelae. Another 5 to 17% are silently infected at birth but suffer late neurologic sequelae, most commonly nerve deafness (31). There is no accepted preventive or therapeutic measure for this most serious public health problem caused by CMV in the immunocompetent population.

So far there have been no results of controlled clinical trials using ganciclovir or any other antiviral in CID or other medical complications of congenital CMV infection. Anecdotal trials of ganciclovir have been reported (117). Results of a phase II trial of ganciclovir in 52 infants were published by the NIAID Collaborative Antiviral Study Group and a placebo-controlled trial is in progress. Doses of 8 or 12 mg/kg twice daily were given for 6 weeks (168). The higher dose was tolerated and reversibly reduced viruria; however viruria returned to near pretreatment levels after cessation of therapy. Hearing improvement or stabilization occurred in 16% of 30 babies 6 months or later, suggesting, but not proving, efficacy.

Prophylactic Strategies

Bone Marrow Transplant Recipients

Immunoglobulin. A number of controlled studies in the 1980s reported that use of immunoglobulin reduced CMV disease, particularly in seronegative recipients, (17, 94, 110, 119, 170). However, this was not found consistently. In an important study of 97 seronegative marrow recipients at the University of Washington, Bowden et al. (17) assigned them to (a) intravenous CMV immunoglobulin and seronegative blood products, (b) seronegative blood products alone, (c) CMV immunoglobulin alone, or (d) neither treatment. CMV infection in the four respective groups was 5, 13, 54, and 40%, respectively. The main conclusion of this study was that among 57 patients with seronegative donors, those who received seronegative blood products had significantly less infection (1 in 32) than those who received the standard blood products (8 of 25; $P < .007$). Immunoglobulin alone had no effect.

This study showed that CMV infection and disease could be prevented in seronegative recipients who had seronegative donors by providing CMV-free blood products. The remaining question was whether immunoglobulin could prevent infection and disease in seronegative recipients with seropositive donors. Bowden et al. (16) showed in a randomized controlled study in 120 such patients (of which 60 were controls) that it could not.

A larger study also from the University of Washington, addressed seropositive recipients (163). Among 308 seropositive recipients evaluated, 22% of control patients and 13% of immunoglobulin recipients developed interstitial pneumonia. The incidence of acute graft-versus-host disease (GVHD) was reduced from 51% in controls to 30% in immunoglobulin recipients. Whether the reduction of pneumonia was a direct effect of immunoglobulin or a secondary effect of the reduction of GVHD by immunoglobulin is unclear. A smaller European study failed to confirm this effect (133).

In summary, while numerous studies showed a beneficial effect of immune globulin in marrow recipients in the 1980s, studies in the 1990s that tested CMV seropositive and seronegative recipients separately did not confirm these results. Hyperimmune globulin does not seem to have a consistent effect against primary infection by CMV in seronegative recipients. Its effect in seropositive recipients is also questionable. Even when effective, its effect may be secondary to a reduction of GVHD.

Antivirals. Patients who are CMV seropositive before marrow transplantation are at greater risk for developing CMV disease after transplantation than seronegative recipients. Regardless of the donor serologic status, the frequency of infection in the first 100 days after transplantation is about 70% (111). This group of patients has been primarily targeted for testing antiviral prophylaxis and therapy.

Meyers et al. (109) found that intravenous acyclovir (500 mg/m^2 given every 8 h starting 5 days before transplantation of CMV seropositive subjects and continued until day 30 thereafter) reduced the incidence of CMV disease from 38 to 22% and the incidence of CMV infection from 75% to 59%. Transplantation-associated mortality was reduced from 54 to 29%. More recently, the European Acyclovir Study Group (128) gave a high intravenous dose (500 mg/m^2 thrice daily) or oral acyclovir for the first 30 days after transplantation and then oral acyclovir or placebo until day 210. The rate of CMV infection, frequency of viremia, and mortality were lower in the group that received intravenous acyclovir. However, the frequency of CMV disease was similar in the two groups. Boeckh et al. (15) evaluated high-dose intravenous acyclovir from 5 days before autologous transplantation to day 100 in a retrospective study. There was no difference in the incidence of CMV disease or pneumonia. Thus intravenous acyclovir regimens were not effective in reducing CMV disease in all reports.

There are two approaches to the use of ganciclovir in CMV seropositive marrow recipients. The first is so-called early treatment; that is, patients identified by recovery of CMV from surveillance cultures are then given ganciclovir. The second approach is to administer ganciclovir after engraftment to all seropositive patients.

Following the first approach, Schmidt et al. (142) performed bronchoalveolar lavage (BAL) surveillance cultures at the median day of engraftment (day 22) and enrolled those with CMV-positive cultures. Twenty patients were randomized to the placebo group and 20 to the treatment group, who received ganciclovir from day 35 after transplantation to day 120. CMV pneumonia was reduced from 70 to 25%. Of the 55 patients who were not positive by BAL (and thus not eligible for the study), 22% developed CMV pneumonia. Goodrich et al. (63) selected patients for prophylaxis by screening for positive CMV cultures from blood, throat washes, or urine. Patients received either ganciclovir until day 100 after transplantation or placebo. Results were obtained on 102 patients. CMV disease was reduced from 43% (15 of 35) in the placebo group to 3% (1 of 37 patients) in the treatment group during the first 100 days after transplantation. CMV infection was reduced from 56% in the placebo group to 15% in the ganciclovir group by the end of 1 week. After 3 weeks, no patient in the ganciclovir group was culture positive, but 12% of patients had CMV disease in the absence of positive surveillance cultures. These studies show that the surveillance methods did not identify all patients who eventually became ill from CMV, although ganciclovir did reduce CMV disease in those who were identified. The other major problem with ganciclovir administration is neutropenia, which occurred in about 30% of those who received the drug in both studies.

Following the second approach, Goodrich et al. (62) gave ganciclovir to all 33 patients, from engraftment to 100 days after transplantation; 45% of the placebo recipients (14 of 31) developed CMV infection 100 days after transplantation compared with 1 (3%) ganciclovir recipient. Neutropenia occurred in 30% of the ganciclovir recipients. Mortality did not differ between the two groups. Winston et al. (169) gave ganciclovir for 1 week before marrow infusion and then starting after engraftment until day 100 after transplantation. CMV infection was similarly reduced from 56 to 24%.

The studies cited above show that ganciclovir is effective in reducing CMV disease if administered *(a)* routinely to all patients or *(b)* selectively to those found to be positive by surveillance cultures. But if one avoids excess toxicity by restricting administration to patients at higher risk, there is the danger of missing those who become ill without positive surveillance cultures. At the moment there is no perfect solution to this problem. Improvement will come with either methods of surveillance with better sensitivity and specificity for CMV disease or development of less toxic antivirals. Antigenemia or some quantitative PCR or DNA amplification method may eventually provide better surveillance.

Solid Organ Transplant Recipients

Immunoglobulin. Using hyperimmune CMV immunoglobulin, Snydman et al. (150) studied 59 seronegative kidney recipients; 24 were treated with 150 mg/kg within 72 h of transplantation, 100 mg/kg at weeks 2 and 4, and 15 mg/kg at weeks 6, 8, 12, and 16. The remainder were controls. CMV infection was not significantly affected, but treatment reduced CMV disease from 60 to 21%, compared with controls, and mortality from 14 to 4%. This result could not be confirmed using a different immune globulin (91). On the basis of this study, CMV immunoglobulin was licensed for use after renal transplantation.

Snydman et al. (148) later used the same CMV immunoglobulin preparation used in the renal transplant study (150), in 69 seronegative and seropositive liver recipients, who were compared with 72 placebo controls. In contrast to the renal transplant study (150), primary disease in the seronegative recipient group was not affected, and severe CMV disease in seropositive patients was only reduced from 31 to 19%. A separate later study showed that CMV disease was reduced from 32 to 14% in the seronegative recipients (149). Saliba et al. (139) also reported a reduction in CMV disease using CMV hyperimmunoglobulin, but Cofer et al. (25) found no protection against either primary or secondary CMV disease in seronegative and seropositive liver recipients.

In conclusion, the type of immune globulin and the type of transplant are important variables in determining efficacy. CMV hyperimmunoglobulin is effective in preventing primary disease in seronegative recipients of renal transplantation. Other selected immune globulin may not be effective. Even proven-effective immune globulin could not consistently prevent primary CMV disease after liver transplantation. There are no controlled studies of prophylaxis against CMV disease using hyperimmune globulin in other types of solid organ transplantation.

Antivirals

Acyclovir. Although acyclovir in usual doses does not reach inhibitory levels against CMV in the bloodstream (see "Single Drug Susceptibility," above), Balfour et al. (12) reported that it was effective in preventing CMV disease due to primary and secondary infection in renal transplant recipients. The hypothetical explanation given was that there might be adequate intracellular concentrations of the phosphorylated form of acyclovir, which is the active form of the drug but is not usually measured. Acyclovir (800 mg) was given orally four times daily for 12 weeks beginning 6 h before transplantation. CMV disease was reduced from 29 to 8%, with the difference particularly significant in the subgroup consisting of seronegative recipients with seropositive donors.

Later indications are that acyclovir may not be effective or may only be marginally effective especially in liver transplantation (140, 162). Singh et al. (145) saw comparable virus shedding in patients who received oral acyclovir and those who did not (25 vs. 22%), and 29% of the acyclovir group developed CMV disease. Numerous reports attest to its inferiority to ganciclovir in efficacy (11, 102, 171).

Ganciclovir. Since intravenous ganciclovir was shown effective in the treatment of CMV disease, it is not surprising to see it used as a prophylactic agent after organ transplantation. Its main defects are toxicity (particularly neutropenia), the requirement for intravenous access, and cost. Merigan et al. (108) treated 76 heart recipients with 5 mg/kg of ganciclovir intravenously twice daily for 14 days, then 6 mg/kg 5 days a week until day 28 after transplantation; 73 patients served as controls. Among 37 seronegative recipients, 35% of ganciclovir-treated patients developed CMV disease, versus 25% in the placebo group. It had no effect. On the other hand, CMV disease in the 56 seropositive recipients was reduced, compared with that in the 56 controls (9 vs. 46%). Thus in this study of heart recipients, ganciclovir prophylaxis was only effective in secondary infection and was ineffective in primary infection, which poses the greater risk for severe disease. Aguado et al. (2) similarly reduced secondary CMV disease in heart recipients from 40 to 6%.

Rondeau et al. (135) studied 39 renal transplant recipients and showed no change in primary infection and disease after 28 days of intravenous ganciclovir after transplantation.

Cohen et al. (27) gave ganciclovir to 65 seropositive and seronegative liver recipients for 14 days during the third and fourth posttransplant weeks. No difference in the amount of CMV disease was seen. Possibly, the treatment was too late or too short. Winston et al. (171) also studied seropositive and seronegative recipients and compared ganciclovir with acyclovir controls. Ganciclovir 6 mg/kg was given once daily on days 1 through 30 then for 5 days a week through day 100. Acyclovir was given for the same duration. CMV infection and disease decreased in the ganciclovir group (0.8 vs. 10%).

Duncan et al. (42) studied 25 seropositive and seronegative lung recipients; 13 patients received ganciclovir 5 mg/kg 4 times daily for 2 weeks starting on day 7, then 5 mg/kg daily for 1 week, and 5 mg/kg/day for 5 days/week to day 90. The control group of 12 patients received ganciclovir 5 mg/kg 4 times daily for 2 weeks starting on day 7, then 5 mg/kg daily for 1 week, then acyclovir 800 mg 4 times daily through day 90. There was a reduction in CMV disease in the group on ganciclovir through day 90 from 25 to 0%. There was also decreased CMV infection.

In summary, these studies show intravenous ganciclovir to be superior to acyclovir in reducing both CMV infection and disease (102, 116). Given in high doses, ganciclovir, beginning immediately after transplantation and continuing up to 3 months, may reduce or eliminate disease due to both primary and secondary CMV infection. However, if not started immediately or not given long enough, disease may only be delayed, or primary disease may not be reduced at all.

One method of avoiding toxicity and other problems with prophylactic agents (including intravenous ganciclovir) while retaining efficacy is to apply so-called preemptive prophylaxis or therapy. This means giving prophylaxis only to those at high risk, such as those who have positive cultures or are undergoing antirejection therapy. Several studies using this strategy have shown success in both kidney and liver recipients.

Singh et al. (145), in a study of 47 seropositive and seronegative recipients, compared acyclovir with ganciclovir given only when surveillance CMV cultures became positive. Ganciclovir (5 mg/kg) was given intravenously twice daily for 7 days. Oral acyclovir (800 mg) was given 4 times daily for 24 weeks. Less CMV disease was seen in the ganciclovir group than in the acyclovir group (29 vs. 4%).

Hibberd et al. (68) treated 64 kidney recipients "preemptively" who had received OKT3 or antilymphocyte globulin. All patients were seropositive for CMV. Ganciclovir 2.5 mg/kg/day was given for the duration of antilymphocyte therapy, and compared with results in 49 patients who received no prophylaxis, CMV disease was decreased from 33 to 14% by ganciclovir.

Oral ganciclovir has been shown to be safe and efficacious in preventing primary and secondary CMV disease in liver recipients (124). Placebo or oral ganciclovir (1 g thrice daily) was given to 304 recipients for 14 weeks after transplantation and assessed at 6 and 12 months. Disease among seropositive recipients was reduced from 14 to 4%, and among seronegative recipients with seropositive donors, disease was reduced from 11 of 25 (44%) to 3 of 21 (14%). Oral ganciclovir has been licensed for this indication.

Prophylaxis in AIDS Patients

The most common and most debilitating form of CMV disease is CMV retinitis, which may eventually lead to blindness despite effective antiviral therapy. CMV retinitis affects 25 to 40% of patients with AIDS, with most patients becoming afflicted when the CD4 count decreases to 50/mm^3 or less (38, 55, 79, 83). The frequency of CMV retinitis is likely to increase as AIDS patients with low CD4 counts survive longer. Thus, prophylaxis for this debilitating and fairly common disease merits consideration.

The situation is complicated during this post-HAART era (after 1996–97) of multiple combinations of multiple anti-HIV nucleoside and nonnucleoside drugs. While such therapy is highly effective in elevating CD4 cell counts, there is suspicion that there may not be commensurate improvement in immunity. Jacobsen et al. (85) reported CMV retinitis in 29 and 14% of patients with CD4 counts above 50 and 100, respectively, following HAART, which is significantly higher than before HAART. Four such patients had counts above 200 cells/mm^3. The functional capacity of recovered CD4 cells may not be optimal (9). This leaves us with the unsettled problem of when to institute prophylaxis for opportunistic infections, such as CMV retinitis, after HAART.

In a placebo-controlled study before HAART, Spector et al. (158) randomized (in a 2:1 ratio) 486 patients who received 1000 mg oral ganciclovir three times daily and 239 controls. Entry criteria were a CD4+ count of 50/mm^3 or less or 100/mm^3. or less and a history of an AIDS-defining event. All patients were infected with CMV but had no history of CMV disease. The median treatment duration was 265 days; the study was then terminated because of the favorable effect of ganciclovir, and all patients were offered open treatment. The incidence of CMV retinitis after 18 months of observation was 39% in the placebo group and 18% in the treated group. Total CMV disease was significantly reduced by treatment (39 vs. 20%), including investigator-reported colitis (13 vs. 4%). One-year mortality rates were not significantly different. Patients in the treated group had more instances of neutropenia, were more frequently on granulocyte colony-stimulating factor, and had more frequent elevations of serum creatinine.

This study suggests that oral ganciclovir effectively reduces CMV retinitis and other significant CMV diseases in advanced AIDS. In view of the complications of ganciclovir and its cost, it may be desirable to restrict its use to patients at greater risk. As in the case of ganciclovir prophylaxis in transplant recipients, there is as yet no accepted sensitive and specific laboratory measure of risk of CMV retinitis and disease except the CD4 T lymphocyte count.

Preliminary results of another controlled study of 994 patients (CPCRA 023, 20) on oral ganciclovir to prevent of CMV retinitis and colitis did not demonstrate efficacy. The study population was less immunosuppressed than that in the Spector study, and preentry criteria did not require examination by an ophthalmologist. Thus, entrants could have had unrecognized CMV retinitis before they were put on prophylaxis. Still, the striking difference between the two studies is of concern.

In conclusion, oral ganciclovir should be considered as a prophylactic agent against CMV retinitis in advanced AIDS. Further studies may better define the population at risk.

ENDPOINTS FOR MONITORING THERAPY
Ganciclovir Toxicity

Ganciclovir use requires monitoring the neutrophil count because neutropenia is the most important of the severe adverse reactions that limit the use of ganciclovir. Neutropenia or an absolute neutrophil count below 1000/μL may occur in 13 to 67% of patients receiving ganciclovir and averages about 30% (52). Severe neutropenia (<500/μL) may be found in 19% of patients. Neutropenia usually resolves with discontinuation of therapy and may be prevented by concomitant administration of granulocyte macrophage colony-stimulating factor (GM-CSF) (see below). Thrombocytopenia is a less common but potentially serious complication of ganciclovir, particularly in patients with AIDS, and further indicates its bone marrow suppressive effect. Other side effects of ganciclovir include rash, nausea, fever, vomiting, anemia, diarrhea, eosinophilia, confusion, seizures, and psychotic reactions in a small number of patients (22).

One of the early problems encountered with ganciclovir was synergistic toxicity with zidovudine, another marrow-suppressive drug (72). No patient could tolerate zidovudine (1200 mg/day) and maintenance intravenous doses of ganciclovir (5 mg/kg/day) without severe hematologic toxicity occurring within weeks. Few patients could tolerate zidovudine (300 mg/day) with maintenance ganciclovir.

The availability of GM-CSF is a major advance in preventing neutropenia caused by ganciclovir. In an ACTG trial, 53 patients with AIDS and CMV retinitis were randomized to receive ganciclovir (5 mg/kg twice daily for 14 days followed by 5 mg/kg/day) with or without GM-CSF (64). The dose (1–8 mg) was adjusted to maintain an absolute neutrophil count between 2500 and 5000 cells/μL. After 16 weeks, zidovudine was given to both groups. Neutropenia developed in 45% of patients who did not receive GM-CSF and 12.5% of those who did. Patients who received GM-CSF missed fewer doses of ganciclovir and tended toward more delayed progression of retinitis. Clearly, GM-CSF effectively reduced the major hematologic toxicity of ganciclovir and may indirectly have contributed to an anti-HIV response.

Foscarnet Toxicity

The major toxicity of foscarnet is renal impairment, which occurs to some degree in most treated patients. Approximately 33% of 189 patients with AIDS and CMV retinitis who received intravenous foscarnet treatment developed impairment manifested as a serum creatinine concentration of 2 mg/dL or higher. Such elevations are usually, but not always, reversed on discontinuation of the drug. Because foscarnet chelates divalent cations, it has also been associated with serum electrolyte imbalance such as hypocalcemia (15%), hypomagnesemia (50%), and hypokalemia (16%). Foscarnet has been associated with seizures in 10% of AIDS patients in five controlled studies. Hypocalcemia may play a role in cases of unexplained seizures or arrhythmia. Anemia has been reported in 33% of patients receiving foscarnet. This has been manageable, and less than 1% required discontinuation of the drug for this reason. Granulocytopenia has been reported in 17% of patients, but only 1% were terminated from studies because of neutropenia. Penile ulceration may result from exposure of the glans penis to unchanged foscarnet in urine (7, 80).

Resistance to Ganciclovir or Foscarnet

Resistance has developed against both ganciclovir and foscarnet after long-term maintenance therapy with either drug. This has been best studied in CMV retinitis. Drew et al. (40) reported that of 13 patients treated with ganciclovir for more than 3 months, 5 (38%) developed resistance. None of 31 patients were excreting CMV resistant to ganciclovir.

Jacobson et al. (84) in ACTG 093 described a phase 2 dose-ranging trial of foscarnet salvage therapy for AIDS patients with CMV retinitis intolerant or resistant to ganciclovir. A total of 156 patients received 60, 90, or 120 mg/kg/day. Time to progression of disease while on ganciclovir was 2 weeks or less, but after shifting to foscarnet, it was extended to a median of 8 weeks. There was no significant difference in the efficacy or toxicity of the different doses. A subsequent study (74) of foscarnet maintenance doses of 90 or 120 mg/kg/day showed the higher dose to be more effective in preserving vision in patients with CMV retinopathy.

Kuppermann et al. (95) studied nine patients with CMV retinitis clinically resistant to either ganciclovir or foscarnet, demonstrated by progression despite induction therapy with either drug at 6 weeks. For induction, they received a combination of ganciclovir (5 mL/kg every 12 h) and foscarnet (60 mg/kg every 8 h). The maintenance combination was ganciclovir 5 mg/kg every 12 to 24 h and foscarnet 90 to 120 mg/kg daily. All patients responded favorably to combination therapy, with complete healing in 12 of 14 eyes and partial healing in the remainder.

While not common, resistance to ganciclovir has also been reported in transplant recipients. Resistance occurred after long-term ganciclovir treatment, and sensitive PCR detected specific resistant mutations at codons 594 and 595 (136). In one patient, however, the resistant mutant (at codon 460) was present prior to therapy (1). With wider application of sensitive PCR methods to detect resistant mutants, the extent and significance of antiviral resistance in all types of CMV infection will become better known.

REFERENCES

1. Alain S, Honderlick P, Grenet D, Stern M, Vadam C, Sanson-LePors MJ, Mazeron MC. Failure of ganciclovir treatment associated with selection of a ganciclovir-resistant cytomegalovirus strain in a lung transplant recipient. Transplantation 1997;63:1533–1536.
2. Aguado JM, Gomez-Sanchez MA, Lumbreras C, Delgado J, Lizasoain M, Otero JR, Rufilanchas JJ, Noriega AR. Prospective randomized trial of efficacy of ganciclovir versus that of anti-cytomegalovirus (CMV) immunoglobulin to prevent CMV disease in CMV-seropositive heart transplant recipients treated with OKT3. Antimicrob Agents Chemother 1995;39:1643–1645.
3. Anand R, Nightingale SD, Fish RH, Smith TJ, Ashton P. Control of cytomegalovirus retinitis using sustained release of intraocular ganciclovir. Arch Ophthalmol 1993;111:223–227.
4. Anderson RD, Griffy KG, Jung D, Dorr A, Hulse JD, Smith RB. Ganciclovir absolute bioavailability and steady-state pharmacokinetics after oral administration of two 3000 mg/d dosing regimens in human immunodeficiency virus- and cytomegalovirus-seropositive patients. Clin Ther 1995;17:425–432.
5. Arribas JR, Storch GA, Clifford DB, Tselis AC. Cytomegalovirus encephalitis. Ann Intern Med 1996;125:577–587.
6. Ashton WT, Karkas JD, Field AK, Tolman RL. Activation by thymidine kinase and potent antiherpetic activity of 2′-nor-2′-deoxyguanosine (2′NDG). Biochem Biophys Res Commun 1982;108:1716–1721.
7. Astra. Foscavir injection: package insert. Physicians desk reference. Oradell, NJ: Medical Economics Co, 1996:547–551.

8. Aukrust P, Farastad IN, Froland SS, Holter E. Cytomegalovirus (CMV) pneumonitis in AIDS patients: the result of intensive CMV replication? Eur Respir J 1992;5:362–364.

9. Autran B, Carcelain G, Li TS, Blanc C, Mathez D, Tubiana R, Katlama C, Debre P, Leibowitch J. Positive effects of combined antiretroviral therapy on CD4+ T cell homeostasis and function in advanced HIV disease. Science 1997;277:112–116.

10. Bach MC, Bagwell SP, Knapp NP, David KM, Hedstron PS. 9-(1,3-Dihydroxy-2-propoxymethyl)guanine for cytomegalovirus infections in patients with the acquired immunodeficiency syndrome. Ann Intern Med 1985;103:381–384.

11. Bailey TC, Ettinger NA, Storch GA, Trulock EP, Hanto DW, Dunagan WC, Jendrisak MD, McCullough CS, Kenzora JL, Powderly WG. Failure of high-dose oral acyclovir with or without immune globulin to prevent primary cytomegalovirus disease in recipients of solid organ transplants. Am J Med 1993; 95:273–278.

12. Balfour HH, Chace BA, Stapleton JT, Simmons RL, Fryd DS. A randomized placebo-controlled trial of oral acyclovir for the prevention of cytomegalovirus disease in recipients of renal allografts. N Engl J Med 1989;320:1381–1387.

13. Berman SM, Kim RC. The development of cytomegalovirus encephalitis in AIDS patients. Am J Med 1994;96:415–419.

14. Blanshard C, Benhamon Y, Dohin E, Lernestedt J-O, Gazzard BG, Katlama C. Treatment of AIDS-associated gastrointestinal cytomegalovirus infection with foscarnet and ganciclovir: a randomized comparison. J Infect Dis 1995;172:622–628.

15. Boeckh M, Gooley TA, Reusser P, Buckner CD, Bowden RA. Failure of high-dose acyclovir to prevent cytomegalovirus disease after autologous marrow transplantation. J Infect Dis 1995; 172:939–943.

16. Bowden RA, Fisher LD, Rogers K, Cays M, Meyers JD. Cytomegalovirus (CMV)-specific intravenous immunoglobulin for the prevention of primary CMV infection and disease after marrow transplant. J Infec Dis 1991;164:483–487.

17. Bowden RA, Sayers M, Flournoy N, Newton B, Banaji M, Thomas ED, Meyers JD. Cytomegalovirus immune globulin and seronegative blood products to prevent primary cytomegalovirus infection after marrow transplantation. N Engl J Med 1986;314:1006–1010.

18. Brodie HR, Broaddus C, Blumenfeld W, Hopewell PC, Moss A, Mills J. Is cytomegalovirus (CMV) a cause of lung disease in patients with AIDS? Clin Res 1985;33:396A.

19. Bronson JJ, Ferrara LM, Hitchcock MHM, Ho HT, Woods KL, Ghazzoufi I, Kern ER, Coike KF. (S)-1-(3-Hydroxy-2-(phosphonylmethoxy)propyl)cytosine (HPMPC): a potent antiherpesvirus agent. In: Lopez C, Mori R, Roizman B, Whitley RJ, eds. Immunobiology and prophylaxis of human herpesvirus infections. New York: Plenum Press, 1991:277–283.

20. Brosgart CL, Craig C, Hillman D, Louis TA, Alston B. A randomized, placebo-controlled trial of the safety and efficacy of oral ganciclovir for prohylaxis of CMV retinal and gastrointestinal mucosal disease in HIV-infected individuals with severe immunosuppression. 35th Interscience Conference on Antimicrobial Agents and Chemotherapy, San Francisco, 17–20 Sept, 1995.

21. Buckner FS, Pomeroy C. Cytomegalovirus disease of the gastrointestinal tract in patients without AIDS. Clin Infect Dis 1993;17:644–656.

22. Buhles WC Jr, Mastre BJ, Tinker AJ, Stranf V, Koretz SH, Syntex Collaborative Ganciclovir Treatment Study Group. Ganciclovir treatment of life- or sight-threatening cytomegalovirus infection: experience in 314 immunocompromised patients. Rev Infect Dis 1988;10:S495–506.

23. Chachoua A, Dieterich D, Krasinski K, Green J, Laubenstein L, Wernz J, Buhles W, Koretz S. 9-(1,3-Dihydroxy-2-propoxymethyl) guanine (ganciclovir) in the treatment of cytomegalovirus gastrointestinal disease with the acquired immunodeficiency syndrome. Ann Intern Med 1987;107:133–137.

24. Christiansen L, Beeman HW, Allen A. Cytomegalic inclusion disease. 1957;57:90–99.

25. Cofer JB, Morris CA, Sutker WL, Husberg BS, Goldstein RM, Gonwa TA, Klintmalm GB. A randomized double-blind study of the effect of prophylactic immune globulin on the incidence and severity of CMV infection in the liver transplant recipient. Transplant Proc 1991;23:1525–1527.

26. Cohen AT, O'Grady JG, Sutherland S, Sallie R, Tan KC, Williams R. Controlled trial of prophylactic versus therapeutic use of ganciclovir after liver transplantation in adults. J Med Virol 1993;40:5–9.

27. Cohen BA, McArthur JC, Grohman S, Patterson B, Glass JD. Neurologic prognosis of cytomegalovirus polyradiculomyelopathy in AIDS. Neurology 1993;43:493–499.

28. D'Alessandro AM, Pirsch JD, Stratta RJ, Sollinger HW, Kalayoglu M, Belzer FO. Successful treatment of severe cytomegalovirus infections with ganciclovir and CMV hyperimmune globulin in liver transplant recipients. Transplant Proc 1989;21:3560–3561.

29. De Gans J, Portegies P, Tiessens G, Troost D, Danner SA, Lange JM. Therapy for cytomegalovirus polyradiculomyelitis in patients with AIDS: treatment with ganciclovir. AIDS 1990:421–425.

30. DeClercq E, Sakuma T, Baba M. Antiviral activity of phosphonylmethoxyalkyl derivatives of purines and pyrimidines. Antiviral Res 1987;8:261–272.

31. Demmler GJ. Summary of a workshop on surveillance for congenital cytomegalovirus disease. Rev Infect Dis 1991;13:315–329.

32. DeRodriguez CV, Fuhrer J, Lake-Bakaar G. Cytomegalovirus colitis in patients with acquired immunodeficiency syndrome. J R Soc Med 1994;87:203–205.

33. Dieterich DT, Kotler DP, Busch DF, Crumpacker C, DuMond C, Dearmand B, Buhles W. Ganciclovir treatment of cytomegalovirus colitis in AIDS: a randomized, double-blind, placebo-controlled multicenter study. J Infect Dis 1993;167:278–282.

34. Dieterich DT, Poles MA, Dicker M, Tepper R, Lew E. Foscarnet treatment of cytomegalovirus gastrointestinal infections in acquired immunodeficiency syndrome patients who have failed ganciclovir induction. Am J Gastroenterol 1993;88:542–548.

35. Dieterich DT, Poles MA, Lew EA, Mendez PE, Murphy R, Addessi A, Holbrook JT, Naughton K, Friedberg DN. Concurrent use of ganciclovir and foscarnet to treat cytomegalovirus infection in AIDS patients. J Infect Dis 1993;167:1184–1188.

36. Dieterich DT, Rahmin M. Cytomegalovirus colitis in AIDS: presentation in 44 patients and a review of the literature. J Acquir Immune Defic Syndr 1991;4:529–35.

37. Dore GJ, Marriott DJ, Duflou JA. Clinico-pathological study of cytomegalovirus (CMV) in AIDS autopsies: under-recognition of CMV pneumonitis and CMV adrenalitis. Aust NZ J Med 1995;25:503–506.

38. Drew WL. Cytomegalovirus infection in patients with AIDS. Clin Infect Dis 1992;14:608–615.

39. Drew WL, Ives D, Lalezari JP, Crumpacker C, Follansbee SE, Spector SA, Benson CA, Friedberg DN, Hubbard L, Stempien MJ. Oral ganciclovir as maintenance treatment for cytomegalovirus retinitis in patients with AIDS. N Engl J Med 1995;333:615–620.

40. Drew WL, Miner RC, Busch DF. Prevalence of resistance in patients receiving ganciclovir for serious cytomegalovirus infection. J Infect Dis 1991;163:716–719.

41. Dummer JS, White LT, Ho M, Griffith BP, Hardesty RL, Bahnson HT. Morbidity of cytomegalovirus infection in recipients of heart or heart-lung transplants who received cyclosporine. J Infect Dis 1985;152:1182–1191.

42. Duncan SR, Grgurich WF, Lacono AT, Burckart GJ, Yousem SA, Paradis IL, Williams PA, Johnson BA, Griffith BP. A comparison of ganciclovir and acyclovir to prevent cytomegalovirus after lung transplantation. Am J Respir Crit Care Med 1994;150:146–152.

43. Duncan SR, Paradis IL, Yousem SA, Similo SL, Grgurick WF, Williams PA, Dauber JH, Griffith BP. Sequelae of cytomegalovirus pulmonary infections in lung allograft recipients. Am Rev Respir Dis 1992;146:1419–1425.

44. Egbert PR, Pollard RB, Gallagher JB, Merigan TC. Cytomegalovirus retinitis in immunosuppressed hosts. II. Ocular manifestations. Ann Intern Med 1980;93;664–670.

45. Emanuel D, Cunningham I, Jules-Elysee K, Brochstein JA, Kernan NA, Laver J, Stover D, White DA, Fels A, Polsky B. Cytomegalovirus pneumonia after bone marrow transplantation successfully treated with the combination of ganciclovir and high-dose intravenous immune globulin. Ann Intern Med 1988;109:777–782.

46. Engstron RE Jr, Holland GN. Perspective: local therapy for cytomegalovirus retinopathy. Am J Ophthalmol 1995;120:376–385.

47. Faulds D, Heel RC. Ganciclovir: a review of its antiviral activity, pharmacokinetic properties and therapeutic efficacy in cytomegalovirus infections. AIDS 1990;39:597–638.

48. Felsenstein D, D'Amico DJ, Hirsch MS, Neumeyer DA, Cederberg DM, deMiranda P, Schooley RT. Treatment of cytomegalovirus retinitis with 9-[2-hydroxy-1-(hydroxymethyl) ethoxymethyl]guanine. Ann Intern Med 1985;103:377–380.

49. Fiala M, Singer EJ, Graves MC, Tourtellotte WW, Stewart JA, Schable CA, Rhodes RH, Vinters HV. AIDS dementia complex complicated by cytomegalovirus encephalopathy. J Neurol 1993;240:223–231.

50. Field AK, Davies ME, DeWitt C, Perry HC, Liou R, Germershausen J, Karkas JD, Ashton WT, Johnston DB, Tolman RL. ([2-Hydroxy-1-(hydroxymethyl)ethoxy]methyl) guanine: a selective inhibitor of herpes group virus replication. Proc Natl Acad Sci USA 1983;80:4139–4143.

51. Fischer SH, Masur H. Editorial response: laboratory monitoring of cytomegalovirus disease—is polymerase chain reaction the answer? Clin Infect Dis 1997;24:841–842.

52. Fletcher CV, Balfour HH. Evaluation of ganciclovir for cytomegalovirus disease. DICP 1989;23:5–12.

53. Foerster HW. Pathology of granulomatous uveitis. Surv Ophthalmol 1959;4:296.

54. Freeman WR, Friedberg DN, Berry C, Quiceno JI, Behette M, Fullerton SC. Risk factors for development of rhegmatogenous retinal detachment in patients with cytomegalovirus retinitis. Am J Ophthalmol 1993;116:713–720.

55. Gallant JE, Moore RD, Chaisson RE. Prophylaxis for opportunistic infections in patients with HIV infection. Ann Intern Med 1994;120:932–944.

56. Gallant JE, Moore RD, Richman DD, Keruly J, Chaisson RE. Incidence and natural history of cytomegalovirus disease in patients with advanced human immunodeficiency virus disease treated with zidovudine. J Infect Dis 1992;166:1223–1227.

57. George MJ, Snydman DR, Werner BG, Dougherty NN, Griffith J, Rohrer RH, Freeman R, Jenkins R, Lewis WD. Use of ganciclovir plus cytomegalovirus immune globulin to treat CMV pneumonia in orthotopic liver transplant recipients. The Boston Center for Liver Transplantation CMVIG Study Group. Transplant Proc 1993;25:22–24.

58. Gerna G, Furione M, Baldanti F, Sarasini A. Comparative quantitation of human cytomegalovirus DNA in blood leukocytes and plasma of transplant and AIDS patients. J Clin Microbiol 1994;32:2709–2717.

59. Gerna G, Zipeto D, Parea M, Revello MG, Silini E, Percivalle E, Zavattoni M, Grossi P, Milanesi G. Monitoring of human cytomegalovirus infections and ganciclovir treatment in heart transplant recipients by determination of viremia, antigenemia, and DNAemia. J Infect Dis 1991;164:488–498.

60. Golden JA. Cytomegalovirus infection or disease. Ann Intern Med 1984;101:882–883.

61. Goodgame RW. Gastrointestinal cytomegalovirus disease. Ann Intern Med 1993;119:924–935.

62. Goodrich JM, Bowden RA, Fisher L, Keller C, Schoch G, Meyers JD. Ganciclovir prophylaxis to prevent cytomegalovirus disease after allogeneic marrow transplant. Ann Intern Med 1993;118:173–178.

63. Goodrich JM, Mori M, Gleaves CA, DuMond C, Cays M, Ebeling DF, Buhles WC, DeArmond B, Meyers JD. Early treatment with ganciclovir to prevent cytomegalvoirus disease after allogeneic bone marrow transplantation. N Engl J Med 1991;325:1601–1607.

64. Hardy D, Spector S, Polsky B, Crumpacker C, van der Horst C, Holland G, Freeman W, Heinemann MH, Sharuk G, Klystra J. Combination of ganciclovir and granulocyte-macrophage colony-stimulating factor in the treatment of cytomegalovirus retinitis in AIDS patients. Eur J Clin Microbiol Infect Dis 1994;13:34–40.

65. Hengge UR, Brockmeyer NH, Malessa R, Ravens U, Goos M. Foscarnet penetrates the blood-brain barrier: rationale for therapy of cytomegalovirus encephalitis. Antimicrob Agents Chemother 1993;37:1010–1014.

66. Henry K, Cantrill H, Fletcher C, Chinnock BJ, Balfour HH. Use of intravitreal ganciclovir (dihydroxy propoxymethyl guanine) for cytomegalovirus retinitis in a patient with AIDS. Am J Ophthalmol 1987;103:17–23.

67. Herry I, Cadranel J, Antoine M. Cytomegalovirus-induced alveolar hemorrhage in patients with AIDS: a new clinical entity? Clin Infect Dis 1996;22:616–620.

68. Hibberd PL, Tolkoff-Rubin NE, Conti D, Stuart F, Thistlethwaite JR, Neylan JF, Snydman DR, Freeman R, Lorber MI, Rubin RH. Preemptive ganciclovir therapy to prevent cytomegalovirus disease in cytomegalovirus antibody-positive renal transplant recipients: a randomized controlled trial. Ann Intern Med 1995;123:18–26.

69. Ho HT, Woods KL, Bronson JJ, DeBoeck H, Martin JC, Hitchcock MJM. Intracellular metabolism of the antiherpes agent (S)-1-[3-hydroxy-2-(phosphonylmethoxy)-propyl]cytosine. Mol Pharmacol 1991;41:197–202.

70. Ho M. Human cytomegalovirus infections in immunosuppressed patients. In: Cytomegalovirus: biology and infection. New York: Plenum Medical, 1991:249–300.

71. Ho M. Virological diagnosis and infections in cells and tissues. In: Cytomegalovirus: biology and infection. New York: Plenum Medical, 1991:75–100.

72. Hochster H, Dieterich D, Bozzette S, Reichman RC, Connor JD,

Liebes L, Sonke RL, Spector SA, Valentine F, Pettinelli, Reichman DD. Toxicity of combined ganciclovir and zidovudine for cytomegalovirus disease associated with AIDS. Ann Intern Med 1990;113:111–117.

73. Holland GN, Gottlieb MS, Yee RD, Schanker HM, Pettit TH. Ocular disorders associated with a new severe acquired cellular immunodeficiency syndrome. Am J Ophthalmol 1982;93:393–402.

74. Holland GN, Levinson RD, Jacobson MA, AIDS Clinical Trials Group Protocol 915 Team. Dose-related difference in progression rates of cytomegalovirus retinopathy during foscarnet maintenance therapy. Am J Ophthalmol 1995;119:576–586.

75. Holland GN, Sakamoto MJ, Hardy D, Sidikaro Y, Kreiger AE, Frenkel LM. Treatment of cytomegalovirus retinopathy in patients with acquired immunodeficiency syndrome. Arch Ophthalmol 1986;104:1794–1800.

76. Holland GN, Sidikaro Y, Kreiger AE, Hardy D, Sakamoto MJ, Frenkel LM, Winston DJ, Gottlieb MS, Bryson YJ, Champlin RE. Treatment of cytomegalovirus retinopathy with ganciclovir. Ophthalmology 1987;94:815–823.

77. Holland NR, Power C, Mathews VP, Glass JD, Forman M, McArthur JC. Cytomegalovirus encephalitis in acquired immunodeficiency syndrome (AIDS). Neurology 1994;44:507–514.

78. Hrebinko R, Jordan ML, Dummer JS, Hickey DP, Shapiro R, Vivas C, Starzl TE, Simmons RL, Hakala TR. Ganciclovir for invasive cytomegalovirus infection in renal allograft recipients. Transplant Proc 1991;23:1346–1347.

79. Jabs DA, Enger C, Bartlett JG. Cytomegalovirus retinitis and acquired immunodeficiency syndrome. Arch Ophthalmol 1989;107:75–80.

80. Jacobson MA. Review of the toxicities of foscarnet [Review]. J Acquir Immune Defic Syndr 1992;1.

81. Jacobson MA. Treatment of cytomegalovirus retinitis in patients with the acquired immunodeficiency syndrome. N Engl J Med 1997;105–114.

82. Jacobson MA, Causey D, Polsky B, Hardy D, Chown M, Davis R, O'Donnell JJ, Kuppermann BD, Heinemann MH, Holland GN. A dose-ranging study of daily maintenance-intravenous foscarnet therapy for cytomegalovirus retinitis in AIDS. J Infect Dis 1993;168:444–448.

83. Jacobson MA, Mills J. Serious cytomegalovirus disease in the acquired immunodeficiency syndrome (AIDS): clinical findings, diagnosis, and treatment. Ann Intern Med 1988;108:585–594.

84. Jacobson MA, Wulfsohn M, Feinberg JE, Davis R, Power M, Owens S, Causey D, Heath-Chiozzi ME, Murphy RL, Cheung TW. Phase II dose-ranging trial of foscarnet salvage therapy for cytomegalovirus retinitis in AIDS patients intolerant of or resistant to ganciclovir (ACTG protocol 093). AIDS Clinical Trials Group of the National Institute of Allergy and Infectious Diseases. AIDS 1994;8:451–459.

85. Jacobson MA, Zegans M, Paven PR, O'Donnell JJ, Sattler F, Rao N, Owens S, Pollard R. Cytomegalovirus retinitis after initiation of highly active antiretroviral therapy. Lancet 1997;349:1443–1445.

86. Jacobson MA, Mills J, Rush J, Peiperl L, Seru V, Mohanty PK, Hopewell PC, Hadley WK, Broadus VC, Leoung G. Morbidity and mortality of patients with AIDS and first-episode Pneumocystis carinii pneumonia unaffected by concomitant pulmonary cytomegalovirus infection. Am Rev Respir Dis 1991;144:6–9.

87. Jazzar A, Cooper DK, Zuhdi N. Cytomegalovirus disease in heart transplant patients. Transplantation 1991;53:1167–1168.

88. Jensen A-MB, Lundgren JD, Benfield T, Nielsen TL, Vestbo J. Does cytomegalovirus predict a poor prognosis in Pneumocystis carinii pneumonia treated with corticosteriods? A note for caution. Chest 1995;108:411–414.

89. Kalayjian RC, Cohen ML, Bonomo RA, Flanigan TP. Cytomegalovirus ventriculoencephalitis in AIDS: A syndrome with distinct clinical and pathologic features. Medicine 1993;72:67–77.

90. Kaplan CS, Petersen EA, Icenogle TB, Copeland JG, Villar HV, Sampliner R, Minnich L, Ray CG. Gastrointestinal cytomegalovirus infection in heart and heart-lung transplant recipients. Arch Intern Med 1989;149:2095–2100.

91. Kasiske BL, Heim-Duthoy KL, Tortorice KL, Ney AL, Odland MD, Venkateswara R. Polyvalent immune globulin and cytomegalovirus infection after renal transplantation. Arch Intern Med 1989;149:2733–2736.

92. Kim YS, Hollander H. Polyradiculopathy due to cytomegalovirus: report of two cases in which improvement occurred after prolonged therapy and review of the literature. Clin Infect Dis 1993;17:32–37.

93. Kirsch LS, Arevalo F, de la Paz EC, Munguia D, deClercq E, Freeman WR. Intravitreal cidofovir (HPMPC) treatment of cytomegalovirus retinitis in patients with acquired immune deficiency syndrome. Ophthalmology 1995;102:533–543.

94. Kubanek B, Ernst P, Ostendorf P, Schafer U, Wold H. Preliminary data of a controlled trial of intravenous hyperimmune globulin in the prevention of cytomegalovirus infection in bone marrow transplant recipients. Transplant Proc 1985;17:468–469.

95. Kuppermann BD, Flores-Aguilar M, Quiceno JI, Rickman LS, Freeman WR. Combination ganciclovir and foscarnet in the treatment of clinically resistant cytomegalovirus retinitis in patients with acquired immunodeficiency syndrome. Arch Ophthalmol 1993;111:1359–1366.

96. Lalezari JP, Drew WL, Glutzer E, James C, Miner D, Flaherty J, Fisher PE, Cundy K, Hannigan J, Martin JC. (S)-1[3-hydroxy-2(phosphonylmethoxy)propyl]cytosine (Cidofovir): results of a phase I/II study of a novel antiviral nucleotide analogue. J Infect Dis 1995;171:788–796.

97. Lalezari JP, Stagg RJ, Kuppermann BD, Holland GN, KrAm F, Ives DV, Youle M, Robinson MR, Drew WL, Jaffe HS. Intravenous cidofovir for peripheral cytomegalovirus retinitis in patients with AIDS. Ann Intern Med 1997;126:257–263.

98. Lang DJ, Cheung KS. Effectiveness of acycloguanosine and trifluorothymidine as inhibitors of cytomegalovirus in vitro. Am J Med 1982;735:49–53.

99. Ljungman P, Engelhard D, Link H. Treatment of interstitial pneumonitis due to cytomegalovirus with ganciclovir and intravenous immune globulin: experience of European bone marrow. Clin Infect Dis 1992;14:831–835.

100. Manian FA, Smith T. Ganciclovir for the treatment of cytomegalovirus pneumonia in an immunocompetent host. Clin Infect Dis 1993;17:137–138.

101. Martin DF, Parks DJ, Mellow SD, Ferris FL, Walton RC, Remaley NA, Chew EY, Ashton P, David MD, Nussenblatt RB. Treatment of cytomegalovirus retinitis with an intraocular sustained-release ganciclovir implant: a randomized controlled clinical trial. Arch Ophthalmol 1994;112:1531–1539.

102. Martin M, Manez R, Linden P, Estores D, Torre-Cisneros J, Kusne S, Ondick L, Ptachcinski R, Irish W, Kisor D. A prospective randomized trial comparing sequential ganciclovir–high dose acyclovir to high dose acyclovir for prevention of cy-

tomegalovirus disease in adult liver transplant recipients. Transplantation 1994;58:779–785.

103. Masur H, Lane HC, Palestine A, Smith PD, Manischewitz J, Stevens G, Fujikawa L, Macher AM, Nussenblatt R, Baird B. Effect of 9(1,3-dihydroxy-2-propoxymethyl)guanine on serious cytomegalovirus disease in eight immunosuppressed homosexuals. Ann Intern Med 1986;104:41–44.

104. Mayoral JL, Loeffler CM, Fasola CG, KrAm MA, Orrom WJ, Matas AJ, Najarian JS, Dunn DL. Diagnosis and treatment of cytomegalovirus disease in transplant patients based on gastrointestinal tract manifestations. Arch Surg 1991;126:202–206.

105. Mazzulli T, Rubin RH, Ferraro MJ, D'Aquila RT, Doveikis SA, Smith BR, The TH, Hirsch MS. Cytomegalovirus antigenemia: clinical correlations in transplant recipients and in persons with AIDS. J Clin Microbiol 1993;31:2824–2827.

106. McCutchan JA. Cytomegalovirus infections of the nervous system in patients with AIDS. Clin Infect Dis 1995;20:747–754.

107. McGuinness G, Scholes JV, Garay SM, Leitman BS, McCauley DI, Naidich DP. Cytomegalovirus pneumonitis: spectrum of parenchymal CT findings with pathologic correlation in 21 AIDS patients. Radiology 1994;192:451–459.

108. Merigan TC, Renlund DG, Keay S, Bristow MR, Starnes V, O'Connell JB, Resta S, Dunn D, Gamberg P, Ratkovec RM. A controlled trial of ganciclovir to prevent cytomegalovirus disease after heart transplantation. N Engl J Med 1992;326:1182–1186.

109. Meyers JD, Reed EC, Shepp DH, Thornquist M, Dandliker PS, Vicary CA, Flournoy N, Kirk LE, Kersey JH, Thomas ED. Acyclovir for prevention of cytomegalovirus infection and disease after allogenic marrow transplantation. N Engl J Med 1988;318:70–75.

110. Meyers JD, Wade JC, McGuffin RW, Springmeyer SC, Thomas ED. The use of acyclovir for cytomegalovirus infections in the immunocompromised host. J Antimicrob Chemother 1983;12:181–193.

111. Meyers J, Flournoy N, Thomas ED. Risk factors for cytomegalovirus infection after human marrow transplant. J Infect Dis 1986;153:478.

112. Mills J, Jacobson MA, O'Donnell JJ, Cederberg D, Honnand GN. Treatment of cytomegalovirus retinitis in patients with AIDS. Rev Infect Dis 1988;3:S522–531.

113. Miles PR, Baughman RP, Linnemann CC. Cytomegalovirus in bronchoalveolar lavage fluid of patients with AIDS. Chest 1990;97:1072–1076.

114. Morley MG, Duker JS, Ashton P, Robinson MR. Replacing ganciclovir implants. Ophthalmology 1995;102:388–392.

115. Musch DC, Martin DF, Gordon JF, Davis MD, Kuppermann BD. Treatment of cytomegalovirus retinitis with a sustained-release ganciclovir implant. The Ganciclovir Implant Study Group. N Engl J Med 1997;337:83–90.

116. Nakazato PZ, Burns W, Moore P, Garcia-Kennedy R, Cox K, Equivel C. Viral prophylaxis in hepatic transplantation: preliminary report of a randomized trial of acyclovir and ganciclovir. Transplant Proc 1993;25:1935–1937.

117. Nigro G, Scholz H, Bartmann U. Ganciclovir therapy for symptomatic congenital cytomegalovirus infection in infants: a two-regimen experience. J Pediatr 1994;124(2):318–322.

118. O'Brien JS, Campoli-Richards DM. Acyclovir—an updated review of its antiviral activity, pharmacokinetic properties and therapeutic efficacy. Drugs 1989;37:233–309.

119. O'Reilly RJ, Reich L, Gold J, Kirkpatrick D, Dinsmore R, Kapoor N, Candie R. A randomized trial of intravenous hyper-

immune globulin for the prevention of cytomegalovirus (CMV) infections following marrow transplantation: preliminary results. Transplant Proc 1983;15:1405–1411.

120. Orellana J, Teich SA, Lieberman RM, Restrepo S, Peairs R. Treatment of retinal detachments in patients with the acquired immune deficiency syndrome. Ophthalmology 1991;98:939–943.

121. OGEAC. The Oral Ganciclovir European and Australian Cooperative Study Group. Intravenous versus oral ganciclovir: European/Australian comparative study of efficacy and safety in the prevention of cytomegalovirus retinitis recurrence in patients with AIDS. AIDS 1995;9:471–477.

122. Palestine AG, Polis MA, DeSmet MD, Baird BF, Falloon J, Kovacs JA, Davey RT, Zurlo JJ, Zunich KM, Davis M, Hubbard L, Brothers R, Ferris FL, Chew E, Davis JL, Rubin BI, Mellow SD, Metcalf JA, Manischewitz MS, Minor JR, Nussenblatt RB, Masur H, Lane HC. A randomized, controlled trial of foscarnet in the treatment of cytomegalovirus retinitis in patients with AIDS. Ann Intern Med 1991;115:665–673.

123. Patel R, Smith TF, Espy M, Portela D, Wiesner RH, Krom RA, Paya CV. A prospective comparison of molecular diagnostic techniques for the early detection of cytomegalovirus in liver transplant recipients. J Infect Dis 1995;171:1010–1014.

124. Pescovitz M, Gane E, Saliba F, Valdecasas G, O'Grady J, Behrend M, Pruett T, Hockerstedt K, Walker M, Robinson C. Efficacy and safety of oral ganciclovir in the prevention of cytomegalovirus (CMV) disease in liver transplant recipients. Abstracts of the 36th Interscience Conference on Antibiotics and Chemotherapy, 1996:163.

125. Peterson PK, Balfour HH, Marker SC, Fryd DS, Howard RJ, Simmons RL. Cytomegalovirus disease in renal allograft recipients: a prospective study of the clinical features, risk factors and impact on renal transplantation. Medicine 1980;59:283–300.

126. Polis MA, Spooner KM, Baird BF, Manischewitz JF, Jaffe HS, Fisher PE, Falloon J, Davey RT Jr, Kovacs JA, Walker RE. Anticytomegaloviral activity and safety of cidofovir in patients with human immunodeficiency virus infection and cytomegalovirus viruria. Antimicrob Agents Chemother 1995;39:882–886.

127. Pollard RB, Egbert PR, Gallagher JG, Merigan TC. Cytomegalovirus retinitis in immunosuppressed hosts. I. Natural history and effects of treatment and adenine arabinoside. Ann Intern Med 1980;93:655–664.

128. Prentice HG, Gluckman E, Powles RL, Ljungman P, Milpied N, Fernandez, Ranada JM, Mandelli F, Kho P, Kennedy L, Bell AR. Impact of long-term acyclovir on cytomegalovirus infection and survival after allogeneic bone marrow transplantation. Lancet 1994;343:749–753.

129. Price TA, Digioia RA, Simon GL. Ganciclovir treatment of cytomegalovirus ventriculitis in a patient infected with human immunodeficiency virus. Clin Infect Dis 1992;15:606–608.

130. Reed EC. Treatment of cytomegalovirus pneumonia in transplant patients. Transplant Proc 1991;23:8–12.

131. Reed EC, Bowden RA, Dandliker PS, Lilleby KE, Meyers JD. Treatment of cytomegalovirus pneumonia with ganciclovir and intravenous cytomegalovirus immunoglobulin in patients with bone marrow transplants. Ann Intern Med 1988;109:783–788.

132. Reed EC, Wolford JL, Kopecky KJ, Lilleby KE, Dandliker PS, Tolaro JL, McDonald GB, Meyers JD. Ganciclovir for the treatment of cytomegalovirus gastroenteritis in bone marrow transplant patients. Ann Intern Med 1990;112:505–510.

133. Ringden O, Pihlstedt P, Volin L, Nikoskelainen J, Lonnqvist B, Ruutu P, Ruutu T, Toivanen A, Wahren B. Failure to prevent

cytomegalovirus infection by cytomegalovirus hyperimmune plasma: a randomized trial by the Nordic Bone Marrow Transplantation Group. Bone Marrow Transplant 1987;2:299–305.

134. Roizman B. Herpesviridae: a brief introduction. In: BN Fields, DM Knipe, eds. Virology. New York: Raven Press, 1990: 1787–1794.

135. Rondeau E, Bourgeon B, Peraldi MN, Lang P, Buisson C, Schulte KM, Weill B, Sraer JD. Effect of prophylactic ganciclovir on cytomegalovirus infection in renal transplant recipients. Nephrol Dial Transplant 1993;8:858–862.

136. Rosen HR, Benner KG, Flora KD, Rabkin JM, Orloff SL, Olyaei A, Chou S. Development of ganciclovir resistance during treatment of primary cytomegalovirus infection after liver transplantation. Transplantation 1997;63:476–478.

137. Roullet E, Assueurs V, Gozlan J, Ropert A, Said G, Baudrimont M, el Amrani M, Jacomet C, Duvivier C, Gonzales-Canali G. Cytomegalovirus multifocal neuropathy in AIDS: analysis of 15 consecutive cases. Neurology 1994;44:2174–2182.

138. Salazar A, Podzamczer D, Rene R, Santin M, Perez JL, Ferrer I, Fernandez-Viladrich P, Gudiol F. Cytomegalovirus ventriculoencephalitis in AIDS patients. Scand J Infect Dis 1995;27: 165–169.

139. Saliba F, Arulnaden JL, Gugenheim J, Serves C, Samuel D, Bismuth A, Mathieu D, Bismuth H. CMV hyperimmune globulin prophylaxis after liver transplantation: a prospective randomized controlled study. Transplant Proc 1989;21:2260–2262.

140. Saliba F, Eyraud D, Samuel MF, David MF, Arulnaden JL, Dussaix E, Mathiew D, Bismuth H. Randomized controlled trial of acyclovir for the prevention of cytomegalovirus infection and disease in liver transplant recipients. Transplant Proc 1993;25:1444–1445.

141. Stanat SC, Reardon JE, Erice A, Jordan MC, Drew WL, Biron KK. Ganciclovir-resistant cytomegalovirus clinical isolates: mode of resistance to ganciclovir. Antimicrob Agents Chemother 1991;35:2191–2197.

142. Schmidt GM, Horak DA, Niland JC, Duncan SR, Forman SJ, Zaia JA. A randomized, controlled trial of prophylactic ganciclovir for cytomegalovirus pulmonary infection in recipients of allogeneic bone marrow transplants. N Engl J Med 1991;324: 1005–1011.

143. Schulman LL, Reison DS, Austin JH, Rose EA. Cytomegalovirus pneumonitis after cardiac transplantation. Arch Intern Med 1991;151:1118–1124.

144. Shuster EA, Beneke JS, Tegtmeier GE, Pearson GR, Gleaves CA, Wold AD, Smith TF. Monoclonal antibody for rapid laboratory detection of cytomegalovirus infections: characterization and diagnostic application. Mayo Clinic Proc 1985;60: 577–585.

145. Singh N, Yu VL, Mieles L, Wagener MM, Miner RC, Gayowski T. High-dose acyclovir compared with short-course preemptive ganciclovir therapy to prevent cytomegalovirus disease in liver transplant recipients: a randomized trial. Ann Intern Med 1994;120:375–381.

146. Small PM, McPhaul LW, Sooy CD, Wofsy CB, Jacobson MA. Cytomegalovirus infection of the laryngeal nerve presenting as hoarseness in patients with acquired immunodeficiency syndrome. Am J Med 1989;86:108–110.

147. Smith TJ, Pearson PA, Blandford DL, Brown JD, Goins KA, Hollins JL, Schmeisser ET, Glavinos P, Baldwin LB, Ashton P. Intravitreal sustained-release ganciclovir. Arch Ophthalmol 1992;110:255–258.

148. Snydman DR, Werner BG, Dougherty NN, Griffith J, Rubin RH, Dienstag JL, Rohrer RH, Freeman R, Jenkins R, Lewis WD. Cytomegalovirus immune globulin prophylaxis in liver transplantation. A randomized, double-blind, placebo-controlled trial. The Boston Center for Liver Transplantation CMVIG Study Group. Ann Intern Med 1993;119:984–991.

149. Snydman DR, Werner BG, Dougherty NN, Griffith J, Rohrer RH, Freeman R, Jenkins R, Lewis WD, O'Rourke E. A further analysis of the use of cytomegalovirus immune globulin in orthotopic liver transplant patients at risk for primary infection. Transplant Proc 1994;26:23–27.

150. Snydman DR, Werner BG, Heinze-Lacey B, Berardi VP, Tilney NL, Kirkman RL, Milford EL, Cho SI, Bush HL Jr, Levey AS. Use of cytomegalovirus immune globulin to prevent cytomegalovirus disease in renal transplant recipients. N Engl J Med 1987;317:1049–1054.

151. SOCA. Studies of Ocular Complications of AIDS Research Group with the AIDS Clinical Trials Group. Mortality in patients with the acquired immunodeficiency syndrome treated with either foscarnet or ganciclovir for cytomegalovirus retinitis. N Engl J Med 1992;326:213–220.

152. SOCA. Foscarnet-ganciclovir cytomegalovirus retinitis trial IV: visual outcomes. Studies of Ocular Complications of AIDS Research Group in collaboration with the AIDS Clinical Trials Group. Ophthalmology 1994;101:1250–1261.

153. SOCA. Studies of Ocular Complications of AIDS Research Group with the AIDS Clinical Trials Group. Morbidity and toxic effects associated with ganciclovir or foscarnet therapy in a randomized cytomegalovirus retinitis trial. Arch Intern Med 1995;155:65–74.

154. SOCA. Studies of Ocular Complications of AIDS Research Group in collaboration with the AIDS Clinical Trials Group. Combination foscarnet and ganciclovir therapy vs monotherapy for the treatment of relapsed cytomegalovirus retinitis in patients with AIDS. Arch Ophthalmol 1996;114:23–33.

155. SOCA, Studies of Ocular Complications of AIDS Research Group in Collaboration with the AIDS Clinical Trials Group. Parenteral cidofovir for cytomegalovirus retinitis in patients with AIDS: the HPMPC peripheral cytomegalovirus retinitis trial. Ann Intern Med 1997;126:264–274.

156. Sommadossi JP, Bevan R, Ling T, Lee F, Mastre B, Chaplin MD, Nerenberg C, Koretz S, Buhles WC Jr. Clinical pharmacokinetics of ganciclovir in patients with normal and impaired renal function. Rev Infect Dis 1988;10:S507–514.

157. Spector SA, Busch DF, Follensbee S, Squires K, Lalezari JP, Jacobson MA, Connor JD, Jung D, Shadman A, Mastre B. Pharmacokinetic, safety and antiviral profiles of oral ganciclovir in persons infected with human immunodeficiency virus: a phase I/II study. J Infect Dis 1995;171:1431–1437.

158. Spector SA, McKinley GF, Lalezari JP, Samo T, Andruczk R, Follansbee S, Sparti PD, Havlir DV, Simpson G, Buhles W, Wong R, Stempien M. Oral ganciclovir for the prevention of cytomegalovirus disease in persons with AIDS. N Engl J Med 1996;334:1491–1497.

159. Spector SA, Weingeist T, Pollard RB, Dieterich DT, Samo T, Benson CA, Busch DF, Freeman WF, Montague P, Kaplan HJ, Kellerman L, Crager M, DeArmond B, Buhles W, Feinberg J, AIDS Clinical Trials Group, and Cytomegalovirus Cooperative Study Group. A randomized, controlled study of intravenous ganciclovir therapy for cytomegalovirus peripheral retinitis in patients with AIDS. J Infect Dis 1993;168:557–563.

160. Stanat SC, Reardon JE, Erice A, Jordan MC, Drew WL, Biron KK. Ganciclovir-resistant cytomegalovirus clinical isolates:

Mode of resistance to ganciclovir. Antimicrob Agents Chemother. 1991;35:2191–2197.

161. Stover DE, White DA, Romano PA, Gellene RA, Robeson WA. Spectrum of pulmonary diseases associated with the acquired immune deficiency syndrome. Am J Med 1985;78:429–437.

162. Stratta RJ, Shaefer MS, Cushing KA, Markin RS, Reed EC, Langnas AN, Pillen TJ, Shaw BW Jr. A randomized prospective trial of acyclovir and immune globulin prophylaxis in liver transplant recipients receiving OKT3 therapy. Arch Surg 1992; 127:55–64.

163. Sullivan KM, Kopecky KJ, Jocom J, Fisher L, Buckner CD, Meyers JD, Counts GW, Bowden RA, Peterson FB, Witherspoon RP. Immunomodulatory and antimicrobial efficacy of intravenous immunoglobulin in bone marrow transplantation. N Engl J Med 1990;323:705–711.

164. Sullivan V, Biron KK, Talarico C, Stanat SC, Davis M, Pozzi M, Coen DM. A point mutation in the human cytomegalovirus DNA polymerase gene confers resistance to ganciclovir and phosphonylmethoxyalkyl derivatives. Antimicrob Agents Chemother 1993;37:19–25.

165. Sullivan V, Coen DM. Isolation of foscarnet-resistant human cytomegalovirus patterns of resistance and sensitivity to other antiviral drugs. J Infect Dis 1991;164:781–784.

166. Wallace JM, Hannah J. Cytomegalovirus pneumonitis in patients with AIDS. Chest 1987;92:198–203.

167. Weinberg DV, Murphy R, Naughton K. Combined daily therapy with intravenous ganciclovir and foscarnet for patients with recurrent cytomegalovirus retinitis. Am J Ophthalmol 1994; 117:776–782.

168. Whitley RJ, Cloud G, Gruber W, Storch GA, Demmler GJ, Jacobs RF, Dankner W, Spector SA, Starr S, Pass RF, Stagno S, Britt WJ, Alford C Jr, Soong S-J, Zhou X-J, Sherrill L, FitzGerald JM, Sommadossi J-P, NIH/NIAID Collaborative Antiviral Study Group. Ganciclovir treatment of symptomatic congenital cytomegalovirus infection: results of a phase II study. J Infect Dis. 1997;175:1080–1086.

169. Winston DJ, Ho WG, Bartoni K, DuMond C, Ebeling DF, Buhles WC, Champlin RE. Ganciclovir prophylaxis of cytomegalovirus infection and disease in allogeneic bone marrow transplant recipients: results of a placebo-controlled, double-blind trial. Ann Intern Med 1993;118:179–184.

170. Winston DJ, Ho WG, Lin CH, Bartoni K, Budinger MD, Gale RP, Champlin RE. Intravenous immune globulin for prevention of cytomegalovirus infection and interstitial pneumonia after bone marrow transplantation. Ann Intern Med 1987;106: 12–18.

171. Winston DJ, Wirin D, Shaked A, Busuttil RW. Randomized comparison of ganciclovir and high-dose acyclovir for long-term cytomegalovirus prophylaxis in liver-transplant recipients. Lancet 1995;346:69–74.

Epstein-Barr Virus and Human Herpesvirus-8

●

Fred Wang

GENERAL DESCRIPTION

Epstein-Barr virus (EBV; human herpesvirus-4) and human herpesvirus-8 (HHV-8; Kaposi's sarcoma herpesvirus) are human herpesviruses belonging to the gamma herpesvirus subgroup. Herpesviruses in this subgroup have tropism for lymphocytes with predilection for latent, rather than lytic, infection. EBV and HHV-8 replicate during lytic infection by mechanisms common to all herpesviruses, and nucleoside analogues such as acyclovir, ganciclovir, and foscarnet have antiviral activity against lytic infection with these gamma herpesviruses. However, diseases induced by EBV and HHV-8 are frequently associated with latent infection; therefore, nucleoside analogues active against lytic replication may not be effective clinically. Currently, treatment of diseases associated with EBV and HHV-8 is more often directed against virus-induced tumors or disease symptoms than against viral replication. Pharmacologic intervention in pathways important for latent infection and vaccines to prevent infection or attenuate disease are potential areas for therapeutic development.

Microbiology and Pathogenesis

Epstein-Barr virus is associated with a variety of clinical disorders arising from different pathogenic mechanisms (reviewed in (50) and (24)). Primary EBV infection usually begins with lytic infection in the oropharynx leading to latent infection of peripheral blood B cells. Infectious virus is produced during lytic infection, and EBV replication is mechanistically similar to that of other herpesviruses. In contrast, during latent EBV infection there is no active viral replication, the viral genome persists as a circular episome, only a limited repertoire of latent viral genes is expressed, and these latent viral genes can cause uncontrolled cell growth. The sudden appearance of latent EBV-infected, growth-transformed B cells stimulates a vigorous humoral and cellular immune response that can result in the characteristic clinical syndrome of infectious mononucleosis. Many aspects of this clinical syndrome (e.g., fever, lymphadenopathy, splenomegaly, atypical lymphocytosis) are due to the vigorous T cell proliferation and cytokine response of the immune system rather than direct viral infection, replication, and cytolysis.

After resolution of the acute syndrome, EBV persists for life as a latent infection in B cells and as a lytic infection in the oropharynx. Persistent EBV infection is controlled by a virus-specific immune response and is asymptomatic in most humans. However, immunosuppression associated with HIV infection, transplantation, or congenital immunodeficiencies can result in uncontrolled latent infection with oligoclonal or monoclonal B cell proliferation or uncontrolled lytic infection in the oropharynx manifested as oral hairy leukoplakia. Persistent, latent EBV infection is also associated with development of Burkitt's lymphoma, nasopharyngeal carcinoma, and certain types of Hodgkin's disease. Determining how latent EBV genes function to affect cell growth is an active area of investigation that may provide novel opportunities for pharmacologic intervention in EBV latent infection and associated malignancies.

The pathogenesis of HHV-8 associated diseases is not as well defined. Infection with HHV-8 in the general population does not appear to be as ubiquitous as infection with EBV and other human herpesviruses (12, 14, 32, 55). Serologic and pathologic studies provide strong epidemiologic evidence for association of HHV-8 with development of Kaposi's sarcoma (KS) in HIV-infected and noninfected patients (11, 21, 29). Latent HHV-8 infection has also been closely associated with certain types of body cavity B cell lymphomas (BCBL) (4, 5) in AIDS patients and with Castleman's disease (57). The importance of more recent reports of HHV-8 infection in multiple myeloma and prostate tissue (26, 34, 49) remains to be determined.

How HHV-8 infection might contribute to development of KS, Castleman's disease, and BCBL is an equally vigorous area of investigation. The HHV-8 genome has been fully cloned and sequenced (52). The identity and function of latency-associated HHV-8 transcripts expressed in B cell lymphomas and KS spindle cells is just beginning to emerge. Like other viruses, HHV-8 also encodes for homologues of cellular genes that can modulate cell growth and host immunity (40). A unifying concept for the natural history of HHV-8 infection and viral pathogenesis in KS and other malignancies remains to be developed. Existing data suggest that HHV-8 is not a transforming virus sufficient for development of KS. It is most likely that other factors act in combination with HHV-8 to result in malignant conversion, not unlike the role of EBV in Burkitt's lymphoma and nasopharyngeal carcinoma. Thus, antiviral agents that inhibit HHV-8 replication can be identified in vitro using virus-infected cell lines, but whether these agents will be clinically effective requires a better understanding of viral pathogenesis and clinical evaluation. Vaccination, immunomodulation, or pharmacologic intervention of important cell-signaling pathways usurped by viral gene products might provide more effective therapeutic strategies against gamma herpesvirus–associated malignancies than traditional antiviral drugs designed to block viral replication.

SUSCEPTIBILITY IN VITRO AND IN VIVO

Because gamma herpesvirus infection typically results in latent infection rather than lytic infection associated with plaque formation, EBV and HHV-8 sensitivity to antiviral drugs cannot be assayed by conventional plaque reduction assays. In-stead, latently infected cell lines are used in which a fraction of cells can be induced to lytic viral replication in the presence or absence of potential antiviral agents. Antiviral activity is measured by quantifying viral DNA and is expressed as the concentration of drug required to inhibit 50% of induced viral DNA replication (IC_{50}). Using these types of assays, acyclovir has an IC_{50} of 0.3 μM for EBV and 60 to 80 μM for HHV-8, and ganciclovir has an IC_{50} of 0.05 μM for EBV and 2.7 to 4 μM for HHV-8 (7, 23, 27). The anti-HHV-8 activity of the newer, clinically approved nucleoside analogues foscarnet and cidofovir has been reported to be 80 to 100 μM and 0.5 to 1 μM, respectively (23).

While it was originally hypothesized that acyclovir was effective against EBV in the absence of an EBV-specified thymidine kinase (TK) (42), EBV does encode a TK (BXLF1), which was belatedly discovered because of the difficulties of inducing EBV lytic replication in vitro (28). The EBV TK shares approximately 50% amino acid similarity with the HSV TK and can use acyclovir and ganciclovir as substrates. Similarly, the EBV DNA polymerase (BALF5) shares approximately 70% amino acid similarity with the HSV DNA polymerase, reflecting the common heritage of lytic replication mechanisms. The HHV-8 sequence reveals both TK (ORF21) and DNA polymerase (ORF9) genes with similar degrees of homology (52). The conserved mechanisms of lytic replication among herpesviruses suggests that other antiviral drugs developed against herpes simplex or cytomegalovirus replication may have activity against EBV and HHV-8.

Despite the effectiveness of acyclovir against EBV lytic replication, acyclovir has no inhibitory activity on replication of the episomal EBV genomes present in latent infection. Thus, acyclovir inhibits production of linear genomes in the minority of cells entering lytic infection in an EBV-infected B cell line, but episomal DNA is replicated by cell DNA polymerases and is unaffected by acyclovir in the majority of EBV-infected B cells that are latently infected. Once removed, lytic replication can resume from the latent EBV genomes (6, 42). Thus, immortal B cell growth induced by latent EBV infection is unaffected by acyclovir treatment in vitro; these in vitro studies are consistent with the clinical experience that nucleoside analogues have little effect on EBV-induced malignancies associated with latent EBV infection.

The potential efficacy of nucleoside analogues against HHV-8-associated KS was considered retrospectively by the Multicenter AIDS Cohort Study (13). While this study found that acyclovir, ganciclovir, or foscarnet use during HIV infection did not significantly reduce the risk of KS, it did not exclude the possibility of a clinical role for nucleoside analogues in HHV-8 infection, since treatment regimens may not have been sufficiently stringent to provide adequate prophylaxis against HHV-8 infection. Additional clinical studies are required to define a role for nucleoside analogues in prevention of HHV-8 infection or treatment of established HHV-8-infected malignancies in which the role of viral replication in malignant pathogenesis is unknown.

The issue of whether nucleoside analogues might be effective during primary gamma herpesvirus infection in which viral replication is more likely to play an important pathogenic role has been extensively studied in infectious mononucleosis. In 6 different studies involving a total of approximately 320 patients, oral or intravenous acyclovir therapy consistently reduced or eliminated lytic EBV infection during therapy as detected by virus shedding in oropharyngeal secretions but had no effect on clinical outcome, duration of symptoms, or establishment of persistent infection in the oropharynx or peripheral blood B lymphocytes (1, 2, 44, 63, 64, 66). Thus, acyclovir can effectively inhibit lytic EBV replication in vivo, but acyclovir treatment initiated after the onset of symptoms has no clinical benefit in infectious mononucleosis, most likely because latent infection has already been established, and the vigorous host immune response to virus infection responsible for the majority of symptoms has been triggered.

ANTIMICROBIAL THERAPY

Treatment of EBV-associated diseases is closely linked to the underlying pathogenesis of the disease. A simple and rapid means of diagnosing HHV-8 infection and the indications for treating HHV-8 infection remain to be defined. The usual treatment for EBV- or HHV-8-associated malignancies is based on cancer chemotherapy and radiation therapy rather than on antiviral strategies, and these options are not discussed here.

Infectious Mononucleosis

Supportive treatment is generally indicated since more than 95% of infectious mononucleosis cases resolve uneventfully without specific therapy. Aspirin or acetaminophen can be used to reduce fever. Use of concomitant antibiotics for possible bacterial pharyngitis should be judicious and supported by positive culture results because of the high incidence of allergic reactions to antibiotics such as ampicillin during acute infectious mononucleosis.

The use of corticosteroids for uncomplicated infectious mononucleosis is still controversial. Corticosteroids have been shown to reduce fever and shorten the duration of constitutional symptoms (3, 8, 25, 46, 54). However, adverse drug complications can arise from even short courses of corticosteroid use (8, 65), and corticosteroid use is probably best avoided for routine, a self-limited disease (30). Corticosteroid use is generally reserved for infectious mononucleosis complicated by potential airway obstruction from enlarged tonsils, severe thrombocytopenia, or severe hemolytic anemia (9, 46, 56). These complications result from the excessive immune response to virus infection rather than uncontrolled viral infection, and a short course of corticosteroids at 1 mg/kg/day of prednisone with tapering over 1 to 2 weeks can be effective in treating the excessive tonsillar proliferation or autoimmune symptoms. Corticosteroids might also be used for other autoimmune complications rarely associated with infectious mononucleosis such as central nervous system involvement, myocarditis, or pericarditis (30).

As described above, acyclovir provides no significant clinical benefit for treatment of uncomplicated infectious mononucleosis. The combination of acyclovir and corticosteroids for uncomplicated infectious mononucleosis still inhibits oral viral replication but provides no clinical benefit (63). In rare, complicated cases of primary EBV infection and infectious mononucleosis in which the patient is immunosuppressed or severely ill, acyclovir or ganciclovir treatment may be rational, given the safety profile of this drug, its ability to inhibit EBV replication in vitro and in vivo, and anecdotal reports of clinical response in unusual cases in which excessive EBV replication may have been pathogenic (10, 22, 41, 53).

Chronic Active EBV Infection/Chronic Fatigue Syndrome

Rare patients have an unusual clinical course following infectious mononucleosis with severe illness and evidence of chronic active EBV infection. These patients typically have extremely high antibody responses to EBV early antigens, lack antibodies to EBNA-1, and have severe disease with end-organ involvement or evidence of increased viral load in affected tissues (31, 53, 59). Both clinical responses and failures with acyclovir or corticosteroids have been noted in anecdotal reports of these unusual patients with chronic active EBV infection (53, 60).

EBV infection has also been implicated as a cause of the much more common chronic fatigue syndrome. However, seroepidemiologic studies have argued against a pathogenic role for EBV in chronic fatigue syndrome (19, 20). In addition, a placebo-controlled study with acyclovir showed no efficacy for patients with chronic fatigue syndrome (61).

Oral Hairy Leukoplakia

Oral hairy leukoplakia is an unusual lesion of the tongue found in HIV-infected patients. Vigorous EBV lytic replication occurs in the excessively proliferating epithelium. This is the only instance in which disease appears to be a direct consequence of lytic EBV replication, and oral acyclovir therapy (3.2 g/day) can temporarily reverse the lesions (48). However, since latent EBV infection persists in the basal epithelial cells and nucleoside analogues have no effect on latent EBV infection, lytic EBV replication and oral hairy leukoplakia frequently reoccur when therapy is withdrawn.

EBV-Induced Lymphoproliferations Associated with Immunosuppression

EBV-infected monoclonal or polyclonal B cell proliferations can arise during immunosuppression associated with congenital immunodeficiencies, transplantation, or HIV infection. Since latent EBV infection is responsible for driving uncontrolled B cell growth, nucleoside analogues generally are not effective against these malignant proliferations. While there are case reports that early, polyclonal EBV-induced B cell proliferations may respond to nucleoside analogues (17, 18), more aggressive or monoclonal EBV-induced B cell lymphoproliferations are generally not responsive to acyclovir (17, 18, 58). Some have suggested that a more active nucleoside analogue such as ganciclovir might be more effective against EBV-induced B cell lymphoproliferations. However, there is no good evidence to support this hypothesis, and it is counterintuitive to the underlying pathogenesis of latent EBV infection. There are no currently available agents effective against latent EBV infection.

If possible, the treatment of choice is to reduce the level of immunosuppression (16, 58). Recently, investigators have successfully treated EBV-induced lymphoproliferative disease by augmenting the host's immune response through adoptive transfer of EBV-specific cytotoxic T cells grown in vitro (45, 51). In these cases, the patient's T cells (or donor T cells in the case of bone marrow transplantation) are harvested prior to transplantation and stimulated in vitro with the autologous EBV-infected B cell line. Cytotoxic T cells specific for EBV antigens are stimulated and expanded in vitro. After transplantation, patients are monitored for EBV viral load by polymerase chain reaction for viral DNA in peripheral blood lymphocytes. If the viral load begins to increase beyond acceptable levels or if EBV-infected tumors are detected, the EBV-specific CTLs are infused. Adoptive transfer of EBV-specific CTLs has been shown to reduce the incidence of EBV-associated lymphoproliferative disease and to induce regression of established EBV-infected lymphoproliferations (45, 51).

EBV-Associated Malignancies (Burkitt's Lymphoma, Nasopharyngeal Carcinoma, Hodgkin's Disease)

There is no effective antiviral therapy for Burkitt's lymphoma, nasopharyngeal carcinoma, and Hodgkin's disease associated with EBV infection, and treatment is usually based upon cancer chemotherapy. Adoptive transfer of EBV-specific CTLs may also be useful for treating these types of EBV-associated malignancies, such as Hodgkin's disease. Novel pharmacologic approaches against latent EBV infection may be another approach for treating these diseases. Antisense oligonucleotides may be used to disrupt specific essential latent gene functions, such as EBNA-1 binding and maintenance of the latent EBV episome (43). Delineation of the cell signaling pathways used by EBV latent genes, such as the tumor necrosis factor receptor pathway by LMP1 (38), may provide unique opportunities to block virus-induced cell proliferation or to induce apoptosis of virus-infected cells.

VACCINES

Strategies for vaccination against HHV-8 infection will require better understanding of HHV-8 genes, biology, and epidemiology. Potential strategies for EBV vaccination include prophylactic approaches (to prevent infection or attenuate morbidity associated with primary infection/infectious mononucleosis), postinfection approaches (to reduce or eliminate persistent EBV infection and risk of EBV-associated malignancies), and therapeutic approaches (to treat established EBV-infected malignancies). Most work has focused on the EBV major membrane glycoprotein, gp350, as a potential prophylactic EBV vaccine (37). EBV binding to the cellular receptor, CD21, is mediated by gp350 (62), and a gp350 subunit vaccine can prevent development of lymphomas after injection of EBV in a cotton-top tamarin animal model for EBV infection (35, 36, 47). A recombinant gp350 vaccinia virus vaccine can induce EBV neutralizing antibodies in human volunteers; however, 3 of 9 vaccinated volunteers with neutralizing antibody were subsequently infected with EBV by natural routes of transmission (15). More studies will be required to determine the relative roles of humoral and cellular

immunity, the importance of mucosal immunity, the optimal adjuvant and delivery system for gp350 vaccines, and whether a gp350 vaccine will provide sufficient protection against EBV infection or significant attenuation of infectious mononucleosis. It remains to be shown whether gp350 represents the optimal candidate for an EBV vaccine. Vaccines that induce cytotoxic T cell activity against EBV latent genes have also been proposed as a potentially effective vaccine strategy and remain to be evaluated (39). The recent discovery of an animal model in rhesus monkeys that reproduces the natural route of oral transmission and other aspects of acute and persistent EBV infection should be useful for development of effective EBV vaccine strategies (33).

REFERENCES

1. Andersson J, Britton S, Ernberg I, Andersson U, Henle W, Skoldenberg B, Tisell A. Effect of acyclovir on infectious mononucleosis: a double-blind, placebo-controlled study. J Infect Dis 1986;153:283–290.
2. Andersson J, Skoldenberg B, Henle W, Giesecke J, Ortqvist A, Julander I, Gustavsson E, Akerlund B, Britton S, Ernberg I. Acyclovir treatment in infectious mononucleosis: a clinical and virological study. Infection 1987;15(Suppl 1):S14–20.
3. Bender CE. The value of corticosteroids in the treatment of infectious mononucleosis. JAMA 1967;199:529–531.
4. Cesarman E, Chang Y, Moore PS, Said JW, Knowles DM. Kaposi's sarcoma-associated herpesvirus-like DNA sequences in AIDS-related body-cavity-based lymphomas. N Engl J Med 1995;332:1186–1191.
5. Cesarman E, Moore PS, Rao PH, Inghirami G, Knowles DM, Chang Y. In vitro establishment and characterization of two acquired immunodeficiency syndrome-related lymphoma cell lines (BC-1 and BC-2) containing Kaposi's sarcoma-associated herpesvirus-like (KSHV) DNA sequences. Blood 1995;86:2708–2714.
6. Colby BM, Shaw JE, Datta AK, Pagano JS. Replication of Epstein-Barr virus DNA in lymphoblastoid cells treated for extended periods with acyclovir. Am J Med 1982;73:77–81.
7. Colby BM, Shaw JE, Elion GB, Pagano JS. Effect of acyclovir [9-(2-hydroxyethoxymethyl)guanine] on Epstein-Barr virus DNA replication. J Virol 1980;34:560–568.
8. Collins M, Fleisher G, Kreisberg J, Fager S. Role of steroids in the treatment of infectious mononucleosis in the ambulatory college student. J Am Coll Health 1984;33:101–105.
9. Copeman H. Infectious mononucleosis with severe thrombocytopenic purpura. Med J Aust 1956;43:925–927.
10. Dellemijn PL, Brandenburg A, Niesters HG, van den Bent MJ, Rothbarth PH, Vlasveld LT. Successful treatment with ganciclovir of presumed Epstein-Barr meningo-encephalitis following bone marrow transplant. Bone Marrow Transplant 1995;16:311–312.
11. Dupin N, Grandadam M, Calvez V, Gorin I, Aubin JT, Havard S, Lamy F, Leibowitch M, Huraux JM, Escande JP, et al. Herpesvirus-like DNA sequences in patients with Mediterranean Kaposi's sarcoma. Lancet 1995;345:761–762.
12. Gao SJ, Kingsley L, Hoover DR, Spira TJ, Rinaldo CR, Saah A, Phair J, Detels R, Parry P, Chang Y, Moore PS. Seroconversion to antibodies against Kaposi's sarcoma-associated herpesvirus-related latent nuclear antigens before the development of Kaposi's sarcoma. N Engl J Med 1996;335:233–241.

13. Glesby MJ, Hoover DR, Weng S, Graham NM, Phair JP, Detels R, Ho M, Saah AJ. Use of antiherpes drugs and the risk of Kaposi's sarcoma: data from the Multicenter AIDS Cohort Study. J Infect Dis 1996;173:1477–1480.

14. Gompels UA, Kasolo FC. HHV-8 serology and Kaposi's sarcoma. Lancet 1996;348:1587–1588.

15. Gu SY, Huang TM, Ruan L, Miao YH, Lu H, Chu CM, Motz M, Wolf H. First EBV vaccine trial in humans using recombinant vaccinia virus expressing the major membrane antigen. Dev Biol Stand 1995;84:171–177.

16. Hanto DW, Frizzera G, Gajl-Peczalska J, Purtilo DT, Klein G, Simmons RL, Najarian JS. The Epstein-Barr virus (EBV) in the pathogenesis of posttransplant lymphoma. Transplant Proc 1981;13:756–760.

17. Hanto DW, Frizzera G, Gajl-Peczalska KJ, Sakamoto K, Purtilo DT, Balfour HH, Simmons RL, Najarian JS. Epstein-Barr virus-induced B-cell lymphoma after renal transplantation: acyclovir therapy and transition from polyclonal to monoclonal B-cell proliferation. N Engl J Med 1982;306:913–918.

18. Hanto DW, Gajl-Peczalska KJ, Frizzera G, Arthur DC, Balfour HH Jr, McClain K, Simmons RL, Najarian JS. Epstein-Barr virus (EBV) induced polyclonal and monoclonal B-cell lymphoproliferative diseases occurring after renal transplantation. Clinical, pathologic, and virologic findings and implications for therapy. Ann Surg 1983;198:356–369.

19. Holmes GP, Kaplan JE, Stewart JA, Hunt B, Pinsky PF, Schonberger LB. A cluster of patients with a chronic mononucleosis-like syndrome. Is Epstein-Barr virus the cause? JAMA 1987;257:2297–2302.

20. Horwitz CA, Henle W, Henle G, Rudnick H, Latts E. Long-term serological follow-up of patients for Epstein-Barr virus after recovery from infectious mononucleosis. J Infect Dis 1985;151:1150–1153.

21. Huang YQ, Li JJ, Kaplan MH, Poiesz B, Katabira E, Zhang WC, Feiner D, Friedman-Kien AE. Human herpesvirus-like nucleic acid in various forms of Kaposi's sarcoma. Lancet 1995;345:759–761.

22. Ishida Y, Yokota Y, Tauchi H, Fukuda M, Takaoka T, Hayashi M, Matsuda H. Ganciclovir for chronic active Epstein-Barr virus infection. Lancet 1993;341:560–561.

23. Kedes DH, Ganem D. Sensitivity of Kaposi's sarcoma-associated herpesvirus replication to antiviral drugs. Implications for potential therapy. J Clin Invest 1997;99:2082–2086.

24. Kieff E. Epstein-Barr virus and its replication. In: Knipe D, Fields B, Howley P, eds. Virology. Philadelphia: Raven Press, 1996:2343–2396.

25. Klein EM, Cochran JF, Buck RL. The effects of short-term corticosteroid therapy on the symptoms of infectious mononucleosis pharyngotonsillitis: a double-blind study. J Am Coll Health Assoc 1969;17:446–452.

26. Lin JC, Lin SC, Mar EC, Pellett PE, Stamey FR, Stewart JA, Spira TJ. Is Kaposi's-sarcoma-associated herpesvirus detectable in semen of HIV-infected homosexual men? Lancet 1995;346:1601–1602.

27. Lin JC, Smith MC, Pagano JS. Prolonged inhibitory effect of 9-(1,3-dihydroxy-2-propoxymethyl)guanine against replication of Epstein-Barr virus. J Virol 1984;50:50–55.

28. Littler E, Zeuthen J, McBride AA, Trost Sorensen E, Powell KL, Walsh-Arrand JE, Arrand JR. Identification of an Epstein-Barr virus-coded thymidine kinase. EMBO J 1986;5:1959–1966.

29. Marchioli CC, Love JL, Abbott LZ, Huang YQ, Remick SC, Surtento-Reodica N, Hutchison RE, Mildvan D, Friedman-Kien AE, Poiesz BJ. Prevalence of human herpesvirus 8 DNA sequences in several patient populations. J Clin Microbiol 1996;34:2635–2638.

30. McGowan JE Jr, Chesney PJ, Crossley KB, LaForce FM. Guidelines for the use of systemic glucocorticosteroids in the management of selected infections. Working Group on Steroid Use, Antimicrobial Agents Committee, Infectious Diseases Society of America. J Infect Dis 1992;165:1–13.

31. Miller G, Grogan E, Rowe D, Rooney C, Heston L, Eastman R, Andiman W, Niederman J, Lenoir G, Henle W, Sullivan J, Schooley R, Vossen J, Strauss S, Issekutz T. Selective lack of antibody to a component of EB nuclear antigen in patients with chronic active Epstein-Barr virus infection. J Infect Dis 1987;156:26–35.

32. Miller G, Rigsby MO, Heston L, Grogan E, Sun R, Metroka C, Levy JA, Gao SJ, Chang Y, Moore P. Antibodies to butyrate-inducible antigens of Kaposi's sarcoma-associated herpesvirus in patients with HIV-1 infection. N Engl J Med 1996;334:1292–1297.

33. Moghaddam A, Rosenzweig M, Lee-Parritz D, Annis B, Johnson RP, Wang F. An animal model for acute and persistent Epstein-Barr virus infection. Science 1997;276:2030–2033.

34. Monini P, de Lellis L, Fabris M, Rigolin F, Cassai E. Kaposi's sarcoma-associated herpesvirus DNA sequences in prostate tissue and human semen. N Engl J Med 1996;334:1168–1172.

35. Morgan AJ, Finerty S, Lovgren K, Scullion FT, Morein B. Prevention of Epstein-Barr (EB) virus-induced lymphoma in cottontop tamarins by vaccination with the EB virus envelope glycoprotein gp340 incorporated into immune-stimulating complexes. J Gen Virol 1988;69:2093–2096.

36. Morgan AJ, Mackett M, Finerty S, Arrand JR, Scullion FT, Epstein MA. Recombinant vaccinia virus expressing Epstein-Barr virus glycoprotein gp340 protects cottontop tamarins against EB virus-induced malignant lymphomas. J Med Virol 1988;25:189–195.

37. Morgan AJ, Wilson DA. Epstein-Barr virus Gp350 vaccines. Epstein-Barr Virus Rep 1997;4:33–39.

38. Mosialos G, Birkenbach M, Yalamanchili R, VanArsdale T, Ware C, Kieff E. The Epstein-Barr virus transforming protein LMP1 engages signaling proteins for the tumor necrosis factor receptor family. Cell 1995;80:389–399.

39. Moss DJ, Schmidt C, Elliott S, Suhrbier A, Burrows S, Khanna R. Strategies involved in developing an effective vaccine for EBV-associated diseases. Adv Cancer Res 1996;69:213–245.

40. Neipel F, Albrecht JC, Fleckenstein B. Cell-homologous genes in the Kaposi's sarcoma-associated rhadinovirus human herpesvirus 8: determinants of its pathogenicity? J Virol 1997;71:4187–4192.

41. Oettle H, Wilborn F, Schmidt CA, Siegert W. Treatment with ganciclovir and Ig for acute Epstein-Barr virus infection after allogeneic bone marrow transplantation. Blood 1993;82:2257–2258.

42. Pagano JS, Datta AK. Perspectives on interactions of acyclovir with Epstein-Barr and other herpes viruses. Am J Med 1982;73:18–26.

43. Pagano JS, Jimenez G, Sung NS, Raab-Traub N, Lin JC. Epstein-Barr viral latency and cell immortalization as targets for antisense oligomers. Ann NY Acad Sci 1992;660:107–116.

44. Pagano JS, Sixbey JW, Lin JC. Acyclovir and Epstein-Barr virus infection. J Antimicrob Chemother 1983;12(Suppl B):113–121.

45. Papadopoulos EB, Ladanyi M, Emanuel D, Mackinnon S, Boulad F, Carabasi MH, Castro-Malaspina H, Childs BH, Gillio AP, Small TN, Young JW, Kernan NA, O'Reilly RJ. Infusions of donor leukocytes to treat Epstein-Barr virus-associated lym-

phoproliferative disorders after allogeneic bone marrow transplantation. N Engl J Med 1994;330:1185–1191.

46. Prout C, Dalrymple W. A double-blind study of eighty-two cases of infectious mononucleosis treated with corticosteroids. J Am Coll Health Assoc 1966;15:62–66.

47. Ragot T, Finerty S, Watkins PE, Perricaudet M, Morgan AJ. Replication-defective recombinant adenovirus expressing the Epstein-Barr virus (EBV) envelope glycoprotein gp340/220 induces protective immunity against EBV-induced lymphomas in the cottontop tamarin. J Gen Virol 1993;74:501–507.

48. Resnick L, Herbst JS, Ablashi DV, Atherton S, Frank B, Rosen L, Horwitz SN. Regression of oral hairy leukoplakia after orally administered acyclovir therapy. JAMA 1988;259:384–388.

49. Rettig MB, Ma HJ, Vescio RA, Pold M, Schiller G, Belson D, Savage A, Nishikubo C, Wu C, Fraser J, Said JW, Berenson JR. Kaposi's sarcoma-associated herpesvirus infection of bone marrow dendritic cells from multiple myeloma patients. Science 1997;276:1851–1854.

50. Rickinson AB, Kieff E. Epstein-Barr virus. In: Knipe D, Fields B, Howley P, eds. Virology. Philadelphia: Raven Press, 1996: 2397–2446.

51. Rooney CM, Smith CA, Ng CY, Loftin S, Li C, Krance RA, Brenner MK, Heslop HE. Use of gene-modified virus-specific T lymphocytes to control Epstein-Barr-virus-related lymphoproliferation. Lancet 1995;345:9–13.

52. Russo JJ, Bohenzky RA, Chien MC, Chen J, Yan M, Maddalena D, Parry JP, Peruzzi D, Edelman IS, Chang Y, Moore PS. Nucleotide sequence of the Kaposi sarcoma-associated herpesvirus (HHV8). Proc Natl Acad Sci USA 1996;93:14862–14867.

53. Schooley RT, Carey RW, Miller G, Henle W, Eastman R, Mark EJ, Kenyon K, Wheeler EO, Rubin RH. Chronic Epstein-Barr virus infection associated with fever and interstitial pneumonitis. Clinical and serologic features and response to antiviral chemotherapy. Ann Intern Med 1986;104:636–643.

54. Schumacher H, Jacobson W, Bemiller C. Treatment of infectious mononucleosis. Ann Intern Med 1963;58:217–228.

55. Simpson GR, Schulz TF, Whitby D, Cook PM, Boshoff C, Rainbow L, Howard MR, Gao SJ, Bohenzky RA, Simmonds P, Lee C, de Ruiter A, Hatzakis A, Tedder RS, Weller IV, Weiss RA, Moore PS. Prevalence of Kaposi's sarcoma associated herpesvirus infection measured by antibodies to recombinant capsid protein and latent immunofluorescence antigen. Lancet 1996; 348:1133–1138.

56. Smith J. Complications of infectious mononucleosis. Ann Intern Med 1956;44:861–873.

57. Soulier J, Grollet L, Oksenhendler E, Cacoub P, Cazals-Hatem D, Babinet P, d'Agay MF, Clauvel JP, Raphael M, Degos L, Sigaux F. Kaposi's sarcoma-associated herpesvirus-like DNA sequences in multicentric Castleman's disease. Blood 1995;86: 1276–1280.

58. Starzl TE, Nalesnik MA, Porter KA, Ho M, Iwatsuki S, Griffith BP, Rosenthal JT, Hakala TR, Shaw BW Jr, Hardesty RL, Atchison RW, Jaffe R, Bahnson HT. Reversibility of lymphomas and lymphoproliferative lesions developing under cyclosporin-steroid therapy. Lancet 1984;1:583–587.

59. Straus SE. The chronic mononucleosis syndrome. J Infect Dis 1988;157:405–412.

60. Straus SE, Cohen JI, Tosato G, Meier J. NIH conference. Epstein-Barr virus infections: biology, pathogenesis, and management. Ann Intern Med 1993;118:45–58.

61. Straus SE, Dale JK, Tobi M, Lawley T, Preble O, Blaese RM, Hallahan C, Henle W. Acyclovir treatment of the chronic fatigue syndrome. Lack of efficacy in a placebo-controlled trial. N Engl J Med 1988;319:1692–1698.

62. Tanner J, Whang Y, Sample J, Sears A, Kieff E. Soluble gp350/220 and deletion mutant glycoproteins block Epstein-Barr virus adsorption to lymphocytes. J Virol 1988;62:4452–4464.

63. Tynell E, Aurelius E, Brandell A, Julander I, Wood M, Yao QY, Rickinson A, Akerlund B, Andersson J. Acyclovir and prednisolone treatment of acute infectious mononucleosis: a multicenter, double-blind, placebo-controlled study. J Infect Dis 1996;174:324–331.

64. van der Horst C, Joncas J, Ahronheim G, Gustafson N, Stein G, Gurwith M, Fleisher G, Sullivan J, Sixbey J, Roland S, Fryer J, Champney K, Schooley R, Sumaya C, Pagano J. Lack of effect of peroral acyclovir for the treatment of acute infectious mononucleosis. J Infect Dis 1991;164:788–792.

65. Waldo RT. Neurologic complications of infectious mononucleosis after steroid therapy. South Med J 1981;74:1159–1160.

66. Yao QY, Ogan P, Rowe M, Wood M, Rickinson AB. The Epstein-Barr virus: host balance in acute infectious mononucleosis patients receiving acyclovir anti-viral therapy. Int J Cancer 1989;43:61–66.

Hepatitis Viruses
(HAV, HEV, HBV, HCV, HDV, HGV)

Mang M. Ma, Graham A. Tipples, Karl P. Fischer, and David L. J. Tyrrell

Viral hepatitis is a common disease and major public health problem. Failure to alter human risk behaviors, poor public hygiene in some communities, inadequacy of vaccination program implementation, and the lack of effective vaccines for some of the hepatitis viruses contribute to the spread of hepatitis viruses. Over the last 30 years, 6 human hepatitis viruses have been characterized: hepatitis A, B, C, D, E, and G viruses (Fig. 1). Their transmission, infectivity, molecular biology,

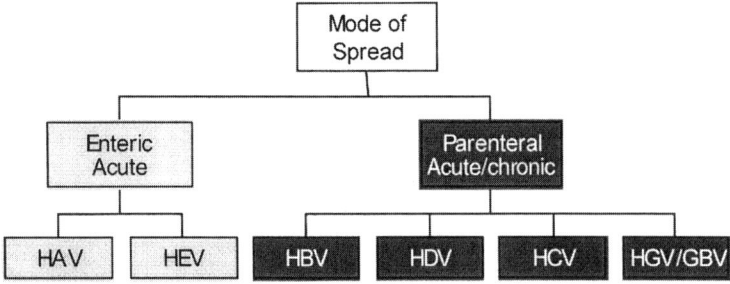

FIGURE 1. Clinical classification of hepatitis viruses.

and natural history have been elucidated. Acute hepatitis can be severe, but patients usually recover. Chronic viral infection can develop, however, in patients infected with hepatitis B, C, D, or G viruses and chronic hepatitis can progress to cirrhosis or end-stage liver disease. Hepatocellular carcinoma is also associated with chronic hepatitis B and C virus and it is a common cancer in parts of the world where hepatitis B virus is pandemic.

The treatment of viral hepatitis has lagged behind our understanding of hepatitis viruses. Currently, antiviral treatment is still at a primitive stage, but effective vaccines do exist for hepatitis A and B viruses. Attempts to cure chronic viral hepatitis have produced many therapeutic challenges and new issues. Because chronic hepatitis B and C infections are common and can progress to end-stage liver disease, much attention has focused on these two viruses. In this chapter, we briefly review the basic molecular biology and natural history of hepatitis viruses. The main emphasis is on prevention and current and prospective therapies for hepatitis viruses.

ENTERICALLY TRANSMITTED HEPATITIS VIRUSES
Hepatitis A Virus (HAV)

General Description

Molecular Biology. Hepatitis A virus (HAV) was conclusively identified by immune electron microscopy in the early seventies (82). HAV belongs to the family *Picornaviridae*, genus *Hepatovirus*. HAV contains a 7478 nucleotide (+) sense, single-stranded, linear RNA genome (Fig. 2). Virus replication occurs in the host cell cytoplasm. The (+) RNA genome serves as the mRNA for translation to synthesize the polyprotein, which can potentially be co- and posttranslationally cleaved into 11 proteins that are essential for viral replication (183). Genomic replication occurs via the synthesis of a complementary (−) RNA intermediate using the viral proteins VPg (primer protein) and 3D (RNA polymerase). The capsid proteins VP1 and VP3 make up the highly conserved dominant neutralizing epitope resulting in a single human HAV serotype. The presence of this conserved neutralizing epitope is a key factor in the successful development of a vaccine for HAV.

Epidemiology. HAV infection is common, and 1.4 million cases are reported in the world each year. Evidence of previous infection can be detected in 30 to 40% of the population in developed countries and 90% of the population in developing countries (240, 264). HAV is usually transmitted by the fecal-oral route. Fecal contamination of water or food supplies causes outbreaks of HAV infection. The virus is present in the stool of patients during the prodrome or preicteric phase until about 2 weeks after the onset of jaundice. Person-to-person spread can cause sporadic cases. Parenteral transmission is rare but has been reported in intravenous drug users. The brief period of viremia present during acute disease can be the source of virus for parenteral transmission.

The infection is most common in the younger age groups. In developing countries, most children have been exposed to the virus. They have very mild symptoms during the acute infection and develop lifelong immunity to HAV. In countries with good sanitation, more symptomatic hepatitis A infection is seen in older patients because they have no immunity to HAV from lack of exposure to the virus during childhood (225). The overall case-fatality is low; children less than 5 years of age have a case-fatality rate of 1.5 per 1000, and patients over the age of 50 have a case-fatality rate of 27 per 1000 (45).

Clinical Manifestation. An HAV infection usually causes mild-to-moderate acute hepatitis. The incubation period is usually 4 weeks and is rarely longer than 6 weeks. Acute hepatitis lasts 2 to 3 weeks and is followed by recovery with lifelong immunity to the virus (Fig. 3). Most patients suffer flu-like symptoms with malaise, fatigue, anorexia, and fever during acute infection. Mild-to-moderate jaundice usually occurs. Infection can also present as a gastrointestinal illness, which may cause a missed diagnosis. Atypical presentations such as prolonged cholestasis occur infrequently. Occasionally, patients with severe hepatitis need hospital admission for supportive care and monitoring for development of fulminant liver failure, which has been reported to cause death or require liver transplantation in elderly patients and patients with underlying chronic liver disease (122, 177).

There is no evidence for a chronic carrier state or development of chronic liver disease. Both IgM and IgG antibodies to the virus (anti-HAV) can be detected, with elevated IgM antibody indicating recent infection. While the IgM response usually becomes undetectable at 6 months, the IgG response persists for life (235, 236).

Susceptibility in Vitro and in Animal Models

As HAV causes acute infection only and the illness tends to be self-limited, there is little interest in establishing the in vitro or animal models required for studying anti-HAV treatment.

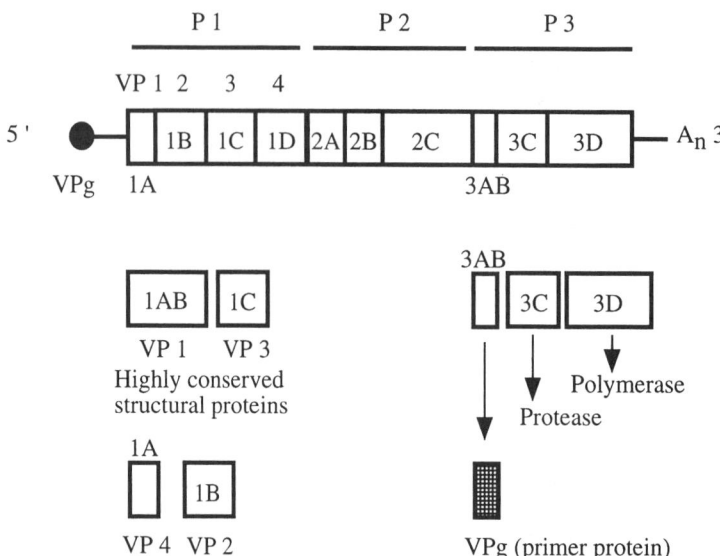

FIGURE 2. HAV genome. The *P1* region contains the structural proteins. *VP1* and *VP3* make up the highly conserved epitope resulting in a single human HAV serotype. The epitope allows development of a successful vaccine.

Chimpanzee and marmoset can be infected with HAV, and they have been used to study immunoglobulin therapy and vaccine prevention (75, 207). HAV can also be propagated in cell culture (197). Using fetal rhesus monkey kidney continuous cell line to support HAV propagation, 20 potential antiviral compounds were screened for anti-HAV activity (274). Only amantadine and ribavirin demonstrated a moderate HAV inhibition without causing severe cytotoxic effects. It is not known whether treatment of acute HAV infection with amantadine or ribavirin would alter its clinical course.

Antiviral Therapy

Immunoglobulin. Immunoglobulin was demonstrated to be effective in preventing "infectious" hepatitis over 50 years ago, prior to the identification of HAV. Immunoglobulin was used to prevent hepatitis during an epidemic of infectious hepatitis in a summer camp for boys and girls in 1945 (237). Since then, multiple studies have confirmed the effectiveness of immunoglobulin in preventing hepatitis A (56, 267). However immunoglobulin recipients can develop IgM antibody to HAV and abnormal levels of transaminases following exposure to the virus (143, 192, 219). These studies suggest that subclinical infections and a form of passive-active immunization can occur in patients who receive immunoglobulin post-HAV exposure.

The minimum level of anti-HAV antibody required for prophylaxis is unknown. Immunoglobulin has an efficacy of 80 to 90% when given before or immediately after exposure (273). After immunoglobulin administration, very low levels of anti-HAV antibody are detected in the recipients (236). It appears that a very small amount of neutralizing antibody (10–20 mIU/mL) is required for protection. With an injection of 5 mL of immunoglobulin, the geometric mean anti-HAV titer was 96 mIU/mL, and this geometric mean titer declined to the minimum protective level of 10 mIU/mL in approximately 3

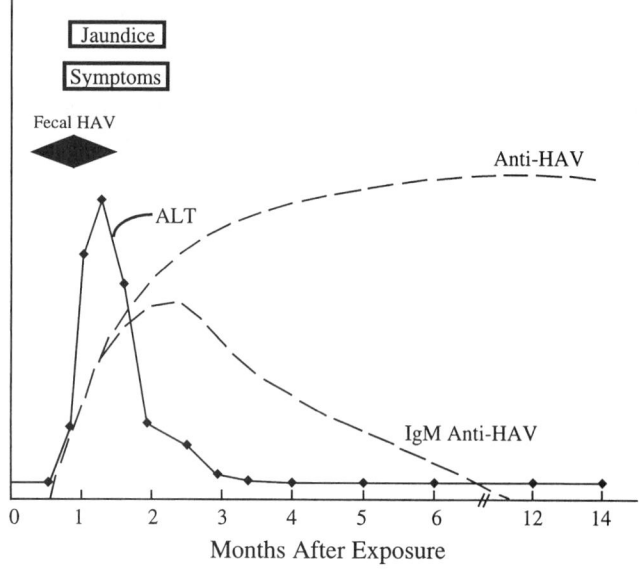

FIGURE 3. Natural history of HAV infection.

months (281). The current recommended dose of immunoglobulin effective for short-term prophylaxis and to prevent symptomatic hepatitis after exposure to hepatitis A virus is 0.02 to 0.06 mL/kg body weight.

Who should receive immunoglobulin for HAV prophylaxis? During an outbreak, both immunoglobulin and HAV vaccine should be used to prevent hepatitis A infection. Close contacts of patients with HAV infection and persons who will be traveling to pandemic areas less than 4 weeks after HAV immunization should be treated with immunoglobulin. Immunoglobulin is also recommended for children under 2 years old traveling to endemic areas (Table 1).

Recipients	Dose
Postexposure	0.02 mL/kg intramuscularly
Close contacts	
During outbreaks	
Traveling to endemic areas	0.06 mL/kg
Children under 2 years	
Patients allergic to vaccine	
Travelers have vaccine <4 weeks	

Prophylaxis and HAV Vaccine

HAV vaccine. Immunoglobulin does not offer long-term HAV prophylaxis. Furthermore, there has been concern that immunoglobulin (especially the intravenous form) can potentially transmit hepatitis C virus (15, 27). For these reasons, there is a demand for safe HAV vaccine and both live attenuated and inactivated HAV vaccine have been studied extensively. Live attenuated vaccine has several disadvantages over inactivated vaccines. The attenuated virus can potentially revert to wild-type virus and cause symptomatic infection. The vaccine recipient could become a public hazard by excreting attenuated virus. Attenuated virus vaccine recipients can develop transiently abnormal liver enzyme levels. For these reasons, formalin-inactivated HAV vaccine has been preferred. The Havrix vaccine (SmithKline Beecham) and VAQTA (Merck Frosst) have been approved by the FDA, and several other inactivated HAV vaccines are currently being assessed.

Results of three placebo-controlled clinical trials studying the efficacy of the inactivated HAV vaccine have been published (114, 167, 270). Most of the participants were children. The vaccination schedules differed in each of these studies. All of the schedules appeared to provide high anti-HAV antibody titers and good efficacy against HAV infection, but the immunogenicity of the vaccine is dose dependent. With a lower dose of inactivated hepatitis A vaccine (360 EU, 720 EU), 90% of recipients developed a protective antibody level after one injection. With a higher dose of vaccine (1440 EU), all recipients developed a protective antibody level after one injection. However, with two injections (primary and booster doses), all recipients of vaccine developed protective antibody regardless of the dose of vaccine administered (271).

Although the vaccine has a high efficacy in preventing symptomatic hepatitis A infection, it does not offer instant protection. Immunoglobulin would have to be given with HAV vaccine after acute exposure to provide instant protection. Simultaneous active and passive immunization against HAV has been studied, and some inhibition of antibody production was reported when immunoglobulin was given with vaccine (265, 281). The geometric titer for the combination group was 30 to 60% lower than the titer in the vaccine-only group; however, the geometric mean titer with the combination treatment was high enough to provide protection. For persons who want to travel immediately to HAV endemic countries or during an outbreak, immunoglobulin treatment could offer short-term prophylaxis while the vaccine provides long-term immunity.

Adverse Effects of HAV Vaccine. The vaccine is well tolerated; no severe adverse effect was reported in any of these studies. The most frequent adverse effect is pain (10–20%) at the site of injection; reactions including fever, headache, and swelling at the injected site have been reported to be less frequent. There are no data regarding the safety of the vaccine in children less than 1 year of age or in pregnant women.

Indication and Dose Schedule for HAV Vaccination. Who should receive the HAV vaccine? Vaccination should be offered to any persons over 1 year of age who are planning to travel to endemic areas, persons living in frequent outbreak areas, military personnel, employees of day-care centers, food handlers, persons for whom hepatitis A is an occupational hazard (sewage workers, health care workers), persons at increased risk because of their sexual practices, and intravenous drug users (Table 2).

It has been recommended that two doses (720 EU each) of Havrix (SmithKline Beecham) be administered intramuscularly in the deltoid muscle region 1 month apart. A booster dose should be given 6 to 12 months after the initial injection, to ensure long-term immunity. If the higher dose of 1440 EU is used, two doses at least 6 months apart are adequate. The VAQTA (Merck Frosst) vaccine should be given as a primary dose and booster dose at least 6 months apart (Table 3).

Adjunctive Therapy

There is no specific antiviral therapy for acute hepatitis A. The illness is self-limited, and regular activities should be encouraged. Strenuous exercise has not been associated with adverse outcome

TABLE 2 • **Indications for HAV Vaccination**

Recipients
Close contacts with person with acute HAV
Travelers to endemic or outbreak areas
Residents of community with outbreaks
Military personnel
Day-care staffs
Health professionals
Health care staffs at chronic care and mental care facilities
Residents of chronic care facilities
Sewage workers
Food handlers
Persons engaging in high-risk sexual activity
Hemophiliacs
Intravenous drug users

TABLE 3 • **HAV Vaccines**

Products	Age of Recipient	Dose	Schedule (month)
Havrix 720 Junior	1–18 years	720 EU	0, 6–12
Havrix (low dose)	Adult	720 EU	0, 1, 6–12
Havrix (high dose)	Adult	1440 EU	0, 6–12
VAQTA	2–17 years	0.5 mL (25 U)	0, 6–12
	Over 18 years	1 mL (50 U)	0, 6–12

during acute hepatitis (76, 204). Some patients with severe acute hepatitis might require hospital support and monitoring.

Once the diagnosis is made, information regarding hygienic measures and immunoprophylaxis should be provided to family members or persons with close contacts with the patients (47). This is important to prevent the spread of the hepatitis. All household members and sexual contacts should receive 0.02 mL/kg of immunoglobulin. HAV vaccine can also be given with the immunoglobulin. If the patient is a child, day-care center members should be considered for immunoglobulin prophylaxis.

Hepatitis E Virus (HEV)

General Description

Molecular Biology. HEV is an RNA virus with an undetermined classification. Electron microscopy shows HEV to be a 32- to 34-nm icosahedral nonenveloped virus that is similar in physical structure to Norwalk virus of the *Caliciviridae* family (132). Nucleotide sequence analysis of the RNA genome indicates three overlapping open reading frames (ORFs) (Fig. 4). Comparison of the protein sequence coded by ORF1 with proteins of other (+) RNA viruses allows identification of five putative functional domains of the nonstructural polyprotein: *(a)* RNA-dependent RNA polymerase, *(b)* RNA helicase, *(c)* methyltransferase, *(d)* unknown functional domain, and *(e)* protease. The ORF2 toward the 3′ end of the genome codes for structural proteins. The structural viral capsid proteins of ORF2 contain neutralizing epitopes that show cross-reactivity between strains, indicating a single HEV serotype or common specific epitopes. This might become the key factor for vaccine development.

Epidemiology. Hepatitis E virus or enteric non-A, non-B hepatitis virus is spread by fecal-oral transmission (1, 36). The illness occurs primarily in developing countries with inadequate sanitation. Outbreaks have been reported from Asia, Africa, and Central America, and fecal contamination of the water supply has led to many of these outbreaks (116, 253). Sporadic infections have occurred. The mode of transmission in sporadic cases has been difficult to identify, but fecal contamination of food has been suggested to be the most common cause, and person-to-person spread is suspected in close-contact situations (208). In developed countries, HEV infection is rare and most HEV cases are imported from travel in endemic countries (105, 233).

Hepatitis E infection in children and young adults accounts for more than half of the cases of acute hepatitis in developing countries (81, 276). The disease tends to be mild. The overall case-fatality ratio is similar to that of hepatitis A and is estimated to be 0.5 to 4% (35, 161). However, morbidity and mortality for hepatitis E infection in pregnant women in the second or third trimester are significantly higher (123, 199, 252) because of the higher incidence of fulminant liver failure (34).

Clinical Manifestation. HEV infection causes self-limited hepatitis with a clinical course quite similar to that of HAV infection (Fig. 5). The incubation period is estimated to be 3 to 8 weeks. The illness has three phases: prodromal, icteric, and convalescent. Fever, malaise, and nausea are common in the preicteric or prodromal phase, which lasts 1 to 10 days (81). The prodromal phase is followed by the icteric phase, lasting 7 to 12 days, in which malaise, fever, nausea, vomiting, anorexia, abdomen discomfort, headaches, and fatigue are common symptoms (81, 253). Physical findings are

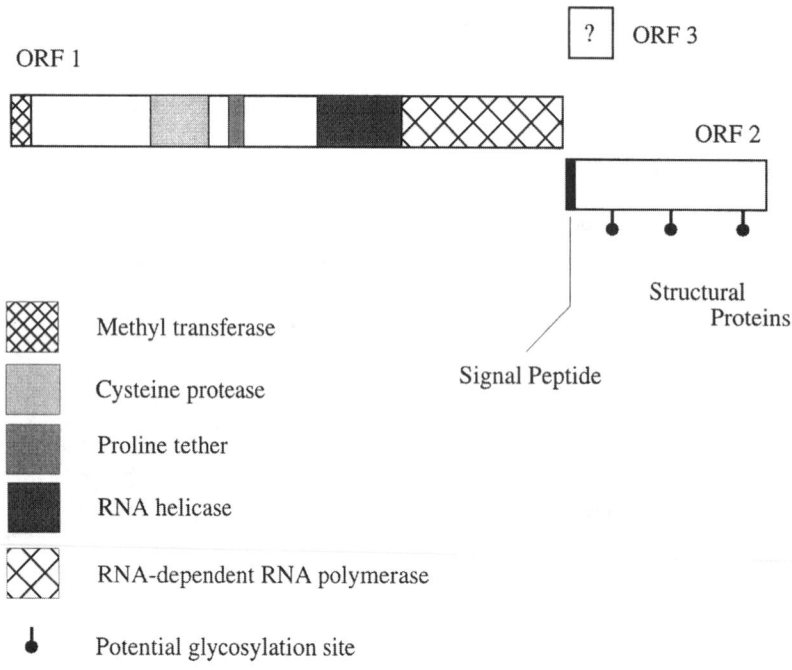

FIGURE 4. HEV genome. HEV genome consists of three open reading frames *(ORF)*. *ORF 1* encodes for structural proteins such as RNA-dependent RNA polymerase. *ORF 2* codes for structural proteins that have similar epitopes in different HEV strains. *ORF 3* has unknown function.

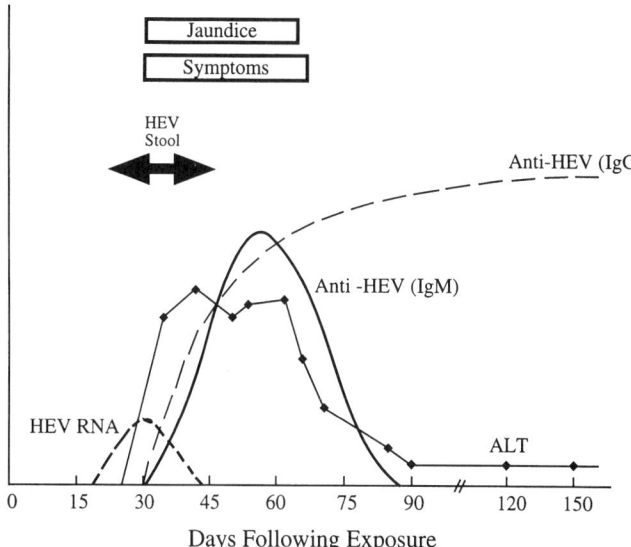

FIGURE 5. Natural history of HEV infection.

uncommon but may include jaundice, hepatomegaly, splenomegaly, abdomen discomfort, and dark-colored urine (253). The overall illness lasts 1 to 2 months. Subclinical infection occurs and is likely very common, but the exact incidence is not known. HEV does not cause chronic hepatitis.

Clinical diagnosis is based on a history of exposure to fecal-oral transmission and the exclusion of HAV, HBV, or HCV infection. Serologic assay and polymerase chain reaction (PCR) for confirmation are available from some reference laboratories. The IgM antibody response to hepatitis E can be demonstrated in the icteric phase of infection. This is rapidly followed by the IgG response, and the IgG titer against HEV remains high for several years (63). It is not clear whether this immune response provides lifelong immunity.

Susceptibility in Vitro and in Animal Models
There is no in vitro culture system to study HEV or its treatment. An animal model using rhesus monkeys is established (172), which would be useful to study HEV vaccine.

Antiviral Therapy
Treatment of Hepatitis E.   Antiviral treatment for HEV infection is not available. Most patients do not require treatment because the disease is usually mild, with a self-limited course. For those rare patients with severe symptoms, temporary hospitalization for close observation and supportive care might be indicated. Although liver transplantation is a treatment for fulminant liver failure (even during pregnancy), this option is not available in most developing countries.

Prevention and Prophylaxis.   The immunoglobulin produced in developed countries appears to be ineffective for HEV prophylaxis, as the preparation contains little or no anti-HEV antibody. It is not clear whether immunoglobulin from developing countries would be more effective. As there is no immune prophylaxis against HEV, travelers to endemic countries should be advised not to consume any uncooked food or untreated water. Safe practices, such as handwashing prior to eating and no swimming in polluted water, decrease the risk of contracting HEV infection. These recommendations are particularly important for pregnant travelers because of the possibility of fulminant liver failure with HEV infection.

Currently there is no vaccine against hepatitis E. Molecular analysis of HEV shows that the structural viral capsid proteins of ORF2 contain neutralizing epitopes that have cross-reactivity between strains. This suggests that HEV might have a single serotype, which might be a key factor for successful vaccine development.

PARENTERALLY TRANSMITTED HEPATITIS VIRUSES
Hepatitis B Virus (HBV)

General Description
Molecular Biology.   Hepatitis B virus (HBV) is an enveloped DNA virus that is the prototype virus of the *Hepadnaviridae* family. The 3.2-kbp circular genome is partially double-stranded and is encapsidated by the core (C) protein to form the nucleocapsid. Surrounding the nucleocapsid is the lipid envelope, which contains small, medium, and large viral surface proteins (HBsAg). The viral polymerase (P) protein has RNase H activity, has reverse transcriptase/polymerase activity, and also provides a terminal protein for priming of DNA synthesis, which is covalently attached to the negative strand of DNA in the nucleocapsid (173). Most of the HBV genome consists of overlapping open reading frames or genes (Fig. 6). Therefore, a mutation in one viral gene often results in a mutation in an overlapping gene, thereby restricting the number of viable mutant viruses. However, HBV variants do occur, and their presence might alter the clinical presentation and disease course (29).

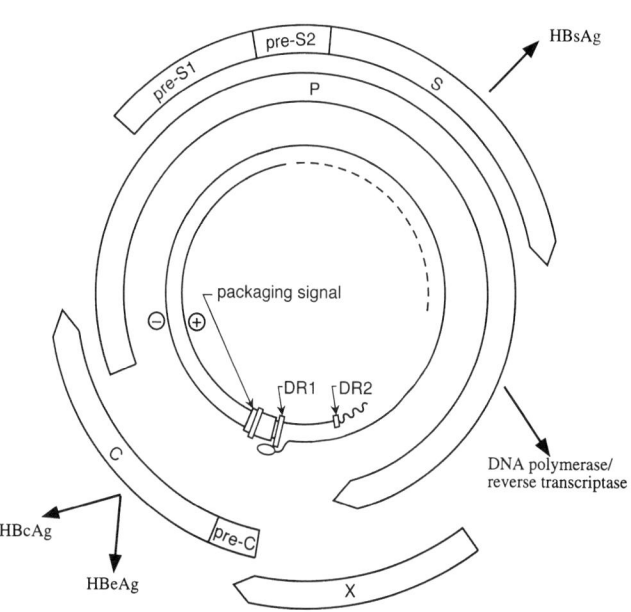

FIGURE 6. HBV genome.

Upon attachment to and entry into the cell, the virus is uncoated, and the viral genome is translocated to the nucleus. The viral genome is then converted to covalently closed circular DNA (ccc-DNA) by the host DNA polymerase. The host RNA polymerase II uses the ccc-DNA as a template for transcription. Four viral transcripts are produced from internal promoters and are 5′ capped and 3′ polyadenylated. The greater-than-genome-length (3.5 kb) pregenomic transcript is used as a template for the viral RNA-dependent DNA polymerase (reverse transcription) to produce the minus DNA strand. Subsequent RNase H and DNA-dependent DNA polymerase activities of the viral polymerase produce the partially double-stranded progeny genomes. The pregenomic transcript is also translated into the preC/C open reading frame products as well as the polymerase protein. The C open reading frame codes for the nucleocapsid or core protein. The preC/C open reading frame codes for a secreted protein termed the e antigen (HBeAg). The function of HBeAg is not fully understood, and the significance of mutant viruses that do not produce HBeAg is not clear (29). The large surface protein is produced via the 2.4-kb preS1 transcript, and the medium and small surface proteins are produced via the 2.1-kb preS2/S transcript. A fourth 0.9-kb transcript is translated into the X protein (HBx). The function of HBx is not entirely clear, but it has been associated with transactivation activity of a number of cellular proteins (211).

The major immunogenic response to HBV is to a highly conserved surface-exposed region of HBsAg called the "a" determinant. All strains of HBV share this conserved epitope. In addition to the "a" determinant, there are other epitopes, d/y and w/r, which result in the existence of four main serotypes (adw, ayw, adr, ayr). Variation within these serotypes results in a total of 9 subtypes. Because the major "a" determinant exists in all strains, an effective vaccine has been developed to prevent infection.

Epidemiology. In the world, there are over 300 million HBV carriers, and the infection is a major cause of end-stage liver disease and hepatocellular carcinoma. In endemic countries, HBV infection frequently occurs in infants and children at a young age through maternal-newborn or child-to-child transmission (21). Infants infected at birth have a 90% chance of developing chronic infection (250). This risk of chronic infection declines to 1 to 5% for older children and adults. In the United States, there are over 1 million HBV carriers (154). Although the incidence of HBV has declined since 1985, the Centers for Disease Control and Prevention (CDC) has estimated that there are still 200,000 to 300,000 persons infected with HBV annually in United States. At present, HBV infection occurs primarily in adolescents and young adults because of sexual activity and experimentation with intravenous drug use (13).

The presence of HBeAg or HBV DNA in blood indicates active viral replication and high infectivity. Percutaneous or mucous membrane exposures to infectious blood or body fluids can lead to acute infection. The primary risk factors for HBV infection include sharing needles for injection of drugs, unprotected sexual activity, hemodialysis, and contacts with contaminated sharp instruments during tattooing or body piercing. Transmission of HBV through needle-stick injuries has declined since the establishment of a vaccination program for hospital personnel. Perinatal transmission of the virus from HBsAg-positive mothers to their newborns has also declined with the introduction of screening programs for HBV infection and immune prophylaxis for newborns. HBV infection from blood transfusion has been almost completely eliminated by routine screening and the use of volunteer blood donors. In United States, the most common route of HBV transmission is heterosexual activity; however, approximately 30% of patients do not have any identifiable risk factors (45).

Clinical Manifestation. HBV is a highly infectious agent, and infection occurs frequently after exposure (8, 193). The clinical course of primary HBV infection can be acute or chronic, and the outcome is frequently age dependent. In adults, the infection is usually self-limited and resolves in less than 6 months. Most infections in adults are subclinical; only one-third of infected adults develop clinical hepatitis (165). A small number of HBV-infected adults develop chronic hepatitis (147). In contrast, HBV infection in the first few months of life seldom causes clinical illness and almost always leads to persistent infection (165, 185).

During acute symptomatic HBV infection, patients may have fever, malaise, fatigue, weakness, anorexia, abdominal discomfort, jaundice, and elevated transaminases. The diagnosis of acute HBV infection is based on history, transaminase profiles, and HBV antigen-antibody detection (Fig. 7). After an incubation period of 4 to 8 weeks, HBsAg can be detected in blood. HBeAg and HBV DNA occurring at the same time indicate active viral replication. Loss of HBeAg is usually associated with a marked decrease in HBV DNA. Some patients seroconvert to HBeAg but remain HBV DNA positive with ac-

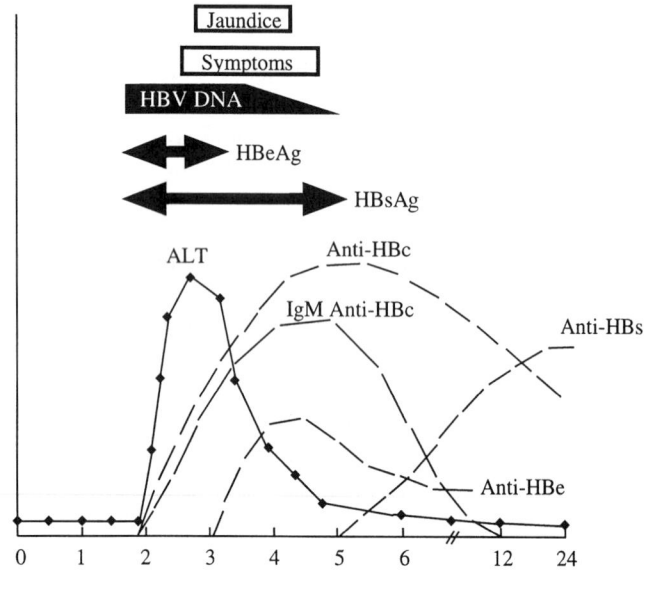

FIGURE 7. Acute HBV infection.

tive liver disease. These patients have the "e" mutant variant or precore mutant of the virus (42). IgM specific anti-HBcAg antibody develops early during infection and is followed by anti-HBs antibody as the patient improves. Most patients recover within 6 months of illness onset, and the transaminases return to normal.

Persistence of HBsAg 6 months after onset of hepatitis illness indicates that the HBV infection has become chronic (Fig. 8). Spontaneous remission or disappearance of HBsAg occurs in a small number of chronic HBV carriers each year (176). Chronic carriers are the principal reservoirs of HBV, and many develop progressive chronic liver disease. Approximately 20% of chronic carriers die from cirrhosis or hepatocellular carcinoma. The immune complexes of HBsAg and antibodies can cause extrahepatic diseases including serum sickness syndrome, polyarteritis nodosa, glomerulonephritis, and cryoglobulinemia.

Hepatocellular carcinoma has been associated with chronic HBV infection. In developing countries, hepatocellular carcinoma causes an estimated 1 to 2 million deaths each year. In the United States, hepatocellular carcinoma is uncommon, and less than one-third of the hepatocellular carcinoma cases are associated with chronic HBV infection (46, 279). This difference in hepatocellular carcinoma rate is likely due to the different epidemiology of HBV infections in developing countries and industrialized countries. Before universal vaccination, mother-to-infant transmission was the most common mode of transmission in developing countries. In industrialized countries, HBV infection occurs primarily through sexual contact and intravenous drug use. The disease course and duration of carrier states differ significantly, which may account for the different rates of hepatocellular carcinoma in developing and industrialized countries.

Susceptibility in Vitro and in Animal Models

The *Hepadnaviridae* family includes viruses affecting ducks, herons, woodchucks, and ground squirrels as well as humans. Antiviral agents have been studied extensively in the duck hepatitis B virus (DHBV) and the woodchuck hepatitis B virus (WHV) systems. The duck system offers the advantages of being relatively inexpensive and readily available, whereas the woodchuck model is more expensive and less readily available. However, the woodchuck model is particularly useful because it is a mammalian virus, and chronic infection in the woodchuck leads to hepatocellular carcinoma within 2 to 3 years (155).

Two cell culture systems have been used extensively to detect compounds with antiviral activity for HBV. Primary duck hepatocytes prepared from congenitally infected ducklings were first described by Suzuki et al. (239). Many laboratories have adopted this system to screen compounds. Another system that has proven very useful for screening compounds against HBV is human liver cells transfected with greater-than-genome-length HBV DNA (222, 238). Korba and Milman (129) optimized the cell line established by Sells et al. (known as 2.2.15 cells) for screening for antivirals against HBV. These two in vitro cell culture systems have been used to identify many compounds with antiviral activity for HBV. A number of these compounds have been studied in vivo in

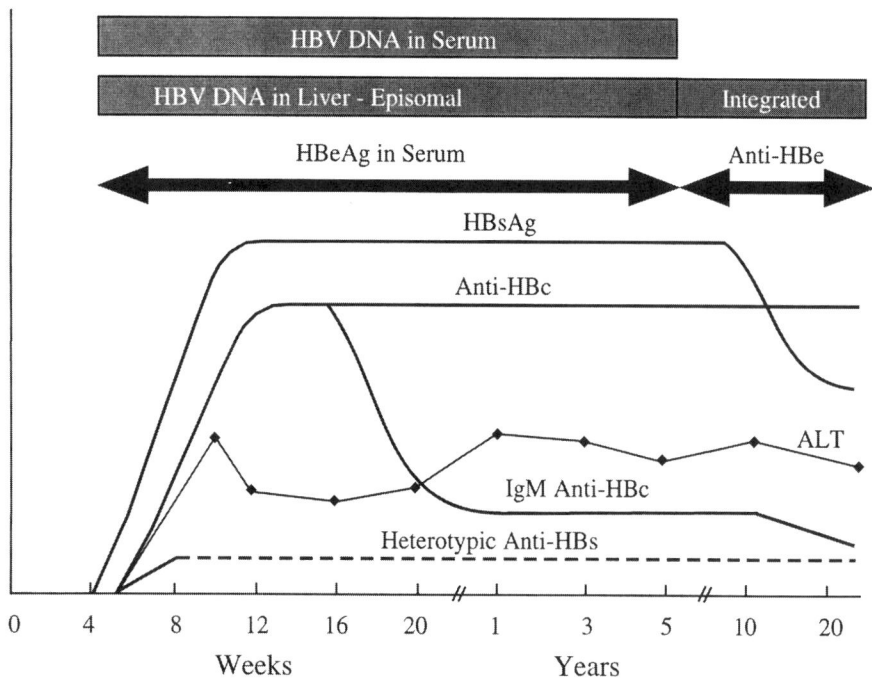

FIGURE 8. Chronic HBV infection.

ducks, woodchucks, or occasionally chimpanzees carrying HBV. Four compounds, famciclovir, lamivudine, lobucavir, and adefovir, are in phase II or II clinical trials.

Famciclovir, an oral prodrug of penciclovir, has been shown to be active against DHBV in primary hepatocytes, with a 50% inhibitory concentration (IC_{50}) of 0.7 μM (226). In 2.2.15 cells, the concentration required to inhibit extracellular virus production by 50% (EC_{50}) was 0.2 μM (128). However, Innaimo et al. (113) reported that penciclovir was inactive against HBV, with an EC_{50} above 100 μM. Famciclovir has also shown activity in vivo in the duck (148, 254). Penciclovir selectively blocks protein priming of the negative strand of viral DNA synthesis (285).

Lamivudine [($-$)-2′,3′-dideoxy-3′-thiacytidine] is a potent in vitro inhibitor of both duck (223) and human hepadnaviruses (48) as well as human immunodeficiency viruses HIV-1 and HIV-2 (54). Lamivudine is a very effective inhibitor of DHBV in ducks and HBV in chimpanzees (256, 257) and is moderately active against WHV in woodchucks. This agent is known to block hepadnaviral DNA synthesis by chain termination (223).

Lobucavir, another guanosine analogue, has broad-spectrum antiviral activity against HBV and herpesviruses. It has an EC_{50} of approximately 2.5 μM in 2.2.15 cells (113). The carbocyclic analogue of 2′-deoxyguanosine (2′-CDG) is an effective inhibitor of DHBV, both in vivo and in vitro (89). Another carbocyclic 2′-deoxyguanosine analogue, BMS 200475, is a very potent and selective inhibitor of HBV with an EC_{50} of 0.00375 μM (113).

The inhibitory effects of 9-(2-phosphonylmethoxyethyl)adenine (PMEA) on DHBV and HBV have been demonstrated in vitro and in vivo (104). This compound is being developed as Adefovir and is in phase II clinical trials. A large number of nucleoside analogues have been reported to have antiviral activity against hepadnaviruses, but many of these compounds are toxic or not very effective clinically, such as foscarnet, ganciclovir, acyclovir, adenine arabinoside, ddC, ddI, or AZT.

The cell culture systems have been used to explore the potential of using combination of antiviral agents for hepadnaviruses. Synergy was observed when lamivudine was used in combination with penciclovir in the primary duck hepatocyte system (55). Lamivudine showed synergy when used with either interferon or penciclovir in the 2.2.15 cell system carrying HBV (127).

The cell culture systems and animal models have yielded a new array of potent antiviral agents against hepatitis B. Given the very encouraging results of using combination chemotherapy in other chronic infectious diseases such as tuberculosis and AIDS, it is very likely that new trials of combination chemotherapy and possibly chemotherapy with immunomodulatory therapy will be initiated. At this time, no meaningful trials have been reported using combination chemotherapy in the treatment of HBV.

Antiviral Therapy

Hepatitis B virus infection can be acute or chronic, asymptomatic to fatal. Most acute HBV infections clear completely,

leaving no evidence of long-term hepatic injury. Therefore, the primary target for antiviral therapy is chronic infection. The goals of therapy are to eradicate replicating virus and prevent chronic inflammation that may lead to cirrhosis. Early intervention with antiviral therapy in chronic HBV infection may also decrease the risk of developing hepatocellular carcinoma. Several studies have shown that patients who lose HBV DNA and seroconvert HBeAg in response to therapy have improved clinical outcomes (151, 174).

Drug of Choice: Interferon-α Treatment of Chronic HBV. Interferon-α is a cytokine produced by monocytes and B cells in response to viral infection. The cytokine has antiviral and immune-system-modulating properties. Interferon-α binds to cellular receptors and activates secondary messengers so as to initiate production of multiple proteins critical to the defense of the cell against viruses. The antiviral effects include degradation of viral mRNA, inhibition of viral protein synthesis, and prevention of viral infection of cells. The immunomodulating effects include enhancement of foreign antigen presentation by HLA I and II to the immune system, activation of NK cells and other immune cells, and increased cytokine production.

Multiple types of recombinant interferon-α have been developed to treat viral hepatitis. While there is at least one report of a short-term regimen of interferon benefiting a patient with acute hepatitis B (115), most studies to date have been placebo-controlled trials studying the efficacy of interferon-α in the treatment of chronic hepatitis B infection. The dose and duration of interferon-α treatment varied in these studies. The dose of interferon-α ranged from 1 to 10 million units 3 times weekly for 3 to 6 months. Patients were usually followed for 6 to 12 months after completion of interferon therapy. The best-designed studies were summarized in a recent meta-analysis (277). Interferon-α is more effective than placebo in suppressing viral replication and terminating the carrier state (Table 4). About one-third of treated patients have a sustained response characterized by HBeAg seroconversion and loss of HBV DNA. Most patients remain carriers of HBsAg. The data show that a high dose of interferon is more effective than a low dose, and the 3- to 4-month interferon treatment protocol is as effective as 6 months of therapy. Responders tend to have elevated aminotransferases approximately 2 months after initiation of interferon treatment, and the aminotransferases return

TABLE 4 • Meta-analysis[a] of Chronic HBV Treatment with Interferon-α

	IFN	Placebo
Loss of HBV DNA	37%	17%
Loss of HBeAg	33%	12%
Loss of HBsAg	8%	2%

Data from Wong DK, Cheung AM, O'Rourke K, Naylor CD, Detsky AS, Heathcote J. Effect of alpha-interferon in patients with hepatitis B e antigen-positive chronic hepatitis B. A meta-analysis. Ann Intern Med 1993;119:312–323.

[a] Fifteen randomized placebo-controlled trials involving 837 patients were used in the analysis. Patients were followed for at least 6 months after cessation of therapy.

to normal as HBV DNA or HBeAg is cleared. In nonresponders, such changes are not normally seen. The predictors of a favorable response listed in Table 5 provide useful guidance for deciding whether interferon treatment is warranted or not in chronic HBV carriers. The recommended treatment is interferon-α 10 million units 3 times weekly for 4 months.

Prednisone pretreatment to enhance the response to interferon offers little benefit over interferon treatment without prednisone (187, 203, 283). Prednisone treatment and subsequent withdrawal can lead to a flare of hepatitis that may be sufficiently severe to cause hepatic decompensation in patients with advanced liver disease. In addition, prednisone has significant adverse effects.

Most of the clinical studies did not follow patients long term after interferon therapy. However, in an early study that followed interferon responders for 3 to 7 years, 3 of 23 patients relapsed with HBV viremia within 1 year of stopping therapy. More encouragingly, 13 of 23 patients became negative for HBsAg (130). In a more-recent long-term follow-up study of interferon-treated patients, patients with HBeAg clearance after interferon treatment had a better clinical outcome than nonresponders or patients who did not receive interferon (174). The risks of death from liver failure, cirrhosis, and the requirement for liver transplant were higher in the group who did not clear HBeAg after interferon therapy (Table 6).

In general, patients with advanced hepatitis B liver diseases do not tolerate interferon treatment well. Interferon treatment can precipitate liver failure. However, use of low-dose or titrated doses of interferon has been found to benefit some patients with chronic hepatitis (188). In patients with HBV-associated cirrhosis and Child's class A or B status, interferon therapy should be administered by physicians who are experienced in treating patients with advanced liver disease. The starting dose of 0.5 million units 3 times weekly should be increased slowly according to the patient's tolerance.

Patients with relapses of HBV infection several months after cessation of interferon treatment may respond to retreatment with interferon. These patients usually respond to a second course of interferon, and some have a sustained response. Patients who fail to normalize aminotransferases or lose HBeAg after a second full course of interferon are unlikely to respond to further interferon treatment.

Interferon has significant adverse effects that tend to be dose dependent (Table 7). Nearly all patients have "flulike" symptoms after the first few doses of interferon. Acetaminophen helps relieve these symptoms, and these early adverse effects tend to subside or improve after the first or second week of treatment. Late adverse effects are less common but more problematic. Myelosuppression with neutropenia and thrombocytopenia can develop during treatment. Clinically significant depression and autoimmune thyroid diseases are also common. The interferon dose may have to be reduced or discontinued with these side effects. Close monitoring and supervision are necessary during treatment.

Antiviral Chemotherapy for Chronic HBV Infection

Fialuridine.   Fialuridine (FIAU) was used in a phase II clinical trial at 0.1 and 0.25 mg/kg/day. Fialuridine had been shown to be a very potent inhibitor of HBV in cell cultures and of WHV in vivo. Unfortunately, 7 of 15 patients treated developed hepatic failure, with 5 deaths and 2 patients requiring liver transplantation. Patients on therapy developed lactic acidosis, pancreatitis, myopathy, and neuropathy (164). The toxicity associated with the racemic mixture of FIAU results from mitochondrial uptake of the D isomer of FIAU triphosphate, which inhibits mitochondrial DNA synthesis (59, 146). The tragedy of this event has resulted in very close monitoring for mitochondrial toxicity associated with nucleoside analogue use in patients.

Lamivudine.   There are many phase II and phase III studies of lamivudine in chronic HBV and HBV DNA-positive patients undergoing liver transplantation. The initial placebo-controlled trial of lamivudine use in chronic HBV indicated that lamivudine at 100 mg or more given orally once daily effectively suppressed HBV DNA in serum (258). In a 3-month study reported by Dienstag et al. (69), lamivudine at 100 or 300 mg orally once daily resulted in HBV DNA levels (by Abbott liquid hybridization assay) becoming undetectable in all patients treated for 3 months. Six patients had sustained loss of HBV DNA when lamivudine was discontinued. However, when lamivudine was discontinued, viral replication recurred in most patients treated for 4 or 12 weeks (133). Leung et al. (145) reported that lamivudine (100 mg/day orally) normalized ALT in 72% of patients, versus 24% normalization in placebo-treated patients. Analysis of pre- and post-treatment biopsy specimens showed histological improvement in 67% of lamivudine-treated

---

TABLE 5 • **Factors Predictive of Responsiveness/ Nonresponsiveness of Chronic HBV Infection to Interferon-α Treatment**

Likely Responders	Likely Nonresponders
Adult acquired infection	Neonatally acquired infection
Short duration of infection (<2 years)	Patients with decompensated cirrhosis
Active liver disease (AST > 2–5×)	HBeAg positive with normal AST
Low HBV DNA	High HBV DNA
Immunocompetent	Immunosuppressed
Absence of HDV infection	Coinfection of HDV infection
Female	Male
HBeAg positive	HIV positive

TABLE 6 • **Long-Term Follow-up of HBeAg-Positive Patients after Interferon Therapy**

	IFN + HBeAg	IFN − HBeAg	Control Group
Death (liver failure)	12%	0%	6%
Cirrhosis	14%	2%	15%
Liver transplant	4%	0%	2%

Data adapted from Niederau C, Heintges T, Lange S, et al. Long-term follow-up of HBeAg-positive patients treated with interferon alfa for chronic hepatitis B. N Engl J Med 1996;334:1422–1487.

TABLE 7 • Adverse Effects of Interferon	
Early and Common	**Late and Less Common**
Fever and chills	Psychiatric symptoms
Myalgia and back pain	Depression
Fatigue	Irritability
Headaches	Insomnia
Anorexia and weight loss	Myelosuppression
Gastrointestinal symptoms	Neutropenia
Abdominal discomfort	Thrombocytopenia
Irritability and poor concentration	Autoimmune diseases
Insomnia	Thyroid diseases
Alopecia	Hepatitis
	Autoantibodies
	Retinopathy

patients, compared with 30% of placebo-treated patients. Progression to fibrosis was slowed to 3% in lamivudine-treated patients compared with 15% in placebo-treated patients (145).

With lamivudine administration for 1 year, seroconversion rates for HBeAg ranged from 16 to 33% (70, 145). Long-term therapy has improved liver histology and suppressed viral markers of ongoing replication (107). Side effects have been relatively few but fatigue, headaches, gastrointestinal upset, musculoskeletal discomfort, dizziness, and numbness have been reported in both placebo- and lamivudine-treated patients. Lamivudine has good bioavailability (>80%) and is excreted in the urine unchanged. There is no evidence of mitochondrial toxicity with prolonged use (108).

Lamivudine will likely be approved for use in 1998, and the most likely recommendation will be 100 mg/day orally. Since lamivudine and 3TC are chemically identical, side effects reported with 3TC use in HIV-positive patients may be expected in chronic HBV patients receiving lamivudine. The most serious side effect seen primarily in HIV-positive patients is rare cases of severe pancreatitis (190). Marked elevations of transaminases were reported in some patients discontinuing lamivudine after therapy for 6 months or more.

Famciclovir. While intravenous ganciclovir has shown some promise clinically as an antihepadnaviral agent (100), its use has been superseded by famciclovir, an orally administered precursor of penciclovir. Famciclovir is well absorbed and rapidly converted to penciclovir by enzymatic hydrolysis. A large placebo-controlled multicenter study showed that famciclovir at doses of 500, 250, or 150 mg given orally three times daily rapidly suppressed HBV DNA and reduced ALT levels. The medication was well tolerated, with side effects similar to placebo (251). However, suppression of HBV DNA in patients has been variable. Use of famciclovir in recurrent HBV after liver transplantation reduced HBV DNA in only 50% of those treated (198). Similarly, only four of seven patients with decompensated liver disease responded to famciclovir (24). HBV DNA does not appear to be as consistently or completely suppressed in patients receiving famciclovir as in those treated with lamivudine. Famciclovir has an excellent

safety profile, and its status as an antiviral for chronic HBV remains unclear.

Lobucavir. Lobucavir is a guanosine analogue with broad-spectrum antiviral activity. It was used in a phase II trial of 22 patients receiving 200 mg twice daily, 200 mg four times daily, or placebo. Treatment was for 4 weeks, and both doses of lobucavir reduced HBV DNA levels by 2 to 4 logs. Within 4 weeks of completing lobucavir treatment, HBV DNA returned to pretreatment levels in all but one patient. No significant toxicity was observed in 4 weeks of treatment (28). It is too early to predict the future of lobucavir in the treatment of chronic HBV.

Adefovir. Adefovir dipivoxil (bis-POM PMEA) is a broad-spectrum antiviral nucleoside analogue that is active against HBV, HIV, and herpesviruses. In a phase I/II trial of adefovir dipivoxil, 125 mg/day for 28 days reduced HBV DNA by 2 logs. Three of 15 patients experienced liver transaminase elevations of more than 300 U/L while on therapy (98). Further studies with lower doses and longer durations of therapy can be expected.

Resistance of HBV to Nucleoside Analogues. Development of mutants resistant to effective antiviral agents is a significant concern. HIV develops resistance to 3TC (220, 248). 3TC-resistance in HIV most commonly results from a mutation in the YMDD motif of the reverse transcriptase (33). Hepadnaviral polymerases contain a similar YMDD motif. The duck model was used to produce lamivudine-resistant DHBV in vitro by mutation of the methionine to valine (86). The prediction of lamivudine resistance with mutations at the YMDD motif was quickly confirmed by reports of lamivudine-resistant HBV mutants in patients on therapy (70, 149, 247). These mutations were localized to the methionine residue of the YMDD motif as predicted from the duck model. Lamivudine-resistant mutants occur more frequently and rapidly in patients receiving lamivudine to suppress HBV in liver transplantation than in those receiving lamivudine for chronic HBV. Lamivudine-resistant HBV in patients treated for chronic HBV has been reported to be 4% at 36 weeks and 14% at 52 weeks of treatment (134). In liver transplant patients, 14 of 68 lamivudine-treated patients had resistant virus after 7 months (189). Famciclovir-resistant mutants of HBV have been described, but the mutations are not localized to the YMDD motif as for lamivudine-resistant mutants (17). Famciclovir-resistant mutants often respond to lamivudine therapy.

Resistance develops more slowly in the treatment of chronic HBV infections with monotherapy but is analogous to resistance to monotherapy in the treatment of HIV. The markedly improved responses in HIV-infected patients receiving combination chemotherapy suggests that combination chemotherapy for chronic HBV will produce more suppression or eradication of the virus and slow the development of resistance. The mechanisms of action of anti-HBV nucleoside analogues differ: lamivudine acts by chain termination (223), and some of the purine analogues block protein priming (111, 239, 286). Possibly, combination chemotherapy of chronic HBV with an antiviral that inhibits chain elongation (e.g., lamivudine) and a purine nucleoside antiviral agent that blocks protein priming of HBV

DNA synthesis may be more effective than monotherapy and slow the development of resistance.

Prevention with Passive and Active Immunization against HBV

Immunoglobulin. Immunoglobulin administered after exposure to HBV can protect against infection. Two different preparations may be used: hepatitis B immunoglobulin (HBIG) is prepared from pooled plasma to yield a product with an anti-HBs titer above 1:100,000, and standard immunoglobulin has an anti-HBs titer of approximately 1:100. A randomized, double-blind trial comparing HBIG with immune serum globulin in patients with needle-stick exposure found clinical hepatitis in 1.4% of HBIG recipients and 5.9% of standard immunoglobulin recipients. Subsequent seroconversion to positive anti-HBs occurred in 5.6% of HBIG recipients and 20.7% of immunoglobulin recipients (261). Without immune prophylaxis, the infection rate after HBV exposure is 20 to 40% (163). HBIG prophylaxis is more effective than standard immunoglobulin in preventing HBV infection after exposure.

Infants born to HBeAg-positive mothers or mothers with acute hepatitis during the third trimester are at a high risk of acquiring the infection. In a small nonrandomized study to assess the efficacy of HBIG in preventing HBV transmission from mothers with acute hepatitis B to their infants, HBIG given to infants at birth was effective in preventing HBV infection (170). In a randomized double-blind placebo-controlled trial to study HBIG prevention of perinatal transmission, infants from HBeAg-carrier mothers received either placebo, three 0.5-mL doses of HBIG, or a 1-mL single dose of HBIG. HBV carrier rates of these infants were 92, 26, and 54%, respectively (22). Although HBIG is useful in preventing perinatal transmission of HBV, it is not a perfect preventive measure; a significant number of infants will still become HBV carriers. This has led to studies using HBIG and HBV vaccine simultaneously; the combination has yielded protection rates above 90%.

HBV Vaccine. Plasma-derived vaccine containing HBsAg first became available in 1981. This inactivated vaccine has been replaced by recombinant HBsAg vaccines. Currently there are two approved recombinant HBV vaccines; both are safe and have very few serious adverse effects. Fever and injection site reaction are common, with anaphylaxis and Guillain-Barré syndrome reported as rare adverse events in recipients.

After a complete course of vaccination (Table 8), 95 to 99% of immunocompetent individuals develop protective anti-HBs titers of 10 mIU/mL (77, 200). After two doses of vaccine, adults usually develop a protective anti-HBs titer (241). The third dose is important to increase anti-HBs antibody titers and the duration of protection. An accelerated schedule of three doses of vaccine can induce more-rapid antibody protection at the expense of lower peak anti-HBs antibody titers (117). Response rates are lower in immunocompromised patients such as those with AIDS, diabetes mellitus, renal failure, increased age, or poor nutrition status. Many who do not develop anti-HBs antibodies after the initial three-dose series develop antibodies with additional doses (103). If the immunization program starts at an early age, the incidence of child carriers can be decreased in areas of high HBV prevalence (272). Many communities have a universal vaccination program for infants or children prior to the age when they might experience the high-risk activities of illicit drug use or sexual activity. Vaccine is also recommended for any persons at risk of acquiring HBV infection (Table 9).

Is a booster dose of HBV vaccine necessary? After completion of HBV vaccination, the level of anti-HBs declines with time. In 10 to 15% of adult responders, the level of anti-HBs decreases below protective titers by 5 years. A similar decline in anti-HBs titer is seen in children who have received active-passive immunization at birth. At 5 years of age, only 86% of the children maintain a protective antibody titer (64). When these patients are challenged with a booster dose of vaccine, immunologic memory can be demonstrated. However, the response time is 4 days (275), a delay that might allow HBV infection of hepatocytes. For high-risk groups and immunocompromised individuals, it might be important to maintain the anti-HBs titer above the protective level with a booster dose of vaccine. Routine booster immunization is not necessary in low-risk immunocompetent persons since current evidence shows continuing protection (266).

Endpoints for Monitoring Therapy

Patients with chronic HBV infection commonly have progressive liver disease and are at risk of developing cirrhosis or hepatocellular carcinoma. The primary goal of antiviral therapy for chronic HBV infection is elimination of virus from all host cells, and the ideal response to therapy would be loss of all HBV markers with the appearance of HBsAb. This has proven to be a difficult but not impossible challenge. An alternative approach may be to control HBV replication and prevent progression of liver disease. Antiviral therapy may result in loss of HBV DNA and HBeAg and normalization of transaminases without clearance of HBsAg. HBV DNA can integrate into the

---

TABLE 8 • Dosages and Administration Schedules for HBV Vaccines

Group	Schedule	Recombivax (Merck)	Energix-B (SmithKline)
Infants	0, 1–2, 6 months	2.5μg	10 μg
Infants (HBsAg mother)	HBIG + 0, 1–2, 6 months	5 μg	10 μg
Children	0, 1–2, 6 months	2.5 μg	10 μg
Adults (healthy)	0, 1–2, 6 months	10 μg	20 μg
Adults (immunocompromised)	0, 1, 6 months	40 μg	40 μg

TABLE 9 • **Candidates for HBV Vaccinations**

High-Risk Groups for HBV Infection
Persons with occupational risks
Heterosexual persons with multiple partners
Sexually active homosexual or bisexual males
Intravenous drug users
Hemophiliacs
Inmates of long-term correctional institutions
Residents and staffs of institutions for developmentally challenged
Intimate contacts of HBV carriers
Hemodialysis patients
International travelers to highly endemic areas

host cell DNA and may continue HBsAg production without producing infectious virus. Integrated HBV DNA is not likely to be eliminated by antiviral therapy.

Adjunctive Therapy

Patient Counseling. It is important to provide counseling to the patients to help prevent the spread of the infection among their close contacts. Close contacts should be tested for HBV infection. If they have not developed HBV infection or immunity to HBV, they should receive HBIG and HBV vaccine.

Liver Transplantation. Liver transplantation is a treatment option for end-stage liver disease. However, cirrhosis associated with chronic HBV infection is a controversial indication for liver transplantation because of the very high reinfection rate of the hepatic allograft and rapid progressive liver disease in the allograft (137, 138). Patients with HBeAg or HBV DNA at the time of liver transplantation are particularly at risk, and the incidence of reinfection of hepatic graft is over 90%. With HBV reinfection of the hepatic graft, the 1-year survival is 68% and 3-year survival is 44% (214), rates significantly below those for patients transplanted for other liver diseases. The clinical course of HBV infection in the hepatic graft is accelerated, and liver failure can occur in a short period of time (249). An unusual form of rapidly progressive liver injury characterized by very high levels of hepatitis B antigen expression in hepatocytes, with marked cholestasis and fibrosis of the transplanted liver develops in 10 to 20% of patients. This condition, known as fibrosing cholestatic hepatitis or cytolytic hepatitis, is virtually 100% fatal (60, 140, 152); patients do not respond to interferon therapy, and retransplantation is rarely of benefit (58). For these reasons, many liver transplant centers do not consider patients with HBV-induced cirrhosis with ongoing viral replication to be suitable candidates for transplantation.

Some transplant centers have used HBIG to prevent HBV infection of hepatic allograft after liver transplantation. The initial experience was disappointing, as the dose of HBIG used was too low. With more effective doses of HBIG, HBV reinfection of the hepatic allograft can be controlled (142, 213). Patients receive 100 mL of HBIG intravenously during the ahepatic phase, and 5 mL of HBIG daily for 1 week after liver

transplantation. During the initial few months posttransplantation, anti-HBs titers should be maintained in the 300 to 500 IU/mL range. With this high level of anti-HBs, HBsAg often disappears from the blood. HBIG treatment has to be continued indefinitely, and 5 mL of HBIG should be given whenever the anti-HBs titer declines to 100 IU/mL. HBIG treatment adds substantial cost to the liver transplantation procedure. HBsAg mutants can develop during maintenance HBIG treatment (N. Terrault, personal communication) and occur more commonly with monoclonal HBIG immunoprophylaxis (166).

Recently a number of centers have used lamivudine pre- and posttransplantation in an attempt to prevent infection of the hepatic allograft. Patients receive lamivudine to lower HBV DNA to undetectable levels prior to liver transplantation. Lamivudine treatment significantly decreases the possibility of allograft reinfection but, unfortunately, lamivudine-resistant mutants do arise in liver transplant patients, with one report of more than 20% of patients at 7 months posttransplant (18, 19, 189). HBV isolates from these patients have mutations in the YMDD motif. Liver transplant recipients with active HBV replication prior to liver transplantation may do better with both lamivudine and HBIG treatment or combination antiviral therapy when additional antiviral agents of proven safety and efficacy become available.

Hepatitis D Virus (HDV)

General Description

Molecular Biology. Hepatitis delta virus (HDV) was discovered in 1977 (205). It is a satellite virus in that it requires concurrent HBV (helper virus) infection. It is presently classified in its own family, *Deltaviridae*. The HDV RNA genome is approximately 1700 bases, single-stranded, circular, and highly base paired. Three genotypes have been discovered in the 14 HDV isolates sequenced so far (44). In addition to the genotypic variation, HDV in a particular patient appears to be slightly heterogeneous and exists as a quasispecies.

The RNA genome and the hepatitis delta antigen (HDAg) constitute the nucleocapsid, which is enclosed by an HBV surface antigen (HBsAg) envelope. The role of HBV as helper virus for HDV infection appears to be production of HBsAg. The only HDV viral protein known is HDAg and is found in the nuclei of HDV-infected hepatocytes. RNA replication likely follows a double rolling circle mechanism that generates greater-than-genome-length antigenomic RNA that is self-cleaved by HDV ribozyme activity to form circular antigenomic RNA monomers (23). This antigenomic RNA is subsequently used as template for production of progeny genomic RNA. The RNA-dependent RNA polymerase activity likely involves the host cell DNA-dependent RNA polymerase II, although the exact mechanism remains to be determined (135).

Epidemiology. As stated above, HDV is a defective RNA virus that requires HBV as a helper for replication. HDV infection occurs either as a coinfection with HBV or as a superinfection of chronic HBV. The epidemiology of HDV is therefore quite similar to that of HBV; both viruses have similar modes of transmission involving parenteral exposures (206). In low endemic countries such as the United States, the predominate mode of HDV transmission involves intravenous drug use (169); sexual transmission of HDV occurs less frequently (144). Patients with hemophilia who require clotting factors prepared from large donor pools also have a relatively high prevalence of chronic HDV infection. There are an estimated 70,000 patients with chronic HDV infection in the United States (11).

HDV and HBV are endemic in Mediterranean and Middle East countries such as Italy and Kuwait (194). However, Southeast Asia has a high prevalence of HBV carriers but a low prevalence of HDV infection. These differences in prevalence may be explained by differences in HBV transmission. In Southeast Asia, HBV infection is frequently acquired through vertical transmission from mother to infant or early in childhood. Southeast Asian mothers have a low prevalence of HDV infection. In countries where HDV is transmitted with HBV, transmission of these viruses frequently results from high-risk activities such as intravenous drug use. Measures taken to prevent AIDS and HBV vaccination have decreased HBV and HDV infection rates.

Clinical Manifestation. The clinical presentation of HDV coinfection with HBV differs from that of HDV superinfection with HBV (Figs. 9 and 10). The initial presentation in both cases is that of acute hepatitis or a "flare" of hepatitis. The subsequent course of disease is markedly different. Severe hepatitis can occur in patients with coinfection, and the incidence of fulminant liver failure is higher than that in HBV infection alone (234). However, most of these patients recover from the HDV and HBV infection. Only 2% of patients with acute coinfection become chronic HDV carriers with progression of liver disease (41). Thus HDV and HBV coinfections usually have a benign course similar to that of acute HBV infection. In contrast, chronic HDV infection occurs in almost all HBV carriers superinfected with HDV (41). Most of these patients de-

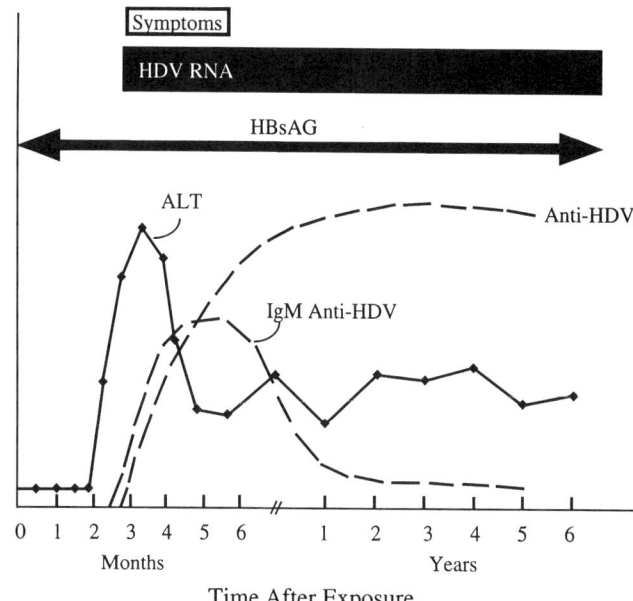

FIGURE 10. Superinfection with HBV and HDV.

velop chronic hepatitis with progressive liver disease more severe than that with chronic HBV infection alone. Cirrhosis with liver failure occurs in 25%, and hepatocellular carcinoma occurs in 35% of these patients (31, 234).

HDV infection should be considered if a patient with acute HBV has severe hepatitis or fulminant hepatitis or a patient with chronic HBV infection has a flare of hepatitis. The diagnosis of HDV infection requires detection of HDV antigen, anti-HDV, or HDV RNA. The HDV antigen can be detected by Western blotting; however this test is not widely available. IgM anti-HDV serology is the most commonly used test. In acute coinfection with HBV and HDV, HBsAg, IgM anti-HBc, and IgM anti-HDV are positive. In acute superinfection with HDV, HBsAg and IgM anti-HDV are positive, but IgM anti-HBc is negative. In chronic HDV infection, HBsAg and IgG anti-HDV are positive, the titer of anti-HDV is persistently high, and HDV RNA is present (246). HDV RNA can be detected by slot blot hybridization or with reverse transcription and PCR, but these are not routinely available.

Antiviral Therapy

Interferon/Ribavirin. Interferon-α is the treatment that has been studied the most extensively (Table 10). Most of the published randomized controlled trials using interferon-α to treat chronic HDV infection involved small numbers of patients, as chronic HDV infection is uncommon, and most of these patients tended to have poor compliance. Interferon therapy appears to be useful in treating chronic HDV infection. The results of one recent trial showed a satisfactory biochemical response with an aminotransferase response rate of 70% during high-dose interferon treatment (9 million units three times weekly) (80). When the interferon was given at 3 million units 3 times weekly, the aminotransferase response rate dropped significantly, from 70 to 29% (80). In all these studies, HDV in-

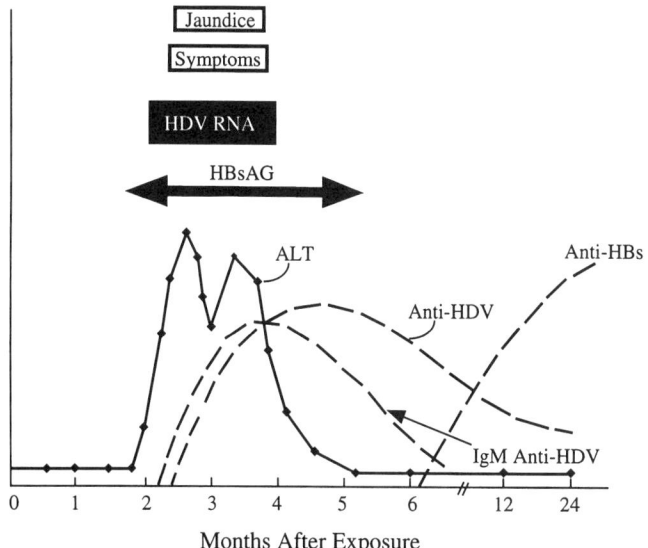

FIGURE 9. Coinfection with HBV and HDV.

TABLE 10 • Interferon Treatment of HDV Infection

Reference	IFN Dose	End of Treatment		Follow-up	
		ALT N[a]	HDV-RNA Neg.	ALT N[a]	HDV-RNA Neg.
Farci 1994	9 MU TIW × 48 weeks	71%	50%	36%	0
	3 MU TIW × 48 weeks	29%	21%	0	0
	Controls	8%	0	0	0
Gaudin 1995	5 MU/m² TIW × 4 months, then 3 MU/m² TIW × 8 months	36%	77%	9%	22%
	Controls	0	12%	0	0
Rosina 1991	As above	26%	N.D.[b]	3%	N.D.
	Controls	7%	N.D.[b]	0	N.D.

[a] N, normal.
[b] N.D., not done or no result was given.

fection relapsed after cessation of interferon therapy in almost all treated patients unless they cleared HBsAg. In the minority of patients who lost HBsAg with interferon treatment, HDV RNA became undetectable in blood and liver (20). At present, interferon is not recommended for routine treatment of chronic HDV because of frequent relapse and the lack of demonstrable long-term benefit in most patients.

A study using ribavirin monotherapy (15 mg/kg/day for 16 weeks) to treat nine patients with chronic hepatitis D infection showed no significant antiviral effects and was not effective in reducing the biochemical markers of liver inflammation and necrosis (95).

Lamivudine.   There is a single report of use of lamivudine in HDV-infected patients. At the end of therapy, all patients remained positive for HDV RNA. Lamivudine monotherapy does not appear to be of value in the treatment of HDV (109).

Prevention.   Persons who are at risk for HBV infection are also at risk for HDV infection. As HDV infection depends on the presence of HBV, HBV vaccination prevents coinfection of HDV and HBV.

Chronic HBV carriers who have acquired their disease through high-risk behavior are at risk of HDV superinfection. Lifestyle counseling to avoid high-risk behavior is important to prevent HDV superinfection in these HBV carriers.

Adjunctive Therapy

Liver Transplantation.   Chronic HDV infection frequently leads to cirrhosis and liver failure, and liver transplantation is an option for these patients. The main concern, however, is recurrence of HBV and HDV infection after liver transplantation. Reinfection of the hepatic graft by HBV can lead to poorer outcomes than liver transplantation for many other liver diseases (178, 249). Reinfection of the hepatic graft by HDV is common after liver transplantation (152, 182, 215). However, the outcome of liver transplantation for patients with both HDV and HBV appears better than that for patients transplanted for cirrhosis induced by HBV alone (65, 74). HDV coinfection of the hepatic graft appears to provide some protection against rapid hepatic graft loss from HBV infection (178).

Anti-HBs immunoglobulins are effective in preventing HBV reinfection of the hepatic graft (212). With anti-HBs immunoglobulin treatment, hepatic graft reinfection with HBV

and HDV occurred in only 13% of transplanted patients (212, 214). The 5-year actuarial survival for liver transplantation in HDV-induced cirrhosis was 88% in this study. Therefore, anti-HBs immunoglobulins should be used with liver transplantation in HDV-infected patients with cirrhosis.

Hepatitis C Virus (HCV)

General Description

Molecular Biology.   Hepatitis C virus was identified by molecular cloning in 1989 (53). HCV is a 40- to 50-nm spherical enveloped virus that contains a (+) sense single-stranded RNA genome. The virus is classified in its own genus in the family *Flaviviridae* on the basis of its genomic organization (110, 259). The approximately 9500-nucleotide (+) sense RNA genome codes for a single 3010–amino acid polyprotein with the structural proteins at the N terminus and the non-structural proteins toward the C terminus: NH_2-C-E1-E2-NS2-NS3-NS4A-NS4B-NS5A-NS5B-COOH (Fig. 11). The polyprotein requires processing by both host and viral proteases. The capsid (C) protein is conserved, while the other two structural proteins, E1 and E2 (envelope glycoproteins) are much more variable. A hypervariable region at the N terminal end of the envelope protein E2 results in HCV existing as a heterogeneous population (quasispecies).

The error-prone replication of HCV via RNA-dependent RNA polymerase activity is due to the absence of proofreading ability. This results in genetic heterogeneity of HCV (38). The heterogeneous population of HCV within an infected individual is called a quasispecies; the variations between separate HCV isolates give rise to genotypes. The accepted genotyping system is based on nucleotide sequence homology of the NS-5 region (230, 231). This system has 6 types and 11 subtypes. Specific genotypes have been found to be associated with different geographic regions and variability in response to antiviral therapy and degree of disease severity (38, 230, 284).

Epidemiology.   HCV has worldwide distribution. It is an important cause of chronic hepatitis and cirrhosis. In the United States, HCV infection accounts for 21% of acute viral hepatitis. The CDC has estimated that there are 150,000 new cases of HCV annually in United States. The overall prevalence of HCV infection in the general population is approximately 1%; however there is great variability among different

Hepatitis C Virus

RNA

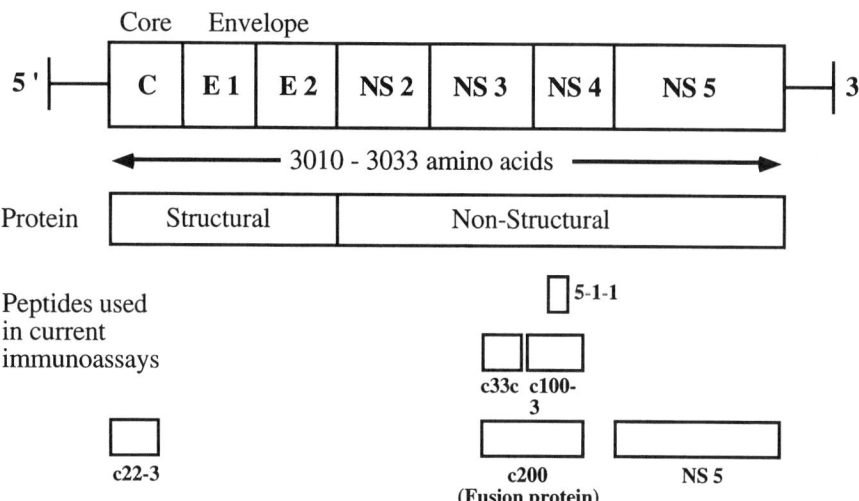

FIGURE 11. HCV genome.

subgroups, with hemophilia patients having a prevalence rate as high as 90%.

The principal mode of HCV transmission is parenteral exposure to the virus. Intravenous drug use is the major cause of HCV infection in the general population, and blood transfusion accounts for 4% of reported cases (9). Nonparenteral transmission through sexual or intimate contact and maternal-infant exposure has been reported but is uncommon (269, 282). Other risk factors include body piercing and intranasal cocaine use (57). A significant percentage of patients with HCV infection has no identifiable risk factors.

The enzyme immunoassay (EIA) for antibody against HCV is the initial test in assessing for possible hepatitis C infection. The latest generation of EIA tests are sensitive and specific for hepatitis C antibody. However, detection of antibody against hepatitis C virus does not distinguish acute, chronic, or past infection. Tests based on HCV nucleic acid detection (branched DNA signal amplification assay or PCR) are important supplementary tests for diagnosis of ongoing HCV infection.

Clinical Manifestation. Acute HCV infection usually causes a milder disease than does HBV infection. The incubation period for HCV is 4 to 10 weeks, and the acute illness usually lasts 2 to 6 weeks. During acute infection, only 25 to 35% develop symptoms including malaise, nausea, anorexia, low-grade fever, and fatigue. Most patients have abnormal liver enzyme levels during acute infection. Rarely, fulminant liver failure results from acute HCV infection (79).

Most patients (80–90%) with acute HCV infections become chronic carriers, many with elevated aminotransferases (12, 224). Patients with chronic HCV infection have minimal symptoms and the level of aminotransferases can fluctuate (Fig. 12). HCV-infected patients with normal transaminases can have

chronic hepatitis on liver biopsy (171). Genotyping of HCV is also useful because severe liver disease is more commonly associated with genotype 1b infection (125, 196). Anti-HCV antibodies do not prevent progression of chronic hepatitis to cirrhosis. More than 20% of patients go on to develop cirrhosis in 20 years. HCV-associated cirrhosis has become one of the most common indications for liver transplantation.

There is also a strong association between chronic HCV infection and development of hepatocellular carcinoma (232). Hepatocellular carcinoma usually occurs late (2–3 decades) in the course of the HCV liver disease. Cryoglobulinemia, porphyria cutanea tarda, aplastic anemia, and membranoproliferative glomerulonephritis are other diseases associated with chronic HCV infection (101).

Susceptibility in Vitro and in Animal Models

It is difficult to introduce and propagate HCV in cell cultures. This has become a stumbling block to study of HCV replication and anti-HCV treatment. Human bone marrow–derived B-cell line CE was infected by HCV and supported production of HCV (25). This appears to be a promising in vitro model for HCV, and its usefulness needs to be established.

Chimpanzees are the only established nonhuman model for HCV. There is a lot of interest in developing alternate animal models to facilitate study of HCV therapy and make such studies less costly. The HCV genome has been transiently expressed in rat liver following liposome-mediated gene transfer (243), and HCV viremia can be obtained transiently by transplanting HCV-infected liver fragments into BNX (beige, nude, X-linked immunodeficient) mice reconstituted with SCID mouse bone marrow cells (92). None of these nonchimpanzee animal models can consistently support propagation of HCV to allow evaluation of anti-HCV drugs.

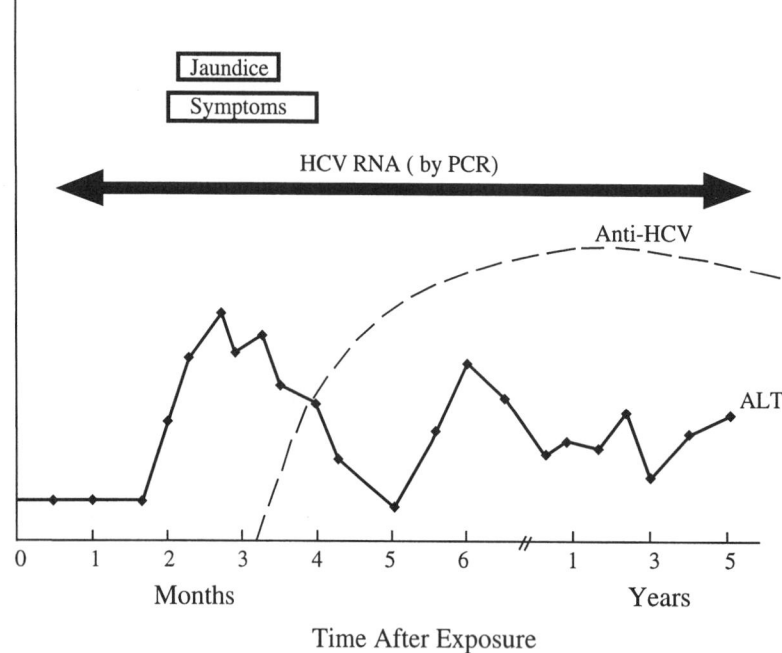

FIGURE 12. Natural history of HCV infection.

Antiviral Therapy

Interferon Treatment of Acute HCV. There are suggestions that treating acute HCV infection with interferon might decrease the frequency of establishment of the chronic carrier state. Three clinical trials have been done in patients with acute posttransfusion HCV infections. Interferon-α (3 million units three times per week for 12 weeks) has been compared with placebo. While these studies involved a small number of patients, they consistently showed interferon to be beneficial in treating acute HCV infection (Table 11).

Two additional studies of patients with posttransfusion and nontransfusion cases of acute HCV studied the effects of interferon-β on progression of acute hepatitis to chronic hepatitis (181, 242). In the first study, patients were treated with interferon-β 3 million units for 5 consecutive days in the first week and the same dose of interferon-β 3 times a week for an additional 3 weeks. At 3-year follow-up, 10 of 11 treated patients were negative for HCV RNA, while only 1 of 14 control patients was negative for HCV RNA (181). The second study examined the effect of dose and duration of interferon-β therapy on acute HCV (242). Patients treated with 6 million units of interferon-β daily had a 90% sustained response at 6 months posttherapy, versus 18% in the patients who received 0.3 million units of interferon β. Interferon-β is not as potent as interferon-α in treating HCV (186).

A meta-analysis that combined randomized and nonrandomized trials of interferon treatment in acute HCV infections from posttransfusion and nontransfusion causes shows that a course of interferon treatment is beneficial for viral clearance and prevention of chronic hepatitis (39). A long-term prospective controlled trial for further study of the optimum dose and duration of interferon therapy in acute HCV infections might be valuable.

At present, interferon therapy should be considered for acute symptomatic HCV. A significant number of these patients clears the virus with interferon treatment. A reasonable treatment schedule is 3 to 6 million units of interferon three times a week for 3 to 6 months (227).

Interferon Treatment for Chronic HCV. Only interferon-α has been approved for treatment of chronic HCV infection. The first randomized controlled trial used 3 million units of interferon three times per week to treat chronic HCV infection. The results showed normalization of transaminases in almost half of the patients receiving interferon, compared with 8% of untreated patients (61). During follow-up, relapse occurred in half of the patients who had normalized transaminases levels during treatment. Corticosteroid priming prior to interferon therapy did not improve the response rate over that with interferon treatment alone (49).

Many controlled trials have studied the effects of dosage and duration of interferon treatment on chronic HCV infection. Most interferon treatment protocols use 28 weeks of therapy; however, several recent studies showed that 12 or 18 months of treatment improves the sustained response rate. In a study from Japan, the sustained response rate was 54% for 52 weeks of treatment, compared with 33% for 28 weeks of treatment. However prolonged treatment did not improve the outcomes of nonresponders (121). In another study, all patients were treated with interferon 3 million units three times per week for 6 months and then divided into three groups receiving (a) 3 million units of interferon three times per week, (b) 1 million units of interferon three times per week, or (c) no further treatment, for an additional 12 months. The patients who received 3 million units of interferon three times per week for 18 months had a 45% sustained response rate, compared with a 27% response

TABLE 11 • Interferon Treatment of Posttransfusion Acute HCV

Reference	Normal Transaminase at End of Therapy		Normal Transaminase at 12–18 Month Follow-up		HCV RNA at 18 Months	
	IFN	Control	IFN	Control	IFN	Control
Viladomiu 1994 (176)	73%	38%	53%	31%	—	—
Hwang 1994 (177)	81%	35%	56%	38%	—	—
Lampertico 1994 (178)	73%	44%	59%	37%	39%	0

rate in the low-dose interferon group and 30% in the no-further-treatment group (195). A schedule of 6 million units of interferon for 4 months followed by a maintenance dose of interferon 3 million units three times per week for 8 months was reported to give a sustained response rate of 49% (51).

Viremia clears in 60 to 80% of sustained responders who received prolonged interferon treatment (51, 216), and interferon retreatment can lead to a sustained response in 40% of patients who have a relapse of HCV infection after interferon therapy (97). Escalating doses of interferon do not improve the total sustained response (153).

Even with prolonged treatment, approximately a third of treated patients do not respond to interferon (121). If there is no biochemical response in 3 months, interferon therapy should be stopped because these patients are unlikely to respond to longer treatment. Retreatment or treatment with a higher dose of interferon might improve transaminase levels without improving the sustained response (32). Some patients experience reactivation or breakthrough of HCV infection during interferon therapy (71). In one study, high titers of neutralizing interferon antibodies seemed to be associated with responders who exhibited breakthrough (209).

Several predictors are associated with a good response to interferon (Table 12). A comparison of interferon treatment in patients with and without cirrhosis shows that noncirrhotic patients have a sustained response rate of 40% after 12 months of therapy versus a response rate of 5% in cirrhotic patients (118). Pretreatment viral titers and genotypes are also important in determining the outcome of interferon treatment. Low pretreatment levels of viral RNA and the non-1b genotypes are associated with a favorable interferon response (3, 160, 184). Early loss of serum HCV RNA after 1 to 2 weeks of therapy also predicts sustained response (120). Other favorable factors include female sex, younger age, shorter duration of infection, and low hepatic iron concentrations (51, 180).

A sustained response to interferon therapy is presumed to translate into decreased end-stage liver disease or hepatocellular carcinoma in chronic HCV carriers. To date, only one study has shown improved long-term results. Treatment of patients with HCV-related cirrhosis with interferon decreased the incidence of hepatocellular carcinoma from 38 to 4% (175), but these results are controversial because the incidence of hepatocellular carcinoma was unusually high in the control group during a relatively short follow-up of 2 to 7 years. It remains to be proven that interferon responders have better long-term outcomes than nonresponders.

TABLE 12 • Predictors of a Good Sustained Response to Interferon Treatment in Patients with HCV Infection

Predictors
Short duration of chronic infection
Young patients
Abnormal ALT
Absence of cirrhosis
Low level of HCV RNA
Not genotype 1b
Low hepatic iron

Chronic hepatitis C patients who have extrahepatic manifestations such as mixed cryoglobulinemia should receive the same treatment as other HCV-infected patients. Essential mixed cryoglobulinemia and glomerulonephritis might improve with interferon therapy (101).

The goals of therapy are to eradicate the virus infection and arrest progression of chronic hepatitis to cirrhosis. Both the National Institutes of Health and the Canadian Association for the Study of Liver Diseases have recommended that the dose and schedule of interferon-α be 3 million units of interferon, three times per week for 12 months to obtain a good sustained response. Patients who have relapse of HCV should receive another course of interferon treatment.

Combination Antiviral Therapy for Chronic HCV. Interferon is only moderately effective in the treatment of HCV infections. Other antiviral agents are used in combination with interferon in the attempt to improve the sustained response. Many of these clinical trials are still ongoing.

Ribavirin, a guanosine nucleoside analogue, has been used to treat chronic HCV infections. Ribavirin has the advantage of being an oral therapy that is relatively free of side effects. Transaminase levels decrease significantly during ribavirin treatment for chronic HCV infection; however they become abnormal again after cessation of therapy (201). Although ribavirin therapy can improve or normalize transaminase levels, the HCV RNA level does not change during treatment (30, 68, 72). In a pilot study, interferon (3 million units three times per week) with ribavirin (1–1.2 g/day) improved the sustained response rate in patients who relapsed or in whom interferon therapy failed (221). Another study showed a 40% sustained response rate 2 years after cessation of interferon-ribavirin combination therapy (136). For interferon nonresponders, combination treatment had a sustained biochemical and virologic response rate of 40% (37). A meta-analysis of European center experience showed a sustained response to combination treatment of 51%, which was two to three times the rate with interferon therapy alone (217). Ribavirin (1000–1200 mg/day) thus appears to be a promising drug that can enhance interferon therapy for chronic HCV infection. It is likely that ribavirin will be approved for use in combination with interferon to treat chronic HCV infection.

Other agents or therapies used in combination with interferon include ursodeoxycholine (124, 245), nonsteroidal anti-inflammatory drugs (14, 255), granulocyte colony-stimulating factor (158), granulocyte macrophage colony-stimulating factor (43, 260), pentoxylline, thymosine, and phlebotomy. These agents add some benefits to interferon therapy, but none of these agents is better than ribavirin in combination with interferon for treating chronic HCV infection.

Immune Prophylaxis and Vaccine Development for HCV. There are currently no data to support the use of immunoglobulin for prevention of HCV infection after exposure. The presence of antibodies to HCV does not mean immune protection from HCV infection. In a chimpanzee study, rechallenge of a convalescent chimpanzee with HCV from the same or different strains resulted in recurrence of hepatitis (78). The genetic heterogeneity of HCV appears to increase as the liver disease progresses (106). The ability of HCV to form quasispecies may allow it to escape host immune responses and establish persistent chronic infection (38). The degree of diversity of HCV quasispecies also correlates inversely with the responsiveness of the virus to interferon treatment (126).

A good antibody response to E1 and E2 envelope glycoproteins of HCV is likely to be required to neutralize the virus and prevent infection. E1 and E2 envelope glycoproteins reside in the hypervariable region of the HCV genome. Under immunologic selection pressure, HCV evolves to escape host immune responses. The ability of HCV to generate quasispecies raises concern about the possibility of developing an effective HCV vaccine. At present, there are at least 9 genotypes of HCV, and a vaccine would have to be effective against all HCV genotypes and their quasispecies.

E1 and E2 proteins have been purified from recombinant vaccinia expression vectors and used in a chimpanzee study (52). The vaccine was given intramuscularly with a variable schedule of at least three doses. The results showed that chimpanzees with high antibody titers were protected from infection during challenge with a similar strain of HCV. However chimpanzees with low antibody titers developed viremia. Further studies are required to examine the protective immunity against heterologous strains or quasispecies.

Cytotoxic T lymphocytes specific for core and envelope proteins of HCV have been identified in patients who have chronic hepatitis from HCV infections (131). The cell-mediated immune response from these patients was not potent enough to eliminate the HCV-infected cells. This raises the question of whether a vaccine augmenting cell-mediated immune response against HCV could be used to prevent infection or as a therapy. Vaccine development for HCV is still in the early stages of animal studies. An effective vaccine for HCV is unlikely in the near future.

Endpoints for Monitoring Therapy
Early studies of interferon in HCV treatment used normalization of transaminase levels to mark response to treatment. Clearly, normalization of transaminase levels during interferon therapy does not correspond to sustained response or clearance of HCV. In the transaminase responders who have relapses, HCV RNA can be detected in serum and liver during and after cessation of therapy (62). Normal transaminase levels and no HCV RNA in serum correlate more closely with a persistent response (202, 229). The duration of follow-up is also important, as HCV viremia can recur many months after completion of therapy. Thus the ideal definition of a sustained response should include normal transaminases and negative HCV RNA 6 to 12 months after cessation of therapy.

Adjunctive Therapy
Patient Counseling. After the diagnosis of chronic HCV infection is made, counseling is important. Sexual transmission of HCV is uncommon but has been reported (4). Condoms should be used during the acute phase of the illness and indefinitely by patients who are immunocompromised. In a new relationship, couples should consider barrier contraception if one partner is a HCV carrier. Couples in a monogamous relationship in which one partner is chronically infected with HCV, should be advised of the risk and encouraged to make their own decision in regard to condom use. Vertical transmission from chronic HCV-carrier mother to newborn is rare (179); however the risk of vertical transmission is much higher if the mother has been infected by HIV (99). As chronic HCV infection can progress to cirrhosis and development of hepatocellular carcinoma, treatment options should be discussed with patients.

Liver Transplantation. The only treatment for HCV-induced end-stage liver disease is liver transplantation. In the last several years, HCV-related cirrhosis has become one of the most common indications for liver transplantation (26). In 1995, 27% of liver transplants at our center were for HCV-related cirrhosis. The short-term outcome of liver transplantation in these patients is excellent.

If HCV viremia is present before liver transplantation, viremia will persist after transplantation, and HCV RNA levels can increase dramatically posttransplantation (50). The diagnosis of recurrent HCV in hepatic grafts can be difficult to make, as the histologic changes can be similar to those of rejection or ischemic injury to the hepatic graft (84). Approximately one-half of patients with HCV viremia do not have biochemical hepatitis (268, 278). Chronic hepatitis is commonly found on liver biopsy of patients with recurrent HCV viremia and abnormal transaminases (278). The hepatitis is usually mild and does not progress rapidly in the first 2 years (84, 228). The 1-, 2-, and 3-year survival for patients with HCV infection and liver transplantation are 94, 89, 87%, respectively (16). These results are comparable to those for patients with liver transplantation for other liver diseases.

Although most posttransplantation HCV infection is mild, rapidly progressive hepatitis has been reported (159). Severe, progressive, cholestatic hepatitis occurs in less than 10% of patients transplanted for HCV end-stage liver disease (218). HCV genotype 1b appears to cause progressive liver damage more frequently than other genotypes (93). The prognosis of these patients is poor, and retransplantation is required.

Interferon has been used to treat HCV infection after liver transplantation. In one study, although 60% of patients had a partial response with a decrease of more than 50% in transaminase or HCV RNA levels, only 1 patient of 14 had a sustained response after cessation of interferon treatment (83). During interferon treatment in this study, 35% of the patients developed chronic rejection.

In a pilot study, ribavirin (1.2 g/day) was used to treat recurrence of HCV infection after liver transplantation. There were biochemical and histologic improvements during ribavirin treatment; however, HCV RNA remained in all patients (94). Hemolysis was common during ribavirin treatment, and dose adjustment was frequently required.

Interferon and ribavirin combination therapy could be used in treating liver transplant patients with progressive liver disease due to HCV infection. Although the risk of hepatic graft rejection appears small, close supervision should be provided during therapy.

Hepatitis G Virus (HGV/GBV-C)

General Description
Molecular Biology. HGV and GBV-C are considered different isolates of the same virus and represent a new genus in the *Flaviviridae* family (5). HGV contains a 9.4-kb RNA genome that codes for a 2900–amino acid polyprotein. The HGV genome contains 5′-coded nonstructural proteins and 3′-coded structural proteins. Identification of putative eukaryotic cleavage sites in HGV suggests that proteolytic cleavage of the polyprotein requires both host and viral proteases, similar to what occurs in HCV. The polyprotein contains highly conserved motifs indicating the presence of a putative helicase, protease, and RNA-dependent RNA polymerase. The RNA polymerase synthesizes a negative-sense RNA through production of a replicative intermediate of partially double-stranded RNA. The negative-sense RNA is used as a template for production of viral genomic RNA. HGV RNA can be detected by reverse transcription–PCR (RT-PCR). Two other similar viruses, GBV-A and B, have also been identified from tamarins infected with blood from a surgeon with hepatitis. While GBV-C (HGV) can infect humans, GBV-A and B are believed to be tamarin viruses and are not found in humans.

Epidemiology
The existence of other hepatitis viruses was predicted because posttransfusion hepatitis can develop even though there is no evidence of HAV, HBV, or HCV infection (6). HGV has been found in association with acute, chronic hepatitis and posttransfusion hepatitis. HGV has worldwide distribution and has been detected in healthy volunteer blood donors (150). The exact prevalence of HGV infection in the general population is not known. In a recent study using RT-PCR to study HGV infection, HGV RNA was detected in 0.9% of healthy blood donors and 3.1% of patients on hemodialysis in Japan (162). In Europe and North America, HGV has a much higher prevalence in persons who have frequent parenteral exposure to blood or blood products. For individuals on hemodialysis or hemophiliacs, the frequency is 20 to 30% (5, 88). In the United States, the prevalence of HGV in voluntary blood donors has been reported to be 1 to 2% (5). It appears that HGV infection is relatively common and that the virus is transmitted by transfusion of blood products (2, 162). Mother-to-baby transmission has also been documented (87, 168, 262).

HGV infection is also associated with other viral hepatitis infections (119). HGV is present in 35% of intravenous drug users, and almost all of these patients are coinfected with HCV (66). Among patients with HCV infections, 10 to 15% have HGV RNA in the blood (67). HGV RNA is present in 17% of patients with HBV infections (157). These high associations suggest that HGV and other parenterally transmitted hepatitis viruses have similar modes of transmission and are likely transmitted together.

Clinical Manifestation. Although HGV viremia can be detected in patients with acute and chronic hepatitis, it remains to be seen whether HGV is a real pathogen. In Italy, the prevalence of HGV in acute and chronic non-A to E hepatitis is 35 and 39%, respectively, suggesting that HGV might be a cause of hepatitis (85). However, in France and in the United States there is no significant association of HGV infection with non-A to E chronic hepatitis (7, 40). Most HGV-infected transfusion recipients have no clinical or biochemical evidence of liver disease (5). In the few patients who appear to have biochemical hepatitis, the hepatitis is usually very mild and does not affect the health of the infected individuals (7, 10). Hemodialysis patients with HGV infection do not have more frequent chronic liver disease (88). Infants who acquired HGV infection from the mother do not have clinical hepatitis (262). Kidney or liver transplant recipients with HGV infection do not have chronic viral hepatitis (73, 91, 102, 191). The virus appears to cause persistent infection in over 75% of patients without causing significant liver injury in most patients. Superinfection of chronic HCV-infected patients with HGV does not affect the clinical course of the HCV infection (90, 156, 244, 280).

Antiviral Therapy
There is very little information regarding the response of HGV to interferon therapy. Most of the HGV treatment studies are uncontrolled and are reported in patients treated for HGV and HCV coinfection. HGV is sensitive to interferon treatment, and preliminary results show that the response of HGV to interferon treatment is similar to that of HCV (90, 244). However, only a small number of patients have a sustained response after interferon discontinuation (119, 141). Ribavirin can improve the transaminase level without affecting the HGV RNA level (157). It remains to be seen whether combination treatment with interferon and ribavirin offers a better sustained response rate, as has been observed with HCV treatment. It is

not known whether chronic HGV infection has any long-term health consequences. In prospective monitoring of these patients, persistent HGV infections do not appear to cause progressive liver disease (10). At present, there is no indication that chronic HGV infection needs to be treated.

Conclusion

This chapter highlights the current state of knowledge of the hepatitis viruses, with emphasis on the treatment of infection through vaccination, passive immunization, and antiviral agents. However, while most hepatitis infections are preventable, they continue to be a profound worldwide health problem. Education, behavior modification, and public health issues (e.g., sanitation) also need to be addressed if global eradication of hepatitis viruses is to succeed. In the interim, continued research on the molecular biology and immunology of hepatitis virus infections is necessary to provide useful new avenues for vaccine development and rational drug design. The recent isolation of hepatitis E and G viruses similarly reinforces the need for continued vigilance in etiologic determination in cases of acute and chronic hepatitis that have no discernible markers of infection by currently identified hepatitis viruses.

REFERENCES

1. Aggarwal R, Naik SR. Faecal excretion of hepatitis E virus. Lancet 1992;340:787.
2. Aikawa T, Sugai Y, Okamoto H. Hepatitis G infection in drug abusers with chronic hepatitis C. N Engl J Med 1996;334:195–196.
3. Aiyama T, Yoshioka K, Hirofuji H, Kusakabe A, Yamada M, Tanaka K, Kakumu S. Changes in serum hepatitis C virus RNA titer and response to interferon therapy in patients with chronic hepatitis C. Dig Dis Sci 1994;39:2244–2249.
4. Akahane Y, Kojima M, Sugai Y, Sakamoto M, Miyazaki Y, Tanaka T, Tsuda F, Mishiro S, Okamoto H, Miyakawa Y, Mayumi M. Hepatitis C virus infection in spouses of patients with type C chronic liver disease. Ann Intern Med 1994;120:748–752.
5. Alter HJ. The cloning and clinical implications of HGV and HGBV-C. N Engl J Med 1996;334:1536–1537.
6. Alter HJ, Bradley DW. Non-A, Non-B hepatitis unrelated to hepatitis C virus (non ABC). Semin Liver Dis 1995;15:110–120.
7. Alter HJ, Nakatsuji Y, Melpolder J, Wages J, Wesley R, Shih JW, Kim JP. The incidence of transfusion-associated hepatitis G virus infection and its relation to liver disease. N Engl J Med 1997;336:747–754.
8. Alter HJ, Seeff LB, Kaplan PM, McAuliffe VJ, Wright EC, Gerin JL, Purcell RH, Holland PV, Zimmerman HJ. Type B hepatitis: the infectivity of blood positive for e antigen and DNA polymerase after accidental needlestick exposure. N Engl J Med 1976;295:909–913.
9. Alter MJ. Epidemiology of hepatitis C in the West. Semin Liver Dis 1995;15:5–14.
10. Alter MJ, Gallagher M, Morris TT, Moyer LA, Meeks EL, Krawczynski K, Kim JP, Margolis HS. Acute non A-E hepatitis in the United States and the role of hepatitis G virus infection. N Engl J Med 1997;336:741–746.
11. Alter MJ, Hadler SC. Delta hepatitis and infection in North America. In: Hadziyannis SJ, Taylor JM, Bonio F, eds. Hepati-

12. tis delta virus: molecular biology, pathogenesis, and clinical aspects. New York: Wiley-Liss, 1993:243.
12. Alter MJ, Margolis HS, Krawczynski K, Judson FN, Mares A, Alexander WJ, Pin Ya Hu, Miller JK, Gerber MA, Sampliner RE, Meeks EL, Beach MJ. The natural history of community-acquired hepatitis C in the United States. N Engl J Med 1992;327:1899–1905.
13. Alter MJ, Mast EE. The epidemiology of viral hepatitis in the United States. Gastroenterol Clin North Am 1994:23:437–455.
14. Anderson FH, Zeng L, Yoshida EM, Rock NR. Failure of ketoprofen and interferon combination therapy to improve interferon-resistant chronic hepatitis C. Can J Gastroenterol 1997;11:294–297.
15. Anonymous 1994. Outbreak of hepatitis C associated with intravenous immunoglobulin administration: United States, October 1993–June. MMWR 1994:505–509.
16. Ascher NL, Lake JR, Emond J, Roberts J. Liver transplantation for hepatitis C virus-related cirrhosis. Hepatology 1994;20(1 Pt 2):24S–27S.
17. Aye TT, Bartholomeusz A, Shaw T, Bowden S, Breschkin A, McMillan J, Angus P, Locarnini S. Hepatitis B virus polymerase mutations during antiviral therapy in a patient following liver transplantation. J Hepatol 1997;26:1148–1153.
18. Bain VG, Kneteman NM, Ma MM, Gutfreund K, Shapiro JA, Fischer K, Tipples G, Lee H, Jewell LD, Tyrrell DL. Efficacy of lamivudine in chronic hepatitis B patients with active viral replication and decompensated cirrhosis undergoing liver transplantation. Transplantation 1996;62:1456–1462.
19. Bartholomew MM, Jansen RW, Jeffers LJ, Reddy KR, Johnson LC, Bunzendahl H, Condreay LD, Tzakis AG, Schiff ER, Brown NA. Hepatitis-B-virus resistance to lamivudine given for recurrent infection after orthotopic liver transplantation. Lancet 1997;349:20–22.
20. Battegay M, Simpson LH, Hoofnagle JH, Sallie R, Di Bisceglie AM. Elimination of hepatitis delta virus infection after loss of hepatitis B surface antigen in patients with chronic delta hepatitis. J Med Virol 1994;44:389–392.
21. Beasley RP, Hwang LY, Lin CC, Leu ML, Stevens CE, Szmuness W, Chen KP. Incidence of hepatitis B virus infections in preschool children in Taiwan. J Infect Dis 1982:146:198–204.
22. Beasley RP, Hwang LY, Szmuness W, Stevens CE, Lin CC, Hsieh FJ, Wang KY, Sun TS. HBIG prophylaxis for perinatal HBV infections—final report of the Taiwan trial. Dev Biol Stand 1983;54:363–375.
23. Been MD. Cis- and trans-acting ribozymes from a human pathogen, hepatitis delta virus. Trends Biochem Sci 1994;19:251–256.
24. Benner KG, Rosen HR, Flora KD. Famciclovir treatment of decompensated HBV cirrhosis. Hepatology 1996;24:282A.
25. Bertolini L, Iacovacci S, Ponzetto A, Gorini G, Battaglia M, Carloni G. The human bone-marrow-derived B-cell line CE, susceptible to hepatitis C virus infection. Res Virol 1993;144:281–285.
26. Bismuth H, Samuel D, Castaing D, Adam R, Chiche L, Johann M, Azoulay D, Farges O, Feray C, Rucay P. The Paul Brousse liver transplant series 1989 to 1992: new trends in the last four years. Clin Transplant 1992:161–166.
27. Bjoro K, Froland SS, Yun Z, Samdal HH, Haaland T. Hepatitis C infection in patients with primary hypogammaglobulinemia after treatment with contaminated immune globulin. N Engl J Med 1994;331:1607–1611.
28. Bloomer J, Chan R, Sherman M, Ingraham P, DeHertogh D. and

the -008 Study Group. A preliminary study of lobucavir for chronic hepatitis B. Hepatology 1997;26:428A.

29. Blum HE. Variants of hepatitis B, C and D viruses: molecular biology and clinical significance. Digestion 1995;56:85–95.

30. Bodenheimer HC Jr, Lindsay KL, Davis GL, Lewis JH, Thung SN, Seeff LB. Tolerance and efficacy of oral ribavirin treatment of chronic hepatitis C: a multicenter trial. Hepatology 1997;26: 473–477.

31. Bonino F, Negro F, Baldi M, Brunetto MR, Chiaberge E, Capalbo M. The natural history of chronic delta hepatitis. In: Rizzetto M, Gerin JL, Purcell RH, eds. The hepatitis delta virus and its infection. New York: Alan R Liss, 1987:145–152.

32. Bonkovsky HL, Clifford BD, Smith LJ, Allan C, Banner B. High-dose interferon-alpha 2b for retreatment of nonresponders or relapsing patients with chronic hepatitis C. A controlled randomized trial. Dig Dis Sci 1996;41:149–154.

33. Boucher CA, Cammack N, Schipper P, Schuurman R, Rouse P, Wainberg MA, Cameron JM. High-level resistance to (−) enantiomeric 2′-deoxy-3′-thiacytidine in vitro is due to one amino acid substitution in the catalytic site of human immunodeficiency virus type 1 reverse transcriptase. Antimicrob Agents Chemother 1993;37:2231–2234.

34. Bradley DW. Enterically-transmitted non-A, non-B hepatitis. Br Med Bull 1990, 46:442–461.

35. Bradley DW. Hepatitis E: epidemiology, aetiology and molecular biology. Rev Med Virol 1992;2:19–28.

36. Bradley DW, Krawczynski K, Cook EH Jr, McCaustland KA, Humphrey CD, Spelbring JE, Myint H, Maynard JE. Enterically transmitted non-A, non-B hepatitis: serial passage of disease in cynomolgus macaques and tamarins and recovery of disease-associated 27 to 31 nm virus like particles. Proc Natl Acad Sci USA 1987;84:6277–6281.

37. Brillanti S, Garson J, Foli M, Whitby K, Deaville R, Masci C, Miglioli M, Barbara L. A pilot study of combination therapy with ribavirin plus interferon alfa for interferon alfa-resistant chronic hepatitis C. Gastroenterology 1994;107:812–817.

38. Bukh J, Miller RH, Purcell RH. Genetic heterogeneity of hepatitis C virus: quasispecies and genotypes. Semin Liver Dis 1995;15:41–63.

39. Camma C, Almasio P, Craxi A. Interferon as treatment for acute hepatitis C. A meta analysis. Dig Dis Sci 1996;41:1248–1255.

40. Carbonell N, Thiers V, Pol S, Charlotte F, Perrin M, Thibault V, Ait Arkoub Z, Lunel F, Breschot C, Poynard T, Opolon P. Non A-E chronic hepatitis (CH): natural History, HGV prevalence. Hepatology 1996;24(4 Pt 2):493A.

41. Caredda F, Antinori S, Re T, Pastecchia C, Moroni M. Course and prognosis of acute HDV infection. In: Rizzetto M, Gerin JL, Purcell RH, eds. The hepatitis delta virus and its infection. New York: Alan R Liss, 1987:267–276.

42. Carman WF, Jacyna MR, Hadziyannis S, Karayiannis P, McGarvey MJ, Makris A, Thomas HC. Mutation preventing formation of hepatitis B e antigen in patients with chronic hepatitis B infection. Lancet 1989;2:588–591.

43. Carreno V, Parra A, Navas S, Quiroga JA. Granulocyte-macrophage colony-stimulating factor as adjuvant therapy for interferon alpha treatment of chronic hepatitis C. Cytokine 1996; 8:318–322.

44. Casey JL, Brown TL, Colan EJ, Wignall FS, Gerin JL. A genotype of hepatitis D virus that occurs in northern South America. Proc Natl Acad Sci USA 1993;90:9016–9020.

45. Centers for Disease Control and Prevention. Hepatitis surveillance report no. 54, 1992.

46. Centers for Disease Control and Prevention. Summary on workshop on screening for hepatocellular carcinoma. MMWR 1990; 39:619–621.

47. Centers for Disease Control. Recommendation of the Immunization Practices Advisory Committee. Recommendations for protection against viral hepatitis. Ann Intern Med 1985;103:391.

48. Chang CN, Doong SL, Zhou JH, Beach JW, Jeong LS, Chu CK, Tsai CH, Cheng YC, Liotta D, Schinazi R. Deoxycytidine deaminase-resistant stereoisomer is the active form of (+/−)-2′,3′-dideoxy-3′-thiacytidine in the inhibition of hepatitis B virus replication. J Biol Chem 1992;267:13938–13942.

49. Chayama K, Tsubota A, Kobayashi M, Hashimoto M, Miyano Y, Koike H, Kobayashi M, Koida I, Arase Y, Saitoh S, Murashima N, Ikeda K, Kumada H. A pilot study of corticosteroid priming for lymphoblastoid interferon alfa in patients with chronic hepatitis C. Hepatology 1996;23:953–957.

50. Chazouilleres O, Kim M, Combs C, Ferrell L, Bacchetti P, Roberts J, Ascher NL, Neuwald P, Wilber J, Urdea M, Quan S, Sanchez-Pescador R, Wright TL. Quantitation of hepatitis C virus RNA in liver transplant recipients. Gastroenterology 1994; 106:994–999.

51. Chemello L, Bonetti P, Cavalletto L, Talato F, Donadon V, Casarin P, Belussi F, Frezza M, Noventa F, Pontisso P, Benvegnu L, Casarin C, Alberti A. and the TriVeneto Viral Hepatitis Group. Randomized trial comparing three different regimens of alpha-2a-interferon in chronic hepatitis C. Hepatology 1995; 22:700–706.

52. Choo Q-L, Kuo G, Ralston R, Weiner A, Chien D, Van Nest G, Han J, Berger K, Thudium K. Kuo C, Kansopon J, McFarland J, Tabrizi A, Ching K, Moss B, Cummins LB. Houghton M, Muchmore E. Vaccination of chimpanzees against infection by the hepatic C virus. Proc Natl Acad Sci USA 1994;91:1294–1298.

53. Choo QL, Kuo G, Weiner AJ, Overby LR, Bradley DW, Houghton M. Isolation of a cDNA clone derived from a bloodborne non-A, non-B viral hepatitis genome. Science 1989;244: 359–363.

54. Coates JA, Cammack N, Jenkinson HJ, Jowett AJ, Jowett MI, Pearson BA, Penn CR, Rouse PL, Viner KC, Cameron JM. (−)-2′-deoxy-3′-thiacytidine is a potent, highly selective inhibitor of human immunodeficiency virus type 1 and type 2 replication in vitro. Antimicrob Agents Chemother 1992;36:733–739.

55. Colledge D, Locarnini S, Shaw T. Synergistic inhibition of hepadnaviral replication by lamivudine in combination with penciclovir in vitro. Hepatology 1997;26:216–225.

56. Conrad ME, Lemon SM. Prevention of endemic icteric viral hepatitis by administration of immune serum gamma globulin. J Infect Dis 1987;156:56–63.

57. Conry-Cantilena C, VanRaden M, Gibble J, Melpolder J, Shakil AO, Viladomiu L, Cheung L, DiBisceglie A, Hoofnagle J, Shih JW, Kaslow R, Ness P, Alter HJ. Routes of infection, viremia, and liver disease in blood donors found to have hepatitis C virus infection. N Engl J Med 1996;334:1691–1696.

58. Crippin J, Foster B, Carlen S, Borcich A, Bodenheimer H Jr. Retransplantation in hepatitis B—a multicenter experience. Transplantation 1994;57:823–826.

59. Cui L, Yoon S, Schinazi RF, Sommadossi JP. Cellular and molecular events leading to mitochondrial toxicity of 1-(2-deoxy-2-fluoro-1-beta-D-arabinofuranosyl)-5-iodouracil in human liver cells. J Clin Invest 1995;95:555–563.

60. Davies SE, Portmann BC, O'Grady JG, Aldis PM, Chaggar K, Alexander GJ, Williams R. Hepatic histological findings after transplantation for chronic hepatitis B virus infection, including

a unique pattern of fibrosing cholestatic hepatitis. Hepatology 1991;13:150–157.

61. Davis GL, Balart LA, Schiff ER, Lindsay K, Bodenheimer, Jr HC, Perrillo RP, Carey W, Jacobson IM, Payne J, Dienstag JL, Van Thiel DH, Tamburro C, Lefkowitch J, Albrecht J, Meschievitz C, Ortego TJ, Gibas A. and the Hepatitis Interventional Therapy Group. Treatment of chronic hepatitis C with recombinant interferon-alfa: a multicenter randomized, controlled trial. N Engl J Med 1989;321:1501–1506.

62. Davis GL, Lau JY. Choice of appropriate end points of response to interferon in chronic hepatitis C virus infection. J Hepatol 1995;22 (Suppl 1):110–114.

63. Dawson GJ, Mushahwar IK, Chau KH, Gitnick GL. Detection of long-lasting antibody to hepatitis E virus in a U.S. traveller to Pakistan. Lancet 1992;340:426–427.

64. Delage G, Remy-Prince S, Montplaisir S. Combined active-passive immunization against the hepatitis B virus: five year follow up of children born to hepatitis B surface antigen-positive mothers. Pediatr Infect Dis J 1993;12:126–130.

65. Devlin J, Smith HM, O'Grady JG, Portmann B, Tan KC, Williams R. Impact of immunoprophylaxis and patient selection on outcome of transplantation for HBsAg-positive liver recipients. J Hepatol 1994;21:204–210.

66. Diamantis I, Bassetti S, Erb P, Ladewig D, Gyr K, Battegay M. Hepatitis G virus in HCV infected IV drug addicts: high prevalence but no influence on hepatitis outcome. Hepatology 1996;24(4 Pt 2):228A.

67. Di Bisceglie AM. Hepatitis G virus infection: a work in progress. Ann Intern Med 1996;125:772–773.

68. Di Bisceglie AM, Conjeevaram HS, Fried MW, Sallie R, Park Y, Yurdaydin C, Swain M, Kleiner DE, Mahaney K, Hoofnagle JH. Ribavirin as therapy for chronic hepatitis C: a randomized, double-blind, placebo-controlled trial. Ann Intern Med 1995;123:897–903.

69. Dienstag JL, Perrillo RP, Schiff ER, Bartholomew M, Vicary C, Rubin M. A preliminary trial of lamivudine for chronic hepatitis B infection. N Engl J Med 1995;333:1657–1661.

70. Dienstag JL, Schiff ER, Mitchell M, Gitlin N, Lissoos T, Condreay L, Garrett L, Rubin M, Brown N. Extended lamivudine re-treatment for chronic hepatitis B [Abstract]. Hepatology 1996;24:188.

71. Diodati G, Bonetti P, Noventa F, Casarin C, Rugge M, Scaccabarozzi S, Tagger A, Pollice L, Tremolada F, Davite C, Realdi G, Ruol A. Treatment of chronic hepatitis C with recombinant human interferon-alfa 2a: results of a randomized controlled clinical trial. Hepatology 1994;19:1–5.

72. Dusheiko G, Main J, Thomas H, Reichard O, Lee C, Dhillon A, Rassam S, Fryden A, Reesink H, Bassendine M, Norkrans G, Cuypers T, Lelie N, Telfer P, Watson J, Weegink C, Sillikens P, Weiland O. Ribavirin treatment for patients with chronic hepatitis C: results of a placebo-controlled study. J Hepatol 1996;25:591–598.

73. Dussol B, Charrel R, De Lamballerie X, Berthezene P, Brunet P, De Micco P, Raoult D, Berland Y. Prevalence of hepatitis G virus infection in kidney transplant recipients. Transplantation 1997;64:537–539.

74. Eason JD, Freeman Jr. RB, Rohrer RJ, Lewis WD, Jenkins R, Dienstag J, Cosimi AB. Should liver transplantation be performed for patients with hepatitis B? Transplantation 1994;57:1588–1593.

75. Ebert JW, Maynard JE, Bradley DW, Lorenz D, Krushak DH. Experimental infection of marmosets with hepatitis A virus. Primates Med 1978;10:295–299.

76. Edlung A. The effect of defined physical exercising in the early convalescence of viral hepatitis. Scand J Infect Dis 1971;3:189–196 .

77. Engerix-B. Package insert. Philadelphia: SmithKline Beecham Pharmaceuticals, 1995.

78. Farci P, Alter HJ, Govindarajan S, Wong DC, Engle R, Lesniewski RR, Mushahwar IK, Desai SM, Miller RH, Ogata N, Purcell R. Lack of protective immunity against reinfection with hepatitis C virus. Science 1992;258:135–140.

79. Farci P, Alter HJ, Shimoda A, Govindarajan S, Cheung LC, Melpolder JC, Sacher RA, Shih JW, Purcell RH. Hepatitis C virus-associated fulminant hepatic failure. N Engl J Med 1996;335:631–634.

80. Farci P, Mandas A, Coiana A, Lai ME, Desmet V, Van Eyken P, Gibo Y, Caruso L, Scaccabarozzi S, Criscuolo D, Ryff J-C, Balestrieri A. Treatment of chronic hepatitis D with interferon alfa-2a. N Engl J Med 1994;330:88–94.

81. Favorov MO, Fields HA, Purdy MA, Yashina TL, Aleksandrov AG, Alter MJ, Yarasheva DM, Bradley DW, Margolis HS. Serologic identification of hepatitis E virus infections in epidemic and endemic settings. J Med Virol 1992;36:246–250.

82. Feinstone SM, Kapikian AZ, Purcell RH. Hepatitis A: detection by immune electron microscopy of a virus-like antigen associated with acute illness. Science 1973;182:1026–1028.

83. Feray C, Samuel D, Gigou M, Paradis V, David MF, Lemonnier C, Reynes M, Bismuth H. An open trial of interferon alfa recombinant for hepatitis C after liver transplantation: antiviral effects and risk of rejection. Hepatology 1995;22:1084–1089.

84. Ferrell LD, Wright TL, Roberts J, Ascher N, Lake J. Hepatitis C viral infection in liver transplant recipients. Hepatology 1992;16:865–876.

85. Fiordalisi G, Zanella I, Mantero G, Bettinardi A, Stellini R, Paraninfo G, Cadeo G, Primi D. High prevalence of GB virus C infection in a group of Italian patients with hepatitis of unknown etiology. J Infect Dis 1996;174:181–183.

86. Fischer KP, Tyrrell DL. Generation of duck hepatitis B virus polymerase mutants through site-directed mutagenesis which demonstrate resistance to lamivudine [(−)-beta-L-2′,3′-dideoxy-3′-thiacytidine] in vitro. Antimicrob Agents Chemother 1996;40:1957–1960.

87. Fischler B, Lara C, Chen M, Sonnerborg A, Nemeth A, Sallberg M. Genetic evidence for mother-to-infant transmission of hepatitis G virus. J Infect Dis 1997;176:281–285.

88. Forns X, Fernandez-Llama P, Costa J, Lopez-Labrador FX, Ampurdanes S, Olmedo E, Saiz JC, Guilera M, Lopez-Pedret J, Sanchez-Tapias JM, Darnell A, Jimenez de Anta MT, Ordinas A, Rodes J. Hepatitis G infection in a haemodialysis unit: prevalence and clinical implications. Neph Dial Transplant 1997;12:956–960.

89. Fourel I, Saputelli J, Schaffer P, Mason WS. The carbocyclic analog of 2′-deoxyguanosine induces a prolonged inhibition of duck hepatitis B virus DNA synthesis in primary hepatocyte cultures and in the liver. J Virol 1994;68:1059–1065.

90. Francesconi R, Giostra F, Ballardini G, Manzin A, Solforosi L, Lari F, Deschovich C, Ghetti S, Grassi A, Zauli D, Clementi M, Bianchi FB. Clinical implications and virological follow up of HGV infection in patients with HCV-related chronic hepatitis. Hepatology 1996;24(4 Pt 2):231A.

91. Fried MW, Khudyakov YE, Smallwood GA, Cong M, Nichols B, Diaz E, Siefert P, Gutekunst K, Gordon RD, Boyer TD, Fields HA. Hepatitis G virus co-infection in liver transplantation recipients with chronic hepatitis C and nonviral chronic liver disease. Hepatology 1997;25:1271–1275.

92. Galun E, Burakova T, Ketzinel M, Lubin I, Shezen E, Kahana Y, Eid A, Ilan Y, Rivkind A, Pizov G, Shouval D, Reisner Y. Hepatitis C virus viremia in SCID → BNX mouse chimera. J Infect Dis 1995;172:25–30.

93. Gane EJ, Naoumov NV, Qian KP, Mondelli MU, Maertens G, Portmann BC, Lau JY, Williams R. A longitudinal analysis of hepatitis C virus replication following liver transplantation. Gastroenterology 1996;110:167–177.

94. Gane EJ, Tibbs CJ, Ramage JK, Portmann BC, Williams R. Ribavirin therapy for hepatitis C infection following liver transplantation. Transplant Int 1995;8:61–64.

95. Garripoli A, Di Marco V, Cozzolongo R, Costa C, Smedile A, Fabiano A, Bonino F, Rizzetto M, Verme G, Craxi A, Rosina F. Ribavirin treatment for chronic hepatitis D: a pilot study. Liver 1994;14:154–157.

96. Gaudin JL, Faure P, Godinot H, Gerard F, Trepo C. The French experience of treatment of chronic type D hepatitis with a 12-month course of interferon alpha-2B. Results of a randomized controlled trial. Liver 1995;15:45–52.

97. Gerken G, Teuber G, Goergen B, Meyer zum Buschenfelde KH. Interferon-alpha retreatment in chronic hepatitis C. J Hepatol 1995;11(1 Suppl):118–121.

98. Gilson RJC, Chopra K, Murray-Lyon I, Newell A, Nelson M, Tedder RS, Toole J, Jaffe HS, Hellmann N, Weller IVD. A placebo-controlled phase I/II study of adefovir dipivoxil (bis-POM PMEA) in patients with chronic hepatitis B infection. Hepatology 1996;24:281A.

99. Giovannini M, Tagger A, Ribero ML, Zuccotti G, Pogliani L, Grossi A, Ferroni P, Fiocchi A. Maternal infant transmission of hepatitis C virus and HIV infections: a possible interaction. Lancet 1990;335:1166.

100. Gish RG, Lau JY, Brooks L, Fang JW, Steady SL, Imperial JC, Garcia-Kennedy R, Esquivel CO, Keeffe EB. Ganciclovir treatment of hepatitis B virus infection in liver transplant recipients. Hepatology 1996;23:1–7.

101. Gumber SC, Chopra S. Hepatitis C: A multifaceted disease. Review of extrahepatic manifestations. Ann Intern Med 1995;123:615–620.

102. Haagsma EB, Cuypers HT, Gouw AS, Sjerps MC, Huizenga JR, Slooff MJ, Jansen PL. High prevalence of hepatitis G virus after liver transplantation without apparent influence on long-term graft function. J Hepatol 1997;26:921–925.

103. Hadler SC, Francis DP, Maynard JE, Thompson SE, Judson FN, Echenberg DF, Ostrow DG, O'Malley PM, Penley KA, Altman NL, Braff E, Shipman GF, Coleman PJ, Mandel EJ. Long-term immunogenicity and efficacy of hepatitis B vaccine in homosexual men. N Engl J Med 1986;315:209–214.

104. Heijtink RA, De Wilde GA, Kruining J, Berk L, Balzarini J, De Clercq E, Holy A, Schalm SW. Inhibitory effect of 9-(2-phosphonylmethoxyethyl)-adenine (PMEA) on human and duck hepatitis B virus infection. Antiviral Res 1993;21:141–153.

105. Herrera JL. Hepatitis E as a cause of acute non-A, non-B hepatitis. Arch Intern Med 1993;153:773–775.

106. Honda M, Kaneko S, Sakai A, Unoura M, Murakami S, Kobayashi K. Degree of diversity of hepatitis C virus quasi-species and progression of the liver disease. Hepatology 1994;20:1144–1151.

107. Honkoop P, de Man RA, Zondervan PE, Schalm SW. Histological improvement in patients with chronic hepatitis B virus infection treated with lamivudine. Liver 1997;17:103–106.

108. Honkoop P, Niesters HG, deMan RA, Osterhaus AD, Schalm SW. Lamivudine resistance in immunocompetent chronic hepatitis B. Incidence and patterns. J Hepatol 1997;26:1393–1395.

109. Honkoop P, deMan RA, Niesters HGM. Heijtnik RA, Schalm SW. Lamivudine treatment in patients with chronic hepatitis delta infection. Hepatology 1997;26:433A.

110. Houghton M. Hepatitis C virus. In: Fields BN, Knipe DM, Howley PM, eds. Fields virology. 3rd ed. Philadelphia: Lippincott-Raven 1996:1035–1058.

111. Howe AY, Robins MJ, Wilson JS, Tyrrell DL. Selective inhibition of the reverse transcription of duck hepatitis B virus by binding of 2′,3′-dideoxyguanosine 5′-triphosphate to the viral polymerase. Hepatology 1996;23:87–96.

112. Hwang SJ, Lee SD, Chan CY, Lu RH, Lo KJ. A randomized, controlled trial of recombinant interferon alpha-2b in the treatment of Chinese patients with acute post-transfusion hepatitis C. J Hepatol 1994;21:831–836.

113. Innaimo SF, Seifer M, Bisacchi GS, Standring DN, Zahler R, Colonno RJ. Identification of BMS-200475 as a potent and selective inhibitor of hepatitis B virus. Antimicrob Agents Chemother 1997;41:1444–1448.

114. Innis BL, Snitbhan R, Kunasol P, Laorakpongse T, Poopatanakool W, Kozik CA, Suntayakorn S, Suknuntapong T, Safary A, Tang DB, Boslego JW. Protection against hepatitis A by an inactivated vaccine. JAMA 1994;271:1328–1334.

115. Iwarson S, Norkrans G, Nordenfelt E, Hagberg R. Interferon treatment in acute hepatitis B infection with prolonged course. Scand J Infect Dis 1980;12:233–234.

116. Jameel S, Durgapal H, Habibullah CM, Khuroo MS, Panda SK. Enteric non-A, non-B hepatitis. Epidemics, animal transmission, and hepatitis E virus detection by the polymerase chain reaction. J Med Virol 1992;37:263–270.

117. Jilg W, Schmidt M, Deinhardt F. Vaccination against hepatitis B: comparison of three different vaccination schedules. J Infect Dis 1989;160:766–769.

118. Jouet P, Roudot-Thoraval F, Dhumeaux D, Metreau JM. Comparative efficacy of interferon alfa in cirrhotic and noncirrhotic patients with non-A, Non-B, hepatitis. Gastroenterology 1994;106:686–690.

119. Karayiannis P, Hadziyannis SJ, Kim J, Pickering JM, Piatak M, Hess G, Yun A, McGarvey MJ, Wages J, Thomas HC. Hepatitis G virus infection: clinical characteristics and response to interferon. J Viral Hepatit 1997;4:37–44.

120. Karino Y, Toyota J, Sugawara M, Higashino K, Sato T, Ohmura T, Suga T, Okuuchi Y, Matsushima T. Early loss of serum hepatitis C virus RNA can predict a sustained response to interferon therapy in patients with chronic hepatitis C. Am J Gastroenterol 1997;92:61–65.

121. Kasahara A, Hayashi N, Hiramatsu N, Oshita M, Hagiwara H, Katayama K, Kato M, Masuzawa M, Yoshihara H, Kishida Y, Shimizu Y, Inoue A, Fusamoto H, Kamada T. Ability of prolonged interferon treatment to suppress relapse after cessation of therapy in patients with chronic hepatitis C: a multicenter randomized controlled trial. Hepatology 1995;21:291–297.

122. Keeffe EB. Is hepatitis A more severe in patients with chronic hepatitis B and other chronic liver diseases? Am J Gastroenterol 1995;90:201–205.

123. Khuroo MS, Duermeyer W, Zargar SA. Acute sporadic non-A, non-B hepatitis in India. Am J Epidemiol 1983;118:360–364.

124. Kiso S, Kawata S, Imai Y, Tamura S, Inui Y, Ito N, Matsuzawa Y. Efficacy of ursodeoxycholic acid therapy in chronic viral hepatitis C with high serum gamma-glutamyltranspeptidase levels. J Gastroenterol 1996;31:75–80.

125. Kobayashi M, Tanaka E, Sodeyama T, Urushihara A, Matsumoto A, Kiyosawa K. The natural course of chronic hepatitis C: a comparison between patients with genotypes 1 and 2 hepatitis C viruses. Hepatology 1996;23:695–699.

126. Koizumi K, Enomoto N, Kurosaki M, Murakami T, Izumi N, Marumo F, Sato C. Diversity of quasispecies in various disease stages of chronic hepatitis C virus infection and its significance in interferon treatment. Hepatology 1995;22:30–35.

127. Korba BE. In vitro evaluation of combination therapies against hepatitis B virus replication. Antiviral Res 1996;29:49–51.

128. Korba BE, Boyd MR. Penciclovir is a selective inhibitor of hepatitis B virus replication in cultured human hepatoblastoma cells. Antimicrob Agents Chemother 1996;40:1282–1284.

129. Korba BE, Milman G. A cell culture assay for compounds which inhibit hepatitis B virus replication. Antiviral Res 1991; 15:217–228.

130. Korenman J, Baker B, Waggoner J, Everhart JE, Di Bisceglie AM, Hoofnagle JH. Long-term remission of chronic hepatitis B after alpha-interferon therapy. Ann Intern Med 1991;114: 629–634.

131. Koziel MJ, Dudley D, Wong JT, Dienstag J, Houghton M, Ralston R, Walker BD. Intrahepatic cytotoxic T lymphocyte specific for hepatitis C virus in persons with chronic hepatitis. J Immunol 1992;149:3339–3344

132. Krawczynski K. Hepatitis E. Hepatology 1993;17:932–941.

133. Lai CL, Ching CK, Tung AK, Li E, Young J, Hill A, Wong BC, Dent J, Wu PC. Lamivudine is effective in suppressing hepatitis B virus DNA in Chinese hepatitis B surface antigen carriers: a placebo-controlled trial. Hepatology. 1997;25:241–244.

134. Lai Cl, Liaw YF, Leung NWY, Deslauriers M, Barnard J, Sanathanan L, Gray DF, Condreay LD. Genotypic resistance to lamivudine in a prospective, placebo-controlled multicentre study in Asia of lamivudine therapy for chronic hepatitis B infection: incidence, kinetics of emergence, and correlation with disease parameters. Hepatology 1997;26:259A.

135. Lai MM. The molecular biology of hepatitis delta virus. Annu Rev Biochem 1995;64:259–286.

136. Lai MY, Kao JH, Yang PM, Wang JT, Chen PJ, Chan KW, Chu JS, Chen S. Long-term efficacy of ribavirin plus interferon alfa in the treatment of chronic hepatitis C. Gastroenterology 1996; 111:1307–1312.

137. Lake JR. Changing indications for liver transplantation. Gastroenterol Clin North Am 1993;22:213–229.

138. Lake JR, Wright TL. Liver transplantation for patients with hepatitis B: have we learned from our results? Hepatology 1991; 13:796–799.

139. Lampertico P, Rumi M, Romeo R, Craxi A, Soffredini R, Biassoni D, Colombo M. A multicenter randomized, controlled trial of recombinant interferon alpha-2b in patients with acute transfusion associated hepatitis C. Hepatology 1994;19:19–22.

140. Lau JY, Bain VG, Davies SE, O'Grady JG, Alberti A, Alexander GJ, Williams R. High level expression of hepatitis B viral antigens in fibrosing cholestatic hepatitis. Gastroenterology 1992;102:956–962.

141. Lau JY, Qian K, Detmer J, Collins ML, Orito E, Kolberg JA, Urdea MS, Mizokami M, Davis GL. Effect of interferon-alpha and ribivirin therapy on serum GB virus C/hepatitis G virus (GBV-C/HGV) RNA levels in patients chronically infected with hepatitis C virus and GBV-C/HGV. J Infect Dis 1997;176:421–426.

142. Lauchart W, Muller R, Pichlmayr R. Long-term immunoprophylaxis of hepatitis B virus (HBV) reinfection in recipients of human liver allografts. Transplant Proc 1987;19:4051–4053.

143. Lednar WM, Lemon SM, Kirkpatrick JW, Redfield RR, Fields ML, Kelley PW. Frequency of illness associated with epidemic hepatitis A virus infections in adults. Am J Epidemiol 1985; 122:226–233.

144. Lettau LA, McCarthy JG, Smith MH, Hadler SC, Morse LJ, Ukena T, Bessette R, Gurwitz A, Irvine WG, Fields HA, Grady GF, Maynard JE. Outbreak of severe hepatitis due to delta and hepatitis B viruses in parenteral drug abusers and their contacts. N Engl J Med 1987;317:1256–1262.

145. Leung NWY, Lai CL, Liaw YF, Chang TT, Guan R, Tai DI, Ng KY, Wu PC, Barber J, Dent JC, Gray DF. Lamivudine (100 mg od) for 1 year significantly improves neuro-inflammatory activity and reduces progression to fibrosis stage: results of a placebo-controlled multicentre study in Asia of lamivudine for chronic hepatitis B infection. Hepatology 1997;26:357A.

146. Lewis W, Levine ES, Griniuviene B, Tankersley KO, Colacino JM, Sommadossi JP, Watanabe KA, Perrino FW. Fialuridine and its metabolites inhibit DNA polymerase gamma at sites of multiple adjacent analog incorporation, decrease mtDNA abundance, and cause mitochondrial structural defects in cultured hepatoblasts. Proc Natl Acad Sci USA 1996;93:3592–3597.

147. Liaw YF, Tai DI, Chu CM, Chen TJ. The development of cirrhosis in patients with chronic type B hepatitis: a prospective study. Hepatology 1988;8:493–496.

148. Lin E, Luscombe C, Wang YY, Shaw T, Locarnini S. The guanine nucleoside analog penciclovir is active against chronic duck hepatitis B virus infection in vivo. Antimicrob Agents Chemother 1996;40:413–418.

149. Ling R, Mutimer D, Ahmed M, Boxall EH, Elias E, Dusheiko GM, Harrison TJ. Selection of mutations in the hepatitis B virus polymerase during therapy of transplant recipients with lamivudine. Hepatology 1996;24:711–713.

150. Linnen J, Wages J Jr, Zhang-Keck ZY, Fry KE, Krawczynski KZ, Alter H, Koonin E, Gallagher M, Alter M, Hadziyannis S, Karayiannis P, Fung K, Nakatsuji Y, Shih JW, Young L, Piatak M Jr, Hoover C, Fernandez J, Chen S, Zou JC, Morris T, Hyams KC, Ismay S, Lifson JD, Hess G, Foung SK, Thomas H, Bradley D, Margolis H, Kim JP. Molecular cloning and disease association of hepatitis G virus: a transfusion-transmissible agent. Science 1996;271:505–508.

151. Lok AS, Chung HT, Liu VW, Ma OC. Long-term follow-up of chronic hepatitis B patients treated with interferon alpha. Gastroenterology 1993;105:1833–1838.

152. Lucey MR, Graham DM, Martin P, Di Bisceglie A, Rosenthal S, Waggoner JG, Merion RM, Campbell DA, Nostrant TT. Appelman HD. Recurrence of hepatitis B and delta hepatitis after orthotopic liver transplantation. Gut 1992;33:1390–1396.

153. Marcellin P, Pouteau M, Martinot-Peignoux M, Degos F, Duchatelle V, Boyer N, Lemonnier C, Degott C, Erlinger S, Benhamou JP. Lack of benefit of escalating dose of interferon alfa in patients with chronic hepatitis C. Gastroenterology 1995;109:156–165.

154. Margolis HS, Alter MJ, Hadler SC. Hepatitis B: evolving epidemiology and implications for control. Semin Liver Dis 1991;11:84–92.

155. Marion PL. Use of animal models to study hepatitis B virus. Prog Med Virol 1988;35:43–75.

156. Marinot M, Marcellin P, Boyer N, Detmer J, Pouteau M, Castelnau C, Degott C, Auperin A, Collins M, Kolberg J, Wilber J, Benhamou JP, Erlinger S. Influence of hepatitis G virus on the severity of liver disease and response to interferon-alpha in patients with chronic hepatitis C. Ann Intern Med 1997;126:874–881.

157. Marrone A, Shih JWK, Nakatsuji Y, Alter HJ, Lau D, Herion D, Vergalla J, Hoofnagle JH. Lack of effect of ribavirin on serum levels of hepatitis C virus (HCV) and hepatitis G virus (HGV) RNA. Hepatology 1996;24(4 Pt 2):225A.

158. Martin J, Navas S, Quiroga JA, Carreno V. Recombinant human granulocyte colony-stimulating factor reduces hepatitis C virus replication in mononuclear cells from chronic hepatitis C patients. Cytokine 1996;8:313–317.

159. Martin P, Munoz SJ, Di Bisceglie AM, Rubin R, Waggoner JG, Armenti VT, Moritz MJ, Jarrell BE, Maddrey WC. Recurrence of hepatitis C virus infection after orthotopic liver transplantation. Hepatology 1991;13:719–721.

160. Martinot-Peignoux M, Marcellin P, Pouteau M, Castelnau C, Boyer N, Poliquin M, Degott C, Descombes I, Le Breton V, Milotova V, Benhamou JP, Erlinger S. Pretreatment serum hepatitis C virus RNA levels and hepatitis C virus genotypes are the main and independent prognostic factors of sustained response to interferon alfa therapy in chronic hepatitis C. Hepatology 1995;22:1050–1056.

161. Mast EE, Krawczynski K. Hepatitis E: an overview. Annu Rev Med 1996;42:257–266.

162. Masuko K, Mitsui T, Iwano K, Yamazaki C, Okuda K, Meguro T, Murayama N, Inoue T, Tsuda F, Okamoto H, Miyakawa Y, Mayumi M. Infection with hepatitis GB virus C in patients on maintenance hemodialysis. N Engl J Med 1996;334:1485–1490.

163. Maynard JE. Passive immunization against hepatitis B: a review of recent studies and comment on current aspects of control. Am J Epidemiol 1978;107:88–86.

164. McKenzie R, Fried MW, Sallie R, Conjeevaram H, Di Bisceglie AM, Park Y, Savarese B, Kleiner D, Tsokos M, Luciano C, Pruett T, Stotka JL, Straus SE, Hoofnagle JH. Hepatic failure and lactic acidosis due to fialuridine (FIAU), an investigational nucleoside analogue for chronic hepatitis B. N Engl J Med 1995;333:1099–1105.

165. McMahon BJ, Alward WL, Hall DB, Heyward WL, Bender TR, Francis DP, Maynard JE. Acute hepatitis B virus infection: relation of age to the clinical expression of disease and subsequent development of the carrier state. J Infect Dis 1985;151: 599–603.

166. McMahon G, Ehrlich PH, Moustafa ZA, McCarthy LA, Dottavio D, Tolpin MD, Nadler PI, Ostberg L. Genetic alterations in the gene encoding the major HBsAg: DNA and immunological analysis of recurrent HBsAg derived from monoclonal antibody-treated liver transplant patients. Hepatology 1992;15:757–766.

167. McMahon BJ, Williams J, Bulkow L, Snowball M, Wainwright R, Kennedy M, Krause D. Immunogenicity of an inactivated hepatitis A vaccine in Alaska native children and native and non-native adults. J Infect Dis 1995;171:676–679.

168. Moaven LD, Tennakoon PS, Bowden DS, Locarnini SA. Mother- to-baby transmission of hepatitis G virus. Med J Aust 1996;165:84–85.

169. Monjardino JP, Saldanha JA. Delta hepatitis: the disease and the virus. Br Med Bull 1990;46:399–407.

170. Nair PV, Weissman JY, Tong MJ, Thursby MW, Paul RH, Henneman CE. Efficacy of hepatitis B immune globulin in prevention of perinatal transmission of the hepatitis B virus. Gastroenterology 1984;87:293–298.

171. Naito M, Hayashi N, Hagiwara H, Hiramatsu N, Kasahara A, Fusamoto H, Kamada T. Serum hepatitis C virus RNA quantity and histological features of hepatitis C virus carriers with persistently normal ALT levels. Hepatology 1994;19:871–875.

172. Nanda SK, Panda SK, Durgapal H, Jameel S. Detection of the negative strand of hepatitis E virus RNA in the livers of experimentally infected rhesus monkeys; evidence for viral replication. J Med Virol 1994;42:237–240.

173. Nassal M, Schaller H. Hepatitis B virus replication. Trends Microbiol 1993;223:221–228.

174. Niederau C, Heintges T, Lange S, Goldmann G, Niederau CM, Mohr L, Haussinger D. Long-term follow-up of HBeAg-positive patients treated with interferon alfa for chronic hepatitis B. N Engl J Med 1996;334:1422–1487.

175. Nishiguchi S, Kuroki T, Nakatani S, Morimoto H, Takeda T, Nakajima S, Shiomi S, Seki S, Kobayashi K, Otani S. Randomized trial of effects of interferon-alpha on incidence of hepatocelluar carcinoma in chronic active hepatitis C with cirrhosis. Lancet 1995;346:1051–1055.

176. Norkrans G, Nordenfelt E, Hermodsson S, Iwarson S. Long-term follow-up of chronic hepatitis patients with HBsAg, HBeAg and Dane particle associated with DNA polymerase. Scand J Infect Dis 1980;12:159–160.

177. O'Grady J. Management of acute and fulminant hepatitis A. Vaccine 1992;10(Suppl 1):S21–23.

178. O'Grady JG, Smith HM, Davies SE, Daniels HM, Donaldson PT, Tan KC, Portmann B, Alexander GJ, Williams R. Hepatitis B reinfection after orthotopic liver transplantation: serological and clinical implications. J Hepatol 1992;14:104–111.

179. Ohto H, Terazawa S, Sasaki N, Sasaki N, Hino K, Ishiwata C, Kako M, Ujie N, Endo C, Matsui A, Okamoto H, Mishiro S, and the Vertical Transmission of Hepatitis C Virus Collaborative Group. Transmission of hepatitis C virus from mothers to infants. N Engl J Med 1994;330:744–750.

180. Olynyk JK, Reddy KR, Di Bisceglie AM, Jeffers LJ, Parker TI, Radick JL, Schiff ER, Bacon BR. Hepatic iron concentration as a predictor of response to interferon alfa therapy in chronic hepatitis C. Gastroenterology 1995;108:1104–1109.

181. Omata M, Yokosuka O, Takano S, Kato N, Hosoda K, Imazeki F, Tada M, Ito Y, Ohto M. Resolution of acute hepatitis C after therapy with natural beta interferon. Lancet 1991;338:914–915.

182. Ottobrelli A, Marzano A, Smedile A, Recchia S, Salizzoni M, Cornu C, Lamy ME, Otte JB, De Hemptinne B, Geubel A, Grendele M, Colledan M, Galmarini D, Marinucci G, Di Giacomo C, Agnes S, Bonino F, Rizzetto M. Patterns of hepatitis delta virus reinfection and disease in liver transplantation. Gastroenterology 1991;101:1649–1655.

183. Palmenberg AC. Proteolytic processing of picornaviral polyprotein. Annu Rev Microbiol 1990;44:603–623.

184. Pawlotsky JM, Roudot-Thoraval F, Bastie A, Darthuy F, Remire J, Metreau JM, Zafrani ES, Duval J, Dhumeaux D. Factors affecting treatment responses to interferon-alpha in chronic hepatitis C. J Infect Dis 1996;174:1–7.

185. Pearce N, Milne A, Moyses C. Hepatitis B virus: the importance of age at infection. NZ Med J 1988;101:188–190.

186. Perez R, Pravia R, Artimez ML, Giganto F, Rodriguez M, Lombrana JL. Rodrigo L. Clinical efficacy of intramuscular human interferon-beta vs interferon-alpha 2b for the treatment of chronic hepatitis C. J Viral Hepatit 1995;2:103–106.

187. Perrillo RP, Schiff ER, Davis GL, Bodenheimer HC Jr, Lindsay K, Payne J, Dienstag JL, O'Brien C, Tamburro C, Jacobson IM, Sampliner R, Feit D, Lefkowitch J, Kuhns M, Meschievitz C, Sanghvi B, Albrecht J, Gibas A, and the Hepatitis Interventional Therapy Group. A randomized, controlled trial of interferon alfa-2b alone and after prednisone withdraw for the treatment of chronic hepatitis B. N Engl J Med 1990;323:295–301.

188. Perrillo R, Tamburro C, Regenstein F, Balart L, Bodenheimer

H, Silva M, Schiff E, Bodicky C, Miller B, Denham C, Brodeur C, Roach K, Albrecht J. Low dose, titratable interferon alfa in decompensated liver disease caused by chronic infection with hepatitis B virus. Gastroenterology 1995;109:908–916.

189. Perrillo R, Rakela J, Martin P, Levy G, Schiff E, Wright T, Dienstag J, Gish R, Villeneuve JP, Caldwell S, Brown N, Self P. Long term lamivudine therapy of patients with recurrent hepatitis B post liver transplantation. Hepatology 1997;26:177A.

190. Perry CM, Faulds D. Lamivudine. A review of its antiviral activity, pharmacokinetic properties and therapeutic efficacy in the management of HIV infection. Drugs 1997;53:657–680.

191. Pessoa MG, Terrault NA, Ferrell LD, Kim JP, Kolberg J, Detmer J, Collins ML, Yun AJ, Viele M, Lake JR, Roberts JP, Ascher NL, Wright TL. Hepatitis G virus in patients with cryptogenic liver disease undergoing liver transplantation. Hepatology 1997;25:1266–1270.

192. Pierce PF, Cappello M, Bernard KW. Subclinical infection with hepatitis A in Peace Corps volunteers following immune globulin prophylaxis. Am J Trop Med Hyg 1990;42:465–469.

193. Polish LB, Shapiro CN, Bauer F, Klotz P, Ginier P, Roberto RR, Margolis HS, Alter MJ. Nosocomial transmission of hepatitis B virus associated with the use of a spring-loaded finger stick device. N Engl J Med 1992;326:721–725.

194. Ponzetto A, Forzani B, Parravicini PP, Hele C, Zanetti A, Rizzetto M. Epidemiology of delta virus (HDV) infection. Eur J Epidemiol 1985;1:257–263.

195. Poynard T, Bedossa P, Chevallier M, Mathurin P, Lemonnier C, Trepo C, Couzigou P, Payen JL, Sajus M, Costa JM. A comparison of three interferon alfa-2b regimens for the long-term treatment of chronic non-A, non-B hepatitis. N Engl J Med 1995;332:1457–1462.

196. Pozzato G, Moretti M, Franzin F, Croce LS, Tiribelli C, Masayu T, Kaneko S, Unoura M, Kobayashi K. Severity of liver disease with different hepatitis C viral clones. Lancet 1991;338:509.

197. Provost PJ, Hillemann MR. Propagation of hepatitis A virus in cell culture in vitro. Proc Soc Exp Biol Med 1979;160:213–221.

198. Rabinovitz M, Dodson F, Rakela J. Famciclovir for recurrent hepatitis B (HBV) infection after liver transplantation (OLTx). Hepatology 1996;24:282A.

199. Ramalingaswami V, Purcell RH. Waterborne non-A, non-B hepatitis. Lancet 1988;1:571–573.

200. Recombivax HB. Package insert. West Point, PA: Merck, 1995.

201. Reichard O, Andersson J, Schvarcz R, Weiland O. Ribavirin treatment for chronic hepatitis C. Lancet 1991;337:1058–1061.

202. Reichard O, Glaumann H, Fryden A, Norkrans G, Schvarcz R, Sonnerborg A, Yun ZB, Weiland O. Two-year biochemical, virological and histological follow-up in patients with chronic hepatitis C responding in a sustained fashion to interferon alpha-2b treatment. Hepatology 1995;21:918–922.

203. Reichen J, Bianchi L, Frei PC, Male PJ, Lavanchy D, Schmid M, and the Swiss Association for the Study of Liver. Efficacy of steroid withdrawal and low-dose interferon treatment in chronic active hepatitis B. Results of a randomized multicenter trial. J Hepatol 1994;20:168–174.

204. Repsher LH, Freebern RK. Effects of early and vigorous exercise on recovery from infectious hepatitis. N Engl J Med 1969; 281:1393–1396.

205. Rizzetto M, Canese MG, Arico S. Immunofluorescence detection of a new antigen/antibody system (delta/anti-delta) associated to the hepatitis B virus in the liver and the serum of HBsAg carriers. Gut 1977;18:997–1003.

206. Rizzetto M, Purcell RH, Gerin JL. Epidemiology of HBV asso-

ciated delta agent: geographical distribution of anti-delta and prevalence in polytransfused HBsAg carriers. Lancet 1980;1: 1215–1218.

207. Robertson BN, D'Hondt EH, Spelbing J, Tian H, Krawczynski K, Margolis H. Effect of postexposure vaccination in a chimpanzee model of hepatitis A virus infection. J Med Virol 1994; 43:249–251.

208. Robson SC, Adams S, Brink N, Woodruff B, Bradley D. Hospital outbreak of hepatitis E. Lancet 1992;339:1424–1425.

209. Roffi L, Mels GC, Antonelli G, Bellati G, Panizzuti F, Piperno A, Pozzi M, Ravizza D, Angeli G, Dianzani F, Mancia G. Breakthrough during recombinant interferon alpha therapy in patients with chronic hepatitis C virus infection: prevalence, etiology and management. Hepatology 1995;21:645–649.

210. Rosina F, Pintus C, Meschievitz C, Rizzetto M. A randomized controlled trial of a 12-month course of recombinant human interferon-alpha in chronic delta(type D) hepatitis: a multicenter Italian study. Hepatology 1991;13:1052–1056.

211. Rossner MT. Review: hepatitis B virus X-gene product: a promiscuous transcriptional activator. J Med Virol 1992;36: 101–117.

212. Samuel D, Bismuth H, Benhamou JP. Liver transplantation in cirrhosis due to hepatitis D virus infection. J Hepatol 1993; 17(Suppl 3):S154–156.

213. Samuel D, Bismuth A, Mathieu D, Arulnaden JL, Reynes M, Benhamou JP, Brechot C, Bismuth H. Passive immunoprophylaxis after liver transplantation in HBsAg-positive patients. Lancet 1991;337:813–815.

214. Samuel D, Muller R, Alexander G, Fassati L, Ducot B, Benhamou JP, Bismuth H. Liver transplantation in European patients with the hepatitis B surface antigen. N Engl J Med 1993;329:1842–1847.

215. Samuel D, Zignego A-L, Reynes M, Feray C, Arulnaden JL, David MF, Gigou M, Bismuth A, Mathieu D, Gentilini P, Benhamou JP, Brechot C, Bismuth H. Long-term clinical and virological outcome after liver transplantation for cirrhosis caused by chronic delta hepatitis. Hepatology 1995;21:333–339.

216. Saracco G, Rosina F, Abate ML, Chiandussi L, Gallo V, Cerutti E, Di Napoli A, Solinas A, Deplano A, Tocco A, Cossu P, Chien D, Kuo G, Polito A, Weiner AJ, Houghton M, Verme G, Bonino F, Rizzetto M. Long-term follow-up of patients with chronic hepatitis C treated with different doses of interferon-alfa 2b. Hepatology 1993;18:1300–1305.

217. Schalm SW, Hansen BE, Chemello L, Bellobuono A, Brouwer JT, Weiland O, Cavalletto L, Schvarcz R, Ideo G, Alberti A. Ribavirin enhances the efficacy but not the adverse effects of interferon in chronic hepatitis C. Meta-analysis of individual patient data from European centers. J Hepatol 1997;26:961–966.

218. Schluger LK, Sheiner PA, Thung SN, Lau JY, Min A, Wolf DC, Fiel I, Zhang D, Gerber MA, Miller CM, Bodenheimer HC Jr. Severe recurrent cholestatic hepatitis C following orthotopic liver transplantation. Hepatology 1996;23:971–976.

219. Schneider AJ, Mosley JW. Studies of variations of glutamic-oxaloacetic transaminase in the serum in infectious hepatitis. Pediatrics 1959;24:367–377.

220. Schuurman R, Nijhuis M, Van Leeuwen R, Schipper P, De Jong D, Collis P, Danner SA, Mulder J, Loveday C, Christopherson C, Kwok S, Sninsky J, Boucher CAB. Rapid changes in human immunodeficiency virus type 1 RNA load and appearance of drug-resistant virus populations in persons treated with lamivudine (3TC). J Infect Dis 1995;171:1411–1419.

221. Schvarcz R, Yun ZB, Sonnerborg A, Weiland O. Combined

treatment with interferon alpha 2b and ribavirin for chronic hepatitis C in patients with a previous non-response or non-sustained response to interferon alone. J Med Virol 1995;46: 43–47.

222. Sells MA, Chen ML, Acs G. Production of hepatitis B virus particles in Hep G2 cells transfected with cloned hepatitis B virus DNA. Proc Natl Acad Sci USA 1987;84:1005–1009.

223. Severini A, Liu XY, Wilson JS, Tyrrell DL. Mechanism of inhibition of duck hepatitis B virus polymerase by (−)-beta-L-2′,3′-dideoxy-3′-thiacytidine. Antimicrob Agents Chemother 1995;39:1430–1435.

224. Shakil AO, Conry-Cantilena C, Alter HJ, Hayashi P, Kleiner DE, Tedeschi V, Krawczynski K, Conjeevaram HS, Sallie R, Di Bisceglie AM. Volunteer blood donors with antibody to hepatitis C virus. Clinical, biochemical, virologic and histologic features. Ann Intern Med 1995;123:330–337.

225. Shapiro CN, Margolis HS. Worldwide epidemiology of hepatitis A virus infection. J Hepatol 1993;18(Suppl 2):S11–14.

226. Shaw T, Amor P, Civitico G, Boyd M, Locarnini S. In vitro antiviral activity of penciclovir, a novel purine nucleoside, against duck hepatitis B virus. Antimicrob Agents Chemother 1994;38: 719–723.

227. Sherman M, CASL Hepatitis Consensus Group. Management of viral hepatitis: clinical and public health perspective—a consensus statement. Can J Gastroenterol 1997;11:407–416.

228. Shiffman ML, Contos MJ, Luketic VA, Sanyal AJ, Purdum PP 3rd, Mills AS, Fisher RA, Posner MP. Biochemical and histologic evaluation of recurrent hepatitis C following orthotopic liver transplantation. Transplantation 1994;57:526–532.

229. Shindo M, Arai K, Sokawa Y, Okuno T. Hepatic hepatitis C virus RNA as a predictor of a long-term response to interferon alpha therapy. Ann Intern Med 1995;122:586–591.

230. Simmonds P. Variability of hepatitis C virus. Hepatology 1995; 21:570–583.

231. Simmonds P, Alberti A, Alter HJ, Bonino F, Bradley DW, Brechot C, Brouwer JT, Chan S-W, Chayama K, Chen D-S, Choo Q-L, Colombo M, Cuypers HTM, Date T, Dusheiko GM, Esteban JI, Fay O, Hadziyannis SJ, Han J, Hatzakis A, Holmes EC, Hotta H, Houghton M, Irvine B, Kohara M, Kolberg JA, Kuo G, Lau JYN, Lelie PN, Maertens G, McOmish F, Miyamura T, Mizokami M, Nomoto A, Prince AM, Reesink HW, Rice C, Roggendorf M, Schalm SW, Shikata T, Shimotohno K, Stuyver L, Trepo C, Weiner A, Yap PL, Utdea MS. A proposed system for the nomenclature of hepatitis C viral genotypes. Hepatology 1994;19:1321–1324.

232. Simonetti RG, Camma C, Fiorello F, Cottone M, Rapicetta M, Marino L, Fiorentino G, Craxi A, Ciccaglione A, Giuseppetti R, Stroffolini T, Pagliaro L. Hepatitis C virus infection as a risk factor for hepatocellular carcinoma in patients with cirrhosis. A case control study. Ann Intern Med 1992;116:97–102.

233. Skidmore SJ, Yarbough PO, Gabor KA, Tam AW, Reyes GR, Flower AJ. Imported hepatitis E in UK. Lancet 1991;337:1541.

234. Smedile A, Farci P, Verme G, Caredda F, Cargnel A, Caporaso N, Dentico P, Trepo C, Opolon P, Gimson A, Vergani D, Williams R, Rizzetto M. Influence of delta infection on severity of hepatitis B. Lancet 1982;2:945–947.

235. Stapleton JT. Host immune response to hepatitis A virus. J Infect Dis 1995;171(Suppl 1):S9–14.

236. Stapleton JT, Jansen R, Lemon SM. Neutralizing antibody to hepatitis A virus in immune serum globulin and in the sera of human recipients of immune serum globulin. Gastroenterology 1985;89:637–642.

237. Stokes J Jr, Neefe JR. The prevention and attenuation of infectious hepatitis by gamma globulin: preliminary note. JAMA 1945;127:144–145.

238. Sureau C, Romet-Lemonne JL, Mullins JI, Essex M. Production of hepatitis B virus by a differentiated human hepatoma cell line after transfection with cloned circular HBV DNA. Cell 1986;47:37–47.

239. Suzuki S, Lee B, Luo W, Tovell D, Robins MJ, Tyrrell DL. Inhibition of duck hepatitis B virus replication by purine 2′,3′-dideoxynucleosides. Biochem Biophys Res Commun 1988; 156:1144–1151.

240. Szmuness W, Dienstag JL, Purcell RH, Stevens CE, Wong DC, Ikram H, Bar-Shany S, Beasley RP, Desmyter J, Gaon JA. The prevalence of antibody to hepatitis A antigen in various parts of the world: a pilot study. Am J Epidemiol 1977;106:392–398.

241. Szmuness W, Stevens CE, Zang EA, Harley EJ, Kellner A. A controlled clinical trial of the efficacy of the hepatitis B vaccine (Heptavax): a final report. Hepatology 1981;1:377–385.

242. Takano S, Satomura Y, Omata M. Effects of interferon beta on non-A, non-B acute hepatitis: a prospective, randomized, controlled-dose study. Japan Acute Hepatitis Cooperative Study Group. Gastroenterology 1994;107:805–811.

243. Takehara T, Hayashi N, Miyamoto Y, Yamamoto M, Mita E, Fusamoto H, Kamada T. Expression of the hepatitis C virus genome in rat liver after cationic liposome-mediated in vivo gene transfer. Hepatology 1995;21:746–751.

244. Tanaka E, Alter HJ, Nakatsuji Y, Shih JW, Kim JP, Matsumoto A, Kobayashi M, Kiyosawa K. Effect of hepatitis G virus infection on chronic hepatitis C. Ann Intern Med 1996;125: 740–743.

245. Tanaka K, Kondo M, Sakaguchi T, Saito S, Arata S, Ikeda M, Kitamura T, Morimoto M, Sekihara H. Efficacy of ursodeoxycholic acid in combination with interferon-alpha in treating chronic hepatitis C: results of a long-term follow-up trial. J Gastroenterol Hepatol 1996;11:1155–1160.

246. Tang JR, Cova L, Lamelin JP, Baginski I, Vitvitski L, Gaudin JL, Hantz O, Trepo C. Clinical revelance of the detection of hepatitis delta virus RNA in serum by RNA hybridization and polymerase chain reaction. J Hepatol 1994;21:953–960.

247. Tipples GA, Ma MM, Fischer KP, Bain VG, Kneteman NM, Tyrrell DL. Mutation in HBV RNA-dependent DNA polymerase confers resistance to lamivudine in vivo. Hepatology 1996;24:714–717.

248. Tisdale M, Kemp SD, Parry NR, Larder BA. Rapid in vitro selection of human immunodeficiency virus type 1 resistant to 3′-thiacytidine inhibitors due to a mutation in the YMDD region of reverse transcriptase. Proc Natl Acad Sci USA 1993;90: 5653–5656.

249. Todo S, Demetris AJ, Van Thiel D, Teperman L, Fung JJ, Starzl TE. Orthotopic liver transplantation for patients with hepatitis B virus-related liver disease. Hepatology 1991;13:619–626.

250. Tong MJ, Thursby M, Rakela J, McPeak C, Edwards VM, Mosley JW. Studies on the maternal-infant transmission of the viruses which cause acute hepatitis. Gastroenterology 1981;80: 999–1004.

251. Trepo C, Jezek P, Atkinson GF, Boon RJ. Efficacy of famciclovir in chronic hepatitis B: results of a dose finding study. Hepatology 1996;24:188A.

252. Tsega E. Viral hepatitis during pregnancy in Ethiopia. East Afr Med J 1976;53:268–277.

253. Tsega E, Krawczynski K, Hansson BG, Nordenfelt E, Negusse Y, Alemu W, Bahru Y. Outbreak of acute hepatitis E virus. In-

fection among military personnel in northern Ethiopia. J Med Virol 1991;34:232–236.

254. Tsiquaye KN, Slomka MJ, Maung M. Oral famciclovir against duck hepatitis B virus replication in hepatic and nonhepatic tissues of ducklings infected in ovo. J Med Virol 1994;42: 306–310.

255. Tsutsumi M, Takada A, Takase S, Sawada M. Effects of combination therapy with interferon and ofloxacin on chronic type C hepatitis: a pilot study. J Gastroenterol Hepatol 1996;11: 1006–1011.

256. Tyrrell DLJ, Fischer K, Cameron J. 2′3′-dideoxy-3′-thiacytidine (Lamivudine) treatment of chimpanzees chronically infected with hepatitis B virus (HBV) resulted in a rapid suppression of HBV DNA in sera. The 8th Triennial Congress of the International Symposium on Viral Hepatitis and Liver Disease. Tokyo, Japan, May 10–14, 1993.

257. Tyrrell DLJ, Fischer K, Sayani K, Tan W, Jewell L. Treatment of chimpanzees and ducks with lamivudine ((−)-2′,3′-dideoxy-3′-thiacytidine) results in a rapid suppression of hepadnaviral DNA in sera. Clin Invest Med 1993;(Suppl 4):B77.

258. Tyrrell, DLJ, Mitchell MC, de Man RA, Schalm SW, Main J, Thomas HC, Fevery J, Nevens F, Beranek P, Vicary C. Phase II clinical trial of lamivudine for chronic hepatitis B infection. Hepatology 1993;18:112A.

259. van Doorn LJ. Review: molecular biology of the hepatitis C virus. J Med Virol 1994;43:345–356.

260. Van Thiel DH, Friedlander L, Kania RJ, Molloy PJ, Hassanein T, Faruki H. A preliminary experience with GM-CSF plus interferon in patients with HBV and HCV resistant to interferon therapy. J Viral Hepatol 1997;4(Suppl 1):101–106.

261. Veterans Administration Cooperative Study. Type B hepatitis after needle-stick injury exposure: prevention with hepatitis B immune globulin. Final report of the Veterans Administration Cooperative Study. Ann Intern Med 1978;88:283–293.

262. Viazov S, Riffelmann M, Sarr S, Ballauff A, Meisel H, Roggendorf M. Transmission of GBV-C/HGV from drug-addicted mothers to their babies. J Hepatol 1997;27:85–90.

263. Viladomiu L, Genesca J, Esteban JI, Allende H, Gonzalez A, Lopez-Talavera JC, Esteban R, Guardia J. Interferon-alpha in acute postransfusion hepatitis C: a randomized, controlled trial. Hepatology 1992;15:767–769.

264. Villarejos VM, Provost PJ, Ittensohn OL, McLean AA, Hilleman MR. Seroepidemiologic investigations of human hepatitis caused by A, B, and a possible third virus. Proc Soc Exp Biol Med 1976;152:524–528.

265. Wagner G, Lavanchy D, Darioli R, Pecoud A, Brulein V, Safary A, Frei PC. Simultaneous active and passive immunization against hepatitis A studied in a population of travellers. Vaccine 1993;11:1027–1032.

266. Wainwright RB, McMahon BJ, Bulkow LR, Parkinson AJ, Harpster AP. Protection provided by hepatitis B vaccine in a Yupik Eskimo population—seven-year results. Arch Intern Med 1991;151:1634–1636.

267. Weiland O, Niklasson B, Berg R, Lundbergh P, Tidestrom L. Clinical and subclinical hepatitis A occurring after immunoglobulin prophylaxis among Swedish UN soldiers in Sinai. Scand J Gastroenterol 1981;16:967–972.

268. Weinstein JS, Poterucha JJ, Zein N, Wiesner RH, Persing DH, Rakela J. Epidemiology and natural history of hepatitis C infections in liver transplant recipients. J Hepatol 1995;22(1 Suppl):154–159.

269. Weinstock HS, Bolan G, Reingold AL, Polish LB. Hepatitis C virus infection among patients attending a clinic for sexually transmitted diseases. JAMA 1993;269:392–394.

270. Werzberger A, Mensch B, Kuter B, Brown L, Lewis J, Sitrin R, Miller W, Shouval D, Wiens B, Calandra G, Ryan J, Provost P, Nalin D. A controlled trial of a formalin-inactivated hepatitis A vaccine in healthy children. N Engl J Med 1992;327:453–457.

271. Westblom TU, Gudipati S, DeRousse C, Midkiff BR, Belshe RB. Safety and Immunogenicity of an inactivated hepatitis A vaccine: effect of dose and vaccination schedule. J Infect Dis 1994;169:996–1001.

272. Whittle HC, Maine N, Pilkington J, Mendy M, Fortuin M, Bunn J, Allison L, Howard C, Hall A. Long term efficacy of continuing hepatitis B vaccination in infancy in two Gambian villages. Lancet 1995;345:1089–1092.

273. Winokur PL, Stapleton JT. Immunoglobulin prophylaxis for hepatitis A. Clin Infect Dis 1992;14:580–586.

274. Widell A, Hansson BG, Oberg B, Nordenfelt E. Influence of twenty potentially antiviral substances on in vitro multiplication of hepatitis A virus. Antiviral Res 1986;6:103–112.

275. Wismans PJ, van Hattum J, Mudde GC, Endeman HJ, Poel J, de Gast GC. Is booster injection with hepatitis B vaccine necessary in healthy responders? A study of the immune response. J Hepatol 1989;8:236–240.

276. Wong DC, Purcell RH, Sreenivasan MA, Prasad SR, Pavri KM. Epidemic and endemic hepatitis in India: evidence for a non-A, non-B hepatitis virus aetiology. Lancet 1980;2:876–879.

277. Wong DK, Cheung AM, O'Rourke K, Naylor CD, Detsky AS, Heathcote J. Effect of alpha-interferon in patients with hepatitis B e antigen-positive chronic hepatitis B. A meta-analysis. Ann Intern Med 1993;119:312–323.

278. Wright TL, Donegan E, Hsu HH, Ferrell L, Lake JR, Kim M, Combs C, Fennessy S, Roberts JP, Ascher NL, Greenberg HB. Recurrent and acquired hepatitis C viral infection in liver transplant recipients. Gastroenterology 1992;103:317–322.

279. Yarish RL, Werner BG, Blumberg BS. Association of hepatitis B virus infection with hepatocellular carcinoma in American patients. Int J Cancer 1980;26:711–715.

280. Yashina TL, Favorov MO, Khudyakov YE, Fields HA, Znoiko OO, Shkurko TV, Bonafonte T, Sevall JS, Agopian MS, Peter JB. Detection of hepatitis G virus (HGV) RNA: clinical characteristics of acute HGV infection. J Infect Dis 1997;175: 1302–1307.

281. Zaaijer HL, Leentvaar-Kuijpers A, Rotman H, Lelie PN. Hepatitis A antibody titres after infection and immunization: implications for passive and active immunization. J Med Virol 1993;40:22–27.

282. Zanetti AR, Tanzi E, Paccagnini S, Principi N, Pizzocolo G, Caccamo ML, D'Amico E, Cambie G, Vecchi L. Mother-to-infant transmission of hepatitis C virus. Lombardy Study Group on Vertical HCV Transmission. Lancet 1995;345:289–291.

283. Zarski JP, Causse X, Cohard M, Cougnard J, Trepo C. A randomized, controlled trial of interferon alpha-2b alone and with simultaneous prednisone for the treatment of chronic hepatitis B. French Multicenter Group. J Hepatol 1994;20:735–741.

284. Zein NN, Persing DH. Hepatitis C genotypes: current trends and future implications. Mayo Clin Proc 1996;71:458–462.

285. Zoulim F, Dannaoui E, Trepo C. Inhibitor effect of penciclovir on the priming of hepadnavirus reverse transcription [Abstract 182]. Abstracts of the 35th Interscience Conference on Antimicrobial Agents and Chemotherapy, Washington, DC: American Society for Microbiology, 1995.

286. Zoulim F, Seeger C. Reverse transcription in hepatitis B viruses is primed by a tyrosine residue of the polymerase. J Virol 1994;68:6–13.

Herpes Simplex Virus

●

Stephen L. Sacks

GENERAL DESCRIPTION
Virology

Herpes simplex virus (HSV) type 1 and type 2 infections are among the most common infections affecting humans. The neurotropism of this virus allows latent infection in dorsal root ganglia, with recurrent infections at skin sites marking the terminus of sensory nerve distributions. HSV-1 is the usual cause of herpes labialis, adult herpes encephalitis, and keratoconjunctivitis. HSV-2 causes most cases of genital, sacral, buttocks, and lower extremity herpes.

A key feature of the herpesviruses is their ability to establish lifelong latency in human tissue. Clinical disease is often characterized by primary infection followed by periodic activation (recurrences). However, viral type does determine recurrence patterns, in part. Recurrences of HSV strictly adhere to the anatomic distribution of the sensory neurons, emanating from the site of ganglionic latency. The trigeminal ganglion is relatively preferred for HSV-1, whereas the sacral site is relatively preferred for HSV-2. Furthermore, there may be additional biologic predispositions to recurrence. Certainly, viral type does not determine the site of inoculation. HSV-1 causes primary genital herpes 15 to 30% of the time. In immunocompromised individuals, HSV produces more severe and chronic mucocutaneous disease and can infect viscera, including esophagus, liver, and lung, by either contiguous or hematogenous spread. There is a large degree of homology between the genomes of HSV-1 and HSV-2, with about 50% of the sequences being highly conserved (13).

Epidemiology

Although 80 to 90% of people over 50 are seropositive for HSV-1, only 20 to 40% of the population experience herpes simplex labialis: vesicular herpetic lesions on the lips or around the mouth caused by type-1 virus (76). Adult HSV-2 seroprevalence ranges from 10 to 40% (58). The incidence of genital herpes has continued to increase to pandemic proportions. A recent serosurvey indicated that 21.7% of adults in the United States have HSV-2 antibodies; a 31% increase in the last decade (29). Nearly 90% of individuals who develop an initial episode will develop recurrent episodes (7), with an average recurrence rate of four per year (12).

Diagnosis

The gold standard laboratory test used to diagnose genital HSV is now the type-specific serologic assay, the Western blot. Growth of virus in tissue culture that results in HSV-specific cytopathic effects after 24 to 96 h is also definitive but requires the presence of active infection. Sensitivity of the culture test depends greatly on lesion stage of the infection, with wet vesiculoloulcerative lesions yielding the highest rate of isolation. Infected epithelial cells scraped with a Dacron-tipped plastic swab from the base of ulcers or vesicles preopened with a sterile needle are transported in a virus-supportive transport medium supplied by the clinical laboratory. Generally, asymptomatic swabs are not taken from patients, since the yield is quite low (<1%). Accurate and sensitive type-specific serologic tests to detect HSV-2-specific glycoprotein G can be performed. The Western blot test for HSV-2 antibody, for example, is about 99% sensitive 4 to 6 months after primary infection.

Some newer rapid antigen detection techniques have variable sensitivity, and a non-type-specific EIA called Herpchek is very sensitive. All patients should have at least one episode typed to provide information about route of transmission and prognosis.

The polymerase chain reaction (PCR) can detect viral DNA from lesions that are culture negative (11). However, because of its extreme sensitivity, clinicians have been plagued by positives that occur even when the virus is not active. PCR diagnosis may find its greatest use when extreme sensitivity is required, such as detecting asymptomatic shedding and in the early diagnosis of viral encephalitis.

Serology has been in limited use until recently. As a result, serology that is non-type-specific is used in conjunction with a positive culture to verify whether an episode is a true primary infection.

SUSCEPTIBILITY IN VIVO AND IN VITRO

Various susceptibility assays are currently in use for HSV. All use the same fundamental principle of subjecting infected cell cultures to varying concentrations of the antiviral agent being evaluated and then assessing inhibition of viral replication. A major stumbling block to interpretation of results is lack of standardization, which precludes direct comparisons between laboratories, even when using the same technique. Indeed, the measured susceptibility values vary markedly depending on the assay method used.

The most commonly used assay is plaque reduction (PRA), which quantifies the ability of an antiviral agent to inhibit formation of viral plaques. A standard inoculum of virus is added to multiwell culture plates and subsequently overlaid with media containing incremental concentrations of the antiviral agent. After an appropriate time (usually 2–3 days) for plaque development, the plates are stained, and the number of plaques per well counted. A dose-response curve is then generated, and the 50% inhibitory concentrations (IC_{50}) is calculated, representing the concentration of drug required to inhibit plaque numbers by 50% compared with drug-free control wells.

The dye uptake assay (DU) is based on spectophotometric quantitation of a vital dye (most commonly neutral red) by viable cells protected from cytopathic effect by the antiviral agent. This method generates up to tenfold higher values for IC_{50} compared with plaque reduction, possibly because of a requirement for a higher viral inoculum (25). Both the PRA and DU assays suffer from time delays caused by the need to prepare titered viral stocks prior to assay performance (6 and 8 days, respectively).

Another approach has been quantifying inhibition of HSV DNA replication using hybridization techniques. In this assay, the monolayer is lysed and the released DNA is adsorbed onto filters that are then incubated in a solution containing HSV DNA probes labeled with iodine-125. Viral DNA is then quantitated by measuring bound radioactivity to generate an IC_{50}. This method can be used with crude clinical specimens, eliminating the need for pretitering virus and tedious plaque counting, but it is far more expensive than plaque reduction, requires specialized equipment, and is still time consuming (8 days) (81).

The emergence of acyclovir-resistant strains of HSV has given rise to the development of several newer assays designed to be of greater utility in the clinic. Recently, a rapid screening test with a turnaround time of 3 days that does not require pretitered virus has been reported (61). A 4-day microplate enzyme-linked immunosorbent assay (MISE) has also been developed, with clinical correlation similar to that achieved by PRA, DU, and the DNA hybridization assay (34, 62). However, the PRA is still considered the gold standard and is recommended by NCCLS as the assay of choice.

The greatest challenge in developing animal models for the study of antiherpetic agents has been establishing sufficient similarity to human infections. The rabbit eye is the most commonly used model to test antiviral agents against herpetic keratitis (53). Mice and guinea pigs are useful for the study of cutaneous infections, which are usually induced by cutaneous inoculation of HSV on the back, lumbrosacral, or orofacial regions. Neonatal, suckling, or weanling animals are used to approximate neonatal herpes. Intravaginal inoculation of the mouse or guinea pig with HSV provides a reasonable model for genital herpes, and herpetic encephalitis is usually induced by injection of HSV intraperitoneally or intracerebrally. Endpoints are commonly mortality rate or survival time. Explanted guinea pig or mouse ganglia are commonly used to study latency and reactivation (32, 53).

Drugs Active against Herpes Simplex

Mechanisms

All of the current commercially available antiviral medications effective against HSV direct their activities against the viral DNA polymerase. Foscarnet does this directly by acting as a pyrophosphate analogue (14). The antiviral nucleosides acyclovir and penciclovir must be triphosphorylated to compete with guanosine triphosphate and inhibit DNA elongation (84). While acyclovir is an "obligate" chain terminator because it lacks a 3' hydroxyl group, both agents are potent chain terminators. Acyclovir triphosphate is approximately 100 times more potent against viral DNA polymerase than penci-

clovir triphosphate. However, penciclovir is phosphorylated to a much greater extent than acyclovir by the key step in drug activation, viral thymidine kinase (TK). This step is rate limiting, viral specific, and substrate selective. This activation step is what provides the high degree of selectivity of these agents. Penciclovir triphosphate is made in great excess and persists in infected cells up to 20 times as long as acyclovir triphosphate, a difference that is largely offset by acyclovir's increased potency against the polymerase.

Deletion of TK is the key change that confers resistance in most situations of acyclovir resistance (26). Without TK, selectivity is lost and along with it, the potency of either compound. Approximately 50% of TK mutations occur in homopolymer runs of guanosines or cytosines, and the other 50% are random changes that generally cause short or dysfunctional peptides. However, mutations can also yield altered TK that maintains enzyme activity for some or all of the naturally occurring nucleosides with reduced phosphorylation of one or another antiviral. These are somewhat more worrisome mutations, since TK activity is tied to virulence and reactivation potential to some extent. Fortunately, these mutations are very uncommon. Even less commonly, HSV can develop mutations in DNA polymerase that alter the effects of the nucleoside triphosphates at the final step. Such mutations may affect acyclovir and penciclovir differently.

The nucleosides acyclovir and penciclovir may be given intravenously or topically. However, both drugs have poor bioavailability. Indeed, penciclovir's bioavailability is too low to be clinically practical. Acyclovir's bioavailability is low, but this often does not interfere with its clinical efficacy. However, the prodrugs, valaciclovir and famciclovir, have bioavailabilities of 55 and 77%, respectively, and are rapidly converted in gut and/or liver to the active nucleoside antiviral compounds (48, 49).

Cidofovir is a nucleotide analogue of cytosine monophosphate. The nucleotide bypasses the need for monophosphorylation by TK and thus remains effective against organisms that have lost TK activity (27). Indeed, because of reduced formation of competing triphosphorylated nucleoside precursors of DNA, cidofovir's activity may even be enhanced by TK deletion. However, this action reduces cidofovir's selectivity to some extent, and persistence of the diphosphate form that inhibits DNA replication can lead to nonspecific cellular cytotoxicity.

Susceptibility Studies (Single Drug and Combination)

Acyclovir

In Vitro Studies. In the early 1960s, two pyrimidine nucleosides, 5-iododeoxyuridine (idoxuridine) and 5-trifluoromethyldeoxyuridine (trifluridine), were found to be active against HSV-1, but both were highly toxic at therapeutic levels in both animals and humans (17). This led to the development of other nucleoside analogues that were limited by either inefficacy or toxicity (e.g. vidarabine, ganciclovir, bromovinyldeoxyuridine (BVDU), 2'-fluoro-5-iodoarabinosylcytosine (FIAC)). A breakthrough occurred in the mid-1970s with the discovery of acyclovir, the first compound to exhibit high potency and low toxicity against HSV-1 and -2 and lesser potency against varicella zoster virus (VZV), Epstein-Barr virus (EBV), and cytomegalovirus (CMV).

As discussed in two comprehensive reviews of acyclovir (45, 53), in vitro susceptibility studies of acyclovir may provide a general picture of potential clinical utility, but they cannot predict the effects of drug penetration, inactivation at the site of infection, and viral multiplicity in vivo and so do not clearly indicate therapeutic efficacy. This is particularly true in immunocompromised individuals, where in vitro susceptibility to acyclovir does not correlate on a 1:1 basis with clinical efficacy (10, 85). There is also variability between in vitro studies, depending on cell type and age, quantity of virus in the inoculum, media pH, length of incubation, and assay method. In general, studies of acyclovir in human herpes simplex cell cultures show greater potency against HSV-1 than HSV-2 (45).

Most of the studies reviewed by Richards et al. show the ID_{50} of acyclovir to be in the range of 0.01 to 0.7 mg/L for HSV-1 and 0.01 to 3.2 mg/L for HSV-2. These studies used African green monkey kidney cells (Vero or GMK strains), human fetal lung fibroblasts, primary rabbit kidney cells, or rabbit corneal cells. Acyclovir in vitro is more potent than idoxuridine and trifluridine, considerably more potent than vidarabine, but less potent than FIAC and ganciclovir.

In Vivo Studies. Similar in nature to in vitro data, studies of acyclovir in animal models are only moderate predictors of clinical response. Differences in animal species, virus strain, inoculum size, route of administration, extent of infection, and dosing make comparison between studies difficult, and their predictive value in humans is tentative at best. Unless indicated otherwise, the data below are derived from the two reviews cited above.

Early studies using acyclovir ointment in the HSV-1 rabbit eye keratitis model showed efficacy at drug concentrations of 1% and above. In several trials, acyclovir 3% ointment applied up to five times a day was equivalent to ointment plus acyclovir intravenously or intramuscularly (50 mg/kg/day). Furthermore, the ointment alone was more effective than intravenous administration alone. Average time to healing (disappearance of lesions) was 4 days. Several comparative studies also indicated that 3% acyclovir ointment was at least as effective as idoxuridine 0.5% and trifluridine 3% ophthalmic ointments and more effective than vidarabine 3% ophthalmic ointment.

Studies using the cutaneous herpes simplex mouse model indicate that acyclovir administered topically (as 3 or 5% gel, ointment, or dimethylsulfoxide solution), subcutaneously (40–60 mg/kg/day) or intraperitoneally (20 or 50 mg/kg/day) within 1 to 2 days of inoculation of virus, decreased mortality rates, severity of lesions, and duration of viral shedding from lesions. Acyclovir combined with topical or intravenous vidarabine was significantly more effective than either agent alone, with the combination preventing ulceration and mortality completely after 2 weeks.

Topical acyclovir (1, 3, or 5% in polyethylene glycol) applied four times daily within 2 days of inoculation caused greater healing of lesions and decreased virus titers in guinea pigs infected with HSV-1. However, acyclovir 5% was less ef-

fective than phosphonoacetic acid 3% and edoxudine 5% but more effective than recombinant interferon-α. One of the great challenges with topical antiherpes treatments has been developing a vehicle that preserves the stability of the active agent and allows efficient drug delivery to the infected site. In animal models, dimethylsulfoxide and modifed aqueous creams exhibit better drug delivery than polyethylene glycol vehicles.

Studies of genital herpes in the murine or guinea pig model have shown acyclovir to be effective in reducing lesion severity, viral titers, mortality, or neurologic sequelae, depending on the mode of application, dose, and time of application. In one study, 2 or 5% acyclovir intravaginal aqueous solution combined with oral administration of approximately 400 mg/kg/day for 4 days significantly reduced mortality in HSV-2 infected mice. In another study, 1 and 5% intravaginal ointments applied up to 72 h after infection and 15.6 to 135 mg/kg/day oral acyclovir given 24 h after inoculation were effective in reducing viral titers. Although combinations of acyclovir (50 mg/kg/day for 4 days), vidarabine (125 mg/kg/day for 6 days), and a low-dose interferon inducer (poly IC(LC)—5 mg/kg on 4 alternate days), showed synergy after intraperitoneal administration 2 days postinoculation in HSV-infected mice, toxicity was reported. Monotherapy with acyclovir was superior to the other two compounds in protecting against symptom onset or death. Oral, intraperitoneal, subcutaneous, or topical acyclovir administered shortly before viral inoculation in guinea pigs was significantly better at reducing lesion severity and neurologic sequelae than acyclovir given 72 h postinfection.

Several animal studies show HSV-2 to cause more severe disease than HSV-1. Effective doses of acyclovir in guinea pigs range from 15 to 45 mg/kg/day intramuscularly, 125 mg/kg orally (given twice daily), and 5% acyclovir in polyethylene glycol (given 4 times daily) when given within 48 h of inoculation. Fifty or 100 mg/kg injected intraperitoneally daily beginning 72 h postinfection decreased the incidence of paralysis and death and healed lesions more rapidly than placebo in guinea pigs with HSV-2 genital infection.

Intraperitoneal, subcutaneous, and oral acyclovir was effective in several studies in decreasing mortality rates and increasing survival times in mice inoculated intracerebrally with HSV-1 or -2. In addition, the drug prevented mortality or reduced central nervous system (CNS) involvement in animal models of secondary encephalitis caused by ocular, genital, or cutaneous HSV infection. Comparative studies have shown equimolar acyclovir to be less potent than ganciclovir and 2'-fluoro-5-methylarabinosyluracil (FMAU) in HSV-1 centrally infected mice but equivalent to VaraU (100 mg/kg/day) and BrVaraU (200 mg/kg/day) when administered at 100 mg/kg/day. In the treatment of HSV-2 centrally infected mice, intraperitoneal or oral acyclovir was superior to VaraU and phosphonoformic acid, of similar potency to vidarabine, but less potent than 2'-fluoro-5-iodoarabinosylcytosine (FIAC) and FMAU.

Combination studies have shown synergy against HSV-2 encephalitis when acyclovir is combined with vidarabine, FIAC, or FMAU in molar ratios of 1:1, 1:1, and 1:8, respectively. The combination of acyclovir with passive immunization with human immune globulin has also shown synergy in several studies of HSV-1-infected mice; however, early immunotherapy was necessary for benefit. Studies in immunocompromised mice showed less effect.

Intraperitoneal acyclovir (50–120 mg/day for 5–10 days) in HSV-2-infected newborn or weanling mice and neonatal rabbits has yielded statistically significant reductions in mortality when administered within 2 days of viral inoculation. Although acyclovir was about 20% better than vidarabine in the neonatal herpes mouse model, the combination was synergistic when treatment was initiated 30 h after infection. The combination of acyclovir and human interferon-α proved toxic.

Famciclovir/Penciclovir

Famciclovir is the prodrug of penciclovir; therefore, most in vitro studies of these agents compare penciclovir with acyclovir. As indicated above, results have been variable depending on cell line, multiplicity of infection, media pH, length of incubation, and assay method.

Although the mechanisms of action of acyclovir and penciclovir are grossly similar, there are some qualitative differences. Penciclovir, like acyclovir, is rapidly phosphorylated to the active form, penciclovir triphosphate, in virus-infected cells only, by viral TK and other cellular enzymes (8, 84). However, penciclovir and acyclovir differ in their rates of phosphorylation, intracellular stabilities of nucleoside triphosphate, and their affinities for viral DNA polymerase (83). Although plasma half-lives for the antiviral nucleosides are essentially identical for both compounds (2.5 h), penciclovir triphosphate is much more extensively phosphorylated and then enjoys a very prolonged intracellular half-life in infected cells (7–20 h vs. 0.7–1 h for acyclovir triphosphate) (58). On the other side of the equation, penciclovir triphosphate is somewhat less active against HSV DNA polymerase.

In Vitro Studies.   The preclinical data concerning famciclovir was extensively reviewed by Perry and Wagstaff (48). Acyclovir and penciclovir, in general, show comparable potencies in in vitro studies. In plaque reduction assays comparing penciclovir and acyclovir in isolates of HSV-1 and -2, mean concentrations of penciclovir producing IC_{50} were 0.4 to 0.6 mg/L and 1.5 mg/L, respectively, whereas for acyclovir they were 0.2 to 0.5 mg/L and 0.6 to 1.3 mg/L (8, reviewed in 48). These figures indicate that HSV-1 is more susceptible to penciclovir than is HSV-2.

In a study using four different assays in HSV-1 and -2 infected MRC-5 cells, penciclovir had greater potency than acylovir in the 24-h viral DNA inhibition assay (IC_{50}, 0.01 vs. 0.06 mg/L) and the 24-h virus yield reduction assay (IC_{50}, 0.06 vs. 1.1 mg/L) but similar activity in the plaque reduction and viral antigen inhibition assays. Although the activity of penciclovir in the virus yield reduction and antigen inhibition assays was inversely related to the multiplicity of infection, it had considerably less effect on the inhibition of viral DNA synthesis (6).

In one study, HSV-1 viral replication in cells was suppressed following exposure to penciclovir, even when the compound was removed from the media (8). Such persistent

activity was not seen with acyclovir. These findings suggest that therapeutic concentrations of serum penciclovir may not be prerequisite for the clinical efficacy of the compound against HSV (48).

Combinations of penciclovir with acyclovir or ganciclovir displayed additive activity against HSV-1 and -2 in cell culture, and combinations of penciclovir with human interferon-α, interferon-β, interferon-γ, or foscarnet showed synergy (80).

In Vivo Studies.   In contrast to earlier in vivo studies on acyclovir, most animal studies of famciclovir have adequately predicted the clinical utility of this compound in humans. Oral famciclovir and various administrations of penciclovir have shown good activity against both HSV-1 and -2 in mouse and guinea pig models of cutaneous, genital, and systemic HSV infection (reviewed in 48). Famciclovir has shown efficacy equivalent to that of acyclovir against genital HSV-2 infection in mice, and one dose of famciclovir was significantly more effective than four doses of acyclovir in HSV-1-infected mice (5).

Intermittent once-daily penciclovir was more effective than acyclovir in an HSV-1 and -2 mouse encephalitis model, as measured by longer survival time; however, continuous dosing of either drug was similarly efficacious. Topical penciclovir was significantly more effective than topical acyclovir against cutaneous HSV-1 infection in mice when treatments were started 72 h postinfection (79).

Two studies recently compared the effects of famciclovir and valaciclovir on HSV-1 and HSV-2 in murine models of immunosuppression and infection (20, 82). In both studies, the compounds were administered for 5 days after infection. Although both compounds reduced viral replication in infected tissues, only the animals treated with valaciclovir experienced a rebound of virus replication in the dorsal root or trigeminal ganglia, ear pinna, or brainstem after cessation of treatment. In mice infected with HSV-2, 60% of the valaciclovir-treated group yielded virus from explanted ganglia 6 weeks later, whereas none of the famciclovir-treated mice showed any sign of latent infection. It is possible that sustained levels of penciclovir triphosphate in HSV-infected cells after treatment may have prevented recurrence in the famciclovir-treated animals, but this awaits confirmation through further study.

Valaciclovir was compared with famciclovir and brivudin (BVDU) in a juvenile mouse model of HSV-1 necrotic hepatitis (92). Necrotic hepatitis was significantly reduced by treatment with 50 mg/kg/day of either famciclovir, acyclovir, or valaciclovir. Treatment with famciclovir (50 mg/kg/day), acyclovir (100 mg/kg/day), or valaciclovir (200 mg/kg/day) was equivalent in reducing mortality in mice.

Cidofovir

Cidofovir (HPMPC, GS 504, 1-[(S)-(3-hydroxy-2-(phosphonylmethoxy)propyl)cytosine was identified from a series of phosphate nucleotide analogues as a potent broad-spectrum antiviral agent, with activity against HSV-1, HSV-2, TK-negative HSV-1, VZV, CMV, EBV, and human papillomaviruses. Unlike acyclovir or ganciclovir, which require intracellular activation by virally encoded enzymes, cidofovir is already a nucleotide, which is converted to the active antiviral anabolite, cidofovir diphosphate independently of virus infection. Cidofovir diphosphate (analogous to another antiviral nucleoside triphosphate) targets viral DNA polymerase. It inhibits HSV-1 and HSV-2 DNA polymerases at concentrations 50- to 600-fold lower than that needed to inhibit human DNA polymerase. In mice and rats, cidofovir was more active than acyclovir in the topical or systemic treatment of HSV-1 or HSV-2 infection and more active than ganciclovir in systemic treatment of CMV infection (15, 36, 42, 43, 68, 78). In an experimental genital herpes model, cidofovir topical gel completely prevented HSV transmission. A single treatment of 0.3, 1, or 3% gel 24 h after inoculation significantly reduced viral replication and lesion development. Continuing treatment past the first dose added only marginal improvement. Accordingly, studies have begun using cidofovir as a single dose against recurrent genital HSV in the immunocompetent host.

ANTIVIRAL THERAPY
Herpes Labialis

Oral-labial herpes infections continue to present a difficult challenge in antiviral management. Primary infection causing acute gingivostomatitis in children has been treated with acyclovir for 5 days with a significant decrease in pain and hypersalivation (16). A controlled trial of 10 days of therapy with an acyclovir suspension also showed a significant effect on drooling, gum swelling, lesion healing, new lesion formation, and viral shedding (4).

Recurrences of herpes labialis have proven much more difficult to treat, in part because of the brief duration, but also because maximal severity is achieved within 8 h of onset, and the inflammatory response contributes markedly to the clinical course (75). Studies with acute, episodic oral acyclovir in this disease demonstrated statistically significant (albeit small) benefit, along with a need for early treatment (52, 73). Topical acyclovir studies have shown generally negative or inconsistent results. The ointment formulation has shown little benefit (18, 69, 72, 50, 51), although the aqueous cream formulation, which has shown mixed clinical results in small trials, has gained approval and success in the marketplace in Europe (19, 51, 64). A large, recent study using topical penciclovir 1% cream for recurrent oral-labial herpes showed clear clinical benefits. Patients in this trial had significant reductions in duration of viral shedding, time to loss of pain, and time to complete healing of lesions (71). The *Medical Letter* has chosen penciclovir cream as the treatment of choice for recurrences of herpes labialis (1). It is applied for 4 days, every 2 h while awake, and used at the first symptom of reactivation. However, delayed treatment in this trial was not associated with a reduced effect. Patients who suffer from frequent recurrences of oral-labial herpes infections, those who wish to suppress their outbreaks for cosmetic or occupational reasons, and those who know their trigger in advance of exposure (e.g., sun exposure skiing or sunbathing) will benefit from chronic suppression with oral acyclovir and use of sun-blocking agents (41, 54, 70, 77). Oral acyclovir suppression is generally given at the same dose range as for genital herpes (200–400 mg two to three times daily). This approach may also benefit patients who suffer severe clinical consequences of oral-labial herpes, (e.g., secondary infections, scarring, eczema herpeticum, or immune-mediated disease such as erythema multiforme) (23, 35, 44). It is likely, albeit unproven, that chronic suppression with valaciclovir or famciclovir would have similar benefits.

Herpes Genitalis

Proper management of genital herpes with antiviral medication must consider the nature of the infection and its presentation, its impact or potential impact upon the patient and possibly the partner, the patient's ability to pay for the medication, and the lifestyle choices of the individual. The impact of genital herpes upon an individual varies widely and must be taken into account in deciding with the patient upon the ideal management. Unlike other diseases, genital herpes causes many people to worry more about their lack of symptoms than about relieving discomfort. The safety of the three available drugs is excellent, and much of the choice regarding which drug, if any, an individual should use, should be left to the individual who understands best what aspect of this disease they are dealing with.

Three drugs have shown clear efficacy in the acute treatment of both first episode and recurrent genital herpes in the immunocompetent host: acyclovir, valaciclovir, and famciclovir. Acyclovir shortens the duration of first episodes of genital herpes—especially primary infections (37, 39). It reduces new lesion formation and shortens shedding of virus from cervix and external lesions. In one study, acyclovir also reduced the duration of painful lymphadenopathy and dysuria (9). Accordingly, all first episodes of genital herpes should be treated with an oral antiviral agent. Valaciclovir and famciclovir are equivalent in efficacy to acyclovir, although far more conveniently dosed for this indication. Famciclovir is given 250 mg three times daily, while studies with valaciclovir used 1000 mg twice daily. This is the approved dose in the United States, although several other countries have approved valaciclovir 500 mg twice daily for first episodes, in keeping with its pharmacokinetic profile. Acyclovir therapy shortens the duration of recurrences by about a day or so. It further reduces the duration of viral shedding and appears to reduce the duration of pain, although demonstrating this effect required very large studies. The usual dose of acyclovir is 200 mg five times daily.

The CDC STD treatment guidelines recommend a dose of 400 mg thrice daily, although this dose has never been tested in clinical trials. Valaciclovir has been tested at doses of 500–1000 mg twice daily. Against placebo, valaciclovir reduces the durations of viral shedding, lesions, and pain. In a large trial, valaciclovir increased the proportion of individuals not developing full-blown vesiculoulcerative lesions from 21% (placebo) to 31% (valaciclovir 500 mg twice daily) (74). Against acyclovir, valacyclovir was equivalent, albeit dosed more conveniently at twice daily (21, 47). Famciclovir studies in recurrent genital herpes compared 125, 250, and 500 mg twice-daily doses (38). Virtually all efficacy parameters were identical among the doses, and 125 mg twice daily has been the approved dose for acute, episodic treatment. Famciclovir reduces the chance of viral reactivation after the prodrome (compared with placebo) and also reduces the duration of viral shedding; time to complete healing; times to cessation of vesicle, ulcer, and crust; time to cessation of pain; and all symptoms, including moderate-to-severe symptoms. Treatment with all drugs is for 5 days, although shorter-duration therapy may be possible and is under investigation.

In general, clinicians are moving away from episodic therapy for genital herpes and more toward chronic suppressive therapy. The latter has the advantage of reducing the frequency of both symptomatic and asymptomatic episodes. With acute, episodic therapy, the patient generally sustains a symptomatic episode with some reduction of discomfort. This approach does not address asymptomatic shedding. The choice needs to be individualized for each patient. If a patient is in a relationship in which both partners have herpes, asymptomatic shedding may be entirely irrelevant. For others, knowing that asymptomatic shedding is reduced may be enough for them to choose chronic suppression, even though transmission prevention data are not yet available. Acyclovir (400 mg twice daily or 200 mg thrice daily), valaciclovir (250 mg twice daily or 1000 mg/day), and famciclovir (250 mg twice daily) are all effective suppressive regimens in genital herpes. In a dose-ranging trial, the subpopulation of patients with fewer than 10 recurrences per year were also equivalently suppressed with valaciclovir (500 mg/day) (74). The choice of drug and dosing regimen for an individual patient depends upon cost, convenience, recurrence frequency, and need for immediate efficacy. Once-daily regimens have not been tested against asymptomatic shedding of virus. To date, both acyclovir and famciclovir have been shown to reduce asymptomatic shedding to less than 0.5% of days. Valaciclovir will almost certainly do the same, although data have not yet been presented. Suppressive therapy can add a great deal of support to a patient who is concerned about recurrences — whether symptomatic or asymptomatic. There is no specific rule that makes clinical sense about frequency rate minimums to trigger suppressive therapy. The choices have to make sense in accordance with what the data show, but the safety records of these drugs are very good, and chronic therapy is often appropriate and less often invoked.

Ocular Herpes

HSV infections of the eye can present in a variety of ways and each presentation is differently managed. Corneal infections classically present with a linear dendritic ulcer but may be punctate or geographic. Deeper stromal involvement tends to appear in some patients with recurrent attacks (disciform keratitis) and is often immune mediated. While topical and systemic steroids and/or immunosuppressive agents can clearly precipitate recurrences in the corneal epithelium and enhance viral replication in corneal lesions, some of these agents are commonly used when immune-mediated phenomena are likely. Iridocyclitis can complicate keratitis or may occur in the absence of keratitis. Indeed, HSV-1 and HSV-2 are known to be possible causes of acute retinal necrosis, although this is relatively rare in the immunocompetent host.

The mainstay of treatment of herpes keratitis remains the topical approach. Both topical trifluorothymidine (trifluridine) and topical acyclovir have been used successfully. There is no evidence of superiority of one over the other. Trifluridine may cause allergic blepharoconjunctivitis and/or corneal epithelial erosions (91). Less commonly invoked are topical idoxuridine or vidarabine. Topical ganciclovir 0.15% gel was shown to be as effective as topical acyclovir 3% ointment against keratitis; both drugs were used five times daily (28). Use of oral acyclovir as adjunctive therapy to prevent stromal keratitis or iritis following keratitis was recently tested. In this study, patients were treated with acyclovir (400 mg five times daily) or placebo for 3 weeks, along with topical trifluridine. Acyclovir provided no benefit, although it was observed that patients who had previous stromal involvement or iritis were more likely to develop this recurrently. Overall, only 10 or 11% of patients developed the complication (1).

Iridocyclitis caused by HSV is generally treated with a combination of antiviral agents and steroid medications. In a recent 10-week treatment study of acyclovir (400 mg five times daily) versus placebo, both patient groups received topical trifluridine and corticosteroids (2). Treatment failure was common (50% for acyclovir and 68% for placebo-recipients). However, the study failed to recruit adequate numbers to prove efficacy. Neither does oral acyclovir added to topical antiviral/antiinflammatory regimens appear to prevent epithelial keratitis following treatment of stromal keratitis or iridocyclitis (91). However, long-term oral acyclovir therapy did appear to reduce the rate and duration of infectious herpetic keratitis in a small (13 patients) uncontrolled trial using doses above 800 mg/day (67). Use of oral acyclovir suppression to reduce the frequency of virus-mediated herpetic keratitis is almost certainly effective and can be an important adjunct to episodic therapy.

Herpes Encephalitis

HSV encephalitis may occur in the neonatal period as a result of infection with either HSV-1 or HSV-2. Treatment and prophylaxis of this syndrome is discussed in the section on neonatal herpes. After the neonatal period, however, encephalitis may occur sporadically. Its presentation does not correlate with mucocutaneous reactivation, and it may represent either primary or recurrent infection. The gold standard of diagnosis is now PCR on cerebrospinal fluid, although treatment should begin at first clinical suspicion. Reactivation through the olfactory temporal pathway is the most likely mechanism of pathogenesis. Acyclovir is superior to vidarabine in this syndrome and reduces mortality to 18% at 3 months, compared with 50% for vidarabine. In one study, 38% of patients who were treated with acyclovir regained apparently normal CNS function (89). However, those with reduced levels of consciousness at presentation, those over age 30, and those with symptoms for more than 4 days before start of therapy had poor outcomes. The dose is 10 mg/kg IV every 8 hours for 14–21 days. Encephalitis in mice appears to respond more quickly and favorably to famciclovir than to valaciclovir, but this has never been tested in humans. The possibility that there may be differences in penetration of the CNS or persistence in the CNS of the active triphosphate moiety between nucleosides raises the question of whether other drugs could have a more favorable result. Unfortunately, the resources now required to answer the question for this relatively uncommon disease reduce the likelihood of a future comparative trial.

Neonatal Infection

HSV infections of the newborn generally occur several days postpartum and may be protean in clinical onset. Less often, newborns are already afflicted at the time of birth following in utero infection. Prevention is the mainstay of management; however, recent data suggest that the clinical presentation of the pregnant woman is not adequate to determine herpes in the infants at risk. Most affected newborns are born to women who have acquired symptomatic or asymptomatic first-episode genital herpes infections in the last 3 to 4 months of pregnancy. Only demonstration of type-specific serologic discordance between partners can hope to result in effective prevention. Nevertheless, cesarean section delivery is still standard medical practice for an infant whose mother is infected with active, symptomatic, recurrent herpes.

Recent studies have suggested that it may be useful to offer mothers prophylaxis with acyclovir in late pregnancy as a means of avoiding this surgical intervention. It is logical that acyclovir will lower the frequency of symptomatic recurrences in women with frequent infection, and this intervention is likely to reduce the chance of symptomatic reactivation. This is not a proven approach, but it has become standard practice in some communities. The safety of acyclovir in pregnancy is probably high, although unproven. Congenital anomalies are not found more frequently in women treated with acyclovir in pregnancy. The effect of acyclovir suppression in pregnancy on the newborn has not been determined. Studies have generally tested the standard dose of acyclovir (400 mg twice daily) for suppression during the last 4 weeks of pregnancy. Because of the physiologic elevation of glomerular filtration rate in late pregnancy, 200 mg of acyclovir every 4 h is appropriate for this purpose. No specific dose has been established, and further, properly controlled trials need to be performed. Ironically, most data support avoidance of cesarean section for recurrent genital herpes reactivations. Accordingly, this will be a very difficult area in which to demonstrate a clear clinical benefit to the newborn.

Once infected with HSV, the infant may develop skin, eye, or mucocutaneous disease, encephalitis, or dissemination. The latter two may present in the absence of skin lesions. As soon as the diagnosis is suspected, infants should be treated with acyclovir intravenously (10 mg/kg every 8 hours). Patients with localized disease have a 98% chance of developing normally at 2 years with acyclovir therapy, although effective therapy still results in death for 18% of those with infection of the CNS and 55% of those with disseminated infection. Those with CNS infection have only a 43% chance of developing normally at 2 years, while those with dissemination have a 57% chance (88). Every possible

attempt at aggressive diagnosis should be made. The prodrugs have not been tried in this setting. Infants with HSV-2 infection often suffer from relapses of disease, and subtle CNS infections may become more clinically important with time. Accordingly, chronic suppressive therapy with acyclovir syrup (300 mg/m^2/dose given either twice or three times per day for 6 months) is appropriate in surviving infants with skin, eye, or mucocutaneous infections. Based on historical controls, this approach appeared efficacious. However, clinically insignificant neutropenia was observed. Furthermore, one infant developed acyclovir resistance, and another shed HSV by PCR in the cerebrospinal fluid during therapy (31). Accordingly, it is not possible to recommend this approach routinely, but not using suppressive therapy in this setting is also a difficult clinical choice pending the outcome of more definitive studies.

Herpes Simplex Reactivation in the Immunocompromised Host

The immuncompromised host is especially prone to reactivation with HSV infections. This may include mucocutaneous disease (HSV-1 and HSV-2) or in severely immunocompromised states may lead to dissemination or contiguous spread to viscera (e.g., pneumonitis, esophagitis). The compromised host is also uniquely vulnerable to prolonged infection that may become clinically and/or virologically resistant to standard therapy. HSV-seropositive organ or bone marrow transplant patients are vulnerable to reactivation of HSV, especially in the early posttransplant period. Acyclovir has been proven effective in both treatment and prophylaxis against mucocutaneous herpes simplex reactivations in the compromised host (40, 65, 66, 86, 90). Most experts would recommend prophylaxis during the acute period of risk (e.g., the first 30 days after allogeneic bone marrow transplant). Because the degree of immunosuppression correlates with risk, not all types of transplant patients require prophylaxis. Patients with inborn immunodeficiency states and those with HIV disease are also at risk of progressive disease. Risk is inversely related to the CD4 count. Because of this and suggestions from the basic science literature that HSV reactivation may upregulate HIV, many patients are given prophylaxis with antivirals. The immunocompromised host should be treated for acute disease and/or provided with prophylaxis during the periods of highest risk.

Both valacyclovir and famciclovir are effective in managing immunocompromised patients and are equivalent in efficacy with oral acyclovir, albeit more conveniently dosed. Valaciclovir (500 mg twice daily and 1000 mg once daily) tested in this setting compared favorably with acyclovir (400 mg twice daily). Famciclovir (500 mg twice daily for 7 days) used as acute treatment in the compromised host showed efficacy identical to that with acyclovir (400 mg five times daily) (22). Acute intravenous therapy of HSV disease in immunocompromised patients was also studied with penciclovir, the nucleoside metabolite of famciclovir. This study showed equivalence of intravenous acyclovir (5 mg/kg every 8 h) with penciclovir (5 mg/kg given either every 8 or 12 h) for oncology/transplant patients with mucocutaneous HSV infections (33). Prophylaxis with famciclovir (500 mg twice daily) was compared with placebo in HIV-positive persons with genital herpes and was found to reduce both the frequency of asymptomatic viral shedding and reported clinical reactivation in this population (63). These doses are also equivalent in efficacy to acyclovir suppression (400 mg five times daily or 400 mg three times daily). This patient population is uniquely susceptible to developing resistance to antiviral therapy.

Resistance to acyclovir can be successfully managed with intravenous foscarnet therapy (40 mg/kg every 8 h) (57, 60). Foscarnet directly inhibits viral DNA polymerase, thereby avoiding the need for activation by viral TK, the most common site for acyclovir resistance. Cidofovir gel (0.3% and 1% once daily for 5 days) has been used successfully for genital herpes resistant to acyclovir, although this has not been approved by the FDA. An expanded access program is available, however. A less effective alternative is trifluorothymidine applied topically in a 1% ophthalmic solution (30). A topical foscarnet cream preparation may also be effective in patients with acyclovir resistance (24), although foscarnet is not effective in immunocompetent patients (56). Acyclovir has low and variable bioavailability, which can be an important issue in patients who are seriously ill. Furthermore, clinically resistant herpes is not always truly resistant in vitro, and resistant disease often spreads slowly and contiguously. Therefore, it is reasonable in some settings to try one of the prodrugs before hospitalizing a patient for foscarnet therapy and its attendant adverse effects (59). If there is no response after a few days, it is reasonable to assume that true acyclovir resistance is present and switch to foscarnet. However, malabsorption problems or other pharmacokinetic issues have led to lack of clinical response, and some patients may respond to valaciclovir or famciclovir.

ADJUNCTIVE THERAPY

Selected patients may require adjunctive therapy for encephalitis, because of cerebral edema. Although it is generally best to hydrate patients well when using intravenous acyclovir, this may not be the best approach for encephalitis. When cerebral edema is suspected, intravenous mannitol and/or dexamethasone is often used in conjunction with antiviral therapy. Another setting in which adjunctive therapy is indicated is erythema multiforme, for which topical and/or systemic immunosuppressive agents may be indicated.

Patients with herpes genitalis or labialis rarely develop secondary bacterial infections. Those who do are usually clinically evident because of fever, cellulitis, or impetiginous changes. When secondary infection is considered, antibiotic coverage for staphylococcal and/or streptococcal skin infection should be added to antiviral therapy.

CONTROVERSIES

Valaciclovir, the new prodrug of acyclovir, has 55% bioavailability. As a result, a higher C_{max} can be achieved with oral valaciclovir than with acyclovir. However, acyclovir has a half-life of approximately 2.5 h regardless of the C_{max}. Nevertheless, dose-ranging trials of valaciclovir showed valaciclovir (1000 mg once daily) to be effective in reducing recurrent infections at about the same rate as twice-daily regimens. Even with this high dose, however, acyclovir levels in the plasma are undetectable for approximately 4 to 6 h/day. When recurrence rates are relatively low (<10/year), genital herpes may be suppressed with only 500 mg of valaciclovir once daily. Should this approach be used as the first line?

Some individuals want the convenience of once-daily dosing and should be provided that opportunity. However, once-daily valaciclovir means dosing very close to every 24 h, because of the prolonged trough levels. Furthermore, studies have not yet been conducted to show that once-daily therapy reduces asymptomatic shedding as effectively as twice-daily therapy. If patients taking valaciclovir have a susceptible partner, they may wish to stay with twice-daily dosing until further data are available (250 mg twice daily is equivalent to 400 mg of acyclovir twice daily). Twice-daily therapy should be chosen for patients who need to have their dosing frequency reduced because of difficulty in coping with the infection.

For those who understand pharmacokinetics and want the convenience of once-daily dosing, there is now such a therapeutic option. Famciclovir is not as effective given once daily, although study designs between famciclovir and valaciclovir have been very different. Comparative data are not yet available. The dose of famciclovir is 250 mg twice daily for suppression.

Famciclovir has been studied in mice early after initial inoculation. These animal studies suggest the famciclovir is significantly superior to valaciclovir in reducing both the brainstem viral burden and the quantum of latency in the trigeminal ganglia of the animals. Accordingly, the sponsor has designed a trial to determine whether treatment of first episodes of HSV-2 might possibly reduce subsequent recurrence rates after treatment of the first episode is ended. There is no real clinical evidence to support this approach as yet, although studies are under way. It is not reasonable to assume or advise that any antiviral agent cures this infection until clinical data exist to back up that claim. On the other hand, the in vivo evidence is compelling and provides an excellent rationale for clinical studies now under way.

Both acyclovir and famciclovir have been shown to reduce asymptomatic shedding. Acyclovir was studied in a small crossover design in 34 women with early postprimary disease (87). In this setting, placebo recipients experienced subclinical shedding nearly 7% of days, and acyclovir reduced this to under 0.4%. In a large, parallel group placebo-controlled randomized trial, famciclovir suppressed asymptomatic shedding to similar levels from a placebo background rate of about 4% (55). Data on valaciclovir are pending. Does this translate to reduced transmission? The answer is unknown, but it is important to note that most transmission episodes of genital herpes occur during asymptomatic periods of infection. It is therefore prudent to advise patients of this effect on asymptomatic shedding, even though it is not possible to advise them with certainty that transmission will be prevented or reduced. Studies are under way to determine this. Nevertheless, because of the excellent safety records of all of these antiviral agents, many patients may wish to choose suppressive therapy while awaiting the outcome of the clinical transmission trials.

It is impossible to compare acyclovir, valaciclovir, and famciclovir with each other adequately to declare one or another superior. In general, acyclovir remains an excellent drug with a long safety record that has become very inexpensive because of its recent classification as a generic drug. Because of poor bioavailability, however, it suffers from frequent dosing in active therapy of disease and fails entirely in relatively uncommon situations because of poor absorption. Patients do not like to take genital herpes drugs five times daily while at work—not only because it is difficult to remember but also because it is potentially embarrassing. However, acyclovir is easily dosed twice daily for suppression. Studies of valaciclovir for first episodes of genital herpes likely used a dose that was higher than necessary, leading to U.S. approval at a dose twice that of other countries. Famciclovir was not approved for treatment of first episodes of genital herpes despite three multinational studies clearly showing equivalence with acyclovir. For first episodes, either valaciclovir 500 mg twice daily or famciclovir 250 mg thrice daily would be good choices.

There have been no trials comparing prodrugs for active treatment of recurrent infections. Valaciclovir is equivalent to acyclovir, but dosing is more convenient. One study suggests that classical vesiculoulcerative lesions may be reduced by about 10% if valaciclovir is taken early. However, the famciclovir trials were not powered to look for this and instead showed that viral shedding could be prevented in a high proportion of patients taking active drug. Furthermore, the famciclovir results in reducing all of the lesion components and each of the uncomfortable symptoms are robust. Since patients who use episodic therapy will require therapy several times, it may be most reasonable to allow each patient to try each drug to determine which is the best for them. The key issue with episodic therapy is that it is too often used in lieu of suppression. Patients with frequent episodes and many others who suffer from psychologic sequelae or concerns about asymptomatic shedding may wish to take chronic suppressive therapy. In this setting, each drug seems about equivalent in efficacy (again there are no comparative trials available yet). Most individuals will find twice-daily suppression convenient and effective. For those who do not, careful selection for once-daily valaciclovir is reasonable.

We still need a good topical drug for herpes genitalis and a good systemic drug for herpes labialis. Many individuals with herpes labialis would welcome a systemic alternative for active or suppressive therapy. Further studies are warranted. It is unfortunate that cidofovir gel did not receive approval for use in HIV-positive patients with resistant herpes genitalis. Even though the numbers were small, the potential clinical advantage of a drug that does not require hospitalization for administration in this patient population is huge. For now, intravenous foscarnet remains the only real alternative for true resistance. This drug is straightforward to give, but it can have a high incidence of important metabolic and renal toxicities, and thus, patients on this drug need to be monitored.

REFERENCES

1. Anonymous. Topical penciclovir for herpes labialis. Med Lett Drugs Ther 1997;39:57–58.
2. Anonymous. A controlled trial of oral acyclovir for iridocyclitis caused by herpes simplex virus. The Herpetic Eye Disease Study Group. Arch Ophthalmol 1996;114:1065–1072.
3. Anonymous. A controlled trial of oral acyclovir for the prevention of stromal keratitis or iritis in patients with herpes simplex virus epithelial keratitis. The Epithelial Keratitis Trial. The Herpetic Eye Disease Study Group. Arch Ophthalmol 1997;115:703–712.
4. Aoki FY, Law BJ, Hammond GW, Cheang M, Boucher FD, Fast M, Sitar DS, Embree J, Williams T, The Acyclovir-Gingivostomatitis Research Group. Acyclovir (ACV) suspension for treatment of acute herpes simplex virus (HSV) gingivostomatitis in children: a placebo (PL)-controlled, double-blind trial [Abstract 1530]. 33rd Interscience Conference on Antimicrobial Agents and Chemotherapy, New Orleans; 17–20 Oct, 1993.
5. Ashton RJ, Abbott KH, Smith GM, Sutton DJ. Antiviral activity of famciclovir and acyclovir in mice infected intraperitoneally with herpes simplex virus type 1 SC16. Antimicrob Chemother 1994;34:287–290.
6. Bacon TH, Howard BA, Spender LC, Boyd MR. Activity of penciclovir in antiviral assays against herpes simplex virus. J Antimicrob Chemother 1996;37:303–313.
7. Benedetti J, Corey L, Ashley R. Recurrence rates in genital herpes after symptomatic first-episode infection. Ann Intern Med 1994;121:847–854.
8. Boyd MR, Bacon TH, Sutton D, Cole M. Antiherpesvirus activity of 9-(4-hydroxy-3-methybut-1-yl)guanine (BRL 39123) in cell culture. Antimicrob Agents Chemother 1987;31:1238–1242.
9. Bryson YJ, Dillon M, Lovett M, Acuna G, Taylor S, Cherry JD, Johnson BL, Wiesmeier E, Growdon W, Creagh-Kirk T, Keeney R. Treatment of first episodes of genital herpes simplex virus infection with oral acyclovir. A randomized double-blind controlled trial in normal subjects. N Engl J Med 1983;308:916–921.
10. Christophers J, Sutton RNP, Noble RV, Anderson H. Clinical resistance to acyclovir of herpes simplex virus infections in immunocompromised patients. J Antimicrob Chemother 1986;18(Suppl B):121–125.
11. Cone RW, Hobson AC, Palmer J, Remington M, Corey L. Extended duration of herpes simplex DNA in genital lesions as detected by the polymerase chain reaction. J Infect Dis 1991;164:757–760.
12. Corey L, Adams HG, Brown ZA, Holmes KK. Genital herpes simplex virus infections: clinical manifestations, course and complications. Ann Intern Med 1993;98:958–972.
13. Corey L, Spear PG. Infections with herpes simplex viruses. N Engl J Med 1986;314:686–691.
14. Crumpacker CS. Mechanism of action of foscarnet against viral polymerases. Am J Med 1992;92(Suppl 2A):3S–7S.
15. De Clerq E, Holy A, Efficacy of (S)-2-(3-hydroxy-2-phosphonylmethoxypropyl) cytosine in various models of herpes simplex virus infection in mice. Antimicrob Agents Chemother. 1991;35:701–706.
16. Ducoulombier H, Cousin J, Dewilde A, Lancrenon S, Renaudie M, Steru D, Wattre P. La stomato-gingivite herpetique de l'enfant:

essai controle aciclovir versus placebo. Ann Pediatr (Paris) 1988; 35:212–216.

17. Elion GB. Acyclovir: discovery, mechanism of action, and selectivity. J Med Virol 1993(Suppl 1):2–6.

18. Fiddian AP, Ivanyi L. Topical acyclovir in the management of recurrent herpes labialis. Br J Dermatol 1983;109:321–326.

19. Fiddian AP, Yeo JM, Stubbings R, Dean D. Successful treatment of herpes labialis with topical acyclovir. Br Med J 1983;286: 1699–1701.

20. Field HJ, Tewari D, Sutton D, Thackray AM. Comparison of efficacies of famciclovir and valaciclovir against herpes simplex virus type 1 in a murine immunosuppression model. Antimicrob Agents Chemother 1995;39:1114–1119.

21. Fife K, The International Valaciclovir HSV Study Group. Valaciclovir or acyclovir for the treatment of first episode genital herpes [Abstract H11]. 35th Interscience Conference on Antimicrobial Agents and Chemotherapy, San Francisco, 17–20 Sept, 1995.

22. Frechette G, Romanowski B, Famciclovir Study Group. Efficacy and safety of famciclovir for the treatment of HSV infection in HIV+ patients [Abstract 301]. 6th Canadian Conference on HIV/AIDS Research. Can J Infect Dis 1997;8(Suppl A):44A.

23. Green JA, Spruance SL, Wenerstrom G, Piepkorn MW. Postherpetic erythema multiforme prevented with prophylactic oral acyclovir. Ann Intern Med 1985;102:632–633.

24. Hardy, et al. IIIrd Conf Retroviruses, Washington, 1996.

25. Harmenberg J, Wahren B, Oberg B. Influence of cells and virus multiplicity on the inhibition of herpesviruses with acycloguanosine. Intervirology 1980;14:239–244.

26. Hill EL, Hunter GA, Ellis MN. In vitro and in vivo characterization of herpes simplex virus clinical isolates recovered from patients infected with human immunodeficiency virus. Antimicrob Agents Chemother 1991;35:2322–2328.

27. Ho HT, Woods KL, Bronson JJ, De Boeck H, Martin JC, Hitchcock MJM. Intracellular metabolism of the antiherpes agent 1-[3-hydroxy-2-(phosphonylmethoxy)propyl]cytosine. Mol Pharmacol 1992;41:197–202.

28. Hoh HB, Hurley C, Claoue C, Viswalingham M, Easty DL, Goldschmidt P, Collum LM. Randomised trial of ganciclovir and acyclovir in the treatment of herpes simplex dendritic keratitis: a multicentre study. Br J Ophthalmol 1996;80:140–143.

29. Johnson R, Lee F, Hadgu A, McQuillan G, Aral S, Kesling S. US genital herpes trends during the first decade of AIDS: prevalence increases in young whites and elevated in blacks [Abstract 22]. Annual meeting of the International Society for STD Research, Helsinki, Finland, Aug 29, 1993.

30. Kessler HA, Hurwitz S, Farthing C, Benson CA, Feinberg J, Kuritzkes DR, Bailey TC, Safrin S, Steigbigel RT, Cheeseman SH, McKinley GF, Wettlaufer B, Owens S, Nevin T, Korvick JA. Pilot study of topical trifluridine for the treatment of acyclovir-resistant mucocutaneous herpes simplex disease in patients with AIDS (ACTG 172). AIDS Clinical Trials Group. J Acquir Immune Defic Syndr Hum Retrovirol 1996;12:147–152.

31. Kimberlin D, Powell D, Gruber W, Diaz P, Arvin A, Kumar M, Jacobs R, Van Dyke R, Burchett S, Soong SJ, Lakeman A, Whitley R. Administration of oral acyclovir suppressive therapy after neonatal herpes simplex virus disease limited to the skin, eyes and mouth: results of a phase I/II trial. Pediatr Infect Dis J 1996; 15:247–254.

32. Kirchner H. Immunobiology of infection with herpes simplex virus. In: Melnick JL, ed. Monographs in virology, vol 13. Basel: Karger, 1982:13–21.

33. Lazarus H, Belanger R, Candon A, Aolin M, Jurewicz R, Lynch S, Boon R, Marks L, PCV IC study group. Efficacy and safety of penciclovir (PCV) for the treatment of HSV infections in immunocompromised (IC) patients [Abstract H72]. 37th Interscience Conference on Antimicrobial Agents and Chemotherapy, Toronto, Ontario, 28 Sept–1 Oct, 1997.

34. Leahy BJ, Christiansen KJ, Shellam G. Standardisation of a microplate in situ ELISA (MISE-test) for the susceptibility testing of herpes simplex virus to acyclovir. J Virol Methods 1994; 48:93–108.

35. Lemak MA, Duvic M, Bean SF. Oral acyclovir for the prevention of herpes-associated erythema multiforme. J Am Acad Dermatol 1986;15:50–54.

36. Maudgal PC, de Clerq E. Effects of phosphonylmethoxy-6-alkyl-purine and pyrimidine derivatives on TK and TK-HSV-1 keratitis in rabbits. Antiviral Res 1991;16:93–100.

37. Mertz GJ, Critchlow CW, Benedetti J, Reichman RC, Dolin R, Connor J, Redfield DC, Savoia MC, Richman DD, Tyrrell DL. Double-blind placebo-controlled trial of oral acyclovir in first-episode genital herpes simplex virus infection. JAMA 1984;252: 1147–1151.

38. Mertz GJ, Loveless MO, Kraus SJ, Tyring SK, Fowler, Collaborative Famciclovir Genital Herpes Research Group. Famciclovir for suppression of genital herpes [Abstract 11]. 34th Interscience Conference on Antimicrobial Agents and Chemotherapy, Orlando, FL, 4–7 Oct, 1994.

39. Mertz GJ, Reichman R, Dolin R, Richman DD, Oxman M, Large K, Tyrell D, Portnoy, Corey L. Double blind placebo controlled trial of oral acyclovir for first episode genital herpes [Abstract]. 22nd Interscience Conference on Antimicrobial Agents and Chemotherapy, Miami, FL, 4–6 Oct, 1982.

40. Meyers JD. Treatment of herpesvirus infections in the immune-compromised host. Scand J Infect Dis 1985;47(Suppl):128–136.

41. Meyrick Thomas RH, Dod HJ, Yeo JM, Kirby JD. Oral acyclovir in the suppression of recurrent non-genital herpes simplex virus infection. Br J Dermatol 1985;113:731–735.

42. Neyts J, Balzarin J, Naesens L, de Clerq E. Efficacy of (S)-1-(3-hydroxy-2-phosphonyl-methoxypropyl)cytosine and 9-(1,3-dihydroxy-2-propoxymethyl)guanine for the treatment of murine cytomegalovirus infection in severe combined immunodeficiency mice. J Med Virol 1992;37:67–71.

43. Neyts J, Balzarini J, De Clerq E. Efficacy of (S)-1-(3-hydroxy-2-phosphonyl-methoxypropyl) cytosine [HPMPC] against intraperitoneal and intracerebral murin cytomegalovirus infections [Abstract 167]. Antiviral Res 1991;(Suppl 1):133.

44. Nimura N, Nishikawa J. Treatment of eczema herpeticum with oral acyclovir. Am J Med 1988;85(Suppl 2A):49.

45. O'Brien JJ, Campoli-Richards DM. Acyclovir: an updated review of its antiviral activity, pharmacokinetic properties and therapeutic efficacy. Drugs 1989;37:233–309.

46. Palmer J, Vogt PE, Kern ER. Prevention and treatment of experimental genital herpes simplex virus type 2 (HSV-2) infections with topical HPMPC [Abstract]. 8th International Conference on Antiviral Research, Santa Fe, NM, 1995.

47. Patel R, Delehanty J, International Valaciclovir HSV Study Group. Valaciclovir for the treatment of first episode genital herpes. 1st European Congress of Antimicrobial Chemotherapy, Glasgow, Scotland, 14–17 May, 1996.

48. Perry CM, Wagstaff AJ. Famciclovir: a review of its pharmacological properties and therapeutic efficacy in herpesvirus infections. Drugs 1995;50:396–415.

49. Perry PM, Faulds D. Valaciclovir: a review of its antiviral activ-

ity, pharmacokinetic properties and therapeutic efficacy in herpesvirus infections. Drugs 1996;52:754–772.

50. Raborn GW, McGaw WT, Grace M, Houle L. Herpes labialis treatment with acyclovir 5 per cent ointment. Can Dent Assoc J 1989;55:135–137.

51. Raborn GW, McGaw WT, Grace M, Percy J, Samuels S. Herpes labialis treatment with acyclovir 5% modified aqueous cream: a double-blind, randomized trial. Oral Surg Oral Med Oral Pathol 1989;67:676–679.

52. Raborn GW, McGaw WT, Grace M, Tyrrell LD, Samuels SM. Oral acyclovir and herpes labialis: a randomized, double-blind, placebo-controlled study. J Am Dent Assoc 1987;115:38–42.

53. Richards DM, Carmine AA, Brogden RN, Heel RC, Speight TM, Avery GS. Acyclovir: a review of its pharmacodynamic properties and therapeutic efficacy. Drugs 1983;26:378–438.

54. Rooney JF, Mannix ML, Dumois J, Wohlenberg CR, Alling D, Straus SE, Notkins AL. Suppression of frequently recurrent herpes labialis by daily oral acyclovir [Abstract]. Clin Res 1992; 40:319A.

55. Sacks SL, Aoki FY, Diaz-Mitoma F, Sellors J, Shafran SD. Patient-initiated, twice-daily oral famciclovir for early recurrent genital herpes. A randomized, double-blind multicenter trial. Canadian Famciclovir Study Group. JAMA 1996;276:44–49.

56. Sacks SL, Portnoy J, Lawee D, Schlech W III, Aoki F, Tyrrell DL, Poisson M, Bright C, Kaluski J, The Canadian Cooperative Study Group. Clinical course of recurrent genital herpes and treatment with foscarnet cream: results of a Canadian multicenter trial. J Infect Dis 1987;155:178–186.

57. Sacks SL, Wanklin RJ, Reece DE, Hicks KA, Tyler KL, Coen DM. Progressive esophagitis from acyclovir-resistant herpes simplex: clinical roles for DNA polymerase mutants and viral heterogeneity? Ann Intern Med 1989;111:893–899.

58. Sacks SL. Genital herpes simplex virus infection and treatment. In: Sacks SL, Straus SE, Whitley RJ, Griffiths PD, eds. Clinical management of herpes viruses. Oxford: IOS Press, 1995:55–74.

59. Sacks SL. Treatment-resistant viruses: mechanisms, monitoring, and management [Abstract]. 37th Interscience Conference on Antimicrobial Agents and Chemotherapy, Toronto, Ont, 28 Sept–1 Oct, 1997.

60. Safrin S, Crumpacker C, Chatis P, Davis R, Hafner R, Rush J, Kessler HA, Landry B, Mills J. A controlled trial comparing foscarnet with vidarabine for acyclovir-resistant mucocutaneous herpes simplex in the acquired immunodeficiency syndrome. The AIDS Clinical Trials Group. N Engl J Med 1991;325:551–555.

61. Safrin S, Elbeik, Mills J. A rapid screen test for in vitro susceptibility of clinical herpes simplex virus isolates. J Infect Dis 1994;169:879–882.

62. Safrin S, Phan L, Elbeik T. A comparative evaluation of three methods of antiviral susceptibility testing of clinical herpes simplex virus isolates. Clin Diagn Virol 1995;4:81–91.

63. Schacker T, Shaughnessy M, Barnum G, Selke S, Zeh J, Corey L. Efficacy of famciclovir for suppressing HSV-2 infections among HIV+ persons [Abstract 13]. 3rd Conference on Retroviruses and Opportunistic Infection, Washington, DC. 28 Jan–1 Feb, 1996.

64. Shaw M, King M, Best JM, Banatvala JE, Gibson JR, Klaber MR. Failure of acyclovir cream in treatment of recurrent herpes labialis. Br Med J 1985;291:7–9.

65. Shepp DH, Dandliker PS, Flournoy N, Meyers JD. Sequential intravenous and twice-daily oral acyclovir for extended prophylaxis of herpes simplex virus infection in marrow transplant patients. Transplantation 1987;43:654–657.

66. Shepp DH, Newton BA, Dandliker PS, Flournoy N, Meyers JD. Oral acyclovir therapy for mucocutaneous herpes simplex virus infections in immunocompromised bone marrow transplant recipients. Ann Intern Med 1985;102:783–785.

67. Simon AL, Pavan-Langston D. Long-term oral acyclovir therapy. Effect on recurrent infectious herpes simplex keratitis in patients with and without grafts. Ophthalmology 1996;103: 1399–1404(discussion:1404–5).

68. Soike KF, Huang JL, Zhang JY, Bohm R, Hitchcock MJM, Martin JC. Evaluation of infrequent dosing regimens with (S)-1-[3-hydroxy-2-(phosphonyl-methoxy)-propyl] cytosine (S-HPMPC) on simian varicella infection in monkeys. Antiviral Res 1991;16: 17–28.

69. Spruance SL, Crumpacker CS, Schnipper LE, Kern ER, Marlow S, Arndt KA, Overall JC Jr. Early, patient-initiated treatment of herpes labialis with topical 10% acyclovir. Antimicrob Agents Chemother 1984;25:553–555.

70. Spruance SL, Hamill ML, Hoge WS, Davis LG, Mills J. Acyclovir prevents reactivation of herpes labialis in skiers. JAMA 1988;260:1597–1599.

71. Spruance SL, Rea TL, Thoming C, Tucker R, Saltzman R, Boon R. Penciclovir cream for the treatment of herpes simplex labialis. A randomized, multicenter, double-blind, placebo-controlled trial. Topical Penciclovir Collaborative Study Group. JAMA 1997;277:1374–1379.

72. Spruance SL, Schnipper LE, Overall JC Jr, Kern ER, Wester B, Modlin J, Wenerstrom G, Burton C, Arndt KA, Chiu GL, Crumpacker CS. Treatment of herpes simplex labialis with topical acyclovir in polyethylene glycol. J Infect Dis 1982;146: 85–90.

73. Spruance SL, Stewart JCB, Rowe NH, McKeough MB, Wenerstrom G, Freeman DJ. Treatment of recurrent herpes simplex labialis with oral acyclovir. J Infect Dis 1990;161:185–190.

74. Spruance SL, Tyring SK, DeGregorio B, Miller C, Beutner K. A large-scale, placebo-controlled, dose-ranging trial of peroral valaciclovir for episodic treatment of recurrent herpes genitalis. Valaciclovir HSV Study Group. Arch Intern Med 1996;156: 1729–1735.

75. Spruance SL, Wenerstrom G. Pathogenesis of herpes simplex labialis: IV. Maturation of lesions within 8 hours after onset and implications for antiviral treatment. Oral Surg Oral Med Oral Pathol 1984;58:667–671.

76. Spruance SL. Herpes simplex labialis. In: Sacks SL, Straus SE, Whitley RJ, Griffiths PD, editors. Clinical management of herpes viruses. Oxford: IOS Press, 1995:3–42.

77. Spruance SL. Prophylactic chemotherapy with acyclovir for recurrent herpes simplex labialis. J Med Virol 1993;41(Suppl 1):27–32.

78. Stals FS, de Clerq E, Bruggeman CA. Comparative activity of (S)-1-(3-hydroxy-2-phosphonyl methoxy propyl) cytosine and 9-(1,3-dihydroxy-2-propoxymethyl) guanine against rat cytomegalovirus infection in vitro and in vivo. Antimicrob Agents Chemother 1991;35:2262–2266.

79. Sutton D, Ashton RJ, Bacon TH. Activity of famciclovir and penciclovir in HSV-infected animals [Abstract]. 6th International Congress for Infectious Diseases. Prague, Czech Republic, 26–30 Apr, 1994.

80. Sutton D, Taylor J, Bacon TH. Activity of penciclovir in combination with azido-thymidine, ganciclovir, acyclovir, foscarnet and human interferons against herpes simplex virus replication in cell culture. Antiviral Chem Chemother 1992;3:85–94.

81. Swierkosz EM, Scholl DR, Brown JL, Jollick JD, Gleaves CA. Improved DNA hybridisation method for detection of

acyclovir-resistant herpes simplex virus. Antimicrob Agents Chemother 1987;31:1465–1469.

82. Thackray AM, Field HJ. Comparison of effects of famciclovir and valaciclovir on pathogenesis of herpes simplex virus type 2 in a murine infection model. Antimicrob Agents Chemother 1995; 40:846–851.

83. Vere Hodge RA, Cheng Y-C. The mode of action of penciclovir. Antiviral Chem Chemother 1993;4(Suppl 1):13–24.

84. Vere Hodge RA. Famciclovir and penciclovir: the mode of action of famciclovir including its conversion to penciclovir. Antiviral Chem Chemother 1993;4:67–84.

85. Wade JC, McLaren C, Meyers JD. Frequency and significance of acyclovir-resistant herpes simplex virus isolated from marrow transplant recipients receiving multiple courses of treatment with acyclovir. J Infect Dis 1983;148:1077–1082.

86. Wade JC, Newton B, Flournoy N, Meyers JD. Oral acyclovir for prevention of herpes simplex virus reactivation after marrow transplantation. Ann Intern Med 1984;100:823–828.

87. Wald A, Zeh J, Barnum G, Davis LG, Corey L. Suppression of subclinical shedding of herpes simplex virus type 2 with acyclovir. Ann Intern Med 1996;124(1 pt 1):8–15.

88. Whitley R, Arvin A, Prober C, Burchett S, Corey L, Powell D, Plotkin S, Starr S, Alford C, Connor J. A controlled trial comparing vidarabine with acyclovir in neonatal herpes simplex virus infection. Infectious Diseases Collaborative Antiviral Study Group. N Engl J Med 1991;324:444–449.

89. Whitley RJ, Alford CA, Hirsch MS, Schooley RT, Luby JP, Aoki FY, Hanley D, Nahmias AJ, Soong SJ. Vidarabine versus acyclovir therapy in herpes simplex encephalitis. N Engl J Med 1986;314:144–149.

90. Whitley RJ, Levin M, Barton N, Hershey BJ, Davis G, Keeney RE, Whelchel J, Diethelm AG, Kartus P, Soong SJ. Infections caused by herpes simplex virus in the immunocompromised host: natural history and topical acyclovir therapy. J Infect Dis 1984;150:323–329.

91. Wilhelmus KR, Dawson CR, Barron BA, Bacchetti P, Gee L, Jones DB, Kaufman HE, Sugar J, Hyndiuk RA, Laibson PR, Stulting RD, Asbell PA. Risk factors for herpes simplex virus epithelial keratitis recurring during treatment of stromal keratitis or iridocyclitis. Herpetic Eye Disease Study Group. Br J Ophthalmol 1996;80:969–972.

92. Wutzler P, Ulbricht A, Farber I. Antiviral efficacies of famciclovir, valaciclovir, and brivudin in disseminated herpes simplex virus type 1 infection in mice. Intervirology 1997;40:15–21.

Human Herpesvirus-6 and Human Herpesvirus-7

Nina Singh and Donald R. Carrigan

HUMAN HERPESVIRUS-6
General Description

In 1986, a novel human herpesvirus was isolated from the peripheral blood of six patients with lymphoproliferative disorders; two of these patients were infected with the human immunodeficiency virus (HIV) (30). The herpesvirus was originally designated human B-lymphotropic virus. Subsequent studies, however, established that the virus was primarily T-cell lymphotropic; it was therefore renamed human herpesvirus-6 (HHV-6). HHV-6 is an enveloped virion with an icosahedral nucleocapsid of 162 capsomers, and it contains a large double-stranded DNA genome. HHV-6 is antigenically distinct from other human herpesviruses, such as cytomegalovirus (CMV), herpes simplex virus types 1 and 2, varicella zoster virus, and Epstein-Barr virus (23). Its closest phylogenetic relative is CMV; nucleotide sequencing has shown 66% DNA sequence homology between CMV and HHV-6 (23).

Primary HHV-6 infection has been shown to cause roseola (exanthema subitum), a febrile illness of early childhood (36). In immunocompetent adults, the virus has been associated with EBV-like mononucleosis syndrome, autoimmune disorders (e.g., Sjögren's disease), non-Hodgkin's and Hodgkin's lymphomas, necrotizing lymphadenitis, and encephalitis (3, 22, 26). Recent evidence suggests that HHV-6 may also play a central role in the pathogenesis of multiple sclerosis; active HHV-6 infection has been detected in association with plaques that are a characteristic pathologic feature of multiple sclerosis (10, 11). HHV-6 is also proposed to be a cofactor in the pathogenesis of AIDS; HIV and HHV-6 can coinfect the same CD4+ lymphocytes (21, 25). HHV-6 can upregulate CD4 receptors on CD8+ T lymphocytes and natural killer cells, thus rendering these cells more susceptible to infection with HIV (25).

In organ transplant recipients, HHV-6 has been associated with idiopathic marrow suppression, interstitial pneumonitis, and fatal encephalitis (32). HHV-6 is a strongly neurotrophic virus, and its propensity to cause central nervous system disease has been noted both in immunocompetent patients, patients with HIV infection, and bone marrow transplant recipients (15, 20, 26).

On the basis of genomic DNA sequences, cell tropism, and protein expression, two distinct variants of HHV-6, designated as the A (HHV-6A) and B (HHV-6B) variants, have been described. The two variants also differ in a number of biologic properties including antiviral susceptibilities. HHV-6A is more frequently isolated from patients with HIV; HHV-6B is isolated predominantly from transplant recipients and children with exanthema subitum (17, 21). HHV-6A induces production of tumor necrosis factor–α (TNF-α) and other proinflammatory cytokines (16, 18), whereas strains of HHV-6B do not. Finally, HHV-6A strains appear to be more susceptible to acyclovir than HHV-6B strains (Carrigan DR and Knox KK, unpublished observation).

In Vitro Susceptibility

Antiviral susceptibilities to HHV-6 are determined in tissue culture systems. Only limited data exist in the literature on in vitro sensitivitives of HHV-6 that must be interpreted in the context of variations in cell culture assays and the HHV-6 strains used for testing. For example, there are fewer than 10 independently obtained strains of HHV-6A worldwide to our knowledge, and two of these (HHV-6A$_{Gs}$ and HHV-6A$_{U1102}$) have been passaged innumerable times in T leukemia cell lines in culture. Such passaging can introduce cell culture artifacts that tend to make a strain less representative of wild-type strains. Such artifacts may also be responsible for the reported resistance of HHV-6A$_{Gs}$ to most antiviral agents (6, 9). Clinical isolates that have received little or no cell passage would be optimal for screening antiviral agents. The type of cell used in the cell culture system may also influence the susceptibility results. For example, most of the testing for HHV-6A strains has involved T cell leukemia lines that are frequently susceptible to drug toxicity and may have abnormal nucleotide kinase expression.

In general, antiviral susceptibilities of HHV-6 resemble those of CMV; that is, HHV-6 is very sensitive to ganciclovir and foscarnet and less so to acyclovir.

Acyclovir

Existing data suggest that HHV-6A and HHV-6B have different sensitivities to acyclovir; HHV-6A strains being more susceptible to acyclovir than the HHV-6B strains. The mean 50% inhibitory concentrations (IC$_{50}$) of HHV-6A strains in the reported studies was approximately 20 μM, with some strains demonstrating greater sensitivity (4, 5, 9). Strains of HHV-B are less sensitive to acyclovir, with a mean IC$_{50}$ of 37 μM (8, 13, 29).

Serum acyclovir levels (1.8–3.6 μg/mL) following low-dose oral acyclovir (200 mg) are inadequate to suppress HHV-6. However, high-dose oral acyclovir (800 mg) can achieve plasma concentrations of approximately 1.6 μg/mL, which may at least partially suppress HHV-6A strains. While these concentrations appear to be ineffective in suppressing HHV-6B, some strains of HHV-6B may also be sensitive to acyclovir (e.g., IC$_{50}$ of 4.4 μM for HHV6B$_{oc}$) (19).

Ganciclovir

Ganciclovir is highly active against HHV-6A and B in vitro. Peak serum concentrations following intravenous ganciclovir (5 mg/kg) average 31 to 43 μM and should be adequate to suppress HHV-6. The IC$_{50}$ of ganciclovir for HHV-6A strains ranged between 1.1 and 25 μM (Table 1). The IC$_{50}$ of HHV-6 for ganciclovir ranges from 1.0 to 2.5 μM (4, 8, 31). For 14 clinical iso-

lates of HHV-6B, the mean IC$_{50}$ $\pm$ 1 SD was 5.9 $\pm$ 3.0 μM (range, 2.2–13.5 μM) (Carrigan, unpublished observation).

Foscarnet

The IC$_{50}$ of foscarnet for HHV-6 ranges from 49 to 67 μM (4, 8, 31). For 14 clinical isolates of HHV-6B tested, the IC$_{50}$ was 67 μM $\pm$ 22 μM (range, 21 μM–117 uM) (Carrigan, unpublished observation). Following infusion of 90 mg/kg/day of foscarnet, peak serum concentrations range between 240 and 650 μM, exceeding the IC$_{50}$ of all but a rare isolate of HHV-6 (Table 2). Furthermore, foscarnet does not possess the potential marrow toxicity associated with ganciclovir.

Other Antiviral Agents

After oral administration, the L-valine ester of acyclovir, valaciclovir, is rapidly and almost completely converted to acyclovir, achieving peak plasma levels of 22 and 38 μM after 100 and 200 mg of valaciclovir, respectively. These levels

TABLE 1 • **Susceptibility of HHV-6A to Inhibition by Currently Available Antiviral Compounds**

Antiviral Compound	50% Inhibitory Concentration (IC$_{50}$)	Virus Strain
Acyclovir	59 μM	HHV-6A$_{GS}$
Acyclovir	27 μM	HHV-6A$_{SIE}$
Acyclovir	30 μM	HHV-6A$_{SIE}$
Acyclovir	7 μM	HHV-6$_{U1102}$
Ganciclovir	25 μM	HHV-6A$_{GS}$
Ganciclovir	1.1 μM	HHV-6A$_{SIE}$
Ganciclovir	2 μM	HHV-6A$_{SIE}$
Ganciclovir	2 μM	HHV-6A$_{U1102}$
Ganciclovir	14 μM	HHV-6A$_{GS}$
Foscarnet	49 μM	HHV-6A$_{GS}$
Foscarnet	2.7 μg/mL	HHV-6A$_{SIE}$
Foscarnet	8.7 μM	HHV-6A$_{SIE}$
Foscarnet	25 μM	HHV-6A$_{U1102}$
Foscarnet	>150 μM	HHV-6A$_{GS}$
Interferon-α	40 IU/mL	HHV-6$_{U1102}$
Interferon-β	16 IU/mL	HHV-6A$_{U1102}$
Zidovudine	>200 μM	HHV-6A$_{GS}$
Zidovudine	>8 μM	HHV-6A$_{SIE}$

Data from references 4, 5, 6, 9, and 10.

TABLE 2 • **Susceptibility of HHV-6B to Inhibition by Antiviral Agents**

Antiviral Agent	IC$_{50}$ (50% inhibitory concentration)
Acyclovir	37 μM (mean)
Ganciclovir	5.9 μM (mean)[a]
Ganciclovir	1.0–2.5 μM[b]
Foscarnet	21–117 μM[a]
Foscarnet	49–67 μM[b]

[a] HHV-6A-infected HSB-2 cells were cultured in the presence of varying concentrations of acyclovir, foscarnet, and ganciclovir. Four days after infection, the infected cells were stained by indirect immunofluorescence for a structural protein of the virus (gp106), and the percentage of viral antigen–positive cells in each culture was determined by direct cell counts. The ID$_{50}$s obtained were 59 μM, >150 μM, and 14 μM for acyclovir, foscarnet, and ganciclovir, respectively. Carrigan DR, Folger K, unpublished observations.

[b] Data from references 4, 8, 13, 29, and 31.

of acyclovir would be effective against most strains of HHV-6A. Other drugs with in vitro activity against HHV-6 are a guanosine analogue (9-[-4 hydroxy-2-(hydroxymethyl)butyl]) guanine, ampligen, and kutapressin (1, 6).

Antimicrobial Therapy

Only a limited number of studies have reported the efficacy of antiviral therapy for HHV-6. Drobyski et al. reported four bone marrow transplant recipients with marrow suppression and viremia due to HHV-6 who were treated with ganciclovir or foscarnet (14). Viremia and neutropenia resolved in all patients, but HHV-6 infection recurred in one patient who eventually died (14). A liver transplant recipient with disseminated invasive HHV-6 infection was successfully treated with ganciclovir (34). Cytopenia resolved in two liver transplant recipients with marrow suppression who were treated with foscarnet (33). A bone marrow transplant recipient with late graft failure and aplastic marrow was successfully treated with foscarnet and retransplantation (28).

Indications for Therapy and Drug of Choice

Transplant Recipients

Because of the latent and ubiquitous nature of HHV-6, the criteria for initiating treatment should include documentation of active or replicative infection, and presence of symptoms or signs attributable to HHV-6 pathogenicity. We propose using the criteria listed in Table 3 to determine which patients should be treated for HHV-6 after transplantation (32). The superiority of either ganciclovir or foscarnet over the other has not been established in clinical studies. However, of 20 bone marrow transplant recipients with CMV viremia, 7 also had HHV-6 detectable in the peripheral blood mononuclear cells by PCR; all 3 patients who received foscarnet became HHV-6 negative, compared with only 1 of the 4 who received ganciclovir (35). Other clinical circumstances such as renal failure or degree of marrow suppression may also dictate whether ganciclovir or foscarnet is used as therapy for HHV-6. For ex-

---

TABLE 3 • Criteria for Initiating Treatment for Human Herpesvirus-6 Infection in Transplant Recipients

Documentation of an active infection by a positive result using one of the following tests
—Isolation of HHV-6 in cell culture from blood, body fluid, or tissue
—Positive polymerase chain reaction assay result for HHV-6 DNA using an acellular specimen such as cerebrospinal fluid, bronchoalveolar lavage fluid, bone marrow plasma, or serum
Positive immunohistochemical staining of a tissue biopsy specimen of cytologic preparation using an antiserum or monoclonal antibody reactive with viral structural proteins indicating productive infection (e.g., p101 or gp82)
Positive sample by rapid shell vial assay that requires passage of infection from the patient's sample to target cell (e.g., MRC-5 fibroblasts)
Presence of one of the three documented clinical manifestations of HHV-6: bone marrow suppression, encephalitis, or pneumonitis

Reproduced with permission from reference 32.

---

ample, ganciclovir may be preferable in patients with renal dysfunction, since foscarnet is potentially nephrotoxic. On the other hand, foscarnet may be preferable in patients with marrow suppression because it does not possess the myelosuppressive effect of ganciclovir.

Other Patients

HHV-6 is generally a self-limited infection in children with exanthema subitum, and therapy is not recommended. The indications and efficacy of antiviral therapy likewise have not been established or proven for HHV-6 infections in other immunocompetent hosts or patients with HIV infection. Antiviral therapy for HHV-6 may be potentially useful in patients with multiple sclerosis (7); clinical trials demonstrating efficacy in this setting are awaited.

Prophylaxis

Since HHV-6 is associated with considerable morbidity and even mortality in transplant recipients (particularly bone marrow transplant recipients), prophylaxis for HHV-6 is a reasonable goal in the transplant setting. The optimal time of initiation, duration, and efficacy of prophylaxis for HHV-6 infection after transplantation remains to be defined. Intravenous ganciclovir and foscarnet could clearly achieve serum concentrations high enough to provide effective prophylaxis against HHV-6. The role of oral ganciclovir remains undetermined. Administration of 1000 mg of ganciclovir orally three times daily resulted in a maximum serum concentration of 4.7 μM (product monograph, Cytovene, Roche Laboratories, Palo Alto, CA). While these levels may suppress some strains of HHV-6, they may not be adequate for all strains. High-dose acyclovir was associated with a significantly lower incidence of HHV-6 in a study in bone marrow transplant recipients (35). Other studies have documented active HHV-6 infection despite high-dose acyclovir (14).

HUMAN HERPESVIRUS-7
General Description

Human herpesvirus-7 (HHV-7), like HHV-6, is a member of the beta *Herpesviridae*. First isolated in 1990 from CD4+ T cells of a healthy individual, HHV-7 bears close homology with HHV-6 (1, 24). HHV-7, however, is more cell associated, less lytic, and slower growing than HHV-6 (2).

The seroepidemiologic prevalence rate of HHV-7 exceeds 85% in the U.S. population, whereas lower prevalence rates (60%) have been reported from Japan (1, 37). Primary infection due to HHV-7 is believed to be acquired later in life than HHV-6. Currently, HHV-7 has not been conclusively linked to any human disease. HHV-7 has been proposed to be one of the causative agents of roseola (exanthema subitum), particularly the second attack of roseola. Viremia due to HHV-7 (detection of HHV-7 DNA by PCR of peripheral blood mononuclear cells) was demonstrated in 57% of bone marrow and 39% of renal transplant recipients (27, 35). HHV-7 selectively uses CD4 as a cellular membrane receptor and is a powerful inhibitor of HIV in cells of mononuclear phagocytic lineage (12). The clinical relevance of these observations remains to be defined.

Antiviral Susceptibility

Reports of in vitro or clinical efficacy of antiviral agents against HHV-7 are lacking at the current time. Clearance of HHV-7 DNA from the blood (detected by PCR) was demonstrated in 1 of 2 bone marrow transplant recipients who received ganciclovir and in 2 of 2 who received foscarnet (35).

REFERENCES

1. Ablashi DV, Berneman ZN, Kramarsky B, Asano Y, Choudhury S, Pearson GR. Human herpesvirus-7. In Vivo 1994;8:549–554.
2. Ablashi DV, Berneman ZN, Lawyer C, Kramarsky B, Ferguson DM, Komaroff AL. Antiviral activity in vitro of Kutapressin against human herpesvirus-6. In Vivo 1994;8:581–586.
3. Agut H. Puzzles concerning the pathogenicity of human herpesvirus-6 [Editorial]. N Engl J Med 1994;329:203–204.
4. Agut H, Aubin JT, Huraux JM. Homogeneous susceptibility of distinct human herpesvirus 6 strains to antivirals in vitro [Letter]. J Infect Dis 1991;163:1382–1383.
5. Agut H, Collandre H, Aubin JT, Guetard D, Favier V, Ingrand D, Montagnier L, Huraux JM. In vitro sensitivity of human herpesvirus 6 to antiviral drugs. Res Virol 1989;140:219–228.
6. Akesson-Johasson A, Harmenberg J, Wahren B, Linde A. Inhibition of human herpesvirus 6 replication by 9-[4-hydroxy-2-(hydroxymethyl)butyl] guanine (2HM-HBG) and other antiviral compounds. Antimicrob Agents Chemother 1990;34:2417–2419.
7. Braun DK, Dominguez G, Pellett PE. Human herpesvirus 6. Clin Microbiol Rev 1997;10:521–567.
8. Burns WH, Sandford GR. Susceptibility of human herpesvirus 6 to antivirals in vitro. J Infect Dis 1990;162:634–637.
9. Carrigan DR, Folger K. Unpublished observations, 1996.
10. Carrigan DR, Harrington D, Knox KK. Subacute leukoencephalitis caused by CNS infection with human herpesvirus-6 manifesting as acute multiple sclerosis. Neurology 1996;47: 145–148.
11. Challoner PB, Smith KT, Parker JD. Plaque associated expression of human herpesvirus 6 in multiple sclerosis. Proc Natl Acad Sci USA 1995;92:7440–7444.
12. Crowley RW, Secchiero P, Zella D, Cara A, Gallo RC, Lusso P. Interference between human herpesvirus 7 and HIV-1 in mononuclear phagocytes. J Immunol 1996;156:2004–2008.
13. DiLuca D, Katsafanas G, Schirmer EC, Balachandran N, Frenkel N. The replication of viral and cellular DNA in human herpesvirus 6 infected cells. Virology 1990;175:199–210.
14. Drobyski WR, Dunne WM, Burd EM, Knox KK, Ash RC, Horowitz MM. Human herpesvirus-6 infection in allogeneic bone marrow transplant recipients: evidence of a marrow suppressive role for HHV-6 in vivo. J Infect Dis 1993;167:735–739.
15. Drobyski WR, Knox KK, Majewski D, Carrigan DR. Brief report: fatal encephalitis due to variant B human herpesvirus-6 infection in a bone marrow transplant recipient. N Engl J Med 1994;330:1356–1360.
16. Flamand L, Gosselin J, Stefanescu I, Ablashi D, Menezes J. Immunosuppressive effect of human herpesvirus 6 on T-cell functions: suppression of interleukin-2 synthesis and cell proliferation. Blood 1995;85:1263–1271.
17. Frenkel N, Katsafanas GC, Wyatt LS, Yoshikawa T, Asano Y. Bone marrow transplant recipients harbor the B variant of human herpesvirus 6. Bone Marrow Transplant 1994;14:839–843.
18. Gosselin J, Flamand L, D'Addario M, Hiscott J, Stefanescu I, Ablashi DV. Modulatory effects of Epstein-Barr, herpes simplex and human herpesvirus-6 viral infections and coinfections on cytokine synthesis: a comparative study. J Immunol 1992;149: 181–187.
19. Kikuta H, Lu H, Matsumoto S. Susceptibility of human herpesvirus 6 to acyclovir. Lancet 1989;2:861.
20. Knox KK, Carrigan DR. Active human herpesvirus (HHV-6) infection of central nervous system in patients with AIDS. J Acquired Immune Defic Syndr Hum Retroviral 1995;9:69–73.
21. Knox KK, Carrigan DR. Active HHV-6 infection in the lymph nodes of HIV infected patients: in vitro evidence that HHV-6 can break HIV latency. J Acquired Immun Defic Syndr Hum Retrovirol 1996;11:370–378.
22. Krueger GR, Klueppelberg U, Hoffman A, Ablashi DV. Clinical correlates of infection with human herpesvirus-6. In vivo. In Vivo 1994;8:457–485.
23. Lawrence GL, Chee M, Craxton MA, Gompels UA, Honess RW, Barrell BG. Human herpesvirus-6 is closely related to human cytomegalovirus. J Virol 1990;64:287–299.
24. Luppi M, Torelli G. The new lymphotrophic herpesvirus (HHV-6, HHV-7, HHV-8) and hepatitis C virus in human lymphoproliferative diseases: an overview. Haematologica 1996;81: 265–281.
25. Lusso P, Gallo RC. Human herpesvirus-6 in AIDS. Immunol Today 1995;16:67–71.
26. McCullers JA, Lakeman FD, Whitley RJ. Human herpesvirus 6 is associated with focal encephalitis. Clin Infect Dis 1996;21: 571–576.
27. Osman HKE, Peiris JSM, Taylor CE, Warwicker P, Jarrett RF, Madeley CR. Cytomegalovirus disease in renal allograft recipients: is human herpesvirus-7 a cofactor for disease progression? J Med Virol 1996;48:295–301.
28. Rosenfeld CS, Rybka WB, Weinbaum D, Carrigan DR, Knox KK, Andrews DF. Late graft failure due to dual bone marrow infection with variants A and B of human herpesvirus-6. Hematology 1995;23:626–629.
29. Russeler SK, Tapper MA, Carrigan DR. Susceptibility of human herpesvirus-6 to acyclovir and ganciclovir. Lancet 1989;2:382.
30. Salahuddin SZ, Ablashi DV, Markham PD, Josephs SF, Sturzenegger S, Kaplan M. Isolation of a new virus, HBLV, in patients with lymphoproliferative disorders. Science 1986;234: 596–601.
31. Shiraki K, Okuno T, Yamanishi K, Takahashi M. Phosphonoacetic acid inhibits replication of human herpesvirus-6. Antiviral Res 1989;12:311–318.
32. Singh N, Carrigan DR. Human herpesvirus-6 in transplantation: an emerging pathogen. Ann Intern Med 1996;124:1065–1071.
33. Singh N, Carrigan DR. Human herpesvirus-6 in liver transplantation: documentation of pathogenicity. Transplantation 1997;64:674–678.
34. Singh N, Carrigan DR, Gayowski T, Singh J, Marino IR. Variant B human herpesvirus-6 associated febrile dermatosis with thrombocytopenia and encephalopathy in a liver transplant recipient. Transplantation 1995;60:1355–1357.
35. Wang FZ, Dahl H, Linde A, Brytting M, Ehrnst A, Ljugman P. Lymphotrophic herpesviruses in allogeneic bone marrow transplantation. Blood 1997;88:3615–3620.
36. Yamanishi K, Okuno T, Shiraki K, Takashi M, Kondo T, Asano Y, et al. Identification of human herpesvirus-2 as a causal agent for exanthem subitum. Lancet 1988;1:1065–1067.
37. Yoshikawa T, Asano Y, Kobayashi I, Nakashima T, Yazaki T, Suga S, Ozaki T, Wyatt LS, Frenkel N. Seroepidemiology of human herpesvirus 7 in healthy children and adults in Japan. J Med Virol 1993;41:319–323.

Human Immunodeficiency Virus

●

Lauri Welles and Robert Yarchoan

The therapy of HIV infection has undergone rapid evolution ever since the observation in 1985 that certain dideoxynucleoside reverse transcriptase inhibitors (RTIs) inhibit viral replication in vitro (132, 136). Since that time, therapeutic strategies have expanded from treatment with one drug to combination therapy with three drugs from two different classes of antiretrovirals and also, in some ongoing studies, a biologic response modifier. This strategy of triple-drug combination therapy has now entered widespread clinical practice and represents state-of-the-art treatment for certain patients with HIV infection.

A growing understanding of viral replication, kinetics, and the host immune response has contributed to an increasingly rational approach to drug design and therapy (89, 93, 171, 205). This chapter attempts to give an overview of current therapeutic options and approaches and provide a basis for understanding potential future strategies.

HIV STRUCTURE AND LIFE CYCLE

HIV is a complex retrovirus whose structure and life cycle have been subject to intense analysis over the past few years. A number of discrete stages in the replication of HIV have been identified and the steps in processing immature particles into infectious virions are being elucidated. A number of these stages are actual or potential targets for specific antiretroviral therapy (Table 1).

HIV-1 is a single-stranded RNA virus. The RNA-dependent DNA polymerase, reverse transcriptase, which replicates the RNA genome through a double-stranded DNA intermediate, is contained within the virion. The virion is surrounded by a bilayered lipid envelope that is derived from the host cell during budding (79).

The viral genome consists of two positive-strand RNA molecules in a 70S complex, bound on either end by long terminal repeat (LTR) sequences that direct and regulate genomic expression (137). HIV contains three genes common to all replication-competent retroviruses: *gag* (group antigen, encoding the core and matrix proteins, p24 and p17), *pol* (polymerase, encoding the enzymatic proteins, reverse transcriptase, RNAse, protease and integrase), and *env* (encoding the envelope and transmembrane glycoproteins, gp 120 and gp41). The products of these genes are polyprotein precursors, two of which, Gag and Gag-Pol, are cleaved by the viral protease during the maturation process. The product of *env*, the third gene, is cleaved by a cellular enzyme. In addition to these three genes, there are at least six regulatory or auxiliary genes—*vif, vpr, vpu, tat, rev,* and *nef*—some of which are critical to the viral life cycle and pathogenesis.

Some details of the viral life cycle have not yet been elucidated and a full description of the known elements is beyond the scope of this chapter. Nevertheless, a brief description of those that are known may provide a framework for understanding the physiologic basis of current and future antiretroviral therapies.

The first step in the viral life cycle is binding of the gp120 protein on the outside of an infectious virion to the CD4 receptor of its cellular target. A second cellular coreceptor also appears to be necessary, and two proteins that serve this function, including CXCR4 (previously called fusin) and CCR5 (previously known as CKR5), have recently been described (52, 55, 156, 206). Both CXCR4 and CCR5 are GTP-binding protein (G-protein-coupled) receptors for chemokines. CXCR4 is a heterotrimeric G-protein that appears to comediate (with CD4) the binding and fusion of T-cell tropic HIV isolates. CCR5, by contrast, is a fusion co-receptor for macrophage-tropic HIV strains. Recently, individuals have been reported with homozygous mutant genes for CCR5 who are resistant to infection with HIV (52) (possibly because monocytes/macrophages or related cells are the initial target cells for HIV). This new information suggests an exciting area for potential therapeutic intervention.

Binding of HIV to its target may induce a conformational change in the viral envelope that ultimately reveals gp41, the transmembrane glycoprotein that anchors the envelope complex to the virus surface and is involved in fusion and viral entry (137). Once inside the cell, the virus is uncoated and releases the viral RNA genome as a nucleoprotein complex. At this point, replication of the viral genome can begin. Reverse transcriptase initiates transcription of a complementary strand of genomic DNA. The RNA template of this RNA-DNA hybrid is degraded by RNase H, and reverse transcriptase then also catalyzes transcription of the second (positive) DNA strand. This double-stranded DNA form of the HIV genome (provirus) migrates to the cellular nucleus. Within the nucleus, incorporation of the provirus into the cellular DNA can be mediated by another *pol* product, integrase. After a variable latency period, depending largely on the state of activation of the target cell, proviral DNA is transcribed to mRNA by host polymerases. A complex interplay of cellular and viral elements (including the six unique viral genes described above) is necessary for viral transcription and translation. As noted above, viral mRNA is largely translated into polyprotein precursors that are then cleaved by the HIV protease and cellular enzymes. In the absence of such cleavage, mature virions cannot be produced, and particles that are produced are not infectious. Viral proteins also undergo other changes such as myris-

TABLE 1 • Potential or Actual Anti-HIV Targets and Interventions

Life Cycle Stage or Target	Intervention (if known)
Binding to host cell	Inhibition of CD_4 receptor and co-receptors (CCR5, CXCR4) by modified ligands or antibodies
Fusion (gp41 fusogenic domain)	Inhibitor of gp41 (investigational: pentafuside[a])
Entry, uncoating, genome release	Bicyclams and hypericin may be inhibitors
Reverse transcriptase	Nucleoside and nonnucleoside reverse transcriptase inhibitors (RTIs)
RNA degradation by RNase H	Inhibitor not identified
Migration of viral DNA to nucleus	Target/intervention not yet identified
Integration (mediated by integrase)	Inhibitor (investigational: zintevir[b])
Transcription and translation	Inhibitors of tat or rev, tar decoys, antisense oligonucleotides
Enhancement by cellular factors	Inhibitors of TNF-α, such as thalidomide, pentoxyphylline, rolipram
Ribosomal frameshifting	Inhibitors may be identified
Gag-pol polyprotein cleavage by protease	HIV protease inhibitors
Myristoylation and glycosylation	Castanospermine and other inhibitors of glycosylation
Assembly and packaging	Zinc finger inhibitors
Viral budding, release	Interferon or interferon inducers

[a] From Lambert D, Johnson M, Barney S. Antiviral activity and pharmacokinetics of T-20 (pentafuside), an amphipathic helical peptide derived from gp41. XIth International Conference on AIDS, Vancouver, Canada. 3. 1996:68.

[b] From Kahn J, Graham E, Cossum P. (1996). Phase I study of AR-177 (zintevir), an HIV-1 inhibitor with significant activity against integrase protein: safety, pharmacokinetics and virologic activity. XIth International Conference on AIDS, Vancouver, Canada, 1996:21.

toylation and glycosylation (mediated by cellular enzymes), and then are assembled into infectious, fully processed virions at the cell surface. Finally, these mature virions are released into the extracellular environment by budding through the cellular membrane and go on to infect other target cells of the HIV virus (137).

DIAGNOSIS

Infection with HIV-1 is generally diagnosed by analysis of relevant serum antibodies using an enzyme-linked immunoabsorbent assay (ELISA) with a Western blot for confirmation; both must be positive for the diagnosis to be made. The sensitivity of these two examinations exceeds 99%. Indeterminate or false-negative results may occur in individuals who *(a)* are in the window period that precedes elaboration of anti-HIV antibodies and lasts for approximately 3 to 6 months after acute infection; *(b)* are infected with subtype O of HIV-1 (which is very rarely seen outside west Africa and appears to occur only in individuals with strains that originated in Cameroon); *(c)* have agammaglobulinemia; or *(d)* are infected with an antigenically distinct but clearly related virus, HIV-2. Infection with HIV-2 alone does not generally result in positive screening examination results for HIV-1 (25). A quantitative test measuring circulating virion-associated plasma HIV RNA by polymerase chain reaction (commonly called RNA PCR) or HIV p24 antigen can detect the virus shortly after acute infection and thus, earlier than the ELISA and Western blot. In the case of indeterminate results, this test may be performed.

Sensitivity testing of viral strains to antiretroviral drugs is not routinely done, although some patients are infected de novo with resistant strains prior to receiving any antiretroviral treatment (61). Experimental techniques for sensitivity testing are becoming available and may, in the future, play a role in therapeutic decision making.

After a positive diagnosis, a physical examination and routine laboratory tests should be performed, including those needed to assess a patient's immune status, such as CD4 cell counts. The patient's viral load should be measured by quantitative plasma HIV-1 RNA PCR to guide decisions about when to initiate or alter an antiretroviral regimen. Ideally, two measurements should be taken at important decision points in a patient's evaluation and treatment. These measurements should be taken at least 1 or 2 weeks apart, utilizing the same laboratory and assay. HIV RNA PCR, which measures the portion of a patient's viral load that is detectable in plasma, adds substantially to the CD4 cell count as an indicator of a patient's disease status and prognosis (125, 146). A variability (from both biologic fluctuation and assay imprecision) of approximately 0.3 to 0.5 $\log_{10}$ (up to threefold) in the measurement of plasma HIV RNA levels is observed. Plasma HIV RNA levels up to 5000 to 10,000 copies/mL are generally thought to represent relatively low viral loads, while 30,000 to 50,000 copies/mL or more are considered evidence of more active HIV infection (171).

INDICATIONS FOR THERAPY

In 1997, an International AIDS Society–USA Panel recommended that therapy begin early in the course of HIV infection, preferably before irreversible immune system damage has occurred, and that regimens that can maximally suppress the virus be chosen (19) (Table 2). Based upon the best current knowledge, these regimens would generally consist of a minimum of three antiretroviral agents with nonoverlapping patterns of resistance and toxicity. This is discussed in greater detail below. Other panels, including one convened by the U.S. Public Health Service, are also in the process of issuing recommendations at this time that may differ slightly from those of the International AIDS Society–USA Panel.

TABLE 2 • **Indications for Treatment As Recommended by the International AIDS Society–USA Panel, 1997**

Antiretroviral therapy is recommended[a]

For all patients with plasma HIV RNA levels above 5000–10,000 copies/mL

For all patients with symptomatic HIV disease (any CD4 cell count or HIV RNA PCR level)

Antiretroviral therapy may be deferred for patients with stable, high CD4 cell counts (>500 cells/mm³) and low plasma HIV RNA levels (<5000 copies/mL); such patients should be reevaluated every 3 to 6 months

From Carpenter C, Fischl M, Hammer S, Martin S, Jacobsen D, Katzenstein D, Montaner J, Richman D, Yeni P, Volberding P. Antiretroviral therapy for HIV infection in 1997. JAMA 1997;277:1962–1969.

[a] For suggested initial regimens, see Table 3 adapted from Carpenter C, Fischl M, Hammer S, et al. Antiretroviral therapy for HIV infection in 1997, updated recommendations of an international panel. JAMA 1997;277:1962–1969.

The panel recommended therapy for all patients with HIV RNA levels above 5000 to 10,000 copies/mL and advised that it should be considered for all HIV-infected patients with detectable levels of HIV RNA in plasma. Therapy may be deferred for those relatively early in the course of infection, with reproducibly stable, high CD4 cell counts (>500 cells/mm³) and low HIV RNA PCR levels, with the patient reevaluated every 3 to 6 months. The panel recommended explaining the importance of strict adherence to the regimen to all patients. As was previously standard practice, the international panel recommended antiretroviral therapy for all symptomatic patients, regardless of CD4 cell counts or viral load. (Symptoms may include hairy leukoplakia, recurrent thrush, night sweats, weight loss, or unexplained fevers.)

This set of recommendations is an attempt to grapple with the additional information provided by RNA-PCR assessment of viral load and is discussed in greater detail below in the section on approaches to HIV therapy. The clinician should remain alert for new information and new sets of recommendations as more information is obtained over the next few years.

REVERSE TRANSCRIPTASE INHIBITORS

The first antiretroviral agents to enter the clinical armamentarium were members of a family of nucleoside analogues called dideoxynucleosides. These agents can strongly inhibit wild-type HIV RT, but their long-term activity may be limited by resistance. Moreover, as a result of prior mutations, even in the absence of drugs, patients with HIV infection contain, at any one time, a large number of HIV quasispecies, some of which are believed to be already resistant to certain anti-HIV drugs (33). Under selective pressure of nucleoside agents, resistance may emerge rapidly, especially in patients with advanced HIV disease, who characteristically have high viral loads and replication rates (164).

In the face of therapy with nucleosides, mutations generally accumulate in an ordered pattern. Three mutations can confer

partial resistance to zidovudine (192), and high-level resistance is generally seen in strains with three or more of the five most common *pol* substitutions. However, the degree of resistance is not strictly proportional to the number of mutations, as specific patterns of mutations can affect HIV replication differently and may interact with one another. The observation that specific sets of mutations can also be mutually antagonistic provides a rational basis for therapy with certain combinations of nucleosides. Didanosine generally induces a specific mutation, L74V, that induces partial didanosine resistance but can restore sensitivity to zidovudine in previously zidovudine-resistant strains (184). Monotherapy with lamivudine induces a mutation at codon 184 (M184V) that rapidly confers high-level resistance to the drug in wild-type HIV and correlates clinically with rapid and substantial loss of drug efficacy when administered as a single agent (176, 192). However, this mutation also restores sensitivity to zidovudine in previously resistant strains (13, 192), and combination therapy with zidovudine and lamivudine has demonstrated substantial benefit to patients.

Certain mutations can induce cross-resistance among dideoxynucleosides. A mutation at codon 65 (K65R) of HIV-1 RT confers partial resistance to several such drugs. More strikingly, a novel set of five mutations in the polymerase domain of RT (at codons 62, 75, 77, 116 and 151) found in isolates obtained from some patients receiving combination nucleoside therapy confers high-level resistance to most nucleosides (97, 177, 178). It has also been reported that specific mutations or patterns of mutations may increase RT fidelity and sensitivity to RTIs, as has been proposed with the mutation at codon 184 induced by lamivudine (203), or that virus exposed simultaneously to multiple antiretroviral agents could be hobbled by mutations so that it becomes somewhat weakened. Finally, there is recent evidence that substantial suppression of HIV replication, as can be seen with a combination of nucleoside RTIs and protease inhibitors, may greatly reduce the rate of resistance development (125). Overall, the profound ability of HIV to develop resistance is one reason for the continued need to develop new antiretroviral drugs and treatment strategies.

Zidovudine (AZT, AZDV)

The first dideoxynucleoside to be developed as an anti-HIV drug was zidovudine. Originally synthesized as a potential anticancer agent (95), zidovudine was subsequently found to have activity against a broad range of retroviruses, including HIV-1, HIV-2, HTLV, and murine retroviruses (133, 136).

The drug is well absorbed from the gut, with an average bioavailability of 60%, which may be reduced somewhat if zidovudine is taken with high-fat meals (195, 212). While the serum half-life of zidovudine is 1.1 h (12, 107, 212), the intracellular half-life of AZT-TP is approximately 2 h longer (75), which allows activity even with thrice-daily dosing of the drug. Zidovudine has been found in saliva and semen (91, 168), and it penetrates into the cerebrospinal fluid (CSF), where concentrations approximately 60% of simultaneous serum concentrations have been found 1 h after administration of zidovudine (107, 211, 212). Zidovudine is thus relatively active in HIV-related central nervous system (CNS) disease (15, 175, 218). It can also decrease HIV-related thrombocytopenia (159) and significantly reduces perinatal transmission of the virus (40).

Zidovudine is primarily metabolized by the liver to an inactive glucuronide, which is then excreted by the kidneys (12). The drug is also, to a lesser extent, directly excreted by the kidneys in its unmetabolized form and can, if necessary, be cleared by hemodialysis (180). Advanced hepatic disease or renal failure may reduce zidovudine clearance, and patients with either of these conditions should be followed closely for signs of toxicity.

In 1986, Yarchoan et al. reported results of a phase I trial of zidovudine conducted at the National Cancer Institute and Duke University which demonstrated that 15 of 19 patients treated with zidovudine had increased CD_4 cell counts (212). Subsequent trials demonstrated a survival advantage over 1 year in asymptomatic patients with advanced HIV infection (69, 163), as well as decreased disease progression in patients who were treated with zidovudine monotherapy (201). However, the multicenter French-British Concorde trial (36) of zidovudine monotherapy in asymptomatic patients over 3 years failed to demonstrate any such benefit over administration of therapy later in the disease process. Also, there was no survival benefit to early therapy in this study. The lack of benefit at 3 years may have, in part, reflected the development of drug resistance. Thus, although the early large-scale studies of previously untreated patients with advanced disease showed a survival advantage to zidovudine monotherapy in those with CD4 cell counts below 200 cells/mm³, and a decreased short-term rate of disease progression among patients with CD4 cell counts below 500 cells/mm³, the benefits of early zidovudine monotherapy were generally not sustained in patients with 200 to 500 CD4 cells/mm³.

However, more-recent studies have shown that combination therapy with zidovudine and other RTIs can yield superior clinical results and a survival advantage over zidovudine monotherapy. Zidovudine has been observed to be synergistic with didanosine in vitro, and as noted above, these agents have antagonistic resistance patterns (184). In addition, other studies showed that long-term activity could be obtained with didanosine monotherapy (145), with the combination of zidovudine and didanosine (35, 157, 213) or with the combination of zidovudine and zalcitabine (126).

Partly on the basis of this information, two very large, multicenter trials were initiated: ACTG (AIDS Clinical Trial Group) 175, an American trial, and Delta, an international, European-Australian study (54, 87, 102). In ACTG 175, disease progression was significantly slowed by treatment with either didanosine monotherapy or a combination regimen of zidovudine/didanosine or zidovudine/zalcitabine, compared with zidovudine monotherapy (87, 102).

The Delta trial demonstrated significantly increased survival among zidovudine-naive patients on a combination regimen of zidovudine and either didanosine or zalcitabine compared with those on zidovudine monotherapy. Among patients with prior zidovudine therapy, a significant increase in survival was observed only in those receiving the zidovudine-didanosine combination (54).

Results of a third large study that compared zidovudine monotherapy with these same combination regimens in patients with advanced HIV infection were somewhat more equivocal (173). This study focused on patients with advanced HIV infection. The population as a whole did not appear to benefit more from these combinations of drugs than from zidovudine monotherapy. However, a subset analysis of individuals with less than 12 months of prior treatment with zidovudine demonstrated a small survival advantage and slowed disease progression in the cohort that received combination therapy.

Thus, the optimal use of zidovudine is in combination with other agents, and zidovudine monotherapy is not recommended. Zidovudine is preferentially phosphorylated in replicating cells, which provides a rationale for using it in combination therapy with such drugs as didanosine, zalcitabine, or lamivudine, which are more active in resting cells (76, 77, 149). In addition, the antagonistic resistance patterns observed with didanosine (184) or lamivudine (13, 192) provide another reason to favor the use of zidovudine with those drugs.

The recommended dosage of zidovudine (administered either in combination or as monotherapy) is 600 mg daily, most commonly given in divided doses of 200 mg every 8 h. If there is excessive toxicity, the dose may be reduced to 100 mg every 8 h. The drug is available in three formulations: capsules, an intravenous formulation, and a raspberry-flavored syrup.

The most common dose-limiting toxicity of zidovudine is myelosupression (67, 68, 201, 212), most frequently manifested as a macrocytic anemia (58, 67). Neutropenia and thrombocytopenia have also been observed, especially in patients with advanced disease. This toxicity is, to some extent, dose dependent and can be mitigated by dose reduction (67) or use of hematopoietic growth factors such as erythropoietin for the anemia (66) and filgrastim for the neutropenia (116, 154).

Zidovudine can also cause a reversible myopathy that is attributed to its effect on the mitochondria of myocytes (44, 131). The myopathy may be difficult to distinguish from that caused by HIV itself and is characterized by insidious onset of proximal muscle weakness and exercise-induced myalgias, sometimes with elevated creatinine phosphokinase levels. Damage to mitochondria in hepatocytes is thought to cause a rare, potentially lethal condition similar to Reye's syndrome that has been described predominantly in female patients with good nutritional status and consists of lactic acidosis and macrovesicular hepatic steatosis (26, 74, 126).

As noted above, zidovudine undergoes hepatic glucuronidation and is then secreted by the kidneys. Drugs that interfere with the hepatic metabolism or renal clearance of zidovudine (e.g., probenecid) should be administered with caution (51, 90, 110). Although there are insufficient data to recommend dose adjustment in patients with impaired liver function, such individuals should be followed closely. In patients with end-stage renal disease, recommended dosing of zidovudine is 100 mg every 6 or 8 h (17).

There is also laboratory evidence that certain drugs may inhibit the antiretroviral activity of zidovudine. Ribavirin, for example, may inhibit the phosphorylation of zidovudine, so these drugs should probably not be administered together outside the setting of a clinical trial (7, 200). Also, as discussed below, there is some evidence that the product of the first step in the phosphorylation of zidovudine, AZT-5-monophosphate, blocks the activity of thymidylate kinase (75) and thus can inhibit phosphorylation of stavudine. This inhibition has been demonstrated clinically.

Patients requiring drugs that have toxicity profiles similar to that of zidovudine should also be monitored closely. For example, individuals with HIV and cytomegalovirus (CMV) infection often experience severe myelosuppression when treated concurrently with ganciclovir and zidovudine. In such patients, foscarnet or cidofovir, alternate drugs approved for treatment of CMV that have relatively little bone marrow toxicity, may be considered. Alternatively, filgrastim may added to the regimen.

Didanosine (ddl)

Didanosine is a purine dideoxynucleoside that inhibits HIV-1 and HIV-2 replication in human lymphocytes and macrophages (132, 134, 149). It is efficiently phosphorylated to its active moiety in resting cells, a property that it shares with zalcitabine and lamivudine (76, 77, 149). By contrast, zidovudine, stavudine, and other nucleosides that are phosphorylated by thymidine kinase are preferentially phosphorylated in actively replicating cells. These differences provide an additional rationale for a judicious combination of drugs from each of these two groups.

Another notable contrast between zidovudine and didanosine is that the in vitro activity of didanosine is not reversed by its physiologic 2'-deoxynucleoside counterparts, 2'-deoxyinosine or 2'-deoxyadenosine (135). Recently, it was reported that the in vitro anti-HIV activity of didanosine is potentiated by agents such as hydroxyurea that deplete intracellular pools of dATP, which competes directly with ddATP for reverse transcriptase as well as for incorporation into proviral DNA (76, 118).

Didanosine is acid labile, which renders it unstable in the acidic gastric environment and reduces its absorption (88). Because of this, it is formulated with a buffer. Currently available formulations of buffered didanosine have an oral bioavailability of about 30 to 40% (8, 88, 109).

The plasma half-life of didanosine is relatively short, 0.5 to 1.5 h (88, 109, 215, 216); however, the intracellular half-life of the active form, ddATP, is much longer, 12 to 24 h or more (4). This relatively long half-life allows once- or twice-daily dosing of the drug. In patients with end-stage renal failure (creatinine clearance <5 mL/min), the half-life can increase up to threefold, as renal excretion accounts for 30 to 50% of the drug's disposition (88). However, the drug can be removed by hemodialysis (181). Didanosine can cross the placental barrier (155) and has been found to penetrate the CSF, although to a lesser extant than does zidovudine. CSF levels after a dose of didanosine were found to be 20% of simultaneous serum levels (88).

An initial phase I trial initiated in 1988 demonstrated that didanosine could induce virologic, immunologic, and clinical improvement in adult patients with HIV disease (88, 215, 216). Similar results were obtained in two other phase I studies, one of which used once-daily dosing (39, 41, 114). In some patients, improved CD4 cell counts have been found to persist for up to 5 years (145). In randomized trials, didanosine monotherapy was slightly inferior to zidovudine in treatment-naive patients, but it was superior in patients with as few as 8 weeks of prior zidovudine therapy (56, 101). Subsequently, trials of combination therapy with zidovudine demonstrated a substantial and prolonged benefit in some patients (35, 158, 213). On the basis of these results, the large-scale, multicenter ACTG 175 and Delta trials discussed above were initiated. As noted, didanosine alone or in combination with zidovudine was both conferred a significant survival advantage and slowed disease progression in patients with CD4 cell counts between 200 and 500 cells/mm^3, while only the combination regimen benefited patients with more advanced disease (54, 87, 102).

There appear to be two principal reasons for the substantial activity of zidovudine in combination with didanosine. One is that the drugs act preferentially in different cells; zidovudine has more activity in dividing cells, while didanosine is more active in resting cells (76, 77, 148). Thus, the combination simultaneously targets both cell populations. Also, the L74V mutation that confers resistance to didanosine actually restores sensitivity to zidovudine-resistant strains with a mutation at codon 215 (184). Thus, these drugs have antagonistic patterns of resistance, and it is relatively difficult for HIV to become resistant to both agents simultaneously.

The most common dose-limiting toxicities of didanosine are painful peripheral neuropathy and pancreatitis (114, 115, 215, 216). The neuropathy presents most commonly in the distal lower extremities and is generally reversible. The pancreatitis is less frequent but can be life threatening in some patients (56). Hematologic toxicity is not generally seen with didanosine (101).

Coadministration of other drugs known to cause peripheral neuropathy or pancreatitis may increase the risk of these complications; for example, simultaneous administration of systemic pentamidine, which can cause pancreatitis, should generally be avoided. Also, H$_2$ blockers such as cimetidine, ranitidine, or famotidine, which may themselves induce pancreatitis and could, theoretically, increase absorption of didanosine should be used cautiously (207). Agents that require an acidic gastric environment for absorption, such as ketoconazole and dapsone, are best administered at least 2 h prior to didanosine to avoid having their absorption decreased by the buffered preparations in the didanosine (130). Although the protease inhibitor indinavir does not specifically require an acidic gastric environment, its absorption is reduced in the nonfasting state, and the buffer in didanosine may interfere with its absorption. Therefore, this drug should also be taken either 1 h before or 1.5 h after didanosine. This is also true for ciprofloxacin, as the magnesium-aluminum cations in the tablet formulation of didanosine may reduce ciprofloxacin bioavailability (172).

The adult dosing of didanosine is as follows: in tablet form, the doses are 200 mg twice a day for adults weighing more than 60 kg and 125 mg twice daily for those weighing less. In the powder (sachet) form, which is not absorbed quite as well as the tablets, the doses are 250 mg twice daily for adults weighing more than 60 kg and 167 mg twice daily for those weighing less.

Zalcitabine (ddC)

Zalcitabine is a dideoxynucleoside analogue of 2'-deoxycytidine in which the 3'-hydroxy group of the sugar ring is replaced by a hydrogen atom (132). Following oral administration, zalcitabine is well absorbed from the gut, with an average oral availability of approximately 70 to 80% (108, 217). Peak plasma concentrations are generally observed within 0.5 to 2 h (108, 208). Zalcitabine penetrates the CSF less well than does zidovudine. The CSF concentration ranges from 9 to 37% of serum concentrations following an intravenous dose (217). The plasma half-life of zalcitabine in HIV-infected adults averages 1.2 to 2 h (85, 108, 217), while the in vitro intracellular half-life of ddC-5'-triphosphate, the active moiety of zalcitabine, is approximately 2.6 h (185). Some 75% of a dose of zalcitabine is cleared by the kidney, and renal impairment may prolong its elimination half-life (108, 208).

Early phase I studies demonstrated that zalcitabine could induce virologic and immunologic improvement in patients with HIV infection (128, 217). A subsequent trial demonstrated a small but statistically significant survival advantage to didanosine therapy in zidovudine-experienced patients (2). Partly on the basis of these results, the Food and Drug Administration (FDA) approved zalcitabine monotherapy at a dose of 0.75 mg every 8 h in patients with advanced HIV disease who have failed, or are intolerant of, zidovudine.

Zidovudine and zalcitabine have different toxicity profiles (see below), and trials using the two drugs in combination began relatively early (217). Indeed, these were among the first trials of combination therapy in HIV infection. In 1987 and 1988, several studies of alternating therapy with zidovudine and zalcitabine trials demonstrated a sustained anti-HIV effect and suggested that the cumulative tolerable dose of each of the drugs given on an alternating schedule exceeded that of either drug given continuously alone (this effect was more striking in the case of zalcitabine toxicity) (152, 182, 217). These and subsequent trials of zidovudine/zalcitabine therapy showed substantial and sustained increases in patients' CD4 cell counts and also suggested that certain subsets of patients had less disease progression on the zalcitabine/zidovudine combination than on zidovudine alone (126, 142, 152, 182, 217).

Subsequently, the large-scale, multicenter Delta and ACTG 175 trials discussed above demonstrated that the combination zidovudine/zalcitabine regimen could offer a significant reduction in disease progression and a survival advantage compared with zidovudine monotherapy in patients with moderate immunosuppression (54, 87, 102).

Several mutations have been reported to be associated with zalcitabine resistance, including T69D, K65R, and M186V (70, 81). The latter two mutations are also associated with cross-reactive resistance to lamivudine, didanosine, and (in the case of K65R) PMEA (72, 82, 183). However, only partial resistance is associated with these mutations.

The principal dose-limiting toxicity of zalcitabine is a painful glove-and-stocking peripheral neuropathy (59, 128, 217), similar to that seen with didanosine and hypothesized to be due to the effects of ddC-5'-triphosphate on DNA polymerase (14, 214). It generally improves slowly after zalcitabine is discontinued but can worsen for 2 to 4 weeks before beginning to improve. Pancreatitis is infrequent but can be life threatening (217). Caution should be used in administering zalcitabine concomitantly with other drugs capable of causing peripheral neuropathies or pancreatitis. Similarly, drugs that could alter the renal clearance of zalcitabine (e.g., amphotericin, foscarnet, and aminoglycosides) should also be used with care, as decreased clearance could lead to elevated serum levels of zalcitabine and increase adverse events.

Stavudine (d4T)

Stavudine is a thymidine analogue with a mechanism of antiretroviral activity similar to that of the other nucleosides described above (9, 86, 117). Like zidovudine, it is preferentially phosphorylated and exerts more potent anti-HIV activity in activated cells than in resting cells (76, 77, 149). However, unlike zidovudine (in which the monophosphate inhibits thymidylate kinase), neither stavudine nor any of its metabolites inhibit the enzymes responsible for its own phosphorylation (94). As a result of this relative lack of effect on cellular kinases, less perturbation of cellular nucleotide pools has been observed with stavudine than with zidovudine, which may, in part, explain why stavudine carries somewhat less marrow toxicity than does zidovudine.

Stavudine has good oral bioavailability. Maximum drug concentrations are generally attained within 0.5 to 1.5 h and then rapidly decline. The overall plasma half-life is 1.22 h $\pm$ 0.09 (range, 0.7–2.2 h) (16).

Early clinical trials of stavudine monotherapy for individuals with AIDS or ARC demonstrated virologic and immunologic improvement in these patients (16, 143). Preliminary results from an ongoing, randomized, blinded, phase III trial that compared continued treatment with zidovudine with treatment with stavudine in zidovudine-experienced patients demonstrated virologic and immunologic improvement only in the stavudine-treated group (165). Partly on the basis of these results, stavudine received FDA approval.

The principal dose-limiting toxicity of stavudine is a peripheral sensory neuropathy (16, 143 , 150, 179). Neuropathy resolves or symptoms diminish with discontinuation of the drug, and some patients can continue treatment at reduced dosages without progression of symptoms. For this reason, however, patients receiving combination therapy with stavudine and either zalcitabine or didanosine (both of which can also cause neuropathy) should be followed closely for signs of toxicity.

Lamivudine (3TC)

Lamivudine, a dideoxynucleoside, is the ($-$) enantiomer of 2'-dideoxy-3'-thiacytidine. In 1995, lamivudine was approved by the FDA for use only in combination with zidovudine.

Lamivudine is absorbed rapidly following oral administration, with a mean t_{max} of 1 h and 82% oral bioavailability. Food may delay absorption, but it does not alter the mean oral bioavailability. The mean elimination half-life of lamivudine is 2.5 h. Most of the drug given (approximately 70%) is excreted unchanged in the urine (197).

Transient virologic and immunologic improvements have been observed with administration of lamivudine as a single agent, particularly at doses of 8.0 mg/kg/day or above, but these improvements were generally not sustained (153, 197). In vitro and in vivo studies have demonstrated rapid emergence of resistance to lamivudine, associated with a mutation at codon 184 (M184I or M184V) of the HIV-1 RT (176, 192). Other mutations have also been described, including a lysine-to-arginine substitution at codon 65 (K65R) of HIV-1 RT that confers partial resistance to lamivudine, as well as zalcitabine, didanosine, and PMEA (72, 80–82, 183). As noted above, the 184 mutation induced by exposure to lamivudine restores viral sensitivity to zidovudine in strains that are zidovudine resistant on the basis of a mutation at codon 215 (13, 192). This, as well as the differential phosphorylation of the two drugs in different target cell populations, provides a strong rationale for administering these two agents together. It was recently reported that HIV strains with the 184 mutation may have increased RT fidelity (i.e., a decreased ability to mutate) (202). Although it has been hypothesized that lamivudine administration may thus delay the ability of HIV to mutate under the pressure of other RTIs or patients' immunologic responses, this remains to be proven clinically.

In clinical trials, significantly greater increases in CD4 cell counts and greater decreases in HIV-1 RNA PCR have been observed with the combination of zidovudine and lamivudine than with either one as a single agent (64). The antagonistic resistance pattern observed with zidovudine and lamivudine (13, 192) has not been found in other nucleoside combinations involving lamivudine, and additional studies are needed to clarify the role of each combination. Nevertheless, preliminary results suggest that the combination of stavudine and lamivudine is active in patients (34).

At the recommended dose of lamivudine (150 mg twice daily), the toxicity profile compares favorably with that of other nucleoside agents, which is one of the attractive features of this drug. Reported toxicities are a peripheral neuropathy as well as mild and transient episodes of headache, insomnia, fatigue, and abdominal symptoms, with a general downward trend in neutrophil counts at higher doses (153, 197).

Nonnucleoside Reverse Transcriptase Inhibitors (NNRTIs)

A number of nonnucleoside agents have been found to be noncompetitive inhibitors of the HIV RT (NNRTIs). These drugs are highly specific for HIV-1 but are generally inactive against HIV-2, SIV, and other retroviruses (47, 49, 129). Two such agents, nevirapine and delavirdine, have gained FDA approval, and other NNRTIs are in development.

While nevirapine was highly active against HIV in vitro, only transient antiretroviral activity could be attributed to this drug alone. However, more-sustained activity was found when it was administered in combination with nucleoside antiretroviral agents (43), and the FDA approved nevirapine for use in such combinations. Nevirapine should not be given as monotherapy, however, as any clinical and virologic improvements are limited by rapid emergence of high-level resistance. Combination therapy with nevirapine and zidovudine does not substantially delay emergence of resistance to nevirapine, although the RT mutation pattern differs from that seen with nevirapine monotherapy (162). Mutations associated with resistance to nevirapine also confer cross-resistance to other NNRTIs (49).

Nevirapine has a bioavailability of more than 90%, which is not affected by coadministration with nucleoside RTIs. It is metabolized by, and induces, hepatic P-450 isoforms, and therefore can potentially interact with other drugs metabolized by this system (62, 169). Metabolites of nevirapine are primarily excreted by the kidney. Nevirapine is thought to induce its own metabolism, which results in a fall in the serum half-life from 43 h at the beginning of therapy to 23 h 2 weeks later (62). Consistent with this, a reduced rate of adverse events is reported when nevirapine dosing is initiated at 200 mg/day for the first 2 weeks of therapy and then increased to twice-daily dosing of 200 mg (400 mg/day) for the balance of therapy (21).

The most common toxicities associated with nevirapine therapy are headache (30%), somnolence (30%), mouth ulcers (30%), a morbilliform rash (29%), fever (27%), and abnormal hepatic transaminases (8%) (43, 169). The abnormal transaminases are usually asymptomatic but have (occasionally) been associated with clinical hepatitis. The rash induced by nevirapine can be severe in up to 3% of patients, with 0.4% progressing to a potentially fatal Stevens-Johnson syndrome. One death due to this syndrome has been reported. This rash is usually seen within 7 to 28 days of the start of therapy but may occur up to 8 weeks later. As noted above, there is potential for drug interactions with other agents metabolized by P-450 cytochromes, so patients on regimens containing these drugs should be followed closely (169).

The other NNRTI to receive FDA approval is delavirdine. This is a bisheteroarylpiperazine (BHAP) NNRTI that, like other members of this class of agents, is highly specific for HIV-1 and inactive against HIV-2 and animal retroviruses (46, 47, 49, 129, 151). As with nevirapine, modest synergistic antiretroviral activity has been attributed to delavirdine when used with a nucleoside RTI in a two-drug regimen, and greater and more-sustained activity was seen when delavirdine was one component of a triple antiretroviral drug combination (46).

A mutation at codon 236 (P236L) of the HIV-1 RT confers high-level resistance to delavirdine (65). Other mutations that confer resistance to additional NNRTIs have also been observed (151), and resistance to delavirdine develops rapidly in monotherapy. Resistance appears to be somewhat delayed when delavirdine is used in combination with nucleoside RTIs (30, 46), particularly in patients who are antiretroviral naive. In one trial, a mutation at codon 215 of the reverse transcriptase gene (as can be induced by prior therapy with zidovudine) independently predicted a poorer response to single-agent or combination therapy with delavirdine, as did a syncytium-inducing phenotype (46).

Delavirdine is metabolized by cytochromes CYP3A and CYP2D6 of the P-450 system of the liver (46, 151). It interacts extensively with other drugs that undergo hepatic metabolism and should generally not be administered to patients receiving certain of these drugs (151). Prescribing information should be consulted for details of such interactions (also see Table 7). Drugs that have increased plasma concentrations when coadministered with delavirdine include protease inhibitors, dapsone, and clarithromycin. Other agents such as rifampin substantially reduce systemic exposure to delavirdine, so delavirdine and rifampin should not be administered together. Coadministration of rifabutin and delavirdine is also contraindicated, as rifabutin decreases the plasma concentration of delavirdine, while delavirdine increases the plasma concentration of rifabutin (151).

The most frequent adverse effect of delavirdine is a rash, which generally persists for less than 2 weeks and does not require altering delavirdine dosing (46, 151). However, such patients should be closely observed, as there have been rare reports of erythema multiforme and Stevens-Johnson syndrome (151). In studies that compared monotherapy with didanosine or delavirdine with combination therapy with delavirdine and either zidovudine or didanosine, there were no significant differences in laboratory abnormalities, except for less neutropenia with the delavirdine-zidovudine combination than with zidovudine monotherapy (151). However, administration of saquinavir with delavirdine has resulted in hepatic transaminase elevations, and such elevations may occur with other protease inhibitors (151). Patients receiving both classes of drugs should therefore be monitored closely.

The recommended dose of delavirdine is 400 mg administered three times daily (151). It may be taken with or without food but should not be taken at the same time as either antacids or didanosine (151). Delavirdine should not be prescribed as monotherapy.

DMP 266–903 (efivirenz) is an NNRTI that is specific for the HIV-1 reverse transcriptase. The terminal half-life after single doses is 52 to 76 h. Meals have no appreciable effects on the drug's bioavailability, but a high-fat diet increased bioavailability by 50%. Two toxicities of interest with DMP 266–903 are rash (which is common with other NNRTIs) and CNS symptoms (dizziness, lightheadedness, and dysphoria). CNS symptoms were infrequent in patients receiving 200 mg and appeared to be more common in patients receiving the higher doses of efivirenz. The CNS symptoms usually occurred after administration of the first dose and lasted for several hours after dosing. These symptoms generally resolved spontaneously after a few days or weeks, but some mild symptoms have continued for longer periods.

Preliminary results suggest that a viral load (measured by quantitative assessment of HIV-RNA levels) is adequately suppressed in most patients for up to 1 year. Preliminary unblinded data from Study DMP 266–903 indicate that efavirenz in combination with indinavir provides a statistically significant reduction in HIV-RNA levels and an increase in CD4 counts.

Other Reverse Transcriptase Inhibitors

Adefovir dipivoxil (bis-POM-PMEA) is an orally bioavailable prodrug of 9-(2-phosphonylmethoxyethyl)adenine (PMEA), a monophosphated acyclic nucleotide analogue that has activity against a broad spectrum of retroviruses and herpesviruses, including CMV, HIV types 1 and 2, and CMV (10, 48, 50, 73). Adefovir dipivoxil is also active against hepatitis B. Its active intracellular metabolite, PMEA diphosphate (PMEApp) is a potent inhibitor of retroviral reverse transcriptase. PMEA has somewhat less activity in vitro in lymphocytes than does zidovudine, but it has more activity in monocytes/macrophages. PMEA appears to be more potent in certain animal systems than are other RTIs. In a primate model, an analogue of PMEA, PMPA, was shown to block initial infection by the HIV analogue, SIV (194). After prolonged in vitro exposure of HIV to PMEA, minimal mutations in codon 65 or 70 of HIV reverse transcriptase have been described (72, 82, 183), but it is unclear if this occurs in patients. Adefovir dipivoxil is now being tested in clinical trials.

Other RTIs are in development. Among these is 2′-β-fluoro-2′,3′-dideoxyadenosine (F-ddA), a nucleoside RTI with an in vitro activity profile similar to that of didanosine (99, 121). However, because F-ddA contains a a fluorine in the 2′-"up" position of purine, it is resistant to acid degradation (121) and does not require administration with buffers. Because of this, the drug may be better tolerated orally than didanosine. An even more interesting feature of F-ddA is that in vitro, it has activity against strains of HIV that have the multidrug resistance mutation at codon 151, as well as other resistance-conferring mutation patterns (M. Tanaka, H. Mitsuya, et al., unpublished observation). A phase I trial of F-ddA is now under way in the National Cancer Institute, and additional studies are anticipated.

Another investigational nucleoside RTI is 1592U89 succinate, a potent guanosine nucleoside analogue that is not metabolized by the liver. It is well absorbed orally and has 18% CSF penetration. This agent has shown in vitro synergy with other antiretroviral agents and is active against zidovudine-resistant strains of HIV (170).

Additional promising nucleoside and nonnucleoside RTIs are in development and offer the potential to expand the range of therapeutic options available to HIV-infected individuals. Indeed, because of the substantial potential of HIV to develop resistance, increasing the number of active drugs is likely to optimize the possibility for long-term control of the disease.

PROTEASE INHIBITORS

The second class of antiretroviral agents to receive FDA approval targets the HIV protease. This enzyme cleaves the long polypeptide products of the viral *gag* and *gag-pol* genes (p55 and p160) to form structural proteins of the virion core (p17, p24, p9, and p7) as well as the essential viral enzymes reverse transcriptase, integrase, RNase, and the protease itself (63, 112, 124). This processing takes place in the late stages of HIV replication and is critical to production of mature, infectious virions.

The development of protease inhibitors was based on knowledge of the substrate sequence and the structure of the protease (144, 167, 204, 210). This information permitted rational development of peptidomimetic and other drugs that could effectively compete with substrate for binding sites. The protease is a C_2-symmetric homodimer (Fig. 1) with a single active site—a hydrophobic substrate-binding pocket located along its central axis at the dimer interface. Each 99–amino acid monomer contributes to the formation of eight enzyme subsites that make up the substrate-binding pocket. There are also two highly conserved aspartic acid residues at the active site, each supplied by one of the component monomers, and two flexible "flaps"—β-hairpin structures that cover the active site and undergo conformational changes during the binding and release of protease substrates. Identification of these structures has proven critical to the design of protease inhibitors.

Despite the potential of protease as a unique antiretroviral target, there were several obstacles to development of clinically useful HIV protease inhibitors (190, 191). First, most of the candidate compounds were hydrophobic peptides, and such non-water-soluble compounds generally have poor bioavailability. Another difficulty was their short plasma half-life due to rapid degradation, hepatic metabolism, and biliary excretion of the drugs. Finally, many of these compounds are structurally complex and difficult (and quite expensive) to synthesize. Nevertheless, a number of protease inhibitors soon entered preclinical testing.

By mid-1997, four HIV protease inhibitors, saquinavir, ritonavir, indinavir, and nelfinavir had received FDA approval (Table 6). In early-phase clinical trials, reduced viral loads were demonstrated in patients receiving these drugs as single agents. However, viral resistance to these inhibitors often emerged during monotherapy, and it became apparent that the optimal use of these agents is in combination regimens. Certain mutations are driven by specific protease inhibitors but can nevertheless result in cross-resistance to additional inhibitors (138, 193). Mutations to protease inhibitors do not confer cross-resistance to nucleoside antiretroviral agents, nor do viral strains with resistance to the nucleosides have decreased susceptibility to the protease inhibitors.

As with the RTIs, the factors influencing emergence of resistant strains include the activity of the drug at the doses used, the degree of resistance afforded by one or more mutations, and the viral load. The greater the rate of replication and consequent viral titer, the higher the likelihood of mutations. But the number of potential mutations does not appear to be infinite, and certain mutations may reduce the ability of a viral strain to replicate (84, 166). Resistance can develop quite rapidly under pressure from certain very active agents. In general, the more mutations required to induce phenotypic resistance, the slower the process. Similarly, the process can be slowed by combinations of antiretroviral agents that substantially reduce viral loads (37). This is one reason for the recent enthusiasm about triple-drug combinations, which reduce the viral loads of some patients below detectable levels (11, 83, 187, 189). However, suboptimal dosing of protease inhibitors may increase the probability of resistance developing rapidly by incompletely inhibiting viral replication while the virus is exposed to drug. This may occur if drugs have partial activity at recommmended doses, if patients take the drugs at less than the recommended dosages, or if patients take them irregularly. However, abrupt cessation of dosing does not enhance de novo emergence of resistance because there is then no selective drug-induced pressure.

Clinical trials have demonstrated that protease inhibitors can be extremely active agents. In some individuals, viral titers have been reduced to undetectable levels and remained undetectable for relatively sustained periods, especially when the drugs are used in combination with nucleoside analogues (11, 83, 187, 189). Additional protease inhibitors are in development, such as 141W94, KNI-272, and others.

The protease inhibitors developed to date fall into broad structural categories. Saquinavir contains transition-state inserts in place of the dipeptidic cleavage sites of the natural substrates (42, 167). Indinavir is an isoteric transition-state substrate analogue of the protease cleavage site and contains a hydroxylaminepentanamide moiety (57, 196). The design of twofold (C_2) symmetric inhibitors, such as ritonavir, is based on the three-dimensional symmetry of the protease active site (105). Novel, nonpeptidic protease inhibitors, such as nelfinavir, have also been formulated (31). Intracellular conversion of the parent compound is not required for activity of any of the protease inhibitors.

The various protease inhibitors have somewhat different toxicity profiles, so if a patient has difficulty tolerating one of the drugs, another agent can be tried. However, as noted above, one protease inhibitor may confer cross-resistance to others. Indeed, an understanding of the cross-resistance pattern of these agents may provide guidance for further treat-

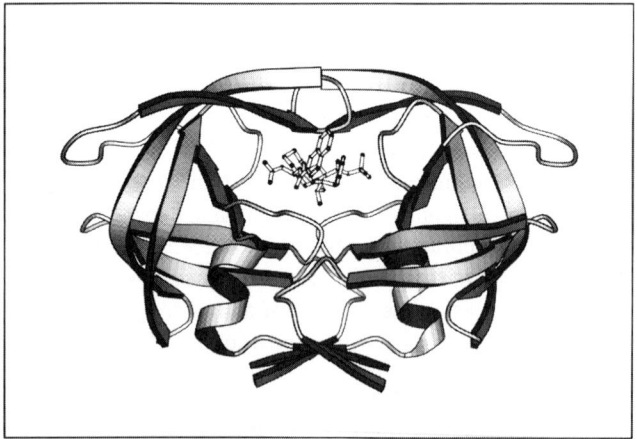

FIGURE 1. View of a complex of synthetic HIV-1 protease with a substrate-based inhibitor at 2.3 Å resolution, from the coordinates determined by Miller M, Schneider J, Sathyanarayana BK, et al. Structure of a complex of synthetic HIV-1 protease with a substrate-based inhibitor and 2.3 Å resolution. Science 1989;246:1149–1152. Figure provided by Dr. Alex Wlodawer.

ment strategies. Also, since resistance develops more slowly in patients whose viral load is substantially suppressed by the combination of protease inhibitors and nucleoside analogues (37), it is hoped that capitalizing on this principle will enable development of even more effective and durable treatment regimens.

Saquinavir

The first protease inhibitor to become widely available was saquinavir. This drug received FDA approval in late 1995 for administration in thrice-daily doses of 600 mg (1800 mg/day total) in combination with a nucleoside analogue. The drug is a transition-state analogue of a protease cleavage site and a highly specific inhibitor of both HIV-1 and HIV-2 (42, 167). It was approved under an expedited process on the basis of three major double-blind studies that demonstrated improvement in surrogate markers of HIV infection.

Saquinavir is poorly absorbed and undergoes extensive first-pass metabolism (53, 106, 141, 174). Bioavailability of the drug when taken with meals is thus only about 4%; in the fasting state, it is lower. Substantial binding of saquinavir to plasma proteins may limit penetration into tissues, and penetration into CSF is negligible. More than 90% of the drug is metabolized by the isozyme CYP3A4 of the hepatic P-450 cytochrome system, and therefore, care should be taken if it is administered with other drugs metabolized by the same system (Table 7).

Saquinavir monotherapy has been studied in doses ranging from 25 mg to 7200 mg daily in divided doses, with the greatest and most sustained improvements in viral load and CD4 cell counts seen at the highest dose (174, 198). By contrast, substantially smaller improvements in these surrogate markers of HIV infection were seen at the approved dose of 1800 mg daily, and no clear benefit was observed in patients administered saquinavir monotherapy at daily doses below 1800 mg. Greater improvements in surrogate markers were observed when saquinavir was administered with one or more antiretroviral nucleoside analogues than when these agents were administered as monotherapy (174, 198), and the triple-drug combination offered the most-sustained benefit.

Resistance to saquinavir has been observed both in vitro and in vivo (98, 174). Mutations at sites that would confer cross-resistance to ritonavir and indinavir are not generally seen, although cross-resistance between saquinavir and nelfinavir may occur (28, 38, 193). However, more studies are needed to clarify the patterns and frequencies of cross-resistance that may develop with different dosing strategies. Interestingly, a lower frequency of mutations was observed in viral isolates from patients receiving 7200 mg/day than in isolates from patients receiving the approved dose of 1800 mg daily (174).

The principal side effects of saquinavir are diarrhea, nausea, and abdominal discomfort. Mild decreases in neutrophil numbers and increases in liver function tests have been reported, although it is not clear that these changes were due to saquinavir. Other serious adverse effects reported in the course of studies of saquinavir include rare occurrences of confusion, ataxia, acute myeloblastic leukemia, hemolytic anemia, seizures, cutaneous reactions, and clinical hepatitis (174, 198). There are

also reports of bleeding episodes in hemophiliacs receiving protease inhibitors, including saquinavir.

As noted above, saquinavir weakly inhibits and is metabolized by the hepatic CYP3A4 system and there is the potential for drug interactions (209). Concomitant administration of drugs that induce these enzymes, such as phenobarbital, phenytoin, dexamethasone, or carbamazepine, may reduce plasma concentrations of saquinavir, whereas the concentrations of drugs that are potent inhibitors of this system may be elevated. These include terfenadine, astemizole, ketoconazole, or itraconazole, as well as substrates of related isozymes, such as calcium channel blockers, dapsone, clindamycin, quinidine, and triazolam (Table 7). Therefore patients receiving both saquinavir and one of these other agents should be closely monitored for toxicity. Recent studies indicate that the area under the time-concentration curve (AUC) of saquinavir can be greatly enhanced by coadministration with ritonavir, and preliminary results indicate that the viral load can be substantially reduced with this combination (18, 92).

The new, soft-gel preparation of saquinavir, Fortovase, has better bioavailablity than the hard-gel formulation, Invirase. Following multiple dosing of Fortovase, the mean steady-state AUC at 3 weeks was 7249 ng·h/L for Fortovase versus 866 ng·h/L for Invirase. Saquinavir soft gel has recently received FDA approval for use in combination with other antiretroviral agents for the treatment of HIV infection.

Ritonavir

Ritonavir is a C_2-symmetric peptide analogue whose structure was designed to optimize antiretroviral activity and bioavailability (63, 103, 105, 210). It is a highly selective and potent reversible competitive inhibitor of the HIV protease, with specific activity against HIV-1 and (to a lesser extent) HIV-2.

Ritonavir has good oral bioavailability, with peak plasma concentrations attained within 2 to 4 h and a plasma half-life of 3 to 5 h (23, 45, 120). The drug is commercially available in both capsule and liquid formulations. The capsule formulation is better and more rapidly absorbed when taken with a meal; the liquid formulation is best taken in the fasting state. In clinical trials, the trough plasma concentrations in patients treated with 600 mg of ritonavir in either dosage form every 12 h (the recommended dose) exceeded the IC_{90} of the virus, and the two formulations are considered generally bioequivalent (103).

Ritonavir is metabolized by the liver (113). Five metabolites have been identified, one of which (the principal metabolite) also has antiretroviral activity. The microsomal P-450 CYP3A isozymes account for most metabolism, with CYP2D6 playing a smaller role. Ritonavir is excreted primarily in the stool, both as unchanged drug and metabolites. Renal clearance accounts for only a small amount of the drug. Following oral administration of 600 mg of the oral solution, 86.4% is excreted in stool (33.8% as unchanged drug), while 11.3% is excreted in the urine (3.5% as unchanged drug) (120).

Resistance to ritonavir has been produced in vitro, and a similar pattern of mutations has been observed in viral strains isolated from patients treated with the drug (28, 38, 138, 193).

These mutations may also confer cross-resistance to indinavir and certain other protease inhibitors, although cross resistance to saquinavir has not been described (166).

Ritonavir has been studied as monotherapy and in combination with nucleosides and was approved for both these uses. Both disease progression and mortality were significantly reduced when ritonavir was added to nucleoside regimens of patients with advanced AIDS (1, 123). Ritonavir was also studied in combination with other protease inhibitors and was shown to inhibit the metabolism of those drugs because of its inhibition of the hepatic P-450 cytochrome isozymes. This effect was most striking in the case of saquinavir. As noted above, several small pilot studies showed that coadministration of ritonavir and saquinavir substantially increases the AUC of saquinavir but has no effect on the plasma concentration of ritonavir (18, 96, 104).

The most frequent adverse effects associated with ritonavir monotherapy have been gastrointestinal. In one clinical study, 23.1% of patients experienced nausea; 12.8%, emesis; 12.8%, diarrhea; 10.3%, taste perversion; and 3.4%, abdominal pain. The most frequently reported laboratory abnormalities have been elevations in hepatic transaminases, triglycerides, CPK, and uric acid (1). There is also evidence that diabetes mellitus can develop in patients using protease inhibitors, including ritonavir.

Clinically significant drug interactions may occur when ritonavir is administered concomitantly with other agents metabolized by the cytochrome P-450 system (Table 7) (1). These include certain agents commonly prescribed to HIV-infected patients such as rifabutin, which should not be administered to patients receiving ritonavir because coadministration of these two drugs can lead to 25-fold increases in the C_{max} of rifabutin and substantial hepatic toxicity (22). Special attention should be given to drugs with narrow therapeutic margins, such as anticoagulants or immunosuppressants. Also, as formulations of ritonavir contain alcohol, patients should not be treated with disulfiram metronidazole or other drugs that may cause disulfiram-like reactions (1).

Indinavir

Indinavir, an isoteric transition-state substrate analogue of the HIV protease cleavage site, is active against both HIV-1 and HIV-2 (57, 196). In the fasting state, indinavir is rapidly absorbed, with time to peak plasma concentrations ranging from 0.5 to 1.1 h. Consumption of a high-fat, high-protein meal reduces peak plasma concentrations by 84% and the AUC by 77%, but consumption of a light meal, such as dry toast and coffee, has little to no effect on the oral pharmacokinetics (57, 196).

As with the other protease inhibitors, indinavir is metabolized by the CYP3A4 isozyme of the hepatic P-450 cytochrome system and thus may interact with drugs metabolized by these isozymes (Table 7) (6, 104, 127). Patients with hepatic insufficiency should be dosed with caution (127).

Indinavir has been extensively evaluated in clinical trials (11, 29, 60, 83, 122, 186189), and additional trials are under way. In one randomized, double-blind phase II study, serum HIV-1 RNA levels were below the level of detection in 91% of patients on a triple-drug combination consisting of indinavir and two nucleosides, while none of the patients on a combination of two nucleoside agents had undetectable serum HIV-1 RNA.

Resistance to indinavir has been observed both in vitro and in vivo (28, 38, 193). More than one mutation is needed for development of high-level resistance, and these mutations may confer resistance to other protease inhibitors such as ritonavir. Also, patients previously treated with ritonavir may have cross-resistance to indinavir (138). In clinical trials comparing monotherapy with indinavir at doses up to 2.4 g daily with combination therapy with indinavir at the same doses and zidovudine at 600 mg daily, the least resistance was seen with the combination regimen containing 2.4 g of indinavir daily, while the highest frequency of resistance was seen among patients treated with indinavir monotherapy at doses below 2.4 g/day (127).

The most serious adverse effect reported to date is nephrolithiasis, which was seen in 5 to 6% of patients and was more likely to occur at doses above 2.4 g/day (127, 186). Nephrolithiasis typically presented with flank pain with or without hematuria and responded to drug cessation and vigorous hydration; its incidence may be reduced by hydration with 1 to 2 L of water daily. Indirect hyperbilirubinemia has been reported in more than 10% of patients but was rarely associated with symptoms or with elevations in hepatic transaminases and does not generally require cessation of drug (188).

Significant drug interactions may occur if patients are treated concurrently with indinavir and other drugs metabolized by the CYP3A4 isozyme (Table 7), although fewer interactions have been reported than in the case of ritonavir (127). In pharmacokinetic studies, significant drug interactions were observed with ketoconazole, rifabutin, and rifampin.

The antiretroviral nucleoside didanosine contains a buffer that may impair absorption of indinavir. Therefore, patients on a combination regimen that contains both these drugs should take indinavir 1 h before or 1 h after didanosine (127). It is generally recommended that indinavir be taken in a fasting or near-fasting state, at least 1 h before or 1.5 h after meals, at doses of 800 mg three times daily. Indinavir should not be taken with grapefruit juice, as a 26% decrease in the AUC was reported after administration of a 400-mg dose of indinavir with grapefruit juice (127).

Nelfinavir

Nelfinavir is a nonpeptidic protease inhibitor that is active against both HIV-1 and HIV-2. It has been approved by the FDA for use in both adult and pediatric populations (3).

The oral absorption of nelfinavir is enhanced by the presence of food, with the maximum AUC increased two- to threefold. Peak plasma levels are reached within 2 to 4 h. Nelfinavir is metabolized by multiple isoenzymes of the hepatic P-450 system, including CYP3A (3).

Nelfinavir received FDA approval on the basis of improvements in surrogate markers in both adult and pediatric HIV-infected populations. Decreases in plasma HIV RNA levels exceeding one log were seen at 24 weeks in patients administered nelfinavir in combination with one or two nucleoside RTIs (3). It is recommended that protease inhibitors be administered in combination with nucleoside analogues because of the increased likelihood of sustained antiviral activity with such a combination.

Although early in vitro studies showed that nelfinavir does not confer cross-resistance to saquinavir, ritonavir, indinavir, or 141W94, resistance to nelfinavir has been demonstrated in isolates from patients previously receiving ritonavir (3). Indinavir, which can be cross-resistant with ritonavir, may also induce reduced viral sensitivity to nelfinavir. This pattern of cross-resistance may be a consideration in the sequence of protease inhibitors administered to patients.

The major adverse effect of nelfinavir is diarrhea (3, 78, 140), which can generally be controlled with over-the-counter antidiarrheal medications (3). There is also potential for interactions with other agents metabolized by hepatic P-450 isoenzymes (Table 7), with those metabolized by the CYP3A isoform of particular concern. Therefore, coadministration of nelfinavir with terfenadine, astemizole, cisapride, triazolam, midazolam, or rifampin is generally contraindicated (3). The dose of rifabutin should be reduced by one-half if coadministered with nelfinavir (3). Other interactions of potential clinical significance may occur with coadministration of oral contraceptives, certain anticonvulsants, and the HIV protease inhibitors indinavir and ritonavir (3). To date, no substantial interaction has been observed when nelfinavir is administered with saquinavir (3). Clinicians are advised to consult the prescribing information prior to administering the drug.

The recommended dose of nelfinavir is 750 mg three times daily, which is best absorbed if taken with a meal or light snack (3). Nelfinavir may be taken at the same time as most other antiretroviral agents (3), with the sole exception of didanosine, because that drug requires administration on an empty stomach.

IMMUNOTHERAPY

While a combination of the two classes of antiretroviral agents may substantially decrease measured HIV-1 RNA levels, CD4 cell counts generally do not return to normal in patients with advanced AIDS, and the improvements that are seen are often transient. Even in clinical trials involving triple-drug therapy in which patients' HIV-1 RNA fell below the limits of detection, not all patients had sustained or substantial increases in CD4 cell counts. Despite undetectable HIV-1 RNA levels, such patients remain immunocompromised and at risk for opportunistic infections and malignancies.

A potential problem with immunomodulatory therapy in AIDS has been that stimulation of immune cells can increase HIV replication. However, development of more potent antiretroviral regimens has provided a means of controlling this problem and thus has spurred interest in approaches using immunotherapy. Promising surrogate marker results were recently reported in a study of interleukin-2 (IL-2) administered to 60 HIV-infected patients with more than 200 CD4 cells/mm^3 (111). In this trial, IL-2 was administered intravenously for 5 days every 2 months at doses of 18 million IU/day, in combination with chronic therapy with one to three nucleoside antiretroviral agents. This was compared with therapy with the antiretroviral agents alone in a control group of patients. After 12 months, CD4 cells in patients in the IL-2 group increased from mean baseline counts of 428 ± 25 cells/mm^3 to 916 ± 128 cells/mm^3, whereas CD4 cell counts in the control group decreased from a mean baseline of 406 ± 29 cells/mm^3 to 349 ± 41 cells/mm^3 ($P < .001$). Although there were transient increases in HIV-1 RNA after IL-2 administration, no substantial differences were observed in HIV-1 RNA levels or p24 antigen over the 12-month period. IL-2 therapy was limited principally by constitutional symptoms such as fever, malaise, or fatigue (27% of patients) or asymptomatic hyperbilirubinemia above 2.5 mg/dL (10% of patients). Additional studies are under way to test this approach in combination with established antiretroviral therapy regimens that include a protease inhibitor and RTIs. However, it is not clear at this time whether the CD4 cell increases observed with IL-2 therapy are associated with improved immunologic function and clinical course.

Other immunomodulatory agents are under investigation. Among these is interleukin-12 (IL-12), a cytokine that has multiple immunomodulatory effects that could benefit HIV-infected patients. These include potentiation of the growth and differentiation of T_H1 cells and concomitant inhibition of T_H2 cell activity, with consequent restoration of cell-mediated immune responses demonstrated ex vivo in T cells from HIV-infected patients (32). IL-12 also activates cytotoxic T cells and NK cells (27) and is a potent antiangiogenic agent (199), which may make it useful for patients with HIV-associated Kaposi's sarcoma or other malignancies. Increased HIV replication was reported in peripheral blood mononuclear cells from HIV-infected patients treated in vitro with IL-12, but this effect is minor and can be blocked by antiretroviral agents (71). While substantial toxicity has been reported with certain regimens in phase I and II trials of IL-12, less-toxic regimens and the potential utility of IL-12 in different diseases are currently being explored. IL-12 continues to be of great interest as potential therapy for HIV-infected individuals.

OVERALL APPROACHES TO HIV THERAPY

A substantial body of data demonstrates a continuum of increasing risk of disease progression as viral loads rise and CD4 cell counts decline. Available virologic, immunologic, and clinical data suggest that the most potent regimens today probably consist of combination therapy with two nucleoside analogues and at least one protease inhibitor (11, 83, 187, 189). Several panels have recently convened to assess these new data and to make recommendations for antiretroviral therapy. These recommendations have often been made with incomplete data utilizing surrogate markers, and they are likely to be modified as new information becomes available. Recommendations of one of these groups, the International AIDS Society–USA Consensus Panel were recently issued (19), and others have been proposed in draft form. There was substantial agreement among the recommendations, and we will review those of the International AIDS Society-USA Panel.

This panel suggested that triple drug regimens may be used at all timepoints in a patient's treatment, including initial therapy (19), since such regimens can suppress viral replication to undetectable levels for prolonged periods (Table 3). The panel also recommended an alternative initial regimen consisting of two nucleosides and one NNRTI, but they noted that this combination may be less potent than one containing a protease inhibitor, and it is generally not recommended as initial therapy for patients with advanced HIV disease. Other multidrug combinations may also substantially suppress viral replication, but there are fewer studies supporting their use as first-line combinations.

Initial Therapy

The choice of initial therapy may be guided by emerging data on cross-resistance between agents, toxicity profiles, and the patient's clinical status and history (19, 20). Indeed, the most important consideration may be how best to avoid simultaneous development of resistance and toxicity. Regimens to which resistance develops relatively slowly are preferred, as there appear to be a limited number of resistance-conferring mutations induced by RTIs and protease inhibitors, and cross-resistance can develop within each class of drug. In this regard, data suggest that emergence of resistance may be slowed by using strategies that substantially suppress HIV (174), preferably to undetectable levels. Resistant mutations are only selected under pressure from active agents. Some patients and physicians have the misconception that once protease inhibitors are started, they cannot ever be stopped or resistance will develop. But when dosing is completely stopped, there is no evolutionary pressure for resistance to develop. By contrast, reducing or skipping doses of drug can create conditions of partial suppression that permit more-rapid emergence of resistance. Thus it is important to maintain continuous dosing at the optimal dose level with protease inhibitors. If toxicity develops with one of these agents, it is generally better to discontinue the drug rather than reduce the dose (19, 20).

Indications for Changing Therapy

The decision to change regimens should be approached with careful consideration of several complex factors. A regimen may fail for many reasons, including initial viral resistance to one or more agents, altered absorption or metabolism of the drug, multidrug pharmacokinetics that adversely affect therapeutic drug levels, and poor patient adherence to a regimen. If a change in therapy is deemed necessary on the basis of drug intolerance, it is appropriate to substitute one or more alternative drugs of the same potency and from the same class of agents as the agent suspected of causing the toxicity.

According to the guidelines of the Panel on Clinical Practices for the Treatment of HIV convened by the Department of Health and Human Services and Henry J. Kaiser Family Foundation (6a), three different populations of patients should be considered with regard to a change in therapy: (a) individuals receiving incompletely suppressive antiretroviral therapy, such as single or double nucleoside therapy, with detectable of undetectable plasma viral load; (b) those who have been on potent combination therapy including a protease inhibitor and whose viremia was initially suppressed to undetectable levels but has again become detectable; and (c) individuals who have been on potent combination therapy including a protease inhibitor whose viremia was never suppressed below detectable limits. While these groups of individuals should have treatment regimens changed to maximize the chances of durable, maximal viral RNA suppression, the first group may have more treatment options, as they are protease-inhibitor naive.

According to the panel (6a), specific criteria that should prompt consideration for changing therapy include

1. Less than a 0.5 to 0.7 log reduction in plasma HIV RNA by 4 weeks following initiation of therapy, or less than a 1 log reduction by 8 weeks.
2. Failure to suppress plasma HIV RNA to undetectable levels within 4 to 6 months of initiating therapy. In this regard, the degree of initial decrease in plasma HIV RNA and the overall trend in decreasing viremia should be considered. For example, a patient with 10^6 viral copies/mL prior to therapy who stabilizes after 6 months of therapy at an HIV RNA level that is detectable but below 10,000 copies/mL may not warrant an immediate change in therapy.
3. Repeated detection of virus in plasma after initial suppression to undetectable levels, suggesting development of resistance.
4. Any reproducible, significant increase (defined as 3-fold or greater) from the nadir of plasma HIV RNA not attributable to intercurrent infection, vaccination, or test methodology except as noted above.

TABLE 3 • Initial Treatment Regimens As Recommended by the International AIDS Society–USA Panel, 1997

Regimen	Comments

1. Two nucleoside RTIs and one protease inhibitor
  a. Recommended nucleoside combinations:
    Zidovudine + lamivudine, didanosine, or zalcitabine
    Stavudine + lamivudine or didanosine
	If HIV RNA levels are not reduced to undetectable levels, consider alternative combination

b. Recommended protease inhibitors: Nelfinavir, indinavir, or ritonavir	Current formulation of saquinavir not recommended due to low bioavailability
2. Two nucleoside RTIs and one NNRTI	May not be as potent as a regimen that contains protease inhibitor; not recommended as initial therapy for patients with low CD_4 cell counts or high HIV RNA levels

Adapted from Carpenter C, Fischl M, Hammer S, et al. Antiretroviral therapy for HIV infection in 1997, updated recommendations of an international panel. JAMA 1997;277:1962–1969.

TABLE 4 • **FDA-Approved Reverse Transcriptase Inhibitors and Their Dosages in Adults**

Drug	Oral Dosage (Adults)	Comments
Nucleosides		
Zidovudine (AZT, ZDV, Retrovir)	100 mg every 4 h (frequently given as 200 mg three times daily)	60% CNS penetration; drug of choice for HIV CNS disease
Didanosine (ddl, Videx)	Tablet form: >60 kg: 200 mg twice daily, <60 kg: 125 mg twice daily; sachet form: >60 kg: 250 mg twice daily, <60 kg: 167 mg twice daily	Antagonistic resistance pattern with AZT (restores viral sensitivity to AZT)
Zalcitabine (ddC, HIVID)	0.75 mg three times daily	Like ddl, ddC and 3TC, more active in resting cells
Stavudine (d4T, Zerit)	>60 kg: 40 mg twice daily <60 kg: 30 mg twice daily	Like AZT, more active in replicating cells
Lamivudine (3TC, Epivir)	150 mg twice daily	Potent in combination with AZT; high level resistance develops within 2–4 weeks in partially suppressive regimens
NNRTIs		
Nevirapine (Viramune)	200 mg daily for 2 weeks, then 400 mg daily	Approved for use in combination with nucleosides
Delavirdine (Rescriptor)	400 mg three times daily	Approved for combination antiretroviral therapy

5. Patients currently receiving two nucleoside RTIs who have achieved the goal of no detectable virus have the option of continuing this regimen or having it modified according to the guidelines in Table 3. Most patients on double-nucleoside therapy are likely to have eventual virologic failure.
6. Persistently declining CD4+ T cell numbers as measured on at least two separate occasions.
7. Clinical deterioration.

A final consideration in the decision to change therapy is recognition of the still limited choice of available agents; clinical trials have shown that partial suppression of virus is superior to no suppression of virus.

Choices of alternative regimens depend upon both the prior regimen and the reason for changing it. Toxicity problems should guide the clinician to a regimen with a different toxicity profile. If there is evidence of treatment failure or a patient's current therapy is suboptimal, a regimen with greater potency, different mechanisms of activity, and non-cross-resistant patterns of resistance should be sought. If possible, the consensus panel recommended that all patients be on regimens that include at least two nucleosides and one protease inhibitor. An NNRTI may be added to such a regimen or, if necessary, substituted for one of the other components, although there have been few studies directly comparing triple-drug combinations containing either a protease inhibitor or an NNRTI. NNRTIs should never be used without concomitant administration of at least one nucleoside antiretroviral agent, to prevent rapid development of strains with high-level resistance. If a patient is unable to tolerate more than one of the available nucleosides, consideration may be given to a regimen consisting of one nucleoside and two protease inhibitors, such as ritonavir and saquinavir, but such combinations also require further evaluation.

TABLE 5 • **Principal Drug Toxicities of Approved Reverse Transcriptase Inhibitors**

Drug	Principal Toxicities
Zidovudine (AZT, ZDV)	Bone marrow suppression: neutropenia and anemia Myositis Nausea, malaise
Didanosine (ddl)	Pancreatitis Peripheral neuropathy
Zalcitabine (ddC)	Peripheral neuropathy Stomatitis
Stavudine (d4T)	Peripheral neuropathy Elevation of hepatic transaminases
Lamivudine (3TC)	Peripheral neuropathy Pancreatitis in children
Nevirapine	Rash Potential interactions with drugs metabolized by hepatic P-450 cytochromes (Table 7)
Delavirdine	Rash Interactions with some drugs metabolized by hepatic P-450 cytochromes (Table 7)

Studies using combinations of other protease inhibitors are currently in progress. These include indinavir and nelfinavir in a twice-daily regimen (89a), ritonavir and indinavir (32a), nelfinavir and ritonavir (75a), nelfinavir and soft-gel saquinavir (112a, 146a), and indinavir with an investigational protease inhibitor, abacavir (125a)

In all cases, an attempt should be made to administer regimens that have been shown to suppress viral replication below detectable levels in most patients for relatively prolonged periods. While such (multidrug) regimens are quite expensive and may also yield substantial cumulative toxicity that could make later use of these agents more difficult, there is evidence that they can be of great benefit to many patients. However, the long-term durability of such benefits has yet to be determined, and many patients will likely require modifications of therapy in the course of their disease. Thus, there is a continuing need for development of additional therapeutic options and improved understanding of the pathophysiology of HIV infection.

Treatment of Primary Infection

Some investigators have recently hypothesized that antiretroviral therapy that reduces viral loads to undetectable levels for sustained periods might potentially be curative if initiated soon after infection (147). However, this has never been proven, and other investigators have suggested that the existence of long-lived memory T cells with integrated HIV, potential viral sanctuary sites such as the brain, and the development of quasispecies with resistant mutations even before therapy is initiated (33) all combine to make this unlikely with current technologies. Nevertheless, because there may be other substantial benefits to very early suppression of viral replication, the panel recommended that patients with primary infection (the period 4 to 7 weeks after exposure, when HIV RNA can be detected in plasma by PCR) be treated with one of the recommended initial-treatment regimens. They recommended that this therapy continue well beyond the time that virus is reduced below undetectable levels, although a specific period has not been defined. Also, all such individuals should be enrolled in ongoing clinical trials, whenever possible.

For postexposure prophylaxis, the panel recommended that therapy with maximally suppressive regimens begin as soon as possible after exposure. Individuals with occupational exposure should be enrolled in an anonymous registry sponsored by the Centers for Disease Control (CDC) of the U.S. Public Health Service and several pharmaceutical companies. The use of at least two drugs that had not been used in the source patient was suggested. However, no firm recommendations were made about the duration of therapy. Previously, it was recommended that therapy should be administered for 4 to 6 weeks, but the panel felt that this was based upon an outmoded understanding of the biology of HIV disease. They noted that new guidelines are being developed by the CDC and should be available shortly.

Finally, for patients beyond primary infection, the panel recommended against discontinuing antiretoviral therapy except, perhaps, for some patients with very advanced disease or those completely intolerant of all available therapeutic modalities.

PREVENTION OF VERTICAL TRANSMISSION OF HIV

In ACTG 076, antiretroviral therapy with zidovudine during the antepartum and infrapartum period and for the newborn for 6 weeks after birth reduced vertical transmission of HIV from 24.9 to 7.8% (40). In 1994, on the basis of early analyses of that study, the CDC recommended that all pregnant HIV-infected women be administered zidovudine (100 mg five times daily) beginning at 14 to 34 weeks of gestation and continuing throughout pregnancy (24). The CDC also recommended that zidovudine be administered during labor (intravenously at 2 mg/kg for 1 h, followed by 1 mg/kg until delivery) and that newborns be given zidovudine syrup (2 mg/kg every 6 h) starting 8 to 12 h after birth and continuing for 6 weeks. The consensus panel, in addition, suggested that HIV-infected women be encouraged to bottlefeed their infants, if possible, as HIV can be transmitted in breast milk (20). The panel recommended that women already taking effective combination antiretrovirals be continued on those regimens.

Preliminary results of some long-term animal toxicity studies have become available. These studies found that some mice exposed to zidovudine in utero subsequently developed lung, liver, and reproductive tract malignancies (100). To date, there has been no indication that zidovudine exposure during the perinatal period presents an increased risk of carcinogenesis for other species, but all women undergoing testing for HIV during pregnancy should be fully informed of the risks of HIV transmission and the risks (and demonstrated benefits) of antiretroviral prophylaxis. Additional studies are under way or are being planned to evaluate other regimens in both zidovudine-experienced and zidovudine-naive HIV-infected pregnant women and in newborns.

FUTURE DIRECTIONS

Development of new and non-cross-resistant reverse transcriptase and protease inhibitors is a very active area of inves-

---

TABLE 6 • FDA-Approved HIV Protease Inhibitors and Their Dosages in Adults

Drug	Oral Dosage	Principal Toxicities[a]/Comments
Saquinavir (Invirase)	600 mg three times daily (with meals)	Gastrointestinal (nausea, bloating, diarrhea); poor bioavailability; approved only for use with nucleosides
Ritonavir (Norvir)	600 mg twice daily (with meals)	Significant interactions with drugs metabolized by hepatic CYP3A P-450 isoenzymes[a]; toxicities include elevated hepatic transaminases, gastrointestinal (including nausea, vomiting, diarrhea), taste perversion, peripheral and circumoral paresthesias
Indinavir (Crixivan)	800 mg three times daily (fasting)	Nephrolithiasis; asymptomatic hyperbilirubinemia; gastrointestinal (include nausea, bloating, diarrhea)
Nelfinavir (Viracept)	750 mg three times daily (with meals)	Diarrhea

[a] All approved protease inhibitors may have interactions with drugs metabolized by the hepatic P-450 cytochromes (see Table 7), but this is most significant with ritonavir.

TABLE 7 • **Potential Drug Interactions with HIV Protease Inhibitors**[a,b]

Some drugs metabolized by hepatic P-450 cytochromes (AUC of drug may be altered)

Alpha blockers	Beta blockers	Immunosuppressants
Antiarrhythmics	Calcium channel blockers	Isoniazid, Rifampin
Antidepressants	Cimetidine	Methyphenidate
Antiemetics[c]	Cisapride	Metoclopramide
Antifungals (incl. disulfiram metronidazole)[c]	Clarithromycin[c]	Narcotic analgesics
	Clofibrate	Pentoxifylline
Antihyperlidemics	Corticosteroids	Phenothiazines
Antimalarials	Diazepams	Rifabutin[c]
Antineoplastics, esp. anthracyclines	Diphenoxylate	Sedatives/hypnotics
Astemizole	Erythromycin	Terfenadine
Atovaquone[c]	Estrogens	Warfarin

[a] See prescribing information for individual protease inhibitors. Also note protease inhibitors may interact with each other if administered concomitantly.

[b] Also potential interactions with nevirapine and delavirdine. See prescribing information.

[c] Drugs used with high frequency in HIV-infected patients.

tigation and a number of such agents are already in the pipeline. But entirely novel approaches to antiretroviral therapy are also being investigated. As noted above (Table 1), the process of HIV replication offers multiple potential targets for novel drug therapies.

An example of an alternative strategy for inhibiting HIV replication under investigation is the use of agents such as thalidomide, pentoxifylline, or rolipram that directly or indirectly inhibit tumor necrosis factor–α (TNF-α) (5, 119, 139). TNF-α activates proviral HIV and promotes the later steps of HIV replication. Thus, inhibitors of this cytokine may be useful in combination with other treatment modalities in a long-term strategy for therapy of HIV disease.

The HIV-1 nucleocapsid protein zinc fingers are among the more novel targets for antiretroviral therapy. These structural components necessary for both acute infection and virion assembly are of particular interest because they are highly conserved and thus may be relatively mutationally intolerant (160). In vitro studies of several disulfide-substituted benzamides (DIBAs) that inhibit the HIV-1 nucleocapsid zinc fingers have demonstrated significant anti-HIV activity, with both acute and chronic infection inhibited (161).

An entirely different approach to therapy focuses on the stimulation of specific immune responses directed against HIV, in combination with antiretroviral therapy, as discussed above. Vaccines, which may prevent primary infection or assist the host response against established infection, are also being studied, as is the feasibility of autologous bone marrow transplant or some modification thereof.

An intriguing new development is the possibility of being able to exploit other host factors, such as CCR5, the HIV coreceptor for monocytotropic strains (52, 55, 156, 206). The fact that initial infection with HIV may be prevented by mutation to the gene that encodes this receptor and that individuals with this mutation may be naturally resistant to HIV makes CCR5

a very attractive target for antiretroviral therapy. Potential strategies exploiting this discovery may involve the techniques of gene manipulation, construction of antisense oligoclonal nucleotides, modification or inhibition of the chemokines or other ligands that bind to this receptor, or allogeneic bone marrow transplantation from donors who have a homozygous CCR5 deletion that makes them naturally resistant to infection by monocytotropic HIV strains.

As more is learned about the disease process initiated by infection with HIV, it is likely that other approaches to therapy will emerge. The advances seen during the past few years, however, are substantial. Available strategies have clearly reduced the morbidity of the disease and prolonged survival. They also offer the potential to customize therapy on the basis of a particular patient's disease status, history of drug toxicity, and viral resistance patterns. Thus, not only have some patients lives been extended, but the quality of their lives has improved, and we have begun to see the transformation of HIV infection from an acute process into a chronic disease. Perhaps most heartening is the fact that these therapeutic advances were based upon the practical application of rational drug design. Indeed, the success of this approach to development of new treatments may be the greatest cause for optimism about the future of antiretroviral therapy.

REFERENCES

1. Abbott Laboratories. Norvir (ritonavir) capsules and oral solution prescribing information (package insert). North Chicago, IL: Abbott Laboratories, 1996.
2. Abrams DI, Goldman AI, Launer C, Korvick JA, Neaton JD, Crane LR, Grodesky M, Wakefield S, Muth K, Kornegay S, Cohn DL, Hallen A, Luskin-Hawk R, Markowitz N, Sampton JH, Thompson M, Deyton L, the Terry Beirn Community Programs for Clinical Research on AIDS. A comparative trial of didanosine or zalcitabine after treatment with zidovudine in pa-

tients with human immunodeficiency virus infection. N Engl J Med 1994;330:657–662.

3. Agouron Pharmaceuticals. Viracept (nelfinavir) prescribing information for tablets and oral powder. La Jolla, CA: Agouron Pharmaceuticals, 1997.

4. Ahluwalia G, Johnson MA, Fridland A, Cooney DA, Broder S, Johns DG. Cellular pharmacology of the anti-HIV agent 2′,3′-dideoxyadenosine. New Orleans. 1988:345.

5. Angel JB, Saget BM, Walsh SP, Greten TF, Dinarello CA, Skolnik PR, Endres S. Rolipram, a specific type IV phosphodiesterase inhibitor, is a potent inhibitor of HIV-1 replication. AIDS 1995; 9:1137–1144.

6. Anonymous. New drugs for HIV infection. Med Lett Drugs Ther 1996;38:35–38.

6a. Anonymous. Guidelines for the use of antiretroviral agents in HIV-infected adults and adolescents. U.S. Department of Health and Human Services (DHHS). BETA, June 1997;11:22.

7. Baba M, Snoeck R, Pauwels R, De Clercq E. Sulfated polysaccharides are potent and selective inhibitors of various enveloped viruses, including herpes simplex virus, cytomegalovirus, vesicular stomatitis virus, and human immunodeficiency virus. Antimicrob Agents Chemother 1988;32:1742–1745.

8. Balis FM, Pizzo RA, Butler KM, Hawkins M, Brouwers P, Husson R, Jacobsen F, Blaney S, Gress J, Jarosinski P. Clinical pharmacology of 2′,3′-dideoxyinosine in human immunodeficiency virus-infected children. J Infect Dis 1992;165:99–104.

9. Balzarini J, Kang G-J, Dalal M, Herdewijn P, de Clercq E, Broder S, Johns DG. The antiHTLVIII (anti-HIV) and cytotoxic activity of 2′,3′-didehydro-2′,3′-dideoxynucleosides: a comparison with their parental 2′,3′-dideoxynucleosides. Mol Pharmacol 1987;32:162–167.

10. Balzarini J, Naesens L, Slachmuylders J, Niphuis H, Rosenberg I, Holy A, Schellekens H, De Clerq E. 9-(2-Phosphonylmethoxethyl)adenine (PMEA) effectively inhibits retrovirus replication in vitro and simian immunodeficiency virus infection in rhesus monkeys. AIDS 1991;5:21–28.

11. Berry P, Kahn J, Cooper R, Chung M, Massari P, Chodakewitz J. Antiretroviral activity and safety of indinavir alone and in combination with zidovudine in zidovudine-naive patients with CD4 cell counts of 50–250 cells/mm³. XIth International Conference on AIDS, Vancouver, Canada, 1996:26.

12. Blum MR, Liao SH, Good SS, P. dM. Pharmacokinetics and bioavailability of zidovudine in humans. Am J Med 1988;85 (Suppl 2A):189–194.

13. Boucher CA, Cammack N, Schipper P, Schurrman R, Rouse P, Wainberg M, Cameron J. High-level resistance to (2)enantiomeric 2′-deoxy-3′-thiacytidine in vitro is due to one amino acid substitution in the catalytic site of human immunodeficiency virus type 1 reverse transcriptase. Antimicrob Agents Chemother 1993;37:2231–2234.

14. Broder S. Pharmacodynamics of 2′,3′-dideoxycytidine: an inhibitor of human immunodeficiency virus. Am J Med 1990; 88(Suppl 5B):2S–7S.

15. Brouwers P, Moss H, Wolters P, Eddy J, Balis F. Effect of continuous-infusion zidovudine therapy on neuropsychologic functioning in children with symptomatic human immunodeficiency virus infection. J Pediatr 1990;117:980–985.

16. Browne MJ, Mayer KH, Chafee SBD, Dudley MN, Posner MR, Steinberg SM, Graham KK, Geletko SM, Zinner SH, Denman SL, Dunkle LM, Kaul S, McLaren C, Skowron G, Kouttab NM, Kennedy TA, Weitberg AB, Curt G. 2′,3′-Didehydro-3′-

deoxythymidine (d4T) in patients with AIDS or AIDS-related complex: a phase I trial. J Infect Dis 1993;167:21–29.

17. Burroughs-Wellcome. Retrovir (zidovudine), capsules and syrup. Package insert. Research Triangle Park, NC: Burroughs-Wellcome Co., 1987.

18. Cameron W, Sun E, Markowitz M, Farthing C, NcMahon D, Poretz D, Follansbee S, Cohen C, Ho D, Mellors J, Hsuu A, Granneman G, Maki R, Salgo M, Couty J, Leonard P. Combination use of ritonavir and saquinavir IN HIV-infected patients: preliminary safety and activity data. XIth International Conference on AIDS, Vancouver, Canada. 3. 1996:20.

19. Carpenter C, Fischl M, Hammer S, Martin S, Jacobsen D, Katzenstein D, Montaner J, Richman D, Yeni P, Volberding P. Antiretroviral therapy for HIV infection in 1997. JAMA 1997; 277:1962–1969.

20. Carpenter C, Fischl M, Hammer S, Volberding P. Antiretroviral therapy for HIV infection in 1996, recommendations of an international panel. JAMA 1996;276:146–154.

21. Carr A, Cooper D. Antimicrobial chemotherapy 4. New York: Plenum, 1996:200–304.

22. Cato A, Cavanaugh J, Shi H, Hsu A, Granneman G, Leonard J. Assessment of multiple doses of ritonavir on the pharmacokinetics of rifabutin. XIth International Conference on AIDS, Vancouver, Canada. 1. 1996:89.

23. Cato A, Hsu A, Granneman R. Assessment of the pharmacokinetic interaction between the HIV-1 protease inhibitor ABT-538 and zidovudine. ICAAC Proceedings, San Francisco, 1995.

24. Centers for Disease Control. Antiretroviral therapy to prevent vertical transmission of HIV. MMWR 1994;43:1.

25. Centers for Disease Control. HIV testing. MMWR 1996;45:181.

26. Chattha G, Arieff AI, Cummings C, Tierney LM Jr. Lactic acidosis complicating the acquired immunodeficiency syndrome. Ann Intern Med 1993;118:37–39.

27. Chemini J, Valiente N, Trinchieri G. Enhancing effect of IL-12 on cell-mediated cytotoxicity against tumor-derived and virus-infected cells. Eur J Immunol 1993;23:1826–1830.

28. Chen Z, Li Y, Schock H. Three-dimensional structure of a HIV protease displaying resistance to all protease inhibitors in clinical trials. J Biol Chem 1995;270:21433–21436.

29. Chodakewitz J, Leavitt R, Massari F, Hildebrand C, Arcuri K, Gilde L, Nessly M, Meibohm A, Ghosg K, Radkowski R, Getson A, Rockhold F. Crixivan: summary of 24-week experience with Crixivan at 2.4 g/d in phase II trials. XIth International Conference on AIDS, Vancouver, Canada. 1. 1996:79.

30. Chong K, Pagano P. Synergistic inhibition of human immunodeficiency virus type 1 in vitro by two and three-drug combination of delavardine, lamivudine and zidovudine. XIth International Conference on AIDS, Vancouver, Canada. 1996:72.

31. Chong U, McGee L, Erickson J. Discovery of potent, orally bioavailable, non-peptidic, cyclic sulfones as HIV protease inhibitors. XIth International Conference on AIDS, Vancouver, Canada. 1. 1996:67.

32. Clerici M, Lucey DR, Berzofsky JA, Pinto LA, Wynn TA, Blatt SP, Dolan MJ, Hendrix CW, Wolf SF, Shearer G. Restoration of HIV-specific cell-mediated immune responses by interleukin-12 in vitro. Science 1993;262:1721–1724.

32a. Clumeck N, Colebunders B, Vandercam B, Kabeya K, Cassano P, Sommereijins B, DeWit S, Picasso Trial Group. Randomized comparative outcome trial of indinavir and ritonavir in protease inhibitor (PI) naive HIV patients with CD4 below 100 cells/μl.

5th Conference on Retrovirus and Opportunistic Infections. Chicago, Feb 1–5, 1998;386.

33. Coffin J. HIV population dynamics in vivo: implications for genetic variation, pathogenesis, and therapy. Science 1995;267: 483–489.

34. Cohen C, Shalit P, Conant M, Scott R, Wong T, Campbell K, Smith J, Frost K. Lamivudine (3TC) and stavudine (d4T) combination therapy: HIV viral load and CD4 changes in a retrospective study of 330 patients. Fourth Conference on Retroviruses and Opportunistic Infections, Washington, DC, 1997:167.

35. Collier AC, Coombs RW, Fischl MA, Skolnik PR, Northfelt D, Boutin P, Hooper CJ, Kaplan LD, Volberding PA, Davis LG, et al. Combination therapy with zidovudine and didanosine compared with zidovudine alone in HIV-1 infection. Ann Intern Med 1993;119:786–793.

36. Concorde Coordinating Committee. Concorde: MRC/ANRS randomised double-blind controlled trial of immediate and deferred zidovudine in symptom-free HIV infection. Lancet 1994; 343:871–881.

37. Condra J, Holder D, Schief W, Chodakewitz J, Massari F, Blahy O, Yang T, Emini E. Bi-directional inhibition of HIV-1 drug resistance selection by combination therapy with indinavir and reverse transcriptase inhibitors. XIth International Conference on AIDS, Vancouver, Canada. 3. 1996:19.

38. Condra JH, Schleif WA, Blahy OM, Gabryelski LJ, Graham DJ, Quintero J, Rhodes A, Robbins HL, Roth E, Shivaprakash M. In vivo emergence of HIV-1 variants resistant to multiple protease inhibitors. Nature 1995;374:569–571.

39. Connolly KJ, Allan JD, Fitch H, Jackson-Pope L, McLaren C, Canetta R, Groopman JE. Phase I study of 2′,3′-dideoxyinosine (ddI) administered orally twice daily to patients with AIDS or AIDS-related complex and hematologic intolerance to zidovudine. Am J Med 1991;91:471–478.

40. Connor E, Mofenson L. Zidovudine for the reduction of perinatal human immunodeficiency virus transmission: pediatric AIDS Clinical Trials Group Protocol 076—results and treatment recommendations. Pediatr Infect Dis J 1995;14:536–541.

41. Cooley TP, Kunches LM, Saunders CA, Ritter JK, Perkins CJ, Colin M, McCaffrey RP, Liebman HA. Once-daily administration of 2′,3′-dideoxyinosine (ddI) in patients with the acquired immunodeficiency syndrome or AIDS-related complex. N Engl J Med 1990;322:1430–1435.

42. Craig J, Duncan I, Hockley D, Grief C, Roberts N, Mills J. Antiviral properties of Ro 31–8959, an inhibitor of HIV proteinase. Antiviral Res 1991;16:295–305.

43. D'Aquila R, Hughes M, Hirsch M. Nevirapine, zidovudine, and didanosine compared with zidovudine and didanosine in patients with HIV-1 infection. Ann Intern Med 1996;124:1019–1030.

44. Dalakas MC, Illa I, Pezeshkpour GH, Laukaitis JP, Cohen B, Griffin JL. Mitochondrial myopathy caused by long-term zidovudine therapy. N Engl J Med 1990;322:1098–1105.

45. Danner S, Carr A, Leonatd J. A short-term study of the safety, pharmacokinetics and efficacy of ritonavir, an inhibitor of HIV-1 protease. N Engl J Med 1995;333:1528–1533.

46. Davey RJ, Chaitt D, Reed G, Freimuth W, Herpin B, Metcalf J, Eastman P, Falloon J, Kovacs J, Polis M, Walker R, Masur H, Boyle J, Coleman S, Cox S, Wathen L, Daenzer C, Lane H. Randomized, controlled phase I/II, trial of combination therapy with delavirdine (U-90152S) and conventional nucleosides in human immunodeficiency virus type 1-infected patients. Antimicrob Agents Chemother 1996;40:1657–1664.

47. De Clercq E. Basic approaches to anti-retroviral treatment. J Acquir Immune Defic Syndr 1991;4:207–218.

48. De Clercq E. Broad-spectrum anti-DNA virus and anti-retrovirus activity of phosphonylmethoxyalkylpurines and -pyrimidines. Biochem Pharmacol 1991;42:963–972.

49. De Clercq E. Non-nucleoside reverse transcriptase inhibitors (NNRTIs) for the treatment of human immunodeficiency virus type 1 (HIV-1) infections: strategies to overcome drug resistance development. Med Res Rev 1996;16:125–157.

50. De Clercq E, Yamamoto N, Pauwels R. Marked in vivo anti-retrovirus activity of 9-(2-phosphonylmethoxy-ethyl)adenine, a selective anti-human immunodeficiency virus agent. Proc Natl Acad Sci USA 1989;86:332–336.

51. de Miranda P, Good SS, Yarchoan R, Thomas RV, Blum MR, Myers CE, Broder S. Alteration of zidovudine pharmacokinetics by probenecid in patients with AIDS or AIDS-related complex. Clin Pharmacol Ther 1989;46:494–500.

52. Dean M, Carrington M, O'Brien S. Genetic restriction of HIV-1 infection and progression to AIDS by a deletion allele of the CKR5 structural gene. Science 1996;273:1856–1862.

53. Delfraissy J, Sereni D, Brun-Vezinet F, Dormont J. A phase I-II dose ranging study of the safety and activity of Ro 31–8959 on previously zidovudine-treated HIV-infected individuals. IXth International Conference on AIDS, Berlin, Germany, 1993.

54. Delta Coordinating Committee. DELTA: a randomized double-blind controlled trial comparing combinations of zidovudine plus didanosine or zalcitabine with zidovudine monotherapy in individuals with HIV infection. Lancet 1996;348:293–291.

55. Deng H, Liu R, Ellmeier W, Choe S, Littman D, Landau N. Identification of a major co-receptor for primary isolates of HIV-1. Nature 1996;381:661–666.

56. Dolin R, Amato D, Fischl M, Liou S-H, Smaldone L, Pettinelli C, the ACTG of the NIAID. Efficacy of didanosine (ddI) versus zidovudine (ZDV) in patients with no or <16 weeks of prior ZVD therapy. IX International Conference on AIDS, Berlin. 1. 1993:67.

57. Dorsey B, Levin R, McDaniel S. L-735,524: The design of a potent and orally bioavailable HIV protease inhibitor. J Med Chem 1994;37:3443–3451.

58. Dournon E, Matheron S, Rozenbaum W, Gharakhanian S, Michon C, Girard PM, Perronne C, Salmon D, de Truchis P, LePort C, Bouvet E, Dazza MC, Lavacher M, Regnier B, the Claude Bernard Hospital AZT Study Group. Effects of zidovudine in 365 consecutive patients with AIDS or AIDS-related complex. Lancet 1988;2:1297–1302.

59. Dubinsky RM, Yarchoan R, Dalakas M, Broder S. Reversible axonal neuropathy from the treatment of AIDS and related disorders with 2′,3′-dideoxycytidine (ddC). Muscle Nerve 1989; 12:856–860.

60. Emini E, Condra J, Chodakewitz J. Maintenance of long-term virus suppression in patients treated with the HIV-1 protease inhibitor Crixivan (indinavir). XIth International Conference on AIDS, Vancouver, Canada, 1996:18.

61. Erice A, Mayers DL, Strike DG, Sannerud KJ, McCutchan FE, Henry K, Balfour HH. Primary infection with zidovudine-resistant human immunodeficiency virus type 1. N Engl J Med 1993; 328:1163–1165.

62. Erickson D. Induction of drug-metabolizing enzymes in rat liver by BI-RG-587. Nevirapine investigator's brochure. 1994:24–31.

63. Erickson J, Neidhart DJ, VanDrie J, Kempf DJ, Wang XC, Norbeck DW, Plattner JJ, Rittenhouse JW, Turon M, Wideburg N, Kohlbrenner WE, Simmer R, Helfrich R, Paul DA, Knigge M.

Design, activity, and 2.8 Å crystal structure of a C_2 symmetric inhibitor complexed to HIV-1 protease. Science 1990;249: 527–533.

64. Eron J, Benoit S, Jemsek J, MacArthur R, Santana J, Quinn J, Kuritzkes D, Fallon M, Rubin M, Party TNAW. Treatment with lamivudine, zidovudine, or both in HIV-positive patients with 200 to 500 CD4 cells per cubic millimeter. N Engl J Med 1995; 333:1662–1669.

65. Fan N, Evans D, Rank K, Thomas R, Tarpley W, Sharma S. Mechanism of resistance to U-90152S and sensitization to L-697,661 by a proline to leucine change at residue 236 of human immunodeficiency virus type 1 (HIV-1) reverse transcriptase. FEBS Lett 1995;359:233–238.

66. Fischl M, Galpin JE, Levine JD, Groopman JE, Henry DH, Kennedy P, Miles S, Robbine W, Starrett B, Zalusky R, Abels RI, Tsai HC, Rudnick SA. Recombinant human erythropoietin for patients with AIDS treated with zidovudine. N Engl J Med 1990;322:1488–1493.

67. Fischl M, Parker C, Pettinelli C, Wulfsohn M, Hirsch MS, Collier AC, Antoniskis D, Ho M, Richman DD, Fuchs Z, Merigan TC, Reichman RC, Gold J, Steigbigel N, Leoung GS, Rasheed S, Tsiatis A, Group tACT. A randomized controlled trial of a reduced daily dose of zidovudine in patients with acquired immunodeficiency syndrome. N Engl J Med 1990;323:1009–1014.

68. Fischl M, Richman DD, Hansen N, Collier AC, Carey JT, Para MF, Hardy D, Dolin R, Powderly WG, Allan JD, Wong B, Mergian TC, McAuliffe VJ, Hyslop NE, Rhame FS, Balfour HH, Spector SA, Volberding P, Petinelli C, Anderson J, Group tACT. The safety and efficacy of zidovudine (AZT) in the treatment of subjects with mildly symptomatic human immunodeficiency virus type I (HIV) infection. A double-blind, placebo controlled trial. Ann Intern Med 1990;112:727–737.

69. Fischl MA, Richman DD, Grieco MH, Gottlieb MS, Volberding PA, Laskin OL, Leedon JM, Groopman JE, Mildvan D, Schooley RT, Jackson GG, Durack DT, King D, the AZT Collaborative Working Group. The efficacy of azidothymidine (AZT) in the treatment of patients with AIDS and AIDS-related complex: a double-blind, placebo-controlled trial. N Engl J Med 1987;317:185–191.

70. Fitzgibbon JE, Howell RM, Haberzettl CA, Sperber SJ, Gocke DJ, Dubin DT. Human immunodeficiency virus type 1 *pol* gene mutations which cause decreased susceptibility to 2′,3′-dideoxycytidine. Antimicrob Agents Chemother 1992;36:153–157.

71. Foli A, Saville M, Baseler M, Yarchoan R. Effects of the TH1 and Th2 stimulatory cytokines interleukin-12 and interleukin-4 on human immunodeficiency virus replication. Blood 1995;85: 2114–2123.

72. Foli A, Sogocio K, Anderson B, Kavlick M, Saville M, Wainberg M, Gu Z, Cherrington J, Mitsuya H, Yarchoan R. In vitro selection and molecular characterization of human immunodeficiency virus type 1 with reduced sensitivity to 9-[2-(phosphonomethoxy) ethyl]adenine (PMEA). Antiviral Res 1996;32:91–98.

73. Foster SA, Cerny J, Cheng Y. Herpes simplex virus-specified DNA polymerase is the target for the antiviral action of 9-(2-phosphonylmethoxyethyl)adenine. J Biol Chem 1991;266: 238–244.

74. Freiman JP, Helfert KE, Hamrell MR, Stein DS. Hepatomegaly with severe steatosis in HIV-seropositive patients. AIDS 1993;7:379–385.

75. Furman PA, Fyfe JA, St Clair M, Weinhold K, Rideout JL, Freeman GA, Nusinoff Lehrman S, Bolognesi DP, Broder S, Mitsuya H, Barry DW. Phosphorylation of 3′-azido-3′-deoxythymidine

and selective interaction of the 5′-triphosphate with human immunodeficiency virus reverse transcriptase. Proc Natl Acad Sci USA 1986;83:8333–8337.

75a. Gallant JE, Heath-Chiozzi M, Raines C, Anderson R, Katz T, Fields C, Flexner C. 5th Conference on Retrovirus and Opportunistic Infections. Chicago, Feb 1–5, 1998;394a.

76. Gao W, Agbaria R, Driscoll JS, Mitsuya H. Divergent anti-human immunodeficiency virus activity and anabolic phosphorylation of 2′,3′-dideoxynucleoside analogs in resting and activated human cells. J Biol Chem 1994;269:12633–12638.

77. Gao W-Y, Shirasaka T, Johns DG, Broder S, Mitsuya H. Differential phosphorylation of azidothymidine, dideoxycytidine, and dideoxyinosine in resting and activated peripheral blood mononuclear cells. J Clin Invest 1993;91:2326–2333.

78. Gathe J. A randomized phase II study of Viracept, a novel HIV protease inhibitor. XI International Conference on AIDS, Vancouver, Canada. 1. 1996:25.

79. Greene W. The molecular biology of HIV-1 infection. N Engl J Med 1991;324:308–317.

80. Gu Z, Arts EJ, Parniak MA, Wainberg MA. Mutated K65R recombinant reverse transcriptase of human immunodeficiency virus type 1 shows diminished chain termination in the presence of 2′,3′-dideoxycytidine 5′-triphosphate and other drugs. Proc Natl Acad Sci USA 1995;92:2760–2764.

81. Gu Z, Gao Q, Fang H, Salomon H, Parniak MA, Goldberg E, Cameron J, Wainberg M. Identification of a mutation at codon 65 in the IKKK motif of reverse transcriptase that encodes human immunodeficiency virus resistance to 2′,3′-dideoxycytidine and 2′,3′-dideoxy-3′-thiacytidine. Antimicrob Agents Chemother 1994;38:275–281.

82. Gu Z, Salomon H, Cherrington JM, Mulato AS, Chen MS, Yarchoan R, Foli A, Sogocio KM, Wainberg MA. K65R mutation of human immunodeficiency virus type 1 reverse transcriptase encodes cross-resistance to 9-(2-phosphonylmethoxyethyl)adenine. Antimicrob Agents Chemother 1995;39:1888–1891.

83. Gulick R, Mellors J, Havlir D, Eron J, Emini E, Chodakewitz J. Potent and sustained antiretroviral activity of indinavir (IDV) in combination with zidovudine (ZDV) and lamivudine (3TC). Third Conference on Retroviruses and Opportunistic Infections, Washington, DC, 1. 1996:162.

84. Gulnik S, Suvorov L, Lie B, Yu B, Anderson B, Mitsuya H, Erickson J. Kinetic characterization and cross-resistance patterns of HIV-1 protease mutants selected under drug pressure. Biochemistry 1995;34:9282–9287.

85. Gustavson LE, Fukuda EK, Rubio FA, Dunton AW. A pilot study of the bioavailability and pharmacokinetics of 2′,3′-dideoxycytidine in patients with AIDS or AIDS-related complex. J Acquir Immune Defic Syndr 1990;3:28–31.

86. Hamamoto Y, Nakashima H, Matsui T, Matsuda A, Ueda T, Yamamoto N. Inhibitory effect of 2′,3′-didehydro-2′,3′-dideoxynucleosides on infectivity, cytopathic effects, and replication of human immunodeficiency virus. Antimicrob Agents Chemother 1987;31:907–910.

87. Hammer S, Katzenstein D, Hughes M, Schooley R, Hirsch M, Merigan T, ACTG 175 Study Team. A trial comparing nucleoside monotherapy with combination therapy in HIV-infected adults with CD4 cell counts from 200 to per cubic millimeter. N Engl J Med 1996;335:1081–1090.

88. Hartman NR, Yarchoan R, Pluda JM, Thomas RV, Marczyk KS, Broder S, Johns DG. Pharmacokinetics of 2′,3′-dideoxyadenosine and 2′,3′-dideoxyinosine in patients with severe HIV infection. Clin Pharmacol Ther 1990;47:647–654.

89. Havlir D, Richman D. Viral dynamics of HIV: implications for drug development and therapeutic strategies. Ann Intern Med 1996;124:984–994.

89b. Havlir DV, Riddler S, Squires K, et al. Co-adminstration of indinavir (IDV) and nelfinavir (NFV) in a twice daily regimen: preliminary safety, pharmacokinetic, and antiviral activity results. 5th Conference on Retrovirus and Opportunistic Infections. Chicago, Feb 1–5, 1998;983.

90. Hedaya MA, Elmquist WF, Sawchuk RJ. Probenecid inhibits the metabolic and renal clearances of zidovudine (AZT) in human volunteers. Pharm Res 1990;7:411–417.

91. Henry K, Chinnock BJ, Quinn RP, Fletcher CV, De Miranda P, et al. Concurrent zidovudine levels in semen and serum determined by radioimmunoassay in patients with AIDS or AIDS-related complex. JAMA 1988;259:3023–3026.

92. Hirschel B, Rutschmann O, Overbeck I. Treatment of advanced HIV infection with ritonavir plus saquinavir. XIth International Conference on AIDS, Vancouver, Canada. 3. 1996:28.

93. Ho D, Neumann A, Perelson A, Chen W, Leonard J, Markowitz M. Rapid turnover of plasma virions and CD4 lymphocytes in HIV-1 infection [see comments]. Nature 1995;373:123–126.

94. Ho HT, Hitchcock MJ. Cellular pharmacology of 2′,3′-dideoxy-2′,3′-didehydrothymidine, a nucleoside analog active against human immunodeficiency virus. Antimicrob Agents Chemother 1989;33: 844–849.

95. Horwitz JP, Chua J, Noel M. Nucleosides. V. The monomesylates of 1-(2′-deoxy-β-D-lyxofuranosyl)thymidine. J Org Chem 1964;29:2076–2078.

96. Hsu A, Granneman G, Leonard J. Assessment of single- and multiple-dose interactions between ritonavir and saquinavir. XIth International Conference on AIDS, Vancouver, Canada. 3. 1996:30.

97. Iversen A, Shafer R, Wehrly K, Winters M, Mullins J, Chesebro B, Merigan T. Multidrug-resistant human immunodeficiency virus type 1 strains resulting from combination antiretroviral therapy. J Virol 1996;70:1086–1090.

98. Jacobbsen H, Yasargil K, Duncan I. Characterizaton of HIV-1 mutants with decreased sensitivity to proteinase inhibitor Ro 31–8959. Virology 1995;206:527–534.

99. Johns DG, Driscoll J. 2-B-Fluoro-2′,3′-dideoxyadenosine (F-DDA): a new anti-HIV clinical drug candidate. XIth International Conference on AIDS, Vancouver, Canada. 1. 1996:68.

100. Johnson S. NIH panel examines consequences of AZT in pregnancy. GMHC Treatment Issues 1997;11:4–5.

101. Kahn JO, Lagakos SW, Richman DD, Cross A, Pettinetti C, Liou S-H, Brown M, Volberding PA, Crumpacker CS, Beall G, Sacks HS, Merigan TC, Beltangady M, Smaldone L, Dolin R, Group tNACT. A controlled trial comparing continued zidovudine with didanosine in human immunodeficiency virus infection. N Engl J Med 1992;327:581–587.

102. Katzenstein D, Hammer S, Hughes M. The relation of virologic and immunologic markers to clinical outcomes after nucleoside therapy in HIV-infected adults with 200–500 CD4 cells per cubic millimeter. N Engl J Med 1996;335:1091–1098.

103. Kempf D, Marsh K, Denissen J. ABT-538 is a potent inhibitor of human immunodeficiency virus protease and has high oral bioavailability in humans. Proc Natl Acad Sci USA 1995;92: 2484–2488.

104. Kempf D, Marsh K, Denissen J, Norbeck D. Coadministration with ritonavir enhances the plasma levels of HIV protease inhibitors by inhibition of cytochrome p450. Third Conference on Retroviruses and Opportunistic Infections, Washington, DC, 1996:79.

105. Kempf D, Norbeck D, Codacovi L. Structure-based C2 symmetric inhibitors of HIV protease. J Med Chem 1990;33: 2687–2689.

106. Kitchen V, SAkinner C, Weber J. Safety and activity of saquinavir in HIV infection. Lancet 1995;345:952–955.

107. Klecker RW Jr, Collins JM, Yarchoan R, Thomas R, Jenkins JF, Broder S, Myers CE. Plasma and cerebrospinal fluid pharmacokinetics of 3′-azido-3′-deoxythymidine: a novel pyrimidine analog with potential application for the treatment of patients with AIDS and related diseases. Clin Pharmacol Ther 1987; 41:407–412.

108. Klecker RW Jr, Collins JM, Yarchoan R, Thomas R, McAtee N, Broder S, Myers S. Pharmacokinetics of 2′,3′-dideoxycytidine in patients with AIDS and related disorders. J Clin Pharm 1988;28:837–842.

109. Knupp CA, Shyu WC, Dolin R, Knupp C, Shyu W, Dolin R, Valentine F, McLaren C, Martin R, Pittman K, Barbhaiya R. Pharmacokinetics of didanosine in patients with acquired immunodeficiency syndrome or acquired immunodeficiency syndrome-related complex. Clin Pharmacol Ther 1991;49: 523–535.

110. Kornhauser DM, Petty BG, Hendrix CW, Woods AS, Nerhood LJ, Bartlett JG, Lietman PS. Probenecid and zidovudine metabolism. Lancet 1989;2:473–475.

111. Kovacs J, Vogel S, Albert J, Lane C. Controlled trial of interleukin-2 infusions in patients with the Human Immunodeficiency Virus. N Engl J Med 1996;335:1350–1356.

112. Kramer RA, Schaber MD, Skalka AM, Ganguly K, Wong SF, Reddy EP. HTLV-III gag protein is processed in yeast cells by the virus pol-protease. Science 1986;231:1580–1584.

112a. Kravcik S, Farnsworth A, Patick A, Duncan I, Hawley-Foss N, Anderson R, Brostow N, Salgo M, Cameron DW. Long-term follow up of combination protease inhibitor therapy with nelfinavir and saquinavir (soft gel) in HIV infection. 5th Conference on Retrovirus and Opportunistic Infections. Chicago, Feb 1–5, 1998;394c.

113. Kumar G, Rodriguez A, Buko A. Cytochrome p450-mediated metabolism of the HIV-1 protease inhibitor ritonavir (ABT-538) in human liver microsomes. J Pharmacol Exp Ther 1996; 227:423–431.

114. Lambert JS, Seidlin M, Reichman RC, Plank CS, Laverty M, Morse GD, Knupp C, McLaren C, Pettinelli C, Valentine FT, Dolin R. 2′,3′-Dideoxyinosine (ddI) in patients with the acquired immunodeficiency syndrome or the AIDS-related complex. A Phase I trial. N Engl J Med 1990;322:1333–1340.

115. Lambert JS, Seidlin M, Valentine FT, Reichman RC, Dolin R. Didanosine: long term follow-up of patients in a phase I study. Clin Infect Dis 1993;16:S40–44.

116. Levine JD, Allan JD, Tessitore JH, Falcone N, Galasso F, Israel RJ, Groopman JE. Recombinant human granulocyte-macrophage colony-stimulating factor ameliorates zidovudine-induced neutropenia in patients with acquired immunodeficiency syndrome (AIDS)/AIDS-related complex. Blood 1991;78: 3148–3154.

117. Lin T-S, Schinazi RF, Prusoff WH. Potent and selective in vitro activity of 3′-deoxythymidin-2′-ene (3′-deoxy-2′,3′-didehydrothymidine) against human immunodeficiency virus. Biochem Pharmacol 1987;36:2713–2718.

118. Lori F, Malykh A, Cara A, Sun D, Weinstein JN, Lisziewicz J, Gallo RC. Hydroxyurea as an inhibitor of human immunodeficiency virus-type 1 replication. Science 1994;266:801–805.

119. Makonkawkeyoon S, Limson-Pobre RN, Moreira AL, Schauf

V, Kaplan G. Thalidomide inhibits the replication of human immunodeficiency virus type 1. Proc Natl Acad Sci USA 1993; 90:5974–5978.

120. Markowitz M, Saag M, Powderly W. A preliminary study of ritonavir, an inhibitor of HIV-1 protease. N Engl J Med 1995; 333:1534–1539.

121. Marquez VE, Tseng CK-H, Driscoll JS, Mitsuya H, Broder S, Roth JS, Kelly JA. 2',3'-Dideoxy-2'-fluoro-ara-A. An acid-stable purine nucleoside active against human immunodeficiency virus (HIV). Biochem Pharmacol 1987;36:2719–2722.

122. Massari F, Conant M, Mellors J, Steigbigel R, Mildvan D, Greenberg R, Carpenter C, Murphy R, Squires K, Rigsby M, Drusano G, McKinley G, Gilde L, Nessly M. A phase II open-label, randomized study of the triple combination of indinavir, zidovudine(ZDV) and didanosine (ddI) versus indinavir alone and zidovudine/didanosine in antiretroviral naive patients. Third Conference on Retroviruses and Opportunistic Infections, Washington, DC, 1996:90.

123. Mathez D, De Truchis P, Gorin I, Katlama C, Pialoux G, Saimot A, Tubiana R, Chauvin J, Bagnarelli P, Clementi M, Leibowitch J. Ritonavir, AZT, ddC as a triple combination in AIDS patients. Third Conference on Retroviruses and Opportunistic Infections, Washington, DC, 1996:106.

124. Meek TD, Lambert DM, Dreyer GB, Carr TJ, Tomaszek TA Jr, Moore ML, Strickler JE, Debouck C, Hyland LJ, Matthews TJ, Metcalf B, Petteway SR. Inhibition of HIV-1 protease in infected T-lymphocytes by synthetic peptide analogues. Nature 1990;343:90–92.

125. Mellors J, Rinaldo C, Phalguni G, White R, Todd J, Kingsley L. Prognosis of HIV-1 infection predicted by the quantity of virus in plasma. Science 1996;272:1167–1170.

125a. Mellors J, Lederman M, Haas D, et al. Antiretroviral effects of therapy combining abacavir (1592) with HIV protease inhibitors. 5th Conference on Retrovirus and Opportunistic Infections. Chicago, Feb 1–5, 1998;4.

126. Meng T-C, Fischl MA, Boota AM, Spector SA, Bennett D, Bassiakos Y, Lai S, Wright B, Richman DD. A phase I/II study of combination therapy with zidovudine and dideoxycytidine in subjects with advanced human immunodeficiency virus (HIV) disease. Ann Intern Med 1992;116:13–20.

127. Merck. Crixivan (indinavir sulfate) capsules prescribing information. 1996; West Point, PA.

128. Merigan TC, Skowron G, Bozzette SA, Richman D, Uttamchandani R, Fischl M, Schooley R, Hirsch M, Soo W, Pettinelli C, Schaumburg H, the ddC Study Group of the AIDS Clinical Trials Group. Circulating p24 antigen levels and responses to dideoxycytidine in human immunodeficiency virus (HIV) infections. Ann Intern Med 1989;110:189–194.

129. Merluzzi VJ, Hargrave KD, Labadia M, Grozinger K, Skoog M, Wu J, Shih C-K, Eckner K, Hattox S, Adams J, Rosenthal AS, Faanes R, Eckner RJ, Koup RA, Sullivan JL. Inhibition of HIV-1 replication by a nonnucleoside reverse transcriptase inhibitor. Science 1990;250:1411–1413.

130. Metroka CE, McMechan MF, Andrada R, Laubenstein LJ, Jacobus DP. Failure of prophylaxis with dapsone in patients taking dideoxyinosine [Letter]. Lancet 1991;325:737.

131. Mhiri C, Baudrimont M, Bonne G, Geny C, Degoul F, Marsac C, Roullet E, Gherardi R. Zidovudine myopathy: a distinctive disorder associated with mitochondrial dysfunction. Ann Neurol 1991;29:606–614.

132. Mitsuya H, Broder S. Inhibition of the in vitro infectivity and cytopathic effect of human T-lymphotropic virus type III/lymphadenopathy virus-associated virus (HTLV-III/LAV) by 2',3'-dideoxynucleosides. Proc Natl Acad Sci USA 1986;83:1911–1915.

133. Mitsuya H, Dahlberg JE, Spigelman Z, Matsushita S, Jarrett RF, Matsukura M, Currens MJ, Aaronson SA, Reitz MS, McCaffrey RS, Broder S. 2',3'-Dideoxynucleosides: broad spectrum antiretroviral activity and mechanism of action. In: Bolognesi D, ed. Human retroviruses, cancer, and AIDS. Approaches to prevention and therapy. New York: Alan R Liss, 1988:407–421.

134. Mitsuya H, Jarrett RF, Matsukura M, di Marzo Veronese F, deVico AL, Sarngadharan MG, Johns DG, Reitz MS, Broder S. Long-term inhibition of human T-lymphotropic virus type III/lymphadenopathy-associated virus (human immunodeficiency virus) DNA synthesis and RNA expression in T cells protected by 2',3'-dideoxynucleosides in vitro. Proc Natl Acad Sci USA 1987;84:2033–2037.

135. Mitsuya H, Matsukura M, Broder S. Rapid in vitro systems for assessing activity of agents against HTLV-III/LAV. In: Broder S, ed. AIDS: modern concepts and therapeutic challenges. New York: Marcel Dekker, 1987:303–333.

136. Mitsuya H, Weinhold KJ, Furman PA, St Clair MH, Nusinoff Lehrman S, Gallo RC, Bolognesi D, Barry DW, Broder S. 3'-Azido-3'-deoxythymidine (BW A509U): an antiviral agent that inhibits the infectivity and cytopathic effect of human T-lymphotropic virus type III/lymphadenopathy-associated virus in vitro. Proc Natl Acad Sci USA 1985;82:7096–7100.

137. Mitsuya H, Yarchoan R, Broder S. Molecular targets for AIDS therapy. Science 1990;249:1533–1544.

138. Molla A, Korneyeva M, Kempf D. Ordered accumulation of mutations in HIV protease confers resistance to ritonavir. Nature Med 1996;2:760–766.

139. Moreira AL, Weiguo Y, Shen Z, Johnson B, Corral L, Kaplan G. Thalidomide reduces HIV-1 production in acutely infected human monocytes in vitro. Third Conference on Retroviruses and Opportunistic Infections, Washington, DC, 1996:111.

140. Moyle G, Youle M, Kobler N. Extended follow-up of safety and activity of Agouron's proteinase inhibitor AG1343 (Viracept) in virological responders from the UK phase I/II dose finding study. XIth International Conference on AIDS, Vancouver, Canada. 1. 1996:18.

141. Muirhead G, Shaw T, Williams P. Pharmacokinetics of the HIV-proteinase inhibitor Ro 31–8959 after single and multiple oral doses in healthy volunteers. Br J Clin Pharmacol 1992; 34:170–171.

142. Murphy R. Clinical aspects of human immunodeficiency virus disease: clinical rationale for treatment. J Infect Dis 1995;171 (Suppl 2):S81–87.

143. Murray HW, Squires KE, Weiss W, Sledz S, Sacks HS, Hassett J, Cross A, Anderson RE, Dunkle LM. Stavudine in patients with AIDS and AIDS-related complex: AIDS clinical trials group 089. J Infect Dis 1995;171(Suppl 2):S123–130.

144. Navia M, Fitzgerald P, McKever B, Navia M, Fitzgerald P, McKeever B, Leu C, Heimbach J, Herber W, Sigal I, Darke P, Springer J. Three dimensional structure of aspartyl protease from HIV-1. Nature 1989;377:615–620.

145. Nguyen B-Y, Yarchoan R, Wyvill KM, Venzon DJ, Pluda JM, Mitsuya H, Broder S. Five-year follow-up of a phase I study of didanosine in patients with advanced human immunodeficiency virus infection. J Infect Dis 1995;171:1180–1189.

146. O'Brien W, Hartigan P, Martin D, Esinhart J. Changes in plasma HIV-1 RNA and CD4-lymphocyte count relative to

treatment and progression to AIDS. N Engl J Med 1996;334: 426–431.

146a. Opravil M, on behalf of the Spice Study Team. Study of protease inhibitor combination in Europe (Spice); saquinavir soft gelatin capsule (SQV-SGC) and nelfinavir in HIV-infected individuals. 5th Conference on Retrovirus and Opportunistic Infections. Chicago, Feb 1–5, 1998;394b.

147. Perelson A, Essunger P, Markowitz M, Ho D. How long should treatment be given if we had an antiretroviral regimen that completely blocks HIV replication. XIth International Conference on AIDS, Vancouver, Canada. 1996:18.

148. Perno C-F, Cooney DA, Gao W-Y, Hao Z, Johns DG, Foli A, Hartman NR, Calio R, Broder S, Yarchoan R. Effects of bone marrow stimulatory cytokines on human immunodeficiency virus replication and the antiviral activity of dideoxynucleosides in cultures of monocyte/macrophages. Blood 1992;80: 995–1003.

149. Perno CF, Yarchoan R, Cooney DA, Hartman NR, Gartner S, Popovic M, Hao Z, Gerrard TL, Wilson YA, Johns DG, Broder S. Inhibition of human immunodeficiency virus (HIV-1/HTLV-III$_{Ba-L}$) replication in fresh and cultured human peripheral blood monocytes/macrophages by azidothymidine and related 2′,3′-dideoxynucleosides. J Exp Med 1988;168:1111–1125.

150. Petersen EA, Ramirez-Ronda CH, Hardy WD, Schwartz R, Sacks HS, Follansbee S, Peterson DM, Cross A, Anderson RE, Dunkle L. Dose-related activity of stavudine in patients infected with human immunodeficiency virus. J Infect Dis 1995;171(Suppl 2):S131–139.

151. Pharmacia and Upjohn Company. Rescriptor (delavirdine) prescribing information for tablets. Kalamzoo, MI: Pharmacia and Upjohn Company, 1997.

152. Pizzo PA, Butler K, Balis F, Brouwers P, Hawkins M, Eddy J, Einloth M, Falloon J, Husson R, Jarosinski P, Meer J, Moss H, Poplack D, Santacroce S, Weiner L, Wolters P. Dideoxycytidine alone and in an alternating schedule with zidovudine (AZT) in children with symptomatic human immunodeficiency virus infection. J Pediatr 1990;117:799–808.

153. Pluda JM, Ruedy J, Levitt N, Cooley T, Becard P, Rubin M, Yarchoan R. Phase I/II study of 3TC in patients with advanced ARC or AIDS. Abstracts of the VIII International Conference on AIDS/III STD World Congress 1992:B91.

154. Pluda JM, Yarchoan R, Smith PD, McAtee N, Shay LE, Oette D, Maha M, Wahl SM, Myers CE, Broder S. Subcutaneous recombinant granulocyte-macrophage colony-stimulating factor used as a single agent and in an alternating regimen with azidothymidine in leukopenic patients with severe human immunodeficiency virus infection. Blood 1990;76:463–472.

155. Pons JC, Boubon MC, Taburet AM, Singlas E, Chambrin V. Fetoplacental passage of 2′,3′-dideoxyinosine. Lancet 1991; 337:732.

156. Premack B, Schall T. Chemokine receptors: gateways to inflammation and infection. Nature Med 1996;2:1174–1178.

157. Ragni M, Amato D, LoFaro M, DeGruttola V, Van Der Horst C, Eyster M, Kessler C, Gjerset G, Ho M, Parenti D. Randomized study of didanosine monotherapy and combination therapy with zidovudine in hemophilic and nonhemophilic subjects with asymptomatic human immunodeficiency virus-1 infection. Blood 1995;85:2337–2346.

158. Ragni M, Dafni R, Amato DA, Korvick J, Merigan TC. Combination zidovudine and dideoxyinosine in asymptomatic HIV(−) patients. VIII International Conference on AIDS/III STD World Congress, Amsterdam. 1. 1992:Mo15.

159. Rarick MU, Espina B, Montgomery T, Easley A, Allen J. The long-term use of zidovudine in patients with severe immune-mediated thrombocytopenia secondary to infection with HIV. AIDS 1991;5:1357–1361.

160. Rice WG, Schaeffer CA, Harten B, Villinger F, South TL, Summers MF, Henderson LE, Bess JW, Arthur LO, McDougal JS, Orloff SL, Mendeleyev J, Kun E. Inhibition of HIV-1 infectivity by zinc-ejecting aromatic C-nitroso compounds. Nature 1993;361:473–475.

161. Rice WG, Supko JG, Malspeis L, Buckheit RW Jr, Clanton D, Bu M, Graham L, Schaeffer CA, Turpin JA, Domagala J, Gogliotti R, Bader JP, Halliday SM, Coren L, Sowder RC, II, Arther LO, Lenderson LE. Inhibitors of HIV nucleocapsid protein zinc fingers as candidates for the treatment of AIDS. Science 1995;270:1194–1197.

162. Richman D, Havlir D, Corbeil. Nevirapine resistance mutations of HIV selected during therapy. J Virol 1994;68:1660–1666.

163. Richman DD, Fischl MA, Grieco MH, Gottlieb MS, Volberding PA, Laskin OL, Leedom JM, Groopman JE, Mildvan D, Hirsch MS, Jackson GG, Durack DT, Nusinoff-Lehrman S, Group TACW. The toxicity of azidothymidine (AZT) in the treatment of patients with AIDS and AIDS-related complex: a double-blind, placebo-controlled trial. N Engl J Med 1987; 317:192–197.

164. Richman DD, Grimes J, Lagakos S. Effect of stage of disease and drug dose on zidovudine susceptibilities of isolates of human immunodeficiency virus. J Acquir Immune Defic Syndr 1990;3:743–746.

165. Riddler SA, Anderson RE, Mellors JW. Antiretroviral activity of stavudine (2′,3′-didehydro-3′-deoxythymidine, D4T). Antiviral Res 1995;27: 189–203.

166. Ridky T, Leis J. Development of drug resistance to HIV-1 protease inhibitors. J Biol Chem 1995;270:29621–29623.

167. Roberts NA, Martin JA, Kinchington D, Broadhurst AV, Craig JC, Duncan IB, Galpin SA, Handa BK, Kay J, Krohn A, Lambert RW, Merrett JH, Mills JS, Parkes KEB, Redshaw S, Ritchie AJ, Taylor DL, Thomas GJ, Machin PJ. Rational design of peptide-based HIV proteinase inhibitors. Science 1990;248: 358–361.

168. Rolinski B, Wintergerst U, Matuschke A, Fuessl H, Goebel FD, Roscher A, Belohradsky B. Evaluation of saliva as a specimen for monitoring therapy in HIV-infected patients. AIDS 1991;5: 858–888.

169. Roxane Laboratories. Viramune (nevirapine) package insert, 1996.

170. Saag M. Preliminary data on the safety and antiviral effect of 1592U89, alone and in combination with zidovudine. XI International Conference on AIDS, Vancouver, Canada. 2. 1996: 225.

171. Saag M, Holodniy M, Kuritzkes D, O'Brien W, Coombs R, Poscher M, Jacobsen D, Shaw G, Richman D, PA V. HIV viral load markers in clinical practice. Nature Med 1996;2:625–629.

172. Sahai J, Gallicano K, Oliveras L, Khaliq S, Hawley-Foss N, Garber G. Cations in the didanosine tablet reduce ciprofloxacin bioavailability. Clin Pharmacol Ther 1993;53:292–297.

173. Saravolatz L, Winslow D, Collins G, Hodges J, Pettinelli C, Stein D, Markowitz N, Reves R, Loveless M, Crane L, Thompson M, Abrams D. Zidovudine alone or in combination with didanosine or zalcitabine in HIV-infected patients with the acquired immunodeficiency syndrome or fewer than 200 CD4 cells per cubic millimeter. N Engl J Med 1996;335: 1099–1106.

174. Schapiro J, Winters M, Stewart F, Efron B, Norris J, Kozal M, Merigan T. The effect of high-dose saquinavir on viral load and CD4 T-cell counts in HIV-infected patients. Ann Intern Med 1996;124:1039–1050.

175. Schmitt FA, Bigley JW, McKinnis R, Logue PE, Evans RW, Drucker JL, the AZT Collaborative Working Group. Neuropsychological outcome of zidovudine (AZT) treatment of patients with AIDS and AIDS-related complex. N Engl J Med 1988;319:1573–1578.

176. Schuurman R, Nijhuis M, van Leeuwen R, Schipper P, de Jong D, Collis P, Danner SA, Mulder J, Loveday C, Christopherson C. Rapid changes in human immunodeficiency virus type 1 RNA load and appearance of drug-resistant virus populations in persons treated with lamivudine (3TC). J Infect Dis 1995;171:1411–1419.

177. Shafer R, Iversen A, Winters M, Aguiniga E, Katzenstein D, Merigan TC. Drug resistance and heterogeneous long-term virologic responses of human immunodeficiency virus type 1-infected subjects to zidovudine and didanosine combination therapy. J Infect Dis 1995;172:70–78.

178. Shirasaka T, Kavlick MF, Ueno T, Gao WY, Kojima E, Alcaide ML, Chokekijchai S, Roy BM, Arnold E, Yarchoan R, Mitsuya H. Emergence of human immunodeficiency virus type 1 variants with resistance to multiple dideoxynucleosides in patients receiving therapy with dideoxynucleosides. Proc Natl Acad Sci USA 1995;92:2398–2402.

179. Simpson DM, Tagliati M. Nucleoside analogue-associated peripheral neuropathy in human immunodeficiency virus infection. J Acquir Immune Defic Syndr Hum Retrovirol 1995;9:153–161.

180. Singlas E, Pioger J-C, Taburet A-M, Colin J-N, Fillastre J-P. Zidovudine disposition in patients with severe renal impairment: influence of hemodialysis. Clin Pharmacol Ther 1989;46:190–197.

181. Singlas E, Taburet AM, Borsa LF, Parent D, Curzon O, Sobel A, Chauveau P, Viron B, Al KR, Poignet JL, Mignon F. Didanosine pharmacokinetics in patients with normal and impaired renal function: influence of hemodialysis. Didanosine pharmacokinetics in patients with normal and impaired renal function: influence of hemodialysis 1992;36:1519–1524.

182. Skowron G, Bozzette SA, Lim L, Pettinelli CB, Schaumberg HH, Arezzo J, Fischl MA, Powderly WG, Gocke DJ, Richman DD, Pottage JC, Antoniskis D, McKinley GF, Hyslop NE, Ray G, Simon G, Reed N, LoFaro ML, Uttamchandani RB, Gelb LD, Sperber SJ, Murphy RL, Leedom JM, Grieco MH, Zachary J, Hirsch MS, Spector SA, Bigley J, Soo W, Merigan TC. Alternating and intermittent regimens of zidovudine and dideoxycytidine in patients with AIDS or AIDS-related complex. Ann Intern Med 1993;118:321–330.

183. Sogocio KM, Foli A, Anderson B, Kavlick M, Saville W, Wainberg M, Cherrington JM, Mitsuya H, Yarchoan R. HIV-1 develops reduced sensitivity to 9-(2-phosphonylmethoxyethyl) adenine (PMEA) in vitro through acquisition of K65R. Bethesda, MD: AIDS Research and Human Retroviruses, 1995:S164.

184. St. Clair MH, Martin JL, Tudor-Williams G, Bach MC, Vavro CL, King DM, Kellam P, Kemp SD, Larder BA. Resistance to ddI and sensitivity to AZT induced by a mutation in HIV-1 reverse transcriptase. Science 1991;253:1557–1559.

185. Starnes MC, Cheng Y-C. Cellular metabolism of 2′,3′-dideoxycytidine, a compound active against human immunodeficiency virus in vitro. J Biol Chem 1987;262:988–991.

186. Steigbigel R, Berry P, Mellors J. Efficacy and safety of the HIV protease inhibitor indinavir sulfate at escalating dose. Third Conference on Retroviruses and Opportunistic Infections, Washington, DC, 1996:80.

187. Stein D, Fish D, Bilello J, Preston S, Martineau G, Drusano G. A 24-week open-label phase I/II evaluation of the HIV protease inhibitor MK-639 (indinavir). AIDS 1996;10:485–492.

188. Stein D, Fish D, Chodakewitz J. Followup data from an open label phase I evaluation of the HIV protease inhibitor MK-639. Third Conference on Retroviruses and Opportunistic Infections, Washington, DC, 1996:80.

189. Suleiman J, Lewi D, Motti E, Leavitt R. Antiretroviral activity and safety of indinavir alone and in combination with zidovudine in zidovudine-naive patients with CD4 cell counts of 50–250 cells/mm³. XIth International Conference on AIDS, Vancouver, Canada. 3. 1996:25.

190. Thaisrivongs S, Janakiraman M, Chong K, Tomich P, Dolak L, Turner S, Strohbach J, Lynn J, Horng M, Hinshaw R, Watenpaugh K. Structure-based design of novel HIV protease inhibitors: sulfonamide-containing 4-hydroxycoumarins and 4-hydroxy-2-pyrones as potent non-peptidic inhibitors. J Med Chem 1996;39:1400–1410.

191. Thaisrivongs S, Watenpaugh K, Howe W, Tomich P, Dolak L, Chong K, Tomich C, Tomasselli A, Turner S, Strohbach JW. Structure-based design of novel HIV protease inhibitors: carboxamide-containing 4-hydroxycoumarins and 4-hydroxy-2-pyrones as potent nonpeptidic inhibitors. J Med Chem 1995;38:3624–3637.

192. Tisdale M, Kemp SD, Parry NR, Larder BA. Rapid in vitro selection of human immunodeficiency virus type 1 resistant to 3′-thiacytidine inhibitors due to a mutation in the YMDD region of reverse transcriptase. Proc Natl Acad Sci USA 1993;90:5653–5656.

193. Tisdale M, Myers R, Maschera B. Cross-resistance analysis of HIV-1 variants individually selected for resistance to five different protease inhibitors. Antimicrob Agents Chemother 1995;39:1704–1710.

194. Tsai C-C, Follis KE, Sabo A, Beck TW, Grant RF, Bischofberger N, Benveniste RE, Black R. Prevention of SIV infection in macaques by (R)-9-(2-phosphonylmethoxypropyl)adenine. Science 1995;270:1197–1199.

195. Unadkat JD, Collier AC, Crosby SS, Cummings D, Opheim KE, et al. Pharmacokinetics of oral zodivudine (azidothymidine) in patients with AIDS when administered with and without a high-fat meal. AIDS 1990;4:229–232.

196. Vacca J, Dorsey B, Schleif W. L-735,524: an orally bioavailable HIV-1 protease inhibitor. Proc Natl Acad Sci USA 1994;91:4096–4100.

197. van Leeuwen R, Lange JMA, Hussey EK, Donn KH, Hall ST, Harker AJ, Jonker P, Danner SA. The safety and pharmacokinetics of a reverse transcriptase inhibitor, 3TC, in patients with HIV infection: a phase I study. AIDS 1992;6:1471–1475.

198. Vella S. Clinical experience with saquinavir. AIDS 1995;9 (Suppl 2):S21–25.

199. Voest E, Kenyon B, O'Reilly M, Truitt G, D'Amato R, Folkman J. Inhibition of angiogenesis in vivo by interleukin 12. J Natl Cancer Inst 1995;87:581–586.

200. Vogt MW, Hartshorn KL, Furman PA, Chou T-C, Fyfe JA, Coleman LA, Crumpacker C, Schooley RT, Hirsch MS. Ribavirin antagonizes the effect of azidothymidine on HIV replication. Science 1987;235:1376–1379.

201. Volberding PA, Lagakos SW, Koch MA, Pettinelli C, Myers

MW, Booth DK, Balfour HH, Reichman RC, Bartlett JA, Hirsch MS, Murphy RL, Hardy WD, Soeiro R, Fischl MA, Bartlett JG, Merigan TC, Hyslop NE, Richman DD, Valentine FT, Corey L, the AIDS Clinical Trials Group of the National Institute of Allergy and Infectious Diseases. Zidovudine in asymptomatic human immunodeficiency virus infection. A controlled trial in persons with fewer than 500 CD4-positive cells per cubic millimeter. N Engl J Med 1990;322:941–949.

202. Wainberg M, Drosopoulos W, Prasad V. Enhanced fidelity of 3TC-selected mutant HIV-1 reverse transcriptase. Science 1996;271:1282–1285.

203. Wainberg MA. Biological and enzymatic studies on the fidelity of wild-type and mutated HIV-1 reverse transcriptase. AIDS Res Hum Retroviruses 1995;11(Suppl 11):S169.

204. Weber I, Miller M, Jaskolski M, Leis J, Skalka A, Wlodawer A. Molecular modeling of the HIV-1 protease and its substrate binding site. Science 1989;243:928–931.

205. Wei X, Ghosh S, Taylor M. Viral dynamics in human immunodeficiency virus type 1 infection. Nature 1995;373: 123–126.

206. Weiss R, Clapham P. Hot fusion of HIV. Nature 1996;381: 647–648.

207. Whitcup SM, Butler KM, Caruso R, de Smet MD, Rubin B, Husson RN, Lopez JS, Belfort R, Pizzo PA, Nussenblatt RB. Retinal toxicity in human immunodeficiency virus-infected children treated with 2′,3′-dideoxyinosine. Am J Ophthalmol 1992;113:1–7.

208. Whittington R, Brogden RN. Zalcitabine: a review of its pharmacology and clinical potential in acquired immunodeficiency syndrome. Drugs 1992;44:656–683.

209. Williams P, Madigan M, Mitchel A. A single dose, randomized cross-over study of the absolute and relative bioavailability of Ro 31–8959 in healthy volunteers. Roche Research Report 1992.

210. Wlodawer A, Miller M, Jaskolski M, Sathyanarayana B, Baldwin E, Weber I, Selk L, Clawson L, Schneider J, Kent S. Conserved folding in retroviral proteases: crystal structure of a synthetic HIV-1 protease. Science 1989;245:616–621.

211. Yarchoan R, Broder S. Strategies for the pharmacological intervention against HTLV-III/LAV. In: S. Broder, ed. AIDS: modern concepts and therapeutic challenges. New York: Marcel Dekker, 1987:335–360.

212. Yarchoan R, Klecker RW, Weinhold KJ, Markham PD, Lyerly HK, Durack DT, Gelmann E, Lehrman SN, Blum RM, Barry DW, Shearer GM, Fischl MA, Mitsuya H, Gallo RC, Collins JM, Bolognesi DP, Myers CE, Broder S. Administration of 3′-azido-3′-deoxythymidine, an inhibitor of HTLV-III/LAV replication, to patients with AIDS or AIDS-related complex. Lancet 1986;1:575–580.

213. Yarchoan R, Lietzau JA, Nguyen B-Y, Brawley OW, Pluda JM, Saville MW, Wyvill KM, Steinberg SM, Agbaria R, Mitsuya H, Broder S. A randomized pilot study of alternating or simultaneous zidovudine and didanosine therapy in patients with symptomatic immunodeficiency virus infection. J Infect Dis 1994;169:9–17.

214. Yarchoan R, Mitsuya H, Myers CE, Broder S. Clinical pharmacology of 3′-azido-2′,3′-dideoxythymidine (zidovudine) and related dideoxynucleosides. N Engl J Med 1989;321: 726–738.

215. Yarchoan R, Mitsuya H, Pluda J, Marczyk KS, Thomas RV, Hartman NR, Brouwers P, Perno C-F, Allain J-P, Johns DG, Broder S. The National Cancer Institute phase I study of ddI administration in adults with AIDS or AIDS-related complex: analysis of activity and toxicity profiles. Rev Infect Dis 1990;12(Suppl 5):S522–S533.

216. Yarchoan R, Mitsuya H, Thomas RV, Pluda JM, Hartman NR, Perno C-F, Marczyk KS, Allain J-P, Johns DG, Broder S. In vivo activity against HIV and favorable toxicity profile of 2′,3′-dideoxyinosine. Science 1989;245:412–415.

217. Yarchoan R, Perno CF, Thomas RV, Klecker RW, Allain J-P, Wills RJ, McAtee N, Fischl MA, Dubinsky R, McNeely MC, Mitsuya H, Pluda JM, Lawley TJ, Leuther M, Safai B, Collins JM, Myers CE, Broder S. Phase I studies of 2′,3′-dideoxycytidine in severe human immunodeficiency virus infection as a single agent and alternating with zidovudine (AZT). Lancet 1988;1:76–81.

218. Yarchoan R, Thomas RV, Grafman J, Wichman A, Dalakas M, McAtee N, Berg G, Fischl M, Perno CF, Klecker RW, Buchbinder A, Tay S, Larson SM, Myers CE, Broder S. Long-term administration of 3′-azido-2′,3′-dideoxythymidine to patients with AIDS-related neurological disease. Ann Neurol 1988;23 (Suppl):S82–S87.

Influenza Viruses

●

John Treanor

GENERAL DESCRIPTION
Microbiology and Pathogenesis

The influenza viruses are classified into three distinct types, influenza A virus, influenza B virus, and influenza C virus, based on major antigenic differences in the nucleoprotein and matrix proteins. In addition, there are significant differences in genetic organization, structure, host range, epidemiology, and clinical characteristics between the three influenza virus types. However, all three viruses share certain characteristics that are fundamental to their biologic behavior, including the presence of a host-cell-derived envelope, envelope glycoproteins of critical importance in virus entry and egress from cells, and a segmented genome of negative-sense (i.e., opposite of message sense) single-stranded RNA. The standard nomenclature for influenza viruses includes the influenza type, place of initial isolation, strain designation, and year of isolation. For example, the current influenza A virus vaccine strain initially isolated in Nanchang, China, in 1996 and given strain designation 933 is designated as the influenza A/Nanchang/933/96 virus.

Several features of influenza virus replication are relevant to development of vaccines and antiviral agents. First, influenza A and B virions attach to susceptible cells through the interaction of the hemagglutinin (HA) with cell surface glycoproteins that contain terminal sialic acid. Virus enters the cell by fusion of the virion envelope with the cell membrane, a process that is also mediated by the HA, which must have previously undergone proteolytic cleavage for this event to occur. Transcription and replication of the viral genome takes place in the nucleus (66). In the nucleus, mRNA is synthesized, some mRNAs are spliced, and the genome is replicated by the viral polymerase, a complex of three proteins (PB1, PB2, and PA) (13, 32). The newly synthesized daughter virion RNAs are transported back to the nucleus where the daughter ribonucleoproteins (RNPs) are formed. Envelope proteins are synthesized, undergo a variety of posttranslational modifications, and are inserted in the cell membrane. The progeny viruses are then assembled and released from the cell by budding.

Epidemiology

Influenza epidemics are regularly associated with excess morbidity and mortality in adults (49), and both influenza A and B can be associated with severe illness (11). During interpandemic years, influenza is usually associated with a "U-shaped" epidemic curve. Attack rates are generally highest in the young, while mortality is generally highest in the elderly (49, 50). Excess morbidity and mortality are particularly high in those with certain "high-risk" medical conditions—adults and children with cardiovascular and pulmonary conditions (including asthma) or those requiring regular medical care because of chronic metabolic disease, renal dysfunction, hemoglobinopathies, or immunodeficiency (3, 18). For this reason, these groups are targeted for special efforts toward prevention and therapy.

Influenza and other RNA viruses are increasingly recognized causes of lower respiratory tract disease in immunocompromised individuals. Influenza may result in more severe disease with prolonged virus shedding in those infected with human immunodeficiency virus (HIV) (129). Pneumonitis in recipients of bone-marrow transplantation has been reported with parainfluenza, respiratory syncytial, and influenza virus infection (128). Influenza infection of these individuals is frequently nosocomially acquired (150).

Clinical Manifestations

The onset of influenza is typically abrupt, and the illness is characterized by the predominance of systemic symptoms, including fever, prostration, myalgias, and malaise. Respiratory symptoms may be relatively minimal, particularly early in the course, and include nasal complaints, sore throat, hoarseness, and nonproductive cough. Involvement of tracheal epithelium in infection may lead to complaints of burning throat and sub-

sternal pain. Other than fever, there are usually few findings on physical examination. Affected individuals may exhibit rhinitis, pharyngitis, conjunctival injection, and tracheal tenderness. The chest is usually clear in uncomplicated cases. Most acute symptoms resolve in 3 to 5 days, but complete recovery may take weeks. The clinical features of influenza A and B virus infection are similar.

Influenza is also an important cause of acute febrile illness in children during epidemics. Generally symptoms of influenza are similar to those in adults, although children may have higher fever with febrile seizures. Influenza is associated with otitis media (65), and influenza virus can be isolated from middle ear fluid in affected children (20). Influenza A viruses are an important cause of croup (acute laryngotracheobronchitis) during influenza epidemics (70, 74), with relatively more severe disease than with other viral causes (70).

Pneumonia represents the most severe complication of influenza virus infection in both normal and compromised hosts (81). Primary influenza viral pneumonia is seen predominantly in those with prior cardiac disease. The patient presents with typical features of acute influenza but experiences a rapid progression of dyspnea, cough and cyanosis, and development of adult respiratory distress syndrome. Chest roentgenographs reveal bilateral interstitial infiltrates, sputum production is scanty, and Gram stain reveals few organisms. Secondary bacterial pneumonia may present 1 to 2 weeks after apparent recovery from an acute influenza episode, with recurrence of fever and signs and symptoms of typical lobar pneumonia (130).

Pulmonary function abnormalities are frequently demonstrated in otherwise healthy, nonasthmatic young adults with uncomplicated (nonpneumonic) acute influenza. Demonstrated defects include diminished forced flow rates, increased total pulmonary resistance, and decreased density-dependent forced flow rates consistent with generalized increased resistance in airways less than 2 mm in diameter (57, 80), as well as increased responses to bronchoprovocation (80). In addition, abnormalities of carbon monoxide diffusing capacity (68) and increases in the alveolar-arterial oxygen gradient (71) have been seen. Pulmonary function defects can persist for weeks after clinical recovery.

Diagnostic Tests and Susceptibility

The constellation of typical clinical symptoms during periods of significant influenza epidemic activity highly suggests influenza. Isolation of virus in cell culture from samples of respiratory secretions such as nasopharyngeal (NP) swabs, washes, or throat gargles remains the gold standard of specific viral diagnosis. Renal epithelial cells, such as Madin-Darby canine kidney (MDCK) or rhesus monkey kidney (RhMK) cells are generally used; alternatively, virus can be isolated in embryonated hen's eggs. Virus isolation and identification requires 3 to 5 days.

A variety of techniques have been used to speed this process. Centrifuging samples directly onto cells in shell vials, with detection of viral antigen production by immunofluorescence (IF) or enzyme immunoassay (ELISA) can reduce the time needed to detect virus to 1 or 2 days (40). Viral antigen can be rapidly detected directly in respiratory secretions by a variety of techniques including IF (30), time-resolved immunofluorescence (TRFIA) (146), radioenzyme immunoassay (28), and ELISA (58). The most rapid ELISAs can produce results in less than 1 h, with sensitivity and specificity approaching that of cell culture under optimal conditions. Available formats include filter immunoassays (Directigen flu A) (147) and microtiter plate assays (Enzygnost A and B) (36). The sensitivity of such tests may be higher with NP washes and swabs than with other samples (126). Recently, polymerase chain reaction (PCR) techniques have been described for rapid detection of influenza virus RNA in clinical samples (21, 112).

Due to the relative dearth of available antiviral agents for influenza virus infection and the need to initiate therapy rapidly if it is to be successful, susceptibility testing is not routinely done and is not available in clinical laboratories. As described below, susceptibility of influenza A virus isolates to the antiviral effects of the two clinically available agents, amantadine and rimantadine, can be predicted from the sequence of the membrane-spanning domain of the M2 protein, generally determined by PCR. This testing is available through the CDC and should be performed on isolates of influenza A virus obtained from persons while they are receiving therapy (19). Detection of resistant virus may have clinical implications in closed settings where prophylaxis of contacts is being considered.

SUSCEPTIBILITY IN VITRO AND IN IN VIVO

Both in vitro cell culture and small-animal models of influenza infection are widely available and are used to demonstrate antiviral activity. Traditionally, influenza viruses are propagated in the laboratory in the amniotic or allantoic cavity of embryonated hen's eggs. However, influenza can also be grown in cell culture in a variety of cell lines of epithelial origin; the most commonly used include MDCK cells, RhMK cells, and primary chick kidney cells. Antiviral susceptibility in these cell lines can be demonstrated by plaque reduction assays or virus yield assays. Among small-animal models, the ferret is very attractive because it has a respiratory tract similar to that of humans and develops respiratory disease with fever upon infection with either influenza A or B viruses. Mice have also been used frequently to demonstrate antiviral effects of candidate agents, although they are not a natural host of influenza and generally do not develop illness unless infected with mouse-adapted strains of virus. In certain circumstances, nonhuman primates and porcine and avian models have also been used.

The use of these models has resulted in identification of myriad candidate antivirals, but only amantadine and rimantadine have reached licensure as antiviral drugs for the prevention and treatment of influenza. These compounds are primary symmetric amines with an unusual "bird cage"–like structure (Fig. 1) (34). Both drugs are active against all strains of influenza A virus in a variety of cell culture systems and animal models (33). In cell culture, inhibitory levels for influenza A

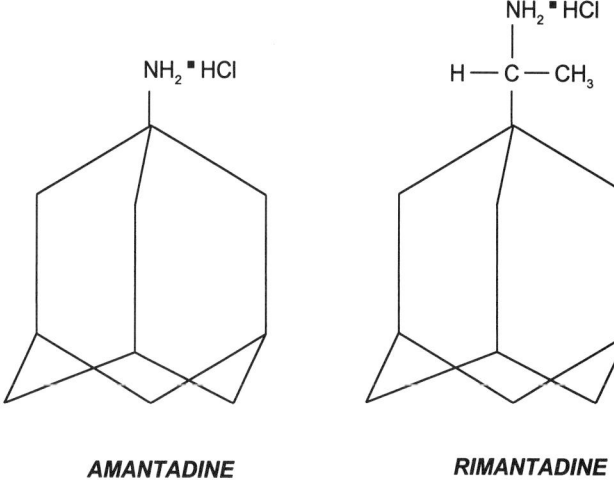

FIGURE 1. Chemical structures of amantadine and rimantadine.

virus range from 0.2 to 0.4 μg/mL for amantadine and from 0.1 to 0.4 μg/mL for rimantadine (37).

Cell culture models, as well as analysis of viral strains resistant to amantadine, have been used to determine that the antiviral activity of these drugs is due to their effects on the M2 protein of susceptible viruses. After entry into the cell, the viral RNPs, containing viral RNA, nucleoprotein, and polymerase proteins, must be transported to the nucleus (84). Cytoplasmic to nuclear transport of the RNPs requires disruption of the association between the M1 protein and the RNPs within the virion, a process referred to as "uncoating." The M2 protein plays a critical role in this process, with the low pH of the endosome triggering the pH-dependent ion channel activity of the influenza A virus M2 protein (111), resulting in transport of H[+] ions into the virion and lowering of the intravirionic pH. The lower intravirionic pH in turn disrupts the RNP-M1 interaction and allows transport of the RNPs to the nucleus (15). It is now known that amantadine and rimantadine bind to the M2 protein of influenza A viruses and interfere with the function of M2 as an ion channel. This effect, then, is primarily seen in cell culture as inhibition of virus uncoating (16, 120, 121, 124). Regulation of the pH of the Golgi apparatus by the M2 protein is also critical in preventing a premature (and irreversible) conformational change of the HA during maturation of this protein to a low pH form that cannot bind to cells (132, 136). Thus amantadine and rimantadine also affect maturation of the HA, although this effect has mostly been documented for avian influenza viruses. The roles of the M2 protein and potential sites of inhibition by rimantadine and amantadine are shown in Figure 2. Similar ion channels have been described for influenza B (BM2) (14, 134) and influenza C (CM2) virus (67). However, amantadine and rimantadine specifically bind only the M2 protein of influenza A viruses and are therefore only active against influenza A at clinically achievable levels.

A variety of other antiviral agents have shown activity against influenza in these model systems. The most promising

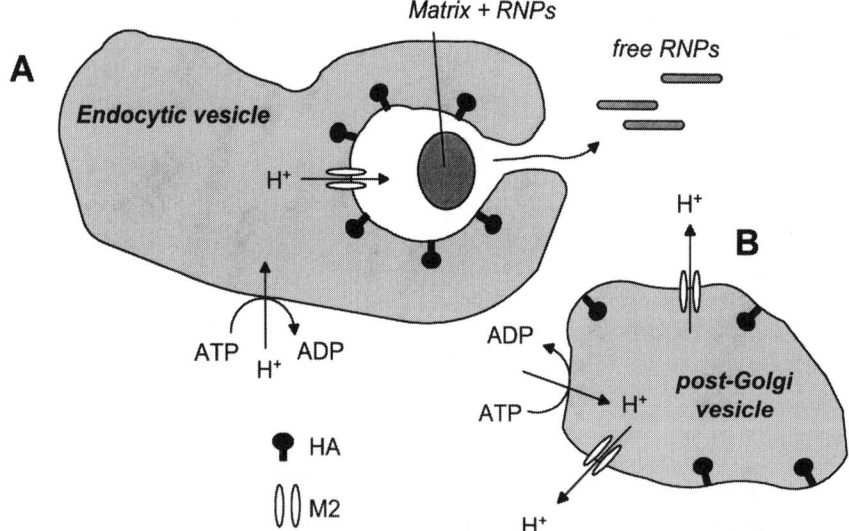

FIGURE 2. The mechanism of action of amantadine involves inhibition of the *M2* protein. M2 is an ion channel thought to be important in two events during virus replication. **A.** Virus enters the cell in an *endocytic vesicle,* the interior of which is acidified by proton pumps. The low pH of the endosome activates the ion channel activity of the M2, and H$^+$ ions enter the interior of the virion, lowering the intravirionic pH. This in turn disrupts the interaction between the M1 protein and the viral *RNPs,* allowing them to be transported into the nucleus. **B.** Acidification of the *post-Golgi vesicle* by cellular proton pumps is countered by M2 to protect the native HA against low pH-induced conformational transition.

agents have been those that inhibit the function of the influenza virus neuraminidase. This enzyme cleaves terminal sialic acid from sialic acid–containing glycoproteins that serve as host cell receptors for attachment of influenza viruses (Fig. 3). As virus replication proceeds within the cell, neuraminidase is synthesized and transported to the cell surface, where it removes the sialic acid from these cell surface glycoproteins. Destruction of these receptors by the neuraminidase allows newly formed viruses to leave the cell and spread to other cells. Studies with mutant neuraminidase-deficient viruses have shown that in the absence of a functional neuraminidase, virus remains attached to the host cell and to other virions (47, 89). In addition, neuraminidase may be important in facilitating the penetration of virus through secretions in the respiratory tract, which are rich in sialic acid–containing macromolecules (27).

Sialic acid analogues are competitive inhibitors of neuraminidase, but early inhibitors, such as Neu5AcEn, were nonspecific and were not effective antivirals (105). The determination of the crystal structure of neuraminidase complexed with sialic acid (144) facilitated development of analogues that strongly and selectively inhibited the neuraminidases of influenza A and B viruses (145). Two such compounds are currently in active clinical development and are likely to become available within the next several years.

Zanamivir (4-guanidino-Neu5Ac2en, GG167) has significant antiviral activity against a wide variety of laboratory and clinical influenza A and B isolates in cell culture and in the mouse and ferret models (145, 153). The drug is not orally bioavailable and is not effective when administered parenterally in animals, apparently because therapeutic levels are not achieved in respiratory secretions (125). Therefore, effective use of this agent requires local administration.

Considerable efforts to develop other neuraminidase inhibitors with potential oral activity are currently under way (93). Recently, a carbocyclic transition state–based inhibitor of influenza virus neuraminidase, GS4071, has been described (73). GS4071 has both neuraminidase-inhibiting and plaque inhibiting activity in vitro against both influenza A and B viruses and potency approximately equal to that of Zanamivir (73). An ester prodrug of this compound, GS4104, is orally bioavailable and active in prevention and treatment of influenza A when administered orally in small animal models. Clinical trials of both Zanamivir and GS4104 are currently in progress. The basic structures of these neuraminidase inhibitors are shown in Figure 3.

Other approaches currently in development include inhibitors of the viral polymerase, the use of bispecific monoclonal antibodies (42), or potential interruption of recently described interactions between the NP (102) and NS1 (152) proteins and cellular proteins, which are probably critical to replication of these viruses.

ANTIVIRAL THERAPY
Drug of Choice

Both amantadine and rimantadine are active in the treatment of experimentally induced and naturally acquired influenza A, and most studies showing lower clinical symptom scores, more rapid reduction of fever, and lower levels and duration of virus shedding than with placebo (Table 1). Amantadine was found to be slightly more effective than aspirin in reducing clinical symptoms of naturally acquired influenza A in young adults (157). In addition, treatment with amantadine results in significantly more rapid improvement in small airways dysfunction in healthy adults with uncomplicated influenza

N-acetyl neuraminyl (α, 2 → 3) lactose

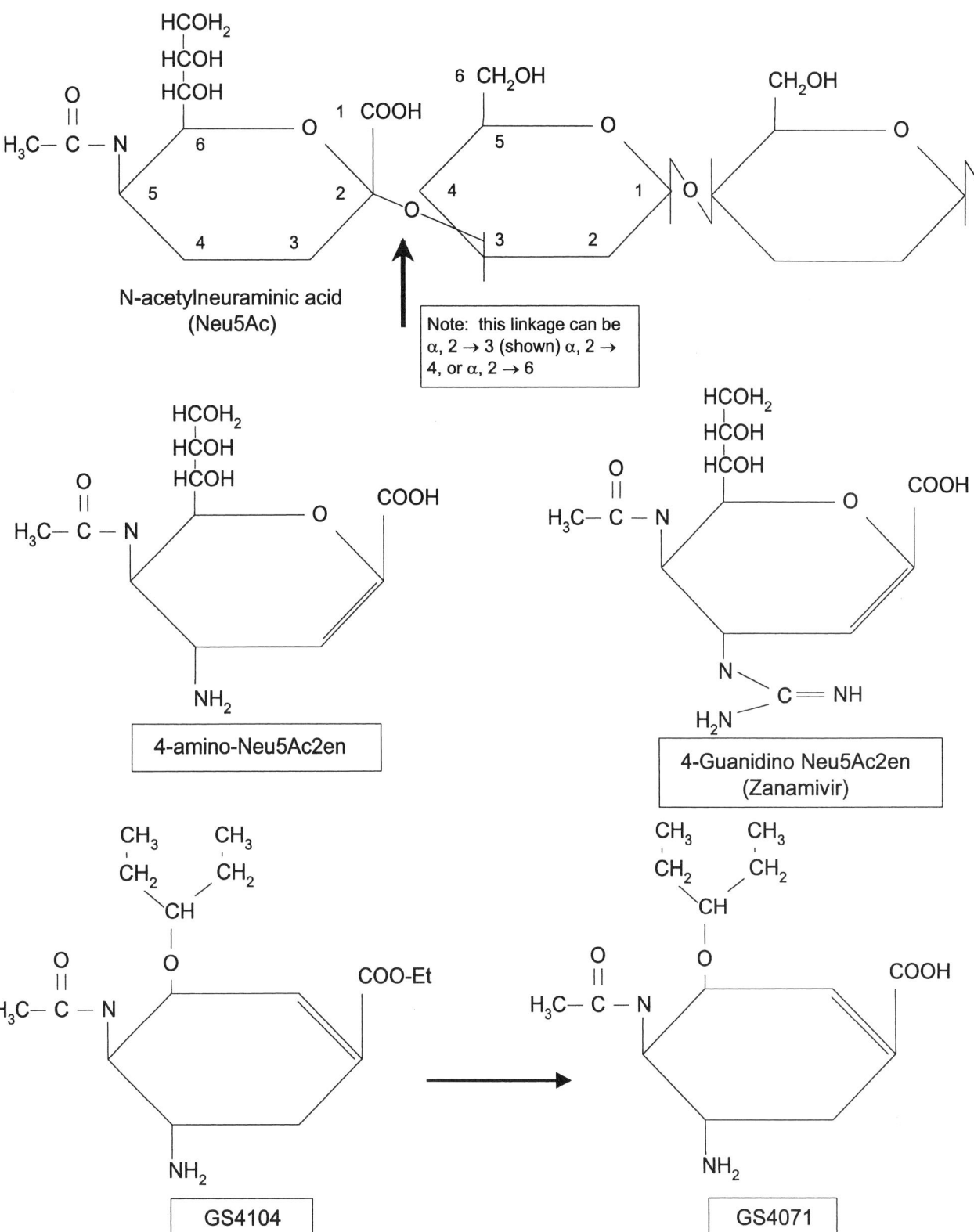

FIGURE 3. Sialic acid is an N-substituted neuraminic acid. In nature, sialic acid is found linked by a ketosidic linkage to D-galactose, D-galactosamine, or possibly other sugars. Sialic acid is always terminal (i.e., the last residue on the chain). The nature of the ketosidic linkage can influence the attachment of HA to the receptor. *4-Amino-Neu5Ac2en,* and *4-guanidino Neu5Ac2en* (Zanamivir) are analogues of sialic acid that are highly potent and specific inhibitors of the neuraminidase by virtue of interactions of the 4-substituted groups with critical residues on this enzyme. *GS4071* is a cyclohexene transition state analogue that also inhibits NA; *GS4104* is an ester prodrug that is active when administered orally.

TABLE 1 • Studies of Amantadine and Rimantadine Therapy

Study	Year	Drug	Study Design	Population	Challenge Virus	Result
H1N1 viruses						
Van Voris et al. (143)	1977	Amantadine	Field trial	Adults	A/USSR/77	Improved symptoms at 48 h and decreased temperature at 24 h vs. placebo; fewer subjects shedding virus at 48 h; very slightly better than rimantadine at 200 mg/day
Van Voris et al. (143)	1977	Rimantadine	Field trial	Adults	A/USSR/77	Improved symptoms at 48 h and decreased temperature at 24 h vs. placebo; fewer subjects shedding virus at 48 h; very slightly worse than amantadine at 200 mg/day
Younkin et al. (151)	1981	Amantadine	Field trial	Adults	A/Brazil/78	Amantadine was associated with more-rapid decrease in symptoms than aspirin or placebo; no difference in virus shedding; 100 mg/day was as effective as 200 mg/day
Thompson et al. (137)	1983	Rimantadine	Field trial	Children	Not specified	Significant decrease in virus shedding on days 1 and 2 following therapy; increase in virus shedding on day 4; no significant differences in symptoms or fever between rimantadine and acetaminophen groups, but very mild illness
H2N2 viruses						
Togo et al [138]	1967	Amantadine	Field trial	Inmates	A/Hong Kong/68	Therapy resulted in 24-h decrease in duration of fever and more subjects considered rapid resolvers; no change in proportion of subjects shedding virus
Hornick et al. (69)	1968	Amantadine	Field trial	Inmates	A/Hong Kong/68	Amantadine was associated with reduction in duration of fever from 88 to 64 h and in increased frequency of "rapid resolution"; no effect on virus shedding or antibody responses
Knight et al. (75)	1969	Amantadine	Field trial	Inmates	A/Hong Kong/68	Subjects who were ill for less than 48 h had more-rapid decrease in cough, sore throat, nasal obstruction, and fever; trend toward decreased virus at 10 h, no effect on antibody response
Galbraith et al. (45)	1969	Amantadine	Field trial	Adults and children	A/Hong Kong/68	Treated subjects had 24-h reduction in duration of fever (75 to 47 h) but no change in symptoms; antibody responses were not affected by therapy.
Hayden and Monto (61)	1983	Rimantadine	Field trial	Adults	A/Bangkok/1/79	Reduced virus shedding; decreased fever and symptom scores on days 2 and 3
Hall et al. (56)	1986	Rimantadine	Field trial	Children	Not specified	Reductions in symptom scores and fever on days 2 and 3; reduced virus on days 2 and 3 with slight increase in titer shed on day 7 relative to acetaminophen; resistant virus shed
Betts et al. (10)	1986	Rimantadine	Field trial	Elderly	Not specified	24-h more rapid return to asymptomatic and afebrile; no significant differences in virus titers
Hayden et al. (63)	1988	Rimantadine	Family	Adults and children	Not specified	Number of days to 50% or greater reduction in symptoms reduced by 2.5 days; no effect on virus shedding; rimantadine recipients shed resistant virus

(79, 80). Rimantadine was also evaluated in the treatment of influenza A in children and shown to reduce the level of virus shedding early in infection, compared with acetaminophen (56, 137). Effects on clinical symptom scores have been more variable; one study showed lower scores and fever than with acetaminophen (56), and the other, in which illness was relatively mild, showed no significant difference (137). In both studies, virus shedding was relatively prolonged in those receiving rimantadine, and resistant virus was shed late in the course of illness. Illness associated with shedding of resistant virus was similar to that associated with drug-sensitive virus. Comparative studies of the efficacy of amantadine or rimantadine in the treatment of more complicated influenza infection (e.g., in hospitalized patients or those with pneumonia) have not been reported. However, most authorities would support the use of amantadine in the treatment of complicated influenza A virus infection, even late in the course of illness (38).

Antiviral drug resistance can result from point mutations at any one of a number of residues within the transmembrane region of M2 (Fig. 4) (7, 59, 82). A single point mutation can cause complete resistance to both drugs, and amantadine- and rimantadine-resistant viruses emerge fairly frequently in treated individuals (60, 63). Resistant virus can be transmitted to, and cause disease in, susceptible contacts (31, 60, 63), and drug-resistant virus retains full pathogenic potential in experimental animals (4, 135). Although resistant virus is seen infrequently in unexposed individuals (6), concern about potential development of resistance has been one factor limiting widespread use of these drugs (91). It has been suggested that combined use of vaccination and amantadine could decrease generation and transmission of resistant viruses (148, 149). The M2 protein remains an attractive target for development of antiviral agents because it is so specific for influenza virus and because highly accurate in vitro screening assays are available (142).

Therapeutic use of these drugs could be considered early in the course of influenza A infection. In deciding to use these drugs therapeutically it is important to consider that they are only active against influenza A virus, so usage should probably be restricted to periods of influenza A virus activity in the community or when accurate rapid viral diagnosis is available. In addition, therapeutic efficacy has only been shown in healthy individuals treated within 48 h of the onset of symptoms, and the possible effects of amantadine or rimantadine therapy on preventing complications among individuals at high risk or in the treatment of more severe disease such as viral pneumonia are unknown. Also, because of the limited available data in children, rimantadine is approved for prophylaxis but not treatment of influenza in children.

Most studies of rimantadine and amantadine have been conducted in healthy adults and have used doses of 200 mg/day given orally in two divided doses. At this dosage, both drugs are associated with mild central nervous system (CNS) side effects: nervousness, difficulty concentrating, and insomnia. These side effects are reversible when drug is discontinued and often disappear on continued use. The rates of CNS side effects appear to be lower in individuals taking rimantadine. More-serious CNS side effects, such as behavioral changes, delirium, and seizures, have been seen in elderly subjects taking amantadine at a dose of 200 mg/day. Thus, a maximum dose of 100 mg/day of amantadine is recommended for individuals over 65. The need to reduce dosage of rimantadine is less clear-cut; currently, it is recommended that nursing home residents receive 100 mg/day, while relatively healthy adults over 65 can receive 200 mg/day with close observation.

More than 90% of amantadine is excreted unchanged, while rimantadine undergoes extensive metabolism. However, both drugs are ultimately excreted by the kidneys, and dosage should be modified for renal dysfunction. Amantadine dosage should be reduced for individuals with a creatinine clearance of 50 mL/min or less, and rimantadine reduced at a creatinine clearance of 10 mL/min or less. In addition, clearance of rimantadine may be reduced in individuals with severe liver disease, and dosage of rimantadine should be reduced in this situation. Because the frequency of seizures with use of these drugs is higher in those with a history of seizure disorder, the drugs should be used with caution in such individuals.

Special Situations

Since there are relatively few options for specific antiviral therapy of influenza, the main clinical decision is whether to use therapy at all. Antiviral therapy has only been shown to be useful when administered early in the course of disease, and it is likely that late complications of influenza, which may occur after the bulk of viral replication has ceased, would not be likely to respond, even to a very effective antiviral agent. For this reason, the primary modality for control of influenza will undoubtedly remain vaccination.

Alternative Therapy

Intranasal Zanamivir was effective in the prophylaxis and therapy of influenza when relatively susceptible young adults were experimentally infected by intranasal drops containing the

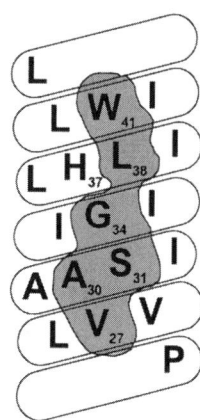

FIGURE 4. Helical net projection of the postulated α-helix of the M2 protein transmembrane region. Mutations associated with decreased antiviral susceptibility to amantadine are shown in *gray*. (Adapted from Holsinger LJ, Nichani D, Pinto LH, Lamb RA. Influenza A virus M2 ion channel protein: a structure-function analysis. J Virol 1994;68:1551–1563.)

A/Texas/36/91 (H1N1) virus. Zanamivir was 82% effective in preventing infection and 95% effective in preventing febrile illness when administered beginning 4 h before virus challenge. In addition, both early treatment (beginning 26–32 h after challenge) and late treatment (beginning 50 h after challenge) reduced virus shedding compared with placebo, and early treatment also reduced symptom scores (64). Preliminary results of treatment of healthy subjects with early, uncomplicated, naturally acquired influenza have also been encouraging (86). Inhaled or combined inhaled and intranasal Zanamivir was associated with a 1 day earlier cessation of symptoms in young adults with naturally acquired influenza who presented within 48 h of the onset of symptoms. Importantly, this study demonstrated potential benefit in healthy adults infected with either influenza A or influenza B; thus these agents represent the first antivirals with clear-cut clinical benefit for influenza B virus in humans (62). Recently, the orally available drug GS4104 was also found effective both for prophylaxis and treatment of infection with influenza A/Texas/91 (H1N1) virus in the human challenge model described above, and further studies of this compound are in progress.

Because these inhibitors interact with highly conserved residues within the influenza virus neuraminidase, it was hoped that antiviral resistance would be relatively limited compared with amantadine and rimantadine. In fact, truly resistant viruses have not been isolated from humans treated with these inhibitors in clinical trials to date. Viruses resistant to the in vitro antiviral activity of GG167 have been isolated after passage in cell culture. Most of these viruses remain sensitive to the neuraminidase-inhibiting activity of GG167, and infections with such viruses remain susceptible to treatment in animal models. Genetic analysis suggests that such pseudoresistant viruses may contain altered HAs with relatively decreased affinity for sialic acid–containing receptors (55). Such mutant viruses may be less dependent on neuraminidase for release from cells. After further passage in the presence of GG167, it is possible to isolate viruses that are resistant to the neuraminidase-inhibiting activity of the drug, associated with a point mutation (Glu-119-Ala) in the NA gene (55). Thus, development of antiviral resistance to GG167 may require prolonged exposure to the inhibitor.

A number of other antiviral drugs have been tested in humans. Ribavirin is active against influenza A and B virus in human challenge models when administered by small particle aerosol (48, 151). However, the relatively limited efficacy of the drug (8) and the cumbersome method of administration have limited its utility in this situation. Intravenous ribavirin has been reported to be useful for the treatment of influenza virus-associated acute myocarditis (116). Intranasal interferon 2, administered as a large-particle aerosol, decreased virus replication and clinical symptoms scores in young adults challenged with influenza A virus (139). However, drug administration was associated with significant local toxicity, which has limited further development of this approach.

Combination Therapy

Combination therapy of influenza in humans has not been evaluated in detail. However, the development of additional safe and effective agents will no doubt lead to studies of this nature. The goal of such a strategy would mainly be to reduce the development of antiviral drug resistance among treated strains. Of note, the combination of vaccination and antiviral therapy was shown to reduce the incidence of isolation of amantadine-resistant viruses in treated birds (149).

Prophylactic Strategies in High-Risk Subjects

Amantadine and rimantadine are effective in the prophylaxis of both experimentally induced and naturally acquired influenza A, with an efficacy of approximately 70 to 90% (Table 2). However, rimantadine is associated with fewer side effects. For example, when both drugs were compared in healthy adults at doses of 200 mg/day versus placebo during an epidemic of predominantly H1N1 influenza A virus, amantadine and rimantadine were equally effective in preventing laboratory-documented influenza A, but withdrawal rates, primarily due to minor CNS side effects, were significantly higher among amantadine recipients (Fig. 5) (35). Amantadine has been shown to be effective in prophylaxis of experimental influenza A (H1N1) in young adults when administered at 100 mg/day (131), with decreased CNS side effects. Relatively less is known about the effectiveness of these drugs in preventing influenza in high-risk subjects. However, preliminary data suggest that rimantadine is effective in preventing influenza A in the elderly or other high-risk individuals and that the protective effect is additive to that provided by inactivated influenza vaccine (10).

To avoid the need to administer drug to large numbers of subjects for prolonged periods, the use of amantadine in prophylaxis of family contacts of index cases during influenza outbreaks has also been evaluated. In one trial, in which both the index case and family members were treated with amantadine, there was no evidence of protection against influenza A (H3N2) (46). In contrast, in a second study performed by the same investigators, but in which the index case was not treated, the rate of laboratory-documented influenza A (H3N2) in household contacts was reduced by 63% (44). More recently, a similar study was performed in which rimantadine was administered to both index cases and family members during outbreaks of H1N1 and H3N2 influenza A. However, the rates of laboratory-documented influenza A infection in family contacts receiving rimantadine did not differ from those in contacts receiving placebo (60). The failure of rimantadine under these circumstances appeared to result from selection of rimantadine-resistant viruses in the treated individuals, which could then spread to family contacts who were receiving rimantadine prophylaxis (60). Illness caused by resistant virus was clinically similar to that caused by sensitive virus.

Amantadine is currently recommended for use during institutional outbreaks of influenza A, a situation that has been compared with an outbreak in a large family (91). While no placebo-controlled, randomized trials have been done to evaluate the use of amantadine under these circumstances, retrospective analyses of such outbreaks support this recommendation (1, 2). These studies have suggested efficacy of amantadine during nosocomial outbreaks among high-risk patients in hospitals as well as

TABLE 2 • **Studies of Amantadine and Rimantadine Prophylaxis**

Study	Year	Drug	Study Design	Population	Challenge Virus	Result
H1N1 viruses						
Monto et al. (93)	1978	Amantadine	Field trial	Adults	A/USSR/77	70.7% reduction in laboratory-confirmed influenza; 39.4% reduction in infection determined serologically
Dolin et al. (35)	1981	Amantadine	Field trial	Adults	A/Brazil/78	Protective efficacy against laboratory-documented influenza A was 91%, but side effects were higher than in those receiving rimantadine
Dolin et al. (35)	1981	Rimantadine	Field trial	Adults	A/Brazil/77	85% protection against laboratory-documented influenza A; less toxic than amantadine
Clover et al. (25)	1984	Rimantadine	Family	Children	Not specified	100% protection against laboratory-documented influenza A; adults also protected
Reuman et al. (119)	1985	Amantadine	Challenge	Adults	A/Bethesda/85	Protective efficacy against illness was 66, 74, and 82%, against infection was 20, 32, and 40%; the lowest dose suppressed serum antibody, higher doses suppressed both nasal and serum antibody responses
Sears and Clements (131)	1986	Amantadine	Challenge	Adults	A/Texas/1/85	Low-dose amantadine provided 78% efficacy against influenza illness; virus shedding was slightly reduced; antibody responses were not affected.
H2N2 viruses						
Quilligan et al. (114)	1964	Amantadine	Field trial	Children	A/Los Angeles64	Approximately 90% reductions in rates of laboratory-confirmed illness while on medication; no significant effect on antibody
Bloomfield et al. (12)	1965	Amantadine	Challenge	Adults	A/Rockville/65	100% protection against laboratory-documented influenza; decreased but not absent antibody responses
Finklea et al. (43)	1965	Amantadine	Field trial	Children	A/AA/1/65	90% reduction in laboratory-documented influenza A
H3N2 viruses						
Oker-Blom et al. (101)	1969	Amantadine	Field trial	Adults	A/Hong Kong/68	68% protection against laboratory-documented influenza, 52% against serologic response
Galbraith et al. (46)	1969	Amantadine	Family	Adults and children	A/Hong Kong/68	No protection, as index case was also treated
Galbraith et al. (44)	1969	Amantadine	Family	Adults and children	A/Hong Kong/68	Protection
Dolin et al. (unpublished)	1983	Rimantadine	Field trial	Elderly	Not specified	Protection against laboratory-documented influenza was 77%
Crawford et al. (29)	1985	Rimantadine	Family	Children	Not specified	60% reduction in laboratory-documented influenza A ($P = .14$)
Hayden et al. (60)	1987	Rimantadine	Family	Adults and Children	Not specified	Rimantadine was not associated with protection because of transmission of resistant virus when the index case is treated

in multiple outbreaks in nursing homes. However, amantadine-resistant virus has also been isolated under these circumstances, with transmission to others (31, 85).

Current recommendations for the use of these drugs have been recently summarized (19). For prophylactic use, amanta-dine and rimantadine should be considered in high-risk individuals and close contacts who have not been vaccinated, who have absolute contraindications to vaccination, or who are expected to have an inadequate antibody response to influenza vaccination because of immunodeficiency. When these drugs

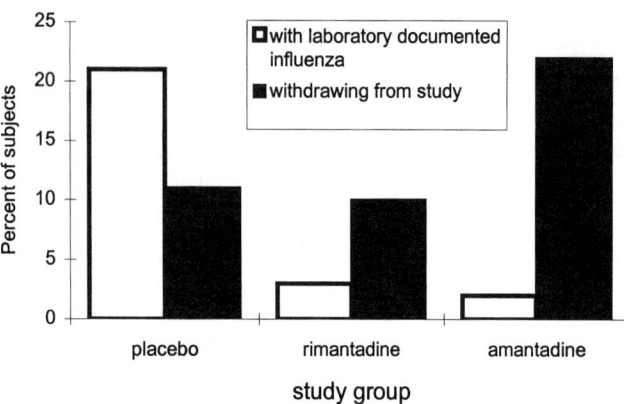

FIGURE 5. Prophylaxis of influenza with amantadine and rimantadine. Both rimantadine and amantadine prevented laboratory-documented influenza, but rimantadine was associated with significantly fewer side effects. (Adapted from Dolin R, Reichman RC, Madore HP, Maynard R, Linton PN, Webber-Jones J. A controlled trial of amantadine and rimantadine in the prophylaxis of influenza A in humans. N Engl J Med 1982;307:580–584.)

are used for seasonal prophylaxis, they should be administered throughout the entire influenza season. Influenza vaccine can still be administered during influenza epidemics; if amantadine or rimantadine are being used to "cover" such a person until vaccine becomes effective, a 2-week course is probably adequate. For control of outbreaks within institutions, these drugs should be administered to both vaccinated and unvaccinated high-risk individuals as soon as possible when a confirmed or suspected outbreak of influenza A is detected. Drug should be administered for 2 weeks, or for 1 week after the outbreak has been terminated. Because of the possibility of spread of drug-resistant virus, efforts should be made to prevent contact between individuals who are receiving the drug therapeutically and those receiving drug prophylaxis within institutions.

COMMERCIALLY AVAILABLE VACCINES

Epidemiologic and experimental observations in humans have shown that infection with influenza virus results in long-lived resistance to reinfection with the homologous virus (99). Influenza viral infection induces both systemic and local antibody, as well as cytotoxic T cell responses, each of which plays a role in recovery from infection and resistance to reinfection.

Two types of vaccines are commercially available or likely to be commercially available within the next several years. Because influenza A (H1N1), A (H3N2), and influenza B viruses cocirculate, both vaccines are administered as a trivalent preparation containing one example of each (sub)type, with specific strains selected for inclusion in the vaccine on the basis of current epidemiologic trends and characterization of antigenic variants.

Inactivated influenza vaccines are designed to induce primarily serum antibody to the hemagglutinin and neuraminidase. The selected viruses are grown in embryonated hens' eggs, and the virions are chemically inactivated. Either whole virus, detergent-treated "split-product," or subunit vaccines can be used. In contrast, the primary goal of live-virus vaccines is induction of mucosal antibody in the respiratory

tract, which appears to play a critical role in preventing influenza infection (118). These vaccines are generated by genetic reassortment between circulating wild-type strains and cold-adapted, attenuated master donor viruses (83). The reassortment vaccine viruses are also grown in embryonated hens' eggs and administered as allantoic fluid.

Indications

Influenza vaccine, the primary modality for preventing influenza, can be used in any individual who wishes to reduce his or her risk of developing this disease. Current recommendations for groups in whom special efforts at vaccination should be targeted are published each year by the US Public Health Service and are summarized in Table 3.

Doses and Schedule

After much trial and error, the dose of inactivated influenza vaccine has been standardized at approximately 15 μg of each hemagglutinin (HA) antigen per 0.5-mL dose, administered by intramuscular injection. This dose appears to give an acceptable combination of immunogenicity, lack of side effects, and reasonable cost of production. Children 35 months of age or younger should receive only 0.25 mL (i.e., 7.5 μg of each HA). The final dose to be chosen for cold-adapted vaccine is still being decided but will likely be on the order of 10^7 to $10^{7.5}$ $TCID_{50}$ per dose, regardless of age. The vaccine is currently being administered as a nasal spray of 0.25 mL to each naris (total 0.5 mL).

Both inactivated and cold-adapted vaccines should be administered in the fall, to provide the greatest potential protection against influenza during the wintertime influenza epidemic season. Inactivated vaccine should be administered as a single dose given annually. However, unprimed individuals

---

TABLE 3 • Target Groups for Influenza Vaccination

Groups at increased risk for influenza related complications:
　Persons 65 years of age
　Residents of chronic care facilities
　Adults and children with chronic pulmonary or cardiovascular disorders
　Adults and children with chronic metabolic disease (including diabetes), renal dysfunction, hemoglobinopathies, or immunosuppression
　Children and adolescents receiving long-term aspirin therapy
Groups that can transmit influenza to high-risk persons defined above:
　Physicians, nurses, and other health care workers
　Employees of hospitals and chronic care facilities
　Providers of home care to high-risk persons
　Household contacts of high-risk persons
In addition, vaccination should be considered in
　Pregnant women
　Individuals with human immunodeficiency virus (HIV) infection
　Individuals who provide essential community services
　Individuals who wish to reduce their chance of acquiring influenza infection

Adapted from 19. CDC. Prevention and control of influenza: recommendations of the Advisory Committee on Immunization Practices (ACIP). MMWR 1996;45(RR-5):1–24.

such as previously unvaccinated children less than 9 years of age or all individuals in the event of antigenic shift should receive a two-dose schedule, with the doses separated by at least 1 month (154, 156). Inactivated vaccine can generally be given safely with other vaccines, such as pneumococcal vaccine.

The most convincing data for efficacy for cold-adapted vaccines in children come from studies using a two-dose regimen (5). Thus, it is anticipated that these vaccines will be recommended for use as a two-dose schedule in children, with the doses separated by approximately 6 weeks. Not enough data exist on the use of these vaccines with other vaccines to make strong recommendations. In adults, a single dose schedule is likely.

No studies on the protective efficacy of cold-adapted vaccine alone have been conducted in the elderly, because of the possibly reduced immunogenicity of the vaccine in this age group. However, the combination of local-live-attenuated influenza vaccine and parenteral inactivated vaccine administered together resulted in approximately 60% fewer cases of laboratory-confirmed influenza in an elderly nursing home population than with inactivated vaccine alone (141). Thus, the strategy for use of these vaccines in the elderly may be simultaneous administration of a single-0.5 mL dose of inactivated vaccine intramuscularly and a 0.5-mL dose of cold-adapted vaccine by intranasal spray each year.

Adverse Effects

Randomized, placebo-controlled trials have shown inactivated influenza vaccines to be well tolerated in all age groups. Mild local reactions occur in a minority of subjects, and systemic symptoms (e.g., malaise, headache, or myalgias) occur at a low rate similar to that with placebo (17, 115, 154). Both whole-virus and split-product vaccines are well tolerated at current doses in adults (78), but whole-virus vaccines are associated with fever in children (156) and should not be used in those under 12 years of age.

Cold-adapted vaccine viruses have also been evaluated in young adults, children, and elderly subjects and found to be reliably attenuated and immunogenic (reviewed in reference 94). Safety has also been demonstrated in high-risk individuals who would not be able to tolerate even minor lower respiratory tract inflammation (e.g., individuals with cystic fibrosis or asthma) (54, 90). Genetic reversion to virulence has not been demonstrated, even in seronegative young children. In addition, there has been no evidence of transmission of cold-adapted vaccine from immunized individuals to unimmunized susceptible contacts, even when vaccine is administered to young children in the day-care setting (155).

Efficacy

Inactivated influenza vaccine was effective in preventing influenza A in several randomized or semirandomized controlled studies conducted in young adults, with levels of protection of 70 to 90% when a good antigenic match existed between vaccine and epidemic viruses (87, 88, 122). Vaccination of young adults also decreases absenteeism from work or school and carries significant cost saving (96). Relatively few

prospective trials of protective efficacy have been conducted in high-risk populations. In one recent randomized, placebo-controlled trial in an elderly population, inactivated vaccine was approximately 58% effective in preventing laboratory-documented influenza (51). In addition, numerous retrospective case-control studies have documented the effectiveness of inactivated influenza vaccines in these individuals (3, 9, 52, 107–109, 123, 127). Vaccine protects against influenza- and pneumonia-related hospitalization in the elderly and is accompanied by a decrease in all-cause mortality (41). It has been estimated that among elderly persons living in the community, influenza vaccination is associated with a direct savings of $117 per year per person vaccinated (97).

Several groups of adults with potentially decreased response to inactivated influenza vaccine have been identified. Individuals with chronic renal disease may respond less well to influenza vaccine (103) and diminished immune responses to vaccination may occur in renal transplant recipients (77, 104, 133). The responsiveness to influenza vaccination in HIV-infected individuals is related to the degree of immunosuppression (95). It has been suggested that the immune activation associated with influenza immunization may transiently stimulate HIV replication (100), but the clinical significance of these observations is unclear. Most patients with chronic lung disease respond reasonably well to vaccination, and steroids at doses commonly used to treat reactive airways disease do not appear to preclude vaccine responses (76, 106). Decreased antibody responsiveness to inactivated influenza vaccine is also seen in older individuals (26, 98, 113, 115, 117, 140).

Studies on the immunogenicity of cold-adapted reassortant vaccines have been carried out in children, adults, and the elderly. Replication of cold-adapted vaccines in the upper respiratory tract and hence the immunogenicity of the vaccine are influenced by the susceptibility of the host at the time of vaccination. The frequency of immune responses to vaccination is thus highest in young children and lowest in elderly subjects who have been repeatedly infected with influenza viruses throughout their lifetimes. Generally, cold-adapted vaccines are more effective than parenterally administered inactivated influenza vaccine at inducing nasal HA-specific IgA, while inactivated vaccine usually induces higher-titered serum HAI- and HA-specific IgG antibody.

Limited field trial evaluations have demonstrated the protective efficacy of cold-adapted reassortant influenza vaccines in children, adults, and the elderly. As expected, the efficacy of these vaccines is particularly good in children less than 6 years of age and may actually exceed that of inactivated vaccine (39, 53, 110). In a recently completed pivotal efficacy trial of trivalent cold-adapted influenza vaccine in 1602 children between 18 and 75 months of age, a two-dose vaccine schedule provided 96% protection against illness associated with isolation of influenza A (H3N2) and 90% protection against illness associated with influenza B (5).

In adults, a recently completed randomized, double-blind trial conducted in 5210 individuals over 5 years showed monovalent cold-adapted vaccine to be approximately equal to inactivated vaccine in preventing laboratory-confirmed influenza illness (39). In addition, the protective efficacy of cold-adapted vaccines in adults is supported by the results of extensive studies of monovalent cold-adapted vaccines in the human challenge model (22, 23) and B (24, 72) with protection at least equaling and sometimes exceeding that provided by inactivated vaccines.

ENDPOINTS FOR MONITORING THERAPY

Individuals being treated with amantadine or rimantadine should be monitored closely for adverse events, and a dosage reduction to 100 mg/day should be considered in the event of early CNS side effects, particularly among elderly patients and those with renal dysfunction. This becomes especially important when these drugs are used for prolonged periods as antiviral prophylaxis. Viral isolates should be obtained from individuals with clinical worsening during therapy or from those who become ill despite prophylaxis, to evaluate for possible antiviral drug resistance, as described above.

REFERENCES

1. Arden NH, Patriarca PA, Fasano MB, Lui K-J, Harmon MW, Kendal AP, Rimland D. The roles of vaccination and amantadine prophylaxis in controlling an outbreak of influenza A(H3N2) in a nursing home. Arch Intern Med 1988;148:865–868.
2. Atkinson WL, Arden NH, Patriarca PA, Leslie N, Lui K-J, Gohd R. Amantadine prophylaxis during an institutional outbreak of type A (H1N1) influenza. Arch Intern Med 1986;146:1751–1756.
3. Barker WH, Mullooly JP. Impact of epidemic type A influenza in a defined adult population. Am J Epidemiol 1980;112:798–813.
4. Bean WJ, Threlkeld SC, Webster RG. Biologic potential of amantadine-resistant influenza A virus in an avian model. J Infect Dis 1989;159:1050–1056.
5. Belshe R, Iacuzio D, Mendelman P, Wolff M. Efficacy of a trivalent live attenuated intranasal influenza vaccine in children. Infectious Diseases Society of America 35th annual meeting, San Francisco, CA, 1997.
6. Belshe RB, Burk B, Newman F, Curruti RL, Sim I. Resistance of influenza A virus to amantadine and rimantadine: results of one decade of surveillance. J Infect Dis 1989;159:430–435.
7. Belshe RB, Smith MH, Hall CB, Betts R, Hay AJ. Genetic basis of resistance to rimantadine emerging during treatment of influenza virus infection. J Virol 1988;62:1508–1512.
8. Bernstein DI, Reuman PD, Sherwood JR, Young EC, Schiff GM. Ribavirin small-particle aerosol treatment of influenza B virus infection. Antimicrob Agents Chemother 1988;32:761–764.
9. Betts RF, Dolin R, Treanor JJ, Roth FK, O'Brien D, Erb S. Inactivated influenza vaccine reduces frequency and severity of illness in the elderly, 24th Interscience Conference on Antimicrobial Agents and Chemotherapy. Washington, DC: American Society for Microbiology, 1984.
10. Betts RF, Treanor J, Braman P, Bentley D, Dolin R. Antiviral agents to prevent or treat influenza in the elderly. J Respir Dis 1987;8:S56–S59.
11. Blaine WB, Luby JP, Martin SM. Severe illness with influenza B. Am J Med 1980;68:181–189.
12. Bloomfield SS, Gaffney TE, Schiff GM. A design for the evaluation of antiviral drugs in human influenza. Am J Epidemiol 1970;91:568–574.
13. Braam J, Ulmanen I, Krug RM. Molecular model of a eukaryotic transcription complex: functions and movement for influenza P proteins during capped RNA-primed transcription. Cell 1983;34:609–618.
14. Brassard DL, Leser GP, Lamb RA. Influenza B virus NB glycoprotein is a component of the virion. Virology 1996;220:350–360.
15. Bui M, Whittaker G, Helenius A. Effect of M1 protein and low pH on nuclear transport of influenza virus ribonucleoproteins. J Virol 1996;70:8391–8401.
16. Bukrinskaya AG, Vorkunova NK, Kornilayeva GV, Narmanbetova RA, Vorkunova GK. Influenza virus uncoating in infected cells and effect of rimantadine. J Gen Virol 1982;60:49–59.
17. Cate TR, Couch RB, Parker D, Baxter B. Reactogenicity, immunogenicity, and antibody persistence in adults given inactivated influenza virus vaccines—1978. Rev Infect Dis 1983;5:737–747.
18. CDC. Prevention and control of influenza: recommendations of the Immunization Practices Advisory Committee (ACIP). MMWR 1992;41:1–17.
19. CDC. Prevention and control of influenza: recommendations of the Advisory Committee on Immunization Practices (ACIP). MMWR 1996;45(RR-5):1–24.
20. Chonmaitree T, Howie V, Truant A. Presence of respiratory viruses in middle ear fluids and nasal wash specimens from children with acute otitis media. Pediatrics 1986;77:698–702.
21. Class ECJ, Sprenger MJW, Kleter GEM, van Beek R, Quint WGV, Masurel N. Type-specific identification of influenza viruses A, B, and C by the polymerase chain reaction. J Virol Methods 1992;39:1–13.
22. Clements ML, Betts RF, Murphy BR. Advantage of live attenuated cold-adapted influenza A virus over inactivated vaccine for A/Washington/80 (H3N2) wild-type virus infection. Lancet 1984;1:704–708.
23. Clements ML, Betts RF, Tierney EL, Murphy BR. Resistance of adults to challenge with influenza A wild-type virus after receiving live or inactivated virus vaccine. J Clin Microbiol 1986;23:73–76.
24. Clements ML, Snyder MH, Sears SD, Maassab HF, Murphy BR. Evaluation of the infectivity, immunogenicity, and efficacy of live cold-adapted influenza B/Ann Arbor/1/86 reassortant virus in adult volunteers. J Infect Dis 1990;161:869–877.
25. Clover RD, Crawford SA, Abell TD, Ramsey CL Jr, Glezen WP, Couch RB. Effectiveness of rimantadine prophylaxis of children within families. Am J Dis Child 1986;140:706–709.
26. Coles FB, Balzano GJ, Morse DL. An outbreak of influenza A(H3N2) in a well immunized nursing home population. J Am Geriatr Soc 1992;40:589–592.
27. Colman PM, Ward CW. Structure and diversity of influenza virus neuraminidase. Curr Top Microbiol Immunol 1985;11:177–255.
28. Coonrod JD, Betts RF, Linnemann Jr CC, Hsu LC. Etiologic diagnosis of influenza A virus by enzymatic radioimmunoassay. J Clin Microbiol 1984;19:361–365.
29. Crawford SA, Clover RD, Abell TD, Ramsey CL Jr, Glezen WP, Couch RB. Rimantadine prophylaxis in children: a follow-up study. Pediatr Infect Dis J 1988;7:379–383.
30. Daisy JA, Lief FS, Friedman HW. Rapid diagnosis of influenza A infection by direct immunofluorescence of nasopharyngeal aspirates in adults. J Clin Microbiol 1979;9:688–692.
31. Degelau J, Somani SK, Cooper SL, Guay DRP, Crossley KB. Amantadine-resistant influenza A in a nursing facility. Arch Intern Med 1992;152:390–392.
32. Detjen BM, St. Angelo C, Katze MG, Krug RM. The three influenza virus polymerase (P) proteins not associated with viral

nucleocapsids in the infected cell are in the form of a complex. J Virol 1987;61:13–22.

33. Dolin R. Antiviral chemotherapy and chemoprophylaxis. Science 1985;227:1296–1303.

34. Dolin R. Amantadine and rimantadine. Antimicrob Agents Ann 1988;3:361–370.

35. Dolin R, Reichman RC, Madore HP, Maynard R, Linton PN, Webber-Jones J. A controlled trial of amantadine and rimantadine in the prophylaxis of influenza A in humans. N Engl J Med 1982;307:580–584.

36. Doller G, Schuy W, Tjhen KY, Stekeler B, Gerth H-J. Direct detection of influenza virus antigen in nasopharyngeal specimens by direct enzyme immunoassay in comparison with quantitating virus shedding. J Clin Microbiol 1992;30:866–869.

37. Douglas RL Jr. Prophylaxis and treatment of influenza. N Engl J Med 1990;322:443–450.

38. Douglas RL Jr. Treatment of influenza [Letter]. N Engl J Med 1992;322:1–53.

39. Edwards KM, dupont WD, Westrich MK, Plummer WDJ, Palmer PS, Wright PF. A randomized controlled trial of cold-adapted and inactivated vaccines for the prevention of influenza A disease. J Infect Dis 1994;169:68–76.

40. Espy MJ, Smith TF, Harmon MW, Kendal AP. Rapid detection of influenza virus by shell vial assay with monoclonal antibodies. J Clin Microbiol 1986;24:677–679.

41. Fedson DS, Wajda A, Nicol JP, Hammond GW, Kalser DL, Roos LL. Clinical effectiveness of influenza vaccination in Manitoba. JAMA 1993;270:1956–1961.

42. Fernandez-Sesma A, Schulman JL, Moran TM. A bispecific antibody recognizing influenza A virus M2 protein redirects effector cells to inhibit virus replication in vitro. J Virol 1996;70: 4800–4804.

43. Finklea JF, Hennessy AV, Davenport FM. A field trial of amantadine prophylaxis in naturally occurring acute respiratory illness. Am J Epidemiol 1967;85:403–412.

44. Galbraith AW, Oxford JS, Schild GC. Protective effect of 1-adamantanamine hydrochloride on influenza A2 in the family environment. Lancet 1969;2:1026–1028.

45. Galbraith AW, Oxford JS, Schild GC, Potter CW, Watson GI. Therapeutic effect of 1-adamantanamine hydrochloride in naturally occurring influenza A2/Hong Kong infection. Lancet 1971;1:113–115.

46. Galbraith AW, Oxford JS, Schild GC, Watson GI. Study of 1-adamantanamine hydrochloride used prophylactically during the Hong Kong influenza epidemic in the family environment. Bull WHO 1969;41:677–682.

47. Garcia-Sastre A, Palese P. The cytoplasmic tail of the neuraminidase protein of influenza A virus does not play an important role in the packaging of this protein into viral envelopes. Virus Res 1995;37:37–47.

48. Gilbert BE, Wilson SZ, Knight V, Couch RB, Quarles JM, Dure L, Hayes N, Willis G. Ribavirin small-particle aerosol treatment of infections caused by influenza virus strains A/Victoria/7/83 (H1N1) and B/Texas/1/84. Antimicrob Agents Chemother 1985; 27:309–313.

49. Glezen WP. Serious morbidity and mortality associated with influenza epidemics. Epidemiol Rev 1982;4:24–44.

50. Glezen WP, Keitel WA, Taber LH, Piedra PA, Clover RC, Couch RB. Age distribution of patients with medically-attended illnesses caused by sequential variants of influenza A/H1N1: comparison to age-specific infection rates, 1978–1989. Am J Epidemiol 1991;133:296–304.

51. Govaert TM, Thijs CT, Masurel N, Sprenger MJ, Dinant GJ, Knottnerus JA. The efficacy of influenza vaccination in elderly individuals. A randomized double-blind placebo-controlled trial. JAMA 1994;270:1956–1961.

52. Gross PA, Quinnan GV, Rodstein M, LaMontagne JR, Kaslow RA, Saah AJ, Wallenstein S, Neufeld R, Denning C, Gaerlan P. Association of influenza immunization with reduction in mortality in an elderly population: a prospective study. Arch Intern Med 1988;148:562–565.

53. Gruber WC, Belshe RB, King JC, Treanor JJ, Piedra PA, Wright PF, Reed GW, Anderson E, Newman F. Evaluation of live attenuated influenza vaccines in children 6–18 months of age: safety, immunogenicity, and efficacy. J Infect Dis 1996;173: 1313–1319.

54. Gruber WC, Campbell PW, Thompson JM, Reed GW, Roberts B, Wright PF. Comparison of live attenuated and inactivated influenza vaccines in cystic fibrosis patients and their families: results of a 3-year study. J Infect Dis 1994;169:241–247.

55. Gubareva LV, Bethell R, Hart GJ, Murti KG, Penn CR, Webster RG. Characterization of mutants of influenza A selected with the neuraminidase inhibitor 4-guanidino-Neu5Ac2en. J Virol 1996;70:1818–1827.

56. Hall CB, Dolin R, Gala CL, Markovitz DM, Zhang YQ, Madore PH, Disney FA, Talpey WB, Green JL, Francis AB, Pichichero ME. Children with influenza A infection: treatment with rimantadine. Pediatrics 1987;80:275–282.

57. Hall WJ, Douglas RL Jr, Hyde RW, Roth FK, Cross AS, Speers DM. Pulmonary mechanics after uncomplicated influenza A infection. Am Rev Respir Dis 1976;113.

58. Harmon MW, Pawlik KM. Enzyme immunoassay for direct detection of influenza type A and adenovirus antigens in clinical specimens. J Clin Microbiol 1982;15:5–11.

59. Hay AJ, Wolstenholme AJ, Skehel JJ, Smith MH. The molecular basis of the specific anti-influenza action of amantadine. EMBO J 1985;4:3021–3024.

60. Hayden FG, Belshe RB, Clover RD, Hay AJ, Oakes MG, Soo W. Emergence and apparent transmission of rimantadine-resistant influenza A virus in families. N Engl J Med 1989;321:1696–1702.

61. Hayden FG, Monto AS. Oral rimantadine hydrochloride therapy of influenza A virus H3N2 subtype infection in adults. Antimicrob Agents Chemother 1986;29:339–341.

62. Hayden FG, Osterhaus ADME, Treanor JJ, Fleming DM, Aoki FY, Nicholson KG, Bohnen AM, Hirst HM, Keene O, Wightman K. Efficacy and safety of the neuraminidase inhibitor GG167 (Zanamivir) in the treatment of influenza virus infections. N Engl J Med 1997;337:874–880.

63. Hayden FG, Sperber SJ, Belshe RB, Clover RD, Hay AJ, Pyke S. Recovery of drug-resistant influenza A virus during therapeutic use of rimantadine. Antimicrob Agents Chemother 1991; 35: 1741–1747.

64. Hayden FG, Treanor JJ, Betts RF, Lobo M, Esinhart JD, Hussey EK. Safety and efficacy of the neuraminidase inhibitor GG167 in experimental human influenza. JAMA 1996;275:295–299.

65. Henderson FW, Collier AM, Sanyal MA, Watkins JM, Fairclough DL, Clyde WA, Jr, Denny FW. A longitudinal study of respiratory viruses and bacteria in the etiology of acute otitis media with effusion. N Engl J Med 1982;306:1377–1383.

66. Herz C, Stavnezer E, Krug RM, Gurney TJ. Influenza virus, an RNA virus, synthesizes its messenger RNA in the nucleus of infected cells. Cell 1981;26:391–400.

67. Hongo S, Sugawara K, Muraki Y, Kitame F, Nakamura K. Characterization of a second protein (CM2) encoded by RNA segment 6 of influenza C virus. J Virol 1997;71:2786–2792.

68. Horner GJ, Gray FL Jr. Effect of uncomplicated, presumptive influenza on the diffusing capacity of the lung. Am Rev Respir Dis 1973;108:866–869.

69. Hornick RB, Togo Y, Mahler S, Iezzoni D. Evaluation of amantadine hydrochloride in the treatment of A2 influenzal disease. Bull WHO 1969;41:671–676.

70. Howard JB. Influenza A2 virus as a cause of croup requiring tracheostomy. J Pediatr 1972;81:1148–1150.

71. Johanson WGJ, Pierce AK, Sanford JP. Pulmonary function in uncomplicated influenza. Am Rev Respir Dis 1969;100: 141–146.

72. Keitel WA, Couch RB, Cate TR, Six HR, Baxter BD. Cold-recombinant influenza B/Texas/1/84 virus vaccine: attenuation, immunogenicity, and efficacy against homotypic challenge. J Infect Dis 1990;161:22–26.

73. Kim CU, Lew W, Williams MA, Liu H, Zhang L, Swaminathan S, Bischofberger N, Chen MS, Mendel DB, Tai CY, Laver WG, Stevens RC. Influenza neuraminidase inhibitors possessing a novel hydrophobic interaction in the enzyme active site: design, synthesis, and structural analysis of carbocyclic sialic acid analogues with potent anti-influenza activity. J Am Chem Soc 1997; 119:681–690.

74. Kim HW, Brandt CD, Arrobio JO, Murphy B, Chanock RM, Parrott RH. Influenza A and B virus infection in infants and young children during the years 1957–1976. Am J Epidemiol 1979;109:464–479.

75. Knight V, Fedson D, Baldini J, Douglas RL Jr, Couch RB. Amantadine therapy of epidemic influenza A2 (Hong Kong). Infect Immun 1970;1:200–204.

76. Kubiet MA, Gonzalez-Rothi RJ, Cottey R, Bender BS. Serum antibody response to influenza vaccine in pulmonary patients receiving corticosteroids. Chest 1996;110:367–370.

77. Kumar SS, Ventura AK, VanderWerf B. Influenza vaccination in renal transplant recipients. JAMA 1978;239:840–842.

78. LaMontagne JR, Noble GR, Quinnan GV, Curlin GT, Blackwelder WC, Smith JI, Ennis FA, Bozeman FM. Summary of clinical trials of inactivated influenza vaccine—1978. Rev Infect Dis 1983;5:723–736.

79. Little J, Hall W, Douglas RGJ, Hyde RW, Speers DM. Amantadine effect on peripheral airways abnormalities in influenza. Ann Intern Med 1976;85:177–182.

80. Little JW, Hall WJ, Douglas RL Jr, Mudholkar GS, Speers DM, Patel K. Airway hyperreactivity and peripheral airway dysfunction in influenza A infection. Am Rev Respir Dis 1978;118:295–303.

81. Louria DB, Blumenfeld HL, Ellis JT, Kilbourne ED, Rogers DE. Studies on influenza in the pandemic of 1957–1958. II. Pulmonary complications of influenza. J Clin Invest 1959;38: 213–265.

82. Lubeck MD, Schulman JL, Palese P. Susceptibility of influenza A viruses to amantadine is influenced by the gene coding for the M protein. J Virol 1978;28:710–716.

83. Maassab HF, DeBorde DC. Development and characterization of cold-adapted viruses for use as live virus vaccines. Vaccine 1985;3:335–369.

84. Martin KAH. Transport of incoming influenza virus nucleocapsids into the nucleus. J Virol 1991;65:232–244.

85. Mast EE, Harman MW, Gravenstein S, Wu S-P, Arden NH, Circo R, Tyska G, Kendal AP, Davis JP. Emergence and possible transmission of amantadine-resistant viruses during nursing home outbreaks of influenza A(H3N2). Am J Epidemiol 1991; 134:988–997.

86. Matsumoto K, Nerome K, Numasaki Y, Oguri K, Fukuda T. Inhaled and intranasal GG167 in the treatment of influenza A and B: preliminary results. In: Bron LE, Hampson AW, Webster RG, eds. Options for the control of influenza III. Amsterdam: Elsevier, 1996:713–717.

87. Meiklejohn G. Viral respiratory disease at Lowry Air Force Base in Denver, 1952–1982. J Infect Dis 1983;148:775–783.

88. Meiklejohn G, Eickhoff TC, Graves PIJ. Antigenic drift and efficacy of influenza virus vaccines, 1976–1977. J Infect Dis 1978;138:618–624.

89. Mitnaul LJ, Castrucci MR, Murti KG, Kawaoka Y. The cytoplasmic tail of influenza A virus neuraminidase (NA) affects NA incorporation into virions, virion morphology, and virulence in mice but is not essential for virus replication. J Virol 1996;70: 873–879.

90. Miyazaki C, Nakayama M, Tanaka Y, Kusuhara K, Okada K, Tokugawa K, Ueda K, Shibata R, Nishima S, Yamane N, Maassab HF. Immunization of institutionalized asthmatic children and patients with psychomotor retardation using live attenuated cold-adapted reassortment influenza A H1N1, H3N2, and B vaccines. Vaccine 1993;11:853–858.

91. Monto AS, Arden NH. Implications of viral resistance to amantadine in control of influenza A. Clin Infect Dis 1992;15: 362–367.

92. Monto AS, Gunn RA, Bandyk MG, King CL. Prevention of Russian influenza by amantadine. JAMA 1979;241:1003–1007.

93. Murakami M, Ikeda K, Achiwa K. Chemoenzymatic synthesis of neuraminic acid analogs structurally varied at C-5 and C-9 as potential inhibitors of the sialidase from influenza virus. Carbohydrate Res 1996;280:101–110.

94. Murphy BR. Use of live, attenuated cold-adapted influenza A reassortant virus vaccines in infants, children, young adults, and elderly adults. Infect Dis Clin Pract 1993;2:176–181.

95. Nelson KE, Clements ML, Miotti P, Cohn S, Polk BF. The influence of human immunodeficiency virus (HIV) infection on antibody responses to influenza vaccines. Ann Intern Med 1988;109:383–388.

96. Nichol KL, Lind A, Margolis KL, Murdoch M, McFadden R, Hauge M, Magnan S, Drake M. The effectiveness of vaccination against influenza in healthy, working adults. N Engl J Med 1995;333:889–893.

97. Nichol KL, Margolis KL, Wuorenma J, Von Sternberg T. The efficacy and cost effectiveness of vaccination against influenza among elderly persons living in the community. N Engl J Med 1994;331:778–784.

98. Nicholson KG, Baker DJ, Chakraverty P, Parquhar A, Hurd D, Kent J, Litton PA, Smith SH. Immunogenicity of inactivated influenza vaccine in residential homes for elderly people. Age Ageing 1992;21:182–188.

99. Noble GR. Epidemiologic and clinical aspects of influenza. In: Beare AS, ed. Basic and applied influenza research. Boca Raton, FL: CRC Press, 1982:1–79.

100. O'Brien WA, Ferbas-Grovit K, Namazi A, Ovcak-Derzic S, Wnag H-J, Park J, Yermian C, Mao S-H, Zack JA. Human immunodeficiency virus–type 1 replication can be increased in peripheral blood of seropositive patients after influenza vaccination. Blood 1995;86:1082–1089.

101. Oker-Blom N, Hovi T, Leinikki P, Palosuo T, Pettersson R, Suni J. Protection of man from natural infection with influenza A2 Hong Kong virus by amantadine: a controlled field trial. Br Med J 1970;3:676–678.

102. O'Neill RE, Palese P. NPI-1, the human homolog of SRP-1, interacts with influenza virus nucleoprotein. Virology 1995;206: 116–125.

103. Pabico RC, Douglas RG Jr, Betts RF, McKenna BA, Freeman RB. Influenza vaccination of patients with glomerular diseases: effects on creatinine clearance, urinary protein excretion, and antibody response. Ann Intern Med 1974;81:171–177.

104. Pabico RC, Douglas RG Jr, Betts RF, McKenna BA, Freeman RB. Antibody response to influenza vaccination in renal transplant patients: correlation with allograft function. Ann Intern Med 1976;85:431–436.

105. Palese P, Schulman JL. Inhibitors of the viral neuraminidase as potential antiviral drugs. In: Oxford JS, ed. Chemoprophylaxis and viral infections of the respiratory tract, vol 1. Boca Raton, FL: CRC Press, 1977:189–205.

106. Park CL, Frank AL, Sullivan M, Jindal P, Baxter BD. Influenza vaccination of children during acute asthma exacerbation and concurrent prednisone therapy. Pediatrics 1996;98:196–200.

107. Patriarca PA, Weber JA, Parker RA, Hall WN, Kendal AP, Bregman DJ, Schonberger LB. Efficacy of influenza vaccine in nursing homes: reduction in illness and complications during an influenza A (H3N2) epidemic. JAMA 1985;253:1136–1139.

108. Patriarca PA, Weber JA, Parker RA, Orenstein WA, Hall WN, Kendal AP, Schonberger LB. Risk factors for outbreaks of influenza in nursing homes: a case-control study. Am J Epidemiol 1986; 124:114–119.

109. Paul WS, Cowan J, Jackson GG. Acute respiratory illness among immunized and nonimmunized patients with high-risk factors during a split season of influenza A and B. J Infect Dis 1988;157:633–639.

110. Piedra PA, Glezen WP. Influenza in children: epidemiology, immunity, and vaccines. Semin Pediatr Infect Dis 1992;2:140–146.

111. Pinto LH, Holsinger LJ, Lamb RA. Influenza virus M2 protein has ion channel activity. Cell 1992;69:517–528.

112. Pisareva M, Bechtereva T, Plyusnin A, Dobretsova A, Kisselev O. PCR-amplification of influenza A virus specific sequences. Arch Virol 1992;125:313–318.

113. Powers DC, Belshe RB. Effect of age on cytotoxic T lymphocyte memory as well as serum and local antibody responses elicited by inactivated influenza vaccine. J Infect Dis 1993;197:584–592.

114. Quilligan JJ, Harayama M, Baernstein HL Jr. The suppression of A2 influenza in children by the chemoprophylactic use of amantadine. J Pediatrics 1966;69:572–575.

115. Quinnan GV, Schooley R, Dolin R, Ennis FA, Gross P, Gwaltney JL Jr. Serologic responses and systemic reactions in adults after vaccination with monovalent A/USSR/77 and trivalent A/USSR/77, A/Texas/77, B/Hong Kong/72 influenza vaccines. Rev Infect Dis 1983;5:748–757.

116. Ray CG, Icenogle TB, Minnich LL, Copeland JG, Grogan TM. The use of intravenous ribavirin to treat influenza virus-associated acute myocarditis. J Infect Dis 1989;159:829–836.

117. Remarque EJ, van Beek WC, Ligthart GJ, Borst RJA, Nagelkerken L, Palache AM, Sprenger MJW, Masurel N. Improvement of the immunoglobulin subclass response to influenza vaccine in elderly nursing-home residents by the use of high-dose vaccines. Vaccine 1993;11:649–654.

118. Renegar KB, Small PAJ. Passive transfer of local immunity to influenza virus by IgA antibody. J Immunol 1991;146:1972–1978.

119. Reuman PD, Bernstein DI, Keefer MC, Young EC, Sherwood JR, Schiff GM. Efficacy and safety of low dosage amantadine hydrochloride as prophylaxis for influenza A. Antiviral Res 1989;11:27–40.

120. Richman DD, Hostetler KY, Yazaki PJ, Clark S. Fate of influenza A virion proteins after entry into subcellular fractions of LLC cells and the effect of amantadine. Virology 1986;151:200–210.

121. Richman DD, Yazaki P, Hoestetler KY. The intracellular distribution and antiviral activity of amantadine. Virology 1981;112:81–90.

122. Ruben FL. Prevention and control of influenza: role of vaccine. Am J Med 1987;82:31–33.

123. Ruben FL, Johnston F, Streiff EJ. Influenza in a partially immunized population: effectiveness of killed Hong Kong vaccine against infection with the England strain. JAMA 1974;230:863–866.

124. Ruigrok RWH, Hirst EMA, Hay AJ. The specific inhibition of influenza A virus maturation by amantadine: an electron microscopic examination. J Gen Virol 1991;72:191–194.

125. Ryan DM, Ticehurst J, Dempsey MH, Penn CR. Inhibition of influenza virus replication in mice by GG167 (4-guanidino-2,4-dideoxy-2,3-dehydro-N-acetylneuraminic acid) is consistent with extracellular activity of viral neuraminidase (sialidase). Antimicrob Agents Chemother 1994;38:2270–2275.

126. Ryan-Pourier KA, Katz JM, Webster RG, Kawaoka Y. Application of directagen FLU-A for the detection of influenza A virus in human and non-human specimens. J Clin Microbiol 1992;30:1072–1075.

127. Saah AJ, Neufeld R, Rodstein M, La Montagne JR, Blackwelder W, Bross P, Quinnan G, Kaslow R. Influenza vaccine and pneumonia mortality in a nursing home population. Arch Intern Med 1986;146:2353–2357.

128. Sable CA, Hayden FG. Orthomyxoviral and paramyxoviral infections in transplant recipients. Infect Transplant 1995;9:987–1003.

129. Safrin S, Rush JD, Mills J. Influenza in patients with human immunodeficiency virus infection. Chest 1990;98:33–37.

130. Schwarzmann SW, Adler JL, Sullivan RFJ, Marine WM. Bacterial pneumonia during the Hong Kong influenza epidemic of 1968–1969. Arch Intern Med 1971;127:1037–1041.

131. Sears SD, Clements ML. Protective efficacy of low-dose amantadine in adults challenged with wild-type influenza A virus. Antimicrob Agents Chemother 1987;31:1470–1473.

132. Shimbo K, Brassard DL, Lamb RA, Pinto LH. Ion selectivity and activation of the M2 ion channel of influenza virus. Biophys J 1996;70:1335–1346.

133. Stiver HG, Graves P, Meiklejohn G, Schroter G, Eickhoff TC. Impaired serum antibody response to inactivated influenza A and B vaccine in renal transplant recipients. Infect Immun 1977;16:738–741.

134. Sunstrom NA, Premkumar LS, Premkumar A, Ewart G, Cox GB, Gage PW. Ion channels formed by NB, an influenza B protein. J Membrane Biol 1996;150:127–132.

135. Sweet C, Hayden FG, Jakeman KJ, Grambas S, Hay AJ. Virulence of rimantadine-resistant human influenza A(H3N2) viruses in ferrets. J Infect Dis 1991;164:969–972.

136. Takeuchi K, Lamb RA. Influenza virus M2 protein ion channel activity stabilizes the native form of fowl plague virus hemagglutinin during intracellular transport. J Virol 1994;68:911–919.

137. Thompson J, Fleet W, Lawrence E, Pierce E, Morris L, Wright P. A comparison of acetaminophen and rimantadine in the treatment of influenza A infection in children. J Med Virol 1987;21:249–255.

138. Togo Y, Hornick RB, Felitti VJ, Kaufman ML, Dawkins AL Jr, Kilpe VE, Claghorn JL. Evaluation of the therapeutic efficacy of amantadine in patients with naturally occurring A2 influenza. JAMA 1970;211:1149–1156.

139. Treanor J, Dolin R, Betts RF, Erb S, Roth F, Reichman RC. Intranasal interferon as prophylaxis against experimentally induced influenza in humans. J Infect Dis 1987;156:379–383.

140. Treanor J, Dumyati G, O'Brien D, Riley MA, Riley G, Erb S, Betts R. Evaluation of cold-adapted, reassortant influenza B virus vaccines in elderly and chronically ill adults. J Infect Dis 1994;169:402–407.

141. Treanor JJ, Mattison HR, Dumyati G, Yinnon A, Erb S, O'Brien D, Dolin R, Betts RF. Protective efficacy of combined live intranasal and inactivated influenza A virus vaccines in the elderly. Ann Intern Med 1992;117:625–633.

142. Tu Q, Pinto LH, Luo G, Shaughnessy MA, Mullaney D, Kurtz S, Krystal M, Lamb RA. Characterization of inhibition of M2 ion channel activity by BL-1743, an inhibitor of influenza A virus. J Virol 1996;70:4246–4252.

143. Van Voris LP, Betts RF, Hayden FG, Christmas WA, Douglas RL Jr. Successful treatment of naturally occurring influenza A/USSR/77 H1N1. JAMA 1981;245:1128–1131.

144. Varghese JN, Laver WG, Colman PM. Structure of the influenza glycoprotein antigen neuraminidase at 2.9A resolution. Nature 1983;303:35–40.

145. von Itzstein M, Wu W-Y, Kok GB, Pegg MS, Dyason JC, Jin B, Phan TV, Smythe ML, White HF, Oliver SW, Colman PM, Varghese JN, Ryan DM, Woods JM, Bethell RC, Hotham VJ, Cameron JM, Penn CR. Rational design of potent sialidase-based inhibitors of influenza virus replication. Nature 1993; 363:418–423.

146. Walls HH, Johansson KH, Harmon MW, Halonen PE, Kendal AP. Time-resolved fluoroimmunoassay with monoclonal antibodies for rapid diagnosis of influenza infections. J Clin Microbiol 1986;24:907–912.

147. Waner JL, Todd SJ, Shalaby H, Murphy M, Wall LV. Comparison of directigen FLU-A with viral isolation and direct immunofluorescence for the rapid detection and identification of influenza A virus. J Clin Microbiol 1991;29:479–482.

148. Webster RG, Kawaoka Y, Bean WJ. Vaccination as a strategy to reduce the emergence of amantadine- and rimantadine-resistant strains of A/Chick/Pennsylvania/83 (H5N2) influenza virus. J Antimicrobial Chemother 1986;18:157–164.

149. Webster RG, Kawaoka Y, Bean WJ, Beard CW, Brugh M. Chemotherapy and vaccination: a possible strategy for the control of highly virulent influenza virus. J Virol 1985;55:173–176.

150. Whimbey E, Eling LS, Couch RB, Lo W, Williams L, Champlin RE, Bodey GP. Influenza A virus infection among hospitalized adult bone marrow transplant recipients. Bone Marrow Transplant 1994;13:437–440.

151. Wilson SZ, Gilbert BE, Quarles JM, Knight V, McClung HW, Moore RV, Couch RB. Treatment of influenza A (H1N1) virus infection with ribavirin aerosol. Antimicrob Agents Chemother 1984;26:200–203.

152. Wolff T, O'Neill RE, Palese P. Interaction cloning of NS1-I, a human protein that binds to the nonstructural NS1 proteins of influenza A and B viruses. J Virol 1996;70:5363–5372.

153. Woods JM, Bethell RC, Coates JAV, Healy N, Hiscox SA, Pearson BA, Ryan DM, Ticehurst J, Tilling J, Walcott SM, Penn CR. 4-Guanidino-2,4-dideoxy-2,3-dehydro-N-acetylneuraminic acid is a highly effective inhibitor both of the sialidase (neuraminidase) and of growth of a wide range of influenza A and B viruses in vitro. Antimicrob Agents Chemother 1993;37:1473–1479.

154. Wright PF, Cherry JD, Foy HM, Glezen WP, Hall CB, McIntosh K, Monto AS, Parrott RH, Protnoy B, Taber LH. Antigenicity and reactogenicity of influenza A/USSR/77 virus vaccine in children—a multicentered evaluation of dosage and toxicity. Rev Infect Dis 1983;5:758–764.

155. Wright PF, Johnson PR, Karzon DT. Clinical experience with live, attenuated vaccines in children. In: Kendal AP, Patriarca PA, eds. Options for the control of influenza. New York: Alan R Liss, 1986:243–253.

156. Wright PF, Thompson J, Vaughn WT, Folland DS, Sell SHW, Karzon DT. Trials of influenza A/New Jersey/76 virus vaccine in normal children: an overview of age-related antigenicity and reactogenicity. J Infect Dis 1977;136:S731–S741.

157. Younkin SW, Betts RF, Roth FK, Douglas RL Jr. Reduction in fever and symptoms in young adults with influenza A/Brazil/78 H1N1 infection after treatment with aspirin or amantadine. Antimicrob Agents Chemother 1983;23:577–582.

Molluscum and Other Poxviruses

Gregory W. Hammond

POXVIRUSES

Humans can be infected by four distinct genera of poxviruses (14). The morphology of three of these (orthopoxviruses, yatapoxviruses, and molluscipox), appears similar by negative-stain electron microscopy, resembling a brick-shaped structure. Ovipox genus viruses are ovoid and have a criss-crossed appearance on negative-stain electron microscopy. Molluscum are considered separately from the other three genera, which are grouped together.

ORTHOPOXVIRUSES, YATAPOXVIRUSES AND OVIPOXVIRUSES
General Description

Poxviruses are the largest animal viruses (220–450 by 140–260 nm), and contain over 100 structural proteins. The virus gene is very large with double-stranded linear DNA ranging from 140 to 210 kbp. The virus genome may rearrange during replication, which occurs in the cell cytoplasm. The genome contains regions that are closely homologous to genes that regulate cell activity. Because of its many virus-encoded genes, its replication is relatively independent of host cell enzymatic activity and products.

Variola (smallpox) is now a historical curiosity. The last human case was diagnosed in 1977, and in 1980 the World Health Organization declared smallpox eradicated. A simple and inexpensive immunization with live attenuated vaccines produced from vaccinia virus, produces lifelong immunity. The last remaining stocks of variola virus exist in laboratories in Atlanta and Moscow. With the exception of molluscipoxvirus (12) discussed below, the remaining poxvirus infections are all zoonoses, a result of contact transmission from animals. Monkeypox is an orthopoxvirus with a mortality rate of up to 17% and no known treatment. Cases usually result from contact with primates in westcentral Africa. Members of the yatapoxvirus genus can be transmitted by direct contact with monkeys (yabapox) or blood-sucking insects transmitting viruses from primates (tanapox) in westcentral Africa. Aside from fever, the infection results in localized, firm, and elevated skin lesions, which become necrotic and heal spontaneously after 2 to 4 weeks.

Members of the parapoxvirus genus include viruses transmitted from domestic animals including orf (which produces painful ulcerative lesions accompanying lymph node enlargement and fever) and milker's nodule lesions, which are up to 2 cm in size, papular, vascular, nonulcerated, and nonpainful and resolve after 6 weeks. Orf is spread from direct contact with sheep, goats, and reindeer and may be found in exposed individuals who work in livestock-related occupations, abattoir workers and occasionally those who work with wild animals. Milker's nodule may occur in dairy cattle handlers. Patients with milker's nodule may develop erythema multiforme–type localized eruption. Both infections are found worldwide.

Susceptibility Data

No susceptibility data are published for poxviruses.

Antiviral Therapy

There was no known effective antiviral therapy for systemic infection with vaccinia virus, although generic methisazone (1-methylisatin, 3-thiosemicarbazone, or Marboran) has been used (1). Prophylactic treatment of smallpox contacts with methisazone had some success (1). Treatment of milker's nodule is generally curettage followed by cautery (15).

Vaccines

Smallpox vaccine at 10-year intervals is recommended for laboratory workers in the United States who work with vaccinia virus in a laboratory level 2 setting (22). However, vaccinia virus immunization of laboratory workers in the United Kingdom is not a routine requirement (2). Disseminated or progressive vaccinia virus infections can occur in individuals who are immunocompromised. Local reactions to vaccinia virus were not uncommon, but even in individuals with a normal immune system, occasionally more severe disseminated infections led to encephalitis, or in individuals with eczema, lesions called exzema vaccinatum developed. There was no known ef-

fective antiviral therapy for systemic infection of vaccinia virus, although Marboran has been used (1).

Poxviruses as Vaccine Vectors

There are a number of reasons why poxviruses are candidate vectors of potential human vaccines for infectious diseases, cancer, or immunotherapy (19, 22, 25, 26). These viruses are very large and can incorporate large genomic fragments of foreign DNA. They minimize any effects on the host cell genome because they replicate entirely within cellular cytoplasm. There is also a great deal of experience using poxviruses as vaccines for humans, and the major side effects were rare enough to allow widespread use of the vaccine in the general public. Further attenuated strains of vaccinia virus have been developed that have even less virulence. NYVAC is highly attenuated by specific deletion of 18 genes of the Copenhagen strain of vaccinia virus and is therefore more desirable as a potential vaccine vector (19).

Other potential poxvirus vaccine vectors are those derived from other species, such as an avipoxvirus, canarypox virus, which does not replicate in mammalian species but expresses protein from inserted genes. A cloned isolate of canarypox called ALVAC can produce effective immunization as a recombinant vaccine (19). Both NYVAC and ALVAC have been used to immunize humans and have acceptable safety records (19). Recombinant vaccinia viruses that express genes of other microorganisms have been used to immunize animals in experimental studies when it was particularly difficult to purify the microorganism's protein antigen. Recombinant vaccinia vectors have also been used to infect autologous or MHC-matched cells, which can be challenged with chromium-labeled effector lymphocytes to determine the target site of cellular immunity (22).

Human Vaccines with Recombinant Poxvirus Vaccines

Recombinant vaccinia virus has been used to express the envelope gene of human immunodeficiency virus type 1 (HIV-1). In phase one clinical trials, no serious adverse effects developed in healthy individuals who received inoculations percutaneously (6, 13). Individuals who had been previously immunized with vaccinia virus vaccines had lower cellular and humoral immune responses than vaccinia-naive subjects (6). Higher antibody titers to HIV-1 envelope were detected in recipients of vaccinia/envelope recombinant vaccines followed by a boost with rpg 160 than with either alone (6, 13). An Epstein-Barr virus membrane glycoprotein has been expressed in recombinant vaccinia virus given to infants and young children in China. Natural infection was prevented or delayed over a 16-month period. Rabies glycoprotein from canarypox virus vectors has been expressed in immunized humans, and the antibody titers reached levels considered protective but were not as high as those with a licensed rabies vaccine (5). Another recombinant canarypox virus vaccine that expressed HIV-1 glycoprotein did not produce measurable cellular and humoral immunity initially (28). However, priming was thought to have occurred because the rgp 160 booster injection produced both humoral and cellular immunity. Use of a nonreplicating live vector such as recombinant canarypox virus enhances the safety of poxvirus vaccines in humans (28).

Poxvirus Vectors for Antitumor Therapy

Poxvirus vectors such as NYVAC and ALVAC recombinants produce effective cellular immunity. Strong cellular immunity is thought to be more important in host defense against tumors than humoral immunity (26). Recombinant vaccines for tumor immunotherapy could be produced by expressing tumor associated antigens from the host's tumors. Immune responses might be further enhanced by incorporation of genes for biologic response modifiers such as cytokines to boost tumor immunity (19, 26). Other approaches using poxvirus vaccines could be for adoptive immunotherapy, in which mononuclear cells are expanded and stimulated ex vivo via the recombinant vaccine and reintroduced into the patient. Alternatively, active immunotherapy has been produced using cancer cells that have been genetically modified by recombinant viruses to stimulate host immunity. Studies examining these concepts have been conducted in animal models (19, 25, 26). In summary, highly attenuated replication-deficient poxviruses as well as strains that are restricted by host-range requirements (such as canarypox virus) have been shown effective in immunizing humans. There is great therapeutic potential in these virus vectors for protective immunization or boosting the host's immune response to a wide variety of infectious, malignant, and immune-related diseases.

MOLLUSCIPOX VIRUS
General Description

Molluscum contagiosum virus (20, 30,) is a natural infection of humans with a worldwide distribution (12). The virus is transmitted by direct human-to-human contact, including genital contact, by fomites in the environment such as towels, or through invasive procedures such as tattooing (20). Infections with molluscum contagiosum are more common in children; 31 of 6424 (0.48%) children with cancer treated at St. Jude Children's Hospital had molluscum contagiosum virus infections (17). This rate of infection appears no higher than the rate in children without cancer. Cases usually occur in individuals, but occasional outbreaks have been described (24). The incubation period is 2 weeks to 3 months. Two genotypes of molluscum contagiosum virus have been described (7), and type 1 appears more common. The appearance of lesions does not differ between type 1 and type 2, although type 2 is thought to be more common in individuals past adolescence. In one study, molluscum contagiosum virus type 2 was not detected in children under 15 years of age (29). There is no anatomic preference for either type in genital or nongenital lesions (29).

The genome of molluscum contagiosum virus major subtype 1 has recently been sequenced (34); 103 of its predicted 163 genome products have homology to smallpox virus, but 59 predicted molluscum contagiosum virus genome products are uncharacterized. Based upon similarities to known genomic sequences, many of these predicted molluscum contagiosum virus gene products encode for proteins that may interfere with the host immune response. These include homologues to major histocompatibility complex class I antigens, chemokines, and glutathione peroxidase. These three gene products may thus be expected to interfere with presentation of molluscum contagiosum virus–specific peptides, reduce inflammation through antagonism to chemokines, and protect from host oxidative damage, respectively.

Clinical Appearance

The clinical appearance of molluscum contagiosum varies, depending upon the immune state of the host. In a nonimmunocompromised individual, the lesions tend to be smaller and have a more limited clinical course. Typical lesions are small (2–5 mm in diameter) raised, and dome-shaped with central umbilication. They are usually flesh colored, although they may be whitish. Some patients may have surrounding erythema (molluscum dermatitis) or the lesions themselves may be inflammatory. Most lesions are asymptomatic and painless, although some may be itchy. Lesions may be distributed anywhere, although palms and soles are rare locations. Adults may exhibit lesions in the genital area, which may reflect sexual transmission. Spontaneous resolution is the usual clinical course, which occurs over a period of several months and may take longer. A biopsy may be required to differentiate molluscum from other lesions. In immunocompromised individuals, the lesions tend to be larger, more widespread, progressive, difficult to treat, and often recurrent. Molluscum contagiosum has been described in a wide variety of immunocompromised individuals, including patients with HIV infection and AIDS (27, 33), common variable hypogammaglobulinemia accompanied by cell-mediated immunity impairment (3), immunosuppression from transplantation, following corticosteroid and methotrexate therapy, selective IgM deficiency (21), and sarcoidosis (27). Molluscum contagiosum virus lesions in HIV-infected individuals tend to be larger than normal and have an atypical location, mainly on the face, neck, and scalp (27). Eyelid lesions may cause keratoconjunctivitis (31). Molluscum contagiosum lesions in immunocompromised patients have proven very difficult to treat, and a biopsy should be done in these patients to confirm the diagnosis prior to beginning therapy (11).

Susceptibility In Vitro and In Vivo

No information is available on antiviral susceptibility for molluscipox viruses, primarily because molluscum contagiosum virus cannot be cultivated in artificial systems (30).

Antiviral Treatment

Most lesions in healthy individuals resolve spontaneously. However, treatment may be indicated primarily for cosmetic reasons and to reduce the possibility of autoinoculation to other sites and potential spread to other individuals. In hosts with normal immunity, the general principle has been mechanical removal of the molluscum lesion. Physical removal of the molluscum lesion is the most common approach, usually by scraping with curettage, although there do not appear to be controlled clinical trials on the best way to remove molluscum lesions mechanically. Another approach uses cryotherapy with liquid nitrogen. CO_2 laser treatment has also been used, but in one report, four of six individuals were left with keloid scars as a result of this modality (9). Following removal of the lesion, a variety of usually chemical means are used to cause desquamation of the remaining molluscum lesion and surrounding skin. These chemical agents are usually caustic and include 1% tincture of iodine, trichloroacetic acid, or podophyllin (23). Electrodesiccation is a mechanical means of desquamation that may be combined with curettage or used alone for small lesions.

To make mechanical removal of these lesions more comfortable for children, one randomized double-blind placebo-controlled study showed that EMLA cream (eutectic mixture of local anesthetics), a mixture of 2.5% lidocaine and 2.5% prilocaine anesthetic cream, given 15 to 60 min prior to curettage provides almost complete pain relief, contrasted with placebo (8). This confirmed an earlier open trial (32). On rare occasions, general anesthesia may be needed before mechanical removal of multiple molluscum lesions (18).

Other combination treatment involves simple mechanical expression of the cheesy material that makes up the molluscum lesions followed by electrodesiccation or a caustic agent, including silver nitrate, carbolic acid, tincture of iodine, podophyllin, phenol, or the other caustic agents mentioned above (12).

Topical chemical treatment to the top surface with a pointed cotton-tipped applicator alone has been used to treat small molluscum lesions. Chemicals used have included cantharidin applied topically in an equal mixture of collodion and acetone in a 0.9% solution (10). A weaker solution of 0.5% collodion was not effective. Regimens have included treating alternate lesions at 7-day intervals. For lesions larger than 2 mm or when initial response to cantharidin was poor, the edges of the lesion were also treated to help lesion removal (10).

Another chemical treatment uses tretinoin (retinoic acid, or topical vitamin A acid) (35), which thought to act through inflammatory response of the skin to this compound, which stimulates release of proteolytic and hydrolytic enzymes (35). Concentrations of vitamin A acid ranging from 0.05% to 0.1% applied twice daily or once at night have been effective.

Systemic treatment has been confined to a small range of compounds, one of which is methisazone (1-methylisatin, 3-thiosemicarbazone), which has been used in treatment of other poxvirus infections (1). An early study showed no benefit from methisazone for three patients with molluscum (1). Methisazone may have helped a single individual with multiple lesions and atopic dermatitis who had failed earlier treatment with curettage, electrodesiccation, and CO_2 cryotherapy. The initial dose of methisazone was 1.5 g, then 700 mg every 6 h for 8 doses, all given orally. This treatment appeared to prevent formation of new lesions. Existing lesions were not initially affected but were eliminated after follow-up topical treatment with 1% tincture of iodine applied to molluscum lesions that were opened and removed (4). A high rate of vomiting in early smallpox trials, resulted in the conclusion that methisazone should not be used for "trivial conditions" (1).

Treatment of immunocompromised individuals, especially those with severe cellular immune defects, is largely ineffective. No local or systemically effective therapy exists for molluscum contagiosum lesions in severely immunocompromised

patients such as HIV-infected patients (33). One study of seven patients reported treatment of HIV-infected patients with skin peels produced by trichloroacetic acid topically in concentrations from 25 to 50%, repeated every 2 weeks as needed (11). This did reduce lesion count an average of 40.5% in the seven patients, but usually the lesions slowly recurred. There were no complications of dissemination of new lesions, scarring, local infection, or delayed healing. The authors believed this treatment might be a useful adjunct for atypical lesions or when other therapies failed.

Zidovudine (200 mg orally every 4 h) was held responsible for improvement in a single HIV-infected patient (2). This patient with 105 CD_4 cells/mm^3 had multiple facial papules that had not responded to repeated curettage, electrodessication, and topical retinoic acid. His response to zidovudine was part of a general overall improvement, and his skin lesions disappeared within 1 month (2). Another example of improvement of molluscum contagiosum virus lesions after antiretroviral therapy was reported, associated with use of ritonavir (16). The report postulated that the improvement was due to improved immunologic function following the use of ritonavir plus zidovudine and lamivudine.

Control of molluscum contagiosum virus lesions in some patients with T-lymphocyte counts below 200 cells/mL^3 was achieved using cantharidin for up to 24 h for the treatment of body and facial lesions, or curettage for more persistent lesions or lesions of the eyelid. This was supplemented with tretinoin cream to a concentration that could be tolerated, applied nightly to the involved facial areas. Interferon treatment (1×10^6 units intravenously daily then 2×10^6 units intravenously three times per week for 5 weeks) was ineffective for disseminated molluscum contagiosum virus lesions in a child with IgM deficiency and heterogenous for other immunologic disorders (21). However, the author cites a Japanese report of cure of molluscum contagiosum virus lesions with local treatment of interferon (21).

Further studies are needed for effective chemotherapy of molluscum contagiosum virus lesions, especially in immunocompromised individuals in whom treatment remains very difficult and successful outcomes very elusive.

Vaccines

No vaccines exist for molluscipox viruses.

Endpoints for Monitoring Therapy

Patients should have follow-up evaluation approximately 6 weeks after initial treatment, as this corresponds to the incubation period for new lesion formation. When sexually active individuals have genital lesions, their sexual partners should be examined to prevent reinfection and to rule out other possible sexually transmitted diseases. Molluscum lesions in the genital area of young children may raise questions of possible sexual abuse, although they may result from autoinoculation by the child.

REFERENCES

1. Bauer DJ. Clinical experience with the antiviral drug marboran. Ann NY Acad Sci 1965;130:110–117.

2. Betlloch I, Pinazo I, Mestre F, Altés J, Villalonga C. Molluscum contagiosum in human immunodeficiency virus infection: Response to zidovudine. Int J Dermatol 1989;28:351–352.

3. Ben-Amitai D, Metzker A, Hodak E, Cohen I, Garty BZ. Molluscum contagiosum in a patient with common variable hypogammaglobulinemia. Isr J Med Sci 1994;30:707–709.

4. Blattner RJ. Molluscum contagiosum: eruptive infection in atopic dermatitis. J Pediatr 1967;70:997–999.

5. Cadoz M, Strady A, Meignier B, Taylor J, Tartaglia J, Paoletti E, Plotkin S. Immunization with canarypox virus expressing rabies glycoprotein. Lancet 1992;339:1429–1432.

6. Cooney, EL, McElrath MJ, Corey L, Hu S-L, Collier AC, Arditti D, Hoffman M, Coombs RW, Smith GE, Greenberg PD. Enhanced immunity to human immunodeficiency virus (HIV) envelope elicited by a combined vaccine regimen consisting of a priming with a vaccinia recombinant expressing HIV envelope and boosting with gp 160 protein. Proc Natl Acad Sci USA 1993; 90:1882–1886.

7. Darai G, Reisner H, Scholz J, Schnitzler P, Lorbacher, de Ruiz H. Analysis of the genome of molluscum contagiosum virus by restriction endonuclease analysis and molecular cloning. J Med Virol 1986;18:29–39.

8. de Waard-van der Spek FB, Oranje AP, Lullieborg S, Hop WCJ, Stolz E. Treatment of molluscum contagiosum using a lidocaine/prilocaine cream (EMLA) for analgesia. J Am Acad Dermatol 1990;4:685–688.

9. Friedman M, Gal D. Keloid scars as a result of CO_2 laser for molluscum contagiosum. Obstet Gynecol 1987;70:394–396.

10. Funt TR. Cantharidin treatment of molluscum contagiosum. Arch Dermatol 1961;83:504–505.

11. Garrett SJ, Robinson JK, Roenick HH. Trichloroacetic acid peel of molluscum contagiosum in immunocompromised patients. J Dermatol Surg Oncol 1992;18:855–858.

12. Gottleib SL, Myskowski PL. Review. Molluscum contagiosum. Int J Dermatol 1994;33:453–461.

13. Graham BS, Matthews TJ, Belshe RB, Clements ML, Dolin R, Wright PF, Gorse GJ, Schwartz PH, Keefer MC, Bolognesi DP, Corey L, Stablein DM, Esterlitz JR, Hu S-L, Smith GE, Fast PE, Koff WC. Augmentation of human immunodeficiency virus type 1 neutralizing antibody by priming with gp 160, recombinant vaccinia and boosting with rgp 160 in vaccinia-naive adults. J Infect Dis 1993;167:533–537.

14. Hammond GW. Poxviridae. In: Long SS, Pickering LK, Prober, CG, eds. Pediatric infectious diseases. New York: Churchill Livingstone, 1997:1129–1133.

15. Hansen SK, Mertz H, Krogdahl A, Veien K. Milker's nodule — a report of 15 cases in the county of North Jutland. Acta Derm Venereol (Stockh) 1995;76:88.

16. Hicks CB, Myers SA, Giner J. Resolution of intractable molluscum contagiosum in a human immunodeficiency virus-infected patient after institution of anti-retroviral therapy with ritonavir. Clin Infec Dis 1997;24:1023–1025.

17. Hughes WT, Parham DM. Molluscum contagiosum in children with cancer or acquired immunodeficiency syndrome. Pediatr Infect Dis J 1991;10:152–156.

18. Kaye JW. Problems in therapy of molluscum contagiosum. Arch Dermatol 1966;94:454–455.

19. Limbach KJ, Paoletti E. Non-replicating expression vectors: applications in vaccine development and gene therapy. Epidemiol Infect 1996;116:241–256.

20. Mark R, Buller L, Palumbo GJ. Poxvirus pathogenesis. Microbiol Rev 1991;55:80–122.

21. Mayumi M, Yamaoka K, Tsutsui T, et al. Selective immunoglobulin M deficiency associated with disseminated molluscum contagiosum. Eur J Pediatr 1986;145:99–103.

22. Moss B. Genetically engineered poxviruses for recombinant gene expression, vaccination and safety. Proc Natl Acad Sci USA 1996;93:11341–11348.

23. Olansky S, Clair A. How we treat molluscum contagiosum. Postgrad Med 1970;47:259–260.

24. Oren B, Wende SO. An outbreak of molluscum contagiosum in a kibbutz. Infection 1991;3:159–161.

25. Paoletti E. Application of pox virus vectors to vaccination: an update. Proc Nat Acad Sci USA 1996;93:11349–11353.

26. Perkus ME, Tartaglia J, Paoletti E. Poxvirus based vaccine candidates for cancer, AIDS and other infectious diseases. J Leukocyte Biol 1995;58:1–13.

27. Petersen CS, Gerstoff J. Molluscum contagiosum in HIV-infected patients. Dermatol 1992;184:19–21.

28. Pialoux G, Excler J-L, Rivière Y, Gonzalez-Canali G, Feuillie V, Couland P, Gluckman JC, Matthews TJ, Meignier B, Kieny MP, Gonnet P, Diaz I, Meric C, Paoletti E, Tartaglia J, Salamon H, Plotkin S. A prime-boost approach to HIV preventive vaccine using a recombinant canarypox virus expressing glycoprotein 160 (MN) followed by a recombinant glycoprotein 160 (MN/LAI). AIDS Res Hum Retroviruses 1995;11:373–381.

29. Porter CD, Blake NW, Archard LC, Muhlemann MF, Rosedale N, Cream JJ. Molluscum contagiosum virus types in genital and non-genital lesions. Br J Dermatol 1989;120:37–41.

30. Postlethwaite R. Molluscum contagiosum; a review. Arch Environ Health 1970;21:432–452.

31. Robinson MR, Udell IJ, Garber PF, Perry HD, Streeten BW. Molluscum contagiosum of the eyelids in patients with acquired immune deficiency syndrome. Opthalmology 1992;99:1745–1747.

32. Rosdahl I, Edmar B, Gisslén H, Nordin P, Lillieborg S. Curettage of molluscum contagiosum in children: analgesia by topical application of a lidocaine/prilocaine cream (EMLA). Acta Derm Venereol (Stockh) 1988;68:149–153.

33. Schwartz JJ, Myskowski PL. Molluscum contagiosum in patients with human immunodeficiency virus infection. A review of twenty-seven patients. J Am Acad Dermatol 1992;27: 583–588.

34. Senkevich TG, Bugert JJ, Sisler JR, Koonin EV, Darai G, Moss B. Genomic sequence of a human tumorigenic poxvirus: prediction of specific host response-evasion genes. Science 1996;273: 813–816.

35. Thomas JR III, Doyle JA. The therapeutic uses of topical vitamin A acid. J Am Acad Dermatol 1981;4:505–513.

Norwalk Virus

●

Jason Rosé and Harry Greenberg

GENERAL DESCRIPTION
Virology

Norwalk virus, a member of the family *Caliciviridae,* is identified as a small (27–32 nm) spherical particle in stool samples, with an amorphous surface morphology. The viral particle contains one major structural protein surrounding a single positive-stranded polyadenylated genomic RNA. A number of small round structured viruses (SRSVs) that display morphologic characteristics similar to those of Norwalk virus have been identified in outbreaks of diarrheal illness. Many, but not all, of these SRSVs have been sequenced and shown to be human caliciviruses, of which Norwalk virus is the prototype. Norwalk and related viruses cannot yet be grown in tissue culture.

Epidemiology

Norwalk virus has classically been associated with food- and waterborne outbreaks of acute nonbacterial gastroenteritis in adults and older children. Transmission of Norwalk and related viruses in food appears to be a major route of infection, with as many as 90% of nonbacterial food-related gastroenteritis outbreaks having been associated with these viruses (3). This virus is not associated with a significant number of severe infections of young children, but that seroprevalence rises dramatically in older children and adults. Serologic studies indicate that Norwalk infections have year-round occurrence and are responsible for approximately 35 to 40% of all outbreaks of acute viral gastroenteritis.

Clinical Manifestations

Norwalk illness is generally mild and self-limited, with symptoms lasting only 2 to 3 days after a mean incubation period of 24 h. In adult volunteer studies, the illness was characterized by sudden onset of vomiting and diarrhea. Nausea and abdominal cramping were common, and a significant number of infected individuals also reported fever and chills. In acute outbreaks, diarrhea predominates in children, while more adults experience vomiting (9). Virus shedding during disease peaked at 3 days postinfection, although sensitive detection methods could detect virus up to 7 days after infection (4).

Pathogenesis

Volunteer studies have also provided considerable data on pathologic changes associated with Norwalk infection. Examination of the proximal small intestine showed broadening and blunting of villi, along with lengthening of crypts and infiltration of round cells into the lamina propria (1). Norwalk infection is associated with transient malabsorption of fat, D-xylose, and lactose, as well as decreased gastric motor function. This last effect may be responsible for the high incidence of nausea and vomiting in infected individuals (11).

Laboratory Diagnosis

Norwalk and related viruses cannot be cultured from infected individuals and are excreted in low enough levels in stool that immunoelectron microscopy (IEM) is required to detect viral particles. Provisional diagnosis of Norwalk infection can be made in the setting of an epidemic of gastroenteritis if bacterial pathogens are not present, vomiting occurs in more than 50% of individuals, and the duration of illness and mean incubation period fall within the periods described above.

Polymerase chain reaction (PCR) and reverse transcriptase (RT)-PCR methods have been established that allow sequencing of genes from Norwalk and other SRSVs. The use of PCR primers has permitted characterization of many of these particles as caliciviruses and allowed them to be placed into distinct genogroups (12). PCR and sequencing methods have proven more sensitive than IEM for identification and classification of these agents. New ELISA methods using recombinant Norwalk capsid protein have been developed that are more sensitive than PCR methods and are specific for detection of Norwalk virus (4, 5). These assays remain largely the province of research laboratories and are not yet widely available.

SUSCEPTIBILITY IN VIVO

Despite attempts to infect a number of animal species with Norwalk virus, no species has been identified that displays clinical symptoms after inoculation. Chimpanzees do develop a serologic response after inoculation and shed detectable levels of Norwalk antigen in their stool (13). Most studies on the pathogenesis of Norwalk have come from human volunteer studies or from examining the effects of porcine or bovine calicivirus infection in piglets and calves, respectively (8). Inoculation of calves with these agents leads to weight loss and diarrhea within 2 to 4 days. Lesions in the intestines of cattle resemble those seen in human volunteers, suggesting that infection of the appropriate hosts with these viruses could be useful for studying the pathophysiology of Norwalk and other caliciviruses in human.

ANTIMICROBIAL CHEMOTHERAPY

At this time no specific antiviral agent is available.

VACCINES

Vaccination strategies for Norwalk virus have so far focused on the use of nonreplicating vaccines. It was recently reported that viruslike particles of Norwalk virus could be generated by expressing the capsid protein (6), although little is currently known about the role or long-term effectiveness of T- or B-cell-mediated immunity in protection from Norwalk infection. Some questions have been raised about the usefulness of a Norwalk vaccine for preventing illness. Volunteer studies showed that individuals with a high preinfection titer of anti-Norwalk antibodies were not significantly protected from infection. In fact, in a number of surveys, a higher preinfection antibody titer against Norwalk was associated with more significant illness than in individuals with low or nonexistant titers (2, 4, 7). Studies suggest that there is a short-term, serotype-specific immunity to Norwalk for up to 3 to 6 weeks postinfection, which may not protect against challenges at later times. Because of these findings, the precise role of antibody in Norwalk immunity is unclear, and it is uncertain whether a vaccine would be able to protect individuals from infection. Experiments with recombinant capsid protein immunization (10) may reveal a more detailed picture of Norwalk immunity.

REFERENCES

1. Agus SG, Dolin R, Wyatt RG, Tousimis AJ, Northrup RS. Acute infectious nonbacterial gastroenteritis: intestinal histopathology. Histologic and enzymatic alterations during illness produced by the Norwalk agent in man. Ann Intern Med 1973;79:18–25.
2. Farstad IN, Halstensen TS, Lazarovits AI, Norstein J, Fausa O, Brandtzaeg P. Human intestinal B-cell blasts and plasma cells express the mucosal homing receptor integrin $\alpha_4\beta_7$. Scand J Immunol 1995;42:662–672.
3. Gastroenteritis PWPo. Foodborne viral gastroenteritis: an overview (with a brief comment on hepatitis A). PHLS Microbiol Dig 1988:69–75.
4. Graham DY, Jiang X, Tanaka T, Opekun AR, Madore HP, Estes
5. Green KY, Lew JF, Jiang X, Kapikian AZ, Estes MK. Comparison of the reactivities of baculovirus-expressed recombinant Norwalk virus capsid antigen with those of the native Norwalk virus antigen in serologic assays and some epidemiologic observations. J Clin Microbiol 1993;31:2185–2191.
6. Jiang X, Wang M, Graham DY, Estes MK. Expression, self-assembly, and antigenicity of the Norwalk virus capsid protein. J Virol 1992;66:6527–6532.
7. Johnson PC, Mathewson JJ, Dupont HL, Breenberg HB. Multiple-challenge study of host susceptibility to Norwalk gastroenteritis in US adults. J Infect Dis 1990;161:18–21.
8. Kapikian AZ, Estes MK, Chanock RM. Norwalk group of viruses. In: Fields BN, Knipe DM, Howley PM, eds. Fields virology, vol 1. Philadelphia: Lippincott-Raven Publishers, 1996:783–810.
9. Kaplan JE, Gary GW, Baron RC, Singh N, Schonberger LB, Feldman R, Greenberg HB. Epidemiology of Norwalk gastroenteritis and the role of Norwalk virus in outbreaks of acute nonbacterial gastroenteritis. Ann Intern Med 1982;96:756–761.
10. Mason HS, Ball JM, Shi J-J, Jiang X, Estes MK, Arntzen CJ. Expression of Norwalk virus protein in transgenic tobacco and potato and its oral immunogenicity in mice. Proc Natl Acad Sci USA 1996;93:5335–5340.
11. Meeroff JC, Schreiber DS, Trier JS, Blacklow NR. Abnormal gastric motor function in viral gastroenteritis. Ann Intern Med 1980;92:370–373.
12. Moe CL, Gentsch J, Grohmann G, Monroe SS, Jiang X, Wang J, Estes MK, Seto Y, Humphrey C, Stine S, Glass RI. Application of PCR to detect Norwalk virus in fecal specimens from outbreaks of gastroenteritis. J Clin Microbiol 1994;32(3):642–648.
13. Wyatt RG, Greenberg HB, Dalgard DW, Allen WP, Sly DL, Thornhill TS, Chanock RM, Kapikian AZ. Experimental infection of chimpanzees with the Norwalk agent of epidemic viral gastroenteritis. J Med Virol 1978;2:89–96.

MK. Norwalk virus infection of volunteers: new insights based on improved assays. J Infect Dis 1994;170:34–43.

Parainfluenza Virus

●

John Treanor

GENERAL DESCRIPTION
Microbiology

Parainfluenza viruses are pleomorphic enveloped viruses with a linear single-stranded RNA genome of negative polarity (2). Four distinct human serotypes are recognized: types 1, 2, 3, and 4. Viral envelope glycoproteins include HN, which serves as both the viral hemagglutinin and neuraminidase, and F, which mediates fusion of the viral envelope with the cell membrane. As is true of respiratory syncytial (RS) virus, formation of infectious virus requires posttranslational cleavage of F by host-cell proteases.

Antibody to both the HN and F proteins plays a role in resistance to infection. Antibody to either HN or F neutralizes infectivity but only antibody to F prevents cell-to-cell fusion. Passive transfer of monospecific antisera to either F or HN can protect animals, and vaccinia viruses expressing either F or HN induce protective immunity in experimental animals.

Clinical Features

The predominant manifestation of infection with parainfluenza virus (PIV) is croup, or viral laryngotracheobronchitis, a clinically distinct illness affecting children under the age of 3. The illness typically begins with upper respiratory tract symptoms of rhinorrhea and sore throat (11), often with a mild cough. After 2 or 3 days, the cough deepens and develops a characteristic brassy, barking quality, similar to a seal's bark. Fever is usually present, generally between 38 and 40°C (12). The child may appear apprehensive and most comfortable sitting forward in bed. The respiratory rate is elevated but usually not over 50; this contrasts with bronchiolitis, in which more-severe tachypnea is often seen. Chest wall retractions, particularly in the supraclavicular and suprasternal areas, may be observed. Children with this finding on presentation have a higher risk of hospitalization or of requiring ventilatory support (24).

The characteristic physical finding of croup is inspiratory stridor. Inspiration is prolonged, and in very severe cases, some degree of expiratory obstruction may also be seen. Rales, rhonchi, and wheezing, reflecting the characteristic involvement of the lower respiratory tract, may be heard on physical examination. These signs, including the barking cough and inspiratory stridor, arise mostly from inflammation occurring in the larynx and trachea (21), which is greatest at the subglottic level, the least distensible part of the airway. Involvement of the lower respiratory tract is integral to the pathophysiology of croup. Inflammatory changes are noted throughout the respiratory tract (21), and hypoxemia is detected in about 80% of children hospitalized with croup (18). A fluctuating course is typical for viral croup, and the child may appear to worsen or improve within an hour. The typical duration of croup is 3 to 4 days

Diagnostics Including Susceptibility

Parainfluenza viruses can be isolated in a variety of readily available cell lines and are generally identified in cell culture by hemadsorption, followed by immunofluorescence. Because there are no currently available antiviral agents, susceptibility testing is not an issue.

ANTIVIRAL THERAPY

There are currently no available antiviral agents with proven effectiveness against parainfluenza virus. Ribavirin is active against parainfluenza viruses in vitro and would theoretically be expected to be active in vivo as well, but there have been no randomized controlled trials in humans to date. Treatment of a child with severe combined immunodeficiency and chronic PIV3 infection with ribavirin aerosol resulted in resolution of fever and virus shedding; however, these returned each time the drug was stopped (10). Multiple additional antiviral agents are active in cell culture and to some extent in animal models (26) but have not been evaluated in humans. However, the potential benefit of the use of antiviral agents in the typical self-limited course of croup would likely be limited.

VACCINES

Initial attempts to develop vaccines for prevention of parainfluenza viruses involved use of formalin-inactivated virus. However, these vaccines failed to provide protection in field trials carried out in the 1960s, despite being modestly immunogenic (6, 7). However, in contrast to RSV vaccines, use

of formalin-inactivated PIV vaccine was not associated with enhanced disease upon subsequent infection. One suggested reason for the lack of protection was that the formalin-inactivated vaccine induced relatively little antibody to the F protein, which may be crucial for complete protection in systems with fusion-induced cell-to-cell spread of virus (17). Several approaches have been explored subsequently to develop an effective parainfluenza vaccine, including use of subunit vaccines and development of live attenuated viruses as potential PIV vaccines, however none of these vaccines are likely to be available in the near future.

ADJUNCTIVE THERAPY

Because most hospitalized children are hypoxic, oxygen is the mainstay of treatment for severe disease and should be given to all hypoxemic patients. Humidified air, or mist therapy, is commonly used and has several potential roles. Desiccation of the inflamed epithelial surfaces is decreased, and the viscosity of the exudate is reduced. However, the value of mist therapy has not been proven, and water from the standard home-use vaporizer cannot reach the lower respiratory tract because of the large particle size (13). In addition, removal of the child from the parents and placement in a mist tent can be more distressing to the child than beneficial (13).

Administration of nebulized racemic epinephrine generally gives rapid, symptomatic relief in croup (19), and several randomized trials have demonstrated rapid benefit on airway obstruction (5, 22, 25). The onset of action is rapid, often within minutes, but the duration of relief is also limited, lasting 2 h or less. Therefore, treated subjects should be observed closely for clinical deterioration. While symptomatic relief is considerable, use of epinephrine is not associated with improvements in oxygenation, probably because the defect in oxygen is associated with ventilation perfusion mismatching due to lower respiratory tract involvement. In addition, tachycardia may occur. Thus, inhaled epinephrine is generally reserved for children who fail to respond to more conservative management, although some centers use it routinely (3). Recommended doses are 0.25 mL of a 2.25% solution of racemic epinephrine for children less than 6 months of age and 0.5 mL for older children (4).

Use of antiinflammatory agents such as adrenocorticosteroids is a logical therapeutic modality, since such agents could theoretically reduce airway inflammation and edema and hence obstruction. Recent studies using well-defined entry criteria and study endpoints have demonstrated that adrenocorticosteroids are beneficial in moderate-to-severe croup. A single injection of dexamethasone at a dose of 0.6 mg/kg was effective in reducing the overall severity of disease, as assessed by symptom scores within the first 24 h after hospitalization (16, 20). Oral steroids are also effective in this illness. Prednisolone given by nasogastric tube reduces the duration of intubation in severely ill children intubated for croup (23); oral dexamethasone at doses as low as 0.15 mg/kg is also effective (8). Aerosolized budesonide has reduced severity in moderate-to-severe croup (14). Inhaled steroids have the advantage of more rapid onset of action and potential for decreased side effects, although side effects of short-term systemic steroids are minimal in healthy children. When compared head to head, oral and aerosolized steroids appeared equally effective (9).

Use of steroids in less severe cases is more controversial. In a recent report, a randomized double-blind trial compared nebulized budenoside versus saline in children aged 3 months to 5 years with mild croup who came to the emergency room but did not require admission. Steroid use was associated with more rapid clinical improvement (15). Therefore, for children with moderately severe to severe croup (i.e., those who are sick enough to be hospitalized), steroid use is reasonable and may result in clinical improvement and decreased risk of intubation. However, because the disease is generally self-limited, routine use of steroids is probably not indicated in mild cases, and nebulized dexamethasone in outpatient care does not appear to be effective in reducing the risk of hospitalization or in altering the clinical outcome at 24 h in such patients (1).

REFERENCES

1. American Academy of Pediatrics. Parainfluenza virus infections. In: Peter G, ed. 1997 Red book: report of the Committee on Infectious Diseases. Elk Grove Village, IL: American Academy of Pediatrics, 1997:443–447.
2. Chanock RM, McIntosh D. Parainfluenza viruses. In: Fields BN, Knipe DM, eds. Virology, vol. 1. New York: Raven Press, 1990:963–988.
3. Cherry JD. Croup (laryngitis, laryngotracheitis, spasmodic croup, and laryngotracheobronchitis). In: Feigin RD, Cherry JD, eds. Textbook of pediatric infectious diseases. Philadelphia: WB Saunders, 1992:209–220.
4. Cressman WR, Myer CM. Diagnosis and management of croup and epiglottitis. Pediatr Clin North Am 1994;41:265–276.
5. Fogel JM, Berg IJ, Gerber MA, Sherter CB. Racemic epinephrine in the treatment of croup: nebulization alone versus nebulization with intermittent positive pressure breathing. J Pediatr 1982;25:1028–1031.
6. Fulginiti VA, Eller JJ, Joyner JW, Askin P. Parainfluenza virus immunization. Am J Dis Child 1967;114:26–28.
7. Fulginiti VA, Sieber OF, John TJ, Askin P, Umlauf HJ. Parainfluenza virus trivalent vaccines. Pediatr Res 1967;1:50–58.
8. Geelhoed GC, Macdonald BWG. Oral dexamethasone in the treatment of croup: 0.15 mg/kg versus 0.3 mg/kg versus 0.6 mg/kg. Pediatr Pulmonol 1995;20:362–368.
9. Geelhoed GC, Macdonald WBG. Oral and inhaled steroids in croup: a randomized, placebo-controlled trial. Pediatric Pulmonology 1995;20:365–361.
10. Gelfand EW, McCurdy D, Rao DP. Ribavirin treatment of viral pneumonitis in severe combined immunodeficiency disease. Lancet 1983;2:732–783.
11. Hall CB. Acute laryngotracheobronchitis (croup). In: Mandell GL, Bennett JE, Dolin R, eds. Principles and Practice of Infectious Diseases. New York: Churchill Livingstone, 1995: 573–579.
12. Hall CB, Geiman JM, Breese BB, Douglas RG Jr. Parainfluenza viral infections in children: Correlation of shedding with clinical manifestations. Journal of Pediatrics 1977;91:194–198.
13. Henry R. Moist air in the treatment of laryngotracheitis. Archives of Diseases of Childhood 1983;58:577.
14. Husby S, Agertoft L, Mortensen S, Pedersen S. Treatment of croup with nebulised steroid (budesonide): a double blind, placebo controlled study. Archives of Diseases of Children 1992;68:352–355.
15. Klassen TP, Feldman ME, Watters LK, Sutcliffe T, Rowe PC. Nebulized budesonide for children with mild-to-moderate croup. New England Journal of Medicine 1994;331:285–289.
16. Kuusela AL, Vesikari T. A randomized double-blind, placebo-controlled trial of dexamethasone and racemic epinephrine in the treatment of croup. Acta Pediatrica Scandinavica 1988;77: 99–104.
17. Merz DC, Scheid A, Choppin PW. Immunological studies of the functions of paramyxovirus glycoproteins. Virology 1981;109: 94–105.
18. Newth CJ, Levison H, Bryan AC. The respiratory status of children with croup. Journal of Pediatrics 1972;81:1068–1072.
19. Skolnik NS. Treatment of croup: a critical review. American Journal of Diseases of Childhood 1989;143:1045–1049.
20. Super DM, Cartelli NA, Brooks LJ, Lembo RM, Kumar ML. A prospective randomized double-blind study to evaluate the effect of dexamethasone in acute laryngotracheitis. Journal of Pediatrics 1989;115:323–329.
21. Szpunar J, Glowacki J, Laskowski A. Fibrinous laryngotracheobronchitis in children. Acta Otolaryngologica 1971;93: 173–178.
22. Taussig LM, Castro O, Beaudry PH, Rox WW, Bureu M. Treatment of laryngotracheobronchitis (croup). American Journal of Diseases of Childhood 1975;129:790–793.
23. Tibballs J, Shann FA, Landau LI. Placebo-controlled trial of prednisolone in children intubated for croup. Lancet 1992;340: 745–748.
24. Wagener JS, Landau LI, Olinsky A, Phelan PD. Management of children hospitalized for laryngotracheobronchitis. Pediatric Pulmonology 1986;2:159–162.
25. Westley CR, Cotton EK, Brooks JG. Nebulized racemic epinephrine by IPPB for the treatment of croup. American Journal of Diseases of Childhood 1978;132:484–487.
26. Wyde PR, Ambrose MW, Meyer HL, Zolinski CL, Gilbert BE. Evaluation of the toxicity and antiviral activity of carbocyclic 3-deazadenosine against respiratory syncytial and parainfluenza type 3 viruses in tissue culture and cotton rats. Journal of Antiviral Research 1990;14:215–222.

Rabies Virus

●

Cherie L. Drenzek and Charles E. Rupprecht

GENERAL DESCRIPTION

From antiquity to the present, rabies has been regarded as one of the most terrifying zoonotic diseases, especially in the context of virus transmission from man's historic companion animal, the dog. The earliest known reference to human rabies resulting from the bite of a dog is in the Eshnunna Code of Babylon, dating from the 23rd century BC (34). The saliva of rabid dogs was recognized as infectious centuries ago and was described historically using the Latin word *virus,* meaning poison or slimy liquid (33). The history of rabies as a cause of human mortality is closely associated with the domestication of the dog, but it is also well established that rabies virus reservoirs occur in many sylvatic species, such as bats, foxes, mongooses, raccoons, and skunks (25).

In developed areas of the world, rabies is no longer a significant cause of human mortality, in large part because of stray animal control programs, widespread canine vaccination campaigns, and availability of safe and effective biologics for human postexposure prophylaxis (PEP) (Table 1). However, the disease remains a threat in the developing and undeveloped world, causing an estimated excess of 35,000 human deaths annually (36). The economic costs associated with establishing and maintaining rabies control programs (primarily in canine populations) for ultimate prevention of human disease can approach $300 million annually and be prohibitive in developing countries whose public health infrastructure must contend with a variety of epidemic diseases. Thus, although human rabies is preventable, these economic considerations often render it unpreventable in many parts of the world.

Virology and Pathogenesis

Rabies virus is classified taxonomically as a member of the family *Rhabdoviridae,* genus *Lyssavirus.* The distinct bullet-shaped virion contains a single-stranded, nonsegmented, negative-sense RNA genome that encodes five structural proteins: a transcriptase, a nucleocapsid protein, a phosphoprotein, a matrix protein, and a glycoprotein. The first three structural proteins are associated with the genomic RNA; the matrix protein forms the inner aspect of the lipid outer envelope of the virion, and the glycoprotein forms the surface peplomers and contains the epitopes against which neutralizing antibodies are directed (37). Monoclonal antibodies directed against both nucleocapsid and glycoprotein antigens have been developed and used to demonstrate that antigenically unique variants of rabies virus circulate in various geographic areas and are usually associated with a primary reservoir species of carnivore or bat (30). In addition, classification of rabies viruses into specific variants or genotypes on the basis of genetic sequencing

of the nucleocapsid protein has permitted detailed analysis of enzootic maintenance cycles of specific virus variants in the United States and provided information regarding variability of the virus itself (31).

The pathogenesis of rabies virus infection remains incompletely understood. After virus transmission (usually transdermally via penetration of skin by teeth), a region of the rabies virus glycoprotein attaches to the plasma membrane of cells; a putative receptor has been identified as the nicotinic acetylcholine (ACh) receptor (10). The virus may remain at the local wound site for prolonged periods (6), perhaps replicating in skeletal muscle cells near the site of inoculation (26) prior to entering peripheral nerves through unmyelinated motor and sensory axon terminals at the myoneuronal junction. Long-term retention of rabies virus within myocytes has been suggested as a mechanism responsible for the long incubation periods observed in human and animal rabies (10); however, direct viral entry into the peripheral nervous system without prior local myocyte replication has also been observed in a mouse model (28). After nervous system entry, the virus is sequestered from the immune system and the progression of infection cannot be stopped via passive and/or active vaccination. The virus then spreads by retrograde axoplasmic flow at 12 to 24 mm/day until it reaches the central nervous system (CNS) at the level of the spinal ganglia. At this point, the first specific symptoms of disease (e.g., pain or paresthesias at the original wound site) may be evident (11). The virus disseminates rapidly in the CNS, leading to development of a progressive encephalitis. This is followed by centrifugal spread of the virus along the peripheral nerves throughout the body, most strikingly in the salivary glands, which leads to salivary viral excretion.

Epidemiology

Rabies is a zoonosis and the epidemiology of human rabies is ultimately linked to cycles of rabies virus transmission in animals. Although rabies virus can potentially infect any mammal, four terrestrial mammals (raccoons, foxes, skunks, and coyotes) and bats are the dominant wildlife reservoirs of rabies in the United States. Eight genetically distinct rabies virus variants are recognized within broad geographic regions of the United States in these hosts. These include variants in raccoons *(Procyon lotor)* in the eastern United States, in red foxes *(Vulpes vulpes)* and Arctic foxes *(Alopex lagopus)* in Alaska and New England, in gray foxes *(Urocyon cinereoargenteus)* in Arizona and Texas, in coyotes *(Canis latrans)* in southern Texas, and in skunks (primarily *Mephitis mephitis*) in California, the north central states, and the south central states. Besides the terrestrial reservoirs, multiple independent rabies reservoirs exist in several species of insectivorous bats in the United States. Cases of bat rabies have been reported in more than 30 different species from all 48 contiguous states. Bats are increasingly implicated as significant wildlife reservoirs for variants of rabies virus transmitted to humans. From 1980 to 1997, 21 (58.3%) of the 36 cases of human rabies diagnosed in the United States were associated with insectivorous bats, and in only 2 of these cases was there a reported history of a bat bite (25).

Current epidemiologic patterns associated with human and animal rabies in the United States can be summarized: *(a)* the annual reports of rabies in wildlife far exceed those in domestic animals (25); *(b)* although bats are responsible for a relatively small proportion of nationally reported animal rabies cases in the United States, bat rabies variants are associated with a disproportionately large number of human rabies infections acquired in the United States; *(c)* most other human rabies cases diagnosed in the United States can be attributed to infections acquired in areas of enzootic canine rabies outside the United States; and *(d)* most human rabies cases originating in the United States have no history of animal bite or other event typically associated with rabies virus transmission and nearly a third were diagnosed postmortem (15).

Clinical Presentation

The clinical presentation of rabies is often characterized as either "furious" or "paralytic/dumb" (23), the former indicating derangement of cerebral functions while the latter describes impairment of spinal cord and peripheral nerve functions. However, the clinical distinction between these two forms is often unclear, as patients with rabies can exhibit signs and symptoms suggesting either category. The clinical presentation of human rabies may, in fact, reflect inherent host factors rather than animal species source or virus virulence, since different persons exposed to the same rabid animal source can exhibit both "furious" or "dumb" rabies (11).

Despite variations in clinical presentation, human rabies infection generally progresses through a series of five clinical phases: incubation, prodrome, acute neurologic period, coma, and either death or recovery (21). The length of the incubation period is quite variable and depends upon several factors such as the site of the virus inoculation (as well as its relative innervation), the quantity of virus introduced into the wound (evidenced by the severity of the bite), and the age and relative immune status of the bite victim (23). Incubation periods as short as 5 days and as long as 19 years have been reported (18), but the usual period of incubation of rabies ranges from 30 to

90 days. In those instances of either extremely short or extremely long incubation periods, the possibility of unknown or unrecognized exposure cannot be excluded.

The prodromal phase of illness follows the subclinical incubation period and is characterized by nonspecific symptoms such as fever, sore throat, chills, malaise, headache, nausea, vomiting, and cough. Local paresthesias or pain at the site of virus inoculation may also be evident during this time. These symptoms indicate viral presence in the dorsal root ganglia and CNS and are not pathognomonic for rabies. In fact, they often direct a clinician's initial diagnostic efforts away from rabies; in a study of 32 cases of human rabies diagnosed in the United States during the period from 1980 to 1996, rabies was included in the differential diagnosis for only 6 (19%) of the 32 patients at the time of hospital admission (27). The duration of the prodromal phase ranges from several hours to several days.

The neurologic phase begins when disturbances in CNS function are the predominant clinical feature; this typically lasts 2 to 7 days. Clinical manifestations include extreme agitation, restlessness, hyperactivity, and autonomic instability, including hypersalivation, hypertension, and tachycardia. Hydrophobia, aerophobia, and dysphagia are common among patients diagnosed with rabies and result from exaggerated respiratory tract irritant reflexes due to CNS dysfunction. These signs may be precipitated by the mere proximity of water or liquid or the threat of being touched by air, especially on the face. Clinical deterioration continues rapidly until sudden death (due to respiratory or cardiac arrest) or coma (in which CNS dysfunction results in generalized paralysis) results.

A less common clinical picture among human rabies patients includes prolonged ascending paralysis, similar to Guillain-Barré syndrome (3, 21). In contrast to the hyperactive presentation, here the patient's mental status remains intact until much later in the clinical course, and the average period of survival is longer. However, the end result remains unchanged as the patient gradually deteriorates into disorientation, stupor, coma, and finally death (20). No epidemiologic or molecular differences have been described among human rabies patients with this paralytic clinical presentation.

Death follows coma within hours to days and most commonly results from complications of hypoxemia, cardiac arrhythmias, cerebral edema, and hypotension (21). Among the 32 cases of human rabies diagnosed in the United States between 1980 and 1996, the median duration of illness from onset of clinical symptoms until death was 16 days, with a range of 7 to 42 days (27). The literature records only four instances of recovery from clinical rabies; in all four cases the patient received either preexposure or postexposure prophylaxis with duck embryo vaccine or suckling mouse brain vaccine prior to the onset of clinical illness (1, 19). It has been suggested that these individuals may, in fact, have experienced postvaccinial encephalomyelitis rather than clinical rabies (23). None of the 32 human rabies patients diagnosed in the United States from 1980 to 1996 received PEP prior to clinical onset; all received intensive medical management, yet none survived (27). A factor contributing to the lack of PEP in these patients may be the inability of both the patients and their consulting medical providers to recognize potential exposure to rabies, perhaps because of the continuing trend of human deaths due to bat-associated rabies virus variants in the United States.

Diagnosis

In most areas of the world, the vast majority of human rabies cases reported to the World Health Organization (WHO) are diagnosed solely on the basis of clinical presentation. Common differential diagnoses include herpesvirus and arbovirus encephalitides, Guillain-Barré syndrome, tetanus, poliomyelitis, delirium tremens, psychosis, cerebrovascular accident, and postvaccinial encephalomyelitis. Differentiating these conditions from clinical rabies is critical in focusing treatment efforts and minimizing potential rabies exposure among attending health care personnel.

Only 20 (63%) of the 32 cases of human rabies reported in the United States from 1980 to 1996 were diagnosed prior to death, as opposed to 28 of 38 cases (74%) from 1960 to 1979 (27). This trend is strongly influenced by at least two factors. First, a history of animal contact relevant to a rabies exposure was either not remembered by the patient or attending friends and family members or not elicited by medical personnel. Careful attention to this detail by medical personnel early in the clinical course may result in earlier rabies diagnoses and reduce the number of PEP regimens administered to medical providers. A recent history of foreign travel to, or immigration from, areas in which canine rabies is endemic is an extremely important risk factor that may help medical personnel arrive at a more timely differential diagnosis of rabies among clinically suspect individuals. A second factor is a low level of suspicion of rabies by clinical attendants because of the rarity of the disease in the United States. Any patient who presents with an encephalopathy of unknown etiology should be considered a potential rabies case, even in the absence of known rabies exposure through animal bite.

Once the clinical diagnosis of rabies is considered, laboratory confirmation may be established via standard serologic, antigen detection, virus isolation, or reverse transcription/polymerase chain reaction (PCR) methodologies, discussed in detail below (32). There are no laboratory tests available to diagnose rabies in humans prior to onset of clinical illness. Aspects of rabies pathogenesis limit the design and success of antemortem tests for evidence of rabies infection, so a battery of the following diagnostic tests is recommended to confirm the diagnosis of rabies.

Serology

Two different tests are used to detect rabies antibody. The rapid fluorescent focus inhibition test measures neutralizing antibody that reacts with rabies virus glycoprotein. An antibody titer of 1:5, defined by the reciprocal of the serum or cerebrospinal fluid (CSF) dilution that reduces the challenge virus by 50%, is considered positive. Antibody binding to the rabies virus ribonucleoprotein in infected cell cultures is detected by an indirect immunofluorescence assay using patient serum or CSF. Antibody in serum is considered diagnostic if no vaccine or antirabies serum was administered to the patient; antibody

in the CSF, regardless of the rabies immunization history, indicates rabies virus infection. Positive results by either serologic method is considered diagnostic confirmation of rabies. Serum samples taken early in the clinical course are unlikely to be useful for diagnosis except as a baseline for subsequent samples.

Virus Isolation

Suspensions of brain or saliva samples are added to mouse neuroblastoma cells and cultured for 24 and 48 h. Culture slides are then examined by direct immunofluorescent assay methods for evidence of infection with rabies virus.

Antigen Detection

Rabies virus antigen is detected by direct immunofluorescent assay of serial frozen sections of nuchal biopsy specimens (obtained from the base of the neck or scalp where the density of hair follicles is high) and touch impressions of corneal epithelial cells and fresh brain material. A positive test result with these specimens confirms the diagnosis of rabies, but a negative finding does not necessarily exclude the diagnosis. For optimal postmortem diagnosis of rabies, direct immunofluorescent assay testing should be performed on samples of the hippocampus, cerebellum, and brainstem/spinal cord.

RNA Detection

Nucleic acids are extracted from samples of undiluted saliva and fresh or paraffin-embedded fixed samples of brain, followed by reverse transcription of RNA and cDNA amplification by PCR with rabies-specific oligonucleotide primers derived from a sequence of the N protein gene. This test has the added advantage of obtaining DNA fragments that can be sequenced and analyzed using databases of known rabies virus variants; however, the specialized equipment and expense of reagents may limit use of this technique to research or reference laboratories.

SUSCEPTIBILITY IN VITRO AND IN VIVO

There is a paucity of data demonstrating rabies virus susceptibility to antiviral agents in vitro or in animal models. Some information about the environmental stability of the virus exists, however; the virus is inactivated at extreme pH levels (<3, >11) and by desiccation, ultraviolet irradiation, sunlight, trypsin, β-propiolactone, ether, and detergents (18).

ANTIVIRAL THERAPY

Specific chemotherapy for clinical rabies does not exist, and treatment consists of intensive medical management, in particular maintaining cardiovascular and respiratory support. The most important clinical complications appear to be hypoxia, hypotension, cerebral edema, increased intracranial pressure, fluid imbalance, and cardiac arrhythmias. Intensive supportive therapy is costly and nearly always futile, but it can prolong the overall clinical progression. However, appropriate isolation procedures must be instituted to protect attending medical personnel from contact with the patient's saliva, CSF, tears, and centrifuged urine. Blood and feces are not considered infectious (22). The risk of rabies exposure (and thus the necessity for administration of PEP) among persons caring for human rabies patients is very low, unless the caretaker is bitten or there is direct mucous membrane contamination with the patient's saliva (e.g., via intubation or mouth-to-mouth resuscitation).

Neither interferon nor antiviral drugs such as intravenous and intrathecal ribavirin, vidarabine, tribavirin, adenosine arabinoside, and inosine pranobex have proven successful in the treatment of human rabies infections (23). Similarly, vaccine and immunoglobulin administration initiated after the onset of clinical disease have shown no positive effect in altering the clinical course of rabies (16). Ten (31%) of the 32 patients diagnosed with rabies in the United States from 1980 to 1996 received antiviral therapy, including interferon, ribavirin, adenine arabinoside, or acyclovir (as herpesvirus infection was a frequently considered diagnosis). Among the patients receiving antiviral therapy, the median duration of illness was 19 days (range, 7–28 days), which did not differ significantly from that in patients not receiving antiviral therapy (median, 15.5 days; range, 7–32 days). Three patients were also given immunoglobulin during the course of their illness; the median duration of illness among them was also 19 days (range, 11–42 days) (15, 27).

VACCINES
General

Although the case:fatality ratio of human rabies approaches unity, it is a completely preventable disease when exposure is recognized and appropriate PEP (i.e., local wound care, immunoglobulin, and vaccine) is administered before the onset of clinical symptoms. In addition, concomitant control of rabies in animals (especially domestic species) by effective vaccination programs, restriction of movement, and ordinances to control stray animals forms the foundation for human rabies prevention.

The first vaccine for antirabies treatment was developed a century ago by Louis Pasteur in the 1880s. It consisted of a modified live rabies virus strain that was developed by intracerebral passage in rabbits (5). Modifications of this original nerve tissue vaccine were introduced during the next 50 years, but problems with low immunologic potency and a high rate of postvaccinial neurologic complications (encephalomyelitis, peripheral neuropathy) were widespread (35). These Semple-type animal nerve tissue vaccines are still frequently used in the developing world because they are inexpensive and relatively easy to produce. The late 1950s brought the development of two new antirabies vaccines (suckling mouse brain vaccine and duck embryo vaccine) that were free of myelin basic proteins believed to be responsible for the immune-mediated neurologic complications observed with nerve tissue vaccines. Duck embryo vaccine was used in the United States from 1958 to 1980; however, low immunologic potency and resultant treatment failures were commonplace (18).

The revolutionary introduction of a safe and potent antirabies vaccine followed the successful adaptation of rabies virus to human diploid cell culture (24). The efficacy of the new human diploid cell vaccine (HDCV) along with adminis-

tration of mule immune serum was demonstrated in 1976 among 45 persons severely bitten by rabid dogs and wolves in Iran; all developed rabies-neutralizing antibodies, and none succumbed to disease (5). Besides HDCV, two other cell culture vaccines, rabies vaccine adsorbed (RVA) and purified chick embryo culture vaccine (PCEC), are currently licensed and available in the United States for both pre- and postexposure rabies prophylaxis.

Indications

Modern rabies PEP consisting of immediate local wound care, administration of human rabies immunoglobulin (HRIG), and vaccine (HDCV, RVA, or PCEC) has proven essentially 100% effective; most human rabies fatalities now occur in people who fail to seek medical treatment, usually because they do not recognize a risk in the animal contact leading to the infection.

In deciding whether to administer PEP to a person who may have been exposed to rabies, a physician should first determine whether an exposure indeed occurred and then assess the probability that the animal involved in the exposure was rabid. Rabies can be transmitted only when the virus is introduced into open cuts or wounds in skin or mucous membranes, which is defined as an exposure. If there has been no exposure, then PEP is not necessary. The likelihood of rabies infection varies with the nature and extent of exposure. Two categories of exposure (bite and nonbite) are considered (Table 2). Any penetration of the skin by teeth constitutes a bite exposure. Bites to the face and hands carry the highest risk, but the site of the bite should not influence the decision to begin PEP. Scratches, abrasions, open wounds, or mucous membranes contaminated with saliva or nervous tissue from a rabid animal constitute nonbite exposures. These exposures usually carry a lower risk than bite exposures. Other contact such as petting a rabid animal or contact with the blood, urine, or feces of a rabid animal does not constitute an exposure and is not an indication for PEP (9).

Guidelines for administration of PEP to persons exposed, or potentially exposed, to rabies by either domestic animals or wild animals have been established (Table 2), but the decision itself is not black and white and must take into account the circumstances surrounding the bite, the disposition of the animal, and the epidemiology of rabies in the area. In virtually all of the United States, a healthy domestic dog, cat, or ferret that bites a person should be confined and observed for 10 days in lieu of immediate PEP administration, since the pathogenesis, clinical signs of rabies, and viral shedding period are well established for these animals. If the dog, cat, or ferret was rabid at the time of the exposure, the animal will become clinically ill and expire during the 10-day period. At this time, if the animal tests positive for rabies infection, then PEP is administered.

On the other hand, since the incubation period, shedding period, and clinical signs of rabies cannot be interpreted reliably in wildlife, PEP is recommended for humans with bite, scratch, or mucous membrane exposure to any wild mammal (especially the five sylvatic reservoirs of rabies in the United States—bats, raccoons, skunks, foxes, and coyotes) unless the animal is available for testing and is negative for rabies virus

TABLE 2 • Rabies Postexposure Prophylaxis (PEP) Recommendations, United States

Animal Type	Evaluation and Disposition of Animal	Type of Exposure	PEP Recommendations
Dogs, cats, ferrets	Healthy, available for 10-day observation period	Bite[a]	No PEP unless animal develops signs of rabies[c]
		Nonbite[b]	No PEP unless animal develops signs of rabies[c]
	Rabid or suspected rabid	Bite	Immediate treatment (HRIG + vaccine)
		Nonbite	Immediate treatment (HRIG + vaccine)
	Unknown or escaped	Bite	Consult public health officials about the epidemiology of rabies in the area
		Nonbite	Consult public health officials
Bats, foxes, raccoons, skunks, woodchucks, and most terrestrial carnivores	Considered rabid unless geographic area is known to be free of rabies or until animal proven negative by laboratory testing[d]	Bite	Immediate treatment (HRIG + vaccine)
		Nonbite	Immediate treatment (HRIG + vaccine)
Livestock, rodents, and lagomorphs	Consider individually	Bite or nonbite	Consult public health officials. Bites of squirrels, hamsters, mice, rats, gerbils, chipmunks, guinea pigs, rabbits, and hares almost never require PEP

Adapted from Centers for Disease Control and Prevention. Rabies prevention—United States, 1991, Recommendations of the Immunizations Practices Advisory Committee (ACIP). MMWR 1991;40:1–19.

[a] Penetration of the skin by teeth.

[b] Scratches, abrasions, open wounds, or mucous membranes contaminated with saliva or nervous tissue. Blood, urine, and feces are considered noninfectious.

[c] Begin PEP (HRIG + vaccine) immediately if a dog, cat, or ferret shows signs considered typical of rabies during the 10-day observation period. The ill animal should be euthanized and tested for rabies virus infection at once.

[d] Wild animals should not be held for observation. They should be euthanized and tested for rabies virus infection as soon as possible after the human exposure. PEP regimen can be discontinued if immunofluorescence test results are negative.

infection. Rodents and lagomorphs are rarely found to be infected with rabies virus, and exposures to such animals constitute a very low risk of rabies virus transmission, with the exception of woodchucks in areas of the United States affected by the raccoon rabies epizootic (due to spillover from infected raccoons). Indirect human exposures, such as caring for wounds inflicted by a wild animal to a pet dog or cat, do not constitute a high risk of exposure to rabies by the caregiver and have never resulted in a documented human fatality. In unclear cases, the state or local health department should be consulted to assist in the decision to recommend PEP to an individual (9).

Bats are increasingly implicated as significant wildlife reservoirs for variants of rabies virus transmitted to humans. Recent epidemiologic data suggest that rabies virus may be transmitted by minor or seemingly insignificant bites from bats. The limited injury inflicted by a bat bite (in contrast to lesions caused by terrestrial carnivores) and an often inaccurate recall of the exact exposure history may limit the ability of health care providers to determine the risk of rabies resulting from an encounter with a bat. In all instances of potential human exposures involving bats, the bat in question should be safely collected, if possible, and submitted for rabies diagnosis. PEP is recommended for all persons with bite, scratch, or mucous membrane exposure to a bat, unless the bat is available for testing and is negative for evidence of rabies. PEP may be appropriate even in the absence of demonstrable bite, scratch, or mucous membrane exposure, when there is reasonable probability that such exposure may have occurred (e.g., a sleeping individual awakes to find a bat in the room, or an adult witnesses a bat in the room with a previously unattended child, mentally challenged person, intoxicated individual). The likely effectiveness of PEP in this setting needs to be balanced against the low risk such exposures appear to present. This recommendation, used in conjunction with current Advisory Committee on Immunization Practices (ACIP) guidelines, should maximize a provider's ability to respond to situations in which accurate exposure histories may not always be obtainable, while still minimizing inappropriate PEP.

Doses and Schedule

The PEP regimen recommended by the ACIP includes immediate local wound care (soap and water) and administration, over a 28-day period, of 5 doses of vaccine (HDCV, RVA, or PCEC) and one dose of HRIG (Table 3). The vaccine is administered intramuscularly in the deltoid (or in the upper thigh in very young children) on days 0, 3, 7, 14, and 28. HRIG is administered only once, at the beginning of antirabies prophylaxis (day 0). If anatomically feasible, the full dose of HRIG (20 IU/kg body weight) should be infiltrated in and around the site of the bite wound; if this is not possible, the dose should be administered intramuscularly at a site distant from the vaccine administration site. HRIG should never be administered in the same syringe or at the same anatomic site as vaccine. If HRIG administration is delayed for some reason, it can be

TABLE 3 • Rabies Postexposure Prophylaxis Schedule Recommended in the United States

Vaccination Status	Treatment	Regimen[a]
Not previously vaccinated	Local wound	Immediate cleansing of wound(s) with soap and water
	HRIG	20 IU/kg body weight; if anatomically feasible, the **full** dose of HRIG should be infiltrated in the area around and into the wound(s); any remaining volume should be administered intramuscularly at a site distant from the vaccine inoculation
	Vaccine	HDCV, RVA, or PCEC, 1.0 mL i.m. (deltoid)[b], one injection each on days 0, 3, 7, 14, and 28
Previously vaccinated[c]	Local wound	Immediate cleansing of wound(s) with soap and water
	HRIG	HRIG should not be administered
	Vaccine	HDCV, RVA, or PCEC, 1.0 mL i.m. (deltoid)[b], one injection each on days 0, 3 only

Adapted from Centers for Disease Control and Prevention. Rabies prevention—United States, 1991, Recommendations of the Immunizations Practices Advisory Committee (ACIP). MMWR 1991;40:1–19.

Abbreviations: HRIG, human rabies immunoglobulin; HDCV, Human diploid cell vaccine; RVA, rabies vaccine adsorbed; PCEC, purified chick embryo culture vaccine

[a] Applicable for all age groups, including children.

[b] The deltoid is the preferred site of vaccination for adults and older children; the outer aspect of the thigh may be used for very young children. Vaccine should never be administered in the gluteal area or in the same anatomic site as HRIG was given.

[c] Any person with a prior history of either preexposure or postexposure vaccination with HCDV, RVA, or PCEC or with previous vaccination with other types of rabies vaccines and a documented history of adequate antibody response to the previous vaccination.

given until day 7 following the initial vaccine dose; HRIG administration is contraindicated after this time because of potential interference with normal immune responses. HRIG provides immediate passive antibodies until the patient responds to the vaccine by actively producing virus-neutralizing antibodies. This regimen is recommended for all types of potential rabies exposure (9). Pregnancy or infancy are not considered reasons to withhold PEP (12).

Strict adherence to recommended PEP protocols is critical. Although there have been no postexposure treatment failures in the United States since HDCV was licensed in 1980, 13 persons outside the United States have contracted rabies following the PEP regimen. In each of these instances, there was some deviation from the recommended protocol (e.g., no local wound treatment, no HRIG administration, administration of vaccine in the gluteal area rather than the deltoid) (29).

Outside the United States, the WHO has approved the use of two abbreviated PEP regimens designed to reduce the cost of postexposure prophylaxis in developing nations. One of the most widely used regimens employs 0.1-mL doses of purified Vero-cell rabies vaccine, given intradermally in two different sites on days 0, 3, and 7, followed by two additional intradermal booster doses given on days 30 and 90 (12).

Preexposure prophylaxis (Table 4) is recommended for persons whose vocational or avocational pursuits lead to increased risk of frequent or unrecognized exposure to rabies, such as veterinarians, animal handlers, rabies laboratory workers, or persons spending more than 30 days in countries where canine rabies is endemic. Two preexposure prophylaxis regimens are approved in the United States. One consists of a series of three 1.0-mL doses of HDCV, RVA, or PCEC administered intramuscularly in the deltoid area on days 0, 7, and 21 or 28. The other approved regimen includes a series of three 0.1-mL doses of HDCV administered intradermally over the

deltoid area, on days 0, 7, and 21 or 28. In addition, single booster doses of vaccine are recommended for some individuals who have received the preexposure regimen if their serum antibody titer falls below 1:5 and their continuous or frequent risk of exposure to rabies remains an issue (Table 4). Preexposure vaccination does not eliminate the need for wound treatment and vaccination after exposure; however, the requirement for HRIG administration is obviated, and the post-exposure series is reduced to two 1.0-mL intramuscular doses of vaccine, on days 0 and 3 (Table 3).

An important consideration in preexposure prophylaxis, relevant to those traveling in countries where canine rabies is endemic, is the deleterious effect of concurrent administration of antimalarial drugs (e.g., chloroquine phosphate) on the development of antibody response after vaccination. This potential can be avoided by using the preexposure prophylaxis regimen with intramuscular administration of vaccine rather than the intradermal regimen (8).

Adverse Effects

Reactions after vaccination with HDCV, RVA, and PCEC are less serious and less common than with previously available vaccines. Nevertheless, reported adverse reactions among recipients of HDCV, RVA, and PCEC worldwide include local pain, redness, swelling, itching, and induration at the site of vaccination; systemic effects such as nausea, fever, vomiting, malaise, and lymphadenopathy have also been noted. Local reactions occurred in 19 to 74% of vaccinees, while systemic effects were reported in 5 to 40% (2). These mild local and systemic reactions are treated symptomatically, if at all, and do not justify discontinuing the PEP regimen in exposed individuals.

There have been four reports of a Guillain-Barré-like neurologic syndrome temporally associated with HDCV administration, although a definitive causal relationship was not es-

TABLE 4 • Rabies Preexposure Prophylaxis Schedule Recommended in the United States

Type of Vaccination	Route	Regimen
Primary series	Intramuscular	HDCV, RVA, or PCEC, 1.0 mL (deltoid), one injection on days 7, 21 or 28
	Intradermal	HDCV, 0.1 mL administered into the dermis over the deltoid area, one injection on days 0, 7, 21, or 28
Booster dose	Intramuscular	HDCV, RVA, or PCEC, 1.0 mL (deltoid), day 0 only
	Intradermal	HDCV, 0.1 mL administered into the dermis over the deltoid area, day 0 only

Adapted from Centers for Disease Control and Prevention. Rabies prevention—United States, 1991, Recommendations of the Immunizations Practices Advisory Committee (ACIP). MMWR 1991;40:1–19.

Abbreviations: HRIG, human rabies immunoglobulin; HDCV, human diploid cell vaccine; RVA, rabies vaccine adsorbed; PCEC, purified chick embryo culture vaccine.

tablished; all affected individuals recovered without sequelae (7). Also, an immune complex–like reaction was reported in approximately 6% of persons receiving booster doses of HDCV; these patients begin to experience generalized urticaria, arthralgia, angioedema, nausea, and vomiting approximately 2 to 21 days after administration of the booster dose of vaccine (14). This reaction appears to be associated with development of IgE antibodies to a component of the vaccine acting as an allergen (β-propiolactone-altered human serum albumin) (4). None of these reported illnesses has been life threatening.

When a person with a history of serious hypersensitivity to rabies vaccine must be revaccinated, antihistamines may be given, and epinephrine should be readily available to counteract potential anaphylactic reactions. These individuals should receive vaccination in a location that permits careful observation and monitoring following administration (e.g., an emergency room).

In general, corticosteroids should not be administered to treat adverse effects of vaccination. Steroids have been reported to increase rabies mortality among experimentally infected animals and to decrease immune response to vaccination (17). Similarly, it is recommended that immunosuppressed persons receiving either pre- or postexposure rabies prophylaxis have serum samples tested for rabies-neutralizing antibody titer 3 to 4 weeks after the last vaccine dose to ensure that an adequate antibody response has developed.

ADJUNCTIVE THERAPIES

Experimental treatment modalities such as immunosuppressive drugs (to lessen the degree of myocarditis due to T cell response), competitive antagonist drugs such as ganglioside preparations capable of selectively blocking excitotoxicity, oligonucleotide therapeutics to inhibit the activity of viral genes, and cellular administration of polyclonal or monoclonal antibodies directed against internal virus proteins have also been unsuccessful to date (23).

FUTURE CONSIDERATIONS

Although HDCV and HRIG have revolutionized modern rabies postexposure treatment, issues of cost and availability remain matters of tremendous concern and impact. Clearly, the need for human rabies vaccines and immunoglobulin replacements that are potent, safe, and inexpensive is a priority

throughout the world. In addition, increased effort to eliminate rabies virus infection in animal reservoirs (both wild and domestic) is the ultimate strategy to prevent human rabies. These goals are best attained by continued basic and applied studies of rabies virus pathobiology and immunoprotective mediators specific for rabies virus in both human and animal populations.

REFERENCES

1. Alvarez L, Fajardo R, Lopez E, Pedroza R, Hemachuda T, Kamolvarin N, Cortes G, Baer GM. Partial recovery from rabies in a nine-year-old boy. Pediatr Infect Dis J 1994;13:1154–1155.
2. Anderson LJ, Winkler WG, Hafkin B, Keenlyside RA, D'Angelo LJ, Deitch MW. Clinical experience with a human diploid cell rabies vaccine. JAMA 1980:244:781.
3. Anderson LJ, Nicholson KG, Tauxe RV, Winkler WG. Human rabies in the United States, 1960 to 1979: epidemiology, diagnosis, and prevention. Ann Intern Med 1984;100:728.
4. Anderson MC, Baer H, Frazier DJ, Quinnan GV. The role of specific IgE and beta-propiolactone in reactions resulting from booster doses of human diploid cell rabies vaccine. J Allergy Clin Immunol 1987;80:861.
5. Bahmanyar M, Fayaz A, Nour-Salehi S, Mohammadi M, Koprowski H. Successful protection of humans exposed to rabies infection. JAMA 1976;236:2751.
6. Baer GM, Cleary WF. A model in mice for the pathogenesis and treatment of rabies. J Infect Dis 1972;125:520.
7. Bernard KW, Smith PW, Kader FJ, Moran MJ. Neuroparalytic illness and human diploid cell rabies vaccine. JAMA 1982;248:3136.
8. Bernard KW, Fishbein DB, Miller KD, Parker RA, Waterman S, Sumner JW, Reid FL, Johnson BK, Rollins AJ, Oster CN. Preexposure rabies immunization with human diploid cell vaccine: decreased antibody responses in persons immunized in developing countries. Am J Trop Med Hyg 1985;34:633.
9. Centers for Disease Control and Prevention. Rabies prevention—United States, 1991, Recommendations of the Immunizations Practices Advisory Committee (ACIP). MMWR 1991;40:1–19.
10. Charlton KM. The pathogenesis of rabies and other lyssaviral infections: recent studies. Curr Top Microbiol Immunol 1994;187:95.
11. Chopra JS, Banerjee AK, Murthy JMK, Pal SR. Paralytic rabies—a clinicopathologic study. Brain 1980;103:789.
12. Chutivongse S, Wilde H, Supich C, Baer GM, Fishbein DB. Postexposure prophylaxis for rabies with antiserum and intradermal vaccination. Lancet 1990;335:896.

13. Chutivongse S, Wilde H, Benjavongkulchai M, Choncey P, Punthawong S. Postexposure rabies vaccination during pregnancy: effect on 202 women and their infants. Clin Infect Dis 1995;20:818–820.
14. Dreesen DW, Bernard KW, Parker RA, Deutsch AJ, Brown J. Immune complex-like disease in 23 persons following a booster dose of rabies human diploid cell vaccine. Vaccine 1986;4:44–45.
15. Drenzek CL, Noah DL, Smith JS, Krebs JW, Rupprecht CE, Fekadu M, Childs JE. Human rabies in the United States, 1980 to 1996: epidemiologic and clinical features. Presented at the VII annual international meeting of Advances Towards Rabies Control in the Americas, Atlanta, GA, Dec 9–13, 1996.
16. Dutta JK, Dutta TK. Treatment of clinical rabies in man: drug therapy and other measures. Int J Clin Pharmacol Ther 1994;32:594–597.
17. Enright JB. The effects of corticosteroids on rabies in mice. Can J Microbiol 1974;16:667.
18. Fishbein DB. Rabies in humans. In: Baer GM, ed. The natural history of rabies. 2nd ed. Boca Raton, FL: CRC Press, 1991:526.
19. Hattwick MAW, Weiss TT, Stechsulte CJ, Baer GM, Gregg MP. Recovery from rabies: a case report. Ann Intern Med 1972;77: 931–942.
20. Hattwick MAW. Human rabies. Public Health Rev 1974; 3:229–244.
21. Held JR, Tierkel ES, Steele JH. Rabies in man and animals in the United States, 1946–1965. Public Health Rep 1967;82:1009–1018.
22. Helmick CG, Tauxe RV, Vernon AA. Is there a risk to contacts of patients with rabies? Rev Infect Dis 1987;9:511–518.
23. Hemachudha T. Human rabies: clinical aspects, pathogenesis, and potential therapy. Curr Top Microbiol 1995;187:121–143.
24. Kissling RE. Growth of rabies virus in non-nervous tissue culture. Proc Soc Exp Biol Med 98:1958;223–225.
25. Krebs JW, Smith JS, Rupprecht CE, Childs JE. Rabies surveillance in the United States during 1996. J Am Vet Med Assoc 1997;211:1525–1539.
26. Murphy FA, Bauer SP. Early street virus infection in striated muscle and later progression to the central nervous system. Intervirology 1974;3:256–268.
27. Noah DL, Drenzek CL, Smith JS, Orciari L, Yager P, Shaddock J, Sanderlin D, Whitfield S, Rupprecht CE, Krebs JW, Fekadu M, Childs JE. The epidemiology of human rabies in the United States, 1980 to 1996. Ann Intern Med, 1998;128:922–930.
28. Shankar V, Dietzchold B, Koprowski H. Direct entry of rabies virus into the central nervous system without prior local replication. J Virol 1991;65:2736–2738.
29. Shill M, Baynes RD, Miller SD. Fatal rabies encephalitis despite appropriate postexposure prophylaxis: a case report. N Engl J Med 1987;316:1257–1258.
30. Smith JS, Reid-Sanden FL, Roumillat LF, Trimarchi C, Clark K, Baer GM, Winkler WG. Demonstration of antigenic variation among rabies virus isolates by using monoclonal antibodies to nucleocapsid proteins. J Clin Microbiol 1986;24:573–580.
31. Smith JS, Orciari LA, Yager PA. Molecular epidemiology of rabies in the United States. Semin Virol 1995;6:387–400.
32. Smith JS. Rabies virus. In: Murray PR, ed. Manual of clinical microbiology. Washington DC: American Society for Microbiology Press, 1995:997–1003.
33. Steele JH, Fernandez PJ. History of rabies and global aspects. In: Baer GM, ed. The natural history of rabies. 2nd ed. Boca Raton, FL: CRC Press, 1991:1–24.
34. Tierkel ES. Rabies. Adv Vet Sci 1959;5:183–226.
35. Wiktor TJ. Historical aspects of rabies treatment. In: Koprowski H, Plotkin S, eds. World's debt to Pasteur. New York: Alan R Liss, 1985:141–151.
36. World Health Organization. Report of the symposium on rabies control in Asian countries. Geneva: World Health Organization, 1993.
37. Wunner WH, Larson JK, Dietzschold B, Smith CL. The molecular biology of rabies viruses. Rev Infect Dis 1988;10(Suppl 4):S771–S784.

Respiratory Syncytial Viruses

John Treanor

GENERAL DESCRIPTION
Microbiology and Pathogenesis

Respiratory syncytial (RS) virus is an enveloped virus with a nonsegmented, linear, single-stranded, negative-sense RNA genome. The RS genome encodes 10 distinct proteins, including the envelope glycoproteins F and G. The G, or attachment, protein mediates binding of the virus to the host cell, while the F, or fusion protein, allows entry of the virus into the cell and promotes cell-to-cell spread (1). Formation of infectious virus depends on posttranslational cleavage of the F protein into F_1 and F_2 subunits by host cell proteases.

Only the F and G viral surface glycoproteins appear to play a role in induction of neutralizing antibody. Monoclonal antibodies to both the F and G protein neutralize infectivity in vitro, but while most monoclonal antibodies to F neutralize virus, only a small proportion of G monoclonal antibodies do so. Antibody to F, but not G, also inhibits fusion, and antibody directed against the F protein appears to be more protective than antibody to G in animal models (2, 3).

Two antigenic subgroups of RS virus, denoted A and B, have been recognized on the basis of reactivity with panels of monoclonal antibodies. This is primarily due to differences in the G glycoprotein between subgroup A and B; the F glycoprotein is relatively well conserved between subgroups (4). Both subgroups circulate in the population, with some indication of a general predominance of one or the other in alternate years. It has been suggested that infections with subgroup A viruses may be somewhat more severe, with more hospitalizations with RS virus in years in which subgroup A viruses predominate than in those with subgroup B (5).

Clinical Manifestations

The major manifestation of RSV infection in young children is bronchiolitis. Incidence peaks between 2 and 6 months of age, with over 80% of cases occurring in the first year of life.(6). The presenting symptoms are dominated by the major pathophysiologic defect, obstruction to expiratory air flow (7). The onset of lower respiratory symptoms is usually preceded by rhinitis, often with nasal congestion and discharge. More-severe symptoms characteristically appear 2 to 3 days later, but in some cases are concurrent with the onset of upper respiratory symptoms (8, 9). In many instances, there may be a history of exposure to an adult or sibling with a cold or other minor respiratory illness or history of exposure to other cases of bronchiolitis in the day-care setting (8).

The hallmark of disease is wheezing, which can be quite marked, with flaring of the nostrils and use of accessory muscles of respiration. Cough may or may not be prominent initially, and when cough is present, it may be paroxysmal. Slight cyanosis is often observed, but the presence or absence of cyanosis does not reliably indicate the degree of oxygenation or severity of disease (10). Physical findings are generally confined to musical or moist rales. Fever is common at the beginning of the illness, but one-third or more of hospitalized infants are afebrile (11). The hospital course is variable, but most infants show improvement in 3 to 4 days (12, 13).

The risk of hospitalization and severe bronchiolitis is particularly high in infants with congenital heart disease, chronic lung disease, or immunodeficiency (14–16). In addition, infants born prematurely and those who are less than 6 weeks of age at the time of presentation are also at risk (17, 18). More-severe disease has also been documented in children with a family history of asthma (18) and those exposed to cigarette smoke in the family setting (19).

Diagnosis

RSV and other viral agents responsible for bronchiolitis can be isolated from nasopharyngeal secretions in cell culture. Generally, several cell lines are inoculated to detect the spectrum of potential agents, including Hep-2, RhMk, and HFF cell lines. Specific viral diagnosis can be made more rapidly by identification of viral antigens in nasopharyngeal secretions (20, 21). This technique has found wide applicability for the detection of RSV. Both immune-based assays, such as immunofluorescence or ELISA techniques, and nucleic acid–based techniques, such as hybridization or PCR, have been developed. Immune-based techniques are generally preferable for routine diagnostic purposes, and several kits are commercially available. The sensitivity of such techniques depends on the quality of the nasopharyngeal specimen, with nasopharyngeal aspirates superior to brushings or swabs (22). The sensitivity of such tests in adults, who shed lower quantities of virus, is significantly lower. In transplant

patients with suspected RSV pneumonia, samples of the lower respiratory tract obtained by bronchoalveolar lavage are more sensitive than throat swabs for detection of RSV antigens (23).

SUSCEPTIBILITY IN VITRO AND IN VIVO

Both cell culture and animal model systems have been used to evaluate antiviral agents for potential activity against RSV. These studies have included plaque reduction or other assays in the cell lines described above as well as studies in the cotton rat and hamsters, the most widely used animal models. The most promising agent to emerge from these studies has been ribavirin (1-β-d-ribofuranosyl-1,2,3-triazole-3-carboxamide) (Fig. 1), a broad-spectrum antiviral agent with in vitro antiviral activity against influenza and parainfluenza viruses as well. The exact mechanism of the antiviral activity of ribavirin is unclear but appears to be related to the structural similarities between ribavirin and guanosine (24).

A large number of additional antiviral agents have been evaluated for activity against RSV. The broad-spectrum antiviral agents pyrazofurin and 3-deazaguanine are active against RSV in cell culture, with a higher selective index than that of ribavirin (25). Pyrazofurin has also been effective in cotton rats; however, toxicity was also seen in this system (26). A very promising compound is carbocyclic 3-diazaadenosine (Cc3-Ado), an inhibitor of S-adenosylhomotransferase, an enzyme involved in mRNA capping. Cc3-Ado is highly active against both RSV and parainfluenza virus in cell culture and was effective when given either orally or intraperitoneally after infection of cotton rats with RSV (27). Other drugs that appear to have some activity against RSV in vitro or in animal models include norakin (28), 1,3,4-thiadiazol-2-yl-cyanamide (LY253963) (29), and tricyclo-decan-9-yl-xanthogenate (D609) (30). SP-303, a polyphenolic plant polymer derived from an *Euphorbiaceae* shrub, was reported to have broad-spectrum antiviral activity in vitro, and to have some efficacy in the treatment of RSV infection in cotton rats when administered intraperitoneally (31) or via small particle aerosol (32). Further studies to evaluate these drugs in humans have not yet been reported.

Antiviral Therapy

General Drug of Choice

Several randomized placebo-controlled trials of ribavirin small-particle aerosol in naturally occurring RSV lower respiratory tract disease were conducted in normal infants (33–37) or in infants with high-risk underlying disease (38). While there were differences in the measures used to assess outcome in these studies, each indicated some benefit of the drug on both virus shedding and clinical illness. Ribavirin also benefited infants requiring mechanical ventilation, who had a markedly decreased total duration of ventilation and hospitalization compared with infants receiving placebo (39) (Fig. 2).

The total number of patients in these controlled studies is small, and the results were not confirmed by larger nonrandomized studies of ribavirin in clinical practice (40). A second randomized study, in which a saline, rather than water, placebo

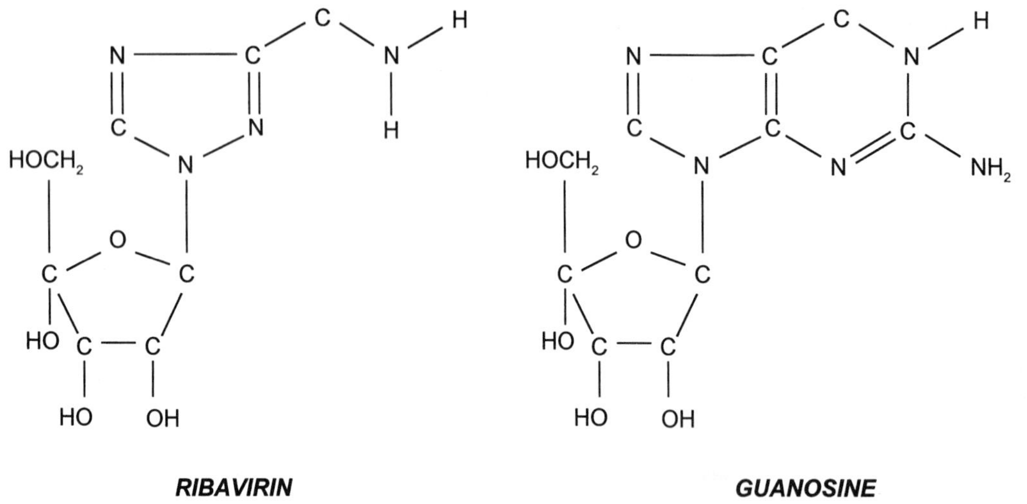

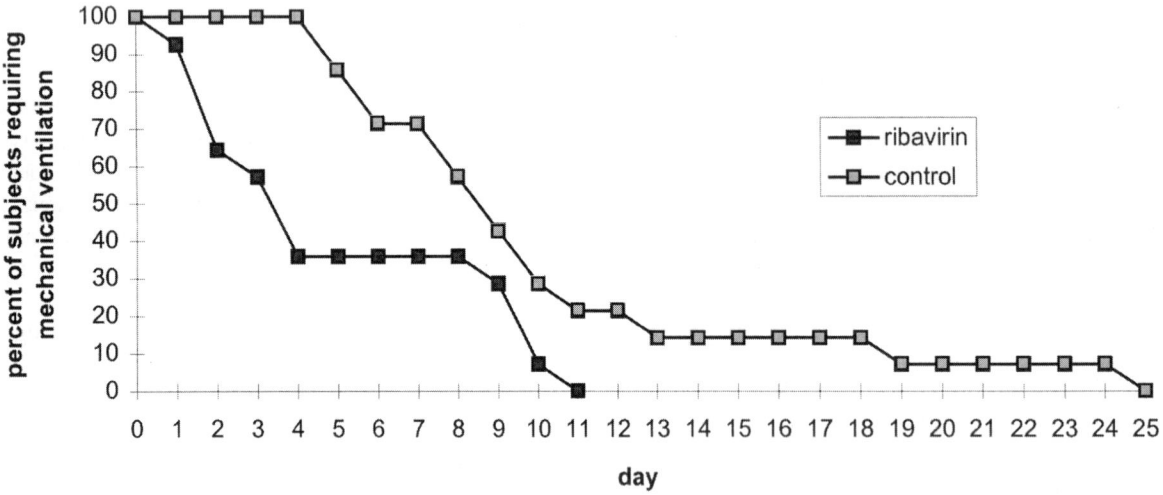

FIGURE 1. The chemical structure of ribavirin resembles that of guanosine.

FIGURE 2. Ribavirin decreases the duration of mechanical ventilation in previously healthy infants with serious lower respiratory tract disease due to respiratory syncytial virus. (From Smith DW, Frankel LR, Mathers LH, et al. A controlled trial of aerosolized ribavirin in infants receiving mechanical ventilation for severe respiratory syncytial virus infection. N Engl J Med 1991;325:24–29, with permission.)

was used for comparison, did not demonstrate a benefit in infants receiving mechanical ventilation (41). These findings, the expense of the drug, and the concern regarding potential environmental exposure of health care workers to the aerosolized drug, has prompted reconsideration of recommendations for use of this drug (42). Ribavirin should be considered for use in selected infants and young children who are at high risk for serious RSV disease (43). These recommendations are summarized in Table 1.

Other supportive care should also be used. Mist tents are generally not useful (8), although oxygen should be humidified. Fluid intake and electrolyte concentrations should be carefully monitored in all infants with severe bronchiolitis, as hyponatremia and SIADH may occur (44). Response to bronchodilators is generally poor, but it is reasonable to attempt use, in part to differentiate allergic disease from bronchiolitis (8). Systemic

corticosteroids also have failed to demonstrate therapeutic effects in this disease (45, 46). However, recent studies in animals suggest that locally applied antiinflammatory drugs in combination with antivirals may be of benefit (47).

Special Situations

While RSV has its greatest impact on infants and small children, adults are frequently reinfected throughout life. For most healthy adults, such RSV reinfections result in symptoms of the common cold, although on occasion, apparently healthy adults seek medical attention for lower respiratory tract disease in association with RSV. As such individuals can be expected to recover spontaneously, specific antiviral therapy is generally not indicated. More-significant illness may be seen in elderly adults, particularly in nursing homes and among individuals with chronic cardiac or pulmonary conditions, in

TABLE 1 • **Infants Hospitalized with Lower Respiratory Tract Disease Caused by RSV Who Should Be Considered for Treatment with Ribavirin**

Infants at high risk for severe or complicated RSV infection
   Congenital heart disease
   Bronchopulmonary dysplasia
   Cystic fibrosis
   Other chronic lung conditions
   Premature infants and those less than 6 weeks of age
   Infants with immunodeficiency or on immunosuppressive
     medication
Infants who are severely ill
   Infants with a $PaO_2 < 65$ mm Hg
   Infants with increasing $PaCO_2$ concentrations
Infants with other considerations
   Increased risk of progression (e.g., <6 weeks of age)
   Underlying condition in which prolonged illness might be
     detrimental

Adapted from American Academy of Pediatrics. Respiratory syncytial virus. In: Peter G, ed. 1997 Red book: report of the Committee on Infectious Diseases. Elk Grove Village, IL: American Academy of Pediatrics, 1997:443–447.

whom an influenza-like syndrome may be produced (48, 49). However, mortality rates in these groups remain low, and trials of antiviral therapy have not been reported in this group. However, ribavirin therapy could be considered in selected patients with severe disease. It might be more practical for most elderly patients in this situation to attempt to deliver ribavirin by intermittent high-dose aerosol (50) rather than by continuous aerosol.

Much more severe disease is being recognized with increasing frequency among immunocompromised adults such as leukemics and particularly after bone marrow or solid organ transplantation (51, 52). In contrast to RSV infections in other adults, the mortality in transplant patients is quite high, approaching 100%. Further, although these individuals are immunocompromised and very ill, the amount of virus present in lower respiratory tract secretions is still at least 1000-fold lower than that in healthy RSV-infected infants (23). Thus, there may be limited room for antiviral agents to operate. Also, a significant proportion of cases are nosocomial (53), and a concerted program of infection control, including the use of mask and gloves, may have a measurable impact on rates of disease (54).

There have been no controlled trials of the use of ribavirin therapy in immunocompromised adults, but both intravenous and inhaled ribavirin have been evaluated in uncontrolled cases series. Although some patients appear to have a rapid symptomatic response to ribavirin aerosol, use of ribavirin (generally given at a dose of 6 g/day diluted in 300 mL of distilled water and administered by continuous aerosol by mask or endotracheal tube for 18–24 h/day) has been associated with only a 30% survival rate (52, 55). Similarly, only 2 of 10 bone marrow transplant recipients with clinically significant RSV pneumonia treated with intravenous ribavirin (25 mg/kg/day) survived (56). Results were not improved when combined intravenous (15–20 mg/kg/day) and inhaled (6 g/day) therapy

was given (57). Results are particularly poor after development of infiltrates on chest x-ray and after intubation.

Alternative Therapy

In a small study, conducted several years ago, intravenous administration of an IVIG preparation containing high titers of antibody against RSV to infants and young children with RSV pneumonia or bronchiolitis significantly reduced RSV shedding and increased oxygenation at 24 h (58). More recently, a randomized, placebo-controlled study of treatment of children with bronchopulmonary dysplasia, congenital heart disease, or premature gestation who were hospitalized with RSV lower respiratory tract disease, showed no significant differences between RSVIG-treated and placebo-treated infants in the mean duration of hospitalization or adjusted symptom scores (59). There were also no differences between the RSVIG and placebo groups in the duration of intensive care unit stay for RSV, mechanical ventilation, or supplemental oxygen.

Combination Therapy

Studies in cotton rats performed several years ago suggested that combination therapy with ribavirin and RSV immune globulin might be more effective than either modality alone (60). This observation led to interest in the use of combined antiviral and immunoglobulin therapy of RSV in immunocompromised adults. In one recent study, treatment with a combination of aerosolized ribavirin (20 mg/mL aerosol for 18 h/day) and selected lots of commercial IVIG with high titers of RSV antibodies (500 mg/kg every other day) was associated with a 78% survival rate (61). In another small study, two patients with RSV pneumonia after bone marrow transplantation did well following treatment with ribavirin and a single dose (1.5 g/kg) of IVIG with high levels of RSV neutralizing activity (62). These studies suggest that use of combined therapy may be of some benefit to transplant patients. However, it is difficult to make firm recommendations for use of this combined therapy considering the apparent lack of efficacy of RSVIG in treatment of high-risk children. Decisions regarding such therapy must be individualized and should be made after consideration of the high mortality of these infections in immunosuppressed individuals and the expense, potential side effects, and availability of potential agents.

Prophylactic Strategies

Passively transferred antiviral antibody may also be useful for prevention of lower respiratory tract infection with RS and parainfluenza viruses (63). Passive transfer of human and rat hyperimmune globulin protects the lower respiratory tract in animal models of RSV infection (64–66). In humans, immunoglobulin with high titers of RSV-neutralizing antibody (RSV-IGIV) (67) prevented lower respiratory tract disease due to RSV when administered prophylactically to infants with prematurity, congenital heart disease, or bronchopulmonary dysplasia (68). This product has been approved for prevention of RSV disease in children less than 24 months of age with bronchopulmonary dysplasia or with a history of premature birth. RSV-IVIG should be administered at a dose of

15 mL/kg (750 mg/kg) once per month just prior to and during the RSV season. Usage should be considered in infants and children with bronchopulmonary dysplasia who are receiving or have recently received oxygen therapy, and in selected premature infants without bronchopulmonary dysplasia. However, because of the volume load, RSV-IGIV should not be used in those with cyanotic congenital heart disease (43).

One drawback of this approach is that the volumes of IVIG required to provide adequate titers of antibody can be large. Two approaches have been attempted to circumvent this problem. Locally applied antibody given as nasal or intratracheal drops is also effective in animal models, at approximately 100-fold lower doses in cotton rats (69) and in owl monkeys (70). A system for aerosolizing antibody has also been developed, and aerosolized IVIG was more active than ribavirin when administered to cotton rats on day 3 after infection (71). Thus, use of aerosolized immunoglobulins may provide a more efficient means of passive immunotherapy for RSV. An additional approach has been to generate humanized monoclonal antibodies with very high RSV-neutralizing titers (72). Clinical trials using such monoclonals administered systemically or locally are in progress.

VACCINES

Initial attempts to develop a vaccine for RSV involved use of formalin-inactivated virus. However, this vaccine failed to provide protection in field trials carried out in the 1960s, despite inducing high levels of RSV antibodies. Instead, subjects who received vaccine experienced enhanced disease upon subsequent RSV infection, compared with others who received control vaccines (73–75). The mechanism of this enhancement remains unknown, although an unbalanced immune response in which most immunity is directed against nonprotective and/or denatured epitopes generated by the inactivation process is currently the most widely held hypothesis (76). Multiple alternative approaches to RS vaccine development have therefore been tried. However, there is currently no commercially available vaccine for prevention of RSV, although several are in clinical development. These include the use of purified viral glycoprotein subunit vaccines (77) and proteins expressed in insect cells using a baculovirus vector (78). Live, attenuated RSV is also being developed (79). Recently, important progress toward the goal of generating infectious virus clones of RSV from cDNA has been reported (80, 81), which may lead the way toward new generations of live attenuated RSV.

REFERENCES

1. McIntosh K, Chanock RM. Respiratory Syncytial Viruses. In: Fields BN, Knipe DM, eds. Virology. New York: Raven Press, 1990.
2. Stott EJ, Taylor G, Ball LA, Anderson K, Young KK, King AMQ, Wertz GW. Immune and histopathologic responses in animals vaccinated with recombinant vaccinia viruses that express individual genes of human respiratory syncytial virus. J Virol 1987;61:3855–3861.
3. Sullender WM, Anderson K, Wertz GW. The respiratory syncytial virus subgroup B attachment glycoprotein: analysis of sequence, expression from a recombinant vector, and evaluation as an immunogen against homologous and heterologous subgroup virus challenge. Virology 1990;178:195–203.
4. Johnson PR, Olmsted RA, Prince GA, Murphy BR, Alling DW, Walsh EE, Collins PL. Antigenic relatedness between the glycoproteins of human respiratory syncytial virus subgroups A and B: evaluation of the contributions of the F and G glycoproteins to immunity. J Virol 1987;61:3163–3166.
5. Hall CR, Walsh EE, Schnabel KC, Long CE, McConnochie KM, Hildreth SW, Anderson LJ. Occurrence of groups A and B of respiratory syncytial virus over 15 years: associated epidemiologic and clinical characteristics in hospitalized and ambulatory children. J Infect Dis 1990;162:1283–1290.
6. Parrott RH, Kim HW, Arrobio JO. Epidemiology of respiratory syncytial virus infection in Washington, D.C. Am J Epidemiol 1973;98:289–300.
7. Wohl MEB, Chernick V. Bronchiolitis. Am Rev Respir Dis 1978;118:759–781.
8. Welliver RC, Cherry JD. Bronchiolitis and infectious asthma. In: Feigin RD, Cherry JD, eds. Textbook of pediatric infectious diseases. Philadelphia: WB Saunders, 1992:245–254.
9. Welliver JR, Welliver RC. Bronchiolitis. Pediatr Rev 1993;14: 134–139.
10. Downes JJ, Wood DW, Striker TW, Haddad C. Acute respiratory failure in infants with bronchiolitis. Anesthesiology 1968; 29:426–434.
11. Hall CB, Powell KR, Schnabel KC, et al. Risk of secondary bacterial infection in infants hospitalized with respiratory syncytial viral infection. J Pediatr 1988;113:266–271.
12. Hall CB, Douglas RG Jr, Geiman J. Quantitative shedding patterns of respiratory syncytial virus in infants. J Infect Dis 1975; 132:151–156.
13. Hall CB, Hall WJ, Speers DM. Clinical and physiological manifestations of bronchiolitis and pneumonia: outcome of respiratory syncytial virus. Am J Dis Child 1979;133:798–302.
14. MacDonald NE, Hall CB, Suffin SC, Alexson C, Harris PJ, Manning JA. Respiratory syncytial virus infection in infants with congenital heart disease. N Engl J Med 1982;307:397–400.
15. Hall CB, Powell KR, MacDonald NE, Gala CL, Menegus ME, Suffin SC, Cohen HJ. Respiratory syncytial viral infection in children with compromised immune function. N Engl J Med 1986;315:77–81.
16. Stretton M, Ajizian SJ, Mitchell I, Newth CJ. Intensive care course and outcome of patients infected with respiratory syncytial virus. Pediatr Pulmonol 1992;13:143–150.
17. Anas N, Boettrich C, Hall CB, Brooks JG. The association of apnea and respiratory syncytial virus infection in infants. J Pediatr 1982;101:65–68.
18. Lebel MH, Gauthier M, Lacroix J, Rousseau E, Buithieu M. Respiratory failure and mechanical ventilation in severe bronchiolitis. Arch Dis Child 1989;64:1431–1437.
19. McConnochie KM, Roghmann KJ. Parental smoking, presence of older siblings, and family history of asthma increase risk of bronchiolitis. Am J Dis Child 1986;140:806–812.
20. Ahluwalia G, Embree J, McNicol P, Law B, Hammond GW. Comparison of nasopharyngeal aspirate and nasopharyngeal swab specimens for respiratory syncytial virus diagnosis by cell culture, indirect immunofluorescence assay, and enzyme-linked immunosorbent assay. J Clin Microbiol 1987;25:763–767.
21. Waner JL, Whitehurst NJ, Todd SJ, Shalaby H, Wall LV. Comparison of directigen RSV with viral isolation and direct im-

munofluorescence for the identification of respiratory syncytial virus. J Clin Microbiol 1990;28:480–483.

22. Barnes SD, Leclair JM, Forman MS, Townsend TR, Laughlin GM, Charache P. Comparison of nasal brush and nasopharyngeal aspirate techniques in obtaining specimens for detection of respiratory syncytial viral antigen by immunofluorescence. Pediatr Infect Dis J 1989;8:598–601.

23. Englund JA, Piedra PA, Jewell A, Patel K, Baxter BB, Whimbey E. Rapid diagnosis of respiratory syncytial virus infections in immunocompromised adults. J Clin Microbiol 1996;34: 1649–1653.

24. Couch RB. Respiratory diseases. In: Galasso GJ, Whitley RJ, Merigan TC, eds. Antiviral agents and viral diseases of man. New York: Raven Press, 1990:327–372.

25. Kanawa F, Shigeta S, Hosoya M, Suzuki H, DeClercq E. Inhibitory effects of antiviral compounds on respiratory syncytial virus replication in vitro. Antimicrob Agents Chemother 1987; 31:1225–1230.

26. Wyde PR, Gilbert BE, Ambrose MW. Comparison of the anti-respiratory syncytial virus activity and toxicity of papaverine hydrochloride and pyrazofurin in vitro and in vivo. Antiviral Res 1989;11:15–26.

27. Wyde PR, Ambrose MW, Meyer HL, Zolinski CL, Gilbert BE. Evaluation of the toxicity and antiviral activity of carbocyclic 3-deazadenosine against respiratory syncytial and parainfluenza type 3 viruses in tissue culture and cotton rats. J Antiviral Res 1990;14:215–222.

28. Mentel R, Schroeder C, Dohner L. Effects of norakin on respiratory syncytial virus in tissue culture and in mice. Acta Virol 1989;33:162–166.

29. Wyde PR, Ambrose Mw, Meyer HL, Gilbert BE. Toxicity and antiviral activity of LY253963 against respiratory syncytial and parainfluenza type 3 viruses in tissue culture and in cotton rats. J Antiviral Res 1990;14:237–247.

30. Villanueva N, Navarro J, Cubero E. Antiviral effects of xanthate D609 on the human respiratory syncytial virus growth cycle. Virology 1991;181:101–108.

31. Wyde PR, Ambrose MW, Meyerson LR, Gilbert BE. The antiviral activity of SP-303, a natural polyphenolic polymer, against respiratory syncytial and parainfluenza type 3 viruses in cotton rats. Antiviral Res 1993;20:145–154.

32. Gilbert BE, Wyde PR, Wildon SZ, Meyerson LR. SP-303 small-particle aerosol treatment of influenza A virus infection in mice and respiratory syncytial virus infection in cotton rats. Antiviral Res 1993;21:37–45.

33. Hall CB, McBride JT, Walsh EE, Bell DM, Gala CL, Hildreth S, Ten Eyck LG, Hall WJ. Aerosolized ribavirin treatment of infants with respiratory syncytial viral infection: a randomized double-blind study. N Engl J Med 1983;308:1443–1447.

34. Taber LH, Knight V, Gilbert BE, McClung HW, Wilson SZ, Norton HJ, Thruson JM, Gordon WH, Atmar RL, Schlaudt WR. Ribavirin aerosol treatment of bronchiolitis associated with respiratory syncytial virus infection in infants. Pediatrics 1983;72: 613–618.

35. Barry W, Cockburn F, Cornall R, Price JF, Sutherland G, Vardag A. Ribavirin aerosol for acute bronchiolitis. Arch Dis Child 1986;61:593–597.

36. Conrad DA, Christenson JC, Waner JL, Marks MI. Aerosolized ribavirin treatment of respiratory syncytial virus infection in infants hospitalized during an epidemic. Pediatr Infect Dis J 1987;6:152–158.

37. Rodriguez WJ, Kim HW, Brandt CD, et al. Aerosolized ribavirin

in the treatment of patients with respiratory syncytial virus diseases. Pediatr Infect Dis J 1987;6:159–163.

38. Hall CB, McBride JT, Gala CL, Hildreth SW, Schnabel KC. Ribavirin treatment of respiratory syncytial viral infection in infants with underlying cardiopulmonary disease. JAMA 1985;254: 3047–3051.

39. Smith DW, Frankel LR, Mathers LH, Tang ATS, Ariagno RL, Prober CG. A controlled trial of aerosolized ribavirin in infants receiving mechanical ventilation for severe respiratory syncytial virus infection. N Engl J Med 1991;325:24–29.

40. Wheeler JG, Wofford J, Turner RB. Historical cohort evaluation of ribavirin efficacy in respiratory syncytial virus infection. Pediatr Infect Dis J 1993;12:209–213.

41. Meert KL, Sarnaik AP, Gelmini MJ, Lich-Lai MW. Aerosolized ribavirin in mechanically ventilated children with respiratory syncytial virus lower respiratory tract disease: a prospective, double-blind, randomized trial. Crit Care Med 1994;22: 566–572.

42. American Academy of Pediatrics. Reassessment of the indications for ribavirin therapy in respiratory syncytial virus infections. Pediatrics 1996;97:137–140.

43. American Academy of Pediatrics. Respiratory syncytial virus. In: Peter G, ed. 1997 Red book: report of the Committee on Infectious Diseases. Elk Grove Village, IL: American Academy of Pediatrics 1997:443–447.

44. Rivers RPA, Forsling ML, Olver RP. Inappropriate secretion of antidiuretic hormone in infants with respiratory infections. Arch Dis Child 1981;56:358–363.

45. Stecenko AA. Treatment of viral bronchiolitis: do steroids make sense? Contemp Pediatr 1987;4:121–130.

46. Springer C, Bar-Yishay E, Uwayyed K, Avital A, Vilozni D, Godfrey S. Corticosteroids do not affect the clinical or physiologic status of infants with bronchiolitis. Pediatr Pulmonol 1990;9:181–185.

47. Prince GA, Porter DD. Treatment of parainfluenza virus type 3 bronchiolitis and pneumonia in a cotton rat model using topical antibody and glucocorticosteroid. J Infect Dis 1996;173: 598–608.

48. Falsey AR, McCann RM, Hall WJ, Tanner MA, Criddle MM, Formica MA, Irvine CS, Kolassa JE, Barker WH, Treanor JJ. Acute respiratory tract infection in daycare centers for older persons. J Am Geriatr Soc 1995;43:30–36.

49. Falsey AR, Walsh EE, Betts RF. Serologic evidence of respiratory syncytial virus infection in nursing home patients. J Infect Dis 1990;162:568–569.

50. Englund JA, Piedra PA, Ahn YM, Gilbert BE, Hiatt P. High-dose, short-duration ribavirin aerosol therapy compared with standard ribavirin therapy in children with suspected respiratory syncytial virus infection [see comments]. J Pediatr 1994;125:635–641.

51. Englund JA, Sullivan CJ, Jordan MC. Respiratory syncytial virus infection in immunocompromised adults. Ann Intern Med 1988;109:203–208.

52. Hertz MI, Englund JA, Snover D, Bitterman PB, McGlave PB. Respiratory syncytial virus-induced acute lung injury in adult patients with bone marrow transplants: a clinical approach and review of the literature. Medicine 1989;68:269–281.

53. Englund JA, Anderson LJ, Rhame FS. Nosocomial transmission of respiratory syncytial virus in immunocompromised adults. J Clin Microbiol 1991;29:115–119.

54. Garcia R, Raad I, Abi-Said D, Bodey G, Champlin R, Tarrand J, Hill LA, Umphrey J, Neumann J, Englund J, Whimbey E. Nosocomial respiratory syncytial virus infections: prevention and

control in bone marrow transplant patients. Infect Control Hosp Epidemiol 1997;18:412–416.

55. Harrington RD, Hooton RD, Hackman RC, et al. An outbreak of respiratory syncytial virus in a bone marrow transplant center. J Infect Dis 1992;165:987–993.

56. Lewinsohn DM, Bowden RA, Mattson D, Crawford SW. Phase I study of intravenous ribavirin treatment of respiratory syncytial virus pneumonia after marrow transplantation. Antimicrob Agents Chemother 1996;40:2555–2557.

57. Sparrelid E, Ljungman P, Ekelof-Andstrom E, Aschan J, Ringden O, Winiarski J, Wahlin B, Andersson J. Ribavirin therapy in bone marrow transplant recipients with viral respiratory tract infections. Bone Marrow Transplant 1997;19:905–908.

58. Hemming VG, Rodriguez W, Kim HW, Brandt CD, Parrott RH, Burch B, Prince GA, Baron P, Fink RJ, Reaman G. Intravenous immunoglobulin treatment of respiratory syncytial virus infections in infants and young children. Antimicrob Agents Chemother 1987;31:1882–1886.

59. Rodriguez WJ, Gruber WC, Welliver RC, Groothuis JR, Simoes EA, Meissner HC, Hemming VG, Hall CB, Lepow ML, Rosas AJ, Robertsen C, Kramer AA. Respiratory syncytial virus (RSV) immune globulin intravenous therapy for RSV lower respiratory tract infection in infants and young children at high risk for severe RSV infections: Respiratory Syncytial Virus Immune Globulin Study Group [see comments]. Pediatrics 1997;99:454–461.

60. Gruber WC, Wilson SZ, Throop BJ, Wyde PR. Immunoglobulin administration and ribavirin therapy: efficacy in respiratory syncytial virus infection of the cotton rat. Pediatr Res 1987;21: 270–274.

61. Whimbey E, Champlin RE, Englund JA, Mirza NQ, Piedra PA, Goodrich JM, Przepiorka D, Luna MA, Morice RC, Neumann JL, Elting LS, Bodey GP. Combination therapy with aerosolized ribavirin and intravenous immunoglobulin for respiratory syncytial virus disease in adult bone marrow transplant recipients. Bone Marrow Transplant 1995;16:393–399.

62. De Vincenzo JP, Leombruno D, Soiffer RJ, Siber GR. Immunotherapy of respiratory syncytial virus pneumonia following bone marrow transplantation. Bone Marrow Transplant 1996; 17:1051–1056.

63. Hemming VG, Prince GA, Groothuis JR, Siber GR. Hyperimmune globulins in prevention and treatment of respiratory syncytial virus infections. Clin Microbiol Rev 1995;8:22–33.

64. Hemming VG, Prince GA, Horswood RL, London WT, Murphy Br, Walsh EE, Fishcer GW, Weisman LE, Baron PA, Chanock RM. Studies of passive immunotherapy for infections of respiratory syncytial virus in the respiratory tract of a primate model. J Infect Dis 1985;152:1083–1087.

65. Walsh EE, Schlesinger JJ, Brandriss MW. Protection from respiratory syncytial virus infection in cotton rats by passive transfer of monoclonal antibodies. Infect Immun 1984;43:756–758.

66. Prince GA, Hemming VA, Horswood RL, Chanock RM. Immunoprophylaxis and immunotherapy of respiratory syncytial virus infection in the cotton rat. Virus Res 1985;3:193–206.

67. Siber GR, Leszczynski J, Pena-Cruz V, Ferren-Gardner C, Anderson R, Hemming VG, Walsh EE, Burns J, McIntosh K, Gonin R, Anderson LJ. Protective activity of a human respiratory syncytial virus immune globulin prepared from donors screened by microneutralization assay. J Infect Dis 1992;165:456–463.

68. Groothuis JR, Simoes EAF, Levin MJ, Hall CB, Long CE, Rodriguez WJ, Arrobio J, Meissner HC, Fulton DR, Welliver RC, Tristram DA, Siber BR, Prince GA, Van Raden M, Hemming VG. Prophylactic administration of respiratory syncytial virus immune globulin to high-risk infants and young children. N Engl J Med 1993;329:1524–1530.

69. Prince GA, Hemming VG, Horswood RL, Baron PA, Chanock RM. Effectiveness of topically administered neutralizing antibodies in experimental immunotherapy of respiratory syncytial virus infection in cotton rats. J Virol 1987;61:1851–1854.

70. Hemming VG, Prince GA, London WT, Baron PA, Brown R, Chanock RM. Topically administered immunoglobulin reduces pulmonary respiratory syncytial virus shedding in owl monkeys. Antimicrob Agents Chemother 1988;32:1269–1270.

71. Piazza FM, Johnson SA, Ottolini MG, Schmidt HJ, Darnell MER, Hemming VG, Prince GA. Immunotherapy of respiratory syncytial virus infection in cotton rats (Sigmodon fulviventer) using IgG in a small-particle aerosol. J Infect Dis 1992;166:1422–1424.

72. Crowe JE, Murphy BR, Chanock RM, Williamson RA, Barbas CF, Burton DR. Recombinant human respiratory syncytial virus (RSV) monoclonal antibody Fab is effective therapeutically when introduced directly into the lungs of RSV-infected mice. Proc Natl Acad Sci USA 1994;91:1386–1390.

73. Kapikian AZ, Mitchell RH, Chanock RM, Shvedoff RA, Stewart CE. An epidemiologic study of altered clinical reactivity to respiratory syncytial (RS) virus infection in children previously vaccinated with an inactivated RS virus vaccine. Am J Epidemiol 1968;89:405–421.

74. Kim HW, Canchola JG, Brandt CD. Respiratory syncytial virus disease in infants despite prior administration of antigenic inactivated vaccine. Am J Epidemiol 1969;89:422–434.

75. Fulginiti VA, Eller JJ, Sieber OF, Joyner JW, Minamitani M, Meiklejohn G. Respiratory virus immunization. I. A field trial of two inactivated respiratory virus vaccines: an aqueous trivalent parainfluenza virus vaccine and an alum-precipitated respiratory syncytial virus vaccine. Am J Epidemiol 1969;89:435–448.

76. Murphy BR, Prince GA, Walsh EE, W KH, Parrot RH, Hemming VG, Rodriguez WJ, Chanock RM. Dissociation between serum neutralizing and glycoprotein antibody responses of infants and children who received inactivated respiratory syncytial virus vaccine. J Clin Microbiol 1986;24:197–202.

77. Tristram DA, Welliver RC, Mohar CK, Hogerman DA, Hildreth SW, Paradiso P. Immunogenicity and safety of respiratory syncytial virus subunit vaccine in seropositive children 18–36 months old. J Infect Dis 1993;167:191–195.

78. Wathen MW, Brideau RJ, Thomsen DR. Immunization of cotton rats with the human respiratory syncytial virus F glycoprotein using a baculovirus vector. J Infect Dis 1989;159:255–264.

79. Crowe JE, Bui PT, London WT, Chanock RM, Davis AR, Murphy BR. Live cold-passaged temperature-sensitive mutants of human respiratory syncytial virus (RSV) are highly attenuated, genetically stable, immunogenic, and efficacious against wild-type challenge in seronegative chimpanzees. 12th Annual meeting of the ASV, Davis, CA, 1993.

80. Collins PL, Mink MA, Stec DS. Rescue of synthetic analogs of respiratory syncytial virus genomic RNA and effect of truncations and mutations on the expression of a foreign reporter gene. Proc Natl Acad Sci USA 1991;88:9663–9667.

81. Collins PL, Mink MA, Hill MGI, Camargo E, Grosfeld H, Stec D. Rescue of a 7502-nucleotide (49.3% of full-length) synthetic analogue of respiratory syncytial virus genome RNA. Virology 1993;195:252–256.

Rhinoviruses

●

John Treanor

GENERAL DESCRIPTION
Microbiology

Rhinoviruses are members of the picornavirus family of viruses, nonenveloped viruses with a linear, single-stranded genome of positive polarity (reviewed in reference 10). Rhinoviruses are differentiated from the related enteroviruses by their relative acid lability and thermal stability. In addition, rhinoviruses replicate most efficiently in cell culture at low temperature (33°C). Humans are the only known natural host. To date, over 100 distinct neutralization serotypes of rhinovirus have been identified. This antigenic diversity results from amino acid sequence variation in four recognized antigenic sites that surround a 25-Å deep canyon in the VP1 protein that has been shown to be the receptor-binding site (42). Although the structure of the canyon is well conserved among rhinovirus serotypes, it is sterically inaccessible to antibody.

A recent advance in our understanding of these viruses was identification of the receptor for rhinovirus attachment to cells. Monoclonal antibodies directed against cell surface proteins were generated that could block rhinovirus attachment in vitro and were used to immunoprecipitate the receptor protein. A partial amino acid sequence of the protein was then determined and used to generate probes for cloning the gene encoding the receptor. Nucleotide sequence analysis of the cDNAs and subsequent confirmatory tests have established that most human rhinoviruses use intracellular adhesion molecule-1 (ICAM-1) as the receptor (23, 48, 49). This "major binding group" accounts for 91 of 102 known rhinovirus serotypes (53).

Rhinovirus serotypes that do not bind to ICAM-1 and are not inhibited by monoclonal antibodies to the major group receptor are referred to as the minor receptor group viruses (53). The minor group receptor has not been identified but appears to be a glycoprotein with an apparent molecular mass of 450 kDa (37). Binding of HRV to the minor group receptor was sensitive to treatment with trypsin and sulfhydryl-modifying agents but not neuraminidase (37). Manipulation of these receptor proteins has been explored as a potential control measure for rhinovirus infection (see below).

Clinical Manifestations

Common colds, familiar to most adults, consist of symptoms of rhinitis with variable degrees of pharyngitis. Predominant associated symptoms include nasal stuffiness, sneezing, runny nose, and sore throat (26, 44). Patients often report chills, but true fever is unusual. Cough and hoarseness are variably present, but other lower respiratory tract signs and symptoms indicate a possible complication. Headache and mild malaise

may be reported. Although a multitude of viruses may be associated with this syndrome, the pattern of symptoms associated with colds does not appear to vary significantly between agents (52). Physical findings are nonspecific and most commonly include nasal discharge and pharyngeal inflammation (26). More-severe disease with higher fever may be seen in children. Colds are generally self-limited, with a total duration of illness of approximately 7 days in adults. Complications of colds include secondary bacterial infections of the paranasal sinuses and middle ear and exacerbations of asthma, chronic bronchitis, and emphysema.

Colds are frequently associated with involvement of the middle ear, and changes in middle ear pressures have been documented following both experimentally induced and naturally occurring rhinovirus and influenza virus infection (8, 16, 19). These abnormalities are likely due to eustachian tube dysfunction and probably account for the frequency with which otitis media complicates colds. Colds are associated with symptomatic otitis media in approximately 2% of cases in adults (13) and in a higher proportion in young children (32). Rhinoviruses and other common cold viruses have been detected in middle ear fluids in approximately 20 to 40% of cases of otitis media with effusion in children (4, 9). Infection with respiratory syncytial virus, influenza virus, and adenoviruses are associated with a higher risk of otitis media (32).

Colds are also associated with detectable abnormalities of the paranasal sinuses that may or may not be evident clinically. Mucosal thickening and/or sinus exudates have been observed in as many as 77% of patients with acute colds (27, 50). These abnormalities are transient and resolve within 21 days in uncomplicated cases (27). However, clinically manifest acute sinusitis is seen in a small (0.5–5%) proportion of individuals with naturally occurring colds (54).

In general, the numbers of rhinovirus-infected cells in the nasopharynx appears to be quite limited, even in fairly symptomatic individuals (5). There is no clear correlation between the level of virus replication or the number of cells infected and the level of symptomatology (5, 14, 51). These results have suggested that virus-induced cellular injury is not the direct cause of symptoms in rhinovirus colds and that inflammatory mediators play an important role. Analysis of the mucosal exudate during rhinovirus colds suggests that nasal secretions during the initial response to rhinovirus infection result predominantly from increased vascular permeability, as demonstrated by elevated levels of plasma proteins in nasal secretions (34, 40). Glandular secretions (lactoferrin, lysozyme, and secretory IgA) predominate late in colds (34). Similar observations have been made in allergic rhinitis. However, in contrast to the situation in allergic rhinitis, where histamine is clearly involved in inducing increased vascular permeability (39), histamine does not appear to play a role in inducing symptoms in colds, as nasal histamine levels do not increase, and therapy with selective H1 antihistamine is not effective (18, 21, 40, 43).

Nasal secretion kinin levels do correlate with symptoms in natural and experimental colds (40). In addition, intranasal administration of bradykinin mimics the induction of signs and symptoms in the common cold, including increased nasal vascular permeability, rhinitis, and sore throat (43, 45). Additional support for the hypothesis that inflammatory mediators are important in induction of symptoms comes from the observation of reduction in cold symptoms by administration of antiinflammatory compounds with no antiviral activity (24, 47). Enhanced synthesis of proinflammatory cytokines and cell adhesion molecules in the middle ear may also contribute to the pathogenesis of otitis media associated with colds (41).

Diagnosis

Specific viral diagnosis is generally not attempted in individuals with colds, except in research settings. However, if such a diagnosis is needed, the mainstay remains isolation of the etiologic agent in cell culture. In general, rhinoviruses are best isolated in cell lines of human origin. By using specific primers, rhinoviruses can be detected in nasal secretions by the polymerase chain reaction (PCR) technique (6, 35). Currently, use of such techniques is limited to the research setting.

ANTIVIRAL THERAPY

Currently no antiviral therapy for rhinovirus infection is clinically available, although a variety of agents with activity in cell culture have been tested in human trials (46). Recombinant interferon-α was effective when administered as early treatment in community- or family-based studies (15, 30, 33). However, long-term use was associated with significant nasal irritation, manifested by development of bleeding and nasal mucosal ulcers associated with lymphocytic infiltration (31).

Agents that bind to a hydrophobic pocket located in the floor of the receptor-binding canyon in the β-barrel structure of the VP1 protein have also been evaluated intensively in humans, with variable results (7). Capsid-binding agents evaluated in humans include dichloroflavone (DCF) (3), chalcone (Ro 09–0410 and derivatives) (2), and pyridazines (R-61837 and derivatives) (1). Only R-61837 showed efficacy these trials (1), but drug-resistant virus is isolated readily from treated subjects (11). Thus despite promising in vitro activity, results in vivo have been disappointing. Since the structural characteristics of these agents and their mechanism of action are so well characterized, further manipulation of these molecules may result in more-active agents or agents with pharmacokinetic properties that result in greater clinical efficacy.

Recent studies show that rhinoviruses exhibit considerably less diversity in their choice of cell receptor than in serotypes. Thus, there has been considerable interest in receptor blockade as a potential strategy for control of rhinovirus infection. High doses of intranasally administered murine receptor-blocking monoclonal antibody administered intranasally modified infection and illness after challenge of normal adults with HRV 39, although the effect was not clinically significant (29). Soluble ICAM-1 (sICAM-1) inhibited CPE by 10 representative major receptor group HRVs at EC_{50}s of 0.1 to 7.9 μg/mL but was not effective against serotypes that use a different receptor (36). Studies with this approach in humans have not been reported.

VACCINATION

Infection of adults generally results in production of specific antisera, and homologous immunity of variable duration develops after infection. In addition, nonspecific heterotypic resistance has been described after rhinovirus infection but is transient (20). However, because of the large variety of serotypes and the fact that it is not possible to identify serotypes with particular importance as causes of disease, development of an effective vaccine does not appear to be a feasible goal (38).

ADJUNCTIVE THERAPY

Treatment of colds in clinical practice is largely symptomatic. Topical application of vasoconstrictors such as phenylephrine or ephedrine relieves nasal obstruction but may be associated with a rebound of symptoms upon discontinuation if used for more than a few days (25). It has been suggested that some analgesic agents, such as aspirin and acetaminophen, may be associated with prolonged virus replication and diminished immune responses in experimental rhinovirus infections (22). However, nonsteroidal antiinflammatory drugs such as naproxen effectively antagonize the symptoms of rhinovirus infection (47). Symptomatic therapy with systemic anticholingergic drugs or anticholinergic-sympathomimetic combinations has not been shown to confer any benefit and is associated with significant side effects (17). However, topical application of ipratropium, a quarternary anticholinergic agent that is minimally absorbed across biologic membranes, reduces rhinorrhea significantly in naturally occurring colds (12). In a recent trial in 411 healthy adults with acute colds, treatment with intranasal ipratropium was associated with reduced subjective complaints of rhinorrhea but also with higher rates of blood-tinged mucus and nasal dryness (28). This agent probably exerts its major effect on the parasympathetic regulation of mucous and seromucous glands. Finally, it has been suggested that the most effective therapy for rhinovirus colds may require the use of a combination of antiviral and antimediator agents (24).

REFERENCES

1. al-Nakib W, Higgins PG, Barrow GI, Tyrrell DAJ, Andries K, Vanden Busshe G, Taylor N, Janssen PAJ. Suppression of colds in human volunteers challenged with rhinovirus by a new synthetic drug (R-61837). Antimicrob Agents Chemother 1989;33: 522–525.
2. al-Nakib W, Higgins PG, Barrow I, Tyrrell DAJ, Lenox-Smith I, Ishitsuka H. Intranasal chalcone Ro 09–0410, as prophylaxis against rhinovirus infection in human volunteers. J Antimicrob Chemother 1987;20:887–892.

3. al-Nakib W, Willman J, Higgins PG, Tyrrell DAJ, Shepherd WM, Freestone DS. Failure of intranasally administered 4′6-dichloroflavan to protect against rhinoviruses in man. Arch Virol 1987;92:255–260.

4. Arola M, Ziegler T, Ruuskanen O, Mertsola J, Nanto-Salonen K, Halonen P. Rhinovirus in acute otitis media. J Pediatr 1988;113:693–695.

5. Arruda E, Boyle TR, Winther B, Pevear DC, Gwaltney JM Jr, Hayden FG. Localization of human rhinovirus replication in the upper respiratory tract by in situ hybridization. J Infect Dis 1995;171:1329–1333.

6. Arruda E, Hayden FG. Detection of human rhinovirus RNA in nasal washings by PCR. Mol Cell Probes 1993;7:373–379.

7. Badger J, Minor I, Kremer MJ, Oliveira MA, Smith TJ, Griffith JP, Guerin DM, Krishnasamy S, Luo M, Rossmann MG. Structural analysis of a series of antiviral agents complexed with human rhinovirus 14. Proc Natl Acad Sci USA 1988;85:3304–3308.

8. Buchman CA, Doyle WJ, Skoner DP, Post JC, Alper CM, Seroky JT, Anderson K, Preston RA, Hayden FG, Fireman P, Ehrlich GD. Influenza A virus-induced acute otitis media. J Infect Dis 1995;172:1348–1351.

9. Chonmaitree T, Howie V, Truant A. Presence of respiratory viruses in middle ear fluids and nasal wash specimens from children with acute otitis media. Pediatrics 1986;77:698–702.

10. Couch R. Rhinoviruses. In: Fields BN, Knipe DM, eds. Virology, vol 1. New York: Raven Press, 1990:607–630.

11. Dearden C, al-Nakib W, Andries D, Woesternborghs R, Tyrrell DA. Drug resistant rhinoviruses from the nose of experimentally treated volunteers. Arch Virol 1989;109:71–81.

12. Diamond L, Dockhorn RJ, Grossman J, Kisicki JC, Posner M, Zinny MA, Koker P, Korts D, Wecker MT. A dose-response study of the efficacy and safety of ipratropium bromide nasal spray in the treatment of the common cold. J Allergy Clin Immunol 1995;95:1139–1146.

13. Dingle JH, Badger GF, Jordan WS Jr. Illness in the home: study of 25,000 illnesses in a group of Cleveland families. Cleveland: Press of Case Western University, 1964.

14. Douglas RG Jr, Cate TR, Gerone PJ, Couch RB. Quantitative rhinovirus shedding patterns in volunteers. Am Rev Respir Dis 1966;94:159–167.

15. Douglas RM, Moore BW, Miles HB, Davies LM, Graham NMH, Ryan R, Worswick DA, Albrecht JK. Prophylactic efficacy of intranasal alpha$_2$-interferon against rhinovirus infections in the family setting. N Engl J Med 1986;314:65–70.

16. Doyle WJ, McBride TP, Swarts JD, Hayden FG, Gwaltney JM Jr. The response of the nasal airway, middle ear, and eustachian tube to experimental rhinovirus infection. Am J Rhinol 1988;2:149–154.

17. Doyle WJ, Riker DK, McBride TP, Hayden FG, Hendley JO, Swarts JD, Gwaltney JM Jr. Therapeutic effects of an anticholinergic-sympathomimetic combination in induced rhinovirus colds. Ann Otol Rhinol Laryngol 1993;102:521–527.

18. Eggleston PA, Hendley JO, Gwaltney JM Jr. Mediators of immediate hypersensitivity in nasal secretions during natural colds and rhinovirus infection. Acta Otolaryngol (Stockholm) 1984;413(Suppl):25–35.

19. Elkhatieb A, Hipskind G, Woerner D, Hayden FG. Middle ear abnormalities during natural rhinovirus colds in adults. J Infect Dis 1993;168:618–621.

20. Fleet WJ, Couch RB, Cate TR, Knight V. Homologous and heterologous resistance to rhinovirus common cold. Am J Epidemiol 1965;82:185–196.

21. Gaffey MJ, Kaiser DL, Hayden FG. Ineffectiveness of oral terfenadine in natural colds: evidence against histamine as a mediator of common cold symptoms. Pediatr Infect Dis J 1988;7:215–242.

22. Graham NMH, Burrell CJ, Douglas RM, Debelle P, Davies L. Adverse effects of aspirin, acetaminophen, and ibuprofen on immune function, viral shedding, and clinical status in rhinovirus-infected volunteers. J Infect Dis 1990;162:1277–1282.

23. Greve JM, Davis G, Meyer AN, Forte CP, Yost SC, Marlor CW, Kamark ME, McClelland A. The major human rhinovirus receptor is ICAM-1. Cell 1989;56:839–847.

24. Gwaltney JM Jr. Combined antiviral and antimediator treatment of rhinovirus colds. J Infect Dis 1992;166:776–782.

25. Gwaltney JM Jr. The common cold. In: Mandell GL, Bennett JE, Dolin R, eds. Principles and practice of infectious diseases. New York: Churchill Livingstone, 1995:561–566.

26. Gwaltney JM, Hendley JO, Simon G, Jordan WS Jr. Rhinovirus infections in an industrialized population. II. Characteristics of illness and antibody response. JAMA 1967;202:158–164.

27. Gwaltney JM Jr, Phillips CD, Miller RD, Riker DK. Computed tomographic study of the common cold. N Engl J Med 1994;330:25–30.

28. Hayden FG, Diamond L, Wood PB, Korts DC, Wecker MT. Effectiveness and safety of intranasal ipratropium bromide in common colds: a randomized, double-blind, placebo-controlled trial. Ann Intern Med 1996;125:89–97.

29. Hayden FG, Gwaltney JM Jr, Colonno RJ. Modification of experimental rhinovirus colds by receptor blockade. Antiviral Res 1988;9:233–247.

30. Hayden FG, Kaiser DL, Albrecht JK. Intranasal recombinant alpha-2b interferon treatment of naturally occurring common colds. Antimicrob Agents Chemother 1988;32:224–230.

31. Hayden FG, Winther G, Donowitz GR, Mills SE, Innes DJ. Human nasal mucosal responses to topically applied recombinant leukocyte A interferon. J Infect Dis 1987;156:64–72.

32. Henderson FW, Collier AM, Sanyal MA, Watkins JM, Fairclough DL, Clyde WA Jr, Denny FW. A longitudinal study of respiratory viruses and bacteria in the etiology of acute otitis media with effusion. N Engl J Med 1982;306:1377–1383.

33. Herzog C, Berger R, Fernex M, Friesecke K, Havas L, Just M, Dubach UC. Intranasal interferon (rIFN-αA, Ro 22–8181) for contact prophylaxis against common cold: a randomized, double-blind and placebo-controlled field study. Antiviral Res 1986;6:171–176.

34. Igarashi Y, Skoner DP, Doyle WJ, White MV, Fireman P, Kaliner MA. Analysis of nasal secretions during experimental rhinovirus upper respiratory infections. J Allergy Clin Immunol 1993;92:722–731.

35. Johnston SL, Sanderson G, Pattemore PK, Smith S, Bardin PG, Bruce CB, Sambden PR, Tyrrell DA, Holgate ST. Use of polymerase chain reaction for diagnosis of picornavirus infection in subjects with and without respiratory symptoms. J Clin Microbiol 1993;31:111–117.

36. Marlin SD, Staunton DE, Springer TA, Stratowa C, Sommergruber W, Merluzzi VJ. A soluble form of intercellular adhesion molecule-1 inhibits rhinovirus infection. Nature 1990;344:70–72.

37. Misthak H, Neubauer C, Kuechler E, Blaas D. Characteristics of the minor group receptor of human rhinoviruses. Virology 1988;163:19–25.

38. Monto AS, Bryan ER, Ohmit S. Rhinovirus infections in Tecumseh, Michigan: frequency of illness and number of serotypes. J Infect Dis 1987;1 1993;31:111–117.

39. Naclerio RM, Meier HL, Atkinson NF, et al. In vitro demonstration of inflammatory mediator release following nasal challenge with antigen. Am Rev Respir Dis 1984;128:597–602.

40. Naclerio RM, Proud D, Kagey-Sobotka A, Lichtenstein LM, Hendley JO, Gwaltney JM Jr. Kinins are generated during experimental rhinovirus colds. J Infect Dis 1988;157:133–142.

41. Okamoto Y, Kudo K, Ishikawa K, Ito E, Togawa K, Saito I, Moro I, Patel JA, Ogra PL. Presence of respiratory syncytial virus genomic sequences in middle ear fluid and its relationship to expression of cytokines and cell adhesion molecules. J Infect Dis 1993;168:1277–1281.

42. Olson NH, Kolatkar PR, Oliveira MA, Cheng RH, Grove JM, McClelland A, Baker TS, Rossmann MG. Structure of a human rhinovirus complexed with its receptor molecule. Proc Natl Acad Sci USA 1993;90:507–511.

43. Proud D, Reynolds CJ, Lacapra S, Kagey-Sobotka A, Lichtenstein LM, Naclerio RM. Nasal provocation with bradykinin induces symptoms of rhinitis and sore throat. Am Rev Respir Dis 1988;137:613–616.

44. Rao SS, Hendley JO, Hayden FG, Gwaltney JM. Symptom expression in natural and experimental rhinovirus colds. Am J Rhinol 1995;9:49–52.

45. Rees GL, Eccles R. Sore throat following nasal and orophayrngeal bradykinin challenge. Acta Otolaryngol 1994;114:311–314.

46. Sperber SJ, Hayden FG. Chemotherapy of rhinovirus colds. Antimicrob Agents Chemother 1988;32:409–419.

47. Sperber SJ, Hendley JO, Hayden FG, Riker DK, Sorrentino JV, Gwaltney JM Jr. Effects of naproxen on experimental rhinovirus colds. A randomized, double-blind, controlled trial. Ann Intern Med 1992;117:37–41.

48. Staunton De, Merluzzi VJ, Rothlein R, Barton R, Marlin SD, Springer TA. A cell adhesion molecule, ICAM-1, is the major surface receptor for rhinoviruses. Cell 1989;56:849–853.

49. Tomassini JE, Graham D, DeWitt CM, Lineberger DW, Rodkey JA, Colonno RJ. cDNA cloning reveals that the major group rhinovirus receptor on HeLa cells is intercellular adhesion molecule 1. Proc Nat Acad Sci USA 1989;86:4907–4911.

50. Turner BW, Cail WS, Hendley JO, Hayden FG, Doyle WJ, Sorrention JV, Gwaltney JM Jr. Physiologic abnormalities in the paranasal sinuses during experimental rhinovirus colds. J Allergy Clin Immunol 1992;90:474–478.

51. Turner RB, Hendley JO, Gwaltney JM Jr. Shedding of infected ciliated epithelial cells in rhinovirus colds. J Infect Dis 1982;145:849–853.

52. Tyrrell DAJ, Cohen S, Schlarb JE. Signs and symptoms in common colds. Epidemiol Infect 1993;111:143–156.

53. Uncapher CR, DeWitt CM, Colonno RJ. The major and minor group receptor families contain all but one human rhinovirus serotype. Virology 1991;180:814–817.

54. Wald ER, Guerra N, Byers C. Upper respiratory tract infections in young children: duration of and frequency of complications. Pediatrics 1991;87:129–133.

Rotaviruses

●

Jason Rosé and Harry Greenberg

GENERAL DESCRIPTION
Virology

Rotaviruses, of the family *Reoviridae,* are icosahedral viruses approximately 75 nm in diameter that comprise three protein layers, giving them a distinct wheellike appearance under the electron microscope. The viral capsid encloses 11 segments of double-stranded RNA, each of which codes for a single viral protein, except for gene 11, which is bicistronic. Five major rotavirus groups (A–E) have been identified on the basis of genetic relatedness and immunologic reactivity of the inner capsid protein VP6. Group A and C rotaviruses can be grown in culture, but no system has been developed for culturing group B viruses.

Epidemiology (Table 1)

Only rotavirus groups A, B, and C have been found to be pathogens in the human population. Group A rotaviruses account for 25 to 50% of the diarrheal illnesses found in both the developing and the developed world (6, 12, 41). In the United States, infections predominate in children between 6 months and 2 years old, while in the developing world, illness is frequently reported in children younger than 6 to 12 months. Maternal antibodies are generally believed to protect neonates from infection, but this protection wanes after the third month. Rotavirus displays a seasonal cycle of infection in temperate climates, with most infections occurring in the winter months. In Washington DC, for example, as many as 60 to 65% of all hospital visits for diarrheal illness in January and February, over an 8-year period, were due to rotavirus infection (6). This same pattern of seasonal distribution of infections is not observed in countries within 10° of the equator, where rotavirus infections occur year-round (23), with a slight increase during the rainy season. Group A viruses are spread predominantly through the fecal-oral route, facilitated by crowding and poor sanitation, which further increase the risks for rotavirus infection in developing countries.

Although less prevalent than group A, the group B and group C viruses are significant pathogens in the human population. Group B rotaviruses were originally identified after an epidemic outbreak of waterborne diarrhea in China in 1982–1983 that affected more than 12,000 adults (39). Unlike

TABLE 1 • Epidemiologic Characteristics of Diarrheal Viruses

	Rotavirus	Enteric Adenovirus	Norwalk Virus	Astrovirus
Population affected	Children (A, C) and adults (B)	Children	Children, epidemic illness in adults	Children, elderly patients, adult epidemics, immuno-compromised
Transmission	Fecal-oral, water	Fecal-oral	Fecal-oral, water, shellfish	Fecal-oral, water, shellfish
Seasonality	Winter/rainy season	Year-round	Year-round	Winter/rainy season

group A viruses, group B viruses produce considerable illness in the adult population, with 85% of infected individuals being over 15 years of age. Group C rotavirus infections occur sporadically and appear to primarily infect older children, between 4 and 7 years of age. Recent preliminary studies have provided evidence linking group C rotavirus infection with primary biliary atresia of neonates (35).

Pathogenesis

Rotaviral illness is characterized by a relatively short incubation period (1–3 days) followed by a symptomatic illness with a 5- to 7-day duration (Table 2). Onset of illness is associated with watery diarrhea, fever, and vomiting, with severe fever ($>39°C$) and severe diarrhea (>10 times per day) occurring with high frequency. Although diarrheal illness persists through the length of the infection, vomiting and fever usually remit within 2 to 3 days after onset. Dehydration is very common in rotavirus illness and is the primary cause of rotavirus-associated mortality in the developing world where access to appropriate rehydration therapy is frequently lacking. Asymptomatic illness is fairly common, especially among neonates and older children and adults.

In most cases, rotavirus infection is restricted to the villus enterocytes in the small intestine and spreads from the proximal small bowel to the ileum. The histopathology of rotavirus infection in humans has not been extensively studied (19). Viral destruction of villus tip cells is thought to result in a loss of absorptive capacity for water and sodium, with the resulting imbalance producing characteristic watery diarrhea. Transient deficiencies in intestinal lactase have also been observed after rotavirus infection (29). Recently, the product of rotavirus gene 10, NSP4, has been implicated as an enterotoxin in animal models and may potentially be responsible for some of the diarrhea occurring during infect-ion (2).

Group B rotavirus displays a slightly different pattern of infection than group A and C viruses. This virus has been found to infect primarily the distal small intestine rather than the proximal small intestine. In addition, group B viruses cause syncytia in the epithelial layer, which can damage large contiguous portions of infected epithelium and may play an additional role in producing diarrheal illness.

Laboratory Diagnosis

Rotavirus infection is associated with large quantities of virus shed in the stool, making the virus easy to detect by electron microscopy, enzyme-linked immunosorbent assay (ELISA), or direct visualization of viral genomic RNA in fecal extracts. Double-stranded RNA is highly stable and can be extracted, separated by polyacryamide gel electrophoresis (PAGE), and stained with silver or ethidium bromide. Polymerase chain reaction (PCR) of the genes encoding VP7 and VP4 has been widely used to identify the serotype of the virus present during infection (17). Solid-phase immunoassays have been particularly useful for identifying the group A rotaviruses, and a number of immunoassay kits are available for rapid identification of subgroup and serotypes of virus in fecal samples (9). These kits, however, do not detect non–group A viruses. In outbreaks of group B rotaviruses in China, classical RNA visualization and electron microscopy both determined that a rotavirus was present and that the genomic structure differed significantly from that of standard group A viruses (39). Recently, a recombinant protein-based ELISA was developed to detect group B rotavirus, but it is not yet widely available (27). Commercial antigen detection tests for group C rotavirus are also not currently available.

SUSCEPTIBILITY IN VIVO

Identifying model systems for studying viral gastroenteritis has been a key step in the identification of mechanisms of immunity and has provided systems in which to study potential vaccination or other therapeutic protocols. Development of animal models has been assisted by the fact that many species harbor viruses that are closely related to human agents. This has been crucial, because in most cases, human viruses are restricted in growth in nonhuman species.

Because rotaviruses are ubiquitous in mammalian species, a number of animal rotaviruses have been identified and used to generate models of human group A rotavirus infection. Although studies of rotavirus infection have been conducted in gnotobiotic lambs and calves, extensive study of the immunologic response, including vaccination studies, has been limited to mice, rabbits, and gnotobiotic pigs.

Infection of mice with murine rotaviruses results in a diarrheal illness only when mice are less than 15 days old, but adult mice generate a full range of protective immune responses (44). Mice are semipermissive for infection by some heterologous (nonmurine) rotaviruses, although disease can only be spread from mouse to mouse when homologous viruses are used. The mouse model has proven useful for studying passive transfer of

TABLE 2 • **Clinical Presentation of Viral Illness**

	Rotavirus[a]	Enteric Adenovirus[a]	Norwalk Virus[b]	Astrovirus[c]
Symptomatic patients studied (N)	168 children	32 children	36 adults	44 children
Diarrhea (%)	98 (21% severe)	97 (22% severe)	66	100
Nausea (%)	NA[d]	NA	75	71
Vomiting (%)	87	78	44	61
Fever (%)	84 (42% severe)	44 (3 severe)	25	80
Dehydration (%)	55	37	NA	5
Abdominal pain (%)	18	25	75	58
Blood in stools (%)	1	3	NA	7
Mucus in stools (%)	17	19	NA	55
Respiratory (%)	33	19	NA	NA
Durations:				
Incubation period	1–3 days	7 days	1–2 days	3–4 days
Diarrhea	5.9 days	10.8 days	15–55 h	5–6 days
Vomiting	2.5 days	3.2 days	23–31 h	NA

[a] From reference (41).

[b] From reference (25).

[c] From reference (4).

[d] NA, not available.

immunity to pups from immunized dams through serum or milk. The availability of many genetic knockout mice has been key in assisting detailed study of the cellular and antibody-mediated immune response to rotavirus.

Rabbits can be productively infected by homologous rotaviruses up to 1 year of age. Natural infections in the field appear to be associated with diarrhea and classic histopathologic lesions (shortening of villi, mononuclear infiltration, vacuolation). Although rabbits can be infected by heterologous viruses, neutralizing antibody responses are lower than those observed with homologous infection (8).

Gnotobiotic pigs are the most convenient model for studying disease as well as viral infection. Piglets can be infected with rotaviruses and develop diarrheal illness up to 6 weeks of age, whether porcine or human virus strains are used. Because the disease parameters and immune response in pigs resemble those observed in humans, this model is the only one in which the impact of immunization on disease, as well as viral infection, can be studied. The cost, however, makes it less generally useful than the rabbit and mouse models of infection.

Group B rotaviruses have been identified as causing epidemics of diarrhea in rats and pigs, and both of these animals have been found to be good models of rotavirus illness after inoculation with group B viruses from the homologous species. Experimentally infected animals develop diarrheal disease that can be transmitted, although they shed lower levels of virus than animals infected with group A viruses. Because no culture system exists for group B viruses, these systems are the only ones available for studying and propagating these viruses.

THERAPY

At present, development of chemotherapeutic agents for treating gastrointestinal viruses has made little headway. Although a number of investigations have been carried out in tissue culture models of rotavirus replication, no agents are currently in clinical trials. Ribavirin, a broad-spectrum antiviral, was originally identified as having antirotavirus activity in tissue culture but no measurable effect in the mouse model of viral infection (37, 38). Isoprinosine and a number of other modified nucleoside analogues have shown an ability to prevent viral RNA and protein synthesis in tissue culture, but no experiments in animal models have been reported (24, 25, 32).

Although experimental, some efforts have been made to treat rotaviral illness by passively transferring antibodies. Human serum immunoglobulin administered orally to immunodeficient children with chronic rotavirus infection was able to associate with rotavirus in the gut, resulting in formation of large immune complexes rather than free virus (26). Antigen shedding was significantly reduced after antibody therapy, although the virus was not eliminated in all cases. In a recent study, bone marrow transplant recipients with severe rotavirus illness were able to eliminate the virus and resolve diarrheal symptoms after receiving oral immunoglobulin for 3 days (16).

Antibody administration protocols have preventative efficacy in normal children as well. A single dose of a human immunoglobulin preparation that had a high titer against rotavirus (1:800–1:3,200) significantly speeded the rate of virus clearance and recovery from diarrhea in children infected with rotavirus (11). Bovine immunoglobulin against rotavirus has been produced by hyperimmunizing cattle with human and simian rotaviruses. Either the milk of hyperimmunized cattle (13) or serum immunoglobulins resuspended in milk formula (40) significantly reduced the incidence of rotavirus illness in children from 3 to 7 months old when orally administered. Children receiving immunoglobulins had no symptoms or significantly diminished symptoms upon becoming infected, compared with children receiving placebo formula.

An alternative means of producing antirotavirus immunoglobulins is to harvest specific immunoglobulins from the yolks of eggs laid by chickens immunized with rotavirus. Egg yolks contain large quantities of specific immunoglobulin following intramuscular immunization of hens, and the antibody is stable for long periods of time (20). Oral dosing of mice and calves with these immunoglobulins significantly reduces overall disease (20, 21). In mice, this protection was directly associated with reduced rotavirus antigen distribution within the intestinal tract, suggesting that replication of the virus had been inhibited. A comprehensive summary of passive immunization literature can be found in a recent review by Bogstedt et al. (5).

A number of recent reports have suggested that bacteria may be useful in the treatment of rotavirus-induced gastroenteritis. Feeding two bacterial strains, *Bifidobacterium bifidum* and *Streptococcus thermophilus,* to hospitalized infants aged 5 to 24 months reduced the incidence of diarrheal illness and rotavirus shedding, suggesting that some mechanism of protection from infection was in operation (36). Feeding another bacterial strain, *Lactobacillus casei* strain GG, to infected children appears to shorten diarrheal illness, presumably by restoring the microflora of the intestine and reversing intestinal osmotic and chemical imbalances (14). In addition, when administered in the acute diarrheal phase, *L. casei* appears to stimulate the immune response to rotavirus, particularly the production of IgA, and may significantly enhance protective immunity to subsequent infection (15).

Because immunotherapy is relatively expensive and the opportunity to treat quite brief, it remains to be seen what the practical utility of these interventions is. Obviously, in the rare cases of chronic rotavirus infection in severely immunocompromised individuals, passive immunotherapy may play a bigger role in treatment.

VACCINES

Because no specific therapies have been developed for rotavirus and because it is endemic throughout the world, major efforts aimed at treating rotavirus diarrhea have focused on developing vaccines to prevent infection. Studies on rotavirus in particular are well advanced because of the existence of animal models, the availability of tissue culture systems to manipulate the virus, and the frequency and severity of the clinical illness in children. It is hoped that the lessons learned in developing an effective rotavirus vaccine will be applicable to developing vaccines for other viral diarrheal agents mentioned elsewhere in this volume.

Replicating Vaccines

Because natural infection with rotavirus does not efficiently protect against repeat infection and mild disease, the goal of vaccination is not to prevent rotavirus infection, but rather to reduce the incidence of severe diarrheal illness during the first 2 years of life. Natural rotavirus infection often provides only partial protection against disease upon subsequent reinfection. Vaccination efforts are currently aimed at group A viruses, as they represent the major cause of severe diarrheal illness. Group A viruses are subdivided into serotypes on the basis of their ability to be neutralized by antibodies to the two major outer capsid proteins, VP4 and VP7. Fourteen serotypes have been identified based on reactivity to VP7 (G serotypes), 8 of which are found in humans. Of these, serotypes G1–G4 represent 80 to 95% of

the viruses that are found in the human population, and all four serotypes can be present at any given time and location, although serotype G1 tends to predominate in most parts of the world. Neutralization studies based on reactivity with VP4 (P serotype) have identified at least 13 distinct P serotypes, but serologic reagents are not as readily available for their identification. While 19 distinct genotypes have been identified by DNA sequence analysis of VP4 sequences, serotype and genotype do not always correlate directly, and viruses are often characterized by VP4 genotype rather than P serotype.

Studies in animal models of rotavirus infection indicated that the most important correlate of protective immunity was a strong local antibody response, rather than a serum antibody response (10). To provide the best chance for presenting rotavirus antigens locally, a Jennerian vaccination strategy was proposed. In this strategy, humans would be inoculated with animal viruses that would present antigen to the gut but not be able to replicate sufficiently to induce clinical symptoms. At least three Jennerian vaccine strains have been tested: RIT 4237, a tissue culture–adapted bovine virus (G6); RRV, a virus isolated from a young rhesus monkey (G3); and WC3, a bovine virus displaying a lower degree of attenuation than RIT 4237. In clinical trials, results have been mixed but generally positive. Although RIT 4237 protected 50% of vaccinees in Finland against infection and 80 to 90% against severe illness (42), it had very little reported efficacy in other areas of the world (Africa, Arizona). The second bovine strain, WC3, was able to protect 100% of children in American trials from severe serotype 1 diarrhea (7), but efficacy in other countries ranged from 0 to 48%. The efficacy of the WC3 and RIT vaccines did, however, demonstrate that cross-serotypic protective responses could be generated. The RRV strain of virus induced a mild-to-moderate symptomatic temperature elevation in some vaccinees and generated a highly serotype-specific G3 antibody response.

Due to the random circulation of all four human serotypes and assuming that immunity was G serotype–specific, an effective vaccine would need to be able to generate a heterotypic or multiple serotype–specific response to protect against the major human strains. (G1–G4). To address this, a modified Jennerian approach was studied in which the gene coding for the VP7 protein in animal viruses (RRV or WC3) was exchanged (reassorted) with genes from three or four human serotypes. The product of this study was the RRV-tetravalent vaccine (RRV-TV). This vaccine contains a mix of RRV (serotype G3) and RRV reassortants containing G1, G2, or G4 VP7 genes. This vaccine has undergone clinical trials in the United States, Finland, and Venezuela and is continuing to undergo clinical trials in other areas. In the United States trials, the tetravalent vaccine sometimes induced a higher incidence of fever after vaccination than a serotype 1 monoreassortant (RRV-S1), although this was not always significant (3, 34). Significant diarrhea and vomiting were not reported, and shedding of the vaccine strain in the stool was detected at a low level. Children receiving RRV-TV displayed a measurable but relatively low type-specific response to serotypes 1 to 4, while RRV-S1 recipients had measurable responses to serotype 1 only. The tetravalent vaccine provided significant protection (65–77%) against disease induced by serotype 3 virus, whereas the monovalent vaccine provided variable protection (0–45%). Thus, although overall protection by the tetravalent vaccine against severe illness caused by all serotypes was only 57%, it provided consistent heterotypic protection that may be necessary for efficacy in areas where serotype prevalence varies. The most significant finding was that RRV-TV vaccination prevented 82% of dehydrating illness associated with gastroenteritis relative to placebo recipients (34). Recent studies in Finland and Venezuela (31) with the RRV-based tetravalent vaccine have confirmed its substantial efficacy against moderate-to-severe diarrhea and support the proposition that this vaccine should be licensed for general use among young children.

Nonreplicating Vaccines

With the application of molecular biology to the vaccine problem, a number of alternatives to live-attenuated vaccines have been developed. All of these alternative candidates are still experimental and have only been evaluated in animal models of disease.

Subunit Vaccines

Using recombinant viral proteins to induce an antirotavirus immune response has focused on the VP4 and VP7 proteins. Expression of recombinant VP7 on the surface of cells by use of a vaccinia virus construct has resulted in an immunogenic protein that can provide passive protection in suckling mice (1). VP4 is efficiently expressed in baculovirus, and immunization of mice with recombinant protein can provide lactogenic immunity to virus challenge (28).

Viruslike Particles

Viruslike particles have been generated by simultaneous expression of viral structural proteins in insect cells, and their potential for vaccination tested in animal models. Viruslike particles are thought to display outer capsid proteins in more nativelike conformations and are stable under a variety of physical conditions. In the mouse model, vaccination of dams with rotavirus viruslike particles conferred significant lactogenic passive protection to viral infection in suckling mice (33).

Encapsulation

A third effort to enhance local immunity is to microencapsulate rotavirus proteins or whole viruses for more effective delivery to mucosal surfaces. Studies in mice have shown that microencapsulated virus is more efficiently absorbed and delivered to gut-associated lymphoid tissue after oral inoculation than free virus, and that the local immune response is greatly enhanced by this mode of presentation (18, 30).

ADJUNCTIVE THERAPY

Due to the absence of pharmaceutical agents to treat rotavirus and the self-limiting nature of the viral infection of the gastrointestinal tract in most normal individuals, the key therapeutic goal is to prevent severe dehydration leading to elec-

trolyte imbalance, shock, and death. Dehydration and complications arising from dehydration are most prevalent in rotavirus infection and are the major cause of mortality in infected children. Rehydration can be performed orally or, in patients with severe vomiting or in shock, by intravenous fluid administration. For oral rehydration, the WHO recommends a standard oral rehydration solution containing 3.5 g of sodium chloride, 2.5 g of sodium bicarbonate, 1.5 g of potassium chloride, and 20 g of glucose per liter. An alternative formulation that contains less sodium (40–60 vs. 90 meq/L) is available in the United States. Intravenous rehydration can be achieved using standard saline solutions containing glucose and potassium. In addition to rehydration therapy, it is recommended that efforts be made to improve the nutritional condition of the patient, as malnutrition exacerbates symptoms and slows recovery from diarrheal illness.

COMMENTS

With regard to rotavirus vaccines, the issue of serotype specificity and immunity has raised considerable interest. The current perception is that immunity is rarely cross-reactive, suggesting that protection from many serotypes of rotavirus could only be induced through the modified Jennerian approach. Although modified Jennerian vaccines do provide cross-serotype protection, protection may not depend entirely on the serotype match between vaccines and strains circulating in the population. In one study, the RRV-tetravalent vaccine was more effective than the serotype 1 monovalent vaccine at preventing diarrheal disease, despite the fact that the major circulating viral strain was serotype 1 (3). This suggests that the immunogenicity of the vaccine may have been more important than the serotype match. A Finnish study also demonstrated that G2 and G1 serotype reassortants were equally effective at preventing diarrheal disease despite the fact that the circulating wild-type viruses in the season studied were G1 (43). Since neutralizing antibody responses to human VP7 proteins do not always correlate with efficacy rates, the indication is that G type-specific antibodies may not provide the whole story in explaining vaccine efficacy.

A complicating factor in drawing conclusions from vaccination trials is the variability in response that occurs in different countries. The RRV-TV vaccine conferred a good level of protection against severe disease in the United States and Venezuela, but different results were obtained in a trial in Lima, Peru. Here, a standard three-dose regimen resulted in only a moderate level of vaccine protection against severe rotavirus diarrhea (35–66%) compared with the previous trials. In approximately 40% of diarrheal illnesses during this trial, bacterial pathogens were associated with rotavirus diarrhea, and in these cases, the vaccine did not protect against severe illness (22). Although it is unclear why the vaccine did not fare well in this trial, preexisting antibody levels in young children and the presence of other enteric pathogens at the time of vaccination and evaluation might have played major roles, or the dose of vaccine administered in the trial may not have been optimal. These situations are more likely to arise in developing than developed countries and may limit the ability of vaccination to provide high-level protection against rotavirus diarrhea.

REFERENCES

1. Andrew ME, Boyle DB, Coupar BEH, Reddy D, Bellamy AR, Both GW. Vaccinia-rotavirus VP7 recombinants protect mice against rotavirus-induced diarrhoea. Vaccine 1992;10: 189–191.
2. Ball JM, Tian P, Zeng CQ, Morris AP, Estes MK. Age-dependent diarrhea induced by a rotaviral nonstructural glycoprotein. Science 1996;272:101–104.
3. Bernstein DI, Glass RI, Rodgers G, Davidson BL, Sack DA. Evaluation of rhesus rotavirus monovalent and tetravalent reassortant vaccines in US children. JAMA 1995;273(5):1191–1196.
4. Blacklow NR, Herrmann JE. Astrovirus gastroenteritis. Trans Am Clin Climat Assoc 1994;106:58–66.
5. Bogstedt AK, Johansen K, Hatta H, Kim M, Casswall T, Svensson L, Hammarström L. Passive immunity against diarrhoea. Acta Paediatr 1996;85:125–128.
6. Brandt CD, Kim HW, Rodriguez WJ, Arrobio JO, Jeffries BC, Stallings EP, Lewis C, Miles AJ, Chanock RM, Kapikian AZ, Parrott RH. Pediatric viral gastroenteritis during eight years of study. J Clin Microbiol 1983;18:71–78.
7. Clark HF, Borian FE, Bell LM, Modesto K, Gouvea V, Plotkin SA. Protective effect of WC3 vaccine against rotavirus diarrhea in infants during a predominantly serotype 1 rotavirus season. J Infect Dis 1988;158:570–587.
8. Conner ME, Estes MK, Graham DY. Rabbit model of rotavirus infection. J Virol 1988;62:1625–1633.
9. Dennehy PH, Gauntlett DR, Tente WE. Comparison of nine commercial immunoassays for the detection of rotavirus in fecal samples. J Clin Microbiol 1988;26:1630–1634.
10. Feng N, Burns JW, Bracy L, Greenberg HB. Comparison of mucosal and systemic humoral immune responses and subsequent protection in mice orally inoculated with a homologous or heterologous rotavirus. J Virol 1994;68:7766–7773.
11. Guarino A, Canani RB, Russo S, Albano F, Canani MB, Ruggeri FM, Donelli G, Rubino A. Oral immunoglobulins for treatment of acute rotaviral gastroenteritis. Pediatrics 1994;93:12–16.
12. Herrmann JE, Blacklow NR, Peron-Henry DM, Clements E, Taylor DN, Echeverria P. Incidence of enteric adenoviruses among children in Thailand and the significance of these viruses in gastroenteritis. J Clin Microbiol 1988;26:1783–1786.
13. Hilpert H, Brüssow H, Mietens C, Sidoti J, Lerner L, Werchau H. Use of bovine milk concentrate containing antibody to rotavirus to treat rotavirus gastroenteritis in infants. J Infect Dis 1987;156:158–166.
14. Isolauri E, Kaila M, Mykkänen H, Ling WH, Salminen S. Oral bacteriotherapy for viral gastroenteritis. Dig Dis Sci 1994;39: 2595–2600.
15. Kaila M, Isolauri E, Saxelin M, Arvilommi H, Vesikari T. Viable versus inactivated lactobacillus strain GG in acute rotavirus diarrhoea. Arch Dis Child 1995;72:51–53.
16. Kanfer EJ, Abrahamson G, Taylor J, Coleman JC, Samson DM. Severe rotavirus-associated diarrhoea following bone marrow transplantation: treatment with oral immunoglobulin. Bone Marrow Transplant 1994;14:651–652.
17. Kapikian AZ, Chanock RM. Rotaviruses. In: Fields BN, Knipe DM, Howley PM, eds. Fields virology, 3rd ed. Philadelphia: Lippincott-Raven, 1996:1657–1708.
18. Khoury CA, Moser CA, Speaker TJ, Offit PA. Oral inoculation

19. Kohler VT, Erben U, Wiedersberg H, Bannert N. Histological findings in the small intestinal mucosa in children with rotavirus infection. Kinderarztl Prax 1990;58:323–327.
20. Kuroki M, Ikemori Y, Yokoyama H, Peralta RC, Icatlo FC Jr, Kodama Y. Passive protection against bovine rotavirus-induced diarrhea in murine model by specific immunoglobulins from chicken egg yolk. Vet Microbiol 1993;37:135–146.
21. Kuroki M, Ohta M, Ikemori Y, Peralta RC, Yokoyama H, Kodama Y. Passive protection against bovine rotavirus in calves by specific immunoglobulins from chicken egg yolk. Arch Virol 1994;138:143–148.
22. Lanata CF, Midthun K, Black RE, Butron B, Huapaya A, Penny ME, Ventura G, Gil A, Jett-Goheen M, Davidson BL. Safety, immunogenicity, and protective efficacy of one and three doses of the tetravalent rhesus rotavirus vaccine in infants in Lima, Peru. J Infect Dis 1996;174:268–275.
23. LeBaron CW, Lew J, Glass RI, Weber JM, Ruiz-Palacios GM. Rotavirus study group. Annual rotavirus epidemic patterns in North America. JAMA 1990;264:983–988.
24. Linhares REC, Lagrota MHC, Nozawa CM. The in vitro antiviral activity of isoprinosine on simian rotavirus (SA-11). Braz J Med Biol Res 1989;22:1095–1103.
25. Linhares REC, Rebello MA, Nozawa CM. Effect of isoprinosine on rotavirus replication in vitro. Braz J Med Biol Res 1996; 29:219–222.
26. Losonsky GA, Johnson JP, Winkelstein JA, Yolken RH. Oral administration of human serum immunoglobulin in immunodeficient patients with viral gastroenteritis. J Clin Invest 1985;76: 2362–2367.
27. Mackow ER. Group B and C rotaviruses. In: Blaser MJ, Smith PD, Ravdin JI, Greenberg HB, Guerrant RL, eds. Infections of the gastrointestinal tract. New York: Raven Press, 1995: 983–1008.
28. Mackow ER, Vo PT, Broome R, Bass D, Greenberg HB. Immunization with baculovirus-expressed VP4 protein passively protects against simian and murine rotavirus challenge. J Virol 1990;64:1698–1703.
29. Noone C, Menzies IS, Banatvala JE, Scopes JW. Intestinal permeability and lactose hydrolysis in human rotaviral gastroenteritis assessed simultaneously by non-invasive differential sugar permeation. Eur J Clin Invest 1986;16:217.
30. Offit PA, Khoury CA, Moser CA, Clark HF, Kim JE, Speaker TJ. Enhancement of rotavirus immunogenicity by microencapsulation. Virology 1994;203:134–143.
31. Perez-Schael I, Guntinas MJ, Perez M, Pagone V, Rojas AM, Gonzalez R, Cunto W, Hoshino Y, Kapikian AZ. Efficacy of the rhesus rotavirus-based quadrivalent vaccine in infants and young children in Venezuela. N Engl J Med 1997;337: 1181–1187.
32. Pizarro JM, Pizarro JL, Fernández J, Sandino AM, Spencer E. Effect of nucleotide analogues on rotavirus transcription and replication. Virology 1991;184:768–772.
33. Redmond MJ, Ijaz MK, Parker MD, Sabara MI, Dent D, Gibbons E, Babiuk LA. Assembly of recombinant rotavirus proteins into virus-like particles and assessment of vaccine potential. Vaccine 1993;11:273–281.
34. Rennels MB, Glass RI, Dennehy PH, Bernstein DI, Pichichero ME, Zito ET, Mack ME, Davidson BL, Kapikian AZ. Safety and efficacy of high-dose rhesus-human reassortant rotavirus

vaccines—report of the national multicenter trial. Pediatrics 1996;97:7–13.

35. Riepenhoff-Talty M, Gouvea V, Evans MJ, Svensson L, Hoffenberg E, Sokol RJ, Unhoo I, Greenberg SJ, Schakel K, Zhaori G. Detection of group C rotavirus in infants with extrahepatic biliary atresia. J Infect Dis 1996;174:8–15.

36. Saavedra JM, Bauman NA, Oung I, Perman JA, Yolken RH. Feeding of *Bifidobacterium bifidum* and *Streptococcus thermophilus* to infants in hospital for prevention of diarrhoea and shedding of rotavirus. Lancet 1994;344:1046–1049.

37. Schoub BD, Prozesky OW. Antiviral activity of ribavirin in rotavirus gastroenteritis of mice. Antimicrob Agents Chemother 1977;12:543–554.

38. Smee DF, Sidwell RW, Clark SM, Barnett BB, Spendlove RS. Inhibition of rotaviruses by selected antiviral substances: mechanisms of viral inhibition and in vivo activity. Antimicrob Agents Chemother 1982;21:66–73.

39. Tao H, Changan W, Zhaoying F, Zinyi C, Xuejian C, Xiaoquang L, Guangmu C, Henli Y, Tungxin C, Weiwe Y, Shuasen D, Wei-

cheng C. Waterborne outbreak of rotavirus diarrhoea in adults in China caused by a novel rotavirus. Lancet 1984;1:1139–1142.

40. Turner RB, Kelsey DK. Passive immunization for prevention of rotavirus illness in healthy infants. Pediatr Infect Dis J 1993; 12:18–22.

41. Unhoo I, Olding-Stenkvist E, Kreuger A. Clinical features of acute gastroenteritis associated with rotavirus, enteric adenoviruses, and bacteria. Arch Dis Child 1986;61:732–738.

42. Vesikari T, Isolauri E, D'Hondt E, Delem A, Andre FE, Zissis G. Protection of infants against rotavirus diarrhoea by RIT4237 attenuated bovine rotavirus strain vaccine. Lancet 1984;1:977–981.

43. Vesikari T, Ruuska T, Green KY, Flores J, Kapikian AZ. Protective efficacy against serotype 1 rotavirus diarrhea by live oral rhesus-human reassortant rotavirus vaccines with human rotavirus VP7 serotype 1 or 2 specificity. Pediatr Infect Dis J 1992; 11: 535–542.

44. Ward RL, McNeal MM, Sheridan JF. Development of an adult mouse model for studies on protection against rotavirus. J Virol 1990;64:5070–5075.

Varicella-Zoster Virus

Ann M. Arvin and Martin J. Wood

GENERAL DESCRIPTION
Virology

Varicella-zoster virus (VZV) is an alphaherpes virus that has an icosahedral nucleocapsid, tegument, and lipid envelope (3). The intact VZV particle is 180 to 200 nm in diameter. It has a linear, double-stranded DNA genome of about 125,000 base pairs with at least 69 open reading frames. It is highly temperature sensitive and depends upon envelope proteins for infectivity. No distinct subtypes have been identified, although epidemiologically unrelated viruses have differences in restriction endonuclease digest patterns.

Pathogenesis

During primary VZV infection, the virus is inoculated at mucous membrane sites and is presumed to spread to regional lymph nodes and cause a primary viremia (3). A secondary viremia occurs 4 or 5 days before onset of symptoms and persists for 1 to 2 days after. VZV is lymphotropic for CD4+ as well as CD8+ T lymphocytes. Infected T cells are presumed to transfer the virus to skin cells. VZV replicates in epidermal and dermal cells to produce the characteristic vesicular rash. The virus has the pathogenic potential to cause disseminated infection involving lungs, liver, central nervous system (CNS), and other organs if the T-cell viremia is not terminated by the host response.

One property of herpesviruses is an ability to establish latent infections without replication in their hosts. During the primary infection, VZV is thought to pass centripetally along the sensory nerve fibers from the skin to the corresponding sensory ganglia. Within the ganglia, VZV establishes latency in neuronal and/or satellite cells. The virus then remains quiescent but reactivates sporadically and infrequently to cause herpes zoster (88). The molecular mechanisms that establish and maintain VZV latency are not fully understood, but reactivation of the virus is clearly related to declining VZV-specific cell-mediated immunity (CMI). CMI to VZV declines markedly in immunocompromised patients and in the elderly (64). Levels of VZV-specific CMI also correlate with development of herpes zoster in leukemic children after live varicella vaccine administration (47).

During reactivation, VZV replication is extensive within the ganglion, causing severe neuronal necrosis and inflammation. VZV then spreads down the sensory nerve to infect the skin, producing the characteristic dermatomal vesicles of herpes zoster.

Epidemiology

Varicella occurs in a worldwide geographic distribution. Annual epidemics are more common in temperate climates than in tropical areas. Cases of varicella or herpes zoster are a source of transmission to susceptible close contacts. VZV is transmissible by the respiratory route from individuals with varicella. The attack rate among household contacts is 80 to 90%.

Although herpes zoster can occur in any individual who has previously been infected with VZV, it is classically a disease of the elderly or those whose CMI is depressed because of disease or immunosuppressive drugs. Epidemiologic data from the United States and United Kingdom suggest that overall, there are between 1.3 and 4.2 cases of herpes zoster per 1000 persons per year (48, 61, 75). Herpes zoster can occur at any age, but the incidence increases dramatically after middle age, and approximately 1% of those over 80 years old develop herpes zoster annually. It is estimated that approximately one-fifth of the population of the developed world will develop herpes zoster at some stage during their lifetime (48, 75). Although the incidence of herpes zoster is highest among those over 75 years of age, population demographics in developed countries mean that most cases of herpes zoster are seen in females in the sixth and seventh decades of life. Children or adolescents who acquired primary VZV infection in utero or in the first year of life have a relative risk up to 20.9 times greater than others of developing herpes zoster before the age of 20 years (7, 14, 44).

Patients with lymphoma or leukemia have a fivefold greater incidence of herpes zoster than the general adult population (66, 75), with the highest incidence in those with Hodgkin's disease (34). Between 30 and 50% of adults and 25% of children develop herpes zoster in the year following bone marrow transplantation (BMT), typically from the third month onward, and herpes zoster occurs in about 10 to 15% of solid organ transplant recipients, usually in the first 6 months after transplantation. Herpes zoster occurs at all stages of HIV, and in HIV-positive individuals, the annual incidence of herpes zoster is increased 10- to 20-fold over the rate in the general population (15, 76). Herpes zoster is less common among vaccinated leukemic children (2%) than in those naturally infected with wild type VZV (15%) (47).

Clinical Manifestations

Varicella. Varicella may be associated with a prodrome of fever, malaise, headache and abdominal pain, occurring 24 to 48 h before rash (4). These symptoms are more common in older children and adults. Varicella is usually diagnosed clinically by the appearance of the rash, which is often initially observed on the face, scalp, or trunk. The lesions are pruritic, erythematous macules that evolve rapidly to vesicles; ulcerative lesions are noted on mucous membranes in many patients. Without treatment, new lesions appear for 1 to 7 days. The number of lesions varies from fewer than 10 to more than 1500, with a usual range of 100 to 300. The rash is more extensive in older children, in secondary household cases, and in patients with skin trauma, such as sunburn. Varicella is usually accompanied by lymphopenia and granulocytopenia in the acute phase, and slightly elevated liver function tests are common. Secondary bacterial infections, usually due to *Staphylococcus aureus* or *Streptococcus pyogenes* (group A β-hemolytic streptococcus), are the most common complication of varicella.

Varicella pneumonia is almost never observed in healthy children but complicates primary VZV infection in up to 5% of adults, with about 1 in 400 adults requiring hospitalization (33). Fever, cough, dyspnea, and hemoptysis develop within a few days of the onset of the rash, and chest radiographs usually show ill-defined diffuse infiltrates (33). Untreated, there is a mortality of about 10%. Neurologic complications include meningoencephalitis, which is associated with direct infection of the CNS, and cerebellar ataxia, which is probably not (54). Encephalitis is usually transient, resolving within 24 to 72 h, and permanent sequelae are rare; cerebellar ataxia often persists for days or weeks but also usually resolves completely (91, 97). Hemorrhagic complications may result from hepatitis and thrombocytopenia and may progress to disseminated intravascular coagulopathy.

Populations at high risk for complications of varicella include patients with lymphoproliferative malignancies or solid tumors, recipients of organ or bone marrow transplantation, patients receiving high-dose or chronic steroid therapy, patients with congenital cellular immunodeficiency disorders, and newborn infants whose mothers have varicella just before or after delivery. Varicella is usually not life threatening in children with HIV infection, but these patients may have unusual hyperkeratotic varicella. Immunosuppressive therapy given during the incubation period and an absolute lymphocyte count below 500 cells at the onset of rash are associated with an increased risk of disseminated varicella. Without antiviral therapy, varicella in high-risk populations is associated with prolonged new lesion formation, increased numbers of lesions, and risk of dissemination, with pneumonia, hepatitis, encephalitis, and disseminated intravascular coagulopathy. Pneumonia occurs within 3 to 7 days and is the primary reason for mortality. Fulminant hepatitis and disseminated intravascular coagulopathy are also associated with high mortality rates.

Herpes Zoster. Herpes zoster is almost always unilateral, affecting one or two adjacent dermatomes. The most frequently affected dermatome is that of the trigeminal nerve, particularly the ophthalmic branch, which is involved in 10 to 15% of all cases. Otherwise, each dermatome is affected at a similar rate of 3 to 4%. About 50% of herpes zoster involves the trunk as a result of reactivation of one or more of the thoracic dermatomes. The pathologic changes of VZV reactivation start in the relevant sensory ganglion, and pain and paresthesias within the affected dermatome often precede the rash by several days. Since it can mimic a wide range of other conditions, the cause of the pain is usually not recognized until the rash appears. The rash of herpes zoster begins as erythematous maculopapules that develop into vesicles, 0.5 to 2 cm in diameter, within 12 h or so. After 3 to 4 days, pustules form that gradually dry and crust over the next 7 to 10 days. New lesions continue to appear for a mean of less than 2 days and for more than 96 h in only 10 to 15% of normal individuals (16). Virus can generally be cultured from the vesicles for 3 or 4 days, although in 15% it is recoverable from lesions for 1 week (18).

Herpes zoster in the immunocompromised is often more extensive than in normal persons, involving the dermis and having hemorrhagic and necrotic lesions. Some cutaneous dissemination is very common, and in 20 to 30% of cases, there is viremic spread with widespread cutaneous and visceral dissemination (59). In advanced HIV-related disease, herpes zoster can be severe, disseminated, and atypical. There is a higher risk of multidermatomal herpes zoster (29) and or recurrent episodes (15, 21), and there are many reports of the skin lesions becoming indolent, hyperkeratotic, and verrucous; there is an association between such chronic lesions and in vitro resistance to acyclovir (49, 58).

Although most cases of herpes zoster in the immunocompetent host are self-limiting and resolve completely, 15 to 20% experience one or more complications. The major complication and cause of morbidity after herpes zoster in the immunocompetent host is continuing pain or postherpetic neuralgia. Postherpetic neuralgia is an arbitrarily defined term, and no definition conveys any important information about the pathophysiology or prognosis of the condition. Pain persists for more than 4 weeks after resolution of the rash in 10 to 15% of adult patients with herpes zoster, but only 30 to 50% of these are still in pain after 3 months, and 25 to 30% after 12 months (16, 48, 75). Prolonged pain is more common in the elderly, and at 1, 3, and 6 months after the illness, 50 to 61%, about 25%, and 9 to 13%, respectively, of patients over 60 years of age are still in pain (62, 72). The pathogenesis of postherpetic neuralgia is poorly understood, but recent research suggests that increased transmission of nociceptive impulses during the period of acute neuronitis induces central sensitization and hyperexcitability of spinal neurons, which is then maintained by changed peripheral input and by excitotoxic damage in the dorsal horn of the spinal cord (42, 102).

Involvement of the eye is commonly seen in patients with ophthalmic herpes zoster (26). Conjunctivitis is the most frequent problem, but anterior uveitis and keratitis are of greater significance. A variety of neurologic complications, including motor paralysis (predominantly in herpes zoster involving the trigeminal nerve or upper cervical dermatomes—the Ramsay Hunt syndrome—other cervical and lumbosacral dermatomes), encephalitis, and myelitis are uncommon complications of herpes zoster in otherwise healthy patients.

A similar wide range of neurologic complications, including myelitis, chronic progressive encephalitis, and Guillain-Barré syndrome, has been reported in patients with AIDS (43, 90). Only two-thirds of these patients have had concomitant or previous cutaneous herpes zoster lesions (60), but the role of VZV in these neurologic complications is indicated by finding VZV antigens and VZV DNA (2) and culturing the virus from cerebrospinal fluid (51).

Acute retinal necrosis, in both otherwise healthy and immunocompromised persons, has been caused by VZV (38). The syndrome is characterized by retinal vasculitis, confluent retinal necrosis, and acute vitritis and produces devastating visual loss. Acute retinal necrosis may occur concurrently or follow herpes zoster, but many cases caused by VZV in HIV-positive patients are not accompanied by any cutaneous lesions. The syndrome of rapidly progressive outer retinal necrosis has been described only in patients with AIDS. It is similar to acute retinal necrosis, but there is an absence of pain

and intraocular inflammation, early involvement of the macula, and a rapidly progressive (often bilateral) course (36).

Diagnostics

Diagnosis of varicella does not require laboratory confirmation in healthy children. Rapid diagnosis may be required to guide decisions about antiviral therapy in immunocompromised children. Direct detection is done by staining cells from the base of a cutaneous vesicle with antibody reagents that bind to VZV proteins or by testing vesicular fluid for viral antigens with enzyme immunoassay methods (39). VZV can be isolated in tissue culture cells to confirm diagnoses made with rapid antigen-detection methods. VZV DNA can also be detected by in situ hybridization or polymerase chain reaction. VZV IgG and IgM antibodies are present at the onset of varicella in some individuals and in almost all patients by 3 days; titers increase more than fourfold during convalescence. Serologic tests for VZV immune status are useful to assess susceptibility of exposed individuals.

The diagnosis of herpes zoster is also generally clinical. In the preeruptive phase, the pain may be confused with that of any localized condition, but once the rash, appears the diagnosis is usually obvious. Routine serology alone is not useful in establishing reactivation of VZV. Virologic confirmation can be made by the same methods as for varicella. Neurologic infection with VZV can be confirmed by PCR amplification of VZV DNA extracted from cerebrospinal fluid (77). Evidence of local production of specific antibodies within the cerebrospinal fluid might also be obtained. To determine the etiology of acute retinal necrosis or progressive outer retinal necrosis, the causative virus can be detected within the affected eye by culture of the vitreous (22); viral DNA may be detected in either vitreous or aqueous fluid by PCR, or intraocular specific antibody production can be detected (23).

SUSCEPTIBILITY IN VITRO AND IN IN VIVO
Single-Drug Susceptibility

In vitro, VZV is susceptible to several antiviral drugs. The activity depends to some extent on the viral strain and the cells used for tissue culture. The ID_{50} of acyclovir for VZV is 3.5 to 18 μmol, and a virtually identical range of values has been determined for penciclovir (31). Both drugs are phosphorylated by a VZV-coded thymidine kinase. Sorivudine (BVaraU), a much more potent inhibitor of VZV replication in cell culture, has an ID_{50} about 2000 to 5000 times lower than acyclovir. It, too, is converted to its monophosphate by VZV thymidine kinase, but it is then further phosphorylated to the diphosphate by additional virally encoded thymidylate kinase activity.

Foscarnet is a pyrophosphate analogue that directly inhibits viral DNA polymerase and has a ID_{50} for VZV of 50 to 90 μM (57). Since it does not depend upon thymidine kinase for activation, foscarnet may be used for VZV strains that are resistant to acyclovir and penciclovir because of thymidine kinase deficiency. Cidofovir is a nucleotide agent that may be used for such resistant strains because it is already phosphorylated and its activity does not depend on virus-encoded enzymes (24).

Combination Drugs

There are no data on combinations of drugs in vitro.

ANTIVIRAL THERAPY
Drug of Choice

Varicella

Oral acyclovir is now licensed for the treatment of varicella in healthy children and adults, on the basis of clinical efficacy and safety demonstrated in placebo-controlled studies. Antiviral therapy with this agent diminishes the clinical symptoms of varicella in otherwise healthy children, adolescents, and adults when given within 24 h after appearance of the initial cutaneous lesions (10, 27, 84). The dose for children, 2 to 12 years old, is 20 mg/kg four times a day for 5 days (maximum, 800 mg/dose). Treatment reduces fever, pruritus, the number of days of new lesion formation, and the total number of cutaneous lesions, compared with placebo (27). Since varicella is a self-limited infection in healthy children, the clinical benefit is essentially limited to converting all cases of varicella to the mildest form of the illness that occurs without treatment. Children treated within 24 h after onset can be expected to have fever for less than 24 to 48 h, new lesion formation for less than 72 h, and fewer than 300 total lesions. Drug efficacy is demonstrated regardless of age, but treatment may have more clinical impact in children who are 5 to 12 years old or are secondary household cases because the illness is more likely to be somewhat more severe. Whether antiviral therapy alters varicella complications in healthy children has not been determined because of the low incidence of these events.

Oral acyclovir reduces the severity of varicella in healthy adolescents, ages 13 to 18 years, and adults (10, 84). The dosage is 800 mg/dose, four times a day for 5 days. Treatment within 24 h of onset reduces the duration of fever, new lesion formation, and total number of lesions. Since varicella is more severe in older individuals, oral acyclovir should be given when it is possible to begin treatment within 24 h. Early antiviral therapy in this age group can potentially reduce the risk of varicella pneumonia.

Oral acyclovir treatment started after the appearance of the cutaneous lesions of varicella does not block acquisition of immunity to VZV. The American Academy of Pediatrics recommends that acyclovir be considered for patients with varicella who have chronic cutaneous or pulmonary diseases or diseases requiring chronic salicylate therapy or who are being treated with short or intermittent courses of steroids or aerosolized corticosteroids (1). Otherwise healthy patients who develop varicella pneumonia, hepatitis, thrombocytopenia, or encephalitis should be treated with intravenous acyclovir, 10 mg/kg/dose ($500 mg/m^2$/dose) every 8 h, for 7 days. The overall mortality for VZV pneumonitis in immunocompromised and immunocompetent hosts treated with intravenous acyclovir ranges from 0 to 20%, with a higher rate in pregnant women and those with respiratory failure at the start of therapy (41, 45, 79). Adults with tachypnea, cough, increasing dyspnea, or hemoptysis and with pulmonary infiltrates should be started on intravenous acyclovir.

Herpes Zoster

The currently available data suggest that oral acyclovir (800 mg five times daily for 7 days), famciclovir (250 mg (in Europe) and 500 mg (U.S.) every 8 h for 7 days), and valacyclovir (1000 mg every 8 h for 7 days) have very similar clinical efficacy in herpes zoster in immunocompetent patients if started within 72 h of onset of the rash. A choice between them may depend on costs and convenience of administration (Table 1).

Randomized placebo-controlled studies have shown that oral acyclovir (800 mg 5 times daily for 7 or 10 days) reduces the duration of new lesion formation and significantly accelerates rash healing in the normal host with herpes zoster (95). In the largest such study, the time to full crusting of skin lesions was reduced by more than 36 h by the use of acyclovir (100). Pain during the acute phase was also improved, but conflicting results were obtained in the individual studies regarding the effect of acyclovir on the incidence of postherpetic neuralgia. Recently, a meta-analysis of all the placebo-controlled data has confirmed that the licensed dose of acyclovir does reduce the duration of pain associated with herpes zoster, however the pain is defined or assessed (99). Extending acyclovir therapy beyond 7 days provides no additional benefit (98).

The L-valine ester of acyclovir, valacyclovir, has improved oral bioavailability and is rapidly converted to acyclovir after oral administration. An oral dose of 1000 mg valacyclovir yields plasma concentrations of acyclovir comparable with those observed with intravenous acyclovir (28). Valacyclovir (1000 mg every 8 h) significantly shortened the duration of zoster-associated pain compared with a standard course of oral acyclovir in immunocompetent individuals over the age of 50 years with herpes zoster of less than 72 hours' duration, although the incidence of pain at various time points after the acute phase of the illness was not significantly reduced (11). The time to rash resolution was also similar for the two drugs. Penciclovir is another acyclic nucleoside with anti-VZV activity equivalent to that of acyclovir, and in a similar fashion, an oral prodrug, famciclovir, has been developed to provide therapeutic plasma concentrations (28). A placebo-controlled trial showed that famciclovir (500 or 750 mg every 8 h) was highly effective for lesion healing, particularly in patients recruited within 48 h of rash onset (83). Resolution of the acute pain in uncomplicated herpes zoster was also statistically significant for the 500 mg every 8 h dose but not for the higher dose when all patients were considered (83). In another study comparing the drug with acyclovir in patients enrolled within 72 h of rash onset, famciclovir given as either 500 mg every 8 h (the dosage licensed in the U.S.) or 250 mg tid (the dosage licensed in Europe) produced similar rates of healing of the rash, duration of VZV shedding, and loss of pain during the period of rash healing (25). When zoster-associated pain was assessed, data showed that for patients treated within 48 h of rash onset, famciclovir at all doses resolved pain significantly faster than acyclovir.

Although there are no controlled clinical trials, early case reports suggested a good response of herpes zoster encephalitis to intravenous acyclovir (10 mg/kg or $500 mg/m^2$ per dose, given 8-hourly for 14–21 days), (13, 19, 30, 52, 67, 81, 82, 94),

TABLE 1 • Comparison of Acyclovir, Famciclovir and Valaciclovir in the Treatment of Herpes Zoster in Normal Immunocompetent Adults

Parameter	Acyclovir	Famciclovir	Valaciclovir
Dosage	800 mg five times daily for 7 days	250 mg[a] or 500 mg[b] q. 8 h[c] for 7 days	1000 mg q. 8 h for 7 days
Healing of rash	Better than placebo	Equivalent to acyclovir	Equivalent to acyclovir
Duration of acute pain	Better than placebo in some studies (20, 50)	Equivalent to acyclovir	Not reported
Postherpetic neuralgia	Lower incidence than with placebo in some studies (46, 50, 65); duration reduced in meta-analysis (99)	Shorter duration with 500-mg dose than with placebo (250-mg dose not studied) (83); not reported in comparison with acyclovir (25)	Shorter duration than with acyclovir (11)
Duration of zoster-associated pain	Reduced in some studies and in meta-analysis (99)	Shorter than with acyclovir (with 500-mg dose only) (25); reduced for 250-mg dose and 500-mg dose for subset treated within 48 h of rash onset (25)	Reduced compared with acyclovir (11)
Efficacy against ocular complications	Reduced compared with placebo (20)	Not studied	Not studied[d]
Experience with drug	Extensive	Limited	Limited[d]
Cost of 7-day course (U.K.)	£82.77	£107.35	£98.50

Data from references 11, 20, 25, 46, 50, 65, 83, 99, 100.

[a] Licensed dose in U.K. and Europe.

[b] Licensed dose in U.S.

[c] 750 mg q. 24 h or 500 mg q. 12 h licensed in some European countries. These doses have not been studied for effects on pain beyond the first month of illness.

[d] Likely to be equivalent to acyclovir, since drug is completely converted to acyclovir after oral administration.

and a review of such data showed a statistical trend toward lower mortality in patients treated with acyclovir (71).

Special Situations

Varicella

Intravenous acyclovir is indicated for treatment of varicella in high-risk patients (74). Those at risk for progressive varicella include patients receiving immunosuppressive therapy for malignancy, organ transplantation, bone marrow transplantation, autoimmune diseases, or other chronic diseases. Newborn infants who are born from 4 days before to 2 days after the onset of maternal varicella and develop varicella at 5 days of age or later are also considered at risk for disseminated infection (73). Acyclovir therapy compensates for impaired host response and terminates viremia and viral replication in skin lesions. Early antiviral therapy reduces the mortality of varicella in immunocompromised patients primarily by reducing the risk or severity of varicella pneumonia. In a controlled trial of acyclovir and vidarabine in children with cancer and varicella, there was no evidence of VZV pneumonitis after 2 days of acyclovir therapy, whereas 30% of the vidarabine recipients developed pneumonitis (35). The dosage of intravenous acyclovir for varicella in high-risk patients is 10 mg/kg/dose (500 mg/m²/dose) every 8 h, with administration continuing for 7 days or in milder cases, until no new lesions have appeared for 48 h. Intravenous acyclovir therapy should be initiated within the first 24 to 72 h after the onset of the rash, because visceral

dissemination occurs within this interval. Treatment later in the course is also beneficial, to inhibit the infection while the host response develops and to treat varicella complications. In immunocompromised patients who do not clinically respond to 8-hourly doses of intravenous acyclovir, continuous infusion of a higher dose (2 mg/kg/h) may be successful (53).

Herpes Zoster

Ophthalmic Zoster. Oral acyclovir (800 mg five times daily) is the drug of choice for patients with herpes zoster ophthalmicus, since in such patients, it has a highly significant effect on those ocular complications such as stromal keratitis and anterior uveitis that tend to occur some time after the acute episode (20, 46). In one study, these benefits were obtained even though patients with rash present for up to 7 days were included in the trial (20). Topical acyclovir has little proven value in acute keratitis accompanying herpes zoster ophthalmicus. There is no reason to believe that valacyclovir would be any less effective, but although patients with ophthalmic zoster were included in the valacyclovir herpes zoster trial (11), no specific data about ocular complications were obtained. There are, as yet, no published reports of famciclovir treatment of ophthalmic herpes zoster.

Immunocompromised Patients. Intravenous acyclovir (10 mg/kg every 8 h or 500 mg/m² every 8 h in children) is the standard therapy for severely immunocompromised patients with localized herpes zoster. Therapy should continue until there have been no fresh cutaneous lesions for 3 days (usually a 5- to 7-day course). Such intravenous acyclovir, although it had no proven effects upon cutaneous resolution or acute pain, significantly decreased the number of patients with cutaneous or visceral dissemination of the disease (8), and a further study (80) conclusively showed acyclovir to be more effective than vidarabine at preventing dissemination of the disease. Cases of multifocal leukoencephalitis caused by VZV have been described in immunocompromised patients (with or without recent cutaneous herpes zoster). One such case, in a 13-year-old child with acute lymphoblastic leukemia, was successfully treated with high-dose (20 mg/kg every 8 h) acyclovir given for 10 weeks (17).

Oral acyclovir may be used in selected patients with minimal immunosuppression and localized herpes zoster. For uncomplicated herpes zoster in HIV-infected patients, oral acyclovir 800 mg five times daily should also suffice. Penciclovir/famciclovir and valacyclovir have not yet been evaluated in immunocompromised patients. Oral sorivudine has value in treating herpes zoster in patients with HIV infection, (12, 28, 87) but is not yet licensed for use.

Acute Retinal Necrosis/Progressive Outer Retinal Necrosis. No randomized trials of therapy have been conducted in acute retinal necrosis. Acyclovir treatment of acute retinal necrosis (10 mg/kg or 500 mg/m^2 given intravenously three times daily for 7–10 days and often followed by oral acyclovir 800 mg five times daily for 12 weeks) speeds resolution of retinal lesions and decreases the risk of disease in the fellow eye (69) but does not prevent retinal detachment and other ocular complications in the initially affected eye.

Monotherapy with acyclovir or ganciclovir is of little or no benefit in progressive outer retinal necrosis, and the outlook for vision is grave. Some success has been claimed for combination therapy with ganciclovir and foscarnet (37).

The optimal therapy for VZV infection in patients with HIV/AIDS is unknown, but by extrapolation from other immunocompromised patients, acyclovir is generally given in high doses intravenously for severe cases and orally for less severe cutaneous herpes zoster.

Alternative Therapy

Vidarabine and interferon were used for varicella and herpes zoster in immunocompromised patients in early clinical trials but have been replaced by acyclovir because it is less toxic and easier to administer (63, 89, 92). Sorivudine (40 mg once daily for 5 days) was statistically superior to placebo in shortening the time to crusting of lesions, new lesion formation, and VZV shedding in varicella in otherwise healthy adults (85). Sorivudine is also effective for HIV-infected adults with acute cutaneous herpes zoster. In the latter study, oral sorivudine (40 mg once daily) was compared with oral acyclovir, both taken for 7 days. Sorivudine significantly shortened the duration of new vesicle formation, and there were fewer recurrences of herpes zoster in sorivudine recipients, but no differences were seen in the incidence and duration of pain (12). Bromovinyl uracil (BVU), a metabolite of sorivudine, inhibits the metabolism of 5-fluorouracil (5-FU). Deaths from 5-FU toxicity have oc-

curred when sorivudine and 5FU were given concomitantly, and the development of sorivudine has been halted in the United States because of concerns about inadvertent administration with 5-FU.

Treatment with intravenous foscarnet (40 mg/kg/day in divided doses every 8 h) is recommended for the thymidine-kinase-deficient, acyclovir-resistant strains of VZV that are sometimes cultured from the chronic lesions of herpes zoster in patients with AIDS (9). Foscarnet has been used successfully to treat VZV pneumonitis in AIDS patients with acyclovir-resistant VZV (78).

Combination Therapy

There is no indication for combination therapy with acyclovir for varicella or herpes zoster. Continued viral replication during primary VZV infection is due to impaired host responses and has not been attributed to emergence of resistance to acyclovir.

Prophylaxis

Varicella-zoster immune globulin (VZIG) is prepared from high-titer immune human serum. In the United States, VZIG is distributed by the American Red Cross Blood Services; the dosage is one vial/10 kg body weight given intramuscularly (1). VZIG reduces the attack rate of primary VZV infection and should be given to susceptible high-risk patients within 96 h, and if possible, within 48 h, after a close exposure to an individual with varicella or herpes zoster. VZIG is ineffective if given after the onset of varicella. VZIG prophylaxis is recommended for immunocompromised children, seronegative pregnant women, and newborn infants exposed to maternal varicella. High-dose intravenous normal immune globulin (100–400 mg/kg) also provides high titers of VZV IgG antibodies. VZIG prophylaxis does not always prevent varicella in high-risk patients. Patients should be followed for breakthrough infection and treated with antiviral therapy if symptoms occur.

Oral acyclovir has been given to children during the incubation period for varicella in uncontrolled studies (6), but it is not recommended because of limited information about its safety and efficacy as prophylaxis. It is possible that treatment before appearance of the cutaneous lesions interferes with development of immunity.

In most patients, reactivation of VZV is very infrequent, and prophylaxis is not appropriate. In patients with AIDS, however, recurrent and relapsing disease is frequent, and after the second or third recurrence (or earlier for severe, relapsing infection), acute therapy could be followed by lifelong oral acyclovir prophylaxis at high dosage (VZV neurologic disease has been reported in AIDS patients receiving oral acyclovir at lower dosages as prophylaxis for HSV (60)). Such long-term prophylaxis with oral acyclovir in an attempt to prevent recrudescence of chronic cutaneous VZV infection in HIV-infected patients has been effective in some, but acyclovir-resistant VZV has emerged in others, and clinical disease has reappeared while on acyclovir prophylaxis (49, 58, 68). Most acyclovir-resistant strains of VZV are thymidine-kinase-negative mutants and thus also resistant to ganciclovir and sorivudine.

VACCINES

The live attenuated varicella vaccine made from the Oka strain of VZV has been licensed for clinical use in several countries (5). It is recommended for universal subcutaneous administration to children 12 to 15 months of age in the United States (1, 55). Alternative regimens recommended in other countries focus on immunization of susceptible adolescents and adults. The vaccine induces high rates of protection against household exposure to varicella in healthy children (5, 55, 86). Seroconversion rates exceed 95% with a single dose of vaccine in children 12 years old or younger; adolescents and adults require two doses to achieve equivalent protection. Mild breakthrough infections occur after immunization of some healthy children and adults, but the disease is modified to fewer than 50 cutaneous lesions without associated fever in most cases. With current vaccine preparations, immunity persists for up to 6 years. The Oka/Merck varicella vaccine has been given to children with acute leukemia in remission, reducing the attack rate following household exposure to 13%, but it is not licensed for this indication.

The vaccine virus can replicate to cause a varicella-like illness in immunocompromised children. Reactivation of the vaccine virus, causing herpes zoster, has occurred but appears to be less common than reactivation of wild-type VZV. The vaccine virus can be transmitted to susceptible contacts from vaccinees who develop vaccine-associated rash. The vaccine virus is inhibited by acyclovir, so episodes of vaccine-related varicella-like illness or herpes zoster can be treated with antiviral therapy if necessary.

Concerns about universal immunization against varicella include questions about the persistence of immunity, whether decreasing the frequency of exogenous reexposures to varicella will affect long-term protection, the possibility that more adolescents and adults will be susceptible to varicella, and uncertainty about the incidence of herpes zoster following vaccination.

Development of herpes zoster is related to declining cellular immunity in an individual previously infected with VZV, and this might be prevented by boosting this immunity with the live attenuated Oka strain vaccine. When this vaccine was given to seropositive elderly adults (mean age, 67 years), most individuals had their VZV-specific cellular immunity boosted significantly, to a level similar to that in a normal 40-year old, a group with a relatively low risk of herpes zoster, and the boost lasted several years (56). The effect of such vaccination of elderly persons on the frequency and severity of herpes zoster remains to be tested in a controlled prospective clinical trial.

ENDPOINTS FOR MONITORING THERAPY

The efficacy of acyclovir treatment of varicella is assessed by cessation of new lesion formation and recovery of the function of involved organs when infection is disseminated. Immunocompromised patients may exhibit new lesion formation shortly after antiviral therapy for varicella is stopped. Retreatment may be required in some cases.

The efficacy of treatment in herpes zoster may be judged by cessation of new lesion formation, by the speed of healing of cutaneous lesions, and by resolution of pain. Attempts have been made to measure the duration of acute pain and postherpetic neuralgia independently, but this can be misleading (96, 101). Patients are unable to determine when acute neuritis stops or when the central pain mechanisms begin and merely recognize that they are in pain. For this reason and because there are statistical difficulties inherent in analyzing only some of the patients initially randomized, it is more appropriate (and probably more clinically relevant) to measure in any individual the duration of painful sensations following initiation of therapy.

ADJUNCTIVE THERAPY

Aspirin is contraindicated in varicella because of risk of Reye syndrome. Oxygen therapy and assisted ventilation are required for some patients with varicella pneumonia. The role of corticosteroids in treatment of severe VZV pneumonitis remains controversial, although there are anecdotal reports of improvement in severe pneumonitis following corticosteroids (33).

Hemorrhagic complications associated with varicella hepatitis, thrombocytopenia, and disseminated intravascular coagulopathy require standard supportive measures to reduce bleeding and maintain blood pressure. Varicella encephalitis may progress to severe neurologic impairment and coma, requiring management in an intensive care unit.

The optimal approach to management of herpes zoster includes appropriate analgesics to control the acute pain. Administration of corticosteroids during the acute phase had some effect on the acute pain of herpes zoster in large double-blind studies (32, 93, 98). Studies that added prednisolone to oral acyclovir showed that pain was reduced during the first few days of the illness, but there was no effect on the incidence, duration, or severity of postherpetic neuralgia (32, 98). A placebo-controlled study that independently analyzed the effects of acyclovir and prednisolone (93) again showed no benefit from steroids on the chronic pain, but patients given prednisolone had significantly less acute pain and returned to work and normal activity more rapidly. Administration of corticosteroids is not without potential hazards, however, especially in an elderly population with other chronic disorders, and caution should be exercised in their use (40).

Topical corticosteroids aid resolution of stromal keratitis and dendritiform keratitis in herpes zoster ophthalmicus (70). Systemic corticosteroids are usually also prescribed in acute retinal necrosis, but their role is unclear.

CONTROVERSIES

The indications for using oral acyclovir to treat varicella in otherwise healthy young children are debated. The pharmacokinetics of the newer nucleoside analogues that inhibit VZV have not been evaluated in children. Since oral acyclovir has not been evaluated in clinical trials among high-risk children, its use should be considered only in selected patients with minimal immunosuppression, with careful follow-up during the illness.

The role of oral valaciclovir and famciclovir in the therapy of herpes zoster in the immunocompromised host has not been determined, but they may remove the need for intravenous therapy in some instances. The debate concerning the use of corticosteroids continues, but any benefits on acute pain need to be weighed against their dangers.

REFERENCES

1. American Academy of Pediatrics Committee on Infectious Diseases. Varicella-zoster virus. Pediatrics 1997.

2. Amlie-Lefond C, Kleinschmidt-DeMasters BK, Mahalingam R, Davis LE, Gilden DH. The vasculopathy of varicella-zoster virus encephalitis. Ann Neurol 1995;37:784–790.

3. Arvin A. Varicella-zoster virus. In: Fields BN, Knipe DM, Chanock R, Hirsch M, Melnick J, Monath T, eds. Virology. 3rd ed. Philadelphia: Lippincott-Raven Press, 1995:2547–2586.

4. Arvin AM. Varicella-zoster virus. In: Long S, Prober C, Pickering L, eds. Principles and practice of pediatric infectious diseases. Philadelphia: Lippincott-Raven Press, 1997.

5. Arvin AM, Gershon AA. Live attenuated varicella vaccine. Annu Rev Microbiol 1996:59–100.

6. Asano Y, Yoshikawa T, Suga S, Kobayashi I, Nakashima T, Yazaki T, Ozaki T, Yamada A, Imanishi J. Postexposure prophylaxis of varicella in family contact by oral acyclovir. Pediatrics 1993;92:219–222.

7. Baba K, Yabuuchi H, Takahashi M, Ogra P. Increased incidence of herpes zoster in normal children infected with varicella zoster virus during infancy; community-based follow-up study. J Pediatr 1986;108:372–377.

8. Balfour HH Jr, Bean B, Laskin OL, Ambinder RF, Meyers JD, Wade JC, Zaia JA, Aeppli D, Kirk LE, Segreti AC, Keeney RE, the Burroughs Wellcome Collaborative Acyclovir Study Group. Acyclovir halts progression of herpes zoster in immunocompromised patients. N Engl J Med 1983;308:1448–1453.

9. Balfour HH Jr, Benson C, Braun J, Cassens B, Erice A, Friedman-Kien A, Klein T, Polsky B, Safrin S. Management of acyclovir-resistant herpes simplex and varicella-zoster virus infections. J Acquir Immun Defic Syndr 1994;7:254–260.

10. Balfour HH Jr, Rotbart HA, Feldman S, Dunkle LM, Feder HM Jr, Prober CG, Hayden GF, Steinberg S, Whitley RJ, Goldberg L, McGuirt PV, the Collaborative Acyclovir Varicella Study Group. Acyclovir treatment of varicella in otherwise healthy adolescents. J Pediatr 1992;120:627–633.

11. Beutner KR, Friedman DJ, Forszpaniak C, Andersen PL, Wood MJ. Valaciclovir compared with acyclovir for improved therapy for herpes zoster in immunocompetent adults. Antimicrob Agents Chemother 1995;39:1546–1553.

12. Bodsworth NJ, Boag F, Burdge D, Généreux M, Borleffs JCC, Evans BA, Modai J, Colebunders R, Thomas M, DeHertogh D, Pacelli L, Thomis J, the Multinational Sorivudine Study Group. Evaluation of sorivudine (BV-araU) versus acyclovir in the treatment of acute localized herpes zoster in human immunodeficiency virus-infected adults. J Infect Dis 1997;176:103–111.

13. Bowman RV, Lythall DA, deWytt CN. A case of herpes zoster associated encephalitis treated with acyclovir. Aust NZ J Med 1985;15:43–44.

14. Brunell PA, Kotchmar GS. Zoster in infancy: Failure to maintain virus latency following intrauterine infection. J Pediatr 1981;98:71–76.

15. Buchbinder SP, Katz MH, Hessol NA, Liu JY, O'Malley PM, Underwood R, Holmberg SD. Herpes zoster and human immunodeficiency virus infection. J Infect Dis 1992;166:1153–1156.

16. Burgoon CF, Burgoon JS, Baldridge GD. The natural history of herpes zoster. JAMA 1957;164:265–269.

17. Carmack MA, Twiss J, Enzmann DR, Amylon MD, Arvin AM. Multifocal leukoencephalitis caused by varicella-zoster virus in a child with leukemia: successful treatment with acyclovir. Pediatr Infect Dis J 1993;12:402–406.

18. Cevenini R, Donati M, Rumpianesi F, Moroni A, Tosti A, Patrizi A, Varotti C, Negosanti M. Virological course of herpes zoster in otherwise normal hosts. J Med Microbiol 1983;16:303–308.

19. Cheesbrough JS, Finch RG, Ward MJ. A case of herpes zoster associated encephalitis with rapid response to acyclovir. Postgrad Med J 1985;61:145–146.

20. Cobo LM, Foulks GN, Liesegang T, Lass J, Sutphin JE, Wilhelmus K, Jones DB, Chapman S, Segreti AC, King DH. Oral acyclovir in the treatment of acute herpes zoster ophthalmicus. Ophthalmol 1986;93:763–770.

21. Colebunders R, Mann JM, Francis H, Bila K, Ilwaya M, Kakonde N, Quinn TC, Piot P. Herpes zoster in African patients: a clinical predictor of human immunodeficiency virus infection. J Infect Dis 1988;157:314–318.

22. Culbertson WW, Blumenkranz MS, Pepose JS, Stewart JA, Curtin VT. Varicella zoster virus is a cause of the acute retinal necrosis syndrome. Ophthalmol 1986;93:559–569.

23. de Boer JH, Luyendijk L, Rothova A, Baarsma GS, de Jong PTVM, Bollemeijer J-G, Rademakers AJJM, Van der Lelij A, Zaal MJW, Kijlstra A. Detection of intraocular antibody production to herpesviruses in acute retinal necrosis syndrome. Am J Ophthalmol 1994;117:201–210.

24. De Clercq E. Therapeutic potential of HPMPC as an antiviral drug. Rev Med Virol 1993;3:85–96.

25. Degreef H, Famciclovir Herpes Zoster Clinical Study Group. Famciclovir, a new oral antiherpes drug: results of the first controlled clinical study demonstrating its efficacy and safety in the treatment of uncomplicated herpes zoster in immunocompetent patients. Int J Antimicrob Agents 1994;4:241–246.

26. deLuise VP. Ocular involvement in herpes zoster. In: Watson CPN, ed. Herpes zoster and postherpetic neuralgia. Amsterdam: Elsevier, 1993:87–96.

27. Dunkle LM, Arvin AM, Whitley RJ, Rotbart HA, Feder HM Jr, Feldman S, Gershon AA, Levy ML, Hayden FG, McGuirt PV, Harris J, Balfour HH Jr. A controlled trial of acyclovir for chickenpox in normal children. N Engl J Med 1991;325:1539–1544.

28. Easterbrook P, Wood MJ. Clinical experience with new drugs for the treatment of herpesviruses, particularly varicella-zoster virus. Rev Med Virol 1995;5:51–57.

29. Edelstein H. Multidermatomal herpes zoster in an AIDS patient. Clin Infect Dis 1994;19:975.

30. Ehrensaft DV, Safani MM. Acyclovir and disseminated varicella zoster and encephalitis. Ann Intern Med 1985;100:421.

31. Ertl P, Snowden W, Lowe D, Miller W, Collins P, Little E. A comparative study of the in vitro and in vivo antiviral activities of acyclovir and penciclovir. Antivir Chem Chemother 1995;6:89–97.

32. Esmann V, Geil JP, Kroon S, Fogh H, Peterslund NA, Petersen CS, Ronne-Rasmussen JO, Danielsen L. Prednisolone does not prevent post-herpetic neuralgia. Lancet 1987;2:126–129.

33. Feldman S. Varicella-zoster virus pneumonitis. Chest 1994;106 (Suppl 1):22S–27S.

34. Feldman S, Hughes WT, Kim HY. Herpes zoster in children with cancer. Am J Dis Child 1973;126:178–184.

35. Feldman S, Lott L. Varicella in children with cancer: impact of antiviral therapy and prophylaxis. Pediatrics 1987;80:465–472.

36. Forster DL, Dugel PU, Frangieh GT, Liggett PE, Rao NA.

Rapidly progressive outer retinal necrosis in acquired immune deficiency syndrome. Am J Ophthalmol 1990;110:341–348.

37. Galindez OA, Sabates NR, Whitacre MM, Sabates FN. Rapidly progressive outer retinal necrosis caused by varicella zoster virus in a patient with human immunodeficiency virus. Clin Infect Dis 1996;22:149–151.

38. Garweg J, Bohnke M. Varicella-zoster virus is strongly associated with atypical necrotizing herpetic retinopathies. Clin Infect Dis 1996;24:603–608.

39. Gershon AA, Steinberg SP, Schmidt NJ. Varicella-zoster virus. In: Balows A, Hauseler WJ, Herrman KL, Isenberg HD, Shadomy HJ, eds. Manual of clinical microbiology. Washington, DC: American Society for Microbiology, 1991.

40. Gill KS, Wood MJ. The value of steroids in the treatment of herpes zoster. Exp Opin Invest Drugs 1994;3:791–797.

41. Gogos CA, Bassaris HP, Vagenakis AG. Varicella pneumonia in adults. A review of pulmonary manifestations, risk factors and treatment. Respiration 1992;59:339–343.

42. Gracely RH, Lynch SA, Bennett GJ. Painful neuropathy: altered central processing, maintained dynamically by peripheral input. Pain 1993;51:175–194.

43. Gray F, Bélec L, Lescs MC, Chrétien F, Ciardi A, Hassine D, Flament-Saillour M, de Truchis P, Clair B, Scaravilli F. Varicella-zoster virus infection of the central nervous system in the acquired immune deficiency syndrome. Brain 1994;117:987–999.

44. Guess HA, Broughton DD, Melton LJ III., Kurland LT. Epidemiology of herpes zoster in children and adolescents: a population-based study. Pediatrics 1985;76:512–517.

45. Haake DA, Zakowski PC, Haake DL, Bryson Y. Early treatment with acyclovir for varicella pneumonia in otherwise healthy adults: retrospective controlled study and review. Rev Infect Dis 1990;12:788–798.

46. Harding SP, Porter SM. Oral acyclovir in herpes zoster ophthalmicus. Curr Eye Res 1991;10(Suppl):177–182.

47. Hardy IB, Gershon A, Steinberg S, LaRussa P, NIAID Varicella Vaccine Collaborative Study Group. The incidence of zoster after immunization with live attenuated varicella vaccine. A study in children with leukemia. N Engl J Med 1991;325:1545–1550.

48. Hope-Simpson RE. The nature of herpes zoster: a long-term study and a new hypothesis. Proc R Soc Med 1965;58:9–20.

49. Hoppenjans WB, Bibler MR, Orme RL, Solinger AM. Prolonged cutaneous herpes zoster in acquired immunodeficiency syndrome. Arch Dermatol 1990;126:1048–1050.

50. Huff JC, Bean B, Balfour HH Jr, Laskin OL, Connor JD, Corey L, Bryson YJ, McGuirt P. Therapy of herpes zoster with oral acyclovir. Am J Med 1988;85(Suppl 2A):84–89.

51. Jemsek J, Greenberg SB, Taber L, Harvey D, Gershon A, Couch RB. Herpes zoster-associated encephalitis: clinicopathologic report of 12 cases and review of the literature. Medicine 1983;62:81–97.

52. Johns DR, Grees DR. Rapid response to acyclovir in herpes zoster associated encephalitis. Am J Med 1987;82:560–562.

53. Kakinuma H, Itoh E. A continuous infusion of acyclovir for severe hemorrhagic varicella. N Engl J Med 1997;336:732–733.

54. Kennedy PGE, Barrass JD, Graham DI, Clements GB. Studies on the pathogenesis of neurological diseases associated with varicella-zoster virus. Neuropathol Appl Neurobiol 1990;16:305–316.

55. Krause P, Klinman DM. Efficacy, immunogenicity, safety and use of live attenuated chickenpox vaccine. J Pediatr 1995;127:518–525.

56. Levin MJ, Murray M, Zerbe GO, White CJ, Hayward A. Immune responses of elderly persons 4 years after receiving a live attenuated varicella vaccine. J Infect Dis 1994;170:522–526.

57. Lietman PS. Clinical pharmacology: foscarnet. Am J Med 1992;92(Suppl 2A):8S–11S.

58. Linnemann CC, Biron KK, Hoppenjans WB, Solinger AM. Emergence of acyclovir-resistant varicella zoster virus in an AIDS patient on prolonged acyclovir therapy. AIDS 1990;4:577–579.

59. Locksley RM, Flournoy N, Sullivan KM, Meyers JD. Infection with varicella zoster virus after marrow transplantation. J Infect Dis 1985;152:1172–1181.

60. Manian FA, Kindred M, Fulling KH. Chronic varicella-zoster virus myelitis without cutaneous eruption in a patient with AIDS: report of a fatal case. Clin Infect Dis 1995;21:986–988.

61. McGregor RM. Herpes zoster, chickenpox and cancer in general practice. Br Med J 1957;1:84–87.

62. McKendrick MW, McGill JI, Wood MJ. Lack of effect of acyclovir on postherpetic neuralgia. Br Med J 1989;298:431.

63. Merigan TC, Rand KH, Pollard RB, Abdullah PS, Jordan GW, Fried RP. Human leukocyte interferon for the treatment of herpes zoster in patients with cancer. N Engl J Med 1978;298:981–987.

64. Miller AE. Selective decline in cellular immune response to varicella zoster in the elderly. Neurology 1980;30:582–587.

65. Morton P, Thomson AN. Oral acyclovir in the treatment of herpes zoster in general practice. NZ Med J 1989;102:93–95.

66. Novelli VM, Brunell PA, Geiser CF, Narkewicz S, Frierson L. Herpes zoster in children with acute lymphocytic leukemia. Am J Dis Child 1988;142:71–72.

67. Ophir O, Siegman-Igra Y, Vardinon N, Liron M. Herpes zoster encephalitis: isolation of virus from cerebrospinal fluid. Isr J Med Sci 1984;230:1189–1192.

68. Pahwa S, Biron K, Lim W, Swenson P, Kaplan MH, Sadick N, Pahwa R. Continuous varicella-zoster virus infection associated with acyclovir resistance in a child with AIDS. JAMA 1988;260:2879–2882.

69. Palay DA, Sternberg P, Davis J, Lewis H, Holland GN, Mieler WF, Jabs DA, Drews C. Decrease in the risk of bilateral acute retinal necrosis by acyclovir therapy. Am J Ophthalmol 1991;112:250–255.

70. Palestine AG. Ocular manifestations of varicella-zoster virus. In: Sacks SL, Straus SE, Whitley RJ, Griffiths PD, eds. Clinical management of herpes viruses. Amsterdam: IOS Press, 1995:245–252.

71. Peterslund NA. Herpes zoster associated encephalitis: clinical findings and acyclovir treatment. Scand J Infect Dis 1988;20:583–592.

72. Peterslund NA, Seyer-Hansen K, Ipsen J, Esmann V, Schönheyder H, Juhl H. Acyclovir in herpes zoster. Lancet 1981;ii:827–830.

73. Prober CG, Gershon AA, Grose C, McCracken GH Jr, Nelson JD. Consensus: varicella-zoster infections in pregnancy and the perinatal period. Pediatr Infect Dis J 1990;9:865–869.

74. Prober CG, Kirk RE, Keeney RE. Acyclovir therapy for chickenpox in immunosuppressed children—a collaborative study. J Pediatr 1982;101:622–625.

75. Ragozzino MW, Melton LJ III, Kurland LT, Chu CP, Perry HO. Population-based study of herpes zoster and its sequelae. Medicine 1982;61:310–316.

76. Rogues A-M, Dupon M, Ladner J, Ragnaud J, Pellergrin J, Dabis F, Groupe d'Epidémiologie Clinique du SIDA en Aquitaine.

Herpes zoster and human immunodeficiency virus infection: a cohort study of 101 coinfected patients. J Infect Dis 1993; 168:245.

77. Rozenberg F, Lebon P. Amplification and characterization of herpesvirus DNA in cerebrospinal fluid from patients with acute encephalitis. J Clin Microbiol 1991;17:2412–2417.

78. Safrin S, Berger TG, Gilson I, Wolfe PR, Wofsy CB, Mills J, Biron KK. Foscarnet therapy in five patients with AIDS and acyclovir-resistant varicella-zoster virus infection. Ann Intern Med 1991;115:19–21.

79. Schlossberg D, Littman M. Varicella pneumonia. Arch Intern Med 1988;148:1630–1632.

80. Shepp DH, Dandliker PS, Meyers JD. Treatment of varicella-zoster virus infection in severely immunocompromised patients. A randomized comparison of acyclovir and vidarabine. N Engl J Med 1986;23:208–212.

81. Steele RW, Keeney RE, Bradsher RW, Moses EB, Soloff BL. Treatment of varicella-zoster meningoencephalitis with acyclovir: demonstration of virus in cerebrospinal fluid by electron microscopy. Am J Clin Pathol 1983;80:57–60.

82. Traverso F, Romagnoli P, Bacigalup F. Uso dell'acyclovir nella zoster-encephalite. Clin Ther 1985;115:79–81.

83. Tyring S, Barbarash RA, Nahlik JE, Cunningham A, Marley J, Heng M, Jones T, Rea T, Boon R, Saltzman R, the Collaborative Famciclovir Herpes Zoster Study Group. Famciclovir for the treatment of acute herpes zoster: effects on acute disease and postherpetic neuralgia. Ann Intern Med 1995;123:89–96.

84. Wallace MR, Bowler WA, Murray NB, Brodine SK, Oldfield EC, III. Treatment of adult varicella with oral acyclovir: a randomized, placebo-controlled trial. Ann Intern Med 1992;117:358–363.

85. Wallace MR, Chamberlin CJ, Sawyer MH, Arvin AM, Harkins J, LaRocco A, Colopy MW, Bowler WA, Oldfield EC III. Treatment of adult varicella with sorivudine: a randomized, placebo-controlled trial. J Infect Dis 1996;174:249–255.

86. White CJ. Varicella-zoster virus vaccine. Clin Infect Dis 1997; 24:753–763.

87. Whitley RJ. Sorivudine: a promising drug for the treatment of varicella-zoster virus infection. Neurology 1995;45(Suppl 8): S73–S75.

88. Whitley RJ. Varicella zoster virus infections. In: Galasso G, Whitley R, Merigan T, eds. Antiviral agents and viral diseases of man. Philadelphia: Lippincott-Raven, 1997:279–304.

89. Whitley RJ, Ch'ien LT, Dolin R, Galasso GJ, Alford CA Jr, the Collaborative Study Group. Adenine arabinoside therapy of herpes zoster in the immunosuppressed: NIAID collaborative antiviral study. N Engl J Med 1976;294:1193–1199.

90. Whitley RJ, Gnann JW Jr. Editorial response: Herpes zoster in patients with human immunodeficiency virus infection—an ever-expanding spectrum of disease. Clin Infect Dis 1995;21:989–990.

91. Whitley RJ, Schlitt M. Encephalitis caused by herpesviruses, including B virus. In: Scheld WM, Whitley RJ, Durack DT, eds. Infections of the central nervous system. New York: Raven Press, 1991:41–86.

92. Whitley RJ, Soong S, Dolin R, Betts R, Linnemann C Jr, Alford CA Jr, the NIAID Collaborative Antiviral Study Group. Early vidarabine therapy to control the complications of herpes zoster in immunosuppressed patients. N Engl J Med 1982;307: 971–975.

93. Whitley RJ, Weiss H, Gnann JW Jr, Tyring S, Mertz GJ, Pappas PG, Schleupner CJ, Hayden F, Wolf J, Soong S, the NIAID Collaborative Antiviral Study Group. Acyclovir with and without prednisolone for the treatment of herpes zoster. Ann Intern Med 1996;125:376–383.

94. Whyte MKB, Ind PW. Effectiveness of intravenous acyclovir in immunocompetent patient with herpes zoster encephalitis. Br Med J 1986;293:1536–1537.

95. Wood MJ. Treatment of zoster. Rev Med Microbiol 1995;6: 165–174.

96. Wood MJ. How to measure and reduce the burden of zoster-associated pain. Scand J Infect Dis 1996;(Suppl 100):55–58.

97. Wood MJ, Anderson M. Neurological infections. London: WB Saunders, 1988.

98. Wood MJ, Johnson RW, McKendrick MW, Taylor J, Mandal BK, Crooks J. A randomized trial of acyclovir for 7 days or 21 days with and without prednisolone for treatment of acute herpes zoster. N Engl J Med 1994;330:896–900.

99. Wood MJ, Kay R, Dworkin RH, Soong S, Whitley RJ. Oral acyclovir therapy accelerates pain resolution in patients with herpes zoster: a meta-analysis of placebo-controlled trials. Clin Infect Dis 1996;22:341–347.

100. Wood MJ, Ogan PH, McKendrick MW, Care CD, McGill JI, Webb EM. Efficacy of oral acyclovir treatment of acute herpes zoster. Am J Med 1988;85(Suppl 2A):79–83.

101. Wood MJ, the Herpes Zoster Clinical Trials Consensus Group. How should zoster trials be conducted? J Antimicrob Chemother 1995;36:1089–1101.

102. Woolf CJ, Thompson SWN. The induction and maintainance of central sensitization is dependent on N-methyl-D-aspartic acid receptor activation: implications for the treatment of post-injury pain hypersensitivity states. Pain 1991;44:293–299.

Amantadine, Rimantadine, and Related Agents

—————•—————

Frederick G. Hayden and Fred Y. Aoki

Amantadine was synthesized in 1941 from adamantane, a hydrocarbon in which the carbon atoms are arranged as in a diamond crystal. In 1960, Eleanor Neumayer recognized that a related molecule, octachloroadamantane, had antiinfluenza activity in an antiviral screening program at Stine Laboratories (E.I. Dupont). Structure-activity studies led to synthesis of 1-aminoadamantane, or amantadine, which was reported to have anti–influenza A activity in 1964 (42). Amantadine was quickly shown to have clinically useful antiviral activity (96) and was initially approved for prevention of influenza A due to H2N2 subtype viruses in 1966 in the United States. Ten years later, the indications were extended for prevention and therapy of infections due to all influenza A subtypes. The therapeutic benefit of amantadine in Parkinson's disease was serendipitously discovered during use for influenza prophylaxis (160), and this constituted its principal use for many years. Rimantadine was shown to have clinically relevant antiinfluenza activity in 1968 (43) and subsequently received extensive study and use in the former Soviet Union (212). Rimantadine (Flumadine, Forest Laboratories) was approved for influenza indications in 1993 in the United States. However, these agents differ in their effects on the central nervous system. When substituted for amantadine during treatment of Parkinson's disease, rimantadine is ineffective (161).

CLASS
Structure

Amantadine (1-adamantanamine hydrochloride) is composed of a unique tricyclic 10-carbon ring structure with a primary amine group on the superior pole (Fig. 1). It is a semisynthetic petroleum hydrocarbon derivative that displays pronounced lipophilicity, a property that facilitates passage across cell membranes. Rimantadine (α-methyl-1-adamantanemethylamine hydrochloride) is a closely related derivative that shares the same hydrocarbon structure but incorporates a carbon with a methyl group between the nitrogen and adamantane ring (Fig. 2). Both drugs are water-soluble, white, crystalline powders that are acid salts of weak bases with a pK_a of approximately 10. Slow oral absorption may be expected, since the predominant species is charged at the pH range of the gastrointestinal tract. Urinary alkalinization slows excretion (132), and acidification may enhance elimination in an overdose setting.

Amantadine is approximately 65%, and rimantadine 40%, bound to plasma proteins. Levels are usually determined by gas chromatographic–mass spectrophotometric methods and are not routinely available. Amantadine binds to red blood cells (41), so whole blood concentrations are 40% or more above plasma concentrations.

Structure-Activity Relationships

Many cogeners and other related amines have been synthesized and tested for antiinfluenza activity (2). In general, replacement of the amino group abolishes activity and N-mono- and dialkyl derivatives are no more active than amantadine. However, N-alkyl substitutions increase behavioral activity assessed by motor stimulation in a murine model (51). Addition of substituents at one or more of the tertiary positions adversely affects antiviral activity. Studies of cyclic alkylamines indicate that the size of the aliphatic ring is important; thus cyclooctylamine possesses antiviral potency comparable to amantadine, cyclopentylamine is inactive, and the heptyl and hexyl moieties show intermediate activity (74).

Rimantadine, unlike amantadine, is asymmetric, but the enantiomers are essentially equipotent with the racemic compound (2). Rimantadine undergoes metabolism with production of various hydroxylated and glucuronidated derivatives. In cell culture–based assays, the antiviral activity of o-hydroxy-rimantadine is about 10-fold less than that of the parent drug (14). The m-hydroxy metabolite is about 100-fold less active, and the activity of the p-hydroxy metabolite lies between the other two.

By screening for inhibitors of M2 protein activity (see below), a spirene-containing compound, designated BL-1743 {2-[3-azaspiro (5,5)undecanol]-2-imidazoline}, with antiinfluenza activity and cross-resistance similar to those of amantadine has been identified (183). Several other compounds have shown activity in experimental human influenza. The adamantane derivative, 1'-methyl spiro (adamantane-2,3'-pyrrolidine) maleate, partially reduces virus shedding and illness frequency following experimental challenge (13). A cyclononane containing a primary amine and resembling amantadine (ICI 130,685) provides dose-related antiviral effects and protection against illness but is associated with central nervous system and gastrointestinal side effects (1).

Tromantadine (N-1-adamantyl-N-[2-(dimethylamine) ethoxy]acetamide hydrochloride), an amantadine derivative with antiherpesvirus activity, is approved for topical treatment of herpes simplex virus (HSV) infections in certain countries outside the United States. In vitro, tromantadine acts at both early and late steps in HSV replication (94). One placebo-controlled clinical trial found no clinical benefit in treating genital herpes in men (139).

ANTIVIRAL ACTIVITY
Spectrum

In Vitro

Amantadine and rimantadine specifically inhibit in vitro replication of influenza A viruses at low concentrations (≤1 μg/mL) achievable in blood and respiratory secretions after oral administration in humans (see below). The inhibitory concentrations for influenza viruses vary with the assay method, inoculum, and virus strain. Amantadine concentra-

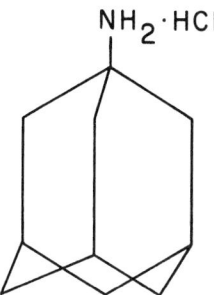

FIGURE 1. Chemical structure of amantadine hydrochloride.

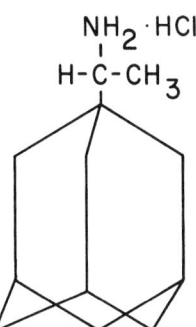

FIGURE 2. Chemical structure of rimantadine hydrochloride.

tions that inhibit plaque formation in Madin-Darby canine kidney cells by 50% range from 0.2 to 0.4 μg/mL for clinical isolates of influenza A viruses including H1N1, H2N2, and H3N2 subtypes (24, 80). Rimantadine shows comparable or greater activity in plaque assays but is 4 to 8 times more active in yield reduction assays in ferret tracheal rings (27) and up to 10 times more active in enzyme immunoassays (14).

The initial steps in replication of many viruses are pH dependent and can be affected by higher amantadine concentrations. Most viruses inhibited by higher amantadine concentrations are enveloped RNA-containing ones that undergo receptor-mediated endocytosis; most DNA and nonenveloped RNA viruses are resistant (39, 65). Depending on the assay method, concentrations of 10 to 50 μg/mL have variable in vitro inhibitory activity against influenza B, rubella and other togaviruses, paramyxoviruses (parainfluenza 1–3, respiratory syncytial, measles), arenaviruses, and rabies (Table 1) (35, 42, 127, 157). Amantadine at 31 μg/mL inhibits acute, but not chronic, rubella virus replication in vitro, and concentrations of 50 μg/mL or more are usually required for inhibition of paramyxoviruses (35). Amantadine concentrations of 50 μg/mL are usually cytotoxic, and those of 100 μg/mL or more are consistently toxic for most cell types after several days of in vitro exposure. Furthermore, these concentrations are too high to be clinically achievable.

Amantadine also possesses activity against nonviral pathogens, in part because of its lysosomotropicity and effects on pH. Although inactive alone, amantadine increases the activity of doxycycline against *Coxiella burnetii* (116). Amantadine inhibits intraerythrocyctic growth of *Plasmodium falciparum* and potentiates the activity of certain antimalarial agents (52, 53).

Animal Models

Both prophylactic and therapeutic activities of amantadine have been demonstrated in experimental influenza A virus infection of animals (reviewed in reference 75). Studies in animals indicate that delivery of amantadine directly to the respiratory tract in aerosol form is more efficacious than systemic administration (55, 189). In several animal model studies, rimantadine showed somewhat greater antiviral activity than

TABLE 1 • In Vitro Antiviral Spectrum of Amantadine and Rimantadine for Human Pathogenic Viruses

Susceptable (≤1 μg/mL)	Intermediate (1–50 μg/mL) or Inconsistent	Resistant (≥50 μg/mL)
Influenza A	Arena (Pichinde, LCM)	Influenza B
	Toga (rubella, dengue)	Mumps
	Parainfluenza 1–3	Corona
	Respiratory syncytial	Picorna (polio)
	Rubeola (measles)	Rubeola (measles)
		Herpes simplex
		Vaccinia
		Papilloma
		Human immunodeficiency
		Rota

Data from references 39, 65, 106, 182, 92.

amantadine against influenza A viruses (159, 182). In mice, rimantadine administration reduces mortality, pulmonary viral titers, and the ability of mice to transmit infection to uninfected cage mates more than comparable doses of amantadine. The pharmacokinetics of amantadine and rimantadine are species dependent, and the pharmacodynamics of these drugs are not well characterized in relevant animal models.

In murine studies, amantadine is not active against influenza B, polio, vesicular stomatitis, Semliki Forest, mouse hepatitis, pseudorabies, herpes simplex, yellow fever, rabies, or vaccinia viruses (28, 208). Intraperitoneal rimantadine does not protect against intracranial dengue virus infection in mice (101). Amantadine slightly reduces *Pneumocystis carinii* lung titers in immunosuppressed rats (191).

Human Infections

Amantadine provides no protection against experimental parainfluenza type 1 virus infection or illness (164). Neither amantadine nor rimantadine provides protection against influenza B virus infection in adults or children (33, 46). Neither drug influences the humoral response to live measles vaccine (46). In patients with chronic hepatitis C, a 6-month course of amantadine is reported to decrease transaminase and hepatitis C virus RNA levels (165), and further studies in combination with other agents are in progress.

Combinations

Rimantadine and amantadine exhibit additive or synergistic antiviral effects when combined with ribavirin, interferon, or zanamivir in vitro (78, 87, 112). Combinations of amantadine and ribavirin given orally, by aerosol, or by intraperitoneal injection show variably enhanced antiviral activity and increased survival over that with monotherapy in experimental murine influenza (61, 76, 202). This combination has been administered to individual patients with severe influenza. It has not been determined whether combinations of antivirals can prevent development of resistance to the antiinfluenza action of amantadine and rimantadine.

MECHANISM OF ACTION

The antiviral mechanism of these drugs has been extensively studied but remains incompletely characterized (reviewed in reference 73). The specific anti–influenza A effect of low amantadine or rimantadine concentrations, which is directed against the M2 protein, inhibits two different stages of viral replication, depending on the influenza subtype. Timing-of-addition studies indicate that amantadine must be present at the time of cell infection for maximal antiviral effect (208). The drugs inhibit an early stage in viral replication, uncoating of the viral genome (97). Amantadine blocks dissociation of the viral M1 (matrix) and ribonucleoproteins (RNPs) and thereby prevents transport of RNPs into the nucleus (114). No effect on virus attachment and penetration, release from cells, or viral RNA-dependent RNA polymerase activity has been found. Rimantadine shares the same mechanism of action and also appears to inhibit release of M1 protein from viral RNPs and prevent their import into the cell nucleus (26). These drugs

also exert a second inhibitory effect on late replication events, related to inhibition of virus maturation and release, with certain avian H7 subtype influenza strains (74, 154).

High concentrations, generally in the millimolar range, of amantadine and other amines raise endosomal-lysosomal pH, which may inhibit virus-mediated membrane fusion events required for replication (73, 74). For arenaviruses such as lymphocytic choriomeningitis virus, this effect may account for concentration-related inhibition of both virion penetration and release of virus from infected cells (194). Although amantadine accumulates intracellularly in lysosomes, its antiinfluenza effect is rapidly lost upon removal from cell culture medium (151). This indicates that most of the cell-associated amantadine probably does not contribute to its antiinfluenza action. Amantadine concentrations exerting selective antiinfluenza activity are generally two orders of magnitude lower than those known to elevate endosomal pH substantially (114).

Genetic studies and characterization of drug-resistant mutants (see below) indicate that amantadine sensitivity is principally mediated by the M gene (segment 7) encoding the M (matrix) and M2 proteins, although the HA gene affects the sensitivity of certain strains (74, 110, 158). The specific target of low amantadine and rimantadine concentrations (≤ 1 μg/mL) is the M2 protein. This 97–amino acid integral membrane protein is expressed as a homotetramer in the plasma membranes of influenza A, but not influenza B, virus-infected cells and is incorporated in low numbers in influenza A virions. M2 functions as an pH-regulated cation channel required for acidification of the virus interior during replication (reviewed in reference 72) (32, 72, 73). During endocytosis, M2 mediates an influx of protons from the acidic endosome into the virion, which in turn causes weakening of protein-protein interactions and dissociation of viral RNPs from the M1 protein. This blocks entry of the RNPs into the nucleus and initiation of transcription. In addition, M2 is needed later in replication, when it removes protons from the trans-Golgi network during intracellular transport of viral HA and other proteins. For some influenza viruses, this effect is essential in maintaining the HA in a pH-neutral form. Inhibition by amantadine results in expression of the low-pH form of HA and inhibits release of infectious virus (154).

The mechanism of the drug-induced M2 block remains controversial. Irreversible binding of one drug molecule per channel complex appears to occur (192), but the exact site of binding is unclear. Neutron diffraction studies suggest that amantadine interacts directly with the transmembrane domain of M2 in a location between Val 27 and Ser 31, findings consistent with formation of a steric block within the channel (50). However, expression of M2 in different cell or lipid bilayer systems suggests that amantadine exerts an allosteric blocking effect (73, 192).

RESISTANCE

Resistance to these drugs is readily achieved by serial passage of influenza A virus strains in the presence of the drug in vitro or in vivo (73, 77). Resistant variants exist as subpopulations in non-drug-exposed virus pools at levels of approximately

10^{-4}. Resistance is high, with 30-fold or greater reductions in vitro susceptibility, and is associated with essentially complete loss of susceptibility. Resistant variants show cross-resistance to amantadine, rimantadine, and related compounds. Consequently, higher drug doses or alternative drugs with the same antiviral target cannot overcome this problem.

Mechanisms of Resistance

Resistant viruses have point mutations in their M gene and corresponding single amino-acid substitutions in the transmembrane domain of the M2 protein at positions 26, 27, 30, 31, or 34 (73). These changes essentially eliminate the inhibitory effects of the drugs on ion channel function. This abolishes the amantadine-induced block of channel function and allows acidification of the virus interior and uncoating of the viral RNPs to proceed. In the absence of drug, some of these changes also reduce the channel activity of certain M2 proteins. In vitro development of resistance corresponds to the complete loss of drug effectiveness in vivo (12). The frequency with which different mutations emerge is strain and subtype dependent. Human H3N2 subtype–resistant variants show a preponderance of position 31 serine to asparagine mutations.

In addition, the loss of drug susceptibility of certain avian viruses may be due to changes in the viral HA and reflect an altered requirement for the function of M2 during intracellular transport of HA (see above) rather than acquisition of resistance mutations in M2 (175). In such viruses, amino acid substitutions in the HA increase acid stability, so that inhibition of M2 function by amantadine does not lead to expression of the low pH form. At present, this mechanism of resistance has not been recognized in human influenza viruses.

Significance of Resistance

Antiviral drug resistance is a relevant clinical issue during use of amantadine and rimantadine. All contemporary pandemic strains of influenza A and over 99% of viruses recovered from non-drug-exposed persons remain susceptible to amantadine and rimantadine (reviewed in reference 77). However, resistant variants are detectable as early as 2 to 3 days after initiating treatment of influenza and emerge in up to 30% of treated children and adults (69, 79, 88). Limited evidence suggests that recovery from illness may be somewhat slower in those developing resistant virus (69). Immunocompetent persons generally stop shedding resistant variants within 10 days, but prolonged shedding has been documented in highly immunocompromised persons (99).

In chickens experimentally infected with an avian influenza virus, amantadine treatment is associated with rapid selection of drug-resistant virus that remains infectious and lethal for contact birds receiving amantadine, although simultaneous administration of inactivated vaccine and amantadine to contact birds is protective (193). In this system, resistant variants do not differ from their drug-susceptible parents in replication capacity, transmissibility in the absence of selective drug pressure, or virulence (12). Similarly, resistant human isolates retain virulence in the ferret (178) and cause typical illness in humans (79). No obvious genotype-related differences in the biologic characteristics of resistant variants have been recognized as yet.

Transmission of resistant viruses from treated persons to close contacts in households or nursing homes has caused failures of drug prophylaxis (79, 93, 115). In the nursing home setting, appropriate isolation of treated ill patients appears to reduce the risk of transmission (44). The frequency of resistance transmission in such epidemiologic circumstances is incompletely defined. Similarly, the potential for epidemic spread of resistant variants and the degree of selective drug pressure necessary to induce such an event are uncertain.

PHARMACOKINETICS

Knowledge of the clinical pharmacokinetic characteristics of amantadine and rimantadine in oral syrup formulations and aerosols, amantadine in oral capsules, and rimantadine in tablets remains incomplete (6, 196, 205).

Absorption

The absolute bioavailability of amantadine and rimantadine oral formulations have not been described. Indirect measures of amantadine absorption, including urinary excretion and absence of drug in feces suggest that it is relatively completely absorbed from oral formulations, independent of dose. Mass balance studies with ^{14}C-rimantadine suggest the same.

Amantadine absorption determined from recovery of unchanged drug in urine of young healthy adults and elderly subjects given a single dose of 25 mg up to 4 mg/kg or the same doses twice daily for up to 15.5 days ranges from 66 to 100%, indicating good-to-excellent oral bioavailability (Table 2). Amantadine in tablet and syrup formulations appears equally bioavailable. Mild renal insufficiency appears not to affect the relative oral bioavailability of amantadine in syrup (91). Rimantadine absorption cannot easily be assessed by recovery of drug from urine because it undergoes extensive metabolism (see below). However, rimantadine oral absorption appears comparable to that of amantadine, ranging from 75 to 93%, based on a mass balance study using a single 200-mg dose containing ^{14}C-labeled rimantadine in young adults (85, 153).

Less than 1 mg of amantadine from a single 100-mg oral dose was recovered in feces collected over 72 h from eight patients with chronic renal insufficiency and six normal controls (210), suggesting that amantadine urine excretion data are a valid reflection of its absorption. Less than 1% of an oral dose of ^{14}C-rimantadine was recovered in feces (196).

Relative oral bioavailability of rimantadine or amantadine has not been described in children.

The rates of amantadine and rimantadine absorption appear to be similar between young and elderly healthy subjects and relatively rapid, based on measurement of time to attain peak drug concentration in plasma (T_{max}) and absorption half-life (T_{abs}) data (Table 3). However, mean T_{max} was more than twice as long for rimantadine (4.6 h) than amantadine (2.1 h) in the young subjects (85). Mean rimantadine T_{max} was 5 to 6 h in young adults after a single 100-mg dose and was independent of formulation (oral solution, capsule, or syrup) (199).

TABLE 2 • **Amantadine Recovery in Urine after Oral Administration**

Subjects	No. of Subjects	Dose	Percentage Recovered in Urine after Administration As			Reference
			Unknown	Tablet	Capsules or Syrup	
Young healthy	5	2–4 mg/kg once	86 ±9[a]	—	—	Bleidner 1965 (19)
	6	200 mg once	—	75%[b]	—	Hayden 1985 (85)
Elderly healthy	2	25 mg once	—	—	90%	Aoki 1985 (5)
	4	50 mg once	—	—	84%	Aoki 1985 (5)
	1	75 mg once	—	—	88%	Aoki 1985 (5)
	1	200 mg once	53%	—	—	Montanari 1975 (120)
	6	200 mg once	—	68%[b]	—	Hayden 1985 (85)
Young, renal insufficiency	6	300 mg once	—	—	52 ± 13%	Horadam 1981 (91)
Elderly, renal insufficiency	1	300 mg once	—	—	104%[b]	Horadam 1981 (91)
Young healthy	4	25 mg b.i.d., 9 days	—	—	100%, 58–468%[c]	Aoki 1979 (7)
	1	100 mg b.i.d., 9 days	92%	—	—	Bleidner 1965 (19)
	4	100 mg b.i.d., 15.5 days	—	—	102%, 72–243%[c]	Aoki 1979 (7)
	5	150 mg b.i.d., 15.5 days	—	—	66%, 11–102%[c]	Aoki 1979 (7)
Elderly healthy	3	25 mg b.i.d., 10.5 days	—	—	88%, 49–107%[c]	Aoki 1985 (5)
	5	50 mg b.i.d., 10.5 days	—	—	84%, 58–111%[c]	Aoki 1985 (5)
	2	75 mg b.i.d., 10.5 days	—	—	78%, 58–88%[c]	Aoki 1985 (5)
	2	200 mg b.i.d., 9 days	59%	—	—	Montanari 1975 (120)

[a] Mean ± SD.

[b] Calculated to determine complete recovery over 5 half-lives.

[c] Median and range.

TABLE 3 • T_{max} **and** T_{abs} **as Indirect Indicators of Amantadine and Rimantadine Oral Absorption (median, range)**

Subjects	Parameter	Amantadine	References	Rimantadine	Reference
Young healthy adults	T_{max}[a]	3.0 (1–8 h) N = 24 (0.41–5.0 mg/kg)	Bleidner 1965 (19) Aoki 1979 (7) Hayden 1985 (85)	4.9 (2.0–6.6 h) N = 6 (2.08–3.33 mg/kg)	Hayden 1985 (85)
Elderly healthy adults	T_{max}	4.5 (0.8–8 h) N = 14 (0.3–3.28 mg/kg)	Aoki 1985 (5) Hayden 1985 (85)	3.3 (1.4–10 h) N = 10 (2.31–3.28 mg/kg)	Hayden 1985 (85)
Young healthy adults	T_{abs}[b]	0.4 (0.2–1.2 h) N = 6 (2.08–3.33 mg/kg)	Hayden 1985 (85)	1.0 (0.4–7.3 H) N = 6 (2.08–3.33 mg/kg)	Hayden 1985 (85)
Elderly healthy adults	T_{abs}	0.6 (0.4–11.9 h) N = 6 (2.47–2.94 mg/kg)	Hayden 1985 (85)	1.3 (0.4–8.5 h) N = 10 (2.31–3.28 mg/kg)	Hayden 1985 (85)

[a] T_{max}, time (h) after ingestion to peak plasma concentration.

[b] T_{abs}, absorption half-life (h)

In 15 women 31 to 62 years of age on neuroleptic drugs for a variety of psychiatric disorders as well as anticholinergic drugs (which might delay absorption), mean T_{max} at steady state after administration of 200 mg of amantadine as capsules was 6 ± 2 h (mean ± SD) (130). In eight infants 1 to 10 months of age given a single daily dose of rimantadine syrup (3.0 mg/kg) for 5 to 9 days, T_{max} ranged from 2.5 to 6.0 h (125), and in 10 children 5 to 8 years of age given a single dose of 6.6 mg/kg rimantadine as syrup, T_{max} was 5.7 ± 0.5 h (mean

± SD) (3). These data are similar to results in adults and suggest that both drugs are relatively rapidly absorbed, independent of dose or age of the subject. Concurrent anticholinergic drug therapy did not appear to retard the speed of absorption of amantadine.

Amantadine peak Cp (C_{max}) in healthy young and elderly adults increases linearly as a function of a single dose from 0.30 to 5.0 mg/kg administered as tablets or syrup ($r = 0.79$ and 0.93), in the two age groups, respectively) (5, 7,19, 85), and in young healthy adults as a function of repeated doses from 0.39 to 2.80 mg/kg at steady state ($r = 0.91$) (7). Amantadine C_{max} is 1.6 to 1.8 times greater in healthy elderly men than in young healthy adults ingesting 25- and 200-mg single doses, reflecting the smaller volume of distribution (Vd) at a given dose in elderly individuals (5, 7, 85). Amantadine C_{max} data reflect modest increments in Vd as amantadine dose increases (6). Collectively, the data parallel other indirect measures of absorption, indicating relatively good dose- and formulation-independent absorption of amantadine in young and elderly healthy adults. The effect of disease on absorption has not been extensively studied. Rimantadine C_{max} is similar in healthy young and elderly subjects given the same dose (85) and increases in proportion to increments in single doses (Table 4), with no consistent differences between formulations. In these two age groups, twice-daily doses produce mean C_{max} levels that are 400 to 500% greater than those observed after single doses, respectively, as predicted from calculations of the accumulation factor, $R = 1/1 - e^{-kT}$. Amantadine C_{max} doubles as predicted from calculation of R in young adults (7). Mean amantadine C_{max} exceeds rimantadine C_{max} by 213% in healthy young subjects and by 320% in older subjects after a single 200-mg dose (85), which reflects the fact that the Vd of amantadine is smaller than that of rimantadine at a given dose.

In eight infants 1 to 10 months of age, median rimantadine C_{max} after a daily dose of 3 mg/kg for 5 to 9 days is 366 ng/mL and ranges from 100 to 574 ng/mL (125). This is within the range observed in young and elderly healthy adults who ingest the currently recommended dose of 200 mg/day (an average of 2.5 (85) and 2.7 mg/kg/day (181) with C_{max} (mean ± SD) of 240 ± 70 and 250 ± 50 ng/mL, respectively). In 10 children aged 5 to 8 years given a single oral dose of rimantadine (6.6 mg/kg), plasma rimantadine concentration 6 h postdose is 657 ± 180 ng/mL (mean + SD) (3).

Rimantadine AUC data in Table 4 suggest that doubling the dose from 100 to 200 mg, ingested once, produces a proportionate doubling in AUC in both young and elderly adults. Data in elderly adults also show that repeated 12-hourly doses of 100 mg produce a 5-fold increase in AUC as predicted from calculation of rimantadine's accumulation factor (see above) (181). For amantadine, AUC after a single dose increases linearly over the dose range 25 to 150 mg in young healthy adults ($r = 0.91$) (7) and over the dose range 25 to 75 mg in elderly healthy subjects ($r = 0.61$) (5). Thus, overall, AUC estimates suggest comparable relative rimantadine and amantadine oral bioavailability.

Amantadine and rimantadine in recommended doses yield similar $AUC_{0-\tau}$ values over 12 h at steady state. In young adults receiving 100 mg of amantadine or rimantadine twice daily, mean $AUC_{0-\tau}$s are 4144 (7) and 4320 (200) ng · h/mL, respectively. The similar results in young adults parallel the comparable results observed in the only trial in which the efficacy of currently recommended doses of amantadine and rimantadine were directly compared (48). In healthy elderly subjects receiving 100 mg/day amantadine, mean AUC_{0-12h} is 6108 ng · h/mL (5) and in similar individuals receiving 200 mg/day rimantadine, 4190 ng · h/mL (181).

The gastrointestinal site(s) of amantadine and rimantadine absorption are not known, nor are the effects of gastrointestinal diseases or other drugs on their absorption characteristics except as cited above. The effect of food on amantadine absorption has not been reported, but rimantadine absorption appears not to be affected (198).

Distribution

Anatomic

Knowledge of the distribution of amantadine and rimantadine within the organs of the body and within cellular compart-

---

TABLE 4 • Rimantadine Relative Oral Bioavailability by AUC and C_{max}

| Subjects | No. of Subjects | Dose | AUC^a/C_{max}^b (mean ± SD) after Ingestion of Rimantadine in | | | Reference |
			Solution	Tablets	Syrup	
Young Healthy Adults	20	100 mg once	3020/70	3540/86	2910/70	Wills 1987 (199)
	12	100 mg once	—	4140/109		Wills 1987 (201)
	12	100 mg once	—	3500/78		Wills 1987 (200)
	12	100 mg once	—	3060/76		Wills 1987 (200)
	6	200 mg once	—		6480 ± 1560/179 ± 41	Capparelli 1988 (30)
	6	200 mg once	—	6180/114		Wills 1987 (198)
	6	200 mg once	—	9800 ± 4500/240 ± 70		Hayden 1985 (85)
	19, 20	200 mg once	—	11917 ± 4421/310 ± 99	11160 ± 3950/319	Anderson 1987 (3)
	12	100 mg daily for 10 days	—	3260/181	± 103	Wills 1987 (200)
	12	100 mg twice daily for 10 days	—	4320/416		Wills 1987 (200)
Healthy elderly	18	100 mg once	—	3530 ± 1250/94 ± 20		Tominack 1988 (181)
	10	200 mg once	—	11500 ± 3900/250 ± 50		Hayden 1985 (85)
	18	100 mg twice daily for 9.5 days	—	—	4190 ± 1070/447 ± 108	Tominack 1988 (181)

[a] $AUC_{0-\infty}$ after single dose and AUC_{0-T} (T = dose interval [h] after multiple doses; ng·h/mL)

[b] C_{max} ng/mL.

ments is incomplete. However, studies of their distribution in the organs of mice and studies of their clinical pharmacokinetic distribution characteristics indicate that they are widely distributed through the body and highly concentrated within some organs; within cells, they are probably sequestered in acidic intracellular organelles.

In mice, amantadine is concentrated in liver, kidney, lung, and heart in descending order (184). Rimantadine concentration in mouse brain is four times that in plasma (171). In rats, rimantadine is transported into brain at 10 times the rate of amantadine (171). Transport of both amantadine and rimantadine across the blood-brain barrier of rats is mediated by a specific carrier mechanism that is 90% inhibited by diphenhydramine but at a concentration (2500 ng/mL) that is 25 times therapeutic blood concentrations (50–100 ng/mL) (163). Other weak bases like propranolol would also be expected to inhibit amantadine and rimantadine transport into brain. The relevance of these observations in rats to patients is uncertain relative to the therapeutic effect of amantadine in Parkinson's disease, the neurotoxic adverse effects of amantadine and rimantadine, and a possible effect of concurrent therapy with drugs such as propranolol in mitigating amantadine or rimantadine neurotoxicity.

Plasma protein binding of amantadine and rimantadine is approximately 67% (109) and 40% (196), respectively. Since amantadine and rimantadine are both highly ionized cations at physiologic pH, it would be expected that they would be primarily bound to α_1, acid-glycoprotein in plasma. However, this has not yet been reported.

In patients, amantadine concentration in cerebrospinal fluid is 52 to 96% of concurrent levels in serum, both at therapeutic doses (22, 103) and at toxic levels, as were observed following ingestion of an overdose of 2.8 g in a suicide attempt (54). In brain tissue of patients treated chronically with amantadine at a median dose of 200 mg/day, the drug was uniformly distributed throughout the brain at a mean concentration of 30,548 ng/mL of tissue (103). Rimantadine distribution and levels in human brain have not been described but may exceed those of amantadine if rimantadine transport across the blood-brain barrier of man exceeds that of amantadine as has been reported in rats (see above).

Amantadine concentrations in saliva of volunteers given it by mouth were reported to equal those in blood, but no levels were provided (19). In nasal mucus of healthy subjects, rimantadine concentrations average 1.5 times those in plasma (85, 181), whereas amantadine concentrations are on average only 0.5 times as great (85). Since amantadine and rimantadine appear to be equieffective in preventing influenza at the same dose (48), the relevance of these observations to antiviral effect is unclear. Amantadine and rimantadine concentrations in nasal mucus of individuals with acute influenzal illness have not been reported.

Rimantadine small-particle aerosol produces concentrations in nasal washings at the end of a well-tolerated 12-h inhalation 100 times those achieved with a 200-mg oral dose (11). Amantadine aerosol generated from a solution containing 10 mg/mL is well tolerated for 30 min twice daily for 8

days (83). Mean nasal wash amantadine concentrations are 91,000 ng/mL 1 h after completion of aerosol treatment. This exceeds mean C_{max} concentrations (20 ng/mL) by more than 400-fold (83) and exceeds levels observed after oral administration of 200 mg (150 ng/mL) by 500-fold (85).

Kinetic

The Vds of both amantadine and rimantadine in man are large and consistent with animal data showing the drugs are concentrated in many tissues relative to the plasma compartment. Vds calculated after single and repeated doses of amantadine and rimantadine and an intravenous dose of amantadine (64) range from 3.6 to 5.1 L/kg for amantadine and 11.6 to 12.4 L/kg for rimantadine. Amantadine Vd is weakly inversely related to dose (6) and may be greater in elderly females than in males. In dialysis-dependent patients, the mean amantadine Vd is similar to that in healthy individuals (170). The large Vd of both molecules accounts in part for their poor dialyzability (30, 91).

Smoking appears to be associated with an increased amantadine Vd. The average Vd is greater (6.05 ± 0.86 L/kg; mean $\pm$ SD) in smokers than in nonsmokers (4.87 ± 0.85) (206), a difference that might be partly due to a nicotine- or cotinine-induced competitive accumulation of amantadine in renal tubular epithelial cells as was observed in studies in rat kidney (207). Comparable studies have not been reported with rimantadine.

The distribution half-lives (T_α) of amantadine and rimantadine do not differ in young healthy adults and in healthy elderly volunteers (85). Tα data indicate rapid net movement out of the plasma compartment and sequestration in extravascular tissues independent of age. Amantadine accumulates within erythrocytes with an erythrocyte:plasma ratio of 2.66 ± 0.49 (mean $\pm$ SD) in normal healthy males, 1.44 ± 0.21 in patients with renal insufficiency, and 1.76 ± 0.17 in hemodialysis patients ($P < .001$ between groups) (41). The rimantadine erythrocyte:plasma ratio is 1.06 (192).

Routes of Elimination

Metabolism

Metabolism of rimantadine (but not amantadine) contributes significantly to its elimination in man. In humans, amantadine undergoes N-acetylation, N-methylation, and formation of Schiff bases and N-formiates (102). *N*-Acetylamantadine is the principal metabolite. In one study it accounted for 5 to 15% of drug in urine after therapeutic doses (102), but in another, only 0.1 to 1.5% of drug excreted (90). No correlation was observed between NAT-2 acetylator phenotype and amantadine acetylation (90). The site of acetylation is not known.

Rimantadine undergoes extensive metabolism by hydroxylation, conjugation, and glucuronidation prior to renal excretion (153). From 8.3 to 43% of an oral dose is recovered in urine as parent compound (153, 198). The proportion of a rimantadine dose undergoing metabolism is not lower in patients with chronic stable liver disease than in normal controls (198).

Rimantadine and amantadine clearance estimates suggest indirectly that rimantadine metabolism (but not amantadine metabolism) is reduced in patients with severe renal failure.

Renal amantadine clearance averages 79 ± 5% (mean ± SEM) of systemic amantadine clearance both in patients with renal insufficiency and in normal volunteers studied concurrently (210). Rimantadine plasma clearance declines as creatinine clearance falls (197) from 483 ± 76 (mean ± SD) mL/h/kg to 297 ± 87 in patients with dialysis-dependent renal failure (30). This difference in systemic clearance persists even after the contribution of renal clearance (74 ± 21 mL/h/kg) is considered, suggesting that renal glucuronidation also contributes to rimantadine plasma clearance.

The 40% reduction in rimantadine systemic clearance in patients with dialysis-dependent renal failure has led to the current reduced dose recommendation for such patients. Less marked renal failure is not felt to necessitate rimantadine dose reductions (197).

Renal Excretion

Amantadine and rimantadine clearance determinations suggest that rimantadine undergoes renal elimination by glomerular filtration, whereas amantadine is eliminated by both glomerular filtration and renal tubular secretion. The median ratio of amantadine clearance to plasma clearance approaches unity (7), although others observed that renal clearance only accounts for 79 ± 5% (mean ± SEM) of total body clearance (210). Renal amantadine clearance correlates highly with creatinine clearance (210). Renal amantadine clearance is 23.85 L/h (median; range, 6.70–41.63) (7) and 21.60 ± 7.84 L/h (mean ± SD) (85) in young healthy volunteers and 7.71 L/h (median; range, 4.08–22.49) (5) and 12.30 ± 3.24 L/h (mean ± SD) (85) in healthy elderly volunteers. These renal clearance values are much greater than corresponding endogenous creatinine clearance rates as a measure of glomerular filtration rate. A high ratio of amantadine:creatinine clearance (median, 4.2; range, 1.35–14.96) is observed in young healthy adults and a lower ratio (median, 2.07; range, 0.64–4.20) in older healthy men (5). These data suggest that amantadine renal tubular secretion declines out of proportion to its excretion by glomerular filtration with advanced age.

Renal clearance of unchanged rimantadine (74 ± 21 mL/h/kg; mean ± SD) is similar to creatinine clearance (88 ± 18) in healthy adults, suggesting that it is eliminated into urine by glomerular filtration without renal tubular secretion (30). The renal clearance of rimantadine metabolites is reduced in patients with renal failure, but their accumulation does not appear to cause adverse effects (197).

Renal clearance of amantadine is inversely related to urine pH (63). At pH 5.0 to 5.5, 6% (range, 4.5–7%) of a single dose of amantadine was excreted per hour, and at pH 7.0 to 8.0, 1% (range, 0.5–1.2%). These observations are consistent with expectations for a molecule with pK_a 10.1. Renal elimination of amantadine is also affected by gender and concurrent ingestion of some drugs. Mean amantadine renal clearance is approximately 50% higher in healthy young males than in females (62, 206). Quinine and quinidine significantly inhibited renal amantadine clearance in males only, renal clearance being reduced from an average 13.2 ± 5.8 L/h (mean ± SD) to 9.7 ± 4.8 L/h by quinine and 8.9 ± 4.0 L/h by quinidine (62). The cation

nicotine and its metabolite cotinine increase accumulation of amantadine in rat renal tubular epithelial cells in vitro at concentrations commonly observed in the blood of smokers (207). However, chronic tobacco smoking did not alter amantadine renal clearance in young healthy subjects (206).

Plasma Elimination Half-Life

The plasma elimination $t_{1/2}$ values for amantadine and rimantadine in healthy individuals and others with chronic renal and hepatic disease are presented in Table 5. Renal disease with creatinine clearance from 10 to 50 mL/min is linearly related to plasma $t_{1/2}$ ($r = -0.62$). Mean plasma rimantadine $t_{1/2}$ plasma is prolonged by 60% in patients with dialysis-dependent chronic renal failure; it is not known whether lesser degrees of renal dysfunction affect rimantadine kinetics.

DOSAGE REGIMENS

Amantadine and rimantadine clinical pharmacokinetic characteristics in young and healthy individuals show relatively large interindividual variation (Table 6) and sample sizes for several parameters are small. The therapeutic range data represent plasma concentrations associated with currently recommended doses. However, their validity as target concentrations which ought to be achieved in patients remains to be confirmed.

Optimal amantadine dose regimens for prevention and treatment of influenza A virus infection have been established by clinical trials only for young healthy adults. In this group, amantadine 200 mg/day has been repeatedly demonstrated to be efficacious and generally well tolerated. This dose is associated with a median trough steady-state plasma concentration of 300 ng/mL (range, 258–310 ng/mL) and a calculated mean plasma concentration throughout the 12-h dose interval of 324 ng/mL (median; range, 275–467 ng/mL) (7). Optimal doses of amantadine for individuals with age- or disease-related reductions in renal function or body weight that vary markedly from that of the young healthy adults (median, 73 kg; range, 58–96 kg) whose data were used to determine the regression of Cp on dose (7, 85) will differ from 200 mg/day because of the effects of diminished renal function on amantadine elimination and altered body weight on Vd, the two critical determinants of drug clearance. Moreover, amantadine Vd varies inversely as a function of dose (6), further complicating dose calculation.

Doses have been determined for individuals in whom amantadine pharmacokinetic characteristics differ from those in young healthy adults by calculating regimens that attempt to simulate target plasma concentrations observed in young healthy adults ingesting 200 mg/day. Target concentrations have ranged from trough levels of 300 (5) to 490 to 700 ng/mL (91). Data demonstrating an increased frequency of side effects and serum amantadine levels above 1000 ng/mL in small, elderly, frail women (mean weight, 57 kg) (45) who were given the dose (100 mg/day) calculated from kinetic data in healthy elderly men (median weight, 72 kg) underscored the need for vigilance in monitoring all patients receiving amantadine. None of the pharmacokinetically derived regimens has been rigorously validated for safety, efficacy, or ability to attain the target plasma concentration of amantadine. Currently

TABLE 5 • **Elimination $t_{1/2}$ of Amantadine from Plasma**

Subjects	Amantadine			Rimantadine		
	No. of Subjects	$t_{1/2}$ (h) Mean ± SD	References	No. of Subjects	$t_{1/2}$ (h) Mean ± SD	Reference
Young healthy adults	19	14.8 ± 6.2	Bleidner 1965 (19) Aoki 1979 (7) Hayden 1985 (85)	46	29.1 ± 9.7	Wills 1987 (198–201) Capparelli 1988 (30) Atmar 1990 (11)
Mild-to-moderate chronic renal insufficiency, adults	20	$y = 99.7 - 1.53x$ $y = t_{1/2}$ (h) $x = Cl_{cr}$ 10–50 mL/min	Horadam 1981 (91) Wu 1982 (210)	—	—	—
Dialysis-dependent renal failure, adults	4	200 ± 36	Horadam 1981 (91)	8	47.1 ± 13.4	Capparelli 1988 (30)
Chronic stable liver disease, adults	—	—	—	6	38.7 ± 17.5	Wills 1987 (198)
Elderly healthy adults	15	26.1 ± 9.7	Aoki 1985 (5) Hayden 1985 (85)	10	36.5 ± 14.5	Hayden 1985 (85)
Children 5–8 years, healthy	—	—	—	10	24.8 ± 9.4	Anderson 1987 (3)

TABLE 6 • **Clinical Pharmacokinetic Characteristics of Amantadine and Rimantadine in Healthy Adults**

	Amantadine		Rimantadine	
	Young	Elderly	Young	Elderly
Relative oral bioavailability (%)	62–93[19]	53[120]–100[5]	75–93[85,153]	N/A[a]
Vd_{ss} (L/kg) at 200 mg/day	6.1 ± 2.1[7,85]	3.6 ± 1.1[85]	18.4 ± 9.6[30,85,198]	11.5 ± 2.9[85]
Plasma protein binding (%)	67[109]	N/A	40[196]	N/A
Clearance (mL/min/kg)				
• Plasma or total	5.0 ± 2.1[7,85]	2.0 ± 0.9[5,85]	6.1 ± 1.9[30,85]	4.7 ± 2.0[85]
• Renal	6.4 ± 3.7[7]	2.0 ± 1.1[5]	1.2 ± 0.4[30]	N/A
• Nonrenal	0[7]	0[5]	6.4 ± 1.4[30]	N/A
Urinary excretion of unchanged drug (%)	62–93[19]	53[120]–100[5]	8.3[198]–43[153]	N/A
Plasma $t_{1/2}$[b] (h)	14.8 ± 6.2	26.1 ± 9.7	29.1 ± 9.7	36.5 ± 14.5
Therapeutic range (ng/mL)				
$C_{max, ss}$				
• 200 mg/day	475 ± 110[7]	—	416 ± 108[200]	447 ± 108[181]
• 100 mg/day	—	362 ± 158[5]	—	—
$C_{trough, ss}$				
• 200 mg/day	302 ± 80[8]	—	300 ± 75[200]	310 ± 87[181]
• 100 mg/day	—	301 ± 75[5]	—	—

[a] N/A, not available

[b] See Table 5.

recommended amantadine doses for children are supported in part by studies that demonstrate the safety of a dose of 6.0 mg/kg/day in 153 children with cystic fibrosis (209) but an increased risk of seizures in others with convulsive disorders (10). No prospective studies describe the safety and efficacy of the current recommended dose for pediatric patients (5 mg/kg/day) or the associated Cp. Currently recommended dose schedules of amantadine based on kinetic calculations and clinical use are presented in Tables 7 and 8. Recommended rimantadine dose schedules are detailed in Tables 9 and 10.

In patients with hepatic disease, amantadine dose reduction is not likely to be needed. In subjects with marked obesity, lean body weight should likely be used for dose calculation for both drugs. No data are available on the need for dose adjustment in patients with wasting or different body builds, ascites or edema, diarrhea, or possible malabsorption.

Monitoring Requirements

Although monitoring the plasma amantadine concentration has been advocated as a means of optimizing amantadine doses (91), the usefulness of maintaining plasma concentration at a target level has not been tested. Moreover, the tedious nature of available assays makes the proposal impractical. Emphasis should be placed on clinical monitoring for adverse effects.

Other Formulations

An intravenous infusion of amantadine sulfate has been used in short-term investigational treatment of parkinsonian patients (29).

TABLE 7 • Amantadine Dosage Regimens for Healthy Individuals

Age (years)	Regimen
Children	
<1	No data available
1–9	5 mg/kg/day to a max. 150 mg/day in 2 individual doses
10–17	1.4 mg/kg to a max. 100 mg twice daily
Adults	
18–64	1.4 mg/kg to a max. 100 mg twice daily
≥65	1.4 mg/kg to a max. 100 mg/day

TABLE 8 • Amantadine Dosage Regimens for Patients with Renal Insufficiency

Children[a]	5 mg/kg/day to a max. 150 mg/day in 2 divided doses reduced in proportion to the reduction in creatinine clearance (mL/min) from normal: age 1–2 years 90 mL/min age >2 years 115 mL/min
Adults[b]	1.4 mg/kg lean body weight to be repeated at the following intervals for creatinine clearance (mL/min): ≥80, 12 h 79–35, every 1 day 34–25, every 2 days 24–15, every 3 days <15, every 7 days

[a] Data from reference 117.

[b] Adapted from reference 210.

TABLE 9 • Rimantadine Dosage Regimens for Healthy Individuals

Children	
<10 years	5 mg/kg once daily to a max. 150 mg
10–17 years	100 mg twice daily
Adults	
> 18 years	100 mg twice daily
Frail elderly	100 mg/day

TABLE 10 • Rimantadine Dosage Regimens for Adults with Marked Renal or Hepatic Dysfunction

Renal insufficiency with Cl_{cr} ≤10 mL/min	100 mg/day
Marked hepatic dysfunction	100 mg/day

ADVERSE EFFECTS
Preclinical Toxicology

Preclinical testing indicates that these drugs lack antiinflammatory and antipyretic effects (187). Amantadine demonstrates indirect activity on the adrenergic nervous system by affecting synthesis, release, and reuptake of catecholamines in the central and peripheral nervous systems (188). The dopaminergic and possibly N-methyl-D-aspartate receptor inhibiting effects of amantadine are probably the basis for its antiparkinsonian activity (103, 185). In dopamine-primed dogs, amantadine causes a dose-related pressor response, whereas rimantadine has a depressor effect (66, 67). Ventricular irritability occurs in animals given high doses of intravenous or oral amantadine. In vitro studies have found that very high concentrations (25–50 μg/mL) of amantadine can inhibit lymphocyte transformation responses to mitogen and specific antigens (113, 147), but no nonspecific immunosuppressive effects have been recognized in clinical trials.

Teratogenicity

Amantadine is teratogenic in rodents, in which high doses cause limb and bone abnormalities, but not rabbits (187). The safety of neither drug has been established during pregnancy or lactation. Isolated instances of cardiac malformation and bone abnormalities have been reported in infants exposed in utero, but the risk of congenital anomalies appears to be low (131, 152).

Human Tolerance

The principal adverse reactions associated with these drugs involve the gastrointestinal tract and central nervous system (CNS). No serious renal, hepatic, or hematopoietic toxicity has been recognized. Relatively common adverse events include nervousness, lightheadedness, difficulty concentrating, insomnia, fatigue, slurred speech, loss of appetite, and nausea. More serious CNS adverse effects include hyperexcitability, confusion, depression, tremors, mood disturbance, ataxia and gait disturbance, hallucinations, psychosis, and coma (68). Long-term amantadine ingestion, primarily in the treatment of Parkinson's disease, has been associated with livedo reticularis and peripheral edema, which resolve on discontinuation of the drug (161). Uncommon or rare adverse effects are listed in Table 11. Orthostatic hypotension, congestive heart failure, leukopenia, and sudden vision loss have been reported in isolated cases (132, 136). Patients with preexisting seizure disorders develop an increased frequency of major motor seizures during amantadine (10) and uncommonly with rimantadine use (169). Dose reductions are probably indicated in those with underlying seizure disorders. Schizophrenic subjects may experience decompensation when amantadine is added to their drug regimen (126). Neuroleptic malignant syndrome has been temporally associated with amantadine withdrawal (20).

Amantadine-associated side effects are related to dose (133) and influenced considerably by renal function. Daily doses of 300 mg are poorly tolerated by healthy adults and decrease performance on psychomotor tests measuring sustained attention and problem-solving ability (81). Doses of 200 mg/day are inconsistently associated with changes in psychomotor or academic performance (25, 81, 119, 137). When used for long-term prophylaxis at the usual dosage of 200 mg/day, adverse complaints have occurred in 5 to 33% of subjects, and excess withdrawals because of drug side effects in 6 to 11% (25, 48, 121). Complaints typically develop within the first week of administration, often resolve despite continued

TABLE 11 • **Uncommon Acute Adverse Reactions to Amantadine or Rimantadine**

Reference	Event	Drug
Atkinson 1986 (10), Soo 1989 (169)	Seizures	Amantadine, rimantadine
Nestlebaum 1986 (126)	Psychotic decompensation in stable schizophrenia	Amantadine
Rego 1989 (148)	Mania, aggression, delirium	Amantadine
Macchio 1993 (111)	Coma	Amantadine
McNamara 1991 (118)	Pathologic jealousy ("Othello syndrome")	Amantadine
Postma 1975 (143), Harper 1973 (70)	Visual hallucinations, lilliputian hallucinations	Amantadine
Blanchard 1990 (18), Fraunfelder 1990 (57), Pearlman 1977 (136)	Visual loss, corneal edema, subepithelial corneal opacities	Amantadine
Pfeiffer 1996 (141)	"Vocal" myoclonus	Amantadine
Fahn 1971 (54), Pimentel 1991 (142), Snoey 1990 (168), Hartshorne 1995 (71)	Ventricular arrhythmias, urinary retention, acid base disturbance, death	Amantadine overdosage
Bower 1994 (20)	Neuroleptic malignant syndrome	Amantadine withdrawal
Lammers 1993 (105)	Hyponatremia	Amantadine

ingestion, and are promptly reversible on discontinuation of the drug. In elderly nursing home residents receiving lower prophylactic doses of 100 mg/day, the frequency of adverse effects ranges up to 41%, and cessation of drug is necessary in 5 to 37% of recipients (45, 138, 173, 174). The risk of falls and need for physical restraints also increase occur in amantadine recipients (68). An increasing number of underlying diagnoses and low body mass (<50 kg) appear to be additional risk factors in the elderly (173). An amantadine dose of 50 mg/day is better tolerated in such patients but does not reliably provide plasma levels associated with protection (155).

Rimantadine causes qualitatively similar adverse effects but is associated with a lower risk of CNS reactions than amantadine. Rimantadine doses of 300 or 400 mg/day in young adults causes excess CNS and gastrointestinal side effects as well as sleep disturbance and tremulousness (137). At doses of 200 mg/day in young adults, the frequency of CNS adverse effects is significantly lower than with amantadine and generally no different from placebo. One 6-week prophylaxis study at this dosage found that withdrawals due to adverse CNS effects were more than twice as frequent with amantadine (13%) than with rimantadine (6%) or placebo (4%) (48). In contrast to amantadine, daily doses of 300 mg of rimantadine do not significantly affect psychomotor performance (81). Gastrointestinal side effects occur at similar frequencies in rimantadine and amantadine recipients, which suggests that different mechanisms may account for the CNS and gastrointestinal toxicities of these drugs. Overall, in adults ingesting rimantadine doses of 200 mg/day, the frequencies of CNS (8.5 vs. 6.0%) and gastrointestinal side effects (3.1 vs. 1.2%) are slightly higher than with placebo (169).

In elderly nursing home residents, long-term administration of rimantadine (200 mg/day) is associated with higher plasma concentrations (mean, 1.2 μg/mL) than observed in young adults and with an approximate 30% excess frequency of anxiety and nausea (134). One prophylaxis study in nursing homes found no differences in reported side effects between rimantadine 100 mg/day, rimantadine 200 mg/day, or placebo for up to 8 weeks (122). However, the risk of adverse health events and study withdrawals in group receiving rimantadine 200 mg was approximately twice that with placebo, and both rimantadine groups had an unexplained excess mortality. A similar nursing home study found excess withdrawals (3–4% vs. placebo), but no differences in mortality in rimantadine recipients (16).

Risk Factors

The risk of adverse effects is related to dose, conditions that alter drug disposition, and to a limited extent blood concentrations for both drugs. In previously healthy adults, significant but low correlations exist between plasma drug concentration and the occurrence of side effects (84, 149), and there is considerable overlap in concentrations that do and do not elicit adverse CNS complaints. Pharmacokinetic differences between the drugs appear to account for the increased frequency of CNS adverse effects seen with amantadine. When matched for particular plasma drug levels, amantadine and rimantadine do not differ substantially in their potential for causing CNS adverse effects (84). Approximately 25% of healthy volunteers with plasma drug concentrations between 1.0 and 1.5 μg/mL develop moderate or marked CNS side effects. An increased seizure frequency was observed in children on anticonvulsants who took an amantadine dosage (6.6 mg/kg/day) that resulted in average serum levels of 2.0 μg/mL (10). Amantadine concentrations above 0.450 μg/mL are associated with adverse CNS effects in elderly nursing home residents (9). Patients with impaired renal function who develop plasma concentrations from 1.0 to 5.0 μg/mL have experienced confusion, delirium, hallucinations, seizures, and other signs of neurotoxicity (95). One pediatric patient with renal failure experienced loss of hallucinations when plasma levels fell below 0.795 μg/mL (177). Delirium progressing to coma has been observed at an amantadine plasma concentration of 1.6 μg/mL (111). It appears that trough plasma concentrations above 0.450 μg/mL and peak ones over 1.0 μg/mL should be avoided (49).

Adverse Drug Interactions

The potential for CNS adverse effects with amantadine appears to be increased by concomitant ingestion of antihistamines or anticholinergic drugs (119). Combined administration with anticholinergics, especially in elderly parkinsonian patients, may be associated with toxic delirium and visual hallucinations (70, 143). Psychosis related to combined amantadine and phenylpropanolamine use has been reported (176).

Pharmacokinetic drug-drug interactions are relevant for amantadine. A diuretic combination of triamterene and hydrochlorothiazide was associated with CNS toxicity and a 50% increase in plasma amantadine concentration due to decreased renal clearance in one case (203). Trimethoprim-sulfamethoxazole has also been associated with amantadine toxicity, probably because of trimethoprim-induced inhibition of tubular secretion (172). Other cationic drugs that undergo active tubular secretion, such as cimetidine and procainamide, could theoretically alter excretion. No clinically important drug-drug interactions have been observed between rimantadine and aspirin, cimetidine, or acetaminophen (197).

Overdosage

Drug overdosage has been associated with severe CNS reactions including toxic delirium, psychosis, hallucinations, and coma as well as acid-base disturbances and complex ventricular arrhythmias (54, 111, 142, 168). Although anticholinergic effects are lacking in animals, clinical observations of dry mouth, pupillary dilation, toxic psychosis, and urinary retention in acute amantadine overdose suggest this activity is present in humans. Fatalities in adults have occurred with ingestion of more than 2 g (36, 156). In doses up to 600 mg daily, amantadine has no significant effect on blood pressure or cardiac rhythm in humans (132). Malignant ventricular arrhythmia after amantadine overdose has been described; lidocaine may be suppressive (156). One study found rimantadine (300 mg/day) to be associated with slight slowing of the heart rate (137). Serious neurotoxic reactions may be transiently reversed by physostigmine administration (15, 31). Activated charcoal and charcoal hemoperfusion have been suggested for serious overdoses but are of uncertain benefit.

CLINICAL INDICATIONS

Immunization using inactivated virus remains the mainstay of influenza prevention, but vaccine efficacy is incomplete, and the vaccine is underutilized. Chemoprophylaxis and chemotherapy with amantadine and rimantadine are useful adjunctive strategies. The potential advantages of using these antiviral agents include (a) antiviral activity independent of the frequent antigenic changes of the virus; (b) rapid onset of protective action during outbreaks; (c) prophylactic activity supplementary to immunoprophylaxis; and (d) therapeutic activity in established illness.

Prophylaxis

The clinical usefulness of amantadine and rimantadine as antiviral agents is limited to the prevention and treatment of influenza A virus infections, and generally no effects on influenza B or noninfluenza respiratory illness are found during drug prophylaxis. In experimentally challenged volunteers, prophylactic administration of amantadine is 15 to 40% effective in reducing the frequency of infection and 50 to 90% effective in reducing the frequency of influenza A virus illness (43, 43, 149, 162, 212). Prophylaxis also reduces measures of viral replication (peak titers, duration of sheddding) and influenza-specific antibody responses in blood and nasal secretions (149, 150). Protection has been demonstrated against challenge with H1N1, H2N2, and H3N2 subtype viruses. No clear dose-related antiviral effects are found over a dose range of 50 to 200 mg/day, but amantadine doses of 100 mg/day provide approximately 75% protection against illness (149, 162).

Seasonal Prophylaxis

Controlled studies have established the protective activity of these drugs against naturally occurring influenza A virus infections due to H1N1, H2N2, and H3N2 subtype viruses (Table 12). When taken daily for seasonal prophylaxis in open populations of children and adults, protective efficacy against epidemic illness ranges from 70 to 100%. The reasons for these variable protection rates have not been determined. Protection is additive to that provided by increasing levels of specific antibody from prior natural infection or immunization (60, 145, 166). Termination of prophylaxis before influenza activity has ceased is sometimes associated with early posttreatment failures of drug prophylaxis (123, 135). Rimantadine is comparable to amantadine in preventing influenza A virus infection and illness under experimental or field conditions (195, 212). One comparative 6-week seasonal prophylaxis trial in students found that at equivalent doses (100 mg twice daily), amantadine had a 91% protective efficacy and rimantadine an 85% protective efficacy against illness due to influenza A virus (48).

Protection has also been found in seronegative populations experiencing infection by new influenza A viruses (121, 124, 140, 167). Protection against pandemic influenza is generally somewhat lower, and efficacy averages approximately 60 to 70% across studies (Table 12). Efficacy against laboratory-documented infection is lower in both epidemic and pandemic influenza, such that a substantial portion of recipients experiences mild or subclinical infections demonstrable by serologic testing. Because such individuals develop humoral immune responses, they would be expected to be protected against reinfection by the same strain. Prophylaxis can have indirect epidemiologic benefits. Seasonal prophylaxis given to school-aged children has reduced the frequency of influenza A virus infection in other family members by 73% (40).

TABLE 12 • Representative Controlled Studies with Amantadine or Rimantadine for Prevention of Natural Influenza

Study	Year of Trial	No. of Subjects	Virus (subtype)[a]	Drug	Dose (mg)[b]	Duration	Population	Efficacy (%) Illness[c]	Efficacy (%) Infection[d]	Comments
Seasonal prophylaxis/open populations										
Oker-Blom 1970 (129)	1969	391	A/HongKong/68(H3N2)[a]	Amantadine	100 b.i.d.	30 days	Adults	59	52	Excess CNS adverse effects (6%) headache (5%) in amantadine
Nafta 1970 (124)	1969	215	A/HongKong/68(H3N2)[a]	Amantadine	100 b.i.d.	20 days	Adults	100	49	Excess dropout rate (6%) in amantadine
Monto 1979 (121)	1978	286	A/USSR/77(H1N1)[a]	Amantadine	200 q.d.	7 weeks	Adults	71	39	
Pettersson 1980 (140)	1978	192	A/USSR/77(H1N1)[a]	Amantadine	100 b.i.d.	3 or 5 weeks	Adults		37	Excess dropout rate (9%) in amantadine
Quarles 1981 (144)	1978	444	A/USSR/77(H1N1)[a]	Amantadine Rimantadine	100 b.i.d. 100 b.i.d.	6 weeks	Adults	31 27	19 9	
Dolin 1982 (48)	1981	450	A/Brazil/78(H1N1) A/Bangkok/79(H3N2)	Amantadine Rimantadine	100 b.i.d. 100 b.i.d.	6 weeks	Adults	91 85	74 66	Excess dropout rate (11%) and CNS adverse effects (9%) in amantadine
Clover 1986 (33)	1984	145	A(H1N1)	Rimantadine	5/kg/day[b]	5 weeks	Children	100	91	Reduced infection rate in adult contacts
Brady 1990 (21)	1988	228	A/Leningrad/87(H3N2)	Rimantadine	100 q.d.	6 weeks	Adults	86	66	
Crawford 1988 (40)	1985	110	A(H3N2)	Rimantadine	5/kg/day[b]	6 weeks	Children	100	77	

Postcontact prophylaxis/households

Reference	Year	n	Virus strain	Drug	Dose	Duration	Population	[c]	[d]	Comments
Galbraith 1969 (59)	1967–68	202	A/England/67(H2N2)	Amantadine	100 b.i.d.[b]	10 days	Adults and children >2 years	100	62	
Galbraith 1969 (60)	1969	107	A/HongKong/68(H3N2)[a]	Amantadine	100 b.i.d.[b]	10 days	Adults and children >2 years	20	0	Index cases also treated
Hayden 1989 (79)	1987–68	115	A(H1N1) A(H3N2)	Rimantadine	200 q.d. 5/kg/day[b]	10 days	Adults and children	3	12	Index cases also treated; Excess GI adverse effects (6%) in adults on rimantadine
Bricaire 1990 (23)	1988–9	301	A(H1N1)	Rimantadine	200 q.d. 5/kg/d[b]	10 days	Adults and children	69[e]		Excess adverse effects (8%) in rimantadine

Nosocomial/Institutional prophylaxis[f]

Reference	Year	n	Virus strain	Drug	Dose	Duration	Population	[c]	[d]	Comments
Quilligan 1966 (145)	1964	200	A/Los Angeles/64(H2N2)	Amantadine	2.6–3.8/kg/day	8+12 weeks	Children	90		
Finklea 1967 (56)	1965	299	A/AnnArbor/65(H2N2)	Amantadine	1.0–2.5/kg/day	18 weeks	Children	90		
Smorodintsev 1970 (166)	1969	6,383	A/HongKong/68(H3N2)[a]	Amantadine	100 q.d.	30 days	Adults	63	28	
O'Donoghue 1973 (128)	1972	171	A(H3N2)	Amantadine	100 b.i.d.	hospital stay (~2 weeks)	Adults	100	80	
Payler 1984 (135)	1983	606	A(H1N1)	Amantadine	100 q.d.	14 days	Teenagers	90		75% protection against illness in vaccinees
Dolin 1987 (47)	1983	105	A(H3N2)	Rimantadine	100 b.i.d.	6 weeks	Elderly	55		

[a] P, pandemic strain.
[b] Pediatric dosing adjustment.
[c] Reduction in laboratory-documented influenza virus illness compared with placebo or no treatment.
[d] Reduction in laboratory-documented influenza virus infection (based on virus isolation and/or rise in specific antibody titers) compared with placebo or no treatment.
[e] Clinical Influenza
[f] Includes studies in hospitals, chronic care facilities, boarding schools.

The minimally effective dose for preventing natural influenza illness has not been determined for either drug. In adults, doses of 100 mg/day of amantadine (135) or rimantadine (21) appear to be effective for prevention and also reduce the risk of drug toxicity. Amantadine at 100 mg/day provided 63% protection against illness during the A/Hong Kong/68(H3N2) pandemic in one trial (167). Other studies in the former Soviet Union suggest that a rimantadine dose of 50 mg/day for up to 30 days is safe and effective prophylactically (212).

Preseason immunization is the principal means of prevention in groups having the highest morbidity and mortality from influenza (4). Seasonal prophylaxis with amantadine is an alternative if the vaccine (a) cannot be administered because of toxicity or allergy (rare), (b) may be ineffective because the epidemic strain differs substantially from the antigens represented in the vaccine, or (c) is unlikely to induce an adequate immune response, as in patients with primary or acquired immunodeficiencies. Because of the additive effect of antibody-associated protection and that provided by these drugs, combined use of preseason vaccine and chemoprophylaxis during an outbreak provides optimal protection for particularly high-risk patients. Chemoprophylaxis needs to continue for the duration of the exposure risk, generally 4 to 8 weeks in a particular community, because premature discontinuation of prophylaxis can result in loss of protection. Because these drugs do inhibit formation of protective antibodies in response to inactivated vaccine, concurrent administration of vaccine and antiviral prophylaxis provides protection in unimmunized individuals, if an outbreak has already begun. The duration of chemoprophylaxis can be shortened to 2 weeks, by which time an adequate response to the vaccine can be anticipated.

Nosocomial/Institutional Prophylaxis

Several controlled trials of closed population prophylaxis have shown protection against illness in hospitals, chronic care facilities, and nursing homes (Table 4). Mass chemoprophylaxis in institutional outbreaks has been temporally associated with cessation of influenza activity in many reports (9). Amantadine administration to patients hospitalized during a community outbreak provided complete protection against nosocomial influenza in one study (128). In immunized elderly nursing home residents, administration of rimantadine (100 mg twice daily) during an outbreak significantly improved protection against illness (75% efficacy) compared with placebo (195).

Several uncontrolled studies suggest that mass chemoprophylaxis may be effective in shortening nosocomial outbreaks in progress. Administration to both patients and staff should be considered in such circumstances (4). Because of the short duration (1–3 weeks) of such outbreaks and delays in recognition, early intervention is difficult to attain unless preseason outbreak plans including medication orders are in place, and rapid diagnostic techniques are used. Because of its lower risk of CNS adverse effects and lesser dependence on renal function for elimination, rimantadine would be preferred to amantadine in elderly patients.

Postexposure Prophylaxis

Studies of postexposure prophylaxis indicate that the drugs are useful in limiting the spread of infection within households (Table 12). When taken by family contacts after onset of illness in an index case, amantadine and rimantadine significantly reduce the risk of influenza A illness (23, 59). In contrast, no significant protection of contacts has been observed in two studies involving concurrent treatment of ill index cases and in one trial, pandemic influenza (60, 79). Prophylaxis failure probably due to transmission of drug-resistant virus from treated index cases to household contacts has been documented. This approach is practical only if amantadine or rimantadine is readily available.

Treatment

Adults

Most studies of amantadine and rimantadine treatment have been conducted in acute uncomplicated influenza in previously healthy young adults (86, 88, 186, 211). If begun within 48 h of symptom onset, doses of 200 mg/day reduce the duration of fever and systemic complaints by 1 to 2 days and, in some studies, the quantity of virus shed in upper respiratory secretions and duration of functional limitation (Table 13). One study comparing the effectiveness of aspirin and amantadine treatment (100 or 200 mg/day) of influenza found that aspirin-treated patients became afebrile more rapidly but experienced significantly higher rates of drug-related side effects (tinnitus, gastrointestinal upset) and slower overall symptomatic improvement than amantadine recipients (211). Another therapy trial comparing equivalent doses (100 mg twice daily for 5 days) in young adults with acute A/USSR/77 (H1N1) illness found that amantadine-treated patients tended to improve more rapidly than rimantadine-treated patients over the first 24 h of treatment (186). By 48 h, both drug groups had significantly less fever, greater symptomatic improvement, lower frequencies of viral shedding, and better functional status than did placebo recipients. Similar therapeutic benefit in regard to resolution of fever and symptoms occurs in elderly adults treated with rimantadine (17). Because of its low initial concentration and slow time to steady-state plasma concentrations, rimantadine regimens that give patients 400 to 500 mg over the first 24 h may provide more rapid antiviral and clinical effects (86, 88, 204).

In acute influenza due to H3N2 subtype viruses, measures of peripheral airway flow (but not bronchial hyperreactivity) improve more rapidly in amantadine-treated patients than in those receiving placebo (107, 108). Such studies have not been conducted with rimantadine. Antiviral treatment generally does not reduce the humoral immune response to influenza or affect the in vitro function of lymphocytes or natural killer cells. However, influenza virus–specific nasal IgG and IgA responses may be reduced, perhaps because of lower antigenic stimulation (34).

Although advocated for patients with serious or life-threatening influenza infections, such as croup in infants or primary viral pneumonia, no controlled studies have been conducted to determine if amantadine prevents or treats the pulmonary com-

TABLE 13 • **Representative Controlled Studies of Treatments of Acute, Uncomplicated Influenza Illness in Adults with Amantadine and Rimantadine**

Study	Year of Trial	No. of Subjects	Virus (subtype)[a]	Drug	Dose (mg)[b]	Duration (days)	Population	Significant Reduction in			Comments
								Viral Titers	Symptoms	Fever	
Rabinovich 1969 (146)	1967	22	A(H2N2)	Rimantadine	150 b.i.d.	10	Adults	ND	Day 2	Yes	
Walters 1970 (190)	1967–68	35	A(H2N2)	Amantadine	100 b.i.d.	10	Elderly	ND	No	Yes	1 death in placebo and 1 in amantadine
Togo 1970 (180)	1968	102	A/Texas/68(H2N2)	Amantadine	100 b.i.d.	10	Adults	ND	Yes	Yes	No effect on viral shedding duration
Wingfield 1969 (204)	1968	95	A/Virginia/68 (H2N2)	Amantadine	100 b.i.d.	10	Adults	ND	Days 2 & 3	Yes	Fever duration 23 (amantadine) vs 19 (rimantadine) vs. 45 (placebo) h; ~1 day reduction in 50% improvement time
				Rimantadine	150 b.i.d			ND	Days 2 & 3	Yes	
Knight 1970 (100)	1969	26	A/HongKong/68 (H3N2)[a]	Amantadine	100 b.i.d.	≥6	Adults	Day 1	Yes	Yes	Fever duration 45 vs. 71 h
Galbraith 1971 (58)	1969–70	153	A/HongKong/68 (H3N2)[a]	Amantadine	100 b.i.d.[b]	7	Adults and children >2 years	ND	No	Yes	Fever duration 47 vs. 75 h
Van Voris 1981 (186)	1978	45	A/USSR/77(H1N1)[a]	Amantadine	100 b.i.d.	5	Adults	Day 2	Yes	Yes	More rapid function recovery (days 2 & 3) and ~1 day reduction in 50% improvement time in drug groups
				Rimantadine	100 b.i.d.			Day 2	Yes	Yes	
Younkin 1983 (145)	1981	47	A/Brazil/78(H1N1)	Amantadine	100 q.d. 200 q.d.	5	Adults	No	Days 2 & 3	No	Fever duration 10 (aspirin) vs. 22 (amantadine 100) vs. 24 (amantadine 200) h
Hayden 1986 (86)	1983	14	A/Bangkok/79 (H3N2)	Rimantadine	200 q.d.	5	Adults	Days 2–4	Days 3 & 4	Yes	Fever duration 31 vs. 68 h
Betts 1987 (17)	1987	83	A	Rimantadine	100 b.i.d.	7	Elderly	Day 2	Days 2–4	Yes	1 death in placebo and 2 in rimantadine
Hayden 1991 (88)	1988	56	A(H3N2)	Rimantadine	200 q.d. 5/kg/day[b]	10	Adults and children >1 year	ND	Day 3–9	Yes	Fever duration decreased 1.6 days; decreased days of missed school/work

[a] P, pandemic strain.

[b] Pediatric dosing adjustment

Note: days refer to days of treatment.

ND, not determined.

plications of influenza. An uncontrolled study using high amantadine doses (400–550 mg/day) found a 55% survival rate in 11 patients with primary influenza viral pneumonia (37).

Intermittent aerosol administration of amantadine or rimantadine has been associated with modest therapeutic benefit in uncomplicated influenza (82, 89). Both drugs cause mucous membrane irritation; a regimen using prolonged aerosol exposure with low rimantadine concentrations is better tolerated and associated with high nasal drug concentrations (11).

Children

In children with influenza A H3N2 subtype infection, rimantadine treatment (6.6 mg/kg/day, up to 150 mg/day for those <9 years and 200 mg/day for older) for 5 days results in lower symptom burden, fever, and viral titers during the first 3 days of treatment than acetaminophen administration (69). However, rimantadine-treated children have more-prolonged shedding of influenza virus by an average of 1 day, and up to 45% of those positive for virus after 4 days shed resistant virus. Another study involving 49 children with either H3N2 or predominately H1N1 subtype infection found reduced frequencies of viral shedding after the first 2 days of treatment but no significant clinical benefit of rimantadine over acetaminophen (179). Amantadine treatment (50–150 mg/day for 7 days) of children with influenza A H3N2 infection is also associated with shorter duration of fever than with placebo (98). Treatment of ill index cases in the household, usually children, appears to decrease the risk of transmitting infection to close contacts by approximately 30% (38). In contrast, antiviral treatment of ill children combined with prophylaxis for their household contacts has been associated with prophylaxis failures due to apparent transmission of drug-resistant viruses (79). The optimal duration of therapy in children is uncertain. While treatment for 5 days is effective in adults and adolescents (Table 13), it remains to be determined whether shorter courses of treatment provide therapeutic benefit and possibly reduce the frequency of drug-resistant virus emergence.

Other Uses

Amantadine continues to be used in treating parkinsonian and drug-induced extrapyramidal symptoms and has been studied in a variety of other neurologic disorders. Its use has recently been associated with improved survival in Parkinson's disease (185) and ameliorating fatigue in multiple sclerosis patients (104). Amantadine has been used to treat persistent hiccups and zoster-associated neuralgia.

REFERENCES

1. Al-Nakib W, Higgins PG, Willman J, Tyrrell DA, Swallow DL, Hurst BC, Rushton A. Prevention and treatment of experimental influenza A virus infection in volunteers with a new antiviral ICI 130,685. J Antimicrob Chemother 1986;18:119–129.
2. Aldrich PE, Hermann EC, Meier WE, Paulshock M, Prichard WW, Snyder JA, Watts JC. Antiviral agents. 2. Structure-activity relationships of compounds related to 1-adamantanamine. J Med Chem 1971;14:535–543.
3. Anderson EL, Van VLP, Bartram J, Hoffman HE, Belshe RB. Pharmacokinetics of a single dose of rimantadine in young adults and children. Antimicrob Agents Chemother 1987;31:1140–1142.
4. Anonymous. Prevention and control of influenza: recommendations of the Advisory Committee on Immunization Practices (ACIP). MMWR 1997;46(RR-9):1–25.
5. Aoki FY, Sitar DS. Amantadine kinetics in healthy elderly men: implications for influenza prevention. Clin Pharmacol Ther 1985;37:137–144.
6. Aoki FY, Sitar DS. Clinical pharmacokinetics of amantadine hydrochloride. [Review]. Clin Pharmacokinet 1988;14:35–51.
7. Aoki FY, Sitar DS, Ogilvie RI. Amantadine kinetics in healthy young subjects after long-term dosing. Clin Pharmacol Ther 1979;26:729–736.
8. Aoki FY, Stiver HG, Sitar DS, Boudreault A, Ogilvie RI. Prophylactic amantadine dose and plasma concentration-effect relationships in healthy adults. Clin Pharmacol Ther 1985;37:128–136.
9. Arden NH, Patriarca PA, Fasano MB, Lui KJ, Harmon MW, Kendal AP, Rimland D. The roles of vaccination and amantadine prophylaxis in controlling an outbreak of influenza A (H3N2) in a nursing home. Arch Intern Med 1988;148:865–868.
10. Atkinson WL, Arden NH, Patriarca PA, Leslie N, Lui KJ, Gohd R. Amantadine prophylaxis during an institutional outbreak of type A (H1N1) influenza. Arch Intern Med 1986;146:1751–1756.
11. Atmar RL, Greenberg SB, Quarles JM, Wilson SZ, Tyler B, Feldman S, Couch RB. Safety and pharmacokinetics of rimantadine small-particle aerosol. Antimicrob Agents Chemother 1990;34:2228–2233.
12. Bean WJ, Threlkeld SC, Webster RG. Biologic potential of amantadine-resistant influenza A virus in an avian model. J Infect Dis 1989;159:1050–1056.
13. Beare AS, Hall TS, Tyrrell DA. Protection of volunteers against challenge with A-Hong Kong-68 influenza virus by a new adamantane compound. Lancet 1972;1(759):1039–1040.
14. Belshe RB, Burk B, Newman F, Cerruti RL, Sim IS. Resistance of influenza A virus to amantadine and rimantadine: results of one decade of surveillance. J Infect Dis 1989;159:430–435.
15. Berkowitz CD. Treatment of acute amantadine toxicity with physostigmine. J Pediatr 1979;95:144–145.
16. Bernstein JM, Betts RF, Demmler RW, Schwartz R. Safety and tolerance of rimantadine in elderly patients. J Respir Dis 1989;10(Suppl)(12A):S38–S41.
17. Betts RF, Treanor JJ, Graman PS, Bentley DW, Dolin R. Antiviral agents to prevent or treat influenza in the elderly. J Respir Dis 1987;8(Suppl)(11A):S56–S59.
18. Blanchard DL. Amantadine caused corneal edema [Letter]. Cornea 1990;9:181.
19. Bleidner WE, Harmon JB, Hewes WE, Lynes TE, Hermann EC. Absorption, distribution and excretion of amantadine hydrochloride. J Pharmacol Exp Ther 1965;150:484–490.
20. Bower DJ, Chalasani P, Ammons JC. Withdrawal-induced neuroleptic malignant syndrome [Letter]. Am J Psychiatry 1994;151:451–452.
21. Brady MT, Sears SD, Pacini DL, Samorodin R, DePamphilis J, Oakes M, Soo W, Clements ML. Safety and prophylactic efficacy of low-dose rimantadine in adults during an influenza A epidemic. Antimicrob Agents Chemother 1990;34:1633–1636.
22. Brenner M, Haass A, Jacobi P, Schimrigk K. Amantadine sulphate in treating Parkinson's disease: clinical effects, psychometric tests and serum concentrations. J Neurol 1989;236:153–156.
23. Bricaire F, Hannoun C, Boissel JP. [Prevention of influenza A. Effectiveness and tolerance of rimantadine hydrochloride] [French]. Presse Med 1990;19:69–72.

24. Browne MJ, Moss MY, Boyd MR. Comparative activity of amantadine and ribavirin against influenza virus in vitro: possible clinical relevance. Antimicrob Agents Chemother 1983;23:503–505.

25. Bryson YJ, Monahan C, Pollack M, Shields WD. A prospective double-blind study of side effects associated with the administration of amantadine for influenza A virus prophylaxis. J Infect Dis 1980;141:543–547.

26. Bukrinskaya AG, Vorkunova NK, Kornilayeva GV, Narmanbetova RA, Vorkunova GK. Influenza virus uncoating in infected cells and effect of rimantadine. J Gen Virol 1982;60(Pt 1):49–59.

27. Burlington DB, Meiklejohn G, Mostow SR. Anti-influenza A virus activity of amantadine hydrochloride and rimantadine hydrochloride in ferret tracheal ciliated epithelium. Antimicrob Agents Chemother 1982;21:794–799.

28. Bussereau F, Picard M, Blancou J, Sureau P. Treatment of rabies in mice and foxes with antiviral compounds. Acta Virol 1988;32:33–49.

29. Buttner T, Kuhn W, Muller T, Patzold T, Przuntek H. Color vision in Parkinson's disease: missing influence of amantadine sulphate. Clin Neuropharmacol 1995;18:458–463.

30. Capparelli EV, Stevens RC, Chow MS, Izard M, Wills RJ. Rimantadine pharmacokinetics in healthy subjects and patients with end-stage renal failure. Clin Pharmacol Ther 1988;43:536–541.

31. Casey DE. Amantadine intoxication reversed by physostigmine [Letter]. N Engl J Med 1978;298:516.

32. Chizhmakov IV, Geraghty FM, Ogden DC, Hayhurst A, Antoniou M, Hay AJ. Selective proton permeability and pH regulation of the influenza virus M2 channel expressed in mouse erythroleukaemia cells. J Physiol 1996;494(Pt 2):329–336.

33. Clover RD, Crawford SA, Abell TD, Ramsey CNJ, Glezen WP, Couch RB. Effectiveness of rimantadine prophylaxis of children within families. Am J Dis Child 1986;140:706–709.

34. Clover RD, Waner JL, Becker L, Davis A. Effect of rimantadine on the immune response to influenza A infections. J Med Virol 1991;34:68–73.

35. Cochran KW, Maassab HF, Tsunoda A, Berlin BS. Studies on the antiviral activity of amantadine hydrochloride. Ann NY Acad Sci 1965;130:432–439.

36. Cook PE, Dermer SW, McGurk T. Fatal overdose with amantadine. Can J Psychiatry—Rev Can Psychiatrie 1986;31:757–758.

37. Couch RB, Jackson GG. Antiviral agents in influenza—summary of Influenza Workshop VIII. J Infect Dis 1976;134:516–527.

38. Couch RB, Kasel JA, Glezen WP, Cate TR, Six HR, Taber LH, Frank AL, Greenberg SB, Zahradnik JM, Keitel WA. Influenza: its control in persons and populations. J Infect Dis 1986; 153:431–440.

39. Couch RB, Six HR. The antiviral spectrum and mechanism of action of amantadine and rimantadine. In: Mills J, Corey L, eds. Antiviral chemotherapy: new directions for clinical application and research. New York: Elsevier; 1986:50–57.

40. Crawford SA, Clover RD, Abell TD, Ramsey CNJ, Glezen P, Couch RB. Rimantadine prophylaxis in children: a follow-up study. Pediatr Infect Dis J 1988;7:379–383.

41. Daugirdas JT, Ing IL, Cheng PJ, Wu MJ, Klawans HL, Soung LS. Binding of amantadine to red blood cells. Ther Drug Monit 1984;6:399–401.

42. Davies WL, Grunert RR, Haff RF, McGahen JW, Neumayer EM, Paulshock M, Watts JC, Wood TR, Hermann EC, Hoffmann CE. Antiviral activity of 1-adamantanamine (amantadine). Science 1964;144:862

43. Dawkins ATJ, Gallager LR, Togo Y, Hornick RB, Harris BA. Studies on induced influenza in man. II. Double-blind study designed to assess the prophylactic efficacy of an analogue of amantadine hydrochloride. JAMA 1968;203:1095–1099.

44. Degelau J, Somani SK, Cooper SL, Guay DR, Crossley KB. Amantadine-resistant influenza A in a nursing facility. Arch Intern Med 1992;152:390–392.

45. Degelau J, Somani SK, Cooper SL, Irvine PW. Occurrence of adverse effects and high amantadine concentrations with influenza prophylaxis in the nursing home. J Am Geriatr Soc 1990;38:428.

46. Dickinson PC, Chang TW, Weinstein L. Effects of amantadines on influenza B and measles virus infection in children. Antimicrob Agents Chemother 1966;6:521–526.

47. Dolin R. Studies of antiviral agents for influenza in geriatric patients. J Respir Dis 1987;8(Suppl)(11A):S67–S72.

48. Dolin R, Reichman RC, Madore HP, Maynard R, Linton PN, Webber-Jones J. A controlled trial of amantadine and rimantadine in the prophylaxis of influenza A infection. N Engl J Med 1982;307:580–584.

49. Douglas RGJ. Prophylaxis and treatment of influenza [Review; see comments]. N Engl J Med 1990;322:443–450.

50. Duff KC, Gilchrist PJ, Saxena AM, Bradshaw JP. Neutron diffraction reveals the site of amantadine blockade in the influenza A M2 ion channel. Virology 1994;202:287–293.

51. Dunn JP, Henkel JG, Gianutsos G. Pharmacological activity of amantadine: effect of N-alkyl substitution. J Pharm Pharmacol 1986;38:353–356.

52. Evans SG, Havlik I. In vitro drug interaction between amantadine and classical antimalarial drugs in Plasmodium falciparum infections. Trans R Soc Trop Med Hyg 1994;88:683–686.

53. Evans SG, Havlik I. Effect of pH on in vitro potency of amantadine against Plasmodium falciparum. Am J Trop Med Hyg 1996;54:232–236.

54. Fahn S, Craddock G, Kumin G. Acute toxic psychosis from suicidal overdosage of amantadine. Arch Neurol 1971;25:45–48.

55. Fenton RJ, Bessell C, Spilling CR, Potter CW. The effects of peroral or local aerosol administration of 1-aminoadamantane hydrochloride (amantadine hydrochloride) on influenza infections of the ferret. J Antimicrob Chemother 1977;3:463–472.

56. Finklea JF, Hennessy AV, Davenport FM. A field trial of amantadine prophylaxis in naturally-occurring acute respiratory illness. Am J Epidemiol 1967;85:403–412.

57. Fraunfelder FT, Coster DJ, Drew R, Fraunfelder FW. Ocular injury induced by methyl ethyl ketone peroxide. Am J Ophthalmol 1990;110:635–640.

58. Galbraith AW, Oxford JS, Schild GC, Potter CW, Watson GI. Therapeutic effect of 1-adamantanamine hydrochloride in naturally occurring influenza A2-Hong Kong infection. A controlled double-blind study. Lancet 1971;2(716):113–115.

59. Galbraith AW, Oxford JS, Schild GC, Watson GI. Protective effect of 1-adamantanamine hydrochloride on influenza A2 infections in the family environment: a controlled double-blind study. Lancet 1969;2(629):1026–1028.

60. Galbraith AW, Oxford JS, Schild GC, Watson GI. Study of 1-adamantanamine hydrochloride used prophylactically during the Hong Kong influenza epidemic in the family environment. Bull WHO 1969;41:677–682.

61. Galegov GA, Pushkarskaya NL, Obrosova-Serova NP, Zhdanov

VM. Combined action of ribovirin and rimantadine in experimental myxovirus infection. Experientia 1977;33:905–906.

62. Gaudry SE, Sitar DS, Smyth DD, McKenzie JK, Aoki FY. Gender and age as factors in the inhibition of renal clearance of amantadine by quinine and quinidine. Clin Pharmacol Ther 1993;54:23–27.

63. Geuens HF, Stephens RL. Influence of the pH of the urine on the rate of excretion of 1-adamantanamine. 5th International Congress of Chemotherapy, Vienna 1967:703–713.

64. Gill MJ, Sitar DS, Aoki FY. Initial pharmacokinetic evaluation of amantadine hydrochloride administered intravenously to young healthy volunteers [Abstract]. Clin Invest Med 1982;5:5B.

65. Glushakova SE, Lukashevich IS. Early events in arenavirus replication are sensitive to lysosomotropic compounds. Arch Virol 1989;104:157–161.

66. Grelak RP, Clark R, Stump JM. Amantadine, rimantadine, catecholamine release and parkinsonism. Am Soc Pharmacol Exp Ther 1970;12:235.

67. Grelak RP, Clark R, Stump JM, Vernier VG. Amantadine-dopamine interaction: possible mode of action in parkinsonism. Science 1970;169(941):203–204.

68. Guay DRP. Amantadine and rimantadine prophylaxis of influenza A in nursing homes. Drugs Aging 1994;5:8–18.

69. Hall CB, Dolin R, Gala CL, Markovitz DM, Zhang YQ, Madore PH, Disney FA, Talpey WB, Green JL, Francis AB. Children with influenza A infection: treatment with rimantadine. Pediatrics 1987;80:275–282.

70. Harper RW, Knothe BU. Coloured lilliputian hallucinations with amantadine. Med J Aust 1973;1:444–445.

71. Hartshorne NJ, Harruff RC, Logan BK. Unexpected amantadine intoxication in the death of a trauma patient. Am J Forensic Med Pathol 1995;16:340–343.

72. Hay AJ. The action of adamantanamines against influenza A viruses: inhibition of the M2 ion channel protein. Semin Virol 1992;3:21–30.

73. Hay AJ. Amantadine and rimantadine—mechanisms. In: Richman DD, ed. Antiviral drug resistance. New York: John Wiley & Sons, 1996:43–58.

74. Hay AJ, Wolstenholme AJ, Skehel JJ, Smith MH. The molecular basis of the specific anti-influenza action of amantadine. EMBO J 1985;4:3021–3024.

75. Hayden FG, Zak O, Sande MA. Animal models of influenza virus infection for evaluation of antiviral agents. Hayden FG, Zak O, Sande MA, eds. Experimental models in antimicrob chemotherapy. London: Academic Press, 1986:353–371.

76. Hayden FG. Combinations of antiviral agents for treatment of influenza virus infections. J Antimicrob Chemotherapy 1986;18 (Suppl B):177–183.

77. Hayden FG. Amantadine and rimantadine—clinical aspects. In: Richman DD, ed. Antiviral drug resistance. New York: John Wiley & Sons, 1996:59–77.

78. Hayden FG. Combination antiviral therapy for respiratory virus infections. Antiviral Res 1996;29:45–48.

79. Hayden FG, Belshe RB, Clover RD, Hay AJ, Oakes MG, Soo W. Emergence and apparent transmission of rimantadine-resistant influenza A virus in families. N Engl J Med 1989;321: 1696–1702.

80. Hayden FG, Cote KM, Douglas RGJ. Plaque inhibition assay for drug susceptibility testing of influenza viruses. Antimicrob Agents Chemother 1980;17:865–870.

81. Hayden FG, Gwaltney JMJ, Van dCRL, Adams KF, Giordani B. Comparative toxicity of amantadine hydrochloride and rimanta-

dine hydrochloride in healthy adults. Antimicrob Agents Chemother 1981;19:226–233.

82. Hayden FG, Hall WJ, Douglas RGJ. Therapeutic effects of aerosolized amantadine in naturally acquired infection due to influenza A virus. J Infect Dis 1980;141:535–542.

83. Hayden FG, Hall WJ, Douglas RG Jr, Speers DM. Amantadine aerosols in normal volunteers: pharmacology and safety testing. Antimicrob Agents Chemother 1979;16:644–650.

84. Hayden FG, Hoffman HE, Spyker DA. Differences in side effects of amantadine hydrochloride and rimantadine hydrochloride relate to differences in pharmacokinetics. Antimicrob Agents Chemother 1983;23:458–464.

85. Hayden FG, Minocha A, Spyker DA, Hoffman HE. Comparative single-dose pharmacokinetics of amantadine hydrochloride and rimantadine hydrochloride in young and elderly adults [published erratum appears in Antimicrob Agents Chemother 1986;30:579]. Antimicrob Agents Chemother 1985;28:216–221.

86. Hayden FG, Monto AS. Oral rimantadine hydrochloride therapy of influenza A virus H3N2 subtype infection in adults. Antimicrob Agents Chemother 1986;29:339–341.

87. Hayden FG, Schlepushkin AN, Pushkarskaya NL. Combined interferon-alpha 2, rimantadine hydrochloride, and ribavirin inhibition of influenza virus replication in vitro. Antimicrob Agents Chemother 1984;25:53–57.

88. Hayden FG, Sperber SJ, Belshe RB, Clover RD, Hay AJ, Pyke S. Recovery of drug-resistant influenza A virus during therapeutic use of rimantadine. Antimicrob Agents Chemother 1991;35: 1741–1747.

89. Hayden FG, Zlydnikov DM, Iljenko VI, Padolka YV. Comparative therapeutic effect of aerosolized and oral rimantadine HCl in experimental human influenza A virus infection. Antiviral Res 1982;2:147–153.

90. Hoff HR, Sitar DS, Aoki FY. Acetylator phenotype does not predict acetylation of amantadine in man. Manitoba Med 1991;61: 164–168.

91. Horadam VW, Sharp JG, Smilack JD, McAnalley BH, Garriott JC, Stephens MK, Prati RC, Brater DC. Pharmacokinetics of amantadine hydrochloride in subjects with normal and impaired renal function. Ann Intern Med 1981;94:454–458.

92. Hosoya M, Shigeta S, Nakamura K, De Clercq E. Inhibitory effect of selected antiviral compounds on measles (SSPE) virus replication in vitro. Antiviral Res 1989;12:87–98.

93. Houck P, Hemphill M, LaCroix S, Hirsh D, Cox N. Amantadine-resistant influenza A in nursing homes. Identification of a resistant virus prior to drug use. Arch Intern Med 1995;155:533–537.

94. Ickes DE, Venetta TM, Phonphok Y, Rosenthal KS. Tromantadine inhibits a late step in herpes simplex virus type 1 replication and syncytium formation. Antiviral Res 1990;14:75–85.

95. Ing TS, Daugirdas JT, Soung LS, Klawans HL, Mahurkar SD, Hayashi JA, Geis WP, Hano JE. Toxic effects of amantadine in patients with renal failure. Can Med Assoc J 1979;120:695–698.

96. Jackson GG, Muldoon RL, Akers LW. Serological evidence for prevention of influenzal infection in volunteers by an anti-influenzal drug adamantanamine hydrochloride. Antimicrob Agents Chemother 1963;3:703–707.

97. Kato N, Eggers HJ. Inhibition of uncoating of fowl plague virus by l-adamantanamine hydrochloride. Virology 1969;37:632–641.

98. Kitamoto O. Therapeutic effectiveness of amantadine hydrochloride in naturally occurring Hong Kong influenza. Jpn J Tuberc Chest Dis 1971;17:1–17.

99. Klimov AI, Rocha E, Hayden FG, Shult PA, Roumillat LF, Cox NJ. Prolonged shedding of amantadine-resistant influenzae A

viruses by immunodeficient patients: detection by polymerase chain reaction-restriction analysis. J Infect Dis 1995;172: 1352–1355.

100. Knight V, Fedson D, Baldini J, Douglas RG, Couch RB. Amantadine therapy of epidemic influenza A2-Hong Kong. Antimicrob Agents Chemother 1969;9:370–371.

101. Koff WC, Pratt RD, Elm JLJ, Venkateshan CN, Halstead SB. Treatment of intracranial dengue virus infections in mice with a lipophilic derivative of ribavirin. Antimicrob Agents Chemother 1983;24:134–136.

102. Koppel C, Tenczer J. A revision of the metabolic disposition of amantadine. Biomed Mass Spectrom 1985;12:499–501.

103. Kornhuber J, Quack G, Danysz W, Jellinger K, Danielczyk W, Gsell W, Riederer P. Therapeutic brain concentration of the NMDA receptor antagonist amantadine. Neuropharmacology 1995;34:713–721.

104. Krupp LB, Coyle PK, Doscher C, Miller A, Cross AH, Jandorf L, Halper J, Johnson B, Morgante L, Grimson R. Fatigue therapy in multiple sclerosis: results of a double-blind, randomized, parallel trial of amantadine, pemoline, and placebo. Neurology 1995;45:1956–1961.

105. Lammers GJ, Roos RA. Hyponatraemia due to amantadine hydrochloride and L-dopa/carbidopa [Letter]. Lancet 1993;342 (8868):439.

106. Leibowitz JL, Reneker SJ. The effect of amantadine on mouse hepatitis virus replication. Adv Exp Med Biol 1993;342: 117–122.

107. Little JW, Hall WJ, Douglas RGJ, Hyde RW, Speers DM. Amantadine effect on peripheral airways abnormalities in influenza. A study in 15 students with natural influenza A infection. Ann Intern Med 1976;85:177–182.

108. Little JW, Hall WJ, Douglas RGJ, Mudholkar GS, Speers DM, Patel K. Airway hyperreactivity and peripheral airway dysfunction in influenza A infection. Am Rev Respir Dis 1978;118: 295–303.

109. Liu P, Cheng PJ, Ing TS, Daugirdas JT, Jeevanandhan R, Soung LS, Galinis S. In vitro binding of amantadine to plasma proteins. Clin Neuropharmacol 1984;7:149–151.

110. Lubeck MD, Schulman JL, Palese P. Susceptibility of influenza A viruses to amantadine is influenced by the gene coding for M protein. J Virol 1978;28:710–716.

111. Macchio GJ, Ito V, Sahgal V. Amantadine-induced coma. Arch Phys Med Rehabil 1993;74:1119–1120.

112. Madren LK, Shipman CJr, Hayden FG. In vitro inhibitory effects of combinations of anti-influenza agents. Antiviral Chem Chemother 1995;6:109–113.

113. Mardiney MRJ, Bredt AB. The immunosuppressive effect of amantadine upon the response of lymphocytes to specific antigens in vitro. Transplantation 1971;12:183–188.

114. Martin K, Helenius A. Nuclear transport of influenza virus ribonucleoproteins: the viral matrix protein (M1) promotes export and inhibits import. Cell 1991;67:117–130.

115. Mast EE, Harmon MW, Gravenstein S, Wu SP, Arden NH, Circo R, Tyszka G, Kendal AP, Davis JP. Emergence and possible transmission of amantadine-resistant viruses during nursing home outbreaks of influenza A (H3N2). Am J Epidemiol 1991;134:988–997.

116. Maurin M, Benoliel AM, Bongrand P, Raoult D. Phagolysosomal alkalinization and the bactericidal effect of antibiotics: the Coxiella burnetii paradigm. J Infect Dis 1992;166: 1097–1102.

117. McCrory W. Developmental nephrology. In: Quantitative measurement of renal function during growth in infancy and childhood. Cambridge, MA: Harvard University Press; 1972:79.

118. McNamara P, Durso R. Reversible pathologic jealousy (Othello syndrome) associated with amantadine. J Geriatr Psychiatry Neurol 1991;4:157–159.

119. Millet VM, Dreisbach M, Bryson YJ. Double-blind controlled study of central nervous system side effects of amantadine, rimantadine, and chlorpheniramine. Antimicrob Agents Chemother 1982;21:1–4.

120. Montanari C, Ferrari P, Bavazzano A. Urinary excretion of amantadine by the elderly. Eur J Clin Pharmacol 1975;8: 349–351.

121. Monto AS, Gunn RA, Bandyk MG, King CL. Prevention of Russian influenza by amantadine. JAMA 1979;241:1003–1007.

122. Monto AS, Ohmit SE, Hornbuckle K, Pearce CL. Safety and efficacy of long-term use of rimantadine for prophylaxis of type A influenza in nursing homes. Antimicrob Agents Chemother 1995;39:2224–2228.

123. Muldoon RL, Stanley ED, Jackson GG. Use and withdrawal of amantadine chemoprophylaxis during epidemic influenza A. Am Rev Respir Dis 1976;113:487–491.

124. Nafta I, Turcanu AG, Braun I, Companetz W, Simionescu A, Birt E, Florea V. Administration of amantadine for the prevention of Hong Kong influenza. Bull WHO 1970;42:423–427.

125. Nahata MC, Brady MT. Serum concentrations and safety of rimantadine in paediatric patients. Eur J Clin Pharmacol 1986; 30:719–722.

126. Nestelbaum Z, Siris SG, Rifkin A, Klar H, Reardon GT. Exacerbation of schizophrenia associated with amantadine. Am J Psychiatry 1986;143:1170–1171.

127. Neumayer EM, Haff RF, hoff, Hoffmann CE. Antiviral activity of amantadine hydrochloride in tissue culture and in ovo. (30191). Virology 1965;119:393–396.

128. O'Donoghue JM, Ray CG, Terry DWJ, Beaty HN. Prevention of nosocomial influenza infection with amantadine. Am J Epidemiol 1973;97:276–282.

129. Oker-Blom N, Hovi T, Leinikki P, Palosuo T, Pettersson R, Suni J. Protection of man from natural infection with influenza A2 Hong Kong virus by amantadine: a controlled field trial. Br Med J 1970;3(724):676–678.

130. Pacifici GM, Nardini M, Ferrari P, Latini R, Fieschi C, Morselli PL. Effect of amantadine on drug-induced parkisonism: relationship between plasma levels and effect. Br J Clin Pharmacol 1976;3:883–889.

131. Pandit PB, Chitayat D, Jefferies AL, Landes A, Qamar IU, Koren G. Tibial hemimelia and tetralogy of Fallot associated with first trimester exposure to amantadine [see comments]. Reprod Toxicol 1994;8:89–92.

132. Parkes D. Amantadine. In: Harper NJ, Simmonds AB, eds. Advances in drug research. London: Academic Press, 1974:11–73.

133. Parkes JD, Zilkha KJ, Marsden P, Baxter RC, Knill-Jones RP. Amantadine dosage in treatment of Parkinson's disease. Lancet 1970;1(657):1130–1133.

134. Patriarca PA, Kater NA, Kendal AP, Bregman DJ, Smith JD, Sikes RK. Safety of prolonged administration of rimantadine hydrochloride in the prophylaxis of influenza A virus infections in nursing homes. Antimicrob Agents Chemother 1984;26: 101–103.

135. Payler DK, Purdham PA. Influenza A prophylaxis with amantadine in a boarding school. Lancet 1984;1(8375):502–504.

136. Pearlman JT, Kadish AH, Ramseyer JC. Vision loss associated with amantadine hydrochloride use [Letter]. JAMA 1977;237: 1200.

137. Peckinpaugh RO, Askin FB, Peirce WE, Edwards EA, Johnson DP, Jackson GG. Field studies with amantadine: acceptability and protection. Ann NY Acad Sci 1970;173:62–73.

138. Peters NL, Oboler S, Hair C, Laxson L, Kost J, Meiklejohn G. Treatment of an influenza A outbreak in a teaching nursing home. Effectiveness of a protocol for prevention and control. J Am Geriatr Soc 1989;37:210–218.

139. Petersen CS, Weismann K, Avnstorp C, Rasmussen LP, Fogh H, Tikjob G. Topical tromantadine in the treatment of genital herpes. A double-blind placebo controlled study. Dan Med Bull 1993;40:506–507.

140. Pettersson RF, Hellstrom PE, Penttinen K, Pyhala R, Tokola O, Vartio T, Visakorpi R. Evaluation of amantadine in the prophylaxis of influenza A (H1N1) virus infection: a controlled field trial among young adults and high-risk patients. J Infect Dis 1980;142:377–383.

141. Pfeiffer RF. Amantadine-induced "vocal" myoclonus [Letter]. Movement Disord 1996;11:104–106.

142. Pimentel L, Hughes B. Amantadine toxicity presenting with complex ventricular ectopy and hallucinations. Pediatr Emerg Care 1991;7:89–92.

143. Postma JU, Tilburg WV. Visual hallucinations and delirium during treatment with amantadine (Symmetrel). J Am Geriatr Soc 1975;23:212.

144. Quarles JM, Couch RB, Cate TR, Goswick CB. Comparison of amantadine and rimantadine for prevention of type A (Russian) influenza. Antiviral Res 1981;1:149–155.

145. Quilligan JJ, Hirayama M, Baernstein HDJ. The suppression of A2 influenza in children by the chemoprophylactic use of amantadine. J Pediatr 1966;69:572–575.

146. Rabinovich S, Baldini JT, Bannister R. The therapeutic efficacy of rimantadine HCl in a naturally occurring influenza A2 outbreak. Am J Med Sci 1969;257:328–335.

147. Rawls WE, Melnick JL, Olson GB, Dent PB, Good RA. Effect of amantadine hydrochloride on the response of human lymphocytes to phytohemagglutinin. Science 1967;158(800):506–507.

148. Rego MD, Giller EJ. Mania secondary to amantadine treatment of neuroleptic-induced hyperprolactinemia. J Clin Psychiatry 1989;50:143–144.

149. Reuman PD, Bernstein DI, Keefer MC, Young EC, Sherwood JR, Schiff GM. Efficacy and safety of low dosage amantadine hydrochloride as prophylaxis for influenza A. Antiviral Res 1989;11:27–40.

150. Reuman PD, Bernstein DI, Keely SP, Young EC, Sherwood JR, Schiff GM. Differential effect of amantadine hydrochloride on the systemic and local immune response to influenza A. J Med Virol 1989;27:137–141.

151. Richman DD, Yazaki P, Hostetler KY. The intracellular distribution and antiviral activity of amantadine. Virology 1981;112:81–90.

152. Rosa F. Amantadine pregnancy experience [Letter; comment]. Reprod Toxicol 1994;8:531.

153. Rubio FR, Fukuda EK, Garland WA. Urinary metabolites of rimantadine in humans. Drug Metab Dispos 1988;16:773–777.

154. Ruigrok RW, Hirst EM, Hay AJ. The specific inhibition of influenza A virus maturation by amantadine: an electron microscopic examination. J Gen Virol 1991;72(Pt 1):191–194.

155. Salma K, Degelau J, Cooper SL, Guay DR, Ehresman D, Zaske D. Comparison of pharmacokinetic and safety profiles of amantadine 50- and 100-mg daily doses in elderly nursing home residents. Pharmacotherapy 1991;11:460–466.

156. Sartori M, Pratt CM, Young JB. Torsade de pointe. Malignant cardiac arrhythmia induced by amantadine poisoning. Am J Med 1984;77:388–391.

157. Schild GC, Sutton RNP. Inhibition of influenza viruses in vitro and in vivo by 1-adamantanamine hydrochloride. Br J Exp Pathol 1965;46:263–273.

158. Scholtissek C, Faulkner GP. Amantadine-resistant and -sensitive influenza A strains and recombinants. J Gen Virol 1979;44:807–815.

159. Schulman JL. Effect of 1-amantadine hydrochloride (amantadine HCl) and methyl-1-adamatanethylamine hydrochloride (rimantadine HCl) on transmission of influenza virus infection in mice (33222). Proc Soc Exp Biol Med 1968;128(1173).

160. Schwab RS, England ACJ, Poskanzer DC, Young RR. Amantadine in the treatment of Parkinson's disease. JAMA 1969;208:1168–1170.

161. Schwab RS, Poskanzer DC, England ACJ, Young RR. Amantadine in Parkinson's disease. Review of more than two years' experience. JAMA 1972;222:792–795.

162. Sears SD, Clements ML. Protective efficacy of low-dose amantadine in adults challenged with wild-type influenza A virus. Antimicrob Agents Chemother 1987;31:1470–1473.

163. Simons KJ, Watson WT, Martin TJ, Chen XY, Simons FE. Diphenhydramine: pharmacokinetics and pharmacodynamics in elderly adults, young adults, and children. J Clin Pharmacol 1990;30:665–671.

164. Smith GB, Purcell RH, Chanock RM. Effect of amantadine-hydrochloride on parainfluenza type 1 virus infections in adult volunteers. Am Rev Respir Dis 1967;95:689–690.

165. Smith JP. Treatment of chronic hepatitis C with amantadine-hydrochloride [Abstract]. Gastroenterology 1996;110:A1330.

166. Smorodintsev AA, Karpuchin GI, Zlydnikov DM, Malysheva AM, Shvetsova EG, Burov SA, Chramtsova LM, Romanov YA, Taros LY, Ivannikov YG. The prospect of amantadine for prevention of influenza A2 in humans (effectiveness of amantadine during influenza A2/Hong Kong epidemics in January-February, 1969 in Leningrad). Ann NY Acad Sci 1970;173:44–61.

167. Smorodintsev AA, Karpuhin GI, Zlydnikov DM, Malyseva AM, Svecova EG, Burov SA, Hramcova LM, Romanov JA, Taros LJ, Ivannikov JG. The prophylactic effectiveness of amantadine hydrochloride in an epidemic of Hong Kong influenza in Leningrad in 1969. Bull WHO 1970;42:865–872.

168. Snoey ER, Bessen HA. Acute psychosis after amantadine overdose. Ann Emerg Med 1990;19:668–670.

169. Soo W. Adverse effects of rimantadine: summary from clinical trials. J Respir Dis 1989;10(Suppl)(12A):S26–S31

170. Soung LS, Ing TS, Daugirdas JT, Wu MJ, Gandhi VC, Ivanovich PT, Hano JE, Viol GW. Amantadine hydrochloride pharmacokinetics in hemodialysis patients. Ann Intern Med 1980;93:46–49.

171. Spector R. Transport of amantadine and rimantadine through the blood-brain barrier. J Pharmacol Exp Ther 1988;244:516–519.

172. Speeg KV, Leighton JA, Maldonado AL. Toxic delirium in a patient taking amantadine and trimethoprim-sulfamethoxazole. Am J Med Sci 1989;298:410–412.

173. Stange KC, Little DW, Blatnik B. Adverse reactions to amantadine prophylaxis of influenza in a retirement home. J Am Geriatr Soc 1991;39:700–705.

174. Staynor K, Foster G, McArthur M, McGeer A, Petric M, Simor AE. Influenza A outbreak in a nursing home: the value of early diagnosis and the use of amantadine hydrochloride [see comments]. Can J Infect Control 1994;9:109–111.

175. Steinhauer DA, Wharton SA, Skehel JJ, Wiley DC, Hay AJ.

Amantadine selection of a mutant influenza virus containing an acid-stable hemagglutinin glycoprotein: evidence for virus-specific regulation of the pH of glycoprotein transport vesicles. Proc Natl Acad Sci USA 1991;88:11525–11529.

176. Stroe AE, Hall J, Amin F. Psychotic episode related to phenylpropanolamine and amantadine in a healthy female [Letter; comment]. Gen Hosp Psychiatry 1995;17:457–458.

177. Strong DK, Eisenstat DD, Bryson SM, Sitar DS, Arbus GS. Amantadine neurotoxicity in a pediatric patient with renal insufficiency. DICP 1991;25:1175–1177.

178. Sweet C, Hayden FG, Jakeman KJ, Grambas S, Hay AJ. Virulence of rimantadine-resistant human influenza A (H3N2) viruses in ferrets. J Infect Dis 1991;164:969–972.

179. Thompson J, Fleet W, Lawrence E, Pierce E, Morris L, Wright P. A comparison of acetaminophen and rimantadine in the treatment of influenza A infection in children. J Med Virol 1987;21: 249–255.

180. Togo Y, Hornick RB, Felitti VJ, Kaufman ML, Dawkins ATJ, Kilpe VE, Claghorn JL. Evaluation of therapeutic efficacy of amantadine in patients with naturally occurring A2 influenza. JAMA 1970;211:1149–1156.

181. Tominack RL, Wills RJ, Gustavson LE, Hayden FG. Multiple-dose pharmacokinetics of rimantadine in elderly adults. Antimicrob Agents Chemother 1988;32:1813–1819.

182. Tsunoda A, Maassab HF, Cochran KW, Eveland WC. Antiviral activity of alpha-methyl-1-adamantanemethylamine hydrochloride. Antimicrob Agents Chemother 1965;5:553–560.

183. Tu Q, Pinto LH, Luo G, Shaughnessy MA, Mullaney D, Kurtz S, Krystal M, Lamb RA. Characterization of inhibition of M2 ion channel activity by BL-1743, an inhibitor of influenza A virus. J Virol 1996;70:4246–4252.

184. Uchiyama M, Shibuya M. Distribution and excretion of 3H-amantadine HCl. Chem Pharm Bull 1969;17:841–843.

185. Uitti RJ, Rajput AH, Ahlskog JE, Offord KP, Schroeder DR, Ho MM, Prasad M, Rajput A, Basran P. Amantadine treatment is an independent predictor of improved survival in Parkinson's disease. Neurology 1996;46:1551–1556.

186. VanVoris LP, Betts RF, Hayden FG, Christmas WA, Douglas RGJ. Successful treatment of naturally occurring influenza A/USSR/77 H1N1. JAMA 1981;245:1128–1131.

187. Vernier VG, Harmon JB, Stump JM, Lynes TE, Marvel JP, Smith DH. The toxicologic and pharmacologic properties of amantadine hydrochloride. Toxicol Appl Pharmacol 1969;15: 642–665.

188. VonVoigtlander PF, Moore KE. Dopamine: release from the brain in vivo by amantadine. Science 1971;174:408–410.

189. Walker JS, Stephen EL, Spertzel RO. Small-particle aerosols of antiviral compounds in treatment of type A influenza pneumonia in mice. J Infect Dis 1976;133(Suppl):A140–A144.

190. Walters HE, Paulshock M. Therapeutic efficacy of amantadine HCl. Mo Med 1970;67:176–179.

191. Walzer PD, Foy J, Steele P, Kim CK, White M, Klein RS, Otter BA, Allegra C. Activities of antifolate, antiviral, and other drugs in an immunosuppressed rat model of Pneumocystis carinii pneumonia. Antimicrob Agents Chemother 1992;36:1935–1942.

192. Wang C, Takeuchi K, Pinto LH, Lamb RA. Ion channel activity of influenza A virus M2 protein: characterization of the amantadine block. J Virol 1993;67:5585–5594.

193. Webster RG, Kawaoka Y, Bean WJ, Beard CW, Brugh M. Chemotherapy and vaccination: a possible strategy for the control of highly virulent influenza virus. J Virol 1985;55:173–176.

194. Welsh RM, Trowbridge RS, Kowalski JB, O'Connell CM, Peau CJ. Amantadine hydrochloride inhibition of early and late stages of lymphocytic choriomenigitis virus-cell interactions. Virology 1971;45:679–686.

195. WHO. Current status of amantadine and rimantadine as anti-influenza-A agents: memorandum from a WHO meeting. Bull WHO 1985;63:51–56.

196. Wills RJ. The clinical pharmacokinetics of rimantadine. J Respir Dis 1987;8(Suppl)(11A):S39–S44

197. Wills RJ. Update on rimantadine's clinical pharmacokinetics. J Respir Dis 1989;10(Suppl)(12A):S20–S25

198. Wills RJ, Belshe R, Tomlinson D, De GF, Lin A, Wells S, Milazzo J, Berry C. Pharmacokinetics of rimantadine hydrochloride in patients with chronic liver disease. Clin Pharmacol Ther 1987;42:449–454.

199. Wills RJ, Choma N, Buonpane G, Lin A, Keigher N. Relative bioavailability of rimantadine HCl tablet and syrup formulations in healthy subjects. J Pharm Sci 1987;76:886–888.

200. Wills RJ, Farolino DA, Choma N, Keigher N. Rimantadine pharmacokinetics after single and multiple doses. Antimicrob Agents Chemother 1987;31:826–828.

201. Wills RJ, Rodriguez LC, Choma N, Oakes M. Influence of a meal on the bioavailability of rimantadine.HCl. J Clin Pharmacol 1987;27:821–823.

202. Wilson SZ, Knight V, Wyde PR, Drake S, Couch RB. Amantadine and ribavirin aerosol treatment of influenza A and B infection in mice. Antimicrob Agents Chemother 1980;17: 642–648.

203. Wilson TW, Rajput AH. Amantadine-dyazide interaction. Can Med Assoc J 1983;129:974–975.

204. Wingfield WL, Pollack D, Grunert RR. Therapeutic efficacy of amantadine HCl and rimantadine HCl in naturally occurring influenza A2 respiratory illness in man. N Engl J Med 1969;281: 579–584.

205. Wintermeyer SM, Nahata MC. Rimantadine: a clinical perspective [Review; 87 refs]. Ann Pharmacother 1995;29: 299–310.

206. Wong LT, Sitar DS, Aoki FY. Chronic tobacco smoking and gender as variables affecting amantadine disposition in healthy subjects. Br J Clin Pharmacol 1995;39:81–84.

207. Wong LT, Smyth DD, Sitar DS. Interference with renal organic cation transport by (−)− and (+)− nicotine at concentrations documented in plasma of habitual tobacco smokers. J Pharmacol Exp Ther 1992;261:21–25.

208. Wood TR. Methods useful in evaluating 1-adamantanamine hydrochloride—a new orally active synthetic antiviral agent. Ann NY Acad Sci 1965;130:419–431.

209. Wright PF, Khaw KT, Oxman MN, Shwachman H. Evaluation of the safety of amantadine-HC1 and the role of respiratory viral infections in children with cystic fibrosis. J Infect Dis 1976;134:144–149.

210. Wu MJ, Ing TS, Soung LS, Daugirdas JT, Hano JE, Gandhi VC. Amantadine hydrochloride pharmacokinetics in patients with impaired renal function. Clin Nephrol 1982;17:19–23.

211. Younkin SW, Betts RF, Roth FK, Douglas RGJ. Reduction in fever and symptoms in young adults with influenza A/Brazil/78 H1N1 infection after treatment with aspirin or amantadine. Antimicrob Agents Chemother 1983;23:577–582.

212. Zlydnikov DM, Kubar OI, Kovaleva TP, Kamforin LE. Study of rimantadine in the USSR: a review of the literature [Review; 91 refs]. Rev Infect Dis 1981;3:408–421.

Antiretroviral Agents: Lamivudine

John E. Fuchs and Richard B. Pollard

CHEMICAL STRUCTURE AND STRUCTURAL ACTIVITY RELATIONSHIPS

Lamivudine is the (−)-enantiomer of 2′-deoxy 3′-thiacytidine and has potent activity against human immunodeficiency virus (HIV)-1, HIV-2 and hepatitis B virus (HBV) (Fig. 1). Although somewhat unusual among nucleoside analogues, the (+)-enantiomer is also active against HIV-1, but it is 20 to 100 times more toxic to human lymphocyte cells and is therefore not used clinically (10).

MECHANISM OF ACTION
HIV-1 and HIV-II

The mechanism by which lamivudine inhibits the replication of HIV is similar to that of other nucleoside analogues. Lamivudine, a cytosine dideoxynucleoside analogue, crosses cell membranes by a nonfacilitated passive diffusion process to inhibit the HIV reverse transcriptase enzyme. Lamivudine must be converted intracellularly to the triphosphate before it is active against HIV. Lamivudine triphosphate competes with cytosine triphosphate for incorporation into the developing viral DNA strand. This step results in chain termination of viral DNA replication (50).

The triphosphate metabolite represents about 40% of the total intracellular metabolic pool and has an intracellular half-life between 10.5 and 13 h in HIV-1 infected cells (13).

Hepatitis B Virus (HBV)

Lamivudine inhibits HBV replication by interfering with DNA synthesis. HBV is a DNA virus that replicates via an RNA template and reverse transcription (15). HBV DNA polymerase is lamivudine's target for interrupting HBV growth (41).

ANTIVIRAL ACTIVITY
HIV-I and HIV-II

Lamivudine is a potent inhibitor of both HIV-I and HIV-2. This has been shown in vitro against a wide variety of HIV strains and in a number of different human cell lines and peripheral blood mononuclear cells (PBMCs) (11). Unlike zidovudine and stavudine, it is more active against quiescent human cell cultures than in replicating cells. The MIC_{50} of HIV-1 has been reported to be 0.67 μM in MT4 cells and 0.0025 μM in PBMCs. In vitro data in PBMCs using both zidovudine-sensitive and -resistant viruses indicate that lamivudine is either additive or synergistic in combination with zidovudine, stavudine, saquinavir, and neviripine (36). Lamivudine has additive anti-HIV-1 activity in vitro when combined with either zalcitabine or didanosine (8). Additionally, 10 combinations of antiretroviral drugs were tested for their ability to prevent

HIV-induced cytopathic changes in human T-lymphoblastoid cells. The combinations included various triple drug regimens that contained protease inhibitors and nonnucleoside reverse transcriptase inhibitors. The most consistent and potent combination was lamivudine combined with zidovudine and didanosine, with which the MIC_{50} of zidovudine was reported to be reduced between 25- and 200-fold (43).

Hepatitis B Virus

The in vitro MIC_{50} for HBV has been reported to range up to 0.1 μmol (9), and HBV replication ceases completely at 0.5 μmol (15). Although lamivudine causes substantial reductions in HBV-transfected 2.215 cell lines, it cannot eliminate intracellular DNA completely. Withdrawal of lamivudine has been reported to result in the reappearance of active HBV replication in both laboratory (2) and clinical isolates (6).

VIRAL RESISTANCE
HIV-1 and HIV-II

Several studies have demonstrated that laboratory strains and clinical isolates of HIV rapidly develop resistance to lamivudine in vitro (38). The mutation most often reported occurs at the M184V codon of the reverse transcriptase enzyme. Although lamivudine resistance due to mutation at the M184V codon has been demonstrated in clinical isolates, persistent clinical effect has been reported with both lamivudine monotherapy (7) and the combination with zidovudine (39). Persistence of clinical effect is greater with zidovudine and lamivudine in combination, which may be due to continued inhibition of a subpopulation of wild-type HIV that remains sensitive to lamivudine. Suggested reasons for the continued effect include an enhanced fidelity of reverse transcriptase that produces a variant that is eradicated by the immune system (51) and reversal of phenotypic resistance to other nucleoside analogues (31, 32).

The mutation at M184V was suggested to be responsible for a loss of response in 20 patients with mildly symptomatic HIV treated with lamivudine monotherapy (42). In this group of patients, a dramatic reduction in plasma HIV RNA (70%) from baseline occurred by the third day, but a subsequent loss of response occurred between 4 and 6 weeks. This loss of response coincided with the appearance of the mutation at M184V and an increase in the MIC_{50} to more than 100 μmol in all patients after 20 weeks. Although plasma RNA levels remained below baseline at 20 weeks, a 20% increase in viral load was reported.

A virologic substudy in 54 patients of protocol NUCA 3001 evaluated resistance to lamividine monotherapy versus lamivu-

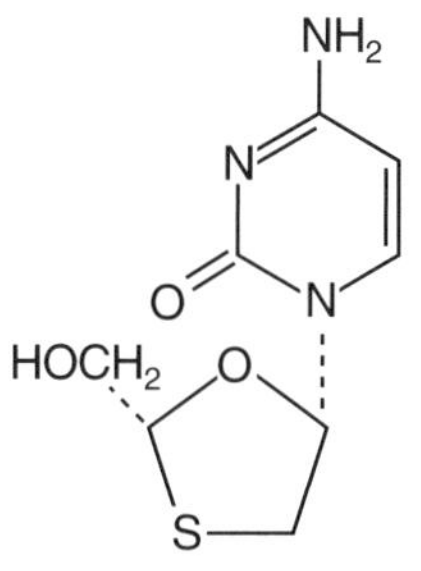

FIGURE 1. Lamivudine structure.

dine in combination with zidovudine (31). In the monotherapy arm at 12 weeks, 70% of the isolates contained a genotypic mutation at the 184 codon, and phenotypic resistance was detected in 87% of patients. The median MIC_{50} for lamivudine at study entry was 0.044 μmol and at week 12 had increased to 44.46 μmol in the lamivudine monotherapy arm. Lamivudine resistance was defined as an MIC_{50} of 1.0 μmol or above. By contrast, median MIC_{50}s at 12 weeks for the lamivudine and zidovudine combination were 4.25 and 14.62 μmol for the high-dose (600 mg/day) and low-dose (300 mg/day) lamivudine treatment arms, respectively. Additionally, it was reported that an early developing resistance mutation to zidovudine, K70R, was reduced from 44 to 9% in the presence of the M184V mutation to lamuvidine, thus enhancing the sensitivity of the isolate to zidovudine. This trial suggested that despite the occurrence of rapid resistance to lamivudine, the combination of lamivudine and zidovudine resulted in a greater reduction in plasma RNA level than zidovudine monotherapy and that prevention of zidovudine resistance contributes to the sustained activity of the combination.

Cross-resistance with lamivudine, didanosine, and zalcitabine is linked with the mutation at codon M184V. Although each of these drugs have been reported to induce a mutation at this site, onset is delayed (months to years) with zalcitabine and didanosine compared with lamivudine (weeks to months). Mutations at this site have been reported to produce high-level resistance to lamivudine (1000-fold reduced sensitivity) and moderate resistance (4- to 8-fold reduced sensitivity) to either didanosine or zalcitabine (19, 35). The clinical relevance of cross-resistance among these drugs is unknown. Whether there is an ideal approach to their sequencing or use in combination therapy to overcome potential cross-resistance awaits the conclusion of ongoing clinical trials.

HBV Infections

Clinical isolates from 5 patients with chronic HBV were reported to have mutations in the YMDD locus of the polymerase gene (3, 34). In each case, an initial response to lamivudine therapy was measured by a significant reduction in HBV DNA but was followed by an increase in HBV DNA titers in 9 or 10 months despite continued therapy. Similar mutations were found in the polymerase gene in all patients. MIC_{50} data was reported for one patient (3). In this patient, the

pretreatment MIC_{50} for lamivudine was about 0.01 μmol and increased to 0.45 μmol after the virus reappeared. The mutation reported in HBV is similar to the YMDD locus associated with resistance to HIV-1 (46, 47).

The combination of lamivudine and penciclovir has been investigated for treatment modalities for HBV. In vitro systems using duck hepatocyte cultures have clearly shown the combination to have a synergistic effect against the virus without increasing cellular toxicity (12). The mechanism for this superior effect is unclear; however it appears that the two drugs have different resistant sites on the HBV DNA polymerase. Clinical trials are currently under way to evaluate this promising combination.

EFFECTS ON HUMAN CELLS

In vitro cytotoxicity of lamivudine has been reported to be low in both monocyte and macrophage cell lines (13, 24). Additionally, no effect on mitochondrial DNA was reported when high concentrations (100 times MIC) of lamivudine was introduced to cell cultures containing HBV (15).

It has been suggested that the minimal effect on mitochondrial DNA is due to the unimpaired function of the 3',5'-exonuclease enzyme that prevents phosphorylated metabolite accumulation in nuclear material (22). In vitro data suggest that lamivudine minimally inhibits mammalian DNA polymerase, and clinical trials have demonstrated that the drug has a low incidence of hematologic abnormalities and peripheral neuropathy (24).

PHARMACOKINETICS
Absorption

Lamivudine tablets, capsules, and oral solution dosage forms were compared. In addition to being rapidly and well absorbed in adults, each of the dosage forms were found to be bioequivalent with a 90% confidence interval (52). The mean T_{max}, C_{max}, and bioavailability from a 100-mg oral dose from tablets, capsules or oral solution have been reported to be 0.9 h, 1.03 μ/mL, and 87% (range, 53–105%), respectively (1, 52).

Distribution

The volume of distribution of lamivudine is approximately 1.3 L/kg (48, 52). Lamivudine cerebrospinal fluid (CSF) concentration was examined in 6 patients (49). Spinal fluid in these patients was collected approximately 2 h after the dose. The CSF concentration of lamivudine ranged between 0.41 and 1.43 μmol (0.094–0.328 μg/mL), resulting in a CSF:serum ratio of 0.06. These data indicate a lower mean CSF:serum ratio than for zidovudine, didanosine, zalcitabine, and stavudine, which have been reported as 0.4, 0.2, 0.2, and 0.2, respectively (16). However, more recent data indicate that the lamivudine CSF:serum ratio may be somewhat higher at 0.12 (18). In this report, the impact on CSF viral load of two antiretroviral combinations (AZT/3TC vs. D4T/3TC) were compared in 10 patients. The results of this trial indicated that each combination was equivalent in which the plasma and CSF viral loads for both regimens was reduced by approximately 1.3 $\log_{10}$ copies/mL. In summary, these data suggest that lamivudine used in combination with zidovudine or stavudine might be expected to have activity in HIV-related central nervous system disease.

Protein binding of lamivudine is less than 36% (21). There is no data describing the extent of lamivudine distribution in breast milk, however preliminary data indicates that concentrations are similar when measured in maternal circulation, umbilical chord blood, and neonatal circulation (29).

Metabolism

Approximately 5.2% of lamivudine is recovered in the urine as a *trans*-sulfoxide metabolite in humans. The significance of the low yield of this metabolite is unknown (21).

Clearance

The total body clearance of lamivudine has been reported to be approximately 400 mL/min in patients with normal renal function. Also in patients with normal renal function, the average half life is about 8.5 h (25, 39, 52). Some 70% of lamivudine is excreted unchanged in the urine, and it has a renal clearance of approximately 340 mL/min, indicating active tubular secretion (48, 52). The half-life is markedly prolonged in patients with varying degrees of renal dysfunction. In patients with creatinine clearance between 10 and 40 mL/min, the half life is prolonged to approximately 14.1 h. When the creatinine clearance is below 10 mL/min, the half-life is prolonged to approximately 20.7 h (25). Dosage adjustments are therefore necessary in patient with renal insufficiency (see "Dosage in Renal Failure," below).

Pediatric Pharmacokinetics

Pharmacokinetics were studied in 53 pediatric patients whose ages ranged from 3 months to 17 years (33). Absorption was rapid and fairly complete. The average time to peak level was 1.5 h, and bioavailability was 67%. The average half-life was reported to be 1.85 h, significantly less than the 8.5 h reported in adults. The total body clearance was reported to be 238 mL/min. Lamivudine concentration was determined in CSF from 44 of these patients. The amount of lamivudine in CSF varied in direct proportion to the dose. Doses of 4, 8, 12, and 20 mg/kg resulted in CSF concentrations of 0.23, 0.31, 0.59, and 0.99 μmol, respectively, corresponding to CSF:serum ratios ranging from 0.1 to 0.17.

DOSING REGIMENS
Adults

Lamivudine is not recommended for use as monotherapy. The usual adult dose of lamivudine for the treatment of HIV-I is 150 mg orally every 12 h. The usual adult dose of lamivudine for the treatment of HBV is 100 mg orally once daily. See dosing schedules in Table 1.

Pediatrics

The usual dose of lamivudine in children aged 3 months to 12 years is 4 mg/kg twice daily up to a maximum of 150 mg twice daily. See dosing schedules in Table 1.

Postexposure Prophylaxis

It is recommended that lamivudine be combined with zidovudine as postexposure prophylaxis for individuals at moderate risk of HIV infection following HIV exposure (20). For individuals considered to be at high risk of HIV transmission or if highly resistant HIV is suspected, lamivudine and zidovudine should be combined with a protease inhibitor and preferably should be instituted within 1 to 2 h after exposure. These drugs should be prescribed in the usual doses and continued for 4 weeks.

Dosage in Renal Failure

Since lamivudine is primarily eliminated unchanged by the kidney, dosing alterations are necessary for patients with reduced renal function. For adult patients with creatinine clearance between 30 and 49 mL/min, the maintenance dose should be reduced to 150 mg once daily. Accordingly, for creatinine clearances between 15 and 29 mL/min, 5 and 14 mL/min, and less than 5 mL/min, the maintenance dose should be reduced to 100, 50, and 25 mg once daily in adults. Although dosing guidelines for patients on hemodialysis are not available, clinical practice suggests that lamivudine should be administered as 50 mg orally once daily after dialysis (see Table 1).

TABLE 1 • Dosing Regimens

	Creatinine Clearance (mL/min)	Maintenance Dose >50 kg	Maintenance Dose <50 kg
Adults			
HBV	>50	100 mg once daily	100 mg once daily
	15–49	50 mg once daily	50 mg once daily
HIV-1	>50	150 mg twice daily	100 mg twice daily
	30–49	150 mg once daily	100 mg once daily
	15–29	100 mg once daily	75 mg once daily
	5–14	50 mg once daily	25 mg once daily
	<5	25 mg once daily	25 mg once daily
Hemodialysis (suggested)		50 mg once daily (after dialysis)	25 mg once daily (after dialysis)
Children (3 months–12 years)	>50	4 mg/kg twice daily	

Dosage in Hepatic Insufficiency

Specific guidelines for dosage alterations for lamivudine are not available.

Pregnancy Effects

The FDA has placed lamivudine in pregnancy category C. No controlled studies have been performed with lamivudine in pregnant women (21).

Nursing Mothers

It is not known if lamivudine is excreted in human breast milk. Therefore, mothers should not breastfeed while receiving lamivudine (21).

ADVERSE REACTIONS
Adults

Phase I, phase II, and phase III clinical trials reported that lamivudine is well tolerated (5, 17, 39, 44). The most common side effects reported are nausea, diarrhea, and headache. There appears to be a relationship between the dose and frequency at which gastrointestinal toxicities occur. Gastrointestinal side effects were reported to occur in 15% of patients who receive 300 mg twice daily, compared with 5% with a dose of 150 mg twice daily (5). Peripheral neuropathy, myalgias, and pancreatitis occur infrequently. Although the number of hematologic reactions reported with lamivudine is low, there is a trend toward a higher frequency of severe neutropenia with doses above 150 mg twice daily and when lamivudine is combined with zidovudine (5, 30, 39, 44).

Pediatrics

Lamivudine was reported to be well tolerated in one series of pediatric patients when doses were kept below 8 mg/kg/day (33). Of concern however, was the occurrence of pancreatitis in seven patients (8%). Most of these patients however, did have other risk factors for pancreatitis, including advanced HIV and a lamivudine dose equal to or exceeding 8 mg/kg/day. Additional information is needed to determine the relationship of lamivudine to pancreatitis in the pediatric population.

DRUG INTERACTIONS
Lamivudine-Zidovudine

It has been reported that concurrent administration of lamivudine and zidovudine does not affect the pharmacokinetics of either agent (27). Dosage adjustments are therefore not required with either drug when combined.

Lamivudine-Zalcitabine

In vitro data indicate that lamivudine reduces the intracellular phosphorylation of zalcitabine by 38%; however, lamivudine phosphorylation is unaffected by zalcitabine (51). This interaction is thought to be due to competition for the enzyme deoxycytidine kinase, which is responsible for the initial phosphorylation step of both drugs.

One clinical trial examined the combination of lamivudine and zalcitabine. In this study, 45 patients with at least 6 months of treatment with zidovudine and zalcitabine were randomized to receive one of three open-label regimens: arm I, continued zidovudine-zalcitabine; arm II, zidovudine-lamivudine; or arm III, zidovudine-zalcitabine-lamivudine. Although arm III showed the greatest reduction in viral load at 6 months (-0.45 $\log_{10}$ copies/mL), additional studies would better characterize the beneficial effects of a regimen containing lamivudine and zalcitabine (40).

Lamivudine-Trimethoprim

Trimethoprim (TMP) was reported to reduce the renal clearance of lamivudine by 40 to 50% in laboratory animals (45). This potential pharmacokinetic interaction was also evaluated in 14 human volunteers (37). In a crossover design, the area under the curve (AUC) of lamivudine was found to be increased by 43% and the renal clearance was reduced by 35%. No changes in the kinetic parameters of sulfamethoxazole (SXT)-TMP were observed. These investigators and others (28), suggested that the interaction between lamivudine and TMP or SXT-TMP does not require dosage adjustment of lamivudine.

Drug-Food Interactions

Food was reported to reduce the maximum peak concentration and delay the time to peak serum concentrations of lamivudine but not to alter the AUC (1, 52). Lamivudine can be given without regard to meals.

CLINICAL TRIALS
Adult HIV-I (Monotherapy Trials)

Phase I/II clinical trials have examined the efficacy and safety of lamivudine monotherapy in patients with HIV-1 disease (39, 42, 48, 49). Dose escalations in these trials ranged from 0.5 to 20 mg/kg/day to determine the minimally effective and maximally tolerated doses. Overall, these clinical trials have yielded similar results: significant reductions in plasma RNA levels and increases in CD4 cells occurred during the first few weeks of treatment. However, most of the beneficial results were reversed by week 24, indicating that lamivudine monotherapy had potent, but short-lived, anti-HIV-1 activity. Additionally, these trials indicated that in adults, 8 mg/kg/day was the most efficacious and 20 mg/kg/day was associated with a higher side effect profile.

Combination Trials

Several phase III trials compared the efficacy of zidovudine as monotherapy with combinations of lamivudine with zidovudine or zalcitabine (5, 17, 30, 44). Three trials evaluated lamivudine in both a low-dose (150 mg twice daily) and high-dose (300 mg twice) combination with zidovudine versus zidovudine monotherapy. One trial compared the combination of lamivudine and zidovudine with the combination of zidovudine and zalcitabine. Overall, the results of these trials indicated that the combination of lamivudine and zidovudine is superior to either zidovudine monotherapy or zidovudine combined with zalcitabine. These studies also shoed that a significant response could occur in patients heavily pretreated with zidovudine. Specifically, CD4 cells increased between 30 and 55 cells/mm³ and plasma HIV RNA decreased between 0.5 and 0.9 logs. These changes in surrogate markers were reported to persist for 48 weeks with the lamivudine and zidovudine combination. No significant differences were detected between the high- and low-dose arms of lamivudine.

Ongoing clinical trials reported on the use of lamivudine in combination with protease inhibitors (4, 23, 26). Preliminary results in the form of abstracts indicate that lamivudine combined with zidovudine and a protease inhibitor elicits a potent and durable anti-HIV response. In these reports, plasma HIV RNA levels have been reduced up to 2 $\log_{10}$ copies/mL, and the average increase in CD4 cells is 100. Additionally, a high percentage of patients receiving these combinations have HIV RNA levels that remain below the limits of detection for at least 24 weeks. Current clinical practice suggests that low viral loads can persist much longer than 24 weeks if patients adhere faithfully to medication regimens.

Pediatric HIV-1

Ninety children, aged 3 months to 17 years, were randomized to receive lamivudine at doses ranging from 0.5 to 10 mg/kg/day (33). Patients were stratified into two groups: group 1 included patients with less than 6 weeks of prior zidovudine and group 2 included those with and without clinical AIDS progression despite prior treatment or drug intolerance to zidovudine. At the end of 24 weeks, the CD4 count was 30 less than baseline after an initial increase to 19 above baseline at week 4. The group that did not have AIDS at the beginning of the trial showed the greatest increase (+82) in CD4 cell numbers by the end of the study. Plasma HIV RNA was reduced by 0.68 logs by the end of the study in the non-AIDS arm and 0.4 logs in the AIDS arm. It was concluded that lamivudine as monotherapy did not have an important advantage in pediatric use and that future regimens would likely require lamivudine in combination with other antiretroviral drugs.

Hepatitis B Virus

Lamivudine was used to treat 32 patients with chronic HBV infection (14), some of whom had previously not responded to subcutaneous regimens of interferon. Lamivudine was administered as 25, 100, or 300 mg once daily for 12 weeks. The patients were subsequently followed for an additional 12 weeks. HBV DNA fell to undetectable levels at week 12 in 70% of the patients receiving 25 mg/day and in 100% of those receiving either 100 or 300 mg/day. Six patients (19%) had sustained undetectable levels at 24 weeks. In most patients however, HBV DNA reappeared after therapy with lamivudine was discontinued.

Forty patients coinfected with HIV and HBV were prospectively treated with lamivudine for 12 months. The patients were randomized to receive either 300 mg twice daily for 12 months or 300 mg twice daily for 9.5 months followed by 150 mg twice daily for 2.5 months (6). Patients were retrospectively analyzed in two groups: high virus replication (HBV DNA above 5 pg/mL) and low virus replication (HBV DNA below 5 pg/mL). Some 96% of patients in the high replication group responded, with HBV DNA levels reduced below 5

pg/mL with a hybridization technique, but PCR (a more sensitive test) detected HBV DNA in 11.5% of these patients. In the low replication group, 60% of patients were reported to have undetectable HBV DNA by PCR. Although lamivudine treatment at the lower dose was only used for about 2.5 months in one arm, there was no change in HBV serology.

REFERENCES

1. Angel JB, Hussey EK, Hall ST, et al. Pharmacokinetics of 3TC administered with and without food to HIV-infected patients. Drug Invest 1993;6:70–74.
2. Ashman C, Larkin D, Cammack N. Lamivudine inhibition of HBV production in HBV transfected cell lines 2.2.15 [Abstract]. 6th International Symposia on Viral Hepatitis, Madrid: International Symposium on Viral Hepatitis, 1994:65.
3. Bartholomew MM, Jansen RW, Jeffers LJ, Reddy KR, Johnson LC, Bunzendahl H, Condreay LD, Tzakis AG, Schiff ER, Brown NA. Hepatitis-B-virus resistance to lamivudine given for recurrent infection after orthotopic liver transplantation. Lancet 1997; 349:20–22.
4. Baruch A, Mastrodonato-Delora P, Schnipper CP. Efficacy and safety of triple combination therapy with saquinavir, lamivudine, and zidovudine in HIV infected patients [Abstract]. 11th International Conference on AIDS. Vancouver, 1996.
5. Bartlett JA, Benoit RN, Johnson VA, Quinn JB, Sepulveda GE, Ehmann WC, Tsoukas C, Fallon MA, Self PL, Rubin M. Lamivudine plus zidovudine compared with zalcitabine plus zidovudine in patients with HIV Infections. Ann Intern Med 1996;125: 161–172.
6. Benhamou Y, Katlama C, Lunel F, Coutellier A, Dohin E, Hamm N, Tubiana R, Herson S, Poynard T, Opolon P. Effects of lamivudine on replication of hepatitis B virus in HIN-infected men. Ann Intern Med 1996;125:705–712.
7. Boucher CAB, Cammack N, Schipper P, Schuurman R, Rouse P, Wainberg MA, Cameron JM. High level resistance to (−)-2′ deoxy 3′-thiacytidine in vitro is due to one amino acid substitution in the catalytic site of HIV type 1 reverse transcriptase. Antimicrob Agents Chemother 1993;37:2231–2234.
8. Bridges EG, Dutschman GE, Gullen EA, Cheng YC. Favorable interaction of beta-L-nucleoside analogs with clinically approved anti-HIV nucleoside analogs for the treatment of human immunodeficiency syndrome. Biochem Pharm 1996;51:731–736.
9. Cameron GM, Collis P, David M. Lamivudine. Drugs Forum 1993;18:319–323.
10. Coates JV, Cammack N, Jenkinson HJ, Mutton IM, Pearson BA, Storer R, Cameron JM, Penn CR. The separated enantiomers of 2′deoxy 3′-thiacytidine (BCH 189) both inhibit HIV replication in vitro. Antimicrob Agents Chemother 1992;36:202–205.
11. Coates JV, Cammack N, Jenkinson HJ, Jowett AJ, Jowett MI, Pearson BA, Penn CR, Rouse PI, Viner KC, Cameron JM. (−)-2′Deoxy 3′-thiacytidine is a potent, highly selective inhibitor of HIV type 1 and type 2 replication in vitro. Antimicrob Agents Chemother 1992;36:733–739.
12. Colledge D, Locarnini S, Shaw T. Synergistic inhibition of hepadnaviral replication by lamivudine in combination with penciclovir in-vitro. Hepatology 1997;26:216–225.
13. Commack N, Rouse P, Marr CL, Reid PJ, Boehme RE, Coates JV, Penn CR, Cameron JM. Cellular metabolism of (−)-enantiomeric-2′ deoxy 3′-thiacytidine. Biochem Pharm 1992; 43:2059–2064.
14. Dienstag JL, Perillo RP, Schiffe ER, Bartholomew M, Vicary C,

Rubin M. A preliminary trial of lamivudine for chronic hepatitis B infections. N Engl J Med 1995;333:1657–1661.

15. Doong SL, Tsai CH, Schinazi RF, Liotta DC, Cheng YC. Inhibition of the replication of hepatitis-B virus in vitro by 2'deoxy 3'-thiacytidine and related analogs. Proc Natl Acad Sci 1991;88: 8495–8499.

16. Dudley MN. Clinical pharmacokinetics of nucleoside anti-retroviral agents. J Infect Dis 1995;171(S2):S99–112.

17. Eron JJ, Benoit RN, Jemsek J, MacArthur RD, Santana J, Quinn JB, Kuritzkes DR, Fallon MA, Rubin M. Treatment with lamivudine, zidovudine, or both in HIV-positive patients with 200 to 500 CD4 cells per cubic millimeter. N Engl J Med 1995;333: 1662–1669.

18. Foudraine N, De Wolf F, Hoetelmans R, Portegies P, Maas J, Lange J. CSF and serum HIV-RNA during AZT/3TC and D4T/3TC treatment [Abstract]. 4th Conference on Retrovirus and Opportunistic Infections, Washington, DC, 1997.

19. Gao Q, Guz X, Parniak MA, Cameron J, Cammack N, Boucher C, Wainberg M. The same mutation that encodes low-level human immunodeficiency-1 resistance to didanosine and zalcitabine confers resistance to lamivudine. Antimicrob Agents Chemother 1993;37:1390–1392.

20. Geberding JL. Prophylaxis for occupational exposure to HIV. Ann Intern Med 1996:497–501.

21. Glaxo-Wellcome. Lamivudine prescribing information. Research Triangle Park, NC: Glaxo-Wellcome Inc., 1996.

22. Gray NM, Marr CLP, Penn CR, Cameron JM, Bethell RC. Intracellular phosphorylation of lamivudine. Biochem Pharmacol 1995;50:1043–1051.

23. Gulick R, Mellors J, Havlir D. Potent and sustained antiretroviral activity of indinavir, zidovudine, and lamivudine [Abstract]. 11th International Conference on AIDS. Vancouver, 1996.

24. Hart GJ, Orr DC, Penn CR, Figueiredo HT, Gray NM, Boehme RE, Cameron JM. Effects of (−)-2' deoxy 3'-thiacytidine 5'triphosphate on HIV reverse transcriptase and mammalian DNA polymerases alpha, beta, and gamma. Antimicrob Agents Chemother 1992;36:1688–1694.

25. Heald AE, Hsyu PH, Yuen GJ, Robinson P, Mydlow P, Bartlett JA. Pharmacokinetics of lamivudine in human immunodeficiency virus-infected patients with renal dysfunction. Antimicrob Agents Chemother 1996;40:1514–1519.

26. Hirsch M, Meibohm A, Rawlins S, Leavill R. Indinavir in combination with zidovudine and lamivudine in zidovudine-experienced patients with CD4 cell counts less than 50 [Abstract]. 4th Conference on Retrovirus and Opportunistic Infections, Washington, DC, 1997.

27. Horton CM, Yuen G, Milolic DM. Pharmacokinetics of oral lamivudine administered alone and with oral zidovudine in asymptomatic patients with HIV [Abstract]. 96th Annual Meeting American Society Clinical Pharmacology and Therapeutics, 1994:198.

28. Hudson M, Nash C. Effect of trimethoprim/sulphamethoxazole on lamivudine bioavailability. JAMA 19xx;276:1140.

29. Johnson MA, Goodwin C, Yuen GJ. The pharmacokinetics of lamivudine administration to HIV-1 infected women (prepartum during labor and post-partum) and their offspring [Abstract]. 11th Int. Conference on AIDS. Vancouver, 1996:249.

30. Katlama C, Ingrand D, Loveday C, Clumeck N, Mallolas J, Staszewski S, Johnson M, Hill AM, Pearce G, McDade H. Safety and efficacy of lamivudine-zidovudine combination therapy in antiretroviral-naive patients. A randomized controlled comparison with zidovudine monotherapy. Lamivudine European HIV Working Groups. JAMA 1996;276:118–125.

31. Kuritzkes DR, Quinn JB, Benoit SL, Shugarts DL, Griffin A, Bakhtiari M, Poticha D, Eron JJ, Fallon MA, Rubin M. Drug resistance and virologic response in NUCA 3001, a randomized trial of lamivudine versus zidovudine versus zidovudine plus lamivudine in previously untreated patients. AIDS 1996;10:975–981.

32. Larder BA, Kemp SD, Harrigan PR. Potential mechanisms for sustained antiretroviral efficacy of AZT-3TC combination therapy. Science 1995;269:696–699.

33. Lewis LL, Venzon D, Church J, Farley M, Wheeler S, Keller A, Rubin M, Yuen G, Mueller B, Sloas M, Wood L, Balis F, Shearer GM, Brouwers P, Goldsmith J, Pizzo PA. Lamivudine in children with HIV infections: a phase I/II study. J Infect Dis 1996; 174:16–25.

34. Ling R, Mutimer D, Ahmed M, Boxall, EH, Elias E, Dusheiko GM, Harrison TJ. Selection of mutations in hepatitis B virus polymerase during transplant of recipients treated with lamivudine. Hepatology 1996;24:711–713.

35. Mayes D. Rational approach to resistance: nucleoside analogs. AIDS 1996;10(S-1):S9–13.

36. Merrill DP, Moonis M, Chou TC, Hirsch MS. Lamivudine or stavudine in 2 and 3 drug combinations against HIV-1 replication in vitro. J Infect Dis 1996;173:355–364.

37. Moore KH, Yuen GJ, Raasch RH, Eron J, Martin D, Hussey E. Pharmacokinetics of lamivudine administered alone and with trimethoprim-sulphamethoxazole. Clin Pharm Toxicol 1996;59: 550.

38. Moyle G. Activity and role of lamivudine in the treatment of adults with HIV-1 infections: a review. Expert Opin Invest Drug 1996;5:913–924.

39. Pluda JM, Cooley TP, Montaner JSG, Shay LE, Reinhalter NE, Warthan SN, Ruedy J, Hirst HM, Vicary CA, Quinn JB, Yuen GJ, Wainburg MA, Rubin M, Yarchoan R. A phase I/II study of 2'deoxy 3'-thiacytidine in patients with advanced HIV infections. J Infect Dis 1995;171:1438–1448.

40. Ruiz L, Romen J, Martinez-Picado J, Schmit JC, Vandamme AN, Balague M, Cabrera C, Puig T, Tural C, Segura A, Sirera G, DeClercq E, Clotet B. Efficacy of triple combination therapy with zidovudine plus zalcitabine plus lamivudine versus double (ZDV plus 3TC) combination therapy in patient previously treated with zidovudine and zalcitabine. AIDS 1996;10:F61–66.

41. Schalm SW. Clinical implications of lamivudine resistance by HBV. Lancet 1997;349:20–22.

42. Schurman R, Nijhuis M, van Leeuwon R, Schipper P, de Jong D, Collis P, Danner SA, Mulder J, Loveday C, Christopherson C, Kwok S, Swinsky J, Boucher CA. Rapid change in HIV-1 RNA load and appearance of drug resistant virus population in persons treated with lamivudine. J Infect Dis 1995;171:1411–1419.

43. St Clair MH, Pennington KN, Rooney J, Barry DW. In-vitro comparison of selected triple drug combinations for suppression of HIV-1 replication: the Inter-Company collaboration Protocol. J AIDS Hum Retrovirus 1995;10(S2):S83–91.

44. Staszewski S, Loveday C, Picazo JJ, Dellamonica P, Skinhof P, Johnson KMA, Danner SA, Harrigan PR, Hill AM, Verity L, McDade VH. Safety and efficacy of lamivudine-zidovudine combination therapy in zidovudine-experienced patients: a randomized controlled comparison with zidovudine monotherapy. JAMA 1996;276:111–117.

45. Sweeney KR, Hsyu PH, Statkevich P, Taft DR. Renal disposition of 2'deoxy 3'-thiacytidine in the isolated perfused rat kidney. Pharm Res 1995;12:1958.

46. Tipples GA, Ma MM, Fischer KP, Bain VG, Kneteman NM, Tyrrell DL. Mutation in HBV RNA-dependent, DNA-polymerase confers resistance to lamivudine in vivo. Hepatology 1996;24:714–717.

47. Tisdale M, Kemp SD, Parry N. Rapid in vitro selection of HIV-1 resistance to lamivudine inhibition due to a mutation in YMDD region of reverse transcriptase. Proc Natl Acad Sci USA 1993; 90:5653–5656.

48. van Leeuwen R, Lange JMA, Hussey KH, Donn KH, Hall ST, Harker AJ, Jonker P, Danner SA. The safety and pharmacokinetics of a reverse transcriptase inhibitor, 3TC, in patients with HIV infections: a phase I study. AIDS 1992;6:1471–1475.

49. van Leeuwen RC, Katlama C, Kitchen V, Boucher CAB, Tubiana R, McBride M, Ingrand D, Weber J, Hill A, McDade H, Danner SA. Evaluation of safety and efficacy of lamivudine in

50. Yarchoan JA, Mitsuya H, Myer CE, Broder S. Clinical pharmacology of 3′-azido-2′3′dideoxythymidine and related dideoxynucleosides. N Engl J Med 1989;321:726–738.

51. Veal GJ, Hoggard PG, Barry MG, Khoo, S, Back DJ. Interaction between 3TC and other nucleoside analogs for intracellular phosphorylation. AIDS 1996;10:546–548.

52. Yuen GJ, Morris DM, Mydlow PK, Haidar S, Hall ST, Hussey EK. Pharmacokinetics, absolute bioavailability, and absorption characteristics of lamivudine. J Clin Pharmacol 1995;35: 1174–1180.

53. Wainberg MA, Drosopoulos WC, Salomon H, Hsu M, Borkow G, Parniak M, Gu Z, Song Q, Manne J, Islam S, Castriota G, Prasad VR. Enhanced fidelity of 3TC-reverse transcriptase. Science 1996;271:1282–1285

patients asymptomatic or mildly symptomatic HIV: a phase I/II study. J Infect Dis 1995;171:1166.

Antiretroviral Agents: Nonnucleoside Analogues

●

Susan Swindells and Courtney V. Fletcher

CLASS
Chemical Structure

Discovered in 1990, nonnucleoside reverse transcriptase inhibitors are a structurally diverse group of compounds with potent and selective in vitro activity against the human immunodeficiency virus (HIV)-1 (3–5, 21, 22, 31, 32, 46, 53, 54, 76). A collection of chemically distinct agents, nonnucleoside reverse transcriptase inhibitors include dipyridodiazepinones (e.g., BIRG-587 or nevirapine), pyridinone derivatives (e.g., L-697,661), tetrahydroimidazobenzodiazepinone derivatives, bis(heteroaryl)piperazine compounds (e.g., atervidine (U-87201E) and delavirdine (U-90152)), benzoxamines (e.g., DMP-266), and α-anilinophenylacetamide derivatives (e.g., loviride). The chemical structures of several nonnucleoside reverse transcriptase inhibitors are shown in Figure 1.

Several nonnucleoside reverse transcriptase inhibitors are in clinical development; two are currently FDA approved: nevirapine and delavirdine. L-697–661, the first nonnucleoside reverse transcriptase inhibitor to be examined, will not be developed further because of disappointing early clinical trial results (62, 68). Atervidine, the first-generation bis(heteroaryl)piperazine compound will similarly not be developed further largely because of the increased potency of the second-generation drug delavirdine (22). DMP-266, the lead compound of the benzoxamine derivatives, and loviride are both in clinical trials (45, 69). Loviride is primarily being developed in Europe. This review focuses on nevirapine and delavirdine because a significant amount of data from human studies is available. Both compounds will continue to be developed and

offer utility to the practicing clinician treating HIV-infected individuals.

Structure/Activity Relationship

Despite the diverse molecular compositions of nonnucleoside reverse transcriptase inhibitors, they share a common relationship between chemical structure and antiviral activity. Unlike nucleoside reverse transcriptase inhibitors, which are incorporated into viral DNA, all nonnucleoside reverse transcriptase inhibitors inhibit HIV-1 by binding directly to the reverse transcriptase molecule. Reverse transcriptase directs polymerization of DNA from viral RNA, an essential step in viral replication. Nonnucleoside reverse transcriptase inhibitors appear to inhibit polymerization allosterically by altering the position of critical amino acids within the catalytic site of the reverse transcriptase enzyme. The description of the crystal structure of reverse transcriptase by Kohlstaedt et al. in 1992 helped demonstrate the binding of nonnucleoside reverse transcriptase inhibitors to the enzyme complex (38). The structure of reverse transcriptase is analogous to that of a right hand, with the p66 subdomain folded into several separate regions often referred to as "fingers," "palm," and "thumb." Nonnucleoside reverse transcriptase inhibitors bind into a deep pocket that lies between the "palm" and the base of the "thumb." This suggests a mechanism in which the inhibitors act like sand in the gears of a machine, altering molecular movement essential for viral replication. The chemical reaction catalyzed by reverse transcriptase is significantly slowed in the presence of nonnucleoside reverse transcriptase in-

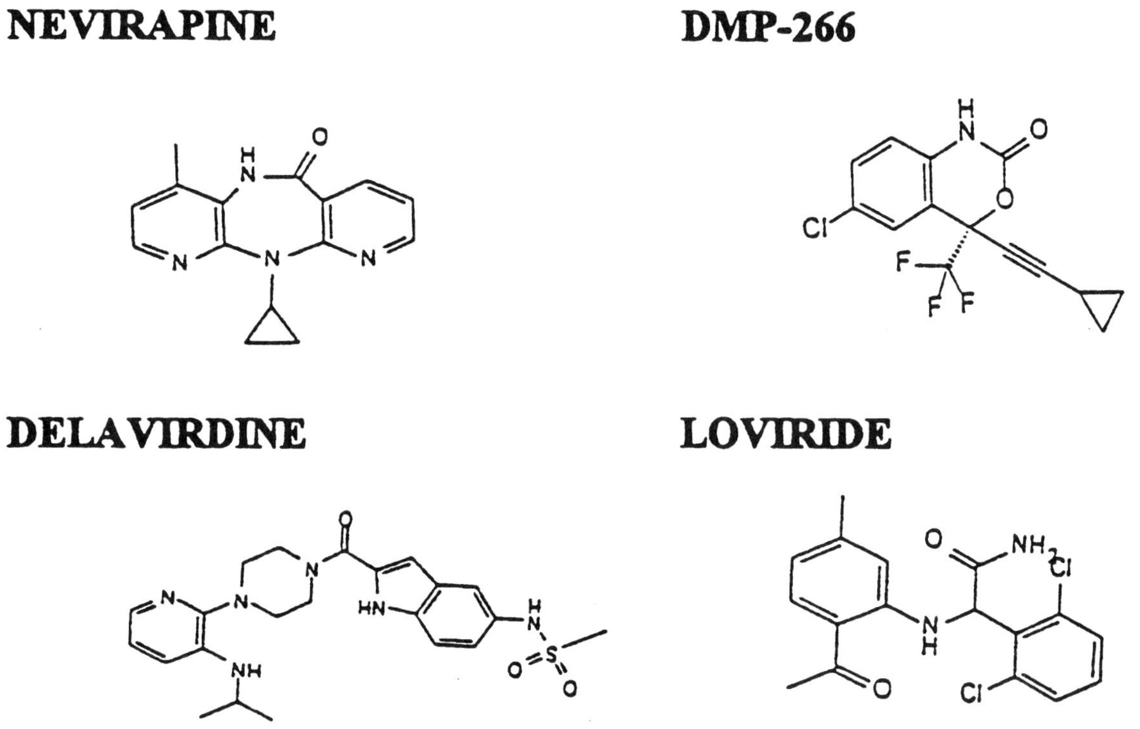

NEVIRAPINE

DMP-266

DELAVIRDINE

LOVIRIDE

FIGURE 1. Structural formulae of nevirapine, delavirdine, DMP-266, and loviride.

hibitors (6, 20, 66). This structure/activity relationship also explains the high degree of specificity of these agents for HIV-1 reverse transcriptase.

ANTIVIRAL ACTIVITY
Spectrum Including in Vitro MICs

The antiviral activity of all nonnucleoside reverse transcriptase inhibitors is highly selective for HIV-1. The compounds do not exhibit activity against other viruses, including HIV-2 or other animal lentiviruses (39). Nonnucleoside reverse transcriptase inhibitors are highly potent antiretroviral drugs in vitro (3–5, 21, 22, 31, 32, 46, 53, 54, 76). Reverse transcriptase inhibition by nanomolar concentrations has been reported, with minimal cytotoxicity in a variety of cell lines. Synergy has been observed in vitro between nonnucleoside reverse transcriptase inhibitors and nucleoside analogues (8, 57). Nonnucleoside reverse transcriptase inhibitors are also active against some nucleoside-resistant strains; for example, nevirapine is active against zidovudine-resistant HIV-1 in vitro (34). Inhibitory activities of L-697–661, nevirapine, delavirdine, and loviride in a variety of cell lines in are shown Table 1. The nucleoside analogues zidovudine and didanosine are also shown for comparison.

Pharmacodynamic Effects

Nevirapine

In vitro, nevirapine is active against HIV-1, including strains that are resistant to zidovudine, and is synergistic with zidovudine, didanosine, stavudine, lamivudine, and saquinavir (61). The in vitro 50% inhibitory concentration (IC_{50}) ranges from

TABLE 1 • **Inhibitory Activities of Nucleoside and Nonnucleoside RT Inhibitors in a Variety of Cell Lines**

Compound	IC_{50} (μM)[a]	Reference
Zidovudine	0.027	41
Didanosine	0.05	22
L-697–661	0.019	31
Nevirapine	0.010–0.040	39
Delavirdine	0.066	22
Loviride	0.013	54

[a] IC_{50} corresponds to the drug concentration required to inhibit HIV-1 replication and cytopathicity by 50% in culture.

0.01 to 0.1 μM. To achieve 95 and 100% inhibition in vitro, nevirapine concentrations of approximately 1 and 10 μM, respectively, are necessary (57). The relationship between in vitro inhibitory values and concentration in the plasma necessary to achieve sustained inhibition of HIV-1 replication is not known. For example, nevirapine was administered in daily doses of 12.5, 50, and 200 mg to 62 HIV-infected persons with CD4 counts below 400 cells/μL. Steady-state trough concentrations at 12.5, 50, and 200 mg/day were 0.9, 4, and 7 μM, respectively, indicating that at the lowest dose, trough concentrations were essentially above the in vitro IC_{50} at all times and were 70 times above at the highest dose. Yet, no patient achieved a sustained virologic response, and all patients in the study had nevirapine-resistant HIV strains within 8 weeks of therapy initiation (12).

Clinical information on relationships between the plasma concentration of nevirapine and anti-HIV effect are sparse and conflicting. Eighteen HIV-infected adults received 400 mg/day of nevirapine and were evaluated for virologic response, defined as at least a 50% reduction in ICD p24 antigen from baseline, sustained for 8 weeks. Ten patients remained in the study for 8 weeks or more and were available for response analysis: eight were classified as responders. The median trough nevirapine concentration was higher in responders than in nonresponders (18 vs. 12 μM, $P = .02$) (35). A phase I evaluation of nevirapine in children found that trough concentrations tended to be higher in responders than in nonresponders (10 vs. 8 μM), but the difference was not statistically significant, and considerable overlap in concentrations existed between the two groups (44). Further work is necessary to establish a relationship between plasma concentration and the anti-HIV effect of nevirapine. Additionally, for nevirapine, delavirdine, and all other antiretroviral drugs, the correlation between in vitro susceptibility values, including which index (IC_{50}, IC_{90}) is the most relevant, and target plasma concentration needs to be elucidated.

Delavirdine Mesylate

Delavirdine belongs to a class of compounds known as bis(heteroaryl)piperazines that have shown in vitro activity against HIV-1 reverse transcriptase. Like other nonnucleoside reverse transcriptase inhibitors including nevirapine, delavirdine has no activity against the reverse transcriptase of HIV-2. The in vitro IC_{50} of delavirdine for HIV-1 averages 0.26 μM (22). Delavirdine is highly selective for HIV-1 reverse transcriptase in that concentrations 2000-fold higher are required to inhibit normal cellular polymerases pol-α and pol-β in vitro. As with nevirapine, the relationship between concentrations required to inhibit HIV-1 replication in vitro and that necessary in the plasma to achieve sustained inhibition is not known. The typical adult dose of 400 mg thrice daily produces average trough concentrations of approximately 16 μM, although there is considerable interpatient variability (28). While this trough considerably exceeds the average IC_{50}, when adjusted for the high degree of binding to plasma proteins (average 98%), the free concentration of delavirdine would only be approximately 0.32 μM. Available data do support some clinical anti-HIV activity of delavirdine mesylate at the dose of 1200 mg daily. However, the effect appears quite weak and perhaps not equivalent, when combined with zidovudine, to a nucleoside combination of zidovudine plus didanosine (17). One potential explanation for this weak antiretroviral effect may be the low ratio of free-drug plasma concentration to in vitro inhibitory concentration.

MECHANISM OF ACTION

Treatment for HIV infection has thus far focused on suppression of viral replication by inhibition of essential viral enzymes. HIV-1 reverse transcriptase remains an attractive target for antiretroviral therapy because there is no related cellular homologue for reverse transcriptase, and the enzyme is essential for viral replication. Reverse transcriptase controls multiple activities and is required prior to provirus production early in the viral life cycle. Clinical benefit has been demonstrated using the five licensed nucleoside analogues, zidovu-dine, didanosine, zalcitabine, stavudine, and lamivudine (9). All have exhibited the ability to suppress HIV-1 replication to varying degrees in vitro and in human studies.

As mentioned above, the mechanism of action of nonnucleoside reverse transcriptase inhibitors differs from that of the nucleoside analogues, which constrain HIV replication by incorporation into the elongating strand of viral DNA, causing chain termination. Nonnucleoside reverse transcriptase inhibitors inhibit HIV-1 replication directly in a unique fashion by binding noncompetitively to HIV-1 reverse transcriptase (29, 60, 67, 74). The drugs bind to a hydrophobic pocket in the enzyme-DNA complex, close to the active-site catalytic residues (67). The mechanism of action of nonnucleoside reverse transcriptase inhibitors does not interfere with nucleotide binding. Unlike nucleoside analogues, nonnucleoside reverse transcriptase inhibitors do not inhibit human DNA polymerases. With their unique specificity for HIV-1, these agents are not active against other viruses, including HIV-2.

MECHANISM OF RESISTANCE

HIV-1 develops in vitro and in vivo resistance to nonnucleoside reverse transcriptase inhibitors readily. For example, resistance to nevirapine has been observed after only a few passages of infected cells in the presence of the drug, both in tissue culture and also in clinical trials (58, 59). Viral isolates resistant to nonnucleoside reverse transcriptase inhibitors have shown some cross-resistance with other nonnucleoside analogues but not with nucleoside reverse transcriptase inhibitors (18). Emergence of resistant mutants has been observed with most nonnucleoside reverse transcriptase inhibitors studied to date when the drugs are used in monotherapy, which limits their utility as single antiretroviral agents.

As with all antiretroviral agents, resistance of HIV-1 to nonnucleoside reverse transcriptase inhibitors develops by genetic mutation in the viral genome. Suppression of wild-type virus permits the outgrowth of minority populations of drug-resistant variants. Most mutations of the reverse transcriptase gene that confer reduced susceptibility to nonnucleoside reverse transcriptase inhibitors are located in the nonnucleoside binding pocket of the enzyme where the inhibitors physically interact (21, 31, 38, 74). However, each compound appears to have a distinct set of mutations that engender viral resistance, and these do not overlap completely. More important, there is little overlap with mutations that confer resistance to nucleoside analogues or HIV-1 protease inhibitors. The spectrum of mutations in the reverse transcriptase gene associated with drug resistance to nevirapine and delavirdine is summarized in Table 2.

Reduced in vitro susceptibility has been observed to varying degrees with each codon mutation. IC_{50} values for some commonly selected mutations are compared with wild-type virus in Table 3.

Mutation at codon 236 in the reverse transcriptase gene, developed by selective pressure from delavirdine, actually increases in vitro susceptibility to nevirapine (23). This suggests intriguing possibilities with regard to tailoring antiretroviral therapy in individual patients, though this concept has yet to be examined in a clinical trial.

TABLE 2 • Spectrum of Mutations in the RT Gene Associated with Drug Resistance to Nevirapine and Delavirdine

	HIV-1 RT Codons Associated with Drug Resistance										
Compound	103K	106K	108V	135I	181I	188Y	190	228	236P	273	Reference
NVP	x	x	x		x	x	x				49
DLV					x			x	x	x	29

Methods to Overcome and Prevent Resistance

As with other antiretroviral agents, methods to prevent resistance have centered around using drugs in combination. Several clinical trials of nonnucleoside reverse transcriptase inhibitors in combination with nucleoside analogues have been performed. Three phase II combination placebo-controlled clinical trials with nevirapine have been completed (BI 1037: #51, ACTG 241: #24, and INCAS: #14) and three more are in progress. Three major combination clinical trials with delavirdine are either completed or in progress (0021: #27, 0017: #28, and ACTG 261: #55). Some preliminary clinical trial data concerning combinations of nevirapine and delavirdine and protease inhibitors are available (15, 25, 26, 30, 33, 40, 64), and more of the latter studies are in progress. Although genetic mutations associated with development of viral resistance to nonnucleoside reverse transcriptase inhibitors have been observed in combination-therapy clinical trials, there is evidence that development of resistant isolates is delayed, and persistent surrogate marker responses have been observed (12, 27).

Overcoming viral resistance is traditionally approached by changing antiretroviral therapy. In the absence of mutant analyses, clinical decision making about when and which drugs to use encompasses knowledge of prior antiretroviral exposure, adverse effects, and drug interaction profiles (9). However, several nonnucleoside reverse transcriptase inhibitors have demonstrated antiviral activity at concentrations 10,000 to 100,000 times lower than cytotoxic dosages (12, 18, 29). These broad therapeutic indices and the good bioavailability of the compounds may permit plasma levels of drug to be sustained above the concentration required to inhibit viral replication. Despite the rapid emergence of viral resistance to nonnucleoside reverse transcriptase inhibitors, persistent antiviral activity has been observed in some clinical trials (35). Twenty-one patients with 400 CD4 cells/mm^3 or less were treated for 24 weeks with nevirapine (400 mg/day). Eleven patients with measurable serum HIV RNA showed a rapid and persistent decrease in viral load. HIV isolates obtained at baseline were all susceptible to nevirapine, though by 8 weeks, isolates obtained from all subjects displayed a rapid reduction in susceptibility to nevirapine, and mutations associated with nevirapine resistance emerged. The nevirapine plasma trough level exceeded the IC$_{50}$ of nevirapine-resistant virus in all but one patient. On average, plasma trough concentrations were twice the mean IC$_{50}$ of the resistant virus, which indicates the need for further investigation of the correlation between in vitro susceptibility assays and plasma levels.

In the Upjohn 0021 study, 1200 subjects with 200 to 500 CD4 cells/mm^3 were randomized to zidovudine alone or in

TABLE 3 • In Vitro Sensitivities of Mutant RT to Nevirapine (NVP) and Delavirdine (DLV)

RT mutant	IC$_{50}$ (μM) of NVP[a]	IC$_{50}$ (μM) of DLV[b]
Wild type	0.04	0.04–0.26
103	0.70	7.7
181	2.3	8.32
188	>25	
236	0.085	18.0

[a] Data from Murphy RL, Montaner J. Nevirapine: a review of its development, pharmacological profile and potential for clinical use. Exp Opin Invest Drugs 1996;5:1183–1199.

[b] Data from Freimuth WW. Delavirdine mesylate, a potent non-nucleoside HIV-1 reverse transcriptase inhibitor. Adv Exp Med Biol 1996;394:279–289.

combination with delavirdine at 200, 300 or 400 mg thrice daily. In a randomly selected sample of 190 patients, delavirdine sensitivity in 88% of isolates evaluated from subjects receiving zidovudine and delavirdine at 400 mg thrice daily remained below median trough levels (8.3 μM) of delavirdine achieved in those patients (73). These data suggest that sufficiently high serum levels, which are achievable with nonnucleoside reverse transcriptase inhibitors, may be useful in overcoming viral resistance.

Considerable debate remains concerning when and how to initiate antiretroviral therapy. Although there has been a clear trend toward early initiation and use of combination therapy throughout the course of HIV disease, precisely how early and which combinations remains controversial. Preventing emergence of resistant isolates is a key factor in this issue. The fact that nonnucleoside reverse transcriptase inhibitors do not engender resistance to nucleoside analogues or protease inhibitors facilitates their use at various stages of HIV disease. Moreover, in a phase II delavirdine plus zidovudine trial with zidovudine-experienced patients, viral isolates demonstrated resensitization to zidovudine during the first 6 months of therapy, with an average 85-fold decrease in the zidovudine IC$_{50}$ (73). These preliminary data suggest that combination of zidovudine with delavirdine may increase or maintain sensitivity to zidovudine.

PHARMACOKINETIC DISPOSITION
Nevirapine

Nevirapine is well absorbed after oral administration. Absolute bioavailability appears to exceed 90%, and maximum concentrations are generally achieved by 4 h after an oral dose. Absorption is not affected by concomitant administration of a high-fat breakfast, antacids, or didanosine (61). Nevirapine is widely distributed in humans; it is highly lipophilic, essentially not ionized at physiologic pH, and approximately 60% bound to plasma proteins. Nevirapine concentrations in the cerebrospinal fluid (CSF) of six individuals were 45% ± 5% of corresponding plasma values: this ratio is approximately equivalent to the unbound fraction in plasma (75). Nevirapine is found in breast milk and crosses the placenta. Seven HIV-infected women received a single oral dose of nevirapine (200 mg) during labor; the median cord blood concentration in the eight term infants was 4.2 μM (47).

Nevirapine is extensively metabolized by the cytochrome P-450 system, principally by isozymes from the cytochrome 3A family. In a mass balance study in healthy volunteers, more than 90% of a radiolabeled dose was recovered, mostly from urine (81%) as glucuronidated metabolites (61). Renal excretion contributes little to elimination of the parent compound. Nevirapine also induces cytochrome P-450 enzymes, including those associated with its own metabolism. This autoinduction is characterized by a decrease in the terminal elimination half-life from approximately 45 h after a single dose to 25 to 30 h after 14 days of multiple doses, a 1.5 to 2-fold increase in apparent oral clearance, and a fall in trough concentrations (11, 35). Available data do not indicate either sex-related or race-related differences in the oral clearance of nevirapine (61). Pharmacokinetic studies of nevirapine in children do indicate that oral clearance is higher in children than in adults. Children receiving multiple doses of nevirapine at 120 to 240 mg/m^2/day had an oral clearance of approximately 0.08 mL/kg/day, a value twice that for adults (43).

Delavirdine mesylate

Delavirdine mesylate is a weak base with very low solubility at pH > 3. While the drug is usually rapidly absorbed after oral administration, reaching maximum concentrations within 1.5 h following a dose, absorption can be delayed and reduced by an increase in gastric pH (2, 29). For example, simultaneous administration with an antacid reduced the delavirdine area under the concentration curve (AUC) by 48% (29). Food and didanosine also appear to delay and reduce delavirdine absorption, although, under steady-state conditions, these interactions do not appear to be clinically significant, and patients can take delavirdine with a meal and with didanosine (15, 48). In general, however, gastric hypoacidity or therapeutic agents that raise gastric pH should be expected to decrease delavirdine absorption and reduce plasma concentrations; delavirdine administration under these conditions should be avoided until proven otherwise.

Delavirdine is highly (98%) protein bound (52), which restricts systemic distribution. The penetration of delavirdine into CSF appears quite low and likely clinically insignificant; in five adults, CSF concentrations were 0.4% of corresponding plasma concentrations (17, 55). Delavirdine is extensively metabolized, and renal clearance of unchanged drug is a negligible route of elimination. The cytochrome P-450 system and isozymes of the 3A family are a significant pathway of metabolism for delavirdine. Delavirdine is not only a substrate for this enzyme system, but is also an inhibitor. Thus, delavirdine

(and/or its metabolites) can actually inhibit its own metabolism, which appears responsible for the nonlinearities observed in delavirdine pharmacokinetics (13). These nonlinearities are characterized by decreased oral clearance, increased terminal elimination half-life, and a greater than proportional increase in plasma concentrations with higher doses of delavirdine. For example, steady-state plasma concentrations at 600 mg/day average 9.2 and 2.3 μM for maximum and minimum, respectively. A twofold increase in dose to 1200 mg daily produced a fourfold increase in maximum concentrations to 36 μM and a sevenfold increase in minimum values to 16 μM (29). Furthermore, delavirdine pharmacokinetics are highly variable between patients. For example, delavirdine trough concentrations in patients receiving 1200 mg daily appear to range from less than 5 μM to approximately 50 μM, a more than tenfold difference. This high degree of variability in delavirdine pharmacokinetics is consistent with known inter-patient differences in cytochrome P-450 activity.

Delavirdine pharmacokinetics have not been studied in individuals under 16 or over 65 years of age. The median delavirdine AUC was shown to be 31% higher in 12 females than in 55 males receiving the standard dose of 400 mg thrice daily (55). At this time, dosing recommendations are the same for females and males. No significant racial difference in delavirdine trough concentrations has been reported.

Pharmacologic parameters of nevirapine and delavirdine are shown in Table 4.

DOSAGE REGIMENS

The usual adult doses of nevirapine and delavirdine are shown in Table 5; neither drug is approved for use in children. While the safety and efficacy of nevirapine in children have not been established, some preliminary pharmacokinetic data are available (43, 61). It appears that oral clearance of a suspension formula is approximately twice that in adults. Dosing recommendations cannot be made at this time; however, clinical evaluations of nevirapine in combination with other antiretroviral agents are under way in children. There are no data on the use of delavirdine in children to date.

The pharmacokinetics of nevirapine and delavirdine in disease states including renal and hepatic dysfunction have not been evaluated. Significant hepatic insufficiency would be expected to decrease the oral clearance of both nevirapine and delavirdine. From a pharmacokinetic standpoint, weight does not appear to affect dosing requirements of nevirapine for adults (49). There are no data on the influence of pregnancy on the pharmacokinetics of nevirapine or delavirdine. The effect of ascites or edema on pharmacokinetic disposition has also not been evaluated for either drug. In patients experiencing significant diarrhea and/or malabsorption, although there are no available data, a reduction in the amount of drug absorbed is a possibility. It is not known whether malnutrition alters the pharmacokinetics of nevirapine or delavirdine.

ADVERSE EFFECTS

The most common adverse effects seen with nevirapine treatment have been rash, liver enzyme elevation, and (rarely) hep-

TABLE 4 • **Pharmacologic Parameters of Nevirapine and Delavirdine**[a]

Drug	In Vitro Susceptibility (Range, μM)	F (%)	Vd/F (L/kg)	$T_{1/2}$ (h)	CL/F (L/kg/h)	Adult Dose	Approximate Plasma C_{max}/C_{min} (μM)
Nevirapine	0.01–0.1	90	1.4	25	0.04	200 mg b.i.d.	27/16
Delavirdine	0.001–0.69	NA[b]	1.0	7	0.07	400 mg t.i.d.	36/16

[a] Abbreviations: F, bioavailability; Vd/F, apparent steady-state distribution volume; $T_{1/2}$, elimination half-life; CL/F, oral clearance; C_{max}, maximum plasma concentration; C_{min}, minimum plasma concentration.

[b] NA, not available.

atitis. Fever, headache, nausea, fatigue, and somnolence have also been reported. With the exception of rash, the incidence of adverse effects in nevirapine recipients in clinical trials has been similar to that seen in non-nevirapine-treated patients.

Rash occurs in 17% of patients receiving nevirapine therapy (49). The rash is most commonly maculopapular and mild to moderate. Although the precise mechanism is unclear, skin biopsy specimens have demonstrated nonspecific inflammatory changes and some have shown perivascular infiltration consistent with a drug eruption. Immune complex deposition has not been observed. Rash typically occurs within 6 weeks of initiation of treatment. In general, the rashes are self-limiting and rarely require treatment, although antihistamines and topical steroid therapy can be used. Severe rashes requiring drug discontinuation have been reported with an incidence of 6%, and Stevens-Johnson syndrome occurs in 0.5% of patients (8 of 1752 participants in clinical trials) (49). One fatality was reported from toxic epidermal necrolysis, possibly due to nevirapine (7). No clear risk factors for development of rash associated with nevirapine have been identified, and the incidence of rash associated with nevirapine has not been shown to correlate with plasma levels of drug. However, lead-in dosing with 200 mg/day for 2 to 4 weeks resulted in better tolerance of 200 mg twice daily and decreased the incidence of rash in participants of ACTG 164/168 (10). This finding has led to dosing recommendations of 200 mg/day for 2 weeks, then 200 mg twice daily when initiating therapy with nevirapine. Because the death due to toxic epidermal necrolysis occurred in a patient who experienced rash during the lead-in period but continued to escalate the dose of nevirapine, new guidelines have been developed. If rash occurs during the 2-week lead-in period, escalation from 200 mg/day to 200 mg twice daily should not occur until the rash resolves. Nevirapine should be discontinued in all patients with severe rash, and rechallenge should not be attempted.

Like nevirapine, the most common adverse effect observed to date with delavirdine has been rash, with an overall incidence around 33% (29). The rash associated with delavirdine is also maculopapular, occurring between 7 and 15 days after initiating treatment. The occurrence, but not severity, of the rash appears to correlate with CD4+ T-cell count and occurs more frequently in patients with less than 100 CD4 cells/mm³. As with nevirapine, the incidence of rash appears unrelated to delavirdine dose or blood level. Pruritus occurs in one-third of patients who develop rash, though other symptoms have not been observed. Clinical trial experience has demonstrated that continuing treat-

TABLE 5 • **Usual Adult Doses of Nevirapine and Delavirdine**

Drug	Usual Adult Dose
NVP	200 mg bid after 200 mg/day lead in for 2 weeks
DLV	400 mg t.i.d.

ment is possible in more than 85% of those who develop rash (29). Dosing through the rash with medication for symptomatic relief or dose interruption and resumption at a lower dose increased over 2 weeks have both been successful. Three clinical trial participants developed buccal mucosa involvement, and one other episode of Stevens-Johnson syndrome described as mild to moderate with complete recovery has been reported (29). As with nevirapine-associated rash, skin biopsy specimens have revealed changes consistent with a drug eruption.

Headache, fatigue, and gastrointestinal complaints have also been reported in clinical trial participants receiving delavirdine therapy. All these adverse effects were generally mild. Two subjects on delavirdine monotherapy developed transient and reversible elevations in liver enzymes. No other serious medical events or laboratory abnormalities have been clearly associated with delavirdine therapy.

Overdose

No overdoses with delavirdine have been reported. No acute toxicities or sequelae were reported for one patient who ingested 800 mg of nevirapine for 1 day (61). There are no known antidotes for overdosing with delavirdine or nevirapine.

MONITORING REQUIREMENTS

Monitoring liver function is prudent for patients receiving treatment with delavirdine or nevirapine, although precise guidelines have not been established. Therapy should be interrupted for patients who develop moderate or severe abnormalities of liver function until these tests return to baseline. Monitoring plasma concentrations of drugs known to interact with delavirdine or nevirapine is recommended when such tests are available (see below).

DRUG INTERACTIONS

Both nevirapine and delavirdine have the potential to cause clinically significant drug interactions. Nevirapine induces hepatic cytochrome P-450 3A; maximal induction seems to occur within 2 to 4 weeks of multiple dosing. Thus, nevirapine can potentially decrease concentrations of other agents metabolized by these isozymes. For example, nevirapine was shown to decrease saquinavir maximum concentrations by 29% and the AUC by 27%, and this combination should be avoided (64). The effect of nevirapine on the pharmacokinetics of indinavir has been evaluated in 24 HIV-infected persons. The indinavir AUC was 28% lower, peak concentration 11% lower, and trough concentration 38% lower when administered with nevirapine (61). These results appear consistent with the known ability of nevirapine to induce the hepatic cytochrome enzyme 3A. An increase in the dose of indinavir to 1000 mg every 8 h is recommended if indinavir and nevirapine are to be coadministered. However, the clinical safety, tolerance, and antiviral effect of this combination has not been evaluated. The effect of nevirapine on the pharmacokinetics of ritonavir has also been evaluated. This combination was studied in 24 HIV-infected persons, although only 14 had evaluable data. Results show the ritonavir AUC to be 11% less, peak concentrations 10% lower, and trough concentrations 9% lower when given with nevirapine. These differences were not statistically significant, and no changes in the ritonavir dosing regimen are recommended (7). Neither indinavir or ritonavir affected the pharmacokinetics of nevirapine. The AUC of nelfinavir may also be reduced, necessitating an increased nelfinavir dose, but clear guidelines are lacking for these combinations.

As an inducer of metabolism, nevirapine can theoretically decrease the plasma concentrations of oral contraceptive agents and increase the risk of contraceptive failure. No clinical data are presently available, but physicians are advised not to administer nevirapine concomitantly with oral contraceptives (61). Nevirapine can reduce zidovudine plasma concentrations by approximately 25% (24). The authors have attributed this interaction to an effect of nevirapine on the bioavailability of zidovudine; induction of glucuronyl transferase activity by nevirapine cannot be excluded, however. Nevirapine has had no effect on the pharmacokinetics of either didanosine or zalcitabine (61).

Nevirapine is extensively metabolized by the cytochrome P-450 system and is a substrate for isozymes from the 3A family. Thus, the metabolism of nevirapine can potentially be increased by inducers or decreased by inhibitors of these enzymes. Rifampin and rifabutin are well-known enzyme inducers that have been shown to reduce steady-state nevirapine trough concentrations by 37 and 16%, respectively (61). Coadministration of nevirapine with these compounds should be avoided. Ketoconazole is an enzyme inhibitor that was shown to inhibit nevirapine metabolism in in vitro experiments (61). However, pharmacokinetic studies in 11 patients receiving nevirapine and ketoconazole found no apparent inhibition of nevirapine metabolism. These contradictory findings seem to warrant additional clinical investigation, especially because cimetidine and macrolide antibiotics have both been shown to inhibit nevirapine metabolism and increase trough concentrations by 21 and 12%, respectively (61).

Like nevirapine, delavirdine's metabolism is mediated by hepatic cytochrome enzymes including those of the 3A family. Thus, the clearance of delavirdine can potentially be affected by inducers or inhibitors of these isozymes. Concomitant administration of delavirdine with rifabutin decreased delavirdine concentrations 5-fold, while administration with rifampin decreased concentrations 27-fold (29). Neither rifabutin or rifampin should be coadministered with delavirdine. Fluconazole and clarithromycin inhibit hepatic drug metabolism. Clinical investigations found that fluconazole did not affect delavirdine metabolism, and that there was no overall significant interaction between delavirdine and clarithromycin. However, clarithromycin does have some ability to inhibit delavirdine metabolism and some patients may be particularly susceptible to this interaction. While there is no apparent contraindication to concomitant administration of these two agents, careful clinical monitoring of delavirdine tolerance is recommended.

Delavirdine, in contrast to nevirapine, is a potent inhibitor of hepatic metabolism. In healthy volunteers, delavirdine increased the AUC of indinavir by approximately 70 to 90% (26). On the basis of these data, the dose of indinavir would need to be reduced from the 800 mg every 8 h presently recommended if delavirdine and indinavir are given as combination therapy; an indinavir dose of 400 or 600 mg every 8 h has been suggested, but clinical safety and efficacy data in HIV-infected patients are lacking. Delavirdine also inhibits the metabolism of saquinavir, increasing the steady-state concentration an average of sixfold (16). There appears to be considerable interpatient variability in the magnitude of this interaction, however, as individual trough saquinavir concentrations were increased from 2- to 15-fold. Delavirdine was not shown to inhibit the metabolism of ritonavir, nor did ritonavir affect the metabolism of delavirdine in a study in healthy volunteers (25). No data are available on the combination of delavirdine and nelfinavir. Perhaps the most serious potential interactions with delavirdine exist in concomitant use with certain nonsedating antihistamines, such as terfenadine and astemizole, and other cytochrome P-450 3A substrates such as cisapride. Combinations of these agents and other inhibitors of cytochrome P-450 3A have led to significant arrhythmias that can be fatal (37, 56). The mechanism of this interaction is inhibition of metabolism of the parent drug, which leads to accumulation of the parent drug, which can be cardiotoxic. Delavirdine is contraindicated for concomitant use with these agents.

CLINICAL INDICATIONS

Treatment for HIV infection has thus far focused on inhibiting the essential viral enzymes. For example, HIV-1 reverse transcriptase remains an attractive target for antiretroviral therapy. However, clinical benefit from currently available nucleoside analogue reverse transcriptase inhibitors in monotherapy is of limited duration (1, 70). Combination antiviral therapy produces greater suppression of HIV replication, increased CD4+ T cell counts, and delayed clinical progression than monotherapy (9). Used in combination with other antiretroviral agents, nonnucleoside reverse transcriptase inhibitors have shown promising results in clinical trials by decreasing viral burden and promoting sustained increases in CD4+ T lymphocyte counts (14, 24, 27, 28, 51, 55). These studies are discussed in more detail below. More recent studies of reverse transcriptase and protease inhibitors in combination have demonstrated more dramatic surrogate marker responses, although long-term efficacy remains to be established (19). With 11 antiretroviral compounds currently licensed for treatment of HIV infection, multiple combinations are possible. Several more combinations are in clinical trials. The question remains, which drugs should be combined? Issues of drug toxicity, viral resistance, and cost further complicate decision making for physician and patient. Results of major clinical trials with nevirapine and delavirdine are given below.

Nevirapine

Also known as BIRG-587, this dipyridodiazepinone compound developed by Boehringer Ingelheim has been studied in a number of different protocols, and several studies are still in progress. ACTG 164, a phase I dose-escalation study, examined 54 subjects with fewer than 400 CD4+ T cells/mm^3 randomized to different doses of nevirapine alone. Despite an initial decrease in p24 antigen levels, titers rose again rapidly in most subjects, with the exception of a subset on high-dose nevirapine (400 mg/day). High-level resistance was observed in most subjects, which correlated with a loss of in vitro viral activity (59). Some subjects on high-dose nevirapine experienced rash, which was occasionally severe, but the drug was otherwise well tolerated. ACTG 168, a follow-up trial, examined nevirapine in combination with zidovudine in 65 subjects with fewer than 400 CD4 cells/mm^3 who were randomized to different doses of nevirapine and zidovudine. Results similar to those in ACTG 164 were seen, and combination therapy did not prevent emergence of viral resistance (35).

In BI1009, addition of nevirapine to preexisting nucleoside therapy was examined (62). Substantial decreases in viral load were seen, and plasma viral RNA fell approximately 15-fold. Patients who failed therapy had viral strains that rapidly developed resistance to nevirapine, with mutations at reverse transcriptase codons 181, 188, and 190. To examine whether higher levels of nevirapine could produce sustained antiviral activity, nevirapine at 400 mg/day in monotherapy was studied in 21 heavily pretreated patients with advanced HIV disease (35). Although viral load was rapidly reduced, nevirapine-resistant isolates developed in all patients by 12 weeks. However, the mean plasma trough level of nevirapine exceeded the mean IC$_{50}$ of resistant virus, and immune complex–dissociated (ICD) p24 antigen and HIV RNA were suppressed for up to 24 weeks.

Three phase II combination placebo-controlled clinical trials with nevirapine have been completed (BI 1037: #51, ACTG 241: #24, and INCAS: #14), and three more are in progress. BI 1037 was a randomized, double-blind, placebo-controlled trial of nevirapine with zidovudine versus zidovudine monotherapy in patients with CD4 counts of 200 to 500 cells/mm^3 (median, 367) and 3 to 24 months (median, 8) of prior zidovudine therapy (51). After the first 24 weeks, all subjects received open-label nevirapine at 400 mg/day. CD4 cell

counts increased in the combination group through week 28, with a maximum increase of 56 cells/mm^3. Initially, HIV-1 RNA decreased by more than 1.5 log$_{10}$ copies/mL, compared with no decrease in the zidovudine monotherapy group.

ACTG 241 examined nevirapine with other combinations in 400 subjects with fewer than 350 CD4 cells/mm^3 who were randomized to receive zidovudine, didanosine and nevirapine, or zidovudine and didanosine (24). The triple combination of zidovudine, didanosine, and nevirapine was superior to the double combination of zidovudine and didanosine, both by CD4+ T cell count and viral load over 48 weeks in patients with extensive (>6 months) prior nucleoside therapy. Nevirapine/zidovudine/didanosine recipients had greater increases in CD4 cell counts and greater maximal decreases in HIV-1 RNA levels (which remained below baseline for more than a year) than zidovudine/didanosine recipients. Patients with more than 200 CD4 cells/mm^3 had the best antiviral response. No significant difference in clinical endpoints between the two groups was observed; however, the study was not powerful enough to detect such differences. Seventeen patients (9%) developed rash; six of these had severe rash associated with fever, and four of these six patients also had oral ulcerations.

The INCAS study (BI 1046) compared zidovudine plus didanosine with or without nevirapine or zidovudine plus nevirapine in 151 subjects with 200 to 600 CD4 cells/mm^3 (mean, 376) who were naive to antiretrovirals (14). At 28 weeks, increase in CD4 cell count over baseline was 120 to 175 cells/mm^3 in the nevirapine/zidovudine/didanosine and zidovudine/didanosine groups, versus a 10-cell increase in nevirapine/zidovudine recipients. Mean change in HIV-1 RNA from baseline to 28 weeks was 1.7 log$_{10}$ for nevirapine/zidovudine/didanosine recipients and 1.3 log$_{10}$ for zidovudine/didanosine recipients. The proportion of subjects with RNA levels below the limit of detection (200 copies/mL) was significantly larger in the nevirapine/zidovudine/didanosine treated group (67%) than in the zidovudine/didanosine group (29%) or nevirapine/zidovudine group (0%) for at least 52 weeks. These responses are comparable to results seen in studies of combinations of nucleoside analogues and protease inhibitors. Moreover, emergence of nevirapine resistance was observed in isolates from only 2 of 47 compliant recipients of the triple combination studied for at least a year (71).

On the basis of this and other studies, other combination trials are in progress. ACTG 193A, a large clinical trial in patients with advanced HIV-1 disease (<50 CD4 cells/mm^3), was recently completed. Subjects were randomized to (a) zidovudine with zalcitabine, (b) zidovudine with didanosine, (c) alternating zidovudine and didanosine, or (d) zidovudine with didanosine and nevirapine. Preliminary analysis demonstrated increased survival in the zidovudine/didanosine/nevirapine arm compared with zidovudine alternating with didanosine or zidovudine with zalcitabine, but not with zidovudine and didanosine (P = .25) (36).

Nevirapine crosses the blood-brain and placental barriers (65, 75); the clinical implications of both are still to be determined. Safety and pharmacokinetics of nevirapine in children and neonates have been examined (43, 47). At doses of 240 mg/m²/day or above, 5 of 10 children studied experienced durable suppression of plasma p24 antigen. Eight infants aged 2.5 to 16 months born to HIV-infected mothers were administered nevirapine, didanosine, and zidovudine (44). A 1.5-log reduction in HIV-1 RNA was observed over the first 2 to 4 weeks in seven of the eight infants, with 0.5- to 3.0-log reductions at 6 months, including two infants in whom RNA levels fell below 10 copies/mL. These data in conjunction with seronegativity in the two infants suggest long-term control of viral replication, and the study is continuing. Studies of nevirapine for prevention of perinatal transmission of HIV-1 are in progress. The potency, rapid onset of action, and less-frequent dosing requirements of nevirapine hold promise in this setting, and possibly in the setting of occupational exposure to HIV.

Some preliminary clinical trial data concerning combinations of nevirapine and protease inhibitors are available (30, 33, 40, 64). Preliminary data indicate that drug interactions do occur but that nevirapine can be used in combination with protease inhibitors, although indinavir dosage needs to be adjusted to 1 g thrice daily. Surrogate marker or clinical benefit in patients has not been determined.

Delavirdine

Three major combination clinical trials with delavirdine are either completed or in progress (0021: #27, 0017: #28, and ACTG 261: #55). In study 0021, patients with 200 to 500 CD4 cells/mm³ and 0 to 6 months prior zidovudine therapy were randomized to zidovudine with delavirdine at varying doses or zidovudine alone. Approximately 200 patients per group with an average CD4 count of 320 to 330 cells/mm³ were randomized. In an interim analysis of the first 800 patients, an increase of about 20 CD4 cells above baseline was observed in the combination arms for more than 1 year, particularly in patients randomized to high-dose delavirdine (400 mg thrice daily) (27). At 60 weeks, many participants had CD4+ T cell counts 35 to 70 cells above baseline values. After 4 weeks of therapy, delavirdine-treated patients experienced a one log decrease in viral burden, and combination therapy with 300 mg thrice daily or 400 mg thrice daily of delavirdine plus zidovudine produced a 0.5-log or greater diminution in viral load, compared with the monotherapy group. The immunologic and virologic responses in naive patients are more profound, but surrogate marker responses have been observed in zidovudine-experienced patients. Because of recent data suggesting that zidovudine monotherapy is no longer optimal treatment, the study was revised to include lamivudine in both arms. Lamivudine and zidovudine have been shown to have in vitro synergy (41). Moreover, as observed with the combination of zidovudine and lamivudine, delavirdine may delay emergence of resistance to zidovudine, and vice versa, in both naive and experienced patients (72, 73). Analysis of the 0021 study is still in progress.

Patients with advanced HIV disease, CD4 counts of 0 to 300 cells/mm³, and prior zidovudine experience were studied in protocol 0017 (28). Subjects were randomized to didanosine plus placebo versus didanosine plus delavirdine at 400 mg thrice daily. An interim analysis of the first 870 patients found

CD4 cell counts 5 to 20/mm³ above baseline during the first 40 weeks, and plasma viral load reductions of approximately 0.5 log for the first 60 weeks in the combination arm. Although less dramatic than results from the 0021 study, subjects who achieved higher plasma concentrations of drug (trough levels above 7.5 μM) had increases in CD4+ T lymphocytes of 10 to 25 cells/mm³ and decreases in viral load above 0.5 log for at least 1 year. Despite these surrogate marker changes, the interim analysis found no difference in clinical efficacy (defined as time to AIDS or death) in an intent-to-treat analysis. The protocol was closed on the recommendation of the Data Safety and Monitoring Board.

ACTG 261 was a phase II double-blind study of delavirdine in combination with zidovudine or didanosine versus the combination of zidovudine and didanosine in approximately 600 patients with CD4 counts between 100 and 500 cells/mm³ with 6 months or less of prior cumulative monotherapy with either zidovudine or didanosine. Enrollment was closed on 1 January 1996, with 549 subjects enrolled. Preliminary results indicate that triple therapy produced the largest CD4 cell count changes, but they did not differ significantly from those with zidovudine and didanosine (55). No statistically significant differences in plasma HIV-1 RNA levels were seen for the three drug combinations compared with the combination of zidovudine and didanosine.

Trials of delavirdine with all three approved protease inhibitors have been performed in healthy volunteers. Delavirdine (400 mg thrice daily) with saquinavir (600 mg thrice daily) resulted in saquinavir concentrations approaching those achieved with saquinavir 7200 mg/day (16). No pharmacokinetic interactions occurred with ritonavir (300 mg twice daily) and delavirdine (400 or 600 mg daily) (25). Delavirdine (400 mg thrice daily) with indinavir (400 or 600 mg thrice daily) achieved concentrations that equaled or exceeded those achieved with indinavir at 800 mg thrice daily (26). Further studies of various dosing regimens in HIV-1 infected patients are planned.

CONCLUSIONS

In the recent excitement surrounding results from protease inhibitor studies, nonnucleoside reverse transcriptase inhibitors have been somewhat overlooked. The antiviral potency, rapid onset of action, and relative lack of toxicity of these drugs will likely make them a useful addition, although their role in the management of HIV disease is not entirely clear. Rapid development of viral resistance to nonnucleoside reverse transcriptase inhibitors limits their utility, and their clinical benefit remains undetermined. Current recommendations for antiretroviral therapy include initiating therapy with a regimen most likely to reduce and maintain plasma HIV RNA levels below the level of detection (400–500 copies/mL, depending on the assay) (9). Although a three-drug regimen with two nucleoside analogues and a protease inhibitor is preferred because of antiviral potency, this may not be practical for every patient. The recommended alternative is a combination of two nucleoside analogues and a nonnucleoside reverse transcriptase inhibitor. Such combinations with clinical trial results available are nevirapine with zidovudine and didanosine, or delavirdine with zidovudine and didanosine or with zidovudine and lamivudine. Studies have been performed with both antiretroviral-naive and -experienced patients. The combination of nevirapine, zidovudine, and didanosine is under study in children. Lamivudine has not been evaluated in combination with nevirapine, and zalcitabine and stavudine have not been evaluated with either nevirapine or delavirdine.

Not all patients can tolerate protease inhibitor therapy for a variety of reasons (19). For example, in the experience of the author and others, HIV-infected hemophiliacs who take protease inhibitors develop more spontaneous bleeding and often more serious bleeding episodes. The mechanism for this has not been elucidated. Moreover, some patients must take essential medications that interact with protease inhibitors and the complex combinations create management difficulties. These medications include antiarrhythmics, anticonvulsants, anticoagulants, analgesics, and oral contraceptives. Overall, nonnucleoside reverse transcriptase inhibitors are better tolerated with fewer interactions than protease inhibitors, so the drugs have an important role if use of protease inhibitor therapy is deferred or if patients are unable or unwilling to take protease inhibitor therapy. Used in combination with nucleoside analogues, nonnucleoside reverse transcriptase inhibitors appear generally less potent than protease inhibitors, although head-to-head trials comparing the two classes have not been performed. In antiretroviral-naive patients with early HIV disease, nonnucleoside reverse transcriptase inhibitors used in combination have produced potent and sustained suppression of viral replication (14). Predicting which patients will obtain the most long-term benefit from such combinations is difficult and requires careful consideration from the prescribing physician. This approach may be significantly less effective in persons previously treated with nucleoside analogues (24, 28). As with protease inhibitor therapy, compliance with the chosen regimen is critical to its success. The only combination with nonnucleoside reverse transcriptase inhibitors shown to suppress plasma viremia to undetectable levels is zidovudine with didanosine and nevirapine in previously untreated subjects. Combination therapy with nonnucleoside reverse transcriptase inhibitors is therefore not recommended for patients with advanced disease (i.e., those with low CD4 counts and/or high plasma RNA levels).

Nonnucleoside reverse transcriptase inhibitors also have an emerging role when antiretroviral therapy fails. Recently revised treatment guidelines recommend changing at least two drugs in a failing regimen and preferably changing to an entirely new regimen. Two new nucleoside analogues with a nonnucleoside reverse transcriptase inhibitor are recommended as alternatives for patients failing triple-drug regimens that included protease inhibitors, although not for those failing double nucleoside reverse transcriptase inhibitor therapy (9). Changing from nevirapine to delavirdine is not recommended, since cross-resistance is likely (29, 49). Combination regimens including nonnucleoside reverse transcriptase inhibitors and protease inhibitors for salvage therapy are being evaluated.

Other specific settings in which the tolerability, antiviral potency, and rapid onset of action of nonnucleoside reverse transcriptase inhibitors present an attractive option include treatment of primary HIV disease, prevention of perinatal transmission, and postexposure prophylaxis for health care workers. Tolerance is especially important when administering antiretroviral agents to healthy, uninfected individuals. The rapid and potent antiviral activity of nonnucleoside reverse transcriptase inhibitors give them an ideal profile as prophylactic agents to prevent HIV transmission. The excellent absorption and tissue penetration of nevirapine, including CSF penetrance, offers potential for use in treating primary HIV infection. Studies in these areas are in progress.

REFERENCES

1. Aboulker J-P, Swart AM. Preliminary analysis of the Concorde trial. Lancet 1993;341:889–890.
2. Akbari B, Shelton MJ, Adams JM, Hewitt RG, Morse GD. Effects of Helicobacter pylori treatment on gastric pH and delavirdine mesylate pharmacokinetics in HIV+ patients with gastric hypoacidity [Abstract A56]. Program and abstracts of the 36th Interscience Conference on Antimicrobial Agents and Chemotherapy, New Orleans, LA, Sept 15–18, 1996.
3. Baba M, De Clercq E, Iida S, Tanaka H, Nitta I, Ubasawa M, Takashima H, Sekiya K, Umezu K, Nakashima H, Shigeta S, Walker RT, Miyasaka T. Anti-human immunodeficiency virus type 1 activities and pharmacokinetics of novel 6-substituted acyclouridine derivatives. Antimicrob Agents Chemother 1990; 34:2358–2363.
4. Baba M, De Clercq E, Tanaka H, Tanaka H, Ubasawa M, Takashima H, Sekiya K, Nitta I, Umezu K, Walker RT, Mori S. Highly potent and selective inhibition of human immunodeficiency virus type 1 by a novel series of 6-substituted acyclouridine derivatives. Mol Pharmacol 1991;39:805–810.
5. Baba M, De Clercq E, Tanaka H, Ubasawa M, Takashima H, Sekiya K, Nitta I, Umezu K, Nakashima H, Mori S. Potent and selective inhibition of human immunodeficiency virus type 1 by 5-ethyl-6-phenylthiouracil derivatives through their interaction with the HIV-1 reverse transcriptase. Proc Natl Acad Sci USA 1991;88:2356–2360.
6. Bacolla A, Shih CK, Rose JM, Piras G, Warren TC, Grygon CA, Ingraham RH, Cousins RC, Greenwood DJ, Richman D. Amino acid substitutions in HIV-1 reverse transcriptase with corresponding residues from HIV-2: effect on kinetic constants and inhibition by non-nucleoside analogs. J Biol Chem 1993;268:16571–16577.
7. Boehringer Ingelheim Pharmaceuticals, Inc, Letter to Investigators, 1997.
8. Campbell TB, Young RK, Eron JJ, D'Aquila RT, Tarpley WG, Kuritzkes DR. Inhibition of human immunodeficiency virus type 1 replication in vitro by the bisheteroarylpiperazine atervidine (U-87201E) in combination with zidovudine or didanosine. J Infect Dis 1993;168:318–326.
9. Carpenter CCJ, Fischl MA, Hammer SM, Hirsch MS, Jacobsen DM, Katzenstein DA, Montaner JSG, Richman DD, Saag MS, Schooley RT, Thompson MA, Vella S, Yeni PG, Volberding PA, for the International AIDS Society–USA. Antiretroviral therapy for HIV infection in 1998. JAMA 1998;280:78–86.
10. Cheeseman SH, Murphy RL, Saag MD, Havlir D, and ACTG 164/168 Study Team. Safety of high dose nevirapine (NVP) after 200 mg/d lead-in [Abstract PO-B26–2109]. Program and abstracts of the International Conference on AIDS, Berlin, June 6–11, 1993.

11. Cheeseman SH, Hattox SE, McLaughlin MM, Koup RA, Andrews C, Bova CA, Pav JW, Roy T, Sullivan JL, Keirns JJ. Pharmacokinetics of nevirapine: initial single-rising-dose study in humans. Antimicrob Agents Chemother 1993;37:178–182.

12. Cheeseman SH, Havlir D, McLaughlin MM, Greenough TC, Sullivan JL, Hall D, Hattox SE, Spector SA, Stein DS, Myers M, Richman DD. Phase I/II evaluation of nevirapine alone and in combination with zidovudine for infection with human immunodeficiency virus. J Acquir Immune Defic Syndr 1995;8:141–151.

13. Cheng CL, Smith DE, Cox SR, Watkins PB, Blake DS, Carver PL, Kauffman CA, Meyer K, Amidon GL, Stetson PL. Steady-state pharmacokinetics of DLV in HIV+ patients: in vivo effect of DLV on the erythromycin breath test [Abstract A57]. Program and abstracts of the 36th Interscience Conference on Antimicrobial Agents and Chemotherapy, New Orleans, LA, Sept 15–18, 1996.

14. Conway B, Montaner JSG, Cooper D. Randomized, double-blind one-year study of the immunological and virological effects of nevirapine, didanosine and zidovudine combinations among antiretroviral-naive, AIDS-free patients with CD4+ cell counts of 200–600/μL [Abstract OP7.1]. Program and abstracts of the Third International Congress on Drug Therapy in HIV Infection, Birmingham, England, Nov 3–7, 1996.

15. Cox SR, Cohn SE, Greisberger C, Reichman RC, Della-Coletta AA, Freimuth WW, Morse GD. Evaluation of the steady-state pharmacokinetic interaction between didanosine and DLV mesylate in HIV+ patients [Abstract I31]. Program and abstracts of the 35th Interscience Conference on Antimicrobial Agents and Chemotherapy, New Orleans, LA, Sept 17–20, 1995.

16. Cox SR, Batts DH, Stewart F, Buss N, Brown A, Chambers JH, Carel BJ, Carberry PA. Evaluation of the pharmacokinetic (PK) interaction between saquinavir (SQV) and delavirdine (DLV) in healthy volunteers. Program and abstracts of the Fourth Conference on Retroviruses and Opportunistic Infections, Washington, DC, Jan 22–26, 1997.

17. Davey RT, Chaitt DG, Reed GF, Freimuth WW, Herpin BR, Metcalf JA, Eastman PS, Falloon J, Kovacs JA, Polis MA, Walker RE, Masur H, Boyle J, Coleman S, Cox SR, Wathen L, Daenzer CL, Lane HC. Randomized, controlled phase I/II trial of combination therapy with delavirdine (U-90152S) and conventional nucleosides in human immunodeficiency virus type-1 infected patients. Antimicrob Agents Chemother 1996;40:1657–1664.

18. De Clercq E. Chemotherapy of the acquired immunodeficiency syndrome (AIDS); non-nucleoside inhibitors of the human immunodeficiency virus type 1 reverse transcriptase. Int J Immunopharmacol 1991;13(Suppl 1):83–89.

19. Deeks SG, Smith MD, Holodniy M, Kahn JO. HIV-1 protease inhibitors. JAMA 1997;277:145–153.

20. Ding J, Das K, Moereels H, Koymans L, Andries K, Janssen PA, Hughes SH, Arnold E. Structure of HIV-1 RT/TIBO R 86183 complex reveals similarity in the binding of diverse nonnucleoside inhibitors. Nature Struct Biol 1995;2:407–415.

21. Dueweke TJ, Kezzdy FJ, Waszak GA, Deibel JR, Tarpley WG. The binding of a novel bisheteroarylpiperazine mediates inhibition of human immunodeficiency virus type 1 reverse transcriptase. J Biol Chem 1992;267:27–30.

22. Dueweke TJ, Poppe SM, Romero DL, Swaney SM, So AG, Downey KM, Althaus IW, Reusser F, Busso M, Resnick L, Mayers DL, Lane J, Aristoff PA, Thomas RC, Tarpley WG. U-90152, a potent inhibitor of human immunodeficiency virus type 1 replication. Antimicrob Agents Chemother 1993;5:1127–1131.

23. Duweke TJ, Pushkarskaya T, Poppe S, Swaney SM, Zhao JQ, Chen IS, Stevenson M, Tarpley WG. A mutation in reverse transcriptase of bis(heteroaryl)piperazine-resistant human immunodeficiency virus type 1 that confers increased sensitivity to other nonnucleoside inhibitors. Proc Natl Acad Sci USA 1993;90:4713–4717.

24. D'Aquila RT, Hughes MD, Johnson VA, Fischl MA, Sommadossi JP, Liou SH, Timpone J, Myers M, Basgoz N, Niu M, Hirsch MS, and the National Institute of Allergy and Infectious Diseases AIDS Clinical Trials Group Protocol 241 Investigators. Nevirapine, zidovudine, and didanosine compared with zidovudine and didanosine in patients with HIV-1 infection. Ann Intern Med 1996;124:1019–1030.

25. Ferry JJ, Schneck DW, Carlson GF, Carberry PA, Della-Coletta AA, Gulotti BR, Cox SR. Evaluation of the pharmacokinetic (PK) interaction between ritonavir (R) and delavirdine (DLV) in healthy volunteers. Program and abstracts of the Fourth Conference on Retroviruses and Opportunistic Infections, Washington, DC, Jan 22–26, 1997.

26. Ferry JJ, Herman BD, Cox SR, Carlson GF, Carberry PA. Delavirdine (DLV) and indinavir (IDV): a pharmacokinetic (PK) drug-drug interaction study in healthy adult volunteers. Program and abstracts of the Fourth Conference on Retroviruses and Opportunistic Infections, Washington, DC, Jan 22–26, 1997.

27. Freimuth WW, Wathen LK, Cox SR, Chuang-Stein CJ, Greenwald CA, Daenzer CL, Wang Y, and Delavirdine Team, Pharmacia & Upjohn, Inc. Delavirdine (DLV) in combination with zidovudine (ZDV) causes sustained antiviral and immunological effects in HIV-1 infected individuals [Abstract LB8]. Program and abstracts of the 3rd Conference on Retroviruses and Opportunistic Infections, Washington, DC, Jan 28–Feb 1, 1996.

28. Freimuth WW, Chuang-Stein CJ, Greenwald CA, Cox SR, Edge-Padbury BA, Carbery PA, Wathen LK and Delavirdine Team, Pharmacia & Upjohn, Inc. Delavirdine (DLV) + didanosine (ddI) combination therapy has sustained surrogate marker response in advanced HIV-1 population [Abstract LB8]. Program and abstracts of the 3rd Conference on Retroviruses and Opportunistic Infections, Washington, DC, Jan 28–Feb 1, 1996.

29. Freimuth WW. Delavirdine mesylate, a potent non-nucleoside HIV-1 reverse transcriptase inhibitor. Adv Exp Med Biol 1996;394:279–289.

30. Gagnier P, Myers M, Lamson M, Greguski R, Love J, Chodakewitz J. Effect of nevirapine (NVP) on pharmacokinetics (PK) of indinavir IDV in HIV-1 patients. Fourth Conference on Retroviruses and Opportunistic Infections, Washington, DC, Jan 22–26, 1997.

31. Goldman ME, Nunberg JH, O'Brien JA, Quintero JC, Schleif WA, Freund KF, Gaul SL, Saari WS, Wai JS, Hoffman JM, Anderson PS, Hupe DJ, Emini EA, Stern AM. Pyridinone derivatives: specific human immunodeficiency virus type 1 reverse transcriptase inhibitors with antiviral activity. Proc Natl Acad Sci USA 1991;88:6863–6867.

32. Goldman ME, O'Brien JA, Ruffing TL, Nunberg JH, Schleif WA, Quintero JC, Siegl PKS, Hoffman JM, Smith AM, Emini EA. L-696,229 specifically inhibits human immunodeficiency virus type 1 reverse transcriptase and possesses antiviral activity in vitro. Antimicrob Agents Chemother 1992;36:1019–1023.

33. Harris M, Durakovic C, Conway B, Fransen S, Shillington A, Montaner JSG, BC Centre for Excellence in HIV/AIDS–Vancouver, BC. A pilot study of indinavir, nevirapine and 3TC in patients with advanced HIV disease [Abstract #234]. Program and abstracts of the Fourth Conference on Retroviruses and Opportunistic Infections, Washington, DC, Jan 22–26, 1997.

34. Havlir D. Antiretroviral therapy: update on nonnucleoside re-

verse transcriptase inhibitors (NNTRI) [Abstract 279]. Program and abstracts of the 34th Interscience Conference on Antimicrobial Agents & Chemotherapy, Oct 4–7, 1994.

35. Havlir D, Cheeseman SH, McLaughlin M, Murphy R, Erice A, Spector SA, Greenough TC, Sullivan JL, Hall D, Myers M, Lamson M, Richman DD. High-dose nevirapine: safety, pharmacokinetics and antiviral effect in patients with human immunodeficiency virus infection. J Infect Dis 1995;171:537–545.

36. Henry K, Tierney C, Kahn J, Jiang Q, Kmack A, Fischl M for the ACTG 193A Study Team. A randomized, double-blind, placebo-controlled study comparing combination nucleoside and triple therapy for the treatment of advanced HIV disease (CD4 $\leq$50/mm^3). Programs and abstracts of the Fourth Conference on Retroviruses and Opportunistic Infections, Washington, DC, Jan 22–26, 1997.

37. Honig PK, Wortham DC, Zamani K, Conner DP, Mullin JC, Cantilena LR. Terfenadine-ketoconazole interaction: pharmacokinetic and electrocardiographic consequences. JAMA 1993;269:1513–1518.

38. Kohlstaedt LA, Wang J, Friedman JM, Rice PA, Steitz TA. Crystal structure at 3.5 Å or resolution of HIV-1 reverse transcriptase complexed with an inhibitor. Science 1992;256:1783–1790.

39. Koup RA, Merluzzi VJ, Hargrave KD, Adams J, Grozinger K, Eckner RJ, Sullivan JL. Inhibition of human immunodeficiency virus type 1 (HIV-1) replication by the dipyridodiazepinone (BI-RG-587). J Infect Dis 1991;163:966–970.

40. Lamson M, Gagnier P, Greguski R, Myers M, Leonard J, Lauva I, Hsu A, Boehringer Ingelheim, Ridgefield CT; Abbott, Abbott Park IL. Effect of nevirapine (NVP) on pharmacokinetics (PK) of ritonavir (RTV) in HIV-1 patients. Program and abstracts of Fourth Conference on Retroviruses and Opportunistic Infections, Washington, DC, Jan 22–26, 1997.

41. Larder BA, Kemp SD, Purifoy DJ. Infectious potential of human immunodeficiency virus type 1 reverse transcriptase mutants with altered inhibitor sensitivity. Proc Natl Acad Sci USA 1989;86:4803–4807.

42. Larder BA, Kemp SD, Harrigan PR, Kinghorn I, Kohi A, Bloor S. Antiviral potency of AZT + 3TC combination therapy supports virological observations [Abstract LB33]. Presented at Second National Conference on Human Retroviruses and Related Infections, Washington, DC, Jan 1995.

43. Luzuriaga K, Bryson Y, McSherry G, Robinson J, Stechenberg B, Scott G, Lamson M, Cort S, Sullivan JL. Pharmacokinetics, safety, and activity of nevirapine in human immunodeficiency virus type 1-infected children. J Infect Dis 1996;174:713–721.

44. Luzuriaga K, Bryson Y, Krogstad P, Robinson J, Stechenberg B, Lamson M, Cort SP, Sullivan JL. Triple combination therapy in early vertical HIV-1 infection: potential for eradication of infection. Program and abstracts of the Fourth Conference on Retroviruses and Opportunistic Infections, Washington, DC, Jan 22–26, 1997.

45. Mayers D, Riddler S, Stein D, Bach M, Havir D, Kahn J. A double-blind pilot study to evaluate the antiviral activity, tolerability and pharmacokinetics (PK) of DMP 266 alone and in combination with indinavir (IDV) [Abstract Lb8A]. Program and abstracts of the 36th Interscience Conference on Antimicrobial Agents and Chemotherapy, New Orleans, LA, Sept 15–18, 1996.

46. Merluzzi VJ, Hargrave KD, Labadia M, Grozinger K, Skoog M, Wu JC, Shih CK, Eckner K, Hattox S, Adams J, Rosenthal AS, Faanea R, Eckner RJ, Koup RA, Sullivan JL. Inhibition of HIV-1 replication by a nonnucleoside reverse transcriptase inhibitor. Science 1990;250:1411–1413.

47. Mirochnick M, Sullivan J, Gagnier P, Fenton T, Sperling R. Safety and pharmacokinetics of nevirapine in neonates born to HIV-1 infected women [Abstract 723]. Programs and abstracts of the Fourth Conference on Retroviruses and Opportunistic Infections, Washington, DC, Jan 22–26, 1997.

48. Morse GD, Fischl MA, Cox SR, Thompson L, Della-Coletta AA, Freimuth WW. Effect of food on the steady-state pharmacokinetics of delavirdine mesylate in HIV+ patients [Abstract I30]. Program and abstracts of the 35th Interscience Conference on Antimicrobial Agents and Chemotherapy, San Francisco, Sept 17–20, 1995.

49. Murphy RL, Montaner J. Nevirapine: a review of its development, pharmacological profile and potential for clinical use. Exp Opin Invest Drugs 1996;5:1183–1199.

50. Murphy R, Gagnier P, Lamson M, Lamson M, Dusek A, Ju W, Hsu A. Effect of nevirapine (NVP) on pharmacokinetics (PK) of indinavir (IDV) in HIV-1 patients [Abstract 374]. Programs and abstracts of the Fourth Conference on Retroviruses and Opportunistic Infections, Washington, DC, Jan 22–26, 1997.

51. Paar D, Pollard R, Hall D, Myers M, Robinson P & Study 1037 Team. Nevirapine (NVP) in combination with zidovudine (ZDV) vs ZDV nucleoside experienced patients [Abstract #383]. Programs and abstracts of the Infectious Diseases Society of America 33rd annual meeting, San Francisco, Sept 16–18, 1995.

52. Para M, Morse G, Fischl M, and the ACTG 260 Study Team. Plasma protein binding of delavirdine in HIV-infected patients in ACTG 260. Programs and abstracts of the XIth International Conference on AIDS, Vancouver, British Columbia, Jul 7–12, 1996.

53. Pauwels R, Andries K, Desmyter J, Schols D, Kula MJ, Breslin HJ, Raeymaeckers A, van Gelder J, Woestenborghs R, Heykants J, Schellekens K, Janssen MAC, DeClerq E, Janssen PA. Potent and selective inhibition of HIV-1 replication by a novel series of TIBO derivatives. Nature 1990;343:470–474.

54. Pauwels R, Andries K, Debyser Z, VanDaele P, Schols D, Stoffels P, DeVreese K, Woestenborghs R, Vandamme AM, Janssen CGM, Anne J, Cauwenbergh G, Desmyter J, Heykants, J, Janssen MAC, DeClercq E, Janssen PAJ. Potent and highly selective human immunodeficiency virus type 1 (HIV-1) inhibition by a series of alpha-anilinophenylacetamide derivatives targeted at HIV-1 reverse transcriptase. Proc Natl Acad Sci USA 1993; 90:1711–1715.

55. Pharmacia & Upjohn Company. Rescriptor (delavirdine). April 1997.

56. Pohjola-Sintonen S, Viitasalo M, Toivonen L, Neuvonen P. Torsades de pointes after terfenadine-itraconazole interaction. Br Med J 1993;306:186.

57. Richman D, Rosenthal AS, Skoog M, Eckner RJ, Chou TC, Sabo JP, Merluzzi VJ. BI-RG-587 is active against zidovudine-resistant human immunodeficiency virus type 1 and synergistic with zidovudine. Antimicrob Agents Chemother 1991;35:305–308.

58. Richman D, Shih CK, Lowy I, Rose J, Prodanovich P, Goff S, Griffin J. Human immunodeficiency virus type 1 mutants resistant to non-nucleoside inhibitors of reverse transcriptase arise in tissue culture. Proc Natl Acad Sci USA 1991;88:11241–11245.

59. Richman DD. Loss of nevirapine activity associated with the emergence of resistance in clinical trials [Abstract B183]. Abstracts of the XIIIth International Conference on AIDS/STD World Congress, Amsterdam, Jul 19–24, 1992.

60. Romero DL, Busso M, Tan CK, Reusser F, Palmer JR, Poppe SM, Aristoff PA, Downey KM, So AG, Resnick L, Tarpley WG. Nonnucleoside reverse transcriptase inhibitors that potently and

specifically block HIV-1 replication. Proc Natl Acad Sci USA 1991;88:8806–8810.

61. Roxane Laboratories, Inc. Viramune (nevirapine). 1996.

62. Saag MS, Emini EA, Laskin OL, Douglas J, Lapidus WI, Schleif WA, Whitley RJ, Hildebrand C, Byrnes VW, Kappes JC, Anderson KW, Massari FE, Shaw GM, the L-697,661 Working Group. A short-term clinical evaluation of L697,661, a nonnucleoside inhibitor of HIV-1 reverse transcriptase. N Engl J Med 1993;329:1065–1072.

63. Saag M, Johnson V, Wei X, Sommadossi JP, Myers M, Cort S, Hall D, Piatak M, Lifson J, Shaw G, and the BI1009 Working Group. Clinical, pharmacokinetic, and virologic results in adults treated with nevirapine (Nev) in combination with AZT/ddC, AZT/ddI or ddI alone: final report of the BI1009 study [Abstract M16]. Programs and abstracts of the 34th Interscience Conference on Antimicrobial Agents and Chemotherapy, Orlando, FL, Oct 4–7, 1994.

64. Sahai J, Cameron W, Salgo M, Stewart F, Myers M, Lamson M, Gagnier P. Drug interaction study between saquinavir (SQV) and nevirapine (NVP) [Abstract 614]. Program and abstracts of the Fourth Conference on Retroviruses and Opportunistic Infections, Washington, DC, Jan 22–26, 1997.

65. Silverstein H, Riska P, Johnstone JN, Richter I, Norris S, Hattox S, Grob P. Nevirapine, a nonnucleoside reverse transcriptase inhibitor, freely enters the brain and crosses the placental barrier [Abstract TuB2325]. Programs and abstracts of the XI International Conference on AIDS, Vancouver, British Columbia, Jul 7–12, 1996.

66. Smerdon SJ, Jager J, Wang J, Kohlstaedt LA, Chirino AJ, Friedman JM, Rice PA, Steitz TA. Structure of the biding site for nonnucleoside inhibitors of the reverse transcriptase of human immunodeficiency virus type. Proc Natl Acad Sci USA 1994;26: 3911–3915.

67. Spence RA, Kati WM, Anderson KS, Johnson KA. Mechanism of inhibition of HIV-1 reverse transcriptase by nonnucleoside inhibitors. Science 1995;267:988–993.

68. Staszewski S, Emini E, Massari F, Hoffstedt B, Durr-Kihn S, Stille W. A double-blind randomized trial for safety, clinical efficacy, biological activity and susceptibility testing in 120 HIV positive patients treated with L,697,661, AZT and combinations of both drugs [Abstract WS-B26–4]. Program and abstracts of the IXth International Conference on AIDS, Berlin, Jun 6–11, 1993.

69. Staszweski S, Miller V, Rehmet S, Stark T, Stille W, Peeters M, DeBrabander M, DeCree J, Stoffels P, Harvey G, VanDen-Broeck R, Janssen PAJ. A triple combination study with zidovudine, lamivudine (3TC) and loviride (R89439) in p24 posi-

tive HIV-1 infected patients. An interim analysis [Abstract I158]. Programs and abstracts of the 34th Interscience Conference on Antimicrobial Agents and Chemotherapy, Orlando, FL, Oct 4–7, 1994.

70. Volberding PA, Lagakos SW, Grimes JM, Stein DS, Balfour HH, Reichman RC, Bartlett JA, Hirsch MS, Phair JP, Mitsuyasu RT, Fischl MA, Soeiro R, for the AIDS Clinical Trials Group of the National Institute of Allergy and Infectious Diseases. The duration of zidovudine benefit in persons with asymptomatic HIV infection: prolonged evaluation of protocol 019 of the AIDS Clinical Trial Group. JAMA 1994;272:437–442.

71. Wainberg MA, Birch C, for the Boehringer-Ingelheim 1046 Study Team (INCAS Trial). Phenotypic and genotypic resistance emergent in naive HIV-1 patients treated with combinations of reverse transcriptase inhibitors [Abstract OP7.2]. Program and abstracts of the Third International Congress on Drug Therapy in HIV Infection, Birmingham, England, Nov 3–7, 1996.

72. Wathen LK, Freimuth WW, Batts DH, Cox SR. Phenotypic and genotypic characterization of HIV-1 viral isolates from patients treated with combined AZT and delavirdine mesylate (DLV) therapy. Third International Workshop on HIV Drug Resistance, Kauai, Hawaii, Aug 2–5, 1994.

73. Wathen LK, Freimuth, Cox SR, Daenzer CL, Peel BG, Roberts CR, Mahrer JM, Batts DH, Pharmacia & Upjohn Company, Kalamazoo, MI and SRA Technologies, Rockville, MD. Phenotypic sensitivity of HIV-1 viral isolates during combination delavirdine + zidovudine therapy. Program and abstracts of the Fourth Conference on Retroviruses and Opportunistic Infections, Washington, DC, Jan 22–26, 1997.

74. Wu JC, Warren TC, Adams J, Proudfoot J, Skiles J, Raghavan P, Perry C, Potocki I, Farina PR, Grob PM. A novel, dipyridodiazepinone inhibitor of HIV-1 reverse transcriptase acts through a non-substrate binding site. Biochemistry 1991;30:2022–2026.

75. Yazdanian M, Ratigan S, Joseph D, Silverstein H, Riska P, Johnstone JN, Richter I, Norris S, Hattox S. Nevirapine, a nonnucleoside RT inhibitor, readily permeates the blood brain barrier [Abstract 567]. Programs and abstracts for the Fourth Conference on Retroviruses and Opportunistic Infections, Washington, DC, Jan 22–26, 1997.

76. Young SD, Britcher SF, Tran LO, Payne LS, Lumma WC, Lyle TA, Huff JR, Anderson PS, Olsen DB, Carroll SS, Pettibone DJ, O'Brien JA, Ball RG, Balani SK, Lin JH, Chen I-W, Schleif WA, Sardana VV, Long WJ, Byrnes VW, Emini EA. L-743726 (DMP-266): a novel, highly potent nonnucleoside inhibitor of the human immunodeficiency virus type 1 reverse transcriptase. Antimicrob Agents Chemother 1995;39:2602–2605.

Antiretroviral Agents: Protease Inhibitors

Rebecca L. Coleman

The introduction of HIV (human immunodeficiency virus) protease inhibitors in 1996–1997 had a significant impact on the treatment of HIV infection, offering the first alternative to nucleoside antiretrovirals (zidovudine, didanosine, zalcitabine, stavudine, and lamivudine) and changing the management of HIV infection from a model emphasizing palliation for a rapidly terminal disease to one of chronic disease management. While these drugs have had a dramatic impact on the disease course in many individuals, their long-term effectiveness and tolerability remains to be determined. Four competitive inhibitors of HIV protease have been approved by the United States Food and Drug Administration (FDA) for the treatment of HIV infection.

CHEMISTRY

The development of HIV protease inhibitors was aided by structure-based computational analysis of the protease enzyme. HIV protease is a large dimer with its active site located in the cleft created by the two identical halves. Following computer-assisted characterization of the crystalline structure of the enzyme and its active binding site, compounds were identified that would compete for occupation of the site. Chemical structures of these drugs are presented in Figure 1.

MECHANISM OF ACTION

HIV protease inhibitors interfere with the cleavage of polyproteins, an essential step late in the intracellular portion of the HIV life cycle that precedes assembly of immature virus proteins into particles (6). These assembled particles later bud from the cell as mature, infectious virions. Protease inhibitors compete for the active cleavage site on the protease enzyme, blocking cleavage of the polyproteins and maturation of new viral particles (Fig. 2).

MICROBIOLOGY

In addition to activity against HIV-1, some of these agents are active against HIV-2 and simian immunodeficiency virus (SIV) (Table 1). Like HIV-1, HIV-2 causes disease in humans, but the onset and velocity of the disease course tend to be less aggressive.

IN VITRO ANTI-HIV ACTIVITY

Comparative in vitro testing of the anti-HIV activity of the protease inhibitors has not been published. The 50% inhibitory concentrations (IC_{50}s) for saquinavir and ritonavir are reported to be 1 to 30 nM and 3.8 to 153 nM, respectively; 95% inhibitory concentrations (IC_{95}s) for indinavir and nelfinavir are reported to be 25 to 100 nM and 7 to 196 nM, respectively (13–16).

EVALUATION OF CLINICAL EFFECTIVENESS

CD4+ lymphocyte counts have been used to characterize the clinical course of HIV disease and to document the effectiveness of many of the currently available treatment regimens. Improvement in CD4+ lymphocyte count was the basis for licensure of the nucleoside agents. CD4+ lymphocyte counts continues to provide relevant information for the clinical management of patients; however these counts reflect virus activity rather than directly measure virus. The development of PCR-based diagnostics in the mid-90s enabled direct measurement of virus in clinical specimens, and quantitative measure of HIV (viral load) is currently recognized as the most accurate way to evaluate clinical effectiveness of antiretroviral therapy. Evaluation of plasma HIV-1 RNA and CD4+ lymphocyte changes during initiation of antiretroviral therapy with nucleoside reverse transcriptase inhibitors and with combinations of nucleoside and nonnucleoside reverse transcriptase inhibitors has demonstrated the prognostic value of these measures. CD4+ lymphocyte count continues to provide useful information for the clinician and can be used in combination with viral load to predict disease prognosis (4, 5, 8–12, 18).

CLINICAL STUDIES

Until comparative studies are completed, only a limited basis exists for determining the relative clinical efficacy of the HIV protease inhibitors. Differences in study population, assay methods, and analysis detract from the reliability of cross-study comparisons.

Saquinavir

Saquinavir was the first protease inhibitor approved for human use. The current formulation of the drug suffers from poor absolute bioavailability (4%) but is generally well tolerated. A new formulation should improve bioavailability. The existing formulation has been studied as a single agent, in combination with nucleoside antiretrovirals and, in an effort to capitalize on the pharmacokinetic interactions of these drugs, in combination with other protease inhibitors.

Saquinavir, in combination with one or two nucleoside reverse transcriptase inhibitors, has been studied in 302 patients with a median of 27 months of previous exposure to zidovudine (AIDS Clinical Trials Group study 229). Patients were randomly assigned to receive (a) saquinavir (600 mg thrice daily) plus zidovudine (200 mg thrice daily) plus zalcitabine (0.75 mg thrice daily), (b) saquinavir (600 mg thrice daily) plus zidovudine (200 mg thrice daily), or (c) zidovudine (200 mg thrice daily) plus zalcitabine (0.75 mg thrice daily). In this study of patients with a median baseline CD4+ lymphocyte count of 156

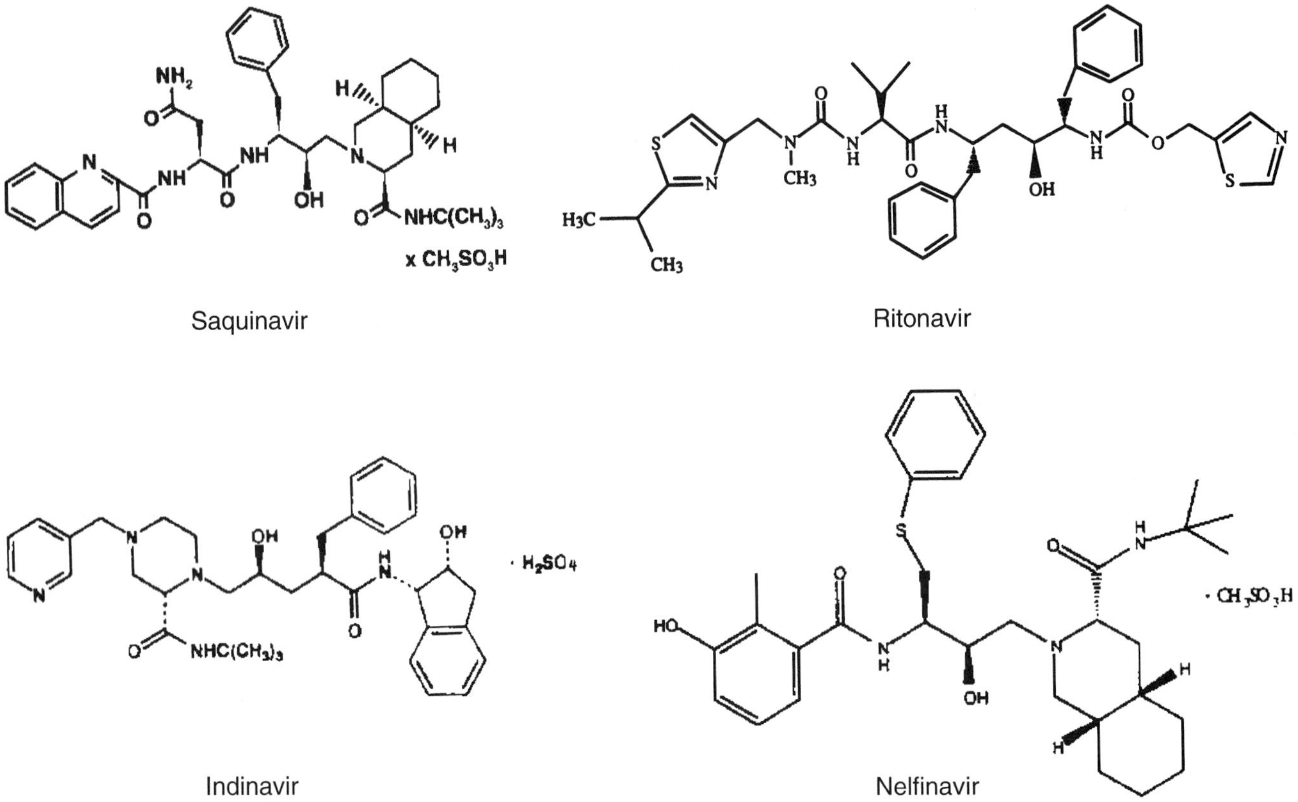

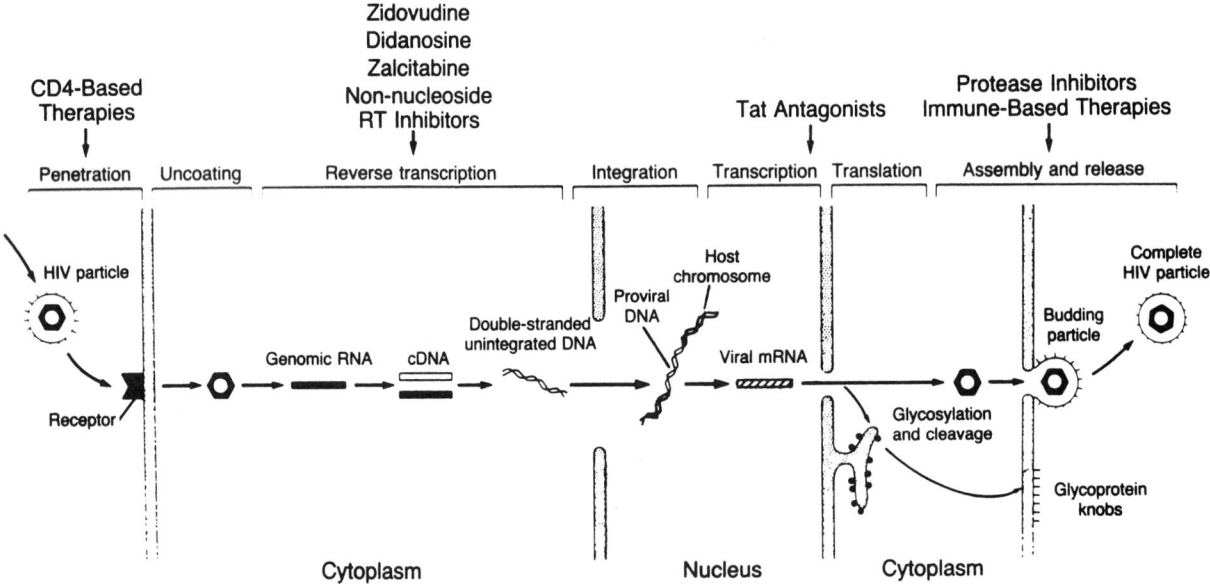

FIGURE 1. Chemical structures of saquinavir, ritonavir, indinavir, and nelfinavir.

FIGURE 2. Life cycle of HIV, focusing on protease enzyme role. (From Hirsch MS, D'Aquila RT. Therapy for human immunodeficiency virus infection. N Engl J Med 1993;328:1686–1695.)

cells/mm³ (range, 25–394), the three-drug combination significantly improved both viral load and CD4+ lymphocyte counts compared with either two-drug combination (2).

A second study compared saquinavir (600 mg thrice daily) plus zalcitabine (0.75 mg thrice daily) with monotherapy using saquinavir (600 mg thrice daily) or zalcitabine (0.75 mg thrice daily). In this study population (median CD4+ lymphocytes, 160–180 cells/mm³), there was significantly greater increase in CD4+ lymphocytes ($P < .001$) and a significantly greater decrease ($P = .001$) in viral load in the three-drug therapy group

TABLE 1 • Antiviral Spectrum (PIs)	
Viruses	
Saquinavir	HIV-1, HIV-2, SIV
Ritonavir	HIV-1, HIV-2
Indinavir	HIV
Nelfinavir	HIV-1, HIV-2

than in either monotherapy group. Further, in analysis of clinical endpoints, three-drug therapy was more beneficial than either monotherapy in time to first AIDS-defining event or death ($P = .0002$) or time to death alone ($P = .002$) (7, 19).

Ritonavir

Approval of ritonavir marked the availability of more potent protease inhibitors for the treatment of HIV infection. The effectiveness of this drug has, however, been compromised in some patients by treatment-limiting adverse effects and a greater potential for significant drug interactions. An algorithm for initiation of the drug based on its pharmacokinetic profile has improved tolerance in the early stages of treatment, and widespread promotion of the need for careful evaluation of the potential for drug interactions has limited the number of clinically significant misadventures involving ritonavir. The initial approval for use in adults was expanded to include children in 1997. Ritonavir has been studied as a single agent, in combination with nucleoside antiretrovirals, and in combination with other protease inhibitors.

One of the ritonavir clinical studies (Abbott Laboratories study 247) documented the first survival benefit secondary to antiretroviral therapy with protease inhibitors. Some 1090 patients with late-stage AIDS (CD4+ cell counts ≤ 100) were randomized to receive placebo or ritonavir (600 mg twice daily) in addition to existing nucleoside antiretroviral therapy. The group with ritonavir added to their therapy had significant improvement in several measures including increased CD4 counts, decreased viral load over the first 16 weeks, disease progression (17 vs. 34%), and mortality (5.8 vs. 10.1%).

A second study (Abbott 245) examined the effect of ritonavir in 356 treatment-naive patients with CD4+ cell counts averaging 364 who were randomized to receive ritonavir (600 mg twice daily), zidovudine (200 mg thrice daily), or ritonavir (600 mg twice daily) plus zidovudine (200 mg thrice daily). All three groups showed improved CD4+ cell counts and viral load. The two groups receiving ritonavir had greater increases in CD4+ cell counts and decreases in viral load than the group receiving zidovudine monotherapy.

Indinavir

Release of indinavir closely followed release of ritonavir, offering an alternative for patients unable to tolerate ritonavir. In general, indinavir is well tolerated but requires more attention to dosing because the drug must be taken every 8 hours and at least 1 hour away from meals. Indinavir has been studied in several HIV-postitive populations evaluating the drug in combination with one or more nucleoside antiretroviral agents. In

each study, those receiving indinavir showed significant improvement over controls.

Merck study 028 evaluated 244 antiretroviral treatment-naive patients with a mean CD4+ cell count of 145. Patients were randomly assigned to receive indinavir (800 mg every 8 h alone), indinavir (800 mg every 8 h) plus zidovudine (200 mg thrice daily), or zidovudine (200 mg thrice daily) alone. After 24 weeks, the groups receiving indinavir alone or indinavir plus zidovudine had significant and sustained increases in CD4+ cell counts (average increase, >100 cells) and significant and sustained decreases in HIV viral load averaging more than one log. The zidovudine-treated group had an initial increase in CD4+ cells averaging about 50, which returned toward baseline by 24 weeks. Viral load decrease in the zidovudine-treated group averaged less than 0.5 log and was sustained at approximately 0.25 log less than baseline by 24 weeks.

Merck study 033 likewise evaluated antiretroviral treatment-naive patients randomized to the same three treatments used in study 028; 266 patients with a mean CD4+ cell count of 254 were randomized into the three groups. Again, after 24 weeks, the two groups receiving indinavir alone or indinavir plus zidovudine had significant and sustained responses measured as an increase in CD4+ cell count and a decrease in HIV viral load, compared with the group receiving zidovudine alone.

In study 035, 96 zidovudine-experienced patients (mean, 31 months) with CD4+ cell counts averaging 175 were randomized to one of three groups: (a) indinavir (800 mg every 8 h) alone, (b) indinavir (800 mg every 8 h) plus zidovudine (200 mg thrice daily) plus lamivudine (150 mg twice daily), or (c) zidovudine (200 mg thrice daily) plus lamivudine (150 mg twice daily). As might be expected in a study in which every patient received at least one new drug, all three groups had positive responses in terms of CD4+ cell count elevation and viral load decrease.

Additional trials have demonstrated the safety and effectiveness of indinavir in combination with stavudine and didanosine.

Nelfinavir

Nelfinavir was the fourth protease inhibitor to gain FDA approval. The drug was unique among this class of agents in gaining indications for both adults and children simultaneously.

Two pivotal studies using nelfinavir were conducted in adults infected with HIV. The first evaluated two doses of nelfinavir (500 or 750 mg thrice daily) in combination with stavudine with stavudine alone in 308 patients with a median CD4+ lymphocyte count of 279 and a mean HIV RNA level of 141,369 copies/mL ($\log_{10} = 4.86$). Previous zidovudine experience ranged from none (20% of subjects) to a mean duration of 32 months in those with any zidovudine experience. An analysis of data through 24 weeks showed that CD4+ lymphocyte counts in the two nelfinavir plus stavudine groups increased significantly more than those in the stavudine-alone group, and HIV RNA decreased significantly more in the combination groups than in the stavudine-alone group.

The second study evaluated 297 patients receiving (a) nelfinavir (500 mg thrice daily) plus zidovudine plus lamivudine, *(b)* nelfinavir (750 mg thrice daily) plus zidovudine plus lamivudine, or *(c)* zidovudine plus lamivudine. The mean baseline CD4+ lymphocytes count was 288 cells/mm³, and the baseline plasma HIV RNA level was 153,044 copies/mL ($\log_{10}$ = 4.86) in these patients with no previous exposure to antiretroviral therapy. After 24 weeks, most subjects in both of the three-drug combination groups (but not in the two-drug group) had HIV RNA levels of 1200 copies or less, the lower limit of detection for the assay used.

Combination Protease Inhibitor Therapy

The rationale for administering two protease inhibitors parallels the basis for most combination therapies, the desire for increased efficacy, minimal toxicity, or avoidance of a factor that compromises efficacy, such as development of resistance or tolerance. Combinations of the current protease inhibitors may increase efficacy without increasing toxicity, because their side effect profiles do not overlap, for the most part. The potent inhibition of CYP-450 3A4 exerted by ritonavir and to a lesser extent by the other protease inhibitors may be exploited to increase the serum concentration of the added drug, enabling dose reduction, or to adjust the dosing schedule to improve patient acceptance.

To evaluate the effects of higher serum levels of saquinavir, the combination of ritonavir and saquinavir was studied. Cytochrome P-450 3A4 is responsible for 90% of the metabolism of saquinavir. Ritonavir, a potent inhibitor of CYP3A4, was selected because of its ability to block metabolism of drugs requiring CYP3A4. The two drugs have independent antiviral activity, nonoverlapping toxicities, and different mutational patterns. In the evaluation of ritonavir and saquinavir, serum concentrations of saquinavir were greatly enhanced by administration with ritonavir (600 mg twice daily), resulting in levels several times those obtained with saquinavir administered alone. Both viral load decrease and CD4 count increase were documented in this small pilot study. Increased side effects were noted, proportional to the increased exposure to saquinavir, but were not treatment limiting. Definition of long-term effects, including any alterations in the development of mutations, awaits further study.

The strategy of combining nelfinavir and saquinavir has been studied. Patients used the new formulation of saquinavir (800 mg thrice daily) and nelfinavir at the approved dose of 750 mg thrice daily. As in the study of combination ritonavir/saquinavir, the saquinavir AUC was five times greater when administered with nelfinavir, because of inhibition of CYP3A4 by nelfinavir. Patients tolerated the combination well and demonstrated increased CD4+ cell counts and decreased viral loads. Further studies of protease combinations that take advantage of the opportunity to alter hepatic metabolism are under way.

RESISTANCE

Both clinical and laboratory isolates with reduced sensitivity have been found for each of the HIV protease inhibitors. While some genotypic changes reliably predict alterations in sensitivity, not all phenotypic changes documented in resistance assays correlate with identification of genotypic changes (Tables 2 and 3).

The clinical implications of genotypic mutations identified to date is the source of much debate, as are the various treatment strategies that claim to take advantage of differences in the mutation patterns associated with these drugs. Further information is required before resistance testing is a useful clinical tool for managing HIV protease therapy.

PHARMACOKINETICS

See Tables 4 to 7.

DOSE

See Tables 8 to 11. No formal dosing adjustments are recommended at this time for differences in body composition (lean vs.

TABLE 2 • Resistance Mutations Selected In Vitro		
	Mutations	**Mutations Conferring Resistance**[a]
Saquinavir	G48V, L90M, I54V, I84V, A71V	G48V, L90M, I84V
Ritonavir	I84V, V82F, A71V, M46I	I84V, V82F
Indinavir		V32I, M46I, A71V, V82
ANelfinavir		

[a] Data from Schinazi RF, Larder BA, Mellors JW. Mutations in HIV-1 reverse transcriptase and protease associated with drug resistance. Int Antiviral News 1996;4:95–107.

TABLE 3 • Resistance Mutations Selected In Vivo		
	Mutations (PIs)	**Mutations Conferring Resistance**[a] **(20)**
Saquinavir	L90M, G48V	L90M, G48V
Ritonavir	V82P/A, I54V, A71V/T, I36L	
Indinavir		L10R, M46I, L63P, V82T, I84V
Nelfinavir	30, 35, 36, 46, 71, 77, 88	

[a] Data from Schinazi RF, Larder BA, Mellors JW. Mutations in HIV-1 reverse transcriptase and protease associated with drug resistance. Int Antiviral News 1996;4:95–107.

TABLE 4 • Absorption

	T_{max} (h)	C_{max}	C_{trough}	Food Effect	Bioavailability (range)	Comments
Saquinavir (hard-gel formulation) (600 mg t.i.d.)	2.4 (fasting) 3.8 (nonfasting)	253.3 ng/mL		High-fat meal increases absorption	4 (1–9) single 4600-mg dose	Greater bioavailability in HIV-infected than in healthy subjects; dose disproportionate (higher doses = higher levels than predicted based on lower doses)
Ritonavir (600 mg q. 12 h)	2 (fasting) 4 (nonfasting)	11.2 ± 3.6 μg/mL	3.7 ± 2.6 μg/mL	15% higher with food		Possible alteration in clearance with continued dosing, AUC is less than predicted from single doses
Indinavir (800 mg q. 8 h)	0.8 ± 0.3	12,6 17 ± 4037 nM	251 ± 178 nM	High fat, calories, and protein decreased AUC by 77% ± 8%; lighter meals had no effect		Dose disproportionate across 200–1000 mg range (higher doses = higher levels than predicted based on lower doses)
Nelfinavir	2–4 (single or multiple doses of 500 or 750 mg)	3–4 μg/mL (750 mg t.i.d.)	1–3 μg/mL (750 mg t.i.d.)	High-fat meal results in 2–3 times higher levels		Dose disproportionate with single doses; not seen with multidosing (higher doses = greater levels than predicted based on lower doses)

TABLE 5 • Distribution

	AUC	Vdss	Protein Binding	CNS Penetration
Saquinavir (hard-gel formulation)	757.2 ng·h/mL	700 L	98 (15–700 ng/mL)	Negligible levels
Ritonavir	129.5 ± 47.1 μg·h/mL (cap) 129 ± 39.3 μg·h/mL (soln)	98–99 (0.01–30 μg/mL)		
Indinavir	30,691 ± 11,407 nM·h		60 (81–16,300 nM)	
Nelfinavir		2–7 L/kg	>98	

TABLE 6 • Metabolism

	Presence in Plasma	Metabolism
Saquinavir	Plasma (p.o.) unchanged 13% (i.v.) unchanged 66% Extensive 1st pass metabolism	CYP3A4 (90%); several mono- and dihydroxylated metabolites; all inactive compounds
Ritonavir	Nearly all in plasma is unchanged; low levels of major metabolite	CYP 3A4, 2D6, 2C9, 2C19, 2A6, 1A2, and 2E1; 5 metabolites, major active metabolite—isopropylthiazole oxidation (M-2)
Indinavir		CYP3A4; 7 metabolites, 1 glucuronide, 6 oxidative metabolites
Nelfinavir	82–86% unchanged	CYP3A4 primarily; several metabolites; one major active metabolite

fat) or in the presence of ascites, edema, diarrhea, malabsorption, decreased plasma proteins, malnutrition, or wasting. Caution should be used in treating patients with these presentations.

ADVERSE EFFECTS

With the exception of the mechanism for the nephrolithiasis noted with indinavir therapy, mechanisms for most common adverse effects associated with the use of HIV protease inhibitors are not known. Indinavir-associated nephrolithiasis is apparently related to the urinary excretion of this agent. Some stones recovered from patients have contained indinavir.

Ramped-dosing initiation, defined as beginning treatment with a low dose and escalating to full dose, has been used successfully to limit the gastrointestinal effects associated with ritonavir therapy. The recommended algorithm initiates dosing at 300 mg twice daily, with 200 mg/day increases every few days to a full dose of 600 mg twice daily after 10 to 14 days.

TABLE 7 • Elimination

	Total Cl	Urine (%)	Feces (%)	Half-Life (h)	Renal Cl
Saquinavir	1.14 L/h/kg	1–3	81–88	7 (mean residence time)	
Ritonavir		11.3 ± 2.8	86.4 ± 2.9		
		Unchanged	Unchanged	3–5	<0.1 L/h
		3.5 ± 1.8%	33.8 + 10.8		
Indinavir		19 ± 3	83 ± 1	1.8 ± 0.4	
		Unchanged	Unchanged		
		19.1%	9.4		
Nelfinavir		1–2	87 Metabolites	3.5–5	
			78 Unchanged		
			22		

TABLE 8 • Adult Dosage Regimens

	Adult Dosage
Saquinavir (hard-gel formulation)	600 mg daily with meals
Ritonavir	600 mg b.i.d. with meals
Indinavir	800 mg q. 8 h, 1 h before or 1 h after meals
Nelfinavir	750 mg t.i.d. with meals

TABLE 9 • Pediatric Dosage Regimens

	Pediatric Dosage
Saquinavir (hard-gel formulation)	Safety not established in children < 16 years
Ritonavir	400 mg/m² twice daily
Indinavir	Safety and effectiveness not established
Nelfinavir	20–30 mg/kg thrice daily

TABLE 10 • Dosing in Renal Dysfunction

	Dosage
Saquinavir (hard-gel formulation)	Pharmacokinetics not studied in renal insufficiency, but renal excretion is negligible
Ritonavir	Pharmacokinetics not studied in renal insufficiency, but renal excretion is negligible
Indinavir	Pharmacokinetics not studied in renal insufficiency
Nelfinavir	Pharmacokinetics not studied in renal insufficiency, but renal excretion is negligible

TABLE 11 • Dosing in Hepatic Failure

	Dosage
Saquinavir (hard gel formulation)	Pharmacokinetics not studied in hepatic insufficiency—no recommendation
Ritonavir	Pharmacokinetics not studied in hepatic insufficiency—no recommendation
Indinavir	Reduce dose to 600 mg every 8 h in mild-to-moderate hepatic insufficiency due to cirrhosis
Nelfinavir	Pharmacokinetics not studied in hepatic insufficiency—no recommendation

Protease inhibitor therapy for patients experiencing treatment-limiting adverse effects should be stopped rather than adjusted downward, to avoid exposing the patient to subtherapeutic doses and increasing the risk for development of resistance (Table 12).

LABORATORY MONITORING

For evaluation of drug effectiveness, measurement of viral load is recommended prior to initiation of new or altered antiretroviral treatment and then approximately 4 weeks later. Follow-up testing is recommended every 3 to 6 months (3). Therapeutic drug monitoring is not currently available for clinical monitoring of protease inhibitor therapy. Safety testing including blood chemistry should be checked at baseline and periodically during therapy.

TABLE 12 • Adverse Effects

	Adverse Effect
Saquinavir	Diarrhea
	Abdominal discomfort
	Nausea
Ritonavir	Nausea
	Diarrhea
	Vomiting
	Anorexia
	Abdominal pain
	Taste perversion
	Circumoral and peripheral paresthesias
Indinavir	Nephrolithiasis
	Asymptomatic hyperbilirubinemia
	Hepatitis
Nelfinavir	Diarrhea

TABLE 13 • Drug Interactions

	Interacting Drugs	Effect	Mechanism
Indinavir (Crixivan)	Ketoconazole (Nizoral)	↑ Indinavir AUC (68% ± 48%); consider indinavir dose reduction to 600 mg every 8 h	CYP3A4 induction by ketoconazole
	Rifabutin (Mycobutin)	↑ Rifabutin AUC (204% ± 142%); reduce rifabutin dose by 50% ↓ indinavir AUC (32% ± 19%)	CYP3A4 inhibition by indinavir
	Rifampin	Possible ↓ in indinavir plasma concentrations **Do not coadminster**	CYP3A4 induction by rifampin
	Terfenidine (Seldane) Astemizole (Hismanal) Cisapride (Propulsid) Pimozide (Orap)	↑ Antihistamine, cisapride serum levels; potential for serious and/or life-threatening arrhythmias **Do not coadminister**	CYP3A4 inhibition by indinavir
	Delavirdine (Rescriptor)	No significant effect on delavirdine, indinavir AUC ↑	CYP3A4 inhibition by delavirdine
	Nevirapine (Viramune)	↓ Indinavir AUC (28%); ↓ nevirapine AUC (<10%)	CYP450 3A induction by nevirapine
	Nelfinavir (Viracept)	Indinavir AUC ↑ (51%); Nelfinavir AUC ↑ (83%)	CYP3A4 inhibition by indinavir and nelfinavir
	Midazolam (Versed) Triazolam (Halcion)	↑ Benzodiazepine serum levels; potential for prolonged sedation	Competition for CYP3A4
Nelfinavir (Viracept)	Terfenidine (Seldane) Astemizole (Hismanal) Cisapride (Propulsid) Pimozide (Orap)	↑ Antihistamine, cisapride serum levels; potential for serious and/or life-threatening arrhythmias **Do not coadminister**	CYP3A4 inhibition by nelfinavir
	Ethinyl estradiol (birth control pills)	↓ Plasma concentrations of ethinyl estradiol—possible failure of birth control	Glucuronyl transferase induction by nelfinavir (?)
	Ketoconazole (Nizoral)	↑ Nelfinavir AUC	CYP3A4 inhibition by ketoconazole
	Rifampin	↓ Nelfinavir AUC	CYP3A4 induction by rifampin
	Ritonavir (Norvir)	Nelfinavir AUC ↑ (152%); effect on nelfinavir AUC not yet known	CYP3A4 inhibition by ritonavir
	Indinavir (Crixivan)	Indinavir AUC ↑ (51%); nelfinavir AUC ↑ (83%)	CYP3A4 inhibition by indinavir and nelfinavir
Ritonavir (Norvir)	Amiodarone (Cordarone) Astemizole (Hismanal) Bepridil (Vascor) Bupropion (Wellbutrin) Cisapride (Propulsid) Clozapine (Clozaril) Dihydroergotamine (DHE 45) Encainide (Enkaid) Ergotamine (Ergostat, Wigraine, Cafergot, Ercaf, Cafatine, Caretrate) Flecanide (Tambocor) Loratadine (Claritin) Meperidine (Demerol) Piroxicam (Feldene) Propafenone (Rythmol) Propoxyphene (Darvon, Darvocet) Quinidine Rifabutin (Mycobutin) Terfenidine (Seldane) Pimozide (Orap)	↑ Plasma concentrations of drug in second column; potential for serious toxicities **Do not coadminister**	
	Alprazolam (Xanax) Clorazepate (Klonopin) Diazepam (Valium) Estazolam (ProSom) Flurazepam (Dalmane)	↑ Plasma concentrations of drug in second column; potential for extreme sedation and respiratory depression **Do not coadminister**	

continued

TABLE 13 • **Drug Interactions—*continued***

Interacting Drugs	Effect	Mechanism
Midazolam (Versed) Triazolam (Halcion) Zolpidem (Ambien) Alfentanil (Alfenta) Amlodipine (Norvasc) Carbamazepine (Tegretol) Clonazepam (Klonopin) Cylcosporine (Sandimmune) Dexamethasone Diltiazem (Cardiazem) Disopyramide (Norpace) Dronabinol (Marinol) Erythromycin Ethosuximide (Zarontin) Etoposide Fentanyl (Duragesic) Felodipine (Plendil) Isradipine (DynaCirc) Lidocaine Lovastatin (Mevacor) Nefazodone (Serzone) Nicardipine (Cardine) Nifedipine (Procardia, Adalat) Nimodipine (Nimotop) Nisoldipine (Sular) Ondansetron (Zofran) Paclitaxel (Taxol) Pravastatin (Pravachol) Prednisone Quinine Rifampin Saquinavir (Invirase) Sertraline (Zoloft) Tamoxifen (Nolvadex) Tacrolimus (Prograf) Trazodone (Desyrel) Verapamil (Calan, Isoptin) Vinblastine Vincristine Warfarin, *R*-enantiomer (Coumadin)	>3× ↑ AUC of drug in second column; coadminister with caution; monitor drug levels when possible	CYP3A4 inhibition by ritonavir
Amitriptyline (Elavil) Chlorpromazine (Thorazine) Clomipramine (Anafranil) Desipramine (Norpramin, Pertofrane) Fluoxetine (Prozac) Haloperidol (Haldol) Hydrocodone (Hycodan) Imipramine (Tofranil) Maprotiline (Ludiomil) Methamphetamine (Desoxyn) Metoprolol (Lopressor) Mexiletine (Mexitil) Nortriptyline (Aventyl, Pamedor) Oxycodone (Percocet, Percodan) Paroxetine (Paxil)	1.5–3× ↑ AUC of drug in second column	CYP2D6 inhibition by ritonavir

continued

TABLE 13 • Drug Interactions—*continued*

Interacting Drugs	Effect	Mechanism
Perphenazine (Trilafon)		
Pindolol (Visken)		
Propranolol (Inderal)		
Risperidone Risperdal)		
Thioridazine (Mellaril)		
Timolol (Blocadren)		
Tramadol (Ultram)		
Venlafaxine (Effexor)		
Diclofenac (Cataflam, Voltaren)	1.5–3× ↑ or ↓ in AUC of drug in second column; monitor need for increased dose or toxicity	CYP2C9/19 competition
Glipizide (Glucotrol)		
Glyburide		
Iboprofen		
Indomethacin		
Lansoprazole (Prevacid)		
Omeprazole (Prilosec)		
Losartan (Cozaar)		
Phenytoin (Dilantin)		
Proguanil		
Tolbutamide		
Warfarin, *S*-enantiomer (Coumadin)		
Acebutolol (Sectral)	Possible ↑ AUC of drug in second column; monitor drug levels when possible	Unknown
Albendazole		
Betaxolol (Kerlone)		
Chloroquine		
Cimetidine		
Cyclophosphamide		
Daunorubicin		
Digoxin		
Doxazosin (Cardura)		
Doxepin (Sinequan)		
Doxorubicin		
Fluvastatin (Lescol)		
Fluvoxamine (Luvox)		
Gemfibrozil (Gemcor, Lopid)		
Itraconazole (Sporonax)		
Ketoconazole (Nizoral)		
Miconazole (Monistat)		
Methadone		
Methylphenidate (Ritalin)		
Metronidazole (Flagyl)		
Nabumetone (Relafen)		
Penbutolol (Levatol)		
Pentoxifylline (Trental)		
Phenobarbital		
Prazosin (Minpress)		
Primaquine		
Prochlorperazine (Compazine)		
Promethazine (Phenergan)		
Pyrimethamine		
Simvastatin (Zocor)		
Sulindac (Clinoril)		
Tocainide (Tonocard)		
Terazosin (Hytrin)		
Disulfiram (Antabuse)	Possible disulfiram reaction	Both capsule and solution preparation contain ethanol
Atovaquone (Mepron)	Possible ↓ AUC of drug in second column; monitor need for increased dose	Increased glucuronidation
Clofibrate (Atromid-S)		
Codeine		

continued

TABLE 13 • Drug Interactions—*continued*

	Interacting Drugs	Effect	Mechanism
	Diphenoxylate (Lomotil)		
	Divalproex (Depakote)		
	Hydromorphone (Dilaudid)		
	Ketoprofen (Orudis)		
	Ketorolac (Tramadol)		
	Lamotrigine (Lamictel)		
	Lorazepam (Ativan)		
	Metoclopramide (Reglan)		
	Morphine		
	Naproxen (Naprosyn)		
	Oxazepam (Serax)		
	Propofol (Diprivan)		
	Temazepam (Restoril)		
	Theophylline		
	Theophylline	↓ AUC of theophylline (43%)	Induction of CYP1A2
	Ethinyl estradiol (birth control pills)	↓ AUC of ethinyl estradiol (41%)	Induction of glucuronyl transferase
Saquinavir (Invirase)	Ketoconazole (Nizoral)	↑ Saquinavir AUC; no adjustment necessary	CYP3A inhibition
	Terfenidine (Seldane)	↑ Antihistamine, cisapride serum	CYP3A inhibition
	Astemizole (Hismanal)	levels; potential for serious and/or	
	Cisapride (Propulsid)	and/olife-threatening arrhythmias	
	Pimozide (Orap)	**Do not coadminister**	
	Rifampin	↓ Saquinavir AUC by 80%	CYP3A induction
		Do not coadminister	
	Ritonavir (Norvir)	>3× ↑ AUC of saquinavir;	CYP3A inhibition by ritonavir,
	Delavirdine (Rescriptor)	coadminster with caution	delavirdine

DRUG INTERACTIONS

Hepatic metabolism of the protease inhibitors involves cytochrome P-450 3A4 (CYP3A4). Ritonavir is also a substrate for CYP 2D6, 2C9, 2C19, 2A6, 1A2, and 2E1 (in order of decreasing influence). These drugs also inhibit CYP 3A4 in approximately the following rank from most to least effective: ritonavir > indinavir ≥ nelfinavir > saquinavir. Other metabolic enzymes are affected by the protease inhibitors such as glucuronyl transferases (Table 13).

Only limited clinical evaluations have been completed examining the potential for drug interactions involving protease inhibitors. Caution should guide the use of protease inhibitors in combination with any drug that undergoes hepatic metabolism, particularly those with narrow therapeutic indexes. Appropriate monitoring for increased toxicity should be used. Antiretroviral regimens combining protease inhibitors with the nonnucleoside reverse transcriptase inhibitors delavirdine or nevirapine can be prescribed with caution. Delavirdine, also a CYP3A4 inhibitor, increases the AUC of both saquinavir and indinavir, but has little effect on ritonavir or nelfinavir. While increased exposure to saquinavir is desirable, the toxicities associated with indinavir are proportional to exposure and thus the dose of indinavir should be reduced to 400 or 600 mg thrice daily when prescribed in combination with delavirdine. Nevirapine, a CYP3A4 inducer, can be prescribed in combination with ritonavir, indinavir, or nelfinavir without dose adjustment. Administration of nevirapine and saquinavir results in a reduction in saquinavir AUC of approximately 28%. While this is not usually considered a significant reduction when evaluating interactions, the marginal exposures achieved with the currently available formulation of saquinavir require careful consideration of possible alternatives, including increasing the prescribed dose of saquinavir. Interactions between the protease inhibitors and nucleoside agents (zidovudine, didanosine, zalcitabine, stavudine, and lamivudine) have not been encountered.

CLINICAL INDICATIONS

Indinavir and nelfinavir are FDA-approved for "treatment of HIV infection when antiretroviral therapy is warranted." Saquinavir has the same indication but is limited to use in combination with nucleoside analogues. Ritonavir has FDA approval for use as a single agent (monotherapy) and in combination with nucleosides. Demonstration that combinations of antiretroviral agents are more efficacious than single agents has resulted in the recommendation that monotherapy not be used and that changes in therapy include switching all agents. In particular, addition of a protease inhibitor should be accompanied by a switch in the nucleoside drugs being prescribed. Recently released guidelines for the treatment of patients with HIV infection recommend the use of ritonavir, indinavir, or nelfinavir in combination with two nucleoside analogues when an aggressive regimen is desired for the treatment of individuals with plasma viral RNA levels above 5000 copies/mL (1) or 10,000 copies/mL (3). Saquinavir (in the currently available hard gel formulation) is considered less likely to achieve the desired result of undetectable plasma viral RNA levels.

Patients who fail to respond or who experience clinical failure while receiving therapy containing a protease inhibitor may benefit from switching to a combination. There is limited experience with patients receiving treatment with ritonavir and saquinavir subsequent to treatment with a regimen including a single protease inhibitor. Unfortunately, there is growing evidence that exposure to any of the protease inhibitors is associated with reduced response to either a second protease inhibitor or to combinations of protease inhibitors, measured either as a lack of initial response or decreased durability of response.

REFERENCES

1. Carpenter CC, Fischl MA, Hammer SM, Hirsch MS, Jacobsen DM, Katzenstein DA, Montaner JS, Richman DD, Saag, MS, Schooley RT, Thompson MA, Vella S, Yeni PG, Volberding PA. Antiretroviral therapy for HIV infection in 1997. JAMA 1997;277:1962–1969.
2. Collier AC, Coombs RW, Schoenfeld DA, Bassett RL, Timpone J, Baruch A, Jones M, Facey K, Whitacre C, McAuliffe VJ, Friedman HM, Merigan TC, Reichman RC, Hooper C, Corey L, for the AIDS Clinical Trials Group. Treatment of human immunodeficiency virus infection with saquinavir, zidovudine, and zalcitabine. N Engl J Med 1996;1334:1011–1017.
3. DHHS and Henry J. Kaiser Family Foundation Panel on Clinical Practices for Treatment of HIV Infection. Guidelines for the use of antiretroviral agents in HIV-infected adults and adolescents, 1997.
4. Hughes MD, Johnson VA, Hirsch MS, Bremer JW, Elbeik T, Erice A, Kuritzkes DR, Scott WA, Spector SA, Basgoz N, Fischl MA, D'Aquila RT. Monitoring plasma HIV-1 RNA levels in addition to CD4+ lymphocyte count improves assessment of antiretroviral therapeutic response. Ann Intern Med 1997;126:929–938.
5. Katzenstein DA, Hammer SM, Hughes MD, Gundacker H, Jackson JB, Fiscus S, Rasheed S, Elbeik T, Reichman R, Japour A, Merigan TC, Hirsch MS for the AIDS Clinical Trials Group Study 175 Virology Study Team. The relation of virologic and immunologic markers to clinical outcomes after nucleoside therapy in HIV-infected adults with 200 to 500 CD4 cells per cubic millimeter. N Engl J Med 1996;335:1091–1098.
6. Kohl NE, Emini EA, Scheif WA, Davis LJ, Heimbach JC, Dixon RAF, Scolnick EM, Sigal IS. Active human immunodeficiency virus protease is required for viral infectivity. Proc Natl Acad Sci USA 1988;85:4686–4690.
7. Lalezari J, Haubrich R, Burger HU, Beattie D, Doonatuacci L,

Salgo MP and the NV 14256 Study Team. Improved survival and decreased progression of HIV in patients treated with saquinavir plus HIVID [Abstract]. Presented at the Eleventh International Conference on AIDS, Vancouver, British Columbia, July 7–12, 1996.
8. Mellors JW, Kingsley LA, Rinaldo CR, Todd JA, Goo BS, Kokka RP, Gupta P. Quantitation of HIV-1 RNA in plasma predicts outcome after seroconversion. Ann Intern Med 1995;122: 573–579.
9. Mellors JW, Rinaldo CR, Gupta P, White RM, Todd JA, Kingsley LA. Prognosis in HIV-1 infection predicted by the quantity of virus in plasma. Science 1996;272:1167–1170.
10. Mellors JW, Munoz A, Giorgi JV, Margolick JB, Tassoni CJ, Gupta P, Kingsley LA, Todd JA, Saah AJ, Detels R, Phair JP, Rinaldo CR. Plasma viral load and CD4+lymphocytes as prognostic markers of HIV-1 infection. Ann Intern Med 1997;126: 946–954.
11. O'Brien WA, Hartigan PM, Martin D, Esinhard J, Hill A, Benoit S, Rubin M, Simberkoff MS, Hamilton JD, and the Veterans Affairs Cooperative Study Group on AIDS. Changes in plasma HIV-1 RNA and CD4+ lymphocyte counts and the risk of progression to AIDS. N Engl J Med 1996;334:426–431.
12. O'Brien WA, Hartigan PM, Daar ES, Simberkoff MS, Hamilton JD, and the VA Cooperative Study Group on AIDS. Changes in plasma HIV RNA levels and CD4+ lymphocyte counts predict both response to antiretroviral therapy and therapeutic failure. Ann Intern Med 1997 126;939–945.
13. Product Information, Invirase (saquinavir mesylate). Nutley, NJ: Roche Laboratories, January, 1997.
14. Product Information, Norvir (ritonavir). North Chicago, IL: Abbott Laboratories, March, 1997.
15. Product Information, Crixivan (indinavir sulfate). West Point, PA: Merck & Co., March, 1996.
16. Product Information, Viracept (nelfinavir mesylate). La Jolla, CA: Agouron Pharmaceuticals, March 21, 1997.
17. Saag MS, Holodnie M, Kuritzkes DR, O'Brien WA, Coombs R, Poscher ME, Jacobsen DM, Shaw GM, Richman DD, Volberding PA. HIV viral load markers in clinical practice. Nature Med 1996;2:625–629.
18. Saag MS. Use of HIV viral load in clinical practice: back to the future. Ann Intern Med 1997;126:983–985.
19. Salgo MP, Beattie D, Bragman K, Donatacci L, Jones M, Montgomery L, the NV14256 Study Team. Saquinavir (Invirase, SQV) vs. HIVID (zalcitibine, ddC) vs. combination as treatment for advanced HIV infection in patients discontinuing/unable to take Retrovir (zidovudine, ZDV) [Abstract]. Presented at the Eleventh International Conference on AIDS, Vancouver, British Columbia, July 7–12, 1996.
20. Schinazi RF, Larder BA, Mellors JW. Mutations in HIV-1 reverse 1996;4:95–107.

Antiretroviral Agents: Stavudine

John E. Fuchs, Jr. and Richard B. Pollard

CHEMICAL STRUCTURE AND STRUCTURAL ACTIVITY RELATIONSHIPS

Stavudine is a 2',3'-didehydro, 3'-deoxythymidine analogue of thymidine. Unlike thymidine, stavudine lacks a 3'-hydroxyl group on the pentose ring but contains a double bond between the 2'- and 3'-carbons on that ring. Zidovudine, also a thymidine analogue, differs from stavudine in containing a 3'-NH3 group without the 2'-3' double bond. With both zidovudine and stavudine, absence of the 3'-hydroxyl group on the pentose ring prevents the critical formation of 3',5'-phosphodiesterase linkage during DNA replication.

MECHANISM OF ACTION

Stavudine must be converted to a triphosphate metabolite before it is active against HIV. Stavudine enters HIV-infected cells by a nonfacilitated diffusion process (2, 10), and intracellular accumulation of stavudine is proportional to its extracellular concentration (3). The rate-limiting step for conversion to the active metabolite is monophosphorylation by cellular thymidine kinase (15, 60). Stavudine monophosphate is converted rapidly and completely to the triphosphate metabolite, so the mono- and diphosphate metabolite do not accumulate intracellularly. This lack of accumulation has been suggested to be partly responsible for stavudine's minimal bone marrow toxicity (60). Once formed, stavudine 5'-triphosphate interferes with the HIV life cycle by competing with thymidine 5'-triphosphate, an essential nucleotide used by the reverse transcriptase enzyme during transcription of viral RNA to DNA. As mentioned above, because stavudine-5'-triphosphate lacks a 3'-hydroxyl group, the critical 3'-5'phosphodiesterase linkage on the RNA template is not made, which results in chain termination of developing viral DNA (57). Additionally, extracellular concentrations of stavudine are proportional to its in vitro antiviral activity in human peripheral blood mononuclear cell (PBMC) and human T cell tissue cultures (37, 42).

Animal models and in vitro drug sensitivities are considered less than ideal in evaluating in vivo result for managing HIV. Most data on drug sensitivities, however, are derived from in vitro human T cells and PBMCs with replicating HIV. Stavudine and zidovudine both have greater activity in replicating human cells than in quiescent ones because of the greater activity of thymidine kinase (55). Therefore data derived from in vitro studies with these drugs may not indicate in vivo response, since both activated and quiescent cells are infected with HIV (16, 56a). Nonetheless, pooled data indicate an MIC_{50} (minimal inhibitory concentration for 50% of isolates) between 0.011 and 0.112 µg/mL (32). These and most data are derived from measuring the extracellular concentrations of stavudine in super-natant media containing human PBMC and T cells. It has been suggested that the intracellular concentrations of HIV reverse transcriptase and the phosphorylated metabolites of stavudine might provide a better measure of in vivo activity; however, such assays are difficult to perform (59).

The suggested dosing regimens of stavudine (every 12 h) are derived from the intracellular stavudine 5'-triphosphate half-life of 3.5 h rather than the plasma half-life, 1.5 h (59). Stavudine has not been shown to have significant activity against other viruses and bacteria (22, 58).

MECHANISMS OF RESISTANCE

Resistance to anti-HIV drugs is associated with disease progression and death (9, 39, 40). Therefore, extensive studies have been performed and are ongoing to identify the resistance patterns to various agents and to devise strategies to minimize the emergence of resistance.

Low levels of resistance to stavudine have been noted occasionally in clinical isolates of HIV-1. The resistance mutation most commonly, but not consistently, identified at codon 75 of the reverse transcriptase enzyme may be associated with decreased sensitivity (19, 31), and this mutation can produce cross-resistance to other dideoxynucleoside analogues including didanosine, lamivudine, and zalcitabine (17).

HIV isolates from a clinical trial that included 13 patients were tested for resistance. These patients had received stavudine at dosages between 0.25 and 2.0 mg/kg/day for more than 18 months (34). Isolates from two patients demonstrated an 8- and 12-fold decrease in sensitivity to stavudine. About half of the isolates demonstrated 9- to 176-fold resistance to zidovudine, and cross-resistance was demonstrated with didanosine. Of equal concern, however, are mutations at other sites on the reverse transcriptase enzyme. A mutation at codon 151 is especially bothersome, since it produces broad cross-resistance to all available nucleoside analogues, including stavudine (26). In general, however, stavudine resistance is moderate and has been relatively difficult to demonstrate in clinical samples. In fact, no consistent mutation that produces decreased sensitivity to stavudine has been identified.

EFFECT ON HUMAN CELLS

Studies evaluating the selective index (concentration required to kill 50% of human cells/concentration producing 50% viral inhibition) indicate that stavudine has good selectivity for HIV. HIV reverse transcriptase has about a 10,000-fold greater affinity for stavudine 5'-triphosphate than most human cellular DNA polymerases (60). Stavudine does interfere with mitochondrial DNA of various cell types, which may be related to some of stavudine's delayed toxicity, but this does not occur to the same extent as with didanosine or zalcitabine (6, 33). Additionally, stavudine is less toxic to in vitro human granulocyte-macrophage and erythroid progenitor cells than zalcitabine or zidovudine (14, 54, 60).

PHARMACOKINETICS
Absorption

Stavudine is rapidly and well absorbed from the gastrointestinal tract. Table 1 summarizes the average pharmacokinetic parameters for both adults and children. Peak serum levels occur about 1 h after an oral dose in adults and about 55 min in children (11, 28). Bioavailability is 99% in adults and 78% in children. The lower bioavailability in children may account for the higher dose requirement in the pediatric population (24, 28). Peak serum level and AUC increase proportionally over a dose range from 0.67 to 4 mg/kg, and stavudine does not accumulate after multiple dosing when it is administered at either 8- or 12-h intervals. The average peak serum level of stavudine is 1.2 μg/mL when blood is sampled 1 h after an oral dose of 0.67 mg/kg.

Distribution

The volume of distribution ranges from 0.54 to 0.69 L/kg in adults and is 9.3 L/mm^3 in children (11, 20, 24, 28), suggesting that stavudine is distributed into both extracellular and intracellular compartments. Limited human data have been published indicating that stavudine distributes into the cerebrospinal fluid

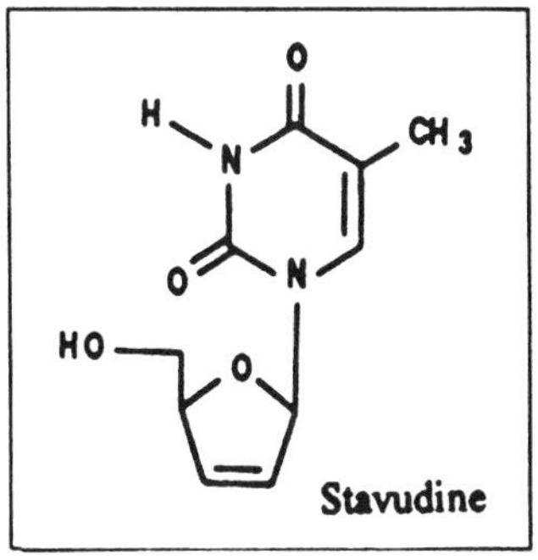

FIGURE 1. Stavudine structure.

(CSF) in clinically significant quantities (11). Stavudine CSF levels in two patients who were receiving chronic therapy with either 1.33 mg/kg or 4 mg/kg every 8 h, were 0.08 and 0.48 μg/mL at 0.5 and 5.0 h after the dose, respectively. CSF levels evaluated in six children were reported to average 55% of the corresponding plasma level (28). The levels of stavudine in CSF in both adults and children are comparable to zidovudine levels, which suggests that stavudine should have activity in HIV-associated central nervous system disease.

Stavudine is not bound to plasma proteins (4).

Metabolism

The metabolic fate of stavudine has not been fully determined in humans. Early animal research indicated that stavudine was not extensively metabolized. In humans, however, it was reported that only about half of an administered dose can be recovered as the parent compound (55). This implies metabolism, and stavudine has been reported to be metabolized to its base form of thymine in nonhuman primates. The thymine metabolite was shown to further convert to β-aminoisobutyric acid (8). These two metabolites represent about 9% of the total metabolites recovered to date. The relevance of these findings is unknown.

Clearance

The total body clearance of stavudine in patients with normal renal function is 515 mL/min (12). The average half-life in patients with normal renal function is 1.5 h. Human studies indicate that approximately 40% of a dose can be recovered as unmetabolized drug in urine and that the half-life is prolonged in patients with renal insufficiency, thus requiring dose alterations. Additionally, low interpatient variability in total clearance was observed in a pharmacokinetic evaluation of 81 patients (24). Because of the low variability in stavudine clearance and the excellent bioavailability (99%), these authors suggested that dosage alterations were probably unnecessary for adults weighing between 40 and 100 kg.

ADVERSE REACTIONS
Peripheral Neuropathy

Peripheral neuropathy is reported to be the most common treatment-limiting adverse effect of stavudine (5, 41, 44, 53).

TABLE 1 • Stavudine Pharmacokinetics

Reference	Dose (mg/kg)	Cmax (μg/mL)	Vd (L/kg)	AUC (mg/h $\times$ h)	CLt (L/h)	$t_{1/2}$ (h)	F (%)
11	0.6	1.19	1.06	1.73	29.4	1.6	
	1.33	1.56	0.88	2.32	30.4	1.0	
	2.62	3.49	0.92	4.81	34.6	1.2	
	4.0	4.19	0.90	6.63	40.7	1.1	82
24	0.25–4.0		68.9 L		30.9		99
27a	10 mg	0.25		0.49		1.77	
	20 mg	0.47		0.98		1.67	
	40 mg	0.89		1.95		1.66	
52	40 mg	0.60		1.25		1.56	
	40 mg + DDI	0.71		1.31		1.68	
	100 mg						
28	1.0	0.44		0.63		1.11	78
	2.0	1.10		1.63		1.13	

Clinical trials have shown a clear relationship between the dose and the occurrence of peripheral neuropathy (Table 2). To summarize these data, peripheral neuropathy is more prevalent when a single dose of stavudine equals or exceeds 1 mg/kg. Onset of neuropathy occurs from 1 to 66 weeks after initiation of therapy and resolves within 1 week to several months after discontinuation. The median time to complete resolution is 17 days. One-third to one-half of patients tolerate stavudine if rechallenged with half of the previous dose. It is advised that patients be rechallenged only after neuropathy symptoms have completely resolved. Additional factors favoring development of neuropathy include a prior history of neuropathy and a CD4 cell count below 100. Two clinical trials in pediatric patients, one with stavudine in combination with didanosine and one with stavudine alone, reported no cases of peripheral neuropathy with doses ranging between 0.125 and 4 mg/kg/day (28, 29). Data collected from clinical trials suggest that didanosine and stavudine used in combination do not increase the risk of peripheral neuropathy (13, 27, 46, 47).

Hematologic Toxicity

Stavudine and zidovudine have different tendencies toward bone marrow suppression. Zidovudine is well known to suppress bone marrow function and cause neutropenia, anemia, and thrombocytopenia in humans; stavudine has been shown both in in vitro testing and clinical trials to rarely suppress the bone marrow. Stavudine may be less toxic to bone marrow for two reasons. First, in vitro data indicate that 50 to 100 times less stavudine is incorporated into human bone marrow cells than zidovudine (55). Second, stavudine 5'-monophosphate does not accumulate significantly intracellularly. On the other hand, zidovudine is associated with significant accumulation of zidovudine 5'-monophosphate, which interferes with the ability of the 3'-5' exonuclease to excise the phosphorylated zidovudine metabolite from human bone marrow DNA.

Additive bone marrow suppression with concurrent administration of zidovudine and stavudine was described on a molecular level, which could have clinical implications (23, 38). It has been suggested that zidovudine 5'-monophosphate accumulation could reduce the ability of 3',5'-exonuclease to excise both zidovudine and stavudine from bone marrow DNA, thus potentially producing an additive suppression of bone marrow. This would appear most likely to occur in zidovu-

dine-experienced patients concurrently treated with stavudine and zidovudine or after concurrent therapy with these drugs for an extended period of time. Completion of ongoing trials should help determine whether this combination produces greater hematologic abnormalities.

Hepatotoxicity

Most clinical trials have indicated a trend toward raising liver function tests; however, severe hepatotoxicity has not been reported as a side effect of stavudine.

DOSAGE AND ADMINISTRATION
Adult Dosing

Stavudine is approved for the treatment of adults with HIV-1 infections. Most clinical trials indicate that it is effective for patients with advanced HIV-1 infections, in patients with immunologic deterioration, and in patients intolerant of previous drug regimens. The role of stavudine as monotherapy in antiretroviral therapy–naive patients is currently being evaluated in the ACTG 298 protocol.

Stavudine dose depends on both body weight and renal function. For adults with normal renal function, the dose is 40 mg twice daily in patients over 60 kg and 30 mg twice daily for patients under 60 kg. However, it has been suggested that dose adjustment may be unnecessary for body weights between 40 and 100 kg (24). No specific guidelines have been suggested for patients under 40 or above 100 kg. Clinical practice resembles the latter dosing guidelines because of the excellent overall safety profile and reversibility of dose-related peripheral neuropathy.

Pediatric Dosing

Stavudine is currently not approved by the FDA for use in children. However, several clinical trials have shown favorable responses in surrogate markers and have reported a lower incidence of new opportunistic infections in the patients treated with stavudine.

The optimal pediatric dose for safety and effectiveness has not been established. However, clinical trials to date suggest that in patients with normal renal function, 2 mg/kg/day in two divided doses (administered every 12 h) is a reasonable starting dose. Table 3 summarizes the usual dosage for stavudine for both pediatric and adult patients.

Food Effects

Stavudine can be taken without regard to meals and should be taken at 12-h intervals.

Pregnancy Effects

The FDA has placed stavudine in pregnancy category C (4). There have been no controlled studies performed with stavudine in pregnant women.

Nursing Mothers

Although it is not known if stavudine is excreted in breast milk, it is recommend that nursing mothers discontinue breastfeeding while receiving stavudine (4).

TABLE 2 • Peripheral Neuropathy		
Reference	Dose	% Patients with PN
5	<2 mg/kg/day>	43
	2 mg/kg/day	65
41	<2 mg/kg/day>	38
	2 mg/kg/day	60
37	40 mg twice daily	12
44	0.1 mg/kg/day	6
	0.5 mg/kg/day	17
	2.0 mg/kg/day	37
1	20 mg twice daily	15
	40 mg twice daily	21

TABLE 3 • Dosing Regimens

	Creatinine Clearance (mL/min)	Weight > 60 kg	Weight < 60 kg
Adults	>50	40 mg twice daily	30 mg twice daily
	26–49	20 mg twice daily	15 mg twice daily
	10–25	20 mg once daily	15 mg once daily
	<10	20 mg every other day	15 mg every other day
	Hemodialysis	20 mg once daily (after dialysis)	15 mg once daily (after dialysis)
Children	>50	2 mg/kg/day in divided doses (every 12 h)	2 mg/kg/day in divided doses (every 12 h)

Renal Insufficiency and Dialysis

Since a large portion of stavudine is eliminated unchanged by glomerular filtration, a decline in renal function to below 50 mL/min results in stavudine accumulation. Therefore, dosage modifications are required in patients with renal insufficiency, to avoid serum level–related adverse effects. Table 3 summarizes the dose modifications for renal insufficiency and dialysis.

Twelve patients on chronic hemodialysis were evaluated. The half-life, total clearance, and AUC were shown to be similar to those for patients with a creatinine clearance below 25 mL/min, and approximately 30% of stavudine is removed by dialysis. Therefore, it is recommended that stavudine be administered after completion of dialysis and at the same time of day on nondialysis days (4, 18).

Hepatic Insufficiency

The half-life of stavudine in patients with cirrhosis is slightly longer (2.2 vs. 1.8 h) than in those without cirrhosis (45). However, the AUC, C_{max}, and total clearance are not significantly different, and accumulation does not occur. Thus, there are no guidelines for dosage adjustment in patients with impaired hepatic function.

DRUG INTERACTIONS
Stavudine-Zidovudine

It has been proposed that stavudine and zidovudine are antagonistic when administered in combination to patients with HIV-1 infections, based on molecular experiments (23), in vitro isolates in PBMCs (38), and data derived from clinical trial ACTG 290. This drug interaction is based on the possibility that the drugs compete for cellular thymidine kinase, which is responsible for initial phosphorylation of both drugs. However, stavudine reportedly has a 600-fold lower affinity for this enzyme, and zidovudine monophosphate accumulation further decreases enzyme activity (23). The net effect would be to reduce the intracellular concentrations of stavudine triphosphate and hence reduce stavudine's therapeutic effect.

In vitro data in PBMCs indicate that stavudine-zidovuding combination is either additive or synergistic against zidovudine-sensitive HIV isolates (38, 56). When tested against zidovudine-resistant isolates, however, the combination has antagonistic effects (38). Some clinical data demonstrate both a survival benefit and a reduced number of opportunistic infections with this combination (36). The completion of ongoing clinical trials will determine whether the drug interaction between stavudine and zidovudine is clinically significant. To date, an arm of ACTG 290 that combined stavudine and zidovudine in zidovudine-experienced patients was prematurely discontinued because of decreasing CD4 levels. Enhanced hematologic abnormalities have been demonstrated in in vitro models with this combination; however ongoing clinical trials may help define the significance of this interaction (see "Hematologic Toxicity" for more detail).

Stavudine-Didanosine

The pharmacokinetics of coadministered stavudine (40 mg) and didanosine (100 mg twice daily) for 5 days was evaluated in 10 HIV-seropositive patients (52). No changes in didanosine kinetics were reported. However, the average maximal plasma concentrations of stavudine increased approximately 20%, and the AUC increased approximately 6.5%. It was concluded that coadministered stavudine and didanosine did not interact pharmcokinetically and that the two drugs could be administered concurrently.

CLINICAL INDICATIONS
Phase I/II Dose-Ranging Studies

The efficacy of stavudine has demonstrated in a number of trials, which have been extensively reviewed (32, 48). Although most of the earlier trials used surrogate markers as endpoints, influence on development of new opportunistic infections and survival data have also been reported. Using dose escalation to toxicity followed by dose deescalation to the minimum effective dose (dose range, 0.1–12 mg/kg/day), these trials determined that the minimum effective dose with clinically significant activity was 0.5 mg/kg/day and the maximum tolerated dose was 2 mg/kg/day. Also, peripheral neuropathy was shown to be dose-limiting. Compared with zidovudine, stavudine produced a clinically significant increase in CD4 levels, reduced p24 antigen, increased body weight, and produced less hematologic toxicity. None of the trials used a placebo control. In the largest trial to date, a parallel-track program indicated little difference in survival rate between 20 and 40 mg twice daily, but surrogate markers were clinically superior with 40 mg twice daily regimen (1).

Comparative or Combination Trials

The BMS 019 trial enrolled 822 patients to receive either stavudine (40 mg twice daily) or continued zidovudine (200

TABLE 4 • Summary of Recent Clinical Investigations Involving Stavudine

Reference	Dosage Regimen	No. Patients	Duration	Mean CD4 Response	Mean VL Response	Other/Comments
36	D4t vs. AZT + D4t	40	10 months			AZT/D4t combination lived longer and had fewer OIs
46	D4t + DDI	86	12 months	+60	−1.4 logs	2/67 PN requiring drug d/c
27	D4t + DDI	13	20 weeks	+52	−2.9 logs	3/12 PN requiring drug d/c
13	D4t + DDI	25	24 weeks	+38	−0.7 logs	3/25 PN requiring drug d/c
47	D4t + DDI	51	22 weeks	+74	−1.0 logs	46% >1.0 log reduction in 54%; 19% ND VL at week 24; 2/51 PN
50	D4t + 3TC	48	8 weeks	NR	−0.97 logs	ARV-naive and pts with higher pretreatment had greater response
7	D4t + 3TC (retrospective)	330	NR	NR	−1.18 logs	Only 0.4 log reduction seen in pts with previous ART
49	D4t + DDI + hydroxyurea	12	12 weeks	+48	−1.9 logs	2-fold reduction in TNF-α; 4/12 developed reversible neutropenia to hydroxyurea combination
43	D4t + DDI + nelfinavir	22	8 weeks	+218	−2.1 logs	3/8 ND VL; mild GI toxicity; 1 allergic rxn to nelfinavir
51	D4t + DDI + ritonavir	33	12 weeks	+138	−2.06 logs	ART naive; 41% ND infectious PBMC; 70% ND HIV-RNA

mg thrice daily) for at least 1 year (37). All patients who entered the trial had previously received zidovudine. This trial found a lower incidence of treatment failure, including death, and a longer time to treatment failure in the stavudine arm.

Stavudine and didanosine combination therapy was evaluated in 86 patients (46). In this double-blind trial, patients were randomized to receive one of several dose combinations that included one-half the usual dose of didanosine and one-fourth the usual dose of stavudine. The mean CD4 cell count at entry was 330, and the mean virus load, 44,000 copies/mL. Data were analyzed after 1 year of therapy. Approximately 60% of the patients had their virus load reduced by 1 $\log_{10}$ copies/mL and 30% had it reduced by 2 $\log_{10}$ copies/mL. The CD4 count increased an average of 70 cells. The greatest response tended to occur in the groups receiving full doses of each drug. Also of clinical significance, only two patients (2.3%) developed peripheral neuropathy that required discontinuing study medications. One of these patients was successfully treated for an additional 6 months following rechallenge with both drugs at half the original dose.

Numerous clinical trials have explored a variety of nucleoside analogue and protease inhibitor combination regimens that include stavudine. Most of the information is published as abstracts of data presented at scientific meetings. Table 4 summarizes the preliminary findings of these trials. At the time of this writing, two AIDS clinical trials are ongoing that involve stavudine. ACTG 290 includes zidovudine-experienced patients. This trial has four arms: stavudine monotherapy, didanosine monotherapy, zidovudine plus didanosine, and zidovudine plus stavudine, and interim analysis indicated a higher incidence of decreased CD4 cells in the zidovudine plus stavudine arm. Another study, ACTG 298, is evaluating stavudine in antiretroviral-naive patients. This trial has three arms:

stavudine monotherapy, stavudine plus zidovudine, and zidovudine plus lamivudine.

Pediatric Clinical Trials

The efficacy and safety of stavudine was examined in two trials in children; one involves stavudine as monotherapy (28), and one used stavudine in combination with didanosine (29). These trials determined the pharmacokinetics of stavudine in children and found that the combination of stavudine and didanosine provided positive effects on surrogate markers and was well tolerated. The patients enrolled in the combination study all had advanced disease, and the duration was 24 weeks. Although the number of patients in these trials was low, the results indicate that the combination of stavudine and didanosine should be further examined in longer controlled trials in patients with less-advanced disease.

A double-blind, randomized trial comparing stavudine with zidovudine was conducted in 216 patients between 3 months and 6 years of age (30). Patients received either stavudine (1 mg/kg twice daily) or zidovudine (180 mg/m^2). Preliminary results of this trial suggest that stavudine and zidovudine are largely comparable in terms of tolerance, but 15% of those receiving zidovudine developed grade 3 or 4 neutropenia, compared with 5% receiving stavudine. Considering efficacy, stavudine patients had a marginally better weight gain, and CD4 cell counts were better maintained.

REFERENCES

1. Anderson RE, Dunkle LM, Smaldone L, Adler M, Wirtz C, Kriesel D, Cross A, Martin RR. Design and implementation of the stavudine parallel-track program. J Infect Dis 1995;171(Suppl 2):118–122.

2. August EM, Birks EM, Prusoff WH. 3′-Deoxythymidine-2′-ene permeation of human lymphocyte H9 cells by non-facilitated diffusion. Mol Pharmacol 1991;39:246–249.

3. Balzarini J, Herdewijn P, De Clercq E. Differential patterns of intracellular metabolism of 2′-3′-didehydro-2′3′-dideoxythymidine and 3′azido-2′3′-dideoxythymidine, two potent anti-human immunodeficiency virus compounds. J Biol Chem 1989;264:6127–6133.

4. Bristol-Meyer Squibb. Product package information. Princeton, NJ: Bristol-Meyer Squibb, 1996.

5. Browne MJ, Mayer KH, Chafee SBD, Dudley MN, Posner MR, Steinberg SM, Graham KK, Geletko SM, Zinner SH, Denman SL, Dunkle LM, Kaoul S, McLaren C, Skowron G, Kouttab NM, Kennedy TA, Weitberg AN, Curt GA. 2′,3′-Didehydro-3′-deoxythymidine in patients with AIDS or AIDS-related complex: a phase I trial. J Infect Dis 1993;167:21–29.

6. Chen C-H, Vazque-Padua M, Cheng Y-C. Effect of anti-human immunodeficiency virus nucleoside analogs on mitochondrial DNA and its implication for delayed toxicity. Mol Pharmacol 1991;39:625–628.

7. Cohen CJ, Shalit P, Conant M, Scott RC, Wong T, Campbell, Smith J, Frost KR. Lamivudine and stavudine combination therapy: HIV viral load and CD4 changes in a retrospective study of 330 patients [Abstract]. Fourth Conference on Retroviruses and Opportunistic Infections, Washington, DC, Jan 1997.

8. Cretton EM, Zhou Z, Kidd LB, McClure HM, Karl S, Hitchcock JMJ, Sommadossi JP. In vitro and in vivo disposition and metabolism of 3′-deoxy-2′,3′-didehydrothymidine. Antimicrob Agents Chemother 1993;37:1816–1825.

9. D'Aquila R, Johnson VA, Welles SL, Japour AJ, Kuritzkes DR, DeGrattola V, Reichelderfer PS, Coombs RW, Crumpacker CS, Kahn J, Richman DO. Zidovudine resistance and HIV-1 disease progression during antiretroviral therapy. Ann Intern Med 1995;122:401–408.

10. Domin BA, Mahoney WB, Zimmerman TP. 2′3′-Dideoxythymidine permeation of the human erythrocyte membrane by nonfacilitated diffusion. Biochem Biophys Res Commun 1988;154:825–831.

11. Dudley MN, Graham KK, Kaul S, Geletko S, Dunkle L, Browne M, Mayer K. Pharmacokinetics of stavudine in patients with AIDS or AIDS-related complex. J Infect Dis 1992;166:480–485.

12. Dudley MN. Clinical pharmacokinetics of nucleoside antiretroviral agents. J Infect Dis 1995;171(Suppl 2):S99–112.

13. Durant J, Rahelinirina V, Dupre F, Carmagnolle MF, Halfon P, Ngo Van P, Dellamonica P. A pilot study of the combination of stavudine and didanosine in patients with less than 350 CD4 and who are not eligible for a treatment with zidovudine [Abstract]. Fourth Conference on Retroviruses and Opportunistic Infections, Washington, DC, Jan 1997.

14. Faraj A, Fowler DA, Bridges EG, Sommadossi JP. Effects of 2′3′-dideoxynucleosides on proliferation and differentiation of human pluripotent progenitors in liquid culture and their effects on mitochondrial DNA synthesis. Antimicrob Agents Chemother 1994;38:924–930.

15. Furman PA, Fyfe JA, St Clair MH, Weinhold K, Rideout JL, Freeman GA, Lehrman SN, Bolognesi DP, Broden S, Mitsuya H, Barry DW. Phosphorylation of 3′-azido-3′deoxythymidine and selective interaction of the 5′-monophosphate with human immunodeficiency virus reverse transcriptase. Proc Natl Acad Sci USA 1986;83:8333–8337.

16. Gao W-Y, Agbaria R, Driscoll JS, Mitsuya H. Divergent anti-human immunodeficiency virus activity and anabolic phosphorylation of 2′3′-dideoxynucleoside analogs in resting and activated human cells. J Biol Chem 1994;269:12633–12638.

17. Gao Q, Gu Z, Salomon H, Parniak MA, Wainberg MA. Generation of multiple drug resistance by sequential in vitro passage of the human immunodeficiency virus type 1. Arch Virol 1994;136:111–122.

18. Grasela D, Christofalo B, Raymond R. Safety and pharmacokinetics of stavudine in subjects with mild, moderate or severe renal impairment [Abstract]. 2nd National Conference on Human Retroviruses and Related Infections, Jan 29, 1995:145.

19. Gu Z, Gao Q, Fang H, Parniak MA, Brenner BG, Wainberg M. Identification of novel mutations that confer drug resistance in the human immunodeficiency virus polymerase gene. Leukemia 1994(Suppl 1):166–169.

20. Gustavason LE, Fukuda EK, Rubio FA, Dunton AW. A pilot study of the bioavailability and pharmacokinetics of 2′,3′ dideoxycytidine in patients with AIDS or AIDS-related complex. J Acquir Immune Defic Syndr 1990;3:28–31.

21. Harper CY. Personal communication. Bristol-Meyers Squibb, 1997.

22. Hitchcock M. 2′,3′-Didehydro-2′,3′-dideoxythymidine—an anti-HIV agent. Antiviral Chem Chemother 1991;30:1270–1278.

23. Ho H-T, Hitchcock KJ. Cellular pharmacology of 2′,3′-dideoxy 2′,3′-didehydrothymidine, a nucleoside analog active against human immunodeficiency virus. Antimicrob Agents Chemother 1989;33:844–849.

24. Horton CM, Dudley MN, Kaul S, Mayer KH, Squires K, Kunkle L, Anderson R. Population pharmacokinetics of stavudine in patients with AIDS or advanced AIDS-related complex. Antimicrob Agents Chemother 1995;39:2309–2315.

25. Huang P, Farquhar D, Plunkett W. Selective action of 2′,3′–dideoxy 2′,3′-didehydrothymidine triphosphate on human immunodeficiency virus reverse transcriptase and human DNA polymerases. J Biol Chem 1992;267:2817–2822.

26. Iversen A, Shafer R, Wehrly K, Winters MA, Mullins JI, Chesebro B, Merigan TC. Multidrug-resistant human immunodeficiency virus type 1 strains resulting from combination antiretroviral therapy. J Virol 1996;70:1086–1090.

27. Kalathoor S, Sinclair J, Andron L, Sension MG, High K. Combination therapy with stavudine and didanosine. [Abstract]. Fourth Conference on Retroviruses and Opportunistic Infections, Washington, DC, Jan 1997.

27a. Kaul S, Mummaneni V, Barbhaina RH. Dose proportionality of stavudine in HIV seropositive asymptomatic subjects: application to bioequivalence assessment of various capsule formulations. Biopharm Drug Dispos 1995;16:125–136.

28. Kline MW, Dunkle L, Church, J, Goldsmith JC, Harris AT, Federici ME, Schultze ME, Woods L, Loewen DF, Kaul S, Cross A, Rutkiewicz VL, Rosenblatt HM, Hanson IC, Shearer WT. A phase I/II evaluation of stavudine in children with human immunodeficiency virus infection. Pediatrics 1995;96:247–252.

29. Kline MW, Fletcher C, Federici M, Harris AT, Evans KD, Rutkiewicz VL, Shearer WT, Dunkle LM. Combination therapy with stavudine and didanosine in children with advanced human immunodeficiency virus infection: pharmacokinetic properties, safety, and immunologic and virologic effects. Pediatrics 1996;97;886–890.

30. Kline MW, Lindsey JC, Culnane M, Van Dyke RB. A randomized comparative trial of zidovudine versus stavudine in children with HIV infection. ACTG 240 [Abstract]. Fourth Conference on Retroviruses and Opportunistic Infections, Washington, DC, Jan 1997.

31. Lacey SF, Larder BA. Novel mutation (V75T) in human immunodeficiency virus type 1 reverse transcriptase confers resistance to 2′3′-didehydro 2′3′-dideoxythymidine in cell culture. Antimicrob Agents Chemother 1994;38:1428–1432.

32. Lea AP, Faulds D. Stavudine: a review of its pharmacodynamic and pharmacokinetic properties and clinical potential in HIV infections. Drugs 1996;51:846–864.

33. Lewis W, Dalakos MC. Mitochondrial toxicity of antiviral drugs. Nature Med 1995;1:417–422.

34. Lin P-F, Samanta H, Rose RE, Patick AK, Trimble J, Bechtold CM, Revie DR, Khan NC, Federici ME, Li H, Lee A, Anderson RE, Colonno RJ. Genotypic and phenotypic analysis of human immunodeficiency virus type 1 isolated from patients on prolonged stavudine therapy. J Infect Dis 1994;170:1157–1164.

35. Lin T-S, Schinazi RF, Prusoff WH. Potent and selective in vitro activity of 3'-deoxythymidine-2'ene against human immunodeficiency virus. Biochem Pharmacol 1987;36:2713–2718.

36. Mars ME, Gensollen S, Ravaux L. Association between AZT and D4T in HIV infected patients: a pilot study comparison with D4T, AZT, and AZT + D4T. [Abstract]. 35th Interscience conference on Antimicrobial Agents and Chemotherapy, 1995:226.

37. Mellors J, Stool E, BMS-019 Study Group. Safety and tolerability of stavudine versus zidovudine in HIV-infected adults with less than 500 CD4 cells after at least 6 months ACV treatment [Abstract]. 35th Interscience Conference on Antimicrobial Agents and Chemotherapy, San Francisco, 1995.

38. Merrill DP, Moonis M, Chou T-C, Hirsch MS. Lamivudine or stavudine in two- and three-drug combinations against human immunodeficiency type 1 replication in vitro. J Infect Dis 1996;173:355–364.

39. Montaner JSG, Singer J, Schechter MT, Rabound JM, Tsoukas C, O'Shanghuessy M, Ruedy J, Nagai K, Salomon H, Spira B, Wainberg M. Clinical correlated of invitro HIV-1 resistant to zidovudine. Results of the Multicentre Canadian AZT trial. AIDS 1993;7:189–196.

40. Montaner, JSG, Schechter MT, Rachlis A, Gill J, Beaulieu R, Tsoukas C, Babaud J, Cameron B, Salomon H, Dunkle L, Smaldone L, Wainberg M. Didanosine compared with continued zidovudine therapy for HIV-infected patients with 200 to 500 CD4 cell/mm^3. Ann Intern Med 1995;123:561–571.

41. Murray H, Squires K, Weiss W, Sledz S, Sacks HS, Hassett J, Cross A, Anderson RE, Dunkle LM. Stavudine in patients with AIDS and AIDS-related Complex: AIDS Clinical Trials Group 089. J Infect Dis 1995;171(Suppl 2):S123–130.

42. Nakashima H, Balzarini J, Pauwels R, Schols D, Desmyter J, DeClerq E. Anti-HIV-1 activity of antiviral compounds, as quantitated by a focal immunoassay in CD4 HeLa cells and a plaque assay in MT-4 cells. J Virol Methods 1990;29:197–208.

43. Pedneault L, Elion R, Adler M, Anderson R, Kelleher T, Knupp C, Kaul S, Kerr B, Cross A, Dunkle L. Stavudine, didanosine, and nelfinavir combination therapy in HIV-infected subjects: antiviral effect and safety in an ongoing pilot study [Abstract]. Fourth Conference on Retroviruses and Opportunistic Infections, Washington, DC, Jan 1997.

44. Petersen E, Ramirez-Ronda C, Hardy W, Schwartz R, Sacks HS, Follansbee S, Peterson DM, Cross A, Anderson RE, Dunkle LM. Dose-related activity of stavudine in patients infected with human immunodeficiency virus. J Infect Dis 1995;171(Suppl 2): S131–139.

45. Petty B, Grasela D, Schaad H. Safety and pharmacokinetics of stavudine in hepatic impairment [Abstract]. 2nd National Conference on Human Retroviruses and Related Infections, Jan 29, 1995:146.

46. Pollard RB, Peterson D, Hardy D, Pedneault L, Rutkiewicz V, Pottage J, Murphy R, Gathe J, Beall G, Skovronski J, Cross A, Dunkle L. Stavudine and didanosine combination therapy in HIV-infected subjects: analysis of antiviral effect and safety in a randomized double-blind study [Abstract]. Tenth International Conference on Antiviral Research, Atlanta, GA, April 1997.

47. Raffi F, Auger S, Billaud E, Besnier JM, Chennebault JM, Michelet C, Perre P, Lafeuillade A, May T, Arvieux C, Paillant C, Barin F, Billaudel S. Antiviral effect and safety of didanosine-stavudine combination therapy in HIV-infected subjects: interim results of a pilot trial [Abstract]. Fourth Conference on Retroviruses and Opportunistic Infections, Washington, DC, Jan 1997.

48. Riddler, S, Anderson R, Mellors A. Antiretroviral activity of stavudine. Antiviral Res 1995;27:189–203.

49. Rossero R, Nokta M, Andron L, Pollard RB. Open label combination therapy with stavudine didanosine and hydroxyurea in nucleoside experienced HIV-1 patients [Abstract]. Fourth Conference on Retroviruses and Opportunistic Infections, Washington, DC, Jan 1997.

50. Rouleau D, Montaner JSG, Conway B, Raboud J, Rae S, Shillington A, Fransen S. Predictors of viral load response in a pilot-open label study of stavudine in combination with lamivudine [Abstract]. Fourth Conference on Retroviruses and Opportunistic Infections, Washington, DC, Jan 1997.

51. Saimot PTAG, Landman R, Damond F, Detruchis P, Gaudebout C, Girard PM, Gorin I, Mathez D, Michon C, Prevot MH, Tubiana R. Ritonavir, stavudine, didanosine as a triple combination treatment in antiretroviral-naive patients [Abstract]. Fourth Conference on Retroviruses and Opportunistic Infections, Washington, DC, Jan 1997.

52. Seifert RD, Stewart MB, Sramek JJ, Conrad J, Kaul S, Cutler NR. Pharmacokinetics of co-administered didanosine and stavudine in HIV-seropositive male patients. Br J Clin Pharmacol 1994:38:405–410.

53. Skowron G. Biologic effect and safety of stavudine: overview of phase I and II clinical trials. J Infect Dis 1995;171(Suppl 2):S113–117.

54. Sommadossi J-P, Zhu Z, Carlisle R, Xie MY, Weidner DA. Pharmacologic studies on nucleosides active against the human immunodeficiency virus. Ann NY Acad Sci 1990;616:356–366.

55. Sommadossi J-P. Comparison of metabolism and invitro antiviral activity of stavudine versus other 2',3'-dideoxynucleoside analogues. J Infect Dis 1995;171(Suppl 2):S88–92.

56. Sorensen AM, Nielsen C, Mathiesen LR, Nielsen JO, Hansen JE. Evaluation of the combination effect of different antiviral compounds against HIV in vitro. Scand J Infect Dis 1993;25:365–371.

56a. Watson A, Wilburn W, Ho H-T. The inhibition of HIV-1 proviral DNA synthesis in resting PBL by nucleosides [Abstract WA 1027]. VII International Conference on AIDS, Florence, Italy, 1991.

57. Yarchoan JA, Mitsuya H, Myers CE, Broder S. Clinical pharmacology of 3'-azido-2'3'dideoxythymidine and related dideoxynucleosides. N Engl J Med 1989;321:726–738.

58. Yokota T, Mochizuki S, Konno K, Mori S, Shigeta S, DeClerq E. Inhibitory effects of selected antiviral compounds on human hepatitis B virus DNA synthesis. Antimicrob Agents Chemother 1992;35:394–397.

59. Zhu Z, Ho H-T, Hitchcock MJ, Somadossi JP. Cellular pharmacology of 2'3'-didehydro-2'3'-dideoxythymidine in human peripheral blood mononuclear cells. Biochem Pharmacol 1990;39:R15–19.

60. Zhu Z, Hitchcock MJ, Sommadossi JP. Metabolism and DNA interaction of 2'3'-didehydro-2'3'-dideoxythymidine in human bone marrow cells. Mol Pharmacol 1991;40:838–845.

Antiretroviral Agents: Zidovudine, Didanosine, and Zalcitabine

●

Margaret A. Fischl and Gene D. Morse

BACKGROUND

Nucleoside reverse transcriptase inhibitors (NRTIs) were the first antiretroviral agents approved for the treatment of patients with HIV infection (Fig. 1). Zidovudine (ZDV), didanosine (ddI), and zalcitabine (ddC) were initially approved as monotherapy and then as combination regimens, either ZDV/ddI or ZDV/ddC. Early studies demonstrated clinical and survival benefits in patients with symptomatic disease and those with asymptomatic disease who had fewer than 500 CD4 cells/mm^3. Durable benefits were limited, partly because of incomplete suppression of HIV replication and emergence of viral resistance. At present, these NRTIs remain as part of three- and four-drug regimens along with other NRTIs (stavudine and lamivudine), HIV-1 protease inhibitors, and nonnucleoside reverse transcriptase inhibitors (NNRTIs).

ZIDOVUDINE

ZDV, a thymidine analogue, was the first antiretroviral agent approved for treatment of HIV infection. ZDV was initially approved for treatment of advanced disease and later for early disease, including asymptomatic patients. ZDV remains an effective antiretroviral agent when used in combination regimens.

Mechanism of Action

ZDV passively diffuses into host lymphocytes and is phosphorylated to ZDV monophosphate (ZDV-MP) by thymidine kinase. ZDV-MP is converted to ZDV diphosphate (ZDV-DP) and then to ZDV triphosphate (ZDV-TP), which has an intracellular half-life of 3 to 4 h (37). ZDV-TP competes with endogenous nucleotides to inhibit HIV reverse transcriptase but also acts as a chain terminator by incorporation into growing strands of DNA or RNA (Fig. 2). The intracellular phosphor-ylated ZDV derivatives are in dynamic equilibrium with intracellular and extracellular ZDV. Excessive accumulation of ZDV-MP may decrease conversion of the host cell thymidine monophosphate to thymidine diphosphate (Michaelis-Menton constant (K_m) = 4 mM) and thus lead to cellular toxicity. There has been an increasing effort to measure intracellular zidovudine anabolites, with earlier attempts to develop assay approaches recently translated into clinical observations (35, 73, 81, 85–87).

Mechanisms of Resistance

Specific mutation sites on the HIV-1 *pol* gene, which codes for the reverse transcriptase, will confer viral resistance to several nucleoside analogues, including ZDV (Fig. 4). Viral resistance to ZDV is associated with a stepwise decrease in susceptibility with mutations (amino acid substitutions) at sites 41, 67, 70, 215, and 219, with sites 41, 70, and 215 being the most important sites of mutations (8, 72). The rate of change in susceptibility of viral isolates to ZDV is associated with the stage of HIV disease (72). After approximately 12 months of ZDV monotherapy, 31% of viral isolates from patients with early HIV disease are resistant, and nearly all isolates from patients with advanced disease are resistant. Although most viral isolates from treatment-naive patients are susceptible to ZDV, resistant strains have been transmitted between sexual partners (29) and from mother to child during pregnancy (36). High-level resistance is an independent risk factor for disease progression and compromises therapeutic regimens (19). For the most part, isolates with decreased susceptibility to ZDV remain sensitive to other nucleoside analogues such as ddI and ddC (74). Multiple resistance to nucleoside analogues has been described after long-term combination therapy. Mutations at amino acid residues 75, 77, 116, 62, and especially 151 impart multiple resistance to ZDV, ddI, ddC, and stavudine.

Pharmacokinetic Disposition

ZDV is well absorbed and subjected to first-pass hepatic glucuronidation, with peak serum concentrations occurring at 0.5 to 1.0 h in the fasted state (7, 54). Although T_{max} is fairly consistent, peak plasma concentrations and AUC can vary (35, 62). Food does not appear to influence total exposure (AUC) (58, 75). The bioavailability (F) of an oral solution (5 mg/kg) of ZDV is about 0.63 ± 0.10, and a capsule dosage form has yielded F values of 0.64 ± 0.10. Data obtained in pediatric patients (solution and capsules) and in hemophilia patients (capsules) are similar but more variable (F = 0.68 ± 0.25) (4, 27, 64).

Following intravenous administration, ZDV serum concentrations decay in a biexponential pattern with a rapid O phase and a β phase half-life of 0.9 to 1.4 h (7, 54). The rapid clearance of ZDV from serum most likely reflects its distribution into blood components and extravascular sites (tissue accumulation and hepatocellular uptake, with subsequent glucuronidation). ZDV distributes throughout body water and tissues, with a distribution volume (Vd$_{ss}$) of 1.6 ± 0.6 L/kg; however, a population pharmacokinetic analysis of ZDV found a Vd$_{ss}$ of 3 to 3.9 L/kg (39). In contrast to high-pressure liquid chromatography (HPLC) analysis, radioimmunoassay analysis detected a more prolonged elimination phase (25, 40, 65).

ZDV diffuses across the blood-brain barrier as noted from analysis of ZDV cerebrospinal fluid (CSF) following continuous intravenous infusion (children) or intermittent intravenous

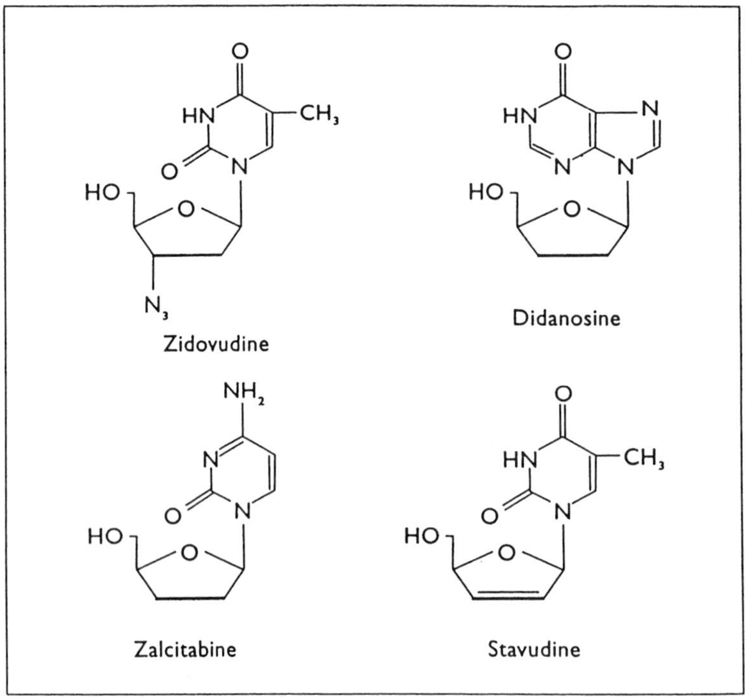

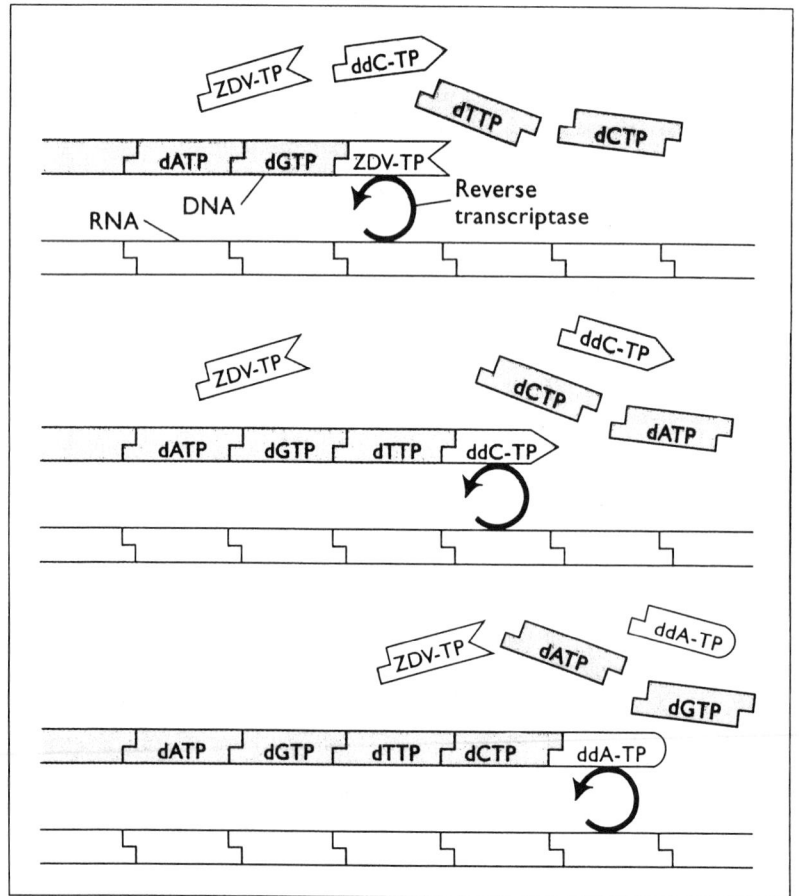

FIGURE 1. Chemical structure of naturally occurring nucleoside analogues (adenosine, thymidine, cytidine, guanine) and the systemic antiviral nucleoside analogues, zidovudine, didanosine, zalcitabine. (Adapted from Atlas of infectious diseases, AIDS, vol I.)

FIGURE 2. The dideoxynucleosides exert anti-HIV activity against the reverse transcriptase level. (Adapted from Atlas of infectious diseases, AIDS, vol I.)

or oral administration (adults) (5, 54). In children, the CSF:serum ratio is 0.28; in adults, the ratio ranges from 0.15 to 1.35. The mean CSF ZDV concentrations in children ranges from 0.31 ± 0.1 to 0.87 ± 0.3 mM/L over a dosage range of 0.5 to 1.8 mg/kg/h. In adults, the CSF concentration ranges from 0.14 to 2.3 mM over a dosage range of 2 to 15 mg/kg. The variability noted among adults may be partially due to the time dependence of ZDV diffusion into CSF. The distribution of ZDV into the CSF also reflects its low protein binding (20%) (14, 67).

Data obtained in monkeys and mice indicate that ZDV is present in breast milk and crosses the placental membrane (89). A report in humans confirmed these data and indicated that fetal glucuronidation of ZDV is impaired (38). ZDV is also detected in semen. The semen:serum ratio ranges from 1.3 to 20, but the reason for this accumulation remains unclear (49).

ZDV is eliminated from plasma by uptake into human cells and conversion to ZDV-TP, by hepatic glucuronidation (GZDV), and by renal excretion of the parent compound. Both GZDV and ZDV are eliminated renally. The total clearance (following intravenous administration of 1–5 mg/kg) ranges from 1.0 to 1.8 L/h/kg in adults, indicating a pattern of high clearance (7, 54). Similar values (641 ± 161 mL/min/m^2) have been noted in children (4). Overall, $18 \pm 5\%$ of an intravenous ZDV dose is excreted unchanged, while $60 \pm 10\%$ is eliminated as GZDV. After oral dosing, recovery in the urine comprises $14 \pm 3\%$ of ZDV and $75 \pm 15\%$ as GZDV. The mean urinary recovery ratio of GZDV/ZDV after oral dosing is about 5.7 and 6.9 (7, 22, 64). Renal clearances in patients with normal renal function (creatinine clearance, 102 ± 29 mL/min) are 188 ± 65 mL/min for ZDV and 293 ± 46 mL/min for GZDV (22). Tubular secretion contributes to the renal excretion of both ZDV and GZDV. Determination of GZDV and ZDV renal excretion during probenecid administration indicates that decreased tubular secretion of GZDV contributes to a higher GZDV AUC, while the ZDV AUC is increased by decreased hepatic glucuronidation and decreased renal clearance caused by probenecid (22, 57). The apparent renal clearance of ZDV decreases to 17 ± 2 mL/min in seronegative uremic patients (mean creatinine clearance, 18 ± 2 mL/min) (23, 79). In anuric seronegative patients, hemodialysis clearance does not contribute to the removal of

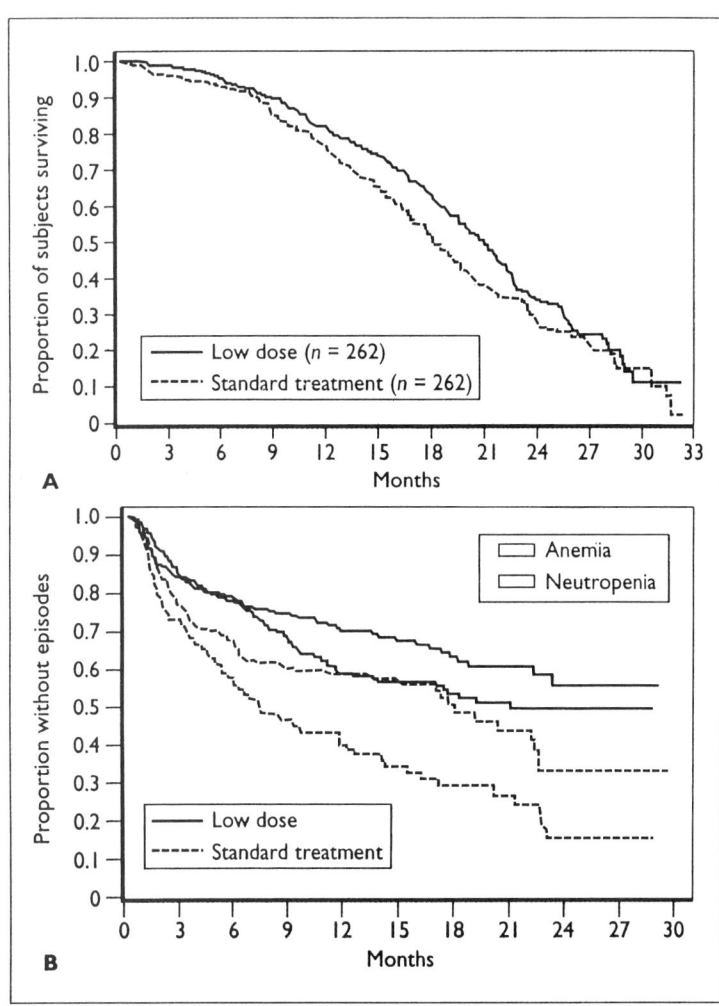

FIGURE 3. **A.** Proportion of patients surviving after receiving two doses of zidovudine (standard dose, 1500 mg/day vs. low dose, 600 mg/day). **B.** Proportion of patients with anemia or neutropenia receiving either the initial standard dose (1500 mg/day) or low dose (600 mg/day) of zidovudine. (Adapted from Atlas of infectious diseases, AIDS, vol I.)

ZDV; however, GZDV is efficiently removed, with interdialytic $t_{1/2}$ and dialysis $t_{1/2}$ values of 52 ± 11 h and 1.7 ± 0.1 h. Dialysis patients may not tolerate the recommended daily dose of ZDV and may require dosage reduction or interval prolongation (100–200 mg every 8–12 h).

The initial ZDV dosing regimen used in clinical studies was 200 mg every 4 h. This regimen was selected on the basis of a rapid terminal elimination half-life of about 1 h and a target serum concentration of 1 mM (37). Subsequent studies using lower daily doses (100 mg five or six times daily) demonstrated equivalent efficacy with less toxicity (31) (Fig. 3). With an estimated intracellular half-life for ZDV-TP of 3 to 4 h, ZDV dosing has been converted to 200 mg thrice daily and most recently to 300 mg twice daily. However, lower doses may not reach effective concentrations in the CSF.

NNRTIs/Zidovudine

ZDV plasma concentrations are decreased 25% by concurrent nevirapine use. This is accompanied by an increase in GZDV, reflecting the hepatic induction capacity of nevirapine. Combined therapy with delavirdine does not appear to alter ZDV disposition.

Adverse Effects

Common toxicities seen with ZDV include anemia, neutropenia, headache, fatigue, nausea, and myalgia (Table 2). Initial symptoms are typically mild and can be managed symptomatically. However, in a small percentage of patients, particularly those receiving three- and four-drug regimens, persistent symptoms may require substitution with another nucleoside analogue such as stavudine. Anemia and neutropenia are more prominent in advanced disease (7 and 37%, respectively) than in early disease (1% and up to 8%, respectively). Macrocytosis with an elevated mean corpuscular volume is common and is not typically associated with anemia. Long-term use of ZDV may be associated with nail pigmentation and muscle toxicity. Progressive muscle wasting, weakness, and elevated serum creatine kinase have been described, as well as rare cases of cardiomyopathy. Elevated liver enzymes have also been noted and in a subset of patients may be associated with severe steatosis, lactic acidosis, and death. Systemic symptoms may be more prominent and less tolerable in early disease, while hematologic side effects may be more evident in patients with advanced disease. ZDV should be cautiously administered with other drugs known to cause bone marrow toxicity.

Drug Interactions

ZDV disposition is minimally affected by concurrent saquinavir, ritonavir, indinavir, and nelfinavir. Ritonavir induces glucuronidation and reduces the ZDV AUC by approximately 25%.

Clinical Indications

ZDV has been used alone and in various combination regimens for the treatment of patients with acute infection, symptomatic infection, and asymptomatic infection. Because of improved clinical outcomes with combination regimens (45) and the decreased risk for viral resistance, ZDV monotherapy for treatment of HIV infection is no longer recommended. ZDV has also been used (a) to decrease the risk of HIV transmission when administered to HIV-infected pregnant women (15) or uninfected individuals following occupational exposure (12), (b) to improve platelet counts in patients with HIV-related thrombocytopenia, and (c) to improve cognitive function in patients with AIDS dementia (41).

ZDV was the first antiretroviral agent to show that intervention can improve outcome in HIV disease. For advanced HIV disease, the probability of disease progression over 24 weeks was significantly lower for zidovudine recipients than for placebo recipients (0.23 vs. 0.43; $P < .001$) (30). In addition, the risk of disease progression was decreased more than

				CD4 Responses (cells/mm³)	Viral Responses (log₁₀)	Clinical Outcome

TABLE 1 • Combination Studies with Zidovudine and other Nucleoside Reverse Transcriptase Inhibitors

Study	Design	Patient Population	Treatment	CD4 Responses (cells/mm³)	Viral Responses ($\log_{10}$)	Clinical Outcome
ACTG 175 (Naive and Experienced)	Placebo-controlled	Early disease: CD4 200–500	ZDV 600/d with ddC 2.25/d or ddI 400/d		ZDV: $-.26$ + ddI: $-.93$ + ddC: $-.89$ at 8 wks	ZDV:ZDV/ddI (HR .54, P<0.001) (ZDV:ZDV/ddC: (HR .54, P<0.001)
Delta 1 Naive	Placebo-controlled	Late disease: CD4 < 350	ZDV 600/d with ddI 400/d pr ddC 2.25/d	ZDV: $+30$ + ddI: $+80$ + ddC: $+67$ at 8 wks		ZDV:ZDV/ddI (HR .64) ZDV:ZDV/ddC (HR .83) Global P=0.001
Delta 2 Experienced	Placebo-controlled	Late disease: CD4 < 350	ZDV 600/d with ddI 400/d or ddC 2.25/d	ZDV: -12 + ddI: $+20$ + ddC: $+3$ at 8 wks		ZDV:ZDV/ddI (HR .95) ZDV:ZDV/ddC (HR .94) Global P=0.87
NUCA 3001	Placebo-controlled	Early disease: CD4 200–500	ZDV: 600/d with 3TC 300/d or 3TC 600/d at 24 wks	ZDV 16.6 + 3TC 300/d; 54.9 +3TC 600/d: 44.9 at 24 wks	ZDV: $-.31$ + 3TC 300/d: -1.12 + 3TC 600/d: -1.15	

TABLE 2 • Toxicities Associated With Nucleoside Analogues

	ZDV	DDI	DDC
Constitutional			
Fever	+	+	++++
Malaise	++++	++++	++++
Myalgias	++++	+	+
Headache	++++	++++	++++
Fatigue	++++	++++	+
Altered taste	+	++++	+
Insomnia	++++	NR	NR
Gastrointestinal			
Nausea	++++	++++	+
Vomiting	+	+	+
Diarrhea	+	++++	+
Abdominal pain	+	++++	+
Pancreatitis	NR	++++	+
Elevated transaminase	++++	++++	+
Stomatitis	NR	NR	++++
Hematologic			
Anemia	++++	+	+
Neutropenia	++++	+	+
Thrombocytopenia	NR	+	+
Neuromuscular			
Myopathy	++++	+	+
Peripheral neuropathy	NR	++++	++++
Metabolic			
Hyperuricemia	NR	++++	NR
Hypertriglyceridemia	NR	++++	NR
Hyperamylasemia	NR	++++	+
Allergic			
Rash	+	+	++++
Fever	+	+	++++

+ = rare; ++++ = more common; NR = not reported.

threefold over placebo by 18 months for patients with symptomatic disease (3.23; P = .0002) (32) and by 12 months for patients with asymptomatic disease (3.1; P = .005) (91).

ZDV has been combined with other nucleoside analogues (ddI, ddC, and lamivudine) and shown to be safe and effective (Table 1). The only direct comparison of nucleoside combinations has been between ZDV and either ddI or ddC. For treatment-naive patients, ZDV/ddC provided better clinical outcome than ZDV/ddI (HR = 0.49 vs. 0.61) (45) and a slightly better survival advantage (HR = 0.59 vs. 0.61). In treatment-experienced patients, ZDV/ddI provided a better clinical outcome (HR = 0.65 vs. 0.91) and a better survival advantage (HR = 0.52 vs. 0.81). The combination of ZDV and lamivudine appears to be the most potent of the current nucleoside combinations that include ZDV. In a meta-analysis, a 66% reduction in disease progression was noted with ZDV and lamivudine, compared with other treatments (84). The combination of ZDV and stavudine in either treatment-experienced or treatment-naive patients proved to be antagonistic, with a detrimental effect on immunologic and virologic responses, and they should not be used together (1).

Greater virologic and immunologic benefit is noted with increasingly potent combination regimens. In general, three-drug regimens appear more potent than two-drug regimens, and three-drug regimens containing HIV-1 protease inhibitors appear to be the most potent (43). Most regimens appear less effective in patients with advanced HIV disease and prior treatment experience. Patients with advanced HIV disease, particularly those with 50 CD4 cells/mm^3 or less, have a higher incidence of incomplete suppression of viral replication and are at greater risk for viral resistance and eventual drug failure (46).

ZDV has been shown to be effective and safe in children. Since ZDV/ddI provided less growth failure, opportunistic infection, neurologic or neurodevelopmental deterioration, and death than ZDV alone, ZDV monotherapy is no longer recommended. ZDV administration during pregnancy decreases maternal-fetal transmission of HIV. In one study, the rate of transmission was 7.6% with ZDV and 22.6% with placebo (P < .0001) (15).

DIDANOSINE

ddI was the second antiretroviral agent approved for the treatment of HIV infection. ddI has several potential advantages: activity against ZDV-resistant strains of HIV, a long intracellular half-life, and minimal bone marrow suppression.

Mechanism of Action

ddI penetrates lymphocytes by a passive process, where it exhibits a complex intracellular disposition (59). Initially, ddI is converted to the monophosphate (ddIMP) by 5'-nucleotidase (18, 51). ddIMP is converted to dideoxyadenosine monophosphate (ddAMP) via adenylosuccinate synthetase and lyase, and subsequently ddAMP is converted to dideoxyadenosine diphosphate (ddADP) and dideoxyadenosine triphosphate (ddATP) (50). The intracellular half-life of ddATP varies from 12 to 24 h, depending on the presence of its natural nucleoside. In the presence of 2'-deoxyadenosine, higher concentrations of ddATP are achieved, but they persist for a shorter time (a half-life of 8–15 vs. 24 h) (2). The prolonged intracellular half-life of ddATP was the rationale for once- and twice-daily dosing regimens used in phase I clinical trials. However, the dosages used in once-daily regimens exceeded the absorption capacity and did not provide adequate antiviral benefit (16, 28). ddI is also a substrate for purine nucleoside phosphorylase, an enzyme that catalyzes cleavage of the dideoxyribose sugar moiety from ddI to form hypoxanthine. Hypoxanthine may be used to generate endogenous nucleotides or be further metabolized to, and excreted as, uric acid.

Mechanisms of Resistance

A number of amino acid residue changes (65, 74, and 184) have been described after prolonged ddI therapy (42, 82). Mutations in general appear more slowly than with ZDV. High-level resistance has not been well described.

Pharmacokinetic Disposition

ddI is susceptible to acid hydrolysis of the C-N bond that links the purine base (hypoxanthine) to the deoxyribose sugar; in the presence of acid, hypoxanthine and deoxyribose are liberated. The absence of hydroxy groups at the 2' and 3' positions of the deoxyribose ring is theorized to stabilize formation of a carbonium intermediate, facilitating acid hydrolysis. An estimated 10% of ddI present at 37°C and pH < 3 is degraded in less than 2 min (3). Various formulations that neutralize gastric pH directly or concurrent antacid administration are used to allow

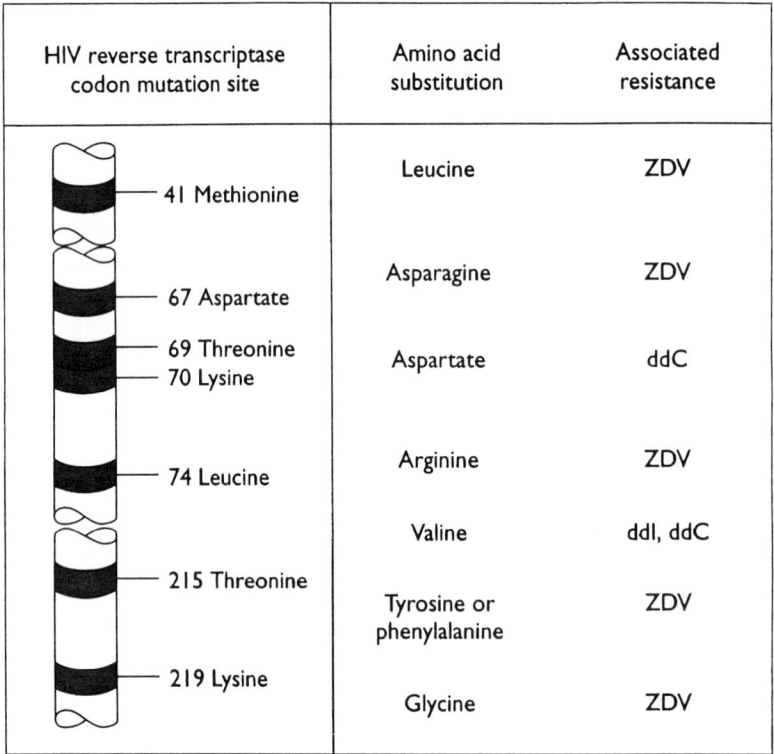

FIGURE 4. Specific mutation sites on the *pol* gene, which codes for the reverse transcriptase and confers resistance to zidovudine (ZDV), didanosine (ddI), and zalcitabine (ddC). (Adapted from Atlas of infectious diseases, AIDS, vol I.)

chronic oral dosing. New enteric formulations are currently being tested to avoid the need for a buffered dosage form.

Most patients in phase I studies of ddI were studied in the fasting state immediately after ingestion of 30 mL of aluminum hydroxide or aluminum/magnesium hydroxide antacid suspensions; bioavailability assessments ranged from 20 to 40% (48). The lower bioavailability observed with higher doses suggests a dose-related absorption, possibly resulting from degradation in the stomach or saturation of an intestinal transport mechanism (28, 56).

ddI is currently measured in plasma by radioimmunoassay (24). The maximum serum concentration (C_{max}) decreased from 2789 ± 1032 mM in the fasting state to 1291 ± 539 mM in the fed state (78). The AUC was also reduced from 21 to 11% of the administered dose. Other pharmacokinetic parameters, including the absorption rate and T_{max}, were unaffected by food. Shyu et al. speculated that increased gastric acid content in the postprandial state or prolonged contact time because of food-induced decreases in gastric emptying may account for these decreases. While food-induced reductions in C_{max} have been seen (58, 90), these effects are likely related to the rate of absorption.

Absorption of ddI appears to be quite variable. Factors such as food ingestion, gastric abnormalities (achlorhydria or HIV enteropathy), and the use of various formulations contribute to this variability (76). Bioavailability may have a significant impact on the determination of both efficacy and safety. For example, systemic exposure (AUC) demonstrates a better corre-

lation with clinical outcome parameters than did actual administered dose in children. Patients with higher AUC values experienced greater improvement in their intelligence quotient score and were more likely to demonstrate a drop in p24 antigen concentration (11).

ddI is rapidly absorbed (k_a = 1.4 h^{-1}), with steady-state C_{max} and $AUC_{(0-12h)}$ demonstrating a linear relationship to dose over the range of 0.8 to 10.2 mg/kg (47, 56). Extrapolated peak serum concentrations for the currently recommended dose of the buffered powder for oral solution approximate in vitro inhibitory concentrations for HIV (5–10 mM). Total body clearance of ddI is approximately 1.0 ± 0.1 L/kg/h, 30 to 50% of which is renal and an unclear percentage of which is metabolism or biliary excretion. Because renal clearance of ddI exceeds that of endogenous creatinine, active tubular secretion most likely contributes to the amount of drug recovered in the urine (10–40%). Neither total nor renal clearance was significantly changed when first-dose pharmacokinetics were compared with those at steady state. ddI pharmacokinetics in four uremic patients on hemodialysis indicate a prolonged half-life (3.3 ± 0.3 h) and reduced clearance (508 ± 182 mL/min, approximately 0.4 L/kg/h) (80). The dialysis extraction ratio was 43 ± 18%, and the hemodialysis clearance was 86 ± 33 mL/min (approximately 0.07 L/h/kg). While the manufacturer recommends considering dosage reduction for patients with renal or hepatic dysfunction, there are insufficient data at present to make specific recommendations.

The steady-state volume of distribution (V_{ss}) ranges from

0.76 to 1.2 L/kg, indicating less tissue distribution than with ZDV (V_{ss} = 1.6 ± 0.6 L/kg) (54). Differences in lipid solubility between ddI and ZDV may contribute to this discrepancy. CSF penetration of ddI was estimated to be 21% of the serum concentration 1 h after an intravenous dose in two patients (56). The serum half-life of ddI is 0.8 to 1.9 h after a single dose and 1.1 to 2.7 h after multiple dosing. In vitro plasma protein binding has been estimated to be below 5%.

ddI pharmacokinetics were evaluated in two patients who were 21 and 24 weeks pregnant (71). Pharmacokinetic parameters following single oral doses of 375 mg did not differ from reported values, but fetal blood concentrations were 14 and 19% of maternal serum concentrations, respectively. Minimal amounts of ddI were found in the amniotic fluid of one patient, and amniotic fluid concentration was similar to that of fetal blood in the other. ddI pharmacokinetics were evaluated in 48 children ranging in age from 8 months to 18 years (11). ddI was administered as a single intravenous dose (20–180 mg/m²) followed by the same dose administered orally every 8 h; oral doses were administered in the fasting state after ingestion of 10 to 20 mL of antacid suspension. Pharmacokinetic parameters were comparable to those obtained from adult patients with the exception of lower bioavailability (mean, 19%; range, 2–89%). Furthermore, the mean bioavailability decreased with increasing dose (21% at 20 mg/m² vs. 14% at 180 mg/m²), although this difference did not achieve significance. The currently approved pediatric dose is approximately 100 mg/m² twice daily. Although this regimen was not examined in the above study, single oral doses of 90 and 120 mg/m² yielded peak serum concentrations of 1.8 and 2.4 mM, respectively. While ddI was undetectable in 17 of 20 CSF samples, approximately 16 to 19% of estimated serum concentrations were detected in 3 CSF samples from patients receiving high doses.

Adverse Effects

ddI therapy is associated with peripheral neuropathy, pancreatitis, hyperamylasemia, hyperuricemia, and gastrointestinal complaints (Table 2). Hepatic toxicity, rare cases of electrolyte imbalance, and cardiac arrhythmias have been noted. Dry mouth, altered taste, decreased palatability, and nausea were particularly prominent with original tablet formulation.

Pancreatitis is the most serous toxicity associated with ddI therapy and in rare cases may lead to death. Abdominal pain, nausea, or vomiting may be the first signs of pancreatitis. Elevations in serum amylase and lipase levels are not uncommon. Asymptomatic elevation in serum amylase is also seen, which may be related to salivary gland toxicity and in some cases lead to xerostomia. Increases in serum amylase may also reflect pancreatic dysfunction, despite lack of a consistent clinical picture for pancreatitis. A painful sensorimotor peripheral neuropathy has been described during ddI administration. Development of peripheral neuropathy appears to be dose related and typically resolves with interruption of therapy or reduction in dose.

Drug Interactions

Drug interactions with ddI have focused primarily on the ability of the buffered formulation to reduce absorption of other drugs. Lower peak concentrations occur for delavirdine; but steady-state studies have yielded less effect on C_{max} and AUC (66). When possible, ddI should be separated from drugs that are optimally absorbed at normal gastric pH (delavirdine, indinavir, ketoconazole).

Clinical Indications

ddI has been used alone and in various combination regimens for the treatment of patients with HIV infection. ddI is approved for use in HIV-infected patients who are unable to tolerate ZDV due to adverse effects or who experience clinical or immunologic deterioration while receiving ZDV. ddI has also been used alone and in combination with either ZDV or stavudine for patients with early HIV disease who have not received prior antiretroviral therapy.

ddI was the first antiretroviral agent to show that switching therapy to another agent can improve clinical and survival benefits in the face of ZDV intolerance or failure. For patients with advanced HIV disease (≤300 CD4 cells/mm³) who had tolerated ZDV for an average of 14 months, switching to ddI provided a threefold decrease in disease progression compared with continuing ZDV (RR = 1.39, CI = 1.06–1.82, P = .0015) (52). However, for patients with advanced HIV disease and no or minimal prior ZDV therapy, ZDV provided a greater than twofold decrease in disease progression compared with ddI (RR = 1.43, IC = 1.02–2.00) (26).

ddI has been combined with other nucleoside analogues (ZDV and stavudine) and shown to be effective and safe. For patients with early HIV infection (200–500 CD4 cells/mm³) and varying amounts of prior ZDV therapy, a smaller proportion had disease progression who were receiving ddI alone (22%; P < .001) or ddI/ZDV (18%; P < .001) than ZDV alone (32%) (45) (Fig. 5). Among treatment-experienced patients, ddI/ZDV provided better clinical and survival outcomes than ddC/ZDV (45). In another large clinical trial, ddI/ZDV decreased risk of mortality by 42% compared with 32% for ddC/ZDV recipients among treatment-naive patients and by 23% compared with 9% for ddC/ZDV recipients among treatment-experienced patients (21). The combination of varying doses of ddI and stavudine in patients with early HIV infection (200–500 CD4 cells/mm³) and no prior antiretroviral therapy resulted in a mean decrease in plasma HIV RNA of 1.2 to 1.4 log_{10} and a mean increase in CD4 cell counts of 42 to 112 cells/mm³ after approximately 6 months of therapy (70).

Based on preliminary data, adding ddI to lamivudine in patients with early HIV disease with no prior antiretroviral therapy did not appear to increase the proportion with plasma HIV RNA levels below the limit of detection (<500 copies/mL) at weeks 20/24 compared with ddI alone (47 vs. 44%) (1). In addition, there was no evidence that ddI in combination with lamivudine differed with respect to the proportion with plasma HIV RNA levels below the limit of detection by weeks 20/24 compared with ZDV in combination with lamivudine (47 vs. 42%). ddI has not been combined with ddC due to concerns about excessive neurologic toxicity.

Preliminary data are available for ddI in three- and four-drug regimens (Table 1). ddI in combination with ZDV and

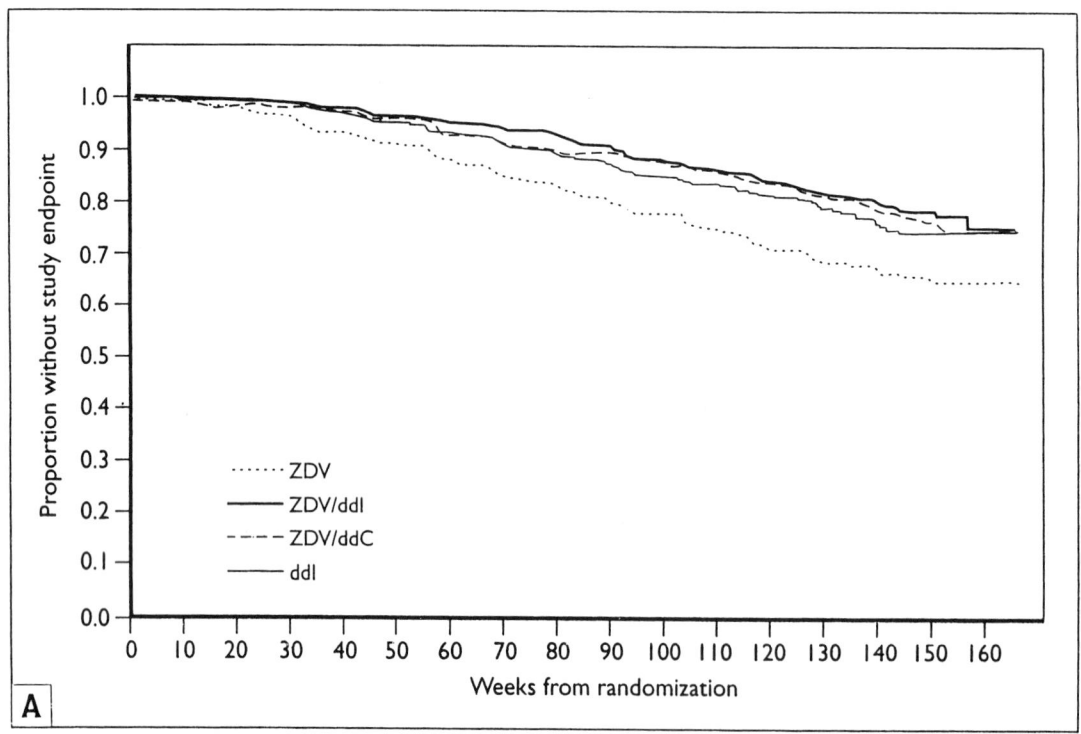

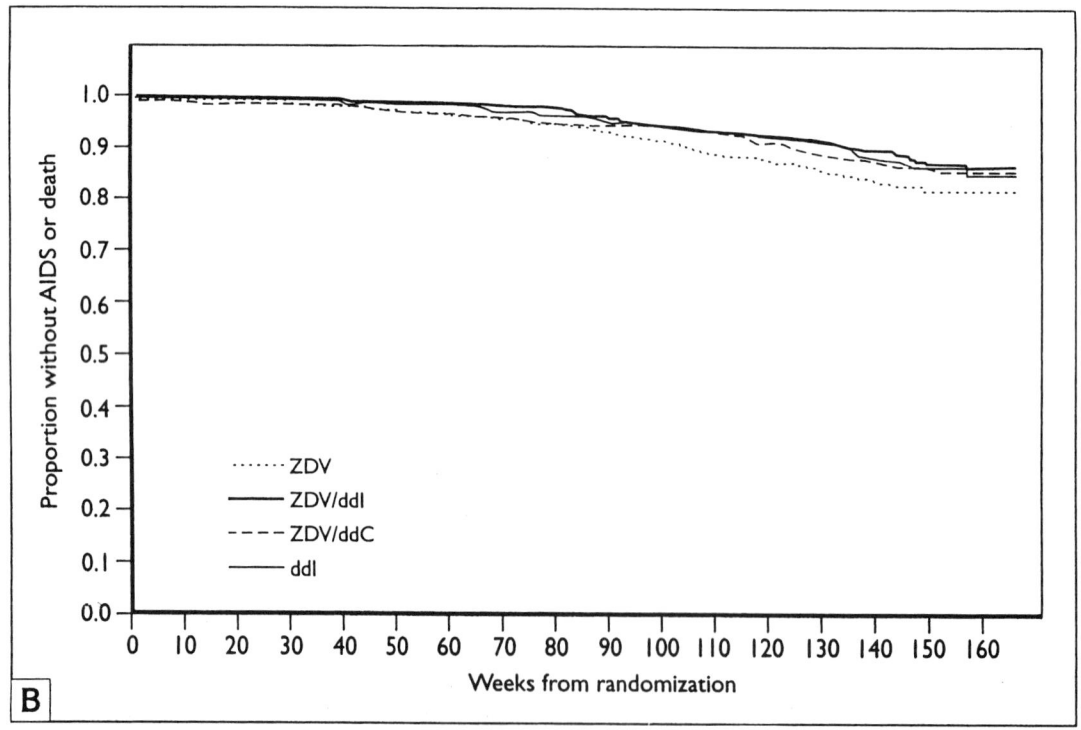

FIGURE 5. Proportion without disease progression (A), including deterioration in CD4 cell count and cumulative disease-free survival (B) among patients receiving combination therapy with zidovudine (ZDV) and either didanosine (ddI) or zalcitabine (ddC) or didanosine or zidovudine alone. (Adapted from Atlas of infectious diseases, AIDS, vol I. 2nd ed.)

nevirapine was evaluated in several clinical trials and shown to provide greater virologic and immunologic benefits. Among patients with advanced HIV disease (≤350 CD4 cells/mm³) and prior nucleoside therapy, the three-drug regimen resulted in less CD4 cell decline than with ddI/ZDV (15 vs. 33%) and

a 0.25 $\log_{10}$ greater decrease in plasma HIV-1 RNA at week 48 (20). ddI in combination with either ZDV or stavudine was also evaluated with HIV-1 protease inhibitors and shown to be safe and effective. However, more prominent gastrointestinal toxicity has been noted with several combinations.

Drug interactions with ddI have been reported. ddI may impair the absorption of indinavir, itraconazole, and ketoconazole. If ddI is to be given with indinavir, the doses should be separated by at least 1 h. Coadministration of oral ganciclovir may increase the ddI concentrations by as much as 70%, requiring a reduction in the dose of ddI.

ZALCITABINE

Zalcitabine (ddC) is a thymidine analogue with potent activity against HIV and minimal toxicity to bone marrow cells. ddC is used in combination regimens, particularly for treatment-naive patients.

Mechanism of Action

In vitro studies, using high viral inocula, have demonstrated complete inhibition of HIV replication in ATH8 cells, a human helper/inducer T-cell line, at a concentration of 0.5 mM ddC (61). ddC appears to enter various cell lines by both nucleoside carrier-mediated and non-carrier-mediated mechanisms (69, 88). Similar to other nucleoside analogues, sequential phosphorylation of ddC to its triphosphorylated form, ddC triphosphate (ddC-TP), is thought to be required to inhibit HIV DNA polymerase (reverse transcriptase). Preferential binding of ddCTP to reverse transcriptase over host cell DNA polymerase is likely to be responsible for ddC's selectivity. However, binding of ddCTP to human DNA polymerase may be related to its neurologic toxicity. HIV-infected and uninfected cells appear equally capable of phosphorylating ddC (9, 17).

ddC is initially phosphorylated to ddC-monophosphate (ddC-MP) via the cellular enzyme, dCyd kinase. However, this enzyme has a lower affinity for ddC ($K_m = 180$ mM) than for dCyd ($K_m = 3$ mM) (93). The K_m values for mitochondrial dCyd kinase are 22 mM and 120 mM, respectively (83). While exact metabolic pathways have yet to be delineated, ddC-MP is further phosphorylated to its di- and triphosphate forms, possibly via cellular kinase enzyme pathways used by dCyd. While dCyd inhibits phosphorylation of ddC (9, 17), deoxythymidine (dThd) enhances its phosphorylation (6). As ddC-TP levels increased, a concomitant decrease in dCyd-TP concentrations occurred, indicating feedback inhibition of dCyd kinase by high levels of dCyd-TP. The three major human DNA polymerases (α, β, and Δ) vary in their susceptibility to inhibition by ddC-TP. DNA polymerase α, involved in DNA replication, is by far the most resistant with a K_i for ddC-TP more than 100 times its K_m for dCyd ($K_m/K_i = 0.008$). DNA polymerase β and Δ, involved in DNA repair and mitochondrial DNA generation, respectively, are more sensitive with reversed K_m/K_i ratios above 1 (1.7 for β and 19 for Δ) (9, 83). Delayed cytotoxicity and selective loss of mitochondrial DNA occurred in Molt-4F cells (a human T lymphoblastic cell line) continuously exposed to 0.1 or 0.2 mM ddC, possibly indicating a mechanism for ddC-associated neurotoxicity (13).

Mechanisms of Resistance

Resistance to ddC related to specific mutations and cross-resistance with ddI have been described (34, 82).

Pharmacokinetic Disposition

Following oral administration as a tablet or oral solution, ddC is 70 to 80% bioavailable (53, 55, 60). The time to maximum serum concentration is about 1 to 2 h. Like most other nucleoside analogues, ddC is rapidly eliminated, with a serum half-life of 1.2 ± 0.6 h and mean total body clearance of 227 ± 86 mL/m^2/min (0.2 L/h/kg). The inadequate sensitivity of the HPLC assay has limited analysis in at least one study because of the relatively low dose of ddC that was given (0.5 mg) (44). Radioimmunoassay is more sensitive and can be used to study ddC disposition (10, 77). The V_{ss} of ddC was found to be 0.54 ± 0.22 L/kg in 10 adult patients and 0.2 L/kg in pediatric patients. ddC concentrations in the CSF range from 9 to 37% of concomitant serum concentrations 2 to 3.5 h after initiation of an intravenous dose (93).

As indicated by the high urinary recovery of unchanged ddC (approximately 75%), renal mechanisms are the predominant clearance pathway for ddC. Total body clearance of ddC is 0.2 to 0.3 L/h/kg determined after single and multiple doses of ddC (44, 55). Lower clearance values of about 150 mL/min/m^2 were found in a pediatric population (68).

Adverse Effects

The dose-limiting toxicity for ddC is a painful sensorimotor peripheral neuropathy predominantly involving the lower extremities. The daily dose and cumulative dose of ddC correlate with the risk of peripheral neuropathy. Approximately 10 to 25% of patients receiving 2.25 mg/day of ddC develop peripheral neuropathy. Symptoms include pain or discomfort in the feet, followed by burning and numbness. Loss of deep tendon reflexes may be an early important sign of peripheral neuropathy. Motor abnormalities are uncommon but may occur if ddC is continued in the face of symptoms consistent with peripheral neuropathy. Other side effects may include gastrointestinal complaints, allergic reactions, anemia, and neutropenia. Rare cases of hepatitis, heart failure, glucose abnormalities, and pancreatitis have been described.

Clinical Indications

ddC was found less effective than ZDV monotherapy and for the most part has been used in various combination regimens for the treatment of patients with HIV infection. Like ddI, ddC is approved for use in patients with HIV infection who have clinical and immunologic deterioration while receiving ZDV or ddI or who are intolerant to either ZDV or ddI. ddC has limited use in treatment-experienced patients. ddC was the first antiretroviral drug to receive accelerated approval by the FDA; initial approval was based on improvements in immunologic and virologic responses. ddC was also the first drug to be approved in a combination regimen (ZDV/ddC). In patients with advanced HIV disease and little or no prior ZDV therapy, ZDV provided a 1.5-fold decrease in disease progression compared with ddC. Estimated 1-year survival rates were 85% for ddC recipients and 92% for ZDV recipients ($P = .007$). ddC monotherapy is therefore not recommended.

ddC has been evaluated in combination with ZDV in

several studies with varying results. Among patients with prior ZDV experience, one study showed no overall difference among patients receiving ddC, ddC in combination with ZDV, or ZDV alone (33); however, patients with CD4 cell counts of 150 CD4 cells/mm³ or above who received ddC/ZDV had better clinical outcomes. In two large studies, ddC in combination with ZDV provided better clinical outcomes than ZDV alone. However, this advantage was less evident among treatment-experienced patients than treatment-naive patients.

REFERENCES

1. ACTG 306 executive summary, 1997.
2. Ahluwalia G, Cooney DA, Mitsuya H, Fridland A, Flora KP, Hao Z, Dalal M, Broder S, Johns DG. Initial studies on the cellular pharmacology of 2′, 3′ dideoxyinosine, an inhibitor of HIV infectivity. Biochem Pharmacol 1987;36:3797–3800.
3. Anderson BD, Wugant NB, Xiang T, Waugh WA, Stella VJ. Preformulation solubility and kinetic studies of 2′,3′-dideoxypurine nucleosides: potential anti-AIDS agents. Int J Pharmacokinet 1988;45:27–37.
4. Balis FM, Pizzo PA, Murphy RF, Eddy T, Jarosinski PF, Falloon J, Broder S, Poplack DG. The pharmacokinetics of zidovudine administered by continuous infusion in children. Ann Intern Med 1989;110:279–285.
5. Balis FM, Pizzo PA, Eddy J, Wilfert C, McKinney R, Scott G, Murphy RF, Jarosinski PF, Falloon J, Poplack DG. Pharmacokinetics of zidovudine administered intravenously and orally in children with human immunodeficiency virus infection. J Pediatr 1989;114:880–884.
6. Balzarini J, Cooney D, Dalal M, Kang GJ, Cupp JE, DeClercq E, Broder S, Johns DG. 2′,3′-dideoxycytidine: regulation of its metabolism and anti-retroviral potency by natural pyrimidine nucleosides and by inhibitors of pyrimidine nucleotide synthesis. Mol Pharmacol 1987;32:798–806.
7. Blum MR, Liao SHT, Good SS, de Miranda P. Pharmacokinetics and bioavailability of zidovudine in humans. Am J Med 1988;85(Suppl 2A):189–194.
8. Boucher C, O'Sullivan E, Mulder J, Ramautarsing C, Kellam P, Darby G, Lange JM, Goudsmit J, Larder BA. Ordered appearance of zidovudine resistance mutations during treatment of 18 human immunodeficiency virus-positive subjects. J Infect Dis 1992;165:105–110.
9. Broder S. Pharmacodynamics of 2′,3′-dideoxycytidine: an inhibitor of human immunodeficiency virus. Am J Med 1990;88 (Suppl 5B):2S–7S.
10. Burger DM, Rosing H, ten Napel CHH, Duyts T, Meenhorst PL, Mulder JW, Koksch CH, Bult A, Beijnen JH. Application of a radioimmunoassay for determination of levels of zalcitabine (ddC) in human plasma, urine, and cerebrospinal fluid. Antimicrob Agents Chemother 1994;38:2763–2767.
11. Butler KM, Husson RN, Balis FM, Brouwers P, Eddy J, el-Amin D, Gress J, Hawkins M, Jarosinski P, Moss H. Dideoxyinosine in children with symptomatic human immunodeficiency virus infection. N Engl J Med 1991;324:137–144.
12. CDC. Case-control study of HIV seroconversion in health-care workers after percutaneous exposure to HIV-infected blood—France, United Kingdom, and United States, January 1988–August 1994. MMWR 1995;44:929–933.
13. Chen CH, Cheng YC. Delayed cytotoxicity and selective loss of mitochondrial DNA in cells treated with the anti-human im-

munodeficiency virus compound 2′,3′-dideoxycytidine. J Biol Chem 1989;264:11934–11937.
14. Collins JM, Unadkat JD. Clinical pharmacokinetics of zidovudine: an overview of current data. Clin Pharmacol 1989;17:1–9.
15. Connor EM, Sperling RS, Gelber R, Kiselev P, Scott G, O'Sullivan MJ, Van Dyke R, Bey M, Shearer W, Jacobson RL. Reduction of maternal-infant transmission of human immunodeficiency virus type 1 with zidovudine treatment. N Engl J Med 1994;331:1173–1180.
16. Cooley TP, Kunches LM, Saunders CA, Ritter JK, Perkins CJ, McLaren C, McCaffrey RP, Liebman HA. Once-daily administration of 2′3′-dideoxyinosine (ddI) in patients with the acquired immunodeficiency syndrome or AIDS-related complex. Results of a phase I trial. N Engl J Med 1990;322:1340–1345.
17. Cooney DA, Dalal M, Mitsuya H, McMahon JB, Nadkarni M, Balzarini J, Broder S, Johns DG. Initial studies on the cellular pharmacology of 2′,3′-dideoxycytidine, an inhibitor of HTLV-III infectivity. Biochem Pharmacol 1986;35:2065–2068.
18. Cooney DA, Ahluwalia G, Mitsuya H, Fridland A, Johnson M, Hao Z, Dalal M, Balzarini J, Broder S, Johns DG. Initial studies on the cellular pharmacology of 2′,3′-dideoxyadenosine, an inhibitor of HTLV-III infectivity. Biochem Pharmacol 1987;36:1765–1768.
19. D'Aquila RT, Johnson VA, Welles SL, Japour AJ, Kuritzkes DR, DeGruttola V, Reichelderfer PS, Coombs RW, Crumpacker CS, Kahn JO. Zidovudine resistance and HIV-1 disease progression during antiretroviral therapy: AIDS Clinical Trials Group Protocol 116B/117 Team and the Virology Committee Resistance Working Group. Ann Intern Med 1995;122:401–408.
20. D'Aquila RT, Hughes MD, Johnson VA, Fischl MA, Sommadossi JP, Liou SH, Timpone J, Myers M, Basgoz N, Niu M, Hirsch MS. Nevirapine, zidovudine, and didanosine compared with zidovudine and didanosine in patients with HIV-1 infection. A randomized, double-blind, placebo-controlled trial. Ann Intern Med 1996;124:1019–1030.
21. Delta Coordinating Committee. Delta: a randomized double-blind controlled trial comparing combinations with zidovudine plus didanosine or zalcitabine with zidovudine alone in HIV infected individuals. Lancet 1996;348:283–291.
22. deMiranda P, Good SS, Yarchoan R, Thomas RV, Blum MR, Myers CE, Broder S. Alteration of zidovudine pharmacokinetics by probenecid in patients with AIDS or AIDS-related complex. Clin Pharmacol Ther 1989;46:494–500.
23. Deray G, Diquet B, Martinez F, Vidal AM, Petitclerc T, Ben Hmida M. Pharmacokinetics of zidovudine in a patient on maintenance hemodialysis. N Engl J Med 1988;319:1606–1607.
24. DeRemer MD, D'Ambrosio RD, Morse GD. Didanosine measurement by radioimmunoassay. Antimicrob Agents Chemother 1996;40:1331–1334.
25. DeRemer M, D'Ambrosio R, Bartos L, Cousins S, Morse GD. Radioimmunoassay of zidovudine: extended use and potential application. Ther Drug Monit 1997;19:195–200.
26. Dolin R, Amato DA, Fischl MA, Pettinelli C, Beltangady M, Liou SH, Brown MJ, Cross AP, Hirsch M, Hardy WD. Zidovudine compared with didanosine in patients with advanced HIV type 1 infection and little or no previous experience with zidovudine. Arch Intern Med 1995;155:961–974.
27. Drew RH, Weller S, Gallis HA, Walmer KA, Bartlett JA, Blum MR. Bioequivalence assessment of zidovudine (Retrovir) syrup, solution, and capsule formulations in patients infected with human immunodeficiency virus. Antimicrob Agents Chemother 1989;33:1801–1803.

28. Drusano GL, Yuen GJ, Morse G, Cooley TP, Seidlin M, Lambert JS, Liebman HA, Valentine FT, Dolin R. Impact of bioavailability on determination of the maximal tolerated dose of a 2′,3′-dideoxyinosine in phase I trials. Antimicrob Agents Chemother 1992;36:1280–1283.

29. Erice A, Mayers DL, Strike DG, Sannerud KJ, McCutchan FE, Henry K, Balfour HH Jr. Primary infection with zidovudine-resistant human immunodeficiency virus type 1. N Engl J Med 1993;328:1163–1165.

30. Fischl MA, Richman DD, Grieco MH, Gottlieb MS, Volberding PA, Laskin OL, Leedom JM, Groopman JE, Mildvan D, Schooley RT. The efficacy of azidothymidine [AZT] in the treatment of patients with AIDS and AIDS-related complex: a double-blind, placebo-controlled trial. N Engl J Med 1987;317:185–191.

31. Fischl MA, Parker CB, Pettinelli C, Wulfsohn M, Hirsch MS, Collier AC, Antoniskis D, Ho M, Richman DD, Fuchs E. A randomized controlled trial of a reduced daily dose of zidovudine in patients with the acquired immunodeficiency syndrome. N Engl J Med 1990;323:1009–1014.

32. Fischl MA, Richman DD, Hansen N, Collier AC, Carey JT, Para MF, Hardy WD, Dolin R, Powderly WG, Allan JD. The safety and efficacy of zidovudine (AZT) in the treatment of subjects with mildly symptomatic human immunodeficiency virus type I (HIV) infection. A double-blind placebo-controlled trial. Ann Intern Med. 1990;112:727–737.

33. Fischl MA, Stanley K, Collier AC, Arduino JM, Stein DS, Feinberg JE, Allan JD, Goldsmith JC, Powderly WG. Combination and monotherapy with zidovudine and zalcitabine in patients with advanced HIV disease. Ann Intern Med 1995;122:24–32.

34. Fitzgibbon JE, Howell RM, Haberzettl CA, Sperber SJ, Gocke DJ, Dubin DT. HIV-1 pol gene mutations which cause decreased susceptibility to 2′,3′-dideoxycytidine. Antimicrob Agents Chemother 1992;36:153–157.

35. Fletcher CV, Kawle SP, Page LM, Remmel RP, Acosta EP, Henry K, Erice A, Balfour HH. Intracellular triphosphate concentrations of antiretroviral nucleosides as a determinant of clinical response in HIV-infected patients. Programs and abstracts of the 4th Conference on Retroviruses and Opportunistic Infections, Washington, DC, January 23, 1997.

36. Frenkel LM, Wagner LE, Demeter LM, Dewhurst S, Coombs RW, Murante BL, Reichman RC. Effects of zidovudine use during pregnancy on resistance and vertical transmission of human immunodeficiency virus type 1. Clin Infect Dis 1995;20:1321–1326.

37. Furman PA, Fyfe JS, St. Clair MH, Weinhold K, Rideout JL, Freeman GA, Lehrman SN, Bolognesi DP, Broder S, Mitsuya H. Phosphorylation of 3′-azido-3′-deoxythymidine and selective interaction of the 5′-triphosphate with human immunodeficiency virus reverse transcriptase. Proc Natl Acad Sci USA 1986;83:833–837.

38. Gillet JY, Garraffo R, Abrar D, Bongain A, Lapalus P, Dellamonica P. Fetoplacental passage of zidovudine. Lancet 1989;i:269–270.

39. Gitterman SR, Drusano GL, Egorin MJ, Standford HC. Population pharmacokinetics of zidovudine (AZT). Clin Pharmacol Ther 1990;48:161–167.

40. Good SS, Reynolds DJ, deMiranda P. Simultaneous quantification of zidovudine and its glucuronide in serum by high-performance liquid chromatography. J Chromatogr 1988;431:123–133.

41. Gray F, Belec L, Keohane C, De Truchis P, Clair B, Durigon M, Sobel A, Gherardi R. Zidovudine therapy and HIV encephalitis: a 10-year neuropathological survey. AIDS 1994;8:489–493.

42. Gu Z, Gao Q, Li X, Parniak MA, Wainberg MA. Novel mutation in the human immunodeficiency virus type 1 reverse transcriptase gene that encodes cross-resistance to 2′,3′-dideoxyinosine and 2′,3′-dideoxycytidine. J Virol 1992;66:7128–7135.

43. Gulick RM, Mellors JW, Havlir D, et al. Treatment with indinavir, zidovudine and lamvidine in adults with human immunodeficiency virus infection and prior antiretroviral therapy. N Engl J Med 1997;337:734–739.

44. Gustavson LE, Fukuda EK, Rubio FA, Dunton AW. A pilot study of the bioavailability and pharmacokinetics of 2′,3′-dideoxycytidine in patients with AIDS or AIDS-related complex. J Acquir Immune Defic Syndr 1990;3:28–31.

45. Hammer SM, Katzenstein DA, Hughes MD, Gundacker H, Schooley RT, Haubrich RH, Henry WK, Lederman MM, Phair JP, Niu M, Hirsch MS, Merigan TC. A trial comparing nucleoside monotherapy with combination therapy in HIV-infected adults with CD4 cell counts from 200 to 500 per cubic millimeter. N Engl J Med 1996;335:1081–1090.

46. Hammer SM, Squires KE, Hughes MD, et al. A controlled trial of two nucleoside analogues plus indinavir in persons with human immunodeficiency virus infection and CD4 cell counts of 200 per cubic millimeter or less. N Engl J Med 1997;337:725–733.

47. Hartman NR, Yarchoan R, Pluda JM, Thomas RV, Marczyk KS, Broder S, Johns DG. Pharmacokinetics of 2′,3′-dideoxyadenosine and 2′,3′-dideoxyinosine in patients with severe acquired immunodeficiency syndrome. Clin Pharmacol Ther 1990;47:647–654.

48. Hartman NR, Yarchoan R, Pluda JM, Thomas RV, Wyvill KM, Flora KP, Broder S, Johns DG. Pharmacokinetics of 2′,3′-dideoxyinosine in patients with severe human immunodeficiency virus infection. II. The effects of different oral formulations and the presence of other medications. Clin Pharmacol Ther 1991;50:278–285.

49. Henry K, Chinnock BJ, Quinn RP, Fletcher CV, deMiranda P, Balfour HH Jr. Concurrent zidovudine levels in semen and serum determined by radioimmunoassay in patients with AIDS or AIDS-related complex. JAMA 1988;259:3023–3026.

50. Johnson MA, Ahluwalia G, Connelly MC, Cooney DA, Broder S, Johns DG, Fridland A. Metabolic pathways for the activation of the antiretroviral agent 2′,3′-dideoxyadenosine in human lymphoid cells. J Biol Chem 1988;263:15354–15357.

51. Johnson MA, Fridland A. Phosphorylation of 2′,3′-dideoxyinosine by cytosolic 5′-nucleotidase of human lymphoid cells. Mol Pharmacol 1989;35:291–295.

52. Kahn JO, Lagakos SW, Richman DD, Cross A, Pettinelli C, Liou SH, Brown M, Volberding PA, Crumpacker CS, Beall G. A controlled trial comparing continued zidovudine with didanosine in human immunodeficiency virus infection. N Engl J Med 1992;327:581–587.

53. Kelley JA, Litterst CI, Roth JS, Vistica DT, Poplack DG, Cooney DA, Nadkarni M, Balis FM, Broder S, Johns DG. The disposition and metabolism of 2′,3′-dideoxycytidine, an in vitro inhibitor of human T-lymphotrophic virus type III infectivity, in mice and monkeys. Drug Metab Dispos 1987;15:595–601.

54. Klecker RW, Collins JM, Yarchoan R, Thomas R, Jenkins JF, Broder S, Myers CE. Plasma and cerebrospinal fluid pharmacokinetics of 3′-azido-3′-deoxythymidine: a novel pyrimidine analog with potential application for the treatment of patients with AIDS and related diseases. Clin Pharmacol Ther 1987;41:407–412.

55. Klecker RW, Collins JM, Yarchoan RC, Thomas R, McAtee N, Broder S, Myers CE. Pharmacokinetics of 2′,3′-dideoxycytidine in patients with AIDS and related disorders. J Clin Pharmacol 1988;28:837–842.

56. Knupp CA, Shyu WC, Dolin R, Valentine FT, McLaren C, Martin RR, Pittman KA, Barbhaiya RH. Pharmacokinetics of didanosine in patients with acquired immunodeficiency syndrome or acquired immunodeficiency syndrome complex. Clin Pharmacol Ther 1991;49:523–535.

57. Kornhauser DM, Petty BG, Hendrix CW, Woods AS, Nerhood LJ, Bartlett JG, Lietman PS. Probenecid and zidovudine metabolism. Lancet 1989;Aug:473–475.

58. Lotterer E, Ruhnke M, Trautmann M, Beyer R, Bauer FE. Decreased and variable systemic availability of zidovudine in patients with AIDS if administered with a meal. Eur J Clin Pharmacol 1991;40:305–308.

59. McGowan JJ, Tomaszdewski JE, Cradock J, Hoth D, Grieshaber CK, Broder S, Mitsuya H. Overview of the preclinical development of an antiretroviral drug, 2′3′-dideoxyinosine. Rev Infect Dis 1990;12(Suppl 5):S513–S521.

60. Merigan TC, Skowron G, Bozette SA, Richman D, Uttamchandani R, Fischl M, School R, Hirsch M, Soo W, Pettinelli C. Circulating p24 antigen levels and responses to dideoxycytidine in human immunodeficiency virus infections: a phase I study. Ann Intern Med 1989;110:189–194.

61. Mitsuya H, Broder S. Inhibition of the in vitro infectivity and cytopathic effect of human T-lymphotropic virus type III/lymphadenopathy-associated virus (HTLV-III/LAV) by 2′,3′-dideoxynucleosides. Proc Natl Acad Sci USA 1986;83: 1911–1915.

62. Morse GD, Olson J, Portmore A, Taylor C, Plank C, Reichman RC. Pharmacokinetics of orally administered zidovudine among patients with hemophilia and asymptomatic human immunodeficiency virus infection. Antiviral Res 1989;11:57–66.

63. Morse GD, Portmore A, Olson L, Taylor C, Plank C, Reichman RC. Multiple-dose pharmacokinetics of oral zidovudine in hemophilia patients with human immunodeficiency virus infection. Antimicrob Agents Chemother 1990;34:394–397.

64. Morse GD, Portmore A, Olson J, Taylor C, Plank C, Reichman RC. Renal excretion of zidovudine and zidovudineglucuronide during multiple dosing [Abstract]. Clin Pharmacol Ther 1990; 47:177.

65. Morse GD, Shelton M, O'Donnell A. Comparative pharmacokinetics of antiviral nucleoside analogs. Clin Pharmacokinet 1993;24:101–123.

66. Morse GD, Fischl MA, Cox SR, Shelton MJ, Driver M, Freimuth WW. Reduced delavirdine absorption during concurrent didanosine administration. Antimicrob Agents Chemother 1997;41:169–174.

67. O'Donnell A, Bartos L, Morse GD. Zidovudine distribution into blood components [Abstract]. Pharmacotherapy 1991:P-39.

68. Pizzo PA, Butler K, Balis F, Brouwers E, Hawkins M, Eddy J, Einloth M, Falloon J, Husson R, Jarosinski P. Dideoxycytidine alone and in an alternating schedule with zidovudine in children with symptomatic human immunodeficiency virus infection. J Pediatr 1990;117:799–808.

69. Plagemann PGW, Woffendi C. Dideoxycytidine permeation and salvage by mouse leukemia cells and human erythrocytes. Biochem Pharmacol 1989;38:3469–75.

70. Pollard R, Peterson D, Hardy D, Pedneault L, McLaren C, Skovronski J, Connaughton E, Grosso R, Reynolds L, Rutkiewicz V, Cross A, Dunkle L, Smaldone L. Antiviral effect and safety of stavudine (d4T) and didanosine (ddI) combination therapy in HIV-infected subjects in an ongoing pilot randomized double-blind trial [Abstract 197]. Program and abstracts of the Third Conference on Retroviruses and Opportunistic Infections, Washington, DC, Jan 28–Feb 1, 1996.

71. Pons JC, Boubon MC, Taburet AM, Singlas E, Chambrin V, Frydman R, Papiernik E, Delfraissy JF. Fetoplacental passage of 2′,3′-dideoxyinosine. Lancet 1991;337:732.

72. Richman DD, Grimes JM, Lagakos SW. Effect of stage of disease and drug dose on zidovudine susceptibilities of isolates of human immunodeficiency virus. J Acquir Immune Defic Syndr 1990;3:743–746.

73. Robbins BL, Rodman J, McDonald C, Srivivas RV, Flynn PM, Fridland A. Enzymatic assay for measurement of zidovudine triphosphate in peripheral blood mononuclear cells. Antimicrob Agents Chemother 1994;38:115–121.

74. Rooke R, Parniak MA, Tremblay M, Soudeyns H, Li XG, Gao Q, Yao XJ, Wainberg MA. Biological comparison of wild-type and zidovudine-resistant isolates of human immunodeficiency virus type 1 from the same subjects: susceptibility and resistance to other drugs. Antimicrob Agents Chemother 1991;35: 988–991.

75. Shelton MJ, Portmore A, Blum MR, Sadler BM, Reichman RC, Morse GD. Prolonged, but not diminished, zidovudine absorption induced by a high-fat breakfast. Pharmacotherapy 1994; 14:671–677.

76. Shelton MJ, Adams JM, Hewitt RG, Steinwandel C, DeRemer M, Cousins S, Morse GD. Effects of spontaneous gastric hypoacidity on the pharmacokinetics of zidovudine and didanosine. Pharmacotherapy 1997;17:438–444.

77. Shelton MJ, Adams JM, Hewitt RG, DeRemer M, D'Ambrosio R, Grasela TH, Morse GD. Zalcitabine population pharmacokinetics: application of radioimmunoassay. Antimicrob Agents Chemother 1998;42:409–413.

78. Shyu WC, Knupp CA, Pittman KA, Dunkle L, Barbhaiya RH. Food-induced reduction in bioavailability of didanosine. Clin Pharmacol Ther 1991;50:503–507.

79. Singlas E, Pioger JC, Taburet AM, Colin JN, Fillastre JP. Zidovudine disposition in patients with severe renal impairment: influence of hemodialysis. Clin Pharmacol Ther 1989;46: 190–197.

80. Singlas E, Parent O, Taburet A-M, et al. Pharmacokinetics of dideoxyinosine in patients with normal and impaired renal function [Abstract 1352]. Programs and abstracts of the 31st Interscience Conference on Antimicrobial Agents and Chemotherapy, Chicago, Sep 29–Oct 2, 1991.

81. Slusher JT, Kuwahara SK, Hamzeh FM, Lewis LD, Kornhauser DM, Lietman PS. Intracellular zidovudine (ZDV) and ZDV phosphates as measured by a validated combined high-pressure liquid chromatography–radioimmunoassay procedure. Antimicrob Agents Chemother 1992;36:2473–2477.

82. St Clair M, Martin J, Tudor-Williams G, Bach MC, Vavro CL, King DM, Kellam P, Kemp SD, Larder BA. Resistance to ddI and sensitivity to AZT induced by a mutation in HIV-1 reverse transcriptase. Science 1991;253:1557–1559.

83. Starnes MC, Cheng YC. Cellular metabolism of 2′,3′-dideoxycytidine, a compound active against human immunodeficiency virus in vitro. J Biol Chem 1987;262:988–991.

84. Staszewski K, Hill AM, Barlett J, Eron JJ, Katlama C, Johnson J, Sawyer W, McDade H. Reductions in HIV-1 disease progression for zidovudine/lamivudine relative to control treatments: a meta-analysis. AIDS 1997;11:477–483.

85. Stretcher BN, Pesce AJ, Frame PT, Greenberg KA, Stein DS. Correlates of zidovudine phosphorylation with markers of HIV disease progression and drug toxicity. AIDS 1994;8:763–769.

86. Stretcher BN, Pesce AJ, Hurtubise PE, Frame PT. Pharmacokinetics of zidovudine phosphorylation in patients infected with the human immunodeficiency virus. Ther Drug Monit 1992;14:281–285.

87. Stretcher BN, Pesce AJ, Hurtubise PE, Vine WH, Frame PT. Concentrations of phosphorylated zidovudine in patient leukocytes do not correlate with ZDV dose or plasma concentrations. Ther Drug Monit 1991;13:325–331.

88. Ullman B, Coons T, Rockwell S, McCartan K. Genetic analysis of 2′,3′-dideoxycytidine incorporation into cultured human T lymphoblasts. J Biol Chem 1988;263:12391–12396.

89. Unadkat JD, Lopez AA, Schumann L. Transplacental transfer and the pharmacokinetics of zidovudine (ZDV) in the near term pregnant macaque. Proceedings of the 28th Interscience Conference on Antimicrobial Agents and Chemotherapy, Los Angeles, 1988:372.

90. Unadkat JD, Coller AC, Crosby SS, Cummings D, Opheim KE, Corey L. Influence of a high-fat meal on zidovudine pharmacokinetics. AIDS 1990;4:229–232.

91. Volberding PA, Lagakos SW, Koch MA, Pettinelli C, Myers MW, Booth DK, Balfour HH Jr, Reichman RC, Bartlett JA, Hirsch MS. Zidovudine in asymptomatic human immunodeficiency virus infection: a controlled trial in persons with fewer than 500 CD4-positive cells per cubic millimeter. N Engl J Med 1990;322:941–949.

92. Yarchoan R, Perno CF, Thomas RV, Klecker RW, Allain JP, Wills RJ, McAtee N, Fischl MA, Dubinsky R, McNeely MC. Phase I studies of 2′,3′-dideoxycytidine in severe human immunodeficiency virus infection as a single agent and alternating with zidovudine (AZT). Lancet 1988;1:76–81.

93. Yarchoan R, Mitsuya H, Thomas RV, Pluda JM, Hartman NR, Perno CF, Marczyk KS, Allain JP, Johns DG, Broder S. In vivo activity against HIV and favorable toxicity profile of 2′,3′-dideoxyinosine. Science 1989;245:412–415.

Ganciclovir

●

John F. Flaherty, Jr. and Clyde S. Crumpacker

Ganciclovir occupies a special place in the early development of antiviral therapy. An analogue of acyclovir, ganciclovir is the first antiviral agent with demonstrable efficacy against human cytomegalovirus (CMV) (5, 53, 57). The development of ganciclovir provides a clear example of the way in which chemists can creatively modify an antiviral molecule such as acyclovir once the chemical structure is known. Ganciclovir was synthesized in two pharmaceutical companies (Syntex Inc. and Merck Sharpe and Dohme) and one university (McGill University in Canada) at about the same time, in 1982. In addition, chemists at Burroughs Wellcome Inc., as an extension of their acyclovir patent, synthesized an identical compound known as BW759. Following its synthesis, ganciclovir was quickly recognized to have the ability to inhibit all of the herpes viruses and to inhibit transformation of normal cord-blood lymphocytes by Epstein-Barr virus (13, 34, 70). Commercial development of the intravenous form of ganciclovir has had a major impact on the treatment and prevention of CMV disease. Recently developed additional dosage forms (e.g., oral capsules and an intraocular implant device) have greatly expanded the clinical utility of this antiviral agent.

CLASS

Ganciclovir is a nucleoside analogue of guanosine and a homologue of acyclovir (Fig. 1). Scientists at Syntex, who are credited with the earliest patent of the drug, synthesized a compound called 2,3-dihydroxy-9-promethyl guanosine (DHPG)

(13). Researchers at Merck, Sharpe and Dohme synthesized a compound known as 2′-nor-2′-deoxyguanosine (2′ NDG), while chemists at Mc Gill University prepared the compound 9-{2-hydroxy-1-(hydroxymethyl)ethyoxy]methyl}guanine] (BIOLOF 62) (34, 70). These three compounds were found to be identical in structure and later described as ganciclovir.

Unlike acyclovir, which contains only one hydroxyl group in its chemical configuration, ganciclovir possesses hydroxyl groups at both the 3′ and 5′ positions of its sugar moiety (58). This slight structural modification is responsible for the enhanced activity of ganciclovir against CMV, compared with acyclovir, and likely explains the differences in pharmacokinetic disposition and tolerability exhibited between these two compounds.

ANTIVIRAL ACTIVITY

In tissue culture, ganciclovir has excellent activity against nearly all herpesviruses. Ganciclovir is 50 times more active than acyclovir against the laboratory strain (AD 169) of human CMV (HCMV) and as much as 100 times more active than acyclovir against some clinical isolates of HCMV (82, 50). Against clinical isolates of CMV, ganciclovir is 30 to 100 times more active than foscarnet and twofold less active than cidofovir (14, 28). Ganciclovir inhibits plaque formation by laboratory strains and clinical isolates of CMV in concentrations ranging from 0.1 to 1.6 µg/mL (19, 50, 60, 82). A multicenter study evaluating the activity of ganciclovir against 54

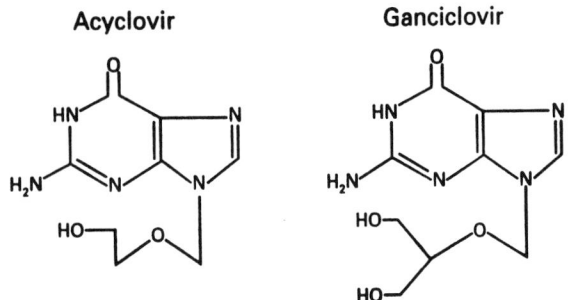

FIGURE 1. Chemical structures of the antiviral drugs acyclovir and ganciclovir. (Adapted from Oliver S, Bubley G, Crumpacker CS. Inhibition of HSV-transformed murine cells by nucleoside analogs, 2'NDG and 2'-nor-cGMP: mechanism of inhibition and reversal by exogenous nucleosides. Virology 1985;145:84–93, with permission.)

clinical isolates of CMV obtained in Boston, Philadelphia, and San Francisco, found 90% of strains to be inhibited by 6 μM (1.5 μg/mL) of ganciclovir (60). There were no obvious differences in ganciclovir sensitivity among study strains when evaluated by geographic location or patient source (e.g., renal transplant recipients, patients with CMV mononucleosis, infants with congenital CMV, or homosexual men). In a study that included 130 isolates of CMV obtained from patients infected with HIV who had not yet received ganciclovir therapy, all isolates but one were inhibited by a concentration (ID_{50}) of 5 μM or less ($\leq$1.25 μg/mL); the mean ID_{50} was 1.94 μM (0.49 μg/mL) (28).

The combination of ganciclovir with foscarnet is synergistic in tissue culture. Mean IC_{50} values for ganciclovir and foscarnet alone were 2.25 μg/mL and 33.25 μg/mL, respectively. When ganciclovir and foscarnet were combined, a concentration-dependent reduction in IC_{50} was demonstrated (49). In another investigation, combination of ganciclovir and cidofovir (HPMPC) synergistically inhibited growth of CMV in human embryo lung cells in vitro (71).

The activity of ganciclovir is similar to that of acyclovir against herpes simplex virus type 1, herpes simplex virus type 2, and varicella-zoster virus (22, 34, 70). Ganciclovir is also active against Epstein-Barr virus (EBV) and inhibits EBV-induced cell transformation that results in establishment of continuous lymphoblastoid cell lines (34). Ganciclovir is very active against human herpesvirus-6 (HHV-6), whereas acyclovir shows very little activity against this virus (1). While ganciclovir is active against adenovirus type 2, it has little activity against vaccinia virus, human papilloma virus, or RNA viruses such as influenza A (70, 81).

MECHANISM OF ACTION

As with other nucleosides such as acyclovir, ganciclovir must be phosphorylated and converted to the triphosphate form before it can exert antiviral activity. Ganciclovir triphosphate inhibits DNA polymerases, including those of herpes simplex virus and CMV, by competitively inhibiting incorporation of deoxyguanosine triphosphate into elongating DNA. After the

release of pyrophosphate, ganciclovir monophosphate is incorporated into the end of a growing chain of viral DNA, slowing replication (13). Unlike acyclovir, ganciclovir is not an obligate chain terminator; rather, short subgenomic CMV DNA fragments continue to be synthesized in the presence of ganciclovir (39). These DNA fragments are not packaged into virions and are therefore not considered infectious.

The mechanism whereby ganciclovir is phosphorylated in CMV-infected cells has been elucidated (46, 80). It was previously demonstrated that ganciclovir is actively phosphorylated to the monophosphate form by herpes simplex virus thymidine kinase in cells infected with HSV (8, 34). Conversion to the di- and triphosphate forms of ganciclovir is accomplished by cellular guanosine monophosphate synthetase. Thymidine kinase–deficient mutants of herpes simplex are thus not inhibited by ganciclovir (22). Human CMV does not possess a thymidine kinase homologue, and the complete nucleotide sequence of the CMV genome indicates no open reading frame that is a likely candidate for a nucleotide kinase such as a virally encoded "guanosine kinase" or "ganciclovir kinase." Instead, an enzyme with putative protein kinase activity capable of phosphorylating ganciclovir has been identified that originates from the UL97 region of the CMV genome (46, 80). The CMV UL97 gene product has strong homology with other known herpesviral protein kinases as well as with the aminoglycoside phosphotransferase of *Escherichia coli* (10).

In MRC-5 cells infected with the AD 169 strain of CMV, the intracellular half-life of ganciclovir triphosphate was estimated to be 16.5 h, compared with an intracellular half-life of 2.5 h for acyclovir triphosphate (8). On a molar basis, ganciclovir triphosphate is not as effective an inhibitor of CMV DNA polymerase as is acyclovir triphosphate (50). The intracellular concentration of the triphosphate form of ganciclovir in CMV-infected cells, however, is 10 times that of acyclovir, and ganciclovir triphosphate persists in cells much longer than acyclovir triphosphate. This explains why ganciclovir is far superior to acyclovir in inhibiting replication of CMV (82).

MECHANISMS OF RESISTANCE

After passaging the AD 169 strain of CMV in the presence of increasing concentrations of ganciclovir, a mutant was selected exhibiting a high level of resistance to ganciclovir (7). This mutant was also resistant to acyclovir but retained sensitivity to foscarnet. Further characterization of this strain revealed that it was unable to induce phosphorylation of ganciclovir in CMV-infected cells to the level seen with the wild-type strain (7). Nucleotide sequence analysis of ganciclovir-resistant mutants reveal that point mutations in the CMV DNA polymerase can confer significant resistance to ganciclovir (47, 79). The other region of the CMV genome that could transfer the resistance marker corresponds to the open reading frame designated UL97 (48, 80). Four amino acid deletions in the UL97 gene product were responsible for selection of this CMV mutant that was unable to phosphorylate ganciclovir. Mutation producing an inability to phosphorylate ganciclovir is the most common mechanism of resistance in the laboratory and the clinic (Fig. 2) (48, 75).

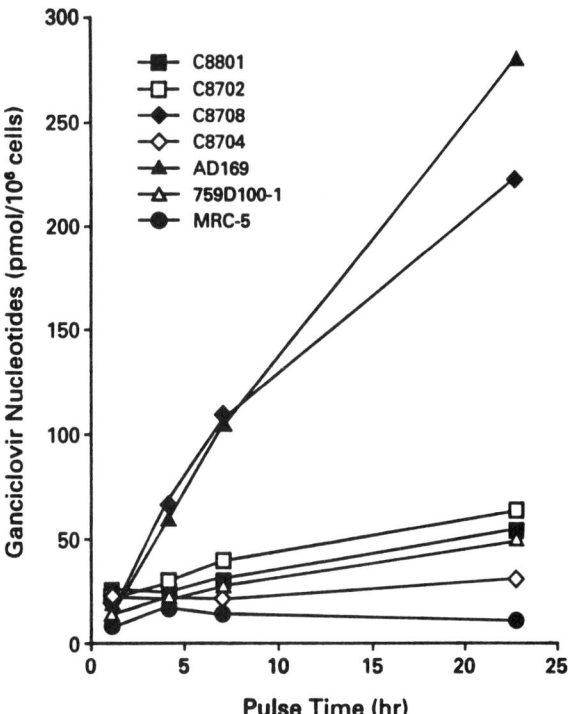

FIGURE 2. Intracellular phosphorylation of ganciclovir by clinical isolates. Infected and uninfected MRC-5 cells were pulse-labeled on day 3 with 12.5 μg of [^{14}C]ganciclovir per milliliter for the times indicated, and phosphorylation was measured by cation-exchange chromatography. Patient isolates C8801 and C8702 were resistant to ganciclovir in vitro. An early-therapy isolate (C8708) was susceptible to ganciclovir, and a late isolate (C8704) from the same patient was resistant. 759D100–1 is a ganciclovir-resistant mutant of AD169. (From Stanat SC, Reardon JE, Erice A, et al. Ganciclovir-resistant cytomegalovirus clinical isolates: mode of resistance to ganciclovir. Antimicrob Agents Chemother 1991;35:2191–2197, with permission.)

The mutations in UL97 that confer resistance to ganciclovir alter codons 460 and 520 and residues between 590 and 596 (6, 15, 21, 86). Isolates containing only UL97 point mutations exhibit a lower level of resistance to ganciclovir (IC$_{50}$ > 6–8 μM); such strains are usually sensitive to foscarnet and cidofovir (48). Resistance mutations arising early in the course of ganciclovir therapy (i.e., >3 months) tend to contain primarily UL97 mutations. Resistant strains possessing mutations in both UL97 and DNA polymerase often exhibit a higher level of resistance (IC$_{50}$ > 30 μM). While these strains retain sensitivity to foscarnet, some are cidofovir resistant (47, 79). CMV isolates containing resistance mutations in both the UL97 gene and DNA polymerase are more likely to appear after long-term (i.e., >9 months) ganciclovir therapy. The CMV isolates that have mutations in the UL97 gene and DNA polymerase exhibit high-level resistance to ganciclovir and are cross-resistant to cidofovir (68). Recently, a rapid diagnostic test based on restriction enzyme analysis has been developed that can reliably detect mutation of the UL97 gene in most (>80%) resistant clinical isolates (15, 16).

Estimation of the precise incidence of CMV resistance in patients treated with ganciclovir has been difficult. Three immunocompromised patients with CMV disease resistant to ganciclovir were described in 1989 (32). In all three cases, CMV disease progressed despite therapy, viral cultures remained positive, and the patients died. One of the three patients had an isolate resistant to ganciclovir prior to starting therapy. In the second patient, susceptibility to ganciclovir of the CMV isolated from serial cultures decreased significantly. Restriction fragment analysis revealed that the serial isolates arose from the same strain. In the third individual, resistance emerged by virtue of infection with a different strain of CMV acquired during treatment with ganciclovir. Thus, this report illustrates the three possible scenarios for clinical development of resistance to ganciclovir (32). In a study of 72 patients with CMV retinitis, 80% of the CMV-infected patients became culture negative after 3 months of ganciclovir therapy. Of those remaining culture positive on therapy, 38% had resistant CMV isolated, for an overall incidence of 8.7% (27). These authors observed that patients shedding resistant virus also experience clinical disease progression; however, retinitis progression also occurred in individuals shedding ganciclovir-sensitive virus (27). The incidence of ganciclovir-resistant CMV in patients receiving ganciclovir treatment for AIDS-related CMV retinitis has been reported to be as high as 42% (69). The real clinical significance of ganciclovir-resistant CMV in patients has not been defined, and this remains a high priority of current research efforts.

PHARMACOKINETIC DISPOSITION
Absorption

Intravenous Administration

Following intravenous administration, the disposition of ganciclovir is best described by a two-compartment pharmacokinetic model. Maximum serum concentrations increase in a linear fashion following intravenous doses over a range of 1 to 5 mg/kg body weight (33, 51). Intravenous administration of a single 5 mg/kg dose infused over 1 h results in a mean peak ganciclovir concentration in serum (C$_{max}$) of 8.3 μg/mL, declining below 0.05 μg/mL at 24 h (Fig. 3) (2). Steady-state peak serum concentrations following multiple doses of ganciclovir are similar to values observed in single-dose studies, suggesting little drug accumulation in individuals with normal renal function (33, 51). The typical regimen of 7.5 to 10 mg of ganciclovir per kilogram per day given intravenously in two or three divided doses results in C$_{max}$ in serum of 4.5 to 10 μg/mL and a C$_{min}$ of 0.8 μg/mL (24).

Oral Administration

Oral absorption of ganciclovir has been evaluated in patients with HIV infection and to a more limited extent in transplant recipients. In a phase I/II evaluation in HIV-infected individuals, C$_{max}$ values of ganciclovir ranged from 0.47 to 0.55 μg/mL following single oral doses of 500 to 2000 mg. Absolute bioavailability was found to be lower with a 2000-mg dose than with a 500-mg single oral dose (2.6 vs. 5.6%) (73). Following multiple doses of 1000 mg or 2000 mg adminis-

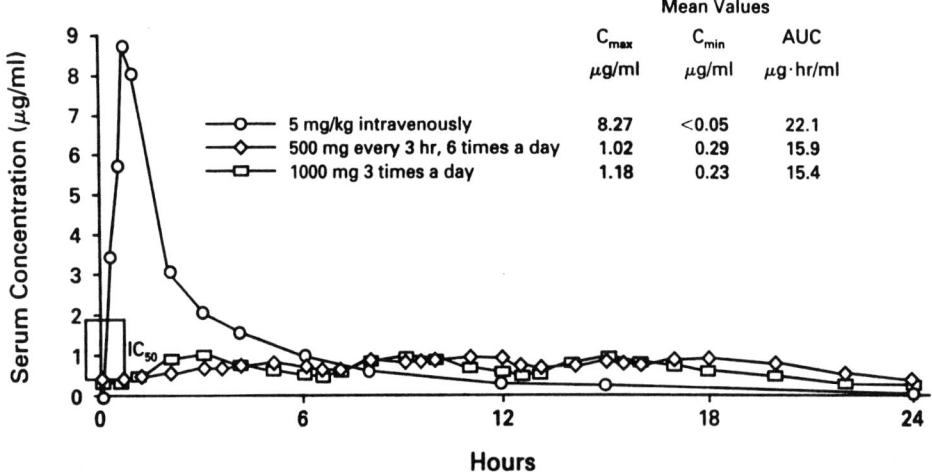

FIGURE 3. Pharmacokinetics of oral and intravenous ganciclovir in normal subjects. The same 16 subjects were included in all studies. C_{max} denotes the maximal concentration after a dose, C_{min} the minimal concentration after a dose, AUC the area under the curve for serum concentration plotted against time, and IC_{50} the concentration of drug that inhibits 50% of CMV in a plaque-reduction assay. (From Anderson RD, Griffy KG, Jung D, et al. Ganciclovir absolute bioavailability and steady-state pharmacokinetics after oral administration of two 3000-mg/d dosing regimens in human immunodeficiency virus- and cytomegalovirus-seropositive patients. Clin Ther 1995;17:425–432, with permission.)

tered every 8 h, C_{max} values of 1.11 and 1.16 µg/mL were observed, respectively.

Ganciclovir absorption was characterized in a three-way crossover study involving 18 HIV-infected patients. Study subjects each received a single 5 mg/kg intravenous dose of ganciclovir, oral ganciclovir 500 mg every 3 h (given 6 times daily) for 3 days, and ganciclovir 1000 mg administered orally thrice daily for 3 days. Absolute bioavailability of the two oral regimens was similar, averaging approximately 8.5% (2). Mean maximum (C_{max}) and minimum (C_{min}) serum concentrations were 1.02 and 0.29 µg/mL and 1.18 and 0.23 µg/mL for the 500 mg six times daily and 1000 mg three times daily regimens, respectively (Fig. 3). Total daily area under the curve (AUC_{0-24h}) averaged 15.9 µg-h/mL and 15.4 µg-h/mL for the 500 mg six times daily and 1000 mg thrice daily regimens, respectively. These results were lower than the AUC_{0-24h} of 22.1 µg-h/mL observed with the intravenous dose of ganciclovir. Although much higher C_{max} values are achieved following intravenous administration of standard doses, orally administered ganciclovir produces serum levels that are more sustained over the course of the day and reside within the IC_{50} range for most clinical isolates of CMV (Fig. 3). Given the similar absorption profiles of the two oral dosing schemes and the greater convenience associated with the 1000 mg thrice daily regimen, the latter has become the preferred regimen for maintenance therapy in patients with CMV retinitis.

Intraocular Administration

Limited information exists regarding the intravitreal concentrations of ganciclovir achieved following intraocular administration. When ocular concentrations were determined in one patient receiving 200-µg doses of ganciclovir administered by intravitreal injection five times over a 15-day period, an intravitreal concentration of 16 µg/mL was measured immedi-

ately after injection (42). The mean intravitreal concentration of ganciclovir was 2.0 µg/mL in 7 of 11 eyes of AIDS patients with CMV retinitis treated with the intraocular implant device. In this study, the mean rate of ganciclovir release from the implant was calculated to be 1.9 µg/h (4).

Distribution

Ganciclovir concentrations were determined in tissues and plasma obtained at autopsy from six patients with acute leukemia who died while undergoing treatment for CMV pneumonia (66). Concentrations of ganciclovir in lung, liver, and testes were roughly equivalent to heart blood concentrations. Higher levels were measured in kidney tissue, suggesting accumulation in this organ. Brain tissue concentrations averaged 38% of simultaneous blood levels (66). The concentration of ganciclovir in four CSF samples obtained from two bone marrow transplant patients ranged from 0.50 to 0.68 µg/mL when collected 0.25 to 6.7 h after the initiation of a 2.5 mg/kg infusion (35). CSF penetration was estimated to be 24 to 67% when these CSF concentrations were compared with simultaneous plasma concentration values predicted from a two-compartment pharmacokinetic model.

The intravitreal penetration of ganciclovir was determined in 53 eyes of patients with AIDS and CMV retinitis undergoing pars plana vitrectomy for retinal detachment (3). Intravitreal concentrations averaged 1.19 ± 0.37 and 0.82 ± 0.46 µg/mL when obtained 1.5 to 72 h after the last induction (n = 23) or maintenance (n = 30) dose of ganciclovir, respectively. Simultaneously obtained plasma concentrations were lower than those measured in the vitreous fluid in 78% of patients. Similar results were reported in another study (44). A mean intravitreal concentration of 0.96 µg/mL was determined an average of 12 h following the ganciclovir dose in 23 eyes of 22 patients with AIDS receiving a mean dose of 6 mg/kg/day. Taken together, these data suggest that standard induction and maintenance doses of ganciclovir result in vitreal concentrations within the range of ID_{50} values for many, but not all, clinical isolates of CMV.

The plasma protein binding of ganciclovir is negligible (<2%), and the drug is passively transported across the placenta (33, 51). The mean steady-state volume of distribution (Vd_{ss}) of ganciclovir has been reported to range between 32.8 and 44.5 L/1.73 m^2 (35, 84), the mean apparent volume of distribution (Vd) in patients with normal renal function is 1.17 ± 0.54 L/kg (72).

Elimination

The kidneys are the primary route of elimination for ganciclovir. In various studies, over 90% of an intravenous dose of ganciclovir is excreted unchanged in the urine (35, 66, 84). Little if any extrarenal elimination occurs. The total clearance of ganciclovir correlates well with creatinine clearance and exceeds this parameter by a factor of 2.4, suggesting that tubular secretion contributes to the elimination of ganciclovir. The total clearance has been reported to average 208 mL/min/1.73 m^2 (35), or 4.2 mL/min/kg (72). The elimination half-life of ganciclovir in individuals with normal renal function ranges between 2 and 4 h.

Renal disease profoundly influences the elimination of ganciclovir, and a dose reduction is mandatory to minimize or avoid toxicity. Ganciclovir total clearance and elimination half-life in 8 patients with mild-to-moderate renal insufficiency (serum creatinine values, 1.5–4.6 mg/dL) averaged 1.2 mL/min/kg and 11.5 h, respectively. Linear regression analysis of ganciclovir clearance (CL) versus creatinine clearance (CL_{cr}) generated the following equation:

$$CL = (1.25 \times CL_{cr}) + 8.57$$

($R = 0.923$) (72). Limited data exist regarding the pharmacokinetic disposition of ganciclovir in patients with severe renal disease, but elimination half-life values of 28 to 40 h have been reported (45, 72). Hemodialysis removes approximately 50% of a ganciclovir dose during a typical 4-h session (45, 72). In three anuric heart transplant patients undergoing continuous venovenous hemodialysis (CVVHD), the mean elimination half-life was 18.9 h, with an average dosage fraction removed of 89.7% (9). This suggests that higher doses than those recommended for patients with end-stage renal disease may be required for critically ill patients undergoing this form of dialysis.

When determined in one patient, the intravitreal half-life of ganciclovir was estimated to be 13 h (42). The pharmacokinetics of ganciclovir were recently characterized in 27 neonates with congenital CMV infections, with results comparable to those of adults (83). Following a single 4 mg/kg intravenous dose, the mean total clearance and elimination half-life of ganciclovir were 189 mL/hr/kg and 2.4 h, respectively.

DOSAGE REGIMENS

Dosing recommendations for ganciclovir therapy in various settings are summarized in Table 1 (20). The recommended dose for induction therapy is 5 mg/kg, administered as a constant intravenous infusion over 1 h every 12 h for 2 to 3 weeks. Intramuscular or subcutaneous injection produces severe tissue irritation because of the alkalinity (pH = 11) of ganciclovir in solution. Oral ganciclovir is not recommended for induction therapy. Maintenance therapy in AIDS patients with CMV retinitis can be accomplished with either daily administration of 5 mg/kg intravenously or orally at a dosage of 1000 mg (four 250-mg capsules) thrice daily (26, 76). Oral ganciclovir should always be taken immediately after a meal or snack to enhance ab-

TABLE 1 • Recommended Doses of Intravenous and Oral Ganciclovir for CMV Infections

Setting	Induction Therapy	Maintenance Therapy
Treatment		
Retinitis	5 mg/kg q. 12 h i.v. for 2 to 3 weeks	5 mg/kg/day i.v. or 1000 mg 3 times a day orally
Gastrointestinal disease	5 mg/kg q. 12 h i.v. for 3 weeks	No recommendation at this time
Neurologic disease	5 mg/kg q. 12 h i.v. for 3 weeks	No recommendation at this time
Pneumonia	5 mg/kg q. 12 h i.v. for 3 weeks, combined with CMV immune globulin	No recommendation at this time
Prophylaxis		
AIDS and CD4 < 100/mm^3	—	1000 mg 3 times a day orally
Bone marrow transplantation	—	5 mg/kg/day or 6 mg/kg 5 days/week i.v. from time of engraftment to day 100–120 posttransplantation
Heart transplantation	5 mg/kg q. 12 h i.v. for 2 weeks	5 mg/kg/day or 6 mg/kg 5 days/week i.v. for 2 weeks
Liver transplantation	6 mg/kg/day i.v. for 30 days 5 mg/kg/day i.v. for 2 weeks	6 mg/kg 5 days/week i.v. until day 100 Acyclovir 800 mg 4 times a day orally through week 12
Preemptive treatment		
Bone marrow transplantation	5 mg/kg q. 12 h i.v. for 2 weeks	5 mg/kg/day or 6 mg/kg 5 days/week i.v. to day 100–120 posttransplantation
Liver and kidney transplantation	—	2.5 or 5 mg/kg/day i.v. during treatment with OKT3 or antilymphocyte antibiotics or for 7 days

Modified from Crumpacker CS. Ganciclovir. N Engl J Med 1996;335:721–729.

sorption (2). Until more information is available regarding immune reconstitution with protease inhibitor–containing regimens, maintenance therapy for CMV retinitis in AIDS should be lifelong. Patients who relapse during maintenance therapy can usually be given a second course of induction therapy before having to switch to an alternative agent. AIDS patients with CMV retinitis progression can be placed on a higher maintenance regimen (10 mg/kg/day) following reinduction (78). Such high-dose regimens often require concomitant filgrastim (G-CSF) or sargramostin (GM-CSF) for management of neutropenia (40). When used as primary prophylaxis for CMV retinitis in patients with AIDS, ganciclovir should be given orally at 1000 mg thrice daily (73).

For intravitreal therapy of CMV retinitis, an induction dose of 400 μg of ganciclovir given two to three times a week followed by 400 μg weekly for maintenance therapy is recommended (17). With surgical placement of the ganciclovir ocular implant, most patients will not require replacement of the device until at least 6 months following insertion (63).

Dosing recommendations for ganciclovir used as preventive therapy in transplant recipients vary according to the type of transplant procedure and whether the agent is used preemptively or prophylactically (Table 1) (20, 30, 33, 41, 54, 61, 62, 64, 65, 67, 85). In most instances, the intravenous form of ganciclovir is used. Oral ganciclovir has recently gained Food and Drug Administration (FDA) approval for prevention of CMV disease in solid organ transplant recipients as an alternative to intravenous drug.

Ganciclovir dosage must be reduced in individuals with impaired renal function (Table 2). Because of its high propensity to cause marrow suppression and other serious adverse effects, serum creatinine must be regularly monitored, and the dosage of ganciclovir adjusted according to the patient's estimated creatinine clearance. Individuals with end-stage renal disease can be treated with thrice-weekly ganciclovir. Patients maintained on hemodialysis should receive ganciclovir after completion of the procedure, because dialysis can reduce ganciclovir concentrations in serum by 50% (33, 45, 72).

ADVERSE EFFECTS

The main dose-limiting adverse effect of ganciclovir is bone marrow suppression, resulting in granulocytopenia and thrombocytopenia. Following an induction course and maintenance therapy with ganciclovir for CMV retinitis, approximately 40% of patients develop a granulocytopenia of less than 1000

cells/mm^3 (12, 26, 76). Severe neutropenia (absolute neutrophil count < 500 cells/mm^3) has been noted in approximately 20% of AIDS patients maintained on long-term (>3 months) therapy (26). A significant thrombocytopenia of less than 50,000 cells/mm^3 has also been noted in up to 15% of patients (12). Granulocytopenia and thrombocytopenia are usually reversible upon discontinuation of ganciclovir; however, one patient reported to have developed irreversible neutropenia while receiving ganciclovir later died of pseudomonal sepsis (12). Anemia may also develop with prolonged ganciclovir therapy (12, 26). Granulocytopenia due to ganciclovir can be prevented or reversed with concomitant filgrastim or sargramostin. Patients who received these factors experienced fewer episodes of neutropenia than those who received ganciclovir alone (40).

Elevations in serum creatinine values to more than 2.5 mg/dL has been observed in 20% of bone marrow transplant patients during a 120-day course of ganciclovir therapy (64). Similar findings were observed in a placebo-controlled trial in heart transplant recipients (54). The serum creatinine elevations were often transient, occurring intermittently during these studies. Most of the patients enrolled in these trials were also receiving concomitant cyclosporine, a known nephrotoxin.

In studies comparing oral and intravenous ganciclovir for maintenance therapy of CMV retinitis, diarrhea and nausea were observed in 40 and 25% of patients, respectively (26). The incidence of adverse gastrointestinal effects did not differ when oral ganciclovir was compared with intravenous drug. Adverse neurologic effects (neuropathy, paresthesias) have been noted in 10% or less of patients enrolled in clinical trials. Fever and rash occur in approximately 5% of treated patients.

In experimental dog studies using prolonged therapy with ganciclovir in doses higher than those used to treat CMV disease in humans, a severe, irreversible loss of spermatogenesis was noted. Pathologic examination revealed marked atrophy and destruction of Leydig cells. There have been no clear studies demonstrating decreased testosterone synthesis as a result of ganciclovir therapy (20). Testicular endocrine function has not been shown to be affected. Animal data indicate that suppression of fertility may occur in women treated with ganciclovir. Since ganciclovir has been shown to be carcinogenic and teratogenic in animal studies, it is designated as pregnancy category C by the FDA. Because ganciclovir may possibly be excreted in breast milk, mothers should be instructed to discontinue nursing if they are receiving ganciclovir therapy. The safety and efficacy of ganciclovir have not been sufficiently

TABLE 2 • **Ganciclovir Dosing in Individuals with Impaired Renal Function**

Creatinine Clearance (mL/min)	IV Induction Regimen	IV Maintenance Regimen	Oral Maintenance Regimen
≥70	5 mg/kg q. 12 h	5 mg/kg q. 24 h	1000 mg three times a day
50–69	2.5 mg/kg q. 12 h	2.5 mg/kg q. 24 h	500 mg three times a day
25–49	2.5 mg/kg q. 24 h	1.25 mg/kg q. 24 h	500 mg twice a day
10–24	1.25 mg/kg q. 24 h	0.625 mg/kg q. 24 h	500 mg/day
<10	1.25 mg/kg three times per week following hemodialysis	0.625 mg/kg three times per week following hemodialysis	500 mg three times per week following hemodialysis

established in children. Given the potential for long-term carcinogenicity or reproductive problems, ganciclovir therapy should not be undertaken in children without carefully considering these risks.

Intravitreal administration of ganciclovir has been associated with conjunctival hemorrhage, bacterial endophthalmitis, cataract formation, and retinal detachment (17). Complications surrounding surgical placement of the intraocular implant of ganciclovir include a transient reduction in visual acuity and vitreous hemorrhage. Bacterial endophthalmitis has also been described. In a trial comparing the intraocular implant of ganciclovir with standard intravenous therapy, retinal detachments were noted in 12% of patients receiving implants versus 5% of those receiving systemic therapy.

MONITORING REQUIREMENTS

Close hematologic monitoring is essential in all patients receiving ganciclovir, to reduce the risk of severe bone marrow suppression. The complete blood count and platelet count should be monitored at regular intervals in all patients receiving systemic therapy. Ganciclovir therapy should be interrupted if the absolute neutrophil count (ANC) falls below 500 cells/mm^3 or if the platelet count is below 25,000/mm^3. Concomitant use of colony-stimulating factors may be required in some individuals to keep ANC values above 500 cells/mm^3 during maintenance therapy. Serum creatinine should be checked regularly to screen for increases in this laboratory parameter and to ensure that the ganciclovir dosage is properly adjusted for renal function. Intravenous catheter-related infections have been known to occur in patients on long-term maintenance therapy with intravenous ganciclovir; careful monitoring for this complication is essential.

To derive the most benefit from therapy with oral ganciclovir, patients must be instructed to adhere to the prescribed regimen. All patients prescribed ganciclovir by the oral route should be regularly assessed for gastrointestinal tolerance and compliance with therapy.

DRUG INTERACTIONS

Use of ganciclovir at full dosage with other drugs capable of inducing bone marrow toxicity can be dangerous and should be avoided. In a well-controlled study of 40 patients, 82% required dose reduction because of the overlapping hematologic toxicity of ganciclovir and zidovudine (43). Probenecid and other agents with active tubular secretion as a component of their elimination reduce ganciclovir renal clearance and increase plasma concentrations of the drug (51). Seizures have been reported in patients receiving imipenem and ganciclovir. Although the mechanism of this interaction is unknown, these two agents should not be used concomitantly without careful consideration of the potential risks (51).

CLINICAL INDICATIONS
Treatment of CMV Disease

CMV Retinitis
Intravenous Ganciclovir. CMV retinitis is a frequent sight-threatening infection in patients with AIDS. Since the first reports of its efficacy in treating CMV retinitis in 1985,

ganciclovir has remained one of the most important agents for treatment of this potentially devastating condition. When ganciclovir was administered at a dose of 5 mg/kg every 12 h for 14 days, CMV retinitis stabilized and healed in over 85% of patients (12). Without treatment, sight-threatening infection progresses to blindness in most patients in 6 to 8 weeks. Following initial induction therapy, continuous maintenance therapy is required to reduce the risk of disease progression. Without maintenance therapy, relapse of retinitis occurs within 20 to 30 days after stopping therapy. Maintenance doses below 20 mg/kg/week are associated with relapse rates comparable to those found with no treatment (12).

Retinal hemorrhage is common in patients with CMV retinitis, and detachment of the retina occurs in roughly 15% of patients, usually before ganciclovir therapy is begun (36). Treatment with ganciclovir leads to stabilization of retinal lesions in 2 weeks, while a month is usually required for complete response to therapy (36). Ganciclovir treatment of CMV retinitis is associated with a clearing of CMV viremia in 7 to 8 days (12) and clearing of CMV DNA from the buffy coat of infected blood in 8 days (23). Intravenous ganciclovir was approved for treatment of CMV retinitis in 1989 without a properly controlled trial because most patients become blind in 4 months without therapy.

A multicenter randomized, open-label clinical trial comparing ganciclovir with foscarnet in the treatment of CMV retinitis in patients with AIDS found no difference in the rate of progression of retinitis (76, 77). However, the mortality rate was higher in patients assigned to ganciclovir treatment, with median survival of 8.5 months in the ganciclovir group and 12.6 months in the foscarnet group. Compared with the foscarnet group, patients assigned to receive ganciclovir received less antiretroviral therapy, but the survival difference could not be attributed to the difference in anti-HIV therapy. A follow-up comparative study in AIDS patients with relapsed CMV retinitis revealed no difference in survival among treatment groups; however, the combination of ganciclovir and foscarnet was superior to either agent alone (even when given in higher than usual doses) for retinitis therapy (78). Among patients with reduced renal function, foscarnet therapy was associated with increased mortality. Results from these studies reveal that the two drugs are equally efficacious for CMV retinitis and that the combination of both drugs was superior for retinitis treatment, particularly when a relapse has occurred. Neither therapy appears to provide a clear survival advantage.

Oral Ganciclovir. Oral ganciclovir has been approved as an alternative to intravenous drug for maintenance therapy of CMV retinitis. It has also been approved to prevent CMV infections in solid organ transplant recipients. In a multicenter randomized, open-label, comparative clinical trial in 123 AIDS patients with CMV retinitis, oral and intravenous ganciclovir were similarly effective for maintenance therapy (26). All study subjects received induction therapy with intravenous ganciclovir over 3 weeks before randomization. When retinitis progression was assessed by serial retinal photographs evaluated by a person masked to treatment assignment, the mean times to first progression were 62 and 57 days for patients receiving intravenous and oral maintenance therapy, respectively ($P = .63$). When progression was assessed funduscopically by study ophthalmologists, patients receiving intravenous therapy were found to have a longer mean time to retinitis progression (96 vs. 68 days; $P = .03$; relative risk, 1.68). Both groups showed a marked decrease in the number of patients with urine culture positivity for CMV, indicating decreased viral replication. Patients assigned to oral ganciclovir had a lower incidence of neutropenia, and fewer patients in this group experienced intravenous catheter-related sepsis.

Intraocular Ganciclovir. Ganciclovir has also been successful in treating CMV retinitis when administered by intravitreal injections (17). Long-term success with intravitreal injections is limited by the relatively frequent need to readminister drug (once weekly for maintenance therapy) and the potential for serious complications including retinal detachments, intravitreous hemorrhages, and endophthalmitis. Results from one of the largest series of patients also revealed an 8-week relapse rate of 53%, development of retinitis involving the contralateral eye in 11%, and extraocular CMV disease in 16% of patients (17).

An intraocular sustained-release implant containing ganciclovir has allowed many of the drawbacks of intravitreal injections to be avoided. Following surgical placement into the vitreous cavity, ganciclovir is released at a constant rate for a period of 5 to 8 months (average, 6 months) (52, 56, 63). A randomized controlled trial was conducted to assess the safety and efficacy of an implant delivering 1 µg of ganciclovir per hour versus deferred therapy in 26 patients (30 eyes) with AIDS and peripheral CMV retinitis (52). The median time to progression was 15 days in the deferred-therapy group and 226 days with the implant ($P < 0.00001$). In a randomized clinical trial of 188 patients with AIDS and newly diagnosed CMV retinitis, two implants (1 and 2 µg/h) were compared with treatment with intravenous ganciclovir (56). Similar median times to retinitis progression were found with the two implants (211 days with the 1-µg/h and 191 days with the 2-µg/h implant), and the implant devices were superior to intravenous therapy in slowing progression (71 days; $P < .001$). Development of retinitis in the uninvolved eye and extraocular CMV infections were less likely in the intravenous group. The commercially approved intraocular implant (Vitrasert) consists of a sterile pellet containing 4.5 mg of ganciclovir that releases drug at a constant rate of 1 µg/h for approximately 6 months. By combining oral ganciclovir with the intraocular implant, many of the above limitations can be overcome while still avoiding the intravenous route. In many cities, the standard of care is becoming oral ganciclovir and an intraocular implant.

Gastrointestinal Infections

CMV can cause a variety of gastrointestinal-related infections, including esophagitis, gastritis, cholecystitis, and colitis (59). CMV colitis is associated with watery diarrhea, and the diagnosis is established by demonstration of inclusion bodies in a biopsy sample or by positive immunostaining, immunofluorescence, or specific in situ hybridization for CMV. In a placebo-controlled trial of treatment of CMV colitis in AIDS patients, a significantly greater reduction in CMV-infected colonic or urinary cultures was seen in patients receiving 14

days of intravenous ganciclovir (10 mg/kg/day in two doses), and colonoscopy scores improved more with ganciclovir than with placebo. The frequency of diarrhea did not differ between study groups. Importantly, extracolonic CMV disease developed in 9% of ganciclovir-treated patients and 23% of placebo recipients ($P = .03$) (25). Although these results are promising, they may indicate that a 14-day course of ganciclovir treatment is inadequate for the colon to heal and for diarrhea to resolve. In bone marrow transplant recipients who had fecal CMV cultures collected on a regular basis, cultures reverted to negative more often in patients given ganciclovir than in those given placebo; however, gastrointestinal symptoms improved at the same rate in both groups. These results show that 2 weeks of ganciclovir treatment does not produce any appreciable clinical or endoscopic improvement in CMV gastroenteritis in bone marrow transplant patients. There is also no evidence that maintenance therapy is useful in preventing relapse of CMV colitis in immunocompromised patients.

Pneumonia

Ganciclovir treatment of primary CMV pneumonia has been most successful in renal transplant patients, and in this patient population, the drug can be lifesaving (41). In bone marrow transplant recipients, however, attempts to treat CMV pneumonia with antiviral therapy alone, including ganciclovir, have been either unsuccessful or had limited success (23, 66). In the first seven patients given intravenous ganciclovir in doses of 7.5 to 15 mg/kg/day for CMV pneumonia, four died of respiratory failure before completing 14 days of therapy, and the three patients who completed the course of therapy died of pulmonary failure within 7 weeks (66). In three uncontrolled trials in bone marrow transplant patients with CMV pneumonia treated with ganciclovir and high-dose intravenous CMV immune globulin, 52 to 69% of patients survived (30, 61, 65). The combination of ganciclovir and high-titer CMV immune globulin is the currently recommended therapy for CMV pneumonia in bone marrow transplant patients.

Infection of the Nervous System

CMV is associated with a progressive polyradiculopathy in patients with AIDS (18, 29). This syndrome usually begins as low back pain with radicular or perianal radiation, followed in 1 to 6 weeks by progressive flaccid paraparesis. Pathologic changes occur in the cauda equina and lumbosacral nerve roots with mononuclear cell infiltrates, axonal destruction, and CMV inclusion bodies in Schwann cells and epithelial cells (29). A few patients have experienced improvement in this polyradiculopathy when treated early in the disease with ganciclovir alone or ganciclovir with foscarnet, but treatment is usually disappointing (18, 55). Use of the polymerase chain reaction to detect CMV DNA in CSF may aid in early diagnosis (87).

Mononeuritis multiplex and painful peripheral neuropathy have also been described in patients with AIDS and have been attributed to CMV (37). In some cases, ganciclovir was given although the benefits of treatment are uncertain. Combination therapy with ganciclovir and foscarnet has been tried in a few patients with CMV meningoencephalitis (31).

Prevention of CMV Disease

CMV Retinitis

Oral ganciclovir has been studied for primary prevention of CMV retinitis in AIDS patients with CD4 counts below 100 cells/mm^3 and seropositivity for CMV (11, 74). A study comparing oral ganciclovir (1000 mg thrice daily) with placebo revealed CMV disease in 26% of placebo recipients (n = 239) but only 14% of patients randomized to receive ganciclovir (n = 486; $P < .001$) (74). The prevalence of CMV-positive urine cultures was also significantly lower in ganciclovir recipients, confirming the clinical benefit. Neutropenia and use of colony-stimulating factors both occurred more often in ganciclovir recipients. Another study of 994 patients failed to show any difference in the incidence of CMV disease with oral ganciclovir or placebo (11). The reason for the differences in results from these trials in unclear; however, in the study showing a lack of benefit, patients enrolled had a higher mean CD4 count, and retinal examinations were not performed on a regular basis.

CMV in Transplant Patients

Prevention of CMV pneumonia or other manifestations of CMV disease with ganciclovir in solid organ and bone marrow transplant recipients was clearly demonstrated in four independent studies (38, 54, 64, 85). The most effective approach to preventing CMV disease was found to be initiation of ganciclovir in response to a positive CMV culture from any site at any time after bone marrow transplantation (prophylaxis) (38), compared with initiating ganciclovir only when the bronchoalveolar fluid obtained at day 35 was culture positive for CMV (preemptive therapy) (64). The efficacy of ganciclovir in preventing CMV pneumonia or death was 97% with prophylactic therapy compared with 75% when preemptive therapy was used. In cardiac transplant patients who were seropositive for CMV and received ganciclovir or placebo for 28 days following surgery, the incidence of CMV disease in the 120 days following transplantation was reduced from 46 to 9% in the ganciclovir group, compared with placebo, and the incidence of CMV infection at day 60 was 56% in the placebo group, but only 19% in the ganciclovir group (54). CMV infection occurred in 38% of patients receiving acyclovir prophylaxis following liver transplantation but only 5% of patients treated with ganciclovir during a follow-up period of 120 days (85). A short course (7 days) of ganciclovir given preemptively when surveillance cultures were positive for CMV was compared with high-dose oral acyclovir given prophylactically following liver transplantation in 47 patients (67). Short-course ganciclovir therapy was associated with a markedly lower incidence of CMV disease than acyclovir (4 vs. 29%; $P < .05$). Although the criteria used in these studies to determine when to begin ganciclovir and to define CMV disease differed, the results clearly demonstrate that ganciclovir is of significant benefit in preventing CMV disease in transplant recipients. Oral ganciclovir has been approved for prevention of CMV disease in solid organ transplant recipients.

REFERENCES

1. Agut H, Huraux JM, Collandre H, Montagnier L. Susceptibility of human herpes virus 6 to acyclovir and ganciclovir. Lancet 1989;2:626.

2. Anderson RD, Griffy KG, Jung D, Dorr A, Hulse JD, Smith RB. Ganciclovir absolute bioavailability and steady-state pharmacokinetics after oral administration of two 3000-mg/d dosing regimens in human immunodeficiency virus- and cytomegalovirus-seropositive patients. Clin Ther 1995;17:425–432.

3. Arevalo JF, Gonzalez C, Capparelli EV, Kirsch LS, Garcia RF, Quiceno JI, Connor JD, Gambertoglio J, Bergeron-Lynn G, Freeman WR. Intravitreous and plasma concentrations of ganciclovir and foscarnet after intravenous therapy in patients with AIDS and cytomegalovirus retinitis. J Infect Dis 1995;172: 951–956.

4. Ashton P, Brown JD, Pearson PA, Blandford DL, Smith TJ, Anand R, Nightingale SD, Sanborn GE. Intravitreal ganciclovir pharmacokinetics in rabbits and man. J Ocul Pharmacol 1992; 8:343–347.

5. Ashton WT, Karkas JD, Field AK, Tolman RL. Activation by thymidine kinase and potent antiherpetic activity of 2′-nor-2′-deoxyguanosine (2′NDG). Biochem Biophys Res Commun 1982;108:1716–1721.

6. Baldanti F, Underwood MR, Stanat SC, Biron KK, Chou S, Sarasini A, Silini E, Gerna G. Single amino acid changes in the DNA polymerase confer foscarnet resistance and slow-growth phenotype, while mutations in the UL97-encoded phosphotransferase confer ganciclovir resistance in three double resistant human cytomegalovirus strains recovered from patients with AIDS. J Virol 1996;70:1390–1395.

7. Biron KK, Fyfe JA, Stanat SC, Leslie LK, Sorrell JB, Lambe CU, Coen DM. A human cytomegalovirus mutant resistant to the nucleoside analog 9-{[2-hydroxy-1-(hydroxy]methyl) ethoxymethyl} guanine (BW B759U) induces reduced levels of BW759U triphosphate. Proc Natl Acad Sci USA 1986;83: 8769–8773.

8. Biron KK, Stanat SC, Sorrell JB, Fyfe JA, Keller PM, Lambe CU, Nelson DJ. Metabolic activation of the nucleoside analog 9-{[2-hydroxy-1-(hydroxymethyl)ethoxy]methyl} guanine in human diploid fibroblasts infected with human cytomegalovirus. Proc Natl Acad Sci USA 1985;82:2473–2477.

9. Boulieu R, Bastien O, Bleyzac N. Pharmacokinetics of ganciclovir in heart transplant patients undergoing continuous venovenous hemodialysis. Ther Drug Monit 1993;15:105–107.

10. Brenner S. Phosphotransferase sequence homology. Nature 1987; 329:21–25.

11. Brosgart CL, Craig C, Hillman D, Louis TA, Alston B, for Terry Bern Community Programs for Clinical Research on AIDS (CPCRA). A randomized, placebo-controlled trial of the safety and efficacy of oral ganciclovir for prophylaxis of CMV retinal and gastrointestinal mucosal disease in HIV-infected individuals with severe immunosuppression [Abstract]. Program and abstracts of the 35th Interscience Conference on Antimicrobial Agents and Chemotherapy (San Francisco). Washington, DC: American Society for Microbiology, 1995.

12. Buhles WC, Mastre BJ, Tinker AJ, Strand V, Koretz SH, and the Syntex Collaborative Ganciclovir Treatment Study Group. Ganciclovir treatment of life- or sight-threatening cytomegalovirus infections: experience in 314 immunocompromised patients. Rev Infect Dis 1988;10(Suppl 3):S495–S503.

13. Cheng YC, Huang ES, Lin J, Mar EC, Pagano JS, Dutschman GE, Grill SP. Unique spectrum of activity of 9-[(1,3-hydroxy-2-propoxy)methyl] guanine against herpesviruses in vitro and its mode of action against herpes simplex virus type 1. Proc Natl Acad Sci USA 1983;80:2767–2770.

14. Cherrington JM, Miner R, Hitchcock MJM, Lalezari JP, Drew WL. Susceptibility of human cytomegalovirus to cidofovir is

unchanged after limited in vivo exposure to various regimens of drug. J Infect Dis 1996;173:987–992.

15. Chou S, Erice A, Jordan MC, Vercellotti GM, Michels KR, Talarico CL, Stanat SC, Biron KK. Analysis of the UL97 phosphotransferase coding sequence in clinical cytomegalovirus isolates and identification of mutations conferring ganciclovir resistance. J Infect Dis 1995:171:576–583.

16. Chou S, Guentzel S, Michels KR, Miner RC, Drew WL. Frequency of UL97 phosphotransferase mutations related to ganciclovir resistance in clinical cytomegalovirus isolates. J Infect Dis 1995;172:239–242.

17. Cochereau-Massin I, Lehoang P, Lautier-Frau M, Zazoun L, Marcel P, Robinet M, Matheron S, Katalama C, Gharakhanian S, Rozenbaum W, Ingrand D, Gentilini M. Efficacy and tolerance of intravitreal ganciclovir in cytomegalovirus retinitis in acquired immune deficiency syndrome. Ophthalmology 1991; 98:1348–1353.

18. Cohen BA, McArthur JC, Grohman S, Patterson B, Glass JD. Neurologic prognosis of cytomegalovirus polyradiculomyelopathy in AIDS. Neurology 1993;43:493–499.

19. Cole NL, Balfour HH Jr. In vitro susceptibility of cytomegalovirus isolates from immunocompromised patients to acyclovir and ganciclovir. Diagn Microbiol Infect Dis 1987;6: 255–261.

20. Crumpacker CS. Ganciclovir. N Engl J Med 1996;335:721–729.

21. Crumpacker CSE. Drug resistance in cytomegalovirus: current knowledge and implications for patient management. J Acquir Immune Defic Syndr 1996;12(Suppl 1):S6–S7.

22. Crumpacker CS, Kowalsky PN, Oliver SA, Schnipper LE, Field AK. Resistance of herpes simplex virus to 9-{[2-hydroxy-1-(hydroxymethyl)ethoxy]methyl} guanine: physical mapping of drug synergism within the viral DNA polymerase locus. Proc Natl Acad Sci USA 1984;81:1556–1560.

23. Crumpacker CS, Marlowe S, Zhang JL, Abrams S, Watkins P, Ganciclovir Bone Marrow Transplant Treatment Group. Treatment of cytomegalovirus pneumonia. Rev Infect Dis 1988;10 (Suppl 3):S538–S546.

24. DeArmond B. Future directions in the management of cytomegalovirus infections. J Acquir Immune Defic Syndr 1991;4 (Suppl 1):S53–S56.

25. Dieterich DT, Kotler DP, Busch DF, Crumpacker C, Du Mond C, Dearmand B, Buhles W. Ganciclovir treatment of serious cytomegalovirus colitis in AIDS: a randomized, double-blind, placebo-controlled multicenter study. J Infect Dis 1993;167: 278–282.

26. Drew WL, Ives D, Lalezari JP, Crumpacker C, Follansbee SE, Spector SA, Benson CA, Friedberg DN, Hubbard L, Stempien MJ, Shadman A, Buhles W, for the Syntex Cooperative Oral Ganciclovir Study Group. Oral ganciclovir as maintenance treatment for cytomegalovirus retinitis in patients with AIDS. N Engl J Med 1995;333:615–620.

27. Drew WL, Miner RC, Busch DF, Follansbee SE, Gullett J, Mehalko SG, Gordon SM, Owen WF Jr, Matthews TR, Buhles WC, DeArmond B. Prevalence of resistance in patients receiving ganciclovir for serious cytomegalovirus infection. J Infect Dis 1991;163:716–719.

28. Drew WL, Miner R, Saleh E. Antiviral susceptibility testing of cytomegalovirus: criteria for detecting resistance to antivirals. Clin Diagn Virol 1993;1:179–185.

29. Eidelberg D, Sorrel A, Vogel H, Walker P, Kleefield J, Crumpacker CS III. Progressive polyradiculopathy in acquired immune deficiency syndrome. Neurology 1986;36:912–916.

30. Emanuel D, Cunningham I, Jules-Elysee K, Brochstein JA, Kerman NA, Laver J, Stover D, White DA, Fels A, Polsky B, Castro-Malaspina H, Peppard JR, Bartus P, Hammerling U, O'Reilly RJ. Cytomegalovirus pneumonia after bone marrow transplantation successfully treated with the combination of ganciclovir and high-dose intravenous immune globulin. Ann Intern Med 1988;109:777–782.

31. Enting R, de Gans J, Reiss P, Jansen C, Portegies P. Ganciclovir/foscarnet for cytomegalovirus meningoencephalitis in AIDS. Lancet 1992;340:559–560.

32. Erice A, Chou S, Biron KK, Stanat SC, Balfour JJ Jr, Jordan MC. Progressive disease due to ganciclovir-resistant cytomegalovirus in immunocompromised patients. N Engl J Med 1989;320:289–293.

33. Faulds D, Heel RC. Ganciclovir: a review of its antiviral activity, pharmacokinetic properties and therapeutic efficacy in cytomegalovirus infections. Drugs 1990;39:597–638.

34. Field AK, Davies ME, DeWitt C, Perry HC, Liou R, Germershausen J, Karkas JD, Ashton WT, Johnston DBR, Tolman RL. 9-{[2-hydroxy-1-(hydroxymethyl)ethoxy]methyl}guanine: a selective inhibitor of herpes group virus replication. Proc Natl Acad Sci USA 1983;80:4139–4143.

35. Fletcher C, Sawchuk R, Chinnock B, de Miranda P, Balfour HH Jr. Human pharmacokinetics of the antiviral drug DHPG. Clin Pharmacol Ther 1986;40:281–286.

36. Freeman WR, Henderly DE, Wan WL, Causey D, Trousdale M, Green RL, Rao NA. Prevalence, pathophysiology, and treatment of rhegmatogenous retinal detachment in treated cytomegalovirus retinitis. Am J Ophthalmol 1987;103:527–536.

37. Fuller GN. Cytomegalovirus and the peripheral nervous nervous system in AIDS. J Acquir Immune Defic Syndr 1992;5(Suppl 1):S33–S36.

38. Goodrich JM, Mori M, Gleaves CA, Du Mond C, Cays M, Ebeling DF, Buhles WC, De Armond B, Meyers JD. Early treatment with ganciclovir to prevent cytomegalovirus disease after allogeneic bone marrow transplantation. N Engl J Med 1991;325: 1601–1607.

39. Hamzeh FM, Lietman PS. Intranuclear accumulation of subgenomic noninfectious human cytomegalovirus DNA in infected cells in the presence of ganciclovir. Antimicrob Agents Chemother 1991;35:1818–1823.

40. Hardy WD. Combined ganciclovir and recombinant human granulocyte-macrophage colony-stimulating factor in the treatment of cytomegalovirus retinitis in AIDS patients. J Acquir Immune Defic Syndr 1991;4(Suppl):S22–S28.

41. Hecht DW, Snydman DR, Crumpacker CS, Werner BG, Heinze-Lacey B, Boston Renal Transplant CMV Study Group. Ganciclovir for treatment of renal transplant-associated primary cytomegalovirus pneumonia. J Infect Dis 1988;157:187–190.

42. Henry K, Cantrill H, Fletcher C, Chinnock BJ, Balfour HH Jr. Use of intravitreal ganciclovir (dihydroxy propylmethyl guanine) for cytomegalovirus retinitis in a patient with AIDS. Am J Ophthalmol 1987;103:17–23.

43. Hochster H, Dieterich D, Bozzette S, Reichmann RC, Connor JD, Liebes L, Sonke RL, Spector SA, Valentine F, Pettinelli C, Richman DD. Toxicity of combined ganciclovir and zidovudine for cytomegalovirus disease associated with AIDS. Ann Intern Med 1990;113:111–117.

44. Kuppermann BD, Quiceno JI, Flores-Aguilar M, Connor JD, Capparelli EV, Sherwood CH, Freeman WR. Intravitreal ganciclovir concentration after intravenous administration in AIDS patients with cytomegalovirus retinitis: implications for therapy. J Infect Dis 1993;168:1506–1509.

45. Lake KD, Fletcher CV, Love KR, Brown DC, Joyce LD, Pritzker MR. Ganciclovir pharmacokinetics during renal impairment. Antimicrob Agents Chemother 1988;32:1899–1900.

46. Littler E, Stuart AD, Chee MS. Human cytomegalovirus UL97 open reading frame encodes a protein that phosphorylates the antiviral nucleoside analogue ganciclovir. Nature 1992;358: 160–162.

47. Lurain NS, Thompson KD, Holmes EW, Read GS. Point mutations in the DNA polymerase gene of human cytomegalovirus that result in resistance to antiviral agents. J Virol 1992;66: 7146–7152.

48. Lurain NS, Spafford LE, Thompson KD. Mutation in the UL97 open reading frame of human cytomegalovirus strains resistant to ganciclovir. J Virol 1994;68:4427–4431.

49. Manischewitz JF, Quinnan GV Jr, Lane HC, Wittek AE. Synergistic effect of ganciclovir and foscarnet on cytomegalovirus replication in vitro. Antimicrob Agents Chemother 1990;34: 373–375.

50. Mar EC, Cheng YC, Huang ES. Effect of 9-(1,3-dihydroxy-2-propoxymethyl)guanine on human cytomegalovirus replication in vitro. Antimicrob Agents Chemother 1983;24:518–521.

51. Markham A, Faulds D. Ganciclovir: an update of its therapeutic use in cytomegalovirus infection. Drugs 1994;48:455–484.

52. Martin DF, Parks DJ, Mellow SD, Ferris FL, Walton RC, Remaley NA, Chew EY, Ashton P, Davis MD, Nussenblatt RB. Treatment of cytomegalovirus retinitis with an intraocular sustained-release ganciclovir implant. Arch Ophthalmol 1994; 112:1531–1539.

53. Martin JC, Dvorak CA, Smee DF, Matthews TR, Verheyden JPH. 9-[(1,3-dihydroxy-2-propoxy)methyl]guanine: a new potent and selective antiherpes agent. J Med Chem 1983;26: 759–761.

54. Merigan TC, Renlund DG, Keay S, Bristow MR, Starnes V, O'-Connell JB, Resta S, Dunn D, Gamberg P, Ratkovec RM, Richenbacher WE, Millar RC, Du Mond C, De Armond B, Sullivan V, Cheney T, Buhles W, Stinson EB. A controlled trial of ganciclovir to prevent cytomegalovirus disease after heart transplantation. N Engl J Med 1992;326:1182–1186.

55. Miller RG, Storey JR, Greco CM. Ganciclovir in the treatment of progressive AIDS-related polyradiculopathy. Neurology 1990;40:569–574.

56. Musch DC, Martin DF, Gordon JF, Davis MD, Kuppermann BD, and the Ganciclovir Implant Study Group. Treatment of cytomegalovirus retinitis with a sustained-release ganciclovir implant. N Engl J Med 1997;337:83–90.

57. Ogilvie UK, Cheriyan UD, Radatus BK, Smith KO, Gallaway KS, Kennell WL. Biologically active acyclonucleoside analogues. II. The synthesis of 9-[[2-hydroxy-1-(hydroxymethyl)ethoxy] methyl] guanine (BIOLF-62). Can J Chem 1982;60:3005–3010.

58. Oliver S, Bubley G, Crumpacker CS. Inhibition of HSV-transformed murine cells by nucleoside analogs, 2′NDG and 2′-nor-cGMP: mechanism of inhibition and reversal by exogenous nucleosides. Virology 1985;145:84–93.

59. Pape JW. Treatment of gastrointestinal infections. AIDS 1988;2 (Suppl 1):S161–S167.

60. Plotkin SA, Drew WL, Felsenstein D, Hirsch MS. Sensitivity of clinical isolates of human cytomegalovirus to 9-(1,3-dihydroxy-2-propoxymethyl) guanine. J Infect Dis 1985;152:833–834.

61. Reed EC, Bowden RA, Dandliker PS, Lilleby KE, Meyers JD. Treatment of cytomegalovirus pneumonia with ganciclovir and intravenous cytomegalovirus immunoglobulin in patients with bone marrow transplants. Ann Intern Med 1988;109:783–788.

62. Reed EC, Wolford JL, Kopecky KJ, Lilleby KE, Dandliker PS, Todaro JL, McDonald GB, Meyers JD. Ganciclovir for the treatment of cytomegalovirus gastroenteritis in bone marrow transplant patients. Ann Intern Med 1990;112:505–510.

63. Sanborn GE, Anand R, Torti RE, Nightingale SD, Cal SX, Yates B, Ashton P, Smith T. Sustained-release ganciclovir therapy for treatment of cytomegalovirus retinitis: use of an intravitreal device. Arch Ophthalmol 1992;110:188–195.

64. Schmidt GM, Horak DA, Niland JC, Duncan SR, Forman SJ, Zaia JA, and the City of Hope-Stanford-Syntex CMV Study Group. A randomized, controlled trial of prophylactic ganciclovir for cytomegalovirus pulmonary infection in recipients of allogeneic bone marrow transplants. N Engl J Med 1991;324: 1005–1011.

65. Schmidt GM, Kovacs A, Zaia JA, Horak DA, Blume KG, Nademanee AP, O'Donnell MR, Snyder DS, Forman SJ. Ganciclovir/immunoglobulin combination therapy for the treatment of human cytomegalovirus-associated interstitial pneumonia in bone marrow allograft recipients. Transplantation 1988;46: 905–907.

66. Shepp DH, Dandliker PS, de Miranda P, Burnette TC, Cederberg DM, Kirk LE, Meyers JD. Activity of 9-{[2-hydroxy-1-(hydroxymethyl)ethoxy]methyl}guanine in the treatment of cytomegalovirus pneumonia. Ann Intern Med 1985;103:368–373.

67. Singh N, Yu VL, Mieles L, Wagener MM, Miner RC, Gayowski T. High-dose acyclovir compared to short-course preemptive ganciclovir therapy to prevent cytomegalovirus disease in liver transplant recipients. Ann Intern Med 1994;120:375–381.

68. Smith IL, Cherrington JM, Jiles RE, Fuller MD, Freeman WR, Spector SA. High-level resistance of cytomegalovirus to ganciclovir is associated with alterations in both UL97 and DNA polymerase genes. J Infect Dis 1997;176:69–77.

69. Smith IL, Flores-Aguilar M, Taskintuna I, Jiles RE, Freeman WR, Spector SA. Cytomegalovirus resistance is associated with clinical failure in AIDS patients receiving ganciclovir treatment for retinitis [Abstract]. Program and abstracts of the 36th Interscience Conference on Antimicrobial Agents and Chemotherapy (New Orleans). Washington, DC: American Society for Microbiology, 1996.

70. Smith KO, Galloway KS, Kennell WL, Ogilvie KK, Radatus BK. A new nucleoside analog 9-{[2-hydroxy-1-(hydroxymethyl) ethoxy]methyl}guanine highly active in vitro against herpes simplex virus types 1 and 2. Antimicrob Agents Chemother 1982; 22:55–61.

71. Snoeck R, Andrei G, Schols D, Balzarini J, De Clercq E. Activity of different antiviral drug combinations against human cytomegalovirus replication in vitro. Eur J Clin Microbiol Infect Dis 1992;11:1144–1155.

72. Sommadossi JP, Bevan R, Ling T, Lee F, Mastre B, Chaplin MD, Nerenberg C, Koretz S, Buhles WC Jr. Clinical pharmacokinetics of ganciclovir in patients with normal and impaired renal function. Rev Infect Dis 1988;10(Suppl 3):S507–S514.

73. Spector SA, Busch DF, Follansbee S, Squires K, Lalezari JP, Jacobson MA, Connor JD, Jung D, Shadman A, Mastre B, Buhles W, Drew WL, AIDS Clinical Trials Group, and Cytomegalovirus Cooperative Study Group. Pharmacokinetic, safety, and antiviral profiles of oral ganciclovir in persons infected with human immunodeficiency virus: a phase I/II study. J Infect Dis 1995;171:1431–1437.

74. Spector SA, McKinley GF, Lalezari JP, Samo T, Andruczk R, Follansbee S, Sparti PD, Havlir DV, Simpson G, Buhles W, Wong R, Stempien MJ, for the Roche Cooperative Oral Ganciclovir Study

Group. Oral ganciclovir for the prevention of cytomegalovirus disease in persons with AIDS. N Engl J Med 1996;334: 1491–1497.

75. Stanat SC, Reardon JE, Erice A, Jordan MC, Drew WL, Biron KK. Ganciclovir-resistant cytomegalovirus clinical isolates: mode of resistance to ganciclovir. Antimicrob Agents Chemother 1991;35:2191–2197.

76. Studies of Ocular Complications of AIDS Research Group, in Collaboration with the AIDS Clinical Trials Group. Mortality in patients with the acquired immunodeficiency syndrome treated with either foscarnet or ganciclovir for cytomegalovirus retinitis. N Engl J Med 1992;326:213–220.

77. Studies of Ocular Complications of AIDS Research Group, in Collaboration with the AIDS Clinical Trials Group. Foscarnet-ganciclovir cytomegalovirus retinitis trial. 4. Visual outcomes. Ophthalmology 1994;101:1250–1261.

78. Studies of Ocular Complications of AIDS Research Group, in Collaboration with the AIDS Clinical Trials Group. Combination foscarnet and ganciclovir therapy vs monotherapy for treatment of relapsed cytomegalovirus retinitis in patients with AIDS. Arch Ophthalmol 1996;114:23–33.

79. Sullivan V, Biron KK, Talarico C, Stanat SC, Davis M, Pozzi LM, Coen DM. A point mutation in the human cytomegalovirus DNA polymerase gene confers resistance to ganciclovir and phosphonylmethoxyalkyl derivatives. Antimicrob Agents Chemother 1993;37:19–25.

80. Sullivan V, Talarico CL, Stanat SC, Davis M, Coen DM, Biron KK. A protein kinase homologue controls phosphorylation of ganciclovir in human cytomegalovirus-infected cells. Nature 1992;358:162–165.

81. Taylor DL, Jeffries DJ, Taylor-Robinson D, Parkin JM, Tyms AS. The susceptibility of adenovirus infection to the anti-cytomegalovirus drug, ganciclovir (DHPG). FEMS Microbiol Lett 1988;49:337–341.

82. Tocci MJ, Livelli TJ, Perry HC, Crumpacker CS, Field AK. Effects of nucleoside analog 2'nor-2'-deoxyguanosine on human cytomegalovirus replication. Antimicrob Agents Chemother 1984;25:247–252.

83. Trang JM, Kidd L, Gruber W, Storch G, Demmler G, Jacobs R, Danker W, Starr S, Pass R, Stagno S, Alford C, Soong SJ, Whitley RJ, Sommadossi JP, and the NIAID Collaborative Antiviral Study Group. Linear single-dose pharmacokinetics of ganciclovir in newborns with congenital cytomegalovirus infections. Clin Pharmacol Ther 1993;53:15–21.

84. Weller S, Liao SHT, Cederberg DM, de Miranda P, Blum MR. The pharmacokinetics of ganciclovir in patients with cytomegalovirus (CMV) infections [Abstract]. J Pharm Sci 1987; 76:S120.

85. Winston DJ, Wirin D, Shaked A, Bussuttil RW. Randomised comparison of ganciclovir and high-dose acyclovir for long-term cytomegalovirus prophylaxis in liver transplant recipients. Lancet 1995;346:69–74.

86. Wolf DG, Smith IL, Lee DJ, Freeman WR, Flores-Aguilar M, Spector SA. Mutations in human cytomegalovirus UL97 gene confer clinical resistance to ganciclovir and can be detected directly in patient plasma. J Clin Invest 1995;95:257–263.

87. Wolf DG, Spector SA. Diagnosis of human cytomegalovirus central nervous system disease in AIDS patients by DNA amplification from cerebrospinal fluid. J Infect Dis 1992;166: 1412–1415.

Interferons

●

Marion G. Peters and Sandra J. Burgess

CLASS
Chemical Structure

Interferons (IFNs) are small secreted glycoproteins and members of the cytokine family. There are three IFNs, which vary structurally, biochemically, and antigenically (36, 45, 58) (Table 1). Multiple highly homologous IFN-α genes are clustered on chromosome 9. Preproteins are produced that are cleaved at the N terminus to form secreted proteins of 165 to 166 amino acids (62). At least 16 IFN-α proteins exist. The molecular mass of IFN-α varies from 16 to 27 kDa depending upon the degree of glycosylation. IFN-α used in clinical practice is recombinant proteins, IFN-α_{2a} and IFN-α_{2b}, lymphoblastoid IFN-α (not licensed in the United States), and consensus IFN-α. These IFNs appear to have similar actions and potency, although some differences are discussed in the treatment sections. Lymphoblastoid IFN-α is derived from a cell line, Namalwa, and contains IFN-α and IFN-β. Consensus IFN is a synthetic IFN-α that uses the most common amino acids from 11 IFN-α gene products. IFN-β and IFN-γ are encoded by single genes. IFN-α and IFN-β are generally acid stable, while IFN-γ is acid labile. The protein structure of IFN-α is 65% α-helix and less than 20% β-sheet content (61). Most IFNs have four cysteine residues involved in disulfide bonding. IFN-β has 30% structural homology to IFN-α (42).

Structure-Activity Relationships

Table 1 lists structural, chemical, and cell of origin of the three IFNs. Human IFNs include IFN-α, IFN-β, and IFN-γ. All share antiviral, antiproliferative, and immunomodulatory properties: IFN-α and IFN-β are predominantly antiviral, and IFN-γ is predominantly immunomodulatory (36, 37). IFNs are induced early in response to foreign antigens. Different bio-

TABLE 1 • Comparison of Human Interferons

	IFN-α	IFN-β	IFN-γ
Number of genes	23	1	1
Gene location	9 short arm	9 short arm	12 long arm
Number of introns	0	0	3
Molecular weight	20,000	23,000	17–25 kDa
N-Linked glycosylation	+	+	2 sites
Amino acids	166	166	143
Cell source	Monocytes, B cells	Fibroblasts	T cells, NK cells
Inducers	Virus	ds RNA, poly IC, virus	Antigen, mitogen
Receptor location: Gene	21	21	6 (21)
Signaling: JAK-activated	JAK-1, tyk-2	JAK-1, tyk-2	JAK-1, JAK-2
Signaling: STAT used	STAT 1, STAT 2	STAT 1, STAT 2	STAT 1

logic stimuli induce IFNs, including pathogens (viral, bacterial, and protozoal) and cytokines. Like other cytokines, they may act in an autocrine or paracrine manner on the cell of production or other cell types.

VIRAL ACTIVITY
Spectrum

IFNs have activity against the following viruses: hepatitis B (HBV), HCV, HDV, human papilloma virus (HPV), herpes simplex viruses (HSV) 1 and 2, cytomegalovirus (CMV), vesicular stomatitis virus (VSV), human immunodeficiency virus (HIV), poliovirus, rhinoviruses, adenoviruses, coronaviruses, and vaccinia. IFN-α is used to treat chronic hepatitides, AIDS-related Kaposi's sarcoma, HPV, hairy cell leukemia, and Philadelphia chromosome–positive CML. It also is used as an adjuvant in chemotherapy and HIV infection. IFN-γ does not have a clinical role as an antiviral agent.

Pharmacodynamic Effects

IFNs have profound immunomodulatory properties: they induce cell surface proteins including class I (all IFNs) and class II (IFN-γ only), $β_2$-microglobulin, growth factors and receptors, the Fc family of receptor proteins, and complement components (36, 37). They also enhance natural killer cell function and T lymphocyte and macrophage activation. They are cytokines and are involved in complex interactions with other cytokines. IFN-γ is produced characteristically by TH1 helper cells, and this appears essential for clearance of some viruses. The immune response to IFN-α appears to be critical for clearance of hepatitis B and C infection, perhaps by altering the type of cytokines produced and thus stimulating a cytotoxic T cell response instead of a predominantly B cell response (53).

MECHANISM OF ACTION
IFN Signaling

IFNs are short-lived proteins that have a rapid onset of action (30 min) after receptor-ligand interaction (56). This is achieved through tyrosine phosphorylation by Janus-activated kinases (JAK) of latent intracytoplasmic proteins named signal transducers and activators of transcription (STATs) (12). STATs do not require protein synthesis for activity as they are constitutively present in the cytoplasm; hence, the rapidity of the cytokine response. After phosphorylation, STATs translocate to the nucleus where they bind to IFN-stimulated response elements (ISREs) in the 5′ untranslated region of cytokine-responsive genes and induce gene transcription. IFN-α and IFN-γ share one JAK and one STAT; their response elements are different but have overlapping sequences (34, 46, 57) (Table 1). Although IFNs share many effects, some are distinct because some genes do not have IFN-α ISREs but do have IFN-γ response elements (named GAS for γ-activated site). Many other cytokines share JAKs and STATs, which explains the redundancy of the cytokine cascade.

Antiviral Effects

IFNs induce transcription of many genes including those for 2′,5′-oligoadenylate synthetase (2′,5′-OAS), double-strand (ds) RNA–dependent protein kinase, and Mx proteins (36). IFN is important in early stages of viral infection, limiting duration of viremia and spread of infection by inhibiting varying stages of viral replication including entry, uncoating, mRNA synthesis, and protein synthesis. 2′,5′-OAS is induced by all IFNs and is activated by dsRNA (i.e., viral RNA). It converts ATP into small oligoadenylates that activate RNase L, a cellular ribonuclease. RNase L then promotes viral RNA degradation (48). dsRNA activates a dsRNA-dependent protein kinase (P68 kinase, P1 eIF-2 kinase). This leads to phosphorylation of the eukaryotic peptide chain initiation factor 2 (eIF-2). Phosphorylation inactivates eIF-2, inhibiting protein synthesis. The role of other proteins, including Mx protein in humans, is unclear.

MECHANISM OF RESISTANCE
Commonly Resistant Organisms

Only 20% of HCV patients respond to IFN-α, although this increases with addition of ribavirin (41). IFN nonresponsiveness has been suggested to be due to IFN-response elements in the HCV genome but may also be related to the type and strength of the host immune response (16, 22, 53). HBV has a higher response rate (50%), and response is often associated with a "flare" in serum aminotransferases, suggesting T cell–mediated cytolysis of hepatocytes (24). For more details see the chapter on hepatitis viruses.

Mechanisms of Resistance

In many chronic infections, viruses evade the immune response by mutations in viral peptides that can bind HLA and T lymphocyte receptor but do not activate the T cell. These altered peptides have been shown for HVB but not as yet for HVC (3). Multiple mechanisms for viral evasion of host defense have been documented, including viral production of host proteins, such as cytokines and their receptors; myxoma virus encodes a IFN-γ receptor (55). Viruses inhibit transcriptional activation of IFN-induced cells; adenovirus type 5 E1A oncogene and HBV decrease STATs, inhibiting IFN signaling (17,26); HBV can inhibit transcription of IFN-β (54).

Some viruses can inhibit the effect of IFN-inducible proteins: HSV produces nonfunctional 2′,5′-OAS (50); adenovirus, HIV, and Epstein-Barr virus (EBV) bind protein kinase and inhibit activity; vaccinia and reovirus bind dsRNA; influenza virus activates a kinase inhibitor; poliovirus enhances proteolysis of the kinase; and HSV inactivates RNAse-L and inhibits complement factors and antibody responses (11, 20, 25, 27). DNA viruses are less sensitive than RNA viruses to the effect of protein kinase activity.

Methods to Overcome and Prevent Resistance

Higher doses of IFN have been used with limited success to overcome resistance. Longer duration improves sustained long-term responses to IFN in hepatitis C but not in hepatitis B (41). Limited data suggest that consensus IFN (CIFN) may have an increased effect in patients with cirrhosis (52). Addition of ribavirin to IFN-α greatly enhances the initial and sustained responses in hepatitis C, especially in patients who respond and then relapse (7, 9).

PHARMACOKINETICS
Absorption

IFNs are poorly absorbed by the oral route because of degradation of the protein structure by enzymes in the gastrointestinal tract. IFN-α is well absorbed after subcutaneous or intramuscular administration, with a bioavailability exceeding 80% (59) (Table 2). Recombinant IFN-αs are stable in saline or water solution at 4°C for prolonged periods. Intravenous administration of IFN-α provides more rapid, higher serum concentrations than intramuscular or subcutaneous administration, and subcutaneous administration results in lower and slower peak serum concentrations than intramuscular administration (59, 60). Few pharmacokinetic data exist regarding CIFN; however, the manufacturer reports that peak serum levels occurred 1 to 4 h after subcutaneous administration in animal models. In humans, CIFN has not been detected in plasma after subcutaneous administration of 1 to 9 μg, however levels of 2′,5′-OAS and β_2 microglobulin were maximal 24 and 24 to 36 h after dosing, respectively. The subcutaneous route is used for treatment of viral hepatitis, although multiple routes of administration have been used. The route of administration does not alter the side effect profile. IFNs are not well absorbed orally and are probably proteolytically degraded by gastrointestinal enzyme activity. IFN-α is filtered through the glomerulus and proteolytic degradation in the renal tubules

---

TABLE 2 • Pharmacokinetic Properties of IFN-α

Absorption
  Oral: Poor
  IM: Bioavailability >80%; T_{max} 3.8 h (1–8); C_{max} 2,020 pg/mL[a]
  SC: Bioavailability >80%; T_{max} 7.3 h (6–8); C_{max} 1,730 pg/mL[a]
  IV: —; —; C_{max} 13,900 pg/mL[a]
Distribution
  Vd: 31 L or 0.4 L/kg in healthy volunteers
  Concentration: may concentrate in kidney, lymph, tumor tissue
  CSF: Poor penetration
  Placenta: unknown whether crosses placenta in humans
  Breast milk: unknown whether excreted in human breast milk; excreted in milk in mice
Metabolism and elimination
  Metabolism: catabolism and excretion by kidneys; minimal hepatic metabolism
  Clearance: total body clearance exceeds GFR; mean 2.79 mL/min/kg after i.v. infusion
  Half-life: 2.3–3.5 h after i.m. or s.c. administration
  Dialysis: not removed by hemodialysis

[a] After administration of 36 MIU to healthy volunteers.

---

follows proximal tubular reabsorption (5). Renal catabolism is related directly to IFN concentration. Little or no drug is excreted into the urine, and hepatic metabolism is deemed minor. IFN-α distributes into the cerebrospinal fluid (CSF) at doses of 50 million units or above; this does not explain the known neurotoxicity of IFNs (60). The specific activity in recombinant IFN and purified human IFN-α is about 1×10^8 IU/mg, based on antiviral activity assays. The clinical significance of serum antibodies to IFN-α is unclear (32, 40).

Distribution

After intravenous administration, serum IFN-alpha concentrations decline in a biexponential manner, with a rapid distribution phase followed by a terminal elimination phase (59). The volume of distribution has been reported to range from 12–40L, with a mean of 31L or 0.4L/kg in healthy volunteers (60) (Table 2). Studies in animal models suggest that recombinant IFN-alpha may concentrate in the kidney, tumors, and lymph tissue. IFN does not appear to penetrate the CSF to an appreciable extent (60), and it is unknown whether it crosses the placenta in humans or is excreted in human breast milk. It has been noted to be excreted in milk in mice according to the product information. The volume of distribution varies from 20–60% of body-weight. The plasma elimination half-lives of IFNs are short: 4–16 hours for IFN-α and 1–2 hours for IFN-β.

Metabolism and Elimination

Total body clearance is nearly two times the glomerular filtration rate, suggesting active tubular secretion, renal catabolism, or extrarenal elimination (5, 59). IFN-α undergoes glomerular filtration and tubular reabsorption, with rapid degradation at the brush border or in the lysosomes of the tubular epithelium during reabsorption. Decreased clearance was noted in nephrectomized rabbits and rats. There is minimal reabsorption of intact IFN, and negligible amounts are recovered in urine. Hepatic metabolism and subsequent biliary excretion play only a minor role in IFN clearance. The half-life of IFN-α was noted to be a mean of 5.1 h after intravenous infusion and 2.3 to 3.5 h after intramuscular or subcutaneous administration, respectively, in healthy volunteers (60). Serum concentrations were undetectable by 16 h after intramuscular or subcutaneous administration in healthy volunteers. The half-life of CIFN was reported as 1.3 to 3.4 h after subcutaneous administration in hamsters and monkeys. IFN does not appear to be removed by hemodialysis (23).

DOSING AND ADMINISTRATION
Normal
Chronic Hepatitis C

The recommended dose of IFN-$_{\alpha 2a}$ or IFN-$_{\alpha 2b}$ is 3 million units (MIU) subcutaneously or or intramuscularly thrice weekly for 12 months (Table 3). Longer courses of treatment (18 months) may be beneficial (18, 41). A reduction in serum ALT with loss of HCV RNA from the serum after 3 months of treatment indicates a response; if there is no response at 3 months, IFN should be discontinued. For patients who relapse after responding to an initial course of therapy, a second course may be administered at 3 MIU or 6 MIU thrice weekly for 6 to 12 months. If patients experience serious adverse effects, the dose should be decreased by 50% or the drug should be temporarily discontinued and restarted at a lower dose after the adverse effect resolves.

The recommended dose of CIFN is 9 μg subcutaneously thrice weekly for 6 months. Patients who do not respond or those who relapse after discontinuation of CIFN may receive a subsequent course (15 μg subcutaneously thrice weekly for 6 months), if tolerated. The manufacturer recommends a dose reduction to 7.5 μg or temporary discontinuation for patients who experience intolerable adverse effects with higher doses.

TABLE 3 • **Dosing and Administration of INF-α for Chronic Viral Hepatitis**

Hepatitis C
  Initial course: 3 million units (MIU) s.c. or 9 μg 3 times weekly × 12 months; consider discontinuation after 3 months if no response
  Relapse: 6 MIU or 15 μg 3 times weekly for 12 months
Hepatitis B
  Adult: 5 MIU/day or 10 MIU 3 times weekly s.c. or i.m. × 16 weeks
  Pediatric: 6 MIU/m² s.c. 3 times weekly has been used; start at 2 MIU/m² and increase to 6 MIU over 3–7 doses
Monitoring patients during treatment

	Pretreatment	During	Treatment end
CBC[a]	+	+ (1 week, month)	+ +
LFTs[b]	+	monthly	+
TSH[c]	+	3-monthly	
Liver biopsy	+		6 months after end

[a] CBC, complete blood count.

[b] LFTs, liver function tests.

[c] TSH, thyrotropin-stimulating hormone.

Chronic Hepatitis B

The recommended dose of IFN-$_{\alpha 2b}$ for chronic hepatitis B in adults is 5 MIU subcutaneously or intramuscularly daily or 10 MIU thrice weekly for 4 months. For pediatric patients, recombinant IFN-$_{\alpha 2b}$ has been administered at a dose of 6 MIU/m² subcutaneously thrice weekly for 4 to 6 months (35). Therapy was initiated at 2 MIU/m² and increased to 6 MIU/m² over three to seven doses to minimize side effects (21). Lymphoblastoid IFN (not available in the U.S.) has been given at a dose of 5 MIU/m² intramuscularly daily for 5 days, then thrice weekly for 11 weeks; however 84% of patients required a dose reduction due to flulike symptoms (15). The safety and efficacy of CIFN in pediatric patients has not been evaluated.

Special Populations

No dosage adjustment is necessary in patients with renal or hepatic dysfunction (23). Elderly patients may be more susceptible to the central nervous system and cardiac side effects from IFN, and dose adjustment may be necessary to ameliorate these effects. Pediatric patients are usually dosed in IU per m². There are no data regarding dosage adjustments in patients with obesity or ascites or in pregnant patients (29). Obese patients may require higher doses (39). IFN-α and CIFN are rated in pregnancy category C; there are no controlled studies in humans, but the drugs have abortifacient properties when administered in high doses in animal models.

Condylomata Acuminata

The recommended dose of IFN-α is 250,000 units (0.05 mL) per wart twice weekly for up to 8 weeks (4). Maximal recommended dose per treatment session is 2.5 MIU (0.5 mL). Inject into the base of each wart using a 30-gauge needle. Large warts may be injected at several points around the periphery using a total dose of 0.05 mL/wart. After the initial 8-week course, do not give further therapy for 3 months to allow time for complete resolution. The recommended dose of IFN-β is 1 MIU thrice weekly for 3 weeks.

Genital Herpes

The recommended dose of IFN-α is 6 MIU subcutaneously, although dosages range from 6 to 18 MIU over 1 to 3 days (10).

AIDS-Related Kaposi's Sarcoma

The recommended dose of IFN-α is 36 MIU/day or 30 MIU/m² for 10 to 12 weeks subcutaneously or until there is no further evidence of tumor. Dosage may be started lower and slowly increased over 9 days. Some patients cannot tolerate the maximal dose because of side effects or severe opportunistic infections.

ADVERSE EFFECTS

See Table 4.

Flulike Syndrome

Most patients treated with IFN-α or CIFN develop a flulike syndrome characterized by fever (40–98%), fatigue or malaise (50–95%), myalgia (30–75%), chills (40–65%),

TABLE 4 • Adverse Effects of IFN-α

Common	Less Common
Flulike syndrome	Altered mental
Myelosuppression,	status/confusion/stupor
especially neutrophils	Other neuropsychiatric effects
Fatigue/malaise/myalgia	Cardiotoxicity
Headache	Proteinuria, nephrotoxicity
Anorexia	Rash, dry skin
Irritability/depression/anxiety	Hyperglycemia, hyperlipidemia
Alopecia	Hepatotoxicity
Immune effects	
ANA	
Hyper- or hypothyroidism	

headache (20–70%), and arthralgia (5–24%) (43). Fever, thought to be mediated by an increase in hypothalamic prostaglandin E_2 (PGE_2) production or release or by an increase in interleukin-1 production, often reaches 38 to 40°C within 6 h, may persist for up to 12 h, and may be accompanied by chills or rigors (14). Acetaminophen or nonsteroidal antiinflammatory agents can be administered concomitantly with the first few does of IFN. It tends to be self-limiting after the first few weeks of treatment but may persist as a low-grade fever. Fatigue can be dose limiting, and the drug may be better tolerated with alternate-day dosing or bedtime administration. Tolerance may develop to the flulike effects after several weeks, particularly with daily dosing. If the interval between doses exceeds 3 days, symptoms tend to recur with each dose.

Hematologic

In general, hematologic toxicity with IFN therapy tends to be dose dependent and mild. It is more common in patients with underlying malignancy or those receiving high systemic doses than in patients receiving intralesional therapy for anogenital warts. Dose-dependent leukopenia occurs in 3 to 69% of patients and is thought to be due to inhibition of the release of cells from bone marrow or sequestration of circulating cells (15, 63). Neutropenia may develop within hours of exposure, tends to stabilize within 1 to 3 weeks, and may be dose limiting. After discontinuing the drug, the white blood cell count returns to baseline within a few days (15). Thrombocytopenia occurs in up to 42% of patients. It develops over several weeks, is usually mild and asymptomatic, and resolves within a few days after discontinuation of IFN. Normochromic, normocytic anemia can develop in up to 69% of patients. Recovery may take several weeks to months, suggesting altered erythropoiesis. Immunologically mediated thrombocytopenia and hemolytic anemia have been reported and can be severe. They resolve after discontinuation of the drug. Granulocyte colony-stimulating factor has been given to increase neutrophil counts. Caution should be used here, as these patients are usually neutropenic because of hypersplenism and may be unable to tolerate IFN because of poor hepatic reserve and thrombocytopenia.

Nervous System

IFN-α and CIFN commonly cause mild central nervous system disturbances such as fatigue, headache, irritability, anxiety, and dizziness (43). While these effects are mild and reversible, they may impair the patient's ability to concentrate and affect interpersonal relationships; improvement is noted after a reduction in dose or interruption of therapy. Fatigue occurs in up to 95% of patients and is often accompanied by fever, lack of drive, and weakness. It develops in the first few weeks of therapy and may necessitate a dose reduction, since patients often do not develop tolerance. Resolution of severe fatigue may take several weeks after withdrawal of IFN. Depression occurs in up to 28% of patients and can be severe. It improves within a few days to weeks after dose reduction or discontinuation of IFN and may respond to antidepressants. Other neuropsychiatric effects include irritability, anxiety, emotional lability, delirium, confusion, psychosis, difficulty concentrating, nervousness, and tearfulness; anxiolytics can be useful. Circumoral or peripheral paresthesia occurs in up to 21% of patients and is more common in patients who received vinca alkaloids in the past or concurrently with IFN. Decreased tendon reflexes, motor neuropathy, polyradiculopathy, abnormalities on EEG, and seizures have been reported and are rare. More-severe disturbances can occur such as delirium, severe neuropsychiatric effects, or stupor. High doses of IFN, advanced age, and underlying psychiatric or central nervous system disorders may predispose patients to adverse effects of IFN. Patients with major psychiatric disorders should not be given IFN.

Gastrointestinal

Nausea and vomiting occur in 6 to 50% of patients. Diarrhea can develop in 20 to 45% of patients and may require the use of antidiarrheal agents or dosage reduction. Anorexia and weight loss occur in 19 to 65% and up to 25% of patients, respectively, and may be dose limiting. Dysgeusia, hypogeusia, abdominal pain, dry mouth, gingivitis, and eructation can also occur.

Cardiovascular and Respiratory

Edema, hypotension, hypertension, tachycardia, chest pain, flushing, and diaphoresis have been reported. Cardiac arrhythmias, usually supraventricular, as well as acute myocardial infarction, cardiomyopathy, and congestive heart failure have occurred rarely in patients receiving IFN. Patients with underlying cardiac disease may be at higher risk of developing cardiotoxicity during IFN therapy. Cough, dyspnea, dry mouth, pharyngitis, nasal congestion, and rhinorrhea have been reported in 2 to 34% of patients.

Hepatic

Patients receiving IFN for the treatment of chronic HBV infection should display an acute rise in aminotransferases, particularly ALT, as immune-mediated destruction of infected hepatocytes occurs. Patients who do not demonstrate an acute increase in ALT often do not respond to therapy. Elevations in bilirubin, alkaline phosphatase, and LDH are less common.

Treatment with IFN may lead to a severe exacerbation of liver disease in patients with autoimmune chronic active hepatitis; thus this diagnosis must be ruled out before initiating therapy. This adverse effect is related to the immunologic effects of IFNs, which enhance immune recognition (increased HLA) and stimulate effector cells to exacerbate autoimmune diseases. IFN can cause a reversible, dose-dependent increase in serum transaminase levels in up to 80% of cancer patients. Fatty liver and hepatocellular necrosis have been reported.

Renal and Genitourinary

Proteinuria can develop in 15 to 25% of patients, though protein loss usually does not exceed 1 g/day (13). Serum creatinine and blood urea nitrogen levels increase in up to 10% of patients, and hyperuricemia occurs in 15% of patients. Interstitial nephritis, nephrotic syndrome, hemolytic uremic syndrome, crescentic glomerulonephritis, and syndrome of inappropriate antidiuretic hormone secretion (SIADH) have been reported rarely. Impotence may occur in up to 6% of patients. Use of IFN in renal transplant recipients has been associated with allograft rejection through enhanced immune recognition of the foreign graft. Thus use after renal transplantation is not routinely recommended.

Endocrine/Metabolic

Clinically significant hyperthyroidism or hypothyroidism can occur, and are thought to be due to induction of autoimmune events or cross-reactivity of thyrotropin-stimulating hormone (TSH) with membrane receptors for IFN (38). TSH should be measured prior to treatment and every 3 months. Treatment may be required for thyroid dysfunction. IFN therapy can lead to low concentrations of testosterone, estradiol, and progesterone, as well as variability in prolactin, growth hormone, TSH, and insulin levels. Gynecomastia and loss of libido have been reported in fewer than 5% of patients. Hypertriglyceridemia and hyperlipoproteinemia can be severe but are reversible (31). Treatment with IFN can lead to hyperglycemia and exacerbation of diabetes mellitus. Mild hyperkalemia, hyperphosphatemia, and hypocalcemia have been reported.

Dermatologic and Hypersensitivity

Alopecia may occur with prolonged ($\geq$3 months) use. It is usually reversible but may take several months to resolve after discontinuation of therapy. Hair discoloration and change in hair texture may also occur. Rashes can develop—papular, macular, maculopapular, or urticarial, usually intermittent and

transient—and generally do not require dose reduction. Biopsy-proven vasculitis has been reported. IFN may cause dry skin, dermatitis, sweating, exacerbation of psoriasis, new-onset psoriasis, or vitiligo. Local reactions, such as pain, burning, pruritus, erythema, and vesiculation can occur at the injection site.

The use of recombinant and natural IFN products has been associated with development of neutralizing antibodies to IFN. The prevalence has been reported to be 0 to 39%; it may be highest in patients being treated for Kaposi's sarcoma. The clinical relevance of these antibodies is not completely understood, as it is unclear whether they affect the efficacy or adverse effect profile of IFN and whether their development is related to the preparation, dose, or duration of use. Development of antinuclear antibodies and a lupuslike syndrome has also been reported with IFN therapy.

DRUG INTERACTIONS

See Table 5.

Caution is recommended when administering IFN with other myelosuppressive drugs, since the effects on bone marrow may be additive and can lead to more or more-severe leukopenia, thrombocytopenia, or anemia. IFN decreases activity of the hepatic cytochrome P-450 mixed-function oxidase system, possibly via increased degradation, suppressed synthesis, or inhibition of cytochrome P-450. Therefore caution should be taken when coadministering drugs metabolized by this route, since accumulation may result, and patients should be monitored for signs of toxicity of those drugs. IFN-α has been shown to increase serum levels of theophylline, aminophylline, and phenobarbital, presumably because of decreased clearance. Increased hematologic toxicity and hepatic toxicity have been reported when IFN is combined with zidovudine, as well as decreased clearance of zidovudine. IFN may have additive effects with other drugs that have neurotoxic or cardiotoxic effects. Increased neurotoxicity has been reported with concomitant administration of vidarabine or vinca alkaloids. Granulocytopenia has been reported when IFN was coadministered with ACE inhibitors. Coadministration with interleukin-2 may increase the risk of renal failure.

CLINICAL INDICATIONS

IFN-α is used to treat chronic hepatitis, AIDS-related Kaposi's sarcoma, hairy cell leukemia, Philadelphia chromosome–positive CML. It also is used as an adjuvant in chemotherapy. Use in hepatitis B and C was noted above.

TABLE 5 • Drug Interactions with IFN-α

Drug	Effect	Mechanism
Myelosuppressive drugs	Thrombocytopenia, leukopenia, anemia	Additive effects of myelosuppression
Drugs metabolized by CYP450	Increased effects of other drugs	Inhibition of CYP450 enzyme system by IFN
Drugs with CNS or cardiac toxicity	Increased incidence of CNS or cardiac side effects	Additive effects
Theophylline	100% increase in serum theophylline level	Decreased clearance of theophylline
Phenobarbital	Increased serum phenobarbital level	Possibly decreased clearance of phenobarbital
Zidovudine	May increase zidovudine AUC	Decreased clearance of zidovudine

Hepatitis D Infection

IFN-α is used in the treatment of patients with chronic hepatitis D infection (HDV or delta virus), a defective RNA virus that depends upon HBV for replication. HDV uses the protein coat of HBV and is therefore only found in combination with HBV infection. It can present as coinfection with both viruses, either acute or chronic, or as acute HDV in patients with chronic HBV (44). IFN-α induces normalization of serum aminotranferases and transient loss of viremia in half of patients, but relapse is common. Higher doses and longer therapy has yielded better results (18 MIU/day for 3–4 months followed by decreasing doses over 1 year) (30).

HCV Special Situations

IFN has been used also in patients who have acute hepatitis C or positive HCV RNA after exposure to infection (needle stick in health care worker) (1, 8). If a patient is exposed, test hepatitis C antibody at baseline and HCV RNA at 1 month. If negative at baseline and HCV-RNA positive at 1 month, the individual has acquired hepatitis C and has better than an 80% chance of developing chronic disease. Treatment with IFN-α for 12 weeks may eradicate virus before evidence of hepatitis develops. After acquisition of hepatitis B, more than 95% of adults recover, so IFN is not used for acute infection. In addition, hepatitis B immune globulin and vaccine can prevent chronic infection.

Cryoglobulinemia is a vasculitis associated with HCV infection. Some 60% of patients with HCV have measurable serum cryoglobulins; fewer patients have disease (leukocytoclastic vasculitis in skin, sensory neuropathy, Raynaud's phenomenon, membranoproliferative glomerulonephritis). These patients may require long-term IFN-α therapy (3 MIU thrice weekly for 1 year initially, then tapered to least tolerated dose) (33). Some patients who fail to respond to these doses may respond to a combination of prednisone and IFN-α on alternate days. Unfortunately, renal lesions appear to be least responsive to IFN-α.

The role of IFN-α alone in liver transplantation appears to be now restricted to HCV renal disease posttransplant. Patients with renal transplantation have a increased risk of rejection on IFN-α but this does not appear to occur after liver transplantation. IFN-α is not efficacious alone for eradication of HBV or HCV infection after liver transplantation (7). HBV reinfection of the graft is prevented by hepatitis B immune globulin and nucleoside analogues. HCV reinfection of the graft is universal, but some patients do not have clinically significant disease. Active clinical studies are evaluating IFN-α, ribavirin, and other antivirals such as amantadine, including treating patients prophylactically (9). One study showed great success, with 48% of patients losing HCV RNA after 6 months of therapy (6). Side effects are no more common, with the exception of bone marrow suppressive effects, presumably associated with the multidrug combinations (Table 5). At the present time there are no clear recommendations for treatment of patients after transplantation.

IFN-γ does not have a clinical role as an antiviral agent, although it is used in chronic granulomatous disease, in which it decreases bacterial infection at doses of 50 μg/m² thrice weekly for patients with a body surface area above 0.5 m² (2). For smaller patients, 1.5 μg/kg/dose is recommended, subcutaneously thrice weekly. IFN-γ has also been used for furunculosis in HIV-infected patients (51), with antimony in leishmaniasis (47, 49), for severe EBV infection (19), and as an adjuvant in fungal infections (28).

Table 3 lists the recommended monitoring for patients on IFN-α. In addition to these tests, patients should be evaluated for proteinuria and autoimmune diseases with serum glucose and antinuclear antibody. Eye examinations should be performed prior to initiation of treatment for all diabetics and hypertensive patients.

REFERENCES

1. Arai Y, Noda K, Enomoto N, Arai K, Yamada Y, Suzuki K, Yoshihara H. A prospective study of hepatitis C virus infection after needlestick accidents. Liver 1996;16:331–334.
2. Bemiller LS, Roberts DH, Starko KM, Curnutte JT. Safety and effectiveness of long-term interferon gamma therapy in patients with chronic granulomatous disease. Blood Cells Mol Dis 1995;21:239–247.
3. Bertoletti A, Sette A, Chisari FV, Penna A, Levrero M, De Carli M, Fiaccadori F, Ferrari C. Natural variants of cytotoxic epitopes are T-cell receptor antagonists for antiviral cytotoxic T cells. Nature 1994;369:407–410.
4. Beutner KR, Ferenczy A. Therapeutic approaches to genital warts [Review; 63 refs]. Am J Med 1997;102:28–37.
5. Bino T, Madar Z, Gertler A, Rosenberg H. The kidney is the main site of interferon degradation. J Interferon Res 1982;2:301–302.
6. Bizollon T, Palazzo U, Ducerf C, Chevallier M, Elliott M, Baulieux J, Pouyet M, Trepo C. Pilot study of the combination of interferon alfa and ribavirin as therapy of recurrent hepatitis C after liver transplantation [see comments]. Hepatology 1997;26:500–504.
7. Brumage LK, Wright TL. Treatment for recurrent viral hepatitis after liver transplantation [Review; 19 refs]. J Hepatol 1997;26:440–445.
8. Camma C, Almasio P, Craxi A. Interferon as treatment for acute hepatitis C. A meta-analysis. Dig Dis Sci 1996;41:1248–1255.
9. Cattral MS, Krajden M, Wanless IR, Rezig M, Cameron R, Greig PD, Chung SW, Levy GA. A pilot study of ribavirin therapy for recurrent hepatitis C virus infection after liver transplantation. Transplantation 1996;61:1483–1488.
10. Conant MA, Berger TG, Coates TJ, Longo DJ, Robinson JK, Drake LA. Genital herpes: an integrated approach to management [Review; 27 refs]. J Am Acad Dermatol 1996;35:601–605.
11. Constantoulakis P, Campbell M, Felber BK, Nasioulas G, Afonina E, Pavlakis GN. Inhibition of Rev-mediated HIV-1 expression by an RNA binding protein encoded by the interferon-inducible 9–27 gene. Science 1993;259:1314–1318.
12. Darnell JE, Kerr IM, Stark GR. Jak-STAT pathways and transcriptional activation in response to IFNs and other extracellular signaling proteins. Science 1994;264:1415–1420.
13. Dimitrov Y, Heibel F, Marcellin L, Chantrel F, Moulin B, Hannedouche T. Acute renal failure and nephrotic syndrome with alpha interferon therapy [Review; 23 refs]. Nephrol Dial Transplant 1997;12:200–203.
14. Dinarello CA, Bernheim HA, Duff GW, Le HV, Nagabhushan TL, Hamilton NC, Coceani F. Mechanisms of fever induced by recombinant human interferon. J Clin Invest 1984;74:906–913.

15. Dusheiko G. Side effects of alpha interferon in chronic hepatitis C [Review; 112 refs]. Hepatology 1997;26:112S–121S.

16. Enomoto N, Sakuma I, Asahina Y, Kurosaki M, Murakami T, Yamamoto C, Ogura Y, Izumi N, Marumo F, Sato C. Mutations in the nonstructural protein 5A gene and response to interferon in patients with chronic hepatitis C virus 1b infection. N Engl J Med 1996;334:77–81.

17. Foster GR, Ackrill AM, Goldin RD, Kerr IM, Thomas HC, Stark GR. Expression of the terminal protein region of hepatitis B virus inhibits cellular responses to interferons alpha and gamma and double-stranded RNA. Proc Natl Acad Sci USA 1991;88: 2888–2892.

18. Fried MW, Hoofnagle JH. Therapy of hepatitis C [Review; 85 refs]. Semin Liver Dis 1995;15:82–91.

19. Fujisaki T, Nagafuchi S, Okamura T. Gamma-interferon for severe chronic active Epstein-Barr virus [Letter]. Ann Intern Med 1993;118:474–475.

20. Gooding LR. Viruses that counteract host immune defenses. Cell 1992;71:5–7.

21. Gregorio GV, Jara P, Hierro L, Diaz C, De la Vega A, Vegnente A, Iorio R, Bortolotti F, Crivellaro C, Zancan L, Daniels H, Portmann B, Mieli-Vergani G. Lymphoblastoid interferon alfa with or without steroid pretreatment in children with chronic hepatitis B: a multicenter controlled trial. Hepatology 1996;23:700–707.

22. Herion D, Hoofnagle JH. The interferon sensitivity determining region: all hepatitis C virus isolates are not the same. Hepatology 1997;25:769–771.

23. Hirsch MS, Tolkoff-Rubin NE, Kelly AP, Rubin RH. Pharmacokinetics of human and recombinant leukocyte interferon in patients with chronic renal failure who are undergoing hemodialysis. J Infect Dis 1983;148:335.

24. Hoofnagle JH. Therapy of acute and chronic viral hepatitis [Review; 151 refs]. Adv Intern Med 1994;39:241–275.

25. Imani F, Jacobs B. Inhibitory activity for the interferon-induced protein kinase is associated with the reovirus serotype 1 a3 protein. Proc Natl Acad Sci USA 1988;85:7887–7891.

26. Kekule AS, Lauer U, Weiss L, Luber B, Hofschneider PH. Hepatitis B virus transactivator HBx uses a tumour promoter signalling pathway. Nature 1993;361:742–745.

27. Kitajewski J, Schneider RJ, Safer B, Munemitsu SM, Samuel CE, Thimmappaya B, Shenk T. Adenovirus VAI RNA antagonizes the antiviral action of interferon by preventing activation of the interferon-induced elF-2a kinase. Cell 1986;45:195–200.

28. Kullberg BJ. Trends in immunotherapy of fungal infections [Review; 31 refs]. Eur J Clin Microbiol Infect Dis 1997;16:51–55.

29. Lam NP, Pitrak D, Speralakis R, Lau AH, Wiley TE, Layden TJ. Effect of obesity on pharmacokinetics and biologic effect of interferon-alpha in hepatitis C. Dig Dis Sci 1997;42:178–185.

30. Madejon A, Cotonat T, Bartolome J, Castillo I, Carreno V. Treatment of chronic hepatitis D virus infection with low and high doses of interferon-alpha 2a: utility of polymerase chain reaction in monitoring antiviral response. Hepatology 1994;19: 1331–1336.

31. Malaguarnera M, Giugno I, Trovato BA, Panebianco MP, Siciliano R, Ruello P. Lipoprotein(a) concentration in patients with chronic active hepatitis C before and after interferon treatment. Clin Ther 1995;17:721–728.

32. Milella M, Antonelli G, Santantonio T, Currenti M, Monno L, Mariano N, Angarano G, Dianzani F, Pastore G. Neutralizing antibodies to recombinant alpha-interferon and response to therapy in chronic hepatitis C virus infection. Liver 1993;13: 146–150.

33. Misiani R, Bellavita P, Fenili D, Vicari O, Marchesi D, Sironi PL, Zilio P, Vernocchi A, Massazza M, Vendramin G. Interferon alfa-2a therapy in cryoglobulinemia associated with hepatitis C virus [see comments]. N Engl J Med 1994;330:751–756.

34. Muller M, Briscoe J, Laxton C, Guschin D, Ziemiecki A, Silvennoinen O, Harpur AG, Barbieri G, Witthuhn BA, Schindler C, Pellegrini S, Wilks AF, Ihle JN, Stark GR, Kerr IM. The protein tyrosine kinase JAK1 complements defects in interferon-alpha/beta and -gamma transduction. Nature 1993;366:129–135.

35. Narkewicz MR, Smith D, Silverman A, Vierling J, Sokol RJ. Clearance of chronic hepatitis B virus infection in young children after alpha interferon treatment. J Pediatr 1995;127: 815–818.

36. Peters M. Mechanisms of action of interferons. Semin Liver Dis 1989;9:235–239.

37. Peters M. Actions of cytokines on the immune response and viral interactions: an overview. Hepatology 1996;23:909–916.

38. Pittau E, Bogliolo A, Tinti A, Mela Q, Ibba G, Salis G, Perpignano G. Development of arthritis and hypothyroidism during alpha-interferon therapy for chronic hepatitis C [Review; 25 refs]. Clin Exp Rheumatol 1997;15:415–419.

39. Pons JC, Lebon P, Frydman R, Delfraissy JF. Pharmacokinetics of interferon-alpha in pregnant women and fetoplacental passage. Fetal Diagn Ther 1995;10:7–10.

40. Porres J, Carreno V, Ruiz M, Marron J, Bartolome J. Interferon antibodies in patients with chronic HBV infection treated with recombinant interferon. J Hepatol 1989;8:351–357.

41. Poynard T, Leroy V, Cohard M, Thevenot T, Mathurin P, Opolon P, Zarski JP. Meta-analysis of interferon randomized trials in the treatment of viral hepatitis C: effects of dose and duration. Hepatology 1996;24:778–789.

42. Rashidbaigi A, Pestka S. Interferons: protein structure. In: Baron S, ed. The interferon system. Austin: University of Texas Press. 1988:149–168.

43. Renault PF, Hoofnagle JH. Side effects of alpha interferon. Semin Liver Dis 1989;9:273–274.

44. Samuel D, Zignego AL, Reynes M, Feray C, Arulnaden JL, David MF, Gigou M, Bismuth A, Mathieu D, Gentilini P. Long-term clinical and virological outcome after liver transplantation for cirrhosis caused by chronic delta hepatitis. Hepatology 1995; 21:333–339.

45. Sen GC, Lengyel P. The interferon system. A bird's eye view of its biochemistry. J Biol Chem 1992;267:5017–5020.

46. Shuai K, Schindler C, Prezioso VR, Darnell JJE. Activation of transcription by IFN-t: tyrosine phosphorylation of a 91-kD DNA binding protein. Science 1992;258:1808–1812.

47. Squires KE, Rosenkaimer F, Sherwood JA, Forni AL, Were JB, Murray HW. Immunochemotherapy for visceral leishmaniasis: a controlled pilot trial of antimony versus antimony plus interferon-gamma. Am J Trop Med Hyg 1993;48:666–669.

48. Staeheli P. Interferon-induced proteins and the antiviral state. Adv Virus Res 1990;38:147–148.

49. Sundar S, Rosenkaimer F, Lesser ML, Murray HW. Immunochemotherapy for a systemic intracellular infection: accelerated response using interferon-gamma in visceral leishmaniasis. J Infect Dis 1995;171:992–996.

50. Taylor JL, Grossberg SE. Recent progress in interferon research: molecular mechanisms of regulation, action, virus circumvention. Virus Res 1990;15:1–58.

51. Thoma-Greber E, Froschl M, Stolz W, Landthaler M, Plewig G. [Interferon-gamma. Therapy of recurrent furunculosis in HIV infections]. [German]. Hautarzt 1993;44:587–589.

52. Tong MJ, Reddy KR, Lee WM, Pockros PJ, Hoefs JC, Keeffe EB, Hollinger FB, Hathcote EJ, White H, Foust RT, Jensen DM, Krawitt EL, Fromm H, Black M, Blatt LM, Klein M, Lubina J. Treatment of chronic hepatitis C with consensus interferon: a multicenter, randomized, controlled trial. Consensus Interferon Study Group. Hepatology 1997;26:747–754.

53. Tsai SL, Liaw YF, Chen MH, Huang CY, Kuo GC. Detection of type 2-like T-helper cells in hepatitis C virus infection: implications for hepatitis C virus chronicity. Hepatology 1997;25:449–458.

54. Twu JS, Lee CH, Lin PM, Schloemer RH. Hepatitis B virus suppresses expression of human beta-interferon. Proc Natl Acad Sci USA 1988;85:252–256.

55. Upton C, Mossman K, McFadden G. Encoding of a homolog of the IFN-t receptor by myxoma virus. Science 1992;258:1369–1372.

56. Uze G, Lutfalla G, Mogensen KE. Alpha and beta interferons and their receptor and their friends and relations [Review; 191 refs]. J Interferon Cytokine Res 1995;15:3–26.

57. Velazquez L, Fellous M, Stark GR, Pellegrini S. A protein tyrosine kinase in the interferon a/b signaling pathway. Cell 1992;70:313–322.

58. Viscomi GC. Structure-activity of type I interferons [Review; 126 refs]. Biotherapy 1997;10:59–86.

59. Wills RJ, Dennis S, Spiegel HE, Gibson DM, Nadler PI. Interferon kinetics and adverse reactions after intravenous, intramuscular,and subcutaneous injection. Clin Pharm Ther 1984;35:722–727.

60. Wills RJ. Clinical pharmacokinetics of interferons. Clin Pharmacokinet 1990;19:390–399.

61. Zav'yalov VP, Denesyuk AI, Zav'yalova GA. Theoretical analysis of conformation and active sites of interferons. Immunol Lett 1989;22:173–182.

62. Zoon KC, Bekisz J, Miller D. Human interferon alpha family: protein structure and function. In: Baron S, Coppenhaver DH, Dianzani F, Fleischman WR, Hughes TK, Klimpel GR, et al., eds. Interferon: principles and medical applications. Galveston: University of Texas Medical Branch at Galveston, 1992:95–116.

63. Zoumbos NC, Djeu JY, Young NS. Interferon is the suppressor of hematopoiesis generated by stimulated lymphocytes in vitro. J Immunol 1984;133:769–774.

Nucleoside Analogues: Acyclovir, Penciclovir, Valaciclovir, and Famciclovir

Martin J. Wood

CLASS
Chemical Structure

Acyclovir (9-[(2-hydroxyethoxy)-methyl]-guanine) and penciclovir (9-(4-hydroxy-3-hydroxymethbut-1-yl)-guanine) are acyclic analogues of the natural nucleoside 2′-deoxyguanosine. Valaciclovir is the L-valyl ester of acyclovir and after oral absorption is rapidly and extensively converted to acyclovir and L-valine, an essential amino acid (22). Famciclovir is the diacetyl, 6-deoxy ester of penciclovir and, similarly, is an oral prodrug of the parent compound.

Structure-Activity Relationships

Acyclovir and penciclovir triphosphate competitively inhibit the natural nucleoside, deoxyguanosine triphosphate, from binding to viral DNA polymerase. Since acyclovir lacks a 3′-hydroxyl moiety, once it is incorporated into a DNA primer-template, it cannot be removed by the 3′,5′-exonuclease activity of the polymerase and prevents further elongation of the DNA chain.

ANTIVIRAL ACTIVITY
Spectrum

These drugs inhibit replication of the herpes group of DNA viruses (Table 1). Acyclovir does not have in vitro antiviral activity against viruses other than herpesviruses, but penciclovir has some activity against hepatitis B virus (66). In general, herpes simplex type 1 (HSV-1) is the most susceptible herpesvirus to either drug, with progressively less activity against herpes simplex type 2 (HSV-2), varicella zoster virus (VZV), Epstein-Barr virus (EBV), and human cytomegalovirus (CMV) (11, 58). The relative activities of the two drugs are affected by the cell line used to determine sensitivity.

Mixed populations of acyclovir/penciclovir-susceptible and -resistant strains (usually considered to be an $ID_{50} > 3$ mg/L) of HSV have been obtained from patients never exposed to these drugs, suggesting that natural mutation is quite frequent. Between 3 and 4% of HSV isolates from patients with genital herpes before the start of long-term acyclovir suppressive therapy were resistant to acyclovir (ID_{50} (3 mg/L) (48). Another study of more than 1400 HSV isolates from 500 nonrandomly selected patients examined over a 10-year period, found only 3% of isolates with significantly diminished sensitivity (5). Although there have been several reports of acyclovir-resistant VZV in patients with AIDS, there are no data regarding the epidemiology of such resistance (10, 37, 52, 70).

Pharmacodynamic Effects

No relationship has been established between the effective in vitro and in vivo concentrations of these nucleosides, although

TABLE 1 • **Summary of the in Vitro Antiviral Activity (ID_{50})^a of Acyclovir and Penciclovir**

Virus	ID_{50} (mg/L) Acyclovir	Penciclovir
HSV-1	0.02–0.9	0.2–0.6
HSV-2	0.03–2.2	0.3–2.4
VZV	0.8–4	0.9–4
EBV	ca. 1.5	—
CMV	2–>50	52

Data from references 11, 12, and 27.

^{a} ID_{50} is the concentration of drug required for 50% inhibition of viral growth in cell culture.

there is a significant correlation between the ID_{50} of acyclovir for the virus and the clinical response. The ID_{90} or ID_{99} may be better predictors of clinical response when acyclovir is used for prophylaxis (5), since these values reflect the natural presence of the less sensitive viral strains that are associated with breakthrough recurrences (69).

MECHANISM OF ACTION

Selective inhibition of viral replication by acyclovir and penciclovir results from their specific phosphorylation by herpesvirus-coded thymidine kinase (TK) (or, in the case of CMV, by the phosphotransferase encoded by the viral *UL97* gene). These enzymes specifically catalyze the initial phosphorylation of the nucleosides to their monophosphates, which are subsequently converted to di- and triphosphates by cellular enzymes. Acyclovir triphosphate (ACV-TP) and penciclovir triphosphate (PCV-TP) are the active metabolites that act as substrates for, and inhibitors of, viral DNA polymerases. Penciclovir has greater affinity than acyclovir for TK, and so there are much higher concentrations of PCV-TP than ACV-TP within infected cells (75). However, ACV-TP is more than 100 times more potent than PCV-TP as an inhibitor of HSV and VZV DNA polymerase (22, 75), and the two compounds have very similar in vitro activity (Table 1).

Resistance to acyclovir and penciclovir develop through mutations in the TK or DNA polymerase genes of HSV or VZV. Any deletion or alteration in these genes has the potential for conferring resistance. Mutants may be deficient in TK or possess a TK with substrate specificity that enables it to phosphorylate thymidine but not acyclovir and/or penciclovir. TK-deficient mutants occur in normal virus populations, and exposing HSV-infected cultures to suboptimal concentrations of acyclovir selects for these resistant variants (29). The incidence of mutants with other forms of resistance is less well defined, and their selection in vitro requires much more stringent conditions (41).

In most tissues TK-deficient viruses grow normally, but their neurovirulence and ability to establish latent infections in sensory ganglia is often impaired (28). Viruses expressing TK of altered substrate specificity or DNA polymerase variants generally retain the pathogenicity and neurovirulence of wild-type virus (58).

In clinical practice, most HSV and VZV isolates with reduced sensitivity to acyclovir and penciclovir have been isolated from patients with AIDS during prolonged acyclovir therapy. In most cases, the virus isolated was relatively TK-deficient, although strains with alterations in TK (25) or viral DNA polymerase (19, 59) have also been reported. Administration of acyclovir, even as long-term prophylactic (suppressive) therapy, to immunocompetent patients has been associated only infrequently with the emergence of resistant strains (30). However, a correlation appears to exist between the susceptibility of presuppression isolates and the occurrence of breakthrough attacks of genital herpes while receiving acyclovir (69). In severely immunocompromised patients, such as bone marrow transplant recipients or AIDS patients, there have been many instances in which HSV isolates with reduced sensitivity failed to respond to acyclovir therapy (5, 15, 16, 18, 26, 61, 74, 76).

PHARMACOKINETICS

The pharmacokinetics of intravenous acyclovir are independent of dose and best fit a two-compartment open model (45). The mean steady-state peak plasma concentrations of acyclovir after 1 h intravenous administration of 2.5, 5.0, and 10.0 mg/kg every 8 h are 6.7, 9.8, and 22.9 mg/L.

Absorption

Acyclovir is slowly and poorly absorbed from the gastrointestinal tract, and the time to reach peak concentrations is 1.5 to 2 h (23). With multidose administration, steady-state plasma concentrations are achieved by the second day. Bioavailability decreases with increasing doses, so steady-state peak plasma concentrations of oral acyclovir are not dose proportional. After 200, 400, and 800 mg 4-hourly dosage regimens in healthy volunteers, the steady state peak and trough concentrations of acyclovir are 0.83 and 0.46 mg/L, 1.21 and 0.63 mg/L, and 1.61 and 0.83 mg/L, respectively. Absorption is unaffected by food. Systemic absorption of acyclovir after topical use is minimal. Oral penciclovir is even less well absorbed than acyclovir, with an oral bioavailability of 5%, and it is not available in an oral formulation.

After oral administration, valaciclovir is well absorbed via intestinal brush border membranes and undergoes rapid and extensive first-pass intestinal/hepatic metabolism by the enzyme valaciclovir hydrolase to acyclovir and L-valine (14, 79). The absolute bioavailability of acyclovir after oral valaciclovir is 54.2% and is not reduced by food (14). After single 100- to 1000-mg doses of valaciclovir, peak plasma concentrations of acyclovir were almost dose proportional, and after valaciclovir 250 mg qid the daily area under the plasma concentration-time curve (AUC) of acyclovir was similar to that after oral acyclovir 800 mg 4-hourly (79). After 1000 mg valaciclovir qds, the daily AUC of acyclovir (systemic acyclovir exposure over 24 h) is similar to that after intravenous acyclovir 5 mg/kg 8-hourly but with lower peak plasma concentrations (C_{max}, 5 mg/L) (79). Very small concentrations of valaciclovir are detected in the systemic circulation.

Famciclovir is absorbed in the duodenum and is converted to penciclovir by first-pass hepatic (presystemic) metabolism.

Dideacetylation of famciclovir occurs in the blood and, possibly, in the intestinal wall, and then, 6-oxidation of the intermediary metabolite to penciclovir is catalyzed by the enzyme aldehyde oxidase in the liver (17, 33). Following oral administration of famciclovir in single doses of 125 to 750 mg, the peak plasma concentration and AUC of penciclovir increased linearly from 0.84 mg/L and 2.2 mg/h/L, respectively, after the 125-mg dose to 5.1 mg/L and 14.1 mg/h/L after the 750-mg dose (56). The absolute bioavailability of penciclovir after oral famciclovir is 77% (33).

Distribution

Acyclovir is widely distributed into tissues and body fluids including brain, kidney, lung, liver, muscle, spleen, uterus, vaginal mucosa, vaginal secretions, cerebrospinal fluid, and herpetic vesicular fluid. Concentrations in kidney and lung were 10 to 13 times plasma concentrations after multidose therapy, and 25 to 70% of the plasma level was found in brain, spinal cord, and cerebrospinal fluid (Table 2). Transplacental passage of acyclovir occurs at all stages of pregnancy (34, 35).

There are no data regarding the distribution of penciclovir into specific tissues or body fluids, but the high volume of distribution of penciclovir (112 L, or 1.5 L/kg) (32) suggests that it is widely distributed into tissues. Penciclovir is phosphorylated within herpesvirus-infected cells, and PCV-TP has a much longer half-life than ACV-TP (75). It has not been convincingly demonstrated, however, that this enhanced intracellular stability and possible prolonged inhibition of viral replication leads to any clinical advantages.

Elimination

The only significant metabolite of acyclovir is the oxidized 9-(carboxymethoxy)methyl guanine. Another minor metabolite, 8-hydroxy-9-(2-hydroxyethoxymethyl) guanine, can be detected in urine at a concentration below 0.15%. Neither metabolite is pharmacologically active. Less than 2% of administered acyclovir can be recovered from feces, and negligible amounts are eliminated in expired CO_2. After intravenous administration of radiolabeled penciclovir to healthy volunteers, nearly 94% of

TABLE 2 • Distribution of Acyclovir into Body Tissues, Biologic Fluids, etc. (expressed as a percentage of plasma concentrations)

Tissue/Biologic Fluid	Acyclovir
Kidney	1000
Brain/spinal cord	25–70
Cerebrospinal fluid	50
Lung	131
Liver	100–150
Heart	100–150
Aqueous humor	30–50
Breast milk	300–350
Saliva	13
Herpetic vesicles	100

Data from O'Brien JJ, Campoli-Richards DM. Acyclovir—an updated review of its antiviral activity, pharmacokinetic properties and therapeutic efficacy. Drugs 1989;37:233–309. Data for penciclovir are not available.

the radioactivity was eliminated in the urine and 2.9% in the feces (31). After radiolabeled oral famciclovir was administered to volunteers, 73 and 27% of the radioactivity was recovered from the urine and feces, respectively.

Renal excretion is the major route of elimination of acyclovir and penciclovir. Approximately 80% of an administered intravenous dose and 10 to 20% of an orally administered dose of acyclovir (51, 58) and 50 to 60% of penciclovir (given as an oral dose of famciclovir) (33) is recovered unchanged (and about 5% as its 6-deoxy precursor) from the urine. Renal clearance of acyclovir is approximately threefold greater and that of penciclovir four- to fivefold greater than the creatinine clearance, indicating tubular secretion as well as glomerular filtration for both drugs. Probenecid and cimetidine increase the half-life of acyclovir by reducing its renal clearance (42); a similar effect with penciclovir is likely.

Pharmacokinetic Parameters

Pharmacokinetic parameters are summarized in Table 3.
The pharmacokinetics of acyclovir in children over 1 year old are similar to those of adults. In infants less than 3 months of age, the plasma half-life is slightly prolonged to about 3.8 h (36), and clearance is about one-third of that in older individuals. There are, currently, no data available on the pharmacokinetics of famciclovir/penciclovir in children.

Disease States

Acyclovir elimination is reduced in patients with renal insufficiency, and in anuric patients, total body clearance is reduced to 1.8 L/h/1.73 m^2, and the mean terminal plasma half-life is increased to 19.5 h (43). As renal function decreases, a greater percentage of the drug is metabolized to carboxymethoxymethyl guanine. Acyclovir is removed by hemodialysis; the half-life during dialysis is approximately 5 h, resulting in a 60% decrease in plasma concentrations following a 6-h dialysis. Therefore, a supplemental dose of acyclovir should be administered after each dialysis (39, 43). No supplemental dose needs to be given after peritoneal dialysis (8, 65). In patients on hemodialysis, the daily dose of valaciclovir should be administered after the hemodialysis has been performed.

Similarly, with increasing degrees of renal failure, the mean penciclovir clearance decreased and the mean elimination half-life increased very markedly (9). In individuals with severe renal impairment (creatinine clearance = 3–18 L/h/1.73 m^2), the total body clearance was 3.2 L/h/1.73 m^2, and the elimination half-life, 9.9 h. Penciclovir is readily removed from plasma during hemodialysis (33); there is a mean 76% lowering of penciclovir plasma concentrations with a mean plasma clearance of 8.5 L/h. An appropriate dosage interval for famciclovir in patients undergoing hemodialysis would be 48 h, with a further full dose immediately after each dialysis. There are no data regarding removal of penciclovir by peritoneal dialysis.

DOSAGE REGIMENS
Normal

In normal subjects with mucocutaneous HSV or VZV, the dosage of intravenous acyclovir is 5 mg/kg every 8 h. For VZV infections in immunocompromised patients, in herpes simplex encephalitis, and for neonatal HSV and VZV infections, 10 mg/kg should be administered every 8 h.

Oral acyclovir is given in a dosage of 200 to 400 mg five times daily for HSV infections; 800 mg (20 mg/kg for children under 40 kg body weight) qds for varicella, and 800 mg five times daily for herpes zoster. In children over the age of 2 years, the oral dose should generally be the same as for adults, but half the adult dose is given to children under 2 years.

Oral valaciclovir is given in a dosage of 500 mg daily or twice daily for genital herpes and 500 mg daily for suppression, or 500 mg twice daily for therapy, for herpes zoster. Adequate hydration should be maintained in the elderly. No dosage schedules have been recommended specifically for children, but guidelines similar to those for acyclovir are likely to be suitable.

Famciclovir is recommended in a dosage of 125 to 250 mg 8-hourly for genital HSV infections and at dosages varying from 750 mg daily to 250 to 500 mg 8-hourly for herpes zoster.

Renal Failure

The dosage of acyclovir should be reduced in patients with renal disease. Dosage of oral acyclovir for HSV and VZV should be reduced to 200 mg every 12 h or 800 mg every 12 h, respectively, in patients with severe renal impairment (creatinine clearance below 10 mL/min/1.73 m^2). If the creatinine clearance is above this value, normal doses may be given for HSV indications; for VZV infections in patients with a creatinine clearance of 10 to 25 mL/min/1.73 m^2, 800 mg every 8 h should be used. Intravenous dosage of acyclovir should be calculated on the scale shown in Table 4. Ointment and cream may be given in normal doses.

For valaciclovir, dosage reduction is advised in patients with moderate-to-severe renal impairment (although the recommendations differ between the United States and Europe). For patients with a creatinine clearance of 30 to 49 mL/min (United States) or 15 to 30 mL/min (Europe), the 1000-mg dose (for herpes zoster) should be given 12-hourly; at creatinine clearances of 10 to 29 mL/min (United States) or below 15 mL/min (Europe), the interval should be 24 h, and in the United States, those with a creatinine clearance below 10 mL/min are advised to be dosed with 500 mg daily. For genital herpes in a patient with a creatinine clearance below 15 mL/min, the recommended dosage of valaciclovir is 500 mg daily, worldwide.

The pharmacokinetics of penciclovir in renal impairment suggest that the administration interval for famciclovir in patients with a calculated creatinine clearance above 60 mL/min/1.73 m^2 (3.6 L/h/1.73 m^2) should be 8 h, but for those with a creatinine clearance of 30 to 59 mL/min/1.73 m^2 (1.8–3.5 L/h/1.73 m^2), the interval should be 12 h, and for those with a creatinine clearance of 5 to 30 mL/min/1.73 m^2 (0.3–1.7 L/h/1.73 m^2); the interval should be 24 h (9).

Hepatic Failure

No dosage adjustments of acyclovir are needed for patients with hepatic failure. The rate of valaciclovir metabolism to acyclovir is reduced in patients with hepatic impairment, but the extent of metabolism is unaffected, and dosage adjustment of valaciclovir is not required in those with mild-or-moderate cirrhosis (53). Similarly, there is a decrease in the rate of metabolism of famciclovir in hepatic insufficiency, but no dosage adjustment is required for those with well-compensated hepatic impairment (55). Even in patients with advanced cirrhosis, dosage adjustment of either drug is probably unnecessary, but there is a need for more clinical experience.

TABLE 3 • Pharmacokinetic Parameters

Parameter	Acyclovir/Valaciclovir	Penciclovir/Famciclovir
Total clearance	19 L/h/1.73 m^2	32 L/h/1.73 m^2
Renal clearance	15–17 L/h/1.73 m^2	25–32 L/h/1.73 m^2
Nonrenal clearance	2–4 L/h/1.73 m^2	1–6 L/h/1.73 m^2
Vd steady state	46.6 ± 13.5 L/1.73 m^2; (range, 22.5–101 L/m^2)	111.9 L (range, 102–125 L)
Half-life (mean; range)	2.93 h; 1.5–6.3 h.	2.16–2.31 h
Plasma protein binding	15.4% (range, 9–24%)	20%
Urinary excretion	80% unchanged	50–60% unchanged
Bioavailability	Acyclovir: 13–21% Valaciclovir: 54%	Penciclovir: 5% Famciclovir: 77%

Data from references 33 and 54.

TABLE 4 • Dosages of Intravenous Acyclovir for Use with Renal Impairment

	Creatinine Clearance (mL/min/1.73 m^2)		
	25–50	10–25	0–10
Dose for herpes simplex (mg/kg)	5 (12-hourly)	5 (24-hourly)	2.5 (24-hourly)
Dose for varicella-zoster (mg/kg)	10 (12-hourly)	10 (24-hourly)	5 (24-hourly)

ADVERSE EFFECTS

No potentially life-threatening adverse effects of acyclovir or penciclovir have been reported, but 1% or so of patients receiving intravenous acyclovir develop lethargy, obtundation, tremors, confusion, hallucinations, agitation, seizures, or coma, symptoms suggesting an encephalopathy (77). Intravenous acyclovir should hence be used with caution in those who have underlying neurologic abnormalities and those with serious hypoxia or renal, hepatic, or electrolyte abnormalities. Microangiopathic hemolytic anemia and thrombocytopenia were reported in some severely immunocompromised patients receiving 8 g daily of valaciclovir for prolonged periods in clinical trials, but the association between these abnormalities and the drug is unclear.

Increased blood urea and/or creatinine levels are infrequent but well described in patients on intravenous acyclovir therapy (13). They are largely avoidable if the patient is kept well hydrated. Very rarely, acute renal failure has been described. The renal dysfunction is probably due to deposition of drug crystals in renal tubules. Dosage of acyclovir, valaciclovir, or famciclovir should be modified in patients with significant renal disease.

Severe local inflammatory reactions sometimes leading to breakdown of skin have occurred when intravenous acyclovir was inadvertently infused into extravascular tissues (38).

The most frequently reported adverse events during clinical trials of oral acyclovir and valaciclovir were malaise, nausea, vomiting, and headache (73), but similar rates were reported by placebo recipients, and spontaneously reported adverse events are insufficiently common in clinical practice to establish causation. In a trial of very high dosage valaciclovir (2000 mg qds) in patients with advanced HIV disease, many patients were unable to tolerate the gastrointestinal adverse effects of the drug (60). In addition to rises in BUN and serum creatinine concentrations, increases in liver-related enzymes and decreases in hematologic indices have been reported after acyclovir administration but are not thought to be directly related to the drug (44).

Both the cream and ophthalmic ointment may cause transient stinging after application. Erythema or mild drying of the skin has occurred after the use of cream, and the ophthalmic preparation has been associated with punctate keratopathy and blepharitis.

Acute Overdosage

Up to 100 mg/kg of acyclovir in a single intravenous dose has been administered with no adverse effects. No patients are known to have deliberately taken an overdose.

MONITORING REQUIREMENTS
Therapeutic Drug Monitoring

It is not useful to measure plasma concentrations of acyclovir or penciclovir.

Other Laboratory Monitoring

It is important to monitor renal function during treatment with acyclovir, particularly in those receiving higher doses of the drug.

DRUG INTERACTIONS

Combination of acyclovir or penciclovir with other antiviral agents that act independently of viral TK might theoretically reduce the emergence of resistant viral strains. There is no consistent and agreed method of determining synergy, but by various techniques, synergic activity has been shown for combinations of acyclovir and vidarabine against HSV-2 (21, 58) and CMV (71) and for acyclovir and interferon-α against HSV, CMV, and VZV (1) in tissue culture.

CLINICAL INDICATIONS
Disease

Acyclovir has benefited a wide range of manifestations of primary and recurrent HSV and VZV infections in immunocompetent hosts. Ocular (20), mucocutaneous (72), genital (57), and central nervous system (68, 80) HSV infections, chickenpox (4), and herpes zoster (4) may all be treated, and acyclovir has been successful in the prophylaxis of frequently recurrent genital herpes (48). In the immunocompromised, it has been used for treatment and prophylaxis of HSV and VZV infections (2, 50, 78), treatment of EBV infections such as oral hairy leukoplakia (62), and for suppression of CMV infections (3, 49).

Oral valaciclovir enables some of these infections (particularly those caused by VZV) to be treated more conveniently (with less frequent oral doses and somewhat better results (6)) and may enable oral therapy to be used in place of intravenous therapy—in some immunocompromised patients with HSV infections, for example. Famciclovir also has more-convenient dosage schedules than acyclovir and is of similar efficacy. There are, as yet, few manifestations of herpesvirus infections in which famciclovir has been specifically studied and fewer direct comparisons of famciclovir and valaciclovir. It is likely that the clinical results in most indications below will be similar for acyclovir (or its prodrug valaciclovir) and penciclovir/famciclovir. Occasional viral isolates remain sensitive to one compound while resistant to the other, but generally, cross-resistance is found. The potential indications for these drugs are listed below, and the appropriate dosage regimens are in Table 5.

1. Treatment of HSV infections
   Primary and recurrent genital herpes (40)
   Mucocutaneous HSV
     Primary HSV gingivostomatitis (24)
     Herpes labialis (72)
     Herpetic whitlow (46)
   Herpetic ocular disease (64)
     Superficial keratitis
     Stromal keratitis
     Keratouveitis
     Acute retinal necrosis (7)
   Herpes encephalitis (68, 80)
   Disseminated HSV in immunocompromised (58)
   Neonatal HSV infection (81)
2. Treatment of VZV infections
   Varicella (81)
   Herpes zoster (82)

TABLE 5 • Regimens of Acyclovir, Penciclovir, and Their Prodrugs of Established Efficacy in Herpesvirus Infections

Indication	Acyclovir (ACV) or valaciclovir (VCV)	Penciclovir (PCV) or famciclovir (FCV)
Herpes keratitis	ACV ophthalmic ointment 4-hourly until at least 3 days after healing	
Mucocutaneous HSV	1. ACV cream 4-hourly for 5–10 days[a] 2. Oral ACV, 200 mg 4-hourly for 5–10 days 3. VCV 500–1000 mg b.i.d. for 5–10 days	1. PCV cream 2-hourly for 4 days 2. Oral FCV, 125 mg b.i.d. to 250 mg tds for 5 days
HSV in immunocompromised	1. i.v. ACV, 5 mg/kg 8-hourly for 5 days; in children 250 mg/kg tds 2. Oral ACV 400 mg 4 hourly for 5–10 days	
Suppression of frequently recurrent genital herpes	1. ACV 400 mg b.i.d.; alternative regimens have included dosages ranging from 200 mg tds to 200 mg 4-hourly 2. VCV 500 mg daily	
Herpes encephalitis or neonatal HSV	i.v. ACV 10 mg/kg tid for 10–14 days	
Prophylaxis in immunocompromised patients	Oral ACV 200–400 mg qds	
Varicella	1. Oral ACV, over 40 kg: 800 mg qds for 5 days; children under 40 kg: 20 mg/kg qds for 5 days 2. i.v. ACV, 5–10 mg/kg tds for 5–7 days; in children, 500 mg/kg tds	
Herpes zoster	1. ACV: 800 mg five times daily for 7 days 2. VCV: 1 g tds for 7 days	FCV 250–500 mg tds for 7 days

[a] Not approved for orolabial HSV in the United States.

Disseminated VZV in immunocompromised (67)
VZV Ocular disease (51)
    Zoster ophthalmicus
    Acute retinal necrosis
3. Prophylaxis
    Frequently recurrent genital herpes (40)
    Erythema multiforme associated with HSV recurrences (63)
    Prevention of HSV and VZV in immunocompromised (51)
    Prevention of CMV in immunocompromised (3, 49)
4. Others
    Oral hairy leukoplakia (62)
5. Hepatitis B (47)

REFERENCES

1. Baba M, Ito M, Shigeta S, De Clercq E. Synergistic antiviral effects of antiherpes compounds and human leukocyte interferon on varicella-zoster virus in vitro. Antimicrob Agents Chemother 1984;25:515–517.
2. Balfour HH Jr. Intravenous acyclovir therapy for varicella in immunocompromised children. J Pediatr 1984;104:134–136.
3. Balfour HH Jr, Chace BA, Stapleton JT, Simmons RL, Fryd DS. A randomized placebo-controlled trial of oral acyclovir for the prevention of cytomegalovirus disease in recipients of renal allograft. N Engl J Med 1989;320:1381–1387.
4. Balfour HH Jr, Kelly JM, Suarez CS, Heussner RC, Englund JA, Crane DD, McGuirt PV, Clemmer AF, Aeppli DM. Acyclovir treatment of varicella in otherwise healthy children. J Pediatr 1990;116:633–639.
5. Barry DW, Nusinoff-Lehrman S, Ellis MN, Biron KK, Furman PA. Viral resistance, clinical experience. Scand J Infect Dis 1985;(Suppl 47):155–164.
6. Beutner KR, Friedman DJ, Forszpaniak C, Andersen PL, Wood MJ. Valaciclovir compared with acyclovir for improved therapy for herpes zoster in immunocompetent adults. Antimicrob Agents Chemother 1995;39:1546–1553.
7. Blumenkranz MS, Culbertson WW, Clarkson JG, Dix R. Treatment of the acute retinal necrosis syndrome with intravenous acyclovir. Ophthalmology 1986;93:296–300.
8. Boelaert J, Schurgers M, Daneels R, Van Landuyt HW, Weatherley BC. Multiple dose pharmacokinetics of intravenous acyclovir in patients on continuous ambulatory peritoneal dialysis. J Antimicrob Chemother 1987;20:69–76.
9. Boike SC, Pue MA, Freed MI, Audet PR, Fairless A, Ilson BE, Zariffa N, Jorkasky DK. Pharmacokinetics of famciclovir in subjects with varying degrees of renal impairment. Clin Pharmacol Ther 1994;55:418–426.
10. Boivin G, Edelman CK, Pedneault L, Talarico CL, Biron KK, Balfour HH Jr. Phenotypic and genotypic characterization of acyclovir-resistant varicella-zoster viruses isolated from persons with AIDS. J Infect Dis 1994;170:68–75.
11. Boyd MR, Bacon TH, Sutton D, Cole M. Antiherpes activity of 9-(4-hydroxy-3-hydroxymethbut-1-yl)guanine (BRL 39123) in cell culture. Antimicrob Agents Chemother 1987;31:1238–1242.
12. Boyd MR, Safrin S, Kern ER. Penciclovir: a review of its spectrum of activity, selective and cross-resistance pattern. Antivir Chem Chemother 1993;4(Suppl 1):3–11.
13. Brigden D, Rosling AE, Woods NC. Renal function after acyclovir intravenous injection. Am J Med 1982;73(Suppl 1A):182–185.
14. Burnette TC, Harrington JA, Reardon JE, Merrill BM, de Miranda P. Purification and characterization of a rat liver enzyme that hydrolyzes valaciclovir, the L-valyl ester prodrug of acyclovir. J Biol Chem 1995;270:15827–15831.
15. Chatis PA, Crumpacker CS. Resistance of herpesviruses to antiviral drugs. Antimicrob Agents Chemother 1992;36:1589–1595.

16. Christophers J, Sutton RNP, Noble RV, Anderson H. Clinical resistance to acyclovir of herpes simplex virus infections in immunocompromised patients. J Antimicrob Chemother 1986; 18(Suppl B):121–5.

17. Clarke SE, Harrell AW, Chenery RJ. Role of aldehyde oxidase in the in vitro conversion of famciclovir to penciclovir in human liver. Drug Metab Dispos 1995;23:251–254.

18. Collins P. Viral sensitivity following the introduction of acyclovir. Am J Med 1988;85(Suppl 2A):129–134.

19. Collins P, Larder BA, Oliver NM, Kemp S, Smith IW, Darby G. Characterization of a DNA polymerase mutant of herpes simplex virus from a severely immunocompromised patient receiving acyclovir. J Gen Virol 1989;70:375–382.

20. Collum LMT, Logan P, Ravenscroft T. Acyclovir (Zovirax) in herpetic disciform keratitis. Br J Ophthalmol 1983;67:115–118.

21. Crane LR, Milne DA. Comparative activities of combinations of acyclovir, vidarabine or its 5′-monophosphate, and cloned human interferons against herpes simplex virus type 2 in human and mouse fibroblast cultures. Antiviral Res 1985;5:325–333.

22. Crooks RJ, Murray A. Valaciclovir—a review of a promising new antiherpes agent. Antivir Chem Chemother 1994;5(Suppl 1):31–37.

23. de Miranda P, Blum MR. Pharmacokinetics of acyclovir after intravenous and oral administration. J Antimicrob Chemother 1983;12(Suppl B):29–37.

24. Ducoulombier H, Cousin J, Dewilde A, Lancrenon S, Renaudie M, Steru D, Wattre P. La stomato-gingivite herpétique de l'enfant: essai controlé aciclovir versus placebo. Ann Pediatr 1988; 35:212–216.

25. Ellis MN, Keller PM, Fyfe JA, Martin JL, Rooney JF, Straus SE, Lehrman SN, Barry DW. Clinical isolate of herpes simplex virus type 2 that induces a thymidine kinase with altered substrate specificity. Antimicrob Agents Chemother 1987;31: 1117–1125.

26. Erlich KS, Mills J, Chatis P, Mertz GJ, Busch DF, Follansbee SE, Grant RM, Crumpacker CS. Acyclovir-resistant herpes simplex virus infections in patients with the acquired immunodeficiency syndrome. N Engl J Med 1989;320:293–296.

27. Ertl P, Snowden W, Lowe D, Miller W, Collins P, Little E. A comparative study of the in vitro and in vivo antiviral activities of acyclovir and penciclovir. Antivir Chem Chemother 1995;6: 89–97.

28. Field H, Darby G. Pathogenicity in mice of strains of herpes simplex virus which are resistant to acyclovir in vitro and in vivo. Antimicrob Agents Chemother 1980;17:209–216.

29. Field H, Darby G, Wildy P. Isolation and characterization of acyclovir-resistant mutants of herpes simplex virus. J Gen Virol 1980b;49:115–124.

30. Fife KH, Crumpacker CS, Mertz GJ, Hill EL, Boone GS, the Acyclovir Study Group. Recurrence and resistance patterns of herpes simplex virus following cessation of >6 years of chronic suppression with acyclovir. J Infect Dis 1994;169: 1338–1341.

31. Filer CW, Allen GD, Brown TA, Fowles SE, Hollis FJ, Prince WT, Ramji JV. Metabolic and pharmacokinetic studies following oral administration of 14C-famciclovir to healthy subjects. Xenobiotica 1994;24:357–368.

32. Fowles SE, Pierce DM, Prince WT, Staniforth D. The tolerance to and pharmacokinetics of penciclovir (BRL 39, 123A), a novel antiherpes agent, administered by intravenous infusion to healthy subjects. Eur J Clin Pharmacol 1992;43:513–516.

33. Gill KS, Wood MJ. The clinical pharmacokinetics of famciclovir. Clin Pharmacokinet 1996;31:1–8.

34. Greffe BS, Dooley SL, Deddish RB, Krasny HC. Transplacental passage of acyclovir. J Pediatr 1986;108:1020–1021.

35. Haddad J, Simeoni U, Messer J, Willard D. Transplacental passage of acyclovir. J Pediatr 1987;110:164.

36. Hintz M, Connor JD, Spector SA, Blum MR, Keeney RE, Yeager AS. Neonatal acyclovir pharmacokinetics in patients with herpes virus infections. Am J Med 1982;73(Suppl 1A):210–214.

37. Jacobson MA, Berger TG, Fikrig S, Becherer P, Moohr JW, Stanat SC, Biron KK. Acyclovir-resistant varicella zoster virus infection after chronic oral acyclovir therapy in patients with the acquired immunodeficiency syndrome (AIDS). Ann Intern Med 1990;112:187–191.

38. Keeney RE, Kirk LE, Brigden D. Acyclovir tolerance in humans. Am J Med 1982;73(Suppl 1A):176–181.

39. Krasny HC, Liao SH, de Miranda P, Laskin OL, Whelton A, Lietman PS. Influence of hemodialysis on acyclovir pharmacokinetics in patients with chronic renal failure. Am J Med 1982;73 (Suppl 1A):202–204.

40. Kroon S. Genital herpes: clinical disease, antiviral therapy and vaccines. In: Arvin AM, ed. Herpes virus infections. London: Ballière Tindall, 1996;5:391–414.

41. Larder B, Darby G. Selection and characterization of acyclovir-resistant herpes simplex type I mutants inducing altered DNA polymerase activities. Virology 1985;146:262–271.

42. Laskin OL, de Miranda P, King DH, Page DA, Longstreth JA, Rocco L, Lietman PS. Effects of probenecid on the pharmacokinetics and elimination of acyclovir in humans. Antimicrob Agents Chemother 1982a;21:804–807.

43. Laskin OL, Longstreth JA, Whelton A, Krasny HC, Keeney RE, Rocco L, Lietman PS. Effect of renal failure on the pharmacokinetics of acyclovir. Am J Med 1982b;73(Suppl 1A):210–214.

44. Laskin OL, Saral R, Burns WH, Angelopulos CM, Lietman PS. Acyclovir concentrations and tolerance during repetitive administration for 18 days. Am J Med 1982c;73(Suppl 1A):221–224.

45. Laskin OL. Clinical pharmacokinetics of acyclovir. Clin Pharmacokinet 1983;8:187–201.

46. Laskin OL. Acyclovir and suppression of frequently recurring herpetic whitlow. Ann Intern Med 1985;102:494–495.

47. Main J, Brown JL, Howells C, Galassini R, Crossey M, Karayiannis P, Georgiou P, Atkinson G, Thomas HC. A double-blind, placebo-controlled study to assess the effect of famciclovir on virus replication in patients with chronic hepatitis B virus infection. J Viral Hepatitis 1996;3:211–215.

48. Mertz GJ, Jones CC, Mills J, Fife KH, Lemon SM, Stepleton JT, Hill EL, Davis G. Long-term acyclovir suppression of frequently recurring genital herpes simplex infection. JAMA 1988;260: 201–206.

49. Meyers JD, Reed EC, Shepp DH, Thornquist M, Dandliker PS, Vacary CA, Flournoy N, Kirk LE, Kersey JH, Thomas ED, Balfour HH Jr. Acyclovir for the prevention of cytomegalovirus infection and disease in allogenic marrow transplantation. N Engl J Med 1988;318:70–75.

50. Meyers JD, Wade JC, Mitchell CD, Saral R, Leitman PS, Durack DT, Levin MJ, Segretti AC, Balfour HH Jr. Multicenter collaborative trial of intravenous acyclovir for treatment of mucocutaneous herpes simplex virus infection in the immunocompromised host. Am J Med 1992;73A:229–235.

51. O'Brien JJ, Campoli-Richards DM. Acyclovir—an updated review of its antiviral activity, pharmacokinetic properties and therapeutic efficacy. Drugs 1989;37:233–309.

52. Pahwa S, Biron K, Lim W, Swenson P, Kaplan MH, Sadick N, Pahwa R. Continuous varicella-zoster virus infection associated

with acyclovir resistance in a child with AIDS. JAMA 1988;260: 2879–2882.

53. Perry CM, Faulds D. Valaciclovir: a review of its antiviral activity, pharmacokinetic properties and therapeutic efficacy in herpesvirus infections. Drugs 1996;52:754–772.

54. Pue MA, Benet LZ. Pharmacokinetics of famciclovir in man. Antivir Chem Chemother 1993;4(Suppl 1):47–55.

55. Pue MA, Boike SC, Freed MI, Audet PR, Fairless A, Ilson B, Zariffa N, Jorkasky DK. Pharmacokinetics of penciclovir in subjects with hepatic insufficiency following oral famciclovir [Abstract]. Br J Clin Pharmacol 1994;37:494P

56. Pue MA, Pratt SK, Fairless AJ, Fowles S, Laroche J, Georgiou P, Prince W. Linear pharmacokinetics of penciclovir following administration of single oral doses of famciclovir 125, 250, 500 and 750 mg to healthy volunteers. J Antimicrob Chemother 1994;33:119–127.

57. Reichman RC, Badger GJ, Mertz GJ, Corey L, Richman DD, Connor JD, Redfield D, Savoia MC, Oxman MN, Bryson Y, Tyrell DL, Portnoy J, Creagh-Kirk T, Keeney RE, Ashikaga T, Dolin R. Orally administered acyclovir in the treatment of recurrent herpes genitalis. JAMA 1984;251:2103–2107.

58. Richards DM, Carmine AA, Brogden RM, Heel RC, Speight TM. Acyclovir: a review of its pharmacodynamic properties and therapeutic efficacy. Drugs 1983;26:378–438.

59. Sacks SL, Wanklin RJ, Reece DE, Hicks KA, Tyler KL, Coen DM. Progressive esophagitis from acyclovir-resistant herpes simplex. Clinical roles for DNA polymerase mutants and viral heterogeneity. Ann Intern Med 1989;111:893–899.

60. Sacks SL, Alrabiah F. Novel herpes treatment: a review. Exp Opin Invest Drugs 1996;5:169–183.

61. Schinazi RF, del Bene V, Taylor Scott R, Dudley-Thorpe JB. Characterization of acyclovir-resistant and -sensitive herpes simplex viruses isolated from a patient with an acquired immune deficiency. J Antimicrob Chemother 1986;17(Suppl B):127–134.

62. Schofer H, Ochsendorf F, Helm F, Milbradt R. Treatment of oral hairy leukoplakia in AIDS patients with vitamin A (orally) or acyclovir (systemically). Dermatologica 1987;174:150–151.

63. Schofield JK, Tatnall FM, Leigh IM. Recurrent erythema multiforme clinical features and treatment in a large series of patients. Br J Dermatol 1993;128:542–545.

64. Schwab IR. Oral acyclovir in the management of herpes simplex ocular infections. Ophthalmology 1988;95:423–429.

65. Shah GM, Winer RL, Krasny HC. Acyclovir pharmacokinetics in a patient on continuous ambulatory peritoneal dialysis. Am J Kidney Dis 1986;7:507–510.

66. Shaw T, Amor P, Civitico G, Boyd M, Locarnini S. In vitro antiviral activity of penciclovir, a novel purine nucleoside, against duck hepatitis B virus. Antimicrob Agents Chemother 1994;38: 719–723.

67. Shepp DH, Dandliker PS, Meyers JD. Treatment of varicella-zoster virus infection in severely immunocompromised patients. A randomized comparison of acyclovir and vidarabine. N Engl J Med 1986;23:208–212.

68. Sköldenberg B, Forsgren M, Alestig K, Bergstrom T, Burman L, Dahlqvist E, Forkman A, Fryden A, Lovgren K, Norlin K, Norrby R, Olding-Stenkvist E, Stiernstedt G, Uhnoo I, De Vahl K. Acyclovir versus vidarabine in herpes simplex encephalitis.

Randomised multicentre study in consecutive Swedish patients. Lancet 1984;2:707–711.

69. Smith DW, Goodwin CS. The use of in-vitro sensitivity testing to predict clinical response of recurrent herpes simplex to suppressive oral acyclovir. J Antimicrob Chemother 1988;21: 657–664.

70. Snoeck R, Gérard M, Sadzot-Delvaux C, Andrei G, Balzarini J, Reyman D, Piette J, Rentier B, Clumeck N, De Clercq E. Meningoradiculoneuritis due to acyclovir-resistant varicella-zoster virus in a patient with AIDS. J Infect Dis 1993;168: 1330–1331.

71. Spector SA, Kelley E. Inhibition of human cytomegalovirus by combined acyclovir and vidarabine. Antimicrob Agents Chemother 1985;27:600–604.

72. Spruance SL, Stewart JCB, Rowe NH, McKeough MB, Wenerstrom G, Freeman DJ. Treatment of recurrent herpes simplex labialis with oral acyclovir. J Infect Dis 1990;161:185–190.

73. Spruance SL, Tyring SK, DeGregorio B, Miller C, Beutner K, the Valaciclovir HSV Study Group. A large-scale, placebo-controlled, dose-ranging trial of peroral valaciclovir for episodic treatment of recurrent herpes genitalis. Arch Intern Med 1996; 156:1729–1735.

74. Straus SE, Takiff HE, Seidlin M, Bachrach S, Lininger L, DiGiovanna JJ, Western KA, Smith HA, Lehrman SN, Creagh-Kirk T, Alling DW. Suppression of frequently recurring genital herpes: a placebo-controlled double blind trial of oral acyclovir. N Engl J Med 1984;310:1545–1550.

75. Vere Hodge RA, Cheng YC. The mode of action of penciclovir. Antivir Chem Chemother 1993;4(Suppl 1):13–24.

76. Wade JC, Newton B, McLaren C, Flournoy N, Keeney RE, Meyers JR. Intravenous acyclovir to treat mucocutaneous herpes simplex virus infection after marrow transplantation: a double blind trial. Ann Intern Med 1982;96:265–269.

77. Wade JC, Meyers JD. Neurological symptoms associated with parenteral acyclovir treatment after marrow transplantation. Ann Intern Med 1983;98:921–925.

78. Wade JC, Day LM, Crowley J, Meyers JD. Recurrent infection with herpes simplex virus after marrow transplant: role of the specific immune response and acyclovir treatment. J Infect Dis 1984;149:750–756.

79. Weller S, Blum MR, Doucette M, Burnette T, Cederberg DM, de Miranda P, Smiley ML. Pharmacokinetics of the acyclovir pro-drug valaciclovir after escalating single- and multiple-dose administration to normal volunteers. Clin Pharmacol Ther 1993;54:595–605.

80. Whitley RJ, Alford CA, Hirsch MS, Schooley RT, Luby JP, Aoki FY, Hanley D, Nahmias AJ, Soong S-J, the NIAID Collaborative Antiviral Study Group. Vidarabine versus acyclovir therapy in herpes simplex encephalitis. N Engl J Med 1986; 314:144–149.

81. Whitley RJ, Arvin A, Prober C, Burchett S, Corey L, Powell D, Plotkin S, Start S, Alford C, Connor J, Jacobs RF, Nahmias AJ, Soong S, the NIAID Collaborative Antiviral Study Group. A controlled trial comparing vidarabine with acyclovir in neonatal herpes simplex virus infection. N Engl J Med 1991;324: 444–449.

82. Wood MJ. Treatment of zoster. Rev Med Microbiol 1995; 6:165–174.

INDEX

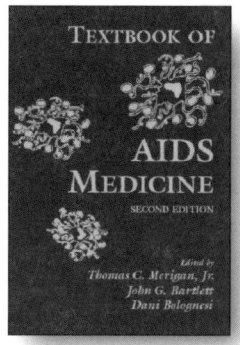
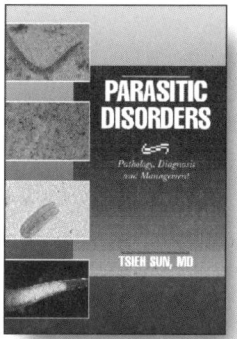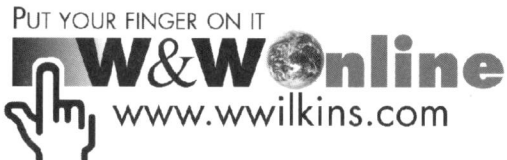